PATHOPHYSIOLOGY
The Biologic Basis for Disease in Adults and Children

KATHRYN L. McCANCE, RN, PhD
Associate Professor,
College of Nursing,
University of Utah,
Salt Lake City, Utah

SUE E. HUETHER, RN, PhD
Associate Professor,
College of Nursing,
University of Utah,
Salt Lake City, Utah

with **979** illustrations

THE C. V. MOSBY COMPANY
St. Louis • Baltimore • Philadelphia • Toronto   1990

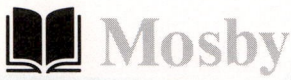

Editor William Grayson Brottmiller
Senior developmental editor Sally Adkisson
Project managers Patricia Gayle May, Lin A. Dempsey
Layout Jeanne Genz
Designer Candace F. Conner

Printed in the United States of America

The C. V. Mosby Company
11830 Westline Industrial Drive, St. Louis, Missouri 63146

Library of Congress Cataloging-in-Publication Data

McCance, Kathryn L.
    Pathophysiology: the biologic basis for disease in adults
and children / Kathryn L. McCance, Sue E. Huether.
        p.   cm.
    Includes bibliographical references.
    ISBN 0-8016-3360-5
    1. Physiology, Pathological.   2. Nursing.   I. Huether, Sue E.
II. Title.
    [DNLM: 1. Disease—nurses' instruction.
2. Pathology—nurses' instruction.   3. Physiology—
nurses' instruction.   QZ 4 M478p]
    RB113.M35   1990
    616.07—dc20   89-13523
                                                      CIP

C/VHP/VHP   9 8 7 6 5 4 3 2

CONTRIBUTORS

Margaret M. Andrews, RN, PhD
Chair, Department of Nursing,
Nazareth College,
Rochester, New York

Barbara J. Boss, RN, PhD
Professor of Nursing,
School of Nursing,
University of Mississippi Medical Center,
Jackson, Mississippi

Marjorie Cengiz Budd, RN, MS
Former Director of Nursing, Critical Care,
Latter Day Saints Hospital;
Clinical Associate Professor,
College of Nursing
University of Utah,
Salt Lake City, Utah

Pamela F. Cipriano, RN, MN
Director of Nursing Development,
Medical University of South Carolina,
Charleston, South Carolina

Katharine M. Donohoe, RN, MS
Doctoral Candidate, School of Nursing;
Clinician, Department of Neurology,
University of Rochester,
Rochester, New York

D. Patricia Gray, RN, PhD
Associate Professor,
Department of Adult Health Nursing,
Georgia State University,
Atlanta, Georgia

Deborah L. Greener, CNM, PhD
Assistant Professor,
Johns Hopkins,
Department of Obstetrics and Gynecology,
Baltimore, Maryland

Sandra W. Haak, RN, MS
Clinical Assistant Professor,
Doctoral Student,
College of Nursing,
University of Utah,
Salt Lake City, Utah

Joleen Heath, RN, MS
Neurology Clinical Nurse Specialist,
Salt Lake Veterans Administration Medical Center,
Salt Lake City, Utah

Katherine Hoare, RN, DNSC
Assistant Director of Nursing,
Nursing Systems,
Quality Assurance and Research,
Santa Clara Valley Medical Center,
San Jose, California

Lynn B. Jorde, PhD
Associate Professor,
Department of Human Genetics,
School of Medicine,
University of Utah,
Salt Lake City, Utah

Melva Kravitz, RN, PhD
Director of Nursing,
Shriners Burn Center,
Galveston, Texas

Patti Ludwig-Beymer, RN, PhD
Systems Coordinator,
Elmhurst College,
Deicke Center for Nursing Education,
Elmhurst, Illinois

Kathleen Hardin Mooney, RN, PhD
Associate Professor,
College of Nursing,
University of Utah,
Salt Lake City, Utah

Pamela D. Parker-Cohen, RN, MS, FNPC
Medical Student,
Thomas Jefferson Medical College,
Philadelphia, Pennsylvania

Stephanie J. Richardson, RN, MS
Instructor and Doctoral Student,
College of Nursing,
University of Utah,
Salt Lake City, Utah

Lee K. Roberts, PhD
Skin Biology Research,
Senior Principal Scientist,
Schering/Plough,
Memphis, Tennessee

Neal S. Rote, PhD
Professor and Chairman, Applied Immunology
    Program,
University of Southern Maine,
Portland, Maine;
Director, Reproductive Immunology Laboratory,
Foundation for Blood Research,
Scarborough, Maine

Mary Schoessler, RN, MS
Assistant Director, Education,
Providence Medical Center,
Portland, Oregon

Sharon L. Sims, RN, PhD
Assistant Professor and Coordinator,
    Nurse Practitioner Program,
College of Nursing,
University of Utah,
Salt Lake City, Utah

Peter M. Sunderland, RN, MS
Clinical Specialist, Division of Neurosurgery,
University of Utah Health Sciences Center;
Doctoral Student, College of Nursing,
University of Utah,
Salt Lake City, Utah

Mary Suzanne Tarmina, RN, PhD
Clinical Associate Professor,
College of Nursing,
University of Utah,
Salt Lake City, Utah

Roger R. Williams, MD
Professor of Medicine,
Director, Cardiovascular Genetics Research Clinic,
School of Medicine,
University of Utah,
Salt Lake City, Utah

REVIEWERS

Sr. Rose Terese Bahr, RN, PhD, FAAN
Professor of Nursing and Chair,
Division of Community Health Nursing,
School of Nursing,
Catholic University of America,
Washington, DC

Jane Ball, RN, CPNP, DrPH
Trauma Services,
Children's Hospital National Medical Center,
Washington, DC

Beverly Bartlett, RN, PhD
Assistant Professor,
College of Nursing,
University of Rhode Island,
Kingston, Rhode Island

Carroll Conner Bouman, RN, MS
Clinical Nurse Specialist in Cardiopulmonary Nursing;
Faculty Member and Doctoral Candidate,
School of Nursing,
University of Rochester,
Rochester, New York

John Carey, MD, MPH
Associate Professor,
Chief, Division of Medical Genetics,
School of Medicine,
University of Utah,
Salt Lake City, Utah

Miguel da Cunha, PhD
Associate Professor,
University of Texas Health Sciences Center
at Houston,
Houston, Texas

Joyce Dains, RN, DrPH
Assistant Professor,
School of Nursing,
University of Texas Health Sciences Center
at Houston,
Houston, Texas

Carol DeMoss, RN, MN, CS
Clinical Nurse Specialist,
Visiting Nurse Association of Allegheny County,
Pittsburgh, Pennsylvania

Dorothy Doughty, RN, MN, CETN
Program Director,
Emory University,
Enterostomal Therapy Nursing Education Program,
Atlanta, Georgia

Harmon J. Eyre, MD
Professor of Medicine,
Division of Hematology/Oncology,
School of Medicine,
University of Utah,
Salt Lake City, Utah

Mikel Gray, PhD Candidate, CURN
Clinical Urodynamics,
Henrietta Egelston Hospital for Children,
   Scottish Rite Children's Hospital,
   Shepherd Spinal Center,
Atlanta, Georgia

Judith Hall, RN, PhD
Assistant Professor,
School of Nursing,
University of Texas at Arlington,
Arlington, Texas

Laurel Halloran, RN, MSN
Assistant Professor;
Clinical Nurse Specialist, Doctoral Candidate,
Department of Nursing,
Western Connecticut State University,
Danbury, Connecticut

K.C. Hayes, DVM, PhD
Director, Foster Biomedical Research Center;
Professor and Chairman, Biology Department,
Brandeis University,
Waltham, Massachusetts

Mary Beth Hayward, RN, MSN
Associate Professor,
School of Nursing,
Medical College of Ohio,
Toledo, Ohio

Ruthellyn Hinton, RN, MS, MN
Associate Professor,
Department of Nursing,
Pittsburg State University,
Pittsburg, Kansas

Linda Jones, RN, MS, CS, OCN
Assistant to the Associate Director
   for Nursing Oncology,
University of Rochester Cancer Center;
Assistant Professor of Clinical Nursing,
University of Rochester School of Nursing,
Rochester, New York

Sr. Joan Klemballa, RN, MA
Associate Professor,
Division of Nursing Education,
University of District of Columbia,
Washington, DC

Helene J. Krouse, RN, C, PhD
Assistant Professor,
School of Nursing,
Boston College,
Chestnut Hill, Massachusetts

Mary Lentz, RN, PhD
Assistant Professor,
School of Nursing,
University of Pittsburgh,
Pittsburgh, Pennsylvania

Stacey Levine, RN, PhD
Associate Professor,
University of Alberta,
Clinical Sciences Department,
Edmonton, Alberta, Canada

Patricia Maybee, RN, MS, CCRN
College of Nursing,
Clemson University,
Department of Instruction,
Clemson, South Carolina

Mary Beth McDowell, RN, MN
Assistant Professor,
College of Allied Health and Nursing,
Eastern Kentucky University,
Richmond, Kentucky

Mary Ellen McMorrow, RN, EdD, CCRN
The College of Staten Island,
School of Nursing,
Staten Island, New York

Diane Melancon, RN, MSN
Associate Professor of Nursing Education,
San Antonio College,
San Antonio, Texas

Kenneth Morgan, PhD
Associate Professor,
Department of Epidemiology and Biostatistics,
McGill University,
Montreal, Canada

Leona Mourad, RN, MS
Associate Professor Emeritus,
College of Nursing,
Ohio State University,
Columbus, Ohio

Christine Mudge-Grout, RN, MS
Clinical Nurse Specialist, Nephrology/Transplant,
Department of Nursing,
University of California at San Francisco,
San Francisco, California

Virginia J. Neelon, RN, PhD
Associate Professor,
School of Nursing,
University of North Carolina at Chapel Hill,
Chapel Hill, North Carolina

Donna Patterson, RN, MSN
Assistant Professor,
Villanova University,
College of Nursing,
Villanova, Pennsylvania

Ann Peterson, RN, BS, BSN
Endocrine Clinical Nurse Specialist,
Nursing Department,
National Institutes of Health,
Bethesda, Maryland

Nancy Redeker, RN, C, MSN, PhD
Instructor,
Rutgers University,
College of Nursing,
Newark, New Jersey

Gayle Reiber, RN, PhD
Associate Professor,
College of Nursing,
University of North Carolina at Charlotte
Charlotte, North Carolina

Linda L. Robertson, RN, PhD
Assistant Professor,
School of Nursing,
University of Pittsburgh,
Pittsburgh, Pennsylvania

Connie Robinson, RN, MN
Assistant Professor,
School of Nursing,
University of California at San Francisco,
San Francisco, California

David B. Roll, PhD
Professor of Medicinal Chemistry,
College of Pharmacy,
University of Utah,
Salt Lake City, Utah

Amy Perrin Ross, RN, MSN, CNRN
Neuroscience Clinical Nurse Specialist,
Loyola University Medical Center,
Maywood, Illinois;
Triton College,
Continuing Education Center for Health Professionals,
River Grove, Illinois

Phyllis Russo, RN, EdD
Chairperson, Undergraduate Nursing,
College of Nursing,
Seton Hall University,
South Orange, New Jersey

Ann Sedore, RN, PhD
Associate Professor,
College of Nursing,
Syracuse University,
Syracuse, New York

Janice Selekman, RN, DNSc
Associate Professor,
Generic Baccalaureate Program Director,
Department of Nursing,
Thomas Jefferson University,
Philadelphia, Pennsylvania

Mary Ann Siefert, RN, MS
Primary Childrens Hospital,
Salt Lake City, Utah

Barbara Peterson Sinclair, RN, MN
Director, OB/GYN Nurse Practitioner Program,
School of Nursing,
California State University,
Los Angeles, California

Lydia DeCastro-Svetich, RN, MS
Associate Professor,
Orvis School of Nursing,
University of Nevada, Reno,
Reno, Nevada

Arthur Vander, PhD
Department of Physiology,
University of Michigan,
Ann Arbor, Michigan

Filomena Varvaro, RN, PhD
Assistant Professor,
School of Nursing,
University of Pittsburgh,
Pittsburgh, Pennsylvania

Sharon Wahl, RN, MSN, EdDc
Assistant Professor,
Department of Nursing,
San Jose State University,
San Jose, California

Eleanor A. Walker, BSN, MS
Assistant Professor,
School of Nursing,
Catholic University of America,
Washington, DC

Lin C. Weeks, RN, MS, CNAA
Administrative Director,
Hospital Education,
Hermann Hospital,
Houston, Texas

Raymond L. White, PhD
Professor and Co-Chairman, Human Genetics
    Department,
Investigator of Howard Hughes Medical Institute,
School of Medicine,
University of Utah,
Salt Lake City, Utah

Gail M. Wilkes, RN, MS, OCN
Clinical Nurse Specialist in Oncology,
Boston City Hospital,
Boston, Massachusetts

Maxwell Wintrobe, MD, BSc (Med), PhD, DSc (Hon. Manitoba), DSc (Hon. Utah), DSc (Hon. Wisc.), MACP, MD (Hon. Athens)
Late Distinguished Professor of Internal Medicine,
School of Medicine,
University of Utah,
Salt Lake City, Utah

To John Wolfer, for keeping the *balance* and *adventure* in my life,
"Here's lookin' at you kid!"

and

To my parents
Dot and Don
with love and affection

KLM

To Suzi, Molly, Courtney, Melissa, Christina, and Mary
my hope for the next generation

SEH

PREFACE

Few subjects of scientific inquiry have been studied in the past few years so intensively as pathophysiology, the study of human diseases and the mechanisms that govern them. Recent discoveries in genetics, gene-environment interaction, immunology, neuroimmunology, cancer, and aging have revolutionized our understanding of basic biology. Without the advances that have taken place in molecular and cell biology—advances so remarkable that the phrase "new biology" has been coined to describe them—less progress would have occurred in the understanding and treatment of human diseases. That is why this new book is subtitled *The Biologic Basis for Disease*.

We had three broad objectives in offering a new textbook on pathophysiology. First, and most important, we have provided a comprehensive presentation of the underlying principles common to all disease processes. Second, we have included consistent coverage of disease processes in all age groups, with separate chapters in each system unit on alterations in children. Pathophysiology associated with elderly adults is presented within the adult chapters, and normal changes associated with aging are clearly distinguished at the conclusion of each chapter that reviews anatomy and physiology. Finally, we have paid scrupulous attention to make this book an effective learning tool. To this end, we have incorporated an intensive two-color illustration program to facilitate ease of learning.

ORGANIZATION

The book is divided into two parts: Part One, *Central Concepts of Pathophysiology: Cells and Tissues,* and Part Two, *Pathophysiologic Alterations: Organs and Systems.* We believe that all of human physiology—no matter how complex—can be described in terms of physical and chemical laws or cellular events. We have attempted to make these basic facts significant by using them to explain more general and familiar principles and concepts.

Part One, 11 chapters organized within four units, presents the foundation for understanding virtually all human diseases, which are then systematically presented in Part Two. Part One begins with a tour of the cell. This first chapter presents the complex and wonderful workings of the cell in ways that were not understood even a few years ago. Insofar as possible, the tour is a pictorial one, in keeping with our view that microscopic entities have to be presented as graphically as possible for students to understand their intricate workings. For students with prior coursework in general biology, the cell is a familiar and logical place to launch their study of pathophysiology.

Once the normal structure and function of the cell are presented, we proceed to other processes related to cells. These include an extensive review of receptor physiology and mechanisms of genetically transmitted diseases, along with an overview of essential epidemiology and its applications to incidence, prevalence, and risk factors for disease states. We then offer an innovative chapter on concepts of gene-environment interaction, in which mechanisms that may mediate the intricate interplay of familial disorders and environmental influences are reviewed. Part One also presents the mechanisms of immunity and inflammation in separate chapters; provides updated models of neuroimmunology that link stress with disease; details the biology of cancer, with theories of carcinogenesis; and extensively discusses the immunobiology of cancer.

Part Two surveys specific diseases from the traditional systems organization, with some strategic twists. This part begins with the neurologic and endocrine systems. It has been our experience that students who understand the global regulatory influences of the neurologic and endocrine systems have less difficulty later in understanding the body systems with more specific functions. Students gain a deeper appreciation for the functions and altered functions in the organ systems by developing a firm appreciation for how nerves and hormones control and mediate processes in all other systems.

The reproductive unit, which follows the endocrine unit, represents a logical development of endocrine function. An exhaustive chapter on sexually transmitted diseases provides an application of concepts learned earlier while offering authoritative information on a set of dread epidemic diseases frought with fear, distortion, and misinformation.

The hematologic unit is next so that the student has a clear understanding of the composition of blood, hematopoiesis, and the mechanisms of hemostasis prior to their application in the ensuing cardiovascular and pulmonary units. The cardiovascular unit provides detailed coverage of manifestations of heart disease, such as heart failure, dysrhythmias, and types of shock, including impairment of cellular metabolism. In like manner, the pulmonary unit includes novel coverage of the clinical manifestations of pulmonary disease, including dyspnea, abnormal sputum, and cough. The book then proceeds to the renal, digestive, musculoskeletal, and integumentary systems. This final unit includes a comprehensive discussion of thermal injury with excellent illustrations.

Several features are integrated throughout Part Two. First, content on cancer is integrated extensively, including theories of carcinogenesis, epidemiology and risk factors, pathogenesis, and evaluation and treatment. Second, we have made use of physical laws, carefully explained, to aid students in understanding alterations. For example, the law of LaPlace is used to explain blood flow through organs to show how it can be applied to the formation of aneurysms. This strategy is in keeping with our general philosophy that students who can grasp basic laws and principles can then understand *how* alterations occur. Finally, in keeping with the contemporary flavor of this book, we have adopted the current practice of referring to diseases named after individuals without the use of the possessive. Thus, for example, what was formerly known as Down's syndrome is referred to as Down syndrome.

The organization within the units themselves was also carefully constructed. As in many books, each system unit begins with a chapter on the normal anatomy and physiology of the system. The normal chapters were carefully edited after the corresponding alterations chapters were written so that the material on normal function *directly* informs the discussion of the specific diseases that follow. Although the normal anatomy and physiology chapters assume some prior study, they are also designed to review concepts that may have become rusty from disuse, and even students whose knowledge of physiology is fresh or more sophisticated will find something of interest in them. The normal chapters include common diagnostic tests and clearly identify the normal aging processes unique to the system.

The second chapter of each unit presents the physio-logic alterations seen in adults. A consistent format is followed: epidemiology and risk factors, pathophysiology or pathogenesis, clinical manifestations, and evaluation and treatment. Major emphasis is devoted to pathophysiology and clinical manifestations because other references on care and clinical management are readily available to students.

As teachers, we have been frustrated by the lack of material on disease mechanisms in children. We have sought to rectify this shortcoming by including a third chapter on alterations in children in every unit, except the endocrine and reproductive units where the content is integrated and much of the primary content is already on congenital alterations.

Throughout the book, extensive cross-references are made to fully integrate the two parts of the book. For example, a thorough understanding of the normal inflammatory response is necessary to understand the diseases of inflammation such as arthritis and glomerulonephritis. By the same token, many clinical examples are used in the foundational chapters to illustrate how the basic concepts are manifested, partly through the use of a device we call *Clinical Commentaries*. In this way, as students learn about cells and tissues, they are shown repeatedly how these mechanisms function in organs and systems. Throughout the book, we have taken pains to draw the student's attention to theoretical controversies and identify gaps in current understanding.

INTEGRATION OF LIFESPAN CONTENT

Beginning in Chapter 2, we present theories of aging. We make reference to this chapter throughout Part Two as the normal changes associated with aging are presented in the normal anatomy and physiology chapter of each system unit. The pathophysiology of diseases associated with advanced age is discussed in the alterations chapters. In this way, we attempt to make it clear to students that there are physiologic changes related to aging that are normal and healthy, and that old age should not be considered synonymous with sickness and death.

In the same fashion, content related to alterations in children is firmly rooted in Part One of the book, and frequent reference is made to cellular content during the discussion of specific diseases of childhood presented in the systems units in Part Two. Material in Part One includes considerations related to childhood, such as congenital immune deficiencies, genetic disorders, familial diseases, and cancer in children. We take the opportunity in the systems chapters on children in Part Two to summarize, when appropriate, the differences between diseases in adults and children, such as differences in tumors.

DEVELOPMENT OF THE BOOK

The content of pathophysiology is complex and ever expanding. We have, therefore, with the assistance of the publisher, gone to great lengths to ensure that this book is highly readable, well illustrated, and pedagogically sound. For the sake of our students we wanted them to find the book interesting as well as accurate.

The illustrations received intense planning and scrutiny. Nearly 1000 illustrations bring to life concepts and processes that are most often invisible, abstract, or hidden from view. Hundreds were created especially for this book, and a large portion of the illustrations are presented in color to draw attention to their salient points. We wrote detailed legends to accompany the illustrations and made sure that each illustration was strategically tied in with the surrounding text.

Pedagogic features were planned for the text to reinforce learning. Key terms, with page numbers indicating where they were first mentioned and defined, are included at the end of each chapter to provide a convenient means of acquiring the large amount of terminology associated with pathophysiology, as well as an orderly way to review content. We draw particular attention to the chapter summaries. The summaries attempt to extend the content of the chapter, synthesize information, and draw connections that students otherwise may not make.

Finally, we have provided a short essay at the beginning of each unit on some aspect of the history of the subject it previews. The essays were deemed important so that students would have a perspective of how recently or long ago advances have been made. They are accompanied by illustrations from the Victorian Era, which are part of the collection of the National Library of Medicine. We hope this device adds color and interest to an otherwise often sober subject.

We would like this book to serve as a pleasurable but comprehensive presentation of the basic principles of disease. Toward this end we believe this book gives a *state of the art and science* approach.

Kathryn L. McCance
Sue E. Huether

ACKNOWLEDGMENTS

Our first acknowledgment goes to a very special person—Sue Meeks. Sue Meeks typed, retyped, programmed, and reprogrammed our manuscript, and she did so in a professional, eager, and courteous manner. This monumental task became "her baby" and she was as invested in its accuracy and appearance as we were. Thank you, Sue.

Many individuals supported the production of this book, especially our colleagues and friends at the University of Utah College of Nursing. We want to particularly thank Joyce Rathbun and Beth Lambrick for keeping track of the many details related to the transmittal and revision of manuscripts. To Debbie Bachan, we thank you for the tremendous assistance in obtaining figure and table permissions—a tedious task. To our Dean, Linda Amos, we greatly appreciate all the support and genuine interest displayed concerning the overall processing of the manuscript.

Every book has its editorial staff; however, this book benefitted from some truly outstanding editors. First of all, we are very indebted to the sheer genius of Kathy Sterling, our primary developmental editor. Kathy undertook the difficult task of shaping the logical progression, consistency, and readability of the manuscript. Kathy's expertise and tenacity made this book what it is! Thank you, Kathy.

Next, we had the great fortune of having Bill Brottmiller as our managing editor at Mosby. From the onset, Bill shared our vision, expanded it, and managed the editorial development in a creative, professional, and up front style. He skillfully brought us to Mosby and gave us a good home. Thank you, Bill, for everything.

Sally Adkisson was our "in house" developmental editor at Mosby, and she directed the book through production. We are grateful to Sally for perseverance and expedience in managing a million details with grace and humor.

Lin Dempsey coordinated final editing, galley production, and the smooth sailing toward page proofs. This task would overwhelm most people, but Lin's professional manner and easygoing style kept us completely on track. Thank you, Lin. Gayle May was the project manager. She coordinated the illustrations and text and managed the page proofs, including the many changes that were introduced in the final stages. Despite our incessant requests to add "just one last change" reported in the literature, she saw to it that the book is as up to date as we can make it, and she never complained. Thank you, Gayle.

Of major importance to any textbook is the art program. We would like to acknowledge two extremely talented artists—George Wassilchenko and Donald O'Connor. They helped to make the book come alive. Thank you, George and Donald.

Many people were involved in reviewing the manuscript at all phases. We would like to acknowledge the reviewers for their astute comments and for taking time out of very busy schedules to give us feedback. Their recommendations added a significant element of quality to the book.

Contents

PART ONE Central Concepts of
Pathophysiology: Cells and Tissues

UNIT I   The Cell

1 Cellular Biology, 4
Kathryn L. McCance

2 Altered Cellular and Tissue Biology, 48
Kathryn L. McCance

3 The Cellular Environment: Fluids and
Electrolytes, Acids and Bases, 82
Sue E. Huether

UNIT II   Genes and Gene-Environment Interaction

4 Genes and Genetic Diseases, 116
Lynn B. Jorde

5 Genes and Environmental Interaction: Familial
Diseases, 153
Roger R. Williams

UNIT III   Mechanisms of Self-Defense

6 Immunity, 192
Neal S. Rote

7 Inflammation, 217
Neal S. Rote

8 Alterations in Immunity and Inflammation, 249
Neal S. Rote

9 Stress and Disease, 279
Kathryn L. McCance

UNIT IV   Cellular Proliferation—Cancer

10 Tumor Biology, 294
Kathryn L. McCance
Kathleen Hardin Mooney
Lee K. Roberts

11 Theories of Carcinogenesis, 324
Kathryn L. McCance
Lee K. Roberts

PART TWO Pathophysiologic Alterations:
Organs and Systems

UNIT V   The Neurologic System

12 Structure and Function of the Neurologic
System, 352
Peter M. Sunderland

13 Pain, Temperature Regulation, Sleep, and
Sensory Function, 390
Mary Schoessler
Patti Ludwig-Beymer
Sue E. Huether

14 Concepts of Neurologic Dysfunction, 431
Barbara J. Boss

15 Alterations of Neurologic Function, 476
Barbara J. Boss
Joleen Heath
Peter M. Sunderland

16 Alterations of Neurologic Function in Children,
531
Margaret Andrews
Kathleen Hardin Mooney

UNIT VI   The Endocrine System

17 Mechanisms of Hormonal Regulation, 564
D. Patricia Gray

18 Alterations of Hormonal Regulation, 594
D. Patricia Gray
Patti Lugwig-Beymer

UNIT VII   The Reproductive System

19 Structure and Function of the Reproductive
Systems, 646
D. Patricia Gray
Sue E. Huether

20 Alterations of the Reproductive Systems, 677
D. Patricia Gray
Sue E. Huether

21 Sexually Transmitted Diseases, 725
Deborah L. Greener

xx   *Contents*

UNIT VIII   The Hematologic System

22   Structure and Function of the Hematologic
      System, 755
      Kathryn L. McCance

23   Alterations of Erythrocyte Function, 784
      Pamela D. Parker-Cohen
      Kathryn L. McCance

24   Alterations of Leukocyte, Lymphoid, and
      Hemostatic Function, 800
      Pamela F. Cipriano
      Kathryn L. McCance

25   Alterations in Hematologic Function in Children,
      825
      Margaret Andrews
      Kathleen Hardin Mooney

UNIT IX   The Cardiovascular and Lymphatic
               System

26   Structure and Function of the Cardiovascular and
      Lymphatic Systems, 859
      Kathryn L. McCance
      Stephanie J. Richardson

27   Alterations of Cardiovascular Function, 916
      Pamela D. Parker-Cohen
      Stephanie J. Richardson
      Sandra Haak

28   Alterations of Cardiovascular Function in
      Children, 992
      Sharon L. Sims

UNIT X   The Pulmonary System

29   Structure and Function of the Pulmonary System,
      1026
      Marjorie Budd

30   Alterations of Pulmonary Function, 1053
      Marjorie Budd
      Kathryn L. McCance

31   Alterations of Pulmonary Function in Children,
      1096
      Margaret M. Andrews

UNIT XI   The Renal and Urologic Systems

32   Structure and Function of the Renal and
      Urologic Systems, 1112
      Sue E. Huether

33   Alterations of Renal and Urinary Tract Function,
      1135
      Sue E. Huether

34   Alterations of Renal and Urinary Tract Function
      in Children, 1160
      Margaret M. Andrews
      Kathleen Hardin Mooney

UNIT XII   The Digestive System

35   Structure and Function of the Digestive System,
      1174
      Sue E. Huether

36   Alterations of Digestive Function, 1212
      Sue E. Huether
      Kathryn L. McCance
      Mary Suzanne Tarmina

37   Alterations of Digestive Function in Children,
      1267
      Margaret M. Andrews
      Sue E. Huether

UNIT XIII   The Musculoskeletal System

38   Structure and Function of the Musculoskeletal
      System, 1292
      Katherine Hoare
      Katharine M. Donohoe

39   Alterations of Musculoskeletal Function, 1319
      Katherine Hoare
      Katharine M. Donohoe

40   Alterations of Musculoskeletal Function in
      Children, 1360
      Margaret M. Andrews
      Kathleen Hardin Mooney

UNIT XIV   The Integumentary System

41   Structure, Function, and Disorders of the
      Integument, 1390
      Sue E. Huether
      Melva Kravitz

42   Alterations of the Integument in Children, 1439
      Sue E. Huether
      Margaret M. Andrews

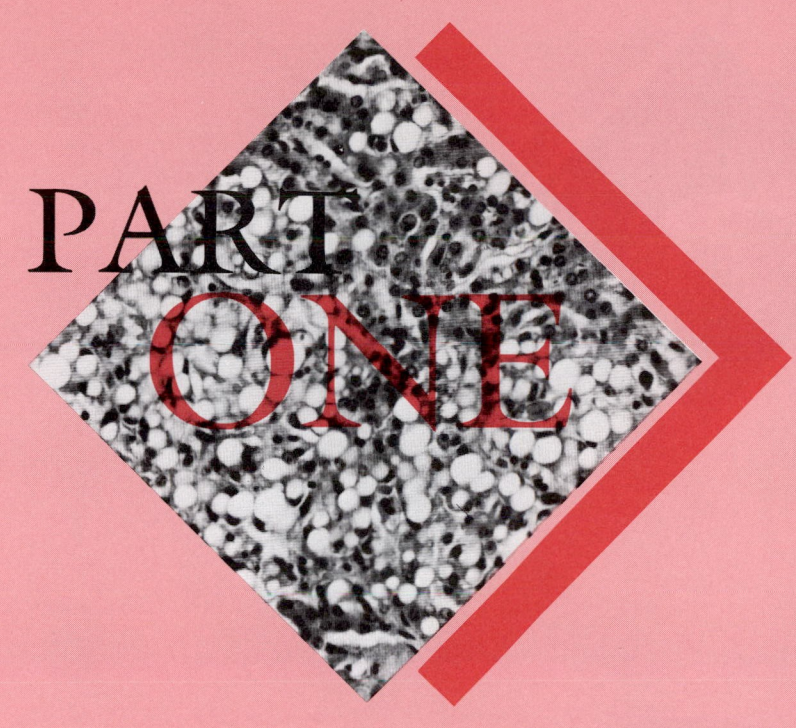

PART ONE

Central Concepts of Pathophysiology: Cells and Tissues

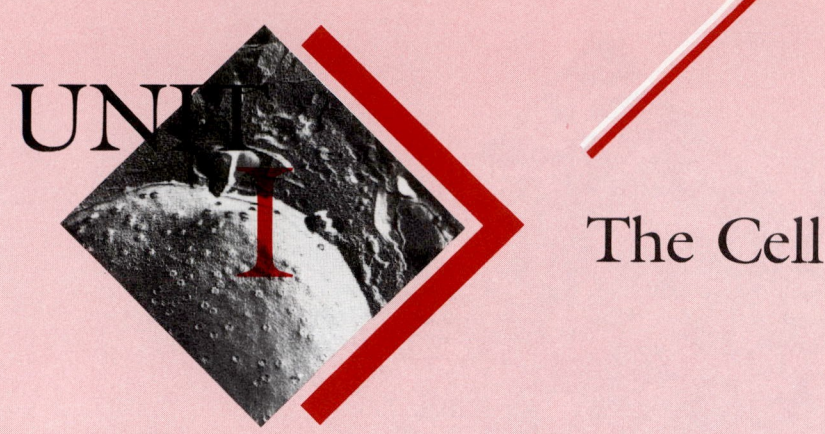

UNIT I

The Cell

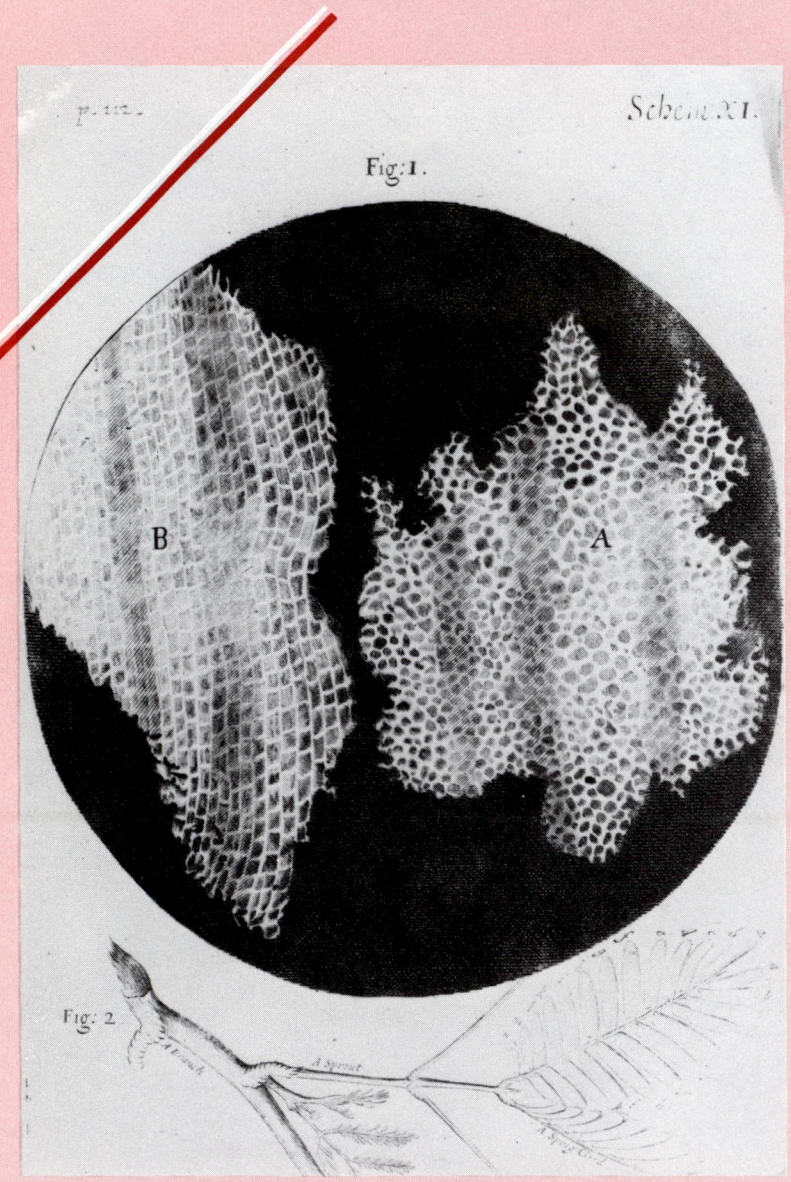

Cork cells. (From Hooke, R: Micrographia. Courtesy National Library of Medicine.)

THE study of cellular biology really began in the seventeenth century, primarily from the discoveries of Englishman Robert Hooke (1635-1723) and Dutchman Anthony van Leeuwenhoek (1632-1723). Hooke was the first to use the term *cell* in biology. He describes in a collection of essays, *Micrographia*, a honeycomb of chambers in cork, which he called "cells." He thought the cells were similar to the veins and arteries of animals, although his microscope did not permit the observation of any intracellular structures.

After improving the microscope lens, Van Leeuwenhoek described a variety of single-celled life forms, including bacteria, in 1683. This was an incredible feat because the dimensions of bacteria are typically about 1 or 2 μm. In 1824, with improved microscopy, R. J. H. Dutrochet noted that all animal and plant tissues are aggregates of cells of various kinds. Although he observed that growth results from an increase in either the size or the number of cells, or both, he did not realize that each cell is capable of reproduction.

Matthias Schleiden and Theodor Schwann, in 1838 and 1839, were the first to argue convincingly that each cell is capable of its own growth and development. Rudolf Virchow (1821-1902), often called the "Pope of Medicine," extended the findings of Schleiden and Schwann by attributing every cell's existence to that of a preexisting cell (*omnis cellula e cellula*—every cell from a cell). The ideas of Schleiden, Schwann, and Virchow became known as the cell theory, or cell doctrine, which states that: (1) all living things are composed of one or more compartments called cells, (2) each cell is capable of maintaining its own unique vitality, and (3) cells can arise only from other cells. The cell theory radically changed the understanding of disease, which could now be studied with respect to alterations in cellular structure and function. Virchow was not a strong supporter of the bacterial theory of disease, but his view that the reactions of the body's cells to invading microorganisms can have more deleterious effects than the invading organism itself is still an essential tenet in the study of disease.

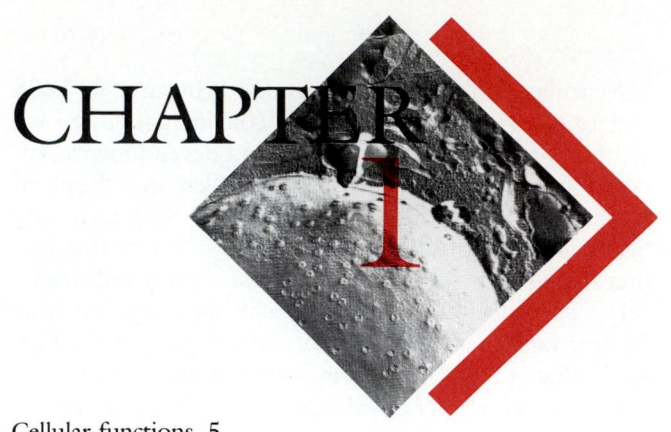

CHAPTER 1

Cellular Biology

Kathryn L. McCance

Cellular functions, 5
Structure and function of cellular components, 5
  Nucleus, 5
  Cytoplasmic organelles, 5
    Ribosomes, 6
    Endoplasmic reticulum, 6
    Golgi complex, 6
    Lysosomes, 8
    Peroxisomes, 10
    Mitochondria, 10
    Cytoskeleton, 10
  Plasma membranes, 12
    Membrane composition, 13
      Lipids, 13
      Proteins, 14
      Carbohydrates, 14
    Membrane fluidity: the fluid mosaic model, 15
  Cellular receptors, 16
Cellular metabolism, 16
  Role of adenosine triphosphate, 17
  Food and the production of cellular energy, 17
  Oxidative phosphorylation, 18
Processes of cellular intake and output, 19
  Movement of water and solutes, 19
    Passive transport, 20
      Diffusion, 20
      Hydrostatic pressure, 20
      Osmosis, 21
    Mediated and active transport, 22
      Mediated transport, 22
      Active transport of Na$^+$ and K$^+$, 23
    Transport by vesicle formation, 25
      Endocytosis and exocytosis, 25
      Receptor-mediated endocytosis, 26
    Movement of electrical impulses: membrane potentials, 28
Cellular reproduction: the cell cycle, 28
  Phases of mitosis and cytokinesis, 29
  Rates of cellular division, 29
Tissues, 31
  Tissue formation, 31
  Intercellular communication, 32
  Types of tissues, 33
    Epithelial tissue, 37
    Connective tissue, 37
    Muscle tissue, 41
    Neural tissue, 41

An understanding of cellular biology is increasingly necessary for an understanding of disease. Recently, an explosion of cellular information has occurred in genetics, tumor biology, immunology, pathology, neurobiology, and clinical therapeutics. A giant, bewildering puzzle is emerging to explain the roles of health habits, personality, cultural and sociologic factors, and aging in cellular alterations. New information on how messages are received, interpreted, and used by the cell has involved the study of acceptor proteins, or receptors, on the surface of the cell. Increased knowledge about the structure and function of cellular membranes has furthered understanding of immune defenses and protection against disease and cellular injury. (The immune response is discussed in Chapter 6.) Information on cellular growth and maturation has enhanced understanding of genetic disorders, tumor development, and aging.

Living cells are generally divided into two major classes, the eucaryotes and procaryotes. The cells of higher animals and plants are eucaryotes, as are the single-celled organisms, fungi, protozoa, and most algae. Procaryotes include cyanobacteria (blue-green algae), bacteria, and rickettsiae. Procaryotes have been significant to the study of human disease because much of what has been learned about the molecular biology of eucaryotic cells has been extrapolated from the study of procaryotic cells.

Eucaryotes (*eu* = good; *karyon* = nucleus) are larger and have more extensive intracellular anatomy and organization than procaryotes. Eucaryotic cells have a characteristic set of membrane-bounded intracellular compartments, called organelles, that includes a well-defined nucleus. The **procaryotes** contain no organelles, and their nuclear material is not encased by a nuclear membrane. Procaryotic cells are characterized by lack of a distinct nucleus.

Besides having structural differences, procaryotic and eucaryotic cells differ in chemical composition and biochemical activity. The "nuclei" of procaryotic cells carry genetic information in a single circular chromosome, and they lack a class of proteins called histones, which in eucaryotic cells bind with deoxyribonucleic acid (DNA) and are involved in the supercoiling of DNA. Eucaryotic cells have several or many chromosomes. Protein production, or synthesis, in the two classes of cells also differs because of major structural differences in ribonucleic acid (RNA) protein complexes. Other distinctions include differences in mechanisms of transport across the outer cellular membrane and in enzyme content.

CELLULAR FUNCTIONS

Cells become specialized through the process of differentiation, or maturation, so that some cells eventually perform one kind of function and other cells perform other functions. Highly developed functions, such as movement, are often associated with the absence of some other property, such as hormone production, which is more highly developed in some other type of specialized cell.

The seven chief cellular functions are the following:

1. *Movement*. Muscle cells can generate forces that produce motion. Muscles that are attached to bones produce limb movements, whereas those that enclose hollow tubes or cavities move or empty contents when they contract. For example, the contraction of smooth muscle cells surrounding blood vessels changes the diameter of the vessels; the contraction of muscles in walls of the urinary bladder expels urine.

2. *Conductivity*. Conduction as a response to a stimulus is manifested by a wave of excitation, an electrical potential, that passes along the surface of the cell to reach its other parts. Conductivity is the chief function of nerve cells.

3. *Metabolic absorption*. All cells can take in and use nutrients and other substances from their surroundings. Cells of the intestine and the kidney are specialized to carry out absorption. Cells of the kidney tubules reabsorb fluids and synthesize proteins. Intestinal epithelial cells reabsorb fluids and synthesize protein enzymes.

4. *Secretion*. Certain cells, such as mucous gland cells, can synthesize new substances from substances they absorb and secrete the new substances to serve as needed elsewhere. Cells of the adrenal gland, testis, and ovary can secrete hormonal steroids.

5. *Excretion*. All cells can rid themselves of waste products resulting from the metabolic breakdown of nutrients. Membrane-bounded sacs (lysosomes) within cells contain enzymes that break down, or digest, large molecules, turning them into waste products that are released from the cell.

6. *Respiration*. Cells absorb oxygen, which is used to transform nutrients into energy in the form of adenosine triphosphate (ATP). Cellular respiration, or oxidation, occurs in organelles called mitochondria.

7. *Reproduction*. Tissue growth occurs as cells enlarge and reproduce themselves. Even without growth, tissue maintenance requires that new cells be produced to replace cells that are lost normally through cellular death. Not all cells are capable of continuous division, and some cells, such as nerve cells, cannot reproduce.

STRUCTURE AND FUNCTION OF CELLULAR COMPONENTS

A "typical" eucaryotic cell is shown in Fig. 1-1. It consists of three components: an outer membrane called the **plasma membrane,** or **plasmalemma;** a fluid "filling," called **cytoplasm,** and the "organs" of the cell—the membrane-bounded intracellular **organelles,** among them the nucleus.

Nucleus

The **nucleus,** which is surrounded by the cytoplasm and is generally located in the center of the cell, is the largest membrane-bounded organelle. Two membranes comprise the **nuclear envelope** (Fig. 1-2, *A*). The outer membrane is continuous with membranes of the endoplasmic reticulum. The nucleus contains the **nucleolus,** most of the cellular DNA, and the DNA-binding proteins, the histones, that regulate its activity. The length of DNA in eucaryotic cells is so great that the risk of breakage is high. Therefore, the histones that bind to DNA cause the folding of DNA into chromosomes (Fig. 1-2, *C*). The wrapping of DNA into tight packages of chromosomes is essential for cell division in eucaryotes.

The primary function of the nucleus is cell division and control of genetic information. Other functions include the replication and repair of DNA and the transcription of the information stored in DNA. Genetic information is transcribed into RNA, which can be processed into messenger, transport, and ribosomal RNA and introduced into the cytoplasm, where it directs cellular activities. Most of the processing of RNA occurs in the nucleolus. (The role of DNA and RNA in protein synthesis is discussed in Chapter 4.)

Cytoplasmic Organelles

Cytoplasm is an aqueous solution (cytosol) that fills the intracellular compartment known as the **cytoplasmic matrix**—the space between the nuclear envelope and the plasma membrane. The organelles suspended in the cytoplasm are enclosed in biologic membranes, which enables them simultaneously to carry out func-

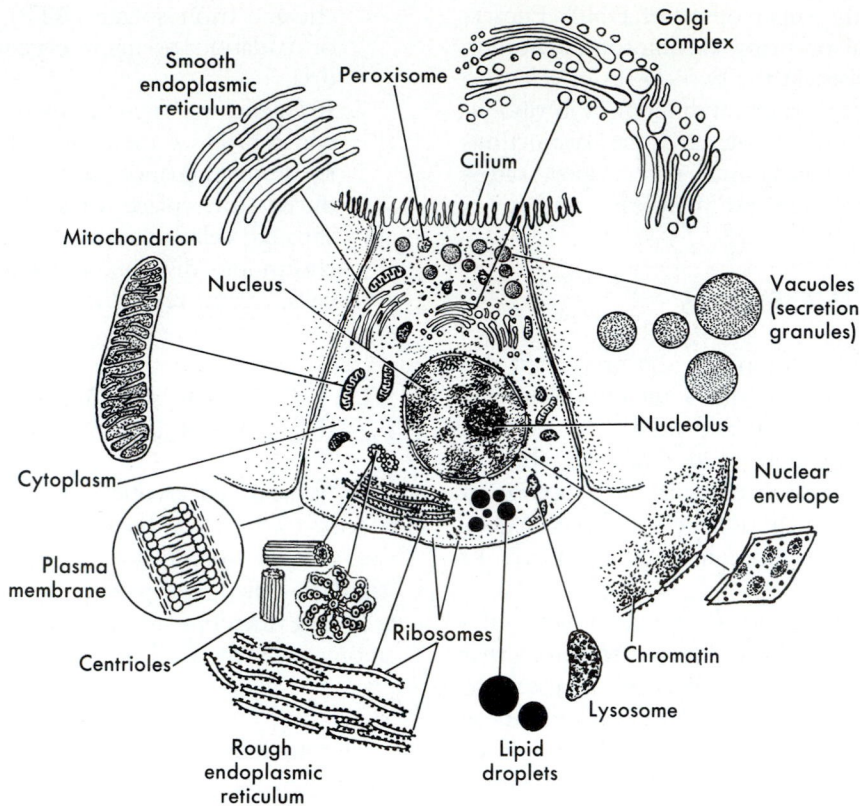

FIG. 1-1. Typical components of a eucaryotic cell.

tions that require different biochemical environments. These functions, many of which are directed by coded messages carried from the nucleus by RNA, include synthesis of proteins and hormones and their transport out of the cell, isolation and elimination of waste products from the cell, metabolic processes, breakdown and disposal of cellular debris and foreign proteins (antigens), and maintenance of cellular structure and motility.

Ribosomes

Ribosomes are RNA-protein complexes (nucleoproteins) that are synthesized in the nucleolus and secreted into the cytoplasm, possibly through pores in the nuclear envelope. These tiny organelles may float free in the cytoplasm or attach themselves to the outer membranes of the endoplasmic reticulum (see Fig. 1-1). Their chief function is to provide sites for cellular protein synthesis.

Endoplasmic Reticulum

The **endoplasmic reticulum** (*endo* = within; *plasm* = cytoplasm; *reticulum* = network) is a membrane factory that specializes in the synthesis and transport of the protein and lipid components of most of the cell's organelles. It consists of a network of tubular or saclike channels (cisternae) that extend throughout the cyto-

plasm and are continuous with the outer nuclear membrane (see Fig. 1-1). The folded membranes that form the cisternae of the endoplasmic reticulum may be rough (granular) or smooth (agranular). The rough endoplasmic reticulum is "rough" because ribosomes and ribonucleoprotein particles are attached to it (Fig. 1-3). Some of the proteins synthesized by these ribosomes remain in the endoplasmic reticulum, and others are used to construct membranes of other organelles (the Golgi complex, lysosomes, peroxisomes, nucleus) and of the cell itself.

Smooth endoplasmic reticulum does not contain ribosomes or ribonucleoprotein particles (see Fig. 1-1). Rather, membranous surfaces of the smooth endoplasmic reticulum contain enzymes involved in the synthesis of steriod hormones and are responsible for a variety of reactions required to remove toxic substances from the cell. The endoplasmic reticulum communicates with the Golgi complex and interacts with other organelles, particularly lysosomes and peroxisomes.

Golgi Complex

The **Golgi complex** (or **Golgi apparatus**) is a network of flattened, smooth membranes and vesicles frequently located near the nucleus of the cell (Fig. 1-4). Proteins from the endoplasmic reticulum are processed

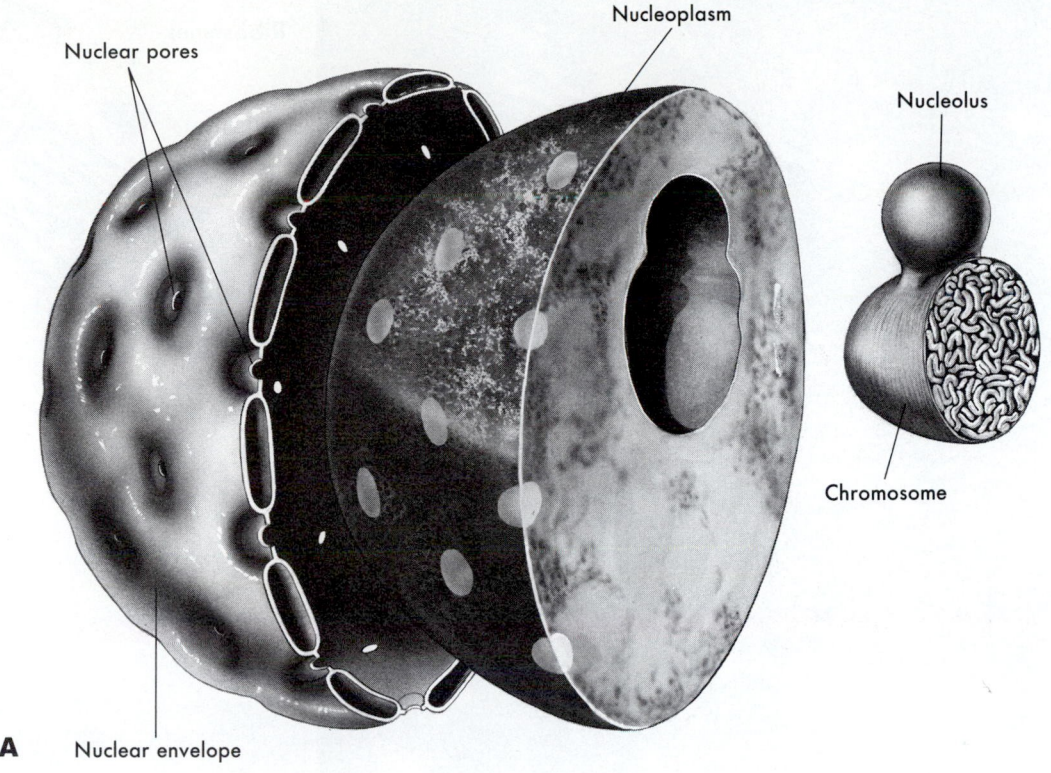

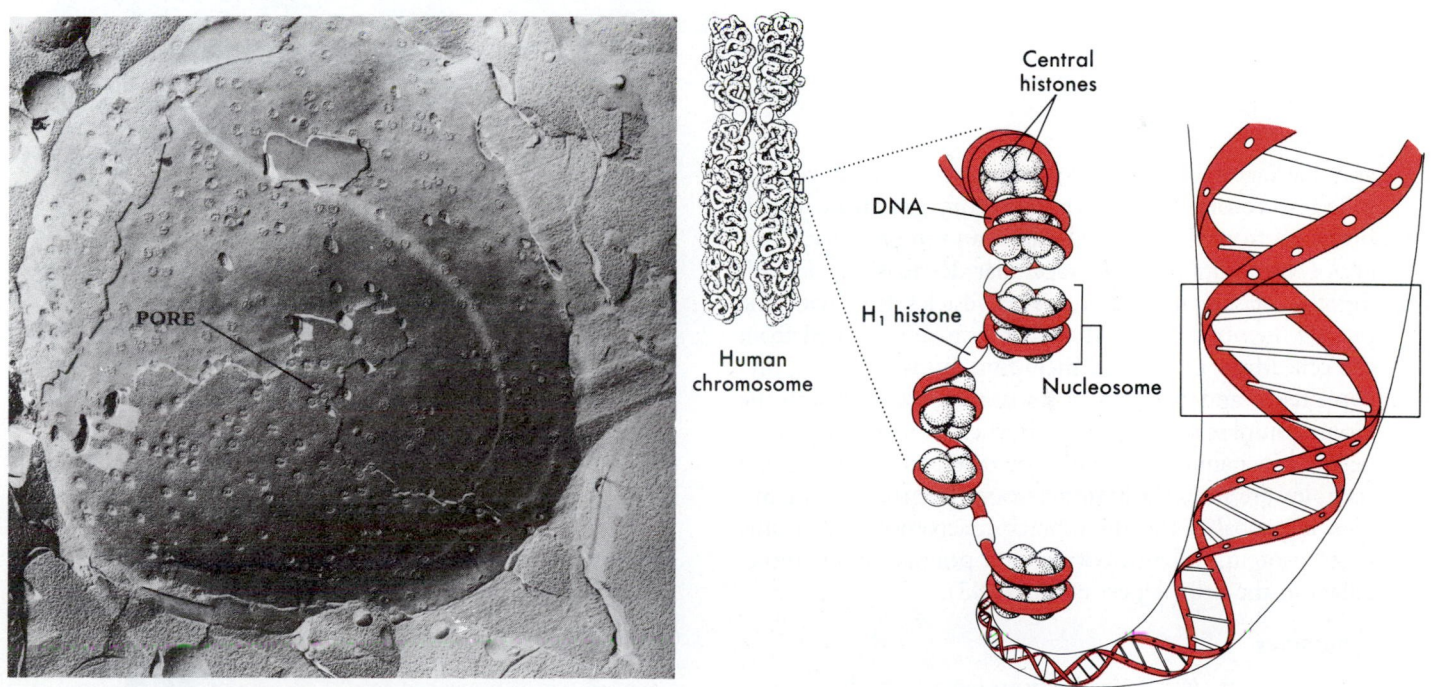

FIG. 1-2. Nucleus. The nucleus is composed of a double membrane, called a nuclear envelope, that encloses the fluid-filled interior, called nucleoplasm. The chromosomes are suspended in the nucleoplasm (here shown much larger than real size to show the tightly packed DNA strands). Swelling at one or more points of the chromosome, shown in **A,** occurs at a nucleolus where genes are being copied into RNA. The nuclear envelope is studded with pores. The pores are visible as dimples in this freeze etch, **B,** of a nuclear envelope. **C,** Histone folding DNA in chromosomes. (From Raven & Johnson, 1986.)

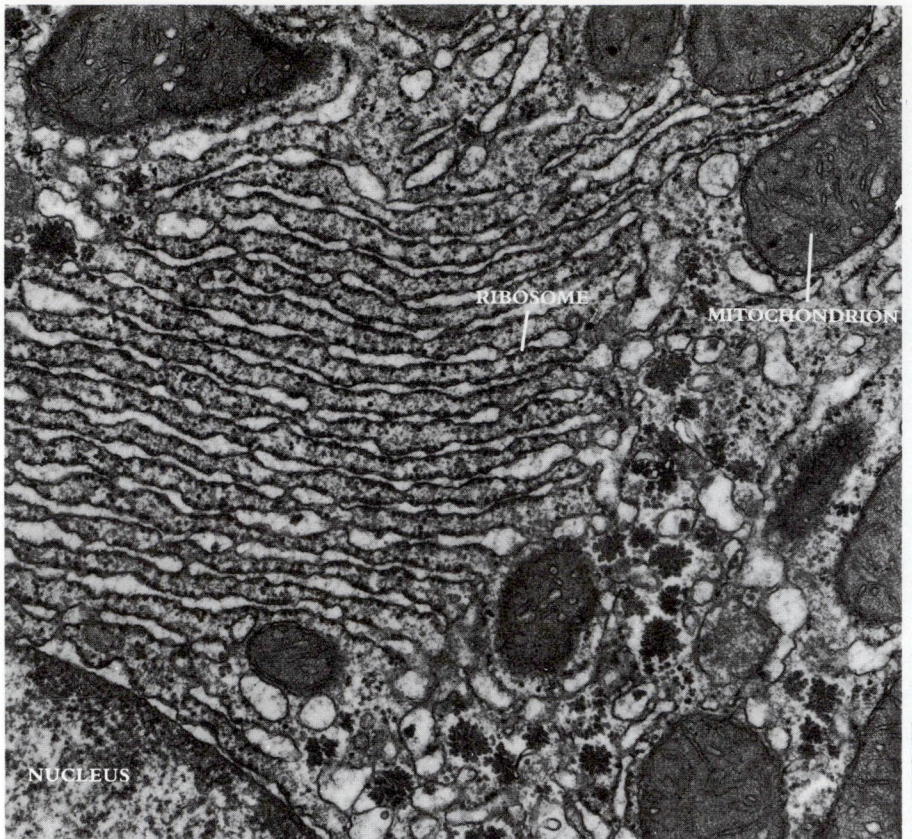

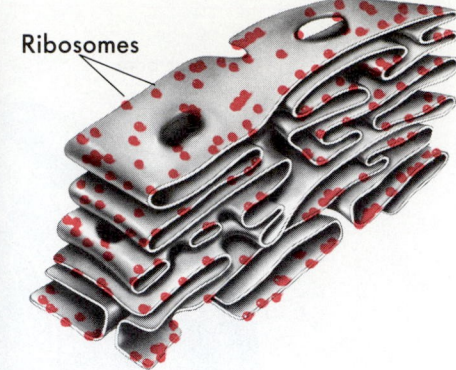

Ribosomes

RIBOSOME

MITOCHONDRION

NUCLEUS

FIG. 1-3. Electron micrograph and diagram of rough endoplasmic reticulum. (From Raven & Johnson, 1986.)

and packaged into small, membrane-bounded vesicles called **secretory vesicles** or **secretory granules,** which break off from the Golgi complex and migrate to a variety of intracellular and extracellular destinations, including the plasma membrane. The vesicles fuse with the plasma membrane, and their contents are released from the cell. Many molecules, including lipids, proteins, glycoproteins, and enzymes of lysosomes, pass through the Golgi complex at some stage in their maturation.

The biochemical changes that take place in the Golgi complex are not clearly understood, but the Golgi complex is probably the director of macromolecular traffic (e.g., protein, polynucleotide, and polysaccharide molecules) in the cell (Alpert et al., 1983).

Lysosomes

Lysosomes (*lyso* = dissolution; *soma* = body) are saclike structures that originate from the Golgi complex (Fig. 1-5; see also Fig. 1-1). They contain over 40 digestive enzymes called hydrolases, which catalyze the hydrolytic cleavage of carbon-oxygen, carbon-nitrogen, carbon-sulfur, and oxygen-phosphorus bonds in proteins, lipids, nucleic acids, and carbohydrates. Lyso-

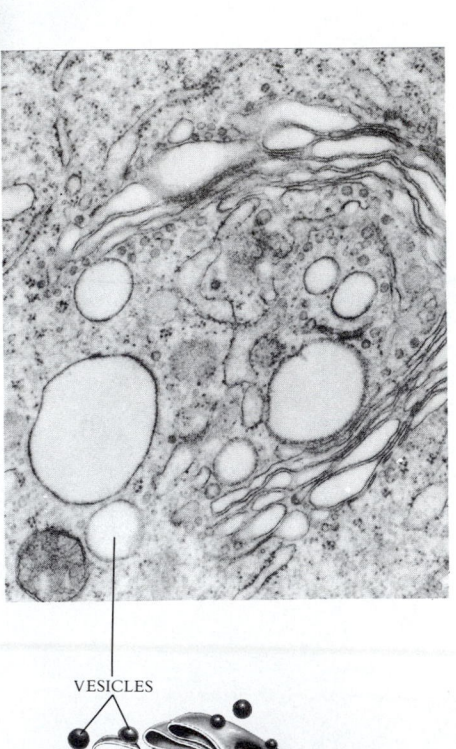

VESICLES

FIG. 1-4. Electron micrograph and diagram of the Golgi complex. (From Raven & Johnson, 1986.)

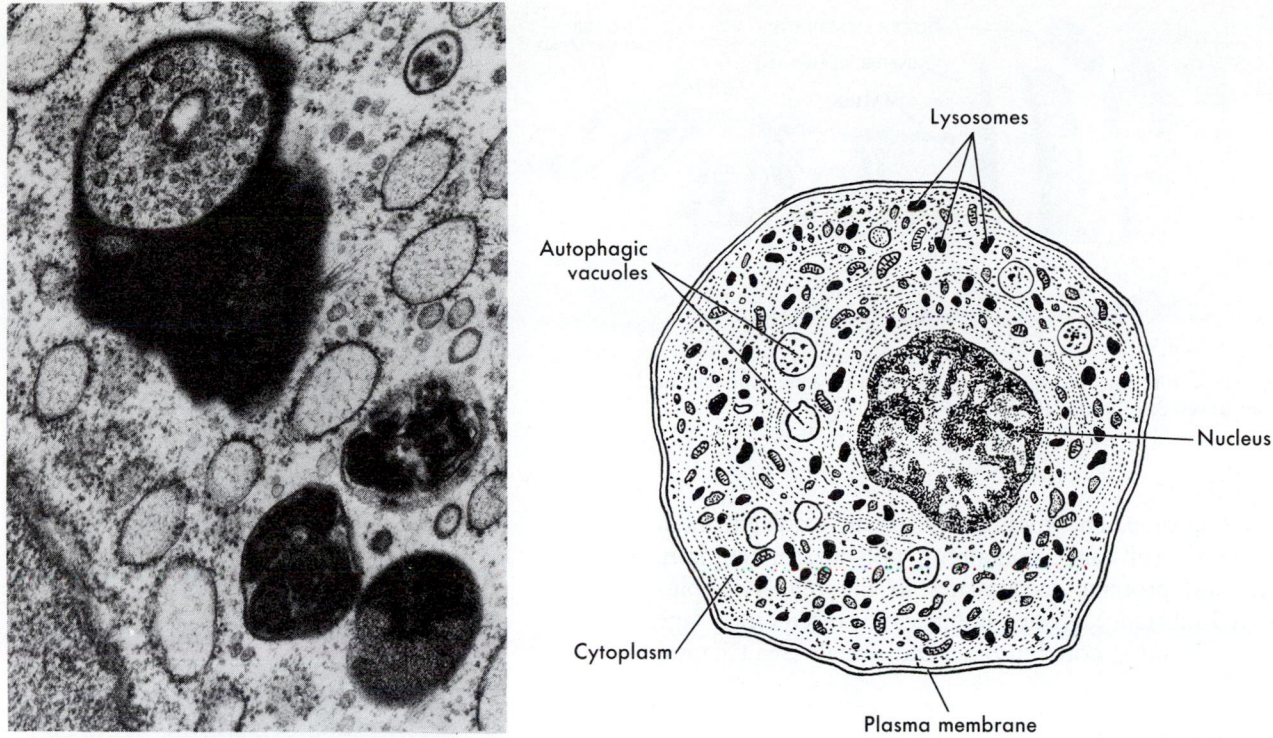

FIG. 1-5. Electron micrograph and diagram of lysosomes in a white blood cell. (Electron micrograph from Kissane, 1985.)

somes function as the intracellular digestive system. Lysosomal enzymes are capable of digesting most cellular constituents down to their basic forms, such as amino acids, fatty acids, and sugars.

The lysosomal membrane acts as a protective shield between the powerful digestive enzymes within the lysosome and the cytoplasm, preventing their leakage into the cytoplasmic matrix. Disruption of the membrane by various treatments or cellular injury leads to a release of the lysosomal enzymes, which can then react with their specific substrates, causing cellular self-digestion. Lysosomal abnormalities are involved in a number of conditions that involve cellular injury and death.

Lysosomal storage diseases may be due to a genetic defect or lack of one or more lysosomal enzymes. For example, the lack of lysosomal alpha-1,4-glucosidase, leads to an accumulation of glycogen in lysosomes known as Pompe disease. Tay-Sachs disease is characterized by an accumulation of GM_2 ganglioside (a lipid) in lysosomes as a result of the deficiency or absence of lysosomal hexosaminidase A. In gout, undigested uric acid accumulates within lysosomes, damaging the lysosomal membrane. Subsequent enzyme leakage results in cell death and tissue injury.

Lysosomes are necessary for normal digestion of cellular nutrients, intracellular debris, and potentially harmful extracellular substances that must be removed from the body. Extracellular substances are taken into the cell and encapsulated in a membrane-bounded vesicle. Lysosomes merge with the vesicle to form a digestive vacuole. Merging releases lysosomal enzymes into the vacuole, and the foreign substance is digested and converted to products that can enter the cytoplasm and be used by the cell. **Primary lysosomes** are lysosomes that have not merged with encapsulated foreign substances and whose enzymes are not as yet involved in the digestive process. **Secondary lysosomes** (digestive vacuoles) are those in which digestion is under way.

As cells complete their life span and die, lysosomes digest the resultant cellular debris. Lysosomes involved in this process, which is called **autodigestion,** are called **autolysosomes.** In living cells, cellular debris is encapsulated within a vesicle that reacts with a lysosome to complete its degradation. This process is called **autophagy.** Autophagy also occurs during starvation, enabling the cell to use a part of its own substance for fuel without doing itself irreparable harm.

Products of autophagy (and of phagocytosis, the ingestion of harmful foreign substances, see Chapter 7) pass out of the lysosome and are reused by the cell. Indigestible material is stored in vesicles called **residual bodies,** whose contents are actively expelled from the cell (see Fig. 1-20). High concentrations of lipids may accumulate within the residual bodies and remain there

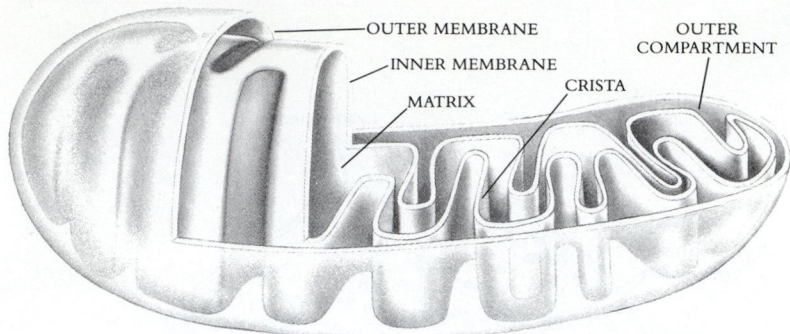

OUTER MEMBRANE
INNER MEMBRANE
MATRIX
CRISTA
OUTER COMPARTMENT

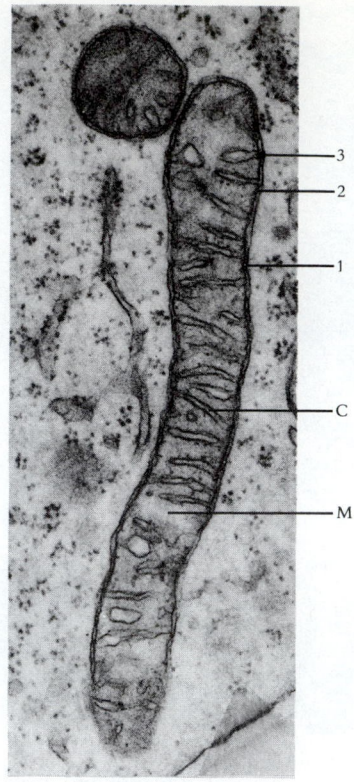

3
2
1
C
M

FIG. 1-6. Electron micrograph and diagram of a mitochondrion. (From Raven & Johnson, 1986.)

for a long time. The lipids are eventually oxidized, and a pigmented substance containing polyunsaturated fatty acids and proteins accumulates in the cell. This pigmented substance, termed lipofuscin, is often called "age pigment" and is noted in older individuals (see Chapter 2).

Peroxisomes

Peroxisomes (microbodies) are similar to lysosomes in microscopic appearance, but they are larger and oval or irregular in shape. Peroxisomes contain several enzymes that either produce or use hydrogen peroxide, for example, the enzyme catalase, which accelerates, or catalyzes, the conversion of two hydrogen peroxides to water and oxygen. Hydrogen peroxide is produced in the peroxisomes by enzymes that oxidize D-amino acids, uric acid, and various 1-hydroxy acids. Beyond their participation in metabolic oxidations involving hydrogen peroxide, the function of peroxisomes is little understood.

Mitochondria

Mitochondria (*mito* = thread; *chondros* = granule) are of much interest because of their role in cellular energy metabolism (see p. 16). These cytoplasmic organelles appear as spheres, rods, or filamentous bodies that are bounded by a double membrane (Fig. 1-6). The outer membrane is smooth and surrounds the mitochondrion itself; the inner membrane is convoluted in the mitochondrial matrix to form partitions called cristae. The inner membrane contains the enzymes of the respiratory chain—the name given to the electron transport chain. These enzymes are essential to the process of oxidative phosphorylation that generates most of the cell's ATP. Metabolic pathways involved in the metabolism of carbohydrates, lipids, and amino acids, and special pathways involving urea and heme synthesis are located in the mitochondrial matrix.

The outer membrane is permeable (passable) to many substances, but the inner membrane is highly selective and contains many transmembranous transport systems. The inner membrane contains a transporter to move electrically charged calcium (calcium ions) (Devlin, 1982). (Membrane transport is discussed on p. 19.)

Cytoskeleton

All eucaryotic cells contain elaborate and specialized internal structures that provide the "bones and muscles" of the cell—the **cytoskeleton.** The cytoskeleton maintains the cell's shape and internal organization, and it permits movement of substances within the cell and of external projections (cilia or microvilli) from the plasma membrane. The internal skeleton is composed of a network of protein filaments, two of the most important of which are microtubules and actin filaments, or microfilaments.

Microtubules are small, hollow, cylindrical, unbranched tubules made of protein. When found together, microtubules exhibit rigidity, unlike the rest of the cytoplasm. Microtubules thus add strength to the cell's structure (Fig. 1-7, *A*). Within the cell, microtubules support and move organelles from one part of the cytoplasm to another, facilitate transport of impulses along nerve cells, and have roles in the inflammatory and immune responses and hormone secretion. Micro-

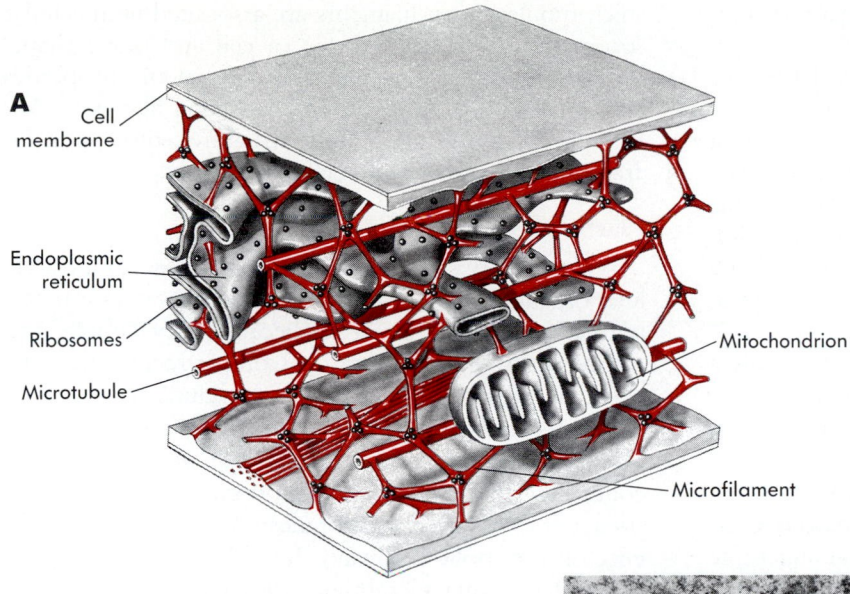

Cell membrane

Endoplasmic reticulum

Ribosomes

Microtubule

Mitochondrion

Microfilament

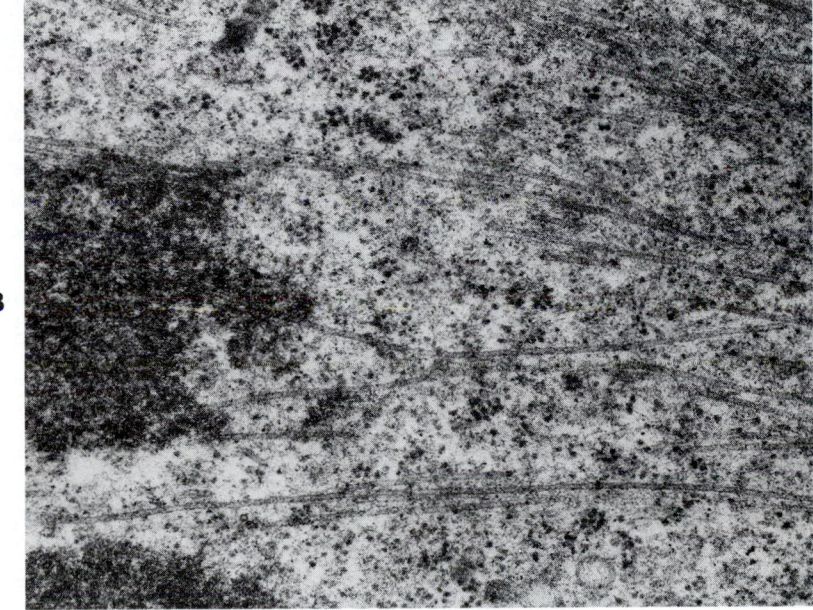

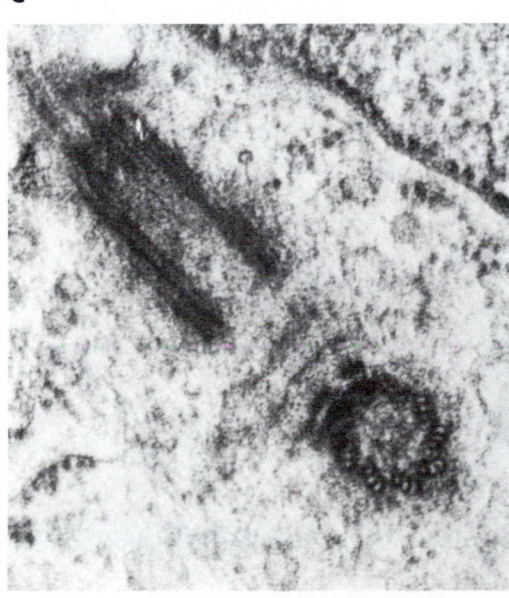

FIG. 1-7. Cytoskeletal organelles. **A,** Network of mitochondria, ribosomes, and endoplasmic reticulum supported by a network of filaments, through which pass microtubules. **B,** Microtubules of mitotic spindle. **C,** Pair of centrioles oriented at right angles to each other. (**A** from Raven & Johnson, 1986. **B** and **C** from Kissane, 1985.)

tubules are also involved in external movement, or motility, of some cells.

Microtubules are arranged in the thickened base, or **basal body,** of a protrusion from the cell's plasma membrane. This arrangement occurs in the basal bodies of sperm flagella and the cilia of certain other cells. The long, whiplike flagella enable sperm cells to move. Cilia usually move substances past the cell, which remains stationary. For example, cilia on cells lining the respiratory tract move together to "beat" mucus toward the throat so that it can be removed by coughing.

While the cell is not in the process of division, only a few microtubules are assembled; cellular division (mitosis) or defense (phagocytosis) does, however, induce a cycle of rapid assembly and disassembly. Microtubules involved in cellular division are arranged as shown in Fig. 1-7, *C.* This arrangement is called a **centriole.** Centrioles always consist of nine bundles containing three microtubules each. During division, the pairs of centrioles split and migrate to opposite poles of the cell (see p. 29).

Alterations of microtubular function are implicated in disease processes. For example, defective protein synthesis has been related to a decreased number of microtubules as a result of increased cellular levels of acetaldehyde (a product of alcohol metabolism) found in chronic alcoholism.

Actin filaments (microfilaments) are smaller fibrils that generally occur in bundles rather than singly. Like microtubules, actin filaments are associated with cellular locomotion and maintenance of cell and tissue shape. Cellular locomotion depends on contractile properties that involve both microtubules and actin filaments. Anesthetic drugs can affect both structures, disrupting intracellular movement and cellular motility.

Plasma Membranes

Whether they surround the cell or enclose an intracellular organelle, membranes are exceedingly important to normal physiologic function because they control the composition of the space, or compartment, they enclose. Membranes can include or exclude a variety of molecules and because of selective transport systems, they can move molecules into or out of the space. By controlling the movement of substances from one compartment to another, membranes exert a powerful influence on metabolic pathways. In addition to these functions, the plasma membrane has an important role in cell-to-cell recognition. For example, protein receptors for hormones and for other chemical signals are associated with the membrane and act as markers that identify a cell to its neighbors. Other functions of the plasma membrane include cellular mobility and the maintenance of cellular shape (Table 1-1).

Plasma membranes are usually thicker than the membranes of intracellular organelles. The outer surfaces of plasma membranes in many cells are not smooth but are studded with cilia or even smaller cylindrical projections

---

TABLE 1-1 Plasma membrane functions

Cellular mechanism	Membrane functions
Structure	Containment of cellular organelles
	Maintenance of relationship with cytoskeleton, endoplasmic reticulum, and other organelles
	Maintenance of fluid and electrolyte balance
Protection	Barrier to toxic molecules and macromolecules (proteins, nucleic acid, polysaccharides)
	Barrier to foreign organisms and cells
Activation of cell	Hormones (regulation of cellular activity)
	Mitogens (cellular division, see Chapter 4)
	Antigens (antibody synthesis, see Chapter 8)
	Growth factors (proliferation and differentiation, see Chapter 10)
Transport	Diffusion and exchange diffusion
	Endocytosis (pinocytosis and phagocytosis)
	Exocytosis (secretion)
	Active transport
Cell-to-cell interaction	Communication and attachment at junctional complexes
	Symbiotic nutritive relationships
	Release of enzymes and antibodies to extracellular environment
	Relationships with extracellular matrix

Adapted from King, Fenoglio, & Lefkowitch, 1983.

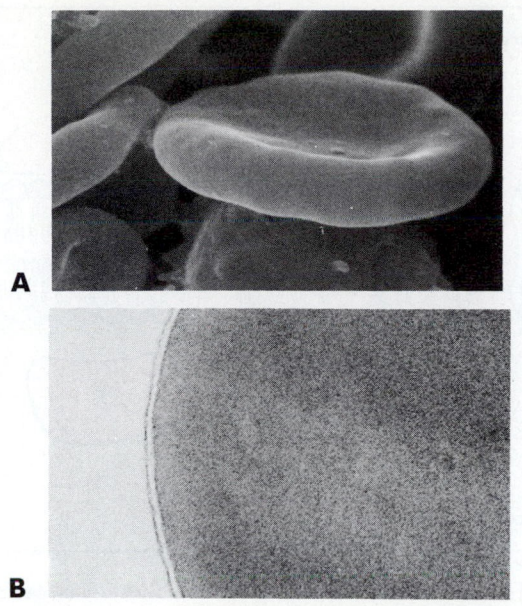

FIG. 1-8. A, Human red blood cell, **B,** is encased with a membrane bilayer, which is clearly visible in the electron micrograph. (From Raven & Johnson, 1986.)

called microvilli, both of which are capable of movement.

Membrane Composition

The major chemical components of all membranes are lipids and proteins, but the percentage of each varies among different membranes. Lipid molecules are the most abundant, but the protein molecules are so large that in total mass these two constituents are roughly equal. The structure of a plasma membrane is shown in Fig. 1-8. Intracellular membranes have a higher percentage of proteins than plasma membranes, presumably because most enzymatic activity occurs within organelles. Carbohydrates are mainly associated with plasma membranes, where they are combined chemically with lipids, forming glycolipids, and, with proteins, forming glycoproteins.

Lipids

The basic component of the plasma membrane is a bilayer of lipid molecules—phospholipids, glycolipids, and cholesterol (respective ratios 70:5:25). The lipids are responsible for the structural integrity of the membrane. Each lipid molecule is said to be polar, or **amphipathic.** An amphipathic molecule is one in which

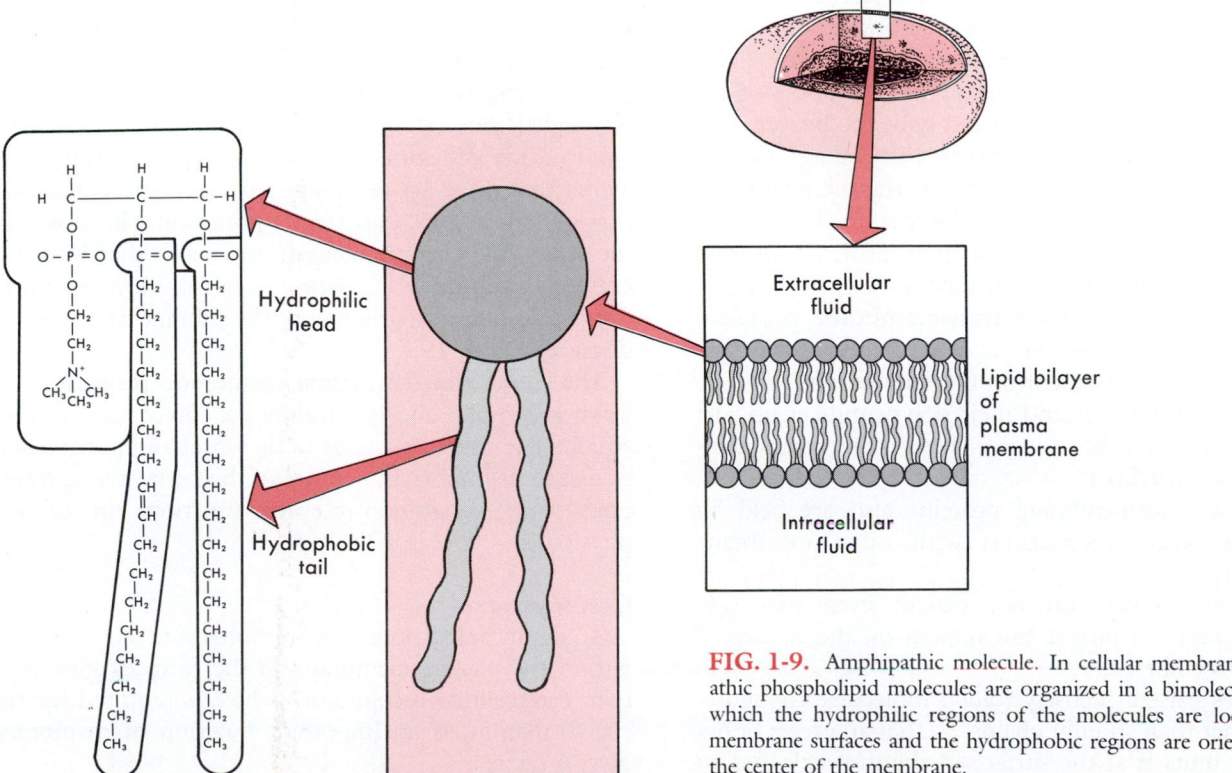

FIG. 1-9. Amphipathic molecule. In cellular membranes, amphipathic phospholipid molecules are organized in a bimolecular layer in which the hydrophilic regions of the molecules are located at the membrane surfaces and the hydrophobic regions are oriented toward the center of the membrane.

one part is hydrophobic (uncharged, or "water hating") and another part is hydrophilic (charged, or "water loving") (Fig. 1-9).

The membrane spontaneously organizes itself into a bilayer because of these two incompatible solubilities. The hydrophobic region (hydrophobic tail) of each lipid molecule is protected from water, whereas the hydrophilic region (hydrophilic head) is immersed in it. The bilayer's structure accounts for one of the essential functions of the plasma membrane: it is impermeable to most water-soluble molecules (molecules that dissolve in water) because they are insoluble in the oily core region. The bilayer serves as a barrier to the diffusion of water and hydrophilic substances, while allowing lipid-soluble molecules, such as oxygen (O_2) and carbon dioxide (CO_2), to diffuse through it readily. Because the bilayer is fluid at temperatures above freezing, components of the cellular environment move slowly and selectively across the membrane all the time. (Components of the cellular environment are discussed in Chapter 3.)

Proteins

Recent research suggests two ways to classify membrane proteins. One way is classification as peripheral or integral proteins (Alpert et al., 1983) (see Fig. 1-12). **Integral membrane proteins** are those embedded in the lipid bilayer, primarily because of hydrophobic interactions with the bilayer. The integral proteins can only be removed from the membrane by detergents that solubilize (dissolve) the lipid. **Peripheral membrane proteins** are not embedded in the bilayer but reside at one surface or the other, bound to an integral protein.

Although the classification of membrane proteins as peripheral or integral is commonly used, it does not describe how proteins are associated with the bilayer. The second mode of classification does so by taking into account the membrane-spanning, or transmembranous, nature of membrane proteins (Alpert et al., 1983) (Fig. 1-10). According to this classification, proteins are associated with the lipid bilayer in four ways:

1. Some proteins, called **transmembrane proteins,** extend across the bilayer and are exposed to an aqueous environment on both sides of it.
2. Some proteins extend their polypeptide chain part way through the bilayer. (These are not transmembrane proteins.)
3. Some transmembrane proteins also are held by noncovalent interactions with other membrane proteins.
4. Some proteins do not extend even part way through the bilayer but remain on the surface of the membrane.

Proteins exist in densely folded molecular configurations rather than straight chains, so that an excess of hydrophilic units is at the surface of the molecule and an

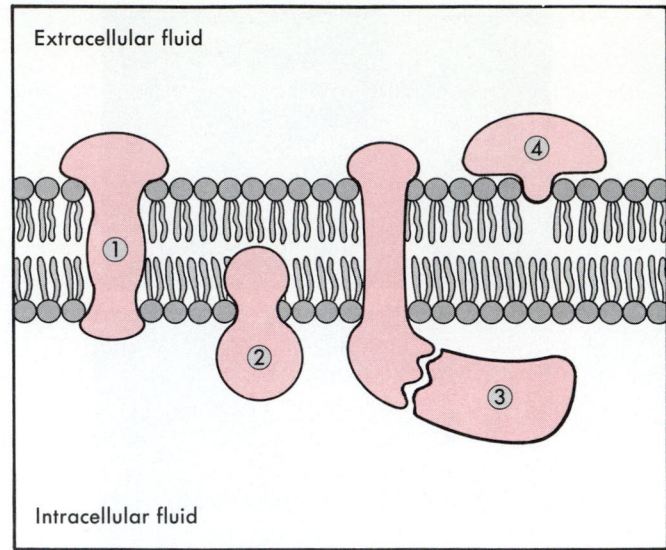

FIG. 1-10. Four ways in which proteins in the lipid bilayer can be associated with the bilayer: (1) some proteins extend across the bilayer; (2) some proteins have one or more covalently attached fatty acid chains that help embed the protein in one layer or the other; (3) some transmembrane proteins are held by noncovalent interactions with other membrane proteins; and (4) some proteins are not embedded in the lipid bilayer at all.

excess of hydrophobic units is inside. Although membrane structure is determined by the lipid bilayer, membrane functions are determined largely by proteins. For example, proteins facilitate transport across membranes by serving as receptors, enzymes, or transporters. Proteins act as (1) recognition and binding units (receptors) for substances moving in and out of the cell, (2) pores or channels for various electrically charged particles called ions or electrolytes, (3) specific carriers for amino acids and monosaccharides, and (4) specific enzymes that drive active pumps that promote concentration of certain ions, particularly potassium (K^+), within the cell, while keeping concentrations of other ions, for example, sodium (Na^+), below concentrations found in the extracellular environment. (Membrane transport is discussed on p. 19.)

The interaction of plasma membrane proteins with lipids is complex and is currently the subject of much research. The role of proteins in the onset and progression of disease is important because of their enzymatic, transport, and recognition-receptor functions in cellular physiology.

Carbohydrates

A significant amount of carbohydrate is contained within the plasma membrane in the form of glycoprotein. Intercellular recognition, which is required for tissue formation, is an important function of membrane glycoproteins.

Membrane Fluidity: The Fluid Mosaic Model

In the 1960s, G. L. Nicholson and S. J. Singer proposed the popular **fluid mosaic model** for biologic membranes (Fig. 1-11). The model, which is continually being modified, presents integral proteins as pieces of a mosaic that float singly or as aggregates in the fluid lipid bilayer. The protein molecules serve to (1) transport other molecules into and out of the cell, (2) facilitate (catalyze) membrane reactions, (3) receive messages, thus acting as receptors for extracellular and intracellular signals, and (4) create structural linkages between the external and internal cellular environments.

The fluid mosaic model accounts for the flexibility of cellular membranes, their self-sealing properties, and their impermeability to many substances. The degree of a membrane's fluidity depends on temperature. At lower temperatures, the lipids are in a gel crystalline state, and at higher temperatures they become highly fluid. These properties are critical for cellular growth, division, and receptor function. Because proteins are free to move within the plasma membranes (like floating icebergs), certain foreign proteins (antigens) may become buried in the bilayer, only to emerge at the surface after injury and attract antibodies (proteins produced by the immune system), that attack host cells. Antigens and antibodies, which are the cause and effect of the immune re-

sponse, are discussed in Chapter 6. The burial and re-emergence of antigens may be one cause of autoimmune disease, which is described in Chapter 8.

In the fluid mosaic model, cellular membranes are dynamic. Not only do lipids and proteins move laterally on the membrane, but ions and other molecules also move through it. The fluid mosaic model is logical in that it describes the entire membrane as existing in a state of change and modulation, which allows the cell to protect itself actively against injurious agents. Hormones, bacteria, viruses, drugs, antibodies, chemicals that transmit nerve impulses (neurotransmitters), and other substances attach to the plasma membrane by means of receptor molecules on its outer layer. The number of receptors present may vary at different times, and the cell is capable of modulating the effects of injurious agents by altering receptor number and pattern (Catt et al., 1979). This aspect of the fluid mosaic model has drastically modified previously held concepts concerning the onset of disease.

The concentration of cholesterol in the plasma membrane affects membrane fluidity. An increased concentration results in less fluidity on the membrane's hydrophilic outer surface and more fluidity at its hydrophobic core. Changes in cholesterol content are factors in some diseases. In cirrhosis of the liver, for example, the cho-

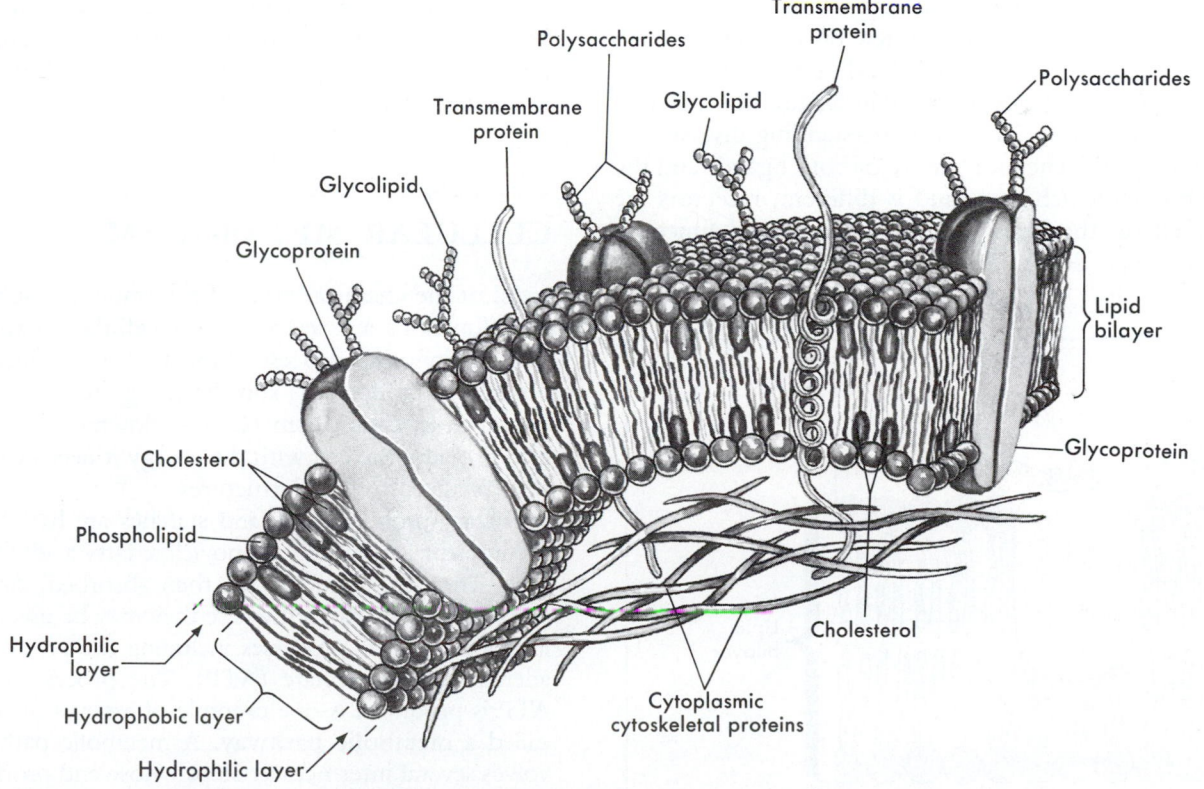

FIG. 1-11. Fluid mosaic model. Schematic, three-dimensional view of the fluid mosaic model of membrane structure. The lipid bilayer provides the basic structure and serves as a relatively impermeable barrier to most water-soluble molecules.

lesterol content of the red blood cell's plasma membrane increases. This causes an overall decrease in membrane fluidity that seriously affects the cell's ability to transport oxygen. The implications of changes in membrane integrity and their role in subsequent disease states are largely unknown. As measurement techniques for studying membrane physiology improve, the pathologic manifestations of many diseases may be explained according to changes in membrane structure and function.

Cellular Receptors

Cellular receptors are protein molecules on the plasma membrane, in the cytoplasm, or in the nucleus that are capable of recognizing and binding with specific smaller molecules called **ligands.** Hormones, for example, are ligands. Recognition and binding depend on the chemical configuration of the receptor and its smaller ligand, which must fit together somewhat like pieces of a jigsaw puzzle.

Plasma membrane receptors are particularly important for cellular uptake of ligands. They protrude from or are exposed at the external surface of the membrane, often attached to integral proteins (Fig. 1-12). Some of these recognition units have all the mobile properties related to membrane fluidity. The ligands that bind with membrane receptors include hormones, neurotransmitters, antigens, complement components, lipoproteins, infectious agents, drugs, and metabolites. The past several years have brought many new discoveries concerning the specific interactions of cellular receptors with their respective ligands. In many instances, this information has provided a basis for understanding disease.

Although the chemical nature of both ligands and the receptors to which they bind is different, receptors are classified on the basis of their location and function. Cellular type determines overall cellular function, but plasma membrane receptors determine which ligands a cell will bind with and how the cell will respond to binding with each. For example, the ability of a hormone or a neurotransmitter to stimulate a cell is regulated by the specificity and number of receptors present on the plasma membrane. Specific processes also control intracellular mechanisms. Hormone binding, for example, depends on special messenger molecules that regulate protein synthesis within the cell (see Chapter 17). Neurotransmitters (discussed in Chapter 12) also operate by causing special messengers to react with specific receptors (Snyder, 1985).

Receptors for different drugs are found on the plasma membrane, in the cytoplasm, and in the nucleus. Membrane receptors have been found for certain anesthetics, opiates, endorphins, enkephalins, antibiotics, cancer chemotherapeutic agents, digitalis, and other drugs. Membrane receptors for endorphins, which are opiate-like peptides isolated from the pituitary gland, are found in large quantities in pain pathways of the nervous system (see Chapter 12). With binding, the endorphins (or drugs like morphine) change the cell's permeability to ions, increase the concentration of molecules that regulate intracellular protein synthesis, and initiate molecular events that modulate pain perception.

Receptors for infectious microorganisms, or antigen receptors, bind bacteria, viruses, and parasites. Antigen receptors on white blood cells (lymphocytes, monocytes, macrophages, and granulocytes) recognize and bind with antigenic microorganisms and activate the immune and inflammatory responses (see Chapters 6 and 7).

CELLULAR METABOLISM

All of the chemical tasks of maintaining essential cellular functions are referred to as **cellular metabolism.** The energy-using process of metabolism is called **anabolism** (*ana* = upward) and the energy-releasing process is known as **catabolism** (*kata* = downward). Metabolism provides the cell with the energy it needs to synthesize (produce) cellular structures.

Dietary proteins, fats, and starches are hydrolized in the intestinal tract into amino acids, fatty acids, and glucose. These constituents are then absorbed, circulated, and taken up by the cell where they may be used for various vital cellular processes including the production of adenosine triphosphate (ATP). The process by which ATP is produced is one example of a series of reactions called a **metabolic pathway.** A metabolic pathway involves several intermediate steps whose end products are not always detectable. A key feature of cellular metabolism is the directing of biochemical reactions by protein catalysts, or enzymes. Most biochemical reactions in a pathway are catalyzed by a specific enzyme. Each en-

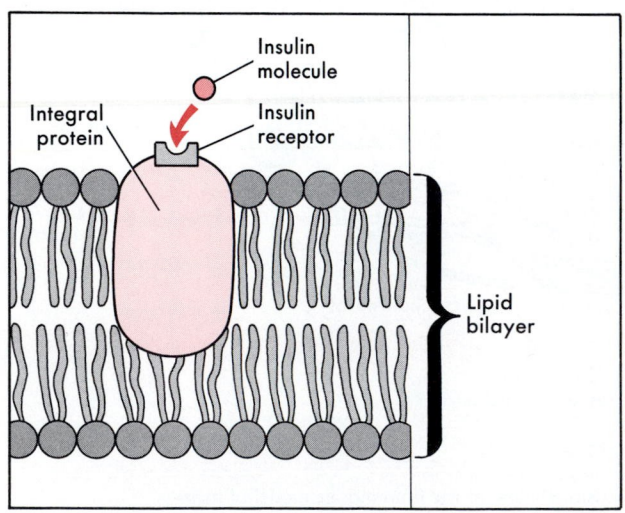

FIG. 1-12. Plasma membrane receptor for a ligand (here, a hormone molecule) on the surface of an integral protein.

zyme has a high affinity for a **substrate**—a specific substance that is converted to a product of the reaction.

Role of Adenosine Triphosphate

For a cell to function, the cell must be able to extract and use the chemical energy contained within the structure of organic molecules. When a mole of glucose is metabolically broken down in the presence of oxygen into carbon dioxide and water, 686 kilocalories (kcal) of energy is released. In a test tube, this energy is released as heat. Because a cell cannot transform heat into work, chemical energy, rather than heat, is created by metabolism. The chemical energy lost by one molecule is transferred to the chemical structure of another molecule by an energy-carrying or transferring molecule, such as ATP. The energy stored in ATP can be used in a variety of energy-requiring reactions and in the process is gen-

erally converted to adenosine diphosphate (ADP) and inorganic phosphate (Pi). The energy available as a result of this reaction is about 7 kcal/mol of ATP. In addition to its use in synthesis (anabolism) of organic molecules, ATP is used by the cell for muscle contraction and active transport of molecules across cellular membranes. The function of ATP is not only to *store* energy but also to *transfer* it from one molecule to another. Energy is stored by molecules of carbohydrate, lipid, and protein, which, when catabolized, transfer energy to ATP.

Food and the Production of Cellular Energy

The process of catabolism of the proteins, lipids, and polysaccharides found in food can be divided into three phases (Fig. 1-13). In phase 1, large molecules are broken down into their smaller subunits—proteins into

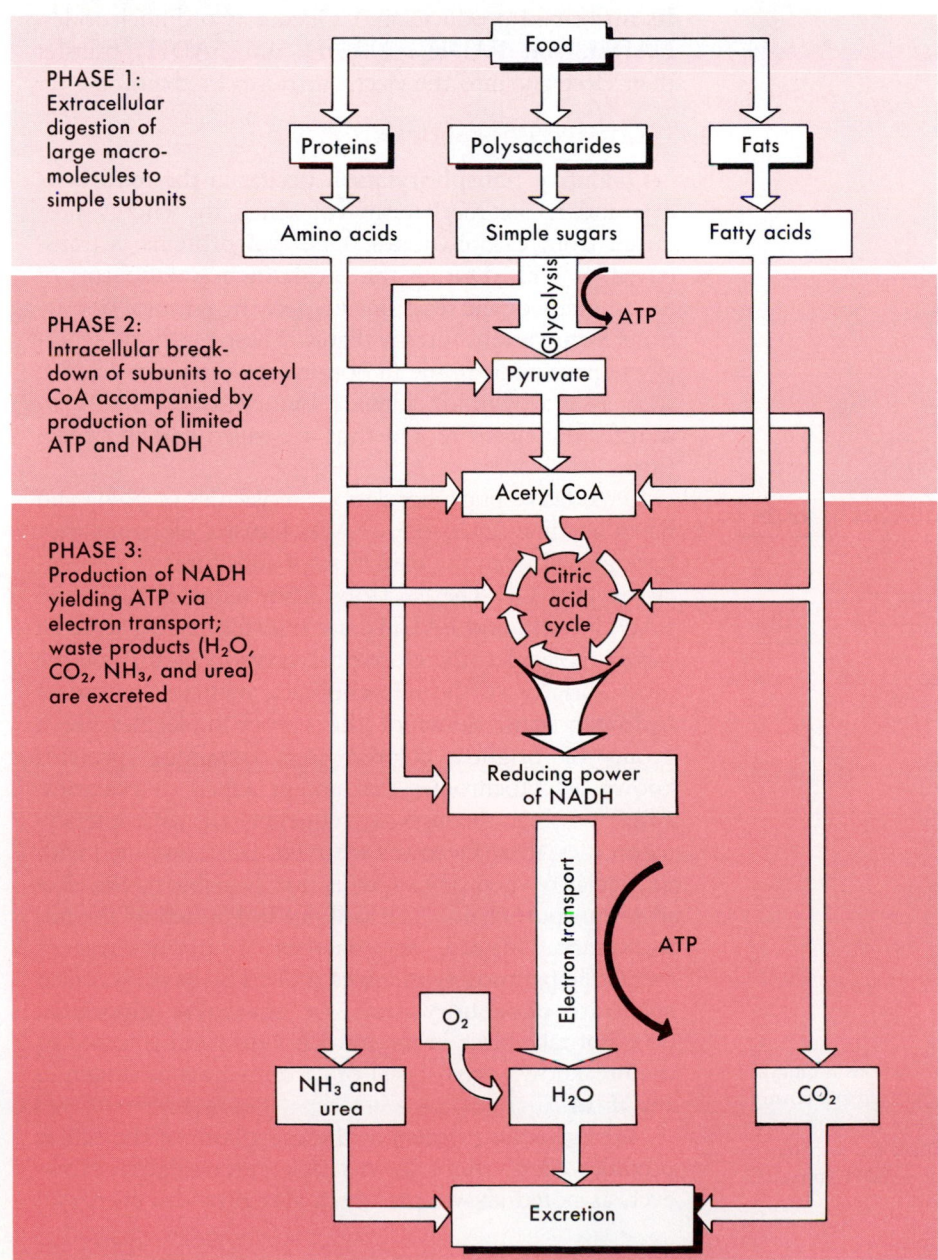

PHASE 1:
Extracellular digestion of large macromolecules to simple subunits

PHASE 2:
Intracellular breakdown of subunits to acetyl CoA accompanied by production of limited ATP and NADH

PHASE 3:
Production of NADH yielding ATP via electron transport; waste products (H_2O, CO_2, NH_3, and urea) are excreted

FIG. 1-13. Three phases of catabolism, which leads from food to waste products. These reactions produce ATP, which is used to drive other processes in the cell. (Adapted from Alpert et al., 1983.)

amino acids, polysaccharides into simple sugars, and fats into fatty acids and glycerol. These processes are called **digestion** and occur outside of the cell by the action of secreted enzymes.

In phase 2, the small molecules enter cells and are further broken down in the cytoplasm. Most of the sugars are converted into pyruvate. Pyruvate then enters mitochondria and is converted to the acetyl groups of acetyl coenzyme A (acetyl CoA). Acetyl CoA, like ATP, releases energy when it is hydrolyzed. The most important part of phase 2 is the lysis (splitting) of glucose, known as **glycolysis** (Fig. 1-14). Glycolysis produces a net of two molecules of ATP per glucose molecule through the process of **oxidation,** or the removal and transfer of a pair of electrons. This process, often called **oxidative**

cellular metabolism, involves nine biochemical reactions. In reactions 1 to 4, glucose is converted to the three-carbon aldehyde (glyceraldehyde 3-phosphate), which requires energy in the form of ATP. In reactions 5 and 6, the aldehyde group of the glyceraldehyde 3-phosphate is oxidized (loses electrons) to carboxylic acid, and the energy from this reaction creates a new high-energy phosphate (ATP) for each molecule of aldehyde. In reactions 7, 8, and 9, a net profit of two molecules of ATP per glucose molecule is produced.

Phase 3 occurs when the acetyl group of acetyl CoA is completely degraded to carbon dioxide (CO_2) and water (H_2O). It is in this final phase that most of the ATP is generated. Phase 3 begins with the **citric acid cycle** (also called the **Krebs cycle,** or the **tricarboxylic acid cycle**) and ends with oxidative phosphorylation. The citric acid cycle accounts for approximately two thirds of the total oxidation of carbon compounds in most cells. Its major end products are CO_2 and two dinucleotides, NADH, and $FADH_2$. NADH and $FADH_2$ transfer their electrons into the electron transport chain.

Oxidative Phosphorylation

Oxidative phosphorylation occurs in the mitochondria and is the mechanism by which the energy produced from carbohydrates, fats, and proteins is transferred to ATP. During the breakdown (catabolism) of foods, many of the reactions involve the removal of electrons from various intermediates. These reactions generally require a coenzyme (a nonprotein carrier molecule), such as nicotinamide adenine dinucleotide (NAD), to transfer the electrons and thus are called **transfer reactions.**

In oxidative phosphorylation, molecules of NAD and flavin adenine nucleotide (FAD) transfer electrons they have gained from the oxidation of substrates to molecular oxygen, O_2. The electrons from reduced NAD and FAD, NADH and $FADH_2$, are transferred to a series of carrier molecules (the **electron-transport chain**), on the inner surfaces of the mitochondria with the release of hydrogen ions. Some of the carrier molecules are a group of brightly colored iron-containing proteins known as cytochromes that accept a pair of electrons. After passing through a sequence of different cytochromes, these electrons are eventually combined with molecular oxygen. If oxygen is not available to the electron-transport chain, ATP will not be formed by the mitochondria. Instead, an anaerobic (without oxygen) metabolic pathway synthesizes ATP. This process, called **substrate phosphorylation,** or **anaerobic glycolysis,** does not take place in the mitochondria and is linked to the breakdown (glycolysis) of carbohydrate as shown in Fig. 1-14.

Since glycolysis occurs in the cytoplasm of the cell, it provides energy for cells that lack mitochondria. However, as noted above, glycolysis also provides energy to

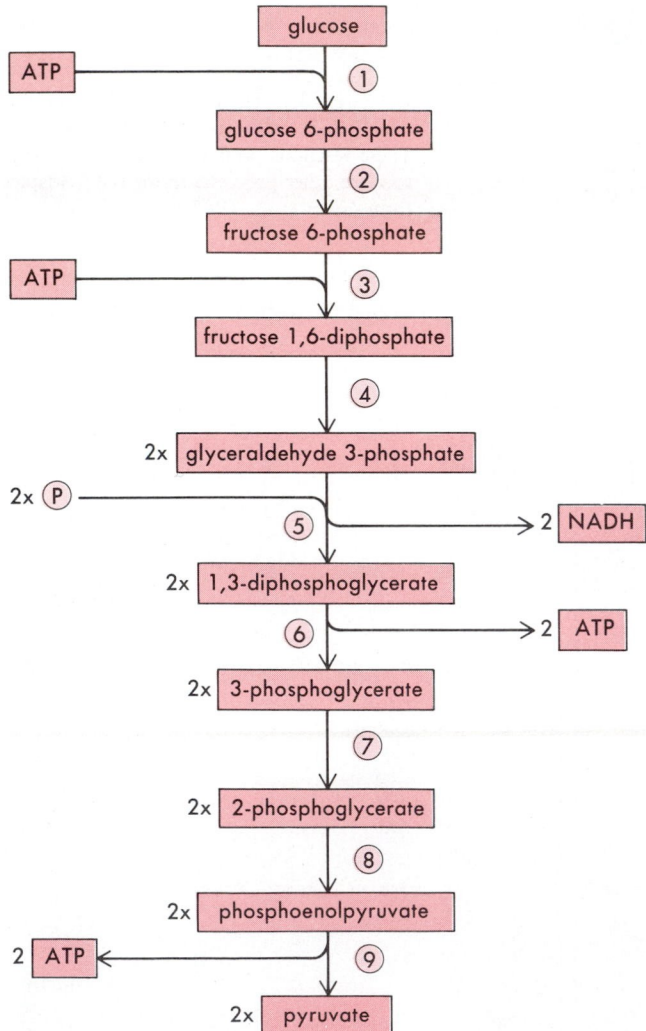

FIG. 1-14. Glycolysis. Each of the numbered reactions is catalyzed by a different enzyme. At step 4, a six-carbon sugar is broken down to give two three-carbon sugars, so that the number of molecules at every step after this is doubled. Reactions 5 and 6 are the reactions responsible for the net synthesis of ATP and NADH molecules. (Adapted from Alpert et al., 1983.)

the cell when oxygen delivery is insufficient or delayed. The reactions in anaerobic glycolysis involve the conversion of glucose to pyruvic acid (pyruvate) with the simultaneous production of ATP. With the glycolysis of one molecule of glucose, two ATP molecules and two molecules of pyruvate are liberated. If oxygen is present, the two molecules of pyruvate move into the mitochondria, where they enter the citric acid cycle. If oxygen is absent, pyruvate is converted to lactic acid and released into the extracellular fluid. The conversion of pyruvic acid to lactic acid is reversible; therefore, once oxygen is restored, lactic acid is quickly converted back to either pyruvic acid or glucose. The anaerobic generation of ATP from glucose, through the reactions of glycolysis, is not as efficient as aerobic generation of ATP. The addition of an oxygen-requiring stage to the catabolic process (stage 3) provides cells with a much more powerful method for extracting energy from food molecules.

PROCESSES OF CELLULAR INTAKE AND OUTPUT

Cells continually take in nutrients, fluids, and chemical messengers from the extracellular environment and expel metabolites or the products of metabolism and end products of lysosomal digestion. Intake and output, or transport, occurs by different mechanisms, depending on the characteristics of the substance to be transported. Water and small, electrically uncharged molecules move easily through pores in the plasma membrane's lipid bilayer. This process, called **passive transport,** will occur naturally through any semipermeable barrier. It is driven by osmosis, hydrostatic pressure, and diffusion, all of which depend on the laws of physics and do not require life. The process is passive in that it does not require any expenditure of energy by the cell.

Other molecules cannot be driven across the plasma membrane solely by forces of diffusion, hydrostatic pressure, or osmosis because they are too large or are ligands that have bound with receptors on the cell's plasma membrane. Some of these molecules are moved into the cell by mechanisms of **active transport,** which requires life, biologic activity, and the expenditure of metabolic energy by the cell. Unlike passive transport, which can be duplicated across any semipermeable barrier in a laboratory, active transport only occurs across living membranes that (1) use energy generated by cellular metabolism and (2) have receptors that are capable of recognizing and binding with the substance to be transported. Large molecules (macromolecules), along with fluids, are transported by means of endocytosis (taking in) and exocytosis (expelling). Water and electrically charged molecules are transported by protein channels embedded in the plasma membrane. Ligands enter the cell by means of receptor-mediated endocytosis.

Movement of Water and Solutes

Cellular membranes are semipermeable and generally allow passage of water and small particles of dissolved substances called **solutes.** The movement of solute molecules through membranes is related to their size, solubility, electrical properties, and concentration on either side of the membrane. Small, lipid-soluble particles, such as oxygen, carbon dioxide, and urea, can readily pass the lipid bilayers of the plasma membrane. Larger, water-soluble particles may pass through pores in the membranes. Although large protein molecules, such as albumin and globulin, pass through membranes by endocytosis, they influence the movement of water by exerting an osmotic effect (see p. 21).

Body fluids are composed of two types of solutes: **electrolytes,** which are electrically charged and dissociate into constituent **ions** when placed in solution, and nonelectrolytes, such as glucose, urea, and creatinine, which do not dissociate. Electrolytes account for approximately 95% of the solute molecules in body water. Electrolytes exhibit **polarity** by orienting themselves toward the positive or negative pole. Ions with a positive charge are known as **cations** and migrate toward the negative pole, or cathode, if an electrical current is passed through the electrolyte solution. **Anions** carry a negative charge and migrate toward the positive pole, or anode, in the presence of electrical current. Anions and cations are located in both the intracellular fluid (ICF) and extracellular fluid (ECF) compartments, although concentration of particular ions varies depending on their location. (Fluid and electrolyte balance between body compartments is discussed in Chapter 3.) For example, sodium (Na^+) is the predominant extracellular cation, and potassium (K^+) is the principal intracellular cation. The difference in ICF and ECF concentrations of these ions is important to the transmission of electrical impulses across the plasma membranes of nerve and muscle cells.

Electrolytes are measured in milliequivalents per liter (mEq/L) or milligrams per deciliter (mg/dl). Milliequivalents per liter indicate the number of electrical charges per unit volume of fluid. The term *milliequivalent* thus indicates the chemical-combining activity of an ion, which depends on the electrical charge, or **valence,** of its ions. In abbreviations, valence is indicated by the *number* of plus or minus signs. Monovalent ions, or ions with one charge, include sodium (Na^+), chlorine (Cl^-), and potassium (K^+). Divalent ions, which have two charges, include calcium (Ca^{++}) and magnesium (Mg^{++}). One millequivalent of any cation can combine chemically with 1 mEq of any anion: one monovalent anion will combine with one monovalent cation. Divalent ions combine more strongly than monovalent ions. To maintain electrochemical balance, one divalent ion will combine with two monovalent ions (e.g., Ca^{++} + $2Cl^-$ = $CaCl_2$).

Passive Transport

Diffusion

Diffusion is the movement of a solute molecule from an area of greater solute concentration to an area of lesser solute concentration. This difference in concentration is known as a **concentration gradient.** Particles in a solution move randomly in any direction. If the concentration of particles in one part of the solution is greater than in another part, the particles distribute themselves evenly throughout the solution. According to the same principle, if the concentration of particles is greater on one side of a permeable membrane than on the other side, the particles diffuse spontaneously from the area of greater concentration to the area of lesser concentration until equilibrium is reached. The higher the concentration on one side, the greater the diffusion rate. The overall effect of diffusion is the passive movement of particles "down" a concentration gradient, that is, from an area of high concentration to an area of low concentration.

The diffusion rate is influenced by differences of electrical potential across the membrane (see p. 28.) Because the pores in the lipid bilayer are often lined with Ca^{++}, other cations (e.g., Na^+ and K^+) diffuse slowly because they are repelled by positive charges in the pores.

The rate of diffusion of a substance depends also on its size (diffusion coefficient) and its lipid solubility (Fig. 1-15). Usually, the smaller the molecule and the more soluble it is in oil, the more hydrophobic or nonpolar it is, and the more rapidly it will diffuse across the bilayer. Oxygen, carbon dioxide, and the steroid hormones are all examples of nonpolar molecules. Water-soluble substances, such as sugars and inorganic ions, diffuse very slowly, whereas uncharged lipophilic ("lipid-loving") molecules, such as fatty acids and steroids, diffuse rapidly. Ions and other polar molecules generally diffuse across cellular membranes more slowly than lipid-soluble substances.

Water readily diffuses through biologic membranes because water molecules are small and uncharged. Although the mechanism is not known with certainty, the dipolar structure of water allows it rapidly to cross the regions of the bilayer containing the lipid head groups. Lipid head groups constitute the two outer regions of the lipid bilayer.

Hydrostatic Pressure

Hydrostatic pressure is the mechanical force of water pushing against cellular membranes. In the vascular system, hydrostatic pressure is the blood pressure generated in vessels by the contraction of the heart. Blood

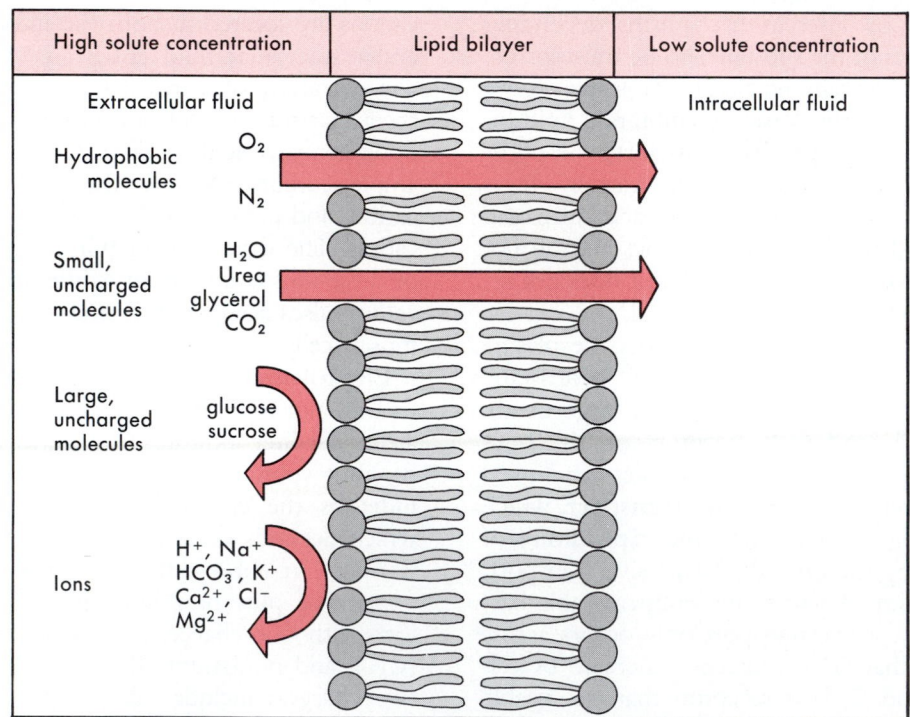

FIG. 1-15. Passive diffusion of solute molecules across the plasma membrane. Oxygen, nitrogen, water, urea, glycerol, and carbon dioxide can diffuse readily down the concentration gradient. Macromolecules are too large to diffuse through pores in the plasma membrane. Ions may be repelled if the pores contain substances with identical charges. If the pores are lined with cations, for example, other cations will have difficulty diffusing because the positive charges will repel one another. Diffusion can still occur, but it occurs more slowly.

reaching the capillary bed has a hydrostatic pressure of 25 to 30 mm Hg, which is sufficient force to push water across the thin capillary membranes into the interstitial space, a process known as *filtration*. Hydrostatic pressure is partially balanced by osmotic pressure: there is a net movement of water out of the capillary partially balanced by osmotic forces that tend to pull water into the capillaries. Water that is not osmotically attracted back into the capillaries moves into the lymph system.

Osmosis

Osmosis is the movement of *water* "down" a concentration gradient; that is, across a semipermeable membrane from a region of higher water concentration to a region of lower water concentration. For osmosis to occur, the membrane must be more permeable to water than to solutes and there must be a greater concentration of solutes so that water moves more easily. Osmosis is directly related to both hydrostatic pressure and solute concentration, but *not* to particle size or weight. For example, particles of the plasma protein albumin are small but more concentrated in body fluids than the larger and heavier particles of globulin. Therefore albumin exerts a greater osmotic force than globulin.

Osmolality controls distribution and movement of water between body compartments. The terms osmolality and osmolarity are often used interchangeably in reference to osmotic activity, but they define different measurements. **Osmolality** is a measure of the number of milliosmoles per kilogram of water, or the concentration of molecules per *weight* of water. **Osmolarity** is a measure of the number of milliosmoles per liter of solution, or the concentration of molecules per *volume* of solution. When solute is added to water, the volume is expanded and includes the original liter of water plus the volume occupied by the solute particles. In measuring osmolarity, the volume of water is therefore reduced by an amount equal to the volume of added solute.

In solutions that contain only dissociable substances, such as sodium and chloride, the difference between the two measurements is negligible. In considering all the different solutes in plasma (proteins, glucose, lipids, etc.), however, the difference between osmolality and osmolarity becomes more significant. In plasma, less of the plasma weight is water, and the overall concentration of particles is therefore greater. The osmolality will be greater than the osmolarity because of the smaller proportion of water. Osmolality is thus the preferred measure of osmotic activity in clinical assessment of individuals.

The normal osmolality of body fluids is 280 to 294 mOsm/kg. The osmolality of intracellular and extracellular fluid tends to equalize and so provides a measure of body fluid concentration and thus the body's hydration status. Hydration is also affected by hydrostatic pres-

sure, since the movement of water by osmosis can be opposed by an equal amount of hydrostatic pressure. The amount of hydrostatic pressure required to oppose the osmotic movement of water is called the **osmotic pressure** of the solution. Factors that determine osmotic pressure are the type and thickness of the plasma membrane, the size of the molecules, the concentration of molecules or the concentration gradient, and the solubility of molecules within the membrane. Examples of the movement of water in relation to hydrostatic and osmotic forces occur in the glomerulus in the kidney (see Chapter 32) and in the capillaries of the microcirculation (see Chapter 26).

Effective osmolality is sustained osmotic activity and depends on the concentration of solutes remaining on one side of a permeable membrane. If the solutes penetrate the membrane and equilibrate with the solution on the other side of the membrane, the osmotic effect will be diminished or lost. For example, urea is a small solute that readily diffuses across cellular membranes. Solutions containing urea rapidly lose their effective osmolality because they rapidly equilibrate. Solutes too large to pass through the membrane thus sustain an effective osmolality, meaning that they enhance osmotic activity. Plasma proteins are examples of molecules that provide effective osmolality because they normally do not cross cellular membranes.

Plasma proteins also influence osmolality because they have a negative charge. The principle by which the plasma protein charge influences osmolality is known as Gibbs-Donnan equilibrium, and it affects the distribution of ions across cellular membranes. Gibbs-Donnan equilibrium occurs when fluid in one compartment contains small diffusable ions such as Na^+ and Cl^-, together with large, nondiffusable charged particles, such as plasma proteins. Because the body tends to maintain an electrical equilibrium, the nondiffusable protein molecules cause asymmetry in the distribution of small ions. Anions such as Cl^- are thus driven out of the cell or plasma, and cations like Na^+ are attracted. The protein-containing compartment will maintain a state of electroneutrality, but the osmolality will be higher. The overall osmotic effect of colloids, such as plasma proteins, is called the **oncotic pressure,** or **colloid osmotic pressure.**

Tonicity describes the effective osmolality of a solution. (The terms *osmolality* and *tonicity* may be used interchangeably.) Solutions, then, have relative degrees of tonicity. An **isotonic solution** (or iso-osmotic solution) has the same osmolality or concentration of particles (285 mOsm) as the ICF or ECF. Examples of isotonic solutions include 5% dextrose in water and normal (0.9%) saline solution. A **hypotonic solution** has a lower concentration and is thus more dilute than body fluids. Water is a hypotonic solution. Consequently, water is osmotically pulled into the cells, causing them to swell or burst. A **hypertonic solution** has a concentration greater than 285 to 294 mOsm/kg. An example of hypertonic solution is 3% saline solution. Water can be pulled out of the cells by a hypertonic solution, so that the cells shrink. The concept of tonicity is important when correcting water and solute imbalances by administering different types of replacement solutions.

Mediated and Active Transport

Mediated Transport

Mediated transport (passive and active) involves integral or transmembrane proteins with receptors having a high degree of specificity for the substance being transported. Inorganic anions and cations (e.g., Na^+, K^+, Ca^{++}, Cl^-, and HCO_3^-) and charged and uncharged organic compounds (e.g., amino acids and sugars) require specific transport systems to facilitate movement through different cellular membranes. Rates at which substances are moved by mediated transport mechanisms have often been measured, yet the specific membrane proteins involved have not been identified. Mediated transport is much faster than simple diffusion.

A **transport protein** is a transmembrane or integral protein that binds with and transfers a specific solute molecule across the lipid bilayer. Each transport protein, or **transporter,** has receptors for a specific solute. When the transporter is saturated—that is, when all receptor sites are occupied by solute molecules—the rate of transport is maximal. Solute binding can be blocked by **competitive inhibitors** that compete for the same receptor site and may or may not be transported by the transport protein. Noncompetitive inhibitors bind elsewhere but can alter the structure of the transporter.

Although the mechanism by which a transport protein functions is not exactly known, it is not likely that the transporter shuttles back and forth across the bilayer. The transporter is probably a transmembrane protein that undergoes a reversible conformational change while transporting the solute molecule across the bilayer (Fig. 1-16). (Transmembrane proteins are illustrated in Figs. 1-10 and 1-11.)

Another model proposed to explain the mechanism of mediated transport is the channel model. In this model the protein transporter creates a channel between the inner and outer sides of the membrane (Fig. 1-17). The channel is controlled by a gate mechanism that determines which receptor-bound solutes can move into the channel that is created after receptor-solute contact. Binding stimulates conformational changes in the protein transporter that move the solute through the channel short distances at a time until it reaches the other side of the membrane. Release of the solute might occur because of lower solute concentrations in the new compartment or because the protein's conformational changes have weakened the receptor's affinity for the solute molecule (Devlin, 1982).

Mediated transport systems can move solute molecules singly or two at a time. Two molecules can be moved simultaneously in one direction (a process called **symport**) or in opposite directions (called **antiport**), or a single molecule can be moved in one direction (called **uniport**) (Fig. 1-18).

In **passive mediated transport,** also called **facilitated diffusion,** the protein transporter moves solute molecules through cellular membranes without expending metabolic energy. The direction of movement is the same as in simple diffusion—down the concentration gradient. Perhaps the most widely referred to passive transport system is that for glucose in erythrocytes (red blood cells). Glucose is transported by a uniport mechanism and demonstrates saturation kinetics; that is, the transport system is saturated when all the glucose-specific receptors on the membrane are occupied and operating at their maximal capacity.

The anions Cl^- and HCO_3^- also undergo passive mediated transport in the erythrocyte. This antiport mechanism allows Cl^- movement in one direction and simultaneous HCO_3^- movement in the opposite direction. The directions of movement depend on the concentration gradients of the ions across the membrane.

In **active mediated transport,** also called active transport, the protein transporter moves molecules against, or up, the concentration gradient. Unlike passive mediated transport, active mediated transport requires the expenditure of energy. Many active mediated transport systems, or pumps, have ATP as their primary energy

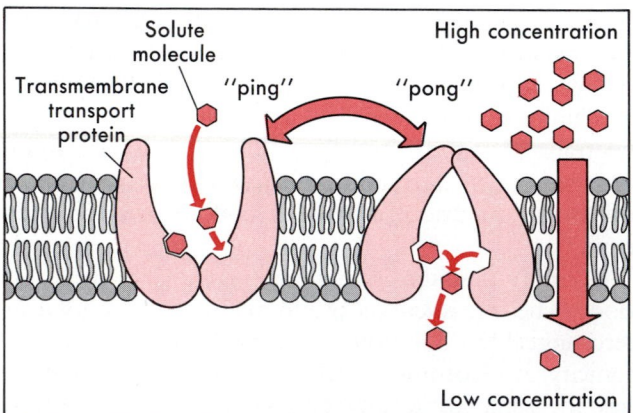

FIG. 1-16. Conformational-change model of mediated transport (facilitated diffusion). The transporter protein has two states, "ping" and "pong." In the ping state, sites for molecules of a specific solute are exposed on the outside of the bilayer. In the pong state, the sites are exposed to the inner side of the bilayer.

source, but not all. Some use the electrochemical gradient of Na^+ across the membrane (Fig. 1-19). Energy in the form of ATP, however, is required for activation of the Na^+ gradient.

A "carrier" mechanism in the plasma membrane mediates the transport of ions, such as Na^+, K^+, H^+, Cl^-, HCO_3^-, and of nutrients, such as glucose and amino acids. Energy supplied by ATP is required to pump ions against a concentration gradient. The best-known pump is the $Na^+ + K^+$-dependent ATPase pump. It continuously regulates the cells' volume by controlling leaks through pores or protein channels and maintains the ionic concentration gradients necessary for cellular excitation and membrane conductivity (see p. 28). The maintenance of intracellular K^+ concentrations is also required for enzyme activity, including that of enzymes involved in protein synthesis.

Active Transport of Na⁺ and K⁺

The active transport system for Na^+ and K^+ is found in virtually all mammalian cells. The Na^+, K^+ antiport system, Na^+ moving out and K^+ moving into the cell, uses the direct energy of ATP to move these cations. The transporter protein is an enzyme, ATPase. ATPase has a requirement for Na^+, K^+, and Mg^{++} ions. The concentration of ATPase in plasma membranes is directly related to Na^+, K^+ transport activity. Approximately 60% to 70% of the ATP synthesized by cells, especially muscle and nerve cells, is used to maintain the Na^+, K^+ transport system. Excitable tissues (e.g., muscle and nerve tissues) have a high concentration of Na^+,K^+ ATPase, as do other tissues that transport significant amounts of Na^+, for example, kidneys and sali-

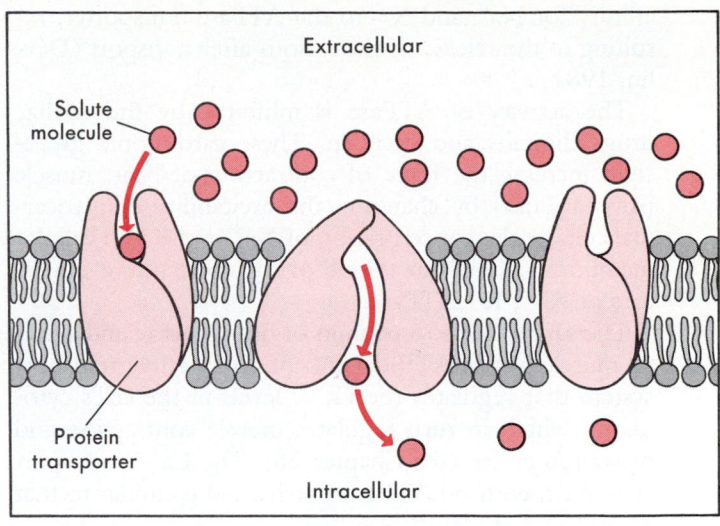

FIG. 1-17. Channel model of mediated transport (facilitated diffusion). The transporter protein in this model binds to the substance on one side of the membrane, which causes a change in the shape of the transporter. The shape change creates a channel through which the substance can move through the transporter to the other side of the membrane.

vary glands. For every ATP molecule hydrolyzed, three molecules of Na^+ are transported out of the cell, whereas only two molecules of K^+ move into the cell. The process leads to an increase in positive charges outside the cell. The exact mechanism for transport of Na^+ and K^+ across the membrane is uncertain. One proposal is that ATPase goes through several conformational changes, causing Na^+ and K^+ to move short distances (see Fig. 1-19). The conformational change creates a lowering of

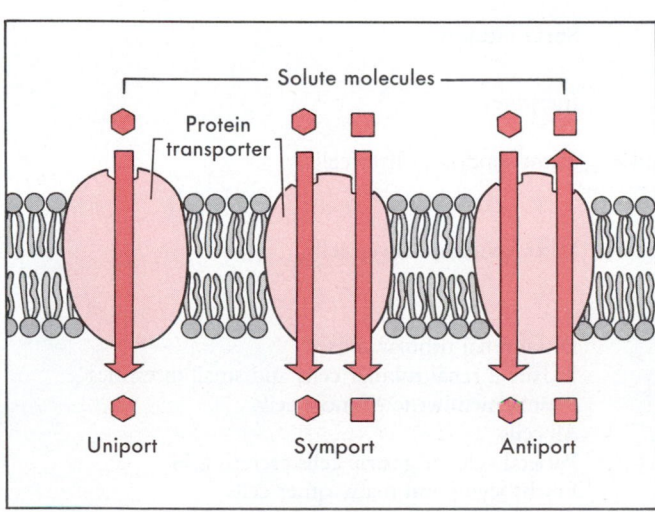

FIG. 1-18. Mediated transport. Simultaneous movement of a single solute molecule in one direction (uniport), of two different solute molecules in one direction (symport), and of two different solute molecules in opposite directions (antiport).

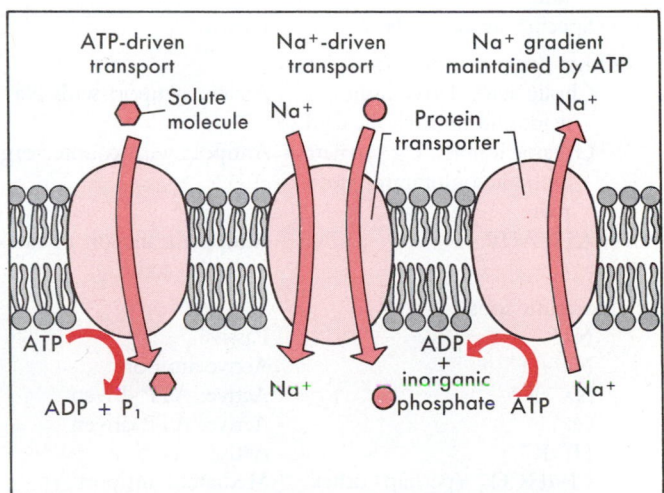

FIG. 1-19. Active mediated transport. Metabolic energy (ATP) controls the active transport of many substances, including Na^+. ATP is necessary for active mediated transport.

affinity for Na$^+$ and K$^+$ to the ATPase transporter, resulting in the release of the cations after transport (Devlin, 1982).

The activity of ATPase is inhibited by the cardiac drugs digitalis and ouabain. These cardiotonic glycosides increase the force of contraction of heart muscle (myocardium) by changing the excitability of myocardial cells or the concentration of Na$^+$ and K$^+$ in cellular membranes. Ouabain is one of the most active inhibitors of Na$^+$, K$^+$ ATPase.

The sarcoplasmic reticulum of heart muscle and skeletal muscle has an ATP-dependent Ca^{++} active transport system that regulates the Ca^{++} levels in the cell's cytoplasm, which in turn regulates muscle contraction and relaxation cycles (see Chapter 26). The Ca^{++} transport system depends on ATPase activity and is similar to that of Na$^+$, K$^+$ ATPase.

The transport of sugars and amino acids across the plasma membrane depends on the simultaneous movement (symport) of Na$^+$ or Na$^+$-dependent transport (see Fig. 1-18). Na$^+$-dependent symport occurs primarily in the plasma membrane of epithelial cells of the kidney tubules and intestines. The transport of glucose is not directly dependent on the hydrolysis of ATP; however, the Na$^+$ gradient is ATP dependent, and thus ATP is indirectly involved in glucose transport. Ouabain can prevent the uptake of glucose by inhibiting the Na$^+$, K$^+$ transporter protein.

The epithelial cells that line the intestines depend on Na$^+$ to transport various amino acids. Similarly, the uptake of Cl$^-$ by the small intestine depends on Na$^+$ symport and antiport mechanisms for the secretion of Ca^{++} from the cell.

Table 1-2 summarizes the major mechanisms of transport through pores and protein transporters in the plasma membranes. Many disease states are caused and/or manifested by loss of these membrane transport systems.

TABLE 1-2 Major transport systems in mammalian cells

Substance transported	Mechanism of transport	Tissues
Sugars		
Glucose	Passive	Most tissues
	Active: symport with Na$^+$	Small intestines and renal tubular cells
Fructose	Passive	Intestines and liver
Amino acids		
Amino acid specific transporters	Active: symport with Na$^+$	Intestines, kidney, and liver
All amino acids except proline	Active: group translocation	Liver
Specific amino acids	Passive	Small intestine
Other organic molecules		
Cholic acid, deoxycholic acid, and taurocholic acid	Active: symport with Na$^+$	Intestines
Organic anions, e.g., malate, alpha-ketoglutarate, glutamate	Antiport with counter-organic anion	Mitochondria of liver cells
ATP-ADP	Antiport transport of nucleotides; can be active	Mitochondria of liver cells
Inorganic ions		
Na$^+$	Passive	Distal renal tubular cells
Na$^+$/H$^+$	Active antiport	Proximal renal tubular cells and small intestines
Na$^+$/K$^+$	Active: ATP driven	Plasma membrane of most cells
Ca^{++}	Active: ATP driven	All cells
H$^+$/K$^+$	Active	Parietal cells of gastric cells secreting H$^+$
Cl$^-$/HCO$_3^-$ (perhaps other anions)	Mediated: antiport	Erythrocytes and many other cells

NOTE: The known transport systems are listed here; others have been proposed. Most transport systems have been studied in only a few tissues, and their sites of activity may be more limited than indicated.
From Devlin, 1982.

Transport by Vesicle Formation
Endocytosis and Exocytosis

Pores and protein transporters cannot move large proteins, polynucleotides, or polysaccharides (macromolecules) across the plasma membrane, yet most cells are able to take in and eject these macromolecules. The active transport mechanisms by which the cells do this are very different from those that mediate small solute and ion transport. Transport of macromolecules involves the sequential formation and fusion of membrane-bounded vesicles.

In **endocytosis,** a section of the plasma membrane enfolds substances from outside the cell, invaginates (folds inward), and separates from the plasma membrane, forming a vesicle that moves into the inside of the cell (Fig. 1-20, *A*). Two types of endocytosis are designated based on the size of the vesicle formed. **Pinocytosis** (cell drinking) involves the ingestion of fluids and solute molecules through formation of small vesi-

cles, and **phagocytosis** (cell eating) involves the ingestion of large particles, such as bacteria, through formation of large vesicles (also called vacuoles).

Since most kinds of cells are continually ingesting fluid and solutes by pinocytosis, the terms *pinocytosis* and *endocytosis* are often used interchangeably. In pinocytosis the vesicle containing fluids, solutes, or both fuses with a lysosome, and lysosomal enzymes digest them for use by the cell. In phagocytosis the large molecular substances are engulfed by the plasma membrane and enter the cell so that they can be isolated and destroyed by lysosomal enzymes (see Chapter 7). Substances that are not degraded by lysosomes are isolated in residual bodies and released by the cell by exocytosis. Both pinocytosis and phagocytosis require metabolic energy and often involve binding of the substance with plasma membrane receptors before membrane invagination and fusion with lysosomes in the cell.

In eucaryotic cells, secretion of macromolecules al-

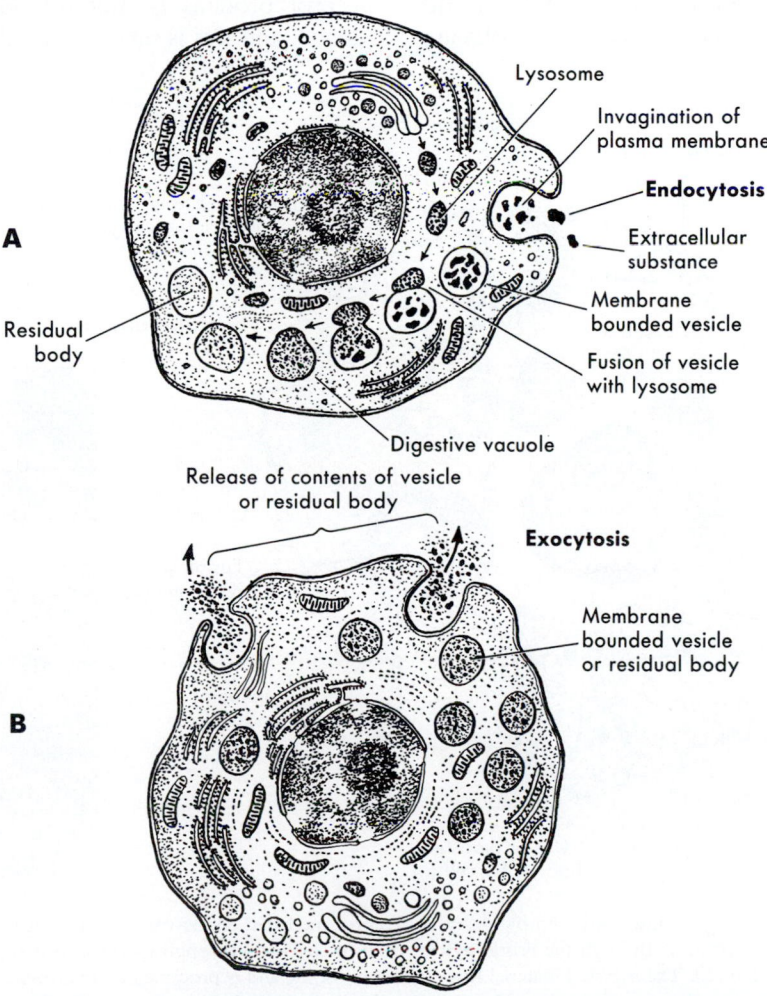

FIG. 1-20. **A,** Endocytosis and fusion with lysosome. **B,** Exocytosis.

most always occurs by **exocytosis** (Fig. 1-20, *B*). For example, to secrete macromolecules of insulin across plasma membranes, insulin-producing cells store and package insulin molecules in intracellular vesicles, which fuse with the plasma membrane and open to the extracellular space, or matrix, releasing the insulin. Not all secreted substances are secreted into the extracellular matrix. Some adhere to the plasma membrane and are thought to replace segments of the membrane lost through endocytosis or diffuse into the blood to nourish or signal other cells. Exocytosis has two main functions: (1) replacement of portions of the plasma membrane that have been removed by endocytosis, and (2) release of molecules synthesized by the cells into the extracellular matrix.

Receptor-Mediated Endocytosis

Ligand binding to plasma membrane receptors leads to clustering, aggregation, and immobilization of the receptors in specialized areas of the membrane called **coated pits** (Fig. 1-21). The pits, which are coated with bristlelike structures (clathrin), deepen and enfold (invaginate), internalizing ligand-receptor complexes and forming a coated vesicle. The clathrin coat or bristles are thought to be responsible for trapping membrane receptors in coated pits. This internalization process, called **receptor-mediated endocytosis,** is rapid and enables the cell to ingest large amounts of specific ligands without ingesting large volumes of extracellular fluid. Inside the cell, the ingested material is processed by lysosomal enzymes.

The cellular uptake of cholesterol, for example, depends on receptor-mediated endocytosis. Cholesterol (a ligand) is primarily carried in blood plasma attached to an acceptor protein. This cholesterol-protein complex is called low-density lipoprotein (LDL). LDL receptors, which bind LDL to the plasma membrane, control the rate at which cholesterol is transferred into the cell. Cholesterol uptake provides cells with the cholesterol needed for membrane synthesis. If cellular uptake is blocked, cholesterol accumulates in the blood and predisposes blood vessel walls to the formation of atherosclerotic plaques (see Chapter 27). After its ingestion by the cell, cholesterol activity is regulated by feedback control. If too much free cholesterol accumulates in the cell, the cell's own synthesis of cholesterol and LDL receptor proteins is shut off. Hence, less cholesterol is made, and less is taken up by the cell.

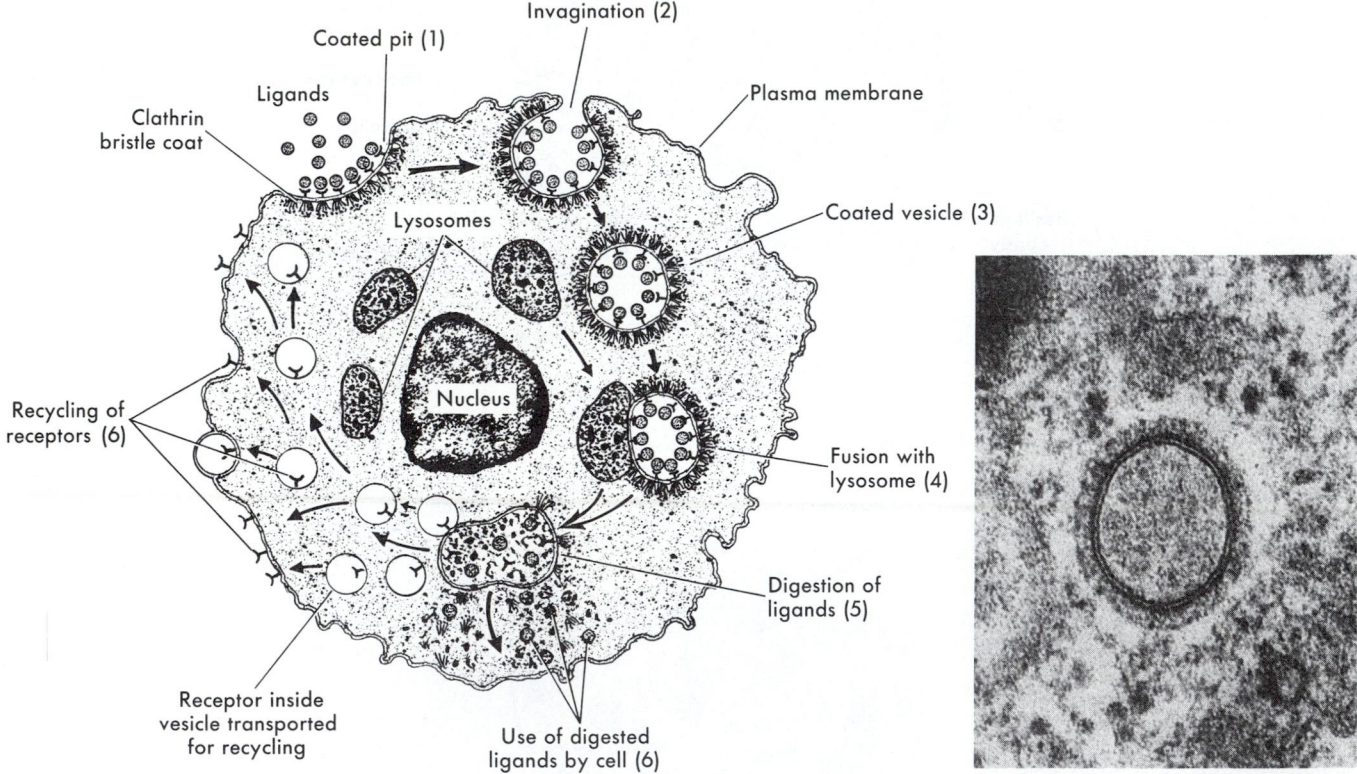

A

B

FIG. 1-21. Ligand internalization by means of receptor-mediated endocytosis. **A,** The ligand attaches to its surface receptor (through the bristle coat or clathrin coat) and through receptor-mediated endocytosis enters the cell. The ingested material fuses with a lysosome and is processed by hydrolytic lysosomal enzymes. Processed molecules can then be transferred to other cellular components. **B,** Electron micrograph of a coated pinocytotic vesicle. (**B** from Kissane, 1985.)

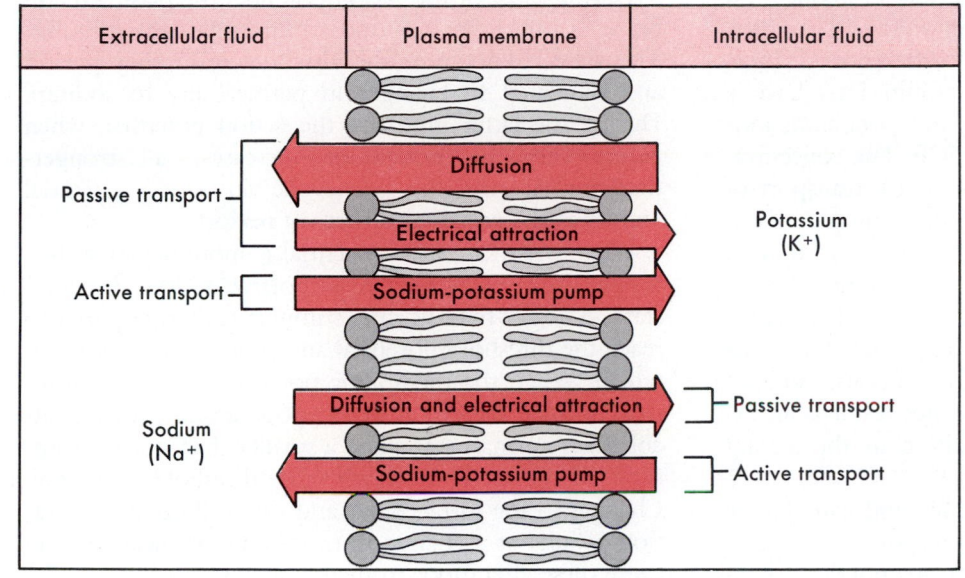

A

| Extracellular fluid | Plasma membrane | Intracellular fluid |

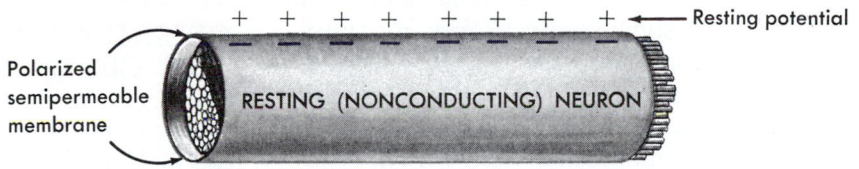

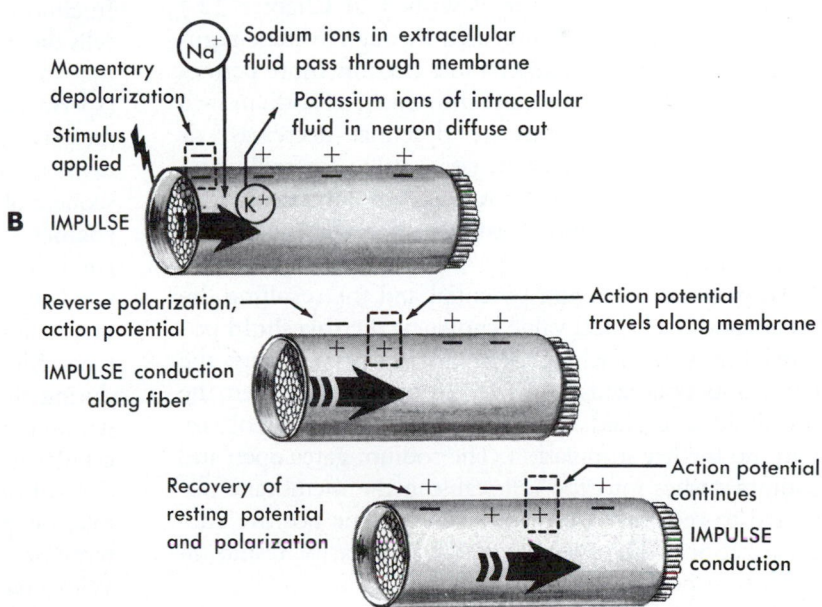

FIG. 1-22. A, Concentration difference of Na$^+$ and K$^+$ intracellularly and extracellularly. The direction of actine transport by the sodium-potassium pump is also shown. **B,** Top diagram represents the polarized state of a neuronal membrane when at rest. The lower diagrams represent changes in sodium and potassium membrane permeabilities with the generation and propagation of an action potential (**B** from Anthony, C.P., & Thibodeau G.A. (1979) *Textbook of anatomy and physiology* (10th ed) C.V. Mosby.)

Movement of Electrical Impulses: Membrane Potentials

All body cells are electrically polarized, with the inside of the cell more negatively charged than the outside. The difference in electrical charge, or voltage, is known as the **resting membrane potential** and is about -70 to -85 millivolts. The difference in voltage across the plasma membrane is a result of the differences in ionic composition of ICF and ECF. Sodium ions have a greater concentration in the ECF, and potassium ions have a greater concentration in the ICF. The concentration difference is maintained by the active transport of Na^+ and K^+, (the sodium-potassium pump), which transports sodium outward and potassium inward (Fig. 1-22). Because the resting plasma membrane is more permeable to K^+ than to Na^+, K^+ can diffuse easily from its area of higher concentration in the ICF to its area of lower concentration in the ECF. Because sodium and potassium are both cations, the net result is an excess of anions inside the cell, resulting in the resting membrane potential.

Nerve and muscle cells are excitable and can change their resting membrane potential in response to electrochemical stimuli. Changes in resting membrane potential convey messages from cell to cell. When a nerve or muscle cell receives a stimulus that exceeds the membrane threshold value there is a rapid change in the resting membrane potential known as the **action potential.** The action potential carries signals along the nerve or muscle cell and conveys information from one cell to another. (Nerve impulses are described in Chapter 12.) When a resting cell is stimulated through voltage-regulated channels, the cell membranes become more permeable to sodium. There is a net movement of sodium into the cell, and the membrane potential decreases, or "moves forward," from a negative value (in millivolts) to zero. This decrease is known as **depolarization.** The depolarized cell is more positively charged, and its polarity is neutralized.

To generate an action potential and the resulting depolarization, a critical value known as the **threshold potential** must be reached. Generally this occurs when the cell has depolarized by 15 to 20 millivolts. When the threshold is reached, the cell will continue to depolarize with no further stimulation. The sodium gates open and sodium rushes into the cell, causing the membrane potential to reduce to zero and then become positive (depolarization). The rapid reversal in polarity results in the action potential.

During **repolarization** the negative polarity of the resting membrane potential is reestablished. As the voltage-gated sodium channels begin to close, voltage-gated potassium channels open. Membrane permeability to sodium decreases, and potassium permeability increases, with an outward movement of potassium ions. The sodium gates close, and with the outward movement of potassium the membrane potential becomes more negative. The Na^+-K^+ pump then returns the membrane to the resting potential by pumping potassium back into the cell and sodium out of the cell.

During most of the action potential the plasma membrane is unable to respond to an additional stimulus. This time is known as the **absolute refractory period** and is related to changes in permeability to sodium. During the latter phase of the action potential, when permeability to potassium increases, a stronger-than-normal stimulus can evoke an action potential known as the **relative refractory period.**

When the membrane potential is more negative than normal, the cell is in a hyperpolarized (less excitable) state. A larger-than-normal stimulus is then required to reach the threshold potential and generate an action potential. When the membrane potential is more positive than normal, the cell is in a hypopolarized (more excitable than normal) state, and a smaller-than-normal stimulus is required to reach the threshold potential. Changes in the intracellular and extracellular concentration of ions or a change in membrane permeability can cause these alterations in membrane excitability.

CELLULAR REPRODUCTION: THE CELL CYCLE

Cells of the human body are subject to wear and tear and most do not last for the lifetime of the individual. In almost all tissues, new cells are created as fast as old cells die. Cellular reproduction is therefore necessary for the maintenance of life. Reproduction of gametes (sperm and egg cells) occurs through a process called meiosis, described in Chapter 4. The reproduction, or division of other body cells (somatic cells), involves two sequential phases: **mitosis,** or nuclear division, and **cytokinesis,** or cytoplasmic division. These two phases occur in close succession, with cytokinesis beginning toward the end of mitosis. Before a cell can divide, however, it must double its mass and duplicate all of its contents. Most of the work of preparing for division occurs during the growth phase, called **interphase.** The alternation between mitosis and interphase in all tissues with cellular turnover is known as the **cell cycle.**

Most of the early work on the cell cycle was limited to microscopic observation of mitosis and cytokinesis. Interphase was considered the "resting stage" of the cell. With recent technologic advances, a considerable amount has been learned about the interphase part of the cell cycle. During interphase many important processes are taking place as the cell produces DNA, RNA, protein, lipids, and other substances and each pair of **chromosomes** (paired organelles that carry genetic information) also make exact copies of themselves.

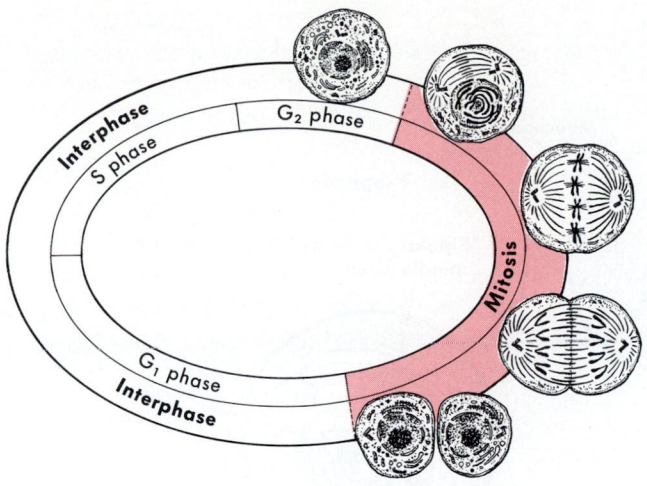

FIG. 1-23. Interphase and the phases of mitosis.

There are four designated phases of the cell cycle (Fig. 1-23). They are (1) the S phase (S = synthesis), in which DNA is synthesized in the cell nucleus; (2) the G_2 phase (G = gap), in which RNA and protein synthesis occurs, the period between the completion of DNA synthesis and the next (M) phase; (3) the M phase (M = mitosis), which includes both nuclear and cytoplasmic division; and (4) the G_1 phase, which is the period between the M phase and the start of DNA synthesis.

Phases of Mitosis and Cytokinesis

Interphase (the G_1, S, and G_2 phases) is the longest phase of the cell cycle. During interphase, chromosomes are not visible under a light microscope. An electron microscope shows that during interphase the chromatin consists of very long, slender rods that are jumbled together in the nucleus. Late in interphase, strands of **chromatin** (the substance that gives the nucleus its granular appearance) begin to coil, causing them to shorten and thicken. This allows the strands to absorb more staining material, so that they become visible as chromosomes under a light microscope. Fig. 1-24 illustrates interphase and the stages of mitosis.

The M phase of the cell cycle, mitosis and cytokinesis, begins with **prophase,** the first appearance of chromosomes. As the phase proceeds, each chromosome is seen as two identical halves called **chromatids,** which lie together and are attached at some point by a spindle attachment site called a **centromere.** (The two chromatids of each chromosome, which are genetically identical, are sometimes called sister chromatids.) The nuclear membrane, which surrounds the nucleus, disappears. **Spindle fibers** are microtubules formed in the cytoplasm. Spindle fibers radiate from two centrioles located at opposite poles of the cell. The role of the spindle fibers is to pull the chromosomes to opposite sides of the cell.

During **metaphase,** the next phase of mitosis and cytokinesis, the spindle fibers begin to pull the centromeres of the chromosomes. The centromeres become aligned in the middle of the spindle, which is called the **equatorial plate** (or **metaphase plate**) of the cell. This is the stage in which chromosomes are easiest to observe microscopically, since they are highly condensed and arranged in a relatively organized fashion in the two-dimensional equatorial plate.

Anaphase begins when the centromeres split and the sister chromatids are pulled apart. The spindle fibers shorten, causing the sister chromatids to be pulled, centromere first, toward opposite sides of the cell. When the sister chromatids are separated, each is considered to be a chromosome. Thus, the cell has 92 chromosomes during this stage. By the end of anaphase, there are 46 chromosomes lying at each side of the cell. Barring mitotic errors, each of the two groups of 46 chromosomes is identical to the original 46 chromosomes present at the start of the cell cycle.

Telophase is the final stage. During telophase, a new nuclear membrane is formed around each group of 46 chromosomes, the spindle fibers disappear, and the chromosomes begin to uncoil. Cytokinesis causes the cytoplasm to divide into roughly equal parts during this phase. At the end of telophase two identical diploid cells, called **daughter cells,** have been formed from the original cell.

Rates of Cellular Division

Although the complete cell cycle lasts from 12 to 24 hours, about 1 hour is generally required for the four stages of mitosis and cytokinesis: prophase, metaphase, anaphase, and telophase. All types of cells undergo mitosis during formation of the embryo, but in many adults cells, such as nerve cells, lens cells of the eye, and muscle cells, they lose their ability to replicate and divide. The cells of other tissues, particularly epithelial cells (e.g., of the intestine, lung, and skin), divide continuously and rapidly, completing the entire cell cycle in less than 10 hours.

The difference between cells that divide slowly and cells that divide rapidly is the length of time spent in the G_1 phase of the cell cycle. Some cells that divide very slowly remain in the G_1 phase for days or even years. Once the S phase begins, however, progression through mitosis takes a relatively constant amount of time. Once a cell has progressed out of the G_1 phase, there is no turning back, it is committed to completing the S, G_2, and M phases. Times associated with the four successive phases differ.

The mechanisms that control the rate of cell division are unknown. Evidently, feedback mechanisms signal cells to divide when new cells are needed. For example, dormant or quiescent liver cells are stimulated to divide

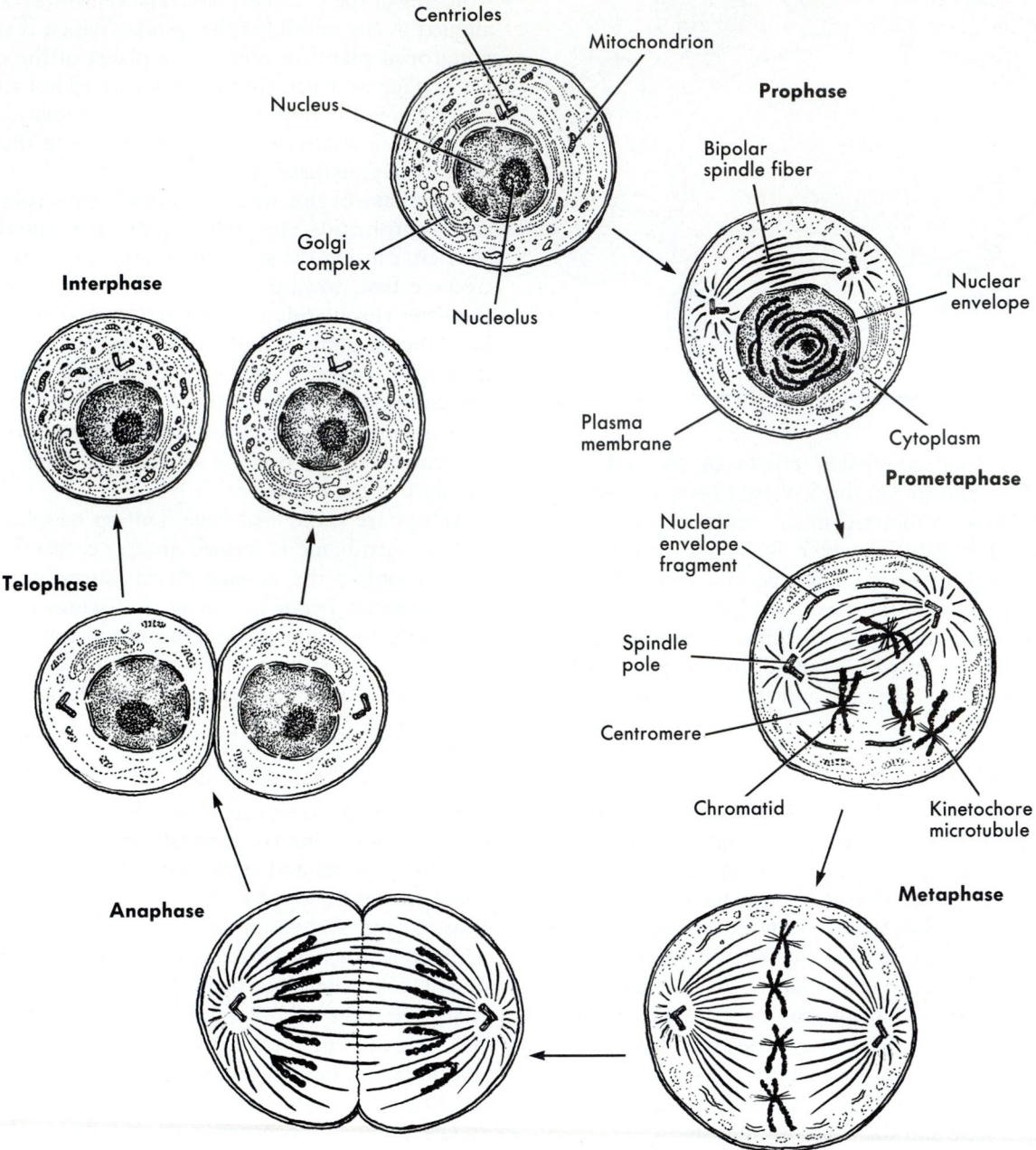

FIG. 1-24. The cell cycle. After the M phase, which includes both nuclear and cytoplasmic division, the two new daughter cells begin interphase of a new cycle. Interphase begins with the G_1 phase. The S phase begins with DNA synthesis and ends when the DNA content in the nucleus doubles and the chromosomes have replicated—causing the development of two identical "sister chromatids." The cell now enters the G_2 phase, which ends when mitosis starts. The M phase begins with mitosis and ends with cytokinesis.

rapidly after part of the liver has been removed, and they cease to divide once the normal liver mass has been restored. This same kind of limited cell division is seen in the skin after injury. Feedback mechanisms that control cell division are necessary to maintain normal structure and function and prevent an abnormal or excessive increase in mitotic rate, as occurs in cancer.

Cells are known to stop dividing when they run out of space or touch one another. This phenomenon is called **contact inhibition.** The term *contact inhibition* is misleading, however, because experiments have shown that it is not cellular contact but the extent to which the cellular mass spreads and the alteration of plasma membrane adhesiveness that stops cellular division. The less cells spread, regardless of contact, the longer their growth cycle. Certain cells are known to require small amounts of specific growth factors (proteins, steroids, or hormones) that stimulate and/or inhibit cell division. For example, epidermal cells (surface cells of the skin) divide only if they are stimulated by an unknown growth factor found between the epidermis and the dermis (the layer of skin beneath the epidermis).

TISSUES

The cells of the body are organized hierarchically: cells of one or more types are organized into tissues, and different types of tissues comprise organs. Finally, organs are integrated to perform complex functions as tracts or systems.

All cells are in contact with a network of extracellular macromolecules known as the **extracellular matrix.** The extracellular matrix not only holds cells and tissues together but also provides an organized latticework within which cells can migrate and interact with one another.

Tissue Formation

To form tissues, cells must exhibit intercellular recognition and adhesion. Specialized cells are thought to form a tissue in one of two different ways. First and simplest is mitosis of one or more **founder cells** (the most basic precursor cell). Founder cells are prevented from "wandering away" by macromolecules in the extracellular matrix and by adherence to one another at specialized junctions on their plasma membranes. Mitosis of founder cells forms, for example, epithelial cell sheets (Fig. 1-25).

The second way in which specialized cells form tissues involves their migration to and subsequent assembly at the site of tissue formation. During embryonic development, for example, cells from the neural crest migrate to several different regions, where they differentiate and as-

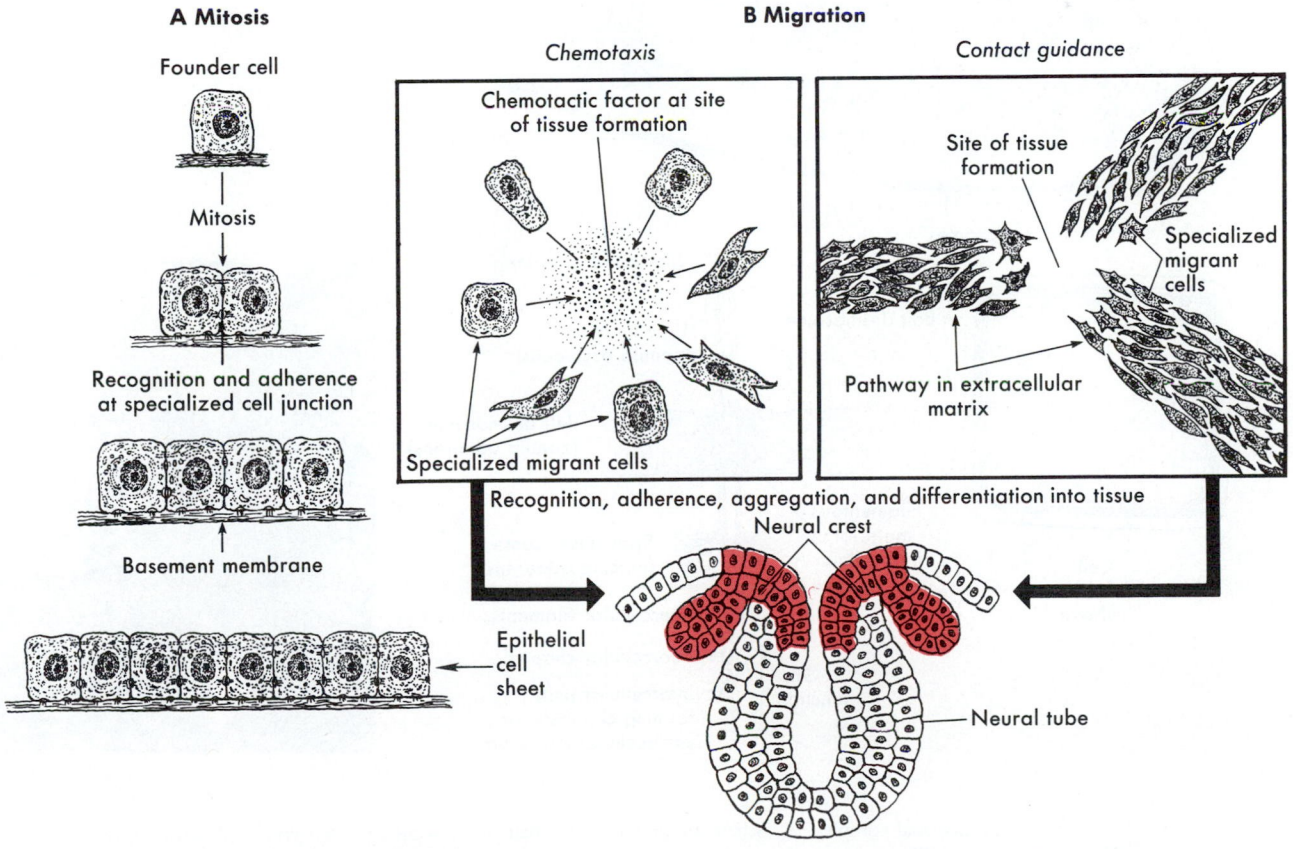

FIG. 1-25. A, Tissue formation by mitosis. Founder cells are kept in place by extracellular matrix and recognition and adherence at cell junctions. **B,** Tissue formation by migration. Specialized cells are attracted to the site of tissue formation by chemotaxis or contact guidance, then aggregate and differentiate into organized tissue.

semble into a variety of tissues, including those of the peripheral nervous system. Migrant cells are thought to arrive at the site of tissue formation through chemotaxis or contact guidance. **Chemotaxis** is movement along a chemical gradient caused by chemical attraction (see Chapter 7). Cells at the migrant cells' destination secrete a chemical, called chemotactic factor, that attracts specific migrant cells. **Contact guidance** is movement along a pathway, or "pavement," in the extracellular matrix (Alpert et al., 1983).

Tissues are not randomly arranged into organs. No matter how tissue is formed, staying together in groups

means that cells must recognize each other and remain distinct from the cells of surrounding tissues. Little is known about the mechanisms involved in these processes.

Intercellular Communication

Cells in direct physical contact with neighboring cells are often linked together at specialized regions of their plasma membranes called **cell junctions.** Cell junctions have two main functions: (1) to hold cells together, and (2) to allow small molecules to pass from cell to cell, allowing coordination of the activities of cells that form

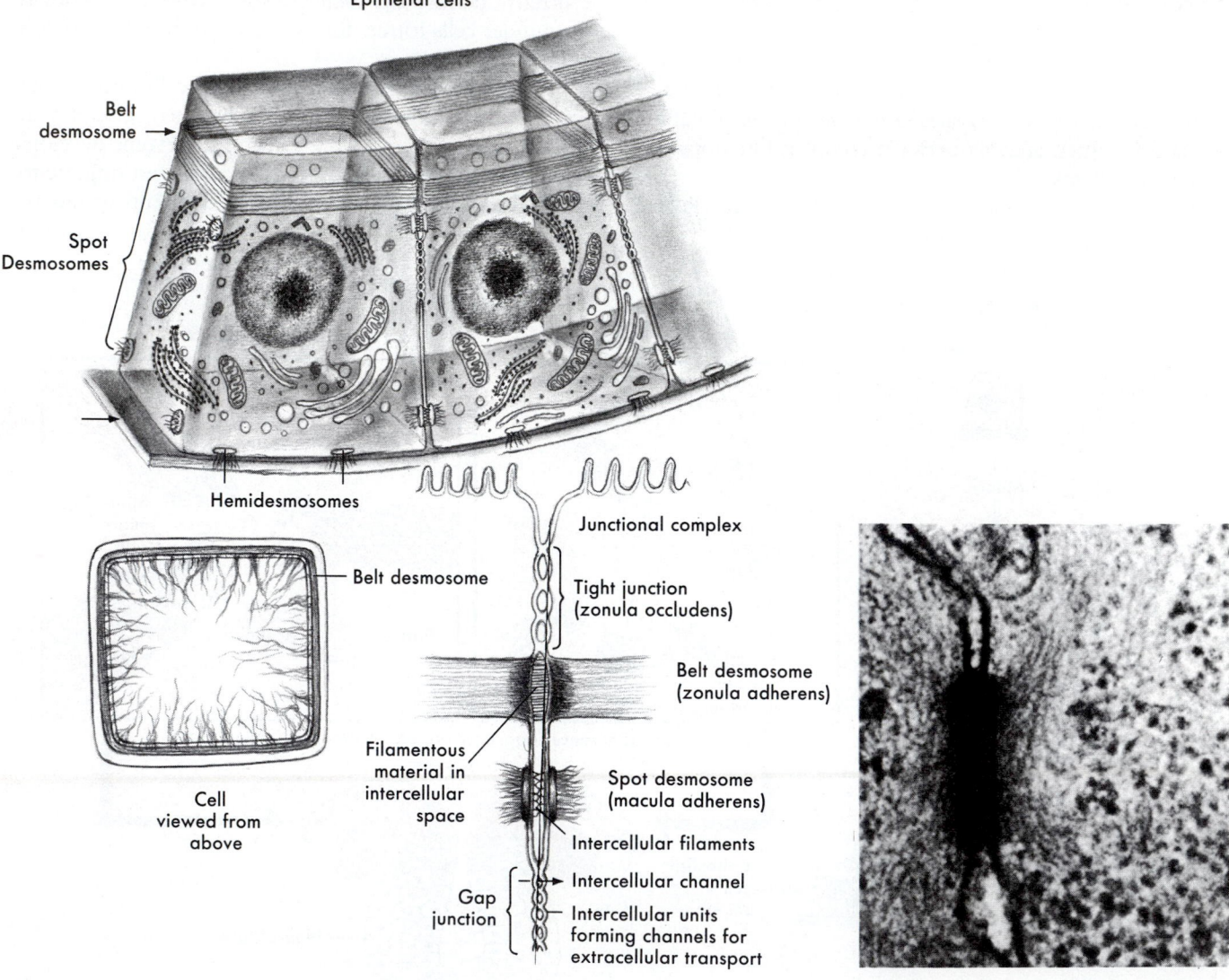

A

B

FIG. 1-26. Junctional complex. **A,** Schematic drawing of a belt desmosome between epithelial cells. This junction, also called zonula adherens, encircles each of the interacting cells. The spot desmosomes and hemidesmosomes, like the belt desmosomes, are adhering junctions. The tight junction is an impermeable junction that holds cells together but seals them in such a way that molecules cannot leak between them. The gap junction as a communicating junction mediates the passage of small molecules from one interacting cell to the other. **B,** Electron micrograph of desmosomes. (From Raven & Johnson, 1986.)

tissues. There are three main types of cell junctions: (1) desmosomes (macula adherens), (2) tight junctions (zonula occludens), and (3) gap junctions (Fig. 1-26). Together they form the **junctional complex. Desmosomes** hold cells together by forming either continuous bands or belts of epithelial sheets or buttonlike points of contact. Desmosomes also act as a system of braces to maintain structural stability. **Tight junctions** serve as a barrier to diffusion, prevent the movement of substances through transport proteins in the plasma membrane, and prevent the leakage of small molecules between the plasma membranes of adjacent cells. **Gap junctions** are clusters of protein channels that allow small ions and molecules to pass directly from the inside of one cell to the inside of another. Cells connected by gap junctions are considered ionically (electrically) and metabolically coupled. Gap junctions coordinate the activities of adjacent cells. They are important, for example, in synchronizing contractions of heart muscle cells through ionic coupling and in permitting action potentials to spread rapidly from cell to cell in neural tissues. The reason that gap junctions occur in tissues that are not electrically active is unknown. Although most gap junctions are associated with junctional complexes, they sometimes exist as independent structures.

The junctional complex is a very permeable part of the plasma membrane. Its permeability is controlled by a process called **gating,** which depends on concentrations of calcium ions in the cytoplasm. Increased cytoplasmic calcium causes decreased permeability at the junctional complex. Gating is an important cellular defense mechanism because it enables uninjured cells to "seal themselves off" from injured neighbors. As damaged cells release calcium, it travels through the junctional complex and increases calcium levels in neighboring cells. (The damaging effects of calcium influx are described in Chapter 2.) This decreases the permeability of the junctional complexes of the neighboring cells, which form a relatively impermeable wall around the injured area.

Types of Tissues

There are four basic types of tissues: epithelial, muscle, nerve, and connective tissues. The structure and function of these four types underlies the structure and function of each organ system.

TABLE 1-3 Characteristics of epithelial tissues

Type of epithelium	Structure	Location	Function
Simple squamous epithelium (Fig. 1-27)	Single layer of cells	Lining of blood vessels	Diffusion and filtration Separation of blood from fluids in tissues
		Lining of pulmonary alveoli (air sacs)	Separation of air from fluids in tissues
		Bowman's capsule (kidney)	Filtration of substances from blood, forming urine

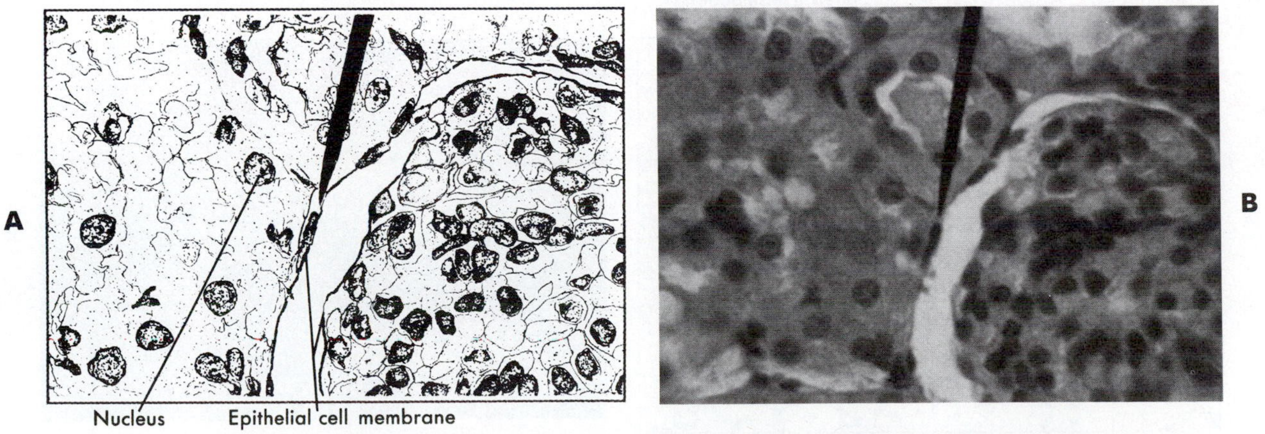

Nucleus   Epithelial cell membrane

FIG. 1-27. A, Simple squamous epithelial cell. **B,** Photomicrograph of simple squamous epithelial cell in parietal wall of Bowman's capsule in kidney. *Arrow* is touching a typical flattened squamous epithelial cell. (×140.) (From Thibodeau, 1987.)

Continued.

TABLE 1-3 Characteristics of epithelial tissues—cont'd

Type of epithelium	Structure	Location	Function
Stratified/squamous epithelium (Fig. 1-28)	Two or more layers, depending on location, with cells closest to basement membrane tending to be cuboidal.	Epidermis of skin Linings of mouth, pharynx, esophagus, anus, vagina	Protection and secretion

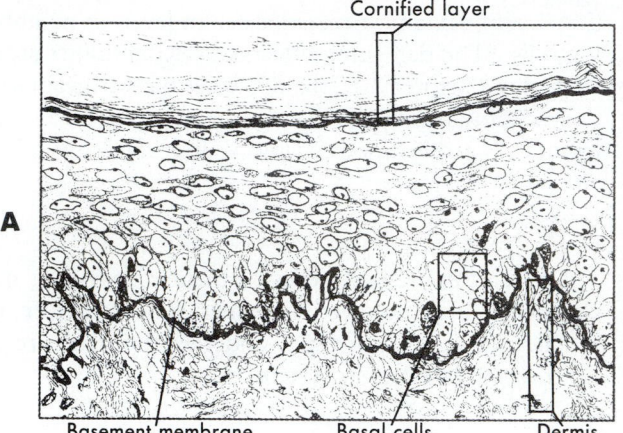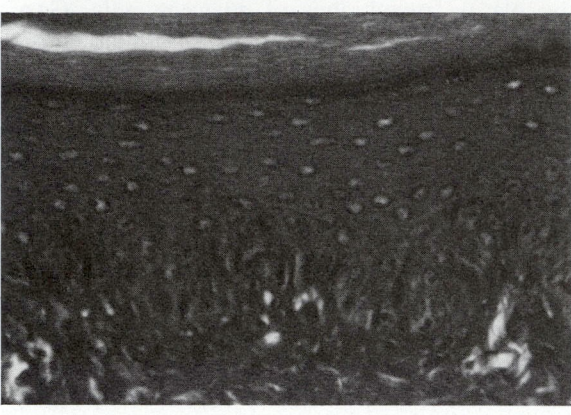

FIG. 1-28. A, Cornified stratified squamous epithelium. **B,** Photomicrograph of stratified squamous epithelium of the skin. (×140.) (From Thibodeau, 1987.)

Transitional epithelium (Fig. 1-29)	Vary in shape from cuboidal to squamous depending on whether basal cells of the bladder are columnar and comprise many layers. When the bladder is full and stretched, the cells flatten and stretch like squamous cells.	Linings of urinary bladder and other hollow structures	Stretching that permits expansion of hollow organs

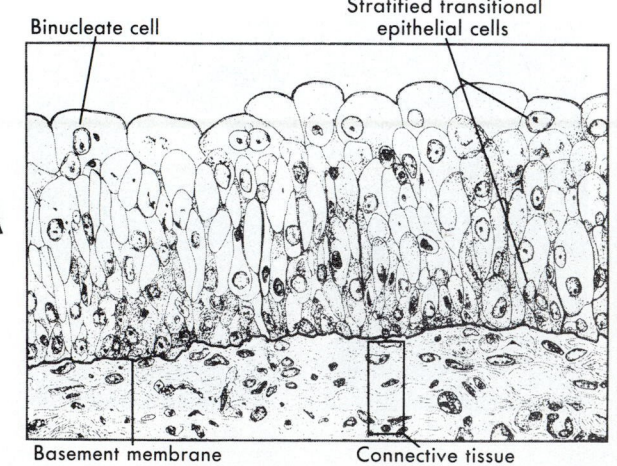

FIG. 1-29. A, Stratified squamous transitional epithelium. **B,** Photomicrograph of stratified squamous transitional epithelium of the vagina. (×140.) (From Thibodeau, 1987.)

TABLE 1-3 Characteristics of epithelial tissues—cont'd

Type of epithelium	Structure	Location	Function
Simple cuboidal epithelium (Fig. 1-30)	Simple cuboidal cells; rarely stratified (layered).	Glands, i.e., thyroid, sweat, and salivary Parts of kidney tubule and outer covering of the ovary	Secretion

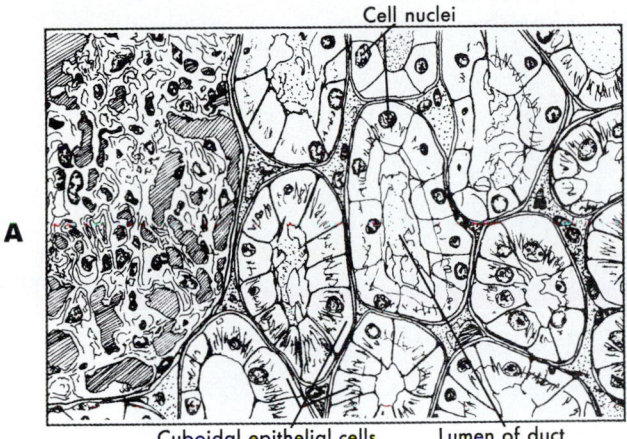
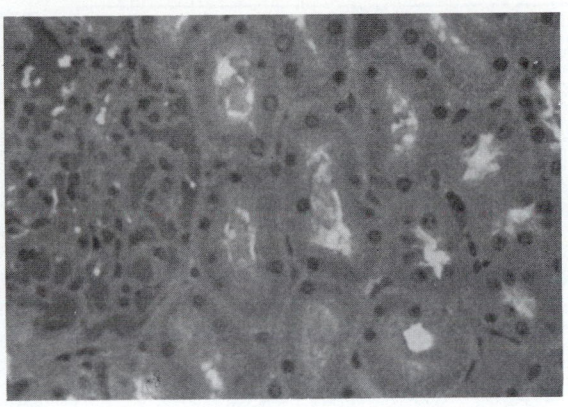

FIG. 1-30. A, Simple cuboidal epithelium. **B,** Photomicrograph of simple cuboidal epithelium of the distal convoluted tubule of the kidney. (×140.) (From Thibodeau, 1987.)

Type of epithelium	Structure	Location	Function
Simple columnar epithelium (Fig. 1-31)	Large amounts of cytoplasm and cellular organelles.	Lining of digestive tube from stomach to anus Ducts of many glands	Secretion and absorption
Ciliated simple columnar epithelium	Same as that of simple columnar epithelium, but ciliated.	Linings of bronchi of the lungs, nasal cavity, and oviducts	Secretion, absorption, and propulsion of fluids and particles

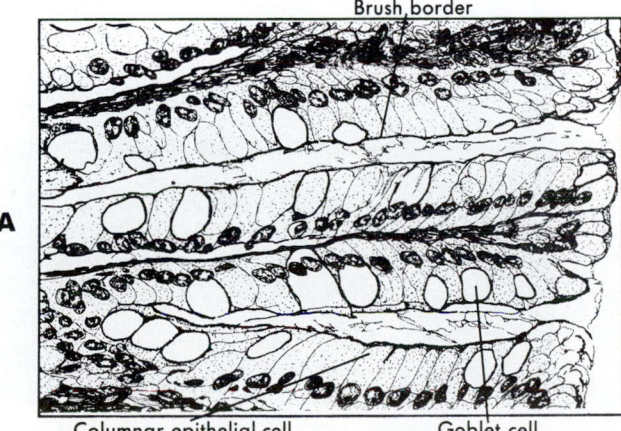
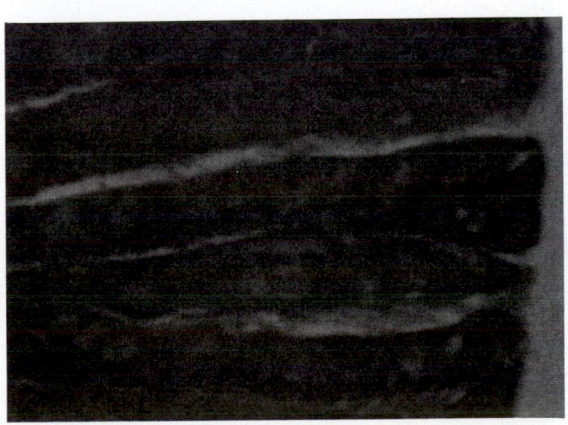

FIG. 1-31. A, Simple columnar epithelium. **B,** Photomicrograph of simple columnar epithelium of the colon. (×140.) (From Thibodeau, 1987.)

Continued.

TABLE 1-3 Characteristics of epithelial tissues—cont'd

Type of epithelium	Structure	Location	Function
Stratified columnar epithelium (Fig. 1-32)	Small and rounded basement membrane (columnar cells do not touch basement membrane).	Linings of epiglottis, part of pharynx, anus, and male urethra	Protection

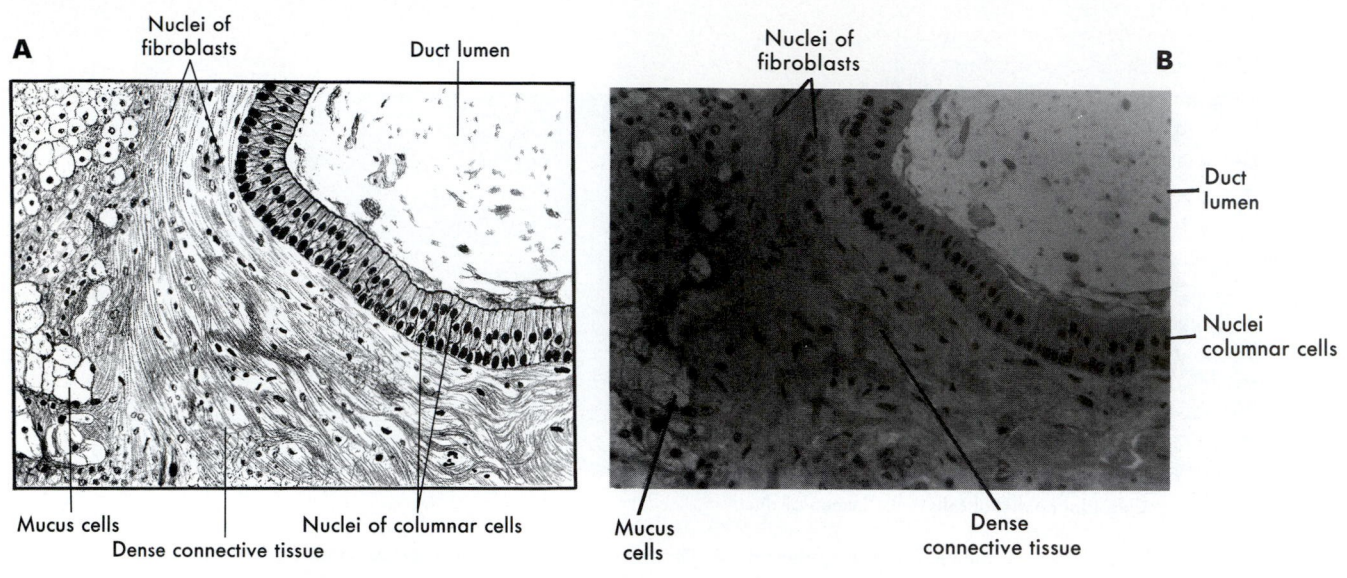

FIG. 1-32. **A,** Stratified columnar epithelium. **B,** Photomicrograph of stratified columnar epithelium of a large duct in the sublingual gland. (×280.) (**A** from Thibodeau, 1987; **B** courtesy Richard Ash, University of Utah.)

Pseudostratified ciliated columnar epithelium (Fig. 1-33)	All cells in contact with basement membrane. Nuclei found at different levels within the cell, giving stratified appearance. Free surface often ciliated.	Linings of large ducts of some glands (parotid, salivary), male urethra, respiratory passages, and eustacian tubes of ears	Transport of substances

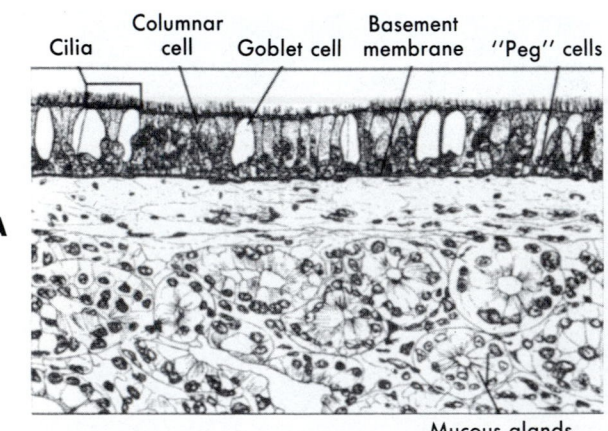

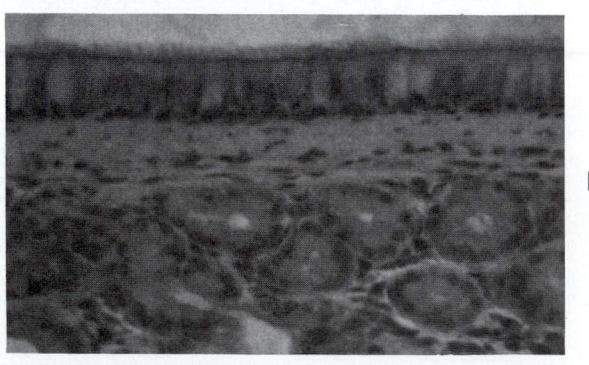

FIG. 1-33. **A,** Pseudostratified ciliated columnar epithelium. **B,** Photomicrograph of pseudostratified ciliated columnar epithelium of the trachea. (×280.) (From Thibodeau, 1987.)

Epithelial Tissue

Epithelial tissue covers most internal and external surfaces of the body. Epithelial cells are closely joined and are attached to a **basement membrane (basement lamina),** which provides a supporting layer and separates the epithelium from underlying connective tissue (see Fig. 1-25, *A*). Because of its variety of locations, epithelial tissue has several diverse functions, including protection, absorption, secretion, and excretion. For example, the epidermis provides a protective barrier between the host and the outside environment, whereas the linings of the internal body organs help absorb substances into the body, excrete waste products, and secrete substances into body cavities.

Epithelial cell surfaces differ according to their location and function. Epithelial cells that line body cavities and blood vessels are smooth, whereas other epithelial cells have tiny cytoplasmic projections called **microvilli** on their free surfaces. Microvilli considerably increase the cell's surface area and are found on cells whose main functions are absorption and secretion, such as the epithelial cells lining the digestive tract. **Cilia,** which are hairlike projections that propel mucus, pus, and dust particles out of the body, are characteristic of cells lining the respiratory passages.

Epithelial tissue is classified in two ways: (1) according to the number and arrangment of cell layers and (2) according to cell shape. Epithelium that is formed by a single layer of cells, all of which are in contact with the basement membrane, is called **simple epithelium.** **Stratified epithelium** has two or more layers of cells, and only the deepest layer is in contact with the basement membrane. Tissue that appears to consist of several cellular layers, but is actually a single layer with all cells contacting the basement membrane, is called **pseudostratified epithelium.**

Three basic cell shapes are found in epithelium: squamous, cuboidal, and columnar. **Squamous cells** are flat and thin; **cuboidal cells** are as high as they are wide and thus appear square in vertical sections; and **columnar cells** are taller than they are wide and appear rectangular in vertical sections. Overall classifications of epithelial tissue, which take into account both the number of cell layers and cell shape, are summarized in Table 1-3.

Connective Tissue

Connective tissue varies considerably in structure and function but is most common as the framework on which epithelial cells cluster to form organs. Other func-

---

TABLE 1-4 Connective tissues

Classification	Structure	Function and location
Loose or areolar tissue (Fig. 1-34)	Unorganized; spaces between fibers Most fibers collagenous, some elastic and reticular Includes many types of cells (fibroblasts and macrophages most common) and large amount of intercellular fluid	Attaches skin to underlying tissue, holds organs in place by filling the spaces between them, supports blood vessels Intercellular fluid transports nutrients and waste products. Fluid accumulation causes swelling (edema).

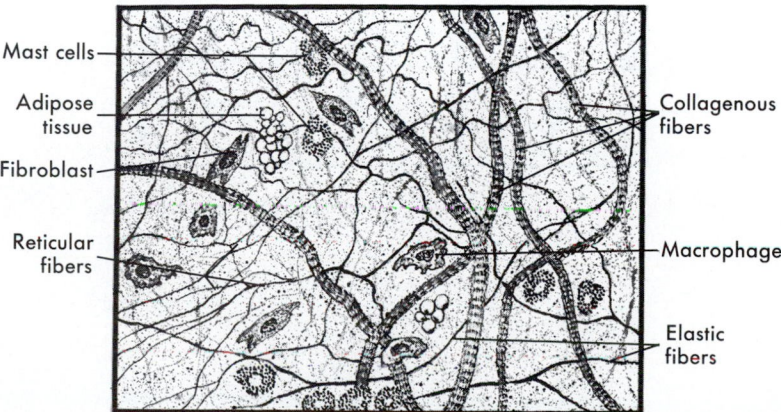

FIG. 1-34. Loose areolar connective tissue.

Continued.

TABLE 1-4 Connective tissues—cont'd

Classification	Structure	Function and location
Dense, irregular tissue (Fig. 1-35)	Dense, compact, and areolar tissue, with fewer cells and more, closely woven collagenous fibers than in loose tissue	Acts as protective barrier; dermis layer of the skin.

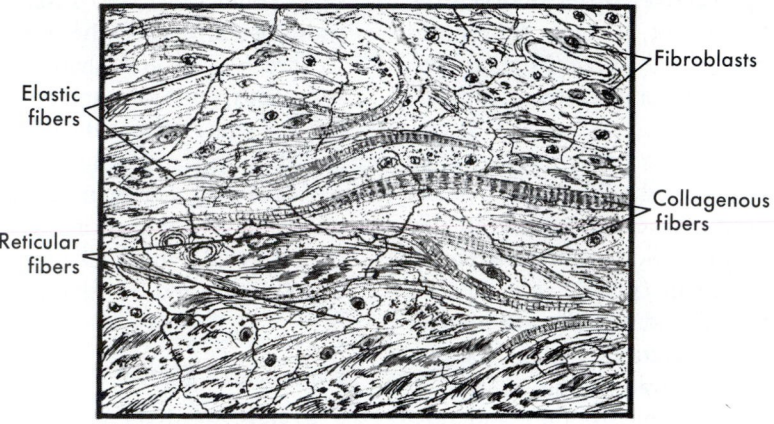

FIG. 1-35. Dense, irregular connective tissue.

Dense, regular (white fibrous) tissue (Fig. 1-36)	Collagenous fibers and some elastic fibers, tightly packed into parallel bundles, with fibroblasts the only cells	Forms strong tendons of muscle, ligaments of joints, some fibrous membranes, fascia that surrounds the organs and muscles.

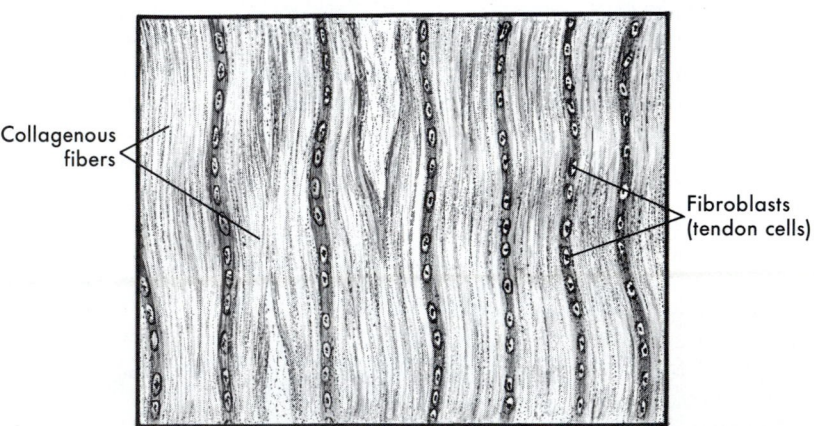

FIG. 1-36. Dense regular (white fibrous) connective tissue.

TABLE 1-4 Connective tissues—cont'd

Classification	Structure	Function and location
Elastic tissue (Fig. 1-37)	Elastic fibers, some collagenous fibers, fibroblasts	Lends strength and elasticity to walls of arteries, trachea, vocal chords, and other structures.

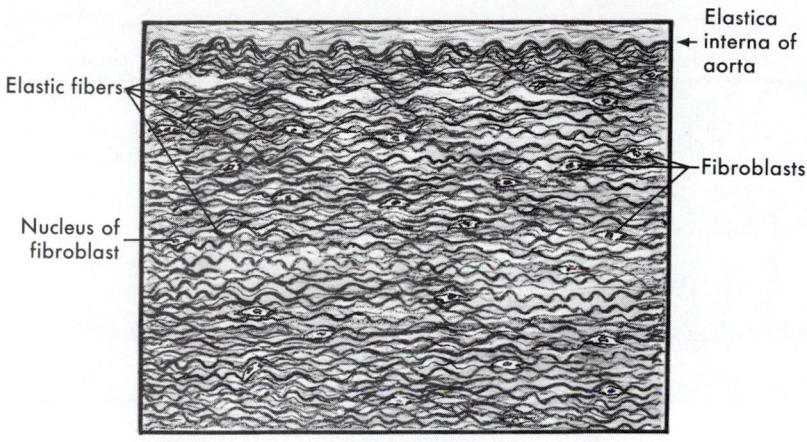

FIG. 1-37. Elastic connective tissue.

Classification	Structure	Function and location
Adipose tissue (Fig. 1-38)	Fat cells dispersed in loose tissue; each cell containing a large droplet of fat flattens nucleus and forces cytoplasm into a ring around cell's periphery.	Stores fat, which provides padding and protection.

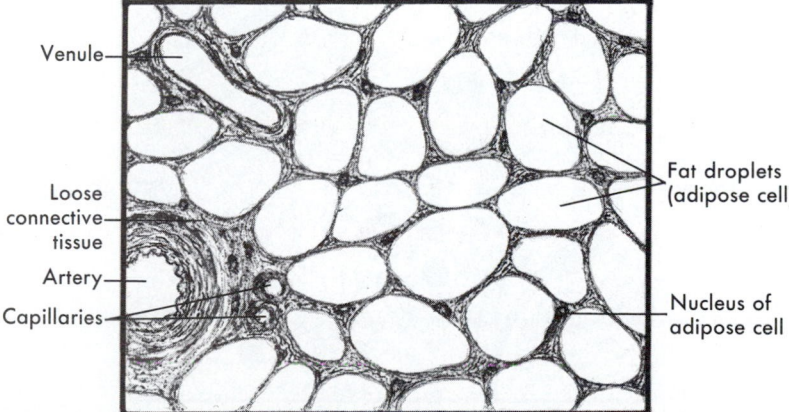

FIG. 1-38. Adipose tissue.

Continued.

TABLE 1-4 Connective tissues—cont'd

Classification	Structure	Function and location
Cartilage (hyaline, elastic, and fibrocartilage) (Fig. 1-39)	Collagenous fibers embedded in a firm matrix (chondrin); no blood supply	Gives form, support, and flexibility to joints, trachea, nose, ear, vertebral disks, embryonic skeleton, and many internal structures.

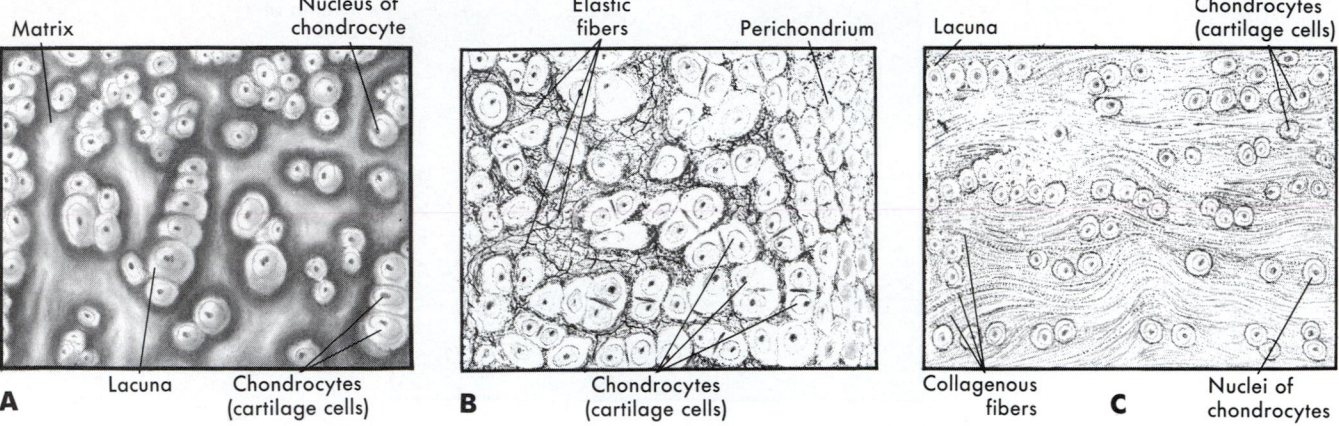

FIG. 1-39. **A,** Hyaline cartilage. **B,** Elastic cartilage. **C,** Fibrous cartilage.

Bone (Fig. 1-40)	Collagenous fibers and inorganic salts called osteoblasts Well supplied by blood vessels (see Chapter 45)	Lends skeleton rigidity and strength.

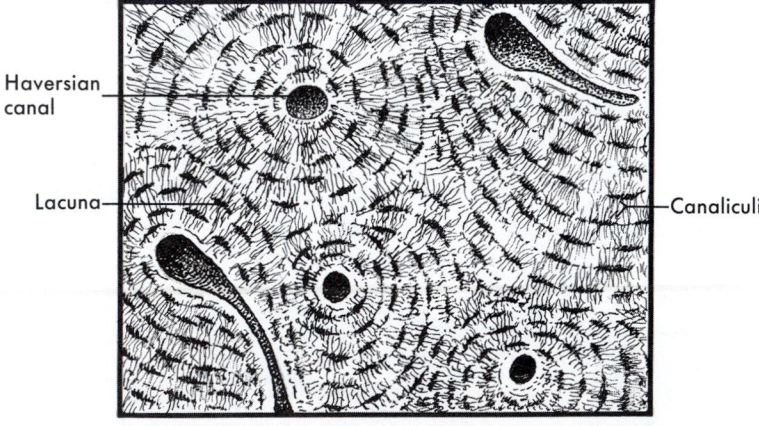

FIG. 1-40. Bone.

Special connective tissues		
Plasma	Fluid	Serves as matrix for blood cells.
Macrophages in tissue, reticuloendothelia, or macrophage system	Scattered macrophages (phagocytes) called Kupffer cells (in liver), alveolar macrophages (in lungs), microglia (in central nervous system)	Facilitate inflammatory response and carry out phagocytosis in loose connective, lymphatic, digestive, medullary (bone marrow), splenic, adrenal, and pituitary tissues.

tions include binding various tissues and organs together, supporting them in their locations, and serving as storage sites for excess nutrients.

In contrast to epithelial tissue, connective tissue is characterized by an abundant extracellular matrix that surrounds few cells. The extracellular matrix is composed of ground substance and fibers. **Ground substance** is a homogeneous mass that varies in consistency from fluid to semisolid gel. Fibers are produced by connective tissue cells (fibroblasts) found within the ground substance. There are three types of fibers: collagenous (white), elastic (yellow), and reticular. **Collagenous fibers** are formed of bundles of smaller fibrils appearing as wavy bands under the microscope. These fibers are composed of the protein collagen and are strong and inelastic. (Collagen synthesis by fibroblasts is described with respect to tissue repair in Chapter 7.) **Elastic fibers** are long, branching fibers composed of a protein called elastin that enables the fibers to return to their original length after stretching. Elastin occurs not only as fibers but also as membranes, particularly the membranes of blood vessels. **Reticular fibers** are thin, short, branching fibers that form an inelastic network made from a collagen-like protein called reticulum. Reticular fibers form the internal framework (stroma) to which the epithelial cells of glands are attached. They are found in loose connective tissue, generally in bone marrow and in the **parenchyma** (that is, the essential substance of an organ rather than its framework) of the liver, spleen, and lymph nodes.

Connective tissues are classified according to the consistency (e.g., as loose, dense) of the ground substance and the type and organization of the fibers within it. Table 1-4 summarizes the characteristics of connective tissues.

Muscle Tissue

Muscle tissue is composed of long, thin, cells or fibers called myocytes. Myocytes are highly contractile. Three different types of muscle tissue are skeletal, cardiac, and smooth (Table 1-5). (Muscles are discussed in detail in Chapter 38.)

Neural Tissue

Neural tissue is composed of highly specialized cells called neurons that receive and transmit electrical impulses very rapidly across junctions called synapses. Synapses are points of functional contact between neurons. At synapses, impulses pass from neuron to neuron or from a neuron to a muscle cell as chemical messengers called neurotransmitters are released (see Chapter 12). The total number of neurons is fixed at birth, and replacement is impossible thereafter.

Different types of neurons have special characteristics that depend on their distribution and function within the nervous system. All neurons, however, are com-

TABLE 1-5 Muscle tissues

Type of muscle	Structural characteristics of cells	Function	Location
Skeletal (striated) muscle (Fig. 1-41)	Long, cylindrical cells that extend throughout length of muscles Striated myofibrils (proteins) Many nuclei on periphery	Voluntary movement of skeleton; maintenance of posture	Attached to bones directly or by tendons

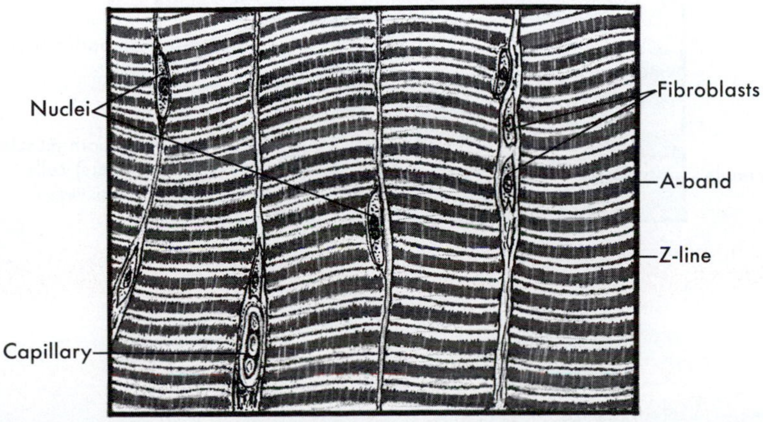

FIG. 1-41. Skeletal (striated) muscle.

Continued.

TABLE 1-5 Muscle tissues—cont'd

Type of muscle	Structural characteristics of cells	Function	Location
Cardiac muscle (Fig. 1-42)	Branching networks throughout muscle tissue Striated myofibrils	Involuntary pumping action of heart	Cells attached end-to-end at intercalated disks; tissue forms walls of heart (myocardium)

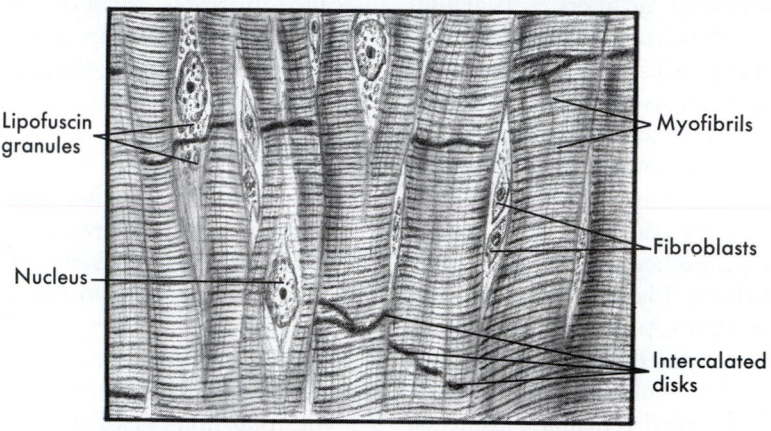

FIG. 1-42. Cardiac muscle.

Smooth (visceral) muscle (Fig. 1-43)	Long spindles that taper to a point Absence of striated myofibrils	Voluntary and involuntary contractions that move substances through hollow structures	Walls of hollow internal structures, such as digestive tract and blood vessels (viscera)

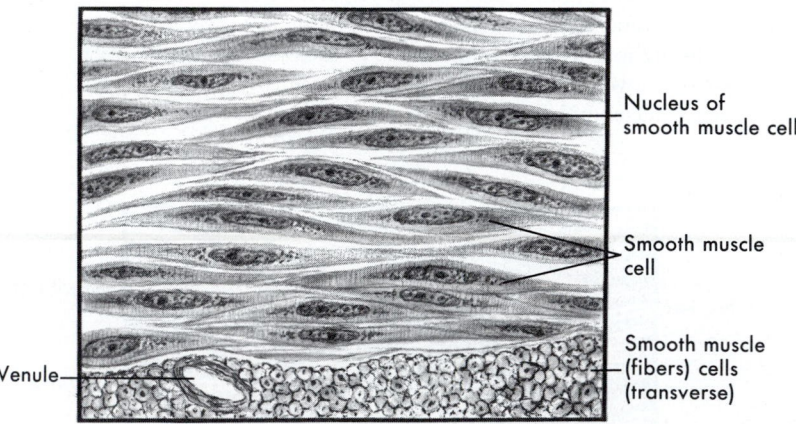

FIG. 1-43. Smooth (visceral) muscle.

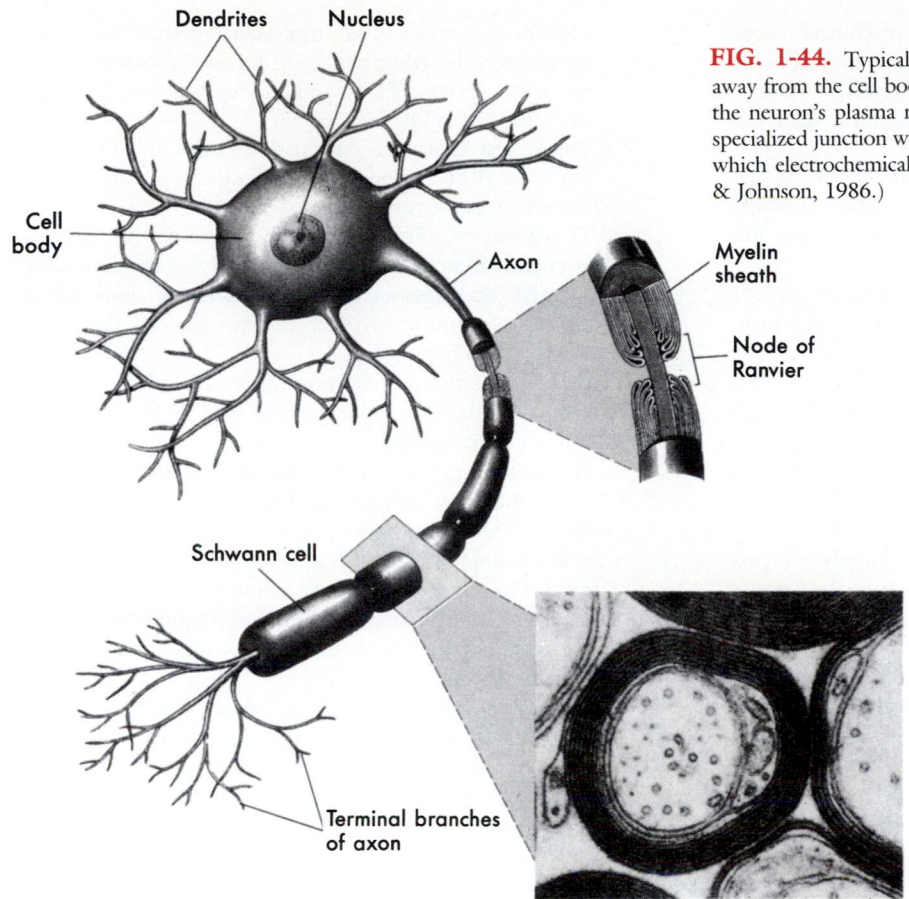

FIG. 1-44. Typical neuron. The axon conducts electrical signals away from the cell body. Signals are produced by a flux of ions across the neuron's plasma membrane. At the synapse, the neuron forms a specialized junction with another neuron (or with a muscle cell) across which electrochemical signals (neurotransmitters) pass. (From Raven & Johnson, 1986.)

Labels on figure: Dendrites, Nucleus, Cell body, Axon, Myelin sheath, Node of Ranvier, Schwann cell, Terminal branches of axon

posed of the following parts: (1) a cell body, (2) a single axon, and (3) one or more dendrites (Fig. 1-44). The cell body contains special cytoplasmic structures, as well as microtubules, actin filaments, Golgi complex, lysosomes, and lipofuscin. The axons and dendrites can be very long. Generally the axon conducts nerve impulses away from the cell body; dendrites conduct nerve impulses toward the cell body. (Neuronal transmission is discussed in Chapter 12).

SUMMARY REVIEW

Cellular Functions

1 Cells become specialized through the process of differentiation or maturation.
2 There are seven specialized cellular functions: movement, conductivity, metabolic absorption, secretion, excretion, respiration, and reproduction.
3 The eucaryotic cell consists of three general components: the plasma membrane, the cytoplasm, and the intracellular organelles.
4 The nucleus is the largest membrane-bounded organelle and is usually found in the cell's center. The chief function of the nucleus is cell division and control of genetic information.

5 Cytoplasm, or the cytoplasmic matrix, is an aqueous solution (cytosol) that fills the space between the nucleus and the plasma membrane.
6 The organelles are suspended in the cytoplasm and are enclosed in biologic membranes.
7 The endoplasmic reticulum is a network of tubular channels (cisternae) that extend throughout the outer nuclear membrane. It specializes in the synthesis and transport of protein and lipid components of most of the organelles.
8 The Golgi complex is a network of smooth membranes and vesicles located near the nucleus. The Golgi complex is responsible for processing and packaging proteins into secretory vesicles that break away from the Golgi complex and migrate to a variety of intracellular and extracellular destinations, including the plasma membrane.
9 Lysosomes are saclike structures that originate from the Golgi complex and contain digestive enzymes. These enzymes are responsible for digesting most cellular substances down to their basic form, such as amino acids, fatty acids, and sugars.
10 Cellular injury leads to a release of the lysosomal enzymes causing cellular self-digestion.
11 Peroxisomes are similar to lysosomes, but contain several enzymes that either produce or use hydrogen peroxide.

12 Mitochondria contain the metabolic machinery necessary for cellular energy metabolism. The enzymes of the respiratory chain (electron transport chain), found in the inner membrane of the mitochondria, generate most of the cell's ATP.

13 The cytoskeleton is the "bone and muscle" of the cell. The internal skeleton is composed of a network of protein filaments including microtubules and actin filaments (microfilaments)

14 The plasma membrane encloses the cell and, by controlling the movement of substances across it, exerts a powerful influence on metabolic pathways.

15 Protein receptors (recognition units) on the plasma membrane enable the cell to interact with other cells and with extracellular substances.

16 The plasma membrane is a bilayer of lipids (phospholipids and glycolipids) and cholesterol, which gives the membrane its structural integrity.

17 Membrane functions are determined largely by proteins. These functions include recognition by protein receptors and transport of substances into and out of the cell.

18 The fluid mosaic model accounts for the fluidity of the lipid bilayer and the flexibility, self-sealing properties, and selective impermeability of the plasma membrane.

19 Cellular receptors are protein molecules on the plasma membrane, in the cytoplasm, or in the nucleus, capable of recognizing and binding smaller molecules, called ligands.

20 The dynamic nature of the fluid plasma membrane enables it to vary the number of receptors on its surface. The cell is, therefore, capable of "hiding" from injurious agents by altering receptor number and pattern.

21 The ligand-receptor complex initiates a series of protein interactions, causing adenylate cyclase to catalyze the transformation of cellular ATP to messenger molecules that stimulate specific responses within the cell.

Cellular Metabolism

1 The chemical tasks of maintaining essential cellular functions are referred to as cellular metabolism. Anabolism is the energy-using process of metabolism, whereas catabolism is the energy-releasing process.

2 Adenosine triphosphate (ATP) functions as an energy-transferring molecule. Energy is stored by molecules of carbohydrate, lipid, and protein, which, when catabolized, transfer energy to ATP.

3 Oxidative phosphorylation occurs in the mitochondria and is the mechanism by which the energy produced from carbohydrates, fats, and proteins is transferred to ATP.

Processes of Cellular Intake and Output

1 Water and small, electrically uncharged molecules move through pores in the plasma membrane's lipid bilayer in the process called passive transport.

2 Passive transport does not require the expenditure of energy; rather it is driven by the physical effects of osmosis, hydrostatic pressure, and diffusion.

3 Larger molecules and molecular complexes (e.g., ligand-receptor complexes) are moved into the cell by active transport, which requires expenditure of energy (by means of ATP) by the cell.

4 The largest molecules (macromolecules) and fluids are transported by the processes of endocytosis (ingestion) and exocytosis (expulsion).

5 Two types of solutes exist in body fluids: (1) electrolytes and (2) nonelectrolytes. Electrolytes are electrically charged and dissociate into constituent ions when placed in solution. Nonelectrolytes do not dissociate when placed in solution.

6 Diffusion is the passive movement of a solute from an area of higher solute concentration to an area of lower solute concentration.

7 Hydrostatic pressure is the mechanical force of water pushing against cellular membranes.

8 Osmosis is the movement of water across a semipermeable membrane from a region of lower solute concentration to a region of higher solute concentration.

9 The amount of hydrostatic pressure required to oppose the osmotic movement of water is called the osmotic pressure of the solution.

10 The overall osmotic effect of colloids, such as plasma proteins, is called the oncotic pressure or colloid osmotic pressure.

11 Mediated transport can be passive or active. Mediated transport includes the movement of two molecules simultaneously in one direction (symport) or in opposite directions (antiport), or the movement of a single molecule in one direction (uniport).

12 Passive mediated transport is also called facilitated diffusion. It does not require the expenditure of metabolic energy.

13 Active mediated transport requires metabolic energy (ATP) to move molecules against the concentration gradient.

14 Active transport also occurs by endocytosis, or vesicle formation, in which the substance to be transported is engulfed by a segment of the plasma membrane, forming a vesicle that moves into the cell.

15 Pinocytosis is a type of endocytosis in which fluids and solute molecules are ingested through formation of small vesicles.

16 Phagocytosis is a type of endocytosis in which large particles, such as bacteria, are ingested through formation of large vesicles, called vacuoles.

17 In receptor-mediated endocytosis, the plasma membrane receptors are clustered, along with bristlelike structures, in specialized areas called coated pits.

18 Endocytosis occurs when coated pits invaginate, internalizing ligand-receptor complexes in coated vesicles.

19 Inside the cell, material ingested by endocytosis is processed and digested by lysosomal enzymes.

20 All body cells are electrically polarized, with the inside of the cell more negatively charged than the outside. The difference in voltage across the plasma membrane is the resting membrane potential.

21 When an excitable (nerve or muscle) cell receives an

electrochemical stimulus, cations enter the cell, causing a rapid change in the resting membrane potential known as the action potential. The action potential "moves" along the cell's plasma membrane and is transmitted to an adjacent cell. This is how electrochemical signals convey information from cell to cell.

Cellular Reproduction: The Cell Cycle

1 Cellular reproduction in body tissues involves mitosis (nuclear division) and cytokinesis (cytoplasmic division).

2 Only mature cells are capable of division. Maturation occurs during a stage of cellular life called interphase (growth phase).

3 The cell cycle is the reproductive process that begins after interphase in all tissues with cellular turnover. There are four phases of the cell cycle: (1) the S phase, during which DNA synthesis takes place in the cell nucleus; (2) the G_2 phase, the period between the completion of DNA synthesis and the next M phase; (3) the M phase, which involves both nuclear (mitotic) and cytoplasmic (cytokinetic) division; and (4) the G phase (growth phase, or interphase), after which the cycle begins again.

4 The M phase (mitosis) involves four stages: prophase, metaphase, anaphase, and telophase.

Tissues

1 Cells of one or more types are organized into tissues, and different types of tissues comprise organs. Organs are organized so as to function as tracts or systems.

2 Specialized cells are thought to form tissue by (1) mitosis of one or more founder cells, or (2) migration of founder cells and their subsequent assembly at the site of tissue formation.

3 Tissue cells are linked at cell junctions, which are specialized regions on their plasma membranes called desmosomes, tight junctions, and gap junctions. Cell junctions attach adjacent cells and allow small molecules to pass between them.

4 The four basic types of tissues are epithelial, muscle, nerve, and connective tissues.

5 Epithelial tissue covers most internal and external surfaces of the body. The functions of epithelial tissue include protection, absorption, secretion, and excretion.

6 Connective tissue binds various tissues and organs together, supporting them in their locations and serving as storage sites for excess nutrients.

7 Muscle tissue is composed of long, thin, highly contractile cells or fibers called myocytes. Muscle tissue that is attached to bones enables voluntary movement. Muscle tissue in internal organs enables involuntary movement, such as the heartbeat.

8 Neural tissue is composed of highly specialized cells called neurons that receive and transmit electrical impulses very rapidly across junctions called synapses.

KEY TERMS

Absolute refractory period, 28

Actin filament (microfilament), 12

Action potential, 28

Active mediated transport, 22

Active transport, 19

Amphipathic molecule, 13

Anabolism, 16

Anaerobic glycolysis, 18

Anaphase, 29

Anion, 19

Antiport, 22

Autodigestion, 9

Autolysosome, 9

Autophagy, 9

Basal body, 12

Basement membrane, 37

Catabolism, 16

Cation, 19

Cell cycle, 28

Cell junction, 32

Cellular metabolism, 16

Cellular receptor, 16

Centriole, 12

Centromere, 29

Chemotaxis, 32

Chromatid, 29

Chromatin, 29

Chromosome, 28

Cilium, 37

Citric acid cycle (Krebs cycle, tricarboxylic cycle), 18

Coated pit, 26

Collagenous fiber, 41

Columnar cell, 37

Competitive inhibitor, 22

Concentration gradient, 20

Contact guidance, 32

Contact inhibition, 30

Cuboidal cell, 37

Cytokinesis, 28

Cytoplasm, 5

Cytoplasmic matrix, 5

Cytoskeleton, 10

Daughter cell, 29

Depolarization, 28

Desmosome, 33

Diffusion, 20

Digestion, 18

Effective osmolality, 21

Elastic fiber, 41

Electrolyte, 19

Electron-transport chain, 18

Endocytosis, 25

Endoplasmic reticulum, 6

Equatorial plate (metaphase plate), 29

Eucaryote, 4

Exocytosis, 26

Extracellular matrix, 31

Fluid mosaic model, 15

Founder cell, 31

Gap junction, 33

Gating, 33

Glycolysis, 18

Golgi complex (Golgi apparatus), 6

Ground substance, 41

Hydrostatic pressure, 20

Hypertonic solution, 22

Hypotonic solution, 21

Integral membrane protein, 14

Interphase, 28

Ion, 19

Isotonic solution, 21

Junctional complex, 33

Ligand, 16

Lysosome, 8

Mediated transport, 22

Metabolic pathway, 16

Metaphase, 29

Microtubule, 10

Microvillus, 37

Mitochondrion, 10

Mitosis, 28

Nuclear envelope, 5

Nucleolus, 5

Nucleus, 5

Oncotic pressure (colloid osmotic pressure), 21

Organelle, 5

Osmolality, 21

Osmolarity, 21

Osmosis, 21

Osmotic pressure, 21

Oxidation, 18

Oxidative cellular metabolism (oxidation), 18

Oxidative phosphorylation, 18

Parenchyma, 41

Passive mediated transport (facilitated diffusion), 22

Passive transport, 19

Peripheral membrane protein, 14

Peroxisome (microbody), 10

Phagocytosis, 25

Pinocytosis, 25

Plasma membrane (plasmalemma), 5

Plasma membrane receptor, 16

Polarity, 19

Primary lysosome, 9

Prophase, 29

Procaryote, 4

Pseudostratified epithelium, 37

Receptor-mediated endocytosis (ligand internalization), 26

Relative refractory period, 28

Repolarization, 28

Residual body, 9

Resting membrane potential, 28

Reticular fiber, 41

Ribosome, 6

Secondary lysosome, 9

Secretory vesicle (secretory granule), 8

Simple epithelium, 37

Solute, 19

Spindle fiber, 29

Squamous cell, 37

Stratified epithelium, 37

Substrate phosphorylation, 18

Symport, 22

Telophase, 29

Threshold potential, 28

Tight junction, 33

Transfer reaction, 18

Transport protein (transporter), 22

Transmembrane protein, 14

Uniport, 22

Valence, 19

REFERENCES

Akera, T. (1977). Membrane adenosinetriphosphatase: A digitalis receptor? *Science, 198,* 569.

Alpert, B., Bray, D., Lewis, J., Raff, M., Roberts K., & Watson, J.K. (1983). *Molecular biology of the cell.* New York: Garland Publishing.

Anthony, C. P. & Kolthoff, N. J. (1975). *Textbook of anatomy and physiology* (9th ed.). St. Louis: C.V. Mosby.

Berne, R. M., & Levy, M. N. (Eds.) 1988. *Physiology.* (2nd ed.). St. Louis: C. V. Mosby.

Berridge, M. J. (1985, October). The molecular basis of communication within the cell. *Scientific American, 253*(4), 142.

Catt, K. J., Harwood, J. P., Aguilera, G., & Dufau, M. L. (1979). Hormonal regulation of peptide receptors and target cell responses. *Nature, 280,* 109-116.

Christensen, H. N. (1975). *Biological transport* (2nd ed.). Reading, PA: Benjamin.

Davies, A. O., & Lefkowitz, R. J. (1981). Regulation of adrenergic receptors. In R. J. Lefkowitz (Ed.), *Receptor regulation* (Series B, Volume 13.). London: Chapman & Hall.

Devlin, T. M (Ed.). (1982). *Textbook of biochemistry: With clinical correlations.* New York: Wiley.

Helmreich, E. J. M., Jenner, H. P., Pfeuffer, T., & Cori, C. F. (1976). Signal transfer from hormone receptor to adenylate cyclase. *Current Topics in Cell Regulation, 10,* 41-87.

Hobbs, A. S., & Albers, R. W. (1980). The structure of proteins involved in active membrane transport. *Annual Review of Biophysics and Bioengineering, 9,* 259-291.

Kaplan, J. (1981). Polypeptide-binding membrane receptors: Analysis and classification. *Science, 212,* 3.

King, D. W., Fenoglio, C. M., & Lefkowitch, J. H. (1983). *General patholoy: Principles and dynamics.* Philadelphia: Lea & Febiger.

Kissane, J. M. (Ed.). (1985). *Anderson's pathology.* (8th ed.). St. Louis: C. V. Mosby.)

Raven, P. H., & Johnson, G. B. (1986). *Biology.* St. Louis: C. V. Mosby.

Singer, S. J. (1977). Thermodynamics: The structure of integral membrane proteins and transport. *Journal of Supramolecular Structure, 6,* 313-323.

Smith, L., & Thier, S. (1981). *Pathophysiology: The biological principles of disease.* Philadelphia: W.B. Saunders.

Snyder, S. H. (1985, October). The molecular basis of communication between cells. *Scientific American, 253,* 4.

Thibodeau, G. A. (1987). *Anatomy and physiology.* St. Louis: Times Mirror/Mosby.

Vick, R. L. (1984). *Contemporary medical physiology.* Menlo Park, CA: Addison-Wesley.

CHAPTER 2

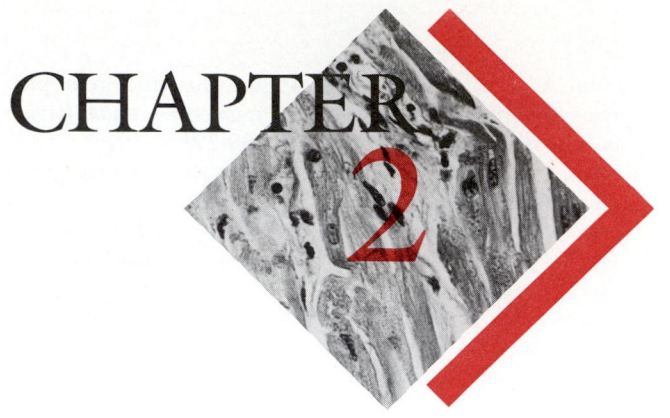

Altered Cellular and Tissue Biology

Kathryn L. McCance

Cellular adaptation, 49
  Atrophy, 50
  Hypertrophy, 50
  Hyperplasia, 50
  Dysplasia, 51
  Metaplasia, 51
Cellular injury, 51
  Hypoxic injury, 52
  Chemical injury, 55
    Mechanisms of chemical injury, 55
    Chemical agents, 56
      Lead, 56
      Gaseous substances, 56
  Infectious injury, 57
    Bacteria, 58
    Viruses, 59
      Viral replication, 59
      Cellular effects of viruses, 61
  Immunologic and inflammatory injury, 61
  Injurious genetic factors, 62
  Injurious nutritional imbalances, 62
  Injurious physical agents, 62
    Temperature extremes, 63
    Changes in atmospheric pressure, 63
    Ionizing radiation, 63
    Illumination, 65
    Mechanical factors, 65
    Noise, 65
    Prolonged vibration, 65
Manifestations of cellular injury, 66
  Cellular manifestations: accumulations, 66
    Water, 66
    Lipids and carbohydrates, 66
    Glycogen, 67
    Proteins, 68
    Pigments, 68
      Melanin, 68
      Hemoproteins, 69
    Calcium, 69
    Hyaline change, 70
  Systemic manifestations, 70
Cellular death, 70

Necrosis, 70
Apoptosis, 72
Aging, 73
  Normal life span, 73
  Theories and mechanisms of aging, 74
    Genetic and environmental factors, 74
    Alterations of cellular control mechanisms, 75
    Degenerative extracellular changes, 75
  Cellular aging, 75
  Tissue and systemic aging, 76
Somatic death, 76

Altered cellular and tissue biology can be due to adaptation, injury, neoplasia, aging, or death. (Neoplasia is discussed in Chapters 10 and 11.) Adaptation occurs in response to both normal, or physiologic, conditions and adverse, or pathologic, conditions. For example, the uterus adapts to pregnancy—a normal physiologic state—by enlarging. Enlargement occurs because of an increase in the size and number of uterine cells. In an adverse condition, such as high blood pressure, myocardial cells are stimulated to enlarge by the increased work of pumping. Like most of the body's adaptive mechanisms, however, cellular adaptations to adverse conditions are usually only temporarily successful. Severe or long-term stressors overwhelm adaptive processes, and cellular injury or death ensues.

Cellular injury can be due to any factor that disrupts cellular structures or deprives the cell of oxygen and nutrients required for survival. Injury may be reversible (sublethal) or irreversible (lethal) and is usually classified as chemical or hypoxic (lack of sufficient oxygen). Cellular injuries from various causes have different clinical and pathophysiologic manifestations.

Cellular death is confirmed by structural changes seen when cells are stained and examined under a microscope. No biochemical indicators of cellular death are universally applicable, however, perhaps because this phenomenon has not received as much attention by researchers as other cellular processes.

Cellular aging causes structural and functional changes that may eventually lead to cellular death or a decreased capacity to recover from injury. Mechanisms explaining how and why cells age are not known, and distinguishing between pathologic changes and physiologic changes that occur with aging is often difficult. Aging clearly causes alterations in cellular structure and function, yet senescence is both inevitable and normal.

CELLULAR ADAPTATION

Cells adapt to their environment to escape and protect themselves from injury. An adapted cell is neither normal nor injured—its condition lies somewhere between these two states. The most significant adaptive changes in cells include atrophy (decrease in cell size), hypertrophy (increase in cell size), hyperplasia (increase in cell number), and metaplasia (reversible replacement of one mature cell type by another, less mature cell

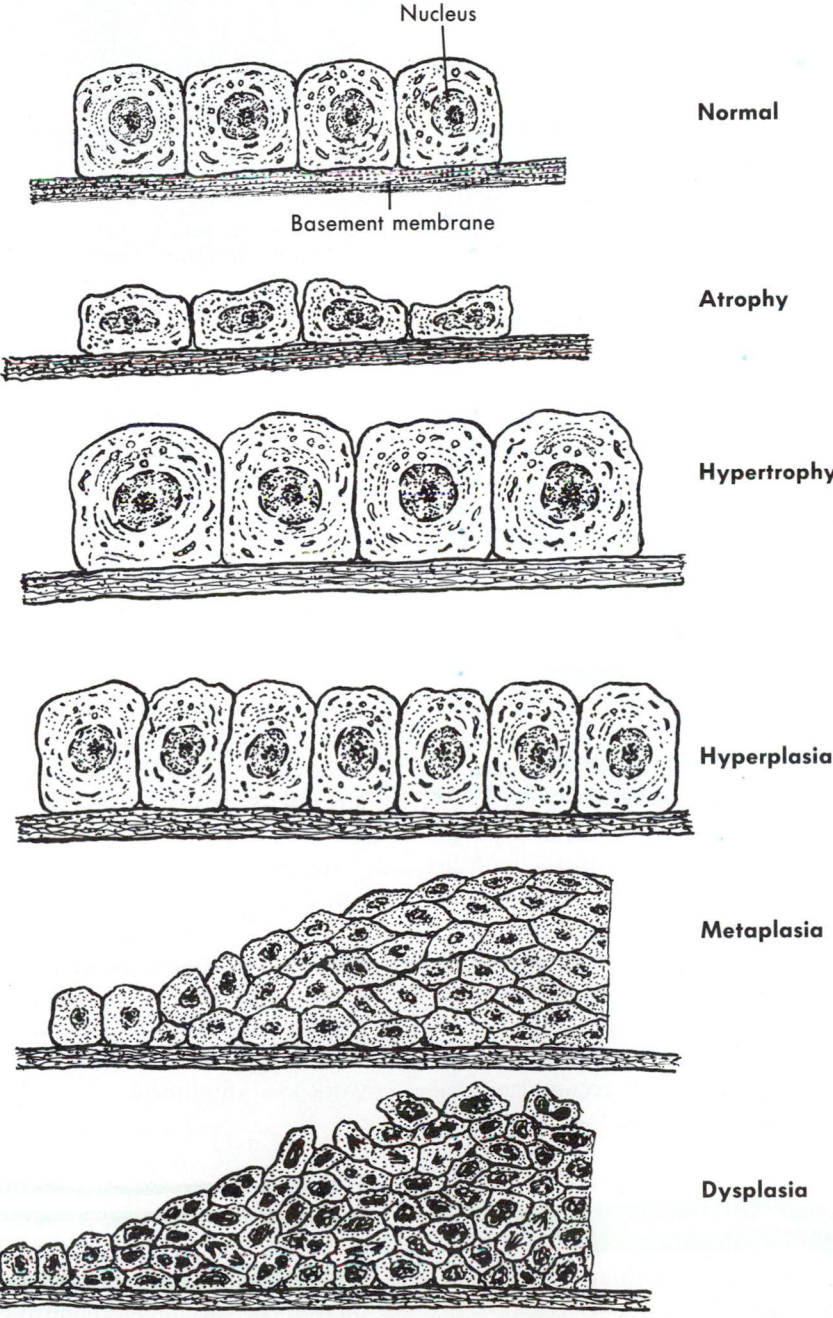

FIG. 2-1. Adaptive alterations in simple cuboidal epithelial cells

type). Dysplasia (deranged cellular growth) is not considered a true cellular adaptation, but rather atypical hyperplasia. These changes are shown in Fig. 2-1.

Atrophy

Atrophy is a decrease or shrinkage in cellular size. If atrophy occurs in a sufficient number of an organ's cells, the entire organ shrinks or becomes atrophic. Atrophy can affect any organ, but it is most common in skeletal muscle, the heart, secondary sex organs, and the brain. The causes of atrophy include decreases in work load, use, blood supply, nutrition, hormonal stimulation, and nervous stimulation. Individuals immobilized in bed for a prolonged time exhibit a type of skeletal muscle atrophy called disuse atrophy. Aging causes brain cells to become atrophic (presumably as arteriosclerosis obstructs the brain's blood supply) and endocrine-dependent organs, such as the gonads, to shrink as hormonal stimulation decreases (Robbins, Cotran, & Kumar, 1984). Whether atrophy is caused by normal physiologic conditions or pathologic conditions, atrophic cells exhibit the same basic changes.

The atrophic muscle cell contains less endoplasmic reticulum and fewer mitochondria and myofilaments (part of the muscle fiber that controls contraction) than the normal cell. In muscular atrophy caused by nerve loss, there is an immediate reduction in oxygen consumption and amino acid uptake. The biochemical changes of atrophy are not well understood, but mechanisms probably include decreased protein synthesis, increased protein catabolism, or both (Goldberg et al., 1980).

Atrophy is often accompanied by an increase in the number of **autophagic vacuoles,** which are membrane-bounded vesicles within the cell that contain cellular debris—small fragments of mitochondria and endoplasmic reticulum—and hydrolytic enzymes. Atrophic change causes a rapid increase in hydrolytic enzymes, which are isolated in autophagic vacuoles to prevent uncontrolled cellular destruction. Thus the vacuoles proliferate as needed to protect the uninjured organelles from the injured organelles and are eventually taken up and destroyed by lysosomes (a process described in Chapter 1). Certain contents of the autophagic vacuole may resist destruction by lysosomal enzymes and persist in membrane-bounded residual bodies. An example of such content are granules that contain **lipofuscin,** the yellow-brown age pigment. Lipofuscin accumulates primarily in liver cells, myocardial cells, and atrophic cells.

Hypertrophy

Hypertrophy is an increase in the size of cells and consequently in the size of the affected organ. The increase in cellular size is associated with an increased accumulation of protein in the cellular components (plasma membrane, endoplasmic reticulum, myofila-

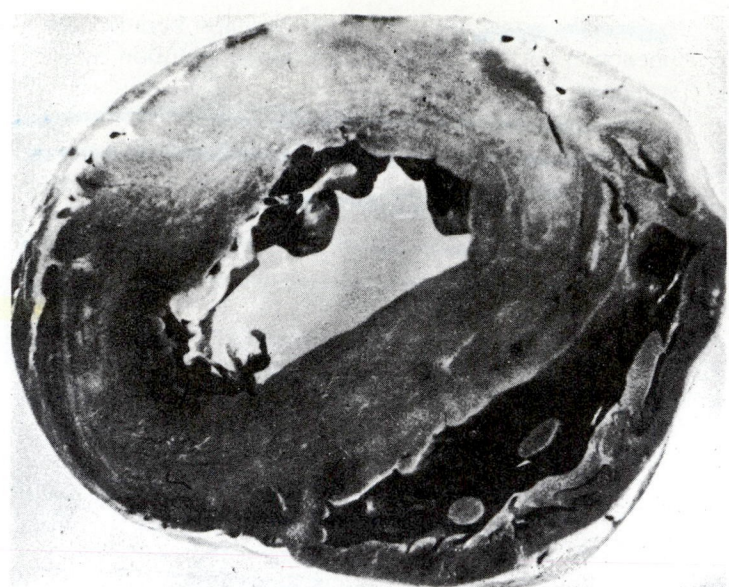

FIG. 2-2. Hypertrophy of the heart. The left ventricle is markedly thickened as an adaptive response to high blood pressure. (From Kissane, 1985.)

ments, and mitochondria), and *not* an increase in cellular fluid. The exact physiologic mechanism of hypertrophy in various cells remains uncertain. Muscular hypertrophy might involve an increase in the rate of protein synthesis, a decrease in the rate of protein degradation, or both. If protein degradation decreases and the rate of protein synthesis is normal or slightly increased, the net effect is an accumulation of cellular protein. In pregnancy, hypertrophy of the uterus is stimulated by estrogenic hormones that bind with estrogen receptors in smooth muscle, resulting in hormone-DNA interactions that increase the synthesis of smooth muscle proteins (Robbins et al., 1984). (Cellular receptors for hormones are discussed in Chapter 17; cellular accumulation of proteins is discussed on p. 68.)

In myocardial hypertrophy, the muscle cells (myocytes) increase in length, diameter, and volume (Smith & Thier, 1981). Myocardial hypertrophy is adaptive in that it permits the heart to meet increased work demands (Fig. 2-2). Eventually, however, advanced hypertrophy can lead to myocardial failure (see Chapter 27). Muscular hypertrophy tends to diminish if the excessive work load diminishes.

Hyperplasia

Hyperplasia is an increase in the number of cells resulting from an increased rate of cellular division (the cell cycle and mitosis are described in Chapter 1). Hyperplasia and hypertrophy often occur together, although the specific mechanism is unknown. Hyperplasia and hypertrophy will both take place if the cells are capable of synthesizing DNA, which enables mitotic division to occur.

Two types of normal, or physiologic, hyperplasia are (1) compensatory hyperplasia and (2) hormonal hyperplasia. **Compensatory hyperplasia** is an adaptive mechanism that enables certain organs to regenerate. For example, removal of part of the liver leads to hyperplasia of the remaining liver cells (hepatocytes) to compensate for the loss. Even with removal of 70% of the liver, regeneration is complete in about 2 weeks. The remarkable regenerating capacity of the liver was even noted by the ancient Greeks. According to the story, Prometheus was chained to a mountain, and his liver was eaten daily by a vulture, only to regenerate every night.

Not all types of mature cells have the same capacity for compensatory hyperplastic growth. Some cells, such as nerve, skeletal muscle, and myocardial cells, and the lens cells of the eye do not regenerate. It is not known why these cells are incapable of self-renewal and hyperplasia. Significant compensatory hyperplasia occurs in epidermal and intestinal epithelia, hepatocytes, bone marrow cells, and fibroblasts, and some hyperplasia is noted in bone, cartilage, and smooth muscle cells. An example of compensatory hyperplasia is a callus, or thickening, of the skin as a result of hyperplasia of epidermal cells in response to a mechanical stimulus (Fig. 2-3).

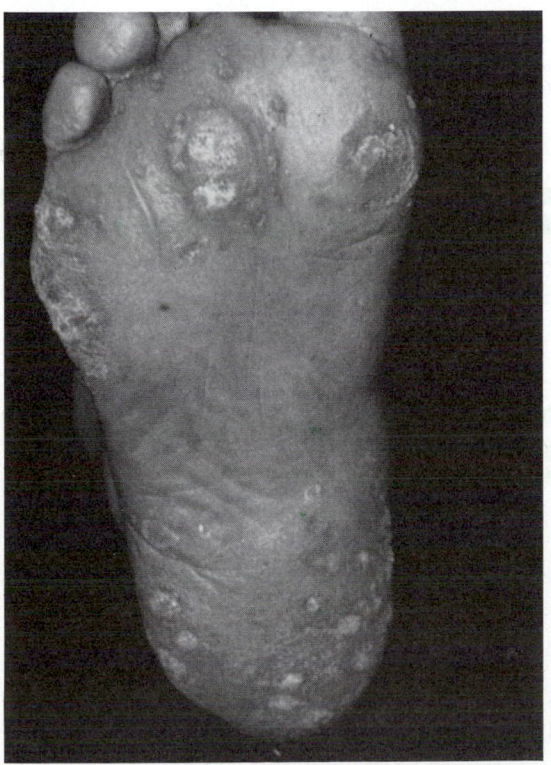

FIG. 2-3. Callus formation and hyperkeratosis or thickening of the skin. (From Thibodeau, 1987.)

Hormonal hyperplasia occurs chiefly in estrogen-dependent organs, such as the uterus and breast. After ovulation, for example, estrogen stimulates the endometrium to grow and thicken for reception of the fertilized ovum. If pregnancy occurs, hormonal hyperplasia, as well as hypertrophy, enables the uterus to enlarge. (Hormone function is described in Chapters 17 and 19.)

Pathologic hyperplasia is the abnormal proliferation of normal cells, usually in response to excessive hormonal stimulation. The most common example is pathologic hyperplasia of the endometrium (which is due to an imbalance between estrogen and progesterone secretion, with oversecretion of estrogen (see Chapter 20). Pathologic endometrial hyperplasia, which causes excessive menstrual bleeding, is under the influence of regular growth-inhibition controls. If these controls fail, hyperplastic endometrial cells can undergo malignant transformation. (Theories of malignant cell transformation are discussed in Chapter 11.)

Dysplasia

Dysplasia refers to abnormal changes in the size, shape, and organization of mature cells. Dysplasia, although not considered a true "adaptive process," is related to hyperplasia and is often called **atypical hyperplasia.** Dysplastic changes are frequently encountered in epithelial tissue of the cervix and respiratory tract, where they are strongly associated with common neoplastic growths and are often found adjacent to cancerous cells. Neoplasia is a term associated with malignant tumors. If the inciting stimulus is removed, dysplastic changes are often reversible.

Metaplasia

Metaplasia is the reversible replacement of one mature cell type by another, sometimes less differentiated, cell type. The best example of metaplasia is replacement of normal columnar ciliated epithelial cells of the bronchial (airway) lining by stratified squamous epithelial cells (Fig. 2-4). The newly formed squamous epithelial cells do not secrete mucus or have cilia, causing loss of a vital protective mechanism (protective mechanisms of the respiratory tract are described in Chapter 29).

Bronchial metaplasia can be reversed if the inducing stimulus, usually cigarette smoking, is removed. With prolonged exposure to the inducing stimulus, however, cancerous transformation can occur.

CELLULAR INJURY

The precise biologic processes responsible for cellular injury are complex, interdependent, and in many cases unknown. In general, cellular injury occurs if the cell is

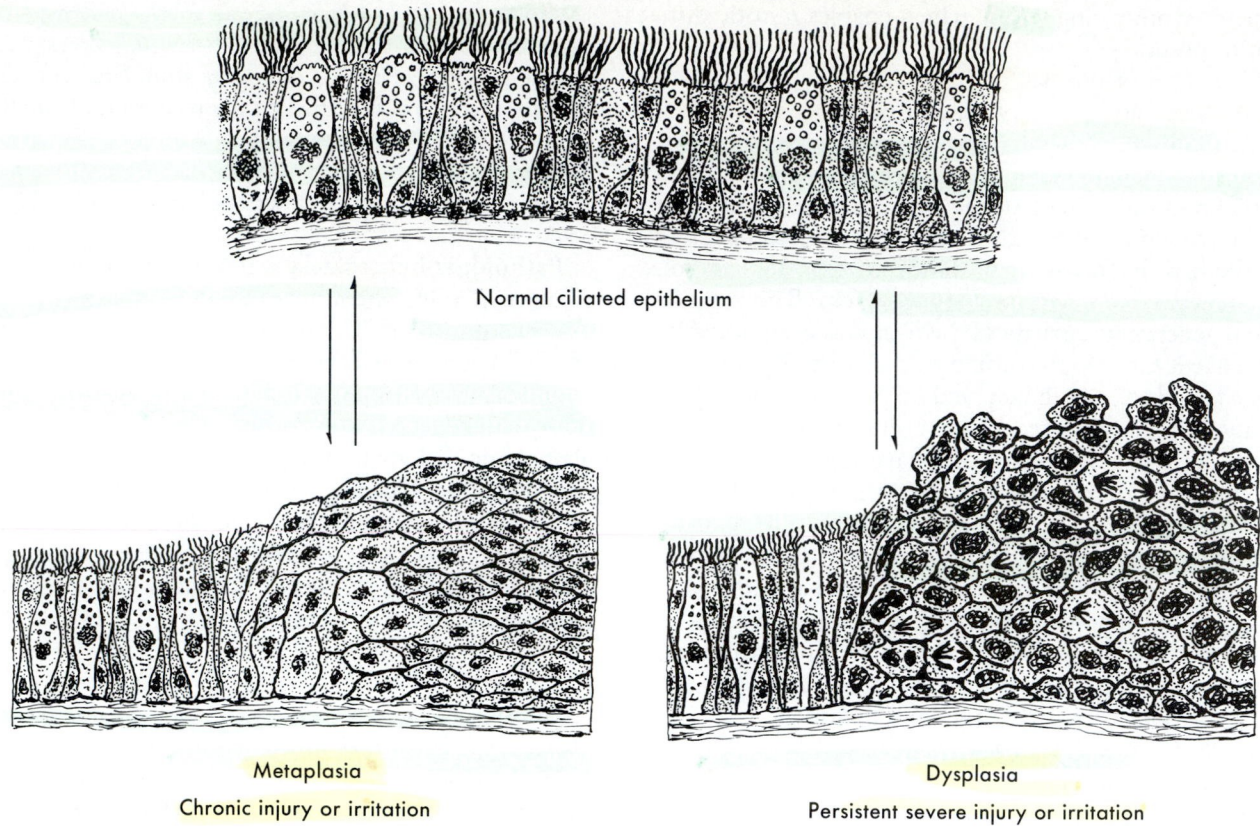

Normal ciliated epithelium

Metaplasia
Chronic injury or irritation

Dysplasia
Persistent severe injury or irritation

FIG. 2-4. Reversible changes in cells lining the bronchi.

unable to maintain homeostasis—a normal or adaptive steady state—in the face of injurious stimuli. Injurious stimuli include chemical agents, lack of sufficient oxygen (hypoxia), infectious agents, physical and mechanical factors, immunologic reactions, genetic factors, and nutritional imbalances.

The mechanisms causing chemical and hypoxic injury are perhaps the best understood. Both of these mechanisms can lead to disruption of selective permeability (i.e., transport mechanisms) of the plasma membrane; reduction or cessation of cellular metabolism; lack of protein synthesis; damage to lysosomal membranes, with leakage of destructive enzymes into the cytoplasm; enzymatic destruction of cellular organelles; cellular death (exhibited by nuclear changes); and phagocytosis of the dead cell by cellular components of the acute inflammatory response (see Chapter 7). The extent of cellular injury depends on the type, state, and adaptive processes of the cell, as well as the type, severity, and duration of the injurious stimulus. Two individuals exposed to an identical stimulus may incur varying degrees of cellular injury. Modifying factors, such as nutritional status, can profoundly influence the extent of injury. The precise "point of no return" that leads to cellular death is a biochemical puzzle, and the exact mechanisms

responsible for the transition from reversible to irreversible cellular damage are currently debated.

Hypoxic Injury

Hypoxia, or lack of sufficient oxygen, is the single most common cause of cellular injury (Fig. 2-5). Hypoxia can result from a decreased amount of oxygen in the air, loss of hemoglobin or hemoglobin function, decreased production of red blood cells, diseases of the respiratory and cardiovascular systems, and poisoning of the oxidative enzymes (cytochromes) within the cells. The most common cause of hypoxia is **ischemia** (reduced blood supply).

Ischemic injury is often caused by gradual narrowing of arteries (**arteriosclerosis**) and complete blockage by blood clots (**thrombos**is). Progressive hypoxia caused by gradual arterial obstruction is better tolerated than the sudden acute **anoxia** (total lack of oxygen) caused by a sudden obstruction, such as can occur with an embolus (a blood clot or other plug in the circulation). An acute obstruction in a coronary artery can cause myocardial cell death (infarction) within minutes if the blood supply is not restored, whereas gradual onset of ischemia usually results in myocardial adaptation. The most common causes of death in the United States, myocardial

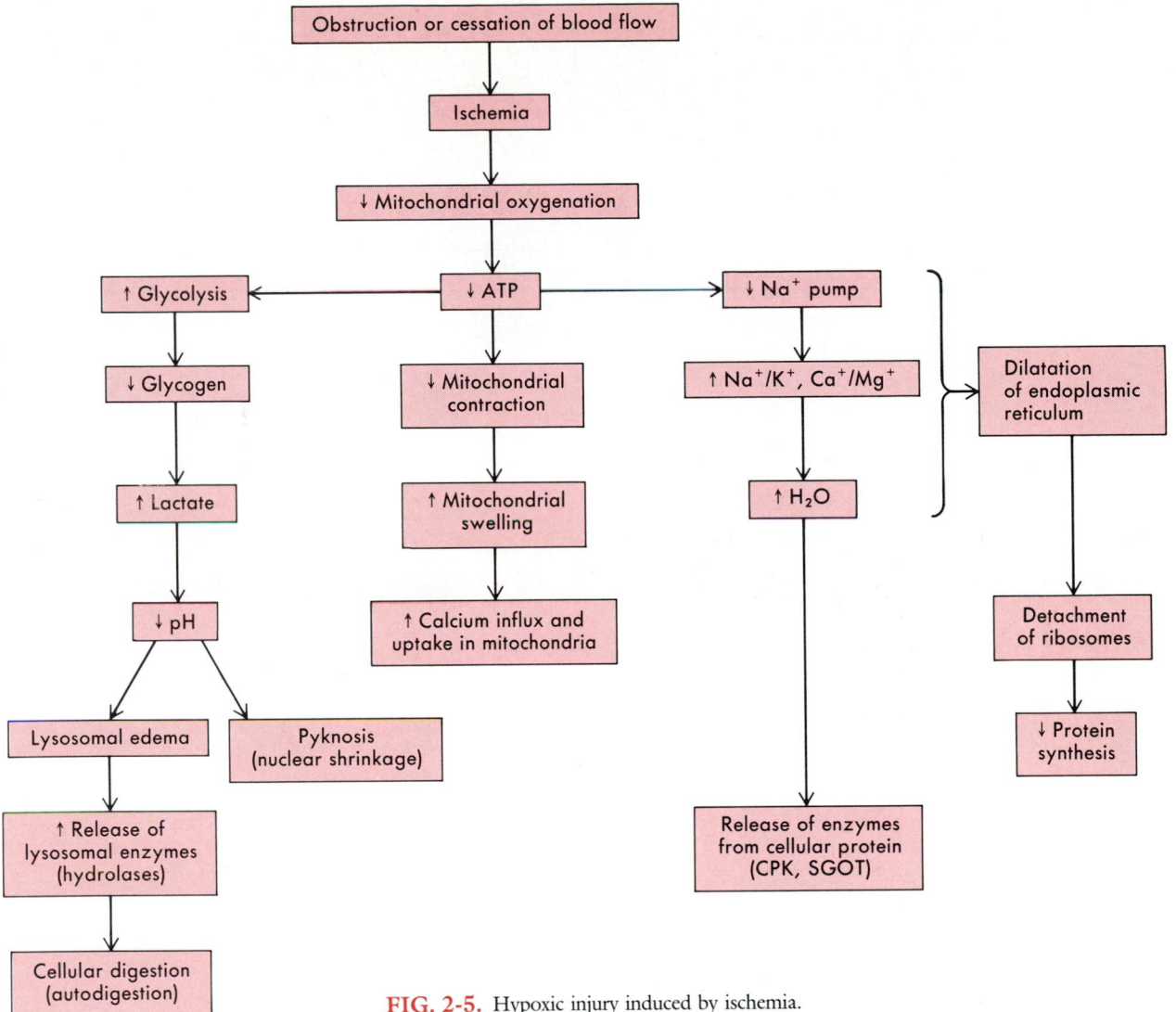

FIG. 2-5. Hypoxic injury induced by ischemia.

infarction and stroke, generally result from atherosclerosis (a type of arteriosclerosis) and consequent ischemic injury. (Vascular obstruction is discussed in Chapter 27.)

Cellular responses to hypoxic injury caused by ischemia have been demonstrated in studies of the heart muscle (Morgan & Neely, 1982; Neely & Morgan, 1974). Within a minute of interruption of blood supply to the myocardium, the heart becomes pale and has difficulty contracting normally. Within 3 to 5 minutes, the ischemic portion of the myocardium ceases to contract. The abrupt lack of contraction is due to a rapid decrease in mitochondrial phosphorylation, which results in insufficient adenosine triphosphate (ATP) production. Lack of ATP leads to an increase in anaerobic metabolism, which generates ATP from glycogen when there is insufficient oxygen. When glycogen stores are depleted, even anaerobic metabolism ceases. (Aerobic and anaerobic cellular metabolism are described in Chapter 1.)

A reduction in ATP levels causes the plasma membrane's sodium-potassium pump to fail, which leads to an intracellular accumulation of sodium and diffusion of potassium out of the cell. (The sodium-potassium pump is discussed in Chapter 1.) Sodium and water can then freely enter the cell, and cellular swelling results. The movement of water and ions into the cell causes early dilation of the endoplasmic reticulum. Dilation causes the ribosomes to detach from the rough endoplasmic reticulum, resulting in reduced protein synthesis. With continued hypoxia, the entire cell becomes markedly swollen with increased concentrations of sodium, water, and chloride, and decreased concentrations of potassium. These disruptions are reversible if oxygen is restored. However, if oxygen is not restored, there is vacuolation (formation of vacuoles) within the cytoplasm and marked swelling of the mitochondria resulting from mitochondrial membrane damage. Structurally, this stage is associated with irreversible cell injury. With

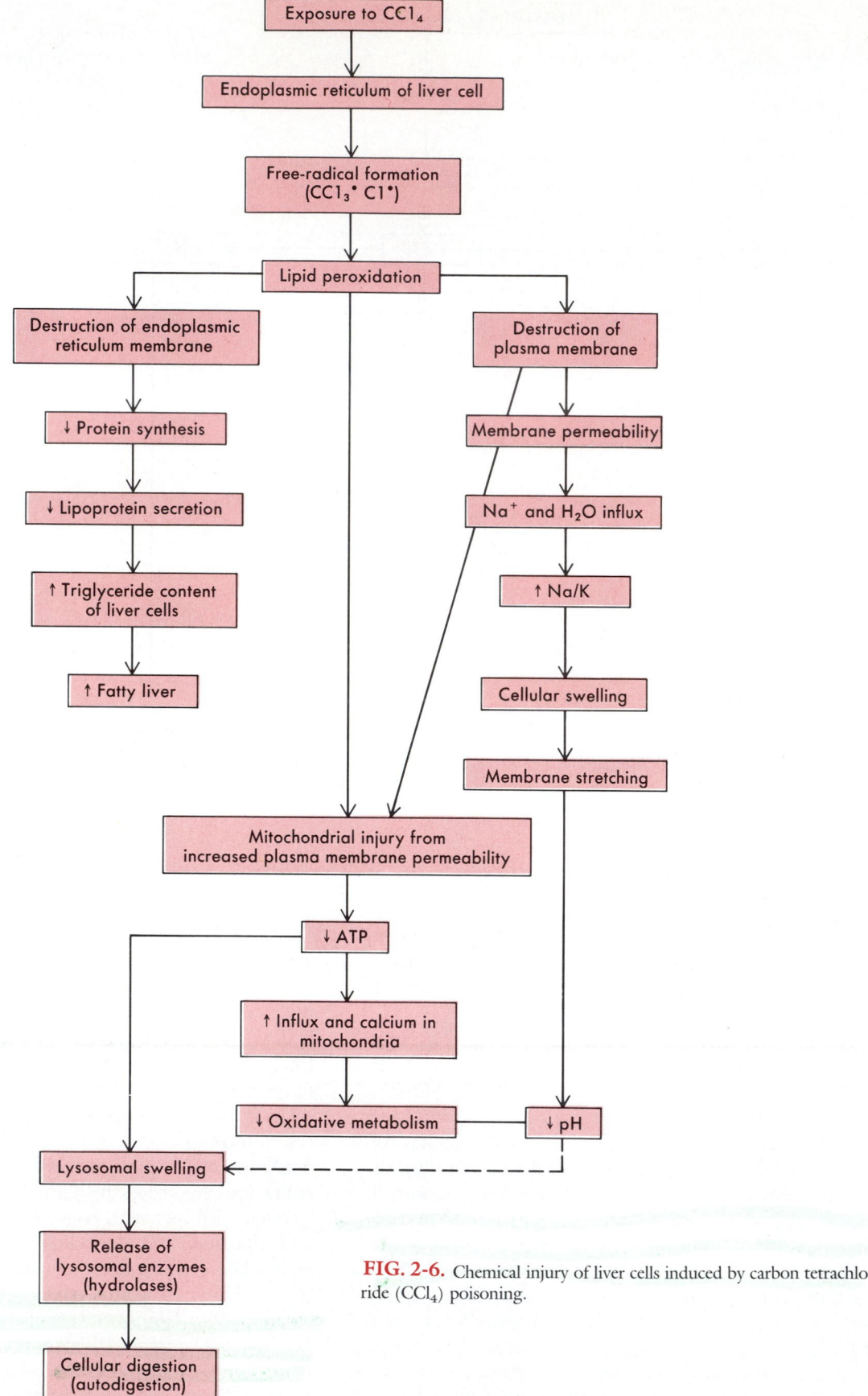

FIG. 2-6. Chemical injury of liver cells induced by carbon tetrachloride (CCl₄) poisoning.

plasma membrane damage, extracellular calcium moves into the cell and accumulates in the mitochondria.

All cells in the body are bathed in a fluid rich in calcium ions. In muscle cells, calcium is necessary for the activation of the contractile proteins, actin and myosin. If the plasma membrane's barrier to calcium ions is eliminated or damaged, calcium readily enters and accumulates in the mitochondria, resulting in mitochondrial swelling and rapid death of the cell (Farber, 1981). Death is due to calcium accumulation compromising ATP production by the mitochondria. In hypoxic injury caused by atherosclerosis, failure of ATP production further deprives the myocardium of the energy needed for contraction.

Chemical Injury
Mechanisms of Chemical Injury

Chemical injury begins with a biochemical interaction between a toxic substance and the cell's plasma membrane, which is ultimately damaged, leading to increased permeability. Not all of the mechanisms causing chemically induced membrane destruction are known.

Because it has been investigated extensively, carbon tetrachloride (CCl_4) injury is a useful example of chemical injury. Carbon tetrachloride, an agent formerly used in dry cleaning, is injurious to cells because an enzyme system in the smooth endoplasmic reticulum of liver cells converts it into CCl_3, a highly toxic free radical. A free radical is an electrically uncharged atom or group of atoms having an unpaired electron that is capable of injurious chemical-bond formation. Free radicals are highly reactive, are difficult to control, and induce chain reactions. The formation of free radicals in biologic materials requires an extreme energy source, such as ioniz-

ing radiation (e.g., x-rays) or interactions with other molecules, such as CCl_4 or oxygen. Free radicals can damage cellular membranes by **lipid peroxidation**, which is the destruction of polyunsaturated lipids (the same process by which fats become rancid). Peroxidation involves the reaction of oxygen-derived free radicals, such as free hydroxyl groups ($\overline{OH}$), and lipids to form free-radical intermediates and moderately stable peroxides (Robbins et al., 1984). These actions can lead to chain reactions, causing autooxidation of the fatty-acid content of lipids in cellular membranes. The formation of free radicals also occurs during phagocytosis as a way of killing bacteria (see Chapter 7).

In CCl_4 injury, newly formed CCl_3 rapidly destroys the endoplasmic reticulum of the liver cell by breaking down the reticulum's lipid component. The next event in CCl_3 injury is an accumulation of lipid molecules within the cytoplasm, starting within cisternae of the endoplasmic reticulum (Fig. 2-6). Fatty liver develops because CCl_4 poisoning blocks the synthesis of **lipid-acceptor proteins (apoproteins)** that normally bind with triglycerides to form lipoproteins, which are transported out of the cell. Blockage of triglyceride (lipoprotein) secretion begins 10 to 15 minutes after CCl_4 exposure. Fat droplets that accumulate in cisternae of the endoplasmic reticulum combine to form larger droplets and fill vacuoles that, in turn, fill the entire cytoplasm (Fig. 2-7). Approximately 10 to 12 hours later, the liver appears grossly enlarged and pale because of the accumulation of fat. (Accumulation of fat is discussed further on p. 67.)

In the meantime, cellular swelling progresses because of alterations in the selective permeability of the plasma membrane. Cellular swelling becomes severe when the

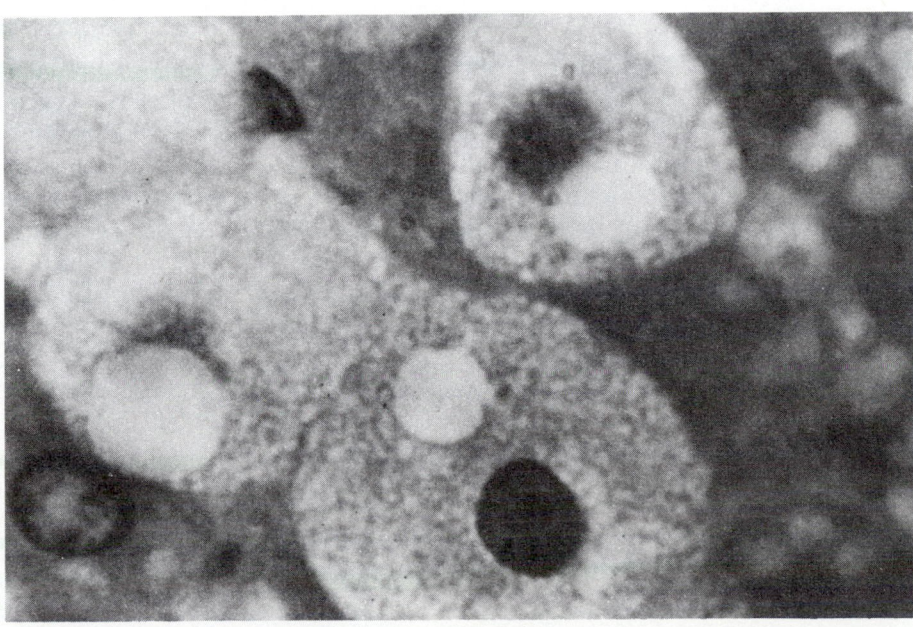

FIG. 2-7. Electron micrograph of liver cells 8 hours after administration of CCl_4. Hepatocytes are large and edematous with a finely granular cytoplasm; clear vacuoles probably represent infiltration of triglycerides. Nuclei appear normal. (From Kissane, 1985.)

plasma membrane loses its ability to prevent the passive inward diffusion of sodium ions and water. The most serious consequence of plasma membrane damage is, as in hypoxic injury, to the mitochondria. An influx of calcium ions from the extracellular compartment and their accumulation in the mitochondria cause the mitochondria to swell, an occurrence that is associated with irreversible cellular injury. The injured mitochondria can no longer generate ATP, but they do continue to accumulate calcium ions. The influx of calcium into the mitochondria interferes with oxidative metabolism (by uncoupling oxidative phosphorylation). Like hypoxic injury, chemical injury causes reduction in ATP, causing failure of the sodium-potassium pump, which results in intracellular accumulation of sodium and diffusion of potassium out of the cell. Sodium and water freely enter the cell and cellular swelling results. As ATP generation fails, the cell loses its capacity for active transport of ions and oxidization of fatty acids, which lowers pH and may lead to further lipid accumulation.

Decreasing cellular pH (caused by the loss of oxidative phosphorylation and ATP), together with fluid and electrolyte imbalances (increased sodium and water and decreased potassium), lead to lysosomal membrane injury, causing a leakage of lysosomal enzymes into the cytoplasm. Enzymatic digestion of cellular organelles, including the nucleus and nucleolus, ensues, halting synthesis of deoxyribonucleic acid (DNA) and ribonucleic acid (RNA) (see Chapter 4.) The leakage of lysosomal enzymes apparently occurs late in chemical injury, well after irreversible lipid accumulation, mitochondrial swelling, and ATP loss. The lysosomal phase of chemical injury is probably similar to that which occurs in hypoxic injury.

Chemical Agents

A number of chemical agents, too numerous to list, cause cellular injury. Highly toxic substances are known as poisons. Minute amounts of some, such as arsenic and cyanide, can rapidly destroy enough cells to cause somatic death (death of the individual). Chronic exposure to air pollutants, insecticides, and herbicides can cause cellular injury. Carbon monoxide, carbon tetrachloride, and social drugs, such as alcohol, can significantly alter cellular function and injure cellular structures. Over-the-counter and prescribed drugs may also cause cellular injury, sometimes leading to death. Accidental or suicidal poisonings by chemical agents cause numerous deaths. The injurious effects of some of these agents—lead, carbon monoxide, hydrogen cyanide, and hydrogen sulfide—exemplify common cellular injuries.

Lead

Heavy metals, such as lead, cause a significant number of childhood poisonings. Lead-based paint, which has a sweet taste, is often ingested by children. Children are particularly vulnerable to lead toxicity because, compared to adults, they absorb lead more readily through the intestines (Chisholm, 1976). If nutrition is compromised, especially if dietary intake of iron, calcium, and vitamin D is insufficient, lead's toxic effects are enhanced.

The organ systems primarily affected by lead include the nervous system, the hematopoietic system (tissues that produce blood cells), and the kidneys. A suggested mechanism by which lead acts on the central nervous system is interference with neurotransmitters, which may cause hyperactive behavior (Fishbein, 1983). Lead inhibits several enzymes involved in red blood cell synthesis (Piomelli, 1981). A significant manifestation of lead toxicity is anemia caused by lysis of red blood cells (hemolysis). Manifestations of brain involvement include convulsions and delirium and, with peripheral nerve involvement, wrist, finger, and sometimes foot paralysis. Renal lesions can cause tubular dysfunction resulting in glycosuria (glucose in the urine), aminoaciduria (amino acids in the urine), and hyperphosphaturia (excess phosphate in the urine). Gastrointestinal symptoms are less severe and include nausea, loss of appetite, weight loss, and abdominal cramping.

Gaseous Substances

Gaseous substances can be classified according to their ability to asphyxiate (interrupt respiration) or irritate. Toxic asphyxiants, such as carbon monoxide, hydrogen cyanide, and hydrogen sulfide, directly interfere with cellular respiration.

Carbon monoxide is odorless, colorless, and undetectable unless it is mixed with a visible or odorous pollutant. It is produced by the incomplete combustion of such fuels as gasoline. Although carbon monoxide is a chemical agent, the ultimate injury it produces is a hypoxic injury, namely oxygen deprivation (Fig. 2-8). Normally, oxygen molecules are carried to tissues bound to hemoglobin in red blood cells (see Chapter 29). Because carbon monoxide's affinity for hemoglobin is 300 times greater than that of oxygen, it quickly binds with the hemoglobin, preventing oxygen molecules from doing so. Minute amounts of carbon monoxide can produce significant percentages of carboxyhemoglobin (carbon monoxide bound with hemoglobin).

Symptoms related to carbon monoxide poisoning include headache, giddiness, tinnitus (ringing in the ears), nausea, weakness, and vomiting. At risk for carbon monoxide exposure are those who (1) breathe air polluted by gasoline engines or defective furnaces, (2) work in such occupations as coal mining, fire fighting, or engine repair, and (3) smoke cigarettes, cigars, or pipes. The fetus is especially at risk from the effects of carbon monoxide because fetal carboxyhemoglobin levels are

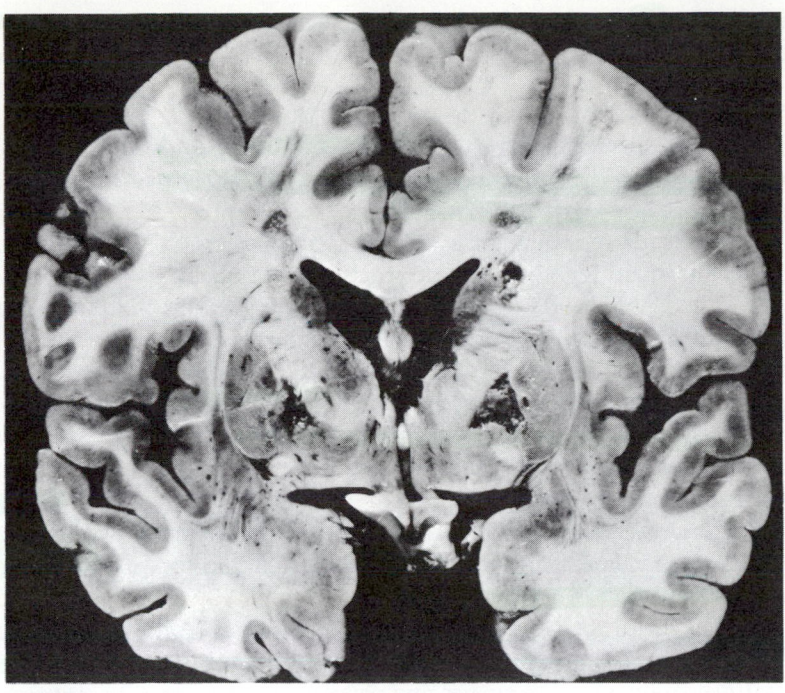

FIG. 2-8. Carbon monoxide poisoning. Bilateral necrosis of globus pallidus in individual who died 42 days after exposure. (From Kissane, 1985.)

likely to be 10% to 15% greater than maternal levels (Holbrook, 1983).

Hydrogen cyanide is an extremely rapid-acting poison that causes somatic death within a few minutes. Once absorbed, cyanide is converted in the body to hydrogen cyanide and the cyanide ion reacts with the ion of cytochrome oxidases, inactivating the enzymes essential for cellular oxygenation. Poisoning from hydrogen cyanide can occur not only from its gas form, which has a sweetish, almondlike odor, but also from its liquid form, which can penetrate the skin. A well-known form of cyanide, amygdalin, is found in the seeds of apricots, peaches, cherries, plums, and apples. This form is used in the controversial cancer drug, Laetrile. Cyanide is also an ingredient in nitroprusside (Nipride), a drug used to treat severe hypertension. If given intravenously in sufficient amounts, nitroprusside can produce mild forms of cyanide poisoning (Kurt, 1983).

Hydrogen sulfide, which has the odor of rotten eggs, interferes with the oxidative enzymes, causing cellular hypoxia. Its odor is extremely pungent, but high concentrations of the gas can produce olfactory fatigue. Therefore, the brief duration or disappearance of odor cannot be taken to mean absence of the gas. Acute, toxic exposure causes altered eye movements and sensitivity to light. Death occurs if the respiratory center of the brain becomes hypoxic, causing respiration to cease. Prolonged or less intense exposure causes headache, loss of energy, and increased mucous membrane secretions. Respiratory problems, such as shortness of breath, bronchitis, pneumonia, and delayed-onset pulmonary edema (fluid accumulation in the lungs), can occur 24

to 72 hours after initial exposure. (These respiratory problems are described in Chapter 30.)

Hydrogen sulfide is present in some natural gas at the wellhead, and toxicities occur as the result of gas-field leaks and accidents. It is also found in coal mines, pools of sewage sludge, liquid manure, sugar beet factories, and breweries (Kurt, 1983).

The three toxic asphyxiants discussed above provide examples of the types of cell injury that can occur from the numerous other asphyxiants in existence. Irritant gases, such as sulfur (SO_2), ammonia (NH_3), chlorine (Cl_2), phosgene ($COCl_2$), bromine (Br), ozone (O_3), and the oxides of nitrogen (NO, NO_2, N_2O_4) cause cellular injury by irritating mucous membranes. Irritation is partially due to the formation of aqueous solutions that are either basic (ammonia) or acidic (bromine, chlorine, phosgene, sulfur dioxide, oxides of nitrogen).

Acute respiratory toxicity from an irritant gas is like a respiratory burn. Initial responses are reflexive glottal and bronchial spasm (inflammation and histamine release causes bronchial constriction), cough, wheezing, and intense tearing. With intense or prolonged exposure, cellular swelling and cell death occur. Scarring from the "burn" may result in the development of bronchiectasis and increased susceptibility to infection.

Infectious Injury

The pathogenicity (virulence) of microorganisms lies in their ability to survive and proliferate in the human body, where they injure cells and tissues. The disease-producing potential of a microorganism depends on its ability to (1) invade and destroy cells, (2) produce toxins, and (3) produce damaging hypersensitivity reactions.

Bacteria

Bacterial survival and growth depend on the effectiveness of the body's defense mechanisms and on the bacterium's ability to resist these defenses (see Chapter 7). One mode of resistance is a coating that protects the bacterium from ingestion and destruction by specialized cells called phagocytes. Such coatings include the thick polysaccharide covering of the pneumococcus, the waxy capsule surrounding the tubercle bacillus, and the M protein cell wall of the streptococcus. Not all virulent extracellular pathogens are encapsulated types. For example, *Mycobacterium tuberculosis* can survive within and be transported by phagocytes.

Bacteria that survive and proliferate in the body produce substances that injure cells and tissues. Some bacteria produce destructive enzymes. For example, a variety of clostridia, *Clostridum perfringens,* produces both collagenases and lecithinases—powerful lytic enzymes that destroy connective tissues and cellular membranes.

Toxins are produced by many microorganisms. Gram-positive bacteria, such as *Corynebacterium diphtheriae, Clostridium tetani,* and *Clostridium botulinum,* produce powerful exotoxins. The term **exotoxin** seems to be a misnomer because exotoxins are toxins contained *within* the bacterium. They are called exotoxins because their toxic effects are produced on their release as metabolic products during bacterial growth.

Exotoxins are proteins and have highly specific effects. For example, the diphtheria toxin produces its effects by inactivating enzymes critical to protein synthesis. *C. tetani* produces a neurotoxin that acts on the central and sympathetic nervous systems by blocking motor inhibition, chiefly in the motor anterior horn cells of the spinal cord. This exotoxin also acts on the respiratory center of the brain, causing spasm or depression of the respiratory muscles, resulting in asphyxia and death. *C. botulinum* produces an exotoxin that causes severe food poisoning. The exotoxin is resistant to gastric digestion and is absorbed into the blood. It interferes with the motor end plates of skeletal muscles and causes paralysis, mainly of the eye orbit, pharynx, larynx, and respiratory muscles.

Bacteria that produce endotoxins are also called pyrogenic bacteria because they activate the inflammatory process and produce fever. (The physiology of fever is discussed in Chapter 13; the inflammatory response is discussed in Chapter 7.) **Endotoxins** are contained in the cell walls of gram-negative bacteria and are released from the phospholipids and polysaccharides of cell walls during lysis, or destruction, of the bacteria. Exotoxins and endotoxins are compared in Table 2-1.

Fever is caused by the release of endogenous pyrogens from macrophages or circulating white blood cells (leukocytes) attracted to the site of injury. Fever is also caused by the release of biochemicals (certain prostaglandins) during the inflammatory response. Endogenous pyrogens are proteins that act on the thermoregu-

---

TABLE 2-1 Properties of exotoxins and endotoxins

Property	Exotoxin	Endotoxin
Bacterial source	Mostly gram-positive bacteria	Almost exclusively gram-negative bacteria
Relation to microorganism	Metabolic product of growing cell	Present in cell wall and released only with destruction of cell
Chemistry	Protein or short peptide	Lipopolysaccharide complex
Heat stability	Unstable; can usually be destroyed at 60°-80° C (except staphylococcal enterotoxin)	Stable; can withstand autoclaving (120° C for 1 hr)
Toxicity (power to cause disease)	High	Low
Toxic effects	Specific for a particular cell structure or function in the host	General, such as fever, weakness, aches, and shock; all produce the same effects
Treatment	Can be converted to toxoids and neutralized by antitoxin	Cannot be converted to toxoids and are not easily neutralized by antitoxin
Lethal dose	Small	Considerably larger
Representative diseases	Gas gangrene, tetanus, botulism, diphtheria, scarlet fever	Bacillary dysentery (shigellosis), epidemic meningitis, and tularemia

From Tortora, Funke, & Case, 1982.

latory centers of the hypothalamus. Mechanisms by which prostaglandins (PGE$_1$ and PGE$_2$) cause fever are not well defined.

Inflammation is the body's response to the presence of the bacteria. The inflammatory response increases capillary permeability, allowing substances involved in bacterial destruction to migrate from the capillaries to the site of infection. Endotoxins increase capillary permeability further through activation of a plasma protein system, the complement cascade (see Chapter 7). Capillary permeability may increase sufficiently to permit escape of large quantities of blood, contributing to the syndrome of disseminated (or diffuse) intravascular coagulation (see Chapter 27) or, in severe cases, cardiovascular shock (see Chapter 27).

The ability to produce hypersensitivity reactions is an important pathogenic mechanism of bacterial toxins. Tissue lesions of many chronic infections are related to the induction of hypersensitivity to the toxin. For example, *M. tuberculosis* causes inflammatory lesions known as granulomas. The inflammatory response to bacterial toxins causes a destructive, or "granulomatous," reaction. Some bacteria alter host tissues so that the tissues evoke self-destructive (autoimmune) reactions. Other bacteria produce substances that "look like" host proteins and cause the body to produce substances (antibodies) that later "recognize" and react with the look-alike host proteins in normal tissues. (Hypersensitivity reactions and autoimmune disease are described in Chapter 8.)

Bacteremia, or septicemia, is the proliferation of microorganisms in the blood. Bacteremia is due to failure of the body's defense mechanisms. The most frequent cause of bacteremia is proliferation of gram-negative bacteria, although a few gram-positive bacteria and fungi are sometimes the cause. (The gram-negative bacteria include *Escherichia coli*, *Serratia marcescens*, *Proteus mirabilis*, *Enterobacter aerogenes*, *Pseudomonas aeruginosa*, and *Bacteriodes* species.) Symptoms of bacteremia are produced by the endotoxins that are released from the cell walls of the bacteria. Once in the blood, endotoxins cause the release of vasoactive peptides that affect blood vessels. One vascular effect is vasodilation that reduces blood pressure, which in turn causes decreased oxygen delivery and subsequent cardiovascular shock (see Chapter 27). Lymphangitis, or inflamed lymphatic vessels, is a manifestation of bacteremia that causes red streaks under the skin of an arm or leg radiating from the infection site.

Viruses

Viruses are intracellular parasites that take over the metabolic machinery of host cells and use it for their own survival and replication. This results in decreased synthesis of macromolecules vital to the host. Viral diseases are the most common afflictions of humans. The common cold affects most people annually. The ubiquitous role of viruses ranges from the "cold sore" of herpes simplex to the causation of cancer (discussed in detail in Chapter 11).

The variable cellular response to viral invasion is poorly understood, but clearly no single mechanism is responsible for altering and destroying the host's cells (Wagner, 1984). Viruses do not produce exotoxins or endotoxins. The protein coat (capsid) that encapsulates most viruses enables them to resist phagocytosis but evokes a very strong immune response. (The role of foreign proteins in stimulating the creation of immunity is described in Chapter 6.) Immunity may protect the individual from an acute exacerbation only or may be sufficiently strong to prevent disease.

Viral Replicaton

Virions, or viral particles, do not possess any of the metabolic organelles that are contained within either procaryotes (e.g., bacteria) or eucaryotes (e.g., human cells) (Fig. 2-9). Thus viruses have no metabolism. Unlike bacteria, viruses are incapable of independent reproduction. Their replication is totally dependent on their ability to infect a permissive host cell—a cell that cannot resist viral invasion and replication. The replication cycle of most viruses can be divided into two distinct phases, infection and integration. Infection begins when a virion binds to receptors on the plasma membrane of a host cell (Fig. 2-10). Specificity of these receptors dictates the range of host cells with which a particular virus can bind (cellular receptors are discussed in Chapter 1). Once bound, the virion enters coated pits to be transferred into cytoplasmic vacuoles (see Figure 1-21). Some virions, like the Sendai virions, enter host cells directly by fusing their coat with the plasma membrane (Bukrinskaya, 1982).

Viruses contain either DNA or RNA and are thus known as DNA or RNA viruses. After uncoating, the viral DNA enters the cell's nucleus, where it becomes incorporated into the host cell's chromosomal DNA. This is the integration phase, during which the viral genome (a complete set of hereditary factors) essentially regulates the metabolic activities of the host cell by directing its own replication. New virions are then released from the cell for transmission of the viral infection to other host cells. The replication of RNA viruses is essentially the same as for DNA viruses, except that different mechanisms of messenger RNA (mRNA) formation occur among different groups of RNA viruses. In all cases, RNA replication is facilitated by specific RNA-dependent RNA polymerase enzymes (replicases) encoded by the viral RNA chromosome. Viral DNA not only replicates in the host cell but also becomes integrated with host DNA and transmitted to the host's

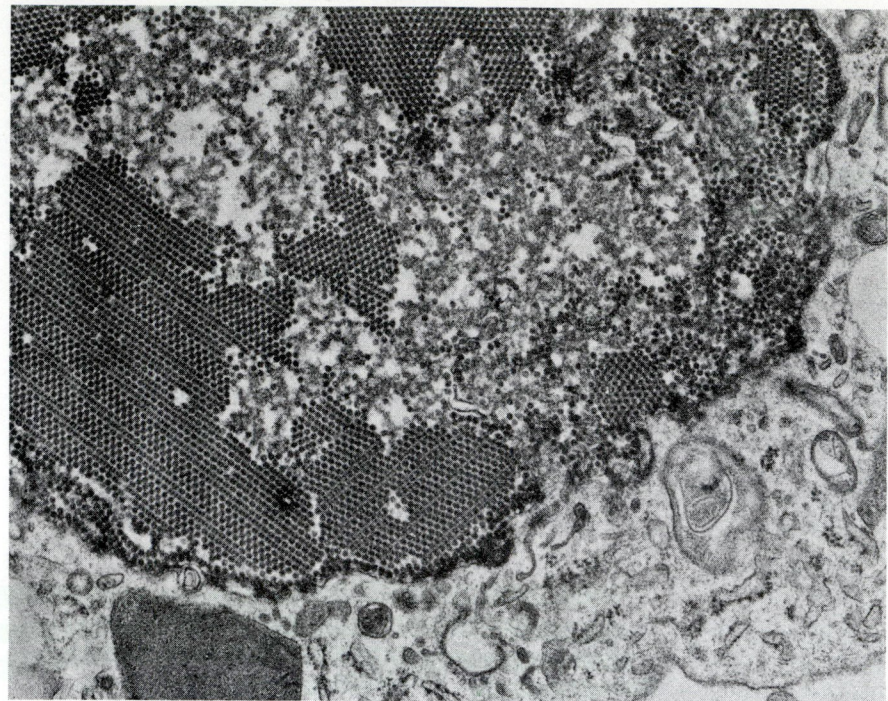

FIG. 2-9. Electron micrograph of virion inclusion in the nucleus of a glial cell. The individual was diagnosed with progressive multifocal leukocephalopathy. (From Kissane, 1985.)

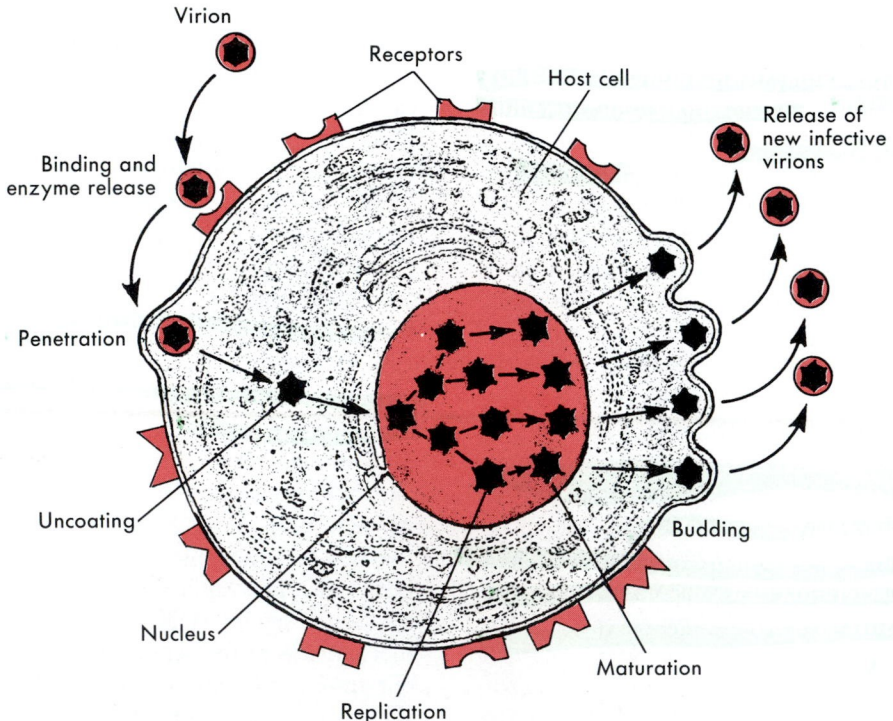

FIG. 2-10. Stages of viral infection of a host cell. The virion *(1)* becomes attached to receptors on the cell's plasma membrane; *(2)* releases enzymes that weaken the membrane and allow it to penetrate the cell; *(3)* uncoats itself; *(4)* replicates; and *(5)* matures and escapes from the cell by budding from the plasma membrane. The infection can then spread to other host cells.

daughter cells during host cell mitosis. By this process, viral genes can become part of the vertically transmitted (inherited) genetic information of the host cell and its progeny. (The process by which DNA transmits genetic information is discussed in Chapter 4.)

Cellular Effects of Viruses

Besides taking over the host cell's metabolic machinery, viral infection can injure cellular structures. In some viral infections, cellular destruction results from plasma membrane damage that occurs when a virion binds with receptors on the host cell and releases enzymes that change the configuration of the membrane's fatty acids, altering the lipid bilayer (see Fig. 2-10). (The lipid bilayer is described and illustrated in Chapter 1.)

Once inside the host cell, virions have many cytopathic effects, including the following:

1. The cessation of protein synthesis. Herpes simplex, for example, stops cell division.
2. Disruption of lysosomal membranes, resulting in release of lysosomal enzymes that can kill the cell (see Chapter 1).
3. Formation of **inclusion bodies** (sites where synthesis of viral nucleic acids or proteins is occurring or has occurred). Some viral infections (e.g., smallpox) are associated with cytoplasmic inclusions.
4. Fusion of host cells, producing multinucleated giant cells. Fusion is seen with measles, influenza, and herpes simplex infections.
5. Alteration of the antigenic properties, or "identity" of the host cell, causing the host's immune system to attack the cell as if it were a foreign protein. (Antigenic properties and autoimmune disease are discussed in Unit III.)
6. Transformation of host cells into cancerous cells, resulting in uninhibited and unregulated growth. The Epstein-Barr virus, for example, is implicated in Burkitt's lymphoma. (The viral theory of cancer is discussed in Chapter 11.)

Human diseases caused by specific viruses are listed in Table 2-2.

Immunologic and Inflammatory Injury

Cellular membranes are injured by direct contact with cellular and chemical components of the immune and inflammatory responses, such as phagocytic cells (lym-

---

TABLE 2-2 Characteristics and pathophysiologic effects of viruses

Virus	Pathophysiologic effects
Papovaviruses (DNA) (papilloma)	Small viruses that induce tumors and cancers in animals, warts (papilloma) in humans.
Adenoviruses (DNA)	Medium-sized viruses that cause various respiratory infections in humans; some cause tumors in animals.
Herpesviruses (DNA) (herpes simplex, herpes zoster)	Medium-sized viruses that cause various diseases in humans, such as fever blisters, chickenpox, shingles, and infectious mononucleosis; implicated in a type of human cancer called Burkitt's lymphoma.
Poxvirus (DNA) (variola, cowpox, vaccinia)	Very large, complex, brick-shaped viruses that cause diseases such as smallpox (variola), molluscum contagiosum (wartlike skin lesions), cowpox, and vaccinia; vaccinia virus gives immunity to smallpox.
Picornaviruses (RNA) (poliovirus, rhinovirus)	Smallest RNA-containing viruses; at least 70 human enteroviruses are known, including the polio-, coxsackie-, and echoviruses; more than 100 rhinoviruses exist and are the most common cause of colds.
Myxoviruses (RNA) (influenza A, B, C)	Medium-sized viruses with a spiked envelope; have the ability to agglutinate red blood cells; cause influenza.
Paramyxoviruses (RNA) (measles, mumps)	Structurally similar to myxoviruses, but generally larger; cause parainfluenza, measles, mumps.
Coronaviruses (RNA)	Associated with upper respiratory tract infections and the common cold.
Retroviruses (RNA)	Tumor-associated viruses; cause leukemia and tumors in animals; some members produce "slow" viral infections, cause of AIDS.
Arenaviruses (RNA) (lassa)	Contain RNA-containing granules; some members produce "slow" viral infections in humans.
Reoviruses (RNA)	Relation to human disease not clear; may be involved in mild respiratory infections and infantile gastroenteritis.

Adapted from Tortora, Funke, & Case, 1982.

phocytes and macrophages) and such substances as histamine, antibodies, lymphokines, complement, and proteases (see Chapter 7). Complement is responsible for many of the membrane alterations that occur during immunologic injury.

Membrane alterations are associated with rapid leakage of K^+ out of the cell and rapid influx of water. Antibodies can interfere with membrane function by binding to and occupying receptor molecules on the plasma membrane. This type of injury is found in certain forms of diabetes mellitus and in myasthenia gravis. Antibodies can also block or destroy cellular junctions, interfering with intercellular communication. (See Chapter 6 for a discussion of antibody binding and Chapter 1 for a description of intercellular junctions and communication.)

Injurious Genetic Factors

Genetic disorders may be the result of genetic factors that alter the cell's nucleus and the plasma membrane's structure, shape, receptors, or transport mechanisms. For example, enzymatic genetic defects can lead to abnormalities in membrane transport. Genetic disorders that cause structural alterations of the red blood cell include sickle cell anemia, Huntington disease, muscular dystrophy, and abetalipoproteinemia. (Mechanisms causing genetic abnormalities are discussed in Unit II.)

Injurious Nutritional Imbalances

Cells require adequate amounts of essential nutrients—proteins, carbohydrates, lipids (fats), vitamins, and minerals—to function normally. If these nutrients are not consumed in the diet and transported to the body's cells, or if excessive amounts of nutrients are consumed and transported, pathophysiologic cellular effects develop.

Proteins, which consist of chains of amino acids, are the major structural units of the cell and participate in many enzymatic and hormonal functions. Protein deficiency causes a decrease in the intestinal mucosal mass decreasing the absorptive function. The integrity of the pancreas is also affected, resulting in diminished exocrine secretion. With starvation or malnutrition the lowered plasma proteins, particularly albumin, causes fluid to move into the interstitium (edema). Protein-calorie malnutrition (PCM) is the predominant worldwide type of malnutrition. Children suffering from malnutrition are very susceptible and often die from infectious diseases. Even with adequate protein intake, cellular injury can occur if amino acid transport mechanisms fail or are defective. In Fanconi syndrome, for example, renal tubular cells may contain accumulated protein droplets that have been absorbed but cannot be transported. (Alterations of renal function are the subject of Chapter 33.)

Glucose is the major carbohydrate obtained from the breakdown of starch (see Chapter 1). Hyperglycemia (excessive glucose in the blood) caused by excessive carbohydrate intake may lead to obesity. Deficiencies of glucose result from starvation or from lack of use, as in diabetes. In both of these conditions, the body compensates by metabolizing fat (lipids). (For details on diabetes, see Chapter 18.)

In lipid deficiency, or **hypolipidemia,** the body compensates by mobilizing fatty acids from adipose tissue. This causes an increase in the production and circulation of ketone bodies, which are acidic by-products of lipid metabolism. The excretion of ketone bodies results in loss of water and electrolytes and causes dehydration and thirst. Severe increases in ketone bodies cause ketoacidosis, coma, and death. **Hyperlipidemia,** or an increase in lipoproteins in the blood, results in deposits of fat in the heart, liver, and muscle.

Vitamins are not sources of energy but are necessary for maintaining normal cellular function. Adequate vitamin intake is necessary because most vitamins are not synthesized by the body. Vitamins are classified as water soluble (thiamine, pyridoxal, cobalamin, ascorbic acid, riboflavin, nicotinic acid, and folic acid) or fat soluble (A, D, E, and K). They are involved in many reactions, including metabolism of visual pigments (vitamin A), calcium and phosphate metabolism (vitamin D), prothrombin synthesis (vitamin K), and antioxidation reactions (vitamin E). Pyridoxal (vitamin B_6) affects amino acid transfer reactions; FAD, FMN, and NAD help the reaction transfer of electrons (see Chapter 1). Deficiencies in vitamin C result in poor wound healing and scurvy. Vitamin D deficiency causes rickets and problems with healing of fractures. Folate deficiency is associated with plasma and membrane changes of the red blood cell and is particularly a problem in individuals with severe liver dysfunction. Vitamin deficiencies are associated with several other disease states.

Alterations in plasma membrane functions can be induced by certain nutritional substances. For example, increases in vitamin A consumption can cause lysis of the plasma membrane, releasing hydrolases that damage lysosomal membranes. With insulin deficiency, glucose cannot cross the plasma membrane to enter the cell, causing energy deficits. Nutritional deficiences are also associated with abnormalities of the chromosomes, nucleus, and DNA synthesis.

Injurious Physical Agents

Injurious physical agents include temperature extremes, changes in atmospheric pressure, radiation, illumination, mechanical factors, noise, and prolonged vibration. Physical injury can result from excessive exposure to many environmental agents, as well as agents used for the diagnosis and treatment of illness.

Temperature Extremes

Chilling or freezing of cells causes **hypothermic injury** directly by creating high intracellular sodium concentrations, which result from the formation and dissolution of ice crystals. Indirect forms of injury occur because of changes in small blood vessels (the microcirculation). Slow chilling can cause vasoconstriction followed by paralysis of vasomotor control, resulting in vasodilation and increased membrane permeability. This causes cellular and tissue swelling. With an abrupt drop in temperature, vasoconstriction and increased viscosity of the blood cause ischemic injury—infarction and necrosis (cellular death) in affected tissues. With continued exposure to freezing temperatures, vasodilation produces severe swelling that causes degenerative changes in the myelin sheath that surrounds peripheral nerves, resulting in sensory and motor disturbances. Thrombosis can also occur and may lead to gangrene of the affected part. (Gangrene is discussed on p. 72.) These conditions are often called frostbite.

Hyperthermic injury (injury caused by excessive heat) varies depending on the nature, intensity, and extent of the injury. A full-thickness burn is an open wound involving skin layers—epidermis, dermis, and subcutaneous layers—and causing extensive loss of fluids and plasma proteins. Cellular regeneration is not possible, so that skin from a donor or from the host must be grafted to the site. Partial-thickness burns result in reddening of the area as a result of dilation of small blood vessels and increased permeability of cellular membranes, with loss of protein-rich fluid, resulting in the typical "burn blister." In surface epithelial cells, membrane permeability increases, causing both cytoplasmic and nuclear swelling. Temperature-sensitive enzymes within certain cells respond to heat by increasing cellular metabolism, with detrimental effects. Intense heat also damages the vascular endothelium and causes coagulation of the blood vessels. (Burns are discussed further in Chapter 41, and other conditions related to temperature changes are discussed in Chapter 13.)

Changes in Atmospheric Pressure

Sudden increases or decreases in atmospheric pressure cause **blast injury,** which can be transmitted by either air (air blast) or water (immersion blast). With sudden increases in pressure, such as in air blast or explosive injuries, tissue injury is due to compressive waves of air impinging upon the body, followed by a sudden wave of decreased pressure. The pressure changes may collapse the thorax, rupture internal solid organs, and cause widespread hemorrhage (Robbins et al., 1984). In increased pressure caused by immersion blast, water pressure is applied suddenly to all sides of the body, forcing the body up out of water. The positive pressure compresses the abdomen and ruptures hollow internal organs, such as the spleen, kidneys, and liver.

With sudden decreases in pressure, carbon dioxide and nitrogen that are normally dissolved in the blood come out of solution and form tiny bubbles called gas emboli. At low atmospheric pressure, such as occurs at altitudes above 15,000 feet, there is a significant decrease in available oxygen. This causes hypoxic injury, and compensatory vasoconstriction shunts blood from the peripheral circulation (in the extremities) to the visceral organs, including the lungs. The combination of increases in pulmonary blood flow and systemic hypoxia causes "high-altitude pulmonary edema" (Roy et al., 1969). (Pulmonary edema is described in Chapter 30.)

Deep sea divers and underwater construction workers who return to the surface too quickly develop a form of gas embolism called **decompression sickness** or **caisson disease** ("the bends"). If water pressure is reduced too rapidly, the gases dissolved in blood bubble out of solution forming emboli. Oxygen is quickly redissolved, but nitrogen bubbles may persist and obstruct blood vessels. Ischemia resulting from gas emboli causes cellular hypoxia, particularly in the muscles, joints, and tendons, which are especially susceptible to changes in oxygen supply. Emboli and interstitial gas accumulate around the joints and skeletal muscles, causing the individual to double up in pain. Tissues of the heart and brain may also be affected by emboli, causing necrosis. The gases can be promptly redissolved in blood by raising the atmospheric pressure. This is accomplished by placing the individual in a decompression chamber. First, pressure is increased until it approximates pressure at the depth to which the diver had descended. This redissolves the gas bubbles in the blood. Then the pressure in the chamber is decreased gradually until it equals pressure at the surface of the water. The slow decrease in pressure slows the gases from bubbling out of solution.

Ionizing Radiation

Ionizing radiation is any form of radiation capable of removing orbital electrons from atoms. Ionizing radiation is emitted by x-rays, gamma rays, alpha and beta particles (which are emitted from atomic nuclei in the process of radioactive decay), and from neutrons, deuterons, protons, and pions (all of which are emitted from cobalt or linear accelerators). Occupational exposure to ionizing radiation is mostly limited to alpha- and beta-particle exposure and exposure to x-rays, gamma rays, and neutrons. Radiant energy from sunlight (solar radiation) can also injure cells.

The most abundant source of exposure to ionizing radiation is the environment. This source includes emissions from radioactive material inside the body, cosmic rays from outer space, and radiation emitted from such substances as soil and building materials. Environmental radioactivity is primarily emitted by uranium, thorium,

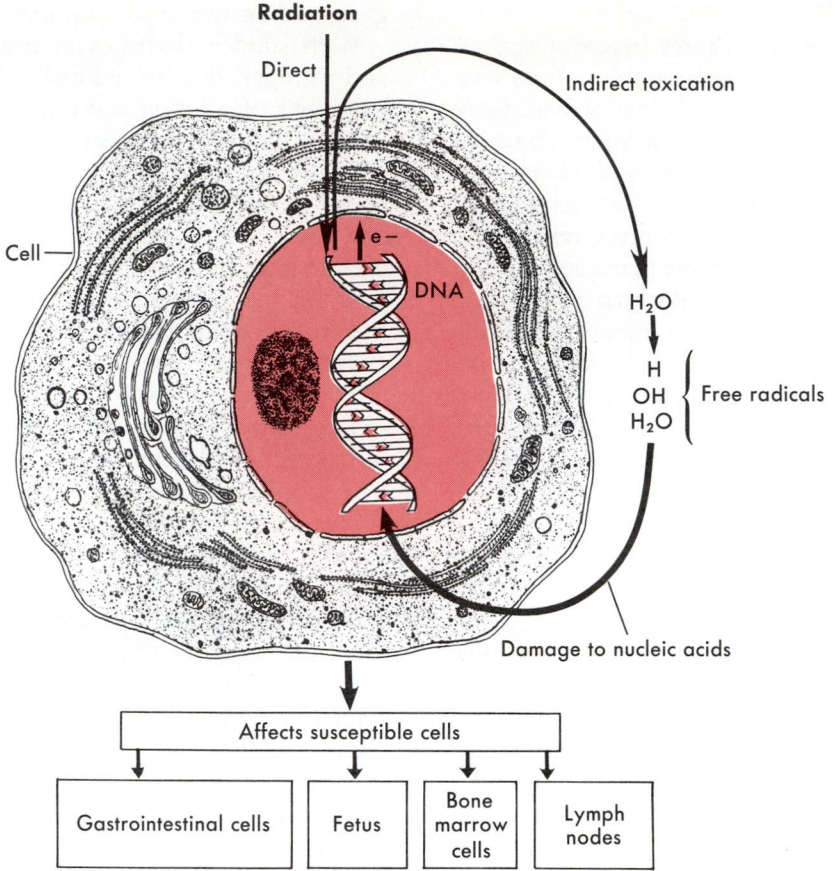

FIG. 2-11. Cellular damage due to ionizing radiation. Radiation can damage macromolecules in two ways: (1) directly, where the micromolecules are ionized; and (2) indirectly, where water is ionized and produces free radicals that in turn damage macromolecules. Cells that are particularly susceptible to damage are those of the gastrointestinal tract, bone marrow, lymph nodes, fetus, and ovarian follicles. (Adapted from King, Fenoglio, & Lefkowitch, 1983.)

and potassium. Other sources are x-rays used for medical diagnosis and treatment, uranium and thorium mines, nuclear weapons, and nuclear reactors that generate electricity.

The mechanism by which ionizing radiation damages cells is shown in Fig. 2-11. DNA is the most vulnerable target of radiation, particularly the bonds within the DNA molecule. Membrane molecules and enzymes are also damaged by radiation. The nuclear changes include nuclear swelling, disappearance of the nuclear membrane, and **pyknosis** (cellular degeneration in which the nucleus shrinks and chromosomes deteriorate). Chromosomal aberrations include breaks, deletions, translocations, and many other structural abnormalities (chromosomal abnormalities are described in Chapter 4). The intensity, duration, and cumulative effects of exposure to ionizing radiation determine the extent of injury.

Not all cells and tissues have the same sensitivity to radiation, although all cells can be affected. Radiosensitivity depends on rate of mitosis and cellular maturity.

Because fetal cells are both immature and undergoing rapid cycling, the fetus is at great risk for injury caused by ionizing radiation. Particularly vulnerable are embryonic germ cells, which are precursors of ova and sperm. Throughout life, cells of the bone marrow, intestinal mucosa, testicular seminiferous epithelium, and ovarian follicles are susceptible to injury because they are always undergoing mitosis, which ensures the presence of vulnerable, immature daughter cells.

The effects of ionizing radiation may be acute or delayed. Acute effects of high doses, such as skin redness, skin damage, or chromosomal aberrations, occur within hours, days, or months. The delayed effects of low doses may not be evident for years. Effects are usually (1) somatic (involving the exposed individual's entire body), for example, leukemia and other cancers; (2) genetic, involving offspring of the exposed individual; or (3) fetal, involving fetuses that are exposed in utero (Wrenn & Mays, 1983). (The carcinogenic effects of radiation are discussed in Chapter 11, and radiation-induced cancers of the thyroid gland, breast, liver, and bone are discussed in Chapters 18, 20, 32, and 39, respectively.)

Illumination

Most discussions about the effects of light and illumination have been limited to questions of occupational safety and efficiency. Researchers have found, however, that illumination has biologic effects related to health (McRee et al., 1979; Neer et al., 1971; Weston, 1948; Wurtman, 1975).

The harmful effects of fluorescent lighting are limited to individuals with certain neurologic problems, such as epilepsy (see Chapter 15). In one study of photosensitive epileptics, seizures occurred when fluorescent tubes were modified to produce flickering and changes in brightness (Binnie, deKarte, & Wisman, 1979). The specific mechanism by which fluorescent light affects neural cells and tissues is unknown. Properly installed and maintained fluorescent bulbs have not been found to harm healthy individuals (Berens & Crouch, 1958).

Damaged sodium and mercury vapor lamps are documented causes of corneal damage. Ultraviolet light emitted by a damaged mercury vapor lamp can cause inflammation of the cornea (Olsen, 1983). The harmful effects of sodium vapor lamps are not well documented, but reports have included color distortion, eye strain, headache, and discomfort caused by glare. So far, no one has documented long-term physical damage caused by insufficient illumination or eye strain.

Mechanical Factors

Mechanical injury is caused by physical impact or irritation. Tight clothing or ill-fitted shoes can irritate epidermal cells, causing local redness or swelling without breaking the skin. More severe injury, ranging from visible abrasion (tearing of epidermal cells) to laceration (a deeper wound, which may extend through the dermis and affect deep tissues or organs), can have serious systemic effects. Such effects can include hemorrhage, disruption of function, shock, and even death. A contusion, or bruise, is caused by broken blood vessels and bleeding beneath the site of a blow to the skin.

The cellular effects of irritation and abrasion are due to the acute inflammatory response (see Chapter 7). Deep wounds also stimulate the inflammatory response, but major injury to cells and tissues is due to gross destruction or lack of blood supply and subsequent hypoxia. A contusion may leave the epidermis intact but cause extensive damage to small blood vessels (e.g., capillaries and venules).

Noise

Noise is sound that has the potential for inflicting bodily harm. The most common pathophysiologic effect of noise is hearing impairment. Noise trauma can be caused by acute loud noise, as well as by the cumulative effects of various intensities, frequencies, and durations of noise.

Two types of hearing loss are associated with noise: (1) acoustic trauma, or instantaneous damage caused by a single sharply rising wave of sound, and (2) noise-induced hearing loss, the most common type, which is due to prolonged exposure to intense sound. Acoustic trauma can rupture the eardrum, displace the ossicles of the middle ear, and damage the organ of Corti in the inner ear.

Noise-induced hearing loss is gradual and painless. In the cochlea sensory hair cells that correspond to certain frequency ranges are damaged, probably because of cochlear ischemia. High-intensity stimulation produces vasoconstriction of capillaries of the cochlea in laboratory animals. This constriction decreases the amount of oxygen and nutrients delivered to the hair cells (Hawkins, 1971; Henderson et al., 1976). It is not uncommon to find distortion or swelling of sensory cells, an increase in lysosomes, and necrotic changes in the outer hair cells (Bohne, 1976). Symptoms of noise-induced hearing loss include loudness recruitment and tinnitus. In loudness recruitment, soft sounds are not heard, but loud sounds are heard normally. Tinnitus is a constant, high-pitched ringing that annoys the individual and contributes to loss of sleep.

Prolonged Vibration

The effects of contact with vibrating machinery are reported widely in the occupational health literature. Persons at risk for the ill effects of long-term exposure to vibration include truck and bus drivers, construction workers, farmers, and workers in occupations that require electric hand tools.

Whole-body vibration, or **resonance,** occurs when body movement equals that of the vibrating machinery. This begins at 5 Hz and chiefly affects the trunk and upper body. Reported alterations include increases in oxygen consumption and pulmonary ventilation, bone deformities, calcification of intervertebral disks, and increases in nerve conduction (Duffner, Hamilton & Schmitz, 1962; Ernstring, 1961; Hood et al., 1966). A disproportionate incidence of bowel, blood, respiratory, and musculoskeletal disorders is also related to whole-body vibration. Exacerbating factors may include body posture, eating habits, and fatigue.

Segmental vibration is exposure of a body part to vibration, often the fingers and hands of operators of such tools as chain saws, pneumatic-hammers, and rotary grinders. The vibratory effects are worsened in cold temperatures and predispose the operator to a condition known as Raynaud's phenomenon, sometimes called "vibration white fingers" or "dead hand." (Raynaud's phenomenon is different from Raynaud's disease, a vasospastic disorder of the small arteries and arterioles, usually in young healthy women.) Raynaud's phenomenon is a secondary disorder associated with exposure to vibrating tools, lead poisoning, arteriosclerosis, and connective tissue diseases. Signs and symptoms of Raynaud's phenomenon include numbness; blanching of the fingers, with some loss of muscular control; and decreased sensitivity to heat and cold with associated pain. Wearing gloves seems to decrease the effects of vibration, especially if it occurs at low frequencies. The exact mechanism that produces the phenomenon is unknown.

MANIFESTATIONS OF CELLULAR INJURY

Cellular Manifestations: Accumulations

Cellular accumulations, also known as **infiltrations,** not only occur in injured cells but also can occur in normal cells. Common accumulations consist of substances that are normally present, such as fluids and electrolytes, triglycerides (lipids), glycogen, calcium, uric acid, proteins, melanin, and bilirubin. Abnormal accumulations of these substances can occur in the cytoplasm (frequently in the lysosomes) or in the nucleus if (1) the normal, endogenous substance is produced in excess or at an increased rate; (2) an endogenous substance (normal or abnormal) is not effectively catabolized, usually because of lack of a vital lysosomal enzyme; or (3) harmful exogenous materials, such as heavy metals, mineral dusts, or microorganisms, accumulate because of inhalation, ingestion, or infection.

In all the storage diseases, the cells attempt to digest, or catabolize, the "stored" substances. As a result, excessive amounts of metabolites (products of catabolism) accumulate in the cells and are expelled into the extracellular matrix, where they are taken up by phagocytic cells called macrophages (see Chapter 7). Some of these scavenger cells circulate throughout the body, while others remain fixed in certain tissues, such as the liver or spleen. As more and more macrophages and other phagocytes migrate to tissues that are producing excessive metabolites, the affected tissues begin to swell. This is the mechanism that causes enlargement of the liver (hepatomegaly) or the spleen (splenomegaly). Enlargement of one of these organs is a clinical manifestation of many of the storage diseases.

Water

Cellular swelling, the most common degenerative change, is caused by the shift of extracellular water into the cells. In hypoxic injury, movement of fluid and ions into the cell is associated with acute failure of metabolism and loss of ATP production. Normally, the pump

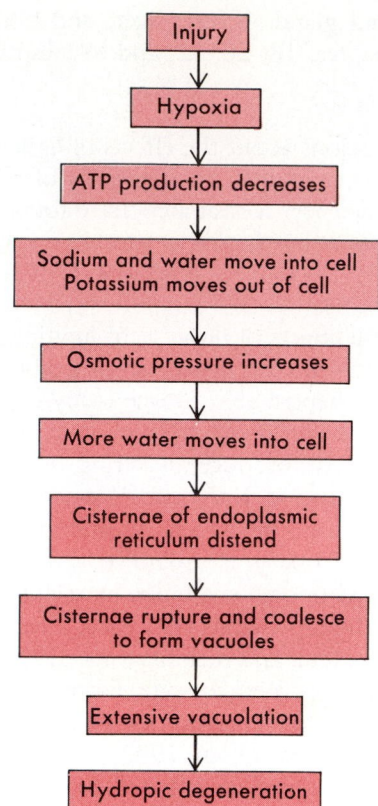

FIG. 2-12. The process of hydropic degeneration.

that transports sodium ions out of the cell is maintained by the presence of ATP and ATPase, the active-transport enzyme. In metabolic failure caused by hypoxia, reduced ATP and ATPase permits sodium to accumulate in the cell, while potassium diffuses outward. The increase of intracellular sodium increases osmotic pressure, which draws more water into the cell (transport mechanisms are described in Chapter 1). The cisternae of the endoplasmic reticulum become distended, rupture, and coalesce to form large vacuoles that isolate the water from the cytoplasm. This process is called **vacuolation.** Progressive vacuolation results in a more serious condition called **hydropic degeneration** (Fig. 2-12). If cellular swelling affects all of the cells in an organ, the organ increases in weight and becomes distended and pale.

Cellular swelling is reversible and is considered to be sublethal. It is, in fact, an early manifestation of almost all types of cellular injury, including severe or lethal cell injury. It is also associated with high fever, hypokalemia (abnormally low concentrations of potassium in the blood; see Chapter 3), and certain infections.

Lipids and Carbohydrates

Certain metabolic disorders result in the abnormal intracellular accumulation of carbohydrates and lipids.

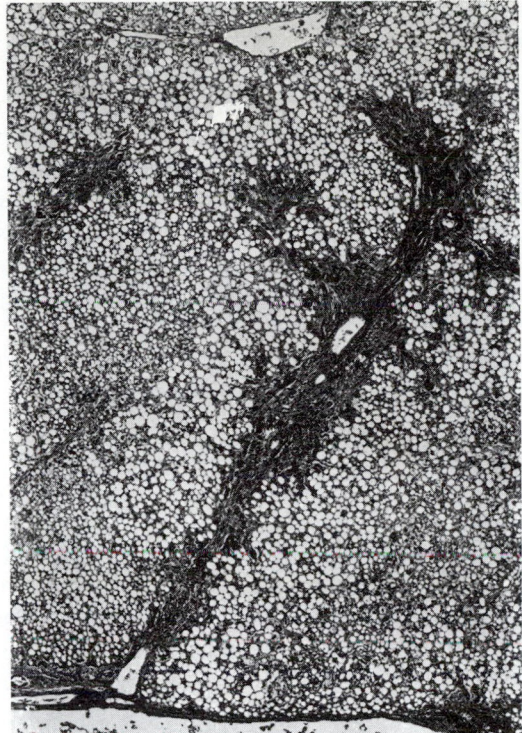

FIG. 2-13. Fatty liver of an alcoholic. The liver is enlarged, swollen, greasy, and yellow. (From Kissane, 1985.)

These substances may accumulate throughout the body, but are found primarily in cells of the spleen, liver, and central nervous system. Accumulations in cells of the central nervous system can cause neurologic dysfunction and severe mental retardation. Lipids accumulate in Tay-Sachs, Neimann-Pick, and Gaucher disease, whereas in the diseases known as mucopolysaccharidoses, the excess is of carbohydrates. The mucopolysaccharidoses are progressive disorders that usually involve multiple organs, including liver, spleen, heart, and blood vessels. The accumulated mucopolysaccharides are found in reticuloendothelial cells, endothelial cells, intimal smooth muscle cells, and fibroblasts throughout the body. These carbohydrate accumulations can cause clouding of the cornea, joint stiffness, and mental retardation (Robbins et al., 1984).

Although lipids sometimes accumulate in heart and kidney cells, the most common site of intracellular lipid accumulation, or **fatty change**, is in liver cells. Because hepatic metabolism and secretion of lipids are crucial to proper body function, imbalances and deficiencies in these processes lead to major pathologic changes. Lipid accumulation in liver cells causes an organic condition known as fatty liver, or fatty change (Fig. 2-13). As lipids fill the cells, vacuolation pushes the nucleus and other organelles aside. Grossly, the liver looks yellowish and greasy.

Lipid accumulation in liver cells occurs after cellular injury sets one or more of the following mechanisms in motion.

1. Increased movement of free fatty acids into the liver. (Starvation, for example, increases breakdown of triglycerides in adipose tissue, releasing fatty acids that subsequently enter liver cells.)
2. Failure of the metabolic process that converts fatty acids to phospholipids, resulting in the preferential conversion of the fatty acids to triglycerides.
3. Increased synthesis of triglycerides from fatty acids. (Increases in an enzyme, alpha-glycerophosphatase, can accelerate triglyceride synthesis.)
4. Decreased synthesis of apoproteins (lipid-acceptor proteins).
5. Failure of lipids to bind with apoproteins and form lipoproteins.
6. Failure of mechanisms that transport lipoproteins out of the cell.

Alcohol abuse is one of the most common causes of fatty liver (see Chapter 36 for a discussion of liver abnormalities). Although the exact mechanism by which alcohol causes fatty change is uncertain, the following defects are implicated: (1) increased movement of free fatty acids into the liver, (2) alternative synthesis of triglycerides, (3) decreased triglyceride use, (4) problems with apoprotein synthesis or lipoprotein transport, and (5) direct damage to the endoplasmic reticulum by free radicals released by alcohol's toxic effects.

Fatty change caused by alcohol can lead to a form of liver fibrosis called cirrhosis. If alcohol intake ceases, the cirrhotic liver can return to a normal size and function. Fatty change from other causes, notably carbon tetrachloride poisoning, is often irreversible.

Glycogen

Intracellular accumulations of glycogen are seen in genetic disorders called glycogen storage diseases and in disorders of glucose and glycogen metabolism. Like water and lipid accumulation, glycogen accumulation results in excessive vacuolation of the cytoplasm.

The most common cause of glycogen accumulation is the disorder of glucose metabolism, diabetes mellitus (see Chapter 18). In diabetes mellitus, glycogen accumulates in the epithelial cells of the proximal convoluted renal tubules, the loop of Henle, liver cells, myocardial cells, and the beta cells of the islets of Langerhans. With the decrease in insulin, glucose concentrations increase in the blood (hyperglycemia) and in the urine (glycosuria) as blood glucose levels rise above the renal threshold. The renal tubular cells reabsorb the excess quantities of glucose and store it as glycogen. With the administration of insulin, glycogen accumulation is reversed, as long as no renal tubular dysfunction is present.

Proteins

Proteins provide cellular structure and constitute most of the cell's dry weight. They are synthesized on ribosomes in the cytoplasm from the essential amino acids lysine, threonine, leucine, isoleucine, methionine, tryptophan, valine, phenylalanine, and histidine. Protein accumulation probably damages cells in two ways. First, metabolites, produced when the cell attempts to digest some proteins, are enzymes that, when released from lysosomes, can damage cellular organelles. Second, excessive amounts of protein in the cytoplasm push against cellular organelles, disrupting organelle function and intracellular communication.

Protein excess accumulates primarily in the epithelial cells of the renal convoluted tubule and in the antibody-forming plasma cells (B lymphocytes) of the immune system (the immune system is described in Chapter 6.) Several types of renal disorders cause excessive excretion of protein molecules in the urine (proteinuria) (see Chapter 33). Normally, little or no protein is present in the urine, and its presence in siginificant amounts indicates cellular injury and altered cellular function. For example, certain renal disorders can cause glomerular damage, which allows proteins to leak across the glomerular membrane and into the glomerular filtrate. The protein then moves into the proximal tubule and is resorbed by the epithelial cells through the process of pinocytosis ("cell drinking"), which is discussed in Chapter 1. The protein-containing pinocytotic vesicles fuse with lysosomes, after which the protein is released into the cytoplasm as a product of lysosomal digestion. Protein accumulations in the cytoplasm of renal tubular cells do not cause direct cellular dysfunction, but they do signify a pathologic process.

Accumulations of protein in B lymphocytes can occur duing active synthesis of antibodies during the immune response. The excess aggregates of protein are called Russell bodies (see Chapter 6). Russell bodies have been identified in multiple myeloma (plasma cell tumor) (see Chapters 24 and 39).

Pigments

Pigment accumulations may be normal or abnormal, endogenous (produced within the body) or exogenous (produced outside the body). Endogenous pigments are derived, for example, from amino acids (e.g., tyrosine, tryptophan). They include melanin and the blood proteins—porphyrins, hemoglobin, and hemosiderin (ferritin). Lipid-rich pigments such as lipofuscin (the aging pigment) give a yellow-brown color to cells undergoing slow, regressive, and often atrophic changes. Exogenous pigments include mineral dusts containing silica and iron particles, lead, silver salts, and dyes for tatoos.

Melanin

Melanin accumulates in epithelial cells (keratinocytes) of the skin and retina. It is an extremely important pigment because it protects the skin against long exposure to sunlight and is considered an essential factor in the prevention of skin cancer (see Chapters 11 and 41). Ultraviolet light (e.g., sunlight) stimulates the synthesis of melanin, which probably absorbs ultraviolet rays during subsequent exposure. Melanin may also protect the skin by trapping the injurious free radicals produced by the action of ultraviolet light on skin.

Melanin is a brown-black pigment derived from the amino acid tryrosine. It is synthesized by epidermal cells called melanocytes, and stored in membrane-bounded cytoplasmic vesicles called melanosomes. Melanosomes are particularly abundant in projections of melanocytic cytoplasm, called dendrites, from which they are transmitted to neighboring keratinocytes, where melanin accumulation occurs (Robbins et al., 1984). (Keratinocytes, which comprise 95% of epidermal cells, are discussed with other skin components in Chapter 41.) The dendritic melanocytes form bridges between neighboring keratinocytes and inject melanosomes into the keratinocytes by an unknown mechanism.

Melanin can also accumulate in melanophores (melanin-containing pigment cells), macrophages, or other phagocytic cells in the dermis. Presumably these cells acquire the melanin from nearby melanocytes or from pigment that has been extruded from dying epidermal cells. This is the mechanism that causes freckles.

Melanin accumulation occurs in the skin of individuals with Addison disease (adrenocortical insufficiency resulting from disorders of the adrenal cortex; see Chapter 18). The increased melaninogenesis (melanin production) seen in Addison disease is due to the loss of feedback control of adrenocorticotrophic hormone (ACTH). Decreased hormonal secretion from the adrenal gland causes increased release of ACTH from the pituitary gland. In Addison disease, the increase in melanin occurs because a segment of the ACTH molecule contains the melanin-stimulating hormone (MSH).

An increase in melanin also occurs in the benign form of "pigmented moles" called nevi (see Chapter 41). Malignant melanoma is a cancerous skin tumor that contains melanin and invades normal tissue early and widely and often leads to death.

A decrease in melanin production occurs in the inherited disorder of melanin metabolism called albinism. Albinism is often diffuse, involving all the skin, the eyes, and the hair. Albinism is also related to phenylalanine metabolism. In classic types, the albino is unable to convert tyrosine to DOPA (3,4-dihydroxyphenylalanine), an intermediate in melanin biosynthesis. Melanin-producing cells are present in normal numbers, but they are unable to make melanin. Coloration in the albino consists of pinks, blues, and yellows, all the result of red blood color seen through a colorless layer of epithelium, and the carotenoid pigments (yellows and oranges) that are produced in normal amounts by most albinos (Jenkins, 1983). Individuals with albinism are very sensitive to sunlight and quickly become sunburned. They are also at high risk for skin cancer.

Hemoproteins

Hemoproteins are among the most essential of the normal endogenous pigments. They include hemoglobin and the oxidative enzymes, the cytochromes. Central to an understanding of disorders involving these pigments is knowledge of iron uptake, metabolism, excretion, and storage (see Chapter 22). Hemoprotein accumulations in cells are caused by excessive storage of iron, which is transferred to the cells from the bloodstream. Iron enters the blood from three primary sources: (1) tissue stores, (2) the intestinal mucosa, and (3) macrophages that remove and destroy dead or defective red blood cells. The amount of iron in blood plasma also depends on the metabolism of the major iron-transport protein, transferrin.

Iron is stored in tissue cells in two forms: as ferritin and, when greater levels of iron are present, as hemosiderin. **Hemosiderin** is a yellow-brown pigment derived from hemoglobin. With pathologic states, excesses of iron cause hemosiderin to accumulate within cells. Accumulation of hemosiderin often occurs in areas of bruising and hemorrhage and in the lungs and spleen after congestion caused by heart failure. With a local hemorrhage, the skin first appears red-blue, then lysis of the escaped red blood cell occurs, causing the hemoglobin to be transformed to hemosiderin. The color changes noted in bruising reflect this transformation.

Hemosiderosis is a condition in which excess iron is stored as hemosiderin in the cells of many organs and tissues. This condition is common in individuals who have received repeated blood transfusions or prolonged parenteral administration of iron. Hemosiderosis is also associated with increased absorption of dietary iron, conditions in which iron storage and transport is impaired, and hemolytic anemia. Excessive alcohol ingestion can also lead to hemosiderosis. Normally, absorption of excessive dietary iron is prevented by an iron-absorption process in the intestines. Failure of this process can lead to total-body iron accumulations in the range of 60 to 80 g, compared to normal iron stores of 4.5 to 5 g (Robbins et al., 1984). Excessive accumulations of iron, such as occurs in hemochromatosis (a genetic disorder of iron metabolism and the most severe example of iron overload) are associated with liver and pancreatic cell damage.

It is debatable whether iron accumulation itself causes cellular injury or whether injury is due to the basic defect that leads to iron storage. The finding that the extent of liver injury (cirrhosis) is related to the extent of iron accumulation (Powell & Kerr, 1975) suggests that excessive iron accumulation does injure cells. Furthermore, with iron removal by repeated phlebotomy (removal of blood) hemosiderin is mobilized, liver fibrosis and cirrhosis begin to dissipate, and liver size and function return to normal (Bomford, Walker, & Williams, 1975).

Bilirubin is a normal, yellow-to-green pigment of bile derived from the porphyrin structure of hemoglobin. Excesses of bilirubin within cells and tissues causes jaundice (icterus), or yellowing of the skin. Jaundice occurs when the bilirubin level exceeds 1.5 to 2 mg/dl of plasma, compared to the normal values of 0.4 to 1 mg/dl. Hyperbilirubinemia occurs with (1) destruction of red blood cells (erythrocytes), such as in hemolytic jaundice; (2) diseases affecting the metabolism and excretion of bilirubin in the liver; and (3) diseases that cause obstruction of the common bile duct, such as gallstones or pancreatic tumors. (For a detailed description of these diseases, see Chapter 36.) Certain drugs can cause the obstruction of normal bile flow through the liver. They are chlorpromazine and other phenothiazine derivatives; estrogenic hormones; and halothane, an anesthetic.

Because unconjugated bilirubin is lipid soluble, it can injure the lipid components of the plasma membrane, but the exact mechanism or mechanisms that produce injury are not clearly known. Albumin, a plasma protein, provides significant protection by binding unconjugated bilirubin in plasma. Albumin-coupled bilirubin has been experimentally shown to be nontoxic to tissue-culture cells (Cowger, 1971). Cowger's experiments demonstrated that unconjugated bilirubin causes two cellular effects—uncoupling of oxidative phosphorylation and a loss of cellular proteins. These two effects could cause structural injury to the various membranes of the cell.

Calcium

Calcium salts accumulate in both injured and dead tissues. An important mechanism of cellular calcification is the influx of extracellular calcium in injured mitochondria (see pp. 52 and 55). Another mechanism that causes calcium accumulation in alveoli (gas-exchange airways of the lungs), gastric epithelium, and renal tubules is the excretion of acid at these sites, leading to the local production of hydroxyl ions. Hydroxyl ions result in precipitation of calcium hydroxide ($Ca[OH]_2$) and hydroxyapatite ($3Ca_3[PO_4]_2^-Ca[OH]_2$), a mixed salt. Damage occurs when calcium salts clump and harden interfering with normal cellular structure and function.

Pathologic calcification can be dystrophic or metastatic. **Dystrophic calcification** is the calcification of dying and dead tissues. This type of calcification occurs in chronic tuberculosis of the lungs and lymph nodes, in

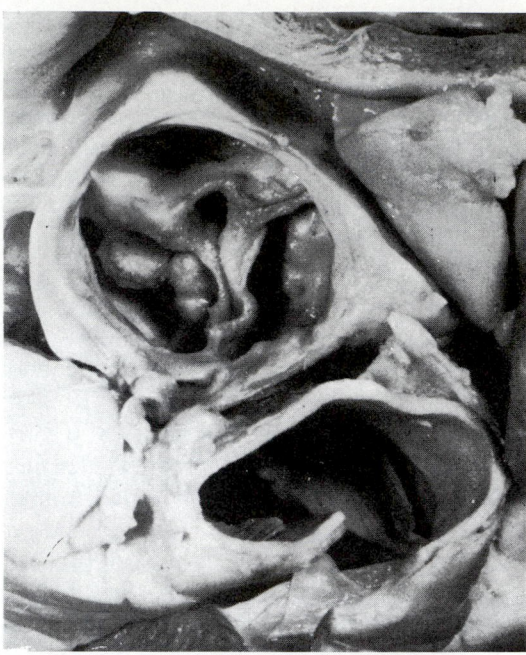

FIG. 2-14. Aortic valve calcification. This aortic valve was unable to close because of calcification caused by rheumatic heart disease. (From Kissane, 1985.)

arteries with advanced atherosclerosis (narrowing as a result of plaque accumulation) and often in injured heart valves (Fig. 2-14). Calcification of the heart valves interferes with opening and closing of the valves, causing heart murmurs (see Chapter 27). Calcification of the coronary arteries predisposes them to severe narrowing and thrombosis, which can lead to myocardial infarction. Another site of dystrophic calcification is the center of tumors. Over time the center is deprived of oxygen supply, dies, and becomes calcified. The calcium salts appear as gritty, clumped granules that can become hard as stone. When several layers clump together, they resemble grains of sand and are called **psammoma bodies.**

The exact pathogenic mechanisms responsible for dystrophic calcification are unknown. A popular hypothesis is that with progressive deterioration of dead cells, the exposed denatured (changed) proteins preferentially bind with phosphate ions. The phosphate ions then react with calcium ions to form deposits of phosphate carbonate precipitates and, sometimes, crystalline formations of calcium phosphate. Dystrophic calcification develops slowly and is an explicit marker for the site of dead cells.

Metastatic calcification consists of mineral deposits that occur in normal tissues as the result of hypercalcemia (an excess of calcium in the blood; see Chapter 3). Conditions that cause hypercalcemia include hyperparathyroidism, toxic levels of vitamin D, hyperthyroidism,

idiopathic hypercalcemia of infancy, Addison disease (adrenal cortical insufficiency), systemic sarcoidosis, milk-alkali syndrome, and the increased bone demineralization that results from bone tumors, leukemia, and disseminated cancers. Hypercalcemia can also occur in some instances of advanced renal failure with phosphate retention, resulting in hyperparathyroidism (Robbins et al., 1984).

Hyaline Change

Hyaline change is the development of a crystalline, glassy, translucent appearance within cells or in the extracellular space. Several mechanisms are known or thought to cause hyaline change. These mechanisms include the flowing:

1. Increased production of basement membrane substances in the walls of arterioles and some arteries, which occurs in uncontrolled hypertension and in diabetes mellitus.
2. Reabsorption of large amounts of protein that have leaked across the glomerular membrane, a process that is associated with changes in the proximal tubular epithelial cells of the kidney.
3. Viral infections, which may cause inclusions of viral nucleoproteins.
4. Extracellular accumulations of glycoproteins in connective tissue.
5. Alterations in the cytoplasm of liver cells, causing changes in the cytoskeleton (microtubules and actin filaments) (see Chapter 1), usually caused by chronic alcoholism.

Systemic Manifestations

Systemic manifestations of cellular injury include a general sense of fatigue and malaise, a loss of well-being, and altered appetite. Fever is frequently present because of biochemicals produced during the inflammatory response (see Chapters 2 and 7). Table 2-3 summarizes the most significant systemic manifestations of cellular injury.

CELLULAR DEATH

Necrosis

Cellular death eventually leads to the process of cellular dissolution, or **necrosis.** Necrosis is the sum of cellular changes following local cell death and the process of cellular self-digestion known as **autodigestion,** or **autolysis** (Fig. 2-15). The structural signs that indicate irreversible injury and progression to necrosis are the dense clumping and progressive disruption of genetic material and disruption of the plasma and organelle membranes. In later stages of necrosis, most organelles are disrupted, and **karyolysis** (nuclear dissolution from

TABLE 2-3 Systemic manifestations of cellular injury

Manifestation	Cause
Fever	Release of endogenous pyrogens (possibly prostaglandins) from bacteria or macrophages; the acute inflammatory response.
Increased heart rate	Increase in oxidative metabolic processes resulting from fever.
Increase in leukocytes (leukocytosis)	With infections there is an increase in the total number of white blood cells; normal is 5000-9000 mm^3. The increase is directly related to the severity of the infection.
Pain	Various mechanisms, such as release of bradykinins, obstruction, pressure.
Presence of cellular enzymes in extracellular fluid	Release of enzymes from cells of tissue*
Lactate dehydrogenase (LDH) (LDH isoenzymes)	Release from red blood cells, liver, kidney, skeletal muscle.
Creatine kinase (CK) (CK isoenzymes)	Release from skeletal muscle, brain, heart.
Aspartate aminotransferase (AST/SGOT)	Release from heart, liver, skeletal muscle, kidney, pancreas.
Alanine aminotransferase (ALT/SGPT)	Release from liver, kidney, heart.
Alkaline phosphatase (ALP)	Release from liver, bone.
Amylase	Release from pancreas.
Aldolase	Release from skeletal muscle, heart

*The rapidity of enzyme transfer is a function of the weight of the enzyme and the concentration gradient across the cellular membrane. The specific metabolic and excretory rates of the enzymes determine how long levels of enzymes remain elevated.

the action of hydrolytic enzymes) is under way. In some cells, the nucleus shrinks and becomes a small, dense mass of genetic material—a process called nuclear pyknosis. The pyknotic nucleus eventually dissolves (by karyolysis) as a result of the action of hydrolytic lysosomal enzymes on DNA.

Different types of necrosis tend to occur in different organs or tissues and can sometimes indicate the mechanism or cause of cellular injury. There are four major types of necrosis: coagulative, liquefactive, caseous, and fatty. Another type, gangrenous necrosis, is *not* a distinctive type of cell death but refers to larger areas of tissue death.

Coagulative necrosis, which occurs primarily in the kidneys, heart, and adrenal glands, commonly results from hypoxia caused by severe ischemia. Another mechanism is hypoxia caused by chemical injury, particularly the ingestion of mercuric chloride. Coagulation is caused by protein denaturation, which causes the protein albumin to change from a gelatinous, transparent state to a firm, opaque state, similar to that of a cooked egg white. The necrotic tissues appear firm and slightly swollen.

Liquefactive necrosis commonly results from ischemic injury to neurons and glial cells in the brain. Dead brain tissue is readily affected by liquefaction necrosis because brain cells are rich in the digestive hydrolytic enzymes and lipids, and the brain contains little connective tissue. As the cells are digested by their own hydrolases, the tissue becomes soft, liquefies, and is walled off from healthy tissue, forming cysts (cyst formation is described in Chapter 7).

Liquefactive necrosis can also result from bacterial infection, particularly by staphylococci, streptococci, and *E. coli.* In this case the hydrolases are released from the lysosomes of neutrophils, which are phagocytes attracted to the infected area to kill the bacteria. (This action is part of the acute inflammatory response, which is discussed in Chapter 7.) Liquefaction of bacterial cells and neighboring tissue cells by neutrophilic hydrolases results in the accumulation of pus.

Caseous necrosis, which commonly results from tuberculous pulmonary infection, particularly by *M. tuberculosis,* is a combination of coagulative and liquefactive necrosis. The dead cells disintegrate, but the debris is not digested completely by hydrolases. Tissues appear soft and granular and resemble clumped cheese, which gives this type of necrosis its name. A granulomatous inflammatory wall encloses areas of caseous necrosis.

Fat necrosis, which occurs in the breast, pancreas,

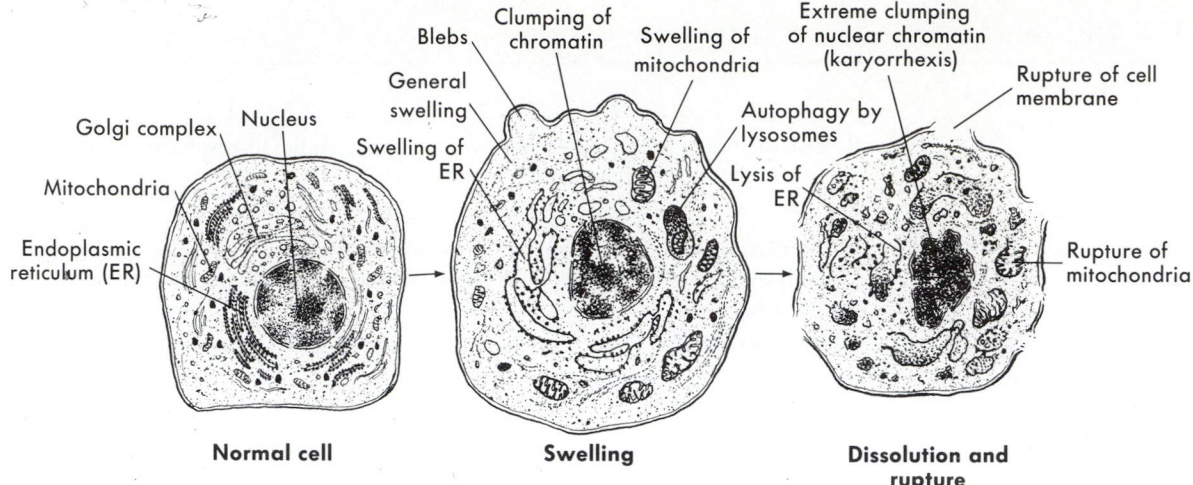

Golgi complex　Nucleus

Mitochondria

Endoplasmic
reticulum (ER)

Blebs

General
swelling

Swelling of
ER

Clumping of
chromatin

Swelling of
mitochondria

Autophagy by
lysosomes

Lysis of
ER

Extreme clumping
of nuclear chromatin
(karyorrhexis)

Rupture of cell
membrane

Rupture of
mitochondria

Normal cell　　　　**Swelling**　　　　**Dissolution and
rupture**

FIG. 2-15. Stages of necrosis.

and other abdominal structures, is a specific type of cellular dissolution caused by powerful enzymes called lipases. Lipases break down triglycerides, releasing free fatty acids, which then combine with calcium, magnesium, and sodium ions, creating soaps (a process known as saponification). The necrotic tissue appears opaque and chalk white.

Gangrenous necrosis refers to death of tissue and results from severe hypoxic injury, commonly occurring because of arteriosclerosis, or blockage, of major arteries, especially in the lower leg. With hypoxia and subsequent bacterial invasion, the tissues can undergo necrosis. **Dry gangrene** is usually due to coagulative necrosis. **Wet gangrene** develops when neutrophils invade the site, causing liquefactive necrosis. In dry gangrene, the skin becomes very dry and shrinks, resulting in wrinkles, and its color changes to dark brown or black (Fig. 2-16). The manifestations of dry gangrene are not as marked as those of rapidly spreading wet gangrene. Red, inflamed tissue creates a visible line of demarcation between wet gangrenous and healthy tissue.

In wet gangrene, which usually occurs in internal organs, the site is cold, swollen, and black. A foul odor produced by the accumulation of pus is usually present. Since the spread of tissue damage is rapid, the line of demarcation is not as pronounced as in dry gangrene. If systemic symptoms become severe, death can ensue.

Gas gangrene, a special type of gangrene, is due to infection of injured tissue by one of many species of Clostridium. These anaerobic bacteria produce hydrolytic enzymes and toxins that destroy connective tissue and cellular membranes, and cause bubbles of gas to form in muscle cells. Gas gangrene can be fatal if enzymes lyse the membranes of red blood cells, destroying their oxygen-carrying capacity. Death is due to shock.

The condition is treated with antitoxins and supplemental oxygen delivered in a hyperbaric (pressurized) chamber.

Apoptosis

Apoptosis is a name recently suggested for an important, distinct type of cell death (Kerr & Searle, 1980) that differs from necrosis in several respects. **Apoptosis** is an active process of cellular self-destruction that is implicated in both normal and pathologic tissue changes. It is the type of cell death responsible for local deletion of cells during normal embryonic development. Recent results have shown that apoptosis plays a major role in endocrine-dependent tissues that are undergoing atro-

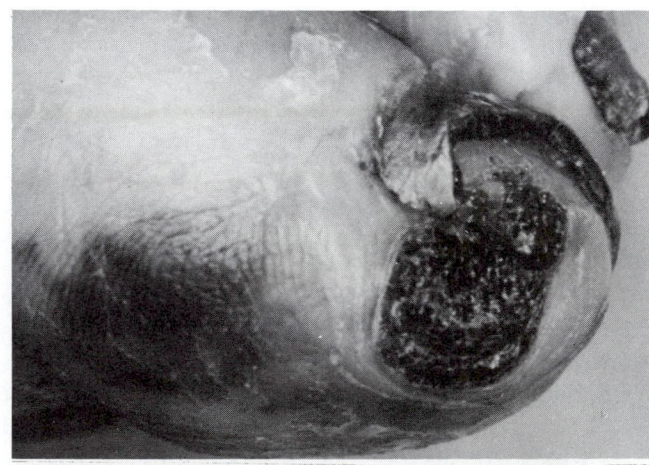

FIG. 2-16. Foot of an individual with gangrene caused by small vessel disease. (From Levin & O'Neal, 1988.)

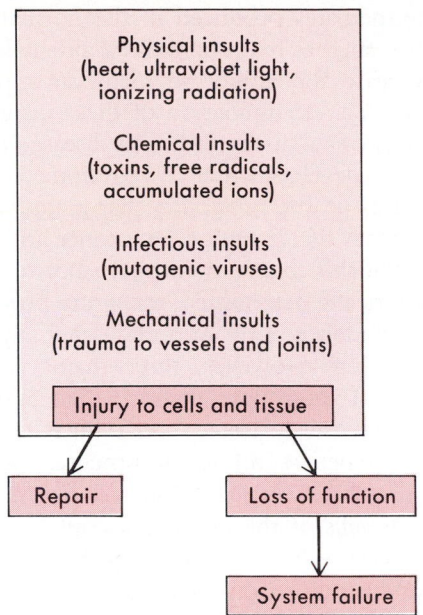

Physical insults
(heat, ultraviolet light,
ionizing radiation)

Chemical insults
(toxins, free radicals,
accumulated ions)

Infectious insults
(mutagenic viruses)

Mechanical insults
(trauma to vessels and joints)

Injury to cells and tissue

Repair   Loss of function

System failure

FIG. 2-17. Microinsults. (Redrawn from Johnson, 1985.)

phic change (Sandford, Searle, & Kerr, 1984). Apoptosis is known to occur spontaneously in malignant tumors and in normal, rapidly proliferating cells treated with cancer chemotherapeutic agents and ionizing radiation (Wyllie, Kerr, & Currie, 1980). Its significance in aging is presently unknown. Necrosis and apoptosis affect tissues differently. Unlike necrosis, apoptosis affects scattered, single cells. Apoptosis is nuclear and cytoplasmic condensation of a cell followed by fragmentation into membrane-bounded fragments and subsequent phagocytosis by neighboring, healthy cells.

The mechanisms of apoptosis are not clear, but they appear to differ from those of necrosis in the following ways:

1. Apoptosis is frequently initiated by normal physiologic stimuli.
2. Apotosis can occur without increases in membrane permeability, and electrolyte balances may remain normal.
3. Intracellular ATP is not necessarily depleted: apoptosis can occur in cells with normal ATP content.
4. Many cell types can undergo apoptosis independent of stimuli.

AGING

Aging is usually defined as a normal physiologic process. Fundamental to the definition of aging is its universal and inevitable nature. To understand the basic mechanisms of aging, one must be able to identify the

irreversible and universal processes at the cellular and molecular level—a very difficult task. It is difficult because it requires the separation of irreversible processes from potentially reversible mechanisms (i.e., those that result from disease or age-related debilities).

Aging has been traditionally excluded from the domain of disease because it is "normal"; disease is usually considered "abnormal." Conceptually, this distinction seems clear until the concept of "injury" is introduced; disease has been defined by some pathologists as the result of injury. Aging has been defined as the time-dependent loss of structure and function that proceeds very slowly and in such small increments that it appears to be due to the accumulation of small, imperceptible injuries—a gradual result of "wear and tear."

Injuries may result from unavoidable and universal microinsults caused by continuous bombardment by ultraviolet light, countless mechanical insults, and reactions to metabolites (Johnson, 1985) (see Fig. 2-17). In this context, the distinction between aging and disease is unclear. For example, some degree of atrophy of the brain is considered "normal" in old age until it proceeds far enough to cause clinically significant disability and is called "disease." Likewise, most human beings have atherosclerosis and the plaques progress with age, but at what point in this progression is it considered abnormal? These conceptual distinctions have given rise to two general categories of theories of aging. The first category proposes that aging is the result of the accumulation of random injuries and events. The second category proposes that aging is the result of a genetically-controlled developmental program, or built-in self-destructive processes.

Normal Life Span

The **maximal life span** of humans is between 80 and 100 years and does not vary among populations significantly. However, individuals with longer life spans were once thought to reside among the Abkhasiz in the Southern Soviet Union, the Andrean Vilcamanda tribe in Ecuador, and the Hunza of Kashmir and were reported to have lived as long as 160 years (Leaf & Lannois, 1973). Recent interviews with the alleged centenarians, however, revealed no significant increases in longevity (Mazess & Forman, 1979; Medvedev, 1974). Few individuals in primitive societies reach the maximal life span; most die in infancy and the early years (Leaf, 1982). In societies with improvements in sanitation, housing, nutrition, and health care, many persons attain the maximal life span. Although the maximal life span has not changed significantly over time, the average life span, or **life expectancy** has increased. In recent years the death rate for people 65 years of age and older has declined significantly. This decline has been largely due to decreases in cardiovascular disease (Brody & Brock, 1985). In each successive age group from 65 and older, women outnumber men; thus women have a greater life expectancy than men. Increases in life expectancy have brought a large elderly population with inherent problems of disability, disease, and socioeconomic hardship.

Theories and Mechanisms of Aging

The theories of aging are multiple and diverse because there is relatively little "indisputable" knowlege on the subject. Table 2-4 presents the historical development of aging research. Many of the theories proposed to explain aging have focused on a single mechanism—the so-called magic bullet approach to arrest aging. It is doubtful that a single theory will explain all the mechanisms of aging. As stated earlier, there are two general categories of theories of aging: (1) that aging is due to the accumulation of injurious events, sometimes called damage-accumulation theories; or (2) that biologic changes of aging are due to a genetically controlled developmental program. In the first category, random accumulation of errors in protein structure, mutations in somatic cells, the accumulation of metabolic waste products, and free-radical mediated damage (from highly re-

active intermediates produced in the normal course of metabolism, such as hydroperoxides, aldehydes, and ketones) decrease the ability to maintain a physiologic steady state. The accumulation of these insults or injuries increases one's susceptibility to disease. The second category, the developmentally programmed theories of aging, focuses on the possibility that aging is the result of certain genes that program senescence and cell death. Supporters of this theory claim that since maximal life span is genetically determined, the aging process is also.

There is evidence both for and against any particular theory of aging. However, three major areas of the mechanisms of aging have retained their appeal and/or have been extensively tested: (1) cellular changes produced by genetic and environmental factors; (2) changes in cellular regulatory, or control mechanisms, especially in cells of the neuroendocrine, immune, and central nervous systems; and (3) degenerative extracellular and vascular alterations (King, Fenoglio, & Lefkowich, 1983; Warner et al., 1987).

Genetic and Environmental Factors

Cellular aging may be the consequence of "wear and tear" that causes functional changes and eventual cellular death. Many investigators propose that cellular damage may occur during replication as a result of factors within the cell, such as DNA and protein mechanisms, or factors outside the cell, such as ionizing radiation. They further propose that cells are already programmed at birth or are injured during life so as to cause errors in mitotic division and in the replication of genetic material that eventually lead either to cellular atrophy or death. Atrophy is common in the thymus, testis, ovary, uterus, and breast of aged individuals, although these organs age differently. For example, the ovary begins to lose function at an average age of 45, whereas the thymus gland begins to atrophy before adolescence.

One of the genetic mechanisms of aging is programmed aging. Regardless of damaging environmental factors, some investigators think that each normal cell may have a finite life span during which it is capable of replication. A classic experiment done by Hayflick (1965) demonstrated that fibroblasts are limited to a finite number of generations (40 to 60 doublings). This phenomenon has not been demonstrated for epithelial cells. Although this theory proposes that human cells have a finite number of replications, its proponents do not propose that aging is the result of cells losing their ability to divide. Rather, they believe that an intrinsic program within the human genome progressively slows or shuts down certain physiologic mechanisms, including mitosis (Russell, 1987).

Another genetic mechanism of aging suggests that mutations in somatic cells cause aging. The **somatic mutation hypothesis** is designed to evaluate DNA

TABLE 2-4 Theories of aging		
Theory	**Year**	**Proponent**
Waste product theory	1923	Carrell & Ebeling
Wear-and-tear theory	1924	Pearl
Rate of living theory[a]	1928	Pearl
Endocrine theory	1947	Korenchevsky & Jones
Free-radical theory	1955	Harman
Collagen theory[b]	1957	Verzar
Metabolic theory[a]	1957; 1961	Carlson et al; Johnson et al.
Somatic mutation theory	1959	Sziliard
Error-catastrophe theory	1963; 1970	Orgel
Cross-linking theory[b]	1968	Bjorksten
Programmed senescence theory	1969	Hayflick
Immunologic theory	1969	Walform

NOTE: Theories with the same superscript may represent the same theory.
From Schneider, 1987.

damage and efficiency of repair, and integrity of DNA synthesis. Most experimental evidence thus far does not support the hypothesis that aging is due to somatic mutation. However, with more sensitive laboratory methods, the future of DNA repair studies appears to be full of promise (Warner et al., 1987).

The **error-prone** or **catastrophic theory** initially proposed by Orgel in 1963, stated that the presence of errors in those enzymes involved in transcription and translation, and thus their own synthesis, leads to an increase in errors and eventually to the death of the cell. The theory was later modified by Orgel in 1970, with the possibility that nongrowing cells may not be subject to error catastrophe if the rate of error production did not increase significantly during protein synthesis. Abnormal forms of some, but not all, cellular proteins do appear during senescence but not as a result of errors in protein synthesis as originally predicted (Dice & Goff, 1987). Rather, the abnormal proteins appear to reflect several types of posttranslational modifications (Dice & Goff, 1987). The error-catastrophe theory has attracted a great deal of interest. Most of the evidence, however, argues against this theory as originally formulated. The accumulation of altered proteins in aging may result from an increased production or decreased ability of aged cells to degrade their cellular proteins, or both.

Alterations of Cellular Control Mechanisms

Many investigators suggest that the overall effects of aging are due to changes in certain cell populations that exert regulatory or control functions, such as cells of the central nervous system, neuroendocrine system, and immune system (Bliznakov et al., 1978; Denckla, 1981; Everitt & Burgess, 1976; Greenberg & Yunis, 1978; Walford, 1980). The **neuroendocrine theory** of aging purports that a genetic program for aging is encoded in the brain and is controlled and relayed to peripheral tissues through hormonal and neural agents. Controversy exists as to what neuroendocrine mechanisms are responsible for aging. Possible mechanisms include (1) increased hormonal degradation, (2) decreased rate of hormonal synthesis and secretion, and (3) decreased target-organ sensitivity related to the number of cellular receptors for hormonal ligands, ligand-receptor binding, or ligand internalization (see Chapter 1). (The neuroendocrine theory of aging is discussed further in Chapter 17.)

Proponents of immune theories of aging believe that the immune system is implicated in aging because (1) immune function declines with age; (2) the decline in immune function is related to certain diseases, such as cancer, and to many other secondary effects; and (3) the number of autoantibodies (antibodies that attack body tissues) increases with age. (Changes in the immune system with age are discussed in Chapter 6.)

Degenerative Extracellular Changes

Extracellular factors that affect the aging process include the binding of collagen; the increase in free radicals' effects on cells; the structural alterations of fascia, tendons, ligaments, bones, and joints; and peripheral vascular disease, particularly arteriosclerosis (King et al., 1983; Kohn, 1985) (see Chapter 27).

Aging affects the extracellular matrix with increased cross-linking (e.g., aging collagen becomes more insoluble, chemically stable but rigid, resulting in a decrease of cell permeability), decreased synthesis, and increased degradation of collagen. These changes, together with the disappearance of elastin and changes in proteoglycans and plasma proteins, cause disorders of the ground substance that result in dehydration and wrinkling of the skin (see Chapter 41). Other age-related defects in the extracellular matrix include skeletal muscle alterations (e.g., atrophy, decreased tone, and loss of contractility), cataracts, diverticula, hernias, and rupture of intervertebral disks.

Free radicals of oxygen that result from oxidative cellular metabolism (e.g., respiratory chain, phagocytosis, prostaglandin synthesis) are thought to damage tissues during the aging process. The oxygen radicals produced include singlet oxygen, superoxide radical, hydroxyl radical, and hydrogen peroxide (free radicals are discussed in Chapter 1). These oxygen products are extremely reactive and can damage nucleic acids, destroy polysaccharides, oxidize proteins, peroxide unsaturated fatty acids, and kill and lyse cells. Investigators have proposed that progressive and cumulative damage from oxygen radicals leads to harmful alterations in cellular function consistent with those of aging (Harman, 1955, 1985). This hypothesis has its foundation from an older theory, the "wear-and-tear" theory of aging, which states that damages accumulate with time, decreasing the organism's ability to maintain a steady state. The hypothesis is controversial because there is no evidence that free radicals increase with aging, nor have higher levels been found in animals with short life spans than in animals with long life spans (Kanugo, 1980; Pryor, 1987).

Of much interest is the relationship between aging and the disappearance or alteration of extracellular substances important for vessel integrity. With aging, lipid, calcium, and plasma proteins are deposited in the walls of vessels. These depositions cause serious basement membrane thickening and alterations in smooth muscle functioning, resulting in arteriosclerosis. Arteriosclerosis is a progressive disease that causes serious problems in the aged individual, including stroke, myocardial infarction, renal disease, and peripheral vascular disease.

Cellular Aging

Cellular changes characteristic of aging include atrophy, decreased function, and loss of cells, possibly caused by apoptosis. Loss of cellular function from any of these causes initiates the compensatory mechanisms of hypertrophy and hyperplasia of remaining cells, which can lead to metaplasia, dysplasia, and neoplasia. All these changes can alter receptor placement and function, nutrient pathways, secretion of cellular products, and neuroendocrine control mechanisms. In the aged cell, DNA, RNA, cellular proteins, and membranes are most susceptible to injurious stimuli. DNA is particularly vulnerable to such injuries as breaks, deletions, and additions. Although DNA generally repairs itself with time, the aged cell's capacity for DNA repair is decreased (King et al., 1983; Setlow, 1987). (The processes of DNA replication and repair are discussed in Chapter 4.) Lack of DNA repair increases the cell's susceptibility to mutations that may be lethal or may promote the development of neoplasia (see Chapter 10).

Tissue and Systemic Aging

It is probably safe to say that every physiologic process can be shown to function less efficiently with increasing age. The most characteristic tissue changes with age is a progressive stiffness or rigidity (Kohn, 1985). The rigidity changes affect many systems including the arterial, pulmonary, and musculoskeletal systems. A consequence of blood vessel and organ stiffness is a progressive increase in peripheral resistance to blood flow. The movement of intracellular and extracellular substances is also usually decreased with age. The diffusion capacity of the lung decreases with each advancing decade (Kohn, 1985). Blood flow through organs decreases, for example, renal plasma flow decreases as a function of age.

Changes in the endocrine and immune systems occur with aging. The thymus atrophies at puberty, causing a decreased immune response to T-dependent antigens (foreign proteins). Later in life, an increase in autoantibodies and immune complexes (antibodies that are bound to antigens) and an overall decrease of immunologic tolerance for the host's own cells further diminishes the effectiveness of the immune system. In women, the reproductive system loses ova, and in men spermatogenesis is decreased. Responsiveness to hormones decreases in the breast and endometrium.

The stomach is affected by a decreased rate of emptying and decreased secretion of hormones and hydrochloric acid. Muscular atrophy diminishes mobility by decreasing motor tone and contractility. The skin of the aged individual is affected by atrophy and wrinkling of the epidermis and alterations in underlying dermis, fat, and muscle.

Total-body changes include a decrease in height; a reduction in circumference of the neck, thighs, and arms; widening of the pelvis; and lengthening of the nose and ears. Several of these changes are due to tissue atrophy

and to decreased bone mass caused by osteoporosis and osteoarthritis. Changes in body weight are mostly related to body fat. Men usually gain weight until about age 50, whereas women gain until about 70 before losing. As fat increases, total-body water decreases. Total-body potassium also decreases because of decreased cellular mass. An increased sodium/potassium ratio suggests that the decreased cellular mass is accompanied by an increased extracellular compartment.

Although some of these alterations are probably inherent in aging, others represent consequences of aging. Advanced age increases susceptibility to disease, and death occurs following an injury or insult because of diminished cellular, tissue, and organic function. To determine that an individual "died of old age" would truly be a monumental task if not an impossible one.

SOMATIC DEATH

Somatic death is death of the entire organism. Unlike the changes that follow cellular death in a live body, **postmortem change** is diffuse and does not involve components of the inflammatory response. Within minutes of death, manifestations of postmortem change appear, eliminating any difficulty in determining that death has occurred. The most notable manifestations are complete cessation of respiration and circulation. The surface of the skin usually becomes pale and yellowish; however, the lifelike color of the cheeks and lips may persist after death from such causes as carbon monoxide poisoning, drowning, and chloroform poisoning (Shennan, 1935).

Body temperature falls gradually immediately after death, then more rapidly (about 1.0° to 1.5° F/hr) until, after 24 hours, body temperature equals that of the environment (Minckler, Anstall, & Minkler, 1971). After death caused by certain infective diseases, body temperature may continue to rise for a short time after death. Postmortem reduction of body temperature is called **algor mortis.**

Blood pressure within the retinal vessels decreases, causing muscle tension to decrease and the pupils to become dilated. The face, nose, and chin become "sharp" or "peaked" looking as blood and fluids drain away (Shennan, 1935). Gravity causes blood to settle in the most dependent, or lowest tissues, which develop a purple discoloration called **livor mortis**. Incisions at this time usually fail to cause bleeding. The skin loses its elasticity and transparency.

Within 6 hours after death, acidic compounds accumulate within the muscles because of the breakdown of carbohydrate and depletion of ATP. This interferes with ATP-dependent detachment of myosin from actin (contractile proteins), and muscle stiffening, or **rigor mor-**

CLINICAL COMMENTARY
Criteria for Somatic Death

Issues involving death and dying are among the most difficult in clinical practice. Contrary to what some law books state as the criterion for death, arrest of the heart is not proof that life has ended because the heart can sometimes be restored to action. If cardiac arrest is not reversed, hypoxic injury to other vital organs ensues. Because of its high oxygen demands, the brain is usually the first such organ to be destroyed. This phenomenon, along with the advent of transplantation procedures requiring viable organs from a donor, has led to the development of criteria for determining "brain death" as proof of somatic death. These criteria are as follows:
1. Coma with cerebral unresponsiveness, including cessation of all brainstem reflexes (pupillary reactions, ocular movement, blinking, and swallowing)
2. Cessation of breathing (no respiratory movement after removal from the respirator for 1 to 2 minutes)
3. Isoelectric ("flat") electroencephalogram (EEG).

---

tis, sets in. The smaller muscles are usually affected first, particularly the muscles of the jaw. Within 12 to 14 hours, rigor mortis usually affects the entire body.

Signs of putrefaction are generally obvious about 24 to 48 hours after death. Rigor mortis gradually diminishes, and the body becomes flaccid in 12 to 14 hours. Putrefactive changes vary depending on the temperature of the environment. The most visible is greenish discoloration of the skin, particularly on the abdomen. The discoloration is thought to be related to the diffusion of hemolyzed blood into the tissues and the production of sulfhemoglobin (Minckler et al., 1971). Slippage or loosening of the skin from underlying tissues occurs at the same time. Following this, swelling or bloating of the body and liquefactive changes occur, sometimes causing opening of the body cavities. At a microscopic level, putrefactive changes are associated with the release of enzymes and lytic dissolution called **postmortem autolysis.**

SUMMARY REVIEW

Cellular Adaptation
1 Cellular adaptation is an alteration that enables the cell to maintain a steady state despite adverse conditions.
2 Atrophy is a decrease in cellular size caused by aging, disuse, or lack of blood supply, hormonal stimulation, or neural stimulation. Amounts of endoplasmic reticulum, mitochondria, and microfilaments are decreased.
3 Hypertrophy is an increase in the size of cells caused by increased work demands or hormonal stimulation. Amounts of protein in the plasma membrane, endoplasmic reticulum, microfilaments, and mitochondria are increased.
4 Hyperplasia is an increase in the number of cells caused by an increased rate of cellular division. Normal hyperplasia is stimulated by hormones or the need to replace lost tissues.
5 Dysplasia, or atypical hyperplasia, is an abnormal change in the size, shape, and organization of mature tissue cells.
6 Metaplasia is the reversible replacement of one mature cell type by another, less mature cell type.

Cellular Injury
1 Cellular injury is caused by lack of oxygen (hypoxia), caustic or toxic chemicals, infectious agents, inflammatory and immune responses, genetic factors, insufficient nutrients, or physical trauma from many causes.
2 Sublethal injury, which does not kill the cell, may result in cellular adaptation. Lethal injury, which does kill the cell, always involves disruption of cellular metabolism.
3 Metabolism cannot occur if the cell's oxygen supply is cut off or if damage to the plasma membrane causes the cell to "drown" in an influx of extracellular fluids and charged solutes. Both insults disable ATP production, which is essential for both metabolism and maintenance of active transport processes that prevent fluid and solute influx.
4 The sequence of events leading to cell death is commonly decreased ATP production, failure of active transport mechanisms (the sodium-potassium pump), cellular swelling, detachment of ribosomes from the endoplasmic reticulum, cessation of protein synthesis, mitochondrial swelling as a result of calcium accumulation, vacuolation, leakage of digestive enzymes from lysosomes, autodigestion of intracellular structures, lysis of the plasma membrane, and death.
5 The initial insult in hypoxic injury is usually ischemia, the cessation of blood flow into vessels that supply the cell with oxygen and nutrients.
6 The initial insult in chemical injury is damage or destruction of the plasma membrane. Chemical agents that cause cellular injury include carbon tetrachloride, lead, carbon monoxide, hydrogen cyanide, and hydrogen sulfide.
7 Bacteria injure cells by producing destructive enzymes, exotoxins, or endotoxins. Enzymes can damage the

plasma membranes of host cells, exotoxins can inactivate enzymes critical to protein synthesis, and endotoxins activate the inflammatory response and produce fever.

8 Bacteremia, or septicemia, is the proliferation of bacteria in the blood. Endotoxins released by blood-borne bacteria cause the release of vasoactive enzymes that increase the permeability of blood vessels. Leakage from vessels causes hypotension that can result in septic shock.

9 Viruses enter host cells and use the metabolic processes of host cells to proliferate.

10 Viruses that have invaded host cells decrease protein synthesis, disrupt lysosomal membranes, form inclusion bodies where synthesis of viral nucleic acids is occurring, fuse with host cells to produce giant cells, alter antigenic properties of the host cell, and transform host cells into cancerous cells.

11 Activation of inflammation and immunity, which occurs after cellular injury or infection, involves powerful biochemicals and proteins capable of damaging normal (uninjured and uninfected) cells.

12 Genetic disorders injure cells by altering the nucleus and the plasma membrane's structure, shape, receptors, or transport mechanisms.

13 Deprivation of essential nutrients (proteins, carbohydrates, lipids, and vitamins) can cause cellular injury by altering cellular structure and function, particularly of transport mechanisms, chromosomes, the nucleus, and DNA.

14 Injurious physical agents include temperature extremes, changes in atmospheric pressure, ionizing radiation, illumination, mechanical factors (such as physical impact or irritation), noise, and prolonged vibration.

Manifestations of Cellular Injury

1 Cellular manifestations of cellular injury include accumulations of water, lipids, carbohydrates, glycogen, proteins, pigments, hemosiderin, bilirubin, and calcium.

2 Accumulations harm cells by "crowding" the organelles and by causing excessive (and sometimes harmful) metabolites to be produced during their catabolism. The metabolites are released into the cytoplasm or expelled into the extracellular matrix.

3 Cellular swelling, the accumulation of excessive water in the cell, is due to the failure of transport mechanisms and is a sign of many types of cellular injury.

4 Accumulations of organic substances—lipids, carbohydrates, glycogen, proteins, and pigments—are due to disorders in which (a) cellular uptake of the substance exceeds the cell's capacity to catabolize (digest) or use it or (b) cellular anabolism (synthesis) of the substance exceeds the cell's capacity to use or secrete it.

5 Dystrophic calcification (accumulation of calcium salts) is always a sign of pathologic change because it only occurs in injured or dead cells. Metastatic calcification, on the other hand, can occur in uninjured cells in individuals with hypercalcemia.

6 Hyaline change is the development of a crystalline, glassy appearance within cells or in the extracellular space. One mechanism of hyaline change is protein excess in cellular structures.

7 Systemic manifestations of cellular injury include fever, leukocytosis, increased heart rate, pain, and serum elevations of enzymes in the plasma.

Cellular Death

1 Cellular death is manifested as cellular dissolution, or necrosis. Necrosis is the sum of the changes after local cell death and includes the process of autolysis, or cellular self-destruction.

2 There are four major types of necrosis: coagulative, liquefactive, caseous, and fat necrosis. Different types of necrosis occur in different tissues.

3 Structural signs that indicate irreversible injury and progression to necrosis are the dense clumping and disruption of genetic material and the disruption of the plasma and organelle membranes.

4 Apoptosis, a distinct type of cellular death, is a process of selective cellular self-destruction, that occurs in both normal and pathologic tissue changes.

5 Gangrenous necrosis, or gangrene, is tissue necrosis due to hypoxia and subsequent bacterial invasion.

Aging

1 It is difficult to determine the physiologic (normal) from the pathologic changes of aging.

2 Humans have an inherent maximal life span (80 to 100 years) that is dictated by currently unknown intrinsic mechanisms.

3 Although the maximal life span has not changed significantly over time, the average life span, or life expectancy, has increased.

4 The physiologic mechanisms of aging are apparently associated with (a) cellular changes produced by genetic and environmental factors, (b) changes in cellular regulatory or control mechanisms, and (c) degenerative extracellular and vascular alterations.

Somatic Death

1 Somatic death is death of the entire organism. Postmortem change is diffuse and does not involve the inflammatory response.

2 Manifestations of somatic death include cessation of respiration and circulation, gradual lowering of body temperature, pupil dilation, loss of elasticity and transparency in the skin, muscle stiffening (rigor mortis), and skin discoloration (livor mortis). Signs of putrefaction are obvious about 24 to 48 hours after death.

KEY TERMS

Algor mortis, 76

Anoxia, 52

Apoptosis, 72

Atrophy, 50

Autolysis, 70

Autophagic vacuole, 50

Bacteremia (septicemia), 59

Bilirubin, 69

Blast injury, 63

Caseous necrosis, 71

Catastrophic (error-prone) theory, 75

Cellular accumulation (infiltration), 66

Cellular swelling, 66

Coagulative necrosis, 71

Compensatory hyperplasia, 51

Decompression sickness (caisson disease), 63

Dry gangrene, 72

Dysplasia (atypical hyperplasia), 51

Dystrophic calcification, 69

Endotoxin, 58

Exotoxin, 58

Fat necrosis, 71

Fatty change, 67

Free radical, 55

Gangrenous necrosis, 72

Gas gangrene, 72

Hemoprotein, 69

Hemosiderin, 69

Hemosiderosis, 69

Hormonal hyperplasia, 51

Hyaline change, 70

Hydropic degeneration, 66

Hyperlipidemia, 62

Hyperplasia, 50

Hyperthermic injury, 63

Hypertrophy, 50

Hypolipidemia, 62

Hypothermic injury, 63

Hypoxia, 52

Inclusion body, 61

Ionizing radiation, 63

Ischemia, 52

Karyolysis, 70

Life expectancy, 73

Lipid-acceptor protein (apoprotein), 55

Lipid peroxidation, 55

Lipofuscin, 50

Liquefactive necrosis, 71

Livor mortis, 76

Maximal life span, 73

Melanin, 68

Metaplasia, 51

Metastatic calcification, 70

Necrosis, 70

Neuroendocrine theory, 75

Noise, 65

Pathologic hyperplasia, 51

Permissive host cell, 59

Postmortem autolysis, 77

Postmortem change, 76

Psammoma body, 70

Pyknosis, 64

Rigor mortis, 76

Segmental vibration, 65

Somatic death, 76

Somatic mutation hypothesis, 74

Vacuolation, 66

Virion (viral particle), 59

Wet gangrene, 72

Whole-body vibration (resonance), 65

REFERENCES

Berens, C., & Crouch, C. L. (Eds.). (1958). Is fluorescent lighting injurious to the eyes? *American Journal of Ophthalmology, 45,* 47.

Binnie, C. D., deKarte, R. A., & Wisman, T. (1979). Flourescent lighting and epilepsy. *Epilepsia, 20,* 725.

Bliznakov, E. G., Wan, Y. P., Chang, D., & Folkers, K. (1978). Partial reaction of impaired immune competence in aged mice by synthetic thymus factors. *Biochemistry/Biophysics Research Communication, 80,* 631-636.

Bohne, B. (1976). Mechanisms of noise damage to the inner ear. In Henderson, D., R. P. Hamerik, D. G. Dosanjh, & J. H. Mills, (Eds.), *Effects of noise on hearing.* New York: Raven Press.

Bomford, A., Walker, R. J., & Williams, R. (1975). Treatment of iron overload, including results in a personal series of 85 patients with idiopathic haemochromatosis. In H. Kief (Ed.), *Iron metabolism and its disorders* (p. 324). New York: American Elsevier.

Brody, J. A., & Brock, D. W. (1985). Epidemiologic and statistical characteristics of the United States elderly population. In C. E. Finch & E. L. Schneider (Eds.), *Handbook of the biology of aging* (2nd ed.). New York: VanNostrand Reinhold.

Bukrinskaya, A. G. (1982). Penetration of viral genetic material into host cell. In M. A. Lauffer, F. B. Bang, K. Mavamorsch, & K. M. Smith (Eds.), *Advances in virus research* (vol. 27). New York: Academic Press.

Chisholm, J. J. (1976). Current status of lead poisoning in children. *Southern Medical Journal, 69,* 529.

Cowger, M. L. (1971). Mechanisms of bilirubin toxicity on tissue culture cells: Factors that affect toxicity reversibility by albumin, and comparison with other respiratory poisons and surfactants. *Biochemical Medicine, 5,* 1-16.

Denckla, W. D. (1981). Aging, dying, and the pituitary. In R. T. Schimke (Ed.). *Biological mechanisms in aging* (NIH Publication No. 81-2 194.). Bethesda, MD: National Institutes on Aging.

Dice J. F., & Goff, S. A. (1987). Molecular determinants of protein half life. *Eucara FASEBJ, Nov 1*(5), 349-357.

Duffner, L. R., Hamilton, L. H., & Schmitz, M. A. (1962). Effects of whole-body vertical vibration on respiration in human subjects. *Journal of Applied Physiology, 17,* 913.

Ernstring, J. (1961). Respiratory effects of whole-body vibration. *I. A. M. report of the Royal Air Force, No. 179.* Farnborough, England: Institute of Aviation Medicine.

Everitt, A. V., & Burgess, J. A. (1976). *Hypothalamus, pituitary, and aging.* Springfield, IL: Charles C Thomas.

Farber, J. L. (1981). Minireview: The role of calcium in cell death. *Life Sciences, 29,* 1289.

Fishbein, A. (1983). Environmental and occupational lead exposure. In W. N. Rom (Ed.), *Environmental and occupational medicine.* Boston: Little, Brown.

Goldberg, A. L., Tischler, M., DeMarhno, G., & Griffin, G. (1980). Hormonal regulation of protein degradation and synthesis in skeletal muscle. *Federation Proceedings, 39,* 31.

Greenberg, L. K., & Yunis, E. J. (1978). Histocompatibility determinants, immune responsiveness, and aging in man. *Federal Proceedings, 37,* 1258.

Harman, D. (1955). Aging: A theory based on free radical and radiation chemistry. *University of California Radiology Lab Report, 3078.*

Harman, D. (1985). Role of free radicals in aging and disease. In H. A. Johnson (Ed.), *Aging: Relations between normal aging and disease* (vol. 28). New York: Raven Press.

Hawkins, J. (1971). The role of vasoconstriction in noise-induced hearing loss. *Transactions of the American Otological Society, 59,* 141.

Hayflick, L. (1965). The limited invitro lifetime of human diploid cell strains. *Experimental Cell Research, 37,* 614.

Hayflick, L. (1980). The biology of human aging. *Advances in Pathobiology, 7,* 80.

Henderson, D., Hamerik, R. P., Dosanjh, D. G., & Mills, J. H. (Eds.). (1976). *Effects of noise on hearing.* New York: Raven Press.

Holbrook, J. (1983). Cigarette smoking. In W. H. Rom (Ed.), *Environmental and occupational medicine.* Boston: Little, Brown.

Hood, W. B., Murray, R. H., Urschel, C. W., Bowers, J. A., & Clark, J. G. (1966). Cardiopulmonary effects of whole-body vibration in man. *Journal of Applied Physiology, 21,* 1725.

Jenkins, J. B. (1983). *Human genetics.* Menlo Park, CA: Benjamin/Cummings.

Johnson, H. A. (Ed.). (1985). Is aging physiological or pathological? In *Relations between normal aging and disease.* New York: Raven Press.

Kanugo, M. S. (1980). *Biochemistry of aging* (pp. 182-192). New York & London: Academic Press.

Kerr, J. F. R., & Searle, J. (1980). Apoptosis: Its nature and kinetic role. In R. E. Meyn & H. R. Withers (Eds.), *Radiation biology in cancer research* (pp. 367-384). New York: Raven Press.

King, D. W., Fenoglio, C. M., & Lefkowich, J. H. (1983). *General pathology principles & dynamics.* Philadelphia: Lea & Febiger.

Kissane, J. M. (Ed.). (1985). *Anderson's pathology* (8th ed.). St. Louis: C. V. Mosby.)

Kohn, R. R. (1985). Aging and age-related diseases: Normal processes. In H. A. Johnson (Ed.), *Relations between normal aging and disease.* New York: Raven Press.

Kurt, T. L. (1983). Chemical asphyxiants. In W. H. Rom (Ed.), *Environmental and occupational medicine.* Boston: Little, Brown.

Leaf, A., (1982). Long-lived populations: Extreme old age. *Journal of the American Geriatric Association, 30,* 485-487.

Leaf, A., & Lannois, J. (1973). Search for the oldest people. *National Geographic, 143,* 93-199.

Levin, M. E., & O'Neal, L. W. (1988). *The diabetic foot* (4th ed.). St. Louis: C. V. Mosby.

Mazess, R. B., & Forman, S. H. (1979). Longevity and age exaggeration in Vilcabamba, Ecuador. *Journal of Gerontology, 34,* 94-98.

McRee, D. I., Elder, J. A., Gage, M. I., Reiter, L. W., Rosenstern, L. S., Shore, M. L., Galloway, W. D., Adey, W. R., & Guy, A. W. (1979). Effects of nonionizing radiation on the central nervous system behavior and blood: A progress report. *Environmental Health Perspective, 30,* 122.

Medvedev, Z. A. (1974). Caucasus and altay longevity: A biological or social problem? *The Gerontologist, 14,* 381-387.

Minckler, J., Anstall, H. B., & Minckler, T. M. (1971). *Pathobiology: An introduction.* St. Louis: C. V. Mosby.

Morgan, H. E., & Neely, J. R. (1982). Metabolic regulation and myocardial function. In J. W. Hurst, R. B. Logue, C. E. Rackley, R. C. Schlant, E. H. Sonnenblick, A. G. Wallace, & N. K. Wenger (Eds.), *The heart arteries and veins* (5th ed.). New York: McGraw-Hill.

Neely, J. R., & Morgan, H. E. (1974). Relationship between carbohydrate and lipid metabolism and energy balance of heart muscle. *Annual Review of Physiology, 36,* 413.

Neer, R. M., Davis, T. R. A., Walcott, A., Koski, S., Schepis, P., Taylor, I., Thonngton, L., & Wurtman, R. J. (1971). Stimulation by artificial lighting of calcium absorption in elderly human subjects. *Nature, 229,* 255.

Olsen, D. M. (1983). Illumination. In W. H. Rom (Ed.), *Environmental and occupational medicine.* Boston: Little, Brown.

Orgel, L. E. (1963). The maintenance of the accuracy of protein synthesis and its relevance to aging. *Proceedings of the National Academy of Sciences, 49,* 517-521.

Orgel, L. E. (1970). The maintenance of the accuracy of protein synthesis and its relevance to aging: A correction. *Proceedings of the National Academy of Sciences, 67,* 1476.

Piomelli, S. (1981). Chemical toxicity of red cells. *Environ Health Perspective, 39,* 65-70.

Powell, L. W., & Kerr, J. F. R. (1975). Pathology of the liver in hemochromatosis. *Pathobiological Annual, 5,* 317.

Pryor, W. A. (1987). The free-radical theory of aging revisited: A critique and a suggested disease-specific theory. In H. R. Warner (Ed.), *Biological theories of aging.* New York: Raven Press.

Robbins, S. L., Cotran, R. S., & Kumar, V. (1984). *Pathologic basis of disease* (3rd ed.). Philadelphia: W. B. Saunders.

Roy, S. B., Gulena, J. S., Khanna, P. K., Manchanda, S. C., Pande, J. N., & Subba, P. S. (1969). Haemodynamic studies in high altitude pulmonary edema. *British Heart Journal, 31,* 52.

Russell, R. L. (1987). Evidence for and against the theory of developmentally programmed aging. In H. R. Warner, R. N. Butler, R. L. Sprott, & E. L. Schneider (Eds.), *Modern biological theories of aging*. New York: Raven Press.

Sandford, N. L., Searle, J. W., & Kerr, J. F. R. (1984). Successive waves of apoptosis in the rat prostate after repeated withdrawal of testostcrone stimulation. *Pathology, 16*(4), 406-410.

Schneider, E. L. (1987). Theories of aging: A perspective. In H. R. Warner, R. N. Butler, R. L. Sprott, & E. L. Schneider (Eds.). *Modern biological theories of aging*. New York: Raven Press.

Searle, J., Kerr, J. F. R., & Bishop, C. (1982). Necrosis and apoptosis: Distinct modes of cell death with fundamentally different significance. *Pathology Annual, 17* (2), 244.

Setlow, R. B. (1987). Theory presentation and background summary. In H. R. Warner, R. N. Butler, R. L. Sprott, & E. L. Schneider (Eds.). *Modern biological theories of aging*. New York: Raven Press.

Shennan, T. (1935). *Postmortems and morbid anatomy* (3rd ed.). Baltimore: William Wood.

Smith, L., & Thier, S. (1981). *Pathophysiology: The biological principles of disease*. Philadelphia: W. B. Saunders.

Thibodeau, G. A. (1987). *Anatomy and physiology*. St. Louis: Times Mirror/Mosby.

Tortora, G. J., Funke, B. R., & Case, C. L. (1982) *Microbiology: An introduction*. Menlo Park, CA: Benjamin Cummings.

Wagner, R. (1984). Cytopathic effects of viruses: A general survey. In H. Fraenkel-Conrat & R. R. Wagner (Eds.), *Comprehensive virology 19*. Chicago: Plenum.

Walford, T. L. (1980). Immunology and aging. *American Journal of Clinical Pathology, 74,* 247.

Warner, H. R., Butler, R. N., Sprott, R. L., & Schneider, E. L. (1987). *Modern biological theories of aging*. New York: Raven Press.

Weston, H. C. (1948). The effects of age and illimination upon visual performance with clore sights. *British Journal of Opthalmology, 32,* 645.

Wrenn, M. E., & Mays, C. W. (1983). Characteristics of ionizing radiation. In W. H. Rom (Ed.) *Environmental and occupational medicine*. Boston: Little, Brown.

Wurtman, R. J. (1975). The effects of light on the human body. *Scientific American, 233,* 68.

Wyllie, A. H., Kerr, J. F. R., & Currie, A. R. (1980). Cell death: The significance of apoptosis. In G. H. Bourne & J. F. Danielli (Eds.), *International Review of Cytology, 68,* 251-306.

CHAPTER 3

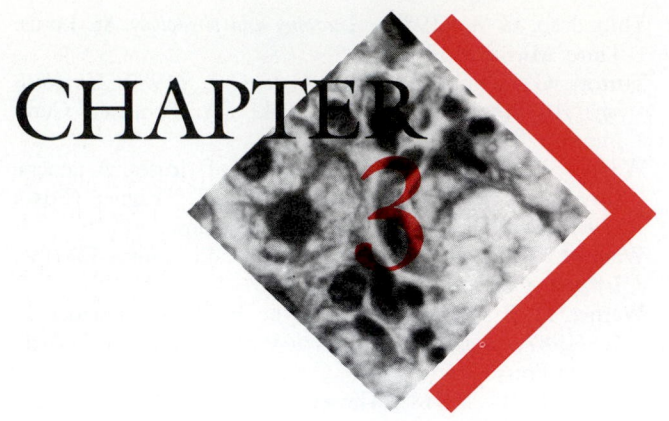

The Cellular Environment: Fluids and Electrolytes, Acids and Bases

Sue E. Huether

Distribution of body fluids, 83
    Water movement between ICF and ECF, 84
    Water movement between plasma and interstitial fluid, 84
Alterations in water movement, 85
    Edema, 85
        Pathophysiology, 85
        Clinical manifestations, 86
        Evaluation and treatment, 87
Sodium, chloride, and water balance, 87
    Water balance, 87
    Sodium and chloride balance, 87
Alterations in sodium, chloride, and water balance, 88
    Isotonic alterations, 89
    Hypertonic alterations, 89
        Hypernatremia, 89
            Pathophysiology, 89
            Clinical manifestations, 89
            Evaluation and treatment, 89
        Water deficit, 90
            Pathophysiology, 90
            Clinical manifestations, 90
            Evaluation and treatment, 90
        Hyperchloremia, 90
    Hypotonic alterations, 91
        Hyponatremia, 91
            Pathophysiology, 91
            Clinical manifestations, 92
            Evaluation and treatment, 92
        Water excess, 92
            Pathophysiology, 92
            Clinical manifestations, 92
            Evaluation and treatment, 92
        Hypochloremia, 92
Alterations in potassium, calcium, phosphate, and magnesium
    balance, 92
    Potassium, 92
    Hypokalemia, 94

        Pathophysiology, 94
        Clinical manifestations, 95
        Evaluation and treatment, 96
    Hyperkalemia, 96
        Pathophysiology, 96
        Clinical manifestations, 97
        Evaluation and treatment, 97
    Calcium and phosphate, 97
    Hypocalcemia, 98
        Pathophysiology, 98
        Clinical manifestations, 99
        Evaluation and treatment, 99
    Hypercalcemia, 99
        Pathophysiology, 99
        Clinical manifestations, 99
        Evaluation and treatment, 99
    Hypophosphatemia, 99
        Pathophysiology, 99
        Clinical manifestations, 99
        Evaluation and treatment, 100
    Hyperphosphatemia, 100
        Pathophysiology, 100
        Clinical manifestations, 100
        Evaluation and treatment, 100
    Magnesium, 100
Acid-base balance, 100
    Hydrogen ion and pH, 100
    Buffer systems, 101
        Carbonic acid–bicarbonate buffering, 102
        Protein buffering, 104
        Renal buffering, 104
        Other buffers, 104
    Acid-base imbalances, 104
        Metabolic acidosis, 105
            Pathophysiology, 105
            Clinical manifestations, 106
            Evaluation and treatment, 107

Metabolic alkalosis, 107
  Pathophysiology, 107
  Clinical manifestation, 107
  Evaluation and treatment, 107
Respiratory acidosis, 108
  Pathophysiology, 108
  Clinical manifestations, 108
  Evaluation and treatment, 109
Respiratory alkalosis, 109
  Pathophysiology, 109
  Clinical manifestations, 110
  Evaluation and treatment, 110

DISTRIBUTION OF BODY FLUIDS

The fluids of the body are distributed among functional compartments, or spaces; and provide a transport medium for cellular and tissue function. The **intracellular fluid (ICF)** comprises all of the fluid contained within cells. The **extracellular fluid (ECF)** is all of the fluid outside the cells and is divided into smaller compartments. The two main ECF compartments are the **interstitial fluid**, or the space between cells and outside the blood vessels (i.e., connective tissue, cartilage, and bone), and the **intravascular fluid**, which is the blood plasma. Other ECF compartments include the lymph and the transcellular fluids such as the synovial, intestinal, cerebrospinal fluid; sweat; urine; and pleural, synovial, peritoneal, pericardial, and intraocular fluids.

The sum of fluids within all compartments comprises the **total body water (TBW)** (Table 3-1). The volume of TBW is usually expressed as a percentage of body weight in kilograms. The standard value for TBW is 60% of a 70 kg adult male, which is equivalent to 42 L of fluid (Table 3-2). The rest of the body weight is made up of fat and fat-free solids, particularly bone.

The distribution of fluid within the body compartments is also represented as a percentage of body weight. Although the amount of fluid within the various compartments is relatively constant, there is exchange of solutes and water between compartments to maintain their unique compositions. Fluid volume is usually measured in liters (L), or milliliters (1 ml = $\frac{1}{1000}$ of a liter). The percent of TBW varies with the amount of body fat and age. Because fat is water repelling (hydrophobic), very little water is contained in adipose cells. Individuals with more body fat will have proportionately less TBW and tend to be more susceptible to fluid imbalances that cause dehydration.

The distribution and amount of TBW change with age (Table 3-2). In newborn infants, TBW is about 75% to 80% of body weight. The percentage of TBW decreases to about 67% of body weight during the first year of life. In the immediate postnatal period there is a physiologic loss of body water amounting to 5% of body weight as the infant adjusts to a new environment. Infants are particularly susceptible to significant changes in TBW, because of their high metabolic rate. The turnover of body fluids in infants is caused by their greater body surface area and by their high metabolic rate. The turnover of body fluid, therefore, is much faster. Loss of fluids from diarrhea can represent a significant proportion of body weight. Renal mechanisms of fluid and electrolyte conservation also may not be mature enough to counter the losses so that dehydration may develop rapidly.

During childhood, TBW slowly falls to 60% to 65% of body weight. At adolescence, the percentage of TBW approaches adult proportions, and sex differences begin to appear. Males eventually have a greater percentage of body water as a function of increasing muscle mass. Females have more body fat and less muscle as a function of estrogens and therefore have less water.

In the elderly, there is a further decline in the percentage of TBW. The decrease is due in part to an increased amount of fat and a decreased amount of muscle and to a reduced ability to regulate sodium and water balance. With age, the kidney becomes less efficient in producing concentrated urine, and the responses for conserving so-

TABLE 3-1 Distribution of body water

	Percentage of body water	Volume (L)
Intracellular fluid (ICF)	40	28
Extracellular fluid (ECF)	20	15
Interstitial	(15)	(12)
Intravascular	(5)	(3)
Total body water (TBW)	60	42

TABLE 3-2 Total body water in relation to body weight

Body build	TBW Adult male (%)	TBW Adult female (%)	TBW Infant (%)
Normal	60	50	70
Lean	70	60	80
Obese	50	42	60

NOTE: TBW is a percentage of body weight.

TABLE 3-3 Normal water gains and losses (70-kg man)

	Daily intake (ml)		Daily output (ml)
Drinking	1400-1800	Urine	1400-1800
Water in food	700-1000	Stool	100
Water of oxidation	300-400	Skin	300-500
		Lungs	600-800
TOTAL	2400-3200		2400-3200

dium become sluggish. The normal reduction of TBW in the elderly becomes clinically important with stress, such as fever or dehydration from any cause; loss of body fluids at such times can be severe and life-threatening.

Although daily fluid intake may fluctuate widely, the body regulates water volume within a relatively narrow range. The primary sources of body water are drinking, ingestion of water in food, and water derived from oxidative metabolism. Normally, the largest amounts of water are lost through renal excretion. Lesser amounts are eliminated through the stool and through vaporization from the skin and lungs (this is insensible water loss) (Table 3-3).

Water Movement between ICF and ECF

The movement of water between ICF and ECF compartments is primarily a function of osmotic forces (osmosis and other mechanisms of passive transport are discussed in Chapter 1). Water moves freely across cell membranes, so that the osmolality of TBW is normally at equilibrium. Sodium is the most abundant ECF ion and is responsible for the osmotic balance of the ECF space. Potassium maintains the osmotic balance of the ICF space. The osmotic force of ICF proteins and other nondiffusable substances is balanced by the active transport of ions out of the cell. Normally, the ICF is not subject to rapid changes in osmolality; but when there are changes in ECF osmolality, a net transfer of water from one compartment to another occurs until osmotic equilibrium is reestablished. A model of the maintenance of osmotic equilibrium is illustrated in Fig. 3-1.

Water Movement between Plasma and Interstitial Fluid

The distribution of water and the movement of nutrients and waste products among the capillary, plasma and the interstitial spaces occurs as a result of changes in hydrostatic pressure and osmotic forces at the arterial and venous ends of the capillary. Because water, sodium, and glucose readily move across the capillary membrane, the plasma proteins maintain the effective osmolality by generating plasma oncotic pressure. Osmotic forces within the capillary are balanced by the hydrostatic pressure, which arises from cardiac contrac-

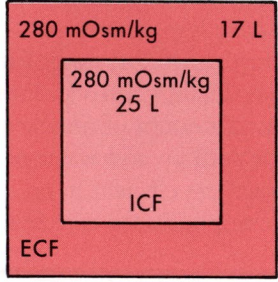

A Normal osmotic equilibrium

280 mOsm/kg   17 L
280 mOsm/kg 25 L
ICF
ECF

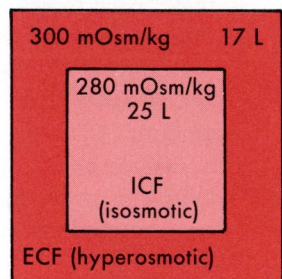

B Addition of solute to ECF osmotic disequilibrium

300 mOsm/kg   17 L
280 mOsm/kg 25 L
ICF (isosmotic)
ECF (hyperosmotic)

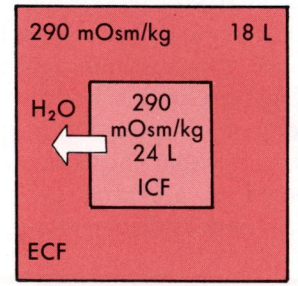

C Reestablishment of osmotic equilibrium

290 mOsm/kg   18 L
H_2O 290 mOsm/kg 24 L
ICF
ECF

Water moves from ICF to ECF according to osmotic gradient. Osmotic equilibrium reestablished with smaller ICF compartment

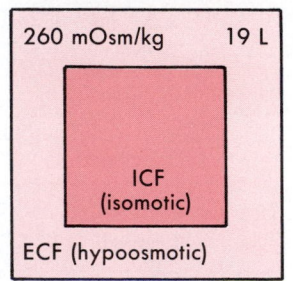

D Addition of free water to ECF osmotic disequilibrium

260 mOsm/kg   19 L
ICF (isosmotic)
ECF (hypoosmotic)

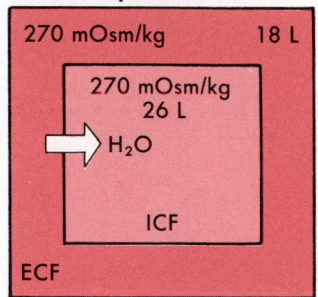

E Reestablishment of osmotic equilibrium

270 mOsm/kg   18 L
270 mOsm/kg 26 L
H_2O
ICF
ECF

Water moves from ECF to ICF according to osmotic gradient. Osmotic equilibrium reestablished with larger ICF and ECF compartments.

FIG. 3-1. Model of osmotic equilibrium.

tion. The movement of fluid back and forth across the capillary wall is called **net filtration** and is best described by **Starling's hypothesis**:

Net filtration = (force favoring filtration) − (forces opposing filtration)

The forces favoring filtration, or movement of water out of the capillary and into the interstitial space, include the capillary hydrostatic pressure and the interstitial oncotic pressure. The forces opposing filtration are the plasma oncotic pressure and the interstitial hydrostatic pressure. Normally, the interstitial forces are negligible, since only a very small percentage of plasma proteins cross the capillary membrane, and interstitial fluid moves into cells or is drawn back into the plasma. Thus the major forces for filtration are within the capillary.

As the plasma flows from the arterial to the venous end of the capillary, changes in the force of hydrostatic pressure facilitate the movement of water across the capillary membrane. Oncotic pressure remains fairly constant because plasma proteins normally do not cross the capillary membrane. At the arterial end of the capillary, hydrostatic pressure is greater than capillary oncotic pressure and water filters into the interstitial space. Because of oncotic forces, there is some movement of water back into the capillary, but the net effect is loss of water from the capillary. The movement of water from the plasma causes the hydrostatic pressure within the capillary to decrease. Thus, at the venous end of the capillary, oncotic pressure exceeds hydrostatic pressure. Fluids are then attracted back into the circulation, balancing the movement of fluids between the plasma and the interstitial space. The overall effect is filtration at the arterial end and reabsorption at the venous end (Fig. 3-2).

An important factor in capillary filtration of fluid is the integrity of the capillary membrane. Changes in membrane permeability may permit the escape of plasma proteins into the interstitial space. The normal relationship defined by Starling's hypothesis is altered with the osmotic movement of water into the interstitial space, causing tissue edema.

ALTERATIONS IN WATER MOVEMENT

Edema

Edema is the accumulation of fluid within the interstitial spaces. It is a problem of fluid distribution and does not necessarily indicate a fluid excess. In some conditions, sequestered fluids can cause both edema and dehydration. The pathophysiologic process is related to an increase in the forces favoring fluid filtration from the capillaries or lymphatic channels into the tissues. The most common mechanisms include increased hydrostatic pressure, decreased plasma oncotic pressure, increased capillary membrane permeability, and lymphatic obstruction (Fig. 3-3).

Pathophysiology

An increase in hydrostatic pressure can result from venous obstruction or salt and water retention. Venous obstruction can cause the hydrostatic pressure of fluid within the capillaries to become great enough to cause fluid to escape into the interstitial spaces. Thrombophlebitis, hepatic obstruction, tight clothing around the extremities, and prolonged standing are common causes of venous obstruction. Congestive heart failure and renal failure are both conditions associated with salt and water retention, which in turn cause volume overload and edema. Additionally, renal failure may be associated with loss of plasma proteins that contributes to the edema of nephrosis.

Losses or diminished production of plasma albumin contributes to a decrease in plasma oncotic pressure. Decreased oncotic attraction of fluid within the capillary causes fluid to move into the interstitial space. Decreased production of plasma protein may occur with liver disease or protein malnutriton. The escape of

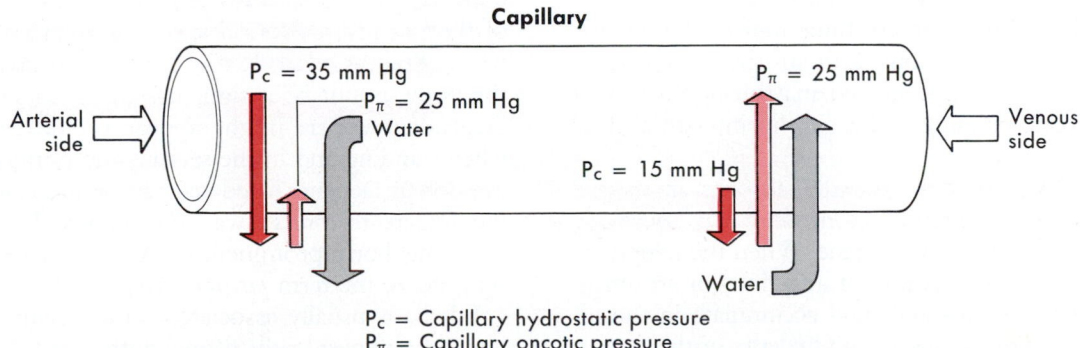

FIG. 3-2. Capillary net filtration forces. P_c, capillary hydrostatic pressure. P_π, capillary oncotic pressure.

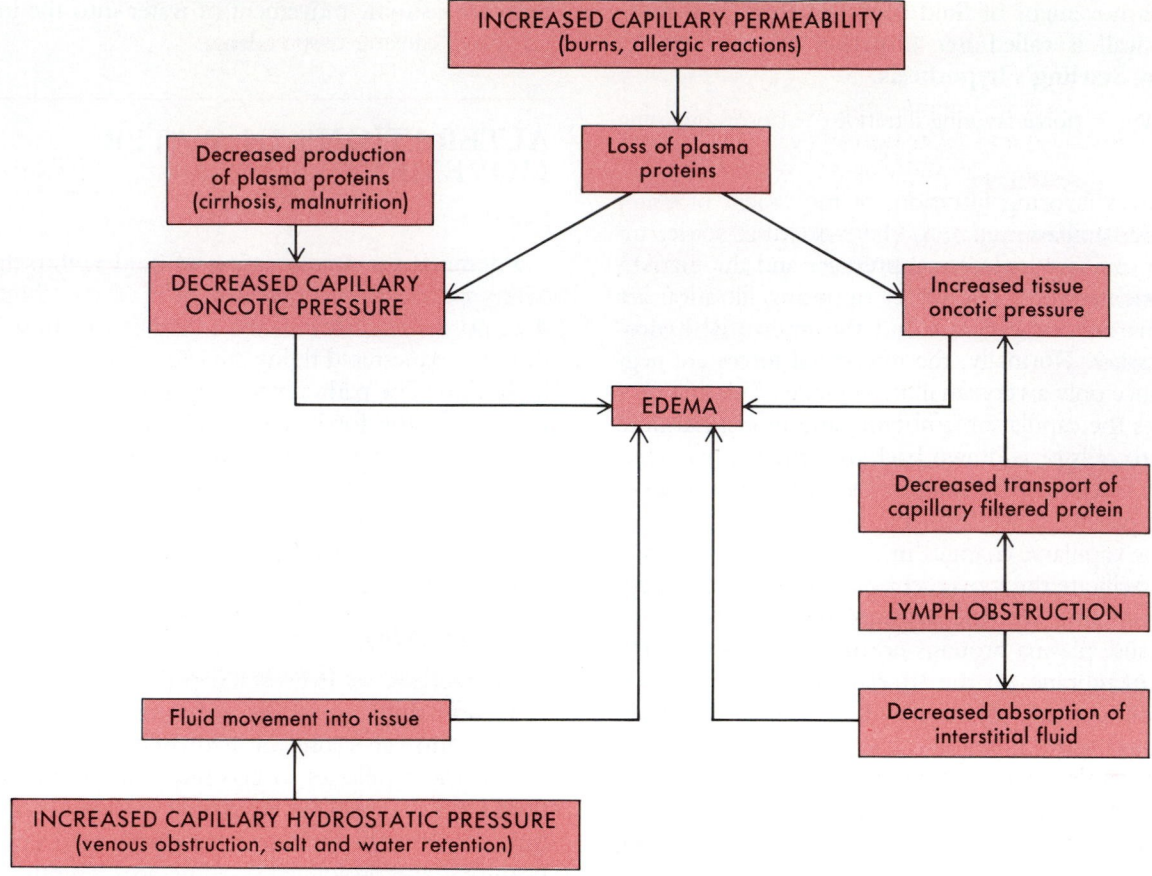

FIG. 3-3. Mechanisms of edema formation.

plasma proteins from the serum into the interstitial space also enhances the movement of water from the plasma into the tissues. Losses of plasma proteins occur with glomerular diseases of the kidney, serous drainage from open wounds, hemorrhage, burns, and cirrhosis of the liver.

Increases in capillary permeability are usually associated with inflammation and the immune response. (Immunity is discussed in Chapter 6; Inflammation is discussed in Chapter 7.) These responses are often due to trauma such as burns or crushing injuries, neoplastic disease, and allergic reactions. Proteins then escape from the vascular bed and produce edema through a loss of capillary oncotic pressure and a gain in interstitial fluid proteins.

The lymphatic system normally absorbs interstitial fluid and the small amount of proteins that normally pass across the capillary membrane. When the lymphatic channels are blocked (because of infection) or are surgically removed, proteins and fluid accumulate in the interstitial space. For example, lymphedema of the arm or leg will occur after surgical removal of axillary and femoral lymph nodes for treatment of carcinoma. Inflamma-

tion or tumors may be a cause of lymphatic obstruction leading to edema.

Clinical Manifestations

Edema may be localized or generalized. Some localized edema is limited to the site of trauma, as in a sprained finger. Another kind of localized edema is the accumulation of fluid within particular organ systems. This includes cerebral edema, pulmonary edema, pleural effusion, pericardial effusion, and ascites (accumulation of fluid in the peritoneal space). Dependent edema, in which fluid acculumates in gravity-dependent areas of the body, might be a sign of more generalized edema. Dependent edema might appear in the feet and legs when standing and in the sacrum and buttocks when lying down. Dependent edema can be identified by using the fingers to press away edematous fluid in tissues overlying bony prominences. A pit will be left in the skin; hence the term *pitting edema.*

Edema is usually associated with weight gain, swelling and puffiness, tight-fitting clothes and shoes, limited movement of the affected area, and symptoms associated with the underlying pathologic condition. The accumulation of fluid increases the distance required for nutrients and waste to move between capillaries and tissues. Increased tissue pressure may diminish capillary blood flow. Therefore wounds heal more slowly, and the risks of infection and formation of pressure sores increase. Edema of specific organs, such as the brain, lung, or larynx, can be life threatening.

Although the accumulation of fluid is excessive, it is trapped in a "third space" and is not available for metabolic processes. A state of dehydration can therefore develop as a result of the sequestering of the edematous fluid. An example of such sequestration occurs with severe burns, in which large amounts of vascular fluid are lost to the interstitial spaces, reducing plasma volume and causing shock (see Chapter 11).

Evaluation and Treatment

Specific conditions causing edema require diagnosis. Edema may be treated symptomatically until the underlying disorder is corrected. Correction measures include elevating edematous limbs, using support stockings, avoiding prolonged standing, restricting salt intake, or taking diuretics.

SODIUM, CHLORIDE, AND WATER BALANCE

Because water follows the osmotic gradients established by changes in salt concentration, sodium and water balance are intimately related. Water balance is primarily regulated by antidiuretic hormone (ADH, also known as vasopressin); sodium is regulated by aldosterone.

Water Balance

Secretion of ADH and perception of thirst are primary factors in the regulation of water balance. Thirst is a sensation that stimulates water-drinking behavior. Thirst is experienced when water loss equals 2% of an individual's body weight or when there is an increase in osmolality. Dry mouth, hyperosmolality, and plasma volume depletion activate osmoreceptors (neurons located in the hypothalamus that are stimulated by increased osmolality). The action of the osmoreceptors then causes thirst. Drinking water dilutes the ECF osmolality and restores plasma volume.

The secretion of ADH is initiated by an increase in plasma osmolality or a decrease in circulating blood volume and a lowered blood pressure. An increase in plasma osmolality occurs with a deficit of water or an excess of sodium in relation to water. The increased osmolality results in decreased extracellular and interstitial fluid volume and stimulates hypothalamic osmoreceptors. In addition to causing thirst, the stimulated os-

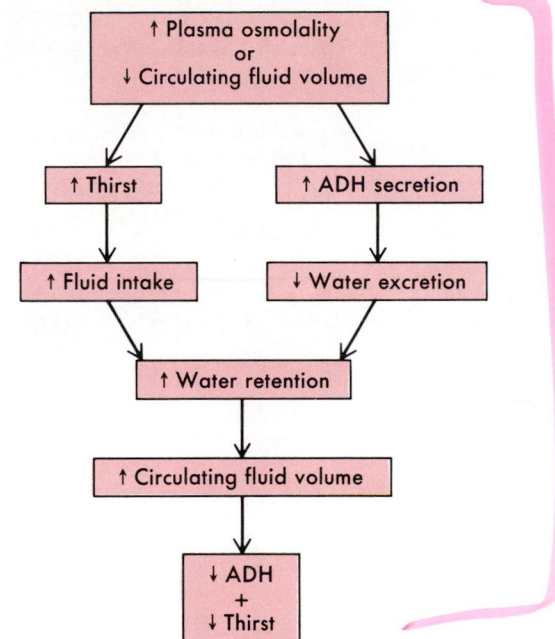

FIG. 3-4. Regulation of thirst and ADH secretion.

moreceptors increase the release of ADH from the posterior pituitary gland. The action of ADH is to increase the permeability of renal tubular cells to water, and water is reabsorbed into the plasma from the distal tubules and collecting ducts of the kidney. Urine concentration increases, and the reabsorbed water decreases plasma osmolality, returning it toward normal. Like most hormones, ADH is regulated by a feedback mechanism as illustrated in Fig. 3-4.

With volume depletion, such as dehydration from vomiting, diarrhea, or excessive sweating, volume-sensitive receptors and baroreceptors (nerve endings that are sensitive to changes in volume and pressure) stimulate release of ADH from the pituitary gland. The volume receptors are located in the right and left atrium and thoracic vessels; baroreceptors are in the aorta and pulmonary arteries, and carotid sinus. Secretion of ADH is also caused by a decrease in atrial pressure, as occurs with decreased blood volume. The reabsorption of water mediated by ADH then promotes the restoration of plasma volume.

Sodium and Chloride Balance

Sodium accounts for 90% of the ECF cations (positively charged ions) and is the most powerful cation in the ECF (the distribution of electrolytes in body compartments is summarized in Table 3-4). As the most abundant ECF cation, along with its constituent anions (negatively charged ions) chloride and bicarbonate, sodium regulates osmotic forces and therefore regulates water balance. Sodium has many important body func-

TABLE 3-4 Distribution of electrolytes in body compartments

	Extracellular fluid (mEq/L)	Intracellular fluid (mEq/L)
Cations		
Sodium	142	10
Potassium	5	156
Calcium	5	4
Magnesium	2	26
TOTALS	154	196
Anions		
Bicarbonate	24	12
Chloride	104	4
Phosphate	2	40-95
Proteins	16	54
Other Anions	8	31-86
TOTALS	154	196

tions including regulation of osmolality (interstitial and intravascular fluid volume), working with potassium and calcium to maintain neuromuscular irritability for conduction of nerve impulses, regulation of acid-base balance (through sodium bicarbonate and sodium phosphate), and participation in cellular chemical reactions.

Chloride is the major anion in the extracellular fluid. It provides electroneutrality, particularly in relation to sodium. The transport of chloride is generally passive and follows the active transport of sodium, so that increases or decreases in chloride are proportional to changes in sodium. Because bicarbonate is the other major anion in the ECF, the concentration of chloride tends to vary inversely with changes in bicarbonate concentration.

The concentration of sodium is maintained within a narrow range (136 to 145 mEq/L) primarily by the kidney in conjunction with neural and hormonal mediators. The average dietary intake of sodium ranges from 5 to 6 g/day; the minimal daily requirement of sodium is 500 mg, although sweating depletes sodium and water volume and increases the body's sodium requirement.

The kidney regulates sodium primarily through renal tubular reabsorption. Under normal rates of sodium intake, the tubules of the kidney function to reabsorb sodium. With an excess or deficit of sodium in relation to water, a combination of hormonal, neural, and renal mechanisms act synergistically to control sodium balance.

The hormonal regulation of sodium balance is mediated by **aldosterone**, a mineralocorticoid synthesized and secreted from the adrenal cortex (see Chapter 17). The secretion of aldosterone is influenced by both circu-

lating blood volume and plasma concentrations of Na^+ and K^+ (i.e., aldosterone is secreted when sodium levels are depressed or potassium levels are increased). The action of aldosterone is to increase the reabsorption of sodium and secretion of potassium by the distal tubule of the kidney. As a result, sodium concentration of the ECF is enhanced, and potassium is excreted with the urine.

When circulating blood volume is reduced, **renin**, an enzyme secreted by the juxtaglomerular cells of the kidney, is released in response to sympathetic nerve stimulation and decreased perfusion of the renal vasculature. Renin stimulates the formation of **angiotensin I**, an inactive polypeptide, which is then converted into **angiotensin II**, which acts as a hormone. Angiotensin II has two major functions. It stimulates the secretion of aldosterone, and it causes vasoconstriction. The aldosterone then promotes sodium and water reabsorption. The vasoconstriction elevates the systemic blood pressure and restores renal perfusion. The restoration of sodium levels, fluid volume, and renal perfusion then inhibits the further release of renin. This mechanism of sodium and water regulation is known as the **renin-angiotensin system** (see Chapter 32).

In addition to sodium regulation by aldosterone, a **natriuretic hormone** (a hormone that promotes urinary excretion of sodium) decreases tubular reabsorption of sodium and causes loss of salt and water. Atrial natriuretic factor is a hormone produced by the atrial muscle of the heart, and one of its functions is renal elimination of sodium for control of sodium and water balance (de Bold, 1982). Natriuretic hormone is sometimes called the "third factor" in sodium regulation. (Increased glomerular filtration rate is thus the "first factor" and aldosterone the "second factor.") The effect of a "third factor" is apparent when there is prolonged elevation of aldosterone from chronic retention of fluid or excessive secretion from an adrenal tumor. In such cases the sodium-retaining action of aldosterone is overcome, and salt is excreted followed by a water diuresis.

ALTERATIONS IN SODIUM, CHLORIDE, AND WATER BALANCE

Alterations in sodium and water balance are closely related. Water imbalances may develop because of changes in osmotic gradients caused by gain or loss of salt. Likewise, sodium imbalances occur with alterations in body water volume. Generally, the alterations can be classified as changes in tonicity, the change in concentration of particles in relation to water (see Chapter 1). Alterations can therefore be classified as isotonic, hypertonic, or hypotonic (Table 3-5).

TABLE 3-5 Water and solute imbalances	
Tonicity	**Mechanism**
Isotonic (isosmolar) imbalance	The gain or loss of ECF resulting in a concentration equivalent to a 0.9% sodium chloride (salt) solution (normal saline). There is no shrinking or swelling of cells.
Hypertonic (hyperosmolar) imbalance	Imbalances that result in an ECF concentration greater than 0.9% salt solution, i.e., water loss or solute gain. Cells shrink in a hypertonic fluid.
Hypotonic (hypoosmolar) imbalance	Imbalance that results in an ECF less than 0.9% salt solution, i.e., water gain or solute loss. Cells swell in a hypotonic fluid.

Isotonic Alterations

Isotonic alterations occur when changes in TBW are accompanied by proportional changes in electrolytes. For example, if an individual loses pure plasma or ECF, fluid volume is depleted, but the number and type of electrolytes and the osmolality remains in a normal range. Excessive amounts of isotonic body fluids can result from excessive administration of intravenous normal saline or oversecretion of aldosterone with renal retention of both sodium and water. Losses of isotonic body fluids include hemorrhage, severe wound drainage, and excessive diaphoresis.

Isotonic volume depletion (isotonic dehydration) causes contraction of the ECF volume with weight loss, dryness of skin and mucous membranes, decresed urine output, and symptoms of hypovolemia. Indicators of hypovolemia include a rapid heart rate, flattened neck veins, and normal or decreased blood pressure. In severe states, hypovolemic shock can occur (see Chapter 27).

Isotonic volume excesses are most commonly due to excessive administration of intravenous fluids, hypersecretion of aldosterone, or the effects of drugs such as cortisone. As the plasma volume expands, symptoms of hypervolemia develop. There will be a decrease in hematocrit and plasma proteins caused by the diluting effect of excess plasma volume. The neck veins may distend, and the blood pressure increases. Increased capillary hydrostatic pressure will lead to edema formation. If the plasma volume is great enough, pulmonary edema and heart failure develop.

Hypertonic Alterations

Hypertonic fluid alterations develop when the osmolality of the ECF is elevated above normal. The most common causes are an increased concentration of ECF sodium (hypernatremia) or a deficit of ECF water. In both instances, the hypertonicity of the ECF attracts water from the intracellular space, causing ICF dehydration. A primary increase in ECF sodium causes an osmotic attraction of water and symptoms of hypervolemia. In contrast, a hypertonic state caused primarily by water loss leads to hypovolemia (Table 3-6).

Hypernatremia

Pathophysiology

Hypernatremia occurs when serum sodium levels exceed 147 mEq/L. Excessive serum sodium may be due to an acute gain in sodium or a loss of water. Sodium gains cause intracellular dehydration; the movement of water to the ECF may cause hypervolemia. With an accompanying water loss, both ICF and ECF dehydration will occur. Hyperosmolality is a common result of hypernatremia.

High amounts of dietary sodium rarely cause hypernatremia. More commonly, high sodium levels occur with inappropriate administration of hypertonic saline solution (e.g., as sodium bicarbonate for treatment of acidosis during cardiac arrest), or sodium levels are high because of over secretion of aldosterone, as in primary hyperaldosteronism, or Cushing syndrome caused by excess secretion of ACTH, which also causes increased secretion of aldosterone.

Increased sodium in relation to water loss is associated with fever or respiratory infections, which increase the respiratory rate and enhance water loss from the lungs. Diabetes insipidus, diabetes mellitus, polyuria, profuse sweating, and also diarrhea cause water loss in relation to sodium. Infants with severe diarrhea are particularly vulnerable. Insufficient water intake can also cause hypernatremia, particulary in individuals who are comatose, confused, or immobilized.

Clinical Manifestations

Water is redistributed to the extracellular space, and intracellular dehydration ensues. Convulsions and pulmonary edema are the most serious symptoms. Thirst, fever, dry mucous menbranes, and restlessness are associated with hypernatremia as a result of water loss. Isotonic increases in both sodium and water cause expansion of ECF volume with weight gain, edema, and hypervolemia.

Evaluation and Treatment

The serum sodium level is usually above 147 mEq/L. If there is water loss, urine specific gravity will be greater than 1.030, and hematocrit and plasma proteins

TABLE 3-6 Causes and consequences of hypertonic imbalances

Cause	Elevated sodium (hypernatremia)	Water deficit	Other factors
Contributing factors	**Excessive administration of hypertonic salt solutions** Intravenous hypertonic sodium Saline-induced abortions Selected infant formulas Near saltwater drownings **Hyperaldosteronism**	**Water deprivation** Confusion or coma Inability to communicate Loss of thirst **Water loss** Watery diarrhea Diabetes insipidus Excessive diuresis Excessive diaphoresis	Hyperglycemia
ECF effects	**Hypervolemia** Weight gain Bounding pulse Increased blood pressure Edema Venous distention **Neuromuscular symptoms** Muscle weakness Seizures	**Hypovolemia** Weight loss Weak pulses Postural hypotension Tachycardia	Initial dilutional hyponatremia Poluria Polydipsia Weight loss Hypovolemia Late hypernatremia

ICF effects	**Intracellular dehydration**	**Intracellular dehydration**
		Thirst
		Fever
		Decreased urine output
		Shrinkage of brain cells:
		  Confusion
		  Coma
		  Cerebral hemorrhage
			Intracellular dehydration

will be elevated. The treatment of hypernatremia is to give an isotonic salt-free fluid (i.e., 5% dextrose in water) until the serum sodium level returns to normal. Hypervolemia and edema require treatment of the underlying clinical condition.

Water Deficit

Pathophysiology

Dehydration is an appropriate term to describe water deficit, but dehydration is also commonly used to indicate both sodium and water loss (isotonic or isoosmolar dehydration). Pure **water deficits** (hyperosmolar or hypertonic dehydration) are rare because most people have access to water. Individuals who are comatose or paralyzed will continue insensible water losses through the skin and lungs with a minimal obligatory formation of urine. Hyperventilation caused by fever may also precipitate water deficit. The most frequent cause of water loss is increased renal clearance of free water as a result of impaired tubular function or inability to concentrate the urine, as with diabetes insipidus (see Chapter 18).

Clinical Manifestations

Marked water deficit is manifested by symptoms of **dehydration**—thirst, dry skin and mucous membranes, elevated temperature, weight loss, and concentrated urine (with the exception of diabetes insipidus). Skin turgor may be normal or decreased. Symptoms of hypovolemia, including tachycardia, weak pulses, and postural hypotension, may be present.

Evaluation and Treatment

An elevated hematocrit and serum sodium concentration are associated with moderate water loss in addition to clinical signs and symptoms.

Treatment is to give water. When intravenous replacement is required, 5% dextrose in water should be used because pure water lyses red blood cells.

Hyperchloremia

Hyperchloremia occurs clinically when there is an excess of sodium or a deficit of bicarbonate. Greater than normal amounts of chloride can be expected with hypernatremia or metabolic acidosis (see p. 105). Inges-

TABLE 3-7 Causes and concequences of hypotonic imbalances

Cause	Decreased sodium (hyponatremia)	Water excess	Other factors
Contributing factors	Inadequate intake, hypoaldosteronism, excessive diuretic therapy Furosemide Ethacrinic acid Thiazides	Excessive pure water intake Excessive administration of hypotonic intravenous solutions Drinking water to replace isotonic fluid losses Tap water enemas Psychogenic polydipsia Renal water retention Syndrome of inappropriate antidiuretic hormone (SIADH)	Isotonic dehydration treated with intravenous D5W. (Glucose in the D5W solution is metabolized, contributing to hyponatremia.)
ECF effects	Hypovolemia (May not be present if there is water excess.)	Hypervolemia (May not be present if fluid trapped in intracellular space.)	
ICF effects	Edema	Edema Brain cell swelling: irritability, depression, confusion Seizures Coma Systemic cellular edema: weakness, anorexia, nausea, diarrhea	Edema

tion of excessive chloride infrequently accompanies the use of an ammonium chloride diuretic. There are no specific symptoms associated with chloride deficit.

Alterations in chloride levels are usually secondary to other pathophysiologic processes. Treatment is therefore usually related to management of the underlying disorder.

Hypotonic Alterations

Hypotonic fluid imbalances occur when the osmolality of the ECF is less than normal. The most common causes are sodium deficit (**hyponatremia**) or water excess. Either of these causes leads to an intracellular overrhydration (edema). When there is a sodium deficit, the osmotic pressure of the ECF decreases, and water moves into the cell, where the osmotic pressure is greater. The plasma volume then decreases, leading to symptoms of hypovolemia. With a water excess, both the ICF and ECF volume increase causing symptoms of hypovolemia (Table 3-7).

Hyponatremia
Pathophysiology

Hyponatremia develops when the serum sodium concentration falls below 135 mEq/L. Sodium deficits usually cause hypoosmolality with movement of water into cells. Several clinical syndromes may cause hyponatremia. These may be caused by sodium loss, inadequate sodium intake, or dilution of the body's sodium level.

Pure sodium deficits are usually caused by extrarenal losses such as vomiting, diarrhea, gastrointestinal suctioning, or burns. **Inadequate intake** of dietary sodium is rare but can occur in individuals on low-sodium diets, particularly among those taking diuretics. **Dilutional hyponatremias** occur when there is an excess of TBW in relation to total body sodium. Replacement of fluid loss with intravenous 5% dextrose in water can also cause a dilutional hyponatremia once the glucose is metabolized, leaving a hypotonic solution with a diluting effect. Excessive sweating may also stimulate thirst and intake of large amounts of water, which dilute sodium. Hyponatremia may also be hypoosmolar or hypertonic. During acute oliguric renal faliure, severe congestive heart failure, or cirrhosis, renal excretion of water is impaired. Both TBW and sodium levels are increased, but TBW exceeds the increase in sodium, producing a hypoosmolar hyponatremia. **Hypertonic hyponatremia** develops with hyperlipidemia, hyperproteinemia, and hyperglycemia. Increases in plasma lipids and proteins displace water volume and decrease sodium concentration. Hyperglycemia increases ECF osmolality and attracts water from the ICF compartment. The osmotic fluid shift to the ECF in turn dilutes the concentration of sodium and other electrolytes.

Clinical Manifestations

Deficits of sodium alter the ability of cells to depolarize and repolarize normally (see Chapter 1). Behavioral and neurologic changes characteristic of hyponatremia include lethargy, confusion, apprehension, seizures, and coma. Pure sodium losses may be accompanied by loss of ECF causing an isotonic **hypovolemia** with symptoms of hypotension, tachycardia, and decreased urine output. Weight gain, edema, ascites, and jugular vein distention are characteristic of dilutional hyponatremias.

Evaluation and Treatment

In hyponatremic states, serum sodium concentration falls below 135 mEq/L. With pure sodium deficits, the hematocrit and plasma protein levels may be elevated. Urine specific gravity is less than 1.010 when renal function is normal because sodium is maximally conserved.

Treatment of hyponatremia is related to the contributing disorder. Losses of sodium and water volume are calculated from the clinical evaluation, and appropriate solutions are then selected for replacement. Restriction of water intake is required in most cases of dilutional hyponatremia because body sodium levels may be normal or increased even though serum levels are low. Hypertonic saline solutions are used cautiously with such severe symptoms as seizures.

Water Excess

Pathophysiology

When the body is functioning normally, it is almost impossible to produce an excess of TBW. Some individuals with psychogenic disorders develop water intoxication from **compulsive water drinking**. Acute renal failure, severe congestive heart failure, and cirrhosis are clinical conditions that can precipitate water excess during intravenous infusion of 5% dextrose in water. **Decreased urine formation** from intrinsic renal disease or decreased renal blood flow contributes to water excess. The overall effect is dilution of the ECF with the movement of water to the intracellular space by osmosis. Water excess produces a hypotonic or hypoosmolar water imbalance.

The **syndrome of inappropriate secretion of ADH (SIADH)** is another circumstance contributing to excess water. The syndrome occurs when factors other than hyperosmolality or hypovolemia stimulate the secretion of ADH. Several clinical conditions associated with stress result in SIADH. These include fear, pain, acute infection, brain trauma, surgery, and drugs such as analgesics and anesthetics. The most common cause is bronchogenic cancer. SIADH is due not to excess water intake but to decreased renal excretion of water. Therefore the presence of SIADH increases the risk of water ex-

cess if intravenous fluids are being administered. Serum sodium and osmolality are reduced. The kidney continues to excrete sodium, and urine specific gravity is elevated, but urine volume is decreased.

Clinical Manifestations

The symptoms of water excess are related to the rate at which water loading has occurred. Acute excesses cause confusion and convulsions. Weakness, nausea, muscle twitching, headache, and weight gain are common symptoms of chronic water accumulation.

Evaluation and Treatment

Serum sodium concentration can be decreased, but this can also occur with a pure sodium deficit. Serum osmolality is decreased as water will be in excess of sodium. The hematocrit is therefore reduced from the dilutional effect of water excess.

Withholding fluid for 24 hours is effective treatment if there are no convulsions. Small amounts of intravenous hypertonic sodium chloride can be given when symptoms are severe.

Hypochloremia

Loss of chloride, **hypochloremia**, is usually the result of hyponatremia or elevated bicarbonate concentration, as in metabolic alkalosis (see p. 107). Hypochloremia develops with vomiting and loss of hydrochloric acid. Sodium deficit related to restricted intake or use of diuretics is accompanied by chloride deficiency. Cystic fibrosis, for example, is also characterized by hypochloremia. As with hyperchloremia, treatment of the underlying condition is required.

ALTERATIONS IN POTASSIUM, CALCIUM, PHOSPHATE, AND MAGNESIUM BALANCE

Potassium

Potassium is the major intracellular electrolyte and contributes to many important cellular functions. Total body potassium content is about 4000 mEq, with most of it located in the cells. Daily dietary intake of potassium is 40 to 150 mEq/day with an average of 1.5 mEq/kg body weight. The ICF concentration of K^+ is 150 to 160 mEq/L; the ECF concentration is 3.5 to 4.5 mEq/L.

The difference in the concentration is maintained by a sodium-potassium active transport system ($Na^+ \cdot K^+$ ATPase pump). The ratio of ECF K^+ to ICF K^+ is the major determinant of the resting membrane potential, which is necessary for the transmission of nerve impulses. (Membrane transport and membrane potentials

TABLE 3-8   Concentration of electrolytes in body fluids

Fluid	Na$^+$ (mEq/L)	K$^+$ (mEq/L)	Cl$^-$ (mEq/L)	HCO$_3^-$ (mEq/L)
Saliva	33	20	34	0
Gastric juice*	60	9	84	0
Bile	149	5	101	45
Pancreatic juice	141	5	77	92
Ileal fluid	129	11	116	29
Cecal fluid	80	21	48	22
Cerebrospinal fluid	141	3	127	23
Sweat	45	5	58	0

From Smith, L.H., & Thier, S.O. (1981). *Pathophysiology: The biological principles of disease.* Philadelphia: W.B. Saunders. Adapted from Arieff, A. In Maxwell, M.H., & Kleeman, C.R. (Eds.). (1972). Clinical disorders of fluid and electrolyte metabolism (2nd ed.). New York: McGraw-Hill.
*The Cl concentration exceeds the Na$^+$, K$^+$ concentration by 15 mEq/L in gastric juice. This largely represents the secretion of H$^+$ by the parietal cells.

are discussed in Chapter 1.) Changes in the ratio of ICF to ECF potassium are responsible for many of the symptoms associated with potassium imbalance.

Potassium is necessary for a variety of metabolic functions. As the predominant ICF ion, it exerts a major influence in the regulation of ICF osmolality and provides the balance for intracellular electrical neutrality in relation to H$^+$ and Na$^+$. Potassium is required for glycogen deposition in liver and skeletal muscle cells. The significant role of potassium in maintaining the resting membrane potential is reflected in transmission and conduction of nerve impulses, maintenance of normal cardiac rhythms, and skeletal and smooth muscle contraction.

Generally, the amount of K$^+$ excreted varies in proportion to the dietary intake (40 to 120 mEq/day). Although potassium is found in most body fluids (Table 3-8), the kidney provides the most efficient regulation of potassium balance. Potassium is freely filtered by the renal glomerulus, and 90% is reabsorbed by the proximal tubule and loop of Henle. The distal tubule secretes potassium and determines the amount of K$^+$ excreted from the body. The transport is passive, so that principles of passive transport govern K$^+$ excretion. Unlike sodium, however, the renal mechanism for conserving K$^+$ is weak, even when total body potassium stores are depleted.

Several factors related to passive transport and aldos-

terone contribute to renal regulation of potassium. These factors include the concentration gradients for potassium at the distal tubule and collecting duct, changes in pH (causing acidosis or alkalosis), changes in electrical potential differences across the distal tubule, and aldosterone levels. (Renal mechanisms are described in more detail in Chapter 32.)

The concentration of potassium in the distal tubular cell is primarily determined by the plasma concentration in the peritubular capillaries. When plasma K$^+$ concentration increases from increased dietary intake or shifts of K$^+$ from the ICF, potassium is secreted into the urine by the distal tubules. Decreases in plasma potassium results in decreased distal tubular secretion, although about 5 to 15 mEq of K$^+$/day will continue to be lost. Changes in the rate of filtrate flow through the distal tubule also influences the concentration gradient for K$^+$ secretion. When the flow rate is high, as occurs with the administration of diuretics, the concentration of potassium in the distal tubular urine will be lower, favoring the secretion of potassium.

Changes in pH and thus in hydrogen ion concentration can also affect K$^+$ balance. Hydrogen ions accumulate in the ICF during states of acidosis. ICF levels of hydrogen are diminished during states of alkalosis. During acidosis, potassium shifts out of the cell to the ECF to maintain a balance of cations across the cell membrane. The decreased ICF K$^+$ results in decreased secretion of K$^+$ by the distal tubular cells, contributing to hyperkalemia. In contrast, alkalosis causes potassium to shift into the cell, so that the distal tubular cells increase their secretion of K$^+$, contributing to hypokalemia.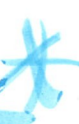

Besides acting to conserve sodium, aldosterone is a major factor in potassium regulation. When potassium concentration is increased, aldosterone is released, stimulating secretion of potassium into the urine by the distal tubules of the kidney. Aldosterone also increases the secretion of K$^+$ from the sweat glands.

Insulin contributes to the regulation of plasma potassium levels by promoting the movement of potassium into liver and muscle cells. Insulin can therefore be used to treat hyperkalemia, and dangerously low levels of plasma potassium can result from the administration of insulin when potassium levels are depressed. Potassium balance is especially significant in the treatment of conditions requiring insulin administration, such as insulin-dependent diabetes.

An interesting aspect of K$^+$ regulation is the ability of the body to adapt to increased levels of potassium intake over a period of time. A sudden increase in potassium may be fatal, but if the intake of potassium is slowly increased by amounts greater than 120 mEq/day, the kidney is able to increase the urinary excretion of potassium and maintain potassium balance. This tolerance to increasing amounts of potassium is known as **potassium adaptation**.

Hypokalemia

Pathophysiology

Potassium deficiency, or **hypokalemia**, develops when the serum potassium concentration falls below 3.5 mEq/L. Because cellular and total body stores of potassium are difficult to measure, changes in potassium balance are described by the plasma concentration, although changes in total body potassium are not always reflected in the plasma potassium concentration. Generally, the lowered serum potassium indicates a loss of total-body potassium. As potassium is lost from the ECF, the change in the concentration gradient favors movement of K^+ from the cell to the ECF. The ICF/ECF concentration ratio is maintained, but total body K^+ is depleted.

ECF hypokalemia can, however, develop without losses of total body potassium. For example, potassium shifts into the cell during states of respiratory or metabolic alkalosis or after administration of insulin. In the event of alkalosis, K^+ shifts into the cell in exchange for H^+ to maintain plasma acid-base balance. Insulin also promotes cellular uptake of K^+, causing a deficit in ECF potassium.

Plasma K^+ levels may be normal or elevated when total body potassium is depleted. In such instances, potassium shifts from the ICF to the ECF. One of the common causes of this problem is diabetic ketoacidosis in which the increased hydrogen ion concentration in the ECF causes H^+ to shift into the cell in exchange for potassium. A normal level of potassium is maintained in the plasma, but potassium continues to be lost in the urine, causing a deficit in total body potassium. Severe, even fatal, hypokalemia may occur if insulin is administered without also providing potassium supplements. Thus total body potassium depletion becomes evident when insulin treatment is initiated.

Potassium loss also occurs through normal body functions without causing hypokalemia. Average daily losses of potassium are as follows:

Location	Daily loss (mEq/L)
Stool	5-10
Sweat	0-20
Kidney	40-120

Factors contributing to the development of hypokalemia include reduced intake of potassium, increased entry of potassium into cells, and increased losses of body potassium. Dietary deficiency of potassium is a rare cause of hypokalemia. It may occur in elderly individuals with both low protein intake and inadequate intake of fruits and vegetables and in those with alcoholism or

anorexia nervosa. Generally, reduced potassium intake becomes a problem when combined with other causes of potassium depletion.

Shifts of potassium from the extracellular to intracellular space cause apparent deficits in total body potassium. Alkalosis, particularly respiratory alkalosis, is the most common clinical problem because potassium and hydrogen exchange corrects the alkalosis by shifting the pH of the ECF. Treatment of pernicious anemia with vitamin B_{12} or folate may also precipitate hypokalemia if the formation of new red blood cells causes enough potassium uptake to cause an extracellular decrease in potassium. Familial hypokalemic periodic paralysis is a rare genetically transmitted disease that also causes potassium to shift into the intracellular space.

Losses of potassium from body stores are most commonly due to gastrointestinal and renal disorders. Diarrhea (from any cause), intestinal drainage tubules or fistulae, and laxative abuse may also result in hypokalemia. Normally, only 5 to 10 mEq of potassium and 100 to 150 ml of water are excreted in the stool each day. With diarrhea, fluid and electrolyte losses can be voluminous with several liters of fluid and 100 to 200 mEq of potassium lost per day. Vomiting or continuous nasogastric suction is frequently associated with potassium depletion, partly because of the potassium lost from the gastric fluid but principally because of renal compensation for volume depletion and the metabolic alkalosis (elevated bicarbonate levels) that occurs from sodium, chloride, and hydrogen ion losses. The loss of fluid and sodium stimulates the secretion of aldosterone, which in turn causes renal losses of potassium. The elevated flow of bicarbonate at the distal tubule contributes to renal excretion of potassium because of increased tubular lumen electronegativity.

Renal losses of potassium are related to increased secretion of potassium by the distal tubule. Use of diuretics, excessive aldosterone secretion, increased distal tubular flow rate, and low plasma magnesium concentration may all contribute to urinary losses of potassium. Many diuretics, including thiazides, furosemide, ethacrynic acid, and osmotic diuretics inhibit the reabsorption of sodium chloride, causing the diuretic effect. The distal tubular flow rate then increases, promoting potassium secretion. If sodium loss is severe, the compensating aldosterone secretion (which causes secondary hyperaldosteronism) may further deplete potassium stores. Primary hyperaldosteronism with excessive secretion of aldosterone from an adrenal adenoma also causes potassium wasting. Many kidney diseases result in a reduced ability to conserve sodium. The disordered sodium reabsorption produces a diuretic effect, and the increased distal tubule flow rate favors the secretion of potassium. Magnesium deficits are also associated with renal potassium losses by some unknown mechanism.

Several antibiotics, including amphotericin B, gentamycin, and carbenicillin, are known to cause hypokalemia.

Clinical Manifestations

A wide range of metabolic dysfunctions may result from potassium deficiency. Carbohydrate metabolism is affected because hypokalemia depresses insulin secretion and alters hepatic and skeletal muscle glycogen synthesis. Renal function is impaired, with a decreased ability to concentrate urine. Polyuria (increased urine) and polydipsia (increased thirst) are associated with decreased responsiveness to ADH. Chronic potassium deficits lasting more than 1 month may damage renal tissue, with interstitial fibrosis and tubular atrophy.

Neuromuscular and cardiac effects of hypokalemia produce the most common symptoms. Neuromuscular excitability is decreased, causing skeletal muscle weakness, smooth muscle atony, and cardiac dysrhythmias. As Chapter 1 describes, the resting membrane potential is primarily determined by the *ratio* of extracellular to intracellular potassium ion concentration. Because the concentration of potassium in the ECF is small, only small changes in ECF potassium are required to influence the resting membrane potential and affect neuromuscular excitability. When extracellular potassium levels drop rapidly and intracellular potassium concentration does not change, the resting membrane potential becomes more negative, and the cell membrane is **hyperpolarized**. If the threshold potential remains stable, the distance between resting membrane potential and threshold potential increases requiring a stronger stimulus to initiate an action potential (Fig. 3-5).

Factors such as calcium concentration and pH also contribute to the changes in neuromuscular excitability associated with hypokalemia. Increases in ECF calcium concentration tend to raise the threshold potential and decrease membrane excitability, potentiating the neuromuscular effects of hypokalemia.

The onset of symptoms is related to the rate of potassium depletion. Because the body can accommodate slow losses of potassium, the decrease in ECF concentration may be slow enough to allow potassium to shift from the intracellular space. The extracellular to intracellular potassium concentration gradient is then restored toward normal, with less severe neuromuscular changes. With acute losses of potassium, changes in neuromuscular excitability are more profound. Skeletal muscle weakness initially occurs in the larger muscles of the legs and arms and ultimately affects the diaphragm and depresses ventilation. Paralysis and respiratory arrest can then occur. Loss of smooth muscle tone is manifested by constipation, intestinal distention, anorexia, nausea, vomiting, and paralytic ileus.

The cardiac effects of hypokalemia are also related to changes in membrane excitability (see Fig. 3-5). Because potassium contributes to the repolarization phase of the action potential, hypokalemia delays ventricular repolarization. A variety of dysrhythmias may occur, including sinus bradycardia, atrioventricular block, and paroxysmal atrial tachycardia. The characteristic changes in the electrocardiogram reflect delayed repolarization. For instance, the amplitude of the T wave is decreased; the amplitude of the U wave is increased; and the S-T segment is depressed (Fig. 3-6). In severe states of hy-

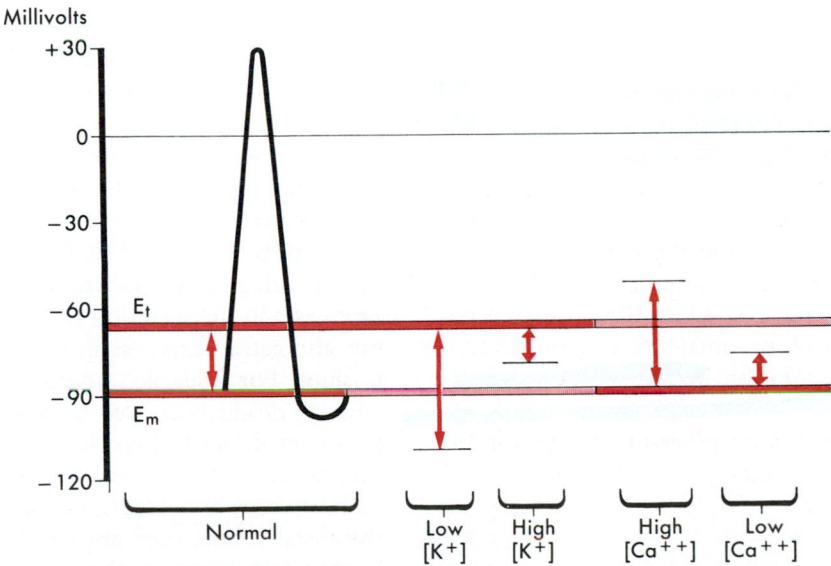

FIG. 3-5. Effects of potassium and calcium on membrane excitability. (Adapted from Leaf & Cotran, 1976.)

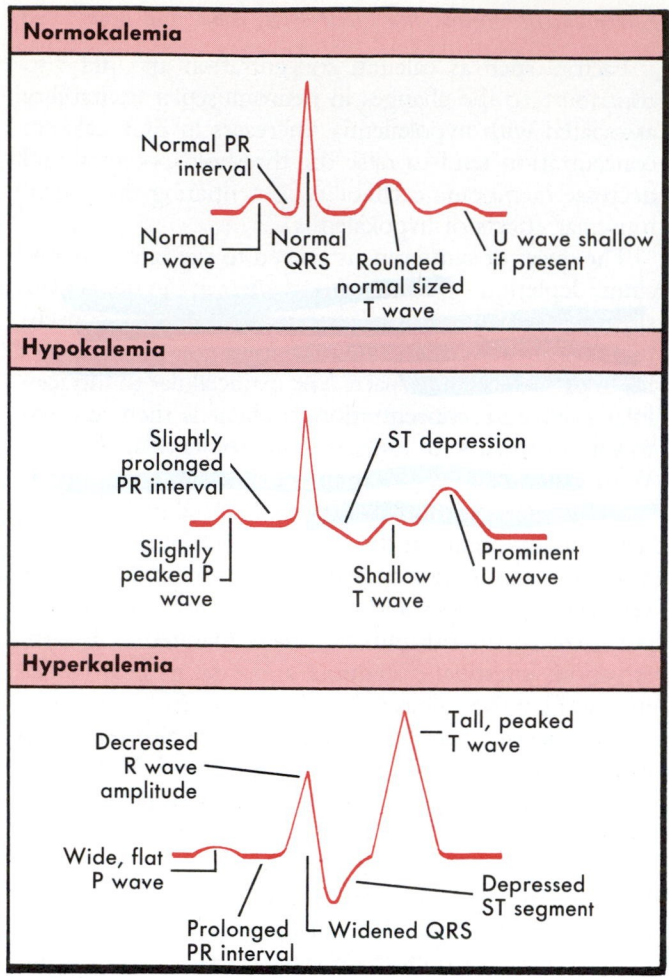

FIG. 3-6. ECG changes with potassium imbalance.

pokalemia, there is peaking of the P waves and prolonging of the QRS complex. Hypokalemia also increases the risk of digitalis toxicity.

Evaluation and Treatment

The diagnosis of hypokalemia is significantly related to the past medical history and the identification of disorders associated with potassium loss. Treatment involves an estimation of total body potassium losses and correction of acid-base imbalances. Further losses of potassium should be prevented, and the individual should be encouraged to eat foods rich in potassium. The maximal rate of oral replacement is 40 to 80 mEq/day if renal function is normal. A maximal safe rate of intravenous replacement is 20 mEq/hr. Because potassium is irritating to blood vessels, a maximal concentration of 40 mEq/L should be used. Serum potassium values can be monitored until normokalemia is achieved.

Hyperkalemia

Pathophysiology

An elevation of ECF potassium *above 5.5 mEq/L* constitutes **hyperkalemia.** Because of efficient renal excre-

tion, increases in total body potassium are relatively rare. Acute increases in serum potassium are handled quickly through an increase in cellular uptake and renal excretion of body potassium excesses. Excretion is partially mediated by the secretion of aldosterone, because it facilitates losses of potassium in the urine.

Excesses of potassium may be caused by increased intake, a shift of potassium from cells to the ECF, or decreased renal excretion. If renal function is normal, slow, chronic increases in potassium intake are usually well tolerated through potassium adaptation, although acute potassium loading can exceed renal excretion rates. Use of stored whole blood and intravenous boluses of penicillin G or replacement potassium can precipitate hyperkalemia, particularly if renal function is impaired. Dietary excesses of potassium are uncommon, but accidental ingestion of potassium salt substitutes can cause toxicity.

Movement of potassium from the ICF to ECF occurs with cell trauma or change in cell membrane permeability, acidosis, insulin deficiency, or cell hypoxia. Burns, massive crushing injuries, and extensive surgeries can cause loss of potassium to the ECF. If renal function is sustained, potassium will be excreted. As cell repair begins, hypokalemia will develop without an adequate intake of potassium.

In states of acidosis hydrogen ions shift into the cells in exchange for ICF potassium and sodium; hyperkalemia and acidosis therefore often occur together. Because insulin promotes cellular entry of potassium, insulin deficits, which occur with such conditions as diabetic ketoacidosis, are accompanied by hyperkalemia. Hypoxia can lead to hyperkalemia by diminishing the efficiency of cell membrane active transport, resulting in the escape of potassium to the ECF. Digitalis overdose may cause hyperkalemia by inhibiting the sodium-potassium ATPase pump, which maintains high intracellular potassium and high extracellular sodium (see Chapter 1).

Decreased renal excretion of potassium is commonly associated with hyperkalemia. Renal failure that results in oliguria (urine output less than 30 ml/hr) is accompanied by elevations of serum potassium. The severity of hyperkalemia is related to the amount of potassium intake, the degree of acidosis, and the rate of cell damage. Decreases in the secretion or renal effects of aldosterone can also cause decreases in the urinary excretion of potassium. For example, Addison's disease results in decreased production and secretion of aldosterone and thus contributes to hyperkalemia. Potassium-sparing diuretics (such as spironolactone, which inhibit sodium reabsorption) and potassium and hydrogen secretion by the distal tubule may also contribute to hyperkalemia. (Frequently, however, these diuretics are used in combination with diuretics that cause potassium wasting in an attempt to balance renal potassium gains and losses.)

Clinical Manifestations

Symptoms of hyperkalemia vary, but common characteristics are muscle weakness or paralysis, and changes in the electrocardiogram. During mild attacks, increased neuromuscular irritability may be manifested as restlessness, intestinal cramping, and diarrhea. Severe hyperkalemia causes muscle weakness, loss of muscle tone, and paralysis. In mild states of hyperkalemia, the more rapid repolarization is reflected in the electrocardiogram as narrow and taller T waves with a shortened Q-T interval. Severe hyperkalemia depresses the S-T segment, prolongs the PR interval, and widens the QRS complex (Fig. 3-6). Bradyarrhythmias are common in hyperkalemia with alterations in cardiac conduction causing ventricular fibrillation or cardiac arrest.

As with hypokalemia, changes in the ratio of intracellular to extracellular potassium concentration contribute to the symptoms of hyperkalemia. If extracellular potassium concentration increases without a significant change in intracellular potassium, the resting membrane potential decreases, and the cell membrane is **hypopolarized** (the inside of the cell becomes less negative or partially depolarized). (Electrical properties of cells are discussed in Chapter 1.) With relatively mild elevations in extracellular potassium, the cell more rapidly repolarizes and becomes more irritable. An action potential is then initiated more rapidly because the distance between the resting membrane potential and the threshold potential has been shortened. With more severe hyperkalemia, the resting membrane potential approaches or exceeds the threshold potential. In this case, the cell will not be able to repolarize and therefore will not respond to excitation stimuli. The most serious consequence is cardiac standstill.

Like the effects of hypokalemia, the neuromuscular effects of hyperkalemia are related to the rate of increase in the ECF potassium concentration and the presence of other contributing factors such as acidosis and calcium balance. Chronic increases in ECF potassium concentration result in shifts of potassium into the cell as the tendency is to maintain a normal ratio of intracellular/extracellular potassium concentrations. Acute elevations of extracellular potassium affect neuromuscular irritability as this ratio is disrupted.

Because calcium influences the threshold potential, changes in extracellular fluid calcium concentration can augment or override the effects of hyperkalemia. Usually, hypocalcemia increases the threshold potential, enhancing the neuromuscular effects of hyperkalemia, and hypercalcemia decreases the threshold potential counteracting the effects of hyperkalemia (Fig. 3-5).

Evaluation and Treatment

Hyperkalemia should be suspected when there is a history of renal disease, massive trauma, insulin defi

ciency, Addison's disease, use of potassium salt substitutes, or metabolic acidosis. The acuity of the onset of symptoms may be related to the underlying cause.

Management of hyperkalemia is related to treating the contributing causes and correcting the potassium excess. Normalizing the extracellular potassium concentration can be achieved with a variety of methods; the treatment chosen is related to the cause and severity of the problem. Calcium gluconate can be administered to restore normal neuromuscular irritability when serum potassium levels are dangerously high. Administration of insulin and glucose facilitates cellular entry of potassium, and sodium bicarbonate corrects metabolic acidosis and lowered serum potassium. Oral or rectal administration of cation exchange resins, which exchange sodium for potassium in the intestine, can be effective. Dialysis effectively removes potassium when there is renal failure.

Calcium and Phosphate

The total body content of calcium is about 1200 g. Most calcium (99%) is located in bone as hydroxyapatite (an inorganic compound that contributes to bone rigidity), and the remainder is in the plasma and body cells. Fifty percent of calcium in plasma is bound to plasma proteins (2.5 mEq/L); about 40% is in the free or ionized form (2.4 mEq/L). The total fraction of calcium circulating in the blood is small (4.5 to 5.5 mEq/L, 8.6 to 10.5 mg/dl). Ionized calcium has the most important physiologic functions.

Calcium is a necessary ion for many fundamental metabolic processes. It is the major cation for the structure of bone and teeth. It serves as an enzymatic cofactor for blood clotting and is required for hormone secretion and the function of cell receptors. Plasma membrane stability and permeability are directly related to calcium ions, as is the transmission of nerve impulses and the contraction of muscles.

Phosphate is found primarily in bone with smaller amounts within the intracellular and extracellular spaces. In the serum, phosphate exists in phospholipids and phosphate esters and as inorganic phosphate, which is the ionized form. The normal serum levels of inorganic phosphate range from 2.5 to 4.5 mg/dl and may be as high as 6.0 to 7.0 mg/dl in infants and young children. Intracellular phosphate has many metabolic forms, including the high-energy structures, creatine phosphate, and adenosine triphosphate (ATP). Phosphate acts as an intracellular and extracellular anion buffer in the regulation of acid-base balance; in the form of ATP it provides energy for muscle contraction.

Calcium and phosphate concentrations are rigidly controlled. They are related by the product of calcium and phosphate, which is a constant ($Ca^{++} \times HPO_4^{=}$ =

K). Thus if the concentration of one ion increases, the other decreases.

Calcium and phosphate balance is mediated by the interaction among three hormones: parathyroid hormone (PTH), vitamin D, and calcitonin. Acting together, these substances determine the amount of dietary calcium and phosphate absorbed from the intestine, the deposition and absorption of calcium and phosphate from the bone, and the renal reabsorption and excretion of calcium and phosphate by the kidney.

The parathyroid glands are sensitive to changes in serum calcium concentrations. The parathyroid glands secrete PTH in response to low serum calcium. PTH initiates renal activation of vitamin D. (The specific actions of PTH in relation to calcium and phosphorus are described in Chapter 17).

The renal regulation of calcium and phosphate balance requires PTH. As PTH secretion is stimulated by low levels of serum calcium, there is increased reabsorption of calcium along the distal part of the nephron and inhibition of phosphate resorption by the proximal segment of the nephron. The net result is an increase in serum calcium and urinary excretion of phosphate. Fig. 3-7 summarizes hormonal regulation of calcium.

Another hormone important to calcium and phosphate regulation is vitamin D. Vitamin D (cholecalciferol) is a fat-soluble steroid ingested in food or synthesized in the skin in the presence of ultraviolet light. Several steps of activation are required before vitamin D can act at target tissues. The first step occurs in the liver; final activation is in the kidney. The renal activation of vitamin D begins when the serum calcium level decreases and stimulates secretion of PTH. PTH then acts to increase calcium reabsorption and enhance renal excretion of phosphate, producing decreased phosphate levels. The combination of low calcium, PTH secretion, and low phosphate thus causes the renal activation of vitamin D. The activated vitamin D then circulates in the plasma and acts to increase absorption of calcium in the small intestine. When there is renal failure, vitamin D will not be activated; serum calcium levels will fall; and phosphate levels will rise.

The exchange of calcium and phosphate between serum and bone is also regulated by hormones. When serum calcium levels are low, PTH and vitamin D stimulate the osteoclasts in bone to resorb bone and release calcium and phosphate into the plasma. As calcium levels increase above 12 mg/dl, the thyroid hormone calcitonin opposes the action of PTH and lowers the serum calcium level by stimulating osteoblasts to deposit calcium and form new bone. When calcium levels are low, the secretion of calcitonin is suppressed.

The fractions of serum calcium that are freely ionized or bound to plasma proteins are influenced by pH. In states of acidosis, there is an increase in levels of ionized calcium. When alkalosis develops, with an increase in pH, there is an increase in protein-bound calcium and a decrease in the physiologically active, ionized calcium. The decreased concentration of ionized calcium may be great enough to cause symptoms of hypocalcemia, such as tetany.

Hypocalcemia

Pathophysiology

Hypocalcemia occurs when serum calcium concentrations are lower than 8.5 mg/dl. Deficits in calcium are related to inadequate intestinal absorption, deposition of ionized calcium into bone or soft tissue, blood administration or decreases in PTH and vitamin D.

Nutritional deficiencies of calcium can occur with inadequate sources of dairy products or green leafy vegetables. Excessive amounts of dietary phosphorus also bind with calcium, so that neither mineral is absorbed. Blood transfusions are also a common cause of hypocalcemia because the citrate solution used in storing whole blood binds with calcium. Pancreatitis causes release of

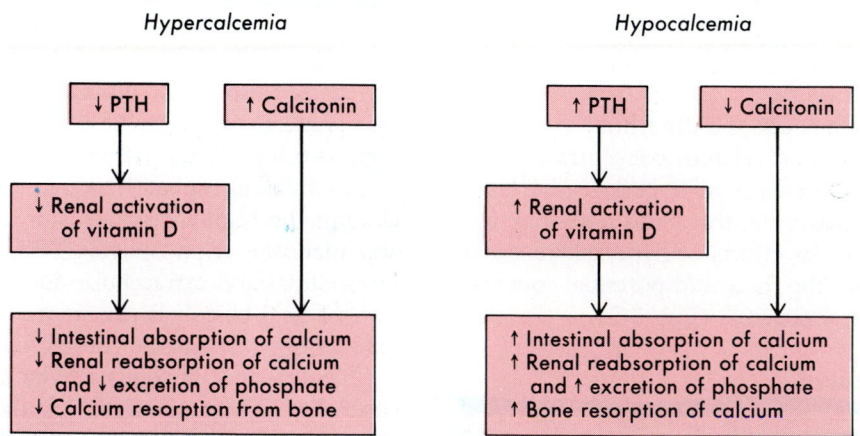

FIG. 3-7. Hormonal regulation of calcium balance.

lipases into soft-tissue spaces, so that the free fatty acids that are formed bind calcium, causing decrease in ionized calcium. Neoplastic bone metastases tend to inhibit bone resorption and increase calcium deposition into bone, thereby decreasing serum calcium levels.

Vitamin D deficiency, which can result from inadequate intake or avoidance of sunlight, causes decreased intestinal absorption of calcium. Malabsorption of fat, including fat-soluble vitamin D, may also contribute to calcium deficiency. Removal of the parathyroid glands with the resulting loss of PTH also causes hypocalcemia. Metabolic or respiratory alkalosis causes symptoms of hypocalcemia as the change in pH enhances protein binding of ionized calcium.

Clinical Manifestations

The clinical manifestations of hypocalcemia are primarly due to an increase in neuromuscular excitability. Calcium deficits cause partial depolarization of nerves and muscle from an increase in the threshold potential. The symptoms include confusion, parasthesias around the mouth and in the digits, carpopedal spasm (muscle spasms in the hands and feet), and hyperreflexia.

Two clinical signs are Chvostek's sign and Trousseau's sign. Chvostek's sign is illicited by tapping on the facial nerve just below the temple. A positive sign is a twitch of the nose or lip. Trousseau's sign is contraction of the hand and fingers when the arterial blood flow in the arm is occluded for 5 minutes.

Severe symptoms include convulsions and tetany, a continuous severe muscle spasm that can interfere with breathing and cause death. The characteristic ECG change is a prolonged Q-T interval indicating prolonged ventricular depolarization. Intestinal cramping and hyperactive bowel sounds may also be present because hypocalcemia affects the smooth muscles of the gastrointestinal tract.

Evaluation and Treatment

The health history may signify underlying pathologic conditions that require further evaluation and treatment. Severe symptoms of hypocalcemia require emergency treatment with intravenous 10% calcium gluconate. Oral calcium replacement should be initiated, and serum calcium levels should be monitored. Decreasing phosphate intake facilitates long-term management of hypocalcemia.

Hypercalcemia

Pathophysiology

Hypercalcemia with serum calcium concentrations exceeding 12 mg/dl can be caused by a number of diseases. The most common among these are hyperparathyroidism; bone metastases with calcium resorption from breast, prostate, and cervical cancer; sarcoidosis;

and excess vitamin D. Many tumors produce PTH and elevate the serum calcium levels. Sarcoidosis appears to increase vitamin D levels.

Clinical Manifestations

Many of the symptoms of hypercalcemia are nonspecific. Because serum calcium levels are increased, a greater amount of calcium is also contained inside the cells. The threshold potential becomes more difficult to reach, and the cell membrane becomes refractory to depolarization. Thus many of the symptoms are related to loss of cell membrane excitability. (Membrane potentials and membrane excitability are discussed in Chapter 1.) Fatigue, weakness, lethargy, anorexia, nausea, and constipation are common. Impaired renal function frequently develops, and kidney stones form as precipitates of calcium salts. A shortened Q-T segment and depressed T waves may also be observed on the electrocardiogram.

Evaluation and Treatment

With elevated serum calcium levels, there is often a reciprocal decrease in serum phosphate values. Specific diagnostic procedures to identify the contributing pathologic condition are required.

Treatment is related to severity of symptoms and the underlying disease. When renal function is normal, oral phosphate administration is effective. When there is acute illness and high calcium levels, intravenous administration of large amounts of normal saline will enhance renal excretion of calcium. Corticosteroids and the cytotoxic drug mithramycin are also used to treat hypercalcemia. Ultimately, the underlying pathologic condition must be treated.

Hypophosphatemia

Pathophysiology

Hypophosphatemia is a serum phosphate level lower than 2.0 mg/dl and is usually an indication of phosphate deficiency. In some conditions, total body phosphate is normal, but serum volumes are low. The most common causes are intestinal malabsorption and increased renal excretion of phosphate. Inadequate absorption is associated with vitamin D deficiency, use of magnesium- and aluminum-containing antacids (which bind with phosphorus), chronic alcohol abuse, and malabsorption syndromes. Respiratory alkalosis can cause severe hypophosphatemia because of cellular use of phosphorus for an accelerated glucose metabolism. Increased renal excretion of phosphorus is associated with hyperparathyroidism.

Clinical Manifestations

The consequences of phosphate deficiency are related to reduced capacity for oxygen transport by red blood cells and to disturbed energy metabolism. Transport and release of oxygen is associated with 2,3-diphosphoglycerate (2,3-DPG) and ATP. When phosphate is depleted, 2,3-DPG and ATP levels become low and diminish release of oxygen to the tissues. The oxyhemoglobin curve shifts to the left (see Chapter 29) and hypoxia can occur.

Leukocyte and platelet dysfunction are also associated with hypophosphatemia. There is greater risk of infection and blood-clotting impairment with potential for hemorrhage. Nerve and muscle function can be affected with derangement in energy metabolism. Irritability, confusion, numbness, coma, and convulsions develop with severe phosphate losses. Muscle weakness may become serious enough to cause respiratory failure, and cardiomyopathies can also develop. In response to low phosphate levels, bone resorption occurs and may lead to rickets or osteomalacia.

Evaluation and Treatment

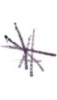

To correct the condition, the underlying cause must be identified and treated. Although serum phosphate levels are below normal, the administration of phosphate salts is dangerous, and low phosphate levels are usually not considered life threatening.

Hyperphosphatemia

Pathophysiology

Hyperphosphatemia, or an elevated serum phosphate level above 4.5 mg/dl, develops with acute or chronic renal failure with significant loss of glomerular filtration. Because most phosphate is located in cells, the cell destruction associated with treatment of metastatic tumors with chemotherapy can release large amounts of phosphate into the serum. Chronic use of phosphate-containing enemas or laxatives may also lead to hyperphosphatemia. Hyperparathyroidism can cause elevated phosphate by increasing renal tubular reabsorption of phosphate.

High levels of serum phosphate also lower serum calcium levels, and increased amounts of phosphate and calcium are deposited in bone and soft tissues. Serum calcium levels may become low enough to cause symptoms of hypocalcemia, including tetany.

Clinical Manifestations

Symptoms of hyperphosphatemia are primarily related to low serum calcium levels and thus are comparable to symptoms of hypocalcemia. With prolonged hyperphosphatemia, calcification of soft tissues will occur in the lungs, kidneys, and joints.

Evaluation and Treatment

To correct the condition, the underlying pathologic condition must be identified and treated. Aluminum hy-

droxide may be administered because it binds phosphate in the gastrointestinal tract and is eliminated. Dialysis is required for management of renal failure.

Magnesium

Magnesium (Mg^{++}) is a major intracellular cation. About 40 to 60% is stored in muscle and bone. Plasma concentration is 1.8 to 2.4 mEq/L with about one third bound to plasma proteins. Regulation of magnesium metabolism is not well understood. Low serum magnesium appears to have a direct effect on the kidney to cause conservation of magnesium. Magnesium is a cofactor in intracellular enzymatic reactions and is a cause of neuromuscular excitability. Calcium and magnesium often interact in reactions at the cellular level.

Hypomagnesemia, a rare condition in which serum magnesium concentration is less than 1.5 mEq/L, increases neuromuscular excitability and can be a cause of tetany. Malnutrition malabsorption syndromes, alcoholism, renal tubular dysfunction, and thiazide diuretics can cause magnesium losses. Symptoms of hypomagnesemia are similar to those of hypocalcemia. Behavioral changes, irritability, increased reflexes, muscle weakness, ataxia, nystagmus, tetany, and convulsions may be observed. Treatment is intramuscular or intravenous administration of magnesium sulfate.

Hypermagnesemia, in which concentration is greater than 2.5 mEq/L, is rare and usually caused by renal failure. Magnesium-containing antacids (e.g., Gaviscon, Gelusil) can potentiate excess magnesium. Excess magnesium depresses skeletal muscle contraction and nerve function. Symptoms include nausea and vomiting, muscle weakness, hypotension, bradycardia, and respiratory depression (Kokko & Tanner, 1986). Treatment is avoidance of magnesium-containing substances and removal by dialysis.

ACID-BASE BALANCE

Hydrogen ion concentration must be regulated within a narrow range for the body to function normally. Slight changes in amounts of hydrogen can significantly alter biologic processes in cells and tissues. Hydrogen ion is necessary to maintain membrane integrity and the speed of enzymatic reactions. Most pathologic conditions disturb acid-base balance, and the degree of severity may be more harmful than the disease process.

Hydrogen Ion and pH

The hydrogen ion concentration $[H^+]$ is commonly expressed as pH, which represents the negative logarithm of hydrogen ions in solution. The logarithmic value means that as the pH changes one unit (e.g., 7.0

to 6.0), the $[H^+]$ changes tenfold. The relationship is commonly expressed as follows:

$$pH = \log \frac{1}{[H^+]}$$

or

$$pH = -\log[H^+]$$

As the $[H^+]$ increases, the pH decreases; likewise, as the $[H^+]$ decreases, the pH increases. The greater the $[H^+]$, the more acidic the solution and the lower the pH. The lower the $[H^+]$, the more basic the solution and the higher the pH. In biologic fluids, a pH of less than 7.4 is defined as acidic and a pH greater than 7.4 is defined as basic.

Different body fluids have different pH values as follows:

Body Fluid	pH
Gastric juices	1.0-3.0
Urine	5.0-6.0
Arterial blood	7.38-7.42
Venous blood	7.37
Cerebrospinal fluid	7.32
Pancreatic fluid	7.8-8.0

Body acids are formed as end products of cellular metabolism. The average person generates 50 to 100 mEq of acid/day from the metabolism of protein, carbohydrates, and fats. To maintain a normal pH, an equal amount of acid therefore must be neutralized or excreted. The lungs, kidneys, and bone are the major organs involved in the regulation of acid-base balance. The systems are interrelated and work together to regulate acute or chronic changes in acid-base status. Body acids exist in two forms: **volatile** and **nonvolatile.** The volatile acid is carbonic acid (H_2CO_3), which is formed from the hydration of carbon dioxide:

$$CO_2 + H_2O \underset{\text{(carbonic anhydrase)}}{\rightleftharpoons} H_2CO_3$$

Carbonic acid is a weak acid, and, in the presence of carbonic anhydrase, it readily dissociates into carbon dioxide. The carbon dioxide is then eliminated by pulmonary ventilation. Sulfuric, phosphoric, and other organic acids are nonvolatile strong acids produced from the metabolism of proteins, carbohydrates, and fats. (Strong acids are those that readily give up their hydrogen; weak acids do not.) Nonvolatile acids are eliminated by the renal tubules. Thus the lungs and kidneys, with the help of body buffer systems, are the prime regulators of acid-base balance.

Buffer Systems

Buffers are substances that can absorb excessive H^+ (acid) or OH^- (base) without a significant change in pH. Although acids are normally added to the body daily, buffers are available to maintain pH within the normal range (7.35 to 7.45). The buffer systems are located in both the ICF and ECF compartments, and they function at different rates. Buffer systems exist as buffer pairs and consist of a weak acid and its conjugate base (Table 3-9). The most important plasma buffer systems are carbonic acid-bicarbonate, protein buffers (hemoglobin), and phosphate ($[HPO_4^=] + H^+ = H_2PO_4^-$).

An important factor for effective buffering is a term known as the *pK value*, which represents the pH at which a buffer pair is half dissociated. Buffer pairs can associate and dissociate. For example:

$$H + HCO_3 \rightleftharpoons H_2CO_3 \rightleftharpoons H_2O + CO_2$$

TABLE 3-9 Buffer systems

Buffer pairs	pK values	Rate
HCO_3/H_2CO_3	6.1	Instantaneous
Hb^-/HHb	7.3	Instantaneous
$HPO_4^-/H_2PO_4^-$	6.8	Instantaneous

Organs	Mechanism	Rate
Lungs	Regulates retention or elimination of CO_2 and therefore H_2CO_3 concentration	Minutes-hours
Ionic shifts	Exchange of intracellular potassium and sodium for hydrogen	2-4 hours
Kidneys	Bicarbonate reabsorption and regeneration, ammonia formation, phosphate buffering	Hours-days
Bone	Exchanges of calcium, phosphate, and release of carbonate	Hours-days

The pK provides a rate constant for the chemical reaction. A buffer system is most effective when the pK for the buffer is close to the pH of the fluid in which the buffer is acting. For the bicarbonate-carbonic acid buffer system, the pK is 6:1. This value is not as high as the pK for other buffer systems (Table 3-9), but this buffer system is still very effective because carbon dioxide is rapidly removed from the blood by the lungs.

The pK value is also a term in the equation used to determine pH. The relationships among pH, pK, and the ratio of bicarbonate/carbonic acid can be expressed as follows by the *Henderson-Hasselbalch equation*:

$$pH = pK + \log \frac{[HCO_3^-]}{[H_2CO_3]}$$

The pH can then be determined when specific values are included in the equation:

$$pH = 6.1 + \log \frac{[HCO_3^-]}{[H_2CO_3]}$$

$$= 6.1 + \log \frac{24}{1.2}$$

$$= 6.1 + \log \frac{20}{1}$$

$$= 6.1 + 1.3$$

$$= 7.40$$

Carbonic Acid–Bicarbonate Buffering

The major buffering system is the carbonic acid–bicarbonate buffer pair, which operates in both the lung and the kidney. The volatile feature of this buffer pair is significant because the amount of carbonic acid formed is a function of the partial pressure of carbon dioxide (P_{CO_2}). The greater the P_{CO_2}, the more carbonic acid is formed. The relationship that exists between carbonic acid (H_2CO_3) and carbon dioxide (P_{CO_2}) can be expressed as follows:

$$H_2CO_3 = 0.03 \times P_{CO_2} \text{ (mm Hg)}$$

The 0.03 represents the soluability coefficient for carbon dioxide. The P_{CO_2} of arterial blood is normally about 40 mm Hg. Therefore the amount of H_2CO_3 is equal to about 1.2 mmol/L (0.03×40). As the amount of carbon dioxide increases or decreases, the amount of H_2CO_3 changes in the same direction.

The relationship between bicarbonate and carbonic acid is usually expressed as a ratio. When the pH is 7.40, this ratio is 20:1 (bicarbonate/carbonic acid). The ratio is defined by the amount of bicarbonate and carbon dioxide (carbonic acid) in the arterial blood. Bicarbonate concentration (HCO_3^-) is normally about 24 mEq/L. Therefore the 20:1 ratio can be developed as follows:

$$\frac{[HCO_3^-] = 24 \text{ mEq/L}}{[H_2CO_3] = (0.03 \times 40 \text{ mm Hg})} = \frac{24}{1.2} = \frac{20}{1}$$

or

$$\frac{[HCO_3^-] = 24 \text{ mEq/L}}{[H_2CO_3] = 1.2 \text{ mmol/L}} = \frac{24}{1.2} = \frac{20}{1}$$

The significance of the ratio is that the values for HCO_3^- and P_{CO_2} (H_2CO_3) can increase or decrease proportionately, but the 20:1 ratio will be maintained.

Another important component of the bicarbonate–carbonic acid buffer system is the renal regulation of bicarbonate. The lungs can decrease the amount of carbonic acid by blowing off CO_2 and leaving water. The kidneys can reabsorb bicarbonate or regenerate new bicarbonate from CO_2 and water. The renal mechanism does not act as rapidly as the lungs, but the two systems are very effective together because acid concentration can be rapidly adjusted by the lungs and bicarbonate is easily reabsorbed or regenerated by the kidneys. Because the lungs and kidneys function at different rates and regulate different components of the bicarbonate–carbonic acid buffer system, the pH equation can be symbolically expressed as:

$$pH = \frac{\text{Renal regulation (slow)}}{\text{Pulmonary regulation (fast)}}$$

or

$$pH = \frac{\text{Base}}{\text{Acid}}$$

or

$$pH = \frac{\text{Metabolic acid} - \text{base function}}{\text{Respiratory acid} - \text{base function}}$$

Changes in either the numerator or the denominator will change the pH. For example, if the amount of bicarbonate is decreased, the pH will also decrease, causing a state of acidosis. The pH can be returned to a normal range if the value of the denominator or the amount of carbonic acid also decreases.

This type of adjustment in pH is known as **compensation**. With compensation, a 20:1 ratio may be achieved, but the actual values for HCO_3^- and H_2CO_3 are not normal. The respiratory system thus compensates for changes in pH by increasing or decreasing ventilation. The renal system compensates by producing more acidic or more alkaline urine. In this example, the respiratory system compensates for metabolic acidosis (Fig. 3-8).

Correction, as a process distinctly different from compensation, occurs when the values for both components of the buffer pair are returned to normal. In this example, pH would be corrected when the bicarbonate and carbonic acid return to their normal concentrations.

FIG. 3-8. Maintenance of HCO_3^-:P_{CO_2} (H_2CO_3) ratio in metabolic acidosis.

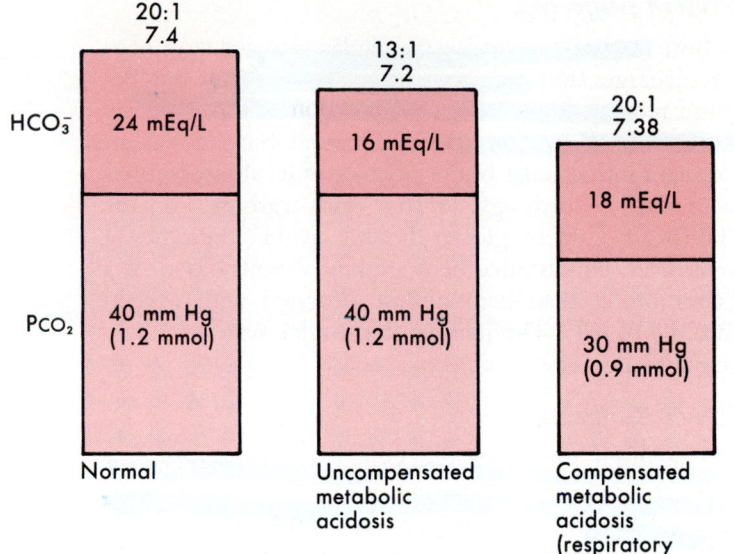

HCO_3^-

PCO₂

20:1
7.4

24 mEq/L

40 mm Hg
(1.2 mmol)

Normal

13:1
7.2

16 mEq/L

40 mm Hg
(1.2 mmol)

Uncompensated
metabolic
acidosis

20:1
7.38

18 mEq/L

30 mm Hg
(0.9 mmol)

Compensated
metabolic
acidosis
(respiratory
buffering response)

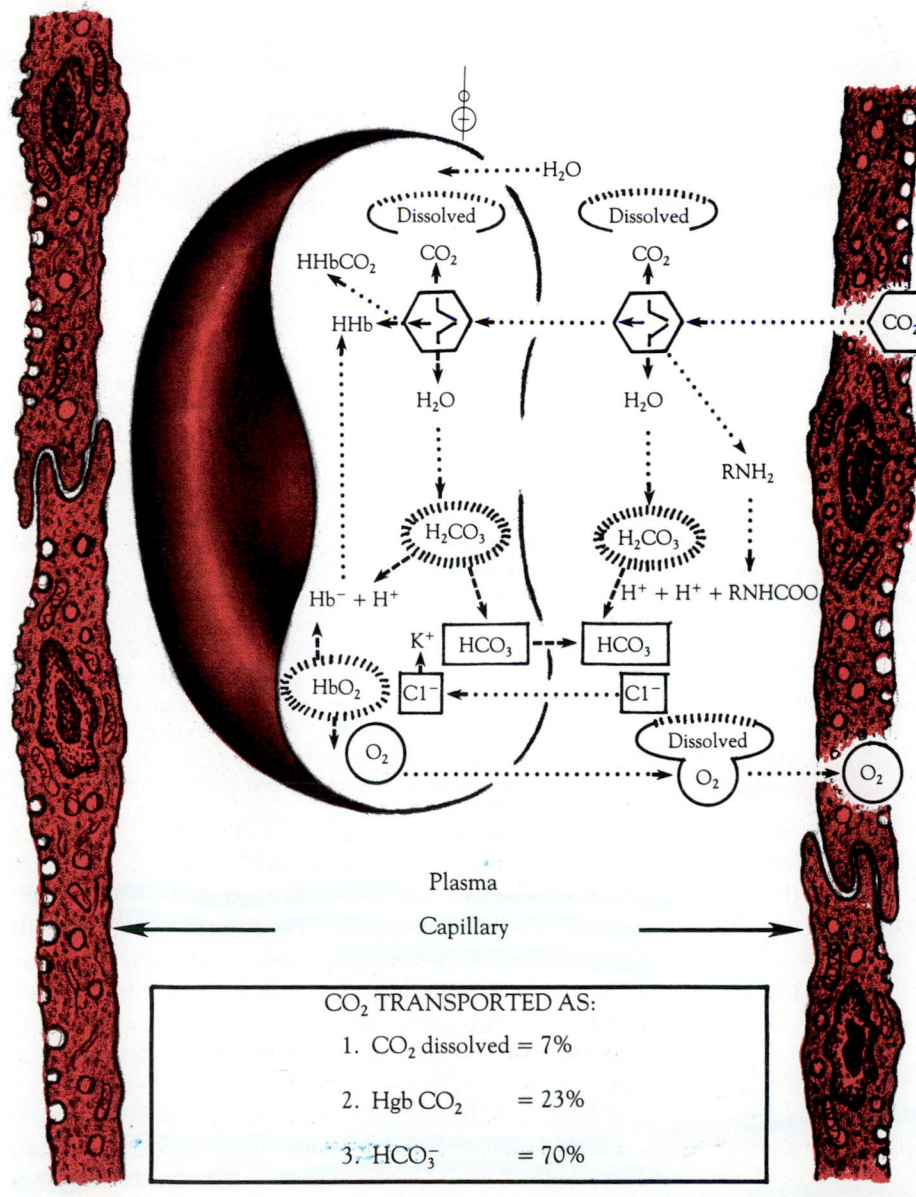

Plasma

Capillary

CO₂ TRANSPORTED AS:

1. CO₂ dissolved = 7%

2. Hgb CO₂ = 23%

3. HCO₃⁻ = 70%

FIG. 3-9. Buffering of hydrogen with hemoglobin and CO_2 transport. CO_2 is produced in tissue cells and diffuses to the plasma *(1)*, where it is transported as dissolved CO_2, or it combines with water to form carbonic acid (H_2CO_3). Most of the CO_2 diffuses into the red blood cell *(2)* and combines with water to form carbonic acid (H_2CO_3) *(3)*. The H_2CO_3 dissociates to form hydrogen (H^+) and bicarbonate (HCO_3^-). Hydrogen combines with hemoglobin that has released its oxygen to form HHb *(4)*, which buffers the hydrogen and makes venous blood slightly more acidic than arterial blood. The HCO_3^- shifts to the plasma, and chloride shifts into the red blood cell *(5)* to maintain electroneutrality. (From Thompson, McFarland, Hirsch, Tucker, & Bowens, 1986.)

Protein Buffering

Both intracellular and extracellular proteins have negative charges and can serve as buffers for H^+, but because most proteins are inside cells, they are primarily an intracellular buffer system. Hemoglobin (Hb) is an excellent intracellular buffer because of its ability to bind with H^+ (forming HHb) and carbon dioxide ($HHbCO_2$). Hemoglobin bound to H^+ becomes a weak acid. Unsaturated hemoglobin (venous blood) is a better buffer than hemoglobin saturated with oxygen (arterial blood). The hemoglobin buffer system is illustrated in Fig. 3-9.

Renal Buffering

The distal tubule of the kidney regulates acid-base balance by secreting hydrogen into the urine and reabsorbing bicarbonate. The maximal acidity that can be achieved in the distal tubular fluid of the kidney is a pH of about 4.4 to 4.7. Buffers in the tubular fluid combine with hydrogen ions, allowing more H^+ to be secreted before the limiting pH value is reached. Dibasic phosphate ($HPO_4^=$) and ammonia (NH_3^-) are two important renal buffers. Dibasic phosphate is filtered at the glomerulus. About 75% is reabsorbed and the remainder is available for buffering H^+. Secreted H^+ combines with $HPO_4^=$ to form monobasic phosphate ($H_2PO_4^-$). The remaining negative charge on the molecule makes it lipid insoluble, and it cannot diffuse back across the tubular cell and into the blood. Thus it is excreted in the urine (see Fig. 3-10).

Ammonia is an important renal buffer. The major source of ammonia (NH_3^-) is derived from the synthesis and enzymatic conversion of glutamine by the renal tubular cells. Ammonia is not ionized (does not carry a charge), and therefore it is lipid soluble and can cross the cell membrane. The presence of NH_3^- in the cell creates a concentration gradient and it diffuses into the tubular fluid where it combines with hydrogen to form ammonium (NH_4). The ionization of NH_4 traps it in the lumen and the hydrogen ion is excreted bound to the buffer (Fig. 3-10).

The renal buffering of hydrogen ions requires the use of CO_2 to form H_2CO_3. The enzyme carbonic anhydrase catalyzes the formation of $H^+ + HCO_3^-$. The hydrogen is secreted from the tubular cell and buffered in the lumen by phosphate and ammonia. The bicarbonate is reabsorbed. The end effect is the addition of new bicarbonate, which contributes to the alkalinity of the plasma, since the hydrogen ion is excreted from the body (Fig. 3-10).

Other Buffers

A cellular ion exchange mechanism is also an important buffering system. The best example is the shift of potassium in exchange for hydrogen during states of ac-

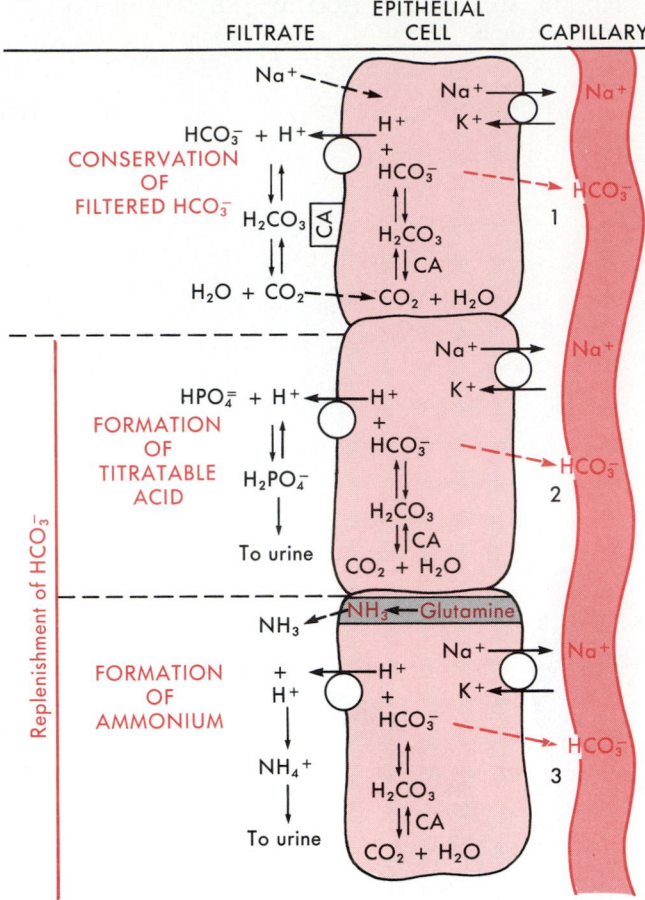

FIG. 3-10. Renal excretion of acid. *1,* Conservation of filtered bicarbonate. Filtered bicarbonate combines with secreted hydrogen in the presence of carbon anhydrase (CA) to form carbonic acid (H_2CO_3), which then dissociates to water (H_2O) and carbon dioxide (CO_2); both diffuse into the epithelial cell. The CO_2 and H_2O combine to form H_2CO_3 in the presence of CA, and the resulting HCO_3^- is converted by reabsorption into the capillary. *2,* Formation of titratable acid. Hydrogen ion is secreted and combines with dibasic phosphate ($HPO_4^=$) to form monobasic phosphate ($H_2PO_4^-$). The secreted hydrogen is formed from the dissociation of H_2CO_3, and the remaining HCO_3^- is reabsorbed into the capillary. *3,* Formation of ammonium. Ammonia (NH_3^-) is produced from glutamine in the epithelial cell and diffused to the tubular lumen, where it combines with H^+ to form ammonium (NH_4). Once NH_4 has been formed, it cannot return to the epithelial cell (diffusional trapping), and the bicarbonate remaining in the epithelial cell is reabsorbed into the capillary. (From Berne & Levy, 1988.)

idosis or alkalosis. During acidosis, potassium tends to leave the intracellular space in exchange for hydrogen. The reverse occurs during alkalosis. Although the ionic shifts facilitate buffering, the changes in intracellular or extracellular potassium concentrations may have serious consequences.

Acid-Base Imbalances

Changes in the concentration of hydrogen ion in the blood lead to acid-base imbalances. **Acidemia** is a state

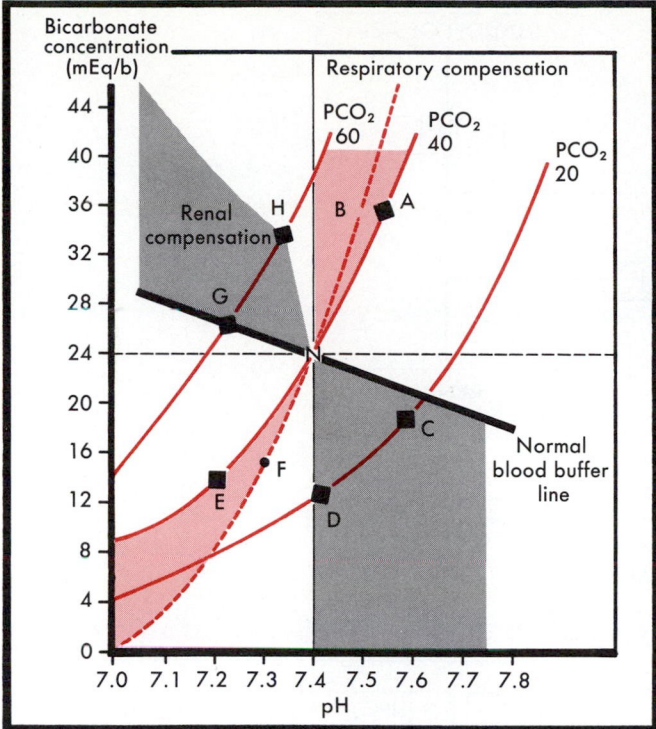

FIG. 3-11. Graph of pH, P_{CO_2} and bicarbonate relationships. *Solid black lines* represent different P_{CO_2} values. *Vertical axis* represents bicarbonate concentration, and *horizontal axis* represents pH values. Thus for any indicated P_{CO_2} there is a corresponding pH and bicarbonate concentration. Any point on the graph predicts the required P_{CO_2}, pH, and bicarbonate values. *Dashed horizontal line* shows behavior of bicarbonate as a pure buffer at 24 mEq/L. The normal blood buffer line represents values that would be obtained if blood were equilibrated at different CO_2 values. Point *N* represents normal values. *A* represents **metabolic alkalosis**, indicated by a normal P_{CO_2} of 40 and pH greater than 7.4. Respiratory compensation is achieved by hypoventilation, which raises the P_{CO_2} to point *B* and decreases the pH. **Respiratory alkalosis** is represented by point *C* and reflects hypocapnia (decreased P_{CO_2}). Renal compensation for respiratory alkalosis is increased renal excretion of bicarbonate to normalize the pH at point *D*. **Metabolic acidosis** at point *E* represents normal P_{CO_2} and a decrease in bicarbonate and pH. Respiratory compensation by hyperventilation is indicated by point *F*. **Respiratory acidosis** at point *G* indicates high P_{CO_2} and low pH values. Renal compensation for chronic high P_{CO_2} values is indicated by point *H*. (Adapted from Berne & Levy, 1988.)

in which the pH of arterial blood is less than 7.35. A systemic increase in hydrogen ion concentration is termed **acidosis**. **Alkalemia** is a state in which the pH of arterial blood is greater than 7.45. A systemic decrease in hydrogen ion concentration is termed **alkalosis**.

An abnormal decrease in bicarbonate concentration or an increase in hydrogen ion concentration is called **metabolic acidosis**. Conversely, an increase in bicarbonate concentration or a decrease in hydrogen ion con-

TABLE 3-10 Primary and compensatory acid-base changes

	Primary disturbance			Compensations		
	pH	P_{CO_2}	HCO_3^-	pH	P_{CO_2}	HCO_3^-
Metabolic acidosis	↓	N	↓	↑-N	↓	↓
Metabolic alkalosis	↑	N	↑	↓-N	↑	↑
Respiratory acidosis	↓	↑	N	↑-N	↑	↑
Respiratory alkalosis	↑	↓	N	↓-N	↓	↓

NOTE: ↑-N, Increase toward normal; ↓-N, decrease toward normal.

centration is known as **metabolic alkalosis.** Changes in the rate of alveolar ventilation produces changes in the P_{CO_2}. When less CO_2 is removed in relation to the amount of CO_2 generated, the P_{CO_2} increases. The resulting condition is known as **respiratory acidosis** because carbonic acid increases. When more CO_2 is removed in relation to the amount of CO_2 generated, the P_{CO_2} decreases. The resulting condition is known as **respiratory alkalosis.** Table 3-10 summarizes changes occurring in pH, P_{CO_2}, and HCO_3^- with respiratory or metabolic acid-base disorders. Fig. 3-11 summarizes the relationships between pH, P_{CO_2}, and bicarbonate during different acid-base alterations.

Metabolic Acidosis

Pathophysiology

Metabolic acidosis can be caused from an increase in noncarbonic acids or loss of bicarbonate from the extracellular fluid (Table 3-11). The development of metabolic acidosis can occur quickly, as in lactic acidosis from poor perfusion, or more slowly, as in renal failure or diabetic ketoacidosis.

The buffer systems compensate for the excess acid and attempt to maintain the arterial pH within a normal range. Buffering by bicarbonate lowers the serum value of this ion. The respiratory system compensates for a metabolic acidosis as the reduced pH stimulates hyperventilation, lowering the Pa_{CO_2} and the amount of H_2CO_3 circulating in the blood. The kidneys excrete the excess acid as NH_4 and titratable acid. When the acidosis is severe, the buffers are unable to compensate for the increasing H^+ load, and the pH continues to fall. The result is a decrease in the 20:1 ratio of bicarbonate to carbonic acid (Fig. 3-12).

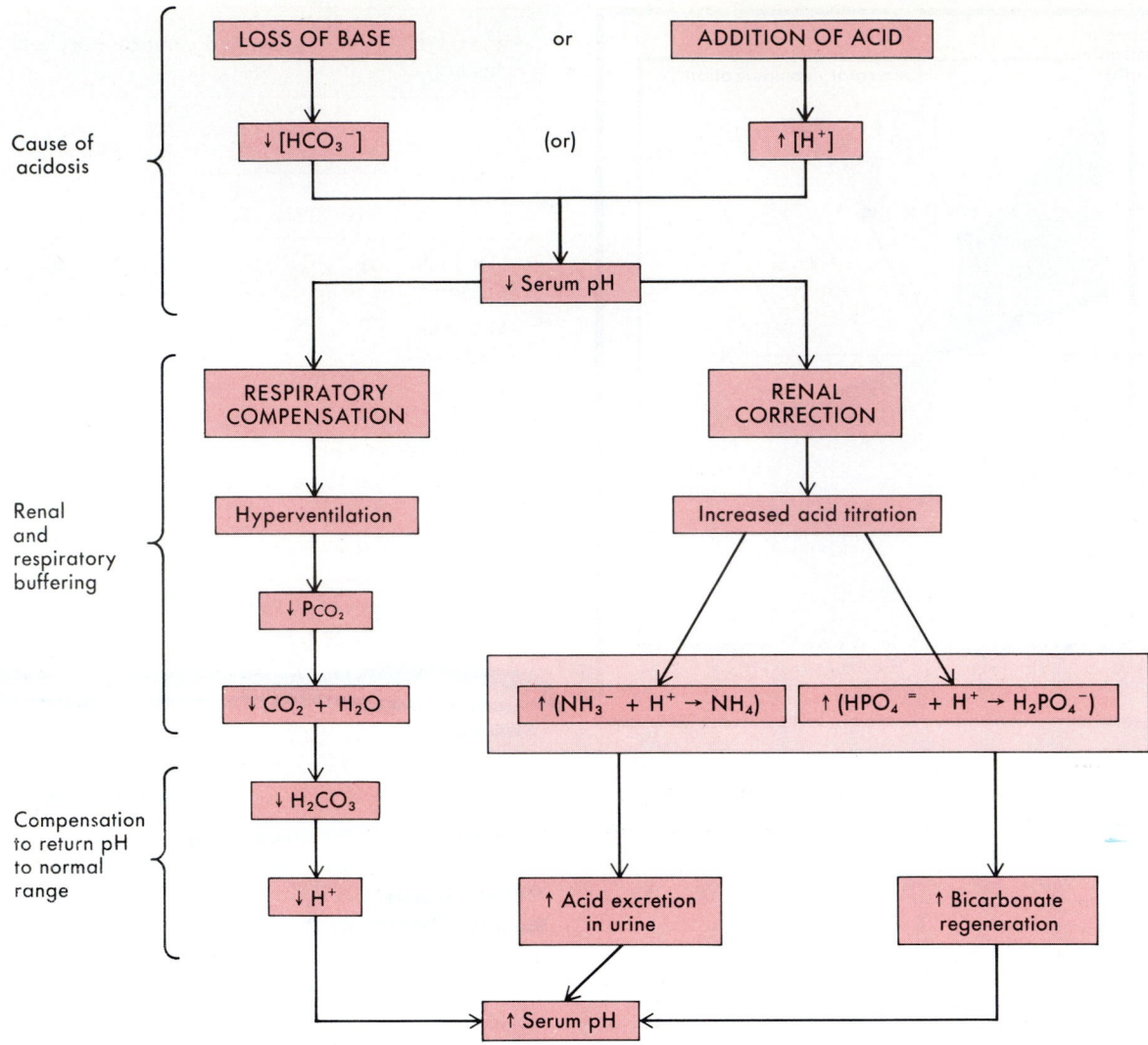

FIG. 3-12. Metabolic acidosis with compensation and correction.

The evaluation of the **anion gap** can be useful for distinguishing different types of metabolic acidosis. Normally, the concentrations of cations and anions in the plasma are equivalent. Some anions, such as protein, sulfates, phosphates, and organic acids, however, are not measured in the common laboratory evaluations of the blood. Therefore the **normal anion gap** represents the **difference between the sum of Na^+ and K^+** and the sum of HCO_3^- and Cl^-, or about 10 to 12 mEq.

Anion gap =
$$[Na^+(140) + K^+(4.0)] - [HCO_3^-(24) + Cl^-(110)]$$
$$= 10-12 \text{ mEq/L}$$

In metabolic acidosis a normal anion gap is characteristic of conditions related to bicarbonate loss with reten-

tion of chloride to maintain an ionic balance. This is called **hyperchloremic metabolic acidosis.** An elevated anion gap is characteristic of acidosis associated with accumulation of anions other than chloride (e.g., lactate and ketoacids) (Table 3-11).

Clinical Manifestations

Metabolic acidosis is manifested by changes in the neurologic, respiratory, gastrointestinal, and cardiovascular systems. Headache and lethargy are early symptoms, which progress to coma with severe acidosis. Deep, rapid respirations (Kussmaul's respirations) are indicative of respiratory compensation. Anorexia, nausea, vomiting, diarrhea, and abdominal discomfort are common. Severe acidosis can compromise ventricular contraction and produce life-threatening dysrhythmias.

TABLE 3-11 Causes of metabolic acidosis

Increased noncarbonic acids (elevated anion gap)	Bicarbonate loss (normal anion gap)
Increased H⁺ load	Diarrhea
Ketoacidosis (e.g., diabetes mellitus, starvation)	Ureterosigmoidoscopy
Lactaic acidosis (e.g., shock)	Renal failure
Ingestions (e.g., ammonium chloride, ethylene glycol, methanol, salicylates, paraldehyde)	Proximal renal tubule acidosis
Decreased H⁺ excretion	
Uremia	
Distal renal tubule acidosis	

Evaluation and Treatment

The diagnosis of metabolic acidosis is established from the health history, clinical symptoms, and laboratory findings. Arterial blood pH is below 7.35, and bicarbonate concentration is less than 24 mEq/L. The underlying condition must be diagnosed to establish effective treatment. During severe acidosis (pH ≤ 7.1), sodium bicarbonate administration is required to elevate the pH to a safe level.

Metabolic Alkalosis

Pathophysiology

Metabolic alkalosis occurs when there is an increase in bicarbonate, usually caused by excessive loss of metabolic acids. Among the conditions that can result in metabolic alkalosis are prolonged vomiting, gastrointestinal suctioning, excessive bicarbonate intake, hyperaldosteronism, and diuretic therapy.

When acid loss is due to vomiting with depletion of ECF and chloride, renal compensation is not very effective because the volume depletion and loss of electrolytes (Na^+, K^+, H^+, and Cl^-) stimulates a paradoxical response by the kidneys. The kidneys increase sodium and bicarbonate reabsorption with excretion of hydrogen. Bicarbonate is reabsorbed because the ECF chloride concentration is decreased. When the potassium concentration is depleted, hydrogen is excreted to maintain an electrochemical balance. The urine is acidic, and the reabsorbed bicarbonate prevents correction of the alkalosis. Correction is achieved when the ECF is expanded with a solution of sodium chloride and potassium. The volume replacement decreases the renal stimulus to reabsorb Na^+. Bicarbonate can then be lost in the urine and hydrogen ion excretion will decrease, correcting the pH.

Hyperaldosteronism has a pathophysiologic process different from the volume depletion that leads to hypochloremic alkalosis. With hyperaldosteronism, the excess aldosterone causes sodium retention and loss of hydrogen and potassium. Mild volume expansion ensues, and bicarbonate is retained with the sodium, causing alkalosis.

Diuretics such as thiazides, ethnacrynic acid, and furosemide produce mild alkalosis by enhancing sodium, potassium, and chloride excretion more than bicarbonate excretion.

Respiratory compensation for metabolic alkalosis occurs when the elevated pH inhibits the respiratory center. The rate and depth of ventilation is decreased, causing retention of carbon dioxide. The ratio of HCO_3^- to H_2CO_3 is reduced toward normal. Respiratory compensation is not very efficient, however, and chronic or severe metabolic alkalosis requires therapeutic intervention (Fig. 3-13).

Clinical Manifestation

Because of the many causes of metabolic alkalosis, the symptoms are varied. Some common symptoms, such as weakness, muscle cramps, and hyperactive reflexes, are related to volume depletion and electrolyte losses. Because alkalosis causes a decrease in ionized calcium, tetany may develop.

Respirations will be slow and shallow to increase carbon dioxide content. Confusions and convulsions occur with severe alkalosis. Atrial tachycardia is a potential problem. The oxyhemoglobin curve is shifted to the left (see Chapter 29), decreasing the dissociation of oxyhemoglobin and increasing the risk of dysrhythmias.

Evaluation and Treatment

The health history provides significant clues to the diagnosis of metabolic alkalosis. The arterial pH is above 7.45, and bicarbonate levels exceed 26 mEq/L. With respiratory compensation, the Pco_2 rises above 40 mm Hg. With hypochloremic alkalosis, serum chloride values are below normal. Potassium levels are usually depleted because hydrogen is released from the cells in exchange for potassium to help regulate the pH level. The K^+ is then secreted from the distal tubule or kidney cells into the urine.

With hypochloremic alkalosis or contraction alkalosis with volume depletion, a sodium chloride solution is required for correction. The renal stimulus to increase ECF volume by retaining Na^+ is diminished, and HCO_3^- can be excreted as $NaHCO_3$ in the urine. The administration of potassium corrects alkalosis caused by hyperaldosteronism or hypokalemia. The potassium causes hydrogen to move back into the ECF and decreases loss of hydrogen from the distal tubule.

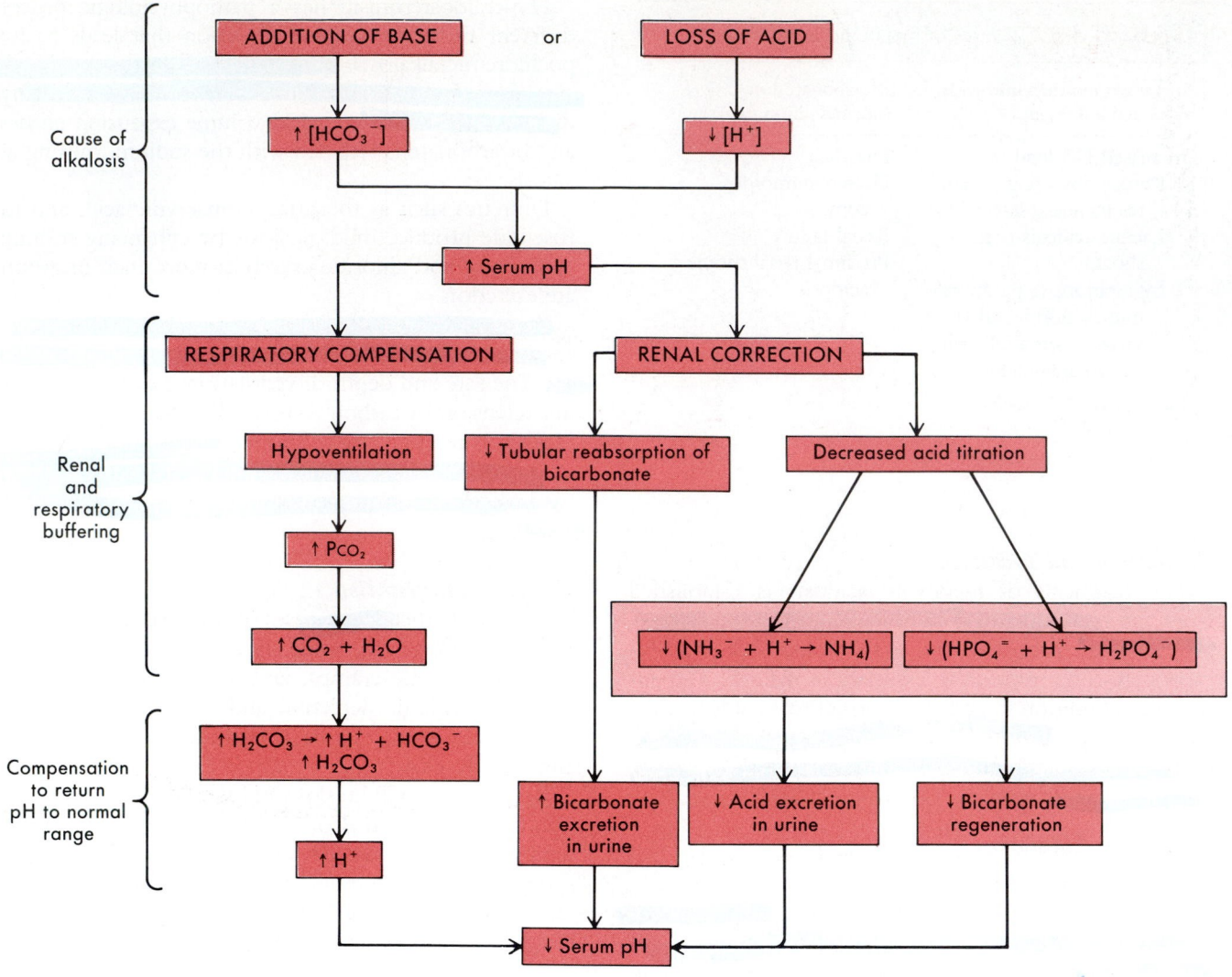

FIG. 3-13. Metabolic alkalosis with compensation and correction.

Respiratory Acidosis

Pathophysiology

Respiratory disorders of acid-base balance are due to increases or decreases of alveolar ventilation in relation to the metabolic production of carbon dioxide. Respiratory acidosis occurs when there is depression of ventilation. Carbon dioxide is retained, increasing $[H^+]$ and producing acidosis. Carbon dioxide excess is called **hypercapnia.** The common causes include depression of the respiratory center (brain stem trauma and oversedation), respiratory muscle paralysis, disorders of the chest wall (kyphoscoliosis, Pickwickian syndrome, and flail chest), and disorders of the lung parenchyma (pneumonia, pulmonary edema, emphysema, asthma, and bronchitis).

Respiratory acidosis may be acute or chronic. Airway obstruction is the most common cause of acute respiratory acidosis. Compensation for respiratory acidosis is not effective because the renal buffer mechanism takes time to function. Furthermore, the protein buffers provide marginal compensation, and HCO_3^- is not a good buffer for CO_2. Acute uncompensated respiratory acidosis is characterized by a decreased pH, elevated P_{CO_2}, and normal or slightly increased bicarbonate level.

Chronic respiratory acidosis is commonly associated with chronic obstructive pulmonary disease and deformities of the chest wall. Renal compensation is effective and is established over several days. The acidosis produced from CO_2 retention stimulates the kidney to secrete hydrogen ion and regenerate bicarbonate. Serum bicarbonate and arterial P_{CO_2} are elevated, and pH will be restored toward normal (Fig. 3-14).

Clinical Manifestations

The symptoms of respiratory acidosis are related to acuity of onset and severity of P_{CO_2} retention. Initial

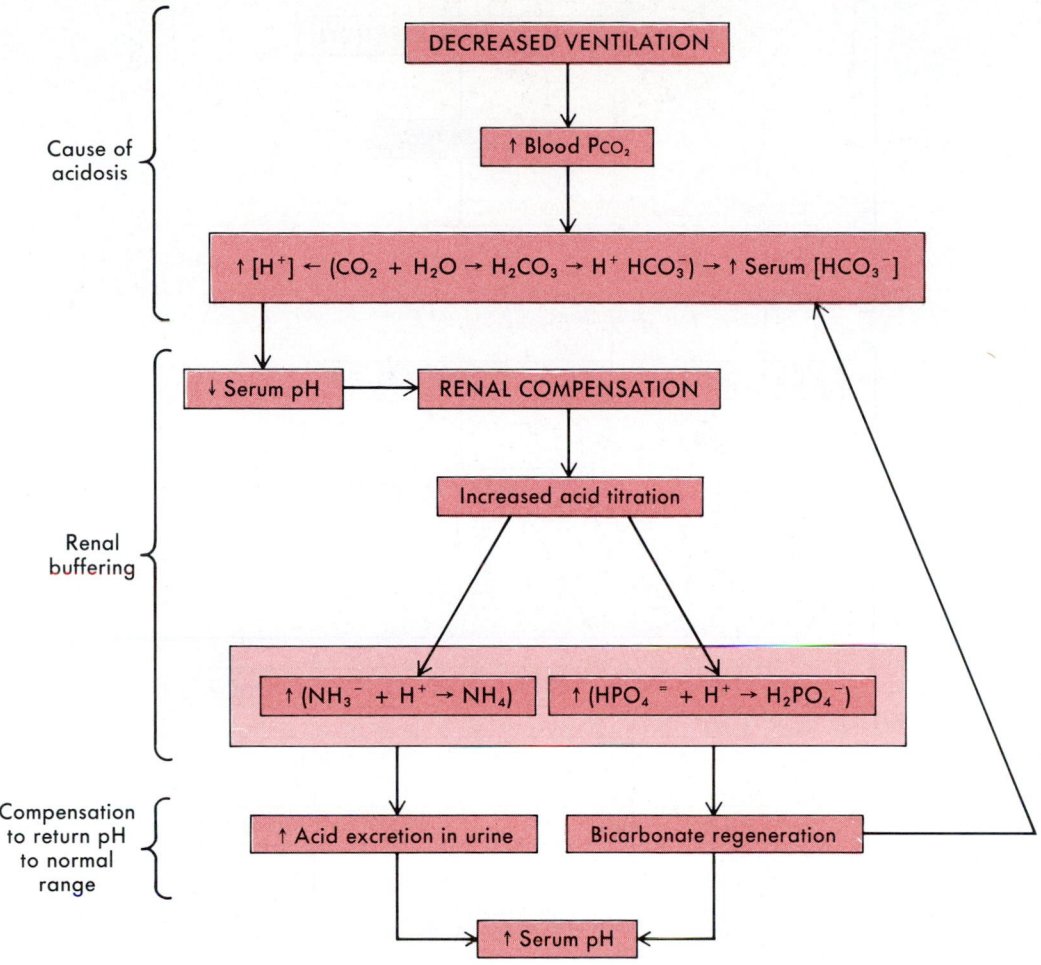

FIG. 3-14. Respiratory acidosis with compensation and correction.

symptoms include restlessness and apprehension followed by lethargy, muscle twitching, tremors, convulsions, and coma. Neurologic symptoms are due to a fall in the pH of cerebrospinal fluid and vasodilation because CO_2 readily crosses the blood-brain barrier. The respiratory rate is rapid at first and gradually becomes depressed because, over time, the respiratory center adapts to increasing levels of CO_2. Cyanosis does not occur unless there is an accompanying hypoxemia, and the skin may instead be pink from vasodilation caused by the acidosis.

Evaluation and Treatment

The primary diagnostic indicators are an arterial pH less than 7.35 and hypercapnia. Acute respiratory acidosis must be distinguished from chronic acidosis, the health history and clinical laboratory data are therefore helpful. With renal compensation, bicarbonate levels are elevated, and the pH is restored toward normal.

The restoration of adequate alveolar ventilation removes excess CO_2. If alveolar ventilation cannot be maintained spontaneously because of drug overdose or neuromuscular disorders, mechanical ventilation is required. The arterial pH, P_{CO_2}, P_{O_2}, and HCO_3^- must be carefully monitored. Rapid reduction of P_{CO_2} can cause respiratory alkalosis with seizures and death.

Renal buffering is usually effective in compensating for uncomplicated chronic respiratory acidosis. The underlying diseases are treated to achieve maximal ventilation. In the presence of hypoxemia and hypercapnia, oxygen can function as a respiratory depressant when the respiratory center is no longer stimulated by the lower pH and elevated P_{CO_2}. Therefore oxygen should be given cautiously.

Respiratory Alkalosis

Pathophysiology

Respiratory alkalosis occurs when there is alveolar hyperventilation and excessive reduction of carbon dioxide (termed **hypocapnia**). Stimulation of ventilation is precipitated by hypoxemia, which may be due to pulmonary disease, congestive heart failure, or high altitudes;

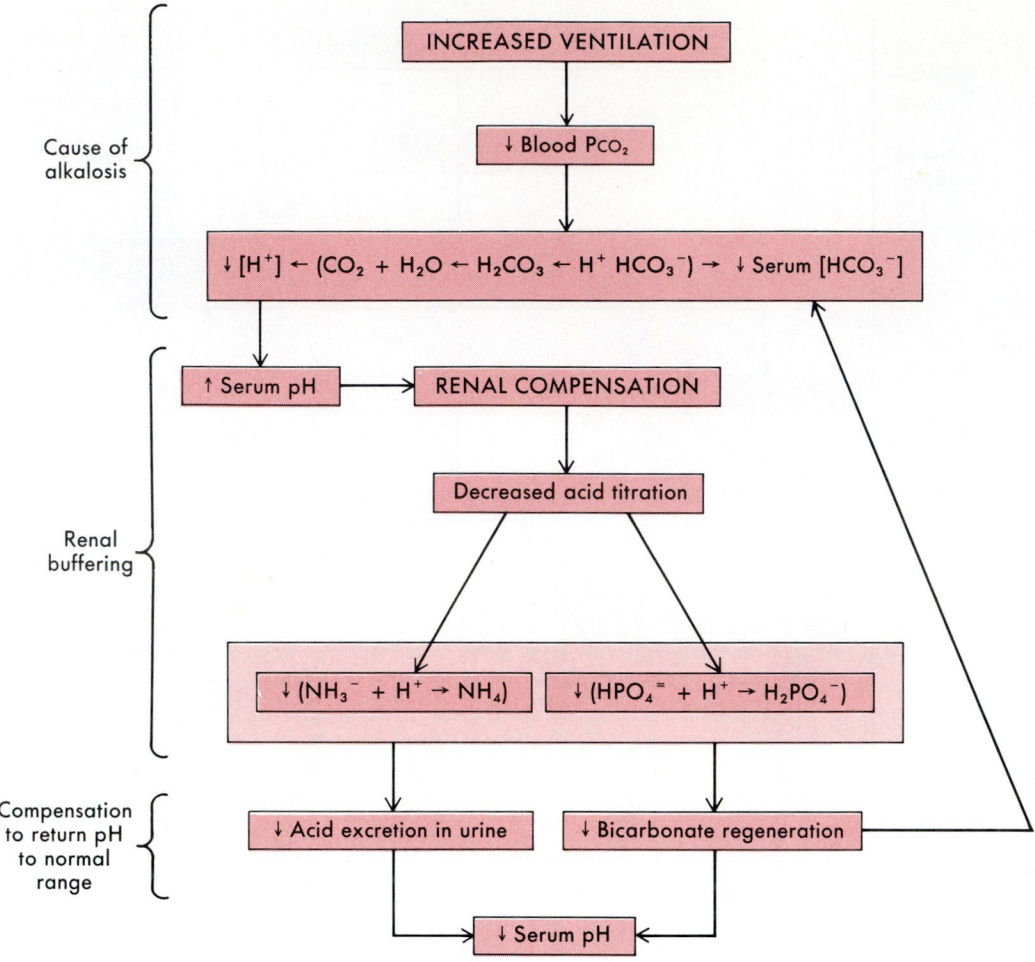

FIG. 3-15. Respiratory alkalosis with compensation and correction.

hypermetabolic states such as fever, anemia, and thyrotoxicosis; early salicylate intoxication; hysteria; cirrhosis; and gram-negative sepsis. Improper use of mechanical ventilators can cause iatrogenic respiratory alkalosis. Secondary respiratory alkalosis may develop from hyperventilation stimulated by metabolic or respiratory acidosis.

The onset of respiratory alkalosis occurs within minutes of hyperventilation. Cellular buffers provide immediate compensation with shifts of H^+ from ICF to ECF. The H^+ shifts are not very effective, however, if there is a significant decrease in P_{CO_2}. When there is chronic respiratory alkalosis, renal compensation restores pH toward normal by decreasing H^+ excretion and bicarbonate absorption (Fig. 3-15).

Clinical Manifestations

Respiratory alkalosis, like metabolic alkalosis, is irritating to the central and peripheral nervous system. Symptoms include dizziness, confusion, tingling of extremities (paresthesias), convulsions, and coma. Carpopedal spasm and other symptoms of hypocalcemia are seen similar to metabolic alkalosis. Deep and rapid respirations (tachypnea) are primary symptoms of respiratory alkalosis.

Evaluation and Treatment

The underlying disturbance must be identified. The arterial pH will be above 7.45, and the P_{CO_2} will be less than 38 mm Hg. In acute states, bicarbonate levels are normal. With chronic respiratory alkalosis, there is a compensatory decrease in the bicarbonate level and the pH is closer to normal.

Treating the underlying disturbance is the most effective treatment. Hypoxemia must be corrected and hypermetabolic states reversed. Symptoms from hysterical hyperventilation can be corrected by rebreathing from a paper bag, which increases the concentration of inspired carbon dioxide and reverses the respiratory alkalosis.

SUMMARY REVIEW

Distribution of Body Fluids

1 Body fluids are distributed among functional compartments and are classified as intracellular fluid (ICF) and extracellular fluid (ECF).
2 The sum of all fluids is the total body water (TBW), which varies with age and amount of body fat.
3 Water moves between the ICF and ECF compartments principally by osmosis.
4 Water moves between the plasma and interstitial fluid by osmosis and hydrostatic pressure, which occur across the capillary membrane.
5 Movement across the capillary wall is called net filtration and is described according to Starling's law.
6 Edema is a problem of fluid distribution that results in accumulation of fluid within the interstitial spaces.
7 The pathophysiologic process that leads to edema is related to an increase in forces favoring fluid filtration from the capillaries or lymphatic channels into the tissues.
8 Edema is caused by arterial dilation, venous obstruction, and increased vascular volume.
9 Edema may be localized or generalized and is usually associated with weight gain, swelling and puffiness, tighter-fitting clothes and shoes, and limited movement of the affected area.

Sodium, Chloride, and Water Balance

1 Sodium and water balance are intimately related; chloride levels are generally proportional to changes in sodium levels.
2 Water balance is regulated by the sensation of thirst and by antidiuretic hormone, which is initiated by an increase in plasma osmolality or a decrease in circulating blood volume.
3 Sodium balance is regulated by aldosterone, which increases reabsorption of sodium by the distal tubule of the kidney.
4 Renin and angiotensin are enzymes that promote or inhibit secretion of aldosterone and thus regulate sodium and water balance.
5 Atrial natriuretic hormone is also involved in decreasing tubular resorption and promoting urinary excretion of sodium.

Alterations in Sodium, Chloride, and Water Balance

1 Alterations in water balance may be classified as isotonic, hypertonic, or hypotonic.
2 Isotonic alterations occur when changes in TBW are accompanied by proportional changes in electrolytes.
3 Hypertonic alterations develop when the osmolality of the ECF is elevated above normal, usually because of an increased concentration of ECF sodium or a deficit of ECF water.
4 Hypernatremia (sodium levels greater than 147 mEq/L) may be caused by an acute increase in sodium or a loss of water.

5 Water deficit, or hypertonic dehydration, is rare but can be caused by lack of access to water, pure water losses, hyperventilation, in arid climates, and increased renal clearance.
6 Hyperchloremia is caused by an excess of sodium or a deficit of bicarbonate.
7 Hypotonic alterations occur when the osmolality of the ECF is less than normal.
8 Hyponatremia (serum sodium concentration less than 135 mEq/L) usually causes movement of water into cells.
9 Hyponatremia may be caused by sodium loss, inadequate sodium intake, or dilution of the body's sodium level.
10 Water excess is rare but can be caused by compulsive water drinking, decreased urine formation, or syndrome of inappropriate secretion of ADH.
11 Hypochloremia is usually the result of hyponatremia or elevated bicarbonate concentrations.

Alterations in Electrolyte Balance

1 Potassium is the predominant ICF ion; it functions to regulate ICF osmolality, maintain the resting membrane potential, and deposit glycogen in liver and skeletal muscle cells.
2 Potassium balance is regulated by the kidney, by aldosterone and insulin secretion, and by changes in pH.
3 A mechanism known as potassium adaptation allows the body to accommodate slowly increased levels of potassium intake.
4 Hypokalemia (serum potassium concentration less than 3.5 mEq/L) indicates loss of total body potassium, although ECF hypokalemia can develop without losses of total body potassium and plasma K^+ levels may be normal or elevated when total body potassium is depleted.
5 Hypokalemia may be caused by reduced potassium intake, increased ICF-to-ECF potassium concentration, loss of potassium from body stores, increased aldosterone secretion (e.g., caused by hypernatremia), and increased renal excretion.
6 Hyperkalemia (potassium levels that are greater than 5.5 mEq/L) may be caused by increased potassium intake, a shift from ICF to ECF potassium, or decreased renal excretion.
7 Calcium is a necessary ion in the structure of bones and teeth, in blood clotting, in hormone secretion and the function of cell receptors, and in membrane stability.
8 Phosphate acts as a buffer in acid-base regulation and provides energy for muscle contraction.
9 Calcium and phosphate concentrations are rigidly controlled by parathyroid hormone (PTH), vitamin D, and calcitonin.
10 Hypocalcemia (serum calcium concentration less than 8.5 mg/dl) is related to inadequate intestinal absorption, deposition of ionized calcium into bone or soft tissue, blood administration, or decreased PTH and vitamin D levels.
11 Hypercalcemia (serum calcium concentration greater than 12 mg/dl) can be caused by a number of diseases,

including hyperparathyroidism, bone metastases, sarcoidosis, and excess vitamin D.

12 Hypophosphatemia is usually caused by intestinal malabsorption and increased renal excretion of phosphate.

13 Hyperphosphatemia develops with acute or chronic renal failure with significant loss of glomerular filtration.

14 Magnesium is a major intracellular cation and is principally regulated by PTH.

15 Magensium functions in enzymatic reactions and often interacts with calcium at the cellular level.

16 Hypomagnesemia (serum magnesium concentrations less than 1.5 mEq/L) may be caused by malabsorption syndromes.

17 Hypermagnesemia (serum magnesium concentrations greater than 2.5 mEq/L) is rare and is usually due to renal failure.

Acid-Base Balance

1 Hydrogen ions, which maintain membrane integrity and the speed of enzymatic reactions, must be concentrated within a narrow range if the body is to function normally.

2 Hydrogen ion concentration is expressed as pH, which represents the negative logarithm of hydrogen ions in solution.

3 Different body fluids have different pH values.

4 The renal and respiratory systems, together with the body's buffer systems, are the principal regulators of acid-base balance.

5 Buffers are substances that can absorb excessive acid or base without a significant change in pH.

6 Buffers exist as acid-base pairs; the principal plasma buffers are carbonic acid-bicarbonate, protein (hemoglobin), and phosphate.

7 Buffer pairs can associate and dissociate; the pK value is the pH at which a buffer pair is half dissociated.

8 The lungs and kidneys act to compensate for changes in pH by increasing or decreasing ventilation and by producing more acidic or more alkaline urine.

9 Correction is a process different from compensation; correction occurs when the values for both components of the buffer pair are returned to normal.

10 Acid-base imbalances are caused by changes in the concentration of H^+ in the blood; an increase causes acidosis, and a decrease causes alkalosis.

11 An abnormal increase or decrease in bicarbonate concentration causes metabolic acidosis or metabolic alkalosis; changes in the rate of alveolar ventilation produce respiratory acidosis or respiratory alkalosis.

12 Metabolic acidosis is caused by an increase in noncarbonic acids or loss of bicarbonate from the extracellular fluid.

13 Metabolic alkalosis occurs with an increase in bicarbonate usually caused by loss of metabolic acids from conditions such as vomiting, gastrointestinal suctioning, excessive bicarbonate intake, hyperaldosteronism, and diuretic therapy.

14 Respiratory acidosis occurs with a decrease of alveolar ventilation and increase in levels of carbon dioxide, which in turn causes hypercapnia.

15 Respiratory alkalosis occurs with alveolar hyperventilation and excessive reduction of carbon dioxide, or hypocapnia.

KEY TERMS

Acidemia, 104

Acidosis, 105

Aldosterone, 88

Alkalemia, 105

Alkalosis, 105

Angiotensin I and II, 88

Aniongap, 106

Baroreceptors, 87

Buffers, 101

Chloride, 88

Compensation, 102

Compulsive water drinking, 92

Correction, 102

Dehydration, 90

Dilutional hyponatremia, 91

Edema, 85

Extracellular fluid, 83

Hypercalcemia, 99

Hypercapnia, 108

Hyperchloremia, 90

Hyperkalemia, 96

Hypermagesemia, 100

Hypernatremia, 89

Hyperphosphatemia, 100

Hyperpolarized, 95

Hypertonic hyponatremia, 91

Hypocalcemia, 98

Hypocapnia, 109

Hypochloremia, 92

Hypokalemia, 94

Hypomagnesemia, 100

Hyponatremia, 91

Hypophosphatemia, 99

Hypovolemia, 92

Inadequate intake, 91

Interstitial fluid, 83

Intracellular fluid, 83

Intravascular fluid, 83

Metabolic acidosis, 106

Metabolic alkalosis, 105

Natriuretic hormone, 88

Net filtration, 85

Nonvolatile, 101

Osmoreceptors, 87

Potassium adaptation, 94

Pure sodium deficits, 91

Renin, 88

Renin-angiotensin system, 88

Respiratory acidosis, 105

Respiratory alkalosis, 105

Starling's hypothesis, 85

Syndrome of inappropriate secretion of ADH (SIADH), 92

Total body water, 83

Volatile, 101

Water deficits, 90

REFERENCES

Berne, R. M., & Levy, M. N. (Eds.) (1988). *Physiology,* (2nd ed.). St. Louis: C. V. Mosby.)

Catehpole, M. (1982, October). Electrolytes, their physiological action and interaction: A review. *Journal of the American Association of Nurse Anesthetists,* 476-481.

Davenport, H. (1974). *The abc of acid-base chemistry* (6th ed.). Chicago: University of Chicago Press.

de Bold, A. J. (1982). Atrial natriuretic factor of the rat heart: Studies on isolation and properties. *Proceedings of the Society for Experimental Bioogy and Medicine, 170,* 133.

DuBose, T. D. (1982, July). Clinical approach to patients with acid-base disorders. *Medical Clinics of North America, 67*(4), 799-813.

Glass, L. B., & Jenkins, C. A. (1983, September). The ups and downs of serum pH. *Nursing 83, 13*(9), 34-41.

Groer, M. W. (1981). *Physiology and pathophysiology of the body fluids.* St. Louis: C. V. Mosby.

Hamilton, H. (Ed.) (1978). *Monitoring fluids and electrolytes precisely.* Horsham, PA: Nursing 78 Books, Intermed Communications.

Janusek, L. W. (1984, July). Metabolic acidosis: Physiology, signs and symptoms. *RN,* 44-45.

Knepil, J. (1983, April). Formation of acids. *Nursing Mirror,* 43-45.

Knepil, J. (1983, April). The buffering and excretion of acids. *Nursing Mirror,* 41-43.

Kokko, J. P., & Tanner, R. L. (1986). *Fluids and electrolytes.* Philadelphia: W. B. Saunders.

Krause, M. V., & Mahan, L. K. (1984). *Food, nutrition, and diet therapy: A textbook of nutritional care* (7th ed.). Philadelphia: W. B. Saunders.

Lane, G., & Poirce, A. G. (1982, January). When persistence pays off: Resolving the mystery of unexplained electrolyte imbalance. *Nursing 82, 12*(1).

Leaf, A., & Cotran, R. (1976). *Renal pathology.* New York: Oxford University Press.

Levy, I. J. (1977, June). Clinical problems in acid-base balance. *Journal of the American Association of Nurse Anesthetists,* 279-289.

Matheny, N. (1981, January). Preoperative fluid balance assessment. *AORN Journal, 33*(1), 51-56.

Maxwell, M. H., & Kleeman, C. (1980). *Clinical disorders of fluid and electrolyte metabolism.* New York: McGraw-Hill.

McBroom, M. J. (1977, February). Fundamentals of acid-base balance. *Journal of the American Association of Nurse Anesthetists,* 23-36.

Menzel, L. K. (1980, September). Clinical problems of electrolyte balance. *Nursing Clinics of North America, 15*(3), 559-576.

Menzel, L. K. (1980, September). Clinical problems of fluid balance. *Nusing Clinics of North America, 15*(3), 549-558.

Methaney, N. M., & Snively, W. D. (1979). *Nurses handbook of fluid balance.* Philadelphia: J. B. Lippincott.

Quinlan, M. (1984, April). Edema: What really causes it, how to control it. *RN,* 55-59.

Rose, D. B. (1977). *Clinical physiology of acid-base and electrolyte disorders.* New York: McGraw-Hill.

Smith, K. (1980). *Fluids and electrolytes: A conceptual approach.* New York: Churchill Livingstone.

Smith, L. H., & Thier, S. O. (1981). *Pathophysiology: The biological principles of disease.* Philadelphia: W. B. Saunders.

Thompson, J. M., McFarland, G. K., Hirsch, J. E., Tucker, S. M., & Bowens, A. C. (1986). *Clinical nursing.* St. Louis: C. V. Mosby.

Urranis, S. T. (1980, September). Physiology of body fluids. *Nursing Clinics of North America, 15*(3), 537-547.

Voda, A. (1970, December). Body water dynamics. *American Journal of Nursing, 70,* 2594-2601.

Winters, R. W. (1982). *Principles of pediatric fluid therapy* (2nd ed.). Boston: Little, Brown.

UNIT

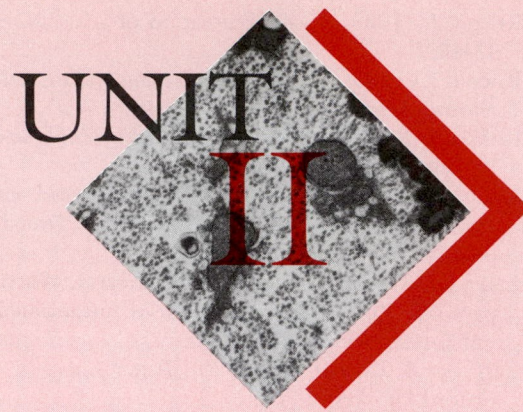

II

Genes and Gene-Environment Interaction

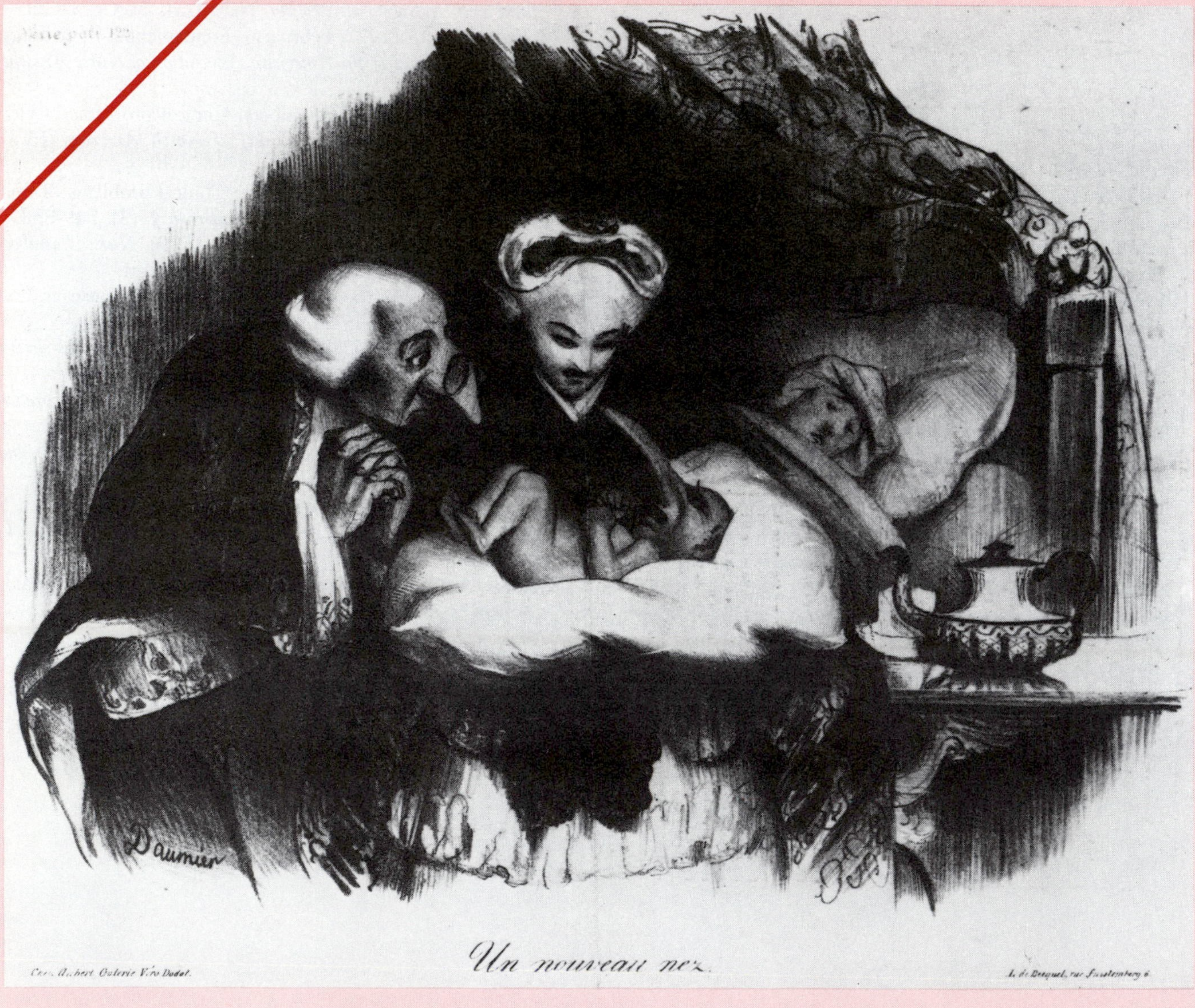

Un nouveau nez.

Caricature on hereditary traits. Courtesy National Library of Medicine.

GREGOR Mendel, an Austrian monk who lived in the nineteenth century, is usually credited as the father of genetics. The ancient Hebrews and Greeks and later scholars of the Middle Ages also observed many important genetic phenomena and proposed theories to account for them, but many of their theories were incorrect. Mendel's great contribution was to formulate several important principles of heredity through careful experimentation with living organisms. His laws of segregation and independent assortment form the foundation of modern genetics. Mendel's findings were published in 1865 in an obscure journal. They remained unnoticed until 1900, when they were simultaneously rediscovered by three scientists working independently in three different countries. One of the great ironies of biologic science is that Charles Darwin, the nineteenth-century founder of the theory of evolution, formulated his theories in complete ignorance of Mendel's discoveries.

The first decade after 1900 saw many important advances in genetics. Landsteiner discovered the ABO blood group in 1900. In 1902 Garrod reported on alkaptonuria, the first recognized "inborn error of metabolism." In 1907 Johannsen coined the term *gene* to denote the basic unit of inheritance.

The next four decades were a time of considerable theoretical work and experimentation. The fruit fly, *Drosophila*, became a mainstay of genetics laboratories and was also used by H. J. Muller to demonstrate the genetic effects of ionizing radiation. Many fundamental concepts of evolutionary genetics were developed by Ronald Fisher, Sewall Wright, and J. B. S. Haldane. The eugenics movement, which sought to "improve" the genetic quality of the human species through differential breeding, gained popularity in the 1920s and 1930s and then rapidly lost favor after the Nazi atrocities. The inheritance patterns of many important hereditary diseases, such as phenylketonuria, cystic fibrosis, and Huntington disease, were elucidated during this period.

The most significant development in genetics during the 1950s was the specification of the physical structure of deoxyribonucleic acid (DNA) by James Watson and Francis Crick (1953). Their work formed the basis for contemporary molecular genetics. Only in 1956, however, was the correct number of human chromosomes (46) identified by cytologists. Until then, it was thought that humans had 48 chromosomes. Three years later, Down syndrome was found to be caused by an extra twenty-first chromosome.

Since 1960 technologic developments in the form of computers and vastly improved laboratory facilities have spurred revolutionary progress in genetics. Laboratory analysis of proteins has demonstrated much more genetic variation in organisms than scientists once thought. Analysis of biochemical pathways involved in genetic diseases has pinpointed much more closely the specific defects responsible for the diseases. Increasing refinement of cytogenetic techniques has enabled researchers to uncover many new types of chromosomal abnormalities. By using elaborate statistical techniques, much has been learned about inheritance patterns of complex genetic diseases and about the interactions of genes and environment (see Chapter 5).

Perhaps the most rapidly progressing area of genetics is molecular genetics. The precise molecular defects involved in several genetic diseases have been discovered, greatly improving prospects for treating, and perhaps curing, those diseases. In addition, new molecular techniques have allowed scientists to identify the locations of many individual genes on each chromosome. This will greatly enhance the already important role of genetics in preventive health care.

CHAPTER 4

Genes and Genetic Diseases

Lynn B. Jorde

DNA, RNA, and proteins: heredity at the molecular level, 117
    DNA, 117
        Composition and structure of DNA, 117
        DNA as the genetic code, 117
        Replication of DNA, 120
        Mutation, 121
    From genes to proteins, 121
        Transcription, 122
        Gene splicing, 123
        Translation, 123
Chromosomes, 124
    X inactivation, 125
    Chromosome aberrations and associated diseases, 126
        Polyploidy, 126
        Aneuploidy, 126
            Autosomal aneuploidy, 128
            Sex chromosome aneuploidy, 129
        Abnormalities of chromosome structure, 131
            Deletions, 132
            Duplications, 132
            Inversions, 132
            Translocations, 133
Elements of population genetics, 133
    Phenotype and genotype, 133
    Dominance and recessiveness, 134
Transmission of genetic diseases, 134
    Autosomal dominant inheritance, 134
        Characteristics of pedigrees, 134
        Recurrence risks, 136
        Delayed age of onset, 136
        Penetrance and expressivity, 137
    Autosomal recessive inheritance, 137
        Characteristics of pedigrees, 137
        Recurrence risks, 138
        Consanguinity, 138
    X-linked inheritance, 139
        Characteristics of pedigrees, 139
        Recurrence risks, 139
        Sex-limited and sex-influenced traits, 139
    Evaluation of pedigrees, 140

Linkage analysis and gene mapping, 141
    Classical pedigree analysis, 141
    Complete human gene map: prospects and benefits, 143
Multifactorial inheritance, 147

In the nineteenth century, microscopic studies of cells led scientists to suspect that the nucleus of the cell contained the important mechanisms of inheritance. They found that chromatin, the substance that gives the nucleus a granular appearance, is observable in nondividing cells. Just before the cell divides, the chromatin condenses to form discrete, dark-staining organelles, which are called chromosomes. (Cell division is discussed in Chapter 1.) With the rediscovery of Mendel's important breeding experiments at the turn of this century, it soon became apparent that the chromosomes contained **genes,** the basic units of inheritance. Chromosomes were the subject of much study, but because of poorly developed laboratory techniques, progress was slow. Since the mid-1950s, however, technologic advances have permitted a rapid increase in scientific knowledge of the form, composition, and function of chromosomes.

The primary constituent of the chromatin is **deoxyribonucleic acid (DNA).** Genes are composed of sequences of DNA. By serving as the blueprints of proteins in the body, genes ultimately influence all aspects of body structure and function. **Structural genes** dictate the makeup of proteins, whereas **regulatory genes** initiate and terminate physiologic processes. Estimates suggest that there are approximately 50,000 structural genes. An error in one of these genes often leads to a recognizable genetic disease.

To date, nearly 4000 genetic conditions have been identified and catalogued (McKusick, 1986a). As infectious diseases come under increasingly effective control, the proportion of beds of pediatric hospitals occupied by children with genetic diseases has risen to one third (Hall et al., 1978). In addition, many common diseases that primarily affect adults, such as hypertension, coronary heart disease, diabetes, and cancer, are now known to have important genetic components. (These diseases are also affected by environmental factors. The interaction between genetic and environmental components is discussed in Chapter 5.)

Great progress is being made in diagnosis of genetic diseases and in the understanding of genetic mechanisms underlying them. With the huge strides being made in molecular genetics, "gene therapy"—the replacement of disease genes with normal ones—is becoming increasingly feasible. Genetics is now one of the most rapidly advancing fields of medicine.

DNA, RNA, AND PROTEINS: HEREDITY AT THE MOLECULAR LEVEL

DNA

Composition and Structure of DNA

Genes are composed of DNA, which has three basic components: the pentose sugar molecule, deoxyribose; a phosphate molecule; and four types of nitrogenous bases. Two of the bases, **cytosine** and **thymine,** are single carbon-nitrogen rings called **pyrimidines.** The other two bases, **adenine** and **guanine,** are double carbon-nitrogen rings called **purines.** The four bases are commonly represented by their first letters: *A, C, T,* and *G.*

One of Watson and Crick's contributions was to demonstrate how these molecules are physically assembled together as DNA. They proposed the now-famous **double-helix** model, in which DNA can be envisioned as a twisted ladder with chemical bonds as its rungs (Fig. 4-1). The two sides of the ladder are composed of the sugar and phosphate molecules, held together by strong phosphodiester bonds. Projecting from each side of the ladder, at regular intervals, are the nitrogenous bases. The base projecting from one side is bound to the base projecting from the other by a weak hydrogen bond. The nitrogenous bases therefore form the rungs of the ladder; adenine pairs with thymine, and guanine pairs with cytosine. Each DNA subunit—consisting of one deoxyribose molecule, one phosphate group, and one base—is called a **nucleotide.**

DNA as the Genetic Code

To serve as the basis of genetic inheritance, DNA must be able to direct the synthesis of all of the body's proteins. Proteins are composed of one or more **polypeptides** (intermediate protein compounds), which are in turn composed of sequences of **amino acids** (organic acids containing NH_2). The body contains 20 different

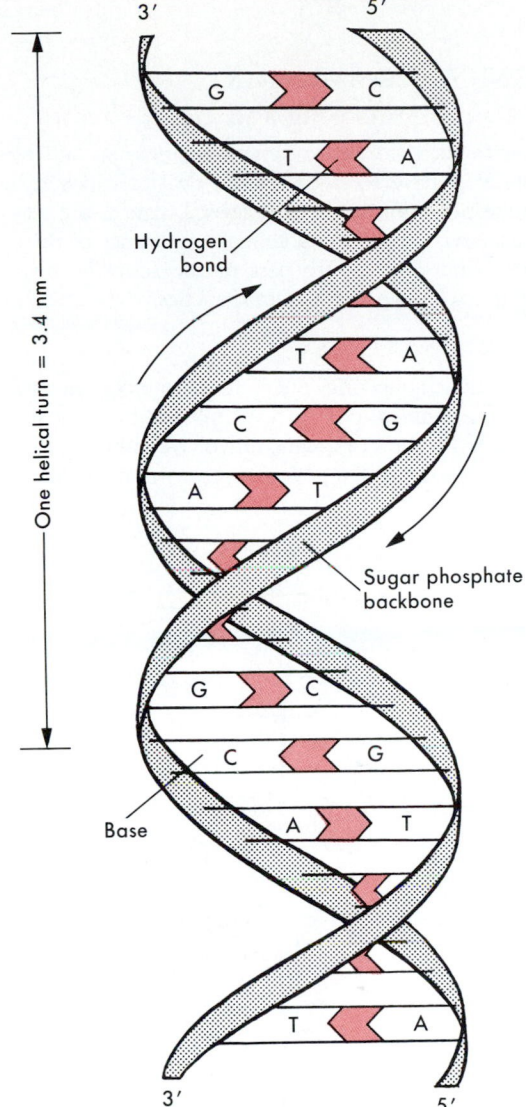

FIG. 4-1. Structure of the double helix that forms the DNA molecule. Sugar-phosphate bonds are the backbones of the two polynucleotide chains. The nitrogenous bases are in the center of the molecule and correspond to the "rungs" in the usual schematic representation of DNA.

types of amino acids, and the amino acid sequences that make up polypeptides must in some way be specified by the DNA molecule.

Because there are 20 possible amino acids and only 4 possible bases, each single nucleotide could not specify an amino acid. Similarly, the amino acids could not be specified by couplets of bases (e.g., adenine-guanine, thyamine-guanine, guanine-cytosine) because there are only 4 times 4, or 16, possible couplets. If series of three bases are translated into amino acids, however, there are 4 times 4 times 4, or 64, possible combinations—more than enough to specify each different amino acid. By manufacturing synthetic nucleotide se-

CLINICAL COMMENTARY

Genetic Engineering and Gene Therapy: The "New Genetics"

Terms such as *cloning, genetic engineering,* and *recombinant DNA* have received a great deal of exposure in the popular press during the past several years as the news media have recognized the potential importance of these techniques. Indeed they are part of the scientific revolution sometimes known as the "new genetics."

RECOMBINANT DNA

Genetic engineering refers to laboratory alteration of genes. Most alterations are accomplished by using recombinant DNA techniques, which involve combining the DNA of two or more different organisms. A number of sophisti-

cated methods have been invented to do this; described here is a common approach that is similar in principle to most other approaches.

Among the key components of recombinant DNA research are bacterial plasmids, small circular pieces of self-replicating DNA that reside in many bacteria but often are not essential to the growth or survival of the bacteria. Plasmids can therefore be extracted from or inserted into bacteria without seriously disrupting bacterial growth or reproduction. Once they are extracted from their bacterial hosts, the plasmids are exposed to restriction endonucleases, which are enzymes that cleave, or cut, the plasmid

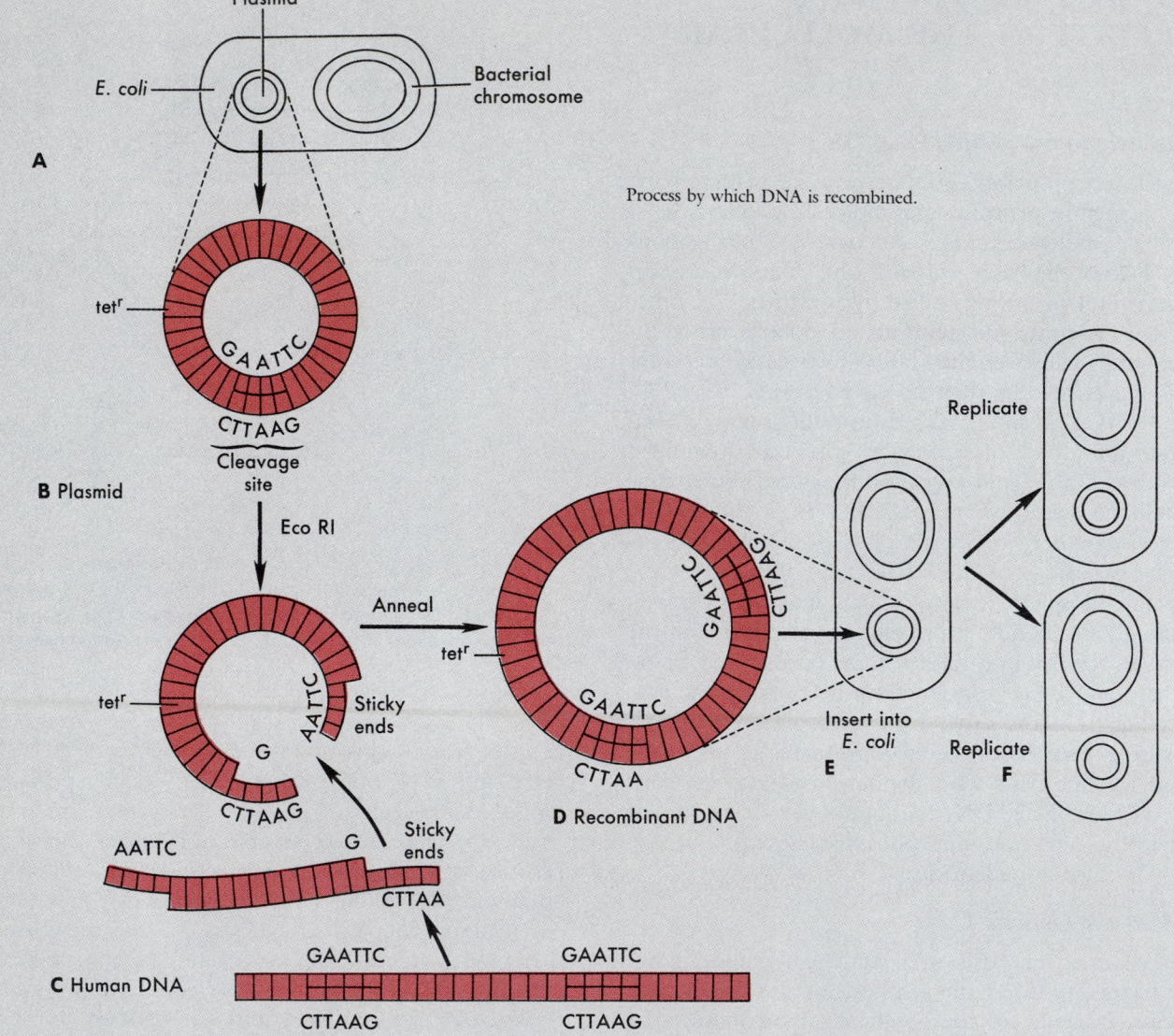

Process by which DNA is recombined.

DNA at a specific nucleotide sequence, called a restriction site.

Different restriction endonucleases have different restriction sites. A commonly used restriction endonuclease is called *Eco*RI (from the bacteria that produce it, *Escherichia coli*). *Eco*RI cleaves DNA only when the sequence GAATTC is found on one DNA strand and the complementary sequence is found on the other strand. The DNA of another organism, such as a human, can also be exposed to *Eco*RI and can be cleaved at the same restriction sites. The resulting human restriction fragments, which are pieces of DNA, have exposed ends that have base sequences complementary to those of the cleaved plasmid DNA. The human and plasmid DNA, if mixed together, undergo complementary base pairing (that is, they recombine).

The result is that the human DNA is incorporated within the plasmid. The plasmids, which now contain human genes in addition to their own, are allowed to reenter bacteria. Selection processes can be applied to pick out the bacteria that contain the desired human genes. These are cultured and allowed to form clones (or genetically identical copies) through normal cell division. Through continued cell division, millions of bacterial clones are formed, all containing the same human gene. Like any other gene, the human gene directs protein synthesis in the bacteria, resulting in the production of human proteins by bacteria.

Because bacteria multiply rapidly, large amounts of a given human protein can be manufactured by using this procedure. It has already been used successfully to produce human insulin in mass quantities. Because the insulin produced this way is actually human insulin, it produces fewer allergic reactions than the insulin taken from animal pancreases. Interferon, a substance that may help the body to fight cancer and viral infections, has also been produced this way, as has human growth hormone, a substance that can be used to cure pituitary dwarfism.

In trying to isolate a particular gene, it is often more convenient to begin work with the mRNA that codes for the gene product. The mRNA can be purified from body cells, and then an enzyme called reverse transcriptase can be used to generate the DNA sequence that is complementary to the mRNA. This complementary DNA (cDNA) can be inserted into plasmids and cloned by using the same recombinant techniques, so that virtually unlimited quantities of the desired gene product can be manufactured.

Recombinant DNA methods have been applied toward the understanding of the single-gene disorder phenylketonuria (PKU), which is the result of a lack of the enzyme phenylalanine hydroxylase. First, mRNA coding for this enzyme was purified from rat liver cells. After attachment of a radioactive "label" to cDNA produced from this mRNA, the cDNA was used as a probe. The probe was exposed to a series of cells that had been manipulated in the laboratory so that each cell line contained only one or a few chromosomes. When the probe hybridized consistently with only the cells containing chromosome 12, it proved that the gene that produces phenylalanine hydroxylase and thus causes PKU is located on this chromosome. Knowing the chromosome location of a gene is a very important step in the diagnosis and understanding of a genetic disease. Ultimately, therapeutic techniques might be developed to correct such disorders by replacing or repairing the abnormal gene.

The advent of this technology has led to fears that organisms that could pose grave threats to the human species might be created. In 1974 a group of molecular geneticists themselves called a moratorium on recombinant DNA research when its implications began to be realized; however, after much study and the introduction of rules regarding laboratory containment, research was resumed. Because of the elaborate precautions taken to prevent inadvertent creation of harmful organisms and because of the very low probability that such organisms could survive outside the laboratory, the possibility of such an event's ever occurring is now considered to be extremely remote.

GENE THERAPY

An area in which recombinant DNA techniques have generated a great deal of controversy is that of gene therapy, which essentially involves replacing defective genes with normal genes. For example, by recombinant DNA methods, a normal gene might be inserted into a human chromosome to counteract the effects of an abnormal or missing gene.

Gene therapy can be applied in two ways. The less controversial approach is somatic cell therapy, which consists of inserting normal genes into the cells of an individual who has a genetic disease. Here a particular tissue, such as bone marrow cells that produce abnormal erythrocytes, would be treated. More controversial is the application of gene therapy very early in embryonic development. By inserting genes into the embryos, all body cells could be altered, including the germ cells. Thus not only would the genetic constitution of the embryo and resulting individual be changed, but all of the descendants of that individual also would have altered genetic constitutions. This procedure is sometimes referred to as germ cell therapy. Neither somatic cell therapy nor germ cell therapy has been practiced successfully in humans, but results in laboratory animals indicate that both approaches may be feasible in the near future. The biologic, legal, and ethical implications of germ cell therapy clearly require careful scrutiny.

quences and allowing them to direct the formation of amino acids in the laboratory, it was proved that amino acids were specified by these triplets of bases, or **codons.**

Of the 64 possible codons, 3 signal the end of a gene and are known as **termination** or **nonsense codons.** The remaining 61 *all* specify amino acids; this means that most amino acids can be specified by more than 1 codon. The genetic code is thus said to be redundant, although each codon can specify only one amino acid.

Another significant feature of the genetic code is that it is universal: *all* living organisms use precisely the same DNA codes to specify proteins. The one known exception to this rule is in mitochondria, cytoplasmic organelles that are the sites of cellular respiration (see Chapter 1). The mitochondria have their own extranuclear DNA. Several codons of mitochondrial DNA code for different amino acids than do the same nuclear DNA codons.

Replication of DNA

In addition to being able to specify amino acid sequences, DNA must be able to replicate itself accurately during cell division if it is to serve as the basic genetic material. DNA replication consists basically of the breaking of the weak hydrogen bonds between the bases, leaving a single strand with each base unpaired. The consistent pairing of adenine with thymine and guanine with cytosine, known as **complementary base pairing,** is the key to accurate replication. The principle of complementary base pairing dictates that the unpaired base will attract a free nucleotide only if the nucleotide has the proper complementary base. Thus a portion of a single strand with a sequence of bases labeled ATTGCT will bond with a series of free nucleotides with the bases TAACGA. When replication is complete, a new double-stranded molecule identical to the original is formed (Fig. 4-2). The single strand is said to be a **template,** or molecule on which a complementary molecule is built, and is the basis for synthesizing the new double strand.

FIG. 4-2. Replication of DNA in which the two chains of the double helix separate and each chain serves as the template for a new complementary chain.

Several different proteins are involved in DNA replication. One protein unwinds the double helix, one holds the strands apart, and others perform other distinct functions. The most important of these proteins is an enzyme known as **DNA polymerase.** This enzyme travels along the single DNA strand, adding the correct nucleotides to the free end of the new strand. In addition to adding the new nucleotides, the DNA poly-

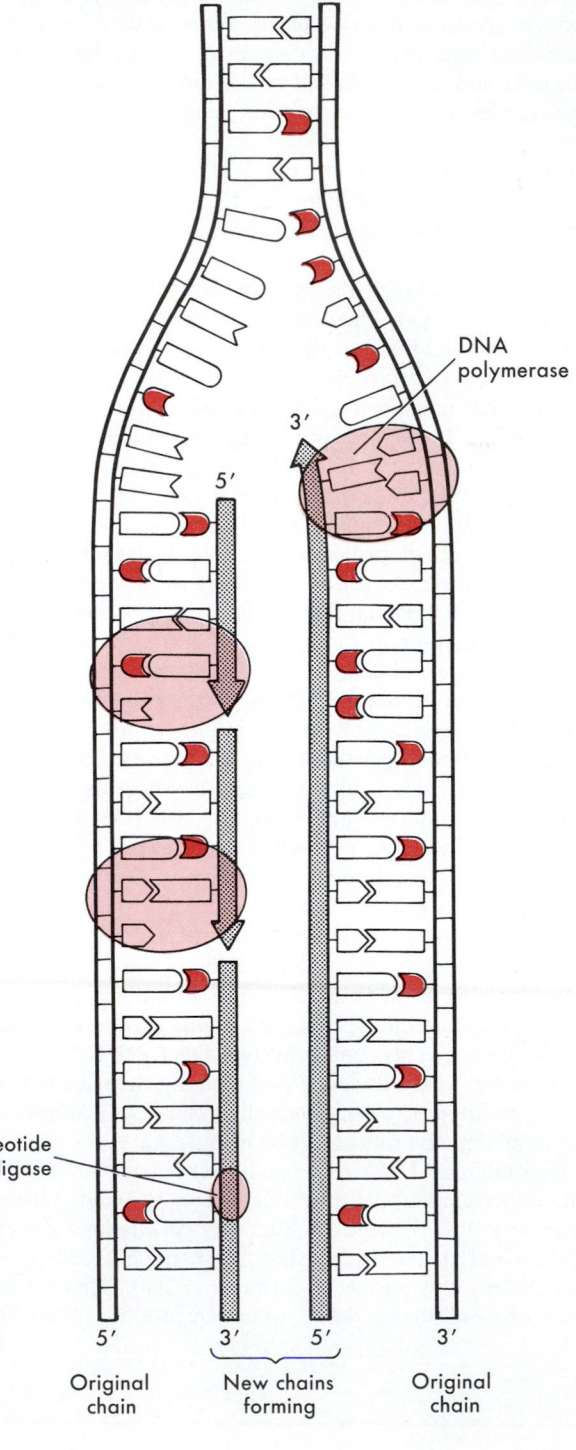

Cytosine

Adenine

Guanine

Thymine

DNA polymerase

Polynucleotide ligase

Original chain   New chains forming   Original chain

merase performs a proofreading procedure. After the new nucleotide is added to the chain, the DNA polymerase checks to make sure that its base is actually complementary to the template base. If it is not, the enzyme excises the incorrect nucleotide and replaces it with a correct one. This procedure, one of the mechanisms of DNA repair, substantially enhances the accuracy of DNA replication.

Mutation

A **mutation** is any inherited alteration of genetic material. Chromosome aberrations that cause congenital defects are examples of mutations. Other mutations are subtle and are not observable as chromosome aberrations. One such mutation is the **base pair substitution,** in which one base pair is replaced by another. This sometimes results in a change in amino acid sequence, but because of the redundancy of the genetic code, many of these mutations have no consequence. Such mutations are often called **silent substitutions.** Profound consequences can result, however, when an amino acid sequence is altered by a base pair substitution. (Many of the serious genetic diseases discussed later are the result of base pair substitutions.)

The second major type of mutation is the **frameshift mutation.** This involves the insertion or deletion of one or more base pairs to the DNA molecule. As Fig. 4-3 shows, these mutations can change the entire "reading frame" of the DNA sequence because codons consist of groups of three base pairs. A frameshift mutation thus can greatly alter the resulting amino acid sequence.

A large number of agents are known to increase the frequency of mutations. These are known collectively as **mutagens.** Radiation, such as that produced by x-rays and nuclear fallout, is an important mutagen and is known to cause cell damage (see Chapter 2). Radiation forms electrically charged ions that can produce chemical reactions that in turn change DNA bases. A variety of chemicals can also induce mutations, often because they are chemically similar to DNA bases. Other chemicals mimic the effects of ionizing radiation, and still others interfere with the process of base pairing. Hundreds of chemicals are now known to be mutagenic in humans and/or laboratory animals. Among these are nitrogen mustard, vinyl chloride, alkylating agents, formaldehyde, sodium nitrite, and saccharin. Some of these, however, are much more potent mutagens than others. Nitrogen mustard, for example, is extremely mutagenic, whereas saccharin is a relatively weak mutagen.

Measurement of the mutation rate in humans is difficult. This is due, in part, to the fact that mutations are very rare events. Current estimates are that the rate of **spontaneous mutation** (mutations that occur in the absence of exposure to known mutagens) in humans is about 10^{-4} to 10^{-7} per gene per generation. This rate appears to vary from one gene to another. Some areas of some chromosomes have particularly high mutation rates and are known as **mutational hot spots.**

From Genes to Proteins

Whereas DNA is formed and replicated in the cell nucleus, protein synthesis takes place in the cytoplasm. The transport of the DNA code from nucleus to cytoplasm and subsequent protein formation involves two basic processes, **transcription** and translation. Both of these processes are mediated by **ribonucleic acid (RNA),** a type of nucleic acid that is chemically very similar to DNA. RNA is also composed of sugar molecules, phosphate groups, and nitrogenous bases. RNA differs from DNA in that the sugar molecule is ribose rather than deoxyribose and in that uracil rather than thymine is one of the four bases. The other bases of RNA, as in DNA, are adenine, cytosine, and guanine. Uracil is structurally very similar to thymine, so it too

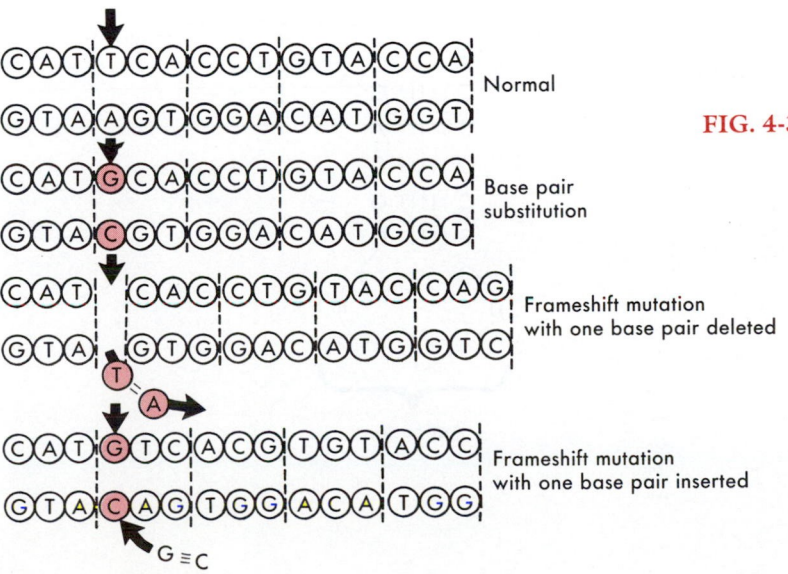

FIG. 4-3. Different kinds of mutations.

DNA chains   RNA chains

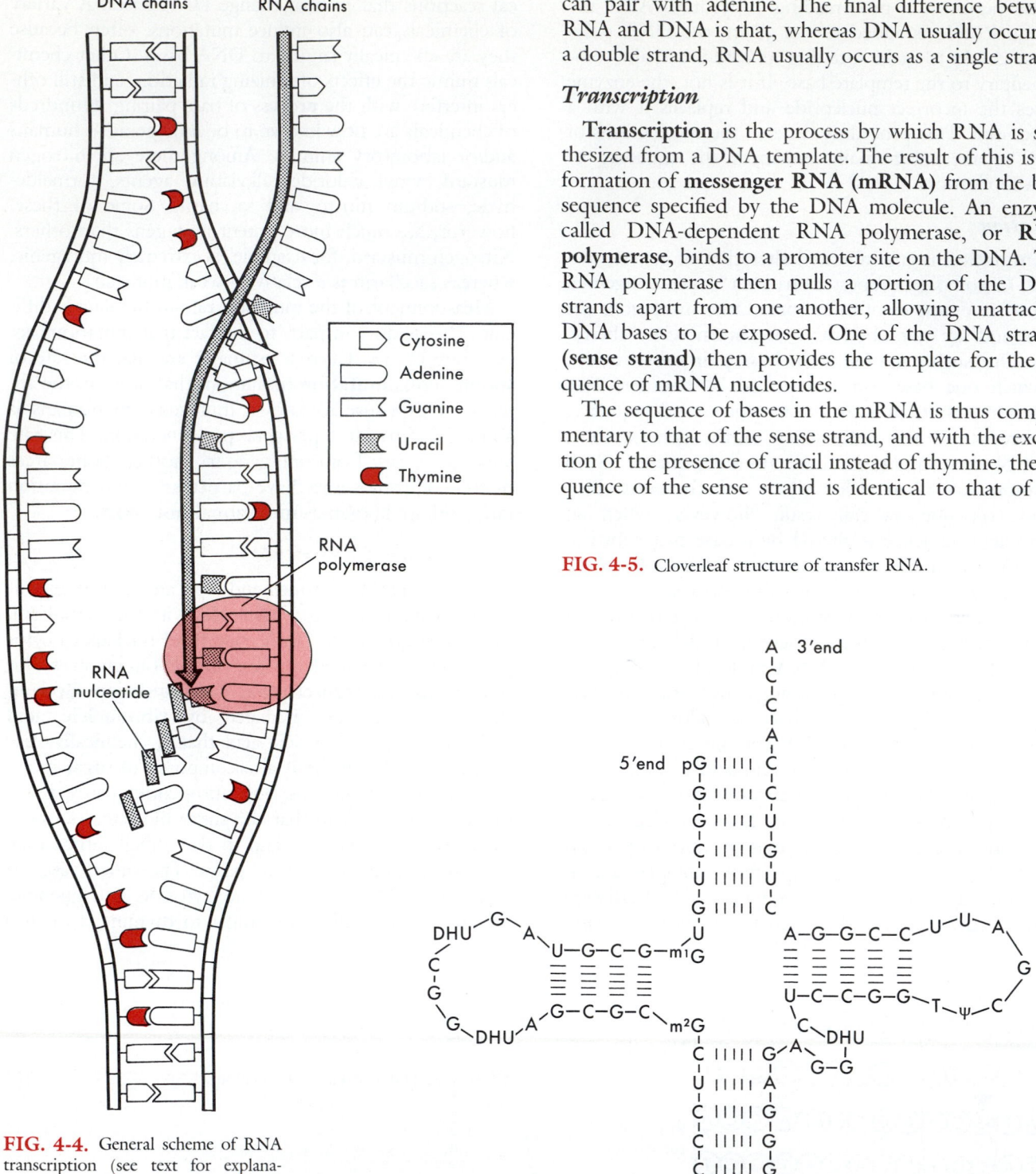

Cytosine

Adenine

Guanine

Uracil

Thymine

RNA polymerase

RNA nucleotide

FIG. 4-4. General scheme of RNA transcription (see text for explanation).

can pair with adenine. The final difference between RNA and DNA is that, whereas DNA usually occurs as a double strand, RNA usually occurs as a single strand.

Transcription

Transcription is the process by which RNA is synthesized from a DNA template. The result of this is the formation of **messenger RNA (mRNA)** from the base sequence specified by the DNA molecule. An enzyme called DNA-dependent RNA polymerase, or **RNA polymerase,** binds to a promoter site on the DNA. The RNA polymerase then pulls a portion of the DNA strands apart from one another, allowing unattached DNA bases to be exposed. One of the DNA strands **(sense strand)** then provides the template for the sequence of mRNA nucleotides.

The sequence of bases in the mRNA is thus complementary to that of the sense strand, and with the exception of the presence of uracil instead of thymine, the sequence of the sense strand is identical to that of the

FIG. 4-5. Cloverleaf structure of transfer RNA.

Anticodon

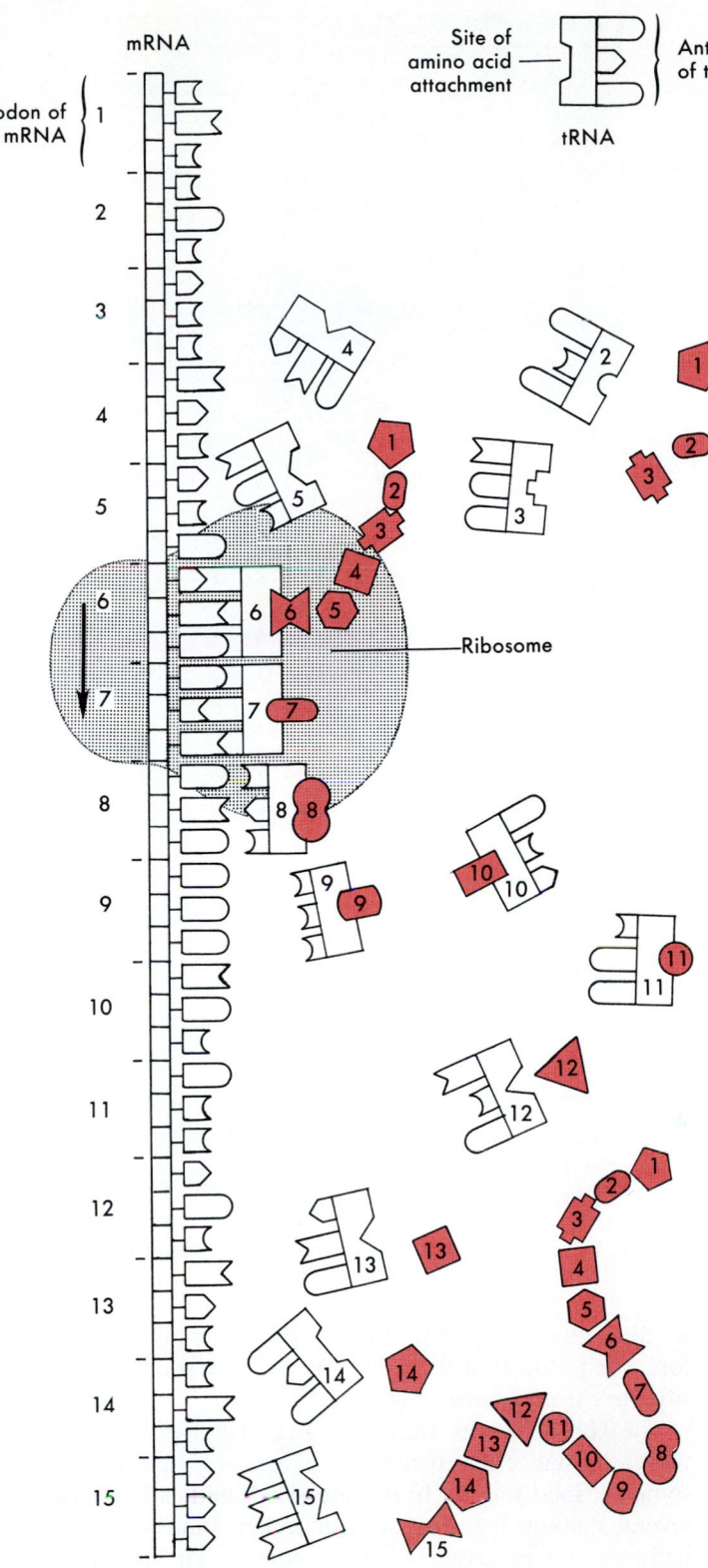

FIG. 4-6. A ribosome "reading" the code of mRNA and assembling a polypeptide chain.

plasm. The process of transcription is summarized in Fig. 4-4.

Gene Splicing

After the mRNA is first transcribed from the DNA template, it reflects exactly the base sequence of the DNA. The RNA in this state is sometimes called **heterogeneous nuclear RNA (hnRNA).** In eukaryotes an important step takes place before this RNA leaves the nucleus. Many of the RNA sequences are removed by nuclear enzymes, and the remaining sequences are spliced together to form the functional mRNA that will migrate to the cytoplasm.

The excised sequences are called **introns,** and the sequences that are left to code for proteins are called **exons.** The function of introns is not yet understood, although they are thought to be involved in the regulation of gene activity (i.e., activating and deactivating certain genes during various stages of the organism's development).

Translation

Translation is the process by which RNA directs the synthesis of a polypeptide. However, mRNA cannot code directly for amino acids. Instead, it interacts with **transfer RNA (tRNA),** a cloverleaf-shaped strand of about 80 nucleotides. As Fig. 4-5 illustrates, the tRNA molecule has a site for the attachment of an amino acid. At the opposite side of the cloverleaf is a sequence of three nucleotides called the **anticodon.** The anticodon undergoes complementary base pairing with an appropriate codon in the mRNA. The mRNA thus specifies the sequence of amino acids by acting through the tRNA.

The site of actual protein synthesis is the **ribosome,** which consists of roughly equal parts of protein and **ribosomal RNA (rRNA).** During translation, depicted in Fig. 4-6, the ribosome first binds to an initiation site on the mRNA sequence. The ribosome then binds the

other DNA strand **(antisense strand).** Transcription continues until a DNA sequence called a **termination sequence** is reached. Then the RNA polymerase detaches from the DNA and the transcribed mRNA is freed to move out of the nucleus and into the cyto-

tRNA to its surface so that base pairing can occur between tRNA and mRNA. The ribosome then moves along the mRNA sequence, codon by codon. As each codon is processed, an amino acid is translated by the interaction of mRNA and tRNA.

In this process the ribosome provides an enzyme that catalyzes the formation of covalent peptide bonds between the adjacent amino acids, resulting in a growing polypeptide. When the ribosome arrives at a termination signal on the mRNA sequence, translation and polypeptide formation cease. The mRNA, ribosome, and polypeptide separate from one another, and the polypeptide is released into the cytoplasm to perform its required function.

CHROMOSOMES

Human cells can be categorized into two types: the **gametes** (sperm and egg cells) and the **somatic cells,** which include all cells other than gametes. Each somatic cell has 46 chromosomes in its nucleus. These are **diploid cells,** meaning that the chromosomes occur in pairs. Thus, each cell actually contains 23 pairs of chromosomes. One member of each pair comes from the individual's mother, and one comes from the father. New somatic cells are formed through mitosis and cytokinesis, through which the cell nucleus and cytoplasm are replicated. (The division process that creates new copies of somatic cells is described in Chapter 1.) Gametes are **haploid cells:** they have only one member of each chromosome pair, giving them a total of 23 chromosomes. The process by which these haploid cells are formed from diploid cells is called **meiosis** and is illustrated in Fig. 4-7.

In 22 of the 23 chromosome pairs, the two members of each pair are virtually identical in microscopic appearance and are thus said to be **homologous** to one another. These 22 chromosome pairs are homologous in both males and females and are termed **autosomes.** The remaining pair of chromosomes, the **sex chromosomes,** consist of two homologous X chromosomes in females and a nonhomologous pair, X and Y, in males.

Fig. 4-8 illustrates a **metaphase spread,** which is a photograph of the chromosomes as they appear in the nucleus during metaphase. A **karyotype** is an ordered display of chromosomes. In Fig. 4-8 the chromosomes in this photograph are cut out and arranged according to size, with the **homologous chromosomes** paired together. The 22 autosomes are numbered according to length, with chromosome number 1 as the longest and chromosome 22 as the shortest. Some natural variation in relative chromosome length can be expected from person to person, however, so it is not always possible

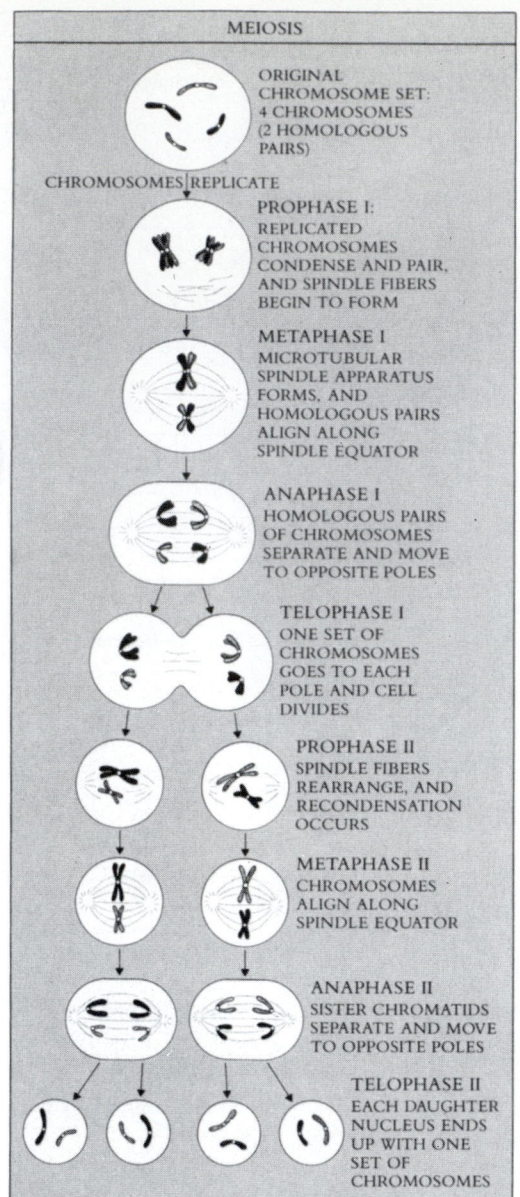

FIG. 4-7. Phases of meiosis. (From Raven & Johnson, 1989.)

to distinguish each chromosome by its length. Therefore, the position of the centromere is also used to classify the chromosomes (Fig. 4-9).

The chromosomes shown in Fig. 4-8 were stained with a substance that penetrates all areas of the chromosome (a "solid stain"). In the late 1960s and early 1970s several staining materials were found to bind preferentially to certain areas of chromosomes. The resulting distinctive **chromosome bands** are evident in various patterns in the different chromosomes, so that each chromosome can be distinguished easily. One of the most commonly used stains is **Giemsa stain.** By using banding techniques, chromosomes can be unambiguously numbered, and individual variation in chromo-

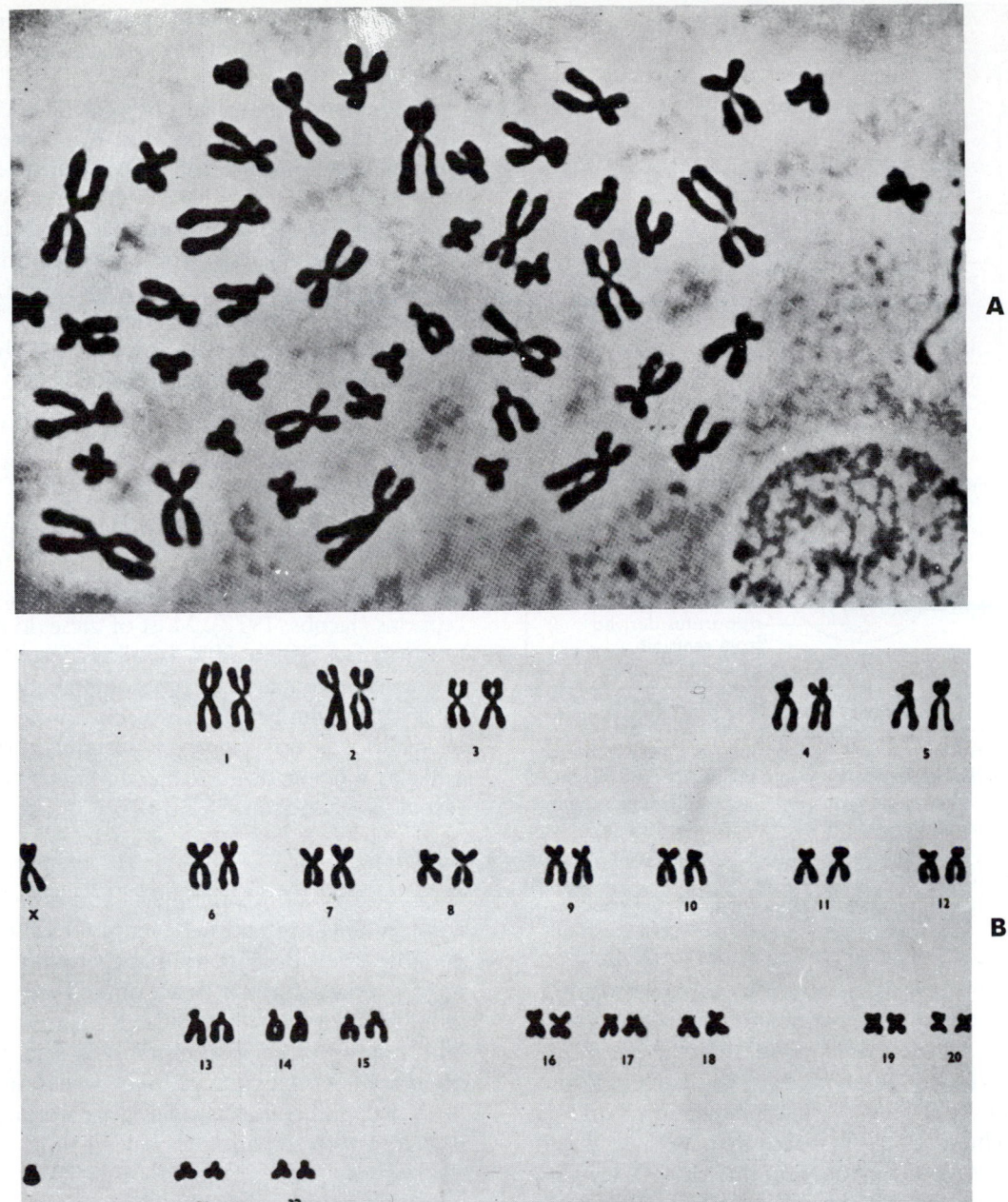

FIG. 4-8. **A,** Chromosomes of normal male (×2000). **B,** Karyotype of chromosomes seen in **A.** Chromosomes were obtained from a leukocyte or white blood cell taken from the blood of a male donor. (From Thibodeau, 1987.)

some composition can be studied. Missing or duplicated portions of chromosomes, which often result in serious diseases, can also be readily identified.

X Inactivation

In the late 1950s Mary Lyon proposed that one X chromosome in the somatic cells of females is permanently inactivated, a process termed X inactivation (Lyon, 1962). This proposal, known as the Lyon hypothesis, explains why most gene products coded by the X chromosome are present in equal amounts in males and females, even though males have only one X chromosome and females have two X chromosomes. This phenomenon is called **dosage compensation.** The inactivated X chromosomes are observable in many interphase cells as highly condensed intranuclear chromatin bodies, termed **Barr bodies** (after Barr and Bertram, who discovered them in the late 1940s). Normal females have one Barr body in each cell, whereas normal males have no Barr bodies.

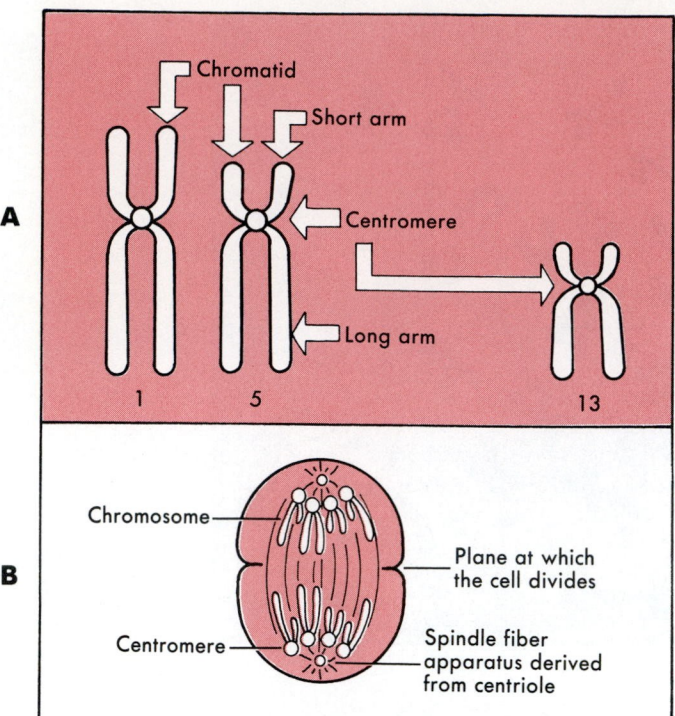

FIG. 4-9. A, Human chromosomes 1, 5, and 13. Each is replicated and consists of two chromatids. Chromosome 1 is a metacentric chromosome because the centromere is close to the middle; chromosome 5 is submetacentric because the centromere is set off from the middle; chromosome 13 is acrocentric because the centromere is at or very near the end. **B,** During mitosis the centromere divides, and the chromosomes move to opposite poles of the cell. At the time of centromere division, the chromatids are designated chromosomes.

The actual process of inactivation occurs very early in embryonic development, sometime after the 16-cell stage. In each somatic cell one of the two X chromosomes is inactivated. In some cells, the X chromosome contributed by the father is inactivated; in others, the maternal X chromosome is inactivated. Because the inactivation process is random, the maternal X chromosome is inactivated in approximately half of the cells, and the paternal X chromosome is inactivated in approximately half of the cells. Once the X chromosome is inactivated in a cell, all of the descendants of that cell have the same chromosome inactivated. Thus, inactivation is said to be *random* but *fixed*.

Some individuals do not have the normal number of X chromosomes in their somatic cells. For example, males with Klinefelter syndrome have at least two X chromosomes and one Y chromosome. These males *do* have one Barr body in each cell. Females whose cell nuclei have three X chromosomes have two Barr bodies in each cell, and females whose cell nuclei have four X chromosomes have three Barr bodies in each cell. Females with Turner syndrome have only one X chromosome and no Barr bodies. Thus the number of Barr bodies is always one less than the number of X chromosomes in the cell. All but one X chromosome is always inactivated.

Persons with abnormal numbers of X chromosomes, such as those with Turner and Klinefelter syndromes, are not physically normal. This presents a puzzle, because they presumably have only one active X chromosome, just like those with normal numbers of chromosomes. One hypothesis is that the abnormal number of chromosomes exerts some influence very early in embryogenesis, before inactivation occurs. Furthermore, the distal part of the short arm of the X chromosome is not inactivated. Thus X inactivation is also known to be *incomplete*.

Chromosome Aberrations and Associated Diseases

Some diseases result from abnormal chromosome number or structure. Estimates indicate that a major chromosome aberration occurs in at least 1 in 12 conceptions (Jacobs, 1977). Most of these do not survive to term; in fact, about 50% of all recovered spontaneous abortuses have major chromosome aberrations (Jacobs, 1977). The number of live births affected by these abnormalities is not, however, insignificant; about 1 in 150 has a major diagnosable chromosome abnormality (Hook & Hamerton, 1977).

Polyploidy

Cells that have a multiple of the normal number of chromosomes are said to be **euploid cells** (Greek *eu* = good or true). Because normal gametes are haploid and most normal somatic cells are diploid, these are both euploid forms. When a euploid cell has more than the diploid number of chromosomes, it is said to be a **polyploid cell.** Several types of body tissues, including liver, bronchial, and epithelial tissues, are normally polyploid. A zygote with somatic cells having three copies of each chromosome rather than the usual two has a form of polyploidy called **triploidy. Tetraploidy,** a condition in which euploid cells have 92 chromosomes, has also been observed. Both of these conditions are incompatible with postnatal survival. Nearly all triploid fetuses are spontaneously aborted or stillborn. A few have survived to term but have died shortly after birth. Tetraploidy has been found primarily in early abortuses, although a very few infants have been born alive. Like triploid infants, however, they do not survive.

Aneuploidy

A somatic cell that does not contain a multiple of 23 chromosomes is an **aneuploid cell.** A cell containing three copies of one chromosome is said to be trisomic (a condition termed **trisomy**) and is aneuploid. **Monosomy,** the presence of only one copy of a given chromo-

CLINICAL COMMENTARY
Prenatal Diagnosis of Chromosome Abnormalities

All of the chromosome abnormalities discussed here can be detected prenatally, using a procedure called *amniocentesis*. At about the sixteenth week of gestation, a sufficient amount of amniotic fluid is available to enable the withdrawal of a small amount of fluid (2 to 20 ml). This fluid contains live skin cells (fibroblasts) shed by the fetus. These cells can be cultured and karyotyped, and chromosome abnormalities can be detected.

Other disorders can be detected with this procedure. These include most neural tube defects, which cause an elevation of α-fetoprotein in the amniotic fluid, and more than 100 diseases caused by mutations of single genes. The procedure involves a risk of losing the fetus, estimated to be between 0.5% and 1%. Thus, amniocentesis is recommended only for pregnancies known to have an elevated risk for a genetic disease. These include pregnancies of women older than 35, in which the risk for Down syndrome and other aneuploidies is elevated, and pregnancies in which parents are known to carry translocations or certain disease genes.

One of the problems with prenatal diagnosis by amniocentesis is that by the time the sixteenth week of gestation is reached and another 2 or 3 weeks to culture the fibroblasts and test for genetic disease elapse, the mother is near the twentieth week of pregnancy. Abortion of an affected fetus at this stage can present serious emotional and personal dilemmas as well as some medical risk. For many parents, abortion would be more acceptable for a fetus at an earlier gestational age. A new technique, *chorionic villi biopsy,* consists of extracting a small amount of villous tissue directly from the chorion. This procedure can be performed at 8 weeks' gestation and does not require in vitro culturing of cells because sufficient numbers are directly available in the extracted tissue. Thus the procedure allows prenatal diagnosis at about 2 months' gestation rather than at nearly 5 months' gestation.

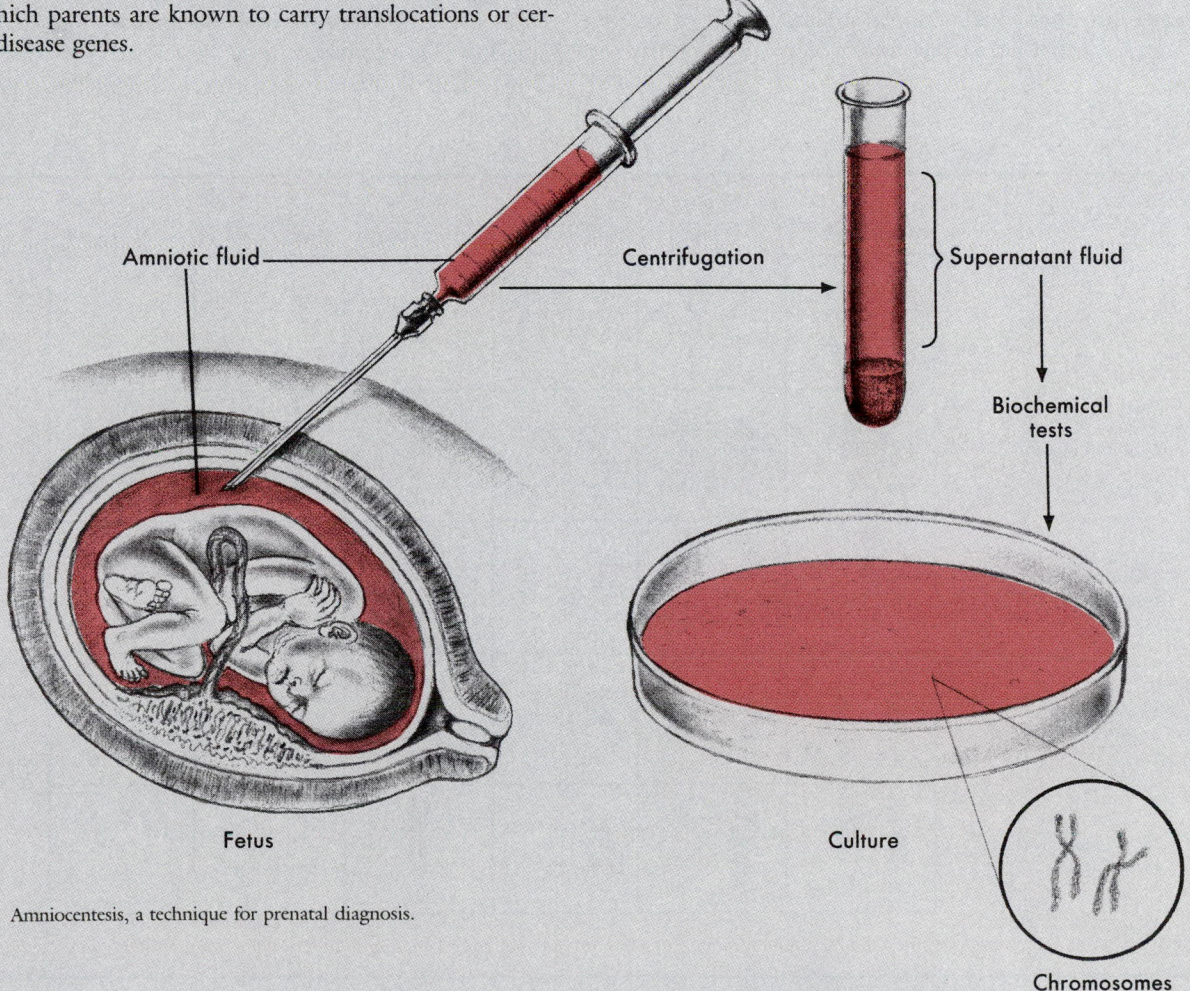

Amniotic fluid

Centrifugation

Supernatant fluid

Biochemical tests

Fetus

Culture

Chromosomes

Amniocentesis, a technique for prenatal diagnosis.

some in a diploid cell, is the other common form of aneuploidy. Among the autosomes, monosomy of any chromosome is lethal, but people with trisomy of some chromosomes can survive. This illustrates an important principle: *in general, loss of chromosome material has more serious consequences than duplication of chromosome material.*

Aneuploidy of the sex chromosomes is less serious than that of the autosomes. For the Y chromosome, this is true because very little genetic material seems to be located on this chromosome. For the X chromosome, inactivation of extra chromosomes largely diminishes their effect. A zygote bearing *no* X chromosome, however, will not survive.

Aneuploidy is the result of **nondisjunction,** an error in which homologous chromosomes or sister chromatids fail to separate normally during meiosis or mitosis (Fig. 4-10). Nondisjunction during either stage of meiosis produces some gametes that have two copies of a given chromosome and others that have no copies of the chromosome. When such gametes unite with normal haploid gametes, the resulting zygote is monosomic or trisomic for that chromosome. Occasionally, a cell can be monosomic or trisomic for more than one chromosome.

Autosomal Aneuploidy

Trisomy can occur for any chromosome, but the only forms seen with an appreciable frequency in live births are trisomies of the thirteenth, eighteenth, or twenty-first chromosomes. Fetuses with most other chromosomal trisomies never survive to term. Trisomy 16, for example, is the most commonly known trisomy among abortuses, but it is not seen in live births (Hassold & Jacobs, 1984).

Partial trisomy, in which only an extra portion of a chromosome is present in each cell, can also occur. As one would expect, the consequences of partial trisomies are not as severe as those of complete trisomies. Trisomies may also occur in only some cells of the body. Such individuals are said to be **chromosomal mosaics,** meaning that the body has two or more different cell lines, each of which has a different karyotype. Mosaics are usually formed by early mitotic nondisjunction. Nondisjunction occurs in one embryo cell but not in others.

The best known example of aneuploidy in an autosome is trisomy of the twenty-first chromosome, which causes trisomy 21 or **Down syndrome** (named after J. Langdon Down, who first described the disease in 1866). This disease was formerly called "mongolism,"

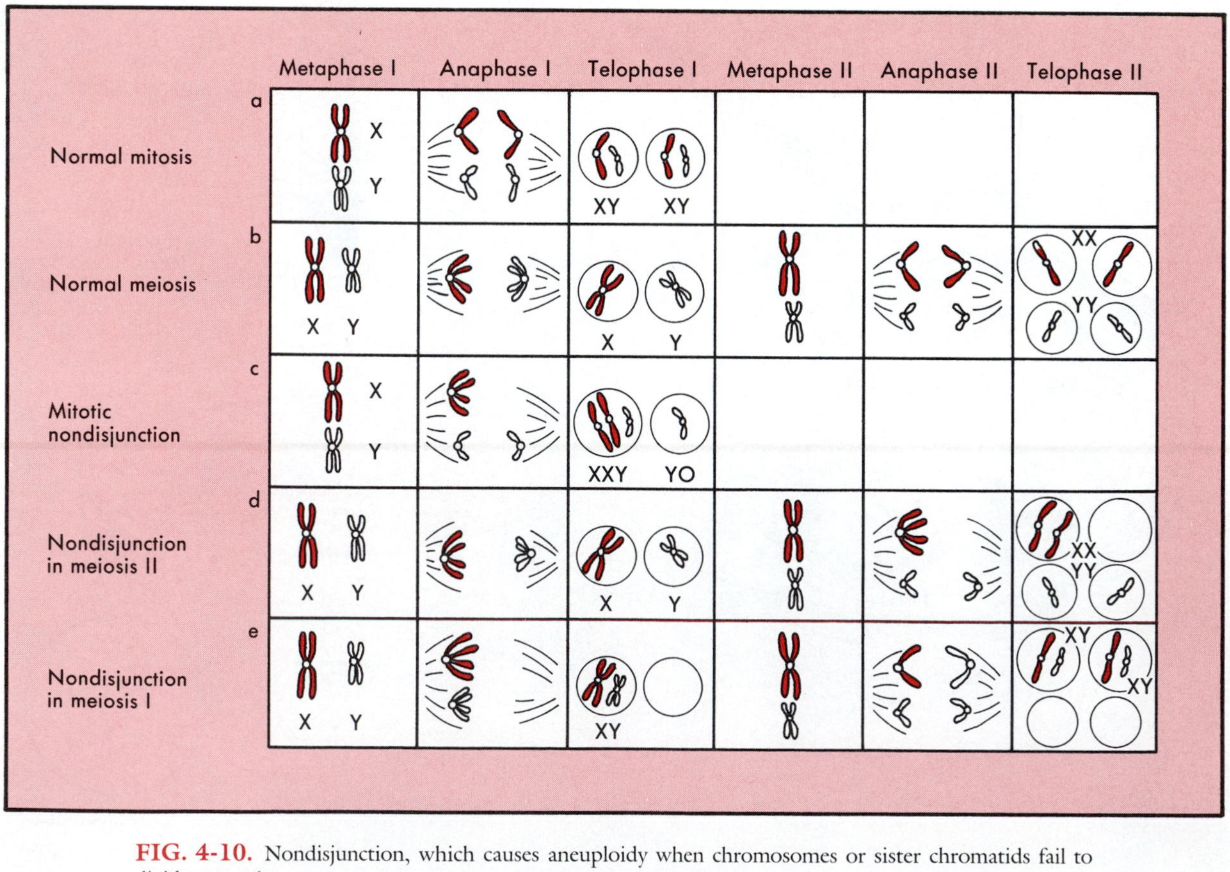

FIG. 4-10. Nondisjunction, which causes aneuploidy when chromosomes or sister chromatids fail to divide properly.

but because of its racist connotations, this term is no longer used. Down syndrome is seen in 1 in 800 live births (Hassold & Jacobs, 1984). Individuals with this disease are mentally retarded, with intelligence quotients (IQs) usually ranging from 25 to 50. The facial appearance is distinctive (Fig. 4-11), with a low nasal bridge, epicanthal folds (which produce the superficially Oriental appearance), protruding tongue, and flat, low-set ears. Poor muscle tone (hypotonia) and short stature are both characteristic. Congenital heart defects affect about one third of live-born children with Down syndrome; a reduced ability to fight respiratory infections and an increased susceptibility to leukemia also contribute to reduced survival rate. About three fourths of fetuses known to have Down syndrome are spontaneously aborted or stillborn. About 20% of babies born with Down syndrome die during their first 10 years of life. Average life expectancy is now a little less than 60 years.

About 97% of Down syndrome cases are due to nondisjunction during the formation of one of the parent's gametes or during early embryonic development. The remaining 3% are due to translocations (discussed later). In approximately three fourths of cases, the nondisjunction occurs in the formation of the mother's egg cell. Paternal nondisjunction is responsible for the other one fourth. Among individuals with Down syndrome, about 1% are known to be mosaics. Because mosaics have a large number of normal cells, the effects of the trisomic cells are attenuated and symptoms are generally less severe.

The risk of having a child with Down syndrome increases greatly with maternal age. As Fig. 4-12 demonstrates, women under the age of 30 have a risk ranging from about 1 in 1000 births to 1 in 2000 births. The risk begins to rise substantially after age 35, and it reaches a figure of 1 in 16 (6%) for women over the age of 45. This dramatic increase in risk may be caused by the age of maternal egg cells, which are held in an arrested state of prophase I from the time they are formed in the female embryo until they are shed in ovulation. Thus, an egg cell formed by a 45-year-old woman is itself 45 years old. This long suspended state may allow for the accumulation of errors leading to nondisjunction. Statistical studies have demonstrated that the age of the father has little, if any, effect on the risk of Down syndrome (Roth et al., 1983).

Sex Chromosome Aneuploidy

The incidence of sex chromosome aneuploidies is fairly high. Among live births, about 1 in 400 males and 1 in 650 females has a form of sex chromosome aneuploidy (Hartl, 1983). Because these conditions are generally less severe than autosomal aneuploidies, all forms except complete absence of an X chromosome allow at least some individuals to survive.

One of the most common sex chromosome aneuploidies, affecting about 1 in 950 newborn females, is trisomy X. Instead of two X chromosomes, these females have three X chromosomes in each cell. Most of them have no overt physical abnormalities, although ste-

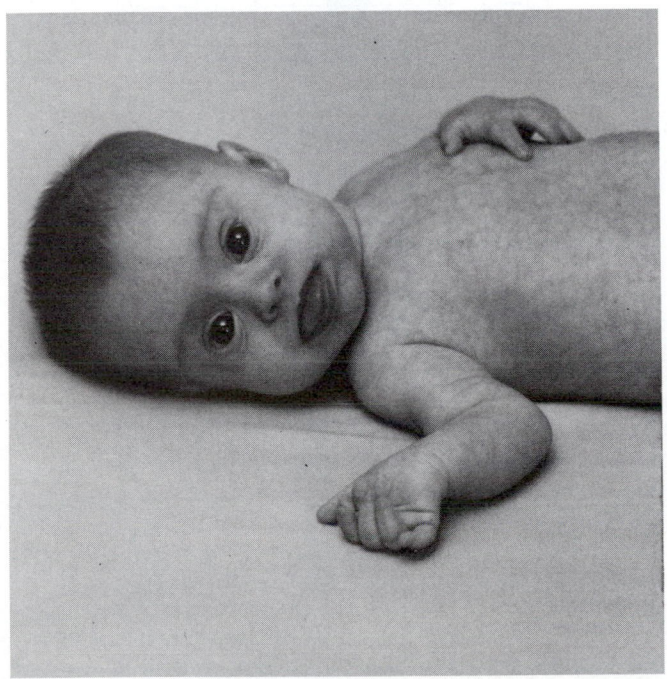

FIG. 4-11. Down syndrome (trisomy 21). (From Whaley & Wong, 1987.)

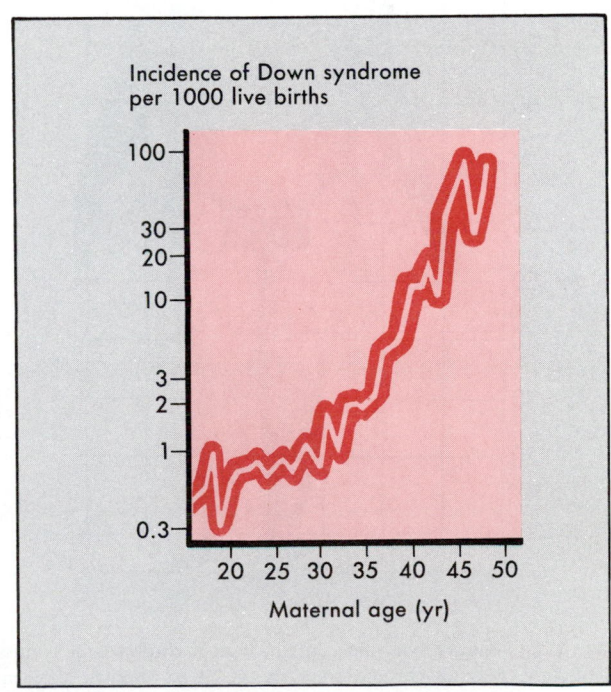

Incidence of Down syndrome per 1000 live births

FIG. 4-12. Rate of Down syndrome per 1000 live births related to maternal age.

rility, menstrual irregularity, or mental retardation are sometimes seen. Some females have four X chromosomes, and they are more often mentally retarded. Those with five or more X chromosomes generally have more severe mental retardation and various physical defects.

A condition that leads to somewhat more serious problems is the presence of a single X chromosome and no homologous X or Y chromosome, so that the individual has a total of 45 chromosomes. The karyotype is usually designated XO, and it causes a set of symptoms known as **Turner syndrome** (Fig. 4-13). Because they have no Y chromosomes, people with Turner syndrome are females. They are sterile, however, and have gonadal streaks rather than ovaries. These streaks of connective tissue are highly susceptible to cancer. Other features of the disorder include short stature, characteristic webbing of the neck, widely spaced nipples, coarctation (narrowing) of the aorta, edema of the feet in newborns, reduced carrying angle at the elbow (cubitus valgus), and sparse body hair. They are not considered retarded, although there is evidence for some impairment of spatial and mathematical reasoning ability. About

three fourths of recognized XO conceptions inherit their X chromosome from their mother. Thus, most cases are due to a **meiotic failure** in the father.

The frequency of Turner syndrome is low compared to that of other sex chromosome aneuploidies: only about 1 in 5000 newborn females is affected (Jacobs, 1977). The XO karyotype is extremely common among conceptions, however, and about 15% to 20% of spontaneous abortions with chromosome abnormalities have this karyotype, making it one of the most common single-chromosome aberrations. Thus the condition is highly lethal during gestation: only about 0.5% of XO conceptions survive to term. The condition may be relatively benign among live-born females because many or most of these individuals are mosaics. Combinations of XO cells with XX, XXX, or XY cells are common among those with Turner syndrome.

Individuals with at least two X chromosomes and a Y chromosome in each cell (XXY karyotype) have a disorder known as **Klinefelter syndrome** (Fig. 4-14). Because of the presence of a Y chromosome, these individuals have a male appearance, but they are sterile, and about half develop femalelike breasts (a condition called gynecomastia). The testicles are small and firm, body hair is sparse, the voice is often somewhat high pitched, and there may be a moderate degree of mental impair-

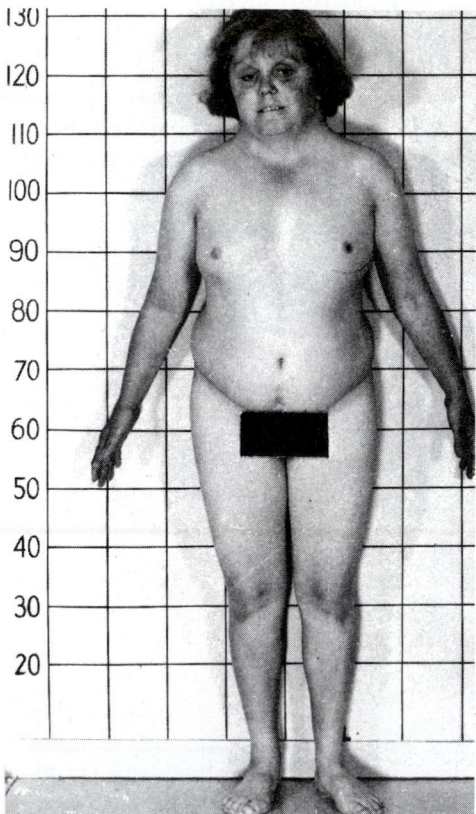

FIG. 4-13. Turner syndrome, in which an X chromosome is missing and the person's chromosomes are XO. Characteristic signs are short stature, female genitalia, webbed neck, shieldlike chest with underdeveloped breasts and widely spaced nipples and imperfectly developed ovaries. (From Goodman & Gorlin, 1977.)

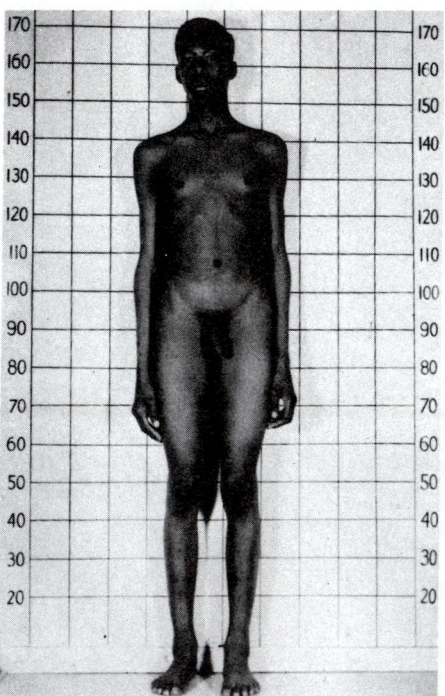

FIG. 4-14. Klinefelter syndrome, in which the person carries an extra X chromosome and is XXY. Characteristic signs are normal male genitalia but with small testicles, sparse body hair, some female breast development, and a rather female body shape. (From Whaley & Wong, 1987.)

ment. Klinefelter syndrome is found in about 1 out of 1000 male births. About two thirds of the cases are due to nondisjunction of the X chromosomes in the mother, and the frequency of the disorder rises with maternal age. Individuals with the XXXY and XXXXY karyotypes are also considered to have Klinefelter syndrome, and the degree of physical and mental impairment increases with each additional X chromosome. Regardless of the number of X chromosomes, however, these individuals have a male appearance. The presence of a single Y chromosome, which causes the undifferentiated gonads to become testes, always produces a male. As in Turner syndrome, mosaicism is fairly common; the most prevalent combination is XXY and XY cells.

Abnormalities of Chromosome Structure

In addition to the loss or gain of whole chromosomes, parts of chromosomes can be lost or duplicated as gametes are formed, and the arrangement of genes on chromosomes can be altered. Unlike aneuploidy and polyploidy, these changes sometimes do not have serious consequences for an individual's health. Some of them can even go entirely unnoticed, especially when very small pieces of chromosomes are involved. Nevertheless, abnormalities of chromosome structure can also produce serious disease in individuals or their offspring.

During meiosis and mitosis, chromosomes usually maintain their structural integrity very well, but **chromosome breakage** does occasionally occur. Mechanisms exist to "heal" these breaks, and generally the break is repaired perfectly with no damage resulting to the daughter cell. Sometimes, however, the breaks remain, or they heal in a fashion that alters the structure of the chromosome. The extent of chromosome breakage is increased in the presence of certain harmful agents, called **clastogens.** Identified clastogens include

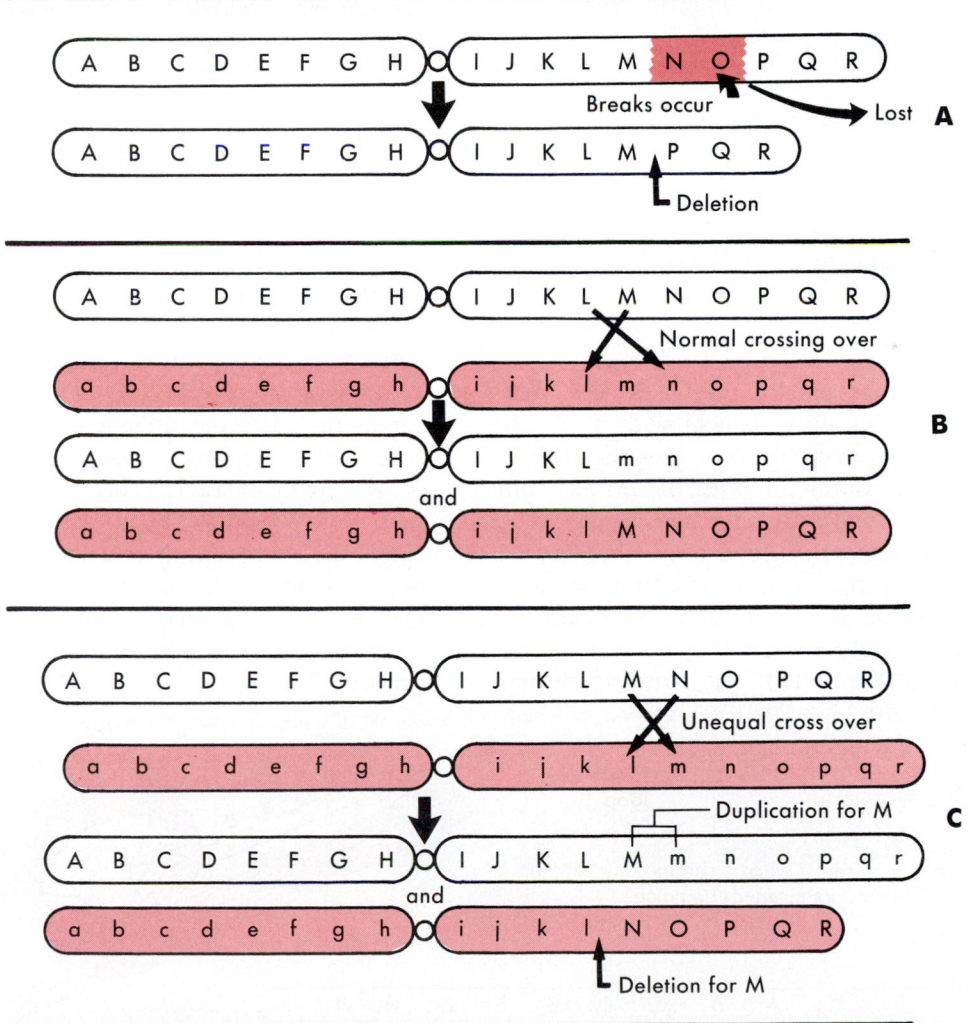

FIG. 4-15. **A,** Deletion occurs when a chromosome segment is lost. **B,** Normal crossing-over. **C,** The generation of duplication and deletion through unequal crossing-over.

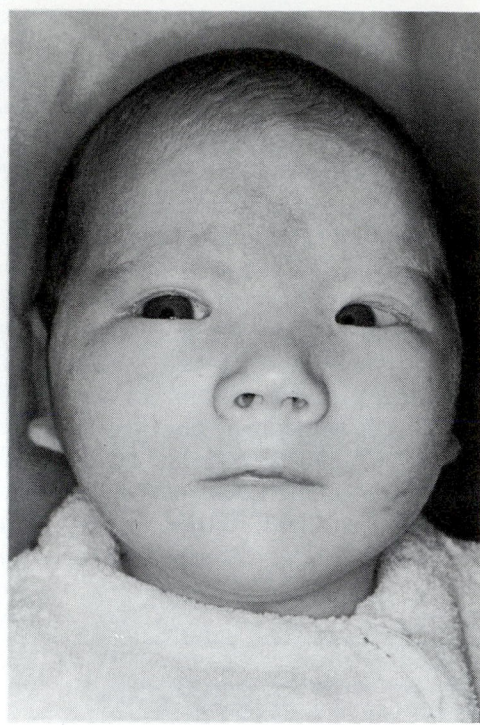

FIG. 4-16. Infant with cri-du-chat syndrome caused by deletion of part of the short arm of chromosome 5. (From Thompson & Thompson, 1986.)

ionizing radiation, some viral infections, and certain chemicals.

Deletions

Broken chromosomes and loss of DNA cause **deletions** (Fig. 4-15). Usually, a gamete with a deletion unites with a normal gamete to form a zygote. The zygote thus has one chromosome with the normal complement of genes and one with some missing genes. Because a fairly large number of genes can be lost in a deletion, serious consequences can result even though one chromosome is normal. The most often cited example of a disease caused by a chromosomal deletion is the **cri-du-chat syndrome** (Fig. 4-16). The term, which literally means "cry of the cat," describes the characteristic cry of the affected child. Other symptoms include low birth weight, mental retardation, microcephaly (smaller than normal head size), heart defects, and the typical facial appearance shown in Fig. 4-16. The disease is caused by a deletion of part of the short arm of chromosome 5.

Duplications

Duplications of chromosome material are, like deletions, a form of chromosome aberration. Because a deficiency of genetic material is more harmful than an excess, duplications usually have less serious consequences than deletions. For example, a deletion of a region of chromosome 5 causes cri-du-chat syndrome, but a duplication of the same region causes mental retardation but physical traits that are nearly normal.

Inversions

An **inversion** is the occurrence of two breaks on a chromosome, followed by the reinsertion of the missing fragment at its original site but in inverted order. Thus, a chromosome symbolized as ABCDEFG might become ABEDCFG after an inversion.

Unlike deletions and duplications, inversions result in no loss or gain of genetic material. They are thus said to be a "balanced" alteration of chromosome structure, and they often have no apparent physical effect. Genes are sometimes influenced by neighboring genes, however, and this **position effect,** a change in a gene's expression caused by its position, does sometimes result in physical defects in persons with inversions.

The serious problems caused by inversions usually occur in the offspring of individuals carrying the inversion. Because chromosomes must line up in perfect order during prophase I, a chromosome with an inversion must form a loop to line up with its normal homologue (Fig. 4-17). Crossing-over within this loop can result in duplications or deletions in the chromosomes of daughter cells. Thus, the offspring of individuals who carry inversions often have chromosome deletions or duplications.

Inversion loop

FIG. 4-17. Inversion loop forms when a chromosome carrying an inversion pairs with a normal (noninverted) homolog.

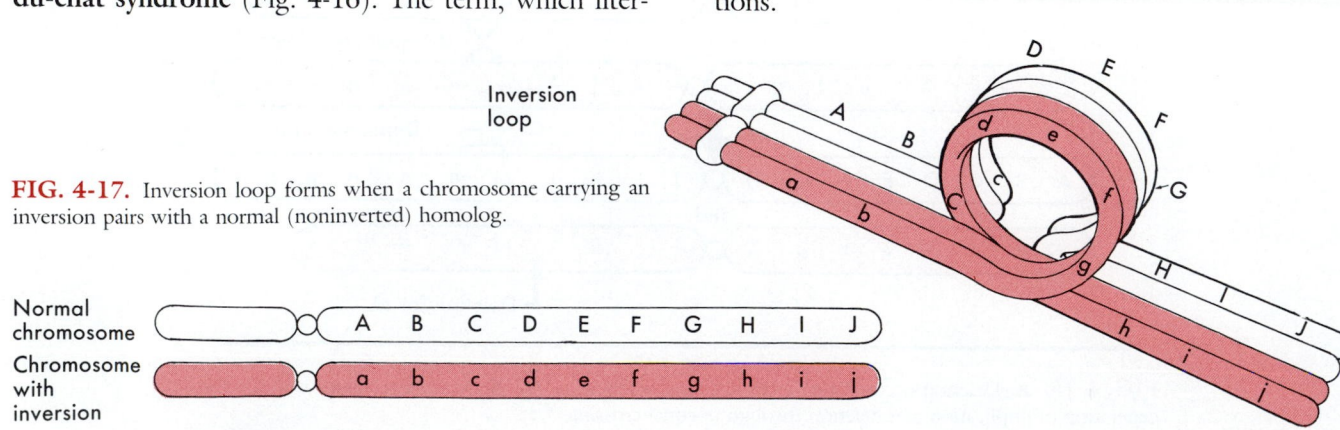

Normal chromosome   A B C D E F G H I J

Chromosome with inversion   a b c d e f g h i j

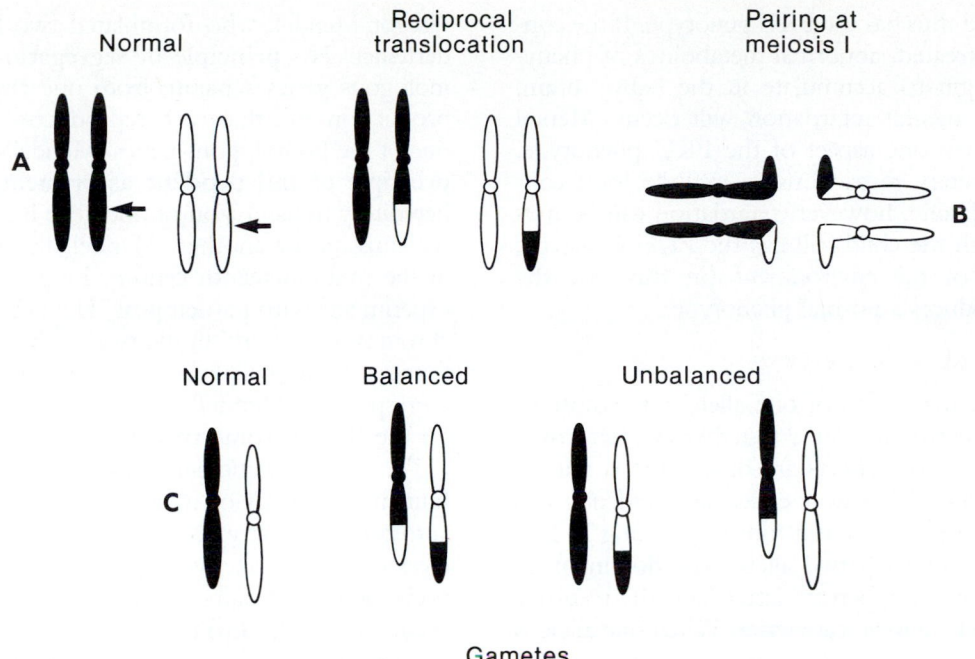

FIG. 4-18. **A,** Normal chromosomes and reciprocal translocation. **B,** Pairing at meiosis. **C,** Consequences of translocation in gametes; unbalanced gametes result in zygotes that are potentially trisomic and partially monosomic and consequently develop abnormally. (From Thompson & Thompson, 1986.)

Translocations

The interchanging of genetic material between nonhomologous chromosomes is called **translocation.** A **reciprocal translocation** occurs when breaks occur in two different chromosomes and the material is exchanged (Fig. 4-18, *A*). As with inversions, the carrier of a reciprocal translocation is usually normal because the individual has a normal complement of genetic material. As Fig. 4-18, *B,* illustrates, however, the carrier's gametes can be normal, can carry the translocation, or can have duplications and deletions.

ELEMENTS OF POPULATION GENETICS

The mechanisms by which an individual's set of paired chromosomes produces traits are the principles of genetic inheritance. Mendel's work with garden peas first defined these principles. Later geneticists have refined Mendel's work to explain patterns of inheritance for traits and diseases that appear in families.

Analysis of traits that occur with defined, predictable patterns has helped geneticists link together the pieces of the human gene map. Current research focuses on assigning genes to specific locations on chromosomes. Eventually, diseases and defects caused by single genes can be traced, and therapies to prevent and treat such diseases can be developed.

Many traits are due to single genes and are often called mendelian traits (after Gregor Mendel). Each gene occupies a position along a chromosome known as a **locus.** The genes at a particular locus can take different forms (i.e., they can be composed of different nucleotide sequences). These different chemical forms are called **alleles.** For example, most people have a type of hemoglobin known as hemoglobin A, whose protein sequence is dictated by a single gene. A few individuals have an alternative form of hemoglobin, termed hemoglobin S, which differs from hemoglobin A by a single amino acid substitution. The genes coding for hemoglobins A and S are thus two different alleles at a locus.

Because humans are diploid organisms, each chromosome is represented twice, with one member of the chromosome pair contributed by the father and one by the mother. At a given locus, an individual has one gene whose origin is paternal and one whose origin is maternal. When the two genes are identical, the individual is **homozygous** at that locus. When the genes are not identical, the individual is **heterozygous** at the locus.

Phenotype and Genotype

The composition of genes at a given locus is known as the **genotype.** The outward appearance of an individual, which is the result of both genotype and environment, is the **phenotype.** For example, a baby who is born with an inability to metabolize the amino acid phenylalanine has the single-gene disorder phenylketonuria (PKU) and thus has the PKU genotype. If the condition is left untreated, abnormal metabolites of phenylalanine will begin to accumulate in the baby's brain, and irreversible mental retardation will occur. Mental retardation is then one aspect of the PKU phenotype. By imposing dietary restrictions to exclude food containing phenylalanine, however, retardation can be prevented. Although the child still has the PKU genotype, a modification of the environment (in this case the child's diet) produces a normal phenotype.

Dominance and Recessiveness

In many loci, the effects of one allele mask those of another when the two are found together in a **heterozygote**. The allele whose effects are observable is said to be **dominant**. The allele whose effects are hidden is said to be **recessive** (from the Latin root for "hiding"). Traditionally, for loci having two alleles, the dominant allele is denoted by an uppercase letter, and the recessive allele is denoted by a lowercase letter. When one allele is dominant over another, the heterozygote genotype, Aa, has the same phenotype as the dominant homozygote, AA. For the recessive allele to be expressed, it must exist in the **homozygote** form, aa.

When the heterozygote is distinguishable from both homozygotes, the locus is said to exhibit either **codominance** or **intermediate inheritance**. For example, in the MN blood group, both alleles, M and N, of the heterozygote are detectable and therefore codominant. Another example is the ABO blood group, in which heterozygotes having the A and B alleles express both of them as A and B antigens on their red cells (forming blood group AB).

A **carrier** is an individual who has a disease gene but is phenotypically normal. The great majority of the genes for a recessive disease occur in heterozygotes who carry one copy of the gene but do not express the disease. Because many recessive genes are lethal in the homozygous state, they are eliminated from the population when they occur in homozygotes. By "hiding" in carriers, however, most recessive genes for diseases survive to be passed on to the next generation.

TRANSMISSION OF GENETIC DISEASES

An important aspect of a genetic disease is the pattern in which it is inherited through the generations of a family, or its **mode of inheritance**. Once the mode of inheritance is known, much can be learned about the disease gene itself, and reliable genetic counseling can be given to members of families in which the disease is present (see Chapter 5).

Modes of inheritance were systematically studied by Gregor Mendel, who formulated two basic laws of inheritance. His **principle of segregation** states that homologous genes separate from one another during reproduction and that each reproductive cell carries only one of the homologous genes. Mendel's second law, the **principle of independent assortment,** states that the hereditary transmission of one gene has no effect on the transmission of another. Mendel discovered these laws in the mid-nineteenth century by performing breeding experiments with garden peas. He had no knowledge of chromosomes. Early in the twentieth century geneticists found that the behavior of chromosomes does basically correspond to Mendel's laws, which now form the basis for the **chromosome theory of inheritance.**

The known single-gene diseases can be classified into four major modes of inheritance: autosomal dominant, autosomal recessive, X-linked dominant, and X-linked recessive. The first two types involve genes known to occur on the 22 pairs of autosomes. The last two types occur on the X chromosome; there is no good documentation of disease genes occurring on the Y chromosome. The number of diseases assigned to each category is growing rapidly. Current catalogs of single-gene traits, which include disease-producing and nonclinical traits (such as attached earlobes), list 1172 known autosomal dominant traits, 610 autosomal recessive traits, and 124 X-linked recessive traits (McKusick, 1983, 1986a, 1986b). In addition, there are 2001 traits whose modes of inheritance are tentatively defined. Only a few diseases are thought to be inherited as X-linked dominant traits.

An important tool in the analysis of modes of inheritance is the **pedigree** chart. The pedigree chart summarizes family relationships and shows which members of a family are affected by a genetic disease (Fig. 4-19). Generally, the pedigree begins with one individual in the family, the **proband,** also termed the **propositus** (males) or **proposita** (females). This individual is usually the first person in the family diagnosed or seen in a clinic.

Autosomal Dominant Inheritance
Characteristics of Pedigrees

Diseases caused by autosomal dominant genes are rare in populations. The most common occur in fewer than 1 in 500 individuals, so that it is uncommon for two individuals both affected by the same autosomal dominant disease to produce offspring together. Fig. 4-20, *A,* illustrates this unusual pattern. More often, affected offspring are produced by the union of a normal parent with an affected heterozygous parent. The diagram (Punnett square) in Fig. 4-20 illustrates this mating. The affected parent can pass either a disease gene or a normal gene to his or her children. Each event has a probability of .5; thus, on the average, half of the chil-

Symbol   **Function**

FIG. 4-19. Symbols commonly used in pedigrees.

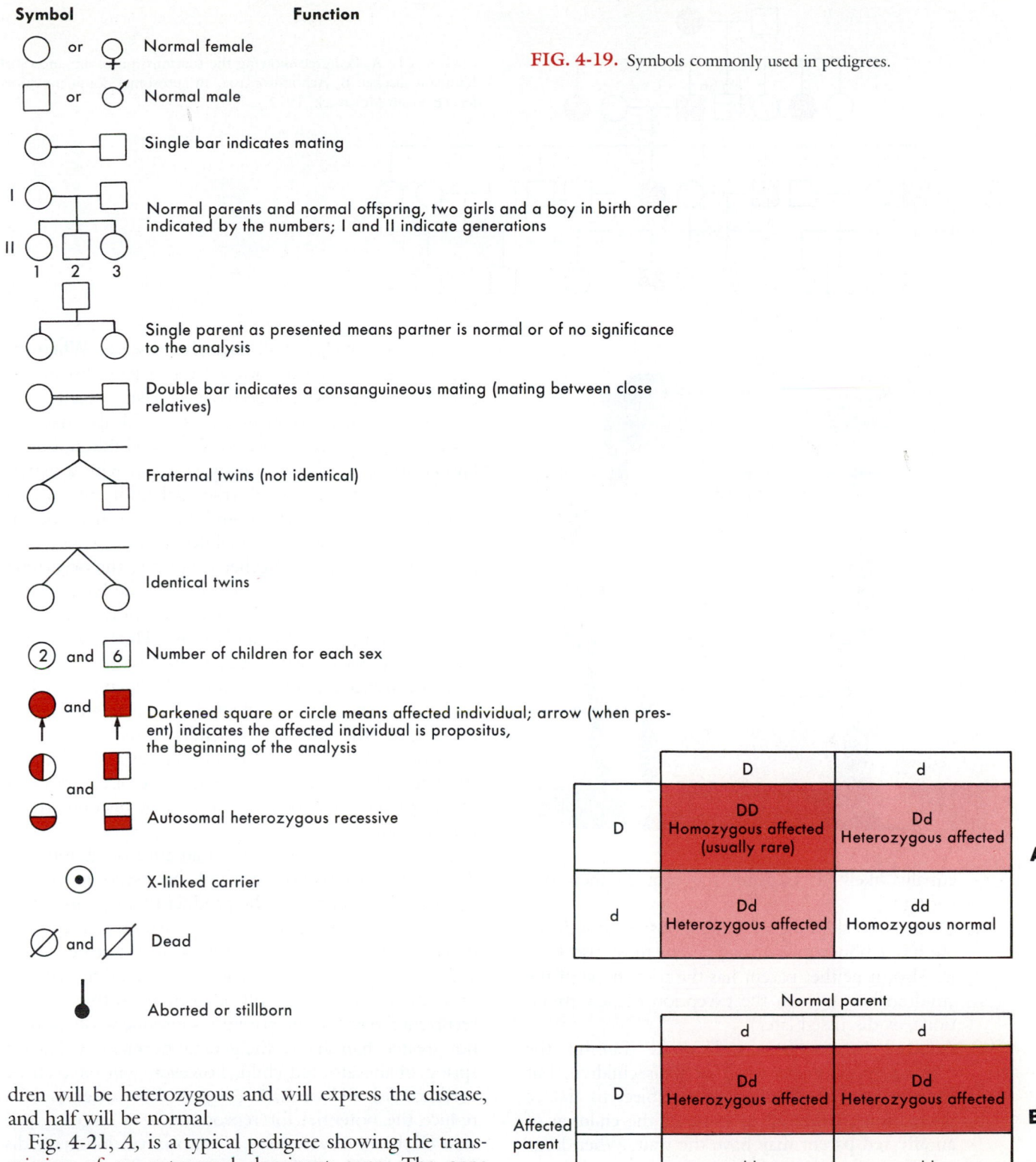

○ or ♀   Normal female

□ or ♂   Normal male

○—□   Single bar indicates mating

Normal parents and normal offspring, two girls and a boy in birth order indicated by the numbers; I and II indicate generations

Single parent as presented means partner is normal or of no significance to the analysis

Double bar indicates a consanguineous mating (mating between close relatives)

Fraternal twins (not identical)

Identical twins

② and ⑥   Number of children for each sex

● and ■   Darkened square or circle means affected individual; arrow (when present) indicates the affected individual is propositus, the beginning of the analysis

◐ and ◪

◓ and ▨   Autosomal heterozygous recessive

⊙   X-linked carrier

⊘ and ⊘   Dead

●   Aborted or stillborn

dren will be heterozygous and will express the disease, and half will be normal.

Fig. 4-21, *A,* is a typical pedigree showing the transmission of an autosomal dominant gene. The gene shown here causes achondroplasia (Fig. 4-21, *B*). Several important characteristics of this pedigree support the conclusion that the trait is due to an autosomal dominant gene:

1. The two sexes exhibit the trait in approximately equal proportions, and males and females are

		D	d
	D	DD Homozygous affected (usually rare)	Dd Heterozygous affected
	d	Dd Heterozygous affected	dd Homozygous normal

A

		Normal parent	
		d	d
Affected parent	D	Dd Heterozygous affected	Dd Heterozygous affected
	d	dd Homozygous normal	dd Homozygous normal

B

FIG. 4-20. **A,** Punnett square for the mating of two individuals with an autosomal dominant gene. Here both parents are affected by the trait. **B,** Punnett square for the mating of a normal individual with a carrier for an autosomal dominant gene.

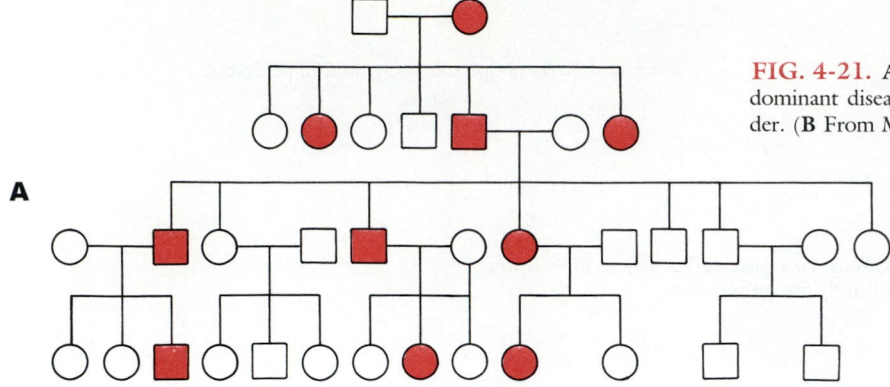

FIG. 4-21. **A,** Pedigree showing the transmission of an autosomal dominant disease. **B,** Achondroplasia, an autosomal dominant disorder. (**B** From McKusick, 1972.)

A

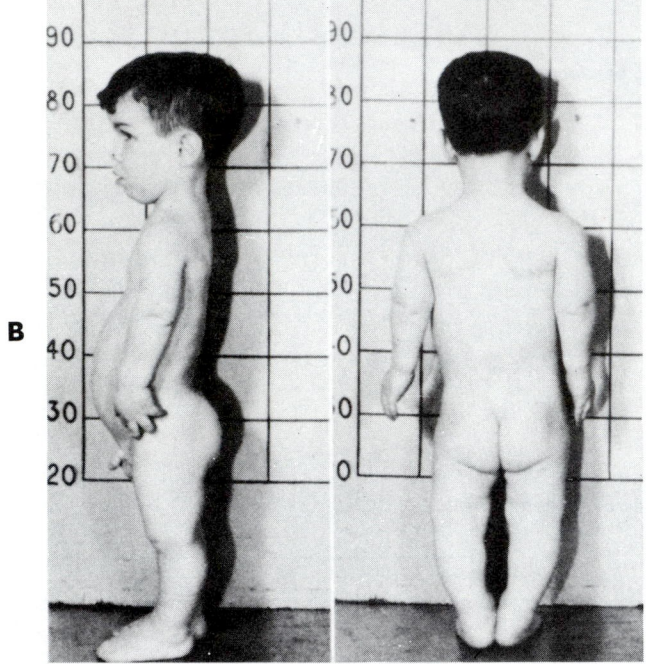

B

equally likely to transmit the trait to their offspring.

2. There is no skipping of generations: if an individual has achondroplasia, one parent must also have it. Also, if neither parent has the trait, none of the children has it (with the exception of new mutations, as discussed later).

3. Affected heterozygous individuals transmit the trait to approximately half of their children, but because gamete transmission is subject to chance fluctuations, either all or none of the children of an affected parent may have the trait. When large numbers of matings of this type are studied, however, the proportion of affected children will closely approach one half.

Recurrence Risks

Parents at risk for producing children with a genetic disease nearly always ask the question, What is the

chance that our child will have this disease? When one child has already been born with a genetic disease, the parents can be given a **recurrence risk,** which is the probability that subsequent children will also have the disease. If the parents have not yet had children, but are known to be at risk for having children with a genetic disease, an **occurrence risk** (the probability that a child will have a specific disease) can be given. When one parent is affected by an autosomal dominant disease (and is a heterozygote) and the other is normal, the occurrence and recurrence risks for each child are one half.

An important principle is that each birth is an independent event, much like a coin toss. Thus even though parents may have already had a child with the disease, their recurrence risk remains one half. Even if they have had several children, all affected (or all unaffected) by the disease, the law of independence dictates that the probability that their next child will have the disease is still one half. Parents' misunderstanding of this principle is one of the most common problems encountered in genetic counseling.

If a child has been born with an autosomal dominant disease and there is no history of the disease in the family, the child is probably the product of a new mutation. The gene transmitted by one of the parents has thus undergone a mutation from a normal to a disease-causing allele. The genes at this locus in most of the parent's other germ cells would still be normal. In this case, the recurrence risk for the parent's subsequent offspring is not greater than that of the general population. The offspring of the affected child, however, will have an occurrence risk of one half. Because these diseases often reduce the potential for reproduction, a large proportion of the observed cases of autosomal dominant diseases are the result of new mutations. For example, approximately seven eighths of all cases of achondroplasia are caused by new mutations.

Delayed Age of Onset

One of the most well-known autosomal dominant diseases is Huntington disease, a neurologic disorder whose main features are progressive dementia and increasingly uncontrollable movements of the limbs (discussed further in Chapter 15). The latter is known as chorea (Greek *khoreia* = dance), and the disease was formerly called Huntington's chorea.

One of the key features of this disease is its **delayed age of onset:** symptoms are not usually seen until age 40 or so. Thus those who develop the disease have often had children before they are aware that they have the gene. If the disease were present at birth, nearly all affected persons would die before reaching reproductive age, and the frequency of the gene in the population would be much lower. From the gene's "point of view," then, a delayed age of onset is quite advantageous. But the individual whose parent has the disease has a 50% chance of developing it during middle age. He or she is thus confronted with a torturous question: Should I have children, knowing that there is a 50-50 chance that I may have this disease gene and pass it to half of my children?

Penetrance and Expressivity

Another important variation seen in some autosomal dominant diseases is reduced penetrance. The **penetrance** of a trait is the percentage of individuals with a specific genotype who also exhibit the expected phenotype. Reduced penetrance means that individuals who have the gene for a disease may not exhibit the disease phenotype at all, even though the gene and the associated disease may be transmitted to the next generation. A pedigree illustrating the transmission of an autosomal dominant gene with reduced penetrance is given in Fig. 4-22. Retinoblastoma, a malignant eye tumor, is one disease that typically exhibits reduced penetrance. About 10% of the individuals who are **obligate carriers** of the gene (i.e., those who have an affected parent and affected children and therefore must themselves carry the gene) do not have the disease. The penetrance of the gene is then said to be **90%.**

A similar complication is variable expressivity. **Expressivity** is the extent of variation in phenotype associ-

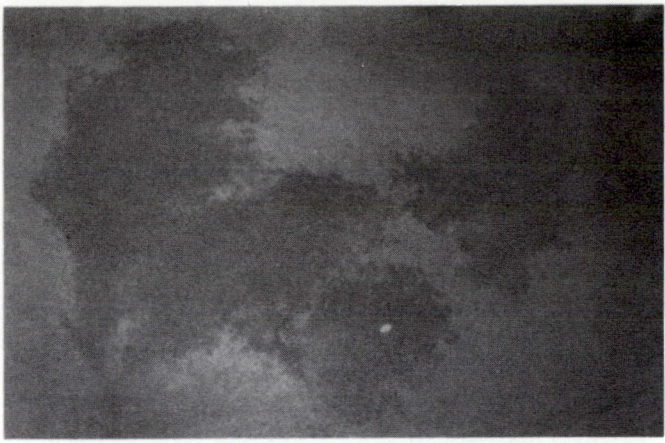

FIG. 4-23. Cafe-au-lait patches suspicious of neurofibromatosis (von Recklinghausen disease). (From Seidel, Ball, Dains, & Benedict, 1987.)

ated with a particular genotype. If expressivity of a disease is variable, the penetrance may be complete, but the severity of the disease can vary greatly. The best known example of variable expressivity in an autosomal dominant disease is neurofibromatosis, or von Recklinghausen disease. This disease has become especially well known as the affliction of the "Elephant Man," the subject of both a play and a movie. The expression of this gene can vary from a few harmless *café-au-lait* spots ("coffee with milk," describing the light-brown color) on the skin to numerous malignant neurofibromas, scoliosis, seizures, gliomas, neuromas, hypertension, and mental retardation (Fig. 4-23).

A parent with mild expression of the disease—so mild that he or she is not aware of it—can transmit the gene to a child, who can then exhibit severe expression of the disease. As with delayed age of onset and reduced penetrance, variable expressivity provides a mechanism by which autosomal dominant genes can be maintained at higher frequencies in populations.

Autosomal Recessive Inheritance
Characteristics of Pedigrees

Like autosomal dominant diseases, diseases caused by autosomal recessive genes are quite rare in populations, although the frequencies of carriers for recessive diseases can be quite high. The most common lethal recessive disease in Caucasian children, cystic fibrosis, occurs in about 1 out of 2000 births. Approximately 1 out of 23 Caucasians carries one copy of the gene for cystic fibrosis (see Chapter 31). Because an individual must be homozygous for a recessive gene to express the disease, the carriers are phenotypically normal. Because most genes for recessive diseases are maintained in normal carriers, they are able to survive in the population from one generation to the next. As with some autosomal dominant

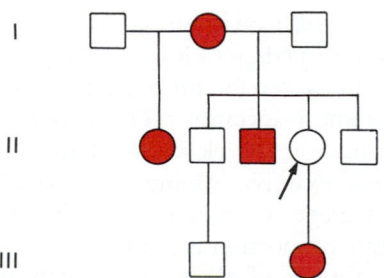

FIG. 4-22. Pedigree for retinoblastoma showing incomplete penetrance. Female with marked arrow in line II must be heterozygous, but she does not express the trait.

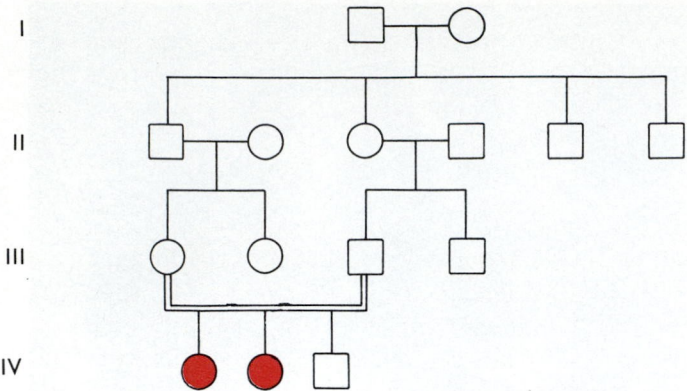

FIG. 4-24. Pedigree for cystic fibrosis.

	D	d
D	DD Homozygous normal	Dd Heterozygous carrier
d	Dd Heterozygous carrier	dd Homozygous affected

FIG. 4-25. Punnett square for the mating of heterozygous carriers typical of most cases of recessive disease.

diseases, some autosomal recessive diseases are characterized by delayed age of onset, reduced penetrance, and variable expressivity.

Fig. 4-24 shows a pedigree for cystic fibrosis. This disease is primarily caused by defects in the secretion of mucus. The digestive organs become obstructed with mucus, causing malnutrition, and the lungs become clogged with mucus. Death from lung disease or heart failure usually occurs before age 25. In the pedigree shown here, the two affected individuals are the offspring of the marriage of two first cousins. Marriage between related individuals, termed **consanguinity** (from the Latin root meaning "common blood"), is often a factor in producing children with recessive diseases because related individuals are more likely to share the same recessive genes.

The important criteria for discerning autosomal recessive inheritance include the following:

1. Males and females are affected in equal proportions.
2. Consanguinity is often present.
3. The disease is seen in siblings but usually not in their parents.
4. On the average, one fourth of the offspring of carrier parents will be affected.

Recurrence Risks

In most cases of recessive disease, the parents of affected individuals are both heterozygous carriers. On the average, one fourth of their offspring will be normal homozygotes, one half will be phenotypically normal carrier heterozygotes, and one fourth will be homozygotes with the disease (Fig. 4-25). Thus the recurrence risk for the offspring of carrier parents is 25%. As before, these are the *average* figures. In any given family, there will likely be chance fluctuations, but a study of a large number of families would yield figures quite close to these proportions.

If two parents have a recessive disease, they each must be homozygous for the disease. Therefore, when two parents are affected by a recessive disease, all of their children must also be affected. This observation helps to distinguish recessive from dominant inheritance, because two parents both affected by a dominant gene are nearly always both heterozygotes, and thus one fourth of their children will be unaffected.

Because carrier parents usually are unaware that they both carry the same recessive gene, they often produce an affected child before knowing of their condition. Increasingly, **carrier detection tests** that can identify heterozygotes by measuring the reduced amount of a critical enzyme are becoming available. The critical enzyme would be totally lacking in a homozygous recessive individual, but an essentially normal phenotype is seen when it is present in a reduced quantity in the carrier. These tests are especially valuable for siblings of known carriers, who may themselves be carriers. Some recessive diseases for which carrier detection tests are now available are PKU, sickle cell disease, and galactosemia.

Consanguinity

Consanguinity and **inbreeding** are sometimes confused. Whereas *consanguinity* refers to the mating of two related individuals, the offspring of such matings are said to be *inbred*. Consanguinity is often an important characteristic of pedigrees for recessive diseases because relatives share a certain proportion of genes received from a common ancestor. The proportion of shared genes depends on the closeness of their biologic relationship. For example, siblings share one half of their genes, on average. With each decreasing degree of relationship, this proportion is reduced by one half. Uncles share one fourth of their genes with nephews and nieces, first cousins share one eighth; first cousins once removed* share one sixteenth; second cousins share one

---

*First cousins once removed are the offspring of one's own first cousins.

thirty-second, and so on. With consanguineous matings there is a significant increase in recessive disorders. Most empirical studies show that the proportion of offspring of marriages of first cousins who are affected by genetic diseases is approximately double that of the general population (Morton, 1961; Stern, 1973). Marriages between first cousins are prohibited in most states of the United States. Marriages between closer relatives (except between double first cousins*) are prohibited throughout the United States.

X-Linked Inheritance

Not all genetic diseases are caused by genes located on the 22 autosomes. Some conditions are instead caused by genes located on the sex chromosomes, so that the mode of inheritance is **sex-linked.** Because the Y chromosome is not yet known to carry any disease-causing genes, the terms **X-linked** and *sex-linked* are sometimes equated. The former, however, is a more specific term. Only a few diseases are known to be inherited as X-linked dominant traits. Because these diseases are so seldom encountered, only the much more common X-linked recessive diseases are discussed here.

Because females receive two X chromosomes, one from the father and one from the mother, they can be homozygous for a disease allele at a given locus, heterozygous, or homozygous for the normal allele at the locus. Males, having only one X chromosome, are said to be **hemizygous** for genes on this chromosome. If a male inherits a recessive disease gene on the X chromosome, he will be affected by the disease because the Y chromosome does not carry a normal allele to counteract the effects of the disease gene. Males are always more frequently affected by X-linked recessive diseases, with the difference becoming more pronounced as the disease becomes rarer.

Characteristics of Pedigrees

X-linked pedigrees show distinctive modes of inheritance. The most striking characteristic is that females are almost never affected. To express an X-linked recessive trait, a female must be homozygous, so that either both of her parents are affected, or her father is affected and her mother is a carrier. Such matings are rare.

The following characteristics define X-linked recessive traits:

1. The trait is seen much more frequently in males than in females.
2. Because a father can give a son only a Y chromosome, the trait is never transmitted from father to son.

3. The gene can be transmitted through a series of carrier females, causing the appearance of a "skipped generation."
4. The gene is passed from an affected father to all of his daughters, who, as phenotypically normal carriers, transmit it to approximately half of their sons, who are affected.

In addition to hemophilia, a number of other well-known diseases and traits are caused by X-linked recessive genes. These include red-green color blindness (caused by either of two X-linked genes, which have a combined frequency of 8% in European males) and Duchenne muscular dystrophy.

Recurrence Risks

The most common mating type involving X-linked recessive genes is the combination of a carrier female and a normal male. On the average, the carrier mother will transmit the disease gene to half of her sons and half of her daughters. As Fig. 4-26, *A,* shows, half of the daughters in such a mating will be carriers, whereas half will be normal. Half of the sons will be normal, whereas half will have the disease. As before, these are probabilities, so that these risks are what can be expected on the *average.*

The other common mating type is an affected father and a normal mother (Fig. 4-26, *B*). Here all of the sons must be normal because the father can transmit only his Y chromosome to them. Because all of the daughters must receive the father's X chromosome, they will all be heterozygous carriers. Because the son *must* receive the Y chromosome and the daughers *must* receive the X with the disease gene, these are predictions and not probabilities. None of the children will inherit the disease.

The final mating pattern, less common than the other two, involves an affected father and a carrier mother (Fig. 4-26, *C*). Here on average half of the daughters will be heterozygous carriers, whereas half will be homozygous for the disease gene and thus affected. Half of the sons will be normal, and half will be affected. Some X-linked recessive diseases, such as Duchenne muscular dystrophy, are fatal or incapacitating before the affected individual reaches reproductive age, so affected fathers are rare or nonexistent.

Sex-Limited and Sex-Influenced Traits

Confusion sometimes exists between traits that are sex-linked and those that are sex-limited or sex-influenced. A **sex-limited trait** is one that can occur in only one of the sexes, often because of anatomic differences. Inherited uterine and testicular defects are two obvious examples.

A **sex-influenced trait** is one that occurs much more frequently in one sex than in the other. A good example

---

*Double first cousins share both sets of grandparents; ordinary first cousins share just one set of grandparents.

CLINICAL COMMENTARY

Hemophilia A and the Russian Revolution

The figure (partial pedigree for descendents of Queen Victoria) is one of the best known disease pedigrees in existence. It shows the transmission of hemophilia A in the European royal families. This disease, often known as "bleeder syndrome," is caused by a defect in one of the blood-clotting factors, factor VIII, and can cause severe hemorrhages. In this pedigree Queen Victoria of England was the first known carrier of the disease, and a number of her male descendants were affected by it. One of the most

historically significant consequences of this pedigree involves the hemophiliac Czarevich Alexis, son of Czar Nicholas II of Russia. Grigori Rasputin, the "mad monk," was reputedly the only person able to prevent the young boy's bleeding episodes and was thus able to gain considerable power over the royal family. His destabilizing influence is thought to have hastened the 1917 Bolshevik revolution.

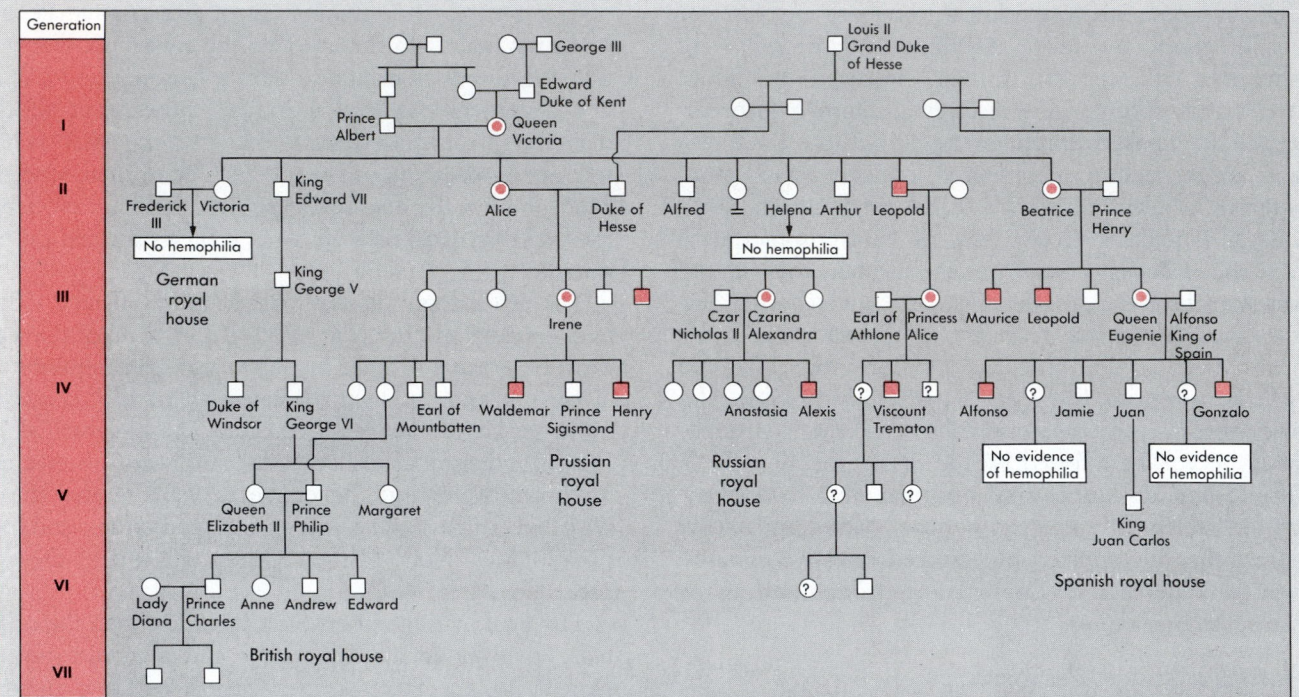

Partial pedigree for descendents of Queen Victoria, showing the appearance of hemophilia A in one of her sons and in his descendants and in the descendants of her daughters and granddaughters. The royal families of Prussia, Hesse, Battenberg (Mountbatten), Russia, and Spain were thus affected with the disease. The present royal family of England, however, is free of the disease, in spite of inbreeding. (From Raven, P. H., & Johnson, G. B. [1986]. St. Louis: C. V. Mosby.)

of a sex-influenced trait is male-pattern baldness, which occurs in both males and females but is much more common in males. In males it is inherited as a dominant trait, whereas in females it is inherited as a recessive trait. Because of their hormonal constitution, females need two copies of the gene to express male-pattern baldness.

Evaluation of Pedigrees

With complications such as incomplete penetrance, variable expressivity, delayed age of onset, and sex-influenced traits, it is not always possible simply to look at a disease pedigree and determine the mode of inheritance. A sophisticated statistical methodology has evolved to deal with such complications. Incorporated into com-

Mother

A

	X_H	X_h
X_H	$X_H X_H$	$X_H X_h$
Y	$X_H Y$	$X_h Y$

Father

FIG. 4-26. A, Punnett square for the mating of a normal male ($X_H Y$) and a female carrier of an X-linked recessive gene ($X_H X_h$). **B,** Punnett square for the mating of a normal female ($X_H X_H$) with a male affected by an X-linked recessive disease ($X_h Y$). **C,** Punnett square for the mating of a female who carries an X-linked recessive gene ($X_H X_h$) with a male who is affected with the disease caused by the gene ($X_h Y$).

Mother

B

	X_H	X_H
X_h	$X_H X_h$	$X_H X_h$
Y	$X_H Y$	$X_H Y$

Father

Mother

C

	X_H	X_h
X_h	$X_H X_h$	$X_h X_h$
Y	$X_H Y$	$X_h Y$

puter programs, these statistical techniques assess the probability of observing a certain pedigree if a certain mode of inheritance (e.g., autosomal dominant with reduced penetrance) is in effect. In addition, environmental factors interact with genetic factors to affect penetrance, expressivity, and age of onset for certain conditions. Analysis of the interaction between genes and environment is discussed in Chapter 5.

LINKAGE ANALYSIS AND GENE MAPPING

Locating genes on chromosomes and on specific areas of chromosomes is one of the most important endeavors in human genetics. The location of a gene can tell much about the function of the gene, its interaction with other genes, and the likelihood that certain individuals will develop a genetic disease.

Classical Pedigree Analysis

Mendel's second law, the principle of independent assortment, states that an individual's genes will be transmitted to the next generation independently of one another. This law is only partly true, however, because genes located close together on the same chromosome *do* tend to be transmitted together to the offspring. Thus Mendel's principle of independent assortment holds true for most pairs of genes but not those that occupy the same region of a chromosome. Such loci demonstrate **linkage** and are said to be linked.

During the first meiotic stage, the arms of homolo-

gous chromosome pairs intertwine and sometimes exchange portions of their DNA (Fig. 4-27) in a process known as **crossing-over.** During crossing-over new combinations of alleles can be formed. For example, two loci on a chromosome have alleles A and a and alleles B and b. Alleles A and B are located together on one chromosome arm, and alleles a and b are located on the other arm. The genotype of this organism is denoted as AB/ab.

As Fig. 4-27, *A* shows, the allele pairs AB and ab would be transmitted together when no crossing-over occurs. But when crossing-over occurs (Fig. 4-27, *B*), all four possible pairs of alleles can be transmitted to the offspring: AB, aB, Ab, and ab. The process of forming such new arrangements of alleles is called **recombination.** Crossing-over does not necessarily lead to recombination, however, because double crossing-over between two loci can result in no actual recombination of the alleles at the loci (Fig. 4-27, *C*).

The rate of crossing-over can be used to infer the distance between two loci on a chromosome, because the

Homologous chromosomes Meiosis gametes

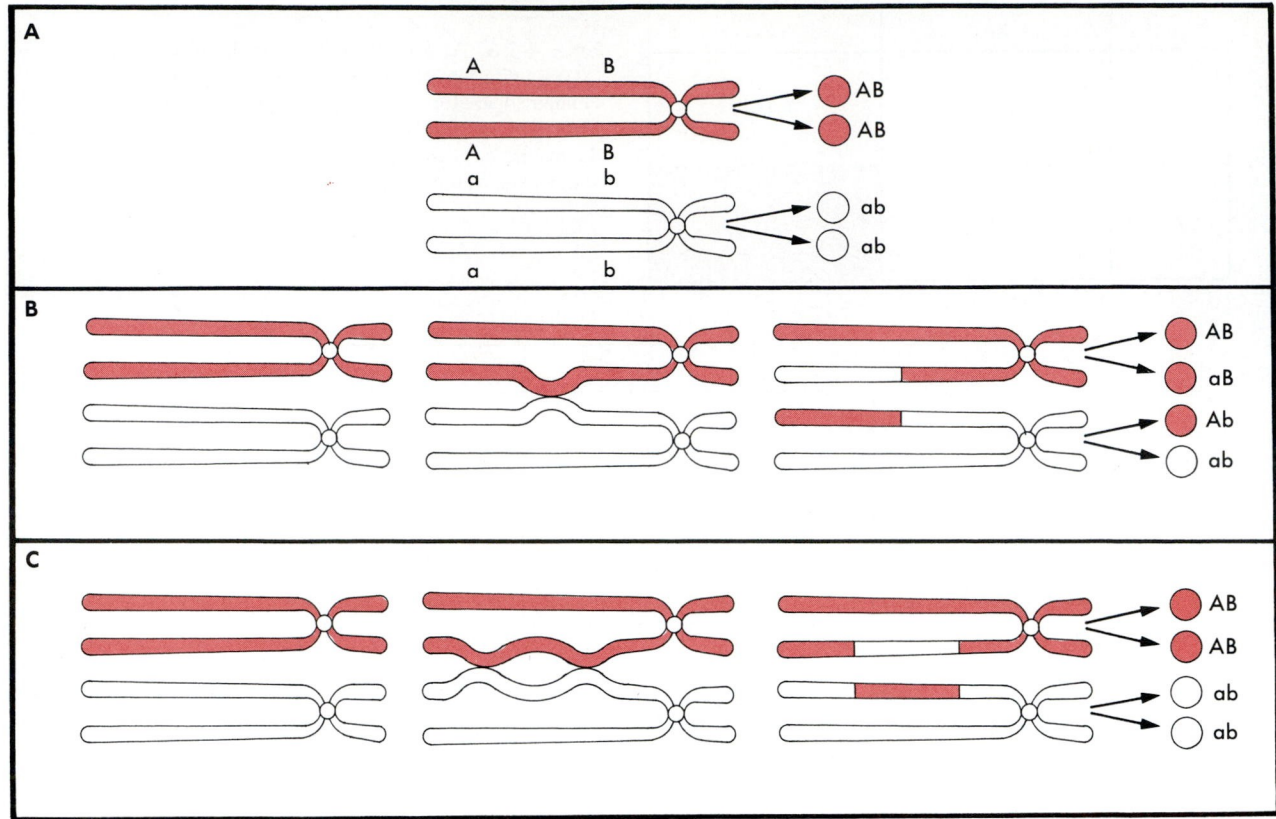

FIG. 4-27. The genetic results of crossing-over. **A,** No crossing-over. **B,** Crossing-over with recombination. **C,** Double crossing-over resulting in no recombination.

probability of crossovers occurring between two loci increases as the loci become more distant. For example, if an organism with genotype AB/ab produces recombinant offspring gametes (composition of Ab and aB) 2% of the time, it is said that the two loci are two map units apart. One **map unit** equals a 1% recombination rate between two loci. When loci on the same chromosome are 50 or more map units apart, they are considered unlinked, because their recombination frequency is just as great as it would be if they were on different chromosomes (where the probability of being transmitted together must equal one half). Because they are on the same chromosome, they are said to be unlinked but **syntenic loci.** Recombination frequencies provide a good estimate of actual physical distance between loci at smaller distances, but because of double crossovers, they tend to yield underestimates at larger distances.

Pedigrees can be used to determine recombination rates between loci. Fig. 4-28 shows a pedigree in which the rare disease nail-patella syndrome (an autosomal dominant disease consisting of malformed patellae and nails) is being transmitted. The individuals in this pedigree have also been typed for the ABO blood group,

whose locus is also located on chromosome 9. Examination of generations one and two shows that the nail-patella gene must be on the same chromosome arm as the gene for blood type A, because the mother, whose blood type was B, was unaffected with the disease. The daughter's genotype would then be AN/Bn, where N indicates the disease allele and n indicates the normal allele. The daughter's husband (individual II-1) must have the genotype On/On. If the loci for nail-patella syndrome and the ABO blood group are linked, the children of this union who are affected with nail-patella syndrome should have blood type A; those who are unaffected should have blood type B. In six out of seven cases we find this to be true. In one case a recombination occurred (individual III-6), indicating a recombination rate of 1/7, or 14%. The two loci are therefore 14 map units apart.

In practice, a much larger sample of families would be used to ensure against statistical artifacts. Also, as with the determination of mode of inheritance, the situation is not always as clear as in Fig. 4-28. Elaborate statistical procedures have been devised to evaluate the probabilities that two loci are linked at a given map distance.

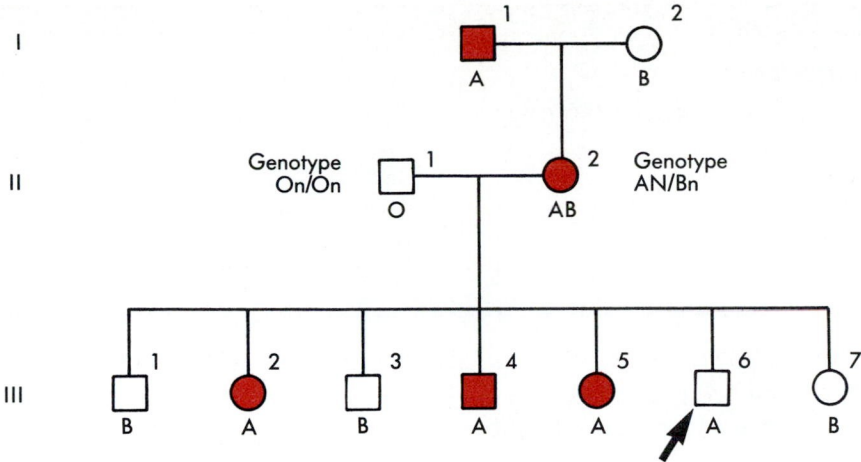

FIG. 4-28. The ABO nail-patella linkage in three generations of a family. Letters below symbols indicate ABO blood groups. Individual III-6 shows recombination.

Once a close linkage is established between a disease locus and a "marker" locus (such as a blood group) and once the alleles of the two loci that are inherited together within a family are determined, reliable predictions of whether a member of a family will develop the disease can be made. If, for example, the recombination rate between a disease locus and a "marker" locus, such as the ABO blood group, is less than 1%, family members can simply have their ABO blood type assayed to find out, with 99% or greater certainty, whether each member carries the disease gene.

This capability is especially important for diseases with delayed age of onset. Linkage has been established between several DNA polymorphisms and the gene for Huntington disease. Determining this kind of linkage means that it will be possible for offspring of an individual with Huntington disease to know whether they also carry the gene and thus could pass it on to their own children. The difficult decision of whether to have children will thus be made easier for these individuals, although, of course, some individuals may prefer to remain uninformed of their genotypes.

For some genetic diseases, prophylactic treatment is available if the condition can be diagnosed in time. An example of this is hemochromatosis, a recessive genetic disease in which excess iron is retained, causing degeneration of the heart, liver, brain, and other vital organs. Diagnosis is usually made at about 40 years of age, after which most individuals survive only a few years. If earlier tests could determine whether an individual had the disease, preventive treatment, consisting of phlebotomies to remove blood and thus excess iron, could be administered before degeneration began. This has recently been made possible by establishing that the gene for hemochromatosis is closely linked to the human leukocyte antigen (HLA) (see Chapter 6) complex on chromosome 6. Individuals at risk for developing the disease can now be determined by assaying their HLA type, and preventive therapy can be given, assuring an ordinary life span. This is one instance in which genetics contributes to preventive medicine in its best sense.

Complete Human Gene Map: Prospects and Benefits

Rapid progress is now being made in assigning genes to their chromosomal locations. A number of important genetic diseases have recently been located on specific areas of individual chromosomes, including Huntington disease, retinoblastoma, Duchenne muscular dystrophy, hemophilia A, cystic fibrosis, PKU, neurofibromatosis, familial Alzheimer disease, and a form of manic-depressive psychosis (Caskey, 1987; Gusella, 1986; Martin, 1987). The development of hundreds of new DNA markers is especially helpful in this effort. Geneticists now talk about a "complete" map of the human genome as a goal achievable within a decade or two. Achievement of this goal will serve several purposes:

1. Marker genes will be available to establish close linkages for many genetic diseases. The biggest single drawback to linkage studies now is the lack of markers distributed throughout the genome. As this is overcome, accurate prediction can be made for the inheritance of many or even most genetic diseases.

2. Knowing the location of genes often yields valuable information about the way genes function and interact with one another. A number of genes with similar functions (e.g., some of the globin genes) are located close to one another on the same chromosome. This characteristic can have important implications for the diseases caused by these genes.

CLINICAL COMMENTARY
Assigning Loci to Specific Chromosomes

GENE MARKERS

Morphologic variations can occasionally be seen microscopically on a chromosome. A good example of such variation is the "uncoiled" appearance of the long arm of chromosome 1, a rare feature that is transmitted in families. Donahue, Bias, Renwick, and McKusick, (1968) first assigned a gene to a specific autosome by studying this variation. Families in which this variant is inherited were typed for a number of blood groups and serum proteins, and it was found that the Duffy blood group locus was closely linked (within 2.5 map units) to the uncoiler locus. Other types of gene markers, such as distinct banding patterns, can also be used in this way.

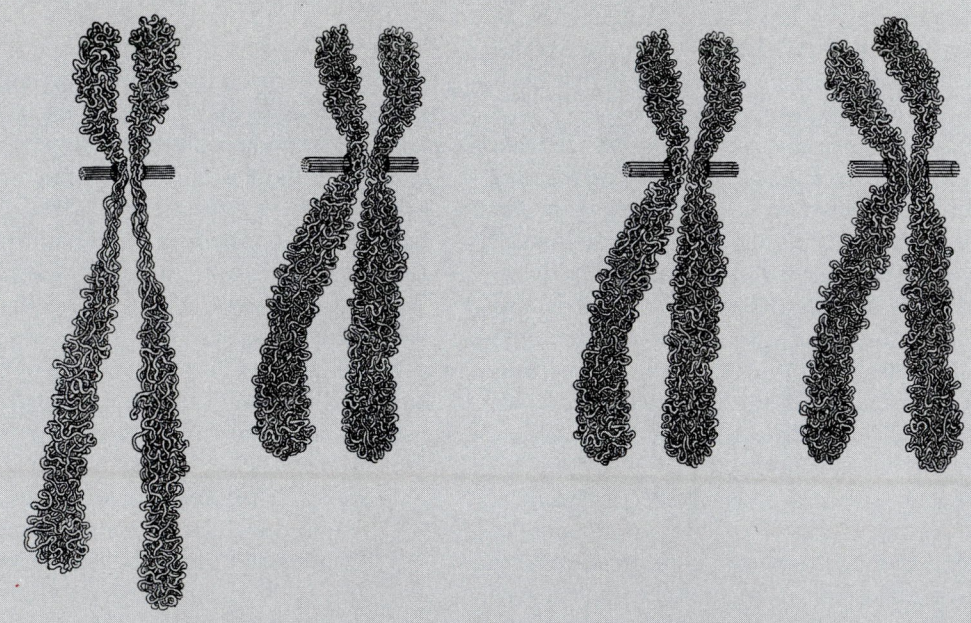

Uncoiled chromosome   **Normal** chromosome   Normal pair

Two pairs of chromosomes. *Left,* From an individual who is heterozygous for the variant "uncoiler" chromosome. *Right,* From a related person who does not carry the variant. (From Donohue, R. P., Bias, W. B., Renwick, J. H., & McKusick, V. A. [1968]. *Proceedings of the National Academy of Sciences, 61.*

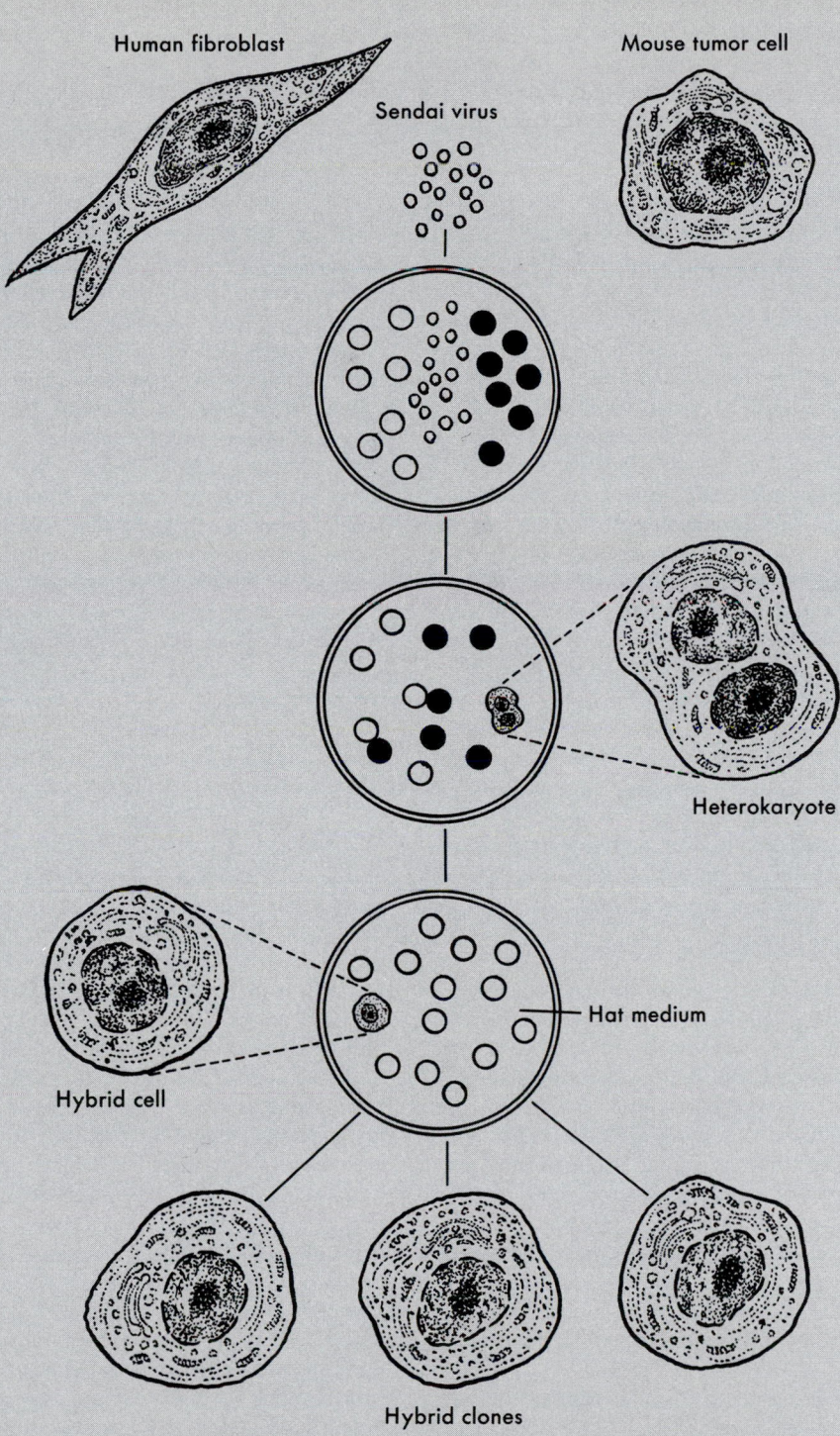

Human fibroblast

Sendai virus

Mouse tumor cell

Heterokaryote

Hat medium

Hybrid cell

Hybrid clones

Somatic cell hybridization. Human fibroblasts are fused to mouse tumor cells that lack either HGPRT or TK enzymes. Sendai viruses promote the fusion. Some of the cells first fuse to produce cells with two nuclei (heterokaryons) and then form true hybrids. The hybrid cells are grown in a selective medium (HAT), where the hybrids thrive at the expense of the nonfused cells. As the hybrid cells divide, they lose human chromosomes randomly, then stabilize into different clones containing different human chromosomes.

Continued.

CLINICAL COMMENTARY
Assigning Loci to Specific Chromosomes, cont'd

GENE DOSAGE ANALYSIS

The amount or dosage of an enzyme associated with a specific gene can sometimes be measured. When a specific portion of a chromosome is deleted, it is sometimes possible to show that only half of the level of an enzyme is present in the organism. If the gene coding for this enzyme is known, the gene can then be associated with the specific area of the chromosome that has been deleted. For example, this method has been used to map the enzymes acid phosphatase (to chromosome 2) and adenylate kinase (to chromosome 9). Assigning loci to chromosomes by analyzing deletions is termed deletion mapping.

The same method can be applied when a portion of a chromosome is duplicated or when an individual has a partial or complete trisomy. When a 150% level of enzyme activity (due to three alleles instead of two) is shown, the amount of enzyme may indicate that a gene coding for the enzyme is located on the duplicated region of the chromosome. For example, superoxide dismutase-1 (SOD-1) has been assigned to the long arm of chromosome 21 in this way. Because individuals with Down syndrome have an additional long arm of this chromosome (trisomy 21), one speculation is that SOD-1 may play a causal role in this disease. Assigning loci to chromosomes by analyzing duplications is called duplication mapping.

SOMATIC CELL HYBRIDIZATION

One of the more astounding biologic discoveries in recent years is that somatic cells from different species, when grown in the same culture, occasionally fuse together to form hybrid cells. This has been done with cells from humans and mice. The resulting hybrid cells contain 86 chromosomes: the 46 human chromosomes together with the 40 mouse chromosomes. The percentage of successful cell fusions can be greatly increased by exposing the cells to certain agents, such as Sendai virus or polyethylene glycol. The cells are then exposed to selective media such as hypoxanthine, aminopterin, and thymidine (HAT) medium to weed out those that do not fuse. The hybrid cells are then cloned, and all clones of a cell necessarily have identical karyotypes.

Because the hybrid cells are unstable, they begin to lose the chromosomes of one of the species as they undergo cell divisions. Eventually cells are left having a full set of mouse chromosomes but only one or a few human chromosomes. The cells are karyotyped to determine which chromosomes remain. These sets of cells can then be studied to determine which enzymes they produce. The mouse and human enzymes are sufficiently different that they can be distinguished from one another. By looking at different cell lines with different groups of human chromosomes, it is possible to establish that a certain chromosome must always be present when a certain enzyme is detected. Thus the gene coding for that enzyme must be located on that chromosome.

Sometimes a gene can be assigned to a specific *segment* of a chromosome by using somatic cell hybridization. Translocations in which only part of a single human chromosome is attached to one of the mouse chromosomes occur infrequently. If a human enzyme is still detectable, then the gene coding for this enzyme must be located on the translocated segment of the human chromosome.

IN SITU HYBRIDIZATION

In situ hybridization involves hybridizing a specific piece of radioactively labeled DNA or RNA (a probe) to fixed metaphase chromosomes. If the radioactive probe matches the DNA of a chromosome segment, it hybridizes and remains at a particular position on the chromosome (hence the term *in situ*). Its position can then be located by autoradiography.

In situ hybridization is often combined with somatic cell hybridization to locate genes on chromosomes. Once the cell lines with different combinations of human chromosomes are created by somatic cell hybridization, they can be exposed to radioactively labeled probes. Consistent hybridization of a probe with cell lines containing a certain chromosome demonstrates that the gene corresponding to the probe is located on that chromosome. In some ways, this approach is superior to the enzyme assay technique described previously, since it does not require the in vitro expression of a phenotype (the enzyme). Somatic cell and in situ hybridization are now the most commonly used techniques for locating genes on chromosomes.

3. Once the location of a disease gene is known, gene therapy becomes more feasible. Although such therapy is not yet possible, the obstacles to some forms of gene therapy are swiftly being overcome.

MULTIFACTORIAL INHERITANCE

Not all traits are produced by single genes; some traits are the result of several genes acting together. These are usually referred to as **polygenic traits.** When environmental factors are also known to influence the expression of the trait (as is usually the case), the term **multifactorial inheritance** is used. Many multifactorial and polygenic traits tend to follow a normal distribution in populations (the familiar "bell-shaped curve)." Fig. 4-29 shows how three loci acting together can cause grain color to vary in a gradual way from white to red, exemplifying multifactorial inheritance. If both the alleles at each of the three loci are "white" alleles, the color is pure white. If most alleles are white but a few are red,

the color is somewhat darker, and if all are red, then the color is dark red.

Other examples of multifactorial traits include height and IQ. Although both height and IQ are determined in part by genes, they are also strongly influenced by environment. For example, the average height of many human populations has increased by 5 to 10 cm since the turn of the century because of improvements in nutrition and health care. Also, IQ scores can be improved dramatically by exposing individuals (especially children) to enriched learning environments. Thus both genes *and* environment contribute to variation in these traits.

A number of diseases do not follow the bell-shaped distribution. Instead they appear to be either present in or absent from an individual. Yet they do not follow the patterns expected of single-gene diseases. Many of these are probably polygenic or multifactorial, but a certain **threshold of liability** must be crossed before the disease is expressed. Below the threshold the individual appears normal; above it the individual is affected by the disease (Fig. 4-30).

One of the best known examples of such a threshold trait is pyloric stenosis, a disorder characterized by a narrowing or obstruction of the pylorus, the area between the stomach and intestine. Chronic vomiting, constipation, weight loss, and electrolyte imbalance can result from the condition, but it is easily corrected by surgery. The prevalence of pyloric stenosis is about 3

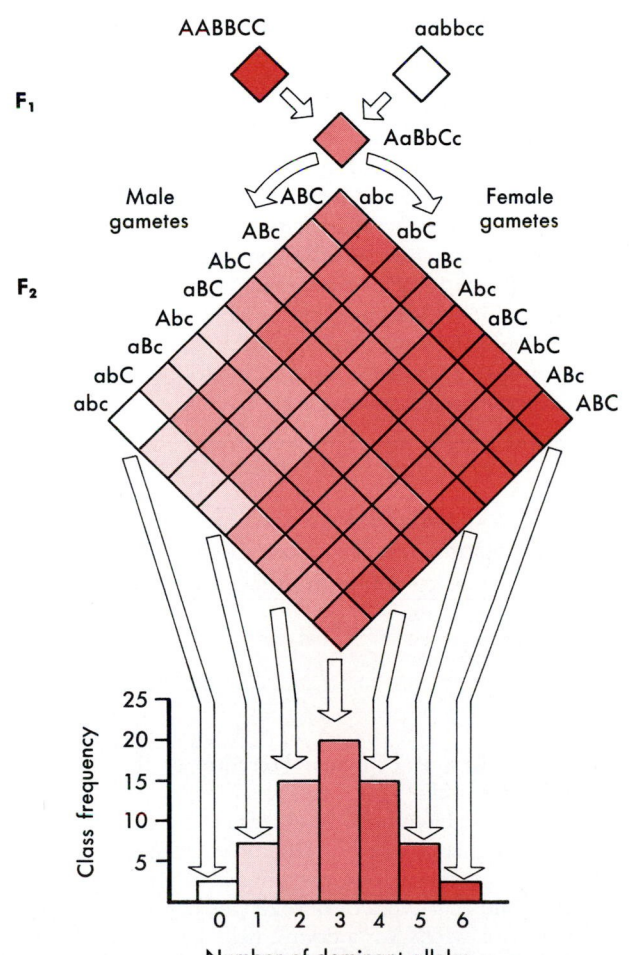

FIG. 4-29. Analysis of mode of inheritance for grain color in wheat. The trait is controlled by three independently assorting gene loci.

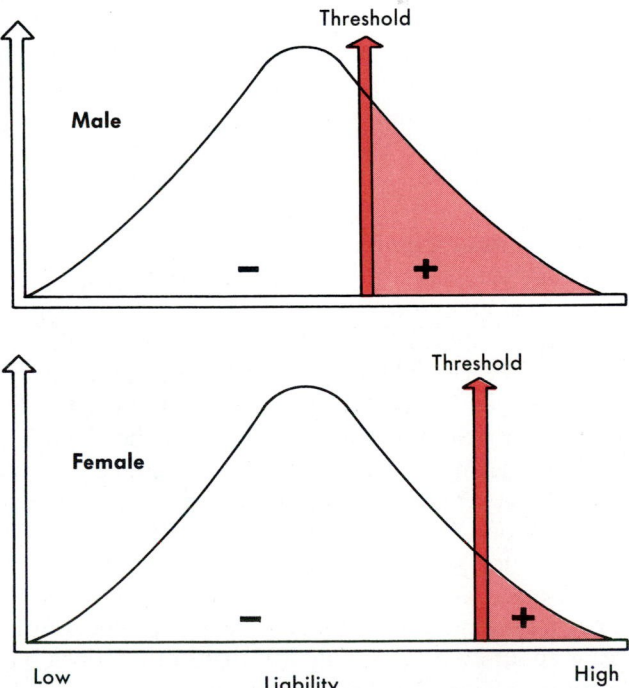

FIG. 4-30. Threshold of liability for pyloric stenosis in males and in females.

TABLE 4-1 The incidence of pyloric stenosis in offspring of patients as compared with the incidence of the general population

Relatives	Risk
Sons of male patients	1 in 18
Daughters of male patients	1 in 42
Sons of female patients	1 in 5
Daughters of female patients	1 in 14

per 1000 live births in Caucasians. It is much more common in males than females, affecting 1 of 200 males and 1 of 1000 females. The reason for this difference is that the threshold of liability is much lower in males than females, as shown in Fig. 4-30. Thus, fewer defective alleles are required to generate the disorder in males. This also means that the offspring of affected females are more likely to have pyloric stenosis, because affected females necessarily carry more disease-causing alleles than do most affected males. Table 4-1 gives the occurrence risks for offspring of males and females with pyloric stenosis, showing a varying threshold of liability.

A number of other common diseases are thought to correspond to this model. They include cleft lip and/or cleft palate, neural tube defects (anencephaly and spina bifida), clubfoot (talipes), and some forms of congenital heart disease.

Although recurrence risks can be given with confidence for single-gene diseases (50% for autosomal dominants, 25% for autosomal recessives, etc.), it is considerably more difficult to do so for multifactorial diseases. The number of genes contributing to the disease is not known, the precise allelic constitution of the parents is not known, and the extent of environmental effects can vary from one population to another. For most multifactorial diseases, **empiric risks** (i.e., those based on direct observation) have been derived. To determine empiric risks, a large population of families in which one child has developed the disease is examined. Then the siblings of each child are surveyed in order to calculate what percentage of them also develop the disease. For example, in Great Britain about 5% of the siblings of children having neural tube defects also have neural tube defects. Thus the recurrence risk for parents who have had one child with a neural tube defect is 5%. Unlike risks for single-gene diseases, those for multifactorial diseases can change from one population to another. The empiric risk for neural tube defects in North America is about 2% to 3%: only half that of the British population.

Another difficulty is distinguishing polygenic or multifactorial diseases from single-gene diseases that have reduced penetrance or variable expressivity. Large data

---

Criteria Used to Define Multifactorial Diseases

1. The recurrence risk becomes higher if more than one family member is affected. For example, the recurrence risk for neural tube defects in a British family increases to 10% if two siblings have been born with the disease. By contrast, the recurrence risk for single-gene diseases remains the same regardless of the number of siblings affected.
2. If the expression of the disease is more severe, the recurrence risk is higher. This is consistent with the liability model; a more severe expression indicates that the individual is at the extreme tail of the liability distribution. Relatives of the affected individual are thus at a higher risk for inheriting disease genes. Cleft lip and/or cleft palate is a disease in which this has been shown to be true.
3. Relatives of probands of the less commonly affected sex are more likely to develop the disease. As with pyloric stenosis, this occurs because an affected individual of the less susceptible sex is usually at a more extreme position on the liability distribution.
4. Generally, if the population frequency of the disease is f, the risk for offspring and siblings of probands is approximately $\sqrt{f}$. This does not usually hold true for single-gene traits.
5. The recurrence risk for the disease decreases rapidly in more remotely related relatives. Although the recurrence risk for single-gene diseases decreases by 50% with each degree of relationship (e.g., a autosomal dominant disease has a 50% recurrence risk for siblings, 25% for uncle-nephew relationship, 12.5% for first cousins), the risk for multifactorial inheritance decreases much more quickly.

---

sets and good epidemiologic data are often necessary to make the distinction. The box above lists criteria that are usually used to define multifactorial diseases.

SUMMARY REVIEW

DNA, RNA, and Proteins: Heredity at the Molecular Level

1 Genes, the basic units of inheritance, are composed of DNA and are located on the chromosomes.
2 DNA is composed of deoxyribose, a phosphate molecule, and four types of nitrogenous bases. The physical structure of DNA is a double helix.
3 The DNA bases code for amino acids, which in turn make up proteins. The amino acids are specified by triplet codons of nitrogenous bases.
4 DNA replication is based on complementary base pair-

ing, in which a single strand of DNA serves as the template for attracting bases that form a new strand of DNA.

5 DNA polymerase is the primary enzyme involved in replication. It adds bases to the new DNA strand and performs proofreading functions.

6 A mutation is an inherited alteration of genetic material (i.e., DNA).

7 Substances that cause mutations are called mutagens.

8 The mutation rate in humans varies from locus to locus and ranges from 10^{-4} to 10^{-7} per gene per generation.

9 Transcription and translation, the two basic processes in which proteins are specified by DNA, both involve ribonucleic acid (RNA). RNA is chemically similar to DNA but it is single-stranded, has a ribose sugar molecule, and has uracil rather than thymine as one of its four nitrogenous bases.

10 Transcription is the process by which DNA specifies a sequence of messenger RNA (mRNA).

11 Much of the DNA sequence is spliced out of the mRNA before the mRNA leaves the nucleus. The excised sequences are called introns, and those that remain to code for proteins are called exons.

12 Translation is the process by which RNA directs the synthesis of polypeptides. This process takes place in the ribosomes, which consist of proteins and ribosomal RNA (rRNA).

13 During translation mRNA interacts with transfer RNA (tRNA), a molecule that has an attachment site for a specific amino acid.

Chromosomes

1 Human cells consist of diploid somatic cells (body cells) and haploid gametes (sperm and egg cells).

2 Humans have 23 pairs of chromosomes. Twenty-two of these pairs are autosomes. The remaining pair consists of the sex chromosomes. Females have two homologous X chromosomes as their sex chromosomes; males have an X and a Y chromosome.

3 A karyotype is an ordered display of chromosomes. They are ordered according to length and the location of the centromere.

4 Various types of stains can be used to make chromosome bands more visible.

5 In each normal female somatic cell, one of the two X chromosomes is inactivated early in embryogenesis.

6 X-inactivation is random, fixed, and incomplete (i.e., only part of the chromosome is actually inactivated).

7 About 1 in 150 live births has a major diagnosable chromosome abnormality.

8 Polyploidy is a condition in which a euploid cell has some multiple of the normal number of chromosomes. Humans have been observed to have triploidy (three copies of each chromosome) and tetraploidy (four copies of each chromosome); both conditions are lethal.

9 Somatic cells that do not have a multiple of 23 chromosomes are aneuploid. Aneuploidy is usually the result of nondisjunction.

10 Trisomy is a type of aneuploidy in which one chromo-

some is present in three copies in somatic cells. A partial trisomy is one in which only part of a chromosome is present in three copies.

11 Monosomy is a type of aneuploidy in which one chromosome is present in only one copy in somatic cells.

12 In general monosomies cause more severe physical defects than trisomies, illustrating the principle that the loss of chromosome material has more severe consequences than the duplication of chromosome material.

13 Down syndrome, a trisomy of chromosome 21, is the best known disease caused by a chromosome aberration. It affects 1 in 800 live births and is much more likely to occur in women over age 35.

14 Most aneuploidies of the sex chromosomes have less severe consequences than those of the autosomes.

15 The most commonly observed sex chromosome aneuploidies are the XXX karyotype, XO karyotype (Turner syndrome), XXY karyotype (Klinefelter syndrome), and XYY karyotype.

16 Abnormalities of chromosome structure include deletions, duplications, inversions, and translocations.

Elements of Population Genetics

1 Mendelian traits are caused by single genes, each of which occupies a position, or locus, on a chromosome.

2 Alleles are different forms of genes located at the same locus on the chromosome.

3 At any given locus in a somatic cell an individual has two genes, one from each parent. An individual may be homozygous or heterozygous for a locus.

4 An individual's genotype is his or her genetic makeup, and the phenotype reflects the interaction of genotype and environment.

5 At a heterozygous locus, a dominant gene's effects mask those of a recessive gene. The recessive gene is expressed only when it is present in two copies.

Transmission of Genetic Diseases

1 Genetic diseases due to single genes usually follow autosomal dominant, autosomal recessive, or X-linked recessive modes of inheritance.

2 Pedigree charts are an important tool in the analysis of modes of inheritance.

3 Recurrence risks specify the probability that future offspring will inherit a genetic disease. For single-gene diseases, recurrence risks remain the same for each offspring, regardless of the number of affected or unaffected offspring.

4 The recurrence risk for autosomal dominant diseases is 50%.

5 Skipped generations are not seen in classical autosomal dominant pedigrees.

6 Males and females are equally likely to exhibit autosomal dominant diseases and to pass them on to their offspring.

7 Many genetic diseases have a delayed age of onset.

8 A gene that is not always expressed phenotypically is said to have incomplete penetrance.

9 Variable expressivity is a characteristic of many genetic diseases.

10 Most commonly parents of children with autosomal recessive diseases are both heterozygous carriers of the disease gene.

11 The recurrence risk for autosomal recessive diseases is 25%.

12 Males and females are equally likely to be affected by autosomal recessive diseases.

13 Consanguinity is often present in families with autosomal recessive diseases, and it becomes more prevalent with rarer recessive diseases.

14 Carrier detection tests for an increasing number of autosomal recessive diseases are available.

15 The frequency of genetic diseases approximately doubles in the offspring of first-cousin matings.

16 X-linked genes are those that are located on the X chromosome. Nearly all known X-linked diseases are caused by X-linked recessive genes.

17 Males are hemizygous for genes on the X chromosome.

18 X-linked recessive diseases are seen much more frequently in males than females, because males need only one copy of the gene to express the disease.

19 Fathers cannot pass X-linked genes to their sons.

20 Skipped generations are often seen in X-linked recessive disease pedigrees because the gene can be transmitted through carrier females.

21 Recurrence risks for X-linked recessive diseases depend on the carrier and affected status of the mother and father.

22 A sex-limited trait is one that occurs only in one of the sexes.

23 A sex-influenced trait is one that occurs more frequently in one sex than in the other.

Linkage Analysis and Gene Mapping

1 During meiosis I, crossing-over occurs. This can cause recombinations of alleles located on the same chromosome.

2 The frequency of recombinations can be used to infer the map distance between loci on the same chromosome.

3 Loci that are on the same chromosome are syntenic.

4 A marker locus, when closely linked to a disease gene locus, can be used to predict whether an individual will develop a genetic disease.

5 A more complete gene map will facilitiate marker studies, studies of gene function and interaction, and gene therapy.

Multifactorial Inheritance

1 Traits that result from the combined effects of several loci are polygenic. When environmental factors also influence the trait, they are multifactorial.

2 Many multifactorial traits have a threshold of liability. Once the threshold of liability is crossed, the disease may be expressed.

3 Empiric risks, based on direct observation of large numbers of families, are used to estimate recurrence risks for multifactorial diseases.

4 Recurrence risks for multifactorial diseases become higher if more than one family member is affected and/or if the expression of the disease in the proband is more severe.

5 If the population frequency of a multifactorial disease is f, the recurrence risk in offspring and siblings is approximately $\sqrt{f}$.

6 Recurrence risks for multifactorial diseases decrease rapidly for more remote relatives.

KEY TERMS

Adenine, 117

Allele, 133

Amino acid, 117

Aneuploid cell, 126

Anticodon, 123

Antisense strand, 123

Autosome, 124

Barr body, 125

Base pair substitution, 121

Carrier, 134

Carrier detection tests, 138

Chromosomal mosaics, 128

Chromosome bands, 124

Chromosome breakage, 131

Chromosome theory of inheritance, 134

Clastogen, 131

Codominance, 134

Codons, 120

Complementary base pairing, 120

Consanguinity, 138

Cri-du-chat syndrome, 132

Crossing-over, 141

Cytosine, 117

Delayed age of onset, 137

Deletions, 132

Deoxyribonucleic acid (DNA), 116

Diploid cells, 124

DNA polymerase, 120

Dominant, 134

Dosage compensation, 125

Double helix, 117

Down syndrome, 128

Duplication, 132

Empiric risk, 148

Euploid cell, 126

Exon, 123

Expressivity, 137

Frameshift mutation, 121

Gamete, 124

Gene, 116

Genotype, 133

Giemsa stain, 124

Guanine, 117

Haploid cell, 124

Hemizygote, 139

Heterogeneous nuclear RNA (hRNA), 123

Heterozygote, 134

Homologous chromosomes, 124

Homozygote, 134

Inbreeding, 138

Intermediate inheritance, 134

Intron, 123

Inversion, 132

Karyotype, 124

Klinefelter syndrome, 130

Linkage, 141

Locus, 133

Map unit, 142

Meiosis, 124

Meiotic failure, 130

Messenger RNA (mRNA), 122

Metaphase spread, 124

Mode of inheritance, 134

Monosomy, 126

Multifactorial inheritance, 147

Mutagen, 121

Mutation, 121

Mutational hot spot, 121

Nondisjunction, 128

Nucleotide, 117

Obligate carrier, 137

Occurrence risk, 136

Partial trisomy, 128

Pedigree, 134

Penetrance, 137

Phenotype, 133

Polygenic trait, 147

Polypeptide, 117

Polyploid cell, 126

Position effect, 132

Principle of independent assortment, 134

Principle of segregation, 134

Proband (propositus/proposita), 134

Purine, 117

Pyrimidine, 117

Recessive, 134

Reciprocal translocation, 133

Recombination, 141

Recurrence risk, 136

Regulatory gene, 116

Ribonucleic acid (RNA), 121

Ribosomal RNA (rRNA), 123

Ribosome, 123

RNA polymerase, 122

Sense strand, 122

Sex chromosome, 124

Sex-influenced trait, 139

Sex-limited trait, 139

Sex-linked, 139

Silent substitution, 121

Somatic cell, 124

Spontaneous mutation, 121

Structural gene, 116

Syntenic loci, 142

Template, 120

Termination or nonsense codon, 120

Termination sequence, 123

Tetraploidy, 126

Threshold of liability, 147

Thymine, 117

Transcription, 121

Transfer RNA (tRNA), 123

Translation, 123

Translocation, 133

Triploidy, 126

Trisomy, 126

Turner syndrome, 130

X-linked inheritance (sex-linked inheritance), 139

REFERENCES

Anderson, W. F. (1984). Prospects for human gene therapy. *Science, 226,* 401.

Bank, A., Mears, J. G., & Ramirez, F. (1980). Disorders of human hemoglobin, *Science, 207,* 486.

Baskin, Y. (1984). *The gene doctors: Medical genetics at the frontier.* New York: William Morrow.

Biggs, R. (1983). Defects in coagulation. In A. E. H. Emery

& D. L. Rimoin (Eds.), *Principles and practice of medical genetics* (Vol. 2.). Edinburgh: Churchill Livingstone.

Boehm, C. D., Antonarakis, S. E., Phillips, J. A., Stetten, G., & Kazazian, H. H. (1983). Prenatal diagnosis using DNA polymorphisms: report on 95 pregnancies at risk for sickle-cell disease or β-thalassemia, *New England Journal of Medicine, 308,* 1054.

Caskey, C. T. (1987). Diasease diagnosis by recombinant DNA complex. *Science, 236,* 1223-1229.

Conneally, P. M. (1984). Huntington's disease: Genetics and epidemiology. *American Journal of Human Genetics, 36,* 506.

Conneally, P. M., & Rivas, M. (1980). Linkage analysis in man. *Advances in Human Genetics, 10,* 209-266.

de Grouchy, J., & Turleau, C. (1984). *Clinical atlas of human chromosomes* (2nd ed.). New York: John Wiley & Sons.

Donahue, R. P., Bias, W. B., Renwick, J. H., & McKusick, V. A. (1968). Probable assignment of the Duffy blood-group locus to chromosome 1 in man. *Proceedings of the National Academy of Science, 61,* 949.

Emery, A. E. H. (1984). *An introduction to recombinant DNA.* New York: Wiley.

Emery, A. E. H. & Rimoin, D. L. (Eds.). (1983). *Principles and practice of medical genetics* (2 vols.). Edinburgh: Churchill Livingstone.

Fraser, F. C. (1976). The multifactorial/threshold concept: Uses and misuses. *Teratology, 14,* 267.

Fuchs, F. (1980). Genetic amniocentesis. *Scientific American, 242,* 47.

Goodman, R. M. & Gorlin, R. J. (1977). *Atlas of the face in genetic disorders* (2nd ed.). St. Louis: C.V. Mosby.

Gusella, J. F. (1986). DNA polymorphism and human disease. *Annual Review of Biochemistry, 55,* 831.

Hall, J. G., Powers, E. K., McIlvaine, R. T., & Ean, V. H. (1978). The frequency and financial burden of genetic disease in a pediatric hospital. *American Journal of Medical Genetics, 1,* 417.

Hartl, D. L. (1983). *Human genetics.* New York: Harper & Row.

Hassold, T. J., & Jacobs, P. A. (1984). Trisomy in man. *Annual Review of Genetics, 18,* 69.

Hook, E. B. & Hamerton, J. L. (1977). The frequency of chromosome abnormalities detected in consecutive newborn studies—differences between studies—results by sex and by severity of phenotypic involvement. *Population cytogenetics: Studies in humans.* New York: Academic Press.

Hook, E. B., & Porter, I. H. (Eds.). (1977). *Population cytogenetics: Studies in humans.* New York: Academic Press.

Jackson, L. G. (1985, March). First-trimester diagnosis of fetal genetic disorders. *Hospital Practice,* 39.

Jacobs, P. A. (1977). Epidemiology of chromosome abnormalities in man. *American Journal of Epidemiology, 105,* 180.

Jenkins, J. B. (1983). *Human genetics.* Menlo Park: Benjamin/Cummings.

Kaufman, S. (1983). Phenylketonuria and its variants. *Advances in Human Genetics, 13,* 217.

Kelly, T. E. (1980). *Clinical genetics and genetics counseling.* Chicago: Year Book Medical Publishers.

Kravitz, K., Skolnick, M., Cannings, C., Carmelli, D., Batg, B., Amos, B., Johnson, A., Mendell, N., Edwards, C., & Cartwright, G. (1979). Genetic linkage between hereditary hemochromatosis and HLA. *American Journal of Human Genetics, 31,* 601.

Lawson, D. (Ed.). (1984). *Cystic fibrosis: Horizons.* New York: Wiley.

Lidsky, A. S., Robson, K. J. H., Thirumalachary, C., Barker, P.E., Ruddle, F. H., Woo, S. L. C. (1984). The PKU locus in man is on chromosome 12. *American Journal of Human Genetics, 36,* 527.

Lyon, M. F. (1962). Sex chromatin and gene action in the mammalian X-chromosome. *American Journal of Human Genetics, 14,* 135.

Martin, J. B. (1987). Molecular genetics: Applications to the clinical neurosciences. *Science, 238,* 765.

McKusick, V. A. (1986a). *Mendelian inheritance in man* (7th ed.). Baltimore: Johns Hopkins University Press.

McKusick, V. A. (1986b). The human gene map. *Clinical Genetics, 29,* 545.

McKusick, V. A. (1972). *Heritable disorders of connective tissues* (4th ed.). St. Louis: C.V. Mosby.

Messer, A., & Porter, I. H. (Eds.). (1983). *Recombinant DNA and medical genetics.* New York: Academic Press.

Morton, N. E. (1961). Morbidity of children from consanguineous marriages. *Progress in Medical Genetics, 1,* 261.

Moser, H. (1984). Duchenne muscular dystrophy: Pathogenetic aspects and genetic prevention. *Human Genetics, 66,* 7.

Pueschel, S. M., & Rynders, J. E. (Eds.). (1982). *Down syndrome: Advances in biomedicine and the behavior sciences.* Cambridge, Mass: Ware Press.

Raven, P., & Johnson, G. (1986). *Biology* (1st ed.). St. Louis: C. V. Mosby.

Riccardi, V. M. (1981). Von Recklinghausen neurofibromatosis. *New England Journal of Medicine, 305,* 1617.

Roth, M. P., Feingold, J., Baumgarten, A., Bigel, P., & Stoll, C. (1983). Re-examination of paternal age effect on Down syndrome. *Human Genetics, 63,* 149.

Ruddle, F. H. (1981). A new era in mammalian gene mapping: Somatic cell genetics and recombinant DNA methodologies. *Nature, 294,* 115.

Seidel, H. M., Ball, M. W., Dains, J. E., & Benedict, G. W. (1987). *Mosby's guide to physical examination.* St. Louis: C. V. Mosby.

Shows, T. B., Sakaguchi, A. Y., & Naylor, S. L. (1982). Mapping the human genome, cloned genes, DNA polymorphisms, and inherited disease. *Advances in Human Genetics, 12,* 341.

Stern, C. (1973). *Principles of human genetics* (3rd ed.). San Francisco: W. H. Freeman.

Thibodeau, G. A. (1987). *Anatomy and physiology.* St. Louis: C. V. Mosby.

Thompson, J. S. & Thompson, M. W. (1986). *Genetics in medicine* (4th ed.). Philadelphia: W. B. Saunders.

Vogel, F. & Motulsky, A. G. (1986). *Human genetics: Problems and approaches* (2nd ed.). Berlin: Springer-Verlag.

Watson, J. D. (1987). *Molecular biology of the gene* (4th ed.). Menlo Park: Benjamin/Cummings.

Watson, J. D. & Crick, F. H. C. (1953). Molecular structure of nucleic acids—A structure for deoxyribosenucleic acid. *Nature, 171,* 737.

Weatherall, D. J. (1985). *The new genetics and clinical practice* (2nd ed.). Oxford: Oxford University Press.

Whaley, L. F. & Wong, D. L. (1987). *Nursing care of infants and children* (3rd ed.). St. Louis: C. V. Mosby.

White, R. L., & Lalouel, J. M. (1987). Investigation of genetic linkage in human families. *Advances in Human Genetics, 16,* 121.

CHAPTER 5

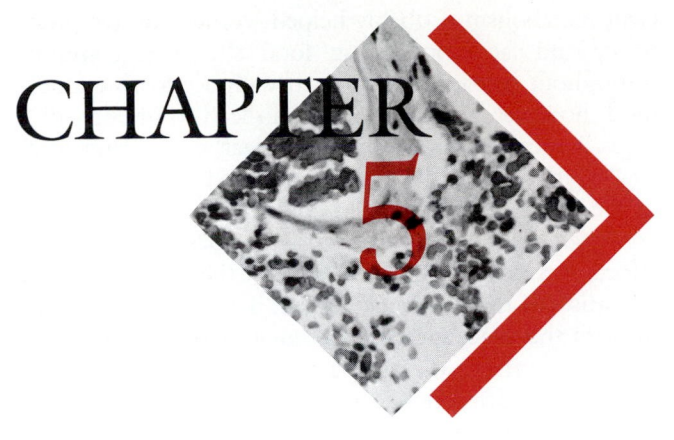

Genes and Environmental Interaction: Familial Diseases

Roger R. Williams

What factors cause disease?, 155
Analyzing disease risk, 158
   Disease rates, 158
   Risk factor analysis, 159
     Analysis with contingency tables, 160
     Analysis with correlation coefficients, 161
Environmental risk factors, 162
   Biologic and immunologic exposures, 162
   Life-style, 162
   Physical and chemical substances, 162
   Psychologic and social factors, 163
Combined effects and interaction among risk factors, 163
   Familial disease tendency, 163
   Aging, 166
Familial diseases and associated risk factors, 168
   Immunologic disorders, 168
   Cancer, 171
     Breast cancer, 171
     Colon cancer, 172
   Endocrine disorders, 173
   Hematologic disorders, 173
   Cardiovascular disorders, 173
     Coronary artery disease, 174
     Hypertension and stroke, 176
   Renal disorders, 178
   Gastrointestinal disorders, 179
     Malabsorption disorders, 179
     Peptic ulcers, 179
     Gallstones, 179
     Obesity, 179
   Neuromuscular disorders, 183
   Psychiatric disorders, 183
The medical family history, 183

Epidemiology is the study of factors governing the occurrence and distribution of disease and disorders in a population. The most significant goal of epidemiology is to acquire the necessary knowledge of causal mechanisms in order to formulate and implement preventive measures against diseases. Almost 2400 years ago, Hippocrates suspected a connection between disease and environment (Hippocrates, republished, 1938). He states, "One should consider attentively the waters which inhabitants use . . .the mode in which the inhabitants live—whether they are fond of drinking and eating to excess or are fond of exercise and labor." Despite this recorded suspicion, virtually no disease-causing characteristics of the environment were discovered in the subsequent 2000 years.

In 1662, John Grant published the first quantitative examination of mortality and birth rates and noted the major impact of the bubonic plague in a defined population. An additional 200 years passed until similar observations led to the beginning of the sustained interest in epidemiology. In 1839, the distribution of cholera was tabulated for England and Wales by William Farr.

In 1855, John Snow published a classic epidemiologic study demonstrating that cholera was caused by water distributed by the Southwark and Vauxhall Water Company in London, which was drawing drinking water from the Thames River at a point heavily polluted by sewage. Two competing water companies supplied water to two different parts of town, causing marked differences in cholera rates and leading to the initial suspicion. Conclusive evidence was found by studying a large portion of London in which the two companies were supplying water to neighboring houses. In this manner, individuals could be matched for socioeconomic status and other characteristics although they had different water supplies. The death rate from cholera was eight times higher among the individuals supplied by the company with polluted water, providing evidence for Snow's hypothesis and eventually leading to a considerable amount of disease prevention.

The studies of Grant, Farr, and Snow were all observational studies. A careful record of disease occurrence in an existing population was correlated with other recorded factors in an effort to determine the cause of a disease. Another test for epidemiologic hypotheses requires intervention to observe whether or not a predicted outcome was associated with a change in a particular environmental factor. Two classic examples include Lind's trying fresh fruit to prevent scurvy (Lind, 1753) and Jenner's trying cowpox vaccination to prevent smallpox (Jenner, 1798).

More current epidemiologic methods have also emphasized common chronic diseases, particularly infectious diseases. The term *epidemic* once meant an outbreak of an infectious disease. The term is now often used by the public and professionals to indicate any disease that seems to have an excessive occurrence. Comparisons between different populations or comparisons of frequencies in different time periods can document changes in disease occurrence. For example, in the United States, coronary atherosclerosis accounts for nearly one third of all deaths, although in some areas of the world it is relatively infrequent. Lung cancer is now over 30 times more common in the United States than it was 50 years ago. Both of these diseases are considered epidemic. Because the rates of occurrence for these diseases have grown relatively slowly, the magnitude of the problem is often not appreciated by the general public. To an American man, the risk of dying of coronary heart disease, for example, equals the risk of major infectious epidemics in past centuries. Current epidemiology also concentrates on unusually low disease frequencies that may provide other clues to what causes and what may prevent disease.

Over the last several decades, epidemiology has rapidly grown into a well-developed discipline. Large observational studies of cardiovascular disease and cancer have involved thousands of investigators, millions of people, and hundreds of millions of dollars. However, even the sophistication of large multicenter, randomized, clinical trials using state-of-the-art biostatistics, laboratory methods, and clinical protocols leaves many important questions unanswered.

Evidence now indicates that many common chronic diseases occur because of a mismatch between genetic and environmental factors. Some inherited traits have helped human beings survive in hostile environments, but these traits now increase susceptibility to chronic disease and early death. For example, genes for an effi-

cient metabolism probably helped women survive pregnancy and lactation during food shortages common throughout history. For women with access to enough food, however, the same genes can lead to obesity, diabetes, hypertension, and stroke. Clearly, environmental factors affect the expression of inherited traits. Scientists of the past generally studied epidemiology and genetics separately. Only within the last 2 decades have scientific efforts increasingly included both of these disciplines in the study of the causes of disease. Today, the goal is to identify the exact genetic and environmental influences that lead to major diseases. This allows individuals with specific susceptibilities to modify environmental factors and avoid tragic consequences. Knowledge of environmental factors should lead to dramatic public health efforts involving screening, identification of high-risk individuals, and effective risk-reduction programs designed to prevent disease.

TABLE 5-1 Environmental factors affecting the occurrence of disease

Type	Examples
Microorganisms and immunologic exposures	Bacteria Viruses Fungi Protozoa Vectors (e.g., insects and animals) Allergens
Personal habits and lifestyle	Smoking Physical exercise Dietary intake
Chemical substances	Toxins Pollutants Medications Solvents, fumes Contaminants
Physical environment	Climate Radiation Physical trauma Geographical location (e.g., sun exposure, altitude) Community (e.g, water and food supplies)
Psychosocial milieu	Family status (e.g., bereavement, loss, status, change) Stress Coping skills Social isolation Ethnic and racial customs Religious customs

WHAT FACTORS CAUSE DISEASE?

Factors causing disease can be simplistically classified as genetic or environmental (Table 5-1). Age and gender play important roles in the development of most diseases. Age often represents the accumulated effects of genetic and environmental factors over time. Sex differences may represent either environmental or genetic factors. Thus, diseases with rates of occurrence that differ between men and women may reflect life-style or environmental differences or anatomic and hormonal differences.

When little is known about the cause of a disease, its occurrence often appears to be a chance or random event. As scientific research identifies more genetic and environmental causes and pathophysiologic mechanisms, however, the number of the diseases that seem to occur at random diminishes. Theoretically, causal factors could be identified for all diseases, so that no disease occurrence could be considered truly random. Furthermore, subtle initiating events, such as mutations or uncommon exposures, might eventually lead researchers to classify all causal factors as either genetic or environmental.

In some cases, of course, the difficulty is in distinguishing between the effects of shared environmental factors and the effects of a genetic background common to a population. Groups of individuals are often reported to have distinctively higher or lower disease rates, either because of shared environmental factors or because of a common gene pool (Carmelli, Williams, & Rissanen, 1982). For example, dietary customs are shared by ethnic groups; genes for some traits are shared by particular racial groups; climate is common to those in shared geographic locations; or health codes shared by religious groups (Table 5-2). Often notable contrasts in disease occurrences are first observed within different populations, leading to the subsequent investigation of possible underlying environmental factors.

Finding and understanding environmental factors that affect the penetrance of specific genes is the single most important concept in preventing chronic familial diseases (see p. 157). For many common chronic diseases, studies suggest that genetic makeup predisposes an individual to the disease but that environmental factors

TABLE 5-2 Populations with shared disease tendencies (due to shared environmental factors, common gene pool, or both)

Disease	Populations	Suggested environmental factors	Shared gene pool
Early coronary heart disease	Very high in Finland (very low in Japan)	Animal fat intake	Genes for high blood cholesterol
Colon cancer	Low in developing countries (e.g., Africa); high in "westernized" countries (USA, Europe)	Dietary fiber and fat intake	
Thalassemia (type of anemia)	High in persons of Mediterranean descent; low in other areas		Major dominant gene for thalassemia
Malaria (many other infectious diseases)	High in some parts of Africa and Asia; low in USA and Europe	Trypanosomes, mosquitoes, disease control measures	
Early type II diabetes and obesity	Native Americans	Change from scarce food supply to plenty	Apparent shared gene pool among various Indian tribes
Lung cancer	Low rates in Mormons and Seventh Day Adventists	Health code against use of tobacco	
Skin cancers	Higher rates among whites than among blacks; higher rates among "sun belt" than in other locations	Ultraviolet light	Inherited level of skin pigmentation

then cause the disease to develop. For example, one hypothesis suggests that genetic predisposition to arterial hypertension is brought out by high salt intake (Williams & Hopkins, 1979). If this theory is true, most of the United States population is exposed to sufficient levels of the environmental factor (high dietary intake of sodium chloride) to allow "salt-sensitive hypertension genes" to be expressed in those who carry them.

Many inherited traits, including some disease states, probably represent the blending of effects of many different genes in which none predominate or stand out. As Chapter 4 explains, these reflect polygenic inheritance; they are therefore termed **polygenic traits.** Environmental influences may then enhance an individual's predisposition to disease, producing a truly multifactorial set of causal factors for any given disease occurrence or observed trait.

Although geneticists often model theories of polygenic traits on the assumption of an infinite number of genes, the wide diversity of genotypes resulting from even three or four loci with two alleles probably ap-

TABLE 5-3 Genetic factors affecting the occurrence of disease

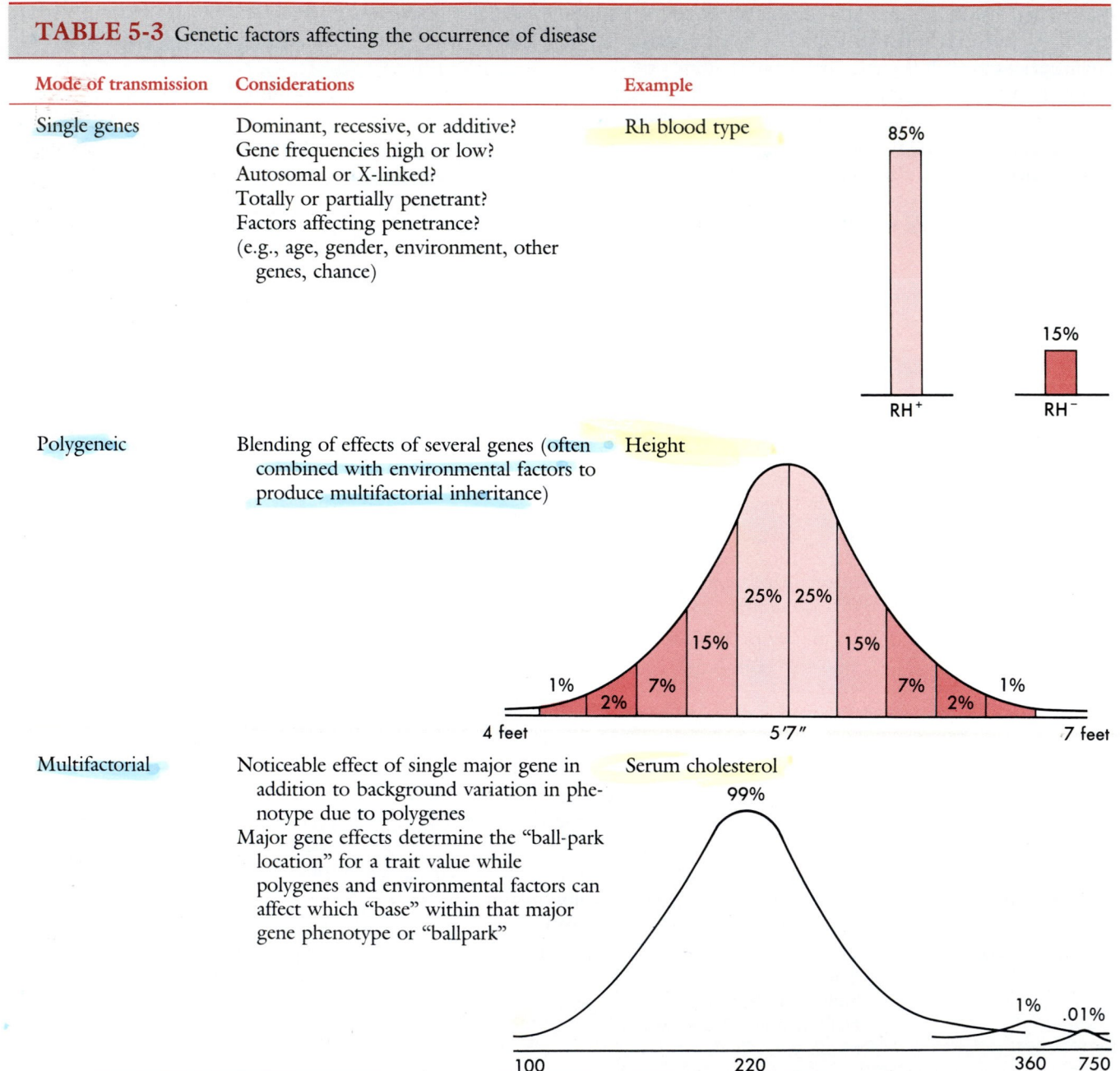

Mode of transmission	Considerations	Example
Single genes	Dominant, recessive, or additive? Gene frequencies high or low? Autosomal or X-linked? Totally or partially penetrant? Factors affecting penetrance? (e.g., age, gender, environment, other genes, chance)	Rh blood type
Polygeneic	Blending of effects of several genes (often combined with environmental factors to produce multifactorial inheritance)	Height
Multifactorial	Noticeable effect of single major gene in addition to background variation in phenotype due to polygenes. Major gene effects determine the "ball-park location" for a trait value while polygenes and environmental factors can affect which "base" within that major gene phenotype or "ballpark"	Serum cholesterol

CLINICAL COMMENTARY
Genetics and Epidemiology: New Applications for Clinical Practice

An ultimate understanding of the causes of disease, of individual susceptibility, and of methods of prevention encompasses the disciplines of genetics and epidemiology together. It also draws on the knowledge of many different disciplines, including pathology, biostatistics, physiology, and numerous subdivisions within each of these disciplines. Epidemiologists identify specific chemicals in the environment thought to induce cancer or cardiovascular disease. Biochemists and molecular physiologists identify cell receptors, the keys to the cellular processes affected by molecules that have been absorbed or manufactured from environmental substances. Biochemists determine the amino acid sequences of cell receptors or enzymes controlling biochemical processes. Population geneticists and clinicians identify specific high-risk families with disorders suspected to involve newly identified biochemical mechanisms, and they obtain ordinary blood samples and important pertinent information about disease occurrence and environmental exposure. Molecular geneticists use this information to develop genetic "probes," extracting DNA from the chromosomes in the nuclei of white blood cells. Like keys in a lock, such probes help to find those individuals in which a "good fit" indicates an inherited predisposition or a specific environmental factor leading to disease.

Although this may sound like science fiction, it is an accurate description of a rapidly evolving technology. Such scientific advances will ultimately lead to the identification and chromosomal location of many genes that cause either susceptibility or resistance to specific diseases. Markers for genetic susceptibility will be developed in conjunction with the identification of the appropriate modifiable environmental variables that work in conjunction with inherited predispositions to cause important chronic disease. Because this field is growing rapidly, a basic understanding of principles needed to understand these applications will be important for health professionals in future decades.

proaches a range of expression similar to the classical polygenic models. Even with only two alleles, two loci produce 9 different genotypes, three loci produce 27 genotypes, and four loci produce 81 genotypes. Even a single locus with three, four, or five alleles will respectively produce 6, 10, or 15 different genotypes. Once environmental influences cause variations in the phenotype for each of these genotypes, a blended spectrum of phenotypes becomes a **multifactorial trait.**

Height is a classic example of a multifactorial trait resulting from many genes with superimposed environmental influences. Heights of individuals in the general population vary across the spectrum from short to tall, although the most common expresssion of the trait is near the middle of the spectrum. Children reach adult status approximately halfway between the height of both parents, after adjustment for females being somewhat shorter than males. With better nutrition, recent generations are also somewhat taller.

The notion of a threshold of liability (defined in Chapter 4) suggests that some disease states may depend on a similar multifactorially determined continuous risk level. A set of multifactorial traits may lead to a varying degree of liability for a disease, but actual expression of the disease occurs only after the liability surpasses some discrete threshold (Cavalli-Storza & Bodner, 1971). For example, serum cholesterol level is a multifactorial trait that is expressed on a continuum. Coronary heart attacks are rarely seen in men with serum cholesterol levels below a threshold of 160 mg/dl and often seen in men above 300 mg/dl.

Even when genetic factors are a primary cause of a condition, other factors might be present as well. With serum cholesterol levels, for example, a major gene may produce strikingly high levels of cholesterol in some individuals, but polygenic inheritance and environmental factors can then cause considerable variation in cholesterol levels among those with this genotype. Many physiologic traits—such as serum cholesterol levels, blood pressure levels, and height—are probably multifactorial traits that result from both polygenic inheritance and environmental factors. The effects of a single gene are observable only when a disease entity emerges, as in the case of striking elevations of cholesterol, high blood pressure, or retarded stature.

Types of genetic factors affecting disease occurrence are described in Table 5-3. Single genes are often expressed as relatively discrete, noticeable phenotypes or as observable genetic defects. The frequency of genetic disease in the general population depends on the gene frequency and the penetrance of a genetic trait (these concepts are defined in Chapter 4). Statistically, dominant genes are more penetrant than recessive genes, but even with genetic predisposition to a specific disorder, individuals with a single dominant gene or with two copies of a recessive gene might not express the genetic disorder. Penetrance can depend on the person's age, gender, environmental factors, and other genes. The effects of these other factors on a particular gene's penetrance are called **interactions** (gene-environment interactions or gene-gene interactions).

ANALYZING DISEASE RISK

Disease Rates

The concepts and terminology used by epidemiologists who assess disease risk provide a foundation for understanding the causes of disease. Several basic rates help to describe the occurrence of disease. All of these rates require accurate surveillance and reporting of disease and a census count of the base population. The **incidence rate** is the number of new cases detected during a given interval (usually 1 year) per number of persons in the population surveyed. The **prevalence rate** refers to the number of persons *living* with the disease (accumulated new and old cases) per number of persons in the population. Thus the prevalance rate is determined by the incidence rate and length of survival for persons with the disease. The **mortality rate** is the number of persons who have died from the disease during a given period (often 1 year) per number of persons in the surveyed population. In 1970, coronary heart disease in American men aged from 50 to 64 showed a prevalence rate of 9.7%, an annual incidence rate of 2.2%, and an annual mortality rate of 0.92% of the base population.

Disease rates can be determined separately in populations with and without exposure to suspected causal factors. If the disease rate is significantly higher in the exposed population, it suggests that the exposure is linked somehow to the disease. In preliminary investigations, most data can only indicate an association or statistical connection between a particular factor and a particular disease. Years of research and a large body of experimental data are often required to determine which disease-associated factors also played a causal role. For example, initial studies showed that lung cancer was most common among cigarette smokers and among men, suggesting that men might have a greater predisposition for developing the disease. Subsequent data, however, showed that the association of male sex with lung cancer is easily explained by the increased level of smoking exhibited by men. Prospective population studies and experimental laboratory investigations have since provided convincing evidence that cigarette smoking causes lung cancer.

FIG. 5-1. Causal and noncausal risk factors associated with lung cancer. Smoking is a causal risk factor for lung cancer. Men and alcohol drinkers have a higher incidence rate for lung cancer because they are also more often smokers. Although construction workers also smoke more, they have more lung cancer even if they are nonsmokers, probably because of exposure to fumes and dust.

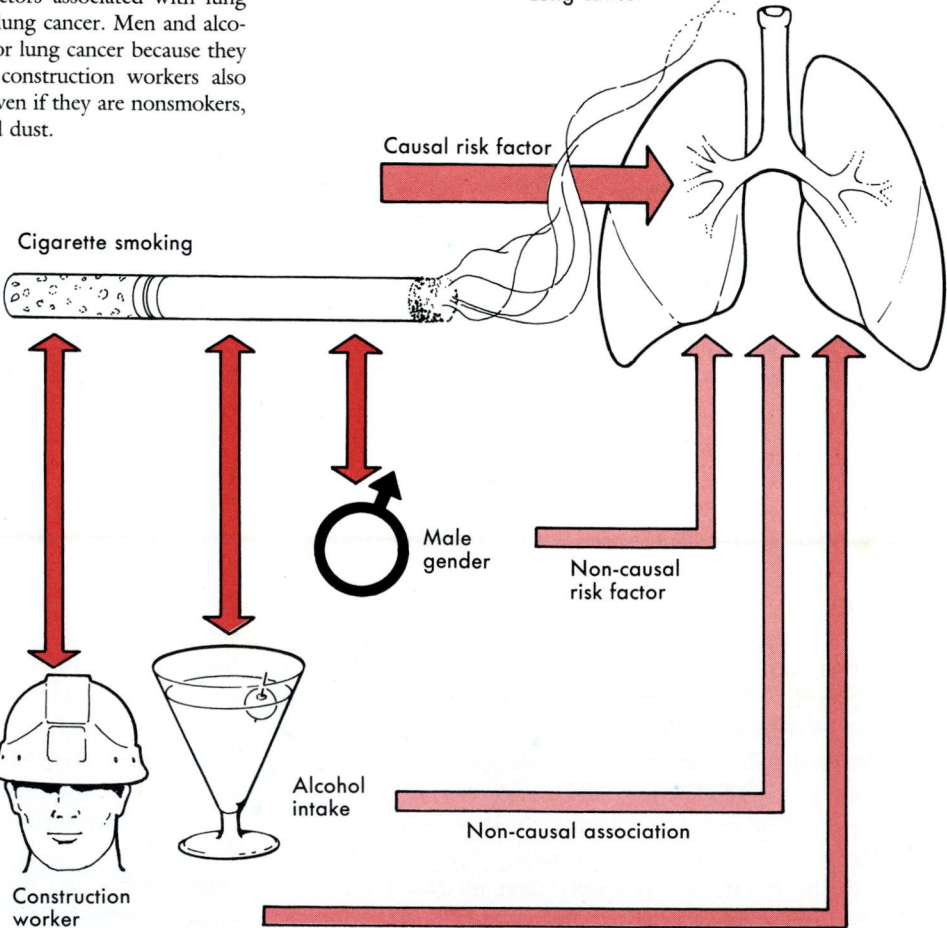

Risk Factor Analysis

Risk factors are indicators of a person's predisposition to developing a disease. A particular risk factor or set of risk factors predicts increased disease rates in a group of individuals (e.g., smokers get more lung cancer than nonsmokers). Risk factors cannot precisely predict whether a specific person will contract or avoid a disease (many smokers do not get lung cancer). As with male sex and lung cancer, risk factors do not always suggest a cause for a disease, but identifying them often provides clues toward identifying the cause of a particular disease.

Sets of risk factors have been developed for many common chronic diseases. Although scientists suspect a causal role for some of these risk factors, solid evidence establishing a causal relationship is lacking for many. The distinction between causal factors and noncausal associations is illustrated in Fig. 5-1. **Causal risk factors** may be identified as those that, when removed or eliminated, will result in the delay or prevention of the disease. **Noncausal risk factors** may be helpful in predicting a person's chances of developing the disease, but they have no direct effect on the underlying cause of the disease.

Cigarette smoking, for example, is a proven causal risk factor leading to lung cancer. Men and alcohol drinkers are more often smokers and, therefore, are also more likely to develop lung cancer. Nonsmoking men and alcohol drinkers do not, however, have an increased risk for lung cancer. Therefore, male gender and alcohol intake are noncausal risk factors for lung cancer. As Fig. 5-1 also shows, the greater incidence of lung cancer among construction workers also suggests a causal association. This may, however, be a result of the dust and

---

TABLE 5-4 Statistical measures used to calculate risk

	Application	Calculation
Contingency table	Lists number of persons according to disease and exposure status	Disease. Exposure: Yes → a, b, m_1 (Exposed persons); No → c, d, m_2 (Nonexposed persons); n_1 Disease cases, n_2 Healthy controls, Grand total
Disease rate (incidence, prevalence, or mortality)	Measures occurrence rate of the disease	$\dfrac{\text{Number of cases, new cases, or deaths}}{\text{Number of persons in the population}}$
Relative risk	Measures the degree of increased disease rate in the exposed population compared to the unexposed population	$\dfrac{\text{Number of exposed cases} \div \text{Number of exposed persons}}{\text{Number of unexposed cases} \div \text{Number of unexposed persons}}$
Population attributable risk (%)*	Measures the percentage of disease cases in a specific population attributable to a specific risk factor	$\dfrac{\left(\begin{array}{c}\text{Number of observed cases} \\ \text{in the exposed} \\ \text{population}\end{array}\right) - \left(\begin{array}{c}\text{Number of expected cases} \\ \text{in the exposed} \\ \text{population}\end{array}\right)}{\text{Total number of cases}} \times 100$
Preventive efficiency	Measures the percentage of exposed persons in a defined population in whom a disease would be prevented if all avoided the causal exposure	$\left(\begin{array}{c}\text{Population-} \\ \text{attributable} \\ \text{risk}\end{array}\right) \times \left(\dfrac{\text{Disease rate}}{\text{Proportion exposed}}\right)$

*Another formula to get same result:

$$\text{Population attributable risk} = \frac{\left(\begin{array}{c}\text{Disease rate} \\ \text{in total} \\ \text{population}\end{array}\right) - \left(\begin{array}{c}\text{Disease rate} \\ \text{in unexposed} \\ \text{population}\end{array}\right)}{(\text{Disease rate in total population})} \times 100$$

fumes associated with construction work (Williams & Horn, 1977; Williams, Stegans, & Goldsmith, 1977).

Analysis with Contingency Tables

The correlation between cigarette smoking and lung cancer also illustrates genetic susceptibility precipitated by environmental exposure. If, as studies indicate, cigarette smoking induces lung cancer more often among individuals who are genetically susceptible (Tokuhata, 1965), the effects of both genetics and environment can be analyzed using **contingency tables.**

The association of a disease with a particular risk factor is often evaluated using 2-by-2 contingency tables illustrated in Table 5-4. The contingency table lists the number of individuals who respectively do or do not have the disease and have or have not experienced exposure to a risk factor. The data that compose the contingency table are then used to calculate various statistical measures.

The **relative risk** of developing the disease is therefore expressed as the ratio of the disease rate among the exposed population to the disease rate in the unexposed population. For lung cancer and cigarette smoking, a relative risk of 13.3 implies a lung cancer rate among smokers that is 13.3 times higher than the rate among nonsmokers. The **population-attributable risk** indicates the percentage of disease cases in the general population that are attributable to a causal risk factor. Although the relative risks and population-attributable risks may be similar measures in susceptible and resistant persons, preventive measures help a higher proportion of people with the genetically susceptible subgroup. This is noted by comparing the **preventive efficiency,** which is the percentage of exposed persons who would be saved from the disease if they all avoided the causal exposure.

In general relative risks show how strongly exposures are linked to specific diseases. Population-attributable risks show which exposures account for the greatest amount of a given disease. Preventive efficiency indicates the cost-effectiveness of prevention programs in specifically defined populations. **High-risk persons** are those exposed to sufficient levels of causal risk factors to increase their disease risk significantly. If they are both

---

TABLE 5-5 Chronic disease rates and relative risks from exposure to risk factors

Risk factor	Possible mechanisms

Genetic predisposition or resistance	Number of different loci promoting or preventing the disease
	Gene frequency of each locus in the population
	Mode of transmission (dominant, polygenic, etc.) of each locus
	Factors increasing or decreasing each gene's survival and effects over generations
	    Death or illness during reproductive years (type I diabetes in past)
	    Heterozygote advantage (e.g., sickle-cell erythrocytes resist malaria)
	    New treatment that improves survival (advances in type I diabetes)
	    Changing environment (e.g., mismatch or "thrifty gene" in Indian tribes surviving for centuries with meager food supply develop obesity and type II diabetes with oversupply of food?)
	Penetrance (sometimes variable depending on interactions with other genes and environmental factors)

Environmental and lifestyle factors that promote or protect	Number and type of exposures or protective factors (e.g., lung cancer and cigarette smoking, and uranium and hydrocarbon fumes) Level of exposure (e.g., packs smoked per day) Duration of exposure (e.g., years of smoking) Potency of exposure (e.g., filtered and nonfiltered cigarettes) Proportion of the general population exposed
Age	Cumulative effects of genes and environment over time Biologic "alarm clock" synchronized to changing metabolism
Gender	X-linked transmission on X chromosome (e.g., hemophilia) Sex-limited expression from hormonal or anatomical differences (e.g., breast cancer) Environmental differences (e.g., men smoke more and have more lung cancer) Combinations (e.g., coronary heart disease and smoking combined with high-density lipoproteins)
Interactions	Combined risk factors (likely present for many familial chronic diseases)

genetically susceptible and exposed to the risk factor, they are at a very high risk of disease. Such individuals are good targets for disease-prevention programs. Factors affecting disease rates and relative risks are summarized in Table 5-5.

Prevention programs must also take into account the difference between cumulative effects leading to disease and acute effects. For example, the accumulated cancer-causing chemicals from cigarette smoking do lead to lung cancer, but the effects require time to develop. Preventing lung cancer thus requires years of smoking avoidance. In contrast, the risk of coronary death seems to be related more to the acute effects of carbon monoxide in cigarette smoke. Even after 20 years of smoking, the risk of coronary death drops to levels similar to those for nonsmokers within 2 years, according to some studies (Feinleib & Williams, 1976).

Analysis with Correlation Coefficients

Sometimes disease characteristics and risk factors can be assessed quantitatively as continuous traits rather than as purely dichotomous (absence or presence) out-comes. In an analysis of disease, **continuous traits** are those that are expressed across a range of severity. Obesity and blood pressure elevation, for example, are related conditions that appear with various degrees of severity. Analyzing obesity as a risk factor in a contingency table requires the choice of numerical dividing lines to obtain simple definition of what constitutes a dichotomous (opposites) classification of subjects into two single groups. Subjects must be either obese or nonobese, hypertensive or normotensive. In such cases quantitative methods may provide greater statistical power for detecting associations between risk factors and disease.

The statistic commonly used to quantify the degree of association between two continuous traits is called the **correlation coefficient** (r). Fig. 5-2 illustrates both a contingency table and a correlation coefficient as methods of analysis applied to simulated data of blood pressure and ideal weight. As Fig. 5-2 shows, each point in the plotted data indicates the blood pressure level and percentage of ideal weight of a single individual. Summarizing the data for many individuals shows graphi-

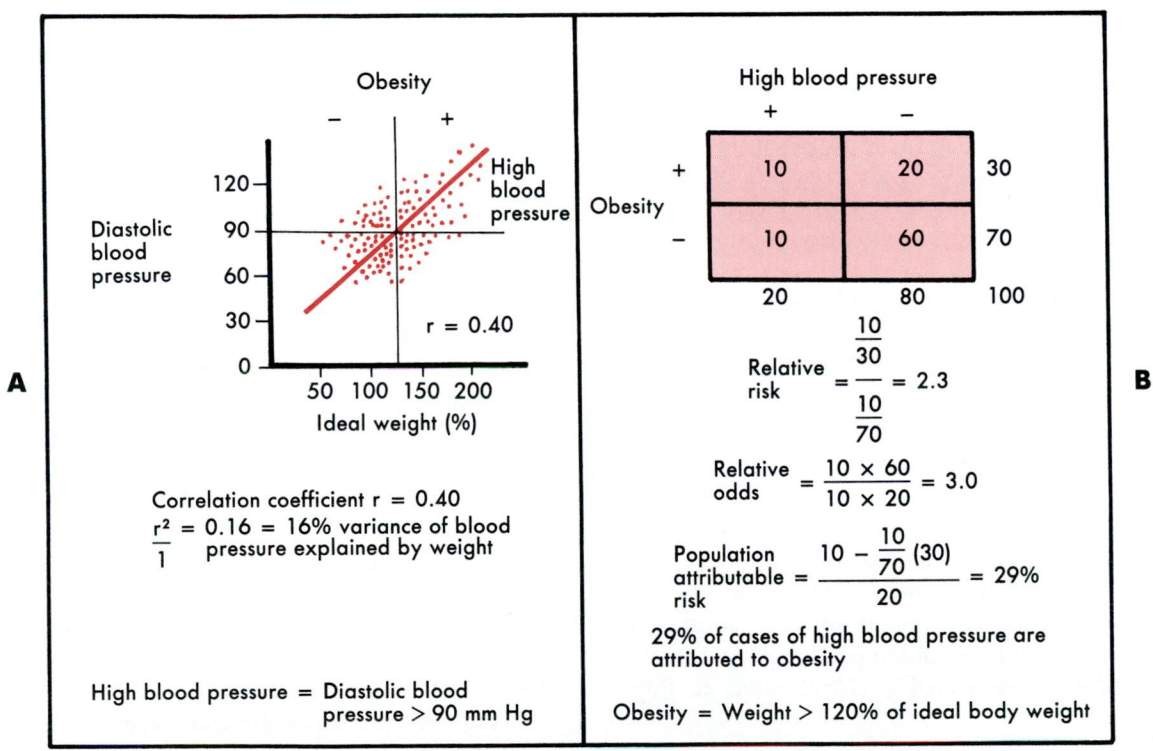

FIG. 5-2. Two methods used to test for an association between specific diseases and causal risk factors for that disease. **A,** Plots and correlation coefficients are used for continuous traits. **B,** A contingency table is used to analyze risk exposure together with the presence or absence of disease. The horizontal line at 90 mm Hg diastolic blood pressure arbitrarily separates points into observations that would be considered to be hypertensive and normotensive individuals. A vertical line at 120% of ideal weight separates individuals arbitrarily into obese and nonobese individuals. These lines thus divide the plotted points into four sections, which correspond to the number of observations tabulated in the contingency table.

cally a general but not perfect correlation between blood pressure values and weight levels. If the correlation between two characteristics were perfect, then all plotted points would fall along a single line, and the correlation coefficient would be 1.00 (this is a positive number for direct relationships and negative for inverse relationships). If there were no correlation, there would be a correlation coefficient of 0.00, and plotted points would show a randomly scattered distribution. The square of the correlation coefficient is also a useful statistic because it indicates the percentage of variation of the dependent variable (in this case diastolic blood pressure) that is explained by the independent test variable (here the percentage of ideal weight).

The same set of data could be analyzed by means of a contingency table by setting a defined point to separate quantitative values for individuals considered obese or nonobese and hypertensive or normotensive. As shown in Fig. 5-2, a contingency table would thus produce a relative risk and a population-attributable risk.

Some statistics can be calculated only when the data are available from the entire general population. For example, disease rates in the exposed and unexposed populations are required for calculations of relative risk and population-attributable risk. To obtain accurate disease rates, surveillance or screening data must be collected from an entire population of mostly healthy people. Large community examination projects such as the Framingham Study (Gordon & Kannel, 1971) or tumor surveillance efforts such as the Third National Cancer Survey (Williams et al., 1977) are examples of such extensive but informative studies. In large-scale studies, a small percentage of subjects are generally found to have the disease of interest.

Initial studies of diseases and risk factors are usually carried out in more cost-efficient, case-control settings. Considerable cost savings result from examining a collection of disease cases and a matched number of healthy controls to see whether the exposure to suspected causal risk factors is more common among disease cases. Although epidemiologists cannot calculate relative risk, studies have shown that for case-control studies, the **relative odds** (or cross-products ratio determined from the data in the contingency table and illustrated in Fig. 5-2) are a reasonable approximation of the relative risk that would be obtained if cross-sectional or population data were available (MacMahon & Pugh, 1970).

For rare diseases and uncommon environmental exposures, the relative odds will be almost identical to the value of the relative risk. When either the disease or the exposure variable becomes common, the relative odds will be inflated, as compared to the relative risk (as it is in the simulated example of two relatively common disorders in Fig. 5-2).

ENVIRONMENTAL RISK FACTORS
Biologic and Immunologic Exposures

Several major types of environmental risk factors known to affect disease occurrence are categorized in Table 5-1. Some of these are environmental pathogens that cause such infectious diseases as pneumonia, tuberculosis, small pox, poliomyelitis, and malaria. Immunologic reactions triggered by microbes and other environmental stimuli also play a prominent role in causing such diseases as asthma, rheumatic heart disease, and probably also type I diabetes and multiple sclerosis. (Immune mechanisms are discussed in Chapter 6.)

Life-style

Personal habits and life-style factors have been found to be associated with some of the most common chronic diseases, including cancer and atherosclerosis. The frequency of this kind of environmental exposure in the general population is often the single most important factor in determining changing disease rates over time. For example, a dramatic increase in the frequency of cigarette smoking from the beginning of the century until the end of World War II was associated with parallel increases in lung cancer and coronary heart disease. Several decades after men began to smoke, greater numbers of women began to increase their cigarette consumption, and similar increases in disease rates were ultimately seen in women. The effects of exposure to smoke can reflect varying degrees of exposure (packs of cigarettes smoked, etc.) or different kinds of environmental exposure, some of which are more potent than others. (For example, cigarette smoking is usually more hazardous than industrial smog.)

Physical and Chemical Substances

Chemical substances introduced into the environment have been associated with diseases ranging from liver damage to rare cancers and cardiac dysrhythmias. Among these exposures are medications, such as chemotherapeutic agents used to treat cancer. These often achieve beneficial effects but sometimes cause adverse effects greater than the ailments they were designed to eliminate (cancer treatment is discussed in Chapter 10). Toxins, pollutants, solvents, fumes, and contaminants in food, air, and water are other examples of disease-causing chemical exposures (see Chapter 2).

Some environmental exposures are identified indirectly. For example, population data show that Mormons develop less lung cancer and myocardial infarction. The association between disease and this group shows that these individuals share some characteristics, one of which is that they avoid cigarette use. Presumably, this is one of the causal risk factors linked to these diseases (Lyon, Klauber et al., 1977; Lyon, Wetzler et al., 1978).

Different components of the physical environment also promote diseases. Climate, for example, is associated with the occurrence of malaria, other infectious diseases, and multiple sclerosis. Different types of radiation exposure lead to disorders ranging from sunburn and heat exhaustion to radiation-induced skin cancer and leukemia (see Chapters 24 and 41). A nuclear holocaust with associated physical trauma, burns, and radiation sickness is the most serious possible environmental exposure, but ordinary burns and lacerations are other illnesses stemming from the physical environment.

Psychologic and Social Factors

Emotional disorders are often associated with other major diseases, either as a contributing cause or as a result of physical illness. Social and psychologic factors have been difficult to define accurately and are challenging to treat. The ill effects of these factors, however, consume a large portion of medical attention.

Increased total mortality and incidence rates of some major cardiovascular diseases and/or cancer have been suggested in studies of several social factors including (1) "type A" hard-driving personality, (2) decreased social supporting networks (friends, relatives, churches), (3) being unmarried (divorced, widowed, or never married), (4) stressful life events (death of a spouse, divorce, bankruptcy), (5) anger, (6) hostility, (7) low self-esteem, and (8) lower socioeconomic status (Chesney & Rosenman, 1985; Hopkins & Williams, 1981). Investigators suggest a significant role for psychologic stress (see Chapter 9), anxiety, and depression in the development and progression of cancers, hypertension, coronary artery disease, and many other chronic illnesses.

COMBINED EFFECTS AND INTERACTION AMONG RISK FACTORS

Unraveling the pathophysiology of many common diseases requires understanding complex combinations and interactions of variables that may be difficult to define. Some risk factors are known and measurable, but other undefined genetic and environmental risk factors also contribute to the disease. When one or more risk factors interact, the individual effects of risk factors may be greatly magnified in a multiplicative or exponential manner, as illustrated in Fig. 5-3. Some factors alone may present little or no risk for disease, but in the presence of another factor, the risk increases substantially. For example, the combined effects of cigarette smoking and oral contraceptives increase the chance of myocardial infarction by approximately eighteenfold in young women (Jick et al., 1978) Either oral contraceptives or cigarette smoking alone has far less effect on coronary disease than the effect of both factors combined.

One of the major goals of current research is to define the **heterogeneity,** or variety of causal factors, of common chronic diseases. When a disease is initially studied in a general population, several different types of the disease with different causes may be combined in a single population of subjects. Careful definition of environmental risk factors, biochemical and genetic markers, and disease characteristics can often lead to the separation of cases into distinctive categories or syndromes with differing pathophysiologic mechanisms. This in turn suggests differing strategies for treatment and prevention. For example, chronic diseases with defined or suspected multiple causes include coronary atherosclerosis, diabetes, essential hypertension, and cancers of the breast and colon. All involve several environmental risk factors and also show familial predispositions in a substantial proportion of cases.

Familial Disease Tendency

Initial assessments of aggregation of disease in families can be made by collecting observations about sets of relatives such as siblings, parents with offspring, spouse pairs, and twin sets. Statistical tests of those observations determine whether pairs of relatives both have a specific disease (or similar test results for continuous traits) more often than two randomly selected individuals from the general population (Hunt, Hasstedt, & Williams, 1986).

Analyses often involve the simple comparison of the outcome of pairs of individuals with a defined relationship. The same statistical methods—correlation coefficients and contingency tables—are used to assess the familial aggregation of the disease, as illustrated in Fig. 5-4. In the first column, height is shown to correlate very highly between identical twin pairs and quite strongly among sibling pairs, suggesting a strong genetic determination. Some detectable correlation at a lower level among spouse pairs might suggest selective mating (i.e., persons tend to marry individuals of similar height).

In the correlation plots in Fig. 5-4, even the two twins who are considered tall and not tall are very close to the boundaries used to separate tall and not tall, indicating a very high degree of correlation and concordance for this trait. In contrast, the lack of similarity of blood pressure in spouse pairs is indicated by plotted points that seem to have a randomly scattered distribution. Significant familial correlations are indicated for blood pressure values in pairs of twins and siblings.

If a point of separation is defined for these continuous traits, the data can be analyzed using contingency tables. Here relative risks and associated levels of statistical significance are objective measures of familial ag-

CLINICAL COMMENTARY
Association Between Cigarette Smoking and Lung Cancer: Data From a Simulated Population

Among both genetically susceptible and genetically resistant individuals, the relative risk and population-attributable risk of cigarette smoking leading to lung cancer are both very high (see below left). If screening methods could be developed to identify genetically susceptible individuals as in the simulated data here, one case of lung cancer would be prevented for each two persons who stopped smoking in this population. In contrast, in the general population one case of lung cancer would be prevented for every 11 persons who stopped smoking.

A lifetime risk summary can be compiled from the simulated data. In the general population an overall risk of ap-

proximately 4% reflects a mixture of smokers with a 10% lifetime risk and nonsmokers with less than 1% risk (see below right). In the simulated data, about half of lung cancers are genetically predisposed. Having only one first-degree relative with lung cancer only indicates a possible positive family history and a somewhat increased risk of lung cancer. A strong family history (indicated by two or more first-degree relatives with disease) increases a person's risk substantially. Because those with strong family histories share half of their genes in common with first-degree relatives, they have a 50-50 chance of having the gene that predisposes them to the disease. Their risk of lung cancer

---

STATISTICAL MEASUREMENT OF SIMULATED DATA

	Total population (N = 3000)	Genetically susceptible subpopulation (N = 300)	Genetically resistant subpopulation (N = 2700)
Contingency table	Lung cancer + − Cigarette + : 100 | 900 | 1000 smoking − : 15 | 1985 | 2000 115 3000	Lung cancer + − Cigarette + : 50 | 50 | 100 smoking − : 10 | 190 | 200 60 300	Lung cancer + − Cigarette + : 50 | 850 | 900 smoking − : 5 | 1795 | 1800 55 2700
Disease rate (lung cancer incidence)	$\frac{115}{3000} \times 100\% = 3.8\%$	$\frac{60}{300} \times 100\% = 20\%$	$\frac{55}{2700} \times 100\% = 2\%$
Relative risk of lung cancer for smokers	$\frac{\frac{100}{1000}}{\frac{15}{2000}} = 13.3$	$\frac{\frac{50}{100}}{\frac{10}{200}} = 10$	$\frac{\frac{50}{900}}{\frac{5}{1800}} = 20$
Population-attributable risk due to smoking	$\frac{100 - \left(\frac{15}{2000}\right)1000}{115} \times 100\%$ $= 80\%$	$\frac{50 - \left(\frac{10}{200}\right)100}{60} \times 100\%$ $= 75\%$	$\frac{50 - \left(\frac{5}{1800}\right)900}{55} \times 100\%$ $= 86\%$
Preventive efficiency for stopping smoking	Eliminate smoking in 1000 persons to prevent 92 cases of lung cancer: $(80\%)\left(\frac{3.8\%}{33\%}\right) = 9\%$	Eliminate smoking in 100 persons to prevent 45 cases of lung cancer: $(75\%)\left(\frac{20\%}{33\%}\right) = 45\%$	Eliminate smoking in 900 persons to prevent 43 cases of lung cancer: $(86\%)\left(\frac{2\%}{33\%}\right) = 5\%$

NOTE: Assumptions for this simulated population:
   3.8% of total population develop lung cancer (115/3000)
   33% of total and subtotal populations smoke (1000/3000; 100/300; 900/2700)
   10% of total population is genetically susceptible (300/3000)
   50% penetrance of lung cancer in smokers who are genetically susceptible.
   The first two assumptions are approximations from actual data. The penetrance and percentage of genetically susceptible individuals are not known but will be discovered in future studies of gene markers.

is, therefore, more than double that of individuals in the general population who have the same smoking status.

If a gene marker could identify exactly those individuals who have a genetic predisposition to lung cancer, then even with a 50% penetrance, individuals could be found who have a 50% probability of developing the disease if they smoke cigarettes. Such individuals, of course, would be ideal targets for intensive risk-reduction programs. Actually, most people who smoke cigarettes do not develop lung cancer, so most of the population would probably fall into the category of individuals who are genetically resistant to smoking-induced lung cancer.

LIFETIME RISK OF LUNG CANCER PREDICTED FROM SIMULATED DATA

Population group or subgroup	Status regarding genetic predisposition	Lifetime lung cancer risk		
		Smokers	Non	Combined
General population	1 of 10 persons carry the gene	10.0%	0.75%	3.8%
Have the gene for lung cancer (found using DNA gene markers)	100% have the gene found using DNA gene marker test (not available now but likely will be within 10 years; see Chapter 6)	50.0%	5.0%	20.0%
Strong positive family history with 2 or more first-degree relatives having lung cancer	½ have the gene (if two relatives with lung cancer cases have gene, ½ of first-degree relatives have it)	25.0%	2.5%	10.0%
Mild positive family history with only one parent or sibling having lung cancer	1 of 4 persons carry the gene (½ of lung cancer cases have the gene; ½ of their first-degree relatives share the gene)	12.5%	1.25%	5.0%
Not genetically susceptible (gene absent in DNA marker test)	0% have the gene	5.5%	0.3%	2.0%

NOTE: Data are based on assumption of a dominant gene for lung cancer with 50% penetrance in cigarette smokers and 5% penetrance in nonsmokers.

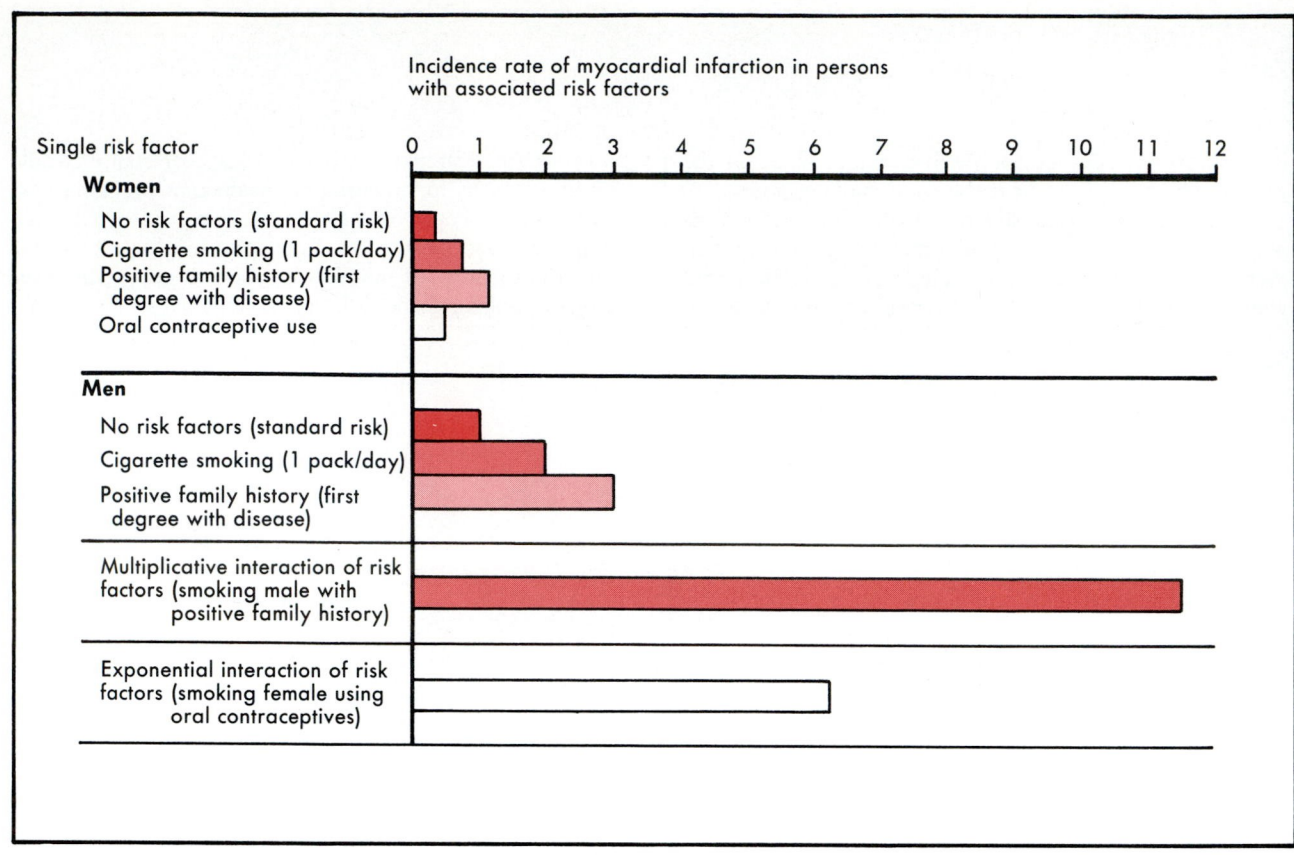

FIG. 5-3. Magnified risks from interactions among risk factors. The rate of myocardial infarction is indicated for 35- to 45-year-old adults in nine different risk settings. Beginning with males and females with standard MI risk, the risk of MI is increased 2 to 3 times each by male gender, smoking, and a positive family history as isolated risk factors. A multiplicative interaction of smoking with a positive family history magnifies the risk well beyond the additive effects of each risk factor alone. Oral contraceptive pill users have little or no increased risk of MI unless they smoke cigarettes too. Their risk is then increased exponentially from that for other women. These data suggest a dramatic reduction in MI risk for high-risk persons who avoid smoking. The data presented are approximations extrapolated from several different reports of actual data (Hopkins & Williams, 1984; Feinlieb & Williams, 1976; Jink, 1976).

gregation of diseases. The concordance rate is a useful descriptive statistic reflecting the degree of familial disease aggregation. It defines the percentage of pairs in which both individuals are affected as a proportion of all pairs in which at least one person is affected.

Familial correlations and contingency table analyses can identify familial aggregation of risk factors, which may be either genetic or shared environmental factors. Contrasting identical and nonidentical twin pairs and related individuals and nonrelated persons living together (such as spouses or adopted children) provide initial impressions of whether or not genetic or environmental factors are responsible for familial disease aggregation.

Definitive understanding of genetic and environmental familial disease aggregations requires sophisticated analyses of many nuclear families or large pedigrees to define gene frequencies, modes of genetic transmission, effects of shared environment, and the factors affecting the penetrance of genetic predispositions. Definitive results often require large and expensive studies with large sample sizes, sophisticated data collection (including DNA markers), and complex mathematical analysis. Unfortunately, few such analyses are currently available for common chronic diseases. Many will likely become available in the future.

Aging

Age is a risk factor for many diseases and may be compared to a clock ticking relentlessly until the alarm goes off and the disease is expressed (Table 5-6). Heart attacks, strokes, cancers, high blood pressure, diabetes, obesity, arthritis, and emotional illness are all more common with increasing age. Because age is accurately

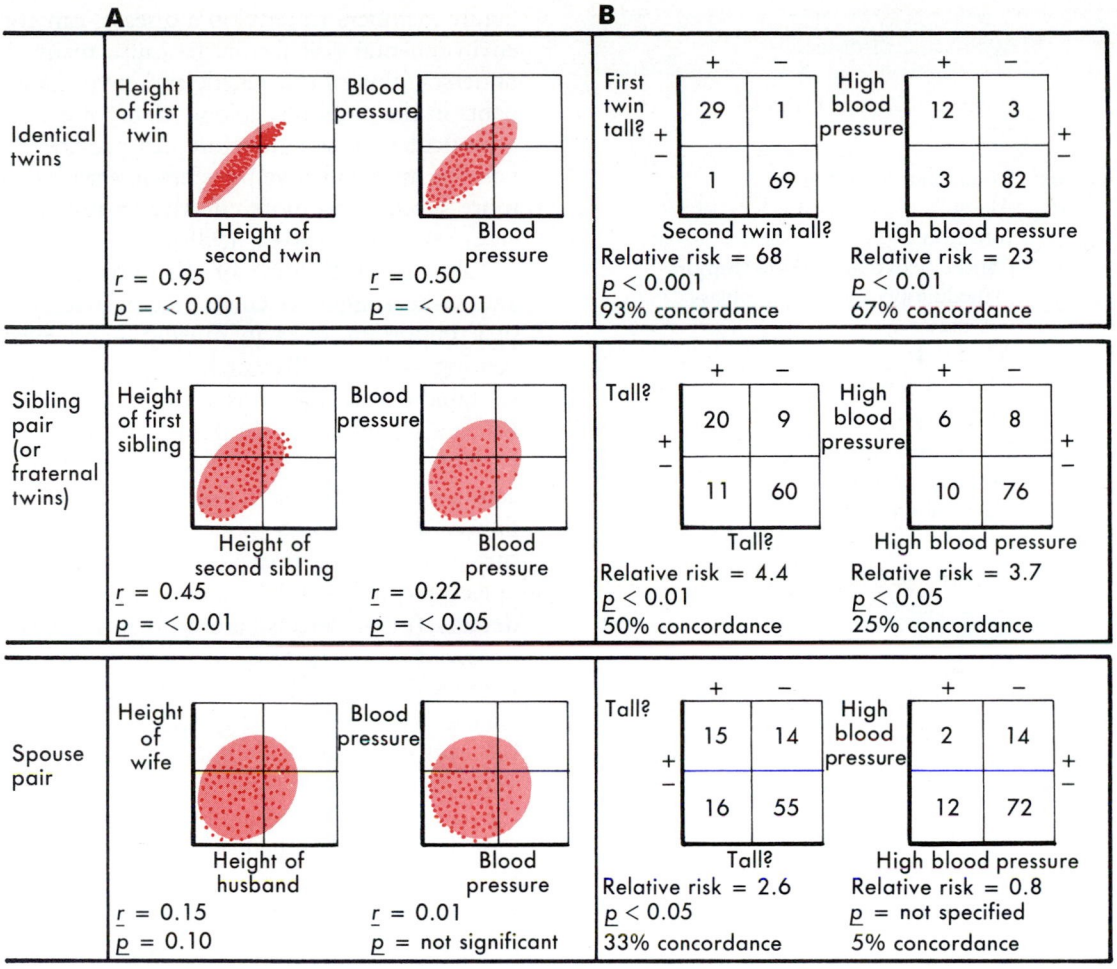

r = Correlation of coefficient; p = probability of occurrence (0.05 or less is considered significant);
Concordance rate = percentage of pairs that share a given trait.

Thirty percent of the general population is defined as tall; 15% of the general population has high blood pressure.

FIG. 5-4. Analysis of familial aggregation of traits and diseases with correlation coefficients and contingency tables. **A,** Horizontal and vertical lines within the correlation plots separate the individual points into four groups corresponding to the number of individuals listed in the four cells of the contingency table to test for familial aggregation or correlation of specific traits or diseases. Each point in the correlation plot represents a pair of relatives. For example, in the top left-hand plot, one point represents the height of the first twin along the vertical axis and the height of the second twin along the horizontal axis. The horizontal and vertical lines arbitrarily divide these twin pairs into individuals who would be considered tall or not tall. **B,** The corresponding contingency table indicates that 29 of these twin pairs were both considered to be tall and 69 were both considered to be not tall, whereas in 2 pairs of twins one individual was considered to be tall and the other considered to be not tall.

determined and is a strong predictor of disease risk, epidemiologists usually test and adjust for the effects of age in their search for the causes of diseases.

Age is not, however, only a confounder and an unmodifiable risk factor. In many cases, age probably represents the accumulating effects of environmental exposures and inherited biochemical processes. Understanding both genetic and environmental causes of disease may eventually lead to "stopping the clock" for some diseases or at least "slowing down the ticking" and de-

laying the age of disease expression. (Theories of aging are discussed in Chapter 2.)

The general degeneration that accompanies aging can also result from deterioration of genetic templates (i.e., malfunction in RNA repair) and loss of immunologic defenses (i.e., against cancer or infection). Tissue integrity is also compromised through changes in elastin, bone matrix, collagen, or through loss of neurons. (The systemic effects of aging are discussed in appropriate units in Part II.)

TABLE 5-6 Age-related disorders

Age	Disorders correlated with age range
Birth-14 years	Congenital disorders Allergy Infection Cancer (leukemia, Wilms' tumor, medulloblastoma, retinoblastoma) Accidents Diabetes (juvenile)
15-30 years	Allergy (asthma) Endocrine Accidents (suicide) Venereal disease
30-40 years	Ulcer Hypertension Breast cancer Homicide Suicide Complications of pregnancy Alcoholism
40-60 years	Heart disease (hypertension, rheumatic, infarction) Kidney disease (glomerular nephritis) Liver disease (cirrhosis) Cancer (lung, colon, breast, ovary)
60-80 years	Cardiovascular Cancer (lung, colon, prostate)
80-100 years	Cancer (leukemia, lymphoma, prostate) Dementia (Alzheimer's, Parkinson's) Osteoporosis Infection Cardiovascular Accidents (fracture)

Adapted from King, Fenoglio, & Lefkowitch, 1983.

FAMILIAL DISEASES AND ASSOCIATED RISK FACTORS

"You can't change your genes, so inherited diseases cannot be prevented, right?" Wrong! Unfortunately, some clinicians and many persons in high-risk families have this misconception and take no steps to avoid the serious consequences of disorders such as early coronary heart disease or breast and colon cancer. A **familial tendency,** of the increased possibility for genetically related family members to develop a disease, can combine with environmental risk factors to cause many diseases. An understanding of the genetic and environmental components in the pathophysiologic chain of events leading to a particular disease therefore can provide a solid rationale for more effective prevention, earlier detection, and more specific and more effective treatment of these diseases (Williams, 1984a, 1988).

Table 5-7 lists some of the known familial diseases and some suggested environmental factors that might play important roles in causing—and eventually preventing—disease. Research in this area is progressing so rapidly that these data cannot be comprehensive. What is significant is the variety of diseases that are apparently familial and the wide variety of potential interacting environmental factors. The promise of more definitive data suggests tremendous opportunities for future detection and prevention of familial disorders.

Recurrence risks for some multifactorial **congenital defects** (birth defects) are estimates based on empiric observations of the frequencies of multiple cases seen in families (Emery & Rimoin, 1983). Some genetic disorders follow well-defined genetic patterns of expression, but even in those disorders that are present at birth, a wide range of expression is evident in relatives sharing the same gene. For example, a proband (the subject or individual being studied) having a neural tube defect expressed as marked deformities of the spinal cord (i.e., spina bifida) might have first-degree relatives with minor defects found on spinal x-ray films but causing no symptoms (a disorder termed spina bifida occulta). Congenital heart defects can be severe or minor in members of the same family. Furthermore, not all congenital disorders are genetically transmitted. Environmental factors such as drugs, radiation, alcohol, and cigarette smoke probably take their toll on the fetus early in pregnancy, perhaps with greater effect among genetically susceptible fetuses.

Factors used in estimating risks for these multifactorial traits include presence of the disease in parents, sibling, or other relatives; severity of the disorder in those already affected; sex-specific predominance for some disorders (e.g., pyloric stenosis occurs five times more often in males); and any environmental factors known. Consanguinity of parents has little effect on the risk of most of these multifactorial disorders. Genetic evaluation and counseling for these birth defects (see Chapter 4) is often quite different from counseling provided for the common chronic diseases that show a familial predisposition.

Immunologic Disorders

Several immunologic diseases seem to have strong familial tendencies (Emery & Rimoin, 1983; Goodman, 1970; Stobo, 1982). Recent developments in identify-

TABLE 5-7 Chronic diseases thought to have genetic predisposition

Disease	Associated pathophysiology or hypothesis	Genetic factors	Environmental factors
Coronary heart disease (especially early disease)(several different syndromes)	Familial hypercholesterolemia	Dominant	Dietary fat, saturated fat, polyunsaturated fat, total fat intake
	LDL receptor defects	Dominant	
	Other high cholesterol?	Unknown	
	Low HDL	Dominant	Exercise, alcohol, diet
	Endothelial factors?	Unknown	Smoking
	Platelet factors?	Unknown	
	Apolipoproteins, etc?	(Apo B dominant?) (Apo A-I recessive) (Lipoprotein [a] codominant)	
	Diabetes I and II	Unknown	
	Hypertension (especially early onset)	Unknown	
	Multiplicative interactions of history and risk factors	Unknown	
Stroke	Hypertension and diabetes	Unknown	
Hypertension	Heterogenous?	Polygenic?	Salt, stress, obesity
	Age at onset?	Major gene?	Polyunsaturated fat, calcium, exercise
	Severity? Etiology?	Quite penetrant?	
Type I diabetes	Islet cell destruction	Recessive?	Viral infection
	Immunologic cause	<50% penetrant	Seasonal variation
		HLA linkage and association with chromosome 6	Complications a function of blood sugar control for years
Type II diabetes	Insulin resistance or decreased production	80%-100% penetrant	Obesity
		Dominant?	Dietary sugar and fiber
		RFLP* association to insulin gene on chromosome 11	Exercise protective Complications a function of blood sugar control and function
Breast cancer	Possibly estrogen related	Some dominant	Age at first birth
	Certain benign tumor precursors	50-90% penetrant in some families	Obesity? Dietary fat? Alcohol? Female hormones
Colon cancer	Several different types of syndromes	Some dominant	Fiber intake
	Often benign polyps are precursors		Dietary fat? (converted by bacteria to carcinogens
Lung cancer	Chemical carcinogens from environment encounter enzymatically susceptible subjects	Known familial aggregation ± smoking	Cigarette smoke Environmental pollutants Radiation exposure
Rheumatic heart disease	Immunologic cross-reactivity to bacteria and heart valves	Familial aggregation	Group A β-strep bacterial infection Penicillin prevents
Asthma and other allergies	Immunologically reactive	Familial aggregation	Many possible allergens—fur, dust, pollen, mold, etc. Avoidance to prevent

*RFLP, Restriction fragment length polymorphism; DNA markers for disease.
†Monozygotic.
‡Dizygotic.

Continued.

TABLE 5-7 Chronic diseases thought to have genetic predisposition—cont'd

Disease	Associated pathophysiology or hypothesis	Genetic factors	Environmental factors
Autoimmune disorders: rheumatic arthritis, Hashimoto thyroiditis and Grave disease, Addison disease, ideopathic thrombocytopenic purpura (ITP), type I diabetes, systemic lupus erythematosis	Autoantibodies to thyroid, adrenal, synovium, platelets	HLA linked on chromosome 6	Viral infections trigger immune responses
Psychiatric disorders: manic–depressive, depression, schizophrenia	Neurochemical disorders in brain tissue	Strongly familial and likely genetic in twin, adoption, and family studies	Uncertain influence Dramatic success with drug treatment for first two
Kidney stones	Mineral-acid-base imbalance	Very familial	Milk? Soda pop? Other fluids?
Gallstones	Fat, cholesterol, bilirubin balance	Quite familial	Dietary fat Obesity?
Obesity (probably very heterogenous)	Less energy wasted? Decreased thermogenesis in brown fat? Other basic energy differences like ATPase pumps? "Thrifty gene?"	Major genes in animals Clusters in families Assortative mating MZ† twins > DZ‡ twins Racial group (American Indians and Polynesians)	Dietary fat, sugar, and total calories Stress, etc., affecting appetite Exercise level Cultural perceptions attractive to be fat or thin
Gout	Several different enzyme defects found	Several autosomal major genes	Dietary intake of meat, etc.
Multiple sclerosis	Autoimmune demyelination of nerve fibers	HLA association Poorly penetrant MZ twins often discordant	Slow virus? Climate dependent
Peptic ulcer disease	Excess acid production and/or decreased mucosal resistance	Biochemical markers of affected Variable penetrance	Stress Diet Dramatic drug Rx
Hemolytic anemia	G6PD deficiency Red cell hemolysis precipitated by exposure to drugs or infections	X-linked recessive	Aspirin Antibiotics Infections
Lactose intolerance	Deficiency of lactase enzyme in intestinal mucosa	Very common in black race	Milk products
Alcoholism	Possible neurochemical origin? Associated with other psychiatric disorders	Quite familial (due to genes and/or family environment?)	Ethyl alcohol intake Social factors
Hemochromatosis	Increased iron absorption	Linked to HLA on chromosome 6 Recessive Quite penetrant	Treat with phlebotomy and prevent organ damage from iron loading

ing cellular markers, such as antigens, have considerably aided the investigation of these disorders (see Chapter 6). These include rheumatoid arthritis, systemic lupus erythematosus, ideopathic Addison disease, thyroid disorders (e.g., autoimmune thyroiditis and Graves disease), and possibly ideopathic thrombocytopenic purpura (ITP). For example, researchers propose that in the case of rheumatoid arthritis, genetically susceptible individuals become sensitive to collagen (Stobo, 1982).

Allergies and asthma also tend to run very strongly in some families (Emery & Rimoin 1983; Goodman, 1970), and here again, interaction with environmental factors is evident. Early exposure to foods in infants and exposure to animal fur, dust, and other pollutants in young children prone to asthma are thought to aid in the progression of allergic diseases. Preventive measures include identifying allergy-prone children and having them avoid exposure to environmental allergens.

Many infectious diseases, such as rheumatic fever, may also involve immunologic susceptibility to severe effects. Furthermore, certain rare and well-defined immunodeficiency syndromes are inherited, and more subtle susceptibilities to viral and bacterial diseases may also run in families, accounting for more common and less severe infectious problems. General susceptibility to cancer may, in some cases, be associated with an inherited decrease in immunologic defenses.

Cancer

Some cancers tend to be familial (Skolnick et al., 1981). Breast, colon, lung, and prostate are the most common sites of cancers with familial aggregation. Ovarian, uterine, and colon cancer in combination also occur in some families. If certain forms of cancer are identified in a family, increased surveillance and special screening procedures can be instituted to help detect cancers at an early and curable stage. (Theories of cancer development are discussed in Chapter 11.)

Perhaps the most preventable familial cancer is lung cancer. As Fig. 5-5 shows, the incidence of lung cancer is strikingly elevated among individuals who have positive family histories and are also cigarette smokers (Tokuhata, 1965). Because of their elevated risk of lung cancer, members of such families should be strongly encouraged to avoid smoking.

Breast Cancer

Breast cancer ranks along with lung cancer as one of the most common cancers in women. As many as one third of the cases of breast cancer involve a familial predisposition, as indicated by a study of 300 women who died of breast cancer in Utah and had at least one other deceased sister (Williams, 1985). Among these women, 30% had a sister who had also died of breast cancer. The relative risk for breast cancer is 2% to 3% for

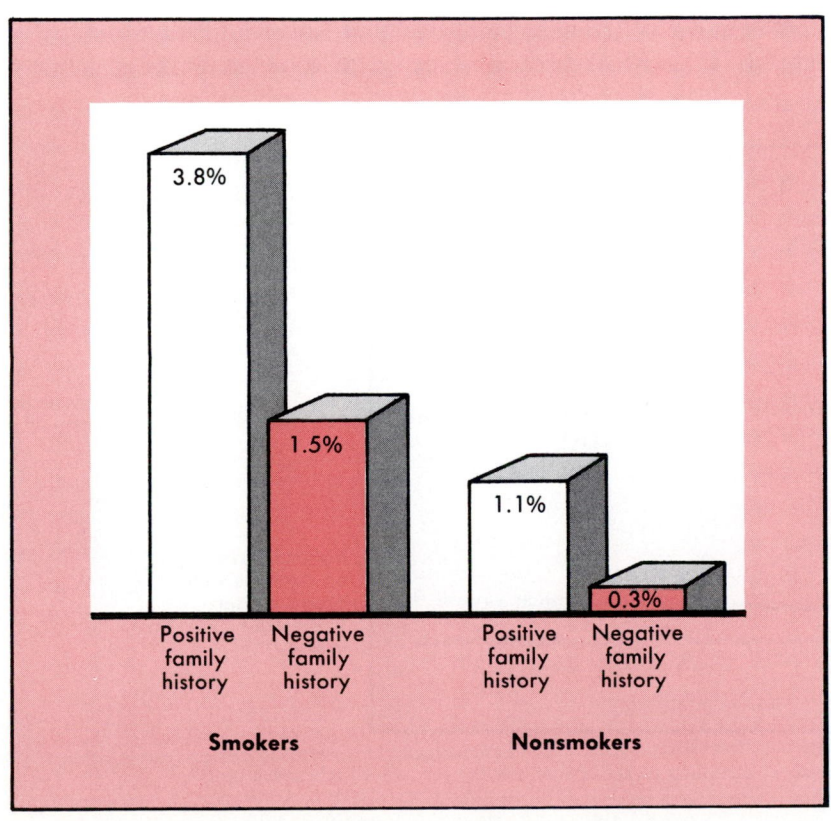

FIG. 5-5. Actual data from a case control study show that the highest rate of lung cancer occurs in smokers with familial prediposition. A familial predisposition was defined as one parent or sibling with lung cancer.

women with an affected sister *or* mother and 14% for women with a mother *and* sister affected (King et al., 1984; Sattins et al., 1985). Preliminary reports of linking the disease to specific genes have not been reproduced yet (King et al., 1980; Skolnick et al., 1984). Markers identifying specific genes will likely be found in the next 5 to 10 years and will greatly facilitate preventive measures for women carrying such genes.

Known risk factors for breast cancer include late age at first delivery, early menarche, late menopause, obesity, benign breast tumors, positive family history, dietary fat intake, and hypothyroidism. Other possible risk factors are alcohol intake, estrogen, medications, and prolactin secretion. Research also indicates that multiparous women and those who have undergone oophrectomies have some measure of protection against breast cancer (MacMahon et al., 1973).

Identified risk factors suggest that gene-environment interactions are sometimes a cause of breast cancer. For example, a late age of first pregnancy is one of the most potential risk factors for breast cancer. As Fig. 5-6 shows, this factor enhances the risk for women already at risk, as indicated by pedigrees comparing them to women without positive family histories of breast cancer (Hunt, 1980). Other studies have suggested that oral contraceptives ordinarily do not increase the risk for breast cancer in the general population but might increase the risk among women with positive family histories (Brinton et al., 1979).

Many well-developed programs are available to help detect breast cancer at a curable stage. Breast self-examination is a procedure that should be taught to all women. Clinical screening and mammography should also be applied conscientiously for all women, especially those at high risk. (Breast cancer is discussed further in Chapter 20.)

Colon Cancer

Colon cancer is one of the most common cancers in both men and women and shows a strong familial tendency in some pedigrees. Familial tendency combined with environmental factors such as low-fiber and high-fat intake may lead to hyperplasia and the development of benign polyps, which eventually undergo malignant degeneration and development of colon cancer.

Some experts dealing with colon cancer in high-risk families are optimistic about their ability to help prevent the spread of disease (Winawer, 1980). With a careful regimen of tests for occult blood, barium enemas, and proctoscopic examinations, benign polyps can often be found and removed before they can undergo malignant degeneration. Some physicians have conscientiously followed this approach for many years and tabulated their own experience, indicating that the occurrence among such carefully surveyed populations is much lower than in the general population (Winawer, 1980).

Certainly, the occurrence of benign colon polyps in association with a positive family history deserves serious and careful attention. Rare families with numerous colon polyps and colon cancer have been known to demonstrate mendelian inheritance (McKusick, 1983). Recently, more common isolated adenomatous polyps have been associated with colon cancer as an inherited

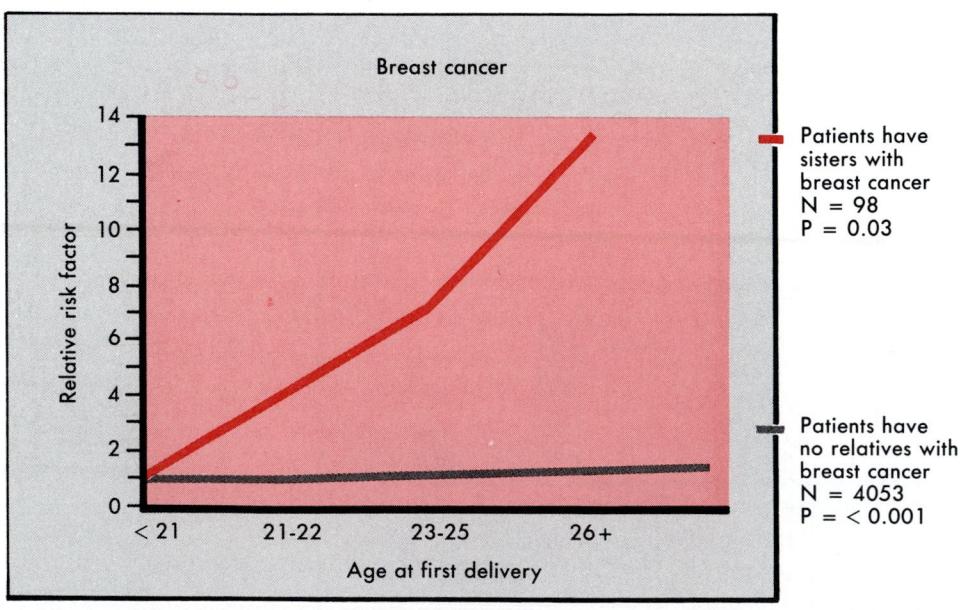

FIG. 5-6. Relative risk of breast cancer according to age of first delivery for women who have no relatives with breast cancer and for women who have a sister with breast cancer.

dominant trait (Burt et al., 1985). Former President Ronald Reagan and his brother were both reported to have cancerous colon polyps removed in 1985, and they too may be an example of a relatively common familial tendency for this disease. Members of such families should be encouraged to have careful periodic screening and to follow a high-fiber diet. (Colon cancer is further discussed in Chapter 36.)

Endocrine Disorders

Diabetes mellitus is a disease that has been extensively studied by both geneticists and epidemiologists (Emery & Rimoin, 1983; Goodman, 1970; McKusick, 1983; Rotter & Rimoin, 1983; West, 1978). The heterogeneity of diabetes and its associated underlying disorders are described in Chapter 18.

Type I diabetes probably occurs because of an immunologic mechanism. Inherited factors probably "cock the trigger," while environmental factors such as some viral insult seem to "pull the trigger" and initiate an autoimmune response that destroys the pancreatic islet cells and leads to total insulin deficiency. Strong association between diabetes and human leukocyte antigen (HLA) indicates that at least some of the genes for this syndrome are carried on chromosome 6. (HLA is discussed in Chapter 6.) Twin studies suggest that the penetrance is less than 40%. In general, the risk of a second sibling's being affected is approximately 11%.

For individuals with positive family histories, the best response at present is reassurance and support. If future advances can help not only to identify individuals who carry the trait but also to develop schemes for preventing the immunologic reaction, immunizations or other preventive techniques might be developed to prevent this disorder altogether. (Type I diabetes is further discussed in Chapter 18.)

Type II diabetes mellitus also shows a strong familial tendency. Identical twin studies show high concordance, suggesting penetrance is near 90%. In some cases, the disease appears to be transmitted as a dominant trait. The age at onset can vary considerably, from the 20s and 30s to elderly ages, which are more common. The age at onset of the disease appears to be somewhat consistent within pedigrees, and manifestations also may follow specific syndromes. One syndrome appears to occur among individuals sharing genes of Native Americans or Pacific island natives (West, 1978; Zimmet, 1979). This type of diabetes has been well documented among the Pima Indians of Arizona and in other Indian groups. Its onset in early adult life, high frequency (40% prevalence in Pimas), associaton with obesity, and hyperinsulinemia are consistent findings in most studies. Some scientists suggest this disorder results from a mismatch of "thrifty genes" and an affluent society (Zimmet, 1979).

Hematologic Disorders

Several hematologic disorders are genetically determined and interact with environmental factors (Emery & Rimoin, 1983; Goodman, 1970; McKusick, 1983). Probably one of the best examples is drug-induced hemolytic anemia associated with glucose-6-phosphate dehydrogenase (G6PD) deficiency. This disorder is found chiefly, but not entirely, among members of the black race; a gene frequency of 11% is found among male American blacks. This enzyme deficiency is also found among Sephardic Jews and other individuals tracing their ethnic origin to the Mediterranean area. Evidence indicates it is inherited as an X-linked recessive trait and leads to hemolysis of red blood cells in the presence of uremia, diabetic ketoacidosis, infection, and a variety of drugs that includes aspirin and some antibiotics.

Hereditary spherocytosis and elliptocytosis are both uncommon autosomal dominant disorders that can also lead to hemolytic anemia. Close relatives should be screened for these disorders, as splenectomy is effective in preventing further hemolytic anemia. (Anemias and related disorders are discussed in Chapter 23.)

Classical hemophilia is a well-known X-linked recessive disorder, but like other well-defined bleeding disorders, it is uncommon. A person with bleeding problems and a positive family history of bleeding disorders should receive screening tests available to distinguish among different types of genetic bleeding disorders. While classical hemophilia is relatively easy to recognize clinically because of the episodes of bleeding into the joints, subtle forms of the disease may be less easy to recognize. For example, women who are heterozygous carriers may have variable levels of clotting factors because of the phenomenon of X-inactivation (see Chapter 4).

Hemochromatosis is a defect that leads to iron collection in tissues and has been identified as a single-gene defect carried on chromosome 6 (linked to HLA haplotypes [Edwards et al., 1977]). (HLA linkage is discussed in Chapter 6.) Hematochromatosis is apparently more common than previously thought. It causes liver disease, heart disease, and diabetes if untreated.

Cardiovascular Disorders

Some forms of cardiovascular disease also show strong familial tendencies (Goodman, 1970). Rheumatic valvular heart disease seems to run strongly in some families. While this could be in part the result of transmission of the streptococcal organism among family members, research suggests that some individuals have an immunologic predisposition to the rheumatic complications of streptococcal infections.

In some pedigrees, a prolonged QT segment (on electrocardiogram) and associated sudden death appear to be caused by a single gene. Several myocardiopathies, including obstructive cardiomyopathy (idiopathic hypertrophic subaortic stenosis) also appear to be caused by single genes in some pedigrees. Probably one of the most common heart abnormalities is prolapsing mitral valve. The exact frequency of occurrence and associated functional problems remain to be defined, but at least some individuals with the disease have symptomatic or even life-threatening arrhythmias. Prolapsing mitral valve also tends to run in some families and may be associated with familial connective tissue disorders. Several forms of congenital heart disease, including atrial and ventricular septal defects, seem to be genetically transmitted, at least in some cases.

As a better understanding of the exact causal mechanisms for these diseases emerge, better detection and more effective screening procedures will help to prevent some of the associated problems. For example, in cases of rheumatic fever, prophylactic penicillin therapy is effective and should be considered for anyone with frequent streptococcal infections and a family history of rheumatic complications. (Cardiovascular diseases are discussed further in Chapter 27.)

Coronary Artery Disease

Early **coronary heart disease** is one of the most common serious chronic diseases with strong familial tendencies. Fig. 5-7 summarizes the major risk factors. Several risk factors are usually associated with early coronary heart disease. Early coronary deaths (men <55, women <65) were associated with two to three risk factors for more than half the cases in one study (Williams, 1980). In evaluations of early coronary diseases, more than half of the affected individuals have strong positive family histories (Hopkins & Williams, 1981; Hopkins, Williams, & Hunt, 1984; Williams, 1979; Williams, Skolnick, Carmelli et al., 1979a).

Studies also suggest several different genetic factors lead to early coronary disease including familial hypercholesterolemia (McKusick, 1983), early severe hypertension (Williams, Dadone, Hunt, & Kuida, 1984), low levels of high-density lipoprotein cholesterol (HDL-cholesterol) (Hasstedt, Ash, & Williams, 1986), low serum apolipoprotein A-I (a protein that attaches to LDL-cholesterol) (Moll et al., 1986), high apolipoprotein B (attaches to LDL-cholesterol) (Hasstedt, Wu, & Williams, 1987), and congenital variations in coronary arteries (Neufeld & Goldbourt, 1983). Platelet factors and the susceptibility to the adverse effects of cigarette smoking may also be inherited mechanisms leading to early familial coronary heart disease. Most of the background risk factors for coronary disease at all ages, including blood pressure and serum lipid and lipoprotein levels, have been found to be multifactorial traits in investigations of the general population with an approximate heritability of 50% (Williams, 1979).

Recent evidence indicates a substantial interaction of genetic predisposition to early coronary disease with environmental risk factors, as illustrated in Fig. 5-7 (Williams, 1984b).

One of the most striking and penetrant examples of familial patterns of coronary disease occurs in males het-

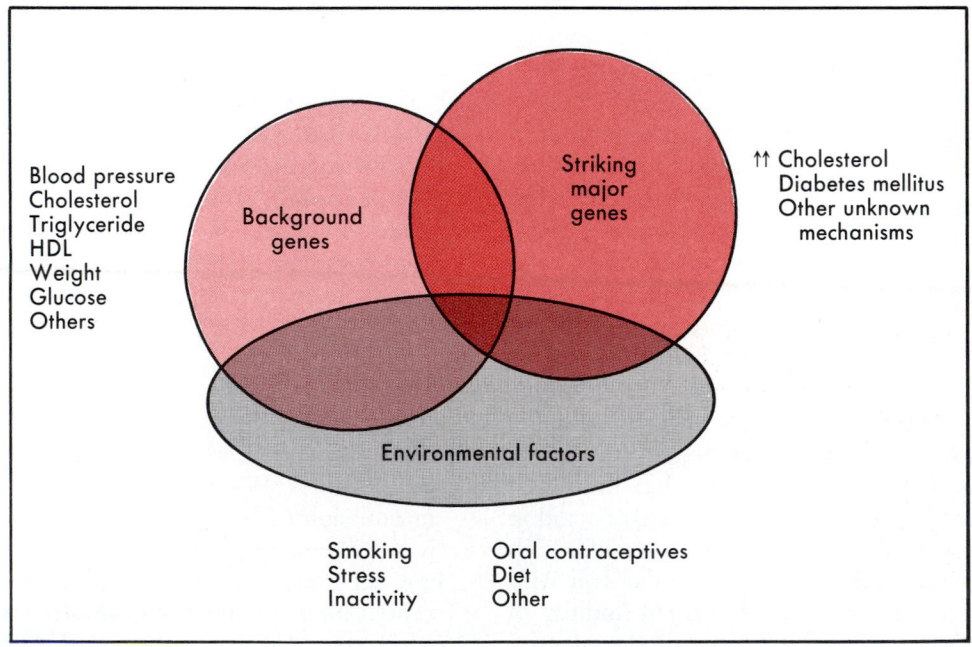

FIG. 5-7. Interacting effects of major genes, background genes, and environmental factors produce the unique coronary risk in given individuals as illustrated.

CLINICAL COMMENTARY
Hypercholesterolemia and Coronary Heart Disease

The gene for hypercholesterolemia is totally penetrant in the last two generations, as illustrated in the pedigree. Four individuals born before 1880 found to be definitely heterozygous for this problem survived respectively to ages 62, 68, 71, and 81, unlike their grandsons and great-grandsons, who died in their 30s, 40s, and 50s because of the same autosomal dominant gene.

The pedigree shows 361 persons in six generations of a pedigree. Dark symbols indicate 40 individuals who carried a gene for early coronary death mediated by very high serum cholesterol levels. Half of the children of affected adults have very high cholesterol levels, and none of them had been screened before their involvement in this study. The founder survived to age 81, but great-grandsons from two different wives show coronary disease usually with onset by age 45. Two of the sons from his first wife and another son from his second wife also had normal life expectancies. Pedigree analysis confirms they carried this dominant gene that led to early coronary death in their grandsons (Williams et al., 1986). This gene has been linked in a DNA marker for LDL receptors on chromosome 19 (Leppert et al., 1986).

Furthermore, variable expression of this gene can be observed in a woman and her two sons in the third and fourth generations of the pedigree. All three were known to have very high serum cholesterol values consistent with heterozygous familial hypercholesterolemia. One of the men was a smoker and died at age 32 of coronary disease; his nonsmoking brother died at age 45 of coronary disease. This suggests approximately 13 years difference in longevity potentially attributable to smoking in these high-risk men. This is in contrast to approximately 2 years difference in the longevity of smokers and nonsmokers in the general population and approximately 7 years difference in longevity between smokers and nonsmokers who die of coronary disease. The mother of these two men was examined at age 67, found to have a cholesterol level of 365, and yet still found to be free of any manifestations of coronary disease by history, physical examination, and electrocardiogram.

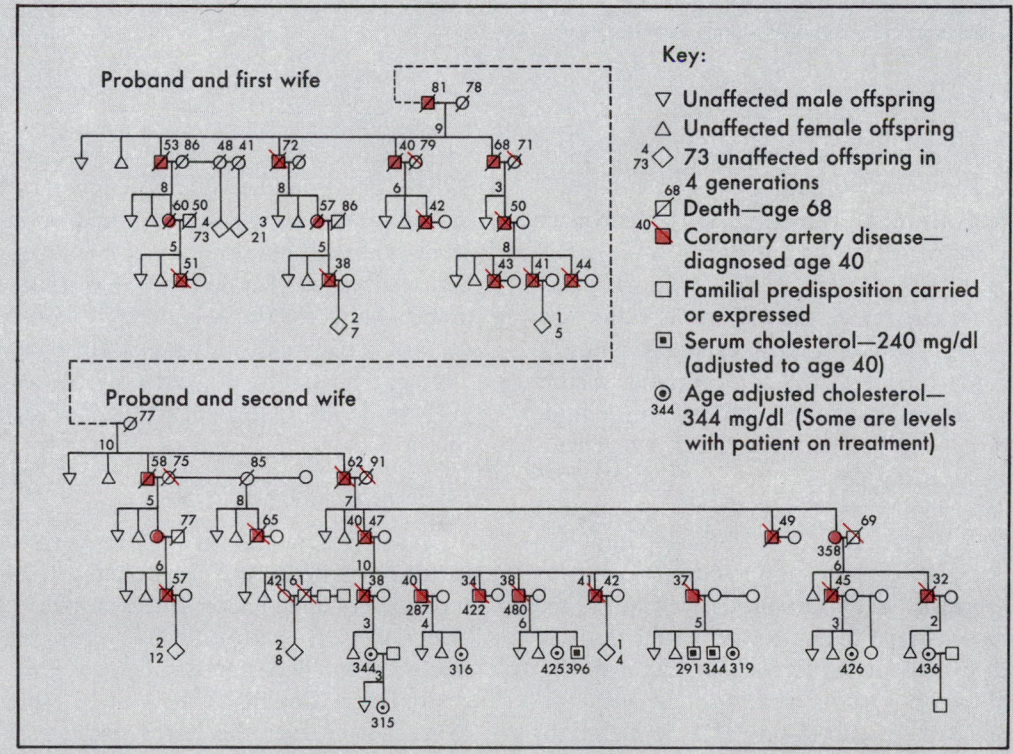

A six-generation pedigree showing patterns of coronary death and high levels of cholesterol.

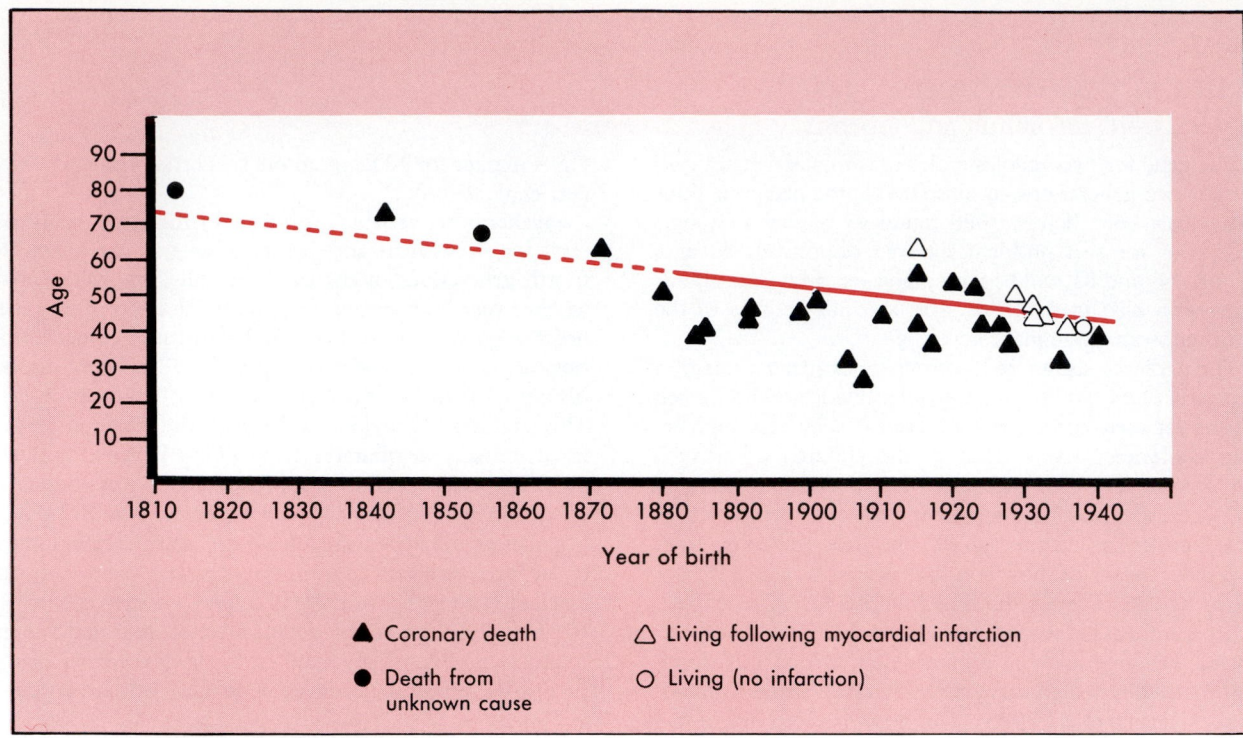

FIG. 5-8. Age and status of men heterozygous for familial hypercholesterolemia show generally early onset of coronary death in current generations with considerable variation and normal life span for four males born before 1880. These data suggest that environmental factors changing over time markedly affect the expression of this potentially lethal gene.

erozygous for familial hypercholesterolemia. Data from one study have shown a distinctive time trend (mid-1800s to present) toward decreasing age at coronary death for affected males as summarized in Fig. 5-8 (Williams, 1984b). This change in the degree of penetrance suggests that environmental factors also affect expression of the trait. Therefore, changes in environmental factors have increased the level of penetrance of this particular gene from essentially unexpressed in the mid-1800s to severe early coronary death in current generations of at least one pedigree.

Population data suggest that many of the risk factors are multiplicative and thus, in any individual at high risk for coronary disease, careful screening and prompt treatment of all risk factors is important. For example, the magnified effects of smoking may be part of the decreasing age at death evident in an analysis of coronary disease. Additional factors such as dietary intake and exercise level with its known effects on HDL levels might also be playing a role. Studies consistently show that women are relatively protected against the effects of hypercholesterolemia.

Current theories of atherogenesis indicate that 10 to 20 years or more of exposure to appropriate risk factors at high enough levels are required for significant coro-

nary artery disease to develop (Hopkins & Williams, 1981). This cumulative effect suggests that the most effective preventive measures should be instituted by late teens and early adult years of life. Exploratory studies and analyses further indicate that lowering serum cholesterol levels for those under age 35 may prevent up to 40% of coronary cases, whereas delaying treatment until after age 55 might prevent only 5% of coronary cases (Whyte, 1975). (Coronary heart disease is discussed further in Chapter 27.)

Hypertension and Stroke

Hypertension and stroke are both strongly familial cardiovascular diseases. Hypertension appears to be the most prominent risk factor for strokes (Kannel & Gordon, 1974). The continually improving detection and treatment of hypertension is probably responsible for the dramatic decline in the United States mortality rate from strokes over the last 3 decades (Williams, Lyon, Brockert, & Maness, 1979). Diabetes is also a significant risk factor for stroke, with a lesser level of possible contribution from hyperlipidemia and smoking (Kannel & Gordon, 1974). Some reported pedigrees have a striking aggregation of stroke and high blood pressure (Williams, Dadone, Hunt, & Kuida, 1984). As Fig. 5-9

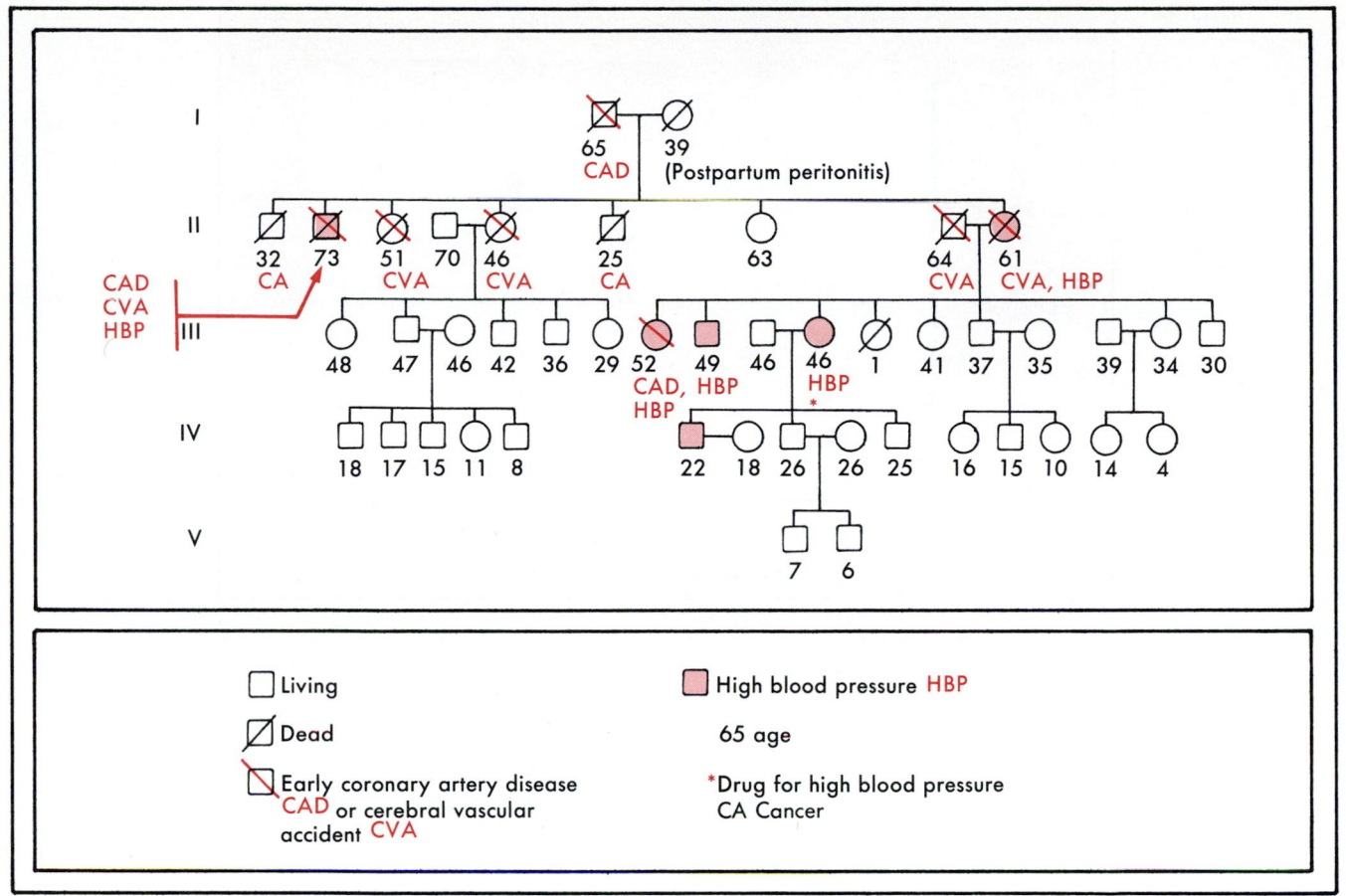

FIG. 5-9. Example of a pedigree in which early strokes, high blood pressure, and early coronary disease occur together. Hypertension is apparently the major underlying risk factor.

indicates, hypertension, coronary disease, and stroke tend to aggregate in some families. Careful detection and treatment of hypertension, therefore, may prevent both strokes and coronary disease in high-risk families (Hopkins et al., 1984; Joint National Committee, 1984).

"Essential hypertension" is one of the most common forms of familial disease. Twin studies and family studies consistently indicate approximately 50% heritability for blood pressure as a continuous trait and show significant coaggregation of hypertension. Essential hypertension demonstrates 85% to 100% concordance in identical twins and approximately 50% concordance in siblings (Feinleib et al., 1975; Hunt, Williams, & Barlow, 1986; Vander Molen et al., 1970; Williams, 1979; Williams, Dadone, Hunt, & Kuida, 1984). International studies have shown a strong correlation between dietary sodium intake and prevalence of hypertension (Fig. 5-10). Studies have also confirmed a strong relationship between obesity and both blood pressure and hypertension (Kannel & Gordon, 1974; Williams, Dadone, Hunt, & Kuida, 1984). The role of environmen-

tal stress, however, has still been poorly defined in the etiology of chronic hypertension. Blacks have repeatedly demonstrated a prevalence of hypertension approximately twice that seen in other populations (Cassel, 1972).

A popular theory that inherited susceptibility to salt-induced hypertension suggests that hypertension can result from high salt intake and inherited inability of kidneys to excrete sodium efficiently without raising arterial blood pressure (Williams, 1979; Williams, Dadone, Hunt, & Kuida, 1984; Williams, Hunt, Dadone, Smith, Ash, & Kuida, 1984). Initially, either low salt intake or absent gene(s) for high blood pressure could prevent hypertension. In some susceptible persons, salt-initiated hypertension may be perpetuated by other mechanisms (such as reset baroreceptors or nephrosclerosis), even on low salt intake.

This long-held theory is now being modified to account for developing evidence for important roles for other factors, including potassium, calcium, magnesium, chloride, and dietary fat intake and metabolism (Kesteloot, 1985; McCarron, 1983; Puska et al., 1983; Smith-

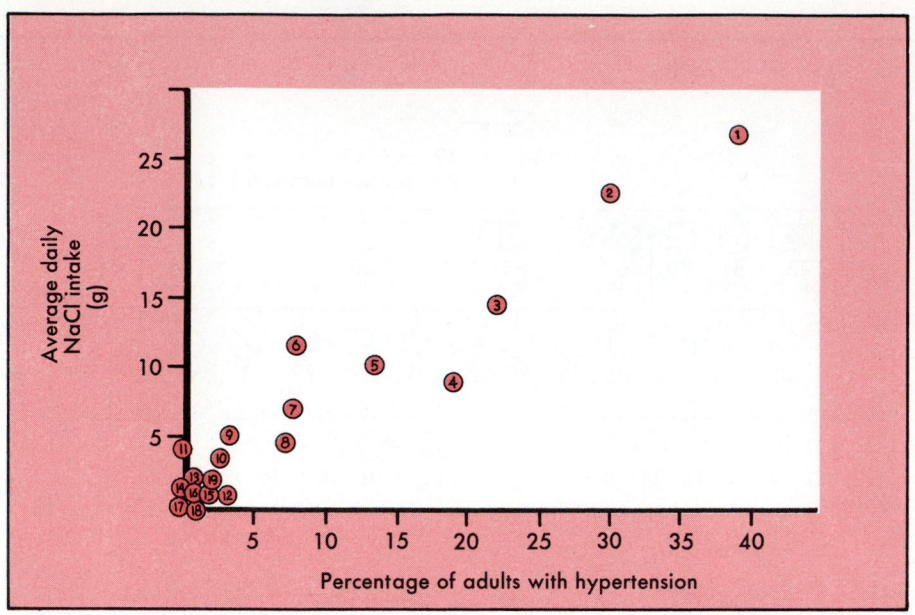

FIG. 5-10. Salt intake versus hypertension in nineteen populations; *r* = 0.96. *p 1,* Japanese, Northern Japan. *2,* Bahama natives, Bahama Islands. *3,* Japanese, Southern Japan. *4,* Rorotongans, Cook Islands. *5,* Americans, United States. *6,* Lau Tribesmen, Solomon Islands. *7,* Marshall Islanders, Pacific. *8,* Chimbu Highlanders, New Guinea. *9,* Hasioi and Nagovisis, Solomon Islands. *10,* Pukapukans, Cook Islands. *11,* Eskimos, Alaska. *12,* Tukisenta natives, New Guinea Highlands. *13,* Aita and Baegu tribesmen, Solomon Islands. *14,* Cuna Indians, Amazon forest, Brazil. *15,* Kwaio tribesmen, Solomon Islands. *16,* Yanomamo Indians, Brazil. *17,* Carajas Indians, Brazil. *18,* Murapins, New Guinea. *19,* Kung Bushmen, Botswana. (Williams, 1979b.)

Barbaro & Pucak, 1983; Whitescarver et al., 1984). Evidence for this theory is as follows:

1. Blood pressure is estimated to be 50% to 80% heritable in studies of twins, with the strong genetic role also supported by family and adoption studies.
2. High blood pressure is practically unknown in countries with diet containing less than 1 g salt daily, and high blood pressure prevalence correlates closely with salt intake in different countries.
3. High blood pressure is often lowered by diuretics, which enhance sodium excretion, or by a low sodium diet.
4. Individual sodium intake correlates with blood pressure level in normotensive persons with family history of high blood pressure but not in persons without hypertensive relatives (some differences between studies).
5. Sodium and potassium flux tested on human erythrocytes suggests altered sodium membrane transport for persons with essential high blood pressure and some of their relatives, compared to rapid sodium transport for normotensive persons without family history of high blood pressure.
6. Certain rat strains are either susceptible or resistant to salt-induced high blood pressure. The inherited susceptibility to high blood pressure can be transplanted with kidneys.

Some biochemical correlates of hypertension related to sodium have been found to be highly heritable, including intraerythrocytic sodium (Dadone, 1987) and sodium-lithium countertransport (Dadone, 1985). These biochemical variables and hypertension also correlate with obesity and plasma lipids (Hunt, Williams, Smith, & Ash, 1986).

Studies of early familial coronary disease have consistently shown that hypertension seems to account for approximately the same magnitude of early coronary disease as hyperlipidemia (Glover et al., 1982; Hopkins & Williams, 1981; Hopkins et al., 1984; Rissanen, 1979; Williams, 1979). More accurate definition of hypertensive syndromes and their expected outcomes should be helpful in allowing clinicians to pinpoint more precisely those individuals who need specific levels of treatment. Ongoing studies attempting to characterize different hypertension syndromes indicate that some new tests may help to distinguish among different types of hypertension (Falkner et al., 1979; Perloff, Sokolow, & Cowan, 1983; Wilson & Meyer, 1981; Wood et al., 1984).

Renal Disorders

Several renal disorders are familial and can be managed quite effectively. For example, gout has been shown to occur with several different types of single-gene enzyme defects (Emery & Rimoin, 1983; Goodman, 1970; McKusick, 1983). Trauma to joints, dietary changes, and other factors are thought to precipitate symptoms by dislodging uric acid crystals (physically or chemically) from the synovial lining of asymptomatic carriers. Medications are available to prevent the accumulation of uric acid crystals in the kidneys and joints of persons with symptoms. Asymptomatic persons with high blood uric acid are at risk for the disorder and can be advised to avoid these precipitating factors and to recognize early symptoms.

Kidney stones commonly occur in some families and recur often in some individuals. Intake of dietary fluids, such as milk or carbonated beverages, are thought to be precipitating environmental factors. Some common dietary recommendations therefore are believed to help prevent stones. (Pathophysiology of kidney stones is discussed in Chapter 33.)

Gastrointestinal Disorders
Malabsorption Disorders

Several relatively common disorders of the digestive system are known or suspected to illustrate underlying interactions of environmental and genetic factors. For example, persons with gluten-sensitive enteropathy (celiac sprue) cannot tolerate gluten contained in wheat. Damaged small bowel lining leads to malabsorption and diarrhea. If symptoms are prolonged without appropriate action, malnutrition and associated medical problems can result. Strict avoidance of wheat and wheat-containing foods produces dramatic improvement. The condition is thought to be inherited as a dominant gene with incomplete penetrance, although the reasons for variable penetrance are not yet understood (Goodman, 1970; McKusick, 1983).

Deficiencies of intestinal disaccharidases have been thought to be genetically transmitted. One example is lactase deficiency (lactose intolerance). A lactose tolerance test has been applied to different populations, indicating that 73% of the black population may have decreased intestinal lactase levels, in contrast to approximately 5% of the adult white population with the same deficiency (Goodman, 1970). Persons symptomatic for the disorder experience abdominal pain and diarrhea after milk consumption; symptoms usually diminish when milk is withdrawn from the diet. Similar symptoms sometimes occur secondarily after other diseases have damaged the intestinal mucosa.

Common inflammatory bowel diseases including ulcerative colitis and Crohn disease are thought to be due in part to genetic predispositions. Markedly increased rates of the disease occur in certain ethnic groups, especially Ashkenazic Jews, as compared to other races and to Sephardic Jews (Goodman, 1970). (Problems in absorption and digestion are discussed further in Chapter 36.)

Peptic Ulcers

Peptic ulcers occur in 5% to 10% of studied general populations and have been established to occur on a familial basis in studies of twins, families, and blood groups. Either duodenal or gastric ulcers can predominate within given families. Further evidence of genetic subtypes shows that approximately one half of individuals with a duodenal ulcer have hyperpepsinogenemia I, as do 50% of the offspring of persons with an ulcer and elevated levels. This biochemical marker is thought to reflect an inherited increase in the mass of acid-secreting cells in the wall of the stomach (Rotter et al., 1979).

Both psychologic stress and cigarette smoking, through their effects on the nervous system and acid secretion, have long been recognized as precipitating or aggravating environmental factors. Cimetidine and other similar drugs that inhibit acid secretion have revolutionized both the treatment and the prevention of serious problems from peptic ulcer disease. (Peptic ulcers are discussed further in Chapter 36.)

Gallstones

Gallstones are eventually found in approximately 30% of all women and 15% of all men during their lifetimes. Cholecystectomy is one of the most common operations performed in North America. Multiple cases occurring among relatives suggest a familial predisposition, although genetic and environmental determinants of gallstones and associated complications remain to be defined in most cases. Some underlying genetic and environmental factors may be shared with obesity, which is commonly associated with gallstones.

Obesity

Perhaps one of the most challenging metabolic disorders is **obesity.** It is associated with hypertension, diabetes, elevated blood lipid levels, and cardiovascular disease (Kannel & Gordon, 1974). Obesity is probably a very heterogeneous group of disorders with multiple etiologies. Significant familial aggregation of obesity has been found in many different kinds of studies, including twin and adoption studies. Single-gene mechanisms have been identified in animal studies, but in humans, shared environmental factors and polygenic determinants probably play important roles in a large proportion of obesity cases.

A growing body of supportive data suggest the possibility that single genes are causal risk factors for such extreme cases as morbid obesity (defined as an excess weight of 100 pounds or weight approximately twice an individual's ideal weight [Williams, 1984c]). This severe form of obesity occurs in less than 1% of the general population but is found quite commonly among relatives of approximately half of morbidly obese individuals. One hypothesis is that basic cell membrane trans-

CLINICAL COMMENTARY

A Hypothetical Model: Genes + Environment = Disease

Research suggests that genetic and environmental factors could combine to produce obesity (Williams, 1984c). To illustrate how this could happen, consider a hypothetical example that two autosomal genes could help to control a person's likelihood of developing obesity. Let us call the first gene the "BAT gene" (BAT signifying brown adipose tissue). The homozygous form of this gene (bb) is assumed to be associated with a marked defect in metabolic pathways that normally buffer excess caloric intake. The expression of this gene could be seen by sampling observations at various points in a chain of events leading from the genotype to expression in obesity.

Obesity could be considered to be a phenotype of this gene, but the condition is at the end of a continuum that is preceded by several intermediate steps. Along the continuum are opportunities for other genes and environmental factors to modify the gene's expression. Obesity might, therefore, be considered to be a "confounded expression"

of this gene because it reflects the genetic effect only partially and also reflects the effect of other undetermined factors.

For this model, the "BAT gene" has a very strong effect, and the only other factors affecting obesity include environmental sugar and caloric intake and another well-defined hypothetical gene we shall call the "tooth gene." The "tooth gene" is manifested by a craving for sugar with its associated tendency toward obesity. The effects of the "tooth gene" are modified by the environmental availability of dietary sugar. It has a mild effect on obesity.

Obesity can be entirely the result of environmental factors, but a higher level of obesity results from a combined effect of environmental factors and the "tooth gene." A striking level of obesity is found to occur when these two factors interact with the "BAT gene." Thus, different levels of obesity depend on the combination of these three variables.

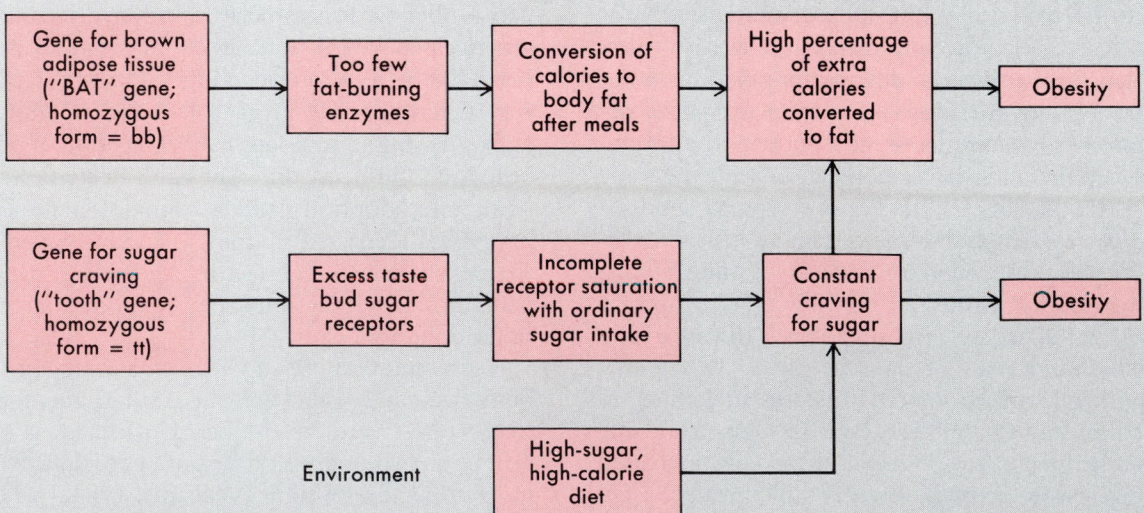

Components of gene-environment interactions in causing obesity.

The phenotype frequency distribution illustrates the principal effect of each of these two genes and the effects of the interaction of these two genes with each other and with the environment. In part *A,* the distribution of persons in the population by weight as a percentage of ideal weight is represented for individuals who have each of the three possible genotypes with respect to the BAT locus: BB (normal), Bb (heterozygous for the abnormal BAT allele), and bb (homozygous for the abnormal BAT allele). Means for individuals with each of these three genotypes are respectively 110%, 140%, and 195% of ideal weight. This range demonstrates the dramatic effect of the homozygous state of this "BAT gene" leading to morbid obesity with a much milder form of obesity seen in heterozygous individuals. A considerable spread within each genotype reflects the influence of other genes, environmental factors, and random variation among individuals.

The considerable overlap between homozygous normal and heterozygous individuals shows the difficulty in distinguishing between the two in the general population. The homozygous affected individuals have a dramatically displaced outcome of morbid obesity with little overlap, making them easier to find in the general population. The single dotted curve in part *A* represents the frequency distribution of all individuals without identification of genotype. The expression of a major gene appears in the form of a "bimodal distribution" (two peaks, one for normal and the other one for those who have the major gene defect).

Part *B* shows the distribution of weight status for different genotypes of the "tooth gene." There is little separation between the means of the three genotypes (98%, 116%, 126%), and there is considerable overlap in the weight status of individuals with all three genotypes. This large spread and overlap is caused primarily by the strong influence of the "BAT gene." The same general phenotype distribution in the entire population is represented by the up-

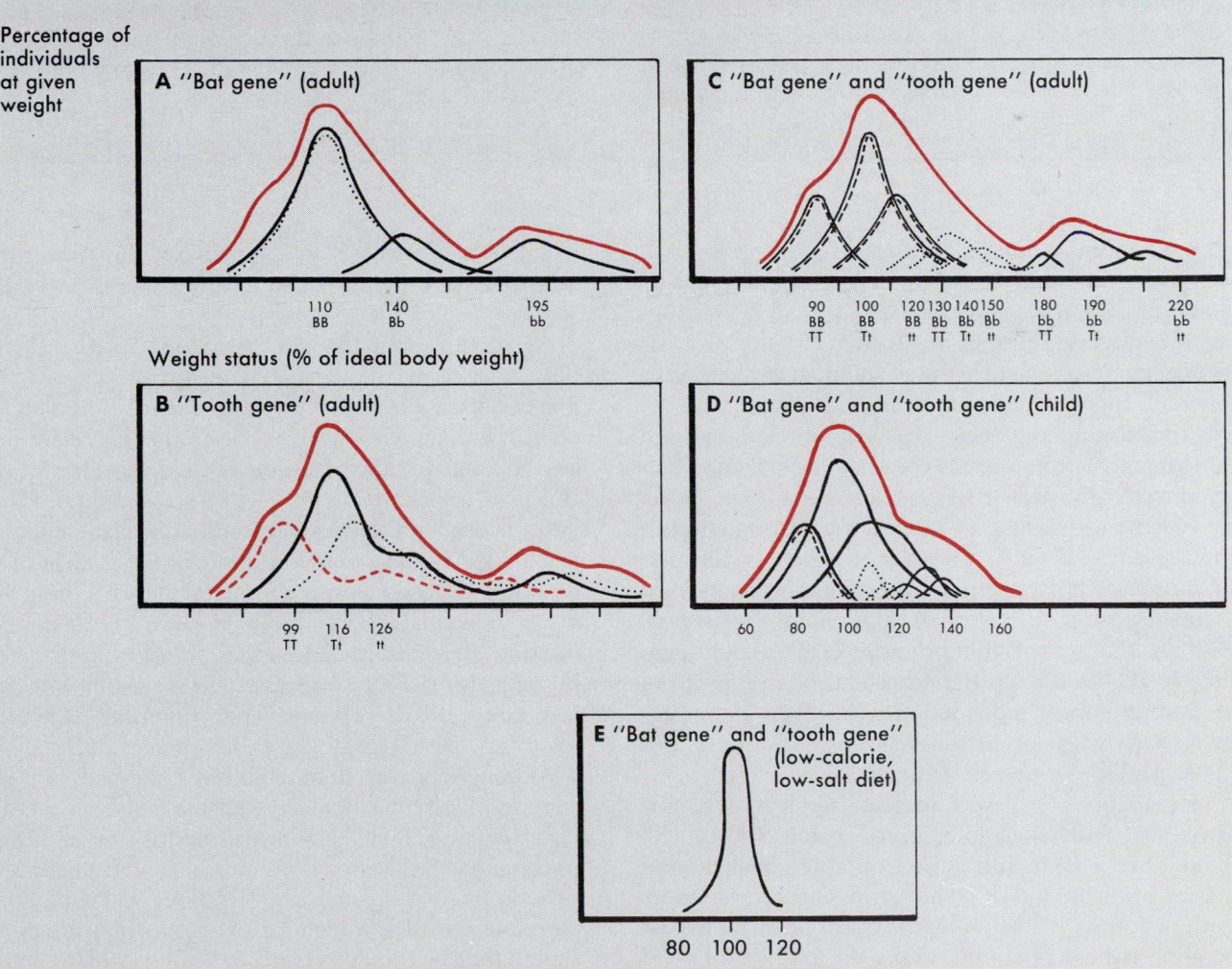

Phenotype frequency and distribution by genotype.

Continued.

per dotted line. Part *B* thus illustrates the difficulty of detecting the mild effects of minor genes when they are confounded by strong effects of major genes or other factors that have not yet been defined.

Part *C* characterizes all subjects according to the genotype of both genes. Nine distinct genotypes are represented by all possible combinations of the two genes. The predominant separation is still attributable to the "BAT gene," but within genotypes for the "BAT gene" is an additional separation according to genotypes for the "tooth gene." Of course, the most striking obesity (220%) is observed in the individuals who are homozygously affected by both genes.

Part *D* illustrates the important role of age. The accumulation of extra calories stored as adipose tissue over time is less prevalent in children than in adults. Less separation in weight status is thus evident in children with the different genotypes. At birth they may show no separation, young children may show a mild separation, and teenagers and adults show a clear separation, as illustrated in Part *C*.

The important roles of dietary calorie and sugar intake are also evident in the phenotype distribution. In an environment completely devoid of excess calories and sugar, there may be no difference in weight status, regardless of genotype, as part *E* shows. An environment abundant with calories and sugar, however, is likely to cause genetic expression of obesity.

An actual understanding of the pathophysiology of obesity requires a more complicated model, and major effects need to be carefully defined before less prominent factors can be detected. Whenever possible, phenotypes close to the genotype should be studied in preference to distant phenotypes influenced by other factors. In a more complex model, other genetic or environmental determinants may include such factors as television advertisements or the absence of taste bud receptors.

Any phenotype that corresponds closely to the genotype can serve as a genetic marker for classifying individuals according to genotype. Then, within genotypes, the different effects of environmental factors might be observed. For example, a high-calorie, high-sugar diet may not lead to obesity in individuals who are normal homozygous with respect to the "BAT gene" and the "tooth gene."

---

port mechanisms might be different in these persons, although the condition is still influenced significantly by dietary caloric intake (Ash et al., 1983). (Metabolic regulation is discussed further in Chapter 35.)

Some interesting biochemical and metabolic studies of obesity indicate that, for some individuals who remain thin throughout their lives despite relatively high caloric intake, factors such as conversion of chemical energy directly into heat energy in brown adipose tissue may buffer excess sugar and fat calories. In one experimental study, volunteer prisoners who were thin and had relatives who were thin were able to consume approximately twice their normal caloric intake for several months without any significant appreciable weight gain (Sims et al., 1973). On the other end of the spectrum are morbidly obese individudals who lose weight very slowly, even when placed on vitamins and intravenous fluids with little or no caloric intake.

For example, after gastric surgery (stapling) for morbid obesity, individuals lose approximately 100 to 150 pounds over a 12-month period on approximately 600 calories of daily intake. This stringent restriction is aided, of course, by the stomach staple, or staple bypass operation, which physically limits the passage of food and consequently helps enforce restricted caloric intake. After approximately 1 year, these indivduals are able to consume approximately 1000 calories/day and seem to maintain a relatively stable weight on this diet, which would result in considerable weight loss by other persons.

Apparently, some people are endowed with a metabolism that can waste consumed energy as heat and thus prevent obesity from developing, whereas others are endowed with an efficient metabolism that may have been an advantage in time of famine but is a considerable detriment in a society saturated with excess calories. Whole body calorimeter studies have indicated that some slender individuals can burn off approximately 25% of excess fat and sugar calories within an hour of a meal; very obese individuals show little or no heat production, indicating they are storing excess calories rather than burning them (Beers & Bassett, 1981; Cioffi, James, & VanItallie, 1981). (Theories concerning the pathophysiology of obesity are discussed in Chapter 36.)

Although proven and established methods for preventing obesity are not yet available, some of the data regarding metabolic factors in obesity suggest several possibilities. Studies of both animals and humans seem to indicate that refined carbohydrates and fat calories contribute to the problem of obesity in individuals and should thus be avoided (Beers & Bassett, 1981; Cioffi et al., 1981). Some suggest that increased physical activity not only consumes calories during the exercise but also has beneficial effects in influencing metabolic processes.

In some families with patterns of obesity, an early onset age seems to be prominent, so that dietary changes and increased activity levels could be promoted among youngsters in obesity-prone families, with the aim of preventing future obesity. Of course, shared environmental factors, such as common family dietary habits, must also contribute to a significant proportion of cases of obesity. Whether the etiology is genetic or environmental, healthful dietary factors and increased physical activity levels remain worthwhile recommendations.

Current studies provide evidence for several different types of obesity syndromes. A more accurate characterization of different syndromes of obesity should lead to a better understanding of the underlying pathophysiology of each type. For example, complications such as diabetes may be much more common in some types such as central obesity as opposed to peripheral obesity.

Neuromuscular Disorders

A variety of neuromuscular disorders are known or suspected to have genetic determinants (Emery & Rimoin, 1983; Goodman, 1970; McKusick, 1983). Disorders such as Huntington disease and muscular dystrophy are known to be genetically determined but are not preventable and are currently managed with symptomatic treatment (see Chapter 15).

Multiple sclerosis is a chronic debilitating neuromuscular disease. Association with HLA phenotypes suggests some inherited immunologic predisposition (Haile et al., 1981) (see Chapter 6). The disease appears to have low penetrance. Viruses have been suspected to be the environmental factor involved in the pathophysiology of the disease. Lower disease rates in lower latitudes (e.g., Los Angeles vs Seattle) suggest protective climate factors. Further studies are required to define the exact pathophysiologic steps and better methods for either prevention or treatment of this tragic disorder. (Multiple sclerosis is discussed further in Chapter 15.)

Alzheimer disease is a relatively common cause of tragic dementia. Genetic predisposition in at least some of the cases is suggested by a recent news report of a link to a DNA marker on chromosome 21.

Psychiatric Disorders

Several psychiatric disorders have been shown to have a strong familial occurrence (Egeland & Sussex, 1985; Emery & Rimoin, 1983; Goodman, 1970; Murray & Lewis, 1985). Extensive studies of twins, siblings, and adopted offspring have clearly demonstrated a genetic role in both schizophrenia and manic-depressive, or bipolar psychosis. Heritability estimates from different studies range from 40% to 100%. Concordance rates for identical twins are 50% to 80%, as compared to 5% to 15% for siblings and nonidentical twins (Gregory, 1968). The practical question is whether or not this known familial tendency can lead to preventive or beneficial measures in psychiatric disorders.

For manic-depressive psychoses, screening tests for detecting the disease in early stages are available. Reports suggest this disorder is limited to a DNA marker on chromosome 11. Dramatic results have been obtained from treatment with lithium carbonate. Without treatment the occurrence of the disease leads to irrational behavior that can have devastating effects on the personal lives of the affected individuals and their close relatives. Preserving a normal social life-style using early treatment with lithium carbonate might be accomplished more easily if the individual is diagnosed and treated before the public embarrassment of irrational behavior. This advantage might be achieved by warning close relatives—and especially offspring and siblings—of known manic-depressive individuals that they have an increased risk of developing the disorder. Although this form of genetic counseling raises some ethical question, it might, in some cases, provide more effective prevention. Those at risk or their relatives could therefore arrange for appropriate screening and monitoring to detect and treat the disease at the earliest possible stages.

Schizophrenia appears to be caused by inherited defects in neurochemistry or brain trauma or both (Murray & Lewis, 1985). Differences in levels of monoamine oxidase or its metabolites have been observed in platelets or cerebrospinal fluid of schizophrenics whose disease shows familial tendencies. Birth trauma, prematurity, soft neurologic signs, abnormal electroencephalograms, or abnormal brain CT scans are found in up to one third of all schizophrenics. Evidence indicates that inherited susceptibility and environmental insult combine to produce some schizophrenia.

Some studies have suggested that neuroses, sociopathic behavior, depression, and alcoholism may also be familial and may, in some cases, be associated with more serious psychoses. Strict avoidance of alcohol could be a safe recommendation for close relatives of alcoholics. Suicide and depression logically run in the same pedigrees (Egeland & Sussex, 1985). Persons with strong positive family histories of depression and/or suicide could be warned of familial tendencies. Their spouses could be educated about the availability of good antidepressant medications. This is especially important because most clinicians consider depression to be a treatable disorder and because, when untreated, the effects of the disorder are profound enough to lead to suicide.

THE MEDICAL FAMILY HISTORY

The key to finding high-risk families is collecting a good medical family history. Family histories are generally useful in three clinical settings:

Medical Family History

WHEN?	WHY?

WHEN?

1. *Individual with disease* that is often familial (e.g., male coronary at age 36)

2. Individual *might* have disease but has nondiagnostic symptoms (e.g., 36-year-old man with vague chest discomfort)

3. General Screening Tool (broad family history overview during new patient workup)

HOW? (What data should be collected)

1. *Sex, age, vital status* for *all target relatives and spouse*
   First-degree relatives: parents, siblings, and offspring
   Second-degree relatives: grandparents, aunts, and uncles

2. *Disease and cause of death*
   Age at diagnosis?
   Prescriptions given?

3. *Risk factors*
   Year of exposure?
   Modification and outcome?

WHY?

1. *Identify high-risk families:* If the family history is strongly positive, it will help identify close relatives who can be helped to avoid the same problem

2. *Use like a diagnostic test:* Positive family history increases suspicion. Special tests or monitoring may be justified

3. *Use to focus future attention:* Be alert to family tendencies. Plan future procedures for screening and prevention.

WHAT CAN BE LEARNED?

1. Is the disease familial?

2. How strong a tendency?

3. Affect males and females alike?

4. Usual age at onset?

5. Which risk factors involved?

6. Pathophysiology?

7. Which relatives need help?

8. Age to start screening?

9. Best way to prevent, screen, or treat?

---

1. From an individual known to have a disease that can be familial, so that a positive family history can alert health professionals to help close relatives avoid the disease

2. From an individual being evaluated for the possibility of the disease, so that a positive family history increases clinical suspicion and may help justify further diagnostic tests

3. From a healthy individual, so that a general screening tool will identify a person with a positive family history that needs further attention.

The most efficient use of a medical family history is to chart histories of proband who have familial disease. For example, approximately one half of men with early coronary disease will have strong positive family histories. This positive family history indicates a familial tendency that can often be avoided by appropriately informed and motivated close relatives (see box above).

SUMMARY REVIEW

What Factors Cause Disease?

1 Factors causing disease can be fundamentally classified as genetic or environmental.

2 Finding and understanding environmental factors that affect the penetrance of specific genes is an important concept in preventing chronic familial diseases.

3 A polygenic trait is an inherited trait caused by the blending of effects of many different genes.

4 A multifactorial trait is produced by the blending of multiple genetic and environmental influences.

5 The penetrance of a single gene or number of genes can depend on the person's age, gender, genetic makeup, and environmental factors.

6 The effects of other factors on a single gene's penetrance are called interactions. They may be gene-gene or gene-environment interactions.

7 Environmental factors that can lead to disease in susceptible individuals include personal habits and lifestyles; exposure to chemicals, toxins, pollutants, and medications; psychologic status; and microorganisms or other immunologic stimuli.

Analyzing Disease Risk

1 Statistical measurements important in determining disease risk are the incidence rate, the prevalence rate, and the mortality rate.

2 Risk factors are indicators of a person's predisposition to developing a disease; risk factors may be either causal or noncausal.

3 Risk factors may be statistically measured by using either contingency tables or correlation coefficients.

4 Measurement of the relative risk, population attribut-

able risk, and preventive efficiency for a particular population indicate the degree of familiality and efficiency of targeted intervention among high-risk persons who may be able to avoid disease with appropriate preventive measures.

5 Continuous traits (e.g., obesity) are traits expressed across a range of severity. Such traits can be analyzed with either correlation coefficients or contingency tables, using a threshold that defines an affected person.

Environmental Risk Factors

1 Environmental pathogens are associated with a variety of infectious diseases, including some that involve immunologic reactions triggered by microbes.

2 Personal habits have been associated with some of the most common chronic diseases.

3 Physical and chemical substances can be both causal factors and protective mechanisms in the development of some diseases.

4 Psychologic and social factors may be direct causes of contributing factors in the development of disease.

Combined Effects and Interaction among Risk Factors

1 Interactions and combined effects of causal risk factors are involved in many disease processes.

2 A goal of current research is to define the heterogeneity, or variety of factors that lead to common chronic diseases.

3 Analyzing disease tendencies in families involves collecting data about sets of relatives and identifying patterns of disease and exposure to risk factors.

4 Age is a risk factor for many diseases. It often represents the effects of exposure to various risk factors and inherited physiologic processes that cause human beings to age.

Familial Diseases and Associated Risks

1 A great variety of diseases are known to show a familial tendency, often in combination with some environmental interactions.

2 For many inherited disorders, expression of the trait depends on environmental exposures.

3 Immunologic disorders that show some familial tendency include rheumatiod arthritis, systemic lupus erythematosus, idiopathic Addison disease, autoimmune thyroiditis, Graves disease, and ideopathic thrombocytopenic purpura (IPT).

4 Allergies and asthma also show familial patterns, and susceptibility to certain infections may be an inherited trait.

5 Cancers that show some familial predisposition include cancer of the breast, colon, lung, ovary, uterus, and prostate.

6 Diabetes mellitus, both type I and type II, shows an inherited tendency that is probably expressed because of other causal risk factors.

7 Hematologic disorders that are inherited and expressed because of environmental risk factors include hemolytic anemia, glucose-6-phosphate dehydrogenase (G6PD) deficiency, hereditary spherocytosis and elliptocytosis, hemophilia, and hemochromatosis.

8 Cardiovascular disorders that show a familial tendency include rheumatic valvular heart disease, a prolonged QT segment (on electrocardiogram), myocardiopathies, prolapsing mitral valve, septal defects, coronary heart disease, hypertension, and stroke.

9 Renal disorders that show a familial tendency include gout and kidney stones.

10 Gastrointestinal disorders that show an inherited susceptibility include malabsorptive syndrome (gluten-sensitive enteropathy, lactase deficiency), ulcerative colitis, Crohn disease, peptic ulcers, and obesity.

11 Neuromuscular disorders that have inherited determinants include Huntington disease, muscular dystrophy, and multiple sclerosis.

12 Psychiatric disorders with some familial tendency include schizophrenia and manic-depressive psychosis.

The Medical Family History

1 The medical family history is useful in screening susceptible individuals, indicating the need for more diagnostic evaluation, and identifying those at risk for certain diseases.

2 Patterns of familial diseases in particular families allow health professionals to begin risk reduction efforts to prevent a disease occurrence or to minimize its severity.

3 Methods for collecting data for a family history include brief screening during routine health assessment, self-administered questionnaires, detailed interviews, verification of data about relatives, and screening and examination of selected relatives.

KEY TERMS

Breast cancer, 171

Causal risk factor, 159

Colon cancer, 172

Congenital defect, 168

Contingency table, 160

Continuous trait, 161

Coronary heart disease, 174

Correlation coefficient, 161

Diabetes, 173

Familial tendency, 168

Heterogeneity, 163

High-risk person, 160

Incidence rate, 158

Interaction (gene-environment interaction, gene-gene interaction), 157

Mortality rate, 158

Multifactorial trait, 157

Multiple sclerosis, 183

Noncausal risk factor, 159

Obesity, 179

Polygenic trait, 156

Population-attributable risk, 160

Prevalence rate, 158

Preventive efficiency, 160

Relative odds, 162

Relative risk, 160

Risk factor, 159

Stroke, 176

REFERENCES

Aagaard, G. N. (1984). Hypetension—implications, goals, and potential risks of drug therapy. *Western Journal of Medicine, 141,* 476-480.

Armitage, P. (1973). *Statistical methods of medical research.* (p. 504). New York: John Wiley & Sons (A Halsted Press Book).

Ash, K. O., Smith, J. B., Kemp, J. W., Lynch, M. B., Moody, F. G., Raymond, J. L., McKnight, M. R., & Williams, R. R. (1983). The effect of diet on ouabain binding to erythrocytes from obese subjects. *Clinical Physiology and Biochemistry, 1,* 293-299.

Beers, R. F. & Bassett, E. G. (1981). *Nutritional factors: modulating effects on metabolic processes.* New York: Raven Press, p. 568.

Botstein, D., White, R. L., Skolnick, M., & Davis, R. W. (1980). Construction of a genetic linkage map in man using restriction fragment length polymorphism. *American Journal of Human Genetics, 32,* 314-331.

Brinton, L. A., Williams, R. R., Hoover, R. N., Stegens, N. L., Feinleib, M., & Fraumeni, J. F. (1979). Breast cancer risk factors among screening program participants. *JNCI, 62,* 37-44.

Burt, R. W., Bishop, T., Cannon, L. A., Dowdle, M. A., Lee, R. G., & Skolnick, M. H. (1985, June). Dominant inheritance of adenomatous colonic polyps and colorectal cancer. *The New England Journal of Medicine, 312,* 1540-1544.

Carmelli, D., Williams, R. R., & Rissanen, A. (1982). Contrasting patterns of familiality for cholesterol and triglyceride in Finland according to type of coronary manifestations and locations. *American Journal of Epidemiology, 116,* 617-621.

Cassel, J. C. (1972). Evans' county cardiovascular and cerebrovascular epidemiologic study. *Archives of Internal Medicine, 128,* 883-895.

Cavalli-Storza, L. L. & Bodner, W. F. (1971). *The genetics of human populations.* San Francisco: W. H. Freeman.

Chesney, M. A. & Rosenman, R. H. (1985). *Anger and hostility in cardiovascular and behavioral disorders* (p. 294). New York: Hemisphere Publishing.

Cioffi, L. A., James, W. P. T., & VanItallie, T. B. (1981). *The body weight regulatory system: Normal and disturbed mechanisms* (p. 380). New York: Raven Press.

Dadone, M. M. (1985). Inheritance of sodium lithium countertransport. *American Journal of Medical Genetics.*

Dadone, M. M. (1987). Preliminary evidence for genetic determination of intraerythrocytic sodium concentration in Utah pedigrees. *American Journal of Medical Genetics, 27*(1), 39-44.

Dadone, M. M. (1984). Genetic analysis of sodium lithium countertransport in ten hypertensive prone kindreds. *American Journal of Medical Genetics, 17,* 565-577.

Dinsdale, J. E. & Moss, J. (1980). Plasma catecholamines in stress and exercise. *Journal of the American Medical Association, 243,* 340-342.

Edwards, C. Q., Carroll, M., Bray, P. F., & Cartwright, G. E. (1977). Hereditary hemochromatosis: Diagnosis in siblings and children. *New England Journal of Medicine, 279,* 7-13.

Egeland, J. A. & Sussex, J. N. (1985, August). Suicide and family loading for affective disorders. *The Journal of the American Medical Association, 254*(7).

Eisdorfer, C. (1984). The conceptualization of stress and a model for further study. In M. R. Zales (Ed.), *Stress in health and disease.* New York: Brunner/Mazel.

Emery, A. E. H. & Rimoin, D. L. (1983). *Principles and practice of medical genetics* (p. 1502). New York: Churchill Livingston.

Falkner, B., Onesti, G., Angelakos, E. T., Fernandes, M., & Langman, C. (1979). Cardiovascular response to mental stress in normal adolescents with hypertensive parents. *Hypertension, 1,* 23-30.

Feinleib, M. & Williams. R. R. (1976). Relative risks of myocardial infarction, cardiovascular disease, and peripheral vascular disease by type of smoking. *Proceedings of third world conference on smoking and health.* In E. L. Wynder, D. Hoffman, & G. B. Gori (Eds.), *Smoking and health. I. Modifying the risk for the smoker.* Washington, DC: U. S. Government Printing Office.

Feinleib, M., Garrison, M. D., Barhani, N., Rosenman, R., & Christian, J. (1975). Studies of hypertension in twins. In O. Paul (Ed.), *Epidemiology and control of hypertension.* New York: Stratton.

Fisher, R. A. (1918). The correlation between relatives on supposition of Mendelian inheritance. *Transcripts of the Royal Society, 52,* 399-433.

Fisher, R. A. (1934). *Statistical methods for research workers* (5th ed.). Edinburgh: Oliver & Boyd.

Glover, M. U., Kuber, M. T., Warren, S. E., & Vieweg, W. V. R. (1982). Myocardial infarction before age 36: Risk factor and arteriographic analysis. *American Journal of Cardiology, 49,* 1600-1603.

Goodman, R. M. (1970). *Genetic disorders of man* (p. 995). Boston: Little, Brown.

Gordon, T. & Kannel, W. B. (1971). Section 1: Introduction and general background. *The Framingham study: An epidemiological investigation of cardiovascular disease.* Washington, DC: U.S. Public Health Service.

Grant, J. (1662). *Natural and political observations made upon the bills of mortality.* London. Reprinted in 1939. Baltimore: The John's Hopkins Press

Gregory, I. (1968). *Fundamentals of psychiatry* (p. 647). Philadelphia: W. B. Saunders.

Haile, R. W., Iselius, L., Hodge, S. E., Morton, N. E., & Detels, R. (1981). Segregation and linkage analysis of 40 multiplex multiple sclerosis families. *Human Heredity, 31,* 252-258.

Hasstedt, S. J., Ash, K. O., & Williams, R. R. (1986). A re-examination of major locus hypotheses for high-density lipoprotein cholesterol level using 2170 persons screened in 55 Utah pedigrees. *American Journal of Medical Genetics, 24,* 57-67.

Hasstedt, S. J., Wu, L. L., & Willliams, R. R. (1987). Major locus inheritance of apolipoprotein B in Utah pedigrees. *Genetic Epidemiology, 4*(2), 67-76.

Havlik, R. J., Garrison, J. R., Katz, S. II., Ellison, R. C., Feinleib, M., & Myrianthopoulos, N. C. (1979). Detection of genetic variance in blood pressure of seven-year-old twins. *American Journal of Epidemiology, 109,* 512-516.

Hippocrates. 1938. On airs, waters, and places. Translated and republished in *Medical Classics, 3,* 19-42.

Hopkins, P. N. & Williams, R. R. (1981). A review of 246 suggested coronary risk factors. *Atherosclerosis, 40,* 1-52.

Hopkins, P. N., Williams, R. R., & Hunt, S. C. (1984). Magnified risks from cigarette smoking for coronary prone families in Utah. *Western Journal of Medicine, 141,* 196-202.

Humphreys, N. A. (1885). *Vital statistics: A memorial volume of selections from the reports and writings of William Farr, 1807-1883.* London: The Sanitary Institute of Great Britian.

Hunt, S. C. (1980). The epidemiology of reproductive factors associated with breast cancer. Doctoral dissertation. University of Utah, Salt Lake City, Utah.

Hunt, S. C., Hasstedt, S. J., & Williams, R. R. (1986). Testing for familial aggregation of dichotomous trait. *Genetic Epidemiology, 3,* 299-312.

Hunt, S. C., Williams, R. R., & Barlow, G. K. (1986). A comparison of positive family history definitions for defining risk of future disease. *Journal of Chronic Disease, 39,* 809-821.

Hunt, S. C., Williams, R. R., Smith, J. B., & Ash, K. O. (1986). Association of three erythrocyte cation transport systems with plasma lipids in Utah subjects. *Hypertension, 8,* 30-36.

Jenkins, C. D. (1971). Psychologic and social precursors of coronary disease. *New England Journal of Medicine, 284,* 244-255, 307-317.

Jenner, E. (1798). *An inquiry into the causes and effects of the variolae vaccine.* London: Law.

Jick, N., Dinan, B., Herman, R., & Rothman, K. J. (1978). Myocardial infarction and other vascular diseases in young women. *Journal of the American Medical Association, 240,* 2548-2552.

Jink, H. K. (1976). Cigarette smoking, use of oral contraceptives, and myocardial infarction. *American Journal of Obstetrics and Gynecology, 126,* 301-307.

Johannsen, W. (1909). *Elemente der Exakten Erblichkidtslehre.* Jena, Germany: Fisher.

Joint National Committee on Detection, Evaluation, & Treatment of High Blood Pressure. (1984). The 1984 report. *Archives of Internal Medicine, 144,* 1045-1057.

Kannel, W. B. & Gordon, T. (1974). *The Framingham study. An epidemiological investigation of cardiovascular disease* (Section 30, Eighteen Year Follow-up). Washington, DC: U.S. Government Printing Office [DHEW Publication No. NIH 74-599].

Kesteloot, H. (1985). Epidemiological studies on the relationship between sodium, potassium, and magnesium and arterial blood pressure. *Journal of Cardiovascular Pharmacology, 6,* S192-S196.

King, M. C., Go, R. C. P., Elston, R. C., Lynch, H. T., & Petrakis, N. L. (1980, April). Allele increasing susceptibility to human breast cancer may be linked to the glutamate-pyruvate transaminase locus. *Science, 208,* 406-408.

King, M. C., Lee, G. M., Spinner, N. B., Thompson, G., & Wrensch, M. R. (1984). Genetic epidemiology. *Annual Review of Public Health, 5,* 1-52.

Knapp, P. H., Mathe, A. A., & Vashon, L. (1976). Psychosomatic aspects of broncial asthma. In E. B. Weiss & M. S. Segal (Eds.), *Bronchial asthma: Mechanisms and therapeutics.* Boston: Little, Brown.

Langford, H. G. (1983). Dietary potassium and hypertention: Epidemiologic data. *Annals of Internal Medicine, 98,* 770-772.

Leppert, M. F., Hasstedt, S. J., Holm, J., O'Connell, P., Wu, L., Ash, O., Williams, R. R., & White, R. (1986). A DNA probe for the LDL receptor gene is tightly linked to hypercholesterolemia in a pedigree with early coronary disease. *American Journal of Human Genetics, 39,* 300-306.

Lind, J. (1753). *Treatise of the scurvy.* Edinburgh: Kincaird & Donaldson. Reprinted in 1953, in C. P. Steward & D. Guthrie (Eds.), *Lind's Treatise on Scurvy.* Edingurgh: University Press.

Lyon, J. L., Klauber, M. R., Gardner, J. W., & Smart, C. R. (1977). Cancer incidence in Mormons and non-Mormons in Utah, 1966-1970. *New England Journal of Medicine, 294,* 129-133.

Lyon, J. L., Wetzler, J. P., Klauber, M. R., & Williams, R. R. (1978). Cardiovascular mortality in Mormons and non-Mormons in Utah, 1969-1971. *American Journal of Epidemiology, 108,* 357-366.

MacMahon, B. & Pugh, T. F. (1970). *Epidemiology, principles and methods* (p. 375). Boston: Little, Brown.

MacMahon, B., Cole, P. & Brown, J. (1973). Etiology of human breast cancer: A review. *JNCI, 50,* 21-42.

Mandel, G. (1866). Versuche Uber Pflanzen Hybriden. Reprinted 1951, *Journal of Heredity, 42,* 1-42.

Mason, J. O., Williams, R. R., & Weber, N. (1983). Family health trees: Targeting prevention strategies. *Utah State Medical Association Bulletin, 31,* 14-16.

Mason, J. W. (1971). A reevaluation of the concept of non-specificity in stress theory. *Journal of Psychiatric Research, 8,* 323-333.

Mason, J. W. (1974). Specificity in the organization of neuroendocrine response profiles. In P. Seeman & G. Brown (Eds.), *Frontiers in neurology and neuroscience.* Toronto: University of Toronto.

McCarron, D. A. (1983). Calcium and magnesium nutrition in human hypertension. *Annals of Internal Medicine, 98,* 800-805.

McKusick, V. A. (1983). *Mendelian inheritance in man* (6th ed.). Baltimore: Johns Hopkins Press.

Moll, P. P., Sing, C. F., Williams, R. R., Mao, S. J. T., & Kottke, B. A. (1986). The genetic determinant of plasma apolipoprotein A-I levels measured by radioimmunoassay: A study of high-risk pedigrees. *American Journal of Human Genetics, 38*(3), 361-372.

Murray, R. M. & Lewis, S. W. (1985, May). Towards an aetiological classification of schizophrenia. *The Lancet,* 1023-1026.

Neufeld, H. N. & Goldbourt, M. A. (1983). Coronary heart disease: Genetic aspects. *Circulation, 67*(5), 943-954.

Perloff, D., Sokolow, M., & Cowan, M. (1983). The prognostic value of ambulatory blood pressures. *Journal of the American Medical Association, 3,* 236-240.

Puska, P., Iacono, J. M., Nissinen, A., Korhanen, H. J., Vartiainen, E., Pietinen, P., Dougherty, R., Leino, U., Mutanen, M., Moisio, S., & Huttunen, J. (1983). Controlled randomised trial of the effect of dietary fat on blood pressure. *Lancet, 1,* 1-5.

Rissanen, A. M. (1979). Familial occurrence of cornary heart disease—Effect of age at diagnosis. *American Journal of Cardiology, 44,* 60-66.

Rotter, J. I. & Rimoin, D. L. (1983). Diabetes mellitus. In A. E. N. Emergy & D. L. Rimoin (Eds.), (pp. 1180-1201). *Principles and practice of medical genetics.* New York: Churchill Livingston.

Rotter, J. I., Sones, J. Q., Samloff, I. M., Richardson, C. T., Gurski, J. T., Walsh, J. H., & Rimoin, D. L. (1979). Duodenal ulcer disease associated with elevated serum pepsinogen I, an inherited autosomal dominant disorder. *New England Journal of Medicine, 300,* 63-66.

Sattins, R. W., Rubin, G. L., Webster, L. A., Huezo, C. M., Wingo, P. A., Ory, H. W., Layde, P. M., & The Cancer and Steroid Hormone Study. (1985). Family history and the risk of breast cancer. *The Journal of the American Medical Association, 253*(13), 1908-1913.

Sims, E. A. H., Danforth, E., Horton, E. S., Bray, G. A., Glennon, J. A., & Salans, L. B. (1973). Endocrine and metabolic defects of experimental obesity in man. *Recent Progress in Hormonal Research, 29,* 457-496.

Skolnick, M. H., Bishop, D. T., Carmelli, D., Gardner, E., Hadley, R., Hasstedt, S. Hill, J. R., Hunt, S., Lyon, J. J., Smart, C. R., & Williams, R. R. (1981). A population-based assessment of familial cancer risk in Utah Mormon genealogies. In R. E. Arrighi, P. N. Rao, & E. Stubblefield (Eds.), *Genes, chromosomes, and neoplasia* (pp. 477-499). New York: Raven Press.

Skolnick, M. H., Thompson, E. A., Bishop, D. T., & Cannon, L. A. (1984). Possible linkage of a breast cancer-susceptibility locus to the ABO locus: Sensitivity of LOD scores to a single new recombinant observation. *Genetic Epidemiology, 1,* 363-373.

Smith-Barbaro, P. A. & Pucak, G. J. (1983). Dietary fat and blood pressure. *Annals of Internal Medicine, 98,* 828-831.

Snow, J. (1855). *On the mode of communication of cholera* (2nd ed.). London: Churchill. Reprinted in 1936, in *Snow on Cholera,* New York: Commonwealth Fund; Reprinted in 1965, New York: Hafner.

Stobo, J. D. (1982). Rheumatoid arthritis—From rubens to restriction maps. *Western Journal of Medicine, 137,* 109-115.

Terman, G. W., Shanit, Y., Lewis, J. W., & Cannon, J. T. (1984, December). Mechanisms of pain inhibition: activation by stress. *Science, 226,* 1271-

Tokuhata, G. K. (1965). Familial factors in lung cancer and smoking. In J. V. Neal, M. W. Shaw, & W. J. Schull (Eds.), *Genetics and the epidemiology of chronic diseases* (pp. 339-353).

Washington, DC: Public Health Service Publication No. 1163.

Vander Molen, R., Brewer, G., Honeyman, M. S., Morrison, J., & Hoobler, S. W. (1970). A study of hypertension in twins. *American Heart Journal, 79,* 454-457.

Ward, M. M., Mefford, I. N., Parker, S. D., Chesney, M. A., Taylor, B., Keegan, D. L., & Barchas, J. (1983). Epinephrine and norepinephrine responses in continuously collected human plasma to a series of stressors. *Psychosomatic Medicine, 45,* 471-485.

West, K. M. (1978). *Epidemiology of diabetes and its vascular lesions.* New York: Elsevier.

Whitescarver, S. A., Cobern, E. O., Jackson, E. A., Gutherie, G. P., & Kotchen, T. A. (1984). Salt-sensitive hypertension: Contribution of chloride. *Science, 233,* 1430-1432.

Whyte, H. M. (1975). Potential effects of coronary heart disease morbidity of lowering the blood cholesterol. *Lancet, 1,* 906.

Williams, R. R. (1979). The role of genes in coronary atherosclerosis. In J. W. Hurst (Ed.), *Update IV: The heart.* (pp. 89-118). New York: McGraw-Hill.

Williams, R. R. (1980). A population perspective for early and familial coronary heart disease. *Proceedings of conference on human health data from defined populations: Banbury report 4.* (pp. 333-350). New York: Cold Spring Harbor Laboratory.

Williams, R. R. (1984a). Understanding genetic and environmental risk factors in susceptible persons. *The Western Journal of Medicine, 141,* 799-806.

Williams, R. R. (1984b). Population-based perspectives of the genetic epidemiology of *early* coronary disease in Framingham and Utah. In D. C. Rao, R. C. Elston, L. H. Kuller, M. Feinleib, C. Carter, & R. Havlik (Eds.), *Genetic epidemiology of coronary heart disease: Past, present, and future* (pp. 89-91). New York: Alan R. Liss, Inc.

Williams, R. R. (1984c). The role of genetic analysis in characterizing obesity. *International Journal of Obesity, 8,* 551-559.

Williams, R. R. (1985). Unpublished data.

Williams, R. R. (1988). Nature, nurture, and family predisposition. *New England Journal of Medicine, 318*(12), 767-771.

Williams, R. R. & Hopkins, P. N. (1979). Salt, hypertension, and genetic-environmental interaction. In C. F. Sing & M. Skolnick (Eds.), *The genetic analysis of common diseases* (pp. 183-194). New York: Alan R. Liss, Inc.

Williams, R. R. & Horn, J. W. (1977) Association of cancer sites with tobacco and alcohol consumption and socioeconimic status: Patient interview study from the third national cancer survey. *Journal of the National Cancer Institute, 58,* 525-546.

Williams, R. R. (1984c). The role of genetic analysis in characterizing obesity. *International Journal of Obesity, 8,* 551-559.

Williams, R. R., Dadone, M., Hunt, S. C., & Kuida, H. (1984). The genetic epidemiology of hypertension: A review of past studies and current results in 948 persons in 48 Utah pedigrees. In D. C. Rao, R. C. Elston, L. H. Kuller, M. Feinleib, C. Carter, & R. Havli, (Eds.), *Genetic epidemiology of coronary heart disease: Past, present, and future* (pp. 420-444). New York: Alan R. Liss, Inc.

Williams, R. R., Hasstedt, S. J., Wilson, D. E., Ash, K. O., Yanowitz, F. G., Reiber, G. E., & Kuida, H. (1986). Evidence that man with familial hypercholesterolemia can avoid early coronary heart disease: An analysis of 77 gene carriers in four Utah pedigrees. *Journal of the American Medical Association, 255,* 219-224.

Williams, R. R., Hunt, S. C., Dadone, M. M., Smith, J. B., Ash, K. O. & Kuida, H. (1984). Cation flux and other possible biological markers of genetically predisposed hypertension. In L. J. Filer & R. M. Lauder (Eds.), *Children's blood pressure, report of the eighty-eighth Ross conference on pediatric research.* (pp. 100-123). Columbus, Ohio: Ross Laboratories.

Williams, R. R., Lyon, J. L., Brockert, J. E., & Maness, A. T. (1979). Decine in coronary mortality rates: Utah vs. U. S. *Proceedings of NHLBI conference of the decline of coronary heart disease* (48-57).

Williams, R. R., Skolnick, M., Carmelli, D., Maness, A. T., Hunt, S. C., Hasstedt, S., Reiber, G. E., & Jones, R. K. (1979a). Utah pedigree studies: Design and preliminary data for premature male CHD deaths. In C. F. Sing & M. Skolnick (Eds.), *The genetic analysis of common diseases.* (pp. 711-721). New York: Alan R. Liss, Inc.

Williams, R. R., Stegens, N. L. & Goldsmith, J. R. (1977). Industries and occupations associated with cancer sites from the TNCS interview study. *Journal of the National Cancer Institute, 59,* 1147-1185.

Wilson, N. V. & Meyer, B. M. (1981). Early prediction of hypertension using exercise blood pressure. *Preventive Medicine, 10,* 62-68.

Winawer, S. J. (1980). Screening for colorectal cancer: An overview. *Cancer, 45,* 1093-1098.

Wood, D. L., Sheps, S. G., Elveback, L. R., & Schirger, A. (1984). Cold pressor test as a predictor of hypertension. *Hypertension, 6,* 301-306.

Zimmet, P. (1979). Epidemiology of diabetes and its macrovascular manifestations in Pacific populations, the medical effects of social progress. *Diabetes Care, 2,* 144-153.

UNIT
III

Mechanisms of Self-Defense

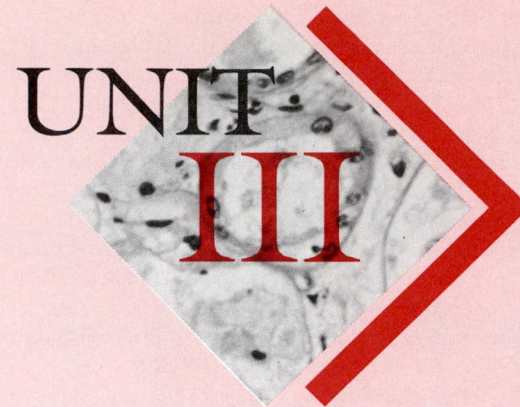

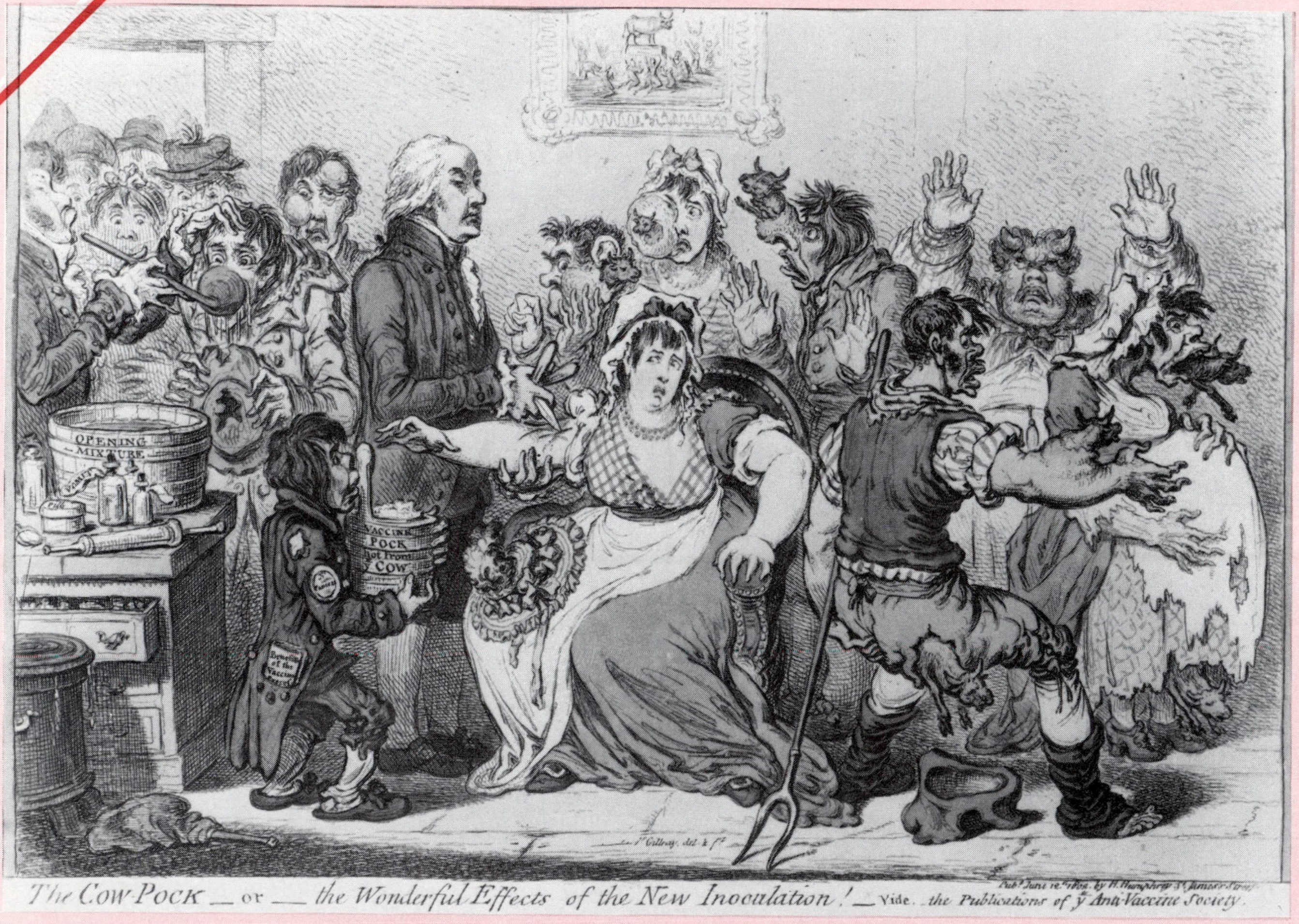

The cow-pock or the wonderful effects of the new inoculation. Courtesy National Library of Medicine.

IMMUNOLOGY is a relatively new science, yet anecdotal evidence shows that people in ancient times were aware of mysterious phenomena that are recognized today as basic concepts of immunology. The ancient Egyptians drew hieroglyphics that represented inflammation. The Greeks, even as far back as the fifth century BC, recognized that individuals who survived a disease seldom contracted the disease a second time. These observations of immune and inflammatory processes were made before the discovery that infectious agents, such as bacteria and viruses, even existed.

The accidental and serendipitous application of immunologic principles ended in the late nineteenth century, when the investigative study of immunology began with the work of an English physician, Edward Jenner. Jenner performed the first experiment in the science that was to become immunology (Jenner, 1798). There are many stories about Jenner's experiment, many fanciful. It is known that Jenner recognized that milkmaids were protected from smallpox if they had developed cowpox, a bovine equivalent of smallpox that causes only mild disease in humans. Jenner took material from a cowpox pustule on the hand of an infected milkmaid (reputed to be named Sarah Nelmes in some stories) and injected it into the arm of James Phipps, an 8-year-old boy. After the boy's initial inflammatory reaction to the injection subsided, Jenner injected him with material from a smallpox pustule. Fortunately the experiment was a success, because Jenner is reported to have reinjected smallpox bacteria into the boy at least 20 times. In 1798 Jenner used the term *vaccination* (*vacca* = cow) to describe his technique.

Knowledge about immunity has resulted from carefully planned, well-executed, and well-interpreted experiments as well as serendipity and chance.

The earliest debates among researchers raged around the relative importance of serum (humoral) factors and cellular factors in immune function. It took years to identify the role of humoral factors—the plasma proteins—in the development of immunity. In 1890 Emile von Behring and Shibasaburo Kitasato injected animals with diphtheria toxin, causing the animals to produce antitoxin that could be identified in sera withdrawn for examination (von Behring & Kitasato, 1890). Rodolf Kraus later demonstrated that the antitoxin, which he called a precipitin, could cause diphtheria toxin to precipitate out of solution in vitro (Kraus, 1897). Other workers showed that the contents of sera from immunized animals could also lyse (dissolve) bacteria (the bacteriolysins) (Pfeiffer, 1894), and agglutinate (clump) bacteria (the agglutinins) (von Gruber & Durham, 1896). In the 1930s researchers finally learned that each of these functions could be attributed to one of the plasma proteins, which became known as antibody.

The role of cells in immune function was also investigated for the first time late in the nineteenth century. In the 1880s the Russian zoologist Elie Metchnikoff studied large, amoeboid white blood cells (macrophages) in starfish and concluded that their function was to accumulate at a site of inflammation and ingest invaders (Metchnikoff, 1883). Later proponents of the cellular theory of immunity proposed that the role of antibody was to prepare (opsonize) the invader for ingestion by the macrophages. The role of other white blood cells (lymphocytes) was suggested in the 1890s by Robert Koch, during his study of tuberculosis. Koch was the first to describe the tuberculin reaction (Koch phenomenon) in which lymphocytes interact with the tuberculin bacillus (Koch, 1891).

In the 1950s extensive research by many scientists led to the realization that antibody and lymphocytes are both effectors of the same immune response. One of the most important breakthroughs was the recognition that discrete lymphoid organs are responsible for the development of these two effectors. Bruce Glick identified the lymphoid organ responsible for the development of antibody-producing cells (Glick, Chang, & Jaap, 1956). He observed that when the bursa of Fabricius (an organ that opens into the terminal portion of the digestive tract of chickens) was removed, the birds lost the ability to produce antibody in response to injected microorganisms. It was later observed that these birds retained cell-mediated immunity. When Glick and his co-workers attempted to publish a paper reporting their findings, it was reportedly rejected by editors of prestigous medical journals and was finally published in *Poultry Science*.

The lymphoid tissue responsible for the development of cellular, or cell-mediated, immunity—the thymus—was identified in the 1960s by Jacques Miller (Miller, 1961) and Robert Good (Good et al., 1962). They observed that experimental animals that had had the thymus removed at birth could not elicit a cell-mediated immune response; that is, their non-antibody-producing lymphocytes did not react to the introduction of infectious agents. They could, however, produce fairly good antibody responses. As a result of the work of these and many other researchers, the study of immunology has risen from a fledgling science in the nineteenth century to what is perhaps the most exciting, diverse, and rapidly advancing discipline in medicine today.

CHAPTER 6

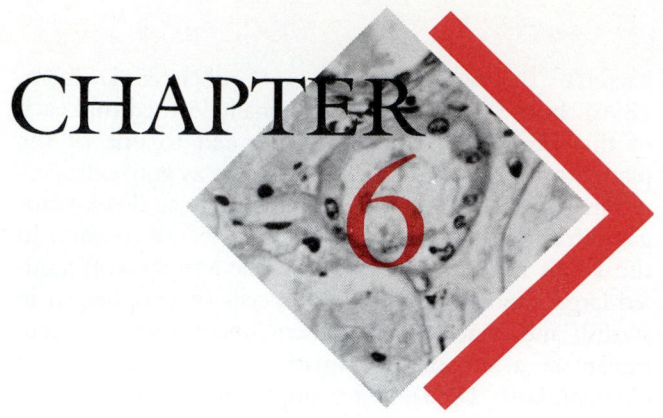

Immunity

Neal S. Rote

Characteristics of the immune response, 193
    Natural versus acquired immunity, 194
    Primary and secondary immune responses, 194
    Humoral versus cell-mediated immunity, 195
Induction of the immune response, 196
    Antigens and immunogens, 196
    Histocompatibility antigens, 198
      The HLA complex, 198
      Role of HLA antigens, 198
    Blood group antigens, 198
      The Rh system, 198
      The ABO system, 199
The humoral immune response, 200
    B lymphocytes, 200
    Immunoglobulins, 202
      Structure of immunoglobulin molecules, 202
      Function of antibodies, 205
        Neutralization of bacterial toxins, 205
        Neutralization of viruses, 206
        Opsonization of bacteria, 206
        Activation of inflammatory processes, 206
      Classes of immunoglobulins, 206
      Monoclonal antibodies, 207
    The secretory immune system, 207
The cell-mediated immune response, 209
Cellular interactions in the immune response, 209
Fetal and neonatal immune function, 212
Immune function in the elderly, 213

The body's first lines of defense are anatomic barriers: the skin and mucous membranes lining the respiratory, gastrointestinal, and genitourinary tracts. These surfaces are biochemical barriers as well. Sebaceous glands in the skin secrete antibacterial and antifungal fatty and lactic acids. Perspiration, tears, and saliva contain an enzyme (lysozyme) that attacks the cell walls of gram-positive bacteria. As a result of these glandular secretions, the surface of the skin is acidic (pH 3 to 5), making it inhospitable to most bacteria.

If an injurious chemical, foreign body, or microorganism penetrates these defenses, the body attempts to eliminate it by mechanical clearance. It may be sloughed off with skin, caught in respiratory mucus and coughed up, vomited, or flushed from the urinary tract by urine. Auxiliary defenses are present in the form of the body's normal population of bacteria, or flora, which produce metabolites (products of metabolism) that inhibit the growth of some invading bacteria. All of these defenses are both external and nonspecific; that is, they protect the host as needed against any and all invaders.

Once external barriers have been compromised, permitting harmful chemicals, foreign bodies, or microorganisms to penetrate cells and tissues, the **inflammatory response,** or **inflammation,** occurs. This response, which begins within seconds of injury or invasion, is also nonspecific. It begins with the immediate marshaling of resources by vascular structures at the site of invasion. The affected tissues are soon surrounded by cells and fluids that are equipped to isolate, destroy, and remove the invaders, and thereby to promote healing.

The third and last line of defense is the **immune response,** or **immunity.** It occurs much more slowly than the inflammatory response and is specific in that it can confer permanent or long-term protection against specific microorganisms. It can also be induced by vaccination or inoculation. Unlike inflammation, which involves many different plasma systems and cell types, immunity is effected by one type of serum protein (immunoglobulin, or antibody) and one type of blood cell (lymphocyte). The many defenses against microorganisms are summarized in Table 6-1.

The inflammatory and immune responses complement one another and interact in complex ways. Because many inflammatory processes are triggered or affected by simultaneous immune processes, an understanding of the immune response is necessary for an understanding of many aspects of inflammation. Therefore, the chapters in this unit will be presented in the sequence of immunity, inflammation, and diseases of immunity and inflammation. Chapter 6 will discuss normal immunity, including the role of antibodies and lymphocytes in protection against infectious organisms. Chapter 7 will discuss normal inflammation, including

TABLE 6-1   Defenses against infection

Type of defense	Specific mechanism
Surface defenses	Physical barriers: skin, conjunctivae, mucous membranes Mechanical removal: desquamation of skin, tears, mucus, ciliary action, coughing, salivation, swallowing, urination, defecation Normal bacterial flora: antibacterial factors Chemical inhibitors: gastric acid, lactic acid, fatty acids, spermine, lactoperoxidase, bile salts Antimicrobial substances: lysozyme, secretory IgA
Nonspecific resistance factors	Fever, interferons, complement, lysozyme, C-reactive protein (reacts with bacterial surface polysaccharides and activates complement), lactoferrin (binds and removes iron as a bacterial nutrient), α-1-antitrypsin (inhibits bacterial enzymes)

Inflammation	Soluble factors
	  Clotting system: Hageman factor (factor XII)
	  Complement system: chemotactic factors, anaphylatoxins
	  Kinin system: bradykinin
	Phagocytes
	  Circulating neutrophils, eosinophils, monocytes, macrophages
	  Fixed cells (of mononuclear phagocyte system) in alveoli, spleen, liver, bone marrow

Immune response	Humoral immune response: B cells, plasma cells, immunoglobulins Cell-mediated immune response: T cells, lymphokines

the interactions of the immune and inflammatory responses. Chapter 8 will discuss medically relevant aberrations in immunity and inflammation, including allergies, diseases that involve unwanted immunologic destruction of healthy tissue, and diseases that are caused by a deficiency in the normal immune or inflammatory responses.

CHARACTERISTICS OF THE IMMUNE RESPONSE

The immune system of the normal adult is continually challenged by a spectrum of chemical substances that it recognizes as foreign, or "nonself." These substances are called **antigens.** Some antigens are infectious agents, such as viruses, bacteria, fungi, or parasites; some are noninfectious substances from the environment, such as pollens, foods, and bee venoms; and others are drugs, vaccines, transfusions, and transplanted tissues.

The body's reaction to antigenic challenges is the immune response, in which physiologic and biochemical interactions cause the maturation and activation of two types of **immunocytes,** or **immunocompetent cells** (Fig. 6-1). The two types of immunocytes, B lymphocytes (B cells) and T lymphocytes (T cells), act in different ways to recognize and destroy specific antigens. They differ from the cells involved in inflammation in two ways. First, they defend the host against specific antigens. The B cells produce antibodies, which incapaci-

tate the antigen, whereas the T cells attack the antigen directly. Second, once the B cells and T cells have been exposed to a particular antigen, some of them, called memory cells, become capable of "remembering" the antigen and of acting even faster should it invade the host again. Thus the immune system possesses memory and specificity and creates long-lasting protection against specific antigens. This process is termed **immunity.**

The immune response can be amplified or suppressed by both exogenous (external) and endogenous (internal) modulators. Some exogenous factors, such as trauma, disease, pollutants, radiation, ultraviolet light, and drugs, have profound effects on the capacity of an individual's immune system to respond to an antigenic challenge. The immune system is also modulated by certain endogenous factors, such as the individual's age, sex, nutritional status, genetic background, and reproductive status. The quality and intensity of the immune response therefore are a sum of the effects of all these factors: antigenic challenge, exogenous modulators, and endogenous factors.

Sometimes the normal immune response does not function in the best interests of the host and must be suppressed. For example, transplanted organs from donors are in danger of rejection as a result of the immune response. One means of lessening the likelihood of rejection is to match host tissues and donor tissues for antigenic compatibility, or histocompatibility. The other means is pharmacologic suppression of the immune response.

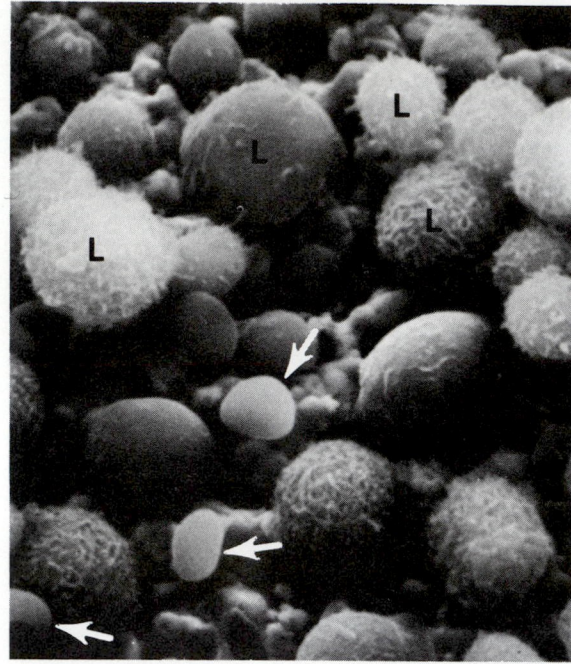

FIG. 6-1. This scanning electron micrograph shows a mixed population of B and T lymphocytes; arrow designates red blood cells. (From King, Fenoglio, & Lefkowitch, 1983.)

Another example of a functioning but detrimental immune response is an allergic reaction. Allergies are detrimental immune responses in which the host's immune system "overreacts," or is hypersensitive, to the antigenic properties of certain substances, such as house dust, animal danders, and certain foods. (Immune deficiency diseases, autoimmune diseases, and allergic hypersensitivity are the subject of Chapter 8.)

Natural versus Acquired Immunity

Natural immunity, also called native or innate resistance, is not produced by the immune response. One type of natural immunity, which is present at birth, is species-dependent. Human beings are naturally immune to some of the infectious agents that cause illness in other species. For example, humans do not contract canine distemper or, as Jenner observed, serious cases of cowpox. The other type of natural immunity is host-dependent and involves the individual's characteristics that play some role in the development of specific diseases. (Analysis of risk factors, as described in Chapter 5, has identified some of these characteristics.)

Acquired immunity is gained after birth as a result of the immune response. Acquired immunity can be either active or passive, depending on whether the components of the immune response have been produced by the host or by a donor. **Active acquired immunity** is produced by the host after either natural exposure to an antigen or immunization. **Passive acquired immunity** does not involve the host's immune response. Rather, preformed antibodies or T lymphocytes are transferred to the recipient. This can occur naturally, as in the passage of maternal antibodies to the fetus, or artificially as in a clinical treatment. Clinically preformed antibodies from a donor (human or animal) are administered in the form of immune serum, which is antibody-containing blood from which the clotting factors and cells have been removed. Passive immunity is temporary and is used in the treatment of such clinical emergencies as rabies exposure, tetanus, and snakebite.

Primary and Secondary Immune Responses

The immune response to antigenic challenge has classically been divided into two phases, the primary and secondary (or anamnestic) responses. These phases can be demonstrated by serologic tests that measure plasma concentrations of antibody over time (Fig. 6-2). The initial administration of (or exposure to) most antigens is followed by a latent period, during which mature B cells (called plasma cells) produce no detectable antibodies (immunoglobulin, [Ig]). After approximately 5 days one class of antibody (IgM) can be detected in the circulation. This marks the beginning of the initial or **primary immune response,** which is usually dominated by IgM, with very little IgG (another class of immunoglobulin). With no further exposure to the antigen the circulating antibody is catabolized (broken down) and measurable quantities fall. The individual's immune system, however, has been primed. A second challenge by the same antigen results in the **secondary immune response,** which is characterized by the production of a more rapid and larger amount of antibody than the primary response. The rapidity of the secondary immune response is due to the presence of memory cells. The quantity of IgM produced in the secondary response is about the same as that produced in the primary response. IgG is the predominant antibody class of the secondary response and is frequently present in concentrations several times those of IgM. The greatest differences between the primary and secondary responses are in the amount of IgG that is produced and the rapidity with which antibody appears after antigen challenge.

The primary and secondary responses confer active acquired immunity. When an antigen, such as a varicella (chickenpox) virus, enters the host for the first time, the primary immune response is activated. Antibody titers are not high, and the host becomes ill but recovers. If the host is exposed to varicella later in life, the secondary response occurs: antibody levels rise immediately, and the virus is neutralized (disabled) before it can cause active infection.

The same thing happens as a result of immunization, except that the antigen is made less infectious (attenuated) or otherwise altered before administration so that

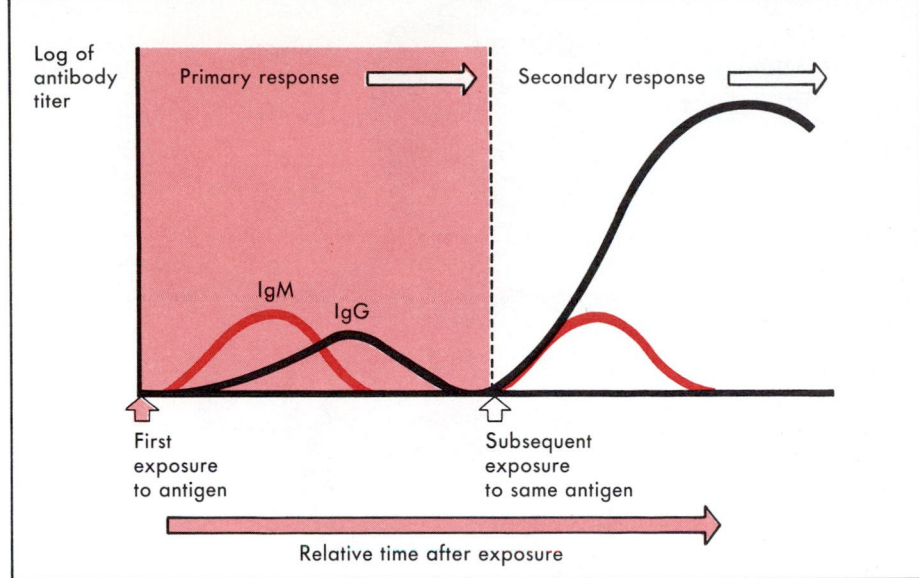

FIG. 6-2. Primary and secondary immune responses. The introduction of antigen induces a response dominated by two classes of immunoglobulins, IgM and IgG. IgM predominates in the primary response, with some IgG appearing later. After the host's immune system is primed, another challenge with the same antigen induces the secondary response, in which some IgM and large amounts of IgG are produced.

it is strong enough to elicit the primary immune response but not strong enough to cause illness. Later exposure to the same antigen elicits the secondary immune response, preventing illness. In Jenner's experiment the cowpox and smallpox antigens were sufficiently similar that the cowpox antigen functioned as an altered, or attenuated, smallpox antigen. The antibodies and lymphocytes sensitized to recognize and destroy cowpox were also able to recognize smallpox bacteria, thereby protecting the immunized child against smallpox.

Humoral versus Cell-Mediated Immunity

The primary immunocyte of the immune response is the lymphocyte (Fig. 6-3). The mature **lymphocyte** is a small, round, white blood cell approximately 6 to 10 microns in diameter.

Lymphocytes originate in the liver and spleen of the fetus and the bone marrow of the child or adult as lymphocyte precursors or stem cells. (Lymphocyte precursors are described in Unit 9.) They are not capable of implementing the immune response. To become immunocompetent, they must migrate through the lymphatics and blood vessels, then through lymphoid tissues in various parts of the body (Fig. 6-4). While passing through these tissues, they mature and undergo changes that commit them to one of two cellular lineages. The lymphocytes that migrate through one set of lymphoid tissues become **B lymphocytes,** or **B cells.** When B cells encounter antigens, they are stimulated to mature into plasma cells that produce antibodies. B cells are ultimately responsible for **humoral immunity** (see p. 200).

The lymphocytes that migrate through the thymus gland become **T lymphocytes,** or **T cells.** T cells are ca-

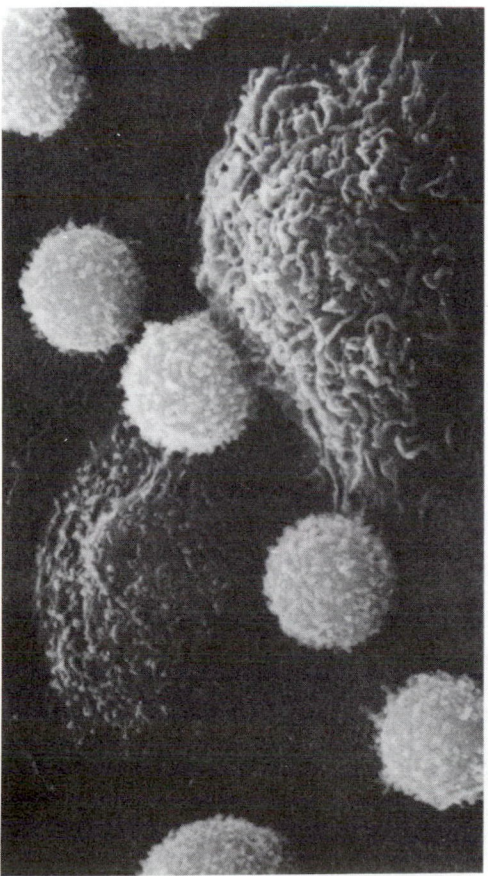

FIG. 6-3. Scanning electron micrograph of a lymphocyte and macrophages. The lymphocytes are small and spherical; the macrophages are larger and more irregular in shape. (From Raven & Johnson, 1986.)

FIG. 6-4. Lymphoid tissues: sites of B cell and T cell differentiation. Immature lymphocytes migrate through central lymphoid tissues: the bone marrow (probable central lymphoid tissue for B lymphocytes) and the thymus (central lymphoid tissue for T lymphocytes). Mature lymphocytes later reside in the T and B lymphocyte-rich areas of the peripheral lymphoid tissues.

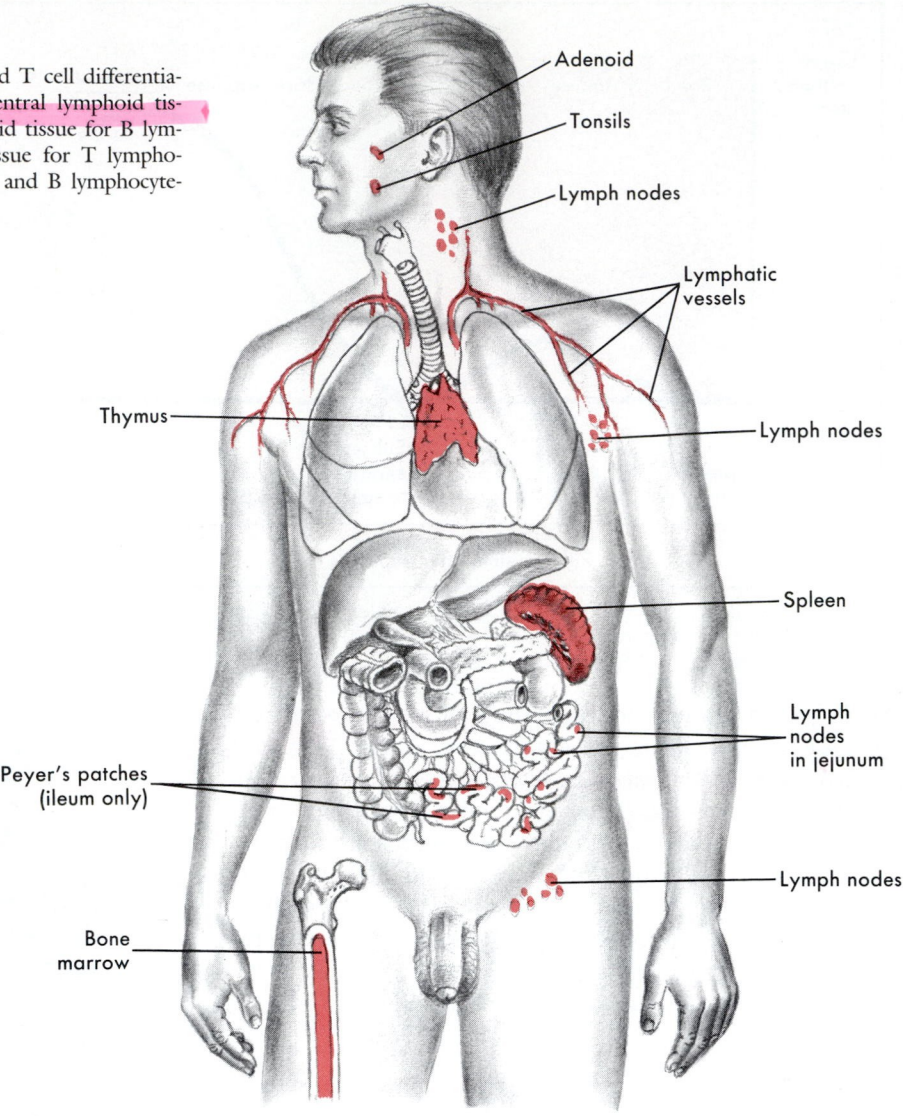

pable of becoming sensitized to and recognizing specific antigens, which they then attack directly. They are responsible for **cell-mediated immunity** (see p. 209).

The success of the immune response depends on the interaction between the humoral and cell-mediated responses, which share some components and processes. Differentiation (maturation) of T cells and B cells is shown in Fig. 6-5.

INDUCTION OF THE IMMUNE RESPONSE

Antigens and Immunogens

Although the terms *antigen* and *immunogen* are used as synonyms, some technical differences between them are significant. An **antigen** is a molecule or molecular complex that reacts with preformed components of the immune system, such as lymphocytes and antibodies. Antigenicity is the molecule's innate capacity *to react with* those preformed components and is determined by the chemical structure of the antigen molecule. An **immunogen** is an antigen that can also *induce the formation of* components of the immune system (i.e., maturation of T and B lymphocytes and production of antibodies). Therefore, a substance may be antigenic—able to react with existing antibodies and mature lymphocytes—yet not immunogenic, that is, not able to induce the immune response.

A molecule is not antigenic unless at least a portion of its chemical structure can be recognized by and bound to specific (matching) receptors on a lymphocyte or antibody molecule. (Receptor function is described in Chapter 1.) The portion of the antigen molecule that is

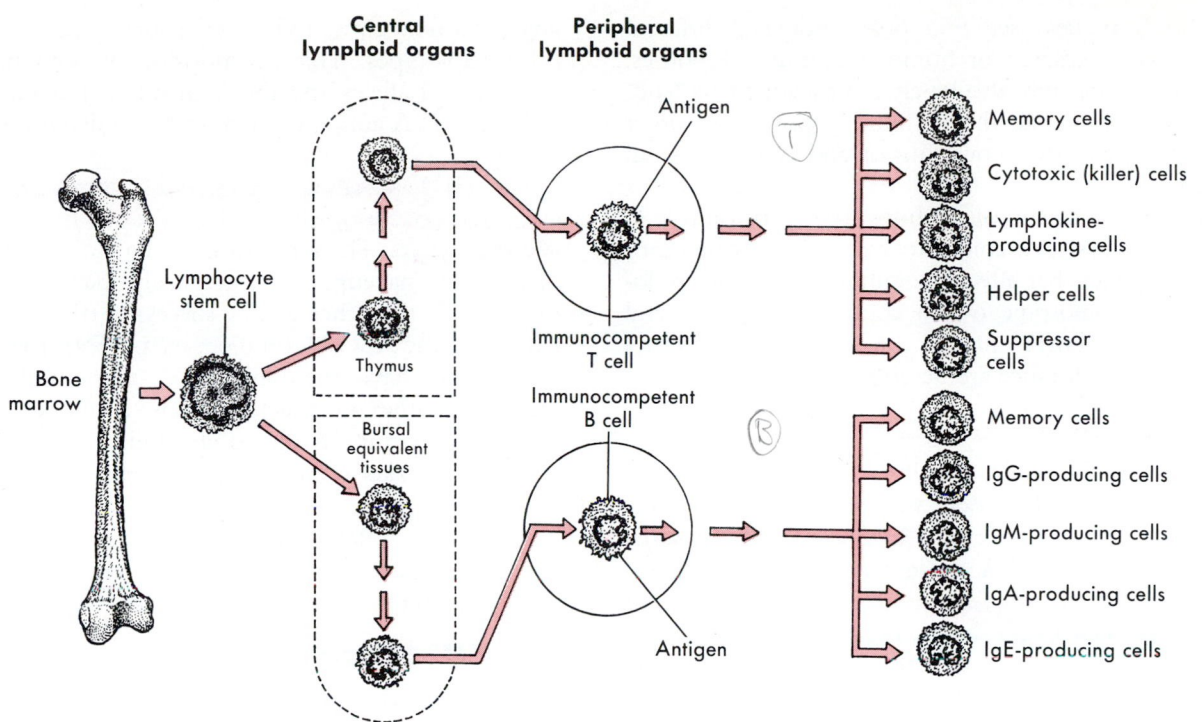

Central lymphoid organs

Peripheral lymphoid organs

Lymphocyte stem cell

Bone marrow

Thymus

Bursal equivalent tissues

Antigen

Immunocompetent T cell

Immunocompetent B cell

Antigen

Memory cells

Cytotoxic (killer) cells

Lymphokine-producing cells

Helper cells

Suppressor cells

Memory cells

IgG-producing cells

IgM-producing cells

IgA-producing cells

IgE-producing cells

FIG. 6-5. Outcome of T (thymus-derived) and B (bursal-derived) pathways of lymphocyte maturation. Mature cells of the T cell lineage which have different functions usually develop from separate immature T cells. Mature B cells, on the other hand, may directly progress through the production of different classes of antibody against the same antigen. IgD is not shown because it does not circulate in the blood.

configured for recognition and binding is called an **antigenic determinant,** or **epitope.** The matching receptor on the lymphocyte or antibody is sometimes referred to as an antigen-binding, or antigen-combining, site, or **paratope.**

To be immunogenic, the antigen molecule also must be (1) sufficiently foreign to the host, (2) sufficiently large, (3) sufficiently complex, and (4) present in sufficient amounts. In addition, the antigen's determinant sites must be accessible. Even if an antigen fulfills all these criteria, its ability to act as an immunogen may be affected by its route of entry into the host and by the host's endogenous characteristics, particularly genetic makeup.

Foremost among the criteria for immunogenicity is the antigen's foreignness. The immune system has the exquisite ability to distinguish self (**self-antigens**) from nonself (foreign antigens). Under normal conditions the immune system does not recognize self-antigens. This is the reason that the immune system is normally tolerant of the host's tissues but is able to reject foreign tissues and destroy infectious agents. **Tolerance,** once thought to be a state of nonresponsiveness in which the immune system passively allowed self-antigens to persist, is now known to be part of the active immune response. Rather than merely tolerating self-antigens, the immune

system prevents their recognition by lymphocytes and antibodies. The response to self-antigens is active suppression of the immune system by specialized T lymphocytes called **suppressor T cells,** abbreviated **Ts** (see Fig. 6-5). Therefore, an antigen that fulfills the criteria of foreignness, size, complexity, and quantity will be immunogenic, whereas a self-antigen, which fulfills all the criteria *except* foreignness, will be **tolergenic.**

Molecular size also contributes to an antigen's immunogenicity. In general, large molecules (those greater than 10,000 daltons), such as proteins, polysaccharides, and nucleic acids, are most immunogenic. Low—molecular weight molecules, such as amino acids, monosaccharides, fatty acids, and the purine and pyrimidine bases, tend to be unable to induce the immune response. Many molecules in this size range can function as **haptens:** antigens that are too small to be immunogens by themselves but become immunogenic in combination with larger molecules.

The route and vehicle of entry or administration to the host are critical to the immunogenicity of some antigens. This has important clinical implications. The most common routes for clinical administration of antigen are the intravenous, intraperitoneal, subcutaneous, intranasal, and oral routes. Each route preferentially stimulates a different set of lymphocyte-containing (lymphoid) tissues (see Fig. 6-4), inducing different types of cell-mediated or humoral immune responses. Immunogenicity may also be altered by adjuvants (substances that stimulate the immune response) or other agents that alter the processing of and response to an antigen.

The genetic makeup of the host plays a critical role in the immune system's ability to respond to many antigens. The genes that affect the immune response are located on chromosome 6 and control the quality and quantity of the host's immune response. (Chromosomes and genetic inheritance are described in Chapter 4.)

Histocompatibility Antigens

How does the body actually recognize that a substance is foreign? The "code" that brings about this recognition consists of the major **histocompatibility antigens** (also called **HLA antigens** or **HLA determinants**), which are proteins found on the surface of nearly every cell in the body. HLA antigens not only play a role in defending the body against infection, but also in distinguishing each individual's tissue from the tissues of others.

The HLA Complex

The major group of genes producing the HLA antigens is known as the **HLA complex,** or the **major histocompatibility complex (MHC).** This complex consists of four closely linked loci located on the short arm of chromosome 6. They are labeled A, B, C, and D/DR. The antigens produced by the A, B, and C loci (class I antigens) are found on the surfaces of virtually all cells except erythrocytes (red blood cells), and they are involved in the rejection of foreign tissue. The D/DR antigens (class II antigens), on the other hand, are confined mostly to B lymphocytes, certain forms of macrophages and antigen-presenting cells, some epithelial cells, and transiently to subpopulations of stimulated T lymphocytes.

Each HLA locus has many alleles: at least 17 at A, 32 at B, 8 at C, 12 at D, and 10 at DR. With so many alleles at each HLA locus, many possible allele combinations exist, making it unlikely that two unrelated individuals will have the same HLA composition.

The specific alleles at the four HLA loci on one chromosome are termed the haplotype. Each individual has two HLA haplotypes, one for each chromosome. Because the loci are closely linked, the haplotypes are not usually disrupted by recombination and are thus transmitted intact to the offspring. Each parent passes one HLA haplotype to his or her offspring. The offspring then share one haplotype with each parent, and, on the average, they share one haplotype with one half of their siblings, both haplotypes with one fourth of their siblings, and no haplotypes with one-fourth of their siblings. Monozygotic twins, of course, have identical HLA haplotypes. This coexpression of both maternal and paternal alleles and the tremendous polymorphism make the HLA antigen system useful in determining paternity.

The HLA complex is particularly important, however, in determining the success of tissue grafts and organ transplants. The more similar two individuals are in their HLA makeup, the more likely that a transplant from one to the other will be successful (they must also have the same ABO blood type; see p. 199). Even when two people have the same HLA makeup, however, grafts sometimes are rejected because a number of other loci also determine tissue compatibility, although their effects are weaker than those of the HLA system. Thus it is always preferable to obtain a graft or transplant from a closely related individual, such as a sibling, because of a greater chance that a sibling will have the same histocompatibility antigens other than HLA.

Role of HLA Antigens

Although a certain degree of HLA matching is necessary for survival of grafted tissue in recipients, the function of the gene products of the major histocompatibility complex remains a partial puzzle. Obviously these products have not evolved to confound transplanters of kidneys or hearts.

One function of class I and II antigens appears to be distinguishing of self from nonself. Many of the cellular interactions of the immune system require the recognition of foreign antigens in the context of self-antigens, primarily class I and II antigenic determinants.

Genetic loci within the HLA complex also control the quality and quantitiy of an immune response. These are referred to as **immune response genes,** or **Ir genes.**

Blood Group Antigens

The HLA antigens are not found on the surfaces of erythrocytes, but a number of other antigens that determine compatibility are found there. These are known collectively as the **blood group antigens.** More than 80 different red cell antigens are grouped into several dozen blood group systems, each determined by a different locus or set of loci. The most important of these, because they provoke the strongest humoral immune response, are the ABO and Rh systems.

The Rh System

The **Rh blood group** (named after the rhesus monkey, the animal in which it was first discovered), with its high degree of polymorphism, is an antigen system second in complexity only to the HLA system. At least five major antigens and a large number of rare variants have been identified and are expressed only on erythrocytes (Rote, 1982). It appears to consist of three very tightly

CLINICAL COMMENTARY
Detection of HLA Antigens

Different methods are used to detect class I and II antigens. Class I antigens are identified by using an antibody-mediated, complement-dependent cytotoxicity assay devised by Terasaki and McClelland (Terasaki & McClelland, 1964). Lymphocytes are used as target cells because they are rich in HLA determinants and are easily obtained. The typing sera used are human sera obtained from either recipients of blood transfusions who have begun to produce antibodies against the leukocytes or multiparous women who have begun to produce antibodies against the HLA antigens of their mates.

Class II antigens have been detected by two different techniques. Originally, differences were determined by the mixed lymphocyte reaction (MLR). In the MLR lymphocytes from two individuals are mixed under tissue-culture conditions. HLA-D antigens expressed on the surface of B lymphocytes from one donor (stimulator cells) stimulate T lymphocytes from the other donor (responder cells). Lymphocyte stimulation is usually measured by incorporating a radioactive precursor, tritiated thymidine, into newly forming DNA. Other measures of proliferation, including increased cell number and formation of new RNA or protein, could also be used. In a two-way MLR, both donors' lymphocytes are allowed to respond and proliferation is measured as the sum of both responses. More commonly, one-way MLRs, in which the lymphocytes of one donor are prevented from responding by preincubation with metabolic inhibitors, such as mitomycin C, or by preirradiation, are performed.

Panels of sera that identify molecules that appear to be identical with or very closely associated with the D antigens are now available. These serologically determined markers are termed HLA-DR, DP, and DQ.

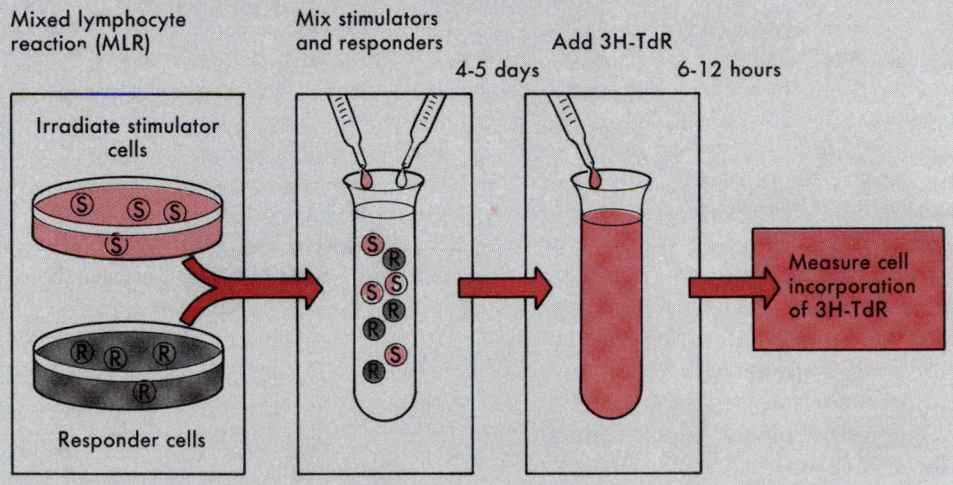

Mixed lymphocyte reaction (MLR). The MLR measures the proliferation of responding T lymphocytes to HLA-D antigenic differences expressed on stimulator cells. Stimulator cells are initially inactivated by irradiation or by incubation with metabolic inhibitors to prevent their uptake of tritiated thymidine.

linked genetic loci, labeled C, D, and E. Each locus has two alleles labeled C and c, D and d, or E and e. Distinct antigens are expressed by C, c, E, e, and D, whereas no distinct antigen has been observed for d. Therefore, d is considered a lack of D. The locus of greatest interest is the D locus, more commonly expressed as $Rh_o(D)$, because it is responsible for Rh maternal-fetal incompatibility and the resulting hemolytic disease of the newborn (see Chapter 25). Persons who have the DD or Dd genotype have the Rh antigen on their erythrocytes and are called Rh-positive. The recessive homozygotes, with genotype dd, are Rh-negative and do not have the Rh antigen. About 85% of North Americans are Rh-positive and about 15% are Rh-negative.

The ABO System

Human blood transfusions were carried out as early as 1818, but they were often unsuccessful. After some transfusions the recipient's red blood cells would clump together, blocking the capillaries, and sometimes causing death. In 1901 Karl Landsteiner reported that this reaction was due to the ABO antigens located on the erythrocyte plasma membranes.

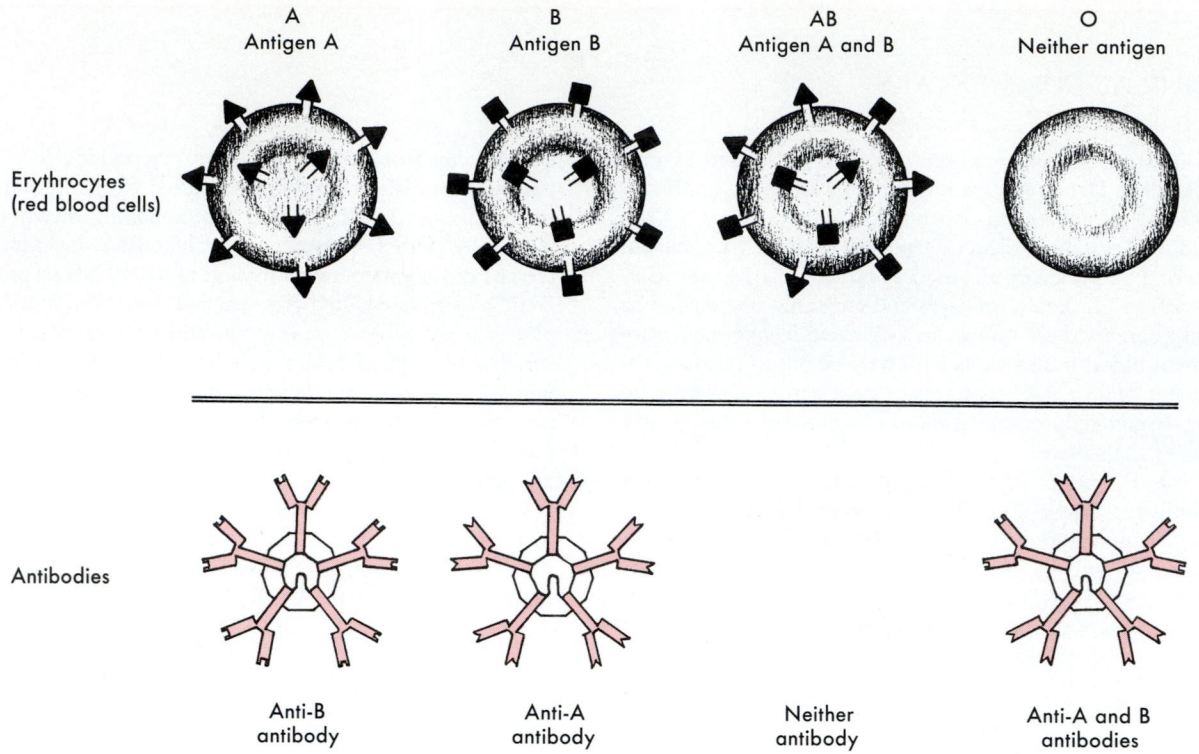

FIG. 6-6. The relationship of antigens and antibodies involved in the ABO blood group system.

The **ABO blood group** consists of two major antigens, labeled A and B (Fig. 6-6). These appear to be codominant, so that individuals can have one of four blood types. Individuals with blood type A carry the A antigen on their erythrocytes; individuals with blood type B carry the B antigen; those with blood type AB carry both A and B; those with type O carry neither antigen. A person with "type A blood" also has anti-B antibodies in the blood. If this person receives blood containing B antigens (i.e., blood from a type AB or B individual), a severe antibody reaction occurs. Similarly, a type B individual (whose blood contains anti-A antibodies) cannot receive blood from a type A or AB donor. Type O individuals, who have neither antigen but have both anti-A and anti-B antibodies, cannot accept blood from any of the other three types. These naturally occurring antibodies are immunoglobulins of the IgM class and are called **isohemagglutinins.**

Because individuals with type O blood lack both types of antigens, they can be "universal donors" and anyone can accept small volumes of their blood. Similarly type AB individuals are "universal recipients," because they lack both anti-A and anti-B antibodies. When large volumes of blood are transfused, however, the donor's antibodies can bind to antigenic determinants on the recipient's erythrocytes. This reaction causes clumping of erythrocytes in the blood. Clumping (agglutina-

tion) or lysis are the causes of harmful transfusion reactions, which can only be prevented by complete and careful ABO matching between donor and recipient.

THE HUMORAL IMMUNE RESPONSE

B Lymphocytes

In birds, an organ called the bursa of Fabricius is responsible for the maturation of B lymphocytes (Glick, Chang, & Japp, 1956). Humans have no discrete bursa but do have tissues (probably the bone marrow) that make up the so-called **human bursal equivalent** (see Fig. 6-4). Lymphocytes destined to become B cells circulate through the bursal equivalent, where they undergo hormonally directed proliferation that enables them to react with antigen and generate diverse antibodies (immunoglobulins) that protect the host against infection (see Fig. 6-5). B cell precursors cannot react with antigen, whereas postbursal B cells produce plasma membrane-bound antibodies of the IgM class, which can bind antigen.

It has been suggested that as many as 10^8 different antigenic determinants may be recognized by the immature B cells. Several theories have been generated to explain how such recognition occurs (Jerne, 1955; Bur-

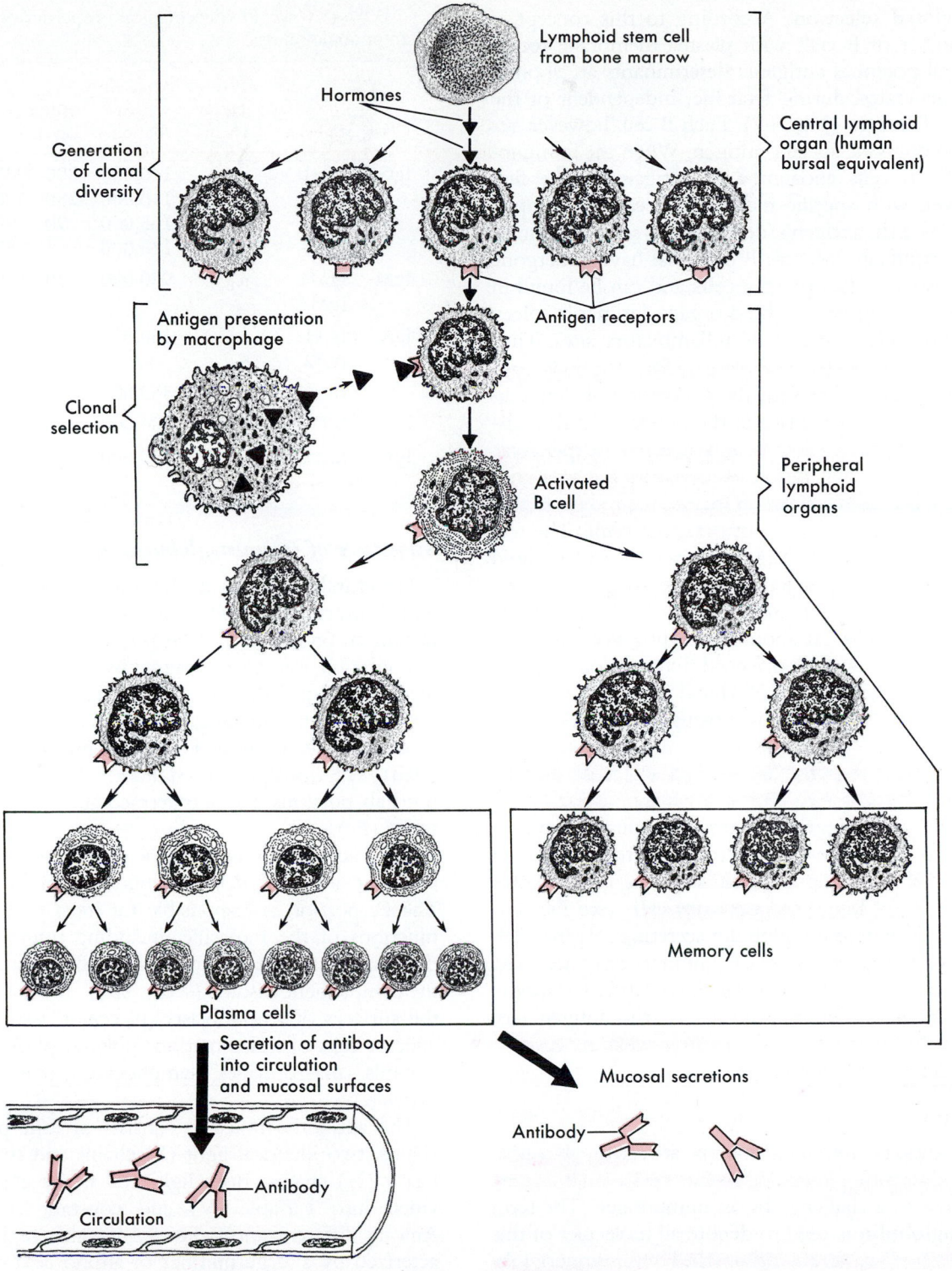

FIG. 6-7. Generation of clones of antigen-specific B lymphocytes (B cells). Under the control of hormones and without antigen, B lymphocyte precursors undergo cellular division in the central lymphoid organs (bursal-equivalent tissues, probably bone marrow) and generate receptors against all possible antigens that may be encountered in the host's adult life. Later, primarily in the peripheral lymphoid organs (spleen and lymph nodes), antigen presented by macrophages (phagocytic cells of inflammation) reacts with the clone of B cells having appropriate receptors on their surfaces, causing those cells to proliferate and produce antibody.

net, 1959). The one most commonly held as correct is that of **clonal selection.** According to this concept, a large number of B cells with plasma membrane receptors for all potential antigenic determinants are spontaneously generated during fetal life, independent of the presence of antigen (Fig. 6-7). Each B cell, however, responds to only one specific antigen. When the immunocompetent B cells encounter an antigen for the first time, those with specific membrane receptors complementary to that antigen's determinant sites are stimulated to proliferate. Mature B cells that have undergone this process are called **plasma cells** and can be found in the blood, secondary lymphoid organs (primarily spleen and lymph nodes), and some inflammatory sites. Thus two proliferative steps take place before antibody production can occur. The first, the generation of clonal diversity, probably takes place in the bursal-equivalent tissues, is hormonally driven and antigen-independent, and results in the generation of immature but immunocompetent B cells with plasma membrane receptors that can recognize virtually any antigenic molecule. The second, clonal selection, occurs in the peripheral lymphoid organs, is antigen-specific and antigen-driven, and results in the proliferation and maturation of antibody-secreting plasma cells. At about the eighth week of gestation in humans, antigen-driven differentiation may begin, although generation of clonal diversity probably continues in the bone marrow throughout most of adult life.

The immune response is initiated when an antigen binds and interacts with receptors on the surface of the immature B cell, triggering it into a sequence of proliferation and differentiation that results in the production of (1) mature immunoglobulin-secreting plasma cells and (2) a set of long-lived **memory cells** (see Fig. 6-5 and 6-7). The immunoglobulin-secreting plasma cells are active during the primary immune response. The memory cells are responsible for the secondary response that occurs upon future exposure to the antigen (see Fig. 6-2). In other words, the memory cells are responsible for long-term immunity.

Immunoglobulins

Antibodies, or immunoglobulins, are serum glycoproteins produced by plasma cells (mature B lymphocytes) in response to a challenge by an immunogen. The term **immunoglobulin** is used to denote all molecules of this type. **Antibodies,** on the other hand, are immunoglobulins known to have specificity for a particular antigen. The five molecular classes of immunoglobulins are IgG, IgA, IgM, IgE, and IgD. These classes are characterized by antigenic, structural, and functional differences (Table 6-2). Within the classes are several distinct subclasses, including four subclasses of IgG and two subclasses each of IgA and IgM.

TABLE 6-2 Physicochemical properties of the immunoglobulins

Class	Subclass	Heavy chain	Molecular weight (daltons)	Adult serum levels (mg/dl)
IgG	IgG1	γ_1	146,000	800–900
	IgG2	γ_2	146,000	280–300
	IgG3	γ_3	165,000	90–100
	IgG4	γ_4	146,000	50
IgM	IgM1	μ_1	970,000	120–150
	IgM2	μ_2		
IgA	IgA1	α_1	160,000	280–300
	IgA2	α_2		50
	sIgA	α_1, α_2	385,000	5
IgD	IgD	δ	184,000	3
IgE	IgE	ϵ	190,000	0.03

Structure of Immunoglobulin Molecules

Structural analysis of the immunoglobulins began with Porter's early studies on the effects of the enzyme papain on IgG (Porter, 1959). Limited papain digestion cleaved IgG into three fragments, two of which were identical (Fig. 6-8). The two identical fragments were found to retain the antigen-binding activity of the molecule and were termed **antigen-binding fragments (Fab).** The third piece crystallized when separated from the Fab portions and was termed the **crystalline fragment (Fc).**

The Fab portions contain the recognition sites (receptors) for antigenic determinants and confer specificity. The Fc portion is responsible for most of the biologic functions of the molecule, including interactions with the nonspecific effector systems of inflammation, such as the complement cascade (see p. 222), and for binding to the surfaces of trophoblasts (placental tissues) and the effector cells of inflammation (polymorphonuclear neutrophils, macrophages, lymphocytes, mast cells, and platelets).

The antibody molecule consists of four polypeptide chains, two identical light (L) chains and two identical heavy (H) chains. Both light and heavy chains are divided into variable (V) and constant (C) regions. Among different antibodies the variable region is characterized by a large number of amino acid differences. The light chains of an antibody molecule are of either the kappa or lambda type and also consist of a variable (VL) and a constant (CL) region. Within the same molecule, the two heavy chains and two light chains are identical. Each class of antibody has a unique type of heavy chain: gamma (IgG), mu (IgM), alpha (IgA), epsilon (IgE), or delta (IgD) (Fig. 6-9). The light and

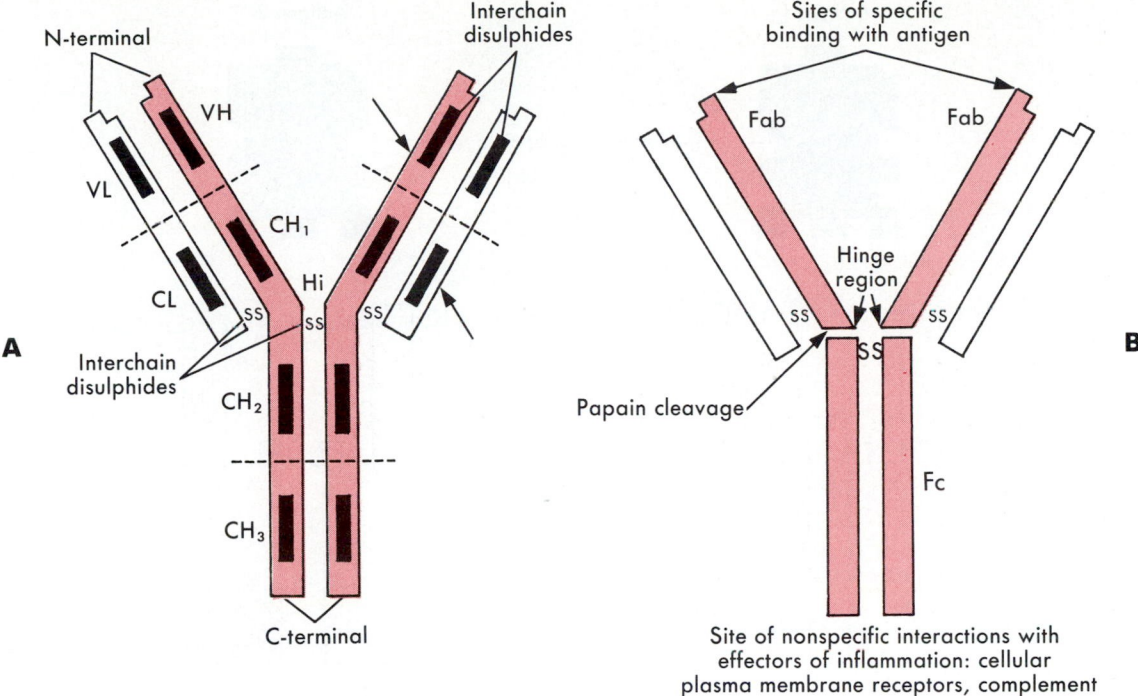

FIG. 6-8. A, Basic molecular structure of an antibody. The molecule consists of four chains, two light *(L)* and two heavy *(H),* held together by intra- and interchain disulfide linkages. The molecule can be divided into regions with variable *(V)* and relatively constant *(C)* amino acid structures (CH₁, CH₂, and CH₃ on the heavy chain). Between the CH₁ and CH₂ regions is the flexible hinge region (Hi). **B,** Experimental fragmentation of IgG into its functional components by limited papain digestion.

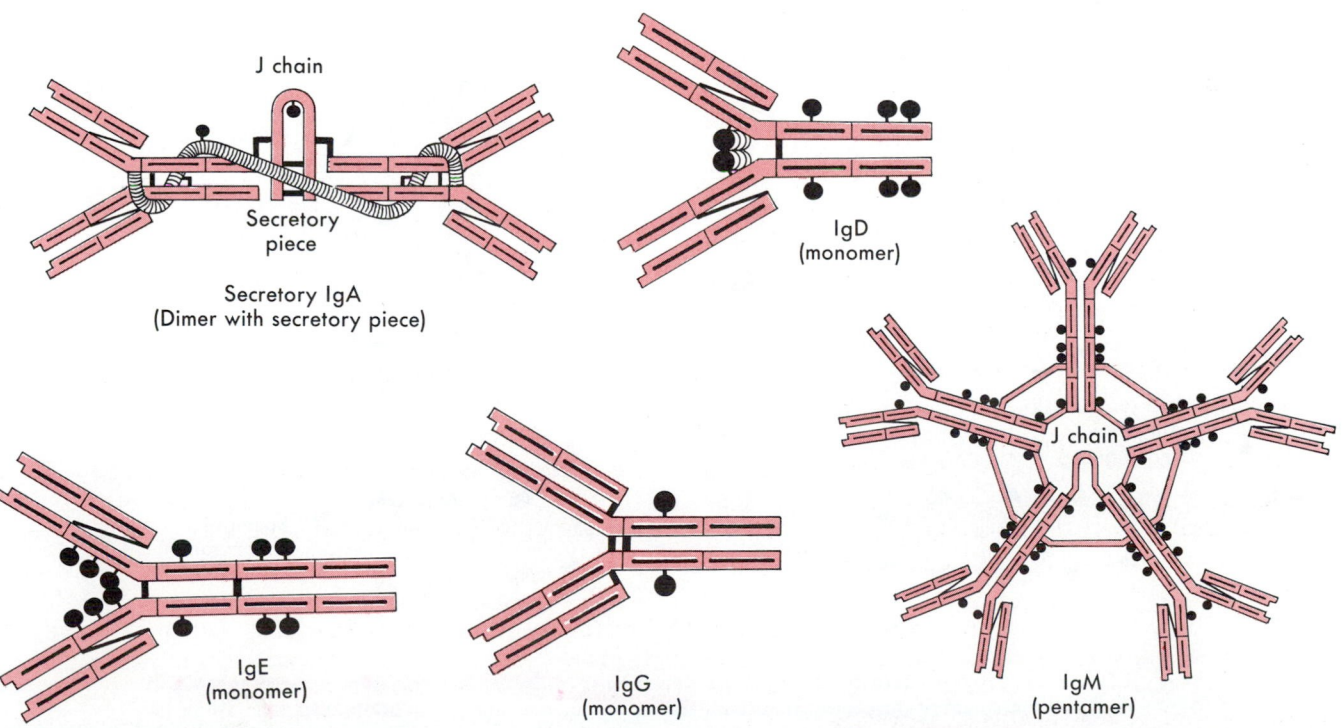

FIG. 6-9. Structure of immunoglobulins. Secretory IgA, IgD, IgE, IgG, and IgM.

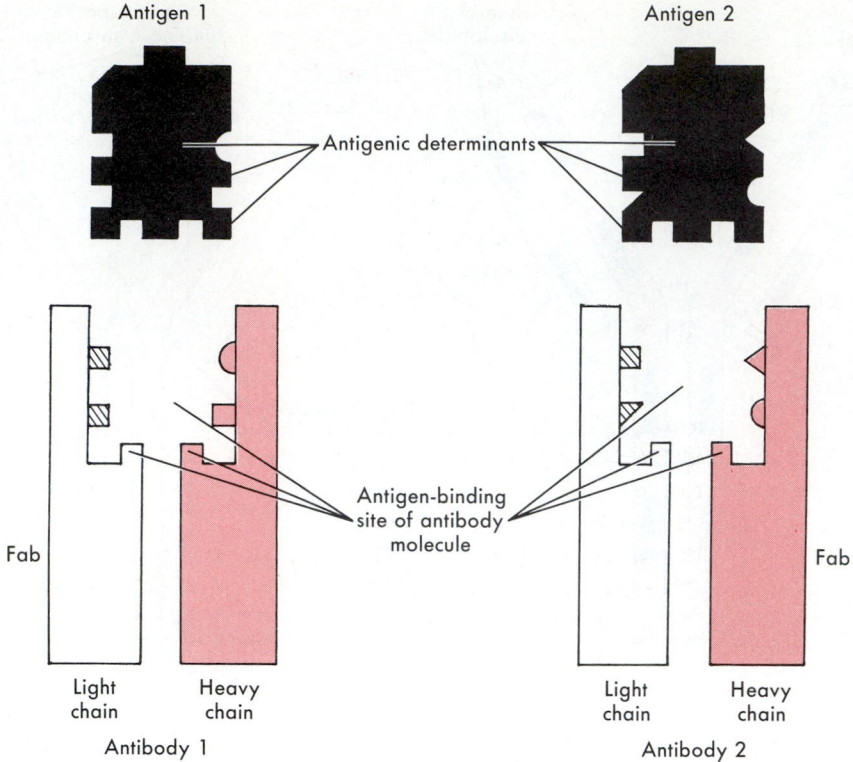

FIG. 6-10. The specificity required for antibody binding with an antigen is determined by the shape of the combining site on the antibody.

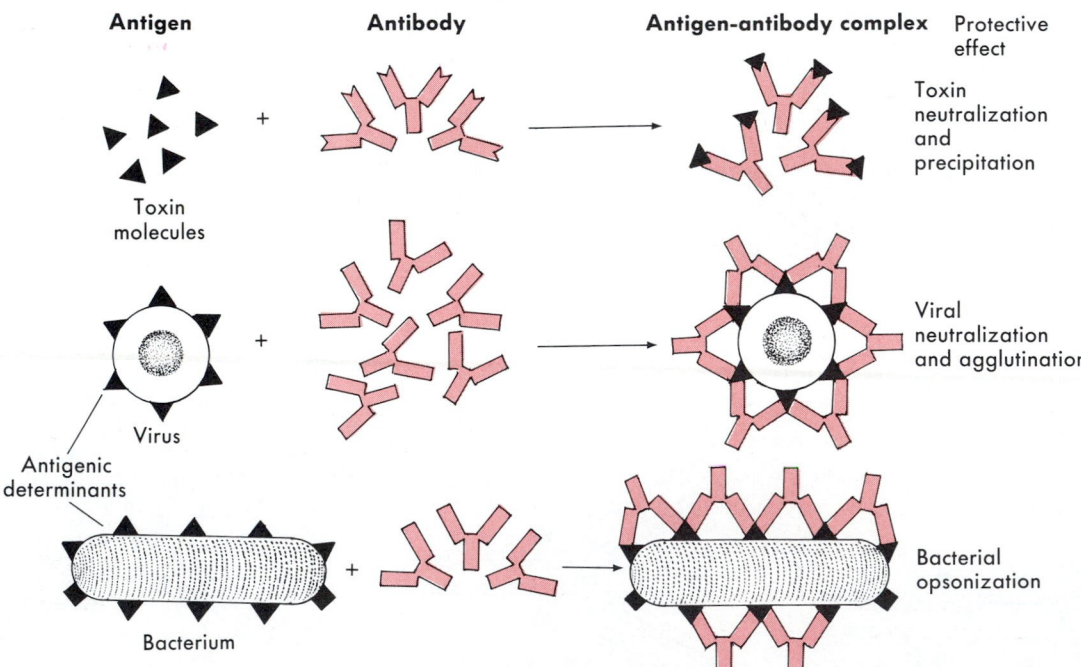

FIG. 6-11. Protective activities of antibodies: neutralization of bacterial exotoxins, neutralization of viruses and prevention of their interactions with cellular membranes, and opsonization of bacteria. All of these mechanisms are followed by removal of the antigen by phagocytosis, drainage along with body fluid, or both.

heavy chains are held together by two major forces: noncovalent bonds and disulfide linkages.

The interaction of the variable region's amino acid sequences on both the heavy and light chains determines the conformation of the antigen-combining site and therefore the antigenic specificity of the immunoglobulin molecule (Fig. 6-10). In some cases the substitution of a single critical amino acid may have a significant effect on the shape of the combining site and specificity of the antibody molecule. The antigen fits into this binding site like a key into a lock and is held there by noncovalent chemical interactions.

Function of Antibodies

The chief functions of antibodies are to protect the host by (1) neutralizing bacterial toxins, (2) neutralizing viruses, (3) opsonizing bacteria (i.e., promoting phagocytosis [see p. 229]), and (4) activating components of the inflammatory response (Fig. 6-11 and Table 6-3).

Normally an antibody circulates in the blood or is suspended in body secretions in an inactive form until it encounters and binds to its appropriate antigen. At that time the antibody may play two roles: (1) it may have a direct effect on the antigen and (2) it may have an indirect effect on other mechanisms of self-defense. Directly, the antibody may produce **agglutination** (cause to clump together), **precipitation** (cause to fall out of solution), or **neutralization** (inactivate) the antigen. Which of these occurs is determined by the class of antibody and the characteristics of the antigen. Protection always begins with antigen-antibody binding. The antibody molecule's Fab portions bind with antigenic determinant sites on the antigen. Binding results in **antigen-antibody complexes,** also called **immune complexes.** Antigen-antibody binding may directly affect the antigen by occupying its antigenic determinant sites, rendering them unable to bind with receptors on host cells. For example, viruses that are neutralized in this way are unable to infect cells because the first step in penetrating a host cell is binding with receptors on the cell's plasma membrane.

The indirect effects of antibodies also involve the binding of antigen into antigen-antibody complexes. Once bound, however, it is the Fc portion of the antibody molecule that confers indirect protection. Indirect protection consists of (1) enhancement of phagocytosis and (2) activation of plasma proteins that are capable of destroying the antigen. Both of these activities involve components of the inflammatory response: phagocytes (see p. 229) and proteins of the complement cascade (see p. 222).

Neutralization of Bacterial Toxins

Many bacteria produce toxins that enhance their pathogenic effects and harm the host in a variety of ways. (The injurious effects of bacterial toxins are described in Chapter 2.) Fortunately for the host, bacterial toxins are immunogens and are capable of initiating the humoral immune response. One of the principal roles of the antibodies subsequently produced is to function as antitoxins that neutralize bacterial toxins.

The mechanism of neutralization is the formation of

TABLE 6-3 Biologic properties of the immunoglobulins

Subclass	Complement activation		Binding to Fc receptors on				Placental transfer	Presence in secretions	Induction of agglutination
	Classical	Alternate	Macrophages	PMNs	Mast cells	Platelets			
IgG1	++	−	+	+	−	+	+++	±	+
IgG2	+	−	−	−	−	+	+	±	+
IgG3	+++	−	+	+	−	+	+++	±	+
IgG4	−	−	−	±	+	+	++	±	+
IgM1	++++	−	−	−	−	−	−	+	+++
IgM2	++++	−	−	−	−	−	−	+	+++
IgA1	−	+	−	±	−	−	−	+	−
IgA2	−	+	−	±	−	−	−	+	−
sIgA	−	−	−	−	−	−	−	++++	−
IgD	−	±	−	−	−	−	−	−	−
IgE	−	±	?	−	+++	−	−	+	−

NOTE: Minus sign, lack of activity; plus sign, relative degree of activity; PMN, polymorphonuclear neutrophil. (Complement activation and the function of monocytes, PMNs, mast cells, and platelets are described in the section on inflammation, beginning on p. 222.)

antigen-antibody complexes (in this case, toxin-antitoxin complexes), which is the result of antigen-antibody binding (see Figs. 6-10 and 6-11). Simply stated, the antibodies "capture" the toxin molecules by occupying their antigenic determinant sites. This prevents the toxins from binding to tissue cells and exerting their harmful effects. Once the antigen-antibody complexes are formed, they may precipitate out of solution in body fluids or be removed from the body by **phagocytosis** (ingestion by phagocytic cells; see p. 229 for a discussion of phagocytosis).

Detection of the presence of specific antitoxins can aid in the diagnosis of specific diseases. For example, laboratory tests that detect anti-streptolysin O or anti-DNAse B measure antibodies produced against those toxins and can be very useful in the diagnosis of group A streptococcal infections.

Actively induced immunity against many pathogens can be achieved by immunization (vaccination) with their toxins. To prevent harming the recipient, the toxins are chemically inactivated, resulting in a toxoid that has few toxic properties but retains immunogenicity. Vaccines against such diseases as diphtheria and tetanus are toxoids.

Neutralization of Viruses

Antibodies protect the host against some viral infections by preventing the attachment and entrance of viruses into host cells. The mechanism of viral neutralization is shown schematically in Fig. 6-11. Neutralized viral particles may agglutinate or be ingested and removed by phagocytes.

Many viruses (e.g., measles, herpes) are usually inaccessible to antibody because they do not circulate in the bloodstream. Instead they remain in extravascular tissue cells and tend to spread by direct cell-to-cell contact. Antibodies against these viruses are most effective in preventing the initial infection and usually play a minor role in recovery from a primary (initial) infection or in preventing recurrent infection. Other viruses, such as polio and influenza, spread from cell to cell through the blood and are more susceptible to the effects of circulating antibodies. These viruses can be controlled by antibodies even after the initial infection.

Protection against many viral infections, such as rubella, mumps, and chickenpox, can be elicited effectively by vaccination with inactivated viruses. Levels of circulating IgG are usually a good indication of the degree of protection. Because antibody protects against reinfection, some vaccines have been designed to induce antibody production at the site of viral entrance into the body. For example, both oral and injected polio vaccines prevent systemic infection in the recipient, but only the oral preparation readily protects against the carrier state by inducing a secretory IgA response at the usual site of viral entry, which is the gastrointestinal tract.

Opsonization of Bacteria

An **opsonin** is a substance that renders bacteria susceptible to phagocytosis. Antibodies themselves are opsonins; antibodies also induce opsonization by complement component C3b (see p. 222). **Opsonization,** the process of opsonin attachment to bacterial antigenic determinants, is necessary because many bacteria have an outer capsule that resists phagocytosis.

Activation of Inflammatory Processes

One function of an antibody is essentially translation: it acts as a bridge that lends specificity to the inflammatory response. One end of the immunoglobulin molecule, Fab, specifically binds to antigens, and the other end, Fc, informs the nonspecific amplifiers of the inflammatory response, both molecular and cellular, that an unwanted substance has invaded the body, either from the outside (e.g., infectious agents) or from within the body (e.g., a malignancy). Antigens are usually complex and bind several antibodies so that when an antigen reacts with the Fab regions of antibody, the Fc portions are held in close proximity to other Fc regions. The clustering of Fc regions results in (1) the binding to and activation of the complement cascade (see p. 222) and (2) the recognition of and binding to receptors (Fc receptors) on the surfaces of inflammatory cells.

Classes of Immunoglobulins

Fig. 6-9 illustrates the structure of the immunoglobulins. IgG constitutes 80% to 85% of the circulating immunoglobulins. The biologic activities attributed to the IgG subclasses are summarized in Table 6-3. IgG is the major class of immunoglobulin in the immune response and is responsible for most of the antibody functions, such as precipitation, agglutination, and complement activation. As a result of selective transport across the trophoblast, maternal IgG is also the major antibody found in fetal blood.

IgA has two subclasses, IgA1 and IgA2. The predominant antibody in normal body secretions is secretory IgA, which is predominantly IgA2. IgA in the blood is predominantly IgA1. The secretory piece is attached to IgA dimers in the mucosal cells and may protect the molecule against degradative enzymes in secretions. (The biologic role of IgA is discussed on p. 208.)

IgM is the largest immunoglobulin and has 10 theoretical antigenic binding sites, although only 5 are functional. It is the first antibody produced during the initial, or primary, response to antigen (see Fig. 6-2). IgM is synthesized early in neonatal life, and its synthesis may be increased as a response to infection in utero.

The trophoblast lacks Fc receptors for IgM; therefore, the molecule does not cross the placenta under normal conditions.

Information on the role of IgD is very limited. It is found in very low concentrations in the blood and is primarily located on the surfaces of developing B lymphocytes.

IgE is the least concentrated of any of the immunoglobulins in the circulation (see Table 6-3). It is also the principal antibody in the allergic response (see Chapter 8) and in the prevention of parasitic infections.

Monoclonal Antibodies

Most humoral immune responses are polyclonal: that is, a mixture of antibodies is produced from multiple clones of B lymphocytes (see Fig. 6-7). This occurs because most immunogens have multiple antigenic determinants and may stimulate a spectrum of B lymphocytes to proliferate. Each clone secretes antibody that differs slightly from that secreted by other clones, even though all the B cells were stimulated to proliferate by the same immunogen. The antibodies are heterogeneous in immunoglobulin class, amino acid sequence, specificity, and function, and some react more strongly with the antigen than others.

In 1975 César Milstein and Georges Kohler produced an antibody, called a **monoclonal antibody,** that would (1) act against a single specific antigen and (2) be produced by a single clone of B cells that could be maintained indefinitely in the laboratory. Monoclonal antibody was produced by hybridizing B cells from the spleens of mice that had been injected with a specific antigen and "immortal" plasma cells (B cells) from a plasma cell tumor (malignant myeloma). The result was a **hybridoma:** a B-cell clone that was both antigen-specific and capable of indefinite proliferation. The hybridoma produced monoclonal antibodies. The advantages of monoclonal antibodies over conventional antisera (antibody-containing sera from a donor) are that (1) a single antibody of known antigenic specificity is generated rather than a mixture of different antibodies; (2) monoclonal antibodies have a single, constant binding affinity; (3) monoclonal antibodies can be diluted to a constant titer (concentration in fluid) because the actual antibody concentration is known; and (4) the antibody can be purified to homogeneity.

The generation of monoclonal antibodies is creating new therapeutic and diagnostic possibilities, particularly in the treatment of cancer and early detection of viral infections. Detection of viral infections thus far has been limited to verification that a particular virus is the cause of disease because any antibody that is produced immediately reacts with circulating antigen and therefore cannot be detected by routine serologic tests. Monoclonal antisera, on the other hand, can be selected against specific antigenic determinants of the virus, produced in large quantities, and used in tests for elevations in circulating viral antigen that appears early in the disease. Over the next 10 years and as a result of hybridoma technology, the clinician will be able to order tests for viral antigens that are specific and diagnostic and detect the disease early in its course.

The Secretory Immune System

The immune system within the body is called the **systemic immune system.** A distinct set of lymphoid tissues make up another, and partially independent, immune system at the external surfaces of the body, the **secretory immune system.** Most humoral immune responses occur when antibodies or B cells encounter antigens in the blood, but sometimes this encounter occurs in other body fluids. Some antibodies are present in secretions such as tears, sweat, saliva, mucus, and breast milk, where they can protect the body (or the neonate) against antigens that have not yet penetrated the skin or mucous membranes.

Although antibodies in both blood and secretions are produced by B cells that have matured into plasma cells, antibodies in blood are produced by cells of the so-called systemic immune system, whereas antibodies in secretions are produced by cells of the **secretory (mucosal) immune system.** The B cells of these two systems follow a different pattern of migration once they leave the bone marrow and enter the lymphatics. Lymphocytes of the systemic immune system travel through the spleen and most lymph nodes (see Fig. 6-4). Lymphocytes of the secretory immune system travel through a different group of lymphoid tissues (Fig. 6-12); the lacrimal (tear-producing) and salivary glands, and lymphoid tissues in the breast, bronchi, intestines, and genitourinary tract. Immunoglobulins that are secreted at these sites are called secretory immunoglobulins (hence secretory IgA) and act locally rather than systemically.

Local protection is necessary to combat antigens (chiefly infectious microorganisms) that are inhaled, are swallowed, or otherwise come in contact with external body surfaces. Once they have taken up residence in the external layers of the body, harmful microorganisms can multiply, and the host becomes a carrier. These microorganisms may (1) cause local disease (e.g., cholera); (2) penetrate the skin or mucosa and cause systemic disease (e.g., gram-negative bacterial infection of the blood—septicemia—if the integrity of the gut is disturbed); (3) not cause disease in the carrier (because of effective systemic immunity) but be spread to other individuals; or (4) pass out of the body without any ill effects (e.g., in feces). The major function of the secretory immune system is to halt viral and bacterial invasion before local or systemic disease develops. When secretory

FIG. 6-12. Mucosal-associated lymphoid tissues of the secretory immune system. Lymphocytes from the mucosal-associated lymphoid tissues circulate throughout the body in a pattern separate from other lymphocytes. For example, lymphocytes from the gut-associated lymphoid tissue circulate through the regional lymph nodes, the thoracic duct, the blood, and return to other mucosal-associated lymphoid tissues rather than to lymphoid tissue of the systemic immune system.

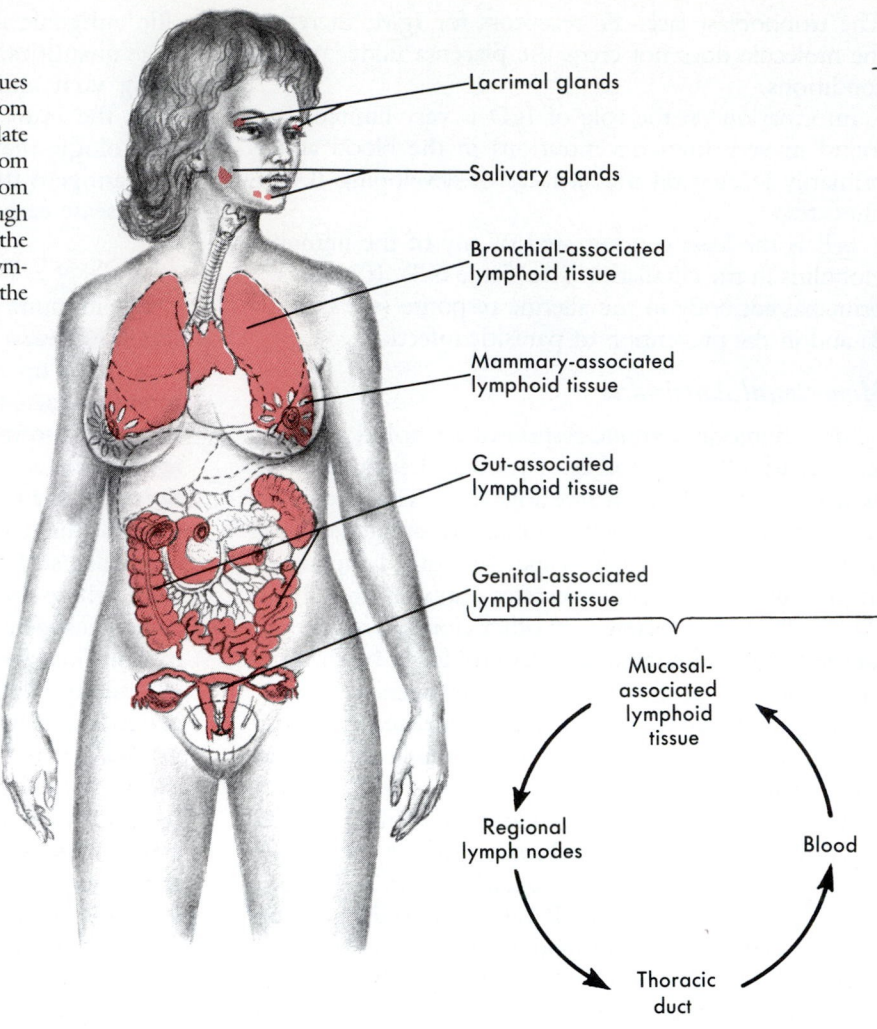

immunoglobulins bind and react with microorganisms, they are unable to attach to and invade mucosal tissue.

IgA is the dominant secretory immunoglobulin, although IgM and IgG are also present in secretions. The primary role of IgA is to prevent the attachment and invasion of pathogens through mucosal membranes, such as those of the gastrointestinal, pulmonary, and genitourinary tracts. In order to induce protective immunity against some pathogens that enter through these routes, providing local immunization seems to be preferable to inducing only systemic immunity. The Sabin vaccine against polio is administered orally as an attenuated live virus. This route causes a transient, limited infection and induces effective systemic immunity and secretory immunity, preventing both the disease and the establishment of a carrier state. The Salk vaccine, on the other hand, consists of killed viruses that are administered intradermally. It induces adequate systemic protection but does not generally prevent an intestinal carrier state.

The breast-associated lymphoid tissue is in the trafficking pattern of cells of the secretory immune system, so that most antigens to which the mother has been exposed gastrointestinally induce sensitized lymphocytes that migrate to the breast and secrete IgA, IgM, and IgG into the milk. Antibodies against infectious disease agents are found in the milk and may provide protection to the newborn against those pathogens, such as polio, that invade through the gut. Colostral antibodies do not cross the newborn's gut after the first 24 hours of life and do not have a role in the newborn's systemic immunity.

The mechanisms of antigen-antibody binding are the same in the secretory and systemic immune systems; that is, binding neutralizes or opsonizes the antigen, preventing it from harming the host. The major differences between the two systems are that

1. their lymphocytes follow different paths of migration and pass through different lymphoid tissues;
2. the secretory immune response is one of the body's first lines of defense, whereas the systemic response is the body's final defense; and
3. the secretory response occurs locally and externally

(in body secretions), whereas the systemic response occurs systemically and internally (in blood and tissues).

THE CELL-MEDIATED IMMUNE RESPONSE

Some lymphocytes are destined to develop into T lymphocytes (T cells), which are responsible for cell-mediated immunity. They are called *T cells* because they are processed through the thymus gland. There are five types of mature T cells, each with a different immune function. **Memory cells** induce the secondary immune response; **lymphokine-producing cells** transfer delayed hypersensitivity (Td) and secrete proteins (lymphokines) that activate other cells such as **macrophages** (see Chapter 8); **cytotoxic (Tc) cells** attack antigens directly and destroy cells that bear foreign antigens, and **helper (Th)** and **suppressor (Ts) cells** control both cell-mediated and humoral processes. (The maturation of T cells is shown in Fig. 6-5.)

The process of T cell proliferation and differentiation shown in Fig. 6-13 is similar to that shown in Fig. 6-7 for B cells. The chief difference is that the generation of clonal diversity takes place in the thymus for T cells and in the human bursal equivalent for B cells.

The role of the thymus in the maturation of the immune system did not become apparent until relatively recently (Miller, 1961; Mitchell & Miller, 1968). Lymphocytes destined to become T cells journey through the thymus, where, under the pressure and guidance of the thymic hormones and without the presence of antigen, they are driven to proliferate and simultaneously generate the capacity to recognize the diversity of antigens that the host will encounter throughout life. They exit the thymus as immature (i.e., inactive) but antigenically committed (immunocompetent) T cells. Immature T cells produce plasma membrane receptors that are not antibody but are related molecules with similar specificity for antigens. The **thymus,** which atrophies at puberty and practically disappears in adulthood, consists of a cortex and a medulla interspersed with connective tissue. Prethymic lymphocytes from the fetal liver, spleen, and bone marrow circulate through the bloodstream and seed the thymus during embryonic life. In the postcapillary venules of the thymic medulla, prethymic lymphocytes interact with thymic endothelial cells and enter the body of the thymus. Entrance into the thymus appears to be highly restricted to lymphocytes and also to be unidirectional. The lymphocytes distribute themselves in the thymic meshwork, where they rapidly proliferate in the cortex of the organ and probably migrate inward to the medulla as they mature into T cells capable of recognizing many different antigens.

The thymic epithelium produces several hormones involved in the maturation of T cells. These include forms of thymosin, thymopoietin, ubiquitin, thymostimulin, and several other hormones. The biologic roles of many thymic hormones are known. Thymic peptide hormones are not only involved in T cell differentiation within the thymus itself but may also diffuse into the bloodstream and influence uncommitted lymphocytes in the bone marrow and peripheral lymphoid tissues to travel to the thymus. In other words, immature precursor lymphocytes may become irreversibly committed to thymic maturation even before entering the thymus.

Antigenically committed but immature T cells exit the thymus through the blood vessels and lymphatics. When immature T cells encounter an antigen they are capable of binding with, they are stimulated to proliferate. This step is different from the proliferation that occurred in the thymus in that (1) all the cells produced are capable of recognizing the same antigen; (2) proliferation is driven by antigen and not dependent on thymic hormones; and (3) subpopulations of the immature T cells produce mature T cells having different functions (cytotoxicity, memory, helper functions, or suppressor functions). Therefore, the end product of antigen-driven proliferation is a large number of T cells capable of acting against the same antigen in a variety of ways.

The major effects of the cell-mediated immune response are the following:

1. *Cytotoxicity*: Cytotoxic T cells mediate the direct, cellular killing of target cells, such as virally infected cells, tumors, or foreign grafts. This function requires cellular contact, binding, and release of toxic substances from the Tc cell.
2. *Delayed hypersensitivity*: The Td cells are involved in the inflammatory response and produce soluble mediators (lymphokines) that influence other cells, such as macrophages.
3. *Memory*: Memory cells are also responsible for the accelerated response to a second antigenic challenge (the secondary immune response).
4. *Control*: Helper T cells facilitate and suppressor T cells inhibit both humoral and cell-mediated immune responses.

CELLULAR INTERACTIONS IN THE IMMUNE RESPONSE

Very few antigens can act alone as immunogens. For example, very few can directly induce immature B lymphocytes to become antibody-producing plasma cells. Antigens that do have this capacity are likely to have repeating antigenic determinants (multiple identical antigenic determinant sites). Because these antigens can

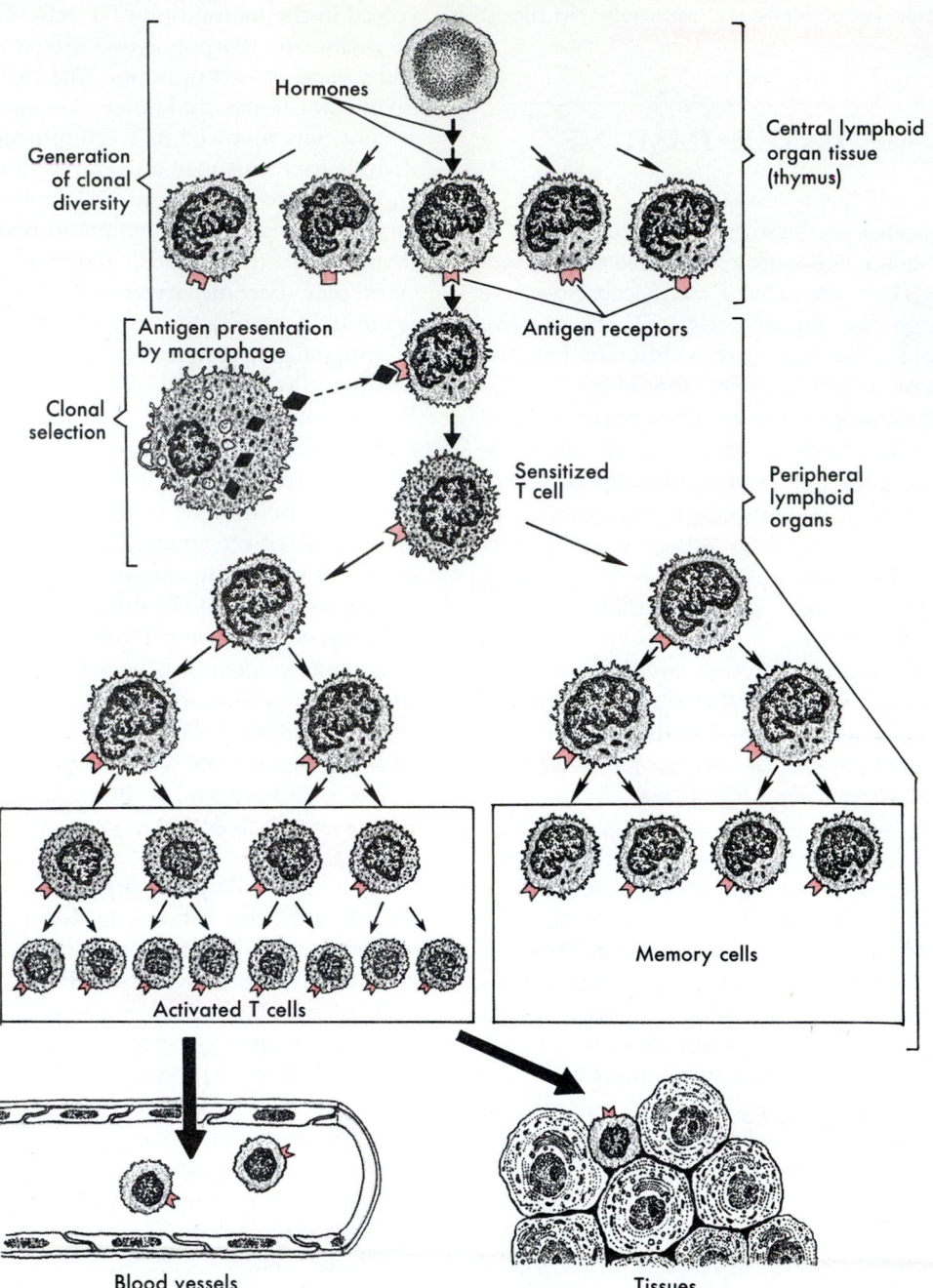

FIG. 6-13. Generation of clones of antigen-reactive T lymphocytes. Under the control of hormones and without antigen, T lymphocyte precursors undergo cellular division in the central lymphoid organ (the thymus) and generate receptors against all possible antigens that may be encountered in the host's adult life. Later, antigen encountered in the peripheral lymphoid organs react with the clones of cells expressing appropriate receptors on their surfaces, causing those cells to proliferate and produce functional T lymphocytes. (Adapted from Tortora, Funke, & Case, 1986.)

stimulate B cells without the help of T cells, they are called T-independent antigens (Fig. 6-14). The repeating antigenic determinants interact with the B cell's membrane receptors at multiple sites, inducing the cross-linking of receptors and the activation of antibody production. Antigens that cannot induce the immune

response independently must first interact with several populations of cells, including T-helper (Th) cells and antigen-presenting cells (usually macrophages; see Fig. 6-7 and 6-13).

When an antigen enters the host, it first equilibrates throughout body fluids. Antigen circulates through the

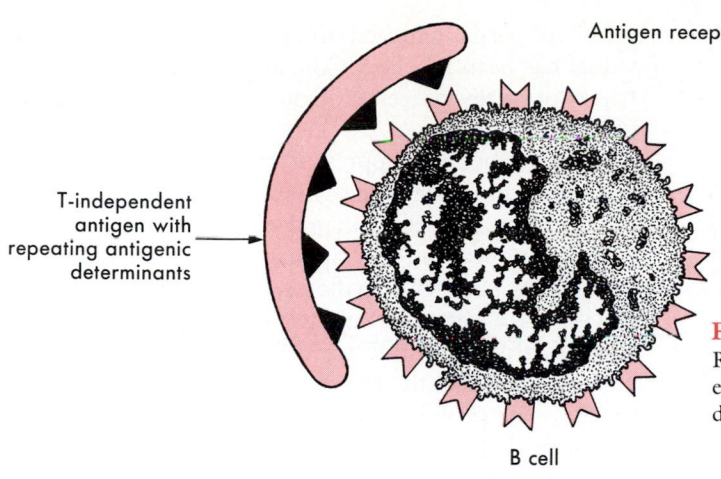

FIG. 6-14. Activation of a B cell by a T cell–independent antigen. Repeating and identical antigenic determinants that interact with several receptors on the surface of the B cell and mainly induce the production of IgM.

spleen if it enters intraperitoneally or intravenously and to the regional draining lymph nodes if it enters by the subcutaneous or gastrointestinal routes. Antigen entering by the bloodstream is usually filtered through the red pulp of the spleen, where it encounters splenic lymphocytes. Antigen entering through the interstitial spaces is usually drained by the afferent lymphatics to the regional lymph nodes, where it enters the sinusoids. These spaces in the lymph node architecture are lined with phagocytic cells that ingest antigen. (Lymph nodes and lymphatic vessels are described in Chapter 26.)

At this point a process known as **antigen processing** occurs (Fig. 6-15). After its ingestion by a macrophage in the lymph node, the antigen is degraded. A portion of the degraded antigen is reexposed, or expressed, on the plasma membrane of the phagocyte, which "presents" it to T or B cells (see Figs. 6-7 and 6-13). In order for Th cells to respond, the antigen must be presented in a complex with class II HLA antigens, those of the HLA-D/DR series. The macrophage also produces a hormone, **interleukin 1,** that helps the T cell to respond. Antigen processing and presentation are necessary for an immune response to occur. Antigen processing can also occur at many other sites including other lymphoid organs, the skin, and mucous membranes.

The development of cytotoxic T cells (Tc), which are responsible for the cell-mediated destruction of such targets as tumor cells or virally infected cells, requires the presentation of foreign antigen in association with class I antigens of the major histocompatibility complex, those of the HLA-A and HLA-B series.

B lymphocytes can also recognize antigen on the surface of antigen-presenting cells, although the particular antigenic determinant recognized may differ from that recognized by the Th cell. This recognition is apparent from studies using carriers and haptens. Haptens are not normally immunogenic. When haptens are covalently bound to high–molecular weight proteins (carriers) and injected into an animal, however, the B lymphocytes fre-

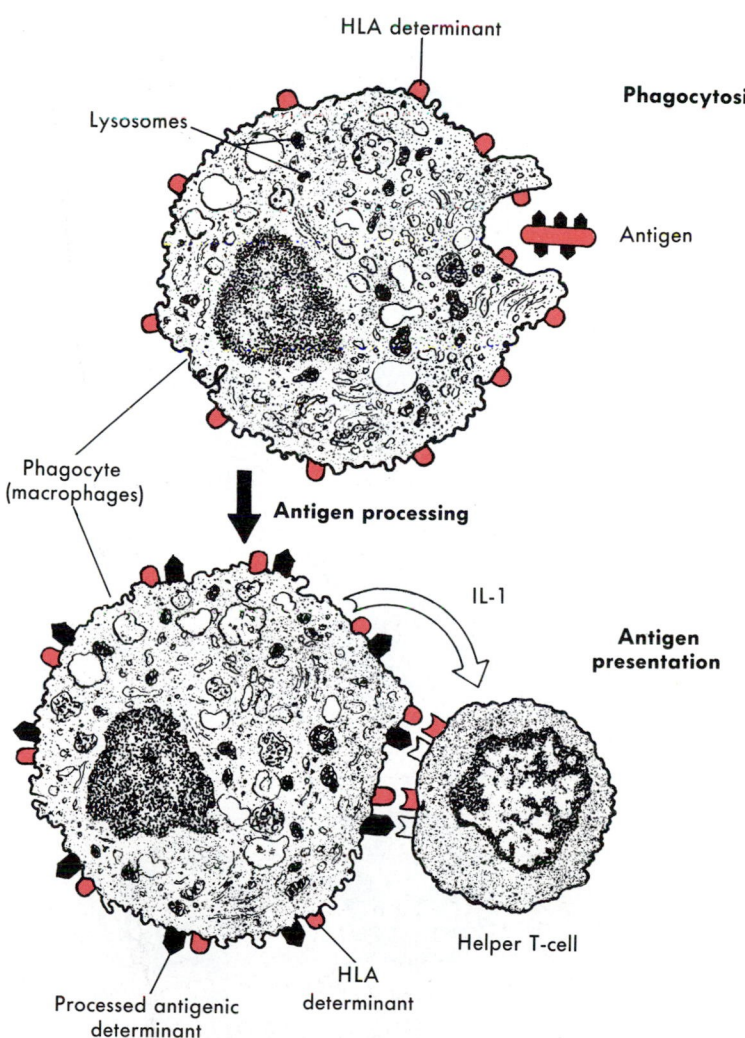

FIG. 6-15. Antigen processing and presentation. Circulating antigen is phagocytosed by macrophages. Remnants of the digested antigen are expressed on the membrane of the phagocyte and, in conjunction with HLA determinants, are presented to lymphocytes to initiate the immune response. The macrophage produces interleukin 1 (IL-1) that helps the T cell to respond to antigen.

quently recognize the hapten, and the Th cell recognizes the carrier portion. The result is the production of antibody against the hapten.

The antibody response of the B lymphocyte is under the control of hormones (interleukin 2 and other interleukins) secreted by the activated Th cell. Some of these hormones probably mimic the effects of antigens with repeating determinants by directly activating the B lymphocytes. Interleukins are not antigen-specific, so that the Th cell activated by one antigen (i.e., the carrier) can produce a factor that facilitates the production of antibody against another antigen (i.e., the hapten).

Like most systems of the body that are activated by outside influences, the immune system is conserved by being activated only during time of need and then completely or partially turned off after the threat to the individual has been repelled. Concurrently the immune system is normally prevented from recognizing and rejecting its own tissue.

Several types of suppressor cells, including Ts cells and some monocytes and macrophages, control both the humoral and cell-mediated activities of the immune system. Suppressor cells appear to vary in specificity, some being antigen-specific and others relatively nonspecific for a particular antigen or specific for only one class of antibody or effector cell (Fig. 6-16). Some suppressor cells affect the recognition of antigen and others suppress the proliferative steps that follow antigen recognition. Tolerance of self-antigens is apparently another suppressor cell function. Although the role of suppressor cells is currently under intense investigation, the degree of their heterogeneity of derivation, function, and specificity is far from determined.

FETAL AND NEONATAL IMMUNE FUNCTION

The normal human infant is immunologically immature at birth. Although cell-mediated immunologic capabilities begin developing early in gestation and are probably completely functional at birth, antibody production, phagocytic activity, and complement activity are clearly deficient. In the last trimester, the fetus appears capable of producing a primary immune response (almost entirely IgM) to antigenic challenge in utero and to infections such as cytomegalovirus, rubella virus, and *Toxoplasma gondii*. The fetus is unable to produce a significant IgG response, however. The capacity to produce IgA is underdeveloped, although some IgA can be detected.

To protect the child against infectious agents in utero and during the first few postnatal months, a system of active transport facilitates the passage of maternal antibodies into the fetal circulation (Fig. 6-17). In the placenta, maternal and fetal blood is separated by a layer of specialized cells termed trophoblasts. Immunoglobulins are too large to diffuse across the trophoblastic layer. The trophoblastic cells actively transport immunoglobulins from the maternal to the fetal circulation. Active transport of maternal IgG is mediated by surface receptors that are specific for the Fc portion of free IgG but not for IgM, IgE, or IgA. Active transport sometimes results in higher antibody titers in umbilical cord blood than in maternal blood. (Active transport mechanisms are discussed in Chapter 1.)

At birth total IgG levels in the umbilical cord are near adult levels. When the source of maternal antibodies is severed at birth, antibody titers in the newborn begin to drop as maternal antibody is catabolized (Fig. 6-18).

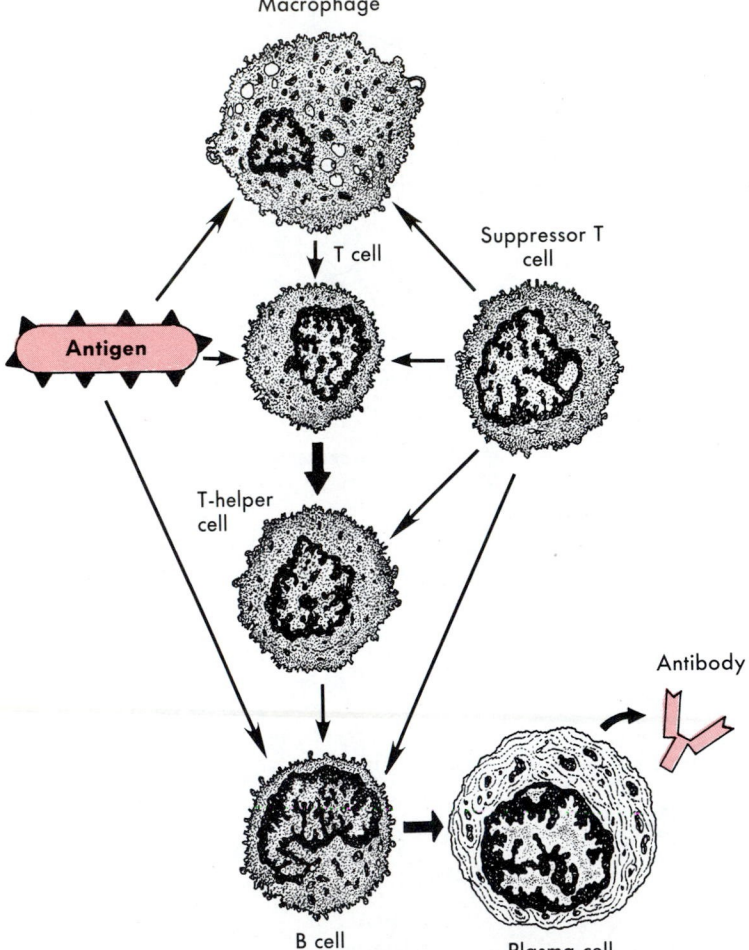

FIG. 6-16. Possible sites of suppressor T lymphocyte *(Ts)* effects on the production of antibody. The effect of one cell on another *(thin arrows)* and the maturation of one cell type into another *(thick arrows)* are represented. The effect of Ts cells appears to be on the early induction or proliferation phases of the immune response. The principal target of soluble suppressor factors is probably the Th cell, although other interactions have not been ruled out.

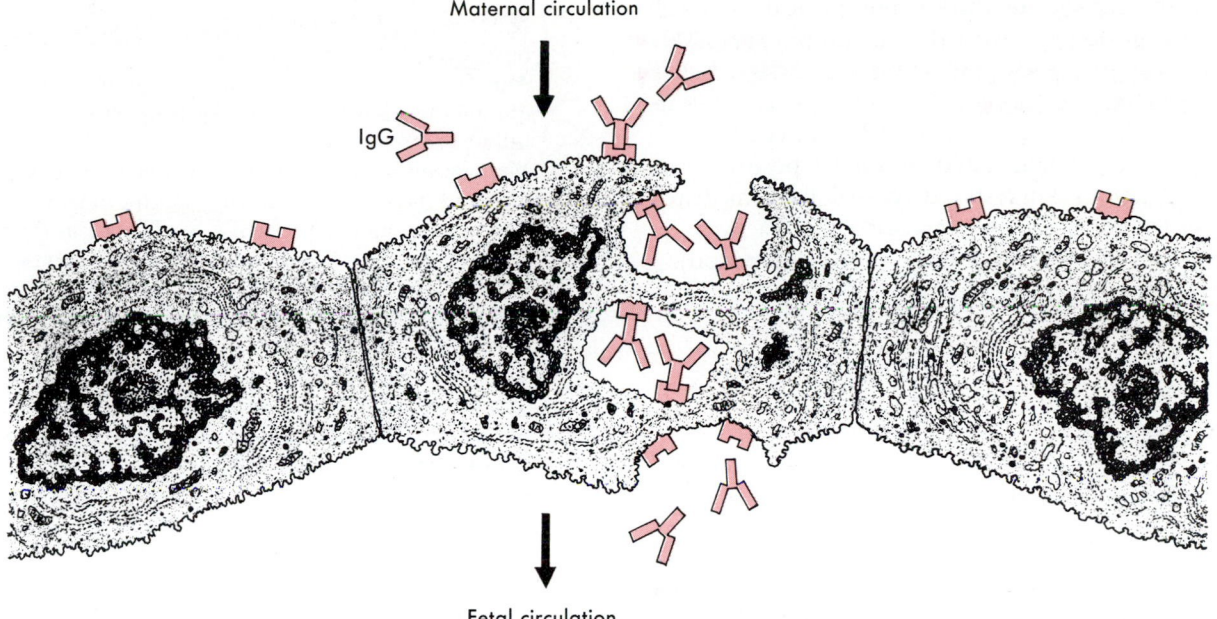

Maternal circulation

IgG

Fetal circulation

FIG. 6-17. Transport of IgG across the trophoblast. The transport of maternal IgG across the tropho-blast and into the fetal circulation is an active process. Maternal IgG binds to Fc receptors on the surface of the trophoblast and is enclosed in vacuoles by the process of endocytosis (see Chapter 1). Receptors on the trophoblast are specific for the Fc portion of IgG and do not bind other classes of immunoglobulins. The interaction of IgG with the receptors protects the antibody from digestion during transport of the vacuole across the cell. On the fetal side, IgG is released into the fetal circulation by exocytosis (see Chapter 1).

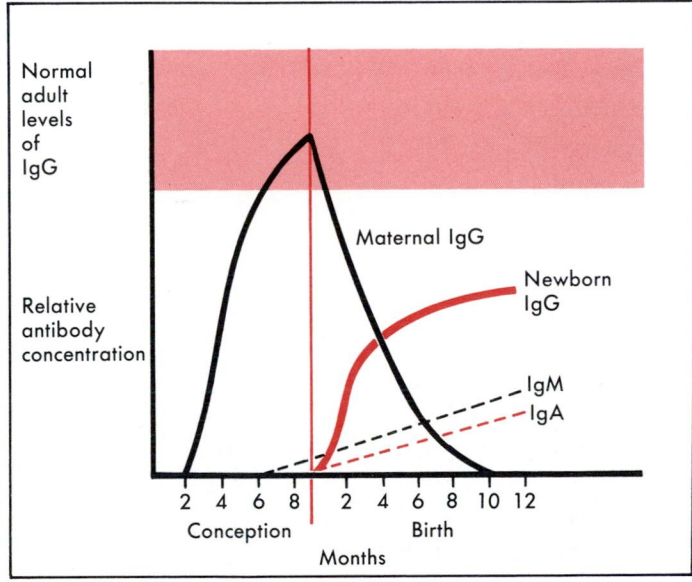

FIG. 6-18. Antibody levels in the umbilical cord blood and neonatal circulation. Early in gestation, maternal IgG crosses the placenta and enters the fetal circulation. At the time of birth, the fetal circulation contains nearly adult levels of IgG, which is almost exclusively maternal, and small amounts of fetal IgM and IgA. After the delivery of the child, maternal IgG is rapidly catabolized while neonatal IgG production increases.

Thus antibody titers drop rapidly even though the neonate's production of IgG is beginning to rise. This occurs because the rate of catabolism is more rapid than the rate of production. Total immunoglobulin levels reach a minimum at 5 to 6 months in the normal child, occasionally causing transient hypogammaglobulinemia (insufficient quantities of circulating immunoglobulins). Many normal infants experience recurrent respiratory tract infections at this time.

IMMUNE FUNCTION IN THE ELDERLY

Immune function decreases in old age. T cell function and specific antibody responses to antigenic challenge diminish, yet there is an increase in levels of circulating autoantibodies (antibodies against self-antigens) and immune complexes. In addition, there is an increased incidence of spontaneous monoclonal antibody production without concurrent B cell malignancy (myeloma).

The central lymphoid organ for T cell development, the thymus, reaches maximum size at sexual maturity and then begins involuting until it is a vestigial remnant by middle age. By age 45 to 50, thymic size is only 15% of its maximum. The level of thymic hormone production and the capacity of the thymus to mediate T cell differentiation decrease with thymic atrophy. Numbers of circulating T cells do not decrease with age, but T cell function may deteriorate. Individuals over 60 years of age generally exhibit decreased delayed hypersensitivity response (as demonstrated by milder positive reactions in tuberculin skin tests), decreased T cell-mediated responses to infections, and decreased T cell activity (as demonstrated by laboratory assays of T cell function).

SUMMARY REVIEW

Normal Immunity

1 Immunity is a state of protection, primarily against infectious agents, characterized by memory and specificity.

2 Antigens are chemical substances that react with preformed components of the immune response. Immunogens are antigens that can also induce an immune response. Haptens are antigens that cannot be immunogenic unless they are bound to larger molecules called carriers.

3 Self-antigens are antigens on host cells. Self-antigens are normally not recognized as immunogenic by the host's immune system, a condition known as tolerance.

4 The immune response is characterized by the activation of two types of immunocytes: B lymphocytes (B cells) and T lymphocytes (T cells). The activities of B cells compose the humoral immune response, those of T cells the cell-mediated immune response.

5 A B cell develops from a stem cell that matures under hormonal control in bursal-equivalent tissues and develops into a mature plasma cell capable of producing antibody against a specific antigen.

6 Antibodies are plasma glycoproteins that can be classified by chemical structure and biologic activity as IgG, IgM, IgA, IgE, or IgD.

7 Antibodies may protect the host from harmful antigens by recognizing and binding with the antigen's antigenic determinant sites. Occupied antigenic determinants on viruses and bacterial toxins are unable to bind with receptors on host cells and are, therefore, unable to have injurious effects.

8 The protective effects of antibodies vary with the identity of the antigen. Antibodies opsonize bacteria, neutralize toxins and viruses, and activate inflammatory processes.

9 Antibodies of the systemic immune system function internally, in the bloodstream and tissues. Antibodies of the secretory, or mucosal, immune system function externally, in the secretions of mucous membranes.

10 A T cell develops from a stem cell that matures under hormonal control in the thymus and develops into a cytotoxic T cell, which can kill target cells directly; a delayed hypersensitivity T cell, which produces lymphokines that affect other cells (especially macrophages); a helper T cell, which induces B cells to produce anti-

body; or a suppressor T cell, which suppresses antibody production and immune function.

11 Antibody production is the final stage of a process requiring the interaction of B cells, helper T cells, and antigen-presenting cells.

12 Mechanisms of self-defense are naturally somewhat deficient in the fetus, the neonate, and the elderly.

13 The primary immune response is adequate in the fetus and neonate, but the secondary immune response does not develop fully until about 6 months of age. Maternal antibodies protect the neonate for the first 6 months, after which they are catabolized.

14 T cell function and antibody production in response to specific antigenic challenge are somewhat deficient in the elderly. The elderly also tend to have increased levels of circulating autoantibodies (antibodies against self-antigens).

KEY TERMS

ABO blood group, 200

Acquired immunity, 194

Active acquired immunity, 194

Agglutination, 205

Antibody, 202

Antigen-binding fragment (Fab), 202

Antigen, 193

Antigen-antibody complexes, 205

Antigenic determinant, 197

Antigen processing, 211

Blood group antigen, 198

B lymphocyte (B cell), 195

Cell-mediated immunity, 196

Clonal selection, 202

Crystalline fragment (Fc), 202

Cytotoxic cell (Tc), 209

Epitope, 197

Hapten, 197

Helper T cell (Th), 209

Histocompatibility antigen (HLA antigen, HLA determinant), 198

HLA complex, 198

Human bursal equivalent, 200

Humoral immunity, 195

Hybridoma, 207

Immune complexes, 205

Immune response (immunity), 192

Immune response gene (Ir gene), 198

Immunity, 193

Immunocyte (immunocompetent cell), 193

Immunogen, 196

Immunoglobulin, 202

Inflammatory response (inflammation), 192

Interleukin 1, 211

Isohemagglutinin, 200

Lymphocyte, 195

Lymphokine-producing cells, 209

Macrophage, 209

Major histocompatiblity complex (MHC), 198

Memory cell, 202

Monoclonal antibody, 207

Neutralization, 205

Opsonin, 206

Opsonization, 206

Paratope, 197

Passive acquired immunity, 194

Plasma cell, 202

Precipitation, 205

Primary immune response, 194

Rh blood group, 198

Secondary immune response (anamnestic response), 194

Secretory (mucosal) immune system, 207

Self-antigen, 197

Suppressor T cell (Ts), 197

Systemic immune system, 207

Thymus, 209

T lymphocyte (T cell), 195

Tolerance, 197

Tolergenic antigen, 197

REFERENCES

Burnet, F. M. (1959). *The clonal selection theory of acquired immunity.* London: Cambridge University Press.

Ballanti, J. (1985). *Immunology III.* Philadelphia: W. B. Saunders.

Bordet, J. (1895). Les leucocytes et les proprietes actives du serum chez les vaccines. *Annals of the Institute of Pasteur, 9,* 462-509.

Dausset, J. (1981). The major histocompatibility complex in man. *Science, 213,* 1469.

Ehrlich, P. (1877). Beitage zur Kenntnis der Anilinfarbungen und Ihrer Verwendung in der Mikroskopischen technik. *Arch Mikr Anat, 13,* 263-277.

Glick, B., Chang, T. S., & Jaap, R. G. (1956). The bursa of fabricius and antibody production. *Poultry Science, 35,* 224-225.

Good, R. A., Dalmasso, A. O., Martinez, C., Archer, O. D., Pierce, J. C., & Papermaster, B. W. (1962). The role of the thymus in development of immunologic capacity in rabbits and mice. *Journal of Experimental Medicine, 116,* 773-796.

Hildemann, W. H., Clark, E. A., & Raison, R. L. (1981). *Comprehensive immunogenetics.* New York: Elsevier.

Jenner, E. (1798). *An inquiry into the causes and effects of the variolae vaccinae: A disease discovered in some of the western counties of England, particularly Gloucestershire, and known by the name of the cow pox.* London: Sampson Low.

Jerne, N. K. (1955). The natural-selection theory of antibody formation. *Proceedings of the National Academy of Sciences, 41,* 849.

King, D. W., Fenoglio, C. M., & Lefkowitch, J. H. (1983). *General pathology: Principles and dynamics.* Philadelphia: Lea & Febiger.

Klein, J. (1982). *Immunology: The science of self-nonself discrimination.* New York: Wiley-Interscience.

Koch, R. (1891). Fortsetzung der Mitteilungen über ein Heilmittel Gegen Tuberkulose. *Deutsche Medizinische Wochenschrift, 9,* 101-102.

Kohler, G., & Milstein, C. (1975). Continuous cultures of fused cells secreting antibody of predefined specificity. *Nature, 256,* 495.

Kraus, R. (1897). Uber spezifische Reaktionen in Keimfreien Flitraten aus Cholera, Typhus, and Pestbouillonculturen, erzeugt durch Homologes Serum. *Weiner Klinische Wochenschrift, 10,* 736-738.

Landsteiner, K. (1901). Uber Aggluanohn-Verschenungen Normaten Menschlichen Blutes. *Weiner Klinishe Wochenschrift, 14,* 1132-1134.

Metchnikoff, E. (1883). Untersuchungen uber die Intracellulare Verdauung bei Wirbellosen Tieren. *Arb Zool Inst Wein und zool station triest, 5,* 141-168.

Milanese, C., Richardson, N. E., & Reinherez, E. L. (1986). Identification of a T helper cell-derived lymphokine that activates resting T lymphocytes. *Science, 231,* 1118-1122.

Miller, J. F. A. P. (1961). Immunological function of the thymus. *Lancet, 2,* 748-749.

Mitchell, G. F., & Miller, J. F. A. P. (1968). Immunological activity of thymus and thoracic duct lymphocytes. *Proceedings of the National Academy of Sciences, 59,* 296.

Nossal, G. J. V. (1987). Current concepts—immunology: The basic components of the immune system. *New England Journal of Medicine, 316,* 1320-1325.

Pfeiffer, R. (1894). Weitere Untersuchungen uber das wesen der Choleraimmunitat und uber specifische Baktericide Prozesse. *Z Hyg Infekt Krankh, 18,* 1-16.

Porter, R. R. (1959). The hydrolysis of rabbit gammaglobulin and antibodies with crystalline papain. *Biochemistry Journal, 73,* 119.

Raven, P. H., & Johnson, G. B. (1986). *Biology.* St. Louis: C. V. Mosby.

Rosenbaum, J. T., & Engleman, E. G. (1982). Histocompatibility antigens and disease susceptibility. In J. J. Twomey (Ed.), *The pathophysiology of human immunologic disorders* (p. 51). Baltimore: Urban and Schwarzenberg.

Rote, N. S. (1982). Pathophysiology of Rh isoimmunization. *Clinical Obstetrics and Gynecology, 25,* 243-254.

Scott, J. R., & Rote, N. S. (1985). *Immunology in obstetrics and gynecology.* Norwalk, Conn.: Appleton-Century-Crofts.

Stiles, D. P., Stobo, J. D., Fudenberg, H. H., & Wells, J. V. (1982). *Basic and clinical immunology.* Los Altos, Calif.: Lange Medical.

Terasaki, P. I. & McClelland, J. D. (1964). Microdroplet assay of human serum cytotoxins. *Nature, 204,* 998.

Terasaki, P. I. (Ed.). (1980). *Histocompatibility testing.* Los Angeles: UCLA Tissue Typing Laboratory.

Tortora, G. J., Funke, B. R., & Case, C. L. (1986.) *Microbiology: An introduction* (p. 450.) (2nd ed.). Menlo Park, CA: Benjamin/Cummings.

von Behring, E., & Kitasato, S. (1890). Uber das Zustandekommen der Diphtherie-immunitat und der Tetanus-immunitat bei Thieren. *Deutsche Medizinishe Wochenschrift, 16,* 1113-1114.

von Gruber, M. & Durham, H. E. (1896). Eine neue Methode zur raschen Erkennung des Choleravibrio und des Typhusbacillus. *Muenchener Medizinische Wochenschrift, 43,* 285-286.

CHAPTER 7

Inflammation

Neal S. Rote

The acute inflammatory response, 218
The mast cell, 220
    Degranulation of vasoactive amines and chemotactic
        factors, 220
    Synthesis of leukotrienes and prostaglandins, 221
Plasma protein systems, 222
    The complement system, 222
      Classical pathway, 223
      Alternative pathway, 225
    The clotting system, 225
    The kinin system, 225
    Control and interaction of plasma protein systems, 225
Cellular components of inflammation, 229
    Function of phagocytes, 229
    Polymorphonuclear neutrophils, 231
    Monocytes and macrophages, 232
    Eosinophils, 233
Cellular products, 235
    Lymphokines, 235
    Interferon, 235
    Interleukins, 236
Systemic manifestations of acute inflammation, 236
Chronic inflammation, 238
Local manifestations of inflammation, 238
Resolution and repair, 239
    Reconstructive phase, 242
    Maturation phase, 243
    Dysfunctional wound healing, 244
      Dysfunction during the inflammatory response, 244
      Dysfunction during the reconstructive phase, 244
        Impaired collagen synthesis, 244
        Impaired epithelialization, 245
        Wound disruption, 245
        Impaired contraction, 245
Aging and mechanisms of self-defense, 246

Inflammation is a biochemical and cellular process that occurs in vascularized tissues. Most of the essential components of the inflammatory process are found in the circulation, and most of the early mediators (facilitators) of inflammation affect the vascular bed so as to increase the movement of plasma and blood cells from the circulation into the tissues surrounding the injury. These substances, known collectively as **exudate,** defend the host against infection and facilitate tissue repair and healing.

As described in antiquity, the superficial hallmarks of inflammation include redness *(rubor),* swelling *(tumor),* heat *(calor),* pain *(dolor),* and loss of function *(functio laesa).* The development of the microscope, however, enabled investigators to detect inflammatory changes at the cellular level. In the nineteenth century, Julius Cohnheim observed three characteristic changes in the microcirculation (arterioles, capillaries, and venules) near the site of an injury. He saw that (1) blood vessels were dilated, increasing blood flow to the area; (2) vascular permeability was increased, resulting in the outward leakage of plasma, which formed an inflammatory exudate; and (3) white blood cells adhered to the inner walls of vessels, then emigrated through vessel walls to the site of injury.

Inflammation and repair can be divided into several phases (Fig. 7-1). The characteristics of the early inflammatory response differ from those of the later response, and each phase involves different biochemical mediators and cells that function together to (1) destroy injurious agents and remove them from the inflammatory site; (2) wall off and confine these agents so as to limit their effects on the host; (3) stimulate and enhance the immune response; and (4) promote healing.

In contrast to the immune system, which is antigen-specific and has memory, the inflammatory response is nonspecific because it takes place in about the same way no matter what the stimulus and occurs in the same manner even on second exposure to the same stimulus. Unlike chronic inflammation, the acute response is self-limiting; that is, it continues only until the threat to the

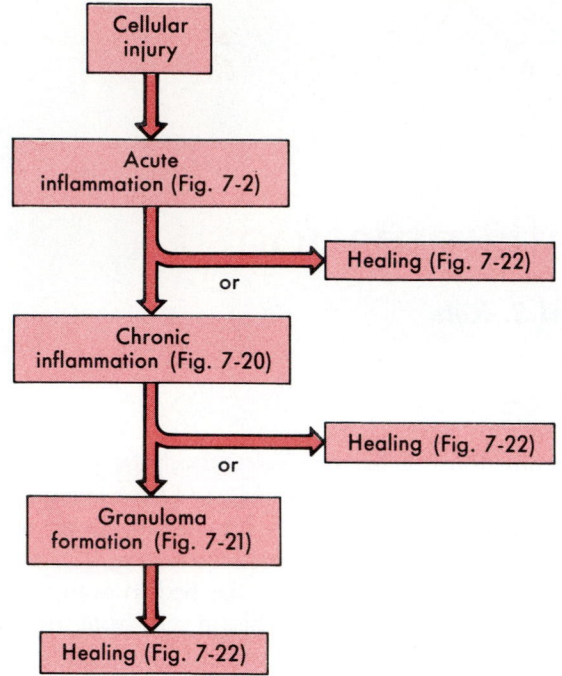

FIG. 7-1. The inflammatory process. Cellular injury leads to acute inflammation, which may result in resolution and healing of the injured site or progress into chronic inflammation. Chronic inflammation, in turn, may either result in healing or progress into the development of a granuloma. The final step of the process is usually healing and reconstruction of the damaged tissue. The figure numbers refer to those in which more detailed information may be found on that portion of the process.

host is eliminated. This usually takes 8 to 10 days, from onset to healing. Inflammation is considered chronic if it persists longer than 2 weeks.

THE ACUTE INFLAMMATORY RESPONSE

The acute inflammatory response begins after lethal or nonlethal cellular injury (Fig. 7-2). Cellular injury may be due to trauma (mechanical forces), oxygen or nutrient deprivation, genetic or immune defects, chemical agents, microorganisms, temperature extremes, or ionizing radiation. (Mechanisms of cellular injury are described in Chapter 2.) Inflammation is also triggered by the presence of dead cells, which may be host cells, microorganisms, or cells of dead parasites.

Unlike the immune response, which takes days to develop, the vascular effects of inflammation are immediate, occurring in seconds. First, arterioles near the site of injury constrict briefly. Vasoconstriction is followed by vasodilation, which increases blood flow to the inflamed site. Arteriolar dilation increases pressure in the microcirculation, which may increase the exudation of plasma and blood cells into the tissues. Exudation causes edema and swelling. As plasma moves outward, blood remaining in the microcirculation flows more slowly and becomes more viscous (thick and sticky). Leukocytes (white blood cells) migrate to vessel walls and adhere there. At the same time biochemical mediators stimulate the endothelial cells that line capillaries and venules to retract, creating spaces at junctions between the cells (Fig. 7-3). (Intercellular junctions are described in Chapter 1.) The leukocytes, which otherwise could not penetrate vessel walls, are able to squeeze out through the spaces created by endothelial retraction.

This state of vascular permeability continues throughout acute inflammation, permitting blood cells and plasma proteins to exude continuously into inflamed tissues. Once in the tissues, these cells and proteins act in concert to (1) stimulate and control subsequent inflammatory processes and (2) interact with components of the immune response.

Neutrophils are the first phagocytic leukocytes to arrive at the inflamed site. They phagocytose (ingest) bacteria, dead cells, and cellular debris, then die and are removed as pus through the epithelium or the lymphatic system. (The lymphatic system is described in Chapter 26.) The next phagocytes on the scene are monocytes and macrophages, which perform many of the same functions as neutrophils but for a longer time and later in the inflammatory response. Other cells that migrate to inflamed tissues are eosinophils, which help to control the inflammatory response and act directly against parasites; basophils, which have a function similar to that of mast cells (described on p. 220); and **platelets,** which are cytoplasmic fragments that stop bleeding if vascular injury has occurred (see Chapter 22).

The cells and platelets carry out their roles with the assistance of three major plasma protein systems (the complement, clotting, and kinin systems) and immunoglobulins. The complement system not only activates and assists inflammatory and immune processes but also plays a major role in the direct destruction of cells (especially bacteria). The clotting system traps bacteria in injured tissues and interacts with platelets to prevent hemorrhage. The kinin system helps to control vascular permeability. Immunoglobulin is the fourth type of plasma protein that participates in inflammatory processes.

All of these cells and protein systems, along with the substances they produce, go to work at the site of tissue injury to kill microorganisms and remove the debris of "battle," including exudate and dead cells. This prepares the lesion for tissue regeneration or repair, the process known as resolution.

Like inappropriate immune processes, inappropriate or exaggerated inflammatory processes have deleterious effects on the host. Even appropriate inflammation can

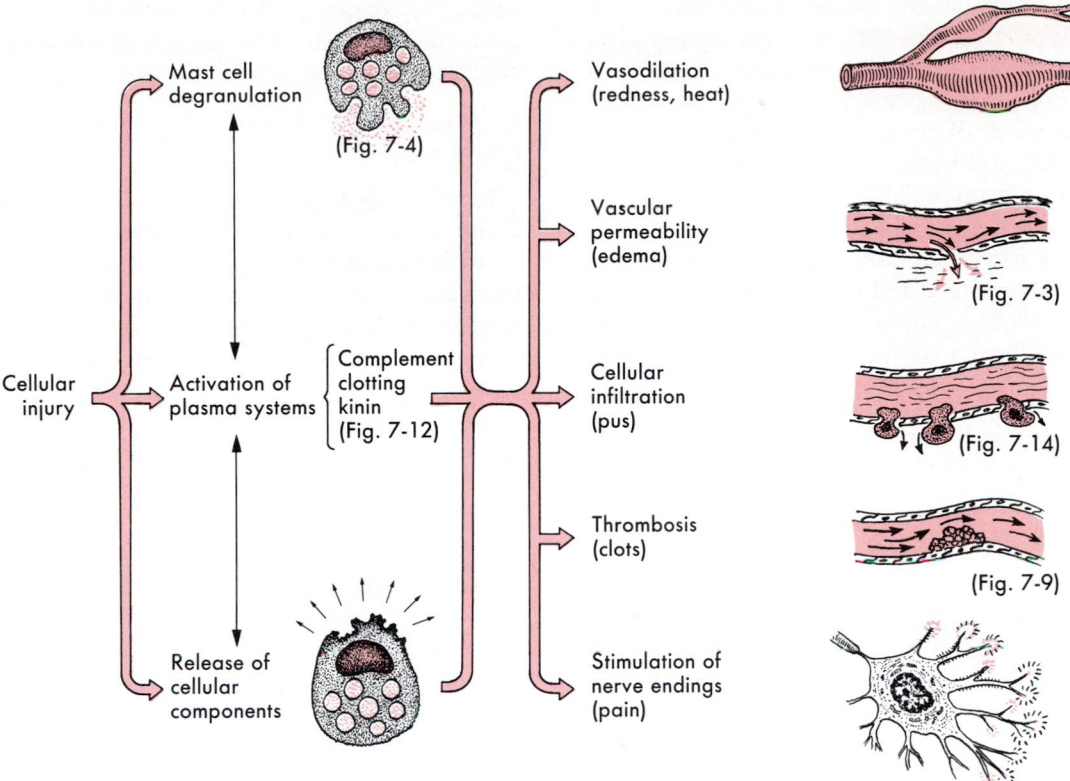

FIG. 7-2. The acute inflammatory response. Inflammation is usually initiated by cellular injury. Mast cell degranulation, the activation of three plasma systems, and the release of subcellular components from the damaged cells occur as a consequence of cellular injury. These systems are interdependent, so that induction of one (e.g., mast cell degranulation) can result in the induction of the other two. The end result is the development of microscopic changes in the inflamed site, as well as characteristic clinical manifestations. The figure numbers refer to those in which more detailed information may be found on that portion of the response.

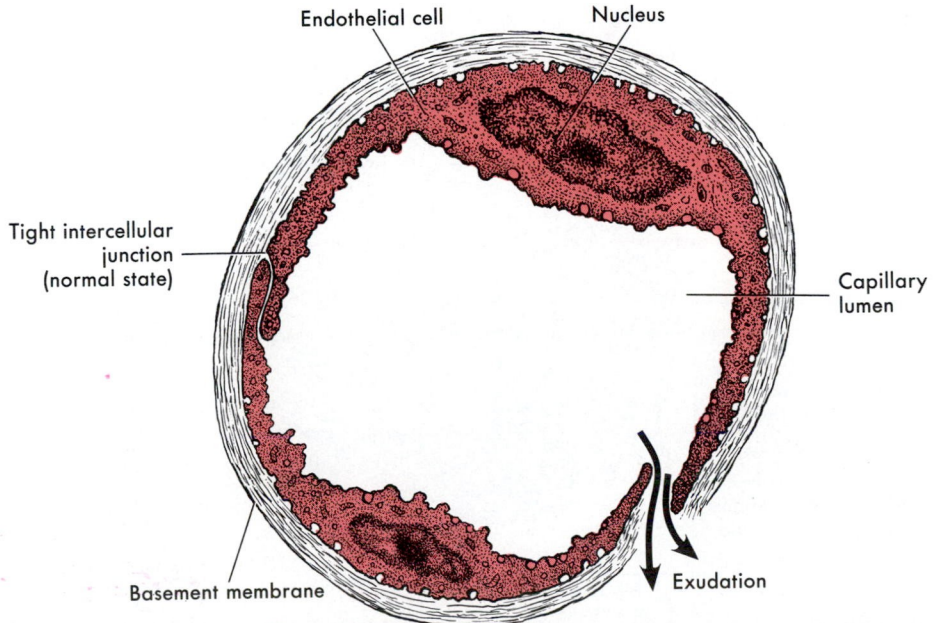

FIG. 7-3. Cross-section of a capillary showing mechanisms of increased vascular permeability. Biochemical mediators cause endothelial cells to retract, leading to opening of intercellular junctions and release (exudation) of plasma and blood cells from the vascular lumen.

be painful and harm healthy tissues. Furthermore, because it is complex, nonspecific, and can be triggered and maintained by a great variety of stimuli, inflammation is often difficult to control with drugs. (See Chapter 8 for a discussion of exaggerated, deficient, or inappropriate immune and inflammatory processes.)

The function of acute inflammation and the stages by which it proceeds are not difficult to understand. The difficulty occurs when one asks, How are the various stages initiated, regulated, and ended? The biochemical mediators and cellular components of the acute inflammatory response form a complex system of interactions that frequently begins with degranulation of mast cells and ends with healing.

THE MAST CELL

The mast cell is probably the most important activator of the inflammatory response (Fig. 7-4). **Mast cells,** first described by Paul Ehrlich in 1877, are cellular bags of granules located in the loose connective tissues close to blood vessels (Ehrlich, 1877). **Basophils** are found in the blood and probably function in the same way as tissue mast cells. Mast cells activate the inflammatory response in two ways. The first is **degranulation,** by

which they release preformed granular contents into the extracellular matrix. The second is synthesis of certain mediators in response to a stimulus.

Degranulation of Vasoactive Amines and Chemotactic Factors

Mast cell degranulation is stimulated by (1) physical injury, such as heat, mechanical trauma, ultraviolet light, or x-rays; (2) chemical agents, such as toxins, snake and bee venoms, tissue proteases (enzymes), dextran, or a cationic protein released from neutrophils; or (3) immunologic means, such as the triggering of IgE-mediated hypersensitivity reactions (see Chapter 8), or direct processes, such as activation of complement components (see p. 222). Preformed biochemical mediators found in the granules, including histamine, neutrophil chemotactic factor, and eosinophil chemotactic factor of anaphylaxis, are released in seconds and exert their effects immediately. Serotonin, another potent mediator, is released by platelets (see p. 229).

Histamine and serotonin are both vasoactive amines. They cause temporary, rapid constriction of the smooth muscle of large vessel walls; dilation of the postcapillary venules, resulting in increased blood flow into the microcirculation; and increased vascular permeability due to retraction of endothelial cells lining the capillaries (Fig. 7-3).

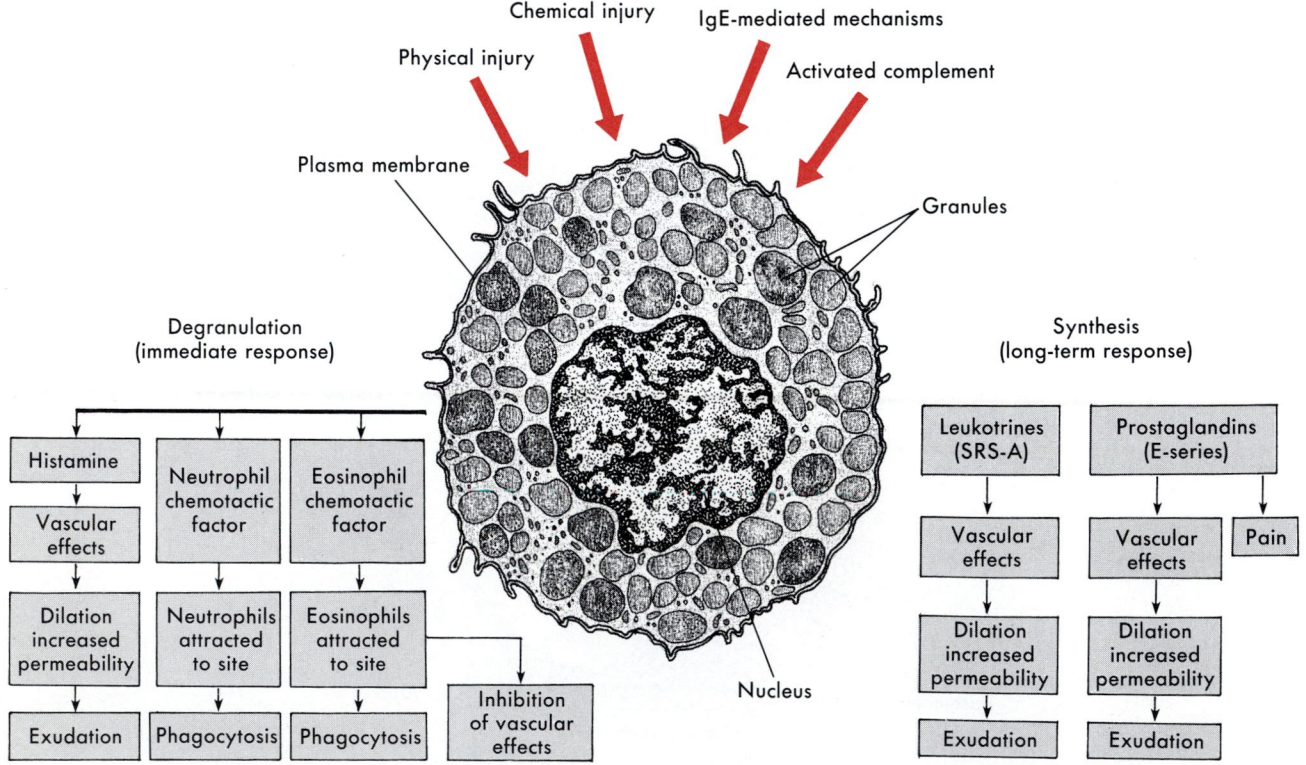

FIG. 7-4. Effects of degranulation *(left)* and synthesis *(right)* by mast cells. The electron micrograph of a tissue mast cell shows darkly stained granules in the cytoplasm (×9200).

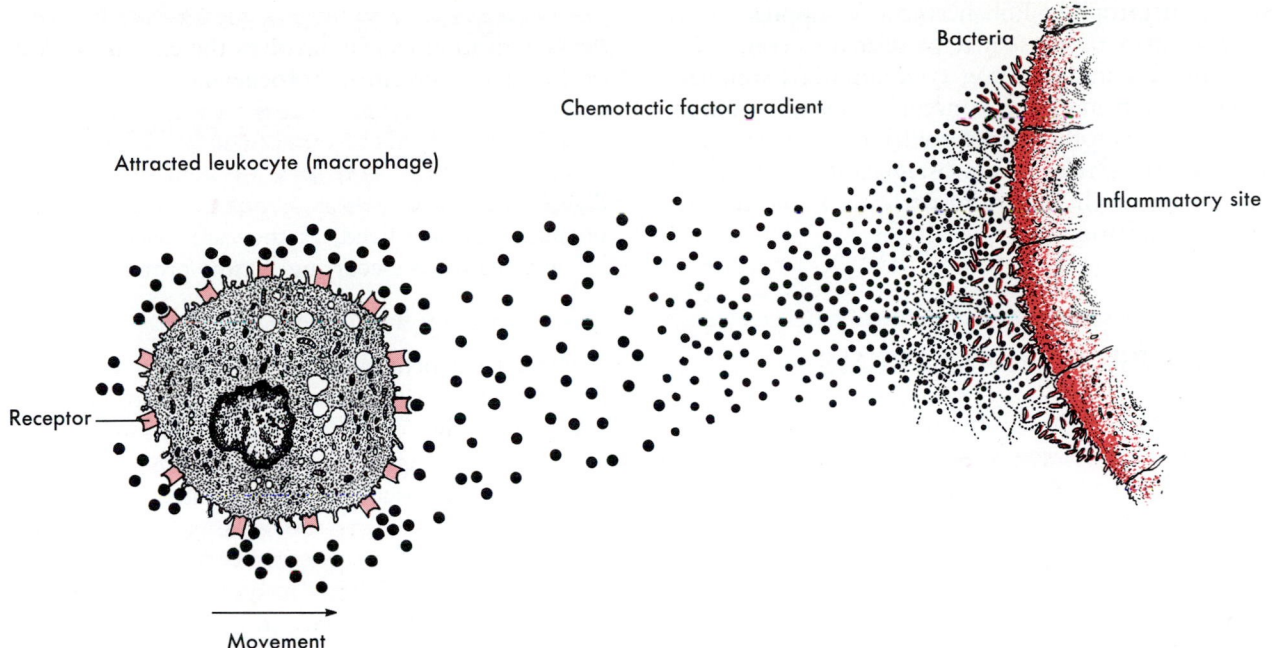

FIG. 7-5. Chemotaxis. Multiple receptors on the leukocyte's plasma membrane sense the area of highest concentration of a chemotactic factor *(dots)*, and the leukocyte (usually a phagocyte) moves toward this area.

Two chemotactic factors, neutrophil chemotactic factor and eosinophil chemotactic factor of anaphylaxis (ECF-A), are also released during mast cell degranulation. A **chemotactic factor** is a biochemical substance that attracts a specific type of leukocyte to the site of inflammation. **Chemotaxis** is directional movement of cells along a chemical gradient formed by a chemotactic factor (Fig. 7-5). Neutrophil chemotactic factor attracts neutrophils to the site of inflammation. Neutrophils are the predominant leukocytes at work during early phases of acute inflammation.

Eosinophil chemotactic factor attracts eosinophils to the inflamed site. Eosinophils are leukocytes that have several functions in the inflammatory response. They are phagocytic and are the body's primary defense against some parasites. Their most important role, however, is to control the mediators of acute inflammation released from mast cells. As with most defense systems of the body, the acute inflammatory response is usually only needed in a circumscribed area and for a limited time. Therefore, control mechanisms are necessary to prevent biochemical mediators from evoking more inflammation than is needed. Eosinophils contain several enzymes that degrade the vasoactive amines, thereby controlling the vascular effects of inflammation. These enzymes include histaminase, which mediates the degradation of histamine, and aryl sulfatase B, which mediates the degradation of leukotrienes.

Synthesis of Leukotrienes and Prostaglandins

Leukotrienes and prostaglandins are mediators synthesized by mast cells (Fig. 7-4). **Leukotrienes (slow-reacting substances of anaphylaxis [SRS-A])** are acidic, sulfur-containing lipids that produce effects similar to those of histamine, namely, smooth muscle contraction, increased vascular permeability, and perhaps neutrophil and eosinophil chemotaxis. Leukotrienes appear to be important in the later stages of the inflammatory response, as they stimulate slower and more prolonged responses than do histamines. Leukotrienes are produced from a lipid, arachidonic acid, that is released from mast cell membranes by an intracellular phospholipase that acts on membrane phospholipids.

The mast cell also synthesizes **prostaglandins,** which, like leukotrienes, cause increased vascular permeability and neutrophil chemotaxis. Prostaglandins also induce pain. Prostaglandins are long-chain, unsaturated fatty acids produced from arachidonic acid by the action of the enzyme cyclooxygenase. They are classified into groups (E, A, F, and B) according to their structure. Prostaglandins E_1 and E_2 probably cause increased vascular permeability and smooth muscle contraction; they appear to act directly on postcapillary venules. They can also inhibit some aspects of inflammation by such actions as suppressing both the release of histamine from mast cells and the release of lysosomal enzymes (enzymes responsible for killing and digesting microorganisms) from neutrophils. Enhancement or suppression of the inflammatory response may be related to concentrations of prostaglandins: lower concentrations stimulating inflammation and larger concentrations inhibiting it. Aspirin and some other nonsteroidal anti-inflammatory agents block the synthesis of prostaglandins of the E series and other arachidonic acid derivatives, thereby inhibiting inflammation.

PLASMA PROTEIN SYSTEMS

Inflammation is mediated by three key plasma protein systems: the complement system, the clotting system, and the kinin system. These systems have several characteristics in common. Each consists of a series of inactive enzymes, or **proenzymes.** When the first proenzyme in the series is converted to an active enzyme, it initiates a cascade in which the substrate of the activated enzyme is the next component of the system. Therefore, the entire

cascade is activated upon activation of the first component. Activation usually involves the enzymatic cleavage of the inactive precursor (proenzyme) into two or more components. The larger one is an active enzyme whose substrate is the next component in the system. The smaller component is usually a potent biochemical mediator of the inflammatory response. Most of these components are short-lived, as they are inactivated rapidly by other naturally occurring plasma proteins.

The Complement System

The complement system consists of at least 10 proteins and makes up 10% of the serum proteins in the circulation (Fig. 7-6). The complement system is perhaps the most important of the plasma protein systems of inflammation because, once activated, its components participate in virtually every inflammatory response. In addition the last few proteins in the complement cascade are capable of killing microorganisms directly.

The complement system can be activated by antigen-antibody complexes, as well as by products released

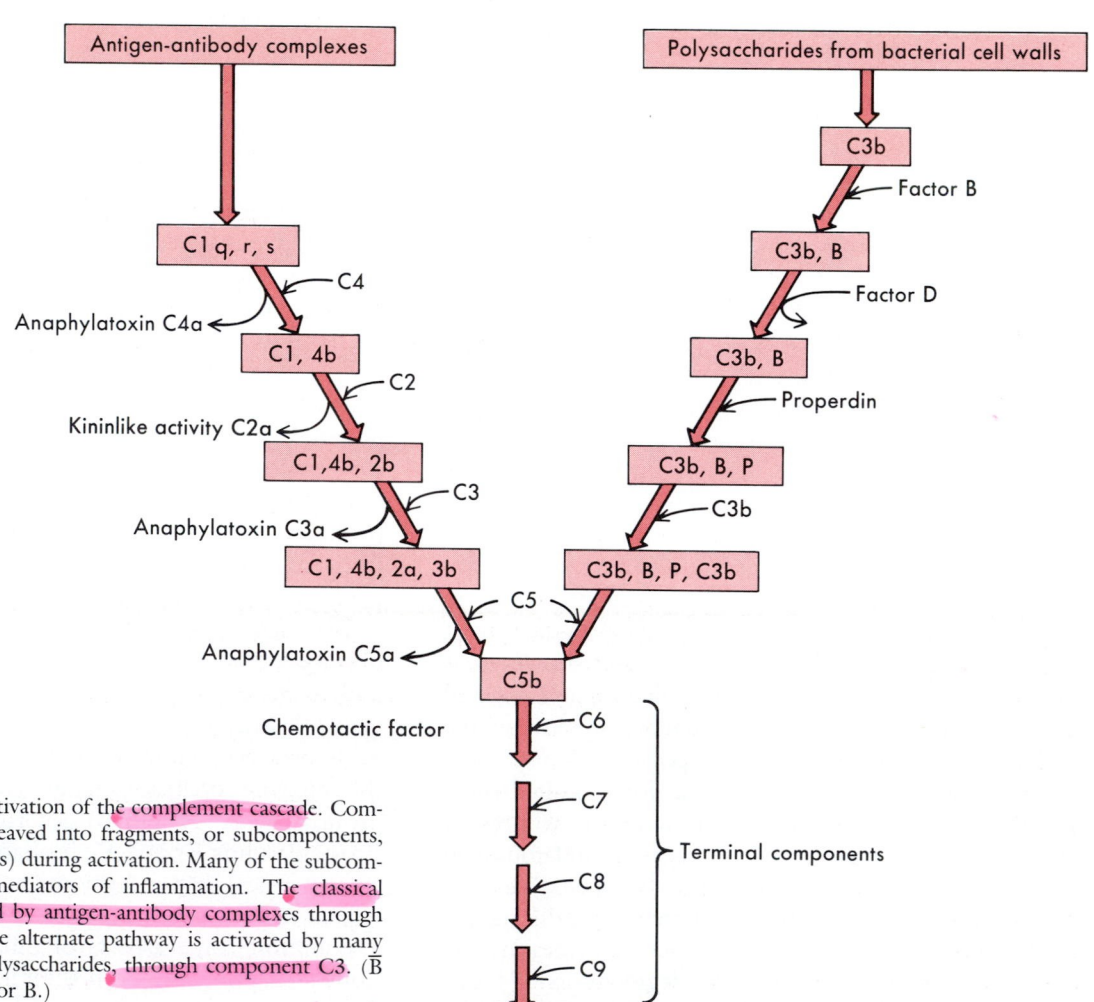

FIG. 7-6. Pathways of activation of the complement cascade. Complement components are cleaved into fragments, or subcomponents, (denoted by lowercase letters) during activation. Many of the subcomponents are biochemical mediators of inflammation. The classical pathway is usually activated by antigen-antibody complexes through component C1, whereas the alternate pathway is activated by many agents, such as bacterial polysaccharides, through component C3. ($\bar{\text{B}}$ is the activated form of factor B.)

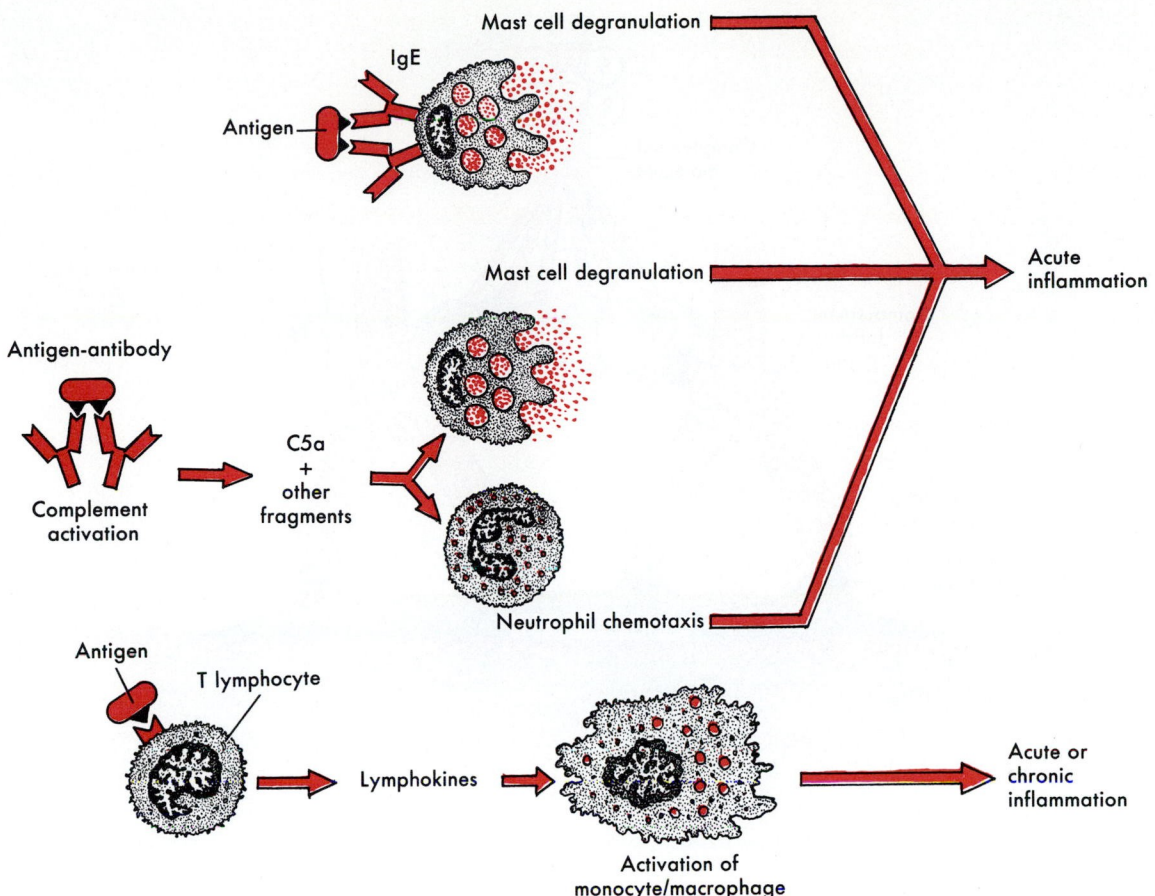

FIG. 7-7. Immunologic mechanisms that activate the inflammatory response. Immunologic factors may affect inflammation through three mechanisms: (1) IgE can bind to the surface of a mast cell and, after binding antigen, induce the cell's degranulation; (2) antigen and antibody can form immune complexes that activate the complement cascade releasing small polypeptide fragments, primarily C5a, that have potent biological activities resulting in mast cell degranulation and neutrophil chemotaxis; and (3) antigen may also react with T lymphocytes resulting in the production of lymphokines that may contribute to the development of either acute or chronic inflammation.

from invading bacteria and by components of the other plasma protein systems (Fig. 7-7). The complement system is a nonspecific mechanism of self-defense. Even when it is activated by a specific mechanism, namely antigen-antibody complexes (the immune system), it mediates inflammation, which is nonspecific. Thus proteins of the complement system (sometimes called complement components) are among the body's most potent defenders against bacterial infection.

The two routes by which the **complement cascade** is activated are shown in Fig. 7-6. The **classical pathway** is activated when an antigen-antibody complex containing IgG or IgM interacts with the first component of the complement cascade, C1. The **alternate pathway** can be activated by several biologic substances, chiefly bacterial and fungal cell wall polysaccharides (especially endotoxin on gram-negative bacteria). (Bacterial endotoxins are described in Chapter 2.)

Activation of components C1 through C5 produces subunits that enhance inflammation by (1) opsonizing bacteria, (2) attracting leukocytes by chemotaxis, and (3) acting as **anaphylatoxins,** that is, inducing degranulation of mast cells. Components C6 through C9 form complexes capable of creating pores in bacterial cell walls. The pores disrupt the bacterium's rigid outer membrane, permitting the influx of water and ions. This causes the bacterium to burst or at least prevents its reproduction. (Cellular injury is discussed in Chapter 2.)

Classical Pathway

Activation of the classical pathway is preceded by formation of an **antigen-antibody complex.** Because antigens tend to be multivalent (to have more than one antigenic determinant), multiple antibodies are bound in the complex. Complement activation occurs as a result of antibody Fc regions being held in close proximity.

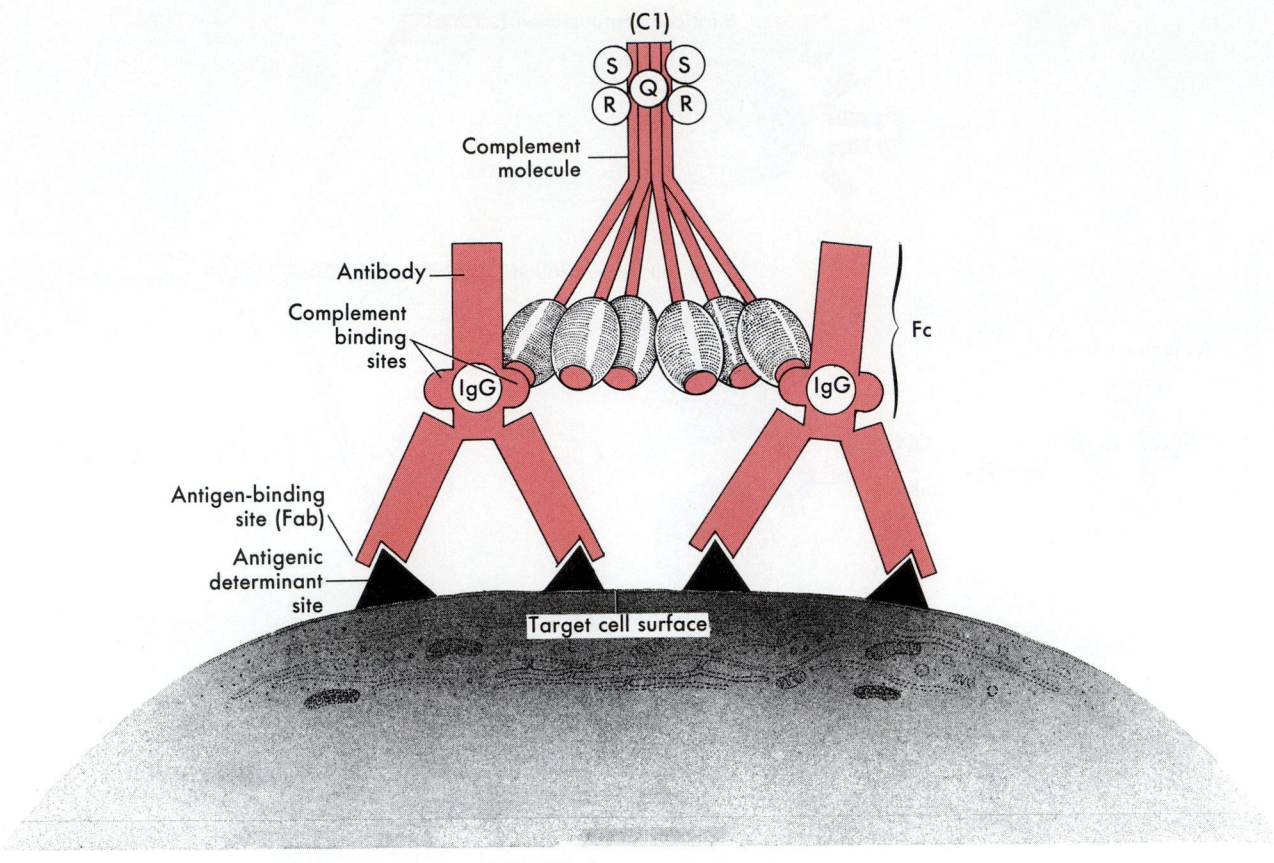

FIG. 7-8. Activation of the first component of complement (Cl). It takes two IgG molecules to activate one complement component. Activation of complement cannot occur unless (1) antigen-antibody binding has occurred, placing two Fc regions of the antibody molecule into close proximity, and (2) the complement component can span the gap between two adjacent Fc portions.

The Fc contains a site that binds Cl. The first component of the classical complement cascade, Cl, has six sites that can bind to the Fc region and is "fixed" to adjacent antibody molecules that are attached to the antigen. The complex formed by antigen-antibody-complement binding is shown in Fig. 7-8.

Activation of Cl results in the sequential enzymatic activation of all other components of the cascade. Although the cascade continues through the terminal components C6, C7, C8, and C9, whose activation results in the lysis of bacteria, the importance of the complement system resides in the activities of the small fragments, or subcomponents, generated during the activation of C4, C2, C3, and C5. C3b, a subcomponent that adheres to the surface of a target cell (e.g., bacterium) is an efficient opsonin. C4a, C2a, C3a, and C5a, which are soluble, low–molecular weight fragments, are potent activators of the acute inflammatory response. C2a affects smooth muscle, causing vasodilation and increased vascular permeability. C3a, C5a, and to a limited extent C4a, are anaphylatoxins; that is, they induce the rapid

degranulation of mast cells, with release of histamine (Fig. 7-4).

The anaphylatoxins C3a and C5a, small polypeptides, are also chemotactic for neutrophils, although C5a is approximately 1000 times more anaphylatoxic and chemotactic than C3a. The dual functions as a chemotaxic factor and an anaphylatoxin are not needed simultaneously or to the same degree. Anaphylatoxic activity is necessary early in inflammation and close to the inflammatory site so as to induce local mast cell degranulation and increase the number of soluble mediators available to enhance vascular permeability. Degranulation of mast cells away from the site of injury would be contrary to the protective nature of the inflammatory response because the substances released would affect healthy neighboring tissues needlessly. Chemotactic activity, on the other hand, is required for a much longer period and distal to the inflammatory site to attract leukocytes from the circulation.

The anaphylatoxic activities of C3a and C5a are inactivated by a naturally occurring enzyme, plasma carboxy-

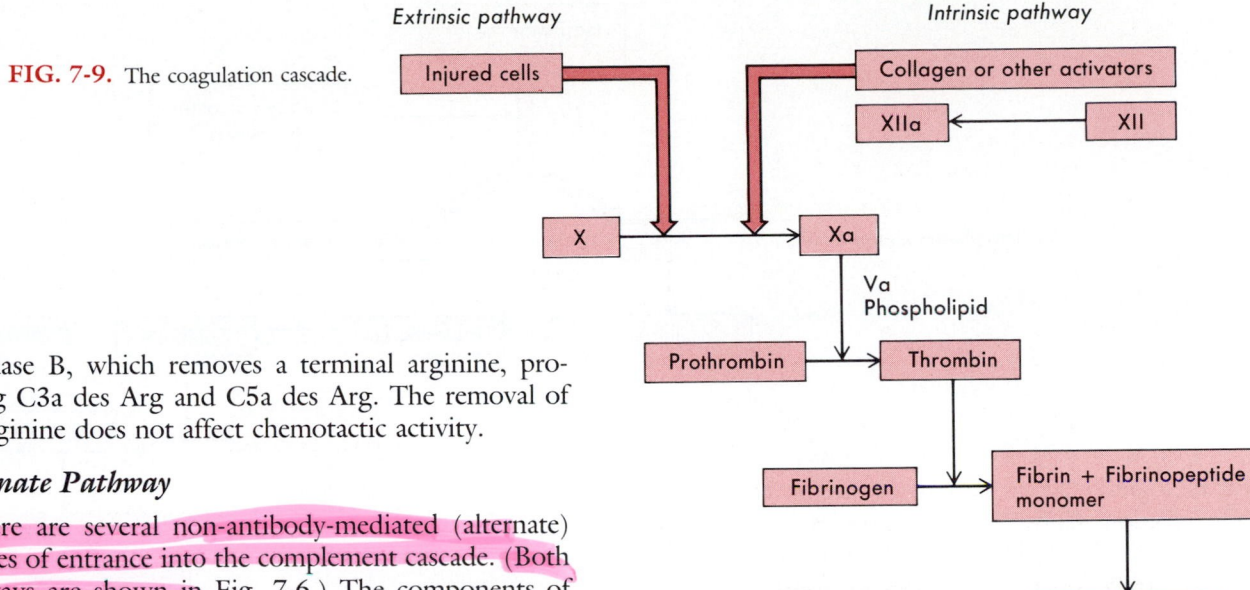

FIG. 7-9. The coagulation cascade.

peptidase B, which removes a terminal arginine, producing C3a des Arg and C5a des Arg. The removal of the arginine does not affect chemotactic activity.

Alternate Pathway

There are several non-antibody-mediated (alternate) avenues of entrance into the complement cascade. (Both pathways are shown in Fig. 7-6.) The components of the alternate pathway include those listed in Fig. 7-6.

The Clotting System

The clotting (coagulation) system is a plasma protein system that forms a fibrinous exudate, or meshwork, at the inflamed site to trap exudates, microorganisms, and foreign bodies. This (1) prevents the spread of infection and inflammation to adjacent tissues, (2) keeps microorganisms and foreign bodies at the site of greatest phagocytic activity, and (3) forms a clot that stops bleeding and provides a framework for future repair and healing. The main substance in this fibrinous mesh is an insoluble protein called fibrin, which is the end product of the coagulation cascade.

Like the complement cascade, the coagulation cascade can be activated through two different pathways that converge at the point where each pathway produces the same substance (Fig. 7-9). In the complement cascade the classical and alternate pathways converge when each has activated C5 (Fig. 7-6). In the coagulation cascade the **extrinsic pathway** and the **intrinsic pathway** converge at factor X. From that point, the cascade proceeds on a common pathway until fibrin is formed. (The coagulation cascade is discussed further and illustrated in Chapter 22.)

The clotting system can be activated by many substances released during tissue destruction and infection, including collagen, proteases, kallikrein, plasmin, and bacterial endotoxins. In addition activation of the clotting cascade produces subcomponents that enhance the inflammatory response. The two low–molecular weight fibrinopeptides released from fibrinogen during fibrin production (especially fibrinopeptide B) are chemotactic for neutrophils and increase vascular permeability by enhancing the effects of bradykinin (formed from the kinin system).

The Kinin System

The third plasma protein system with a role in inflammation is the kinin system. The primary kinin is **bradykinin,** which, at low doses, causes dilation of vessels, acts with prostaglandins to induce pain, causes extravascular smooth muscle contraction, increases vascular permeability, and may increase leukocyte chemotaxis. Bradykinin induces smooth muscle contraction more slowly than histamine and may be more important during the prolonged phase of inflammation. Bradykinin, along with prostaglandins of the E series, is probably responsible for endothelial cell retraction and increased vascular permeability in the later phases of inflammation (endothelial cell retraction is shown in Fig. 7-3).

The kinin system is activated by stimulation of the **plasma kinin cascade** (Fig. 7-10). The conversion of plasma prekallikrein to kallikrein is induced by a subunit, *prekallikrein activator,* that is generated during the activation of Hageman factor (factor XII) by the coagulation cascade. Kallikrein then converts kininogen to kinin, the primary kinin being bradykinin. Another source of kinin is the tissue kallikreins in saliva, sweat, tears, urine, and feces. These kallikreins convert serum kininogens to kallidin (lysylbradykinin), which may be converted to bradykinin by plasma aminopeptidase. Kinins are rapidly degraded and, therefore, controlled by kininases, which are enzymes present in plasma and tissues.

Control and Interaction of Plasma Protein Systems

The activation of the plasma protein systems involved in inflammation produces a large number of very po-

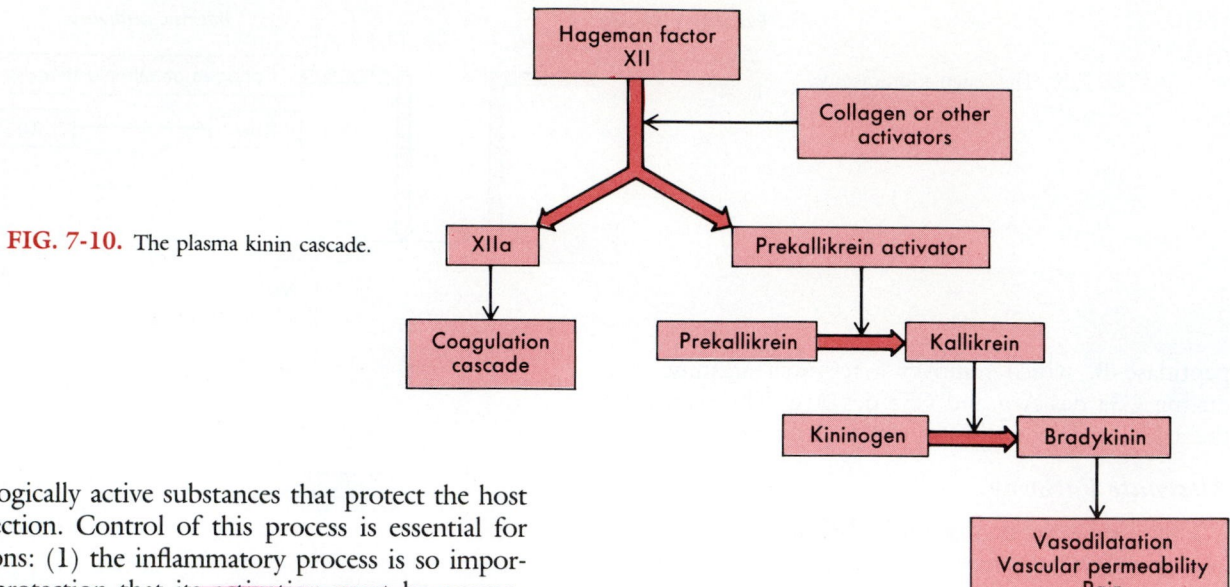

FIG. 7-10. The plasma kinin cascade.

tent, biologically active substances that protect the host from infection. Control of this process is essential for two reasons: (1) the inflammatory process is so important for protection that its activation must be guaranteed; therefore, there are multiple means of assessing inflammation; and (2) the activities of the biochemical mediators generated during this process are so potent and potentially detrimental to the host that their actions must be confined to injured or infected tissues; therefore, multiple mechanisms are available to inactivate or regulate the inflammatory mediators.

Control is apparent at many levels. Many components of inflammation are rapidly destroyed within seconds by enzymes from the plasma. Two components of the complement cascade, C3a and C5a, are inactivated by the plasma enzyme carboxypeptidase, and histamine and leukotrienes are inactivated by the eosinophilic enzymes histaminase and arylsulfatase. Many other natural inhib-

itors are present, including antagonists for histamine, the kinins, the complement components, kallikrein, and plasmin.

Histamine activity is controlled, in part, by histamine receptors on the host's target cells. At least two types of receptors exist for histamine: H1 and H2 receptors (Fig. 7-11). The H1 receptor is responsible for promoting inflammation, whereas inflammation is generally inhibited through the H2 receptor by suppression of leukocyte function and mast cell degranulation. The H1 receptor is thought to be present on cells of smooth muscle, especially those of the bronchi, and to cause

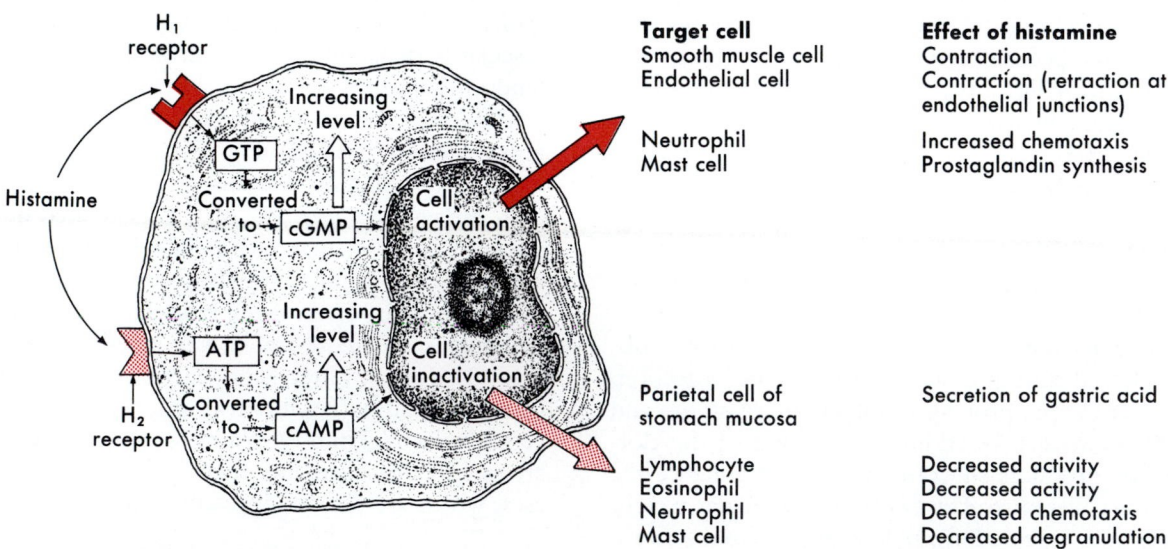

Target cell	Effect of histamine
Smooth muscle cell	Contraction
Endothelial cell	Contraction (retraction at endothelial junctions)
Neutrophil	Increased chemotaxis
Mast cell	Prostaglandin synthesis
Parietal cell of stomach mucosa	Secretion of gastric acid
Lymphocyte	Decreased activity
Eosinophil	Decreased activity
Neutrophil	Decreased chemotaxis
Mast cell	Decreased degranulation

FIG. 7-11. Effects of histamine through H1 and H2 receptors. Effects depend on (1) density and affinity of H1 and/or H2 receptors on the target cell and (2) the identity of the target cell. *GTP,* Guanosine triphosphate; *cGMP,* cyclic guanosine monophosphate; *ATP,* adenosine triphosphate; *cAMP,* cyclic adenosine monophosphate.

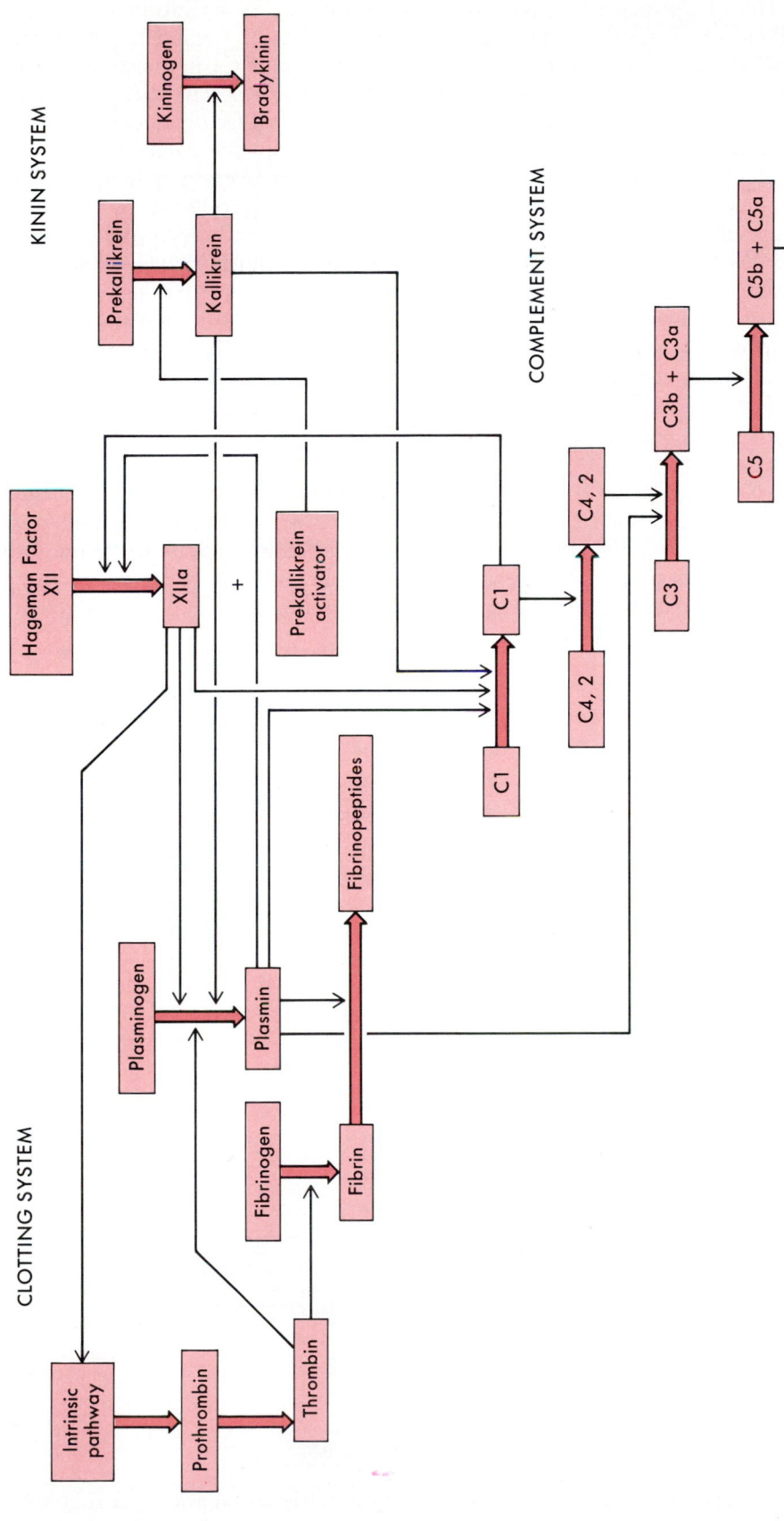

FIG. 7-12. Interaction of the complement, clotting, kinin, and fibrinolytic (plasmin) systems. Bold arrows denote the activation of factors within a system. Thin arrows denote where a particular factor activates another system.

bronchial smooth muscle to contract (bronchoconstriction) when stimulated. The H2 receptor is especially abundant on parietal cells of the stomach mucosa and induces the secretion of gastric acids upon stimulation. The distribution of both types of receptors is variable, and frequently they are present on the same cells and may act in an antagonistic fashion. For instance, both receptors are present on neutrophils. Stimulation of H1 receptors results in the augmentation of chemotaxis, whereas H2 stimulation results in its inhibition. The role of H1 and H2 receptors is discussed further in Chapter 8 (allergic reactions).

Most of the control processes interact, so that the activation or control of one plasma system results in a similar effect on others (Fig. 7-12). Plasmin controls clot formation (by degrading fibrin and fibrinogen) and activates the complement cascade through C1, C3, and C5, as does thrombin. Plasmin also activates the plasma kinin cascade by activating Hageman factor and producing prekallikrein activator. The activation of Hageman factor has four effects: (1) activation of the clotting cascade through factor XI; (2) activation of the fibrinolytic systems through conversion of plasminogen proactiva-

tor to plasminogen activator, resulting in the generation of plasmin; (3) activation of the kinin system by a Hageman factor fragment, prekallikrein activator; and (4) activation of C1 in the complement cascade. Plasmin itself exists as a proenzyme, plasminogen, which is activated by several factors, including plasminogen activator generated from the kallikrein system; thrombin generated from the clotting system; bacterial factors, such as streptokinase (produced by hemolytic streptococci); plasminogen activators produced by endothelial cells; and several cellular enzymes released during tissue destruction.

The interaction of control mechanisms is exemplified by the effects of C1 esterase inhibitor. Hereditary angioneurotic edema is an autosomal dominant disease characterized by a deficiency of C1 esterase inhibitor. In individuals with this disease, emotional stress and other stimuli frequently result in recurrent edema in the gastrointestinal tract, respiratory tract, and skin, with death occurring in some cases because of laryngeal swelling. The mechanism appears to be one of episodic, uncontrolled activation of plasmin, resulting in Hageman factor activation, bradykinin production, and C1 activa-

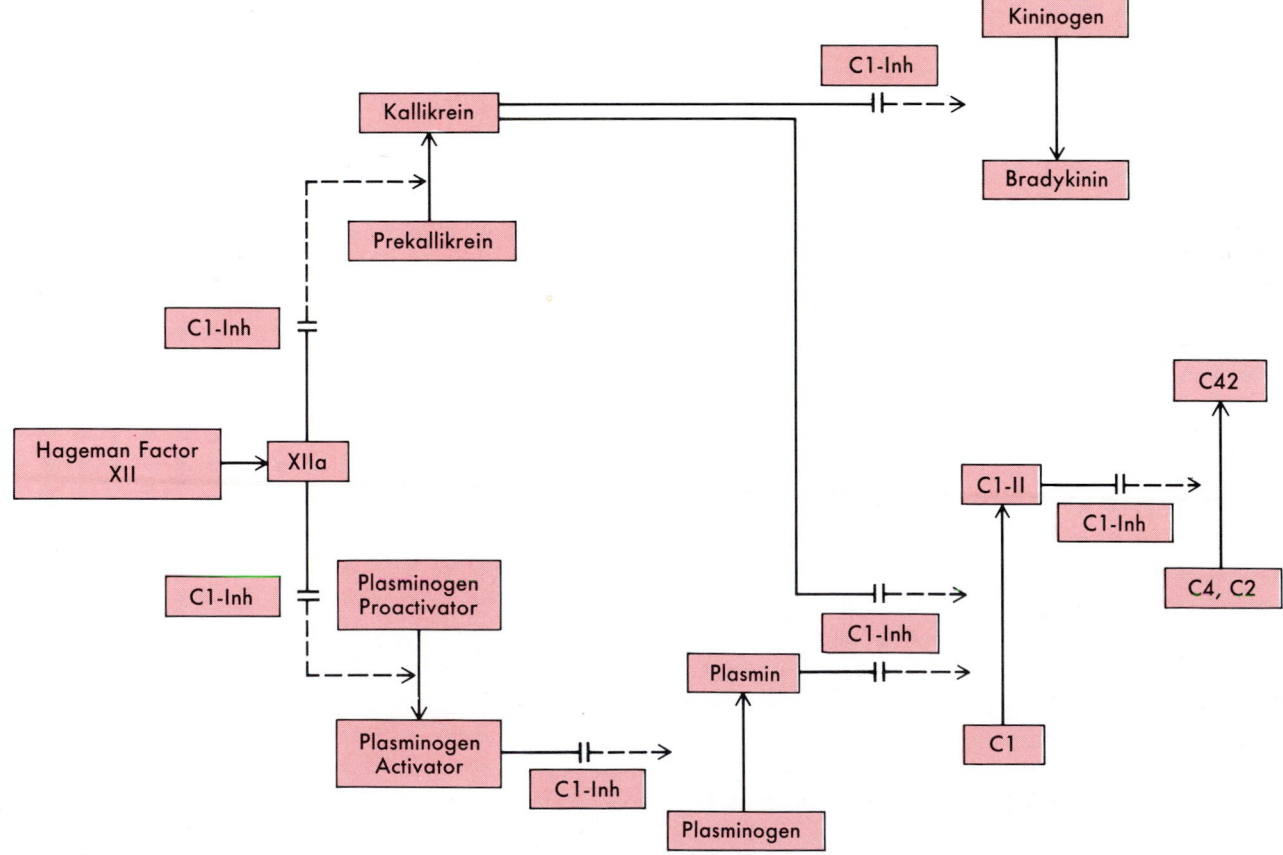

FIG. 7-13. Common control of the complement, clotting, and kinin systems by C1 esterase inhibitor (*C1-Inh*).

tion. Cl esterase inhibitor blocks several steps in the activation of all three cascades, including Cl esterase of the complement system, the effects of activated Hageman factor on the kinin system, and the effects of kallikrein and plasmin, as shown in Fig. 7-13. That activation of plasmin may be the most important single cause of hereditary angioneurotic edema is indicated by the fact that attacks are prevented by v-aminocaproic acid, which prevents the conversion of plasminogen to plasmin.

CELLULAR COMPONENTS OF INFLAMMATION

The two main classes of leukocytes to carry out inflammatory processes are the granulocytes and the monocytes/macrophages. The granulocytes, so called because of the many enzyme-containing lysosomal granules in their cytoplasm, include the neutrophils, eosinophils, and basophils. Monocytes (the immature form in the blood) and macrophages (the mature cell in the tissues) have fewer and larger lysosomes in their cytoplasm than do granulocytes. All of these cells are phagocytes (capable of phagocytosis, the ingestion of unwanted matter), but the most important of the phagocytes are the neutrophils and macrophages. Lymphocytes also participate in inflammation, primarily by producing soluble mediators (see the section on immunity).

The other cellular component important to inflammation is the platelet. Platelets are cytoplasmic fragments that circulate in the bloodstream until vascular injury occurs. After injury platelets (1) interact with components of the coagulation cascade to stop bleeding and (2) degranulate, releasing biochemical mediators, such as serotonin, which has vascular effects similar to those of histamine. Their activation is stimulated by many products of inflammation, including collagen, platelet-activating factor (PAF) released from mast cells, and antigen-antibody complexes. (Platelet function is described in detail in Chapter 22.)

Function of Phagocytes

The neutrophils and macrophages have essentially the same characteristics and functions. Each normally circulates in the bloodstream and is stimulated by inflammation to migrate through vessel walls near an inflammatory lesion. Once in the exudate, each is attracted to the lesion by specific chemotactic factors and kept there by the meshwork formed by fibrinous exudate. Once at the site, each type of cell phagocytoses (ingests) foreign or dead cells until its life span is over. The dead phagocyte then becomes part of the purulent exudate, or *pus,* which leaves the body through the lymphatic system or through the epithelium. Neutrophils and monocytes/

macrophages differ chiefly in (1) the speed with which they arrive at the site, the neutrophils arriving first; (2) the length of time they remain active, the macrophages being longer-lived; (3) the chemotactic factors capable of attracting them; (4) the enzymatic content of their lysosomes, or digestive vacuoles; and (5) their participation in the immune response, the macrophages being involved in antigen processing.

The phagocytes' role begins when the inflammatory response causes them to stick avidly to capillary and venule walls in a process called **margination,** or **pavementing** (Fig. 7-14). Margination is caused by increased stickiness of the phagocytes and increased adsorption by the endothelial cells lining the vessels. This is followed by **diapedesis,** or emigration through the retracting endothelial junctions and the basement membrane and out into the surrounding tissues (see Fig. 7-3).

Once they enter the inflammatory exudate, the phagocytes are attracted to the inflammatory site by chemotaxis. They respond to chemotactic factors because they can detect simultaneously, through chemoreceptors at multiple locations on their plasma membrane, where chemotactic factors are most highly concentrated (see Fig. 7-5). They then migrate in the direction of highest concentration. The primary chemotactic factors for neutrophils, eosinophils, and monocytes include many bacterial products, complement components C5a and C3a, kallikrein and plasminogen activator, fibrinopeptides, products of fibrin degradation, prostaglandins, the activated C567 complex from the complement system, the eosinophil and neutrophil chemotactic factors released from mast cells, and a monocyte chemotactic factor released from the neutrophil. Histamine, though not chemotactic itself, may facilitate chemotaxis. Some bacterial toxins, such as streptococcal streptolysins, inhibit neutrophil chemotaxis.

Phagocytosis, the engulfment and destruction of microorganisms, dead cells, and foreign particles, begins when the phagocytic cell enters the inflammatory site. The process of phagocytosis involves four steps: (1) recognition of the target and its adherence to the phagocyte, (2) engulfment (ingestion, or endocytosis), (3) fusion with lysosomes within the phagocyte; and (4) destruction of the target by lysosomal enzymes (lysosomes are described in Chapter 1). Throughout the process both target and digestive enzymes are isolated within membrane-bounded vesicles. Isolation protects the phagocyte from the harmful effects of target microorganisms and its own enzymes. Phagocytosis of an opsonized bacterium is illustrated in Fig. 7-15.

Most phagocytes can trap and engulf bacteria that have not been "coated" with an opsonin, but the process is slow and inefficient. Opsonization, usually by antibody or complement component C3b, greatly en-

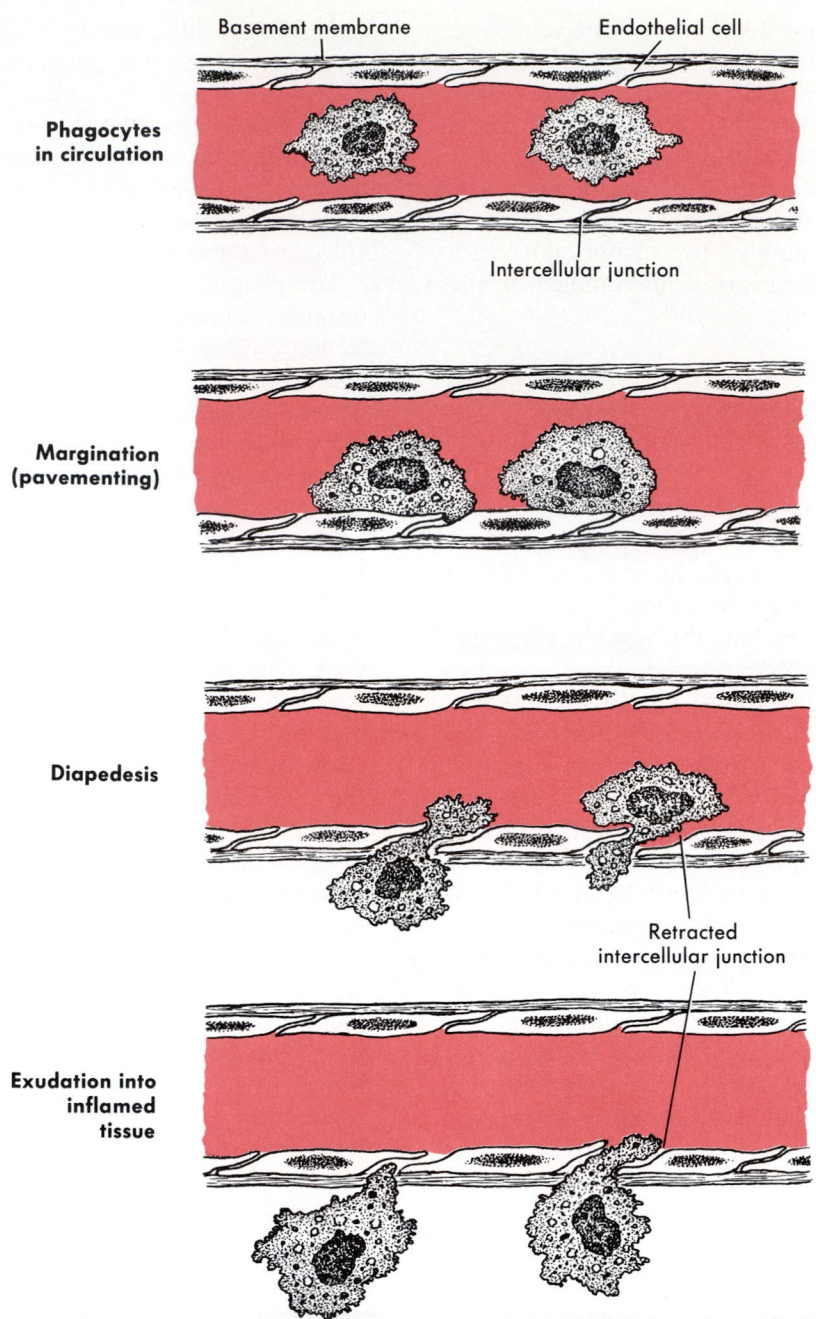

Phagocytes in circulation

Margination (pavementing)

Diapedesis

Exudation into inflamed tissue

Basement membrane Endothelial cell

Intercellular junction

Retracted intercellular junction

FIG. 7-14. Diapedesis of a phagocyte. Phagocytes are capable of ameboid movement, which allows them to squeeze through intercellular junctions and migrate to inflammatory lesions.

hances both recognition and binding (also called *adherence*). Opsonins function as "glue" between the phagocyte and the target cell because receptors on the phagocyte are specific for sites on the opsonin (Fc receptors for antibody, C3b receptors for C3b). This enables the phagocyte to bind opsonized bacteria very tightly to its surface. Although antibody forms a stronger attachment, C3b facilitates phagocytosis to a greater extent.

Engulfment is carried out by small pseudopods that extend from the plasma membrane and surround the adhered microorganism (Fig. 7-16), forming an intracellular phagocytic vacuole, or **phagosome.** The membrane that surrounds the phagosome consists of inverted plasma membrane. After the formation of the phagosome, lysosomes converge, fuse with the phagosome, and discharge their contents, creating a **phagolysosome.** Destruction of the bacterium takes place within the phagolysosome (see Fig. 7-15).

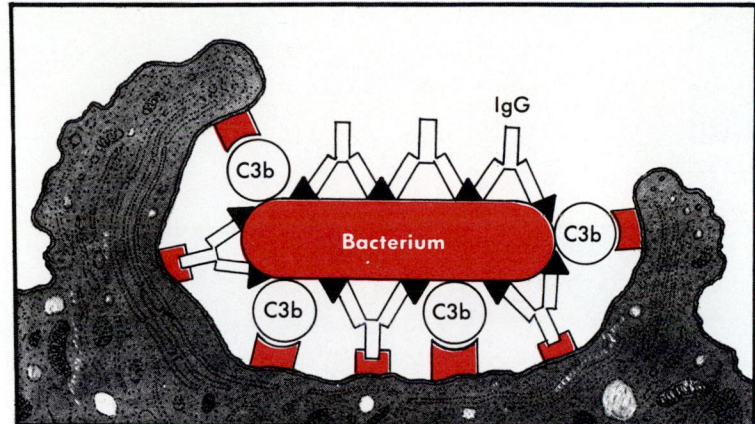

FIG. 7-15. Phases of phagocytosis. Opsonized microorganisms bind to the surface of a phagocyte *(1)* and are ingested *(2)* into a phagocytic vacuole, or phagosome *(3)*. Lysosomes fuse with the phagosome *(4)*, releasing their digestive enzymes into the vacuole. This results in the formation of a phagolysosome *(5)*, within which the microorganism is killed and digested.

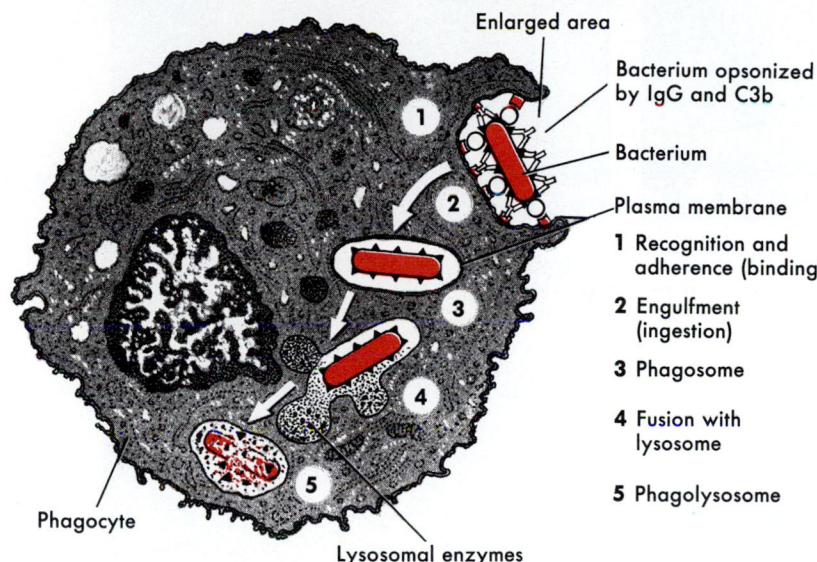

Enlarged area

Bacterium opsonized by IgG and C3b

Bacterium

Plasma membrane

1 Recognition and adherence (binding)

2 Engulfment (ingestion)

3 Phagosome

4 Fusion with lysosome

5 Phagolysosome

Phagocyte

Lysosomal enzymes

Phagocytosis is accompanied by a burst of metabolic activity in the phagocyte, resulting in the production of several oxygen-containing molecules that are reactive and highly damaging to cells. This is known as an oxygen-dependent killing mechanism. The principal oxygen-dependent mechanism of killing is hydrogen peroxide, especially in conjunction with the lysosomal enzyme myeloperoxidase and halide anions(I^-,Cl^-, and Br^-). Myeloperoxidase probably kills by iodination or the formation of toxic chloramines and aldehydes on the target cell's surface. The oxygen-independent mechanisms of killing are (1) acid pH (3.5 to 4.0) of the phagolysosome due to lactic acid production; (2) the cationic proteins, which bind to and damage target cell membranes; (3) lysozyme and elastase, which attack mucopeptides in the target cell wall; and (4) lactoferrin, which inhibits bacterial growth by binding iron.

When the phagocyte dies at the inflammatory site, it lyses (breaks open) and its cytoplasmic contents, including the lysosomal enzymes, are released. Enzymes released from lysosomes can digest the connective tissue

matrix, causing much of the tissue destruction associated with inflammation. α-1-Antitrypsin, a plasma protein produced by the liver, inhibits the destructive effects of many enzymes released by dead phagocytes. An inherited deficiency of α-1-antitrypsin often results in chronic lung damage and emphysema as a result of inflammation. (The pulmonary effects of α-1-antitrypsin deficiency are described in Chapter 30.)

Released lysosomal products contribute to other aspects of inflammation. These include increased vascular permeability, chemotaxis for monocytes, breakdown of connective tissues, and activation of the complement and kinin systems.

Polymorphonuclear Neutrophils

The **neutrophil,** or **polymorphonuclear neutrophil (PMN),** is the predominant phagocytic cell in the early inflammatory response, entering the inflammatory site within 6 to 12 hours after the initial injury. Neutrophils arrive first because they are attracted by the immediately generated chemotactic factors, such as complement sub-

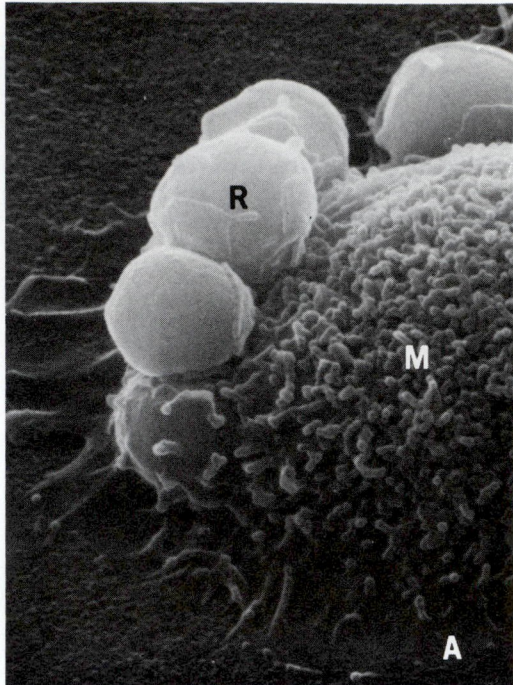

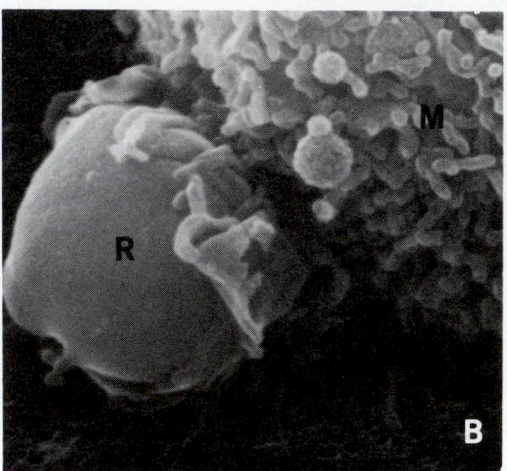

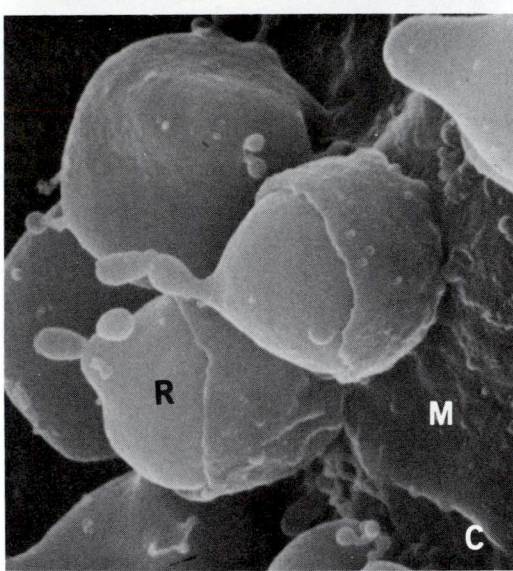

FIG. 7-16. This scanning electron micrograph shows the progressive steps in phagocytosis. **A,** Red blood cells *(R)* attach to the surface of a macrophage *(M).* **B,** Part of macrophage *(M)* membrane starts to enclose the red cell *(R).* **C,** The red blood cells are almost totally engulfed by the macrophage. (From King, Fenoglio, & Lefkowitch, 1983.)

components. Macrophages and lymphocytes, on the other hand, enter the site later, usually after 24 hours, and gradually replace the neutrophils.

Because the neutrophil is a mature cell incapable of division and is sensitive to the acidic environment of inflammatory lesions, it is short-lived in the inflammatory site. The primary roles of the neutrophil are removal of debris in sterile lesions, such as burns, and phagocytosis of bacteria in nonsterile lesions.

Monocytes and Macrophages

The **monocyte** is the largest normal blood cell (14 to 20 µm in diameter). Its single nucleus is usually indented or horseshoe-shaped. It is produced in the bone marrow, enters the circulation, and migrates to the inflammatory site, where it develops into a macrophage. The **macrophage** is generally larger (20 to 40 µm) and is a more active phagocyte than the monocyte (Fig. 7-16). Monocytes that originate in the bone marrow also appear to be the precursors of macrophages that are fixed in tissues (tissue macrophages), including those of the mononuclear phagocytic system (formerly known as the reticuloendothelial system), including Kupffer cells of the liver and alveolar macrophages of the lungs. (Tissue macrophages are discussed in Chapter 6.)

Macrophage and lymphocyte infiltration is characteristic of chronic rather than acute inflammation. Macrophages may appear at the inflammatory site soon after the initial neutrophil infiltration (within 24 hours of injury) but usually arrive 3 to 7 days later. They migrate to the site slowly because (1) many of the chemotactic factors that attract them, such as macrophage chemotactic factor, are released by neutrophils and (2) monocytes, the immature macrophages, move somewhat sluggishly.

Macrophages are better suited than neutrophils to long-term defense against infectious agents because macrophages can survive and divide in the acidic inflammatory site, whereas neutrophils cannot. Macrophages can also fuse into larger cells capable of phagocytosing larger targets.

Macrophages have several roles in inflammation and immunity. They are responsive to the soluble products (lymphokines) secreted by T cells, participate in activating the immune response by processing antigen for presentation to lymphocytes (Figs. 6-8, 6-14, and 6-16), and are a source of a soluble factor (colony-stimulating factor) that stimulates the growth and differentiation of granulocytes and monocytes in the bone marrow. Macrophages also secrete substances that promote regrowth of tissues during wound healing (see p. 229).

Several bacteria can survive and even thrive inside macrophages. Microorganisms such as *Mycobacterium tuberculosis*, *Mycobacterium leprae*, *Salmonella typhi*, *Brucella abortus*, and *Listeria monocytogenes* can remain dormant or multiply inside the phagolysosomes of macrophages. This occurrence is prevented or ameliorated with the help of the immune system, which is active by the time macrophages have infiltrated the inflammatory site (Fig. 7-7). Macrophages are further activated, or "turned on," by lymphokines secreted by T cells. Lymphokines increase the killing capacity of the macrophage by increasing its phagocytic activity, size, plasma membrane area, glucose metabolism, and number of lysosomes (Fig. 7-17).

Failure of macrophages to turn on has been traced to defective T cell responses to certain microorganisms. For example, a form of leprosy called lepromatous leprosy is characterized by the survival of *M. leprae* that have been phagocytosed by macrophages. In individuals with lepromatous leprosy, T cells fail to secrete the lymphokines needed to transform the macrophages into cells more highly dedicated to killing.

Eosinophils

Eosinophils are granulocytes that have large numbers of lysosomes containing (1) biochemical mediators that control the vascular effects of serotonin and histamine (see p. 226) and (2) a caustic protein that is capable of dissolving the surface membranes of parasites. Eosinophils do not phagocytose parasites, many of which are multicellular organisms. Rather they bind to and degranulate onto the parasite, damaging its surface. Degranulation is preceded by the processes shown in Fig. 7-18.

IgE is the chief immunoglobulin involved in allergic hypersensitivity reactions, which are usually detrimental to the host (see Chapter 8). IgE may also mediate normal defenses against some pathogenic organisms (Fig. 7-7). Multicellular parasites, particularly worms, elicit an IgE-mediated allergic response that benefits the host by destroying the parasite. As in allergic reaction, IgE mediates degranulation of mast cells in the presence of soluble antigens. Degranulation releases eosinophil chemotactic factor of anaphylaxis, ECF-A, which attracts eosinophils to the site of parasitic infestation. ECF-A also induces the eosinophil to increase the density of its membrane receptors for two opsonins, complement component C3b and the Fc portion of IgG.

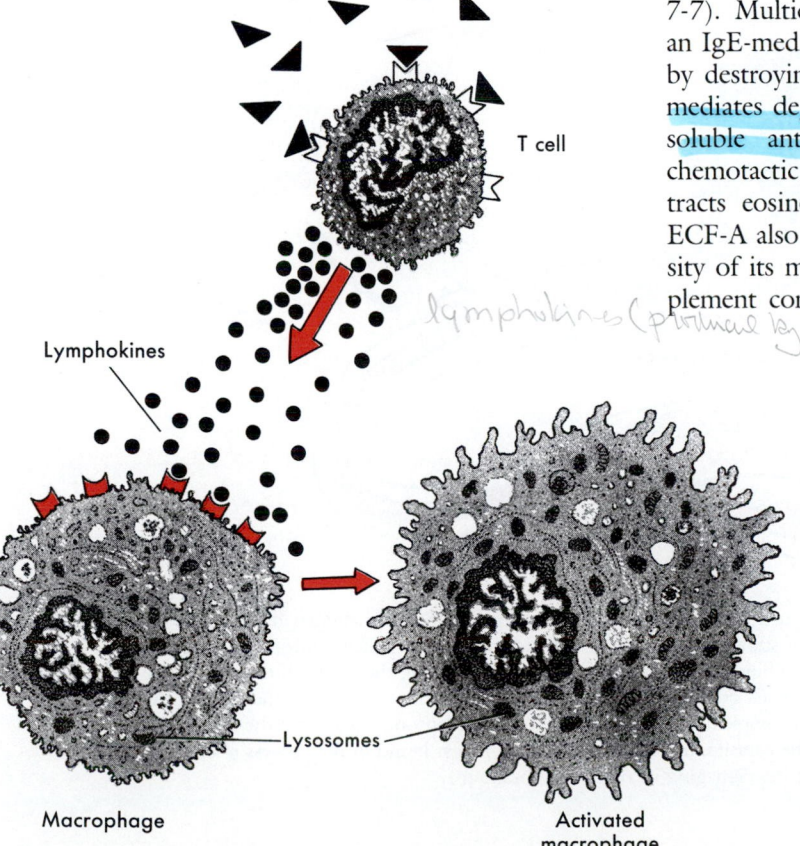

FIG. 7-17. Activation of a macrophage by a lymphokine (macrophage-activating factor, or MAF). Lymphokine is produced by T cells that have been stimulated by an antigen. The ruffled plasma membrane indicates macrophage activation.

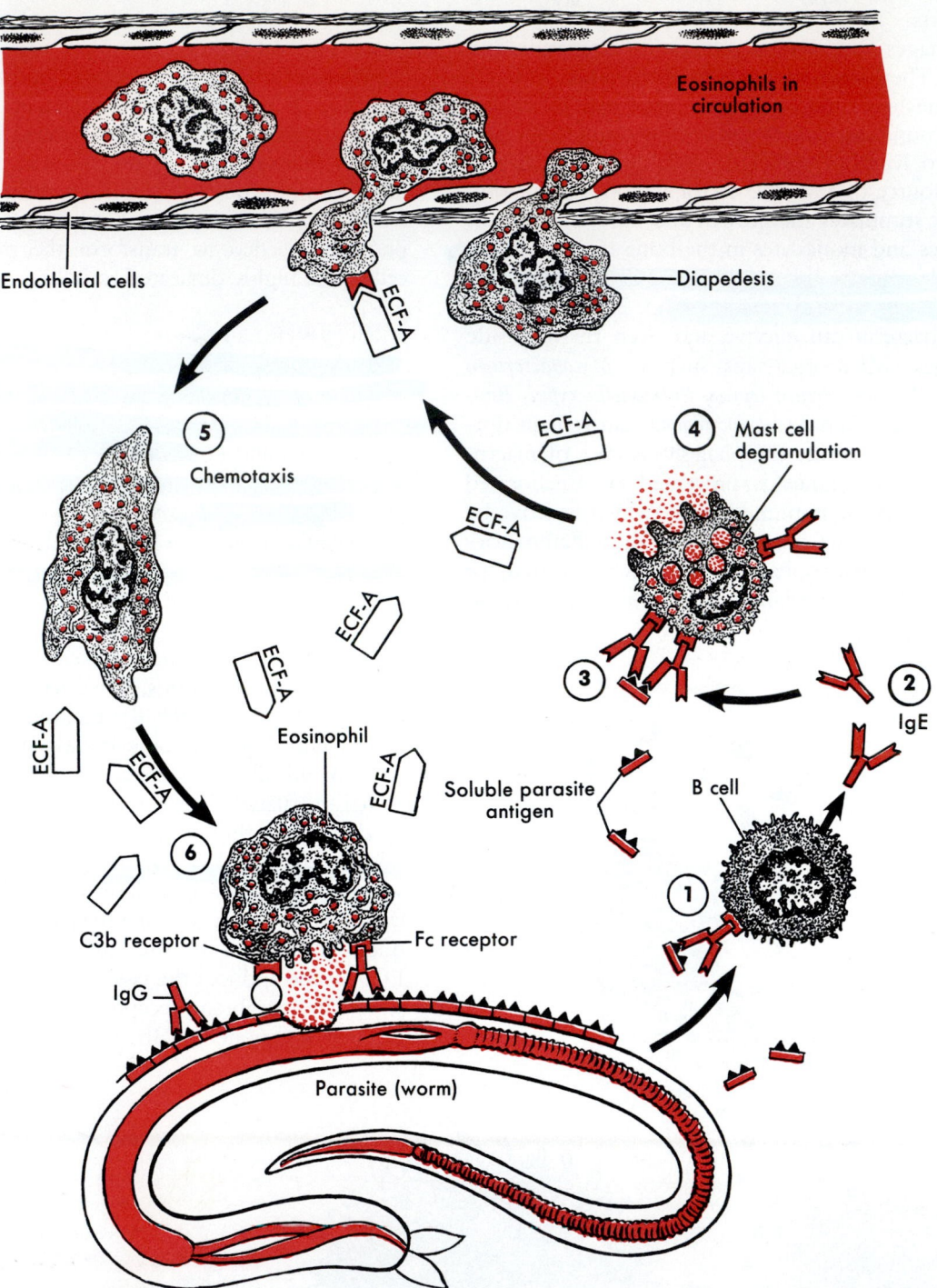

FIG. 7-18. IgE-mediated destruction of a parasite by an eosinophil. Soluble antigen from a parasite binds to an IgE-bearing B cell *(1)*, stimulating the B cell to produce IgE *(2)*, which binds to Fc receptors on a mast cell. Soluble antigen also binds to IgE on the mast cell *(3)*, causing the mast cell to degranulate *(4)*. ECF-A released from the mast cell granules attracts eosinophils out of the circulation and toward the site of inflammation *(5)*. IgG and complement component C3b are the opsonins that bind the eosinophil to the parasite. Once bound to the parasite, the eosinophil tries to ingest it and in the process releases its lysosomal enzymes onto the parasite, damaging its outer membrane *(6)*.

The increased density of receptors for these opsonins enables the eosinophil to bind very tightly to the parasite. The eosinophil is unable to phagocytose the large parasite. Instead of ingesting the organism and enclosing it in a phagolysosome, the eosinophil's lysosomal granules migrate to the surface of the eosinophil and discharge their contents, including highly caustic cationic proteins, onto the parasite's outer membrane. This causes extensive damage to the parasite, and the tight fit between the eosinophil and its target prevents lysosomal contents from damaging neighboring host tissues.

CELLULAR PRODUCTS

Some host cells produce soluble factors that contribute to nonspecific mechanisms of defense by affecting other, neighboring host cells. These factors include lymphokines (produced by T cells involved in delayed hypersensitivity), interferons (produced by many host cells in response to viral infection), and interleukins (produced by phagocytes and lymphocytes). Although some of these factors may be produced in response to specific antigenic stimulation (especially the lymphokines), all of them act in a nonspecific manner to enhance the inflammatory response.

Lymphokines

Lymphokines, which are produced by T cells in response to antigenic stimulation, are biochemical mediators that affect other cells of the immune and inflammatory responses (Fig. 7-7). Although they are produced by cells of the immune system—a specific mechanism of self-defense—lymphokines have nonspecific effects.

Different lymphokines have different effects. One lymphokine, called **migration-inhibitory factor (MIF),** is a glycoprotein that inhibits macrophage migration from the inflamed site. Another, **macrophage-activating factor (MAF)** increases the phagocytic activities of macrophages (Fig. 7-17). At least three other lymphokines affect macrophages by causing chemotaxis, promoting maturation of monocytes into macrophages, enhancing macrophage migration along chemotactic gradients, and stimulating macrophages to aggregate or fuse into giant cells (see p. 238). Some lymphokines are chemotactic for the other phagocytes: neutrophils and eosinophils.

Other lymphokines affect lymphocytes, inducing them to produce more lymphokines, proliferate, or diminish their activities. Lymphokines called lymphotoxins are nonspecific killers of nonlymphocytes. A lymphokine called transfer factor is a ribonucleoprotein that, when extracted from leukocytes and innoculated into another individual, can transfer immunity from an immunocompetent donor to an immunoincompetent recipient and may be involved in the recruiting of other lymphocytes.

Interferon

One of the body's defenses against viral infection is the production of interferon. (Mechanisms of viral infection are described in Chapter 2.) Interferon does not kill viruses, but it can prevent them from infecting healthy cells. **Interferon** consists of small, low–molecular weight proteins produced and released by host cells that have been invaded by a virus. Once released, interferon molecules attach themselves to receptors on neighboring host cells. If a neighboring cell is uninfected, the

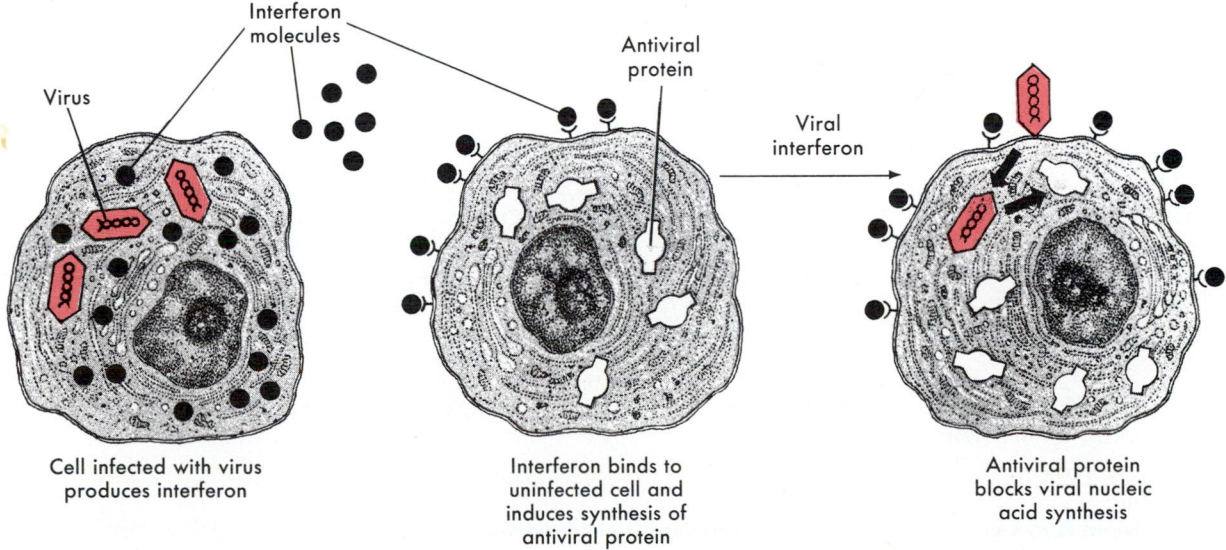

Cell infected with virus produces interferon

Interferon binds to uninfected cell and induces synthesis of antiviral protein

Antiviral protein blocks viral nucleic acid synthesis

FIG. 7-19. The action of interferon.

interferon stimulates it to produce an antiviral protein (Fig. 7-19). Interferon has no effect on a cell that is already infected by the virus.

Slightly different kinds of interferon are produced by different types of cells. All types are host-specific but not virus-specific; therefore, human interferon is only effective in humans, but it is effective against almost all viruses.

Interleukins

The **interleukins (ILs)** are biochemical messengers sent from one leukocyte to another. The seven interleukins described thus far are produced by macrophages or lymphocytes in response to stimulation by an antigen or by products of inflammation (Lachman & Maizel, 1983; Milanese, Richardson & Reinherz, 1986). The function of this series of hormones is to enhance the response of lymphocytes and other cells to antigens and other foreign substances.

Interleukin 1 (IL-1) is produced mostly by phagocytes and antigen-presenting cells that have been stimulated by substances associated with tissue injury, including bacteria, endotoxins (bacterial pyrogens), interferon, antigen-antibody complexes, and antigen. IL-1 is a lymphocyte-activating factor that, among other functions, probably augments antibody production by enhancing the production of IL-2 by T helper cells. Macrophage-produced IL-1 has been shown to promote the growth and function of almost every cell on which it has been tested. It has several effects on neutrophils, including induction of neutrophilia (proliferation that increases the number of circulating neutrophils), chemotaxis, increased hexose-monophosphate shunt activity (i.e., cellular metabolism), and increased lysosomal enzyme activity. Other interleukins, notably IL-2 and IL-4, appear to effect clonal selection and proliferation of antigen-specific clones of B or T cells. This effect speeds up antibody production and increases populations of T cells capable of direct or nonspecific protective responses to the antigen.

SYSTEMIC MANIFESTATIONS OF ACUTE INFLAMMATION

The three primary systemic changes associated with the acute inflammatory response are fever, leukocytosis (a transient increase in circulating leukocytes), and increase in circulating plasma proteins. Fever appears to be induced by a mediator, endogenous pyrogen, which may be identical to interleukin 1 and is released from neutrophils and macrophages. Endogenous pyrogen (a fever-causing chemical) acts directly on the hypothalamus, the portion of the brain that controls the body's thermostat. The release of endogenous pyrogen activity occurs after phagocytosis or after exposure of the cell to bacterial endotoxin or to antigen-antibody complexes. (Mechanisms of temperature regulation are discussed in Chapter 13.)

The generation of a febrile response can be beneficial to the defense of the host because the microorganisms that cause some conditions (e.g., syphilis, gonococcal urethritis) are very sensitive to small increases in body temperature. On the other hand fever may have some harmful side effects, for it may enhance the host's susceptibility to the effects of endotoxins associated with

TABLE 7-1 Circulating levels of acute-phase reactants during inflammation

Increased	Decreased	Function
Fibrinogen Prothrombin Factor VIII Plasminogen	None	Coagulation components
α-1-antitrypsin α-1-antichymotrypsin	Inter-α-antitypsin	Protease inhibitors
Haptoglobin Hemopexin Ceruloplasmin Ferritin	Transferrin	Transport proteins
C1s, C2, C3, C4, C5, C9, factor B, C1 inhibitor	Properdin	Complement components
α-1-acid glycoprotein Fibronectin Serum amyloid A (SAA) C-reactive protein (CRP)	Albumin Prealbumin α-1-lipoprotein β-lipoprotein	Miscellaneous proteins

gram-negative bacterial infections (bacterial toxins are described in Chapter 2).

During many infections numbers of circulating leukocytes, primarily neutrophils, increase. This increase is usually accompanied by a "left shift" in the ratio of immature to mature neutrophils, so that the more immature forms of neutrophils, such as band cells, metamyelocytes, and, occasionally, myelocytes, are present in greater than normal proportions. (See Chapter 22 for a discussion of the development and maturation of blood cells.) Leukocyte production increases because it is stimulated by several products of inflammation, including complement component C3a. Colony-stimulating factors produced by phagocytes also induce granulopoiesis (formation of granulocytes, namely, neutrophils, eosinophils, and basophils) in the bone marrow, primarily by the proliferation of committed precursors of granulocytes and monocytes (see Chapter 22).

Many plasma proteins, most of which are products of the liver, are increased during inflammation; these are referred to as **acute-phase reactants** (Table 7-1). Acute-phase reactants reach maximal circulating levels in 10 to 40 hours. Many are anti-inflammatory proteins whose rate of synthesis is increased in the liver (such as inhibi-

tors of proteases released during inflammation or proteins that are consumed during inflammation). Interleukin 1 may induce synthesis of acute-phase reactants directly by stimulating liver cells. Administration of IL-1 into animals leads to elevation of most acute-phase reactants, including fibrinogen, C-reactive protein, haptoglobin, alpha-1-antitrypsin, and ceruloplasmin.

A major systemic complication of infection is *septicemia,* or bacterial infection of the blood. (Septicemia is described briefly in Chapter 2. Its cardiovascular consequences, which include anaphylactic shock, are described in Chapter 27.)

Acute inflammation can be verified by hematologic tests, which are described in Chapter 22. An increase in blood levels of acute-phase reactants, primarily fibrinogen (see Table 7-1), is usually associated with an increased erythrocyte sedimentation rate. The alteration in plasma proteins probably leads to an enhanced erythrocyte rouleaux formation (stacking of erythrocytes, as in a stack of coins) and increased rates of sedimentation. Although a nonspecific reaction, increased erythrocyte sedimentation is considered a good indicator of an acute inflammatory response.

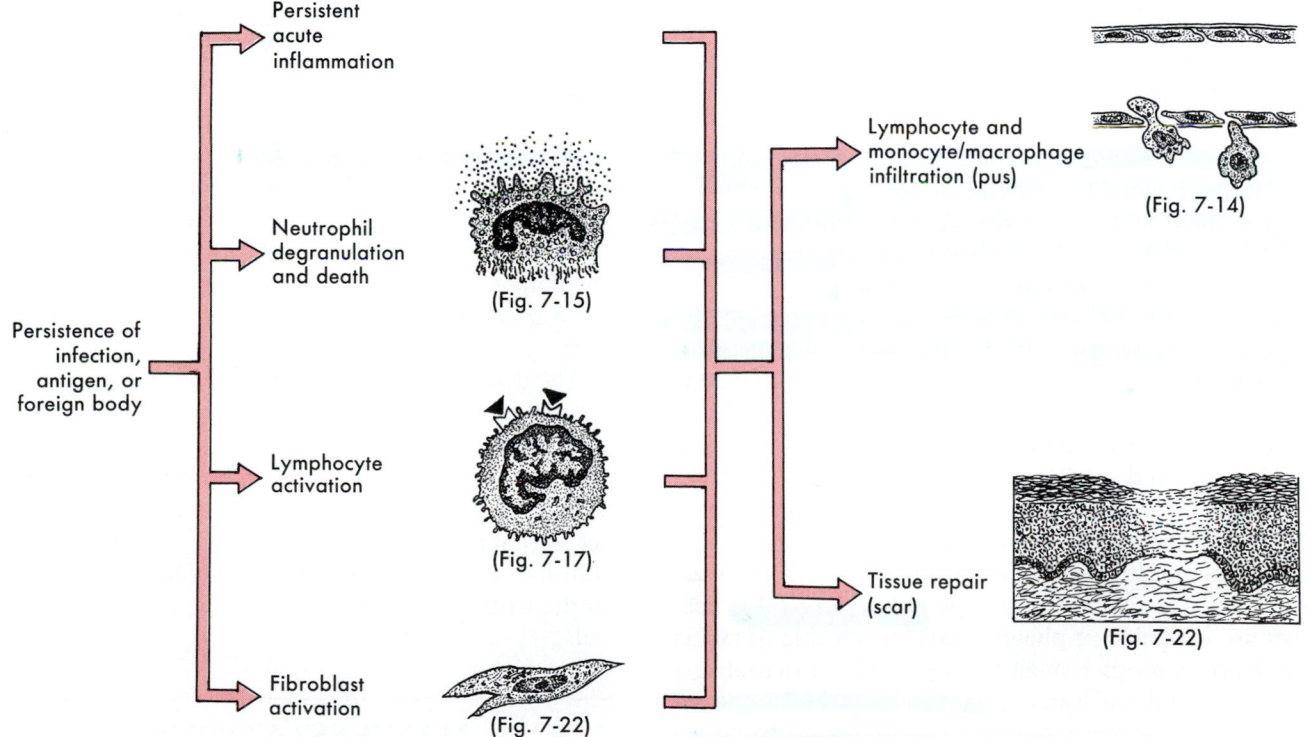

FIG. 7-20. The chronic inflammatory response. Inflammation usually becomes chronic because of the persistence of an infection, an antigen, or a foreign body in the wound. Chronic inflammation is characterized by the persistence of many of the processes of acute inflammation. In addition, large amounts of neutrophil degranulation and death, the activation of lymphocytes, and the concurrent activation of fibroblasts result in the release of mediators that induce the infiltration of more lymphocytes and monocytes/macrophages and the beginning of wound healing and tissue repair. The figure numbers refer to those in which more detailed information may be found on that portion of the response.

CHRONIC INFLAMMATION

Superficially the difference between acute and chronic inflammation is purely one of duration, in that chronic inflammation lasts 2 weeks or longer, regardless of cause. There may also be characteristic histologic and mechanistic differences (Fig. 7-20). Chronic inflammation is sometimes preceded by an unsuccessful acute inflammatory response. For example, if bacterial contamination or foreign objects (e.g., dirt, wood splinter, glass) persist in a traumatic wound, an inflammatory response that is difficult to differentiate from the acute response will continue beyond 2 weeks. Suppuration, pus formation, and incomplete wound healing may characterize this type of chronic inflammation.

Chronic inflammation can also occur as a distinct process without much acute inflammation. Some microorganisms (e.g., mycobacteria) have cell walls with a very high lipid and wax content, making them relatively insensitive to degradation by phagocytes. The persistence of these bacteria continues to stimulate inflammation. Others, such as the microorganisms that cause tuberculosis, leprosy, syphilis, and brucellosis, can survive within the macrophage. In addition some microorganisms produce toxins that stimulate tissue-damaging reactions even after they are killed. Persistent inflammation can also be due to prolonged irritation by chemicals, particulate matter, or physical irritants (e.g., inhaled dusts, wood splinters, or suture material).

Chronic inflammation is characterized by a dense infiltration of lymphocytes and macrophages. If macrophages are unable to protect the host from tissue damage, the body attempts to wall off and isolate the infected site, thus forming a **granuloma** (Fig. 7-21). Granulomas are formed if neutrophils and macrophages are unable to destroy microorganisms during the acute inflammatory response. Infections due to some bacteria (listerosis, brucellosis), fungi (histoplasmosis, coccidiomycosis), parasites (leishmaniasis, shistosomiasis, toxoplasmosis), and perhaps large antigen-antibody complexes (rheumatoid arthritis) result in granuloma formation.

Granuloma formation begins when some of the macrophages differentiate into large **epithelioid cells:** cells that are incapable of phagocytosis but capable of taking up debris and other small particles. Other macrophages fuse into multinucleated **giant cells,** which are active phagocytes and can engulf particles too large to be engulfed by single macrophages. The granuloma itself is usually walled off (encapsulated) by fibrous deposits of collagen and may be hyalinized or calcified by deposits of calcium carbonate and calcium phosphate.

The classic granuloma associated with tuberculosis is characterized by a wall of epithelioid cells surrounding a

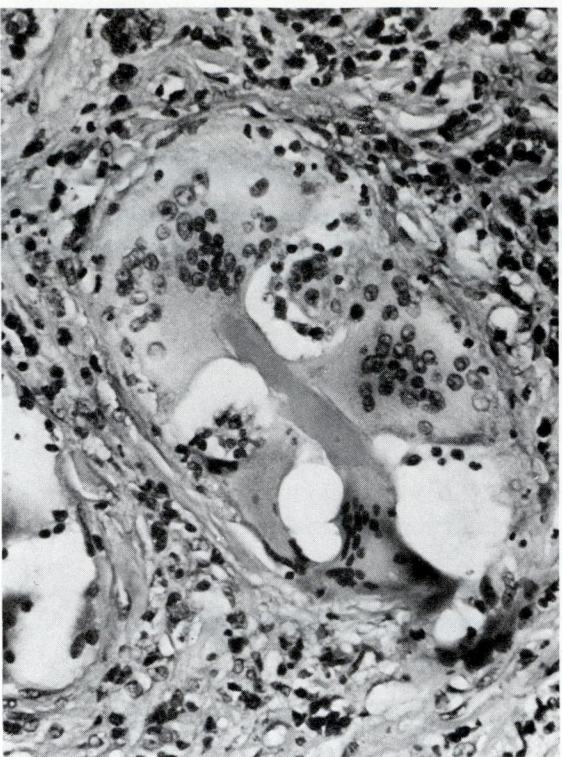

FIG. 7-21. Cross-section of a granuloma. Granulomatous (de Quervain's) thyroiditis. Outside the follicle (lightly shaded) are mononuclear inflammatory cells and fibrosis (×300). (From Kissane, 1985.)

center of dead and decaying tissue (caseous necrosis; see Chapter 2) and mycobacteria. Some of the epithelioid cells fuse into Langhans'-type giant cells, with their nuclei distributed in a horseshoe pattern inside the plasma membrane (see Fig. 7-21). The epithelioid cells persist for 3 to 4 weeks, whereas the giant cells live only a few days.

The decay of cells within the granuloma results in the release of acids and the enzymatic contents of dead phagocytes' lysosomes. In this inhospitable environment the cellular debris is broken down into its basic constituents and a clear fluid (liquefaction necrosis; see Chapter 2) remains in the granuloma. Eventually this fluid diffuses out and leaves a hollow, thick-walled structure in the tissue that may remain for the life of the individual.

LOCAL MANIFESTATIONS OF INFLAMMATION

Because inflammation is a nonspecific defense mechanism, it generally proceeds in the same way, no matter what type of injury has occurred. All the local manifestations of acute inflammation are due to vascular changes and exudation. Swelling occurs as exudate accumulates. Swelling is usually accompanied by pain due to pressure exerted by exudate accumulation and the presence of soluble biochemical mediators, such as prostaglandins and bradykinin. Heat and redness are the result of increased perfusion (increased blood flow through the area).

The function of vascular changes and exudation is to deliver leukocytes, plasma proteins, and their biochemical mediators to the site of injury. Exudate and its contents have three functions: (1) to dilute toxins produced by bacteria and toxic products released by dying cells, (2) to carry plasma proteins (including antibody) and leukocytes (both phagocytes and lymphocytes) to the site, and (3) to carry away bacterial toxins, dead cells, debris, and other products of inflammation. This third function occurs via channels through the epithelium (sinuses) or through lymphatic vessels. Drainage by lymphatic vessels facilitates the immune response because antigens in lymphatic fluid pass through the lymph nodes, where they stimulate B lymphocytes to become antibody-producing plasma cells or T lymphocytes to become effector T cells. (The lymphatic system is described in Chapter 26.)

Exudate varies in composition, depending on the stage of the inflammatory response and, to some extent, the injurious stimulus. In early or mild inflammation the exudate is watery, or a **serous exudate,** with very few plasma proteins or leukocytes, such as fluid in a blister. In more severe or advanced inflammation the exudate may be thick and clotted, or a **fibrinous exudate,** such as in the lungs of individuals with lobar pneumonia. If a large number of leukocytes accumulates, as in persistent bacterial infections, the exudate consists of pus and is called a **purulent suppurative** exudate. Purulent exudate is characteristic of walled-off lesions (**cysts** or **abscesses**). If bleeding occurs, the exudate is filled with erythrocytes and is described as a **hemorrhagic exudate.**

The local manifestations of inflammation can affect all vascularized tissues, but lesions vary, depending on the organ or tissue involved. The lesion resulting from widespread cellular death (necrosis), for example, differs in myocardial (heart muscle), brain, and hepatic (liver) tissue. Cellular death due to myocardial infarction (deprivation of oxygen caused by cessation of blood flow) causes a response that proceeds to replacement of the dead tissue with a fibrinous scar. The same injury to brain tissue is more likely to result in the formation of an abscess filled with necrotic tissue (types of necrosis are described in Chapter 2). Destruction of liver tissue stimulates the regrowth, or regeneration, of liver cells.

Because inflammation can occur only in vascularized and perfused tissues, perforative injuries, such as wounds or ulcers, and gangrene, in which an area of a limb or internal organ is killed by bacteria and lack of perfusion, result in inflammation at the *borders* of the lesion. (Gangrene is discussed in Chapter 2.)

Local manifestations of inflammation also accompany all types of nonlethal cellular and tissue injury, from fractures or strains of musculoskeletal system to burn injuries (see Chapter 2). No matter what the cause or where the lesion, inflammation occurs without fail because without it, healing could not occur. Acute inflammation is so closely tied to healing that it is sometimes called the defense phase of healing.

RESOLUTION AND REPAIR

Destruction of tissue is followed by a period of healing that begins during acute inflammation and may not be complete for as long as 2 years. The most favorable outcome of healing is complete return to normal structure and function. This is possible if damage is minor, no complications occur, or destroyed tissues are capable of **regeneration** (mitotic proliferation of remaining cells; mitosis is described in Chapter 1). Restoration of original structure and physiologic function is called **resolution.**

Factors That Affect Tissue Regeneration

CAPACITY FOR MITOSIS
Not capable of mitosis
   Neurons (nerve cells)
   Myocardium (heart muscle cells)
Capable after biochemical stimulation
   Skeletal muscle
   Bone
   Connective tissue
   Undifferentiated embryonic tissue (mesenchyma)
   Endocrine epithelium
   Lung
   Liver
   Renal tubular epithelium
Capable at all times
   Bone marrow
   Skin
   Gastrointestinal epithelium
   Genitourinary epithelium
   Reproductive epithelium

SYSTEMIC FACTORS
Age
Nutrition
Hormones

LOCAL FACTORS
Site of lesion
Blood supply to area

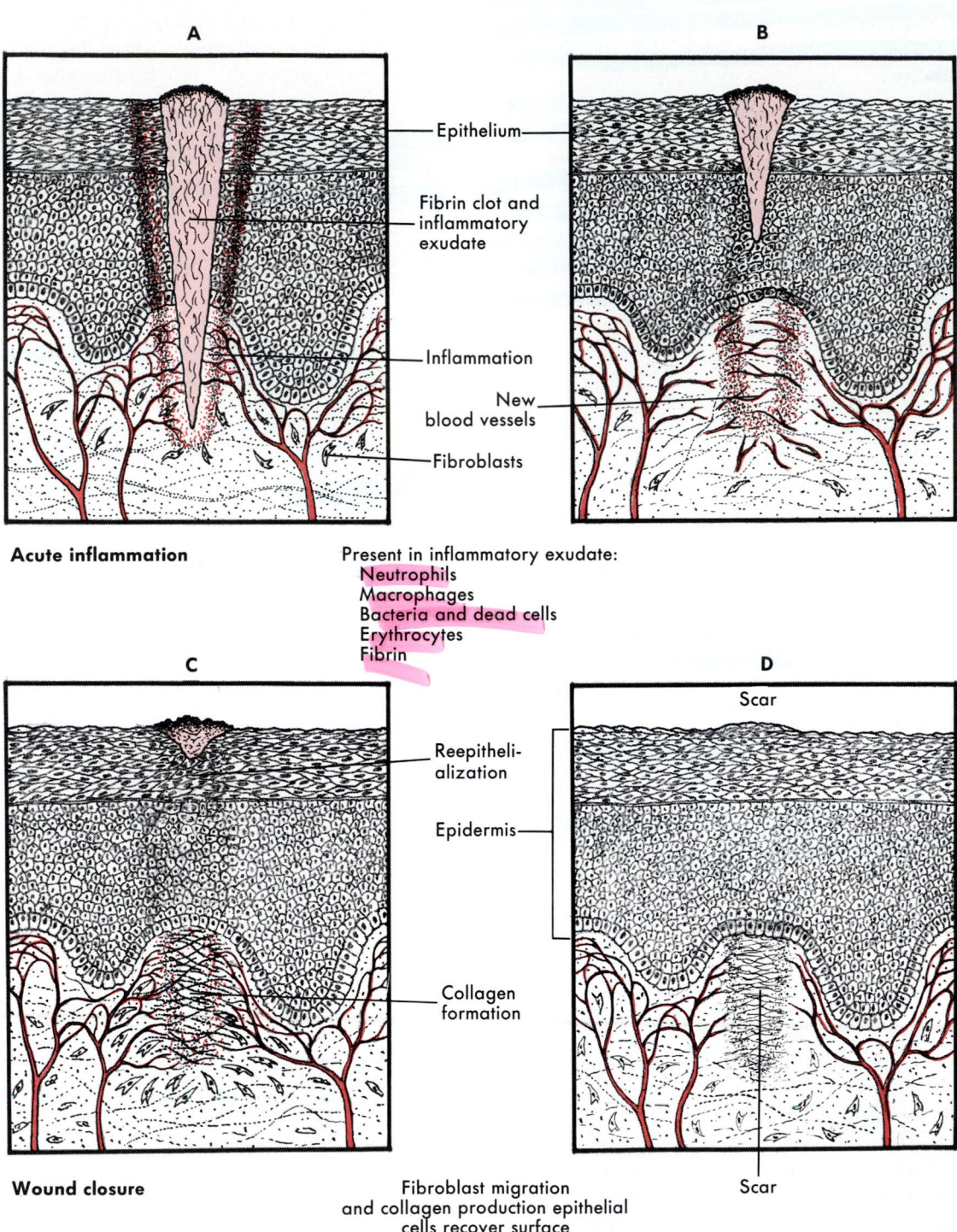

A

Epithelium

Fibrin clot and inflammatory exudate

Inflammation

New blood vessels

Fibroblasts

B

Acute inflammation

Present in inflammatory exudate:
Neutrophils
Macrophages
Bacteria and dead cells
Erythrocytes
Fibrin

C

Reepithelialization

Epidermis

Collagen formation

Scar

D

Scar

Wound closure

Fibroblast migration and collagen production epithelial cells recover surface

FIG. 7-22. Wound repair by primary or secondary intention.

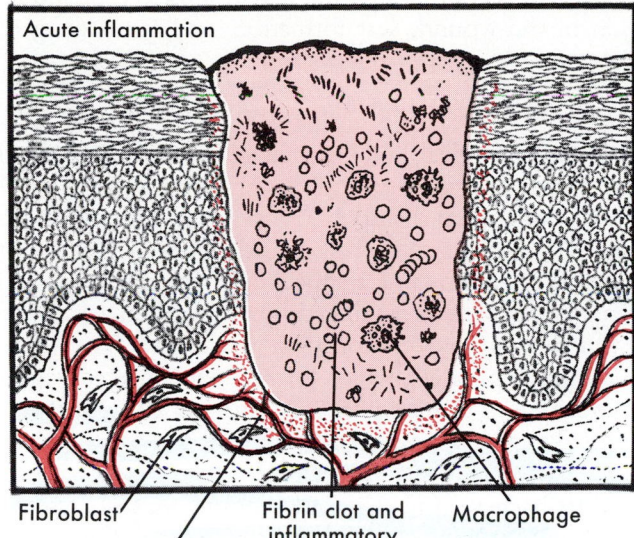

Acute inflammation

Fibroblast

Inflammation

Fibrin clot and inflammatory exudate

Macrophage

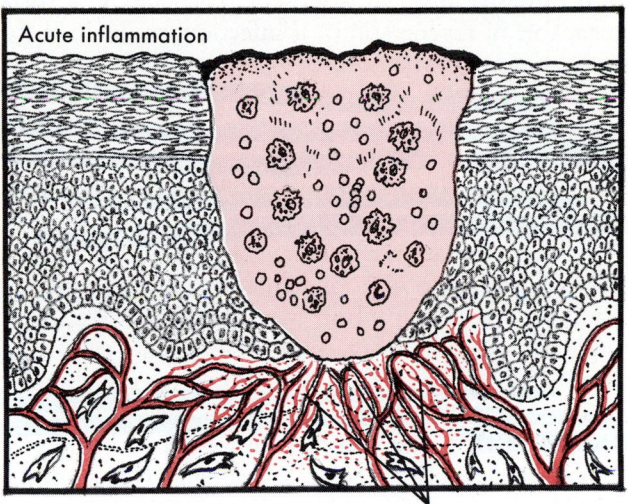

Acute inflammation

New blood vessels

Acute inflammation
Present in inflammatory exudate: neutrophils, macrophages, bacteria, dead cells, and erythrocytes.
Macrophages release (1) angiogenesis factor to attract epithelial cells and vascular endothelial cells (capillary and lymphatic buds) and (2) fibroblast-activating factor to attract fibroblasts.

Reconstructing phase
Epithelialization includes formation of granulation tissue, inward migration of fibroblasts, and the beginning of collagen synthesis and secretion.
Granulation tissue becomes scar tissue, contraction begins, and differentiation begins.

Maturation phase
This phase includes completion of contraction, differentiation, and remodeling of scar tissue, and disappearance of capillaries from scar tissue.

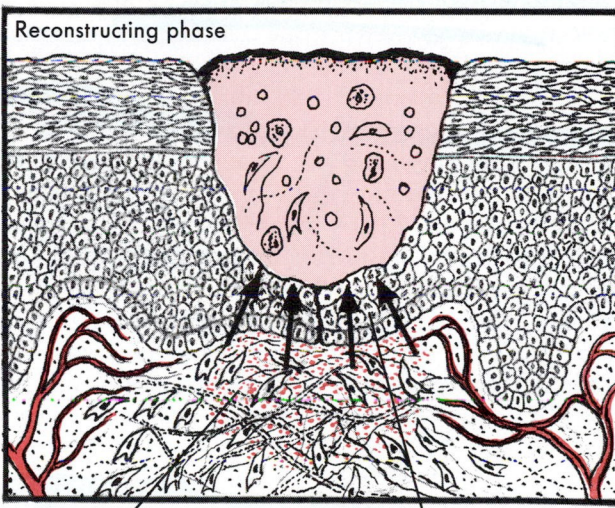

Reconstructing phase

Granulation tissue

Epithelialization

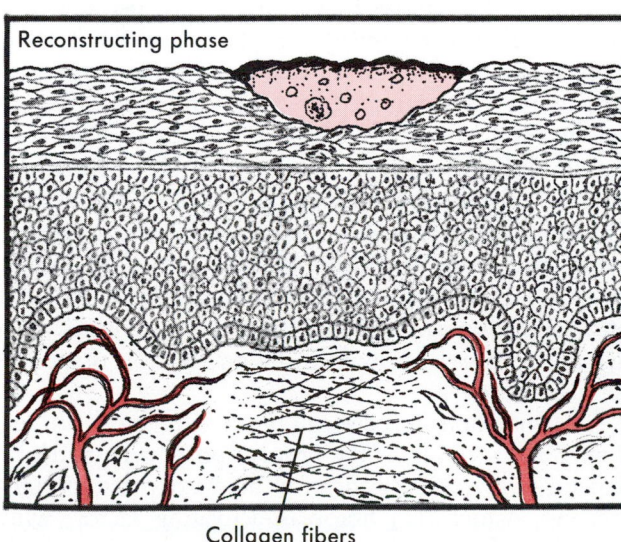

Reconstructing phase

Collagen fibers

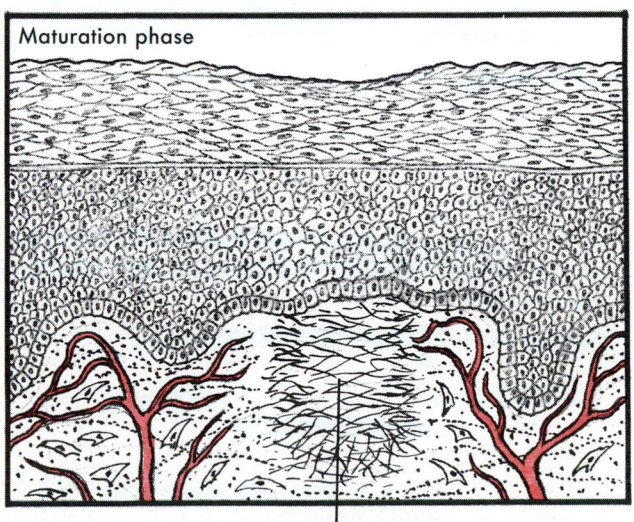

Maturation phase

Scar tissue

Fig 7-22, cont'd.

If extensive damage is present (particularly in tissues incapable of regeneration), if infection results in abscess or granuloma formation, or if fibrin persists in the lesion, resolution is not possible and repair takes place instead. **Repair** is the replacement of destroyed tissue with scar tissue. Scar tissue is composed of **collagen.** It fills in the lesion and restores tensile strength but cannot carry out the physiologic functions of destroyed tissue.

Both regeneration and repair begin during inflammation with phagocytosis of particulate matter in the inflammatory exudate (fibrin from dissolved clots, microorganisms, erythrocytes, and dead tissue cells). This cleanup of the lesion, which also involves dissolution of fibrin clots (or scabs) by fibrinolytic enzymes, is called **débridement.** After débridement, exudate, toxic products, and particulate matter are drained away, and vascular dilatation and permeability are reversed, preparing the lesion for either regeneration or repair.

Repair, which ends in the formation of scar tissue, always involves processes that (1) fill in the wound, (2) cover or seal the wound, and (3) shrink the wound. These common denominators of wound healing vary in importance and duration among different types of wounds. A clean incision, such as a "paper cut" or a sutured surgical wound, heals primarily through the process of collagen synthesis. Because sealing of this type of wound has already been facilitated by minimal tissue loss and apposition (joining) of the wound edges, very little sealing (epithelialization) and shrinkage (contraction) are required for healing. Wounds that heal under conditions of minimal tissue loss are said to heal by **primary intention** (Fig. 7-22).

Other wounds do not heal so neatly and easily. Healing of an open wound, such as a stage IV pressure sore (decubitus ulcer), requires a great deal more tissue replacement than healing of a surgical incision. With an open wound, epithelializaton, scar formation, and contraction takes longer, and healing occurs through **secondary intention** (Fig. 7-22). Healing by either primary or secondary intention may occur at different rates for different types of tissue and for different types of injury.

Resolution and repair occur in two overlapping phases. The first phase, called the **reconstructive phase,** begins 3 to 4 days after the initial injury and continues for up to 2 weeks. This phase is also known as the proliferative, fibroblastic, or connective tissue phase. During the reconstructive phase the lesion is characterized by fibroblast (connective tissue cell) proliferation, which is followed by collagen synthesis by the fibroblasts, epithelialization, and cellular differentiation.

The second phase, the **maturation phase,** begins several weeks post injury and is normally complete within 2 years. The maturation phase is also known as the differentiation, remodeling, or plateau phase. With maturation there is continuing differentiation of cells, contraction of the wound, scar formation, and remodeling of the scar.

Reconstructive Phase

Because surgical and perforative wounds exhibit all the phases of resolution and repair, they are useful models of both normal and abnormal (dysfunctional) healing. The wound is initially sealed off by a blood clot containing fibrin and trapped cells (erythrocytes and leukocytes). The cross-linked mesh of fibrin is created by activation of the coagulation cascade. The fibrin mesh traps platelets, which further seal damaged vessels by forming a platelet plug (see Chapter 22). Most surgical wounds are completely sealed with fibrin several hours after they have been closed. Sealing creates a barrier to bacterial invasion, although it does not always prevent it. The fibrin seal also helps to unite the wound edges. Fibrin provides a framework for the collagen molecules or regenerated tissue cells that will ultimately fill the wound.

For healing to proceed, the fibrin clot must be dissolved and replaced by normal tissue or scar tissue. Enzymatic digestion of the clot usually occurs after activation of the plasma fibrinolytic system (plasmin generation, see Chapter 22) or release of lysosomal enzymes from dead neutrophils. Macrophages invade the dissolving clot and clear away debris and dead cells by phagocytosis. Débridement by macrophages and remaining neutrophils is followed by simple resolution with regeneration of destroyed cells or, if regeneration is not possible, by the process of repair that ends in scar formation (see Fig. 7-22).

Repair begins as tissue called **granulation tissue** grows inward from surrounding healthy connective tissue. Granulation tissue is filled with new capillaries that give it a red, granular appearance and is surrounded by fibroblasts and macrophages. First, capillary buds sprout out of vascular endothelial cells around the wound and extend into the debrided areas. Loops form when the young capillaries join *(anastomose)*. The loops are more fragile and permeable than mature vessels, resulting in a leakage of erythrocytes and neutrophils. The erythrocytes are phagocytosed by macrophages, and the neutrophils participate in further débridement of the inflammatory lesion. Many of the new capillaries differentiate into arterioles and venules as repair continues. New lymphatic vessels grow into the granulation tissue by a similar process.

The macrophage performs several functions in healing. Besides acting as the primary phagocyte of débridement, it secretes biochemical mediators that promote healing, namely (1) fibroblast-activating factor, which stimulates fibroblasts to enter the lesion and synthesize and secrete the collagen precursor, procollagen; (2)

angiogenesis factor, which stimulates vascular endothelial cells to form capillary buds that grow into the lesion; and (3) an unidentified factor that stimulates epithelial cells to grow over and seal the wound's surface. Macrophages also secrete collagenase, which debrides injured collagen fibers in the wound.

As the clot or scab is being dissolved and granulation tissue is being formed, the healing wound must be protected. This is accomplished by **epithelialization,** the process by which epithelial cells grow into the wound from surrounding healthy tissue. Attracted by a factor secreted by macrophages, the epithelial cells migrate under the clot or scab, using proteolytic enzymes to sever the connection between the clot and the wound surface (see Fig. 7-22). Eventually the migrating epithelial cells contact similar cells from all sides of the wound, make contact, and seal the wound, after which migration and proliferation cease. The epithelial cells remain active, however, undergoing differentiation to give rise to the various epidermal layers (see Chapter 41). Epithelialization of a skin wound can be hastened if the wound is kept moist, preventing the fibrin clot from becoming a scab.

Fibroblasts are the most important cells during the reconstructive phase of wound healing because they synthesize and secrete collagen. Fibroblasts are stimulated by fibroblast-activating factor (from macrophages) to proliferate and enter the lesion. The collagen produced by fibroblasts is laid down in debrided areas about 6 days after fibroblasts have entered the lesion.

Collagen is the most abundant protein in the body and is the material of tissue repair. It is present in skin, bones, teeth, blood vessels, tendons, cartilage, and connective tissue. Collagen is produced in fibroblasts as a polypeptide of repeating sequences of the amino acids glycine, proline, hydroxyproline, lysine, and hydroxylysine. Proline and lysine are enzymatically hydroxylated after the polypeptide chain is synthesized, and their hydroxylation is absolutely necessary for collagen polymerization and function. Cofactors that are necessary for hydroxylation include iron, ascorbic acid (vitamin C), α-ketoglutarate (from the Krebs cycle), and molecular oxygen (O_2). Absence of these cofactors results in incomplete wound healing.

Immature collagen, termed **procollagen,** is secreted by the fibroblast as a complex of three polypeptide chains cross-linked by intermolecular bonds. Procollagen must be activated further by the removal of a small polypeptide sequence by a specific protease. As the scar tissue matures, collagen molecules are cross-linked by intramolecular bonds to form collagen fibrils. Cross-linking involves the formation of covalent bonds between lysine residues. At this point, the secreted collagen molecules are still of a gel-like consistency in the wound. With further cross-linking, the fibrils form fibers. This process occurs over a period of several months. The collagen is initially deposited randomly, but during remodeling of the scar tissue that has formed the fibers are dissolved by collagenase and reformed. During this period the fibers reorient along the lines of mechanical stress and further cross-linking adds strength.

Wound **contraction** is the final process of the reconstructive phase of healing. It is necessary for closure of all wounds, but especially of those that heal by secondary intention. Contraction is noticeable 6 to 12 days after injury. In normal healing contraction may amount to inward movement of the wound edge by approximately 0.5 mm per day.

The granulation tissue contains **myofibroblasts,** specialized cells that probably cause wound contraction. As the name implies, myofibroblasts have features of both smooth muscle cells and fibroblasts. Microscopically the myofibroblast appears similar to a fibroblast, but it differs in that its cytoplasm contains bundles of parallel fibers similar to those found in smooth muscle cells. These fibers exert a contractile force within the cell. Wound contraction occurs as structures extending from the plasma membrane of the myofibroblast establish connections with neighboring cells. Once connected, myofibroblasts can exert pull on neighboring cells and anchor themselves to the wound bed, promoting contraction.

Maturation Phase

Collagen deposition, tissue regeneration, and wound contraction all begin during the reconstructive phase. When this phase ends, about 2 weeks after injury, these processes are usually not complete. Therefore, they continue into the maturation phase, which can continue for years. During the maturation phase scar tissue is remodeled. Capillaries disappear, leaving an avascular scar. Within 2 to 3 weeks after maturation has begun, the scar tissue has gained about two thirds of its eventual maximum strength.

Epidermal wounds that heal by secondary intention and unsutured internal lesions are seldom completely restored by healing. At best repaired tissue regains 80% of its original tensile strength. Only epithelial, hepatic (liver), and bone marrow cells are capable of the complete mitotic regeneration known as compensatory hyperplasia (hyperplasia is described in Chapter 2). In fibrous connective tissue, such as joints and ligaments, normal healing results in the replacement of the original tissue, but the new tissue does not have exactly the same structure as the original. Some damaged tissue heals without replacement. For instance, the damage resulting from myocardial infarction heals with a scar composed of fibrous tissue rather than replacing cardiac muscle. Although the composition of healed tissue may differ, the healing process of soft tissues is the same for all wounds.

Dysfunctional Wound Healing

Dysfunctional healing may occur during any phase of the wound-healing process and may involve insufficient repair, excessive repair, or infection. The etiology of dysfunctional healing can be related to a predisposing disorder, such as diabetes mellitus, or to an acquired condition, such as hypoxemia (insufficient oxygen in arterial blood). Numerous drugs and nutrients can also affect wound healing. Wound repair delays healing by reactivating inflammatory processes.

Dysfunction During the Inflammatory Response

Healing may be prolonged if bleeding is not stopped during acute inflammation. Hemorrhage in a damaged area delays healing for several reasons. A clot increases the amount of space that granulation tissue has to fill and serves as a mechanical barrier to oxygen diffusion. The accumulation of excess blood cells resulting from hemorrhage prolongs the inflammatory process, since these cells must be cleared prior to repair. Accumulated blood, which is an excellent culture medium for bacteria, promotes infection and prolongs inflammation by increasing exudation and pus formation. In addition to slowing healing, sepsis can promote excessive scar formation or prevent healing completely.

Excessive amounts of fibrin are also detrimental to healing. The great amount of fibrin that is released in response to injury must eventually be reabsorbed so it will not organize into fibrous adhesions. Adhesions are seldom clinically significant unless they form in the pleural, pericardial, or abdominal cavities. Adhesions in these areas may bind organs together by fibrous bands, the shrinkage of which can distort or strangulate the affected organ.

Many factors may adversely effect the inflammatory process during wound healing. Hypovolemia decreased blood volume inhibits inflammation. The physiologic response to hypovolemia is vessel constriction rather than the dilatation required to deliver inflammatory cells to the site of injury. Anti-inflammatory steroids prevent macrophages from migrating to the site of injury and inhibit their release of collagenase and plasminogen activator (Alvarez et al., 1984). Anti-inflammatory steroids also inhibit fibroblast migration into the wound during the reconstructive phase of healing.

Optimal nutrition is important during all phases of healing because metabolic needs are increased. During inflammation the substances most essential for healing are glucose, oxygen, and protein. Because leukocytes need glucose to produce the adenosine triphosphate 5'(ATP) needed for chemotaxis, phagocytosis, and intercellular killing, the wounds of diabetics who receive insufficient insulin heal poorly, mainly because of infection. Diabetics are at risk for ischemic wounds because they are likely to have both small-vessel diseases that impair the microcirculation and altered (glycosylated) hemoglobin, which has an increased affinity for oxygen and thus does not readily release oxygen in tissues. (Hemoglobin's function as the oxygen-carrying component of blood is described in Chapter 22.) Oxygen delivery is also compromised by hypoxemic states. Ischemic tissue is susceptible to infection, which prolongs inflammation. Hypoproteinemia also prolongs inflammation because it impairs fibroblast proliferation.

Wound sepsis is treated in several ways. Most important is the removal or debridement of necrotic tissue and foreign bodies. Débridement is accomplished by surgery or use of absorbent dressings. Wound irrigation and antibiotic therapy also combat infection.

Dysfunction During the Reconstructive Phase

Impaired Collagen Synthesis

A number of factors may interfere with the production of collagen in healing tissues. Most of these factors are nutritional. Scurvy, for example, is a condition due to lack of ascorbic acid. Ascorbic acid is one of the cofactors required for the hydroxylation of the amino acids proline and lysine. Without hydroxylation these amino acids cannot be incorporated into collagen monomers; therefore, procollagen is not secreted from the fibroblast. The results of scurvy are poorly formed connective tissue and greatly impaired healing.

Other nutrients play a cofactor role in enzyme systems required for collagen synthesis. These include iron, oxygen, α-ketoglutarate, manganese, copper, and calcium. Usually such minute amounts of these substances are required as cofactors that deficiencies are not clinically significant.

Protein is essential for collagen synthesis. Especially important is the amino acid methionine, which is converted to cystine. The role of cystine in collagen synthesis is twofold: (1) it functions as an important cofactor in enzyme systems required for collagen synthesis; and (2) it contains sulfur, which contributes to the formation of strong disulfide bonds in cross-linked collagen fibrils.

Collagen synthesis may be impaired during the processes of polymerization and cross-linking. After procollagen is secreted from the fibroblast, it must be activated by cleavage of its terminal peptides. Cleavage does not occur, for example, in individuals with Ehlers-Danlos syndrome (type VII). This disease prevents formation of normal connective tissue, causing the skin to be thin and fragile. All forms of Ehlers-Danlos syndrome are characterized by defects in collagen cross-linking. (The role of collagen in bone formation is described in Chapter 38.)

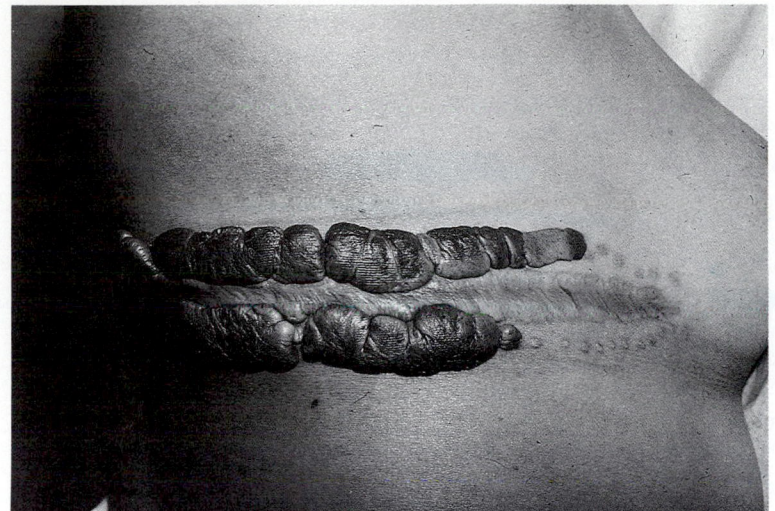

FIG. 7-23. Scar caused by excessive synthesis of collagen. Keloid from suture marks in a black individual. (From Habif, 1984.)

Dysfunctional collagen synthesis may also involve excessive production of collagen. This causes surface overhealing, which is manifested by a keloid or a hypertrophic scar (Fig. 7-23). Both keloid and hypertrophic scars are due to an imbalance between collagen synthesis and collagen lysis in which synthesis is increased and lysis (degradation) is decreased. A **keloid** is a raised scar that extends beyond the original boundaries of the wound. It invades surrounding tissue and is likely to recur after surgical removal. A familial tendency to keloid formation has been observed, with a greater incidence in blacks than whites. A **hypertrophic scar** is raised but remains within the original boundaries of the wound. Hypertrophic scars tend to regress over time.

Impaired Epithelialization

Epithelialization is suppressed by anti-inflammatory steroids, hypoxemia, ionizing radiation, and zinc deficiencies. Wound care technique may greatly influence epithelial cell migration.

External wounds that are draining or healing by secondary intention are often debrided and protected with dressings. The ideal dressing is one that absorbs some drainage without being incorporated into the clot or granulation tissue. Because epithelial cells must migrate across the wound during healing, dressings that debride healthy epithelial cells along with necrotic tissue prolong epithelialization.

Many solutions that have traditionally been used to clean or irrigate wounds are deleterious to the fragile new cells in the wound bed. Normal saline is the most innocuous solution that can be used to cleanse or irrigate a wound that is healing primarily by epithelialization. Solutions such as povidone-iodine and hydrogen peroxide are very desiccating (drying) and subsequently inhibit rather than promote epithelial cell migration.

Wound Disruption

A potential complication of wounds that are sutured closed is **dehiscence,** in which the wound pulls apart at the suture line. The greatest incidence of dehiscence occurs 5 to 12 days after suturing. Paradoxically this is the time when collagen synthesis is at its peak. Approximately 50% of the time dehiscence is associated with wound sepsis. It may also occur when sutures break due to excessive strain. Obesity increases the risk for dehiscence because adipose tissue is difficult to suture. Wound dehiscence is usually heralded by an increase in serous drainage from the wound. Additionally the individual may report a feeling that "something gave way." Prompt surgical attention is required.

Impaired Contraction

Wound contraction is necessary for healing. This process may become pathologic when there is excessive contraction resulting in a deformity or **contracture.** Burns are especially susceptible to the development of contractures. Internal contracture may occur in cirrhosis of the liver. Scar tissue that becomes contracted constricts vascular flow, which may contribute to the development of portal hypertension and esophageal varices. Other types of internal contraction deformity include duodenal strictures due to dysfunctional healing of an ulcer and esophageal strictures due to lye burns.

Proper positioning and range-of-motion exercises and surgery are among the physical means used to overcome myofibroblast pull and prevent contractures. Biochemical means include control of myofibroblast contraction by the administration of smooth muscle inhibitors (e.g., colchicine and triphenamil hydrochloride [Trocinate]) and attempts to inhibit collagen synthesis with drugs that prevent collagen cross-linking or collagenase activity. This treatment is based on the knowledge that collagen can "lock" contracted myofibroblasts into position. Clinical use of pharmacologic methods for control of wound contracture is still largely experimental.

AGING AND MECHANISMS OF SELF-DEFENSE

Besides immature or depressed immune function, neonates frequently have transiently depressed inflammatory function. For example, neutrophils and perhaps monocytes may not be capable of chemotaxis. Insufficient response to chemotactic factors appears to be due to lack of fluidity in the phagocyte's plasma membrane, so that it cannot form pseudopods and migrate. Neonates are prone to infections associated with chemotactic defects, including cutaneous abscesses due to staphylococci and cutaneous candidiasis. Furthermore, neutrophils in neonates stressed by in utero infection or respiratory insufficiency have diminished oxidative and bacterial responses. (Acquired phagocytic defects, which may be induced by a variety of infections, metabolic disorders, nutrition deficiencies, or drugs, are described in Chapter 8.)

Neonates are also partially deficient in complement, especially components of the alternative pathway. They tend to have a relative deficiency of factor B and to develop severe, overwhelming sepsis and meningitis when infected with bacteria against which there is no transferred maternal antibody.

The elderly population is at risk for impaired wound healing. There is no concrete evidence that impaired wound healing is a consequence of normal aging, however. Often impaired healing is associated with chronic illnesses, such as diabetes mellitus or cardiovascular disease. Additionally many elderly persons require medications, such as anti inflammatory steroids, that interfere with healing.

Because of impaired sensation or mobility and physiologic changes in the skin, the elderly are at increased risk for sustaining various wounds. With aging subcutaneous fat is lost, diminishing a layer of protection. Collagen fibers become thicker and less elastic, thus further contributing to loss of protection.

Diminished immune function may interfere with the elderly person's natural ability to ward off infection in a wound. The regenerative capability of the skin is maintained with aging, but the epidermis undergoes some atrophy that includes atrophy of underlying capillaries. The consequent decrease of perfusion makes the elderly more susceptible than others to the adverse effects of hypoxia (insufficient oxygen) in the wound bed.

SUMMARY REVIEW

1 Inflammation is a rapid and nonspecific protective response to cellular injury from any cause. It can occur only in vascularized tissue.

2 The macroscopic hallmarks of inflammation are redness, swelling, heat, pain, and loss of function of the inflamed tissues.

3 The microscopic hallmark of inflammation is an accumulation of fluid and cells at the inflammatory site.

4 The most important activator of the inflammatory response is the mast cell, which initiates inflammation by releasing biochemical mediators (histamine, chemotactic factors) from preformed cytoplasmic granules and synthesizing other mediators (prostaglandins, leukotrienes) in response to a stimulus.

5 Histamine and serotinin are the major vasoactive amines of inflammation. Both cause constriction of vascular smooth muscles, dilation of capillaries, and retraction of endothelial cells lining the capillaries, which increases vascular permeability.

6 Inflammation is mediated by three key plasma protein systems: the complement system, the clotting system, and the kinin system. The components of all three systems are a series of inactive proteins (proenzymes) that are activated in cascade fashion.

7 The complement system can be activated by antigen-antibody reactions (through the classical pathway) or by other products, especially bacterial polysaccharides (through the alternate pathway), resulting in the production of biologically active (anaphylatoxic or chemotactic) fragments and target cell lysis.

8 The cells involved in the inflammatory process include phagocytic leukocytes (neutrophils, macrophages, and eosinophils), platelets, and lymphocytes.

9 Phagocytic cells engulf and destroy microorganisms by enclosing them in phagocytic vacuoles (phagolysosomes), within which toxic products (especially metabolites of oxygen) and degradative lysosomal enzymes kill and digest the microorganisms.

10 Opsonins, such as antibody and complement component C3b, coat microorganisms and make them more susceptible to phagocytosis by binding them more tightly to the phagocyte.

11 The polymorphonuclear neutrophil (PMN), the predominant phagocytic cell in the early inflammatory response, exits the circulation by diapedesis through the retracted endothelial cell junctions and moves to the inflammatory site by chemotaxis.

12 The macrophage, the predominant phagocytic cell in the late inflammatory response, is highly phagocytic, responsive to lymphokines, and responsible for antigen processing and presentation to lymphocytes.

13 Eosinophils release products that control the inflammatory response and are induced by IgE-mediated mechanisms of hypersensitivity to kill parasitic organisms directly.

14 The cells involved in immunity and inflammation stim-

ulate other cells by secreting lymphokines, interferons, or interleukins.

15 Lymphokines are produced by T cells and have their most important effects on macrophages. These effects include chemotaxis, inhibition of migration once the macrophage has entered the inflammatory site, and activation of the macrophage, which makes it a more powerful phagocyte.

16 Interferons are produced by host cells that are already infected by viruses. Once released from infected cells, interferons can stimulate neighboring healthy cells to produce substances that prevent viral penetration.

17 Interleukins are produced by leukocytes that have been stimulated by an antigen. Interleukins stimulate other leukocytes to proliferate or otherwise increase their immune functions. The chief effect of interleukins is to accelerate the immune response.

18 The systemic effects of inflammation are fever and increases in levels of circulating leukocytes and plasma proteins.

19 Local manifestations of inflammation all involve the same hallmarks of inflammation, but types of exudate and necrosis vary with the injury and the tissue or organ affected.

20 Inflammatory lesions proceed to resolution if little tissue has been lost or injured tissue is capable of regeneration. This is called healing by primary intention.

21 Inflammatory lesions that involve extensive damage or tissues incapable of regeneration heal by repair. This process is called healing by secondary intention.

KEY TERMS

Abscess, 239

Acute-phase reactant, 237

Alternative pathway, 223

Anaphylatoxin, 223

Antigen-antibody complex (immune complex), 223

Basophil, 220

Bradykinin, 225

Chemotactic factor, 221

Chemotaxis, 221

Classical pathway, 223

Collagen, 242

Complement cascade, 223

Contraction, 243

Contracture, 245

Cyst, 239

Débridement, 242

Degranulation, 220

Dehiscence, 245

Diapedesis, 229

Eosinophil, 233

Epithelialization, 243

Epithelioid cell, 238

Extrinsic pathway, 225

Exudate, 217

Fibrinous exudate, 239

Fibroblast, 243

Giant cell, 238

Granulation tissue, 242

Granuloma, 238

Hemorrhagic exudate, 239

Hypertrophic scar, 245

Interferon, 235

Interleukin (IL), 236

Intrinsic pathway, 225

Keloid, 245

Leukotriene (slow-reacting substance of anaphylaxis [SRS-A]), 221

Lymphokine, 235

Macrophage, 232

Macrophage-activating factor (MAF), 235

Margination (pavementing), 229

Mast cell, 220

Maturation phase, 242

Migration-inhibitory factor (MIF), 235

Monocyte, 232

Myofibroblast, 243

Neutrophil, 231

Phagocytosis, 229

Phagolysosome, 230

Phagosome, 230

Plasma kinin cascade, 225

Platelet, 218

Polymorphonuclear neutrophil (PMN), 231

Primary intention, 242

Procollagen, 243

Proenzyme, 222

Prostaglandin, 221

Purulent (suppurative) exudate, 239

Reconstructive phase, 242

Regeneration, 239

Repair, 242

Resolution, 239

Secondary intention, 242

Serous exudate, 239

REFERENCES

Alvarez, O. M., Levendorf, K. D., Smerbeck, R. V., Mertz, P. M., & Eaglstein, W. H. (1984). Effect of topically applied steroidal and nonsteroidal anti-inflammatory agents on skin repair and regeneration. *Federation Proceedings, 43,* 2793-2798.

Carrico, T. J., Mehrhof, A. I., & Cohen, I. K. (1984). Biology of wound healing. *Surgical Clinics of North America, 64,* 721-733.

Cohen, I. K., & McCoy, B. J. (1980). The biology and control of surface overhealing. *World Journal of Surgery, 4,* 289-295.

Cohen, I. K., McCoy, B. J., & Diegelmann, R. F. (1979). An update on wound healing. *Annals of Plastic Surgery, 3,* 264-272.

Diegelmann, R. F., Cohen, I. K., & Kaplan, A. M. (1981). The role of macrophages in wound repair: A review. *Plastic and Reconstructive Surgery, 68,* 107-113.

Dinarello, C. A., & Mier, J. W. (1987). Current concepts: Lymphokines. *New England Journal of Medicine, 317,* 940-945.

Ehrlich, P. (1877). Dietbage zur Kenntnis der Anilinsfarb und Ihrer Verwendung nin ungen der Mikroskopichen technik. *Arch Mikr Anat, 13,* 263-277.

Ellis, H. (1980). Internal overhealing: The problem of intraperitoneal adhesions. *World Jounal of Surgery, 4,* 303-306.

Evans, P. (1980). The healing process at cellular level: A review. *Physiotherapy, 66,* 256-259.

Fernandez, A., & Finley, J. M. (1983). Wound healing: Helping a natural process. *Postgraduate Medicine, 74,* 311-317.

Habif, T. P. (1984). *Clinical dermatology.* St. Louis: C. V. Mosby.

Henson, P. M. 1985. Mechanisms of tissue injury produced by immunologic reactions. In J. A. Bellanti (Ed.), *Immunology III.* (p. 251.) Philadelphia: W.B. Saunders.

Hotter, A. N. (1982). Physiologic aspects of clinical implications of wound healing. *Heart & Lung, 11,* 522-531.

Hunt, T. K. (1980). Disorders of wound healing. *World Journal of Surgery, 4,* 271-277.

Hunt, T. K., & Dunphy, J. E. (1979). *Fundamentals of wound management.* New York: Appleton-Century-Crofts.

King, D. W., Fenoglio, C. M., & Lefwitch, J. H. 1983. *General pathology: Principles and Dynamics.* Philadelphia: Lea & Febiger. Courtesy of Jan Orenstein, The George Washington University Center, Washington, D. C.

Lachman, L. B., & Maizel, A. L. (1983). The interleukins: Immunoregulatory molecules. *Clinical Immunology Newsletter, 4,* 113-115.

Malech, H. L., & Gallen, J. I. (1987). Current concepts—immunobiology: Neutrophils in human diseases. *New England Journal of Medicine, 317,* 687-693.

Milanese, C., Richardson, N. E., & Reinherz, E. L. (1986). Identification of a T helper cell-derived lymphokine that activates resting T lymphocytes. *Science, 231*(4742), 1118-1122.

Moncada S., & Vane, J. R. (1984). Prostacyclin and its clinical applications. *Annals of Clinical Research, 16,* 241-252.

Ross, R. (1980). Contraction and control of contraction. *World Journal of Surgery, 4,* 279-287.

Ruberg, R. L. (1984). Role of nutrition in wound healing. *Surgical Clinics of North America, 64,* 705-714.

Serafin, W. E., & Austen, K. F. (1987). Current concepts: Mediators of immediate hypersensitivity reactions. *New England Journal of Medicine, 317,* 30-34.

Taussig, M. J. (1979). *Processes in pathology.* Oxford: Blackwell Scientific Publishers.

Tobin, G. R. (1984). Closure of contaminated wounds. *Surgical Clinics of North America, 64,* 639-652.

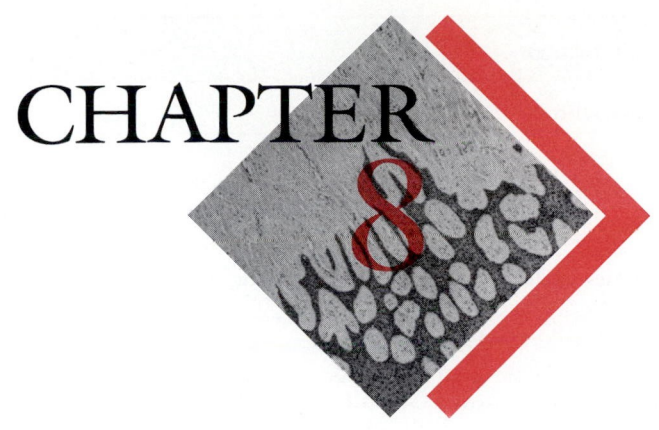

CHAPTER 8

Alterations in Immunity and Inflammation

Neal S. Rote

Hypersensitivity: allergy, autoimmunity, and isoimmunity, 249
  Mechanisms of hypersensitivity, 252
    IgE-mediated reactions, 252
      Role of IgE, 253
      Mechanisms of IgE-mediated hypersensitivity, 253
      Clinical manifestations, 254
      Genetic predisposition, 255
      Tests of IgE-mediated hypersensitivity, 255
      Desensitization, 255
    Tissue-specific reactions, 255
    Immune-complex–mediated injury, 257
      Mechanisms, 257
      Immune-complex disease, 258
        Serum sickness, 258
        Arthus reaction, 258
    Cell-mediated tissue destruction, 258
  Targets of hypersensitivity, 260
    Allergy, 260
    Autoimmunity, 261
      Breakdown of tolerance, 261
        Sequestered antigen, 261
        Neoantigen, 261
        Infectious disease, 261
        Forbidden clone, 261
        Suppressor cell dysfunction, 261
      Original insult, 262
      Genetic factors, 262
    Isoimmunity, 262
  Autoimmune and isoimmune diseases, 263
    Systemic lupus erythematosus, 263
    Graft rejection, 264
Deficiencies in immunity and inflammation, 265
  Congenital immune deficiencies, 266
  Acquired deficiencies, 268
    Nutritional deficiencies, 268
    Iatrogenic deficiencies, 268
    Deficiencies caused by trauma, 269
    Deficiencies caused by stress, 269
    Acquired Immune Deficiency Syndrome (AIDS), 269
      Epidemiology, 269
      Etiology, 270

      Clinical manifestations, 273
      Treatment, 274
  Clinical evaluation of immunity, 274
  Replacement therapies for immune deficiencies, 274
    Gamma globulin therapy, 274
    Transplantation and transfusion, 275

The immune system is a finely tuned network that protects the host against foreign antigens, particularly infectious agents. Sometimes this network breaks down, causing the immune system to react inappropriately. Inappropriate immune responses may be (1) exaggerated against environmental antigens (allergy), (2) misdirected against the host's own cells (autoimmunity), (3) directed against beneficial foreign tissues, such as transfusions or transplants (isoimmunity), or (4) insufficient for protection (immune deficiency). All of these can be serious or life-threatening. Exaggerated immune responses (allergy) are the most common and usually the least life-threatening.

HYPERSENSITIVITY: ALLERGY, AUTOIMMUNITY, AND ISOIMMUNITY

The first three types of inappropriate responses listed above can be collectively classified as **hypersensitivity.** Hypersensitivity is an altered immunologic reactivity to an antigen that results in a pathologic immune response after reexposure. Allergy, autoimmunity, and isoimmunity are differentiated by the source of the antigen against which the hypersensitivity response is directed (Table 8-1). The term **allergy** originally denoted both facets of the immune response: immunity, which is beneficial, and hypersensitivity, which is harmful. Allergy

TABLE 8-1   Relative incidences and examples of hypersensitivity reactions

	Mechanism			
Target antigen	I (IgE- mediated)	II (tissue-specific)	III (immune- complex)	IV (cell- mediated)
Allergy (Environmental antigens)	++++ Hay fever	+ Hemolysis in drug allergies	+ Gluten (wheat) allergy	++ Poison ivy allergy
Autoimmunity (Self-antigens)	± May contribute to some Type III reactions	++ Autoimmune thrombocytopenia	+++ Systemic lupus erythematosus	+ Hashimoto's thyroiditis
Isoimmunity (Other person's antigens)	± May contribute to some Type III reactions	++ Hemolytic disease of the newborn	+ Anaphylaxis to IgA in IV gamma globulin	++ Graft rejection

The frequency of each reaction is indicated in a range from rare (±) to very common (++++). An example of each reaction is given.

has come to mean the deleterious effects of hypersensitivity to environmental (exogenous) antigens, and immunity the protective responses to antigens expressed by disease-causing agents.

Autoimmunity is a disturbance in the immunologic tolerance of self-antigens. A great variety of clinical disorders are associated with autoimmunity and are referred to as **autoimmune diseases** (Table 8-2). Autoimmune diseases occur when the immune system reacts against self-antigens and destroys host tissues. Antibod-

TABLE 8-2   Disorders associated with autoimmunity

System disease	Organ or tissue	Probable self-antigen
ENDOCRINE SYSTEM		
Hyperthyroidism (Graves' disease)	Thyroid gland	Receptors for thyroid-stimulating hormone on plasma membrane of thyroid cells
Autoimmune thyroiditis	Thyroid gland	Thyroglobulin; microsomes
Primary myxedema	Thyroid gland	Microsomes
Insulin-dependent diabetes	Pancreas	Islet cells, insulin, insulin receptors on pancreatic cells
Addison's disease	Adrenal gland	Surface antigens on steroid producing cells; microsomes of adrenal cortex
Premature gonadal failure	Ovary	Interstitial cells; corpus luteum
Male infertility	Testis	Surface antigens on spermatozoa
Orchitis	Testis	Germinal epithelium
Female infertility	Ovary	Zona pellucida
Idiopathic hypoparathyroidism	Parathyroid gland	Surface antigens on chief cells (epithelial cells of gland)
Partial pituitary deficiency	Pituitary gland	Prolactin-producing cells; growth-hormone-producing cells
SKIN		
Pemphigus vulgaris	Skin	Intercellular substances in stratified squamous epithelium
Bullous pemphigoid	Skin	Basement membrane
Dermatitis herpetiformis	Skin	Basement membrane (IgA)
Vitiligo	Skin	Surface antigens on melanocytes (melanin-producing cells)

TABLE 8-2 Disorders associated with autoimmunity—cont'd

System disease	Organ or tissue	Probable self-antigen
NEUROMUSCULAR TISSUE		
Polymyositis (dermatomyositis)	Muscle	Nuclear materials; myosin
Multiple sclerosis	Neural tissue	Unknown
Myasthenia gravis	Neuromuscular junction	Acetylcholine receptors; striations of skeletal and cardiac muscle
Polyneuritis	Nerve cell	Peripheral myelin
Rheumatic fever	Heart	Cardiac tissue (subsarcolemmal membrane); cross-reaction with group A streptococcal antigen
Cardiomyopathy	Heart	Cardiac muscle
Postvaccinal or postinfectious encephalitis	Central nervous system	Central nervous system myelin or basic protein
GASTROINTESTINAL SYSTEM		
Celiac disease (gluten-sensitive enteropathy)	Intestine	Gluten
Ulcerative colitis	Colon	Mucosal cells
Crohn's disease	Ileum	Unknown
Pernicious anemia	Stomach	Surface antigens of parietal cells; intrinsic factor
Atrophic gastritis	Stomach	Parietal cells
Primary biliary cirrhosis	Liver	Mitochondria; cells of bile duct
Chronic active hepatitis	Liver	Surface antigens, nuclei, microsomes, mitochondria or hepatocytes; smooth muscle
CONNECTIVE TISSUE		
Ankylosing spondylitis	Joints	Sacroiliac and spinal apophyseal joint
Rheumatoid arthritis	Joints	IgG, collagen
Systemic lupus erythematosus	Multiple sites	Numerous antigens in nuclei, organelles, and extracellular matrix
Mixed connective tissue disease	Multiple sites	Ribonucleoprotein and numerous others
Polyarteritis nodosa (necrotizing vasculitis)	Arterioles (small arteries)	Unknown
Scleroderma (progressive systemic sclerosis)	Multiple organs	Nuclear antigens; IgG
Felty's syndrome	Joints	IgG
EYE		
Sjögren's syndrome	Lacrimal gland	Antigens of lacrimal gland, salivary gland, thyroid, and nuclei of cells; IgG
Uveitis	Uveal structures	Antigens of the iris, ciliary body, and choroid
RENAL SYSTEM		
Immune-complex glomerulonephritis	Kidney	Numerous immune complexes
Goodpasture's disease	Kidney	Glomerular basement membrane
HEMATOLOGIC SYSTEM		
Idiopathic neutropenia	Neutrophil	Surface antigens on polymorphonuclear neutrophils
Idiopathic lymphopenia	Lymphocytes	Surface antigens on lymphocytes
Autoimmune hemolytic anemia	Erythrocytes	Surface antigens on erythrocytes
Autoimmune thrombocytopenic purpura	Platelets	Surface antigens on platelets
RESPIRATORY SYSTEM		
Goodpasture's disease	Lung	Septal membrane of alveolus

ies against self-antigens, termed **autoantibodies,** are also produced by healthy individuals, particularly the elderly. In fact, part of the aging process may, in part, represent a deterioration of tolerance to self-antigens. Healthy individuals of all ages may produce autoantibodies, without concurrent overt autoimmune disease, in response to tissue damage. Therefore, the presence of low quantities of autoantibodies does not necessarily indicate a disease state.

Isoimmune diseases occur when the immune system of one individual produces an immunologic reaction against tissues of another individual. **Isoimmunity** can be observed during immunologic reactions against transfusions, grafted tissue, or the fetus during pregnancy.

The pathogenesis of hypersensitivity, whether it consists of allergy, autoimmunity, or isoimmunity, is not completely understood. It is generally accepted that genetic, infectious, and possibly environmental factors contribute to hypersensitivity. Most diseases caused by hypersensitivity evolve because of the interactions of at least three variables: (1) an original insult, which alters **immunologic homeostasis** (a steady state of tolerance to self-antigens; more important in autoimmunity than in isoimmunity or allergy); (2) the individual's genetic makeup, which determines susceptibility to the effects of the insult; and (3) an immunologic process that amplifies the insult.

Mechanisms of Hypersensitivity

Diseases due to hypersensitivity are also characterized by immune mechanisms that initiate inflammation and result in the destruction of healthy tissue (Table 8-1). These mechanisms are apparent in most hypersensitivity reactions and have been divided into four distinct types:

(1) type I (IgE-mediated allergic reactions), (2) type II (tissue-specific reactions), (3) type III (immune-complex-mediated reactions), and (4) type IV (cell-mediated reactions) (Gell, Coombs, & Lachman, 1975) (Table 8-3). This classification is artificial and seldom is a particular disease associated with a single mechanism only. The four mechanisms are interrelated and, in most hypersensitivity reactions, several are at work simultaneously. Some of them are secondary to disease, whereas others are pathognomonic (diagnostic of) and the primary cause of tissue destruction.

Hypersensitivity reactions are immediate or delayed, depending on the time required to elicit the secondary immune response (i.e., for the reaction to appear after reexposure to the antigen). Reactions that occur within minutes are termed **immediate hypersensitivity reactions. Delayed hypersensitivity reactions** may take several hours to appear and are at maximum severity days after reexposure to the antigen.

The most rapid immediate hypersensitivity reaction is anaphylaxis. **Anaphylaxis** is a rapid and severe response that occurs within minutes of reexposure to the antigen and can be either systemic (generalized) or cutaneous (localized) (Portier & Richet, 1902). Individuals with systemic anaphylaxis present with itching, erythema, vomiting, abdominal cramps, diarrhea, and breathing difficulties. In severe cases, laryngeal edema and vascular collapse may result in respiratory distress, decreased blood pressure, shock, and death. Cutaneous anaphylaxis causes the less severe symptoms of local inflammation.

IgE-Mediated Reactions

Type I reactions are characterized by the production of antigen-specific IgE after exposure to an antigen.

TABLE 8-3   Immunologic mechanisms of tissue destruction

Type	Name	Rate of development	Class of antibody involved	Principal effector cells involved	Complement participation	Examples of disorders
I	IgE-mediated reaction	Immediate	IgE	Mast cells	No	Seasonal allergic rhinitis
II	Tissue-specific reaction	Immediate	IgG IgM	Macrophages in tissues	Frequently	Autoimmune thrombocytopenic purpura, Graves' disease, Autoimmune hemolytic anemia
III	Immune-complex-mediated reaction	Immediate	IgG IgM	Neutrophils	Yes	Systemic lupus erythematosus
IV	Cell-mediated reaction	Delayed	None	Lymphocytes Macrophages	No	Contact sensitivity to poison ivy and metals

Most common allergic reactions are mediated by IgE and are, therefore, type I reactions. In addition, most type I reactions are against environmental antigens and are, therefore, allergic. Antigens that cause allergic responses are called **allergens.** It is not known why some antigens are allergens and others are not, but most allergens appear to be proteins that enter the host from the environment.

Role of IgE

In some individuals, exposure to an allergen causes IgE production by selected B cells. Repeated exposure to relatively large doses of allergen is usually required to elicit enough IgE so that the person is "sensitized." IgE binds to Fc receptors on the plasma membranes of mast cells (Fig. 8-1). The Fc region of IgE and the subclass IgG4 have binding sites specific for receptors on the mast cell. Antibody that binds to mast cells is termed **cytotropic** (able to bind to cell surfaces). **Reagin,** or skin-sensitizing antibody, has been used interchangeably with the term cytotropic antibody. The Fc receptors on mast cells bind with IgE that has not previously interacted with antigen.

After the individual is sensitized, and with further exposure to the allergen, the allergen's antigenic determinants bind to two molecules of mast-cell-bound IgE, cross-linking two IgE-Fc receptor complexes and initiating degranulation of the mast cell and the release of a plethora of mast cell products (see Chapter 6). Sometimes the IgE-mediated allergic response is beneficial to the host as is the case with IgE-mediated destruction of parasites. (This mechanism is described in Chapter 7 and illustrated in Fig. 7-18.)

Mechanisms of IgE-mediated Hypersensitivity

The products of mast cell degranulation can modulate almost all aspects of an acute inflammatory response. (The effects of biochemical mediators released by mast cells are illustrated in Fig. 7-4.) The most potent mediator of IgE-mediated hypersensitivity is histamine, which has effects on key target cells. Acting through certain histamine receptors (H1 receptors) on target cells in the host tissue, histamine contracts bronchial smooth muscles causing bronchial constriction, increases vascular permeability causing edema, and causes vasodilation increasing blood flow into the affected area (see Fig. 7-11). The interaction of histamine with H2 receptors on target cells results in increased gastric secretion and a decrease of histamine released from mast cells and basophils (basophils are granulocytes in the blood that are thought to be similar to mast cells). The action of histamine through H2 receptors suggests an important negative-feedback loop which stops degranulation. That is, the released histamine inhibits release of additional histamine by interacting with H2 receptors

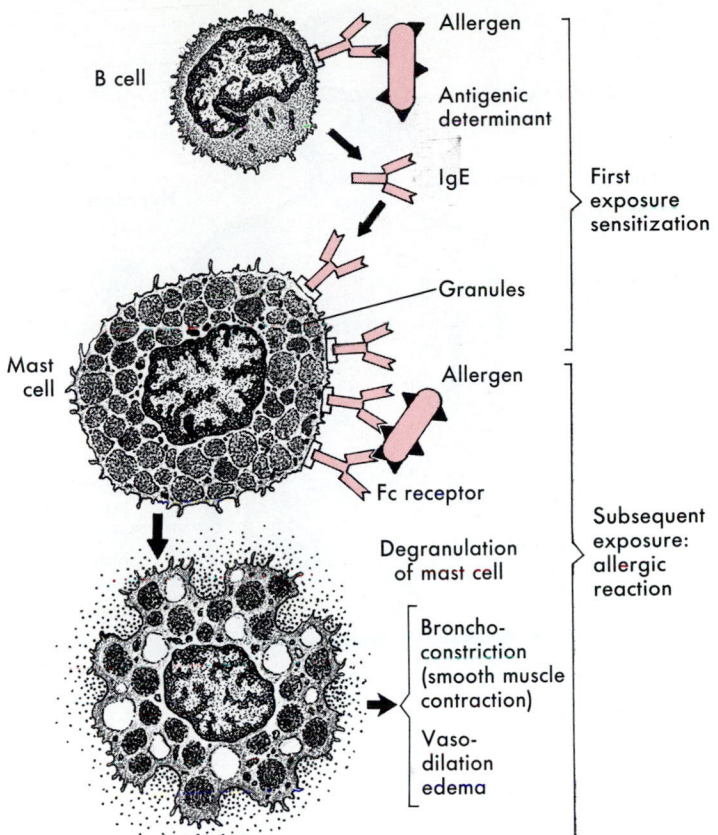

FIG. 8-1. Mechanism of type I IgE-mediated reactions. Initial sensitization to an allergen stimulates B cells to produce IgE. The IgE coats the surface of the mast cell by binding with IgE-specific Fc receptors on the mast cell's plasma membrane. Further exposure to the same allergen cross-links the surface-bound IgE and causes degranulation of the mast cell.

on the mast cells. Histamine may also affect control of the immune response through H2 receptors on most T suppressor cells. Another important activity of histamine is its function as a chemotactic factor for eosinophils. In conjunction with ECF-A, the histamine enhances attraction of eosinophils into sites of allergic inflammatory reactions, and also deactivates and prevents them from migrating out of the inflammatory site. (The role of the eosinophil in inflammation is discussed in Chapter 7.)

Although some control of the allergic response is mediated through histamine receptors, the primary mechanism of control is the autonomic nervous system. The autonomic nervous system includes biochemical mediators (e.g., epinephrine and acetylcholine) that, like the mediators of the inflammatory response, have profound effects on the behavior of target cells in the host tissue. The nervous system mediators bind to appropriate receptors on both mast cells and the target cells of inflammation, thereby controlling (1) release of inflammatory

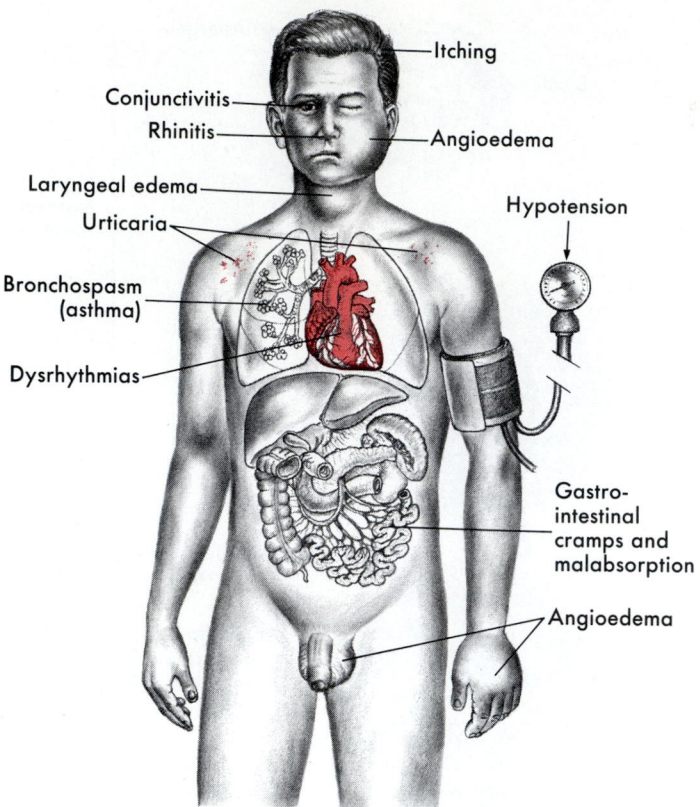

Itching
Conjunctivitis
Rhinitis
Angioedema
Laryngeal edema
Hypotension
Urticaria
Bronchospasm (asthma)
Dysrhythmias
Gastro-intestinal cramps and malabsorption
Angioedema

FIG. 8-2. Local manifestations of allergic reactions as a result of type I hypersensitivity include itching, angioedema (swelling due to exudation), edema of the larynx, urticaria (hives), bronchospasm (constriction of airways in the lungs), hypotension (low blood pressure) and dysrhythmias (irregular heart beat) because of anaphylactic shock, and gastrointestinal cramping due to inflammation of the gastrointestinal mucosa.

mediators from mast cells and (2) the degree to which target cells will respond to inflammatory mediators (see Chapters 1 and 12).

Clinical Manifestations

The clinical manifestations of type I reactions are mostly attributable to the biologic effects of histamine released during mast cell degranulation. The target tissues of the type I response contain large numbers of mast cells and are sensitive to the effects of histamine released from them. These tissues are found in the gastrointestinal tract, the skin, and the respiratory tract (Fig. 8-2 and Table 8-4).

Gastrointestinal allergy is primarily caused by allergens that enter through the mouth, usually foods. Hypersensitivity is frequently manifested by vomiting, diarrhea, or abdominal pain and may be severe enough to result in malabsorption or protein-losing enteropathy. Foods most frequently implicated in gastrointestinal allergies are milk, chocolate, citrus fruits, eggs, wheat, nuts, peanut butter, and fish. When food is the allergen, the active immunogen may be an unidentifiable product of food breakdown by digestive enzymes. Sometimes the allergen is a drug, additive, or preservative in the food. For example, cows treated for mastitis with penicillin yield milk containing trace amounts of this antibiotic. Thus, hypersensitivity apparently caused by milk proteins may instead be the result of an allergy to penicillin.

Urticaria, or **hives,** are a dermal (skin) manifestation of allergic reactions. The underlying mechanism is the localized release of histamines and increased vascular

---

TABLE 8-4   Causes of clinical manifestations of allergy

Typical allergen	Mechanism of hypersensitivity	Clinical manifestation
INGESTANTS		
Foods	Type I	Gastrointestinal allergy
Drugs	Types I, II, III	Urticaria, immediate drug reaction, hemolytic anemia, serum sickness
INHALANTS		
Pollens, dust, molds	Type I	Allergic rhinitis, bronchial asthma
Aspergillus fumigatus	Types I, III	Allergic bronchopulmonary aspergillosis
Thermophilic actinomycetes*	Types III, IV	Extrinsic allergic alveolitis
INJECTANTS		
Drugs	Types I, II, III	Immediate drug reaction, hemolytic anemia, serum sickness
Bee venom	Type I	Anaphylaxis
Vaccines	Type III	Localized Arthus reaction
Serum	Types I, III	Anaphylaxis, serum sickness
CONTACTANTS		
Poison ivy, metals	Type IV	Contact dermatitis

Modified from Bellanti, J.A. 1985. *Immunology III*. Philadelphia: Saunders.
*An order of fungi that is stimulated by warmth to grow and proliferate.

permeability resulting in limited areas of edema. Uticaria are characterized by white fluid-filled blisters (wheals) surrounded by areas of erythema, or redness (flares). The wheal-and-flare reaction is usually accompanied by itching. Not all urticarias are caused by allergic (immunologic) reactions. Some, termed nonimmunologic urticaria, result from exposure to cold temperatures, emotional stress, drugs, systemic diseases, hyperthyroidism, or malignancies (e.g., lymphomas).

Effects of allergens on the mucosa of the eyes, nose, and respiratory tract include conjunctivitis (inflammation of the membranes lining the eyelids), rhinitis (inflammation of the mucous membranes of the nose), and asthma (constriction of the bronchi). Clinical manifestations are caused by vasodilation, hypersecretion of mucus, edema, and swelling of the respiratory mucosa. Because the mucous membranes lining the respiratory tract (accessory sinuses, nasopharynx, and upper and lower respiratory tract) are continuous, they are all adversely affected by the allergic reaction. The degree to which each is affected determines the clinical manifestations of the disease.

The central defect in allergic diseases of the lung, such as asthma, is obstruction of the lumen of the large and small airways (bronchi) of the lower respiratory tract by bronchospasm (constriction of smooth muscle in airway walls), edema, thick secretions, and hyperplasia of smooth muscle and mucus-secreting glands. This leads to ventilatory insufficiency, wheezing, and difficult or labored breathing. Asthma is acute, intermittent, and reversible. Extrinsic asthma is an allergic reaction caused by a known exogenous allergen, whereas intrinsic asthma has no known cause. (Asthma is described further in Chapter 30.)

Genetic Predisposition

Certain individuals appear to be "prone" to allergies, or are **atopic.** Atopic individuals tend to produce higher concentrations of IgE and to have more Fc receptors on their mast cells. Subtle defects in T lymphocyte function (e.g., a deficiency in IgE-specific suppressor cells) may account for heightened IgE production. The airways and the skin of atopic individuals are also more responsive to a wide variety of both specific and nonspecific stimuli than the airways and skin of normal individuals. There appears to be a genetic basis for the state; some individuals are genetically predisposed to become sensitized against allergens. In families in which one parent has an allergy, allergies will develop in about 40% of the offspring. If both parents have atopic disease, the incidence in offspring is approximately 80%. (Principles of genetic inheritance are discussed in Chapter 4.)

Tests of IgE-mediated Hypersensitivity

Allergic reactions can be life-threatening; therefore it is essential that severely allergic individuals be made aware of the specific allergen against which they are sensitized and instructed to avoid contact with that material. Several tests are available to determine the specific allergen. These tests include skin tests with allergens and laboratory tests for total IgE and allergen-specific IgE.

Upon injection of an allergen into (intradermal) or onto (epicutaneous or prick test) the skin of a sensitized individual, a local anaphylactic reaction will occur within a few minutes. It consists of a localized swelling and redness; a **wheal and flare** reaction. The diameter of the flare reaction is usually indicative of the individual's sensitivity to that allergen. In the most severely allergic individuals even the extremely small amounts of allergen used for the skin test may evoke a systemic anaphylaxis.

There are a variety of laboratory tests for the detection of IgE antibodies. **Radioimmunosorbent (RIST) testing** measures circulating levels of total IgE; atopic individuals usually having elevated levels. **Radioallergosorbent (RAST) testing** has been used to measure circulating levels of specific IgE antibodies against many allergens and the amount of IgE has been found to correlate well with the degree of positive skin test and the severity of clinical symptoms.

Desensitization

Clinical desensitization to allergens can be achieved in some individuals. Minute quantities of the allergen to which the person is sensitive are injected in increasing doses over a prolonged period. This procedure may reduce the severity of the allergic reaction in the treated individual. Desensitization may work by inducing the production of large amounts of so-called blocking antibodies. A **blocking antibody** presumably competes in the tissues or in the circulation for binding with antigenic determinants on the allergen. Thus neutralized, the antigen is unable to bind with IgE on mast cells. In serum, blocking antibodies are predominantly IgG. The role of blocking antibodies has not been firmly established. Desensitization injections may also stimulate the generation of clones of suppressor T lymphocytes, which inhibit hypersensitivity by suppressing the production of IgE.

Tissue-Specific Reactions

Type II hypersensitivity reactions are generally characterized by the destruction of a target cell through the action of antibody against an antigen on the cell's plasma membrane. In addition to histocompatibility (HLA) antigens, most tissues have other antigens. These other antigens are generally called **tissue-specific antigens,** because they are only expressed on the plasma membranes of certain cells. Platelets, for example, have groups of self-antigens that are found on no other cells of the body. Because of limited distribution of tissue-specific antigens, type II diseases are limited to those tis-

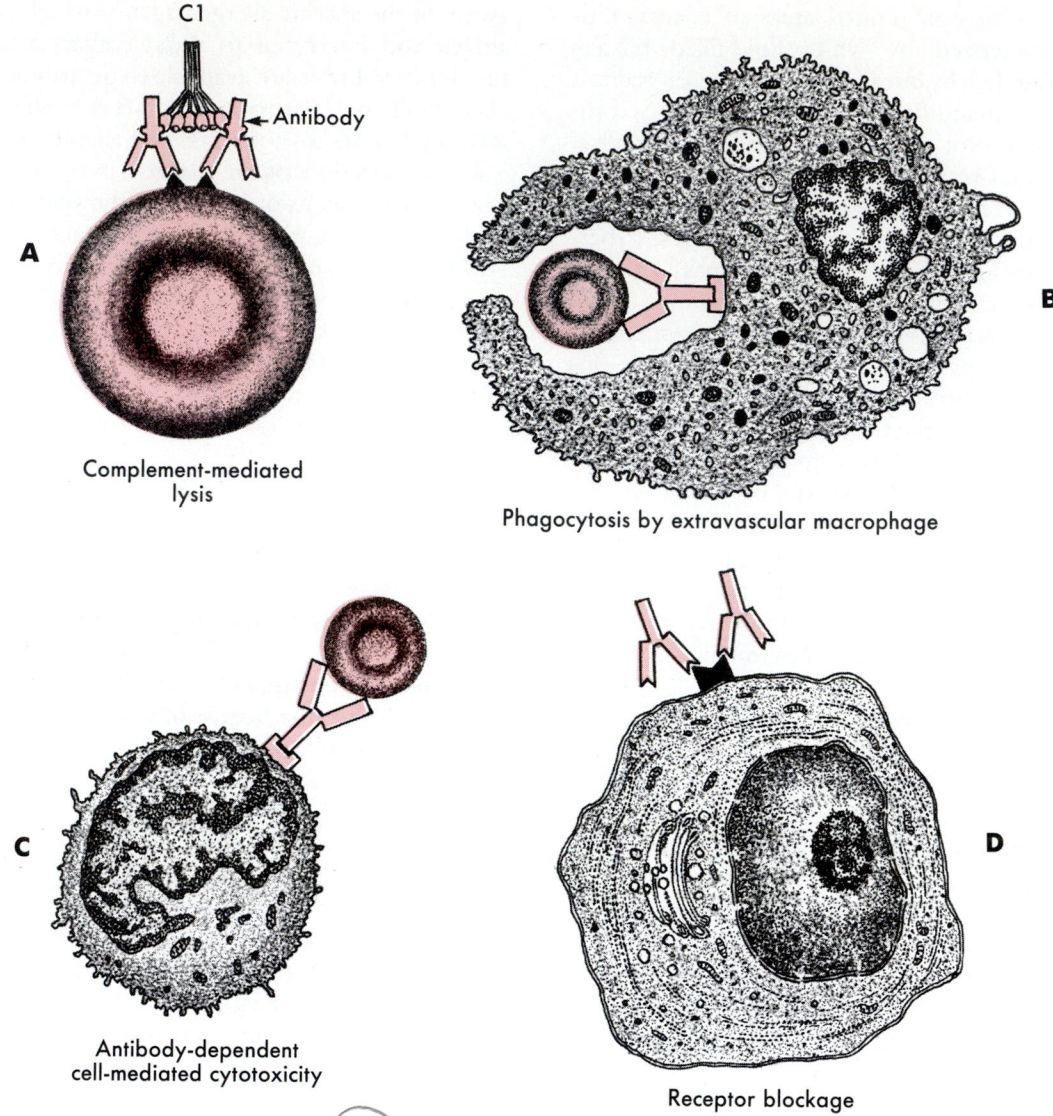

C1

← Antibody

A

Complement-mediated
lysis

B

Phagocytosis by extravascular macrophage

C

Antibody-dependent
cell-mediated cytotoxicity

D

Receptor blockage

FIG. 8-3.   Mechanisms of type II, tissue-specific reactions. Antigens on the target cell bind with antibody and are destroyed or prevented from functioning by **(A)** complement-mediated lysis, **(B)** clearance by macrophages in tissues, **(C)** antibody-dependent cell-mediated cytoxicity (ADCC) or **(D)** the modulation or blockage of receptors on the target cell.

sues or organs that express the particular antigen. Environmental antigens (e.g., drugs or their metabolites) may also bind to the plasma membranes of cells (especially erythrocytes and platelets) and function as targets of type II reactions.

There are four mechanisms by which type II, or tissue-specific, hypersensitivity reactions can destroy or alter cells (Fig. 8-3). All of these mechanisms begin with antibody binding to tissue-specific antigens.

The first mechanism, complement-mediated lysis of cells, occurs by the same mechanism described and illustrated in Chapter 7 for foreign antigens (see Fig. 7-6). Antibody that is bound to the target cell "fixes" complement, initiating the complement cascade and ultimately dissolving (lysing) the plasma membrane of the cell.

Circulating erythrocytes, for example, are destroyed by complement-mediated lysis in individuals with autoimmune hemolytic anemia (see Chapter 23) or isoimmune reactions to transfused blood cells from a donor (see p. 262).

A second mechanism of type II cell destruction is phagocytosis by macrophages of the mononuclear phagocyte system. Fc receptors on the macrophage recognize and bind the antibody on the opsonized cell. Phagocytosis of the target cell follows. (Phagocytosis is illustrated in Fig. 7-15.)

Antibody-dependent   cell-mediated   cytotoxicity (ADCC) is the third mechanism of type II host cell destruction. This mechanism involves cell destruction by a subpopulation of cytotoxic cells, which are not antigen-specific. Antibody on the target cell is recognized by and bound to Fc receptors on the cytotoxic cells, which release toxic substances that destroy the cell.

The fourth mechanism does not destroy the target cell, but rather causes it to "malfunction." In this mechanism of type II injury, the damage is done by antibody binding alone. The antibody binds to the target cell, occupying and altering receptors that would bind with the various molecules (ligands) required for normal cellular function. For example, in hyperthyroidism (excessive thyroid activity) caused by Graves' disease, autoantibody activates receptors for thyroid-stimulating hormone (TSH) (a pituitary hormone that controls the production of the hormone thyroxine by the thyroid). The antibody-activated receptors stimulate the thyroid cells to continue producing thyroxine despite decreasing amounts of TSH (see Chapter 18).

Immune-Complex–Mediated Injury

Mechanisms

Most type III hypersensitivity diseases are caused by antigen-antibody (immune) complexes that are formed in the circulation and deposited later in vessel walls or extravascular tissues (Fig. 8-4). Type III, immune-complex–mediated reactions, therefore, are not organ-specific and symptoms have very little to do with the antigenic target of the antibody (Rote, 1985). In some instances, immune-complex disease begins with the deposition of antigen in the tissues, and is followed by local interactions with antibody and complement. Regardless of whether immune complexes are formed in the circulation or in the tissues, their harmful effects are caused by complement activation, particularly the generation of complement fragments that are chemotactic for neutrophils. The neutrophils attempt to ingest the immune complexes but are frequently unsuccessful because the complexes are bound to the tissues. During the neutrophil's attempts to phagocytose the immune complexes, large quantities of lysosomal enzymes are released into the inflammatory site instead of into phagolysosomes. The attraction of neutrophils and the subsequent release of lysosomal enzymes cause most of the resulting tissue damage.

The fate of circulating immune complexes depends upon the ratio of antigen to antibody and other variables in the components of the immune complex. Other

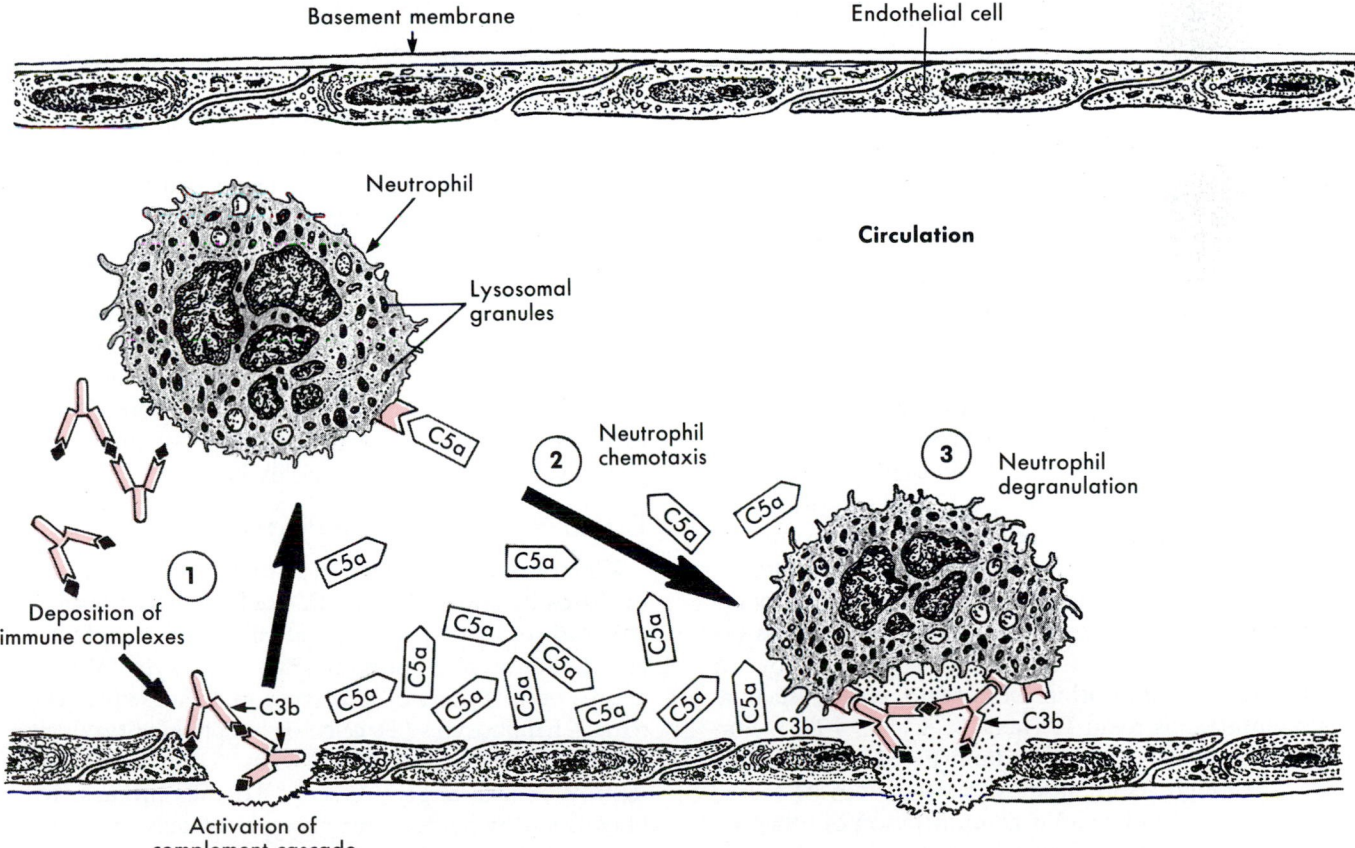

FIG. 8-4. Mechanism of type III, immune-complex-mediated reactions. Immune complex are deposited in the vessels or other healthy tissue, where they activate the complement cascade and generate complement fragments including C5a *(1)*. C5a is chemotactic for neutrophils and attracts many degradative enzymes that destroy healthy tissues *(3)*.

variables that influence immune-complex clearance are the inclusion of complement in the complex, the class or subclass of the antibody, and the nature and size of the antigen. Fairly large immune complexes are rapidly cleared from the circulation by the tissue macrophages of the mononuclear phagocyte system, whereas very small complexes are eventually filtered from blood through the kidneys, without any pathologic consequences. Intermediate-size immune complexes (formed at a ratio of antigen to antibody that has a slight excess of antigen) are likely to be deposited in the tissues, where they have severe pathologic consequences, such as glomerulonephritis or degenerative joint disease (arthritis).

Immune-Complex Disease

The nature of the immune complexes may change and result in changes in severity of the symptoms. Variations in the ratio of antigen to antibody, the class and subclass of antibody, and the quantity and quality of circulating antigen cause the disease activity to be in constant flux.

Because some immune complexes activate complement very effectively and covalently bind some complement components, complement levels in the blood are also in flux. In many conditions in which immune complexes are formed, the individual's blood becomes **hypocomplementemic** (i.e., contains decreased amounts of complement activity). In conditions caused by the other three mechanisms of hypersensitivity (types I, II, and IV) some components of the complement cascade, such as C3, may even be increased. The interaction of complement with some immune complexes results in the dissolution of the complex and an alteration in its harmful effects.

Immune-complex formation is dynamic: immune complexes formed early in a disease may be totally different from those formed later in the disease. At any one time, several types of immune complexes may be present simultaneously. With the tremendous potential heterogeneity of immune complexes, it is not surprising that these diseases are characterized by a variety of symptoms and periods of remission or exacerbation of symptoms.

Serum Sickness   The systemic form of immune-complex–mediated disease is called **serum sickness** because it was initially described as being caused by the therapeutic administration of foreign serum, such as horse antitetanus toxin (Pirquet & Schick, 1905). Foreign serum is generally not administered to individuals today, although serum sickness reactions can be caused by the repeated intravenous administration of other antigens, such as drugs. Serum sickness is caused by the generalized deposition of immune complexes and inflammation. Typically affected are the blood vessels, joints, and kidneys. Other manifestations include fever, enlarged lymph nodes, rash, and pain at sites of inflamma-

tion. Laboratory findings may include decreased levels of circulating lymphocytes, granulocytes, and platelets.

A form of serum sickness is **Raynaud's phenomenon,** an autoimmune condition caused by the temperature-dependent deposition of immune complexes in the peripheral circulation. (Immune complexes that precipitate at temperatures below normal body temperature are called cryoglobulins.) The symptoms of Raynaud's phenomenon are localized pallor and numbness (usually in the fingers and toes), followed by cyanosis (a bluish tinge resulting from oxygen deprivation) and gangrene or by pain and redness. These signs and symptoms are caused by the temperature-dependent precipitation of immune complexes in the capillary beds of the peripheral circulation and the resulting inflammatory processes.

Arthus Reaction   An **Arthus reaction** is an example of a localized immune-complex–mediated inflammatory response (Arthus & Breton, 1903). It is caused by repeated local exposure to exogenous antigen that reacts with preformed antibody in the walls of blood vessels. Symptoms of an Arthus reaction begin within an hour of exposure and peak at 6 to 12 hours later. The lesions are characterized by a typical inflammatory reaction, with increased vascular permeability, an accumulation of neutrophils, edema, hemorrhage, clotting, and tissue damage.

Arthus reactions are observed after injection, ingestion, or inhalation of exogenous antigens. Skin reactions can follow subcutaneous or intradermal inoculation with drugs, fungal extracts, or antigens used in skin tests. Gastrointestinal reactions, such as gluten-sensitive enteropathy (celiac disease), follow ingestion of antigen, usually gluten from wheat products (see Chapter 36). Allergic alveolitis (farmer's lung; pigeon breeder's disease) is an Arthuslike acute hemorrhagic inflammation of the air sacs (alveoli) of the lung (see Chapter 30). Allergic alveolitis is caused by inhalation of fungal antigens, usually particles from moldy hay.

Cell-Mediated Tissue Destruction

Whereas hypersensitivity reactions I, II, and III were mediated by antibody, type IV (cell-mediated) reactions are mediated by specifically sensitized T lymphocytes and do not involve antibody (Fig. 8-5). Type IV mechanisms occur as one of two types involving either cytotoxic T lymphocytes (Tc cells) or lymphokine-producing T cells (Td cells). Cytotoxic T cells (Tc) can attack and destroy cellular targets directly. Td cells produce lymphokines, which affect various types of cells and can recruit and activate phagocytic cells, especially macrophages, at the inflammatory site. Tissue destruction is usually caused by direct killing by toxins from cytotoxic T cells or the release of soluble factors, such as lysosomal enzymes and toxic oxygen products from macrophages.

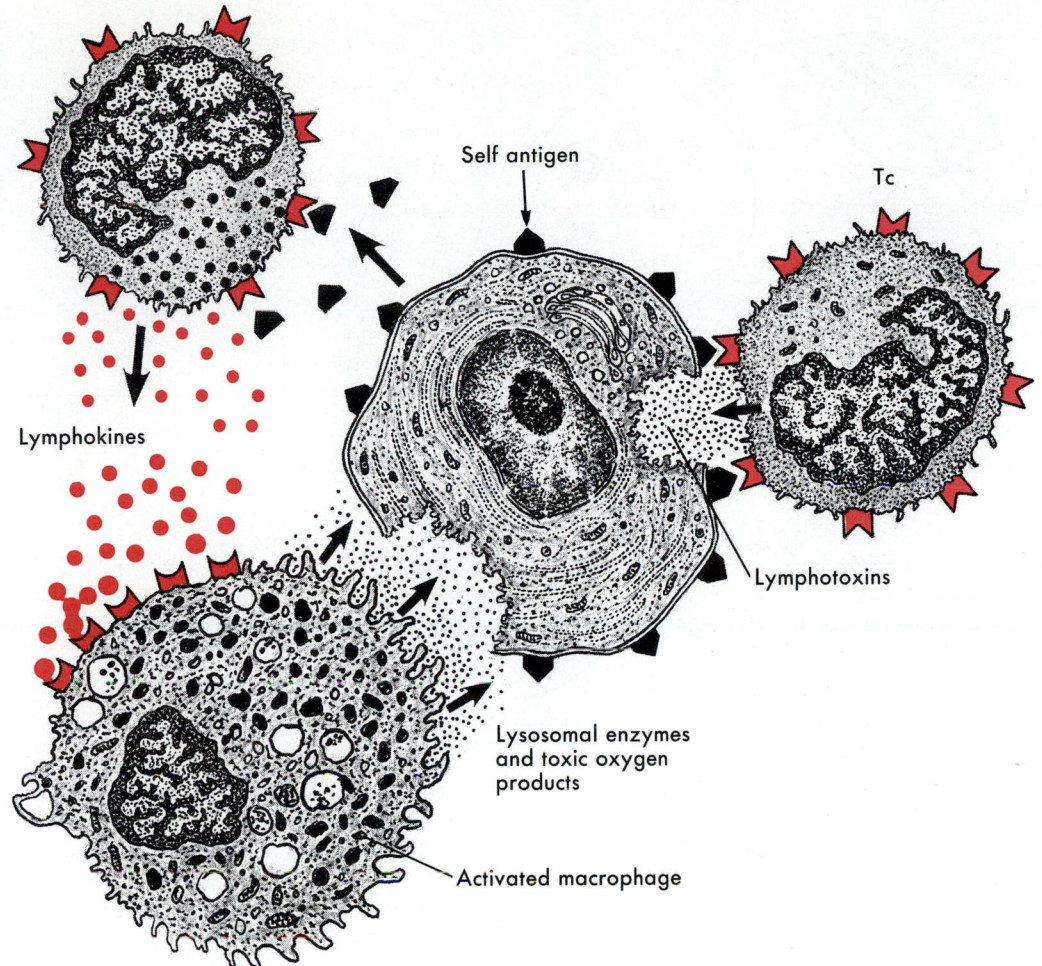

FIG. 8-5. Mechanism of type IV, cell-mediated reactions. Self-antigens from target cells stimulate T cells to produce cytotoxic T cells, *(Tc)*, which have direct cytotoxic activity, and T cells involved in delayed hypersensitivity *(Td)*. Td cells produce lymphokines, some of which attract and activate macrophages. The macrophages and enzymes released by them are responsible for most of the tissue destruction.

Clinical examples of type IV hypersensitivity include graft rejection, tumor rejection, the tuberculin reaction, and allergic reactions resulting from contact with such substances as poison ivy and metals. A type IV component may also be present in many autoimmune diseases such as rheumatoid arthritis, in which the self-antigen is apparently type II collagen (a protein present in joint tissues); autoimmune thyroiditis (Hashimoto's disease), in which the self-antigen is a protein on thyroid cells; and insulin-dependent diabetes mellitus, in which the self-antigen is a protein on the beta cell of the pancreas (the cell that normally produces insulin).

A type IV hypersensitivity in the skin was first thoroughly described in 1891 and led to the development of a diagnostic skin test for tuberculosis (Koch, 1891). The reaction in the skin that follows intradermal injec-

tion of antigen into a suitably sensitized individual is called delayed hypersensitivity because of its slow onset—24 to 72 hours to reach maximal intensity. The reaction site is also infiltrated with T lymphocytes and macrophages. One of the characteristics of delayed hypersensitivity is that it can be transferred to an unreactive recipient by cells but not by antiserum. This demonstrates that type IV hypersensitivity is mediated by lymphocytes rather than by antibody.

Allergic type IV reactions are elicited by some environmental antigens that are too small to be immunogenic by themselves (haptens). (Immunogenicity is described in Chapter 6.) Antigens with a molecular weight of less than 1000 daltons are not usually immunogenic but become so after binding with a carrier protein in the host. In cases of allergic contact dermatitis, the carrier

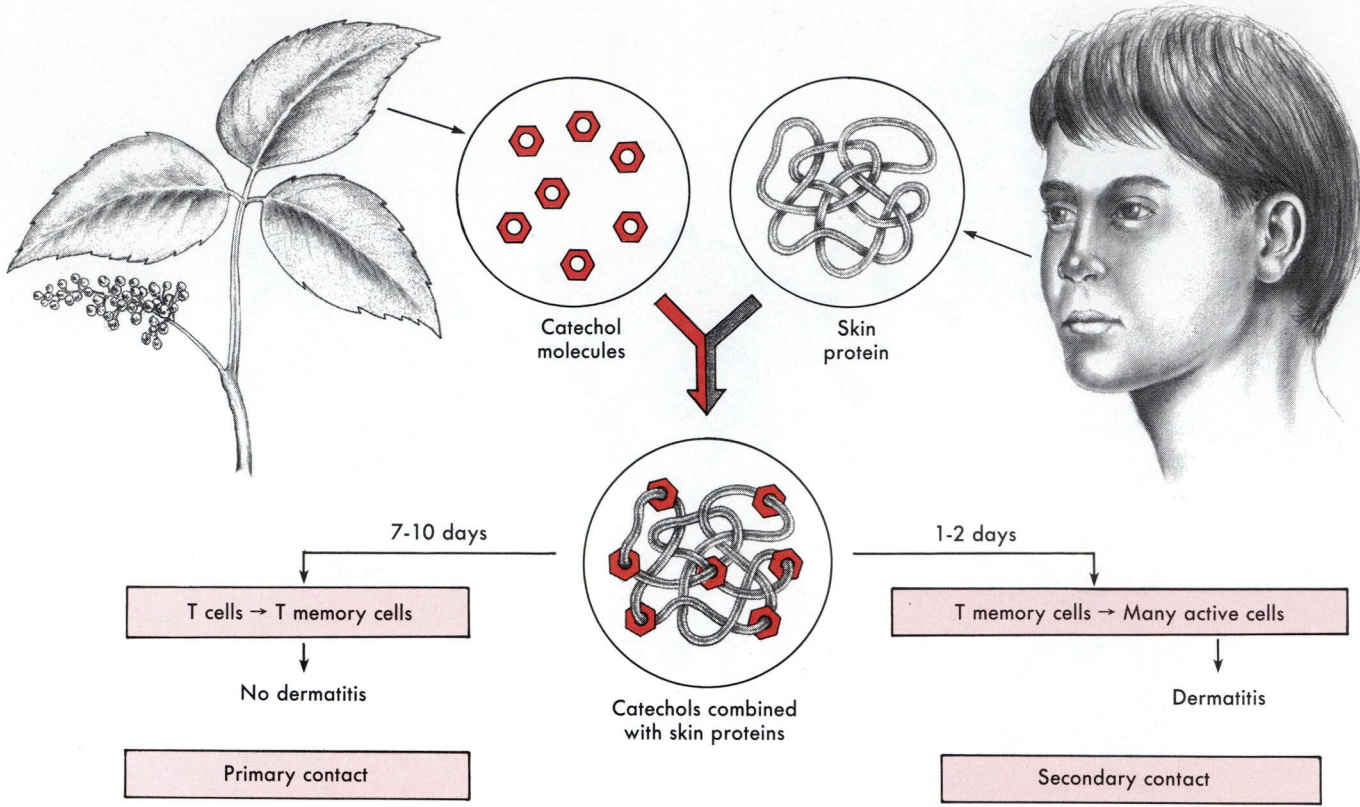

FIG. 8-6. Development of allergic contact dermatitis, a delayed hypersensitivity reaction. Shown here is the development of allergy to catechols from poison ivy. No dermatitis results from the primary contact because the antigens (catechols) are catabolized before any sensitized T cells are produced. Secondary contact, however, quickly activates a type IV, cell-mediated reaction that causes dermatitis.

protein is in the skin of the host. The best known example of allergic contact dermatitis is the delayed reaction caused by contact with poison ivy (Fig. 8-6). The antigen in this instance is a plant catechol, urushiol, that reacts with normal skin proteins and evokes a cell-mediated immune response. Skin reactions to industrial chemicals, cosmetics, detergents, clothing, food, metals, and topical medicines (such as penicillin) are elicited by the same mechanism.

Whether a skin reaction is caused by immediate or delayed hypersensitivity may be determined by the distribution of the lesions. The immediate reaction, termed **atopic dermatitis,** is manifested by widely distributed lesions, whereas **contact dermatitis** consists of lesions only at the site of contact (Fig. 8-7).

Targets of Hypersensitivity
Allergy

Allergens are environmental antigens that cause atypically exorbitant immunologic responses in genetically predisposed individuals. Typical allergens include pollens (e.g., rag weed, timothy), molds and fungi (e.g., *Penicillium notatum*), foods (e.g., milk, eggs, fish), animals (e.g., cat dander, dog dander), cigarette smoke, and components of house dust (e.g., fecal pellets of

house mites). Frequently, the allergen is contained within a particle that is too large to be phagocytosed or is surrounded by a protective nonallergenic coat. The actual allergen is released after enzymatic breakdown (e.g., by lysozyme in secretions) of the larger particle. Most allergens are either haptens that have the capacity to react with proteins or small-molecular-weight immunogenic proteins.

In certain situations an allergen complexes with components of host-tissue. The **neoantigen,** or new antigenic determinant, is recognized as foreign and the tissue is destroyed. This occurs in allergic reactions to drugs (e.g., penicillin, sulfonamides), in which the drug binds to proteins on the plasma membranes of host cells. The drugs, which are usually haptens, become immunogenic after binding to the host cell's proteins. The immune system attacks the neoantigen on the host cell's membrane and destroys the cell as well. In allergic reactions to penicillin, the immunogenic antigen is a metabolite of penicillin catabolism that binds to the plasma membranes of erythrocytes and induces an antibody response that destroys the cells, causing anemia.

The allergens that induce contact hypersensitivity, a type IV allergic reaction, are also haptens (e.g., metals such as nickel, aceylates and chemicals in rubber, resins

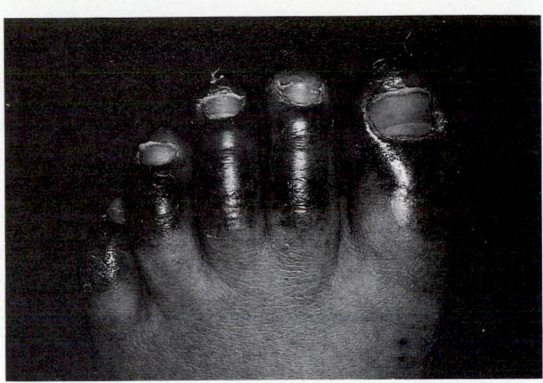

FIG. 8-7. Contact dermatitis caused by a delayed hypersensitivity reaction to shoes. (From Habif, 1985.)

in poison ivy and poison oak), which react with normal self-proteins in the skin. When presented in this fashion, these antigens induce a cell-mediated response.

Autoimmunity

Breakdown of Tolerance

Self-antigens are usually tolerated by the host's own immune system. Immunologic tolerance, or immunologic homeostasis, develops in humans during the embryonic period, during which any autoreactive lymphocytes are either eliminated or suppressed. Autoimmunity is a breakdown of tolerance in which the body's immune system begins to recognize self-antigens as foreign. The mechanisms of breakdown are many and vary among autoimmune disease, though in most such diseases the mechanism is unknown. Some of the mechanisms that have been implicated in the development of autoimmunity include (1) exposure within the body of a previously sequestered antigen, (2) the development of a neoantigen, (3) the complications of an infectious disease, (4) the emergence of a previously controlled or "forbidden" clone of lymphocytes with specificity for self-antigens, and (5) an alteration of suppressor T cell function.

Sequestered Antigen To be tolerated after birth, a self-antigen must be present in the fetus and exposed to the developing fetal immune system. Some self-antigens are not normally encountered in either fetal or adult life. Certain self-antigens, for example, in the cornea of the eye and in the testicles, are in areas of the body that are not drained by the lymphatics. Therefore these self-antigens never encounter antigen-processing cells in the draining lymph nodes or other lymphoid organs. They are sequestered or hidden from the immune system in **immunologically privileged sites,** so named because foreign tissues can be transplanted into these sites without danger of immunologic rejection. Immunologically privileged sites are vascular, however, so that if an immunologic reaction should occur, antibodies and lymphocytes can enter the site and cause immunologic rejection of the tissue. In some situations, especially trauma, the structure of an immunologically privileged site is disturbed and the previously **sequestered antigens** are released from the damaged tissue and enter the lymphatics. The immune system recognizes these antigens as foreign, and a primary immune response occurs that can inflict extensive immunologic damage to the untraumatized site. An example of this occurrence is sympathetic uveitis, an ocular disease in which physical trauma to one eye results in immunologic injury to the other eye.

Neoantigen In certain situations, a neoantigen that induces an allergic reaction may also lead to autoimmunity. Many neoantigens are haptens, which become immunogenic after binding to host proteins. The immune reaction against the neoantigen may lead to an immunologic reaction against the unaltered host protein. Many experimental autoimmune diseases (e.g., experimental autoimmune thyroiditis) can be initiated by this mechanism.

Infectious Disease Foreign antigens from infectious microorganisms can initiate autoimmune disease by (1) forming immune complexes that precipitate in host tissues, causing inflammatory disease; or (2) so closely resembling a particular self-antigen (cross-reacts with the self-antigen) that they stimulate production of antibodies that also recognize the self-antigen as foreign. Group A streptococci are capable of initiating both of these mechanisms, usually as sequelae to streptococcal pharyngitis.

The first mechanism, deposition of immune complexes, is the cause of post-streptococcal glomerulonephritis (inflammation of the kidney). Deposition elicits an inflammatory response that destroys tissues in the glomeruli of the kidney (in Fig. 8-4 this mechanism is illustrated in a blood vessel). The second mechanism, in which the foreign antigen mimics the molecular structure of a self-antigen, occurs in rheumatic fever. In rheumatic fever, streptococcal antigens so closely resemble self-antigens on the heart valve that antibodies produced to incapacitate the streptococci also damage cells of the heart valve.

Forbidden Clone One theory that explains tolerance is that maturing lymphocytes in the central lymphoid organs encounter self-antigen during embryogenesis and, as lymphocytes reactive against self-antigen develop, their clones are prevented, or "forbidden," from maturing. Autoimmunity may result from the survival of a **forbidden clone** and its proliferation later in life. No known autoimmune disease has been shown to be caused by this mechanism, but the pathogenesis of most autoimmune diseases has not yet been discovered.

Suppressor Cell Dysfunction Despite the normal development of tolerance, sometimes clones of lymphocytes against self-antigens develop in healthy adults. One of the roles of suppressor T cells is to suppress the immune responses that these clones activate. Suppressor T cell dysfunction can, therefore, result in autoimmune disease. If a single antigen-specific population of suppressor cells is affected, a tissue-specific autoimmune disease will result. A generalized autoimmune reaction will occur if many suppressor cell populations are dysfunctional. Systemic lupus erythematosus (SLE), which is characterized by the production of a large array of autoantibodies, may be caused by a general breakdown in the suppressor cell network.

Original Insult

The cause of some immune diseases is quite apparent. For example, in drug-induced anemia or thrombocytopenia (decreased numbers of circulating platelets), there is ample evidence that immunologic destruction of erythrocytes or platelets follows the integration of a drug or its metabolite (product of catabolism) into the plasma membranes of the host cells. This causes the immune system to recognize the altered plasma membranes as new and foreign cellular antigens. B cells are stimulated to produce antibody against the drug-cell complex, and immune processes destroy the host cells. Viruses can induce autoimmune reactions by altering the plasma membranes of host cells. In rubella infections, for example, encephalitis can ensue when cells of the nervous system become infected and express virally derived antigens on their plasma membranes. Like the antigenic alterations caused by drug metabolism, virus-induced changes result in the destruction of infected cells by the host's immune system.

The causes of other immune diseases, such as rheumatoid arthritis and SLE, are less clear. Most autoimmune diseases are probably sequelae of preexisting infections that leave no traces to facilitate their identification.

Genetic Factors

Genetic factors that contribute to autoimmunity are easier to identify than pathogenic agents. It is fairly well established that autoimmune diseases are familial. Affected family members may not all develop the same disease, but several members may have different disorders characterized by hypersensitivity.

The association of diseases with specific HLA antigens (see Chapter 6) has been recognized only recently and is a relatively nebulous phenomenon. The HLA types of susceptible and resistant individuals have been analyzed for almost every known disease and, almost universally, individuals with certain diseases are more likely than the general population to have a specific HLA allele or alleles. Some associations are strong, whereas others are more tenuous. The reason why some HLA alleles are associated with inappropriate immune

function is unclear, but it may directly involve the products of the HLA locus or the histocompatibility-complex-linked immune response (Ir) genes. These genes may determine an individual's susceptibility to specific infectious agents or the capacity of that individual to mount an immune response against specific antigens. Therefore, an individual of a specific HLA type may have inappropriate or exaggerated immune responses against a microorganism, resulting in a hypersensitivity reaction.

Isoimmunity

Isoimmunity occurs when an individual's immune system reacts against antigens on the tissues of other members of the same species. There are two clinically relevant examples of this reactivity: (1) transient neonatal diseases (in which the maternal immune system become sensitized against antigens expressed by the fetus) and (2) transplant rejection and transfusion reactions (in which the immune system of a recipient of an organ transplant or blood transfusion reacts against antigens on the donor cells).

Since the fetus is a hybrid between the mother and father, it expresses paternal antigens that are not found in the mother. Occasionally, these fetal antigens will cross the placenta and elicit an immune response in the mother. Maternal antibody may be transported into the fetal circulation to produce isoimmune disease in the fetus. The mother's immune system produces the antibody, but because her cells do not express the target antigen, she has no manifestations of the disease.

Isoimmune disease may be in conjunction with maternal autoimmune diseases. The mother may be producing an IgG autoantibody specific for maternal self-antigens that are found on fetal cells as well. Therefore, symptoms of the same autoimmune disease may affect both mother and child, even though the autoantibody is being produced only by the mother's immune system. This form of disease usually only occurs in association with type II (tissue-specific) reactions. It does not occur in association with IgE-mediated (type I) reactions, immune-complex–mediated (type III) reactions, or cell-mediated (type IV) reactions because the immunologic products of these reactions do not readily cross the placenta and enter the fetal circulation in sufficient quantity.

At birth the source of the antibody in the fetal circulation is removed. Although symptoms of the isoimmune disease may be manifested in utero or immediately after birth and may be fatal to the fetus or neonate, if symptoms are successfully treated at birth the disease will disappear as the maternal antibody is catabolized.

Examples of immunologic diseases in which the child can be affected include such antibody-mediated diseases as the following:

1. Graves' disease, an autoimmune disease in which maternal antibody against the receptor for thyroid-stimulating hormone causes neonatal hyperthyroidism.
2. Myasthenia gravis, an autoimmune disease in which maternal antibody binds with receptors for neural transmitters on muscle cells, causing neonatal muscular weakness (see Chapter 15).
3. Immune thrombocytopenic purpura, in which maternal antiplatelet antibody destroys platelets in the neonate (see Chapter 25).
4. Isoimmune neutropenia, in which maternal antibody against neutrophils destroys neutrophils in the neonate.
5. SLE, in which diverse maternal autoantibodies induce anomalies (e.g., congenital heart defects) in the fetus.
6. Rh and ABO isoimmunization (e.g., erythroblastosis fetalis) in which maternal antibody against erythrocyte antigens induces anemia in the child (see Chapter 25).

Autoimmune and Isoimmune Diseases

Autoimmunity and isoimmunity are exemplified by two disease states, SLE (an autoimmune disease) and transplant rejection (an isoimmune phenomenon). Most of the classic autoimmune diseases, including disorders of the endocrine system (autoimmune thyroiditis and Graves' disease), hematologic system (the hemolytic and pernicious anemias), nervous system (myasthenia gravis), and connective tissue in joints (rheumatoid arthritis) are discussed in Part II of this book.

Systemic Lupus Erythematosus

Systemic lupus erythematosus (SLE), which is a chronic, multisystem, inflammatory disease, is one of the most common, complex, and serious of the autoimmune disorders. SLE is characterized by the production of a large variety of autoantibodies against nucleic acids, erythrocytes, coagulation proteins, phospholipids, lymphocytes, platelets, and many other self-components. The most characteristic autoantibodies produced in SLE are against nucleic acids: single-stranded DNA, double-stranded DNA, histones, ribonucleoproteins, and other nuclear materials.

Deposition of circulating immune complexes containing antibody against host DNA produces tissue damage in individuals with SLE. DNA and DNA-containing immune complexes have a high affinity for glomerular basement membranes and may, therefore, be selectively deposited in the glomerulus (kidney structures are described in Chapter 33). The presence of DNA in the circulation increases from cellular damage in response to trauma, drugs, or infections, and is usually removed in the liver, but removal of circulating DNA is slowed in the presence of immune complexes, thereby increasing the potential for deposition in the kidney. (The liver's role in removing waste products from the blood is discussed in Chapter 35.) Deposition of immune complexes composed of DNA and antibody also cause inflammatory lesions in the renal tubular basement membranes, brain (choroid plexus), heart, spleen, lung, gastrointestinal tract, skin, and peritoneum.

SLE, as with most autoimmune diseases, is seen more frequently in women, especially in the 20- to 40-year-old age group. Blacks are affected more frequently than whites. A genetic predisposition for the disease has been implicated on the basis of increased incidence in twins and the existence of autoimmune disease in the families of individuals with SLE.

A transient lupus-like syndrome that is indistinguishable both clinically and in the laboratory from spontaneously occurring SLE can also develop from the prolonged use of drugs. The drugs most often implicated are hydralazine (an antihypertensive agent) and procainamide (an antiarrhythmic drug). In genetically susceptible individuals, certain environmental agents, such as ultraviolet light, and several infectious agents may trigger lupuslike immune reactions.

Clinical manifestations of SLE include arthralgias or arthritis (90% of individuals), vasculitis and rash (70% to 80% of individuals), renal disease (40% to 50% of individuals), hematologic abnormalities (50% of individuals, with anemia being the most common complication), and cardiovascular diseases (30% to 50% of individuals). As with most autoimmune diseases, SLE is characterized by frequent remissions and exacerbations. Because the signs and symptoms affect almost every body system and tend to come and go, SLE is extremely difficult to diagnose. This has led to the development of a list of eleven clinical findings. The serial or simultaneous presence of at least four of them indicates that the individual has SLE. The eleven findings are as follows (Fritzler & Tan, 1985):

1. Facial rash confined to the cheeks (malar rash)
2. Discoid rash (raised patches, scaling)
3. Photosensitivity (skin rash in sunlight)
4. Oral or nasopharyngeal ulcers
5. Nonerosive arthritis of at least two peripheral joints
6. Serositis (pleurisy, pericarditis)
7. Renal disorder (proteinuria of 0.5 g/day or cellular casts)
8. Neurologic disorders (seizures or psychosis)
9. Hematologic disorders (hemolytic anemia, leukopenia, lymphopenia, or thrombocytopenia)
10. Immunologic disorders (positive LE cell prep, anti-nDNA, anti-Smith (Sm) antigen, or false-positive serologic test for syphilis)
11. Presence of anti-nuclear antibody (ANA)

Graft Rejection

Transplantation of organs is commonly complicated by an immune response against antigens—primarily HLA antigens-on the donated tissue. Most knowledge on the transplantation of organs, and the emphasis here, is from renal transplant studies. The primary mechanism of the rejection of transplanted organs is a type IV, cell-mediated reaction. Two randomly chosen individuals are almost certainly antigenically different to some degree. Organ transplants between them are rejected in approximately 2 weeks without the extensive use of immunosuppressive drugs.

Because HLA antigens are the principle targets of the rejection reaction, HLA matching of donor and recipient greatly enhances the probability of acceptance of the graft. Matching at each HLA locus is of differential importance; matching at the HLA-D/DR locus appears to be the most critical for graft acceptance and at HLA-A, B, and C of lesser importance. (These loci are discussed in Chapter 6.)

Transplant rejection is classified as hyperacute, acute, or chronic, depending on the amount of time that elapses between transplantation and rejection. Hyperacute rejection is immediate and rare. When the circulation is reestablished to the grafted area, the graft may immediately turn white (the so-called white graft) instead of a normal pink color. Hyperacute rejection usually occurs in recipients with preexisting antibody to antigens in the graft. As circulation to the graft is established, antibody binds to the grafted tissue and activates the inflammatory response, including the coagulation cascade, which results in stasis of blood flow into the tissue. (Coagulation is described in Chapters 7 and 22.) Biopsies of the graft frequently show deposits of antibody (IgG and IgM), complement, and neutrophils.

Acute rejection is a cell-mediated immune response that occurs approximately 2 weeks after the transplant. This type of rejection occurs when the recipient develops an immune response against unmatched HLA antigens after transplantation. Immunosuppressive drugs may delay or lessen the intensity of acute rejection. A biopsy of the rejected organ shows an infiltration of lymphocytes and macrophages characteristic of a type IV reaction.

Chronic rejection may occur after a period of months or years of normal function. It is characterized by slow, progressive organ failure. Chronic rejection may be caused by inflammatory damage to endothelial cells lining blood vessels as a result of a weak immunologic reaction against minor histocompatibility antigens on the grafted tissue.

Diseases Caused by Immune Deficiency

PRIMARILY T CELL DEFECTS
Severe combined immune deficiency (SCID)
  Reticular dysgenesis
  Swiss-type SCID
  X-linked SCID
  Adenosine deaminase deficiency
  Nucleoside phosphorylase deficiency
DiGeorge syndrome (thymic aplasia or thymic hypoplasia)
Wiskott-Aldrich syndrome
Ataxia telangiectasia
Chronic mucocutaneous candidiasis
Nezelof syndrome
Hypoxanthine-guanosine phosphoribosyl transferase deficiency
5'nucleotidase deficiency
Biotin-dependent carboxylase deficiency
T cell immune deficiency with short-limbed dwarfism
Cartilage hair hypoplasia
Immune deficiency with thymoma
Immune deficiency with Down syndrome

PRIMARILY B CELL DEFECTS
Bruton's agammaglobulinemia
Common variable immune deficiency
Selective IgA deficiency

Hypogammaglobulinemia with normal IgM
Selective IgM deficiency
Immune deficiency with growth hormone deficiency
Transcobalamin II deficiency
B cell immune deficiency with short-limbed dwarfism
Selective IgE deficiency
Secretory component deficiency

PHAGOCYTIC DEFECTS
Quantitative defects
  Congenital splenic aplasia
  Sickle cell anemia
  Congenital neutropenia
Chemotactic defects
  Lazy leukocyte syndrome
  Hyperimmunoglobulin E
  Chediak-Higashi syndrome
Microbicidal defects
  Chronic granulomatous disease
  Myeloperoxidase deficiency
Related diseases
  Job syndrome
  Tuftsin deficiency

COMPLEMENT DEFECTS
C1q, C1r, C1s, C4, C2, C3, C5, C6, C7, C8, and C9 deficiency Factor B, factor D, and properdin deficiencies

DEFICIENCIES IN IMMUNITY AND INFLAMMATION

Disorders resulting from immune deficiency are the clinical sequelae (results) of impaired function of one or more components of the immune or inflammatory response, including B cells, T cells, phagocytic cells, and complement (see Table 8-5 for defects in phagocytic cells and complement). An **immune deficiency** is the failure of these mechanisms of self-defense to function at their normal capacity. **Congenital (primary) immune deficiency** is caused by a genetic anomaly, whereas **acquired (secondary) immune deficiency** is caused by another illness, such as cancer or viral infection, or by normal physiologic changes, such as aging. Acquired forms of immune deficiency are far more common than the congenital forms.

Whether congenital or acquired, the chief cause of immune deficiency is disruption of lymphocyte function. A stem cell defect may prevent normal lymphocyte development and cause total failure of the immune system, a central lymphoid organ dysfunction may prevent maturation of stem cells into B or T cells, or the final stages of B cell maturation may be disrupted, precluding the production of a specific class of immunoglobulin. Other defects may interfere with intercellular cooperation. For example, hyperactive suppressor T cells may prevent a normal immune response from taking place or

helper T cells may be unable to mediate immune interactions. Sometimes enzymatic defects in lymphocytes cause a general accumulation of toxic metabolites. Alterations in the inflammatory response, particularly the chemotactic and phagocytic activities of neutrophils and macrophages, or the activity of complement, can also result in impaired host resistance.

The clinical hallmark of immune deficiency is a tendency to develop unusual or recurrent, severe infections. Preschool and school-aged children normally have six to twelve infections per year and adults have two to four per year. Most of these are not severe and are limited to viral infections of the upper respiratory tract or recurrent streptococcal pharyngitis. Potential immune deficiencies are considered if the individual has had severe, documented bouts of pneumonia, otitis media, sinusitis, bronchitis, septicemia, or meningitis, or infections with microorganisms that are not normally pathogenic (e.g., *Pneumocystis carinii*). Deficiencies in T cell immune responses are suspected when recurrent infections are caused by certain viruses (e.g., varicella, vaccinia, herpes, cytomegalovirus), fungi and yeasts (e.g., candida, histoplasma), or certain atypical organisms (e.g., *P. carinii*). B cell deficiencies, on the other hand, are suspected if the individual has documented, recurrent infections with microorganisms that require opsonization (e.g., encapsulated bacteria) or viruses against which humoral immunity is normally effective (e.g., rubella).

TABLE 8-5   Congenital defects of phagocytosis and complement function

Type of defect	Characteristic	Clinical manifestation
DEFECTS OF PHAGOCYTOSIS		
Quantitative defects	Neutropenia (decreased granulocyte number)	General increase in bacterial infections
Chemotactic defects	Decreased neutrophil response to chemotactic factors	General increase in bacterial infections
Bacterial killing defects	Decreased bacterial killing because of insufficient H_2O_2 or lysosomal enzymes	Increased bacterial infections—especially with catalase + organisms
COMPLEMENT DEFECTS		
Defects in early classical pathway	Decreased activity of C1, C2, or C4	Mild bacterial infections; SLE-like syndrome
Defects in alternative pathway	Decreased activity of alternative pathway components-especially factor B	Increased infections with encapsulated bacteria
Defects in C3 and C5	Decreased production of C3b and C5a	Severe infections mostly with encapsulated bacteria
Defects in late pathway	Decreased activity of C6, C7, or C8	Recurrent disseminated *Neisseria gonorrhoreae* or *N. meningitidis* infections

Many immune deficiencies are also associated with other defects; some of these appear to be unrelated to the immune defect, yet may be life-threatening by themselves. Examples include eczema and thrombocytopenia (in Wiskott-Aldrich syndrome); cardiac anomalies, low levels of calcium in the blood, and structural anomalies of the face (in DiGeorge syndrome); and a severe lack of muscular coordination and dilation of the small blood vessels (in ataxia telangiectasia). The association of these other symptoms can sometimes clarify the pathophysiology of the disease. For instance, in DiGeorge syndrome the defects are the partial or complete absence of a thymus (resulting in depressed T cell immunity), partial or complete absence of the parathyroid gland (resulting in decreased blood calcium levels), and structural defects in the heart. Each of these anatomic structures originates from the same region in the embryo during the twelfth week of gestation, therefore the defect in DiGeorge syndrome can be traced to an abnormal development at a specific time and in a specific region during embryogenesis.

Routine care of individuals with immune deficiencies must be tempered with the knowledge that the immune system may be totally ineffective. It is unsafe to administer conventional immunizing agents or blood products to many of these individuals because of the risk that the immunizing agent will cause an uncontrolled infection. Uncontrolled infection is particularly a problem when attenuated vaccines that contain live, but weakened, microorganisms are used (e.g., vaccinia virus used for immunization against small pox). Although the virus is attenuated enough to be destroyed by a normal immune system, it can survive, multiply, and cause severe disease in an immune-deficient recipient. Furthermore, even simple procedures, such as penetrating the skin for routine blood tests, may lead to fatal septicemia (bacterial infection of the blood) in the immune-deficient person.

Individuals with immune deficiencies are also at risk for graft-versus-host disease. This occurs if T cells in a graft (e.g., transfused blood) are mature and are therefore capable of the cell-mediated destruction of tissues in the graft recipient. If the recipient's immune system is normal, the grafted T cells are controlled and no tissue destruction occurs. If, however, the recipient's immune system is deficient, the grafted T cells will remain unchecked and attack the recipient's tissues.

Congenital Immune Deficiencies

Congenital, or primary, immune deficiency occurs if lymphocyte development is arrested or disrupted in the fetus or embryo (Fig. 8-8). Defects that occur at different stages of stem cell, T cell, or B cell maturation cause different immune deficiency diseases. Some diseases are primarily caused by a defect in one or the other of the cell lines, though both T and B cell lines may be deficient in some respect. Other congenital immune deficiency diseases affect stem cells of both cell lines, disrupting both cell-mediated and humoral immune processes. A defect in B cell development results in lower levels of circulating immunoglobulin. The condition in which immunoglobulins are present in insufficient amounts is termed **hypogammaglobulinemia.** The condition in which they are totally or nearly absent is termed **agammaglobulinemia.** (Normal lymphocyte development is discussed in Chapter 6.)

Although most congenital immune deficiency diseases are rare, much of our current understanding of the development of the immune system and the interactions of the cells in the immune response was developed by studying congenital immune deficiencies or, as they have been called, "experiments of nature." The immune systems of experimental animals have been studied in the laboratory by specifically altering or removing one component of the system and observing the effect of that manipulation on the remainder of the immune response. Studying congenital immune deficiencies allows us the opportunity to make similar observations in humans.

The role of bone marrow stem cells in the evolution of the immune system was elucidated by studying children with the most severe deficiencies, **severe combined immune deficiencies (SCID).** The most severe form of SCID is **reticular dysgenesis** (failure of blood cells to develop), in which a common stem cell for all white blood cells is absent; therefore, T cells, B cells, and phagocytic cells never develop (Fig. 8-8). Most children with reticular dysgenesis die in utero or very soon after birth.

The common stem cell normally matures into more developed stem cells for individual populations of white blood cells. Most individuals with SCID are deficient only in a stem cell for lymphocyte development and, therefore, have normal numbers of all other white cells and few, if any, detectable lymphocytes. T and B lymphocytes are few or totally absent in both the circulation and secondary lymphoid organs (spleen, lymph nodes). The thymus is usually hypoplastic (underdeveloped) because of the absence of T cells. Immunoglobulin levels, especially of IgM and IgA, are absent or greatly reduced, though IgG levels may be almost normal because of the presence of maternal antibodies.

Stem cells mature in the central or primary lymphoid organs (thymus and bursal equivalence tissue). The importance of these organs was determined by studying children who failed to develop them during embryogenesis. These children presented with either a defective thymus (DiGeorge syndrome) or a defective bursal-equivalent tissue (Bruton's agammaglobulinemia).

DiGeorge syndrome (congenital thymic aplasia or hypoplasia) is caused by the lack, or more commonly

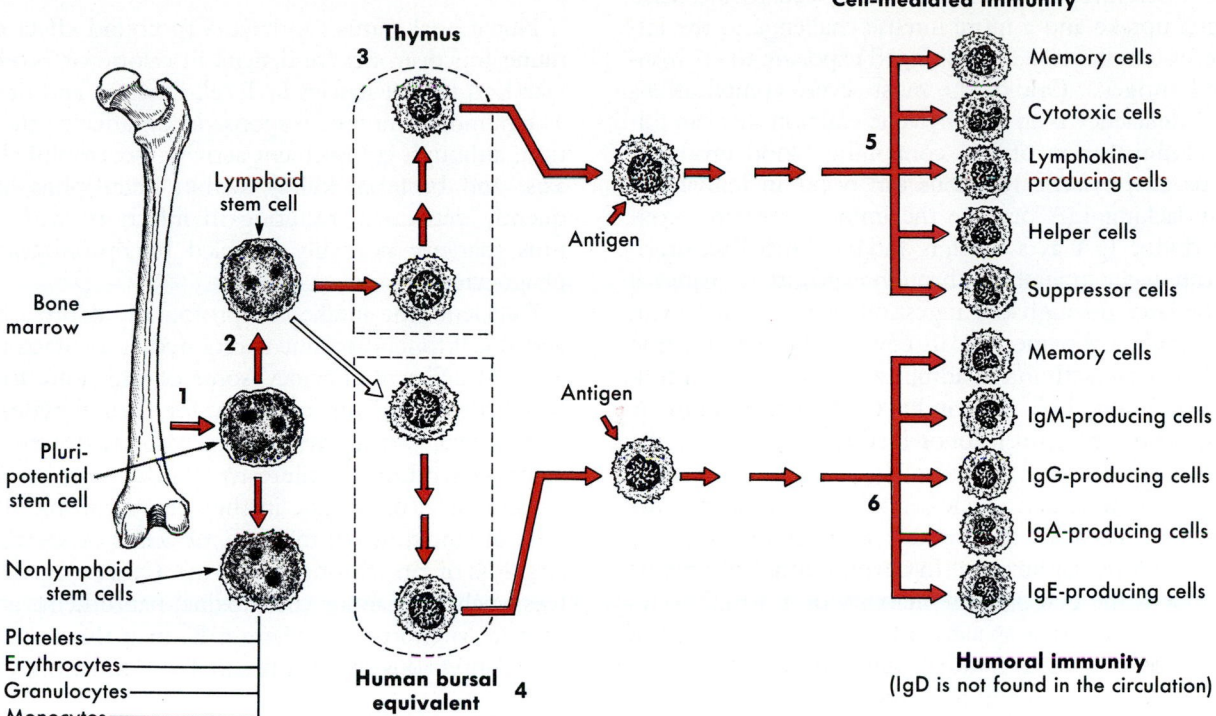

FIG. 8-8. Defects in lymphoctye development that may account for congenital immune deficiencies: *(1)* Reticular dysgenesis, *(2)* severe combined immune deficiency (SCID), *(3)* DiGeorge syndrome, *(4)* Bruton's agammaglobulinemia, *(5)* chronic mucocutaneous candidiasis, and *(6)* selective IgA deficiency.

partial lack, of the thymus, resulting in lymphopenia with greatly decreased T cell numbers and function (DiGeorge, 1968) (Fig. 8-8).

Bruton's agammaglobulinemia is caused by blocked development of B cell precursors into mature B cells because of the lack of normal bursal-equivalent tissue (Fig. 8-8). There are few or no circulating B cells, though T cell number and function are normal. At 6 months, the approximate normal serum concentrations of immunoglobulins are IgG, 400 mg/dl; IgM, 40 mg/dl; and IgA, 30 mg/dl. In 6-month-old children with Bruton's agammaglobulinemia, serum IgG levels are well below 100 mg/dl, and IgM and IgA are almost absent.

Some immune deficiences involve a defect that results in depressed development of a small portion of the immune system and, therefore, provide us with information about the function of that portion. For instance, an individual can be unable to produce a certain class of antibody. An example is **Wiskott-Aldrich syndrome** (an X-linked recessive disorder) in which IgM antibody production is greatly depressed and, therefore, antibody responses against antigens that elicit primarily an IgM response, such as polysaccharide antigens from bacterial cell walls (e.g., of *P. aeruginosa, S. pneumoniae, H. influ-*

enzae, and other microorganisms with polysaccharide outer capsules), are deficient.

Another defect in which a particular class of antibody is affected is **selective IgA deficiency.** This is the most common type of immune deficiency, having an incidence of between 1 in 700 and 1 in 400 individuals. Individuals with selective IgA deficiency are able to produce other classes of immunoglobulins, but fail to produce IgA. This suggests a disruption of terminal processes of differentiation, so that immature B cells that are committed to IgA production fail to mature into IgA-producing plasma cells (Fig. 8-8). Many individuals are asymptomatic, though others manifest a history of severe recurring sinus, lung, and gastrointestinal infections. Individuals with IgA deficiency frequently present with chronic intestinal candidiasis (infection with *C. albicans*). (The secretory, or mucosal, immune system is described in Chapter 6.)

Complications of IgA deficiency include severe atopic disease and autoimmune diseases; selective IgA deficiency is two or three times more common in atopic individuals than in others. As a result of studying these individuals we can conclude that secretory IgA may normally prevent the uptake of allergens from the environment. Therefore, IgA deficiency may lead to increased allergen uptake and a more intense challenge to the immune system because of prolonged exposure to environmental antigens. One of the most severe complications of IgA deficiency is an anaphylactic reaction that can follow administration of IgA-containing blood products. Serious anaphylactic reactions can occur in individuals totally lacking IgA because the immune system recognizes donor IgA as a foreign antigen. Initial sensitization can occur in fetal life through exposure to maternal IgA or later through the ingestion of maternal IgA in breast milk or bovine IgA in cow's milk. Sensitization can also occur with initial administration of blood products containing IgA. The individual's primed immune system then acts against donor IgA upon subsequent exposure.

Other immune deficiencies are characterized by a defect in the capacity to produce an immune response against a particular antigen. In **chronic mucocutaneous candidiasis** the defect is the inability of T lymphocytes to respond against a specific infectious agent, *Candida albicans* (Fig. 8-8). Individuals with chronic mucocutaneous candidiasis usually have mild to extremely severe recurrent Candida infections that involve the mucous membranes and skin. Systemic candidiasis is extremely rare, though infection of the mucosal lining of the esophagus may develop.

Acquired Deficiencies

Acquired, or secondary, immune and inflammatory deficiency develops after birth and is not related to genetic defects. The following physiologic or pathophysiologic conditions are associated with acquired deficiencies:

Pregnancy

Infancy

Infections, such as rubella (congenital), cytomegalovirus (congenital), measles, leprosy, tuberculosis, coccidiomycosis

Down's syndrome

Malignancies, such as Hodgkins disease, acute or chronic leukemia, nonlymphoid malignancy, or myeloma

Stress due to surgery or emotional trauma

Malnutrition due to insufficient intake of protein, calories, iron, or zinc

Aging

Diabetes

Alcoholic cirrhosis

Sickle cell anemia

Immunosuppressive treatment with corticosteroids, cytotoxic drugs, or ionizing radiation

Anesthesia

Nutritional Deficiencies

Nutritional status can have a profound effect on immune function. Severe deficits in calorie or protein intake lead to deficiencies in T cell function and numbers. The humoral immune response is less affected by starvation, although complement activity, neutrophil chemotaxis, and bacterial killing within neutrophils are frequently depressed, resulting in infections with organisms that are normally disabled by opsonization and phagocytosis.

Deficient zinc intake can profoundly depress both T and B cell function. Zinc is required as a cofactor for at least 70 different enzymes, some of which are found in lymphocytes and are necessary for their function. Secondary zinc deficiencies may be associated with malabsorption syndrome (failure to absorb zinc), chronic renal disease (loss of zinc in the urine), chronic diarrhea (loss of zinc through the gut), or burns or severe psoriasis (loss of zinc through the skin). Other enzyme cofactors, such as vitamins (pyridoxine, pantothenic acid, folic acid, vitamin A, or vitamin E) may also result in severe depressions of both B and T cell function.

Iatrogenic Deficiencies

Iatrogenic disorders are caused by some form of medical treatment (e.g., iatrogenic neutropenia is usually caused by drugs). Some drugs (e.g., cancer chemotherapeutic agents) profoundly suppress blood cell formation in the bone marrow. Other drugs induce immunologic responses that destroy mature granulocytes. The list of drugs having this effect is ever-increasing and includes analgesics, antithyroid medications, anticonvulsants, antihistamines, antimicrobial agents, and tranquilizers.

Many drugs also affect B and T cell function, especially against antigens that require the interaction of T helper and B cells for antibody production. These complications have been observed since the advent of potent immunosuppressive (e.g., corticosteroids) and chemotherapeutic drugs as treatment for individuals with transplants, cancer, or autoimmune diseases. Depression of B and T cell formation is manifested as a progressive increase in infections with opportunistic microorganisms (especially *P. carinii*, cytomegalovirus, *C. albicans*, and other fungi), the extent and location of which are unusual.

The immunosuppressive effects of chemotherapeutic drugs are exacerbated by concurrent treatment with ionizing radiation (x-rays). Most cytotoxic drugs and x-rays destroy cells that are proliferating or are in susceptible stages in their cell cycles. Therefore, these therapies mainly suppress the primary immune response, which involves proliferation of clones of B and T cells.

Surgery and anesthesia can also suppress both T and B cell function. Transient, severe lymphopenia is a com mon postoperative condition that can last for up to 1 month. Surgery to remove the spleen (splenectomy) results in a depressed humoral response against encapsulated bacteria (especially *S. pneumoniae, H. influenzae, S. aureus,* the group A Streptococcus, and *N. meningitidis*), depressed serum IgM levels, and decreased levels of opsonins.

Deficiencies Caused by Trauma

Burn victims are susceptible to severe bacterial infections. Thermal burns appear to be associated with decreased neutrophil function (especially chemotaxis), decreased complement levels, decreased cell-mediated immunity, and decreased primary humoral responses, although secondary humoral responses are normal. The mechanism of this immunosuppression may be twofold. Sera from burned individuals contain nonspecific immunosuppressive factors (will suppress all immune responses, regardless of the antigen involved). In addition, burn victims also have increased suppressor cell function, which may increase antigen-specific suppression.

Deficiencies Caused by Stress

The relationship between emotional stress and depressed immune function has recently become an area of intense research interest. For many decades there were anecdotal reports of increased incidence of infection and malignancy associated with periods of both intense stress (e.g., the loss of a loved one, divorce) and relatively minor stress (e.g., final examination periods at colleges and universities). In addition, early studies showed that immune function, as demonstrated by delayed hypersensitivity skin tests results, could be depressed through posthypnotic suggestion.

Only recently have the mechanisms of this interaction begun to be investigated. Many of the lymphoid organs are innervated and can be affected by nerve stimulation. In addition, lymphocytes have receptors for many hormones (i.e., sex hormones, neurotransmitters, and neuropeptides) and can respond to changing levels of these chemicals with increased or decreased function. (Further discussion of the effects of stress on susceptibility to disease can be found in Chapter 9.)

Acquired Immune Deficiency Syndrome (AIDS)

AIDS, or **acquired immune deficiency syndrome,** is currently the best known example of an acquired dysfunction of the immune system. It represents one of the most frightening diseases to appear in modern times because of its extremely high mortality rate (over 90% of individuals who develop the most severe form of the disease die within 4 years of diagnosis); the possibility of transmission by asymptomatic individuals who appar-

ently incubate the disease over a period of years; the rapid increase in the number of clinical cases (more than 70,000 in the United States as of this writing and increasing logarithmically at almost 100% per year); and the relatively uncontrollable modes of transmission (which include transplacental or perinatal routes and blood products or semen transmitted through homosexual and heterosexual contact, intravenous drug abuse, or the medical use of blood or blood products). AIDS is a viral disease that probably arose in central Africa in the 1950s, but is now found throughout the world. As of March 21, 1988, 136 countries or territories have reported 84,256 cases of AIDS and only 37 had reported no cases. Seventy-three percent of reported cases were in the Americas, 13% in Europe, 13% in Africa, and 1% in Asia (Morbidity and Mortality Weekly, 1988, May 13). The virus infects and depletes a portion of the immune system, making the individuals extremely susceptible to life-threatening infections and malignancies.

Epidemiology

The groups at highest risk for developing AIDS include homosexual and bisexual men (about 74% of the reported cases, with only 8% being attributable to intravenous drug users), homosexual and heterosexual abusers of injected drugs (27%), female sexual partners of people in AIDS risk groups (1%), and children born of mothers at risk (<1%) (Fig. 8-9). The incidence of AIDS was approximately 8% in women (52% were intravenous drug abusers and 17% were sexual partners of intravenous drug abusers) and 2% in children under the age of thirteen (Morbidity and Mortality Weekly, 1988). It is estimated that over 50% of homosexual men in some urban areas, such as New York City, are infected (Piot et al., 1988). With increased education, however, the incidence among homosexual men may be stabilizing, whereas in some metropolitan areas the incidence rates among intravenous drug abusers are beginning to surpass those of the homosexual population.

Although the incidence of apparently heterosexual transmission of AIDS is currently rather low (approximately 2% of men and 24% of women), this route is becoming increasingly common in the United States and is currently the most prevalent route in Africa (Adler, 1987). It is estimated that almost 100% of prostitutes in Kenya are infected (Piot et al., 1988). Recipients of blood products or of semen for artificial insemination have also developed AIDS, but AIDS tests for screening donors of these products have greatly reduced this risk. Approximately 3% of AIDS patients have been transfusion recipients or had received blood products for coagulation disorders. The incidence of HIV seropositivity in hemophiliacs is 70% in individuals with hemophilia A (factor VIII deficiency) and 35% in individ-

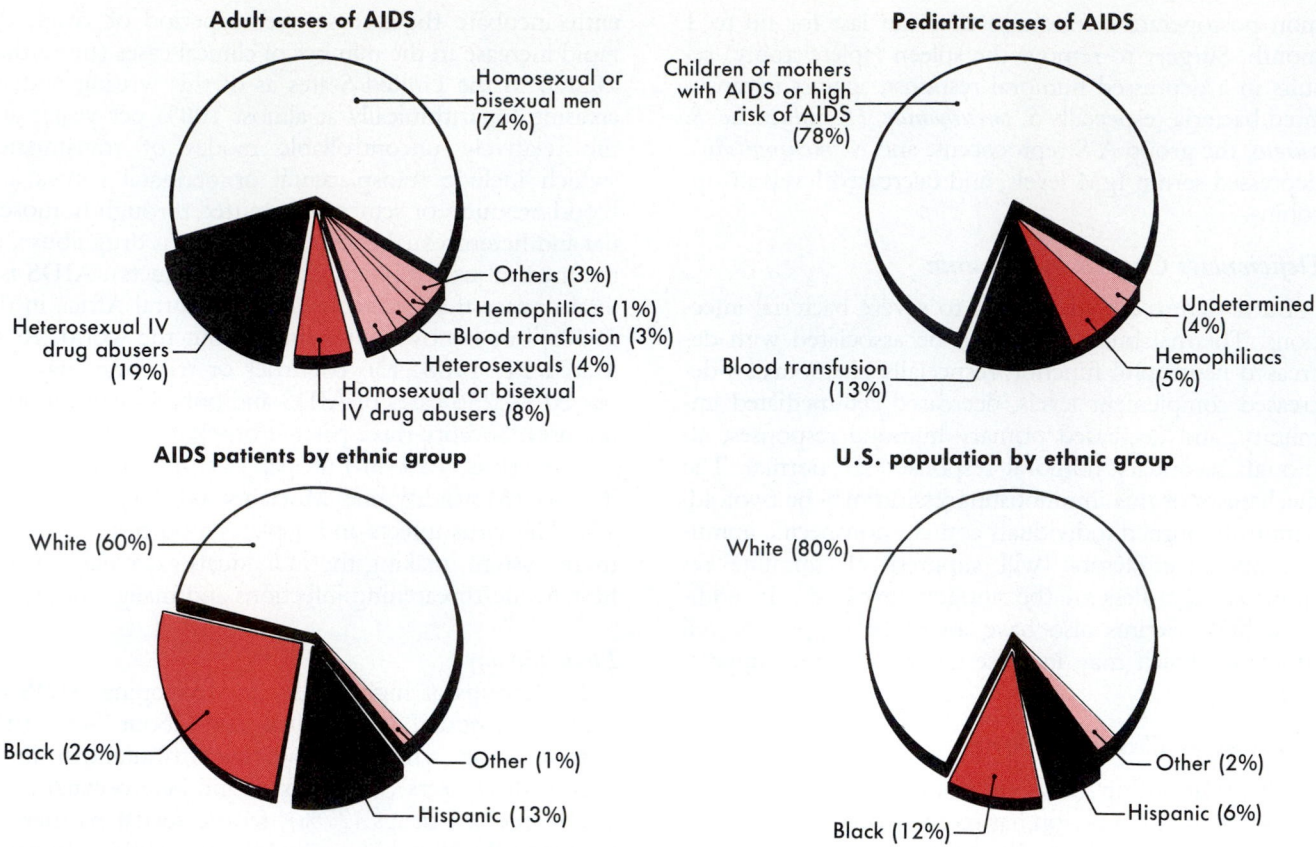

FIG. 8-9. Pie charts of population groups accounting for the adult *(left)* and child *(right)* cases of AIDS as of July 5, 1988. Note homosexual or bisexual men and IV drug abusers together account for 89% of all adult cases. More than three-fourths of the children with AIDS acquired the disease from a mother who either had AIDS or was a member of the group at increased risk for AIDS. (Data from Heyward & Curran, 1989.)

uals with hemophilia B (factor IX deficiency), mostly because of pre-1985 exposure (Morbidity and Mortality Weekly, 1987, December 18).

The disease appears to be especially prevalent in the black and Hispanic communities. As of July 4, 1988, 66,464 AIDS cases had been reported nationally, 60% in non-Hispanic whites, 26% in blacks, and 13% in Hispanics (Morbidity and Mortality Weekly, 1988). Blacks and Hispanics accounted for 70% of cases in heterosexual men, 70% of cases in women, and 75% of cases in children in the United States. Most were associated with intravenous drug abuse.

At least fifteen individuals have been documented to have contracted AIDS through occupational exposure, primarily health care workers who had been accidentally stuck with needles containing virus-contaminated blood or had broken areas of skin exposed to large quantities of contaminated blood. As of March 14, 1988, 2,586 health care workers in the United States have been diagnosed as having AIDS, of which 95% fall into known risk groups; however, most of the remaining 5% are still under investigation. As of December 31, 1987, 901 health care workers had been exposed through sticks

(needles or other sharp objects); of these, 870 were exposed to blood and the rest to other fluids) and four were infected (all through blood), and 169 were exposed through mucous membrane, open wound, or nonintact skin and none were infected. However, more recent reports on health care workers who are infected without other risks include 15 cases in which workers have seroconverted and 7 in which they have not. The seroconverted individuals include four nurses, one home health care provider, one phlebotomist, one technologist, one research laboratory worker, and seven not specified (Morbidity and Mortality Weekly, 1988, April 22). Because of the potential risk, all health care personnel should routinely follow the guidelines published for the Center for Disease Control (Morbidity and Mortality Weekly, 1988, June 24).

Etiology

AIDS is caused by a virus, currently named human immunodeficiency virus or HIV, that has been isolated by researchers at the National Institutes of Health as the human T-lymphotropic virus type III or HTLV-III (Gallo et al., 1984) and the Pasteur Institute as the lym-

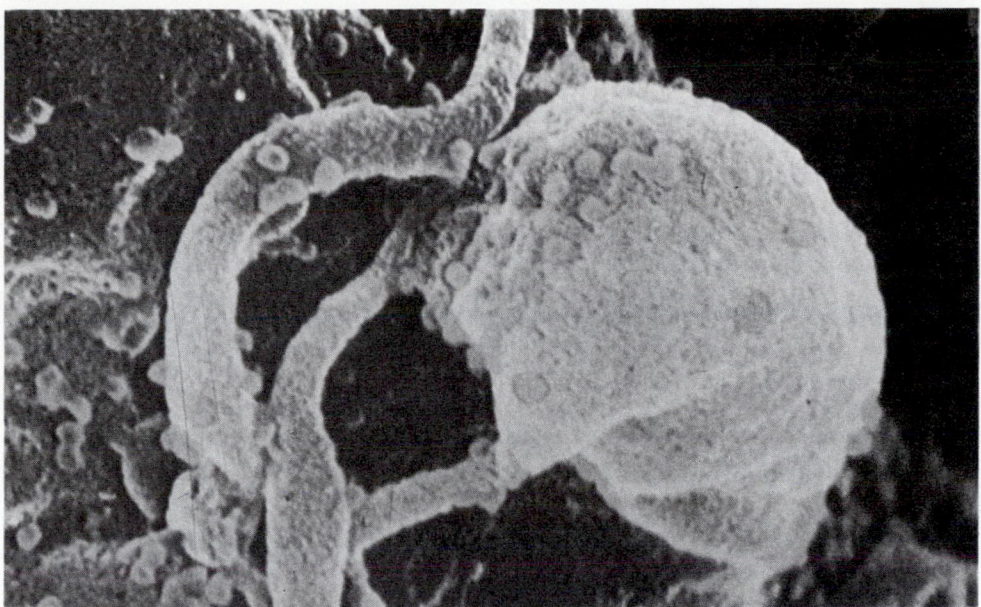

FIG. 8-10. Human immunodeficiency virus released from infected T$_4$ cells (particles spherical in shape) spread over adjacent T$_4$ cells, infecting them in turn. The individual AIDS particles are very tiny, over 200 million would fit on the period at the end of this sentence.

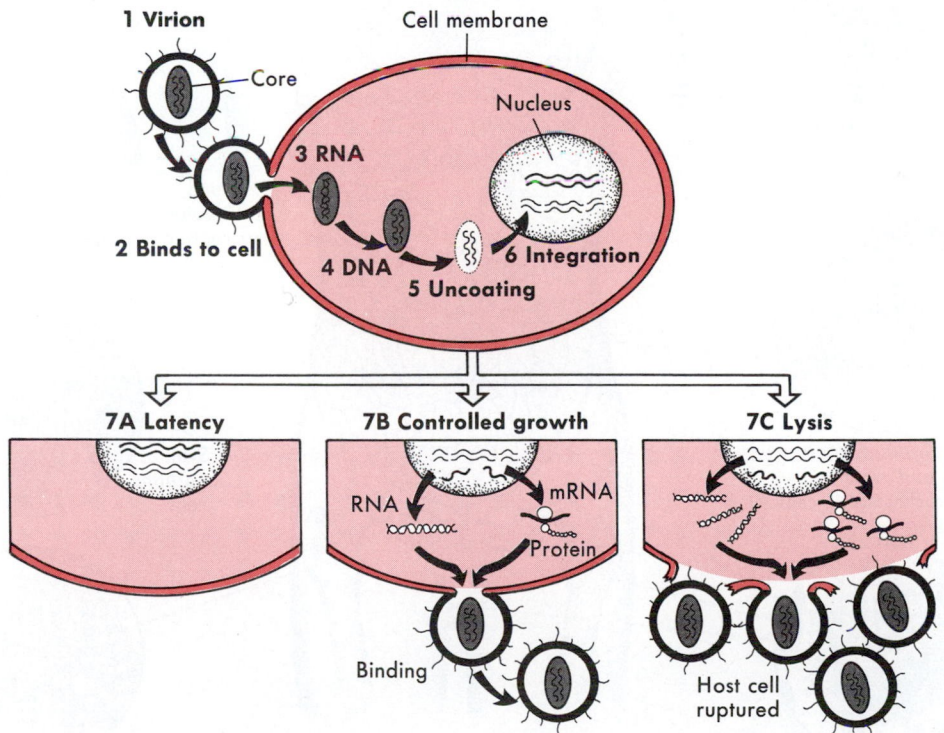

FIG. 8-11. HIV infection begins *(top)* when a virion, or virus particle, binds to the outside of a susceptible cell and fuses with it, injecting the core proteins and two strands of viral RNA. The double-stranded DNA (provirus) migrates to the nucleus and is integrated into the cell's own DNA. The provirus can then do a couple of things: (a) remain latent or (b) activate cellular mechanisms to copy its genes into RNA, some of which is translated into viral proteins or ribosomes. The proteins and additional RNA are then assembled into new virions that bud from the cell. The process can take place slowly, sparing the host cell (b), or so rapidly that the cell is lysed or ruptured (c).

phadenopathy/AIDS virus or LAV (Barre-Sinoussi et al., 1983). At least one other AIDS-virus (HIV-II) has been identified (Clavel et al., 1987).

HIV is a retrovirus carrying genetic information in RNA rather than DNA (Fig. 8-10). Retroviruses infect cells by binding to the surface of a target cell through a receptor and inserting their RNA into the target cell (Fig. 8-11). Through the use of a viral enzyme, reverse transcriptase, the viral RNA is converted to DNA and inserted into the infected cell's genetic material. If the cell is activated, viral proliferation may occur, resulting in the lysis and death of the infected cell. If, however, the cell remains relatively dormant, the viral genetic material is integrated into the infected cell's DNA, may remain dormant for years, and is probably present for the life of the individual (Ho, Pomerantz, & Kaplan, 1987).

CD4 is an antigen on the surface of T-helper cells that acts as a receptor for the HIV. The virus primarily infects CD4-positive T-helper lymphocytes, but may also infect various other cells of the central nervous system

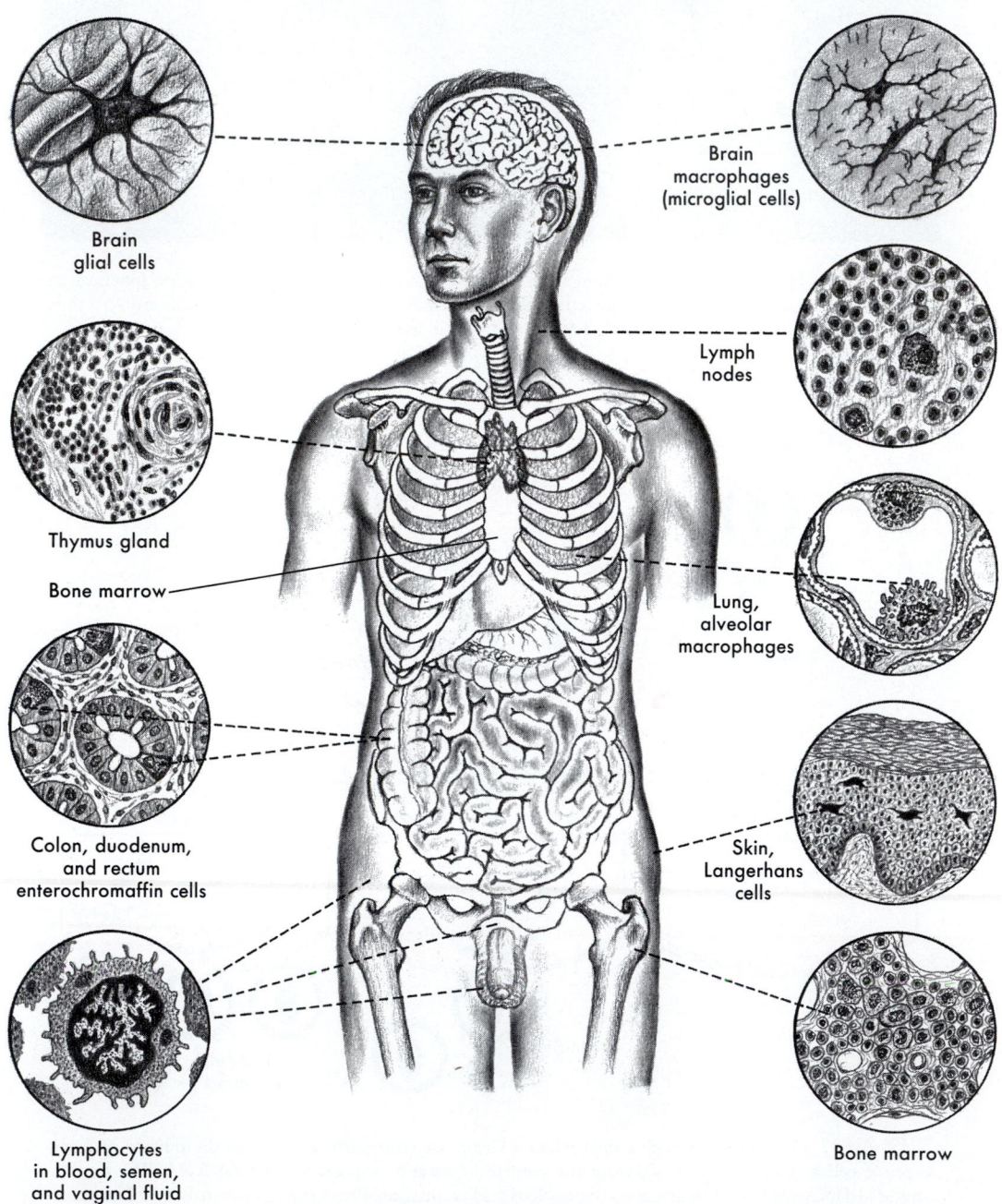

FIG. 8-12. Distribution of tissues that can be infected by the HIV. Infection is closely linked to the presence of CD4 receptors on host tissue, with the possible exceptions of glial cells in the brain and chromaffin cells in the colon, duodenum, and rectum. (Adapted from Weber & Weiss, 1989.)

that also express the CD4 antigen (Funke et al., 1987). Once activated, the virus infects other CD4-positive cells and kills them, causing a marked decrease in CD4 cells.

A second virus, HIV-II, has recently been identified in Africa. The first case of HIV-II in the United States was diagnosed in December 1987 in a recent visitor from West Africa (Morbidity and Mortality Weekly, 1988, April 15).

Clinical Manifestations

At the time of diagnosis, the individual may manifest one of three different conditions: serologically positive but asymptomatic, AIDS-related complex (ARC), or full-blown AIDS. The clinical symptoms of AIDS include persistent lymphadenopathy, weight loss, recurrent fevers, neurologic abnormalities, recurrent pulmonary infiltrates, and the development of opportunistic infections (such as *Pneumocystis carinii* pneumonia) and atypical malignancies (such as Kaposi's sarcoma) (Fig. 8-12). Individuals who have ARC present with relatively mild symptoms that may resemble influenza,

whereas full-blown AIDS is characterized by severe symptoms and an increase in infections and malignancies.

HIV also infects the central nervous system, resulting in AIDS dementia complex in the late stages of the disease (Price et al., 1988). Dementia is present in most individuals because of atrophy of cells of the cerebrum and degeneration of the nerve endings. Symptoms include lack of motor coordination and behavioral changes, including psychosis in the most extreme cases.

The presence of circulating antibody against the AIDS virus apparently indicates infection by the virus, although many of these individuals will be asymptomatic. Antibody appears rather rapidly after infection through blood products, usually within 4 to 7 weeks. After sexual exposure, however, the individual can be infected yet seronegative for 6 to 14 months. In addition, in the late stages of the disease some individuals become seronegative because of a deficient immune system. The incidence of antibody detected in asymptomatic individuals suggests that approximately 1 to 2 million people in the United States are infected at the

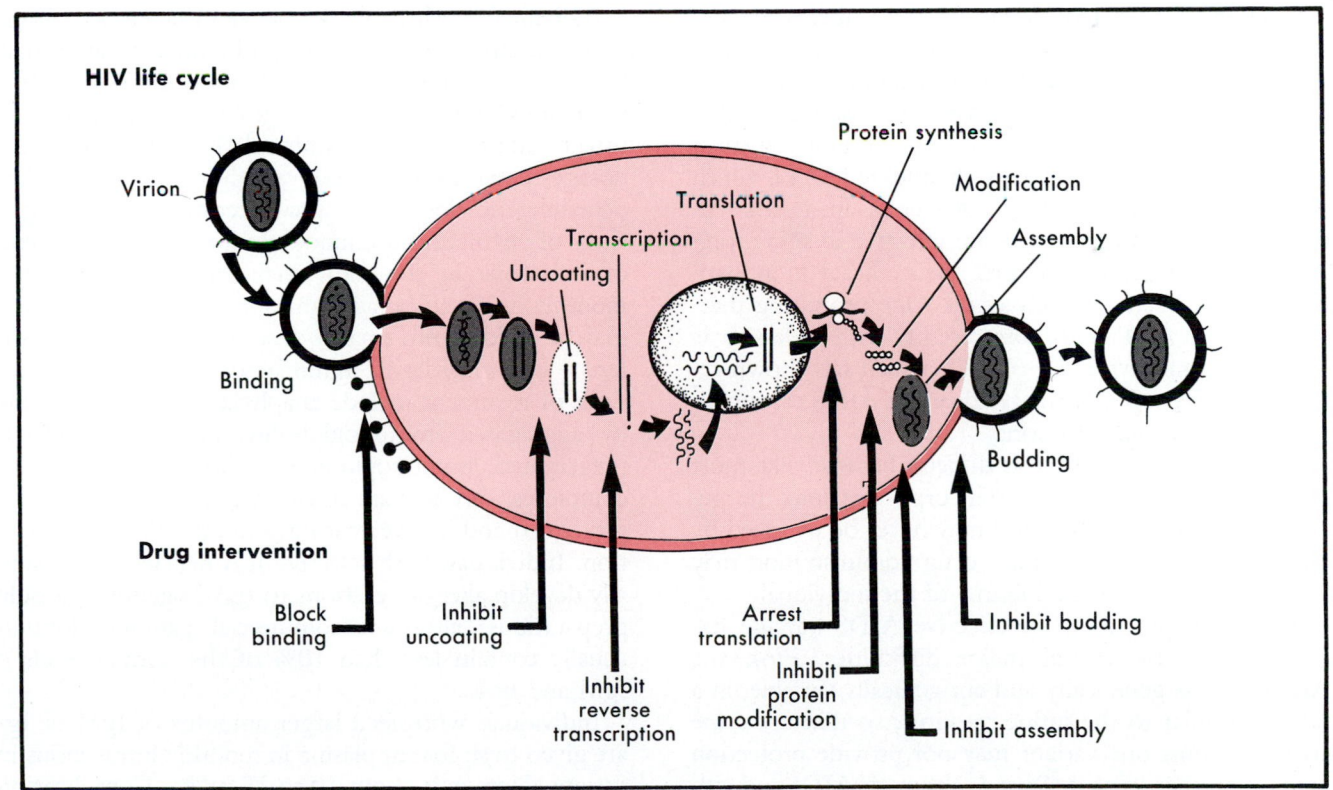

FIG. 8-13. HIV is subject to attack by drugs at several stages. Certain agents could block the binding of the HIV to CD4 receptors on the surface of helper T cells (1). Other agents might keep viral RNA and reverse transcriptase from leaving their protein coat (2). Drugs such as *AZT* and other *dideoxynucleosides* prevent the reverse transcription of viral RNA into viral DNA (3). Later, *antisense oligonucleotides* could block the transulation of mRNA into viral proteins. (4) Certain compounds could interfere with viral assembly by modifying such processes (5) and finally, antiviral agents such as *interferon* could keep the virus from assemblying itself and budding out of the cell. (Adapted from Yarchoan, Metsuya, & Broder, 1989.)

time of this writing and from 500,000 to 3 million people worldwide will develop AIDS by 1992.

The major immunologic finding in AIDS is the striking decrease in the number of T-helper cells (CD4-positive cells). Suppressor cells, which have the CD8 antigen, are usually normal or slightly elevated in number. This results in a reversal of the normal helper-to-suppressor T cell ratio, which is about 1.9. Most individuals with full-blown AIDS have ratios much lower than 0.9 and frequently near 0. In contrast, B cell numbers are usually normal.

Treatment

There are two approaches to treatment for AIDS: restoration of immune function and prevention of viral replication. Restoration of immune function has been attempted with bone marrow transplants, transfusions of white blood cells from healthy donors, and the injection of soluble mediators (e.g., interleuken-2, interferons). Attempts at restoration have met with little or no success because the virus very quickly infects the donor cells.

Several antibiotics have been tried to prevent viral replication (Fig. 8-13). Some of these agents are designed to block reverse transcriptase activity and some have been successful as antibiotics against other viruses or parasites (e.g., suramin against trypanosomiasis; ribavirin against cold and flu viruses; acyclovir against herpes simplex virus; and azidothymidine [AZT], which suppresses retrovirus-induced leukemia in mice). Although most of these agents are effective in preventing AIDS virus replication in vitro, their efficacy in individuals has not been generally good. One promising therapy has been AZT, and more recently with its less toxic analogue cyanothymidine (CNT), which has shown remarkable effects in extremely advanced AIDS cases with recurrent *P. carinii* infections.

Drug therapy for AIDS is difficult because, like most retroviruses, the AIDS virus incorporates into the genetic material of the host and may never be removed by antibiotic therapy. Therefore, drug administration may have to continue for the lifetime of the individual.

The development of an effective AIDS vaccine has been slowed by several major difficulties. *First,* the AIDS virus is genetically and antigenically variable, in a fashion similar to the influenza virus, so that a vaccine created against one variant may not provide protection against another variant. *Second,* although AIDS individuals have high levels of circulating antibodies against the virus, these antibodies do not appear to be protective. Therefore, even if an antibody response can be induced by vaccine, that response might not be effective. *Third,* the AIDS virus is transmitted from cell-to-cell and may initially enter the body in an infected cell. Microorganisms that spread by cell-to-cell contact are usually not susceptible to circulating antibody. *Fourth,* the only good animal model for AIDS experimentation is the chimpanzee, which is a protected species and relatively unavailable for medical research. This means that the efficacy and toxicity of candidate vaccines cannot easily be evaluated.

Clinical Evaluation of Immunity

Individuals with immune deficiencies present to the health provider with one common symptom, recurrent infections. In order to delineate the pathophysiology of a particular deficiency, certain observations and tests of the immune system are made. Significant information on the specific immune deficiency can be obtained by noting certain characteristics of the individual, including the presence of any associated anomalies, age, sex, and the types of infections (bacterial, viral, or fungal, and the specific organisms involved). Laboratory evaluation of immune deficiencies is presented in Table 8-6.

Replacement Therapies For Immune Deficiencies
Gamma Globulin Therapy

Individuals with B cell deficiencies that cause hypogammaglobulinemia or agammaglobulinemia can usually be treated successfully with administration of gamma globulin. Commercial gamma globulin preparations are usually administered intramuscularly once a month at dosages determined by body weight (0.2 to 0.6 ml/kg). Schedule and dosage are also determined according to titers of circulating immunoglobulins and the incidence of infections in the individual. In a 70-kg adult, a monthly dose can be as high as 42 ml, in which case it may be divided into smaller doses injected weekly at different sites in order to minimize discomfort. Complications of treatment include anaphylactic reactions caused by aggregated immunoglobulins in the preparations (aggregated immunoglobulins, though not immune complexes, can activate inflammation as immune complexes do) and inadvertent intravenous (IV) administration. Individuals with selective IgA deficiency occasionally develop allergic reactions to IgA in gamma globulin preparations, although commercial gamma globulins usually contain less than 10% of the normal levels of IgM and IgA.

Individuals who need larger amounts of IgM or IgA are given fresh frozen plasma in monthly intravenous infusions. Dosage is about 10 to 15 ml/kg. Complications associated with plasma therapy include the potential transmission of hepatitis or AIDS. The plasma is irradiated to destroy immunocompetent T cells and avoid graft-versus-host disease in individuals with accompanying T cell deficiencies. Administration of fresh frozen plasma is successful in individuals with Wiskott-Aldrich syndrome (IgM deficient), ataxia telangiectasia (IgA deficient), or complement component deficiencies.

TABLE 8-6 Laboratory evaluation of immune deficiencies

Function tested	Laboratory test	Interpretation of test
TESTS OF HUMORAL IMMUNE FUNCTION		
Antibody production	Total immunoglobulin levels	Presence of antibody producing B cells
	Levels of isohemagglutinins	Capacity to produce specific IgM antibodies
	Levels of antibodies against vaccines—especially diptheria and tetanus toxoids	Capacity to produce specific IgG antibodies
B cell numbers	Numbers of lymphocytes with surface immunoglobulin	Presence of circulating B cells
TESTS OF CELLULAR IMMUNE FUNCTION		
Delayed hypersensitivity skin test	Skin test reaction against previously encountered antigens—especially *C. albicans* or tetanus toxoid	Presence of antigen-responsive T cells and cellular interactions (e.g., lymphokine activity and macrophage function)
T cell numbers	Numbers of T cells forming rosettes with sheep erythrocytes or expressing membrane CD3 or CD11 antigen	Presence of circulating T cells
T cell proliferation in vitro	Proliferative response to nonspecific mitogens (e.g., phytohemaglutinin)	Capacity of all T cells to divide in response to nonspecific stimulation (mitogens)
	Proliferative response to antigens (e.g., tetanus toxoid)	Capacity of antigen-reactive T cells to respond to antigen

Transplantation and Transfusion

In SCID caused by a lack of stem cells, bone marrow is transplanted from a HLA-matched donor. Other diseases involving depletion of the bone marrow (i.e., aplastic anemia, leukemia requiring eradication of tumor cells in the marrow) are also treated by bone marrow transplantation. At least 75% of bone marrow transplants between individuals who are matched for HLA-A, B, C, and DR, and whose lymphocytes are nonstimulatory in one-way mixed lymphocyte reactions (matched at HLA-D), are accepted. Most rejections of HLA-matched transplants are because of recognition of minor histocompatibility antigens by individuals who have received multiple transfusions and are, as a result, sensitized against those antigens, which are not evaluated in tissue typing.

Graft-versus-host (GVH) disease may develop if the recipient's cells express histocompatibility antigens not found on the donor's cells. GVH disease occurs when immunocompetent T lymphocytes in the grafted material recognize foreign antigens in the recipient, initiating a type IV hypersensitivity reaction against the recipient's tissues. The main target tissues of the reaction are the skin, gastrointestinal mucosa, and the liver. Symptoms of a GVH reaction usually appear within 10 to 30 days after the transplant, develop as a skin rash, hepatomegaly, and diarrhea, and may lead to death due to infec-

tions. GVH disease is not a problem when the recipient is immunocompetent; that is, has an immune system that can control the donor's lymphocytes.

Several attempts have been made to prevent GVH disease by removing mature immunocompetent T lymphocytes from grafts. One procedure is to infuse the graft with monoclonal antibody against plasma membrane antigens found only on mature T cells. Another is to use fetal tissue as the graft. For example, fetal liver, which contains stem cells but not immunocompetent lymphocytes, is sometimes grafted in place of bone marrow if a HLA-matched donor cannot be found. Usually, fetal liver transplants are only successful over the short term.

Reconstitution of thymic function is one therapy for deficiency diseases in which the individual lacks a thymus or thymic function (i.e., DiGeorge syndrome, ataxia telangiectasia, or chronic mucocutaneous candidiasis). The procedure is to transplant fetal thymus tissue, which lacks immunocompetent T cells, or thymic epithelial cells (the cells that produce the thymic hormones) from which mature T cells have been removed. In some individuals, transplantation increases the number of circulating mature T cells, but in most cases improvement is only temporary.

Enzymatic defects that cause SCID (e.g., adenosine deaminase deficiency) are sometimes treated successfully with transfusions of glycerol frozen-packed erythrocytes. The donor erythrocytes contain the needed enzyme and can, at least temporarily, provide sufficient enzyme for normal lymphocyte function.

The administration of soluble materials that affect lymphocyte function can restore T cell function, especially in individuals with Wiskott-Aldrich syndrome or chronic mucocutaneous candidiasis. Transfer factor, a low-molecular-weight nucleoprotein prepared from lymphocyte lysates, can confer specific reactivity against certain antigens and has been used successfully in some individuals. Thymosin, a thymic hormone, has also been used, although with limited success.

SUMMARY REVIEW

Hypersensitivity: Allergy, Autoimmunity, and Isoimmunity

1 Hypersensitivity is an inappropriate immune response misdirected against the host's own tissues (autoimmunity); directed against beneficial foreign tissues, such as transfusions or transplants (isoimmunity); or exaggerated responses against environmental antigens (allergy).

2 Mechanisms of hypersensitivity are classified as type I (IgE-mediated) reactions, type II (tissue-specific) reactions, type III (immune-complex-mediated) reactions, and type IV (cell-mediated) reactions.

3 Hypersensitivity reactions can be immediate (developing within seconds or hours) or delayed (developing within hours or days).

4 Anaphylaxis, the most rapid immediate hypersensitivity reaction, is an explosive reaction that occurs within minutes of reexposure to the antigen and can lead to cardiovascular shock.

5 Allergens are antigens that cause allergic responses.

6 Type I (IgE-mediated) reactions are mediated through the binding of IgE to Fc receptors on mast cells and cross-linking of IgE by antigens that bind to the Fab portions of IgE. Cross-linking causes mast cell degranulation and the release of histamine and other inflammatory substances.

7 Type II (tissue-specific) reactions are caused by four possible mechanisms: complement-mediated lysis, opsonization and phagocytosis, antibody-dependent cell-mediated cytotoxicity, and modulation of cellular function.

8 Type III (immune-complex-mediated) reactions are caused by the formation of immune complexes that are deposited in target tissues, where they activate the complement cascade, generating chemotactic fragments that attract neutrophils into the inflammatory site.

9 Immune-complex disease can be a systemic reaction, such as serum sickness or localized, such as the Arthus reaction.

10 Type IV (cell-mediated) reactions are caused by specifically sensitized T cells, which either kill target cells directly or release lymphokines that activate other cells, such as macrophages.

11 Allergies can be mediated by any of the four mechanisms of hypersensitivity.

12 Clinical manifestations of allergic reactions are usually confined to the areas of initial intake or contact with the allergen. Ingested allergens induce gastrointestinal symptoms, air-borne allergens induce respiratory or skin manifestations, and contact allergens induce allergic responses at the site of contact.

13 Atopic individuals are genetically predisposed to the development of allergies.

14 Autoimmunity is a breakdown of immunologic homeostasis, the immune system's tolerance of self-antigens.

15 Autoimmune disease can be caused by the exposure of a previously sequestered antigen, the development of a neoantigen, the complications of infectious disease, the emergence of a forbidden clone of lymphocytes, or an alteration of suppressor T cell function.

16 Isoimmunity is the immune system's reaction against antigens on the tissues of other members of the same species.

17 Isoimmune disorders include transient neonatal disease, in which the maternal immune system becomes sensitized against antigens expressed by the fetus, and transplant rejection and transfusion reactions, in which the immune system of the recipient of an organ transplant or blood transfusion reacts against foreign antigens on the donor's cells.

Immune Deficiency

1 Immune deficiency is the failure of mechanisms of self-defense to function in their normal capacity.

2 Immune deficiencies are either congenital (primary) or acquired (secondary). Congenital immune deficiences are caused by genetic defects that disrupt lymphocyte development, whereas acquired immune deficiencies are secondary to disease or other physiologic alterations.

3 The clinical hallmark of immune deficiency is a propensity to unusual or recurrent severe infections. The type of infection usually reflects the immune system defect.

4 The most common infections in individuals with defects of cell-mediated immune response are fungal and viral, whereas infections in individuals with defects of the humoral immune response or complement function are primarily bacterial.

5 Severe combined immune deficiency (SCID) is a total lack of T cell function and a severe (either partial or total) lack of B cell function.

6 DiGeorge syndrome (congenital thymic aplasia or hypoplasia) is characterized by complete or partial lack of the thymus (resulting in depressed T cell immunity), the parathyroid glands (resulting in hypocalcemia), and cardiac anomalies.

7 Defects in B cell function are diverse, ranging from a complete lack of the human bursal equivalent, the lymphoid organs required for B cell maturation (as in Bruton's agammaglobulinemia), to deficiencies in a single

class of immunoglobulins (e.g., selective IgA deficiency).

8 Defects in phagocyte function, which include insufficient numbers of phagocytes or defects of chemotaxis, phagocytosis, or killing, can result in recurrent, life-threatening infections, such as septicemia and disseminated pyogenic lesions.

9 Acquired immune deficiencies are caused by superimposed conditions, such as malnutrition, medical therapies, physical or psychological trauma, or infections.

10 AIDS is an acquired dysfunction of the immune system caused by a retrovirus (HIV) that infects and destroys T4 positive lymphocytes (helper T cells).

11 Immune deficiency syndromes are usually treated by replacement therapy. Deficient antibody production is treated by replacement of missing immunoglobulins with commercial gamma globulin preparations. Lymphocyte deficiencies are treated with the replacement of host lymphocytes with transplants of bone marrow, fetal liver, or fetal thymus from a donor.

KEY TERMS

Acquired (secondary) immune deficiency, 265

Acquired immune deficiency syndrome (AIDS), 269

Agammaglobulinemia, 266

Allergen, 253

Allergy, 249

Anaphylaxis, 252

Arthus reaction, 258

Atopic dermatitis, 260

Atopic individual, 255

Autoantibody, 252

Autoimmune disease (autoimmunity), 250

Blocking antibody, 255

Bruton's agammaglobulinemia, 267

Chronic mucocutaneous candidiasis, 268

Congenital (primary) immune deficiency, 265

Contact dermatitis, 260

Cytotropic, 253

Delayed hypersensitivity reaction, 252

DiGeorge syndrome, 266

Forbidden clone, 261

Hypersensitivity, 249

Hypocomplementemia, 258

Hypogammaglobulinemia, 266

Immediate hypersensitivity reaction, 252

Immune deficiency, 265

Immunologically privileged site, 261

Immunologic homeostasis (tolerance), 252

Isoimmune diseases, 252

Isoimmunity, 252

Neoantigen, 260

Radioallergosorbent (RAST) testing, 255

Radioimmunosorbent (RIST) testing, 255

Raynaud's phenomenon, 258

Reagin, 253

Reticular dysgenesis, 266

Selective IgA deficiency, 267

Sequestered antigen, 261

Serum sickness, 258

Severe combined immune deficiency (SCID), 266

Systemic lypus erythematosus (SLE), 263

Tissue-specific antigen, 255

Urticaria (hives), 254

Wheal and flare reaction, 255

Wiskott-Aldrich syndrome, 267

REFERENCES

Adler, M. W. (1987). ABC of AIDS: Development of the epidemic. *British Medical Journal, 294,* 1083-1085.

Arthus, M. & Breton, M. (1903). Lesions cutanees produites par les injections de serum. *Compt Rend Soc Biol, 55,* 817-820.

Barnes, D. M. (1987). Research news: AIDS: Statistics but few answers. *Science, 236,* 1423-1425.

Barre-Sinoussi, F., Chermann, J. C., Rey, F., Nugeyre, M. T., Chamaret, S., Gruest, J., Daugquet, C., Axler-Blin, C., Vezinet-Brun, F., Rouzioux, C., Qozenbaum, W., & Montagnier, L. (1983). Isolation of a T-lymphocyte retroviruses from a patient at risk for acquired immune deficiency syndrome (AIDS). *Science, 220,* 868-871.

Bruton, O. C. (1952). Agammaglobulinemia. *Pediatrics, 9,* 722-728.

CDC surveillance summaries: Report on selected racial/ethnic groups. (1988). *Morbidity and Mortality Weekly, 37,* 1-10.

Church, J. A. & Schlegel, R. J. (1985). Immune deficiency disorders. In J. A. Bellanti (Ed.), *Immunology III.* Philadelphia: W.B. Saunders, p. 493.

Clavel, F., Mansinho, K., Chamaret, S., Guetard, D., Favier, V., Nina, J., Santos-Ferreira, M-O, Champalimaud, J-J., & Montagnier, L. (1987). Human immunodeficiency virus type 2 infection associated with AIDS in West Africa. *New England Journal of Medicine, 316,* 1180-1185.

DiGeorge, A. M. (1968). Congenital absence of the thymus and its immunologic consequences. In D. Bergsma & F.A. McKusick (Eds.), *Immunologic deficiency diseases in man.* National Foundation—March of Dimes Original Article Series: Williams & Wilkins.

Frank, M. M. (1987). Current concepts: Complement in the pathophysiology of human disease. *New England Journal of Medicine, 316,* 1525-1530.

Fritzler, M. J. & Tan, E. M. (1985). Antinuclear antibodies and the connective tissue diseases. In A. S. Cohen (Ed.), *Laboratory diagnostic procedures in the rheumatic diseases.* Orlando, FL: Grune and Stratton, Inc., p. 213.

Funke, I., Hahn, A., Reiber, E. P., Weiss, E., & Riethmüller, G. (1987). The cellular receptor (CD4) of the human immunodeficiency virus is expressed on neurons and glial cells in human brain. *Journal of Experimental Medicine, 165,* 1230-1235.

Gallo, R. C., Salahuddin, S. Z., Popovic, M., Shearer, G. S., Kaplan, M., Haynes, B. F., Kaplan, M., Palker, T. J., Redfield, R., Oleske, J., Safai, B. et al. (1984). Frequent detection and isolation of cytopathic retroviruses (HTLV-III) from patients with AIDS. *Science, 224,* 500-503.

Gell, P. G. H., Coombs, R. R. A., & Lachman, P. T. (1975). *Clinical aspects of immunology.* Oxford: Blackwell Scientific Publications.

Habif, T. P. (1985). *Clinical dermatology: a color guide to diagnosis and therapy.* St. Louis: C. V. Mosby.

Heyward, W. L., & Curran, J. W. (1989). The epidemiology of AIDS in the U.S. In *The science of AIDS: readings from Scientific American.* New York: W. H. Freeman.

Ho, D. D., Pomerantz, R. J., & Kaplan, J. C. (1987). Pathogenesis of infection with human immunodeficiency virus. *New England Journal of Medicine, 317,* 278-286.

Human immunodeficiency virus infection in the United States: A review of current knowledge. (1987). *Morbidity and Mortality Weekly, 36,* 1-48.

Koch, R. (1891). Fortsetzung der mitteilungen über ein heilmittel gegen tuberkulose. *Deutsch Med Wochenschr, 9,* 101-102.

Piot, P., Plummer, F. A., Mhalu, F. S., Lamboray, J-L, Chin, J., & Mann, J. M. (1988). AIDS: An international perspective. *Science, 239,* 573-579.

Pirquet, C. & Schick, B. (1905). *Serum sickness.* Leipzig: Franz Denticke.

Portier, P. & Richet, C. (1902). De l'action anaphylactique de certains venins. *CR Soc Biol* (Paris), *54,* 170-172.

Price, R. W., Brew, B., Sidtis, J., Rosenblum, M., Schenk, A. C., & Cleary, P. (1988). The brain in AIDS: Central nervous system HIV-1 infection and AIDS dementia complex. *Science, 239,* 586-592.

Quarterly report to the domestic policy council on the prevalence and rate of spread of HIV and AIDS in the United States. (1988). *Morbidity and Mortality Weekly, 37,* 223-227.

Rote, N. S. (1985). Immune complex disorders and vasculitis. In N. Gleicher (Ed.), *Principles of medical therapy in pregnancy.* New York: Plenum Medical Book Company, pp. 981-989.

Schlegel, R. J., Bernier, G. M., Bellanti, J. A. et al. (1970). Severe candidiasis associated with thymic dysplasia, IgA deficiency, and plasma antilymphocyte effects. *Pediatrics, 45,* 926.

Update: Acquired immunodeficiency syndrome (AIDS) - Worldwide. (1988). *Morbidity and Mortality Weekly, 37,* 286-295.

Update: Acquired immunodeficiency syndrome and human immunodeficiency virus infection among health-care workers. (1988). *Morbidity and Mortality Weekly, 37,* 229-239.

Update: Universal precautions for prevention of transmission of human immunodeficiency virus, hepatitis B virus, and other bloodborne pathogens in health-care settings. (1988). *Morbidity and Mortality Weekly, 37,* 377-388.

Weber, J. N., & Weiss, R. A. (1989). HIV infection: the cellular picture. In *The science of AIDS: readings from Scientific American.* New York: W. H. Freeman.

Yarchoan, R., Mitsuya, H., & Broder, S. (1989). AIDS therapies. In *The science of AIDS: readings from Scientific American.* New York: W. H. Freeman.

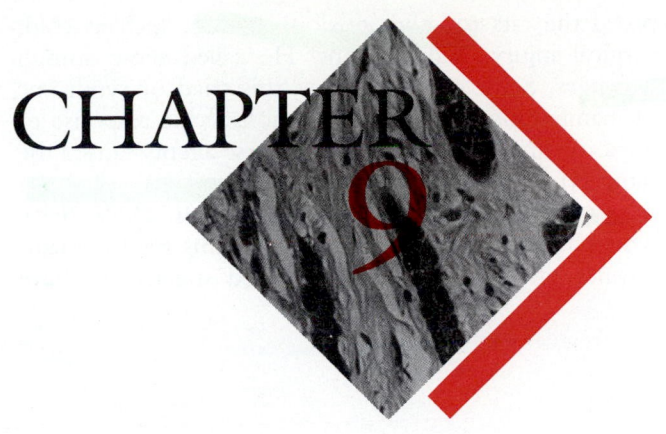

CHAPTER 9

Stress and Disease

Kathryn L. McCance

Concepts of stress, 279
    General adaptation syndrome, 279
    Psychologic mediators and specificity, 282
    Homeostasis as a dynamic steady state, 283
The stress response, 283
    Neuroendocrine regulation, 283
      Catecholamines, 283
      Cortisol, 284
    Other hormones, 286
      Endorphins, 286
      Growth hormone, 286
      Somatotropin, 286
      Prolactin, 286
      Testosterone, 287
    Role of the immune system, 287
Stress, coping, and illness, 288

The notion that prolonged emotional and/or psychologic stress can contribute to or even cause the development of physical illness has a long history. For example, Galen (200 AD) stated that "melancholic" women developed breast cancer more often than did "sanguine" women (Bieliauskas, 1982).

It is often reported that the usage of the term *stress* in a biologic sense began with Hans Selye in 1946. However, in 1914 Walter B. Cannon used the term in both a physiologic and a psychologic sense in a paper reporting his psychoendocrine studies. In his report Cannon used such phrases as "great emotional stress" and "times of stress" (Cannon, 1914). In 1935 Cannon published another paper, called "Stresses and Strains of Homeostasis." In it he applied the engineering concept of stress and strain in a physiologic context (Cannon, 1935). Cannon also thought that stress involved psychologic factors; he stated in his paper that physical as well as emotional stimuli can cause stress. The *popularization* of the term, however, began with Hans Selye's work.

The concept that stress may influence immunity and resistance to disease has been the subject of several investigations since the middle of the century. Studies reporting psychosocial factors to infectious diseases appeared in the literature in the 1950s. Rene Dubos (1955, 1961) emphasized that a multitude of factors cause disease, including prior exposure to a microorganism and development of immunity, nutritional status of the individual, presence of other disease, and many genetic factors.

Meyer and Haggarty (1962) reported that during the course of 1 year, the significant factor that determined whether an individual acquired a respiratory tract infection was acute or chronic family stress. Jacobs and colleagues reported that psychologic stimuli characterized by failure, unresolved role crisis, and social isolation in students were frequently associated with respiratory infections (Jacobs, Spilken, & Norman, 1969; Jacobs, Spilken, Norman, & Andersson, 1970). Overall, studies in the 1970s found that life changes and/or emotions resulting from life changes occurring for a prolonged period of time were associated with decreases in one or more immune functions. These studies, however, are only a beginning and much more research is needed to understand life changes and immune function.

Research in the 1980s provided answers to the biochemical relationships of the central and autonomic nervous systems, the endocrine system, and the immune system. Discoveries of these links have, in fact, created two new fields, neuroimmunomodulation and psychoneuroimmunology (which has a greater emphasis on behavior).

CONCEPTS OF STRESS

The term "stress" has been used persistently and widely in specialities such as biology, health sciences, and social sciences, despite numerous disagreements over its definition. Stress has an indefinite meaning and symbolizes different things to different people, yet historically, the concept of an association between stress and disease has endured.

General Adaptation Syndrome

Selye originally sought to discover a new sex hormone when he discovered the biologic syndrome of stress. In his attempts to discover the new hormone, Selye injected crude ovarian extracts into rats. Repeatedly, he found that the following triad of structural changes occurred: (1) enlargement of the cortex of the adrenal gland, (2) atrophy of the thymus gland and other lymphoid structures, and (3) development of bleeding ulcers of the stomach and duodenal lining. Selye soon discovered that this triad of manifestations was not specific for his ovarian extracts, but also occurred after he exposed the rats to other noxious stimuli, such as cold, surgical injury, and restraint. He called these stimuli **stressors.** Selye concluded that this triad or syndrome of manifestations represented a nonspecific response to noxious stimuli. Because many diverse agents caused the same syndrome, Selye suggested that it be called the **general adaptation syndrome** (GAS). In 1959, Selye wrote: "Specific homeostatic mechanisms for the maintenance of body temperature, blood sugar, etc., have

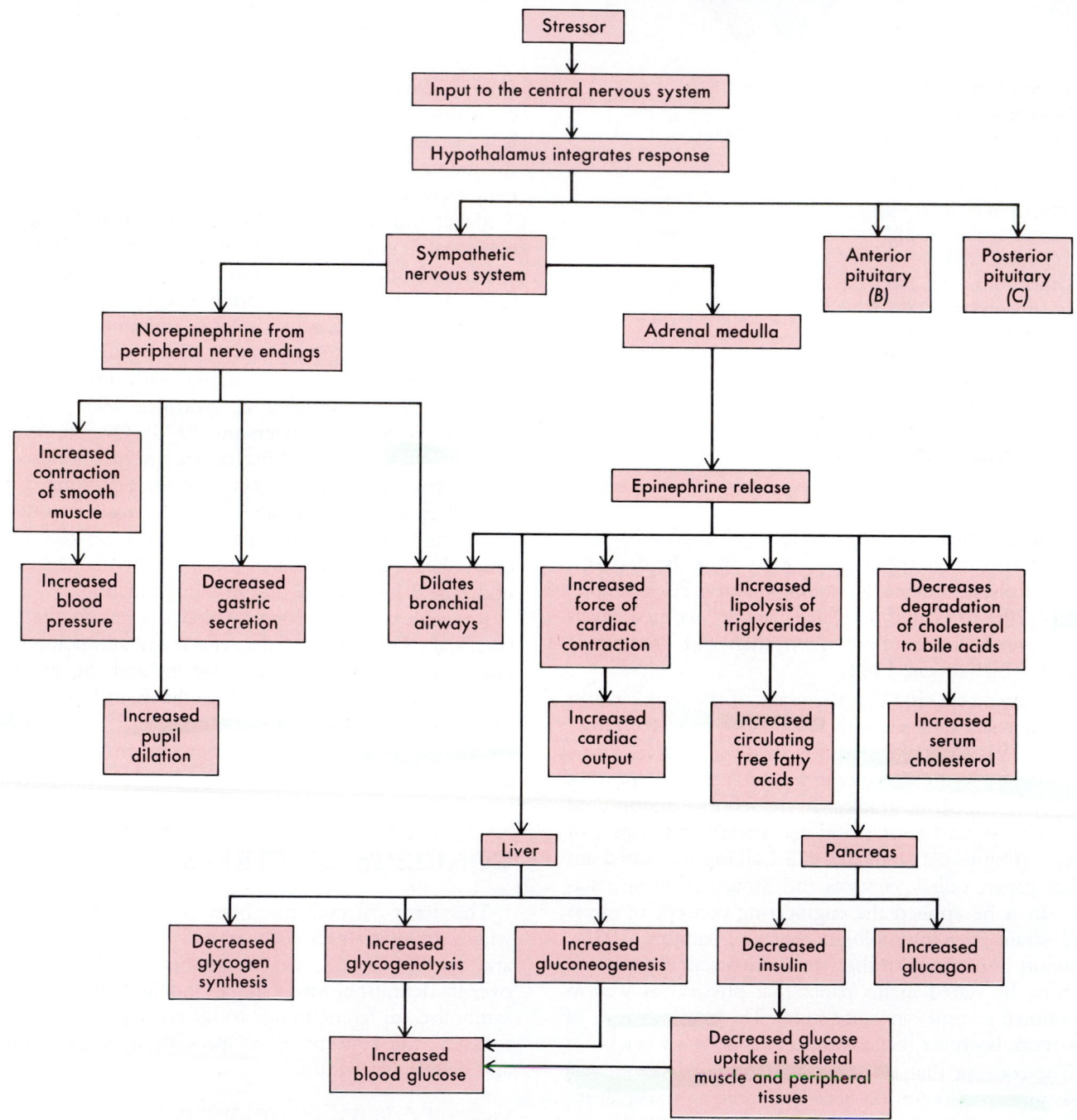

FIG. 9-1. The stress response. See text for explanation of hormone functions.

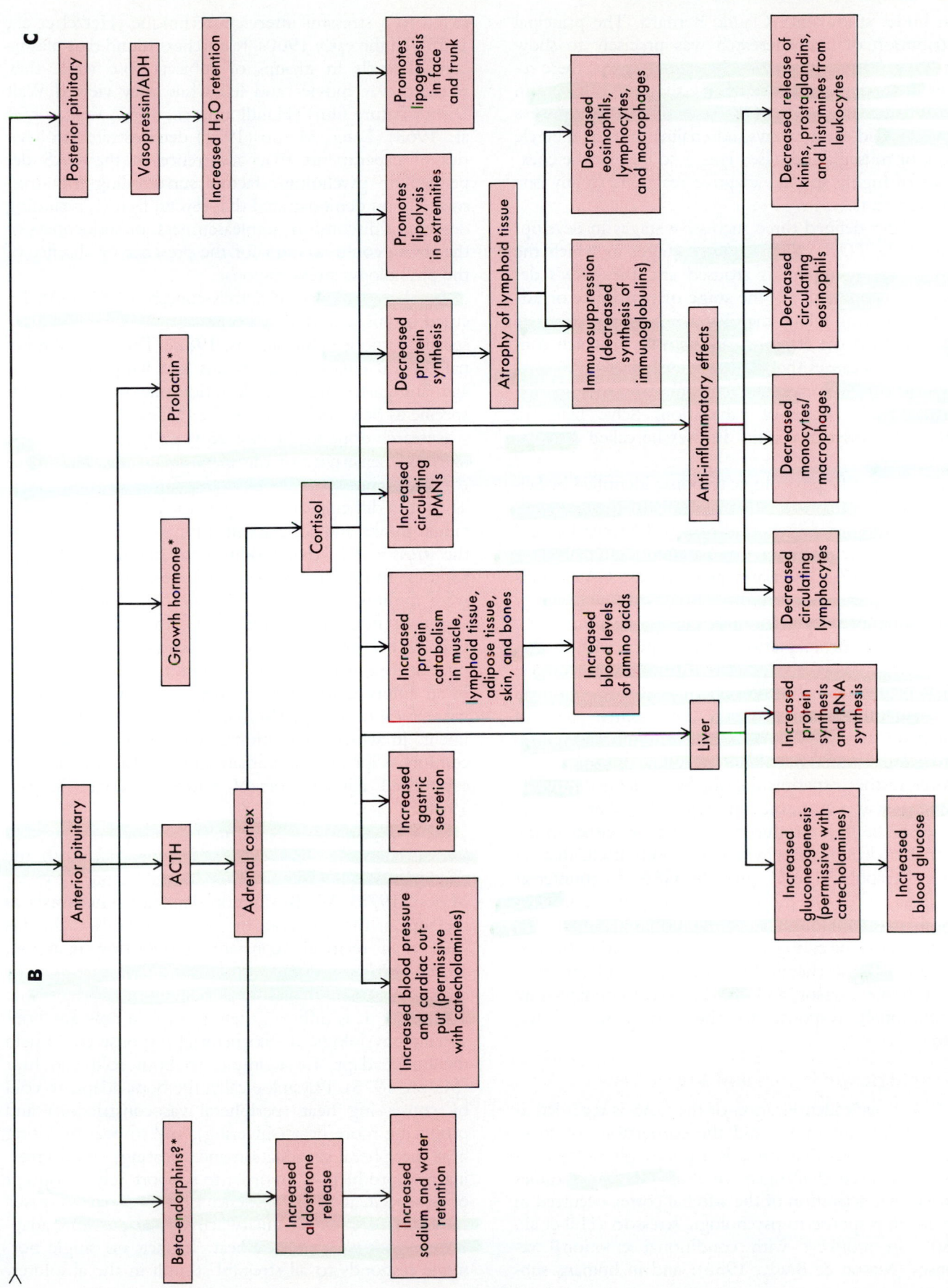

FIG. 9-1. cont'd. The stress response. (?, Unclear if endorphins originate from pituitary gland or CNS; *, explained in text.)

been under study since Claude Bernard. The principal contribution of stress research was precisely to show that if we abstract from three specific reactions, there remains a common residual response that is nonspecific in regard to its cause and can be elicited with such diverse agents as cold, heat, x-rays, adrenalin, insulin, tubercle bacilli, or muscular exercise. This is so despite the coexistence of highly specific adaptive reactions to any one of these agents."

Selye later defined three successive stages in development of the GAS: (1) the **alarm stage,** in which the central nervous system is aroused and the body's defenses are mobilized; (2) the **stage of resistance or adaptation,** during which mobilization leads to "flight or fight;" and (3) the **stage of exhaustion,** in which continuous stress causes the progressive breakdown of compensatory mechanisms (acquired adaptations) and homeostasis. The stage of exhaustion, Selye believed, marked the onset of certain diseases he called **diseases of adaptation.**

The nonspecific physiologic response identified by Selye consists of interaction among the sympathetic branch of the autonomic nervous system (see Chapter 12) and two glands, the pituitary gland and the adrenal gland (see Chapter 17). The alarm phase of the GAS begins when a stressor triggers the actions of the pituitary gland and the sympathetic nervous system (Fig. 9-1). The resistance or adaptation phase begins with the actions of the adrenal hormones cortisol, norepinephrine, and epinephrine. Exhaustion occurs if stress continues and adaptation is not successful. The ultimate signs of exhaustion are impairment of the immune response, heart failure, and kidney failure, leading to death.

After further experimentation, Selye defined **physiologic stress** as a chemical or physical disturbance in the cells or tissue fluid produced by a change, either in the external environment or within the body itself, that requires a response (i.e., begins the GAS) to counteract the disturbance. On the basis of this definition, Selye identified three components of physiologic stress: (1) the exogenous or endogenous stressor initiating the disturbance, (2) the chemical or physical disturbance produced by the stressor, and (3) the body's counteracting (adaptational) response to the disturbance (Selye, 1946).

Psychologic Mediators and Specificity

While Selye's identification of the GAS is regarded as tremendously important and the cornerstone of stress research, the idea that stress is a purely physiologic response has been challenged. In the mid-1950s, studies showed that activation of the adrenal cortex occurred in humans in response to psychologic stressors (Hill et al., 1956); in monkeys with conditional emotional responses (Mason & Brady, 1956); and in humans subjected to a stressful interview technique (Hetzel et al., 1955). In the early 1960s, researchers found that plasma cortisol levels in groups of subjects rose while they watched war movies and fell while they viewed Walt Disney nature films (Handlon et al., 1962; Wadeson et al., 1963). Later, Mason (1971) demonstrated in a series of experiments that occurrence of the GAS depended on psychologic factors surrounding the stressors. Mason demonstrated that several factors, including degrees of discomfort, unpleasantness, or suddenness of the stress, could account for the presence or absence of the physiologic stress response.

Another challenge to Selye's concept of the GAS focused on his idea that stressors cause a general or nonspecific response (Bieliauskas, 1982). The triad of adrenal cortical enlargment, thymus and lymphoid shrinkage, and gastrointestinal ulceration may not be as nonspecific as Selye believed it to be (Mason, 1975).

Research done in the past 25 years has shown the remarkable sensitivity of the pituitary gland and adrenal cortex to emotional, psychologic, and social influences. Thus it is difficult to know when it is the way an individual thinks and feels about a physical stressor and/or the stressor itself that produces the neuroendocrine responses. In experiments in which psychologic reactions were minimized, physical stressors did not appear to stimulate the pituitary or adrenal cortex in a nonspecific fashion. For example, fasting monkeys who were given nonnutritive placebo food to minimize the discomfort of an empty gastrointestinal tract did not secrete adrenal cortical hormones (Mason, 1972). In another experiment, in which precautions were taken to avoid discomfort, exposure of human subjects to heat actually suppressed adrenal cortical hormone levels (Mason, 1974).

Many physiologists resist Selye's concept of nonspecificity because it appears to be incompatible with the principles of physiologic homeostasis (Cannon, 1963; Mason, 1975). W. B. Cannon defined **homeostasis** as the sum of the processes by which the body maintains itself at a relatively constant composition (Cannon, 1935). Adaptive bodily responses are selective and are organized to counteract the specific bodily changes that elicit them. It is difficult, then, to explain how any nonspecific physiologic or biochemical response could help the body adapt, for example, to both cold and heat (Mason, 1975). Physiologically, the body adapts to cold by conserving heat (peripheral vasoconstriction) and producing more heat (shivering), and to heat by losing heat (peripheral vasodilation and sweating) and decreasing heat production. In order to support Selye's concept of nonspecificity, hard evidence is needed that increased adrenal cortical or medullary activity can promote adaptations to both cold and heat. In fact, no single hormone responds to all stressful stimuli in the absolutely nonspecific fashion implied in Selye's definition of the GAS.

Homeostasis as a Dynamic Steady State

Another source of confusion in the literature about stress is the concept of homeostasis. Selye used Cannon's definition of homeostasis (the sum of the processes by which the body maintains itself at a relatively constant composition) and expanded it to mean also that the body's need determines body responses and that adaptive responses are necessary to maintain body stability. Both Cannon's definition and Selye's extrapolation were oversimplified. Research with a variety of radioisotopes has since demonstrated that homeostasis does not mean "constant composition." Much more accurate is the concept of homeostasis as a **dynamic steady state.** For example, the fat or protein content of the body may not vary much from day to day, but the substances that make up the fat and protein—fatty acids and amino acids—can vary widely (Dickman, 1988). The enzymes in a healthy person are constantly synthesizing fat and proteins and also constantly breaking them down. The process of synthesis and breakdown of all bodily substances is known as **turnover.** Homeostasis, then, is more accurately defined as a dynamic steady state representing the net effect of all the turnover reactions.

Stressors cause a series of reactions that alter the dynamic steady state. This alteration may be either short- or long-term. For example, the normal concentration of glucose in the blood is 80 + or - 10 mg/100 ml. The concentration of glucose rises with acute stress, such as a burn injury, and then slowly returns to normal. If blood glucose remains high in the absence of a known stressor, it is diagnosed as a sign of disease—probably diabetes mellitus. Prolonged, unrelenting stress can cause a chronic elevation of glucose levels that leads to diabetes mellitus.

THE STRESS RESPONSE

Neuroendocrine Regulation

Stressors, such as infection, noise, decreased oxygen supply, pain, malnutrition, heat, cold, trauma, prolonged exertion, anxiety, depression, anger, fear, radiation, obesity, old age, excitement, drugs, disease, surgery, and medical treatment can elicit the physiologic stress response. The **stress response** is response initiated by the nervous and endocrine systems, specifically the sympathetic nervous system, the pituitary gland, and the adrenal gland (see Fig. 9-1). Recent evidence is linking the stress response with the immune system (see p. 287). The sympathetic nervous system is aroused during the stress response and causes the medulla of the adrenal gland to release catecholamines (epinephrine, norepinephrine, and dopamine) into the bloodstream. The adrenal medulla is actually an extension of the sympathetic nervous system because preganglionic fibers from the splanchnic nerve terminate in the medulla where they innervate the chromaffin cells that produce the catecholamine hormones. Simultaneously, the pituitary gland is stimulated to release a variety of hormones, including antidiuretic hormone, from the posterior pituitary gland, and prolactin, growth hormone, and adrenocorticotropin hormone (ACTH) from the anterior pituitary gland. ACTH stimulates the cortex of the adrenal gland to release cortisol.

Catecholamines

Epinephrine released from the adrenal medulla goes to the liver and skeletal muscle, but is then rapidly metabolized. Very little adrenal norepinephrine reaches distal tissue, thus, the effects caused by norepinephrine during the stress response are primarily from the sympathetic nervous system (Granner, 1988). Catecholamines cannot cross the blood-brain barrier; hence, they are synthesized locally in the brain (Granner, 1988). Catecholamines circulate in plasma in a loose association with albumin (Granner, 1988).

The catecholamines act by stimulating two major classes of receptors: α-adrenergic receptors and β-adrenergic receptors. These two classes are divided further into two subclasses: (1) α_1 and α_2, and (2) β_1 and β_2. Table 9-1 summarizes the actions of the two subclasses of adrenergic receptors. (A thorough discussion of receptors can be found in Chapters 1, 17, and 26.) Epinephrine binds to and activates both α and β receptors. Norepinephrine at physiologic concentrations primarily binds to α receptors (Granner, 1988).

The circulating catecholamines have essentially the same effects as direct sympathetic stimulation. (Sympathetic function is described in Chapter 12.) Norepinephrine regulates blood pressure because it is the primary constrictor of smooth muscle in all blood vessels. During stress, norepinephrine raises blood pressure by constricting peripheral vessels. It also inhibits gastrointestinal activity and dilates the pupil of the eye (Fig. 9-1).

Epinephrine causes some of the same effects as norepinephrine, yet it has greater influence on cardiac action and is the principal catecholamine involved in metabolic regulation. Epinephrine enhances myocardial contractility (inotropic effect), increases the heart rate (chronotropic effect), and increases venous return to the heart, all of which increase cardiac output and blood pressure. Metabollically, epinephrine causes transient hyperglycemia (high blood sugar) by activating enzymes whose actions promote glucose formation (gluconeogenesis and glycogenolysis in the liver) while inhibiting

TABLE 9-1 Summary of the physiologic actions of the alpha and beta receptors

Receptor	Physiologic actions
Alpha$_1$	Increased glycogenolysis; smooth muscle contraction (blood vessels, genitourinary tract)
Alpha$_2$	Smooth musle relaxation (gastrointestinal tract); smooth muscle contraction (some vascular beds); inhibition of lipolysis, renin release, platelet aggregation, and insulin secretion
Beta$_1$	Stimulation of lipolysis; myocardial contraction (increased rate, increased force)
Beta$_2$	Increased hepatic gluconeogenesis; increased hepatic glycogenolysis; increased muscle glycogenolysis; increased release of insulin, glucagon, and renin; smooth muscle relaxation (bronchi, blood vessels, genitourinary tract, gastrointestinal tract)

From Granner, 1988.

epinephrine → both α & β
norepinephrin → α

TABLE 9-2 Physiologic effects of the catecholamines*

Organ	Process or result
Brain	Increased blood flow
	Increased glucose metabolism
Cardiovascular system	Increased rate and force of contraction
	Peripheral vasoconstriction
Pulmonary system	Increased oxygen supply
	Bronchodilation
	Increased ventilation
Muscle	Increased glycogenolysis
	Increased contraction
Liver	Increased glucose production
	Increased gluconeogenesis
	Increased glycogenolysis
	Decreased glycogen synthesis
Adipose tissue	Increased lipolysis
	Increased fatty acids and glycerol
Skin	Decreased blood flow
Skeleton	Decreased glucose uptake and utilization (decreases insulin release)
Gastrointestinal & genitourinary tracts	Decreased protein synthesis
Lymphoid tissue	Increased protein breakdown (lymphoid tissue shrinks)

From Granner, 1988.
*Some of these responses require glucocorticoids (e.g., cortisol) for maximal activity (see text for explanation).

glucose breakdown. Epinephrine decreases glucose uptake in the muscle and other organs and decreases insulin release from the pancreas. The decrease in insulin release prevents glucose from being taken up by peripheral tissue and thus preserves it for the central nervous system. Epinephrine also mobilizes free fatty acids and cholesterol by stimulating lipolysis, freeing triglycerides and fatty acids from fat stores, and inhibiting the degradation of circulating cholesterol to bile acids. The metabolic actions of epinephrine aid the metabolic actions of cortisol, which are similar. Table 9-2 summarizes other well-known effects of adrenal catecholamines. All of these effects prepare the body to take physical action—to "fight or flee." Stressors commonly associated with catecholamine release by the adrenal medulla include exercise, thermal changes, and acute emotional states.

Cortisol

The adrenal cortex is activated during stress by adrenal corticotropin hormone (Fig. 9-1). Activation increases adrenal cortical secretion of glucocorticoid (steroid) hormones, primarily cortisol. (Cortisol is also known as hydrocortisone.) Cortisol circulates in the plasma, both protein-bound and free. The main plasma-binding protein is called **transcortin** of **corticosteroid-binding globulin.** The unbound, or free, fraction is about 8% of the total plasma cortisol and is the most biologically active fraction of cortisol (Granner, 1988). Cortisol mobilizes substances needed for cellular metabolism. One of the primary effects of cortisol is the stimulation of gluconeogenesis, or the formation of glycogen from noncarbohydrate sources, such as amino or free fatty acids in the liver. In addition, cortisol enhances the elevation of blood glucose promoted by other hormones, such as epinephrine, glucagon, and somatotropic growth hormone. This action by cortisol is said to be **permissive** for the actions of other hormones. Cortisol also inhibits the uptake and oxidation of glucose by many body cells. The overall action of cortisol on carbohydrate metabolism results in an elevation of blood glucose.

Cortisol also affects protein metabolism. It has an anabolic effect, or increases the rate of synthesis, of proteins and RNA in liver, and catabolic effects in muscle, lymphoid tissue, adipose tissue, skin, and bone (Granner, 1988). The overall breakdown effect of proteins results in a negative nitrogen balance and an increase in circulating amino acids. There is some evidence that cortisol depresses transport of amino acids into muscle cells, while enhancing their uptake into the liver, where they are converted to glucose. Cortisol can also promote lipolysis in some areas of the body (the extremities) and lipogenesis in others (the face and trunk). The lipid effects of tissue are specific because not all areas show increased fat deposition or lipolysis (Granner, 1988).

Cortisol acts as an immunosuppressant by suppressing protein synthesis, including synthesis of immunoglobulin. Cortisol also reduces populations of eosinophils, lymphocytes, and macrophages (Fauci, 1975; Granner, 1988; Stein, 1985). Large doses of cortisol are known to promote atrophy of lymphoid tissue in the thymus, spleen, and lymph nodes (Granner, 1988). This action of cortisol could account for the lymphoid atrophy observed by Selye.

Cortisol directly influences immune responses to antibodies (Berne & Levy, 1988). The mechanisms of inhibition of the immune response are multifactorial (Fig. 9-2). When an antigen intrudes into the body, it is picked up by a macrophage. The macrophage presents the antigen to thymus-derived lymphocytes (T cells) and simultaneously produces and releases interleukin 1, a protein lymphokine that activates a subset of T cells with helper function. Likewise, helper T cells secrete interleukin 2, a protein that stimulates the proliferation of still more T cells. These T cells can either activate or suppress bursa-derived lymphocytes (B cells). These B cells then produce antibodies directed against the original invading antigen. Cortisol inhibits the production of both interleukin 1 and macrophages and interleukin 2 by helper T cells, thus decreasing T cell responses. The diminished helper T cells cause a decrease in B cells and antibody production (see Chapter 6). Once antibodies are present, neither their degradation nor their specific reaction with antigen molecules are affected by cortisol (Berne & Levy, 1988).

The ability of cortisol and other glucocorticoids to suppress the inflammatory response is well documented and provides the basis for the major therapeutic use of these steroids. Cortisol decreases the number of circulating lymphocytes, monocytes/macrophages, and eosinophils because these cells are shifted from the vascular compartment to other sites, including the bone marrow, lymphoid tissue, and spleen (Granner, 1988). Cortisol enhances the release of polymorphonuclear leukocytes

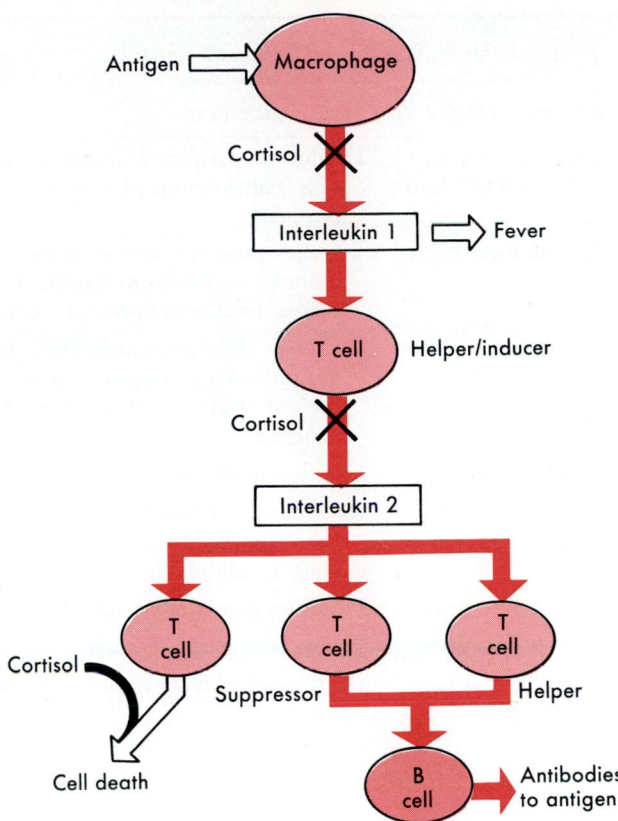

FIG. 9-2. Cortisol effects on cell-mediated immunity. Cortisol inhibits antigen-stimulated production of the peptide interleukin-1 macrophages, decreasing the initial recruitment of T lymphocytes. Cortisol also inhibits production of interleukin-2, reducing secondary proliferation of helper and suppressor T lymphocytes. Depending in part on the ratio of these two cell populations, production of antibody to the original antigen may either be facilitated or retarded. In some species, large doses of cortisol are also lymphocytotoxic, causing cell death. (Adapted from Berne & Levy, 1988.)

from bone marrow, thus increasing their number in blood, although their effectiveness decreases. Glucocorticoids inhibit the accumulation of leukocytes at the site of inflammation and inhibit the release of substances involved in the inflammatory response (e.g., kinins, plasminogen-activating factor, prostaglandins, and histamine) from the leukocytes (Granner, 1988). Cortisol inhibits fibroblast proliferation and function at the site of an inflammatory response. This inhibition accounts for the poor wound healing, increased susceptibility to infection, and decreased inflammatory response that are often seen in individuals with glucocorticoid excess. Glucocorticoids are necessary for the maintenance of normal blood pressure and cardiac output. This is another example of how cortisol maximizes the action of the catecholamines (the "permissive effect").

In the gastrointestinal tract, cortisol promotes gastric secretion. This is opposite to the effect of norepineph-

TABLE 9-3 Physiologic effects of cortisol

Functions affected	Physiologic effects
Carbohydrate and lipid metabolism	Diminishes peripheral uptake and utilization of glucose; promotes gluconeogenesis in liver cells; enhances the gluconeogenic response to other hormones; promotes lipolysis in adipose tissue
Protein metabolism	Increases protein synthesis in the liver and depresses protein synthesis (including immunoglobulin synthesis) in muscle, lymphoid tissue, adipose tissue, skin, and bone; Increases plasma level of amino acids; stimulates deamination in the liver
Inflammatory effects	Decreases circulating eosinophils, lymphocytes, and monocytes; increases release of polymorphonuclear leukocytes from the bone marrow; decreases accumulation of leukocytes at the site of inflammation; delays healing; permissive for vasoconstrictive action of norepinephrine
Lipid metabolism	Lipolysis in the extremities and lipogenesis in the face and trunk
Immune reserve	Decreases the tissue mass of all lymphoid tissues (e.g., decreases protein synthesis); Promotes rapid decrease in circulating lymphocytes, eosinophils, basophils, and macrophages; inhibits the production of interleukin-1 and interleukin-2
Digestive function	Promotes gastric secretion
Urinary function	Enhances urinary excretion
Connective tissue function	Decreases proliferation of fibrinoblasts in connective tissue (thus, delaying healing)

rine, which reduces gastric secretion. Excessive cortisol may stimulate gastric secretion enough to cause ulceration of the gastric mucosa. This could account for the gastrointestinal ulceration observed by Selye.

It is not entirely clear why cortisol secretion during stress is beneficial. It has been suggested that gluconeogenesis promoted by cortisol ensures an adequate source of glucose (energy) for body tissues, and nerve cells in particular. The pooling of amino acids from catabolized proteins may ensure amino acid availability for protein synthesis in certain cells. The redistribution of protein to sites where replacement is critical, such as muscle or cells of damaged tissue, would be beneficial. The biologic effects of cortisol are summarized in Table 9-3.

Other Hormones

Endorphins

β-endorphins (endogenous opiates) are released into the blood as part of the response to stressful stimuli (Guillemin et al., 1977). The secretion of ACTH and β-endorphin is stimulated by corticotropin-releasing factor; it is unclear if β-endorphins come from the pituitary gland or the central nervous system. Evidence is accumulating that β-endorphins can regulate ACTH secretion and, with ACTH, inhibit hypothalamic CRF secretion.

Increased β-endorphin levels are associated with a parallel increase in pain threshold, i.e., stress-induced analgesia (Cohen et al., 1982; Jungkunz et al., 1983).

In a number of conditions or activities in which there is increased endogenous opiate activity, subjects not only experience insensitivity to pain but also report increased feelings of excitement, positive well-being, or euphoria (Rose, 1985). For example, vigorous running increases β-endorphin levels (Colt, Wardlaw, & Franz, 1981). Endorphins may play a role in the excitement and exhilaration produced by dancing, contact sports, and combat. There is little direct evidence, however, documenting the endorphin system in most of these activities.

Growth Hormone

Somatotropin Growth hormone is released from the anterior pituitary gland and affects protein, lipid, and carbohydrate metabolism. Growth hormone levels increase in the blood following a variety of stressful stimuli, such as cardiac catheterization, electroshock therapy, gastroscopy, and physical exercise (Schalach, 1967). Psychologic stimuli associated with increased levels of growth hormone include examinations, viewing of violent or sexually arousing films, anticipation of exhausting exercise, and certain psychologic performance tests. In most circumstances, the increase in growth hormone occurs only with a parallel rise in cortisol secretion.

Prolactin

Prolactin is released from the anterior pituitary gland and is necessary for lactation and breast development

(Shiu & Friesen, 1980). Prolactin levels in plasma increase from a variety of stressful stimuli, including such procedures as gastroscopy, proctoscopy, pelvic examination, and during surgery (Noel et al., 1972). Prolactin also rises during parachute jumping, during motion sickness, and following examinations (Rose, 1985). Unlike growth hormone, prolactin levels show little change after exercise. However, like growth hormone, prolactin appears to require a more intense stimuli than those leading to increases in catecholamine or cortisol levels. Prolactin levels also increase in the plasma following a variety of sexual stimuli, for example, stimulation of the nipple or areola in women.

Testosterone

Testosterone, a hormone secreted by Leydig cells, regulates male secondary sex characteristics and libido. Testosterone levels decrease after stressful stimuli. The decrease in testosterone occurs following such stimuli as ether or anesthesia, surgery, marathon running, and mountain climbing (Matsumoto et al., 1970). The mechanism causing decreased levels of testosterone is unknown.

Psychologic stimuli also lead to a decrease in testosterone levels. Men engaged in rigorous combat training and those engaged in the first several weeks of Officer Candidate School experience significant drops in testosterone levels (Aakvaag et al., 1978; Kreuz, Rose, & Jennings, 1972). Individuals with acute illness, such as respiratory failure, burns, and congestive heart failure, show a marked reduction in plasma testosterone (Rose, 1985).

Role of the Immune System

Many conditions and diseases are associated with stress (Table 9-4). The specific stress-induced mechanisms causing these illnesses are as yet unknown. Recent research is focused on the "regulatory loop" between the immune system and the neuroendocrine system (Blalock & Smith, 1985a; Meyer et al., 1987; Smith & Blalock, 1988; Smith, Harbour, & Blalock, 1987). Evidence so far suggests that the immune and neuroendocrine systems are connected through proteins (immunoreactive hormones) common to both systems (Fig. 9-3). Production of immunoreactive (ir) hormones (e.g., ACTH, endorphins, and thyroid-stimulating hormone [TSH]) by lymphocytes, a signal that the stress response is occurring, represent one direction of the circuit. The ability of ACTH, endorphins, enkephalins, and steroid hormones produced by the neuroendocrine system to modulate immune responses represents a pathway in the opposite direction and completes the loop.

Structurally, the ir ACTH is very similar to pituitary ACTH and ir ACTH also responds to corticotropin-releasing factor (CRF) (Smith et al., 1986). Thus, cells of

TABLE 9-4 Examples of stress-related diseases and conditions

Target organ or system	Disease or condition
Cardiovascular system	Coronary artery disease Hypertension Stroke Disturbances of heart rhythm
Muscles	Tension headaches Muscle contraction backache
Connective tissues	Rheumatoid arthritis (autoimmune disease) Related inflammatory diseases of connective tissue
Pulmonary system	Asthma (hypersensitivity reaction) Hay fever (hypersensitivity reaction)
Immune system	Immunosuppression or deficiency Autoimmune diseases
Gastrointestinal system	Ulcer Irritable bowel syndrome Diarrhea Nausea and vomiting Ulcerative colitis
Genitourinary system	Diuresis Impotence Frigidity
Skin	Eczema Neurodermatitis Acne
Endocrine system	Diabetes mellitus
Central nervous system	Fatigue and lethargy Type A behavior Overeating Depression Insomnia

the immune system resemble pituitary cells in their ability to be regulated by the hypothalamus and adrenal glands. The immune system's primary role in this regulatory circuit may be to detect the presence of a biologic stressor (virus, bacteria, tumors) and transmit this information to the neuroendocrine system through production of an ir hormone. The resulting neuroendocrine response is thought to alter the dynamic steady state (Blalock & Smith, 1985a). Other evidence also supports the regulatory loop between the immune system and the neuroendocrine system. For example, recent studies have found that interleukin 1 (e.g., lymphokine), a protein produced mostly by activated macrophages and monocytes, was found to activate the pituitary-adrenal

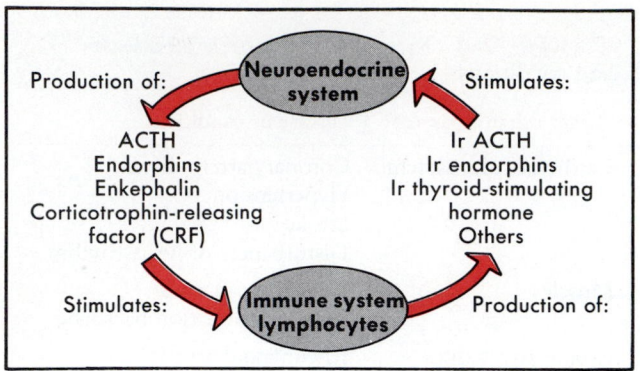

FIG. 9-3. Model illustrating the complete regulatory loop between the immune and neuroendocrine systems. *ACTH*, Adrenocorticotropic hormone; *ir*, immunoreactive.

system in rats. Interleukin 1 helps regulate immune function by stimulating the production of growth factors and activating T cell helper functions. The growth factors act as a chemotactic factor for lymphocytes to assist B cell proliferation and antibody production (delRey et al., 1987). Recent evidence also shows that interleukin 1-induced pituitary-adrenocortical response in rats is mediated by the secretion of corticotropin-releasing factor (CRF) (Berkenbosch et al., 1987). Likewise, corticosteroids from the adrenal gland decrease the ability of macrophages to produce interleukin 1 and the T cells to produce interleukin 2. Interleukin 2 stimulates the proliferation of additionally needed T cells during an immune response (see Fig. 9-2 and "Cortisol" section).

Other links and relationships have been found between the hypothalamic-pituitary-adrenal system and the immune system. In addition to producing peptide hormones, cells of the immune system seem to possess their receptors. T cells, B cells, and monocytes/macrophages all possess receptors for steroids; therefore, steroids can help regulate immune cell activity (Lippmann & Barr, 1977). Cortisol reduces the number of circulating T and B cells in the blood; however, the effect on T cells is greater (Fauci & Dale, 1974). The effect of corticosteroids (e.g., cortisol) on B cell function is complex. At low or moderate blood levels of cortisol, the number of antibody-producing cells, the plasma cells, and the secreted immunoglobulins is increased (Grayson et al., 1981). This increase in antibody production is because the corticosteroids inhibit suppressor T cells. Antibody production is controlled in large part by the level of T cell activity (see Chapter 6). High levels of cortisol decrease antibody production and can actually kill B cells (Grayson et al., 1981). The existence of such a regulatory mechanism would provide a mechanism for neuroendocrine control of the immune responses and may explain the pathophysiology of dis-

eases having immune and neuroendocrine components.

The presence of β-adrenergic receptors on the surfaces of T cells, B cells, and macrophages has prompted the observation that neurotransmitters and/or neuropeptides are involved in modulating immunity. Anatomic studies have provided more evidence of the connections between the autonomic nervous system (ANS) and the immune system by isolating nerve fibers that penetrate the bone marrow, thymus gland, spleen, and other lymphoid tissues (Bullock, 1985). Autonomic nerve innervation of major lymphoid tissues provides some evidence of neural control in the production and function of the lymphocyte.

Much evidence supports a linkage between the neuroendocrine and immune systems. The bidirectional communication involves shared usage of signal molecules and their receptors. In summary, the main findings are (1) cells of the immune system can synthesize biologically active neuroendocrine peptide hormones; (2) immune cells can also possess receptors for many of these peptides; (3) these same neuroendocrine hormones can influence immune function; and (4) lymphokines, like interleukin 1, can influence neuroendocrine tissue (Weingert & Blalock, 1987).

STRESS, COPING, AND ILLNESS

An event or situation can be a stressor for one person and not for another. The studies already described have demonstrated that many stressors, such as fasting or extreme heat, do not necessarily cause a physiologic stress response if psychologic factors are minimized. Therefore, the perception of stressors is instrumental in mediating the physiologic response to stress. The perception of stressors is complex and depends on the context in which the stressor appears to the individual, the individual's previous experience with the stressor, and the individual's ability to cope with the stressor (Bieliauskas, 1982).

For a stimulus to be stressful, it must first be perceived as such. Wolf and Goodell (1968) reported that cultural factors, personal and social factors, and vulnerability all help to determine whether a stimulus is perceived as a stressor. Lazarus (1977) clarified this notion by focusing on the individual's initial appraisal of the stimulus. For example, a mathematician appraising a complex mathematical problem is not likely to perceive solving it as a stressor. Appraisal of the problem by someone without successful previous experience or knowledge of appropriate formulas is, on the other hand, very likely to cause stress.

Once a stimulus is perceived as a stressor, its physiologic effect will depend on the individual's ability to cope with it. Lazarus and Folkman (1984) defined the

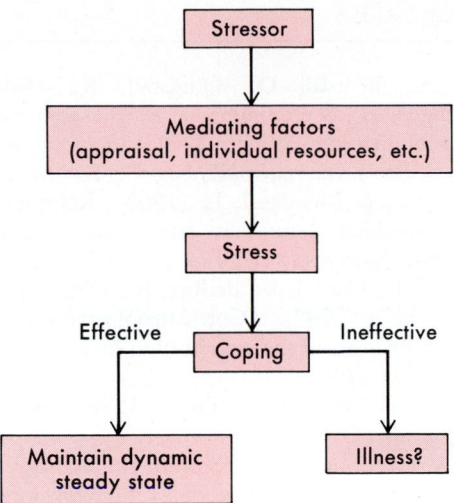

FIG. 9-4. Model of interaction of a stressor, its appraisal, and illness onset.

coping process as the individual's psychologic response to the stressor. The effectiveness of coping determines the risk of maladaptive illness because it also determines whether the physiologic stress response will continue or diminish. For example, Aldrich and Mendkoff (1963) found that the incidence of mortality increased among elderly individuals who were displaced and moved to another living situation, such as a nursing home or their child's home. Actual mortality differed, however, depending on how each individual coped with the displacement; those who reacted with psychosis or depression tended to do poorly, while those who responded angrily or philosophically to the change tended to do better (Bieliauskas, 1982).

Fig. 9-4 depicts a model of the interaction of a stressor, its appraisal, and the reaction to it in terms of illness onset. Although the model cannot fully account for the many interacting factors affecting the response to a stressor or explain the related implications for illness, it illustrates the complexity defining the steps between the onset of a stressor and ensuing illness. Besides appraisal and individual resources, mediating factors, such as social support, personality type, and genetic and biologic makeup, affect the response to a stressor.

SUMMARY REVIEW

Concepts of Stress

1 Hans Selye identified three structural changes in rats subjected repeatedly to noxious stimuli (stressors): enlargement of the cortex of the adrenal gland, atrophy of the thymus gland and other lymphoid tissues, and gastrointestinal ulceration.

2 Selye believed that the three changes were caused by nonspecific physiologic response to any long-term stressor. He called this response the general adaptation syndrome (GAS).

3 The GAS occurs in three stages: the alarm stage, the stage of resistance or adaptation, and the stage of exhaustion. Diseases of adaptation develop if the stage of resistance or adaptation does not restore homeostasis.

4 Selye identified three components of physiologic stress: the stressor, the physiologic or chemical disturbance produced by the stressor, and the body's adaptational response to the stressor.

5 Other investigators have shown that the physiologic stress response also occurs in response to psychologic or emotional stress.

6 There is disagreement on the nonspecific nature of the stress response because different processes occur in response to specific stimuli, such as exposure to cold or heat.

7 W.B. Cannon defined homeostasis as the sum of the processes by which the body maintains itself at a relatively constant composition. This definition has since been modified. Homeostasis is now considered to mean the sum of the processes by which the body maintains itself in a dynamic steady state.

8 The function of the physiologic stress response is to maintain the body's dynamic steady state.

The Stress Response

1 The stress response involves the nervous system (sympathetic branch of the autonomic nervous system), the endocrine system (pituitary and adrenal glands), and the immune system.

2 The stress response is initiated when a stressor is present in the body and/or perceived by the mind.

3 The neuroendocrine response to stress consists of sympathetic stimulation of the adrenal medulla to secrete catecholamines (norepinephrine and epinephrine) and stressor-induced stimulation of the pituitary to secrete adenocorticotropic hormone (ACTH) which, in turn, stimulates the adrenal cortex to secrete steroid hormones, particularly cortisol.

4 In general, the catecholamines prepare the body to act, and cortisol mobilizes energy (glucose) and other substances needed to fuel the action.

5 Epinephrine exerts its chief effects on the cardiovascular system. Epinephrine increases cardiac output and increases blood flow to the heart, brain, and skeletal muscles by dilating vessels that supply these organs. It also dilates the airways, thereby increasing delivery of oxygen to the bloodstream.

6 Norepinephrine's chief effects complement those of epinephrine. Norepinephrine constricts blood vessels of the viscera and skin; this has the effect of shifting blood flow to the vessels dilated by epinephrine. Norepinephrine also increases mental alertness.

7 Cortisol's chief effects involve metabolic processes. By inhibiting the use of metabolic substances while promoting their formation, cortisol mobilizes glucose,

amino acids, lipids, and fatty acids, and delivers them to the bloodstream. Cortisol also suppresses immune and inflammatory function.

8 The neuroendocrine and immune responses are thought to interact through proteins common to both systems: lymphocytes produce immunoreactive hormones (ir), for example, ir ACTH, ir endorphins, ir thyroid-stimulating hormone, and other lymphokines.

9 A regulatory loop is thought to be formed between the immune and endocrine systems as the ir hormones detect the presence of an antigen (e.g., bacterium, virus, or tumor cell) and signal the endocrine mediators of the stress response. These mediators (e.g., ACTH, endorphins, and steroid hormones produced by the adrenal cortex) modulate the stress response, thereby completing the regulatory loop.

10 Other hormones are affected by the stress response and include increased circulating levels of β-endorphins, growth hormone, prolactin, and antidiuretic hormone. Testosterone decreases during the stress response.

Stress, Coping, and Illness

1 The physiologic stress response is affected by the individual's appraisal (perception) of the stressor and his or her ability to cope with the stressor, both physically and psychologically.

2 Coping is mediated by the individual's state of health, genetic makeup, physiologic makeup, personality type, past experiences in coping with stress, and support systems.

KEY TERMS

Alarm stage, 282

Coping process, 289

Corticosteroid-binding globulin, 284

Diseases of adaptation, 282

Dynamic steady state, 283

General adaptation syndrome (GAS), 280

Homeostasis, 282

Immunoreactive hormone (ir hormone), 287

Permissive, 284

Physiologic stress, 282

Stage of exhaustion, 282

State of resistance or adaptation, 282

Stress response, 283

Stressor, 280

Transcortin, 284

Turnover, 283

REFERENCES

Aakvaag, A., Bentdal, O., Quigstad, K., Walstad, P., Rohnningen, H., & Fonnum, F. (1978). Testosterone and testosterone-binding globulin (TeBG) in young men during prolonged stress. *International Journal of Androl, 1,* 22-31.

Aldrich, C. K., & Mendkoff, E. (1963). Relocation of the aged and disabled: A mortality study. *Journal of the American Geriatric Society, 11,* 185-194.

Berkenbosch, F., Oers, J. V., delRay, A., Tilders, F., & Besedovsky, H. (1987). Corticotropin-releasing factor-producing neurons in the rat activated by interleukin-1. *Science, 238,* 524-526.

Berne, R. M., & Levy, M. N. (Eds.). (1988). *Physiology* (2nd ed.). St. Louis: C. V. Mosby.

Besedovsky, H. L., delRay, A., Sorkin, E., & Dinarello, C. A. (1986). Immunoregulatory feedback between interleukin-1 and glucocorticoid hormones. *Science, 233,* 652.

Bieliauskas, L. A. (1982). *Stress and its relationship to health and illness.* Boulder, Colo.: Westview Press.

Blalock, J. E., & Smith, E. M. (1985a, January). A complete regulatory loop between the immune and neuroendocrine systems. *Federation Proceedings, 44*(1), 108-111.

Bullock, K. (1985). Neuroanatomy of lymphoid tissue: A review. In R. Guillemin & M. Cohen (Eds.), *Neural modulation of immunity.* New York: Raven Press.

Cannon, W. B. (1935). Stresses and strains of homeostasis. *American Journal of Medical Science, 189,* 1-14.

Cannon, W. B. (1963). *The wisdom of the body.* New York: W. W. Norton & Co.

Coffey, R. G., & Hadden, J. W. (1985, January). Neurotransmitters, hormones, and cyclic nucleotides in lymphocyte regulation. *Federation Proceedings, 44*(1), 112-117.

Cohen, M. R., Pickar, D., Dubois, M., & Bunney, W. E., Jr. (1982). Stress-induced plasma beta-endorphin immunoreactivity may predict post-operative morphine usage. *Psychiatry Research, 6,* 7-12.

Colt, E. W. D., Wardlaw, S. L., & Franz, A. G. (1981). The effect of running on plasma β-endorphin. *Life Science, 28,* 1637-1640.

Day, S. B. (1986). *Cancer: Stress and death* (2nd ed.). New York: Plenum Medical Book Co.

delRay, A., Besedovsky, H. L., Sorkin, E., & Dinnarello, C. A. (1987). Interleukin-1 and glucocorticoid hormones integrate an immunoregulatory feedback circuit. *Annals of the New York Academy of Science, 496,* 85-89.

Dickman, S. R. (1988). *Pathways to wellness.* Champagne, Ill.: Life Enhancement Publishers.

Fauci, A. S. & Dale, D. C. (1974). The effect of in vitro hydrocortisone on subpopulations of human lymphocytes. *Journal of Clinical Investigation, 53,* 240-246.

Fauci, A. S., (1975). Corticosteroids and circulating lymphocytes. *Transplant Proceedings, 7,* 37-48.

Granner, D. K. (1988). Hormones of the adrenal medulla. In R. K. Murray et al. (Eds.), *Harper's biochemistry* (21st ed.). Lange Medical Books.

Grayson, J., Dooley, N. J., Koski, I. R., & Blaese, R. M. 1981. Immunoglobulin production induced in vitro by glucocorticoid hormones. T-cell-dependent stimulation of immunoglobulin production without B-cell proliferation in cultures of human peripheral lymphocytes. *Journal of Clinical Investigation, 68,* 1539-1547.

Guillemin, R., Vargo, T., Rosier, J., Minick, S., Ling, N., Rivier, C., Valle, W., & Bloom, F. (1977). Beta-endorphin and adrenocorticotropin are secreted concomitantly by the pituitary gland. *Science, 197,* 1367-1369.

Handlon, J. H., Wadeson, R. W., Fishman, J. R., Sachar, E. J., Hamburg, D. A., & Mason, J. W. (1962). Psychological factors in 17-hydroxycorticosteriod concentration. *Psychosomatic Medicine, 24,* 535-542.

Hetzel, B. S., Schottstaedt, W. W., Grace, W. J., & Wolff, H. G. (1955). Changes in urinary 17-hydroxycorticosteroid excretion during stressful life situations in man. *Journal of Clinical Endocrinology, 15,* 1057-1068.

Hill, S. R., Goetz, F. C., Fox, H. M., Murawski, B. J., Krakauer, L. J., Reifenstein, R. W., Gray, S. J., Reddy, W. J., Hedberg, S. E., St. Marc, J. R., & Thorn, G. W. (1956). Studies on adrenocortical and psychological responses to stress in man. *Archives of Internal Medicine, 97,* 269-298.

Jacobs, M. A., Spilken, A., & Norman, M. M. (1969). Relationship of life change, maladaptive aggression, and upper respiratory infection in male college students. *Psychomatic Medicine, 33,* 33-42.

Jacobs, M. A., Spilken, A., Norman, M. M., & Andersson, L. S. (1970). Life stress and respiratory illness, *Psychomatic Medicine, 32,* 233-242.

Jungkunz, G., Engel, R. R., King, U. G., & Kuss, H. J. (1983). Endogenous opiates increase pain tolerance after stress in humans. *Psychiatry Research, 8,* 13-18.

Kreuz, L. E., Rose, R. M., & Jennings, J. R. (1972). Suppression of plasma testosterone levels and psychological stress: A longitudinal study of young men in officer candidate school. *Archives of General Psychiatry, 26,* 479-482.

Lazarus, R. S. (1977). Psychological stress and coping in adaptation and illness. In Z. J. Lipowski, D. R. Lipsih, & P. C. Whybrow (Eds.), *Psychosomatic medicine: Current trends and clinical applications.* New York: Oxford University Press.

Lazarus, R. S., & Folkman, S. (1984). *Stress, appraisal, and coping.* New York: McGraw-Hill.

Lindsay, A. M., & Carrieri, V. K. (1986). Stress response. In A. M. Lindsay, V. K. Carrieri, & C. M. West (Eds.), *Pathophysiological phenomenon in nursing: Human responses to illness.* Philadelphia: W. B. Saunders.

Lippmann, M. E., & Barr, R. (1977). Glucocorticoid receptors in purified subpopulations of human peripheral blood lymphocytes. *Journal of Immunobiology, 118,* 1977-1981.

Mason, J. W. (1971). A reevaluation of the concept of nonspecificity in stress theory. *Journal of Psychiatric Research, 8,* 323-333.

Mason, J. W. (1972). Organization of psychoendocrine mechanisms: A review and reconsideration of research. In N. S. Greenfield & R. A. Steinbach (Eds.), *Handbook of psychophysiology.* New York: Holt, Rinehart, & Winston, pp. 3-91.

Mason, J. W. (1974). Specificity in the organization of neuroendocrine response profiles. In P. Seeman & G. Brown (Eds.), *Frontiers in neurology and neuroscience research.* Toronto, Canada: University of Toronto.

Mason, J. W. (1975, March). A historical view of the stress field. *Journal of Human Stress, 1*(1), 6-12.

Mason, J. W., & Brady, J. V. (1956). Plasma 17-hydroxycorticosteroid changes related to reserpine effects on emotional behaviors. *Science, 124,* 983-984.

Matsumoto, K., Takeyasu, K., Mizutani, S., Hamanaka, Y., & Uozumi, T. (1970). Plasma testosterone levels following surgical stress in male patients. *Acta Endocrinology, 65,* 11-17.

Meyer, R. J. & Haggerty, R. J. (1962). Streptococcal infections in families: Factors altering individual susceptibility. *Journal of Pediatrics, 29,* 539-549.

Meyer, W. J., Smith, E. M., Richards, G. E., Cavallo, A., Morrill, A. C., & Blalock, J. E. (1987). In vivo adrenocorticotropin (ACTH) production by human mononuclear leukocytes from normal and ACTH-deficient individuals. *Journal of Clinical Endocrinology and Metabolism, 64*(1), 98-105.

Noel, G. L., Suh, H. K., Stone, J. G., & Frantz, A. G. (1972). Human prolactin and growth hormone release during surgery and other conditions of stress. *Journal of Clinical Endocrinology and Metabolism, 35,* 840-851.

Ramsey, J. M. (1982). *Basic pathophysiology of modern stress and the disease process.* Menlo Park, Calif.: Addison-Wesley.

Rose, R. M. (1985). Psychoendocrinology. In J. D. Wilson & D. W. Foster (Eds.), *Williams textbook of endocrinology* (7th ed.), Philadelphia: W. B. Saunders.

Schalach, D. S. (1967). The influence of physical stress and exercise on growth hormone and insulin secretion in man. *Journal of Laboratory and Clinical Medicine, 69,* 256-269.

Selye, H. (1946). The general adaptation syndrome and the diseases of adaptation. *Journal of Clinical Endocrinology, 6,* 117-230.

Selye, H. (1959). Perspectives in stress research. *Perspectives in Biology and Medicine, 2*(4), 403-416.

Selye, H. (1975). Confusion and controversy in the stress field. *Journal of Human Stress, 1*(2), 37-44.

Shiu, R. P. C., & Friesen, H. G. (1980). Mechanisms of action of prolactin in the control of mammary gland function. *Annual Review of Physiology, 42,* 83-96.

Smith, E. M., & Blalock, J. E. (1988). A molecular basis for interactions between the immune and neuroendocrine systems. *Journal of Neuroscience, 38,* 455-464.

Smith, E. M., Harbour, D. V., & Blalock, J. E. (1987). Leukocyte production of endorphins. *Annals of the New York Academy of Sciences, 496,* 192-195.

Smith, E. M., Meyer, M. J., Morrill, A. C., & Blalock, J. E. (1986). Corticotropin–releasing factor induction of leukocyte-derived immunoreactive ACTH and endorphins. *Nature, 321,* 881.

Stein, N. (1985). Bereavement, depression, stress, and immunity. In R. Guillemin & M. Cohen (Eds.), *Neural modulation of immunity.* New York: Raven Press, pp. 29-44.

Wadeson, R. W., Mason, J. W., Hamburg, D. A., & Handlon, J. H. (1963). Plasma and urinary 17-OHCS responses to motion pictures. *Archives of General Psychiatry, 9,* 146-156.

Weingert, D. A., & Blalock, J. E. (1987). Interactions between the neuroendocrine and immune systems: Common hormones and receptors. *Immunological Review, 100,* 79-108.

Wolf, S., & Goodell, H. (1968). *Stress and disease.* Springfield, Ill.: Charles C. Thomas.

UNIT IV

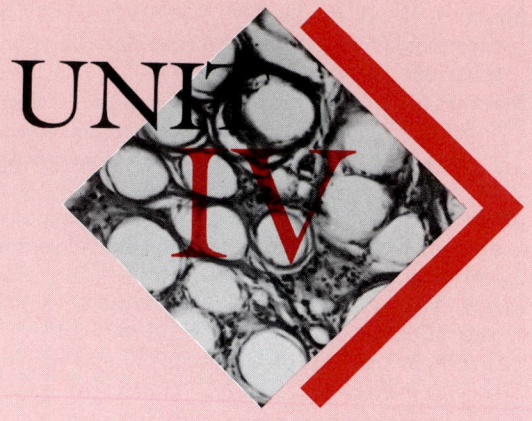

Cellular Proliferation— Cancer

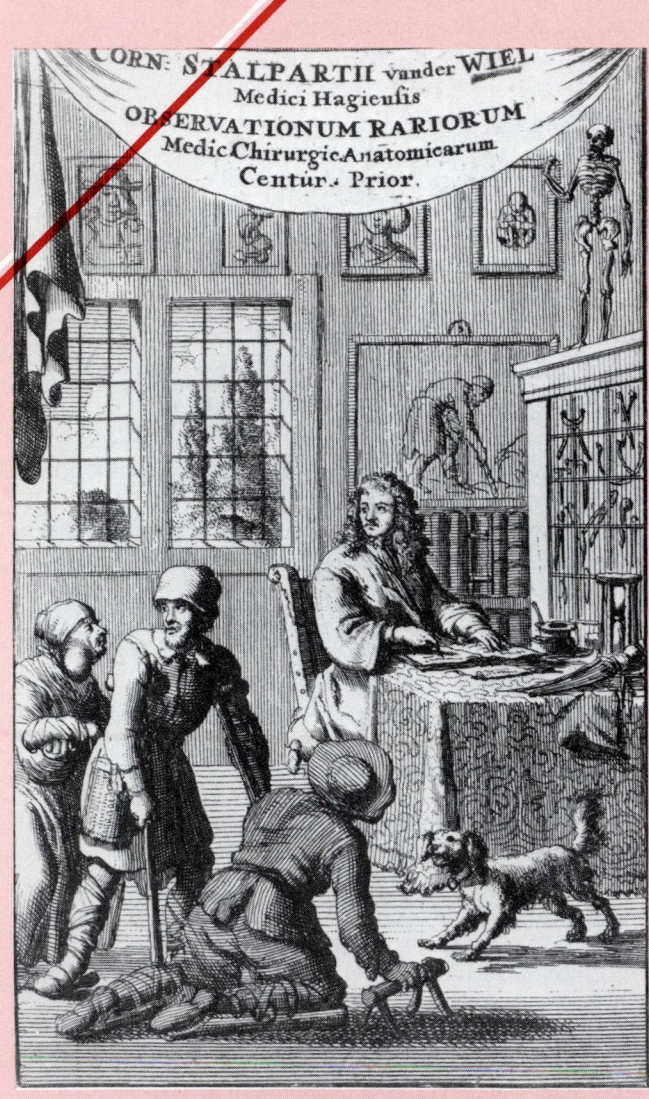

Physician's office. Three patients (patient on left with a tumor) and dog with physician attending. From Stalpart vander Will, C.: *Observationum rariorum,* 1687. Courtesy National Library of Medicine.

CANCER occurs in most if not all multicellular animals—mammals, fish, reptiles, and amphibians. Evidence from fossil records even shows bone cancer in dinosaurs, and sarcomas have been observed in bones from Egyptian mummies (Moodie, 1923). Hippocrates (460-375 BC) is given credit for the term "carcinoma," the Greek word for crab, possibly because of the invasive and spreading nature of the disease.

Theories about the causes of cancer began with a proposal by Galen (131-203 AD) that all tumors were caused by concentrations of black bile. Later, Marcello Malpighi examined cancer tissue with a crude microscope and saw no black bile, but did see large amounts of blood and lymph. This observation led to the "lymph theory": that a drop of cancer lymph caused cancer when it moved to nearby nodes (Rusch, 1983). Not until the nineteenth century did Johannes Peta Muller, Karl Rokitansky, and Rudolf Virchow demonstrate with improved microscopes a cancer cell's emergence from other nonlymphatic cells (Ewing, 1940). With this new cellular knowledge of cancer came several competing hypotheses:

- Excretion from cancer cells produced cancer in normal cells.
- Cells with abnormal membranes permitted uncontrolled epithelial growth.
- Retained embryo cells in the adult were responsible for later malignancy.
- Bacteria and parasites caused cancer.

With the discovery that cancer also develops in animals, transplantation experiments began, and cancer cells were implanted from one animal to another. Because of this significant procedure, investigators learned to induce tumor growth from biologic and chemical stimulation. The testing of chemicals as cancer-producing agents (carcinogens) started long after the dramatically astute observation mady by Sir Percival Pott in 1775 (Pott, 1981). He proposed that scrotal cancer in young chimney sweeps may be caused by "the lodgment of soot in the rugae (folds) of the scrotum" (Pott, 1981). This was the first observation that linked an environmental agent, coal tar, to cancer growth. Not until 1918, however, did the first experiments using chemical derivatives, the polycyclic hydrocarbons, specifically benzo[a]pyrene found in coal tar, demonstrate skin cancer in rats. The first report that an infectious agent could cause cancer was made by Vilhelm Ellerman and Oluf Bang, two investigators from Denmark. In 1908, they reported on the transmission of a blood disease in domestic fowl that resembled human leukemia. Their experiments lead to the observation that the cancer was caused by a virus. In 1911, Peyton Rous established a viral cause for another type of cancer in domestic fowl—sarcoma. The importance of his discovery was recognized 55 years later when he was awarded the Nobel Prize. Since these early studies, a number of cancer-causing viruses (oncogenic viruses) have been identified.

The harmful effects of radiation became known soon after Wilhelm Konrad Roentgen discovered the x-ray in 1896. Roentgen himself developed skin cancer. X-ray calibration procedures were unknown at this time, and proper radiation dosage was determined by taking repeated pictures of the operator's hand. Soon after, the first cancer of the hand was reported from these excessive doses. The most dramatic observation linking radiation and cancer occurred from the increase in leukemias in people exposed to the Hiroshima atomic bomb. Currently, researchers are studying the effects of low-dose ionizing radiation and its potential carcinogenic effects.

In 1932, Lacassagne reported that estrogen injections caused mammary cancer in mice. This stimulated research into the relationship between hormones and cancer. The current emphasis in cancer research is on the role of viruses, genetics, radiation therapy, hormones, the immune system, chemotherapy, and surgery, and on the methods of cancer detection and prevention.

CHAPTER 10

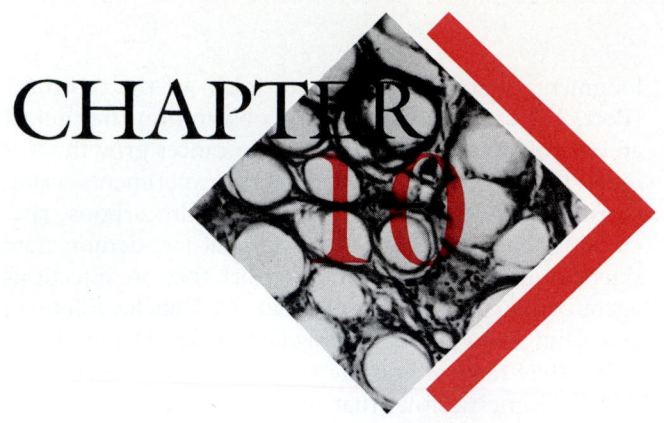

Tumor Biology

Kathryn L. McCance
Kathleen Hardin Mooney
Lee K. Roberts

Tumor classification and nomenclature, 295
Characteristics of cancer cells, 295
　Nuclear and cytoplasmic changes, 297
　Tumor cell markers, 298
　　Hormones, 299
　　Enzymes, 299
　　Tumor antigens, 301
Tumor development, 301
　Growth rates, 302
　Tumor spread, 302
　Local spread, 302
　Metastasis, 303
　　Metastasis by lymphatics and veins, 303
　　Metastasis by implantation, 305
Clinical manifestations of cancer, 305
　Pain, 305
　Cachexia, 306
　Anemia, 306
　Leukopenia and thrombocytopenia, 307
　Infection, 308
Cancer treatment, 308
　Chemotherapy, 308
　Radiation, 308
　Surgery, 309
　Immunotherapy, 310
　　Immunomodulating agents, 310
　　Interferons, 311
　　Antigens, 311
　　Effector cells and lymphokines, 312
　　Monoclonal antibodies, 312
　　Applications and clinical complications of
　　　immunotherapies, 316
Cancer in children, 316
　Types of childhood cancers, 317
　Incidence rates, 317
　Etiology, 317
　　Genetic factors, 317
　　Environmental factors, 319
　　Prenatal exposure, 319
　　Childhood exposure, 319
　Prognosis, 319

Perhaps no other disease causes more concern, fear, and disability than cancer. The human responses to cancer are vast and profound, progressing from shock and disbelief to uncertainty and dread of recurrence, to hope and coping or possible cure. Cancer is, in reality, a variety of disorders with differing pathophysiology. Mechanisms of cancer development vary according to the site of the disease and the precipitating cause. (Current theories of cancer development are discussed in Chapter 11.)

Abnormal growths are classified as **benign tumors,** which do not spread by infiltration of tissue, or **malignant tumors,** which invade or grow at distant sites and destroy host tissue. While the term neoplasm means a new and abnormal formation of tissue, it is most often associated with malignant (or cancer-producing) tumors, which spread through various mechanisms of **metastasis** from primary to distant sites.

Benign tumors usually resemble their tissue of origin and the cells may or may not be in their normal relationship. Benign tumors arise in most tissues, increase in size, but do not invade. They are usually separated from the surrounding normal tissue by a capsule of connective tissue (Franks & Teich, 1986). Benign tumors, however, can cause many pathologic alterations. For example, a benign tumor growing in the lung may obstruct or partially occlude a bronchus, causing difficulty in breathing and risk of infection. Benign tumors are usually surgically removed when discerning a benign from a malignant tumor is difficult, or when the tumor is causing obstructive problems. Table 10-1 summarizes the differences between benign and malignant tumors.

TABLE 10- 1	Differences between benign and malignant tumors	
Characteristic	**Benign tumor**	**Malignant tumor**
Structure and differentiation	Typical of tissue of origin	Atypical
Nuclear membranes	Typical of tissue of origin	Frequently irregular
Mitochondria	Typical of tissue of origin	Decreased in number
Endoplasmic reticulum (ER)	Typical of tissue of origin	Diminished and smooth
Cytoplasm	Typical of tissue of origin	RNA particles often scattered, seen as free from endoplasmic reticulum, unknown particles scattered throughout
Golgi apparatus	Typical of tissue of origin	Diminished or increased
Cell membrane	Typical of tissue of origin	Simplified
Rate of growth	Usually slow	Rapid or very rapid
Mode of growth	Expands (mostly encapsulated)	Usually infiltrates (loosely or not encapsulated)
Vascularity	Slight	Moderate or increased
Metastastes	Absent	Frequently
Necrosis and ulceration	Unusual	Common
Recurrence after surgical removal	Rare	Common
Fatality	Usually does not kill host	Kills host if untreated

From Rubin, Bakemeier, & Krackov, 1984.

TUMOR CLASSIFICATION AND NOMENCLATURE

Tumors are classified on the basis of cell type, tissue of origin, whether benign or malignant, degree of differentiation (well, moderately, or poorly), anatomic site, and function. Tumors are named according to the tissues from which they arise, generally with the suffix "oma." Cancers include those of epithelial tissue (**carcinomas**), connective tissue (**sarcomas**), lymphatic tissue (**lymphomas**), glial cells of the central nervous system (**gliomas**), and blood-forming organs, primarily the bone marrow (**leukemias**). The leukemias usually involve an abnormal growth or proliferation of blood-forming cells that infiltrate and replace normal bone marrow and lymphatic tissue. Table 10-2 presents the nomenclature and classification of tumors.

Carcinoma in situ refers to preinvasive epithelial tumors of glandular or squamous cell origin. These tumors have not broken through basement membranes of the squamous cells. Carcinoma in situ occurs in the cervix, skin, oral cavity, esophagus, and bronchus. In glandular epithelium, in situ lesions occur in the stomach, endometrium, and large bowel. These lesions may erroneously be confused with benign tumors, but both the squamous and glandular cell types show disorganization and atypical changes of epithelium. The time that such lesions remain in situ before becoming invasive is unknown. Some carcinomas of the cervix are known to be preinvasive lesions in situ for several years before they progress to invasive carcinoma.

CHARACTERISTICS OF CANCER CELLS

The dominant theme in cancer production is a cellular defect that causes anaplasia and autonomy. **Autonomy** refers to the cancer cell's independence from normal cellular controls. **Anaplasia** is the loss of differentiation, the process of developing specialized functions, and organization, meaning literally "without form" (see Chapter 1). In general, the cancer cell has lost its ability to function normally and to control its growth and division. Cancer cells become more like embryonic cells and are less differentiated (thus the observation that cancerous tissue resembles embryonic tissue). Any definition applied to *all* cancer cells, however, would be presumptuous. Some tumors retain useful functions and closely mimic normal tissue, whereas others are so disorganized that the tissue of origin is unidentifiable. The following characteristics describes the standard cellular features of cancerous cells:

- Local increase in cell number
- Loss of normal arrangement of cells
- Variation in cell shape and size

TABLE 10-2 Nomenclature and classification of benign and malignant tumors

Tissue of origin	Benign tumor	Malignant tumor
EPITHELIAL TISSUE	Papilloma	Carcinoma
Glandular epithelial	Adenoma	Adenocarcinoma
Epidermoid or squamous epithelial	Squamous papilloma	Squamous epithelium carcinoma
Basal layer of epidermis		Basal cell carcinoma
Hair sheath	Pilomatrixoma	
Melanocytes of basal layer	Nevi (mole)	Malignant melanoma
Epithelium of respiratory tract	Papilloma	Bronchogenic carcinoma
Renal tubular epithelium	Adenoma	Renal cell carcinoma or renal adenocarcinoma
CONNECTIVE TISSUE OR MESENCHYME		
Fibrous tissue	Fibroma	Fibrosarcoma
Adipose tissue	Lipoma	Liposarcoma
Cartilage	Chondroma	Chondrosarcoma
Bone	Osteoma	Osteosarcoma
Blood vessels	Hemangioma	Hemangiosarcoma
Muscle		
smooth	Leiomyoma	Leiomyosarcoma
skeletal	Rhabdomyoma	Rhabdomyosarcoma
HEMATOPOIETIC TISSUE		
Leukocytes		Leukemias
Granular leukocytes and precursors		Granulocytic leukemia Myelocytic leukemias Myelogenous leukemias
Plasma cells		Multiple myeloma
Lymphoid		
Nongranular leukocytes and prelymphocytes		Lymphomas
Proliferating lymphocytes and monocytes		Lymphocytic leukemia
Proliferating immature precursor monocytes		Lymphoblastic leukemia
Solid tumors of lymph tissue (thymus, spleen, lymph nodes)		Lymphoma or lymphosarcoma
NERVE TISSUE		
Nerve cell	Neuroma	
Glial tissue		Glioma or neuroglioma
Nerve sheaths	Neurilemoma	Neurilemic sarcoma
Meninges	meningioma	Meningeal sarcoma
Neuroectoderm	neurocytoma	Neuroblastoma
Retina		Retinoblastoma
ADRENAL MEDULLA	Pheochromocytoma	Pheochromocytoma
MIXED TISSUE		
Breast	Fibroadenoma	Cystosarcoma phyllodes*
Embryonic kidney		Nephroblastoma (Wilms' tumor)

TABLE 10-2 Nomenclature and classification of benign and malignant tumors—cont'd

Tissue of origin	Benign tumor	Malignant tumor
Uterus		Mixed mesodermal, leiomyosarcoma
OTHERS DIFFICULT TO CLASSIFY		
Melanoblasts	Pigmented nevus	Melanoma
Placenta	Hydatiform mole	Choriocarcinoma
Ovary	Granulosa-theca cell tumors	Carcinoma
	Brenner tumor	
	Arrhenoblastoma	
	Gynandroblastoma	
	Hilar cell tumor	
	Sex cord mesenchyme	
Testis	Interstitial cell tumor	Seminoma
		Carcinoma
		Chariocarcinoma
Thymus	Thymoma	Yolksac

From: Rubin, Bakemeier, & Krackov, 1984.

- Increase in nuclear size and density of staining (reflects an increase in total DNA)
- Increase in mitotic activity
- Abnormal mitoses and chromosomes

Two types of disorganization are generally involved. The first is the chaotic nuclear changes and cytoplasmic changes, and second is the disordered relationship of the component cells to each other. Nuclear and cytoplasmic changes are characteristic of cells undergoing **transformation,** the process by which a normal cell becomes a cancer cell. Cancer cells are disordered cells with pronounced cellular proliferation and great variation in size and shape of cells. They divide in an uncoordinated fashion, invading and destroying neighboring tissue, a process termed **progression.** Cancer tumor progression means a worsening in the abnormal biologic properties and *not* necessarily a progression in tumor size. The biologic worsening is related to the tumor's malignant capabilities or its lack of differentiation.

A cancer is, therefore, a delinquent cell mass. Disorganized cellular relationships are caused by differences between the cell surface properties of normal and cancerous cells (see Fig. 10-2). The surfaces of normal cells bind to each other better than do cancer cells. This reduction in adhesiveness that is characteristic of cancer cells has been suggested as the physical basis of malignancy (Bell, 1978). The changes in the cell surface glycoproteins of malignant cells and the poorly developed tight junctions and desmosomes may be important factors in decreasing cellular adhesiveness and in promoting invasion and subsequent metastasis.

These cellular changes can be demonstrated in the laboratory. When two or more normal cells grown in a monolayer culture come in contact with each other, they tend to "stick" together causing movement to stop—a process called contact inhibition—and form a parallel line without piling up on one another. In contrast, cancer cell movement is chaotic and does not stop with contact from other cells. Cancer cells have lost contact inhibition. Thus the cells often pile up in a disorganized fashion and form irregular masses, several layers deep (Fig. 10-1).

Nuclear and Cytoplasmic Changes

The nuclei of malignant cells are often enlarged and have variable shapes (and thus are said to be pleomorphic). Peripheral clumping of chromatin is sometimes noted along the periphery of the nucleus. The nuclear membrane can show several changes, including projections, pockets, blebbing, and an overall diminished number of nuclear pores, which are associated with DNA replication sites. The rate of mitosis is frequently increased in cancerous tissues. Changes in chromosomes include breaks, deletions, ring forms, and abnormal

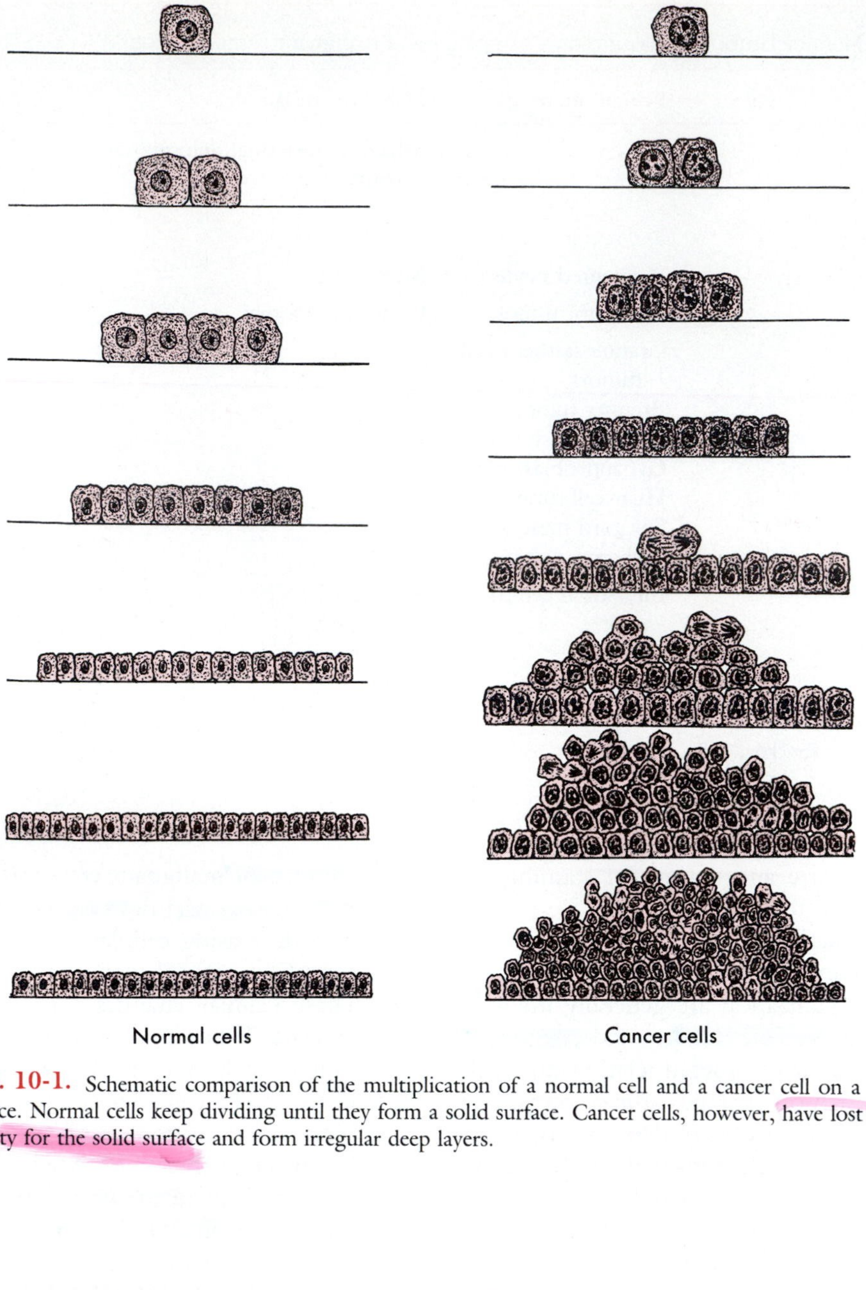

FIG. 10-1. Schematic comparison of the multiplication of a normal cell and a cancer cell on a solid surface. Normal cells keep dividing until they form a solid surface. Cancer cells, however, have lost their affinity for the solid surface and form irregular deep layers.

chromosomal karyotypes. For example, consistent changes are reported in chromosomes 1 and 17 in a number of hematologic cancers. Changes in chromosome 22, where the long arm is translocated to chromosome 9, is well known in chronic granulocytic leukemia and is called the Philadelphia chromosome (see Chapter 24).

Several differences are also evident in the plasma membrane. The plasma membranes of cancer cells have altered surface characteristics, fewer glycolipids, decreased amounts of membrane proteins, altered membrane fluidity, and loss of contact inhibition (Fig. 10-2). Changes in internal membrane function are inferred from transport studies (Chen & Chen, 1977). For example, increased glucose transport is associated with surface alterations in cancer cells.

Tumor Cell Markers

Tumor cell markers are substances produced by cancer cells that are found on tumor plasma membranes or in the blood, spinal fluid, or urine (Berlin, 1981; Franks & Teich, 1986). Biologic markers have been associated

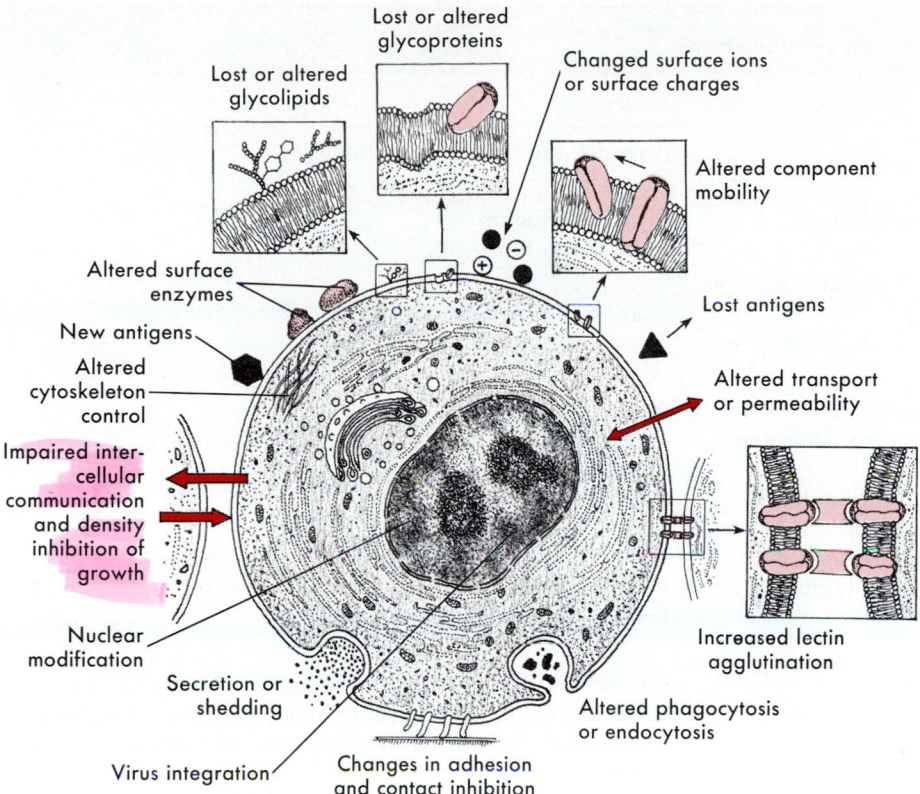

FIG. 10-2. Cell surface changes reported in cancer cells.

with cancer for many decades (McIntire, 1985). Such markers include hormones, enzymes, and antigens. (Characteristics of tumor antigens are described in Chapter 11.) Tumor markers vary with the degree of tumor progression and are products from the cancer cell's genetic material, which is activated during carcinogenesis (Table 10-3).

Tumor cell markers can be used in three ways: (1) to screen and identify individuals at high risk for cancer, (2) to help diagnose the specific type of tumor in individuals with clinical manifestations relating to cancer, and (3) to follow the clinical course of individuals with cancer. A problem in diagnosis of cancer from tumor marker assays is that nonmalignant disease can be associated with the same marker. In fact, the nonmalignant conditions greatly exceed the malignant conditions. The presence of a tumor marker may increase the suspicion of cancer, but should not be used alone as a diagnostic test (Franks & Teich, 1986; McIntire, 1985). The need for tumor cell markers remains a high priority, however, because improvement in cancer therapy will depend on earlier detection and tumor identification.

Hormones

Some tumors inappropriately produce hormones, such as adrenocorticotropic hormone (ACTH), insulin, human chorionic gonadotropin (HCG), parathyroid hormones, and erythropoietin. The term "ectopic hormone production" is used to describe the production of hormones by tumors of nonendocrine origin. Detection of certain tumors occurs through abnormally high serum levels of hormones and substrates produced by the hormone. Human chorionic gonadotropin, for example, is one of the best clinical detectors or tumor markers.

Ectopic ACTH production causes the increased adrenal secretion of cortisol. Cortisol causes muscle weakness, diabetes, peripheral edema, hypertension, bone demineralization, susceptibility to infection, thin and easily bruised skin, and hypokalemic alkalosis (high serum levels of cortisol promote increased renal losses of potassium, which causes hypokalemia).

Enzymes

There are two types of basic abnormalities of expression of enzymes in cancer, (1) the expression of an immature or fetal form of an enzyme, and (2) the ectopic

TABLE 10-3   Tumor-cell markers

Marker	Tumor
Cytology	Aspirates, exudates, urine, brushings
Antigens	
Carcinoembryonic antigen	Many solid tumors
α-fetoprotein	Liver, ovary, testis
Tumor-specific cell-mediated reactions	
Cytotoxicity tests	Many solid tumors
Delayed hypersensitivity reaction to tumor extracts	Many solid tumors
Ectopic hormones	
Human chorionic gonadotropin	Many tumors
Parathormone	Kidney, Lung
Adrenocorticotropic hormone	Lung
Antidiuretic hormone	Lung
Melanin-stimulating hormone	Lung
Thyroid-stimulating hormone	Placenta (choriocarcinoma)
Insulin	Lung
Isoenzymes	
Acid phosphatase	Carcinoma of the prostate, breast cancer
Placental alkaline phosphatase	Choriocarcinoma; carcinomas of ovary, pancreas, colon, breast, uterus, bronchus, testicular cancers, reticulum cell sarcoma, Hodgkin disease; multiple myeloma
Nonplacental alkaline phosphatase	Osteogenic sarcoma; parathyroid carcinoma; cancers metastatic to bone from prostate, breast, multiple myeloma, infiltrative cancers of the liver, leukemia, reticulum cell sarcoma
Galactosyl transferase	Carcinomas of lung, breast, esophagus, stomach, pancreas, colon, gallbladder; chronic lymphocytic leukemia
Aminopeptidases	Carcinomas of pancreas, liver, stomach lining; carcinoma metastatic to liver
Gamma glutamyl transpeptidase	Carcinomas metastatic to liver
Ribonuclease	Carcinoma of pancreas
Sialyl transferase	Carcinomas of breast, colon, lung, prostate; leiomyosarcoma; leukemia; lymphoma; melanoma
Elevated normal substances	
Immunoglobulins	Multiple myeloma
Insulin	Islet cell tumors
Serotonin	Carcinoid tumors
Parathormone	Parathyroid tumors
Prolactin	Pituitary tumors
Gastrin	Islet cell tumors
Human chorionic gonadotropin	Choriocarcinoma
Calcium	Medullary carcinoma (thyroid), parathyroid tumors

Adapted from: King, Fenoglio, & Lefkowitch, 1983; and Moosa, Robson, & Schimpff, 1986.

production of enzymes. Of current interest are isoenzymes (variable forms of an enzyme). A partial listing of isoenzymes is located in Table 10-3.

The extensive research of enzymes and isoenzymes in cancer has clearly shown that cancers do not produce new or unique enzymes. The enzymes or isoenzymes found are normally produced by the noncancerous tissue from which the cancer arises (Moosa, Robson, &

Schimpff, 1986). However, the tumor may cause the production of enzymes in different or abnormal proportions. Decreases and increases in enzymes within a given cell type are *associated* with cancer (Weber, 1977). These enzyme changes occur mainly within the tumor itself and unfortunately are expressed in the circulation only when the tumor is very large or widespread metastases has occurred (Moosa et al., 1986).

Tumor Antigens

Cancer cells express antigens called tumor-associated antigens (TAA). These antigens are not found on their normal, noncancerous cell counterparts. (Tumor antigens are discussed in detail in Chapter 11.)

TUMOR DEVELOPMENT

Tumors grow at different rates, but become malignant when they invade normal tissue and eventually metastasize. **Carcinogenesis** (production of cancer) is influenced by the site, nutritional status, and many other factors in the host. Specific sites of tumor development also vary with the age of the host (Table 10-4). Tumors develop in progressive steps, from normal, initiated (when the DNA is altered), preneoplastic growth to malignant growth.

A current controversy is whether a cancer originates from a single cell that proliferates widely, producing clones, or from several cells that proliferate at the same time (i.e., field origin) (Franks & Teich, 1986; King, Fenoglio, & Lefkowitch, 1983). Evidence from tissue cultures demonstrate that carcinoma of the cervix arises from one cell; experiments in mice reveal that carcinomas of the liver arise from a mosaic of several cells; in humans, multiple bladder carcinomas also can arise simultaneously. Experimental evidence thus suggests that both types of origin, clonal and field, represent valid theories and the origin depends on the type of tissue affected.

Tumors are graded according to structural features that reflect the degree of differentiation (Table 10-5). The better differentiated a tumor is, the more it resembles its tissue of origin. The less the tumor resembles normal tissue, the more undifferentiated or anaplastic the tumor is said to be. Tumor **grading** is thus an evaluation of the tumor's degree of malignancy. It is a process different from **staging**, which determines the extent of disease in an individual.

TABLE 10-4 Cancer sites and relationships to age

Cancer site	Relationship to age
Respiratory system	Among men, rates exceptionally high at ages 45-64 years compared with other cancers; in both sexes rates increase with age through 65-74 years
Digestive system	Low rates under 45 years; large increases extend through very advanced ages
Breast (female)	Rates highest of all cancers among women at ages 25-54 years
Male genital organs	High rates at ages 64 and over; large increases with ages among older men
Female genital organs	Rates are significant at ages 35-54, but rate increases into older ages
Urinary organs	Very low rates under age 55 years; large increases through advanced ages
Leukemia	Compared with other cancers in children, a significant rate, but still a low rate; marked increases in rate starting at 35-44 years
Other lymph and blood tissues	Rare among children and young adults; age gradient starts in middle adult years

From Shapiro, 1983.

TABLE 10-5 Tumor grading: degrees of differentiation

Grade	Tumor characteristics
Grade I: Well differentiated	Tumor closely resembles tissue of origin and thus retains some specialized functions
Grade II: Moderately differentiated	Tumor has less resemblance to tissue of origin; more variation in size and shape of tumor cells; increased mitoses
Grade III: Poorly to very poorly differentiated	Tumor does not closely resemble tissue of origin; much variation in size and shape of tumor cells; greatly increased mitoses
Grade IV: Very poorly differentiated	Tumor has no resemblance to tissue of origin; great variation in size and shape of tumor cells

Adapted from Moosa, Robson, & Schimpff, 1986.

Growth Rates

Tumor growth rates vary and are influenced by vascular supply and tumor integrity. **Angiogenesis** (new growth of blood vessels to vascularize tissues) is critical to the development of solid tumors. This process separates the development of any solid tumor into two phases: the avascular phase and vascular phase. In the avascular phase, tumor cells multiply and form aggregates in the interstitial tissue where nutrients arrive by diffusion. Tumors 1 to 2 mm in diameter are generally attached to the host vascular system. Vascularity does not cause an extremely large growth spurt until the capillaries have penetrated the edge of a tumor.

One measure of tumor growth rate is the **doubling time.** This is the mean length of time for division of all the tumor cells present. It has been calculated that approximately thirty doubling-times are required for a tumor to reach 1 cm in diameter (Rubin, Bakemeier, & Krackov, 1984). The growth process is thought to be increased by growth factors, prostaglandin E_1, proteolytic enzymes, and possibly a tumor angiogenesis factor (TAF) (Gospodarowica, Bailecki, & Thakral, 1979; Guillino, 1981; Taylor & Folkman, 1982). Solid tumors and cancerous cells have been reported to secrete TAF, promoting growth of endothelial cells. Currently, no single agent or TAF has been isolated. However, many agents are thought to be responsible for the angiogenic response (Sporn, Roberts, & Driscoll, 1985). It has been suggested that TAF is the stimulus for increasing the network of blood vessels in the tumor (Fig. 10-3).

Sophisticated mathematical formulas help to predict tumor growth patterns. These are helpful in determining the amount of a drug required to avert the cancer, but, because tumors can include several cell types with only some cells that divide, each with their own proliferation rates, accurate responses to treatment are difficult to predict. A slowing down of tumor growth can occur because of compression of blood vessels, cell division at a slower rate, or cells enter a dormant state (see the Cell Cycle, Chapter 1).

Tumor Spread

Tumor spread throughout the body can take several forms: (1) direct invasion of contiguous organs or local spread, (2) metastasis to distant organs by lymphatics and veins, and (3) metastases by implantation (del Regato, Spjut, & Cox, 1985). Spreading of a tumor depends on its rate of growth, its degree of differentiation, the anatomic presence or absence of barriers and other unknown biologic factors.

Local Spread

Invasion, or local spread, is poorly understood. Four possible mechanisms of invasion, however, are that it occurs as a result of (1) cellular multiplication, (2) mechanical pressure, (3) release of lytic enzymes, and (4) the increased motility of individual tumor cells (Franks & Teich, 1986). These mechanisms are not mutually exclusive and it is likely that in a given tumor any combination of the four may be involved. Invasion depends on the rate of cellular multiplication, which is a function

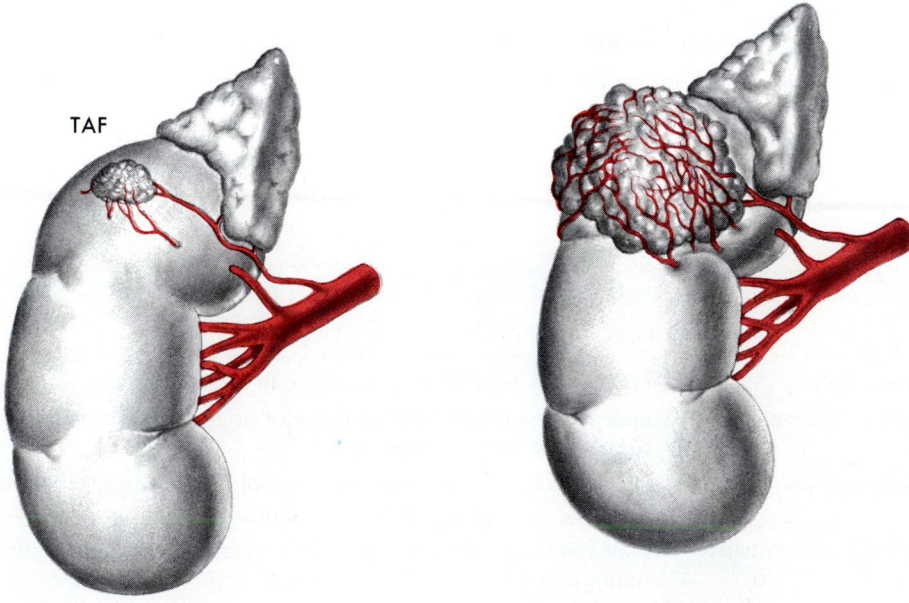

FIG. 10-3. Tumor angiogenesis factor (TAF) and tumor growth.

of the cell generation time (through the cell cycle), the number of cells that are dividing (growth fraction), and the cell loss from the tumor. Cells from malignant lesions thus can divide rapidly, but the tumor may not grow because a number of cells are rapidly dying.

Invasion, according to mechanical pressure, is analagous to the way in which plants force their roots through the soil (i.e., by building up pressure that forces sheets, fingerlike projections, along the lines of least mechanical resistance). Pressure from the growing mass blocks local blood vessels, leading to local tissue death and a reduction in mechanical resistance that further aids the spread (Franks & Teich, 1986).

Areas of normal host tissue adjacent to areas of tumor invasion show considerable amounts of lytic damage. Because many animal and human tumors have higher levels of hydrolases (e.g., proteases and collagenases) than corresponding normal tissue, the concept that malignant tumors produce and secrete lytic enzymes that destroy normal tissue has become firmly established.

Experiments have shown that tumor cells in the body, as in tissue culture, are capable of active movement and migration. To what extent this motility is used in tumor invasion is unknown, but it seems likely that the malignant cells do move through normal tissue by active locomotion (Franks & Teich, 1986).

Movement and direct extension of a tumor is influenced by anatomic location. Certain natural barriers can retard, but not totally prevent tumor extension. For example, periosteum, cartilage, muscle, and dense connective tissues are barriers that retard, but do not totally prevent spread. Tumor extension out of the kidney is also difficult because of its dense surrounding capsules (del Regato et al., 1985).

Normal tissue factors, as well as tumor cell factors, influence tumor invasion of host tissue. For example, normal fibrinolytics and proteolytic enzymes may enhance cancer cell invasion by modifying or destroying surrounding host tissue.

Metastasis

Metastasis, the spread of cancer cells from a primary site of origin to a distant site, is the life-threatening characteristic of malignancy. Local invasion is thought to be a condition of metastases (Moosa et al., 1986). Methods exist for successfully eradicating **primary tumors** (original sites of tumor origin), yet the real challenge for reducing cancer mortality is controlling metastasis because removal of the primary tumor does not affect the proliferating growth at other sites. Often, the primary tumor is not even diagnosed before secondary spread occurs.

Some tumors can grow in any organ, whereas others have preferred sites of growth. For example, carcinoma of the prostate, breast, thyroid gland, and kidney metas-tisize and grow in bone. Metastases and tumor growth do occur frequently in the lungs, bone, brain, and liver, depending on the primary tumor location and route of spread.

Metastasis by Lymphatics and Veins

The process of metastasis involves a series of sequential steps: (1) extension or local invasion of the surrounding tissue; (2) penetration into blood vessels or lymphatics or both, and into body cavities; (3) release into the lymph or blood circulation; (4) transport to a secondary site; and (5) arrest, adherence, and proliferation of cells at the secondary site (Fig. 10-4). Distant cancer spread involves invasion and penetration of tumor cells into blood vessels or lymphatics or both. Lymphatics and thin-walled venules offer relatively little mechanical resistance to penetration by tumor cells. Blood vessels within tumors offer malignant cells direct access into the circulation. Clusters, single cells, and fragments of tumor cells become separated from the primary tumor site and disseminate by these routes. Clumps of cells have a better chance of successful metastasis than do single cells. Those that arise close to a serous surface can invade through that surface, implant, and become distant metastases. These effusions, also known as seeding, occur in the pleural space surrounding the lung and in the peritoneal space surrounding the abdominal cavity.

The most common route for distant metastases is through the lymphatics. Carcinomas, melanomas, and some lymphomas, including Hodgkin disease, tend to metastasize first from the lymphatics and only secondarily from the bloodstream, but this may be an arbitrary division. There are connections between the lymphatics and the blood vessels and radio-labelled circulating tumor cells have been shown to move between these two systems, either through direct veno-lymphatic communications or from the lymphatics into the thoracic duct that empties into the jugular vein and the venous circulation (Franks & Teich, 1986). Tumor cell invasion into host tissue results in the penetration of small lymphatic vessels. This penetration causes the release of tumor cell emboli into these lymphatic vessels and is responsible for lymphatic metastases. Shedding of emboli is influenced by changes in vessel pressure, by turbulent alterations in lymphatic flow, and by movements or manipulation of the tumor during diagnostic tests or surgery.

Lymphatic spread *usually* progresses in an orderly sequence, moving tumor emboli from one node to the next node without bypassing a chain of lymph nodes. This contiguous involvement further indicates that lymph nodes can act as temporary barriers to further spread. Lymph nodes can be skipped, however, if obstructed by inflammation or previous infiltration by cancer cells. Lymph nodes close to the tumor (regional

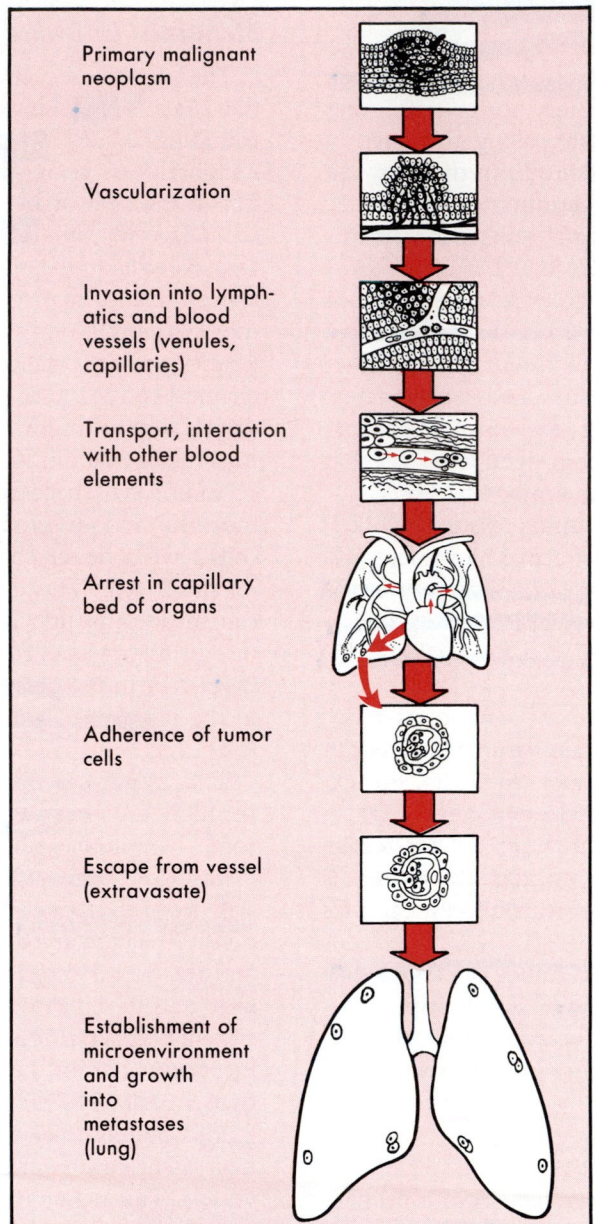

Primary malignant neoplasm

Vascularization

Invasion into lymphatics and blood vessels (venules, capillaries)

Transport, interaction with other blood elements

Arrest in capillary bed of organs

Adherence of tumor cells

Escape from vessel (extravasate)

Establishment of microenvironment and growth into metastases (lung)

FIG. 10-4. Pathogenesis of metastasis. Initial neoplastic transformation of susceptible cells gives rise to a small population of tumor cells. Vascularization of this initial neoplastic lesion allows further proliferation of tumor cells and enlargement of the primary tumor. Malignant cells within the primary tumor next begin to invade the surrounding host tissue(s). Entry of invading tumor cells into lymphatics or blood vessels serves to transport them to distant sites in the body, where they lodge and arrest in the capillary beds of various organs. For illustrative purposes, this figure shows arrest of malignant cells in the lung capillary bed. The arrested cells then exit from capillaries into the surrounding lung parenchyma where, subject to provision of a suitable environment, they proliferate to form metastases. (From Poste & Fidler, 1980.)

nodes) are almost always invaded first, before spread occurs to more distant nodes.

Often the first clinical symptom indicating the presence of cancer is an enlarged lymph node. For example, an enlarged axillary lymph node may signal breast cancer; an enlarged inguinal node may indicate a malignant melanoma; and an enlarged mesenteric node may be caused by cancer of the gastrointestinal tract. Tumor cells may grow in a lymph node, replace the entire lymph node, and enlarge it to as much as 10 cm in diameter.

Determining the number of lymph nodes involved is important for cure. For example, 5-year tumor-free survival in breast cancer may be predicted by the number of lymph nodes involved: with no nodes involved, the survival rate is 80%; with one to three nodes involved, the survival rate is 50%; and with four or more nodes involved, the rate is 25%.

Tumors can grow into veins, form thrombi, and release tumor emboli into the circulation. Such vascular involvement is common for lung cancer. From the lung, tumors often invade the pulmonary veins, travel to the left side of the heart, and thus to the systemic circulation. Thrombi often form in the vascular wall because of wall destruction by the tumor. Significant wall destruction can occur and form a large tumor thrombus, plugging the vessel's lumen.

Of interest is the lack of splenic involvement from circulatory spread. The spleen is a highly vascular, large organ and seems likely to be vulnerable to circulatory spread, yet this is very uncommon for all cancers except Hodgkin disease. Emboli from carcinomas, sarcomas, and melanomas travel to the spleen, but do not usually colonize and grow.

Metastasis by Implantation

Tumor cells can invade and implant themselves into surrounding proximal serous cavities. This route for metastasis is particularly evident in cancers of the ovary that spread to the peritoneal surface. Once tumors reach serous cavities, such as pleural and peritoneal cavities, loose tumor cells are free to implant themselves anywhere in that cavity. During the process of implantation, however, the spreading tumor cells are vulnerable to destruction, so that only a small percentage of circulating tumor cells actually survive to form secondary growths. Implantation is facilitated by tumors that produce mucin (a glycoprotein found in mucus), which drains into lymphathetic channels transporting cancer cells from, for example, the pancreas, stomach, ovary, and gallbladder.

Implantation is also known to occur from the circulating blood because of surgical procedures. The surgeon's scalpel or glove can carry and implant cancer cells in nearby regions, and manipulation of the tumor can increase the number of cancer cells found in the bloodstream (del Regato et al., 1985; Smith & Hilberg, 1955; Spjut et al., 1958). Rough handling of the tumor during surgery, physical examinations, preparation of the skin before surgery, and vasodilation and curretage of the cervix and endometrium can increase the number of cancer cells in the bloodstream. Although this type of spread is infrequent, cautious handling of tissue during surgical procedures is imperative for decreasing mortality and facilitating healing. Undue diagnostic procedures and operative manipulation should always be avoided.

CLINICAL MANIFESTATIONS OF CANCER

Pain

Usually little or no pain is associated with the early stages of malignant disease, but pain does affect 60% to 80% of those who are terminally ill with cancer. Pain is strongly influenced by fear, anxiety, sleep loss, fatigue, and overall physical deterioration. Pain is known to occur through an interaction among psychogenic, cultural, and physiologic components. (The neurophysiology of pain is discussed in Chapter 13.)

General mechanisms causing pain associated with cancer include pressure, obstruction, invasion of a sensitive structure, stretching of visceral surfaces, tissue destruction, and inflammation. The pain may or may not be directly related to the malignancy, but might be the result of other problems, such as infection. A very common cause of pain is bone metastasis, but the pain may be referred away from the involved bone and might, for example, be manifested as back pain. Bone pain can be caused by periosteal irritation, medullary pressure, and pathologic fractures.

Abdominal pain is often caused by severe stretching from the tumor invasion of the hollow viscus. Tumors that obstruct and distend the bowel cause pain. Small-bowel obstructions in individuals with known malignant disease are commonly the result of recurrent cancer, surgical adhesions, or new primary tumors. Surgery is often needed to obtain symptomatic relief. Enlargement of the liver from hepatic malignancies will stretch the liver, resulting in a dull pain or a feeling of fullness over the right upper quadrant of the abdomen.

Tumor compression of nerve endings against a firm surface will create pain. Brain tumors have very little space to grow without compressing blood vessels and nerve endings between the tumor and the cranial vault. Tissue destruction from infection and necrosis can cause pain. A frequent site of infection is the oral area, in which a common cause of pain is ulcerative lesions of the mouth and esophagus.

Cachexia

The syndrome of **cachexia** includes anorexia, early satiety (filling), weight loss, anemia, and asthenia (marked weakness) (Fig. 10-5). Anorexia, or loss of appetite, can frequently be attributed to pain, depression, chemotherapy, or radiotherapy. Alterations in taste can also account for the anorexia of cancer. Reductions in sensitivities to sweet, sour, and salty tastes make ordinary seasoned foods seem bland. Individuals with cancer, especially involving the liver, commonly have an aversion to red meat. Other aversions include coffee and chocolate. The mechanisms producing such aversions are unknown, although several mechanisms have been suggested. These include the following:

1. Poor use of glucose, resulting in an elevation of blood sugar that may depress appetite.
2. A decreased supply of insulin, resulting in and causing an elevation of blood sugar, may depress appetite.
3. Increased mobilization of proteins and elevated amino acid level in the blood stimulates the satiety center, resulting in reduced appetite.
4. Stimulation of visceral receptors from decreased peristalsis caused by surgery and other treatments stimulates the satiety center.
5. A reduction in the emotional pleasures of eating or alterations in smell or taste of food can depress appetite.

Anorexia leads to a protein-energy malnutrition (PEM), which has been classified according to three types: (1) similar to kwashiorkor, (2) marasmus, and (3) a combination of the two. Kwashiorkor is a form of malnutrition that evolves from a protein-deficient diet, in which calories are primarily gained from carbohydrates. Because the onset is usually rapid, anthropometric measurements tend to be normal, but serum proteins (transferrin, albumin) are decreased. This protein serum decrease (hypoalbuminemia) causes the serum colloid osmotic pressure to decrease, so that fluid escapes to the interstium and causes edema. Marasmus is a form of malnutrition resulting from a decreased intake of calories and proteins. It is characterized by decreased anthropometric measurements caused by a prolonged and gradual wasting of muscle mass and normal serum albumin. A combination of kwashiorkor amd marasmus causes hypoalbuminemia, edema, diminished immunologic competence (which depends on normal protein stores), and an overall physical deterioration. (Malnutrition is discussed in detail in Chapter 36.)

Progressive weight loss in the person with cancer occurs despite normal or increased food intake. Starvation usually decreases the basal metabolic rate (BMR), but metabolic rates in persons with cancer are high. The relationship of increased BMR and weight loss resulting in a breakdown of protein and nitrogen loss or negative nitrogen balance is unclear. This increase may be a result of accelerated metabolic activity of the tumor itself. Malignant cells replicate more rapidly than normal cells and require more food for their growth, but at the expense of the normal tissue. The normal tissue, over time, is sacrificed, and the individual begins to waste. Alterations in protein, lipid, and carbohydrate metabolism undoubtedly play a role.

Carbohydrate metabolism is altered, causing a syndrome resembling diabetes mellitus. Hyperinsulinemia is present, and many individuals show insulin resistance, hyperglycemia, and an abnormal glucose tolerance test. The result of these disturbances is an increased gluconeogenesis, which produces glucose from amino acids. In starvation, protein is usually spared to protect vital structures, but in cancer, protein and fatty acids are used for meeting energy needs. Fatty acids are released from the breakdown of adipose tissue.

An unusual and frustrating component of care is the cancer patient's early satiety, or a sense of filling. The individual may initially feel hungry, but after a few mouthfuls of food feels full. One hypothesis is that a humoral factor is responsible for this phenomenon, but little solid evidence concerning humans is available to substantiate this theory.

Anemia

Anemia is a common disorder associated with malignancy. The majority of individuals with cancer usually have a mild anemia, although 20% may have hemoglobin concentrations below 9 g per 100 ml (nl = 15 g/100 ml). Several mechanisms cause anemia in persons with cancer; these include chronic bleeding resulting in iron deficiency, severe malnutrition, medical therapies, or malignancy in blood-forming organs. Chronic bleeding and iron deficiency can accompany colorectal or

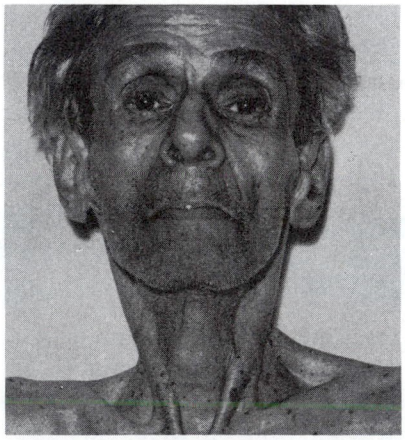

FIG. 10-5. Cachexia. Sunken appearance of the eyes, cheeks, and temporal areas; sharp nose; dry rough skin. (From Seidel, Ball, Dains, and Benedict, 1987).

genitourinary malignancy. Iron is also malabsorbed in individuals with gastric, pancreatic, or upper intestinal cancer. Anorexia can also cause iron deficiency, although folate deficiency is more common with anorexia.

Generally, anemia is not a common consequence of chemotherapy, but normochromic (normal hemoglobin concentration) and normocytic (average red cell size) anemias can occur after prolonged administration of alkylating agents or nitrosoureas, both classes of chemotherapeutic agents. Megaloblastic (large red cell) anemias may develop after treatment with methotrexate, which causes abnormal folate metabolism.

Malignancy of the blood-forming organs is associated with a number of hemolytic anemias. Individuals with chronic lymphocytic leukemia occasionally develop an autoimmune hemolytic anemia. (Anemia associated with leukemia is discussed in Chapter 23.)

Leukopenia and Thrombocytopenia

Direct tumor invasion to the bone marrow causes both leukopenia (a decreased leukocyte count), and thrombocytopenia (a decreased number of platelets). Chemotherapeutic drugs are toxic to the bone marrow, often causing both granulocytopenia and thrombocytopenia. Leukopenia is usually the result of chemotherapy, but radiotherapy of areas of the bone marrow also causes leukopenia. Thrombocytopenia, reduction in number of platelets, is a major cause of hemorrhage in individuals with cancer. It is usually the result of chemotherapy or bone marrow involvement by the malignancy. Thrombocytopenia is an accompanying disorder of disseminated intravascular coagulation, which is found in individuals with acute promyelocytic leukemia (see Chapter 23) and prostate cancer (see Chapter 20).

TABLE 10-6 Factors predisposing cancer patients to infection

Factor	Basis
Age	Many common malignancies occur mostly in older age.
	Immunologic functions decline with age.
	General debility reduces immunocompetence.
	Immobility predisposes to infection.
	Far-advanced cancer often results in immobility and general debility that worsens with age.
	Elderly persons are predisposed to nutritional inadequacies.
	Malnutrition impairs immunocompetence.
Tumor	Can cause nutritional derangements.
	Can create sites and circumstances favorable to growth of microorganisms (obstruction, serous or blood effusion, ulceration).
	Far-advanced disease predisposes to debility and immobility.
	May cause humoral or cellular immune defects.
	Metastasis to bone marrow may cause leukopenia, other defects in immunity.
Leukemias	Inadequate granulocyte production (impaired phagocytosis).
	Thrombocytopenia (bleeding, breaks in skin integrity).
	Late effect: Chronic lung disease from *Pneumocystitis carini* pneumonia during therapy.
Lymphomas and other reticuloendothelial malignancies	Humoral and cellular immune defects (anergy, altered immunoglobin production).
	Late effect: Splenectomy in children: increased susceptibility to infection.
Treatment: surgery	Invasive (interrupts first lines of defense).
	Often radical (removal of large blocks of tissue in lengthy procedures)—hemorrhage, decreased tissue perfusion, creation of dead spaces, devitalization of tissues.
	May be "dirty" surgery (bowel, infected or contaminated areas).
	Often done on older, poorer-risk patients.
	Often done after long preoperative hospitalization.
	Patients may have had previous adrenocorticosteroid therapy.
	Patients may have infections at sites remote from operative area.
	May cause nutritional derangements (especially important in head and neck surgery).
	Lymph node dissection may predispose to local infection, impair containment to area.
	Gynecologic surgery may result in fistulas.
	Lung surgery may cause bronchopleural fistulas.
	May cause debility, immobility.

From Donovan, & Girton, 1984.

Common Microorganisms Causing Infection in Cancer

Organism
E. coli
Pseudomonas
Klebsiella
Staphylococcus
Candida
Streptococcus
Bacteriodes
Proteus
Clostridium

Adapted from Donovan & Girton, 1984.

Infection

Infection is the most significant cause of complications and death in individuals with malignant disease. A reduction in the absolute granulocyte or lymphocyte count increases the risk of infection development and individuals with cancer are very susceptible to infection because of reductions in immunologic functions, debility with advanced disease, and immunosuppression from radiotherapy and chemotherapy. (Factors predisposing individuals to infection are summarized in Table 10-6.) Surgery can also lower resistance to infection because removal of large quantities of tissue, together with hemorrhage, dead spaces, and poor tissue perfusion, create favorable sites for infection. The incidence of hospital-related (nosocomial) infections is increased because of indwelling medical devices, quality of wound care, and the introduction of microorganisms from visitors and other patients (see box above).

Leukopenia from bone marrow radiation dramatically increases the risk of infection. Mucous membranes and other rapidly dividing cells in the radiation field are prone to irritation and ulceration. Radiation can also lead to fistula formation or abnormal passages between tissue cavities. Fistula formations can result from radiation of the cervix, bladder, and intestinal tract. Surgery is often required to repair the fistula and eliminate continuous infectious cross-contaminations.

CANCER TREATMENT

Cancer is treated with chemotherapy, radiotherapy, surgery, immunotherapy, and combinations of these modalities (Table 10-7).

Chemotherapy

Several classes of chemotherapeutic agents are used concurrently to treat different types of cancer tumors (Table 10-8). The mechanism by which each drug acts

---

TABLE 10-7 Examples of treatment of site-specific cancers

Usual treatment	Site
Surgery	Colon
	Breast
	Ovary
	Lung
	Thyroid
	Skin
	Uterus
Chemotherapy	Lymphoma
	Leukemia
	Choriocarcinoma
	Ovary
	Breast
Radiation	Breast (all have been combined with surgery)
	Uterus or cervix
	Lymphomas
	Lung
	Combined with surgery in many sites.
Hormones	Breast
	Prostate
	Endometrium

Adapted from King, Fenoglio, & Lefkowitch, 1983.

to eradicate tumor cells depends largely on its effect on the cell cycle (described in Chapter 1). Malignant tumors have three cellular compartments: (1) cells undergoing mitosis and cytokinesis, (2) cells capable of entering the cell cycle in the G_1 phase (see Fig. 1-23), and (3) cells that do not divide and have irreversibly left the cell cycle (dying malignant cells, differentiated malignant cells, nonmalignant support cells). Cells in compartment 3 will die a natural death without chemotherapy. The specific aim of chemotherapy, therefore, is to kill cells from compartments 1 and 2—cells that are dividing and cells that are in interphase. Table 10-9 summarizes the mechanisms of action of certain common chemotherapeutic drugs.

To be curative, chemotherapy must eradicate enough tumor cells so the body's own defenses can eradicate the remaining cells. Smaller tumors have a faster growth rate and are generally more sensitive to chemotherapy. Few cells in a large tumor are dividing and, as a result, these are largely insensitive to chemotherapy.

Radiation

Ionizing radiation is a common approach to the treatment of malignant disease. The goals are (1) to eradi-

TABLE 10-8 Classes of chemotherapeutic drugs

Class	Drug
Antimetabolites	Methotrexate
	Cytosine arabinoside
	Aminopterin
	Bromouridyldeoxyriboside (BUDR)
	Fluorouridyldeoxyriboside (FUDR)
	Hydroxyurea
	Thymidine
Alkylating agents	Nitrogen mustard
	Cyclophosphamide
	Chlorambucil
	Mechlorethamine
	Melphalan
	Busupfan
Antibiotics	Daunorubican
	Doxorubicin (Adriamycin)
	Actinomycin D
	Bleomycin
	Mitomycin C
Hormones	Estrogens
	Androgens
	Steroids
Mitotic inhibitors	Vincristine
	Vinblastine
	Etoposide
	Teniposide
Nitrosoureas	Lomustine
	Semustine
	Streptozocin

cate cancer without producing excessive toxicity during treatment and (2) to avoid damage to normal structures. The application of radiation therefore requires precision and skillful application.

Ionizing radiation leads to damage of important macromolecules, especially DNA. Damage resulting from radiation is divided into three categories: (1) lethal damage, in which the cell is killed by radiation; (2) potentially lethal damage, in which the cell is so severely affected by radiation that modifications in its environment will cause it to die; and (3) sublethal damage, in which the cell is damaged, but can subsequently repair itself. Cellular compartments with rapidly renewing cells are, in general, more radiosensitive. (Cellular effects of ionizing radiation are discussed in Chapter 2.)

Surgery

Surgical therapy is used when the tumor has not yet spread beyond the limits of surgical excision. Surgeons are generally in agreement that if there is any chance of regional lymph node involvement and there is no evidence of distant disease, the lymph nodes also should be removed. In some circumstances, the removal of adjacent tissues has increased survival and enhanced cure. However, in more than half the cases, there may be evidence of micrometastatic disease at the time of surgery, or solid tumors.

Curative resections are done when there is no evidence of distant metastasis. The goals of palliative surgery (alleviation without cure) are (1) prevention of symptoms that would have occurred if the individual was not treated, and (2) relief of symptoms that are present.

Surgery is also indicated for benign tumors that could progress into malignant tumors. Premalignant and in situ tumors of epithelial tissues, such as skin, mouth, and cervix, are therefore removed.

TABLE 10-9 Mechanisms of action of common chemotherapeutic drugs

Drug	Mechanism
Actinomycin D	Prevents transcription; inhibits tRNA, mRNA synthesis. Inhibits protein synthesis.
Bleomycin	Breaks and fragments single strands of DNA. Damages nonproliferating as well as proliferating cells.
Cytosine arabinoside	Decreases production of DNA replicating units. Inhibits transcription. Prematurely terminates nucleic acid chains.
Adriamycin	Binds to DNA. Uncoils DNA helix. Inhibits DNA-directed RNA polymerase.
Mitomycin	Produces cross-linking of DNA strands.

Immunotherapy

Chemotherapy and radiation treatments are currently two of the most acceptable methods for managing cancer. Although effective in their control of certain types of cancer, these modalities are associated with some inherent drawbacks. In general, both forms of therapy act by eliminating mitotically or metabolically active cells. Within a tumor mass, however, a significant portion of cells is in a part of the cell cycle that is not affected by either metabolic inhibitors or mitotic poisons. In addition, these therapies cause an appreciable amount of discomfort to the individual because they affect the cell populations that, like transformed cells, have high rates of cell division. Cells of the gut epithelium, hair follicles, bone marrow, and gonads are affected by radiation and chemotherapy.

Because cancer is a dynamic disease in which the transformed cells that constitute a tumor mass possess a certain potential for adapting to changes in their environment, a form of cancer therapy that is effective against all types of cancer may not be possible. More specific methods, however, may eventually eliminate transformed cells without damaging normal tissues.

In this regard, immunotherapy holds great promise as an alternative form of cancer treatment, because of the unique properties of the immune system. (The immune system is discussed in detail in Chapter 6.) First, the immune system has specificity for antigen recognition and is highly regulated; thus, anti-tumor immune rejection responses can selectively eliminate cancer cells while sparing normal tissues. Second, immune memory cells are long lived and capable of providing extended protection against the emergence of recurrent primary tumor cells and foci of metastatic cancer cells. Third, there are numerous immunologic mechanisms that are able to cause rejection of various types of cancer. (These tumor-immune mediators are described in Chapter 11.) Although tumor-immune surveillance provides protection against cancer, certain evasive mechanisms allow tumor cells to escape immune rejection. Therefore the current research efforts for establishing effective anti-cancer immunotherapies are focused on characterizing the immunogenic properties of various tumor-associated antigens and developing methods to selectively enhance specific tumor rejection immune responses.

Immunotherapies for the treatment of cancer are generally referred to as **biological response modifiers** (BRMs) (Oldham & Smalley, 1985). BRMs are defined as mammalian gene products, agents, and clinical protocols that affect biologic responses in host-tumor interactions. Three mechanisms describe the activities of BRMs. These are (1) a direct cytotoxic effect on cancer cells; (2) the initiation or augmentation of the host's tumor-immune rejection response; and (3) the modification of cancer cell susceptibility to the lytic or tumor-

static effects of the immune system. The major classifications of BRMs are presented in Table 10-10. The basis of action and clinical applications of specific BRMs, selected from among the major classifications, are briefly discussed in the remainder of this section.

Immunomodulating Agents

Nonspecific stimulation of the immune system by an adjuvant (a substance that enhances the immune response) has been attempted in individuals with a variety of different cancers (Fig. 10-6). This therapy consists of the administration of an adjuvant (a bacterium), such as *C. parvum* or *Bacillus Calmette-Guerin* (BCG), an atten-

---

TABLE 10-10   Classification of biologic response modifiers

Major classification	Specific examples
Immunomodulating agents	Alkyl lysophospholipids
	BCG
	Bestatin
	C. parvum
	Endotoxin
	Levamisole
	Muramyldipeptide
	Picibanil (OK432)
	Tuftsin
Interferons and interferon inducers	Interferons (alpha, beta, and gamma)
	Poly IC-LC
	Brucella abortus
	Viruses
Thymosins	Thymosin alpha-1
	Other Thymosin factors
	Thymosin factor V
Antigens	Tumor- associated antigens
	Hapten-modified tumor- antigens
	Vaccines
Effector cells	Macrophages
	Natural killer cells
	Cytotoxic T cells
	LAK-cells
Lymphokines and cytokines	Colony- stimulating factors (CSF)
	Lymphotoxin
	Interleukins (IL-1, IL-2, IL-3, etc.)
Monoclonal antibodies	Cytotoxic antibodies
	Immunotoxins
	Phototoxins

Adapted from Oldham, & Smalley, 1985.

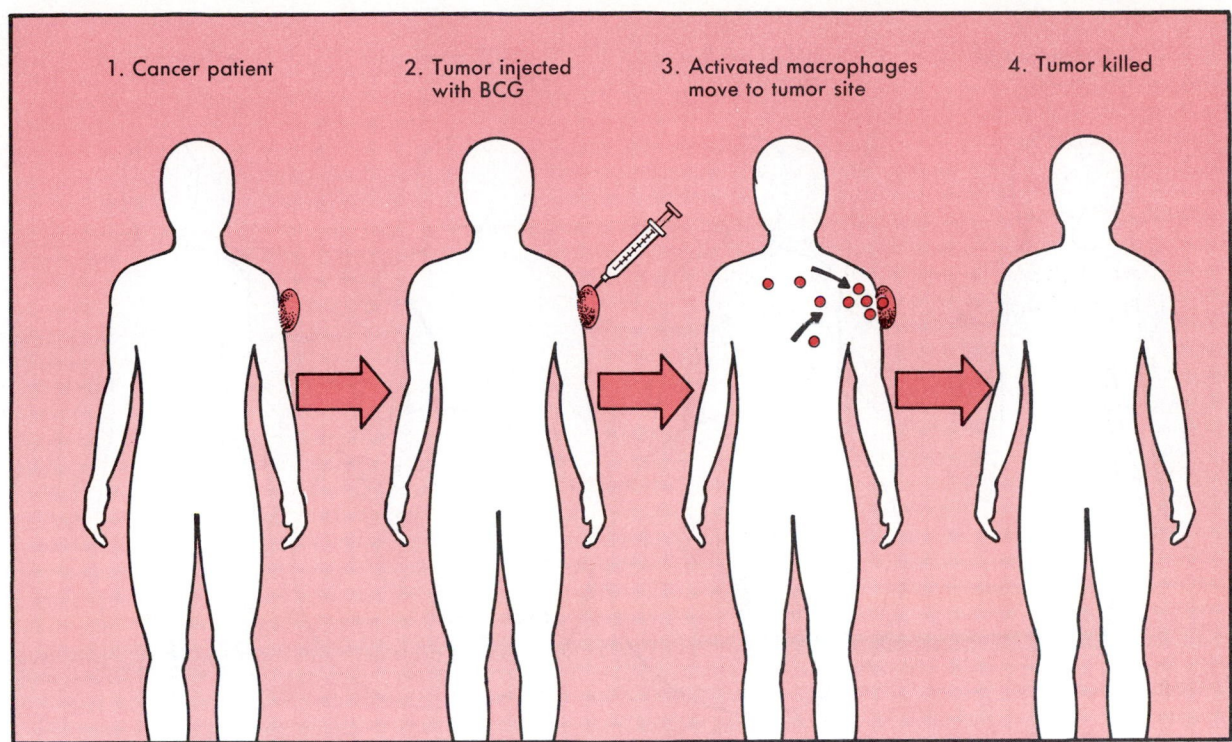

1. Cancer patient   2. Tumor injected with BCG   3. Activated macrophages move to tumor site   4. Tumor killed

FIG. 10-6. Immunostimulation in cancer therapy.

tuated strain of *Mycobacterium bovis*. For this type of treatment, injections of bacterial cell wall extracts, live BCG, or nonviable *C. parvum* are made at the tumor site. Retardation of tumor growth appears to result through the activation of macrophages, augmentation of natural killer cells, or by some degree of antigenic cross-reactivity between the organism (BCG) and the antigen produced by certain human cancers, such as melanomas.

Some success has also been observed in the treatment of genitourinary and lung cancer, usually through combined adjuvant treatments and chemotherapies. The most effective use of this type of immunotherapy, however, has been in the treatment of skin cancers.

Interferons

The interferons are a family of cell-derived proteins that have anti-viral and immune modulating activities. The most successful clinical trials have come from the use of α-interferon. α-interferon is a 20 to 25 kD molecular weight glycoprotein derived from activated leukocytes. In addition to its anti-viral activity, α-interferon has been shown to inhibit tumor growth, enhance natural killer cell activity, and increase cancer cell expression of tumor-antigens, thus making them more immunogenic (i.e., eliciting stronger tumor-immune rejection responses). Used either alone or in combination with other treatment modalities, α-interferon has been effec-

tive in the treatment of hairy-cell leukemia, Kaposi sarcoma (a common cancer of AIDS patients), and renal cell carcinoma. The use of interferons in cancer therapy is greatly enhanced by the ability to produce these biologic agents by recombinant gene-cloning techniques.

Antigens

Some success in causing the elimination of skin tumors has been achieved through the application of contact sensitizing agents (materials that cause a hypersensitivity response in the skin), such as dinitrochlorobenzene (DNCB) (Fig. 10-7). With this approach, the individual is first sensitized to DNCB through topical application to normal skin, and the tumor is subsequently painted with DNCB.

Tumor regression is thought to occur by inducing a contact hypersensitivity response to the DNCB at the tumor site. (Hypersensitivity reactions are discussed in Chapter 8.) Tumor cells are probably killed because DNCB has become associated with their cell surface and functions as an antigen. This type of therapy, however, is restricted to superficial tumors of the skin.

Research efforts are underway to identify tumor-associated antigens (the various types of antigens are described in Chapter 11) that could be used to develop anti-cancer vaccines. Ideally, common tumor-antigens expressed by a wide range of cancers could be developed

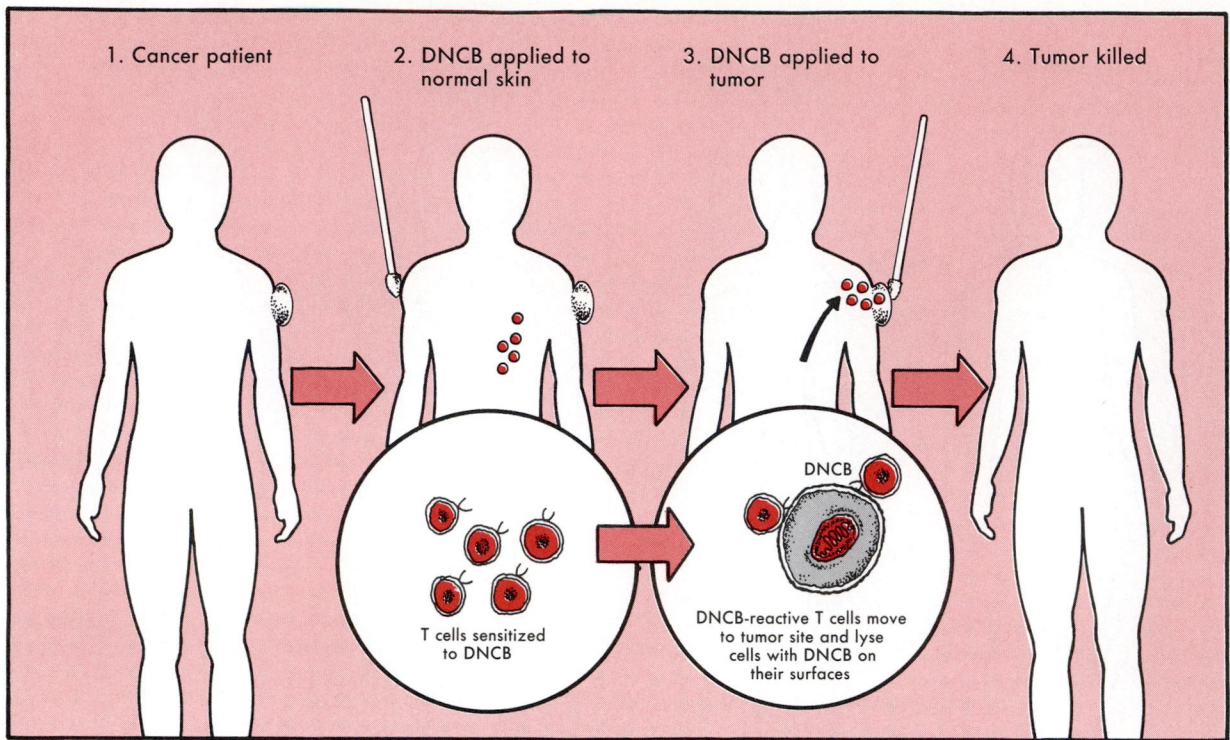

1. Cancer patient
2. DNCB applied to normal skin
3. DNCB applied to tumor
4. Tumor killed

DNCB

T cells sensitized to DNCB

DNCB-reactive T cells move to tumor site and lyse cells with DNCB on their surfaces

FIG. 10-7. Cancer therapy through antigen modification with dinitrochlorobenzene (DNCB).

as vaccines. These vaccines could be used as either immunotherapies to augment the host's immune response against their tumor or preventive techniques to immunize populations at risk to inhibit cancer emergence.

Effector Cells and Lymphokines

Theoretically, the most effective form of cellular immunotherapy would result from the transfer of cytotoxic T cells (Tc cells), which are specific for the antigens expressed by the tumor cells, into the cancer patient (Fig. 10-8). This type of therapy has been attempted by immunizing paired cancer patients against each other's tumors. After the immunization, lymphocytes are exchanged between the two persons. These attempts have not been successful in causing tumor regression, but this lack of success may result from the host's own immune response against the donor cell's histocompatibility antigens, which results in the elimination of the Tc cells. (Histocompatibility antigens are discussed in Chapter 6.) Similar attempts, in which lymphocytes are exchanged between histocompatible twins, have also failed, possibly because the tumor mass in these individuals is too large to be controlled by the number of lymphocytes transferred. Some positive results have been achieved through the reinoculation of the person's own lymphocytes. No long-term cures, however, have resulted.

Because this represents such an attractive form of immunotherapy for cancer, a new treatment protocol has been established and is currently undergoing extensive clinical trials. It is referred to as "LAK-cell therapy," for lymphokine-activated killer cells. The idea is to establish tumor-specific cytotoxic cell lines in tissue culture, that can mediate tumor rejection when injected back into the cancer patient. The procedure takes advantage of the ability to expand LAK-cells in vitro by growing them in tissue culture medium containing interleukin 2, the T cell growth factor. LAK-cells are phenotypically distinct from T-lymphocytes. When fused into the patient, LAK-cells are able to infiltrate into the tumor and mediate lysis of cancer cells. LAK-cell therapy is usually combined with treating the patient with interleukin 2. Treating the patient with interleukin 2 is thought to both maintain LAK-cell activity and enhance other antitumor immune rejection mechanisms. LAK-cell therapy has been used successfully in the treatment of melanoma and renal cell carcinoma.

Monoclonal Antibodies

The development of the monoclonal antibody technology has provided a method to generate highly specific antibody reagents that could not be obtained with traditional antisera. (Monoclonal antibodies are discussed in Chapter 6.) These reagents have a promising future in both the diagnosis and treatment of human cancer (Fig. 10-9).

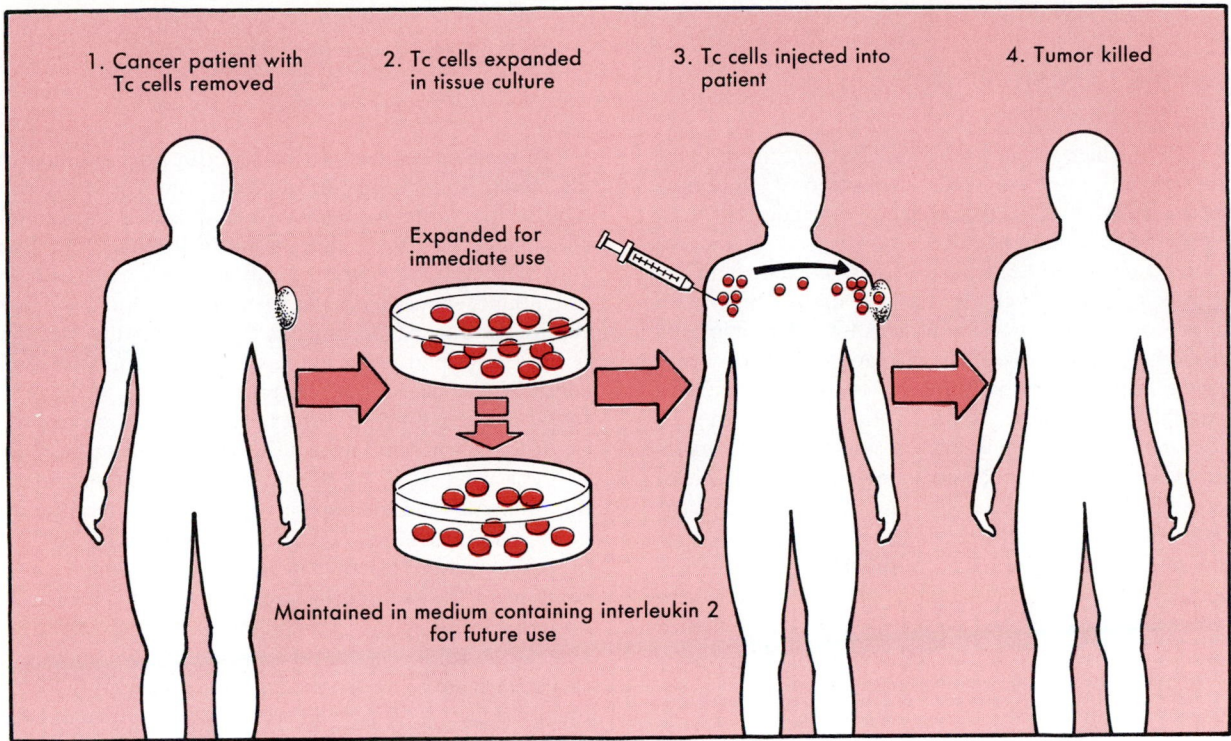

1. Cancer patient with Tc cells removed
2. Tc cells expanded in tissue culture
3. Tc cells injected into patient
4. Tumor killed

Expanded for immediate use

Maintained in medium containing interleukin 2 for future use

FIG. 10-8. Development of cytotoxic T cell (Tc cell) lines for cancer immunotherapy.

In the past, clinicians have relied on a number of methods to diagnose human cancers. For example, in the case of most skin cancers, the diagnosis can be made by visual examination of the lesion. In contrast, the diagnosis of various soft-tissue cancers, such as lung tumors, may require identifying certain clinical signs in the individual (e.g., obstruction, bleeding, pain). Cytologic methods (e.g., Pap smear) or histologic analysis of cells can also be used to diagnose various types of cancer. The diagnoses made by these methods are generally confirmed by tissue biopsies and pathologic evaluations. The major problems associated with these diagnostic methods are that some tests can give false results or may detect only tumor masses that have either become too large to be removed surgically, have invaded and destroyed surrounding tissues and organs, or have already metastasized to secondary sites.

The reason for developing and using monoclonal antibodies as diagnostic reagents for detecting cancer is that their high specificity for antigen could reduce the number of false results. Coupled with the appropriate assay system, monoclonal antibodies may provide methods for earlier detection of neoplastic disease. For example, highly purified monoclonal antibodies could be used to detect circulating tumor antigens and thus provide a method for periodic screening of individudals who are at high risk of developing a specific type of cancer. Monoclonal antibodies, when bound to a radionu-

clide (radioactive material), could also be used for radiologic imaging (a diagnostic process for detecting radioactive deposits in tissues). Such techniques could help in diagnosing both primary tumors, and metastases in individuals suspected of having disease.

Another goal for use of monoclonal antibodies is to develop monoclonal antibodies specific for tumor antigens that would mediate tumor rejection without affecting the normal tissues of the individual. In recent clinical trials, monoclonal antibodies against specific antigens expressed by B-lymphomas (the specific immunoglobulin on the cell surface) have been very effective in causing tumor regression. The ability to couple cytotoxic substances or cell poisons, such as the α chain of ricin (immunotoxins) and porphyrins (phototoxins), to monoclonal antibodies could greatly enhance the efficacy of these reagents as immunotherapy for cancer. The major problems that are currently faced in attempting to use monoclonal antibodies in cancer therapy are: (1) developing functional reagents with the appropriate antigen specificities, (2) overcoming clinical complications to the individual that are associated with injecting large amounts of foreign antibodies (currently, most monoclonal antibodies can only be made in rodents), and (3) controlling immunoregulatory mechanisms that would eliminate their efficacy. Certainly the potential use of monoclonal antibodies, as well as other forms of immunotherapy, has generated new interest in immune sur-

CLINICAL COMMENTARY
Monoclonal antibodies

In 1975, Kohler and Milstein described their method for fusing mouse myeloma cells (transformed antibody-producing cells) with normal antibody-secreting cells from the spleens of immunized mice. The resulting hybridoma cells (fused or "hybridized" cancer cells) possessed characteristics of both the myeloma cells and the B-lymphocytes used for fusion. These hydridoma cells were both immortal (characteristics of the myeloma cells) and capable of secreting antigen-specific antibody (characteristic of the normal B-lymphocyte). Because these hybridoma cells can be cloned (generate a cell line from a single cell) and maintained in tissue culture indefinitely, investigators are able to select individual hybridoma cell lines that produce large amounts of highly specific monoclonal antibody (a single species of antibody protein). Since the development of this technology, the use and potential application of monoclonal antibodies have reached virtually every field of applied science. As a result, Kohler and Milstein received the Nobel Prize in 1984 for their contributions.

The basic monoclonal antibody technology is quite simple. First, animals are immunized with the antigen to which a monclonal antibody is desired. Second, spleen cells (B-lymphocytes) from the immunized animal are fused with HAT-sensitive myeloma cells and grown in HAT (hypoxanthine, aminopterin and thymidine) -containing tissue culture medium. This strategy is based on the fact that: normal B-lymphocytes cannot survive in long-term tissue culture; myeloma cells, selected because they lack the necessary enzyme required for the nucleotide salvage pathway, are killed when cultured in HAT-medium because purine synthesis is blocked; and only hybrid cells (immortalized by the myeloma cells and capable of nucleotide reutilization) grow in HAT-medium. Third, supernatants from the wells of tissue culture plates containing hybridoma cells are screened for antigen-specific antibody activity. Fourth, hybridomas secreting the appropriate antibody are cloned (to generate a homogenous cell line) and large amounts of monoclonal antibody are produced in expanded tissue culture or ascites fluids (i.e., hybridoma cells grown as an ascites tumor in mice). And finally, purified monoclonal antibodies can be obtained for experimental or clinical use. The advantages for developing monoclonal antibodies compared to conventional antiserum are: (1) a single antibody species of known antigen specificity is generated rather than a mixture of different antibody molecules; (2) monoclonal antibodies have a single, constant binding affinity; (3) monoclonal antibodies can be diluted to a constant titer because the actual antibody concentration is known; and (4) the antibody can be purified to homogeneity. The application of monoclonal antibodies for cancer diagnosis and therapy has a potentially great future.

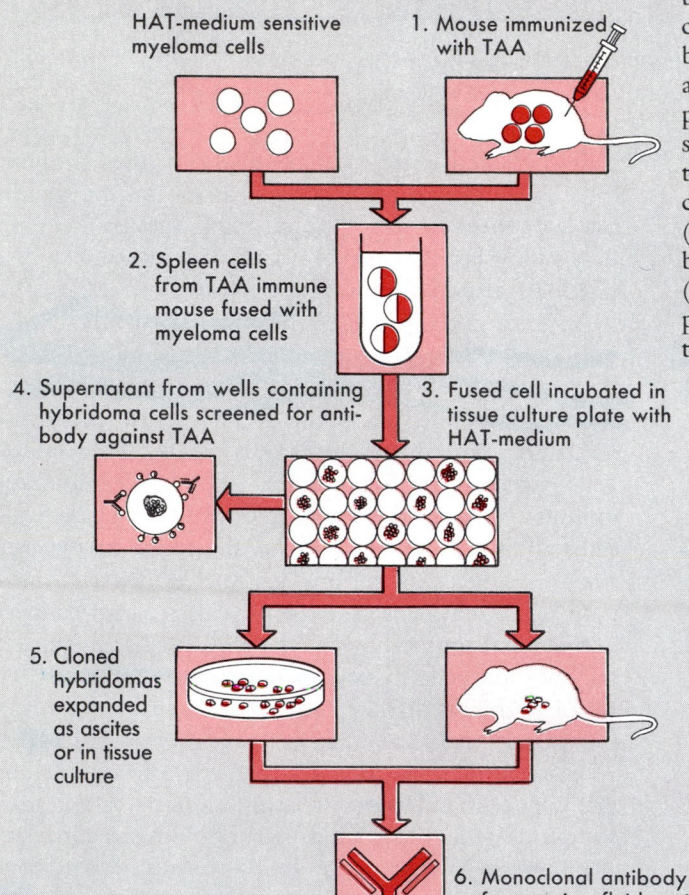

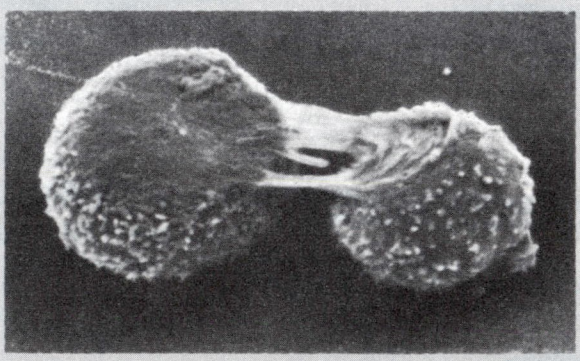

Technique for developing monoclonal antibodies. Inset is a hybridoma dividing. (From Raven supplement.)

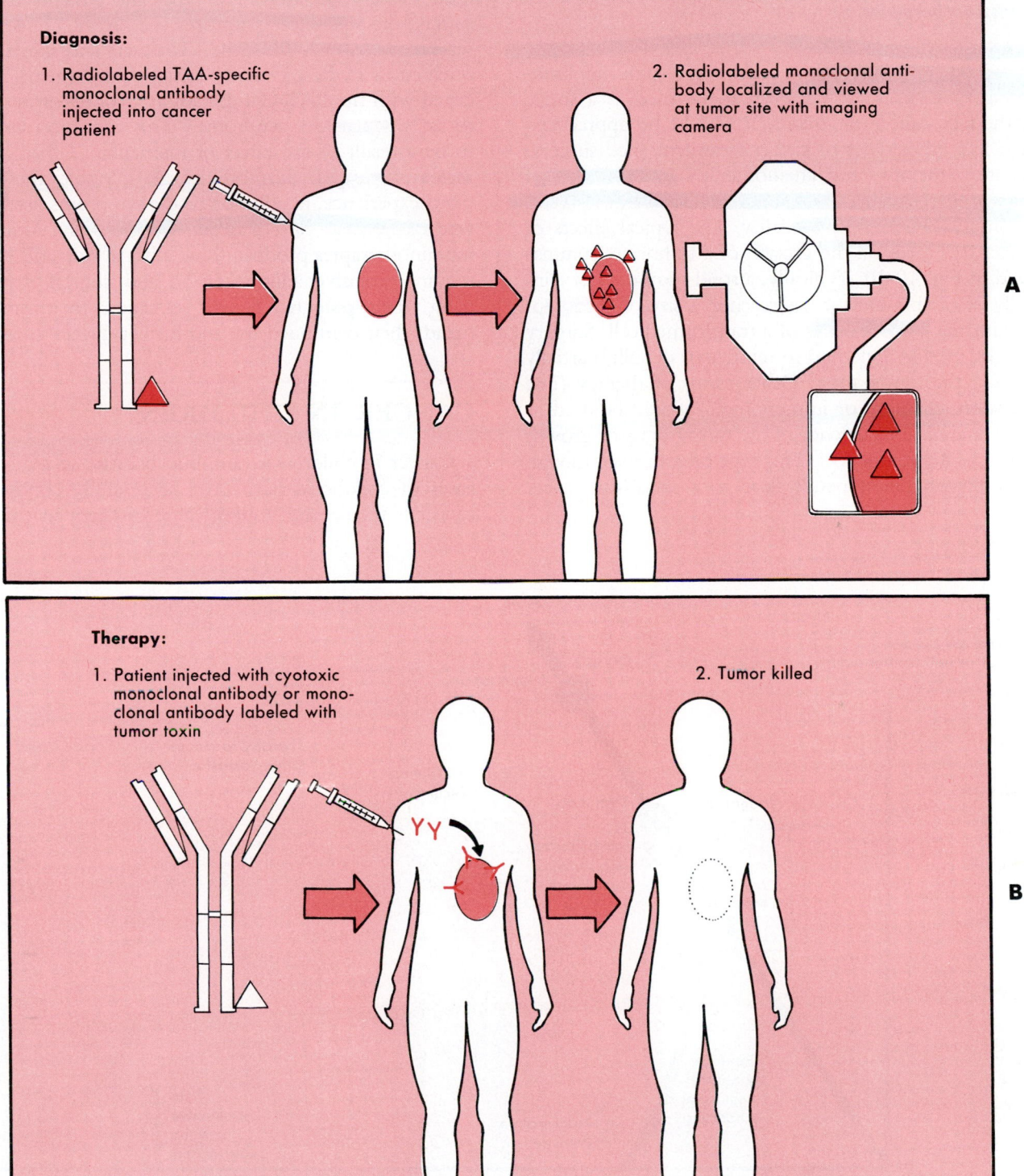

Diagnosis:

1. Radiolabeled TAA-specific monoclonal antibody injected into cancer patient

2. Radiolabeled monoclonal antibody localized and viewed at tumor site with imaging camera

A

Therapy:

1. Patient injected with cyotoxic monoclonal antibody or monoclonal antibody labeled with tumor toxin

2. Tumor killed

B

FIG. 10-9. A, Tumor immunodiagnosis and **B,** cancer immunotherapy with monoclonal antibodies. (*TAA*, tumor associated antigen.)

veillance mechanisms as possible methods for development of immunotherapies for treatment of cancer.

Applications and Clinical Complications of Immunotherapies

Immunotherapy represents the so-called "fourth modality" of cancer treatment. Although some immunotherapy protocols are designed to be used as a single method of cancer treatment, it should be appreciated that, like other types of cancer treatment (i.e., surgery, radiation therapy, and chemotherapy), the efficacy of immunotherapy may be increased when used as part of a combined treatment modality. The typical effects of cancer treatment on the growth of a tumor are summarized in Fig. 10-10. Typically, a solid tumor is not clinically detectable until it has reached a size of 1 cm, approximately 30 doublings of a transformed cell. Surgery is often used as a method to remove or debulk (partially reduce) the tumor mass. Other forms of therapy (i.e., radiation, chemical or immunologic) would be used to prevent clinical recurrence of the tumor mass or growth of metastatic tumor foci. This type of combined modality approach can hopefully lead to a successful cancer cure.

As with other forms of cancer treatment, there are numerous side effects associated with various immunotherapies. In general, during the administration of the immunotherapy (regardless of type) the patients usually suffer from "flu-like" symptoms (i.e., fever, chills, nausea, vomiting, and headache). Urticaria and skin rashes often occur in these patients during the treatment. Associated with the LAK-cell therapy is a condition referred to as "vascular-leak syndrome." This condition appears to be a result of the effect of interleukin 2 that causes increased vascular permeability. As a result, these patients experience, in addition to the symptoms listed, severe edema and cardiovascular hypotension. Although immunotherapies produce some adverse side effects and require extensive administration and clinical management, their potential benefit in cancer treatment demands their continued use and further development.

CANCER IN CHILDREN

Cancer in children is rare, but, because so many diseases of childhood have been successfully conquered, cancer is the second leading cause of death in children

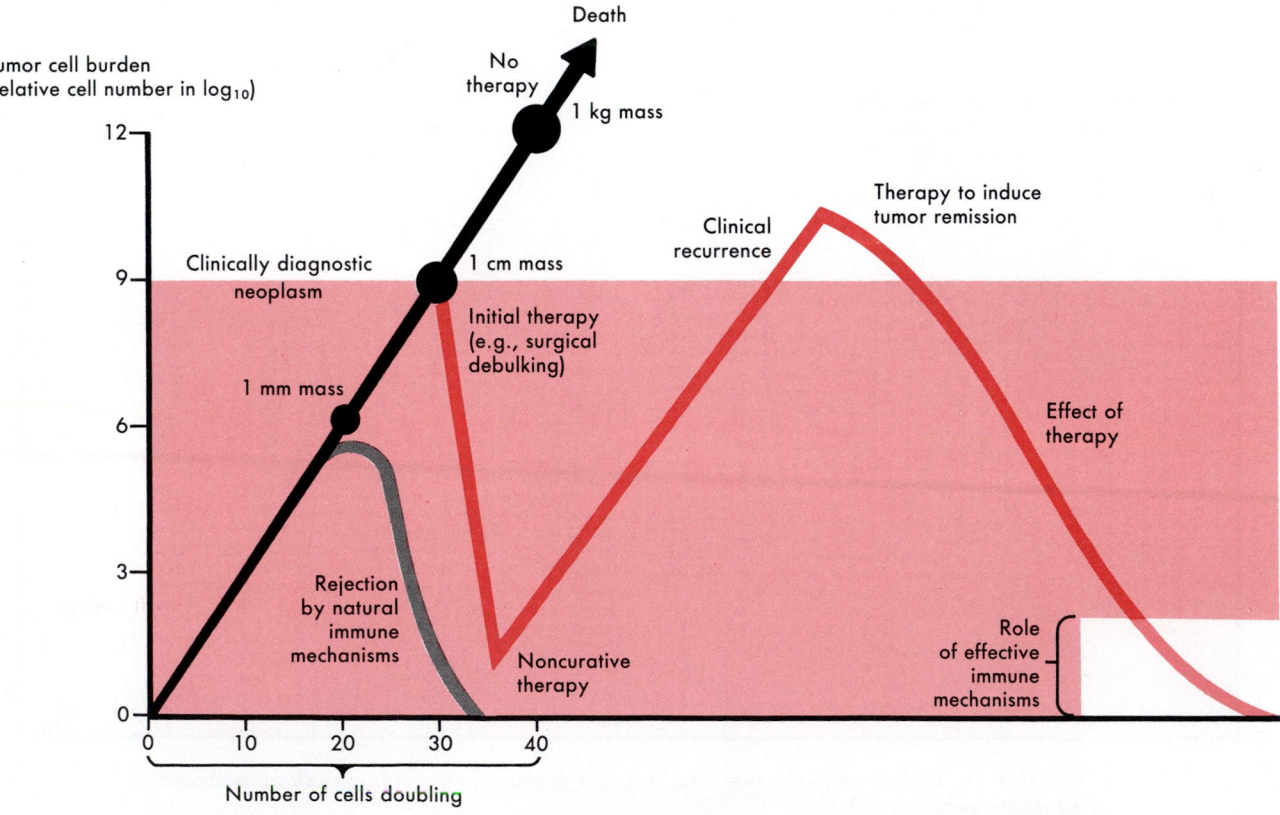

FIG. 10-10. Relationship between tumor cell burden and phases of cancer treatment. (Adapted from Bakemeier, 1978.)

TABLE 10-11 Childhood cancers by age

Site	Percentage of each tumor in three age groups		
	0-5 years	5-10 years	9-15 years
Leukemia	39.6*	35.7	22.1
Lymphoma	3.7	13.3	16.4*
Central nervous system	15.0	27.1*	18.9
Neuroblastoma	13.0*	2.2	0.5
Soft tissue sarcoma	3.7	3.5	6.0*
Wilms tumor	9.2*	6.1	2.0
Bone tumor	0.6	5.0	10.5*
Retinoblastoma	6.4*	1.3	0.0
Other	8.6	5.9	23.7
Total	100.0	100.0	100.0

*Peak incidence for tumor.

who have survived their first year. (Trauma remains the leading killer of children between 1 and 15 years of age.) The unique feature of childhood cancer is the short latent time, a sharp contrast to adult tumors, which usually involve a long latent period of time.

Types of Childhood Cancers

Both the incidence rates and the types of cancer that develop vary between children and adults (Table 10-11). For example, approximately 6,600 new childhood cancers were diagnosed in 1988, whereas approximately 979,000 adults were diagnosed with cancer during the same year (American Cancer Society, 1988). Children are more often affected by leukemias, sarcomas, and embryonic tumors. Embryonic tumors originate during intrauterine life. These tumors contain abnormal cells appearing to be immature embryonic tissue that is unable to mature or differentiate into fully developed functional cells. Embryonic tumors are diagnosed early in life (usually by 5 years of age) and therefore are very rare in adults. Embryonic tumors are often named with the term "blast," which refers to the immature nature of the cells.

Sarcomas and lymphoreticular cancers seen in childhood also occur in adults, but most adult cancers involve epithelial tissue (and are therefore, carcinomas). Carcinomas are almost nonexistent in children because these cancers are most commonly the result of environmental carcinogens and require a long period from exposure to the appearance of the carcinoma. Children have not lived long enough for carcinoma to develop.

By far the most common malignancy in children is leukemia, which accounts for more than one third of childhood cancers. The second most common group of cancers is tumors of the nervous system, primarily brain tumors. All other pediatric malignancies occur much less frequently. Neuroblastoma and Wilms tumor are both embryonic tumors. Neuroblastoma is a tumor of the sympathetic nervous system. Wilms tumor is a malignancy of the kidney (named after Max Wilms, who identified the tumor); the histologic name is nephroblastoma. Rhabdomyosarcoma is a soft-tissue sarcoma of striated muscle. Two major bone tumors also occur in children. These are osteosarcoma and Ewing sarcoma (named after James Ewing, who identified it).

Incidence Rates

Many childhood cancers have a peak incidence before the age of five. Among these are the leukemias and the embryonic tumors: neuroblastomas, Wilms tumor, and retinoblastoma. Central nervous system tumors are more common from ages 5 to 10 years, and bone tumors, soft-tissue sarcomas, and lymphomas are more likely to occur from 10 to 15 years of age.

Although incidence rates indicate only slight variations between white and black children, leukemia is more frequent in white children than in black children (American Cancer Society, 1988; Young & Miller, 1975). Some geographic differences are also found. These include increases in Burkitt's lymphoma in Nigeria, intestinal lymphomas in Israel, Hodgkin's disease in Colombia, and retinoblastoma in India. Childhood cancer is also slightly more common in males than females in the United States. The male to female ratio for childhood cancers is 1.2:1.0, respectively.

Etiology

As in adult cancer, the causes of cancer in childhood are largely unknown. Some environmental and host factors are known to predipose a child to cancer, but causal factors have not been established for most childhood cancers. A number of host factors, many of which are genetic risk factors or congenital conditions, have been implicated in the development of childhood cancer (Table 10-12).

Most childhood cancers do not, however, lend themselves to early cancer warning signs. Certainly the American Cancer Society's seven "Warning Signs of Cancer" do not apply because they describe adult, environmentally caused carcinomas. While host factors are important in identifying populations of children at risk for cancer, most children who are diagnosed with cancer do not demonstrate any predisposing environmental or host factors.

Genetic Factors

Genetic factors may involve chromosome aberrations or single-gene defects. Some congenital malformations

TABLE 10-12 Host factors associated with childhood cancer

Syndrome	Associated Risk Factors
Chromosome alterations	
Down syndrome	Acute leukemia
13q- syndrome	Retinoblastoma
Chromosome instability	
Ataxia-telangiectasia	Lymphoma
Bloom syndrome	Acute leukemia
Faconi anemia	Non-lymphocytic leukemia
Hereditary syndromes	
Beckwith-Wiedemann syndrome	Wilms tumor, sarcoma, brain tumors
Neurofibromatosis	Brain tumors, sarcomas, neuroblastoma, Wilms tumor, non-lymphocytic leukemia
Tuberous sclerosis	Brain tumors
Immune deficiency disorders	
Congenital:	
Agammoglobulinemia (Burton disease)	Lymphoma, leukemia, brain tumors
IgA deficiency	Lymphomas, leukemia, brain tumors
Wiskott- Aldrich syndrome	Leukemia, lymphoma
Acquired:	
Aplastic anemia	Leukemia
Organ transplantation	Leukemia, lymphoma
Congenital malformation syndromes	
Aniridia, hemihypertrophy, hamartoma, genitourinary anomalies	Wilms tumor
Cystorchidism	Testicular tumor
Gonadal dysgenesis	Gonadoblastoma
Family susceptibility	
Twin or sibling with leukemia	Leukemia

herald the onset of pediatric malignancies. For example, certain syndromes involve easily diagnosed abnormalities, and the children can then be carefully followed and screened for tumor development. One of the more recognized syndromes is the association of trisomy 21 (Down syndrome) with an increased susceptibility to acute leukemia. For children with Down syndrome, the risk of developing leukemia is ten to eighteen times greater during the first 10 years of life than the risk in healthy children (Miller, 1970). After a child reaches 10 years of age, the evidence shows no increase in susceptibility.

Wilms tumor (nephroblastoma) is particularly recognized for its association with a number of malformations, including genitourinary anomalies, for example horseshoe kidney, cryptorchidism (undescended testicles), and collecting system malformation; aniridia (congenital absence of the iris of the eye), and hemihypertrophy (muscular overgrowth of one half of the body or face). Approximately 15% of children diagnosed with

Wilms tumor demonstrate one of these congenital abnormalities. Retinoblastoma, a malignant embryonic tumor of the eye, occurs both as an inherited defect and as a mutation. In 2% of individuals with retinoblastoma, the defect involves the deletion of a specific portion of chromosome 13.

More than 150 single-gene defects have been associated with the subsequent development of both childhood and adult cancers (Mulvihill, 1975). For instance, two autosomal recessive diseases involving increased chromosome fragility, Faconi anemia and Bloom syndrome, are risk factors that evidently predispose the child to acute nonlymphocytic leukemia.

The relative ineffectiveness of the immune surveillance system during intrauterine life may be an explanation for embryonic tumors (the immune surveillance system is discussed in Chapter 11). Because this period requires rapid proliferation and differentiation of cells in the developing fetus, cell mutation theoretically could result in embryonic tumors.

Children with immunodeficiencies experience a striking 100-fold increased risk of subsequent cancer than healthy children (Lenarsky, 1983). These conditions may be either congenital, generally involving x-linked recessive inheritance, or acquired, generally caused by therapeutic immunosuppression after organ transplantation or treatment for aplastic anemia.

Although not determined to be genetically transmitted, a few malignancies seem to demonstrate a familial tendency, suggested by the clustering of specific cancers in a particular family. A child who has a sibling with leukemia has a risk for developing leukemia that is four times greater than for children with normal siblings (Strong, 1984). A strong association for subsequent leukemia is also apparent in children with monozygous twins who have leukemia. The degree of risk appears to be age related. If the twin with leukemia was diagnosed at less than 1 year of age, the probability is nearly 100%; if diagnosed between the ages of 1 and 4 years, the risk drops to 15%; after 4 years of age, the risk is equal to that of other siblings.

Environmental Factors

Although many adult cancers are associated with environmental agents, few childhood tumors share that association. Because of the lengthy latent time required between exposure and development of cancer, a child's exposure to carcinogens does not result in a tumor until the child is an adult.

Prenatal Exposure

Prenatal exposure to some drugs and to ionizing radiation have been linked to subsequent cancers. Perhaps the most well-known such drug is diethylstilbestrol (DES), a drug taken to avert early abortion. In 1971, DES was identified as a transplacental chemical carcinogen. A small percentage of the daughters of mothers who had taken DES while pregnant have developed adenocarcinoma of the vagina. Most of these cancers appeared when the daughters were between the ages of 14 and 23. Other potential transplacental carcinogens have been identified, but await further study before any conclusion can be drawn (Strong, 1984).

Intrauterine radiation by obstetric x-rays may increase risk of all childhood cancers. A British study reported a 1.4- to 1.5-fold increase in cancers in children who had experienced x-rays in utero (Bithell & Stewart, 1975). Studies of children who were in utero when their mothers were exposed to atomic fallout, however, showed no increase in childhood cancers (Jablon & Kato, 1970).

Childhood Exposure

Childhood exposures to drugs, ionizing radiation, and viruses have been implicated as risk factors that increase susceptibility to specific cancers. Besides those drug and environmental agents that are known to cause cancer in adults and therefore also are risks for exposure during childhood, a few drugs may particularly increase cancer risk during childhood. These drugs include (1) anabolic androgenic steroids, which are used in the treatment of aplastic anemia or used illegally by teenage athletes for body development and have been associated with subsequent hepatocellular carcinoma, (2) cytotoxic agents used in the treatment of pediatric cancers, which may predispose the child to leukemia in later years, and (3) immunosuppressive agents, particularly those used for transplant surgeries, which have been shown to increase the risk of reticulum cell sarcoma and lymphoma.

Although viruses have been implicated in childhood cancers, research has not yet been able to prove the association. Viruses have been shown to affect cancer development in some animal models, but causal evidence is only suggestive in humans. (The viral theory of carcinogenesis is discussed in Chapter 11.) In children, the strongest carcinogenic relationship has been shown between the Epstein-Barr virus (EBV) and Burkitt lymphoma. Most African children with Burkitt lymphoma have high titers or antibodies against EBV. Up to 50% of American children with Burkitt lymphoma do not, however, have elevated EBV titers (Hirschaut, Cohen, & Stevens, 1974). Therefore, although EBV can induce lymphocyte transformation in laboratory studies, evidence has not yet shown whether the relationship is causal. Investigators are examining the role of viruses in the development of neuroblastomas, Wilms tumor, and osteosarcoma.

Prognosis

Today, childhood cancer should not be considered an inevitably fatal illness. Significant progress has been made in the last 10 years, so that more than 50% of children diagnosed with cancer can now be expected to survive (American Cancer Society, 1988). Overall, children have a more favorable prognosis than adults (American Cancer Society, 1988). Children appear to be both more responsive to available treatments and better able to tolerate the therapies.

Because of the progress made in successful treatment of childhood cancers, health care providers are now grappling with a system to determine length of treatment needed and the point at which cure has been achieved. In adults, a general rule-of-thumb is a 5-year survival rate, although a number of cancers (for example, breast cancer) can recur well after the 5-year time frame. For children, a unique method has been suggested to determine when a cure has been achieved (Sutow, 1984). Because a pediatric cancer could not have been present any longer than the age of the child at diagnosis, plus 9 months of intrauterine life, it could be assumed that, if the cancer were to recur, it would grow to its size at the initial diagnosis in the same amount of time. This time period is called the **period of risk** (Sutow, 1984). This theory does not take into account alterations in the growth curves of tumors caused by the effect of treatment, but other cancer specialists have found the period of risk to be clinically accurate. A clinically practical 2-year period of therapy followed by two disease-free years has also been compared with the period of risk and found to be of equal value for predicting cure (Platt & Linden, 1964). This 2-year disease-free period is useful for older children diagnosed with cancer because a much shorter period of time is required to determine cure than with the period of risk.

Because childhood cancer should be viewed as a chronic disease instead of a fatal illness, the focus of treatment is on the quality of life. Even those cancers that cannot be cured can generally be treated, resulting in a significant period of quality time. But with increasing survival, the long-term effects of treatment are under careful investigation. More effective yet less toxic chemotherapy and radiation treatments must be found. Cured children still face residual and late effects of treatment. Potential effects needing further attention include physical impairments, reproductive dysfunction, soft tissue and bone atrophy, learning disabilities, secondary cancers, and psychological sequelae. More must be learned about the genetic factors associated with childhood malignancies and about the genetic consequences of treatment. Genetic counseling is appropriate for children cured of cancers known to be transmitted genetically (e.g., retinoblastoma).

SUMMARY REVIEW

Characteristics of Cancer Cells

1 Cancer cells are characterized by anaplasia, or loss of differentiation, and autonomy, or independence from normal cellular controls.
2 The degree of disorganization varies among tumors, but disordered nuclear and structural components of cells are common.
3 Loss of contact inhibition, the reduction in adhesiveness of the cell surface, is a factor in cancer development and possibly in cancer spread.
4 Nuclei of malignant cells are often enlarged, and have abnormal shapes, and various chromosomal changes; plasma membranes of cancer cells show altered surface characteristics.
5 Tumor cell markers are substances, such as hormones, enzymes, and antigens, that denote specific tumors.

Tumors

1 Benign tumors are noncancerous growths that do not metastasize; malignant tumors are cancerous growths that invade and destroy host tissue.
2 Tumors are classified on the basis of cell type, tissue of origin, whether benign or malignant, degree of differentiation, anatomic site, and function.
3 Carcinoma in situ is a cancerous tumor of glandular or squamous cell origin that has not broken through basement membranes of the squamous cells.
4 Tumor development is influenced by the site of the tumor and by the nutritional status, age, and other host factors.
5 Tumor growth differs from hyperplasia, although hyperplasia can stimulate the development of cancer.
6 A current controversy is whether cancer originates from a single cell that produces clones or from several cells proliferating together (i.e., clonal origin vs. field origin).
7 Tumor grading is an evaluation of the tumor's growth; tumors are graded according to structural features that reflect the degree of differentiation.
8 Tumor growth rates are influenced by vascular supply and tumor integrity; tumors grow faster once they have developed a vascular system and capillaries have reached the edges of the tumor.
9 Metastasis, the spread of cancer cells, is the life-threatening characteristic of malignancy.
10 Metastasis is a function of the tumor's rate of growth, its lack of cellular adhesion, and the absence of cellular barriers.
11 Routes of metastases include lymphatic, venous, and implantation into serous cavities.

Clinical Manifestations of Cancer

1 Clinical manifestations of cancer include pain, cachexia, anemia, leukopenia, thrombocytopenia, and infection.
2 Pain is generally associated with the late stages of cancer. It may be caused by pressure, obstruction, invasion of a structure sensitive to pain, stretching, tissue destruction, and inflammation.
3 Cachexia (loss of appetite, weakness, and inability to maintain weight) leads to protein-calorie malnutrition and progressive wasting.
4 Anemia associated with cancer usually occurs because of malnutrition, chronic bleeding and resulting iron deficiency, chemotherapy, and malignancies in the blood-forming organs.
5 Leukopenia is usually a result of chemotherapy, which is toxic to bone marrow, or radiation, which kills circulating leukocytes.
6 Thrombocytopenia is usually the result of chemotherapy or malignancy in the bone marrow.
7 Infection may be caused by leukopenia, immunosuppression, or debility associated with advanced disease.

Cancer Treatment

1 Cancer is treated with surgery, radiation therapy, chemotherapy, immunotherapy, and combinations of these modalities.
2 Regimens of chemotherapy are based on the vulnerability of tumor cells in various stages of the cell cycle, theoretically. The goal of chemotherapy is to eradicate enough tumor cells so that the body's natural defenses can eradicate remaining cells.
3 Ionizing radiation causes cell damage, so that the goal of radiation therapy is to damage the tumor without causing excessive toxicity or damage to undiseased structures.
4 Surgical therapy is used for nonmetastatic disease, for which cure is possible by removing the tumor, and as a palliative measure to alleviate symptoms.
5 Immunotherapy is appropriate for cancers than cannot be effectively managed by chemotherapy or radiation, usually because enough tumor cells are inactive and not vulnerable to these modalities.
6 Forms of immunotherapy known as biological response modifiers include immunomodulating agents, interferous antigens, effector cells, lymphokines, and monoclonal antibodies.
7 The use of effector cells and lymphokines is a form of cellular immunotherapy that involves the transfer of cytotoxic T cells (Tc cells) that are specific for tumor cell antigens.
8 The use of immunomodulating agents is the nonspecific stimulation of the immune system by means of an adjuvant; it is most effective in treating skin cancers.
9 The use of antigens causes regression in skin tumors by causing a hypersensitivity response that affects the antigenic properties of the cell surface.
10 Monoclonal antibodies might ultimately be used both as diagnostic reagents for detecting cancer and as a form of cancer therapy in which antibodies specific for tumor antigens would mediate tumor rejection.

Cancer in Children

1 Although childhood cancer is rare, it is still the second leading cause of death in children.
2 The unique feature of childhood cancers is the short period of lateny, which contrasts sharply with the long lateny period common in adults.
3 Common childhood cancers include leukemias, sarcomas, and embryonic tumors that contain immature fetal tissue that has not differentiated into fully developed cells.
4 Embryonic tumors are almost always diagnosed early and are very rare in adults.
5 Because most carcinomas are caused by environmental exposure, these cancers are extremely rare in children, who have not lived long enough to be affected.
6 Host factors are especially important in identifying a child at risk for cancer because environmental risk factors have had less effect on the short life of the child.
7 Genetic factors that place a child at risk for cancer include some congenital malformations that are chromosome aberrations or single-gene defects.
8 A familial tendency is evident for a few childhood cancers, including leukemia.
9 Environmental risk factors associated with childhood cancer include prenatal exposure to some drugs and to ionizing radiation and postnatal exposure to certain drugs (particularly anabolic steroids and some cytotoxic and immunosuppressive agents), to radiation, and possibly to certain viruses.
10 Considerable progress in the treatment and prognosis for childhood cancer now means that health care providers are identifying formulas, such as the period of risk, that define the point at which the child is cured.
11 Improved survival for children with cancer has led to investigations for less toxic treatments that minimize residual effects and for more research into the genetic factors associated with cancer in childhood.

KEY TERMS

Anaplasia, 295

Angiogenesis, 302

Autonomy, 295

Benign tumor, 294

Biological response modifiers, 310

Cachexia, 306

Carcinogenesis, 301

Carcinoma, 295

Carcinoma in situ, 295

Doubling time, 302

Glioma, 295

Grading, 301

Invasion, 302

Leukemia, 295

Lymphoma, 295

Malignant tumor, 294

Metastasis, 294

Neoplasm, 294

Period of risk, 320

Primary tumor, 303

Progression, 297

Staging, 301

Sarcoma, 295

Transformation, 297

Tumor cell marker, 298

REFERENCES

American Cancer Society. 1988. *Cancer facts & figures 1988.* New York: American Cancer Society.

Androphy, E. J., & Lowy, D. R. (1984). Tumor viruses, oncogenes, and human cancer. *Journal of the American Academy of Dermatologists, 10,* 125.

Bakemeier, R. F. (1978). Principles of medical oncology and cancer chemotherapy. In P Rubin (Ed.), *Clinical oncology for medical students and physicians: A multidisciplinary approach.* American Cancer Society, p. 43.

Bell, G. I. (1978). Models for the specific adhesions of cells to cells. *Science, 200*(4342), 618-627.

Berenblum, I., & Shubik, P. (1947). A new quantitative approach to the study of the stages of chemical carcinogenesis in the mouse's skin. *British Journal of Cancer, l,* 383-391.

Berlin, N. I. (1981). Tumor markers in cancer prevention and detection. *Cancer, 47,* 1151.

BIER Committee. (1980). *The effects on populations of exposure to low levels of ionizing radiation: 1980.* Washington, D.C.: National Academy Press.

Bithell, J., & Stewart, A. (1975). Pre-natal irradiation and childhood malignancy: A review of British data from the Oxford survey. *British Journal of Cancer, 31,* 271-287.

Burnet, M. (1970). *Immunological surveillance.* London: Pergamon Press.

Chen, T. S., & Chen, P. S. (1977). *Essential hepatology.* Woburn, MA: Butterworth.

del Regato, J., Spjut, H. J., & Cox, J. D. (1985). *Ackerman and del Regato's cancer: Diagnosis, treatment, and prognosis* (6th ed.). St. Louis: C.V. Mosby.

DeVita, Jr., V., Hellman, S., & Rosenberg, S. (1982). *Cancer principles and practice of oncology.* Philadelphia: J. B. Lippincott.

Doll, R., & Peto, R. (1981). Avoidable risks of cancer. *United States Journal for the National Cancer Institute, 66,* 1191-1308.

Donovan, M. I., & Girton, S. F. (1984). *Cancer care nursing* (2nd ed.). New York: Appleton-Century-Crofts.

Draper, G. (1980). Population studies of incidence, survival and follow-up. In J. Van Eys & M. Sullivan (Eds.), *Status of the curability of childhood cancers.* New York: Raven Press.

Ellerman V., & Bang, O. (1908). Experimentelle leukamie bie huhnern [Abstract]. *Vorlaufige mitteilung. centralbl. f bakerteriol.* 1 Abt. Jena, 1908; xlvi, orig. 4.

Epstein, S. (1978). *The politics of cancer.* San Francisco: Sierra.

Epstein, W. L. et al. (1971). Ultraviolet light, DNA repair and skin carcinogenesis in man. *Federal Proceedings, 30,* 1766-1771.

Ewing, J. (1940). *Neoplastic disease.* Philadelphia: Saunders.

Fisher, B., & Fisher, E. R. (1967). The barrier function of the lymph node to tumor cells and erythrocytes: I. Normal nodes. *Cancer, 20,* 1907.

Fitzpatrick, T., Eisen, A., Wolff, K., Freedburg, I., & Austen, K. F. (1979). *Dermatology in general medicine* (2nd ed.). New York: McGraw-Hill.

Foley, E. J. (1953). Antigenic properties of methylcholanthrene-induced tumors in mice of the strain of origin. *Cancer Research, 13,* 835.

Folkman, J. (1982). Tumor invasion and metastasis. In J. F. Holland & E. Frei (Eds.), *Cancer medicine* (2nd ed.). Philadelphia: Lea & Febiger.

Franks, L. M., & Teich, N. (1986). *Introduction to the cellular and molecular biology of cancer.* New York: Oxford University Press.

Gospodarowicz, D., Bailecki, H., & Thakral, T. K. (1979). The angiogenic activity of the fibroblast and epidermal growth factor. *Experimental Eye Research, 28,* 501-514.

Groer, M., & Shekleton, M. (1979). *Basic pathophysiology: A conceptual approach.* St. Louis: C.V. Mosby.

Gullino, P. M. (1981). Tissue growth factors. In R. Baserga (Ed.), *Handbook of experimental pharmacology.* Berlin: Springer-Verlag, pp. 427-449.

Hannewalt, P. C. (1975). Molecular mechanisms involved in DNA repair. *Genetics* (Supplement) *79,* 179-197.

HEW. (1979). *Report on the work group on exposure reduction. Interagency task force on the health effect of ionizing radiation.* Washington, DC: U.S. Department of Health and Human Services.

Hirschaut, Y., Cohen, N. M., & Stevens, D. A. (1974). Letter: Epstein-Barr virus and Burkitt and lymphoma. *Lancet, 1,* 742.

Hood, L. E., Weissman, I. L., & Wood, W. B. (1978). *Immunology.* Menlo Park, CA: Benjamin/Cummings.

Jablon, S., & Kato, H. (1970). Childhood cancer in relation to prenatal exposure to atomic bomb radiation. *Lancet, 2,* 1000-1003.

Jaffe, N. (1984). Late sequelae of cancer therapy. In W. Sutow, D. Fernbach, & T. Vietti (Eds.), *Clinical pediatric oncology.* St. Louis: C. V. Mosby.

Jordon, C. (1983). Hormones. In B. Kahn, R. Lone, C. Sherman, & R. Chakravarty (Eds.). *Concepts in cancer medicine.* New York: Grune & Stratton.

Kahn, S., Lone, R., Sherman, C., & Chakravorty, R. (Eds). (1983). *Concepts in clinical medicine.* New York: Grune & Stratton.

Karayalcin, G. (1983). Late effects of cancer treatment. In P. Lanzkowsky (Ed.), *Pediatric oncology.* New York: McGraw-Hill.

Kermett, R. H., McKearn, T. J., & Bechtol, K. B. (1980). *Monoclonal antibodies.* New York: Plenum.

King, D. W., Fenoglio, C. M., & Lefkowitch, J. H. (1983). *General pathophysiology: Principles and dynamics.* Philadelphia: Lea & Febiger.

Klein, G., Sjogren, H. O., Klein, E., & Hellstrom, K. E. (1960). Demonstration of resistance against methylcholanthrene-induced sarcomas in the primary autochthonous host. *Cancer Research, 20,* 1561.

Kohler, G., & Milstein, C. (1975). Conhuuais cultures of fused cells secreting antibody of pre-defined specificity. *Nature, 256,* 495.

Koocher, F., & O'Malley, J. (1981). *The damodes syndrome: Psychosocial consequences of surviving childhood cancer.* New York: McGraw-Hill.

Lacassagne, A. (1932). Appartition de cancers de la mamelle dez la souvis male soumis a des injections de folliculine. *Compt. rend. Acad. d. sc., 195,* 630-632.

Lenarsky, C. (1983). Etiology of childhood malignancy. In P.

Lanzkowsky (Ed.), *Pediatric oncology*. New York: McGraw-Hill.

Lokich, J. J. (1978). Tumor markers: Hormone antigen and enzyme in malignant disease. *Oncology, 35,* 54.

Magnus, I. A. (1976). *Dermatological photobiology: Clinical and experimental aspects*. Oxford: Blackwell.

McIntire, K. R. (1985). Tumor markers. In V. T. Devita, S. Hellman, & S. A. Rosenberg (Eds.), *Cancer: Principles and practice of oncology* (vol. 1, 2nd ed.). Philadelphia: J. B. Lippincott.

McKhann, C. (1981). *A guide for patients, family, and friends: The facts about cancer*. Englewood Cliffs, NJ: Prentice Hall.

Miller, R. (1970). Neoplasia and Down syndrome. *Annual New York Academy of Sciences, 171,* 637.

Moodie, R. L. (1923). *Paleopathology*. Urbana: University of Illinois Press.

Moosa, A. R., Robson, M. C., & Schimpff, S. C. (Eds.). (1986). *Comprehensive textbook of oncology*. Baltimore: Williams & Wilkins.

Mulvihill, J. (1975). Congenital and genetic diseases. In J. Fraumeni, Jr. (Ed.), *Persons at high risk of cancer: An approach to cancer etiology and control*. New York: Academic Press.

Oldham, R., & Smalley, R. (1985). Biologicals and biological response modifiers. In V. DeVita, S. Hellman, & S. Rosenberg (Eds.), *Cancer principles and practices of oncology*. Philadelphia: J. B. Lippincott, p. 2224.

Platt, B., & Linden, G. (1964). Wilms' tumor—A comparison of 2 criteria for survival. *Cancer, 17,* 1573-1578.

Porth, C. (1986). *Pathophysiology—Concepts of altered health states* (2nd ed.). Philadelphia: J. B. Lippincott Company.

Poste, G., & Fidler, I. J. (1980). The pathogenesis of cancer metastasis. *Nature, 20,* 139-145.

Pott, P. (Reprinted, 1981). Chirugical observations relative to the cataract, polyps of the nose, the cancer of the scrotum, the different kinds of rupture and the mortification of the toes and feet [London, 1775]. In R. Doll & R. Peto (Eds.), *Causes of cancer*. New York: Oxford University Press.

Prehn, R. T., & Main, J. M. (1957). Immunity to methylcholanthrene-induced sarcomas. *Journal of the National Cancer Institute, 18,* 769.

Roberts, L. K., & Daynes, R. A. (1985). Active immunoregulation toward antigens expressed by ultraviolet radiation-induced skin tumors. *Experimental and clinical photoimmunology* (vol. III). Boca Raton: CRC Press Inc.

Roentgen, W. C. (1896). On a new kind of rays. *Science*. New York & Lancaster, PA, 227-231.

Rous, P. (1911). Sarcoma of the fowl transmissable by an agent separable from tumor cells. *Journal of Experimental Medicine B, 397*.

Rubin, P., Bakemeier, R. F., & Krackov, S. K. (Eds.). (1984). *Clinical oncology for medical students and physicians: A multidisciplinary approach* (6th ed.). American Cancer Society.

Rudden, R. W. (Ed.). (1978). *Biological markers of neoplasia: Basic and applied aspects*. New York: Elsevier.

Rusch, H. P. (1983). History of research on cancer causation. In S. B. Kahn, R. R. Love, C. Sherman, & R. Chakravarty

(Eds.), *Concepts in Cancer Medicine*. New York: Grune & Stratton.

Seidel, H. M., Ball, M. W., Dains, J. E.,.MDSU/ & Benedict, G. W. (1987). *Mosby's guide to physical examination*. St. Louis: C. V. Mosby.

Shapiro, S. (Ed.). (1983). Epidemiology of ischemic heart disease and cancer in Mechanic, D. *Handbook of health, health care, and the health professions*. New York: The Free Press, Collier Macmillan Publishers.

Slamon, D. J., deKernion, J. B., Verma, I. M., & Cline, M. J. (1984). Expression of cellular oncogenes in human malignancies. *Science, 224,* 256.

Smith, L., & Thier, S. (1981). *Pathophysiology: The biological principles of disease*. Philadelphia: W. B. Saunders.

Smith, R. R., & Hilberg, A. W. (1955). Cancer-cell seeding of operative wounds. *Journal of the National Cancer Institute, 16,* 645-657.

Spjut, H. K., Hendrix, V. J., Ramirez, R. A., & Roper, C. L. (1958). Carcinoma cells in pleural cavity washings. *Cancer, 11,* 1222-1225.

Sporn, M. B., Roberts, A. B., & Driscoll, J. S. (1985). Principles of cancer biology: Growth factor and differentiation. In V. T. Devita, S. Hellman, & S. A. Rosenberg (Eds.), *Cancer: Principles and practice of oncology*. Philadelphia: J. B. Lippincott.

Strong, L. (1984). Genetics, etiology, and epidemiology of childhood cancer. In W. Sutow, D. Fernbach, & T. Vietti (Eds.), *Clinical pediatric oncology* (3rd ed.). St. Louis: C. V. Mosby.

Sutherland, B. M. (1974). Photoreactivating enzyme from human leukocytes. *Nature, 248,* 109-112.

Sutow, W. (1984). General aspects of childhood cancer. In W. Sutow, D. Fernbach, & T. Vietti (Eds.), *Clinical pediatric oncology*. St. Louis: C.V. Mosby.

Taylor, S., & Folkman, J. (1982). Protamine in an inhibitor of angiogenesis. *Nature, 297,* 307.

U.S. Public Health Service. (1981). *The health consequences of smoking: The changing cigarette. A report of the surgeon general of the public health service*. Washington, DC: U.S. Government Printing Office.

Uhr, J. W. (1984). Immunotoxins: Harnessing nature's poisons. *Journal of Immunology, 133,* i.

Urback, F. (Ed.). (1964). *National cancer institute monograph, No. 10*. Washington, DC: U.S. Government Printing Office.

Van Eys, J., & Sullivan, M. (Eds.). (1980). *Status of curability of childhood cancers*. New York: Raven Press.

Warren, S. (1931). Chondrosarcoma with intravascular growth and tumor emboli to the lungs. *American Journal of Pathology, 7,* 161-168.

Watson, J. et al. (1987). *Molecular biology of the gene* (4th ed., vol. 1). Menlo Park: W. A. Benjamin, Inc.

Weber, G. (1977). Enzymology of cancer. *New England Journal of Medicine, 296,* 486.

Young, J., Jr., & Miller, R. (1975). Incidence of malignant tumors in U.S. children. *Journal of Pediatrics, 86,* 54.

CHAPTER 11

Theories of Carcinogenesis

Kathryn L. McCance
Lee K. Roberts

The multistage theory: initiation and promotion, 324
   Environmental risk factors, 325
      Personal behaviors, 326
         Tobacco use, 326
         Diet, 326
         Alcohol, 329
         Sexual and reproductive behavior, 329
      Air pollution, 329
      Occupation, 330
      Ultraviolet radiation, 330
         Ionizing radiation, 331
         Carcinogenesis, 332
      Hormones, 332
      Estrogens, 333
      Progesterone and androgens, 333
Carcinogenic pathogens, 333
   Oncogenic viruses, 333
      Classification of oncogenic viruses, 333
         Oncogenic DNA viruses, 334
         Oncogenic RNA viruses, 334
         Oncogenes, 335
      Mechanisms of viral carcinogenesis, 337
         Direct mechanisms, 337
         Indirect mechanisms, 337
Immunobiology of cancer, 337
   The immune surveillance theory, 337
      Tumor antigens, 337
         Viral antigens, 338
         Oncofetal antigens, 339
      Immunologic defense against tumors, 339
         Immune mechanisms for defense against cancer, 340
         Immune surveillance escape mechanisms, 342

Many cancers can be avoided. Of the one out of four Americans afflicted with cancer, half can be cured; consensus among most cancer experts is that many cancers can be prevented. Knowing the mechanisms that lead to cancer should ultimately make prevention and cure possible for most cancers. Two general theories of carcinogenesis are the multistage theory, which defines initiation and promotion as the process by which cells are transformed, and the viral theory, which defines cancer as a disease caused by a pathogenic agent. However, whether cancer results from a multistage or infectious process, carcinogenesis can be influenced by the host's immune response.

Precise pathophysiologic mechanisms are still under investigation. What is known, however, is that most cancers are influenced or caused by environmental factors—some natural, others synthetic—that directly interact with genes.

THE MULTISTAGE THEORY: INITIATION AND PROMOTION

In 1941 Rous and Kidd hypothesized a two-stage mechanism for the development of cancer: an initiation stage followed by a promotion stage by another agent (Rous & Kidd, 1941) (Fig. 11-1). In the late 1940s, Berenblum and Shubik devised a series of experiments that demonstrated the two-stage mechanism for skin cancer (Fig. 11-2). The initiating agent was methylcholanthrene and the promoting agent was croton oil. Neither agent alone would cause carcinogenesis (i.e., the process required both agents). When two such agents promote carcinogenesis, they are called **cocarcinogens.**

Initiation or DNA damage (mutation) is the development of cancer after exposure to the carcinogen; it is an irreversible step. However, the initiated cell may not be considered cancerous until a promoting agent acts on these cells to produce an altered, autonomous phenotype. **Promotion** appears to involve cell proliferation and tumor development, thus accelerating the process by which the initiated cells become cancerous. Initiation and promotion mechanisms have not been experimentally shown for all cancers, but the process is most useful when applied to chemical agents, such as benzo[*a*]pyrene found in coal tar or cigarette smoke. Other carcin

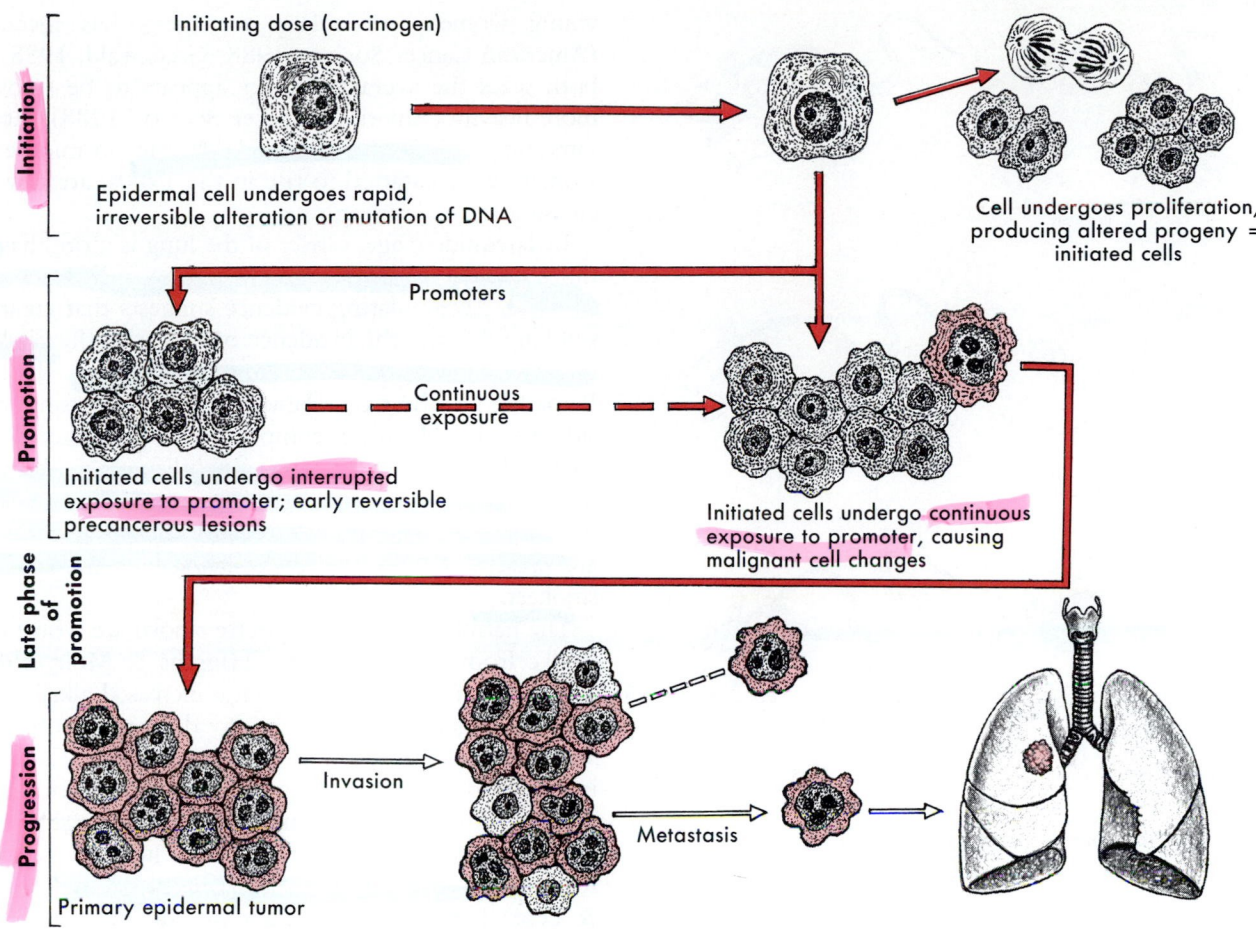

FIG. 11-1. Tumor development according to the multistage theory: initiation, promotion, progression.

ogens are part of the physical environment (e.g., ionizing and nonionizing radiation) or are biologic agents (e.g., viruses or hormones).

Initiators cause alterations in the DNA. The DNA changes can include one or more complete interruptions of the DNA chain, errors in DNA repair, or an elimination of a base pair (pyrimidine or purine) or sugar. (Normal DNA replication is discussed in Chapter 4.) Promoters may affect cell proliferation by altering cell-to-cell communication or by the production of oxygen radicals (Ames, Magaw, & Gold, 1987). Promoters include hormones, drugs, chemicals, plant products, and other environmental factors. These factors induce cells to divide in an initiated tissue (Franks & Teich, 1986). Several agents will induce cell division, but only promoters will induce tumor development. It is suggested that promoting agents may interfere with the process of differentiation, usually after division has occurred (Franks & Teich, 1986). In the early stages of epidermal carcinogenesis the biologic effects of promotion are reversible and are modulated by diet, hormones, and re-

lated factors. Table 11-1 compares initiation and promotion substances.

Boutwell (1964) suggested that progression of a tumor may be a late phase of promotion. (Tumor transformation and progression is discussed in Chapter 10.) The biologic difference between promotion and progression is unknown, but progression is thought to depend on structural changes in the chromosome and, contrarily, promotion may not cause chromosome abnormalities.

Environmental Risk Factors

Because the exact biochemical cause of cancer is unknown, the traditional emphasis (as part of the initiation-promotion theory) is on those factors with suggested pathogenic mechanisms that increase the incidence of different cancerous tumors. (Methods of risk factor analysis are discussed in Chapter 5.)

Table 11-2 summarizes the estimated new cases and deaths by sex for specified sites. Although population trends in incidence rates of cancer are the focus of epi-

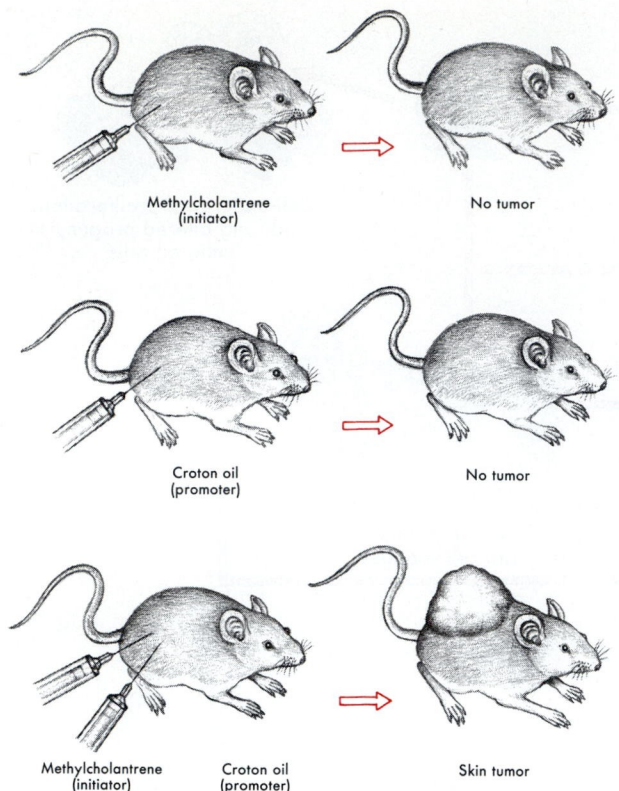

Methylcholantrene
(initiator)

No tumor

Croton oil
(promoter)

No tumor

Methylcholantrene   Croton oil
(initiator)   (promoter)

Skin tumor

FIG. 11-2. Procedure demonstrating initiation and promotion of tumors.

demiologists, laboratory scientists are occupied with experimental approaches to determine the effect and nature of environmental factors as initiators or promoters of carcinogenesis. Laboratory scientists must demonstrate that altered DNA changes occur in response to variable doses of particular agents, a difficult task at best. Thus the relationship between life-style and carcinogenesis is being explored and evaluated from two divergent but equally important approaches: epidemiologic and experimental. Each approach has strengths and weaknesses, and each requires cautionary interpretations. However, these two perspectives do indicate some agreement about particular agents or conditions that either cause cancer or are associated with an increase in cancer incidence rates.

Personal Behaviors

Tobacco Use

Both epidemiologic and experimental data support the conclusion that cigarette smoke is carcinogenic. Between 1920 and 1955, cigarette consumption in the United States increased fourfold for all persons 14 years of age or older. From 1976 to 1985, men smokers (20 years and older) dropped from 42% of the population to 32%, and women smokers decreased from 32% to 28%; however, the amount of cigarettes smoked by young women, particularly teenagers, has increased (American Cancer Society, 1988; Greenwald, 1985). In both sexes the average smoker appears to be smoking more heavily (American Cancer Society, 1988). At the same time, respiratory cancer death rates in middle-age women, which started to rise in the 1960s, are now increasing at an alarming rate.

By late middle age, cancer of the lung is more than 10 times greater in cigarette smokers than in lifelong nonsmokers. Accumulating evidence suggests that cigarette smoking doubles the incidence of cancer of the bladder, pancreas, and to a lesser extent, the kidney (Doll & Peto, 1981). These correlations are not surprising, considering the chemical composition of smoke. These chemicals possess mutagenic capabilities, are absorbed from the lungs into the blood, through their distribution by the circulation gain access to distant organs, and are present in increased concentration in the urine of smokers.

The harmful effects of cigarette smoke are worse than smoke from pipes or cigars (Higgins & Muir, 1982). This difference may be due to the increased alkalinity of pipe and cigar smoke, which may decrease nicotine absorption rates in the blood. Alkaline smoke is also more irritating than cigarette smoke and is therefore less readily inhaled into the lungs. The greatest risk among the numerous causes of cancer of the lung thus appears to be related to the inhalation of tobacco smoke (Doll & Peto, 1981). Low-tar cigarettes do not reduce the risk of lung cancer (American Cancer Society, 1988).

There are hazards for nonsmokers who breathe the smoke of other's cigarettes (American Cancer Society, 1988). A recent study conducted by the American Cancer Society (1988) found an increased risk of lung cancer among nonsmoking wives of cigarette smokers. However, not all studies have found this effect, promoting more investigations in this area.

There has been a recent resurgence in the use of forms of smokeless tobacco—plug, leaf, and snuff. "Dipping snuff" has caused the greatest concern, where a coarse, moist powder is placed between the cheek and gum, and nicotine and other carcinogens are directly absorbed through the oral tissue. Oral cancer occurs more frequently among snuff dippers compared with nontobacco users (American Cancer Society, 1988).

Diet

Perhaps no other area of cancer investigation has proven more difficult than identifying the carcinogenic nature of dietary practices. Reliable information is scarce, particularly about the cancer-causing effects of substances occurring naturally in food or produced during the processes of food storage, cooking, and digestion. Some dietary factors may have anticancer properties (Franks & Teich, 1986; Palmer & Bakshi, 1986).

TABLE 11-1 Initiation and promotion substances

Initiators	Promoters
Single exposure to alter cell	Contact after initiator and requires prolonged exposure
Irreversible process	Reversible during early stage
Metabolically converted to reactants that bind covalently to DNA	Neither metabolic conversion nor covalent binding necessary
High doses carcinogenic	Only weakly carcinogenic without prior treatment of initiator

Adapted from Weinstein, 1976; King, Fenoglio, & Lefkowitch, 1983.

TABLE 11-2 Estimated new cancer cases and deaths by sex for specified sites, 1989

Types of cancer	Estimated new cases			Estimated deaths		
	Total	Female	Male	Total	Female	Male
Oral	30,600	10,000	20,600	8,650	2,875	5,775
Esophagus	10,100	2,900	7,200	9,400	2,500	6,900
Stomach	20,000	8,100	11,900	13,900	5,700	8,200
Pancreas	27,000	14,000	13,000	25,000	12,500	12,500
Colon (large intestine)	107,000	57,000	50,000	53,500	27,500	26,000
Rectum	44,000	21,000	23,000	7,800	3,800	4,000
Lung	155,000	54,000	101,000	142,000	49,000	93,000
Bone	2,100	900	1,200	1,300	600	700
Skin	27,000*	12,500*	14,500*	8,200†	3,000	5,200
Breast	142,900‡	142,000‡	900‡	43,300	43,000	300
Cervix	13,000‡	13,000‡	—	7,000	7,000	—
Corpus, endometrium	34,000	34,000	—	3,000	3,000	—
Ovary	20,000	20,000	—	12,000	12,000	—
Prostate	103,000	—	103,000	28,500	—	28,500
Testis	5,700	—	5,700	350	—	350
Bladder	47,100	12,600	34,500	10,200	3,300	6,900
Brain and central nervous system	15,000	6,800	8,200	11,000	5,000	6,000
Thyroid	11,300	8,300	3,000	1,025	650	375
Leukemias	27,300	12,100	15,200	18,100	8,300	9,800
Hodgkin's disease	7,400	3,200	4,200	1,500	600	900
ALL SITES TOTAL:	1,010,000	505,000	505,000	502,000	236,000	266,000

*Melanoma only.
†Melanoma, 6,000; other skin cancers, 2,200
‡Invasive only.
From American Cancer Society, (1989).

For example, vitamin A and its esters and analogs (retinoids) can block tumor promotion in animals and cancerous transformation in tissue cultures (Bjelke, 1975; Lasnitzki, 1955). Similarly, low levels of serum vitamin A have been reported in the serum of people with cancer.

Diet seems also to function over time to place an individual at risk for cancer (Doll & Peto, 1981; Franks & Teich, 1986; Palmer & Bakshi, 1986; Yang, 1980). Studies have found a consistent relationship between increasing weight in women and the risk of cancer, although this has not been the case for men. Obesity is a consistent risk factor for endometrial cancer, possibly because "overnutrition" causes the excessive exposure to estrogen. After menopause, the only natural estrogens produced are those from adipose tissue, so that more adipose tissue causes more estrogen exposure. High consumption of dietary fat in women has also been linked to endometrial, breast, and colon cancer (Carroll, 1975; Gold, 1984; Hulka et al., 1980). However, recent evidence has suggested that a moderate reduction in fat intake by adult women is unlikely to result in a substantial decrease in the incidence of breast cancer (Willett et al., 1987a) (see Chapter 20).

Much controversy concerns the need to limit the amount of preservatives added to foods. Food preservation is needed because food is grown in one part of the world and eaten in another, sometimes months or even years later. Advocates argue that preservatives allow people more dietary freedom and actually may encourage "better" diets. However, consumers may ingest chemicals unknowingly, unnecessarily, and without judicious knowledge for making responsible choices. Most noteworthy among the preservatives and artificial additives under study are saccharin and nitrites.

Facts concerning saccharin are the following:

- Saccharin has been shown to cause bladder cancer in rats, more clearly in males than females, after very large quantities have been consumed.
- Cancer has not occurred in other organs or in other animals under the same conditions.
- The mechanism of action is unclear and obscure.
- Thus far, studies with humans have failed to show a relationship between cancer and saccharin intake.

Nitrites are used as preservatives in fish and meat and may concentrate in the soil and water of some regions. The reaction of nitrites to other nitro compounds causes cancer of the glandular stomach in animals. Potentially harmful nitrite reactions can occur when foods are cooked. For example, nitrite-cured bacon, when cooked, yields nitrous acid that then reacts with amines (derivative of ammonia present in many foods) in the meat to form dimethylnitrosamine (DMN). This reaction is favored at an acidic pH and therefore occurs when nitrites and secondary amines are ingested and encounter the acidic gastric juice. Dietary salts also seem to enhance this reaction. By decreasing the formation of carcinogenic nitrosamines, vitamins C and E (in lettuce and salad greens) exert a protective effect when ingested at the same time as salt and nitrites (American Cancer Society, 1986). The inhabitants of countries with high rates of gastric cancer (Japan, for example) ingest large quantities of nitrites in staple foods such as mackerel.

Three primary mechanisms whereby dietary factors may affect cancer production are suggested (Doll & Peto, 1981). These are (1) direct-acting carcinogens or their precursors, (2) indirect-acting carcinogens (those that affect the formation of body carcinogens), and (3) dietary factors that affect transport, activation, and deactivation of carcinogens.

Direct-acting carcinogens include dietary substances in natural foodstuffs, carcinogens produced by cooking, and carcinogens produced by microorganisms in stored foods. The thorough search for naturally occurring carcinogenic food substances is incomplete, especially for humans. Compounds, such as hydrazines found in some mushrooms, aflatoxin produced by some food-related fungi, and other substances are known to cause cancer in experimental animals. Aflatoxin is also likely to be carcinogenic for humans because human liver cells contain the enzymes needed to activate the agent metabolically. High intake in the tropics is associated with a high rate of liver cancer, at least among those chronically affected with the hepatitis B virus (Ames et al., 1987). Aflatoxin is found in contaminated peanuts and other staple carbohydrate foods stored in hot and humid climates. This association raises the possibility that other toxins in food may be carcinogenic.

Some carcinogens may be produced by cooking (Spingarn, Slocum, & Weisburger, 1980). Benzo[*a*]pyrene and other polycyclic hydrocarbons are produced when meat or fish is excessively smoked or broiled or when fat is used repeatedly to fry food. However, food must be nearly charred or cooked at very high temperatures to produce these potentially harmful substances.

Indirect-acting carcinogens provide necessary compounds for the formation of carcinogens in the body (e.g., the production of N-nitrosamine compounds). Animal studies have shown these compounds to be powerful carcinogenic agents; their carcinogenic effects in humans have not been verified, although they have been suggested (Palmer & Bakshi, 1986). Nitrosable compounds can occur naturally in many foods such as fish and meat; they may be ingested as pesticide residues or drugs; and they may be formed in the colon from amino acids.

Certain ingested fats might contribute to the production of carcinogens in the body by increasing the amount of bile acids and cholesterol metabolites in the feces. These metabolites, which include deoxycholic and lithocholic acids, are found in greater quantities in populations that ingest a typical Western fatty diet and in whom colorectal cancer is common.

The most significant dietary factor affecting transport is fiber. Much work has been done to characterize the various components of dietary fiber. (Fiber refers to the remnants of the cell wall not hydrolyzed by human digestive enzymes.) Burkitt (1969) observed that the incidence of colon cancer is lower in countries (particularly Africa and India) where dietary consumption is high in fiber. However, research results are very inconsistent regarding the role of fiber and carcinogenesis. Different fiber components are both reported as inhibiting and promoting carcinogenesis (American Cancer Society, 1986; Palmer & Bakshi, 1986).

For many carcinogens, certain intermediate steps must happen before they can cause cellular damage. Some carcinogens must be oxidized, yielding metabolically activated intermediates. These activated metabolites are generated from the mechanisms of oxidation and peroxidation and include the short-lived intermediates, the oxidative free radicals (free radical OH^- and the superoxide radical O_2) (see Chapter 2). The destruction of toxic peroxides or radicals depends on selenium-containing enzymes. Levels of selenium have been found to be lower in individuals with cancer than individuals without cancer (Shamberger, Tytko, & Willis, 1976). High selenium areas in the United States (Western plains regions) have the lowest colon cancer rates (Blott & Fraumeni, 1982).

Alcohol

Incidence rates for cancer of the mouth, pharynx, larynx, and esophagus are higher in individuals who ingest large quantities of both alcohol and smoke (American Cancer Society, 1986, 1989; Pitot, 1985). (These cancers are discussed further in Chapter 36.) Alcohol interacts with smoke, increasing the risk of malignant tumors, possibly by acting as a solvent for the carcinogenic smoke products. No experimental evidence currently indicates that alcohol per se is carcinogenic, yet recent investigations have concluded that a higher risk of breast cancer is associated with even moderate drinking (about three drinks a week) (Schatzkin et al., 1987; Willett et al., 1987b). These studies are considered important because they involved large numbers of women. The mechanisms for increasing the incidence of breast cancer caused by alcohol are unknown; however, suggestions include the liver's inability to rid the body of carcinogens, impairment of the immune system, or increasing the susceptibility of breast tissue to cancer. (Breast cancer is discussed further in Chapter 20.) The relationship between cancer risk and alcohol consumption is difficult to determine because of problems in accurately measuring the amount of alcohol ingested and

in defining other behavioral habits, such as smoking, that further complicate or confound the clinical picture.

Sexual and Reproductive Behavior

The risk of developing cervical cancer is related to the age of first sexual intercourse and to the number of sexual partners (American Cancer Society, 1989). Women who have had one sexual partner are also at risk if that partner has had previous multiple partners. The possible mechanism may be a virus transmitted between partners. A number of viruses have been implicated including herpes simplex virus type 2 (HSV-2) and human papillomavirus (HPV) (Brinton, 1984; Ostrow et al., 1986).

HSV-2 has not been shown to be a causative agent, but antibodies to the virus increase with the severity of cervical dysplasia, and invasive carcinoma is associated with higher antibody titers. The exact relationship between HSV-2 and cancer is questionable because a certain segment of the female population with normal cervical tissue has antibodies to HSV-2.

HPV has been identified as the pathogen present in condyloma acuminata (genital warts) thought to be a precursor of squamous cell carcinoma of the genital tract (Micha, 1984; Ostrow et al., 1986). The risk factors associated with the disorder include sexually active young women, multiple sexual partners, and a sexual partner with multiple partners. The most common cause of abnormal Papanicolaou smears is the HPV virus, followed by cervical dysplasia (Micha, 1984).

The incidence of invasive cervical cancer is two and one-half times greater in black women than white women in the United States (American Cancer Society, 1989). Cervical malignancy is also found more often in women from lower socioeconomic groups (Devesa & Diamond, 1980). Cancers of the breast, ovary, and cervix account for 13% of all cancers and 29% of all female cancer deaths in the United States. (These cancers are discussed further in Chapter 20.)

Pregnancy and childbearing seem to be protective factors against cancers of the endometrium, ovary, and breast. Other factors related to a decreased risk of breast cancer are the onset of menstruation at a later age (especially with undernutrition) and early menopause. An important but not-understood risk factor for breast cancer is the age of first pregnancy (see Chapter 20). The younger the age at first pregnancy, the less the risk for breast cancer development.

Air Pollution

A person inhales about 20,000 L of air in 1 day; thus even modest contamination of the atmosphere can result in inhalation of appreciable doses of pollutants (Ames et al., 1987). Concerns have recently focused on industrial emissions including arsenicals, benzene, chloroform, vinyl chloride, and acrylonitrile. Proximity of residence to certain industries is a recognized cancer risk factor (Epstein & Swartz, 1988). It is difficult, however, to determine cancer risk from outdoor pollution because investigators must accurately control for smoking and radon. One team of investigators estimate that one must breathe Los Angeles smog for 1 year to inhale the same amount of burnt material that a two-pack-per-day smoker inhales in 1 day (Ames, 1983). Other studies that controlled or stratified for smoking demonstrate associations between excess lung cancer rates and heavy metal and aromatic hydrocarbon emissions (Epstein & Swartz, 1981).

Indoor pollution is generally considered worse than outdoor pollution, partly because of cigarette smoke (Ames et al., 1987). Another significant indoor air pollutant may be radon gas. Radon is a natural radioactive gas that is present in soil, trapped in houses, and gives rise to radioactive decay products that are known to be carcinogenic to humans (Ames et al., 1987). Estimated cases of lung cancer attributed to radon pollution in houses is 10% (Ames et al., 1987). The most hazardous houses can be identified and modified to prevent radon contamination.

Occupation

One way of providing useful information (amid an avalanche of information) about occupational practices and exposures to subsequent cancer risk is to identify cancers associated with occupational hazards. Table 11-3 identifies occupational hazards causally associated with cancers in humans.

A substantial percentage of cancers of the upper respiratory passages, lung, bladder, and peritoneum are attributed to occupational factors. One notable occupational factor is asbestos, which may cause as much as 5% of all lung cancers (Doll & Peto, 1981). Carcinoma of the bladder has been linked with the manufacture of dyes, rubber, paint, and aromatic amines, especially β-naphthylamine and benzidine. Benzol inhalation is linked to leukemia in shoemakers and in workers in the rubber cement, explosives, and dyeing industries.

Ultraviolet Radiation

Ultraviolet (UV) sunlight or solar radiation *causes* basal cell carcinoma and squamous cell carcinoma, two common skin cancers found in white individuals. Basal cell carcinoma is commonly located on the head and neck. Individuals with these tumors generally have light

---

TABLE 11-3 Occupational exposures and cancer

Cancer sites (causal agent)	Work or exposure
Lung	
Bischloro- methylether	Ion exchange resins producers
Chromium	Ore and pigment manufacturers
Mustard gas	Poison gas producers
Lung, pleura (asbestos)	Asbestos, miners, insulation, shipyard workers
Lung and skin (arsenic)	Smelter and pesticide workers
Lung and nasal (nickel)	Nickel refiners
Lung and skin (polycyclic hydrocarbons)	Mineral oil and tar workers
Skin (UV light)	Outdoor workers, fishermen
Liver	
Vinyl chloride	Vinyl chloride workers
Alcohol	Brewery workers
Bladder	
Aromatic amines	Dye and rubber workers
Leukemia	
Benzene	Glue and varnish workers
Nasal	
Isopropyl alcohol manufacturers	Isopropyl alcohol
Wood dusts	Furniture workers
Multiple sites	
Ionizing radiation	Radium dial painters, uranium miners

Adapted from American Cancer Society, 1986.

CLINICAL COMMENTARY
Sources of Radiation

Medical and dental procedures in which radiation is used for treatment and diagnosis account for the largest source of *deliberately* generated radiation in North America. It is estimated that more than 300,000 x-ray units (excluding portable units) are used by medical personnel for diagnosis and therapy. Of the total average annual dose of ionizing radiation, half is attributable to medical use.

The units of radiation dose and exposure include roentgen, rad, gray, and rem. Roentgen (R) is a measure of exposure that defines the intensity of a radiation beam or field. Exposure of 1 g of soft tissue or water to 1 R of x-ray results in a dose of around 1 rad, or 100 ergs of energy absorbed per gram of tissue. A millirad corresponds to absorption of 0.1 erg/g. The rem (rad-equivalent-mammal) is a unit accounting for differences in the relative biologic effectiveness of different types of ionizing radiation (1 rem = 1 rad times a correction factor to equalize biologic effects).

Large particle radiations (alpha rays and accelerated protons) are described as high-linear-energy-transfer (LET) radiations, whereas x-rays and gamma rays (electromagnetic radiations) are low-LET radiations. The biologic effects (e.g., a chromosome break) depend on the LET. More cellular damage occurs with high-LET than with low-LET radiation. Of major concern to the general public, however, is the effect of low-LET radiation to which individuals are repeatedly exposed by common x-ray procedures. At present, the specific carcinogenic effects that are produced by low-LET radiation are unclear.

The major overall source of radiation exposure to humans is from natural sources in the environment. These sources come from extraterrestrial or cosmic radiation and terrestrial radiation from radionuclides in the earth. Cosmic radiation (whole-body) exposure, originating from the sun and stars, produces its effects because of the energetic particles that strike the earth. The atmosphere serves as a shield against cosmic radiation—the thinner the shield, the greater the dose-equivalent (DE) rate. Therefore the cosmic radiation DE rate increases with altitude. The earth's magnetic field also modulates the exposure of cosmic rays. The average DE rate per person in North America is 28 mrem per year. Travel in airplanes slightly increases cosmic ray exposure.

Terrestrial radiation exposure varies with the concentration of radionuclides in the soil. People living in areas where foods are grown in soil with extensive deposits of uranium, thorium, or phosphates containing uranium will receive higher radiation doses. Foods grown in areas with high radioactivity will also have increased concentrations of incorporated radionuclides.

The deposition of naturally occurring radionuclides in the human body results from inhalation and ingestion of these substances in air, food, and water. Lung cancer in miners has recently been linked to the inhalation of radon gas in the air of mines. Luminescent instrument dial painters who ingest paint that contains radium and mesothorium (by licking the paint brush to prepare the dials) have an increased incidence of osteogenic sarcomas. Radionuclides that are soluble salts, like radium and strontium, tend to invade bone, such as potassium or iodine, penetrate soft-tissue organs like the thyroid, and can cause cancer. Accidental injection is another mechanism for radionuclides or isotope exposure in an industrial setting.

Carcinogenic effects are associated with the half-lives of different nucleotides. Longer half-lives are associated with longer exposure to radiation and therefore cause greater cellular damage.

---

complexions, light eyes, and fair hair, and they live in areas of high sunlight exposure. In general, these cancers arise on areas of the body that receive the greatest sun exposure, although they are not necessarily always restricted to these cancer sites. Squamous cell carcinoma is found more commonly in men who work outdoors. These tumors are distributed over the head, neck, and exposed areas of the upper extremities (see Chapter 41).

The incidence of melanoma, a malignant pigmented mole, *correlates* with the amount of exposure to UV light. However, although the nonmelanoma skin cancers are related to cumulative exposure to UV radiation, melanoma is related to heavy, blistering overdoses at a young age (American Cancer Society, 1989; Scotto, Fears, & Gori, 1976). The relatively recent worldwide increase in melanoma among white-skinned people is largely attributed to changes in clothing that promote greater exposure. The body areas receiving greater sun exposure vary between the sexes because of clothing differences. Malignant melanomas occur on the upper back and the dorsum of the hands of both sexes and the legs of females.

Xeroderma pigmentosum is a rare autosomal disease characterized by pigmentation abnormalities and malignancies. Persons with this disease demonstrate excessive skin damage caused by sun exposure at very young ages.

Ionizing Radiation

Much knowledge of the effects of radiation and human cancer have stemmed from observations of the Hiroshima and Nagasaki atomic bomb exposures. These unfortunate exposures caused acute leukemias in adults and children and increased frequencies of thyroid and breast carcinomas. Lung, stomach, colon, esophageal, and urinary tract cancers, and multiple myeloma have lately been added to the list. At Nagasaki and Hiroshima, leukemia incidence in individuals 15 years or younger reached its peak 6 to 7 years after the explosions and has steadily declined since 1952. Middle-aged people, 45 years and older at the time of exposure, had a latent period of 20 years before developing acute leukemia. Children conceived after the exposure of their parents to the atomic bombs have surprisingly suffered no increase in any cancer thus far. Human exposure to ionizing radiation includes emissions from x-rays, radioisotopes, and other radioactive sources.

Carcinogenesis. An important effect of ionizing radiation is thought to be inhibition of cell division. Cells of lymphoid tissue, bone marrow, and intestinal epithelium are normally short-lived, rapidly dividing cells. Symptoms and causes of death from exposure to large doses of whole-body radiation are related to the inability of these cells to divide. For example, the suppression of stem cell (primitive precursor cells) division in bone marrow can cause the disappearance of granulocytes and cause the remaining stem cells, if there are any, to repopulate the tissues. Depending on how many cells are lost, repopulation may require days, weeks, or more, which may be too late to reverse the effects.

At low doses of radiation a small percentage of the dividing cells may be damaged, and in some tissues this may lead to no detectable change in function. However, smaller doses can alter the developing fetus (del Regato, Spjut, & Cox, 1985). Organ development occurs early and extremely rapidly during pregnancy; exposure of the fetus to radiation can greatly alter cellular integrity and normal development. These effects depend on the number of stem cells available and the stage of fetal development.

Carcinogenesis can occur from mutation or cell transformation caused by radiation (see Chapter 2). Radiation can cause dominant and recessive mutations in the DNA and chromosome aberrations. To produce a carcinogenic effect, these DNA alterations must survive in cells capable of cell division. Radiation can directly damage macromolecules or carbohydrates, proteins, lipids, and nucleic acids. Indirectly, radiation interacts with substances (generally water) within the cell, producing reactive-free radicals that then interact and damage DNA.

Carcinogenesis can also be the result of gene-environment interactions. Host factors can influence the carcinogenic effects of radiation. For example, although cells can repair some lesions in DNA, some genetic abnor-malities alter the repair mechanism, making the individual sensitive to ionizing radiation. Disturbances in the DNA repair mechanism affect the risk of radiation-induced genetic effects and the risk of cancer.

Many other biologic variables affect responses to radiation, including the part and percentage of the body exposed, the individual's age or developmental stage at time of exposure, hormonal balance (e.g., sex hormones regulate cellular growth), genetic integrity, drugs, and other disease processes. Certain drugs can inhibit the immune response by affecting the surveillance role of the lymphoid cells. In the presence of infections viral nucleoproteins may be introduced into the DNA, rendering the cell susceptible to transformation. Solid tumors caused by whole-body radiation are found in the breasts in women, and the thyroid, the lung, and some digestive organs (Boice & Land, 1982). A latent period occurs between radiation exposure and the development of cancer. Solid tumors seldom appear before 10 years after radiation exposure and continue to appear for 30 years or more after exposure. Leukemia is an exception, appearing within a few years after radiation exposure.

Hormones

The relationship between hormones and human cancer has been extensively studied. Interest began in 1919 when Laek reported that the removal of the ovaries in female mice prevented the development of breast cancer. Because of this observation and the demonstrated carcinogenic effects of estrogens in rodents, some researchers suggest that the clinical use of estrogens may be carcinogenic. However, no strong evidence exists so far.

Much of the present research on hormones and cancer is centered on the direct actions of the sex steroids (estrogens, testosterone, and progesterone). Prolactin, a major pituitary hormone, has a direct role in rat mammary cancer growth but is not believed to be of primary importance in human breast cancer.

Although many investigations have been done to study the relationship of oral contraceptives and cancer risk, findings are inconclusive. Derivatives of the steroid contraceptives given in large doses to laboratory animals are related to cancers of the breast and liver. However, these dosages are far greater than the low levels used for contraception. The most widely used birth control pills are "combination" pills containing both estrogen and progestin. Combination pills may actually decrease the risk of developing some cancers (ovarian and endometrial) (American Cancer Society, 1986, 1989; Centers for Disease Control, 1983a, 1983b).

Male sex hormones, testosterone and its derivative 5, dihydrotestosterone (DHT), stimulate the growth of target tissues, such as the prostate. However, men who take exogenous androgens do not seem to have a higher risk of prostate cancer, whereas women who take estrogens after menopause seem to have a higher risk for development of endometrial cancer.

Three notable types of human cancer—carcinoma of the breast, endometrium, and prostate—occur in target, or hormone-responsive, tissues. (These cancers are discussed further in Unit 20.) The difficulty in understanding the carcinogenic nature of hormones has been the separation of the hormones as modulators of target tissue growth and function from their potential causative carcinogenic effects. More simply, do hormones cause cancer, or do they promote only tumor growth, or do they do both? Most of the evidence thus far supports their role as promoters of carcinogenesis in target tissues rather than as primary carcinogens. The sex steroids produce their actions by way of the receptor mechanism (see Chapters 1 and 19), sensitizing the cell to the carcinogenic insult, promoting the carcinogenic process, and modifying the growth of the established tumor. Hormones thus appear as promoters rather than primary carcinogens.

Estrogens

Estrogen replacement therapy has been prescribed for women to relieve postmenopausal symptoms (e.g., hot flashes) and to prevent osteoporosis. Chronic use of estrogens by these women has been linked to endometrial cancer (American Cancer Society, 1989; Hulka, 1984). The synthetic estrogen diethylstilbestrol (DES) has also been linked to cancer. Daughters of women treated with DES to avert habitual abortion have demonstrated a higher than expected percentage of clear cell adenocarcinomas of the vagina (Buchler, 1983; Herbst, Ulfelder, & Poskanzer, 1971). DES has a low affinity for binding to its transporter protein, plasma steroid-binding globulin, which may in turn result in high free levels of circulating DES that cross the placenta to the fetus.

A major controversy is the role of estrogens in breast cancer. However, the results of current research do not allow clinicians to predict whether women develop breast cancer based solely on the role of estrogens (del Regato et al., 1985). American women, who have a much greater incidence of breast cancer than Asian women, have demonstrated significantly lower estriol ratios to the two main estrogen fractions, estrone and estradiol. The ratio of estriol to estrone and estradiol is also elevated during pregnancy, which may account for the protective effect of childbearing. Estriol itself increases the incidence of mammary tumors in mice (Rudali, Apiou, & Muel, 1975).

Progesterone and Androgens

Controversy exists as to the role of progesterone and its relationship to breast cancer. Lower plasma progesterone levels were reported in premenopausal women at high risk for breast cancer and those with breast cancer

than premenopausal women at low risk (Bulbrook et al., 1978). Contrarily, other studies found no differences between serum progesterone levels or its urinary metabolites in individuals with breast cancer when these levels were compared with controls (Cowan et al., 1981). Androgens such as testosterone and dihydrotestosterone stimulate the growth of such target tissue as the prostate. However, to date no hormonal factors have been firmly established as causes of cancer of the prostate.

CARCINOGENIC PATHOGENS

Oncogenic Viruses

Certain environmental agents, such as chemical carcinogens, x-rays, and UV radiation, are known to cause specific types of cancer. However, many human cancers appear to arise spontaneously (i.e., develop in individuals who are not exposed to any known carcinogenic agent). To explain how these neoplasms arise, it was proposed that cancer, like many other diseases, is caused by either genetic factors inherent in certain individuals or pathogenic agents (infectious bacteria or viruses that cause a disease). Although many infectious agents have been considered as possible carcinogens, it appears that viruses are the most likely pathogenic factors associated with vertebrate neoplasia.

Researchers first isolated viruses from certain types of cancer in the early 1900s. They discovered that these viruses caused cancers when transferred into normal healthy animals. Since these early studies, a number of **oncogenic viruses** (cancer-causing viruses) have been identified, including a few that appear to cause specific forms of neoplasia in humans. The known oncogenic viruses function as true pathogenic agents because each induces only a specific type of malignant or benign tumor in susceptible animals. Studies to identify and characterize oncogenic viruses have been facilitated by the finding that most of these agents are capable of transforming normal tissue culture cell lines in vitro (cells grown outside the animal under tissue culture conditions). Active research is currently in progress to identify all of the possible human oncogenic viruses, to determine how these agents cause cancer, and to evaluate potential therapeutic approaches to inhibit the actions of these viruses. The remainder of this section will focus on the classification of oncogenic viruses, the characterization of oncogenes, and the possible mechanisms of viral carcinogenesis.

Classification of Oncogenic Viruses

Oncogenic viruses are divided into two major groups according to the nucleic acid content (DNA or RNA) of the viral particle (Table 11-4). Both DNA and RNA oncogenic viruses have been identified. Since their dis-

TABLE 11-4 Classification and examples of oncogenic viruses

Viral class	Virus	Species of isolation
ONCOGENIC DNA VIRUSES		
Papovaviruses	Papilloma	Rabbit, human, others
	Polyoma	Mouse
	SV 40	Monkey
Adenoviruses*	Adenovirus 12	Human
Herpes viruses	Epstein-Barr	Human
	Lucke carcinoma	Frog
	Merek's disease	Chicken
ONCOGENIC RNA VIRUSES†		
Acute-acting type	Rous sarcoma	Chicken
	Maloney sarcoma	Mouse
	Harvey/Kirsten sarcoma	Rat
Subacute type	Avian leukosis	Chicken
	Mouse mammary tumor	Mouse
	Bovine leukemia	Cow

Adapted from Ruddon, 1981.
*There are 31 types of adenovirus that have been isolated from man. Three of these (types 12, 18, and 31) are highly oncogenic when inoculated into newborn rodents.
†The oncogenic RNA viruses are divided into two classes. The acute-acting types transform cells in vitro, induce rapid disease in vivo, and carry oncogenes in their genome. The subacute types do not cause cell transformation in vitro, have long latency periods for disease induction in vivo, do not possess oncogenes, and appear to be horizontally transmitted.

covery, a tremendous amount of work has been directed toward establishing the mechanism(s) by which oncogenic viruses are able to cause cell transformation. These studies have led to the development of the "oncogene hypothesis." This hypothesis states that virtually all normal cells possess **oncogenes** (cancer-causing genes) that are similar to the genes of the oncogenic viruses. The activation of these genes in a normal cell is associated with the transformation process. These transformations can result in neoplastic cells that are capable of developing into a benign or malignant tumor. However, it is unknown how oncogenes are activated in normal cells or their role in maintaining the transformed cell phenotype.

Oncogenic DNA Viruses

Three main types of oncogenic DNA viruses are papovaviruses, adenoviruses, and herpesviruses (Table 11-4). DNA viruses penetrate host cells by the action of their coat proteins. The uncoated viral DNA then enters the cell's nucleus where it is inserted (integrated) into the host's DNA. The integrated viral DNA is then transcribed in two "waves" to produce early and late mRNAs (messenger RNAs are described in Chapter 4). The early mRNAs code for viral proteins that are involved in the replication of the viral DNA. Late mRNAs are transcribed after viral DNA replication and code for the viral structural proteins. (Viral replication

is discussed in Chapter 1. RNA transcription is discussed in Chapter 4.)

Oncogenic DNA viruses can cause tumors in a variety of tissues of different animal species. The papovavirus and DNA herpesviruses can cause tumors in humans. The HPV causes benign tumors (warts) in humans and is associated with skin, anal, and genital warts. Papilloma viruses also cause oral and laryngeal papillomas. Recent studies indicate that benign tumors induced by certain types of HPV can convert to maligant tumors (Johnson & Smith, 1986; Ostrow et al., 1986). Humans are subject to infection by five of the herpesviruses: (1) herpes simplex virus 1 (HSV-1), (2) herpes simplex virus 2 (HSV-2), (3) herpes zoster virus, (4) cytomegalovirus, and (5) Epstein-Barr virus (EBV). Of these, EBV appears to be the causative agent of Burkitt's lymphoma (see Chapter 24) and nasopharyngeal carcinoma (human cancers of the B lymphocytes and the squamous cells of the nasopharynx mucous membrane, respectively). HSV-1 and HSV-2 may cause cancers of the uterine cervix and other genitourinary and oropharyngeal tumors.

Oncogenic RNA Viruses

The oncogenic RNA viruses are termed **retroviruses** because they contain the unique enzyme **reverse transcriptase**. This enzyme is required for successful infection by the virus. Before viral replication can occur in

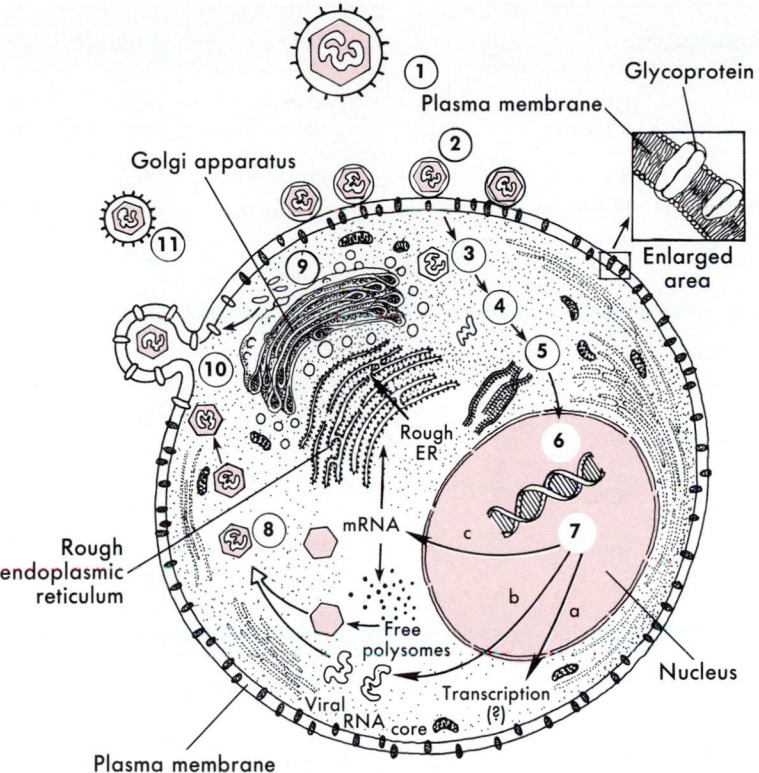

1 Oncogenic retrovirus

2 Absorption—virus binds to cell surface

3 Penetration—virus enters cytoplasm

4 Eclipse—viral RNA freed from core

5 Reverse transcriptase—viral RNA to viral DNA

6 Viral DNA incorporated into host DNA

7 Transcription of host DNA—virus replication
  a. Transcribed v-onc causes transformation
  b. Viral mRNA released to cytoplasm: core protein translated on free polysomes and coat proteins processed on rough endoplasmic reticulum and golgi apparatus

8 Maturation—core and capsid are assembled in cytoplasm

9 Coat proteins are inserted into plasma membrane

10 Release—virus cores bind to coat proteins and "bud" from cell surface

11 Infectious virus particles

FIG. 11-3. Stages of oncogenic RNA viral infection.

the host cell, the viral genome (all the genetic information of the virus) must be transcribed from viral RNA to viral DNA by the reverse transcriptase enzyme (Fig. 11-3). Once the viral genome has been transcribed to viral DNA, it can be integrated into the host's DNA, where it is transcribed and replicated by the host's genetic machinery. A classification of several retroviruses is given in Table 11-4.

Oncogenes

In addition to the genes required by the virus to maintain its integrity as an infectious agent (i.e., the virus core proteins, the envelope glycoproteins, and the reverse transcriptase), the oncogenic retroviruses also possess a specific oncogene(s) termed **v-onc** (identifying it as a viral oncogene). It is the v-onc that causes the transformation to occur. In 1976 Stehelin showed that cellular oncogenes (termed **c-onc**) in normal, nontransformed chicken cells and the v-onc of the avian sarcoma virus had virtually identical nucleic acid sequences. Based on this observation, a number of c-onc and corresponding v-onc have now been characterized (Table 11-5). For example, the active transforming gene present within the Rous sarcoma virus has been given the name

TABLE 11-5 Retroviral oncogenes

Species of isolation	Oncogenic virus	Oncogene acronym
Chicken	Rous sarcoma virus	src
	Avian erythroblastosis virus	erbA
	Avian erythroblastosis virus	erbB
	Y73 sarcoma virus	yes
	Fujinami sarcoma virus	fps
	VR II avian sarcoma virus	ros
	MC 29 myelocytomatosis virus	myc
	Avian myelobastosis virus	myb
	MH2 virus	mil (mht)
	E26 virus	ets
	Avian SKV770 virus	ski
Turkey	Reticuloendotheliosis virus	rel
Mouse	Molony sarcoma virus	mos
	Abelson murine leukemia virus	abl
	FBJ osteosarcoma virus	fos
Rat	Harey murine sarcoma virus	ha-ras
	Kirsten murine sarcoma virus	ki-ras
Cat	ST feline sarcoma virus	fes
	McDonough feline sarcoma virus	fms
	Gardner-Rasheed feline sarcoma virus	fgr
	3611 murine sarcoma virus	far
Wolley monkey	Simian sarcoma virus	sis

Adapted from Land, Parada, & Weinburg, 1983.

NOTE: Various viral oncogenes are listed by the species and virus from which they were originally isolated. V-onc and c-onc are designated by their oncogene acronym (abbreviated name).

v-src, which differentiates it from its cellular counterpart, the *c-src* oncogene.

Studies now show that c-onc are incorporated into the genomes of a variety of different organisms, including humans (Land, Prada, & Weinberg, 1983; Slamon et al., 1984). Since normal, nontransformed cells carry c-onc, a number of conclusions have been drawn concerning the origin and function of these genes.

First, the existence of these c-onc, throughout evolution in a variety of unrelated animal species, suggests

TABLE 11-6 Products of viral oncogenes

Oncogene product	Oncogene	Cellular location of oncogene product
Tryosine kinase	abl	Plasma membrane
	fes	Cytoplasm
	fps	Cytoplasm
	fgr	
	ros	Cytoplasmic membranes
	src	Plasma membrane
	yes	
Tryosine kinase structure without kinase activity	erbB	Plasma membrane
	frbs	Cytoplasm
	raf	Cytoplasm
	mil (mht)	
	mos	
Growth factor	sis	Cytoplasm
Bind GTP	Ha-ras	Plasma membrane
	Ki-ras	Plasma membrane
May bind DNA	fos	Nucleus
	myb	Nuclear matrix
	myc	Nuclear matrix

Adapted from Land, Parada, & Weinburg, 1983.

that they may play an important role in the normal function of the cell (Androphy & Lowy, 1984; Land et al., 1983). The term **proto-oncogene** has been applied to refer collectively to the various c-onc (i.e., proto-oncogenes and c-onc are, in essence, synonymous terms). The term *proto-oncogene* is used to indicate that the c-onc and v-onc represent genes derived from a common prototype gene. This suggests that the proto-oncogenes are both normal genetic components of the cell and encode for a vital product or activity required for cell survival. In this regard, recent studies have identified several proto-oncogenes as having growth hormone functions, growth hormone receptor activities, or cell-growth regulating enzyme properties (Table 11-6) (Androphy & Lowy, 1984; Land et al., 1983). Although their exact function is currently unknown, many of these oncogenes may have originated from normal cellular DNA sequences.

Second, it appears that most v-onc were actually derived from proto-oncogenes that were initially of cellular origin. It is known that certain viruses, especially the retroviruses, can incorporate infected host cell genes into their viral genome during their replication process. In this case the retroviruses act as parasitic agents that carry the oncogenes between different cells. Although this mechanism of transport suggests a number of different possible ways that the oncogenes might become activated in host cells, it alone does not explain the transformation process that leads to the induction of cancer.

Mechanisms of Viral Carcinogenesis

Although it is well established that oncogenic viruses are capable of directly transforming normal cells, the exact process is still unknown. Because these pathogenic agents are intracellular parasites, a number of mechanisms for viral carcinogenesis are proposed. In this section, some examples of these mechanisms will be discussed. It should be appreciated, however, that cancer represents a complex disease process. Like other diseases, the pathogenic agents may have either (1) a direct effect, in which the tumor cells are or were at some stage infected with the oncogenic virus; or (2) an indirect effect, in which the neoplastic cells were not altered by the virus but were stimulated to grow because of the viral infection.

Direct Mechanisms

During the infection process the virus may cause mutations in surviving cells that could lead to neoplastic changes. This "hit and run" process does not cause cellular transformation, although viral genes may persist within the tumor cells. However, these viral genes appear to be incorporated into the host genome in a random manner, suggesting that the viral genes did not cause transformation.

In contrast, most oncogenic viruses cause transformation by a mechanism termed **insertional mutagenesis.** In this process the viral genes are incorporated into the host's genome at specific sites. Insertion of the v-onc within the host genome can lead to activation of the v-onc or c-onc genes that are associated with cell transformation. These inserted genes become an inherited trait of all the cancer cells derived from the original transformed cell.

Indirect Mechanisms

Because viral infections lead to tissue damage, after the infection there is a burst of cell proliferation in the damaged tissue that is associated with the normal repair and healing processes. Actively dividing cells are known to be at higher risk of mutation than resting cells. As a result, these cells would be more susceptible to both spontaneous mutagenesis and transformation by a physical carcinogen. Alternatively, during some viral infections, the host's immune system can become compromised. This reduced immunologic protection can allow neoplastic cells to emerge that would normally be rejected by the host. The role of the immune system in cancer is discussed in more detail in the following section. In conclusion, viral infections may have an indirect effect on carcinogenesis by increasing the individual's risk for neoplasia induced by other means.

IMMUNOBIOLOGY OF CANCER

The Immune Surveillance Theory

One conclusion that can be drawn from the viral theory of carcinogenesis is that the induction of altered or abnormal cell products is not necessarily required for the development of cancer cells. It is conceivable that the only difference between normal and transformed cells is the amount, rather than the type, of cellular components (e.g., enzymes, cell surface receptors, plasma membrane-bound proteins) that each possesses. In this regard the overall structural composition of the plasma membranes of normal and transformed cells may be quite similar, if not identical. Thus any differences between normal and cancer cells may be both subtle and possibly imperceptible by the organism.

The immune system of higher organisms, such as humans, has evolved to recognize antigens that are considered to be "foreign," or "nonself," structures (see Chapter 6). If the immune system is capable of recognizing and rejecting tumors, cancer cells must express "nonself" antigens. The **immune surveillance theory** is based on this assumption.

For some time investigators have been intrigued with the idea that the body could defend itself against the development of cancer. In 1908 Paul Ehrlich, the renowned biologist, proposed that the transformation process was a common event and that as a result cancer cells were constantly arising in normal animals. He went on to propose that most cancer cells express "foreign" antigens that make them susceptible to rejection by their host's immune system.

Since that time, a number of studies have supported Ehrlich's general concept. Based on this work, Sir Macfarlin Burnet formally proposed the immune surveillance theory in 1970. In short, Burnet proposed that cell-mediated cytotoxicity (tumor cell killing by immunologic cells such as lymphocytes) evolved as an immunologic need to act as a primary surveillant for the emergence of cancer cells. Certain experimental and clinical observations form the basis of Burnet's theory; these include the identification of tumor antigens and the demonstration of T cell–mediated cellular immunity (described in Chapter 6).

Tumor Antigens

Tumor associated antigens (TAA) are generally divided into two main groups: (1) tumor-specific transplantation antigens (TSTA), which are unique for each tumor, and (2) cross-reactive tumor-associated transplantation antigens (TATA), which are shared by a number of different tumors (Fig. 11-4).

The TSTA are generally the most immunogenic (i.e., causing the strongest immune response) TAA expressed

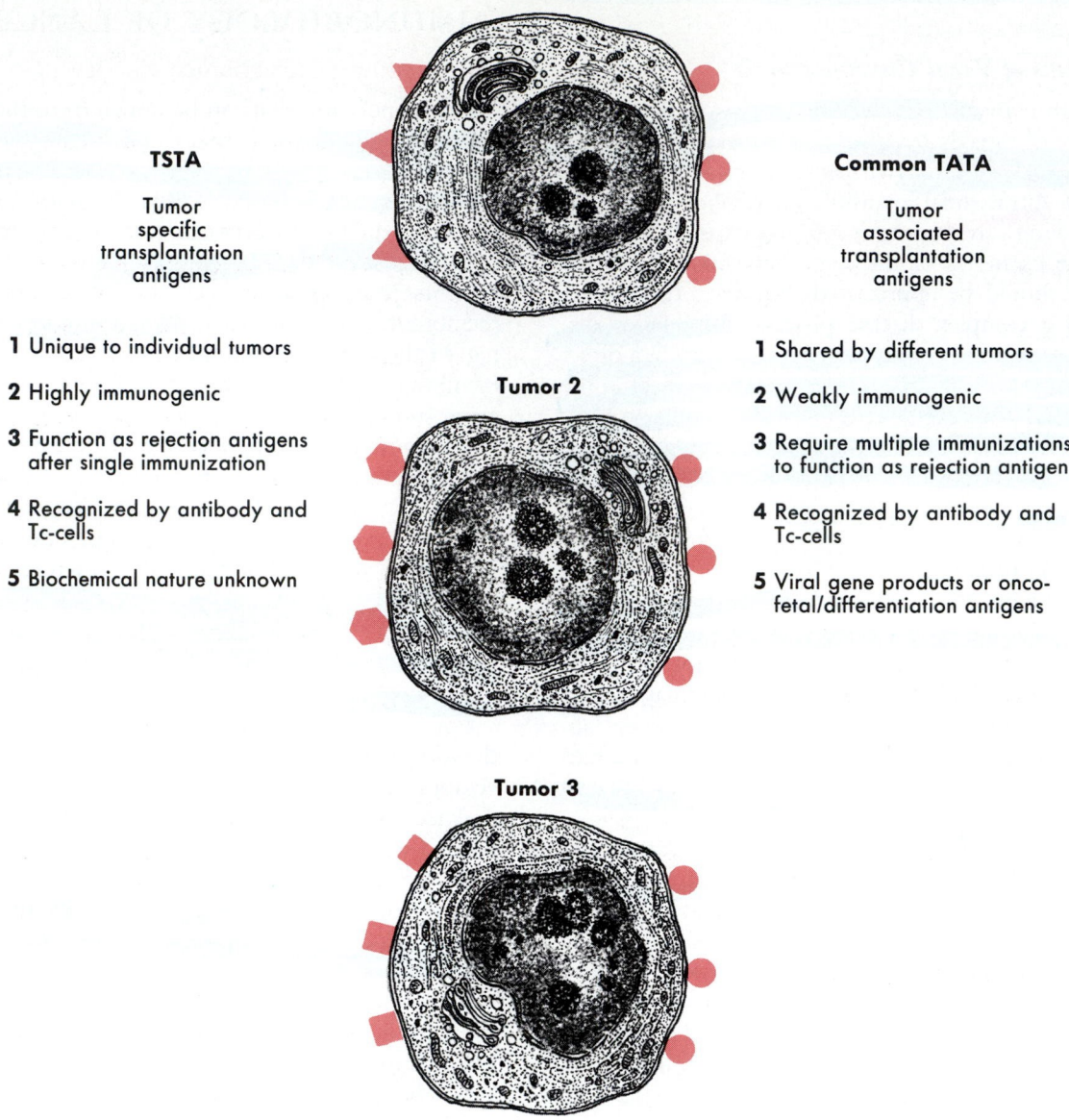

Tumor 1

TSTA

Tumor
specific
transplantation
antigens

1 Unique to individual tumors

2 Highly immunogenic

3 Function as rejection antigens
  after single immunization

4 Recognized by antibody and
  Tc-cells

5 Biochemical nature unknown

Common TATA

Tumor
associated
transplantation
antigens

1 Shared by different tumors

2 Weakly immunogenic

3 Require multiple immunizations
  to function as rejection antigen

4 Recognized by antibody and
  Tc-cells

5 Viral gene products or onco-
  fetal/differentiation antigens

Tumor 2

Tumor 3

FIG. 11-4. Two general classes of tumor-associated antigens (TAA).

by experimentally induced tumors. However, very little is known about the exact biochemical nature of the TSTA that are expressed by either experimental or human tumors. Currently, the best recognized example of TSTA associated with human cancer cells is the immunoglobulin idiotype antigens (unique antigenic determinants associated with the antigen-binding site of immunoglobulins) that are expressed by B lymphomas.

In contrast to the TSTA expressed by various experimentally induced tumors, the cross-reactive TATA appear to be less immunogenic. Although these antigens are less effective in eliciting tumor rejection responses in

syngeneic (identical genotype) hosts, the cross-reactive TATA have been better characterized in human cancers.

Viral Antigens

The **viral antigens** represent products expressed by virally transformed cells that are encoded for by viral genes. These antigens are plasma membrane-bound products of the viral capsid, envelope, core, or v-onc. As such, these antigens are common to all tumors induced by the same virus.

Research suggests that Burkitt's lymphoma and nasopharyngeal carcinoma are caused by EBV. For example, individuals with Burkitt's lymphoma (1) have higher antibody titers to EBV antigens than unaffected individuals of the same age, sex, and geographic location; (2) the tumor cells have copies of the EBV genes incorporated into their genome; (3) EBV transforms human B lymphocytes in vitro; and (4) EBV causes cancer when inoculated into subhuman primates. Further, the antibody titers against EBV in individuals with nasopharyngeal carcinoma correlate with the stage of their disease. This suggests that viral antigens are continually expressed by the tumor cells. (Lymphomas are further discussed in Chapter 24.)

Oncofetal Antigens

The oncofetal antigens represent molecules that are expressed by cells during certain stages of embryonic development but are absent or expressed at very low concentrations by normal adult cells. The two best characterized antigens in this group are alpha-fetoprotein and carcinoembryonic antigen.

The α-fetoprotein (α-FP) is a serum alpha-globulin that is secreted by embryonic liver cells. During the first trimester, α-FP composes about 90% of the total serum globulins in the blood of human embryos. These levels quickly decline after birth. Individuals with hepatic, pancreatic, and embryonal carcinomas (malignant tumors of epithelial cells), have high levels of α-FP in their serum. Although α-FP appears to be associated specifically with these types of tumors, increased α-FP levels in the blood of individuals with non-neoplastic disease, such as acute viral hepatitis, have also been observed.

The carcinoembryonic antigen (CEA) appears to be associated with the mucous coating of the cells of the fetal gut, pancreas, and liver through the sixth month of gestation. Antibody titers to CEA have been found in the serum of individuals with various types of cancer. For example, 70% of colon, 90% of pancreas, and 35% of breast cancer patients have detectable CEA antibody titers, compared with normal individuals (about 5% of the normal human population have CEA reactive antibody titers). As with α-FP, however, serologic titers to CEA have been found in a large percentage of specific groups of normal people (e.g., pregnant women and heavy cigarette smokers) and in individuals with non-cancerous diseases. Because α-FP and CEA antigens are found in a large number of normal individuals, their use as diagnostic tools for cancer screening is not as promising as once thought.

Immunologic Defense Against Tumors

Under conditions in which a developing tumor expresses cell surface TAA, an immunologically competent host possesses the potential for recognizing these antigens and making an appropriate immune response to reject the tumor. Like other types of antigenic stimuli, TAA can elicit a diverse range of immune responses. These responses can be specific or nonspecific and humoral or cell mediated. In any case the appropriate immune response is part of the overall immune surveillance mechanism that protects the individual against the continued growth and spread of newly emerging cancer cells.

A number of clinical observations strongly support the concept of immunologic involvement in the tumor surveillance process. First, early oncologists noted that individuals with draining, abscessed tumors lived longer than those whose tumors did not appear to be inflamed. Second, Berg, in 1959, reported that women with breast cancer tumors that were infiltrated with lymphocytes had a better prognosis than women whose tumors were free of lymphocytes. Third, for certain types of neoplasia there is an increased risk (2% to 20% increase over the normal population) of developing cancer in individuals who are immunologically suppressed. Such individuals (Table 11-7) include (1) children with immunodeficiency diseases, (2) organ transplant recipients whose immune systems are suppressed with drugs (like cyclosporin A to block graft rejection), (3) individuals with cancer for whom cancer therapy results in the suppression of immune responsiveness (many of the current radiation and chemotherapies that are used to treat various forms of cancer depress the immune system, and these individuals have a high risk of developing secondary tumors), and (4) individuals with acquired immune deficiency syndrome (AIDS).

For those with AIDS, there is a great risk of develop-

TABLE 11-7 Correlation between immunodeficiency and cancer risk

Types of cancer	Increase risk over normal population
Lymphomas	14 times greater
Leukemias	6 times greater
Carcinomas	
Skin (low-sun geographic areas)	4-7 times greater
(high-sun geographic areas)	21 times greater
Uterine cervix	13 times greater
Stomach	11 times greater
Urinary bladder	2 times greater

NOTE: There is an increased risk for developing specific types of cancer in individuals with various immunodeficiencies versus that of the normal population. The values presented are generalized to include the various immunodeficient conditions. There is no increased risk in immunodeficient individuals for specific cancers not listed.
Adapted from Penn 1981.

ing a rare type of cancer called Kaposi's sarcoma (a multifocal angiomatosis that localizes in the skin). In fact, Kaposi's sarcoma has become one of the diagnostic signs of AIDS. Evidence still has not shown whether Kaposi's sarcoma develops as a result of the immunodeficiency in these individuals or is associated directly with AIDS, although experimental evidence does suggest that Kaposi's sarcoma and AIDS have a common viral cause. (AIDS is fully described in Chapter 8.) These various clinical observations provide strong support for immune surveillance mechanisms and their role in the development of certain types of human cancer.

Immune Mechanisms for Defense Against Cancer

Like other antigens, TAA can elicit a wide range of immune responses (humoral or cellular, specific or non-

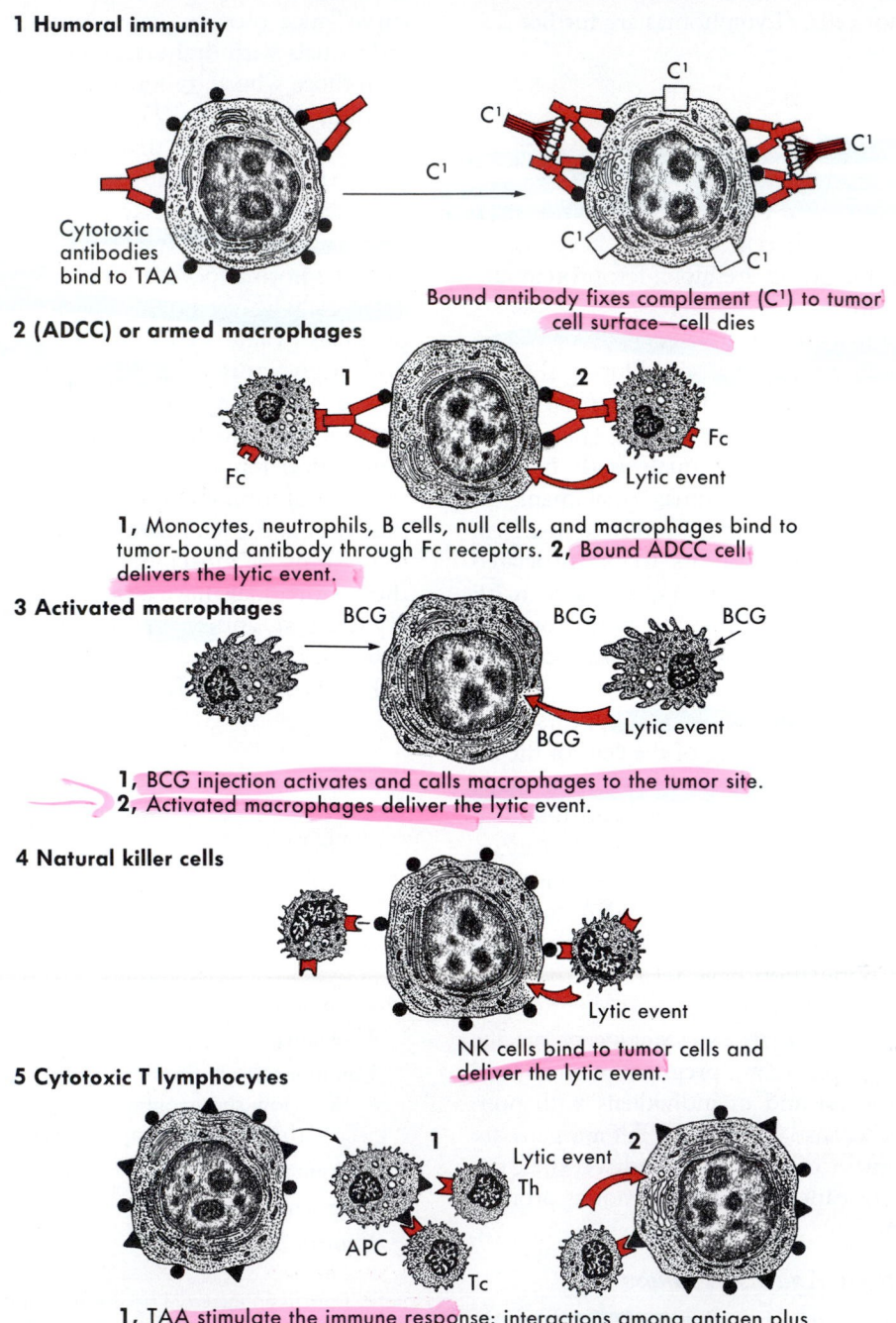

1 Humoral immunity

Cytotoxic antibodies bind to TAA

Bound antibody fixes complement (C¹) to tumor cell surface—cell dies

2 (ADCC) or armed macrophages

Fc

Fc

Lytic event

1, Monocytes, neutrophils, B cells, null cells, and macrophages bind to tumor-bound antibody through Fc receptors. **2,** Bound ADCC cell delivers the lytic event.

3 Activated macrophages

BCG   BCG   BCG

Lytic event

BCG

1, BCG injection activates and calls macrophages to the tumor site.
2, Activated macrophages deliver the lytic event.

4 Natural killer cells

Lytic event

NK cells bind to tumor cells and deliver the lytic event.

5 Cytotoxic T lymphocytes

1   Lytic event   2

Th

APC

Tc

1, TAA stimulate the immune response: interactions among antigen plus antigen-presenting cells plus T helper cells and T cytotoxic cell.
2, Tc cell binds to TAA (specifically) and delivers the lytic event.

FIG. 11-5. Tumor immune surveillance mechanisms.

specific) that can protect the host against tumor growth. Clearly, certain immune responses are potentially more beneficial than others for protecting the individual against cancer. The various types of known cancer defense mechanisms are summarized in Fig. 11-5.

The main involvement of B lymphocytes in a host's defense against cancer is through the production of TAA-specific antibodies. Individuals with cancer can possess natural or spontaneous antibodies in addition to specifically induced antibodies that are capable of reacting with various TAA. Two types of functional antibodies can protect the host against cancer growth. Cytotoxic antibodies are capable of mediating complement killing of tumor cells. Alternatively, TAA-specific antibodies can participate in a cellular mechanism of tumor cell killing called antibody-dependent, cell-mediated cytotoxicity (ADCC) (see Chapter 6).

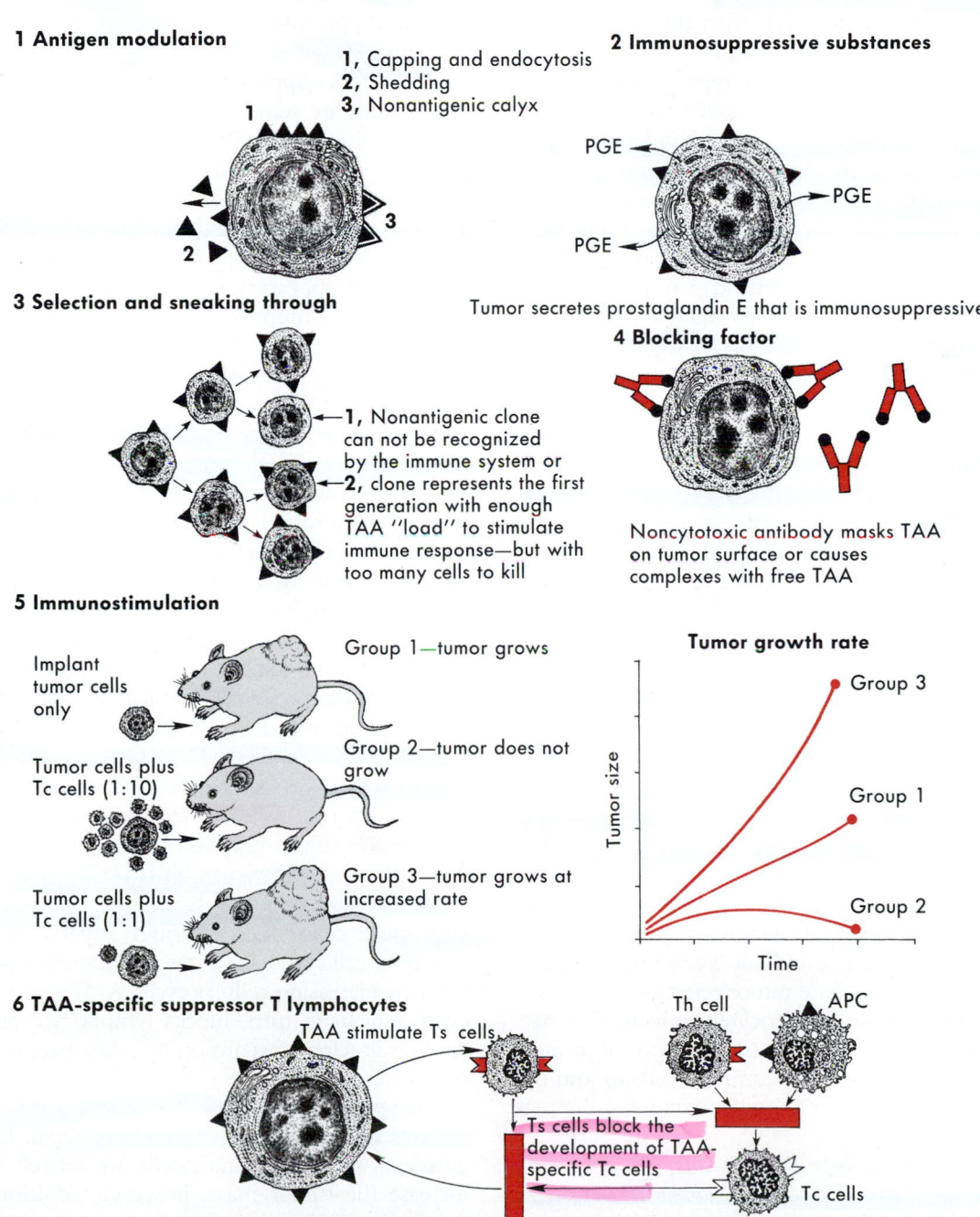

1 Antigen modulation

1, Capping and endocytosis
2, Shedding
3, Nonantigenic calyx

2 Immunosuppressive substances

PGE

PGE

PGE

Tumor secretes prostaglandin E that is immunosuppressive

3 Selection and sneaking through

1, Nonantigenic clone can not be recognized by the immune system or
2, clone represents the first generation with enough TAA "load" to stimulate immune response—but with too many cells to kill

4 Blocking factor

Noncytotoxic antibody masks TAA on tumor surface or causes complexes with free TAA

5 Immunostimulation

Implant tumor cells only

Group 1—tumor grows

Tumor cells plus Tc cells (1:10)

Group 2—tumor does not grow

Tumor cells plus Tc cells (1:1)

Group 3—tumor grows at increased rate

Tumor growth rate

Group 3

Group 1

Group 2

Tumor size

Time

6 TAA-specific suppressor T lymphocytes

TAA stimulate Ts cells

Th cell   APC

Ts cells block the development of TAA-specific Tc cells

Tc cells

FIG. 11-6. Potential immune surveillance escape mechanisms.

ADCC, or armed macrophages, is a cellular mechanism whereby cells that are capable of killing tumor cells gain the ability to recognize TAA by binding antibodies to their cell surfaces. These cells usually bind TAA-specific antibodies by receptors on their cell surface that recognize the Fc portion of the antibody molecule (see Chapter 6). These cells can then use the cell surface-bound antibody to recognize and bind to tumor cells. Once bound, these cells can deliver the tumor cell-killing signal (lytic event). Cells that possess ADCC function are monocytes, neutrophils, B cells, and certain null cells called killer cells, or K cells. When macrophages are the ADCC-mediating cell type, they are usually referred to as "armed macrophages."

Unlike "armed macrophages," a type of nonspecific tumor cell killing is mediated by so-called activated macrophages. Macrophages can be activated and called into an antitumor immune response in several ways. One way is through injection of adjuvant, such as the bacteria *Corynebacterium parvum* and Bacillus Calmette-Guerin (BCG). These agents have been used in immunotherapy (see Chapter 8). A second way that macrophages are extensively activated to kill tumor cells is through the release of specific macrophage-activating factors by immune T lymphocytes. Once activated, these macrophages kill tumor cells in a localized, antigen-non-specific fashion.

Natural killer (NK) and K cells (a population of null cells) may represent the first line of defense against the emergence of cancer cells. NK cells can be identified in normal, cancer-free individuals. Both specific (by the introduction of TAA) and nonspecific (adjuvant) stimulation of the immune system can lead to a rapid, transient increase in NK cell activity that peaks at about 3 days. High levels of NK cell activity in various mouse strains appear to correlate with the relative resistance of these strains to the growth of certain transplantable tumors. In many humans with cancer the level of NK cell activity is below normal.

Cytotoxic T lymphocytes (Tc cells) represent the dominant cell type in mediating tumor rejection. Tc cells are TAA-specific and differentiate from resting T cells after TAA-antigen presentation by macrophages and stimulation by helper T lymphocytes. Once activated, Tc cells can recognize and kill specific tumor cells. Activated Tc cells can mediate tumor rejection by secreting lymphokines (soluble lymphocyte products) that directly lyse tumor cells, inhibit the growth of transformed cells, or stimulate noncommitted cells to join in an antitumor response.

Immune Surveillance Escape Mechanisms

In spite of the immune system's ability to reject cancer cells, individuals with apparently normal immunologic competency develop and eventually succumb to neoplastic disease. Therefore the host-tumor relationship at any given time during tumor emergence and progression is a complex process. Changes in both the host's immunologic potential (i.e., range of antigenic responses) and the characteristics of progressively growing cancer cells (e.g., TAA expression, growth rate, metabolism) are constantly taking place. Unlike most antigens encountered by the immune system, cancer cells must be viewed as parasites capable of bypassing the host's immune surveillance potential. Some possible ways that tumors can escape immunologic rejection include (1) antigenic modulation, (2) tumor secretion of immunosuppressive substances, (3) escape and sneaking through, (4) blocking factor, (5) immunostimulation, and (6) TAA suppressor T lymphocytes. These escape mechanisms are summarized in Fig. 11-6.

It is well recognized that cancer cells can down-regulate their expression of cell surface molecules when grown in the presence of specific antibodies. The term given to such a process is **antigenic modulation.** It is thought to occur by way of patching (antigen-antibody clumps that appear as patches) and capping (the antigen-antibody clumps form a cap on part of the cell surface), which are followed by either endocytosis (uptake of extracellular material, discussed in Chapter 1) or shedding of antigens.

Alternatively, some cancer cells mask their TAA through biochemical modifications. For example, the cell surface can be coated by a glycoprotein calyx that masks the expressed antigens. Human glioma cells (tumors of the central nervous system) have been shown to be surrounded by a hyaluronic acid-rich glycosaminoglycan coat that masks the cell surface antigens. In the presence of an effective antitumor immune response an antigenically modulated tumor, by either shedding its TAA or masking its cell surface, would not be recognized and destroyed.

Some tumors are known to secrete soluble **immunosuppressive substances.** These substances can either interfere with the necessary cellular interactions required for effective tumor rejection or directly inhibit lymphocyte activation. Prostaglandin E (PGE) is an example of an immunosuppressive substance that is secreted by certain cancer cells. PGE, although capable of affecting a variety of cell types, mediates its immunosuppressive activity by increasing cellular cyclic AMP levels in lymphocytes, which, in turn, blocks lymphocyte proliferation. As a result, clonal expansion of TAA-reactive T lymphocytes cannot occur.

Most tumors arise from the transformation of a single cell and are considered to be monoclonal. During progression, where the tumor cells are actively dividing to increase the tumor mass, however, additional changes can occur. Therefore, when a tumor reaches an appreciable size, the transformed cells within it can represent a complex heterogenous mixture of subclones. Such a process can facilitate **escape** from host defense mechanisms, especially under conditions in which daughter cells have the potential to lose or modify the nature of their tumor antigens.

Experiments show that some tumors are rejected when a large number of cells are transplanted into a syngeneic host. When fewer cells of the same tumor are transplanted, however, tumors eventually grow in the syngeneic recipients. This observation led to the theory of **sneaking through.** Because tumors originate from a single transformed cell, it is possible that small amounts of TAA are not immunogenic and that, when a tumor reaches a size where enough antigen is expressed to stimulate an immune response, it is too large (with too many rapidly growing cells) to be eliminated by the immune system.

Blocking factor, or **blocking antibodies,** has been found in the sera of experimental tumor-bearing animals and in some individuals with cancer. These represent antibodies that are TAA specific but are incapable of either functioning in an ADCC response or lysing tumors by fixing complement. Blocking antibodies can inhibit tumor rejection by (1) binding to tumor cells, thus masking TAA; (2) forming antigen-antibody complexes that cannot be processed by the appropriate antigen-presenting cells; and (3) inhibiting Tc cell interaction with the tumor by masking the TAA.

Prehn (1971) has shown that a "little" **immunologic stimulation** can actually enhance tumor cell growth. In his experiments, he found that, when tumor cells were mixed with an optimal number of Tc cells and transplanted to syngeneic hosts, the tumors were rejected. In contrast, when tumor cells were mixed with suboptimal numbers of Tc cells, the tumor implants were not rejected and grew even faster than implants of tumor cells alone. Similar results were obtained with TAA-specific antibodies. From these studies, Prehn concluded that as the immune response develops toward the TAA, the early phases of Tc-cell infiltration into the tumor mass actually stimulate cancer cell growth.

The immune system, with its many types of effector functions, is carefully regulated. Because of the potential for tissue destruction associated with immunologically mediated mechanisms, the evolution of such regulatory processes is essential. One way in which the overall system is controlled is through the induction of **suppressor T lymphocytes** (Ts cells) (Fig.11-6). These Ts cells can be elicited by either the TSTA expressed by progressively growing tumors or by cross-reactive TAA associated with tissues that are altered by environmental insults. The generation of Ts cells is an antigen-specific immune response. The function of Ts cells is to (1) block other types of immune responses, (2) switch off an ongoing immune response, or (3) mediate a modification in the magnitude or type of immune response that is elicited.

The induction of active suppression has been reported to represent an important means by which tumors evade immunologic elimination. The stimulation of such a regulatory mechanism during tumor progression is probably caused by the immune system's inability to determine whether an actively dividing cell is detrimental (as it is in transformed cells) or beneficial (as it is in actively dividing bone marrow cells) to the host. This is a very complex problem because most cell surface molecules present on tumor cells are also expressed by their normal cell counterparts.

In addition to antigen-specific suppressor T lymphocytes, **activated macrophages** have been reported to exert suppressive activity. Suppression of tumor immune response by macrophages is nonspecific, however, and results in a general depression of the immune system. The mechanism of suppression by macrophages is unknown.

In conclusion, it appears that tumor growth or rejection depends on complex interactions between cancer cells and the immune system of their host. In this regard a range of immunologic protective mechanisms have been identified that mediate tumor lysis and tumor growth. In addition, the transformation process itself can select for transformed cells that are capable of evading the immunologic insults of the host and, depending on the carcinogenic agent, can cause an immunosuppressed state that renders the individual susceptible to the growth of neoplasia.

SUMMARY REVIEW

The Multistage Theory—Initiation and Promotion

1 One theory of carcinogenesis suggests that cancer development is a two-stage process: (1) an initiation stage that causes irreversible changes in DNA after exposure to a carcinogen and (2) a promotion stage in which the initiated cells become cancerous.

2 Initiators and promoters include hormones, drugs, environmental agents, and a variety of personal behaviors. Because the precise biochemical cause of cancer is unknown, these are actually risk factors associated with increased incidence of cancer.

3 Personal behaviors associated with increased cancer risk includes smoking and chewing smokeless tobacco, as well as sexual and reproductive behavior.

4 Smoking is associated with cancers of the lung, bladder, and kidney—lung cancer is related to inhalation of tobacco smoke, which contains known carcinogenic compounds.

5 Oral cancer is associated with "dipping snuff."

6 Dietary factors can act as cancer-promoting or cancer-inhibiting agents.

7 Vitamin A is known to block tumor production in animals and cancerous transformation in tissue cultures.

8 Obesity is associated with endometrial cancer, and high-fat diets are associated with endometrial, breast, and colon cancer.

9 Artificial additives and preservatives in food may include some compounds that are carcinogenic; particularly controversial is the use of nitrites, which react to form direct-or indirect-acting carcinogens when food is cooked.

10 Three primary mechanisms by which dietary factors affect cancer production are direct-acting carcinogens or their precursors; indirect-acting carcinogens; and dietary factors that affect transport, activation, and deactivation of carcinogens.

11 Direct-acting carcinogens may occur in natural foodstuffs, may be produced by cooking, and may be produced by microorganisms in stored foods.

12 Indirect-acting carcinogens provide compounds that act to form carcinogens in the body. Compounds currently being studied include nitrites, fats, and cholesterol.

13 Dietary factors that affect transport, activation, or deactivation of carcinogens include dietary fiber, which probably promotes rapid passage of food through the digestive tract, and selenium, which appears to destroy cytotoxic radicals when reacting at low levels.

14 Age at first sexual intercourse and number of sexual partners is related to development of cervical cancer.

15 Herpes simplex virus type 2 and human papillomavirus appear to be related to the development of cervical cancer, although a causal association has not been definitely established.

16 Pregnancy and childbearing seem to be protective factors against cancer of the endometrium, ovary, and breast; other reproductive factors related to decreased risk for breast cancer include late onset of menstruation and early menopause.

17 Air pollution is a concern for causing cancer because of inhalation of emissions including arsenicals, benzene, chloroform, vinyl chloride, and acrylonitrile. Indoor pollution is considered worse than outdoor pollution because of cigarette smoke and possibly radon gas.

18 Cancers of the upper respiratory tract, lung, bladder, and peritoneum are often attributed to occupational exposures, including asbestos, fossil fuels, dyes, rubber, and paint.

19 Ultraviolet sunlight causes basal cell and squamous cell carcinomas, is associated with malignant melanoma, and is also implicated in increasing the severity of xeroderma pigmentosum.

20 Ultraviolet light damages DNA, inhibits cell division, and can lead to cell death. Damaged DNA can cause cancer by misrepairing itself and creating mutagenic cells that are susceptible to tumor development.

21 Exposure to ionizing radiation is caused by emissions from x-rays, radioisotopes, and other radioactive sources, some of which are industry- or occupation-related exposures.

22 Ionizing radiation inhibits cell division, especially in lymphoid tissue, bone marrow, and intestinal epithelium, which contain normally short-lived, rapidly dividing cells.

23 Carcinogenesis can occur from radiation-induced mutations or cell transformations; mutations may be dominant or recessive and may also cause chromosome aberrations.

24 Genetic factors can alter the repair mechanisms for DNA, so that an individual is particularly sensitive to the carcinogenic effects of ionizing radiation.

25 Biologic variables that affect responses to radiation include the part and percentage of the body exposed, the individual's age or stage of development at the time of exposure, genetic integrity, drugs, and other disease processes.

26 Radiation exposure in the neonate, infant, or child can also cause growth retardation; the younger the child, the more vulnerable the child is to the effects of radiation.

27 For cancers that occur in hormone-responsive target tissues, hormones probably act as promoters of carcinogenesis rather than as primary carcinogens.

Immunobiology of Cancer

1 The viral theory of carcinogenesis is based on research showing that when a virus enters a cell, its genetic material can be inserted into host chromosomes.

2 Oncogenic viruses are viruses that cause cancer and are classified according to their nucleic acid (DNA or RNA).

3 The oncogene hypothesis suggests that normal cells possess oncogenes (cancer-causing genes) that are similar to the genes of oncogenic viruses. When activated, oncogenes can transform the cell and cause a tumor to develop.

4 Oncogenic DNA viruses insert viral DNA into the host's DNA, so that the viral DNA is then transcribed with the host's DNA.

5 Oncogenic DNA viruses include papovavirus and herpesvirus, which in some forms can cause malignancies in humans.

6 Oncogenic RNA viruses are called retroviruses because they contain reverse transcriptase, which causes infection in the host by transcribing viral RNA to viral DNA.

7 Retroviruses carry specific oncogenes termed v-onc; normal cells carry oncogenes termed c-onc. Oncogenic viruses appear to have become capable of transforming normal cells because they acquired specific c-onc into their genome during replication within host-infected cells.

8 The c-onc of various animal species are collectively termed proto-oncogenes. Some of these are homogenous with v-onc, and some can be identified in nonvirally induced tumors, suggesting that they are activated during the transformation process by environmental carcinogens.

9 Because c-onc are probably required for the normal functioning of the cell, identifying the biochemical products encoded by these genes should ultimately lead to a better understanding of the cellular transformation process that produces tumors.

10 The immune surveillance theory of carcinogenesis is based on the assumption that cancer cells must express "nonself" antigens that should, in a normally functioning individual, be recognized and rejected by the immune system.

11 Cancer cells express tumor-associated antigens, which are not found on normal, nontransformed cells.

12 Tumor-associated antigens may be caused by synthesis of new molecules, by unmasking of potential tumor-associated antigen, by loss of plasma membrane components, by biochemical modification, or by release of intracellular components.

13 Tumor-associated antigens are generally classified as tumor-specific transplantation antigens (TSTA) or cross-reactive, tumor-associated transplantation antigens (TATA).

14 TSTA are apparently more immunogenic than TATA and therefore produce a stronger immune response.

15 Cross-reactive TATA include viral antigens and oncofetal antigens (alpha-fetoprotein and carcinoembryonic antigen).

16 When a developing tumor expresses TAA, an immunologically competent host can recognize these antigens and produce a range of immune responses to reject the tumor.

17 In spite of the immune system's ability to reject cancer cells, some cancer cells are apparently capable of bypassing the host's immune surveillance and by "escaping" can cause cancer.

18 Proposed "immune surveillance escape mechanisms" include antigenic modulation, secretion of immunosuppressive substances, escape and sneaking through, selective stimulation of suppressor cells, production of blocking antibodies, and immunostimulation.

KEY TERMS

Activated macrophages, 343

α-fetoprotein (α-FP), 339

Antigenic modulation, 342

Blocking antibody, 343

Blocking factor, 343

Carcinoembryonic antigen (CEA), 339

Cocarcinogen, 324

c-onc, 335

Immune surveillance theory, 337

Immunologic stimulation, 343

Immunosuppressive substance, 342

Initiation, 324

Insertional mutagenesis, 337

Oncofetal antigen, 339

Oncogene, 334

Oncogenic virus, 333

Promotion, 324

Proto-oncogene, 336

Retrovirus, 334

Reverse transcriptase, 334

Sneaking through, 343

Suppressor T lymphocyte, 343

Tumor-associated antigen (TAA)

Viral antigen, 338

v-onc, 335

REFERENCES

American Cancer Society. 1986. *Cancer manual* (7th ed.). Boston: The Society.

American Cancer Society. 1989. *Cancer statistics, 1989.* New York: The Society.

American Cancer Society. 1989. *A cancer journal for clinicians.* New York: The Society.

Ames, B. N. (1983). Dietary carcinogens and anticarcinogens. *Science, 221,* 1256.

Ames, B. N., Magaw, R., & Gold, L. S. (1987). Ranking possible carcinogenic hazards. *Science, 236,* 271-280.

Androphy, E. J., & Lowy, D. R. (1984). Tumor viruses, oncogenes, and human cancer. *Journal of the American Academy of Dermatology, 10,* 125.

Armstrong, B., & Doll, R. (1975). Bladder cancer mortality in diabetes in relation to saccharin consumption and smoking habits. *British Journal and Preview of Social Medicine, 30,* 151-157.

Armstrong, B. K., Lea, A. J., Adelstein, A. M., et al. (1976). Cancer mortality and saccharin consumption in diabetics. *British Journal and Preview of Social Medicine, 30,* 151-157.

Bjelke, E. (1975). Dietary vitamin A and human lung cancer. *International Journal of Cancer, 15,* 561-565.

Blott, W. J., & Fraumeni, J. F., Jr. (1982). Geographic epidemiology of cancer in the United States. In D. Schottenfield & J. F. Fraumeni, Jr. (Eds.), *Cancer epidemiology and prevention (pp. 179-193).* Philadelphia: W. B. Saunders.

Boice, J. D., Jr., & Land, C. E. (1982). Ionizing radiation. In D. Schottenfield & J. F. Fraumeni, Jr. (Eds.), *Cancer epidemiology and prevention (pp. 231-253).* Philadelphia: W. B. Saunders.

Boutwell, R. K. (1964). Some biological aspects of skin carcinogenesis. *Progress Experimental Tumor Research, 4,* 207-250.

Brill, B. (Ed.). (1982). *Low-level radiation effects: a fact book.* New York: The Society of Nuclear Medicine.

Brinton, L. A. (1984). Etiologic factors for invasive and noninvasive cervical abnormalities. In E. B. Gold (Ed.), *The changing risk of disease in women: An epidemiologic approach.* Lexington, Mass: The Collamore Press.

Buchler, D. A. (1983). Cervical cancer. In B. S. Kahn et al., (Eds.), *Concepts in cancer medicine*. New York: Grunne & Stratton.

Bulbrook, R. D., Moore, J. W., Clark, G. M. G., Wang, D. Y., Tong, D., & Hayward, J. L. (1978). Plasma oestradiol and progesterone levels in women with varying degrees of risk of breast cancer. *European Journal of Cancer, 14,* 1369-1375.

Burkitt, D. (1969). Related disease: related cause. *Lancet, 2,* 1229-1231.

Burnet, M. (1970). *Immunological surviellance*. London: Pergamon Press.

Carroll, K. K. (1975). Experimental evidence of dietary factors and hormone-dependent cancers. *Cancer Research, 35,* 3374-3383.

Centers for Disease Control. (1983a). Oral contraceptive use and the risk of ovarian cancer. *JAMA, 249,* 1594-1599.

Centers for Disease Control. (1983b). Oral contraceptive use and the risk of endometrial cancer. *JAMA, 249,* 1600-1604.

Cowan, L. D., Gordis, L., Tonascia, J. A., & Jones, G. S. (1981). Breast cancer incidence in women with a history of progesterone deficiency. *American Journal of Epidemiology, 114,* 209-217.

delRegato, J. A., Spjut, H. J., & Cox, J. D. (1985). *Ackerman and del Regato's cancer: Diagnosis, treatment, and prognosis* (6th ed.). St. Louis: The C. V. Mosby Co.

Devesa, S. S., & Diamond, E. L. (1980). Association of breast cancer and cervical cancer incidences with income and education among whites and blacks. *National Cancer Institute, 65,* 515-528.

Doll, R., & Peto, R. (1981). *The causes of cancer*. New York: Oxford University Press.

Epstein, S. S., & Swartz, J. B. (1981). Fallacies of lifestyle cancer theories. *Nature, 289,* 127.

Epstein, S. S., & Swartz, J. B. (1988). Technical comments: Carcinogenic risk estimates. *Science, 240,* 1043-1045.

Fine, D. N., Ross, D., Raunbehler, D. P., et al. (1977). Formation in vivo of volatile N-nitrosamines in man after ingestion of cooked bacon and spinach. *Nature, 265,* 753-754.

Foley, E. J. (1953). Antigenic properties of methlcholanthrene-induced tumors in mice of the strain of origin. *Cancer Research, 13,* 835.

Franks, L. M., & Teich, N. (1986). *Introduction to the cellular and molecular biology of cancer*. New York: Oxford University Press.

Gold, E. B. (Ed.). (1984). *The changing risk of disease in women: an epidemiologic approach*. Lexington, Mass: Collamore Press.

Greenwald, P. (1985). Prevention of cancer. In V. T. Devita, S. Hellman, & S. A. Rosenberg (Eds.), *Cancer: Principles and practice of oncology* (2nd ed.). Philadelphia: J. B. Lippincott.

Hammond, E. C., Selikoff, I. J., & Seidman, H. (1979). Asbestos exposure, cigarette smoking, and death rates. *Annual of the New York Academy of Science, 330,* 473-490.

Herbst, A. L., Ultelder, H., & Poskanzer, D. C. (1971). Adenocarcinomas of the vagina: Association of maternal stilbestrol therapy with tumor appearance in young females. *New England Journal of Medicine, 284,* 878-881.

Higgins, J., & Muir, C. S. (1982). Epidemiology of cancer. In

J. F. Holland & E. Frei (Eds.), *Cancer medicine* (2nd ed.). Philadelphia: Lea & Febiger.

Hood, L. E., Weissman, I. L., & Wood, W. B. (1978). *Immunology*. Menlo Park, Calif: Benjamin/Cummings.

Hulka, B. S., Fowler, W. D., Kaufman, D. G., Grimson, R. C., Greenberg, B. G., Hogue, C. J., Berger, G. S., & Pulliam, C. C. (1980). Estrogen and endometrial cancer: cases and two control groups. *North Carolina American Journal of Obstetrics and Gynecology, 137,* 92-101.

Hulka, B. S. (1984). Estrogens and endometrial cancer. In E. B. Gold (Ed.), *The changing risk of disease in women: an epidemiologic approach*. Lexington, MA:Collamore Press.

Johnson, G. H., & Smith, W. G. (1986). Genital warts. *Gynecological Oncology, 3,* 18-22.

Kahn, H. A. (1966). The dorn study of smoking and mortality among U.S. veterans: Report on eight and one-half years of observation. *National Cancer Institute Monograph, 19,* 1-125.

Kennett, R. H., McKearn, T. J., & Bechtol, K. B. (1980). *Monoclonal antibodies*. New York: Plenum Publishing.

Kessler, I. I. (1970). Cancer mortality among diabetics. *Journal of the National Cancer Institute, 44, 673-686.*

King, D. W., Fenoglio, C. M., & Lefkowitch, J. H. (1983). *General pathology*. Philadelphia: Lea & Febiger.

Kline, G., Sjogren, H. O., Klein, E., & Hellstrom, K. E. (1960). Demonstration of resistance against methylcholanthrene-induced sarcomas in the primary autochthonous host. *Cancer Research, 20,* 1561.

Land, H., Parada, L. F., & Weinberg, R. A. (1983). Cellular oncogenes and multistep carcinogenesis. *Science, 222, 771.*

Lasnitzki, I. (1955). The influence of hyper-vitaminosis on the effect of 20-methylcholanthrene on mouse prostate glands grown in vitro. *British Journal of Cancer, 9,* 438-439.

Linsell, C. A., & Peers, F. G. (1977). Field studies on liver cell cancer. In H. H. Hiah, J. D. Watson, & S. A. Weinsten (Eds.), *Origins of human cancer.(pp. 549-556)*. Cold Spring Harbor, NY: Cold Spring Harbor Laboratory.

Micha, J. P. (1984). Genital warts: Treatable warning of cancer. *The Female Patient, 9,* 31-34.

Miller, E. C., & Miller, J. A. (1979). Naturally occurring carcinogens that may be present in foods. In A. Neuberger & T.H. Jukes (Eds.). *Biochemistry of nutrition on IA*. Baltimore: University Park Press.

Naor, D. (1979). Suppressor cells: permitters and promotors of malignancy? *Advanced Cancer Research, 29,* 45.

Ostrow, R. S., Zachow, K. R., Niimura, M., Okagaki, T., Muller, S., Bender, M., & Faras, A. J. (1986). Detection of papilloma virus DNA in human semen. *Science, 231,* 731-733.

Palmer, S., & Bakshi, K. (1986). Public health considerations in reducing cancer risk: Interim dietary guidelines. *Seminars in Oncology, X(3),* 342-347.

Penn, I. (1981). Depressed immunity and the development of cancer. *Clinical and Experimental Immunology, 46, 459-474.*

Pitot, H. C. (1985). Cancer biology: Chemical carcinogens. In V. T. DeVita, S. Hellman, & S. T. Rosenberg (Eds.), *Cancer: principles and practices of oncology*. Philadelphia: J. B. Lippincott.

Prehn, R. T. (1971). Perspectives on oncogenesis: does immunity stimulate or inhibit neoplasia? *Journal of the Reticuloendothelial Society, 10,* 1.

Prehn, R. T., & Main, J. M. (1957). Immunity to methylcholanthrene-induced sarcomas. *Journal of the National Cancer Institute, 18,* 769.

Public Health Services. (1985). *Cancer rates & risks* (3rd ed.). Washington, DC: U.S. Government Printing Office [NIH No. 85-691].

Robbins, J. H., Kraemer, K. H., Latmer, M. A., et al. (1974). Xeroderma pigmentosum: An inhcrited disease with sun sensitivity, multiple cutaneous neoplasms, and abnormal DNA repair. *Annual of Interim Medicine, 80,* 221-248.

Roberts, L. K., & Daynes, R. A. (1985). Active immunoregulation toward antigens expressed by ultraviolet radiation-induced skin tumors. In *Experimental and clinical photoimmunology* (vol. III). Boca Raton: CRC Press.

Rous, P., & Kidd, J. G. (1941). Conditional neoplasms and subthreshold neoplastic states. *Journal of Experimental Medicine, 73,* 365.

Rudali, G., Apiou, F., & Muel, B. (1975). Mammary cancer produced in mice with estriol. *European Journal on Cancer, 11,* 39-41.

Ruddon, R. (1981). *Cancer biology.* New York: Oxford University Press.

Schatzkin, A., Hoover, R. N., Brinton, L. A., Harvey, E. B., Licitra, L. M., & Larsen, D. B. (1987). Alcohol consumption and breast cancer in epidemiologic follow-up study of the first national health and nutrition examination survey. *New England Journal of Medicine, 316,* 1169-1173.

Scotto, J., Fears, T. R., & Gori, G. B. (1976). *Measurements of ultraviolet radiation in the United States and comparisons with skin cancer data* (DHEW Publication No. NIH 76-1029, pp. 3.1-3.10). Washington, DC: U.S. Government Printing Office.

Selikoff, I. J., Lilis, R., & Nicholson, W. J. (1979). Asbestos disease in United States shipyards. *Annual of the New York Academy of Science, 330,* 295-311.

Shamberger, R. J., Tytko, S. A., & Willis, C. E. (1976). Antioxidants and cancer VI: Selenium and age adjusted human cancer mortality. *Archives of Environmental Health, 31,* 231-235.

Slamon, D. J., deKernion, J. B., Verma, I. M., & Cline, M. J. (1984). Expression of cellular oncogenes in human malignancies. *Science, 224,* 835.

Spingarn, N. E., Slocum, L. A., & Weisburger, J. H. (1980). Formation of mutagens in cooked foods II: foods with high starch content. *Cancer Letters, 9,* 7-12.

Stehelin, D., Varmus, H. F., Bishop, J. M., & Vogt, P. K. (1976). DNA related to the transforming gene(s) of avian sarcoma viruses is present in normal avian DNA. *Nature, 269,* 170-173.

Uhr, J. W. (1984). Immunotoxins: harnessing nature's poisons. *Journal of Immunology, 133,* i.

Weinstein, I. B. (1976). Molecular events in chemical carcinogenesis. *Advanced Pathobiology, 4,* 106.

Willett, W. C., Stampfer, M. J., Colditz, G. A., Rosner, B. A., Hennekens, C. H., & Speizer, F. E. (1987a). Fat and the risk of breast cancer. *New England Journal of Medicine, 316*(1), 22-28.

Willett, W. C., Stampfer, M. J., Colditz, G. A., Rosner, B. A., Hennekins, C. H., & Speizer, F. E. (1987b). Moderate alcohol consumption and the risk of breast cancer. *New England Journal of Medicine, 316,* 1174-1180.

Yamasahi, E., & Ames, B.N. (1977). Concentration of mutagens from wine by absorption with the non-polar resin XAD-2: Cigarette smokers have mutagenic wine. *Proceedings of the National Academy of Sciences, 74,* 3555-3559.

Yang, C. S. (1980) Research on esophageal cancer in China: A review. *Cancer Research, 40,* 2633.

Young, D. (1976). Relationship between cigarette smoking, oral contraceptives, and plasma vitamins. *American Journal of Clinical Nutrition, 29,* 1216-1221.

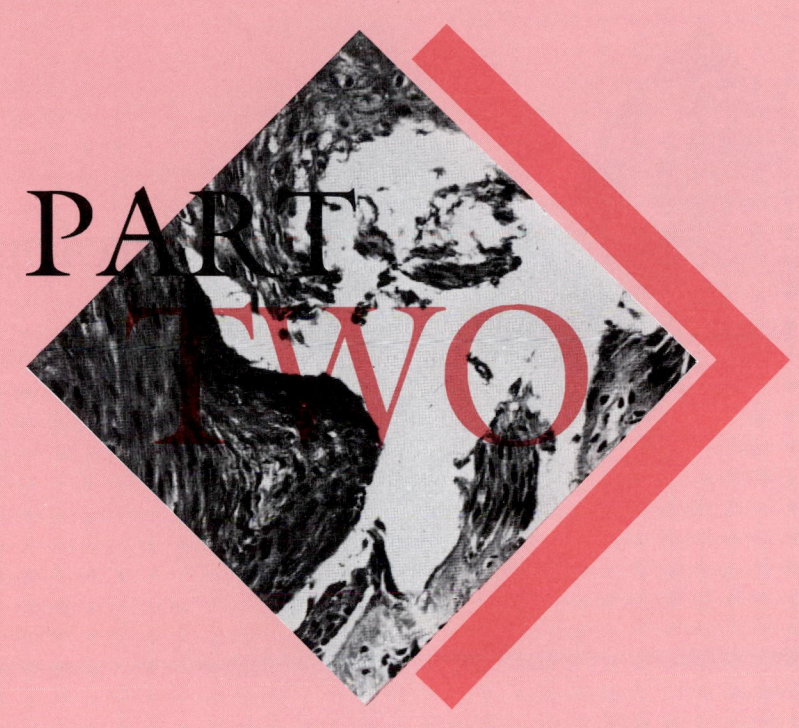

PART TWO

Pathophysiologic Alterations: Organs and Systems

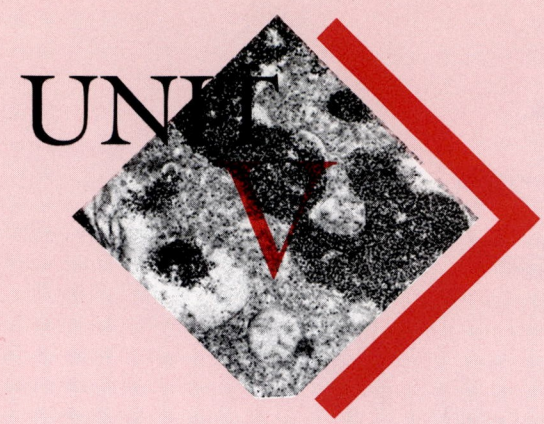

UNIT V

The Neurologic System

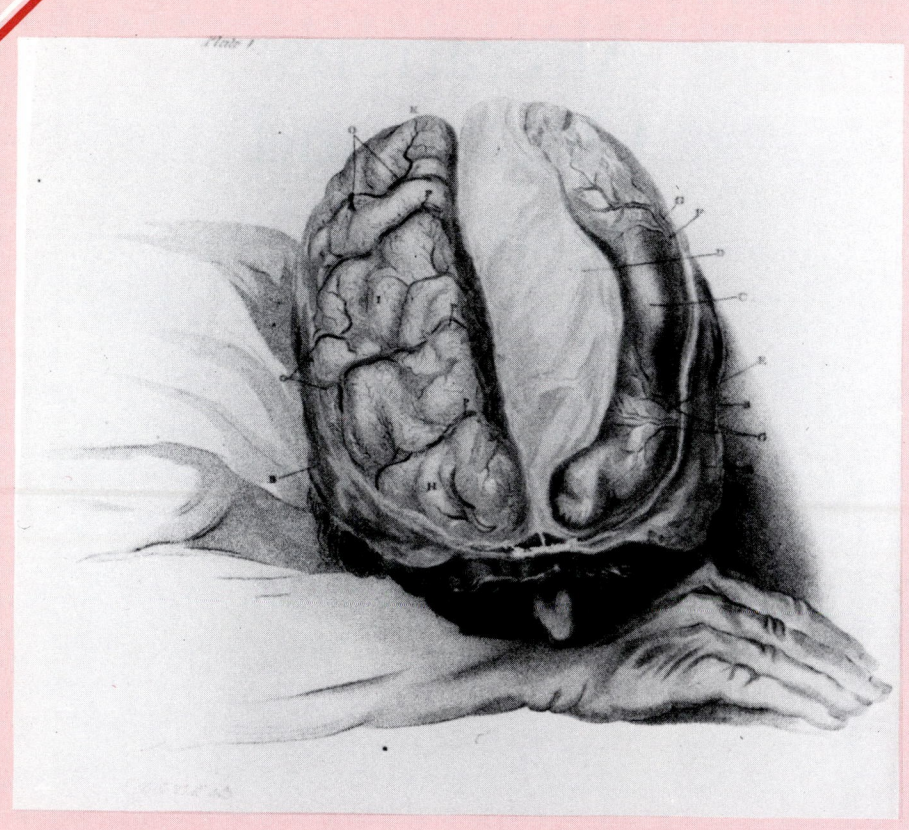

Man's head resting on his right arm, the crown opened to show general anatomy and subdivisions of the brain. (From Bell, Sir Charles: *The anatomy of the brain,* London, 1807. Courtesy National Library of Medicine.)

Treatment of neurologic disease dates back prior to written history. Trephination, the process of cutting away a piece of the skull, dates back to the Neolithic Period (about 7000 to 3000 BC), although no written record exists to provide a rationale for the procedure. Evidence of such procedures have been found in France, Peru, and other widespread geographic areas. The earliest written record of the study and treatment of neurologic disease, known as the Edwin Smith papyrus, consists of 48 hypothetical cases of neurologic disease and dysfunction with prognosis and management; it dates back to 1600 BC and represents a copy of an older work.

Although the Greeks believed the heart was the source of human thought and feelings, and that animal spirit was made in the ventricles and resided there to be distributed by hollow nerve fibers to the body, Hippocrates (born 460 BC) did fairly accurately describe facial paralysis, sciatica, the complex of headache, visual disturbance, and vomiting in his writings. He accurately described signs associated with disorders of the brain, such as aphasia, unconsciousness, pupillary inequality, ophthaloplegia, and respiratory and cardiovascular irregularities. This Greek physician was aware that injury to one side of the head could be followed by convulsions or paralysis of the contralateral extremities, that compression of the spinal cord had functional effects, and that dural lacerations had a poor prognosis. His writings contain the first recorded description of trephination and vertebral dislocation reduction.

Galen, a noted Greek physician of the second century AD, having studied brain structure through animal dissection and brain function and injury while he served as physician to gladiators in Rome, tried to refute the belief that the heart (and not the brain) was the center of human thought, with limited success. Little progress was made for centuries. What would become the fields of neuroanatomy, neurophysiology, and neuropathology began to advance slightly in the fourteenth century when Italian medical schools were permitted to authorize the dissection of human cadavers. Laws gradually became so liberalized that nonphysicians, like Leonardo DaVinci could conduct dissections. Although DaVinci's neurophysiology was wanting (he declared that the first ventricle mediated imagination and common sense, the second ventricle mediated reasoning, and the third mediated memory), his drawings and the drawings of others in Europe and Britian during the 1600s and 1700s were amazingly accurate and detailed. Willis, in 1664, was the man who finally retired the belief that the ventricles were more important than the brain, itself a pivotal point in the emergence of modern neuroscience. The door was opened for study of the localization of function within the nervous system, although this emergence had to wait two centuries while the search for localization of the soul in the brain was pursued and the theory of phenomology overshadowed attempts to study the relationship between neuroanatomy and neural function.

Broca, a general surgeon, initiated the localization work with his basic discovery of the motor speech area named after him in 1861. Neurologists and neurosurgeons, like Wernicke, Foerster, and Penfield, advanced the science of neurophysiology, along with other neuroscientists and histologists.

Neuropathology had its true birth in the latter part of the 1800s and the early 1900s. Charcot is viewed as one of the principal founders of the field. Using simple staining techniques, Charcot established the histologic basis of a number of nervous system diseases. Charcot and his pupils—Marie, Dejerione, and Babinski—established the anatomic and clinical classification of neurologic processes. Cajal, a Spaniard, provided early knowledge of synapses and supported von Waldeyer's Neuron Theory, while German neuroscientists—Nissl, Alzheimer, Spiermeyer, and Weigert—established the basic neurohistopathology of nervous system disorders. The study of the neuropathology of specific diseases and the origin and pathogenesis of specific features, such as ischemia, inflammation, and edema, were clearly launched. Technologic advances in this century, including the electron microscope, histochemistry, computed axial tomography scanning (CT scanning), positron emission tomography (PET), and nuclear magnetic resonance scanning (MRI), are now rapidly advancing the field.

CHAPTER 12

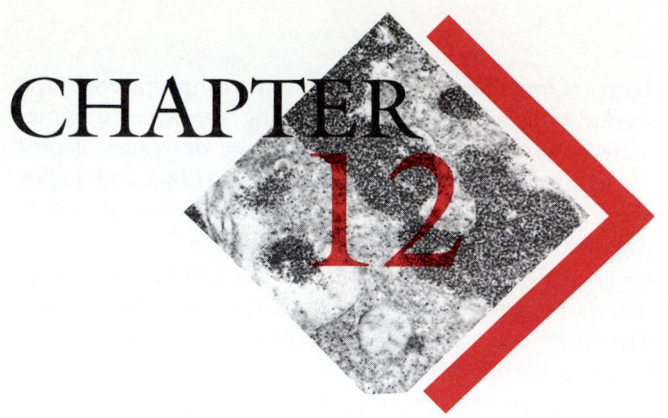

Structure and Function of the Neurologic System

Peter M. Sunderland

Structure and function of the nervous system, 352
Cells of the nervous system, 353
  The neuron, 353
  Neuroglia and Schwann cells, 355
  Nerve injury and regeneration, 356
The nerve impulse, 356
  Synapses, 356
  Neurotransmitters, 357
The central nervous system, 357
  The brain, 357
    Forebrain, 359
      Telencephalon, 359
      Diencephalon, 360
    Midbrain, 361
    Hindbrain, 362
      Metencephalon, 362
      Myelencephalon, 362
  The spinal cord, 362
  Protective structures of the central nervous system, 365
    Cranium, 365
    Meninges, 366
    Cerebrospinal fluid and the ventricular system, 367
    Vertebral column, 367
  Blood supply of the central nervous system, 368
    Blood supply to the brain, 368
    Blood-brain barrier, 370
    Blood supply to the spinal cord, 371
The peripheral nervous system, 371
The autonomic nervous system, 372
  Anatomy of the sympathetic nervous system, 376
  Anatomy of the parasympathetic nervous system, 377
  Neurotransmitters and neuroreceptors, 378
  Functions of the autonomic nervous system, 378
Aging and the nervous system, 380
  Structural changes with aging, 380
  Cellular changes with aging, 382
  Functional changes with aging, 383
Tests of nervous system function, 383
  Skull and spine roentgenograms, 383

Computerized tomography (CT), 383
Magnetic resonance imaging (MRI), 383
Positron emission tomography (PET scan), 385
Brain scan, 385
Cerebral angiography, 385
Myelography, 385
Echoencephalography (ultrasound), 385
Electroencephalography (EEG), 385
Evoked potentials (EVP), 385
Cerebrospinal fluid (CSF) analysis, 385

STRUCTURE AND FUNCTION OF THE NERVOUS SYSTEM

The human nervous system is a remarkable structure responsible for the body's ability to interact with the environment, and for the regulation of activities involving internal organs. The nervous system literally drives the other systems of the body. It is a network composed of complex structures that transmit signals—both electrically and chemically—from the body's many organs and tissues to the brain.

Although the nervous system functions as a unified whole, it contains many divisions. Structurally, the nervous system is divided into the central nervous system (CNS) and the peripheral nervous system (PNS). The **central nervous system** consists of the brain and spinal cord, enclosed within the rigid cranial vault and the bony spine. The **peripheral nervous system** is composed of the **cranial nerves** which communicate with the brain through foramina (openings) in the skull, and the **spinal nerves,** which communicate through the spinal cord. Peripheral nerve pathways are differentiated into **afferent pathways** that carry sensory impulses toward the central nervous system, and **efferent pathways** that innervate skeletal muscle or effector organs by transmitting motor impulses away from the CNS.

Functionally, the peripheral nervous system can be divided into the somatic nervous system and the autonomic nervous system. The **somatic nervous system** consists of pathways regulating voluntary motor control (i.e., skeletal muscle). The **autonomic nervous system** is involved with regulation of the body's internal environment (viscera) through involuntary innervation of organ systems. The autonomic nervous system is further divided into sympathetic and parasympathetic divisions. Organs innervated by specific components of the nervous system are called **effector organs.**

CELLS OF THE NERVOUS SYSTEM

Two basic types of cells comprise nervous tissue, neurons and supporting cells. The **neuron** is the primary cell of the nervous system. Working alone or as units, neurons detect environmental changes and initiate body responses to maintain a dynamic steady state. The supporting cells, such as the **neuroglial cells** of the central nervous system and the **Schwann cells** of the peripheral nervous system, provide structural support and nutrition for the neurons.

The Neuron

The neuronal structure varies markedly, so that each neuron is adapted to perform specialized functions. Neurons share many of the same metabolic activities and constituents as other types of cells. The fuel source for the neuron is predominantly glucose; insulin is not required for cellular glucose uptake in the central nervous system. Neurons also have unique cellular constit-

uents, microtubules, neurofibrils, microfilaments, and nissl substances. **Microtubules, microfilaments,** and **neurofibrils** are believed to be involved in transport of cellular products. **Nissl substances** are involved in protein synthesis. An entire neuron, because it lacks centrosomes, lacks the ability to regenerate. Cell division ceases at the time of birth and the neuron is unable to divide and replace itself.

A neuron (Fig. 12-1) has three components: a cell body (soma) and the thin processes of the cell, the dendrites and the axons. The intracellular organelles within the **cell body** are similar to other cells of the body. They lack, however, the cellular machinery to reproduce themselves. Most cell bodies are located within the central nervous system. Cells bodies located outside the central nervous system, in the peripheral nervous system, are usually found in groups called **ganglia.** The **dendrites** are extensions of the cell body that carry nerve impulses toward the cell body. The **dendritic zone** is the receptive portion of a neuron where an electrical stimulus originates. **Axons** are long, conductive projections from the cell body that carry nerve impulses away from the cell body. The **axon hillock** is the cone-shaped process where the axon leaves the cell body. A typical neuron has only one axon. The axon may be covered with a segmented layer of lipid material called **myelin,** which acts as an insulating substance. The entire membrane is referred to as the **myelin sheath,** while the thin membrane between the myelin sheath and the **endoneurium** is the **neurilemma,** or **Schwann's sheath.** The neurilemma and the myelin sheath are interrupted at regular intervals by the **nodes of Ranvier.** Axons are capable of extensive branching, which occurs at the nodes of Ranvier. The principle of divergence refers to the ability of these branches to influence many different

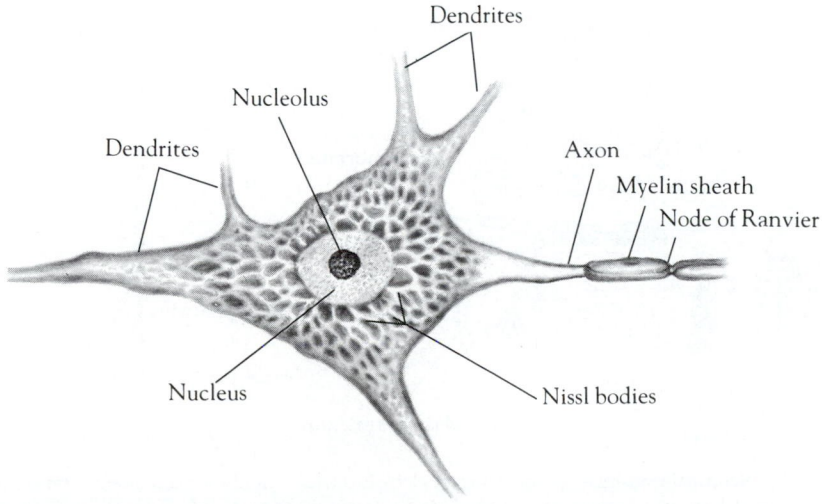

FIG. 12-1. Diagram of neuron with composite parts. (From Rudy, 1984.)

neurons. Convergence is the term applied to branches of various numbers of neurons "converging" on and influencing a single neuron. Exchange of nutrients is not possible through the myelin sheath, although nutrient exchange can occur at the nodes of Ranvier. The presence of myelin is associated with an increase in the velocity of nerve impulses. Myelin acts as an insulator that allows ions to flow between segments rather than along the entire length of the membrane, resulting in this in-

creased velocity. This mechanism is referred to as **saltatory conduction.** Disorders of the myelin sheath (demyelinating diseases), such as multiple sclerosis and Guillian Barré syndrome demonstrate the important role myelin plays in nerve function (see Chapter 14). Besides depending on the myelin coating, conduction velocities also depend on the diameter of the axon. Larger axons transmit impulses at a faster rate.

Neurons are structurally classified on the basis of the

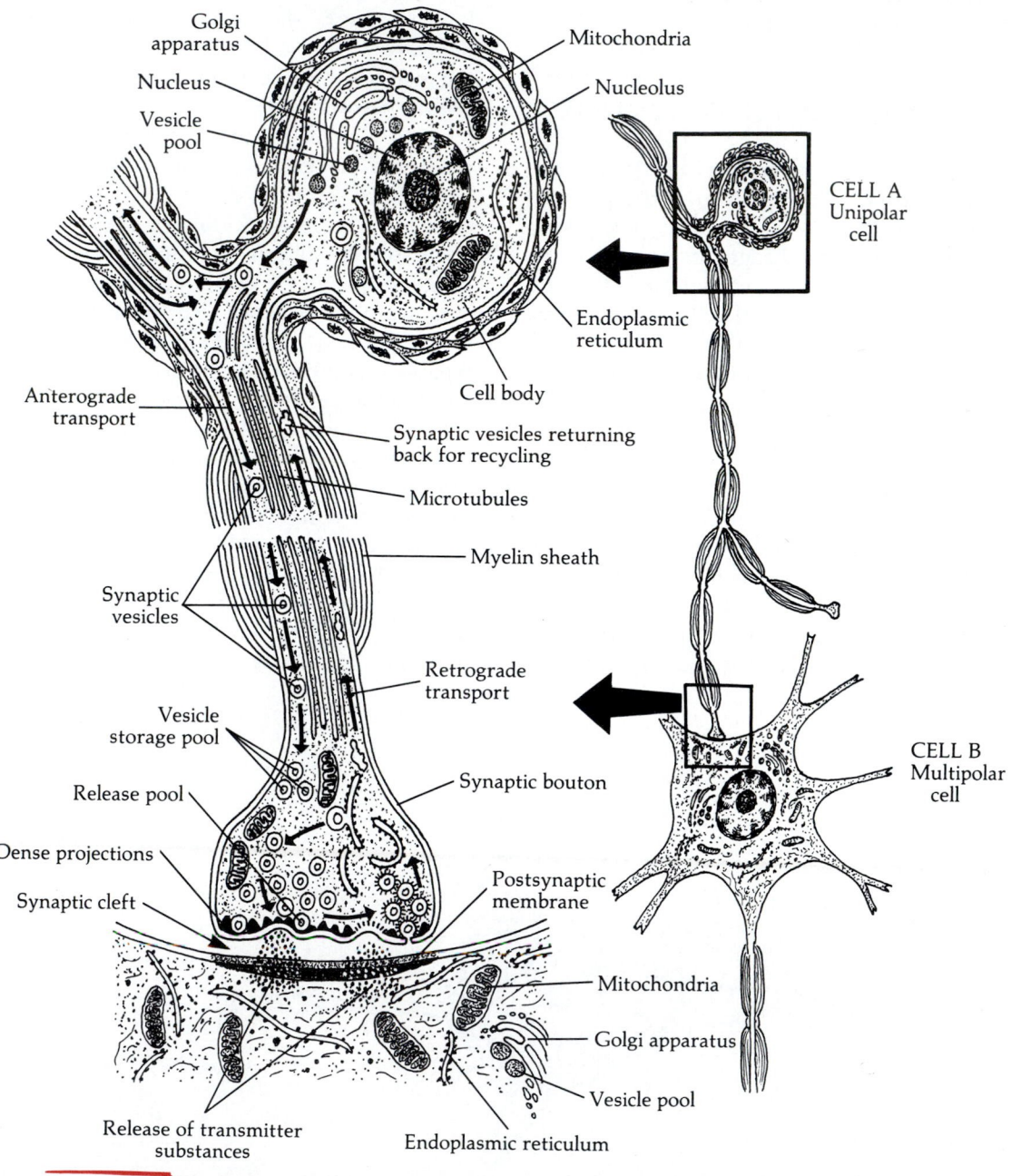

FIG. 12-2. Neuronal transmission and synaptic cleft. Electrical impulse travels along axon of first neuron to synapse. Chemical transmitter is secreted into synaptic space to depolarize membrane (dendrite or cell body) of next neuron in pathway. Cell A represents unipolar cell; cell B represents multipolar cell. (From Thompson et al., 1989.)

number of processes (projections) extending from the cell body. There are three types of projections (1) unipolar, (2) bipolar, and (3) multipolar. **Unipolar neurons** have one process that branches shortly after leaving the cell body. One process extends away from the central nervous system while the other projects into the CNS. Sensory spinal nerves are a good example of unipolar neurons. **Bipolar neurons,** such as rod and cone cells of the retina, have two distinct processes arising from the cell body. **Multipolar neurons** are the most common in the nervous system and have multiple processes capable of branching extensively. A motor neuron is typically multipolar (Fig. 12-2).

Functionally, there are three types of neurons: (1) motor (efferent, multipolar), (2) sensory (afferent, mostly unipolar), and (3) interneuron (association, multipolar). **Motor** neurons transmit impulses away from the central nervous system to an effector. They form a **neuromuscular** or **myoneural junction** with the skeletal muscles they supply. **Sensory** neurons carry impulses from peripheral sensory receptors to the central nervous system. There are five major types of sensory receptors: (1) **nociceptors** (pain), (2) **mechanoreceptors** (touch, pressure, and mechanical deformation), (3) **photochemical** (light on the retina), (4) **chemoreceptors** (flavors, odors, oxygen levels, osmolarity, and carbon dioxide levels), and (5) **thermoreceptors** (heat and cold). **Interneurons** transmit impulses from one neuron to another and are found only in the central nervous system.

Neuroglia and Schwann Cells

Neuroglia ("nerve glue") are the general classification of cells that support the neurons of the central nervous system. They comprise approximately half of the total brain and spinal cord volume and are five to ten times more numerous than neurons. Different types of neuroglia serve different functions. **Astrocytes,** for example, form points of contact between the nervous and circulatory systems; **oligodendroglia** function to deposit mye-

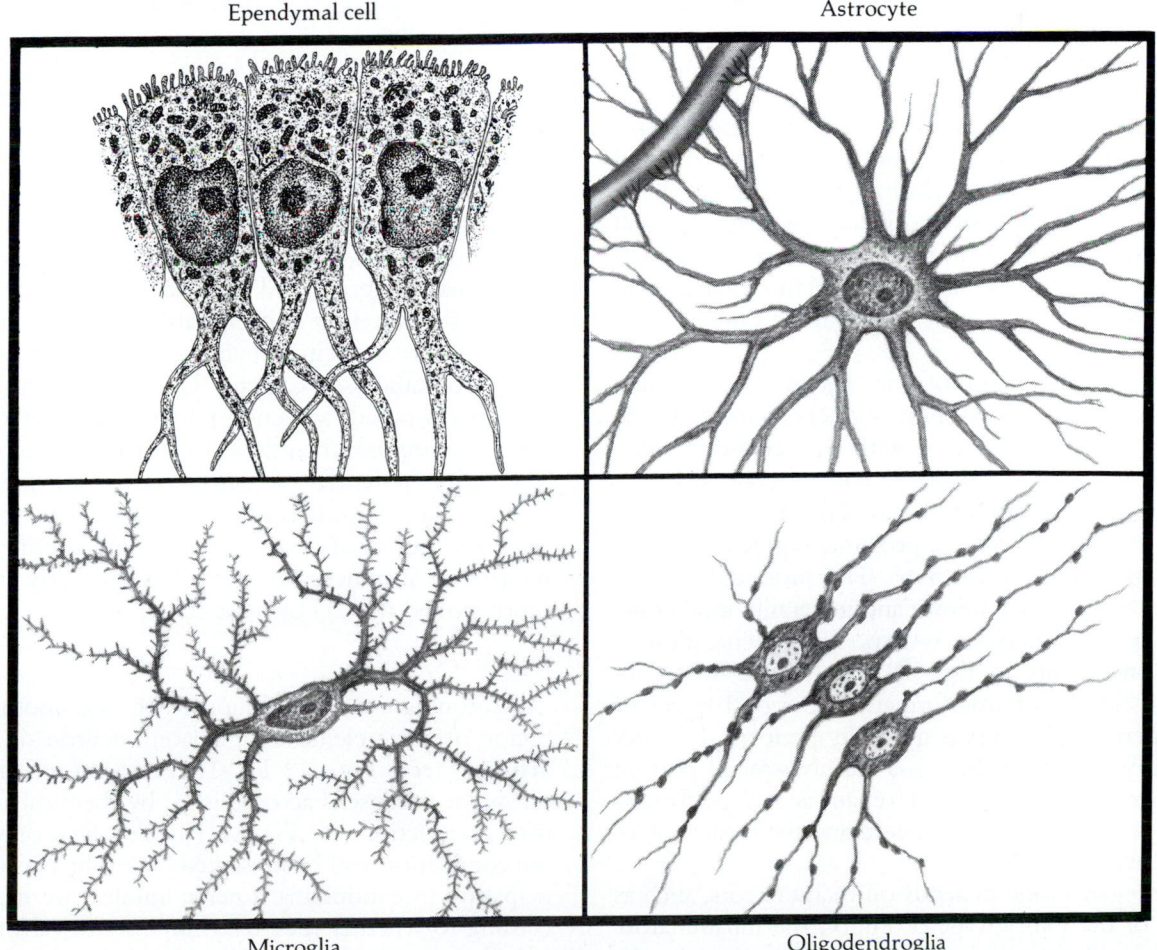

Ependymal cell

Astrocyte

Microglia

Oligodendroglia

FIG. 12-3. Types of neuroglia cells. (From Thompson et al., 1989.)

TABLE 12-1 Support cells of the nervous system	
Cell type	Primary functions
Astrocytes	Form specialized contacts between neuronal surfaces and blood vessels
	Provide for rapid transport for nutrients and metabolites
	Believed to form an essential component of the blood-brain barrier
	Appear to be the scar-forming cells of the CNS, which may be the foci for seizures
	May play a role in segregating postsynaptic receptor surfaces from other regions
Oligodendroglia	Deposition of myelin within the CNS
Schwann cells	Formation of the myelin sheath and neurilemma in the PNS
Microglia	Responsible for clearing cellular debris-phagocytic properties
Ependymal cells	Serve as a lining for the ventricles and choroid plexuses involved in the production of cerebral spinal fluid

lin within the CNS; **ependymal cells** line portions of the CNS. **Schwann cells** are the counterpart of the oligodendroglia in the peripheral nervous system. **Microglia** function as the brain's garbage collectors. (Characteristics of neuroglia and Schwann cells are summarized in Fig. 12-3 and Table 12-1.)

Nerve Injury and Regeneration

When an axon is severed, a typical sequence of events occurs. A characteristic swelling appears at the distal portion of the axon; the neurofilaments hypertrophy; the myelin sheath shrinks and finally disintegrates; and the axon degenerates and finally disappears. The **neurilemma** usually remains intact. **Wallerian degeneration** is the term describing these changes in the distal axon as a result of injury.

At the proximal end of the injured axon similar changes occur, but only a short segment is affected. The cell body responds to trauma with an increase in metabolic activity, protein synthesis, and mitochondrial activity. Approximately 7 to 14 days after the injury, new neurofibrils project from the proximal segment and may enter the remaining neurilemma. This process, however, is limited to myelinated fibers and generally occurs only in the peripheral nervous system. The regeneration of axonal constituents in the CNS is limited by an increased incidence of scar formation. Surgical repair of injured peripheral nerves is generally performed shortly after injury and when there is a cleanly severed portion of the axon to reconnect. If repair is not performed early, degenerative processes begin and the repair is generally delayed.

Nerve regeneration depends on many factors, such as location of the injury, type of injury, the inflammatory responses, and the process of scarring. The closer to the cell body the nerve is injured, the greater the chances that the nerve cell will die and not regenerate. A crushing type of injury, versus a cut that severs the nerve, affects recovery. A crushed nerve may fully recover, whereas a severed or even partially cut nerve quickly forms a connective tissue scar, blocking the regenerating axonal branches.

THE NERVE IMPULSE

The neuron's basic role is the generation and conduction of electrical and chemical impulses. This is accomplished by selectively changing the electrical potential of its plasma membrane and influencing other nearby neurons by the secretion of chemicals (neurotransmitter). A neuron in its unexcited state maintains a resting membrane potential (see Chapter 1). When the membrane potential is raised, an action potential is generated, and the nerve impulse then flows to all parts of the neuron. The action potential of a neuron is not a graded response. The stimulus is either strong enough to induce an action potential or is too weak, and the membrane remains in its unexcited state. This property is sometimes termed the "all or none response."

Synapses

Neurons are not continuous with one another. The region between elements of adjacent neurons is called a **synapse** (see Fig. 12-1). Transmission of impulses across the synapse is accomplished by chemical and electrical conduction (see Fig. 12-13); however, only chemical conduction will be presented here. The neurons participating in conducting a nerve impulse are named according to whether they relay impulses toward the synapse **(presynaptic neurons)** or away from the synapse **(postsynaptic neurons).** Four basic types of connections occur in regions of contact between the presynaptic and postsynaptic neurons. These are between axons (axoaxonic), axon to cell body (axosomatic), axon to dendrite (axodendritic), and dendrite to dendrite (dendodendritic).

Transmission of impulses across the synapse is accomplished by chemical conduction. When an impulse originates in a presynaptic neuron, the impulse reaches the vesicles, where chemicals **(neurotransmitters)** are stored in the terminal end of the axon (called the **synaptic terminal).** Once released from the vesicles, the neurotransmitters diffuse across the **synaptic cleft** (the space between the neurons) and bind to receptor sites on the plasma membrane of the postsynaptic neuron (see Fig. 12-1).

Neurotransmitters

Because the neurotransmitter is stored on one side of the synaptic cleft and the receptor sites are on the other side, chemical synapses operate in only one direction. Action potentials are therefore transmitted along a multineuronal pathway in only one direction. The binding of the neurotransmitter at the receptor site changes the permeability of the postsynaptic neuron and consequently in its membrane potential. Two possible potentials can then follow: (1) the postsynaptic neuron may be either excited (depolarized) or (2) the postsynaptic neuron's plasma membrane may be inhibited (hyperpolarized). These effects on the plasma membrane of the postsynaptic neuron are referred to as **excitatory postsynaptic potentials (EPSPs)** and **inhibitory postsynaptic potentials (IPSPs).**

A single EPSP is not generally capable of inducing a neuron's action potential and the propagation of the nerve impulse. Whether this occurs depends on the number and frequency of potentials the postsynaptic neuron receives. This concept is referred to as **summation. Temporal summation** (time relationship) refers to the effects of successive impulses received at the same synapse. **Spatial summation** (spacing effect) is the combined effects of impulses a single neuron transmits to different synapses at the same time. **Facilitation** is a term referring to the effect of EPSPs on the plasma membrane potential. The plasma membrane is said to be facilitated when summation has brought the membrane closer to the threshold potential and the stimulus required to induce an action potential is then less. The effect that a chemical neurotransmitter has on the plasma membrane potential depends on the balance of these effects. The mechanisms of convergence, divergence, summation, and facilitation allow for the integrative processes of the nervous system.

There are more than 30 substances suspected of being neurotransmitters. Most noted are norepinephrine, acetylcholine, dopamine, and serotonin. Many of these transmitters have more than one function. For example, norepinephrine in the brain is probably involved in the regulation of mood, in dreaming sleep, and in the maintenance of arousal. Several amino acids are thought to be neurotransmitters, including gamma-aminobutyric acid (GABA), glutamic acid, and aspartic acid. Small chains of amino acids are also known to be neurotransmitters, such as enkephalins and endorphins. These neuropeptides are involved in the perception and integration of pain as well as in emotional experiences.

THE CENTRAL NERVOUS SYSTEM

The Brain

The human brain is credited with a multitude of tasks that make reason, intellectual function, personality, mood, and interaction with the environment possible. The brain is characterized as a pinkish gray organ approximately 3 pounds. It receives approximately 15% to 20% of the total cardiac output. The three major divisions of the brain, based on embryologic origin, are (1) the forebrain, which includes the two cerebral hemispheres; (2) the midbrain, including the corpora quadrigemina, tegmentum, and cerebral peduncles, and (3) the hindbrain, which forms the cerebellum pons and the medulla (see Table 12-2). The midbrain, together with the medulla and pons, comprise the **brainstem,** which connects the hemispheres of the brain, cerebellum, and

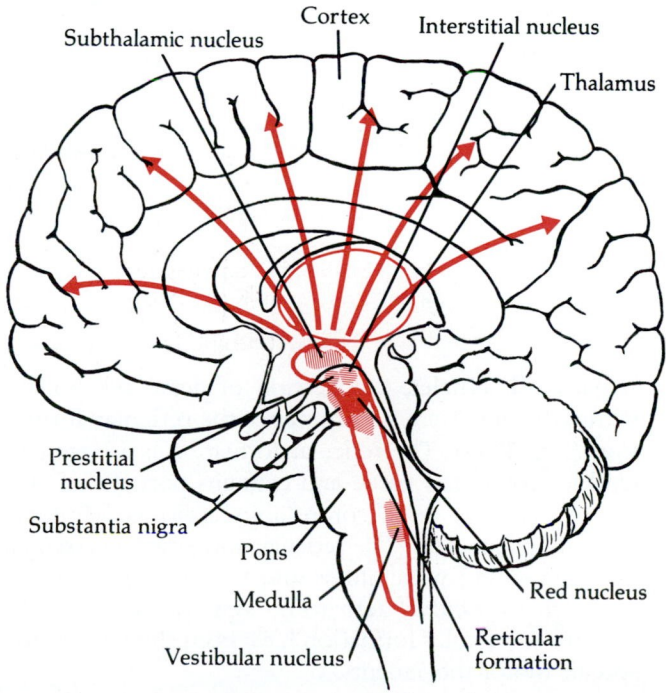

FIG. 12-4. The reticular activating system. (From Rudy, 1984.)

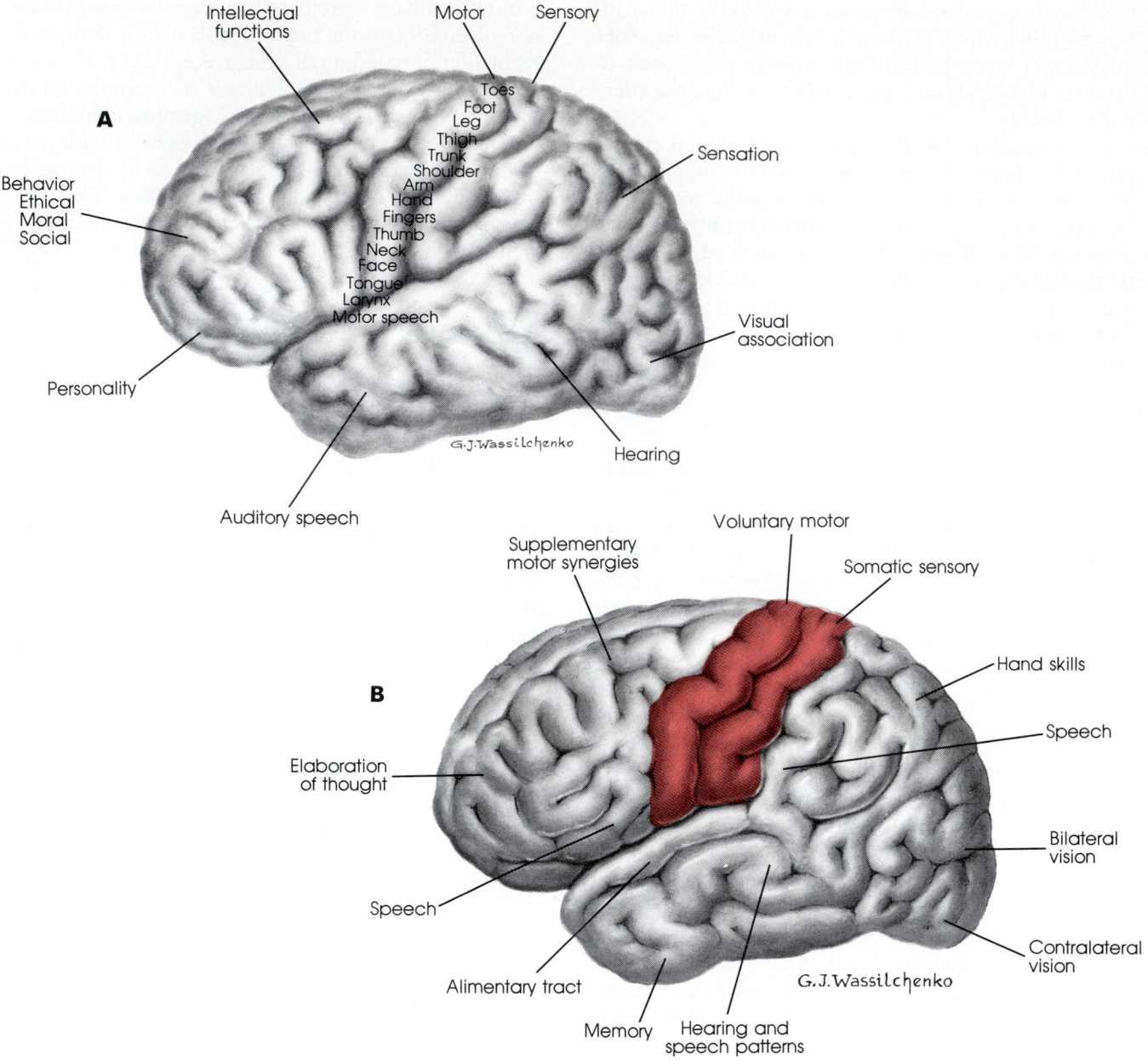

FIG. 12-5. **A,** Principal functional subdivisions of cerebral hemisphere. **B,** Functional areas of specific cortical areas. (From Rudy, 1984.)

spinal cord. **Nuclei,** a collection of nerve cell bodies, within the brainstem also comprise the **reticular formation** (Fig. 12-4). The reticular formation is a large network of connected tissue and contains portions of vital reflexes, such as those controlling cardiovascular function and respiration. The reticular formation is essential for maintaining wakefulness and is, therefore, referred to as the **reticular activating system.** Some nuclei within the reticular formation have been shown to cause specific motor movements.

Divisions of the brain are associated with different functions, but attributing specific functions to definite regions of the brain is not entirely accurate. Many activities may actually be performed in several different regions. Understanding functional destinations is very useful, however, especially when attempting to determine or localize the effects of pathology in various regions.

Many attempts have been made to ascribe function to various regions of the cerebral cortex. A neuropsychiatrist (Brodmann) is credited with postulating various activities to many regions of the cerebral cortex. (Fig. 12-5 illustrates these regions and describes some of the areas.)

TABLE 12-2 Division of the central nervous system

Primary vesicles	Secondary vesicles	Associated structures
Forebrain (Prosencephalon)	Telencephalon	Cerebral hemispheres Cerebral cortex Rhinencephalon Basal ganglia
	Diencephalon	Epithalamus Thalamus Hypothalamus Subthalamus
Midbrain (Mesencephalon)	Mesencephalon	Corpus quadrigemina Tegmentum Cerebral peduncles
Hindbrain (Rhombencephalon)	Metencephalon	Cerebellum Pons
	Myelencephalon	Medulla oblongata
Spinal cord	Spinal cord	Spinal cord

Forebrain

Telencephalon

The **telencephalon** consists of the **cerebrum** (the main portion of the brain), the limbic system, and **basal ganglia** composed of several "nuclei." The surface of the cerebrum is characterized by many convolutions (Fig. 12-6). This irregular structural arrangement increases the surface area in which the nerve cell bodies can lie and thereby maximizes their function. The raised projections on the cerebral surface are termed **gyri,** whereas the grooves are called **sulci.** Deeper grooves are referred to as **fissures.** The **cerebral cortex** (surface of the cerebrum) contains the cell bodies of neurons, a substance termed **gray matter. White matter** lies beneath the ce-

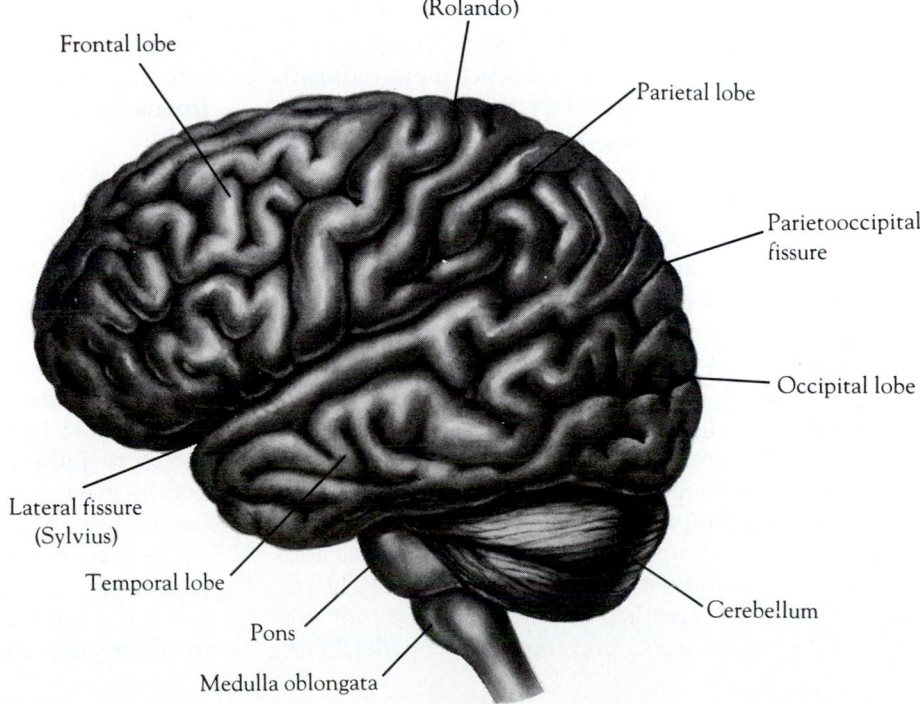

FIG. 12-6. Lateral view of cerebral hemisphere (showing lobes and principal fissures), cerebellum, pons, and medulla oblongata. (From Rudy, 1984.)

rebral cortex (medulla) and is composed of myelinated nerve fibers. Cerebral impulses control function in the opposite side of the body, a phenomenon termed **contralateral control.**

The two cerebral hemispheres are separated by the longitudinal fissure. The surface of each hemisphere is divided into lobes taking their names from the region of the skull under which each of them lies (Fig. 12-6). The **frontal lobe** has its posterior margin on the central fissure, or **fissure of Rolando,** and it borders inferiorly on the lateral fissure, or **sylvian fissure.** The **prefrontal area** is responsible for goal-oriented behavior (i.e., ability to concentrate) and the elaboration of thought. It also exerts an inhibitory influence over the limbic and vegetative areas of the cerebrum. The **premotor area** contains motor programs for fine repetitive motor movements. This area contains the cell bodies that form part of the **extrapyramidal system** (efferent pathways outside the pyramidal pathway that connect the cerebral cortex with spinal nerve pathways). The term *pyramidal* originates from a pyramid-shaped structure in the medulla, where these pathways converge.

The **primary motor area** is located along the **precentral gyrus** and forms the **primary voluntary motor pathway.** The axons traveling from the cell bodies in this region are projection fibers that form the **pyramidal system** that descends into the spinal cord. At the inferior edge of the precentral gyrus (usually in the left hemisphere) is **Broca's speech area.** It is responsible for the motor aspects of speech. Damage to this area, commonly as a result of a cerebrovascular accident (stroke), results in the inability to form words (expressive aphasia) (see Chapter 14).

The **parietal lobe** lies between the borders of the central, parietooccipital, and lateral fissure. This lobe contains the major area for somatic sensory input, primarily located along the **postcentral gyrus,** which is adjacent to the primary motor area. Communication between the motor and sensory areas (and among other regions in the cortex) is provided by **association fibers.** The remainder of this region is involved in sensory association (storage, analysis, and interpretation of sensory stimuli). (Fig. 12-5, *A,* shows the distribution of function associated with both the primary motor area and the primary sensory area of the cerebral cortex.)

The **occipital lobe** lies behind the parietooccipital sulci and above the cerebellum. The primary visual cortex (visual receptive area) is located in this region. The remainder of this lobe is primarily involved in visual association. The **temporal lobe** lies below the lateral fissure. Primary auditory and secondary associational areas account for the primary functional aspects of this region. **Wernicke's area** lies in the superioposterior portion of this region and extends up into the parietal lobe.

This area is responsible for reception and interpretation of speech, and dysfunction may result in receptive aphasia. The temporal lobe is also involved as a major area for memory as well as secondary functions, such as balance, taste, and smell.

Lying directly beneath the longitudinal fissure is a mass of white matter pathways called the **corpus callosum** (transverse or commissural fibers). The corpus callosum connects the two cerebral hemispheres and is essential in the coordination of activities between hemispheres, especially specific tasks that may be present in only one hemisphere (see Fig. 12-14).

The **internal capsule** is a region in which afferent and efferent white matter pathways from the cerebral cortex converge. Located nearby are the basal ganglia, which are composed of corpus striatum, and **amygdala.** In turn, the corpus striatum is composed of the caudate, putamen, and globus pallidus. The **corpus striatum** appears striped because of the connections between its gray matter and the white matter of the internal capsule.

The basal ganglia are considered extensions of the extrapyramidal system. They contain multiple connections to various regions of the CNS and are believed to exert a fine-tuning effect on motor movements. Parkinson disease, and Huntington disease are conditions associated with defects of the basal ganglia. They are characterized by various involuntary or exaggerated motor movements (see Chapters 14 and 15).

The **limbic system** is primarily composed of a group of structures surrounding the corpus callosum, as well as parts of the diencephalon. Its principal effects are believed to be involved with primitive behavioral responses, visceral reaction to emotion, feeding behaviors, biologic rhythms, and the sense of smell. Expression of affect (emotional and behavioral states) are mediated by extensive connections with the limbic system and prefrontal cortex.

Diencephalon

The **diencephalon,** within the cerebrum, is made up of four divisions: **epithalamus, thalamus, hypothalamus,** and **subthalamus** (see Table 12-2 and Fig. 12-7). The epithalamus forms the roof of the third ventricle (a brain cavity) and composes the most superior portion of the diencephalon. It has connections and functions closely associated with those of the limbic system. For example, the hormones of the pineal body have been shown to influence reproductive ability and the secretion of melatonin is associated with circadian rhythms (see Chapter 17).

The largest component of the diencephalon is the thalamus. It borders and surrounds the third ventricle, and it is a major integrating center for afferent impulses to the cerebral cortex. The perception of various sensa-

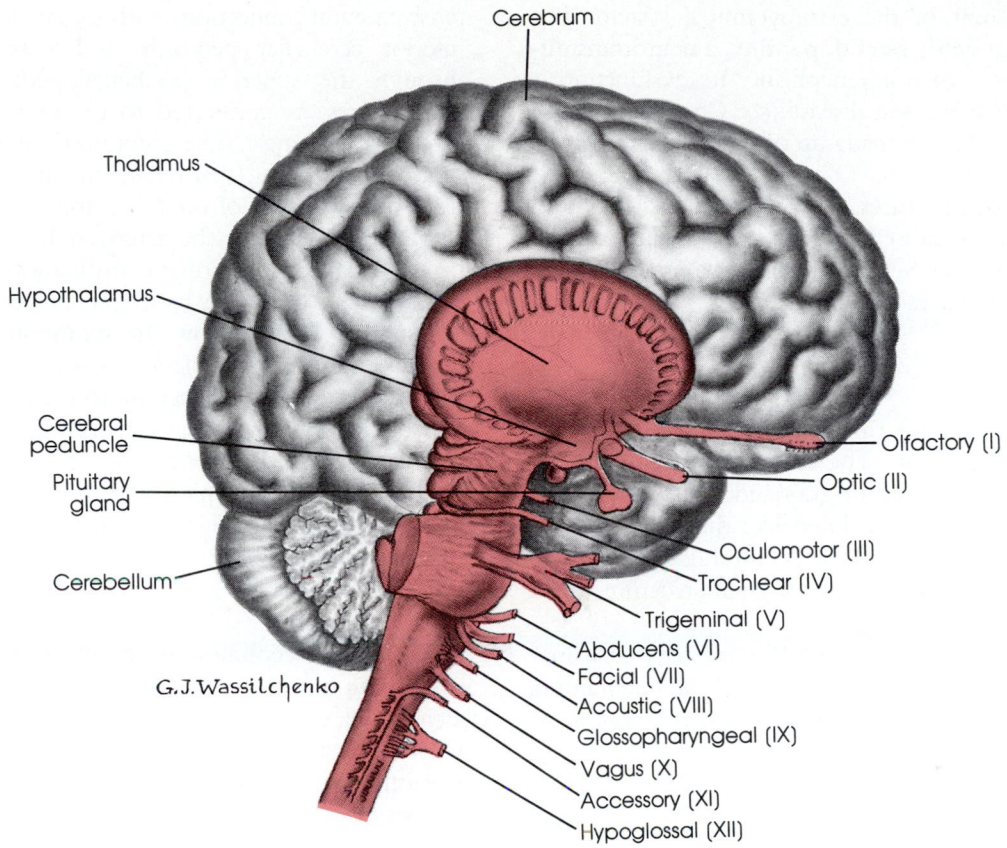

Cerebrum

Thalamus

Hypothalamus

Cerebral peduncle

Pituitary gland

Cerebellum

G.J.Wassilchenko

Olfactory (I)

Optic (II)

Oculomotor (III)

Trochlear (IV)

Trigeminal (V)

Abducens (VI)

Facial (VII)

Acoustic (VIII)

Glossopharyngeal (IX)

Vagus (X)

Accessory (XI)

Hypoglossal (XII)

FIG. 12-7. The diencephalon (thalamus and hypothalamus) and cranial nerves. (From Rudy, 1984.)

tions occurs at this level but requires cortical processing for interpretation. The thalamus also serves as a relay center for information from the basal ganglia and cerebellum that is sent to the appropriate portion of the motor area.

The hypothalamus forms the base of the diencephalon. Hypothalamic function falls into two major areas: (1) maintenance of a constant internal environment and (2) behavioral patterns. Integrative centers control autonomic nervous system function, regulation of body temperature, endocrine function, and regulation of emotional expression. (Temperature regulation is discussed in Chapter 13.) The hypothalamus exerts its influence through the endocrine system as well as neural pathways (see the box at right for a more detailed description). (Endocrine functions of the hypothalamus and pituitary are discussed in Chapter 17.)

The subthalamus flanks the hypothalamus laterally. It serves as an important extrapyramidal center for motor activities.

Midbrain

The midbrain (**mesencephalon**) is composed of three structures: the **corpora quadrigemina** (composed of

the superior and inferior colliculi), the **tegmentum** (containing the red nucleus and substantia nigra), and the cerebral peduncles.

The **superior colliculi** are involved with voluntary and involuntary visual motor movements (e.g., the ability to follow objects). The **inferior colliculi** accomplish similar motor activities but involve movements affecting the auditory system (such as positioning of the head to improve hearing). The **red nucleus** and **substantia ni-**

Functions of the Hypothalamus

Visceral and somatic responses
Affectual responses
Hormone synthesis
Autonomic nervous system activity
Temperature regulation
Feeding responses
Physical expression of emotions
Sexual behavior
Pleasure-punishment centers
Awakeness

gra are extensions of the extrapyramidal system. The substantia nigra synthesizes **dopamine,** a neurotransmitter and precursor of norepinephrine. Its dysfunction is associated with Parkinson disease (see Chapter 15). The **cerebral peduncles** are made up of efferent fibers of the corticospinal tract.

Other notable structures of this region are the nuclei of the third and fourth cranial nerves. The **cerebral aqueduct** (aqueduct of Sylvius), which carries cerebrospinal fluid, also traverses this structure.

Hindbrain

Metencephalon

The major structures of the **metencephalon** are the cerebellum and the pons. The **cerebellum** (see Figs. 12-6 and 12-7) is composed of gray and white matter and its cortical surface is convoluted like the surface of the cerebrum. It is also divided by a central fissure into two lobes that are connected by a midline structure called the **vermis.**

The cerebellum is responsible for reflexive, involuntary fine-tuning of motor control and for maintaining balance and posture. This is accomplished through ex-

tensive neural connections with the medulla through the inferior cerebellar peduncle and with the midbrain through the superior cerebellar peduncle. The two hemispheres are connected to the pons by the middle cerebellar peduncle. These connections allow extensive sampling of visual, vestibular, and proprioceptive data from other regions of the CNS and periphery. Damage to the cerebellum is characterized by a loss of equilibrium, balance, and motor coordination.

The **pons** (bridge) is easily recognized by its bulging appearance. It lies below the midbrain and above the medulla. Its primary function is the transmission of information from the cerebellum to the brainstem and between the two cerebellar hemispheres. The pons is an important center for the control of respiration (i.e., rate and relationship of inspiration to expiration). The nuclei of the fifth through eighth cranial nerves are located in this structure.

Myelencephalon

The **myelencephalon** is usually called the **medulla oblongata** and forms the lowest portion of the brainstem. Reflex activities, such as heart rate, respiration, blood pressure, coughing, sneezing, swallowing, and vomiting, are controlled in this area. The nuclei of cranial nerves IX through XII are also located in this region.

The medulla is the point at which a major portion of the descending motor pathways (i.e., corticospinal tracts) cross to the other side, or decussate (Fig. 12-8). These pathways, together with other areas of decussation in the CNS, are the basis for the phenomenon of contralateral control. Sleep-wake rhythms are also processed by neural influences from lower brain centers and are associated with a complex group of diffuse structures and functions (see Chapter 13). Among these structures is the reticular activating system, a system of cells that receives collateral signals from the afferent sensory pathways and projects the signals to the higher brain centers, thus controlling CNS activity.

The Spinal Cord

The **spinal cord,** an extension of the CNS, lies within the vertebral canal and is surrounded and protected by the **vertebral column.** The spinal cord essentially functions as a large nerve cable that connects the brain and body. It extends from the medulla and ends at the level of the first or second lumbar vertebrae (Fig. 12-9). The end of the spinal cord is cone-shaped and is termed the **conus medullaris.** Spinal nerves continue from the end of the spinal cord and are called the **cauda equina.**

A cross section of the spinal cord (Fig. 12-10) is characterized by a butterfly-shaped inner core of gray matter (containing nerve cell bodies). In the center of this region lies the **central canal,** which extends through the

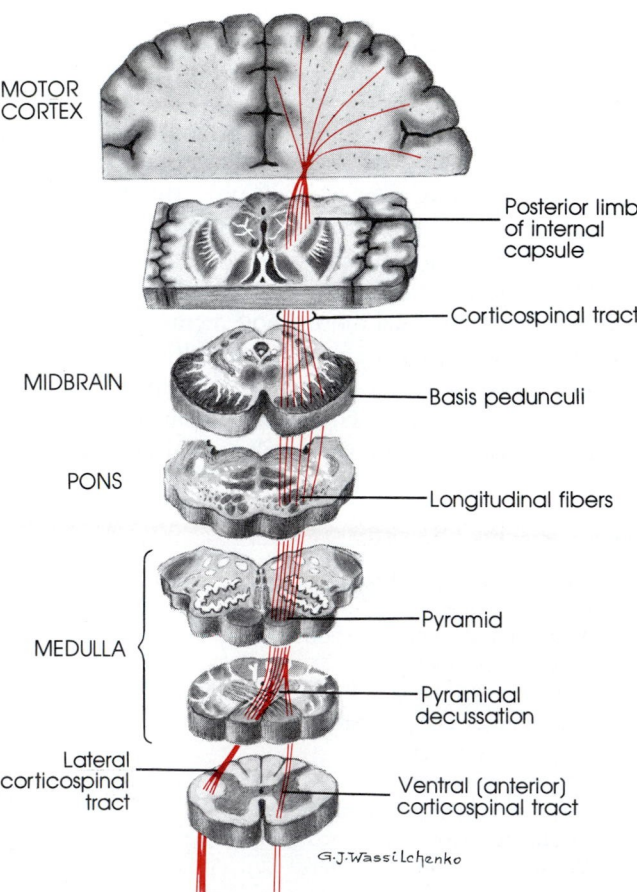

MOTOR CORTEX

Posterior limb of internal capsule

Corticospinal tract

MIDBRAIN

Basis pedunculi

PONS

Longitudinal fibers

Pyramid

MEDULLA

Pyramidal decussation

Lateral corticospinal tract

Ventral (anterior) corticospinal tract

G.J.Wassilchenko

FIG. 12-8. Schematic drawing of decussation of pyramids at level of medulla. (From Rudy, 1984.)

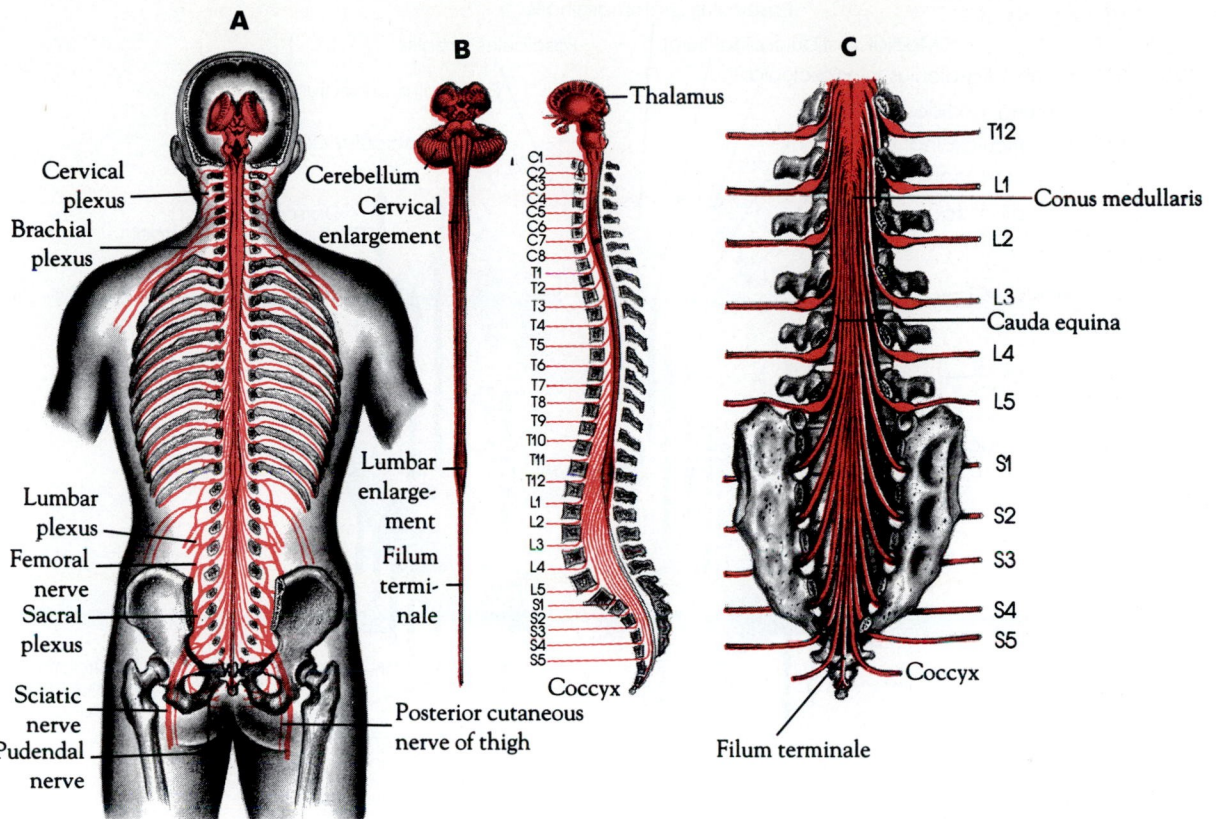

FIG. 12-9. Spinal cord within vertebral canal and exiting spinal nerves. **A,** Posterior view of brainstem and spinal cord in situ with spinal nerves and plexus. **B,** Anterior view of brainstem and spinal cord. **C,** Enlargement of caudal area showing termination of spinal cord (conus medullaris) and group of nerve fibers constituting the cauda equina. (From Rudy, 1984.)

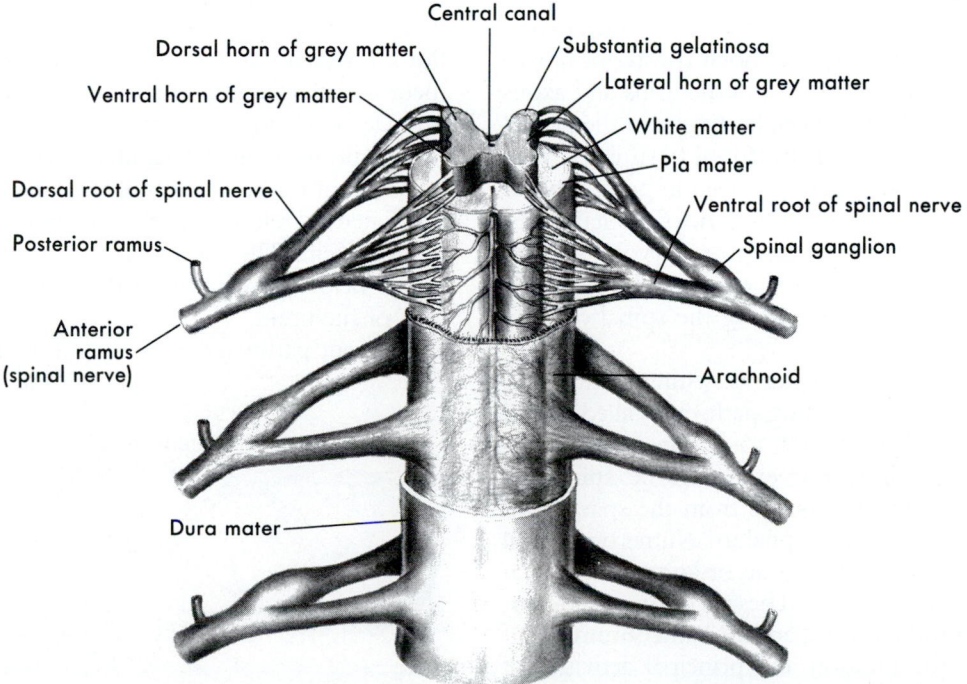

FIG. 12-10. Cross section of spinal cord showing attachments of spinal nerves.

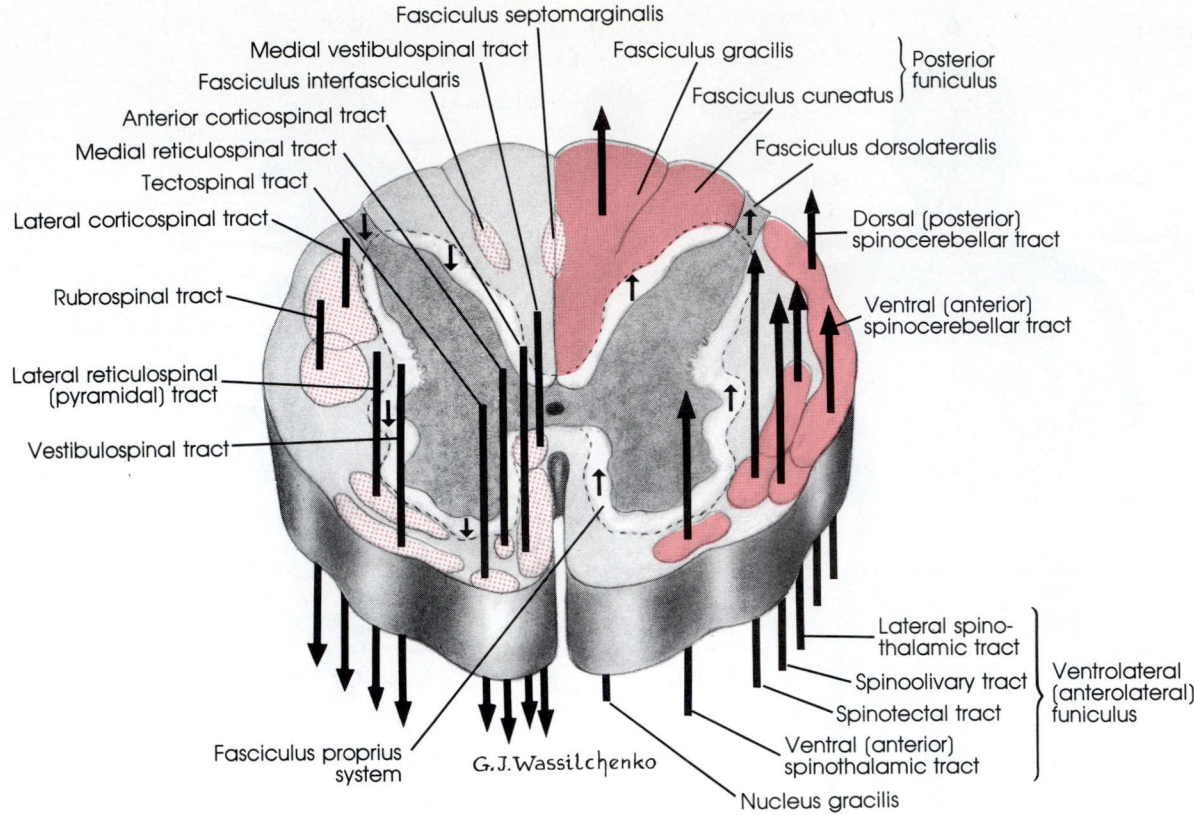

Fasciculus septomarginalis
Medial vestibulospinal tract
Fasciculus interfascicularis
Anterior corticospinal tract
Medial reticulospinal tract
Tectospinal tract
Lateral corticospinal tract
Rubrospinal tract
Lateral reticulospinal (pyramidal) tract
Vestibulospinal tract
Fasciculus proprius system
G.J.Wassilchenko

Fasciculus gracilis
Fasciculus cuneatus
} Posterior funiculus
Fasciculus dorsolateralis
Dorsal (posterior) spinocerebellar tract
Ventral (anterior) spinocerebellar tract
Lateral spino-thalamic tract
Spinoolivary tract
Spinotectal tract
} Ventrolateral (anterolateral) funiculus
Ventral (anterior) spinothalamic tract
Nucleus gracilis

FIG. 12-11. Spinal cord tracts. Cross section of upper thoracic cord. Tracts and their placement at various levels of the cord. (From Rudy, 1984.)

spinal cord from its origin in the fourth ventricle. The gray matter of the spinal cord is divided into three regions and displays specific functional characteristics. These regions include the **dorsal horn** (posterior horn), which is primarily composed of interneurons and axons from sensory neurons whose cell bodies lie in the **dorsal root ganglion.** At the tip of the dorsal horn is the **substantia gelatinosa,** a structure involved in perception of pain (see Chapter 13). The **lateral horn** contains cell bodies involved with the autonomic nervous system. The **ventral horn** (anterior horn) contains the nerve cell bodies for efferent pathways leaving the spinal cord by way of spinal nerves.

Surrounding the gray matter is white matter that forms ascending and descending pathways called **spinal tracts.** Spinal tracts are named to denote their beginning and ending points. For example, the **spinothalamic tract** carries nerve impulses from the spinal cord to the thalamus in the diencephalon. Numerous spinal tracts are grouped into columns according to their location within the white matter. These consist of the **ventral column, lateral column,** and **dorsal column.** (Fig. 12-11 identifies the location and principal activities of the major spinal tracts.)

Neural circuits in the spinal cord, when activated, dis-

play specific sets of motor responses. **Reflex areas** form basic units that respond to stimuli and provide protective circuitry for motor output. Structures mandatory for a **reflex arc** are a receptor, an **afferent** (or sensory) neuron, an **efferent** (motor) neuron, and an effector muscle or gland. A simple reflex arc may contain only two neurons. (Fig. 12-12 illustrates a simple reflex arc.)

Much of the regulation of the internal environment is mediated by reflex activity involving the autonomic nervous system. The motor effects of reflex arcs generally occur before perception of the event in the higher centers of the brain.

Afferent pathways transmit information from periph-

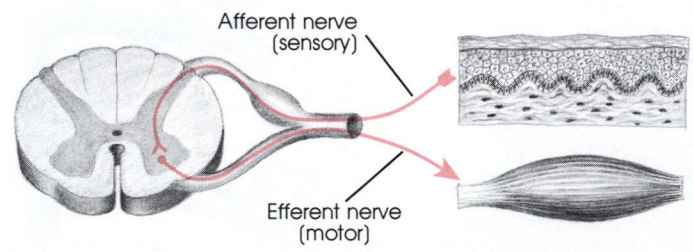

Afferent nerve (sensory)
Efferent nerve (motor)

FIG. 12-12. Cross section of spinal cord showing simple reflex arc. (From Rudy, 1984.)

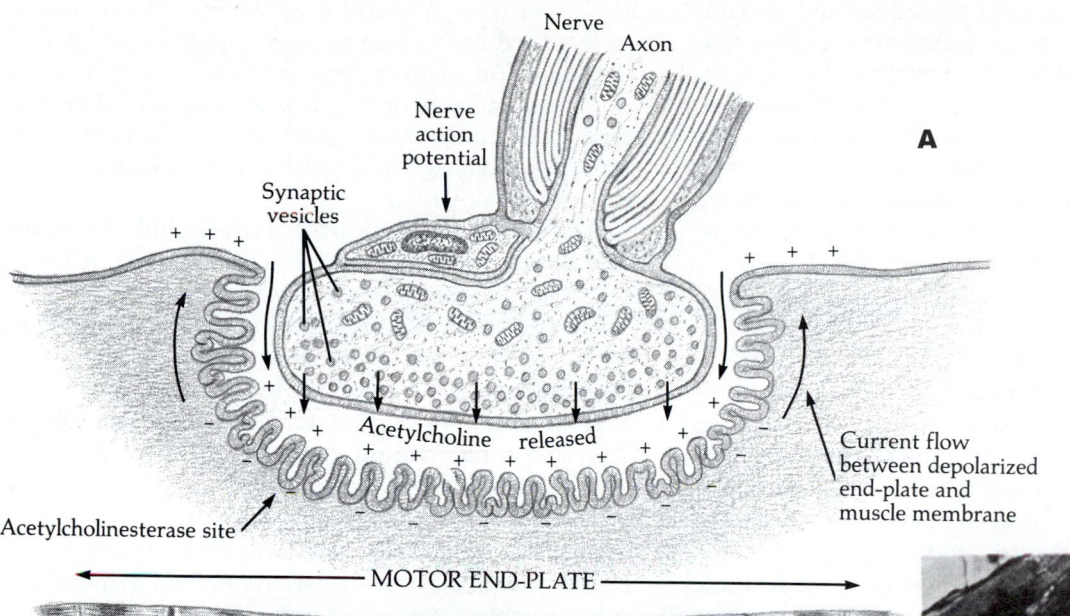

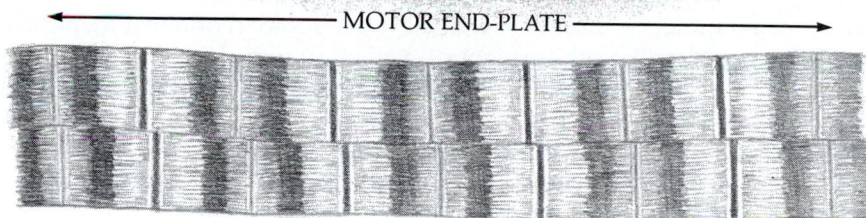

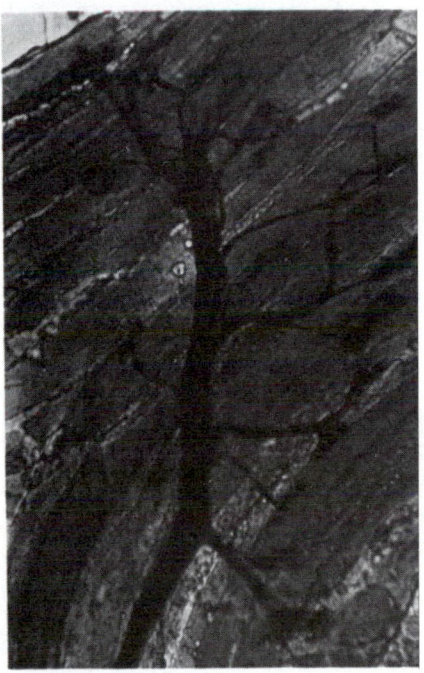

FIG. 12-13. A, Neuromuscular junction. **B,** Neuron axons typically branch as they connect with skeletal muscle as shown here. Each connection at a neuromuscular junction ends in a motor end plate. (**A** from Thompson et al., 1989; **B** from Raven & Johnson, 1986.)

eral receptors and eventually terminate in the cerebral and/or cerebellar cortex. Efferent pathways primarily relay information from the cerebrum to the brainstem or spinal cord. **Upper motor neurons** are the classification of motor pathways completely contained within the CNS. Their primary role is influencing and modifying spinal reflex arcs and circuits. Generally, upper motor neurons form synapses with interneurons, which then form synapses with lower motor neurons before projecting into the periphery. **Lower motor neurons** are responsible for direct influence to muscles. Their cell bodies lie in the gray matter of the spinal cord, but their processes extend out of the CNS.

Muscle activity (i.e., stimulation and contraction) is regulated by nerve impulses. Motor neurons innervate one or more muscle cells, forming **motor units** consisting of a neuron and the skeletal muscles it stimulates. The junction between the axon of the motor neuron and the plasma membrane of the muscle cell is called the **neuromuscular junction** (Fig. 12-13). (Injury to motor neurons is discussed in Chapter 14.)

Protective Structures of the Central Nervous System
Cranium

The cranium is composed of eight bones that fuse early in childhood. The cranial vault functions to enclose and protect the brain and its associated structures.

The **galea aponeurotica** is a thick fibrous band of tissue overlying the cranium between the frontalis and occipitalis muscle and affords added protection to the bony structure of the skull. The subgaleal space has venous connections with the dural sinuses and, with increased intracranial pressure, blood can be shunted to the space, thus reducing pressure in the intracranial cavity. The subgaleal space is also a common site for wound drains after intracranial surgery.

The floor of the cranial vault is irregular and contains many foramina (openings) for cranial nerves, blood vessels, and the spinal cord to exit. The cranial floor is divided into three fossae (depressions). The frontal lobes lie in the **anterior fossa,** temporal lobes and base of the diencephalon in the **middle fossa** (or temporal fossa), and cerebellum in the **posterior fossa.** These terms are commonly used anatomic landmarks to describe the location of intracranial lesions.

Meninges

Surrounding the brain and spinal cord are three protective membranes; the dura mater, the arachnoid membrane, and the pia mater. Collectively they are called the **meninges** (Fig. 12-14). The **dura mater** (meaning literally "hard mother") is composed of two layers, with the venous sinuses formed between them. The outermost layer forms the **periosteum** (endosteal layer) of the skull. The **inner dura** (meningeal layer) is responsible for the formation of rigid plates that serve to support and separate various brain structures.

One of these membranous plates, the **falx cerebri,** dips between the two cerebral hemispheres along the longitudinal fissure. The falx cerebri is anchored anteriorly to the base of the brain at the crista galli of the ethmoid bone. The **tentorium cerebelli** is a membrane that surrounds the brainstem and separates the cerebellum below from the cerebral structures above. The tentorium is also a common landmark used to describe intracranial lesions. For example, supratentorial means above the tentorium and infratentorial means below the tentorium. The tentorium also functions during periods of increased intracranial pressure caused by an injury to the brain. An injury within the cranial cavity tends to shift intracranial contents, and as structures shift, they tend to be compressed against these rigid membranes, resulting in damage or destruction. A common example is tentorial herniation.

Below the dura mater lies the **arachnoid membrane,** characterized by its spongy weblike structure. It loosely follows the contours of the cerebral structures.

The space between the dura and arachnoid membrane is the **subdural space**. Many small bridging veins that have little support traverse the subdural space. Their disruption results in a subdural hematoma (see Chapter 15). The **subarachnoid space** lies between the arachnoid membrane and the pia mater and contains cerebrospinal fluid (see Fig. 12-14). Disruption of intracranial vessels can lead to a condition called a subarachnoid hemorrhage. This occult location of blood frequently results in signs of meningeal irritation.

Unlike the dura mater and arachnoid membrane, the delicate pia mater follows the contours of the brain and spinal cord very closely. It provides support for blood vessels serving brain tissue. The **choroid plexuses,** structures that produce cerebrospinal fluid, arise from the pial membrane (see Fig. 12-14).

The meninges also form potential and real spaces important to understanding functional and pathologic mechanisms. For example, between the dura mater and skull lies a potential space termed the **epidural space** (see Fig. 12-14). The arterial supply to the meninges

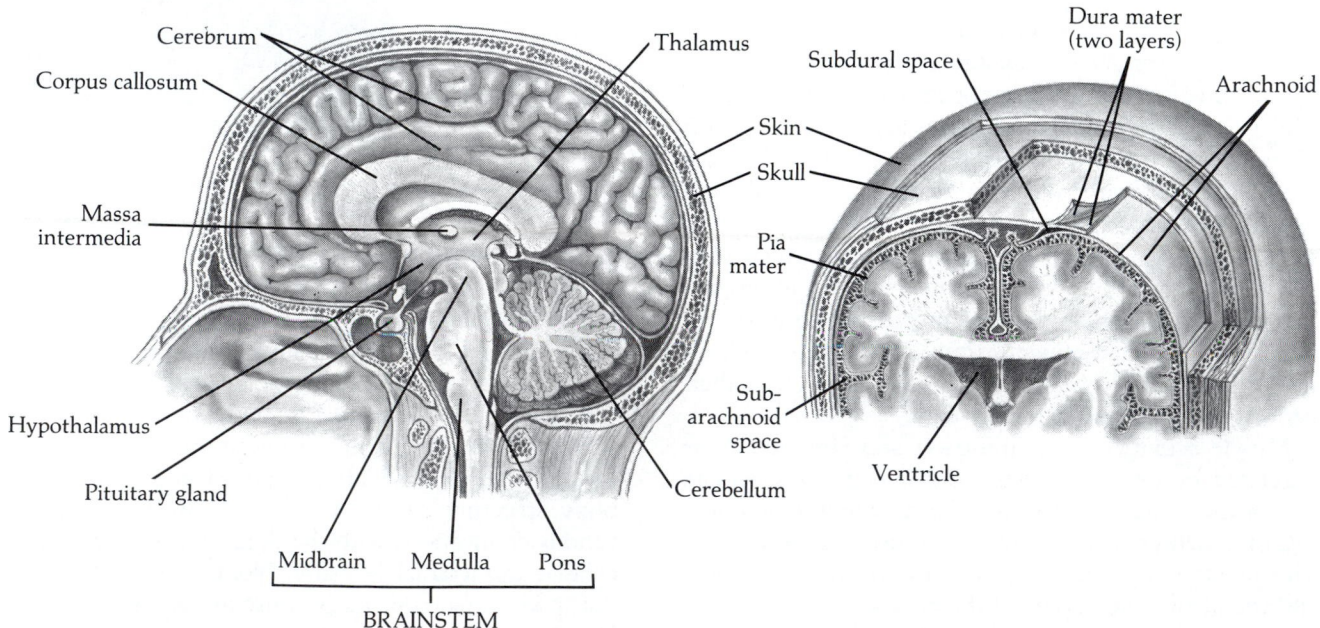

FIG. 12-14. Meninges of brain. (From Thompson et al., 1989.)

consists of blood vessels that lie within grooves in the skull. As a result of trauma, the skull can be fractured and the blood vessels disrupted. The ruptured vessels can lead to an accumulation of blood within the epidural space, called an epidural hematoma (see Chapter 15). An inflammation of the meninges (meningitis) can also have serious implications because of the relative proximity to the brain. (Disorders of the CNS are discussed in Chapter 15.)

Cerebrospinal Fluid and the Ventricular System

Cerebrospinal fluid (CSF) is a clear, colorless fluid similar to that of blood plasma and interstitial fluid. It cushions the central nervous system by protecting soft tissue from jolts and blows. The intracranial and spinal cord structures float in CSF. The CSF's buoyant properties protect the delicate structures of the brain and prevent the brain from tugging on meninges, nerve roots, and blood vessels. (Constituents of CSF are listed in Table 12-3.) Between 125 and 150 ml of CSF is circulating within the **ventricles** (small cavities) and subarachnoid space at any given time. Approximately 600 ml of CSF is produced daily.

The choroid plexuses in the lateral, third, and fourth ventricles produce the major portion of CSF. (Ventricles are illustrated in Fig. 12-14.) These plexuses are characterized by a rich network of blood vessels, supplied by the pia mater, that lie in close contact with the ependymal cells of the ventricles.

The CSF exerts pressure within the brain and spinal cord. With a person in a recumbent position, CSF pressure is approximately 120 to 180 mm of water pressure or 12 mm of Hg pressure. CSF flow is a result of a pressure gradient between the arterial system and the CSF-filled cavities. Beginning in the lateral ventricles, the CSF flows through the **interventricular foramen** (foramen of Monro) into the third ventricle. From the third ventricle it passes through the cerebral aqueduct (aqueduct of Sylvius) into the fourth ventricle. From the fourth ventricle the CSF may pass through either the paired **foramina of Luschka** or **foramen of Magendie** before communicating with the subarachnoid spaces of the brain and spinal cord. The CSF does not, however, accumulate. Instead, it is reabsorbed into the venous circulation through the arachnoid villi. The **arachnoid villi** are structures that protrude from the arachnoid space, through the dura mater, and lie within the blood flow of the venous sinuses. CSF is reabsorbed by means of a pressure gradient between the arachnoid villi and the cerebral venous sinuses. The villi function as one-way valves directing CSF outflow into the blood but preventing blood flow into the subarachnoid space. Thus, CSF is formed from the blood, and after circulating throughout the CNS, it returns to the blood.

Samples of cerebrospinal fluid are withdrawn for diagnostic purposes by inserting a needle between the third and fourth lumbar vertebra into the subarachnoid space—a procedure called **lumbar puncture**—or from an intraventricular catheter. Spinal anesthesias (blocks) are administered in a similar manner.

Vertebral Column

The vertebral column (Fig. 12-15) is composed of 33 vertebrae: 7 cervical, 12 thoracic, 5 lumbar, 5 fused sacral, and 4 fused coccygeal. Between each interspace (ex-

TABLE 12-3 Composition of CSF

Constituent	Normal value
Na^+	148 mM
K^+	2.9 mM
Cl^-	125 mM
HCO_3^-	22.9 mM
Glucose (fasting)	50-75 mg/100 ml
pH	7.3
Protein	15-45 mg/100 ml
Albumin	80%
Gamma globulin	6-10%
Cells	
White (lymphocytes)	0-6 per mm³
Red	0 per mm³

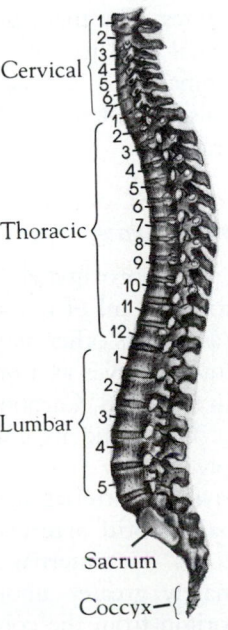

FIG. 12-15. Vertebral column. (From Rudy, 1984.)

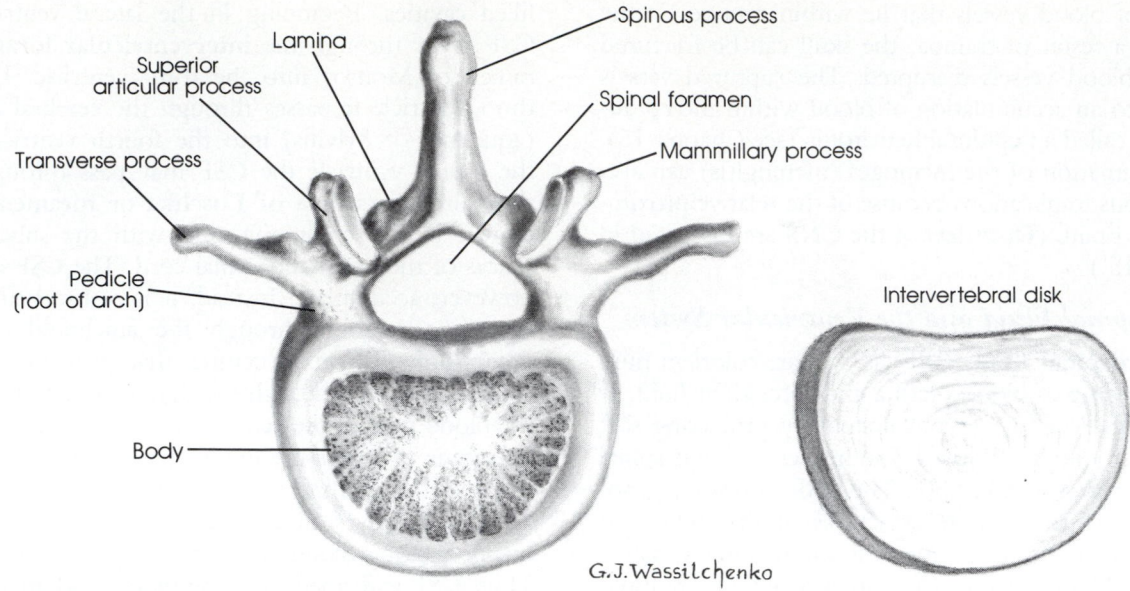

Lamina
Spinous process
Superior articular process
Spinal foramen
Transverse process
Mammillary process
Pedicle (root of arch)
Intervertebral disk
Body

G.J.Wassilchenko

FIG. 12-16. Vertebra and intervertebral disk. (From Rudy, 1984.)

cept the fused sacral and coccygeal vertebrae) is an **intervertebral disk** (Fig. 12-16). At the center of the intervertebral disk is the **nucleus pulposus**, a pulpy mass of elastic fibers. The intervertebral disk functions to absorb shocks, preventing damage to the vertebrae. The intervertebral disk is also a common source of back problems. If too much stress is applied to the vertebral column, the disk may rupture and protrude into the spinal canal, causing compression of the spinal cord or nerve roots.

The spinal cord is anchored to the vertebrae by extensions of the meninges. The meninges continue beyond the end of the spinal cord to the lower portion of the sacrum. Cerebrospinal fluid, contained within the subarachnoid space, also circulates down to about the second sacral vertebrae.

Blood Supply of the Central Nervous System
Blood Supply to the Brain

The brain receives approximately 20% of the cardiac output, or 800 to 1000 ml of blood flow, per minute. Carbon dioxide (as well as other neural input regulating cardiovascular centers) serves as a primary regulator for blood flow within the CNS. Carbon dioxide is a potent vasodilator in the CNS, and its effects ensure an adequate blood supply.

The brain derives its arterial supply from two systems: the **internal carotid arteries** and the **vertebral arteries** (Fig. 12-17). The internal carotid arteries supply a proportionately greater amount of blood flow. They take their origin from the common carotid arteries, enter the cranium through the base of the skull, and

pass through the **cavernous sinus.** After giving off some small branches, they divide into the anterior and middle cerebral arteries. The vertebral arteries originate at the subclavian arteries and pass through the transverse foramina of the cervical vertebrae, and enter the cranium through the foramen magnum. They join at the junction of the pons and medulla to form the **basilar artery.** The basilar artery divides at the level of the midbrain to form paired posterior cerebral arteries. The large arteries on the surface of the brain and their branches are called **superficial arteries** (conducting arteries). The small branches that project into the brain are termed **projecting arteries** (nutrient arteries).

The **circle of Willis** (see Fig. 12-18) is a structure credited with the ability to compensate for reduced blood flow from any one of the major contributors (collateral blood flow). The circle of Willis is formed by the posterior cerebral arteries, posterior communicating arteries, internal carotid arteries, anterior cerebral arteries, and anterior communicating artery. The anterior cerebral, middle cerebral, and posterior cerebral arteries leave the circle of Willis and extend to various brain structures. (Table 12-4 and Fig. 12-19 illustrate structures served, functional relationships, and pathologic consideration related to occlusion of cerebral arteries.)

The venous drainage of the cerebrum is not parallel (side by side) to the arterial supply, whereas the venous drainage of the brainstem and cerebellum is parallel to the arterial supply. The cerebral veins are classified as superficial veins and deep cerebral veins. The veins drain into venous plexuses and dural sinuses (formed between the dural layers) and eventually drain into the internal

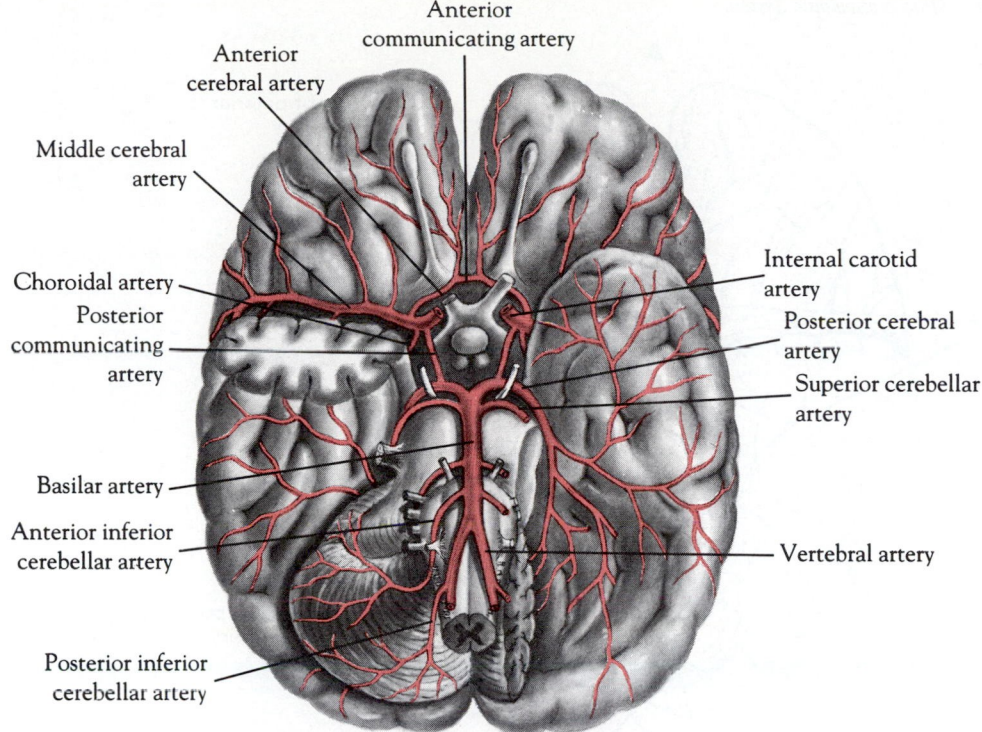

FIG. 12-17. Blood supply of the brain. (From Rudy, 1984.)

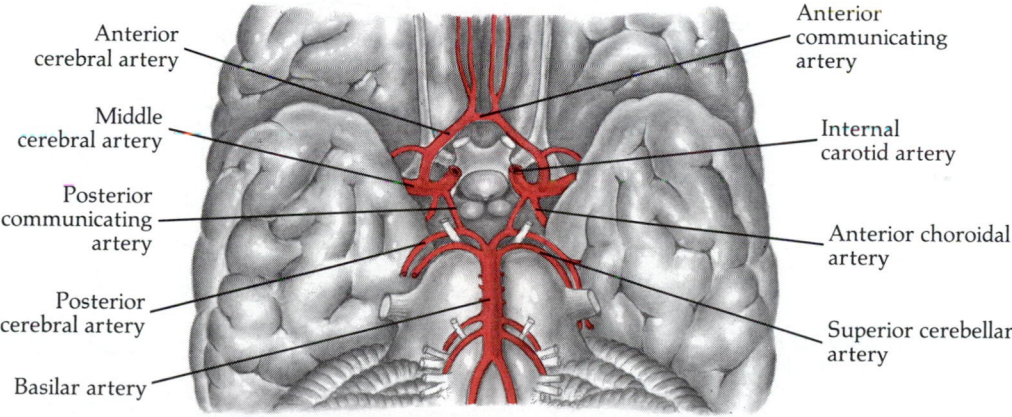

FIG. 12-18. Anatomic diagram of circle of Willis. (From Thompson et al., 1989.)

TABLE 12-4 Arterial systems supplying the brain

Arterial origin	Structures served	Conditions caused by occlusion
Anterior cerebral artery	Basal ganglia; corpus callosum; medial surface of cerebral hemispheres; superior surface of frontal and parietal lobes	Hemiplegia on the contralateral side of the body, greater in the lower than in the upper extremities (see Fig. 12-6)
Middle cerebral artery	Frontal lobe, parietal lobe; temporal lobe (primarily the cortical surfaces)	Aphasia in dominant hemisphere (see Chapter 14)
Posterior cerebral artery	Part of the diencephalon and temporal lobe; occipital lobe	Contralateral hemiplegia greater in the face and upper extremities than in the lower extremities; sensory loss; visual loss

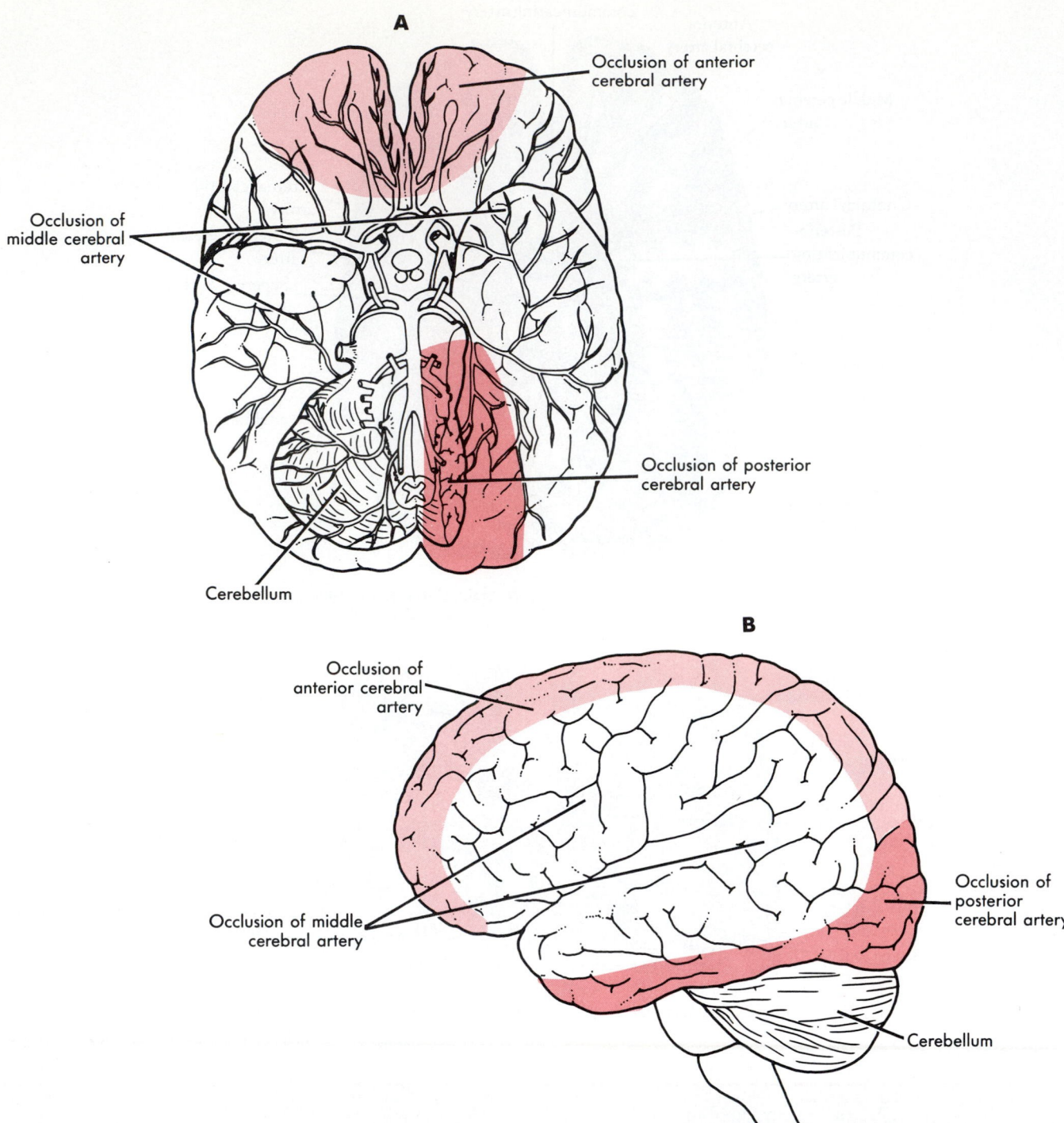

FIG. 12-19. Circulation of the brain from the anterior, middle, and posterior cerebral artery branches. **A,** Cross section. **B,** Lateral view. (From Rudy, 1984.)

jugular veins at the base of the skull (see Fig. 12-20). Adequacy of venous outflow can have a significant effect on intracranial pressure. For example, in individuals with head injury, turning or letting the head fall to the side partially occludes venous return and can increase intracranial pressure.

Blood-Brain Barrier

The **blood-brain barrier** is a term used to describe cellular structures that selectively inhibit certain substances in the blood from entering the interstitial spaces of the brain or CSF. This term emphasizes the impermeability of the nervous system to large and potentially

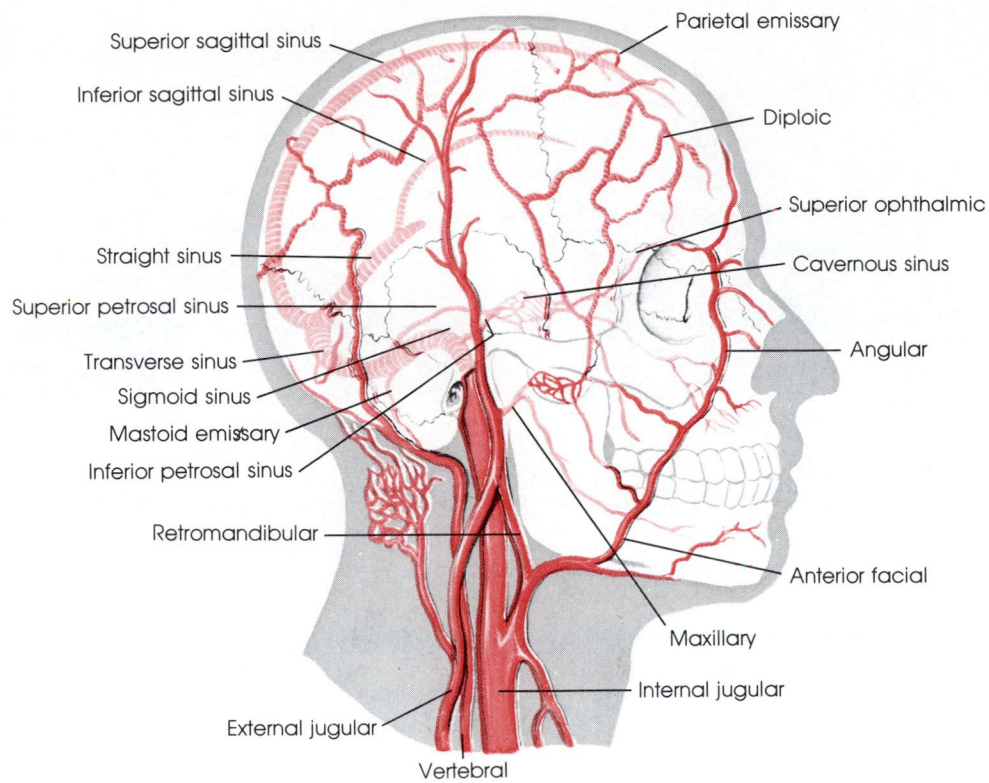

FIG. 12-20. Large veins of the head. Deep veins and dural sinuses are projected on the skull. Note connections (emissary veins) between the superficial and deep veins. (From Rudy, 1984.)

harmful molecules. It is thought that the supporting cells (neuroglia), particularly the astrocytes, and tight junctions between endothelial cells are involved in the formation of the blood-brain barrier. The exact nature of this mechanism is controversial, but it appears that certain metabolites, electrolytes, and chemicals have differing abilities to cross into the brain. This has substantial implications for drug therapy because certain types of antibiotics and chemotherapeutic drugs show a greater propensity than others for crossing the barrier.

Blood Supply to the Spinal Cord

The spinal cord derives its blood supply from branches off the vertebral arteries and from branches from various regions of the aorta (Fig. 12-21). The **anterior spinal arteries** and the paired **posterior spinal arteries** branch off the vertebral artery at the base of the cranium and descend alongside the spinal cord. Arterial branches from vessels exterior to the spinal cord follow the spinal nerve through the intervertebral foramina, pass through the dura, and divide into the anterior and posterior radicular arteries.

The radicular arteries eventually reconnect to the spinal arteries. Branches from the radicular and spinal arteries form plexuses whose branches penetrate the spinal cord, supplying the deeper tissues. Venous drainage parallels the arterial supply closely and drains into venous sinuses located between the dura and periosteum of the vertebrae.

THE PERIPHERAL NERVOUS SYSTEM

The cranial and spinal nerves, including their branches and ganglia, constitute the peripheral nervous system. A peripheral nerve (cranial or spinal) is composed of individual axons wrapped in a myelin sheath. These individual fibers are arranged in bundles called **fascicles** (Fig. 12-22). The coverings supply structural support, a blood supply, and interstitial compartments necessary for the supply of essential electrolytes to support nerve impulse conduction.

The 31 pairs of spinal nerves derive their names from the vertebral level from which they exit. The cervical nerves take their names from the vertebral level below, thus forming eight cervical nerves. From the thoracic region (and inferiorly) nerves correspond to the vertebral level above their exit.

Spinal nerves contain both sensory and motor neu-

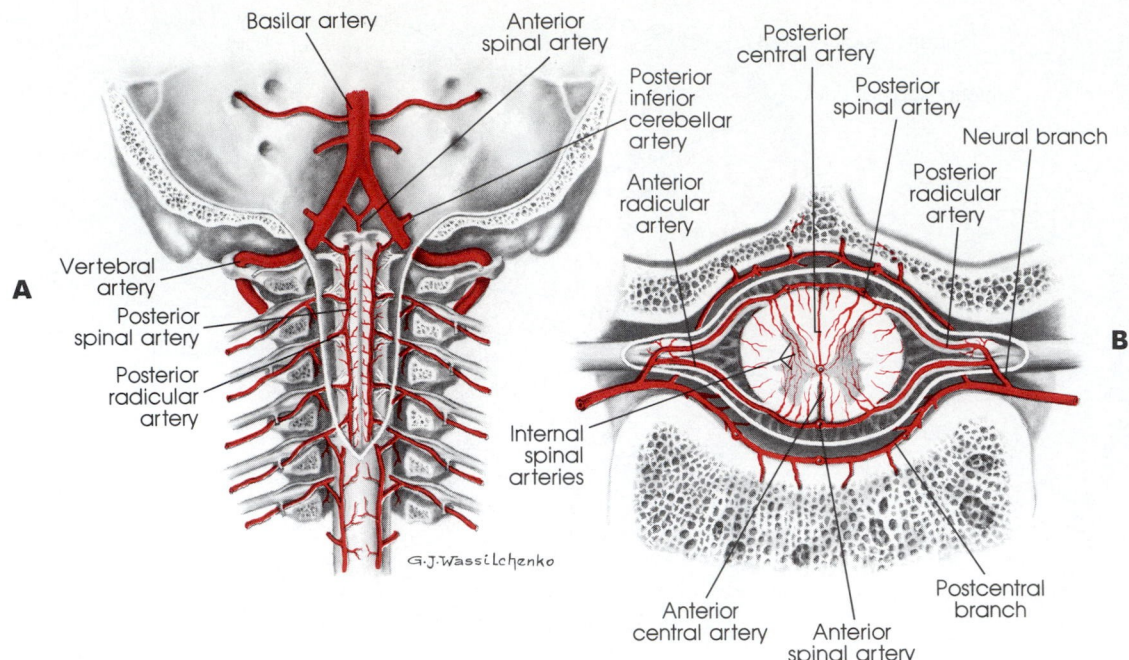

FIG. 12-21. Arteries of the spinal cord. **A,** Arteries of cervical cord exposed from the rear. **B,** Arteries of spinal cord diagrammatically shown in horizontal section. (From Rudy, 1984.)

rons and are called **mixed nerves** that originate as rootlets from the ventral and dorsal horn cells of the spinal cord. The two spinal nerve roots exit the spinal cord and converge to form the spinal nerve trunk. Shortly after converging, the spinal nerve divided into anterior and posterior rami (branches). The anterior rami (except the thoracic) initially form **plexuses** (networks of nerve fibers), which then branch into the peripheral nerves. Instead of forming plexuses, the thoracic nerves pass through the intercostal spaces and innervate regions of the thorax.

The main spinal nerve plexuses innervate the skin and the underlying muscles of the limbs. The **brachial plexus,** for example, is formed by the last four cervical nerves (C_5 to C_8) and the first thoracic nerve (T_1). The brachial plexus extends downward and laterally to innervate the nerves of the arm, wrist, and hand. The **lumbar plexus** and **sacral plexus** contain nerves that innervate the anterior and posterior portions of the lower body, respectively.

The posterior rami of each spinal nerve, with their many processes, are distributed to a specific area in the body. Sensory signals thus arise from specific sites associated with a specific spinal cord segment. Specific areas of cutaneous innervation at these spinal cord segments are called **dermatomes.** The dermatomes of various spinal nerves are distributed in a fairly regular pattern, although adjacent regions between dermatomes can be innervated by more than one spinal nerve.

Like spinal nerves, cranial nerves are categorized as peripheral nerves. Most of these are mixed nerves (like the spinal nerves), although some are purely sensory or purely motor. Cranial nerves arise from surfaces of the brain and brainstem. (Fig. 12-7 illustrates their structure, and Table 12-5 describes structural and functional characteristics.)

THE AUTONOMIC NERVOUS SYSTEM

Components of the autonomic nervous system (ANS) are located in both the peripheral and central nervous system; however, the ANS is considered part of the efferent division of the peripheral nervous system. Many neurons of the ANS travel in the spinal nerves and certain cranial nerves. The widespread activity of this system indicates that its components are distributed all over the body. The peripheral autonomic nerves are mainly efferent fibers, but not purely motor or secretory. The motor component of the ANS is a two-neuron system consisting of **preganglionic** and **postganglionic** neurons. This arrangement contrasts with the somatic nervous system, where a single motor neuron travels from the CNS to the structure innervated.

The ANS coordinates and maintains a steady state among visceral (internal) organs, such as regulation of cardiac muscle and the glands of the body. This system

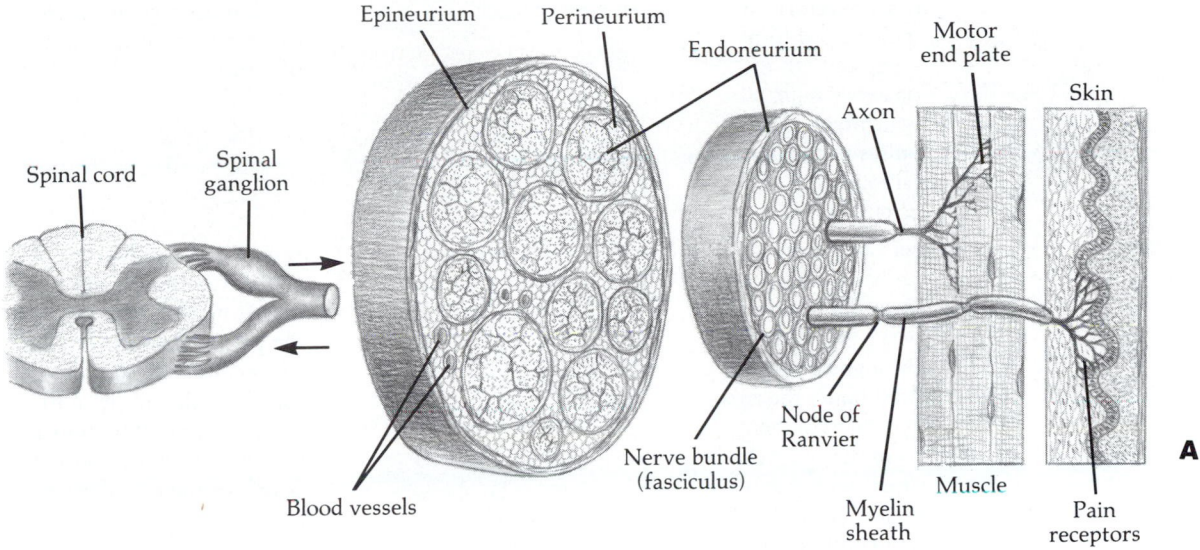

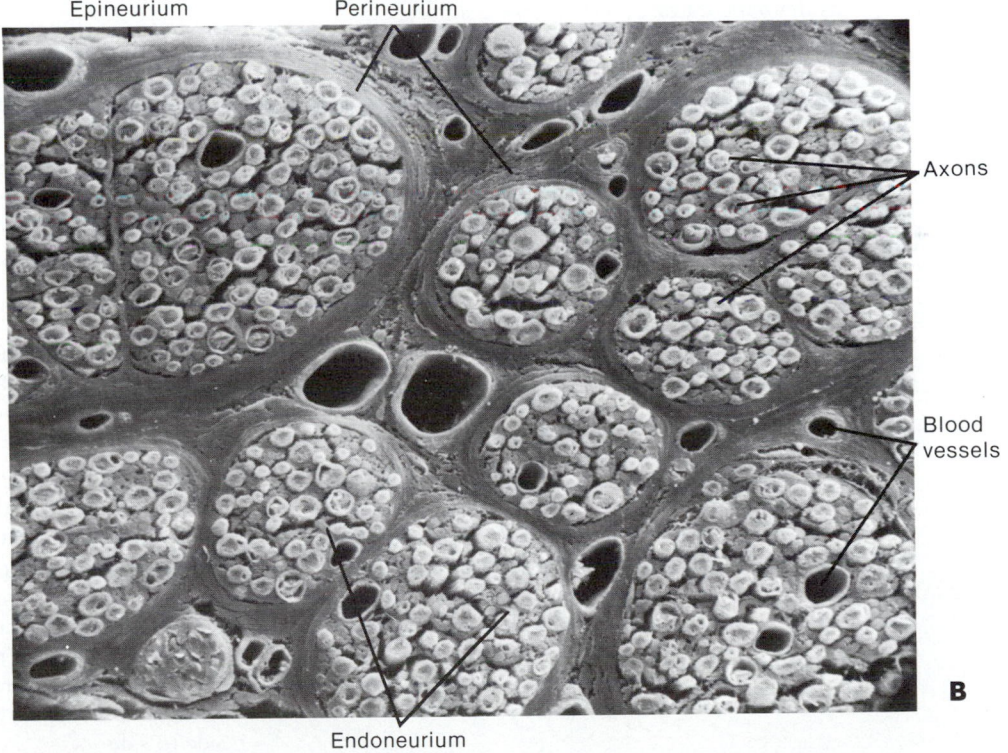

FIG. 12-22. A, Peripheral nerve trunk and coverings. **B,** Scanning electron micrograph of a freeze-fractured preparation of peripheral nerve. (**A** from Thompson et al., 1989; **B** from Nolte, 1988.)

TABLE 12-5 The cranial nerves

Number and Name	Origin and course	Function	How tested
I. Olfactory	Fibers arise from the nasal olfactory epithelium and form synapses with the olfactory bulbs, which transmit impulses to the temporal lobe of the cerebral cortex	Purely sensory; carries impulses for sense of smell	Person is asked to sniff aromatic substances, such as oil of cloves and vanilla, and identify them
II. Optic	Fibers arise from the retina of the eye to form the optic nerve, which passes through the sphenoid bone; the two optic nerves then form the optic chiasma (with partial crossover of fibers) and continue on to the occipital cortex as the optic tracts	Purely sensory; carries impulses for vision	Vision and visual field are tested with an eye chart and by testing the point at which the person first sees an object (finger) moving into the visual field; the inside of the eye is viewed with ophthalmoscope to observe blood vessels of the eye interior
III. Oculomotor	Fibers emerge from midbrain and exit from skull to run to eye	Contains motor fibers to the superior, inferior, and medial rectus muscles that direct the eyeball to the muscles of the eyelid, and to the iris and smooth muscle controlling lens shape; contains proprioceptor fibers from the external eye muscles to the brain	Pupils are examined for size and shape, and equality; pupillary reflex is tested with a penlight (pupils should constrict when illuminated); ability to follow moving objects
IV. Trochlear	Fibers emerge from the midbrain and exit from skull to run to eye	Proprioceptor and motor fibers for superior oblique muscle of the eye (external eye muscle)	Tested in common with cranial nerve III relative to the ability to follow moving objects
V. Trigeminal	Fibers emerge from pons and form three divisions that exit from skull and run to face	Both motor and sensory for face; conducts sensory impulses from mouth, nose, and surface of eyes; also contains motor fibers that stimulate chewing muscles	Sensations of pain, touch, and temperature are tested with safety pin and hot and cold objects; corneal reflex tested with a whisp of cotton; motor branch tested by asking the subject to clench teeth, open mouth against resistance, and move jaw from side to side

TABLE 12-5 The cranial nerves—cont'd

Number and Name	Origin and course	Function	How tested
VI. Abducens	Fibers leave inferior pons and exit from skull to run to eye	Contains motor fibers to lateral rectus muscle and proprioceptor fibers from same muscle to brain	Tested in common with cranial nerve III relative to the ability to move each eye laterally
VII. Facial	Fibers leave pons and travel through temporal bone to reach face	Mixed: (a) Supplies motor fibers to muscles of facial expression and to lacrimal and salivary glands and (b) carries sensory fibers from taste buds of anterior part of tongue	Anterior two thirds of tongue is tested for ability to taste sweet (sugar), salty, sour (vinegar), and bitter (quinine) substances; symmetry of face is checked; subject is asked to close eyes, smile, whistle, and so on; tearing is tested with ammonia fumes
VIII. Vestibulocochlear (acoustic)	Fibers run from inner ear hearing and equilibrium receptors in temporal bone to enter brainstem just below pons	Purely sensory; vestibular branch transmits impulses for sense of equilibrium; cochlear branch transmits impulses for sense of hearing	Hearing is checked by air and bone conduction using a tuning fork
IX. Glossopharyngeal	Fibers emerge from midbrain and leave skull to run to throat	Mixed: (a) Motor fibers serve pharynx (throat) and salivary glands and (b) sensory fibers carry impulses from pharynx, posterior tongue (taste buds), and pressure receptors of the carotid artery	Gag and swallowing reflexes are checked; subject is asked to speak and cough; posterior one third of tongue may be tested for taste
X. Vagus	Fibers emerge from medulla, pass through skull, and descend through neck region into thorax and abdominal region	Fibers carry sensory and motor impulses for pharynx; a large part of this nerve is parasympathetic motor fibers, which supply the smooth muscles of abdominal organs; transmits sensory impulses from the viscera	Same as for cranial nerve IX (IX and X) are tested in common since they both serve muscles of the throat)
XI. Spinal accessory	Fibers arise from medulla and superior spinal cord and travel to the muscles of neck and back	Provides sensory and motor fibers for sternocleidomastoid and trapezius muscles and muscles of soft palate, pharynx, and larynx	Sternocleidomastoid and trapezius muscles are checked for strength by asking subject to rotate head and shrug shoulders against resistance
XII. Hypoglossal	Fibers arise from medulla and exit from skull to travel to tongue	Carries motor fibers to muscles of tongue and sensory impulses from tongue to brain	Subject is asked to stick out tongue, and any position abnormalities are noted

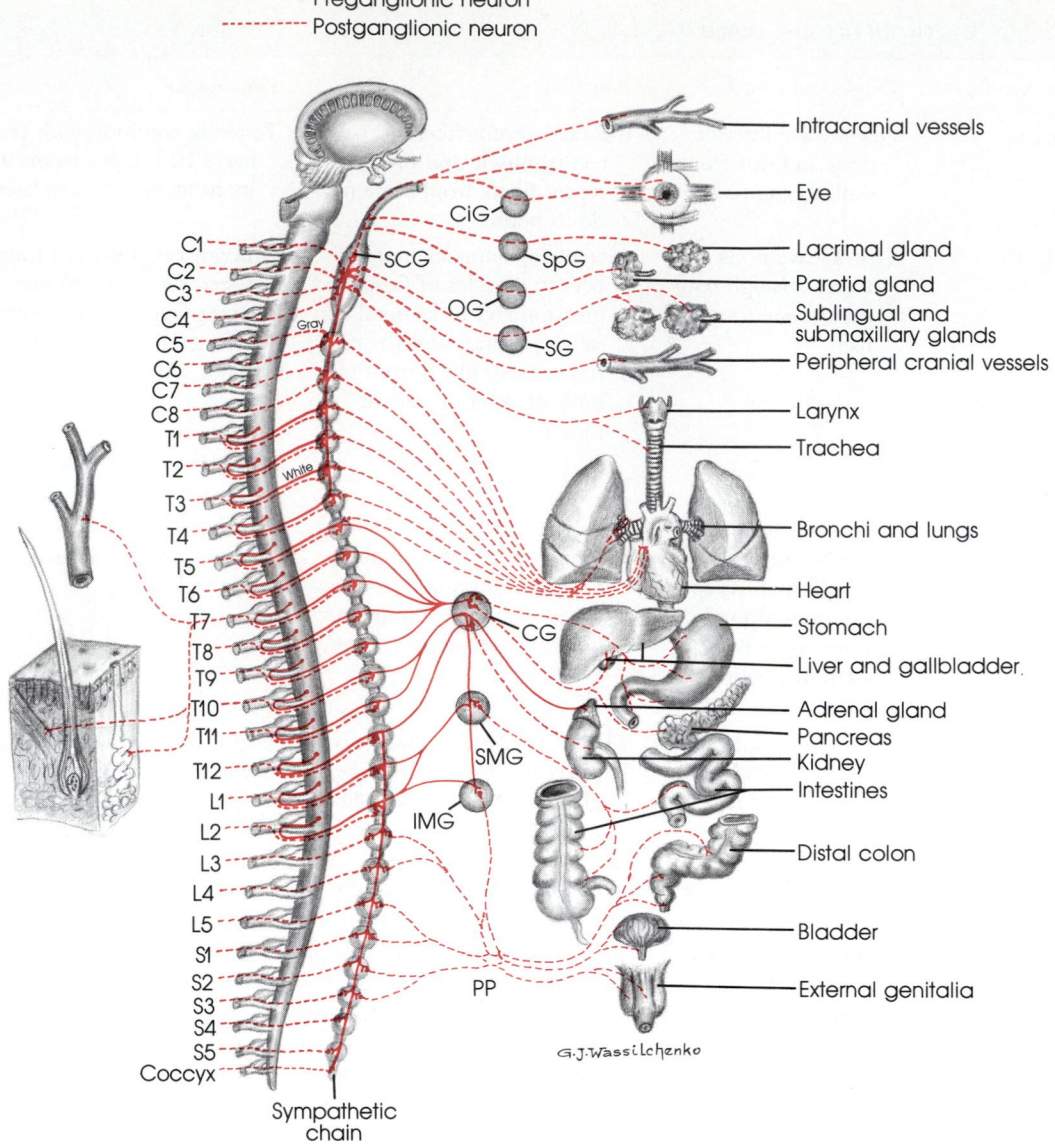

— Preganglionic neuron
---- Postganglionic neuron

FIG. 12-23. Sympathetic division of the autonomic nervous system. *CiG,* Ciliary ganglion; *SpG,* sphenopalatine ganglion; *SCG,* superior cervical ganglion; *OG,* otic ganglion; *SG,* submandibular ganglion; *CG,* celiac ganglion; *SMG,* superior mesenteric ganglion; *IMG,* inferior mesenteric ganglion; *PP,* pelvic plexus. (From Rudy, 1984.)

is mostly an involuntary system, whereby one *generally* cannot "will" these functions to happen. The ANS is separated both structurally and functionally into two divisions: (1) the **sympathetic nervous system** (Fig. 12-23) and (2) the **parasympathetic nervous system** (Fig. 12-24).

Anatomy of the Sympathetic Nervous System

The **sympathetic system** functions to mobilize energy stores in times of need (e.g., in the "fight or flight response") (see Fig. 9-1; see also Chapter 9). The sympathetic division receives its innervation from cell bodies

located from the first thoracic (T1), through the second lumbar (L2) regions of the spinal cord and is therefore called the **thoracolumbar division.** The preganglionic axons of the sympathetic division form synapses shortly after leaving the cord in the **sympathetic (paravertebral) ganglia.** At this point the impulse may travel several ways: (1) directly across the same ganglion level and form a synapse with the cell bodies of the postganglionic neuron, (2) up or down the sympathetic chain before forming synapses with a higher or lower postganglionic neuron, or (3) pass through the chain ganglion without synapsing. Some of the preganglionic ax-

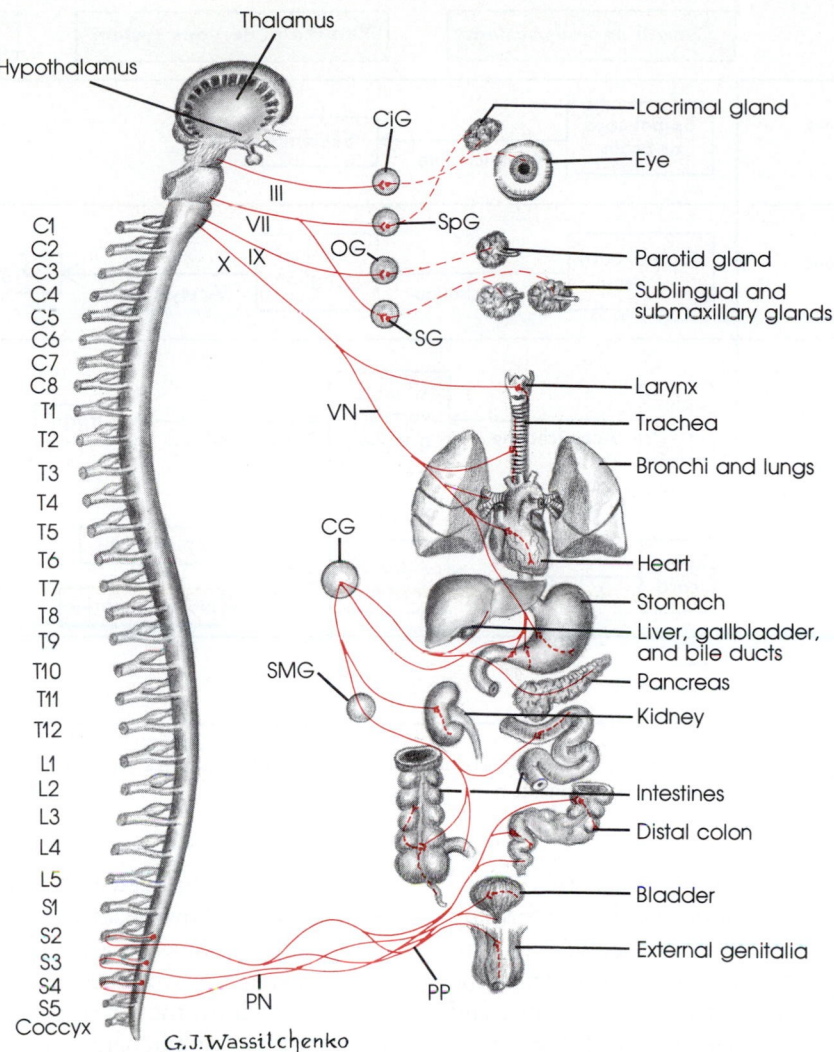

FIG. 12-24. Parasympathetic division of the autonomic nervous system. *CiG,* Ciliary ganglion; *SpG,* sphenopalatine ganglion; *OG,* otic ganglion; *SG,* submandibular ganglion; *VN,* vagus nerve; *CG,* celiac ganglion; *SMG,* superior mesenteric ganglion; *PP,* pelvic plexus; *PN,* pelvic nerve. Fibers of the parasympathetic system pass through the CG and SMG, but these ganglia are not part of the parasympathetic system. (From Rudy, 1984.)

ons form pathways called **splachnic nerves,** which lead to **collateral ganglia** located on the front of the aorta. The collateral ganglia are named according to the branches of the aorta nearest them, the **celiac, superior mesenteric,** and **inferior mesenteric.** The preganglionic neurons synapses with postganglionic neurons within the collateral ganglia. These postganglionic neurons leave the collateral ganglia and innervate the viscera below the diaphragm.

Preganglionic sympathetic neurons that innervate the adrenal medulla also travel in the splachnic nerves and *do not* synapse before reaching the gland. There is no postganglionic sympathetic component to the adrenal medulla, thus it is the only exception to the usual two-neuron chain in the autonomic afferent pathway. Since preganglionic sympathetic fibers are all myelinated, travel to the adrenal medulla is quick, and innervation causes the rapid release of epinephrine and norepinephrine. Epinephrine and norepinephrine are mediators of the "fight or flight response" (see Chapter 9).

Anatomy of the Parasympathetic Nervous System

The **parasympathetic system** functions to conserve and restore energy. The nerve cell bodies of this division are located in the cranial nerve nuclei and in the sacral region of the spinal cord and are therefore called the **craniosacral division.** Unlike the sympathetic branch,

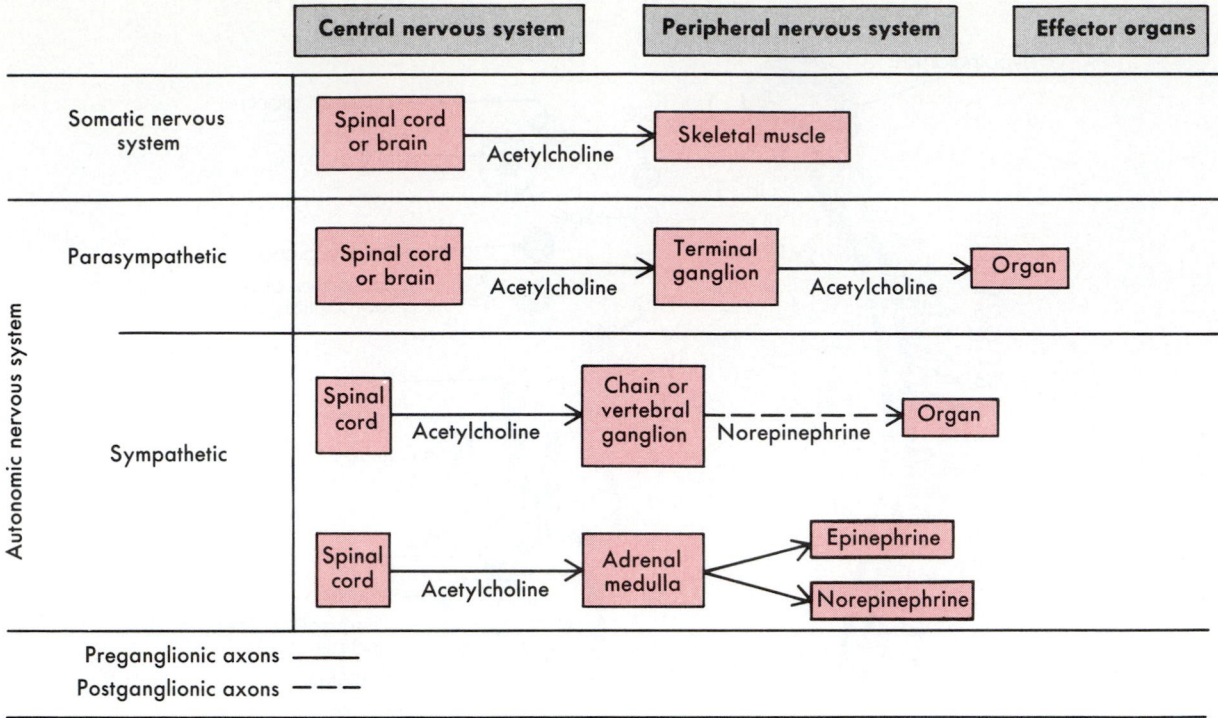

FIG. 12-25. The autonomic nervous system and the type of neurotransmitters secreted by preganglionic and postganglionic fibers. A somatic nerve is used for comparison.

the preganglionic fibers in the parasympathetic division travel close to the organs they innervate before forming synapses with the relatively short postganglionic neurons. Parasympathetic nerves arising from nuclei in the brainstem travel to the viscera of the head, thorax, and abdomen within cranial nerves—including the oculomotor (III), facial (VII), glossopharyngeal (IX), and vagus nerves (X).

Preganglionic parasympathetic nerves that originate from the sacral region of the spinal cord run either separately or together with some spinal nerves. The preganglionic axons join together to form the **pelvic nerve,** which innervates the viscera of the pelvic cavity. These preganglionic axons synapse with postganglionic neurons in terminal ganglia located close to the organs they innervate.

Neurotransmitters and Neuroreceptors

Sympathetic preganglionic fibers and parasympathetic preganglionic and postganglionic fibers release **acetylcholine**—the same neurotransmitter released by somatic efferent neurons (Fig. 12-25). Transmission, therefore, by these fibers is called **cholinergic.** Most postganglionic sympathetic fibers release **norepinephrine** (adrenaline), and this is thus called **adrenergic** transmission. A few postganglionic sympathetic fibers release acetylcholine, such as those that innervate the sweat glands.

The action of catecholamines varies with the type of neuroreceptor stimulated. Remember, catecholamines are also released by the adrenal medulla gland that physiologically and biochemically resembles the sympathetic nervous system. Two types of adrenergic receptors exist, α and β. Cells of the effector organs may have only one or both types of adrenergic receptors. The **α receptors** have been further subdivided according to the action produced. α_1 activity is mostly associated with excitation or stimulation; α_2 activity is associated with relaxation or inhibition. Most of the α receptors on effector organs belong to the α_1 class. The **β receptors** are classified as β_1 receptors (that facilitate increased heart rate and contractility and cause the release of renin from the kidney) and β_2 receptors (that facilitate all of the remaining effects attributed to β receptors (Vick, 1984). Norepinephrine stimulates all α and β_1 receptors and only certain β_2 receptors. The primary response from norepinephrine, however, is stimulation of the α_1 receptors causing vasoconstriction. Epinephrine strongly stimulates all four types of receptors and overall induces vasodilation because of the predominence of β receptors in muscle vasculatures. (Table 12-6 summarizes the effects of neuroreceptors on their effector organs.)

Functions of the Autonomic Nervous System

Many body organs are innervated by both the sympathetic and parasympathetic nervous systems. The two divisions frequently cause opposite responses, for exam-

TABLE 12-6 Actions of the autonomic nervous system on neuroreceptors

Effector organ or tissue	Receptor	Adrenergic effect	Cholinergic effect
Eye, iris			
Radial muscle	α	Contraction (mydriasis)	—
Sphincter muscle	α	—	Contraction (miosis)
Eye, ciliary muscle	β_2	Relaxation (slight)	Contraction
Lacrimal glands	—	—	Secretion
Nasopharyngeal glands	—	—	Secretion
Salivary glands	α	Secretion of ions and water	Secretion of ions and water
	β_2	Secretion of amylase	—
Heart			
SA node	β_1	Increase heart rate	Decrease heart rate
Atria	β_1	Increase contractility	Decrease contractility
AV junction	β_1	Increase automaticity and propagation	Decrease automaticity and
Purkinje system	β_1	velocity	propagation velocity
Ventricles	β_1	Increase automaticity and propagation	—
		velocity	—
		Increase contractility	
Arterioles			
Coronary	α,β_2	Constriction, dilatation	—
Skin	α,β_2	Constriction, dilatation	—
Mucosa	α	Constriction	—
Skeletal muscle	α,β_2	Constriction, dilatation	Dilatation
Cerebral	α	Constriction (slight)	—
Pulmonary	α,β_2	Constriction, dilatation	—
Mesenteric	α	Constriction	—
Renal	α,D^*	Constriction, dilatation	—
Salivary glands	α	Constriction	Dilatation
Veins, systemic	α,β_2	Constriction, dilatation	—
Lung			
Bronchial muscle	β_2	Relaxation	Contraction
Bronchial glands	—	Inhibition (?)	Stimulation
Stomach			
Motility	β_2	Decrease	Increase
Sphincters	α	Contraction	Relaxation
Secretion	—	Inhibition (?)	Stimulation
Liver			
	β_2	Glycogenolysis	—
	$\alpha,\beta_?$	Kalemotropic action	—
Gallbladder and ducts	—	Relaxation	Contraction
Pancreas			
Acini	α	Decreased secretion	Secretion
Islet cells	α,β_2	Decreased secretion, increased secretion	—
Intestine			
Motility	α_2,β_2	Decrease	Increase
Sphincters	α	Contraction	Relaxation
Secretion	—	Inhibition (?)	Stimulation
Adrenal medulla	—	—	Secretion of epinephrine
			and norepinephrine
Kidney	β_1	Secretion of renin	—
Ureter			
Motility	α	Increased	Increased

From Vick, 1984.

*D = dopaminergic.

Continued.

TABLE 12-6 Actions of the autonomic nervous system on neuroreceptors—cont'd			
Effector organ or tissue	Receptor	Adrenergic effect	Cholinergic effect
Urinary bladder			
Detrusor	β_2	Relaxation	Contraction
Trigone and sphincter	α	Contraction	Relaxation
Sex organs, male	α	Ejaculation	Erection
Skin			
Pilomotor muscles	α	Contraction	—
Sweat glands	α	Localized secretion	Generalized secretion
Fat cells	α,β_2	Lipolysis	—
Pineal gland	β_2	Melatonin synthesis	—

ple, sympathetic stimulation of the stomach causes decreased peristalsis, whereas parasympathetic stimulation of the intestine increases peristalsis. In general, sympathetic stimulation promotes responses that are concerned with the protection of the individual. For example, sympathetic activity increases blood sugar levels, temperature, and raises the blood pressure. In emergency situations, there is a generalized and widespread discharge of the sympathetic system. This is accomplished by an increase in the firing frequency of sympathetic fibers and also activation of sympathetic fibers normally silent and at rest (fibers to the sweat glands, pilomotor muscles, and the adrenal medulla, as well as vasodilator fibers to muscle). Regulation of vasomotor tone is considered the single most important function of the sympathetic nervous system. (Fig. 12-26 illustrates some of the most important functions of the sympathetic nervous system; also see Fig. 9-1).

Increased parasympathetic activity promotes rest and tranquility and is characterized by reduced heart rate and enhanced visceral functions leading to digestion. Stimulation of the vagus nerve in the gastrointestinal tract increases peristalsis and secretion, as well as relaxation of sphincters. Activation of parasympathetic fibers in the head, provided by cranial nerves III, VII, and IX, causes constriction of the pupil, tear secretion, and increased salivary secretion. Stimulation of the sacral division of the parasympathetic system contracts the urinary bladder and facilitates the process of genital erection.

The parasympathetic system lacks the generalized and widespread response of the sympathetic system. Specific parasympathetic fibers are activated for the regulation of particular functions. While the actions of the parasypa-

thetic and sympathetic systems are usually antagonistic, there are exceptions. Peripheral vascular resistance, for example, is increased dramatically by sympathetic activation but is not appreciably altered by activity of the parasympathetic system. Most of the blood vessels involved in the control of blood pressure are innervated by sympathetic nerves. To decrease blood pressure, therefore, it is more important to block or paralyze the continuous (tonic) discharge of the sympathetic system than promote parasympathetic activity.

AGING AND THE NERVOUS SYSTEM

The mechanisms involved in the aging process in the central nervous system are extremely complex, and many questions concerning the neurologic effects of aging have yet to be answered. Some of the identified mechanisms associated with aging are pathological, but the distinction between these mechanisms and those that are a part of the normal aging process remain somewhat cloudy.

Structural Changes with Aging

The CNS demonstrates many structural changes during the aging process. The primary mechanism responsible for most of these structural changes is a decrease in the number of neurons. Predominant external features of the aged brain include decreased brain weight and size (primarily the frontal hemispheres), increased adherence of the dura mater to the skull, fibrosis and thickening of the meninges, narrowed gyri, and wid-

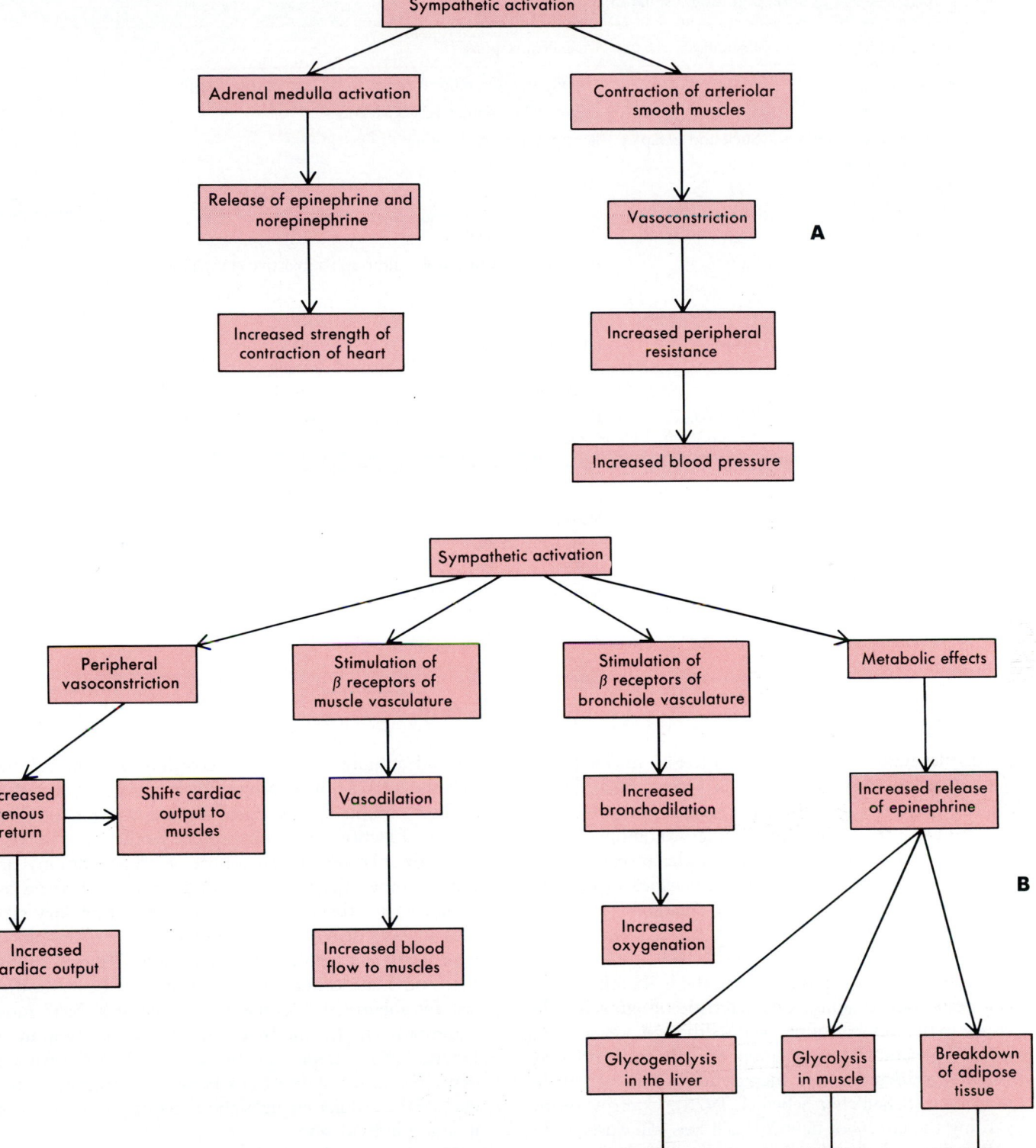

FIG. 12-26. Some important functions of the sympathetic nervous system. **A,** Regulation of vasomotor tone. **B,** Regulation of strenuous muscular exercise ("fight or flight response"). (See also Chapter 9 and Fig. 9-1 for more detail of the stress response.)

TABLE 12-7 Common neurologic signs in aging

Neurologic sign	Examples	Change in response
Reflexes	Ankle reflex	Usually the first tendon reflex to be lost in the elderly
	Superficial reflex	Decreased or absent responsiveness
Primitive reflexes (reflexes seen normally in infancy but that subside with maturity)	Suck and grasp	Reappearance with aging
Sensation	Taste and smell	Progressive deficit
	Pain	Increased pain threshold, although subjective complaints increase
	Vibratory sense	Decreased
	Vision	Decreased visual color sense in a significant percentage of the aged; pupils commonly smaller; slowing of pupillary relaxation and accommodation
Motor function	Physiologic tremor	Exaggeration of normally unnoticeable resting tremor that is present at all ages
	Neuromuscular control	Decreased, resulting in postural effects
	Posture	Stance commonly shows increased flexion of hips and knees; swaying motion while standing in one position more common
	Gait	Shuffling or shortened stride; loss of arm movement with walking
	Muscular atrophy	Age-associated loss of muscle fibers

ened sulci with a corresponding increase in the size of the subarachnoid space (Hirano & Llena, 1983). Dayan and Lewis (1985) cite the basal ganglia and ventricular system as internal structures that commonly reveal changes with aging. The basal ganglia reveals aberrations in vascular structures and the ventricles (primarily the lateral and third ventricles) are enlarged.

Cellular Changes with Aging

Practically every cell type within the CNS reflects specific responses to aging. Characteristic of aging is a decrease in the number of neurons. Although neuronal cell loss is a general feature of aging, the effects are not consistent with deteriorating mental function or age of the individual (Scheibel & Scheibel, 1975). Controversy regarding the effects of neuronal cell loss still exists.

Principal cellular changes associated with aging include dendrite structure, lipofuscin deposition, and presence of neurofibrillary tangles, senile plaques, and Lewy bodies. Hirano and Llena (1983) described a decreased number of dendritic processes and their multiple synaptic connections. Lipofuscin, a yellow-brown fatty pigment, is found to be deposited intracellularly in in-

creased amounts with age. According to Scheibel and Scheibel (1975), increasing intracellular quantities of lipofuscin might be associated with disruption of cytoplasmic function, probably protein synthesis.

Senile plaques (areas of nerve degeneration) are found in the interstitial spaces of the cerebral cortex associated with tissue degeneration. **Neurofibrillary tangles** involve degenerative changes in neural protein fibers. These entities are also common in Alzheimer's disease and some other forms of dementia. **Lewy bodies** are intraneuronal, degenerative structures seen most commonly in the midbrain and brainstem (Dayan & Lewis, 1985). At present, however, little definitive evidence has shown a direct link between quantitative presence of the cellular changes and nervous system function in aging individuals.

Closely paralleling cell function is a selective alteration in neurotransmitter function. One potentially fruitful area of research is correlating the effects of acetylcholine (i.e., cholinergic transmission) and defects of memory and cognitive function associated with aging (Rossor, 1985).

Functional Changes with Aging

Because of integrative processes in the CNS, the consequences of aging have widespread implications for critical steady state, psychologic, and social function. Many theories have been proposed to explain the observations of progressive slowing of neurologic responses seen in the aged (Table 12-7). Studies of changes in brain electrical activity have been helpful in determining alterations in neural function. Timiras (1972, p. 516) described the relationship between transmission of neural signals and slowing of responses observed in the aged: "It is evident that the efficacy of the signals may be disturbed not only by irregularities in the action of cells carrying the signals but also by the amount of random background activity. This background activity is termed 'neural noise'."

TESTS OF NERVOUS SYSTEM FUNCTION

Skull and Spine Roentgenograms

Roentgenograms (x-ray films) of the skull or spine, from multiple angles (views), are used primarily to localize bony defects, bone density, erosion, or calcified structures. X-ray films are likely the most commonly used radiologic studies.

Computerized Tomography (CT)

Computerized tomography (CT) creates two-dimensional reconstructions from multiple radiologic images using computer-assisted analysis. It is capable of demonstrating fine distinctions in densities of a variety of tissues. CT imaging is a safe and noninvasive procedure used in evaluating cranial and spinal structures. A variety of contrast mediums are also commonly used in conjunction with this procedure to aid in enhanced delineation of selected structures.

Magnetic Resonance Imaging (MRI)

A new development in diagnostics is magnetic resonance imaging (MRI). Instead of radiation, it uses a static magnetic field to orient physiologic atomic particles. Disruption of this orientation by excitation of the particles using serial radio-frequency pulsations provides the image data. The specific tissue reaction is computer analyzed to give an image of exquisite detail, similar to that provided by CT. The MRI also provides reconstruction of images in three views at right angles (i.e., axial, sagittal, and coronal) (see Fig. 12-27). The MRI is reported to have no adverse effects: none of the associated side effects of radiation examinations, in particular.

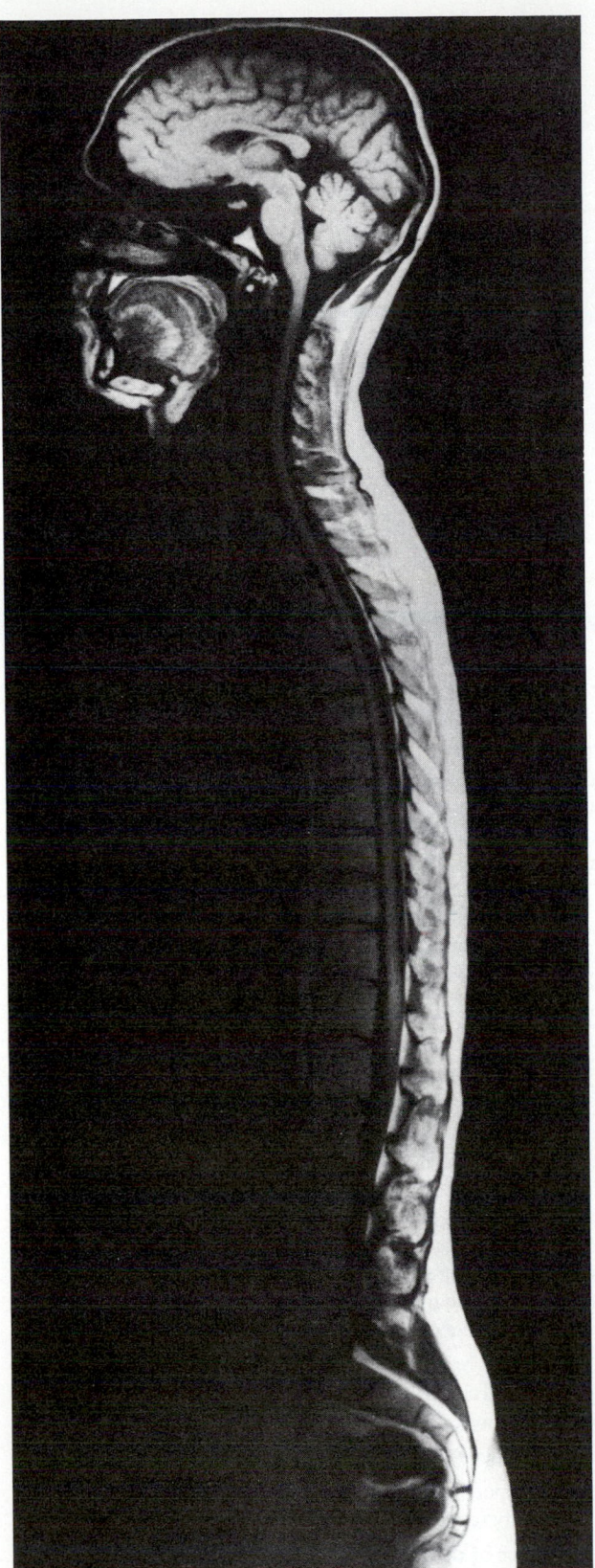

FIG. 12-27. Midsagittal MRI image, demonstrating the extraordinary anatomic detail possible with this technique. (From Nolte, 1988.)

TABLE 12-8 Cerebrospinal fluid analysis

Parameters	Normal	Abnormal	Possible cause
Pressure (initial readings)	75-180 mm H_2O (5-15 mm Hg)	<60 mm	Faulty needle placement Dehydration Spinal block along subarachnoid space Block of foramen magnum
		>200 mm	Muscle tension Abdominal compression Brain tumor Subdural hematoma Brain abcess Brain cyst Cerebral edema (any cause) Hydrocephalus
Color	Clear, colorless	Cloudy	Increased cell count Increased microorganisms
		Yellow	Xanthochromic (due to RBC pigments) High protein content
		Smoky	Presence of RBCs
Red blood cells	None	Blood-tinged	Traumatic tap
		Grossly bloody	Traumatic tap Subarachnoid hemorrhage
White blood cells	0-6 mm³	>10 mm³ (Cell counts range from below 100 to many thousands depending on causative factor; all are abnormal findings.)	Occurs in many conditions: 　Bacterial infections of meninges 　Viral infections of meninges 　Neurosyphilis 　Tuberculous meningitis 　Metastatic neoplastic lesions 　Parasitic infections 　Acute demyelinating diseases 　Following introduction of air or blood into subarachnoid space
Protein*	15-45 mg/100 ml (1% of serum protein)	<10 mg/100 ml	Little clinical significance
		>60 mg/100 ml	Occurs in many conditions: 　Complete spinal block 　Gullain-Barré syndrome 　Carcinomatosis of meninges 　Tumors close to pial or ependymal surfaces, or in cerebellopositive angle 　Acute and chronic meningitis 　Meningeal hemorrhage 　Demyelinating disorders 　Degenerative diseases
Glucose	50-75 mg/100 ml (approximately 60% of blood glucose level)	<40 mg/100 ml	Acute bacterial meningitis Tuberculous meningitis Meningeal carcinomatosis
		>100 mg/100 ml	Diabetes
Chloride	700-750 mg/100 ml; 125 mM	<625 mg/100 ml	Hypochloremia Tuberculous meningitis
		>800 mg/100 ml	Not of neurological significance; correlate with blood levels of chloride

From Rudy, 1984.

*NOTE: If CSF contains blood this will raise the protein level.

Positron Emission Tomography (PET Scan)

The positron emission tomography (PET) scan uses CT imaging to detect the emission of positive electrons from radioactive substances. These substances are injected into the bloodstream or administered as inhaled gases. As they are distributed in tissues, they display characteristic patterns that indicate physiologic and metabolic processes, for example, glucose and oxygen uptake, cerebral blood flow, neural and neurotransmitter function, and the effects of drugs.

Brain Scan

The brain scan images radionuclide substances (technetium [Tc 99 m]) that have been introduced into the bloodstream. For example, visualization of tissue uptake of the radioactive agent provides an indication of blood-brain barrier integrity (increased uptake of the agent indicates disruption). This scanning technique can also identify abnormalities in blood flow dynamics and cellular metabolic function. The brain scan is particularly helpful in detecting abnormal vascularity resulting from the presence of neoplasms, abscesses, and vascular lesions.

Isotope cisternography is another radionuclide imaging technique that uses brain scan imaging to detect cerebrospinal fluid (CSF) flow, CSF resorption, and integrity of CSF pathways. The radionuclide agent in this case is injected directly into the subarachnoid space. Under normal conditions the agent passes over the cortical surface and is resorbed through the arachnoid villi. Demonstration of the agent in the ventricular system after a specific period of time is indicative of CSF obstruction.

Cerebral Angiography

Angiography is a radiologic technique that demonstrates cerebral vascular blood flow. This technique is commonly performed by the introduction of a small catheter into the femoral artery. The catheter is then passed to the level of the cerebral circulation and a contrast dye is injected. Serial x-ray films are then taken. These films demonstrate flow of the dye through the cerebral vasculature and provide information on patency, location, and size of the vessels. Another technique used in cerebral angiography is the retrograde (reverse flow) injection of the dye through catheterization of a brachial, axillary, subclavian, or femoral vein.

Myelography

A myelogram demonstrates intraspinal anatomy by the introduction of a radiographic dye into the lumbar subarachnoid space or the cisterna magna. The dye is allowed to flow in a cephalic direction, as in the case of a lumbar injection, or caudally in a cisterna magna puncture. X-ray films are then obtained. The distribution of the dye delineates spinal cord and nerve root structure and integrity.

Echoencephalography (Ultrasound)

Echoencephalography, or ultrasound, is a safe, noninvasive procedure using sound waves that are deflected at differing rates, depending on the density of the tissue. Information is processed and displayed on an oscilloscope screen. It is useful primarily in the detection of structural characteristics from intracranial space-occupying mass lesions and determination of ventricular dimensions, especially in newborns.

Electroencephalography (EEG)

The electroencephalograph (EEG) is a recording of electrical impulses, arising from the cortical surface of the brain, that is detected by scalp electrodes. The recording of brainwave patterns is analyzed for alterations or localization of specific electrical activity, or both. This test is especially useful in detecting and localizing foci that initiate seizure activity.

Evoked Potentials (EVP)

Evoked potentials (EVPs) is a method of detecting electrical brain activity that results from a stimulus—primarily auditory, visual, or peripheral sensory. Electrical activity is computer formatted to display changes in trends. The primary uses of EVP includes perioperative detection of sensory pathway integrity and disease- or drug-related sensory dysfunction.

Cerebrospinal Fluid (CSF) Analysis

Cerebrospinal fluid (CSF) is generally obtained from the lumbar or cisternal subarachnoid space using a hollow needle that allows passive flow. The lumbar puncture is performed most often at the L3-4 interspace (below the level of the spinal cord at L1-2). Cisternal puncture is performed by the insertion of a needle into the cisterna magna using an approach from the back of the neck in the region of the foramen magnum. CSF pressure is also commonly measured during these procedures. The CSF can also be analyzed for gross characteristics and constituents (color, blood cells, electrolytes, and protein). The CSF may also be cultured for microorganisms (see Table 12-8).

SUMMARY REVIEW

Structure and Function of the Nervous System

1 The divisions of the nervous system are either structural (central nervous system) or functional (peripheral nervous system).

2 The central nervous system is contained within the brain and spinal cord.

3 The peripheral nervous system is composed of cranial and spinal nerves, which carry impulses toward the the CNS (afferent) and away from the CNS (efferent) to target organs or skeletal muscle.

Cells of the Nervous System

1 The neuron and neuroglial cell comprise nervous tissue. The neuron is specialized to transmit and receive electrical and chemical impulses, whereas the neuroglial cell provides supportive functions. The neuron is further divided into unipolar, bipolar, and multipolar, according to their structure and particular mechanics of impulse transmission.

2 The neuron is composed of a cell body, dendrite(s), and an axon. A myelin sheath around selected axons forms an insulation that allows quicker nerve impulse conduction.

The Nerve Impulse

1 The region between the neurons is the synapse and the region between the neuron and muscle is the myoneural junction. Neurotransmitters are responsible for chemical conduction across the synapse and myonerual junction. Nerve impulse is predominantly regulated by a balance of IPSPs and EPSPs, temporal and spatial summation, and convergence and divergence.

The Central Nervous System

1 The brain is contained within the cranial vault and is divided into three distinct regions: (1) forebrain, (2) hindbrain, and (3) midbrain.

2 The forebrain comprises the two cerebral hemispheres and allows conscious perception of internal and external stimuli, thought and memory processes, and voluntary control of skeletal muscles. The deep portion of the forebrain is termed the diencephalon and processes incoming sensory data. The center for voluntary control of skeletal muscle movements is located along the precentral gyrus in the frontal lobe, whereas the center for perception is along the postcentral gyrus in the parietal lobe. Broca's area (inferior edge of the postcentral gyrus) and Wernicke's area (superioposterior temporal lobe) are major speech centers.

3 The hindbrain allows sampling and comparison of sensory data, from the periphery and motor impulses from the cerebral hemispheres, for the purpose of coordination and refinement of skeletal muscle movement.

4 The midbrain is primarily a relay center for motor and sensory tracts, as well as a center for auditory and visual reflexes.

5 The spinal cord contains the majority of nerve fibers connecting the brain with the periphery. Reflex arcs are completed in the spinal cord and influenced by the higher centers in the brain.

6 The central nervous system is protected by the scalp, bony cranium, the spinal cord, and the cerebrospinal fluid. Cerebrospinal fluid is formed from blood components in the choroid plexuses of the ventricles and is reabsorbed in the arachnoid villi (located in the dural venous sinuses) after circulating through the brain and spinal cord.

7 The paired carotid and vertebral arteries supply blood to the brain and connect to form the circle of Willis. The major branches projecting from the circle of Willis are the anterior, middle, and posterior cerebral arteries. Drainage of blood from the brain is accomplished through the venous sinuses and jugular veins.

8 Blood supply to the spinal cord originates from the vertebral arteries and branches arising from the aorta.

The Peripheral Nervous System

1 The peripheral nervous system functions to relay information from the central nervous system to muscle and effector organs through cranial and spinal nerve tracts arranged in fascicles (multiple fascicles bound together form the peripheral nerve).

The Autonomic Nervous System

1 The autonomic nervous system is responsible for the maintenance of a steady state in the internal environment. Two opposing systems comprise the autonomic nervous system: (1) the sympathetic nervous system reponds to stress by mobilizing energy stores and prepares the body to defend itself, and (2) the parasympathetic nervous system conserves energy and the body's resources.

Tests of the Nervous System

1 Tests of nervous system function include x-ray films, computerized tomography, magnetic resonance imaging, positron emission tomography, brain scan, cerebral angiography, myelography, echoencephalography, electroencephalography, evoked potentials, and analysis of the cerebral spinal fluid.

KEY TERMS

Acetylcholine, 378

Adrenergic transmission, 378

Afferent neuron, 364

Afferent pathway (ascending pathway), 352

Amygdala, 360

Anterior fossa, 366

Anterior spinal artery, 371

Arachnoid membrane, 366

Arachnoid villi, 367

Association fiber, 360

Astrocyte, 355

Autonomic nervous system, 353

Axon, 353

Axon hillock, 353

Basal ganglia, 359

Basilar artery, 368

Bipolar neurons, 355

Blood-brain barrier, 370

Brainstem, 357

Brachial plexus, 372

Broca's speech area, 360

Cauda equina, 362

Caudate,

Cavernous sinus, 368

Celiac, 377

Cell body, 353

Central canal, 362

Central nervous system (CNS), 352

Cerebellum, 362

Cerebral aqueduct (aqueduct of Sylvius), 362

Cerebral cortex, 359

Cerebral peduncle, 362

Cerebrospinal fluid, 367

Cerebrum, 359

Chemoreceptors, 355

Cholinergic transmission, 378

Choroid plexus, 366

Cingulate gyrus,

Circle of Willis, 368

Collateral ganglia, 377

Contralateral control, 360

Conus medullaris, 362

Corpus callosum (transverse fibers, commissual fibers), 360

Corpus quadrigemina, 361

Corpus striatum, 360

Cranial nerves, 352

Craniosacral division, 377

Dendrite, 353

Dendritic zone, 353

Dermatome, 372

Diencephalon, 360

Dopamine, 362

Dorsal column, 364

Dorsal horn (posterior horn), 364

Dorsal root ganglion, 364

Dura mater, 366

Effector organ, 353

Efferent neuron, 364

Efferent pathway (descending pathway), 352

Endoneurium, 353

Ependymal cell, 356

Epidural space, 366

Epithalamus, 360

Excitatory postsynaptic potential (EPSP), 357

Extrapyramidal system, 360

Facilitation, 357

Falx cerebri, 366

Fascicle, 371

Fissure, 359

Fissure of Rolando (central fissure), 360

Foramen of Luschka, 367

Foramen of Magendie, 367

Frontal lobe, 360

Galea aponeurotica, 365

Ganglia, 353

Gray matter, 359

Gyri, 359

Hypothalamus, 360

Inferior colliculi, 361

Inferior mesenteric, 377

Inhibitory postsynaptic potential (IPSP), 357

Inner dura (meningeal layer), 366

Internal capsule, 360

Internal carotid arteries, 368

Interneuron, 355

Interventricular foramen (foramen of Monro), 367

Intervertebral disk, 368

Lateral column, 364

Lateral horn, 364

Lewy body, 382

Limbic system, 360

Lower motor neuron, 365

Lumbar plexus, 372

Lumbar puncture, 367

Mechanoreceptors, 355

Medulla oblongata, 362

Meninges, 366

Mesencephalon (midbrain), 361

Metencephalon, 362

Microfilaments, 353

Microglia, 356

Microtubule, 353

Middle fossa (temporal fossa), 366

Mixed nerves, 372

Motor unit, 365

Multipolar neuron, 355

Myelencephalon (medulla oblongata), 362

Myelin, 353

Myelin sheath, 353

Neurilemma, 353

Neurofibrillary tangles, 382

Neuroglia, 355

Neuromuscular junction, 355

Neuron, 353

Neurotransmitter, 357

Nissl substance, 353

Nociceptors, 355

Node of Ranvier, 353

Norepinephrine, 378

Nuclei, 358

Nucleus pulposus, 368

Occipital lobe, 360

Oligodendrocyte (pl. = oligodendroglia), 355

Parasympathetic nervous system, 376

Parietal lobe, 360

Pelvic nerve, 378

Periosteum (endosteal layer), 366

Peripheral nervous system (PNS), 352

Photochemical, 355

Plexus, 372

Pons, 362

Postcentral gyrus, 360

Posterior fossa, 366

Posterior spinal artery, 371

Postganglionic neuron, 372

Postsynaptic neuron, 356

Precentral gyrus, 360

Prefrontal area, 360

Preganglionic neuron, 372

Premotor area, 360

Presynaptic neuron, 356

Primary motor area, 360

Primary voluntary motor pathway, 360

Projective artery (nutrient artery), 368

Pyramidal system, 360

α receptor, 378

β receptor, 378

Red nucleus, 361

Reflex arc, 364

Reflex areas, 364

Reticular activating system, 358

Reticular formation, 358

Sacral plexus, 372

Saltatory conduction, 354

Schwann cell, 353

Senile plaque, 382

Sensory neurons, 355

Schwann's sheath, 353

Somatic nervous system, 353

Spatial summation, 357

Spinal cord, 362

Spinal nerve, 352

Spinal tract, 364

Spinothalamic tract, 364

Splanchnic nerves, 377

Subarachnoid space, 366

Subdural space, 366

Substantia gelatinosa, 364

Substantia nigra, 361

Subthalamus, 360

Sulci, 359

Summation, 357

Superficial artery (conducting artery), 368

Superior colliculi, 361

Superior mesenteric, 377

Sylvian fissure (lateral fissure), 360

Sympathetic (paravertebral) ganglia, 376

Sympathetic nervous system, 376

Synapse, 356

Synaptic cleft, 357

Synaptic terminal, 357

Tegmentum, 361

Telencephalon, 359

Temporal lobe, 360

Temporal summation, 357

Tentorium cerebelli, 366

Thalamus, 360

Thermoreceptors, 355

Thoracolumbar division, 376

Unipolar neuron, 355

Ventral horn (anterior horn), 364

Ventricle, 367

Vermis, 362

Vertebral artery, 368

Vertebral column, 362

Wallerian degeneration, 356

Wernicke's area, 360

White matter, 359

REFERENCES

Brown, D. R. (1980). *Neurosciences for allied health therapies.* St. Louis: C.V. Mosby.

Chusid, J. G. (1985). *Correlative neuroanatomy and functional neurology.* Los Altos, Calif.: Lange Medical Publications.

Conway-Rutkowski, B. L. (1982). *Carini and Owens' neurological and neurosurgical nursing.* St. Louis: C.V. Mosby.

Davis, A. O., & Lefkowitz, R. J. (1981). Regulation of adrenergic receptors. In R. J. Lefkowitz (Ed.), *Receptor regulation* (series B, vol. 13). London: Chapman & Hall.

Dayan, A. D., & Lewis, P. D. (1985). The central nervous system—Neuropathology of aging. In J. C. Brocklehurst (Ed.), *Textbook of geriatric medicine and gerontology.* New York: Churchill Livingston, pp. 268-293.

Department of Neurosciences, University of Florida. (1979). *Neuroanatomy and neurophysiology.* Gainesville, FL: Author.

Eyzaguirre, C., & Fidone, S. J. (1975). *Physiology of the nervous system: An introductory text* (2nd ed.). Chicago, Yearbook Publishers.

Gehrke, M. (1980). Identifying brain tumors. *Journal of Neursurgical Nursing, 12*(2), 90-92.

Gilman, S., & Winans, S. (Eds.). (1987). *Manter and Gatz's essentials of clinical neuroanatomy and neurophysiology* (7th ed.). Philadelphia: Davis.

Hickey, J. V. (1986). *The clinical practice of neurological and neurosurgical nursing* (2nd ed.). Philadelphia: Lippincott.

Hirano, A., & Llena, J. F. (1983). Degenerative diseases of the central nervous system. In R. N. Rosenburg (Ed.), *The clinical neurosciences: Neuropathology.* New York: Churchill Livingstone, pp. 285-324.

Larson, E. (1980). The epidemiology of brain tumors. *Journal of Neurosurgical Nursing, 12*(3), 121-127.

Lindsley, D. F., & Holmes, J. E. (1984). *Basic human neurophysiology.* New York: Elsevier.

Nobeck, C. R., & Demarst, R. J. (1986). *The human nervous system. Basic principles of neurobiology.* New York: McGraw-Hill.

Nolte, J. (1988). *An introduction to its functional anatomy* (2nd ed.). St. Louis: C.V. Mosby.)

Pathy, M. S. (1985). The central nervous system—Clinical presentations and management of neurological disorders in old age. In J. C. Brocklehurst (Ed.), *Textbook of geriatric medicine and gerontology.* New York: Churchill Livingstone, pp. 391-426.

Raven, P. H., & Johnson, G. B. (1986). *Biology.* St. Louis: C.V. Mosby.)

Restak, R. M. (1984). *The brain.* New York: Bantam.

Rossor, M. N. (1985). The central nervous system—Neurochemistry of the aging brain and dementia. In J. C. Brocklehurst (Ed.), *Textbook of geriatric medicine and gerontology.* New York: Churchill Livingstone, pp. 294-308.

Rudy, E. B. (Ed.). (1984). *Advanced neurological and neurosurgical nursing.* St. Louis: C.V. Mosby.

Scheibel, E. S., & Scheibel, B. S. (1975). Structural changes in the aging brain. In H. Brody, D. Harman, & J. M. Ordy (Eds.), *Clinical, morphological, and neurochemical aspects of the aging nervous system.* New York: Raven Press, pp. 11-37.

Snyder, S. H. (1985, October). The molecular basis of communication between cells. *Scientific American, 253,* 4.

Spence, A. P., & Mason, E. B. (1983). *Human anatomy and physiology.* Menlo Park, Calif.: Benjamin Cummings.

Thompson, J. M. et al. (1989). *Mosby's manual of clinical nursing* (2nd ed.). St. Louis: C.V. Mosby.)

Timiras, P. S. (Ed.). (1972). *Development physiology and aging.* New York: Macmillan.

Timiras, P. S., & Vernadakis, A. (1972). Structural, biochemical, and functional aging of the nervous system. In P. S. Timiras (Ed.), *Developmental physiology and aging.* New York: MacMillan, pp. 502-526.

Vick, R. L. (1984). *Contemporary medical physiology.* Menlo Park, Calif.: Addison-Wesley.

Willis, W. D., & Grosman, R. G. (1981). *Medical neurobiology: Neuroanatomical and neurophysiological practices basic to clinical neuroscience* (3rd ed.). St. Louis: C.V. Mosby.

CHAPTER 13

Pain, Temperature Regulation, Sleep, and Sensory Function

Mary Schoessler
Patti Ludwig-Beymer
Sue E. Huether

Pain, 391
    The experience of pain, 391
        Somatic vs. psychogenic pain, 391
        Acute vs. chronic pain, 392
        Pain threshold and pain tolerance, 392
        Age and the perception of pain, 393
    Neuroanatomy of pain, 393
        The role of the afferent and efferent pathways, 394
        The role of the spinal cord, 395
    Neurophysiology of pain, 396
        Theories of pain, 396
        Neuromodulation, 397
    Clinical manifestations of pain, 397
        Acute pain, 397
            Physiologic response, 399
            Psychologic and behavioral response, 399
        Chronic pain, 399
            Physiologic response, 399
            Psychologic and behavorial response, 399
            Chronic pain conditions, 399
Temperature regulation, 400
    Hypothalamic control of temperature, 401
    Mechanisms of heat production, 402
        Chemical reactions of metabolism, 402
        Skeletal muscle contraction, 402
        Chemical thermogenesis, 402
    Mechanisms of heat loss, 402
        Radiation, 402
        Conduction, 402
        Convection, 402
        Vasodilation, 402
        Decreased muscle tone, 403
        Evaporation, 403
        Increased respiration, 403
        Voluntary mechanisms, 403
        Adaptation to warmer climates, 403

Mechanisms of heat conservation, 403
        Vasoconstriction, 403
        Voluntary mechanisms, 403
    Changes in temperature regulation with age, 404
Physiology of fever, 404
    Pathogenesis of fever, 404
    Benefits of fever, 405
Disorders of temperature regulation, 405
    Hyperthermia, 405
        Heat cramps, 405
        Heat exhaustion, 405
        Heatstroke, 405
        Malignant hyperthermia, 406
    Hypothermia, 406
        Accidental hypothermia, 406
        Therapeutic hypothermia, 407
    Trauma, 407
        Central nervous system trauma, 408
        Accidental injuries, 408
        Hemorrhagic shock, 408
        Major surgery, 408
        Thermal burns, 408
Sleep, 408
    Stages of sleep, 409
    Aging and sleep patterns, 410
        Sleep patterns in children, 410
        Sleep patterns of the elderly, 410
    Sleep disorders, 411
        Disorders of initiating sleep—insomnia, 411
        Disorders of excessive somnolence, 411
        Disorders of the sleep-wake schedule, 411
        Dysfunctions of sleep, sleep stages, or partial arousals, 412
            Somnambulism, 412
            Night terrors, 412
            Enuresis, 412
    Relation between sleep and disease, 412

Secondary sleep disorders, 412
Sleep-provoked disorders, 412
The special senses, 413
Vision, 413
The external eye structures, 413
Conjunctivitis, 413
Keratitis, 414
The normal eye, 414
Aging and vision, 415
Visual dysfunction, 415
Alterations in ocular movements, 415
Alterations in visual acuity, 416
Alterations in accommodation, 416
Alterations in refraction, 417
Alterations in color vision, 417
Neurologic disorders causing visual dysfunction, 418
Hearing, 419
The normal ear, 419
Aging and hearing, 420
Auditory dysfunction, 420
Conductive hearing loss, 420
Sensorineural hearing loss, 421
Mixed hearing loss, 421
Functional hearing loss, 421
Olfaction and taste, 421
Aging and olfaction and taste, 422
Olfaction, 422
Taste, 422
Olfactory dysfunction, 422
Taste dysfunction, 423
Somatosensory function, 423
Touch, 423
Proprioception, 423

Alterations in sensory function may involve dysfunctions of the general or special senses. Dysfunctions of the general senses include chronic pain, abnormal temperature regulation, tactile dysfunction, and proprioceptive dysfunction. Dysfunction of the special senses includes visual, auditory, vestibular, olfactory, and gustatory dysfunction.

The special senses of vision, hearing, touch, smell, and taste are the means by which individuals perceive stimuli that are essential in interacting with the environment. Special sensory receptors are connected to specific areas of the cerebral cortex through the afferent pathways of the CNS. Each of the special senses thus involves a connected system of organs and tissues that receive stimuli and portions of the CNS, where sensory stimuli are processed.

All definitions of pain suggest that it is a complex phenomenon composed of sensory experiences that include time, space, intensity, emotion, cognition, and motivation. Pain is an unpleasant phenomenon that is uniquely experienced by each individual; it cannot be adequately defined, identified, or measured by an observer. McCaffery (1980d) defines pain as "whatever the experiencing person says it is, existing whenever he says it does."

Unlike pain, which is a subjective experience without a precise form of measurement, temperature regulation is measured by clearly defined normal limits. Like pain, however, variations in temperature can signal disease. Fever is a common manifestation of dysfunction and is often the first symptom observed in an infectious or inflammatory condition. If the body's temperature regulatory mechanism is out of balance, the result may be death.

Sleep is a normal cyclical process that restores the body's energy and maintains normal functioning. Sleep is so essential to both physiologic and psychologic function that sleep deprivation causes a wide range of clinical manifestations. Prolonged deprivation or disruption of sleep ultimately leads to serious dysfunction.

PAIN

The Experience of Pain

Three systems interact to produce pain. They are the (1) sensory/discriminative system, (2) the motivational/affective system, and (3) the cognitive/evaluative system (Saunders, 1979). The **sensory/discriminative system** processes information about the strength, intensity, and temporal and spacial aspects of pain. These sensations are mediated through afferent nerve fibers, the spinal cord, the brainstem, and the higher brain centers. The **motivational/affective system** determines the individual's approach/avoidance behaviors. These behaviors are mediated through the interaction of the reticular formation, limbic system, and brainstem.

The **cognitive/evaluative system** overlies the individual's learned behavior concerning the experience of pain. The individual's interpretation of appropriate pain behavior is learned in several ways, among them cultural preferences, male and female roles, and past experience. The influence of the cognitive/evaluative system may block, modulate, or enhance the perception of pain.

Somatogenic vs. Psychogenic Pain

Attempts to categorize pain have suggested two common classes: (1) somatogenic and (2) psychogenic. **Somatogenic pain,** such as the pain of a crushed finger or a heart attack, is pain with a cause. In contrast, **psychogenic pain** is pain for which there is no known physical cause. Psychogenic pain, however, is *not* imaginary pain. It may be just as intense as somatogenic pain and just as distressing. The labels somatogenic and psychogenic provide some basis for describing pain, but pain is only *primarily* somatogenic or psychogenic; it is rarely, if ever, purely one type or the other (McCaffery, 1980d).

TABLE 13-1 Comparison of acute and chronic pain

Characteristic	Acute pain	Chronic pain
Experience	An event	A situation, state of existence
Source	External agent or internal disease	Unknown; if known, treatment is prolonged or ineffective
Onset	Usually sudden	May be sudden or develop insidiously
Duration	Transient (up to 6 months)	Prolonged (months to years)
Pain identification	Painful and nonpainful areas generally well identified	Painful and nonpainful areas less easily differentiated; change in sensations becomes more difficult to evaluate
Clinical signs	Typical response pattern with more visible signs	Response patterns vary; fewer overt signs (adaptation)
Significance	Significant (informs person something is wrong)	Insignificant; person looks for significance
Pattern	Self-limiting or readily corrected	Continuous or intermittent; intensity may vary or remain constant
Course	Suffering usually decreases over time	Suffering usually increases over time
Actions	Leads to actions to relieve pain	Leads to actions to modify pain experience
Prognosis	Likelihood of eventual complete relief	Complete relief usually not possible

Adapted from Black, 1975.

Acute vs. Chronic Pain

The pain experience may be functionally divided into acute and chronic types. **Acute pain** is a protective mechanism that alerts the individual to a condition or experience that is immediately harmful to the body. The onset of acute pain is usually sudden, and the pain is relieved when the threatening stimulus is removed. Acute anxiety is always associated with acute pain. Anxiety is a response to the threat inherent in the painful experience, including issues surrounding the cause of pain, its treatment, and prognosis. Hope of recovery is also associated with acute pain. Acute pain mobilizes the individual to prompt action to relieve it (Melzack & Wall, 1983).

Chronic pain is persistent, usually defined as lasting at least 6 months. The cause of chronic pain is often unknown, and if the cause is known, the pain does not respond to usual therapy. The onset may be sudden, but chronic pain often develops insidiously so that the individual generally experiences more suffering over time. Individual behavior is adaptive and directed toward modifying the pain. Chronic pain is very often associated with a sense of hopelessness and helplessness as the cure becomes more elusive and the timeframe protracted. The pain is perceived as meaningless. Depression often results. (**Table 13-1** compares the characteristics of chronic and acute pain.)

Pain Threshold and Pain Tolerance

The **pain threshold** is the point at which a stimulus is perceived as pain. The threshold does not vary significantly among people or in the same person over time. Intense pain at one location may, however, cause an increase in the threshold in another location. For example, a person with severe pain in one knee is less likely to experience chronic back pain that is less intense. This phenomenon is called **perceptual dominance.** Because of perceptual dominance, an individual with many painful sites may report only the most painful one. Then, when the dominant pain is diminished, the individual identifies other painful areas (Berlin, Boodell, & Wolff, 1958).

Pain tolerance is the duration of time or the intensity of pain that an individual will endure before initiating overt pain responses. It is the amount of pain the person will tolerate before outwardly responding to it. Pain tolerance is influenced by the person's cultural prescriptions, expectations, role behaviors, and physical and mental health. Pain tolerance is generally decreased with repeated exposure to pain. Tolerance is also decreased by fatigue, anger, boredom, apprehension, and sleep deprivation. Tolerance may be increased by alcohol consumption, medication, hypnosis, warmth, distracting activities, and strong beliefs or faith (McCaffery, 1980d).

Pain tolerance varies greatly among people and in the same person over time. Because of the body's ability to

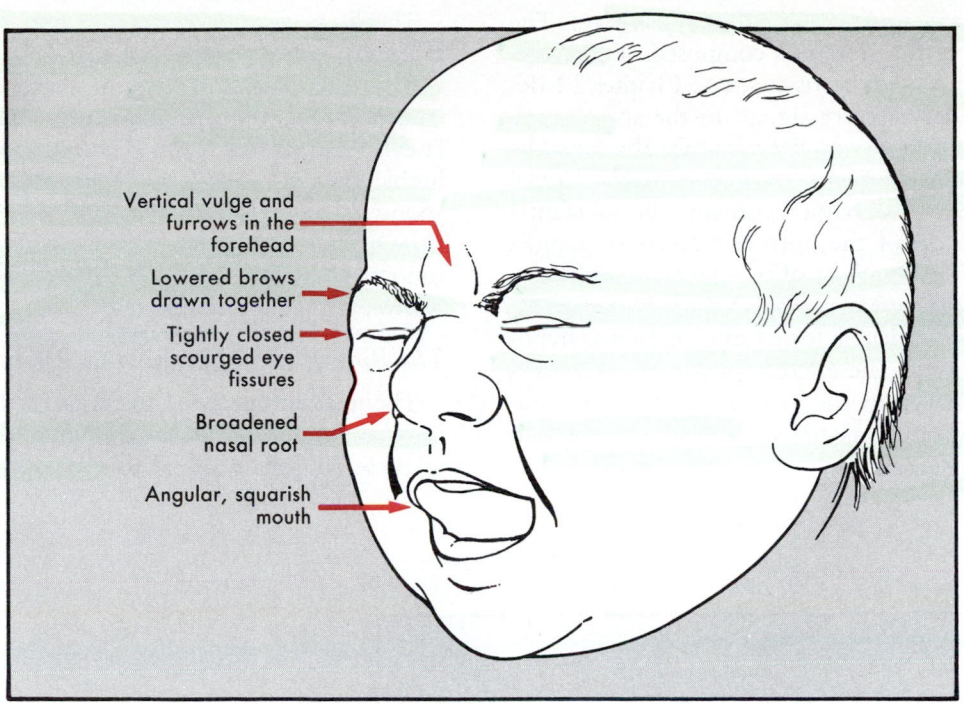

Vertical vulge and
furrows in the
forehead

Lowered brows
drawn together

Tightly closed
scourged eye
fissures

Broadened
nasal root

Angular, squarish
mouth

FIG. 13-1. Painful facial expression of infants two to four months.

respond differently to the noxious stimuli, pain tolerance varies. No direct relationship exists between the intensity of painful stimuli and an individual's perception
of pain or response to pain.

Age and the Perception of Pain

Children and the elderly may experience or express
pain differently than adults. Controversy exists over the
ability of very young infants to feel pain. Although
some authors (Terenius, 1981) believe that infants in
the first 1 to 2 days of life are less sensitive to pain, others (Johnston & Strada, 1986) believe that the young
simply lack the ability to verbalize the pain experience.
Richard, Bernal, and Brackbill (1976) reported that infants who were circumcised without local anesthesia
cried more than those who received anesthesia. The increase in crying lasted for several days. A full behavioral
response to pain is apparent at 3 to 12 months of life
(Terenius, 1981).

Change in facial expression is the most consistent expression of pain in infants 2 to 4 months of age
(Johnston & Strada, 1986). The painful facial expression includes lowered brows drawn together; presence
of a vertical bulge and furrows in the forehead between
the brows; broadened nasal root; tightly closed,
scourged eye fissures; and angular, squarish mouth (Fig.

13-1). Other, less consistent expressions include a drop
in heart rate, long high-pitched cry with subsequent apnea, and rigidity of torso and limbs. Older children, between the ages of 5 and 18 years, tend to have a lower
pain threshold than do adults (Haslam, 1969).

Studies on pain perception in the elderly have yielded
conflicting evidence. Some studies show an increase in
the pain threshold with aging (Sherman & Mitchell,
1974); others show no change (Birren, Shapiro, &
Miller, 1950; Harkins & Warner, 1977). The varied results are probably a function of independent variation in
the sensory/discriminative, motivational/affective, and
cognitive/evaluative components of the pain experience.
In general studies confirm that an increase in the pain
threshold occurs in some elderly people. This change is
probably caused by peripheral neuropathies and changes
in the thickness of the skin (Kenshalo & Hall, 1974).
(Neuropathies are discussed in Chapter 15.) A decrease
in pain tolerance is also evident in the elderly, and
women appear to be more sensitive to pain than men
(Woodrow, Friedman, & Siegelaub, 1972).

Neuroanatomy of Pain

The portions of the nervous system responsible for
the sensation and perception of pain may be divided
into three areas: (1) the afferent pathways, (2) the cen-

tral nervous system, and (3) the efferent pathways. The afferent portion of the system is composed of **nociceptors** (pain receptors) in the tissues. (As Chapter 12 describes, afferent nerves carry signals to the spinal cord, and the spinal cord network that transmits the signal to the brain. Afferent pathways terminate in the dorsal horn of the spinal cord, which contains the substantia gelatinosa at the tip of the horn and layers of ganglia called laminae.) The portions of the central nervous system involved in the interpretation of the pain signals are the limbic system, reticular formation, thalamus, hypothalamus, and cortex. The efferent pathways, composed of the fibers connecting the reticular formation, midbrain, and substantia gelatinosa, are responsible for modulating pain sensation.

The brain first perceives the sensation of pain. The thalamus, cortex, and postcentral gyrus perceive, describe, and localize the pain. Parts of the thalamus, brainstem, and reticular formation identify dull, longer-lasting, and diffuse pain. The reticular formation and limbic system control the emotional and affective response to pain. Because the cortex, thalamus, and brainstem are interconnected with the hypothalamus and autonomic nervous system, the perception of pain is associated with an autonomic response.

The Role of the Afferent and Efferent Pathways

The nociceptors are at the ends of the small unmyelinated and lightly myelinated afferent neurons. The ends of these neurons respond to chemical, mechanical, and

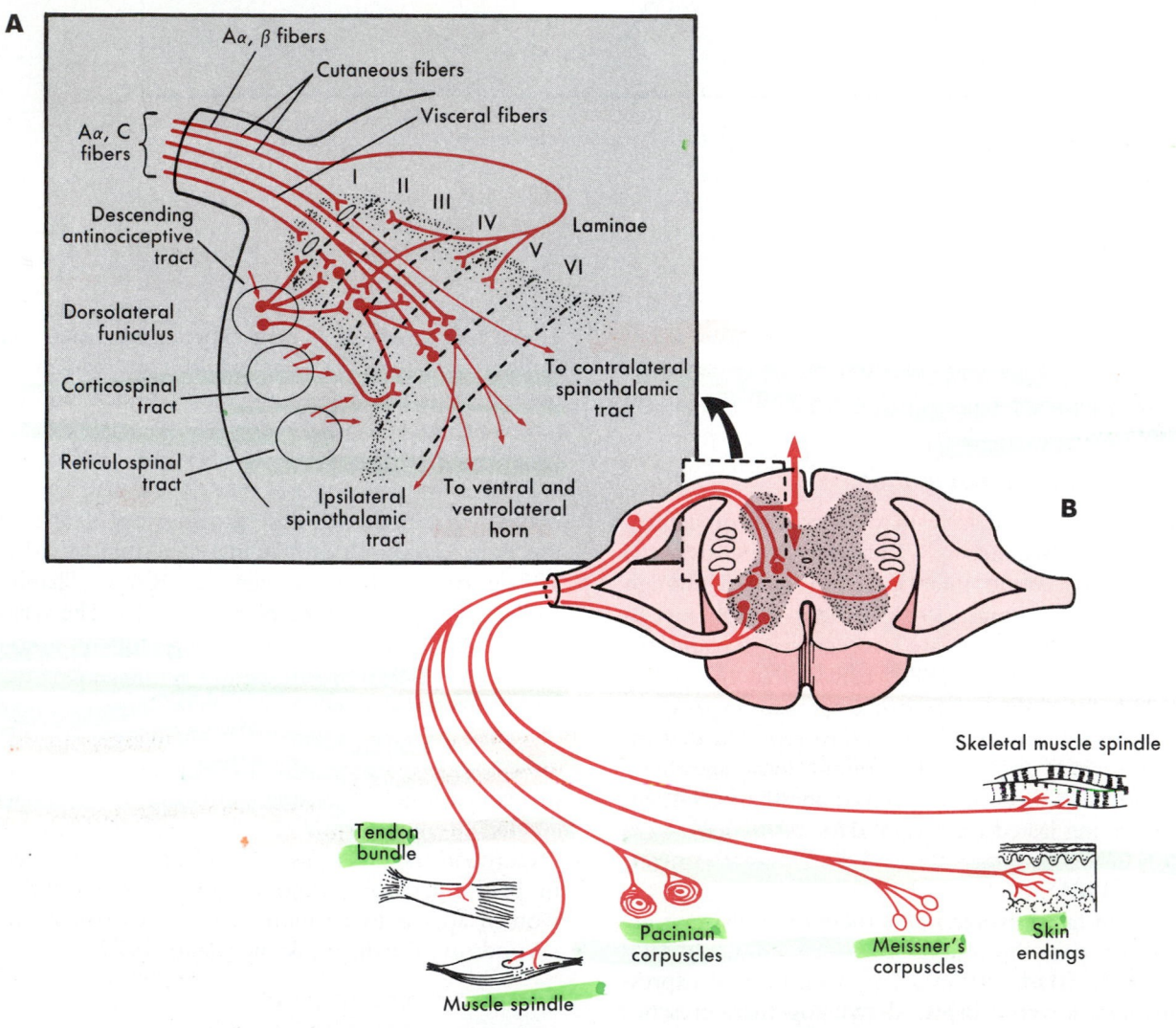

FIG. 13-2. Nociceptors and spinal segment. **A,** Nociceptive and other afferent and efferent pathways in a spinal nerve at the dorsal horn. **B,** Small A-delta and C fibers from synapses primarily with cells in lamina V but also with cells in laminae IV and VI.

thermal stimuli. Mild stimulation, such as gentle touch or warmth, may produce a positive, pleasurable sensation. Deep pressure or extreme heat generally produces pain. The differences in the interpretation of these stimuli are a result of the frequency and amplitude of the afferent signal. In addition to distal stimulation, nociceptors may be activated more proximally as they pass through areas of entrapment in the spinal column. Heat injury and inflammation associated with rheumatic disease appear initially to lower the threshold and increase the intensity of response to additional painful stimuli. However, repeated noxious stimulation to inflamed joints results in an eventual decrease in sensitivity (Smukler, 1985). In some instances, physiologic states, such as increased skeletal muscle tone, enhance excitability of nociceptors (Brena, 1985).

Nociceptors may be found in the muscles, tendons, subcutaneous tissue (as nerve endings termed **pacinian corpuscles**), and epidermis (as **Meissner corpuscles**). They also appear as bare endings in the skin. They are not evenly distributed in the body. For example, the skin has many more nociceptors than the internal structures, and the eye has many more than the arm. This maldistribution of nociceptors affects the relative sensitivity to pain of different areas of the body.

As Fig. 13-2 illustrates, stimulation of nociceptors produces impulses that are transmitted through small A-delta fibers and C fibers to the spinal cord, where they form synapses with neurons in the dorsal horn. From the dorsal horn the nociceptive impulses are transmitted to various parts of the spinal cord and to the rest of the central nervous system.

The small unmyelinated C neurons are responsible for the transmission of diffuse burning or aching sensations. Because of the size of the fiber and the lack of a myelin sheath, transmission through C fibers is relatively slow. Transmission through the slightly larger, myelinated A fibers occurs much more quickly. A fibers carry well-localized, sharp pain sensations. The reflex arc to and from the spinal cord is much faster than the transmission of the pain stimulus. Therefore, the retraction of the injured body part occurs before the individual perceives the pain.

The efferent pathway is responsible for modulation or inhibition of afferent pain signals. Afferent stimulation of the **periaqueductal gray (PAG)** (gray matter surrounding the cerebral aqueduct) in the midbrain stimulates the efferent pathway. Efferent neurons located in the PAG form synapses in the medulla. From there the impulse is transmitted through the spinal cord to the dorsal horn. The dorsolateral funiculus (a cordlike structure lying between the dorsal root ganglion and ventral root ganglion) contains efferent inhibitory fibers that make contact with cells in laminae I, II, and V to impair or block transmission of nociceptive impulses.

The Role of the Spinal Cord

Most afferent pain fibers terminate in the dorsal horn of the spinal segment that they enter. Some, however, extend toward the head or the foot for several segments before terminating. The A fibers terminate in the substantia gelatinosa; some large A-delta fibers and small C fibers terminate in the laminae. The laminae then transmit specific information. For example, lamina I specifically transmits information about burned or crushed skin, and lamina IV transmits information about gentle pressure.

Secondary neurons transmit the impulse from the substantia gelatinosa and laminae through the ventral and lateral horn, crossing, in the same or adjacent spinal segments, to the other side of the cord. From there the impulse is carried through the spinothalamic tracts to the brain (Fig. 13-3). The two divisions of the spinothalamic tract that carry pain information to the

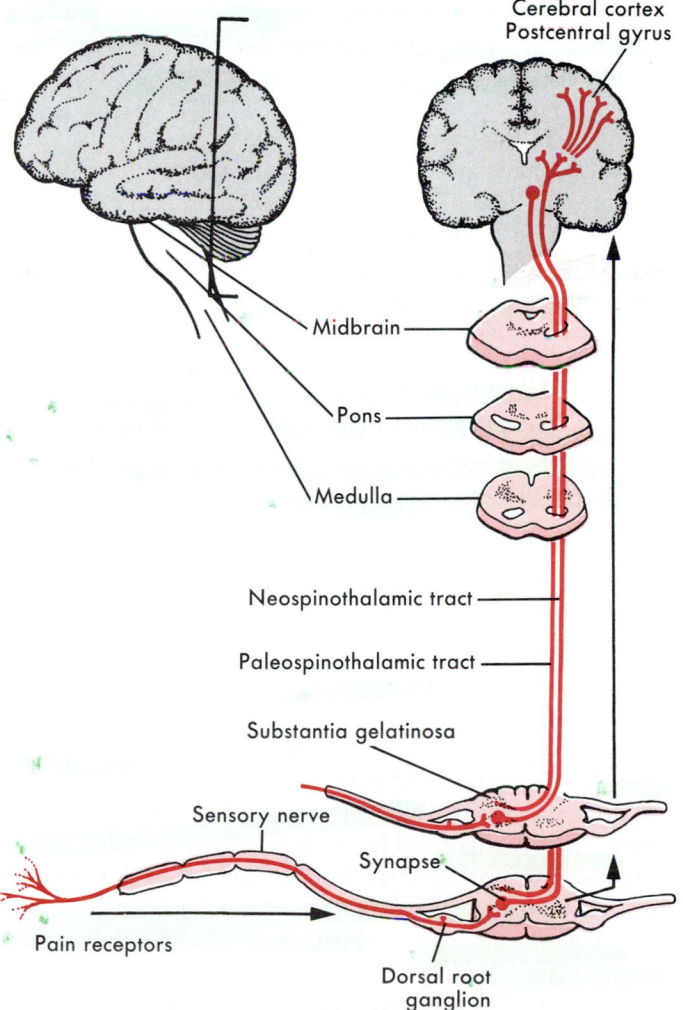

Cerebral cortex
Postcentral gyrus

Midbrain

Pons

Medulla

Neospinothalamic tract

Paleospinothalamic tract

Substantia gelatinosa

Sensory nerve

Synapse

Pain receptors

Dorsal root ganglion

FIG. 13-3. Spinal cord and CNS pathway. Stimuli are transmitted from pain receptors through sensory nerves into the dorsal root ganglia. The impulse enters the spinal cord, forms a synapse, crosses the cord, and rises to the spinothalamic tract.

TABLE 13-2 Stimuli that activate nociceptors (pain receptors)

Location of receptor	Provoking stimuli
Skin	Pricking, cutting, crushing, burning, freezing
Gastrointestinal tract	Engorged or inflamed mucosa, distention or spasm of smooth muscle, traction on mesenteric attachment
Skeletal muscle	Ischemia, injuries of the connective tissue sheaths, necrosis, hemorrhage, prolonged contraction, injection of irritating solutions
Joints	Synovial membrane inflammation
Arteries	Piercing, inflammed
Headache	Traction and displacement of arteries and meningeal structures, arterial pulsation

brain are (1) the neospinothalamic tract and (2) the paleospinothalamic tract. The neospinothalamic tract carries information to the midbrain, postcentral gyrus (where pain is perceived), and cortex. The paleospinothalamic tract carries information to the reticular formation, pons, limbic system, and midbrain.

Neurophysiology of Pain

Nociceptors around the body respond to various "painful" stimuli (Table 13-2). These stimuli produce or are produced by tissue damage. Damaged tissues release proteolytic enzymes that provoke the release of bradykinins, histamines, and prostaglandins. These substances depolarize adjacent nociceptors. The nociceptors then continue to depolarize as long as the painful stimulus is applied. Leukokinin, released from lymphocytes in chronic inflammatory lesions, mimics the action of prostaglandins, histamine, and bradykinins and may be responsible for some types of chronic pain. (Inflammation is discussed in Chapter 7.)

Theories of Pain

Several theories have been proposed to describe the mechanisms of pain. The earliest, the specificity theory, was proposed by Max Von Frey. Later, several theorists (Livingston, Noordenbos, and others) proposed slightly different theories (collectively known as the pattern theory). They claimed that pain is caused by patterns of incoming stimuli. In 1965 Melzak and Wall proposed the gate control theory. The theory was later refined by Melzak and Casey (1968) and Melzak and Wall (1970).

The **specificity theory** proposes four major categories of cutaneous sensation: (1) touch, (2) warmth, (3) cold, and (4) pain. Each cutaneous sensation is the result of stimulation of specific receptor sites on the skin. Stimulation of the nerve endings of the pain receptors precipitates transmission of the painful stimuli (through A-δ and C fibers) to the spinal cord. The pain neurons form synapses in the substantia gelatinosa and cross to the opposite side of the spinal cord, ascending to the brain through the spinothalamic tract. The perception of pain then occurs in special areas of the thalamus and cerebral cortex.

According to the specificity theory there is a direct relationship between the stimulus and the perception of pain. Although this theory postulates the existence of specific skin receptors for pain and explains why actual tissue damage causes pain, it fails to account for adaptation to pain and effects of psychosocial factors on pain perception (Melzak & Wall, 1965).

The **pattern theory** suggests that the perception of pain is the result of stimulus intensity (a function of the length of time and the amount of tissue involved) and the summation of the impulses. According to the pattern theory, nonspecific receptors transmit patterns of nerve impulses from the skin to the spinal cord. Certain patterns of impulses are then perceived as pain. Theorists disagree about where the summation occurs. According to some, summation occurs in the spinal cord; according to others, it occurs in the brain. Although the pattern theories do not account for adaptation to pain, they do allow for the many factors that contribute to pain perception (Melzak & Wall, 1965).

Melzak and Wall proposed the **gate control theory** in 1965 (Fig. 13-4). According to this theory, nociceptive impulses are transmitted from specialized skin receptors to the spinal cord through small A and larger C fibers (Fig. 13-4). These fibers terminate in the substantia gelatinosa, in the dorsal horn of the spinal cord. Cells in the substantia gelatinosa function as a gate, regulating transmission of impulses to the central nervous system. Stimulation of larger fibers causes the cells in the substantia gelatinosa to "close the gate." A closed gate decreases stimulation of trigger cells, decreases transmission impulses, and diminishes pain perception. Persistent stimulation of the large fibers, however, allows adaptation. When adpatation to impulses from large fibers occurs, the result is a relative increase in

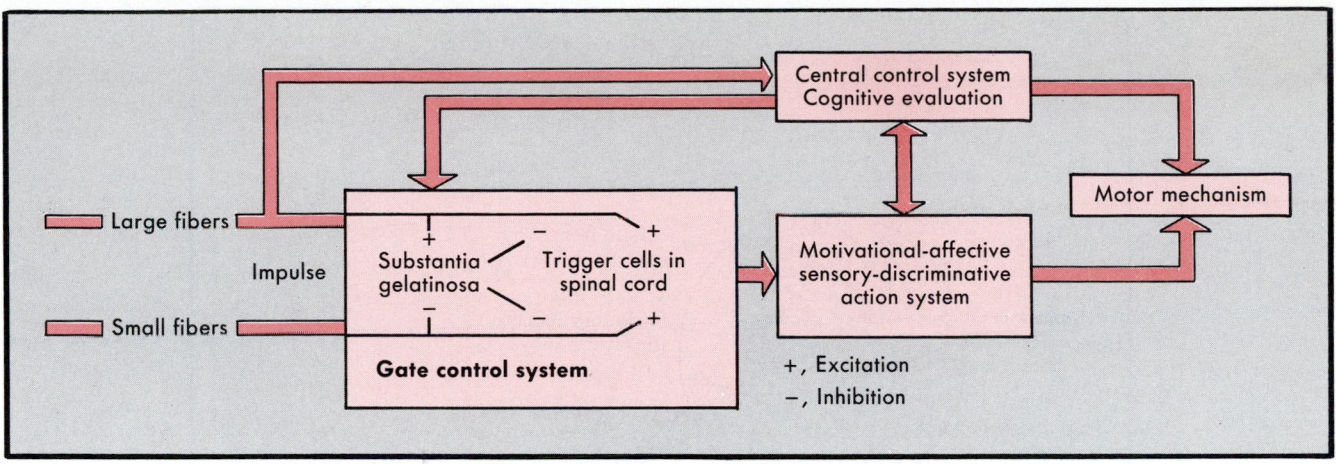

FIG. 13-4. Schematic diagram of the gate control theory of pain mechanism.

small neuron activity. Adaptation to larger fibers may thus "open the gate." Scratching and vibration prevent large neuron adaptation and keep the gate closed over prolonged periods.

Small fiber input inhibits cells in the substantia gelatinosa and opens the gate. An open gate increases the stimulation of trigger cells, increases transmission of impulses, and enhances pain perception. In addition to gate control through large and small fiber stimulation, the central nervous system, through efferent pathways, may close, partially close, or open the gate.

Cognitive functioning may thus modulate pain perception. Interaction of the cognitive/evaluative, motivational/affective, and sensory/discriminative systems determines the individual's pain response (Melzak, 1975; Melzak & Casey, 1968; Melzak & Wall, 1965, 1970).

Neuromodulation

Another group of naturally occurring chemicals called **endorphins** (endogenous morphines) inhibits transmission of the pain impulse (Foley, 1984). Endorphins are present in varying concentrations in neurons in the brain, spinal cord, and gastrointestinal tract. Endorphins in the brain are released in response to afferent noxious stimuli (Snyder, 1977). Endorphins in the spinal cord are released in response to efferent impulses.

Three classifications of endorphins are (1) β-lypotrophin, (2) enkephalin, and (3) dynorphin. **β-lypotrophin** (β-, γ-, and α-endorphin) is a potent endorphin located in the hypothalamus and the pituitary gland. These endorphins may be responsible for general sensations of well-being. **Enkephalin,** found in the neurons of the brain and spinal cord, is a weaker analgesic than other endorphins but is more potent and longer lasting than morphine. **Dynorphin** (a powerful endorphin) is 50 times more potent than β-endorphin. Dynorphin re-

portedly originates in the neural lobe of the pituitary (Henry, 1986).

All endorphins act by attaching to **opiate receptors** on the plasma membrane of the afferent neuron (Fig. 13-5). The combination of the opiate receptor and endorphin inhibits the release of the neurotransmitter, thus blocking the transmission of the painful stimulus. In much the same way exogenous opiates relieve pain by attaching to the opiate receptors and augmenting the natural endorphin response (West, 1981). The enkephalin-endorphin receptors have also been identified as specific cellular attachment sites for morphine and other exogenous narcotic molecules.

Stress, excessive physical exertion, acupuncture, intercourse, and other factors increase the level of circulating endorphins, raising the pain threshold (Henry, 1986). Although still controversial, there is some evidence to suggest that high levels of circulating endorphins may play a role in so-called painless myocardial ischemia and infarction (Van Rijn & Rabkin, 1981; Sheps et al., 1987).

Clinical Manifestations of Pain
Acute Pain

Three types of acute pain are (1) somatic, (2) visceral, and (3) referred. **Somatic pain** is superficial (coming from the skin or close to the surface of the body) and is either sharp and well localized or dull, aching, poorly localized, and accompanied by nausea and vomiting. **Visceral pain** refers to pain in internal organs, the abdomen, or skeleton. It is poorly localized and is associated with nausea and vomiting, hypotension, restlessness, and, in some cases, shock. Visceral pain often radiates (spreads away from the actual site of the pain) or is referred. **Referred pain** is pain that is present in an area removed or distant from its point of origin. The area of

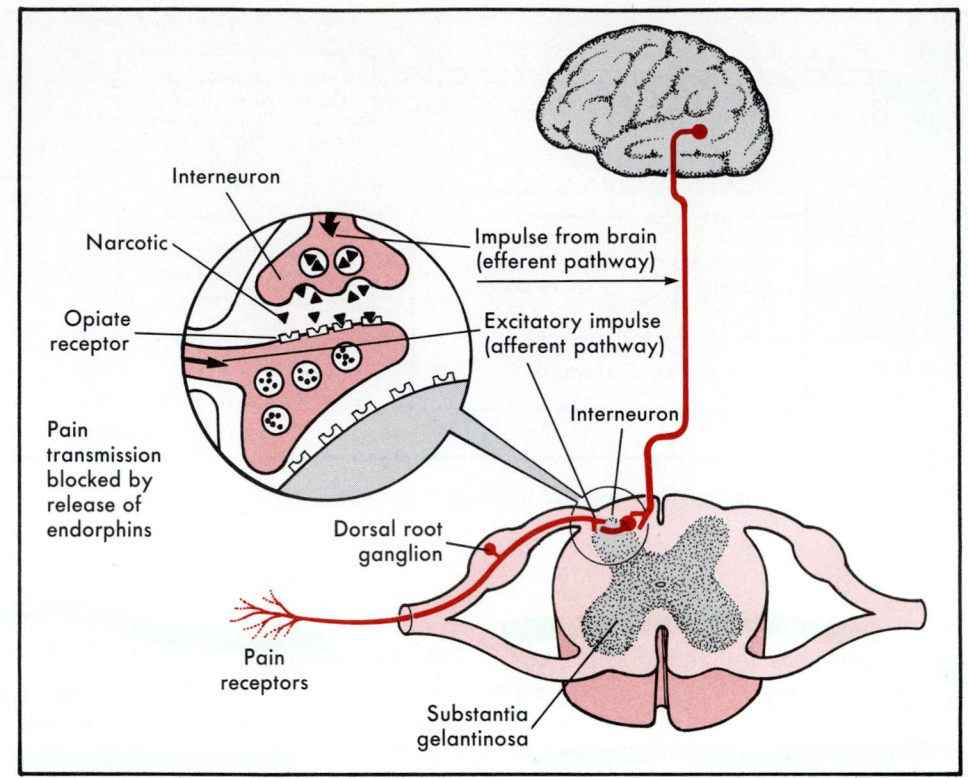

FIG. 13-5. Descending pathway and endorphin response. The biologic receptors of the enkephalins and endorphins are located close to known pain receptors in the ascending and descending pain pathways.

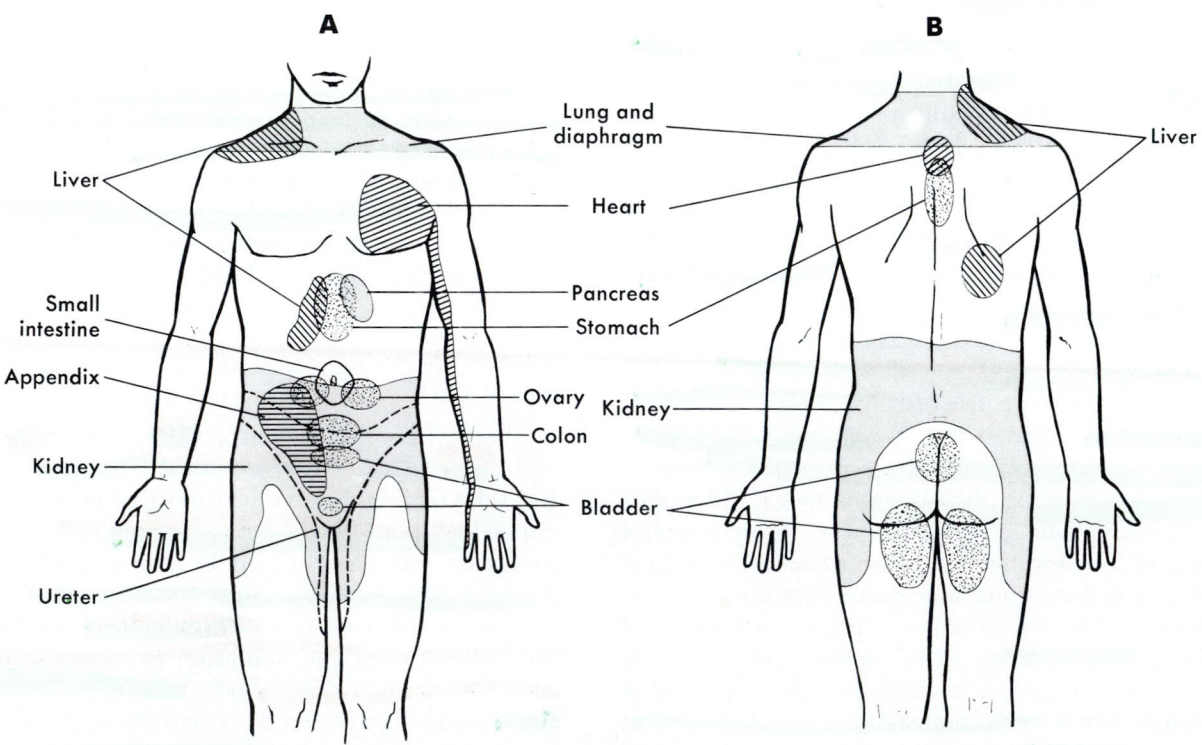

FIG. 13-6. Sites of referred pain. **A,** Front. **B,** Back. (From Phipps, Long, & Woods, 1987.)

referred pain is supplied by the same spinal segment as the actual site of pain (Meinhart & McCaffery, 1983). Convergence of cutaneous and visceral fibers in lamina V in the spinal cord segment is probably the basis for referred pain. Referred pain is regional and predictable. (Common areas of referred pain and their associated sites of origin appear in Fig. 13-6.)

Physiologic Response

Acute pain is a warning of actual or impending tissue injury. Physiologic responses therefore include increased heart rate, increased respiratory rate, elevated blood pressure, pallor or flushing, dilated pupils, and diaphoresis. Blood sugar is elevated; gastric acid secretion and motility are decreased; and blood flow to the viscera and skin is decreased. Nausea occasionally occurs.

Psychologic and Behavioral Response

Individuals often psychologically respond to acute pain with fear (e.g., fear of diagnosis, fear of continued pain), anxiety, and a general sense of unpleasantness or unease. The stress of fear may in turn contribute to the physiologic signs of pain. Individuals do not always discuss their pain. One study, for example, showed that 70% of hospitalized persons with acute pain did not like to discuss it with others, either because of negative social connotations or because they believed their pain to be insignificant when measured against others' problems. More than two thirds of these individuals would not communicate about their pain until it became severe (Jacox, 1979).

Chronic Pain

Chronic pain is prolonged pain that may be persistent (e.g., low back pain) or intermittent (e.g., migraines). Chronic pain may be caused or aggravated by a decreased level of endorphins or a predominance of a C neuron stimulation (Almay et al., 1980). Chronic pain is more difficult to manage or control than acute pain (see Table 13-1).

Physiologic Response

Physiologic responses to chronic pain depend on the persistent or intermittent nature of the pain. Intermittent pain produces a physiologic response similar to acute pain, whereas persistent pain allows for physiologic adaptation. Adaptation produces normal heart and respiratory rates and normal blood pressure. Other physiologic responses to acute pain also become normal, but even though the physiologic responses are normal, the pain is not relieved.

Psychologic and Behavioral Response

Chronic pain produces significant behavioral and psychologic changes. Individuals with chronic pain often are depressed, have difficulty sleeping, and may become preoccupied with the pain (Sternbach, 1974). Living with chronic pain requires constant attention to the earliest signs of pain so that the pain-provoking stimuli can be identified and avoided. Persons with chronic pain generally attempt to keep pain-related behavior to a minimum so that they appear as normal as possible. The need to have someone understand that the pain and the need to hide it are usually conflicting drives for those with chronic pain. They tend not to report pain for fear of being labeled complainers. They often deny pain and sometimes engage in activities that provoke pain so that they can keep up with others. Even in learning to pace themselves through the day's activities, they may aggravate the pain (Strauss & Glasser, 1975).

Chronic Pain Conditions

The most common chronic pain condition is persistent low back pain. This, like many other conditions, is a result of poor muscle tone, inactivity, muscle strain, or sudden vigorous exercise. Other chronic conditions include neuralgias, hyperesthesias, myofascial pain syndrome, and hemiageusias. Chronic pain is associated with cancer in some instances.

Neuralgias are painful conditions that result from an infection or disease that damages a peripheral nerve. Causalgias and reflex sympathetic dystrophies are types of neuralgias. **Causalgia** is a condition causing severe burning pain that may be triggered by normally nonnoxious stimuli such as light touch, sound, or cold. The pain appears 1 to 2 weeks after injury to either the brachial plexus, the median nerves, or the sciatic nerves. The severe, diffuse, and persistent pain occurs in the extremity supplied by the injured nerve. Discoloration and changes in the texture of the skin may appear in the affected area. Excessive nail growth may be noted, and swelling and stiffness of proximate joints may occur.

Reflex sympathetic dystrophies occur after peripheral nerve injury and are characterized by continuous severe, burning pain. The pain is often associated with vasospasm and vasomotor changes. Vasomotor changes usually begin with vasodilation and are followed by vasoconstriction and cool cyanotic and edematous extremities. As muscle wasting occurs, amputation of the involved extremity may be required.

Hyperesthesias are chronic pain conditions characterized by increased sensitivity and decreased pain threshold to tactile and painful stimuli. Stimuli that usually do not produce pain thus become painful. The pain is usually diffuse, modified by fatigue and emotion, and mixed with other sensations. The hyperesthesia may be the result of chronic irritation of the thalamus and other central areas.

Myofascial pain syndromes are the second most common cause of chronic pain. These conditions include myositis, fibrositis, myofibrositis, myalgia, and muscle strain; they involve injury to the muscle and fascia. The pain is a result of muscle spasm, tenderness, and stiffness. These conditions lead to muscle guarding, a behavior that limits muscle motion. In turn limited motion causes muscle weakness, stiffness, tenderness, and spasm, all of which produce more pain. The pain is described as dull and aching and may be mild to disabling. During the early stages of the disorder, the pain is localized, but as the disorder progresses, the pain becomes more generalized.

Hemiagnosia is a loss of ability to identify the source of pain on one side (the affected side) of the body. Application of painful stimuli to the affected side thus produces anxiety, moaning, agitation, and distress but no attempt to withdraw from or push aside the offending stimulus. Individuals report unbearable discomfort but cannot identify the source because they are unable to locate the site through normal sensory pathways. Emotional and autonomic responses to the pain may be intensified. Hemiagnosia is associated with stroke that produces paralysis and a hypersensitivity to pain in the affected side. Application of painful stimuli to the unaffected side produces a normal response.

Phantom limb pain is pain that an individual feels in an amputated limb. The pain persists after the stump has completely healed and is more likely to appear in individuals who experienced pain in the limb before amputation. Phantom limb pain may be influenced by emotions and sympathetic stimulation and may also be associated with trigger points. **Trigger points** are small hypersensitive regions in the muscle or connective tissue. They may be close to or removed from the area of pain, but stimulation of the trigger point produces pain in a specific area.

Cancer is often associated with chronic pain. Studies done at Memorial Sloan-Kettering Cancer Center indicate three major categories of pain syndromes that result in chronic pain in the individual with cancer (Foley, 1984). The categories are (1) pain attributed to the advance of the disease, (2) pain associated with treatment of the disease, and (3) pain attributed to coexisting entities (e.g., osteoarthritis) that are unrelated to the disease.

By far the most common cause of chronic pain in the individual with cancer is that attributed to the advance of the disease (Foley, 1984). Pain can be caused by infection and inflammation, increasing pressure of a growing tumor on nerve endings, stretching of visceral surfaces, and/or obstruction of ducts and intestine. This pain may be acute, intermittent, or continuous. Therapeutic approaches are partially effective in controlling the pain. Pain from tumor infiltration of nerve tissue; trauma or chemical injury to the nerve; damage from radiation, chemotherapy, or surgical sectioning of the nerve produces another form of chronic pain referred to as deafferentation pain. (Deafferentation refers to a loss of sensory input from a portion of the body.) Deafferentation pain is described as a constant dull ache, "viselike," with paroxysms of burning or electrical-shock-like sensations. It may lead to hyperactivity of neurons in the spinal cord and thalamus. Deafferentation pain is poorly controlled by peripheral and epidural analgesia (Foley, 1985; Payne, 1987).

Some individuals experience chronic pain after treatment (see Chapter 10). Chronic postoperative pain occurs in a small percentage of individuals after the following:

1. Thoracotomy, with pain often caused by tumor recurrence or invasion of the chest wall
2. Radical mastectomy, with pain resulting from interruption of the intercostobrachial nerve (which branches from the brachial plexus to the thoracic region)
3. Radical neck dissection, with pain attributable to surgical injury or interruption of the cranial nerves
4. Surgical amputation, which may be followed by phantom limb pain

Chemotherapy, especially treatment with vinca alkaloids, may be associated with a variety of neuropathies producing painful dysthesias (needles and pins sensations) in the feet and hands. Radiation therapy may result in connective tissue fibrosis and secondary nerve injury that produces pain (Foley, 1984).

TEMPERATURE REGULATION

In all homeothermic animals, temperature regulation is achieved through precise balancing of heat production, heat conservation, and heat loss. In humans, body temperature is maintained in a range around 37° C (98.6° F). The normal range is considered to be 36.2 to 37.7° C (96.2 to 99.4° F), but all parts of the body do not have the same temperature. The extremities, for example, are generally cooler than the trunk. The temperature at the core of the body (as measured by rectal temperature) is generally 0.05° C higher than at the surface (as measured by oral temperature). The internal temperature varies normally in response to activity, environmental temperature, and daily fluctuation of **circadian rhythm** (the pattern of each 24-hour day). Oral temperatures generally fluctuate within ± 0.02 to 0.05° C over a 24-hour period. Women tend to have wider fluctuations that follow the menstrual cycle, with a sharp rise in temperature just prior to ovulation. In both sexes the daily fluctuating temperature peaks around 6:00 in the evening and is at its lowest during sleep (Dinarello & Wolff, 1978).

Maintenance of body temperature within the normal

range is necessary for life. **Hyperthermia** (marked warming of core temperature) can produce nerve damage, coagulation of cell proteins, and death. At 41° C (106° F) nerve damage produces convulsions in the adult. At 43° C (109° F) death results. **Hypothermia** (marked cooling of core temperature) produces vasoconstriction, alterations in microcirculation, coagulation, and ischemic tissue damage. In a controlled situation, such as surgical procedure, most tissues can tolerate temperatures as low as 7° C. In severe hypothermia ice crystals forming on the inside of the cell cause cells to rupture and die.

Hypothalamic Control of Temperature

Temperature regulation is mediated hormonally by the hypothalamus. Peripheral thermoreceptors in the skin and central thermoreceptors in the hypothalamus, spinal cord, abdominal organs, and other central locations provide the hypothalamus with information about skin and core temperatures. If these temperatures are low, the hypothalamus responds by triggering heat production and heat conservation mechanisms.

Increased heat production is initiated by a series of hormonal mechanisms involving the hypothalamus and its connections with the endocrine system (see Chapter 17). The heat-producing mechanism begins with a hypothalamic hormone, thyrotropin-stimulating hormone-releasing hormone (TSH-RH). TSH-RH in turn stimulates the anterior pituitary to release thyroid-stimulating hormone (TSH), which acts on the thyroid gland, stimulating release of thyroxine (T_4), one of the thyroid hormones. This hormone then acts on the adrenal medulla, causing the release of epinephrine (a catecholamine and vasopressive hormone) into the bloodstream (see Chapter 17). Epinephrine causes vasoconstriction, stimulates glycolysis, and increases metabolic rates, thus increasing heat production.

The hypothalamus also triggers heat conservation.

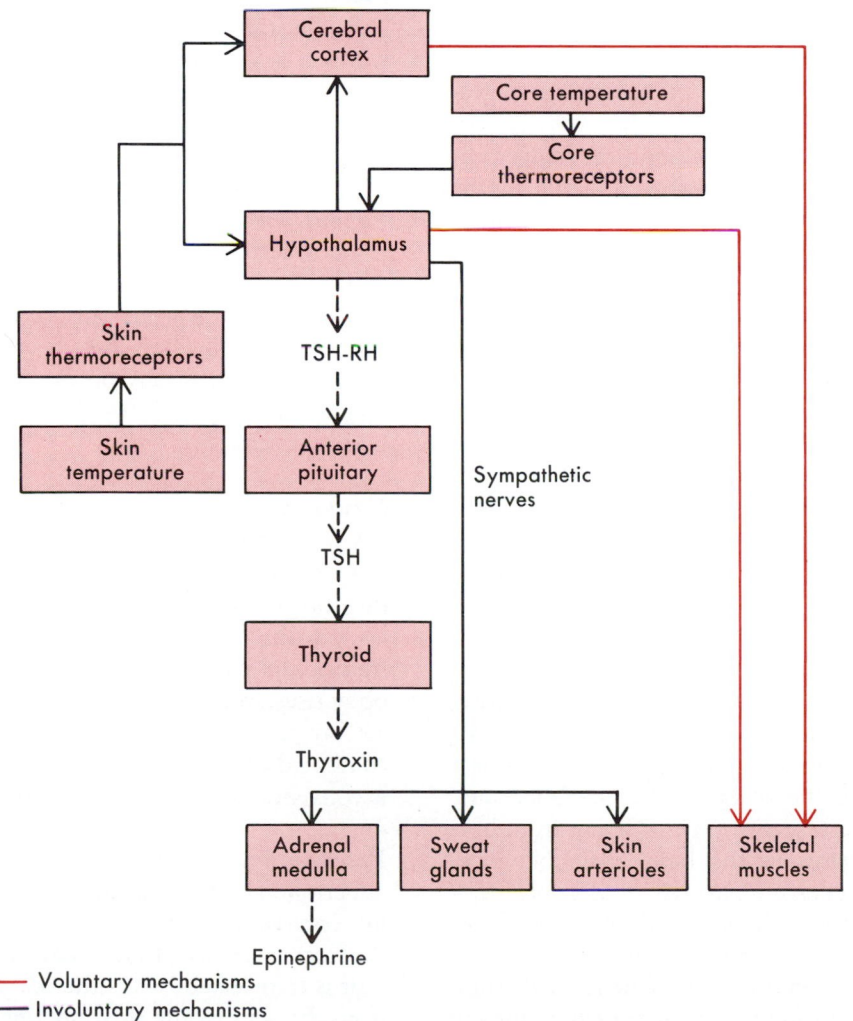

FIG. 13-7. Temperature-regulating mechanisms. The dashed lines are hormonal pathways, which are probably of minor importance in human beings. (Adapted from Phipps & Long, 1983.)

The mechanisms of heat conservation involve stimulating the sympathetic nervous system, which is responsible for stimulating the adrenal cortex, increasing skeletal muscle tone, initiating the shivering response, and producing vasoconstriction. The hypothalamus also functions in raising body temperatures by relaying information to the cerebral cortex. Awareness of cold provokes voluntary responses such as increased body movement.

The hypothalamus responds to warmer core and peripheral temperatures by reversing the same mechanisms. The TSH-RH pathway is shut down. The sympathetic pathway is prompted to produce vasodilation, decreased muscle tone, and increased sweat production. Hypothalamic stimulation of the cerebral cortex provokes voluntary measures to reduce heat production and promote heat loss (Fig. 13-7).

Mechanisms of Heat Production

Body heat is produced by the chemical reactions of metabolism, skeletal muscle tone and contraction, and chemical thermogenesis.

Chemical Reactions of Metabolism

The chemical reactions that occur during the ingestion and metabolism of food and those required to maintain the body at rest (basal metabolism) require energy and give off heat. These processes occur in the body core and are in part responsible for the maintenance of core temperature.

Skeletal Muscle Contraction

Skeletal muscles produce heat through two mechanisms: (1) gradual increase in muscle tone and (2) rapid muscle oscillations (shivering). Both increasing muscle tone and shivering are controlled by the hypothalamus and occur in response to cold. As peripheral temperature drops, muscle tone increases, and shivering begins. Shivering is a fairly effective method for increasing heat production, because no work is performed and all the energy produced is retained as heat.

Chemical Thermogenesis

Chemical thermogenesis, also called nonshivering thermogenesis, results from the release of epinephrine. Epinephrine produces a rapid, transient increase in heat production by raising the body's basal metabolic rate. Chemical thermogenesis seems to be different from hormone-triggered increases in the basal metabolic rate. Chemical thermogenesis—through epinephrine—produces a quick, brief rise in basal metabolic rate, whereas the hormone thyroxine triggers a slow, prolonged rise (Himms-Hagen, 1980). Chemical thermogenesis occurs in brown adipose tissue present mainly in small newborn mammals that have high surface-to-volume ratios. Like other small newborn mammals,

human infants lose more heat through conduction and convection than they are capable of generating through normal metabolic mechanisms. Brown adipose tissue, therefore, plays an important role in maintaining body temperature in the newborn. As with most mammals reared in a temperature-controlled environment, humans gradually lose the capacity for chemical thermogenesis as brown adipose cells dedifferentiate. This can occur as early as 4 weeks after birth (Benito, 1985). Because of the decrease in brown adipose tissue in the adult, the role of this mechanism of heat production in adults is unknown (Heaton, 1972).

Mechanisms of Heat Loss

Heat loss is achieved through several mechanisms: (1) radiation, (2) conduction, (3) convection, (4) vasodilation, (5) decreased muscle tone, (6) evaporation, (7) increased respiration, (8) voluntary measures, and (9) adaption to warmer climates.

Radiation

Radiation refers to heat loss through electromagnetic waves. These waves emanate from surfaces with temperatures higher than the surrounding air. Thus if the temperature of the skin is higher than that of the air, the skin and therefore the body lose heat to the air.

Conduction

Conduction refers to heat loss by direct molecule-to-molecule transfer from one surface to another. Through conduction the warmer surface loses heat to the cooler surface. Thus the skin loses heat through direct contact with cooler air, water, or another surface. In the same manner the core of the body loses heat to the cooler body surface.

Convection

Convection is the transfer of heat through currents of gases or liquids. It greatly aids heat loss through conduction by exchanging warmer air at the surface of the body with cooler air in the surrounding space. Convection occurs passively as warmer air at the surface of the body rises away from the body and is replaced by cooler air, but the process may be aided by fans or wind. (The combined effect of conduction and convection by wind is conventionally measured as the "wind-chill factor.")

Vasodilation

Peripheral vasodilation increases heat loss by diverting core-warmed blood to the surface of the body. As the core-warmed blood passes through the periphery, heat is transferred by conduction to the skin surface and from the skin to the surrounding environment. Because heat loss through conduction depends on the temperature of the surrounding medium, heat loss through conduction is minimal to nonexistent if the surrounding air is warmer than the body surface.

Vasodilation occurs in response to autonomic stimulation under the control of the hypothalamus. It is useful in instances of moderate temperature elevation. As core temperature rises vasodilation increases until maximal dilation is achieved. At that point the body must use additional heat loss mechanisms.

Decreased Muscle Tone

To decrease heat production muscle tone may be moderately reduced and voluntary muscle activity curtailed. These mechanisms explain in part the "washed-out" feeling associated with high temperatures and warm weather. Both decreased muscle tone and reduced activity have a limited effect on decreasing heat production, however, as muscle tone and heat production cannot be reduced below basal body requirements.

Evaporation

Evaporation of body water from the surface of the skin and the linings of the mucous membranes is a major source of heat reduction. Insensible water loss (in the absence of perceptible sweating) accounts for a loss of about 600 ml of water per day. Heat is lost as surface fluid is converted to gas, so that heat loss by evaporation is increased if more fluids are available at the body surface. To speed this process, fluids are actively secreted through the sweat glands. Up to 4 L of fluid per hour may be lost by sweating. Electrolytes are lost with the water. Therefore, loss of large volumes through sweating may result in decreased plasma volume, decreased blood pressure, weakness, and fainting. (Alterations in fluid balance are discussed in Chapter 3.)

Like other heat reduction mechanisms, stimulation of sweating occurs in response to sympathetic neural activity and depends on a favorable temperature difference between the body and the environment. In addition heat loss through evaporation is affected by the relative humidity of the air. If the humidity of the air is low, sweat evaporates quickly, but if the humidity is high, sweat does not evaporate and instead remains on the skin or drips off.

Increased Respiration

Exchanging air with the environment through the normal respiratory process provides some heat loss, although it is minimal. As air is inhaled, the air draws heat from the upper respiratory tract. The air is further warmed in the alveoli by blood in the microcirculation. This warmed air is then exhaled into the environment. This normal process occurs faster at higher body temperatures through an increase in respiratory rates. Thus hyperventilation is associated with hyperthermia. (Normal pulmonary function is discussed in Chapter 29.)

Voluntary Mechanisms

In response to high body temperatures, people typically "stretch out," thereby increasing the body surface area available for heat loss. They also "slow down" or "take it easy," thereby decreasing skeletal muscle work, and they "dress for warm weather." The most efficient dress for warm weather is a light-colored, loose-fitting garment, because light colors reflect heat from the body and loose-fitting garments allow free air movement for convection, conduction, and evaporation to occur.

Adaptation to Warmer Climates

When individuals move from cooler to much warmer climates, their bodies undergo a period of adjustment, a process that takes several days to weeks. At first the individual experiences feelings of lassitude, weakness, and faintness with even moderate activity. Body temperatures rise with any work. Within several days, however, the individual experiences an earlier onset of sweating; the volume of sweat is increased; and the sodium content is lowered. Heart rate is decreased and stroke volume increased so that cardiac output remains unchanged. Extracellular fluid volume increases as does plasma volume. These physiologic adaptations result in improved warm weather functioning and decreased symptoms of heat intolerance. Work output, endurance, and coordination increase, while subjective feelings of discomfort decrease (Yousef, 1987).

Mechanisms of Heat Conservation

The body conserves heat and protects core temperature through two important mechanisms: (1) involuntary vasoconstriction and (2) voluntary mechanisms. To preserve core temperature, the skin and periphery are used as an insulating cover (Yousef, 1987).

Vasoconstriction

By constricting peripheral blood vessels, centrally warmed blood is shunted away from the periphery (where radiation, conduction, and convection would allow heat loss) to the core of the body, where heat can be retained. This mechanism takes advantage of the insulating layers of the skin and subcutaneous fat to protect core temperature.

Voluntary Mechanisms

In response to lower body temperatures, individuals typically "bundle up," "keep moving," or "curl up in a ball." Bundling up involves dressing with several layers of clothes that allow air to be trapped between the skin and the clothing, thus providing an additional layer of insulation. Keeping moving, stamping feet, clapping hands, jogging, and other types of physical activity increase skeletal muscle activity and thus promote heat production. Curling up in a ball decreases the amount of skin surface available for heat loss through radiation, convection, and conduction.

Changes in Temperature Regulation with Age

Infants and the elderly require special attention to maintenance of body temperature. Infants produce sufficient body heat but are unable to conserve heat produced. The poor heat conservation is caused by the infant's small body size and greater ratio of body surface to body weight, which give the infant more surface area for heat loss. Infants also have a very thin layer of subcutaneous fat and thus are not as well insulated as adults (Hammarlund, Stromberg, & Sedin, 1986). The elderly have poor responses to environmental temperature extremes as a result of slowed blood circulation, structural and functional changes in the skin, and overall decrease in heat-producing activities. Other factors affecting thermal regulation in the elderly include decrease in shivering response (delayed onset and decreased effectiveness), slowed metabolic rate, sedentary life-style, decreased vasoconstrictor response, diminished or absent sweating, desynchronization of circadian rhythm, undernutrition, and decreased perception of heat and cold (Collins & Exton-Smith, 1983; Fellows, McDonald, & Bennett, 1985).

Both infants and elderly people have difficulty regulating body heat through physiologic mechanisms of heat production and conservation. Health care providers need to be aware of these particular developmental differences, because infants cannot adjust to the environment to compensate for heat loss, and the elderly, because of decreased peripheral sensation, may not be alerted to the need to do so.

Physiology of Fever

The appearance of fever (temperature elevation) suggests a pathologic process such as viral or bacterial infection. It is triggered by the release of leukocytic **endogenous pyrogens** (fever-producing substances), now called interleukin I (IL-1), primarily from mononuclear phagocytes and other cells (including neutrophils) involved in the immune response, and it is mediated by prostaglandins of the E series. Fever is a symptom of the disease and a normal immunologic mechanism. (The immune response is discussed in Chapter 7. Cellular effects of fever are discussed in Chapter 2).

Pathogenesis of Fever

Fever is not the result of a failure of the normal thermoregulatory mechanism but is thought to be a "resetting of the thermostat" to a higher level. The thermoregulatory mechanisms adjust heat production, conservation, and loss to maintain body core temperature at a normal level. During fever this level is raised so that the thermoregulatory center now adjusts heat production, conservation, and loss to maintain the core temperature at the new, higher temperature, which functions as a new "set point" (Dinarello & Wolff, 1978). Interleukin I and mediating prostaglandins are responsible for elevating the "set point."

The pathophysiology of fever begins with the introduction of exogenous pyrogens (Fig. 13-8). The most frequently encountered exogenous pyrogens include endotoxins, gram-positive bacteria, and viruses. Endotoxins, or bacterial pyrogens, are lipopolysaccharides. They are derived from cell walls of gram-negative organisms, and the lipid part of the molecule is necessary for their pyrogenic actions (Cooper & Veale, 1987). The production and release of IL-1 occur as exogenous bacteria are destroyed and absorbed by phagocytic cells within the host. Interleukin I acts on the brain to cause fever. The precise locus of action in the central system is unknown (Cooper & Veale, 1987). The action of IL-1 appears to be due in part to release of the prostaglandin E series. Other mechanisms are known to be involved but are currently unidentified. As the set point is raised, the hypothalamus signals an increase in heat production and conservation to raise body temperature to the new level. Peripheral vasoconstriction occurs; epinephrine release increases metabolic rate; and muscle tone increases. Shivering may also occur. The individual feels colder, dresses more warmly, decreases body surface area by curling up, and may go to bed in an effort to get warm. Body temperature is maintained at the new level until the fever "breaks."

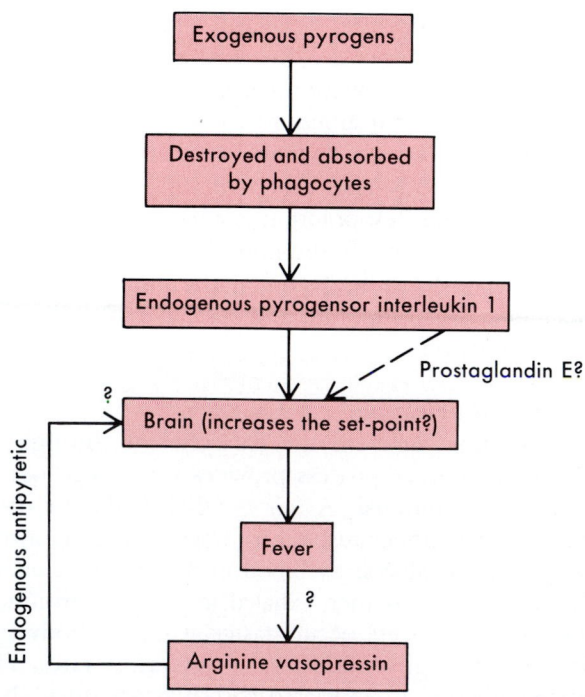

FIG. 13-8. Pathophysiology of fever. (See text for explanation.)

During fever arginine vasopressin (AVP) is released from nerve fibers where it acts as an **endogenous antipyretic,** or helps to diminish the febrile response. This antipyretic effect constitutes a negative feedback loop (Fig. 13-8) (Cooper & Veale, 1987). The antipyretic effect may help to explain fluctuations in the febrile response. When the fever breaks, the set point is returned to normal. The hypothalamus responds by signaling a decrease in heat production and an increase in heat reduction mechanisms. The result is decreased muscle tone, peripheral vasodilation, flushing of the skin, and sweating. The individual feels very warm, replaces warm clothing with cooler clothes, throws off the covers, and stretches out. Once the body has returned to a normal temperature, the individual feels more comfortable, and the hypothalamus adjusts thermoregulatory mechanisms to maintain the new temperature.

Benefits of Fever

Fever production aids responses to infectious processes through several mechanisms (Bernheim, Block, & Atkins, 1979; Cunha, Digamon-Beltran, & Gobbo, 1984). Simple raising of body temperature kills many microorganisms and has adverse effects on the growth and replication of others. Higher body temperatures decrease serum levels of iron, zinc, and copper, all of which are needed for bacterial replication. Increased temperature also causes lysosomal breakdown and autodestruction of cells, thus preventing viral replication in infected cells. Heat increases lymphocytic transformation and motility of polymorphonuclear neutrophils, thus facilitating the immune response. Phagocytosis is enhanced, and production of antiviral interferon may be augmented (Dinarello & Wolff, 1982).

Because fever is a beneficial response to infection, suppression of fever by treatment with antipyrogenic medications should be carefully reviewed. Such treatment should be employed only if the fever produces or is high enough to produce serious side effects such as nerve damage or convulsion (Cunha et al., 1984; Gurevich, 1985.)

Infection and fever responses in the elderly and in children may vary from those in the normal adult. The elderly may have decreased or no fever response to infection. The absence of fever responses to infection and, therefore, the beneficial aspects of fever production may explain the increase in morbidity and mortality seen in the very elderly (Norman, Grahn, & Hoshikawa, 1985). In contrast to the very elderly, children develop higher temperatures than adults for relatively minor infections. Febrile seizures may occur with temperatures above 39° C (102.2° F), although most children do not develop febrile seizures until temperatures are much higher. Febrile seizures are more predominant in male children before the age of 5. Febrile seizures are generally brief and self-limiting, lasting less than 5 minutes in 40% of children and less than 20 minutes in 75% of children. Authorities differ over the significance of febrile seizures. Although in most instances there appears to be no long-term effect on the child, a very few children (1% to 2%) may develop epilepsy (Fruthaler, 1985; Wright, 1987).

Disorders of Temperature Regulation
Hyperthermia

Hyperthermia may be accidental or therapeutic. Therapeutic hyperthermia is a form of local or general body-induced hyperthermia. Its purpose is to destroy pathologic microorganisms and/or tumor cells by facilitating the host's natural immune process through fever production. As a form of treatment, it is generally controversial. The four forms of accidental hyperthermia are (1) heat cramps, (2) heat exhaustion, (3) heatstroke, and (4) malignant hyperthermia.

Heat Cramps

Heat cramps are severe, spasmotic cramps in the abdomen and extremities that follow prolonged sweating and associated sodium loss. Heat cramps usually appear in individuals who are not accustomed to heat or in those who are performing strenuous work in very warm climates. Fever, rapid pulse, and increased blood pressure often accompany the cramps. Treatment involves administration of dilute salt solutions through oral or parenteral routes.

Heat Exhaustion

Heat exhaustion, or collapse, is a result of prolonged high core or environmental temperatures. These high temperatures cause the appropriate hypothalamic response of profound vasodilation and profuse sweating. Over a prolonged period the hypothalamic responses produce dehydration, decreased plasma volumes, hypotension, decreased cardiac output, and tachycardia. The individual feels weak, dizzy, nauseated, and faint. The symptoms of heat exhaustion cause the individual to stop work, lie down, and rest. Ceasing activity decreases muscle work, causing decreased heat production. Lying down redistributes vascular volume. The individual should be encouraged to drink warm fluids to replace fluid lost through sweating.

Heatstroke

Heatstroke is a potentially lethal result of a breakdown in control of an overstressed thermoregulatory center. The brain cannot tolerate temperatures over 40.5° C (105° F). When core temperature reaches or exceeds 40.5° C (105° F) the brain may be preferentially cooled by maximal blood flow through the veins of the head and face, specifically the forehead. Sweat production on the face is maintained even during dehydration.

Evaporation of the sweat cools the blood in the veins of the face and forehead; the blood is then returned to the endocranial venous network and sinus cavernosus, cooling the blood in the cerebral arterial vessels that lie in close proximity. Fanning the face enhances this mechanism. In this way the brain can be temporarily maintained at 40° C (105° F), even when core temperatures are higher (Cabanac & Brinnell, 1987; Yousef, 1987). In instances of very high core temperatures (40 to 43° C(104 to 109.4° F)), the regulatory center may cease to function appropriately. Sweating ceases, and the skin becomes dry and flushed. The individual may be irritable, confused, stuporous, or comatose. Visual disturbances may occur.

As heat loss through the evaporation of sweat ceases, core temperatures rise rapidly. High core temperatures and vascular collapse produce cerebral edema, degeneration of the central nervous system, swollen dendrites, and renal tubular necrosis. Death results unless immediate, effective treatment is initiated (Clowes & O'Donnell, 1974).

Treatment includes removing the person from the warm environment, if possible, and using a cooling blanket or cool water bath. Care must be taken to prevent too rapid cooling of the surface, which causes peripheral vasoconstriction and prevents core cooling. Individuals who recover from heat stroke may have permanent damage to the thermoregulatory center and may thus have difficulty tolerating environmental temperature changes.

Children are more susceptible to heat stroke than adults because (1) they produce more metabolic heat when exercising, (2) they have a greater surface area to mass ratio, and (3) their sweating capacity is less than that of adults (Committee on Sports Medicine, 1982).

Malignant Hyperthermia

Malignant hyperthermia is a potentially lethal complication of an inherited muscle disorder. The condition is precipitated by the administration of volatile anesthetics and neuromuscular blocking agents. About 1 in 200 individuals may be at risk for the muscle disorder. Malignant hyperthermia is caused by either increased calcium release or decreased calcium uptake with muscle contraction. This allows intracellular calcium levels to rise, producing sustained, uncoordinated muscle contractions, which in turn increase muscle work, oxygen consumption, and lactic acid production. As a result of these contractions, acidosis develops and temperature rises (body temperature may rise 1° C [1.8F] every 5 minutes); approximately 20% of those who develop malignant hyperthermia do not survive. Malignant hyperthermia occurs most often in children and young adults immediately after the induction of anesthesia.

Sympathetic responses and acidosis produce tachycar-
dia and cardiac arrhythmias, followed by hypotension, decreased cardiac output, and, eventually, cardiac arrest. Increasing temperature, acidosis, hyperkalemia, and hypoxia produce comalike symptoms in the central nervous system (including unconsciousness, absent reflexes, fixed pupils, apnea, and, sometimes, a flat electroencephalogram [EEG]). Oliguria and aneuria are common, probably resulting from shock, ischemia, and low cardiac output (Rogers & Sturgeon, 1985).

Treatment includes withdrawal of the provoking agents and administration of dantrolene sodium (a skeletal relaxant that inhibits calcium release during muscle contraction). Procainamide (Pronestyl) is used to treat cardiac arrhythmias. Sodium bicarbonate may also be used. Body temperature can be decreased through use of ice bags, cooling blanket, and iced saline lavage (Rogers & Sturgeon, 1985).

Hypothermia

Tissue hypothermia slows the rate of chemical reactions (tissue metabolism), increases the viscosity of the blood, slows blood flow through the microcirculation, facilitates blood coagulation, and stimulates profound vasoconstriction. Hypothermia may be accidental or therapeutic.

Accidental Hypothermia

Accidental hypothermia (i.e., temperature below 35° C [95° F]) is generally the result of sudden immersion in cold water or prolonged exposure to cold environments. At particular risk for accidental hypothermia are the young and the elderly, because thermoregulatory mechanisms are altered in these two groups (Reuler, 1978). Also at risk are individuals with conditions that diminish the ability to generate heat. Such conditions include hypothyroidism, hypopituitarism, malnutrition, Parkinson disease, and rheumatoid arthritis. Other risk factors include chronic increased vasodilation and decreased thermoregulatory control caused by cerebral injuries, ketoacidosis, uremia, and drug overdoses (DeLapp, 1983).

In acute hypothermia peripheral vasoconstriction shunts blood away from the cooler skin to the core in an effort to decrease heat loss. This peripheral vasoconstriction produces peripheral tissue ischemia. Intermittent reperfusion of the extremities (the Lewis phenomenon) helps preserve peripheral oxygenation. Intermittent peripheral perfusion continues until core temperatures drop dramatically.

The hypothalamic center stimulates shivering in an effort to increase heat production. Severe shivering occurs at core temperatures of 35° C (95° F) and continues until core temperature drops to about 30 to 32° C (86 to 89.6° F). Thinking becomes sluggish and coordination is decreased at 34° C (93.2° F). As hypothermia deepens, paradoxical undressing may occur as hypothalamic control of vasoconstriction is lost and vasodilation occurs with loss of core heat to the periphery. The hypothermic individual, therefore, feels suddenly warm and begins to remove clothing (DeLapp, 1983).

At 30° C (86° F) the individual becomes stuporous; heart rate and respiratory rates decline; and cardiac output is diminished. Cerebral blood flow is decreased. Metabolic rate declines, further decreasing core temperature. Sinus node depression occurs with slowing of conduction through the atrioventricular node. In severe hypothermia (core temperature of 26 to 28° C [78.8 to 82.4° F]), pulse and respirations may be undetectable. Acidosis is moderate to severe. Ventricular fibrillation and asystole are common (Cabanac & Brinnel, 1987).

If hypothermia is mild, passive rewarming may be sufficient. Passive rewarming includes provision of warm, dry clothes and warm drinks and performance of isometric exercises to increase heat production and minimize heat loss. Core temperature should be checked as soon as possible.

If core temperature is above 30° C (86° F), active rewarming may also be required. Active rewarming employs warm water baths, warm blankets, heating pads, and warm oral fluids when the individual is fully alert. Active core rewarming is performed when core temperatures have dropped below 30° C (86° F) or when severe cardiovascular abnormalities appear. Core rewarming may be accomplished through administration of warm intravenous solutions, warm gastric lavage, warm peritoneal lavage, inhalation of warmed gases, and, in extreme cases, exchange transfusions, warming blood in a pump oxygenator circuit, and mediastinal lavage (Dean, 1987).

Rewarming generally should proceed at no faster than a few degrees per hour. (Short-term complications of rewarming are listed in Table 13-3.) Long-term complications include congestive heart failure, hepatic and renal failure, abnormal erythropoiesis, myocardial infarction, pancreatitis, and neurologic dysfunctions.

Therapeutic Hypothermia

Therapeutic hypothermia is used to slow metabolism and thus preserve ischemic tissue during surgery or limb reimplantation. The actual mechanism of tissue preservation has been recently debated (Osterman et al., 1984). It was originally believed that the slowed metabolism in hypothermic tissues preserved adenosine triphosphate (ATP), but recent evidence suggests that ATP is not preserved in hypothermia. Regardless of the mechanism, however, it is clear that hypothermic ischemic cells remain viable long after normothermic ischemic cells have died. Survival from accidental hypothermia has been reported in individuals with core temperatures at 16° C (60.8° F) and from therapeutic hypothermia with temperatures at 9° C (48.2° F) (Cabanac & Brinnel, 1987).

The temperature changes of hypothermia place a great deal of stress on the heart. Moderate to severe hypothermia may lead to ventricular fibrillation and cardiac arrest. (This may be the desired outcome in open heart surgery when the heart must be stopped during portions of the surgical procedure [Shaver et al., 1984].) Prolonged hypothermia may precipitate exhaustion of liver glycogen stores by prolonged shivering. Surface cooling may cause burns, frostbite, and fat necrosis.

Trauma

Major body trauma has varying effects on temperature regulation, depending on the body systems involved. Five types of traumatic injury that usually affect temperature regulation are (1) central nervous system trauma (discussed in Chapter 15), (2) accidental injury, (3) hemorrhagic shock, (4) major surgery, and (5) thermal burns.

TABLE 13-3 Accidental hypothermia: complications of Rewarming

Complication	Mechanism
Acidosis	Rewarming stimulates peripheral vasodilation. Peripheral blood, returning to the core from the ischemic peripheral tissues, causes a reduction in the pH of core blood.
Rewarming shock	As rewarming and vasodilation progress, the body is unable to maintain blood pressure because of reduced fluid volume (from "cold diuresis"), catecholamine depletion (prolonged shivering), and myocardial injury.
Deep-ended hypothermia	As colder surface blood is returned to the core, core temperatures may drop. This is also referred to as "after fall" or "after drop."
Dysrhythmia	Rewarming places an additional stress on an already severely stressed myocardium.

Central Nervous System Trauma

Central nervous system (CNS) trauma that causes CNS damage, inflammation, increased intracranial pressures, or intracranial bleeding typically produces a fever of greater than 39° C (102° F). This temperature, often referred to as a "central fever," appears with or without relative bradycardia. The temperature is sustained, does not induce sweating, and is very resistant to antipyretic therapy (Cunha et al., 1984).

Accidental Injuries

Mild accidental injuries may produce a slight elevation in core temperature. Moderate to severe injuries result in peripheral vasoconstriction with decreased surface and core temperatures. Core temperature seems inversely related to the severity of the injury and may be a result of decreased oxygen transport to the tissues. In severe injuries, shivering is absent and some alteration in thermoregulation is evident (Little & Stoner, 1981).

Hemorrhagic Shock

Loss of blood volume in hemorrhage triggers peripheral vasoconstriction and a slight rise in core temperature. Subsequent decreases in core temperature have been demonstrated in individuals with hemorrhagic shock treated with unwarmed volume-expanding solutions and surgical repair. Volume expansion with warmed solutions is recommended to prevent the deleterious effects of hypothermia on cardiac output, cardiac rhythm, and the immune system (Shaver et al., 1984).

Major Surgery

Because many victims of trauma undergo major surgical repair, the effect of the surgical procedure on temperature regulation needs to be considered by health care providers. Major surgery often induces significant hypothermia through exposure of body cavities to the relatively cool operating room environment. Other mechanisms that contribute to intraoperative hypothermia include irrigation of body cavities with room temperature solutions, infusion of room temperature intravenous solutions, use of drugs that impair thermoregulatory mechanisms, and inhalation of unwarmed anesthetic agents (Shaver et al., 1984). Use of warmed irrigating and intravenous solutions may reduce intraoperative hypothermia.

Thermal Burns

Large burn injuries produce significant hypothermia because of the loss of the skin barrier to fluid evaporation and the loss of control of the microcirculation in the skin. Severe burns also compromise the normal insulation of the skin and subcutaneous tissues. (Burns are discussed in Chapter 40.)

SLEEP

Sleep, described by some as a period of relative unconsciousness, is a time in which the body is actively repairing and restoring itself. Sleep is a period in which growth hormone is released and brain synthesis occurs. The restorative, reparative, and growth processes occur during slow-wave sleep (so defined because of the appearance of slow-wave activity on the EEG). Brain synthesis, which appears to organize and "file" the day's activities, occurs during the stage of rapid eye movement sleep (REM sleep).

Sleep serves important recuperative and integrative functions. Sleep deprivation, even for one night, can cause a decrease in the functioning of the awake individual. Prolonged sleep deprivation can cause profound

---

TABLE 13-4 Manifestations of sleep deprivation

Muscle tremor	Deterioration of intellectual capacity*
Lack of muscle coordination	Personality changes* (severe anxiety, depression, jealousy, irrational behavior)
Impairment of speech	
Decreased facial expression	Decreased libido*
Visual distortions*	Loud snoring
Decreased coping strength	Loud snoring interrupted by periods of apnea†
Morning headache	Nocturnal enuresis†
Excessive daytime somnolence	Abnormal motor activity during sleep†
Hypnagogic hallucinations†	
Autonomic behavior* (performance of semiautomatic behaviors without conscious purpose or knowledge and with no after memory)	

*Seen in prolonged sleep deprivation.
†Accompanying disorders of excessive somnolence.

changes in personality and functioning (Kales & Kales, 1970). A variety of signs and symptoms accompany sleep deprivation. Some, such as nocturnal enuresis and loud snoring, appear during sleep and are closely tied to the cause of sleep deprivation. Others, such as lack of muscle coordination and diminished coping ability, appear during the waking hours and are direct results of sleep loss (Table 13-4). Sleep deprivation also causes an increase in creatine phosphokinase and blood glucose and a decrease in plasma iron and cholesterol. In addition heart rate, blood pressure, and oral temperature are lowered by moderate sleep loss.

Stages of Sleep

The waking state is maintained by the afferent portion of the reticular formation in the mesencephalon and brainstem. The reticular formation, at the center core of the brainstem, produces a variety of neurotransmitters and their precursors. The neurotransmitters norepinephrine and dopamine stimulate wakefulness. During the waking state respiration is governed by metabolic and behavioral processes. When a person falls asleep, control of respiration depends on the stage of sleep. Although it is clear that the brain actively generates sleep and that sleep is produced when several neuronal centers in the brain are stimulated, it is not clear which chemical activators trigger drowsiness and sleep. L-tryptophan, serotonin, and adenosine have been implicated (Karnovsky, 1986; Radulovacki, 1987).

As individuals sleep, they progress through several distinct stages. To the observer the most dramatic difference between states is the presence or absence of rapid eye movement (REM). This feature distinguishes two stages of sleep, REM sleep and **non-REM sleep.** With the aid of the electroencephalogram, non-REM and REM sleep can be further subdivided into non-REM stages I, II, III, IV and REM stages tonic and phasic (Table 13-5) (Long, 1982).

Non-REM sleep is initiated by the withdrawal of neurotransmitters from the reticular formation and by the inhibition of arousal mechanisms in the cerebral cortex. During non-REM sleep respiration is controlled by metabolic processes (Phillipson, 1978). The basal metabolic rate is decreased by 10%-15%. Temperature is decreased 0.5 to 1° C (1° F). Heart rate decreases by 10 to 30 beats per minute. Respiration, blood pressure, and muscle tone all decrease. Knee jerk reflexes are absent. Pupils are constricted. During stages I and II cerebral blood flow to the brainstem and cerebellum is decreased. During stages III and IV cerebral blood flow to the cortex is decreased (Sakai et al., 1980). Growth hormone is released during stage IV, and levels of corticosteroids and catecholamines are depressed.

REM sleep, which comprises approximately 20% of total sleep time in the adult, is controlled by mechanisms in the pontine reticular formation. Individuals dream and experience increased autonomic activity. Heart rate becomes irregular; blood pressure is variable; erections may occur in men; and clitoral engorgement may occur in women. Steroids are released in short bursts. The EEG pattern resembles the normal awake pattern.

Respiratory effort is dominated by behavioral systems arising in the cerebral cortex and in the portions of the

---

TABLE 13-5 Stages of sleep

Stage of sleep	Characteristics
Non-REM	
Stage I	Individuals are somewhat aware of their surroundings, feel relaxed and dreamy, and may jump or jerk as they relax. Alpha waves appear in the EEG. Comprises approximately 5% of total sleep time.
Stage II	Individuals are unaware of their surroundings but awaken easily. Spindle waves appear on the EEG. Comprises approximately 50-55% of total sleep time.
Stage III	Individuals are unaware of their surroundings but awaken easily. Delta waves appear on the EEG. Comprises approximately 10% of total sleep time.
Stage IV	Individuals are deeply asleep, difficult to awaken, and exhibit little body movement. Heart rate, respiratory rate, and blood pressure decline. Comprises approximately 10% of total sleep time. Each stage IV cycle lasts 5-15 minutes.
REM	
Tonic	Rapid eye movement is present, but other muscle activity is suppressed.
Phasic	Rapid eye movement is present, and muscle contraction and movement occur.

brain that use the respiratory system to produce speech. During REM sleep respiratory control appears largely independent of metabolic requirements and oxygen homeostasis. Loss of normal voluntary muscle control in the tongue and upper pharynx may produce some respiratory obstruction. Cerebral blood flow to both hemispheres is increased.

While asleep, an individual progresses through REM and non-REM sleep in a predictable cycle. Each cycle lasts approximately 90 to 100 minutes, with the individual's passing through four to five cycles per night. The first cycle of the night begins with stage I. The individual then progresses through stages II, III, IV, III, II, and REM sleep. A new cycle, begining with stage II, follows each REM sleep. With each successive cycle the amount of time spent in stage IV sleep decreases, and the amount of time spent in REM increases (Fig. 13-9). The individual who is awakened begins the next cycle with stage I. Forced awakenings in the middle of the night may result in increased difficulty returning to sleep or alter the normal progression of sleep, or both (Campbell, 1987). If the individual is awakened frequently throughout the night, sleep deprivation can occur (Kales & Kales, 1970). Optimally individuals change body position twice during each sleep cycle: one at the conclusion of stage IV and again at the conclusion of each REM sleep. Too many or too few position shifts contribute to a poor night's sleep (Long, 1982).

Aging and Sleep Patterns
Sleep Patterns in Children

The sleep patterns of the newborn and young child vary from those of the adult in total sleep time, cycle length, and percentage of time spent in each sleep cycle. Newborns sleep about 16 to 17 hours per day. About 53% of that time is spent in active sleep (REM sleep), 23% in quiet sleep (non-REM sleep), and the remainder in an indeterminate phase. The infant sleep cycle is approximately 50 to 60 minutes in length, with 20 minutes of quiet sleep and 10 to 45 minutes of REM sleep, in contrast to the adult sleep cycle. Newborns enter REM sleep immediately upon falling asleep (Anders & Keener, 1985; Keefe, 1987). At about 1 year of age the infant spends approximately 45% of total sleep time in quiet sleep and 41% in REM sleep. Total sleep time decreases slightly from birth to 1 year. In the American culture, where infants are bottle-fed and do not share sleeping space with the mother, infants increase maximum sleep time from 4 to 5 hours to 8 to 10 hours by 4 months of age. They begin to "sleep through the night." In other cultures, where infants are breast fed for up to 2 years of age and share sleeping space with the mother, they continue to sleep in short bouts and waken frequently to nurse (Elias et al., 1986).

In the young child the sleep cycle length is 45 to 60 minutes, in contrast to 90 to 100 minutes in the adult. The child assumes the adult sleep pattern at some point during the first 2 to 5 years of life (Kales & Kales, 1970).

Sleep Patterns of the Elderly

The sleep pattern of the older adult differs from that of the younger adult or child. Total sleep time is decreased, and the older individual takes longer to fall asleep. The elderly awaken earlier in the morning and more frequently during the night. Total REM and stage II time is unchanged, but stage IV sleep decreases by 15 to 30%. On EEG the spindle indicating stage II sleep is less well formed (Guazzelli, Feinberg, & Aminoff, 1986).

These changes in the older adult's sleep pattern may be associated with changes in life-style, physical ailments, lack of daily routine, desynchronization of circadian rhythm, and use of sedatives. The alteration in

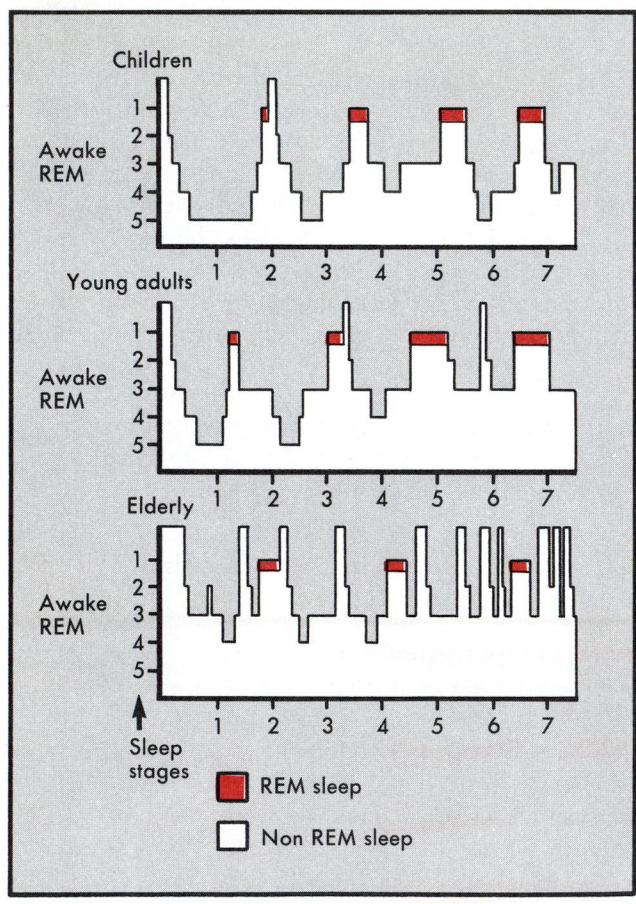

FIG. 13-9. Normal sleep cycles. REM sleep occurs cyclically throughout the night at intervals of approximately nine minutes in all age groups. REM sleep shows little variation in the different age, groups whereas stage IV sleep decreases with age. In addition, the elderly awaken frequently and show a marked increase in total time awake.

sleep pattern typically appears about 10 years later in women than in men. Older adults are less able than younger individuals to tolerate sleep deprivation (Kales & Kales, 1970).

Sleep Disorders

Sleep disorders are classified by their signs and symptoms rather than by their etiology. Four classifications of sleep disorders are (1) disorders of initiating sleep, (2) disorders of excessive somnolence, (3) disorders of the sleep-wake schedule, and (4) dysfunctions of sleep, sleep stages, or partial arousals.

Disorders of Initiating Sleep: Insomnia

Insomnia is defined as the inability to fall or stay asleep. Insomnia is often accompanied by varying sleep spindle production on EEG, increased levels of REM sleep, and decreased sleep efficiency. Heart rate and temperature are increased prior to and during sleep periods. Interestingly, 10% of the insomniacs studied by Mendelson in the sleep laboratory report being awake when "awakened" from EEG certified sleep (Long, 1982).

Insomnia often results from pain, discomfort, fear, depression, changes in presleep routine, or excessive hypnotic therapy with REM-suppressant drugs. Drugs known to produce insomnia include amphetamines, steroids, central adrenergic blockers, bronchodilating agents, and caffeine.

Disorders of Excessive Somnolence

Two disorders of excessive somnolence, or excessive daytime sleepiness, are **pickwickian syndrome** and **hypersomnia sleep apnea (HSA) syndrome.** Substantially more men than women are affected by these syndromes. One hypothesis is that the female hormone progesterone (a respiratory stimulant) may protect premenopausal women from sleep-disordered breathing (Block, 1980). Both pickwickian syndrome and HSA syndrome are associated with periodic breathing and episodes of apnea appearing in stages I, II, and REM sleep. The periodic breathing is associated with decreased arterial oxygen saturation, which eventually produces arousal. Each arousal causes an interruption in the sleep cycle, reducing total sleep time and producing sleep and REM deprivation (Long, 1982).

Sleep apnea (lack of breathing during sleep) results from one of three mechanisms: (1) central apnea, which is apparently the result of altered chemosensitivity and cerebral respiratory control; (2) obstructive apnea, which is caused by partial or complete obstruction of the upper airway during sleep; and (3) mixed apnea, which results from both central and obstructive causes (Guilleminault, Tilkian, & Dement, 1976). In pickwickian syndrome sleep is frequently interrupted by apneic periods lasting 10 seconds or longer. The apneic periods are generally a result of obesity, decreased chemosensitivity to carbon dioxide and oxygen tensions, or upper airway obstruction occurring during sleep. The apnea that results is a combination of central nervous system dysfunction (decreased O_2 and CO_2 sensitivity) and upper airway obstruction. The sleep apnea produces low oxygen saturation and eventually produces polycythemia, pulmonary hypertension, right-sided congestive heart failure, liver congestion, cyanosis, and peripheral edema. Cardiac arrhythmias during sleep are common.

Because the apnea is due in part to an alteration of central nervous control of respiration, daytime hypercapnia also occurs. Individuals exhibit excessive daytime sleepiness, often falling asleep when driving a car, working, or even in the middle of a conversation. Treatment includes weight loss, controlled oxygen therapy, administration of a respiratory stimulant, and treatment of congestive heart failure (Block, 1980).

HSA syndrome is primarily a result of upper airway obstruction occurring during sleep. Persons with HSA syndrome may experience hundreds of apneic episodes each night; these are followed by excessive daytime sleepiness. Their spouses often observe excessive snoring or snorting and thrashing about during sleep. Some individuals may sleepwalk or experience enuresis. Profound personality changes, depression, and impotence can occur. Physiologic changes include polycythemia and right-sided heart failure. Daytime respirations, Po_2, and Pco_2 are normal. Treatment involves relief of the upper airway obstruction during sleep (Block, 1980).

Disorders of the Sleep-Wake Schedule

Common disorders of the sleep-wake schedule include rapid time-zone change (or "jet-lag syndrome"), changing sleep schedule with an advance or a delay of 3 hours or more in sleep time, or a change in total sleep time from day to day. These changes in the timing of established sleep schedules have been shown to desynchronize circadian rhythm. Degree of vigilance, performance of psychomotor tasks, and subjective reports of levels of arousal are markedly depressed after alterations in the sleep-wake schedule. Individuals may experience short sleep episodes called microsleeps without being aware of decreased vigila (Long, 1982).

It is well established that industrial shift workers exhibit a decrease in accuracy and increased accident proneness (Taub & Berger, 1976). For similar reasons persons suffering from jet lag require several days to adapt to the new time zone. Travel across time zones requires 2 days to adjust the sleep-wake schedule, 5 days to adjust the body temperature cycle, and 8 days to adjust cortisol secretion. Transmeridian travel requires up to 10 days to adjust the body clock when traveling from east to west. Czeisler's experiments with timed bright-light stimulation have had some success in retiming or resetting the body clock after time zone shifts (Long, 1982).

Dysfunctions of Sleep, Sleep Stages, or Partial Arousals

Three dysfunctions of sleep are common in children. They are **somnambulism** (sleepwalking), **night terrors** (dream anxiety attacks), and **enuresis** (bedwetting).

Somnambulism

Somnambulism is primarily a disorder of childhood and appears to resolve itself within several years of the onset of the sleepwalking episodes. Sleepwalking occurs in stages III and IV and is therefore not associated with dreaming. During the sleepwalking episode the child functions at a very low level of arousal and has no memory of the event upon awakening.

The greatest concern is for the safety of the child, as some children leave home or in some way injure themselves during sleepwalking episodes. If the child does not "outgrow" the disorder or grave safety risks arise, drugs to suppress stage IV sleep are sometimes administered.

Night Terrors

Night terrors are characterized by "sudden apparent arousals in which the child expresses intense fear or emotion" (Kales & Kales, 1970). The child, however, is not awake and is very difficult to arouse. Once awakened, the child has no memory of the night terror event. Night terrors occur during stage IV sleep and are not associated with the dreams of REM sleep. Although night terrors occur most often in children, adults may experience them as well. Unlike children, however, adults often display corresponding daytime anxiety (Long, 1982).

Enuresis

Enuresis is possibly the most disturbing of the childhood sleep dysfunctions, because of the stress society places on nighttime continence and the misconception that children are bedwetting to act out against parents. Bedwetting incidents are also incorrectly associated with dreaming. Laboratory studies of sleep have demonstrated that very few incidents of bedwetting occur when the child is dreaming and that by far most incidents occur during non-REM sleep and during the first one third of the night when the child is most difficult to arouse (Kales & Kales, 1970). If the bed is not changed, however, the child may incorporate the feeling of wetness with the next REM dream cycle and may therefore incorrectly associate the enuresis with the dream. Children do eventually "outgrow" the enuretic episodes.

Relation Between Sleep and Disease

Sleep and disease are interrelated. Some diseases produce alterations in the quantity and quality of sleep or affect sleep stages. These are referred to as **secondary sleep disorders.** In some instances sleep stages produce alterations in certain disease states. These are referred to as **sleep-provoked disorders.** Other entities, such as sudden infant death syndrome (SIDS) and sudden unexplained noctural death syndrome (SUNDS), produce unexplained death almost exclusively during sleep (Long, 1982).

Secondary Sleep Disorders

The most common causes of secondary sleep disorders are depression, alterations in thyroid hormone secretion (hypo- or hyperthyroidism), pain, and sleep apnea syndromes. Depressed persons have difficulty falling asleep and exhibit less slow-wave sleep, less time spent in REM sleep, and less total sleep time. In addition, depressed individuals move through the sleep stages more quickly than do individuals who are not depressed. Sleep deprivation paradoxically relieves depression (Long, 1982).

Changes in thyroid hormone secretion produce changes in stage III and IV sleep. An increase in thyroid secretion produces an increase in stage III and IV activity, whereas a decrease in thyroid hormone produces a decrease in both stage III and IV sleep.

Chronic pain is a cause of insomnia. Chronic pain inhibits sleep, increases arousals during sleep, and causes prolonged awake intervals during the night. Individuals with chronic pain report not only a decrease in the quantity of sleep but also a decrease in its quality.

Sleep-Provoked Disorders

Some diseases are provoked by sleep. Signs and symptoms of the disease appear during, or are enhanced by, sleep. Diseases that are affected by sleep include coronary artery disease, bronchial asthma, chronic obstructive pulmonary disease (COPD), diabetes, and duodenal ulcers.

Coronary artery disease is most affected during REM sleep. During REM dreams may provoke noctural angina, increased heart rate, and electrocardiogram (ECG) changes. In adults attacks of bronchial asthma may occur at any time during the night. The attacks cause the individual to spend more of the sleep period awake and thus cause a decrease in stage IV sleep. In children bronchial asthma attacks are uncommon during the first one third of the night, when stage IV sleep predominates, and occur more frequently during the final two thirds of the night. Stage IV sleep is decreased overall in the child with bronchial asthma. In addition to these changes asthmatics may experience bronchial spasm during REM sleep (Kales & Kales, 1970).

Persons with COPD experience significantly lowered oxygen tension and increases in carbon dioxide retention during sleep (Calverly et al., 1982). The lowered oxygen tension is most significant in the tonic phase of REM sleep when voluntary neuromuscular control, including intercostal muscle function, is depressed. Pulmonary spasm and transient pulmonary hypertension result. These changes are particularly evident in the so-called blue bloater individual and may contribute to early pulmonary hypertension and cor pulmonale in these individuals (Block, 1981).

Because blood glucose levels vary during sleep, individuals with uncontrolled diabetes may need careful attention to blood sugar levels during sleep. Studies show that people with duodenal ulcers secrete 3 to 20 times more gastric acid during REM sleep than people without duodenal ulcers. This increased gastric acid secretion often produces nocturnal epigastric pain (Kales & Kales, 1970).

Sudden infant death syndrome (SIDS) affects children primarily in the first 2 years of life and may be related to central sleep apnea episodes. (For further discussion of SIDS, see Chapter 31.) Sudden unexplained nocturnal death syndrome (SUNDS) occurs in previously healthy Asian men in the second, third, or fourth decade of life. Postmortem studies have demonstrated abnormalities of the cardiac conduction system and, frequently, left ventricular hypertrophy or cardiomyopathy. The relationship between the SUNDS event and sleep is unclear but may involve cardiac arrhythmias occuring during REM sleep (Kirschner, Eckner, & Baron, 1986; Melles, 1987).

THE SPECIAL SENSES

Vision

Visual dysfunction may be caused by abnormal ocular movements or alterations in visual acuity, refraction, color vision, or accommodation. Visual dysfunction may also be the secondary effect of another neurologic disorder.

The External Eye Structures

The external structures protecting the eye include the eyelids (palpebrae), conjunctiva, and lacrimal apparatus (Fig. 13-10). Infection and inflammatory responses are the most common conditions affecting the supporting structures of the eyes. Blepharitis is an inflammation of the eyelids caused by staphylococcus or seborrheic dermatitis. Redness, edema, and itching are common syndromes. A hordeolum is an infection of the sebaceous glands of the eyelids, and a chalazion is an infection of the meibomian gland. These conditions are treated symptomatically.

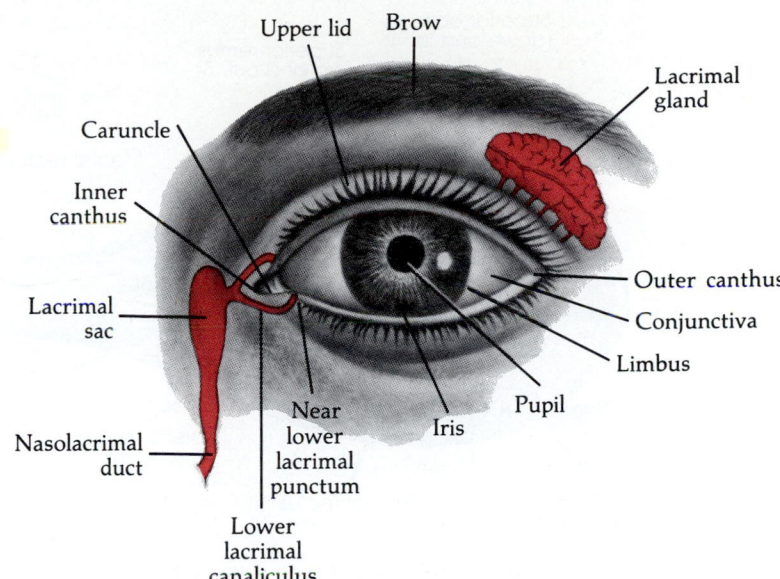

FIG. 13-10. External eye structures. (From Thompson et al., 1989.)

Conjunctivitis

Conjunctivitis is an inflammation of the conjunctiva and can be caused by bacteria, viruses, allergies, or chemical irritations. The inflammatory response produces redness, edema, pain, and lacrimation. Treatment is related to cause.

Acute bacterial conjunctivitis (pinkeye) is highly contagious and can be caused by gram-positive organisms (*Staphylococcus, Haemophilus, Proteus*), although other bacteria may be involved. The onset is acute with both eyes producing a mucopurulent drainage. Preventing spread of the organism with meticulous hand washing and use of separate towels is important. The disease is frequently self-limiting and resolves spontaneously in 10 to 14 days. Antibiotic eyedrops are usually effective.

Viral conjuctivitis is caused by an adenovirus. Symptoms vary from mild to severe. Some strains of virus cause conjunctivitis and pharyngitis (pharynogconjunctival fever), and others cause keratoconjunctivitis. Both diseases are contagious with watering, redness, and photophobia. Treatment is symptomatic.

Allergic conjunctivitis is associated with a variety of antigens, including pollens. There is ocular itching associated with photophobia, burning, and gritty sensations in the eye. Treatment is symptomatic and may include antihistamines, steroids, and vasoconstrictors.

Chronic conjunctivitis is the result of any persistent conjunctivitis. The cause requires identification for effective treatment.

Trachoma (chlamydial conjunctivitis) is caused by *Chlamydia trachomatis*. It is often associated with poor hygiene and is the leading cause of preventable blind-

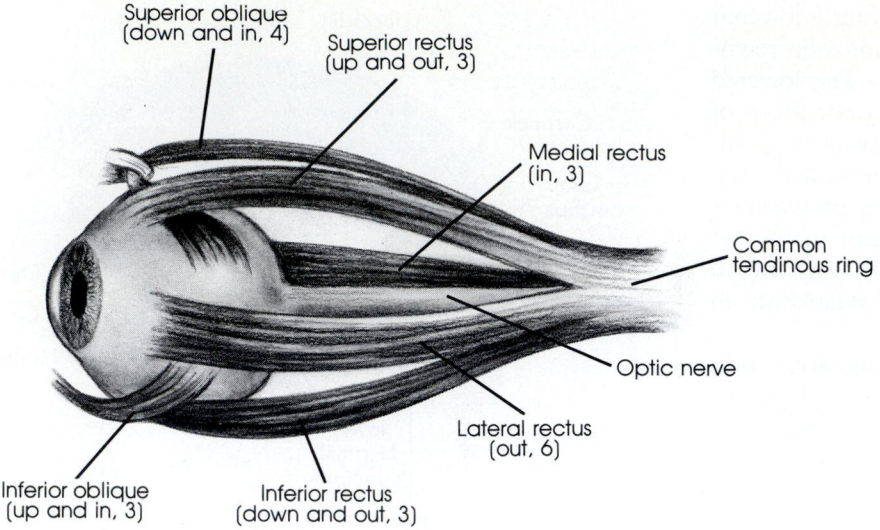

Superior oblique (down and in, 4)

Superior rectus (up and out, 3)

Medial rectus (in, 3)

Common tendinous ring

Optic nerve

Lateral rectus (out, 6)

Inferior oblique (up and in, 3)

Inferior rectus (down and out, 3)

FIG. 13-11. Extraocular muscles. (From Rudy, 1984.)

ness in the world. The common fly is the most probable vector, along with direct human contact. The severity of the disease varies but can involve inflammation and vascularization of the cornea with scarring of the conjunctiva and eyelids, leading to blindness. Chlamydial organisms are sensitive to antibiotics that are usually given locally or systemically. Flies must be eliminated and hygienic conditions improved.

Keratitis

Keratitis is an infection of the cornea that can be caused by bacteria or viruses. Bacterial infections often cause corneal ulceration and require intensive antibiotic treatment. Type I herpes simplex virus can involve both the cornea and conjunctiva. Common symptoms include photophobia, pain, and lacrimation. Severe ulcerations with residual scarring require corneal transplantation.

The Normal Eye

The eye is quite sophisticated, containing 70% of all the sensory receptors in the body. Six extrinsic eye muscles, attached to the outer surface of each eye, allow gross eye movements and permit eyes to follow a moving object (Fig. 13-11).

The wall of the eye is formed of three layers: (1) sclera, (2) choroid, and (3) retina (Fig. 13-10). The **sclera** is the thick, white, outermost layer. It becomes transparent at the **cornea,** the portion of the sclera in the central anterior region that allows light to enter the eye. The **choroid** is the deeply pigmented middle layer that prevents light from scattering inside the eye. The **iris,** part of the choroid, has a round opening, the **pupil,** through which light passes. Smooth muscle fibers control the size of the pupil so that in close vision and

bright light the pupil constricts and in distant vision and dim light the pupil dilates.

The innermost layer of the eye, the **retina,** contains millions of rods and cones, special photoreceptors that convert light energy into nerve impulses. In the retina **rods** mediate peripheral and dim light vision and are densest at the periphery. **Cones,** densest in the center of the retina, are color and detail receptors. The impulses

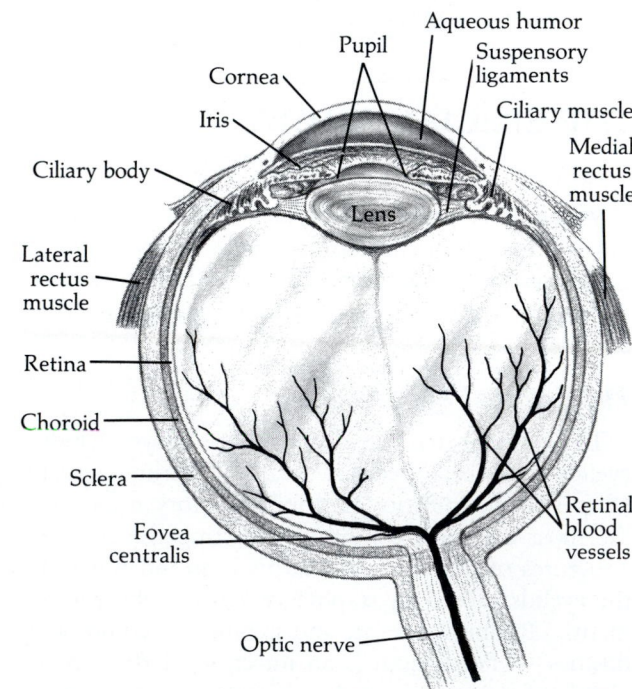

Aqueous humor

Pupil

Cornea

Suspensory ligaments

Iris

Ciliary muscle

Ciliary body

Medial rectus muscle

Lens

Lateral rectus muscle

Retina

Choroid

Sclera

Fovea centralis

Retinal blood vessels

Optic nerve

FIG. 13-12. Internal anatomy of the eye. (From Thompson et al., 1989.)

generated are transmitted to the portion of the cerebral cortex that mediates vision (see Fig. 12-5). The photoreceptive rods and cones are distributed over the entire retina, except where the optic nerve leaves the eyeball. Lack of rods and cones in this area results in the **optic disk,** or blind spot. Lateral to each optic disk is the **fovea centralis,** a tiny area that contains only cones and provides the greatest visual acuity (Fig. 13-12).

Light entering the eye is focused on the retina by the **lens:** a flexible, biconvex crystal-like structure. In youth the lens is transparent and has the consistency of hardened jelly. With age the lens become increasingly hard and opaque. The lens divides the anterior chamber into (1) the aqueous chamber and (2) the vitreous chamber. **Aqueous humor,** which fills the aqueous chamber, helps to maintain the pressure inside the eye and provides nutrients to the lens and cornea. Aqueous humor is constantly secreted by an area of the choroid and is continually reabsorbed into the canal of Schlemm. If drainage is blocked, pressure within the eye increases (as it does with glaucoma). The vitreous chamber is filled with a gel-like substance called **vitreous humor.** Vitreous humor helps to prevent the eyeball from collapsing inward.

Aging and Vision

Changes in the structural components of the eye caused by aging begin at an early age, particularly in the lens of the eye. Changes due to aging are summarized in **Table** 13-6. The combined structural changes result in a decline in visual acuity. The most significant alterations are increases in the opacity and hardness of the lens, producing cataracts and presbyopia (Graham, 1985).

Visual Dysfunction

Alterations in Ocular Movements

Abnormal ocular movements occur as a result of oculomotor, trochlear, and/or abducens nerve dysfunction (see Table 12-6). The three types of eye movement disorders are (1) strabismus, (2) nystagmus, and (3) paralysis of individual extraocular muscles.

Strabismus is the deviation of one eye from the other when the person is looking at an object. The cause is a weak or hypertonic muscle in one of the eyes. The deviation may be upward, downward, inward, or outward. Strabismus in children requires early intervention to prevent the development of **amblyopia** (reduced vision in the affected eye often caused by cerebral blockage of the visual stimuli). The primary symptom of strabismus is **diplopia** (double vision). Strabismus may be caused by a neuromuscular disorder of the eye muscle, diseases involving the cerebral hemispheres, and/or thyroid disease.

Nystagmus is an involuntary unilateral or bilateral rhythmic movement of the eyes. It may be present at rest, or it may occur with eye movement. The two major forms of nystagmus are pendular nystagmus and jerk nystagmus. **Pendular nystagmus** is characterized by a regular to-and-fro movement of the eyes in which both phases of the movement are equal in length. In **jerk nystagmus,** one phase of the eye movement is faster than the other. Nystagmus may be caused by an imbalance in the normally coordinated reflex activity of the inner ear, vestibular nuclei (connecting the vestibular nerve with vestibulospinal tracts), cerebellum, medial longitudinal fascicle (connecting the mesencephalon with the upper portion of the spinal cord), or nuclei of

---

TABLE 13-6 Changes in the eye caused by aging

Structure	Change	Consequence
Cornea	Thicker and less curved	Increase in astigmatism
	Formation of a gray ring at the edge of the cornea (arcus senilus)	Not detrimental to vision
Anterior chamber	Decrease in size and volume caused by thickening of lens	Occasionally exerts pressure on Schlemm canal and may lead to increased intraocular pressure and glaucoma
Lens	Increase in opacity	Decrease in refraction with increased light scattering and decreased color vision (yellow to blue); can lead to cataracts
	Increased firmness and loss of elasticity	Decrease in accommodation for near vision; presbyopia develops by age 50-55 years
Ciliary muscles	Reduction in pupil diameter, atrophy of radial dilation muscles	Persistent constriction (senile miosis); decrease in critical flicker frequency*
Retina	Reduction in number of rods at periphery, loss of rods and associated nerve cells	Increase in the minimum amount of light necessary to see an object

*The rate at which consecutive visual stimuli can be presented and still be perceived as separate.

the oculomotor, trochlear, and abducens nerves (see Table 12-5). Drugs, retinal disease, and diseases involving the cervical cord may also produce nystagmus.

Paralysis of specific extraocular muscles may cause a variety of abnormalities, including limited abduction, abnormal closure of the eyelid, ptosis (drooping of the eyelid), and diplopia. The abnormalities occur as a result of unopposed muscle activity. For example, the oculomotor nerve (cranial nerve III) innervates the eyelid. With paresis or paralysis the eyelid droops. Trauma or pressure in the area of the cranial nerves may cause paralysis of specific extraocular muscles. Diseases such as diabetes mellitus and myasthenia gravis may also affect specific extraocular muscles.

Alterations in Visual Acuity

Visual acuity is the ability to see objects in sharp detail. With advancing age the lens of the eye becomes less flexible and less adjustable. In addition the sclera changes shape, causing light to fall on the macula (an opaque portion of the cornea). Thus visual acuity declines with age. In addition visual acuity may change or diminish for many other reasons. Specific causes of visual acuity changes are (1) amblyopia, (2) scotoma, (3) cataracts, (4) papilledema, (5) local ocular conditions, and (6) dark adaptation.

Amblyopia is a reduction or dimness of vision for unknown reasons. It does not result from a change in refraction (i.e., deviation of light rays) or from any visible changes in the eye. Amblyopia is associated with such diseases as diabetes mellitus, renal failure, and malaria and with toxic substances such as alcohol and tobacco.

A **scotoma** is a circumscribed defect of the central field of vision. It is most often a sequel to **retrobulbar neuritis,** an inflammatory lesion of the optic nerve frequently associated with multiple sclerosis (see Chapter 15). Less common causes include the compression of one optic nerve by a retroorbital tumor, neuromyelitis optica (inflammation of the optic nerve), pernicious anemia, and toxic/metabolic causes such as methyl alcohol poisoning and use of tobacco. The precise mechanisms for these conditions' causing a scotoma are uncertain, but the result is always a serious impairment in visual acuity.

Cataract formation is the development of opacities of the ocular lens. The incidence of cataracts increases with age as the lens enlarges. Cataracts develop because of alterations of metabolism and transport of nutrition within the lens. Although the most common form of cataract is degenerative, cataracts may also occur congenitally as a result of infection, radiation, trauma, drugs, or diabetes mellitus. Cataracts cause decreased visual acuity, blurred vision, glare, and decreased color perception.

Papilledema is edema and inflammation of the optic nerve at its point of entrance into the eyeball. Generally papilledema is caused by some obstruction to the venous return from the retina. An early symptom is distention of the retinal vein. Obliteration of the physiologic cup (a bright area normally located in the center of the optic disc) follows. Later the optic disc becomes raised above the level of the surrounding retina, while the margins become blurred and indistinct. With severe swelling, hemorrhage and patches of white exudate develop around the disc margins. The three principal causes of papilledema are (1) increased intracranial pressure, (2) retrobulbar neuritis, and (3) changes in the retinal blood vessels. Retinal blood vessel changes are especially prevalent in individuals with diabetes mellitus and/or hypertension. Such changes account for a large percentage of individuals newly affected with blindness each year. Typically the blood vessels narrow, and hemorrhages and white exudate appear. Ultimately papilledema occurs.

Dark adaptation also affects visual acuity. Low illumination causes impaired visual acuity, particularly in the elderly. On the average 80-year-olds need over 200 times as much light as 20-year-olds to see equally well. Changes in the quantity and quality of rhodopsin, a substance found in the rods and responsible for low-light vision, are thought to be responsible for reduced dark adaptation in older adults. Vitamin A deficiencies can cause the same phenomenon in individuals of any age.

Glaucoma is characterized by intraocular pressures above the normal pressures of 13 to 22 mmHg maintained by the aqueous fluid. The mechanisms of intraocular fluid accumulation are summarized in Fig. 13-13. Chronic increased intraocular pressure first causes loss of peripheral vision, which is followed by central vision impairment and blindness. Loss of visual acuity results from pressure on the retinal artery with decreased blood flow to the retina. The types of glaucoma are summarized in Table 13-7.

Alterations in Accommodation

Accommodation is the process whereby the lens changes shape (i.e., constricts in response to near objects and light and dilates in response to far objects and dark) to bring about a focused image. Accommodation is needed for clear vision and is mediated through the oculomotor nerve. Pressure, inflammation, and disease of the oculomotor nerve may alter accommodation. Symptoms include diplopia, blurred vision, and headache. Accommodation is also affected by the decreased flexibility of the lens that occurs with aging. By the age of 60, the lens has become so inelastic that accommodation is not possible.

Loss of accommodation in the elderly is termed **pres-**

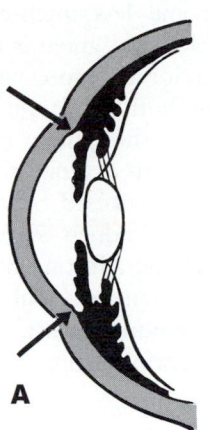
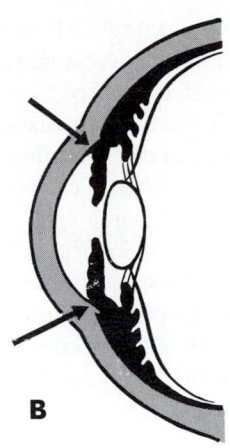

FIG. 13-13. Glaucoma. **A,** Open-angle glaucoma. The obstruction to aqueous flow lies in the trabecular meshwork. **B,** Closed-angle glaucoma. The trabecular meshwork is covered by the root of the iris. (From Stein, Slatt, & Stein, 1988.)

byopia, a condition in which the ocular lens becomes larger, firmer, and less elastic. The major symptom is reduced near vision, causing the holding of reading material at arm's length. Correction is accomplished through reading glasses or bifocal lenses.

Alterations in Refraction

Alterations in refraction are the most common visual problem. The problem exists because of a defect in the refracting media of the eye, which prevents light rays from bending and converging into a single focus on the retina. Defects are due to irregularities of the corneal curvature, the focusing power of the lens, and the length of the eye. The major symptoms of refraction alterations are blurred vision and headache. Three types of refraction alterations are (1) myopia, (2) hyperopia, and (4) astigmatism (Fig. 13-14).

Myopia (nearsightedness) involves the focusing of light rays anterior to the retina when the person is looking at a distinct object. A concave lens is needed for correction. Myopia requires frequent changes of eyeglasses while the eyeball is lengthening in childhood.

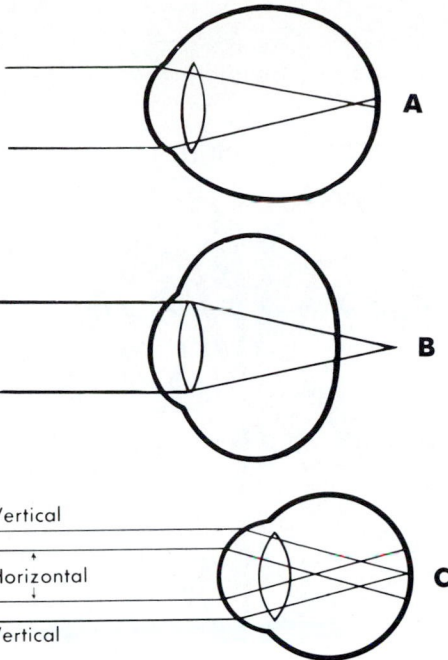

FIG. 13-14. Alterations in refraction. **A,** Myopic eye. Parallel rays of light are brought to a focus in front of the retina. **B,** Hyperopic eye. Parallel rays of light come to a focus behind the retina in the unaccomodative eye. **C,** Simple myopic astigmatism. The verticle bundle of rays is focused on the retina; the horizontal rays are focused in front of the retina. (From Stein, Slatt, & Stein, 1988.)

Hyperopia (farsightedness) involves the focusing of light rays behind the retina when the person is looking at a near object. Hyperopia is corrected with a convex lens. **Astigmatism** is caused by an unequal curvature of the cornea. In astigmatism light rays are bent unevenly and do not come to a single focus on the retina. Astigmatism may coexist with myopia, hyperopia, and/or presbyopia. Correction is accomplished with a cylinder lens.

Alterations in Color Vision

Normal sensitivity to color diminishes with age because of the progressive yellowing of the lens that oc-

---

TABLE 13-7 Types of glaucoma

Type	Mechanism of increased pressure
Open angle glaucoma	Obstruction to the outflow of aqueous humor at the trabecular meshwork or Schlemm canal
Narrow angle glaucoma (angle closure)	Forward displacement of the iris toward the cornea with narrowing of the iridocorneal angle and obstruction to the outflow of aqueous humor from the anterior chamber
Acute angle closure glaucoma	Acute closure of the iridocorneal angle with a sudden rise in intraocular pressure producing nerve pain and visual disturbances

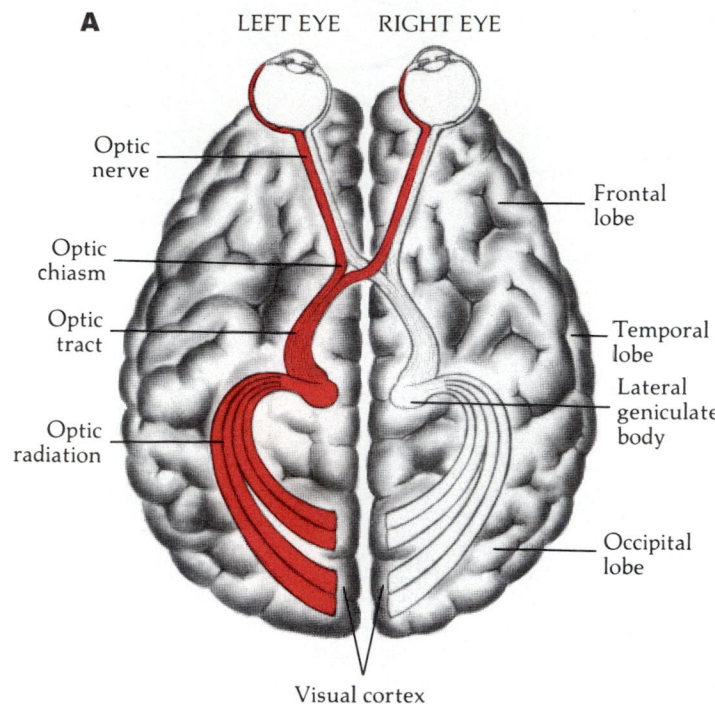

A, LEFT EYE   RIGHT EYE

Optic nerve

Optic chiasm

Optic tract

Optic radiation

Frontal lobe

Temporal lobe

Lateral geniculate body

Occipital lobe

Visual cortex

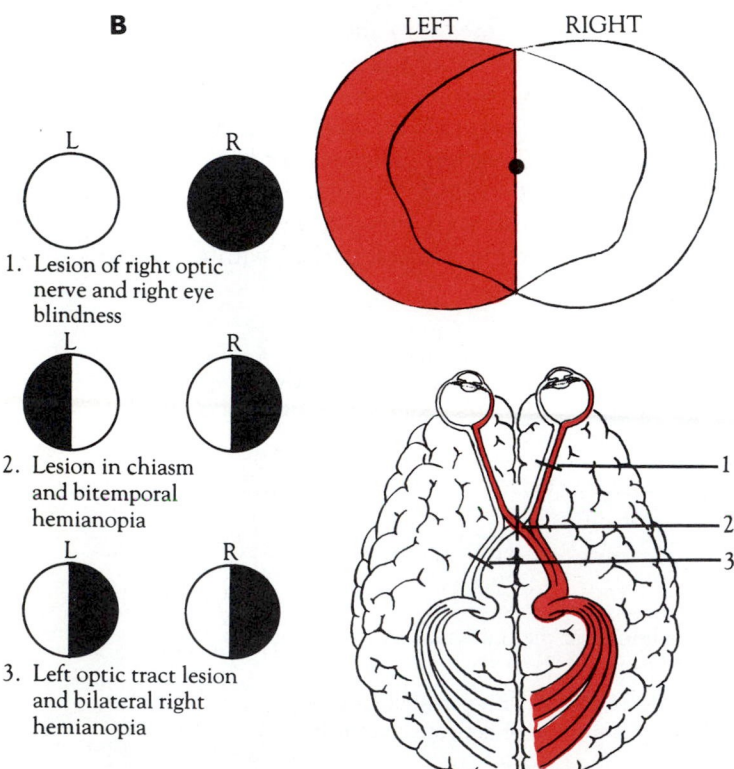

B, LEFT   RIGHT

L   R

1. Lesion of right optic nerve and right eye blindness

L   R

2. Lesion in chiasm and bitemporal hemianopia

L   R

3. Left optic tract lesion and bilateral right hemianopia

FIG. 13-15. A, Visual pathway. **B,** Visual pathway defects. (From Thompson et al., 1989.)

curs with aging. All colors become less intense, although color discrimination for blue and green is most greatly affected. Color vision deteriorates more rapidly for individuals with diabetes mellitus than for the general population. The deterioration is thought to be an accelerated version of senile color vision deterioration.

Abnormal color vision may also be caused by **color blindness,** an inherited trait. Color blindness is generally an X-linked, recessive characteristic affecting 8% of the male population and 0.5% of the female population. Although many forms of color blindness exist, most commonly the affected individual cannot distinguish red from green.

Neurologic Disorders Causing Visual Dysfunction

Various neurologic disorders may cause visual dysfunction. Vision may be disrupted at many points along the visual pathway, causing a variety of defects in fields of vision. Visual changes do not always cause defects or blindness in the entire visual field; **hemianopia** is the term that describes defective vision in half a visual field. (Fig. 13-15 illustrates the many areas along the visual pathway that may be damaged and the associated visual changes.)

Injury to the optic nerve causes ipsilateral (same side) blindness but a normal contralateral (opposite side) visual field. Vision is affected in this manner because of the normal anatomy and physiology of the optic nerve, in which each optic nerve carries information from the eye of the same side. Injury to the **optic chiasm** (the X-shaped crossing of the optic nerves), often caused by atherosclerotic ischemia or external compression from trauma or aneurysm, can cause a variety of defects, depending on the location of injury. These defects vary because at the optic chiasm, nerve fibers from the medial half of each retina separate from the lateral half and enter the opposite optic tract.

Destruction of one optic tract causes **homonymous hemianopia** (complete loss of vision in the inner half of one eye and the outer half of the other). This loss occurs because of the normal structure and function of the visual pathway, in which each optic tract carries the lateral (temporal) field of the same side and the medial (nasal) field of the opposite side. Thus if an injury to the left optic tract occurs, the individual is blind in the right eye's medial (inner) field and the left eye's lateral (outer) field. If the compression of the optic tract is asymmetrical, an incongruous (or uneven) homonymous defect results. Injury to one optic radiation (an ocular pathway in the internal capsule, temporal lobe, or occipital lobe) also causes a homonymous (same field) defect. A major injury in the optic radiation causes homonymous hemianopsia. A lesser injury may cause an upper quadrant homonymous defect. Generally the defects are the same size in both eyes. When the homonymous hemianopsia is caused by an occipital lobe lesion, the area of hemianopia is split. Although visual acuity may remain unimpaired, reading is difficult because of the inability to group words.

Hearing

The external ear is surrounded by the bones of the cranium. Its opening (meatus) is just above the **mastoid process,** which contains air-filled sinuses called **mastoid air cells.** These promote conductivity between the external and the middle ear.

The Normal Ear

The ear is divided into three areas: (1) the external ear, involved only with hearing; (2) the middle ear, involved only with hearing; and (3) the inner ear, involved with both hearing and equilibrium.

The external ear is composed of the **pinna** (auricle), which is the visible portion of the ear, and the **external auditory canal,** a tube that leads to the middle ear (Fig. 13-16). Sound waves entering the external auditory canal hit the **tympanic membrane** (eardrum) and cause it to vibrate. The tympanic membrane separates the external ear from the middle ear.

The middle ear is composed of the **tympanic cavity,** a small chamber in the temporal bone. Three ossicles (small bones) transmit the vibration of the tympanic membrane to the inner ear. The three ossicles are termed the hammer, anvil, and stirrup. When the tympanic membrane moves, the **hammer** moves with it and transfers the vibration to the **anvil,** which passes it on to the **stirrup.** The stirrup presses against the **oval window,** a small membrane of the inner ear. The movement of the oval window sets the fluids of the inner ear in motion (Fig. 3-16).

The **eustachian tube** connects the middle ear with the thorax. Normally flat and closed, the eustachian tube opens briefly when a person swallows and yawns, and it equalizes the pressure in the middle ear with atmospheric pressure. Equalized pressure permits the tympanic membrane to vibrate freely. Through the eustachian tube the mucosa of the middle ear is continuous with the mucosal lining of the throat.

The inner ear is a system of osseous labyrinths (bony, mazelike chambers) filled with a fluid called **perilymph.** The bony labyrinth is divided into the **cochlea,** the **vestibule,** and the **semicircular canals** (see Fig. 13-16). Suspended in the perilymph is a membranous labyrinth that basically follows the shape of the bony labyrinth. The membranous labyrinth is filled with a thicker fluid called **endolymph.**

Within the cochlea is the **organ of Corti,** which contains the **hair cells** (hearing receptors). Sound waves that reach the cochlea through vibrations of the tympanic membrane, ossicles, and oval window set the co-

chlear fluids into motion. Receptor cells on the basilar membrane are stimulated when their hairs are bent or pulled by the movement. Once stimulated, hair cells transmit impulses along the cochlear nerve (a division of the vestibulocochlear nerve) to the auditory cortex of the temporal lobe in the brain (Fig. 13-17). There interpretation of the sound occurs.

The semicircular canals and vestibule of the inner ear contain the **equilibrium receptors.** In the semicircular canals the dynamic equilibrium receptors respond to changes in direction of movement. Within each semicir-

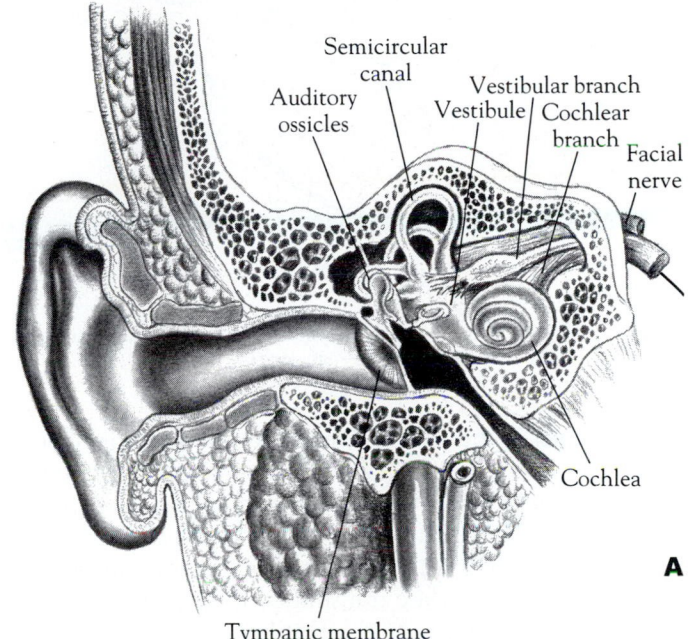

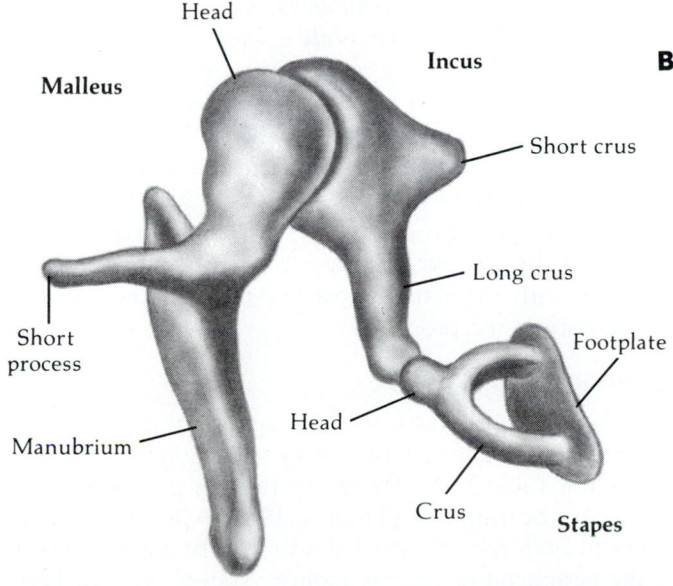

FIG. 13-16. A, Relationship of external, middle, and inner ear. **B,** Ossicles of right middle ear. (From Thompson et al., 1989.)

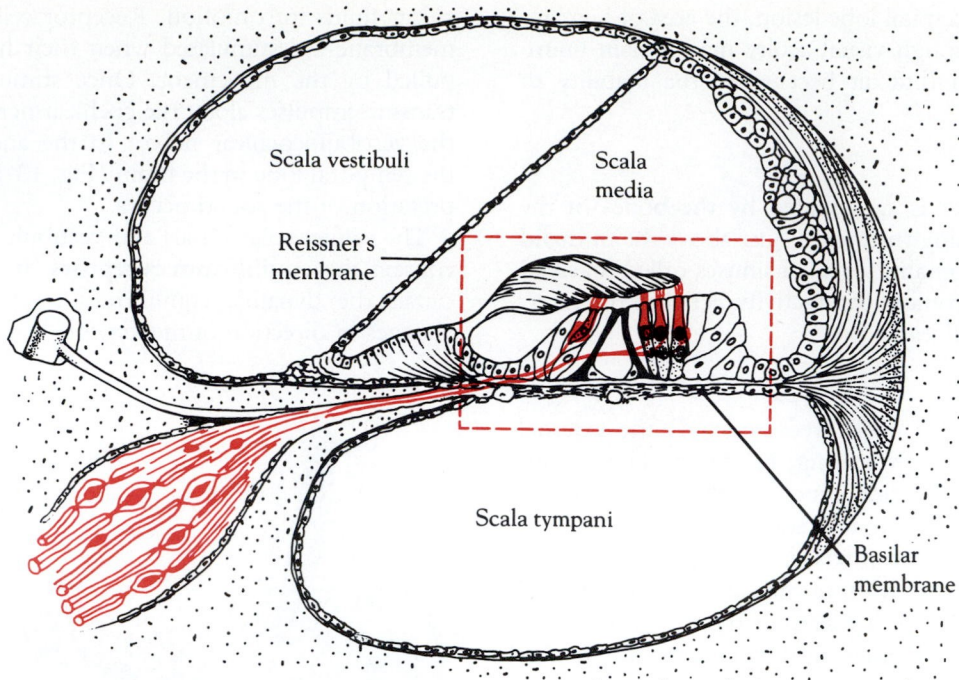

FIG. 13-17. Scalae of the cochlea, separated by Reissner's membrane and basilar membrane. (From Thompson et al., 1989.)

cular canal is the **cristae ampullaris,** a receptor region composed of a tuft of hair cells covered by a gelatinous copula (cap). When the head is rotated, the endolymph in the canal lags behind and moves in the direction opposite to the head's movement. The hair cells are stimulated, and impulses are transmitted through the vestibular nerve (a division of the vestibulocochlear nerve) to the cerebellum.

The vestibule in the inner ear contains **maculae,** receptors essential to the body's sense of static equilibrium. As the head moves, **otoliths** (small pieces of calcium salts) move in a gel-like material in response to changes in the pull of gravity. The otoliths pull on the gel, which in turn pulls on the hair cells in the maculae. Nerve impulses in the hair cells are triggered and transmitted to the brain (Fig. 13-17). Thus the ear not only permits the hearing of a large range of sounds but also assists with maintaining balance through the sensitive equilibrium receptors.

Aging and Hearing

Auditory changes caused by aging are common and incremental. Changes in hearing with aging are summarized in Table 13-8. About one third of people over age 65 have hearing loss (Timiras, 1988). Changes may occur in both the structural and functional components of the peripheral or central auditory system. Loss of hearing for sounds in the high-frequency range (presbycusis) is most common and interferes with understanding speech, particularly consonants, which are high-frequency sounds. Hearing may be lost in both ears but not at the same time. Elderly individuals from rural areas have less hearing loss than those in noisy cities. The ability to discriminate localization of sound varies with high and low frequencies and diminishes with age. In the low-frequency range, sound localization is a function of the timing of sound arrival between the two ears. Localization of high-frequency sounds is a function of sound intensity between the two ears. Since the elderly tend to lose high-frequency hearing first, they may have difficulty localizing high-frequency sounds.

Auditory Dysfunction

Between 5% and 10% of the population have a hearing impairment. The major categories of auditory dysfunction are conductive hearing loss, sensorineural hearing loss, mixed hearing loss, and functional hearing loss. Hearing loss is more common among the elderly, occurring in about 30% of the older population in the United States. Age-related losses are greater for high-toned pitches. Diminished auditory function may occur, however, for a number of reasons.

Conductive Hearing Loss

A **conductive hearing loss** occurs when a change in the outer and/or middle ear impairs the sound from being conducted from the outer to the inner ear. Conductive hearing loss occurs when there is interference in air

TABLE 13-8 Changes in hearing caused by aging

Change in structure	Change in function
Cochlear hair cell degeneration	Inability to hear high-frequency sounds (sensory/neural loss)
Loss of auditory neurons in spiral ganglia of organ of Corti	Inability to hear high-frequency sounds (sensory/neural loss)
Degeneration of basilar (cochlear) conductive membrane of cochlea	Inability to hear at all frequencies but more pronounced at higher frequencies (cochlear conductive loss)
Decreased vascularity of cochlea	Equal loss of hearing at all frequencies (strial loss)
Loss of cortical auditory neurons	Diminished hearing and speech comprehension

conduction. Conditions that commonly cause a conductive hearing loss include impacted cerumen, foreign bodies lodged in the ear canal, benign tumors of the middle ear, carcinoma of the external auditory canal and/or middle ear, eustachian tube dysfunction, otitis media, acute viral otitis media, chronic suppurative otitis media, cholesteatoma, and otosclerosis.

Symptoms of conductive hearing loss include diminished hearing and soft speaking voice. The voice is soft because often the individual hears his or her voice, conducted by bone, as loud. In addition, although the cause is unknown, the individual often hears better in a noisy environment than in a quiet one (a condition called paracusia willisiani). Treatment of the underlying cause generally eliminates the hearing loss. A hearing aid is used if the hearing loss is greater than 40 to 50 decibels.

Sensorineural Hearing Loss

A **sensorineural hearing loss** is due to impairment of the organ of Corti or its central connections. The hearing loss may be gradual or sudden. Conditions that commonly cause sensorineural hearing loss include congenital and hereditary factors, noise exposure, aging, Meniere disease, ototoxicity, and systemic disease (syphilis, Paget disease, collagen diseases, diabetes mellitus). Congenital and neonatal sensorineural hearing loss may be caused by maternal rubella, ototoxic drugs, prematurity, traumatic delivery, erythroblastosis fetalis, and congenital hereditary malfunction. Diagnosis is often made when delayed speech development is noted.

Presbycusis is the most common form of sensorineural hearing loss and is especially common in the elderly. Presbycusis may occur because of atrophy of the basal end of the organ of Corti, a loss in the number of auditory receptors, vascular changes, and/or stiffening of the basilar membranes. Because of the slow progression of hearing loss, onset of symptoms is gradual.

In addition drug ototoxicities (drugs that cause destruction of auditory function) have been observed after exposure to a variety of chemicals. Antibiotics such as streptomycin, neomycin, gentamicin, and vancomycin; diuretics such as ethacrynic acid and furosemide; and chemicals such as salicylate, quinine, carbon monoxide, nitrogen mustard, arsenic, mercury, gold, tobacco, and alcohol are considered ototoxic. Because of increased concentrations of antibiotics in the endolymph, these drugs generally cause damage to the cells of the cristae and maculae (located in the inner ear) and/or the cells of the organ of Corti. The increased concentration of drugs in the endolymph is preferentially toxic to the cells.

Diuretics affect hearing primarily by altering the sodium-potassium balance, causing extracellular fluid accumulation and changes in the microstructure of secretory cells. Quinine, mercury, and lead affect the neural pathways of hearing, including the spinal ganglia, the eighth cranial nerve, and the cochlear nucleus. The site of action for the other chemicals, including alcohol and tobacco, has not yet been determined. In most instances the drugs and chemicals listed previously initially cause **tinnitus** (ringing in the ear), followed by a progressive high-tone sensorineural hearing loss. Care is aimed at prevention of further hearing loss because the loss is usually permanent.

Mixed Hearing Loss

A **mixed hearing loss** is caused by a combination of conductive and sensorineural losses.

Functional Hearing Loss

A **functional hearing loss** occurs for no organic reason. The individual does not respond to voice and appears not to hear. Functional hearing loss is thought to be due to emotional or psychologic factors. It occurs only rarely.

Olfaction and Taste

Olfaction (smell) and taste (gustation) dysfunctions may occur separately or jointly. The strong relationship between smell and taste creates sensation of flavor. If ei-

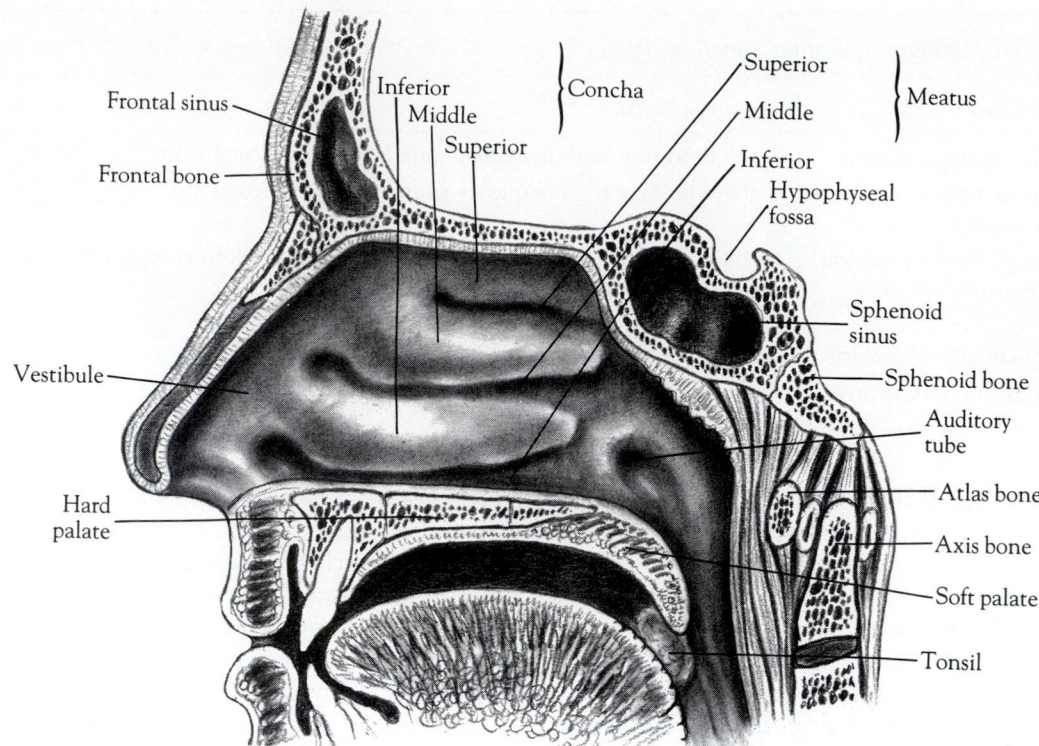

FIG. 13-18. Lateral wall of nose. (From Thompson et al., 1989.)

ther sensation is impaired, the perception of flavor is altered. (Olfactory structures are illustrated in Fig. 13-18.)

Aging and Olfaction and Taste

Olfaction

Sensitivity to odors declines steadily with aging (Stevens & Cain, 1986). A recent study of odor identification indicates an increasing ability from childhood to adolescence and then a decine after age 60 years. The most significant impairments develop after 80 years (Doty et al., 1984). Women generally have better olfactory abilities than men, but the patterns of decline are similar.

The olfactory mucosa covers the walls of the superior nasal cavities. The mucosa consists of neuroepithelium and is intact in the infant but begins to degenerate in the adult with loss of olfactory sensory neurons and loss of cells from the olfactory bulbs (Bhatnagar et al., 1987). Loss of olfactory sensitivity and odor identification may diminish appetite and food selection and thus may lead to malnutrition. (Flavor is thought to be associated with food odors.) Safety may also be compromised with an inability to smell toxic or hazardous gases.

Taste

The decline in taste sensation is more gradual than that of smell. Higher concentrations of flavors are required and the elderly have difficulty differentiating combinations of flavors. The best known changes with aging are the decline in the number of fungiform papillae on the tongue, which decrease by 50% at about 50 years of age (Hans & Coons, 1979). Taste may also be affected by decreased salivary gland secretion. Amylase, contained in saliva, facilitates perception of sweet sensations and is also reduced with aging.

Olfactory Dysfunction

Olfactory dysfunctions include hyposmia, anosmia, hallucinations, and parosmia. **Hyposmia** is the impaired sense of smell, whereas **anosmia** is the complete loss of smell. When hyposmia or anosmia occurs bilaterally, it is usually the result of rhinitis (inflammation of the nasal mucosa), severe coryza (head cold), or excessive smoking. Unilateral hyposmia or anosmia may indicate compression of one olfactory bulb (a bulblike portion of the olfactory nerves) or nerve tract (olfactory nerve pathway), possibly by tumor. **Olfactory hallucinations** arise from hyperactivity in cortical neurons and involve the smelling of odors that are not really present. They are associated with temporal lobe seizures and rarely with schizophrenia. **Parosmia,** an abnormal or perverted sense of smell, may occur with severe depression. The sense of smell normally diminishes only slightly with age.

Taste Dysfunction

The sense of taste can be impaired by injury or by aging. The number of taste buds ordinarily declines after the age of 50. Taste acuity diminishes with age to such an extent that people in their eighties have difficulty distinguishing among sweet, sour, salty, and bitter. An alteration in taste may be due to impairment of smell associated with injury near the hippocampus.

Hypogeusia is the decrease in taste sensation, whereas **ageusia** is the absence of taste. Ageusia affecting the entire tongue may follow head injury. Damage to the glossopharyngeal nerve (cranial nerve IX, which innervates the posterior one third of the tongue) causes the loss of the ability to detect bitterness. This loss occurs because the receptors for bitter are located on the base of the tongue. Damage to the facial nerve (cranial nerve VIII, which innervates the anterior two thirds of the tongue) causes loss of the ability to detect sour, sweet, and salt tastes. Only bitter tastes can be detected. These losses occur because sour, sweet, and salt receptors are located on the anterior portion of the tongue. **Parageusia** is a perversion of taste in which substances possess an unpleasant flavor. Parageusia occasionally develops for no apparent reason in the elderly and also is common in individuals receiving chemotherapy for cancer. In both cases parageusia often leads to anorexia.

SOMATOSENSORY FUNCTION

Touch

Touch is not a uniform sensory experience. The sensation of touch involves the fusion of several qualities, including modality, intensity, location, and duration of the sensory stimulus. Receptors sensitive to touch are present in the skin. Specific sensory input is carried to the higher levels of the central nervous system by the dorsal column of the spinal cord and the anterior spinothalamic tract.

Much of the development of the cutaneous senses takes place before birth, but structural growth of the cutaneous senses continues into early adulthood at a reduced rate. Then a gradual decline occurs. Several studies have documented loss in tactile sensitivity with advancing age. This occurs simultaneously with an increase in the size of pacinian corpuscles and a decrease in the number of corpuscles. Sensitivity to touch then appears to decrease with age.

Abnormal tactile perception may be caused by alterations at any level of the nervous system, from the receptor to the cerebral cortex. Any factor that interrupts or impairs reception, transmission, perception, or interpretation of touch also alters tactile sensation. Trauma, tumor, infection, metabolic changes, vascular changes, and degenerative diseases thus may cause tactile dysfunction, which may involve heightened or diminished tactile perceptions.

In addition, most tactile sensations evoke affective responses that determine whether the sensation is unpleasant, pleasant, or neutral. Cerebral and hypothalamic centers influence this response. Sedative drugs and prefrontal injury, which interrupt connections between the prefrontal cortex and subcortical centers, diminish the interpretation of the sensations.

Proprioception

The perception and awareness of the position of the body and its parts depends on impulses from the inner ear and from receptors in joints and ligaments. The role of muscle, tendon, and cutaneous receptors is indefinite. Sensory data are transmitted to higher centers through the dorsal columns and the spinocerebellar tracts. Comparatively few proprioceptive stimuli are perceived consciously. The stimuli are necessary, however, for the coordination of movements, the grading of muscular contraction, and the maintenance of equilibrium. A progressive loss of proprioception has been reported in the elderly.

Proprioceptive dysfunction may be caused by alterations at any level of the nervous system. As with tactile dysfunction, any factor that interrupts or impairs the reception, transmission, perception, or interpretation of proprioceptive stimuli also alters proprioception. Two frequent causes of proprioceptive dysfunction are vestibular dysfunction and neuropathy.

Specific vestibular dysfunctions are vestibular nystagmus and vertigo. **Vestibular nystagmus** is the constant, involuntary movement of the eyeball caused by ear disturbances. This condition occurs when the semicircular canal system is overstimulated. **Vertigo** is the sensation of spinning that occurs with inflammation of the semicircular canals in the ear. The individual may feel either that he or she is moving in space or that the world is revolving. Vertigo often causes loss of balance. Vertigo and nystagmus may occur in a variety of conditions, including labyrinthitis, vestibular neuritis, acute toxic labyrinthitis, and Meniere disease.

Meniere disease is a vestibular disorder that can cause proprioceptive dysfunction. The pathologic basis of Meniere disease is still unclear. The individual with Meniere disease may experience loss of proprioception during an acute attack, so that standing or walking is impossible.

Peripheral neuropathies can also cause proprioceptive dysfunctions. Neuropathies may be caused by a variety of conditions and are commonly associated with renal disease and diabetes mellitus. Although the exact sequence of events is unknown, neuropathies are thought to be caused by a metabolic disturbance of the neuron itself. The result is a diminished or absent sense of body position or position of body parts. Gait changes often occur. (Neuropathies are further discussed in Chapter 15.)

SUMMARY REVIEW

Pain

1 Pain is a complex phenomenon composed of sensory experiences (time, space, intensity) and emotion, cognition, and motivation.

2 Categories of pain include somatogenic pain (with a known physiologic cause), psychogenic pain (without a physiologic cause), acute pain (signal to the person of a harmful stimulus), and chronic pain (persistence of pain of unknown cause or unusual response to therapy).

3 Pain threshold is the point at which pain is perceived. Pain threshold does not vary significantly among people or within the same person over time.

4 Pain tolerance is the duration of time or the intensity of pain that an individual will endure before initiating overt pain response. Tolerance varies widely among individuals and in the same individual over time.

5 Young children have a lower pain threshold than do adults. Older individuals tend to have a slightly higher pain threshold, probably because of changes in the thickness of the skin and peripheral neuropathies. In all age groups women appear to be more sensitive to pain than men.

6 The portions of the nervous system responsible for the sensation and perception of pain may be divided into three areas: (1) the afferent fibers, (2) the central nervous system, and (3) the afferent pathways.

7 The afferent system is composed of nociceptors, A and C fibers, the dorsal horn of the spinal column, and afferent neurons in the spinothalamic tract.

8 Efferent pathways from the periaqueductal gray are responsible for modulation or inhibition of afferent pain signals.

9 The thalamus, cortex, and postcentral gyrus perceive, describe, and localize pain. The reticular formation and limbic system control the emotional and affective response to pain.

10 The specificity theory of pain proposes that pain is caused by stimulation of nerve endings in the skin, transmission of the painful stimuli through A and C fibers to the spinal cord, and ascent of impulses to the brain, causing a direct relationship between the stimulus and the perception of pain.

11 Endorphins inhibit transmission of the pain impulse. They are present in varying concentration in the neurons in the brain, spinal cord, and gastrointestinal tract.

12 According to the gate control theory, there are specialized cells within the substantia gelatinosa that act as a gate, opening and closing the afferent pathways to transmission of painful stimuli.

13 According to the pattern theory of pain, pain perception is the result of stimulus intensity and summation of the impulses.

14 Acute pain may be (a) somatic (superficial), (b) visceral (internal), or (c) referred (present in an area distant from its origin). The area of referred pain is supplied by the same spinal segment as the actual site of pain.

15 Physiologic responses to acute pain include increased heart rate, respiratory rate, and blood pressure; pallor or flushing; dilated pupils; and diaphoresis. Blood sugar is elevated; gastric secretion and motility are decreased; and blood flow to the viscera and skin is decreased.

16 Psychologic, behavioral, and physiologic responses to chronic pain include depression, difficulty in sleeping, preoccupation with pain, life-style changes, and physiologic adaptation.

17 Chronic pain may be a result of decreased levels of endorphins, predominance of C neuron stimulation, or leukokinin.

18 Chronic pain conditions include lower back pain, neuralgias, reflex sympathetic dystrophies, hyperesthesias, myofascial pain syndrome, pain hemiagnosia, phantom limb pain, and chronic pain associated with cancer.

Temperature Regulation

1 Temperature regulation is achieved through precise balancing of heat production, heat conservation, and heat loss. Body temperature is maintained in a range around 37° C (98.6° F).

2 Temperature regulation is mediated by the hypothalamus. Peripheral thermoreceptors in the skin and central thermoreceptors in the hypothalamus, spinal cord, and abdominal organs provide the hypothalamus with information about skin and core temperatures.

3 Heat is produced through chemical reactions of metabolism, skeletal muscle contraction, and chemical thermogenesis.

4 Heat is lost through radiation, conduction, convection, vasodilation, decreased muscle tone, evaporation of sweat, increased respiration, and voluntary mechanisms.

5 Heat conservation is accomplished through vasoconstriction and voluntary mechanisms.

6 Infants and the elderly require special attention to maintenance of body temperature. Because of their greater body-surface-to-mass ratio and decreased subcutaneous fat, infants do not conserve heat well. The elderly have poor responses to environmental temperature extremes as a result of slowed blood circulation, structural and functional changes in skin, and overall decrease in heat-producing activities.

7 Fever is triggered by the release of pyrogens from leukocytes and other cells involved in the immune response. Fever is both a symptom of a disease and a normal immunologic mechanism.

8 Fever involves the "resetting of the thermostat" to a higher level. When the fever breaks, the "set point" is returned to normal.

9 Fever production aids responses to infectious processes. Higher temperatures kill many microorganisms and decrease serum levels of iron, zinc, and copper that are needed for bacterial replication.

10 Hyperthermia (marked warming of core temperature) can produce nerve damage, coagulation of cell proteins, and death. Forms of accidental hyperthermia include heat cramps, heat exhaustion, heatstroke, and malignant hyperthermia. Heatstroke and malignant hyperthermia are potentially lethal developments.

11 Hypothermia (marked cooling of core temperature) slows the rate of chemical reaction (tissue metabolism), increases the viscosity of the blood, slows blood flow through the microcirculation, facilitates blood coagulation, and stimulates profound vasoconstriction. Hypothermia may be accidental or therapeutic.

Sleep

1 During sleep the body is actively engaged in restoring and repairing itself. Sleep deprivation can cause profound changes in personality and functioning.

2 The restorative, reparative, and growth processes occur during slow wave sleep.

3 Sleep may be divided into REM and non-REM stages, each of which has its own series of stages. While asleep an individual progresses through REM and non-REM sleep in a predictable cycle.

4 Brain synthesis, which organizes the day's activities, occurs during REM sleep.

5 Sleep is initiated by the withdrawal of neurotransmitters from the afferent formation and by the inhibition of arousal mechanisms in the cerebral cortex. REM sleep is controlled by mechanisms in the pontine reticular formation.

6 The sleep patterns of the newborn and young child vary from those of the adult in total sleep time, cycle length, and percentage of time spent in each sleep cycle. The elderly experience a total decrease in sleep time.

7 Sleep disorders include (a) disorders of initiating sleep (insomnia), (b) disorders of excessive somnolence (pickwickian syndrome and hypersomnia sleep apnea syndrome), (c) disorders of the sleep-wake schedule (jet lag, shift work), and (d) dysfunctions of sleep, sleep stages, or partial arousals (somnambulism, night terrors, or enuresis).

8 Ingestion of alcohol and some medications can alter or suppress sleep stages, producing sleep disorders.

9 Sleep and disease are interrelated. Some diseases produce alterations in the quantity and quality of sleep or affect sleep stages. These are referred to as secondary sleep disorders. In some instances sleep stages produce alterations in certain disease states. These are referred to as sleep-provoked disorders.

The Special Senses

1 The eyelids, conjunctiva, and lacrimal apparatus protect the eye. Infections are the most common disorders; they include blepharitis, conjunctivitis, chalazion, and hordeolum.

2 Conjunctivitis can be acute or chronic, bacterial, viral, or allergic. Redness, edema, pain, and lacrimation are common symptoms. Chlamydial conjunctivitis is the leading cause of blindness in the world and is associated with poor sanitary conditions.

3 Keratitis is a bacterial or viral infection of the cornea that can lead to corneal ulceration. Photophobia, pain, and tearing are common symptoms.

4 The wall of the eye has three layers: sclera, choroid, and retina. The retina contains millions of baroreceptors known as rods and cones that receive light through the lens and then convey signals to the optic nerve and subsequently to the visual cortex of the brain.

5 The eye is filled with vitreous and aqueous humor that prevent it from collapsing.

6 The major alterations in ocular movement include strabismus, nystagmus, and paralysis of the extraocular muscles.

7 Alterations in visual acuity can be caused by amblyopia, scotoma, cataracts, papilledema, macular degeneration, and glaucoma.

8 Alterations in accommodation develop with increased intraocular pressure, inflammation, and disease of the oculomotor nerve. Presbyopia is loss of accommodation caused by loss of elasticity of the lens with aging.

9 Alterations in refraction, including myopia, hyperopia, and astigmatism, are the most common visual disorders.

10 Trauma or disease of the optic nerve pathways, or optic radiations, can cause blindness in the visual fields. Homonymous hemianopia is due to damage of one optic track.

11 The ear is composed of external, middle, and inner structures. The external structures are the pinna, auditory canal, and tympanic membrane. The tympanic cavity (containing three bones: the hammer, the anvil, and the stirrup), oval window, eustachian tube, and fluid compose the middle ear and transmit sound vibrations to the inner ear.

12 The inner ear includes the bony and membranous labyrinths that transmit sound waves through the cochlea to the division of the eighth cranial nerve. The semicircular canals and vestibule help maintain balance through the equilibrium receptors.

13 Hearing loss can be classified as conductive, sensorineural, mixed, and functional.

14 Conductive hearing loss occurs when sound waves cannot be conducted through the middle ear.

15 Sensorineural hearing loss develops with impairment of the organ of Corti or its central connections.

16 A combination of conductive and sensorineural loss is a mixed hearing loss.

17 Loss of hearing with no known organic cause is a functional hearing loss.

18 Hyposmia is a decrease in the sense of smell, and anosmia is the complete loss of smell. Inflammation of the nasal mucosa and trauma or tumors of the olfactory nerve lead to diminished smell.

19 Hypogeusia is a decrease in taste sensation, and ageusia is the absence of taste. Loss of taste buds or trauma to the facial or glossopharyngeal nerves decreases taste sensation.

Somatosensory Function

1 Tactile sensation is a function of receptors present in the skin (pacinian corpuscles), and the sensory response is conducted to the brain through the dorsal column and anterior spinothalamic tract.

2 Alterations in touch can result from disruption of skin receptors, sensory transmission, or central nervous system perception.

3 Proprioception is the position and location of the body and its parts. Proprioceptors are located in the inner ear, joints, and ligaments. Proprioceptive stimuli are necessary for balance, coordinated movement, and grading of muscular contraction.

4 Disorders of proprioception can occur at any level of the nervous system with impaired balance and lack of coordinated movement.

KEY TERMS

Acute bacterial conjunctivitis (pink eye), 413

Acute pain, 392

Ageusia, 423

Allergic conjunctivitis, 413

Amblyopia, 415, 416

Anosmia, 422

Anvil, 419

Aqueous humor, 415

Astigmatism, 417

β-Lypotrophin, 397

Cataract, 416

Causalgia, 399

Choroid, 414

Chronic conjunctivitis, 413

Chronic pain, 392

Circadian rhythm, 400

Cochlea, 419

Cognitive/evaluative system, 391

Color blindness, 418

Conduction, 402

Conductive hearing loss, 420

Cone, 414

Convection, 402

Cornea, 414

Cristae ampullaris, 420

Diplopia, 415

Dynorphin, 397

Endogenous antipyretic, 405

Endogenous pyrogen, 404

Endolymph, 419

Endorphin, 397

Enkephalin, 397

Enuresis, 412

Equilibrium receptor, 419

Eustachian tube, 419

External auditory canal, 419

Fovea centralis, 415

Functional hearing loss, 421

Gate control theory, 396

Glaucoma, 416

Hair cell, 419

Hammer, 419

Heat cramps, 405

Heat exhaustion, 405

Heatstroke, 405

Hemianopia, 418

Homonymous hemianopia, 418

Hyperopia, 417

Hyperesthesia, 399

Hypersomnia sleep apnea (HSA) syndrome, 411

Hyperthermia, 401

Hypogeusia, 423

Hyposmia, 422

Hypothermia, 401

Insomnia, 411

Iris, 414

Jerk nystagmus, 415

Lens, 415

Macula, 420

Malignant hyperthermia, 406

Mastoid air cell, 419

Mastoid process, 419

Meissner corpuscles, 395

Meniere disease, 423

Mixed hearing loss, 421

Motivational/affective system, 391

Myofascial pain syndrome, 399

Myopia, 417

Neuralgia, 399

Night terrors, 412

Nociceptor, 394

Non-REM sleep, 409

Nystagmus, 415

Olfactory hallucination, 422

Opiate receptor, 397

Optic chiasma, 418

Optic disk, 415

Organ of Corti, 419

Otolith, 420

Oval window, 419

Pacinian corpuscle, 395

Pain hemiagnosia, 400

Pain threshold, 392

Pain tolerance, 392

Papilledema, 416

Parageusia, 423

Parosmia, 423

Pattern theory, 396

Pendular nystagmus, 415

Perceptual dominance, 392

Periaqueductal gray (PAG), 395

Perilymph, 419

Phantom limb pain, 400

Pickwickian syndrome, 411

Pinna, 419

Presbycusis, 421

Presbyia,

Presbyopia, 416

Psychogenic pain, 391

Pupil, 414

Radiation, 402

Rapid eye movement sleep (REM sleep), 408

Referred pain, 397

Reflex sympathetic dystrophy, 399

Retina, 414

Retrobulbar neuritis, 416

Rod, 414

Sclera, 414

Scotoma, 416

Secondary sleep disorder, 412

Semicircular canal, 419

Sensorineural hearing loss, 421

Sensory/discriminative system, 391

Sleep apnea, 411

Sleep-provoked disorder, 412

Slow-wave sleep, 408

Somatic pain, 397

Somatogenic pain, 391

Somnambulism, 412

Specificity theory, 396

Stirrup, 419

Strabismus, 415

Tinnitus, 421

Trachoma, 413

Trigger point, 400

Tympanic cavity, 419

Tympanic membrane, 419

Vertigo, 423

Vestibular nystagmus, 423

Vestibule, 419

Viral conjunctivitis, 413

Visceral pain, 397

Vitreous humor, 415

REFERENCES

Adams, R., & Victor, M. (1981). *Principles of Neurology.* San Francisco: McGraw-Hill.

Almay, G. L., Johansson, F., Knorring, L., Sedvall, G., & Terenius, L. (1980). Relationships between CSF levels of endorphins and monoamine metabolites in chronic pain patients. *Psychopharmacology, 67,* 139-142.

Anders, T. F., & Keener, M. (1985). Developmental course of nighttime sleep-wake patterns in full-term and premature infants during the first year of life. *Sleep, 8*(3), 173-192.

Benito, M. (1985). Contribution of brown fat to the neonatal thermogenesis. *Biology of the Neonate, 48*(4), 245-249.

Berglund, B., Berglund, U., & Lindvall, T. (1986). Theory and methods for odor evaluation. *Experientia, 42*(3), 280-287.

Berlin, L., Boodell, H., & Wolff, H. G. (1958). Relation of pain perception and central inhibitory effects of noxious stimulation to phenomenon of excitation of pain. *Archives of Neurology, 80,* 533-543.

Berman, D. A. (1979, January-March). Pain relief and acupuncture: The if, why, and how. *American Journal of Acupuncture,* 31-38.

Berne, R. M., & Levy, M. N. (Eds.). (1988). *Physiology* (2nd ed.). St. Louis: C.V. Mosby.

Bernheim, H. A., Block, L. H., & Atkins, E. (1979). Fever: Pathogenesis, pathophysiology, and purpose. *Annals of Internal Medicine, 91,* 261-270.

Bhatnagar, K. P., Kennedy, R. C., Baron, G., & Greenberg, R. A. (1987). Number of mitral cells and the bulb volume in the aging human olfactory bulb: A quantitative morphological study. *Anatomical Record, 218,* 73-87.

Biddle, C. (1986). Hypothermia: Implications for the critical care nurse. *Critical Care Nurse, 5*(2), 34-38.

Birren, J. E., Shapiro, H. B., & Miller, J. H. (1950). The effect of salicylate upon pain sensitivity. *Journal of Pharmacological Experimental Therapy, 100,* 67-71.

Black, R. G. (1975). The chronic pain syndrome. *Surgical Clinics of North America,* 999-1011.

Block, A. J. (1980, November-December). Respiratory disorders during sleep. Part I. *Heart and Lung,* 1011-1024.

Block, A. J. (1981, January-February). Respiratory disorders during sleep. Part II. *Heart and Lung,* 90-96.

Brena, S. F. (1985). Nerve blocks and chronic pain states—an update. *Post Graduate Medicine, 78*(4), 77-86.

Brunner, L., & Suddarth, D. (1984). *Textbook of medical-surgical nursing* (5th ed.). Philadelphia: J. B. Lippincott.

Bullock, T. H., Orkand, R., & Grinnell, A. (1977). *Introduction to nervous systems.* San Francisco: W. H. Freeman.

Cabanac, M., & Brinnel, H. (1987). The pathology of human temperature regulation: Thermiatrics. *Experimentia, 43*(1), 19-27.

Calverly, P. M., Brezinova, V., Douglas, N. J., Catterall, J. R., & Flenley, D. C. (1982). The effect of oxygenation on sleep quality in chronic bronchitis and emphysema. *American Review of Respiratory Disease, 126,* 206-210.

Campbell, S. S. (1987). Evolution of sleep structure following brief intervals of wakefulness. *Electroenchalography and Clinical Neurophysiology, 66*(2), 175-184.

Cauna, N. (1965). The effects of aging on the receptor organs of the human dermis. In N. Montagna (Ed.), *Advances in biology of skin, Vol. VI: aging.* New York: Pergamon Press.

Clowes, G. H., & O'Donnell, T. F. (1974). Heat stroke. *The New England Journal of Medicine, 291,* 564-567.

Cohen, F. L. (1980). Postsurgical pain relief: Patients' status and nurses' medication choices. *Pain,* 265-274.

Collins, K. J., & Exton-Smith, A. N. (1983). Thermal homeostasis in old age. *Journal of the American Geriatrics Society, 31*(9), 519-524.

Committee on Sports Medicine. (1982). Climatic heat stress and the exercising child. *Pediatrics, 69,* 808-809.

Cooper, K. E., & Veale, W. L. (1987). Effects of endotoxins on heat tolerance and exercise performance. In J. R. S. Hales & D. A. B. Richards (Eds.), *Heat stress: Physical exertion and environment.* New York: Elsevier Science Publications.

Corso, J. F. (1981). *Aging sensory systems and perception.* New York: Praeger.

Cummings, D. (1981, January). Stopping chronic pain before it starts. *Nursing 81,* 60-62.

Cunha, B. A., Digamon-Beltran, M., & Gobbo, P. N. (1984). Implications of fever in the critical care setting. *Heart and Lung, 13,* 460-465.

Dawes, C., & Watanabe, S. (1987). The effect of taste adaptation on salivary flow rate and salivary sugar clearance. *Journal of Dental Research, 66*(3), 740-746.

Dean, N. C. (1987). Hypothermia. *Post Graduate Medicine, 82*(8), 48-58.

Dear, T. A. (1987). Controlling noise at its source can help protect worker's hearing. *Occupational Health and Safety, 56*(6), 60, 62, 65.

DeBlasi, M. (1979, January). Using analgesics effectively. *American Journal of Nursing,* 74-78.

DeLapp, T. D. (1983, January). Accidental hypothermia. *American Journal of Nursing,* 63-67.

Devney, A. M., & Kingsbury, B. A. (1972, January). Hypothermia in fact and fantasy. *American Journal of Nursing,* 1424-1425.

Dinarello, C. A., & Wolff, S. M. (1982). Molecular basis of fever in humans. *The American Journal of Medicine, 72,* 799-810.

Dinarello, C. A., & Wolff, S. M. (1978, March). Pathogenesis of fever in man. *New England Journal of Medicine,* 607-612.

Doty, R. L., Shaman, P., Applebaum, S. L., Giberson, R., Sikorski, L., & Rosenberg, L. (1984). Smell identification ability changes with age. *Science, 226,* 1441-1443.

Edelman, I. S. (1974). Thyroid thermogenesis. *Physiology in Medicine, 29*(23), 1303-1308.

Elias, M. F., Nicholson, N. A., Bora, C., & Johnston, J. (1986). Sleep/wake patterns of breast-fed infants in the first 2 years of life. *Pediatrics, 77*(3), 322-329.

Fagerhaugh, S. Y., & Strauss, A. (1980, February). How to manage your patient's pain . . . and how not to. *Nursing 80,* 44-47.

Felig, P., & Wahren, J. (1975, November). Fuel homeostasis in exercise. *New England Journal of Medicine,* 1078-1084.

Fellows, I. W., MacDonald, I. A., & Bennett, T. (1985). The effect of undernutrition on thermoregulation in the elderly. *Clinical Science, 69*(5), 525-532.

Foley, K. M. (1984, Summer). A review of pain syndromes in patients with cancer. *Symposium on the Management of Cancer Pain,* 7-16.

Foley, K. M. (1985). The treatment of cancer pain. *The New England Journal of Medicine, 313,* 84-95.

Fruthaler, G. J. (1985). Fever in children: Phobia vs. facts. *Hospital Practice, 20*(11A), 49-53.

Gildea, J. H., & Quick, T. R. (1977, December). Assessing the pain experience in children. *Nursing Clinics of North America,* 631-637.

Gordon, G. (Ed.). (1978). *Active touch.* Oxford: Pergamon Press.

Graham, P. (1985). The eye. In M. S. S. Pathy (Ed.), *Principles and practice of geriatric medicine* (pp. 833-844), London: Wiley.

Gronert, G. A. (1980). Malignant hyperthermia. *Anesthesiology, 53,* 395-423.

Guazzelli, M., Feinberg, I., & Aminoff, M. (1986). Sleep spindles in the normal elderly: Comparison with young adult patterns and relation to nocturnal awakening, cognitive function, and brain atrophy. *Electroencephalography and Clinical Neurophysiology, 63*(6), 526-539.

Guilleminault, C., Eldridge, F. L., Tilkian, A., Simmons, F. B., & Dement, W. C. (1977, March). Sleep apnea syndrome due to upper airway obstruction. *Archives of Internal Medicine,* 296.

Guilleminault, C., Tilkian, A., & Dement, W. C. (1976). The sleep apnea syndromes. *Annual Review of Medicine,* 465-484.

Gurevich, I. (1985). Fever: When to worry about it. *RN, 48,* 14-19.

Hammarlund, K., Stromberg, B., & Sedin, G. (1986). Heat loss from the skin of preterm and full-term newborn infants during the first weeks after birth. *Biology of the Neonate, 50*(1), 1-10.

Hans, S. S., & Coons, D. H. (Eds.). (1979). *Special senses in aging.* Ann Arbor, Mich.: University of Michigan Institute of Gerontology.

Harkins, S. W., & Warner, M. H. (1977). Age and pain. *Behavioral and Social Sciences,* 121-129.

Haslam, D. R. (1969). Age and the perception of pain. *Psychonomic Science, 15,* 86.

Hayter, J. (1980, March). The rhythm of sleep. *American Journal of Nursing,* 457-461.

Heaton, J. M. (1972). The distribution of brown adipose tissue in the human. *Journal of Anatomy, 112,* 35-39.

Hendler, N., Viernstein, M., Gucer, P., & Long, D. (1979, December). Preoperative screening test for chronic back pain patients. *Psychosomatics,* 801-808.

Henry, J. L. (1986). Role of circulating opoids in the modulation of pain. *Annals of the New York Academy of Sciences, 467,* 169-181.

Himms-Hagen, J. (1980). Current status of nonshivering thermogenesis. In Ross Laboratories, *Assessment of energy metabolism in health and disease: A report of the first Ross conference in medical research.* Columbus, OH: Ross Laboratories.

Institute of Medicine, Division of Mental Health and Behavior Science. (1979). *Sleeping pills, insomnia, and medical practice.* Washington, DC: National Academy of Sciences.

Jacox, A. K. (1979, May). Assessing pain. *American Journal of Nursing,* 895-900.

Johns, M. W. (1971, March). Methods of assessing human sleep. *Archives of Internal Medicine,* 484-492.

Johnson, J. E., et al. (1978). Altering patient's responses to surgery: An extension and replication. *Research in Nursing and Health,* 111-121.

Johnston, C. C., & Strada, M. E. (1986). Acute pain response in infants: A multidimensional description. *Pain, 24*(3), 373-382.

Kales, A., & Kales, J. D. (1970, September). Evaluation, diagnosis, and treatment of clinical conditions related to sleep. *Journal of American Medical Association,* 2229-2235.

Kales, A., & Kales, J.D. (1974, February). Sleep disorders. *The New England Journal of Medicine,* 487-499.

Kales, A., Saldatos, C. R., & Kales, J. D. (1980, August). Taking a sleep history. *American Family Physician,* 101-107.

Kantor, T. G. (1984, Summer). Nonsteroidal anti-inflammatory analgesic agents in management of cancer pain. *Symposium on the Management of Cancer Pain,* 30-34.

Karnovsky, M. L. (1986). Progress in sleep. *New England Journal of Medicine, 315,* 1026-1028.

Keefe, M. R. (1987). Comparison of neonatal nighttime sleep-wake patterns in nursing versus rooming-in environments. *Nursing Research, 36*(3), 140-144.

Kenshalo, D. R., & Hall, E. C. (1974). Thermal thresholds of the rhesus monkey. *Journal of Comparative Physiology Psychology, 86,* 902-910.

Kirschner, R. N., Eckner, F. A., & Baron, R. C. (1986). The cardiac pathology of sudden unexplained nocturnal death in southeast Asian refugees. *Journal of the American Medical Association, 256*(19), 2700-2705.

Little, R. A., & Stoner, H. B. (1981). Body temperature after accidental injury. *British Journal of Surgery, 68,* 221.

Long, M. E. (1982). Sleep. *National Geographic, 172*(6), 786-821.

Malasanos, L., Barkauskas, V., Moss, M., & Stoltenberg-Allen, K. (1985). *Health Assessment.* (3rd ed.). St. Louis: C.V. Mosby.

Marks, R. N., & Sachar, E. J. (1973). Undertreatment of medical patients with narcotic analgesics. *Annals of Internal Medicine, 78,* 173-181.

McCaffery, M. (1980a, December). Relieving pain with noninvasive techniques. *Nursing 80,* 55-57.

McCaffery, M. (1980b, November). How to relieve your patient's pain fast and effectively . . . with oral analgesics. *Nursing 80,* 58-63.

McCaffery, M. (1980c, October). Patients shouldn't have to suffer: How to relieve pain with injectable narcotics. *Nursing 80,* 34-39.

McCaffery, M. (1980d, September). Understanding your patient's pain. *Nursing 80,* 26-31.

McCaffery, M., & Hart, L. L. (1976, October). Undertreatment of acute pain with narcotics. *American Journal of Nursing,* 1586-1591.

McDonnell, D. E. (1980, September). TENS in treating chronic pain. *American Operating Room Nurses' Journal,* 401-409.

McGuire, L. (1981, March). A short, simple tool for assessing your patient's pain. *Nursing 81,* 48-49.

Meinhart, N., & McCaffery, M. (1983). *Pain.* Norwalk, Conn.: Appleton-Century-Crofts.

Melles, R. B. (1987). Sudden, unexplained nocturnal death syndrome and night terrors. *Journal of the American Medical Association, 257*(21), 2918-2919.

Melzak, R. (1975). The McGill pain questionnaire: Major properties and scoring methods. *Pain, 1,* 277-299.

Melzak, R., & Casey, K. L. (1968). Sensory, motivational, and central control determinants of pain: A new conceptual model. In D. Kenshalto (Ed.), *The skin senses.* Springfield, Ill.: Charles C Thomas.

Melzak, R., & Wall, P. (1965). Pain mechanisms: A new theory. *Science, 150,* 971-979.

Melzak, R., & Wall, P. (1970). Psychophysiology of pain. *International Anesthesiology Clinics, 8,* 3-33.

Melzak, R., & Wall, P. (1983). *The challenge of pain.* New York: Basic Books.

Miller, T. W., & Jay, L. L. (1985, January). Cognitive-behavioral and pharmaceutical approaches to sensory pain management. *Topics in Clinical Nursing,* 34-40.

Moses, R. A. (Ed.). (1981). *Adler's physiology of the eye: Clinical application* (7th ed.). St. Louis: C.V. Mosby.

Murphy, T. M., & Bonica, J. J. (1977, July). Acupuncture analgesia and anesthesia. *Archives in Surgery,* 896-902.

Newman, R. Q., & Seres, J. L. (1978, June). A therapeutic milieu for chronic pain patients. *Journal of Human Stress, 4,* 8-12.

Norman, D. C., Grahn, D., & Hoshikawa, T. T. (1985). Fever and aging. *Journal of the American Geriatrics Society, 33,* 859-863.

Oosterveld, W. J. (Ed.). (1983). *Meniere disease: A comprehensive appraisal.* Chichester: John Wiley and Sons

Osterman, A. L., Heppenstall, R. B., Sapega, A. A., Katz, M., Chance, B., & Sokolow, D. (1984). Muscle ischemia and hypothermia: A bioenergetic study using phosphorus nuclear magnetic resonance spectroscopy. *The Journal of Trauma, 24*(9), 811-817.

Payne, R. (1987). Anatomy, physiology, and neuropharmacology of cancer pain. *Medical Clinics of North America, 71*(2), 153-167.

Perry, S. W. (1981, April). Placebo response: Myth and matter. *American Journal of Nursing,* 720-725.

Phillipson, E. A. (1978). State-of-the-art control of breathing during sleep. *American Review of Respiratory Disease, 118,* 909-939.

Phipps & Long, 1983. In Vander, A. J., et al., (Eds.), *Human physiology: The mechanisms of body functions.* New York: McGraw-Hill.

Phipps, W. J., Long, B. C., & Woods, W. F. (1987). *Medical surgical nursing: Concepts and clinical practice* (p. 306). St. Louis: C.V. Mosby.

Prochazka, A. (1986). Proprioception during voluntary movement. *Canadian Journal of Physiology and Pharmacology, 64*(4), 499-504.

Radulovacki, M. (1987). Progress in sleep [letter]. *New England Journal of Medicine, 316*, 1275-1276.

Reuler, R. (1978). Hypothermia: Pathophysiology, clinical settings, and management. *Annals of Internal Medicine, 89*, 519-527.

Richard, M. P. M., Bernal, J. F., & Brackbill, Y. (1976). Early behavioral differences: Gender or circumcision? *Developmental Psychobiology, 9*, 89-95.

Rogers, A. L., & Sturgeon, C. L. (1985). Malignant hyperthermia. *AORN Journal, 41*, 369-374.

Rudy, E. B. (1984). *Advanced neurological and neurosurgical nursing.* St. Louis: C.V. Mosby.

Sakai, F., Meyer, J. S., Karacan, I., Derman, S., & Yamamoto, M. (1980, May). Normal human sleep: Regional cerebral hemodynamics. *Annals of Neurology, 7*(5), 471-478.

Sanders, S. H. (1979). Behavioral assessment and treatment of clinical pain: Appraisal of current status. *Progress in Behavior Modification, 8*, 249-285.

Schmitt, M. (1977, December). The nature of pain with some personal notes. *Nursing Clinics of North America*, 621-629.

Schuknecht, H. F. (1974). *Pathology of the ear.* Cambridge, Mass.: Harvard University Press.

Shaver, J., Camarata, G., Taleisnik, A., & Gazzaniga, A. B. (1984). Changes in epicardial and core temperatures during resuscitation of hemorrhagic shock. *The Journal of Trauma, 24*(11), 957-963.

Sheps, D. S., Adams, K. F., Hinderliter, A., Price, C., Bissette, J., Orlanda, G., Margolis, B., & Koch, G. (1987). Endorphins are related to pain perception in coronary artery disease. *The American Journal of Cardiology, 59*, 523-527.

Sherman, A. D., & Mitchell, C. L. (1974). Effect of morphine on regional levels of gamma hydroxybutyrate in mouse brain. *Neuropharmacology, 13*, 239-243.

Sinclair, D. (1981). *Mechanisms of cutaneous sensation.* New York: Oxford University Press.

Smukler, N. M. (1985). Pain perception. *Bulletin of the Rheumatic Diseases, 35*(1), 1-8.

Snyder, S. H. (1977). Opiate receptors in the brain. *The New England Journal of Medicine, 5*, 266-271.

Sodeman, W., & Sodeman, W. (1974). *Pathologic physiology.* Philadelphia: W. B. Saunders.

Stein, H. A., Slatt, B. J., & Stein, R. M. (1988). *The ophthalamic assistant: Fundamentals in clinical practice.* St. Louis: C. V Mosby.

Sternbach, R. A. (1974). *Pain patients: Traits and treatment.* New York: Academic Press.

Stevens, J. C., & Cain, W. S. (1986). Aging impairs the ability to perceive gas odor. *Chemical Senses and Nutrition, 11*, 679.

Strauss, A. L., & Glasser, B. G. (1975). *Chronic illness and the quality of life.* St. Louis: C.V. Mosby.

Taub, J. M., & Berger, R. J. (1976). The effects of changing the phase and duration of sleep. *Journal of Experimental Psychology: Human Perception and Performance, 2*(1), 30-41.

Terenius, L. (1981). Endorphins and pain. In T. B. van Wimmersma Greidanus, & L. H. Rees (Eds.), *Frontiers of hormone research 8* (pp. 162-177). Basel: S. Karger.

Thompson, J. M., et al. (1989). *Mosby's manual of clinical nursing* (2nd ed.). St. Louis: C.V. Mosby.

Timiras, P. S. (1988). *Physiological basis of geriatrics.* New York: Macmillan, p. 163.

Van Rijn, T., & Rabkin, S. W. (1981). Effect of naloxone, a specific opiod antagonist on exercise-induced angina pectoris. *Circulation, 64* (IV), 149.

West, A. B. (1981, February). Understanding endorphins: Our natural pain relief system. *Nursing 81*, 50-53.

Woodrow, K. M., Friedman, G. D., & Siegelaub, A. B. (1972). Pain tolerance: Differences according to age, sex, and race. *Psychosomatic Medicine, 34*, 548-556.

Wright, S. W. (1987). The child with febrile seizures. *American Family Physician, 36*(5), 163-167.

Yousef, M. K. (1987). Effects of climactic stresses on thermoregulatory processes in man. *Experientia, 43*(1), 14-19.

CHAPTER 14

Concepts of Neurologic Dysfunction

Barbara J. Boss

Alterations in consciousness, 432
  Pathophysiology, 432
  Clinical manifestations and evaluation, 433
    Level of consciousness, 433
    Pattern of breathing, 433
    Pupillary changes, 435
    Oculomotor responses, 436
    Motor responses, 437
    Outcomes, 437
  Acute alterations in content of thought, 440
    Pathophysiology, 441
    Clinical manifestations, 441
    Evaluation and treatment, 442
  Subacute and chronic alterations in consciousness, 442
    Vegetative states, 442
    Types of dementing processes, 442
      Pathophysiology, 443
      Clinical manifestations, 444
      Evaluation and treatment, 444
    Alzheimer disease, 444
      Pathogenesis, 444
      Clinical manifestations, 444
      Evaluation and treatment, 445
  Seizures, 445
    Conditions associated with seizure disorders, 446
    Types of seizure disorders, 446
      Pathophysiology, 447
      Clinical manifestations, 448
      Evaluation and treatment, 451
Alterations in motor function, 451
  Clinical manifestations of motor dysfunction, 451
    Abnormalities in muscle mass, 451
    Abnormalities in muscle strength, 451
    Abnormalities in muscle tone, 451
    Postural abnormalities, 451
    Abnormal movements, 452
      Akinesias, 452
      Hyperkinesia and dyskinesia, 453
  Motor syndromes, 455
    CNS motor syndromes, 455

      Pyramidal motor syndrome, 455
      Extrapyramidal motor syndromes, 457
        Basal ganglia motor syndromes, 457
        Cerebellar motor syndromes, 458
    Motor unit syndromes, 458
      Lower motor neuron syndromes, 458
      Amyotrophies, 459
      Radiculopathies, 460
      Neuropathies, 460
      Neuromuscular junction syndromes, 461
      Myopathies, 461
Alterations in emotions and emotional control, 461
  Pathophysiology, 461
  Clinical manifestations, 462
  Evaluation and treatment, 462
Alterations in unifocal cortical function, 462
  Agnosias, 462
  Dyspraxia, 464
  Dysphasia, 464
Alterations in cerebral homeostasis, 465
  Increased intracranial pressure, 465
  Cerebral edema, 469
  Herniation syndromes, 470
    Supratentorial herniation, 470
    Infratentorial herniation, 470

Neurologic dysfunction often reveals the enormous complexity of the nervous system. Unlike organ systems with unified functions, the nervous system is both a connected system of structures and a series of mechanisms that monitor and regulate all other body systems. Alterations in neurologic function may therefore become evident through a great range of signs and symptoms, some of which are themselves manifestations of specific neurologic disorders (described in Chapter 15).

Some neurologic dysfunction is associated with specific structures in the nervous system. Motor function,

431

for example, is controlled by the central nervous system, and many disorders of movement can be traced to structures that regulate motor activity. Other neurologic dysfunctions, such as consciousness, are multifocal and therefore are associated with the complex interaction among components of the nervous system.

ALTERATIONS IN CONSCIOUSNESS

Consciousness is both a state of awareness of oneself and the environment and a set of responses to that environment. Full consciousness implies that the individual responds to external stimuli. Any decrease in this state of awareness and response is thus a decrease in consciousness. The cerebral hemispheres and reticular formation of the brainstem modulate consciousness. Consciousness has two distinct components, content of thought and level of arousal.

Content of thought encompasses all cognitive functions that embody awareness of self, environment, and affective states (i.e., moods). Content of thought is mediated, for the most part, by the cortical areas of the cerebral hemispheres. **Level of arousal** is the state of awakeness that an individual exhibits. Level of arousal is mediated by the reticular activating system that extends from mid pons to the diencephalon. The reticular activating system provides arousal to the cerebral hemispheres. When cerebral function is lost, the reticular activating system and brainstem can maintain a crude waking state known as a vegetative state. Cognitive cerebral functions, however, cannot occur without a functioning reticular activating system.

Possible causes of an altered level of consciousness with an acute onset may be separated into three major groups: structural, metabolic, and psychogenic. Structural causes are divided according to original location of the pathology: supratentorial (above the tentorium cerebelli), infratentorial (subtentorial, below the tentorium cerebelli), subdural (below the dura mater), extracerebral (outside the brain tissue), and intracerebral (within the brain tissue).

Causes of altered level of consciousness are also grouped according to pathologic process: infectious, vascular, neoplastic, traumatic, congenital (developmental), degenerative, polygenic, and metabolic. Metabolic causes may be further divided into hypoxia, electrolyte disturbances, hypoglycemia, drugs, and toxins (both endogenous and exogenous). All of the systemic diseases that eventually produce nervous system dysfunction are part of this metabolic category.

Pathophysiology

Supratentorial processes produce a decreased level of consciousness by one of three mechanisms: (1) diffuse bilateral cortical dysfunction, (2) bilateral subcortical dysfunction, or (3) localized hemispheric dysfunction. Disease processes may produce diffuse bilateral cortical dysfunction (e.g., encephalitis) and may actually occur in either the cerebral cortex or the underlying subcortical white matter. Bilateral subcortical dysfunction involves destructive pathology that compromises the reticular activating system (e.g., brainstem trauma or cerebral vascular accident) and probably surrounding structures. Localized hemispheric dysfunction is generally caused by masses that directly impinge on deep diencephalic structures or secondarily compress these structures in the process of herniation. Such localized destructive processes directly impair function of the thalamic or hypothalamic activating systems.

Extracerebral disorders can also produce diffuse bilateral cortical dysfunction. Extracerebral disorders include neoplasms, closed-head trauma with subsequent bleeding, and subdural empyema (accumulation of pus). Intracerebral disorders (those within the brain substance) primarily function as masses. These disorders include bleeding, infarcts and emboli, and tumors.

Infratentorial processes produce a reduction in arousal in one of two ways: (1) there may be direct destruction of the reticular activating system and its pathways, or (2) the brainstem may be destroyed either by direct invasion or by indirect impairment of its blood supply. The most common cause of direct destruction is cerebrovascular disease, but demyelinating diseases, neoplasms, granulomas, abscesses, and head injury may also cause brainstem destruction.

Decreased level of consciousness may also be caused by compression of the reticular activating system by a disease process. Compression of the reticular activating system may occur as a result of (1) direct pressure on the pons and mesencephalon producing ischemia and edema of the neurons of the reticular activating system, (2) upward herniation of the cerebellum through the tentorial notch, thus compressing the upper mesencephalon and diencephalon, and (3) downward herniation of the cerebellum through the foramen magnum, compressing and displacing the myelencephalon. Specific causes of compression of the brainstem include hematomas, hemorrhage, and aneurysm; cerebellar hemorrhage, infarcts, abscesses and neoplasms; and demyelinating disorders.

A wide spectrum of diseases may produce a metabolically induced alteration in arousal. With encephalopathies, there is widespread direct or indirect interference with neuronal metabolism throughout much of the brain (see Chapter 15). Psychogenic unresponsiveness, although uncommon, may arise as a sign in general psychiatric disorders. Despite apparent unconsciousness, the person is actually physiologically awake.

TABLE 14-1 Clinical manifestations of metabolic and structural causes of comas

Manifestation	Metabolically induced coma	Structurally induced coma
Blink to threat (cranial nerves II, V)	Equal	Asymmetric
Disks (cranial nerve II)	Flat, good pulsation	Papilledema
Extraocular movement (cranial nerves III, IV, VI)	Roving eye movements; normal doll's eyes and calorics	Gaze paresis, III nerve palsy, MLF syndrome (internuclear ophthalmoplegia)
Pupils (cranial nerves II, III)	Equal and reactive, may be large (i.e., atropine), pinpoint (i.e., opiates), or midposition and fixed (i.e., Doriden)	Asymmetric and/or nonreactive; may be midposition (midbrain injury), pinpoint (pons injury), large (tectal injury)
Corneal reflex (cranial nerve V)	Symmetric response	Asymmetric response
Grimace to pain (cranial nerve VII)	Symmetric response	Asymmetric response
Motor function movement	Symmetric	Asymmetric
Tone	Symmetric	Paratonic, spastic, flaccid, especially if asymmetric
Posture	Symmetric	Decorticate, especially if symmetric; decerebrate, especially if asymmetric
Deep tendon reflexes	Symmetric	Asymmetric
Babinski sign	Absent or symmetric response	Present
Sensation	Symmetric	Asymmetric

Adapted from Heilman, Watson, and Greer, 1977.

Clinical Manifestations and Evaluation

Evaluating an altered level of arousal requires distinguishing between organic and functional causes. A further distinction between metabolic and structural causes then is made (Table 14-1). If the cause is structural, the pathology must be localized.

Patterns of clinical manifestations and their evolution have been identified. The patterns of clinical manifestation are important because they help in determining the extent of brain dysfunction and they serve as indices for identifying increasing or decreasing central nervous system function. The specific clusters of manifestations of abnormal function and their evolution suggest whether the cause of the altered arousal state is supratentorial, infratentorial, metabolic, or psychogenic (Table 14-2). Five categories of neurologic function are critical to the evaluation process. The categories are (1) level of consciousness, (2) pattern of breathing, (3) size and reactivity of pupils, (4) eye position and reflexive responses, and (5) skeletal muscle motor responses.

Level of Consciousness

Level of consciousness is the most critical clinical index of nervous system function or dysfunction. An alteration in consciousness indicates either improvement or deterioration of the individual's condition. An individ-ual who is alert and oriented to self, others, place, and time is considered to be functioning at the highest level of consciousness, which implies that the person has full use of all possessed cognitive capacities.

Because many different terms are used to indicate level of consciousness, definition becomes necessary. The term "unconscious," for example, has no specific clinical definition and signifies different things to different people. From the normal alert state, levels of consciousness diminish in stages, each of which are clinically defined (Table 14-3).

Pattern of Breathing

Several characteristic respiratory patterns are helpful in evaluating level of brain dysfunction and level of coma. Among these characteristics are rate, rhythm, and pattern of breathing. The breathing patterns can be categorized as hemispheric or brainstem breathing patterns (Table 14-4).

With normal breathing, a neural center believed to be located in the cerebrum produces a rhythmic breathing pattern despite lowered arterial carbon dioxide (Pco_2). When neural control at this center is lost as consciousness decreases, the lower brainstem centers regulate the breathing pattern by responding only to changes in

TABLE 14-2 Differential characteristics of states causing sustained unconsciousness

Mechanism	Manifestations
Supratentorial mass lesions compressing or displacing the diencephalon or brainstem	Initiating signs usually of focal cerebral dysfunction Signs of dysfunction progress rostral to caudal Neurologic signs at any given time point to one anatomic area (e.g., diencephalon, mesencephalon, medulla) Motor signs often asymmetrical
Infratentorial mass of destruction causing coma	History of preceding brainstem dysfunction or sudden onset of coma Localizing brainstem signs precede or accompany onset of coma and always include oculovestibular abnormality Cranial nerve palsies usually present "bizarre" respiratory patterns common and usually appear at onset
Metabolic coma	Confusion and stupor commonly precede motor signs Motor signs are usually symmetrical Pupillary reactions are usually preserved Asterixis, myoclonus, tremor, and seizures are common Acid-base imbalance with hyper- or hypoventilation is frequent
Psychiatric unresponsiveness	Lids close actively Pupils reactive or dilated (cycloplegics) Oculocephalic reflexes are unpredictable; oculovestibular reflexes are physiologic (nystagmus is present) Motor tone is inconsistent or normal Eupnea or hyperventilation is usual No pathologic reflexes are present EEG is normal

Adapted from Plum & Posner, 1980.

P_{CO_2} levels. The result is the irregular breathing associated with posthyperventilation apnea (PHVA).

The pathophysiology of Cheyne-Stokes respirations (CSR) involves an increased ventilatory response to CO_2 stimulation, causing hypercapnea and a diminished ventilatory stimulus. The neural center that causes PHVA is thus related to the CSR, as changes in P_{CO_2} produce irregular breathing that contributes to overbreathing when stimulated by CO_2. As a result, the P_{CO_2} level decreases to below normal, and because of the cerebral brain dysfunction, breathing stops until the CO_2 reaccumulates to bring the P_{CO_2} level to normal. In

TABLE 14-3 Levels of consciousness

State	Definition
Confusion	Loss of ability to think rapidly and clearly. Impaired judgment and decision-making.
Disorientation	Beginning loss of consciousness. Disorientation to time followed by disorientation to place and impaired memory. Lost last is recognition of self.
Lethargy	Limited spontaneous movement or speech. Easy arousal with normal speech or touch. May or may not be oriented to time, place, or person.
Obtundation	Mild to moderate reduction in arousal (awakeness) with limited response to the environment. Falls asleep unless stimulated verbally or tactilely. Questions answered with minimum response.
Stupor	A condition of deep sleep or unresponsiveness from which the person may be aroused or caused to respond motorwise or verbally only by vigorous and repeated stimulation. Response is often withdrawal or grabbing at stimulus.
Coma	No motor or verbal response to the external environment or to any stimuli even noxious stimuli such as deep pain or suctioning. No arousal to any stimulus.

TABLE 14-4 Patterns of breathing

Breathing pattern	Description	Location of injury
HEMISPHERIC BREATHING PATTERNS		
Normal	After a period of hyperventilation that lowers the arterial carbon dioxide (Pco_2), the individual continues to breathe regularly but with a reduced depth.	Response of the nervous system to an external stressor—not associated with injury to the CNS.
Posthyperventilation apnea (PHVA)	Respirations stop after hyperventilation has lowered the Pco_2 level below normal. Rhythmic breathing returns when the Pco_2 level returns to normal.	Associated with diffuse bilateral metabolic or structural disease of the cerebrum.
Cheyne-Stokes respirations (CSR)	The breathing pattern has a smooth increase (crescendo) in the rate and depth of breathing (hyperpnea), which peaks and is followed by a gradual smooth decrease (decrescendo) in the rate and depth of breathing to the point of apnea when the cycle repeats itself. The hyperpneic phase lasts longer than the apneic phase.	Bilateral dysfunction of the deep cerebral and/or diencephalic structures, seen with supratentorial injury and metabolically induced coma states.
BRAINSTEM BREATHING PATTERNS		
Central neurogenic hyperventilation (CNH)	A sustained deep rapid, but regular pattern (hyperpnea), with a decreased Pco_2 and a corresponding increase in pH and increased Po_2.	May result from CNS damage or disease that involves the midbrain and upper pons; seen following increased intracranial pressure and blunt head trauma.
Apneusis	A prolonged inspiratory cramp (a pause at full inspiration) occurs. A common variant of this is a brief end-inspiratory pause of 2 or 3 seconds often alternating with an end-expiratory pause.	Indicates damage to the respiratory control mechanism located at the pontine level. Most commonly associated with pontine infarction but documented with hypoglycemia, anoxia, and meningitis.
Cluster breathing	A cluster of breaths having a disordered sequence with irregular pauses between breaths.	Dysfunction in the lower pontine and high medullary areas.
Ataxic breathing	Completely irregular breathing with random shallow and deep breaths and irregular pauses. Often the rate is slow.	Originates from a primary dysfunction of the medullary neurons controlling breathing.
Gasping breathing pattern	A pattern or deep "all-or-none" breaths accompanied by a slow respiratory rate.	Indicative of a failing medullary respiratory center.

cases of opiate or sedative drug overdose, the respiratory center is depressed, and the rate of breathing gradually decreases until respiratory failure occurs.

Certain motor activities related to breathing signify the level of brain dysfunction. Yawning, vomiting, and hiccups are complex reflex-like motor responses that are integrated by neural mechanisms in the lower brainstem. These responses may be produced by compression or diseases that involve tissues in the myelencephalon. Such disorders include infection, neoplasm, or infarct. Similar responses are produced by dysfunction in the lower brainstem through direct stimulation.

Most central nervous system (CNS) disorders produce both nausea and vomiting. Vomiting with no associated nausea indicates direct involvement of the central neural mechanism. Vomiting is particularly associated with CNS injuries that (1) involve the vestibular nuclei (located in the lower pons and myelencephalon) or its immediate projections, particularly when double vision (diplopia) is also present; (2) impinge directly on the floor of the fourth ventricle; or (3) produce brainstem compression secondary to increased intracranial pressure.

Pupillary Changes

Anatomically, brainstem areas controlling arousal are adjacent to areas controlling pupils. Pupillary changes thus are a valuable guide to evaluating the presence and level of brainstem dysfunction (Fig. 14-1).

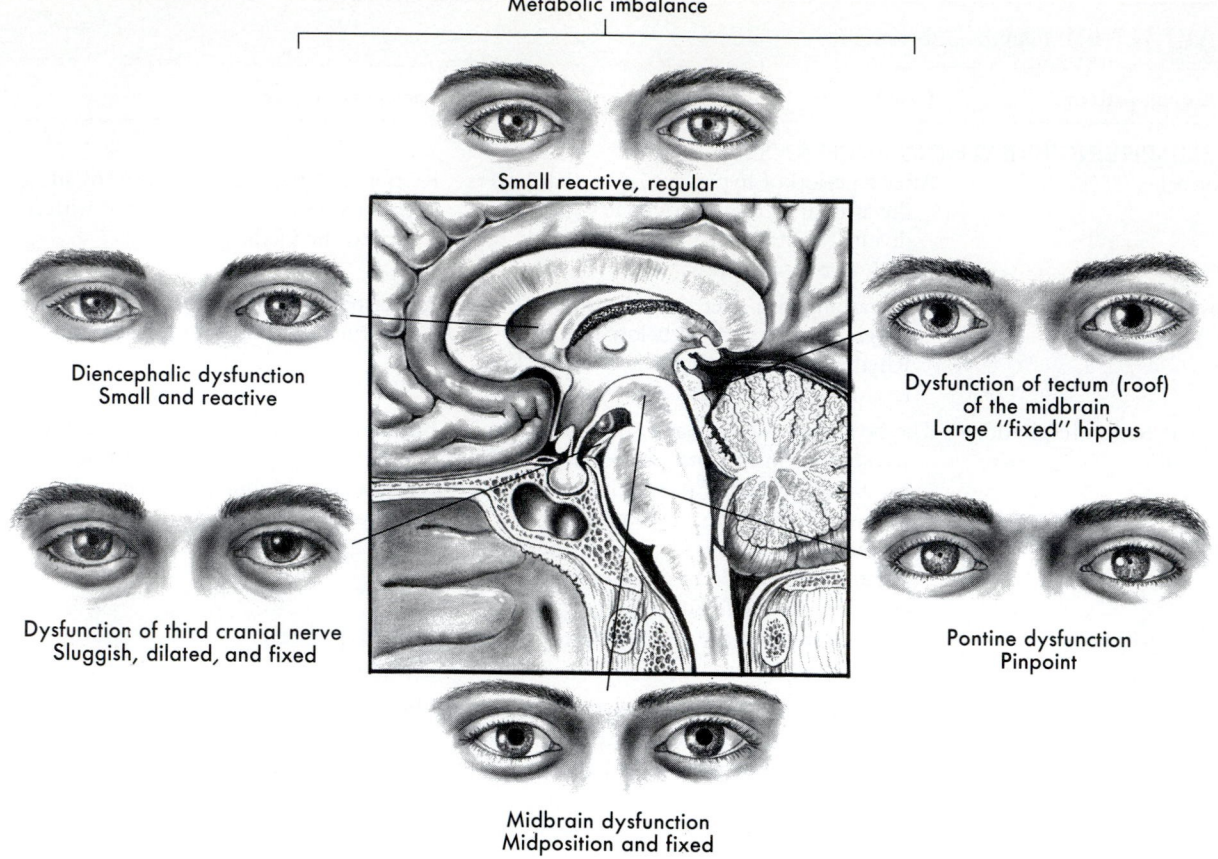

Metabolic imbalance

Small reactive, regular

Diencephalic dysfunction
Small and reactive

Dysfunction of third cranial nerve
Sluggish, dilated, and fixed

Dysfunction of tectum (roof)
of the midbrain
Large "fixed" hippus

Pontine dysfunction
Pinpoint

Midbrain dysfunction
Midposition and fixed

FIG. 14-1. Pupils at different levels of consciousness.

Certain drugs that affect pupils must be considered when evaluating pupillary response in comatose states. Atropine and scopolamine in large concentrations fully dilate and fix pupils. Glutethimide (Doriden) in amounts sufficient to produce a coma cause the pupils to become midposition or moderately dilated (4 to 8 mm in diameter), unequal, and frequently fixed to light. Opiates (heroin and morphine) cause pinpoint pupils. Severe barbiturate intoxication may produced fixed pupils.

Severe ischemia and hypoxia produce bilaterally wide and fixed pupils in most instances. Occasionally, the pupils remain small or midposition even in the presence of profound hypoxia. Hypothermia may also fix pupils.

Oculomotor Responses

Resting, spontaneous, and reflexive eye movements (oculocephalic [doll's head, doll's eyes] and oculovestibular [caloric] reflexes) undergo change at various levels of brain dysfunction (see Table 14-5). Persons with metabolically induced coma, except in cases of barbiturate-hypnotic and phenytoin (Dilantin) poisoning, generally do retain ocular reflexes, however, even when other signs of brainstem damage, such as central neurogenic hyperventilation, are present.

The presence of brisk oculocephalic reflexes, roving eye movements and the failure to elicit nystagmus with instillation of cold or warm water into the external ear canal indicates a decrease in consciousness (loss of cortical influence) but with an intact brainstem (see Figs. 14-2 and 14-3).

Destructive or compressive injury to the brainstem cause specific abnormalities of the oculocephalic and oculovestibular reflexes. For example, a skewed deviation, in which one eye diverges downward and the other looks upward, indicates brainstem dysfunction. Destructive or compressive disease processes that involve an oculomotor nucleus or nerve cause the involved eye to deviate outward, producing a resting dysconjugate lateral position of the eyes. Unilateral abducens paralysis (paralysis of cranial nerve VI) results in an upward deviation of the ipsilateral eye. With bilateral abducens paralysis, the eyes come together (converge).

TABLE 14-5 Changes in oculomotor responses

	Resting and spontaneous eye movements	Reflexive eye movements
Full consciousness	Eyes at rest, still (cortical gaze centers inhibit spontaneous roving eye movements)	Eyes move as the head turns Oculocephalic responses not elicited or inconsistently elicited (frontal gaze centers inhibit brainstem reflexes that fix gaze straight ahead) Oculovestibular (caloric) stimulation produces nystagmus
Cortical dysfunction or disruption of efferent pathways	Roving eye movements may well be present (cortical gaze centers no longer inhibit these brainstem-generated roving eye movements)	Gaze fixed straight ahead regardless of head position—positive Doll's eyes (normal oculocephalic reflexes are no longer inhibited by frontal gaze centers) Nystagmus is no longer induced by caloric stimulation (normally a cold water stimulus produces deviation of the eyes opposite the irrigated ear; a warm water stimulus deviates the eyes to the same [ipsilateral] side) With an injury that depresses cortical gaze center function, the eyes (and often the entire head) will deviate, or appear to look toward the side of the injured hemisphere With an injury that irritates (stimulates) the neurons of the cortical gaze center, the eyes (and often the entire head) will deviate away from the injured hemisphere (all fibers from the frontal gaze centers decussate and therefore control the function of the contralateral pontine gaze center, which moves the eyes in the ipsilateral direction)
Mesencephalon dysfunction	Roving eye movements cease, and the eyes become immobile and directed ahead (roving eye movements require an intact brainstem)	Oculovestibular reflexes become inconsistent and abnormal Loss of Bell's phenomenon (upward deviation of eyes on stimulation) (required intact eye movement pathways from the mesencephalon to pons)
Pontine dysfunction	Loss of spontaneous blinking (requires an intact pons)	

Motor Responses

Motor responses contribute both to evaluating the level of brain dysfunction and to determining the side of the brain that is maximally damaged. The pattern of response is described to be (1) purposeful, a defensive or withdrawal movement to noxious stimuli, (2) inappropriate (i.e., not purposeful), generalized motor movement, grimacing or groaning, and (3) not present (i.e., no motor response).

Motor signs indicating loss of cortical inhibition that are commonly associated with decreased consciousness include contralateral or bilateral (depending on whether the process is localized or diffuse) reflex grasping, reflex sucking, snout reflex, palmomental reflex, and rigidity (paratonia) (see Fig. 14-4). Abnormal flexor and extensor responses in the upper and lower extremities are defined in Table 14-6 and illustrated in Fig. 14-5.

Outcomes

Two forms of neurologic death, cerebral death and brain death, are the result of severe pathology and associated coma. **Cerebral death** (irreversible coma) is death of the cerebral hemispheres exclusive of the brainstem and cerebellum. Brain damage is permanent and sufficiently severe that the individual is unable forever to respond behaviorally in any significant way to the envi-

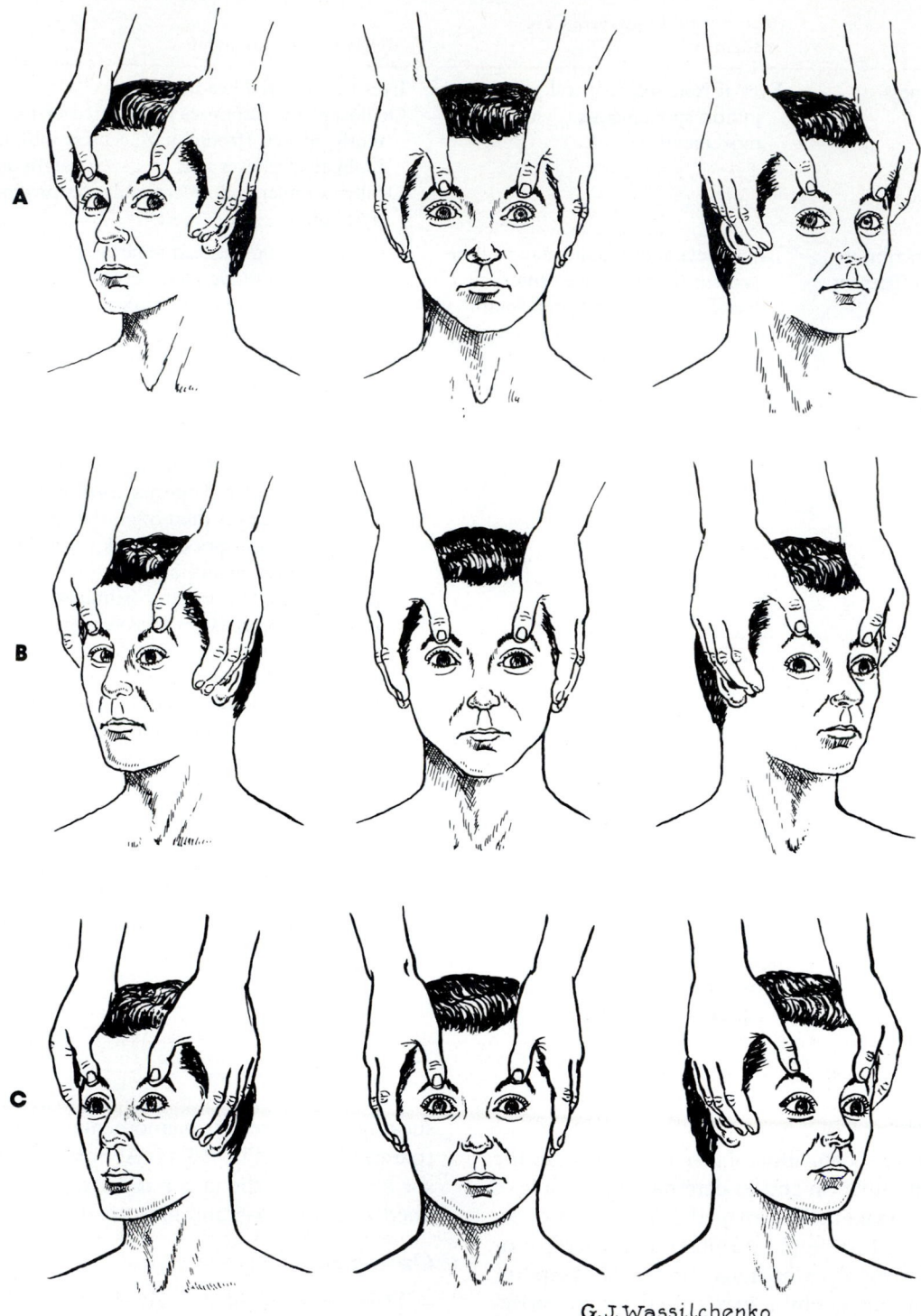

G.J.Wassilchenko

FIG. 14-2. Test for oculocephalic reflex response (doll's eyes phenomenon). **A,** Normal response—eyes turn together to side opposite from turn of head. **B,** Abnormal response—eyes do not turn in conjugate manner. **C,** Absent response—eyes do not turn as head position changed. (From Rudy, 1984.)

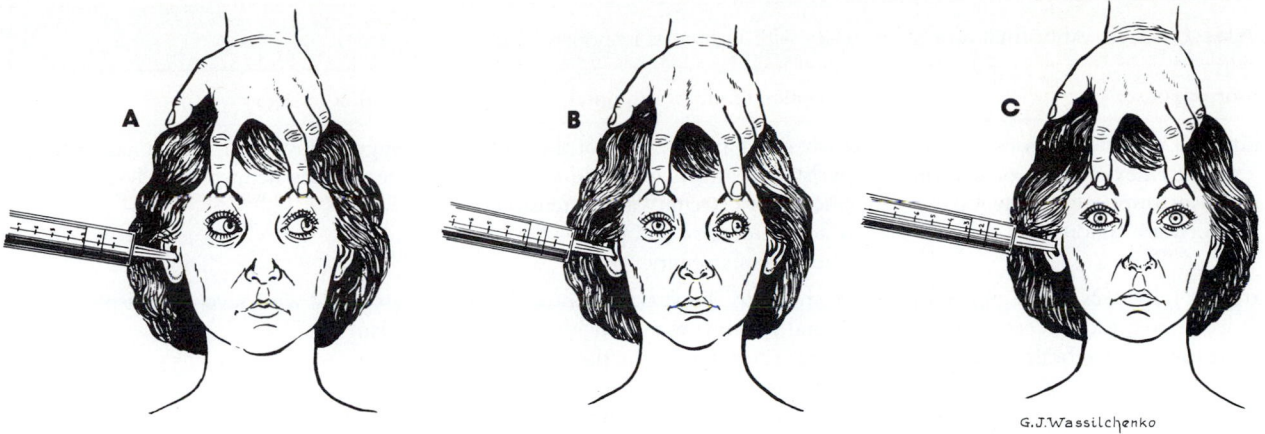

FIG. 14-3. Test for oculovestibular reflex (caloric ice water test). **A,** Normal response—conjugate eye movements. **B,** Abnormal response—dysconjugate or asymmetric eye movements. **C,** Absent response—no eye movements. (From Rudy, 1984.)

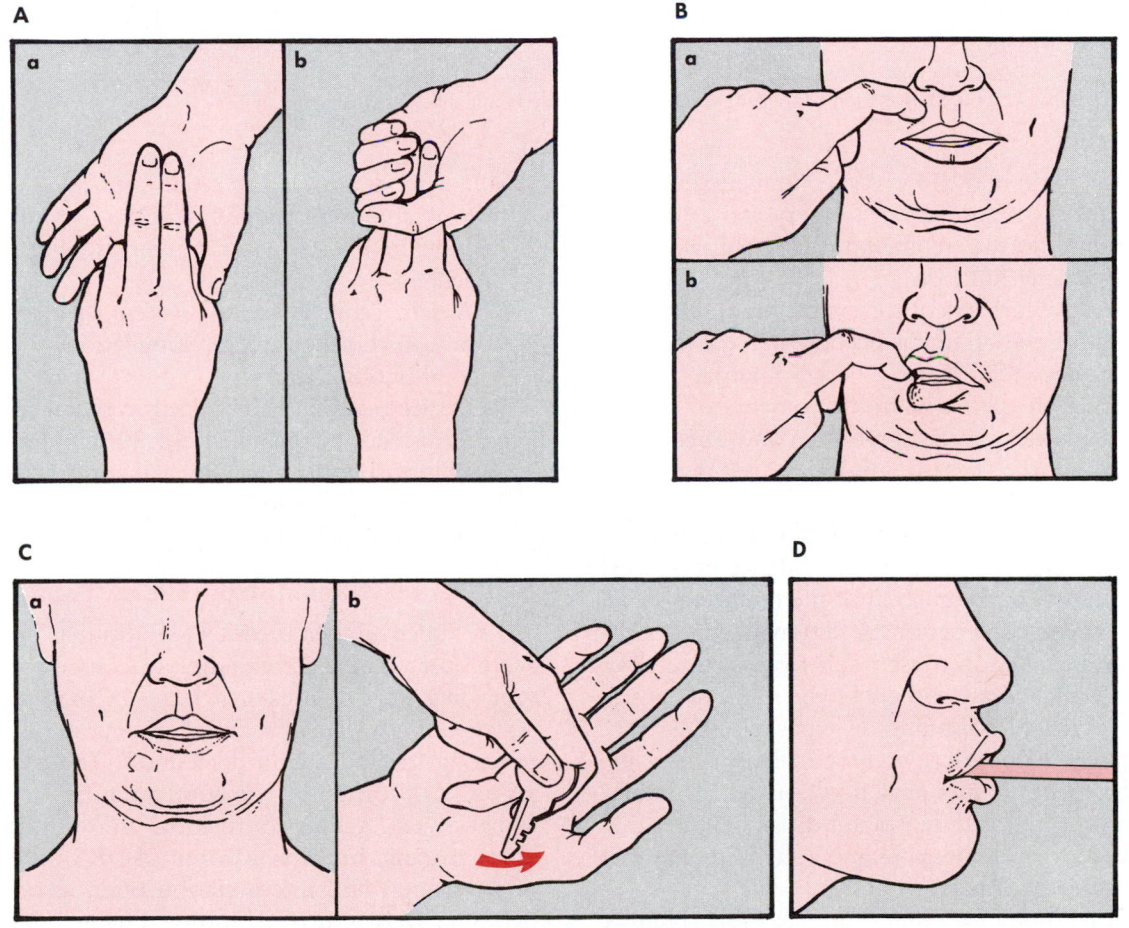

FIG. 14-4. Motor responses to noxious stimulation in unconscious states—decorticate and decerebrate posture.

TABLE 14-6 Abnormal motor responses with decreased responsiveness

Motor responses	Description of motor responses	Location of injury*
Abnormal motor responses, upper extremity flexion with or without extensor responses in the leg (decorticate rigidity)	Slowly developing flexion of the arm, wrist, and fingers with adduction in the upper extremity and extension, internal rotation and plantar flexion of the lower extremity	Suggest mostly cortical damage and less severe hemispheric dysfunction
Extensor responses in the upper and lower extremities (decerebrate posturing, decerebrate rigidity)	Opisthotonus (hyperextension of the vertebral column) with clenching of the teeth; extension, adduction, and hyperpronation of the arms; and extension of the lower extremities In acute brain injury, shivering and hyperpnea may accompany unelicited recurrent decerebrate spasms	Associated with severe hemispheric damage
Extensor responses in the upper extremities accompanied by flexion in the lower extremities		Indicates pontine level dysfunction
Flaccid state with little or no motor response to stimuli		Damage to lower pons and upper myelencephalon

*A less fully developed response has the same localizing significance but reflects a smaller, less-damaging injury.

ronment. The brain may, however, continue to maintain internal homeostasis (normal respiratory and cardiovascular functions, normal temperature control, and normal gastrointestinal function).

Brain death occurs when irreversible brain damage is so extensive that the brain has no potential for recovery and can no longer maintain the body's internal homeostasis. Destruction of the neuronal contents of the intracranial cavity includes the brainstem and cerebellum. On postmortem, the brain is autolyzing (self-digesting) or already autolyzed.

General agreement holds that brain death has occurred when there is no discernible evidence of cerebral hemisphere function or function of the brainstem's vital centers for an extended period. Additionally, the abnormality of brain function must result from structural or known metabolic disease and *not* be the result of depressant drug or alcohol poisoning or hypothermia. An isoelectric, or flat, EEG (electrocerebral silence) for a period of 6 to 12 hours in a person who is not hypothermic and has not ingested depressant drugs indicates that no mental recovery is possible and usually means that the brain is already dead.

The clinical criteria for brain death are these (Plum & Posner, 1980):

1. Completion of all appropriate and therapeutic procedures
2. Unresponsive coma (absence of motor and reflex movements)
3. No spontaneous respiration (apnea)—a P_{CO_2} that rises above 60 mmHg without breathing efforts provides evidence of a nonfunctioning respiratory center
4. Absent cephalic reflexes (no ocular responses to head turning or caloric stimulation) with dilated, fixed pupils
5. Isoelectric (flat) EEG (electrocerebral silence)
6. Persistence of the above for 30 minutes to 1 hour and for 6 hours after onset of coma and apnea
7. Confirming test indicating absence of cerebral circulation (optional)

Acute Alterations in Content of Thought

The states of altered content of thought may have an acute onset. These are clouding of consciousness, delirium, and acute confusional states. **Clouding of consciousness** is a state of reduced awareness, often with alternating irritability and drowsiness. The condition involves less cortical dysfunction than an acute confusional state. **Acute confusional states,** also labeled **acute organic brain syndrome (AOBS),** are disorders of perception and interpretation often associated with delirium. **Delirium** is a disordered mental state of acute onset. Disorientation, disorders of perception, delusions, anxiety, and overactivity of the autonomic nervous system are associated with delirium. Some causes of acute confusional states are associated with stupor and coma rather than delirium, especially those caused

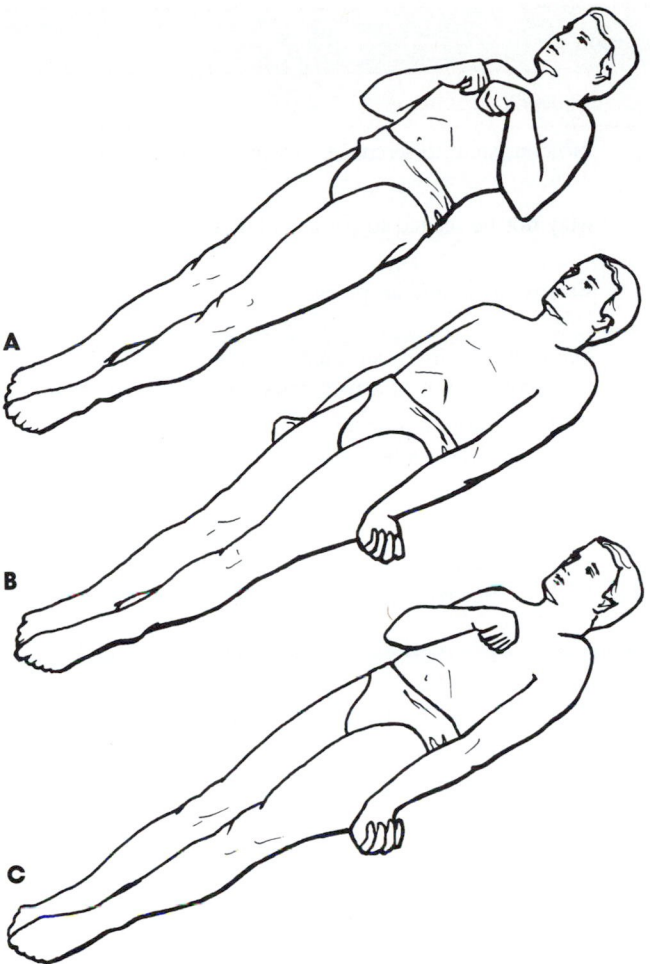

FIG. 14-5. Decorticate and decerebrate responses. **A,** Decorticate response. Flexion of arms, wrists, and fingers with adduction in upper extremities. Extension, internal rotation, and plantar flexion in lower extremities. **B,** Decerebrate response. All four extremities in rigid extension, with hyperpronation of forearms and plantar extension of feet. **C,** Decorticate response on right side of body and decerebrate response on left side of body. (From Rudy, 1984.)

by metabolic derangements associated with hypoxia, hypoglycemia, severe fluid and electrolyte disorders, sepsis, liver or renal failure, or poisons or drug overdoses. Acute behavior and mood disturbances are predominant clinical features of all acute confusional states.

Acute confusional states result from cerebral dysfunction secondary to such causes as drug intoxication or nervous system disease. A common cause of an acute confusional state is withdrawal from alcohol, barbiturate, or other sedative drug ingestion. Acute confusional states of toxic origin may have either sudden or gradual onset, depending on the amount of exposure to the toxin. Acute confusional states often occur with febrile

illnesses, with systemic diseases such as heart failure, following head injury, or after anesthesia.

Pathophysiology

Three pathophysiologic mechanisms probably underly the development of acute confusional states associated with delirium. These are (1) injury to nervous tissue, (2) action of exogenous chemicals on neuronal cells, and (3) overactivity of a previously depressed brain center. Destructive injuries directly affect the nervous tissues and disturb the function of the neurons. In states of intoxication, the direct action of toxins or chemicals on neuronal cells produces dysfunction of the involved cells. In states of withdrawal, the lower brain centers are overactive after the depressant action of the drug wears off, and this overactivity accounts for the development of the acute confusional state.

Clinical Manifestations

The predominant features of an acute confusional state are impaired or lost goal-oriented behavior and impaired short-term memory. Because of dysfunction of the prefrontal cortex (see Fig. 12-6), the ability to sustain attentional focus is seriously impaired or completely lost. The person is highly distractible and unable to concentrate on incoming sensory information or on any one particular mental or motor task.

The onset of an acute confusional state is usually abrupt rather than insidious. Memory impairments, distractibility and disorientation, misperception and misinterpretation of sensory stimuli (illusion), and frank delusions are all manifestations of acute confusional states. Intellectual functioning is also inadequate, and judgment is impaired. Anxiety and restlessness appear, and obsessions, compulsive behavior, and rituals may be evident.

In acute confusional states with associated underactivity, the individual exhibits decreases in mental function. Alertness is decreased, as are attention span, accurate perception, and interpretation of the environment. Forgetfulness is prominent. Reactions to the environment are slowed and indecisive. The individual dozes frequently.

Delirium typically develops over a period of 2 to 3 days. Early clinical manifestations include difficulty in concentrating, restlessness, irritability, insomnia, tremulousness, and poor appetite. Some persons experience seizures. Unpleasant, even terrifying, dreams may occur.

In a fully developed delirium state, the individual is completely inattentive, and perceptions are grossly altered. Misperception and misinterpretation are predominant. Hallucinations may be present. The person appears distressed and often very perplexed. Conversation is incoherent. Frank tremor is evident, and a great deal

TABLE 14-7 Differences between organic and functional confusion

Factor	Organic confusion	Functional confusion
Memory impairment	Recent, more impaired than remote	No consistent difference between recent and remote
Disorientation		
Time	Within own lifetime or reasonably near future	May not be related to patient's lifetime
Place	Familiar place or one where patient might easily be	Bizarre or unfamiliar places
Person	Sense of identity, usually preserved Misidentification of others as familiar	Sense of identity diminished Misidentification of others based on delusion system
Hallucinations	Visual, vivid Animals and insects common	Auditory more frequent Bizarre and symbolic
Illusions	Common	Not prominent
Delusions	Concerns everyday occurrences and people	Bizarre and symbolic
Confused	Spotty confusion Clear intervals mixed with confused episodes Worse at night	More consistent No tendency to become worse at night

From Morris & Rhodes, 1972.

of restless movement is common. Violent behavior may be present. The individual cannot sleep, is flushed, and has dilated pupils, a rapid pulse (tachycardia), temperature elevation, and perfuse sweating (diaphoresis). Delirium typically abates suddenly or gradually in 2 to 3 days, although occasional delirium states persist for several weeks.

Evaluation and Treatment

The initial goal is to establish that the individual is confused, and the cause must be distinguished as organic or functional (Table 14-7). Next, the goal is to determine whether the confusion is delirium, an acute confusional state with associated underactivity, or an underlying dementia. The precise cause of an acute confusional state is established through the complete history and physical examination. Laboratory tests include an electrocardiogram, blood, urine, cerebrospinal fluid, and radiologic studies.

Once the cause is established, treatment is directed at controlling the primary disorder. In an acute confusional state, all drugs that may be contributing to or causing the condition are discontinued unless the problem is due to drug withdrawal. Supportive measures are designed to enhance coping skills and minimize the individual's need for drug-altered cortical function. Supportive management also involves maintaining the person's intact cortical functions by promoting use of these functions.

Subacute and Chronic Alterations in Consciousness

Three states describe subacute and chronic alterations in consciousness. These are dementia, hypersomnia, and the vegetative states (Table 14-8). **Dementia** is a progressive or permanent (chronic) disorder in which content of thought but not level of arousal is reduced. **Hypersomnia** is excessive sleep but without loss of response to stimulation. **Vegetative states** are characterized by lack of cognitive function but not necessarily by reduced level of arousal.

Vegetative States

Cerebral function is lost in the vegetative state but sleep-wake cycles are present. The person's eyes open spontaneously in response to external stimuli such as voice or touch. The individual maintains blood pressure and breathing without support, and brainstem reflexes (pupillary, oculocephalic, chewing, swallowing) are intact. No discrete localizing motor responses are present, and the individual does not speak any comprehensible words or follow commands.

A vegetative state is distinctly different from **locked-in syndrome.** With a locked-in syndrome, both the content of thought and level of arousal are intact, but the efferent pathways are disrupted. Thus, the individual cannot communicate either through speech or through body movement but the person is fully conscious with intact cognitive function. The upper cranial nerves (I through IV) are often preserved, however, so that the person possesses vertical eye movement and blinking as a means of communication.

Types of Dementing Processes

The dementias are characterized by reduction in mental capacity (intellectual function). Mental abilities are impaired in the dementing process. The result may be a decrease in orientation, general knowledge and informa-

TABLE 14-8 States of altered consciousness with a subacute or chronic onset

Term	Definition
Dementia	Progressive or permanent (chronic) reduction in content of thought (cognition, mentation) unaccompanied by a reduction in arousal.
Hypersomnia	Excessive drowsiness characterized by excessive but normal-appearing sleep from which the person readily awakens when stimulated.
Vegetative states	Subacute or chronic states that emerge after severe brain injury where there is a return of wakefulness accompanied by an apparent complete lack of cognitive function.

tion, immediate recall, short-term memory, long-term memory, judgment, insight, and interpretation. Because of declining intellectual ability, the individual exhibits alterations in behavior.

Dementias can be classified according to etiology (i.e., trauma, tumors, vascular disorders, infections) and according to associated clinical and laboratory signs. Most recently dementing processes have been grouped according to types of memory disorders, **attentional dementia** (loss of immediate recall), **amnestic dementia** (loss of short-term memory), **cognitive dementia** (loss of long-term memory), and **intentional dementia** (loss of goal orientation). The culmination of a progressive dementing process is nerve cell degeneration and brain atrophy.

Pathophysiology

Mechanisms in dementing processes include tissue destruction, compression, inflammation, and biochemical imbalances. For example, persons with Alzheimer disease have a lack of acetylcholine, a neurotransmitter, the first biochemical abnormality that has been demonstrated consistently (Sims et al., 1983; Danison, 1986). Acetylcholine is needed for short-term memory at the biochemical level. As the level of acetylcholine is reduced, the individual is able to store less and less information until all short-term memory is lost. The cause for the enzyme system that produces acetylcholine to fail is not known. Slow-growing viruses are probably associated with some unexplained dementias, such as Jacob-Creutzfield disease.

A genetic predisposition is probably a contributing factor to the dementing process. In some instances, a familial history of dementia increases the likelihood of an individual's developing dementia by four times. Environmental influences may also play a role in the pathogenesis of dementia. The exact nature of the influence of environmental factors, such as aluminum, are not clearly understood as yet.

Diseases that cause dementia prevent the acquisition

TABLE 14-9 Clinical manifestations of dementia

Type	Location	Manifestation
Amnestic dementia	Temporal lobe	Difficulty with naming Decreased language comprehension Loss of memory and intellectual function Development of a vegetative state
Intentional dementia	Frontal lobe	Distraction and failure to achieve specific goals Can follow simple commands but not able to carry out sequential intellectual functions Loss of attention span Inability to make decisions or judgments Accident prone Personality changes and inappropriate affect Loss of motor function: wide shuffling gait with small steps, muscle rigidity, flexion posturing, tendency to fall, abnormal reflexes, bowel and bladder incontinence, immobility
Cognitive dementia	Cerebral cortex	Loss of long-term memory Decreased language comprehension Decreased mathematical skill Altered visual-spatial relationships

of new information, interfere with information retrieval, or destroy stored information. (The ability to learn is therefore affected.)

Clinical Manifestations

A summary of the clinical manifestations of the dementias is presented in Table 14-9.

Evaluation and Treatment

Establishing the etiology for a dementing process may be complicated, but all persons evidencing the clinical manifestations of dementia should be evaluated with laboratory and neuropsychologic testing to identify underlying causes that may be treatable.

If a specific treatable cause is identified, the appropriate treatment is initiated. For example, an infectious process requires the appropriate antibiotic, and a potentially resectable mass may require neurosurgery. Nutritional deficiencies are corrected. If the cause is metabolic, the imbalance is corrected and/or the metabolic disorder is treated.

Unfortunately, most progressive dementias have no specific treatment or cure for the process. In such instances, therapy is directed at maintaining and maximizing use of the remaining capacities, restoring functions if possible, and accommodating to lost abilities. Assisting the family to understand the dementing process and to learn ways to assist the demented individual are essential components of supportive management.

Alzheimer Disease

Alzheimer disease is a very commonly occurring neurologic disorder. Formerly believed to occur mostly in persons under 65 years of age, Alzheimer disease has now been demonstrated to be one of the most common causes of severe cognitive dysfunction in older persons (Coyle, Price, & Delong, 1983). Alzheimer disease is found in 2% to 3% of the general population and in 5% to 6% of persons 65 years of age or older (Coyle et al., 1983). Presenile dementia of the Alzheimer type is a rare disorder in which persons, typically in their 50s, develop a rapidly progressing deterioration in cognitive function (Coyle et al., 1983). Senile dementia of the Alzheimer type is the common disorder developing in persons after the age of 65.

Pathogenesis

The exact cause of Alzheimer disease is unknown; several possible causes are currently under investigation. Alzheimer disease has recently been linked to chemical changes—a loss of the enzyme choline acetyltransferase resulting in a selective deficit in acetylcholine in acetylcholine-releasing neurons (Kolata, 1981, 1983). Alzheimer disease has also been recently linked to the uninhibited activity of ribonuclease, an enzyme that breaks

down RNA in neurons. The link between the pathology of Alzheimer disease and aluminum has been established and results from the degenerating neurons releasing detectable amounts of aluminum (Crapper et al., 1980). Researchers have not yet been able to isolate a virus that causes Alzheimer disease (Mozar, Bal, & Howard, 1987), but submicroscopic proteinaceous infectious particles ("prions") have been isolated. These prions have already been linked to at least one other form of degenerative brain disease. Antibrain antibodies may account for Alzheimer disease, and an autoimmune etiology is also being investigated. Regarding a genetic etiology, Alzheimer disease may be due to an autosomal dominant gene (Coyle et al., 1983; McLachlan-Crapper, & Lewis, 1985). An extra copy of a gene on chromosome 21 may be responsible for the production of protein amyloid in cells from both patients with Alzheimer disease and Down syndrome (*Science News,* 1987a). Familial risk appears to be greatest in families affected by the classic early onset of Alzheimer disease (Kolata, 1981). The risk when a sibling develops Alzheimer disease after age 70 does not differ from that of the general population.

Microscopically, the protein in the neurons becomes distorted and twisted forming a tangle called a **neurofibrillary tangle** (Fig. 14-6). There is an accumulation of these bundles of paired helical abnormal protein fibers (filaments) within the neurons. Groups of nerve cells, especially terminal axons, degenerate and coalesce around a fibrous core. These areas of degeneration appear like plaques under microscopy and are, therefore, called **senile plaques.** These plaques disrupt nerve impulse transmission. Senile plaques and neurofibrillary tangles are more concentrated in the cerebral cortex and hippocampus (Coyle et al., 1983). The greater the number of senile plaques and neurofibrillary tangles, the more dysfunction is present (Coyle et al., 1983; Kolata 1983).

Clinical Manifestations

Initial clinical manifestations are insidious and often attributed to forgetfulness, emotional upset, or other illness. The individual becomes progressively more forgetful over time, particularly when related to recent events. Memory loss increases as the disorder advances and the person become disoriented and confused. The ability to concentrate declines. Abstraction, problem-solving, and judgment gradually deteriorate. There is a failure in mathematical calculation ability, language, and visuospatial orientation. Dyspraxias may appear. The mental status changes induce behavioral changes including irritability, agitation, and restlessness. Mood changes also result from the deterioration in cognition. The person may become anxious, depressed, hostile, emotionally labile, and prone to mood swings. Motor changes may

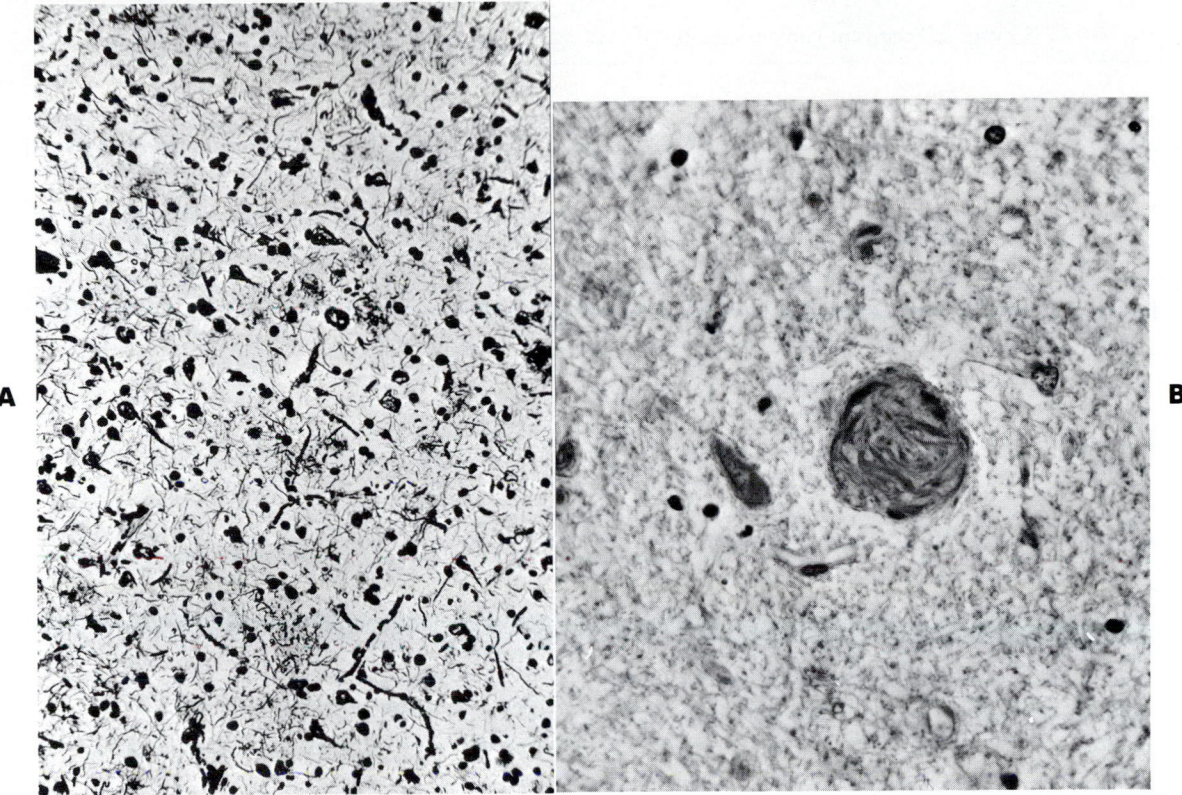

FIG. 14-6. **A,** Neuritic (senile) plaques and neurofibrillary tangles in Alzheimer disease. (Hortega silver carbonate; × 135.) **B,** Neurofibrillary change in cell of locus cureleus in individual with parkinsonism. (Hemotoxylin and eosin; ×600.) (From Kissane, 1985.)

occur if the posterior frontal lobes are involved. The individual exhibits rigidity (paratonia, gegenhalten) with flexion posturing, propulsion, and retropulsion.

Evaluation and Treatment

The diagnosis of Alzheimer disease is made by ruling out other causes of a dementing process. A blood-cell membrane aberration is currently being investigated as a biologic marker for Alzheimer disease (*Science News,* 1987b). The history, including the mental status examination, and the course of the illness are used to diagnose Alzheimer disease. The course of the disorder is highly variable, usually developing over 5 years or more.

The treatment of Alzheimer disease is directed at decreasing the need for the impaired cognitive function by a compensation technique, such as memory aids, maintaining those cognitive functions that are not impaired, and maintaining or improving the general state of hygiene, nutrition, and health. Environmental management, counseling, education, pharmacotherapy, and health promotion measures are the foundation upon which a comprehensive treatment program is built. Tetrahydroaminoacridine (THA), an investigational drug

being studied that was believed to hold some hope for alleviating some of the symptoms (especially in the early stages) of this disease, was suspended in October of 1987 because of liver toxicity (Weiss, 1987).

Seizures

A **seizure** is a sudden, explosive, disorderly discharge of cerebral neurons and is characterized by a sudden, transient alteration in brain function, usually involving motor, sensory, autonomic, or psychic clinical manifestations and an alteration in level of consciousness. Seizure disorders, the second most common neurologic disorder, represent a syndrome, however, and not a specific disease entity.

The term *convulsion,* sometimes applied to seizures, refers to the clonic-tonic (jerky, contract-relax) movement associated with some seizures. The term *epilepsy,* meaning "to be seized by a force from without," is generally applied to conditions in which no underlying correctable cause for the seizures is found so that the seizure activity recurs without treatment. **Epilepsy** is therefore a general term for the primary condition that causes seizures.

TABLE 14-10 Causes of recurrent convulsions in different age groups

Age of Onset (Years)	Probable Cause
Infancy, under 2	Congenital maldevelopment, birth injury, metabolic disorders (hypocalcemia, hypoglycemia), vitamin B deficiency, phenylketonuria.
Childhood, 2-10	Birth injury, trauma, infections, thrombosis of cerebral arteries or veins, beginning of idiopathic epilepsy.
Adolescence, 10-18	Idiopathic epilepsy, trauma, congenital defects.
Early adulthood 18-35	Trauma, neoplasm, idiopathic epilepsy, alcoholism, drug addiction.
Middle age, 35-60	Neoplasm, trauma, vascular disease, alcoholism, drug addiction.
Late life, over 60	Vascular disease, degeneration, tumor.

From Adams, 1977.

Conditions Associated with Seizure Disorders

Any disorder that alters the neuronal environment may cause seizure activity, so that theoretically, any individual may experience a seizure. Some persons, however, have a genetic predisposition toward seizure activity; their "seizure threshold" in neuronal tissues is apparently lower.

A seizure disorder may also be produced by a variety of pathologic processes, including medical diseases, that can extend to involve the nervous system. The onset of a seizure disorder may also indicate the presence of an ongoing primary neurologic disease. Persons with organic brain injury have greater tendencies toward seizure activity than do persons with normal CNS function. Generally etiologies of seizures originate from (1) cerebral lesions, (2) biochemical disorders, (3) cerebral trauma, and (4) epilepsy. Among the causes of seizure activity are

Metabolic defects
Congenital malformation
Genetic predisposition
Perinatal injury
Postnatal trauma
Motor syndromes
Epilepsy
Infection
Brain tumor
Vascular disease

Causes of recurrent seizures are also age related (Table 14-10).

In persons with seizure disorders, seizure activity may be precipitated by hypoglycemia, fatigue or lack of sleep, emotional or physical stress, febrile illness, large amounts of water ingestion, constipation, use of stimulant drugs, withdrawal from depressant drugs (including alcohol), hyperventilation (respiratory alkalosis), and some environmental stimuli such as blinking lights, a poorly adjusted television screen, loud noises, certain music, certain odors, or merely being startled. Females may have increased seizure activity immediately before or during menses.

Types of Seizure Disorders

Seizures are classified in different ways—by clinical manifestations, site of origin, EEG correlates, or response to therapy. A simplified version of the international classification of epileptic seizures is presented in Table 14-11. **Generalized seizures** involve neurons bilaterally, often do not have a local (focal) onset, and usually originate from a subcortical or deeper brain focus. With a generalized seizure, consciousness is always impaired or lost. **Partial seizures (focal seizures)** involve neurons only unilaterally, often have a local (focal) onset, and usually originate from cortical brain tissue, thereby having a superficial focus. Consciousness is usually maintained as long as the seizure activity is limited to one hemisphere, but partial seizures may generalize to involve neurons of the other hemisphere and the deeper brain nuclei. This process is called **secondary generalization.** Consciousness is lost at the point of generalization.

Status epilepticus is the experience of a second, a third, and often subsequent seizures before the person has fully regained consciousness from the preceding seizure. The person is still in a **postictal state** (state that follows a seizure) when the next seizure begins. Status epilepticus most frequently results from abrupt discontinuation of anticonvulsant medications but may also occur in untreated or inadequately treated persons with seizure disorders. The situation is a medical emergency because of the resulting cerebral hypoxia. Mental retardation, dementia, and other brain damage, and even death, are serious threats. Aspiration is also a great risk. (Terminology associated with seizure activity is defined in Table 14-12.)

TABLE 14-11 International classification of epileptic seizures

Traditional terminology	New nomenclature
	I. Partial seizures (seizures beginning locally)
Focal motor; Jacksonian seizures (occasionally become secondarily generalized)	A. Simple (without impairment of consciousness) 1. With motor symptoms 2. With special sensory or somatosensory symptoms 3. With autonomic symptoms 4. With psychic symptoms
Temporal lobe or psychomotor seizures	B. Complex (with impairment of consciousness) 1. Simple partial onset followed by impaired consciousness—with or without automatisms 2. Impaired consciousness at onset—with or without automatisms
	C. Secondarily generalized (partial onset evolving to generalized tonic-clonic seizures)
	II. Generalized seizures (bilaterally symmetrical and without local onset)
Petit mal	A. Absences
Minor motor	B. Myoclonic seizures
Limited grand mal	C. Clonic seizure
	D. Tonic seizure
Grand mal	E. Tonic-clonic seizure
Drop attacks	F. Atonic seizure
	G. Infantile spasms
	III. Unclassified seizures (because of incomplete data)
	IV. Status epilepticus (prolonged partial or generalized seizures without recovery between attacks)

Adapted from Rothner, 1983.

Pathophysiology

An **epileptogenic focus** appears to be a group of neurons that have lost their afferent stimulation. The plasma membranes of neuronal cells appear to be more permeable, making them more easily activated by hyperthermia, hypoxia, hypoglycemia, hyponatremia, repeated sensory stimulation, and certain sleep phases. These neurons are hypersensitive and may even remain in a chronic partially depolarized state.

The firing of involved epileptogenic neurons becomes increasingly greater in frequency and amplitude. When the intensity of the neuronal discharge reaches a threshold point, the discharge spreads to adjacent normal neurons through corticocortical synapses. If uninhibited at this point, the cortical excitation spreads through interhemispheric tracts to the contralateral cortex and through projection pathways to the subcortical areas of the basal ganglia, thalamus, and brainstem. The excita-

TABLE 14-12 Terminology applied to a seizure disorder

Term	Definition
Aura	A peculiar sensation immediately preceding the onset of a seizure that may take the form of gustatory, visual, or auditory experience or a feeling of dizziness, numbness, or just "a funny feeling"
Prodroma	Early clinical manifestations such as malaise, headache, a sense of depression, that may occur hours to a few days before the onset of a seizure
Tonic phase	A state of muscle contraction where there is excessive muscle tone
Clonic phase	A state of alternating contraction and relaxation of muscles
Postictal state	The time period immediately following the cessation of seizure activity

tion spread to the subcortical, thalamic, and brainstem areas corresponds to the **tonic phase** (phase of muscle contraction with increased muscle tone) and is associated with loss of consciousness. Autonomic clinical manifestations may also emerge at this point, and apnea may be present for a few seconds. The excitation is further projected downward to the spinal cord neurons through the corticospinal and reticulospinal pathways.

The **clonic phase** (phase of alternating contraction and relaxation of muscles) begins as inhibitory neurons in the cortex, anterior thalamus, and basal ganglia begin to inhibit the cortical excitation. This inhibition causes an interruption in the seizure discharge, producing an intermittent contract-relax pattern of muscle contractions. The intermittent clonic bursts gradually become more and more infrequent until they finally cease. At this point, the epileptogenic neurons are exhausted, and the neuronal membranes may also be hyperpolarized.

Maintaining seizure activity demands a 250% increase in ATP. Cerebral oxygen consumption is increased by 60%. Although cerebral blood flow also increases approximately 250% during seizure activity, available glucose and oxygen are readily depleted. With a severe sei-

zure, the brain tissue may require more ATP than can be produced by the tissues from the available oxygen and glucose. A deficiency of ATP, phosphocreatine, and glucose then occurs, and lactate accumulates in the brain tissues. Severe seizures may thus produce secondary hypoxia, acidosis, and lactate accumulation, all of which are imbalances that may result in progressive brain tissue injury and destruction. Cellular exhaustion and destruction are consequences of these events.

If a seizure focus is active for a prolonged period of time, a secondary focus, called a **mirror focus,** may develop in normal tissue. This process is apparently caused by the interhemispheric communication, as the mirror focus is located in the contralateral cortical area.

Clinical Manifestations

The clinical manifestations associated with seizure depend on the type of seizure (Table 14-13). Two types of symptoms often signal an impending seizure. These are an **aura,** a peculiar sensation that immediately precedes the onset of a seizure, and a **prodroma,** an early manifestation that may occur hours to days before a seizure (see Table 14-12). Both of these manifestations may be-

TABLE 14-13 Clinical manifestations related to seizure types

Type	Clinical manifestations	Site
I. PARTIAL SEIZURES		
A. Simple		
1. With motor symptoms:		
a. without Jacksonian march (focal motor seizure—the motor movements do not extend into adjacent areas	Motor activity is usually clonic. Motor movement elicited by the seizure activity depends on the anatomic-physiologic portion of the irritated cortex but motor seizures most often begin in the face and hands. Focal seizures begin with slow, repetitive jerking of the body part, which increases in strength and rate over a period of 5 to 15 seconds. The seizure can cease spontaneously, with a gradual decrease in clonic movement.	Primary motor area
b. with Jacksonian march (Jacksonian seizure—the seizure activity spreads in an orderly fashion of adjacent areas)	Seizure activity spreads to adjacent areas after the initial clonic movement increases; motor movements, for example, would begin in the fingers of one side and spread to the hand, wrist, forearm, arm, face, and finally the lower extremity on the same side of the body. After spreading, the jerking movements in all areas would spontaneously stop.	Primary motor area
c. adversive seizure	Turning movement of hand and eyes to the side opposite the irritative focus. Often associated with contractions of the trunk and extremities. May remain local or develop into a generalized seizure.	Frontal lobe anterior to the primary motor area

Adapted from Hickey, 1981.

TABLE 14-13 Clinical manifestations related to seizure types—cont'd

Type	Clinical manifestations	Site
2. With special sensory or somatosensory symptoms (focal sensory seizure); less common than focal motor seizures; any age may be affected	Sensory experience is subjective and confined to the primary sensory modalities (somesthetic, visual, auditory-vestibular, or olfactory).	Sensory cortex
	If sensory seizure begins on the hand area of the sensory cortex, the patient experiences numbness, tingling, or "pins and needles" phenomena. Other sensory experiences including burning, a crawling sensation, or a feeling of movement of the body part.	Postcentral gyrus (parietal lobe) with involvement of the primary sensory area
	Most frequent areas affected include lips, fingers, and toes.	
	May remain local or develop into a generalized seizure.	
B. Complex (temporary lobe or psychomotor seizure)		
1. Simple partial onset followed by impairment of consciousness—with or without automatisms; common seizures found in both children and adults but in most persons occurs before the age of 20	The person is able to interact with the environment with purposeful, although inappropriate, movements; although the body muscles stiffen, the person does not fall and may even continue the complex activity in which he/she was involved, such as driving; the person may appear "wide eyed."	Temporal lobe and its connections
	A wide variety of sensory experiences precede the automatism and include illusions, hallucinations, and primative visceral, olfactory, and gustatory sensations.	
	Most characteristic event of a temporal lobe seizure is the automatism; common examples of automatism are lip-smacking, chewing, facial grimacing, swallowing movements, and patting, picking, or rubbing oneself or one's clothing.	
	Temporal lobe seizures generally last from 1 to 4 minutes and are followed by several minutes of postictal confusion.	
2. Impaired consciousness at onset—with or without automatisms:	See above, under Simple Partial Onset.	
C. Secondarily generalized	Unconsciousness appears.	
	General symptoms are produced.	
II. GENERALIZED SEIZURES		
A. Absences (petit mal seizure), always occurs in children after the age of 4 years and before puberty	Characterized by an abrupt cessation of activity with a momentary arrest of consciousness lasting about 5 to 10 seconds, while a few last 30 seconds; the eyes become vacant and roll or the child may stare straight ahead; the lips may droop or twitch.	Multifocal
	The child is responsive if spoken to during the seizure.	
	The child resumes previous activity after a seizure.	
B. Myoclonic (minor major seizure)	Characterized by sudden, uncontrollable jerking movements of one or more extremities or the entire body.	Multifocal
	Seizures usually occur in the morning.	
	Usually momentary loss of consciousness followed by postictal confusion.	
	Person often violently flung to the ground so that injury is a real possibility.	
	Myoclonic seizures can occur in clusters.	
	If the frequency and amplitude of the seizures are severe, mental retardation can result.	

(Continued.)

TABLE 14-13 Clinical manifestations related to seizure types—cont'd

Type	Clinical manifestations	Site
C. Clonic	Characterized by repetitive clonic jerks of constant amplitude and diminishing frequency.	
D. Tonic (affects infants and children)	Loss of postural tone without evidence of clonicity, with flexion of the upper limbs and extension of the lower limbs. Child assumes an abnormal posture for seconds or minutes without losing consciousness.	
E. Tonic–clonic (grand mal seizure) (affects both children and adults)	A prodromal period of irritability and tension may precede a tonic-clonic seizure by several hours or days; however, in majority of persons, seizures begin without warnings. Characteristically tonic–clonic seizures begin with a sudden loss of consciousness and generalized tonic muscle contractions; the person falls to the ground and the body stiffens in an opisthotonus position with legs and, usually, arms extended; the jaw snaps shut; a shrill cry may be heard due to forceful exhalation of air through the closed vocal cords as the thoracic muscles initially contract; the bladder and, less often, the bowel may evacuate; during the tonic phase, the person is apneic with subsequent cyanosis; pupils are dilated and unresponsive to light. The tonic phase lasts less than 1 minute (average 15 seconds). The clonic phase is characterized by violent, rhythmic, muscular contractions accompanied by strenuous hyperventilation; the face is contorted; the eyes roll, and there is excessive salivation with frothing from the mouth; profuse sweating, and a rapid pulse are evident. The clonic jerking subsides in frequency and amplitude over a period of about 30 seconds. The tonic–clonic seizure lasts from 2 to 5 minutes. After the clonic phase, the person is in a stupor or coma for about 5 minutes; the extremities are limp; breathing is quiet; and the pupils begin to respond to light. When the person awakens, he/she may be confused and disoriented, complains of headache, muscle aching, and fatigue. There is no recollection of the attack. Tonic–clonic seizures may occur at any time of the day or night, whether the person is awake or asleep. The frequency of reoccurrence may vary from hours, weeks, months, or years.	Multifocal
F. Atonic (drop attack, akinetic seizure)	Characterized by sudden loss of postural muscle tone.	Multifocal
G. Infantile spasms (affects 3 month to 2 year age group)	Characterized by flexor spasms of the extremities and the head (have been described as jackknife seizures). Seizure lasts a few seconds and often appears in clusters with several clusters occurring daily. Infantile spasms associated with metabolic, degenerative, or structural illness in 50% of cases; in other 50% no correlation is noted. Majority of victims mentally retarded.	

Adapted from Hickey, 1981.

come familiar to the person experiencing recurrent seizures and so may help in preventing injuries during the seizure.

Evaluation and Treatment

The health history is the most critical aspect in diagnosing a seizure disorder and establishing the cause. The health history is supplemented by the physical examination and laboratory tests of blood and urine (blood glucose, serum calcium, blood urea nitrogens, urine sodium, and creatinine clearance) to identify any systemic diseases known to have seizures as a clinical manifestation. Skull x-ray films, CT scan, and cerebrospinal fluid examination are useful to identify any neurologic diseases associated with seizures. The electroencephalogram is useful in assessing the type of seizure and may help to determine its focus.

Treatment for a seizure disorder is first to correct or control its cause, if possible. If this is not possible, the major means of management is the judicious administration of anticonvulsant medications. The therapeutic goal is complete suppression of seizure activity without intolerable side effects of the drug. Other medical therapies may include prescription of a ketogenic diet, biofeedback, and surgery. In severe cases, psychologic, social, educational, and vocational counseling are often appropriate for the individual and family.

ALTERATIONS IN MOTOR FUNCTION

Movements are complex patterns of activity controlled by the CNS. Movements are influenced by the cerebral cortex, the pyramidal system, the extrapyramidal system, and the motor units. Dysfunction in any of these areas may cause motor dysfunction. General motor dysfunctions may produce changes in muscle mass, muscle strength, muscle tone, postural abnormalities, or abnormal movements.

Clinical Manifestations of Motor Dysfunction
Abnormalities in Muscle Mass

Muscle mass may **atrophy** (shrink) or **hypertrophy** (enlarge), depending on the level of dysfunction (see Chapter 2). Atrophy results from disuse. When muscle fibers are deprived of their nerve supply, they eventually atrophy. Because of the absent nerve impulses, muscles are gradually replaced by connective tissue and fat.

Hypertrophy, in contrast, results from frequent or continual use of a muscle. Some muscle hypertrophy is caused by normal exercise, but severe hypertrophy results from overstimulation of muscle fibers. Overstimulation occurs when the motor unit reflex arc remains intact and functioning but is not inhibited by higher cen-

ters. The loss of inhibition and the constant state of excitation cause continual muscle contraction, resulting in enlargement of the muscle mass.

Abnormalities in Muscle Strength

Muscle strength is quantitatively evaluated on a scale of 0 to 4+, where 4+ is normal and 0 indicates an inability to move against gravity. Degrees of abnormal muscle strength range from **paresis** (weakness) to **paralysis** (inability of a muscle group to overcome gravity). Sites of paresis and paralysis are named in different ways. **Hemiparesis** refers to weakness on one side of the body; **hemiplegia** indicates paralysis on one side of the body. These conditions result from dysfunction, such as a tumor or cerebral vascular accident, in the brain or brainstem.

Paraplegia refers to paralysis of the lower extremities; whereas **quadriplegia** refers to paralysis of all four extremities. Both paraplegia and quadriplegia may be caused by dysfunction of the spinal cord. Upper cord damage results in quadriplegia, and lower cord damage preserves upper extremity function and causes paraplegia (spinal cord injury is discussed in Chapter 15).

Abnormalities in Muscle Tone

Normal muscle tone involves a slight resistance to passive movement. The resistance is smooth, constant, and even throughout the range of motion. The abnormalities of muscle tone are presented in Table 14-14. The abnormalities may range from hypotonia to rigidity.

Postural Abnormalities

An inequality of tone in muscle groups due to a loss of normal postural reflexes results in a posturing of limbs. Many reflex systems govern tone and posture, but the most important factor for controlling posture is the **stretch reflex,** in which stretching of extensor (antigravity) muscles causes increased extensor tone and inhibited flexor tone.

Dystonia is the maintenance of an abnormal posture through muscular contractions. When muscular contractions are sustained for several seconds, they are called **dystonic movements,** such as in choreoathetoid movements associated with high levels of L-dopa; when contractions last for longer periods, they are called **dystonic postures,** such as in torticollis. Dystonic postures may last for weeks, causing permanent fixed contractures. Dystonia has been associated with pathology of the basal ganglia, but the exact pathophysiologic mechanisms are unknown.

Two types of posturing are (1) decerebrate posture and (2) decorticate posture (see Figs. 14-4 and 14-5). **Decerebrate posture** refers to increased tone in extensor muscles and trunk muscles with active tonic neck re-

TABLE 14-14 Abnormalities in muscle tone

Abnormality	Characteristics	Cause
Hypotonia	Passive movement of a muscle mass with little or no resistance	Thought to be caused by decreased muscle spindle activity due to decreased excitability of neurons
Flaccidity	A type of hypotonia in which muscles may be rapidly moved without resistance Associated with limp, atrophied muscles and paralysis	Occurs typically when nerve impulses necessary for muscle tone are lost
Hypertonia	Increased muscle resistance to passive movement May be associated with paralysis May be accompanied by muscle hypertrophy	Results when the lower motor unit reflex arc continues to function but is not mediated or regulated by higher centers
Spasticity	Type of hypertonia characterized by a gradual increase in tone causing increased resistance until tone is suddenly reduced causing clasp-knife phenomenon	Exact mechanism is not clear; appears to arise from an increased excitability of the alpha motor neurons to any input due to absence of the descending inhibition of the pyramidal systems
Rigidity	Type of hypertonia characterized by muscle resistance to passive movement of a rigid limb that is uniform in both flexion and extension throughout the motion The uniform resistance may be interrupted by a series of brief jerks resulting in movements much like a rachet, "cogwheel" phenomenon	Occurs as a result of constant, involuntary contraction of muscle

flexes. When the head is in a neutral position, all four limbs are rigidly extended. The decerebrate posture is caused by severe injury to the brain and brainstem, resulting in overstimulation of the postural righting and vestibular reflexes. **Decorticate posture** (also referred to as **antigravity posture** or **hemiplegic posture**) is characterized by upper extremities flexed at the elbows and held closely to the body and lower extremities that are externally rotated and extended. Decorticate posture is thought to occur when the brainstem, which facilitates the antigravity position, is not inhibited by the motor function of the cerebral cortex.

Abnormal Movements

Movement requires a change in the contractile state of muscles. Abnormal movements may occur when a variety of CNS dysfunctions alter muscular innervation. Movement disorders are not well understood. Present knowledge has come predominantly from neuropharmacology and experimental therapeutics. The neurotransmitter dopamine has an apparent role in motor function. Some movement disorders (such as the akinesias) result from too little dopaminergic activity, whereas others (such as chorea, ballism, and tardive dyskinesia) result from too much dopaminergic activity. Still others are not primarily related to dopamine function. Movement disorders are not necessarily associated with mass, strength, tone, or posture, but are neurologic dysfunc-

tions with either a decreased amount of movement or an excess of movement.

Akinesias

Akinesia is a decrease in associated and voluntary movements. The components of akinesia are **hypokinesia** (decreased associated movements of expression and locomotion) and **bradykinesia** (slowness of voluntary movements). Both components are related to dysfunction of the extrapyramidal system, such as parkinsonism. Pathogenesis is related to either a deficiency of dopamine or a defect of the postsynaptic dopamine receptors, which occurs in parkinsonism (see Chapter 15).

In hypokinesia, the normal, habitually associated movements that provide skill, grace, and balance to voluntary movements are lost. Decreased associated movements accompanying emotional expression cause an expressionless face, a statuesque posture, absence of speech inflection, and absence of spontaneous gestures. Decreased associated movements accompanying locomotion cause reduced arm and shoulder movements, hip swinging, and rotary motion of the cervical spine.

In bradykinesia, all voluntary movements become slow, labored, and deliberate. Bradykinesia consists of (1) difficulty in initiating movements, (2) difficulty in continuing movements smoothly, and (3) difficulty in performing synchronous (at the same time) and consecutive tasks. Difficulty in initiating movements ranges from slight hesitancy to severe **freezing** (transient, help-less immobility). Each intended movement requires ef-fort. Difficulty in continuing motions smoothly causes jerky, irregular, rapid movements, which then decrease in rate and amplitude until they stop. The individual is scarcely aware of the cessation. Difficulty in performing synchronous and consecutive tasks means that each mo-tor act is performed separately. The individual is unable to integrate two acts or to change from one motor pat-tern to the next with a single smooth motion.

Hyperkinesia and Dyskinesia

Hyperkinesia (excessive movements) and **dyskinesia** (abnormal, involuntary movements) represent the sec-ond broad category of abnormal movements. Within this category there are a number of specific dysfunctions (see Table 14-15).

Tremor is a rhythmic, oscillating movement affecting one or more body parts. The movement is due to the regular contraction of opposing groups of muscles. The rate, location, amplitude, and constancy vary depending

TABLE 14-15 Types of hyperkinesias and dyskinesias

Type	Characteristics	Cause
Fasciculations	Rapid muscle contractions involving several motor units; may involve hands and feet, tongue, or entire body Occasionally related to a rare familial muscle dis-order called benign fasciculations	Most cases are evidence of damage to either anterior horn cells or the motor axon as it travels to the motor unit
Clonus	Usually occurs in a severely spastic limb but may occur in any muscle	Repetitive, sustained stretch reflex from overexcite-ment of the muscle
Myoclonus	Series of shock-like contractions that cause throw-ing movements of a limb Usually appear at random but frequently triggered by sudden startle Does not disappear during sleep	Associated with an irritable nervous system and spontaneous electrical discharge of neurons Structures associated with myoclonus include the cerebral cortex, cerebellum, reticular formation and spinal cord
Chorea	Brief, irregular, symmetrical movements present at rest but accentuated by movement Tend to flow from one muscle to another in vari-ous parts of the body	Associated with excess concentration of or a super-sensitivity to dopamine within the synapses of the basal ganglia
Ballism	Gross form of chorea consisting of continuous, irregular contraction of muscles; complex move-ment with violent flinging of extremities Movements are augmented by physical effort or excitement and diminished by rest Ballism is seen most commonly on one side of the body, a condition termed hemiballism Decreased dopamine concentration may reduce or eliminate ballism	Results from injury to subthalamus nucleus (one of the nuclei that comprise the basal ganglia) Thought to be due to reduced inhibitory influence in the nucleus Hemiballism results from injury to the contralateral subthalamic nucleus
Athetosis	Slower, more fluid-like movements than chorea Typically consists of flexion and extension of fin-gers, wrist, and elbows, abduction and adduc-tion of the arm	Occurs most commonly as a result of injury to the basal ganglia in infancy that allows the release of primitive reflex movements Exact pathophysiologic mechanism is now known
Choreathetosis	Involves both chorea and athetosis	Precise pathophysiologic mechanism is not known
Tics	Rapid, occasionally sustained movements that ap-pear in a sequential pattern; the pattern is re-peated at the next occurrence of the tic Movements may be simple or complex Typically preceded by a compulsive urge to carry out the pattern	Have been associated with excess dopamine but structures involved are not conclusively known
Spasm	A strong muscle contraction	Originates locally from muscle or from some level of the nervous system
Hiccup	A spasm	Produced by irritation of the sensory nerves in the stomach or diaphragm or by injuries causing pressure on the myelencephalon

TABLE 14-16 Causes and characteristics of tremors

Type	Cause	Characteristics
TREMOR-AT-REST		
Parkinsonian tremor	Loss of inhibitory influence of dopamine in the basal ganglia, causing instability of basal ganglial feedback circuit with the cerebral cortex	Regular, rhythmical, slow flexion–extension contraction; involves principally the metacarpophalangeal and wrist joints; alternating movements between thumb and index finger described as "pill rolling"; disappears during voluntary movement
POSTURAL TREMOR		
Asterixis (tremor of hepatic encephalopathy)	Exact mechanism responsible unknown; thought to be related to accumulation of products normally detoxified by the liver	Irregular flapping movement of the hands accentuated by outstretching arms
Metabolic tremor	Occurs in conditions associated with disturbed metabolism or toxicity, as in thyrotoxicosis (hyperthyroidism), alcoholism, and chronic use of barbiturates; exact mechanism responsible unknown	Rapid, rhythmic tremor affecting fingers, lips, and tongue; accentuated by extending the body part
Essential (familial) tremor	Not associated with any other neurologic abnormalities; cause unknown	Tremor of fingers, hands and feet; absent at rest, but accentuated by extension of body part, prolonged muscular activity, and stress
Cerebellar tremor	Occurs in disease of the dentate nucleus (one of the cerebellar deep nuclei responsible for efferent output) and the superior cerebellar penduncle (a stalklike structure connected to the pons); caused by errors in feedback from the periphery and errors in preprogramming goal-directed movement	Tremor initiated by movement, maximal toward end of movement
Rubral tremor	Results from lesions involving the dentatorubothalamic tract (a spinothalamic tract connecting the red nucleus in the reticular formation and the dentate nucleus in the cerebellum)	Rhythmic tremor of limbs that originates proximally by movement

on the specific type of tremor and its severity. Tremors are classified as **tremor-at-rest** (present when an individual is sitting or lying), **postural tremor** (present when a body part is held in one position), and **intention tremor** (present upon voluntary movement of a body part). Causes differ according to type (Table 14-16).

In general, a tremor-at-rest is associated with lesions of the dopaminergic nigrostriatal pathway and is characteristic of parkinsonism (see Chapter 15). The structures associated with postural tremors, such as essential tremor or metabolic tremor, are not known. Intention tremor is the result of an injury in the cerebellar efferent pathway and is most common in multiple sclerosis.

Paroxysmal dyskinesias are abnormal, involuntary movements that occur paroxysmally. The type of dyskinesia varies depending on the specific disorder. **Paroxysmal kinesigenic choreoathetosis** is a sudden burst of choreic movement (formerly described) initiated by a sudden body movement. The chorea is brief, usually lasting less than a minute. The cause is unknown. **Paroxysmal dystonia** is the sudden contraction and twisting of muscles which may last several hours. Paroxysmal dystonia is induced by sudden stress, fatigue, or ingestion of alcohol or caffeine and is believed to represent a seizure disorder of the basal ganglia.

Tardive dyskinesia is the involuntary movement of the face, trunk, and extremities. Although the condition

TABLE 14-17 Upper and lower motor neuron syndromes

	Upper motor neuron syndromes*	Lower motor neuron syndromes†
Distribution of affected muscles	Muscle groups are affected; when movement is possible, the proper relationship among agonists, antagonists, synergists, and fixators is preserved	Individual muscles may be affected
	Synkinesias (residual movements) are present; attempts to move paralyzed part causes a variety of associated movements; movements of normal limb may cause imitative or mirror movements in the paralyzed limb	Individual muscles may be affected
Muscle tone	Hypertonia, specifically spasticity	Hypotonia, flaccidity
Tendon reflexes	Hyperreflexia with extensor plantar reflex present	Hyporeflexia, no abnormal reflexes present
Atrophy	Slight, due to disuse	Pronounced atrophy
Fasciculations	Absent	May be present

*Pyramidal motor syndromes.
†All are motor unit syndromes.

occurs occasionally in individuals with Parkinson disease, it usually occurs as a side effect of prolonged phenothiazine drug therapy. The antipsychotic drugs bind to the dopamine receptor, somehow altering the receptor so that it mimics the effect of too much dopamine. The most common symptom of tardive dyskinesia is rapid, repetitive stereotypic movements. Most typically, these movements are continual chewing with intermittent protrusions of the tongue. Stereotypic movements are felt to be a form of excessive dopaminergic activity.

Akathitic movements are partly voluntary. The movements occur because of **akathisia,** a feeling of inner motor restlessness. With akathisia, an individual feels the need to perform an action, and carrying out the movement brings relief from akathisia. Akathisia is a frequent complication of antipsychotic drugs. It may occur when drug therapy is begun (acute akathisia) or with chronic treatment (tardive dyskinesia). The exact mechanism of akathisia is unknown, but the dopamine-rich limbic system is thought to be involved. Akathitic movements may be transiently suppressed.

Motor Syndromes

Any pathologic change in the nervous system causes manifestations that reflect the type and extent of damage. The extent of damage within the nervous system determines which manifestations emerge. The specific manifestations also depend on whether there is destruction or irritation (stimulation) of nervous tissue. If a portion of the nervous system is destroyed, manifestations are caused by two mechanisms: (1) functions normally performed by the affected area are lost and (2) abnormal phenomena appear because of the hyperactivity in areas normally inhibited, opposed, or mediated by

the affected area. If a portion of the nervous tissue system is irritated, the result is an exaggeration of the normal function of the affected area.

Motor syndromes are classified according to level and area of damage. The two general motor syndromes are CNS motor syndromes and motor unit syndromes. Other classifications distinguish upper from lower motor neuron syndromes (Table 14-17). Lower motor neuron syndromes involve dysfunction of some motor units, whereas upper motor neuron syndromes involve dysfunction of the pyramidal system and are thus termed pyramidal motor syndromes (Fig. 14-7).

CNS Motor Syndromes

The two CNS motor syndromes are (1) the pyramidal motor syndrome and (2) the extrapyramidal motor syndromes. These syndromes involve different areas of injury, and individuals therefore exhibit very different clinical manifestations.

Pyramidal Motor Syndrome

The pyramidal motor syndrome is a series of motor dysfunctions that result from interruption of the pyramidal system (Fig. 14-8). The injury may be in the cerebral cortex, the subcortical white matter, the internal capsule, the brainstem, or the spinal cord. The clinical manifestations of a pure pyramidal injury without other damage are not known, but bilateral interruption of the pyramidal system in monkeys causes hypotonic paralysis, although much control of movement eventually returns. In humans, however, injury generally involves more than merely the interruption of the pyramidal system, so that an upper motor neuron paralysis occurs, indicating involvement of several motor pathways.

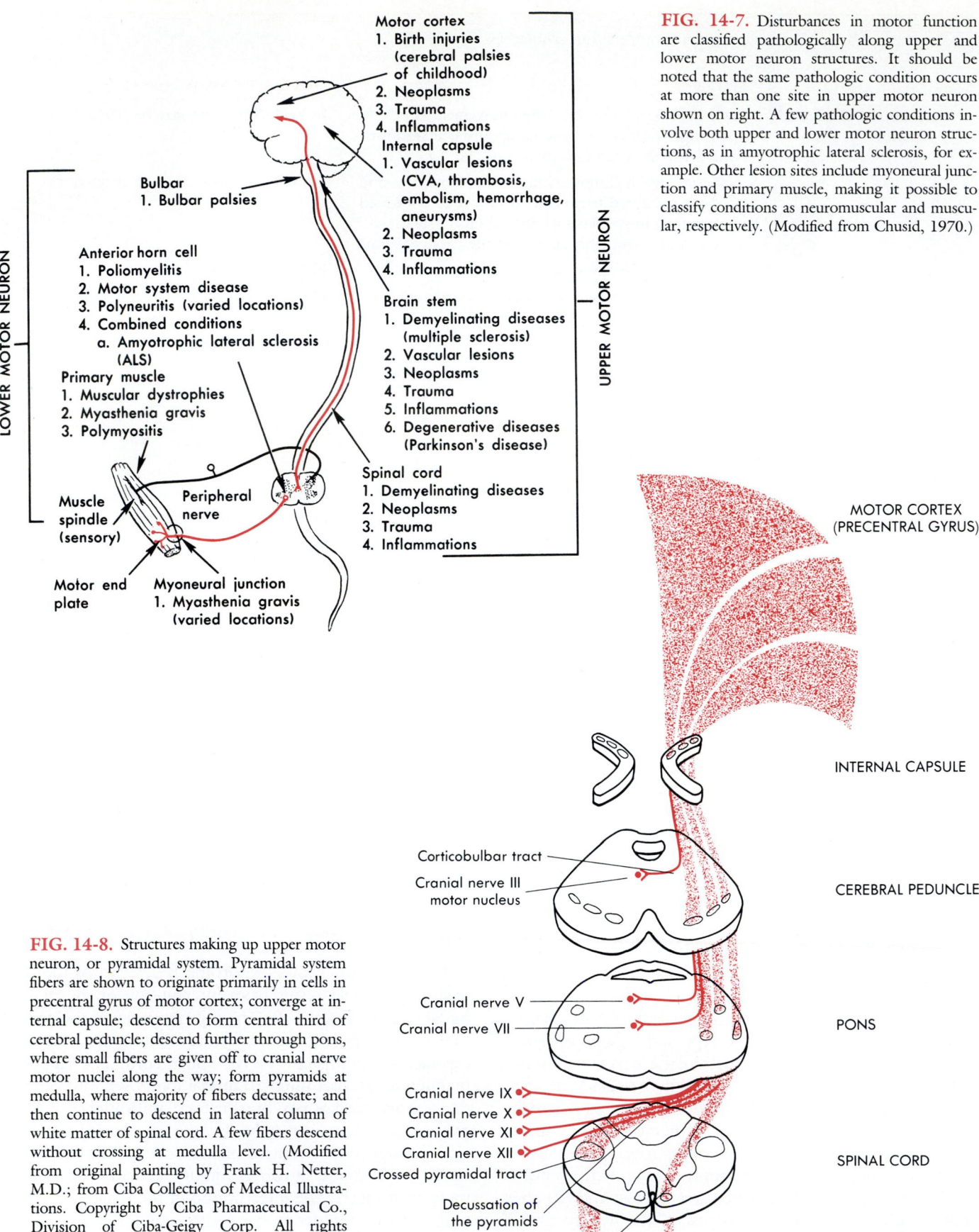

Motor cortex
1. Birth injuries (cerebral palsies of childhood)
2. Neoplasms
3. Trauma
4. Inflammations

Internal capsule
1. Vascular lesions (CVA, thrombosis, embolism, hemorrhage, aneurysms)
2. Neoplasms
3. Trauma
4. Inflammations

Brain stem
1. Demyelinating diseases (multiple sclerosis)
2. Vascular lesions
3. Neoplasms
4. Trauma
5. Inflammations
6. Degenerative diseases (Parkinson's disease)

Spinal cord
1. Demyelinating diseases
2. Neoplasms
3. Trauma
4. Inflammations

Bulbar
1. Bulbar palsies

Anterior horn cell
1. Poliomyelitis
2. Motor system disease
3. Polyneuritis (varied locations)
4. Combined conditions
   a. Amyotrophic lateral sclerosis (ALS)

Primary muscle
1. Muscular dystrophies
2. Myasthenia gravis
3. Polymyositis

Muscle spindle (sensory)

Peripheral nerve

Motor end plate

Myoneural junction
1. Myasthenia gravis (varied locations)

LOWER MOTOR NEURON

UPPER MOTOR NEURON

FIG. 14-7. Disturbances in motor function are classified pathologically along upper and lower motor neuron structures. It should be noted that the same pathologic condition occurs at more than one site in upper motor neuron shown on right. A few pathologic conditions involve both upper and lower motor neuron structions, as in amyotrophic lateral sclerosis, for example. Other lesion sites include myoneural junction and primary muscle, making it possible to classify conditions as neuromuscular and muscular, respectively. (Modified from Chusid, 1970.)

MOTOR CORTEX (PRECENTRAL GYRUS)

INTERNAL CAPSULE

Corticobulbar tract
Cranial nerve III motor nucleus

CEREBRAL PEDUNCLE

Cranial nerve V
Cranial nerve VII

PONS

Cranial nerve IX
Cranial nerve X
Cranial nerve XI
Cranial nerve XII
Crossed pyramidal tract

Decussation of the pyramids

Ventral corticospinal tract

SPINAL CORD

FIG. 14-8. Structures making up upper motor neuron, or pyramidal system. Pyramidal system fibers are shown to originate primarily in cells in precentral gyrus of motor cortex; converge at internal capsule; descend to form central third of cerebral peduncle; descend further through pons, where small fibers are given off to cranial nerve motor nuclei along the way; form pyramids at medulla, where majority of fibers decussate; and then continue to descend in lateral column of white matter of spinal cord. A few fibers descend without crossing at medulla level. (Modified from original painting by Frank H. Netter, M.D.; from Ciba Collection of Medical Illustrations. Copyright by Ciba Pharmaceutical Co., Division of Ciba-Geigy Corp. All rights reserved.)

The distribution of clinical manifestations varies depending upon the location of the lesion, although certain features are constant. Excessive movements such as clonus and spasms occur regularly, much variation exists depending on the suddenness of onset and the age of the individual.

When the pyramidal system is destroyed below the level of the pons, spinal shock occurs. **Spinal shock** is the complete cessation of spinal cord functions below the lesion. It is characterized by complete flaccid paralysis, absence of reflexes, and marked disturbances of bowel and bladder function. The reasons for spinal shock are not fully understood, but a major factor is the sudden destruction of the efferent pathways. If destruction occurs more slowly, spinal shock may not develop (see Chapter 15).

If the pyramidal system is interrupted above the level of the pons, the hand and arm muscles are greatly affected. Paralysis rarely involves all of the muscles on one side of the body, however, even when the hemiplegia results from complete damage to the internal capsule. Bilateral movements, such as those of the eye, jaw, and larynx, are affected only slightly if at all. The limbs are predominantly affected. Because of their bilateral control, trunk muscles are much less influenced.

Paralysis associated with a pyramidal motor syndrome rarely remains flaccid for a prolonged length of time. After a few days or weeks, a gradual return of spinal reflexes marks the end of spinal shock. Reflexes then become hyperactive, and muscle tone is significantly increased, particularly in antigravity muscles. Spasticity is common, although rigidity occasionally occurs. Most often, passive range-of-motion causes the "clasp-knife" phenomenon, probably because of the activation of the two varieties of stretch receptors: (1) the muscle spindles and (2) the Golgi tendon organs. (Muscle function is discussed in Chapter 38.) With pyramidal motor syndrome, the flexors of the arms and extensors of the legs are predominantly affected.

Extrapyramidal Motor Syndromes

Because the extrapyramidal system encompasses all the motor pathways except the pyramidal system, two types of motor dysfunction comprise the **extrapyramidal motor syndromes:** (1) the basal ganglia motor syndromes and (2) the cerebellar motor syndromes. Unlike pyramidal motor syndromes, both of these syndromes result in movement or posture disturbance without significant paralysis, along with other distinctive symptoms (Table 14-18).

Basal Ganglia Motor Syndromes **Basal ganglia motor syndromes** are movement disorders that involve either a paucity or an excess of movements. Stress and nervous tension typically worsen the symptoms, whereas relaxation improves motor performance. Akinesia may occur despite normal strength. Involuntary movements, such as tremor, chorea, ballism, athetosis, and dystonia may also occur and are probably caused by the loss of the normal modulating effects of the corpus striatum and other parts of the basal ganglia.

Basal ganglia motor syndromes are also characterized by alterations in muscle tone and posture. Rigidity, together with the cogwheel phenomenon, is present in all muscle groups but is most prominent in those that maintain flexed position. Postural abnormalities result from the loss of normal postural reflexes and not from defects in proprioceptive, labyrinthine, or visual function. Dysfunctional equilibrium results from the loss of postural stability, as the individual is unable to make the appropriate postural adjustment to tilting or falling and falls down instead. Dysfunctional righting is the inability to right oneself when changing from a lying or crouching to a standing position or when rolling from the supine to the lateral or prone position. Dysfunctional postural fixation is the involuntary flexion of the head and neck, causing difficulty in maintaining an upright trunk position while standing or walking.

The symptomatology of basal ganglia motor syndromes is explained as an imbalance of dopaminergic

---

TABLE 14-18 Pyramidal versus extrapyramidal motor syndrome

Manifestations	Pyramidal motor syndrome	Extrapyramidal motor syndromes
Unilateral movement	Paralysis of voluntary movement	Little or no paralysis of voluntary movement
Tendon reflexes	Increased tendon reflexes	Normal or slightly increased tendon reflexes
Involuntary movements	Absence of involuntary movements	Presence of tremor, chorea, athetosis, or dystonia
Muscle tone	General spasticity in muscles (e.g., clasp-phenomenon) Hypertonia present in flexors of arms and extensors of legs	May have rigidity or intermittent rigidity (cogwheel rigidity)

TABLE 14-19 Cerebellar motor syndromes

Syndrome	Location of dysfunction	Characteristics
Lateral cerebellar	Intermediate and lateral corticonuclear zone of anterior and posterior lobes	Muscles of the extremities on the side of the injury become hypotonic with decreased resistance to passive movement Reflexes hypoactive Ataxia (uncoordination) of extremities is prevalent during voluntary movement causing some degree of gait disturbance Dysmetria (extremity overshooting its target) occurs Intentional and postural tremors present
Medial cerebellar	Medical corticonuclear zone and flocculonodular lobe	Disequilibrium of head and trunk during static posture and locomotion Posture and gait are normal Oculomotor disturbances are common Muscle tone is normal Extremities are not ataxic in voluntary movement

and cholinergic activity in the corpus striatum. A relative excess of cholinergic activity produces akinesia and hypertonia. A relative excess of dopaminergic activity produces hyperkinesia and hypotonia. The precise mechanisms by which imbalances of these striatal neurotransmitters produce specific symptoms is unknown.

Cerebellar Motor Syndromes **Cerebellar motor syndromes** involve the cerebellum and may result in (1) loss of muscle tone, (2) difficulty with coordination of voluntary movements, (3) minor degrees of muscle weakness, tendency toward fatigue and impairment of associated movements, and (4) disorders of equilibrium and gait. Cerebellar effects are chiefly ipsilateral (primarily affecting the same side of the body), so that damage to the right cerebellum generally causes symptoms on the right side of the body. Predominant symptoms depend on the area of damage within the cerebellum. The two cerebellar syndromes are (1) the lateral syndrome and (2) the medial syndrome (see Table 14-19).

Diagnosis of a cerebellar motor syndrome is based on the symptoms, but these may vary because of the individual's attempts at compensation. Furthermore, the nervous system can often operate well despite destruction of parts of the cerebellum, although the mechanisms responsible for this retained function are not fully understood.

Motor Unit Syndromes

Lower Motor Neuron Syndromes

Lower (primary, alpha) motor neurons are the large motor neurons in the anterior (or ventral) horn of the spinal cord, the motor nuclei of the brainstem, and the axons that originate from these nerve cell bodies (to course the anterior spinal roots and the spine or in the cranial nerves to reach skeletal muscles) (Fig. 14-9). Dysfunction in this motor system impairs movement,

both voluntary and involuntary. The degree of paralysis or paresis is proportional to the number of lower motor neurons affected. If only a portion of the motor units supplying a muscle are affected, only partial paralysis (paresis) results. If all the motor units are affected, a complete paralysis results. Other clinical manifestations are also proportional to the degree of dysfunction, but the precise manifestations depend on the location of the dysfunction in the motor unit and in the CNS.

Small motor (gamma) neurons, which function to maintain muscle tone and protect the muscle from injury, are also necessary for normal motor movement. These neurons depend on input from the muscle spindle (arriving through an afferent limb rising to the cord). Dysfunction in this motor system impairs tone and reduces the tendon reflexes, causing hyporeflexia. The muscle is lax and soft with a decrease in normal tone, or hypotonia, which impairs voluntary and involuntary motor movements. The muscles become susceptible to damage from hyperextensibility because the normal protective mechanisms, which prevent muscle fiber injury, are impaired. The degree of tone loss and the loss of tendon reflexes are proportional to the dysfunction in these reflex motor units.

Generally, in a pathologic process the large and small motor neuron systems are equally affected. Therefore, the paresis and paralysis due to a disorder of the lower motor neurons is called a **flaccid paresis/paralysis** because the muscle has reduced or absent tone and is accompanied by hyporeflexia or **areflexia** (loss of tendon reflexes).

A few **gamma neuropathies** (small motor neuron disorders) affect only the gamma motor system. A manifestation of these disorders is a marked reduction in the deep tendon reflexes, which are strikingly out of proportion to the degree of muscle weakness present.

FIG. 14-9. Structures making up lower motor neuron including motor (efferent) and sensory (afferent) elements. Shown on left is anterior horn cell in anterior gray column of spinal cord and its axon terminating in motor end-plate as it innervates extrafusal muscle fibers in quadriceps muscle. Detailed in enlargment are sensory and motor elements of γ-loop system. γ-Efferent fiber is shown innervating polar or end region of muscle spindle (sensory receptor of skeletal muscle). Contraction of muscle spindle fibers stretch central portion of spindle and cause afferent spindle fiber to transmit impulse centrally to cord. Muscle spindle afferent fibers in turn synapse on anterior horn cell and are transmitted by way of γ-efferent fibers to skeletal (extrafusal) muscle, causing it to contract. Muscle spindle discharge is interrupted by active contraction of extrafusal muscle fibers. (Modified from Truex & Carpenter, 1969.) *Human neuroanatomy* [6th ed.]. Baltimore: The Williams & Wilkins, Co.

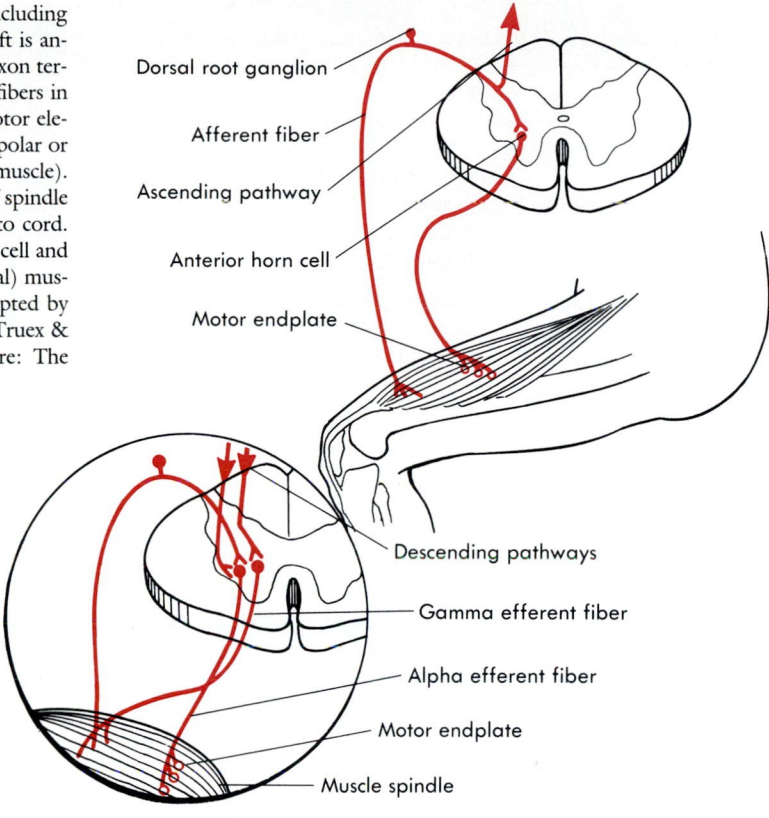

Denervated muscles (i.e., muscles that have lost their nervous system input) undergo atrophy over weeks to months, mostly from disuse. Denervated muscles also demonstrate fasciculations, which are seen as muscle rippling or quivering under the skin. Occasionally, denervated muscles cramp. **Fibrillation** (isolated contraction of a single muscle fiber) also may occur, although this manifestation is not visible clinically.

Amyotrophies

Lower motor neuron syndromes originating in the anterior horn cells or the motor nuclei of the cranial nerves are called **amyotrophies.** Paralytic poliomyelitis is the prototype of these disorders. It involves a severe inflammatory reaction in motor neurons, some of which do not survive, leaving a permanent lower motor neuron syndrome.

Several pathologic processes may give rise to an amyotrophy. A virally induced or postinfectious/postvaccination inflammatory process may injure or destroy anterior horn cells or cranial nerve cell bodies. Most of these inflammatory processes are mild and are followed by rapid cellular recovery.

In the amyotrophies, muscle strength, muscle tone, and muscle bulk are affected in the muscles innervated by the involved motor neurons. The paresis and paralysis associated with anterior horn cell injury is segmental,

but because each muscle is supplied by two or more roots, the segmental character of the weakness may be difficult to recognize. When cranial nerve motor nuclei are affected (these lack nerve roots and have only small rootlets near the point of exit from the brainstem), the distribution of the motor weakness follows that of the peripheral nerve. The weakness may involve distal muscles, proximal muscles, and the muscles of midline structures. Hypotonia and hyporeflexia/areflexia are present.

The atrophy associated with amyotrophy is segmental when the anterior horn cells of the spinal cord are involved and follows the distribution of the peripheral nerve when the cranial nerve(s) motor nuclei are affected. The atrophy may be in distal, proximal, or midline muscles. Fasciculations are particularly associated with primary motor neuron injury, and muscle cramps are common. Mild fatigue is a frequent complaint. If the pathologic process is limited to the primary motor neuron, no sensory changes are evident.

Because degenerative disorders cause loss of nerve cells in the anterior horn or motor nuclei, the surviving cells are small, shrunken, and filled with lipofuscin. Lost neurons are replaced by astrocytes. The roots or rootlets are thin and the muscles show denervation and atrophy.

Several brainstem syndromes involve damage to one or more of the cranial nerve nuclei. These are called **nuclear palsies** (Table 14-20) and may be caused by vas-

TABLE 14-20 Examples of nuclear palsy syndromes

Type of nuclear palsy	Causes	Associated clinical manifestations
Ocular nuclear palsies	Upper brainstem tumor Cerebrovascular disease in the vertebrobasilar system Aneurysm Intramedullary bleed	Other cranial nerve signs Contralateral spastic hemiparesis/plegia Contralateral hyperreflexia Contralateral extensor plantar reflex
Facial nuclear palsy	Pontine tumor Cerebrovascular disease in the vertebrobasilar system	Paresis/paralysis of both the upper and lower facial muscles for both voluntary movement and emotionally induced movement
Vagal nuclear palsy	Intramedullary tumor Cerebrovascular disease in the vertebrobasilar system	Ipsilateral loss of pain and temperature sensations of the face Contralateral spastic arm and leg paresis/plegia Ipsilateral cerebellar signs
Hypoglossal nuclear palsy	Intramedullary tumor Cerebrovascular disease in the vertebrobasilar system	Contralateral loss of position sense and vibration in the arm and leg Contralateral spastic hemispheresis/plegia

cular occlusion, tumor, aneurysm, tuberculosis, or hemorrhage.

The anterior horn cells and the motor nuclei of the cranial nerves may be secondarily affected in many severe pathologic processes that primarily involve the peripheral nerves. The pathology may extend proximally to affect the nerve roots or rootlets and the motor neurons themselves, a process commonly seen, for example, in Guillain-Barré syndrome. If sufficient numbers of motor neurons are destroyed, permanent loss of motor function results because regeneration of the damaged axons requires a living neuronal cell body.

A group of degenerative disorders principally cause progressive motor cell atrophy. One of these is **progressive spinal muscular atrophy** in which the anterior horn cells of the spinal cord are the affected motor neurons. This disorder occurs in adults and closely resembles the familial progressive muscular atrophies that occur in infants and children and are considered inherited metabolic disorders (see Chapter 15). If the motor nuclei of the cranial nerves are affected instead of the anterior horn cells, the disorder is labeled **progressive bulbar palsy,** so named because the myelencephalon was originally called the bulb and a degenerative process causes a progressively more serious condition. When any lower motor neuron syndrome involves the cranial nerves that arise from the bulb (i.e., cranial nerves IX, X, and XII), the dysfunction is called a **bulbar palsy.**

The clinical manifestations of bulbar palsy include paresis or paralysis of the jaw, face, pharynx, and tongue musculature. Articulation is affected, especially articulation of the lingual (r, n, l), labial (b, m, p, f), dental (d, t), and pallatal (k, g) consonants. Modulation is impaired, making the voice rasping or nasal. Pharyngeal reflexes are diminished or lost. Palate and vocal cord movement during phonation is impaired, and chewing and swallowing are affected. The facial muscles are weak, and the face appears to droop. The jaw jerk is decreased. Atrophy eventually becomes apparent, as do fasciculations. All these manifestations become progressively worse, leading to aspiration, malnutrition, possible dehydration, and an inability to communicate verbally.

Radiculopathies

When the ventral root composed of the axons emerging from the anterior horn cells of the spinal cord is affected by a pathologic process, the condition is called a **radiculopathy.** One or many roots may be affected. The strength, tone, and bulk of the muscles innervated by the involved roots are affected. The pattern and distribution of weakness and atrophy are similar to those of the amyotrophies. Tone and deep-tendon reflexes are decreased but rarely absent because the involved muscles usually are innervated by two or more spinal roots. Fasciculations are often present, and mild fatigue may be experienced. Because pathologic processes usually affect both the ventral and dorsal roots, sensory alterations are common. (Specific radiculopathies are discussed in Chapter 15.)

Neuropathies

When the peripheral nerves are affected by a pathologic process, the disorder is called a **neuropathy** or a **neuritis** when an inflammatory process is involved. Many pathologic processes may give rise to neuropathies, and one or many nerves may be involved. Sites of injury include the peripheral nerves formed from the spinal roots, the cranial nerves, or both systems of nerves.

When the axons are affected, muscle strength, muscle tone, and muscle bulk are also affected. Whole muscles or groups of muscles are paretic or paralyzed, and the muscles of the feet and legs are often affected first and more severely. These long, large axons are thought (1) to be more vulnerable to injury because of their size and length, (2) have more Schwann cells available to be injured, and (3) exhibit a "dying back" phenomenon due to the difficulty of nerve cell body in maintaining the terminal portion of the axon. If unchecked, the pathologic process tends to involve the hands and arms because these are the next longest and largest axons.

Tone and the deep tendon reflexes in the affected muscles are generally decreased in a neuropathy. Atrophy is distributed according to the peripheral nerves involved. The degree and distribution of the atrophy probably depends on the extent of the injury. Fasciculation may be present, especially with associated ventral root, motor neuron changes, or both as in Guillain-Barré syndrome, diabetic neuropathy, and porphyric neuropathy. Mild fatigue may be experienced. A few disorders, notably Guillain-Barré syndrome, produce a pattern of paresis and paralysis that involves all limbs, the trunk, and the neck. Peripheral bifacial and other cranial nerve palsies may be seen with a variety of disorders. Tenderness of the nerve trunks and associated sensory alterations help to distinguish neuropathy from amyotrophy. (Specific neuropathies are discussed in Chapter 15.)

Neuromuscular Junction Syndromes

Transmission of the nerve impulse at the neuromuscular junction requires the release of adequate amounts of neurotransmitter from the presynaptic terminals of the axon and effective binding of the released transmitter to the receptors on the membranes of muscle cells (Fig. 12-13). Nutritional deficits, certain drugs (e.g., reserpine or aldomet), and certain disorders that interfere with the synthesis or packaging of the neurotransmitter or its release into the synaptic cleft may result in weakness. Likewise, any pathologic process or drug that interferes with the binding of the neurotransmitter to the receptor may cause weakness.

Marked weakness results from interference with neuromuscular transmission. The distribution of affected muscles is mainly in the bulbar, respiratory, and proximal muscle groups. Botulism toxin has a predilection for the cranial nerves. Eaton-Lambert syndrome affects limb musculature, whereas myasthenia gravis predominantly involves ocular, bulbar, and proximal upper extremity muscles. There is marked fatigability. Muscle tone may be slightly reduced, as may deep tendon reflexes, but the muscle cells are not denervated. Atrophy,

if present, is only mild, probably because the small motor system is intact so that tone is maintained to a large degree. Fasciculations or sensory alterations are not present.

The weakness associated with presynaptic dysfunction, as in botulism or Eaton-Lambert syndrome, and that associated with postsynaptic dysfunction, as in myasthenia gravis, are difficult to distinguish clinically, although theoretically some difference should be evident. (Specific disorders are discussed in Chapter 15.)

Myopathies

Myopathy is the term applied to a primary muscle disorder. Many pathologic processes affect muscles and cause loss of functional muscle cells. Within myopathies, muscle strength, tone, and bulk are affected.

Primary muscle disease is invariably associated with weakness, usually marked weakness. The distribution of the weakness in myopathy is usually symmetrical and proximal, although occasionally, the weakness is predominantly distal, such as in myotonic dystrophy. The weakness is associated with mild fatigue. Tone is decreased as are the tendon reflexes. Atrophy may be present. Some myopathies are associated with muscle hypertrophy as in cretinism and the familial progressive muscular dystrophies of childhood, in which hypertrophied muscles are rubbery and weak. Fasciculations are not present with myopathy because no denervation is present. No sensory changes are found. (Specific myopathies are discussed in Chapter 39.)

ALTERATIONS IN EMOTIONS AND EMOTIONAL CONTROL

Emotions such as anger, hostility, envy, fear, and love all guide behavior and are largely mediated by the limbic system. Alterations in emotions or emotional control arise from dysfunction in the limbic system, in the hypothalamus, which choreographs the behaviors that accompany emotional states, or in the cerebral cortex, especially the neural tracts of the frontal lobes, which project to the limbic system to exert inhibiting and modulating effects. Changes in the physical, chemical, or electrical status of the frontal lobes, limbic system, or hypothalamus may be associated with significant changes in emotions and behavior. Changes in emotions and behavior can result from abscesses, tumors, hemorrhages, metabolic disorders, and intoxication states.

Pathophysiology

Damage to the frontal lobes and frontolimbic tracts that project inhibitory influences to the limbic system free the limbic system and leave it unchecked to generate an array of emotions. Behavior then becomes erratic and unpredictable. Pathology within the limbic system itself may produce a deficiency in emotional response, either a lack of arousability (as in the depressive disorder) or excessive arousability, as in certain psychomotor seizures or acute anxiety states.

Hypothalamic dysfunction may excessively arouse the limbic system by supplying too much epinephrine, the fear-producing hormone and neurotransmitter, to the limbic system, resulting in an acute anxiety state or producing associated behaviors without inducing the feelings. For example, tumors involving the tracts projecting from the hypothalamus are associated with raging behaviors, but the feeling of anger or rage is not present.

Clinical Manifestations

Common among all types of frontal lobe damage is a change in the experience and expression of emotion. The clinical manifestations associated with frontal lobe dysfunction range from excessive, seemingly purposeless activity to spontaneity. Irritability, impulsiveness, mood swings, mood shifts, inability to tolerate frustration, and loss of control are frequent. Clinical manifestations can include depression, mania, hyperactivity, acute anxiety, acute confusional states, and dementia.

Evaluation and Treatment

Evaluation of alterations in emotion include several strategies: physical and psychologic examinations, computerized tomography (CT) scans, magnetic resonance imaging (MRI), electroencephalogram (EEG), and appropriate blood chemistries. Treatment is directed at preventing injury, including suicide, medically or surgically treating the underlying cause, instituting appropriate drug therapy and psychotherapy, and providing support and guidance to the family. Drugs used to achieve symptomatic control alter the levels of neurotransmitters with the brain tissues. For example, diazepam (Valium) and other drugs compete for the receptors ordinarily occupied by epinephrine so that level of arousal is decreased.

ALTERATIONS IN UNIFOCAL CORTICAL FUNCTION

Agnosias

Agnosia is a defect of recognition, a failure to recognize the form and nature of objects. The disorder involves the loss of recognition through one sense, although the object or person may still be recognized by

---

TABLE 14-21 Types of agnosia

Type of agnosia	Definition	Location of injury
Tactile agnosia (astereognosia)	Inability to recognize objects by touch	Parietal lobe
Spatial agnosia	Incapacity to find one's way around familiar places	Parietal lobe
Body image agnosias		
Anosognosia	Ignorance or denial of the existence of the disease	Right parietal lobe
Autotopagnosia	Loss of ability to identify the body, in whole or in part or to recognize relationships between various parts	Right parietal lobe
Prosopagnosia	Inability to recognize human faces	Temporooccipital region
Visual agnosia	Inability to recognize objects and pictures and human faces	Temporoparietooccipital area
Word blindness (alexia)	Inability to recognize written symbols	Left parietotemporal region
Color agnosia	Inability to understand colors as qualities of objects, faulty color concepts, and inability to evoke color images in the absence of color blindness	Occipital lobe; posterior corpus callosum
Auditory agnosia (pure word deafness)	Inability to recognize speech sounds	Superior temporal area
Amusia (music deafness)	Loss of capacity to recognize tones and melodies	Right superior temporal area
Gertsmann syndrome		Left angular gyrus
Finger agnosia	Inability to identify the names of one's fingers	
Right-left confusion	Inability to distinguish right from left	
Agraphia	Inability to write	
Acalculia	Inability to perform math calculations	

other senses. Agnosias may be tactile, visual, or auditory. For example, an individual may be unable to identify a safety pin by touching it with a hand but is able to name it when looking at it. Agnosias may be as minimal as a finger agnosia (failure to identify by name the fingers of one's hand) to as devastating as complete denial of hemiplegia.

Agnosias are produced by dysfunction in the primary sensory area or in the interpretive areas of the cerebral cortex (Fig. 12-5) (The types of agnosias and the associated area that is most commonly involved are presented in Table 14-21.) Although agnosias are most commonly associated with cerebrovascular accidents, ag-

---

TABLE 14-22 The dyspraxias

Types of dyspraxia	Description of dyspraxia	Location of dyspraxia
DYSPRAXIAS DESCRIBING THE COMPONENTS OF A MOTOR ACT		
Ideational dyspraxia	Impairment in ability to comprehend, grasp an idea, or retain the idea of the described act	Diffuse cortical injury
Ideomotor dyspraxia	Impairment in ability to perform a given motor act correctly (but habitual motor acts may be performed spontaneously or repetitiously)	Associated with left hemisphere dysfunction in the posteriosuperior area of temporal lobe and in the inferior areas of parietal and frontal lobes
Motor (limb kinetic) dyspraxia	Impairment in use of kinesthetic memory patterns (engrams) necessary to perform a motor act. Automatic tone and position changes necessary for action do not occur	Associated with premotor area dysfunction
DYSPRAXIAS RELATED TO SPECIFIC TYPES OF MOTOR ACTIVITY		
Constructional dyspraxia	Impairment in ability to draw or use shapes and designs accurately	May occur with visual association area dysfunction and with posterior parietal lobe injury, more severe when right posterior hemisphere is involved rather than left hemisphere because right parietooccipital area controls visual–spatial orientation
Dressing dyspraxia	Impairment in ability to clothe oneself correctly. Agnosia and neglect syndrome contribute to dressing dyspraxia and may be entirely responsible for its occurrence	Associated with right parietal injury
Speech dyspraxia (dyspraxia of speech)	An articulation disorder resulting from impairment of capacity to program positioning of speech musculature and sequencing of muscle movements for volitional production of speech sounds (phonemes). A motor dyspraxia	Associated with dysfunction in Broca's area in left hemisphere
	When involvement is more extensive than just the muscles used in speech articulation, the dysfunction is called facial dyspraxia	Associated with dysfunction in Broca's area and premotor areas controlling the facial muscles
Gait dyspraxia (dyspraxia of gait, frontal lobe ataxia, frontal lobe gait)	Impairment in ability to use extremities effectively and in coordinated manner when ambulating, producing a low, shuffled gait with small and hesitant steps	Associated with loss of integration between cortex and basal ganglion related to stance and locomotion. Not a true dyspraxia because dysfunction is not purely cortical
Callosal dyspraxia	An ideomotor dyspraxia where right arm and leg use is normal but with impairment in ability to perform the same movements with left arm and leg	Associated with anterior corpus callosum injury

nosias may arise from any pathologic process that injures the specific areas of the brain.

Sensory inattentiveness is a mild form of agnosia and may be visual, auditory, or tactile. The person with sensory inattentiveness is able to recognize individual sensory input from the dysfunctional side when called upon to do so but ignores (i.e., neglects, extinguishes) the sensory input from the dysfunctional side when stimulated from both sides. This phenomenon is called **extinction.** The entire complex of denial of dysfunction, loss of recognition of one's own body parts, and extinction is sometimes referred to as the **neglect syndrome.**

Dyspraxia

Dyspraxia, impairment in the execution of a planned motor act in the absence of paresis/paralysis, ataxia, sensory loss, or lack of comprehension may be seen in association with vascular disorders, trauma, tumor, degenerative disorders, infections, and metabolic disorders. Because the performance of any activity is composed of three parts, (1) the development of the idea, (2) the formulation of the plan of execution, and (3) the motor performance of the activity, three types of dyspraxia have been described (Table 14-22).

True dyspraxias arise when the connecting pathways between the left and right cortical areas are interrupted (Fig. 14-10). Dyspraxias may arise from any pathologic process that disrupts the cortical areas necessary for the conceptualization and execution of a complex motor act or the communication pathways within the left hemisphere or between the hemispheres.

Dysphasia

Dysphasia is impairment of comprehension or production of language. With dysphasia, comprehension or use of symbols, in either written or verbal language, is disturbed or lost. **Aphasia** is *loss* of the comprehension or production of language.

Dysphasias are usually associated with cerebrovascular accident involving the middle cerebral artery or one of its many branches. The language disorders may, however, arise from a variety of injuries and diseases—vascular, neoplastic, traumatic, degenerative, metabolic, or infectious. Dysphasia results from dysfunction in the left cerebral hemisphere most commonly in the frontotemporal region, particularly around the insula (see Fig. 14-10 and 14-11, and Fig. 12-5). Most language disorders are due to acute processes that either resolve or cause a

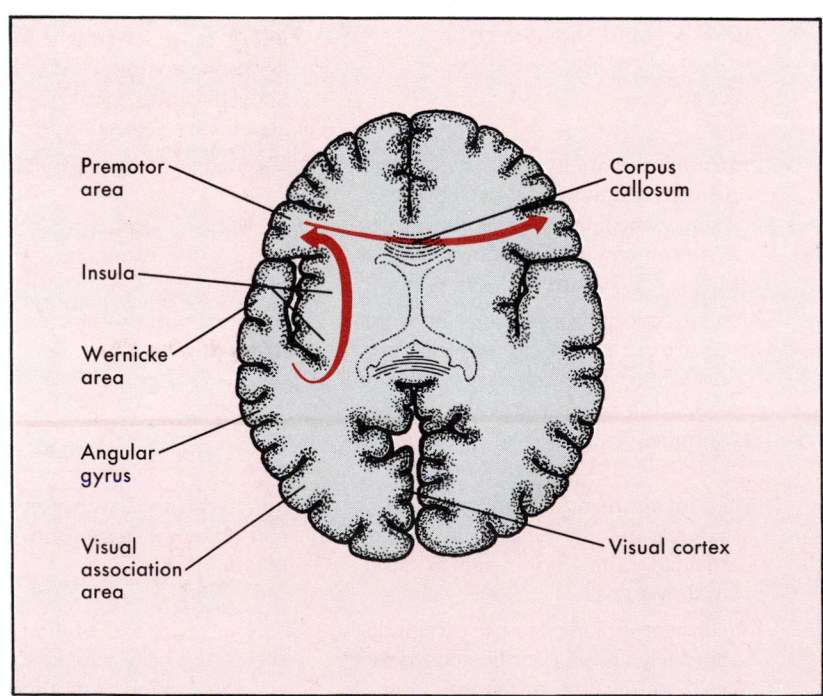

FIG. 14-10. Pathways disrupted in dyspraxias. Formulation of the idea of the motor act is believed to originate in the region of the supramarginal gyrus in the inferior left parietal lobe. This area is connected via associational pathways to the left premotor cortex. The left premotor cortex is connected through the corpus callosum to the right premotor and motor areas. An injury that interrupts the pathways between the left supramarginal gyrus and the premotor region produces a dyspraxia that involves the entire body. An injury that disrupts the callosal pathways produces a dyspraxia of the left side of the body only.

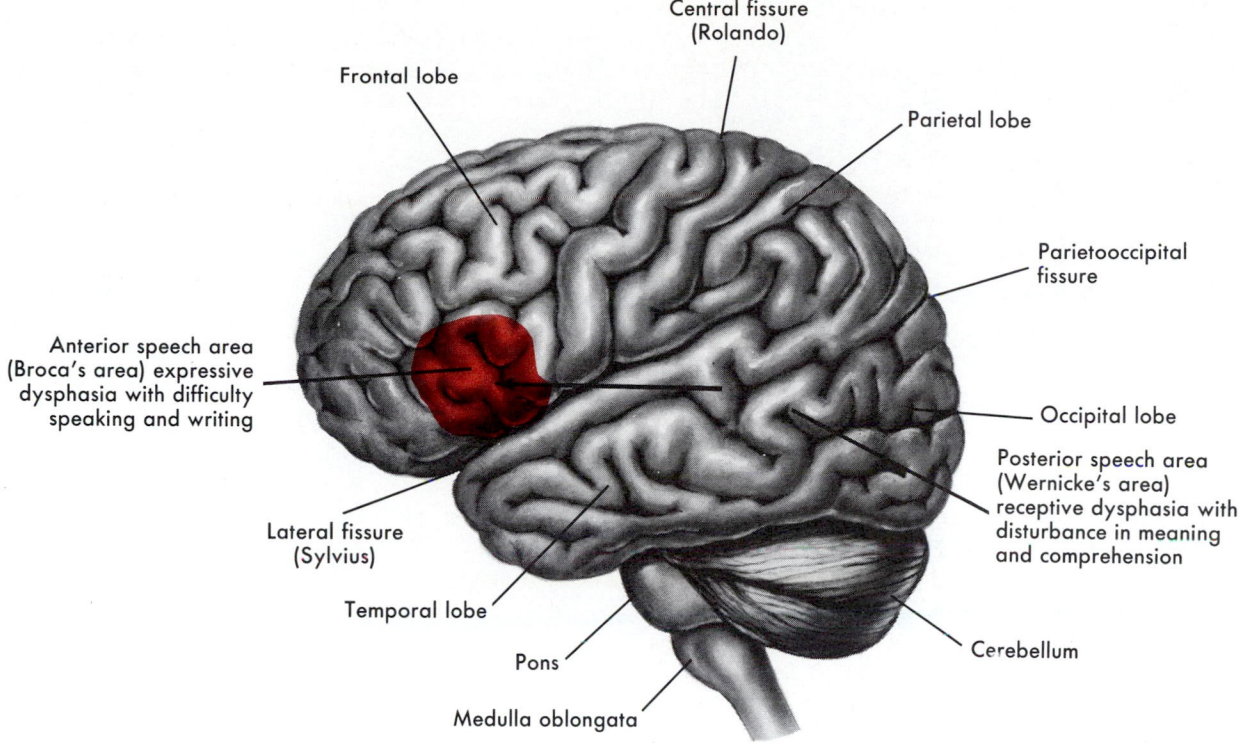

FIG. 14-11. Portion of the left cerebral hemisphere considered most important in the development of dysphasia. Arrow indicates link between two speech areas. (From Thompson, et al., 1989.)

chronic residual deficit. Some language disorders are due to degenerative disorders that make the dysfunction progressive.

Dysphasias have been classified both anatomically and functionally. Other classifications are linguistics and describe fluency, volume, or quantity of speech. Pure forms of any language dysfunction, however, are very rare. **Expressive dysphasias** are primarily characterized by expressive deficits, but a verbal comprehension (auditory-receptive element) deficit may be present. Receptive dysphasias have expressive deficits. (Table 14-23 compares types of dysphasias; Table 14-24 illustrates some of the language disturbances.)

Dysphasias referred to as **transcortical dysphasias (transcortical sensory dysphasia, mixed transcortical dysphasia, isolated speech center)** involve the ability to repeat (called **echolalia**) and to recite. Speech is fluent but with striking paraphrases. The individual is unable to read and write, and comprehension is impaired.

Transcortical dysphasias are caused by hypoxia from prolonged hypotension, carbon monoxide poisoning, or other mechanisms that destroy the border zone (watershed area) between the anterior, middle, and posterior cerebral arteries (Fig. 12-18). Blood supply is marginal in this region. Hypoxia in this area may occasionally isolate the posterior speech areas or all the speech areas from the remainder of the cortex, although both areas remain intact. The sensory and motor speech areas are, therefore, functional, but connections with other sensory or motor areas are impaired. Information from the remaining areas of the cortex cannot be transmitted to Wernicke area to be transformed into language.

ALTERATIONS IN CEREBRAL HOMEOSTASIS

Increased Intracranial Pressure

Intracranial pressure is normally 5 to 15 mm Hg or 60 to 180 cm H_2O. Increased intracranial pressure may result from an increase in intracranial content (as occurs with tumor growth), edema, excess cerebrospinal fluid, or hemorrhage. A rise in intracranial pressure necessitates an equal reduction in volume of the other contents. The most readily displaced content of the cranial vault is cerebrospinal fluid (CSF). After CSF displacement out of the cranial vault, if intracranial pressure still remains high, cerebral blood volume is altered, called stage 1 of intracranial hypertension. Vasoconstriction and external compression of the venous system occurs in an attempt to further decrease the intracranial pressure. Thus, during the first stage of intracranial hypertension, intracranial pressure may not change because of the effective compensatory mechanism. Cerebrospinal fluid is

TABLE 14-23 Major types of dysphasia

	Expression	Verbal Comprehension	Repetition	Name	Reading comprehension	Writing	Location of lesion	Cause of lesion
EXPRESSIVE (Broca's, motor)	Nonfluent; impairment of ability to find words, difficulty in writing	Relatively intact	Impaired	Impaired	Variable	Impaired	Posterior–inferior frontal lobe (Broca's area)	Occlusion of inferior division of left middle cerebral artery
RECEPTIVE (Wernicke's sensory)	Fluent: able to produce verbal language but language is meaningless; words are often inappropriate; words with similar sounds or words with similar meaning are substituted for the correct words; words that are not part of the language may be present; these neologisms may be so extensive as to make the speech entirely incomprehensible; because the person has no means to monitor the language for correctness, errors are not recognized; intonation, accent, cadence, rhythm, and articulation are normal	Impaired (Disturbance in understanding all language)	Impaired	Impaired	Impaired	Impaired	Posterior–superior temporal lobe (Wernicke's area)	
(word deafness or auditory verbal agnosia, sensory)	Fluent; self-initiated speech is normal	Impaired; hears noise rather than language; language has no meaning and is perceived as foreign	Impaired, unable to repeat what is said	Impaired	Intact; able to read	Intact; able to write	Pathways connecting the primary auditory cortex and the auditory association areas in the middle third of the left superior temporal gyrus	Small, superficial injury typically associated with occlusion of a branch of the middle cerebral artery

GLOBAL (sensory–motor, receptive–expressive)	Nonfluent; produces little speech; at best speaks a few words or phrases	Impaired or completely lost; person understands only the simplest things said	Impaired; not able to repeat	Impaired	Impaired or completely lost	Impaired: produces little written language	Frontotemporal lobe; anterior and posterior speech areas extensively impaired	Occlusion of the left middle cerebral artery of left internal carotid artery; tumors, other mass lesions, and hemorrhage may cause
CONDUCTION	Fluence but with paraphrasia in self-initiated speech, writing or reading aloud	Relatively intact	Impaired; not able to repeat	Impaired	Variable	Impaired	Arcuate fasciculus, supramarginal gyrus, disruption of the large bundle of fibers that arise from the temporal lobe and pass posteriorly around the sylvian fissure and then project anteriorly to the premotor area	Typical cause an embolic occlusion of the ascending parietal or posterior temporal branch of the middle cerebral artery
NOMINAL (anomic)	Fluent but impaired ability to name objects, persons, qualities or characteristics; know what wants to say but cannot find words; may even use desired word in another context but still cannot isolate word when needed	Relatively intact; able to recognize word when it is given	Intact	Impaired	Variable	Variable	Angular gyrus posterior–superior temporal lobe	
TRANSCORTICAL MOTOR	Nonfluent	Relatively intact	Intact	Impaired	Variable	Impaired	Anterior presylvian fissure	
TRANSCORTICAL SENSORY	Fluent	Impaired	Intact	Impaired	Impaired	Impaired	Posterior presylvian fissure	

From Mancall, 1981.

TABLE 14-24 Examples of language disturbances

Disorder		Example
Verbal paraphasia	Question:	What did the car do?
	Patient:	The car would spit sweetly down the road. (The car sped swiftly down the road.)
Literal paraphasia	Request:	Say "persistence is essential to success."
	Patient:	Mesastence is instans to success.
Neologism	Question:	What do you call this? (Pointing to a plant.)
	Patient:	It's a logper.
Circumlotion	Question:	What do you call this? (Pointing to a plant.)
	Patient:	Something that grows.
Anomia	Question:	What do you call this? (Pointing to a plant.)
	Patient:	It's - - - - - - - - -
		or
	Question:	What did you do this morning?
	Patient:	Reading.
	Question:	Were you reading a book or a newspaper?
	Patient:	One of those.
Telegraphic Style	Question:	Where is your daughter?
	Patient:	New Orleans . . . home . . . Monday.

From Boss, 1984.

reduced through increased reabsorption. Blood volume is reduced by compression of intracranial veins. Small increases in volume cause a dramatic increase in pressure and the pressure may take longer to return to baseline. Clinical manifestations at this stage are usually subtle and often transient and include episodes of confusion, drowsiness, and slight pupillary and breathing changes.

If intracranial pressure is still high, a state of intracranial hypertension occurs. With continued expansion of the intracranial content, the resulting increase in intracranial pressure may exceed the brain's compensatory capacity to adjust to the increasing pressure. In this state, the pressure begins to compromise neuronal oxygenation and systemic arterial vasoconstriction occurs in an attempt to elevate the systemic blood pressure sufficiently to overcome the increased intracranial pressure. This stage is called stage 2 of intracranial hypertension.

As intracranial pressure begins to approach arterial pressure, the brain tissues begin to experience hypoxia and hypercapnia—the individual rapidly deteriorates. Clinical manifestations include decreasing levels of consciousness, Cheyne-Stokes respirations and/or central neurogenic hyperventilation, pupils that become sluggish and dilated, widened pulse pressure, and bradycardia.

Dramatic sustained rises in intracranial pressure are not seen until all the compensatory mechanisms have been exhausted. Once decompensation begins, dramatic rises in intracranial pressure occur over a very short period of time. Autoregulation, the compensatory alteration in the diameter of the intracranial blood vessels designed to maintain a constant blood flow during changes in cerebral perfusion pressure, is lost with progressively increased intracranial pressure. Accumulating CO_2 may still cause vasodilatation at the local tissue level but now without autoregulation this vasodilatation causes the hydrostatic (blood) pressure in the vessels to drop and blood volume to increase. The brain volume is thus further enhanced and intracranial pressure continues to rise. This is called stage 3 of intracranial hypertension. Small increases in volume cause dramatic increases in intracranial pressure and the pressure takes longer to return to baseline. As the intracranial pressure begins to approach systemic blood pressure, cerebral perfusion pressure falls and cerebral perfusion slows dramatically. The brain tissues experience severe hypoxia and acidosis.

Increased intracranial pressure in one compartment of the cranial vault is not evenly distributed throughout the other vault compartments. In the last stage of intracranial hypertension, called stage 4 of intracranial hypertension, brain tissue shifts (herniates) from the compartment of greater pressure to a compartment of lesser pressure (Fig. 14-12). With this shift in brain tissue, the

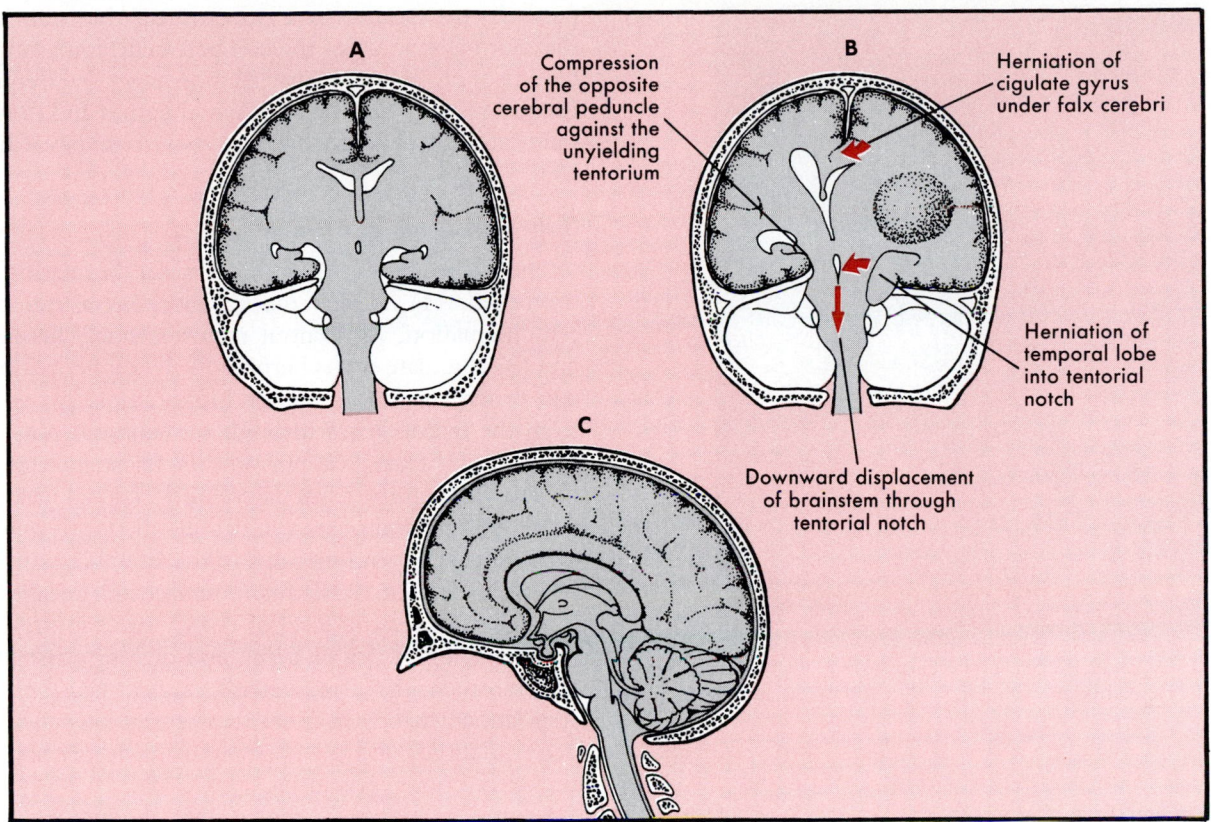

FIG. 14-12. Herniation. **A,** The normal relationship of intracranial structures. **B,** Shift of intracranial structures. **C,** Downward herniation of the cerebellar tonsils into the foramen magnum.

herniating brain tissue's blood supply is compromised causing further ischemia and hypoxia in the herniating tissues. The herniated brain tissues increase the volume of content within the lower pressure compartment exerting pressure on the brain tissue that normally occupies that compartment, thus impairing that tissue's blood supply. Small hemorrhages frequently develop in the involved brain tissue. Obstructive hydrocephalus may develop. The herniation process markedly and rapidly increases intracranial pressure. Mean systolic arterial pressure soon equals intracranial pressure and cerebral blood flow ceases at this point.

Cerebral Edema

Cerebral edema is an increase in the fluid content of brain tissue (Fig. 14-13). Cerebral edema causes an increase in extracellular or intracellular tissue volume after brain insult from trauma, infection, hemorrhage, tumor, ischemia, infarct, or hypoxia. The harmful effects of cerebral edema are caused by the distortion of blood vessels, the displacement of brain tissues, and the eventual herniation of brain tissue from one brain compartment to another.

Four types of cerebral edema are (1) vasogenic edema, (2) cytotoxic (metabolic) edema, (3) ischemic edema, and (4) interstitial edema. Vasogenic edema is clinically the most important type. It is caused by the increased permeability of the capillary endothelium of the brain after injury to the vascular structure. The result is a disruption in the blood-brain barrier. Plasma proteins leak into the extracellular spaces, drawing water to them, and the water content of the brain parenchyma increases. Vasogenic edema starts in the area of injury and spreads with preferential accumulation in the white matter of the ipsilateral side because the parallel myelinated fibers separate more easily. Edema then promotes more edema because of ischemia from increasing pressure.

Clinical manifestations of vasogenic edema include focal neurologic deficits, disturbances of consciousness, and a severe increase in intracranial pressure. Vasogenic edema resolves by slow diffusion.

In cytotoxic (metabolic) edema, toxic factors directly affect the cellular elements of the brain parenchyma (neuronal, glial, and endothelial cells), causing failure of the active transport systems. The cells lose their potas-

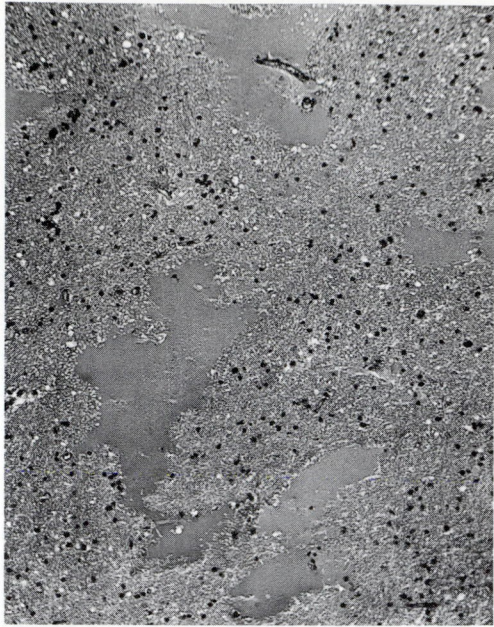

FIG. 14-13. Brain edema. Intercellular lakes of high protein content fluid. (Hematoxylin and eosin; × 90.) (From Kissane, 1985.)

sium and gain larger amounts of sodium. Water follows by osmosis into the cell, so that the cells swell. Cytotoxic edema principally occurs in the gray matter and may enhance vasogenic edema.

Ischemic edema follows cerebral infarction. The ischemia has components of both vasogenic and cytotoxic edema. Soon after the onset of ischemia, the initial edema is confined to the intracellular compartment. During the following hours and then over several days, brain cells begin to undergo necrosis and die, releasing lysosomes. In this autodigestive process, the blood-brain barrier's permeability is increased.

Interstitial edema is most often seen with noncommunicating hydrocephalus (see Chapter 15). The edema is caused by transependymal movement of cerebrospinal fluid from the ventricles into the extracellular spaces of the brain tissues. The brain fluid volume is thus increased predominantly around the ventricles. The hydrostatic pressure within the white matter increases, and the size of the white matter is reduced because of the rapid disappearance of myelin lipids.

Herniation Syndromes

Increased pressure in one compartment of the cranial vault is not evenly distributed among the other brain compartments (Fig. 14-12). Instead, the brain tissues shift (herniate) from the compartment of greater pressure to the compartment of a lower pressure. The herniating brain's blood supply is compromised, producing further ischemia and hypoxia. In addition, the herniated parenchymal tissues exert pressure on the brain tissue that normally occupies the compartment, impairing that blood supply as well. Small hemorrhages are frequently found in the involved parenchymal tissues and noncommunicating hydrocephalus may also occur (see Chapter 15).

Supratentorial Herniation

The three types of supratentorial herniation syndromes are (1) uncal (temporal lobe, lateral transtentorial) herniation, (2) central (transtentorial) herniation, and (3) cingulate gyrus herniation. Uncal herniation occurs when the uncus and/or hippocampal gyrus shifts from the middle fossa through the tentorial notch into the posterior fossa, compressing the ipsilateral third cranial nerve, then the contralateral third cranial nerve, and finally the mesencephalon. Uncal herniation is generally caused by an expanding mass in the lateral region of the middle fossa. The classic manifestations of uncal herniation are a decreasing level of consciousness, pupils that become sluggish before fixing and dilating (first the ipsilateral then the contralateral pupil), Cheyne-Stokes respirations (which later shift to central neurogenic hyperventilation), and the appearance of decorticate, then later decerebrate, posturing.

Central herniation is the straight downward shift of the diencephalon through the tentorial notch. Causes of central herniation are injuries or masses located around the outer perimeter of the frontal, parietal, or occipital lobes, extracerebral injuries around the central apex (top) of the cranium, bilaterally positioned injuries or masses, and unilateral cingulate gyrus herniation. The individual experiencing transtentorial herniation rapidly passes from a conscious to an unconscious state; from Cheyne-Stokes respirations to apnea; from small, reactive pupils to dilated and fixed pupils; and from decortication to decerebration.

Cingulate gyrus herniation occurs when the cingulate gyrus shifts under the falx cerebri. Little is known about the clinical manifestations of this type of herniation.

Infratentorial Herniation

Two types of infratentorial herniation syndromes may occur. In the most common infratentorial herniation syndrome, a cerebellar tonsil(s) shift(s) through the foramen magnum because of increased pressure within the posterior fossa. The clinical manifestations of this downward infratentorial herniation are an arched stiff neck, paresthesias in the shoulder area, decreased consciousness, respiratory abnormalities, and pulse rate variations. Occasionally, the pressure force is such that an upward transtentorial herniation of a cerebellar tonsil or the lower brainstem results. No specific set of clinical manifestations are associated with this infratentorial herniation syndrome.

SUMMARY REVIEW

Alterations in Consciousness

1 Consciousness is an awareness of oneself and the environment with an ability to respond to external stimuli.
2 Decreased level of consciousness occurs by diffuse bilateral cortical dysfunction, bilateral subcortical (reticular formation, brainstem) dysfunction, and localized hemispheric dysfunction.
3 An alteration in breathing pattern and level of coma reflect the level of brain dysfunction.
4 Pupillary changes reflect changes in level of brainstem function, drug action, and response to hypoxia and ischemia.
5 Pathologic eye movements, including nystagmus and divergent gaze, reflect alterations in brainstem function.
6 Level of brain function is manifested by changes in generalized motor responses or no responses.
7 Loss of cortical inhibition associated with decreased consciousness includes abnormal flexor and extensor movements.
8 Cerebral death or irreversible coma represents permanent brain damage with an ability to maintain cardiac, respiratory, and other vital functions.
9 Brain death results from irreversible brain damage with an inability to maintain internal hemeostasis.
10 Clouding of consciousness (decreased awareness), delirium, and acute confusional states result in alterations in thought content and may result from drug intoxication, febrile illness, heart failure, or brain injury.
11 Subacute or chronic alterations in consciousness include dementia, hypersomnia, and vegetative states.
12 Alzheimer disease is a chronic irreversible dementia that may be related to genetic or viral etiologies.
13 Seizures represent a sudden, chaotic discharge of cerebral neurons with transient alterations in brain function. Seizures may be generalized or focal and can result from cerebral lesions, biochemical disorders, trauma, or epilepsy.

Alterations in Motor Function

1 Dysfunction of the cerebral cortex, pyramidal system, or extrapyramidal system causes motor dysfunction.
2 Clinical manifestations of motor dysfunction include muscle atrophy or hypertrophy, paresis, and paralysis.
3 Dystonia and decerebrate or decorticate posturing represents cortical and brainstem abnormalities.
4 Alteration in movements include akinesia, hypokinesia, bradykinesia, hyperkinesia, dyskinesia, and tremors.
5 Two general motor syndromes are CNS motor syndromes and motor unit syndromes.
6 Pyramidal motor syndromes usually involve upper motor neurons, and symptoms relate to location of the lesion.
7 Interruption of the pyramidal tract below the pons results in spinal shock.
8 Extrapyramidal motor syndromes include basal ganglia and cerebellar motor syndromes.

9 Basal ganglia disorders are manifested by alterations in muscle tone and posture, including rigidity, involuntary movements, and loss of postural reflexes.
10 Cerebellar motor syndromes result in loss of muscle tone, difficulty with coordination, and disorders of equilibrium and gait.
11 Lower motor neuron (LMN) syndromes are manifested by impaired voluntary and involuntary movements. Partial paralysis occurs with only partial loss of alpha motor neurons and total paralysis is complete loss of alpha motor units. Loss of gamma motor neurons impairs muscle tone and decreases tendon reflexes.
12 Amyotrophies (i.e., poliomyelitis) is an LMN syndrome involving the anterior horn cells with loss of muscle tone and strength resulting in segmental paresis and hyporeflexia.
13 Nuclear palsies involve damage to the cranial nerve nuclei.
14 Bulbar palsies involve cranial nerves IX, X, and XII.
15 Radiculopathies develop from lesions in the ventral root axons of anterior horn cells with muscle weakness and atrophy.
16 Neuropathies are disorders of peripheral nerves resulting in loss of muscle strength, tone, and bulk with decreased deep tendon reflexes.
17 Interference with transmission of impulses at the neuromuscular junction causes weakness from blockage or inadequate release of neurotransmitters.
18 Primary disorders of muscle with weakness and atrophy are known as myopathies.

Alterations in Emotions and Emotional Control

1 Disorders of the frontal lobes, limbic system, or hypothalamus may be associated with a broad range of changes in emotion and behavior.

Alterations in Unifocal Cortical Function

1 Agnosias are a defect of recognition and may be tactile, visual, or auditory and are due to dysfunction in the primary sensory area or the interpretive areas of the cerebral cortex.
2 Dyspraxia is an impairment of the conceptualization or execution of a complex motor act.
3 Dysphasia is an impairment of comprehension or production of language. Dysphasia may be expressive or sensory.
4 Aphasia is loss of language comprehension or production.
5 Wernicke dysphasia is a disturbance in understanding all language, both verbal and reading comprehension.
6 Conductive dysphasias result from disruption of temporal lobe fibers with a failure to repeat words but an ability to initiate speech, writing, and reading aloud.
7 Anomic dysphasia is an inability to name objects, persons, or qualities.
8 Transcortical dysphasias involve an inability to repeat and recite.
9 Broca dysphasia is an expressive dysphasia of speech and writing but with retention of comprehension.

10 Global aphasia involves both anterior and posterior speech areas with both expressive and receptive aphasia.

Alterations in Cerebral Homeostasis

1 Increased intracranial pressure may result from edema, excess cerebrospinal fluid, hemorrhage, or tumor growth. When intracranial pressure approaches arterial pressure, hypoxia and hypercapnia produce brain damage.
2 Cerebral edema is an increase in the fluid content of the brain resulting from infection, hemorrhage, tumor, ischemia, infarct, or hypoxia.
3 The shifting or herniation of brain tissue from one compartment to another disrupts the blood flow of both compartments and damages brain tissue.
4 Supratentorial herniation involves temporal lobe and hippocampal gyrus shifting from the middle fossa to posterior fossa; transtentorial herniation with a downward shift of the diencephalon through the tentorial notch; and when the cingulate gyrus herniation shifts under the falx.
5 The most common infratentorial herniation is a shift of the cerebellar tonsils through the foramen magnum.

KEY TERMS

Acute confusional state, 440

Acute organic brain syndrome (AOBS), 440

Agnosia, 462

Akathisia, 455

Akathitic movement, 455

Akinesia, 452

Alzheimer disease (senile disease complex), 444

Amnestic dementia, 443

Amyotrophy, 459

Anomic dysphasia, 467

Aphasia, 464

Areflexia, 458

Ataxia, 458

Athetosis, 453

Atrophy, 451

Attentional dementia, 443

Aura, 448

Ballism, 453

Basal ganglia motor syndrome, 457

Benign fasciculation, 453

Bradykinesia, 452

Brain death, 440

Bulbar palsy, 460

Cerebellar motor syndrome, 458

Cerebral death, 437

Chorea, 453

Choreoathetosis, 453

Clasp-knife phenomenon,

Clonic phase, 448

Clonus, 453

Clouding of consciousness, 440

Cognitive dementia, 443

Coma, 434

Confusion, 434

Consciousness, 432

Content of thought, 432

Decerebrate posture, 451

Decorticate posture (hemiplegic posture, antigravity posture), 452

Delirium, 440

Dementia, 442

Disorientation, 434

Dyskinesia, 453

Dysmetria, 458

Dysphasia, 464

Dyspraxia, 464

Dystonia, 451

Dystonic movement, 451

Dystonic posture, 451

Echolalia, 465

Epilepsy, 445

Epileptogenic focus, 447

Expressive dysphasia, 465

Extinction, 464

Extrapyramidal motor syndrome, 457

Fasciculation, 453

Fibrillation, 459

Flaccid paresis/paralysis, 458

Flaccidity, 452

Freezing, 452

Gamma neuropathy, 458

Generalized seizure, 446

Global aphasia,

Hemiballism, 453

Hemiparesis, 451

Hemiplegia, 451

Hiccup, 453

Hyperkinesia, 453

Hypersomnia, 442

Hypertonia, 452

Hypertrophy, 451

Hypokinesia,

Hypotonia, 452

Intentional dementia, 443

Intention tremor, 454

Isolated speech center, 465

Lateral cerebellar syndrome, 458

Level of arousal, 432

Literal paraphasia, 468

Locked-in syndrome, 442

Lower motor neuron syndrome, 458

Medial cerebellar syndrome, 458

Mirror focus, 448

Mixed transcortical dysphasia, 465

Muscle cramp,

Myoclonus, 453

Myopathy, 461

Neglect syndrome, 464

Neuritis, 460

Neurofibrillary tangle, 444

Neuropathy, 460

Nuclear palsy, 459

Obtundation, 434

Paralysis, 451

Paraphasia,

Paraplegia, 451

Paresis, 451

Paroxysmal dyskinesia, 454

Paroxysmal dystonia, 454

Paroxysmal kinesigenic choreoathetosis, 454

Partial seizures (focal seizures), 446

Postictal state, 446

Postural tremor, 454

Prodroma, 448

Progressive bulbar palsy, 460

Progressive spinal muscular atrophy, 460

Pyramidal motor syndrome (upper motor neuron syndrome), 455

Quadriplegia, 451

Radiculopathy, 460

Retained utterance,

Rigidity, 452

Secondary generalization, 446

Seizure, 445

Semicoma,

Senile plaques, 444

Sensory inattentiveness, 464

Spasm, 453

Spasticity, 452

Spinal shock, 457

Status epilepticus, 446

Stretch reflex, 451

Stupor, 434

Synkinesia, 455

Tardive dyskinesia, 454

Tic, 453

Tonic phase, 448

Transcortical dysphasia, 465

Transcortical sensory dysphasia, 465

Tremor, 453

Tremor-at-rest, 454

Vegetative state, 442

REFERENCES

Adams, R. D. (1977). The convulsive state and idiopathic epilepsy. In G. W. Thorn et al. (Eds.), *Harrison's principles of internal medicine*. New York: McGraw-Hill.

Adams, R. D. (1983). Coma and related disturbances of consciousness. In R. G. Petersdorf, R. D. Adams, E. Braunwald, K. J. Isselbacher, J. B. Martin, & J. D. Wilson (Eds.), *Harrison's principles of internal medicine*. New York: McGraw-Hill Book Company.

Adams, R. D., & Ashbury, A. K. (1983). Diseases of the peripheral nervous system. In R. G. Petersdorf, R. D. Adams, E. Braunwald, K. J. Isselbacher, J. B. Martin, & J. D. Wilson (Eds.), *Harrison's principles of internal medicine* (pp. 2156-2169). New York: McGraw-Hill Book Company.

Adams, R. D., & Victor, M. (1983). Delirium and other acute confusional states. In R. G. Petersdorf, R. D. Adams, E. Braunwald, K. J. Isselbacher, J. B. Martin, & J. D. Wilson (Eds.), *Harrison's principles of internal medicine* (pp. 131-136). New York: McGraw-Hill Book Company.

Adams, R. D., & Victor, M. (1985). *Principles of neurology*. New York: McGraw-Hill Book Company.

Amato, I. (1986). Alzheimer's disease: Scientists report research advances. *Science News, 130,* 327.

Armstrong, M. E., Howe, J., Smith, A. P., & Shider, M. J. (Eds.). (1979). *McGraw-Hill Nursing Dictionary*. New York: McGraw-Hill Book Company.

Barlow, H. B., & Mollon, J. D. (Eds.). (1982). *The senses*. Cambridge: Cambridge University Press.

Barnes, D. M. (1987). Defect in Alzheimer's is on chromosome 21. *Science, 235,* 846-847.

Berry, D. R., & Borkan, L. (1985). Biochemistry of Alzheimer's disease: A report. *Psychopharmacology Bulletin, 21*(2), 347-355.

Boss, B. J. (1982). Acute mood and behavior disturbances of neurological origin: Acute confusional states. *Journal of Neurosurgical Nursing, 14*(2), 61-68.

Boss, B. J. (1983). The dementias. *Journal of Neurosurgical Nursing, 15*(2), 87-97.

Boss, B. J. (1984). Dysphasia, dyspraxia, and dysarthria: Distinguishing features, Part I. *Journal of Neurosurgical Nursing, 16*(3), 151-160.

Boss, B. J. (1984). Pathogenesis of acute confusional states. In *Proceedings 1984 NTI* (pp. 183-186). Newport Beach, CA: American Association of Critical-Care Nurses.

Boss, B. J. (1984). The nervous system. In J. Howe, E. J. Dickason, S. A. Jones, M. J. Snider, & M. E. Armstrong

(Eds.), *The handbook of nursing* (pp. 669-788). New York: John Wiley & Sons.

Bradley, W. G., & Adams, R. D. (1983). Other major muscle syndromes. In R. G. Petersdorf, R. D. Adams, E. Braunwald, K. J. Isselbacher, J. B. Martin, & J. D. Wilson (Eds.), *Harrison's principles of internal medicine* (pp. 2198-2201). New York: McGraw-Hill Book Comapny.

Bradley, W. G., & Rebeiz, J. J. (1983). Progressive muscular dystrophy and chronic myopathies. In R. G. Petersdorf, R. D. Adams, E. Braunwald, K. J. Isselbacher, J. B. Martin, & J. D. Wilson (Eds.), *Harrison's principles of internal medicine* (pp. 2188-2193). New York: McGraw-Hill Book Company.

Bradley, W. G., & Salam-Adams, M. (1983). Acute and subacute myopathic paralysis. In R. G. Petersdorf, R. D. Adams, E. Braunwald, K. J. Isselbacher, J. B. Martin, & J. D. Wilson (Eds.), *Harrison's principles of internal medicine* (pp. 2184-2187). New York: McGraw-Hill Book Company.

Buchner, D. M., & Larson, E. B. (1987). Falls and fractures in patients with Alzheimer's type dementia. *Journal of the American Medical Association, 257,* 1492-1495.

Campos, R. J., Dimitrijevic, M. M., Faganel, J., & Sharkey, P. C. (1981). Clinical evaluation of the effect of spinal cord stimulation on motor performance in patients with upper motor neuron lesions. *Applied Neurophysiology, 44*(1-3), 141-151.

Cawson, R. A., McCracken, A. W., & Marcus, P. B. (1982). *Pathologic mechanisms and human disease.* St. Louis: C. V. Mosby.

Chusid, J. G. (1970). *Correlative neuroanatomy and functional neurology* (15th ed.) pp. 793. Los Altos, CA: Lange Medical Publications.

Chusid, J. G. (1985). *Correlative neuroanatomy and functional neurology.* Los Altos, CA: Lange Medical Publications.

Coyle, J. T., Price, D. L., & Delong, M. R. (1983). Alzheimer's disease: A disorder of cortical cholinergic innervation. *Science, 217,* 1184-1189.

Crapper, D. R., Quittkat, S., Krishnan, S. S., Dalton, A. J., & DeBeni, U. (1980). Intranuclear aluminum content in Alzheimer's disease, dialysis, encephalopathy, and experimental aluminum encephalopathy. *Acta Neuropathology, 50,* 19-24.

Danison, A. N. (1986). New concepts in relation to the pathophysiology of Alzheimer's disease. In M. Briley, A. Kato, & M. Weber (Eds.), *New concepts in Alzheimer's disease.* London: Macmillan Press, Ltd.

Fahn, S., & Duffy, P. (1977). Parkinson's disease. In E. S. Goldensohn & S. H. Appel (Eds.), *Scientific approaches to clinical neurology* (pp. 1119-1158). Philadelphia: Lea and Febiger.

Field, W. E., & Ruelke, W. (1973). Hallucinations and how to deal with them. *American Journal of Nursing, 73*(4), 638-640.

Fozard, J. L., Wolf, E., Bell, B., McFarland, R. A., & Podolsky, S. (1977). Visual perception and communication. In J. E. Birren & K. W. Schaie (Eds.), *Handbook of the psychology of aging.* New York: Van Nostrand Reinhold.

Frohlich, E. D. (1984). *Pathophysiology - Altered regulatory mechanisms in disease.* Philadelphia: J. B. Lippincott Company.

Gardner, E. (1975). *Fundamentals of neurology: A psychophysiological approach.* Philadelphia: W. B. Saunders Company.

Gilroy, J., & Holiday, P. L. (1982). *Basic neurology.* New York: Macmillan Publishing.

Grzegorczyk, P. B., Jones, S. W., & Mistretta, C. M. (1979). Age-related differences in salt taste acuity. *Journal of Gerontology, 34*(8), 34-840.

Guyton, A. C. (1986). *Textbook of medical physiology.* Philadelphia: W. B. Saunders Company.

Haase, G. R. (1977). Diseases presenting as dementia. In C. E. Wells (Ed.), *Dementia.* Philadelphia: F. A. Davis Company.

Heilman, D. M., Watson, R. T., & Greer, M. (1977). *Handbook for differential diagnosis of neurologic signs and symptoms.* New York: Appleton-Century-Crofts.

Hickey, J. V. (1981). *The clinical practice of neurological and neurosurgical nursing.* Philadelphia: J. B. Lippincott.

Holmes, G. (1939). The cerebellum of man. *Brain, 62,* 1.

Jankovic, J., & Fahn, S. (1980). Physiologic and pathologic tremors. *Annual Internal Medicine, 93,* 460.

Kissane, J. M. (ed.). (1985). *Anderson's Pathology* (8th ed.). St. Louis: C. V. Mosby.

Kolata, G. B. (1981, March). Clues to the causes of senile dementia. *Science, 211,* 1032-1033.

Kolata, G. B. (1983). Clues to Alzheimer's disease emerge. *Science, 219,* 941-942.

Kroner, K. (1979). Dealing with the confused patient. *Nursing, 9*(10), 91-98.

Lehman, E. (1974). Reality orientation, doing it better. *Nursing, 4*(3), 61-62.

Mancall, E. L. (1981). *Alper's and Mancall's essentials of the neurologic examination.* Philadephia: F. A. Davis Company.

Marieb, E. N. (1984). *Essentials of human anatomy and physiology.* Menlo Park, CA: Addison-Wesley.

Mathews, W. B., & Miller, H. (1975). *Diseases of the nervous system.* Oxford: Blackwell Scientific Publications.

McLachlan-Crapper, D. R., & Lewis, P. N. (1985). Alzheimer's disease: Errors in gene expression. *Canadian Journal of Neurological Science, 12,* 1-5.

Morris, M., & Rhodes, M. (1972). Guidelines for the case of confused patients. *American Journal of Nursing, 72*(9), 1632.

Mozar, H. N., Bal, D. G., & Howard, J. T. (1987). Perspectives on the etiology of Alzheimer's disease. *Journal of the American Medical Association, 257,* 1503-1507.

Noback, C. R., & Demarst, R. J. (1981). *The human nervous system: Basic principles of neurobiology.* New York: McGraw-Hill Book Company.

Nursing skillbook: coping with neurologic problems proficiency. (1979). Horsham, PA: Intermed Communications, Inc.

Phipps, W. J., Long, B. C., & Woods, W. F. (1987). *Medical surgical nursing: Concepts and clinical practice.* St. Louis: C. V. Mosby.

Pitts, D. G. (1982). Visual acuity as a function of age. *Journal of the American Optometrists Association, 532*(a), 117-124.

Plorde, J. J. (1983). Trichinosis. In R. G. Petersdorf, R. D. Adams, E. Braunwald, K. J. Isselbacher, J. B. Martin, & J. D. Wilson (Eds.), *Harrison's principles of internal medicine* (pp. 1212-1214). New York: McGraw-Hill Book Company.

Plum, F., & Posner, J. B. (1980). *The diagnosis of stupor and coma*. Philadelphia: F. A. Davis Company.

Porter, R. (Ed.). (1978). *Studies in neurophysiology*. Cambridge: Cambridge University Press.

Purtilo, D. T. (1978). *A survey of human diseases*. Menlo Park, CA: Addison-Wesley Publishing Co.

Rassman, I. (Ed.). (1979). *Clinical geriatrics* (2nd ed.). Philadelphia: J. B. Lippincott.

Reilly, K. M. et al. (1981). Progressive hearing loss in children: Hearing aids and other factors. *Journal of Speech and Hearing Disorders, 463*(8), 328-334.

Resler, M. M., & Tumulty, G. (1983, May). Glaucoma update. *American Journal of Nursing, 83*, 752-765.

Restak, R. M. (1984). *The brain*. New York: Bantam Books.

Rothner, A.D. (Ed.). (1983). *Recent development in the treatment of epilepsy*. North Chicago: Abbott Laboratories.

Rovee, C. K., Cohen, R. Y., & Shlapak, W. (1975). Life-span stability in olfactory sensitivity. *Developmental Psychology, 11*, 311-318.

Rudy, E. B. (1984). *Advanced neurological and neurosurgical nursing*. St. Louis: C. V. Mosby.

Schmidt, R. F. (Ed.). (1977). *Fundamentals of sensory physiology*. New York: Springer-Verlag.

Science News. (1987a). Alzheimer/down syndrome bond tightens. *Science News, 123*, 188.

Science News. (1987b). Inherited membranes predict Alzheimer's. *Science News, 132*, 301.

Sims, N. R., Bowen, D. M., Allen, S. J., Smith, C. C. T., Neary, D., Thomas, D. J., & Daniston, A. N. (1983). Presynaptic cholinergic dysfunction in patients with dementia. *Journal of Neurochemistry, 40*, 503-509.

Smith, L. H., & Thier, S. O. (1981). *Pathophysiology: The biological principles of disease*. Philadelphia: W. B. Saunders Co.

Summers, W. K., Majonski, L. V., Marsh, G. M., Tachiki, K., & Kling, A. (1986). Oral tetrahydroaminoacridine in long-term treatment of senile dementia, Alzheimer type. *New England Journal of Medicine, 315*, 1241-1245.

Thompson, J. M. et al. (1989). *Mosby's manual of clinical nursing* (2nd ed.). St. Louis: C. V. Mosby.

Toole, J. F. (Ed.). (1977). *Clinical concepts of neurological disorders*. Baltimore: Williams & Wilkins Co.

Torak, R. M., & Gegel, H. M. (1983). Immunopathology of brain aging and senile dementia of the Alzheimer type. In J. Cervos-Navarro & H. I. Sarkander (Eds.), *Brain aging neuropathology and neuropharmacology Vol. 21*. New York: Raven Press.

Trockman, G. (1978). Caring for the confused or delirious patient. *American Journal of Nursing, 78*(9), 1495-1499.

Wassenberg, C. (1981). Common visual disorders in children. *Nursing Clinics of North America, 16*(3), 479-485.

Watson, R. T., & Heilman, K. M. (1979). Dementia. *Continuing Education for the Family Physician, 10*(4), 22-29.

Weiss, R. (1987). THA trials suspended, research probed. *Science News, 132*, 292.

Wells, C. E. (1977). *Dementia*. Philadelphia: F. A. Davis Company.

Wells, C. E. (1978). Geriatric organ psychoses. *Psychiatric Annals, 8*(9), 57-73.

Whitehouse, P. J., Price, D. L., Struble, R. G., Clark, A. W., Coyle, J. T., & Delong, M. R. (1982). Alzheimer's disease and senile dementia: Loss of neurons in the basal forebrain. *Science, 215*, 1237-1239.

Wilson, V. J., & Peterson, B. W. (1978). Peripheral and control substrates of vestibulospinal reflexes. *Physiology Review, 58*, 80.

Wurtman, R. J., & Zeisel, S. H. (1982). Brain choline: Its source and effects on the synthesis and release of acetylcholine. In S. Corkin, J. H. Growdon, K. L. Danis, E. Usdin, & R. J. Wuetman (Eds.), *Alzheimer's disease: A report on progress in research* (vol. 9 [Aging series]) (pp. 303-313) New York: Raven Press.

Zschoche, D. (1981). *Mosby's comprehensive review of critical care* (2nd ed.) St. Louis: C. V. Mosby.)

CHAPTER 15

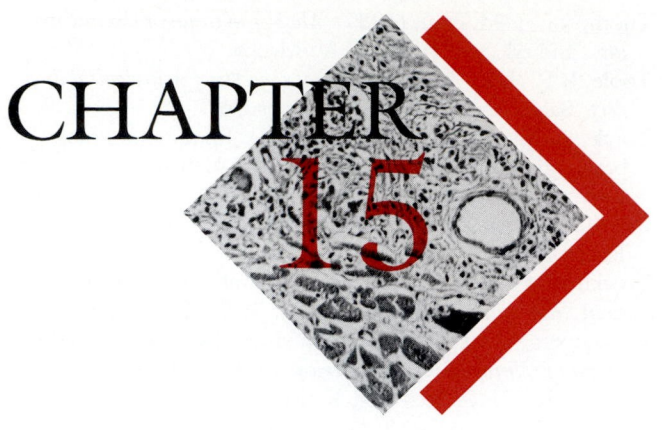

Alterations of Neurologic Function

Barbara J. Boss
Joleen Heath
Peter M. Sunderland

Central nervous system disorders, 477
  Trauma, 477
    Closed-head trauma, 477
      Clinical manifestations, 477
      Concussion, 478
      Contusion and laceration, 480
      Extradural hematoma, 480
      Subdural hematoma, 481
      Intracerebral hematoma, 482
    Open-head trauma, 482
      Compound fracture, 483
    Spinal cord trauma, 483
      Pathophysiology, 485
      Clinical manifestations, 485
      Evaluation and treatment, 488
    Low back pain, 489
      Pathogenesis, 490
      Degenerative disk disease, 490
      Spondylolysis, 491
      Spondylolisthesis, 491
      Spinal stenosis, 491
      Evaluation and treatment, 491
    Herniated intervertebral disk, 491
      Pathophysiology, 491
      Clinical manifestations, 491
      Evaluation and treatment, 491
  Cerebrovascular disorders, 493
    Cerebrovascular accidents, 493
      Pathophysiology, 493
        Thrombotic stroke, 493
        Embolic stroke, 493
        Hemorrhagic stroke, 494
      Clinical manifestations, 494
      Evaluation and treatment, 494
    Intracranial aneurysm, 494
      Pathophysiology, 494
      Clinical manifestations, 496
      Evaluation and treatment, 497
    Arteriovenous malformation, 497
      Pathophysiology. 497
      Clinical manifestations, 497
      Evaluation and treatment, 497
    Subarachnoid hemorrhage, 497
      Pathophysiology, 497

  Clinical manifestations, 498
  Evaluation and treatment, 498
Tumors of the central nervous system, 498
  Primary intracerebral tumors, 499
    Glioblastoma multiforme, 501
    Astrocytoma, 501
    Oligodendroglioma, 502
    Ependymoma, 502
  Primary extracerebral tumors, 503
    Meningioma, 503
    Neurilemmoma, 503
    Metastatic carcinoma, 504
  Spinal cord tumors, 504
    Pathophysiology, 504
    Clinical manifestations, 504
    Evaluation and treatment, 505
Infection and inflammation of the central nervous system,
    505
  Meningitis, 505
    Pathophysiology, 506
    Clinical manifestations, 506
    Evaluation and treatment, 506
  Abscess, 506
    Pathophysiology, 507
    Clinical manifestations, 507
    Evaluation and treatment, 507
  Encephalitis, 507
    Pathophysiology, 508
    Clinical manifestations, 508
    Evaluation and treatment, 508
  Neurosyphilis, 508
  Wernicke disease, 509
    Pathophysiology, 509
    Clinical manifestations, 509
    Evaluation and treatment, 509
Degenerative diseases, 509
  Parkinson disease, 509
    Pathophysiology, 510
    Clinical manifestations, 511
    Parkinsonian tremor, rigidity, and akinesia, 511
    Postural abnormalities, 511
    Autonomic and neuroendocrine systems, 512
    Late symptoms, 513
    Evaluation and treatment, 513

Huntington disease, 513
Pathophysiology, 513
Clinical manifestations, 514
Evaluation and treatment, 514
Multiple sclerosis, 514
Pathophysiology, 515
Clinical manifestations, 516
Corticospinal syndrome, 516
Brainstem syndrome, 516
Cerebellar syndrome, 516
Cerebral syndrome, 517
Evaluation and treatment, 517
Amyotrophic lateral sclerosis, 517
Pathophysiology, 518
Clinical manifestations, 518
Evaluation and treatment, 518
Hydrocephalus, 519
Types of hydrocephalus, 519
Course of the disease, 519
Pathogenesis, 519
Clinical manifestations, 519
Evaluation and treatment, 519
Peripheral nervous system and neuromuscular junction
disorders, 519
Peripheral nervous system disorders, 519
Radiculopathies, 520
Pathophysiology, 520
Clinical manifestations, 520
Evaluation and treatment, 520
Plexus injuries, 520
Neuropathies, 520
Pathophysiology, 520
Clinical manifestations, 521
Evaluation and treatment, 521
Guillain-Barré syndrome, 521
Pathophysiology, 521
Clinical manifestations, 521
Evaluation and treatment, 521
Neuromuscular junction disorders, 521
Botulism, 521
Pathophysiology, 522
Clinical manifestations, 522
Evaluation and treatment, 522
Mysthenia gravis, 522
Pathophysiology, 522
Clinical manifestations, 522
Evaluation and treatment, 523

Alterations in central nervous system function are caused by traumatic injury, vascular disorders, tumor growth, infectious and inflammatory processes, metabolic derangements (including those arising from nutritional deficiencies and drugs/chemicals), and degenerative processes. Alterations in peripheral nervous system function involve the nerve roots (radiculopathies), a nerve plexus, or the nerves themselves (neuropathies). Disorders of the neuromuscular junction also occur.

CENTRAL NERVOUS SYSTEM DISORDERS

Trauma

Motor vehicle accidents are the major cause of traumatic CNS injury. At risk for such injury are children between 6 months and 2 years of age, young school-aged children, young adults involved in sports and recreational activities, persons living in high-crime areas, and elderly adults.

Traumatic injuries may be categorized as **closed-head trauma** (blunt trauma) or **open-head trauma** (penetrating trauma). In both categories neural tissues are damaged by compression that pushes the tissues together, tension that pulls or exerts traction on the tissues, shearing that slides tissues onto other tissues, or a combination of forces. With open-head trauma, tissues are directly damaged.

Closed-Head Trauma

Closed-head trauma, the most frequently encountered traumatic head injury, occurs when the head strikes a hard surface or when a rapidly moving blunt object strikes the head. The trauma may or may not cause a loss in level of consciousness. The dura mater remains intact, and the brain tissues are not exposed to the environment. Brain injury from closed-head trauma may occur through several mechanisms (Fig. 15-1).

The injury site may be the site of impact, where the skull hits the brain. This is called a **coup injury.** The rebound effect of injury on the side opposite from the impact of the brain and skull is called a **contracoup injury.** For example, a blow to the frontal region (coup) causes rebound damage to the occipital region (contracoup) of the brain. Contusion and hemorrhage are the primary effects of trauma. Edema forms secondarily around and in damaged neural tissues. Edema can then cause a rise in intracranial pressure. The maximum effect of the injury occurs about 12 to 24 hours after severe closed-head injury.

Clinical Manifestations

Clinical manifestations associated with brain injury may have an immediate or delayed onset (Fig. 15-2). In mild head injury, the individual may or may not lose consciousness but, if rendered unresponsive, usually regains full consciousness rapidly. With moderate head trauma, consciousness may not be regained for many minutes to a few hours. With moderate head trauma, possible focal signs of dysfunction include paresis or paralysis and cranial nerve palsy. When the individual does not regain a normal level of consciousness in a few hours, a severe head injury has been sustained.

Some individuals who have sustained closed-head

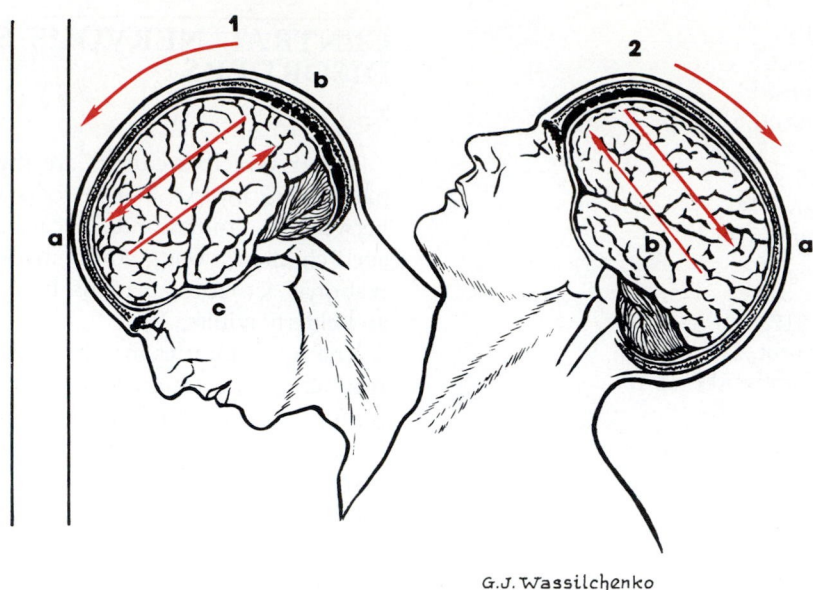

G.J.Wassilchenko

FIG. 15-1 Coup and contrecoup head injury following blunt trauma. **1,** Coup injury: impact against object. **a,** Site of impact and direct trauma to brain. **b,** Shearing of subdural veins. **c,** Trauma to base of brain. **2,** Contrecoup injury: impact within skull. **a,** Site of impact from brain hitting opposite side of skull. **b,** Shearing forces through brain. These injuries occur in one continuous motion—the head strikes the wall (coup), then rebounds (contrecoup). (From Rudy, 1984.)

trauma rapidly recover full consciousness and appear to have sustained a mild trauma, only to deteriorate neurologically hours or days later. The delayed onset of clinical manifestations in severe head trauma is caused by a progressive injury process, such as bleeding into tissues, bleeding into the extradural space, bleeding into the subdural space, and cerebrospinal fluid (CSF) collection in the subdural space.

Mild and moderate head trauma are managed by supportive therapy. In severe head trauma, edema and intracranial pressure must be controlled. (Increased intracranial pressure is discussed in Chapter 14.) Surgical decompression may be necessary.

Concussion

The word **concussion** means "shaken violently." Concussion represents a transient loss of consciousness due to a blow to the head, but no general agreement currently defines what should be included as concussion. A concussion usually involves no structural brain damage and is therefore considered the most benign form of brain injury. Conclusive evidence, however, that all concussions are free of structural injury does not yet exist. Concussions are characterized by the immediate onset of clinical manifestations at the time of injury and the transient nature of these manifestations. The exact pathology and pathophysiologic mechanisms of a concussive state remain unclear. Current theories suggest a disconnection between the cortex and brainstem.

The clinical manifestations of a concussion are immediate loss of consciousness (generally accepted to last no longer than 5 minutes), loss of reflexes with which the individual falls to the ground, transient cessation of respiration, brief period of bradycardia, and fall in blood pressure (lasting 30 seconds to a few minutes). A momentary rise in cerebrospinal fluid pressure and electrocardiographic (ECG) and electroencephalographic (EEG) changes have been demonstrated to occur on impact. Vital signs stabilize to normal values in a few seconds. Reflexes return next, and the person begins to regain consciousness. Returning to full awakeness and alertness takes variable periods of time from minutes to days. Evaluation should include a complete history and physical examination. Skull and spinal x-rays are frequently taken, and a computerized tomography (CT) scan or (MRI) magnetic resonance imaging may be done.

Some of the effects of a concussion may persist for weeks or months, depending on the severity of the injury. A **postconcussive syndrome** that includes headache, nervousness or anxiety, irritability, insomnia, depression, inability to concentrate, forgetfulness, and fatigability may develop.

Treatment entails reassurance and symptomatic relief. A period of 24 hours of close observation by a reliable individual is indicated, so that immediate intervention can be obtained if delayed effects become severe.

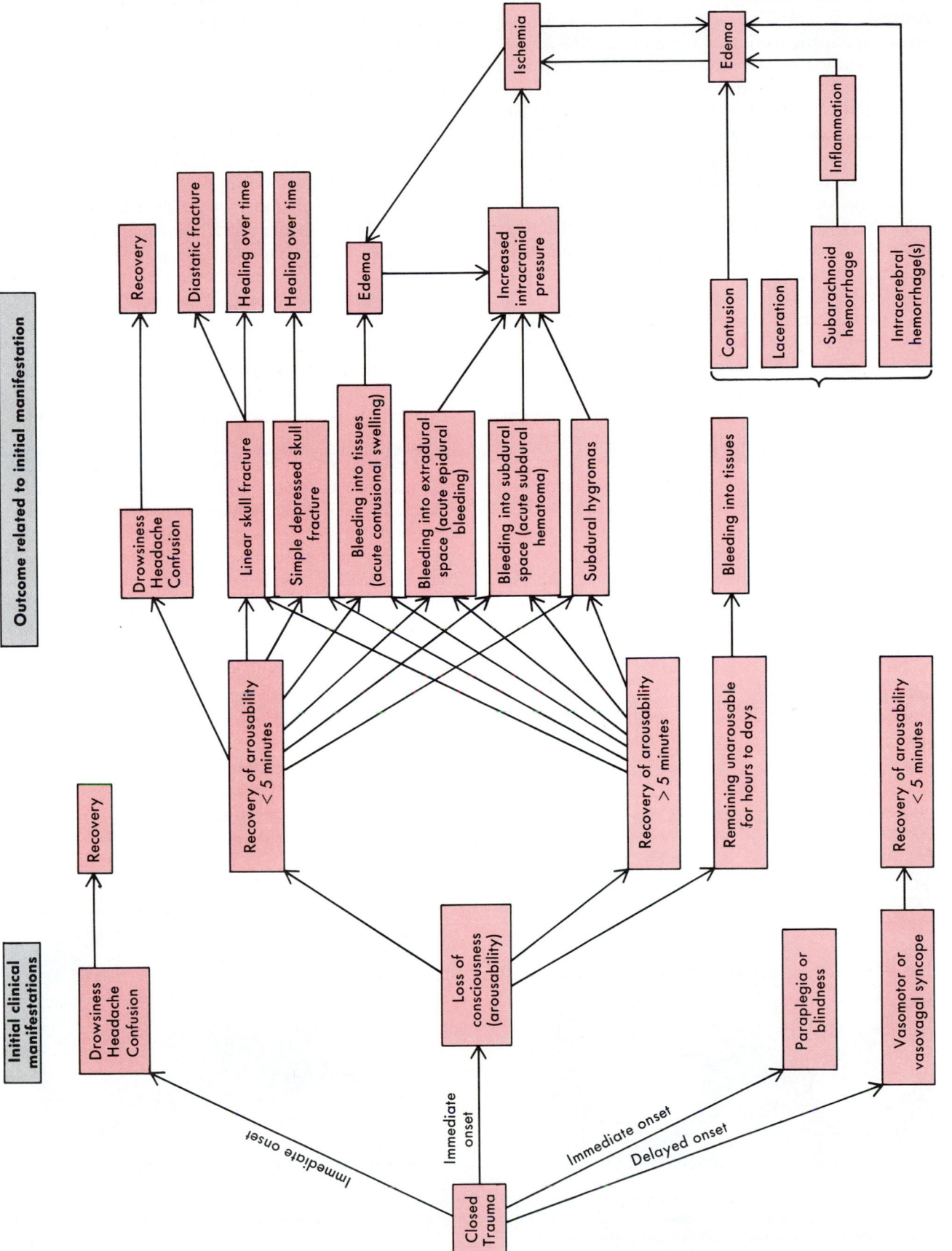

FIG. 15-2. Possible outcomes of closed-head trauma.

Contusion and Laceration

A **contusion** is a bruising of part of the brain. A **laceration** is a traumatic tearing of brain tissue. The severity of the contusion or laceration is associated with the amount of energy transmitted to underlying brain tissue. Contusions and lacerations can occur throughout the brain tissues, as well as under a skull fracture. These injuries are produced by the deformation and bending of the bone at the time of impact, causing shearing forces from the rotational injury. Because of the concentration of the force in a small area, the smaller the area of impact, the greater the severity of injury. The injury may be coup, contracoup, or throughout the brain tissue.

The indirect effects on tissue include edema, bleeding, and subsequent increased intracranial pressure. Within the contused or lacerated areas are infarction and necrosis, hemorrhage, and edema (Fig. 15-3). The tissue has a pulpy quality. Contusion, hemorrhage, and brain swelling are at their peak 12 to 24 hours after injury.

Initial manifestations are similar to those of a concussion. The difference is a slower recovery time. Regaining a full level of consciousness may be extremely slow, and residual deficits may persist. In some persons full level of consciousness never really returns.

Large contusions and lacerations with hemorrhage may be surgically excised. Otherwise treatment is directed at controlling intracranial pressure and managing symptoms.

Extradural Hematoma

Extradural hematoma, also called epidural hematoma or epidural hemorrhage, is an accumulation of blood, most commonly arterial blood, above the dura mater but beneath the skull (Fig. 15-4). Extradural hematomas represent 1% to 2% of major head injuries and are life-threatening. They occur in every age group but are most common in persons 20 to 40 years of age and are found in males four times more often than in females. Of extradural hematomas 85% have an artery as the source of bleeding, but about 15% result from injury to a meningeal vein or dural sinus. The most common site of an extradural hematoma is over the temporal lobe because the middle meningeal artery runs in a groove on the surface of the temporal bone prior to penetrating the skull. Extradural hematomas may occur over the subfrontal and the occipital-suboccipital lobes.

The most common cause of extradural hematomas is motor vehicle accidents, although these injuries are occasionally caused by minor falls and sporting accidents. Aggressive diagnosis and treatment have reduced the mortality rate from extradural hematomas from 50% to 20%.

Individuals with classic temporal extradural hematomas (i.e., over the temporal lobe) have a period of loss of consciousness at the time of injury followed by a lucid period that lasts from a few hours to a few days (if a vein is bleeding). As the hematoma accumulates, a headache of increasing severity, vomiting, drowsiness, confusion, seizure, and hemiparesis may develop. Level of consciousness may be rapidly lost as the temporal lobe herniation begins. Clinical manifestations of temporal lobe herniation also include ipsilateral pupillary dilatation and contralateral hemiparesis.

The diagnosis of an extradural hematoma is usually made with a CT scan or MRI. In some instances diagnosis is made by history and clinical findings, as time for a CT scan or MRI is not available. The prognosis is usually good if intervention is initiated prior to bilateral dilatation of the pupils.

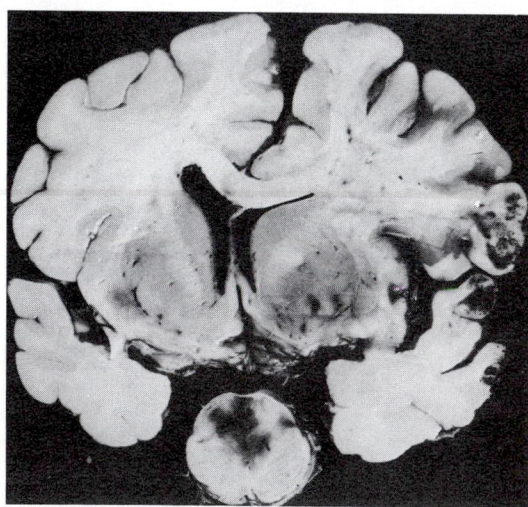

FIG. 15-3. Recent contusions of frontal and temporal lobes. There is displacement of cingulate gyrus and lateral ventricles. Secondary hemorrhages have occurred in lower midbrain and upper pons. (From Kissane, 1985.)

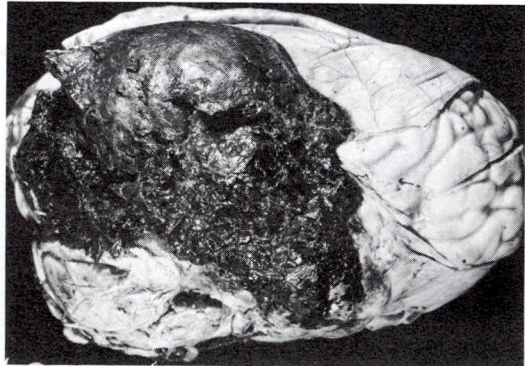

FIG. 15-4. Acute epidural hematoma resulting from skull fracture with tear of middle meningeal artery and vein. (From Kissane, 1985.)

Surgical therapy is evacuation of the hematoma through burr holes, which is followed by ligation of the bleeding vessel(s). Extradural hematomas are almost always medical emergencies.

Subdural Hematoma

A **subdural hematoma** is the collection of blood, usually venous, between the dura mater and the arachnoid membrane (see Figs. 15-5 and 12-14). Approximately 10% to 20% of persons with head injuries develop subdural hematomas. Subdural hematomas are classified as acute, subacute, or chronic. The classification depends on the interval between injury and appearance of clinical manifestations. The diagnosis of subdural hematoma is generally made with CT scan or MRI.

Acute subdural hematomas develop rapidly, usually within hours, although development can take 1 to 2 weeks from the time of injury. Acute subdural hematomas are almost always located over the top of the skull, and 50% are also associated with skull fractures. The most common cause is motor vehicle accidents. Acute subdural hematomas are also associated with massive cerebral and/or brainstem contusions, which contribute to the extremely high mortality rate of 50%.

Acute, rapidly developing subdural hematomas are produced by the tearing of veins. The expanding clots directly compress the brain, giving rise to the clinical manifestations. As the intracranial pressure rises, the bleeding veins are compressed, and thus bleeding is self-limiting, although cerebral compression and displacement of brain tissue can cause temporal lobe herniation.

An acute subdural hematoma classically begins with headache, drowsiness, restlessness or agitation, slowed cognition, and confusion. These symptoms worsen over time and progress to loss of consciousness, respiratory pattern changes, and pupillary dilatation (i.e., the symptoms of temporal lobe herniation). These manifestations are more pronounced than focal manifestations such as dysphasia, dyspraxia, or hemiparesis. Other clinical manifestations may include homonymous hemianopia (defective vision in either the right or the left field), dysconjugate gaze, and gaze palsies.

Subacute subdural hematoma develops more slowly, from 7 days to a few weeks. The mortality figures are considerably lower because of this slow development. The pathophysiology of subacute subdural hematoma is similar to that of acute underlying subdural hematoma. Presentation and clinical manifestations are also similar but progress more slowly.

Chronic subdural hematomas are most commonly found in elderly persons and alcoholics who have some degree of brain atrophy and a subsequent increase in the size of the extradural space. Other individuals at risk are those on long-term anticoagulant therapy and those with blood dyscrasias. The trauma initiating the bleeding may be minor, often just a slight bump to the head.

Chronic subdural hematomas take several weeks to accumulate (Fig. 15-6). Blood gradually fills the existing

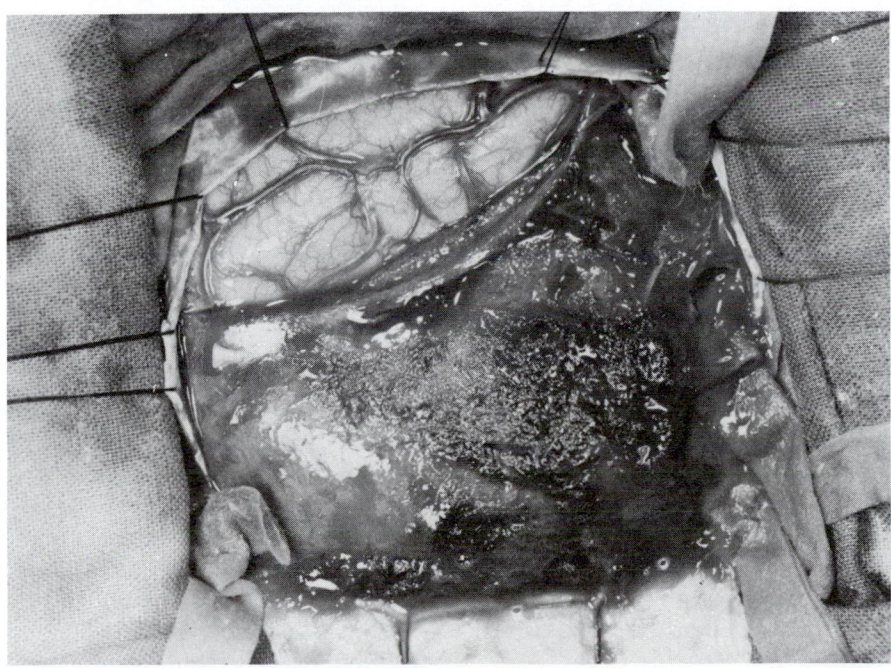

FIG. 15-5. Subdural hematoma. Dura has been reflected downward, exposing neomembrane and hematoma in situ, and normal underlying pia-arachnoid and brain are exposed in upper part of field. (Courtesy Dr. H. G. Schwartz, St. Louis, Mo. From Rosai, 1981.)

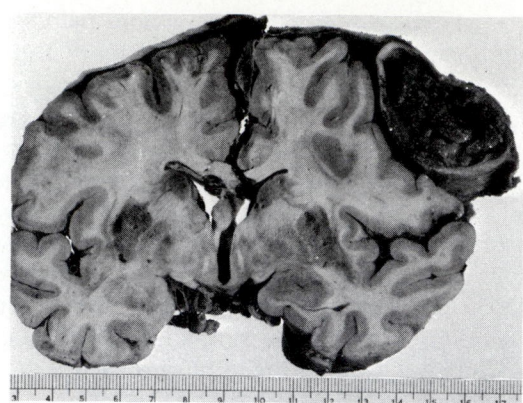

FIG. 15-6. Chronic subdural hematoma with compression of underlying brain and lateral ventricle. Note bone formation in falx and uncal herniation on side of hematoma. (From Kissane, 1985.)

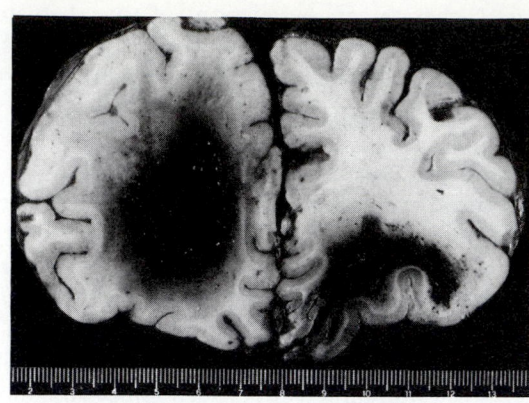

FIG. 15-7. Recent hematomas in frontal lobes, resulting from trauma. (From Kissane, 1985.)

subdural space. Usually in 2 weeks a vascular membrane forms around the hematoma. In some persons the hematoma then enlarges until compressive focal clinical manifestations or generalized manifestations of increased intracranial pressure develop.

Presenting manifestations of chronic subdural hematomas are varied. Of persons affected 80% have chronic headaches and tenderness over the hematoma on percussion. Most persons appear to have a progressive dementia accompanied by generalized rigidity (paratonia).

Whereas most acute and subacute subdural hematomas are treated with clot evacuation through a burr hole, chronic subdural hematomas (and some that are subacute) require a craniotomy to evacuate the gelatinous blood. The membrane around a chronic subdural hematoma is then dissected away from the dura mater and arachnoid membranes. A technique for percutaneous drainage for chronic subdural hematomas has recently proved successful.

Intracerebral Hematoma

Intracerebral hematomas, bleeding into the brain parenchyma, occur in 2% to 3% of head injuries. Intracerebral hematomas may be singular or multiple and are associated with contusions. They are commonly located in the frontal and temporal lobes (Fig. 15-7). Shearing forces traumatize small blood vessels and account for the intracerebral hematomas found deep in the cerebral hemispheres. Intracranial hematomas act as expanding masses causing increased intracranial pressure and compression of brain tissues with resultant edema and further increases in pressure.

A decreasing level of consciousness is associated with an intracerebral hematoma. Coma or a confusional state from other injuries, however, can make the cause of this

increasing unresponsiveness difficult to detect. Contralateral hemiplegia may also occur. As the intracranial pressure rises, clinical manifestations of temporal lobe herniation may appear. In delayed intracerebral hematoma the presentation is similar to that of a hypertensive brain hemorrhage: sudden, rapidly progressive decreased level of consciousness with pupillary dilatation, breathing pattern changes, hemiplegia, and bilateral positive Babinski reflexes.

History and physical examination help to establish the diagnosis. CT scan, MRI, and cerebral angiography confirm the diagnosis. Evacuation of a singular intracerebral hematoma has only occasionally been helpful, mostly for subcortical white matter hematomas. Otherwise treatment is directed at reducing the intracranial pressure and allowing the hematoma to reabsorb slowly.

Open-Head Trauma

An open-head trauma involves a skull fracture with penetration of the dura mater resulting in the exposure of the contents of the cranial vault to the environment. The fracture may lacerate the dura mater, the brain tissue, or both. Bone fragments also may be driven into the dura mater and possibly into the brain tissue as well. Bleeding results from tissue laceration. Edema forms around and in the damaged neural tissue. Intracranial pressure rises, often rapidly.

With open-head injury, most persons lose consciousness. The depth of the coma and the length of the unresponsive state are related to the location of injury, extent of damage, and amount of bleeding.

Open-head injury often requires surgery to debride the traumatized tissues to prevent infection and to remove blood clots to help reduce the intracranial pressure. Intracranial pressure is also managed with steroids, dehydrating agents, osmotic diuretics, or a combination of these drugs. Broad-spectrum antibiotics are administered.

Compound Fracture

A **compound fracture** (perforated fracture) involves a skull fracture that communicates with a scalp laceration, a sinus, or the middle ear cavity. The common mechanism is the creation of a pathway into the intracranial cavity. The fracture may be linear (i.e., a simple break in the continuity of the bone but without a change in alignment of the bone fragments), comminuted (i.e., with bone fragments from multiple linear fractures), or depressed (i.e., with displaced comminuted fragments). A compound fracture is suspected when there are lacerations of the scalp, tympanic membrane, a sinus, eye, and/or mucous membranes. Bone fragments may be clearly visible or felt on cautious palpation.

Compound fractures occur in the cranial vault or at the base of the skull, where they are termed **basilar skull fractures.** Basilar skull fractures most frequently arise as extensions of a linear fracture of the cranial vault. The fracture extends to the base of the skull, particularly in the anterior and middle fossae. The fragility of these bones and the strong adherence of the dura mater account for the frequency of these fractures and the resultant CSF leakage through the dural tear. About 75% of basilar skull fractures involve the temporal bone; an occasional fracture involves the posterior fossa.

In basilar skull fracture the dura mater may be torn; overlying brain tissue, cranial nerves, or blood vessels may be contused and/or lacerated; and a pathway for intracranial infection may be created. If portions of the arachnoid membrane and dura mater become trapped in the fracture edge, a permanent route of leakage for cerebrospinal fluid is formed.

In particular, longitudinal basilar skull fractures along the temporal bone produce a deformity of the external ear canal and/or rupture of the tympanic membrane. Leakage of cerebrospinal fluid from the ear canal (otorrhea) is characteristic. Postauricular swelling and hematoma, called **Battle sign,** become clinically evident 24 to 48 hours after injury.

The diagnosis of a compound fracture is made through physical examination, skull x-ray films, or both. The diagnosis of a basilar skull fracture is made on the basis of clinical findings. Skull x-rays often do not demonstrate the fracture, although intracranial air or air in the sinuses on x-ray film, CT scan, or MRI is indirect evidence of a basilar skull fracture.

A compound linear fracture is debrided nonsurgically in cooperative adults and surgically in children and uncooperative adults. Cranioplasty with insertion of bone or an artificial graft may be necessary. Antibiotics are administered after surgery.

Bed rest and close observation for meningitis and other complications are prescribed for a basilar skull fracture. Use of prophylactic antibiotics is controversial because studies have failed to demonstrate that they reduce the rate of infection.

Spinal Cord Trauma

Each year 5000 to 10,000 persons suffer serious spinal cord injury. Most are men between the ages of 15 and 30 who sustain their injuries from car and motorcycle accidents, sports activities (football, diving), and penetrating injuries (gunshot or stab wounds). The elderly, because of preexisting degenerative vertebral dis-

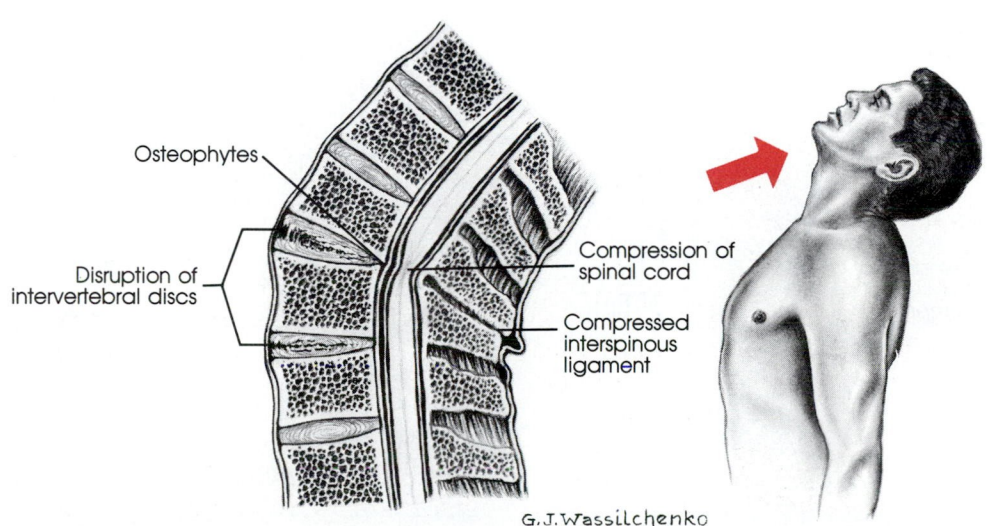

FIG. 15-8. Hyperextension injuries of the spine. (From Rudy, 1984.)

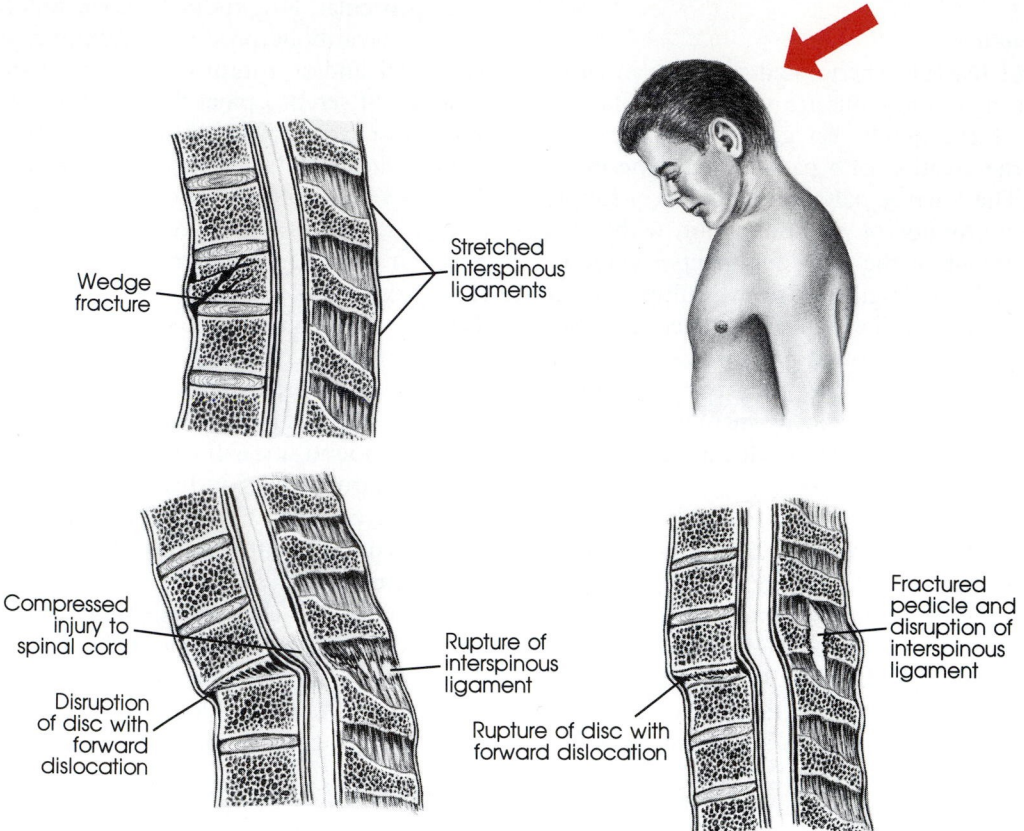

FIG. 15-9. Flexion injury of the spine. (From Rudy, 1984.)

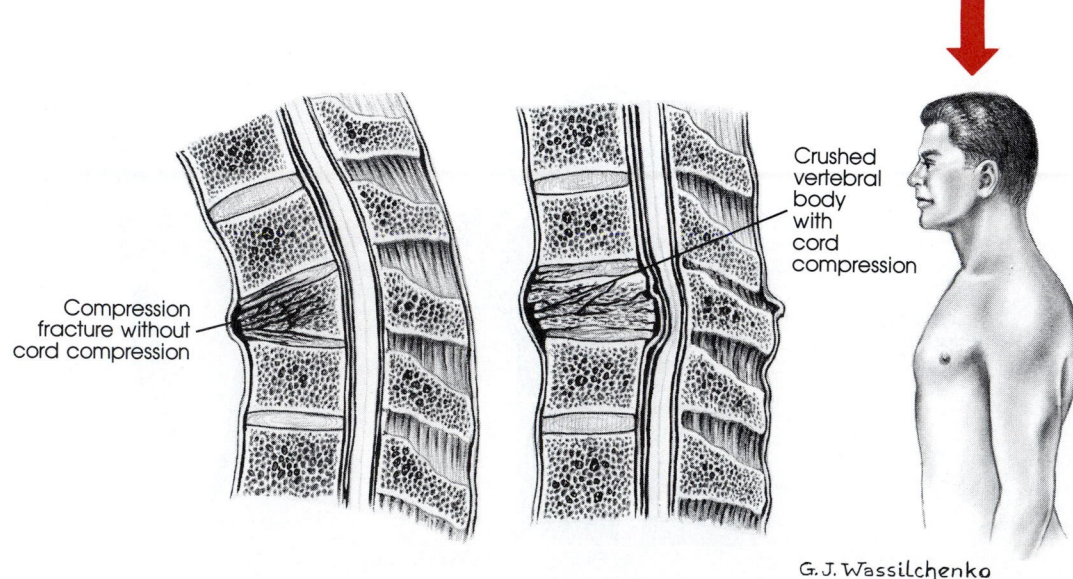

G. J. Wassilchenko

FIG. 15-10. Compression injuries of the spine. (From Rudy, 1984.)

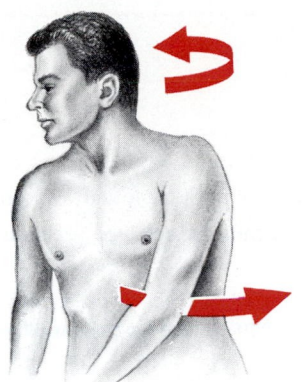

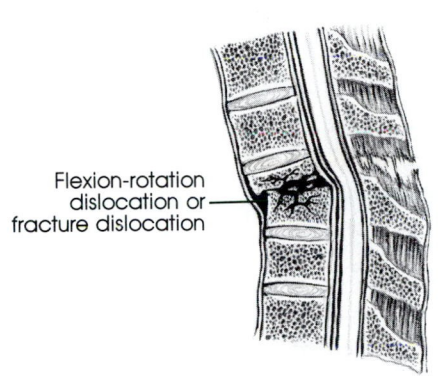

Flexion-rotation
dislocation or
fracture dislocation

FIG. 15-11. Flexion-rotation injuries of the spine. (From Rudy, 1984.)

orders, are particularly at risk for minor trauma resulting in serious spinal cord injury. The most common sites of spinal cord injury are the first and second cervical vertebrae, the fourth to sixth cervical vertebrae, and the eleventh thoracic to second lumbar vertebrae.

Pathophysiology

Spinal cord injuries most commonly occur because of vertebral injuries. They are the result of acceleration, deceleration, or deformation forces most frequently applied at a distance. These forces injure the vertebral and/or neural tissues by compressing the tissue, pulling or exerting a traction (tension) on the tissues, or shearing tissues so that they slide into one another. These forces may be exerted on the vertebral and neural tissues by hyperextension, hyperflexion, vertical compression, and/ or rotation of the spine (Figs. 15-8 to 15-11). The bones, ligaments, and joints of the vertebral column may be damaged. The vertebral column may incur fracture and often compression of one or more elements, dislocation of its elements, or both fracture and dislocation.

The vertebrae fracture readily with both direct and indirect trauma. When the supporting ligaments are torn, the vertebrae move out of alignment and dislocations occur. A horizontal force moves the vertebrae straight forward; if the individual is in a flexed position at the time of injury, the vertebrae are then in an angulated position. Flexion and extension injuries may result in dislocations. (The bone, ligament, and joint injuries are presented in Table 15-1.)

Vertebral injuries occur mostly at the first to second cervical, fourth to sixth cervical, and eleventh thoracic to second lumbar vertebrae (see Fig. 12-15). These are the most mobile portions of the vertebral column. The cord occupies most of the vertebral canal in the cervical and lumbar regions. The size makes the cord in these areas more easily injured. (Injuries to the cord are summarized in Table 15-2).

Edema and microscopic hemorrhages follow injury and are maximal at the level of injury and for two cord segments above and below it. Cord swelling increases the individual's degree of dysfunction, so that distinguishing the functions to be permanently lost from those that are just temporarily impaired becomes difficult. In the cervical region cord swelling may be life-threatening because of the possibility of resulting impairment of the diaphragm function (phrenic nerves exit C_1 to C_4) and vegetative functions mediated by the medulla oblongata.

Clinical Manifestations

Normal activity of the spinal cord cells at and below the level of injury ceases because of loss of the continuous tonic discharge from the brain or brainstem immediately after cord injury, thus causing spinal shock. *Spinal shock* is characterized by a complete loss of reflex

TABLE 15-1 Mechanisms of vertebral injury	
Mechanism of injury	**Vertebral injury**
Hyperextension	Fracture and dislocation of posterior elements such as spinous processes, transverse processes, laminae, pedicles, or posterior ligaments
Hyperflexion	Fracture or dislocation of the vertebral bodies, disks, or ligaments
Vertical compression	Shattering fractures
Rotational forces	Rupture supporting ligaments in addition to producing fractures

TABLE 15-2 Spinal cord injuries

Injury	Description
Cord concussion	Results in a temporary disruption of cord-mediated functions
Cord contusion	Bruising of the neural tissue causing swelling and temporary loss of cord-mediated functions
Cord compression	Pressure on the cord causing ischemia to tissues; must be relieved (decompressed) to prevent permanent damage to the spinal cord
Laceration	Tearing of the neural tissues of the spinal cord; may be reversible if only slight damage sustained by the neural tissues; may result in permanent loss of cord-mediated functions if spinal tracts are disrupted
Transection	Severing of the spinal cord, causing permanent loss of function
Complete	All tracts in the spinal cord completely disrupted; all cord-mediated functions below the transection are completely and permanently lost
Incomplete	Some tracts in the spinal cord remain intact, together with functions mediated by these tracts; has the potential for recovery although function is temporarily lost
Hemorrhage	Bleeding into the neural tissue due to blood vessel damage; usually no major loss of function
Damage or obstruction of spinal blood supply	Causes local ischemia

function in all segments below the level of the lesion. This condition involves all skeletal muscles, bladder, bowel, sexual function, and autonomic control. Severe impairment below the level of the lesion is obvious; it includes paralysis and flaccidity in muscles, absence of sensation, loss of bladder and rectal control, transient drop in blood pressure, and poor venous circulation. The condition also results in disturbed thermal control because the sympathetic nervous system is damaged. This damage causes faulty control of sweating and radiation through capillary dilatation. The hypothalamus cannot regulate body heat through vasoconstriction and increased metabolism. Therefore, the individual assumes the temperature of the air.

Spinal shock may last for 7 to 20 days following onset; it may persist for as short a time as a few days or as long as 3 months. Indications that spinal shock is terminating include the reappearance of reflex activity, hyperreflexia, spasticity, and reflex emptying of the bladder.

Loss of motor and sensory function depends upon the level of injury. All motor, sensory, reflex, and autonomic functions cease below any transected area and may also cease below concussed, contused, compressed, or ischemic areas (Table 15-3). Paralysis of the lower half of the body with both legs involved is termed paraplegia. Paralysis involving all four extremities is termed quadriplegia (tetraplegia). In complete quadriplegia the level of injury is above C_6, and all upper-extremity function is lost. In incomplete quadriplegia function at or above C_6 is preserved, leaving the shoulder, upper arm, and some forearm muscle control intact. With accelera-

tion injuries the greatest stress point is C_{4-5}. With a deceleration force the greatest stress point is at C_{5-6}.

Return of spinal neuron excitability occurs slowly. Either motor, sensory, reflex, and autonomic functions return to normal, or autonomic neural activity in the isolated segment develops, depending on the degree of damage. The sequence of hyperactivity phases, which vary in length, may include (1) minimal reflex activity, (2) flexor spasms, (3) alternation between flexor and extensor spasms, and (4) predominant extensor spasms.

The initial clinical manifestations associated with acute spinal cord injury are rapid loss of (1) voluntary movement in body parts below the level of injury, (2) sensations in the lower extremities and possibly lower trunk (depending on the level of injury), and (3) spinal and autonomic reflexes below the level of injury. The duration of this areflexic state is highly variable. In most persons reflex activity returns in 1 to 2 weeks.

Gradually reflexes return and become increasingly easier to elicit. A pattern of flexion reflexes emerges, first involving the toes and later the feet and legs. Reflex voiding and bowel elimination appear. Flexor spasms accompanied by profuse sweating, piloerection, and automatic bladder emptying (together called a **mass reflex**) may develop. The ability to sweat when overheated may be disrupted, and extensor spasms may develop, usually after full development of flexor spasms. Sometimes after several months episodes of autonomic hyperreflexia are elicited.

Autonomic hyperreflexia (dysreflexia) is a syndrome that may occur at any time after spinal injury. The syn-

TABLE 15-3 Clinical manifestations of spinal cord injury

Stage	Manifestations
SPINAL SHOCK STAGE	
Complete transection	Loss of motor function
	a. Quadriplegia with injuries of the cervical spinal cord
	b. Paraplegia with injuries of the thoracic spinal cord
	Muscle flaccidity
	Loss of all reflexes below the level of injury
	Loss of pain, temperature, touch, pressure, and proprioception below the level of injury
	Pain at the site of injury due to a zone of hyperesthesia above the injury
	Atonic bladder and bowel
	Paralytic ileus with distention
	Loss of vasomotor tone in the lower body parts, low and unstable blood pressure
	Loss of perspiration below the level of injury
	Loss or extreme depression of genital reflexes such as penile erection and bulbocavernous reflex
	Dry and pale skin, possible ulceration over bony prominences
Partial spinal cord transection	Asymmetrical flaccid motor paralysis below the level of injury
	Assymetrical reflex loss
	Preservation of some sensation below the level of injury
	Vasomotor instability less severe than with complete cord transection
	Bowel and bladder impairment less severe than that seen with complete cord transection
	Preservation of ability to perspire in some portions of the body below the level of injury
	Brown-Séquard syndrome (associated with penetrating injuries, arises from a relative hemisection of the cord)
	a. Ipsilateral paralysis or paresis below the level of injury
	b. Ipsilateral loss of touch, pressure, vibration, and position sense below the level of injury
	c. Contralateral loss of pain and temperature sensations below the level of injury
	Central cervical cord syndrome (associated with hyperextension or interruption of blood supply)
	a. Motor deficit in the upper extremities denser than in the lower extremities
	b. Varying degrees of bladder dysfunction
	Anterior cord syndrome (compromise of the anterior spinal artery by occlusion or the pressure effect of bone fragments or disk)
	a. Loss of motor function below the level of injury
	b. Loss of pain and temperature sensations below the level of injury
	c. Touch, pressure, position, and vibration senses intact
	Horner syndrome (injury to preganglionic sympathetic trunk or postganglionic sympathetic neurons of the superior cervical ganglion)
	a. Ipsilateral pupil smaller than contralateral pupil
	b. Sunken ipsilateral eyeball
	c. Ptosis of the affected eyeball
	d. Lack of perspiration on the ipsilateral side of the face
HEIGHTENED REFLEX ACTIVITY STAGE	Emergence of Babinski reflexes, possibly progressing to a triple reflex; possible development of still later flexor spasms
	Reappearance of ankle and knee reflexes, which become hyperactive
	Contraction of reflex detrusor muscle leading to urinary incontinence
	Appearance of reflex defecation
	Mass reflex with flexion spasms, profuse sweating, piloerection, and bladder and occasional bowel emptying may be evoked by an autonomic stimulation of skin or from a full bladder
	Episodes of hypertension
	Defective heat-induced sweating
	Eventual development of extensor reflexes, first in muscles of hip and thigh, later in leg
	Possible paresthesias below the level of transection: dull, burning pain in the lower back, abdomen, buttocks, and perineum

Adapted from Boss, 1984.

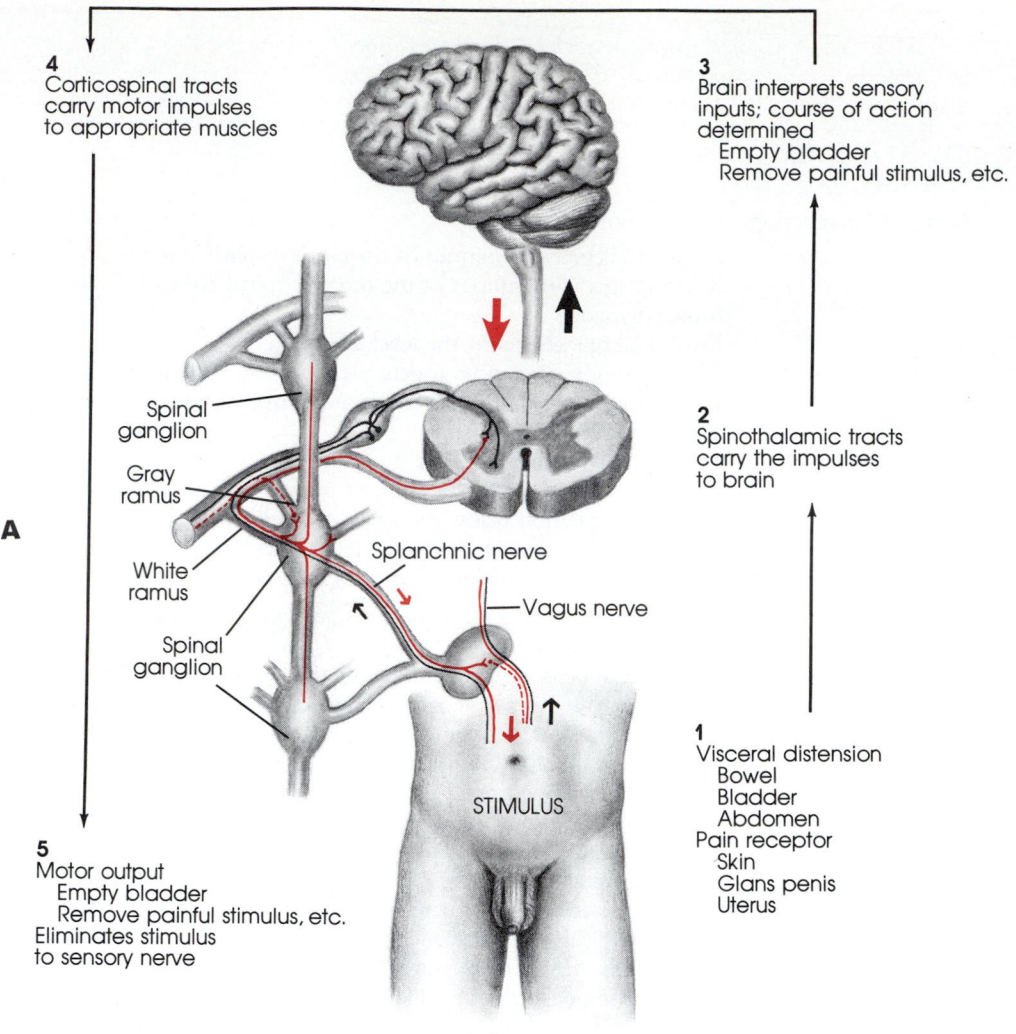

4
Corticospinal tracts
carry motor impulses
to appropriate muscles

3
Brain interprets sensory
inputs; course of action
determined
    Empty bladder
    Remove painful stimulus, etc.

Spinal
ganglion

Gray
ramus

A

White
ramus

Splanchnic nerve

Spinal
ganglion

Vagus nerve

2
Spinothalamic tracts
carry the impulses
to brain

STIMULUS

1
Visceral distension
    Bowel
    Bladder
    Abdomen
Pain receptor
    Skin
    Glans penis
    Uterus

5
Motor output
    Empty bladder
    Remove painful stimulus, etc.
Eliminates stimulus
to sensory nerve

G.J. Wassilchenko

FIG. 15-12. A, Normal response pathway. **B,** Autonomic dysreflexia pathway. (From Rudy, 1984.)

drome is associated with a massive, uncompensated cardiovascular response to stimulation of the sympathetic nervous system (Fig. 15-12). The condition is life-threatening and requires immediate treatment. Individuals most likely to be affected have lesions at the T_7 level or above. Autonomic hyperreflexia is characterized by paroxysmal hypertension (up to 300 mm Hg, systolic), a pounding headache, blurred vision, sweating above the level of the lesion with flushing of the skin, nasal congestion, nausea, piloerection due to pilomotor spasm, and bradycardia (30 to 40 beats per minute). The symptoms may develop singly or in combination (syndrome) and are often associated with a distended bladder or rectum.

Pathophysiology of hyperreflexia involves the stimulation of sensory receptors below the level of the cord lesion. The intact autonomic nervous system reflexively responds with an arteriolar spasm that increases blood pressure. Baroreceptors in the cerebral vessels, the carotid sinus, and the aorta sense the hypertension and stimulate the parasympathetic system. The heart rate de-

creases, but the visceral and peripheral vessels do not dilate because efferent impulses cannot pass through the cord.

The most common precipitating cause is a distended bladder or rectum, but any sensory stimulation can elicit autonomic hyperreflexia. Stimulation of the skin or stimulation of the pain receptors may cause autonomic hyperreflexia. Emptying of the bladder or bowel usually relieves the syndrome, and this may be facilitated by drugs, such as phenoxybenzamine.

Evaluation and Treatment

Diagnosis of spinal cord injury is made on the basis of physical examination, radiologic examination, CT scan, and/or MRI. For a suspected or confirmed verte-

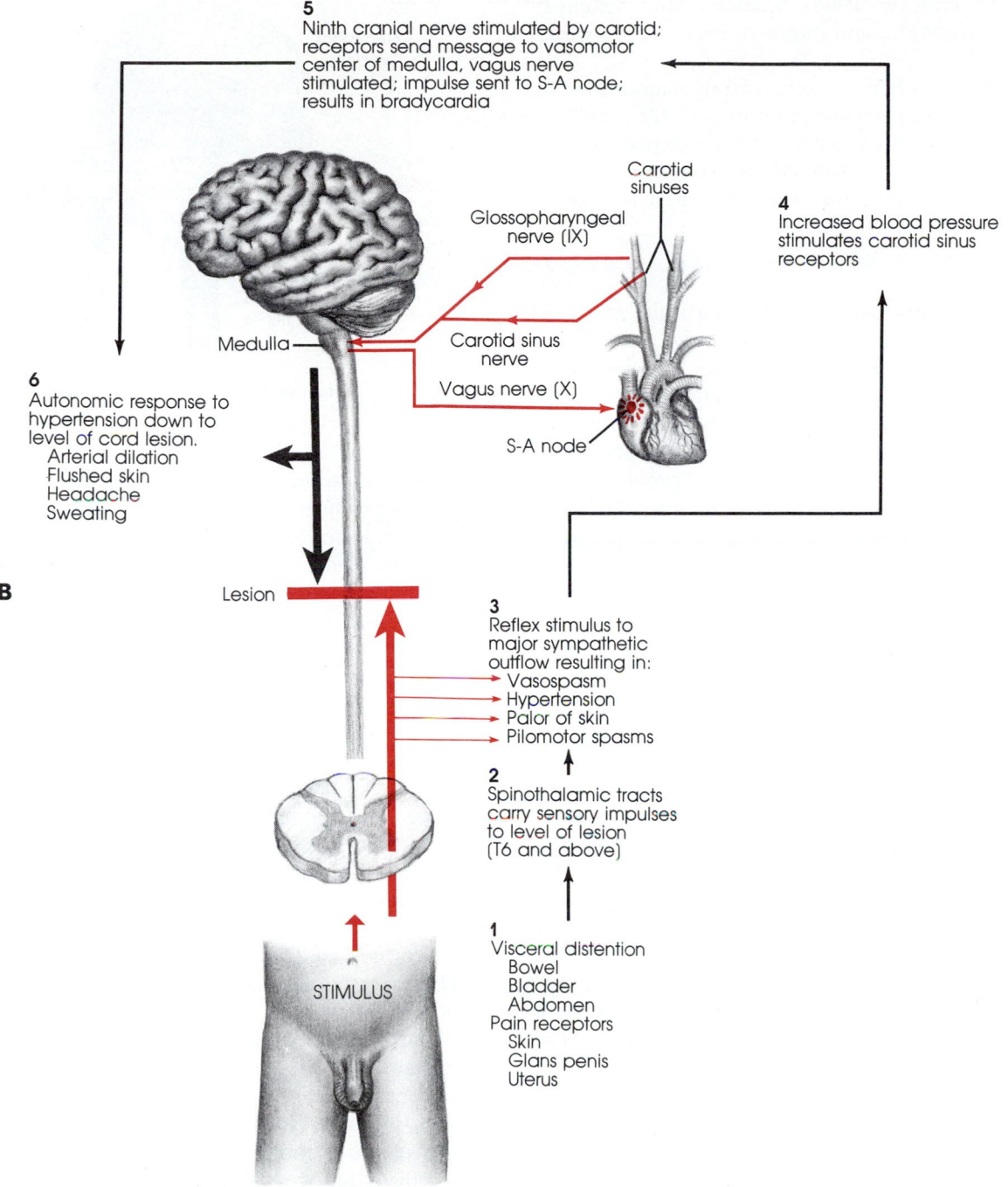

5
Ninth cranial nerve stimulated by carotid; receptors send message to vasomotor center of medulla, vagus nerve stimulated; impulse sent to S-A node; results in bradycardia

Carotid sinuses

Glossopharyngeal nerve (IX)

4
Increased blood pressure stimulates carotid sinus receptors

Medulla

Carotid sinus nerve

Vagus nerve (X)

6
Autonomic response to hypertension down to level of cord lesion.
Arterial dilation
Flushed skin
Headache
Sweating

S-A node

B

Lesion

3
Reflex stimulus to major sympathetic outflow resulting in:
Vasospasm
Hypertension
Palor of skin
Pilomotor spasms

2
Spinothalamic tracts carry sensory impulses to level of lesion (T6 and above)

STIMULUS

1
Visceral distention
Bowel
Bladder
Abdomen
Pain receptors
Skin
Glans penis
Uterus

bral fracture or dislocation, regardless of the presence or absence of spinal cord injury, the immediate intervention is immobilization of the spine to prevent further injury. Decompression and surgical fixation may be necessary. Corticosteroids may be given to decrease cord swelling. Nutrition, lung function, skin integrity, and bladder and bowel management must be addressed. Plans for rehabilitation need early consideration.

In cases of autonomic hyperreflexia intervention must be prompt because cerebrovascular accident is possible.

The head of the bed should be elevated, and the stimulus should be found and removed. Medications may be used if these measures do not effectively reduce blood pressure.

Low Back Pain

Low back pain affects the area between the lower rib cage and gluteal muscles and often radiates into the thighs. About 1% of individuals with acute low back pain have sciatica, pain in the distribution of a lumbar nerve root (Frymoyer, 1988). Sciatica is often accompanied by neurosensory and motor deficits, such as weakness.

The incidence of, or percent of population affected with, low back pain at some point in one's life is 60% to 90% and the annual incidence is 5% (Frymoyer, 1988). Men and women are equally affected; however, women report low back symptoms more often after the age of 60.

Pathogenesis

Most cases of low back pain are idiopathic, and clinicians are unable to provide a precise diagnosis for most individuals suffering from this disorder. The local processes involved in low back pain range from tension caused by tumors or disk prolapse, bursitis, synovitis, rising venous and tissue pressure (found in degenerative joint disease), abnormal bone pressures, problems with spinal mobility, inflammation caused by infection (as in osteomyelitis), bony fractures, or ligamentous sprains to pain referred from viscera or the posterior peritoneum.

General processes resulting in low back pain include bone diseases such as osteoporosis or osteomalacia and hyperparathyroidism (White & Gordon, 1982). The various origins of low back pain have been classified under five general headings: (1) spondylogenic (involving the spinal segment), (2) vascular, (3) neurogenic, (4) viscerogenic, and (5) psychogenic.

Several risk factors have been identified in the pathogenesis of low back pain. They include involvement caused by occupations that require repetitious lifting in the forward bent-and-twisted position, exposure to vibrations caused by vehicles or industrial machinery, and cigarette smoking (Frymoyer, 1988). Osteoporosis increases the risk of spinal compression fractures and may be the reason why elderly women report more symptoms than men. Genetic predispositions of low back pain include isthmic spondylolisthesis (vertebra slides forward or slips in relation to a vertebra below), spinal osteochondrosis, and spinal stenosis associated with achondroplasia. Variations in posture, such as lordosis and scoliosis of less than 60 degrees, do not appear to increase the risk of low back pain or sciatica (Pope et al., 1985; Weinstein, 1986). Differences in weight, height, and leg length are controversial (Pope et al., 1985).

Anatomically, low back pain must come from innervated structures, but deep pain is widely referred and varies from person to person. The nucleus pulposus has no intrinsic innervation, however, when extruded or herniated through a diskal prolapse, it irritates the dural membranes and is responsible for pain referred to the segmental area (Fig. 15-13) (White & Gordon, 1982).

The interspinous bursae can be a source of low back pain between L_3, L_4, L_5, and S_1, but may also affect L_1, L_2, and L_3 spinous processes, depending on the close-

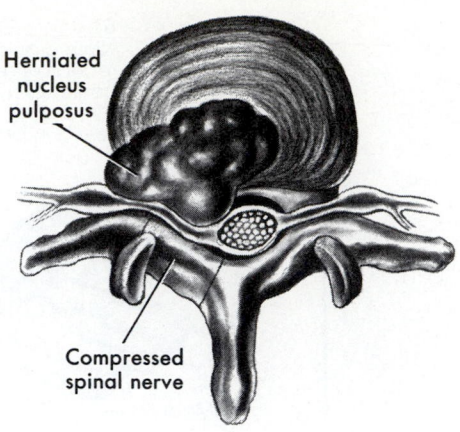

FIG. 15-13. Herniated nucleus pulposus. (From Thompson, 1989.)

ness of the adjacent pair of spines. The anterior and posterior longitudinal ligaments of the spine and the interspinous and supraspinous ligaments are abundantly supplied with pain receptors, as is the ligamentum flavia. All of these ligaments are vulnerable to traumatic tears (sprains) and fracture. The role of muscle injury in the production of low back pain remains uncertain, even though sprains and strains are the most common diagnosis (Frymoyer, 1988). The muscle spasms that are often produced during sieges of low back pain are thought to be produced by as yet unknown sensory or motor-reflex pathways (Frymoyer, 1988). The most commonly encountered causes of low back pain include lumbar disk herniation, degenerative disk disease, spondylolysis, spondylolisthesis, and spinal stenosis. (For a discussion of disk herniation and rupture, see p. 491.)

Degenerative Disk Disease

Degenerative disk disease is a common finding in individuals 50 years of age and older; however, only a small percentage of people with degenerative disk disease have any functional incapacity because of pain (Spengler, 1982). The etiology for degenerative disk disease includes biochemical and biomechanical alterations of tissue comprising the intervertebral disk. Fibrocartilage replaces the gelatinous mucoid material of the nucleus pulposus as the disk changes with aging, and the narrowing disk results in variable segmental instability. The process seems to stablize when segmental fibrosis results and often the incidence of back pain decreases (Spengler, 1982).

Spondylolysis

Spondylolysis is a structural defect of the spine involving the lamina or neural arch of the vertebra. The most common site affected is the lumbar spine. This defect occurs in the portion of the lamina between the superior and inferior articular facets called the pars interarticularis. Mechanical pressure may cause a forward displacement of the deficient vertebra, called spondylolisthesis.

Heredity plays a significant role, and spondylolysis is associated with an increased incidence of other congenital spinal defects. As a result of torsional and rotational "stress," "microfractures" occur at the affected site and eventually cause dissolution of the pars interarticularis.

Spondylolisthesis

Spondylolisthesis is caused when a vertebra slides forward in relation to the vertebra below, commonly occurring at L_5-S_1. Spondylolisthesis is graded from 1 to 4 on the basis of the percentage of slip that has occurred. Individuals with grade 3 or 4 are considered for operative decompression or stabilization, or both. Grades 1 and 2 are usually managed symptomatically and by nonsurgical methods.

Spinal Stenosis

Spinal stenosis may represent several conditions ranging from entrapment of a single nerve root in the lateral recess to diffuse central stenosis involving many roots. It is classified as acquired (more common) or developmental (such as occurs in achondroplastic dwarfs). Surgical decompression is recommended for those with chronic symptoms and those who remain unresponsive to medical management.

Evaluation and Treatment

Diagnosis of low back injury is made on the basis of physical examination, electromyelography, CT, and/or MRI. Most individuals with acute low back pain benefit from a nonspecific short-term treatment regimen including bed rest, analgesic medications, exercises, physical therapy, and education. Surgical treatments may be indicated if individuals do not respond to medical management. Surgical treatments include chemonucleolysis (recently classified as a surgically invasive procedure because of associated complications and morbidity), diskectomy, and spinal fusions. Individuals with chronic low back pain can be treated with anti-inflammatory and muscle relaxant medications and exercise programs. Currently aerobic exercises are a popular treatment and seem to be more effective than traction or low-back exercises (Frymoyer, 1988). Spinal surgery has a limited role in curing chronic low back pain.

Herniated Intervertebral Disk

Herniation of an intervertebral disk is a protrusion of part of the nucleus pulposus (like stepping on an ice cream sandwich) through a tear in the posterior rim of the annulus fibrosus (the fibrous capsule enclosing the gelatinous center of the disk) (see Fig. 15-13). Rupture of an intervertebral disk is usually caused by trauma. Lifting with the trunk flexed and sudden straining when the back is in an unstable position are the most common causes. Most commonly affected are the lumbosacral disks, that is, L_5-S_1 and L_4-L_5. Disk herniation occasionally occurs in the cervical area, usually at C_5-C_6 and C_6-C_7. Herniations at the thoracic level are extremely rare. The injury may have an immediate onset or an onset within a few hours, or the manifestations of injury may take months to years to develop.

Pathophysiology

In a herniated disk the ligament and posterior capsule of the disk are usually torn, allowing the fibrocartilaginous material (the nucleus pulposus) to extrude. This extrusion compresses the nerve root. Occasionally the injury tears the entire disk loose, and it protrudes onto the nerve root or compresses the spinal cord. One or more nerve roots may be compressed. This multiple nerve root compression is especially found at the L_5-S_1 level, where the cauda equina may be compressed. Large amounts of extruded nucleus pulposus or complete disk herniation (that is, of both the capsule and the nucleus pulposus) may compress the spinal cord.

Clinical Manifestations

The location and size of the herniation into the spinal canal, together with the amount of space that exists inside the spinal canal, determine the clinical manifestations associated with the injury (Fig. 15-14). A herniated disk in the lumbosacral area is associated with pain that radiates along the sciatic nerve course over the buttock and into the calf or ankle. The pain occurs with straining, including coughing and sneezing, and usually on straight leg raising. Other clinical manifestations include limited range of motion of the lumbar spine; tenderness on palpation in the sciatic notch and along the sciatic nerve; impaired pain, temperature, and touch sensation in the L_5-S_1 or L_4-L_5 dermatones in the leg and foot; decreased or absent ankle jerk; and mild weakness of the foot.

With the herniation of a lower cervical disk, paresthesias and pain are present in the upper arm, forearm, and hand in the affected nerve root distribution. Neck and nerve root pain may be increased by neck motion and straining, including coughing and sneezing. Neck range of motion is diminished. Slight weakness and atrophy of biceps or triceps may occur; the biceps or triceps reflex may decrease. Occasionally signs of corticospinal and sensory tract impairments appear. These include motor weakness of the lower extremities, sensory disturbances in the lower extremities, and presence of a Babinski reflex.

Evaluation and Treatment

Diagnosis of a herniated intervertebral disk is made through the history and physical examination, spinal x-rays, electromyelography, CT scan, MRI, and nerve conduction studies. Multiple avenues of therapy are

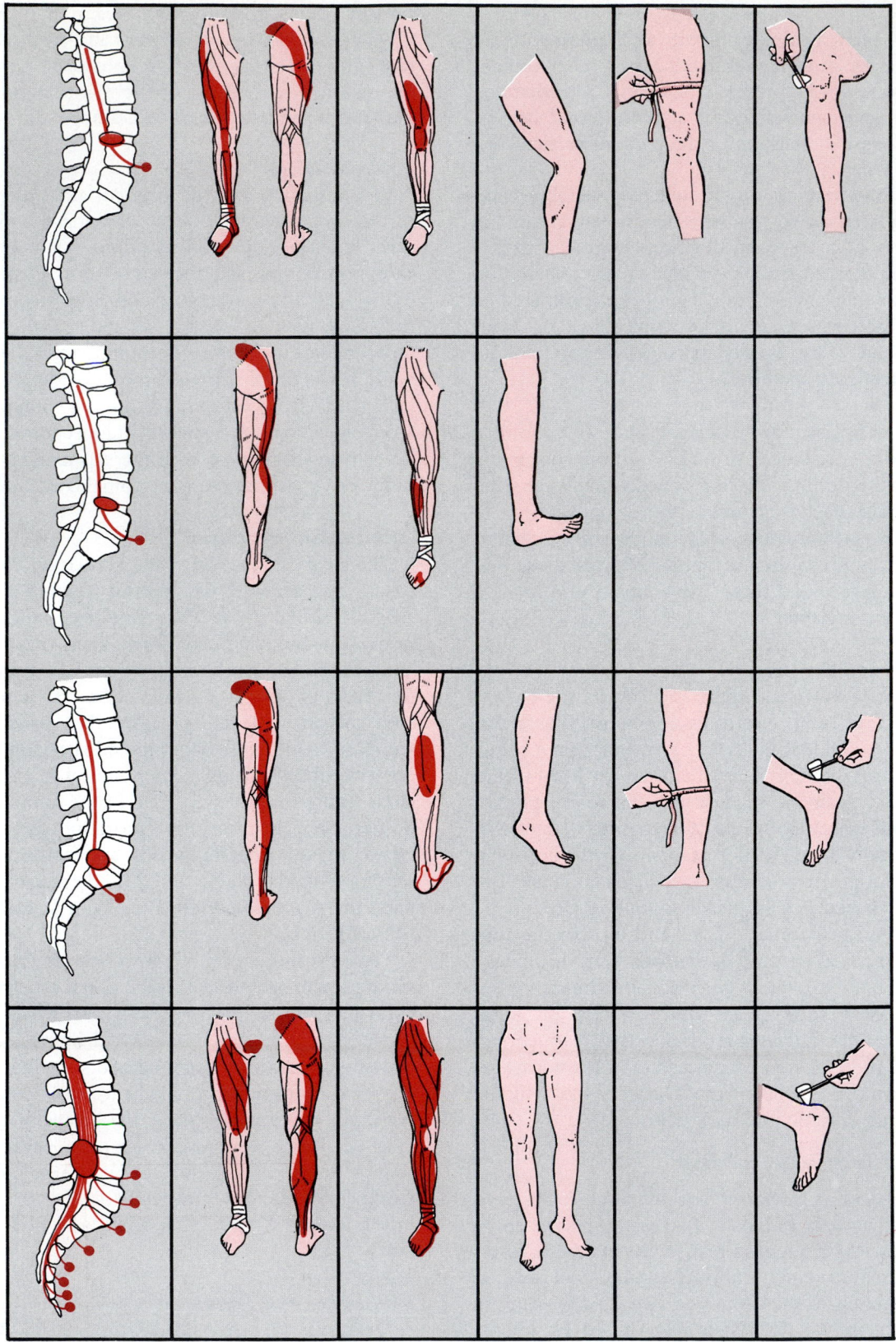

FIG. 15-14. Clinical features of a herniated lumbar nucleus pulposus.

available. The conservative approach comprises traction, bed rest, heat and ice to the affected areas, and an effective analgesic regimen. The surgical approach is indicated if there is evidence of severe compression (weakness, decreased deep tendon reflexes and bladder/bowel reflexes) or if the conservative approach is unsuccessful. The newest therapy is injection of the enzyme chymopapain into the disk to dissolve it. Chymopapain injections, however, are currently being debated in terms of relative effectiveness because they sometimes cause muscle spasms.

Cerebrovascular Disorders

Cerebrovascular disease is the most frequently occurring neurologic disorder. More than 50% of the persons admitted to general hospitals with neurologic problems have cerebrovascular disease. Any abnormality of the brain caused by a pathologic process in the blood vessels is referred to as a cerebrovascular disease. Included in this category are lesions of the vessel wall, occlusion of the vessel lumen by thrombus or embolus, rupture of the vessel, and alteration in vessel permeability such as increased blood viscosity.

The brain abnormalities induced by cerebrovascular disease are of two types: (1) ischemia with or without infarction (death of brain tissues) and (2) hemorrhage. The common clinical manifestation of cerebrovascular disease is a **cerebrovascular accident** (CVA, stroke): a sudden, nonconvulsive focal neurologic deficit.

Cerebrovascular Accidents

Cerebrovascular accidents are the third leading cause of death in the United States. The highest incidence of stroke is among those between 75 and 85 years of age. Strokes, however, do occur in about one out of seven individuals under the age of 65. Stroke tends to run in families and is more frequent in men than women. The incidence is greater in blacks than whites presumably because of the greater incidence of hypertension in blacks. In its mildest form a CVA is so minimal as to be almost unnoticed. In its most severe state, hemiplegia, coma, and death result.

Pathophysiology

Cerebrovascular accidents are classified according to pathophysiology and thus are thrombotic, embolic, or hemorrhagic.

Thrombotic Stroke

Thrombotic strokes arise from arterial occlusions caused by thrombi formed in the arteries supplying the brain or in the intracranial vessels. The risk factors for cerebrovascular occlusive disease are the following:

Arteriosclerosis, which includes the following risk factors: hypertension, cigarette smoking, elevated blood cholesterol and/or triglyceride levels, diabetes mellitus, sedentary life-style

Hypothyroidism
Use of oral contraceptives
Sickle cell disease
Coagulation disorders
Polycythemia vera
Arteritis
Chronic hypoxia
Dehydration, especially when combined with any of the preceding conditions.

The development of a cerebral thrombosis is most frequently attributed to atherosclerosis and inflammatory disease processes that damage arterial walls. Increased coagulation can lead to thrombus formation. Conditions causing inadequate cerebral perfusion (such as dehydration, hypotension, and prolonged vasoconstriction from malignant hypertension) increase the risk of thrombosis. Over 20 to 30 years atheromatous plaques tend to form at branchings and curves in the cerebral circulation. Degeneration or bleeding into the vessel wall may cause endothelial damage. Platelets and fibrin adhere to the damaged wall and delicate clots form. Small thrombi collect over time, with gradual occlusion of the artery. Once the artery is occluded, the thrombus may enlarge both distally and proximally in the vessel.

Thrombotic strokes may be further subdivided on the basis of clinical manifestations into transient ischemic attacks, strokes-in-evolution, and completed strokes. **Transient ischemic attacks** (TIAs) probably represent thrombotic particles causing an intermittent blockage of circulation. In a true transient ischemic attack all the neurologic deficits must be completely clear within 24 hours, leaving no residual dysfunction. Approximately 35% of completed thrombotic strokes are preceded by TIAs.

The symptoms of thrombotic strokes occasionally have an abrupt onset but tend to be slowly progressive, evolving in a step-by-step fashion over minutes to hours. The typical development of thrombotic stroke causes the clinical syndrome known as a **stroke-in-evolution.** An intermittent progression of a neurologic deficit over hours to days is characteristic of thrombotic stroke. The **completed stroke** is a cerebrovascular accident that has reached its maximum destructiveness in producing neurologic deficits, although cerebral edema may not have reached its maximum.

Embolic Stroke

An **embolic stroke** involves fragments that break from a thrombus formed outside the brain, in the heart, aorta, common carotid, or thorax. Emboli infrequently arise from the ascending aorta or common carotid artery. The embolus usually obstructs at a bifurcation or other point of narrowing, thus causing ischemia. An embolus may plug the lumen entirely and remain in place or break into fragments and move up the vessel. Conditions associated with the onset of an embolic stroke include atrial fibrillation, myocardial infarction, endocarditis, rheumatic heart disease, valvular protheses, atrial-septal defects and disorders of the aorta, and carotids, or vertebral-basilar circulation. Less common contributors to embolic stroke are air, fat, and tumors. Fat emboli sometimes develop with fractures of long bones. Air emboli can also develop after certain types of surgery. In persons who experience an embolic stroke, usually a second stroke follows at some point because the source of emboli continues to exist.

Hemorrhagic Stroke

Hemorrhagic stroke (intracranial hemorrhage) is the third most frequent cause of cerebrovascular accident. The most common causes of hemorrhagic stroke are hypertension, ruptured aneurysms or arteriovenous malformation, and hemorrhage associated with bleeding disorders.

A hypertensive hemorrhage usually occurs within the brain tissue. A mass of blood is formed, and its volume increases. Adjacent brain tissue is displaced and compressed. Rupture or seepage into the ventricular system occurs in many of the cases. Hemorrhages are described as massive, small, slit, or petechial. Massive hemorrhages are several centimeters in diameter; small hemorrhages are 1 to 2 cm in diameter; a slit hemorrhage lies in the subcortical area, whereas petechial hemorrhage is the size of a pinhead bleed. The most common sites for hypertensive hemorrhages are in the putamen of the basal ganglia (a portion of the lentiform nucleus), the internal capsule, the thalamus, the cerebral hemisphere, and the pons.

Clinical Manifestations

Because neurons surrounding the ischemic or infarcted areas undergo changes that disrupt plasma membranes, cellular edema results, causing further compression of capillaries. Cerebral edema reaches its maximum in about 72 hours and takes about 2 weeks to subside. Most persons survive an initial hemispheric ischemic stroke unless massive cerebral edema develops. Massive brainstem infarcts, caused by basilar thrombosis or embolism, are almost always fatal however.

Clinical manifestations of thrombotic stroke vary, depending on the artery obstructed. Different sites of obstruction create different occlusion syndromes (see Table 15-4).

With hemorrhagic stroke clinical manifestations vary, depending on the location and size of the bleed. Once a deep unresponsive state occurs, the person rarely survives. The immediate prognosis is grave. If, however, the person survives, recovery of function is frequently possible.

Individuals experiencing intracranial hemorrhage from a ruptured or leaking aneurysm have one of three sets of symptoms: (1) onset of an excruciating generalized headache with an almost-immediate lapse into an unresponsive state, (2) headache but with consciousness maintained, and (3) sudden lapse into unconsciousness. If the hemorrhage is confined to the subarachnoid space there may be no local signs. If bleeding spreads into the brain tissue, hemiparesis/paralysis, dysphasia, or homonymous hemianopia may be present. Warning signs of an impending aneurysm rupture may include headache, transient unilateral weakness, transient numbness and tingling, and transient speech disturbance. Warning signs, however, are often not present.

Evaluation and Treatment

In thrombotic strokes treatment is directed at supportive management to control cerebral edema and increased intracranial pressure. Later surgical intervention to restore blood supply may be indicated. Arresting the disease process by control of risk factors is critical. In embolic strokes treatment is directed at preventing further embolization by instituting anticoagulation therapy and correcting the primary problem. Rehabilitation is indicated in both thrombotic and embolic stroke. Treatment of an intracranial bleed, regardless of cause, is focused on stopping or reducing the bleeding, controlling the increased intracranial pressure, preventing a rebleed, and preventing vasospasm. Occasionally an attempt is made to evacuate or aspirate the blood.

Intracranial Aneurysm

Intracranial aneurysms may result from arteriosclerosis, congenital abnormality, embolus, or trauma. The size may vary from 2 mm to 2 cm to 3 cm. Most aneurysms are located at bifurcations in or near the circle of Willis or in the vertebrobasilar arteries, or within the carotid system (see Fig. 12-17). Aneurysms may be single, but in 20% of the cases, more than one aneurysm is present. In these instances the aneurysms may be unilateral or bilateral.

Pathophysiology

Aneurysms may be classified on the basis of pathophysiology. **Saccular aneurysms** (berry aneurysms) occur frequently (in approximately 2% of the population) and are probably the result of congenital abnormalities in the media of the arterial wall. The sac gradually grows over time. A saccular aneurysm may be (1) round with a narrow stalk connecting it to the parent artery, (2) broad-based without a stalk, or (3) cylindrical (Fig. 15-15). Saccular aneurysms are rare in childhood; their highest incidence of rupturing or bleeding is among persons 35 to 65 years of age (Fig. 15-16).

Fusiform aneurysms (giant aneurysms) occur as a result of diffuse arteriosclerotic changes and are most commonly found in the basilar arteries or terminal portions of the internal carotid arteries (see Fig. 15-15, *B*). They act as space-occupying lesions. **Mycotic aneu-**

I. CVA INVOLVING THE ANTERIOR CERE-
BRAL ARTERY:

Mental status impairments
• Confusion
• Amnesia
• Perseveration
• Personality changes; flat affect, apathy
• Cognitive changes: short attention span, slowness
• Deterioration of intellectual function

Urinary incontinence (long duration)

Contralateral hemiparesis or hemiplegia; sensory impairments; foot and leg deficits greater than arm deficits

Footdrop

Apraxia on affected side

Expressive aphasia (for dominant hemisphere involvement)

Deviation of eyes and head toward affected side

Albulia (inability to make decisions or perform voluntary acts)

Gait dysfunction

II. CVA INVOLVING THE MIDDLE CEREBRAL
ARTERY:

Dysphasia (dominant hemisphere involvement), dyslexia, dysgraphia

Contralateral hemiparesis or hemiplegia

Contralateral hemisensory disturbances

Rapid deterioration in consciousness from confusion
to coma

Vomiting

Homonymous hemianopia

Denial or lack of recognition of a paralyzed extremity

Inability to turn eyes toward affected side

III. CVA INVOLVING THE POSTERIOR CERE-
BRAL ARTERY:

Peripheral signs
• Visual disturbances:
  – Homonymous hemianopia
  – Cortical blindness
  – Lack of depth perception
  – Failure to see objects not centered in the field of
    vision
  – Visual hallucinations
• Memory deficits
• Perseveration
• Dyslexia

Central Signs
• Thalamic or subthalamic nuclei involvement: diffuse
  sensory loss, mild hemiparesis, intentional tremor
• Cerebral peduncle involvement: contralateral hemiplegia, oculomotor nerve deficits
• Brain stem involvement: pupillary dysfunction,
  nystagmus, loss of conjugate gaze (Hickey, 1981)

IV. CVA INVOLVING THE INTERNAL
CAROTID ARTERY:

Contralateral hemiparesis with facial asymmetry

Contralateral sensory deficits, especially paresthesia

Hemianopia

Ipsilateral episodes of visual blurring or amaurosis
fugax (temporary blindness)

Dysphasia (dominant hemisphere involvement)

Carotid bifurcation bruit

Mild Horner syndrome

V. CVA INVOLVING THE VERTEBRAL-
BASILAR SYSTEM:

Dysarthria, dysphagia

Vertigo, nausea, and syncope

Memory loss, disorientation

Ataxic gait

Dysmetria

Visual symptoms: double vision, homonymous
hemianopia

Tinnitus, hearing loss

Ocular signs: nystagmus, conjugate gaze paralysis,
ophthalmoplegia

Akinetic mutism (locked-in syndrome when basilar
artery occlusion occurs)

Numbness of tongue

Facial weakness, alternating motor paresis

Drop attacks

VI. CVA INVOLVING THE ANTERIOR-
INFERIOR CEREBELLAR ARTERY
(INFERIOR LATERAL PONTINE SYN-
DROME):

Contralateral signs
• Horizontal nystagmus
• Sensory impairments, mainly of trunk and limbs

Ipsilateral signs
• Horner syndrome
• Tinnitus and deafness
• Ataxia and nystagmus
• Facial paralysis and loss of tactile sensation

VII. CVA INVOLVING THE POSTERIOR-
INFERIOR CEREBELLAR ARTERY:

Dysarthria, dysphagia, dysphonia

Vertigo, nystagmus, unsteady gait

Ipsilateral Horner syndrome

Sensory changes—ipsilateral face and contralateral
body

Hiccoughs, vomiting

Paralysis of larynx and soft palate

Wallenberg syndrome: sudden onset of:
• Vertigo, horizontal nystagmus, ataxia
• Nausea and vomiting
• Dysphagia
• Horner syndrome (ipsilateral)
• Pain and temperature loss on trunk and limbs
  (contralateral)
• Balance loss on affected side
• Pain and temperature loss on face (ipsilateral)

From Kneisl & Ames, 1986.

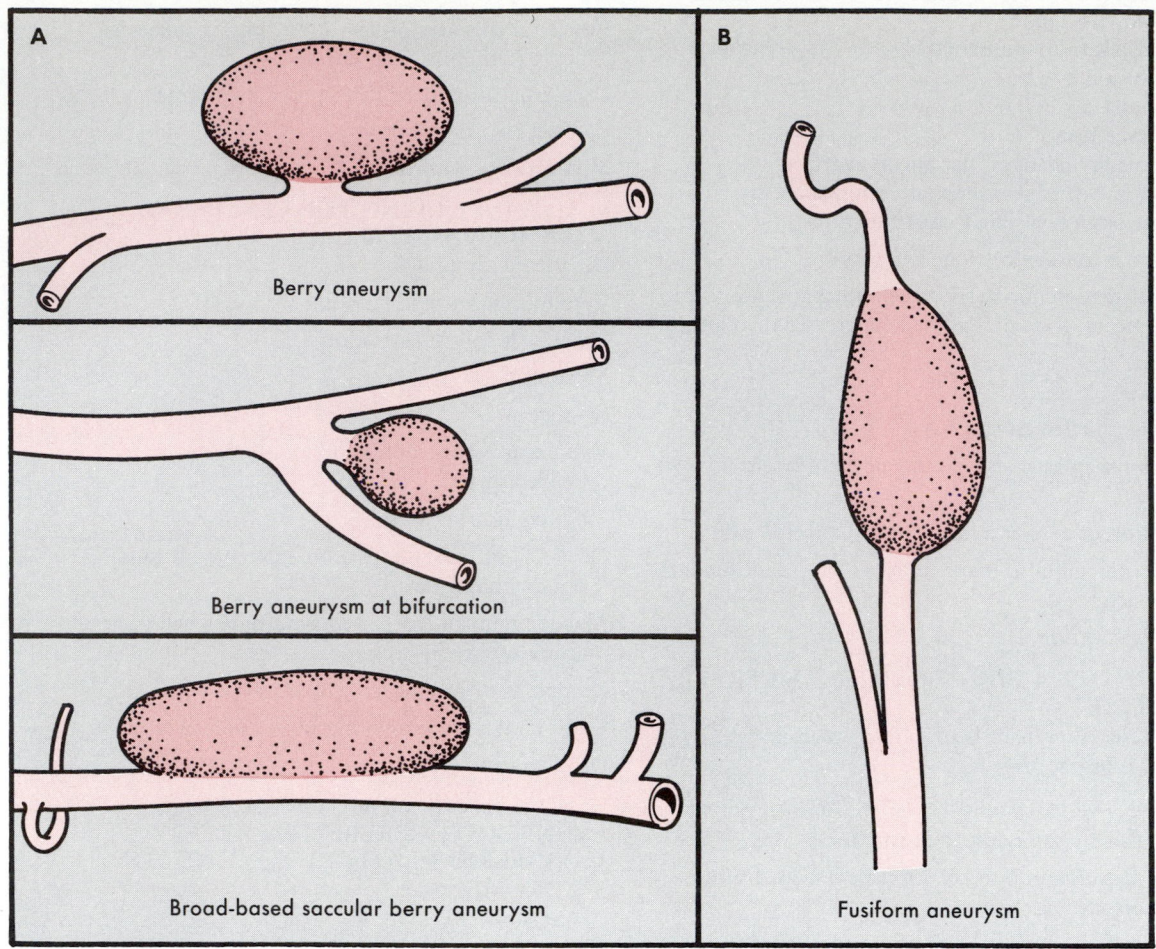

FIG. 15-15. Types of aneurysms.

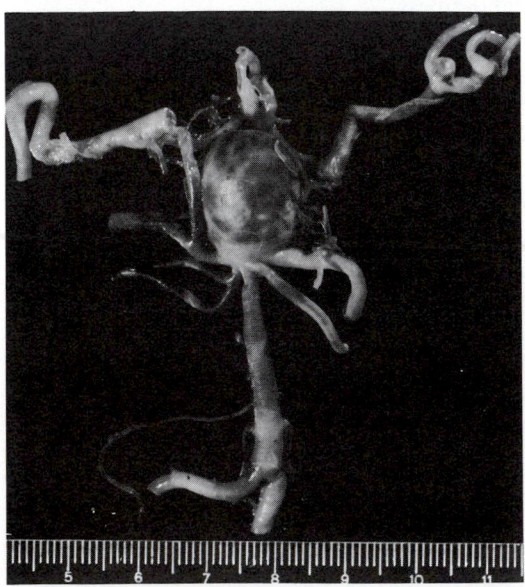

FIG. 15-16. Ruptured berry aneurysms. Larger aneurysm is at terminal portion of basilar artery. Smaller aneurysm is in bifurcation angle of middle cerebral artery on right. (From Kissane, 1985.)

rysms result from arteritis due to bacterial emboli; these aneurysms are uncommon. **Traumatic aneurysms** are caused by a weakening of the arterial wall by a fracture line or a penetrating missile.

Clinical Manifestations

Aneurysms are frequently asymptomatic. Of all persons undergoing routine autopsy 2% are found to have one or more intracranial aneurysms. Clinical manifestations may arise from cranial nerve compression, but the signs vary, depending on the location and size of the aneurysm. Most often, cranial nerves III, IV, V, and VI are affected (see Table 12-5). Unfortunately the most common first indication of the presence of an aneurysm is an acute subarachnoid hemorrhage, intracerebral hemorrhage, or combined subarachnoid-intracerebral hemorrhage (see p. 497).

Ruptured intracranial aneurysms cause two major complications, rebleeding and cerebrovasospasm. Rebleeding is the major cause of death in the unoperated individual. The risk of rebleeding is greatest within 24 hours and again 7 to 10 days after the initial bleed

(Kneisl & Ames, 1986). When the aneurysm first ruptures, a fibrin clot forms, sealing the dome; 7 to 10 days later, the clot undergoes normal lysis, leaving the aneurysm vulnerable to rebleeding.

Vasospasm is thought to occur because of the effects of vasoactive substances, one of which is calcium on the arteries of the subarachnoid space. After injury from the rupture of the cerebral aneurysm, extracellular calcium moves into the lining of the vascular smooth muscle, causing the muscle to become irritable and to constrict. The narrowed vessels are found both adjacent and nonadjacent to the aneurysm. Symptoms of acute vasospasm occur 1 to 3 hours after the initial aneurysm rupture. Chronic vasospasm is slow and insidious, occurring 5 days later or more.

Evaluation and Treatment

Diagnosis prior to a bleeding episode is made through arteriography. After a subarachnoid or intracerebral hemorrhage a tentative diagnosis of an aneurysm is based on clinical manifestations and history. The treatment of choice for an aneurysm is surgical management. The location and size of the aneurysm and the person's clinical status determine whether invasive therapy is feasible.

Arteriovenous Malformation

An **arteriovenous malformation (AVM)** is a tangled mass of dilated blood vessels creating abnormal channels between the arterial and venous systems (arteriovenous fistula). Arteriovenous malformations may occur in any part of the brain. Their size is highly variable, from those of a few millimeters to large malformations that extend from the cortex to the ventricle, and they are usually cone-shaped. The large arteriovenous malformations may also involve the dura mater, including the falx cerebri and the tentorium cerebelli. Arteriovenous malformations occur twice as frequently in males as in females, and they tend to occur in families. Although usually present at birth, arteriovenous malformations exhibit a delayed age of onset, and symptoms most commonly occur between the ages of 10 and 20.

Pathophysiology

Arteriovenous malformations do not have a normal blood vessel structure and are abnormally thin. The involved vessels are thought by some to enlarge over time. The arteriovenous malformation may be fed by one or several arteries. These feeder vessels become tortuous over time and often dilated. With moderate to large AVMs sufficient blood is shunted into the malformation to deprive surrounding tissue of adequate blood perfusion.

Clinical Manifestations

Clinical manifestations vary. Persons with an arteriovenous malformation usually have a characteristic chronic nondescript headache although some experience migraine. Bleeding from an arteriovenous malformation into the subarachnoid space causes clinical manifestations identical to those associated with a ruptured aneurysm. If bleeding is into the brain tissue, focal signs that develop resemble a stroke-in-evolution.

In 20% of persons, headache, dementia, or hemiparesis is evident. The dementia is caused by ischemia or infarction from shunting, compression causing ischemia or infarction, and gliosis (excess glial tissue) resulting from prolonged ischemia. Hemiparesis is usually caused by compression or rupture. Thirty percent of persons experience seizure disorders caused by compression. Initially the seizures tend to be focal or jacksonian; generalization often occurs over time. (Seizures are discussed in Chapter 14). The other 50% suffer an intracerebral, subarachnoid, or subdural hemorrhage. At times noncommunicating hydrocephalus (see p. 519) develops with a large arteriovenous malformation that extends into the ventricle lining.

Evaluation and Treatment

A systolic bruit over the carotid in the neck, the mastoid process, or the eyeball in a young person is almost diagnostic of an arteriovenous malformation. Confirming diagnosis is made by arteriogram. Treatment of choice is surgical management through block dissection or obliteration by ligation of feeders if dissection is not possible. Radiation is used in cases that are surgically unapproachable.

Subarachnoid Hemorrhage

With a **subarachnoid hemorrhage,** blood escapes from a defective or injured vasculature into the subarachnoid space (Fig. 15-17). Individuals at risk for a subarachnoid hemorrhage are those with intracranial aneurysm, intracranial arteriovenous malformation, or hypertension and those who have sustained head injuries. Subarachnoid hemorrhages often recur, especially from a ruptured intracranial aneurysm.

Pathophysiology

When a vessel is leaking, blood oozes into the subarachnoid space. When a vessel tears, blood under pressure is pumped into the subarachnoid space. The blood is extremely irritating to the meningeal and other neural tissues and so produces an inflammatory reaction in these tissues. Additionally the blood coats nerve roots, clogs arachnoid granulations (impairing CSF absorption), and clogs foramina within the ventricular system (impairing CSF circulation). Intracranial pressure rapidly rises. Granulation tissue is formed, and scarring of

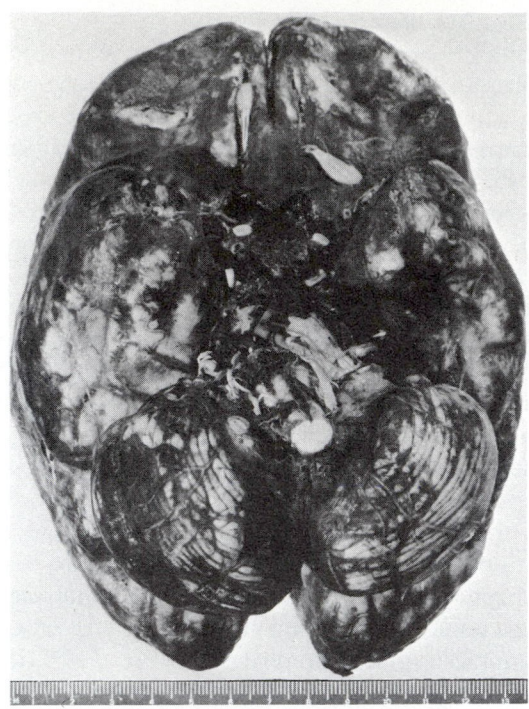

FIG. 15-17. Recent diffuse subarachnoid hemorrhage in individual with massive intracerebral hemorrhage. (From Kissane, 1985.)

the meninges with resulting impairment of CSF reabsorption and secondary hydrocephalus often results.

Clinical Manifestations

Early manifestations associated with leaking vessels are episodic headache, transient changes in mental status, transitory visual or speech disturbances, transient motor weakness, and transitory numbness and tingling. A ruptured vessel is often accompanied by a sudden throbbing, "explosive" headache. The headache is associated with nausea and vomiting, visual disturbances, motor deficits, and loss of consciousness. These signs can all be related to a dramatic rise in intracranial pressure (ICP). Meningeal irritation and inflammation often occur, causing neck stiffness (nuchal rigidity), photophobia, blurred vision, irritability, restlessness, and low-grade fever. A positive **Kernig sign** (in which straightening the knee with the hip and knee in a flexed position produces pain in the back and neck regions) and **Brudzinski sign** (in which passive flexion of the neck produces neck pain and increased rigidity) may appear. No localizing signs are present if the bleed is confined completely to the subarachnoid space.

Vasospasm is a serious complication of a subarachnoid hemorrhage. During the first 2 weeks 30% to 40% of persons with a subarachnoid hemorrhage experience vasospasms in adjacent and sometimes in nonadjacent

vessels. Vasospasm causes ischemia and may produce infarct. The peak time of occurrence is 5 to 7 days after the initial bleed, but vasospasm may persist for several weeks.

Evaluation and Treatment

The diagnosis of a subarachnoid hemorrhage is based on the clinical presentation, a CT scan, MRI, and a lumbar puncture. Arteriography is the definitive diagnostic measure for identifying an aneurysm or arteriovenous malformation. Treatment is directed at control of intracranial pressure, prevention of ischemia and hypoxia of neural tissues, and prevention of rebleeding episodes. Calcium channel blockers, such as verapamil and nifedipine, are used to prevent or reverse vasospasm. A new protocol is to expand blood volume and augment cerebral perfusion by using colloids (albumin) and packed red blood cells to maintain a hematocrit of 33% (Kneisl & Ames, 1986). The primary problem must be diagnosed and corrected as well.

Tumors of the Central Nervous System

Tumors within the cranium can be either primary or metastatic. Primary tumors are classified as primary intracerebral tumors or primary extracerebral tumors. Primary intracerebral tumors originate from brain substance, neuroglia, neurons, cells of the blood vessels, and connective tissue. Primary extracerebral tumors originate outside the substance of the brain and include meningiomas, acoustic nerve tumors, and tumors of the pituitary and pineal glands. Metastatic tumors, or secondary tumors, can be found inside and/or outside the brain substance. Sites of intracranial tumors are illustrated in Fig. 15-18. Central nervous system tumors include both brain and spinal cord tumors.

The incidence of CNS tumors seems to increase up to age 70, then decreases. These tumors represent the second most common group of tumors in children (Fischer, Linggood, & Recht, 1986). Approximately 70% of all intracranial tumors in children are located infratentorially, and in adults 70% are located supratentorially (Robbins, Cotran, & Kumar, 1984). Peripheral nerve tumors are rare in children and common in adults.

CNS tumors cause local and generalized clinical manifestations. The local effects are due to the destructive action of the tumor itself on a particular site in the brain. The effects are varied and include seizures, visual disturbances, unstable gait, and cranial nerve dysfunction.

The generalized effects result from increased ICP (Fig. 15-19). Increased ICP may occur because of obstruction of the ventricular system, hemorrhages occurring in and around the tumor, or cerebral edema caused by tumors (Robbins et al., 1984).

Intracranial brain tumors do not metastasize as readily

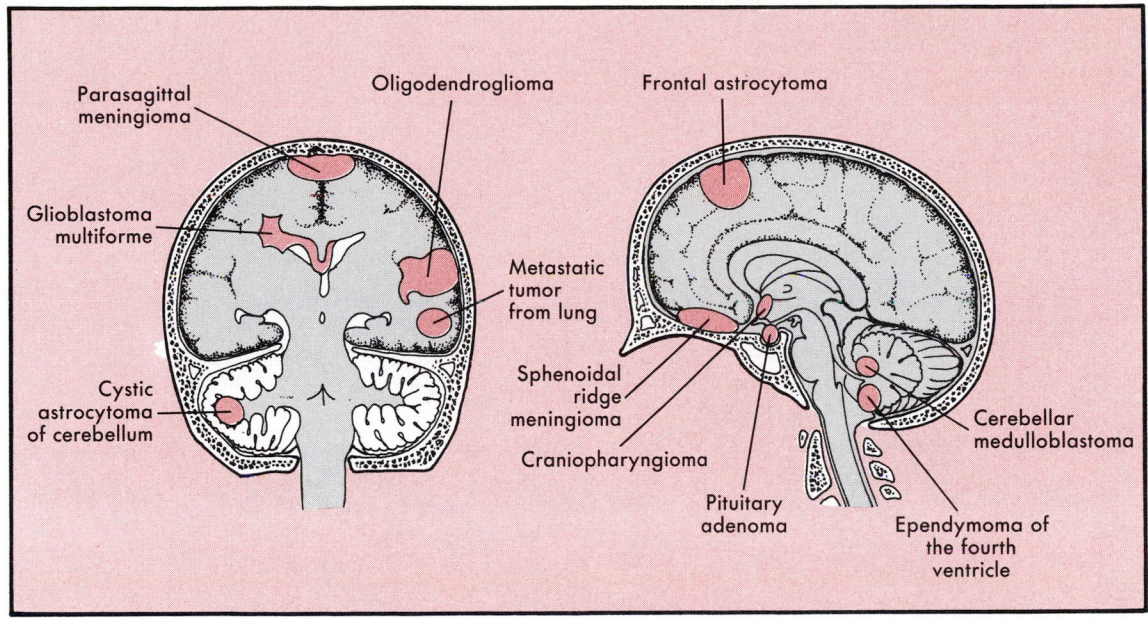

FIG. 15-18. Common sites of intracranial tumors. Tumors metastasize to a variety of locations.

as tumors in other organs because there are no lymphatic channels within the brain substance. If metastasis does occur, it is usually through seeding of the cerebrospinal fluid or through artificial shunts.

Primary Intracerebral Tumors

Primary intracerebral tumors, also called **gliomas,** comprise both encapsulated and nonencapsulated or invasive tumors (Table 15-5). Typically the invasive tumors invade and destroy adjacent normal CNS tissue, whereas more distal neural and vascular tissues are dis-

placed and compressed, causing ischemia, edema, and increased intracranial pressure. Encapsulated tumors do not generally invade adjacent tissues but displace and compress adjacent and distal CNS tissues and vasculature. As with invasive tumors, encapsulated tumors produce ischemia, edema, and increased pressure. Normal function of the neurons is ultimately impaired by the invasion or compression.

The principal treatment for cerebral tumors is surgical excision or surgical decompression if total excision is not possible. Chemotherapy and radiation therapy also

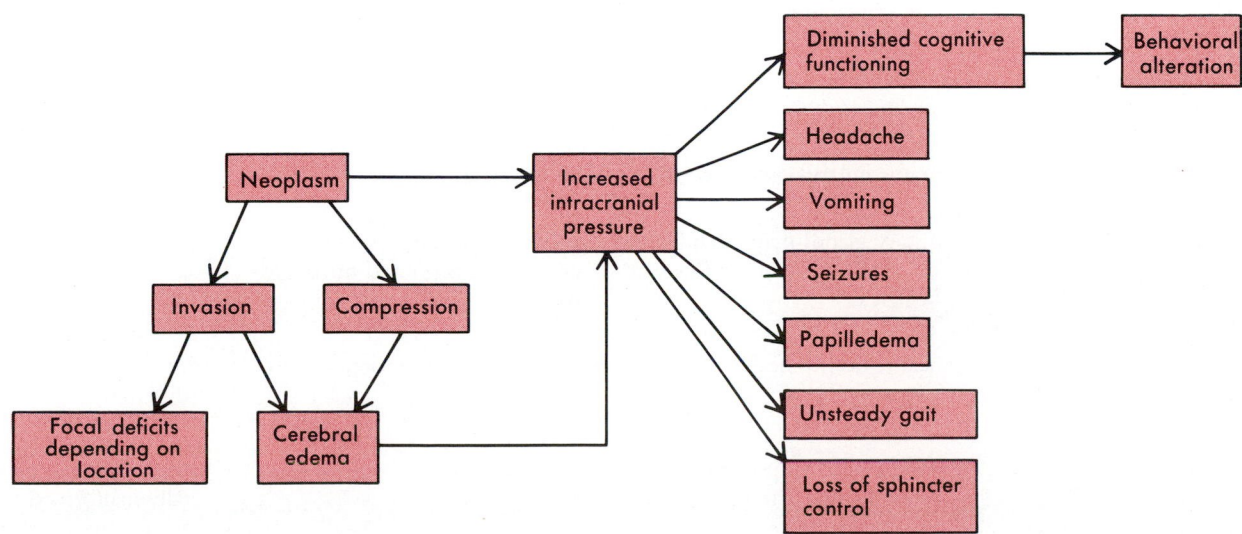

FIG. 15-19. Origin of clinical manifestations associated with an intracranial neoplasm.

TABLE 15-5 Brain and spinal cord tumors

Neoplasm	Location	Characteristics	Cell of origin
Gliomas			
Astrocytoma	Anywhere in brain or spinal cord	Slow-growing, invasive	Astrocytes
Glioblastoma multiforme	Predominantly in cerebral hemispheres	Highly invasive and malignant	Thought to arise from mature astrocytes
Oligodendrocytoma	Most commonly in frontal lobes deep in white matter; may arise in brain stem, cerebellum, and spinal cord	Relatively avascular, tends to be encapsulated; more malignant form called an oligodendroblastoma	Oligodendrites
Ependymoma	Intramedullary: wall of the ventricles; may arise in caudal tail of the spinal cord	More common in children, variable growth rates; more malignant, invasive form is called ependymoblastoma; may extend into the ventricle or invade brain tissue	Ependymal cells
Neuronal cell			
Medulloblastoma	Posterior cerebellar vermis, roof of fourth ventricle	Well-demarcated, rapid-growing, fills fourth ventricle	Embryonic cells
Mesodermal tissue			
Meningioma	Intradural, extramedullary: sylvian fissure region, superior parasagittal surface of frontal and parietal lobes, olfactory groove, wing of sphenoid bone, superior surface of cerebellum, cerebellopontine angle, spinal cord	Slow-growing, circumscribed, encapsulated, sharply demarcated from normal tissues, compressive in nature	Arachnoid cells, may be from fibroblast
Choroid plexus			
Papillomas	Choroid plexus of the ventricular system, lateral ventricle in children, fourth ventricle in adults	Usually benign, slow expansion inducing hemorrhage and hydrocephalus; malignant tumor is rare	Epithelial cells
Cranial nerves and spinal nerve roots			
Neurilemmoma	Cranial nerves (most commonly vestibular division of cranial nerve VIII)	Slow-growing	Schwann cells
Neurofibroma	Extramedullary—spinal cord	Slow-growing	Neurilemma, Schwann cells
Pituitary tumors	Pituitary gland; may extend to or invade floor of the third ventricle	Age-linked, several types slow-growing, macro- and microadenomas	Pituitary cells, pituitary chromophobes, basophils, eosinophils
Pineal region	Pineal region; pineal parenchyma	Several types (germinoma, pineocytoma, teratoma)	Several types with different cell origins
Blood vessel tumors			
Angioma	Predominantly in posterior cerebral hemispheres	Slow-growing	Arising from congenitally malformed arteriovenous connections
Hemangioblastomas	Predominant in cerebellum	Slow-growing	Embryonic vascular tissue

may be used. Supportive treatment is directed at reducing edema. (Cancer treatment is discussed in Chapter 10.)

Glioblastoma Multiforme

Glioblastoma multiforme, now thought to arise from mature astrocytes, comprise approximately 25% of all brain tumors and over 55% of gliomas. The peak age of occurrence is in middle age, and incidence in men is twice that in women. These highly malignant, extensively infiltrative, highly vascular tumors are predominantly located in the cerebral hemispheres. Such tumors may also be located in the brainstem, cerebellum, or spinal cord. The etiology for glioblastoma multiforme is unknown. Genetic factors, trauma, radiation, chemical factors, and viruses have all been implicated.

Glioblastomas are not encapsulated. They may become large enough to extend from the meningeal surface through to the ventricular wall. Of glioblastomas 50% are bilateral or at least occupy more than one lobe at the time of death.

The typical clinical presentation for a glioblastoma multiforme is that of diffuse, nonspecific clinical manifestations such as headache, irritability, and "personality change" that progress to more clear-cut manifestations of increased intracranial pressure such as headache on position change, papilledema, or vomiting. Of persons affected 30% to 40% experience seizure activity. Symptoms may progress to definite focal signs such as hemiparesis, dysphasia, dyspraxia, cranial nerve palsies, and visual field deficits in addition to the generalized signs from the increased intracranial pressure.

Diagnosis most commonly takes from 3 to 6 months from onset of the first clinical manifestations because the person does not recognize the need to consult a health care provider. The treatment of choice is surgical resection, which is more commonly followed by radiation and then chemotherapy. Fewer than one fifth of persons survive 12 to 18 months beyond the onset of clinical manifestations; fewer than 10% live beyond two years. Adding radiation therapy to the conventional surgical regimen has extended mean survival time after surgery from 14 to 36 weeks. Adding chemotherapy to the regimen has increased this mean survival time to 51 weeks.

Astrocytoma

Astrocytomas are slow-growing infiltrative gliomas that tend to form cavities (pseudocysts). Some astrocytomas, however, are firm, noncavitating, avascular, gray-white masses that are difficult to distinguish from normal white matter of the brain. Although these tumors may occur anywhere in the brain or spinal cord, they most commonly are located in the cerebrum, cerebellum, hypothalamus, optic nerve, optic chiasma, and pons (Fig. 15-20).

Approximately one half of persons with astrocytomas experience a focal or generalized seizure. Onset of a focal seizure disorder between the second and sixth decade of life suggests an astrocytoma. Other general or focal neurologic manifestations follow gradually. Headache and increased intracranial pressure are usually late clinical manifestations.

Surgery is the treatment of choice, often followed by radiotherapy. The average survival time from the first

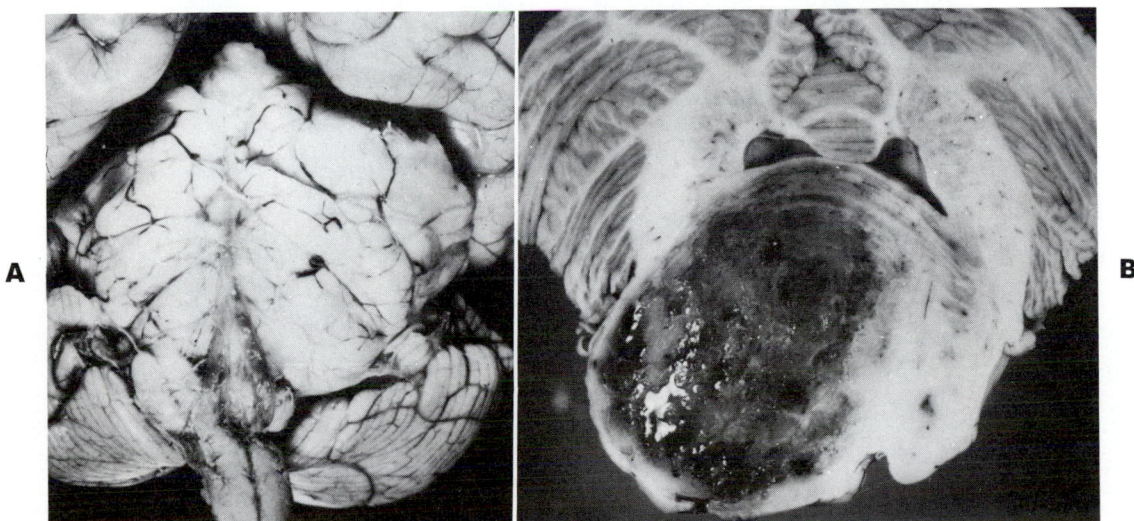

FIG. 15-20. A, External appearance of astrocytoma of pons, illustrating symmetric enlargement of structure often seen in this tumor. **B,** Cross section of astrocytoma of pons, showing hemorrhagic tumor of ill-defined margins partially obliterating fourth ventricle. (Courtesy Dr. J. E. Olivera-Rabiela, Mexico City, Mexico. From Rosai, 1981.)

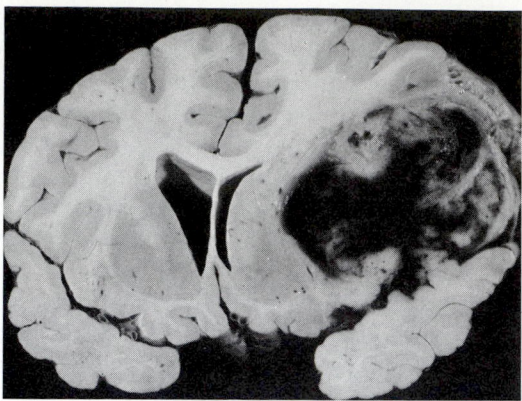

FIG. 15-21. Oligodendroglioma with operative hemorrhage. There is ventricular displacement and cingulate gyrus herniation. (From Kissane, 1985.)

clinical manifestations is over 5 years for cerebral astrocytomas and 7 years for cerebellar astrocytomas.

Oligodendroglioma

A far less commonly occurring glioma is the **oligodendroglioma,** comprising perhaps 5% to 7% of all intracranial gliomas. A typically slow-growing tumor, most oligodendrogliomas are macroscopically indistinguishable from other gliomas (Fig. 15-21). Of oligodendrogliomas 40% to 70% develop in the frontal lobes, often in the deep white matter. They may also be found in other parts of the cerebrum, third ventricle,

brainstem, cerebellum, and spinal cord. About one-half of these tumors generally classified as oligodendrogliomas are actually a mixed type of oligodendroglioma and astrocytoma. Malignant degeneration occurs in about one-third of persons with oligodendrogliomas, and the tumors are then referred to as **oligodendroblastomas.** The tumor rarely becomes a glioblastoma. If there is extension to the pia mater or ependymal wall (see Fig. 12-14), oligodendrogliomas may metastasize to distant CNS sites through the ventriculoarachnoid spaces.

More than 50% of individuals experience a focal or generalized seizure as the first clinical manifestation. Only about one half of persons with an oligodendroglioma have experienced increased intracranial pressure at the time of diagnosis and surgery, and only one third develop any focal manifestations. The time from first clinical manifestation to surgical intervention often ranges from 2 to 6 years. Mean survival time postoperatively is approximately 5 years, and recurrences are common after surgery.

Ependymoma

Ependymomas are gliomas that arise from ependymal cells that form the walls of the ventricles and grow either into the ventricle or into adjacent brain tissue; they are not encapsulated (see Fig. 15-22 and Table 15-5). They comprise about 5% of all intracranial gliomas in adults and 10% to 12% in children. Of ependymomas 70% occur in the fourth ventricle. Other common sites for ependymomas are the third ventricle, lateral

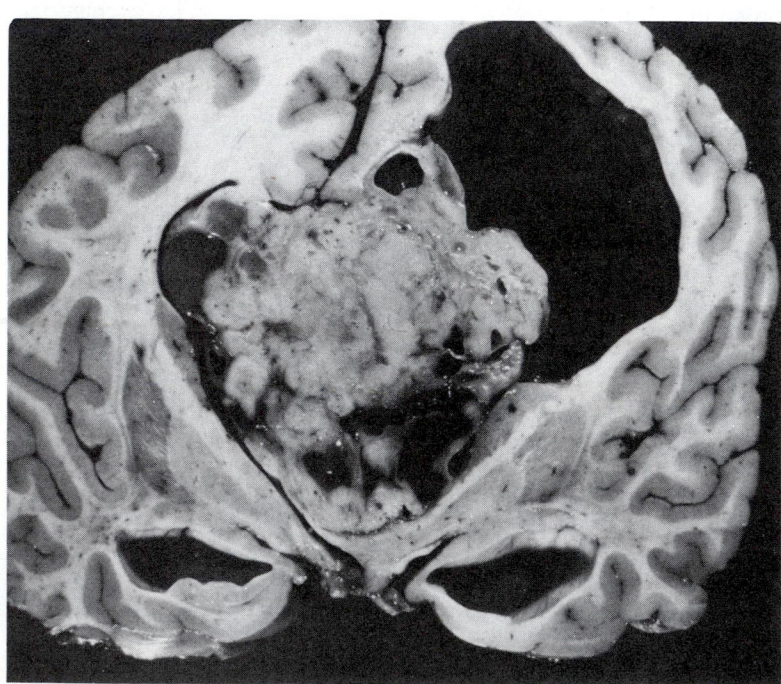

FIG. 15-22. Large septal ependymoma, with secondary hydrocephalus. (Courtesy Dr. J. E. Olivera-Rabiela, Mexico City, Mexico. From Rosai, 1981.)

ventricles, and caudal portion of the spinal cord. About 40% of the infratentorial ependymomas occur in children younger than 10 years of age. Occurrence of cerebral (supratentorial) ependymomas is distributed among all ages.

Ependymomas in the cerebrum resemble other gliomas in their clinical presentation. In approximately one third of persons, seizures occur. In fourth ventricle ependymomas, two thirds of persons have increased intracranial pressure. Other clinical manifestations may include vomiting, vertigo, difficulty swallowing, head tilt, and paresthesias of the extremities.

Clinical manifestations and progression of dysfunction associated with ependymomas may follow a short or long course. The interval between first manifestations and surgery may be as short as 4 weeks with some ependymoblastomas to as long as 7 to 8 years with others.

Surgery is the treatment of choice. Ependymomas are not very radiosensitive. Some persons benefit from a shunting procedure when the ependymoma has caused a noncommunicating hydrocephalus (see p. 519).

Primary Extracerebral Tumors

Meningioma

Meningioma comprises 15% of all intracranial tumors. They are considered benign because they are encapsulated and usually do not invade the surrounding brain (Fig. 15-23). These tumors originate from the dura mater or arachnoid membranes. Rarely do meningiomas arise from arachnoid cells of the choroid plexus of the ventricles. Meningiomas most commonly are located in the olfactory grooves, on the wings of the sphenoid bone (at the base of the skull), in the tuberculum

sella (a structure next to the sella turcica), on the superior surface of the cerebellum, and in the cerebellopontine angle and spinal cord.

Small meningiomas (less than 2.0 cm in diameter) are often found on postmortem examination in middle-aged and elderly individuals who had experienced no clinical manifestations and died of totally unrelated causes. The etiology for meningiomas is unknown.

A meningioma is a sharply circumscribed mass that derives its shape from the space it occupies. A meningioma may extend to the dural surface and erode the cranial bones or produce an osteoblastic reaction. A few meningiomas exhibit malignant, invasive qualities.

Only when meningiomas reach a certain size, where they begin to indent the brain parenchyma, do they begin to produce clinical manifestations. Focal seizures are frequently the first manifestation. Other clinical manifestations depend on the tumor's location. Because of the extremely slow-growing nature of most meningiomas, increased intracranial pressure is less common than with gliomas.

Surgical excision results in a cure if all the tumor and its meningeal stem are accessible. If only partial resection is possible, the tumor recurs.

Neurilemmoma

Neurilemmoma (neuromas, schwannomas) arise from the sheath of Schwann cells surrounding the axons of the cranial nerves. The tumors most commonly affect persons over 50 years of age, and both sexes are affected equally. The vestibular division of cranial nerve VIII is most commonly affected, although neurilemmomas of the acoustic division of cranial nerve VIII, cranial nerve V, and cranial nerve IX are found (Fig. 15-24).

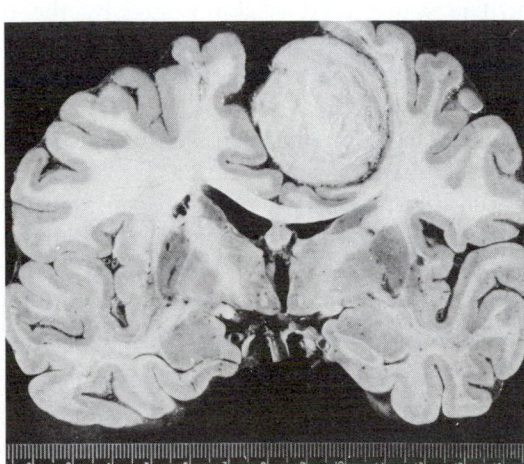

FIG. 15-23. Parasagittal meningioma, fibrous type. There are small, remote anemic infarcts in internal capsules and left putamen. (From Kissane, 1985.)

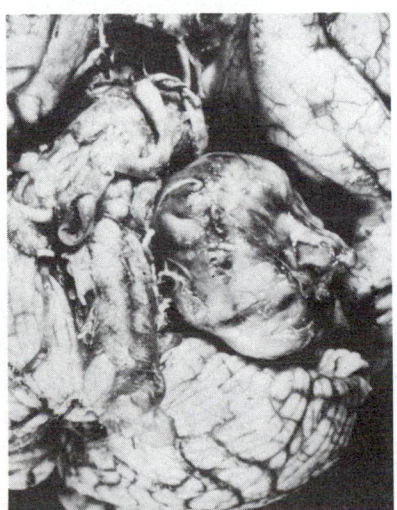

FIG. 15-24. External appearance of neurilemoma of cerebellopontine angle. Tapered end of acoustic nerve on one side and compression of pons and medulla on other are well appreciated. (Courtesy Dr. J. E. Olivera-Rabiela, Mexico City, Mexico. From Rosai, 1981.)

The tumor most commonly originates just distal to the junction between the nerve root and the brainstem. As the tumor grows, it extends into the posterior fossa to occupy the cerebropontine angle and compress adjacent nerves. Eventually the brainstem is displaced, and the CSF flow is obstructed.

Initial clinical manifestations may include headache, tinnitus, hearing loss, impaired balance, unsteady gait, facial pain, and loss of facial sensations. Later, vertigo with nausea and vomiting, a sense of pressure in the ear, and moderate to severe unsteadiness with rapid position changes may appear.

CT scan or MRI can establish the diagnosis. Posterior fossa dye studies may be required. Treatment is by surgical excision of the neurilemmoma. Pituitary tumors are discussed in Chapter 18, and cerebral tumors in children are discussed in Chapter 16.

Metastatic Carcinoma

One third of metastatic brain tumors arise from the lung, approximately one sixth from the breast, and a lesser number from the gastrointestinal tract and kidney. Melanoma and carcinoma of the gallbladder, liver, thyroid, testes, uterus, ovary, and pancreas may also metastasize to the brain. Other tumors besides carcinomas, known to metastasize only occasionally, are rhabdomyosarcomas, Ewing tumor, chorioepithelioma, lymphoma, and carcinoma.

Carcinomas are disseminated to the brain from the circulation. In more than three-fourths of persons, the metastases are multiple and found in both the cerebrum and cerebellum in a scattered distribution. The metastatic tumors are often located in the meninges and near the brain surface in the gray matter and subcortical white matter. These tumors produce little glial cell reaction in the brain tissue but do cause vasogenic edema in the surrounding brain tissue.

The clinical manifestation of a metastatic brain tumor usually resembles that of a glioblastoma although several unusual syndromes do exist. Carcinomatous encephalopathy causes headache, nervousness, depressed mood, trembling, confusion, and forgetfulness. In carcinomatosis of the cerebellum, headache, dizziness, and ataxia are found. Carcinomatosis of the craniospinal meninges (carcinomatous meningitis) manifests with headache, confusion, and manifestations of cranial or spinal nerve root dysfunction.

Metastatic brain tumors carry a very poor prognosis. If a solitary tumor is found, surgery and/or radiation therapy is used, but if multiple tumors exist, symptomatic relief only is pursued.

Spinal Cord Tumors

Spinal cord tumors are named to reflect their cell type, growth rate, and structure of origin. Spinal cord tumors are classified as **intramedullary tumors** (originating within the neural tissues) or **extramedullary tumors** (originating from tissues outside the spinal cord). Extramedullary tumors arise from the meninges or roots (forming **intradural tumors**) or from epidural tissue or vertebral structure (forming **extradural tumors**). About 5% of spinal cord tumors seen in general hospital settings are intramedullary; 40% are intradural-extramedullary; and 55% are extradural.

Metastatic spinal cord tumors are usually carcinomas, lymphomas, or myelomas. Their location is often extradural. Of extradural tumors 50% are metastatic and have spread to the spine through direct extension from tumors of the vertebral structures or from extraspinal sources extending through the interventricular foramen or through the bloodstream.

The most common primary extramedullary spinal cord tumors are neurofibromas and meningiomas. These tumors are intradural more often than extradural. Neurofibromas are found most commonly in the thoracic region. Meningiomas are more evenly distributed through the spine. Other extramedullary tumors in order of frequency of occurrence are sarcomas, vascular tumors, chordomas, and epidermoid and similar tumors. Of intradural-extramedullary tumors 70% are meningiomas, neurofibromas, or sarcomas.

Intramedullary tumors have the same cellular origins as brain tumors. Ependymomas account for 40% of intramedullary spinal cord tumors. Astrocytomas, glioblastomas, oligodendrogliomas, ganglioneuromas, medullablastomas, hemangiomas, and hemangioblastomas are more or less equally distributed in frequency of occurrence.

Pathophysiology

Extramedullary spinal cord tumors produce dysfunction by compression of adjacent tissue, not by direct invasion. The spinal cord is compressed by the tumor from without, and destruction of the white matter tracts occurs. The spinal canal around the cord becomes filled by tumor.

Intramedullary spinal cord tumors produce dysfunction by both invasion and compression. The cord enlarges from the tumor that is enlarging inside the cord. Additionally distortion of adjacent white matter tracts occurs. Metastases from spinal cord tumors occur from seeding through the cerebrospinal fluid; medulloblastomas and ependymomas establish distant implants in this manner.

Clinical Manifestations

The acute onset of clinical manifestations suggests a vascular insult caused by thrombosis of vessels supplying the spinal cord. Clinical manifestations that are gradual and progressive suggest compression. The clinical manifestations associated with spinal cord tumors fall into three major categories: (1) a compressive syndrome (sensorimotor syndrome), (2) an irritative syndrome (radicular syndrome), and (3) rarely, a syringomyelic syndrome.

The **compressive syndrome** is associated with compression and is less frequently caused by invasion and destruction of the spinal cord tracts. Symptoms are usually gradual and progressive, and initial manifestations may be asymmetric. With tumors located in the cervical area, the motor dysfunction usually has the following pattern: ipsilateral arm involvement, followed by ipsilateral and contralateral leg involvement, and finally involvement of the opposite arm. With thoracic tumors the pattern of motor involvement is paresis and spasticity of one leg, followed by involvement of the opposite leg. The sensory clinical manifestations of tingling paresthesias have a similar pattern to that of the motor signs. Pain and temperature dysfunctions are more commonly found than touch, vibration, and proprioceptive changes, although posterior column signs are also frequently found. Pain is less well localized than with an irritative syndrome caused by root involvement. Initially the pain and temperature changes are contralateral to the motor deficit (Brown-Sequard syndrome). Bladder and bowel deficits usually appear when paresis develops in the legs.

The **irritative syndrome** combines the clinical manifestations of a cord compression with radicular pain, which is pain in the sensory root distribution and indicates root irritation. The segmental manifestations associated with root irritation include segmental sensory changes that include paresthesias and impaired pain and touch perception; motor disturbances, including cramps, atrophy, fasciculations, and decreased or absent deep tendon reflexes; and ache in the spine. Tenderness of the spinous processes over the tumor is present in about one-half of persons with extramedullary tumors. The segmental changes may appear months and sometimes years before the clinical manifestations of compression in benign tumors. The compressive clinical manifestations include an asymmetric spastic paresis of the lower extremities with tumors in the thoracic or lumbar region, paresis of the arms and legs with tumors in the cervical area, decreased or absent pain and temperature perception below the tumor site, posterior column signs, and spastic bladder.

Because they involve the central gray matter of the cord, intramedullary spinal cord tumors, notably ependymomas, may be a **syringomyelic syndrome,** or inflammation of the spinal cord. Inflammation results in the development of tubular (syrinx) cavities in the spinal cord. Occasionally an extramedullary tumor may produce the same effect, although the mechanisms are unknown.

Evaluation and Treatment

The diagnosis of a spinal cord tumor is made through spinal x-rays, cerebrospinal fluid studies, CT scan, MRI, myelogram, and spinal angiography. Involvement of specific cord segments is established. Any metastases are also identified.

Treatment varies, depending on the nature of the tumor and the person's clinical status. Intradural-extramedullary tumors are surgically removed or decompressed through laminectomy. Laminectomy with decompression and excision is used for gliomas and is followed by radiotherapy. Extradural metastatic tumors are often managed by radiotherapy, chemotherapy, hormonal therapy, or pain management protocols.

Infection and Inflammation of the Central Nervous System

The CNS may be affected directly by bacteria, viruses, fungi, protozoans, and rickettsia. The resulting infection is pyogenic, or pus-producing. Bacterial toxins may also affect the CNS. The meninges, neural tissues, and vasculature may also be involved in the inflammatory process.

Meningitis

Meningitis (infection of the meninges) may be caused by bacteria, viruses, and fungi. The infections are classified as acute, subacute, or chronic processes, and the pathophysiology, clinical manifestations, and treatment are different for each type of organism.

Bacterial meningitis is primarily an infection of the pia mater and arachnoid and of the fluid in the subarachnoid space. A systemic or bloodstream infection or a direct extension from an infected area is the access route to the subarachnoid space. The ventricles are involved in bacterial meningitis. Meningococcus *(Neisseria meningitidis),* pneumococcus *(Streptococcus pneumoniae),* and *Haemophilus influenzae* are the common causes of bacterial meningitis.

Meningococcus has been identified worldwide. Meningococcal meningitis occurs predominately in males and in the fall, winter, and spring of the year. Epidemics of meningococcal meningitis occur in approximately 10-year cycles. Children and adolescents are predominantly affected. With pneumococcal meningitis, the young and those over 40 years of age are mostly affected. *Haemophilus influenzae* occurs almost exclusively in children 2 months to 7 years of age. Less frequent causes are staphylococcus, streptococcus, gonococcus, and gram-negative bacteria.

Aseptic meningitis (nonpurulent meningitis) is an inflammation believed to be limited to the meninges. Aseptic meningitis produces a variety of symptoms and is caused by a variety of infectious agents, most of which are viruses. Enteroviral viruses (echovirus, cosackievirus, and nonparalytic poliomyelitis), mumps, herpes simplex (type I), adenoviruses, and California virus are the most common causes of aseptic meningitis. Bacterial infections not adequately treated are another cause of aseptic meningitis.

Fungal meningitis is a chronic, much less common condition than bacterial or viral meningitis. The most common fungal infections of the nervous system are cryptococcosis, coccidioidomycosis, mucormycosis, candidiasis, and aspergillosis. Fungal meningitis most frequently occurs in persons with impaired immune responses or alterations in normal body flora. Fungal meningitis develops insidiously, usually over days or weeks.

Pathophysiology

The bacteria that commonly cause bacterial meningitis are common inhabitants of the nasopharynx, but a predisposing factor such as a prior upper respiratory infection must be present before the bacteria become blood-borne. The method of CNS entry is still unclear. The bacteria or their toxins do, however, function as irritants and induce vascular changes, specifically congestion and increased permeability. The meningeal vessels become hyperemic, and blood cells (neutrophils) migrate into the subarachnoid space. An inflammatory reaction is mobilized by the meninges (pia and arachnoid), the CSF, and the ventricles. A purulent inflammatory exudate is formed and increases rapidly, especially around the base of the brain, and extends into the sheaths of the cranial and spinal nerves and into the perivascular spaces of the cortex. The small- and medium-sized subarachnoid arteries, veins, and choroid plexuses undergo inflammatory changes. The cortical neurons also show some changes, including an increase in the number of microglia and astrocytes.

Fungi in the nervous system usually produce a granulomatous reaction with formations of granulomas or gelatinous masses. These usually develop in the meninges at the base of the brain. Fungi may also extend along the perivascular sites in the subarachnoid space and into the brain tissue, producing arteritis with thrombosis, infarction, and communicating hydrocephalus. Meningeal fibrosis develops later in the inflammatory process. Cranial nerve dysfunction, caused by compression, often results from the granulomas and fibrosis.

Clinical Manifestations

The clinical manifestations of a bacterial meningitis that arise from the meningeal inflammation are a generalized throbbing headache that becomes very severe, forceful flexion of the neck onto the chest, causing Brudzinski sign (flexion of the legs and thighs); and Kernig sign (inability to extend the leg with the hip flexed at a right angle). The irritation and damage to the cranial nerve produced by the inflamed sheaths are man-

ifested in photophobia, which becomes extreme; diplopia; and tinnitus. Neck stiffness, pain with nuchal rigidity, and possibly head retraction reflect the irritability of the spinal accessory and cervical spinal nerves. Often the vomiting center is irritated, causing projectile vomiting. Confusion and decreasing responsiveness are evidence of the cortical involvement. Fever is usually present. With meningococcal meningitis, there is a petechial or purpuric rash involving the skin and mucous membranes. As intracranial pressure rises, papilledema may develop and delirium may progress so that the individual reaches an unconscious state.

The clinical manifestations of aspetic meningitis are mild compared to those associated with bacterial meningitis. Mild generalized throbbing headache, mild photophobia, mild neck pain, stiffness, fever, and malaise are all manifestations of aseptic meningitis.

Fungal meningitis develops slowly and insidiously. The first manifestations are often those of dementia (see Chapter 14) or communicating hydrocephalus (see p. 519). The individual is characteristically afebrile.

Evaluation and Treatment

Diagnosis of bacterial meningitis is based on physical examination and cultures of blood and cerebral spinal fluid. Bacterial meningitis and fungal meningitis are treated with appropriate antibiotic therapy and other supportive measures. Aseptic meningitis is sometimes managed pharmacologically with antibiotics, antiviral drugs, and steroids.

Abscess

Abscesses most often originate from infections outside the CNS. The infective sources are the middle ear, mastoid cells, nasal cavity, nasal sinuses, heart, and lungs. Other, less common foci are the pelvic organs, skin, tonsils, abscessed teeth, osteomyelitis in other than cranial bones, and results of intravenous drug abuse. Microbes may be introduced into the CNS by open trauma or neurosurgery. Streptococci, often in combination with anaerobes, are the most common bacteria that cause abscesses, but fungi have also been found in CNS abscesses. The sizes of CNS abscesses are highly variable.

Brain abscesses are classified as extradural or intracerebral. **Extradural brain abscesses** are associated with osteomyelitis in a cranial bone. Unlike **intracerebral brain abscesses,** they rarely arise from a vascular source. **Spinal cord abscesses** are classified as epidural or intramedullary. Individuals with diabetes mellitus show an increased incidence of **spinal epidural abscesses** (which form in the epidural space), whereas debilitated individuals with sepsis more frequently develop **intramedullary spinal cord abscesses** (those within the spinal cord). Epidural spinal abscesses usually originate as osteomyelitis in a vertebra; the infection then spreads into the epidural space. (Osteomyelitis is discussed in Chapter 39.)

Pathophysiology

Organisms gain entrance to the CNS from adjacent sites by direct extension from osteomyelitis or spread along the wall of a vein. Infective emboli carry the organisms from distant sites. Initially a localized inflammatory process develops with exudate formation, septic thrombosis of vessels, and aggregates of degenerating leukocytes. The surrounding tissues are edematous (Fig. 15-25). The veins are filled with fibrin and polymorphonuclear leukocytes (white blood cells [WBCs]). After a few days the intense reaction abates, and the infection becomes delimited with a center of pus and a wall of granular tissue. Abscesses may be encapsulated or free (not encapsulated). Existing abscesses also tend to spread and form daughter abscesses.

Abscesses arising from the ear are frequently located in the middle or inferior temporal lobe or in the anteriolateral cerebellar hemispheres. Abscesses originating from the nasal area most commonly are located in the frontal and temporal lobes. Abscesses from distant foci often occur in multiple numbers in the distal portion of the middle cerebral arteries. In extradural abscesses pus and granulation tissue accumulate in the extradural space.

Clinical Manifestations

Early clinical manifestations of brain abscesses are low-grade fever, headache, neck pain and stiffness with mild nuchal rigidity, confusion, drowsiness, sensory deficits, and communication deficits. Headache is the most frequent early symptom. Later clinical manifestations may include inattentiveness (distractability), memory deficits, decreased visual acuity and narrowed visual fields, papilledema, ocular palsy, ataxia, and dementia. Symptoms depend on the location of the abscess. The development of symptoms may be very insidious, often making an abscess difficult to diagnose.

Extradural brain abscesses are associated with localized pain, purulent drainage from the nasal passages or auditory canal, fever, localized tenderness, and neck stiffness. Occasionally the individual experiences a focal seizure.

Early clinical manifestations of a spinal cord abscess are pain, which is usually severe; spasms of the back muscles; and limiting of vertebral movement caused by pain and spasm. Later signs are of progressive cord compression causing paresis, paralysis, and limited movement.

Evaluation and Treatment

Diagnosis is based on clinical features and CT scans. Antibiotic therapy, surgical drainage, and aspiration are the major therapeutic interventions for brain abscesses. In addition intracranial pressure may have to be managed. Because decompression is necessary, spinal cord abscesses are treated with surgical drainage or aspiration. Antibiotic and supportive therapy is also instituted.

Encephalitis

Encephalitis is an acute febrile illness of viral origin with nervous system involvement. The most common encephalitides are caused by arthropod-borne viruses and herpes simplex, almost exclusively herpes simplex type I (Fig. 15-26). Encephalitis may also occur as a

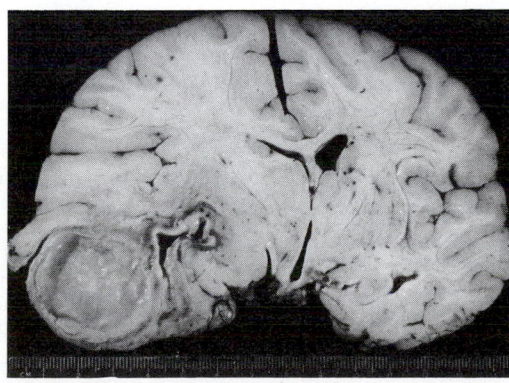

FIG. 15-25. Chronic brain abscesses in temporal lobe and insula. Surrounding brain shows swelling and edema. There are compression and displacement of lateral and third ventricles. Cingulate gyrus and uncal herniations are also present. (From Kissane, 1985.)

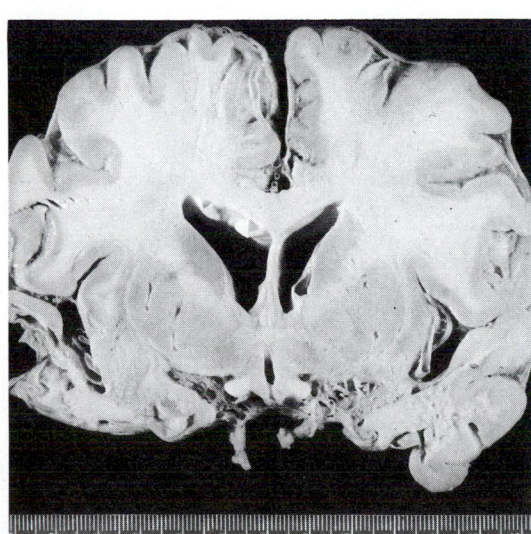

FIG. 15-26. Chronic necrotizing encephalitis caused by herpes simplex. There is necrosis of temporal lobes, insula, and cingulate gyri. (From Kissane, 1985.)

TABLE 15-6 Viral encephalitis

Type	Geographic incidence	Seasonal incidence
Arthropod-borne: Eastern equine encephalitis	Eastern United States	Autumn
Western equine encephalitis	Uniform distribution, throughout the United States	Summer and early fall
St. Louis encephalitis	Widespread distribution; in the far west occurs in rural areas, elsewhere in urban areas	Late summer
Venezuelan equine encephalitis	Southwestern United States	Year round
California virus encephalitis	Midwestern states	Early fall
Herpes simplex encephalitis	No particular geographic distribution	No seasonal incidence
Poliovirus poliomyelitis	Sporadic distribution where non-immunized persons cluster	Summer and early fall
Rabies	Sporadic distribution throughout the United States	Bites more common in late spring and throughout the early fall

From Boss, 1984.

complication of systemic viral diseases such as poliomyelitis, rabies, or mononucleosis, or it may arise after recovery from some viral infection such as rubella or rubeola. Encephalitis also may follow vaccination with a live attentuate virus vaccine, if the vaccine has an encephalitis component. Such vaccines include measles, mumps, and rubella. Typhus, trichinosis, malaria, and schistosomiasis are also associated with encephalitis.

With the exception of the California viral encephalitis, which is endemic, the arthropod-borne encephalitides occur in epidemics, varying in geographical and seasonal incidences (see Table 15-6). Eastern equine encephalitis is the most serious but least common of the encephalitides.

Pathophysiology

Evidence of meningeal involvement appears in all encephalitides. The arthropod-borne viral encephalitides cause widespread nerve cell degeneration. Edema and areas of necrosis with or without hemorrhage develop. Increased intracranial pressure develops and may progress to herniation. Large degenerative injuries are found in Eastern equine encephalitis, whereas the other arthropod-borne viral encephalitides have microscopic areas of injury and degeneration. Herpes simplex type I has a tendency to infect the inferiomedial surfaces of the temporal and frontal lobes and causes hemorrhagic necrosis.

Clinical Manifestations

The dramatic clinical manifestations of encephalitis are fever, delirium, or confusion progressing to unconsciousness, seizure activity, cranial nerve palsies, paresis and paralysis, involuntary movement, and abnormal reflexes. Signs of marked intracranial pressure may be present.

Evaluation and Treatment

Until very recently no definitive treatment was available for the viral encephalitides, but herpes encephalitis is now being treated with antiviral agents such as acyclovir. Supportive therapy is initiated, and measures to control intracranial pressure are paramount.

Neurosyphilis

One fourth of persons with syphilis develop **neurosyphilis,** an infection caused by the organism *Treponema pallidum,* which usually invades the CNS 3 to 18 months after the initial infection. Initially an aseptic meningitis develops. Within 2 to 7 years a symptomatic meningitis or meningovascular syphilis may appear with symptoms of headache, stiff neck, confusion, sensory loss, and language and visual disturbances. Syphilis causes the most chronic form of meningitis, and parenchymal damage results in later years. **Tabes dorsalis,** a degeneration of the dorsal columns of the spinal cord, is characteristic. General paresis, optic atrophy, and meningomyelitis may appear with progressive dementia, hyperreflexia, dysarthria and action tremors, and ataxia. Diagnosis and treatment are the same as for primary syphilis (see Chapter 21).

Wernicke Disease

Wernicke disease (Wernicke encephalopathy) is a nutritional deficiency disease characterized by mental confusion, ataxia of gait, and abducens and conjugate gaze palsies. The disease is caused by thiamine deficiency and is predominantly found in persons who abuse alcohol. Other individuals at risk are the malnourished or starving, those who engage in dietary fads, or those who have a malabsorption syndrome. Males are slightly more affected than females, and onset of the disease is usually between 30 and 70 years of age.

Korsakoff psychosis is usually associated with Wernicke disease in the nutritionally deficient person. **Korsakoff psychosis** (amnesic-confabulatory psychosis, psychosis polyneuritis) refers to a unique memory disorder in which recent memory is rather exclusively and severely impaired. The memory impairment is totally out of proportion to any other impairment of cortical function, and the person is otherwise alert and responsive. Korsakoff psychosis may be a symptom of other neurologic disorders that injure the diencephalon or temporal lobes, such as third ventricle tumors, infarction of the inferiomedial temporal lobe, hypoxic encephalopathy; after herpes simplex encephalitis; and in Alzheimer disease.

Pathophysiology

Thiamine (vitamin B_1) is essential as a coenzyme in the neuron's metabolic pathways. Without an adequate supply of thiamine, neurons cannot maintain their own energy production and other vital functions. In acute Wernicke disease, injury is found in both thalami and the hypothalamus around the ventricles, in the mamillary bodies, in the midbrain around the aqueduct, in the fourth ventricle near the vagus motor nuclei and vestibular division of cranial nerve VIII, and in the superior vermis of the cerebellum (Fig. 15-27).

The injury found in Korsakoff psychosis is similar to that in Wernicke disease. Additional injury areas are found in the medial dorsal nucleus and the posterior nucleus of the thalami.

Clinical Manifestations

The clinical manifestations of Wernicke disease are threefold: (1) a disordered mentation of consciousness,

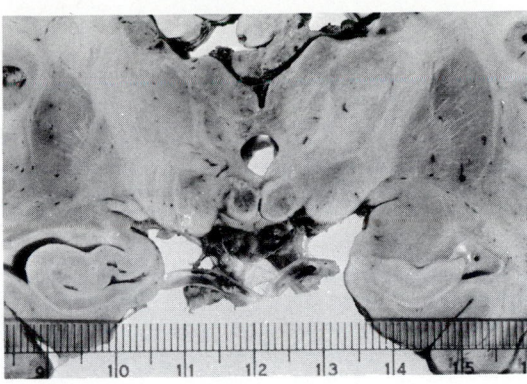

FIG. 15-27. Acute Wernicke disease with involvement of mamillary bodies, hypothalami, and thalami. (From Kissane, 1985.)

(2) an ataxia, and (3) ophthalmoplegia. Any of the three signs may be the initial manifestation. The disordered consciousness most commonly takes the form of a global confusional state. Stupor and coma are rarely initial signs but develop if the person is not treated. Korsakoff psychosis may be early or late in onset but manifests with an anterograde amnesia (a defect in learning new information) and a retrograde amnesia (a disturbance in retrieving past memories). Confabulation (the making up and providing of false information) is not always present. The ataxia involves a wide-based stance and a slow, uncertain, staggering gait. The person may not be able to stand or walk without support. The ocular abnormalities include nystagmus, conjugate gaze palsy, and paresis or paralysis of the external rectus muscles.

Evaluation and Treatment

The initial diagnosis of Wernicke disease is made on the basis of history and physical examination. Any individual in a coma of unknown origin is treated with thiamine.

Wernicke disease is a medical emergency. The individual must be treated with thiamine to prevent progression of the disease and reverse the deficits that have not progressed to structural damage. Early administration of thiamine may prevent Korsakoff psychosis from developing as a residual deficit.

Degenerative Diseases
Parkinson Disease

Parkinson disease is a commonly occurring degenerative disorder of the basal ganglia (corpus striatum) involving the dopaminergic (dopamine-secreting) nigrostriatal pathway. Nigrostriatal disorders produce a syndrome of abnormal movement called **parkinsonism** (Parkinson syndrome, parkinsonian syndrome) (Fig. 15-28).

Etiologic classification of parkinsonism includes pri-

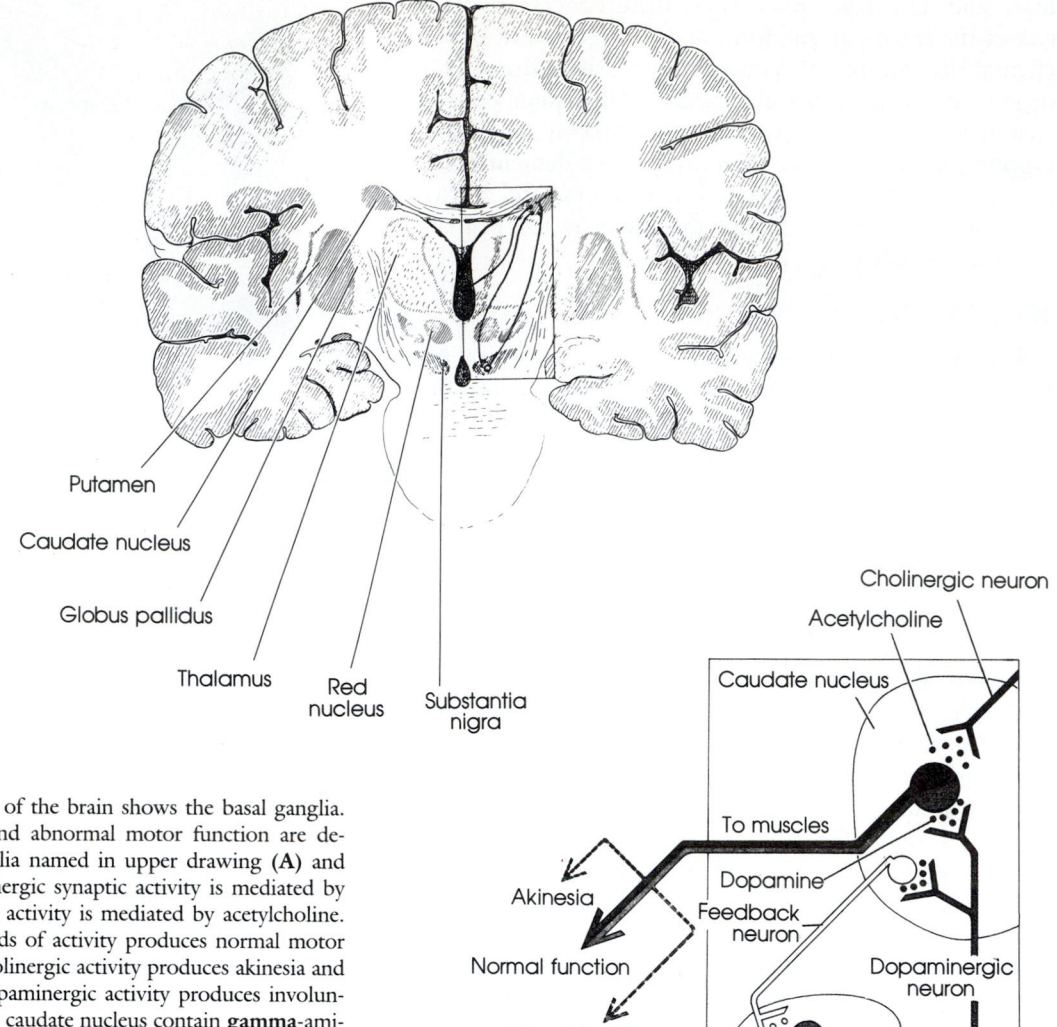

Putamen

Caudate nucleus

Globus pallidus

Thalamus Red nucleus Substantia nigra

Cholinergic neuron

Acetylcholine

Caudate nucleus

To muscles

Akinesia

Dopamine

Feedback neuron

Normal function

Dopaminergic neuron

Hyperkinesia

Substantia nigra

GABA

FIG. 15-28. Coronal section of the brain shows the basal ganglia. Pathways controlling normal and abnormal motor function are depicted in portion of basal ganglia named in upper drawing (**A**) and enlarged at right (**B**). Dopaminergic synaptic activity is mediated by dopamine. Cholinergic synaptic activity is mediated by acetylcholine. A balance between the two kinds of activity produces normal motor function. A relative excess of cholinergic activity produces akinesia and rigidity. A relative excess of dopaminergic activity produces involuntary movements. Neurons in the caudate nucleus contain **gamma**-aminobutyric acid (GABA) and possibly control dopaminergic neurons in the substantia nigra through a feedback pathway. (From Cutler, 1983.)

mary Parkinson disease and secondary parkinsonism. Secondary parkinsonism is parkinsonism caused by disorders other than Parkinson disease (i.e., trauma, infection, neoplasm, drug intoxication). Drug-induced parkinsonism, particularly that caused by phenothiazines, is the most common cause of the secondary form and is usually reversible.

The onset of Parkinson disease is after age 40, with peak age of onset in the early sixties (Duvoisin, 1984). Men and women appear to be equally affected (Duvoisin, 1984). Parkinson disease is one of the most prevalent of the primary CNS disorders (Calne & Eisler, 1979) and a leading cause of neurologic disability in individuals over 60 (Merritt, 1979). The prevalence rate varies between 60 and 120 per 100,000 persons (Gilroy & Holliday, 1982). An estimated half-million persons in the United States are affected.

Pathophysiology

The pathogenesis of Parkinson disease is unknown. The disease does not show a hereditary pattern or familial tendency. Epidemiologic data suggest vascular, viral, and metabolic factors as possible causes. One hypothesis is that age predisposes the nigrostriatal pathway to damage by viruses or toxins.

Atrophy and neuronal loss are found in the cerebral cortex in over one half of individuals with Parkinson disease (Duvoisin, 1984). The principal pathologic feature of Parkinson disease is degeneration of the dopaminergic nigrostriatal pathway, which is composed of neurons of the substantia nigra ("black substance") with fibers synapsing in the caudate and putamen basal ganglia (Fig. 15-28, *A*). Signs of inflammation or infection are absent. The severity of Parkinson disease seems to correlate with the degree of neuronal loss in the substantia nigra. Another pathologic feature is significant reduction in cyclase-linked dopamine receptors (D_1 receptors) in the basal ganglia. The functional import of this change is unknown. It is associated with an increase in neuroleptic-linked dopamine receptors (D_2 receptors) in the brain that is thought to represent a compensatory response to dopaminergic dysfunction in Parkinson disease.

Nigral and basal ganglial depletion of dopamine, an inhibitory neurotransmitter, is the principal biochemical alteration in Parkinson disease (Fig. 15-28, *B*). Symptom development in basal ganglial disorders is explained as an imbalance of dopaminergic (inhibitory) and cholinergic (excitatory) activity in the caudate and putamen basal ganglia. Dopaminergic-cholinergic balance produces normal motor function. In Parkinson disease degeneration of the dopaminergic nigrostriatal pathway causes dopamine depletion in the basal ganglia and relative excess of cholinergic activity in the feedback circuit involving the cerebral cortex, basal ganglia, and thalamus. A relative excess of cholinergic activity in this circuit, as in Parkinson disease, is manifested by hypertonia (tremor and rigidity) and akinesia.

Clinical Manifestations

The classic manifestations of Parkinson disease are tremor at rest (resting tremor), rigidity (muscle stiffness), and akinesia (poverty of movement). They may develop alone or in combination, but as the disease progresses, all three are usually present to at least some degree. There is no true paralysis. The symptoms are always bilateral but usually develop asymmetrically, a characteristic of neurologic degenerative disorders. Because of the insidious onset the beginning of symptoms is difficult to document. In early stages of the disease, reflex, sensory, and mental status are usually normal. Postural abnormalities, autonomic-neuroendocrine symptoms, and, in some cases, dementia are also part of the syndrome.

Parkinsonian Tremor, Rigidity, and Akinesia

Parkinsonian tremor is usually the first symptom to appear. It is an asymmetric, regular, rhythmic, low-amplitude tremor, with slowly alternating flexion-extension contraction (4 to 8 cycles per second). Later the tremor becomes symmetric at 7 to 12 cycles per second. It is a tremor at rest, disappearing briefly during the course of a voluntary movement and reappearing when the limb is held in a stationary position. Intensity and amplitude vary.

Parkinsonian tremor appears to result from instability of feedback from the basal ganglia to the cerebral cortex, a process caused by loss of the inhibitory influence of dopamine in the basal ganglia. The normal feedback cycles of motor outflow, except that from the cerebellum, are illustrated in Fig. 15-29. Oscillation in the feedback circuit when the muscles are at rest produces the tremor. When the individual performs voluntary movements, the tremor becomes temporarily blocked, presumably because other motor control signals arriving in the thalamus override the abnormal basal ganglial signals. As the disorder worsens, tremor may lessen as rigidity supervenes.

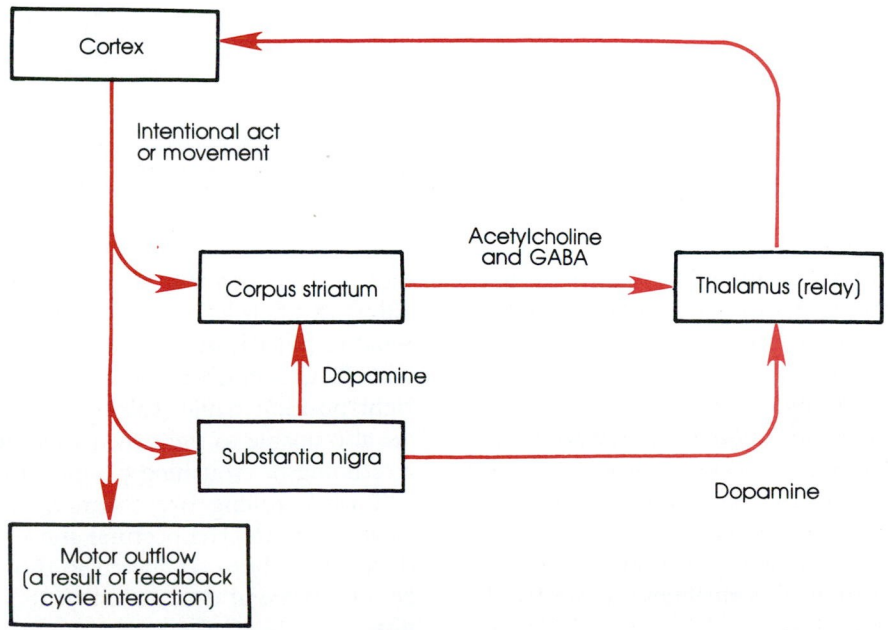

FIG. 15-29. Feedback cycles of motor outflow. (Redrawn from Riley & Massey, 1980; from Rudy, 1984.)

Rigidity, a state of involuntary contraction of all skeletal muscles, impedes active and passive movement. The first symptoms of rigidity may be painful muscle cramps in the toes or hands. More commonly the limb feels stiff, heavy, tired, or aching. Rigidity is felt by the examiner as lead-pipe resistance during passive movement that may be interrupted by brief jerks palpable as a cogwheel sensation. The mechanism underlying rigidity is increased resting muscle activity. In many individuals baseline muscle activity may break up into a rhythmic tremor at rest that is classically named **paralysis agitans.**

Akinesia is poverty of associated and voluntary movements. It is the most prevalent and crippling symptom and is often overlooked in the early stages. All striated muscles—extremity, trunk, ocular, facial—are eventually affected, including muscles of mastication (chewing), deglutition (swallowing), and articulation. Extreme underactivity in the individual with Parkinson disease makes the person appear stiff, even when resistance to passive movement cannot be felt. Akinesia is a separate phenomenon from rigidity and may be severe even in the presence of rigidity. Individuals state that they feel "wooden" as though moving "against resistance" and complain of rapid, severe fatigue. Akinesia is attributed to failure of the mechanism programming movement patterns manifested as a defect in the voluntary production of smooth motions at different speeds.

Akinetic symptoms are hypokinesia and bradykinesia. Hypokinesia, decreased frequency or absence of associated movements, is one of the earliest akinetic symptoms. Individuals with Parkinson disease sit and lie motionless for long periods of time without the little shifts a normal person makes to prevent discomfort and stiffness. Bradykinesia, slowness of voluntary movements, is characterized by difficulty initiating, continuing, or synchronizing movements. Both associated and voluntary movements are interspersed by freezing. Freezing may be precipitated by (1) increasing the effort to move, (2) turning, and (3) initiating certain types of tactile and visual contact.

Postural Abnormalities

Postural abnormalities are caused by a loss of normal postural reflexes. Three types of postural abnormalities occur in individuals with Parkinson disease: (1) disorders of postural fixation, (2) disorders of equilibrium, and (3) disorders of righting.

The disorder of postural fixation associated with Parkinson disease is involuntary flexion of the head and neck. The individual is unable to maintain an upright position of the trunk while standing or walking. The stooped (flexed, forward leaning) posture is characteristic (Fig. 15-30). Postural abnormalities of the hands and feet also occur.

Disorders of equilibrium result from loss of postural stability. The person with Parkinson disease is unable to

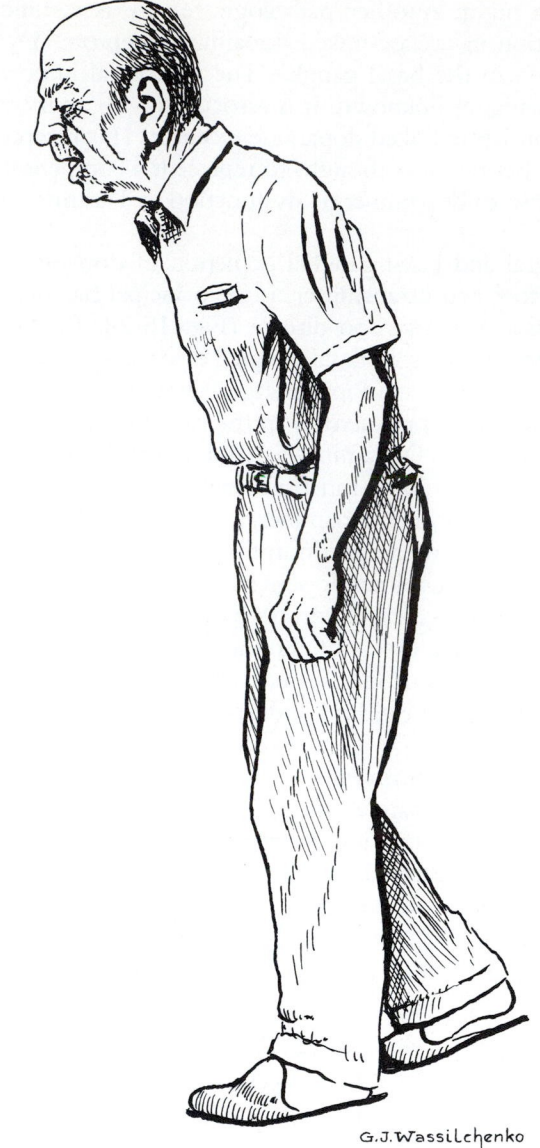

FIG. 15-30. Characteristic shuffling gait of individual with Parkinson's disease. (From Rudy, 1984.)

make the appropriate postural adjustment to tilting or falling and falls like a post when starting to tilt. The festinating gait (short, accelerating steps) of the individual with Parkinson disease is an attempt to maintain an upright position while walking (Fig. 15-30). Individuals are also unable to right themselves when changing from a reclining or crouching position to a standing position and when rolling over from a supine to a lateral or prone position. The postural abnormalities of Parkinson disease have been compared to those produced in monkeys by bilateral destruction of the pallidum basal ganglia.

Autonomic and Neuroendocrine Symptoms

Autonomic and neuroendocrine dysfunctions in Parkinson disease produce symptoms that are distressing but not incapacitating. The basal ganglia influence hypothalamic function (autonomic and neuroendocrine) through pathways connecting the hypothalamus with the basal ganglia and cerebral cortex. Common autonomic symptoms in Parkinson disease include inappropriate diaphoresis, orthostatic hypotension, gastric retention, constipation, and urinary retention. A symptom attributed to neuroendocrine dysfunction is seborrhea. Hypothalamic hypersecretion of hormonal-releasing factors acting on the anterior pituitary causes hypersecretion of androgenotropic hormones. The androgen excess produces sebum hypersecretion by sebaceous glands. The resulting seborrhea is characterized by oily skin with seborrheic dermatitis along the hairline and in chin-nasal creases.

Late Symptoms

Progressive dementia may be associated with the advanced stages of the disease and is manifested on the EEG as diffuse slowing and disorganization. The person's mental status may be further compromised by the side effects of the medication taken to control symptoms.

The combination of all the parkinsonian symptoms gives the individual a characteristic appearance: a wide-eyed, unblinking, staring expression with the facial muscles smoothed out and almost immobile. Saliva frequently drools from the corners of the slightly open mouth. The skin of the face is frequently greasy. The gait is pathognomic: the individual walks with slow, short, shuffling steps; the arms are flexed, adducted, and held stiffly at the side; and the trunk is bent slightly forward. The person may break into a run spontaneously or when pushed forward or backward. Because of the disorder of postural fixation, the tendency is to fall to the side.

Evaluation and Treatment

The diagnosis of Parkinson disease is based on the history and physical examination. Causes of secondary parkinsonism are first excluded. No specific diagnostic tests are available. Treatment of Parkinson disease is symptomatic. Drug therapy includes administration of levodopa (L-dopa), a precursor of dopamine (dopamine does not cross the blood-brain barrier). The drug is used to decrease akinesia. Because of levodopa's troublesome side effects, however, drug therapy is not started until the symptoms become incapacitating. Dysphagia and general immobility are special problems of the person with Parkinson disease requiring preventive, symptomatic, supportive, and rehabilitative management.

Parkinson disease takes a slowly progressive course for 15 to 20 years before producing total invalidism (Duvoisin, 1984). The course shows much variation among individuals. The prognosis is better since the ad-

vent of levodopa, but the disorder still shortens life substantially. Pneumonia is the leading cause of death.

Huntington Disease

Huntington disease (HD), also known as chorea, is a relatively rare, hereditary-degenerative disorder diffusely involving the basal ganglia and cerebral cortex. The onset of Huntington disease is usually between 40 and 50 years of age when the trait may already have been passed to the victim's children. The disorder has a prevalence rate of approximately 6.5 per 100,000 persons and occurs in all races (Gilroy & Holliday, 1982).

Pathophysiology

Huntington disease is inherited as an autosomal dominant trait with high penetrance. (Mechanisms of genetic inheritance are discussed in Chapter 4.) The principal pathologic feature of Huntington disease is severe degeneration of the basal ganglia, particularly the caudate and putamen nuclei, and the frontal cerebral cortex (Fig. 15-31). The basal ganglia normally contain a preponderance of GABAnergic (γ-aminobutyric-acid-secreting) neurons, including the pathway between the basal ganglia and substantia nigra (pallidonigral pathway). Basal ganglia and nigral depletion of GABA, an inhibitory neurotransmitter, is the principal biochemical alteration in Huntington disease. In Huntington disease degeneration of the GABAnergic pallidonigral pathway causes GABA depletion in the substantia nigra with decreased inhibitory GABA activity on dopaminergic neurons in the substantia nigra and relative excess of dopaminergic activity in the basal ganglial feedback circuit with the cerebral cortex. A relative excess of dopa-

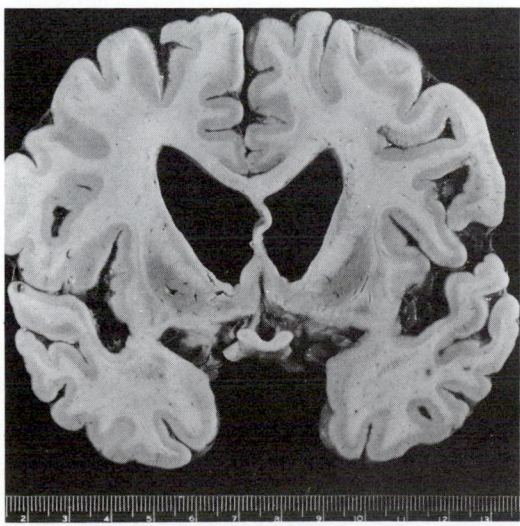

FIG. 15-31. Huntington disease. Atrophy of caudate nuclei and putamina is diagnostic. Cortical atrophy is moderate. There is compensatory internal and external hydrocephalus. (From Kissane, 1985.)

minergic activity in this circuit, as in Huntington disease, is manifested by hypotonia and hyperkinesia (involuntary, fragmentary movements such as chorea).

Clinical Manifestations

The classic manifestations of Huntington disease are abnormal movement and progressive dysfunction of intellectual processes (dementia) and thought processes. Any one of these features may mark the onset of the disease. Chorea is the most common type of abnormal movement affecting individuals with Huntington disease. Choreiform movements begin in the face and arms, eventually affecting the entire body. Consistent signs of intellectual dysfunction are impaired memory and judgment. Individuals with Huntington disease are prone to a wide variety of thought disturbances, including delusions and depressive disorders.

Evaluation and Treatment

The diagnosis of Huntington disease is based on family history and clinical presentation of the disorder. No known treatment is effective in halting the degeneration or progression of symptoms. The discovery in 1983 of the Huntington disease marker, called G8, on chromosome 4 paves the way for presymptomatic diagnosis of

the disorder and isolation of the Huntington disease gene. Recombinant genetic techniques may someday prevent or control the disorder.

Multiple Sclerosis

Multiple sclerosis (MS) is a relatively common degenerative disorder diffusely involving CNS myelin. The peripheral nervous system is not involved. Multiple sclerosis is one of many CNS demyelinating disorders. They are acquired conditions and are characterized by degeneration of previously normal myelin with relative preservation of axons. CNS demyelinating disorders are subclassified as primary and secondary. Multiple sclerosis and its variants are primary demyelinating disorders. In secondary disorders CNS demyelination is caused by disorders other than multiple sclerosis.

The onset of multiple sclerosis is usually between 20 and 40 years of age (Merritt, 1979). Male-to-female ratio is about 1 to 2 (Gilroy & Meyer, 1979). Multiple sclerosis is the most prevalent CNS demyelinating disorder and a leading cause of neurologic disability in early adulthood. The disease is most prevalent in areas far from the equator. In the United States and Canada the prevalence rate ranges from 40 to 60 per 100,000 persons (Berg, Chesanow, & Perensky, 1984). Multiple

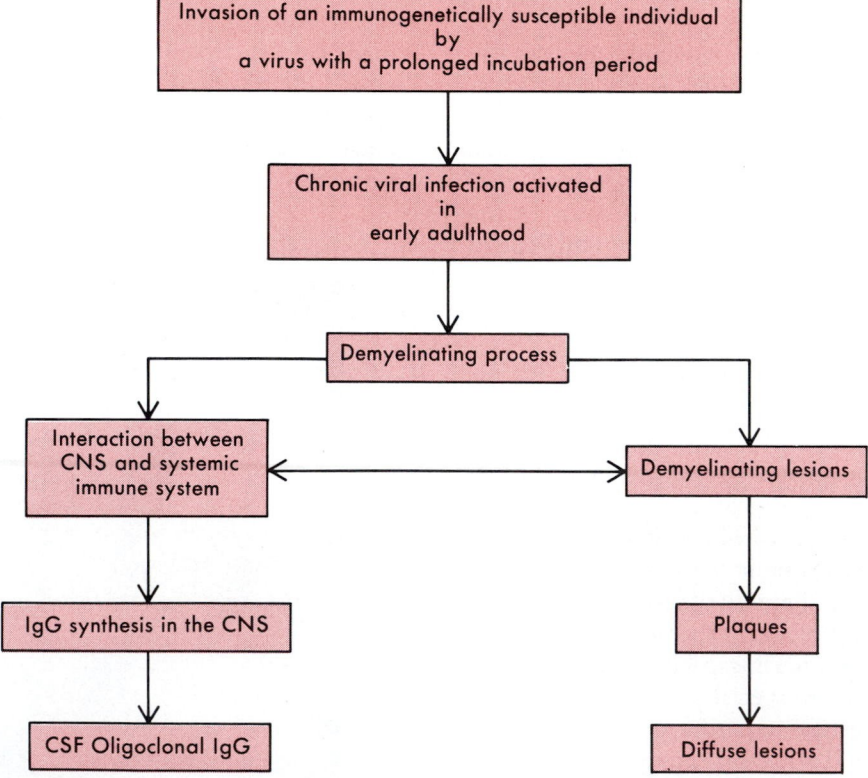

FIG. 15-32. An etiopathogenic model for MS. The initiating or trigger event in MS is presumed to be invasion by a virus with a prolonged incubation period, causing an altered immune response. The resulting chronic viral infection or other environmental insult becomes active in early adulthood, provoking the demyelinating process.

sclerosis occurs in all races, but it is chiefly a disorder of caucasians. Although the disorder does not exhibit a defined inheritance pattern, it is fifteen times more likely to occur in first-degree relatives of affected persons than in the population at large (McAlpine, Lumsden, & Acheson, 1972).

Pathophysiology

The pathogenesis of multiple sclerosis is unknown. (A theoretic pathogenic model is shown in Fig. 15-32). Although controversial, most theories suggest an immunogenetic-viral cause for multiple sclerosis. The disease is associated with a possible genetic predisposition and interaction with environmental risk factors (see Chapter 5). Possible genetically determined susceptibility is suggested by a pattern (haplotype) of histocompatibility antigens (HLA-A3, B7, Bf, Dr2, Dw2) found more frequently in persons with multiple sclerosis than in normal individuals (Stewart & Kirk, 1983). (HLA is discussed in Chapter 6.) According to theory this haplotype is a marker for a multiple sclerosis susceptibility gene of low penetrance that alters the body's immune response to viral infection (Stewart & Kirk, 1983). The central component of the pathogenic model is the demyelinating process. Pathologic features of this process are (1) interaction between the systemic immune system and the CNS and (2) demyelinating lesions (plaques and diffuse lesions) (Fig. 15-33). (The systemic immune system is discussed in Chapter 6.)

The interaction between the systemic immune system and the CNS is a complex and incompletely understood process. An immune response, possibly to chronic viral infection, causes initial and recurring mild inflammatory reactions in the form of a venular vasculitis. The vasculitis causes focal, limited intermittent breakdown of the blood-brain barrier. Some B-lymphocyte clones that migrate into the CNS during the inflammatory episodes of onset and exacerbation are trapped there when the inflammation subsides. In response to constant antigenic stimulation, these B-lymphocyte clones colonize the CNS. Within the brain and spinal cord they form plasma cells that secrete immunoglobulin G (IgG) against unknown virus(es). IgG synthesis against these antigens persists throughout the disease and is increased during exacerbations. Some of the elevated IgG in the CSF, therefore, represents antibodies produced by a restricted number of B-lymphocyte clones specific for the CNS antigen(s). CNS-produced IgG causes an oligoclonal electrophoretic pattern in which several IgG bands in the CSF are not seen in the serum, indicating immunologic activity in the brain. Most of the remainder of the elevated CSF IgG in multiple sclerosis is diffuse and polyclonal (as seen on electrophoresis). Systemic-produced IgG causes a polyclonal electrophoretic pattern in which IgG bands in the CSF correspond with those in the serum, indicating a systemic immune response to the antigen(s). Neither elevated CSF IgG nor oligoclonal IgG bands, however, are specific for multiple sclerosis. These findings are also seen in other conditions, such as neurosyphilis.

The number of T-suppressor cells fluctuates in the peripheral blood during the course of multiple sclerosis. T-suppressor cell count decreases with episodes of onset and exacerbation and becomes progressively more normal thereafter.

The demyelinating lesions (plaques and diffuse lesions) are the second pathologic feature of the demyelinating process. Whether these lesions are a cause or an effect of the interaction between the systemic immune system and the CNS is not known. Virus(es) or other antigens may directly attack the myelin or provoke a hypersensitivity reaction, destroying myelin or the oligodendrogliocytes. In either case immunogenetic defects may be a predisposing factor.

Plaques characteristically involve the CNS white matter, but occasionally they may extend into the adjacent gray matter. They often coalesce into much larger plaques. In established disease the multifocal, multistaged feature of plaques gives rise to the aphorism that the lesions are "scattered in space and time." Symptoms therefore are multiple and variable. Whether plaques are multiple from the onset of the disease is not known. In many individuals the initial symptoms suggest a single lesion. The stages of plaque formation are acute (early) and chronic (late).

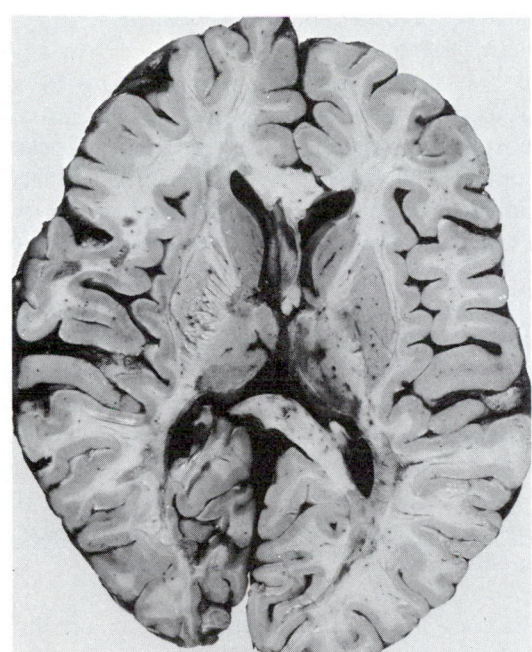

FIG. 15-33. Multiple sclerosis of chronic relapsing type with numerous plaques. Plaques occur in all characteristic areas. (From Kissane, 1985.)

The acute stage of plaque formation is characterized by the process of perivenular demyelination. Most of the neurologic deficits in the acute stage are attributed to inflammatory edema in and around the plaque and to partial demyelination. Symptoms usually remit, partially or completely, weeks after the onset of an early episode (Adams, 1985).

The chronic stage of demyelination and plaque formation is characterized by the process of **gliosis** (glial scarring with late degeneration of axons). Progressive loss of function leads to permanent disability, usually over 20 years or more (Adams & Victor, 1985).

Although plaques are considered diagnostic of multiple sclerosis, diffuse lesions are common pathologic findings in actively progressive cases. Diffuse lesions are small, widespread areas of perivenular demyelination that do not progress through gliosis. These lesions are sometimes accompanied by edema of surrounding normal brain tissue. The relationship of plaques to diffuse lesions is unknown.

Clinical Manifestations

A variety of events occurring immediately before the onset or exacerbation of symptoms are regarded as precipitating factors related to MS. Infection, physical injury, pregnancy, emotional stress, and fatigue are the most important. Most of the pregnancy-related exacerbations occur 3 months postpartum, suggesting a relation to the stresses of labor and the increased fatigue during the puerperium rather than to the pregnancy itself (Adams & Victor, 1985).

The major manifestations of MS are initial syndromes followed by remissions and established syndromes with no remissions. Usually persons with early multiple sclerosis predominantly have one of the initial syndromes—spinal, brainstem, cerebellar, or cerebral—that occur in the order of frequency indicated. The initial syndrome depends on the portion of the CNS that is most involved (see box at right). After about 15 years almost all individuals appear to have established syndromes of mixed involvement (Scheinberg, 1983).

Corticospinal Syndrome

The corticospinal syndrome is most common, chiefly involving the corticospinal tracts and dorsal column. Subjective corticospinal (upper motor neuron) symptoms—stiffness, slowness, weakness—are a component of fatigability. Corticospinal signs are usually symmetrical, with lower limbs more often and more severely affected than upper limbs; spastic paraparesis is probably the most common single neurologic finding in multiple sclerosis.

Bladder and bowel symptoms occur with major spinal cord involvement. Urgency and hesitancy generally precede incontinence. Bladder dysfunction is most often that of a small, spastic bladder, although occasionally a

---

Initial Syndromes of Multiple Sclerosis

Cerebral Syndrome
Optic Neuritis (ON)
Intellectual-emotional changes
Seizures
Hemiparesis, hemisensory loss, dysphasia

Cerebellar Syndrome
Motor Ataxia
Hypotonia
Asthenia

Brainstem Syndrome
Intranuclear ophthalmoplegia (INO)
Nystagmus
Dysarthria

Spinal Syndrome
Spastic paresis
Bowel and bladder dysfunction
Paresthesias

---

large, flaccid bladder may result. Neurogenic impotence is not unusual when sphincter symptoms are present. Bowel incontinence is rare, but constipation is not unusual in severe cases. Subjective dorsal column symptoms are symmetrical paresthesias (tingling and numbness) in an unpredictable pattern, with a predilection for lower extremities over upper extremities. Dorsal column signs are vibration, position, and two-point discrimination deficits. The sensory complaints are often not substantiated by objective findings.

Brainstem Syndrome

The brainstem syndrome reflects lesions of cranial nerves III through XII at the root, nuclear, or corticobulbar (upper motor neuron) level. Intranuclear ophthalmoplegia, nystagmus, and dysarthria are the most common brainstem symptoms, followed by vertigo, tinnitus, facial weakness, and facial sensory deficit. Dysphagia and deafness are uncommon. Intranuclear ophthalmoplegia is lateral gaze paralysis of the medial rectus muscle caused by involvement of the medial longitudinal fasciculus, the brainstem pathway that coordinates eye movement. Diplopia and eyeball pain are the common complaints. Physical examination shows failure of adduction in the ipsilateral eye on lateral conjugate gaze but not on convergence. Nystagmus is seen in the abducting eye. Bilateral intranuclear ophthalmoplegia in a young adult is virtually diagnostic of MS.

Cerebellar Syndrome

Deficits of the cerebellar syndrome are usually symmetrical; four-limb involvement is not uncommon. With combined corticospinal and cerebellar involvement, the individual has a spastic ataxic gait and ataxia of the arms. Pure cerebellar symptoms are those of motor ataxia, hypotonia, and asthenia (weakness). Manifestations of motor ataxia are decomposition of movement, inability to perform rapid alternating movements (dysdiodochokinesia), dysmetria, and Charcot triad (a combination of dysarthria, intention tremor, and nystagmus). Manifestations of hypotonia are decreased resistance to passive movement, hypoactive deep tendon reflexes, and pendular knee jerk.

Cerebral Syndrome

The cerebral syndrome is characterized by optic neuritis, the manifestation of optic nerve demyelination. Although not as common as other symptoms, it is highly suggestive of MS. Involvement may be unilateral or bilateral. Subjective symptoms are impaired central vision (blurring, fogginess, haziness) and impaired color perception. Signs are decreased central visual acuity; central or paracentral scotoma (area of diminished vision); acquired color vision deficit, especially to red and green; and defective pupillary reaction to light. In the acute phase these symptoms may reflect optic papillitis (inflammation and swelling of the optic disk) or retrobulbar neuritis with a normal disk. Later pallor of the temporal half of the disk occurs from demyelination of the papillomacular bundle (a portion of the optic nerve). (Normal visual function is discussed in Chapter 13.)

Intellectual and emotional changes also occur. Depression is more common than euphoria, although euphoria is sometimes associated with dementia. Other less common symptoms of cerebral involvement include seizures, hemiparesis, hemisensory loss, and dysphasia.

Within the overall course of multiple sclerosis short-lived and paroxysmal attacks may occur. Symptoms of the attack tend to subside as the inciting event is removed.

Short-lived attacks are the temporary appearance or worsening of symptoms. The mechanism of these attacks is complete, reversible conduction block in partially demyelinated axons. Conditions that cause short-lived attacks include (1) minor increases in body temperature or serum Ca^{++} concentration and (2) functional demands exceeding conduction capacity. An increase in body temperature or serum Ca^{++} level increases current leakage through demyelinated neurons. Persons with multiple sclerosis may become dramatically worse when body temperature is raised. As with hypoventilation hypercalcemia induced by decreased serum pH may aggravate symptoms of multiple sclerosis. Physical and emotional stress impose functional demands that may exceed conduction capacity of affected neurons.

Paroxysmal attacks are sensory or motor symptoms of abrupt onset and short duration (few seconds or minutes). These symptoms include paresthesias, dysarthria and ataxia, and tonic head turning. The mechanism of paroxysmal attacks is nonsynaptic transmission in which nerve impulses are directly transmitted between adjacent demyelinated axons. These impulses arise focally and spuriously in the cervical portion of the spinal cord or in the brainstem. A common paroxysmal symptom, called Lhermitte sign, is the momentary paresthesia (shocklike or tingling sensation) that shoots down the trunk and/or limbs during active or passive flexion of the neck. Bending the neck evokes nonsynaptic impulses in demyelinated axons of the dorsal column in the spinal cord. A person with multiple sclerosis may have many paroxysmal attacks each day. Inciting events include sensory stimulation, voluntary movement, hyperventilation, and emotional stress. Paroxysmal attacks tend to persist for weeks or months and may be followed by progressive symptoms of multiple sclerosis.

Evaluation and Treatment

The diagnosis of multiple sclerosis (definite, probable, or possible) is based on the history and physical examination supported by findings from CSF examination, evoked response (ER) studies, CT scans of the head, and MRI. Persistently elevated CSF IgG is found in about two thirds of individuals with multiple sclerosis (Adams & Victor, 1977), and oligoclonal IgG bands on electrophoresis are found in more than 90% (Poser, 1985). ER studies aid diagnosis by detecting decreased conduction velocity in visual, auditory, and somatosensory pathways. In the study reported by Kirshner, Tsai, Runge, and Price, positive MRI scans in 27 individuals with "definite" multiple sclerosis suggest that MRI is the most sensitive available method of detecting the disease as compared to oligoclonal banding, ER studies, or CT scanning (Kirshner et al., 1985). MRI, which is not subject to bone artifacts, shows brainstem lesions not detected by CT. Optic nerve and spinal cord lesions, however, are not detected by current MRI techniques. When MRI is normal, ER studies are useful in confirming suspected multiple sclerosis.

No treatment is currently available to alter the overall course of MS. Adrenocorticotropic hormone and prednisone are used to shorten the duration of acute exacerbations. Special problems requiring preventive and symptomatic management are weakness; spasticity; bladder, bowel, and sexual dysfunction; pain; tremor and ataxia; depression; and heat intolerance. Supportive and rehabilitative management is directed toward preventing the complications of immobility, especially pressure sores and infections of the pulmonary and genitourinary systems. Estimates suggest that current therapies and management will permit a normal life span for approximately 85% of individuals (Slater & Yearwood, 1980).

Amyotrophic Lateral Sclerosis

Amyotrophic lateral sclerosis (ALS, sporadic motor neuron disease, or sporadic motor system disease) is a relatively rare degenerative disorder diffusely involving lower and upper motor neurons. The term *amyotrophic* (without muscle nutrition or progressive muscle wasting) refers to the predominant lower motor neuron component of the syndrome. Lateral sclerosis, scarring of the corticospinal tract in the lateral column of the spinal cord, refers to the upper motor neuron component of the syndrome. ALS differs from other motor neuron disorders in that both upper and lower motor neurons are involved.

Classic ALS (Lou Gehrig disease) may begin at any time from the third decade of life; its peak occurrence rate is in the early 50s (Amico & Antel, 1981). Male-to-female ratio is 2 to 1 (Gilroy & Meyer, 1979). The disorder has a prevalence rate of approximately 1 per 100,000 persons (Gilroy & Meyer, 1979), and as many as 10,000 persons in the United States are affected (Merritt, 1979).

Pathophysiology

The pathogenesis of ALS is unknown. Epidemiologic data suggest viral-immune and metabolic (i.e., nutritional, toxic) factors as possible causes. Poliomyelitis and ALS both affect lower motor neurons, suggesting a common etiology. Serum immune complexes are elevated in ALS, but the nature of the complexes is unknown. Presumably multiple and diverse processes underlie the process of motor system degeneration.

The principal pathologic feature of ALS is lower and upper motor neuron degeneration, although without inflammation. There is a reduction in the number of large motor neurons in the spinal cord, brainstem, and cerebral cortex (premotor and motor areas), with ongoing degeneration in the remaining motor neurons. The nuclei of cranial nerves III, IV, and VI are not involved. Death of the motor neuron results in axonal degeneration and secondary demyelination with glial proliferation and sclerosis (scarring).

Lower motor neuron degeneration denervates motor units. Adjacent, still-viable lower motor neurons attempt to compensate by a process of distal intramuscular sprouting, reinnervation, and enlargement of motor units. The initial symptoms of the disease may be related to lower and upper motor neuron dysfunction or to both.

Clinical Manifestations

Weakness may begin in any or all muscles of the body. Muscle weakness in ALS exhibits the following characteristics:

1. Paresis usually begins in a single muscle group.
2. Corresponding muscle groups are asymmetrically affected in a mottled distribution.
3. Gradual involvement occurs in all striated muscles except extraocular muscles and heart and pro-

gresses to paralysis with no remissions.
4. Flaccid and spastic paresis may coexist in a single muscle group; flaccid paresis may mask spasticity, which is usually mild.
5. Urethral and anal sphincter weakness is uncommon.
6. No associated mental, sensory, or autonomic symptoms are present. Normal intellectual and sensory functions are sustained until death.

The lower motor neuron syndrome of flaccid paresis consists of weakness of individual muscles, progressing to paralysis, associated with hypotonia and primary muscle atrophy (i.e., atrophy caused by denervation). Hypotonia is manifested by (1) decreased resistance to passive movement, (2) hypoactive or absent deep tendon reflexes, (3) absent abdominal and cremasteric reflexes, and (4) absent Babinski sign. Primary atrophy is manifested by (1) severe, irreversible muscular wasting; (2) fasciculations; (3) metabolically related changes in the skin and appendages; and (4) specific electromyelographic findings. Fasciculations, along with fibrillations, are prominent features of ALS. Metabolic changes include (1) thinning of the skin, (2) thickening of the nails, (3) loss of body hair, and (4) decreased perspiration.

The upper motor neuron syndrome of spastic paresis consists of weakness of movement patterns, progressing to paralysis, associated with spasticity and, in some cases, atrophy secondary to disuse. Spasticity is manifested by (1) clasp-knife phenomenon, evident with passive movement; (2) hyperactive deep tendon reflexes and clonus with severe spasticity; (3) absent abdominal and cremasteric reflexes; and (4) presence of Babinski sign.

Evaluation and Treatment

The diagnosis of the syndrome is based predominantly on the history and physical examination. Electromyography and muscle biopsy verify lower motor neuron degeneration and denervation. Muscle biopsy usually is not needed to confirm the diagnosis. No treatment is currently available to alter the overall course of the ALS syndrome. Special problems requiring preventive and symptomatic management are communication difficulty caused by dysphonia and dysarthria; dehydration and weight loss resulting from dysmasesis and dysphagia; and dyspnea caused by diaphragmatic and intercostal weakness. Supportive and rehabilitative management is directed toward preventing complications of immobility. Unlike MS, the disorder progresses without remissions and exacerbations. Psychological support of the affected individual and the family is extremely important in this disorder.

The average duration of life is approximately 3 years from the appearance of symptoms, but the course of the disease may run from a few months to 15 years (Merrit, 1979). The 5-year survival rate for all persons with ALS is 40% (Rosen, 1978).

Hydrocephalus

The term **hydrocephalus** refers to a variety of conditions characterized by an excess of fluid within the cranial vault, subarachnoid space, or both. Hydrocephalus occurs because of interference with cerebrospinal fluid flow caused by increased fluid production, obstruction within the ventricular system, or defective reabsorption of the fluid. A papilloma (i.e., epithelial tumor) may, in rare instances, cause overproduction of cerebrospinal fluid.

Types of Hydrocephalus

Obstruction within the ventricular system, called **noncommunicating hydrocephalus** or internal hydrocephalus, may result from congenital abnormalities in the ventricular system or mass lesions such as a tumor that compresses one of the structures of the ventricular system (see Pediatrics [Chapter 16] for additional discussion). Impaired absorption of cerebrospinal fluid from the subarachnoid space occurs when an obstructive process disrupts the flow of cerebrospinal fluid through the subarachnoid space. The fluid is prevented from reaching the convex portion of the cerebrum, where the arachnoid granulations are located.

Hydrocephalus from impaired absorption may be caused by adhesions from inflammation, as with a meningitis or subarachnoid hemorrhage; compression of the subarachnoid space by a mass, such as a tumor; congenital abnormalities of the subarachnoid space; or high venous pressure within the sagittal sinus. This type of hydrocephalus is termed **communicating hydrocephalus.** The most common causes of communicating hydrocephalus are subarachnoid hemorrhage, developmental malformation, and neoplasm.

One form of communicating hydrocephalus is **hydrocephalus ex vacuo,** which arises from cerebral atrophy. Cerebrospinal fluid fills the unoccupied space. The amount of cerebrospinal fluid is increased, but the fluid is not under pressure. Another form of communicating hydrocephalus is **normal-pressure hydrocephalus** (low-pressure, adult, or occult hydrocephalus), which occurs mostly in late middle age. The cause is thought to be arachnoid adhesions that obstruct the subarachnoid space. This form of hydrocephalus is most frequently seen as a complication of head injury and subarachnoid hemorrhage.

Course of the Disease

Hydrocephalus may develop from infancy through adulthood. Congenital hydrocephalus (i.e., ventricular enlargement prior to birth) is rare. Noncommunicating hydrocephalus is more commonly seen in children. The more frequent type of hydrocephalus in adults is the "communicating" type. (Hydrocephalus in children is discussed in Chapter 16.)

Most hydrocephalus develops gradually and insidiously over a period of time. **Acute hydrocephalus,** however, may develop in a couple of hours in persons who have sustained head injuries. Acute hydrocephalus contributes significantly to increased intracranial pressure.

Pathogenesis

The obstruction of cerebrospinal fluid flow associated with hydrocephalus produces dilation of the ventricles proximal to the obstruction. Obstructed cerebrospinal fluid is under pressure causing atrophy of the cerebral cortex and degeneration of the white matter tracts. When excess cerebrospinal fluid fills a defect caused by atrophy, a degenerative disorder, or a surgical excision, this fluid is not under pressure; therefore, atrophy and degenerative changes are not induced.

Clinical Manifestations

The presentation of acute hydrocephalus is one of rapidly developing increased intracranial pressure. The person deteriorates rapidly into a deep coma if not promptly treated. Normal-pressure hydrocephalus has a chronic presentation and develops slowly over time. The individual or family complains of declining memory and cognitive function. An unsteady, broad-based gait with a history of falling is common. Additional clinical manifestations are apathy, inattentiveness, and indifference to self, family, and the environment. Urinary incontinence is present.

Evaluation and Treatment

The diagnosis is made on the basis of physical examination, CT scan, and MRI. A radioisotopic cisternogram may be performed to diagnose normal-pressure hydrocephalus. Hydrocephalus can be treated by draining the ventricles through the use of shunts. Excision or coagulation of the choroid plexus is occasionally needed when a papilloma is present. In normal-pressure hydrocephalus, reduction in cerebrospinal fluid through a diuresis regimen is often used.

PERIPHERAL NERVOUS SYSTEM AND NEUROMUSCULAR JUNCTION DISORDERS

Peripheral Nervous System Disorders

The axons traveling to and from the brainstem and spinal cord neuronal cell bodies may be injured by a multitude of disease processes. Distinct anatomic areas of the axon may be injured, or the spinal nerves may be affected at the spinal roots, at the plexus prior to peripheral nerve formation, or at the peripheral nerves themselves. The cranial nerves do not have roots or plexuses so are only affected within the nerves themselves. Autonomic nerve fibers may be injured as they travel within certain cranial nerves or emerge through the ventral root and plexuses to travel in the peripheral nerves of the body.

Radiculopathies

As the spinal roots emerge from or enter into the vertebral canal, they may be injured or damaged by compression, inflammation, or direct trauma in which the roots are stretched or torn. **Radiculopathies** are disorders of roots of spinal nerves. **Radiculitis** (radiculoneuritis) refers to an inflammatory disorder of the spinal nerve roots.

Pathophysiology

Many different pathologic conditions may cause compression, inflammation, or tearing of nerve roots. Roots may be traumatized by a forceful tearing of a nerve, termed **avulsion,** often associated with injuries to the head and shoulders. An acute intervertebral disk prolapse (herniated disk) or a benign tumor may compress nerve roots. Metastatic tumors of the lung, breast, and gastrointestinal tract may produce a carcinomatous meningitis causing compression and inflammatory changes in nerve roots. Other causes of inflammatory changes in nerve roots are chronic meningitis, neurosyphilis, sarcoidosis, and **inflammatory arachnoiditis** produced by myelography and lumbar punctures.

Clinical Manifestations

Diseases that involve spinal roots typically produce local pain; pain on local percussion; pain and paresthesias in the sensory root distribution (called **radicular pain** and **radicular parethesia**); increased pain with movement, stretching of the root, and manuevers that transiently increase cerebrospinal fluid pressure; sensory loss in a radicular pattern; spasms of the muscles surrounding the vertebral column (i.e., paravertebral muscle spasms); and decreased or lost deep tendon reflexes in the distribution of the affected roots.

Evaluation and Treatment

Diagnostic measures may include spinal films, electromyography, lumbar puncture with cerebrospinal fluid examination, myelography, and biopsy of tumor masses. Treatment is directed at the cause of the injury and may take the form of surgery, antibiotics, removal of the injurious agent, steroids, and radiotherapy and chemo-

therapy. Supportive management may include control of the discomfort, protection from further injury, prevention of complications, and rehabilitation where appropriate.

Plexus Injuries

Plexus injuries involve the nerve plexus distal to the spinal roots but proximal to the formation of the peripheral nerves. Such injuries may be caused by trauma, compression, or infiltration, or they may be iatrogenic, caused by positioning during surgery or by an intramuscular injection. Clinical manifestations include motor weakness, muscle atrophy, and sensory loss of affected areas. Paralysis can occur with complete plexus lesions.

The diagnosis is made on the basis of history and clinical manifestations. Therapeutic treatment is directed at removal of the cause, repair and approximation of nervous tissue, prevention of further injury, control of discomfort, prevention of complications, and rehabilitation where appropriate.

Neuropathies

Where the peripheral nerves themselves are affected, whether cranial nerves, nerves arising from spinal roots and plexuses, or autonomic nervous system fibers, this resulting syndrome is a neuropathy or **neuritis** when an inflammatory process is involved. Most neuropathies are classified as **sensorimotor neuropathies** because motor, sensory, and reflex changes are generally present, although some neuropathies are predominantly motor or sensory. **Sensory neuropathies** are predominantly caused by leprosy, some industrial solvents, chloramphenicol, and hereditary mechanisms. **Motor neuropathies** are predominantly caused by Guillain-Barré syndrome, infectious mononucleosis, viral hepatitis, acute porphyria, lead, mercury, and triorthocresylphosphates (TCP). Autonomic fibers may be involved in either a motor or a sensorimotor neuropathy.

Pathophysiology

Although distinct pathophysiologic processes are recognized in a neuropathy, these are not disease specific and may exist simultaneously in any one neuropathy. Wallerian degeneration, in which the axon and myelin distal to the site of axonal interruption degenerate, may be present (see Chapter 12). This type of degeneration is characteristic of a traumatic nerve injury in which the nerve is severed. In some neuropathies the axon may be spared and only the myelin degenerates. Such polyneuropathies are called **segmental demyelinating neuropathies.** This type of degeneration is especially seen in the early phases of many neuropathies. In **axonal degeneration** distal degeneration of the axon occurs first and is followed by degeneration of the myelin and the axon.

Clinical Manifestations

The neuropathies are characterized by varying degrees of paresis and paralysis, and secondary atrophy may be present. Sensory disturbances may be found. These include paresthesias and dysthesias as well as decreased or absent primary sensations such as temperature, touch, light pain, position sense, or vibratory sense. Ataxia of gait or limb may arise from the loss of position and vibratory sensations (i.e., proprioceptive sensory loss) and may be enhanced by motor weakness. Reflexes may be altered. These include reflex-mediated autonomic nervous system functions such as sweating and pupillary size.

Neuropathies associated with autonomic disturbances include diabetes mellitus, alcoholism and related nutritional neuropathies, amyloidosis, porphyria, Guillain-Barré syndrome, Riley-Day syndrome, and familial sensory neuropathy. In many chronic polyneuropathies the feet, hands, and spine become deformed. Metabolic changes may arise secondary to nerve dysfunction.

Evaluation and Treatment

The diagnostic workup to determine the cause of a neuropathy is often extensive. Early diagnosis and treatment before irreversible neuronal cell damage ensues are of paramount importance. Although axonal regrowth and recovery of function may take months, many neuropathies can be reversed. The therapeutic management is directed first and foremost at elimination of the cause, if possible. At least the primary disorder, such as diabetes mellitus, should be controlled. Further damage to the axon must be prevented by avoiding trauma from too-early demand for reuse of the nerve and accidents that cause tissue damage, and by avoiding hypoxia and ischemia or other deprivation of essential substrates.

Guillain-Barré Syndrome

Guillain-Barré syndrome (idiopathic polyneuritis, acute inflammatory demyelinating polyradiculopathy, postinfectious polyneuritis) is characterized by the acute onset of a motor paralysis usually of an ascending nature. This neurologic disorder, first described by Landry in 1859, occurs throughout the world, affects children and adults of both sexes and all age groups equally, and occurs in all seasons of the year. Precipitating, or at least preceding, events include a mild respiratory or gastrointestinal viral infection 4 to 21 days prior to onset of neurologic manifestations, surgical procedures, viral immunizations, and lymphomatous disease.

Pathophysiology

The neurologic dysfunctions in Guillain-Barré syndrome are caused by a cell-mediated immunologic reaction directed at the peripheral nerves. Lymphocytes migrate into the areas adjacent to the nerve and attack the myelin sheath surrounding the nerve fibers, causing demyelination of nerve segments. As the process continues the axons themselves are interrupted. The muscle innervated by the damaged peripheral nerves undergoes denervation and atrophy.

If the cell body survives, regeneration of the peripheral nerve takes place, and recovery of motor function is likely. If the cell body dies from intense ventral root involvement in the inflammatory-degenerative process, then no regeneration from surviving axons and regenerating axons may take place. In this case motor recovery is less complete, and residual deficits persist.

Clinical Manifestations

Clinical manifestations may vary from paresis of the legs to complete quadriplegia, respiratory insufficiency, and autonomic nervous system instability. The individual may have a symmetrical weakness or paralysis involving the legs, the trunk, and possibly the neck and face. Hypotonia of the involved muscles is present, and the deep tendon reflexes are absent. The person may complain of paresthesias that began in the legs and ascended upward. Position and vibratory sensations may be decreased. Autonomic nervous system dysfunction may be manifested as sinus tachycardia, hypertension, hypotension, and/or loss of sweating. Ventilatory capacity is often decreased, and the individual may complain of shortness of breath. Persons may experience a respiratory arrest or cardiovascular collapse.

Evaluation and Treatment

The individual's clinical history helps to diagnose the disorder. The significant signs include paresthesias, paralysis, and CSF findings. The major diagnostic tests are the examination of the CSF and nerve conduction tests. The CSF findings include an unusually high protein level (750 mg/ml) without cellular abnormality. Ventilatory support and management of the autonomic nervous system dysfunction are two dominant aspects of the therapeutic management. During the acute phase, steroid therapy may be initiated. After the disorder begins to remit, aggressive rehabilitation should be instituted.

Neuromuscular Junction Disorders

The neuromuscular junction is the site of dysfunction for two specific disorders: botulism and myasthenia gravis. Because of their shared site of dysfunction, these disorders have very similar clinical manifestations.

Botulism

Botulism, a form of acute food poisoning, is caused by the ingestion of the exotoxin produced by *Clostrid-*

ium botulinum, an anaerobic, spore-forming gram-negative rod.

Pathophysiology

Toxins block nerve impulse transmission at the neuromuscular junction by interfering with the release of acetylcholine and perhaps by binding it at or near the release sites.

Clinical Manifestations

The severity of the illness may range from mild symptoms to ultimate death. Generally symptoms begin 12 to 48 hours after ingestion of the exotoxin. Earlier appearance of symptoms suggests a more serious illness. Nausea and vomiting occur with some types of botulism. Weakness, lethargy, dizziness, and vertigo may appear early in the course of the disease. Severe dryness of the mouth and throat may be present.

Neurologic symptoms arising from cranial nerve paresis include lid drooping (ptosis); paralysis of extraocular muscles resulting in blurred vision, double vision (diplopia), and difficulty coordinating eye movements (convergence); dilated pupils; difficulty in swallowing (dysphagia); speech dyspraxia; and difficulty in vocalizing (dysphonia). Skeletal muscle weakness of the trunk and extremities follows cranial nerve weakness. The weakness may eventually lead to failure of the respiratory muscles. Autonomic nervous system involvement is manifested in smooth muscle paresis of the bowel and bladder, causing absent bowel sounds with abdominal distention and urinary retention.

Evaluation and Treatment

The diagnosis of botulism is made on the basis of the history, the gastrointestinal signs and symptoms, the predominant motor paresis, and the lack of response to edrophonium chloride (Tensilon), a rapidly acting anticholinesterase. Therapeutic management includes removal of any nonabsorbed exotoxin, administration of a trivalent antiserum, supportive respiratory and fluid and electrolyte therapy, and prevention of infections and secondary complications. Guanidine hydrochloride is sometimes given in an attempt to reverse the weakness.

Myasthenia Gravis

Myasthenia gravis is a disorder of voluntary (striated) muscles characterized by muscle weakness and fatigability. In 15% to 20% of persons with myasthenia gravis, thymic tumors are found. Such tumors are more common in males than in females. Myasthenia gravis is an autoimmune disease associated with an increased incidence of other autoimmune diseases, including systemic lupus erythematosus, rheumatoid arthritis, polymyositis, and thyrotoxicosis. (Autoimmune mechanisms are discussed in Chapter 8.) Transitory signs of myasthenia gravis are present in 10% to 15% of infants born to mothers with myasthenia gravis.

The three types of myasthenia gravis are ocular, generalized, and bulbar myasthenia. **Ocular myasthenia,** which is more common in males, involves muscle weakness that is confined to the eye muscles. **Generalized myasthenia** involves the proximal musculature throughout the body and has several courses: (1) a course with periodic remissions, (2) a slowly progressive course, (3) a rapidly progressive course, or (4) a fulminating course. **Bulbar myasthenia** involves the muscles innervated by cranial nerves IX, X, XI, and XII and tends to be rapidly progressive or fulminating.

Pathophysiology

Myasthenia gravis results from a defect in nerve impulse transmission at the neuromuscular junction. The postsynaptic acetylcholine receptors on the muscle cell's plasma membrane for an unknown reason are no longer recognized as "self" and therefore elicit an antigenic effect. IgG antibody is secreted against the acetylcholine receptors. These antibodies fix onto the receptor sites and block the binding of acetylcholine. Eventually the antibody action causes the destruction of receptor sites and the number of receptors on the plasma membrane is reduced. The destruction of receptor sites causes diminished transmission of the nerve impulse across the neuromuscular junction. Muscle depolarization is not achieved.

The cause of this autosensitization is not known. Evidence supports the autoimmune theory. Clinical and laboratory data show the following:

1. Receptor-binding antibodies are present in 80% to 85% of persons with myasthenia gravis.
2. Passive transfer of myasthenia gravis to animals is possible by injecting serum and IgG from humans with myasthenia gravis.
3. Myasthenia gravis is frequently associated with other autoimmune disorders, such as rheumatoid arthritis and systemic lupus erythematosus.
4. Transitory neonatal myasthenia gravis occurs.
5. A strong association between myasthenia gravis and thymus gland hyperplasia exists.
6. Steroid therapy, antimetabolite drugs, plasma exchange, and thoracic duct drainage all improve the clinical status of the person who has myasthenia gravis.

Clinical Manifestations

Myasthenia gravis typically has an insidious onset. Clinical manifestations may first appear during pregnancy, during the postpartum period, or in conjunction with the administration of certain anesthetic agents. The person often complains of fatigue after exercise and has a recent history of recurring upper respiratory tract infections. The muscles of the eyes, face, mouth, throat, and neck are usually affected first. The extraocular (eye) muscles and the levator muscles are most affected. Manifestations include diplopia, ptosis, and ocular palsies.

The muscles of facial expression, mastication, swallowing, and speech are the next most involved. The results are facial droop and an expressionless face; difficulty chewing and swallowing associated with dietary changes and weight loss; drooling, episodes of choking and aspiration; and a nasal, low-volume but high-pitched monotonous speech pattern.

The muscles of the neck, shoulder girdle, and hip flexors are less frequently affected. When these muscles do become involved, however, the person experiences fatigue and requires periods of rest, weakness of the arms and legs that improves with rest, and difficulty in maintaining head position. The respiratory muscles of the diaphragm and chest wall become weak and ventilation is impaired. Impairment in deep breathing and coughing predispose the individual to atelectasis and congestion. In the advanced stage of the disease all the muscles are weak.

Myasthenic crisis occurs when severe muscle weakness causes extreme quadriparesis or quadriplegia, respiratory insufficiency with shortness of breath and a markedly decreased tidal volume and vital capacity, and extreme difficulty in swallowing. The individual in myasthenic crisis is in danger of respiratory arrest.

Cholinergic crisis may arise from anticholinesterase drug toxicity. The clinical picture is like that of myasthenic crisis, but other symptoms are also present. Intestinal motility increases and is associated with episodes of diarrhea and complaints of cramping; fasciculation, bradycardia, pupillary constriction, increased salivation, and increased sweating are present. These clinical manifestations are caused by the smooth muscle hyperactivity secondary to excessive accumulation of acetylcholine at the neuromuscular junctions and excessive parasympatheticlike activity. As in myasthenic crisis, the individual is in danger of respiratory arrest.

Evaluation and Treatment

The diagnosis of myasthenia gravis is made on the basis of a response to edrophonium chloride (Tensilon) and electromyography (EMG). With the intravenous administration of the drug immediate demonstrable improvement in muscle strength usually persists for several minutes. On EMG the amplitude of the action potentials of stimulated muscles rapidly declines. Mediastinal tomography is used to determine whether a thymoma is present. The progression of myasthenia gravis is highly variable. In some individuals it is mild and spontaneously remits. There is usually a series of relapses with symptom-free intervals ranging from weeks to months. Over time the disease can progress, leading to death.

Ocular myasthenia carries a very good prognosis.

Anticholinergic drugs, steroids, and, occasionally, chemotherapeutic drugs, such as cytoxan, are used to treat myasthenia gravis and myasthenic crisis. Plasmaphoresis is also being tried at some centers. For individuals with cholinergic crisis treatment is to withhold anticholinergic drugs until blood levels fall out of the toxic range, while providing ventilatory support and preventing respiratory complications. Thymectomy is the treatment of choice in individuals with a thymoma.

SUMMARY REVIEW

Central Nervous System (CNS) Disorders

1 Motor accidents are the major cause of traumatic CNS injury. Traumatic injuries are classified as closed-head trauma (blunt) or open-head trauma (penetrating). Closed-head trauma is the more frequent type of trauma.

2 Clinical manifestations associated with brain injury may have an immediate or delayed onset. The individual may temporarily lose consciousness and regain it quickly with mild injury. Consciousness may not be regained for many minutes to a few hours with moderate injury; severe head injury is sustained when arousal is not regained in a few hours.

3 Different types of head injury include concussion (transient loss of consciousness), contusion (bruising of the brain), laceration (tearing of brain tissue), extradural hematoma (accumulation of blood above the dura mater), subdural hematoma (blood between the dura mater and arachnoid membrane), and intracerebral hematoma (bleeding into the brain).

4 Open-head trauma involves a skull fracture with exposure of the cranial vault to the environment. The types of open-head trauma (compound fracture, perforated fracture) are linear, comminuted, compound, and basilar skull fracture (in the cranial vault or at the base of the skull).

5 Spinal cord injuries occur most frequently in men between 15 and 30 years of age who sustain different kinds of injuries (recreational or travel-related) and the elderly because of preexisting degenerative vertebral disorders.

6 Spinal cord injury involves damage to vertebral and/or neural tissues by compressing tissue, pulling or exerting tension on tissue, or shearing tissues so that they slide into one another.

7 Spinal cord injury often causes spinal shock with cessation of all motor, sensory, reflex, and autonomic functions below any transected area. Loss of motor and sensory function depends on the level of injury.

8 Paralysis of the lower half of the body with both legs involved is called paraplegia. Paralysis involving all four extremities is called quadriplegia.

9 Return of spinal neuron excitability occurs slowly. Reflex activity can return in 1 to 2 weeks in most persons

with acute spinal cord injury. A pattern of flexion reflexes emerges, involving first the toes, then the feet and the legs. Eventually reflex voiding and bowel elimination appear, and mass reflex (flexor spasms accompanied by profuse sweating, piloerection, and automatic bladder emptying) may develop.

10 Immobilization of the spine is the immediate intervention for a suspected or confirmed vertebral fracture.

11 Low back pain is pain between the lower rib cage and gluteal muscles and often radiates into the thigh.

12 Low back pain has a high prevalence, affecting 60% to 90% of the population at some point in their lifetime. Sciatica affects about 1% of those with low back pain.

13 Most causes of low back pain are unknown; however, some secondary causes are disk prolapse, tumors, bursitis, synovitis, degenerative joint disease, osteoporosis, fracture, inflammation, and sprain.

14 The role of muscle injury in low back pain remains uncertain; however, muscle spasms often accompany low back pain.

15 Diagnosis of injury to the lower back is made on the basis of physical examination, electromyography, computed tomography, and magnetic resonance imaging.

16 Treatment for low back pain includes bed rest, use of analgesias and anti-inflammatory agents, exercise, physical therapy, education, and surgery.

17 Herniation of an intervertebral disk is a protrusion of part of the nucleus pulposus. Herniation most commonly affects the lumbrosacral disks (L_5-S_1 and L_4-$_5$). The extruded pulposus compresses the nerve root, causing pain that radiates along the sciatic nerve course.

18 The conservative approach to treatment of an intervertebral rupture is traction and bed rest. Surgery is indicated if there is evidence of severe compression (weakness, chronic pain, decreased deep tendon reflexes, and bladder/bowel reflexes).

19 Cerebrovascular disease is the most frequently occurring neurologic disorder. Any abnormality of the blood vessels of the brain is referred to as a cerebrovascular disease.

20 Cerebrovascular disease is associated with two types of brain abnormalities: (a) ischemia with or without infarction and (b) hemorrhage.

21 The most common clinical manifestation of cerebrovascular disease is a cerebrovascular accident (CVA, stroke).

22 Cerebrovascular accidents are classified according to pathophysiology and include thrombotic (arterial occlusions caused by thrombi), embolic (fragments that break from a thrombus outside the brain), and hemorrhagic (intracranial hemorrhage).

23 Treatment for an ischemic CVA includes anticoagulant therapy and supportive management for cerebral edema and increased intracranial pressure. Surgical intervention may be needed to restore blood supply.

24 Intracranial aneurysms result from defects in the vascular wall and are classified on the basis of pathophysiology. They are frequently asymptomatic, but the signs vary, depending on the location and size of the aneurysm.

25 Ruptured cerebral aneurysms have two major complications, rebleeding and cerebrovasospasm. Surgical intervention is the treatment of choice prior to rupture.

26 An arteriovenous malformation (AVM) is a tangled mass of dilated blood vessels. Although sometimes present at birth, AVM exhibits a delayed age of onset.

27 Clinical manifestations of AVM range from headache and dementia to seizures and intracerebral, subarachnoid, or subdural hemorrhage. Surgery is the treatment of choice, if symptomatic.

28 A subarachnoid hemorrhage occurs when blood escapes from defective or injured vasculature into the subarachnoid space. When a vessel tears, blood under pressure is pumped into the subarachnoid space. The blood produces an inflammatory reaction in these tissues.

29 Clinical manifestations of a subarachnoid hemorrhage include headache, changes in mental status, transient motor weakness, and numbness and tingling. Vasospasm is a serious complication and may cause ischemia and infarct. Treatment includes use of calcium channel blockers to prevent or reverse vasospasm, control intracranial pressure, and augment cerebral perfusion by expanding blood volume and packed red blood cells.

30 Two main types of tumors occur within the cranium: primary and metastatic. Primary tumors are classified as intracerebral tumors or extracranial tumors. Metastatic tumors can be found inside or outside the brain substance.

31 CNS tumors cause local and generalized manifestations. The effects are varied and include seizures, visual disturbances, loss of equilibrium, and cranial nerve dysfunction.

32 The principal treatment for cerebral tumors is surgical excision or decompression if total excision is not possible. Chemotherapy and radiation therapy are also used.

33 Spinal cord tumors are classified as intramedullary tumors (within the neural tissues) or extramedullary tumors (outside the spinal cord). Metastatic spinal cord tumors are usually carcinomas, lymphomas, or myelomas.

34 Extramedullary spinal cord tumors produce dysfunction by compression of adjacent tissue, not by direct invasion. Intramedullary spinal cord tumors produce dysfunction by both invasion and compression.

35 The onset of clinical manifestations of spinal cord tumors is gradual and progressive, suggesting compression. Specific manifestations depend on the location of the tumor; for example, there may be paresis and spasticity of one leg with thoracic tumors, followed by involvement of the opposite leg.

36 Spinal cord tumors are treated by surgery, radiotherapy, chemotherapy, and hormonal therapy.

37 Infection and inflammation of the CNS can occur by bacteria, viruses, fungi, protozoans, and rickettsia. The resulting infection of bacterial infections is pus-producing, or pyogenic.

38 Meningitis (infection of the meninges) is classified as bacterial, aseptic (nonpurulent), or fungal. Bacterial meningitis is primarily an infection of the pia mater and arachnoid, and of the fluid of the subarachnoid space. Aseptic meningitis is believed to be limited to the meninges. Fungal meningitis is a chronic, less common type of meningitis.

39 The meningeal vessels become hyperemic and neutrophils migrate into the subarachnoid space with bacterial meningitis. An inflammatory reaction occurs and exudate is formed and increases rapidly.

40 The variety of clinical manifestations depends on the type of meningitis and range from throbbing headache to neck stiffness and rigidity and decreasing responsiveness. Specific cranial nerve dysfunction is a common occurrence.

41 Bacterial meningitis and fungal meningitis are treated with appropriate antibiotic therapy; aseptic meningitis is treated with antibiotics, antiviral drugs, and steroids.

42 Brain abscesses often originate from infections outside the CNS. Organisms gain access to the CNS from adjacent sites or spread along the wall of a vein. A localized inflammatory process develops with exudate formation, thrombosis of vessels, and degenerating leukocytes. After a few days the infection becomes delimited with a center of pus and wall of granular tissue.

43 Clinical manifestations of brain abscesses include headache, nuchal rigidity, confusion, drowsiness, and sensory and communication deficits. Treatment includes antibiotic therapy and surgical drainage.

44 Encephalitis is an acute, febrile illness of viral origin with nervous system involvement. The most common encephalitides are caused by arthropoid-borne viruses and herpes simplex. Meningeal involvement appears in all encephalitides.

45 Clinical manifestations of encephalitis include fever, delirium, confusion, seizures, abnormal and involuntary movement, and increased intracranial pressure.

46 Herpes encephalitis is treated with antiviral agents. No definitive treatment exists for the other encephalitides.

47 Neurosyphilis occurs in about one-fourth of persons with syphilis and is caused by the organism *Treponema pallidum*. An aseptic meningitis initially develops, and a symptomatic meningitis may appear within 2 to 7 years. Syphilis causes a chronic form of meningitis. Tabes dorsalis, a degeneration of the dorsal columns of the spinal cord, may develop. Treatment is the same as that for primary syphilis (see Chapter 21).

48 Parkinson disease is a commonly occurring degenerative disorder of the basal ganglia (corpus striatum) involving degeneration of the dopamine-secreting nigrostriatal pathway. The pathogenesis of Parkinson disease is unknown, but researchers suggest vascular, viral, and metabolic factors as possible causes.

49 Degeneration of the dopaminergic nigrostriatal pathway causes dopamine depletion in the basal ganglia and excess of cholinergic activity in the cortex, basal ganglia, and thalamus. Tremor and rigidity are caused by the excess cholinergic activity. Progressive dementia may be associated with an advanced stage of the disease.

50 Treatment of Parkinson disease is symptomatic, involving levodopa (L-dopa), a precursor of dopamine. The disease takes a slowly progressive course for 15 to 20 years before producing complete invalidism.

51 Huntington disease (chorea) is a rare hereditary disease involving the basal ganglia and cerebral cortex. It is inherited as an autosomal dominant trait and commonly manifests between 40 and 50 years of age.

52 The major pathologic feature of Huntington disease is severe degeneration of the basal ganglia and the frontal cerebral cortex. The basal ganglia and the substantia nigra exhibit a depletion of γ-amino butyric acid (an inhibitory neurotransmitter) secreting neurons. This depletion leads to an excess of dopaminergic activity that causes involuntary, fragmentary movements.

53 No known treatment is effective in halting the degenerative process in Huntington disease.

54 Multiple sclerosis (MS) is a relatively common degenerative disorder involving CNS myelin. Although the pathogenesis is unknown, the demyelination is thought to result from an immunogenetic-viral cause. Viruses or other antigens may directly attack the myelin or provoke a hypersensitivity reaction.

55 The clinical manifestations of MS involve different syndromes: corticospinal (corticospinal tract and dorsal column), brainstem (cranial nerves), cerebellar (corticospinal tract and/or cerebellum), and cerebral (optic neuritis). Persons with early MS usually have one of the initial syndromes; over time individuals eventually have mixed involvement.

56 No treatment is currently available to alter the course of MS. Hormone therapy is used to shorten the duration of acute exacerbations.

57 Amyotrophic lateral sclerosis (ALS) is a rare degenerative disorder diffusely involving lower and upper motor neurons. The pathogenesis of ALS is unknown; however, there is lower and upper motor neuron degeneration.

58 Clinical manifestations of ALS may include weakness in all muscles. Flaccid paresis progressing to paralysis is characteristic of the lower motor neuron syndrome. No treatment is currently available to alter the overall course of the ALS syndrome.

59 Hydrocephalus comprises a variety of disorders characterized by an excess of fluid within the cranial vault, subarachnoid space, or both. Hydrocephalus occurs because of interference with cerebrospinal fluid flow caused by increased fluid production or obstruction within the ventricular system or by defective reabsorption of the fluid.

60 Hydrocephalus can be treated by reducing CSF in the ventricles through the use of shunts and diuretic therapy.

Peripheral Nervous System and Neuromuscular Joint Disorders

1 Radiculopathies are disorders of the roots of spinal cord nerves. The roots may be compressed, inflamed, or torn. Clinical manifestations include local pain and/or paresthesias in the sensory root distribution. Treatment may involve surgery, antibiotics, steroids, radiotherapy, and chemotherapy.

2 Plexus injuries involve the plexus distal to the spinal roots. Paralysis can occur with complete plexus involvement.

3 Neuropathies are the resulting syndrome when the peripheral nerves are affected and involve the inflammatory process. Axon and myelin degeneration may be present. Neuropathies are classified as sensorimotor, sensory, or motor. The neuropathies are characterized by varying degrees of paresis and paralysis, and secondary atrophy may be present.

4 Therapy for the neuropathies is directed at the primary cause, such as diabetes mellitus. Axonal regrowth and recovery of function may take months but many neuropathies can be reversed.

5 Guillain-Barré is a demyelinating disorder caused by a cell-mediated immunologic reaction directed at the peripheral nerves. The clinical manifestations may vary from paresis of the legs to complete quadriplegia, respiratory insufficiency, and autonomic nervous system instability. Steroid therapy may be used during the acute phase and followed by aggressive rehabilitation.

6 Botulism, a form of acute food poisoning produced by *Clostridium botulinum,* blocks nerve impulse transmission at the neuromuscular junction. Symptoms are varied and may include nausea and vomiting, lethargy, dizziness, vertigo, and death.

7 Treatment of botulism involves removal of any unabsorbed exotoxin and supportive therapy.

8 Myasthenia gravis is a disorder of voluntary muscles characterized by muscle weakness and fatigability. It is considered an autoimmune disease and is associated with an increased incidence of other autoimmune diseases.

9 Myasthenia gravis results from a defect in nerve impulse transmission at the neuromuscular junction. IgG antibody is secreted against the "self" acetylcholine receptors and blocks the binding of acetylcholine. The antibody action destroys the receptor sites, causing decreased transmission of the nerve impulse across the neuromuscular junction.

10 Clinical manifestations of myasthenia gravis include weakness of the muscles of the face and throat and may involve muscles of the diaphragm and chest wall.

11 Treatment of myasthenia gravis involves symptom relief. The progression of the disease is highly variable; in some individuals it is mild and spontaneously remits.

KEY TERMS

Acute hydrocephalus, 519

Amyotrophic lateral sclerosis (ALS, sporadic motor system disease, sporadic motor neuron disease), 517

Arteriovenous malformation (AVM), 497

Aseptic meningitis (nonpurulent meningitis), 505

Astrocytoma, 501

Autonomic hyperreflexia (autonomic dysreflexia), 486

Avulsion, 520

Bacterial meningitis, 505

Basilar skull fracture, 483

Battle sign, 483

Botulism, 521

Brain abscess, 506

Brudzinski sign, 498

Bulbar myasthenia, 522

Cerebrovascular accident (CVA, stroke), 493

Cholinergic crisis, 523

Classic ALS (Lou Gehrig's disease), 518

Closed-head trauma (blunt trauma), 477

Communicating hydrocephalus, 519

Completed stroke, 493

Compound fracture (perforated fracture), 483

Compressive syndrome (sensorimotor syndrome), 505

Concussion, 478

Contracoup injury, 477

Contusion, 480

Coup injury, 477

Degenerative disk disease, 490

Embolic stroke, 493

Encephalitis, 507

Encephalopathy,

Ependymoblastoma,

Ependymoma, 502

Extradural brain abscess, 506

Extradural hematoma, 480

Extradural tumor, 504

Extramedullary tumor, 504

Fungal meningitis, 506

Fusiform aneurysm (giant aneurysm), 494

Generalized myasthenia, 522

Glioblastoma multiforme, 501

Glioma, 499

Gliosis, 516

Guillain-Barré syndrome, 521

Hemorrhagic stroke (intracranial hemorrhage), 494

Huntington disease, 513

Hydrocephalus, 519

Hydrocephalus ex vacuo, 519

Inflammatory arachnoiditis, 520

Intracerebral brain abscess, 506

Intracerebral hematoma, 482

Intradural tumor,

Intramedullary spinal cord abscess, 506

Intramedullary tumor, 504

Irritative syndrome (radicular syndrome), 505

Kernig sign, 498

Korsakoff psychosis, 509

Laceration, 480

Lhermitte sign, 517

Mass reflex,

Meningioma, 503

Meningitis, 505

Motor neuropathy, 520

Multiple sclerosis, 514

Myasthenia gravis, 522

Myasthenic crisis, 523

Mycotic aneurysm, 494

Neurilemmoma, 503

Neuritis, 520

Neurosyphilis, 508

Noncommunicating hydrocephalus (internal hydrocephalus), 519

Normal-pressure hydrocephalus, 519

Ocular myasthenia, 522

Oligodendroblastoma, 502

Oligodendroglioma, 502

Open-head trauma (penetrating trauma), 477

Paralysis agitans, 512

Parkinson disease, 509

Parkinsonian tremor, 511

Parkinsonism (Parkinson syndrome, parkinsonian syndrome), 509

Penetrating cranial injury,

Plexus injury, 520

Postconcussive syndrome, 478

Radicular pain, 520

Radicular paresthesia, 520

Radiculitis (radiculoneuritis), 520

Radiculopathy, 520

Saccular aneurysm (berry aneurysm), 494

Segmental demyelination neuropathy, 520

Sensorimotor neuropathy, 520

Sensory neuropathy, 520

Spinal cord abscess, 506

Spinal epidural abscess, 506

Spinal stenosis, 491

Spondylolisthesis, 491

Spondylolysis, 490

Stroke-in-evolution, 493

Subarachnoid hemorrhage, 497

Subdural hematoma, 481

Syringomyelic syndrome, 505

Tabes dorsalis,

Thrombotic stroke (cerebral thrombosis), 493

Transient ischemic attack (TIA), 493

Traumatic aneurysm, 496

Wernicke disease, 509

REFERENCES

Adams, C. W. M. (1975). The onset and progression of the lesion in multiple sclerosis. *Journal of Neurological Science, 25,* 165.

Adams, C. W. M. (1977). Pathology of multiple sclerosis: Progression of the lesion. *British Medical Bulletin, 33,* 15.

Adams, R. D., & Ashbury, A. K. (1983). Diseases of the peripheral nervous system. In R. G. Petersdorf, R. D. Adams, E. Braunwald, K. J. Isselbacher, J. B. Martin, & J. D. Wilson (Eds.), *Harrison's principles of internal medicine.* New York: McGraw-Hill, pp. 2156-2169.

Adams, R. D., & Victor, M. (1985). *Principles of neurology.* New York: McGraw-Hill.

Aita, J. F. (1982). Why patients with Parkinson's disease fall. *Journal of the American Medical Association, 247*(4), 515.

Amico, L. L., & Antel, J. P. (1981). Amyotropic lateral sclerosis—current concepts. *Postgraduate Medicine, 70*(2), 50.

Baum, H. M., & Rothschild, B. B. (1983). Multiple sclerosis and mobility restriction. *Archives Physical Medical Rehabilitation, 64*(12), 591.

Beeson, P. B., McDermott, W., & Wyngaarden, J. B. (Eds.). (1979). *Cecil textbook of medicine* (15th ed.). Philadelphia: W. B. Saunders.

Berg, L., Chesanow, R. L., & Prensky, A. L. (1984). Demyelinating diseases of the nervous system. In S. G. Eliasson, A. L. Prensky, & W. B. Hardin, Jr. (Eds.), *Neurological pathophysiology* (3rd ed.). New York: Oxford University Press.

Bobowick, A. R., & Brody, J. A. (1973). Epidemiology of motor-neuron diseases. *New England Journal of Medicine, 288,* 1047.

Boss, B. J. (1984.) The nervous system. In Howe, J., et al. (Eds.), *The handbook of nursing.* New York: John Wiley & Sons.

Bradley, W. G., & Adams, R. D. (1983). Other major muscle syndromes. In R. G. Petersdorf, Bradley, W. G., & Adams, R. D. (Eds.), *Harrison's principles of internal medicine* (pp. 2198-2201) New York: McGraw-Hill.

Bradley, W. G., & Rebeiz, J. J. (1983). Progressive muscular dystrophy and chronic myopathies. In R. G. Petersdorf, Bradley, W. G., & Rebeiz, J. J. (Eds.), *Harrison's principles of internal medicine* (pp. 2188-2193) New York: McGraw-Hill.

Bradley, W. G., & Salam-Adams, M. (1983). Acute and subacute myopathic paralysis. In R. G. Petersdorf, R. D. Adams, E. Braunwald, K. J. Isselbacher, J. B. Martin, & J. D. Wilson (Eds.), *Harrison's principles of internal medicine* (pp. 2184-2187) New York: McGraw-Hill.

Calne, D. B. (1984). Progress in Parkinson's disease [Editorial]. *New England Journal of Medicine, 310*(8), 523.

Calne, D. B., & Eisler, T. (1979, July). The pathogenesis and medical treatment of extrapyramidal disease. *Medical Clinics of North America, 63*(4), 715.

Chusid, J. G. (1985). *Corrective neuroanatomy and functional neurology.* Los Altos, Calif: Lange Medical Publications.

Cohen, S. R., Brooks, B. R., Herdon, R. M. & McKhaun G. M. (1980). A diagnostic index of active demyelination: Myelin basic protein in cerebrospinal fluid. *Annals of Neurology, 8,* 25.

Conway-Rutkowski, B. L. (1982). *Carini and Owen's neurological and neurosurgical nursing.* St. Louis: C. V. Mosby.

DeLisa, J. A., Mikulic, M. A., Miller, R. M., & Melnick, R. R. (1979). Amyotrophic lateral sclerosis: Comprehensive management. *Americal Family Physician, 19,* 137.

Donovan, W. H. (1982). Comprehensive management of spinal cord injury. *Clinical Symposium, 34*(2), 2-36.

Dovoisin, R. (1976). Parkinsonism. *CIBA Clinical Symposia, 28,* 1.

Duvoisin, R. C. (1984). *Parkinson's disease, a guide for patient and family* (2nd ed.). New York: Raven Press.

Eliasson, S. G., Prensky, A. L., & Hardin, W. B. (Eds.). (1978). *Neurological pathophysiology* (2nd ed.). New York: Oxford University Press.

Engle, W. K., Siddique, T., & Nicoloff, J. T. (1983). Effect on weakness and spasticity in amyotrophic lateral sclerosis of thyrotropin-releasing hormone. *Lancet, 2*(8341), 73.

Esiri, M. M. (1980). Multiple sclerosis: A quantitative and qualitative study of immunoglobulin-containing cells in the central nervous system. *Neuropathy Applied Neurobiology, 6,* 9.

Fink, J. M., & Arnason, B. G. W. (1982). Immunologic aspects of neurological and neuromuscular diseases. *Journal of the American Medical Association, 248*(20), 2710.

Fischer, E. G., Linggood, R. M., & Recht, L. D. (1986). Cancers of the central nervous system. In *Cancer Manual.* Boston, Mass.: American Cancer Society.

Fog, T. (1965). The topography of plaques in multiple sclerosis. *Acta Neurologic Scandinavica Supplementum, 41*(5) 1.

Forster, F. M. (1978). *Clinical neurology* (4th ed.). St. Louis: C. V. Mosby.

Freidman, W. A. (1982). Head injuries. *Clinical Symposia, 35*(4), 2-32.

Frymoyer, J. W. (1988, February). Back pain and sciatica. *New England Journal of Medicine, 318*(5), 291-300.

Gehrke, M. (1980). Identifying brain tumors. *Journal of Neurosurgical Nursing, 12*(2), 90-92.

Gilman, A. G., Goodman, L. S., Rall, T. W., & Murad, F. (1985). *Goodman and Gilman's the pharmacological basis of therapeutics* (7th ed.). New York: Macmillan.

Gilroy, J., & Holliday, P. L. (1982). *Basic neurology.* New York: Macmillan.

Gilroy, J., & Meyer, J. (1979). *Medical neurology* (3rd ed.). New York: Macmillan.

Guyton, A. C. (1986). *Basic human neurophysiology* (3rd ed.). Philadelphia: W. B. Saunders.

Hallpike, J. F., Adams, C. W. M., & Tourtellotte, W. W. (Eds.). (1983). *Multiple sclerosis: Pathology, diagnosis, and management.* Baltimore: Williams & Wilkins.

Hart, R., & Sherman, D. (1983). The diagnosis of multiple sclerosis. *Journal of the American Medical Association, 247,* 498.

Heilman, K. M., Watson, R. T., & Greer, M. (1977). *Handbook for differential diagnosis of neurologic signs and symptoms.* New York: Appleton-Century-Croft.

Herndon, R. M., & Rudick, R. A. (1983). Multiple sclerosis: The spectrum of severity. *Archives of Neurology, 40*(9), 531.

Hickey, J. V. (1986). *The clinical practice of neurological and neurosurgical nursing.* Philadelphia: J. B Lippincott.

Huntington, H. W., & Terry, R. D. (1966). The origin of the reactive cells in cerebral stab wounds. *Journal of Neuropathology and Experimental Neurology, 25,* 646.

Ibrahim, M. Z. M., & Adams, C. W. M. (1965). The relationship between enzyme activity and neuroglia in early plaques of multiple sclerosis. *Journal of Pathological Bacteriology, 90,* 239.

Jane, M. J., Freewater, A. A., Hazel, C., Lindan, R., & Joiner, E. (1982, September). Autonomic dysreflexia: A cause of morbidity and mortality in orthopedic patients with spinal cord injury. *Clinical Orthopedics, 169,* 151-158.

Keim, H. A. (1973). Low back pain. *Clinical Symposia, 24*(3), 2-32.

Kirshner, H. S., Tsai, S. I., Runge, V. M., & Price, A. C. (1985). Magnetic resonance imaging and other techniques in the diagnosis of multiple sclerosis. *Archives of Neurology, 42,* 859.

Kneisl, C. R., & Ames, S. A. (1986). Adult health nursing: A biopsychosocial approach. Reading, Mass.: Addison-Wesley.

Kott, E., Livni, E., Zamir, R., & Kuritzky, A. (1979). Cell-mediated immunity to polio and human leukocyte antigens in amyotrophic lateral sclerosis. *Neurology, 29,* 1040.

Larson, E. (1980). The epidemiology of brain tumors. *Journal of Neurosurgical Nursing, 12*(3), 121-127.

Lumsden, C. E. (1951). Fundamental problems in the pathology of multiple sclerosis and allied demyelinating diseases. *British Medical Journal, 1,* 1035.

Lumsden, C. E. (1971). The immunogenesis of the multiple sclerosis plaque. *Brain Research, 97,* 179.

Mackay, R. P. (1963). Course and prognosis in amyotrophic lateral sclerosis. *Archives of Neurology, 8,* 117.

Mancall, E. L. (1981). *Alper's and Mancall's essentials of the neurologic examination.* Philadelphia: F. A. Davis.

Marsden, C. D., & Fahn, S. (Eds.). (1982). *Movement disorders.* London: Butterworth.

Matthews, B. (1978). *Multiple sclerosis: The facts.* New York: Oxford University Press.

Matthews, W. B., & Miller, H. (1975). *Diseases of the nervous system.* Oxford: Blackwell Scientific Publications.

McAlpine, D., Lumsden, C. E., & Acheson, E. D. (1972). *Multiple sclerosis—a reappraisal* (2nd ed.). Baltimore: Williams & Wilkins.

McDonald, W. I. (1974). Pathophysiology in multiple sclerosis. *Brain, 97,* 179.

Merritt, H. H. (1979). *A textbook of neurology* (6th ed.). Philadelphia: Lea & Febiger.

Morariu, M. A., Wilkins, D. E. & Patch, S. (1980). Multiple sclerosis and serial computerized tomography: Delayed contrast enhancement of acute and early lesions. *Archives of Neurology, 37*(3), 189.

Morse, S. D. (1982, August). Acute central cervical spinal cord syndrome. *Annals Emergency Medicine, 11*(8), 436-439.

Netter, F. H. (1962). *The CIBA collection of medical illustrations. Volume I: Nervous system with a supplement on hypothalamus.* CIBA Pharmaceutical Company, Division of CIBA Corporation.

Newman, R. P., & Calne, D. B. (1984). Diagnosis and management of Parkinson's disease. *Geriatrics, 39*(5), 87.

Nursing skillbook: Coping with neurologic problems proficiently. (1979). Horsham, Penn.: Intermed Communications.

Oppenheimer, D. R. (1978). The cervical cord in multiple sclerosis. *Nueropathology and Applied Neurobiology, 4*:151.

Paylakis, A. J., Siroky, M. B., Goldstein, I., & Krane, R. J. (1983). Neurologic findings in Parkinson's disease. *Journal of Urology, 129*(1), 80.

Petersdorf, R. G., Adams, R. D., Braunwald, E., Isselbacher, K. J., Martin, J. B., & Wilson, J. D. (Eds.). (1983). *Harrison's principles of internal medicine.* New York: McGraw-Hill.

Plorde, J. J. (1983). Trichinosis. In R. G. Petersdorf, Plorde, J. J. (Eds.), *Harrison's principles of internal medicine* (pp. 1212-1214). New York: McGraw-Hill.

Pope, M. H., Bevins, T., Wilder, D. G., & Frymoyer, J. W. (1985). The relationship between anthropometric, postural, muscular, and mobility characteristics of males ages 18-55. *Spine, 10,* 644-648.

Poser, C. M. (1979). Multiple sclerosis: A critical update. *Medical Clinics of North America, 63,* 729.

Poser, C. M. (1985). MRI and CT scan in multiple sclerosis [Letter]. *Journal of the American Medical Association, 253*(22), 3250.

Prineas, J., & Raine, C. S. (1976). Electron microscopy and immunoperoxidase studies of early multiple sclerosis lesions. *Neurology* (Part 2), *26,* 29.

Purtilo, D. T. (1978). *A survey of human diseases.* Menlo Park, Calif.: Addison-Wesley.

Reinhertz, E. L., Weiner, H. L., Hausye, S. L., Cohen, J. A., Distase, J. A., & Schlossman, S.F. (1980). Loss of suppressor T cells in active multiple sclerosis. *New England Journal of Medicine, 303,* 125.

Rhoton, A. L., Jackson, F., Gleave, J., & Rumbaugh, C. T. (1977). Congenital and traumatic intracranial aneurysm. *Clinical Symposia, 29*(4), 2-40.

Riley, T., & Massey, W. (1980). *Postgrad. Med., 68*(86), 268.

Robbins, S. L., Cotran, R. S., & Kumar, V. (1984). *Pathologic basis of disease* (3rd ed.). Philadelphia: W. B. Saunders.

Roos, R. P., Viola, M. V., Wollmann, R., Hatch, M. H., & Antel, J. D. (1980). Amyotrophic lateral sclerosis with antecedent poliomyelitis. *Archives of Neurology, 37,* 312.

Rose, C. (Ed.). (1979). *Neuroimmunology.* London: Medical Society of London.

Rosen, A. D. (1978). Amyotrophic lateral sclerosis: Clinical features and prognosis. *Archives of Neurology, 35,* 638.

Rudy, E. B. (1984). *Advanced neurological and neurosurgical nursing.* St. Louis: C. V. Mosby.

Sadeh, M. (1982). Effects of anticholinergic drugs on memory in Parkinson's disease. *Archives of Neurology, 39*(10), 666.

Schauf, C. L., Antel, J. P., Arnason, B. G. W., Davis, F. A., & Rooney, M. W. (1980). Neuroelectric blocking activity and plasmapheresis in amyotrophic lateral sclerosis. *Neurology, 30*:1011.

Scheinberg, L. C. (Ed.). (1983). *Multiple sclerosis, a guide for patients and their families.* New York: Raven Press.

Schwankhaus, J. D. (1984). Diagnosis of multiple sclerosis. *American Family Physician, 29*(1), 231.

Slater, R. J., & Yearwood, A. C. (1980). MS: Facts, faith, and hope. *American Journal of Nursing, 80,* 276.

Smith, L. H., & Thier, S. O. (1981). *Pathophysiology: The biological principles of disease.* Philadelphia: W. B. Saunders.

Somasundaram, M., Cho, E. S., & Posner, J. B. (1975). Anterior horn cell degeneration as a remote effect of lymphoma. *Transactions of the American Neurological Association, 100,* 144.

Spengler, D. M. (1982). *Low back pain, assessment, and management.* New York: Grune & Stratton.

Stenwig, A. E. (1972). The origin of brain macrophages in traumatic lesions, Wallerian degeneration and retrograde degeneration. *Journal of Neuropathology and Experimental Neurology, 31,* 696.

Stewart, G. J., & Kirk, R. L. (1983). The genetics of multiple sclerosis: The HLA system and other genetic markers. In J. F. Hallpike, C. W. M. Adams, & W. W. Tourtellotte (Eds.), *Multiple sclerosis pathology, diagnosis, and management.* London: Chapman & Hall.

Toole, J. F. (Ed.) (1977). *Clinical concepts of neurological disorders.* Baltimore: Williams & Wilkins.

Vander, A. J., Sherman, J. H., & Luciano, D. S. (1980). *Human physiology: The mechanisms of body function* (3rd ed.). New York: McGraw-Hill.

Vick, N. A. (1976). *Grinker's neurology* (7th ed.). Springfield, Ill.: Charles C Thomas.

Vinken, P. J., & Bruyn, G. W. (Eds.). (1970). *Handbook of clinical neurology.* Amsterdam: North-Holland.

Waksman, B. H. (1983). Rationales of current therapies for multiple sclerosis. *Archives of Neurology, 40*(11), 671.

Weiner, L. P. (1980). Possible role of androgen receptors in amyotrophic lateral sclerosis: A hypothesis. *Archives of Neurology, 37,* 129.

Weiner, M. (1982). Update on antiparkinsonian agents. *Geriatrics, 37*(9), 81.

Weinstein, S. L. (1986). Idiopathic scoliosis: Natural history. *Spine, 11,* 780-783.

White, A. A., & Gordon, S. C. (Eds.). (1982). *American Academy of Orthopaedic Surgeons symposium on idiopathic low back pain.* St. Louis: C. V. Mosby.

Wisneiwski, H. M. (1977). Immunopathology of demyelination in autoimmune diseases and virus infection. *British Medical Bulletin, 33,* 54.

Wolf, J. K. (1980). *Practical clinical neurology.* Garden City, New York: Medical Examination.

CHAPTER 16

Alterations of Neurologic Function in Children

Margaret Andrews
Kathleen Hardin Mooney

Structure and function of the nervous system in children, 532
  Myelin sheath, 533
Normal growth and development, 533
Structural malformations, 535
  Defects of neural tube closure, 535
    Anencephaly, 536
    Encephalocele, 536
      Clinical manifestations, 536
      Evaluation and treatment, 536
    Meningocele, 536
      Clinical manifestations, 536
      Evaluation and treatment, 536
    Myelomeningocele, 536
      Clinical manifestations, 537
      Evaluation and treatment, 538
  Malformations of the axial skeleton, 538
    Spina bifida occulta, 538
    Cranial deformities, 538
      Acrania, 538
      Craniosynostosis, 538
        Pathophysiology, 538
        Clinical manifestations, 539
        Evaluation and treatment, 539
      Microcephaly, 540
      Congenital hydrocephalus, 541
        Pathophysiology, 541
        Clinical manifestations, 541
        Evaluation and treatment, 541
Encephalopathies, 542
  Static encephalopathies, 542
    Cerebral palsy, 542
      Pathophysiology, 543
        Prenatal cerebral hypoxia, 543
        Perinatal trauma, 543
      Clinical manifestations, 543
      Evaluation and treatment, 543
    Inherited metabolic disorders of the CNS, 544
      Defects in amino acid metabolism, 544

Defects in lipid metabolism, 546
Seizure disorders in children, 546
  Generalized seizures, 546
    Tonic-clonic seizures, 546
    Myoclonic seizures, 546
    Infantile spasms, 546
    Atonic and akinetic seizures, 547
  Partial seizures, 547
  Febrile seizures, 547
Acute encephalopathies, 548
  Reye syndrome, 548
    Pathophysiology, 548
    Clinical manifestation, 548
    Evaluation and treatment, 548
  Intoxications of the CNS, 549
  Bacterial meningitis in children, 549
    Pathogenesis, 551
    Clinical manifestations, 551
    Evaluation and treatment, 551
Cerebrovascular disease in children, 551
Childhood tumors, 552
  Brain tumors in children, 552
  Types of brain tumors, 552
  Cause of the disease, 553
    Pathogenesis, 553
    Clinical manifestations, 553
    Evaluation and treatment, 555
  Embryonal tumors, 555
    Neuroblastoma, 555
      Pathogenesis, 556
      Clinical manifestations, 556
      Evaluation and treatment, 556
    Retinoblastoma, 557
      Pathogenesis, 557
      Clinical manifestations, 557
      Evaluation and treatment, 558

Central nervous system malformations are responsible for 75% of fetal deaths and 40% of deaths during the first year of life. During the perinatal period, CNS malformations account for one third of all apparent congenital malformations. Ninety percent of CNS malformations are defects of neural tube closure. Although embryology is a highly complex and often difficult science, the process of embryonic development explains many of the malformations that occur in children.

Environmental influences also play a significant role in nervous system development. Nutrition, hormones, oxygen levels, and external stimulation all affect normal growth. The proper proportions of essential nutrients are necessary for proliferation of the nervous system tissue. Maternal life-style, nutrition, and state of health also have a crucial impact on nervous system development at certain critical periods of development.

STRUCTURE AND FUNCTION OF THE NERVOUS SYSTEM IN CHILDREN

The central nervous system develops from a dorsal thickening of the ectoderm known as the **neural plate.** This plate appears around the middle of the third gestational week and unfolds to form a **neural groove** and **neural folds.** During the fourth gestational week, the neural groove deepens; its folds develop laterally; and it closes dorsally to form the **neural tube,** epithelial tissue that ultimately becomes the CNS. The neural tube closes first in the cervical region and then "zippers" in two directions, cranially and caudally (Fig. 16-1).

In the developmental process, some neuroectodermal cells do not become part of the neural tube but remain between the tube and the surface ectoderm, creating

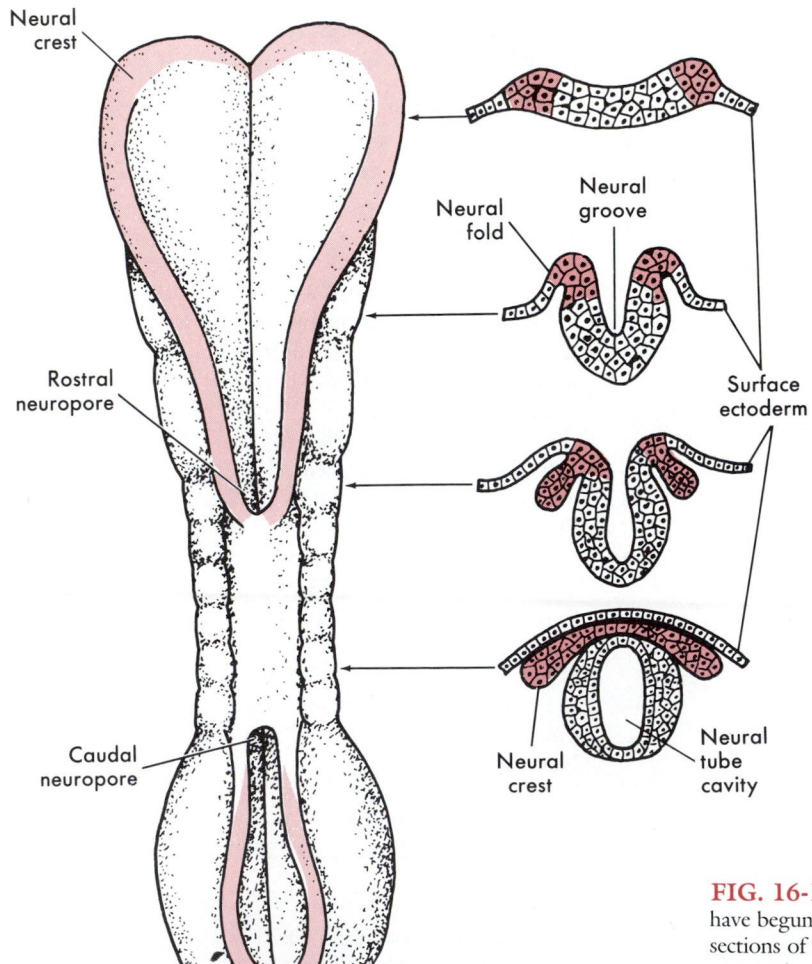

FIG. 16-1. Neural tube at the end of the third week. Neural folds have begun to fuse at the cervical level of the future spinal cord. Cross sections of the neural tube at four different levels shown on the right; at any given level the embryonic CNS goes through a series of stages resembling these four cross sections. Total length of neural tube at this time is about 2.5 mm. (From Nolte, 1988.)

what is called the **neural crest,** a cellular band that develops into the cranial and spinal ganglia. Other structures associated with the nervous system arise from mesoderm **(somite)** and include blood vessels, microglial cells, dura and arachnoid layers of the meninges, capsule of some peripheral sensory nerve endings, and peripheral nerve coverings.

The cranial end of the neural tube forms the brain, and the remainder develops into the spinal cord. The lumen of the neural tube becomes the ventricles of the brain and the central canal of the spinal cord (Fig. 16-2). On either side of the neural tube's inner surface is a longitudinal groove **(sulcus limitans).** Anterior to this region **(basal plate)** the gray matter differentiates into the nuclei of the lower motor neurons. The region posterior to the sulcus **(alar plate)** differentiates into the sensory nuclei of the spinal cord.

Embryonic development of the nervous system occurs in six stages: (1) dorsal (posterior) induction, (2) ventral (anterior) induction, (3) proliferation, (4) migra-

tion, (5) organization, and (6) myelination. (Fig.16-3 summarizes the embryonic development of the nervous system and identifies disorders associated with interference in any of these stages.) Many different events happen simultaneously, and critical periods must pass uninterrupted if the vulnerable fetus is to develop normally.

In the newborn, the bones of the skull are separated, but definite **sutures** (bands of connective tissue) form shortly thereafter. The edges are several millimeters wide to allow for normal growth. At the junctions of the sutures are wider spaces of unossified membranous tissue called **fontanelles.** Sutures and fontanelles close as the skull and brain grow and develop.

By 3 months, the posterior fontanelle is closed. By 6 months fibrous union of suture lines occurs, and serrated edges interlock. By 20 months, the anterior fontanelle is closed (Fig. 16-4). At 8 years, ossification of the cranial bones is complete, and by 12 years the sutures cannot be separated by increased intracranial pressure.

Myelin Sheath

Axons are wrapped in concentric layers of myelin, a lipid-protein sheath (see Chapter 12). Specialized connective tissue cells, that in the peripheral nervous system are called **Schwann cells,** form membranes that wrap around the axon during embryonic development, laying down the lipoprotein lamellae of the myelin sheath. These axons are myelinated, whereas the axons lacking a sheath are thinner, unmyelinated fibers and conduct nerve impulses more slowly. During the first year of life, the presence or absence of various reflexes is indicative of the myelination that has occurred with growth of the infant.

Normal Growth and Development

Human neurologic functioning is primarily at a subcortical level at birth (impulses are handled by the brainstem and spinal cord). Many reflex patterns mediated by brainstem and spinal cord mechanisms are present at birth and disappear at predictable times during infancy. Table 16-1 summarizes the age at which reflexes appear and disappear.

Absence of expected reflex responses at the appropriate age indicates general depression of central or peripheral motor functions. Asymmetric responses may indicate lesions in the motor cortex or may occur with fractures of bones after traumatic delivery or postnatal injury. As the infant matures, the neonatal reflexes disappear in a predictable order as voluntary motor functions supersede them. Abnormal persistence of these reflexes is seen in infants with developmental delays or with central motor lesions.

Several differences between adults and children are helpful in understanding the pathophysiology of the

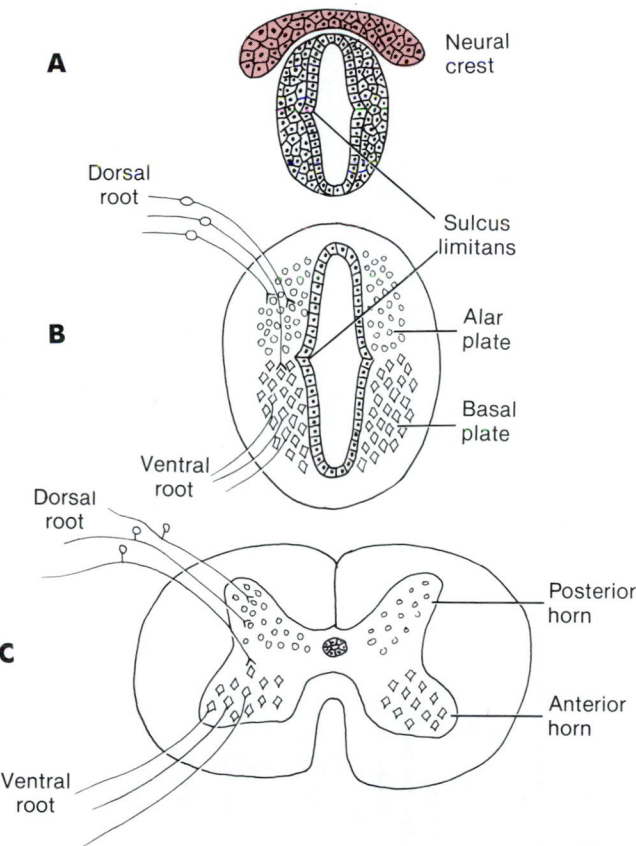

FIG. 16-2. Sulcus limitans and alar and basal plates. **A,** Neural tube during the fourth week. **B,** Embryonic spinal cord during the sixth week; dorsal root ganglion cells, derived from the neural crest, send their central processes into the spinal cord to terminate mainly in alar plate cells; basal plate cells become motor neurons, whose axons exit in the ventral roots. **C,** Adult spinal cord. (From Nolte, 1988.)

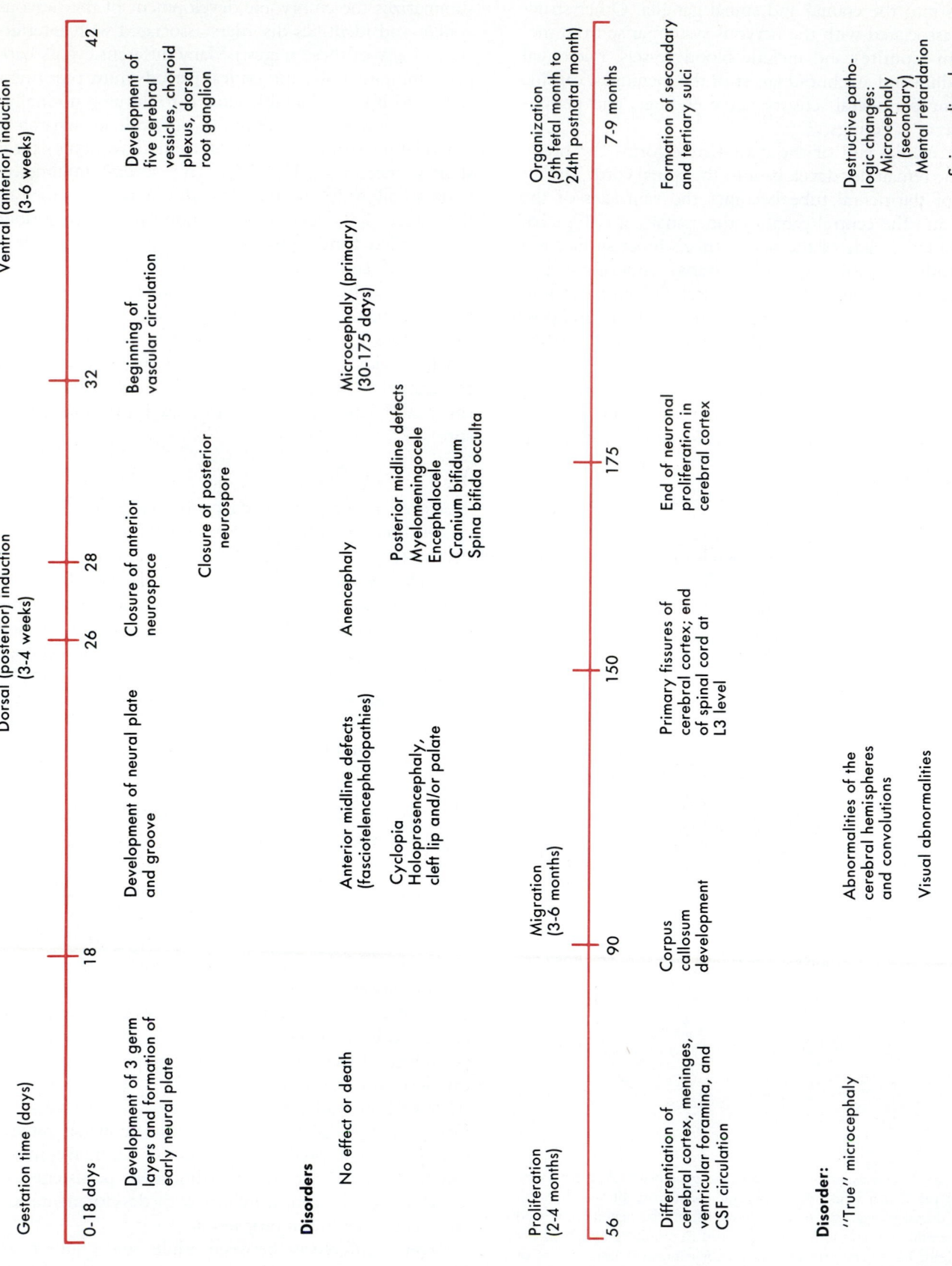

FIG. 16-3. Disorders associated with specific stages of embryonic development.

Myelination
(6 months gestation to adulthood)

6 months   Adulthood
Development of myelin wrapping

Disorder:
Schilder disease
Childhood multiple sclerosis
Leukodystrophies

FIG. 16-3, cont'd. Disorders associated with specific stages of embryonic development.

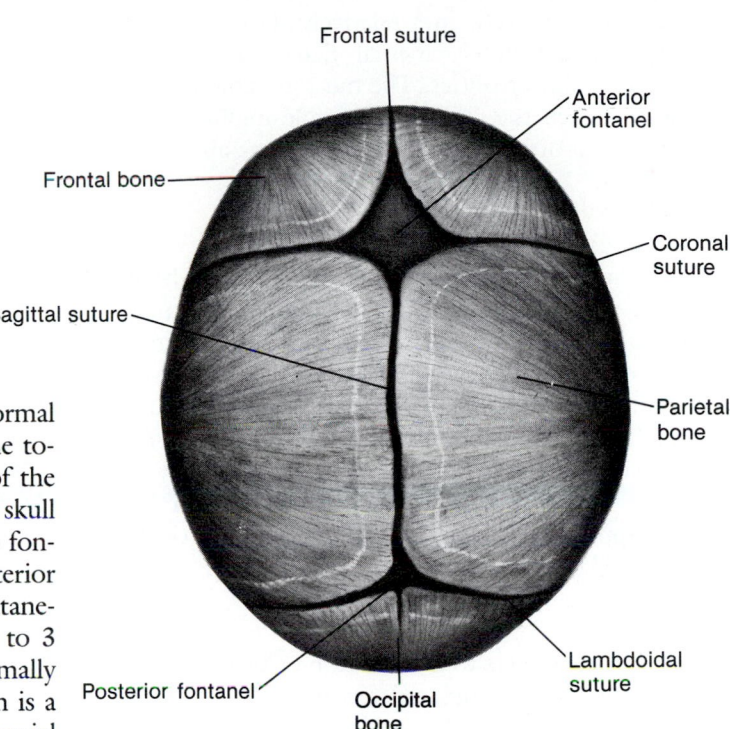

FIG. 16-4. Cranial sutures and fontanelles in infancy. Fibrous union of suture lines and interlocking of serated edges (occurs by 6 months; solid union requires approximately 12 years). (From Whaley & Wong, 1987.)

nervous system in children. First, the head of a normal infant accounts for approximately one fourth of the total height, whereas an adult's head is one eighth of the total body height. Second, the bones of the infant's skull are separated at the suture lines, thus forming two fontanelles or "soft spots," one diamond-shaped anterior fontanelle and one triangular-shaped posterior fontanelle. The posterior fontanelle may be open until 2 to 3 months of age, whereas the anterior fontanelle normally closes by 18 months. Although the adult's cranium is a closed cavity with sutures firmly holding the cranial bones together, the infant's cranium has room for expansion through the fontanelles. An adult's head size will not expand, regardless of intracranial events such as trauma or increased production of cerebrospinal fluid. The infant's head circumference, on the other hand, increases in size as a result of normal growth up to age 5 years. The head is the fastest growing body part during infancy. Abnormal intracranial conditions, such as those characterized by increased intracranial pressure, may also result in an increased head circumference in excess of that expected with normal growth. Health care providers carefully monitor head growth during the first 5 years of life by measuring head circumference and comparing the results with a standardized growth chart.

STRUCTURAL MALFORMATIONS

Defects of Neural Tube Closure

Neural tube defects, which are caused by an arrest of the normal development process, have an incidence rate of 2 per 1000 live births. Defects of neural tube closure are divided into two categories: (1) posterior defects and (2) anterior midline defects.

Posterior defects are more common. These include **anencephaly** (an= without; enkephalos=brain) and a group of disorders collectively referred to as the **myelo-**

TABLE 16-1 Reflexes of infancy

Reflex	Age at appearance of reflex	Age at which reflex should no longer be obtainable
Moro	Birth	3 months
Stepping	Birth	6 weeks
Sucking	Birth	4 months awake 7 months asleep
Rooting	Birth	4 months awake 7 months asleep
Palmar grasp	Birth	6 months
Plantar grasp	Birth	10 months
Tonic neck	2 months	5 months
Neck righting	4-6 months	24 months
Landau	3 months	24 months
Parachute reaction	9 months	Persists for life

dysplasias (dys=bad; plassein=to form). Although my-elodysplasia is defined as a defective formation of the spinal cord, the term is used to refer to anomalies of both the vertebral column and the spine.

Anterior midline defects are less common because the inductive processes occur in a relatively short, 2- to 3-day period. These developmental defects may cause brain and skull abnormalities. The most extreme form is **cyclopia,** in which the child has a single midline orbit and eye with a protruding noselike appendage above the orbit.

Anencephaly

Anencephaly is an anomaly in which the soft, bony component of the skull and part of the brain are missing. This is a relatively common disorder, with an incidence rate of 1 to 6.7 per 1000 live births. When development is arrested early in anterior closure of the neural tube, the cerebral hemispheres, diencephalon, mesencephalon, cerebellum, brainstem, or spinal cord may be affected. At birth, the infant's head, viewed face-on, has a froglike appearance. These infants are stillborn or die within a few days after birth.

Encephalocele

Encelphalocele refers to a herniation or protrusion of brain and meninges through a defect in the skull, resulting in a saclike structure. The incidence rate is 1 in 6500 live births (Conway-Rutkowski, 1982). When the defect contains only meninges, it is referred to as a **cranial meningocele.** Seventy-five precent of encephaloceles occur in the occipital area; the remainder are found in the parietal, frontal, or nasopharyngeal regions (Behrman & Vaughan, 1983).

Clinical Manifestations

Encephalocele is usually seen at birth as a midline skull defect through which a large mass protrudes (Fig. 16-5). If the defect is located in the nasopharynx, no external anomaly is visible, but the child may experience nasal airway obstruction. On examination with a nasal speculum, a smooth, round mass will be visible in the nasal passages. A frontal encephalocele may extend into the orbit of the eye and produce proptosis on the affected side.

Evaluation and Treatment

Diagnosis is made on the basis of clinical manifestations and examination of the meningeal sac. Surgical repair of the defect brings a good prognosis for cranial meningocele with 60% of affected infants having normal intellectual and motor functioning. The prognosis is guarded with occipital encephalocele; there is only about a 10% chance of normal intelligence (Behrman & Vaughan, 1983).

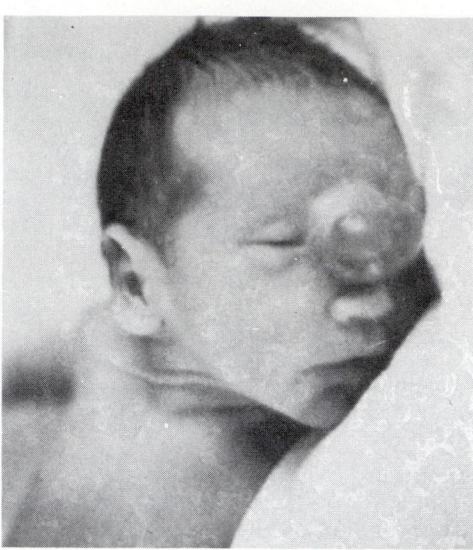

FIG. 16-5. Newborn with frontal, nasal, interocular encephalocele. (Courtesy of Dr. Charles Linder, Medical College of Georgia. From Dyken & Miller, 1980.)

Meningocele

Meningocele is a saclike cyst of meninges filled with spinal fluid that protrudes through a defect in the spine (Fig. 16-6). Like myelomeningocele, meningocele is caused by incomplete closure of the neural tube and vertebral arches; with meningocele, however, neural tissue is not exposed. Meningoceles occur with equal frequency in the cervical, thoracic, and lumbar spine areas.

Clinical Manifestations

Because a meningocele does not contain neural tissue, symptoms and signs of neurologic dysfunction usually are absent. A "minor" neurologic abnormality is present in 40% of children with meningocele. Talipes equinovarus (club foot), gait disturbance, bladder dysfunction, and partial hand paralysis have also been associated with meningocele. A meningocele in the cranial or high cervical area is commonly associated with hydrocephalus.

Evaluation and Treatment

The diagnosis is made from examination of the clinical manifestations and examination of the meningeal sac. Elective surgical closure of the sac after the infant has reached 3 months of age is the preferred treatment. Shunting should precede surgical correction of the meningocele because after surgery the cerebrospinal fluid no longer has an absorption surface equal to cerebrospinal fluid production, thus leading to intracranial pressure.

Myelomeningocele

Myelomeningocele (meningomyclocele; spina bifida cystica) is a hernial protrusion of a saclike cyst

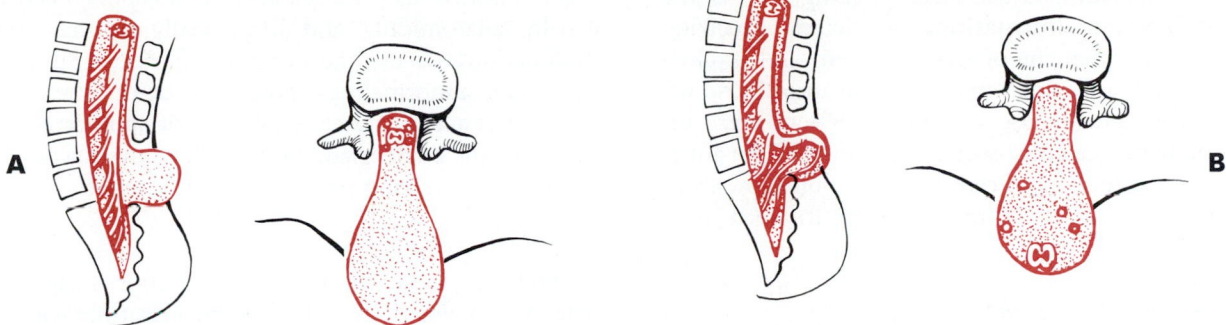

FIG. 16-6. **A,** Meningocele. **B,** Myelomeningocele. (From Whaley & Wong, 1987.)

(containing meninges, spinal fluid, and a portion of the spinal cord with its nerves) through a defect in the posterior arch of a vertebra. Eighty percent of myelomeningoceles are located in the lumbar and lumbosacral regions, the last regions of the neural tube to close. One of the most common developmental anomalies of the nervous system, myelomeningocele has an incidence rate ranging from 0.2 to 0.4 per 1000 live births (Behrman & Vaughan, 1983). The defect may occur with or without encephalocele.

Clinical Manifestations

Myelomeningocele is evident at birth as a skin defect on the infant's back (Figs. 16-6, *B* and 16-7). The bony prominences of the unfused neural arches can be palpated at the lateral border of the defect. The defect is usually covered by a transparent membrane that may

have neural tissue attached to its inner surface. Although cerebrospinal fluid leaks from this membrane at first, the membrane becomes dried from exposure to air and permeability decreases. As cerebrospinal fluid accumulates, the membrane begins to bulge and enlarges into a large sac unless it is surgically closed. The leaking myelomeningocele sac may repair (i.e., seal) itself when granulation tissue is generated as a response to infection. This inflammatory fibrosis, however, may lead to scarring and permanent loss of neural function.

An absence of neurologic function may occur in some infants with myelomeningocele. Function usually may be attained if underlying fluid or pus accumulation is prevented from stretching the neural tissue or if the biochemical alterations do not cause neural tissue to die. Residual neural tissue also may be temporarily lost at birth because of trauma to the tissue during delivery.

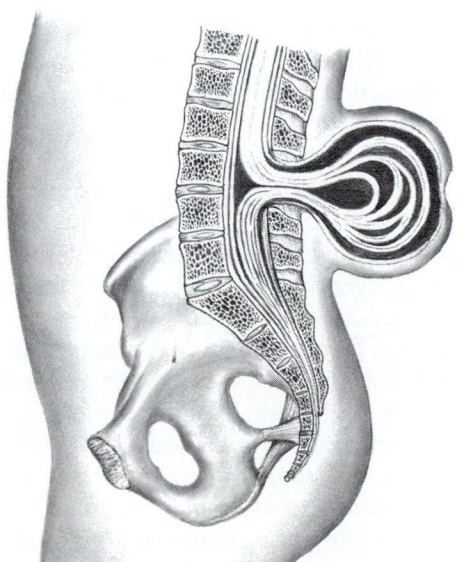

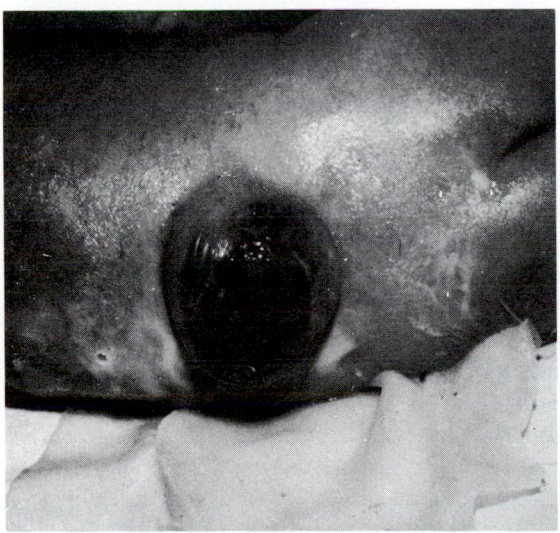

FIG. 16-7. Meningomyelocele before surgery. (Courtesy M. C. Gleason, M. D., San Diego, CA. From Whaley & Wong, 1987.)

Frequently accompanying myelomeningocele is the **Arnold-Chiari malformation,** a defect involving downward displacement of the brainstem and cerebellum through the foramen magnum and into the spinal canal. Hydrocephalus also occurs in 95% of these infants. The hydrocephalus is due to stenosis of the aqueduct or to obstruction of cerebrospinal fluid flow from the fourth ventricle in the region of the foramen magnum.

Evaluation and Treatment

Diagnosis is made on the basis of clinical manifestations and examination of the meningeal sac. Immediate surgical repair of the myelomeningocele sac is indicated. Orthopedic procedures are sometimes helpful to correct the hip and foot deformities that often accompany this disorder.

The prognosis depends on the extent of the motor deficit present at birth, involvement of bladder innervation, and the presence of associated cerebral anomalies. Children with lesser degrees of involvement, especially those with spina bifida and meningocele with evidence of neurologic deficit at birth, have a much more favorable outlook (Behrman & Vaughan, 1983).

Malformations of the Axial Skeleton
Spina Bifida Occulta

When defects of neural tube closure occur, such as meningocele and myelomeningocele, there is an accompanying vertebral defect that allows the protrusion of the neural tube contents. Such a defect is called **spina bifida.** It is also possible for a defect to occur without any visible exposure of meninges or neural tissue. Because the defect is not apparent to the naked eye ("occult" or hidden), the term **spina bifida occulta** is used. In spina bifida occulta, the posterior vertebral laminae have failed to fuse. Extremely common, the defect occurs to some degree in 10% to 25% of infants. Approximately 80% of these vertebral defects are located in the lumbosacral regions, most commonly in the fifth lumbar vertebra and the first sacral vertebra, and may be detected prenatally with ultrasonic scanning and alpha-fetoprotein. About 3% of normal adults have spina bifida occulta of the atlas (cervical vertebra 1).

Certain cutaneous or subcutaneous abnormalities are suggestive of underlying spina bifida. These abnormalities include:

1. Abnormal growth of hair along the spine, which is often either very coarse or very silky
2. A midline dimple with or without a sinus tract
3. A cutaneous angioma, usually of the "port wine" variety
4. A subcutaneous mass, usually representing a lipoma or dermoid cyst

Spina bifida occulta usually causes no serious neurologic dysfunctions. The spinal cord and spinal nerves are usually anatomically and functionally normal. When dysfunctions occur, the common lumbosacral defects cause gait abnormalities, positional deformities of the feet as a result of muscle weakness, or sphincter disturbances of the bladder and bowel. These dysfunctions become evident during periods of rapid growth.

Cranial Deformities

Skull malformations range from minor, insignificant defects to major defects that are incompatible with life.

Acrania

In **acrania,** the cranial vault is almost completely absent and an extensive defect of the vertebral column is often present. Acrania associated with anencephaly (absence of brain and spinal column) occurs in approximately 1 per 1000 live births and is incompatible with life. The malformation results from a failure of the cranial end of the neural tube to close during the fourth gestational week. Subsequently, the cranial vault fails to form.

Craniosynostosis

Craniosynostosis (craniostenosis) is the premature closure during the first 18 to 20 months of one or more of the cranial sutures. The incidence of craniosynostosis is 5 per 10,000 live births. Males are affected twice as often as females. Craniosynostosis prevents normal skull expansion and causes asymmetric skull growth. Premature closure of a suture causes failure of the growth of the bone located at a right angle to the involved suture. Compensatory growth occurs in regions where the sutures are patent, and this causes the various cosmetic deformities. In the absence of adequate sutures, cerebral growth may exceed the space present. Brain growth may be restricted, and compression may cause neurologic dysfunction from brain damage after age 6 months (Fig. 16-8).

Pathophysiology

The exact causes of craniosynostosis are unknown, but the condition does represent more than a single disorder of embryonic development. One possible explanation is a germ layer disturbance involving the mesenchyma (embryonic connective tissue that gives rise to the connective tissues, blood vessels, and lymphatics). This mesenchymal defect may be due to a deficiency in enzyme inhibition of ossification. A number of metabolic disorders are accompanied by premature or delayed ossification of cranial bones, suggesting a metabolic mechanism. A genetic defect of hormonal or mineral metabolism may create ossification centers at abnormal sites. Mechanical factors also appear to play a role in craniosynostosis because secondary premature fusion of sutures occurs in microcephaly and after shunting in hydrocephalus.

Sagittal
suture

Coronal
suture

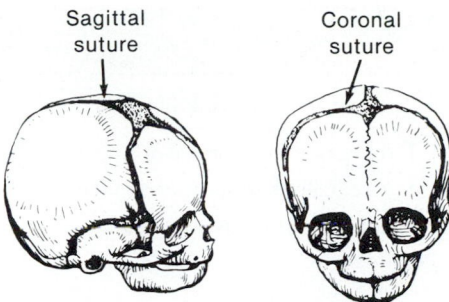

NORMAL SKULL

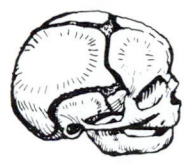 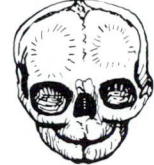

MICROCEPHALY AND CRANIOSTENOSIS

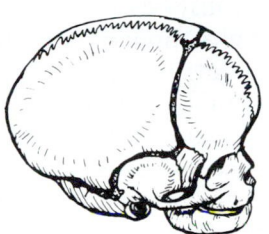 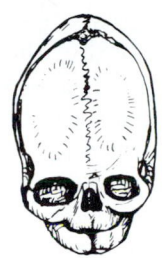

SCAPHOCEPHALY OR DOLICHOCEPHALY

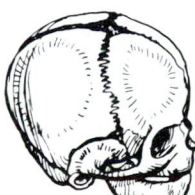 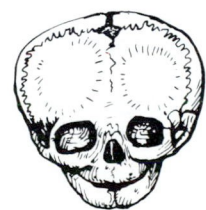

BRACHYCEPHALY

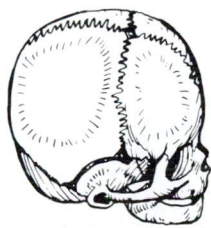 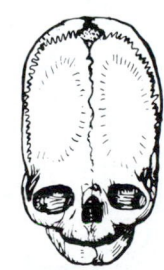

OXYCEPHALY OR ACROCEPHALY

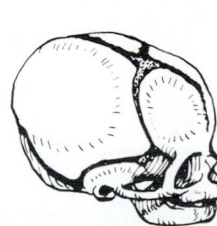 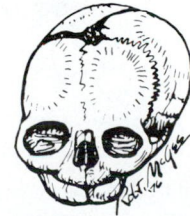

PLAGIOCEPHALY

FIG. 16-8. Craniosynostosis. Abnormal head configuration resulting from premature closing of cranial sutures. *Normal skull:* bones separated by membraneous seams until sutures gradually close. *Microcephaly and craniostenosis:* microcephaly is head circumference more than 2 standard deviations below the mean for age, sex, race, and gestation and reflecting a small brain; craniosynostosis is premature closure of sutures. *Scaphocephaly or dolichocephaly* (frequency 56%): premature closure of sagittal suture resulting in restricted lateral growth. *Brachycephaly:* premature closure of coronal suture resulting in excessive lateral growth. *Oxycephaly or acrocephaly* (frequency 5.8%/12%): premature closure of all coronal and sagittal sutures resulting in accelerated upward growth and small head circumference. *Plagiocephaly* (frequency 13%): unilateral premature closure of coronal suture resulting in asymmetric growth. (From Whaley & Wong, 1987.)

Clinical Manifestations

Craniosynostosis is classified according to head contour or suture involvement. Final skull contour is determined by the sutures that close, the duration and order of closure, and the ability of other sutures to compensate by expansion. (The frequency and types of craniosynostosis are depicted in Fig. 16-9.)

Premature closure of the sagittal suture, the most common form of craniosynostosis, causes elongation of the skull in the anterior-posterior direction. Other anomalies are seen in 25% of these children. When the coronal suture fuses prematurely, the brain expands in a lateral direction. This type of craniosynostosis is associated with a 33% to 66% incidence of associated anomalies. Approximately half of these children are mentally retarded.

Evaluation and Treatment

Diagnosis is made on the basis of physical examination, head circumference measurements, and radiologic examination. Surgical treatment is indicated when clo-

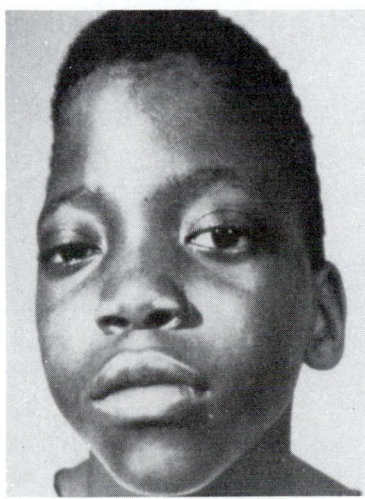

FIG. 16-9. Fourteen-year-old boy with dolichoscaphocephaly, one of the less threatening of the craniosynostoses. (From Siedel, Ball, Dains, & Benedict, 1987.)

TABLE 16-2 Causes of microencephaly

Defects in brain development	Intrauterine infections	Perinatal and postnatal disorders
Hereditary (recessive) microcephaly	Congenital rubella	Intrauterine or neonatal anoxia
Down syndrome and other trisomy syndromes	Cytomegalovirus infection	Severe malnutrition in early infancy
Fetal ionizing radiation exposure	Congenital toxoplasmosis	Neonatal herpesvirus infection
Maternal phenylketonuria	Congenital syphilis	
Seckel dwarfism		
Cornelia de Lange syndrome		
Rubinstein-Taybi syndrome		
Smith-Lemli-Opitz syndrome		
Fetal alcohol syndrome		

Adapted from Behrman & Vaughan, 1983.

sure of multiple sutures causes chronic increased intracranial pressure. Surgery then limits the extent of brain damage. In children with craniosynostosis of one suture, surgery is often performed for cosmetic purposes, to limit the appearance of deformity.

Microcephaly

Microcephaly is a defect in brain growth as a whole (Fig. 16-8). The word microcephaly is derived from the Greek (*mikros* = small; *kephale* = head). Cranial size is significantly below average for the infant's age, sex, race, and gestation. The small size of the skull reflects a small brain, except in infants with premature closure of the sutures. The condition is not treatable.

True (primary) microcephaly may be caused by an autosomal recessive disorder, by a chromosomal abnormality, or by toxin exposure during the period of induction and major cell migration (Table 16-2). Radiation, maternal infection, or chemical exposure may be the initiating factor. Secondary microcephaly is associated with a variety of causes. Infection, trauma, metabolic disorders, and anorexia experienced during the third trimester of pregnancy, the perinatal period, or early infancy may be responsible.

Brain weight may be as low as 25% of normal in the microcephalic brain. Both the number and the size of the cortical gyri may be diminished. Growth of the frontal lobes is severely stunted, and the cerebellum is

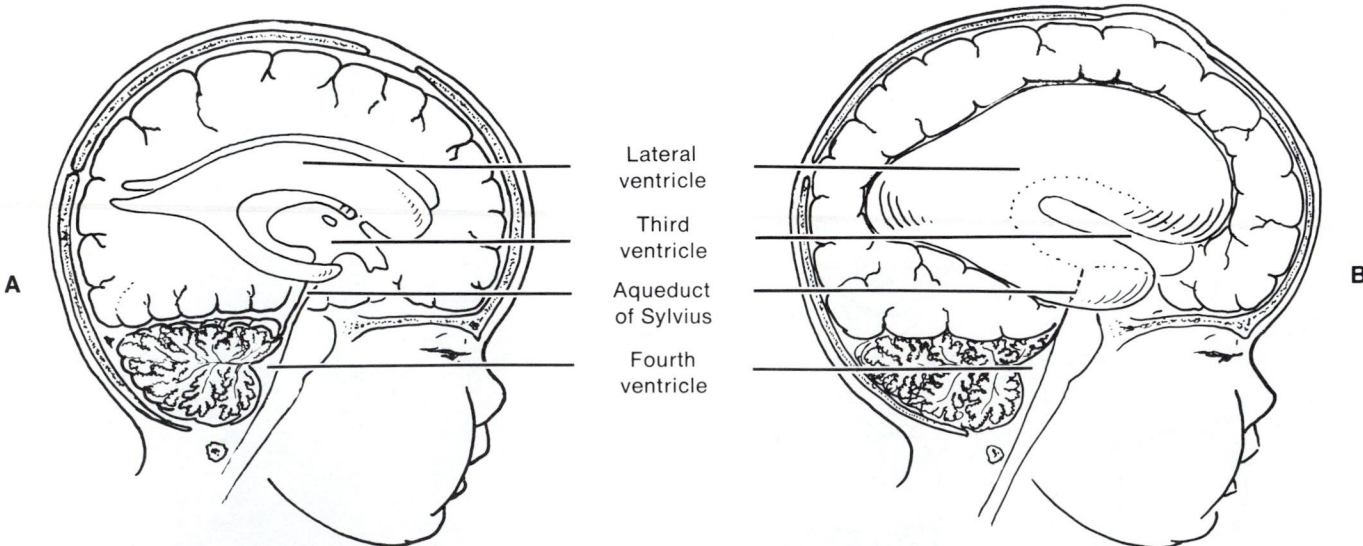

FIG. 16-10. Hydrocephalus: a block in flow of cerebrospinal fluid. **A,** Patent cerebrospinal fluid circulation. **B,** Enlarged lateral and third ventricles caused by obstruction of circulation—stenosis of aqueduct of Sylvius. (From Whaley, & Wong, 1987.)

Lateral ventricle

Third ventricle

Aqueduct of Sylvius

Fourth ventricle

often disproportionately large. In microcephaly caused by perinatal or postnatal disorders, neuronal loss and gliosis may be present in the cerebral cortex. The neurologic manifestations of microcephaly range from a decerebrate position, complete unresponsiveness, and autistic behavior, to mild motor impairment, **mental retardation,** and hyperkinesis.

Congenital Hydrocephalus

Hydrocephalus is characterized by an increased volume of cerebrospinal fluid that either is or has been under pressure (Fig. 16-10). An imbalance in production or a reduced reabsorption causes enlargement of the ventricles. When hydrocephalus develops before fusion of the cranial sutures, the head enlarges. Congenital hydrocephalus, including that associated with myelomeningocele, occurs in approximately 4 per 1000 live births. Other forms of hydrocephalus occur in 1 per 1000 individuals. (Types of hydrocephalus are discussed in Chapter 14.)

Pathophysiology

Obstructive hydrocephalus is most commonly caused by congenital aqueduct stenosis. The cerebral aqueduct is narrowed or replaced by multiple channels, or "forks," that end blindly. In a small number of children, the stenosis is transmitted as an X-linked recessive trait. Occasionally, compression of the aqueduct by a mass posterior to the brainstem occurs. The **Dandy-Walker malformation** is a congenital defect of midline cerebellar structures in which hydrocephalus is caused by atresia (ends in a "blind pouch") of the foramina of Luschka or Magendie, and by brain tumors.

Clinical Manifestations

Congenital hydrocephalus may cause fetal death in utero, or it may require delivery of the infant by cesarean section. Most infants, however, are asymptomatic at birth. During the early weeks of life, the head begins to grow at an abnormal rate. The fontanelles enlarge (Fig. 16-11). The separation of cranial sutures leads to a resonant note when the skull is tapped, a manifestation termed **Macewen sign** or **"cracked-pot" sign.** The eyes may assume a staring expression, with sclera visible above the cornea, a manifestation termed **sunset sign.** The infant may have difficulty holding the head upright. Scalp veins are prominent. The scalp skin is thin and shiny. The large cranial vault and the face are disproportionate. In the Dandy-Walker malformation occipital expansion is seen with transillumination of the skull. This is a result of massive dilation of the fourth ventricle. The infant's cry becomes high-pitched as intracranial pressure rises. Compression of the optic nerves, and optic chiasm occurs in chronic, untreated hydrocephalus. Fortunately these signs of hydrocephalus are rarely seen because of early surgical intervention.

When hydrocephalus develops late in childhood, the head is often not enlarged. Evidence of increased intracranial pressure is present (see Chapter 14).

The relationship between hydrocephalus and mental retardation has been much debated. Any correlation between the degree of hydrocephalus and cognitive dysfunction, however, is unclear.

Evaluation and Treatment

The definitive diagnostic tool for hydrocephalus is computed tomography. In infancy, head circumference measurements are also performed. The treatment is surgical shunting of excess fluid from the ventricle to the peritoneum (V-P shunt). With neurosurgical intervention and follow-up, about 70% of infants with congenital hydrocephalus may be expected to live beyond infancy. Of these, about 40% will have normal cognitive and motor function. The prognosis for infants having both hydrocephalus and meningocele is considerably worse.

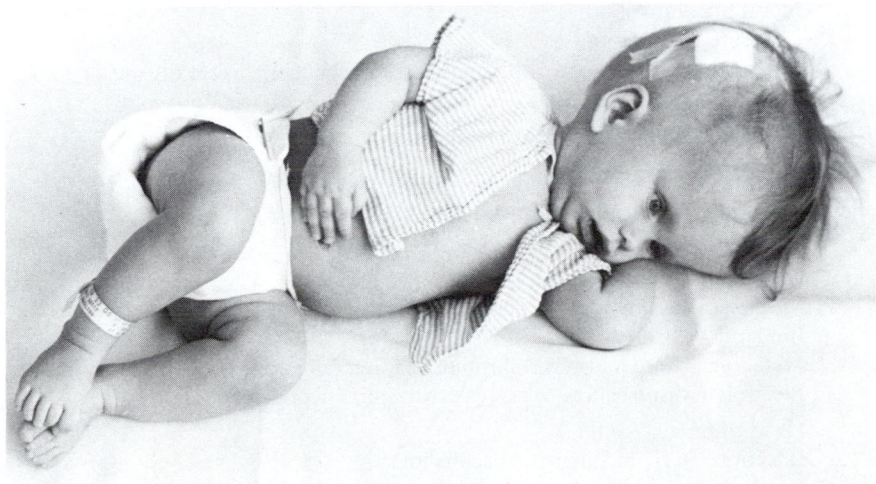

FIG. 16-11. Child with enlarged head caused by hydrocephalus. (From Whaley, & Wong, 1987.)

ENCEPHALOPATHIES

Encephalopathy, a disorder involving the brain, is a general category that includes a number of syndromes and diseases (see Chapter 14). Encephalopathies in children are associated with a great variety of known and suspected causes. These disorders may be acute or chronic and static or progressive.

Static Encephalopathies

Brain injury may occur during gestation, birth, or childhood, causing a static, nonprogressive disorder. The clinical manifestations depend on the site and extent of the injury and on the gestational age at the time of the injury. For example, cerebral palsy results when the motor areas of the brain are injured. Mental retardation or mental deficiency usually follows diffuse cerebral injury, but small areas of injury occurring early in gestation may interfere with normal cerebral maturation and cause cognitive deficit. Brain injury may impair sight and hearing. Seizures most commonly develop from cortical injury.

Prenatal factors affecting the developing nervous system may be endogenous or exogenous. The fetus may be affected by impaired embryo implantation, chromosomal abnormalities, infection, trauma, radiation, and toxic substances. Maternal toxemia and diabetes mellitus can produce neurologic damage in the fetus. The developing nervous system is most susceptible to injury occurring during the first trimester of pregnancy. Anoxia or trauma are the most common factors causing injury to the nervous system in the perinatal period. In the postnatal period, infections, inborn errors of metabolism, trauma, toxins, and vascular disease may injure the nervous system.

Cerebral Palsy

Cerebral palsy is the name given to a diverse group of nonprogressive syndromes affecting the brain and causing motor dysfunction. Although cerebral palsy is by definition nonprogressive, its clinical manifestations change with growth and maturation of the child.

Cerebral palsy is one of the most common crippling disorders of childhood, affecting nearly 300,000 children in the United States alone. Although the exact incidence is unknown, studies suggest that the incidence is 5 to 6 cases per 1000 live births. The prevalence among children at entry into school is 2 cases per 1000 live births (Paneth, 1986). Causes of cerebral palsy are nu-

TABLE 16-3 Cerebal palsy: predisposing factors and known causes

Risk factors	Associated causes
Prenatal factors	
Maternal factors	Maternal metabolic diseases
	Maternal nutritional deficiencies (e.g., anemia)
	Twin or multiple births
	Maternal bleeding
	Toxemia
	Blood imcompatibilities
	Exposure to radiation
	Infection (e.g, rubella, toxoplasmosis, cytomegalic inclusion disease)
	Premature labor
Prematurity	Asphyxia leading to cerebral hemorrhage
Genetic factors	Absence of corpus collosum, aqueductal stenosis, cerebellar hypoplasia
Congenital anomalies of the brain	Unknown causes not evident on clinical examination
Perinatal factors	Anesthesia or analgesia during labor and delivery
	Mechanical trauma during delivery
	Immaturity at birth
	Metabolic disorders (hyperbilirubinemia, hypoglycemia, amino acid disorders, hyperosmolality)
	Electrolyte disturbances (e.g., hypernatremia, hypoglycemia)
Postnatal factors	Head trauma
	Infections (e.g., meningitis, encephalitis)
	Cerebral vascular accidents
	Toxicoses
	Environmental toxins (lead ingestion, methylmercury ingestion from contaminated fish)

merous. Both genetic and environmental factors may be responsible. These factors may occur during the prenatal, perinatal, or postnatal periods (see Table 16-3).

Pathophysiology

Several factors acting solely or in combination may produce brain damage. Physical trauma to the central or peripheral nervous system may occur when the fetal head sustains an injury such as **caput succedaneum** (swelling produced on the presenting part of the fetal head during labor), **cephalohematoma** (a subcutaneous swelling containing blood, often found on the head of an infant several days after birth and associated with forceps delivery), or a skull fracture.

Linear and depressed fractures are seen in newborns when head molding is extreme with resultant hemorrhages and tears of the tentorium or falx cerebri. Tearing of the superficial cerebral veins is a relatively common occurrence and causes a thin layer of blood over the cerebral convexity. Breech deliveries may also cause traumatic injury to the brainstem or spinal cord.

Although physical trauma during the neonatal period contributes significantly to mortality, hypoxia and other metabolic alterations are responsbile for most persistent neurologic dysfunction.

Prenatal Cerebral Hypoxia

Cerebral hypoxia before birth is believed to be responsible for systemic degeneration of incompletely myelinated areas of the brain. Hypoxic injury is almost always bilateral.

Two fundamental types of injury result from cerebral hypoxia: deep (periventricular) injury and superficial (cortical) injury. The gestational age at the time of injury is related to the type of injury. Premature infants (25 to 36 weeks' gestation) suffer deep injury. Term infants sustain superficial injury.

Hypoxia and asphyxia are known to cause edema in the developing brain. Lack of oxygen and the incorporation of amino acids during protein synthesis lead to acidosis. Failure of fetal capillary circulation and an accumulation of carbon dioxide and lactic acid also cause acidosis and osmotic pressure changes. These then contribute to the brain injury.

Perinatal Trauma

In the full-term infant, the most common site of brain damage is in the cortex. Major structural alterations caused by perinatal injury are rarely located in the cerebellum, pons, or brainstem. Infarctions in the cortex are a result of arterial or venous stasis and thromboses. Intracranial hemorrhages can be caused by direct trauma to the brain or by hypoxia. Two types of hemorrhage are intraventricular and subarachnoid. Intraventricular hemorrhage is a common cause of death in newborns; subarachnoid hemorrhage is a condition in which bleeding is circumscribed and relatively minor.

Malformations of the CNS play an important role in brain injury from perinatal trauma. In the premature infant both faulty maturation of the nervous system and a greater vulnerability to perinatal trauma and hypoxia are responsible for the high incidence of neurologic dysfunctions. Hypermyelination and demyelination within the basal ganglia are seen in most infants subjected to perinatal trauma.

Clinical Manifestations

The syndromes associated with cerebral palsy are classified according to the predominant clinical manifestations (as indicated in Table 16-4). Children with cerebral palsy often have associated neurologic syndromes, particularly seizure disorders (25% to 35%) and mental retardation or developmental disability (25% to 75%). Because standard intelligence tests do not allow for the physical handicaps of cerebral palsy, the incidence of associated mental retardation is widely disputed. Children with cerebral palsy do show a high incidence of speech and visual disabilities.

Evaluation and Treatment

Diagnosis of cerebral palsy is made on the basis of neurologic examination and medical history. Additional diagnostic tools include electroencephalography, tomography, screening for metabolic defects, and serum electrolyte analyses. The management of children with cerebral palsy varies with age, type, severity of involvement, presence or absence of seizures, and level of cog-

TABLE 16-4 Types of cerebral palsy

Type	Percentage
Spastic	65.0
Monoplegia	0.4
Involves one limb only	
Paraplegia	35.6
Involves both legs	
Diplegia	3.0
Involves same limbs bilaterally (i.e., both arms or both legs)	
Hemiplegia	40.0
Involves one side of body	
Triplegia	20.0
Involves three extremities, usually both legs and one arm	
Quadriplegia	19.0
Involves all four extremities	
Extrapyramidal	22.0
Mixed	13.0

TABLE 16-5 Inherited metabolic disorders of the CNS

Age of onset	CNS disorders
Neonatal period	Pyridoxine dependency, galactosemia, maple syrup urine disease and its variant, PKU
Early infancy	Tay-Sachs disease and its variants, infantile Gaucher disease, infantile Neimann-Pick disease, Krabbe globoid-body leukodystrophy, Farber lipogranulomatosis, Pelizaeus-Merzbacker and other sudanophilic leukodystrophies, spongy degeneration, Alexander disease, Alper disease, Leigh subacute necrotizing encephalomyelopathy, congenital lactic acidosis, Zellweger encephalopathy, Lowe oculorenalcerebral disease
Late infancy and early childhood	Disorders of amino acid metabolism, metachromatic leukodystrophy, late infantile G gangliosidosis, M1, late infantile Gaucher and Neimann-Pick disease, neuroaxonal dystrophy, mucopolysaccharidosis, mucolipidosis, fucosidosis, mannosidosis, Aspartylglycosaminuria, Battin-Bielschowsky-Spielmeyer-Jansky "ceroid" lipofuscinosis, Cockayne disease
Later childhood and adolescence	Progressive cerebellar ataxias of childhood and adolescence, hepatolenticular degeneration (Wilson disease), Hallervorden-Spatz disease, Lesch-Nyhan syndrome and other uremic states, familial calcification of vessels in basal ganglia and cerebellum, familial polymyoclonias, chronic familial leukodystrophies, homocystinuria, Fabray disease

nitive function. The scope of the child and family therefore includes social and educational intervention and a multidisciplinary team approach.

Although the brain injury is static, the clinical picture may change over time. Spasticity may not become apparent until late in the first year of life. Children with spasticity are prone to contractures, and without proper attention, the dysfunction may increase. Frequent seizures physically disable some children, and repeated asphyxia can further reduce their cognitive function. Functional improvement does occur in some children who are not also mentally retarded.

Inherited Metabolic Disorders of the CNS

A large number of inherited metabolic disorders have been identified, and many are newly discovered. Because these disorders are inherited, they are mostly manifested in infancy and childhood. Typically, these metabolic disorders damage the entire CNS so extensively that these children do not survive to adulthood. The clinical syndromes of the inherited metabolic disorders depend on the nature of the biochemical defect and the stage of nervous system maturation. (Table 16-5 lists some of these inherited metabolic disorders.) Defects in amino acid and lipid metabolism are more common than rarely occurring defects in carbohydrate metabolism.

Defects in Amino Acid Metabolism

Biochemically, defects in amino acid metabolism may be classified as (1) those in which the transport of amino acid is impaired, (2) those involving an enzyme or cofactor deficiency, and (3) those grouped around certain chemical components such as sulfur-containing amino acids (Farmer, 1983). Most of the inherited disorders of amino acid metabolism have been discovered by systemic screening of disabled children. **Phenylketonuria (PKU)** is an inborn error of metabolism characterized by the inability of the body to convert the essential amino acid phenylalanine to tyrosine. With an incidence of 1:14,000 live births, PKU is the most common of the amino acidopathies (Behrman & Vaughan, 1983; Berman et al., 1969; Matson & Breuning, 1983).

Normally, the hepatic enzyme phenylalanine hydroxylase controls the conversion of the essential amino acid phenylalanine to tyrosine. Most natural food proteins contain about 15% phenylalanine, that ordinarily is degraded by way of the tyrosine pathway common to all protein metabolism. In PKU, phenylalanine hydroxylase is absent, causing the accumulation of phenylalanine in the blood and in the urinary excretion of abnormal metabolites called phenyl acids. One of these phenyl acids, phenylpyruvic acid, gives urine a characteristic musty odor and is responsible for the name given to the disorder, phenylketonuria (PKU).

In addition to the accumulating phenylalanine, the amino acid tyrosine is absent. Tyrosine is required for the formation of the pigment melanin and the hormones epinephrine and thyroxin. Because of the lack of tyrosine, children with PKU have a characteristic phenotype that includes blond hair, blue eyes, and fair skin. Children with genetically darker complexions may be red-haired or brunette. (Fig. 16-12 summarizes the interrelationship of the pathophysiology and clinical manifestations of PKU.)

In 1934, a Norwegian biochemist and physician, Asbjorn Folling, discovered that, in the presence of ferric chloride, phenylpyruvic acid turns urine green, and the disorder was in this way identified for the first time. In more recent years it has become apparent that "classic" PKU is at one end of the spectrum of conditions known as **hyperphenylalaninemia**. The less severe forms are variants caused by defects in the phenylalanine hydroxylase system, rather than in phenylalanine hydroxylase itself. These variants are the result of a deficiency in the enzyme dihydropteridine reductase or in the synthesis of dihydropiopterin. The significance of these variant forms lies in the diagnosis and treatment. Although their phenylalanine levels are in the greater-than-normal range, most of these children develop normally on a regular diet. Those with classic PKU must restrict foods with phenylalanine (for example meat and cow's milk).

In PKU, phenylalanine accumulates in the blood and is converted into metabolites that disrupt normal development of the CNS. Among the abnormalities are defective myelination, cystic degeneration of the gray and white matter, and disturbances in cortical layers. Unfortunately, brain damage occurs before the metabolites can be detected in the urine, and damage continues as

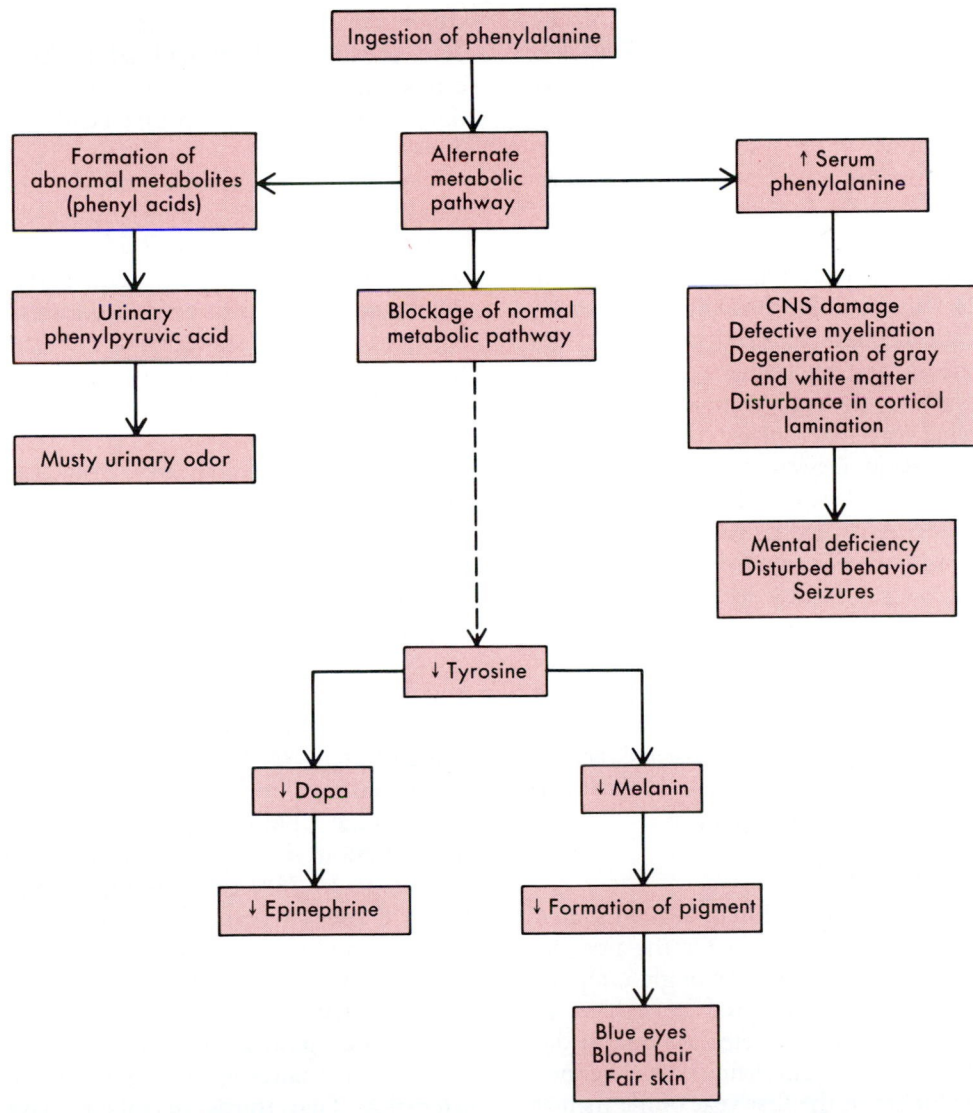

FIG. 16-12. Metabolic pathways and neurologic manifestations associated with phenylketonuria.

long as the phenylalanine level remains high. Clinical manifestations related to CNS damage include bizarre and schizoid behavior patterns such as screaming, banging the head, biting the arm, disorientation, lack of response to strong stimuli, and a catatonic state. Other CNS manifestations may include irritability, hyperactivity, unpredictable and erratic behavior, and seizures.

Defects in Lipid Metabolism

Disorders of lipid metabolism are termed **lysosomal storage diseases** because each of the disorders in this group can be traced to a missing lysosomal enzyme. (Lysosomes, the vesicles within the cell whose primary function is to degrade the breakdown products of cellular metabolism, are discussed in Chapter 1.) An estimated 25 to 30 enzymes within the lysosomes participate in the breakdown of lipids, carbohydrates, proteins, and proteolipids (see Chapter 2). A missing or defective enzyme causes an excessive accumulation of a particular metabolite and impairment of cell function. The enzyme defect may occur in the brain, liver, spleen, bone, and lung, thus involving several organ systems. Therapy has been unsuccessful to date.

Perhaps the best known of the lysosomal storage disorders is **Tay-Sachs disease,** a hereditary, autosomal recessive disorder that occurs primarily in children of Eastern European descent.

In Tay-Sachs disease the pathologic changes predominate in the CNS, but neurons throughout the body contain characteristic changes in the cytoplasm. With time, neurons are lost, and microglial cells, which are also swollen and filled with large granules, proliferate. Changes in the spinal cord, particularly the ventral horn cells, are also characteristic. Defective neurotransmission is related to enzymatic deficiency. The classic clinical manifestations include psychomotor retardation, deterioration after 4 to 6 months of normal development, and a startle response to sound. Muscle weakness, including loss of head control and loss of interest in surroundings, occur as the toxic buildup continues. Little can be done for the affected child, who usually dies by age 3 to 4 years. Genetic counseling programs have been carried out and screening techniques for couples at risk are offered, particularly to those with Ashkenazi Jewish heritage among whom the carrier rate is 1 in 25.

Seizure Disorders in Children

Seizures are common among children, although their frequency is unknown. The incidence for the first decade of life is about 3 per 1000, although rates for childhood seizures have been estimated as high as 20 per 1000. Differences in incidence rates are due to differing epidemiologic methods and definitions. The incidence of seizures is higher in the first year of life than at any other period in life.

Some major differences between the immature and mature nervous systems explain, in part, the changing patterns of clinical seizures with age. For instance, the immature nervous system has an increased seizure threshold and a reduced capacity for sustaining well-organized seizures. Intracortical connections are poorly developed, and cortical-cortical sending of impulses is severely limited. At the cellular level, neurons are less capable of firing in repetitive high-frequency bursts. The excitatory output of a seizure focus is further diminished because affected neurons do not act synchronously. Furthermore, changing levels of neurotransmitters, immaturity of certain cell types, and ongoing postnatal changes at synaptic junctions are other maturational factors that affect seizure susceptibility and expression in children. (Types of seizures are discussed in Chapter 14.)

Generalized Seizures

Generalized seizures occur with greater frequency in children than in adults, representing about 55% of all seizures in childhood. As with adults, generalized seizures can be either convulsive or nonconvulsive, and more than one type is possible in any given child (see Table 13-23).

Tonic-Clonic Seizures

The tonic-clonic seizure (major motor) is the classic attack, although the complete tonic-clonic sequence is rare in infants and young children. Rather, generalized seizures before adolescence tend to take either a predominantly tonic form or a predominantly clonic form. In addition, manifestations are characteristically less intense and the duration and postictal periods are shorter in duration.

Myoclonic seizures

Myoclonic seizures are seen in retarded children with nonprogressive static encephalopathies (e.g., cerebral palsy). On rare occasions, this type of seizure is associated with progressive neurologic syndromes. A **ketogenic diet** (a high-fat, low-protein, low-carbohydrate diet) may be effective in children with myoclonic seizures caused by brain damage. The diet induces ketosis and acidosis and tends to reduce seizure activity, although the mechanism is unknown.

Intermittent or flickering light may provoke myoclonic seizures in children having photosensitive seizures. Some children typically experience seizures during television viewing because of the light flashing on the screen. In 75% of children, the age of onset is between 8 and 19 years. Attempts to eliminate the provoking stimulus and anticonvulsant medications are the usual forms of treatment.

Infantile Spasms

Infantile spasms constitute an age-specific form of generalized seizures with unique clinical and EEG characteristics. Two thirds of infants have spasms by 6 months of age. For the remainder, the onset is the end of the first year. The clinical manifestations are diverse, but **flexor spasm** is best known. In this form, a sudden flexion of the head and trunk occurs simultaneously with flexion and adduction of the limbs. Spasms may be aggravated during the transition between sleep and wakefulness or during various forms of stimulation such as feeding and handling. Eighty percent of the time, infantile spasms are the first manifestation of a seizure disorder.

Fifty percent of children become free of spasms by 2 years of age, and nearly all cease seizure activity by 5 years. Unfortunately, cessation of spasms is accompanied by severe retardation and recurring seizures in about two thirds of surviving children.

Atonic and Akinetic Seizures

Atonic seizures are particularly common in children with static encephalopathies. Often refractory to treatment, these seizures are sometimes successfully treated with a ketogenic diet.

The term **Lennox-Gastaut syndrome** (childhood epileptic encephalopathy) has been applied to a diverse group of children with severe mental retardation, severe seizures, and a characteristic EEG pattern. Seizures usually begin in the first 3 years of life and are characteristically severe and refractory to anticonvulsant medications. Atonic, tonic, and atypical absences are the most common types of seizure seen in younger children, whereas tonic-clonic seizures are seen in older children and adolescents. Mental retardation is present in 80% to 90% of these children.

Partial Seizures

Partial seizures are less common in children than in adults, accounting for 45% of all childhood seizure disorders. As in adults, partial seizures suggest localized cerebral dysfunction, although in children this is unlikely to be due to a definable lesion. In infants, partial seizures may be the presenting sign of a subdural hematoma. Children with congenital heart disease and right-to-left shunts may suffer cerebral emboli that cause a neurologic deficit accompanied by partial seizures. More commonly, partial seizures arise from static lesions acquired early in life. Metabolic disorders such as transient hypocalcemia, hypoglycemia, and water intoxication are often associated with partial seizures.

Febrile Seizures

Febrile seizures occur in 3% to 4% of children under 5 years of age. These seizures are usually brief and self-limited, and they occur most frequently between the ages of 6 months and 3 years. Boys are affected more often than girls.

The criteria used to categorize febrile seizures are (1) a first convulsion associated with a temperature greater than 38° C, (2) a child younger than 6 years of age, (3) no evidence of CNS infection or inflammation, and (4) no acute systemic metabolic disorder. Febrile seizures may be classified as **benign febrile seizures** if they are characterized by a duration less than 15 minutes and do not have focal features. **Complex febrile seizures** are longer and have focal characteristics. They occur in a prolonged series (Rudolph, 1982).

The pathogenesis of febrile seizures is unknown. Higher incidences of febrile seizures, epilepsy, and EEG abnormalities do occur in families of children who have febrile seizures, thus indicating a genetic predisposition to the problem. Factors contributing to susceptibility include age, degree of temperature elevation, nature of the particular fever-inducing illness, genetic predispositions, and rate of fever increase. Unless other factors contribute to the lowering of the seizure threshold (such factors as metabolic and electrolyte shifts, bacterial toxins, and certain therapeutic measures), the seizure occurs during the first hours of the fever while the temperature is rising rapidly. The seizure threshold may be lowered by a variety of medications (e.g., aspirin that may trigger hypoglycemia, large doses of penicillin parenterally that may give rise to seizures, and many decongestants that are potential CNS excitants). It is not proven that these medications lower seizure threshold; however, caution is warranted until further research has been done.

Any disorder producing a high fever may provoke febrile seizures in susceptible children. These include upper respiratory infections, otitis media, pharyngitis, and roseola. Most febrile seizures occur within the first 24 hours of illness. In some children, the seizure is the first sign of illness. The degree of fever is not, however, the key factor in precipitating a seizure. If the fever falls and rises a second time during an illness, the child does not necessarily experience a second seizure, even though the same temperature elevation is reached.

Most children have benign febrile seizures and have only one seizure during a febrile illness. Of those having complex febrile seizures, approximately 80% have a complex seizure as a first episode. Children who are more likely to have complex febrile seizures cannot be identified before the occurrence, but they are more likely to be less than 18 months of age and have a history of neurologic dysfunction or abnormal development.

Reduction of elevated body temperature usually controls febrile seizures without anticonvulsant medication. Although the exact reason for the effect is unknown, the recurrence rate for febrile seizures may be reduced by two thirds with the daily administration of phenobarbital (Fishman, 1987). The recurrence rate for febrile seizures is 25% to 50%, whereas children who have the first seizure at 1 year of age or less have a 65% chance of recurrence. This contrasts to a 35% chance of recurrence in those 1 to 1½ years of age, and 20% recurrence rate when the onset is after 2½ years of age. Approximately two thirds of recurrences take place within 1 year of the first seizure.

Children who have febrile seizures are at increased risk for developing seizures later in life. The degree of risk is influenced by a variety of factors including abnormal neurologic status before the seizure, the occurrence of complex febrile seizures, and a family history of afebrile seizures.

Acute Encephalopathies
Reye Syndrome

Reye syndrome is characterized by encephalopathy and fatty changes in a variety of organs, especially the liver. Reye syndrome is among the 10 major causes of death in children between ages 1 and 10 years. Although this disorder mainly affects children, some cases have been reported in adults. Reye syndrome may affect children between 2 months of age and adolescence. Most commonly, it develops in children between ages 6 and 9 years and 11 and 14 years. Both sexes are affected equally and the mortality rate is 20% to 40%. No natural immunity develops, so a child may contract the disorder more than once.

Pathophysiology

Reye syndrome is usually associated with influenza B or varicella virus infections, although a wide variety of associated viral infections have been reported. A rather distinct clinical syndrome is apparent. The profound hypoglycemia, especially in children under 5 years, hyperammonemia, and an increase in short chain fatty acids in the serum after liver involvement are responsible for the cerebral manifestations. The liver shows diffuse deposits of lipids and absence of any inflammatory reaction or necrosis. Fatty degeneration of the kidneys leads to azotemia (excess urea in the blood). The brain is very edematous.

The cause of Reye syndrome and the pathogenesis are unknown, although five theories have been offered. One theory suggests that prolonged vomiting caused by a viral infection leads to a fasting state. Fasting decreases glycogen stores and mobilizes fatty acids from adipose tissue. These free fatty acids normally are handled by the mitochondria in the liver, but a disturbance in liver metabolism enables the free fatty acids to accumulate as glycerides in the liver, thus causing mitochondrial injury. Free fatty acids may induce coma by inhibiting metabolic processes in the brain.

A second theory attributes the disorder to a defect in the mobilization and excretion of amino acids. Increased amounts of amino acids cause the same damage as the free fatty acids. A third theory suggests that an endogenous or exogenous toxin, such as ammonia, accumulates in the child's body, causing damage to both the liver

and the brain. The fourth theory links the disorder to an interaction between a toxin and a virus. The suggested toxins are environmental chemicals and insecticides that interfere with or suppress the child's natural defenses and thus allow the virus to replicate until a toxic level is reached.

The fifth theory is based on epidemiologic evidence. The increased incidence of Reye syndrome in rural areas, among non-black children, and in siblings suggests a genetic and metabolic predisposition to the illness.

Administration of salicylates (aspirin) has been linked to Reye syndrome. A greater percentage of children who subsequently developed Reye syndrome have been given aspirin during an antecedent illness. Consequently, the Academy of Pediatrics has recommended discretion when using aspirin for children who have varicella or flulike symptoms. There has been a marked decrease in the incidence of Reye syndrome since the warning.

Clinical Manifestations

Typically, Reye syndrome develops in a previously healthy child who is recovering from varicella, influenza B, upper respiratory infection, or gastroenteritis. The manifestations of the various clinical states are as follows:

Stage I	Vomiting, lethargy, drowsiness
Stage II	Disorientation, delerium, aggressiveness, and combativeness, central neurologic hyperventilation (or sometimes shallow breathing), hyperactive reflexes, and stupor
Stage III	Obtundation, coma, hyperventilation, and decorticate rigidity
Stage IV	Deepening coma, decerebrate rigidity, loss of ocular reflexes, large fixed pupils, and divergent eye movements
Stage V	Seizures, loss of deep tendon reflexes, flaccidity, and respiratory arrest

Evaluation and Treatment

Definitive diagnosis of Reye syndrome is established by liver biopsy. Additional diagnostic tools include serum blood and cerebrospinal fluid analyses. Regardless of clinical stage, all children suspected of having Reye syndrome should be admitted to an intensive care unit. Considerable evidence has indicated that cerebral edema plays a vital role in the development of the neurologic picture, although the mechanisms of its production and its relation to liver damage are unclear.

The severity of the disabilities is inversely related to the age of the child at the onset of the illness. Children 1 year of age or younger may be left profoundly retarded. Although mortality may reach as high as 80% to 90%, recently a reduction to 30% to 40% has been

TABLE 16-6 Commonly ingested poisons

Pharmacologic agents	Heavy metals	Venoms	Miscellaneous agents
Acetaminophen	Lead	Snakebite	Botulism
Amphetamines	Acute	Tick paralysis	Carbon monoxide
Anticonvulsants	Chronic		Ethyl alcohol
Antidepressants	Mercury		Organophosphates
Antihistamines	Thallium		Petroleum distillates
Atropine			
Barbiturates			
Methadone			
Phencyclidine			
Salicylates			
Tranquilizers			

From Swaiman & Wright, 1982.

achieved with more intensive care, use of peritoneal dialysis, and exchange transfusion.

Intoxications of the CNS

Accidental poisoning is common among young children. In adolescents with CNS intoxication, substance abuse and suicide must be suspected. (The most commonly ingested poisons are listed in Table 16-6.) About 2 million childhood poisonings that require medical attention occur each year. Approximately 1000 children die each year from poisoning.

In lead poisoning, for example, lead encephalopathy is responsible for the serious and irreversible neurologic damage occurring in the child (Fig. 16-13). Those at greatest risk are 2- to 3-year-olds and those prone to pica. **Pica** is the habitual, purposeful, and compulsive ingestion of nonfood substances, such as clay, dirt, paint chips, paper, pencils, cigarette butts, and matches. The term is derived from the Latin word for magpie, a bird of voracious and indiscriminate appetite.

An estimated 225,000 children in the United States and 4% of children 6 months to 5 years of age have excessive amounts of lead in their blood. Black children have a six times greater incidence of symptoms than white children. The Centers for Disease Control report that adolescents, including Native Americans on reservations, have elevated lead levels from sniffing gasoline.

Bacterial Meningitis in Children

Nearly 70% of all reported cases of bacterial meningitis occur in children younger than 5 years of age. Three organisms account for 84% of all reported cases of bacterial meningitis in the United States: *Hemophilus influenzae, Neisseria meningitidis,* and *Streptococcus pneumoniae.* Despite the availability of antibiotics capable of killing these microorganisms, the general incidence of bacterial meningitis has increased in recent years.

In general, bacterial meningitis affects males more frequently than females and is most prevalent during infancy (Klein, Feigin, & McCracken, 1986). Conditions associated with increased incidence of respiratory infection enhance the incidence of bacterial meningitis.

Hemophilus influenzae type B is the most common bacterial meningitis in children. Its incidence during the first 5 years of life is 35 to 50 cases per 100,000 population. Otitis media or sinusitis may be a precursor. It is almost always associated with a bacterium in the blood.

The second most common organism is **Neisseria meningitidis** (meningococcus). Approximately 2% to 5% of healthy children are carriers of *N. meningitidis.* The risk of meningitis in day care center contacts of children with meningococcal disease is 1 per 1000. During epidemics among military personnel, as many as 90% have *N. meningitidis* present in secretions from the nose and mouth, suggesting a high rate of infectious transmission.

The third organism is **Streptococcus pneumoniae,** which is likely to be found in children with sickle cell disease or splenectomy. The risk is 5 1/2 times greater in blacks than in whites and is not linked to income or population density. One in every 24 children with sickle cell disease develops pneumococcal meningitis by 4 years of age. This incidence is 36 times greater than that found in the black population without sickle cell disease and 314 times greater than in white children. *S. pneumoniae* is associated with meningitis in children older than 5 years of age in whom the infection has extended from its origin in the middle ear, sinuses, or mastoid cells. Meningitis after neurosurgery or skull fracture usually is due to *S. pneumoniae.*

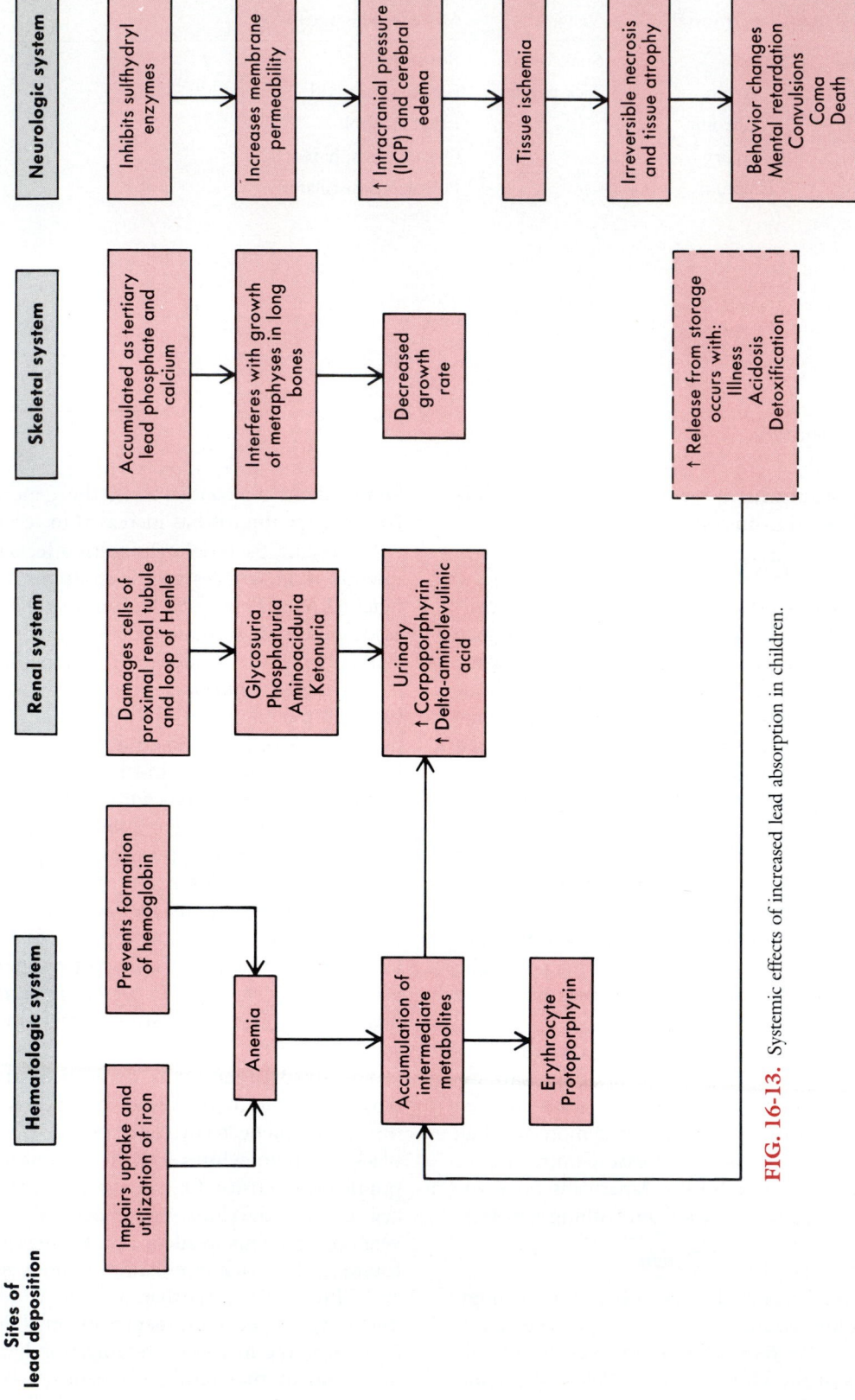

FIG. 16-13. Systemic effects of increased lead absorption in children.

Although a skull fracture through the sinuses may be complicated by meningitis reflecting the respiratory flora, immunosuppressed children may develop gram-negative meningitis from organisms generally considered to be nonpathogenic.

Pathogenesis

The cause of bacterial meningitis is related to the age of the child and to a number of factors that predispose the child to bacterial infection or alter the child's response to an invading microorganism. Any microorganism may, however, be pathogenic under the appropriate circumstances in a given individual.

During the first 2 months of life, the causative organisms are those that reflect the maternal flora or the environment in which the infant has been placed (e.g., gram-negative intestinal bacilli and group B streptococci). Most bacterial meningitis in children 2 months to 12 years of age is due to *H. influenzae* type B, *S. pneumoniae,* or *N. meningitidis.* In children older than 12 years of age, meningitis usually is due to *S. pneumoniae* or *N. meningitidis.* When the child's response has been compromised or when anatomic defects are present, other organisms may be responsible. These include *Pseudomonas,* staphylococci, salmonellae, or Serratia.

Meningitis may follow bacterial infections of the paranasal sinuses or mastoid cells. Bacterial meningitis in children with otitis media generally follows bacteremia. Direct invasion of the meninges is rare. Infection may spread through the blood to the meninges in children with infective endocarditis, pneumonia, or thrombophlebitis.

Direct invasion of the CNS occurs with fracture of the paranasal sinus, dermoid sinus tracts, or myelomeningoceles if direct communication occurs between the skin and meninges. Meningitis also may occur after neurosurgical procedures, particularly those involving cerebrospinal fluid diversion, such as shunting. Infection of the CNS may be caused by environmental contamination or manipulation. The child with cystic fibrosis or with severe burns may develop meningitis caused by *Staphylococcus aureus* or *Pseudomonas aeruginosa.* (For further discussion, see Chapter 15.)

Clinical Manifestations

Acute bacterial meningitis often is preceded by an upper respiratory or gastrointestinal infection. Fever, headache, vomiting, irritability, photophobia, and nuchal and spinal rigidity develop and can progress rapidly to a decreased level of consciousness and seizures. Irritation of the meninges and spinal roots causes pain and resistance to neck flexion (nuchal rigidity), a positive Kernig's sign (resistance to knee extension in the supine position with the hips and knees flexed against the body), and a positive Brudzinski's sign (flexion of the knees and hips when the neck is flexed forward rapidly). With severe meningeal irritation, the child might demonstrate opisthotonic posturing (rigid arching of the back with the head extended). Meningococcal meningitis can produce a characteristic petechial rash.

Increased intracranial pressure is caused by cerebral edema and might be increased further by obstruction to the cerebrospinal fluid circulation. Thickened meninges and fibrous exudate in the subarachnoid space at the base of the brain obstruct the cerebrospinal fluid, resulting in communicating hydrocephalus.

Evaluation and Treatment

A definitive diagnosis is made *only* by examination of the cerebrospinal fluid from a lumbar puncture. The principles of treatment are similar to those followed for adults (see Chapter 14) and are based on the culture results in which the causative organism is identified. The vaccines against *H. influenzae,* however, do not effect antibody production in children younger than 2 years of age.

The factors that influence outcomes are the age of the child (mortality is highest in infants younger than 1 year old), the infective organism (the lowest mortality is in meningococcal meningitis and the highest in meningitis caused by gram-negative enteric organisms), and the duration and extent of inflammation before treatment. Approximately 8% of children with *H. influenzae* meningitis die. Thirty-five percent of the survivors have serious and permanent sensory or motor dysfunction caused by pressure on the peripheral nerves during the early phases of the illness. Approximately 5% of the children who survive meningitis have hearing deficits; 10% to 15% have cerebral damage, hydrocephalus, motor deficits, or sensory impairments.

CEREBROVASCULAR DISEASE IN CHILDREN

Cerebrovascular disease in children differs from that in adults in three ways: (1) predisposing factors, (2) clinical response, and (3) anatomic site of the pathologic condition. Heart disease, cyanotic and congenital, is the most common disorder that becomes complicated by cerebral arterial or venous occlusion. Approximately 11% of children with cyanotic congenital heart disease have evidence of cerebral infarction (blockage in the flow of blood that leads to tissue death).

Excellent collateral circulation in the child's brain allows for more rapid recovery of motor function. The developing brain, however, may suffer more global, long-term effects leading to mental retardation, behavior disorders, and seizures.

The site of the pathologic condition also tends to differ between children and adults. For example, in the adult the cervical portion of the internal carotid artery frequently is the site of occlusion. Children, on the other hand, often show narrowing and occlusion of the intracranial portion of the carotid artery and its immediate branches, the anterior and middle cerebral arteries. Clinical manifestations of cerebral vascular disease in children are sudden hemiplegia in a previously well child, multiple seizures, high fever, coma, and flaccid weakness (2 weeks' duration) leading to spastic hemiparesis, hemianopsia, hemisensory deficit, facial palsy, and temporary aphasia.

CHILDHOOD TUMORS

Brain Tumors in Children

Brain tumors are the most common childhood tumor involving the CNS. Intraspinal tumors do occur, but they are quite rare. Brain tumors are the second most common childhood cancer, exceeded in frequency only by the leukemias. Overall, brain tumors account for nearly 20% of childhood cancers and represent the most common solid tumor of childhood with an annual incidence of 2.4 per 100,000. Approximately 1200 to 1500 new cases are diagnosed each year in the United States (Young & Miller, 1975). Brain tumors occur slightly more frequently in males than females, and the inci-

dence is identical for black and white children in the United States. Although brain tumors occur at all ages during childhood, they are most frequent between the ages of 5 and 10.

The cause of childhood brain tumors is largely unknown, although genetic factors seem to be involved in some tumors. Brain tumors occasionally have been reported to occur with increased frequency in some families. Prenatal defects during organ development are also implicated because of the high incidence of midline CNS tumors in children. This theory suggests that tumors are caused by cells that were "misplaced" during embryonic development, never maturing but later proliferating in this immature form. Other factors investigated in the cause of pediatric brain tumors include radiation, oncogenic viruses, and chemical carcinogens. None of these factors, however, has proven significant.

Types of Brain Tumors

Most childhood brain tumors arise from glial tissue, the supportive tissue of the brain. Less commonly, tumors may arise from other tissue such as nerve cells, cranial nerves, the pineal gland, blood vessels, or neuroepithelium. Brain tumors are classified by the tissue and location from which they arise, but a uniform pathologic nomenclature has not been established, and inconsistencies often are found when comparing reported statistics.

In children, most brain tumors are located below the

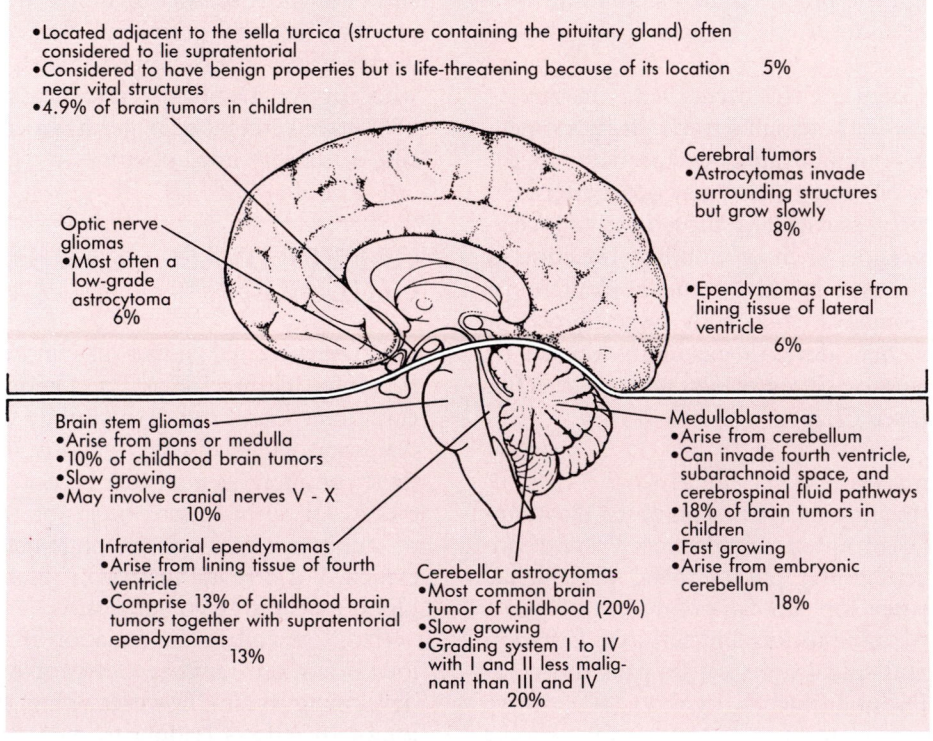

FIG. 16-14. Location of brain tumors in children.

TABLE 16-7 Brain tumors in children

Type	Characteristics
Astrocytoma	Arise from astrocytes often in the cerebellum or lateral hemisphere Slow growing, solid or cystic Often very large before diagnosed Vary in degree of malignancy
Optic nerve gliomas	Arise from optic chiasm or optic nerve Slow-growing, low-grade astrocytoma
Medulloblastoma (infiltrating glioma)	Often located in cerebellum and extends into fourth ventricle and spinal fluid pathway Rapidly growing malignant tumor Can extend outside of CNS
Brain stem glioma	Arise from pons or myencephalon Numerous cell types Compresses cranial nerves V through X
Ependymomas	Arise from ependyma cells lining ventricles Circumscribed, solid, nodular tumors
Craniopharyngiomas	Arise near pituitary gland, optic chiasm, and hypothalamus Cystic and solid tumors that affect vision, pituitary, and hypothalamic functions.

roof of the cerebellum, usually in the cerebellum or brainstem (Fig. 16-14). These tumors are called infratentorial because they are located below the tentorium in the posterior third of the brain. The remaining pediatric brain tumors are located above the cerebellum in the anterior two thirds of the brain. These tumors, lying above the tentorium and generally in the cerebrum, are referred to as supratentorial. The less frequent supratentorial location of brain tumors in children is in direct contrast to adults, where supratentorial tumors are more common. The types and characteristics of childhood brain tumors are summarized in Table 16-7.

Cause of the Disease

Pathogenesis

The actual location of any brain tumor will dictate the type and extent of presenting signs and symptoms. The location is very important in determining how amenable the tumor is to surgical removal and hence how good the prognosis. A number of pediatric brain tumors, such as the **craniopharyngioma,** are histologically considered benign, but because of their location and growth patterns, they are considered to be clinically malignant. Indeed, they can cause significant morbidity and death. As a whole, brain tumors rarely metastasize, and those few that do metastasize usually spread to other areas within the CNS along systemic pathways.

Clinical Manifestations

In addition to tumor location, the rate of growth of a particular tumor is important in determining presenting signs and symptoms. Fast-growing tumors can become symptomatic when they are relatively small, whereas slow-growing tumors can reach enormous size and create tremendous shifts in the anatomic structures before symptoms are apparent. Signs and symptoms of a brain tumor are often subtle in their earliest presentation. Early diagnosis of tumors in young children is particularly problematic because the sutures have not yet closed, allowing large amounts of tumor to accumulate before symptoms emerge. Children are also less likely to report symptoms, such as visual changes or headache, leading to increased delay in prompt diagnosis.

Two major categories of signs and symptoms occur in children: (1) those that are generalized and (2) those that are localized (i.e., specific to the anatomic location and extent of the tumor). Increased intracranial pressure, caused by obstruction of the cerebrospinal fluid pathways, is the most common general symptom and occurs because the tumors are primarily located in the posterior fossa or along the midline. Increased intracranial pressure without additional localized dysfunction may be the only initial finding. When increased intracranial pressure occurs, a tumor of the ventricles or deep midline structures is suspected. Local findings without increased intracranial pressure or with mild elevation in pressure may initially be present. The specific symptoms will determine if the tumor is in the cerebral hemispheres, brainstem, or cerebellum.

The symptoms of increased intracranial pressure include headache, vomiting, and irritability. If a young child complains of a headache, a thorough investigation should take place because headache is an uncommon complaint in young children. The headache is caused by increased intracranial pressure, is most notable in the morning, and gradually improves during the day (when the child is upright and venous drainage is enhanced), only to return the next morning. Initially, the headache is mild and not present every morning, but over time it increases in severity and frequency. A headache related to increased intracranial pressure generally occurs because of expansion of the lateral ventricle and cerebral hemisphere that causes stretching of the pain-sensitive dura mater. Irritability, or possibly apathy and increased somnolence, may also result from increased intracranial pressure. In the infant or toddler, who cannot report headache, irritability and somnolence may be the only presenting symptoms. Like headache, vomiting also occurs more commonly in the morning. It is frequently not preceded by nausea and may become projectile. Unlike a gastrointestinal disturbance, the child may be ready to eat immediately after vomiting.

Other signs that accompany increased intracranial pressure include (1) rapid increase in head circumference and bulging fontanelles (in the child younger than 2 years) as a result of obstruction of the cerebrospinal fluid, producing hydrocephalus; (2) palsies of the sixth cranial nerve from pressure on the nerves that result in a paralytic strabismus, for which children compensate by tilting the head to eliminate double vision; and (3) papilledema, with retinal changes apparent on the optic disc.

Localized findings relate to the degree of disturbance in physiologic functioning in the area where the tumor is located (see Table 14-6). Infratentorial tumors of the cerebellum exhibit localized signs of impaired coordination and balance including loss of balance, ataxia, and wide-based gate. Seizures are not associated with infratentorial tumors. Midline cerebellar tumors, arising from the cerebellar vermis or fourth ventricle, are often associated with truncal ataxia (poor coordination of the muscles of the trunk) and general nystagmus (involuntary rapid movement of the eyeball). **Medulloblastomas** and ependymomas are the two tumors that are most commonly located in the midline. In contrast, cerebellar hemisphere tumors most often cause unilateral limb ataxia (i.e., on the same side of the body as the tumor) and nystagmus when the eyes are turned toward the tumor. Cerebellar hemisphere tumors are generally low-grade astrocytomas.

Brainstem tumors often cause a combination of cranial nerve involvements, cerebellar signs such as ataxia, and corticospinal tract dysfunction. A common clinical pattern would include unilateral paralysis of cranial nerves VI and VII (with contralateral paralysis of the leg and arm), hyperreflexia and extensor plantar re-

sponses, cerebellar signs, and vertical nystagmus. Increased intracranial pressure is generally not present. **Brainstem gliomas** of the pons, myencephalon, and mesencephalon are the most common brainstem tumors of childhood.

Supratentorial tumors of the cerebral hemisphere in children are generally located near the cortical surface or in the deep structures. Tumors near the cortical surface are associated with seizures and focal cerebral dysfunction. In contrast, deep cerebral hemisphere tumors exhibit hemiplegic signs and certain visual field defects. Local cerebral signs depend on the specific lobe involved. Involvement of the frontal lobe may cause few localizing signs, or the child may simply show emotional dullness and apathy. Other findings may include motor weakness, a change in handedness, loss of fluent speech while retaining language comprehension (Broca's aphasia), and seizures characterized as tonic or clonic convulsions of the contralateral extremities.

Occipital lobe tumors can cause a specific type of hemianopia (blindness in half of the visual field). Seizures also occur and often include visual hallucinations. Tumors in the temporal lobe may be seen with an epileptic pattern associated with auditory or olfactory-gustatory hallucinations, déjà vu experiences, or vertigo. Seizures associated with a tumor of the motor cortex may exhibit a secondary generalization, which means they begin with a localized focus and progress to a generalized seizure. The seizure pattern may follow a jacksonian progression (see Table 14-13), which is described as seizure activity "marching up" an extremity, such as movement in the fingers, then the hand, then the lower arm, and so forth.

The area of the sella turcica, the structure containing the pituitary gland, is the site of several childhood brain tumors. These tumors may originate from the pituitary gland or from the hypothalamus. Other tumors include the optic nerve and optic chiasm. An infant exhibiting a tumor in this region occasionally is seen with what is termed the **diencephalic syndrome of infancy** (characterized by anorexia and wasting in an infant who otherwise appears alert and active). Nystagmus, however, is often present. In contrast, the same diencephalic syndrome in the older child is characterized by excess eating and obesity. This syndrome is also associated with autonomic seizures that include episodes of hypertension, tachycardia, and sweating. Tumors involving the optic tract may cause complete unilateral blindness and hemianopia in the other eye. Optic atrophy is a common finding. Childhood tumors located near the sella turcica are commonly craniopharyngiomas, whereas those near the optic nerve are generally **optic nerve gliomas.**

TABLE 16-8 Treatment strategies for childhood brain tumors

Tumor type	Treatment and prognosis
Cerebellar astrocytoma	Surgery, can be curative Radiation and chemotherapy have not proven successful but may delay recurrence 50% to 75% survive more than 5 years; if tumor recurs, it does so very slowly
Medulloblastoma	Surgery, primarily as a partial resection to relieve increased intracranial pressure and "debulk" the tumor Radiation as the primary treatment, may include spinal radiation Chemotherapy showing some promise 35% 5-year survival rate
Brain stem glioma	Surgery, resection occasionally possible Radiation, primarily palliative treatment Chemotherapy not yet proven beneficial, but new protocols being studied 20% to 40% 5-year survival rate
Ependymoma	Tumor possibly indolent for many years Surgery rarely curative and risk of resecting an infratentorial tumor too great Radiation for palliation (current controversy whether local or craniospinal radiation is best) Chemotherapy used for recurrent disease but with disappointing results
Craniopharyngioma	Surgery possibly successful when a complete resection is performed (partial resection usually requires further treatment) Radiation after partial surgical resection Chemotherapy not commonly used 75% to 85% 5-year survival rate
Optic nerve glioma	Initial treatment controversial Surgery used for diagnosis or relief of hydrocephalis Radiation useful, particularly if the tumor not treated by surgery
Cerebral astrocytoma	Surgery used if resection is possible Radiation useful for all grades of astrocytoma Chemotherapy beneficial in higher grade tumors, but further study required

Evaluation and Treatment

A complete workup is warranted when signs and symptoms of a brain tumor are present and should include neurologic, developmental, and ophthalmic examinations. Radiologic studies may include skull x-ray examinations, radioisotope brain scanning, and computed tomography (CT scan) (the most useful procedure). Magnetic resonance imaging (MRI) promises additional aid in the diagnosis of brain tumors. Biopsy provides the definitive diagnosis. In those tumors where surgical biopsy carries a high risk of mortality or serious morbidity, however, biopsy may not be performed and the diagnosis will instead be made on radiologic evidence and clinical manifestations.

The most useful treatment for brain tumors is surgical resection if it can be performed safely. The use of laser technology in surgical procedures may significantly improve surgical outcomes because lasers can destroy tumors located in very delicate areas without undue injury to viable tissues. Astrocytomas, particularly the cystic cerebellar astrocytomas, and medulloblastomas may be entirely resectable. If complete resection is not possible, partial resection or "debulking" may help to control the tumor and also serves as a secondary treatment to radiation or chemotherapy. (Table 16-8 summarizes the most common treatment used for specific childhood tumors.)

Embryonal Tumors
Neuroblastoma

Neuroblastoma is an embryonal tumor that arises from neural crest cells, that normally give rise to the sympathetic ganglia and the adrenal medulla. The primitive neural crest cells (also called sympathogonia) are pluripotential (i.e., they give rise to several cell types). They mature into ganglion cells, pheochromocytes (which are found in the sympathetic nervous system), or neurofibrous tissue. Thus, tumors that develop from neural crest cells reflect the varying degrees of differentiation of the cells. **Ganglioneuroblastomas** are tumors of intermediate level of cellular differentiation. The most differentiated tumor is a **ganglioneuroma,** which is considered benign and does not metastasize.

Because neuroblastoma involves a defect of embryonal tissue, it is most commonly diagnosed in young children and infants. Most tumors are diagnosed during the first 2 years of life, and 75% are found before the age of 5. Occasionally, these tumors have been diagnosed at birth with metastasis apparent in the placenta. In the United States, neuroblastoma is seen more commonly in white children (9.6 per/million) than black children (7 per/million). Although it accounts for 6% to 8% of pediatric malignancies, neuroblastoma causes only 15% of cancer deaths in children.

Pathogenesis

Neuroblastoma is the most primitive, or immature, form of the sympathetic nervous system tumors. Areas of necrosis and calcification are often present in the tumor.

Neuroblastoma, more than any other cancer, has been associated with spontaneous remission, commonly in infants who demonstrate liver, bone marrow, or skin involvement in addition to the primary site. Remission has been estimated to occur in approximately 7% of cases but it may occur much more frequently. Neuroblastoma in situ (i.e., noninvasive tumor) has been found during autopsies of infants who died of other causes.

The cause of neuroblastoma is elusive. The tumor has been associated with a number of conditions, including neurofibromatosis and Hirschsprung disease, but most children with neuroblastoma have neither of these conditions. Familial tendency has been demonstrated for a few individuals, but most children with neuroblastoma demonstrate a nonfamilial or sporadic pattern. The current hypothesis is that the potential to develop neuroblastoma is an autosomal dominant trait (mechanisms of inheritance are discussed in Chapter 4).

Clinical Manifestations

The clinical manifestations of neuroblastoma depend on the location of the tumor. Because neuroblastoma originates where there are elements of sympathetic nervous tissue, the tumor can arise in the sympathetic chain (column of sympathetic ganglia that parallels the spinal column), ganglia of effector organs, peripheral ganglia, adrenal medulla, bladder, and inner genitalia (see Fig. 11-26). The most common location is in the retroperitoneal region (65% of cases) and most frequently the adrenal medulla. The tumor is evident as an abdominal mass and may cause anorexia, bowel and bladder alteration, and sometimes spinal cord compression.

The second most common location of neuroblastoma is the mediastinum (area separating the lungs) (15% of cases). There the tumor may cause dyspnea or infection related to airway obstruction. If it is large, compression of the trachea, bronchi, lymphatic vessels, and mediastinal veins often results. Neck and facial edema may then be caused by superior vena cava syndrome. Less commonly, neuroblastoma may arise from the cervical sympathetic ganglion (3% to 4% of cases). Cervical neuroblastoma often causes Horner's syndrome, which consists of miosis (pupil contraction), ptosis (drooping eyelid), enophthalmos (backward displacement of the eyeball), and anhidrosis (sweat deficiency).

The initial signs and symptoms of neuroblastoma are often related to metastatic disease. Two thirds of children have metastatic disease at the time of diagnosis. Common sites of metastasis include the skin, with characteristic blue or purple nodules; the liver, causing enlargement; bone, causing pain and pathologic fracture; and bone marrow infiltration, occurring in greater than 50% of children. A unique but uncommon site of metastasis is the orbit of the eye, causing an ecchymotic discoloration of the upper and lower eyelids and a "raccoon" eye appearance.

A number of systemic signs and symptoms are also characteristic of neuroblastoma including weight loss, irritability, fatigue, and fever. Intractable diarrhea occurs in 7% to 9% of children and is due to tumor secretion of a hormone called vasoactive intestinal polypeptide.

More than 90% of children with neuroblastoma have increased amounts of catecholamines and associated metabolites in their urine. High levels of urinary catecholamines and serum ferritin are associated with a poorer prognosis.

Evaluation and Treatment

Initial diagnostic studies are dictated by the location of the site of the primary site tumor. Diagnosis begins with a complete physical examination, including a neurologic evaluation. Radiologic examination and computed axial tomography (CT scan) of the primary site, including intravenous pyelogram, provide further information. Investigation of metastatic disease includes skeletal survey, bone scan, liver scan, and bone marrow examination. Urinary catecholamine levels are measured by two metabolites, vanillylmandelic acid (VMA) and homovanillic acid (HVA). Measurement requires a 24-hour urine collection.

The diagnosis of neuroblastoma is confirmed by surgical biopsy. Occasionally, the biopsy may be avoided if bone marrow aspiration shows tumor infiltration and urinary catecholamines are significantly elevated. The primary staging classification of neuroblastoma was proposed by Evans, D'Angio, and Randolph (1971):

1. Stage I represents localized disease that is completely resectable.
2. Stage II represents disease that extends beyond the original site but does not cross the midline.
3. Stage III represents disease extending beyond the midline.
4. Stage IV represents metastatic disease.

A special stage IV-S is used for infants who would otherwise be classified as either stage I or stage II but who also have metastatic disease involving the liver, skin, or bone.

Treatment is based on the extent of the disease. Stages I and II are treated by primary excision of the tumor. Neuroblastoma is a radiosensitive tumor, so postoperative radiation may be given for residual disease. The success of radiation in stages I and II, however, is controversial. Chemotherapy has not proven beneficial for diseases at stages I or II.

Stage III or IV disease is treated by surgical debulking of as much tumor as possible. Radiation is directed at residual disease at the primary site. Systemic chemotherapy is used to control remaining disease, and many drugs have been tried over the past 20 years.

Stage IV-S disease requires very little treatment, primarily because of the high rate of spontaneous regression. Low-dose radiation treatment or single-course chemotherapy may be used to reduce large tumors.

Retinoblastoma

Retinoblastoma is a rare congenital eye tumor of young children that originates in the retina of one or both eyes (Fig. 16-15). One or more separate tumors in the affected eye(s) may be evident at diagnosis. Unilateral disease is most commonly diagnosed in children 2 or 3 years of age. In contrast, bilateral disease is usually diagnosed in infants less than 1 year of age. Retinoblastoma is rarely diagnosed after 5 years of age.

Although retinoblastoma is the most common pediatric intraocular tumor, only 200 children are diagnosed each year in the United States.

Pathogenesis
Recent evidence indicates that a locus (Rb) mapped to the long arm of chromosome 13 confers susceptibility to retinoblastoma (Lee et al., 1987). Mutations affecting this locus may be inherited from a parent, may occur during gametogenesis, or may occur somatically. For retinoblastoma to develop, both members of the chromosome pair must have a mutation at the Rb locus. If a mutation has occurred somatically, a second somatic mutation must occur at the Rb locus in the other member of the chromosome pair *in the same cell* for retinoblastoma to develop. This results in the nonhereditary form of retinoblastoma, which usually affects one eye and is responsible for 60% to 70% of the observed cases of the disease. If a child has inherited a mutation at the Rb locus from a parent, *all* cells of the retina will carry one copy of this mutation. A second somatic mutation in any one of these cells will cause a retinoblastoma to form. Since there are thousands of retinal cells, such a mutation usually does occur. In fact, it generally occurs several times. As a result, most individuals with the hereditary form of retinoblastoma develop multiple tumors in both eyes. However, about 10% of children who inherit the mutation are fortunate enough never to experience the second somatic mutation. Thus retinoblastoma is an example of reduced penetrance in a genetic disease.

Clinical Manifestations
Retinoblastoma grows as one or more tumors in the retina and extends into the vitreous humor. Freefloating, small tumors in the vitreous humor may attach to the surface of the retina in multiple areas and proliferate (Fig. 16-16). The tumor can also invade the optic nerve by infiltrating through the cribriform plate of the ethmoid bone (see Fig. 12-15) or can spread through the sheath around the nerve. In either case the tumor can gain access to the subarachnoid space and CNS. The tumor spreads into the choroid in 25% of children with retinoblastoma. Because the choroid is highly vascular,

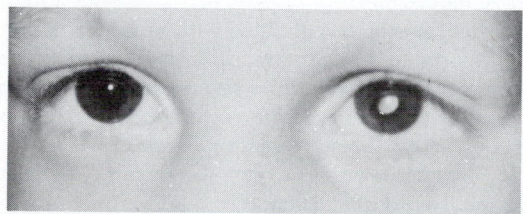

FIG. 16-15. Prominent white reflex present in dilated pupil of left eye owing to retinoblastoma. (From Kissane, 1985.)

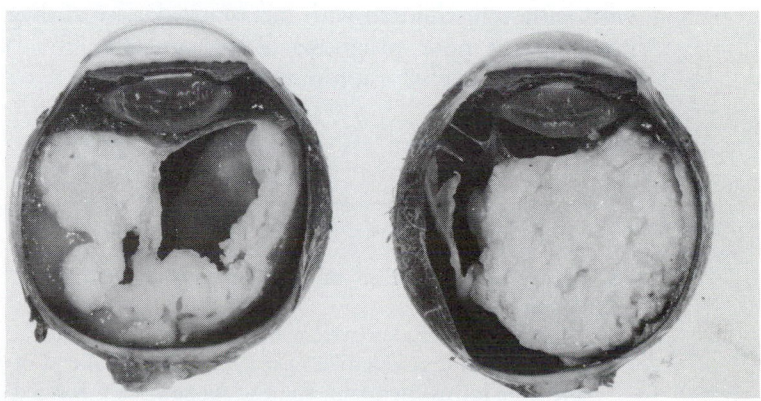

FIG. 16-16. Bilateral retinoblastoma showing presence of white mass consisting of detached retina and neoplastic tissue immediately behind lens in each eye. (From Kissane, 1985.)

metastasis by means of hematogenous spread is possible. When hematogeneous spread occurs, metastatic sites include the bone marrow, long bones, lymph nodes, and liver. Should the tumor invade the orbit, lymphatic spread is possible. Spontaneous regression infrequently occurs with retinoblastoma and may be due to the tumor's outgrowing its blood supply.

The primary sign of retinoblastoma is leukokoria, a white pupillary reflex also called "cat's eye reflex," that is due to the mass behind the lens (Fig. 16-15). At this point, the tumor is large enough that a light shone into the eye is reflected back by the tumor, making the pupil appear white. Other signs and symptoms include strabismus, a red, painful eye, and limited vision. Any of these signs and symptoms in a child younger than 4 years of age warrants careful ophthalmic examination of both eyes. Similarly, any newborn child with a known genetic risk for retinoblastoma should have routine ophthalmologic examinations.

Evaluation and Treatment

Diagnostic evaluation for retinoblastoma includes documentation of family history, complete ophthalmic examination, and metastatic studies that include bone marrow aspiration, lumbar puncture for spinal fluid examination, bone scan, and additional radiologic and CT studies of the orbit and brain. Because of the potential hereditary risk to a child's siblings, all siblings less than the age of 4 should also receive ophthalmologic evaluations.

Because retinoblastoma is a very treatable tumor, dual priorities are saving the child's life and restoring useful vision. Radiation therapy is the primary treatment for small tumors. Large and multiple tumors, indicating more advanced disease, may require enucleation (removal) of the eye. Every attempt is made to preserve useful vision in at least one eye without jeopardizing the survival of the child.

The prognosis for most children with retinoblastoma is excellent and has a greater than 90% long-term survival, although children with metastatic disease at diagnosis have a poor prognosis. Approximately 75% of children have useful vision in the treated eye.

SUMMARY REVIEW

Structure and Function of the Nervous System in Children

1 The central nervous system develops from the neural tube, which is ectodermal in origin. The cranial end of the tube forms the brain, and the spinal cord is formed from the remainder of the tube.
2 The cranial and spinal ganglia form the neural crest.
3 There are six stages to the development of the nervous system and disruption of any of the stages can lead to malfunction of the nervous system.
4 The bones of the skull are joined by sutures, and the wide membranous junctions of the sutures are known as fontanelles that close by 20 months of age.
5 Myelin is a sheath that develops around axons to facilitate speed of nerve impulse conduction. Progressive development of reflexes corresponds to normal maturation of nerve tissue.

Structural Malformation

1 Defects of neural tube closure include anencephaly, encephalocele, meningocele, and myelomeningocele.
2 Failure of the vertebra to close with protrusion of neural tube contents is known as spina bifida occulta.
3 Acrania is nearly complete absence of the cranial vault.
4 Premature closure of the cranial sutures causes craniosynostosis and prevents normal skull expansion and compression of growing brain tissue.
5 Microcephaly is lack of brain growth and retarded mental and motor development.
6 Congenital hydrocephalus results from an imbalance between the production and reabsorption of cerebrospinal fluid.

Encephalopathies

1 Static encephalopathies are nonprogressive disorders of the brain that can occur during gestation, birth, or childhood and can be caused by endogenous or exogenous factors.
2 Cerebral palsy can be caused by prenatal cerebral hypoxia or perinatal trauma with symptoms of mental retardation, seizure disorders, or developmental disabilitites.
3 Inherited metabolic disorders that damage the nervous system include defects in amino acid metabolism (phenylketonuria) and lipid metabolism (Tay-Sachs disease) and result in abnormal behavior, seizures, and deficient psychomotor development.
4 Seizure disorders are associated with numerous nervous system disorders and are more often a generalized rather than a partial type of seizure.
5 Generalized forms of seizures include tonic-clonic, myoclonic, atonic, akinetic, and infantile spasms.
6 Partial seizures suggest more localized brain dysfunction.
7 Febrile seizures are usually limited to the ages of 6 months to 3 years with a pattern of one seizure per febrile illness.
8 Reye syndrome is associated with influenza B and varicella virus and symptoms of hypoglycemia, hyperammonemia, and increased serum short-chain fatty acids. Progressive manifestations include lethargy, stupor, rigidity, seizures, and respiratory arrest.
9 Accidental poisonings from a variety of toxins can cause serious neurologic damage.
10 Bacterial meningitis is commonly caused by *Hemophilus influenza, Neisseria meningitidis,* or *Streptococcus pneumonia* and may result from respiratory or gastrointestinal

infections with symptoms of fever, headaches, photophobia, seizures, rigidity, and stupor.

Cerebrovascular Disease in Children

1 Cyanotic and congenital heart disease can be complicated by cerebrovascular occlusion that causes cerebral infarction and brain damage.

Childhood Tumors

1 Brain tumors are the most common tumors of the nervous system and the second most common cause of childhood cancer.
2 Tumors in children are most frequently located below the tentorial membrane.
3 Fast-growing tumors produce symptoms early in the disease, slow-growing tumors may become very large before symptoms appear.
4 Symptoms of brain tumors may be generalized or localized. The most common general symptom is increased intracranial pressure (headache, irritability, vomiting, somnolence, and bulging of fontanelles).
5 Localized signs of infratentorial tumors in the cerebellum include imparied coordination and balance. Cranial nerve signs occur with tumors near the brainstem.
6 Supratentorial tumors may be located near the cortex or deep in the brain. Symptoms depend on the specific location of the tumor.
7 Neuroblastoma is an embryonal tumor of the sympathetic nervous system and can be located anywhere there is sympathetic nervous tissue. Symptoms are related to tumor location and size of metastasis.
8 Retinoblastoma is a congenital eye tumor that has both a hereditary and nonhereditary form.

KEY TERMS

Acrania, 538

Alar plate, 533

Anencephaly, 535

Arnold-Chiari malformation, 538

Basal plate, 533

Benign febrile seizure, 547

Brainstem glioma, 554

Caput succedaneum, 543

Cephalohematoma, 543

Cerebral palsy, 542

Complex febrile seizure, 547

Cranial meningocele, 536

Craniopharyngioma, 553

Craniosynostosis, 538

Cyclopia, 536

Dandy-Walker malformation, 541

Diencephalic syndrome of infancy, 554

Encephalocele, 536

Encephalopathy, 542

Flexor spasm, 547

Fontanelle, 533

Ganglioneuroblastoma, 556

Ganglioneuroma, 556

Hyperphenylalaninemia, 545

Infantile spasm, 546

Ketogenic diet, 546

Lennox-Gastaut syndrome, 547

Lysosomal storage disease, 546

Macewen sign (cracked-pot sign), 541

Medulloblastoma, 554

Meningocele, 536

Mental retardation, 541

Microcephaly, 540

Myelodysplasia, 535

Myelomeningocele (meningomyclocele, spina bifida cystica), 536

Neisseria meningitidis, 549

Neural crest, 533

Neural fold, 532

Neural groove, 532

Neural plate, 532

Neural tube, 532

Neuroblastoma, 555

Optic nerve glioma, 554

Phenylketonuria (PKU), 544

Pica, 549

Retinoblastoma, 557

Reye syndrome, 548

Schwann cells, 533

Somite, 533

Spina bifida, 538

Spina bifida occulta, 538

Streptococcus pneumoniae, 549

Sulcus limitans, 533

Sunset sign, 541

Suture, 533

Tay-Sachs disease, 546

REFERENCES

Allen, J., et al. (1986). Brain tumors in children: Current cooperative and institutional chemotherapy trials in newly diagnosed and recurrent disease. *Seminars in Oncology, 13*(1), 110-122.

Allen, J., et al. (1985). Childhood brain tumors: Current status of clinical trials in newly diagnosed and recurrent disease. *Pediatric Clinics of North America, 32*(3), 633-651.

Annest, J. L., et al. (1982). Blood lead levels for persons 6 months-74 years of age: U.S., 1976-80. Vital and health statistics, National Center for Health Statistics. *Advance Data, 79,* 1-24.

Avery, G. B. (1981). *Neonatology: Pathophysiology and management of the newborn* (2nd ed.). Philadelphia: JB Lippincott.

Baker, A. B., & Baker, L. H. (1980). *Clinical neurology* (Vol. 3). New York: Harper & Row.

Barabas, G., & Taft, L. T. (1986). Early signs and differential diagnosis of cerebral palsy. *Pediatric Annals, 15*(3), 203-214.

Beckwith, J., & Perrin, E. (1963). In situ neuroblastoma: A contribution to the natural history of neural crest tumors. *American Journal of Pathology, 43,* 1089-1104.

Behrman, R. E., & Vaughan, V. C. (1983). *Nelson textbook of pediatrics* (12th ed.). Philadelphia: WB Saunders.

Bell, W. E., & McCormick, W. F. (1981). *Neurologic infections in children* (2nd ed.). Philadelphia: WB Saunders.

Benenson, A. S. (Ed.). (1980). *Control of communicable diseases in man* (13th ed.). Washington, DC: American Public Health Association.

Berman, J. L., Cunningham, G. C., Day, R. W., Ford, R., & Hsia, D. Y. (1969). Causes for high phenylalanine with normal tyrosine in newborn screening programs. *American Journal of Diseases of Children, 117,* 54-65.

Bray, P. F. (1970). *Neurology in pediatrics.* Chicago: Year Book.

Cleaveland, M. J. (1982). Nursing care in childhood cancer: Brain tumors. *American Journal of Nursing, 82,* 422.

Committee on Infectious Diseases. (1982). Aspirin and Reye's syndrome. *Pediatrics, 62,* 810-812.

Conway-Rutkowski, B. L. (1982). *Carini and Owens' neurological and neurosurgical nursing* (8th ed.). St. Louis: CV Mosby.

Dalgas, P. (1983). Reye's syndrome update. *Maternal Child Nursing, 8,* 345-350.

Damon, J., & Taylor, L. (1980). Brain tumors in children. *Nursing Clinics of North America, 15,* 99.

Dimond, M. (1986). Rehabilitation strategies for the child with cerebral palsy. *Pediatric Annals, 15*(3), 230-236.

Dobbing, J. (Ed.). (1983). *Prevention of spina bifida and other neural tube defects.* New York: Academic Press.

Dolcourt, J.L., et al. (1981). Hazard of lead exposure in the home from recycled automobile storage batteries. *Pediatrics, 68*(2), 225-230.

Donaldson, S. (1982). Retinoblastoma. In A. Levine (Ed.), *Cancer in the young.* New York: Masson Publishing.

Drummond, A. H., Jr. (1981). Lead poisoning in children. *Journal of School Health, 51*(1), 43-47.

Dyment, P., & Jaffe, N. (1983). Retinoblastoma. In P. Lanzkowsky (Ed.), *Pediatric oncology: A treatise for the clinician.* New York: McGraw-Hill.

Evans, A., D'Angio, G., & Randolph, J. (1971). A proposed staging for children with neuroblastoma. *Cancer, 27,* 374-378.

Farmer, T. H. (Ed.). (1983). *Pediatric neurology* (3rd ed.). Hagerstown, MD: Harper & Row.

Fishman, M. A. (1987). Febrile seizures. In A. M. Rudolph (Ed.), J. I. E. Hoffman & S. Axlerod (Coeds.), *Pediatrics* (18th ed.). Norwalk CT: Appleton & Lange.

Healy, M., et al. (1982, March). Lead poisoning: Something in the air. *Nursing Mirror, 31,* 42-44.

Hobdell, E. (1982, August). Hypotonia in infants and children. *Journal of Neurosurgical Nursing, 14,* 170-172.

Holtzhauer, F. J., Campbell, R. J., Hall, L. J., & Halpin, T. J. (1986). Reye's syndrome: an epidemiologic analysis of mild disease. *American Journal of Diseases of Children, 140*(12), 1231-1236.

Kelley, V. C. (1983). *Practice of pediatrics.* New York: Harper Row.

Kissane, J. M. (Ed.). (1985). *Anderson's pathology.* (8th ed.). St. Louis: C.V. Mosby.

Klein, J. O., Feigin, R. D., & McCracken, G. H. (1986). Report of the task force on treatment and management of meningitis. *Pediatrics* (Suppl.), *78*(5), 959-982.

Klein, M., & Festa, R. (1983). Central nervous system malignancies. In P. Lanzkowsky (Ed.), *Pediatric oncology: A treatise for the clinician.* New York: McGraw-Hill.

Knudson, A., Jr. (1971). Mutation and cancer: Statistical study of retinoblastoma. *Proceedings of the National Academy of Sciences, 68,* 425-432.

Knudson, A., Jr. (1978). Retinoblastoma: A prototypic hereditary neoplasm. *Seminars in Oncology, 5,* 57-60.

Knudson, A., Jr., & Strong, L. (1972). Mutation and cancer: Neuroblastoma and pheochromocytoma. *American Journal of Human Genetics, 24,* 514-532.

Lanzkowsky, P. (1983). Neuroblastoma. In P. Lanzkowsky (Ed.), *Pediatric oncology: A treatise for the clinician* (pp. 204-231). New York: McGraw-Hill.

Lee, W. H., Bookstein, R., Hong, F., Young, L. J., Stew, J. Y., & Lee, E. Y. (1987). Human retinoblastoma susceptible gene: Cloning, identification, and sequelae. *Science, 235,* 1394-1399.

Lopez-Ibor, B., & Schwartz, A. (1985). Neuroblastoma. *Pediatric Clinics of North America, 32,* 755-778.

Matson, J. L., & Breuning, S. E. (1983). *Assessing the mentally retarded.* New York: Grune & Stratton.

Menkes, J. H. (1980). *Child neurology.* Philadephia: Lea & Febiger.

Moore, K. L. (1982). *The developing human: Clinically oriented embryology* (3rd ed.). Philadephia: WB Saunders.

Nolte, J. (1988). *The brain—An introduction to its functional anatomy.* (2nd ed.). St. Louis: C.V. Mosby.

Paneth, N. (1986). Etiologic factors in cerebral palsy. *Pediatric Annals, 15*(3), 191-201.

Reye, R. D., et al. (1963, October 12). Encephalopathy and fatty degeneration of the viscera: A disease entity in childhood. *Lancet, 2,* 749-752.

Rudolph, A. M. (Ed.). (1982). *Pediatrics* (17th ed.). Norwalk, CT: Appleton-Century-Crofts.

Seidel, H. M., Ball, J. W., Dains, J. E., & Benedict, G. W. (1987). *Mosby's guide to physical examination.* St. Louis: C.V. Mosby.

Sell, S. H. W. (1984). Long-term sequelae of bacterial meningitis in children. *Pediatric Infectious Diseases, 2,* 90-93.

Silver, L. (1986). Controversial approaches to treating learning disabilities and attention deficit disorders. *American Journal of Diseases of Children, 140*(10), 1045-1052.

Swainman, K. F., & Wright, F. S. (1982). *The practice of pediatric neurology.* St. Louis: CV Mosby.

Tapley, N., Strong, L., & Sutow, W. (1984). Retinoblastoma. In W. Sutow, D. Fernback, & T. Vietti (Eds.), *Clinical pediatric oncology* (3rd ed.). St. Louis: CV Mosby.

Tudor, M. (1981). *Child development.* New York: McGraw-Hill.

VanEys, J. (1984). Malignant tumors of the central nervous system. In W. Sutow, D. Fernbach, & T. Vietti (Eds.), *Clinical pediatric oncology* (3rd ed.). St. Louis, CV Mosby.

Volpe, J. J. (1981). *Neurology of the newborn.* Philadelphia: WB Saunders.

Voute, P. (1984). Neuroblastoma. In W. Sutow, D. Fernbach, & T. Vietti (Eds.), *Clinical pediatric oncology* (3rd ed.) (pp. 559-587). St. Louis: CV Mosby.

Walker, M. (1982). Tumors of the central nervous system. In A. Levine (Ed.), *Cancer in the young.* New York: Masson Publishing.

Warkany, J., Lemire, R. J., & Cohen, M. M. (1981). *Mental retardation and congenital malformations of the central nervous system.* Chicago: Year Book.

Waskerwitz, M., & Ruccione, K. (1985). An overview of cancer in children in the 1980s. *Nursing Clinics of North America, 20,* 5-29.

Wasserman, E., & Gromisch, D. S. (1981). *Survey of clinical pediatrics,* (7th ed.). New York: McGraw-Hill.

Whaley, L. F., & Wong, D. L. (1987). *Nursing care of infants and children.* (3rd ed.). St. Louis: C.V. Mosby.

Wong, D., & Dornan, L. (1982). Nursing care in childhood cancer: Retinoblastoma. *American Journal of Nursing, 82,* 425-431.

Young, J., & Miller, R. (1975). Incidence of malignant tumors in U.S. children. *Journal of Pediatrics, 86,* 254-258.

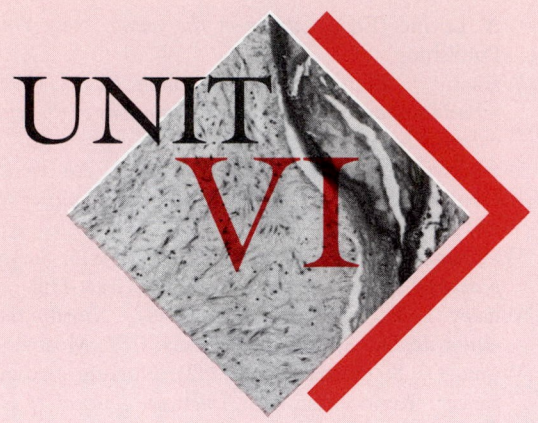

UNIT VI

The Endocrine System

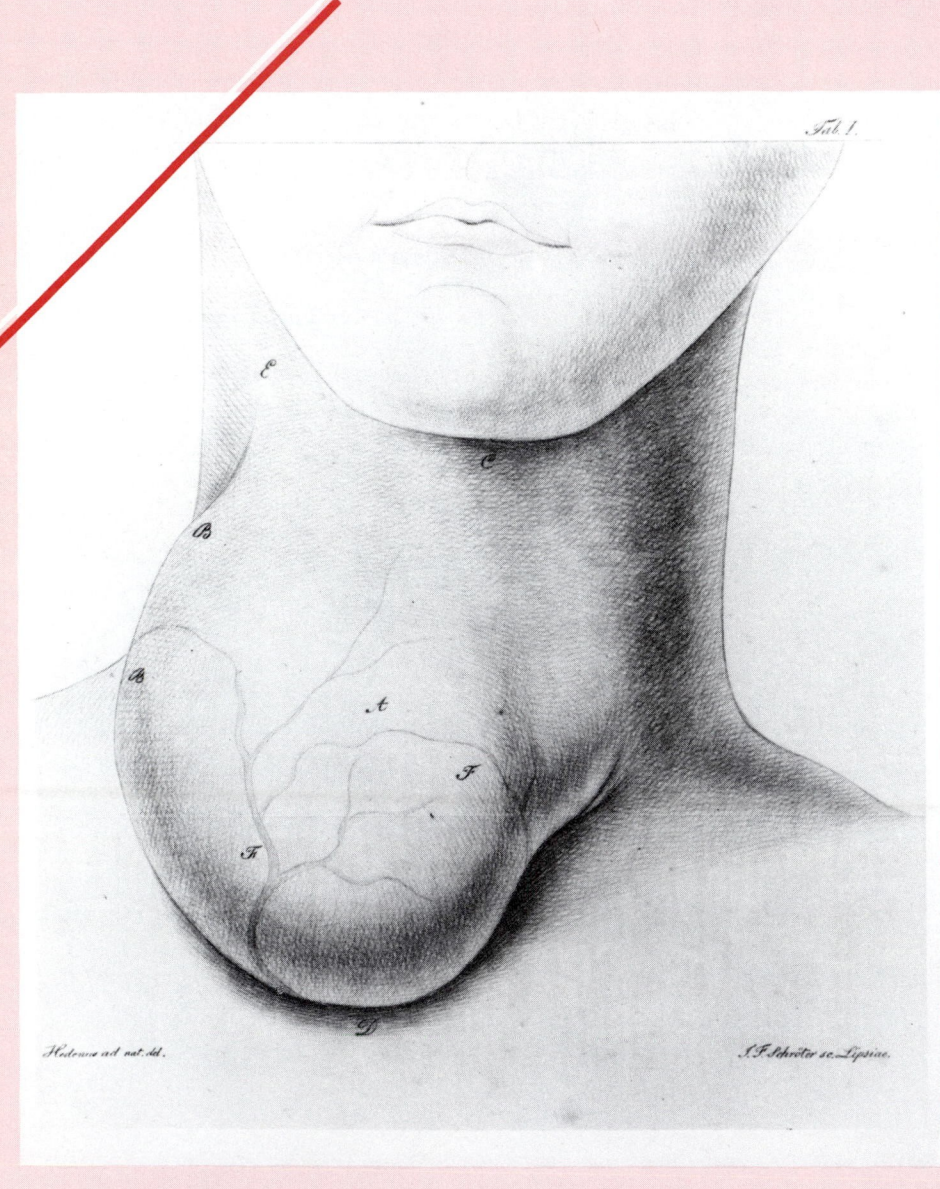

Endocrine diseases. Front view, nose to shoulder, of a male with goiter. (From A. W. Hedenus: Tractatus de glandula thyreoidea, 1822. Courtesy National Library of Medicine.)

THERE are numerous examples that indicate an early awareness of endocrine dysfunction. Goiters were described as far back as the Roman Empire, and it appears that people in early times recognized the anatomic and physiologic effects of castration in males, although the mechanisms for the effects were not understood. An Egyptian papyrus, dated 1500 BC, described a person producing excessive amounts of sweet urine. Despite these descriptions, the surviving written records do not reflect an understanding of the endocrine system as such until the 1700s.

In 1766, A.V. Haller identified the thymus, thyroid, spleen, and glands without ducts that pour special substances into the veins and, thus, into the general secretion. The term *internal secretions* as a descriptor for the special substances was introduced in 1855 by Claude Bernard. The term *hormone* was first used in 1905 by two British physiologists, W.M. Bayliss and E.H. Starling. The word *hormone* is derived from a Greek word meaning "I arouse to activity."

One of the first endocrine deficiencies to be successfully treated was a case of hypothyroidism in 1891. G.R. Murray administered extract from the thyroid gland of a freshly killed sheep to his patient and the symptoms of hypothyroidism subsequently improved. Hyperthyroidism was the first condition described as a result of the overproduction of an endocrine secretion. Surgical removal of the thyroid glands was done in the mid-1800s and resulted in improvement of symptoms. The procedure was neither a common nor a successful treatment until after the development of surgical anesthesia and the implementation of surgical asepsis.

By the late 1890s and early 1900s, several endocrine glands and their functions had been identified. The substances secreted by the endocrine glands were not identified until much later. The parathyroid glands were discovered in 1855; their function was discovered in 1896, but parathyroid hormone was not isolated until 1925. The endocrine functions of the pancreas were identified in 1889; in 1928 insulin was developed in a pure enough form for use in humans. Its amino acid sequence was not established until 1953 by Sanger. The subspecialty of endocrinology was established in the 1930s, with H.D. Rolleston's definition of endocrinology as the clinical and biochemical study of all aspects of the ductless glands. In the 1940s through the 1970s, a number of technologic advances contributed to dramatic advances in knowledge about the endocrine system; the development of paper and column chromatography, completely automated amino acid analyzers, and solid phase peptide synthesis are some examples. Recent advances include the development of assays to determine hormonal levels, including radioimmunoassay and enzyme-linked immunosorbent assays, and genetic engineering techniques to manufacture human insulin. These techniques have contributed to discoveries in the area of endocrinology. The intricate relationships between the endocrine, immunologic, and nervous systems are just beginning to be explored, offering the possibilities for the emergence of many new ideas about endocrine homeodynamics.

CHAPTER 17

Mechanisms of Hormonal Regulation

D. Patricia Gray

Regulation of hormone release, 565
Hormone transport, 565
Cellular mechanisms of hormone action, 568
  Water-soluble hormones, 568
    First messenger, 568
    Second messenger, 569
      Cyclic AMP, 569
      Calcium, 570
  Steroid hormones, 570
Structure and function of the endocrine glands, 570
  The hypothalamic-pituitary system, 570
    Hormones of the posterior pituitary, 573
      Antidiuretic hormone, 573
      Oxytocin, 574
    Hormones of the anterior pituitary, 574
  The thyroid and parathyroid glands, 574
    The thyroid gland, 575
      Regulation of thyroid hormone secretion, 576
      Synthesis of thyroid hormone, 576
    The parathyroid glands, 577
  The endocrine pancreas, 578
    Somatostatin, 578
    Insulin, 580
    Glucagon, 580
  The adrenal glands, 580
    Adrenal cortex, 580
      Glucocorticoids, 582
        Functions of glucocorticoids, 582
        Cortisol, 583
      Mineralocorticoids: aldosterone, 584
      Adrenal estrogens and androgens, 586
    Adrenal medulla, 586
  The neuroendocrine response to stressors, 586
  Tests of endocrine function, 587
Aging and the endocrine system, 588
  Theories about the effects of aging, 588
  Effects of aging on specific glands, 588
    The thyroid gland, 588
    The parathyroid gland, 589
    The adrenal glands, 589
    The posterior pituitary, 589
    The anterior pituitary, 589

The endocrine system, together with the nervous system, acts as the body's communication network. The endocrine system is composed of various glands located throughout the body (Fig. 17-1). These glands are capable of synthesizing and releasing special chemical messengers called **hormones.** The endocrine system has five general functions: (1) differentiation of the reproductive and central nervous systems in the developing fetus; (2) stimulation of sequential growth and development during childhood and adolescence; (3) coordination of the male and female reproductive systems, which makes sexual reproduction possible; (4) maintenance of an optimal internal environment throughout the lifespan; and (5) initiation of corrective and adaptive responses when emergency demands occur.

The endocrine glands respond to specific signals by synthesizing and releasing hormones into the circulation. Although a wide variety of hormones function within the body, they all have certain general characteristics:

1. Hormones have specific rates and patterns of secretion. Three basic secretion patterns are (1) diurnal patterns, (2) pulsatile and cyclic patterns, and (3) patterns that depend on levels of circulating substrates (e.g., calcium, sodium, potassium, or the hormones themselves). Diurnal, pulsatile, and cyclic patterns of hormone release involve consistent patterns of secretion.
2. Hormones operate within feedback systems, either positive or negative, to maintain an optimal internal environment (see p. 565).
3. Hormones affect only cells with appropriate receptors and then act on these cells to initiate specific cell functions or activities.
4. Hormones are all constantly excreted by the kidneys or deactivated by the liver or by other cellular mechanisms.

Hormones may be classified according to structure, gland of origin, effects, or chemical composition. (Table

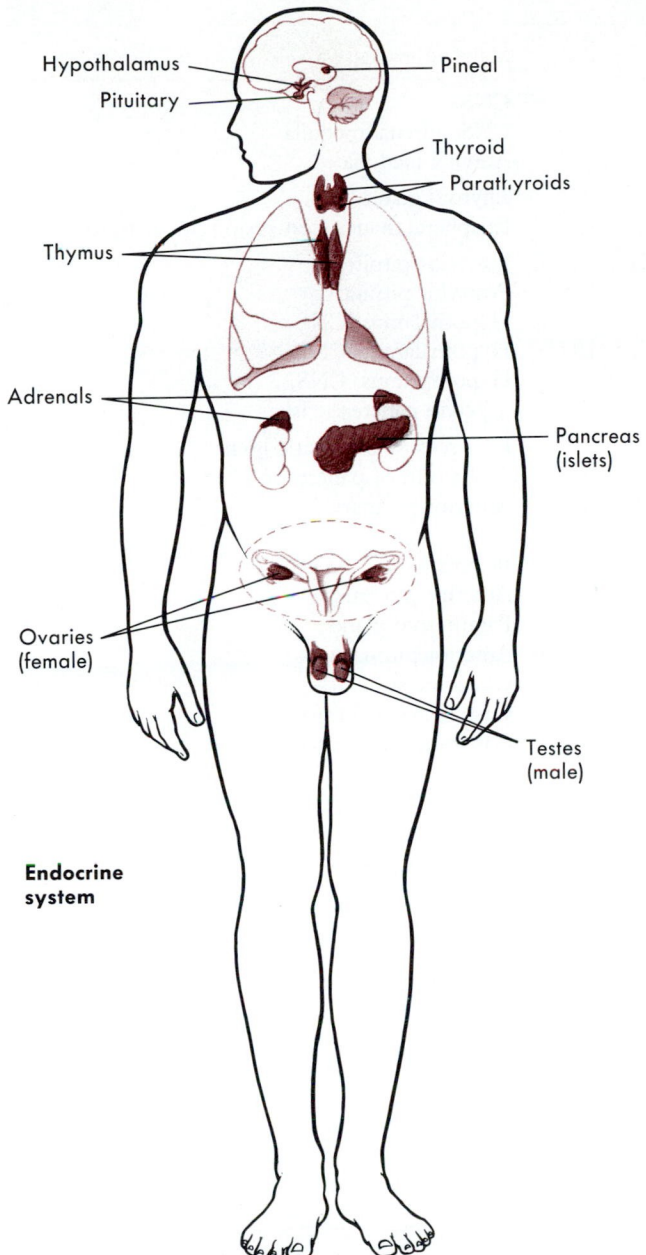

Hypothalamus
Pituitary
Pineal
Thyroid
Parathyroids
Thymus
Adrenals
Pancreas
(islets)
Ovaries
(female)
Testes
(male)

**Endocrine
system**

FIG. 17-1. The endocrine system. (From Thibodeau, 1987.)

mentation of hormone release has led to the identification of physiologic variables that trigger hormone secretion. For example, secretion of certain hormones may be initiated by changes in levels of circulating substances, such as glucose, calcium, potassium, or sodium or by electrical stimulation of an endocrine gland. Hormones themselves may directly regulate their own secretion. This process is called **endocrine regulation.** This process of hormone regulation occurs because some secretory cells are sensitive to hormone concentration in the plasma and secrete enough hormone to maintain a certain level.

Hormone secretion may be regulated by one or several of these regulatory mechanisms. For example, insulin is secreted in response to increased glucose levels (a chemical stimulus); to direct stimulation of the insulin-secreting cells of the pancreas by the autonomic nervous system (an electrical stimulus); and to the secretion of cortisol by the adrenal medulla, a form of endocrine regulation.

Regulation of hormone secretion is achieved by the use of a variety of feedback systems, which provide precise monitoring and control of the cellular environment. **Negative feedback** is the most common feedback system. The feedback is negative because the rising hormone level negates the initiating change that triggered the release of the hormone. For example, if serum calcium levels fall (the initiating change), parathyroid hormone (PTH) secretion is increased. PTH causes an increase in serum calcium. The increase in calcium then serves to decrease PTH secretion, or "turn off" the system. In this manner, serum calcium levels are maintained (Fig. 17-2). **Positive feedback,** which occurs when hormone secretion continues to trigger additional hormone secretion, is rarely seen in the endocrine system.

Feedback is also described in terms of ultra-short, short, and long feedback loops. The feedback loops are used to describe regulation of hormone secretion by hormones themselves (endocrine regulation). (These regulatory systems are diagrammed in Fig. 17-3.)

Hormone Transport

Once hormones are released into the circulatory system by the endocrine glands, they are distributed throughout the body. The protein hormones (insulin and pituitary, hypothalamic, and parathyroid hormone) are water soluble and generally circulate in free, or unbound, forms. This process immediately exposes these water-soluble hormones to physiologic decomposition, giving them an expected half-life of seconds to minutes. Unlike protein hormones, steroid and thyroid hormones are lipid soluble and are primarily transported by carrier or binding proteins, although a small amount is left unbound. The amount of bound hormone is generally de-

17-1 categorizes known hormones by chemical classes.) The secretion and mechanisms of action of hormones represent an extremely complex system of integrated responses. Although much has been learned about these complex systems, many of the specific mechanisms of action are not yet understood.

Regulation of Hormone Release

The release of hormones occurs either in response to an alteration in the cellular environment or in the process of maintaining a regulated level of certain hormones or certain substances. Extensive study and docu-

TABLE 17-1 Chemical classification of hormones

Chemical class	Hormones	Major source
Amines	Dopamine	CNS
	Norepinephrine	CNS, adrenal medulla
	Epinephrine	Adrenal medulla
Iodothyronines	Thyroxine (T_4)	Thyroid gland
	Triiodothyronine (T_3)	Peripheral tissues (conversion site of T_4 to T_3)
Small peptides	Vasopressin (antidiuretic hormone; ADH)	Posterior pituitary
	Oxytocin	Posterior pituitary
	Thyrotrophin-releasing hormone (TRH)	Hypothalamus, CNS
	Gonadotropin-releasing hormone (GnRH, LHRH)	Hypothalamus, CNS
	Somatostatin (SRIF)	Hypothalamus, CNS, pectin pancreatic islets
Proteins	Insulin	Beta cells of pancreatic islets
	Glucagon	Alpha cells of pancreatic islets
	Growth hormone or somatotropin (GH, STH)	Anterior pituitary
	Placental lactogen (PL)	
	Prolactin (PRL)	Placenta
	Parathyroid hormone (PTH)	Anterior pituitary
	ACTH	Parathyroid gland
	Secretin	Anterior pituitary
	Cholecystokinin (CCK)	Gastrointestinal tract
	Gastrin	Gastrointestinal tract
	Gastric-inhibitory peptide (GIP)	Gastrointestinal tract
Glycoproteins	Follicle-stimulating hormone (FSH)	Anterior pituitary
	Luteinizing hormone (LH)	Anterior pituitary
	Chorionic gonadotrophin (CG)	Placenta
	Thyroid-stimulating hormone (TSH)	Anterior pituitary
Steroids (fat soluble)	Estrogens (E_2, E_3)	Ovary, placenta
	Progesterone (P)	Corpus luteum, placenta
	Testosterone (T)	Testis
	Dihydrotestosterone (DHT)	T-sensitive tissues
	Glucocorticoids	Adrenal cortex
	Aldosterone	Adrenal cortex
	Cholecalciferol (vitamin D) metabolites	Liver, kidneys

From Felig et al., 1981.

TABLE 17-2 Binding proteins, their hormones, and variables that affect their circulating levels

Binding protein	Hormone	Factors that increase binding protein	Factors that decrease binding protein
Corticosteroid-binding globulin	Cortisol Progesterone	Estrogen	Liver disease
Sex hormone–binding globulin	Dihydrotesterone Testosterone Estradiol		Androgens Hypothyroidism Liver disease
Thyroid-binding globulin	T_4 T_3	Estrogen Hyperthyroidism	Testosterone Glucocorticoids Liver disease
Albumin	All lipid-soluble hormones	Estrogen	Liver disease Malnutrition Renal disease

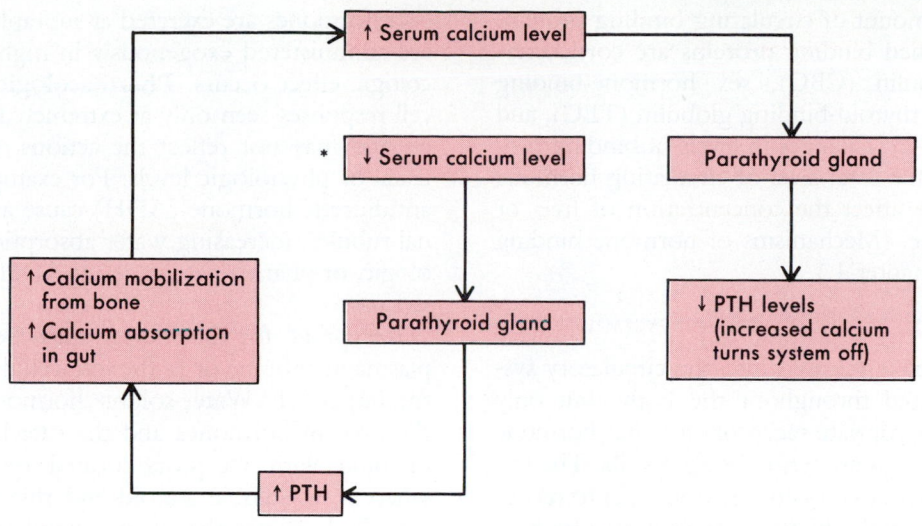

* Start   **FIG. 17-2.** Negative feedback for calcium regulation.

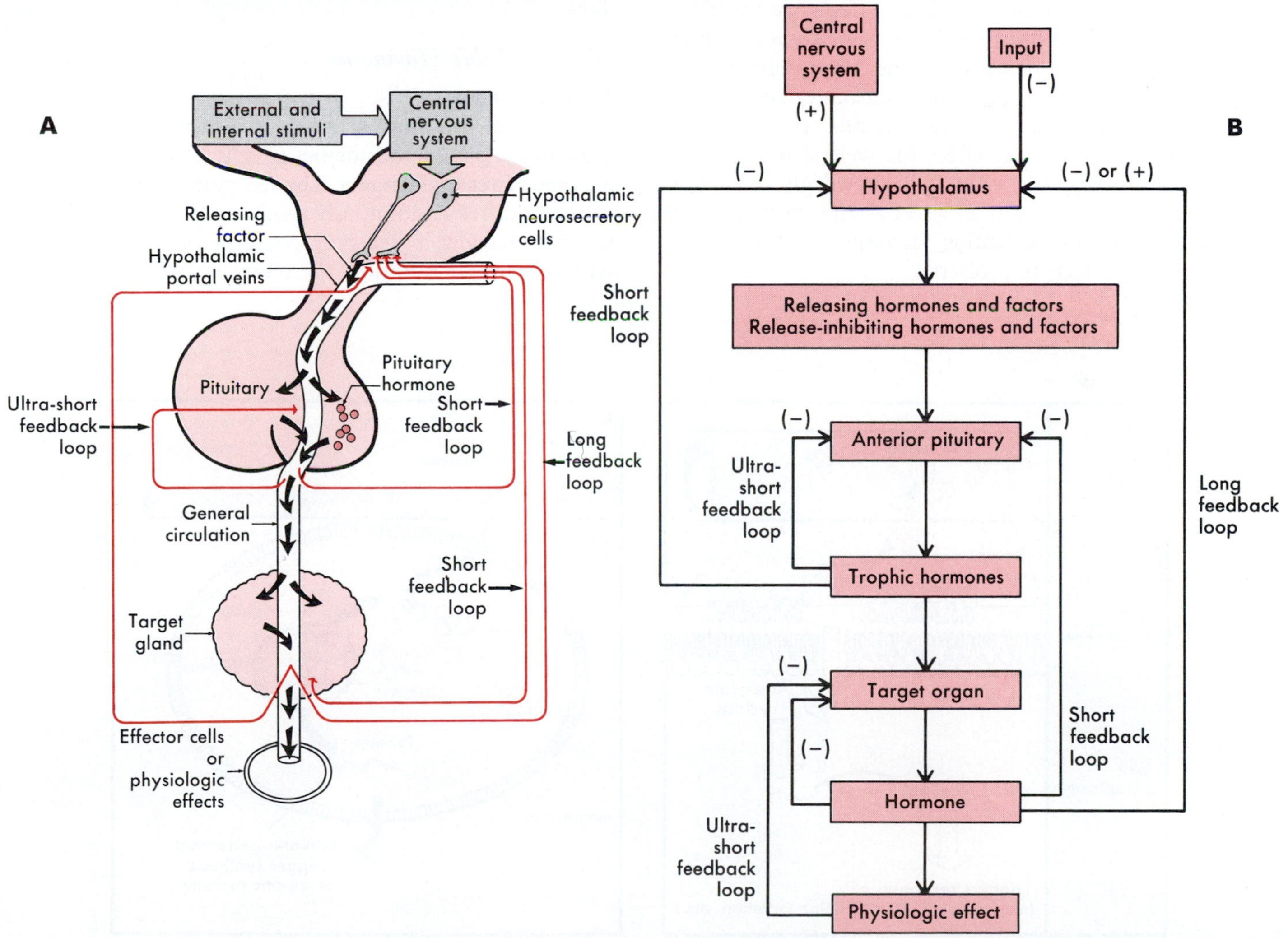

FIG. 17-3. **A,** Endocrine feedback loops involving the hypothalamus-pituitary gland and end organs.
B, General model for control and feedback to hypothalamic-pituitary target organ systems.

termined by the amount of circulating binding protein. Among the identified binding proteins are corticosteroid binding globulin (CBG), sex hormone-binding globulin (SHBG), thyroid-binding globulin (TBG), and albumin (Table 17-2). Changes in levels of binding proteins might affect the total level of circulating hormone but do not usually affect the concentration of free, or unbound, hormone. (Mechanisms of hormone binding are discussed in Chapter 1.)

Cellular Mechanisms of Hormone Action

When a hormone is released into the circulatory system, it is distributed throughout the body, but only those cells with appropriate receptors for that hormone are affected. These cells are termed **target cells.** The target cell receptors have two main functions: (1) to recognize and bind with high affinity to their particular hormones and (2) to initiate a signal to appropriate intracellular effectors.

Hormones have two general types of effects on target cells: direct and permissive. **Direct effects** are the obvious changes in cell function that specifically result from stimulation by a particular hormone. **Permissive effects** are less obvious hormone-induced changes that facilitate the maximal response or functioning of a cell. For example, insulin has a direct effect on skeletal muscle cells with insulin receptors, causing increased glucose transport into these cells. Insulin also has a permissive effect on mammary cells, facilitating the response of these cells to the direct effects of prolactin.

If hormones are excreted at supraphysiologic levels or are administered exogenously in high doses, a pharmacologic effect occurs. **Pharmacologic effects** are those cell responses seen only at extremely high hormone levels and may not reflect the actions of the hormone at usual or physiologic levels. For example, usual levels of antidiuretic hormone (ADH) cause an effect on the renal tubules, increasing water absorption. At supraphysiologic, or pharmacologic, levels ADH acts as a vasoconstrictor.

Receptors for hormones may be located on the plasma membrane or in the intracellular compartment of the target cell. Water-soluble hormones, which include the protein hormones and the catecholamines, interact or bind with receptors located on the cell surface, whereas fat-soluble steroid and thyroid hormones diffuse freely across the plasma membrane and bind with an intracellular receptor (Fig. 17-4). (Types of hormones, their corresponding receptors, and the mechanisms by which they affect the cell are summarized in Table 17-3.)

Water-Soluble Hormones

First Messenger

Receptors for most water-soluble hormones are located in the plasma membranes of cells. These hormones are called **first messengers.** The receptors on the plasma membranes are continuously synthesized and degraded, so that changes in receptor concentration may occur within hours. In addition, the receptor's affinity for the

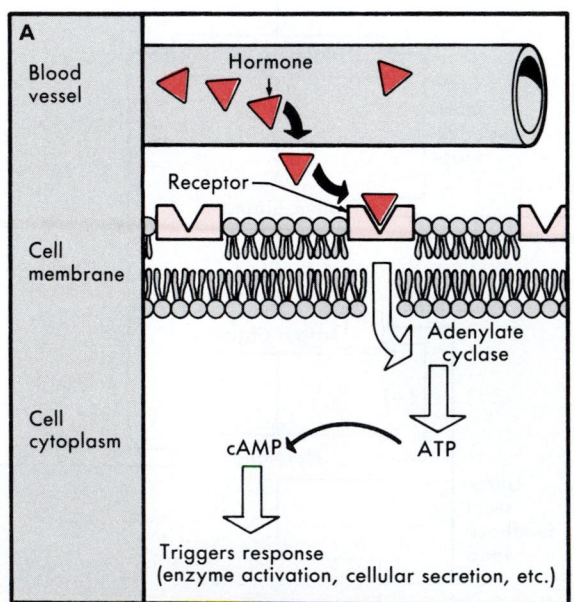
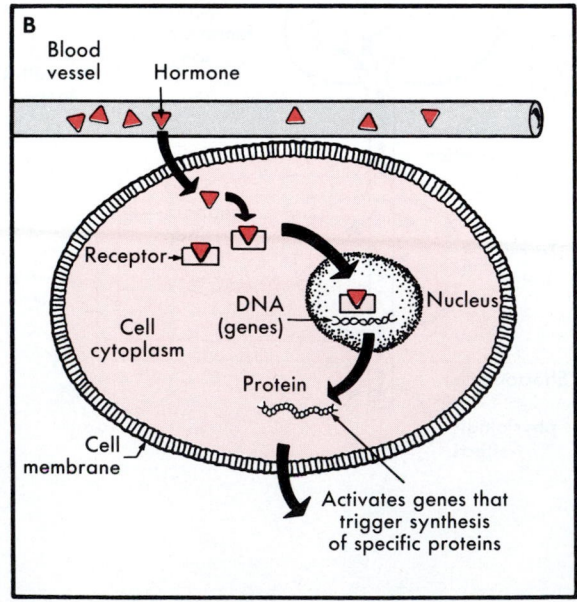

FIG. 17-4. A, Receptors for most water-soluble hormones are located in the plasma membrane of cells. **B,** Receptors for some lipid-soluble (steroid) hormones are located in the intracellular compartment.

TABLE 17-3 Types of hormones, their receptors, and their mechanisms of action

Hormone	Type of receptor	Mechanism of action
WATER-SOLUBLE HORMONES (glycoproteins, amines, small peptides and proteins, except insulin)	Plasma membrane receptors	Second messenger, cAMP, cGMP, Ca^{++}, others
Insulin	Plasma membrane receptors	Second messenger other than cAMP, cGMP, or calcium
LIPID-SOLUBLE HORMONES Steroid hormones	Nuclear receptors	Nuclear translocation and altered genome transcription
Thyroid hormones (iodothyronines)	Nuclear receptors Cystolic receptors	Altered genome transcription

From Lefkowitz, 1982.

hormone may also vary. Both receptor affinity and receptor concentration are regulated by intracellular and extracellular mechanisms, which include the following:

Physiochemical environment
    pH
    Temperature
    Calcium concentration
    Sodium concentration
Urea concentration
    Levels of cyclic AMP (a "second messenger")
Lipid matrix of the plasma membrane
    Cholesterol content
    Saturation of fatty acid side chains
    Polar groups or phospholipids
    Alterations of the plasma membrane
Circulating levels of hormones
Stage of growth and development
Diet
Exercise
Drugs

The receptors for the water-soluble hormones serve first to recognize the hormone on the plasma membrane and then bind with the hormone. Once recognition and binding have occurred, the hormone-receptor complex initiates the transmission of an intracellular signal by way of a "second messenger."

Second Messenger

In 1958, Sutherland and Rall were the first to propose the "second messenger" theory of water-soluble hormone action. They proposed that the signals initiated by hormone-receptor binding were transmitted into the cell by the action of a **second messenger.** In subsequent papers, Sutherland and his colleagues identified cyclic adenosine monophosphate as a second messenger. Sutherland was awarded the Nobel Prize in Physiology in 1971 for this work. The second messen-

ger theory suggests that once the hormone receptor has combined with its first messenger, it is able to bind with a second protein on the inner surface of the plasma membrane. The second protein is then activated by the binding with the receptor. This mechanism, whereby hormone receptors initiate the appropriate intracellular response, is now well accepted.

Second messengers that have been identified include cyclic adenosine monophosphate (cyclic AMP), cyclic guanosine monophosphate (cyclic GMP), calcium, and prostaglandins. The second messengers for insulin, growth hormone, prolactin, and others have yet to be identified. Evidence suggests that second messengers for these hormones do exist. (The hormones and their associated second messengers are listed in Table 17-4.)

Cyclic AMP

Hormone-receptor binding initiates an increase in the intracellular level of the second messenger. For this to occur, a series of interactions within the plasma membrane must take place. For cells having cyclic AMP as a second messenger, the purpose of these interactions is to activate the intracellular cyclic nucleotides, adenylate or guanylate cyclase. Adenylate cyclase is an enzyme that converts adenosine triphosphate (ATP) to cyclic AMP, whereas guanylate cyclase enzymatically converts guanosine triphosphate (GTP) to cyclic GMP.

An example of the function of cyclic AMP as a second messenger can be seen with the action of the hormone, epinephrine. Epinephrine stimulates breakdown of glycogen to glucose in the liver. Once activated by the epinephrine-receptor complex, adenylate cyclase catalyzes the synthesis of cyclic AMP. Cyclic AMP, in turn, activates the enzyme protein kinase, which then catalyzes the phosphorylation (addition of a phosphate group) to yet another enzyme, phosphorylase kinase. Activated phosphorylase kinase phosphorylates (and thus acti-

TABLE 17-4 Second messengers identified for specific hormones

Second messenger	Associated hormones
Cyclic AMP	Adrenocorticotropic hormone (ACTH)
	Luteinizing hormone (LH)
	Human chorionic gonadotropin (HCG)
	Follicle-stimulating hormone (FSH)
	Thyroid-stimulating hormone (TSH)
	Antidiuretic hormone (ADH)
	Thyrotropin-releasing hormone (TRH)
	Parathyroid hormone (PTH)
	Glucagon
Calcium	Angiotensin II
	Gonadotropin-releasing hormone (GNRH)
Unidentified	Insulin
	Growth hormone
	Prolactin

vates) another enzyme that catalyzes the breakdown of glycogen to glucose. Thus an elaborate cascade emerges in which inactive enzymes are converted in sequence to active enzymes, leading to glycogen breakdown.

Calcium

Increasing evidence suggests that calcium ions within the cell, like cAMP, function as a second messenger for certain hormones, such as angiotensin II and gonadotropin-releasing hormone. The specific mechanism of regulation by calcium ions is not clearly understood at present. It is known that hormone-receptor binding results in an influx of calcium ions into the cytoplasm, either from the extracellular fluid or from internal cellular stores. With the rise in intracellular calcium, calcium ions bind with an intracellular regulatory protein, calmodulin. The calcium-calmodulin complex mediates the effects of calcium on intracellular activities. These effects are similar to the actions of the cyclic nucleotides on intracellular protein kinases. The calmodulin-dependent protein kinases are involved in control of intracellular contractile components, alteration of plasma membrane permeability, and regulation of intracellular enzyme activity.

Calcium-calmodulin and the cyclic nucleotides appear to interact in regulating the cell's metabolic and physiologic response to hormonal stimulation. These second messengers may act synergistically with each other or as antagonists to each other in achieving their effects.

Steroid Hormones

The lipid-soluble hormones are classified as steroid hormones (including androgens, estrogens, progestins, glucocorticoids, and mineralocorticoids) and thyroid hormones. Because steroid hormones are relatively small, hydrophobic molecules (synthesized from cholesterol), they can cross the plasma membrane by simple diffusion (see Chapter 1). Some research suggests that steroid hormones also bind to membrane receptors (King, 1984). Once activated by hormones, the receptor is thought to bind to specific sites on the chromatin of the target cell, causing RNA transcription and increased synthesis of specific proteins (discussed in Chapter 4).

STRUCTURE AND FUNCTION OF THE ENDOCRINE GLANDS

The Hypothalamic-Pituitary System

The hormones of the pituitary gland regulate several other endocrine glands and affect a number of diverse body functions. Part of the pituitary gland is directly connected to the brain, and the pituitary gland is also closely related to the nervous system. Some of the hormones secreted by the pituitary gland act directly on organs of the reproductive system (see Unit 7). Other hormones act in conjunction with the thyroid and adrenal glands and with the endocrine pancreas.

The hypothalamic-pituitary unit forms the structural and functional basis for central integration of the neurologic and endocrine systems (Figs 17-5 to 17-7). The hypothalamus, containing special neurosecretory cells and located at the base of the brain, is connected to the pituitary gland by a stalklike structure, the **infundibular stem.** The special cells of the hypothalamus are like other neurons in that they have similar electrical properties, organelles, membranes, and synapses. Neurosecretory cells, however, are able to synthesize and to secrete the hypothalamic-releasing hormones and to synthesize the hormones of the posterior portion of the pituitary gland.

The **pituitary gland** is located in the sella turcica (a saddle-shaped depression on the superior surface of the body). The pituitary gland weighs approximately 0.5 g, except during pregnancy when its weight approaches 1.0 g. It is composed of two distinctly different lobes: (1) the posterior pituitary, or neurohypophysis, and (2) the anterior pituitary, or adenohypophysis. These two lobes differ in their embryonic origins, cell types, and functional relationship to the hypothalamus.

The embryonic posterior pituitary is derived from the hypothalamus and comprises three parts: (1) the median eminence located at the base of the hypothalamus, (2) the infundibular stem, and (3) the infundibular process also known as the pars nervosa or neural lobe. The **median eminence** is composed largely of the nerve endings of axons that arise primarily in the ventral hypothala-

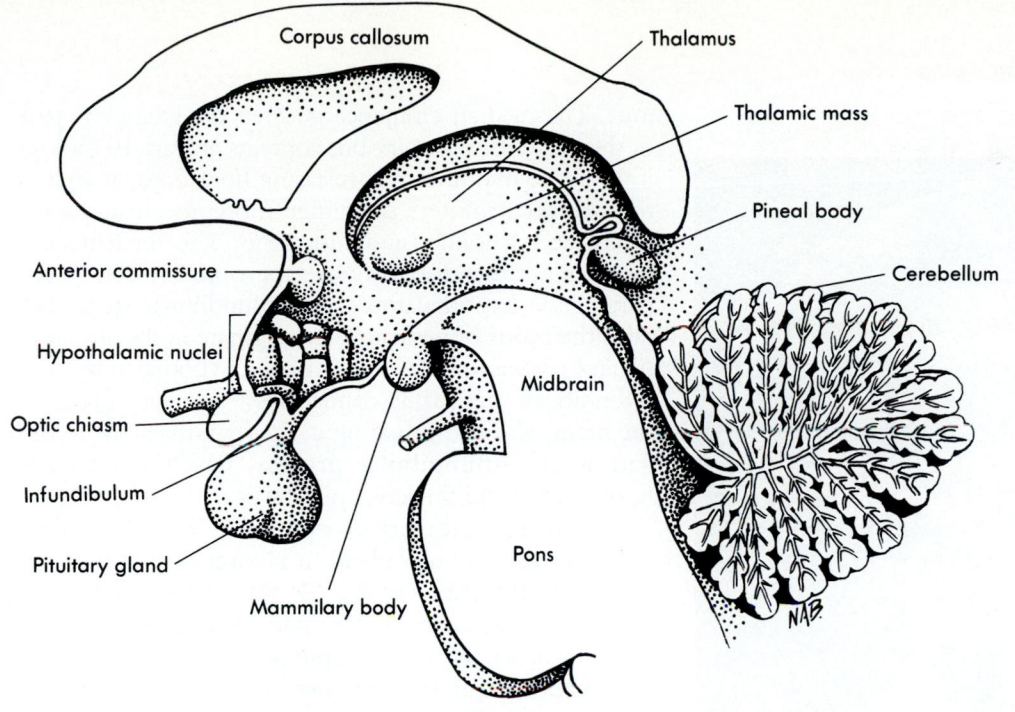

FIG. 17-5. Saggital section through the brain showing the hypothalamic nucleic and pituitary gland. (From Phipps, Long, & Woods, 1987.)

FIG. 17-6. Anterior pituitary hormones and their target organs: adrenocorticotropic hormone (ACTH); thyroid-stimulating hormone (TSH); follicle-stimulating hormone (FSH); leutinizing hormone (LH); male analogue or LH (ICSH); melanocyte-stimulating hormone (MSH). (From Thibodeau, 1987.)

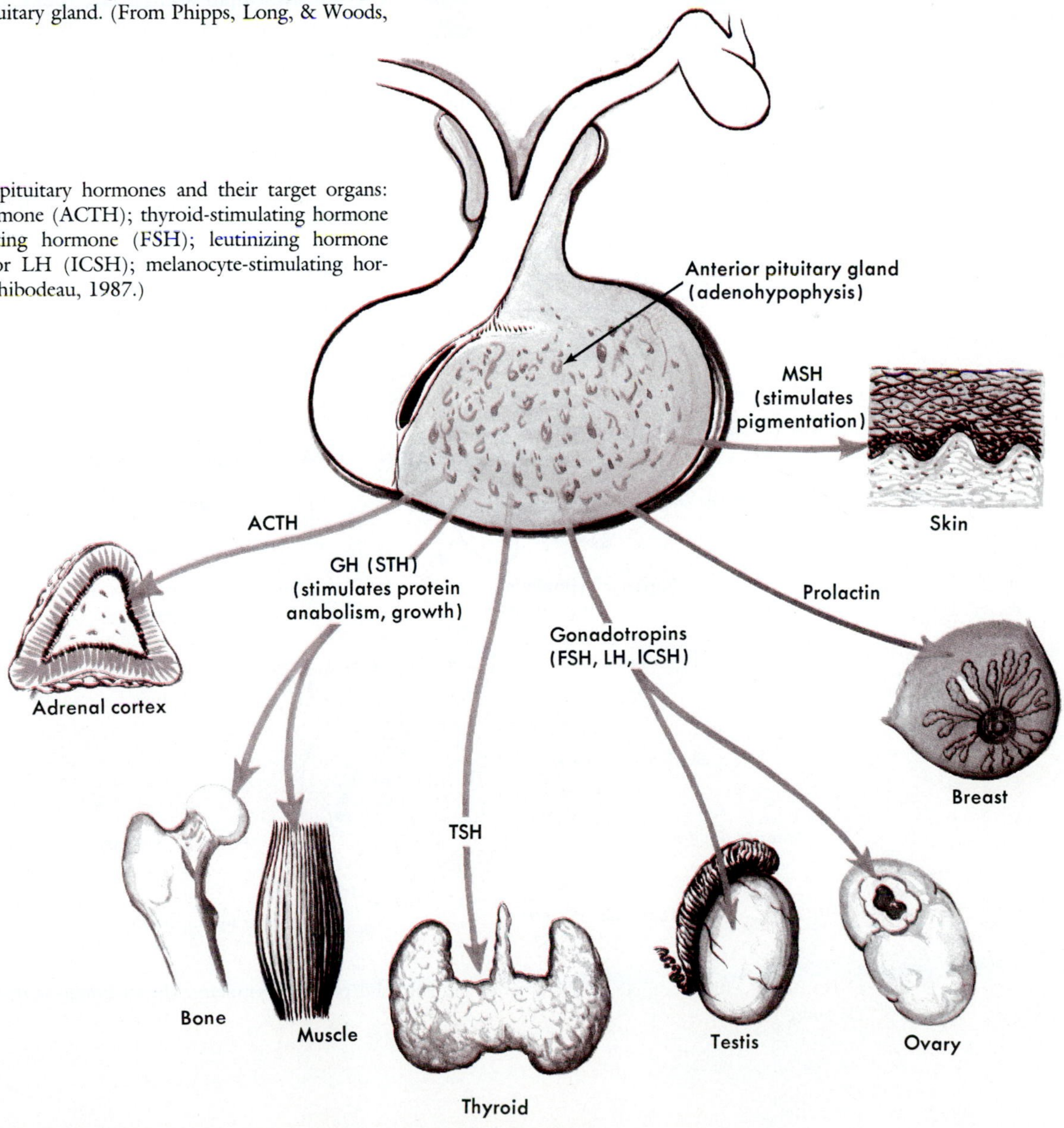

Anterior pituitary gland (adenohypophysis)

MSH (stimulates pigmentation)

Skin

ACTH

GH (STH) (stimulates protein anabolism, growth)

Gonadotropins (FSH, LH, ICSH)

Prolactin

Adrenal cortex

Breast

Bone

Muscle

TSH

Testis

Ovary

Thyroid

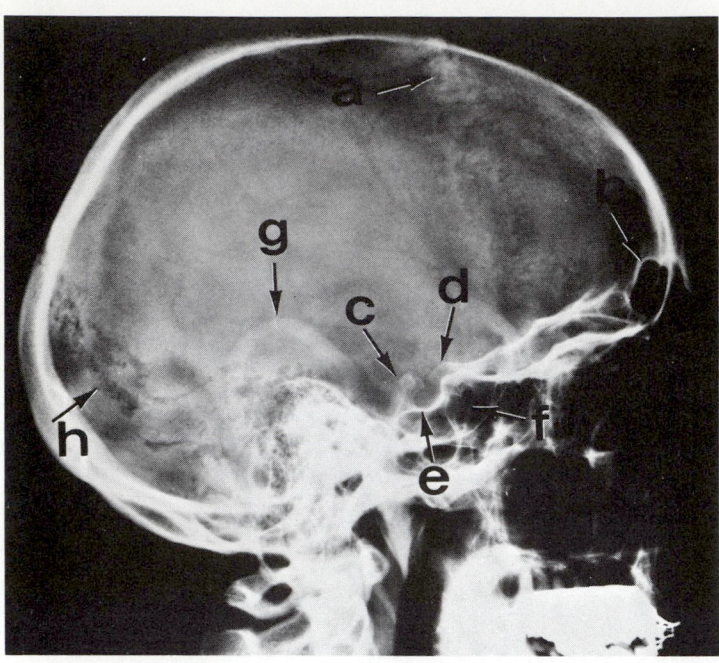

FIG. 17-7. Normal skull, lateral view: *(a)* coronal suture, *(b)* frontal sinus, *(c)* dorsum sellae, *(d)* anteior clinoid process, *(e)* floor of sella tunica (pituitary gland), *(f)* sphenoid sinus, *(g)* shadow of earlobe, *(h)* lamboidal suture. (From Thibodeau, 1987.)

mus. The median eminence is often designated as part of the posterior pituitary but contains at least 10 biologically active hypothalamic-releasing hormones, as well as the neurotransmitters dopamine, norepinephrine, serotonin, acetylcholine, and histamine. The median eminence might therefore be more appropriately considered part of the hypothalamus. The infundibular stem contains the axons of neurons that originate in the supraoptic and paraventricular nuclei of the hypothalamus. The infundibular stem thus connects the pituitary gland to the brain. Axons originating in the hypothalamus terminate in the **infundibular process,** which secretes the hormones of the posterior pituitary.

The anterior pituitary accounts for 75% of the total weight of the pituitary gland. It is composed of three regions: (1) the pars distalis, (2) the pars tuberalis, and (3) the pars intermedia. The **pars distalis** is the major component of the anterior pituitary and the source of the anterior pituitary hormones. The **pars tuberalis** is a thin layer of cells on the anterior and lateral portions of the infundibular stem. The **pars intermedia** lies between the two lobes of the pituitary gland. In the adult, the distinct intermediate lobe disappears and the individual cells are distributed diffusely throughout the pars distalis and neural lobe (Reichlin, 1985).

The pituitary gland receives its blood supply primarily from a special portal system (illustrated in Fig. 17-8). This system of blood flow facilitates communication among the hypothalamus, median eminence, and adenohypophysis.

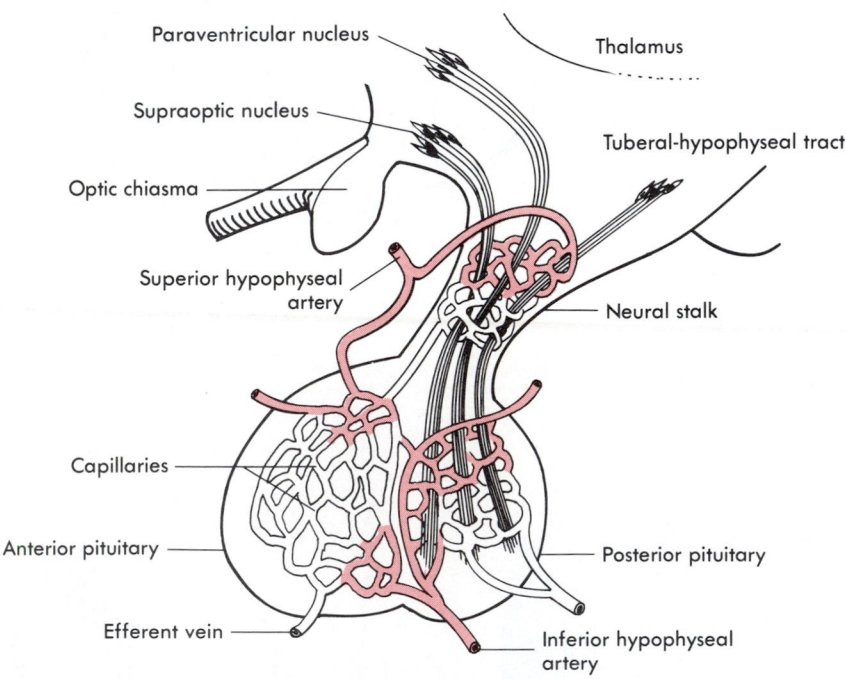

FIG. 17-8. Blood supply to the anterior pituitary and posterior pituitary. (From Phipps, Long, & Woods, 1987.)

TABLE 17-5 Hypothalamic hormones

Hormone	Target site	Action
Thyrotropin-releasing hormone (TRH)	Anterior pituitary	Stimulates release of thyroid-stimulating hormone (TSH) Modulates prolactin secretion
Gonadotropin-releasing hormone (GnRH)	Anterior pituitary	Stimualtes release of follicle-stimulating hormone (FSH) and luteinizing hormone (LH)
Somatostatin	Anterior pituitary	Inhibits release of growth hormone (GH)
	Gastrointestinal tract	Decreases gastric motility, intestinal secretion, and secretion of thyroid-stimulating hormone, parathyroid hormone, renin, glucagon, and insulin
Growth hormone–releasing factor (GRF)	Anterior pituitary	Stimulates release of GH
Corticotropin-releasing hormone (CRH)	Anterior pituitary	Stimualtes release of adrenocorticotropic hormone (ACTH) and beta-endorphin
Substance P	Anterior pituitary	Inhibits synthesis and release of ACTH Stimulates secretion of GH, FSH, LH, and prolactin
Prolactin-inhibiting factor (PIF; possibly dopamine)	Anterior pituitary	Inhibits secretion of prolactin

The hormones—neurotransmitters and releasing factors—secreted by the hypothalamus serve as major regulators of anterior pituitary function. The neurosecretory products released into the portal system are technically termed releasing hormones if their chemical structures have been identified and **releasing factors** if there is evidence of their presence but no definitive chemical identification.

When hypothalamic neurons are stimulated and neurosecretory cells respond by releasing hormones, the neurosecretory products are released into the portal circulation and travel to the anterior pituitary. The neurosecretory products apparently bind to plasma membrane receptors in the anterior pituitary, where their action is mediated by cyclic AMP.

The hypothalamus synthesizes and releases hormones that regulate secretion by other glands. These hormones include **prolactin-inhibiting factor** (PIF), **thyrotropin-releasing hormone** (TRH), **gonadotropin-releasing hormone** (GnRH), **somatostatin, growth hormone–releasing factor** (GRF), **corticotropin-releasing hormone** (CRH), and **substance P.** These hormones are summarized in Table 17-5.

Hormones of the Posterior Pituitary

The posterior pituitary secretes two hormones: (1) **antidiuretic hormone (ADH),** also called vasopressin, and (2) **oxytocin.** These peptide hormones are very similar in structure, differing by only two amino acids. They are synthesized, along with their binding proteins, the neurophysins, in the supraoptic and paraventricular nuclei of the hypothalamus (Fig. 17-9). Once synthesized, the hormones and their carrier proteins are packaged in secretory vesicles. They are moved down the axons of the infundibular stem to the infundibular process for storage. The posterior pituitary can thus be seen as a storage and releasing site for hormones synthesized in the hypothalamus.

The release of ADH and oxytocin is mediated by cholinergic and adrenergic neurotransmitters. Stimulation of the cholinergic receptors by acetylcholine, angiotensin II, and beta-endorphins stimulates the release of ADH and oxytocin, whereas activation of beta-adrenergic receptors inhibits hormone secretion. Before release into the circulatory system, ADH and oxytocin are split from the neurophysins and are secreted in unbound form.

Antidiuretic Hormone

The major homeostatic function of the posterior pituitary is the control of plasma osmolality as regulated by ADH, or vasopressin (see Chapter 3). At physiologic levels, ADH acts to increase the permeability of the distal renal tubules and collecting ducts (see Chapter 32). This increased permeability leads to an increase in water reabsorption and the production of more concentrated urine. These effects may be inhibited by hypercalcemia, prostaglandin E, and hypokalemia. ADH has no direct effect on electrolyte levels.

ADH was originally named vasopressin because in extremely high doses, it does cause vasoconstriction and a resulting increase in arterial blood pressure. These levels

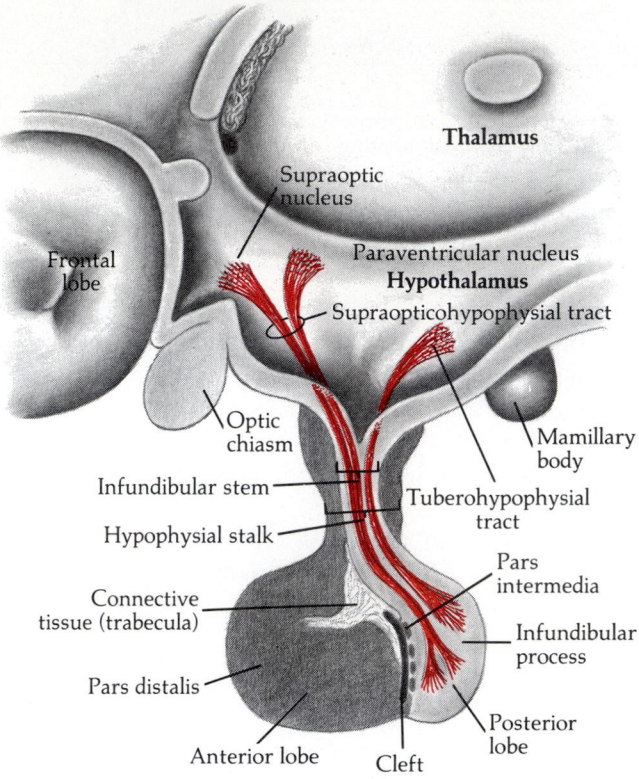

FIG. 17-9. Nerve tracts from hypothalamus to poterior lobe of pituitary gland. (From Thompson et al., 1989.)

are not reached physiologically, but this effect may be achieved pharmacologically. For example, high doses of ADH (as the drug vasopressin) may be administered to achieve hemostasis during hemorrhage.

The secretion of ADH is primarily regulated by the osmoreceptors of the hypothalamus, located near or in the supraoptic nuclei (osmoreceptors are stimulated by increased osmolality). The plasma osmolality is maintained at the mean set point of approximately 280 mOsm/kg. As plasma osmolality increases, the rate of ADH secretion increases.

Other mechanisms affect ADH secretion. ADH secretion is increased by changes in intravascular volume. Intravascular volume changes are monitored by baroreceptors in the right atrium and in the carotid and aortic arches. A volume loss of 7% to 25% acts through these receptors to stimulate ADH secretion. This mechanism for regulating ADH secretion is much less sensitive than that of the osmoreceptors. Stress, trauma, pain, exercise, nausea, nicotine, exposure to heat, and drugs, such as chloroform and morphine, also increase ADH secretion, apparently by activating cholinergic neurotransmitters in the hypothalamus. ADH secretion decreases with a decrease in plasma osmolality, an increase in intravascular volume, hypertension, and alcohol ingestion.

Oxytocin

Oxytocin is responsible for contraction of the uterus and lactation in females and may have a role in sperm motility in males, although this effect has not yet been clearly elucidated. In both men and women, oxytocin has an antidiuretic effect similar to that of ADH. The mechanisms by which this effect is achieved appears similar to those of ADH, but the physiologic significance is not clear. (The function of this hormone is discussed in Chapter 19.)

The release of oxytocin has been studied more extensively in women. In the woman, oxytocin is secreted in response to suckling and mechanical distention of the female reproductive tract. Oxytocin is required for the milk "let down" reflex. Stimulated by sucking, oxytocin binds to its receptors on myoepithelial cells in the mammary tissues and causes contraction of those cells. This results in increased intramammary pressure and milk expression.

Oxytocin also acts on the uterus to stimulate contractions. Its role in initiating labor has been debated, since levels of oxytocin do not increase until near the end of labor. At this stage, oxytocin functions to enhance effectiveness of contractions, to promote delivery of the placenta, and to stimulate postpartum contractions to prevent excessive bleeding (Martin, 1985).

Hormones of the Anterior Pituitary

The anterior pituitary is composed of two main cell types: (1) the **chromophobes,** which appear to be nonsecretory, and (2) the **chromophils,** which are considered the secretory cells of the adenohypophysis. The chromophils are subdivided into six secretory cell types and each cell type secretes specific hormone(s) (Table 17-6).

In general, the regulation of the anterior pituitary hormones is achieved by the following mechanisms: (1) secretion of hypothalamic peptide hormones or releasing factors, (2) feedback effects of the hormones secreted by target glands, and (3) direct effects of other mediating neurotransmitters. (These mechanisms are summarized in Fig. 17-3.)

The hormones secreted by the anterior pituitary include adrenocorticotropic hormone (ACTH), melanocyte-stimulating hormone (MSH), somatotropic hormones (growth hormone and prolactin), and the glycoprotein hormones (follicle-stimulating hormone, luteinizing hormone, and thyroid-stimulating hormone). Each of these hormones affects the physiologic function of specific target organs (see Fig. 17-3 and Table 17-6).

The Thyroid and Parathyroid Glands

The thyroid gland, located in the neck just below the larynx, produces hormones that control the rates of metabolic processes through the body. The parathyroid

TABLE 17-6 Hormones of the anterior pituitary and their functions

Hormone	Secretory cell type	Target organs	Functions
Adrenocorticotropic hormone (ACTH)	Corticotropic	Adrenal gland	Increased steroidogenesis Synthesis of adrenal proteins contributing to maintenance of the adrenal gland
Melanocyte-stimulating hormone (MSH)	Melanotropic	Anterior pituitary	Promotes secretion of melanin and lipotropis by anterior pituitary
Somatomotropic hormones: Growth hormone (GH)	Somatotropic	Muscle, bone, liver	Regulates metabolic processes related to growth and adaptation to physical and emotional stressors including skeletal growth, muscle growth, increased protein synthesis, increased liver glycogenolysis, increased fat mobilization
		Liver	Induces formation of somatomedins, or insulin-like growth factors (IFG) that have actions similar to insulin
Prolactin	Lactotropic	Breast	Lactogenesis
Glycoprotein hormones: Thyroid-stimulating hormone (TSH)	Thyrotropic	Thyroid gland	Increased production and secretion of thyroid hormone Increased iodine uptake
FSH and LH	Gonadotropic	In women: ovarian follicle In men: Leydig cells	Follicular maturation Regulates spermatogenesis

glands are located near the thyroid. The four parathyroid glands function to control serum calcium levels.

The Thyroid Gland

The **thyroid gland** is composed of two lobes that lie on either side of the trachea, inferior to the thyroid cartilage (Fig. 17-10). The lobes are joined by a small band of tissue, the **isthmus,** which crosses the anterior surface of the trachea and larynx at the cricoid cartilage. The normal thyroid gland is not visible on inspection, but it may be palpated on swallowing, which causes upward displacement of the gland.

Microscopically, the thyroid gland is composed of **follicles.** The follicles are composed of follicular cells that surround a viscous substance called colloid. The follicular cells synthesize and secrete some of the thyroid hormones. Neurons terminate on blood vessels within the thyroid gland and on the follicular cells themselves. This anatomic finding suggests that neurotransmitters may directly affect secretory activity of the follicular cells (Ahren, 1986).

Also found in the tissue of the thyroid are parafollicular cells, or **C cells.** The C cells secrete various polypeptides including calcitonin and somatostatin (Ahren, 1986). **Calcitonin,** also called thyrocalcitonin, acts to

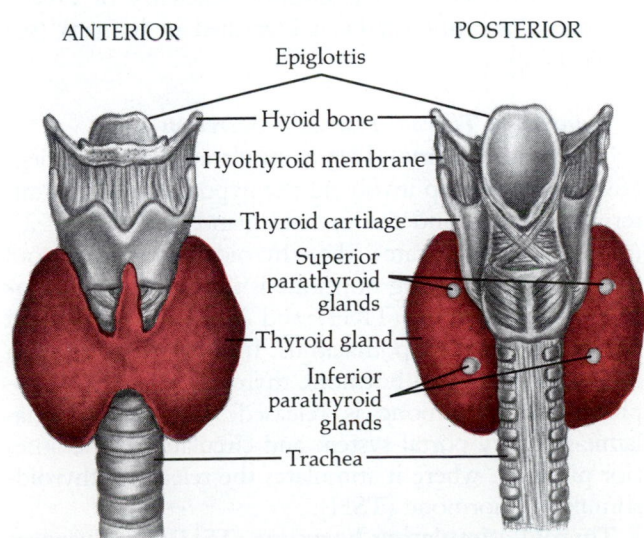

FIG. 17-10. Thyroid and parathyroid glands. Note their location to each other and to the larynx and trachea. (From Thompson et al., 1989.)

TABLE 17-7 Thyroid gland hormones and their regulation and function

Hormone	Regulation	Functions

Thyroxine T_4 and Triiodothyronine (T_3)	T_4 and T_3 levels are controlled by TSH
	Hormones show diurnal variation with a peak during late evening
	Influences on amount secreted
	  Gender
	  Pregnancy
	  Gonadal- and adrenal cortical-increased steroids = ↑ levels
	  Exposure to extreme cold = ↑ levels
	  Nutritional state
	  Chemicals
	    GHIH = ↓ levels
	    Dopamine = ↓ levels
	    Catecholamines = ↑ levels
		Regulates protein, fat, and carbohydrate catabolism in all cells
		Regulates metabolic rate of all cells
		Regulates body heat production
		Insulin antagonist
		Maintains growth hormone secretion, skeletal maturation
		Affects CNS development
		Necessary for muscle tone and vigor
		Mantains cardiac rate, force, and output
		Maintains secretion of GI tract
		Affects respiratory rate and oxygen utilization
		Maintains calcium mobilization
		Affects RBC production
		Stimulates lipid turnover, free fatty acid release, and cholesterol synthesis

Calcitonin	Elevated serum calcium—major stimulant for calcitonin
	Other stimulants
	  Gastrin
	  Calcium-rich foods (regardless of serum Ca^{++} levels)
	  Pregnancy
	Lowered serum calcium—suppresses calcitonin release
		Major function:
		  Lowers serum calcium by opposing bone-resorbing effects of PTH, prostaglandins, and calciferols by inhibiting osteoclastic activity
		  Also lowers serum phosphate levels
		  May also decrease calcium and phosphorus absorption in GI tract

From Phipps, Long, & Woods, 1987.

lower serum calcium by direct, rapid, and significant inhibition of bone resorption and bone-resorbing cells. (Bone resorption is explained in Chapter 21.) The metabolic consequences of calcitonin deficiency or excess, however, have not yet been identified in humans (see Table 17-7).

Regulation of Thyroid Hormone Secretion

Thyroid hormone (TH) is regulated through a negative feedback loop involving the hypothalamus, the anterior pituitary, and the thyroid gland (see Fig. 17-3). (Fig. 17-10 illustrates the thyroid and parathyroid glands.) The initiating hormone is termed **thyrotropin-releasing hormone** (TRH) and it is synthesized and stored within the hypothalamus. In response to a fall in levels of the thyroid hormone thyroxine (T_4), thyrotropin-releasing hormone is released into the hypothalamic-pituitary portal system and circulates to the anterior pituitary, where it stimulates the release of thyroid-stimulating hormone (TSH).

Thyroid-stimulating hormone (TSH) is a glycoprotein hormone synthesized and stored within the anterior pituitary. Once TSH is secreted by the anterior pituitary, it circulates to bind with TSH receptor sites located on the outer side of the thyroid cell's plasma membrane. The effects of TSH on the thyroid include (1) an immediate increase in the release of stored thyroid hormones, (2) an increase in iodine uptake and oxidation, (3) an increase in thyroid hormone synthesis, and (4) an increase in the synthesis and secretion of prostaglandins by the thyroid. Thyroid gland hormones and their regulation and function are summarized in Table 17-7.

When TH is secreted by the thyroid gland, it acts on the thyroid gland, the anterior pituitary, and the median eminence to regulate further TH production. Thyroid hormones have a negative feedback effect and inhibit TRH and TSH, which decreases TH synthesis and secretion.

Synthesis of Thyroid Hormone

The thyroid gland is stimulated to produce thyroid hormone by TSH, by low serum iodide levels, or by drugs interfering with uptake of iodide in the blood by the thyroid gland. The first step in the synthesis of thyroid hormone is the concentration of iodide (an iodine compound) by the thyroid gland. Because there is a iodine concentration gradient of about 30 to 40:1 between the thyroid gland and the blood, iodine is moved by active transport from the extracellular fluid to the thyroid follicular cells. (Mechanisms of active transport are discussed in Chapter 1.) Before using iodide to form TH, however, the iodide must be oxidized to iodine. This reaction is facilitated by the enzyme peroxidase inside the follicular cells. The major naturally occurring source of iodine is seafood; in the United States iodine is added to salt and flour. Approximately 25% of ingested iodine is trapped by the thyroid gland.

For the synthesis of TH to occur, another molecule, thyroglobulin, must also be present. **Thyroglobulin** is a large glycoprotein synthesized within the follicular cell. After its synthesis, the uniodinated thyroglobulin is released into the colloid. Iodine then combines with tyrosine in the thyroglobulin to form iodotyrosines. Two major iodotyrosines are monoiodotyrosine (MIT) with one iodine molecule and diiodotyrosine (DIT) with two iodine molecules. Several hours after the iodotyrosines are formed, coupling of the iodotyrosines takes place to form iodothyronines, two of which are active thyroid hormones. The exact mechanism for this coupling is not clearly understood. The most commonly held view is that two DIT molecules are coupled to form T_4 **(thyroxine),** and one DIT and one MIT molecule are joined to form **triiodothyronine (T_3).** The thyroid gland normally produces 90% T_4 and 10% T_3. In the body tissues, however, T_4 is converted to T_3, and T_3 probably has the greatest metabolic effects. Once released into the circulation, about 99% of T_3 and T_4 is bound by plasma proteins for transport to body tissues.

The Parathyroid Glands

Two pairs of parathyroid glands are normally present. They are small and located behind the upper pole of the thyroid gland and behind the lower pole (Fig. 17-10). The number of parathyroid glands may, however, range from two to six.

The parathyroid glands produce **parathyroid hormone** (PTH), a regulator of serum calcium. PTH is regulated primarily by the level of ionized plasma calcium, although these regulatory mechanisms are not precisely clear. Calcium also increases intraparathyroid destruction of PTH but apparently does not affect the rate of PTH synthesis.

Magnesium and phosphate levels also affect PTH secretion. Hypomagnesemia in individuals with normal calcium levels acts as a mild stimulant to PTH secretion. In hypocalcemic individuals, hypomagnesemia decreases PTH secretion. Hyperphosphatemia leads to hypocalcemia, probably because of calcium-phosphate precipitation in soft tissue and bone. Alterations in serum phosphate levels may therefore indirectly influence PTH secretion by affecting serum calcium levels (Fig. 17-11).

Once the parathyroid gland is stimulated, PTH is secreted. On release, PTH enters the circulation in unbound form. The hormone attaches to plasma membrane receptors in target tissues, where the biologic effects of PTH are primarily mediated by activation of the adenylate cyclase system (see Chapter 1).

PTH is the single most important factor in the regulation of serum calcium levels (Fig. 17-12). To achieve regulation of serum calcium, PTH acts directly on bone

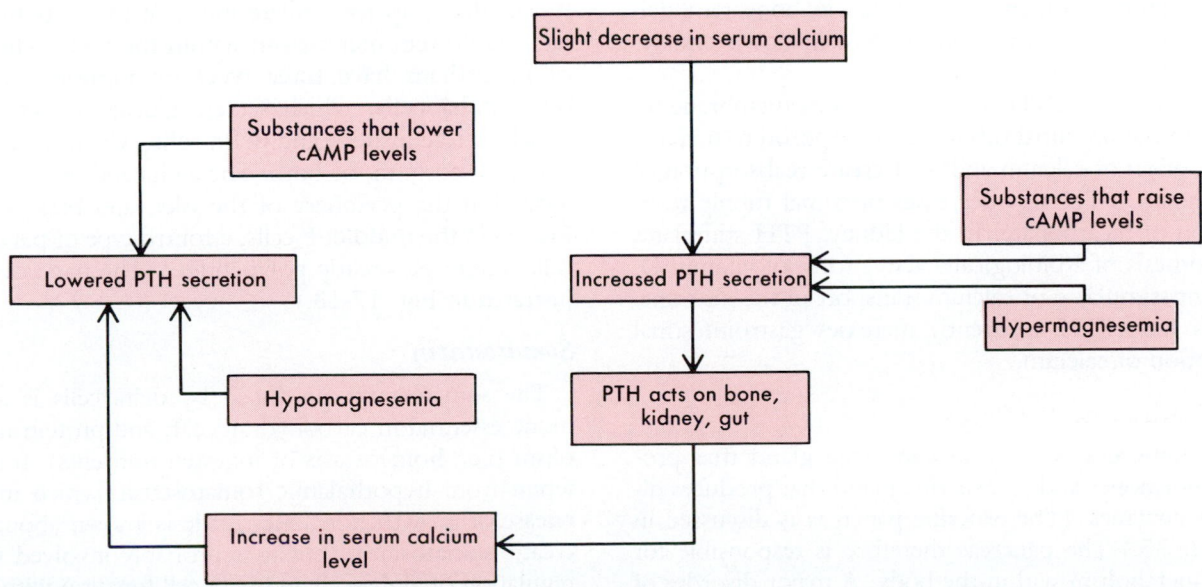

FIG. 17-11. Variables affecting PTH secretion.

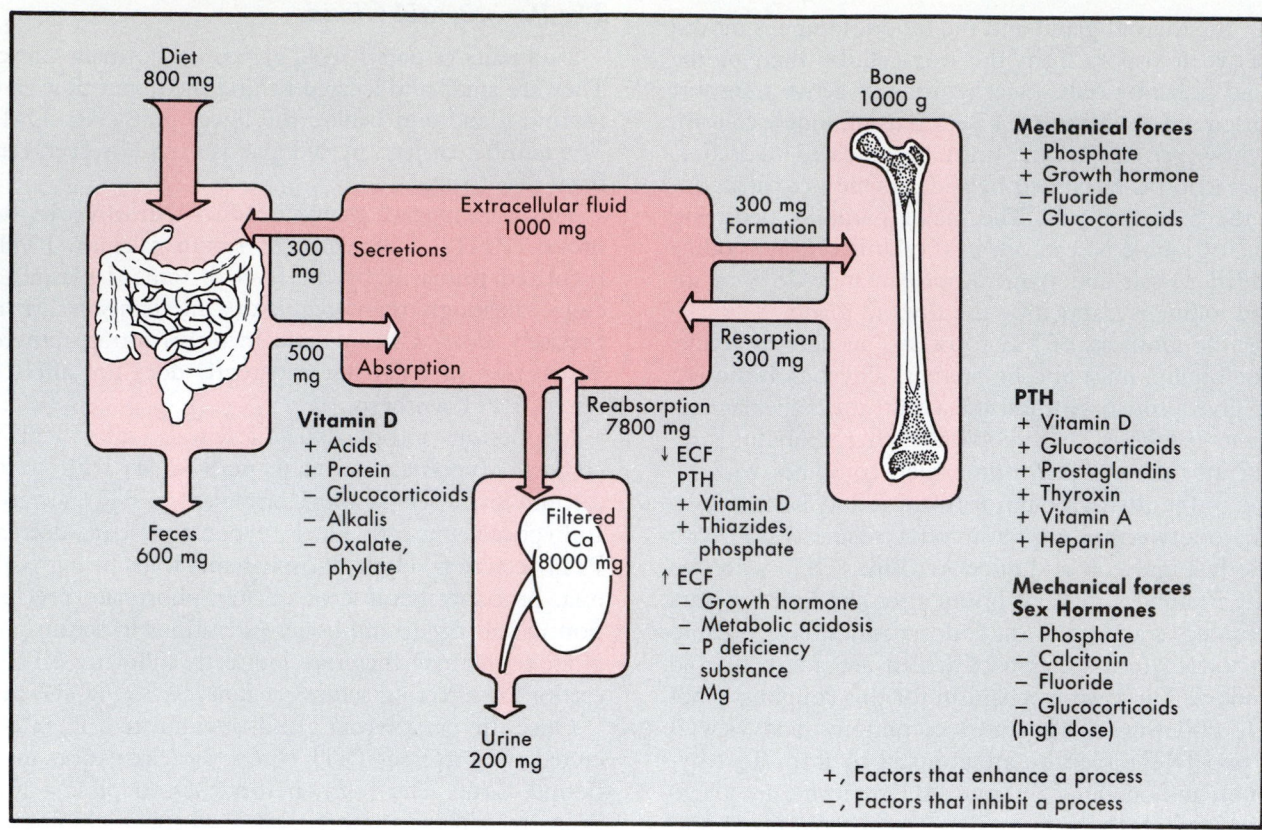

FIG. 17-12. Normal calcium metabolism regulated by PTH. (Adapted from Ezrin, Godden, & Volpe, 1979.)

and on the kidneys. In bone, PTH has at least two effects. The effect of intense acute stimulation involves the breakdown and resorption of bone (see Chapter 21). Chronic stimulation by PTH results in bone remodeling, a process in which bone is broken down and reformed.

In the kidneys, PTH acts on its plasma membrane receptor in the proximal tubule of the nephron to increase reabsorption of calcium and to decrease reabsorption of phosphorus. PTH also decreases proximal tubule reabsorption of bicarbonate. In the kidney, PTH stimulates the synthesis of a biologically active form of vitamin D, a potent stimulator of calcium transport in the intestine. In this way, PTH apparently increases gastrointestinal absorption of calcium.

The Endocrine Pancreas

The **pancreas** is both an endocrine gland that produces hormones and an exocrine gland that produces digestive enzymes. (The exocrine pancreas is discussed in Chapter 35.) The pancreas therefore is responsible for much metabolism within the body. A major disorder of the endocrine pancreas is diabetes mellitus.

The pancreas is located behind the stomach, between the spleen and the duodenum. It houses the **islets of Langerhans,** which secrete **glucagon** and **insulin,** hormones that help to regulate much of the carbohydrate, fat, and protein metabolism within the body. The islets of Langerhans have three types of hormone-secreting cells: **alpha cells,** which secrete glucagon; **beta cells,** which secrete insulin; and **delta cells,** which secrete gastrin, somatostatin, or both. The alpha and delta cells are located at the periphery of the islet, and beta cells are located in the middle. F cells, a fourth type of pancreatic cell, secrete pancreatic polypeptide. (The pancreas is illustrated in Fig. 17-13.)

Somatostatin

The somatostatin produced by delta cells is a hormone essential in carbohydrate, fat, and protein metabolism (i.e., homeostasis of ingested nutrients). It is different from hypothalamic somatostatin, which inhibits release of growth hormone. Little is known about pancreatic somatostatin, but it is probably involved in the regulation of alpha-cell and beta-cell function within the islets. Presumably, somatostatin inhibits both glucagon and insulin secretion.

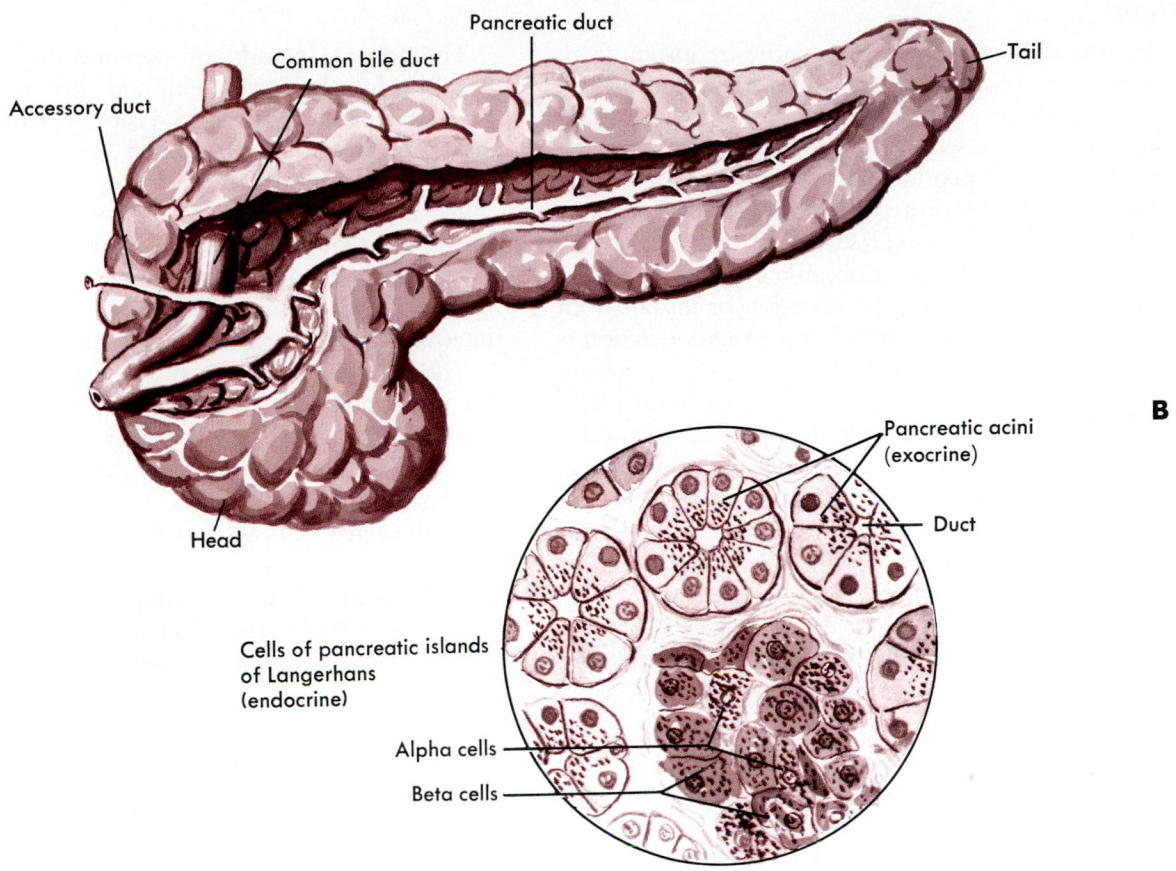

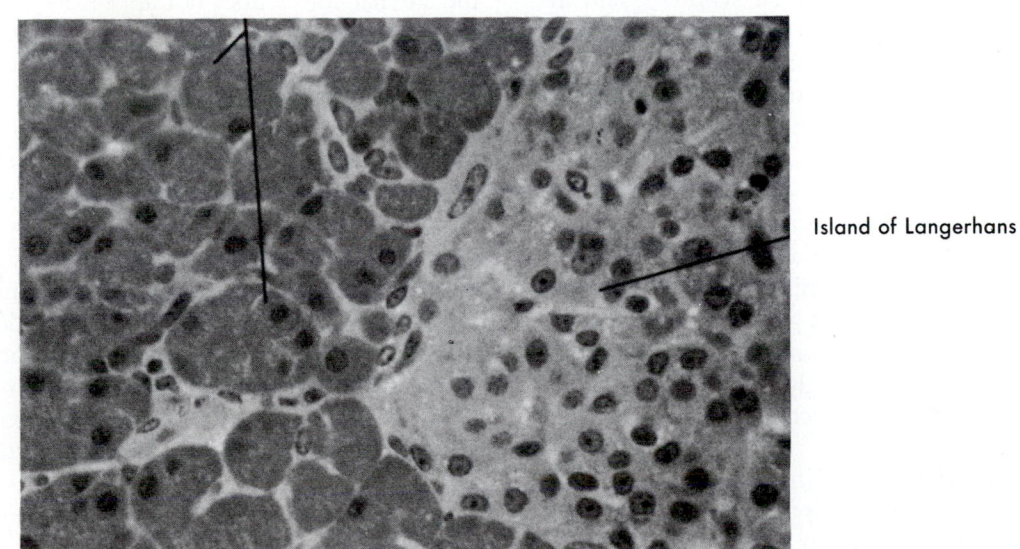

FIG. 17-13. The pancreas. **A,** Pancreas dissected to show main and accessory ducts. **B,** Exocrine and endocrine glandular cells. Alpha endocrine cells secrete glucagon and beta cells secrete insulin. **C,** Photo micrograph of pancreas showing pancreatic islands and adjacent exocrine cells (×150). (From Thibodeau, 1987.)

Insulin

The beta cells of the pancreas synthesize insulin from the precursor, proinsulin. Proinsulin is formed from a larger and earlier precursor molecule, preproinsulin. Proinsulin is composed of an A peptide and a B peptide connected by a C peptide and two disulfide bonds. C peptide is cleaved by proteolytic enzymes, leaving the A and B peptide chain connected by the disulfide bonds. The bonded A and B chains become insulin.

Several factors regulate the secretion of insulin from beta cells in the islets of Langerhans. Insulin secretion is promoted by increased blood levels of glucose, amino acids (arginine and glucagon), and gastrointestinal hormones and by sympathetic stimulation of the beta cells. Insulin secretion diminishes in response to low blood levels of glucose (hypoglycemia), high levels of insulin (through negative feedback to the beta cells), and sympathetic stimulation of the alpha cells in the islets. Prostaglandins also may inhibit insulin secretion (Felig, 1985).

Insulin is an anabolic hormone that promotes the synthesis of proteins, carbohydrates, lipids, and nucleic acids. The major sites of insulin-promoted synthesis are the liver, muscle, and adipose tissue. The brain and red blood cells are not sensitive to insulin. In the liver, insulin increases glucose uptake; stimulates synthesis of glycogen and fatty acids; and inhibits gluconeogenesis (glucose formation), glycogenolysis (the splitting of glycogen to form glucose), and ketogenesis (formation of ketones from fats). In muscle, insulin increases uptake of glucose and amino acids; increases glycogen synthesis, stimulates protein synthesis, and inhibits protein breakdown (proteolysis). In adipose tissue, insulin increases glucose uptake, stimulates fat synthesis, and inhibits fat breakdown (lipolysis). The net effect of insulin in these tissues is to stimulate cellular metabolism. Overall, however, the major consequence of insulin release is to decrease blood glucose. Insulin also facilitates the intracellular transport of potassium.

Glucagon

Glucagon is produced by the alpha cells of the pancreas and by a number of cells lining the gastrointestinal tract. High glucose levels cause glucagon release to be inhibited; low glucose levels promote glucagon release. Amino acids, such as alanine, glycine, and asparagine, serve to stimulate glucagon secretion. A protein-rich meal has the same effect.

Glucagon acts primarily in the liver and increases blood glucose by stimulating glycogenolysis and gluconeogenesis. Glucagon acts as an antagonist to insulin. Much controversy exists regarding the role of glucagon in carbohydrate regulation, both normally and in diabetes mellitus. Glucagon also stimulates lipolysis, which has a ketogenic effect from the metabolism of free fatty acids by the liver.

The Adrenal Glands

The **adrenal glands** are pyramid-shaped organs located behind the peritoneum and close to each kidney. Each gland is surrounded by a capsule, embedded in fat, and well supplied with blood vessels. Each adrenal gland consists of two separate portions—an inner medulla and an outer cortex. These two portions have different embryonic origins, different structures, and different hormonal functions. In effect, each adrenal gland functions like two separate glands, although there are interrelationships between functions of each portion.

The adrenal glands are paired glands; one is located at the upper pole of each kidney. Each gland weighs from 4 to 5 g in the adult. The adrenal glands have an abundant blood supply from the phrenic and renal arteries, the aorta, and other arteries. Venous return on the left is to the renal vein and on the right is to the inferior vena cava.

Each adrenal gland is composed of a cortex and a medulla (Fig. 17-14). The **adrenal cortex,** or outer region of the gland, accounts for 80% of the weight of the adult gland. The cortex is histologically subdivided into three zones. The outer layer, the **zona glomerulosa,** constitutes approximately 15% of the cortex and primarily produces the mineralocorticoid, aldosterone. The middle zona, the **fasciculata** (78% of the cortex) and the inner zona, the **reticularis** (7% of the cortex), secrete the mineralocorticoids, the adrenal androgens and estrogens, and the glucocorticoids. The **adrenal medulla,** accounting for 20% of the gland's total weight, secretes the catecholamines epinephrine, norepinephrine, and dopamine. Both sympathetic and parasympathetic cholinergic fibers innervate the adrenal medulla; the adrenal cortex does not appear to be directly innervated.

Adrenal Cortex

The adrenal cortex secretes several steroid hormones, including the glucocorticoids, the mineralocorticoids, and the adrenal androgens and estrogens. These hormones are all synthesized from cholesterol. The cells of the adrenal cortex must be stimulated by the extraadrenal regulator, **adrenocorticotropic hormone** (ACTH), for cholesterol to be used in steroidogenesis. Steroidogenesis is not totally dependent on ACTH, but there appears to be an ACTH-independent baseline glucocorticoid secretion of 3% to 10% (Neville & O'Hare, 1982). The best known pathway of steroidogenesis involves the conversion of cholesterol to pregnenolone, which is then converted to the major corticosteroids (Fig. 17-15).

Little storage of the steroid hormones occurs in the adrenal gland. The adrenal cortex also contains a high concentration of ascorbic acid and vitamin A; the functional roles within the adrenal glands are not known at present.

FIG. 17-14. Structure of the adrenal gland showing cell layers (zona) of the cortex. Zona glomerulosa secretes aldosterone. Zona fasiculata secretes abundant amounts of glucocorticoids, chiefly cortisol. Zona reticularis secretes minute amounts of sex hormones and glucocorticoids. A portion of the medulla is visible at lower right in the photomicrograph (×35) and at the bottom of the drawing. (From Thibodeau, 1987.)

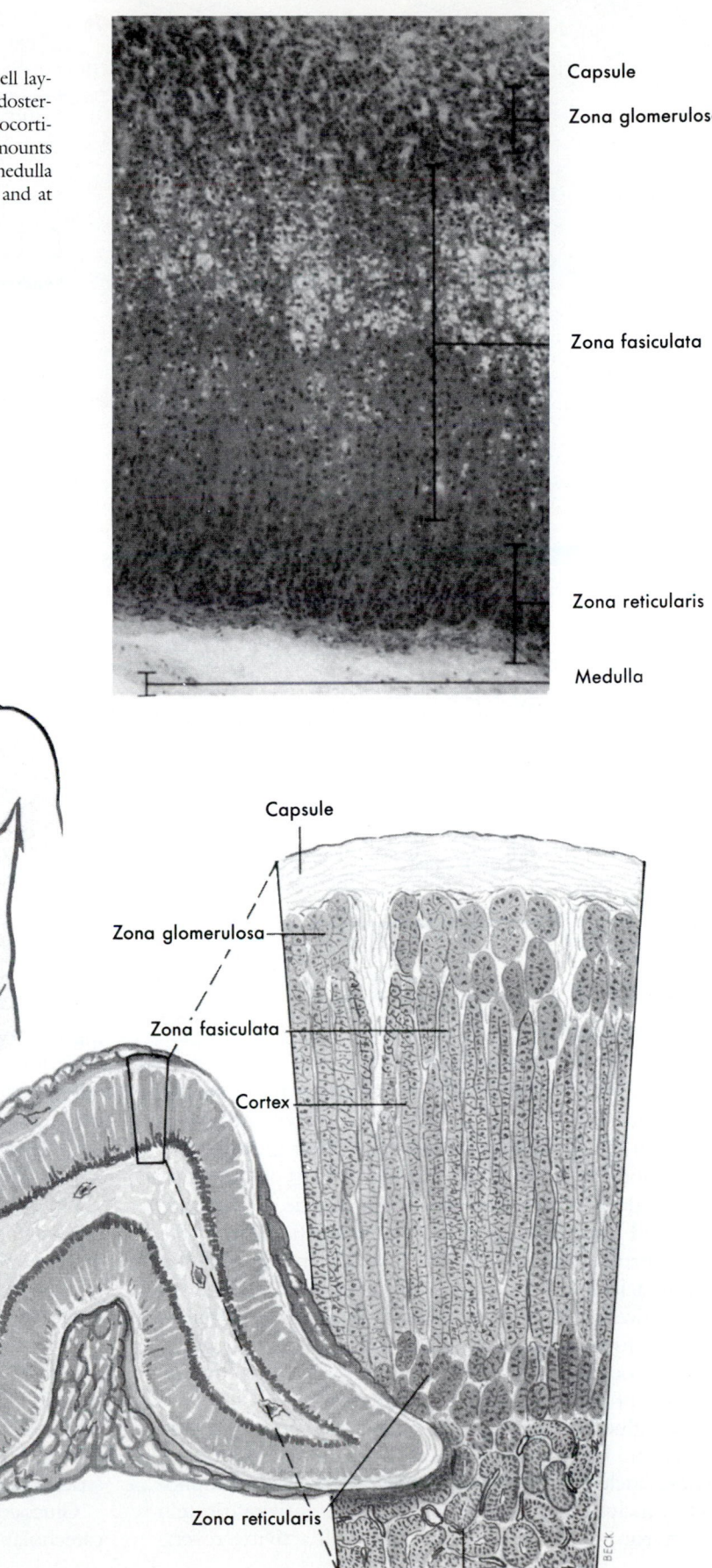

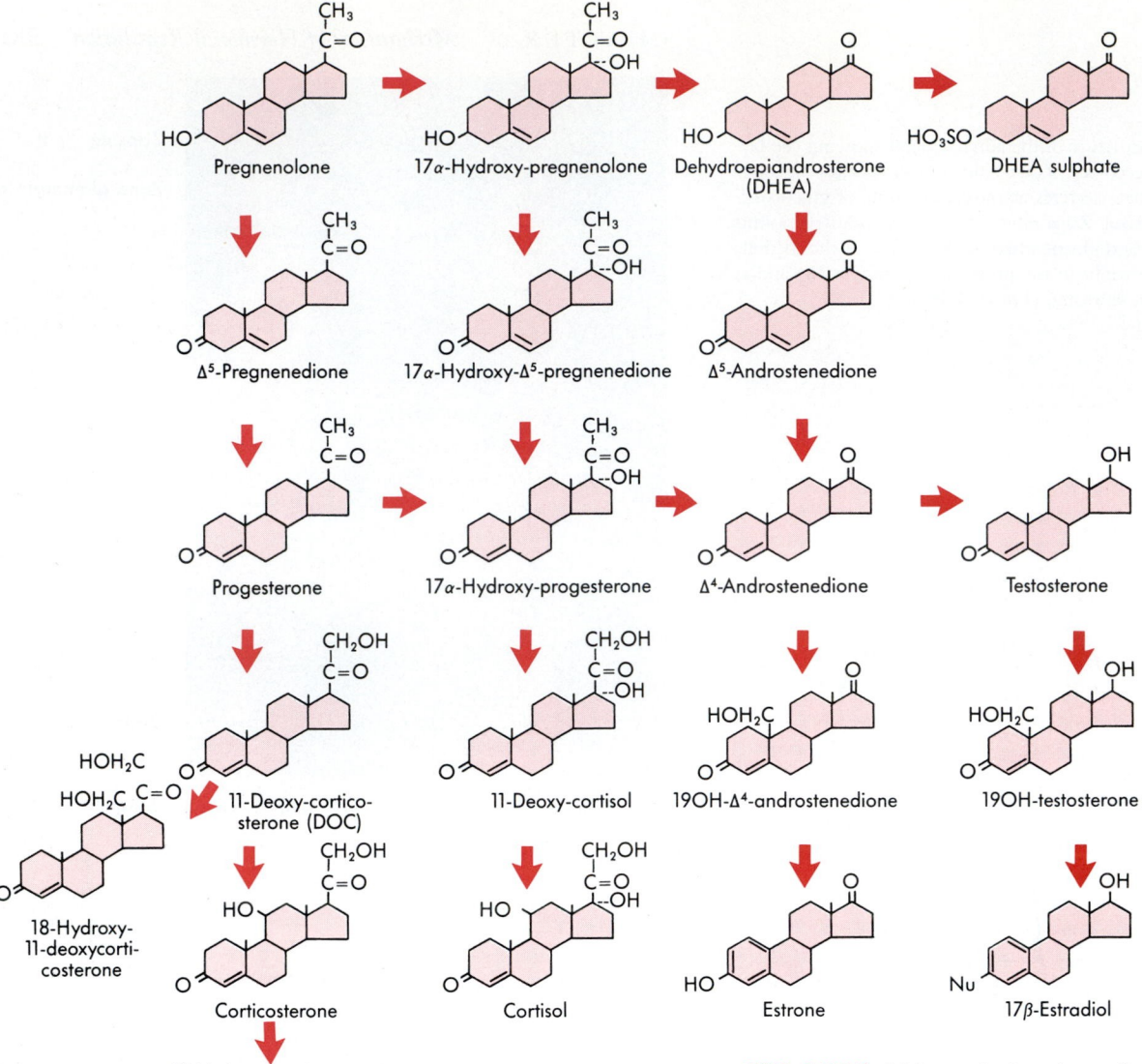

FIG. 17-15. Major synthetic pathways for adrenal steroids.

Pregnenolone • 17α-Hydroxy-pregnenolone • Dehydroepiandrosterone (DHEA) • DHEA sulphate

Δ⁵-Pregnenedione • 17α-Hydroxy-Δ⁵-pregnenedione • Δ⁵-Androstenedione

Progesterone • 17α-Hydroxy-progesterone • Δ⁴-Androstenedione • Testosterone

11-Deoxy-cortico-sterone (DOC) • 11-Deoxy-cortisol • 19OH-Δ⁴-androstenedione • 19OH-testosterone

18-Hydroxy-11-deoxycorti-costerone • Corticosterone • Cortisol • Estrone • 17β-Estradiol

18-Hydroxy-corticosterone

aldosterone

Glucocorticoids

Functions of the Glucocorticoids

The term **glucocorticoid** is applied to those steroid hormones that have direct effects on carbohydrate metabolism. These hormones increase blood glucose concentration by promoting gluconeogenesis in the liver and by decreasing use of glucose in muscle, adipose tissue, and lymphatic tissue. In extrahepatic tissues, the glucocorticoids stimulate protein catabolism and inhibit amino acid uptake and protein synthesis. In hepatic tissue, however, glucocorticoids act primarily to stimulate glucose formation and synthesis of enzymes that mediate glucocorticoid effects. The ultimate effect on the body is protein breakdown (catabolism).

The glucocorticoids act at several sites to inhibit immune and inflammatory reactions (described in Unit 3). These include depressing proliferation of T lymphocytes, including those that produce the antiviral protein interferon; decreasing natural killer cell activity; revers-

ing macrophage activity; and suppressing the synthesis, secretion, and actions of chemical mediators involved in inflammatory and immune responses. These chemical mediators include prostaglandins, leukotrienes, bradykinin, serotonin, and histamine (Munck, Guyre, & Holbrook, 1984).

Other actions of the glucocorticoids include increasing circulating erythrocytes, leading to polycythemia; increasing the appetite; promoting fat deposits in the face and cervical areas; increasing uric acid excretion; decreasing serum calcium levels, possibly by inhibiting gastrointestinal absorption of calcium; suppressing the secretion and synthesis of ACTH; and suppressing growth hormone secretion so that somatic growth is inhibited. The glucocorticoids also have important "permissive" effects, sensitizing arterioles to the vasoconstrictive effects of norepinephrine.

Glucocorticoids appear to potentiate the effects of catecholamines, thyroid hormone, and growth hormone on adipose tissue. It has also been speculated that a metabolite of cortisol may act like a barbiturate and depress nerve cell function in the brain. This may account for the noted effects on mood associated with steroid fluctuation in disease or stress (Tepperman, 1987).

Cortisol

The most potent of the naturally occurring glucocorticoids is **cortisol.** It is the main secretory product of the adrenal cortex and is necessary for the maintenance of life and for protection from stress (see p. 586 and Chapter 9, Fig. 9-1). Cortisol has a biologic half-life of approximately 90 minutes, with the liver primarily responsible for its deactivation.

The secretion of cortisol is regulated primarily by the hypothalamus and the anterior pituitary gland (Fig. 17-16). In the hypothalamus, corticotropin-releasing hormone (CRH) is produced in several nuclei and stored in the median eminence. Once released, CRH travels through the portal vessels to stimulate the production of ACTH, beta-lipotropin, gamma-lipotropin, endorphins, and enkephalins by the anterior pituitary. ACTH is the main regulator of cortisol secretion and adrenocortical growth.

Three factors appear to be primarily involved in regulating the secretion of ACTH: (1) high circulating levels of cortisol and synthetic glucocorticoids suppress both CRH and ACTH, whereas low cortisol levels stimulate their secretion; (2) diurnal rhythms affect ACTH and cortisol levels (in individuals with regular sleep-wake patterns, ACTH peaks 3 to 5 hours after sleep begins and declines throughout the day), and cortisol levels follow a similar pattern; and (3) stress has been shown to increase ACTH secretion, leading to increased cortisol levels. (Neurologic mechanisms regulating sleep are discussed in Chapter 13.) A form of ACTH (e.g., ir ACTH) is also produced by the cells of the immune system. It is detectable through laboratory techniques, and it physiologically appears to exert the usual feedback effects (see Chapter 9). This mechanism may account, in part, for integration of the immune and endocrine systems.

Once ACTH is secreted, it binds to specific plasma membrane receptors on the cells of the adrenal cortex and on other extraadrenal tissues. Since both adrenal and extraadrenal tissues have ACTH receptors, a number of effects result from stimulation by ACTH. (These are summarized in the box on p. 584.) Both adrenal and extraadrenal effects appear to be mediated through the activation of the adenylate cyclase system. The most well-known extraadrenal effect is melanocyte stimulation, which causes increased pigmentation (Franco-Saenz et al., 1986).

Once ACTH stimulates the cells of the adrenal cortex, cortisol synthesis and secretion immediately occur. In the normal individual, the secretory patterns of ACTH and cortisol are nearly identical. After secretion, most cortisol circulates in bound form. Fifteen percent to 30% is bound to albumin, and 55% to 75% is tightly but reversibly bound to a plasma glycoprotein, transcortin, or corticosteroid-binding globulin. Transcortin levels are significantly elevated by increased estrogen levels

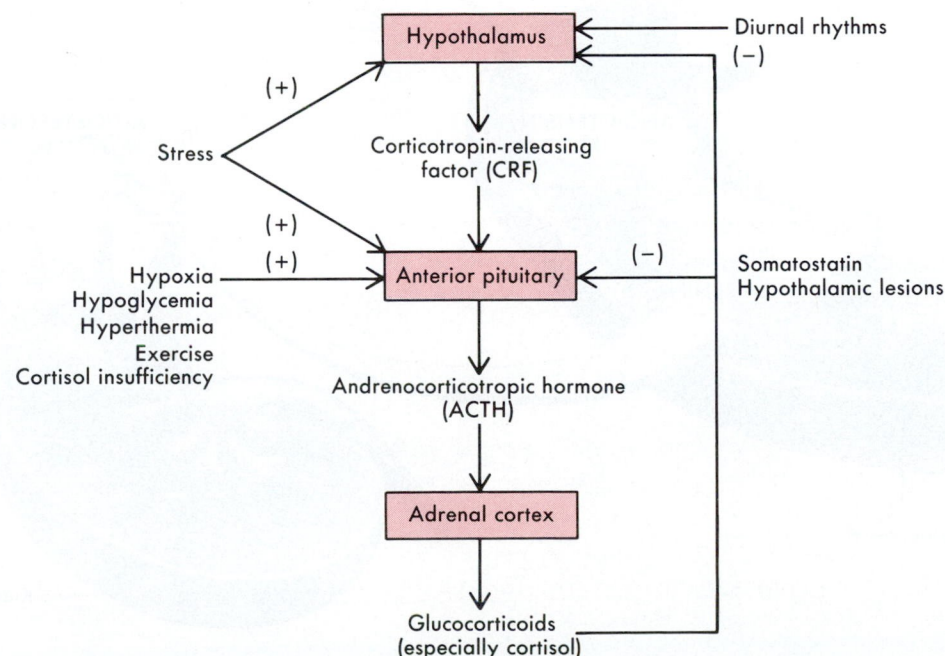

FIG. 17-16. Feedback control of glucocorticoid synthesis and secretion.

Effects of ACTH

ADRENAL
Maintenance of gland size
Depletion of ascorbic acid
Activation of adenylate cyclase
Conversion of cholesterol to pregnenolone
Maintenance of enzymes active in converting
    pregnenolone to other steroids
Accumulation of cholesterol
Secretion of cortisol and adrenal androgens

EXTRAADRENAL
Melanocyte stimulation
Activation of tissue lipase

Mineralocorticoids: Aldosterone

Mineralocorticoid is the term applied to those steroids that directly affect ion transport by epithelial cells, causing sodium retention and potassium and hydrogen loss. **Aldosterone** is the most potent of the naturally occurring mineralocorticoids. The primary role of aldosterone is to conserve sodium. This is accomplished by increasing the activity of the sodium pump of the epithelial cells. (The sodium pump is described in Chapter 1.)

The initial stages of aldosterone synthesis occur in the zona fasciculata and zona reticularis. The final conversion of corticosterone to aldosterone, however, is apparently confined to the zona glomerulosa. Aldosterone synthesis and secretion are primarily regulated by the renin-angiotensin system (described in Chapter 32), although other factors also may be involved. Sodium and potassium levels may directly affect aldosterone secretion, although the mechanisms involved are not understood. ACTH may transiently stimulate aldosterone synthesis but does not appear to be a major regulator of aldosterone secretion.

Aldosterone secretion is stimulated by angiotensin, which is converted by renin to angiotensin I and then to angiotensin II and III (see Chapter 32). Once angioten-

that occur with pregnancy and hormone therapy. Ten percent to 15% of the cortisol secreted circulates unbound. The unbound portion is free to diffuse into cells, but only those cells with specific intracellular glucocorticoid receptors respond to cortisol stimulation. ACTH is rapidly inactivated in the circulation, and the liver and kidneys remove the deactivated hormone.

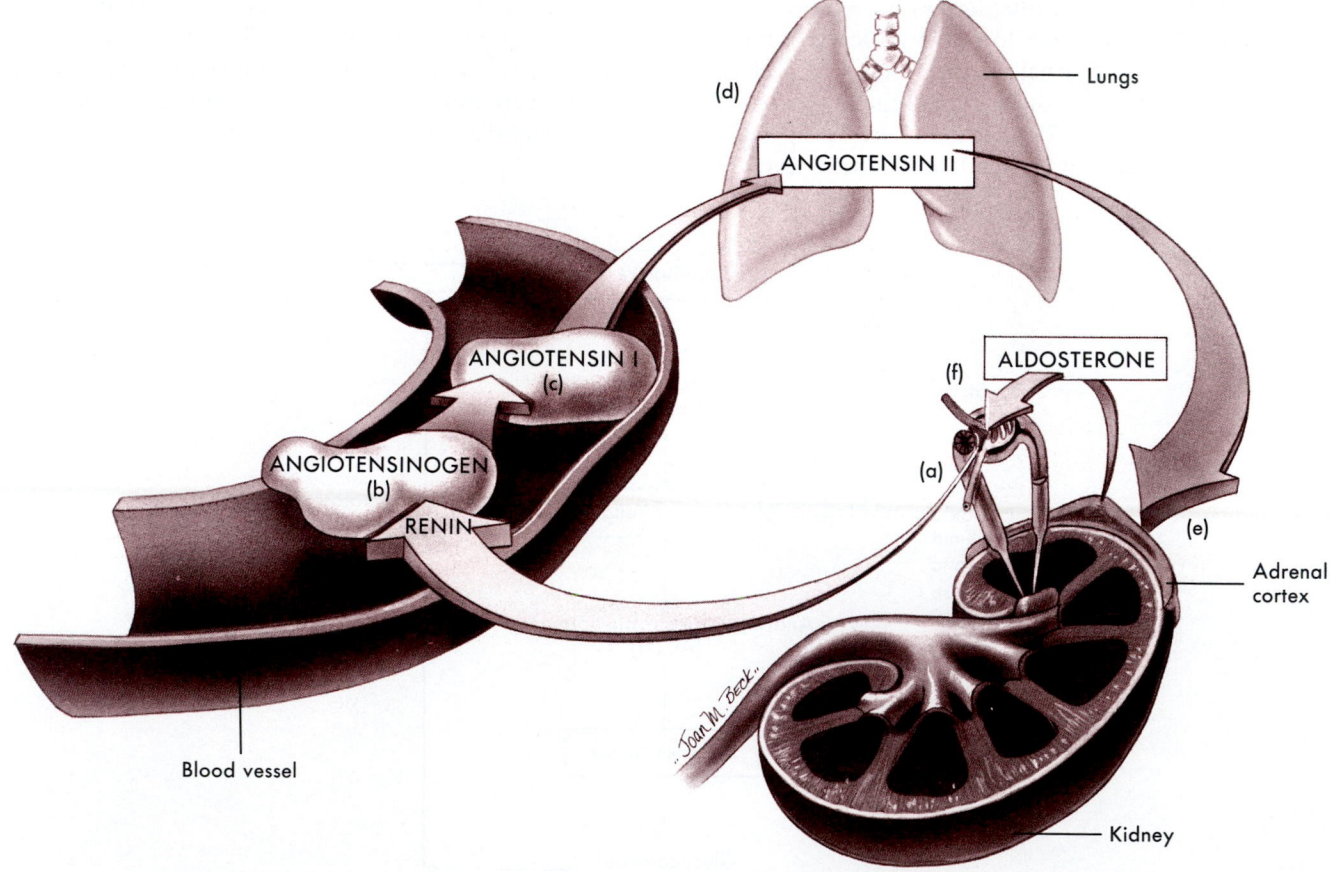

FIG. 17-17. Renin-angiotensin mechanisms for regulating aldosterone secretion. (From Thibodeau, 1987.)

sin II and III are formed, they appear to stimulate aldosterone synthesis (Fig. 17-17). The renin-angiotensin system is primarily activated by sodium and water depletion and a diminished effective blood volume. (The postulated relationships among these factors are summarized in Fig. 17-18.)

When sodium and potassium levels are within normal limits, approximately 50 to 250 mg of aldosterone is secreted daily. Fifty percent to 75% of the secreted aldosterone binds to plasma proteins, including albumin, transcortin, and an alpha₁-acid glycoprotein (AAG). The relatively large proportion of unbound aldosterone contributes to its rapid metabolic turnover in the liver, its low plasma concentration, and its short half-life of approximately 15 minutes. The main site of aldosterone degradation is the liver, with the metabolic end products excreted by the kidney.

The mechanism for aldolsterone action involves, like that of other steroid hormones, binding to a nuclear binding site and acting to alter protein production in the target cell. In the kidney, aldosterone acts on the ascending portion of the loop of Henle, the distal predominantly convoluted tubule, and the collecting ducts to increase sodium ion reabsorption and increase potassium and hydrogen ion excretion. (Kidney function is discussed in Chapter 32.) This renal effect takes 90 minutes to 6 hours to occur after stimulation by aldosterone. Other effects of aldosterone include enhancement

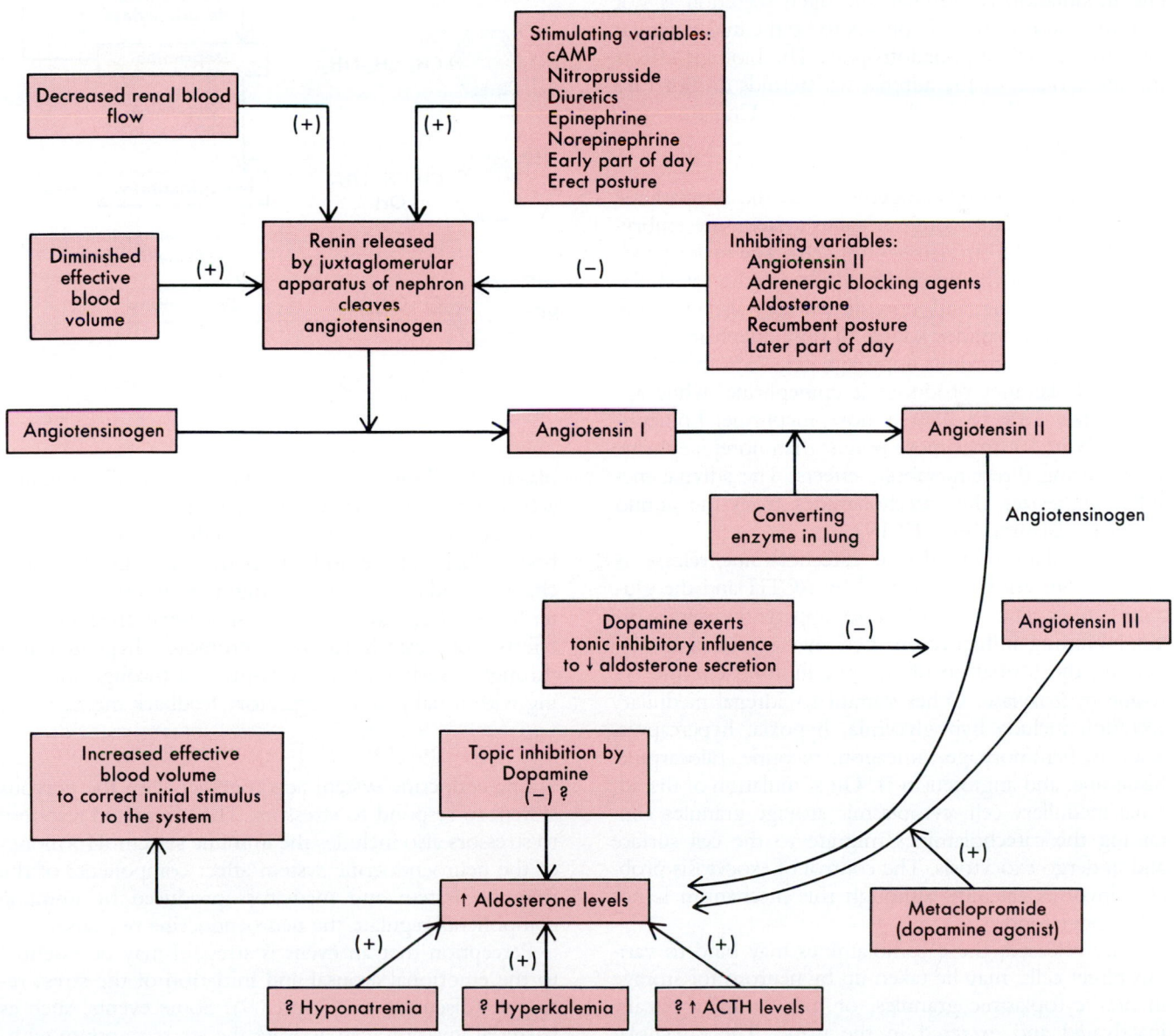

FIG. 17-18. The feedback mechanisms regulating aldosterone secretion.

of cardiac muscle concentration and possible stimulation of ectopic ventricular activity, secondary cardiac pacemakers in the ventricles.

Adrenal Estrogens and Androgens

Estrogen secretion by the normal adrenal cortex is so minimal as to be considered physiologically unimportant. The adrenal cortex also secretes androgens. Some of the weakly androgenic substances secreted by the cortex are then converted by peripheral tissues to stronger androgens, such as testosterone, thus accounting for some androgenic effect initiated by the adrenal cortex. An increased capacity for peripheral conversion of adrenal androgens to estrogens occurs in particular cases, however, including aging, obesity, liver disease, and hyperthyroidism (Genazzani, Thijssen, & Siiteri, 1980). The modulation of adrenal androgen secretion is not well understood. ACTH appears to be the major regulator rather than the gonadotropins. The biologic effects and metabolism of the adrenal sex steroids do not vary from those produced by the gonads (see Unit 7).

Adrenal Medulla

The adrenal medulla, together with the sympathetic divisions of the autonomic nervous system, are embryonically derived from neural crest cells. The major products secreted by the adrenal medulla are the catecholamines epinephrine and norepinephrine, although the medulla is only a minor source of norepinephrine.

In the adrenal medulla approximately 75% to 85% of the catecholamines produced is epinephrine, while approximately 15% to 25% is norepinephrine. Epinephrine is about 10 times more potent than norepinephrine in producing direct metabolic effects. The adrenal medulla synthesizes the catecholamines from the amino acid phenylalanine (Fig. 17-19).

The regulation of adrenal catecholamine release is complex. Secretion is increased by ACTH and the glucocorticoids. The catecholamines apparently exert a direct inhibiting influence on their own secretion by decreasing the formation of the rate-limiting enzyme tyrosine hydroxylase. Other stimuli to adrenal medullary secretion include hypoglycemia, hypoxia, hypercapnia, acidosis, hemmorhage, glucagon, nicotine, pilocarpine, histamine, and angiotensin II. On stimulation of the adrenal medullary cell, cytoplasmic storage granules containing the catecholamines migrate to the cell surface and undergo exocytosis. The control of exocytosis probably involves calcium, although this mechanism is not fully understood.

Once released, the catecholamines may bind to various target cells, may be taken up by neurons for storage in new cytoplasmic granules, or may be metabolically inactivated and excreted in the urine. The catecholamines exert their biologic effects after binding to a

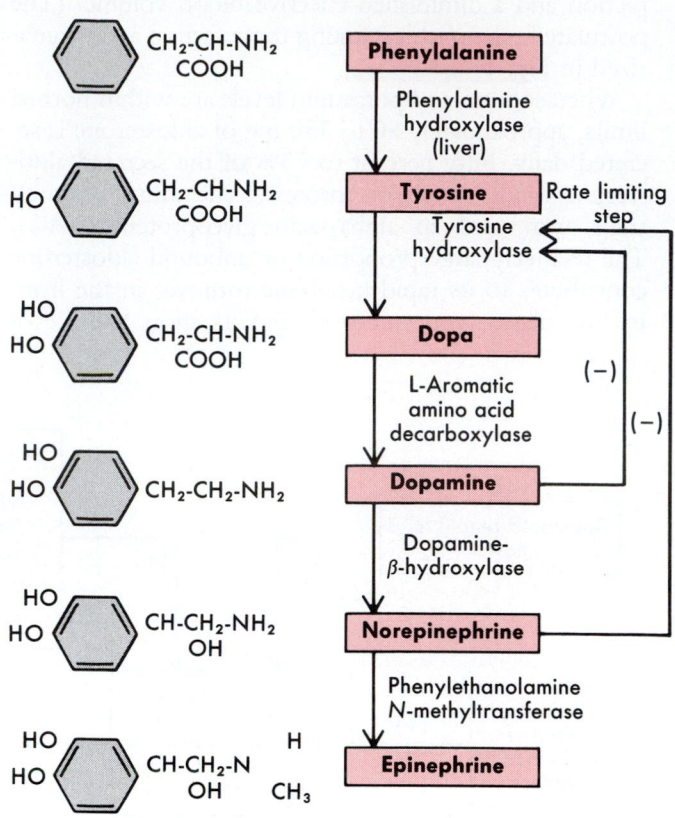

FIG. 17-19. Synthesis of catecholamines.

plasma membrane receptor in target cells. This binding activates the adenylase cyclase system.

Catecholamines have diverse effects on the entire body. Their release and the body's response has been characterized as the "fight or flight" response (see Chapter 9, Fig. 9-1, and Table 9-2). In general, the metabolic effects of catecholamines promote hyperglycemia through a variety of mechanisms and through interfering with usual glucose regulatory feedback mechanisms.

The Neuroendocrine Response to Stressors

The endocrine system acts together with the nervous system to respond to stressors. The integrated response to stressors also includes the immune system. Hormones of the neuroendocrine system affect components of the immune system and mediators produced by immune components regulate the neuroendocrine response.

Perception that an event is stressful may be essential to the emotional arousal and initiation of the stress response (discussed in Chapter 9). Some events, such as bacterial invasion, can activate the stress response without emotional arousal. The hypothalamus receives input from a variety of areas within the brain and ultimately directs the neuroendocrine response to stress. In addition to the neuroendocrine components of the stress response, the gamma motor neuron system is activated to increase skeletal motor tone. The neuroendocrine response to stressors involves two components: (1) activation of the sympathetic division of the autonomic nervous system and (2) activation of the endocrine system, particularly the adrenal cortex.

Activation of the sympathetic nervous system results in immediate release of norepinephrine from adrenergic nerve terminals throughout the body. (The effects of sympathetic stimulation are discussed in Chapter 12.) Because the adrenal gland is directly innervated by the sympathetic nervous system, activation of the sympathetic nervous system results in exocytosis of epinephrine and some norepinephrine from the adrenal medulla, as well as an increase in catecholamine synthesis by medullary cells. The sympathetic effects of nervous system activation are sustained by the release of epinephrine and norepinephrine. Catecholamine release, both locally and systemically, causes activation of alpha 1 and 2 and beta 1 and 2 receptors, generating the "fight or flight" response.

The adrenal cortex is also stimulated through hormones of the hypothalamus and anterior pituitary, causing release of cortisol and aldosterone. Cortisol secretion, which leads to hyperglycemia and immune suppression, appears to be an absolute requirement for mounting an effective response to stressful situations. Cortisol secretion enhances and prolongs the elevation of blood glucose levels, initially achieved by epinephrine and norepinephrine. Other hormones secreted in response to stressors that contribute to hyperglycemia include glucagon and growth hormone. Insulin secretion is decreased as a result of sympathetic stimulation. The maintenance of hyperglycemia is considered adaptive in stressful situations, since glucose provides a ready energy source for the brain, heart, and other vital organs. In prolonged severe stress, however, severe hyperglycemia may cause hyperosmolality (see Chapter 3). Hyperosmolality is considered maladaptive because it adversely affects water and electrolyte balance, as well as brain function.

Increased cortisol secretion is also associated with suppression of the immune system (see Chapter 9). The beneficial effects of immune suppression during the stress response have not been appreciated until recently. In the absence of cortisol, the immune system's response to stressors may "overshoot" the body's need for the inflammatory defense mechanisms of the immune response (see Chapter 6). This overshooting may lead to such adverse effects as tissue destruction, severe vasodilation, and the initiation of an autoimmune reaction. Cortisol prevents overshooting by the immune system

and serves to stabilize the immune response. With long-term stimulation of the adrenal cortex and chronically elevated cortisol levels, however, this adaptive response may become maladaptive, severely suppressing the immune system and increasing the risk for serious infection (Munck et al., 1984). Secretion of aldosterone by the adrenal cortex contributes to increased blood volume by causing increased sodium absorption. Antidiuretic hormone (ADH) secretion by the posterior pituitary enhances renal reabsorption of water, which also increases blood volume.

In addition to the altered secretion patterns of the catecholamines, cortisol, aldosterone, ADH, insulin, growth hormone, and glucagon, secretion of prolactin, testosterone, follicle-stimulating hormone (FSH), and luteinizing hormone (LH) are also affected. Prolactin levels apparently increase, whereas testosterone, FSH, and LH levels decline. The contribution of these changes to the stress response is not clear at present.

The neuroendocrine response to stressful stimuli may vary according to the duration and frequency of the individual's exposure to the stressor. If an individual is exposed to a new stressor for a brief interval, the stress response occurs. This allows the individual to maintain a steady state for the duration of the acute stressor. If an individual is exposed to a chronic, intermittent stressor (that is, a discrete stimulus presented repeatedly but not continuously), the initial response is similar to the response to a new stressor. Within a few days to several weeks, however, an anticipatory response to the stressor develops so that the maximal response occurs before exposure to the stressor. Such a phenomenon may represent adaptation to the stressor. If exposure to the stressor continues, the cortisol response becomes blunted, although the catecholamine responses do not diminish. Exposure to a new stressor in already stressed individuals results in an immediate and supranormal stress response, although the blunted and anticipatory response to the chronic intermittent stressor is maintained. If exposure to a stressor is continuous and unabated, cortisol and catecholamine secretion are maximal until the stressor is removed, until the threat is no longer perceived as stressful, or until exhaustion and death occur.

Tests of Endocrine Function

Tests of the endocrine system involve several general types of clinical evaluation. Measurement of hormone level is accomplished by radioimmunoassay (RIA), enzyme-linked immunosorbent assay (ELISA), and less commonly by bioassay. **Radioimmunoassay (RIA)** is an immunologic technique in which known amounts of antibody and radiolabeled hormone are placed in an assay tube with the unlabeled hormone. The radiolabeled hormone competes chemically with the nonlabeled hormone molecules for binding sites on the antibodies.

When increasing amounts of unlabeled hormones are added to the assay, the limited binding sites of the antibody can bind less of the radiolabeled hormone. Therefore, the higher the concentration of unlabeled hormone, the fewer the number of radioactive "counts," or labeled hormone, that bind to the fixed concentration of antibody. A quantitative value is established by use of standard reference curves.

Enzyme-linked immunosorbent assays (ELISA) are also used to determine circulating hormone levels. The method is similar to that of RIA but is less expensive and easier to conduct. Instead of using radiolabeled hormones, an enzyme-labeled hormone is used. The enzyme activity in either the bound or unbound fraction is determined and related to the concentration of the unlabeled hormone.

A **bioassay** involves using graded doses of hormone in a reference preparation and then comparing the effect of an unkown sample to this reference. Bioassays are used more commonly in investigative endocrinology than in clinical laboratories.

The major problems in evaluating the endocrine system include these: (1) the complexity of the clinical presentation owing to multiple organ system involvement, (2) the nonspecific nature of complaints frequently associated with endocrine dysfunction, and (3) the inappropriate use of interpretation of laboratory tests.

AGING AND THE ENDOCRINE SYSTEM

The precise relationships between aging and the endocrine system are not clear. Perhaps most important, the question of whether changes in endocrine function are a consequence or a cause of aging has yet to be resolved. These relationships have been difficult to identify, in part because of a number of age-related variables that may coexist, such as acute and chronic nonendocrine disease, use of medications, alterations in diet, body composition and weight, and changes in sleep-wake cycles (Blackman, 1987).

Theories about the Effects of Aging

Investigation into the role of the endocrine glands and their interactions in the aging process has generated much data, although the evidence is contradictory. Altered biologic activity of hormones, altered circulating levels of hormones, altered secretory response of the endocrine glands, altered metabolism of hormones, and loss of circadian control of hormone secretion are among the findings.

Theories of cellular damage deal with adverse cellular conditions that produce the biologic effects associated with aging. (These theories are discussed in Chapter 2.)

The endocrine system has not been specifically implicated in any of these theories, particularly as a causative variable. The cellular changes or consequences described by these theories do, however, affect endocrine glands and might contribute to endocrine gland dysfunction or alterations in responsiveness of target organs. For example, the loss of self-regulatory patterns of the immune system leads to an autoimmune phenomenon characterized by either autoimmunity or immunodeficiencies. These mechanisms may account for the onset of type II diabetes mellitus (see Chapter 18).

Theories of stress and adaptation suggest that body structures wear out from overuse or are no longer able to adapt to the cumulative effects of physiologic stress. One such endocrine function that may be affected is the sympathoadrenal axis. Exhaustion of this axis may be associated with an inability of the body to respond effectively to stressors.

Theories of programmed change are concerned with genetic control of cell function. Certain secretory cells may be programmed genetically to secrete hormones for a prescribed length of time. Changes seen with female reproductive function may represent the phenomenon of programmed change.

All changes in cellular activity—as a result of damage, programmed change, or wear and tear—may affect neuroendocrine regulation. Impaired secretion of hypothalamic regulatory factors and hormones or impaired hypothalamic feedback sensitivity may contribute to impaired control of an optimal internal environment. The dynamic equilibrium of the endocrine system may also be affected by altered secretion of neurotransmitters within certain areas of the brain, affecting hypothalamic and pituitary function. Such alterations may include an excess or deficit in secretion of pituitary hormones and loss of appropriate secretory pattern of those hormones. Loss of endocrine steady states may be associated with or contribute to aging.

Effects of Aging on Specific Glands
The Thyroid Gland

Changes in thyroid structure and function occur with aging. Structurally, some glandular atrophy and fibrosis occur with nodularity and increasing inflammatory infiltrates. These infiltrative changes may reflect age-related autoimmune damage (Spaulding, 1987).

Changes relative to TH and its function are more difficult to assess. One difficulty is finding older adults who are free of all systemic and thyroid-related illness, so that the resulting changes can be attributed to aging. Much of the available data is contradictory. Most evidence, however, supports the following age-related changes: (1) T_4 secretion and turnover are decreased; (2) plasma levels of T_3 decline, especially in men; (3) hypothyroidism is seen with increasing frequency as age advances; (4) basal plasma TSH levels are generally higher; and (5) responsiveness of plasma TSH concentration to TRH administration is reduced, especially in men (Ingbar, 1981). Additionally, it appears that the average dose for thyroid hormone replacement appears to be lower in the elderly because the peripheral metabolism of thyroid hormone decreases with age (Spaulding, 1987).

The Parathyroid Gland

An age-related alteration in PTH secretion has been proposed to explain alterations in calcium homeostasis that have been noted in older adults. Such an alteration, however, has not been consistently documented. Calcium intake, especially in women, tends to decrease with aging. The average daily intake of 450 to 500 mg/day causes a negative calcium balance greater than 40 mg/day, and may be related to the absolute bone loss of approximately 1.5% /year. Older adults show decreased intestinal adaptation to variations in calcium intake. Many older adults also have a mild, persistent hypercalciuria, indicating a defective renal mechanism for responding to decreased calcium intake. Decreased circulating levels of vitamin D have also been documented.

The decrease in calcium intake, an age-related decrease in circulating vitamin D, and a blunted response of older individuals to PTH, may explain these changes seen in aging (Korenman, 1982). Additional investigation into these mechanisms is required before the age-associated alterations can be explained.

The Adrenal Glands

The adrenal cortex loses some weight and has more fibrous tissue after the age of 50. Age does not appear to affect the feedback mechanisms involved in maintaining glucocorticoid levels, but the decrease in the metabolic clearance rate of the glucocorticoids is age related.

The metabolic clearance of cortisol decreases with an age-related decline in liver and kidney function. Furthermore, less cortisol appears to be used by the body when aging is accompanied by a loss of lean body mass. Both decreased clearance and reduced use of cortisol contribute to higher circulating cortisol levels. Because feedback mechanisms are intact, the higher cortisol levels cause a decrease in cortisol secretion. Plasma levels of the adrenal androgens, as well as urinary excretion of the metabolic end products, decrease gradually but dramatically with age, to as much as 50% to 70% of the young adult level. This change appears to reflect a decline in the function of the zona reticularis. The effects of decreased secretion are obscured, however, by the effects of aging on gonadal androgen secretion (see Unit 7). Because cortisol secretion does not vary significantly with aging, the decrease in secretion of adrenal androgens is probably independent of ACTH. The mecha-

nism for this decrease is not yet known (Korenman, 1982). Circadian patterns of ACTH and cortisol secretion do not change with aging.

The Posterior Pituitary

Although hyponatremia is a common finding in older people, it appears related to changes in renal function rather than ADH-related mechanisms. Morphologic studies have not shown significant age-related degenerative changes in the neuroendocrine pathways that regulate the synthesis and secretion of ADH. It appears that ADH secretion is augmented when stimulated by changes in osmotic concentration, whereas baroreceptor-mediated ADH secretion is reduced (Blackman, 1987).

The Anterior Pituitary

The anterior pituitary in older people is characterized by a number of morphologic changes including increases in fibrosis, focal necrosis, iron deposits, microadenoma formation, and a moderate decrease in size. The data regarding alterations in the hormones of the anterior pituitary are contradictory (Blackman, 1987).

SUMMARY REVIEW

Mechanisms of Hormonal Regulation

1 The endocrine system has diverse functions, including sexual differentiation, growth and development, and continuous maintenance of the body's internal environment.

2 Hormones are chemical messengers synthesized by endocrine glands and released into the circulation.

3 Hormones have specific negative and positive feedback mechanisms. Most hormone levels are regulated by negative feedback, in which hormone secretion raises the level of a specific hormone, ultimately causing secretion to subside.

4 Endocrine feedback is described in terms of short, long, and ultra-short feedback loops.

5 Water-soluble hormones circulate throughout the body in unbound form, whereas lipid-soluble hormones (i.e., steroid and thyroid hormones) circulate throughout the body bound to carrier proteins.

6 Hormones affect only target cells with appropriate receptors and then act on these cells to initiate specific cell functions or activities.

7 Hormones have two general types of effects on cells: (1) direct effects, or obvious changes in cell function; and (2) permissive effects, or less obvious changes that facilitate cell function.

8 Receptors for hormones may be located on the plasma membrane or in the intracellular compartment of a target cell.

9 Water-soluble hormones act as first messengers, bind-

ing to receptors on the cell's plasma membrane. The signals initiated by hormone-receptor binding are then transmitted into the cell by the action of second messengers.

10 Second messengers that have been identified include cyclic AMP, cyclic GMP, calcium, and prostaglandins.

11 For cells having cyclic AMP as their second messenger, a series of interactions within the plasma membrane must activate the intracellular cyclic nucleotides, converting intracellular substances to active enzymes.

12 For cells having calcium as their second messenger, a rise in intracellular calcium causes calcium to bind with calmodulin, a regulatory protein. This step then initiates other intracellular processes.

13 Lipid-soluble hormones (including steroid and thyroid hormones) may cross the plasma membrane through diffusion. These hormones either bind to cytoplasmic proteins or diffuse directly into the cell nucleus and bind to nuclear receptors.

Structure and Function of the Endocrine Glands

1 The pituitary gland, consisting of anterior and posterior portions, is connected to the CNS through the hypothalamus.

2 The hypothalamus regulates anterior pituitary function by secreting releasing hormones and releasing factors into the portal circulation. Releasing hormones have identified chemical structures; releasing factors have hormonal properties but no definitive chemical identification.

3 Hypothalamic hormones include prolactin-inhibiting factor (PIF), which inhibits prolacting secretion; thyrotropin-releasing factor (TRF), which affects release of thyroid hormones; gonadotropin-releasing hormone (GRH), which facilitates release of adrenocorticotropic hormone (ACTH) and endorphins; and substance P, which inhibits ACTH release and stimulates release of a variety of other hormones.

4 The posterior pituitary secretes antidiuretic hormone (ADH), which is also called vasopressin, and oxytocin.

5 ADH controls serum osmolality, increases permeability of the renal tubules, and causes vasoconstriction when administered pharmacologically in high doses. ADH may also regulate some CNS functions.

6 Oxytocin causes uterine contraction and lactation in women and may have a role in sperm motility in men. In both men and women, oxytocin has an antidiuretic effect similar to that of ADH.

7 Hormones of the anterior pituitary are regulated by (1) secretion of hypothalamic-releasing hormones or factors, (2) negative feedback from hormones secreted by target organs, and (3) mediating effects of neurotransmitters.

8 Hormones of the anterior pituitary include ACTH, melanocyte-stimulating hormone, somatotropic hormones (GH and prolactin), and glycoprotein hormones (FSH, LH, and TSH).

9 The two-lobed thyroid gland contains follicles, which secrete some of the thyroid hormones, and C cells, which secrete calcitonin and somatostatin.

10 Regulation of thyroid hormone (TH) levels is complex and involves the hypothalamus, anterior pituitary, thyroid gland, and numerous biochemical variables.

11 Thyroid hormone (TH) secretion is regulated by thyroid-releasing hormone, through a negative feedback loop involving the anterior pituitary and hypothalamus.

12 Thyroid-stimulating hormone (TSH), which is synthesized and stored in the anterior pituitary, stimulates secretion of TH by activating intracellular processes, including uptake of iodine necessary for the synthesis of TH.

13 Once secreted, TH acts on the thyroid gland, the anterior pituitary, and the median eminence to regulate further TH production.

14 Synthesis of TH depends on the glycoprotein thyroglobulin, which contains a precursor of TH, tyrosine. Tyrosine then combines with iodine to form precursor molecules of the thyroid hormones thyroxine (T_4) and triiodothyronine (T_3).

15 When released into the circulation, T_3 and T_4 are bound by carrier proteins in the plasma, which store these hormones and provide a buffer for rapid changes in hormone levels.

16 Thyroid hormones alter protein synthesis and have a wide range of metabolic effects on proteins, carbohydrates, lipids, and vitamins. TH also affects calorigenesis and cardiac function.

17 The paired parathyroid glands are normally located behind the upper and lower poles of the thyroid. These glands secrete parathyroid hormone (PTH), an important regulator of serum calcium levels.

18 PTH secretion is regulated by levels of ionized calcium in the plasma and by cyclic AMP within the cell. Some other substances—hormones, neurotransmitters, and ions—affect PTH secretion by inhibiting cyclic AMP or by changing calcium levels.

19 In bone, PTH causes bone breakdown and resorption. In the kidney, PTH increases reabsorption of calcium and decreases reabsorption of phosphorus and bicarbonate.

20 The endocrine pancreas contains the islets of Langerhans, which secrete hormones responsible for much of the carbohydrate metabolism in the body.

21 The islets of Langerhans are made up of alpha cells, beta cells, and delta cells.

22 Delta cells secrete somatostatin, which inhibits glucagon and insulin secretion.

23 Beta cells secrete preproinsulin, which is ultimately converted to insulin.

24 Insulin is a hormone that regulates blood glucose concentrations and overall body metabolism of fat, protein, and carbohydrates.

25 Alpha cells produce glucagon, which is secreted inversely to blood glucose concentrations.

26 The paired adrenal glands are situated in the kidneys. Each gland consists of an adrenal medulla, which secretes catecholamines, and an adrenal cortex, which secretes steroid hormones.

27 The steroid hormones secreted by the adrenal cortex are all synthesized from cholesterol. These hormones in-

clude glucocorticoids, mineralocorticoids, and adrenal androgens and estrogens.

28 Glucocorticoids have direct effects on carbohydrate metabolism by increased blood glucose concentration through gluconeogenesis in the liver and through decreased use of glucose. Glucocorticoids also inhibit immune and inflammatory responses.

29 The most potent naturally occurring glucocorticoid is cortisol, which is necessary for the maintenance of life and for protection from stress. Secretion of cortisol is regulated by the hypothalamus and anterior pituitary.

30 Cortisol secretion is related to secretion of adrenocorticotropic hormone (ACTH), which is stimulated by corticotropin-releasing hormone (CRH). ACTH binds with receptors of the adrenal cortex, which activates intracellular mechanisms (specifically cyclic AMP) and leads to cortisol release.

31 Mineralocorticoids are steroid hormones that directly affect ion transport by epithelial cells, causing sodium retention and potassium and hydrogen loss.

32 Aldosterone is the most potent of the naturally occurring mineralocorticoids. Its primary role is to conserve sodium.

33 Aldosterone secretion is primarily regulated by the renin-angiotensin system.

34 Aldosterone acts by binding to a site on the cell nucleus and altering protein production within the cell. Its principal site of action is the kidney, where it causes sodium reabsorption and potassium and hydrogen excretion.

35 Androgens and estrogens secreted by the adrenal cortex act in the same way as those secreted by the gonads.

36 The adrenal medulla secretes the catecholamines epinephrine and norepinephrine. Catecholamines are synthesized from the amino acid phenylalanine. Their release is stimulated by sympathetic nervous system stimulation, ACTH, and glucocorticoids.

37 Catecholamines bind with various target cells, are taken up by neurons, or are excreted in the urine. They cause a range of metabolic effects that are generally characterized as the "flight or fight" response.

38 The endocrine system acts together with the nervous system to respond to stressors.

39 The response to stressors involves (1) activation of the sympathetic division of the autonomic nervous system and (2) activation of the endocrine system.

40 The adrenal glands and the sympathetic neurons that innervate these glands form the sympathoadrenal axis.

41 Activation of the sympathetic neurons causes the activation of an enzymatic pathway that increases catecholamine synthesis, leading to manifestations of the "fight or flight" response, hyperglycemia, and immune suppression.

42 Both hyperglycemia and immune suppression appear to be adaptive responses that are essential in the body's ability to react to stressors.

43 Other hormones that are secreted in response to stress include growth hormone, prolactin, testosterone, ADH, and insulin.

Aging and the Endocrine System

1 Endocrine changes that may be associated with aging include altered biologic activity of hormones, altered circulating levels of hormones, altered secretory responses of endocrine glands, altered metabolism of hormones, and loss of circadian control of hormone release.

2 Cellular damage associated with aging, genetically programmed cell change, and chronic wear and tear may contribute to endocrine gland dysfunction or alterations in responsiveness of target organs.

3 Aging apparently causes atrophy of the thyroid gland and is associated with infiltrative glandular changes. Secretion of thyroid hormones may diminish with age.

4 Aging is associated with alterations in calcium steady states, which may be related to alterations in PTH secretion from the parathyroid glands.

5 Age-related changes in adrenal function include decreased clearance of glucocorticoids and a decrease in levels of adrenal androgens. The effects of these changes, however, are offset by feedback mechanisms that maintain glucocorticoid levels and by gonadal secretion of androgens.

KEY TERMS

Adrenal cortex, 580

Adrenal gland, 580

Adrenal medulla, 580

Adrenocorticotropic hormone (ACTH), 580

Aldosterone, 584

Alpha cell, 578

Antidiuretic hormone (ADH), 573

Beta cell, 578

Bioassay, 588

C cell, 575

Calcitonin, 575

Chromophils, 574

Chromophobes, 574

Corticotropin-releasing hormone (CRH), 573

Cortisol, 583

Delta cell, 578

Direct effect, 568

Endocrine regulation, 565

Enzyme-linked immunosorbent assay (ELISA), 588

Fasciculata, 580

First messenger, 568

Follicle, 575

Glucagon, 578

Glucocorticoid, 582

Gonadotropin-releasing hormone (GnRH), 573

Growth hormone–releasing factor (GRF), 573

Hormone, 564

Infundibular process, 572

Infundibular stem, 570

Insulin, 578

Islet of Langerhans, 578

Isthmus, 575

Median eminence, 570

Mineralocorticoid, 584

Negative feedback, 565

Oxytocin, 573

Pancreas, 578

Parathyroid hormone (PTH), 577

Pars distalis, 572

Pars intermedia, 572

Pars tuberalis, 572

Permissive effect, 568

Pharmacologic effect, 568

Pituitary gland, 570

Positive feedback, 565

Prolactin-inhibiting factor (PIF), 573

Radioimmunoassay (RIA), 587

Releasing factors, 573

Reticularis, 580

Second messenger, 569

Somatostatin, 573

Substance P, 573

Target cell, 568

Thyroglobulin, 577

Thyroid gland, 575

Thyroid hormone (TH), 576

Thyroid-releasing hormone (TRH)

Thyroid-stimulating hormone (TSH), 576

Thyrotropin-releasing hromone (TRH), 573

Thyroxine (T$_4$), 577

Triiodothyronine (T$_3$), 577

Zona glomerulosa, 580

REFERENCES

Adelman, R., & Roth, G. (1982). *Endocrine and neuroendocrine mechanisms of aging.* Boca Raton, FL: CRC Press.

Ahren, B. (1986). Thyroid neuroendocrinology: Neural regulation of thyroid hormone secretion. *Endocrine Reviews, 7*(2), 149-155.

Alperts, B., Bray, D., Lewis,J., Raff, M., Roberts, K., & Watson, J. K. (1983). *Molecular biology of the cell.* New York: Garland Publishing.

Barnes, D. M. (1986). Steroids may influence changes in mood. *Science, 232,* 1344-1345.

Berridge, M. J. (1976). The interaction of cyclic nucleotides and calcium in control of cellular activity. *Advances in Cyclic Nucleotide Research, 6.*

Berridge, M. J. (1985, October). The molecular basis of communication within the cell. *Scientific American, 253*(4), 142.

Blackman, M. (1987). Hormones and aging. *Endocrine & Metabolism Clinics of North America, 16*(4).

Burchfield, S. R. (1979). The stress response: A new perspective. *Psychosomatic Medicine, 41*(8), 661-669.

Catt, K. J., & Dufau, M. L. (1977). Peptide hormone receptors. *Annual Review of Physiology, 39,* 529.

Cooperstein, S. J., & Watkins, D. (1981). *The islets of Langerhans.* New York: Academic Press.

Cuatracasas, P., Hollenberg, M. D., Chang, K. J., & Bennett, V. (1975). Hormone receptor complexes and their modulation of membrane function. *Recent Progress on Hormone Research, 31,* 37.

Ebersole, P., & Hess, P. (1985). *Toward healthy aging* (2nd ed.). St. Louis: CV Mosby.

Ezrin, C., Godden, J. D., & Volpe, R. (1979). *Systematic endocrinology.* (2nd ed.). New York: Harper & Row.

Felig, P. (1985). Diabetic control: Is it worth it? *Transactions of the Association of Life Insurance Medical Directions of America, 68,* 61-65.

Felig, P., Baster, J., Porodus, A., & Frohman, L. (Eds.). *Endocrinology and metabolism.* New York: McGraw-Hill.

Franco-Saenz, R., Atarashi, K., Takagi, M., & Mulrow, P. J. (1986). Effects of atrial natriuretic factor on the renin-angiotensin aldosterone axis. *Journal of Hypertension (Suppl.), 4,* 523-525.

Genazzani, A. R., Thijssen, J. H. H., & Siiteri, P. K. (Eds.). (1980). *Adrenal androgens.* New York: Raven Press.

Goldberg, N. D., & Haddox, M. C. (1977). GMP metabolism and involvement in biological regulation. *Annual Review of Biochemistry, 46,* 823.

Greenblatt, R. B. (1978). Geriatric endocrinology. *Aging* (vol. 5). New York: Raven Press.

Hadley, M. E. (1984). *Endocrinology.* Englewood Cliffs, NJ: Prentice-Hall.

Ingbar, S. H. (1981). The effects of aging on the thyroid hormone economy in man. *Progress in Clinical & Biological Research, 74,* 135-145.

Kasl, S. V. (1984). Stress and health. *Annual Review of Public Health,* (5), 319-341.

King, R. J. B. (1984). Enlightenment and confusion over steroid hormone receptors. *Nature, 312,* 20.

Korenman, S. G. (Ed.). (1982). *Endocrine aspects of aging.* New York: Elsevier.

Lefkowitz, R. J. (1982, August). Biochemical mechanisms of hormone receptor-effector coupling. *Federation Proceedings, 41*(10), 2662-3.

Makara, G. B. (1985). Mechanisms by which stressful stimuli activate the pituitary-adrenal system (Part 2). *Federal Proceedings, 44*(1), 149-153.

Martin, C. R. (1985). *Endocrine physiology.* New York: Oxford Press.

Munck, A., & Foley, R. (1979). Activation of steroid hormone-receptor complexes in intact target cells in physiological conditions. *Nature, 278,* 752.

Munck, A., Guyre, P. M., & Holbrook, N. J. (1984). Physiological functions of glucocorticoids in stress and their relation to pharmacological actions. *Endocrine Reviews, 5*(1), 25-44.

Neville, A. M., & O'Hare, M. J. (1982). *The human adrenal cortex*. New York & Berlin: Springer Verlag.

O'Mally, B. W., Schwartz, R. J., & Schrader, W. T. (1976). A review of regulation of gene expression by steroid hormone receptors. *Journal of Steroid Biochemistry, 7,* 1151.

Phipps, J. W., Long, B. C., & Woods, N. F. (1987). *Medical-surgical nursing: Concepts and clinical practice*. (3rd ed.). St. Louis: C.V. Mosby.

Rasmussen, H., Jensen, P. Lake, W., Friedmann, N., & Goodman, D. B. P. (1975). Cyclic nucleotides and cellular calcium metabolism. In G. L. Drummond et al. (Eds.), *Advances in cyclic nucleotide research* (Vol. 5). New York: Raven Press.

Reichlin, S. (1985). Neuroendocrinology. In J. Wilson & D. Foster, (Eds.), *Williams textbook of endocrinology*. Philadelphia: WB Saunders.

Rose, R. M. (1980). Endocrine responses to stressful events. *Psychiatric Clinics of North America, 3,* 251-276.

Ross, E. M., & Gilman, A. G. (1980). Biochemical properties of hormone sensitive adenylate cyclase. *Annual Review of Biochemistry, 49,* 533.

Sato, R. J., deNicola, A., & Blaquier, J. (Eds.) (1980). *Pathophysiology of endocrine diseases and mechanics of hormone action*. New York: Allan R. Liss.

Spaulding, S. (1987). Age and the thyroid. *Endocrine & Metabolism Clinics of North America, 16*(4).

Stanley, J. C. (1981). Mechanisms of hormone action. *British Journal of Anesthesiology, 53,* 147.

Streeten, D. H. P., Anderson, G. H., Dalakos, T. G., Seeley, D., Mallov, J. S., Eusebio, R., Sunderlin, F. S., Badawy, S. Z., & King, R. B. (1984). Normal and abnormal function of the hypothalamic-pituitary-adrenocortical system in man. *Endocrine Reviews, 5*(3), 371-394.

Sutherland, E. W., & Rall, T. W. (1958). Fractionation and characterization of a cyclic adenine ribonucleotide formed by tissue particles. *Journal of Biological Chemistry, 232,* 1077-1091

Sutterly, D. C., & Donnelly, G. F. (1982). *Coping with stress: A nursing perspective*. Rockville, MD: Aspen.

Tata, J. R. (1980). Thyroid human receptors. In D. Schulster & A. Levitzki (Eds.), *Cellular receptors for hormones and neurotransmitters*. New York: Wiley.

Tepperman, J. (1987). *Metabolic and endocrine physiology: An introductory text* (5th ed.). Chicago: Year Book.

Thibodeau, G. A. (1987). *Anatomy and physiology*. St. Louis: Times Mirror/Mosby.

Thompson, J. M. et al. (1989). *Mosby's manual of clinical nursing* (2nd ed.). St. Louis: C.V. Mosby.

CHAPTER 18

Alterations of Hormonal Regulation

D. Patricia Gray
Patti Ludwig-Beymer

Mechanisms of hormonal alterations, 595
Alterations of the hypothalamic-pituitary system, 596
  Diseases of the posterior pituitary, 597
    Syndrome of inappropriate antidiuretic hormone secretion, 597
      Pathophysiology, 597
      Clinical manifestations, 597
      Evaluation and treatment, 597
    Diabetes insipidus, 598
      Pathophysiology, 598
      Clinical manifestations, 598
      Evaluation and treatment, 598
  Diseases of the anterior pituitary, 599
    Hypopituitarism, 599
      Pathophysiology, 599
      Clinical manifestations, 599
      Evaluation and treatment, 600
    Hyperpituitarism: primary adenoma, 600
      Pathophysiology, 600
      Clinical manifestations, 601
      Evaluation and treatment, 601
    Hypersecretion of growth hormone: acromegaly, 602
      Pathophysiology, 602
      Clinical manifestations, 602
      Evaluation and treatment, 603
Alterations of thyroid function, 603
  Hyperthyroidism, 603
    Course of hyperthyroidism, 603
      Clinical manifestations, 603
      Evaluation and treatment, 603
    Hyperthyroid conditions, 604
      Graves disease, 604
      Nodular goiter, 605
      Thyrotoxic crisis, 605
    Hypothyroidism, 606
      Pathophysiology, 607
      Clinical manifestations, 607
      Evaluation and treatment, 607
    Hypothyroid conditions, 608
      Myxedema coma, 608

Congenital hypothyroidism, 608
Thyroid carcinoma, 608
Alterations of parathyroid function, 609
  Hyperparathyroidism, 609
    Pathophysiology, 609
      Primary hyperparathyroidism, 609
      Secondary hyperparathyroidism, 609
      Tertiary hyperparathyroidism, 610
    Clinical manifestations, 610
    Evaluation and treatment, 611
  Hypoparathyroidism, 611
    Clinical manifestations, 611
    Evaluation and treatment, 611
Dysfunction of the endocrine pancreas: diabetes mellitus, 612
  Types of diabetes mellitus, 612
    Type I diabetes mellitus, 612
      Pathophysiology, 612
      Clinical manifestations, 615
      Evaluation and treatment, 615
        Insulin, 616
        Diet, 616
        Exercise, 616
        Transplantation, 616
    Type II diabetes mellitus, 616
      Pathophysiology, 616
      Clinical manifestations, 617
      Evaluation and treatment, 617
    Gestational diabetes, 618
  Acute complications of diabetes mellitus, 618
    Hypoglycemia, 618
    Diabetic ketoacidosis, 619
      Clinical manifestations, 619
      Evaluation and treatment, 621
    Hyperosmolar hyperglycemic nonketotic coma, 622
      Clinical manifestations, 623
      Evaluation and treatment, 623
    Dawn phenomenon, 623
    Somogyi effects, 624
      Clinical manifestations, 624
      Evaluation and treatment, 624

Chronic complications of diabetes mellitus, 624
  Diabetic neuropathies, 624
  Microvascular disease, 624
    Retinopathy, 625
    Nephropathy, 625
  Macrovascular disease, 626
    Coronary artery disease, 626
    Stroke, 627
    Peripheral vascular disease, 627
  Infection, 627
Alterations of adrenal function, 628
  Disorders of the adrenal cortex, 628
    Hypercortical function (Cushing disease, Cushing
      syndrome), 629
    Pathophysiology, 629
    Clinical manifestations, 629
    Evaluation and treatment, 631
    Hyperaldosteronism, 631
    Pathophysiology, 632
    Clinical manifestations, 633
    Evaluation and treatment, 633
    Hypersecretion of adrenal androgens and estrogens, 633
    Hypocortical functioning, 633
    Pathophysiology, 634
      Idiopathic Addison disease, 634
      Secondary hypocortisolism, 634
    Clinical manifestations, 635
    Evaluation and treatment, 635
  Disorders of the adrenal medulla, 635
  Adrenal medulla hypofunction, 635
  Adrenal medulla hyperfunction, 636
    Pathophysiology, 636
    Clinical manifestations, 636
    Evaluation and treatment, 636

Function of the endocrine system involves complex interrelationships and interactions that maintain dynamic steady states and provide growth and reproductive capabilities. Dysfunction of the endocrine system was initially described in terms of excessive or insufficient function of the endocrine gland with alterations in hormone levels. Alterations in function were thought to be caused by either hyper- or hyposecretion of the various hormones, leading to abnormal hormone concentrations in the blood. Techniques for studying the various components of the endocrine system have improved, and evidence has shown that dysfunction may result from abnormal receptor function or from altered intracellular response to the hormone-receptor complex.

MECHANISMS OF HORMONAL ALTERATIONS

Significantly elevated or depressed hormone levels may result from a variety of causes (Fig. 18-1). Feed-back systems that recognize the need for a particular hormone may fail to function properly or may respond to inappropriate signals (see Chapter 17). Dysfunction of an endocrine gland may involve the gland's failure to produce adequate amounts of biologically free or active hormone forms. This failure may occur when the secretory cells are unable to produce or obtain an adequate quantity of required hormone precursors, or are unable to convert the precursors to the appropriate form. A gland also may synthesize or release excessive amounts of hormone. Once hormones are released into the circulation, they may be degraded at an altered rate, or they may be inactivated by antibodies before reaching the target cell. Ectopic sources of hormones (hormones produced by nonendocrine tissues) may also result in abnormally elevated hormone levels. This mechanism operates without benefit of the normal feedback system for hormone control. In these cases, the ectopic hormone production is said to be autonomous.

Recently, research has been directed toward understanding causes for the failure of the target cell to respond to its hormone. The general types of abnormal target cell responses currently recognized are (1) receptor-associated disorders and (2) intracellular disorders. Receptor-associated disorders have been primarily identified in water-soluble hormones, such as insulin. These types of disorders are usually one of the following: (1) a decrease in the number of receptors, leading to decreased or defective hormone-receptor binding, (2) impaired receptor function resulting in insensitivity to the hormone, (3) presence of antibodies against specific receptors that either reduce available binding sites or mimic hormone action, exaggerating target cell response, or (4) unusual expression of receptor function, as occurs in some tumor cells with abnormal receptor activity.

Intracellular disorders may involve inadequate synthesis of the second messenger, such as cAMP, needed to transduce the hormonal signal into intracellular events. The target cell for water-soluble hormones may have a faulty response to hormone-receptor binding and thus fail to generate the required second messenger. The cell also may have an abnormal response to the second messenger if levels of intracellular enzymes or proteins are altered. (Second messengers for various hormones are listed in Chapter 17, Table 17-4). Both of these pathogenic mechanisms result in failure of the target cell to express the usual hormonal effect.

Pathogenic mechanisms affecting target cell response for lipid-soluble hormones, such as thyroid hormone, either occur less frequently or are recognized less frequently than are those affecting the water-soluble hormones. These mechanisms are not yet precisely understood, although some theories have been proposed. The number of intracellular receptors may be decreased, or

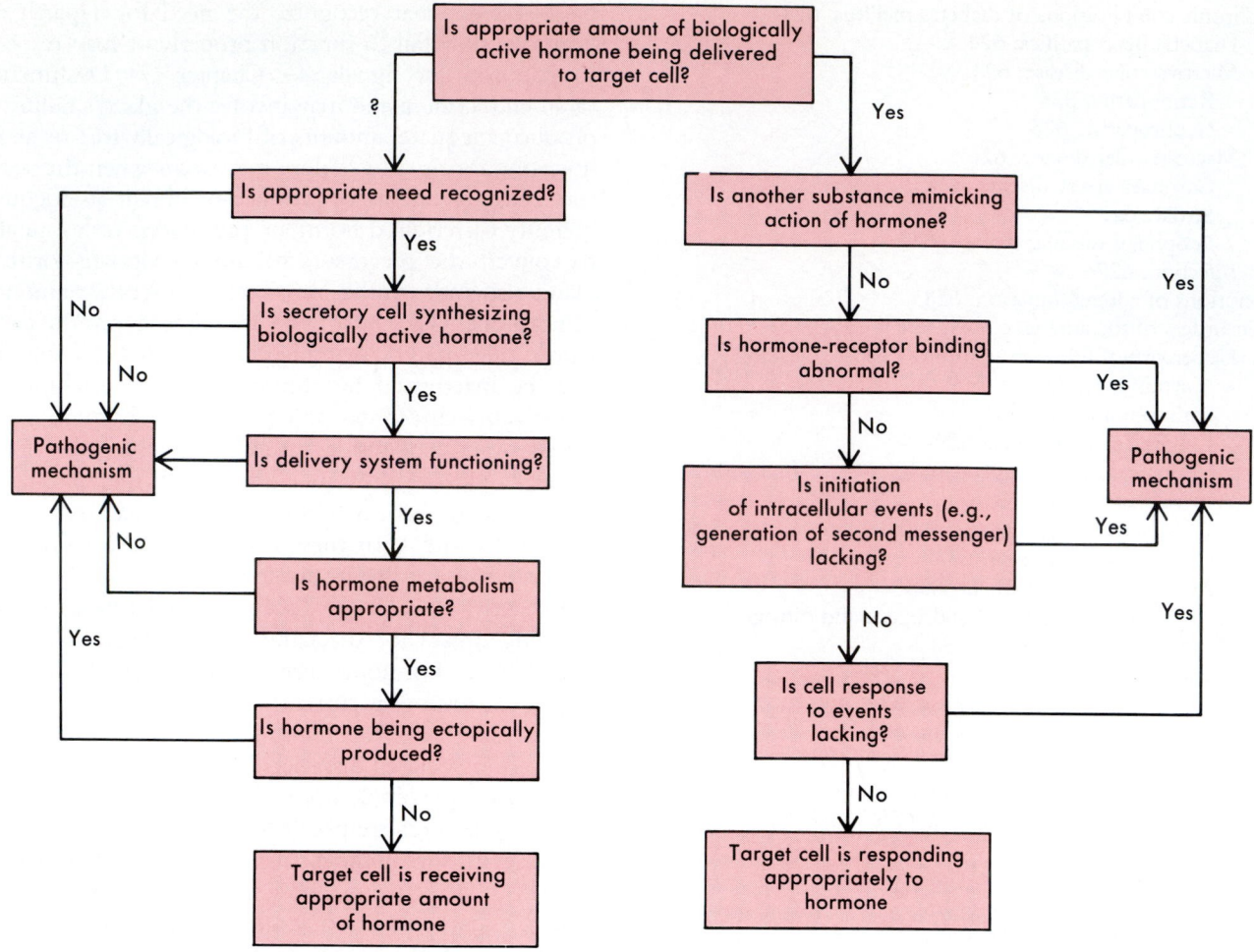

FIG. 18-1. Phases at which pathogenic mechanisms may develop in delivering appropriate amounts of hormone to the cells.

those receptors may have an altered affinity for hormones. Both mechanisms would affect hormone-receptor binding. Alterations in generation of new messenger RNA or absence of substrates for new protein synthesis may also occur, resulting in altered target cell response.

ALTERATIONS OF THE HYPOTHALAMIC-PITUITARY SYSTEM

Because of the relative inaccessibility of the hypothalamic-pituitary unit in the brain and the short half-life and small concentrations of the hypothalamic hormones, documenting abnormal release of hypothalamic-releasing hormones has been difficult. The most common hypothalamic diseases probably result from interruption in the infundibular stem due to destructive lesions of the stem, rupture of the stem after head injury,

surgical transection of the stem, or stem tumor. In these cases, interruption of the physical connections between the hypothalamus and the pituitary causes hypo-hypothalamic disease. For example, diabetes insipidus (antidiuretic hormone insufficiency) may result, depending on the location at which the infundibular stem is interrupted. If the lesion is close to the hypothalamus, diabetes insipidus is likely; the farther away the lesion is from the hypothalamus, the less likely the occurrence of diabetes insipidus.

The absence of hypothalamic hormones (Fig. 18-2) causes a variety of manifestations. In adult women the menses cease and in adult males spermatogenesis is impaired because of the absence of gonadotropin-releasing hormone (GnRH) stimulation of the gonadotropin follicle-stimulating hormone (FSH) and lutenizing hormone (LH). ACTH response to low serum cortisol levels is decreased because of the absence of corticotropic-releasing hormone (CRH). Hypothalamic hypothyroidism is caused by the absence of thyrotropin-

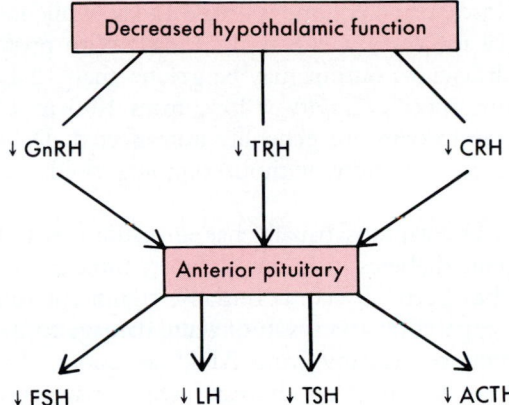

FIG. 18-2. Loss of hypothalamic hormones.

releasing hormone (TRH). Low levels of growth hormone cause the absence of growth hormone regulatory hormones. Hyperprolactinemia is caused by an absence of usual inhibitory controls of prolactin secretion.

Diseases of the Posterior Pituitary
Syndrome of Inappropriate Antidiuretic Hormone Secretion

Diseases of the posterior pituitary that cause clinically observable symptoms are rare. If they do occur, they are usually related to abnormal antidiuretic hormone (ADH/vasopressin) secretion. **Syndrome of inappropriate ADH secretion** (SIADH) is characterized by high levels of ADH in the absence of normal physiologic stimuli for its release.

The most common cause of elevated levels of ADH is ectopically produced ADH. SIADH is associated with some forms of cancer, apparently because of the ectopic secretion of ADH by tumor cells. Tumors that have been reported in association with SIADH include oat cell adenocarcinoma of the lung, carcinoma of the duodenum and pancreas, leukemia, lymphoma, Hodgkin disease, sarcoma, and squamous cell carcinoma of the tongue.

Transient SIADH may follow pituitary surgery, as stored ADH is released in an unregulated fashion. When postoperative fluid volume shifts occur following any type of surgery, ADH secretion is increased for 5 to 7 days. This is apparently related to volume changes within the body and may be considered a normal response to surgery. SIADH may be seen in individuals with a variety of infectious pulmonary diseases. This may be due to the ectopic production of ADH by infected lung tissue (Vorherr et al., 1970) or by increased posterior pituitary secretion of ADH in response to a hypoxia-induced decrease in pulmonary perfusion (Labhart, 1986).

SIADH may be associated with psychiatric disease

and may also occur after treatment with a variety of drugs. These include hypoglycemic medications (thioridazine), barbiturates, general anesthesia, vincristine, nicotine, morphine, diuretics, and synthetic hormones. These drugs serve either to simulate ADH release or to potentiate circulating ADH (Labhart, 986).

Pathophysiology

The main features of SIADH are water retention or increases in total body H_2O; solute loss, particularly Na; and osmotic inactivation of cellular solutes. These features lead to hyponatremia and hypo-osmolality. In SIADH, ADH is released continually. Water retention results from the normal action of ADH on the renal tubules and collecting ducts, increasing their permeability to water and increasing water reabsorption by the kidneys. (Renal function is discussed in Chapter 34.)

An expansion of extracellular fluid volume results, and a dilutional hyponatremia develops. Hyponatremia acts to suppress renin and therefore aldosterone secretion, decreasing proximal tubule reabsorption of sodium. This effect explains renal sodium loss during a hyponatremic state.

Clinical Manifestations

A diagnosis of SIADH requires the following signs: (1) serum hypo-osmolality and hyponatremia, (2) urine hypersomoalarity (that is, the osmolality of the urine is greater than expected for the concomitant serum osmolality), (3) urine sodium excretion that matches sodium intake, (4) improvement in hyponatremia with water restriction, and (5) absence of other causes of decreased diluting ability.

The symptoms of SIADH are primarily the result of hyponatremia. The severity and the sudden onset of the hyponatremia determine the extent of the symptoms. Even if hyponatremia develops slowly, serum sodium levels below 110 to 115 mEq/L are likely to cause severe and sometimes irreversible neurologic damage.

Thirst, impaired taste, anorexia, dyspnea on exertion, fatigue, and dulled sensorium occur when the serum sodium falls rapidly from 140 to 130 mEq/L. Severe gastrointestinal symptoms, including vomiting and abdominal cramps, occur with a drop in sodium from 130 to 120 mEq/L. With a serum sodium level below 115 mEq/L, confusion, lethargy, muscle twitching, and convulsions may occur. Symptoms usually resolve with correction of hyponatremia.

Evaluation and Treatment

Serum electrolyte levels, serum osmolality and urine volume, urine electrolyte levels, and urine osmolality are adequate measures of the presence of SIADH. The treatment of SIADH involves the correction of any underlying causal problems, emergency correction of severe hyponatremia by administration of hypertonic saline, and, most important, fluid restriction to 600 to 800 ml/day. Resolution usually occurs within 3 days with a 2 to 3 kg weight loss and correction of hyponatremia and salt wasting. Phenytoin may be administered, particularly for excessive ADH release by the posterior pituitary. At present, no drug therapy is available to suppress ectopically produced ADH.

Diabetes Insipidus

Diabetes insipidus is related to an insufficiency of ADH leading to polyuria and polydipsia. There are three forms of diabetes insipidus: (1) a neurogenic or central form, (2) a nephrogenic form, and (3) a psychogenic form (Culpepper, Heber, & Andreoli, 1985). The neurogenic form is caused by insufficient amounts of ADH; the nephrogenic form is caused by an inadequate response to ADH. The psychogenic form is caused by extremely large volumes of fluid intake, producing a decreased ADH level.

The neurogenic form of diabetes insipidus occurs when any organic lesion of the hypothalamus, infundibular stem, or posterior pituitary interferes with ADH synthesis, transport, or release. These lesions include primary brain tumors, hypophysectomy, aneurysms, thrombosis, infections, and immunologic disorders. Diabetes insipidus is a well-recognized complication of closed-head trauma.

The nephrogenic form of diabetes insipidus is usually an acquired disorder. An idiopathic form has been documented and is usually genetic. Nephrogenic diabetes insipidus represents end organ failure, with an insensitivity of the renal tubule to ADH. Nephrogenic diabetes insipidus is generally related to disorders and drugs that damage the renal tubules or inhibit the generation of cAMP in the tubules. These disorders include pyelonephritis, amyloidosis, destructive uropathies, polycystic disease, and intrinsic renal disease, all of which lead to irreversible diabetes insipidus. Drugs that may induce a generally reversible form of nephrogenic diabetes insipidus include lithium carbonate, general anesthetics, methoxyflurane, and cemechlocydine.

Pathophysiology

Individuals with diabetes insipidus may have partial to total inability to concentrate urine. This inability apparently results from chronic polyuria causing washout of the renal medullary concentration gradient (see Chapter 32).

Insufficient ADH secretion causes immediate excretion of large volumes of dilute urine, leading to an increase in plasma osmolality. In conscious individuals, the thirst mechanism is stimulated and induces polydipsia. For unknown reasons, the person usually craves cold drinks. The urine output is varied. In about one-half of cases, urine volume is 4 to 8 L/day, while in one-fourth of the cases it is 8 to 12 L/day. With profound ADH deficiency, output may be greater than 12 L/day. The urine specific gravity is low, from 1.00 to 1.005. Serum electrolytes are generally not affected. Dehydration develops rapidly without ongoing fluid replacement.

Diabetes insipidus usually has an acute onset. With neurogenic diabetes insipidus a classic, three-phase syndrome has been observed. Initially, significant diuresis occurs, apparently as a result of acute damage to the hypothalamic centers involving ADH secretion. The second phase is one of antidiuresis, which may represent necrosis of denervated tissue of the posterior pituitary with release of ADH into the circulation. The final phase is one of polyuria and polydipsia reflecting a permanent loss of the ability to secrete adequate amounts of ADH. ADH does not have to be completely absent for polyuria and polydipsia to occur.

Clinical Manifestations

The clinical manifestations of diabetes insipidus are due to the absence of ADH. These signs and symptoms include polyuria, nocturia, continuous thirst, polydipsia, low urine specific gravity, low urine osmolality (Cecil, 1985), and high-normal plasma osmolality (300 mOsm/kg H_2O or more) (Labhart, 1986). Plasma osmolality is always higher than urine osmolality in diabetes insipidus after 8 hours of water deprivation. Individuals with longstanding diabetes insipidus develop a large bladder capacity and hydronephrosis (see Chapter 33).

Evaluation and Treatment

Diabetes insipidus must be distinguished from other polyuric states, including diabetes mellitus, osmotically induced diuresis, and primary polydipsia. Water restriction is a useful test because people without diabetes insipidus respond with a rapid decrease in urine volume (800 mOsm/kg), whereas persons with diabetes insipidus have no decrease in urine volume and maintain a urine osmolality of approximately 100 mOsm/kg. Water deprivation tests, or dehydration testing, should be done with careful monitoring because depriving an individual with diabetes insipidus of water can lead to circulatory collapse or hypertonic encephalopathy. During dehydration tests, if the patient has nothing by mouth for 4 to 18 hours, urine osmolarity, and specific gravity hourly greater than 3% of body weight occurs, the test should be terminated to avoid hypotension. The psychogenic form, compulsive water drinking, of diabetes insipidus is diagnosed when 24-hour urine volume is greater than 18 L/24 hours, random plasma osmolarity is less than 285 mOsm/kg of H_2O, and there is episodic polyuria (Cecil, 1985).

Treatment of neurogenic diabetes insipidus is based

on the extent of the ADH deficiency and on individual variables, such as age, endocrine and cardiovascular status, and lifestyle. Individuals who have a urine output in excess of 9 L/day and a urine osmolality of less than 100 mOsm/kg after a dehydration or water restriction test generally require ADH replacement (Reichlin, 1984).

Replacement therapy for symptomatic central or neurogenic diabetes insipidus includes administration of the synthetic vasopressin analogue DDAVP (Desmopressin) applied intravascularly. Drugs that potentiate the action of otherwise insufficient amounts of endogenous ADH, such as chlorpropamide, may be used in individuals with incomplete ADH deficiency. Clofibrate or carbamazepine are drugs that are used in a limited fashion with mildly to moderately affected individuals (Camargo & Kolb, 1988). They stimulate ADH release from the hypothalamus.

Diseases of the Anterior Pituitary

Disorders of the anterior pituitary may involve either hypofunction or hyperfunction of the gland. **Hypopituitarism** is defined as a range of dysfunction, from the absence of selective pituitary hormones to complete failure of hormonal functions of the anterior pituitary. Pituitary hypofunction may be classified as primary (caused by intrinsic pituitary disease), secondary (caused by hypothalamic disorders), or functional (related to anorexia nervosa or chronic starvation). **Hyperpituitarism** is generally caused by a pituitary adenoma.

Anterior pituitary hypofunction may result from infarction of the gland, removal or destruction of the gland, or space-occupying lesions such as pituitary adenomas or aneurysms that compress otherwise-normal secreting pituitary cells and lead to compromised hormonal output. Growth hormone-secreting cells are most sensitive to pressure. Hyperfunction of the anterior pituitary generally implies an adenoma composed of secretory pituitary cells. Compression of a portion of the gland by an adenoma may lead to hypersecretion of one hormone produced by the adenoma, and hyposecretion of another due to the compression effects of the tumor.

Hypopituitarism

Primary and secondary hypopituitarism are not usually distinguished. Secondary hypopituitarism (resulting from dysfunction of the hypothalamus) is difficult to document because the neurohormonal output of the hypothalamus does not lend itself to measurement.

A cause of hypopituitarism is pituitary infarction. Infarction may be seen in conjunction with Sheehan syndrome (postpartum pituitary necrosis), pituitary apoplexy, shock, sickle cell disease, and diabetes mellitus. Other causes of hypopituitarism are head trauma; infections (such as meningitis, syphilis, and tuberculosis); vascular malformations; surgical ablation related to tu-

mor removal; and, rarely, granulomatous lesions. Hypopituitarism has been studied most frequently in cases of Sheehan syndrome.

Pathophysiology

The pituitary gland is extremely vascular and is therefore extremely vulnerable to infarction. The likelihood of infarction is increased with the increased size and vasculature of the gland, which occurs during pregnancy. Sheehan and Stanfield proposed in 1961 that the primary pathologic mechanism in postpartum pituitary infarction is vasospasm of the artery supplying the anterior pituitary. A frequently identified cause is some event that leads to circulatory collapse and compensatory vasospasm. If vasospasm is sustained for more than several hours, tissue necrosis occurs. The pituitary gland may be particularly susceptible to necrosis because its blood supply, through the portal system, is already partially deoxygenated and, especially in the hyperplastic pituitary of pregnancy, oxygen demands are increased.

Following tissue necrosis, edema occurs. Expansion of the pituitary within the fixed confines of the sella turcica further impedes blood supply to the pituitary. A second mechanism, which may be involved in pituitary infarction in the postpartum woman, is an increased risk for intravascular coagulation. In such individuals excessive fibrin is deposited in the pituitary vessels, predisposing the woman to decreased blood supply and infarction of the pituitary (Sheehan & Davis, 1982).

Clinical Manifestations

The signs and symptoms of hypofunction of the anterior pituitary depend on the affected hormones. If all hormones are absent (a condition termed **panhypopituitarism**), the individual suffers from cortisol deficiency from lack of ACTH, thyroid deficiency from lack of thyroid-stimulating hormone (TSH), diabetes insipidus from lack of ADH, and gonadal failure and loss of secondary sex characteristics from absence of FSH and LH. Growth hormone and, consequently, somatomedin levels are low and may affect children, but these deficiencies do not generally develop into a symptom complex in adults (Fig. 18-3). Additionally, postpartum women are unable to lactate, because of the absence of prolactin.

ACTH deficiency is a potentially life-threatening disorder, because cortisol is required for functional maintenance. ACTH deficiency is usually encountered with generalized pituitary hypofunction; it rarely occurs as an isolated event. Within 2 weeks of the complete absence of ACTH, symptoms of cortisol insufficiency develop. These include nausea, vomiting, anorexia, fatigue, and weakness. The resulting hypoglycemia is caused by increased insulin sensitivity, decreased glycogen reserves, and decreased gluconeogenesis associated with hypo-

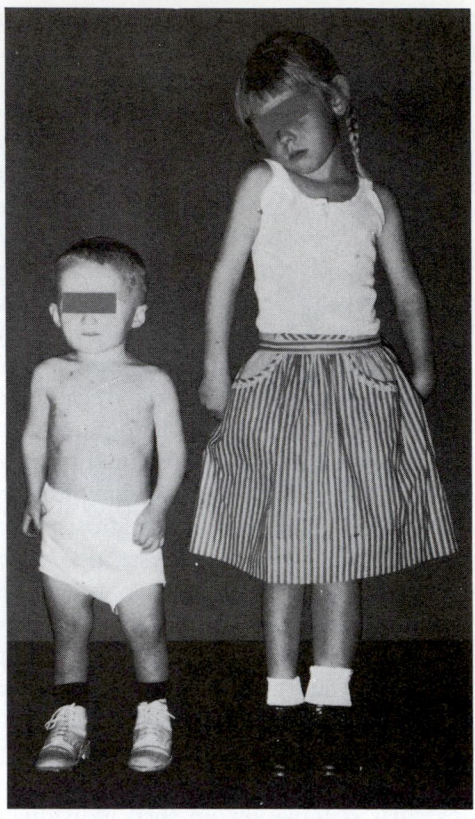

FIG. 18-3. Hypopituitary dwarfism in a 4-year-old boy whose height is 25 inches. Girl is also 4 years old and has a normal height of 39 inches. Dwarf has a normal face, as well as head, trunk, and limbs of approximately normal proportions. (From Brasher & Raney, 1986.)

cortisolism. In women, loss of body hair and decreased libido may be due to decreased adrenal androgen production.

ACTH deficiency also limits maximum aldosterone secretion, although the renin-angiotensin system is capable of stimulating some aldosterone secretion. Glomerular filtration rate is decreased with ACTH deficiency and may explain the decreased urine output. (Renal function is described in Chapter 32.) This may be of some benefit in the individual who has diabetes insipidus, but the polyuria associated with diabetes insipidus worsens after correction of cortisol levels. Frequently, individuals maintain some low level of ACTH secretion, so that cortisol replacement is not necessary. If ACTH is completely absent, however, cortisol replacement is required to maintain life.

TSH deficiency is rarely seen in isolation but frequently occurs in conjunction with other pituitary hormone deficiencies. The effects of decreased TSH levels may become apparent 4 to 8 weeks after the onset of hypothyrotropinemia. Cold intolerance, dryness of skin, mild myxedema, lethargy, and decreased metabolic rate

occur as a result of hypothyroidism induced by decreased TSH levels. The symptoms are usually less severe than those associated with primary hypothyroidism.

The onset of FSH and LH deficiencies in women of reproductive age is associated with amenorrhea and an atrophic vagina, uterus, and breasts. In postpubertal males, atrophy of the testicles and decreased beard growth occur. Both men and women experience a decrease in body hair and diminished libido. FSH and LH deficiencies frequently occur as a result of pressure on the gonadotropes from other sources, such as tumors.

Evaluation and Treatment

The diagnostic tests evaluating hypopituitarism are not definitive but must be interpreted together with the individual's signs and symptoms. In cases of hypopituitarism, the underlying disorder should be corrected as quickly as possible. Frequently, cerebral edema is corrected by the administration of dexamethasone, which also corrects hypocortisolism. Thyroid and cortisol replacement therapy will need to be maintained. Sex steroid replacement therapy may be initiated, depending on the needs and desires of the indivdidual.

Hyperpituitarism: Primary Adenoma

Pituitary adenomas are usually benign, slow-growing tumors that frequently arise from cells of the anterior pituitary. The incidence of pituitary adenomas may be as high as 22%, but most of these adenomas are microscopic and asymptomatic. Most are found only on postmortem examinations. The cause of pituitary adenomas is not known. The mortality associated with pituitary tumors is usually due to alterations in hormone secretion or tissue changes caused by expanding adenomas.

Pathophysiology

Local expansion of pituitary adenomas causes both neurologic and secretory effects. Neurologically, the tumor may impinge on the optic chiasma, particularly if it extends upward from the sella turcica. This causes a variety of visual disturbances, depending upon the portion of the nerve that is compressed. If the tumor is malignant, invasion of the oculomotor and trigeminal nerves occurs, evoking symptoms relative to their function. Extension may also involve the hypothalamus, disturbing hypothalamic control of wakefulness, thirst, appetite, and temperature.

The adenomatous tissue secretes the hormone of the cell type from which it arose, without regard to the needs of the body and without benefit of regulatory feedback mechanisms. Because of the pressure exerted by a tumor growing in the unexpandable skull, those secreting cells of the anterior pituitary that are most sensitive to pressure may also be affected (growth hormone-secreting cells, FSH- and LH-secreting cells). The result of such pressure is hyposecretion of these hormones.

Clinical Manifestations

The clinical manifestations of pituitary adenomas are related to tumor growth and hormone hypersecretion and hyposecretion. Effects from an increase in tumor size include such nonspecific complaints as headache, fatigue, neck pain or stiffness, and seizures. Visual changes produced by pressure on the optic chiasma include visual field impairments (frequently beginning in one eye and progressing to the other) and temporary blindness. If the tumor infiltrates other cranial nerves, neuromuscular function is affected.

The hyposecretion of the pituitary hormones caused by pressure changes results in impaired pituitary function. Hyposecretion of growth hormone almost always occurs, but in adults this is clinically asymptomatic. Gonadotropic hyposecretion frequently results in menstrual irregularity in women, decreased libido, and receding secondary sex characteristics in both men and women. If the tumor exerts sufficient pressure, thyroid and adrenal hypofunction may occur because of lack of TSH and ACTH. These result in the symptoms of hypothyroidism and hypocortisolism. Hypersecretion of hormones secreted by the adenoma, itself, leads to symptoms associated with the particular hormone that is affected.

Evaluation and Treatment

Diagnosis of pituitary adenoma involves physical and laboratory evaluations, including pertinent hormone assays and radiographic examination of the skull. This may be accomplished by computed tomographic scanning used in conjunction with contrast material.

The goal of treatment is to protect the individual from the effects of tumor growth and to control hormone hypersecretion while minimizing damage to appropriately secreting portions of the pituitary. Surgery and radiation therapy are used, depending on the extent of tumor growth and the suitability of the individual for surgery.

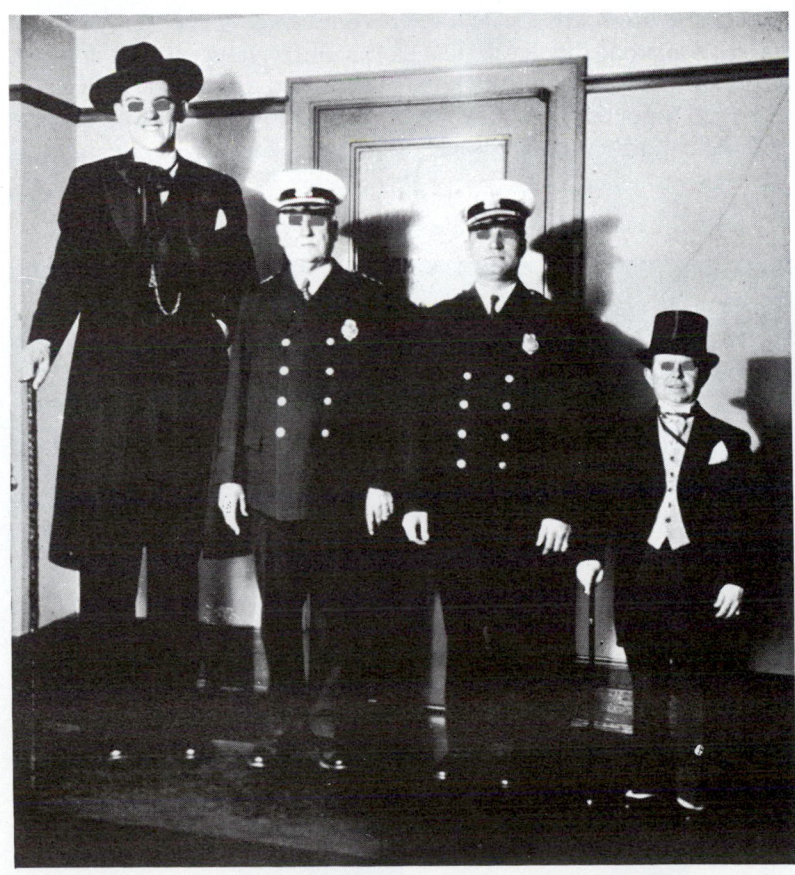

FIG. 18-4. A pituitary giant and dwarf contrasted with normal-sized men. Excessive secretion of growth hormone by the anterior lobe of the pituitary gland during the early years of life produces giants of this type, whereas deficient secretion of this substance produces well-formed dwarfs. (From Thibodeau, 1987.)

Hypersecretion of Growth Hormone: Acromegaly

Acromegaly occurs in adults who are exposed to continuously excessive levels of growth hormone (GH). In children and adolescents whose epiphyseal plates have not yet closed, the effect of increased GH levels is termed **giantism** (Fig. 18-4).

Acromegaly is a relatively uncommon disease, estimated to occur in about 40 cases per million (Imera, 1985). Approximately 15% of all pituitary tumors release excessive GH. The most common cause of acromegaly is a primary autonomous GH-secreting pituitary adenoma. Acromegaly occurs more frequently in women than men and is diagnosed most frequently in adults in their 40s and 50s, although the disease was usually present for years preceding the diagnosis.

Acromegaly is a slowly progressive disease, which, if untreated, is associated with a decreased life expectancy. The increased number of deaths associated with acromegaly are apparently due to an increased occurrence of hypertension and diabetes mellitus.

Pathophysiology

With a GH-secreting adenoma, the usual GH baseline secretion pattern is lost, as are sleep-related GH peaks. A totally unpredictable secretory pattern ensues. With only slight elevations of GH, somatomedin levels increase, stimulating growth. In the adult, epiphyseal closure has occurred, and increased amounts of GH and somatomedins cannot stimulate further long bone growth. Instead these elevations cause connective tissue proliferation and an increase in the cytoplasmic matrix, as well as bony proliferation that results in the characteristic appearance of acromegaly.

GH acts on the renal tubules to increase phosphate reabsorption, leading to mild hyperphosphatemia. The metabolic effects of GH hypersecretion include impaired carbohydrate tolerance and increased metabolic rate. Hyperglycemia may be seen as a result of GH's inhibition of peripheral glucose uptake and increased hepatic glucose production, followed by compensatory hyperinsulinism, and finally, insulin resistance. Diabetes mellitus occurs when the pancreas is unable to secrete enough insulin to offset the effects of GH. Somatotropic tumors are frequently associated with decreased gonadotropin secretion, leading to oligoamenorrhea in women and impotence in men.

Clinical Manifestations

As a result of connective tissue proliferation, individuals with acromegaly have enlarged tongues, interstitial edema, increase in the size and function of sebaceous and sweat glands (leading to increased body odor), and coarse skin and body hair. The course skin condition becomes very apparent when procedures such as inserting an intravenous needle are performed; the skin is very thick and difficult to penetrate (Fig. 18-5). Bony proliferation involves periosteal vertebral growth and enlargement of the facial bones, and the bones of the hands and

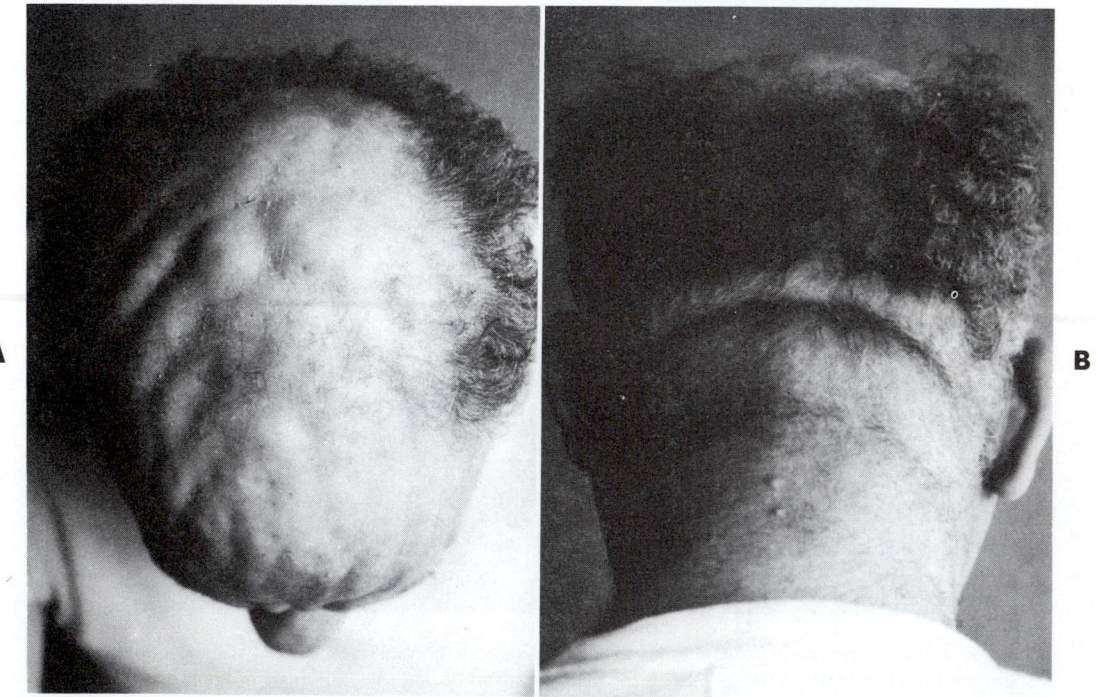

FIG. 18-5. Acromegaly. Note thickening of skin on, scalp **(A)** and posterior surface of neck **(B)**. (From Thibodeau, 1987.)

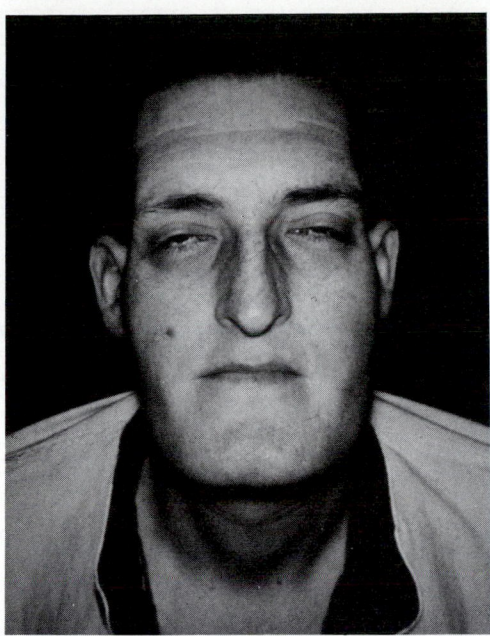

FIG. 18-6. Acromegaly. Note large head, forward projection of jaw, and protrusion of frontal bone. (From Thibodeau, 1987.)

feet (Fig. 18-6). When the bony proliferation is pronounced or advanced, the sinuses become enlarged and the sound of the individual's voice reverberates in the sinuses producing an unusual effect. The associated growth results in protrusion of the lower jaw and forehead and a need for increasingly larger sizes of shoes, hats, rings, and gloves.

Because somatomedins stimulate cartilaginous growth, the increased somatomedin levels cause elongation of ribs at the bone-cartilage junction, leading to a barrel-chested appearance and increased proliferation of cartilage in joints. This in turn causes backache, arthralgia, and arthritis. These are early manifestations of acromegaly. Soft tissue overgrowth is particularly obvious upon examination of the palms of the hands and the soles of the feet. When shaking hands with an individual with acromegaly, one can palpate the large soft tissues. With bony and soft-tissue overgrowth, entrapment of nerves may occur, leading to peripheral nerve damage as manifested by weakness, muscular atrophy, foot drop, and sensory changes in the hands.

Hypertension and congestive heart failure are seen in one third to one half of individuals with acromegaly, although the associated pathophysiology is not understood at present (Ezrin et al., 1980). Headache occurs in 50% to 87% of cases and does not appear related to GH levels, size, or extension of the tumor or presence of hypertension. Because of a space-occupying lesion, central nervous system symptoms of headache, seizure activity, visual disturbances (such as bitemporal hemaniopia from compression of the optic chiasma), papilledema, and compression hypopituitarism may occur.

If compression hypopituitarism does occur, the secretion of the gonadotropins may be affected. This causes amenorrhea in women and impotence in men. The secretion of prolactin-inhibiting factor is impaired in 30% to 40% of individuals with acromegaly. Approximately one third of people with acromegaly have impaired glucose tolerance, and one half of these are diabetic (Ezrin et al., 1980).

Evaluation and Treatment

Diagnosis of GH hypersecretion involves measurement of serum GH by radioreceptor assay or radioimmunoassay at basal conditions and in response to glucose administration. The goals of treatment are to normalize or reduce GH secretion, if possible, allowing normal pituitary function and relieving or preventing complications related to tumor expansion. The treatment of choice in acromegaly is surgical removal of the GH-secreting adenoma. Treatment by radiotherapy may be effective when rapid control of GH levels is not essential, when the individual is not a good surgical candidate, or when hyperfunction persists after subtotal resection.

ALTERATIONS OF THYROID FUNCTION

Hyperthyroidism
Course of Hyperthyroidism

Hyperthyroidism is a condition in which thyroid hormones (TH) exert greater-than-normal responses (Rabin & McKenna, 1982). Hyperthyroidism has a variety of causes. Identifying the cause is important because the treatment and expected outcome vary accordingly. Specific diseases that can cause hyperthyroidism include Graves disease, exogenous hyperthyroidism (iatrogenic, iodine induced), thyroiditis (acute, subacute), toxic nodular goiter, toxic multinodular goiter, and thyroid cancer. Each of these conditions is associated with specific pathophysiology and manifestations, which will be described in the following pages. All forms of hyperthyroidism share some common characteristics.

Clinical Manifestations

The clinical features of hyperthyroidism are due to the metabolic effects of increased circulating levels of thyroid hormones. This usually results in an increased metabolic rate with heat intolerance and an increased tissue sensitivity to stimulation by the sympathetic division of the autonomic nervous system. The major manifestations are summarized in Table 18-1.

Evaluation and Treatment

The diagnosis of hyperthyroidism is related to the symptoms acompanying specific diseases that cause hy-

TABLE 18-1 Systemic effects of hyperthyroidism

System	Manifestations	Mechanisms
Endocrine	Enlarged thyroid gland (97%-99% of cases) systolic or continuous bruit over thyroid; increased cortisol degradation. Hypercalcemia and decreased PTH secretion; diminished sensitivity to exogenous insulin	Hyperactivity of the thyroid gland; excess bone resorption leading to hypercalcemia and a disruption of PTH-regulating mechanisms; increased insulin degradation
Reproductive	Oligomenorrhea or amenorrhea in women, impotence and decreased libido in men; increased serum estradiol and estrone but lower than normal levels of free estradiol and estrone	Menstrual cycle alterations that may be related to hypothalamic or pituitary disturbances; increase in sex hormone-binding globulin
Gastrointestinal	Weight loss and an associated increase in appetite; increased peristalsis leading to less formed and more frequent stools; nausea, vomiting, anorexia, abdominal pain; increased use of hepatic glycogen stores and of adipose and protein stores; decrease in serum lipid levels (including triglycerides, phospholipids, and cholesterol); changes in vitamin metabolism leading to decrease in tissue stores of vitamins	Increased catabolism leading to the body's inability to meet its metabolic needs; malabsorption of fat; increased glucose absorption; increase in cholesterol excretion in feces and cholesterol conversion to bile salts; impaired conversion of B vitamins to their coenzymes, causing increased need for water-soluble and fat-soluble vitamins
Integumentary	Excessive sweating, flushing, and warm skin; heat intolerance; hair fine, soft, and straight; temporary hair loss; nails that grow away from nail beds	Hyperdynamic circulatory state
Sensory	Ocular manifestations including elevated upper eyelid leading to decreased blinking and a staring quality; infiltrative ocular changes associated with Graves disease	Overactivity of Muller's muscle

perthyroidism and associated laboratory findings. Elevated serum T_4, T_3, and radioactive iodine uptake (RAIU) are common in hyperthyroid states.

The treatment of hyperthyroidism is directed at controlling excessive TH production, secretion, or action. The major types of therapy currently used to achieve these goals include drug therapy, radioactive iodine therapy, and surgery.

Antithyroid drugs currently used act either to impair production of thyroid hormones (propylthiouracil) or to block their action (methimazole). Propranolol, a beta-adrenergic blocking agent, may also be given to decrease sympathetic nervous system responses to hyperthyroidism.

Radioactive iodine (I131), administered orally, is concentrated in active thyroid tissue and produces a local destructive effect. This treatment is recommended for permanent control of hyperthyroidism.

A subtotal thyroidectomy is the treatment of choice in children and younger individuals, in persons with severe disease, and in situations in which radioactive iodine is contraindicated or refused by the individual.

Hyperthyroid Conditions

Graves Disease

Graves disease is the most common cause of hyperthyroidism. Although the exact cause of Graves disease is currently unknown, the most accepted theory is that the disease is associated with autoimmune abnormalities (see Chapter 8). Graves disease is a familial disorder, characterized as a multisystem syndrome consisting of one or more of the following: (1) hyperthyroidism, (2) diffuse thyroid enlargement, (3) ophthalmopathy, (4) dermopathy, and (5) effects on the extremities (Farid & Stenzky, 1988).

The pathology of Graves disease indicates that normal regulatory mechanisms are overridden by some abnormal thyroid-stimulating mechanism. Substances termed thyroid-stimulating immunoglobulins (TSI) of the IgG class are found in more than 95% of subjects with Graves disease. The hyperfunction of the thyroid gland leads to suppression of TSH and thyrotropin-releasing hormone (TRH), although these usual feedback mechanisms are ineffective in lowering TH levels. The hyperfunction of the thyroid gland is reflected in a dramatically increased iodine uptake and increased rate of thyroid gland metabolism, which may in turn contribute to the hypervascularity and enlargement of the gland. The disproportionate increase in T_3 production reflects chronic hyperstimulation of the thyroid gland. A decrease in the concentration of thyroid-binding globulin, combined with the increased production of thyroid hormone, causes increased circulating levels of thyroid hormone responsible for many of the thyrotoxic symptoms.

A small number of individuals with Graves disease experience **pretibial myxedema,** characterized by subcutaneous swelling on the anterior portions of the legs, and by indurated and erythematous skin. These manifestations occasionally appear on the hands as well. Because pretibial myxedema is a widespread alteration in a number of disorders, Graves dermopathy has been proposed as a term to replace pretibial myxedema (Ezrin, 1979).

Many individuals with Graves disease experience ocular manifestations (Fig. 18-7). Two categories of ocular manifestations are associated with Graves disease: (1) functional abnormalities resulting from hyperactivity of the sympathetic division of the autonomic nervous system and (2) infiltrative changes involving the orbital contents. Functional abnormalities occur in most individuals with Graves disease. These abnormalities include a lag of the globe on upward gaze or a lag of the upper lid on downward gaze. This manifestation does not appear to affect ocular function and appears to resolve with treatment for hyperthyroidism.

Infiltrative ophthalmopathy may occur with Graves disease, although the ophthalmopathy appears to be a separate disorder. It appears in 50% to 70% of individuals with Graves disease (Rabin & McKenna, 1982), and it is characterized by edema of the orbital contents, protrusion of the globe, paralysis of the extraocular muscles, and damage to the retina and optic nerve, which may lead to blindness. These changes result in exophthalmos, periorbital edema, and extraocular muscle weakness leading to diplopia. The individual may experience irritation, pain, lacrimation, photophobia, and blurred vision. Occasionally, decreased visual acuity, papilledema, visual field impairment, exposure keratosis, and corneal ulceration may occur.

Unfortunately, current treatment for Graves disease does not reverse the infiltrative ophthalmopathy or the pretibial myxedema. Therapy for these problems is palliative, although skin lesions rarely require treatment.

Nodular Goiter

The thyroid gland normally hypertrophies in response to an increased demand for TH which occurs in puberty, pregnancy, and iodine deficiency. The hypertrophy is a compensatory mechanism in response to increased TSH levels. When the condition requiring increased TH resolves, TSH secretion normally subsides and the thyroid gland returns to its original size.

Irreversible changes may, however, have occurred in some follicular cells, so that such cells now function autonomously. Hyperthyroidism may or may not result from these irreversible changes. Autonomously functioning cells may produce less TH than the body requires. The remainder of the gland then functions to supply the remainder of the body's need and a euthyroid state is achieved and maintained. If the autonomously functioning cells produce sufficient or excessive TH for the usual body requirement, the remainder of the gland undergoes involution, becoming normal but inactive tissue. This condition may result in euthyroidism or hyperthyroidism, depending on the amount of TH produced.

Once hyperthyroidism results, the condition is generally termed **toxic nodular goiter.** The manifestations of hyperthyroidism resulting from toxic nodular goiter are similar to those of Graves disease, although infiltrative opthalmopathy and myxedema do not occur. The symptoms usually develop slowly and appear over time.

Thyrotoxic Crisis

Thyrotoxic crisis (thyroid storm) is a dangerous worsening of the thyrotoxic state, in which death occurs within 48 hours without treatment. The condition may develop spontaneously, but it occurs most frequently in individuals who have undiagnosed or partially treated severe hyperthyroidism and who are subjected to excessive stress from other causes. These causes may include infection, pulmonary or cardiovascular disorders, emo-

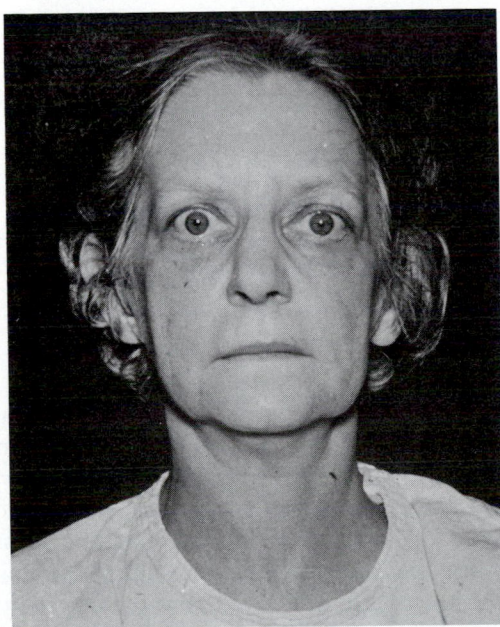

FIG. 18-7. Graves disease. Note large and protruding eyeballs. (From Thibodeau, 1987.)

TABLE 18-2 Systemic manifestations of hypothyroidism

System	Manifestations	Mechanisms
Neurologic	Confusion, syncope, slowed speech and thinking, memory loss; lethargy, headaches, hearing loss, night blindness; slow, clumsy movements. Cerebellar ataxia; slow alpha wave activity and loss of amplitude in EEG; reduced cAMP response to epinephrine, glucagon, and PTH	Decreased cerebral blood flow leading to cerebral hypoxia; reduced intracellular processes caused by decreased beta-adrenergic activity that may be related to a decrease in the number of beta-adrenergic receptor sites
Endocrine	Increased TSH production in primary hypothyroidism; enlarged pituitary thyrotropes, increase in serum prolactin levels with galactorrhea; decreased rate of cortisol turnover but with normal serum cortisol levels.	Impaired TH synthesis or defects in iodide trapping leading to compensatory TSH production; chronic overstimulation of thyrotropes by TRH and by TSH synthesis; stimulation of lactotropes by TRH related to increased prolactin levels; decreased deactivation of cortisol
Reproductive	Decreased androgen secretion in men, increased estriol formation in women; low total hormone values but with increased amounts of unbound hormone; anovulation, decreased libido, and a high incidence of spontaneous abortion in women; impotence, decreased libido, and digospermia in men	Altered metabolism of estrogens and androgens; decreased sex hormone-binding globulin
Hematologic	Decrease in red cell mass leading to normocytic, normochromic anemia; macrocytic anemia associated with vitamin B_{12} deficiency and inadequate folate or iron absorption in the GI tract	Decreased basal metabolic rate and reduced oxygen requirements, decreased production of erythropoietin, possible relationship between TH and optimal hematologic response to vitamin B_{12}.
Cardiovascular	Reduction in stroke volume and heart rate causing lowered cardiac output; increased peripheral vascular resistance to maintain systolic blood pressure; normal response to exercise but with alterations in circulatory system at rest (prolonged circulation time and decreased blood flow to tissues); cool skin and cold tolerance; enlarged heart; decreased intensity of heart sounds and variety of ECG changes (sinus bradycardia, prolonged PR interval, depressed P waves, flattened or inverted T waves, and low-amplitude QRS complexes); cardiac tamponade (although rare)	Decreased metabolic demands and loss of regulatory and rate-setting effects of TH; protein-mucopolysaccharide-rich fluid in the periocardial sac associated with enlarged heart; pericardial effusions associated with heart sounds and ECG changes

tional distress, or inadequate preparation for thyroid surgery.

The symptoms of thyrotoxic crisis include hyperthermia; tachycardia, especially atrial tachydysrhythmias; high-output heart failure; agitation or delirium; and nausea, vomiting, or diarrhea contributing to fluid volume depletion. The treatment is designed to reduce both circulating TH levels by inducing a block of thyroid hormone synthesis and thereby reducing their effects to eliminate the precipitating disorder; and to provide supportive care.

Hypothyroidism

Deficient production of TH by the thyroid gland results in the clinical state termed **hypothyroidism.** Hypothyroidism may be either primary or secondary. Primary causes include (1) congenital defects or loss of thyroid tissue following treatment for hyperthyroidism and (2) defective hormone synthesis resulting from autoimmune (circulating antithyroid antibodies) thyroiditis, endemic iodine deficiency, or antithyroid drugs. Causes of secondary hypothyroidism include (1) insufficient stimulation of the normal gland, causing TSH defi-

TABLE 18-2 Systemic manifestations of hypothyroidism—cont'd

System	Manifestations	Mechanisms
Pulmonary	Dyspnea; myxedematous changes in respiratory muscles leading to hypoventilation and carbon dioxide retention, which contribute to myxedema coma	Pleural effusions associated with dyspnea, although effusions may be asymptomatic
Renal	Reduced renal blood flow and glomerular filtration rate leading to decreased renal excretion of water; increase in total body water and dilutional hyponatremia; reduced production of erythropoietin	Hemodynamic alterations associated with reduced blood flow and filtration; increased total body water related to decreased excretion and mucinous deposits in tissue
Gastrointestinal	Decreased appetite; constipation, weight gain, and fluid retention; decreased absorption of most nutrients; decreased protein metabolism leading to retarded skeletal and soft-tissue growth and slightly positive nitrogen balance; edema; decreased glucose absorption and delayed glucose uptake; increased sensitivity to exogenous insulin; elevated serum lipid values	Reduced intake and reduced peristaltic activity that may progress to fecal impaction; water absorption related to prolonged transit time; fluid retention associated with myxedematous changes; edema associated with high concentrations of exchangeable albumin in the extravascular space caused by increased capillary permeability to proteins; depressed insulin degradation; depressed lipid synthesis and degradation
Musculoskeletal	Muscle aching and stiffness; slow movement and slow tendon jerk reflexes; decreased bone formation and resorption, increased bone density; aching and stiffness in joints.	Decreased rate of muscle contraction and relaxation contributing to slow movement and reflexes
Integumentary	Dry, flaky skin; dry, brittle head and body hair; reduced growth of nails and hair	Reduced sweat and sebaceous gland secretion

ciency from hypothyroidism of the pituitary or hypothalamus and (2) peripheral resistance to TH (Ezrin, 1979; Williams, 1981).

Pathophysiology

In primary hypothyroidism, the loss of thyroid tissue leads to a decreased production of TH. The response is an increased secretion of TSH that leads to goiter. Secondary hypothyroidism is most commonly caused by failure of the pituitary to synthesize adequate amounts of TSH. Postpartum pituitary necrosis and a pituitary tumor are the most frequent causes of secondary hypothyroidism.

Clinical Manifestations

Hypothyroidism generally affects all body systems with the extent of the symptoms closely related to the degree of TH deficiency. The lowered levels of TH result in decreased energy metabolism and heat production. The individual develops a low basal metabolic rate, cold intolerance, and slightly lowered basal body temperature (Table 18-2). A decrease in TH may lead to excessive TSH production and goiter.

The characteristic sign of hypothyroidism is **myxedema,** which is histologically similar to the pretibial myxedema deposits that often occur with Graves disease. Myxedema is a result of an alteration in the composition of the dermis and other tissues. The connective fibers are separated by an increased amount of protein and mucopolysaccharides.

This protein-mucopolysaccharide complex binds water, producing nonpitting, boggy edema, especially around the eyes, hands, and feet and in the supraclavicular fossae (Fig. 18-8). Binding with water is also responsible for thickening of the tongue and the laryngeal and pharyngeal mucous membranes. This results in thick slurred speech and hoarseness, both common in hypothyroidism.

Evaluation and Treatment

In addition to the clinical symptoms of hypothyroidism, a decrease in serum T_4 and free T_4 is nearly always present. When hypothyroidism is caused by pituitary deficiencies, serum TSH levels will be decreased. Hormone replacement therapy is the treatment of choice for hypothyroidism. TH is currently available as

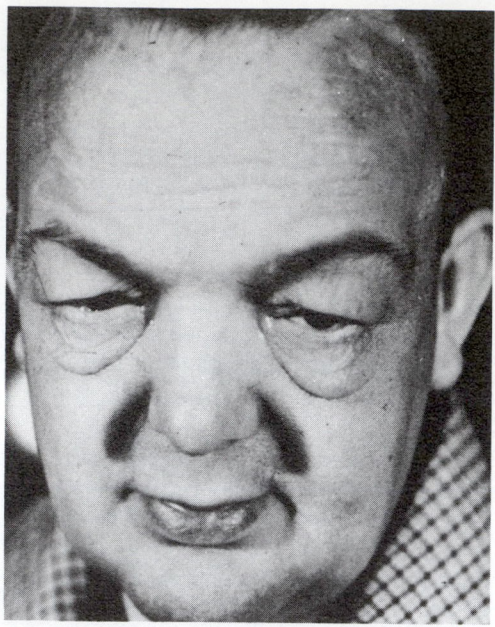

FIG. 18-8. Myxedema. Note the edema around eyes and facial puffiness. (From Thibodeau, 1987.)

a synthetic hormone (levothyroxine or liothyronine) and is generally preferred over the crude extract from animal thyroid glands (desiccated thyroid).

The restoration of normal TH levels should be timed appropriately; a regimen of hormonal therapy depends on the individual's age, the duration and severity of the hypothyroidism, and the presence of other disorders, particularly cardiovascular disorders. The goal is maximal metabolic restoration consistent with the individual's overall well-being.

Hypothyroid Conditions

Hypothyroidism results from three relatively rare disorders, none of which is related to any of the others by etiology, symptoms, management, or outcome. These three conditions are acute thyroiditis, subacute thyroiditis, and autoimmune thyroiditis. **Acute thyroiditis** is caused by a bacterial infection of the thyroid gland. **Subacute thyroiditis** is a non-bacterial inflammation of the thyroid often preceded by a viral infection. Both conditions are accompanied by fever, tenderness, and enlargement of the thyroid. The inflammatory process results in hypothyroidism. **Autoimmune thyroiditis** (Hashimoto disease or chronic lymphocytic thyroiditis) results in destruction of thyroid tissue by circulating thyroid antibodies and infiltration of lymphocytes. Autoimmune thyroiditis may also be caused by an inherited immune defect.

Myxedema Coma

A medical emergency, **myxedema coma** is a diminished level of consciousness associated with severe hypothyroidism. Symptoms include hypothermia without shivering, hypoventilation, hypotension, hypoglycemia, and lactic acidosis. Older patients with severe vascular disease and with moderate or untreated hypothyroidism are particularly at risk for developing myxedema coma. It may also occur after overuse of narcotics or sedatives or after an acute illness in hypothyroid individuals.

Congenital Hypothyroidism

Hypothyroidism in infants occurs as a result of absent thyroid tissue (thyroid dysgenesis) and hereditary defects in thyroid hormone synthesis. Thyroid dysgenesis occurs more frequently in female infants with permanent abnormalities in 1 of every 400 live births (Jubitz, 1985).

Thyroid hormone is essential for embryonic growth, particularly of brain tissue. The infant will be mentally retarded if there is no thyroxine during fetal life, but this can be partially reversed with administration of thyroxine immediately after birth.

Clinical manifestations of hypothyroidism may not be evident until after 4 months of age. Symptoms include difficulty eating, hoarse cry, and protruding tongue due to myxedema of oral tissues and vocal cords; hypotonic muscles of the abdomen with constipation, abdominal protrusion, and umbilical hernia; subnormal temperature; lethargy; excessive sleeping; slow pulse; and cold mottled skin. Skeletal growth is stunted due to impaired protein synthesis, poor absorption of nutrients, and lack of bone mineralization. The child will be dwarfed, with short limbs, if not treated (Fig. 18-9). Dentition is often delayed. Mental retardation is a function of the severity of hypothyroidism and the delay before initiation of treatment.

Cord blood can be examined in the first days of life for thyroxine and TSH levels. Treatment is administration of thyroxine. There is a high probability of normal growth and intellectual function if treatment is started before the child is 3 or 4 months old.

Thyroid Carcinoma

Thyroid carcinoma is relatively rare, accounting for 11,000 new cases annually and approximately 0.5% of all cancer deaths per year (American Cancer Society, 1988). Iodine deficiency, chronic long-term use of goitrogenic drugs, exposure to ionizing radiation, or a combination of these causal factors has been shown to produce thyroid hyperplasia and, ultimately, malignancy in animals. In approximately 10% of cases, hyperplasia of the thyroid gland leads to thyroid carcinoma in humans. The most consistent causal risk factor in the development of thyroid cancer appears to be exposure to ionizing radiation, especially exposure during childhood.

Most individuals with thyroid carcinoma have normal T_3 and T_4 levels and are therefore euthyroid. Thyroid cancer is typically discovered as a small thyroid nodule

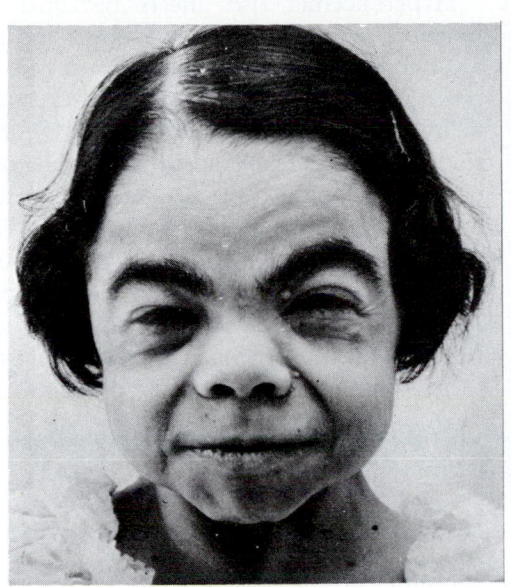
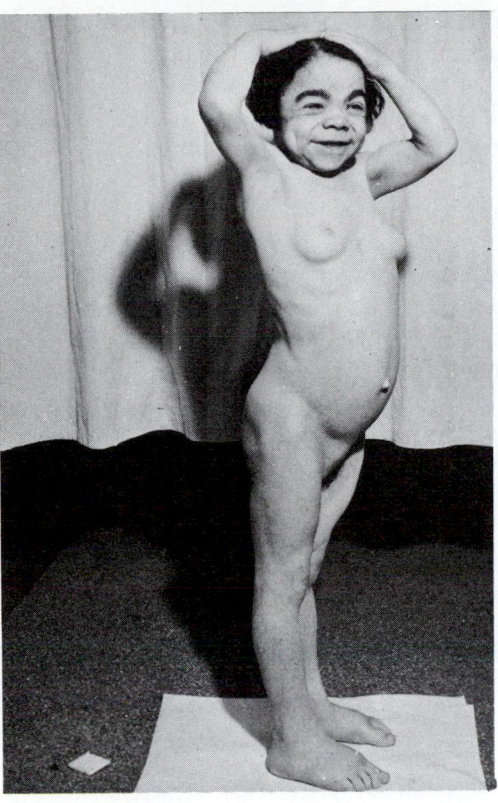

FIG. 18-9. Adult cretin. Note characteristic facial features, dwarfism (44 inches), absent axillary and scant pubic hair, poorly developed breasts, potbelly, and small umbilical hernia. (From Schneeburg, 1970.)

or as a metastatic tumor most commonly occurring in the lungs, brain, or bone. Changes in voice and swallowing and difficulty in breathing are related to tumor growth impinging on the trachea or esophagus. Diagnosing a thyroid cancer involves (1) measurement of serum thyroid levels, (2) radioisotope scanning, (3) ultrasonography, or (4) thyroid biopsy.

Treatment for thyroid carcinoma remains controversial, primarily because of the rarity of the disease, its protracted nature, and the relatively low mortality rate regardless of the method of treatment. Treatment may include partial or total thyroidectomy, TSH suppression therapy (levothyroxine), radioactive iodine therapy (in iodine-concentrating tumors), postoperative radiation therapy, and chemotherapy (especially in anaplastic carcinoma) (Camargo & Kolb, 1988).

ALTERATIONS OF PARATHYROID FUNCTION

Hyperparathyroidism

Hyperparathyroidism is characterized by greater than normal secretion of PTH. Hyperparathyroidism is classified as one of three types: primary, secondary, or tertiary.

Pathophysiology

Estimates suggest that primary hyperparathyroidism occurs in 0.2% to 0.3% of the adult population and occurs twice as often in women. It is generally found in older adults (Braunwald et al., 1987). Because postmenopausal women are a group already at risk for developing osteoporosis, the effects of increased levels of PTH on bone disease can be significant. Most cases of hyperparathyroidism (approximately 80%) are the result of a chief cell adenoma with an increased secretion of parathyroid hormone.

Primary Hyperparathyroidism

In **primary hyperparathyroidism,** the normal regulatory relationship between serum calcium levels and PTH secretion is interrupted so that PTH secretion is autonomous and not under the usual feedback control mechanisms. The increase in gastrointestinal absorption of calcium is presumed to reflect the kidney's increased generation of biologically active vitamin D in response to increased PTH levels (see Chapter 3, Fig. 3-7).

Secondary Hyperparathyroidism

Secondary hyperparathyroidism is a compensatory, although not inevitable, response of the parathyroid glands to chronic hypocalcemia. Chronic hypercalcemia can be associated with decreased renal activation of vitamin D as occurs in renal failure (see Chapters 3 and 35). In secondary hyperparathyroidism, secretion of PTH is elevated but PTH is unable to achieve normal calcium levels due to failure of a target organ, the kidney.

Tertiary Hyperparathyroidism

Hyperplasia of the parathyroid glands and a loss of sensitivity to circulating calcium levels can cause autonomous secretion of PTH, even with normal calcium levels. The condition is then termed **tertiary hyperthyroidism.** Tertiary hyperthyroidism frequently occurs in individuals with chronic renal failure. Signs and symptoms of this syndrome are similar to those of primary hyperparathyroidism.

Clinical Manifestations

Hypersecretion of PTH causes excessive osteoclastic and osteocytic activity, resulting in bone resorption. (Bone resorption is discussed in Chapter 38.) Pathologic bone changes include pathologic fractures, kyphosis of the dorsal spine, and compression fractures of the vertebral bodies. PTH hypersecretion and its resulting hypercalcemia increase the renal filtration load of calcium, leading to hypercalcuria.

Hypercalcemia also affects proximal renal tubular function, causing metabolic acidosis and production of an abnormally alkaline urine. Because calcium and phosphate levels are inversely related, hypercalcemia results in hypophosphatemia (see Chapter 3). Hyperparathyroidism directly results in hyperphosphaturia. The combination of these three variables—hypercalcuria, alkaline urine, and hyperphosphaturia—predisposes the individual to the formation of calcium stones. Kidney stones are frequently formed in the renal pelvis or in the renal collecting ducts and may be associated with infections. Both kidney stones and renal infection may lead to impaired renal function. Hypercalcemia also impairs

---

TABLE 18-3 Manifestations of primary hyperparathyroidism

Symptoms	Responsible derangements	Mechanisms
Renal colic, nephrolithiasis, recurrent urinary tract infections, renal failure	Hypercalcemia, hyperphosphaturia, proximal renal tubular bicarbonate leak, urine pH>6	Calcium phosphate salts precipitate in alkaline urine, in renal pelvis, and in collecting ducts. Calcium oxalate stones also formed.
Abdominal pain, peptic ulcer disease	Hypercalcemia-stimulated hypergastrinemia	Elevated hydrochloric acid secretion
Pancreatitis	Hypercalcemia	Etiology of relationship unknown
Bone disease, osteitis fibrosa and cystica, osteoporosis	PTH-stimulated bone resorption, metabolic acidosis	Osteoporosis now more commonly encountered, but other disorders more specific for hyperparathyroidism
Muscle weakness, myalgia	PTH excess, possible direct effect on striated muscle and on nerves	Characteristic myopathic changes in muscle histology, nerve conduction rate suppressed
Neurological and psychiatric problems	Hypercalcemia	Neuropathy. Electroencephalographic changes present
Polyuria, polydipsia	Hypercalcemia	Direct effect on renal tubule to decrease responsiveness to antidiuretic hormone
Constipation	Hypercalcemia	Decreased peristalsis of gastrointestinal tract
Anorexia, nausea, and vomiting	Hypercalcemia	Central stimulation of vomiting center
Hypertension	Renal disease, direct effect of calcium on arterial smooth muscle, pheochromocytoma	Plasma renin activity elevated or normal
Arthralgia and arthritis	Gout, pseudogout, periarticular classification	Hyperuricemia, chronic renal failure with high calcium X phosphate product

From Rabin, 1982.

the concentrating ability of the renal tubule by decreasing its response to ADH.

Chronic hypercalcemia of hyperparathyroidism is associated with insulin resistance, necessitating increased insulin secretion to maintain normal glucose levels. Hypercalcemia also affects the muscular, nervous, and gastrointestinal systems. (The clinical symptoms of primary hyperparathyroidism are summarized in Table 18-3.)

Evaluation and Treatment

The diagnosis of hyperparathyroidism is generally accomplished by excluding all the other possible causes of hypercalcemia. A definitive diagnosis must then be supported by at least a 6-month history of symptoms associated with hypercalcemia, including kidney stones, hypophosphatemia, hyperchloremia, and increased urinary calcium levels. Tests used to document hyperparathyroidism include measurement of serum calcium, phosphorus, magnesium, bicarbonate, chloride, and pH (urinary pH, calcium, and hydroxyproline); bone x-ray films and densiometry; catheterization of the thyroid veins to document the source of PTH secretion; and radioimmunoassays. Radioimmunoassays for PTH are not generally required for the diagnosis of hyperparathyroidism, and this test currently poses many problems in providing clear-cut evidence of hyperparathyroidism.

The treatment of hyperparathyroidism includes lowering of severely elevated calcium levels, increasing urinary calcium excretion with diuretics, and long-term management of hypercalcemia by use of drugs that decrease resorption of calcium from bone. Definitive treatment for hyperparathyroidism involves the surgical removal of the hyperplastic parathyroid glands.

Hypoparathyroidism

Hypoparathyroidism (abnormally low PTH levels) is most commonly caused by damage to the parathyroid glands during thyroid surgery. Overt postoperative parathyroid failure occurs in approximately 1% of all individuals undergoing thyroid surgery, with the incidence increasing to 10% after repeated neck explorations.

In hypoparathyroidism, a lack of circulating PTH causes a depressed serum calcium level and an increased serum phosphate level. In the absence of PTH, the abilities to resorb calcium from bone and to regulate calcium reabsorption from the renal tubules are impaired. Phosphate reabsorption by the renal tubules is therefore increased, causing hyperphosphatemia.

Hypoparathyroidism appears to result from hypomagnesemia, although the effects of hypomagnesemia on the peripheral metabolism and clearance of PTH are not clearly understood at present. Once serum magnesium levels are returned to normal, however, PTH secretion returns to normal. Hypomagnesemia may be related to chronic alcoholism, malnutrition, malabsorption, increased renal clearance of magnesium caused by the use of aminoglycoside antibiotics or certain chemotherapeutic agents, or prolonged magnesium-deficient parenteral nutritional therapy.

Clinical Manifestations

Symptoms associated with hypoparathyroidism are primarily those of hypocalcemia. Hypocalcemia causes a lowering of the threshold for nerve and muscle excitation so that a nerve impulse may be initiated by a slight stimulus anywhere along the length of a nerve or muscle fiber. This is manifested as muscle spasms, hyperreflexia, clonic-tonic convulsions, laryngeal spasms, and, in severe cases, death from asphyxiation.

Other symptoms of hypocalcemia are caused by mechanisms that are not yet understood. These symptoms include dry skin, loss of body and scalp hair, hypoplasia of developing teeth, horizontal ridges on the nails, cataracts, basal ganglia calcifications (which may be associated with a parkinsonian syndrome), and bone deformities including brachydactyly and bowing of the long bones.

Phosphate retention caused by increased renal reabsorption of phosphate is also associated with hypoparathyroidism. Hyperphosphatemia is associated with inhibition of the renal enzyme necessary for the conversion of vitamin D to its most active form. This tends to depress serum calcium levels further by reducing gastrointestinal absorption of calcium.

Evaluation and Treatment

A low serum calcium and high phosphorus level in the absence of renal failure, intestinal disorders, or nutritional deficiencies is diagnostic of hypoparathyroidism. PTH levels are usually normal in primary hypoparathyroidism.

The treatment of hypoparathyroidism is directed toward the alleviation of hypocalcemia. In acute states, this involves parenteral administration of calcium, which allows correction of serum calcium within minutes. Maintenance of serum calcium is achieved with pharmacologic doses of an active form of vitamin D and oral calcium. The recommended daily dose of calcium is 1 to 3 grams.

Hypoplastic dentition, cataracts, bone deformities, and basal ganglia calcifications do not respond to the correction of hypocalcemia, but the other symptoms of hypocalcemia are reversible. As serum calcium levels return to normal, phosphaturia is usually stimulated. This leads to a return to normal of serum phosphate levels. In some individuals, however, the absence of the phosphaturic effect of PTH causes a persistent hyperphosphatemia.

Significant elevations of phosphorus should be treated

with drugs that inhibit gastrointestinal absorption of phosphate and thus prevent ectopic calcifications. Such calcifications are likely to occur if the mathematical product of the serum calcium and serum phosphate levels exceeds 70 (i.e., $Ca^+ \times PO_4 = 70$). In such instances calcifications can be expected.

DYSFUNCTION OF THE ENDOCRINE PANCREAS: DIABETES MELLITUS

Diabetes mellitus is a complex syndrome that causes a number of physiologic changes, including alterations in carbohydrate, protein, and fat metabolism. The term has been applied to a number of pathogenically heterogeneous disorders, all characterized by a decreased tolerance for carbohydrates. Originally, *diabetes* described a disorder heralded by the passage of sweet urine, excessive urination and thirst, and excessive hunger and weight loss. The disease was recognized in at least two forms, one form that primarily affected the obese and another that was more common among younger, thin individuals. The overall prevalence of diabetes is about 1%.

The term *diabetes mellitus* is now used to describe a syndrome characterized by chronic hyperglycemia and other disturbances of metabolism. The current classification now divides diabetes mellitus into two general types. **Type I diabetes mellitus** is also referred to as insulin-dependent diabetes mellitus (IDDM) and is characterized by an acute onset. **Type II diabetes mellitus,** commonly referred to as non-insulin-dependent diabetes mellitus (NIDDM), generally has a more chronic onset. (Table 18-4 describes terminology and characteristics related to both types.)

The diagnosis of diabetes is based on (1) unequivocal elevation of plasma glucose concentrations in conjunction with classic signs and symptoms, (2) more than one elevated fasting plasma glucose level, or (3) more than one elevated plasma glucose level in response to oral glucose challenge. Because numerous epidemiologic studies have shown severe cardiovascular disease in individuals with only impaired glucose tolerance, early screening and detection is important and may be accomplished in a variety of ways. If urine is to be tested, it should be obtained 2 hours after a large carbohydrate load so that the test is most sensitive and helpful. After an individual reaches age 50, the test's sensitivity diminishes as the renal glucose threshold rises from about 160 mg/100 ml to 250 mg/100 ml, or higher in many elderly individuals. In addition, urine testing is not an accurate reflection of blood glucose levels when renal dysfunction is also present. Because of advances in monitoring blood glucose levels, urine testing is no longer routinely used for self-monitoring in individuals with diabetes.

An oral glucose tolerance test consists of the administration of a glucose load followed by a measurement of glucose in the urine and blood at specified intervals. Intravenous glucose tolerance tests are rarely used because they are generally less sensitive than oral glucose tolerance tests and may cause painful venous thrombosis. Another mechanism, used primarily to identify the plasma glucose concentration over time, is the measurement of glycosylated hemoglobin. In the normal 120-day life span of the red blood cell, glucose molecules join hemoglobin, forming glycosylated hemoglobin. In individuals with poorly controlled diabetes, increases in the quantities of three glycosylated hemoglobins A1A, A1B, and A1C are noted. Once a hemoglobin molecule is glycosylated, it remains that way. A build-up of glycosylated hemoglobin within the red cell reflects the average level of glucose to which the cell has been exposed during its life cycle. By measuring the glycosylated hemoglobin, particularly A1C, long-term glucose levels and the effectiveness of therapy may be monitored.

Types of Diabetes Mellitus
Type I Diabetes Mellitus

Although still controversial, evidence indicates no actual changes in the incidence of type I diabetes (Zimmet, 1983). The lack of standard methodology and diagnostic criteria make global comparisons difficult, but genuine differences in susceptibility to type I diabetes mellitus do appear among races. The disease is more common among whites, but the relation between genetic and environmental factors is not clear. Although the disease may affect older individuals, it is most typical in those under 30 years of age. Type I diabetes has a peak onset between the ages of 11 and 13. (Table 18-5 summarizes the epidemiology of diabetes mellitus.)

Pathophysiology

Before hyperglycemia or other symptoms of diabetes develop, 80% to 90% of the insulin-secreting beta cells in the islets of Langerhans must be destroyed. Several mechanisms contribute to beta cell dysfunction and eventual destruction in type I diabetes. The size and number of islet cells are significantly decreased. The remaining cells are small, atrophic, and fibrotic. Although beta cells are present in the islets at the onset of type I diabetes, they disappear as the disease progresses, and within a year, no beta cells may remain. Therefore no functional insulin is produced in type I diabetes.

The process of cellular destruction is marked by the appearance of **islet cell antibodies (ICA)** of the IgG class. (Classification of antibodies is described in Chapter 6.) ICA occurs in up to 85% of newly diagnosed insulin-dependent diabetics. The functional role of ICA is

TABLE 18-4 Classification and characteristics of diabetes mellitus

Name	Previous synonyms	Characteristics
Type I		
Insulin-dependent diabetes mellitus (IDDM)	Juvenile diabetes Juvenile-onset diabetes Ketosis-prone diabetes Brittle diabetes Idiopathic diabetes	Abrupt onset of symptoms Individual prone to ketoacidosis Insulin dependent Viral etiology, autoimmune basis, genetic importance being investigated Often affects young Decrease in size and number of islet cells
Type II		
Non-insulin-dependent diabetes mellitus (NIDDM)	Adult onset diabetes Maturity onset diabetes Stable diabetes Ketosis-resistant diabetes	Usually not insulin dependent Individual not ketosis prone (but individual may form ketones under stress) Several syndromes, both nonobese and obese Generally occurs in those over the age of 40 Strong familial pattern being investigated
Secondary diabetes	Same	Cause established or strongly suspected May be associated with pancreatic disease, hormonal diseases, drugs and chemical agents, genetic syndromes, or malnutrition
Impaired glucose tolerance (IGT)	Asymptomatic diabetes Chemical diabetes Borderline diabetes Subclinical diabetes Latent diabetes	Show abnormal response to oral glucose tolerance test May revert to normal, remain impaired, or progress to diabetes Many with IGT are obese
Gestational diabetes mellitus (GDM)	Same	Glucose intolerance first recognized during pregnancy Following pregnancy, glucose may normalize, remain impaired, or progress to diabetes mellitus.
Statistical risk class: •Previously abnormal glucose level •Potential abnormal glucose tolerance	Latent diabetes Prediabetes Potential diabetes	Previous abnormality of oral glucose tolerance test or increased risk of developing diabetes because of genetic relationship with a diabetic

unknown, and the antibodies tend to disappear with time after diagnosis. ICA occurs in 5% of individuals with type II diabetes and in 2% of individuals without diabetes mellitus (Fitzgerald & Kilveat, 1985).

A variety of theories explains the etiology of type I diabetes mellitus. These theories propose that type I diabetes involves an immune reaction, a viral disease, or inherited susceptibility combined with environmental factors (see Chapter 5). Evidence suggests that type I diabetes is caused by a gradual process of autoimmune destruction in genetically susceptible individuals (Zimmet, 1983). Although the exact nature of genetic susceptibility is not yet understood, a major factor is HLA-linked. (Human leukocyte antigen [HLA] loci and associated histocompatibility antigens are discussed in Chapter 6.) The strongest association with type I diabetes is with alleles at the HLA-D and HLA-DR loci. The risk of developing type I diabetes increases approximately five times when more specific loci, HLA-DR3 or HLA-DR4, are present. Although the familial tendency is not as strong as in cases of type II diabetes mellitus, the susceptibility to type I diabetes does appear to be inherited.

The cause that triggers autoimmune destruction is uncertain. Although no direct evidence of such a mechanism exists, the stimulus is assumed to be a virus or a group of viruses (Gamble, Taylor, & Cumming, 1973). This theory is somewhat supported by the incidence of type I diabetes. In the northern hemisphere, its highest incidence occurs during autumn and winter, in conjunction with increased viral infections. Investigations linking type I diabetes with coxsackie B4 virus or mumps infections are currently under way.

Regardless of the cause, a disequilibrium of hormones

TABLE 18-5 Epidemiology and etiology of diabetes mellitus

	Type I (IDDM)	Type II (NIDDM)
INCIDENCE		
Frequency	Relatively rare Rates for whites under 18 reported as 8-24/100,000 per year	Accounts for most cases Prevalence rates of 1% or more exist throughout most of the world
Change in frequency	Conflicting data Some studies suggest increased frequency, others no increase	No change in frequency when diagnostic methods, criteria, and age held constant
CHARACTERISTICS		
Age at onset	Peak onset at age 11 to 13 (slightly earlier for girls and later for boys) Rare in children under age 1 and adults over 30	Risk of developing diabetes increases after age 40
Sex	Slightly more common in males in some studies	Conflicting studies (with age adjustment, prevalence most likely higher in males)
Racial distribution	Rates for whites 1.5 to 2 times higher than for non-whites Higher rates for those of Scandinavian descent than for those of central or southern European descent	Certain racial groups may be more likely to develop type II diabetes when exposed to a particular environment Common in migrant groups encountering a different environment (e.g., Polynesians moving from traditional to western lifestyle) Most common among Pima Indians (a Native American tribe), who report 40% of males and 50% of females 45 years of age or older have type II diabetes
Socioeconomic status	Incidence of disease increases with higher social class	In the United States, disease is 3 times more prevalent in adults with lower incomes and less education
Seasonal distribution	More new cases documented during fall and winter in the northern hemisphere	No known association
Childbirth association	No association documented	Increased incidence in women with higher parity
ETIOLOGY		
Common theory	Gradual process of autoimmune destruction in genetically susceptible individuals Strong association with HLA-DR3 and HLA-DR4	Disease results from the action of several genes Associated with long-duration obesity
Heredity	Inherited susceptibility	Inherited susceptibility Familial tendency stronger than for type 1
Presence of antibody	Islet cell antibodies (ICA) reported in newly diagnosed individuals but tend to disappear with time after diagnosis	Islet cell antibodies rare
Insulin resistance	Insulin resistance is rare	Increased insulin resistance due to a decrease in number of cell receptor sites and altered cellular metabolism

TABLE 18-6 Clinical manifestations and rationale for type I diabetes mellitus	
Manifestations	**Rationale**
Polydipsia	Because of elevated blood sugar levels, water is osmotically attracted from body cells resulting in intracellular dehydration and stimulation of thirst in the hypothalamus
Polyuria	Hyperglycemia acts as an osmotic diuretic; the amount of glucose filtered by the glomeruli of the kidney exceeds that which can be reabsorbed by the renal tubules; glycosuria results, accompanied by large amounts of water lost in the urine
Polyphagia	Depletion of cellular stores of carbohydrates, fats, and protein results in cellular starvation and a corresponding increase in hunger
Weight loss	Weight loss occurs because of fluid loss in osmotic diuresis and the loss of body tissue as fats and proteins are used for energy.
Fatigue	Metabolic changes result in poor use of food products, contributing to lethargy and fatigue

produced by the islets of Langerhans occurs in diabetes mellitus. Considerable evidence suggests that both alpha-cell and beta-cell functions are abnormal and that both, a lack of insulin and a relative excess of glucagon (produced by alpha cells), exist in type I diabetes.

Hyperglycemia and hyperketonemia are not possible as a result of insulin deficiency alone; glucagon must be present in relative excess. Thus the full metabolic syndrome is caused by both hormones, a finding that may ultimately provide an entirely new therapeutic approach to the management of diabetes mellitus (Porte & Woods, 1983). Relative hyperglucagonemia occurs in every form of diabetes mellitus. The concentration of glucagon therefore is relatively high in comparison to the relative or absolute deficiency of insulin, and elevated blood glucose levels fail to suppress the production of glucagon. Overproduction of glucose and ketones, as occurs in uncontrolled diabetes mellitus, results from excessive glucagon relative to the amount of effective insulin. The ratio of insulin to glucagon in the portal vein—and not the concentration of each hormone—controls hepatic glucose and fat metabolism.

Clinical Manifestations

Type I diabetes mellitus affects the metabolism of fat, protein, and carbohydrates. Glucose accumulates in the blood and spills into the urine as the renal threshold for glucose is exceeded. In addition, protein and fat breakdown occurs because of the lack of insulin, resulting in weight loss.

Initial clinical manifestations of type I diabetes are generally acute. The individual often has the classic symptoms of polyuria, polydipsia, and polyphagia (Table 18-6). Weight loss and wide fluctuations in blood glucose levels occur.

Ketoacidosis, caused by increased levels of circulating ketones without the inhibiting effects of insulin, is also common. Accumulation of ketone acids causes a drop in pH and triggers the buffering system associated with metabolic acidosis (see Chapter 3). Acetone is then blown off, giving the breath a sweet or "fruity" odor. Occasionally, diabetic coma is the initial symptom of the disease.

Evaluation and Treatment

The diagnosis of diabetes is not difficult when the symptoms of polydipsia, polyuria, polyphagia, weight loss, and hyperglycemia are present in fasting and postprandial states. The diagnosis becomes more difficult in asymptomatic individuals with fasting blood glucose levels that are near normal. A fasting blood glucose value greater than 140 mg/dl documented on at least two occasions is considered abnormal. Table 18-7 summarizes the criteria established by the National Diabetes Data Group (1979), using fasting blood or an oral glucose tolerance test (OGTT). Age, diet, drugs, activity, and presence of disease must be considered when performing and interpreting the OGTT.

The ideal goal of treatment for individuals with type I

TABLE 18-7 Diagnostic criteria for diabetes mellitus in nonpregnant adults		
	Fasting	**OGTT (2 hrs)**
Venous plasma glucose	>140 mg/dl	>200 mg/dl
Venous whole blood glucose	> 120 mg/dl	>180 mg/dl
Capillary blood glucose	>120 mg/dl	>200 mg/dl

diabetes mellitus is the restoration of normal blood glucose levels and correction of all metabolic disorders. Most investigations support the view that most long-term complications are associated with hyperglycemia, wide fluctuations in glucose levels, and other metabolic abnormalities. Thus the more normally the glucose metabolism can be regulated, the more likely it is that complications can be avoided. Management of diabetes mellitus requires individual planning according to type of disease, age, and activity level, but all individuals require some combination of insulin, diet, and exercise.

Insulin Insulin administration is used to normalize blood glucose levels and to avoid or reduce the complications of diabetes. Exogenous insulin has been used only since 1922. Using recombinant DNA techniques, insulin has been recently derived from beef or pork or from synthetic production. The structure of human, porcine, and bovine insulin is fairly similar.

Beef insulin is the least expensive and most readily available of the insulins; however, it is the most immunogenic. Pork insulin more closely resembles human insulin and is therefore less immunogenic. Human insulin is also available. Most types of insulin are available in various strengths and may be treated with zinc or protamine to render it longer lasting.

Insulin is broken down by gastric enzymes and thus may not be given orally. In the management of type I diabetes, insulin is most commonly given subcutaneously one to three times daily. This method does not normalize blood glucose levels throughout the day but instead allows wide fluctuations in both glucose and insulin levels. Insulin may also be administered continually through an open-loop system, which provides a continuous subcutaneous insulin infusion delivered by a small battery-powered infusion pump. Although data are inconclusive because of the short time in which treatment with open-loop insulin administration has been available, several individuals have shown improvement in retinopathy and neuropathy with this form of treatment (Pickup et al., 1979; Pietri, Dunn, & Raskin, 1980).

Although insulin is essential in the treatment of type I diabetes mellitus, it is occasionally associated with a variety of long-term complications. Many of the complications are linked to impurities in the insulin. As insulin purification becomes more advanced, these complications are decreasing.

Diet The individual with type I diabetes mellitus must consume sufficient calories to achieve and maintain normal weight for height and age. Caloric intake should be regulated with consideration of age, activity, and severity of the diabetes. In general, approximately 55% to 60% of the total calories should be derived from carbohydrates, whereas less than 30% should be derived from fats, and 15% to 20% from proteins. Excessive calories are detrimental for all individuals with diabetes and the consistent timing of meals and snacks is essential.

Exercise Individuals with type I diabetes tend to respond to exercise somewhat differently from nondiabetics. Exercise may precipitate severe hypoglycemia after the administration of insulin, particularly in individuals with good blood glucose control. Therefore insulin requirements are diminished with exercise. Further research is needed to formulate exercise programs beneficial for individuals with type I diabetes mellitus.

Transplantation One last treatment used for those with type I diabetes is pancreatic tissue transplant. Transplantation is still experimental and not a common form of treatment. The whole pancreas or isolated islets of Langerhans may be transplanted. As with any transplant, rejection remains a problem, and lifelong immunosuppression is necessary.

Type II Diabetes Mellitus

Type II diabetes mellitus is much more common than type I, and there is compelling evidence of a genetic susceptibility to type II diabetes (Pyke, 1979). The disease is rare in populations not affected by urban modernization. Certain Native American and Pacific Island populations have experienced increased prevalence to epidemic proportions. Findings in Polynesia, for example, reveal a low incidence of type II diabetes among those living in traditional tribal societies, whereas the condition is common in members of the same tribe living in an urban environment. Hypotheses therefore suggest that a genetic susceptibility to type II diabetes mellitus is unmasked by environmental factors (see Table 18-8).

Pathophysiology

Pancreatic changes in individuals with type II diabetes mellitus are nonspecific and have been observed to a lesser degree in nondiabetics. Hyalinization of the islets is a typical lesion of the diabetic pancreas. The process occurs as tissue is converted to an albuminoid substance. Hyalinization is unevenly distributed and consists of a cellular material that may completely replace a large number of islets. It increases with age in both nondiabetic individuals and those with type II diabetes, but it is most pronounced in diabetics.

Liver changes are related to elevated serum lipid levels. Fatty pancreatic and hepatic atrophy, while affecting both those with and without diabetes, occurs with much greater frequency in the individual with type II diabetes. Although tissue atrophies, fat infiltration may increase the overall size of the liver and pancreas, and glycogen vacuoles may be found in the cell nuclei. Ischemia caused by vascular sclerosis may cause the fatty atrophy. One theory holds that these lesions precede diabetes; another posits that the lesions follow or result from the disease (Felig et al., 1987).

TABLE 18-8 Clinical manifestations and rationale for type II diabetes mellitus

Manifestations	Rationale
Recurrent infections (e.g., boils and carbuncles; skin infections) and prolonged wound healing	Growth of microorganisms is stimulated by increased glucose levels; impaired blood supply hinders healing
Genital pruritus	Hyperglycemia and glycosuria favor fungal growth; candidal infections, resulting in pruritus, are a common presenting symptom in women
Visual changes	Blurred vision occurs as water balance in the eye fluctuates because of elevated blood glucose levels; diabetic retinopathy may ensue
Paresthesias	Paresthesias are common manifestations of diabetic neuropathies
Fatigue	Metabolic changes result in poor use of food products, contributing to lethargy and fatigue

A decrease in the weight and number of beta cells generally occurs in type II diabetes, but the cause is unclear. The decrease in beta cells may be the result of progressive deterioration over time. To confuse the issue further, the ratio of alpha cells to beta cells may be completely normal in the individual with type II diabetes, and most individuals with type II diabetes have plasma and pancreatic insulin levels that are not decreased. This latter finding supports the hypothesis that diabetes is a disorder caused by both insulin and glucagon, so that a deficiency of insulin and an excess of glucagon may be either relative or absolute. An inherited secretory deficiency of the beta cells may also play a role (Felig et al., 1987). Type II diabetes is usually caused by some combination of gene-environmental interaction, although the contribution of each component varies under different circumstances. The most powerful risk factor for type II diabetes, identified by the World Health Organization Expert Committee (1980), is obesity. (Risk factor analysis is discussed in Chapter 5.) Excessive caloric intake does appear to predispose an individual to type II diabetes by contributing to obesity.

In the obese, insulin has a decreased ability to influence glucose uptake and metabolism in the liver, skeletal muscles, and adipose tissue. Multiple theories have been presented to explain this phenomenon. One theory postulates that a decreased number of insulin receptors in the plasma membrane causes decreased insulin binding. Another theory holds that postreceptor events in insulin-sensitive cells are responsible for insulin resistance in the obese. A third theory states that hyperinsulinemia, which often occurs in the early stages of type II diabetes, is a compensatory adaptation to insulin resistance in tissues. This theory suggests that elevated levels of circulating insulin are induced by obesity until the pancreas cannot continue to overproduce insulin. Still another theory holds that overeating leads to hyperinsulinemia, which necessitates the development of peripheral insulin resistance to protect against hypoglycemia (Olefsky, 1983). In any event, the mechanism(s) responsible for insulin receptor binding or postreceptor activity may be reversed through weight loss.

Clinical Manifestations

Clinical manifestations of type II diabetes are often nonspecific. Although younger people may develop the condition, it generally affects those over the age of 40. The individual often is overweight and hyperlipidemic. The onset is frequently slow and insidious. The individual with type II diabetes may show some classic symptoms of diabetes but more often will have nonspecific symptoms such as pruritus, recurrent infections, visual changes, and paresthesias (see Table 18-8).

Evaluation and Treatment

The diagnosis of type II diabetes is similar to type I (see p. 612). As with type I diabetes, the goal of treatment for individuals with type II diabetes is the restoration of euglycemia (a normal blood glucose level) and correction of related metabolic disorders. Dietary measures, including the restriction of the total caloric intake, assume primary importance in the overweight individual. As the obese individual loses weight, the body's resistance to insulin often diminishes so that weight loss results in improved glucose tolerance. Nonobese individuals with type II diabetes should consume calories consistent with their ideal weight and pattern of activity. As in type I diabetes, the ratio of fats, carbohydrates, and protein is important, and both cholesterol and saturated fats are restricted.

Although the first approach to treatment of the individual with type II diabetes is an appropriate diet, medication may be needed for optimal management. Sulfonylurea drugs are useful in treating some individuals with type II diabetes and are the only oral hypoglycemic agents approved for clinical use in the United States. Use of sulfonylureas require a pancreas capable of synthesizing insulin. Insulin may also be used in the treatment of some individuals with type II diabetes.

Exercise is as important for the indivdual with type II diabetes as for the individual with type I. Exercise not only reduces postprandial blood glucose levels and diminishes insulin requirement, but also lowers triglyceride and cholesterol levels while increasing the level of high-density lipoprotein (HDL) cholesterol. In addition, exercise is a valuable adjunct to weight loss for the overweight individual.

Gestational Diabetes

The onset of glucose intolerance that has its first onset during pregnancy is termed **gestational diabetes.** Gestational diabetes is most likely to occur during the third trimester when there is an increased demand for glucose regulation. Obese women are at greatest risk. A screening glucose tolerance test performed between the twenty-fourth and twenty-eighth week facilitates a definitive diagnosis. Normal carbohydrate metabolism returns in the immediate postpartum period in about 50% of cases. Treatment is by dietary regulation or diet and insulin. Yearly evaluations are recommended because of the increased risk of carbohydrate intolerance or the development of NIDDM.

Acute Complications of Diabetes Mellitus
Hypoglycemia

Hypoglycemia is a lowered blood glucose level. It may be due to exogenous, endogenous, or functional causes (see Tables 18-9, 18-10, and 18-11 for a summary of etiologies). In general, hypoglycemia occurs when blood glucose levels are below 35 mg/dl in newborns for the first 48 hours of life and 45 to 60 mg/dl in children and adults. Evidence also indicates that some individuals may become symptomatic before glucose levels fall to 50 mg/dl if the decrease is relatively rapid (Lefebvre & Luyckx, 1983). The most frequent hypoglycemia occurs in individuals with diabetes mellitus, particularly those with type I (Table 18-9 lists predisposing factors). Hypoglycemia in diabetes is sometimes called insulin shock, or insulin reaction.

Symptoms result from an adrenergic reaction and from cellular malnutrition. Symptoms frequently vary among individuals but tend to be consistent for each person. An adrenergic reaction occurs when the fall in blood glucose is rapid with tachycardia, diaphoresis, tremors, pallor, and hunger. A typical sympathetic response is probably generated when the hypothalamus senses decreased glucose levels. The neuron receives inadequate supplies of carbohydrates to metabolize and is thus unable to maintain normal function. Cellular malnutrition produces further neurologic symptoms. The symptoms include headache, irritability, confusion, double vision, seizures, or coma. If an individual is receiving a beta-blocking medication, the anatomic symptoms may be absent.

When hypoglycemic symptoms are nonspecific, the safest treatment is to provide some form of glucose, as failure to provide glucose may precipitate convulsions, coma, and death. If the hypoglycemic individual is conscious, ingestion of fast-acting carbohydrate is preferred; if the individual is unconscious, intravenous glu-

---

TABLE 18-9 Exogenous causes of hypoglycemia

Exogenous cause	Predisposing factor	Occurrence
Insulin	Intentional or accidental overdose; may be combined with inadequate food intake, unusually increased exercise, decrease in insulin requirement, or potentiating medications	Most frequent cause of hypoglycemia
Oral hypoglycemia agents	Intentional or accidental overdose; may be combined with inadequate food intake, increased exercise, or potentiating medications	Frequent cause of hypoglycemia
Alcohol	Particularly likely in chronically malnourished or acutely food-deprived individuals	Occurs within 6-36 hours of ingesting moderate to large amounts of alcohol
Other agents	Salicylates, hypoglycins, pentamidine, perhexilin	Common in children under the age of 2
Exercise	Increased duration and intensity of exercise increases glucose uptake, and normally decreases insulin secretion	Occurs with both insulin and sulfonylurea administration and intense exercise, but may be unpredictable in onset

TABLE 18-10 Endogenous causes of hypoglycemia

Endogenous hypoglycemia	Predisposing factors	Occurrence
Organic hypoglycemia	Insulinoma	Uncommon neoplasm of beta cells of islet of Langerhaus
	Nesidioblastosis and beta cell hyperplasia	Rare disease causing persistent hypoglycemia of infancy
Extrapancreatic neoplasms	May be mesenchymal tumors, hepatomas, adrenocortical carcinomas, gastrointestinal tumors, lymphomas, or leukemias	Rare; most common in adults 40-70 years of age
Inborn errors of metabolism	Hereditary fructose intolerance	Rare autosomal recessively inherited inborn error of metabolism
	Fructose-1,6-disphosphatase deficiency	Rare autosomal recessive disease
	Galactosemia	Autosomal recessive disease; hypoglycemia less common than in fructose intolerance
	Phosphoenolpyruvate carboxykinase deficiency	Reported in a few infant cases
	Inborn errors in glycogen metabolism, leucine sensitivity	Reported in von Gierke disease, Hers disease, and type IXb glycogen storage disease

cose, or subcutaneous glucagon administration will reverse the hypoglycemia. Following the crisis, the individual should be observed for a subsequent relapse, and a longer-lasting protein food source should be provided. Prevention of hypoglycemia episodes through proper education, however, should be the goal.

Diabetic Ketoacidosis

Ketoacidosis, a serious complication of diabetes mellitus, is a common cause for hospital admissions, and average mortality rates throughout the United States are 7% to 8%. **Diabetic ketoacidosis** develops when there is an absolute or relative deficiency of insulin and an increase in stress with a hormonal shift to insulin antagonism (Fig. 18-10). The counter-regulatory hormones include glucagon, catecholamines, cortisol, and growth hormone; they all antagonize insulin by increasing glucose production. In addition, catecholamines, cortisol, and growth hormone decrease use of glucose. Ketoacidosis occurs most often in stressful situations such as infections, trauma, surgery, myocardial infarction, or emotional stress (Schade & Eaton, 1978).

Insulin deficiency results in decreased glucose utilization, an increased release of fatty acids and accelerated gluconeogenesis and ketogenesis. Relatively increased glucagon levels are simultaneously responsible for activation of the gluconeogenic (glucose-forming) and ketogenic (ketone-forming) pathways in the liver. Because of the insulin deficiency, hepatic overproduction of beta-hydroxybutyrate and acetoacetic acids causes increased ketone concentrations. Ordinarily, ketones used by the brain or skeletal muscle as an energy source regenerate bicarbonate. This balances the loss of bicarbonate, which occurs when the ketone is formed. Hyperketonemia (increased blood ketone levels) may be a result of impairment in the use of ketones by peripheral tissue, which permits strong organic acids to circulate freely (Kreisberg, 1983). Bicarbonate buffering then does not occur, and the individual develops a metabolic acidosis.

Clinical Manifestations

The signs and symptoms of diabetic ketoacidosis are fairly nonspecific, and an individual rarely progresses to complete coma without intervention today. Polyuria and dehydration result from the osmotic diuresis associated with hyperglycemia. Here the blood glucose level is higher than the individual's renal threshold, allowing much glucose to be lost in the urine. Although the water deficits may reach 100 ml/kg body weight, they are generally not as severe as those experienced by the individual with a type II complication of hyperosmolar nonketotic hyperglycemic coma. Sodium, phosphorus, and magnesium deficits are common. The most important electrolyte disturbance, however, is a marked deficiency in total body potassium. Although the serum potassium may appear normal or elevated because of volume contraction and a shift of potassium from the cell due to metabolic acidosis, total deficiencies may be as large as 10 mEq/kg. Symptoms of diabetic ketoacidosis include Kussmaul respirations (hyperventilation in an attempt

TABLE 18-11 Functional causes of hypoglycemia

Dysfunction	Precipitating factors	Occurrence
Alimentary hypoglycemia	Rapid dumping of carbohydrates into the upper small intestine	Postgastrectomy
Spontaneous reactive hypoglycemia	Syndrome with symptoms such as diaphoresis, tachycardia, tremulousness, headache, fatigue, drowsiness, and irritability	Rarely diagnosed thoughout the world; widely diagnosed in United States, prompting American Diabetes Association and Endocrine Society to issue statement that entity is probably overdiagnosed
Alcohol-promoted reactive hypoglycemia	Drinking on an empty stomach	More common with drinks containing both alcohol and glucose or sacchrin (e.g., beer, gin and tonic, rum and coke, whisky and ginger ale, etc.)
Posthyperalimentation hypoglycemia	Rapid discontinuation of total parenteral alimentation	Easily prevented
Endocrine-deficiency states	Glucocorticoid deficiency	A danger for any person with adrenal insufficiency
	Growth hormone deficiency	Particularly during a prolonged fast
	Catecholamine deficiency	Possible cause in children
Severe liver deficiency	Insufficient glucose output by the liver	Fasting hypoglycemia
Lack of body stores for protein, fat, and carbohydrates	Profound malnutrition	Frequent; also found with relative frequency in kwashiorkor
Prolonged muscular exercise	Metabolism of energy-producing substances	Occurs if exercise is too prolonged or severe or if nutritional intake and carbohydrate stores are insufficient
Functional or transient hypoglycemia in infancy	Transient neonatal hypoglycemia	Occurs in 10% of live births, during 1st 3 days of life
	Maternal diabetes	Due to beta-cell hyperplasia and possibly relative hypoglucagonemia
	Erythroblastosis fetalis	Frequently associated with erythroblastosis fetalis
	Leucine-induced hypoglycemia	Generally in infants under 6 months of age; severe hypoglycemia attacks may occur postprandially or after short periods of fasting
	Ketotic or ketogenic hypoglycemia	One of the most common forms of hypoglycemia in childhood, occurs after food deprivation in children 1-8 years old; generally, spontaneous recovery before age 10
	Maple sugar urine disease	Frequent in those with maple sugar urine disease
	Adrenal hyporesponsiveness	Found in children born small for dates, after complicated pregnancy

Diabetic ketoacidosis

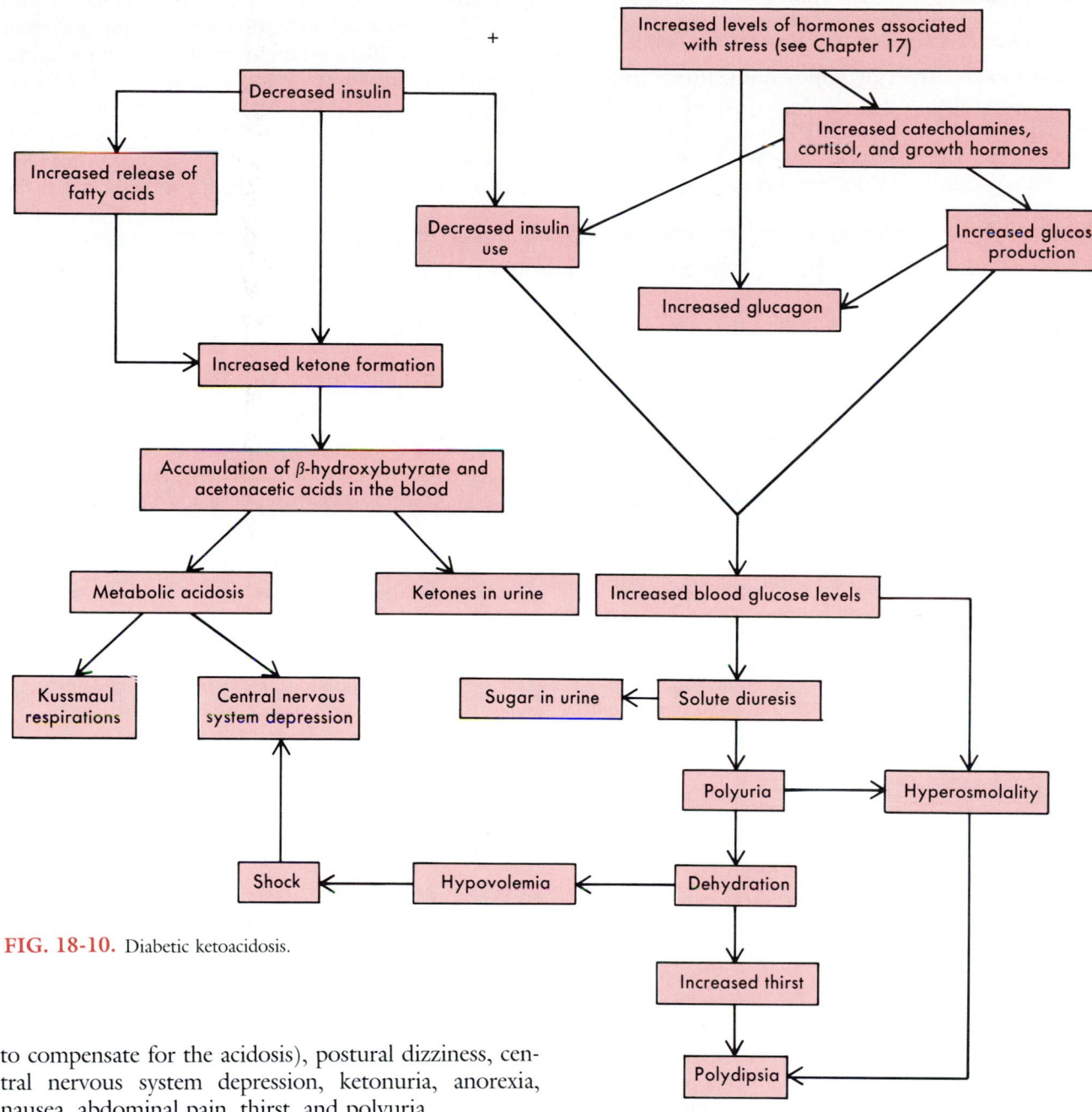

FIG. 18-10. Diabetic ketoacidosis.

to compensate for the acidosis), postural dizziness, central nervous system depression, ketonuria, anorexia, nausea, abdominal pain, thirst, and polyuria.

Evaluation and Treatment

The diagnosis of ketoacidosis is suspected when individuals have symptoms of vomiting, abdominal pain, dehydration, and an acetone odor on the breath. Laboratory findings include blood glucose greater than 200 mg/dl, 4+ glucosuria, strong reaction for urine ketones, $Paco_2 \leq$ to 400 mm Hg, arterial pH less than 7.3, and strong reaction for serum ketones.

Treatment of diabetic ketoacidosis involves continual administration of low-dose insulin to cause glucose levels to drop. Fluids are administered to replace lost fluid

volume, and electrolytes—particularly sodium, potassium, and phosphorus—are administered as needed. Following the administration of insulin, the concentration of beta-hydroxybutyrate promptly begins to decrease and after a slight increase, acetoacetate also begins to fall. A persistent ketonuria may be observed for several days after treatment. Fluid and electrolytes should be closely monitored. Electrolyte deficits become apparent as fluid volume is replaced. Again, as with hypoglycemia, prevention is the goal. Health teaching concerning the predisposing factors and avoidance of diabetic ketoacidosis is an important part of treatment.

Hyperosmolar Hyperglycemic Nonketotic Coma

Hyperosmolar hyperglycemic nonketotic coma (HHNK), also called hyperosmolar hyperglycemia syndrome, was first described in 1886, but even today no satisfactory evidence has explained how HHNK differs pathophysiologically from diabetic ketoacidosis. Levels

of free fatty acids in HHNK are consistently lower than those found in diabetic ketoacidosis. HHNK is also characterized by a lack of ketosis, since insulin is present to some degree. Because the amount of insulin required to inhibit fat breakdown is less than that needed for effective glucose transport, insulin levels are sufficient to prevent excessive lipolysis but not to use glucose properly. Glucose levels are considerably higher in HHNK than in diabetic ketoacidosis. One hypothesis is that the

TABLE 18-12 Common acute complications of diabetes mellitus

Hypoglycemia in the diabetic	Diabetic ketoacidosis	Hyperosmolar hyperglycemic nonketotic coma
SYNONYMS		
Insulin shock, insulin reaction	Diabetic coma syndrome	Hyperosmolar hyperglycemia
THOSE AT RISK		
Individuals with type I diabetes	Individuals with type I	Elderly, individuals with type II, nondiabetics with predisposing factors, those with renal insufficiency, undiagnosed individuals with diabetes
Individuals with rapidly fluctuating blood sugar	Nondiagnosed individuals with diabetes	
Individuals with type II diabetes taking oral agents, especially chloropropamide		
PREDISPOSING FACTORS		
Excessive insulin or hypoglycemic intake, lack of sufficient food intake, excessive physical exercise, abrupt decline in insulin needs (e.g., immediately postpartum, some cases of insulin reaction) simultaneous use of insulin-potentiating agents	Stressful situation such as infection, accident, trauma, emotional stress; omission of insulin; Medications that antagonize insulin	High-carbohydrate diets (e.g., tube feedings; total parenteral nutrition), prolonged mannitol diuresis, peritoneal or hemodialysis with hyperosmolar dialysate, medications antagonizing insulin
TYPICAL ONSET		
Rapid	Slow	Slowest
PRESENTING SYMPTOMS		
Adrenergic reaction: pallor, sweating, tachycardia, palpitations, hunger, restlessness, anxiety	Malaise, dry mouth, headache, polyuria, polydipsia, weight loss, nausea, vomiting, pruritus, abdominal pain, lethargy, shortness of breath, Kussmaul respirations, "fruity" or acetone odor to breath	Polyuria, polydipsia, hypovolemia, dehydration (parched lips, poor skin tugor), hypotension, tachycardia, hypoperfusion, weight loss, weakness, nausea, vomiting, abdominal pain, hypothermia, stupor, coma, increased blood urea nitrogen and creatinine
Neurologic malnutrition: fatigue, irritability, headache, loss of concentration, visual disturbances, confusion, transient sensory or motor defects, convulsions, coma, death		
LABORATORY ANALYSIS		
Blood glucose below 30 mg/dl in newborn (first 2-3 days) and below 55-60 mg/dl in adults	Glucose levels 350-750 mg/dl, reduction in bicarbonate concentration, increased anion gap, increased plasma levels of beta-hydroxybutyrate and acetoacetate (measurements not routinely available), increased levels of acetone (low toxicity when compared to ketones, but easily measured)	Glucose levels 600-4800 mg/dl, lack of ketosis, serum osmolarity above 350 m0sm/L

lack of ketonemia in HHNK permits greater synthesis of glucose and thus more severe hyperglycemia.

Clinical Manifestations

Glycosuria and polyuria in HHNK result from the extreme blood glucose elevation. As much as 19 g of glucose per hour may be lost in diuresis, which also causes severe volume depletion and intracellular dehydration. Water losses are generally between 4.8 and 12.6 L, and although some electrolytes are lost with the fluid, the urine is hypotonic. This, along with increased glucose levels, contributes to the increased serum osmolarity. Neurologic changes, such as stupor, correlate with the degree of hyperosmolarity. Glomerular filtration will also decrease with the hyperosmolality, resulting in further blood glucose increases.

Evaluation and Treatment

The serum ketone concentration is normal or only mildly elevated in HHNK. In addition to the depressed mental state, laboratory findings include blood glucose levels greater than 600 mg/dl, serum osmolarity greater than 310 mOsm, and BUN of 70 to 90 mg/dl. Diabetic ketoacidosis and HHNK show considerable overlap in symptoms and treatment. An important distinction, however, is that the dehydration experienced in HHNK is far more severe than that in diabetic ketoacidosis. Thus fluid replacement, with both crystalloids and colloids, is more rapid. As many as 2000 ml may be given the first hour, together with monitoring of the response to therapy. Potassium deficits may be so extreme in HHNK that more than a week may be needed to correct the total body deficits. Phosphorus and sodium may also be needed. The mortality rate is also considerably higher in HHNK, currently 15% to 20% (Matz, 1983). Thus, although the exact mechanisms are unknown at this time, real differences exist between diabetic ketoacidosis and HHNK. (Table 18-12 compares and contrasts the three acute complications described thus far.)

Dawn Phenomenon

The **dawn phenomenon** is an early morning rise in blood glucose concentration with no hypoglycemia during the night. It may be related to a surge in growth hormone activity, a decrease in insulin sensitivity (Campbell et al., 1985), or a normal circadian variant. Periodic monitoring postprandial of blood glucose values in the morning will ascertain need for additional morning

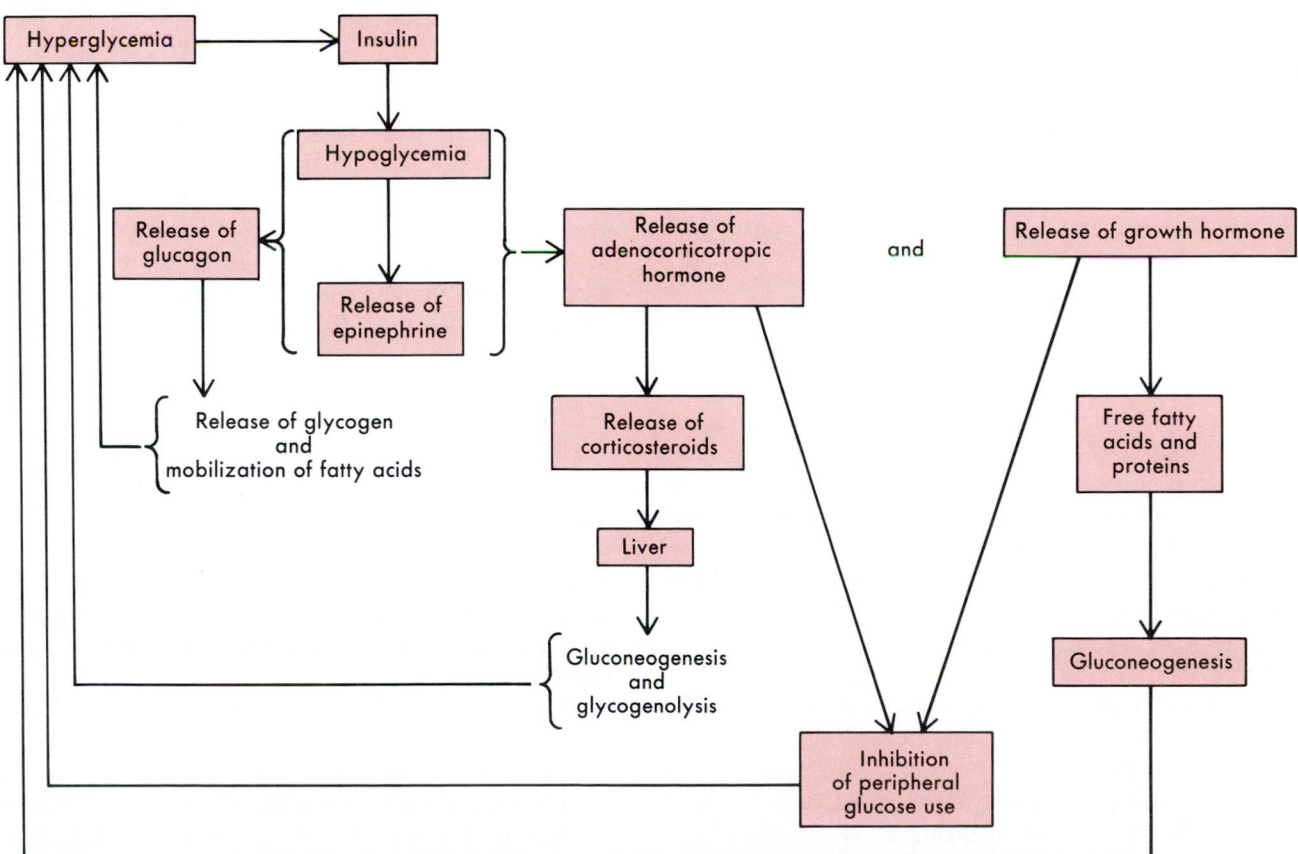

FIG. 18-11. The Somogyi effect.

insulin. Altering the time and dose of insulin manages the problem.

Somogyi Effect

The **Somogyi effect** is a unique combination of hypoglycemia during the night with rebound hyperglycemia in the morning. The problem is more common in individuals with type I diabetes mellitus, particularly in children, and should be suspected whenever fluctuations in blood sugar levels are serious. The Somogyi effect may be caused by an increase in insulin sensitivity, which causes hypoglycemia and a mobilization of the body's counter-regulatory hormones to provide energy sources (Fig. 18-11). Hormones involved include epinephrine, glucagon, cortisol, and growth hormone. These hormones serve to increase blood glucose by gluconeogenesis (formation of glucose from nonglucose sources) and glycogenolysis (breakdown of glycogen into glucose). They mobilize fatty acids and proteins while inhibiting peripheral glucose use.

Clinical Manifestations

In addition to fluctuating glucose levels, subtle symptoms of hypoglycemia occur. The individual often complains of nightmares and early morning headaches. Both symptoms probably reflect a hypoglycemic state. Ketonuria may occur if the mobilization of energy sources overshoots the body's need for glucose and exogenous insulin is depleted.

Evaluation and Treatment

Diagnosis involves the documentation of night time hypoglycemia by several blood sugar analyses at 2:00 A.M., 4:00 A.M., and 7:00 A.M. Treatment consists of a decrease in insulin dose or changing the time of administration.

Chronic Complications of Diabetes Mellitus

Before the discovery of long-term insulin, complications in individuals with diabetes had little significance because the survival time was short, especially for individuals with type I diabetes. Today, long-term survival is the rule. As a result, the problems of neuropathy, microvascular disease, and macrovascular disease have become important in clinical management. Infection also presents difficulties.

Diabetic Neuropathies

Although **diabetic neuropathy** is probably the most common complication in diabetes, it remains poorly understood. The underlying pathologic mechanism may be vascular, metabolic, or a combination of both mechanisms. Currently, diabetic neuropathy is considered to be a form of a "dying back" neuropathy, in which the distal portions of the neurons are initially and eventually more severely affected. The earliest morphologic change in both peripheral nerves and the central nervous system is axonal degeneration that preferentially involves unmyelinated nerve fibers. Schwann cell abnormalities then occur because of changes in the axons they support. Metabolic activity of the Schwann cell is disturbed, causing segmental loss of myelin and the characteristic pattern of demyelination and remyelination observed in long-term diabetic neuropathy. The location of the pathology may include the spinal cord, the posterior root ganglia, or the peripheral nerves. These changes may occur alone or in combination.

Motor nerve conduction velocity, electromyography, and sensory perception have shown abnormalities at the onset of diabetes. Sensory nerve conduction may also be impaired at this stage and is probably the most sensitive index of peripheral neuropathy. These abnormalities have sometimes been restored to normal by good glucose control. While these changes suggest early involvement of the nervous system in individuals with diabetes, they are not generally accompanied by clinical symptomatology.

A number of different diabetic neuropathies occur with varying etiologies, pathogeneses, and clinical backgrounds (Table 18-13). Some of the diabetic neuropathic syndromes are progressive, but many, such as painful peripheral neuropathy, mononeurophy (wrist drop, foot drop), diabetic amyatrophy, diabetic neuropathic cachexia, and visceral manifestations associated with autonomic neuropathy, such as diabetic diarrhea and orthostatic hypotention, are reversible. This suggests that metabolic changes are not completely responsible for the neuropathies. In fact, any neuropathy may occur during periods of good glucose control and may be the initial clinical manifestation of diabetes, even without overt glucose intolerance. Obviously, much investigation regarding diabetic neuropathies remains to be done.

Microvascular Disease

Thickening of the capillary basement membrane is characteristic of diabetic microangiopathy and emerges over a period of 1 to 2 years. The thickening eventually results in decreased tissue perfusion. Although some degree of hyperglycemia is a necessary prerequisite for the vascular changes, no conclusive evidence is available to correlate the basement membrane thickening with the severity of diabetes. The frequency of the lesions appears to be proportional to the duration of the disease.

Although there is no firm evidence that good diabetic care will prevent microvascular changes, there is sufficient indirect evidence to make the attempt worthwhile (Fitzgerald & Kilveat, 1985). Hypoxia and ischemia of various organs may result from microangiopathy. Two areas often affected are the retina and the kidney.

TABLE 18-13 Classification of diabetic neuropathies

Location	Characteristics
SOMATIC (PERIPHERAL) NEUROPATHIES	
Lower extremities	Most commonly bilateral, symmetric, and sensory
Asymptomatic	Paresthesias, progressive and irreversible, underlie the development of neuropathic ulcers and charcot joints
Painful	Pain and paresthesias, particularly nocturnally; anorexia, depression, and irritability; absence of knee and ankle jerk reflexes; the greater the pain, the better the prognosis
Upper extremities	Involves muscle atrophy, asthenia, sensory impairment, and radiculitis
Asymmetric neuropathies	Predominantly motor involvement, absent sensory involvement, sudden onset, severe pain, good prognosis
Diabetic neuropathic cachexia	Profound weight loss with severe pain, spontaneous recovery
VISCERAL NEUROPATHIES (generally occur with peripheral neuropathy)	
Cranial nerves	Involves cranial nerves VII, VIII, and XII as well as pupillary changes
Gastrointestinal tract	Involves esophagus, stomach, and small bowel; spontaneous remission may occur
Genitourinary tract	Insidious and progressive bladder paralysis with urinary retention; sexual dysfunction in males, including retrograde ejaculation and impotence
Autonomic nervous system	Includes cardiovascular reflexes, anhydrosis, and vasomotor instability

Retinopathy

Diabetic retinopathy appears to be a response to retinal ischemia caused by microangiopathy (L'Esperance & James, 1983). The retina is the most metabolically active structure per weight of tissue in the body. Thus, the retina is a vulnerable target for microvascular occlusion in diabetes mellitus. In 1980, diabetic retinopathy accounted for over 23% of all newly reported cases of blindness in the United States (L'Esperance & James, 1983).

There are three stages of retinopathy and they can develop in both type I and type II diabetes (Table 18-14). Nonproliferative retinopathy (Stage I) is characterized by an increase in retinal capillary permeability, vein dilation, microaneurysm formation, and superficial (flame shaped) and deep (blot) hemorrhages. Preproliferative retinopathy (Stage II) is a progression of retinal ischemia with areas of poor perfusion that culminate in infarcts. Proliferative diabetic retinopathy (Stage III) is the result of neovasculization and fibrous tissue formation within the retina or optic disc. Traction of the new vessels on the vitreous humor may cause retinal detachment or hemorrhage into the vitreous humor.

Maculopathy is a progressive process that may accompany the increased retinal capillary permeability, vessel occlusion, and ischemia. If formation of exudates, edema, or ischemia occur near the fovea, serious loss of vision may result.

Nephropathy

Renal glomerular changes can occur early in diabetes mellitus and may occasionally precede the overt manifestation of the disease. Glomerular enlargement and glomerular basement membrane thickening, resulting in diffuse intercapillary glomerulosclerosis, develops during the first few years of diabetes. The Kimmelstiel-Wilson nodule, thickening at the center of the glomerular lobules with thickening of the peripheral basement membrane, is distinctive in individuals with diabetes. Proteinuria is the first manifestation of renal dysfunction.

In type I diabetes, proteinuria is usually first noted routinely after 10 to 15 years of insulin treatment. Continuous proteinuria generally heralds a life expectancy of less than 10 years. Urinary protein losses may reach 10 to 30 g daily. Scanty information is available to explain

TABLE 18-14 Findings in diabetic retinopathy

Type of retinopathy	Pathologic findings
Venous abnormalities	Increased tortuosity, dilation with irregular constriction; frequency increases with increased severity of retinopathy
Microaneurysms	Mostly thin-walled, 15-50 μm in diameter, pathogenesis controversial
Interetinal hemorrhage	Circular and small; may take several months to resorb
Macular edema	Due to serum leakage through incompetent vessel walls, may resorb in several weeks
Hard exudates	Characteristically "hard," exudates with pattern of exudation, irregular in shape, and sharply defined, may appear and disappear over months to years; common with hypertension; "soft" exudates may appear and disappear more frequently; related to increased retinal capillary permeability
Preproliferative diabetic retinopathy	
"Cottonwool" patches	Infarcts of the nerve fiber layer due to retinal ischemia
Intraretinal microvascular shunts	Tortuous shunts between patent and occluded retinal vessels
Proliferative diabetic retinopathy	
Neovascularization	New vessels surrounded by connective tissue; five distinct groups representing different hazards to the eye
Glial proliferation	Often produced to reinforce neovascularization; may occur on optic disk and along vascular arcades
Vitreoretinal traction hemorrhage; retinal detachment	Traction occurring from the vitreous jelly; eventually causes small blood vessels to hemorrhage and retinal detachment to occur

the determinants of proteinuria in diabetic nephropathy. Leakage of albumin into glomerular filtrate results from factors other than increased membrane pore size, although these other factors are not yet defined. As renal failure progresses, extensive vascular and extravascular changes occur.

Before the development of proteinuria, no clinical signs or symptoms of progressive glomerulosclerosis are likely to be evident. Later, hypoproteinemia, reduction in plasma oncotic pressure, fluid overload, anasarca (generalized body edema), and hypertension may occur. As renal function continues to deteriorate, individuals with type I diabetes may experience hypoglycemia, which necessitates a decrease in insulin therapy. The hypoglycemia occurs because the kidney's ability to metabolize insulin is lost along with other renal functions. As the glomerular filtraton rate drops below 10 ml/min, uremic signs such as nausea, lethargy, acidosis, anemia, and uncontrolled hypertension occur (see Chapter 33 for a discussion of renal failure). Impaired kidney function also accelerates retinopathy. Death from renal failure is much more common in individuals with type I diabetes mellitus than those with type II.

Macrovascular Disease

Macrovascular disease is the most prominent, overall cause of morbidity and mortality among individuals with type II diabetes mellitus (Ganda, 1980). Unlike microangiopathy, atherosclerotic disease is unrelated to the severity of diabetes and is often present in those with merely an impaired glucose tolerance. (Atherosclerosis is discussed in Chapter 27.) The current theory of the pathogenesis of atherosclerosis is related to the theory of response to injury (Ross, Bernstein, & Rifkin, 1983). The fibrous plaques of atherosclerosis result from the proliferation of subendothelial smooth muscle in the arterial wall. Other factors in the serum of individuals with diabetes also stimulate this proliferation (Fig. 18-12).

In addition, deposition of lipids in the lesions may also be facilitated in individuals with diabetes. Triglyceride and serum cholesterol elevations are very common. High-density lipoproteins (HDL), which tend to protect vessels, are present in only low concentrations in individuals with diabetes. As in the nondiabetic, the presence of other risk factors increases vulnerability to atherosclerosis. Further work is needed to clarify the complexities of macrovascular complications.

Coronary Artery Disease

The prevalence of coronary artery disease (coronary heart disease) in individuals with diabetes is high, accounting in several studies for 75% of the deaths of individuals with type II diabetes (Fein & Schever, 1983).

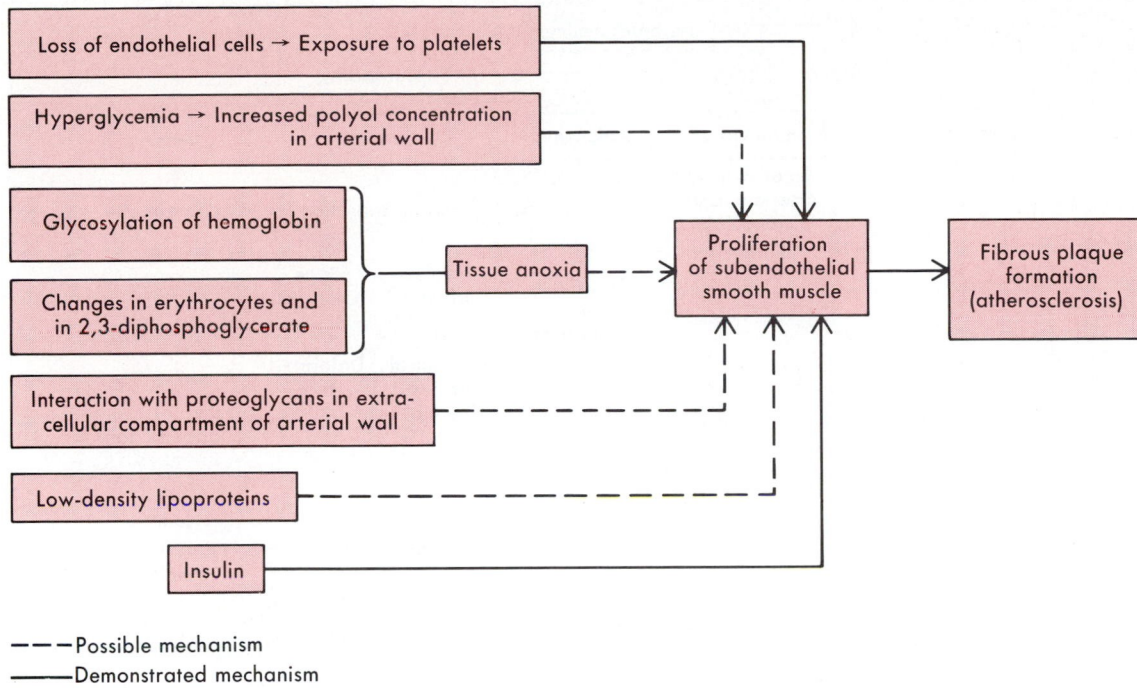

FIG. 18-12. Contributing causes of proliferation of subendothelial smooth muscle in arterial wall, resulting in atherosclerosis.

Whereas the cardiovascular mortality is increased in all age groups, mortality is most marked at or before middle age, particularly in women. In general, the prevalence of coronary artery disease increases with the duration but not the severity of diabetes.

Myocardial infarction (death of heart muscle due to coronary artery occlusion) occurs frequently, and individuals with diabetes mellitus have a higher mortality rate during the acute phase of myocardial infarctions than do nondiabetics. In addition, the incidence of congestive heart failure is higher in the individual with diabetes, even without myocardial infarction. The reason is unclear but may be related to the presence of increased amounts of collagen in the ventricular wall, which reduces the mechanical compliance of the heart during filling. (Heart disease is described in Chapter 27.)

Stroke

The incidence of cerebral atherosclerosis is greater in individuals with type II diabetes than in nondiabetics. The survival rate for an individual with diabetes after a massive stroke is typically shorter than for a nondiabetic. Hypertension is a definite risk factor (see Chapter 15). No data are available to evaluate the effects of blood sugar control on the incidence of stroke. Strokes do, however, account for the death of approximately 15% of men and 20% of women with type II diabetes mellitus (Levin & O'Neal, 1983).

Peripheral Vascular Disease

The increased incidence of peripheral vascular disease, gangrene, and amputation in the individual with diabetes has been documented in many studies, particularly in individuals with type II diabetes (Levin & O'Neal, 1983). To see how foot lesions of diabetes can lead to amputation, see Fig. 18-13. Many individuals with type II diabetes have evidence of peripheral vascular disease at the time of their initial diagnosis. The atherosclerotic process in the individual with diabetes is more common, appears at a younger age, and advances more rapidly than vascular changes in nondiabetics. It occurs equally often in males and females with diabetes.

Because of occlusions of the small arteries and arterioles, most of the gangrenous changes of the lower extremities occur in patchy areas of the feet and toes. Smaller vessels often have more advanced disease than larger vessels in the same individuals. Hospital mortality for individuals with diabetes who undergo major amputation is between 10% and 23%. The survival rate after surgery is only 40% at the end of 5 years (Levin & O'Neal, 1983). The high mortality rate explains why only 3% of the population with diabetes mellitus are amputees at any given time.

Infection

Virtually every organ and system is affected by diabetes mellitus, and the individual with diabetes is at in-

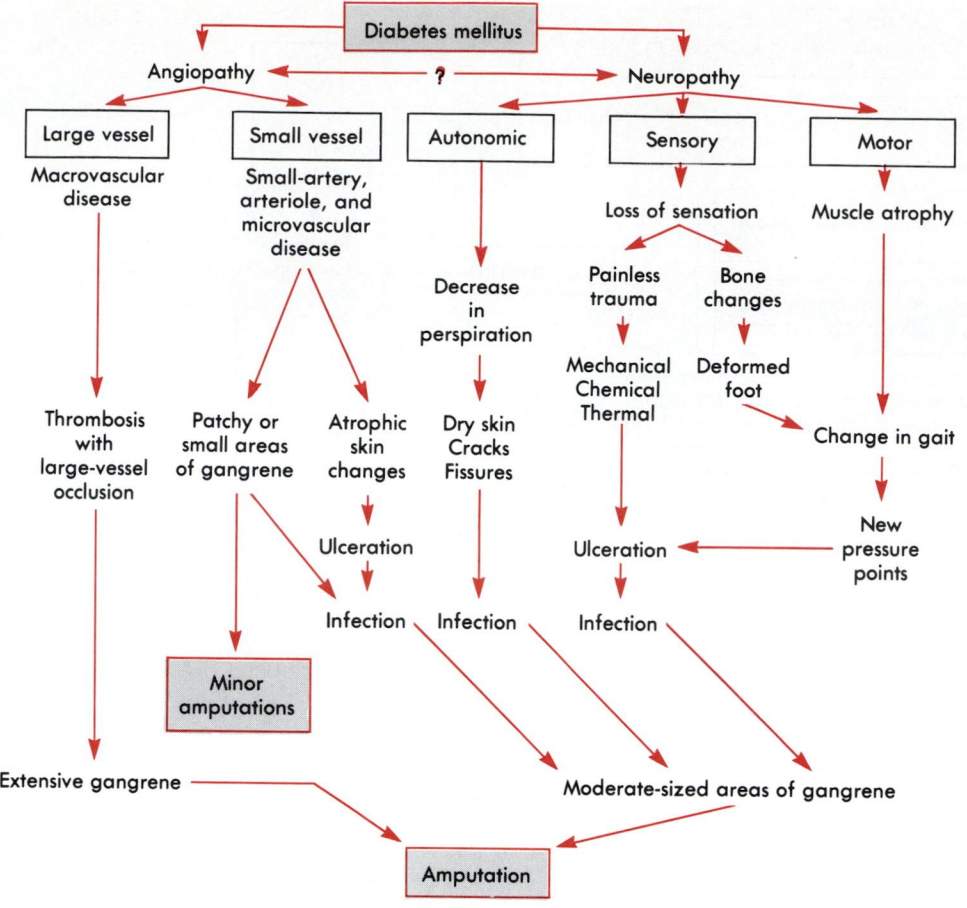

FIG. 18-13. How foot lesions of diabetes can lead to amputation. (From Phipps, Long, & Woods, 1987.)

creased risk for infection throughout the body for a number of reasons. One major reason involves the senses. Impaired vision due to retinal changes and impaired touch due to neuropathy diminish the prevention of breaks in the skin by decreasing the early warning systems. Once breaks in skin integrity occur, tissues may have increased susceptibility to infection because of hypoxia, a second reason for susceptibility to infection. Microvascular and macrovascular complications cause decreased oxygen supply to tissues. In addition, the increased content of glycosylated hemoglobin on the red blood cell impedes the release of oxygen to tissues.

The third general reason for infection in individuals with diabetes is that pathogens are able to multiply rapidly once they have gained access to the tissues. Some pathogens proliferate rapidly because the increased glucose in body fluids provides an excellent source of energy. In addition, the decreased blood supply resulting from vascular changes decreases the supply of white blood cells to the affected area. The fourth reason for susceptibility to infection is that the function of the white cells is impaired. Chemotaxis is abnormal, and

phagocytosis is defective. The cause for all of these mechanisms has not been identified, but the end result is an individual at considerable risk for the development of infections. (Factors that promote healing are described in Chapter 7.) The risk of infection is especially high for individuals undergoing surgery and for those taking immunosuppressant medications.

ALTERATIONS OF ADRENAL FUNCTION

Disorders of the Adrenal Cortex

Disorders of the adrenal cortex are related either to hyperfunction or to hypofunction. Hyperfunction that causes increased levels of circulating cortisol leads to Cushing disease, or Cushing syndrome; that which causes increased secretion of adrenal androgens and estrogens leads to virilizaton or feminization; and that which causes increased levels of aldosterone leads to hyperaldosteronism, which may be primary or secondary.

Hypofunction of the adrenal cortex leads to Addison disease, which has a variety of causal factors.

Hypercortical Function (Cushing Disease, Cushing Syndrome)

Cushing syndrome refers to chronic **hypercortisolism** (excessive levels of circulating cortisol) caused by hyperfunction of the adrenal cortex, with or without pituitary involvement. **Cushing disease** refers specifically to pituitary-dependent hypercortisolism. Additionally, a Cushing-like syndrome may develop as a result of the exogenous administration of cortisone.

ACTH-induced Cushing disease is more common in adults and is two to three times more common in females than in males. Cushing syndrome resulting from ectopic ACTH secretion is more common in older adults, particularly males. Adrenal tumors, rather than pituitary tumors, are more common in children, especially girls. Cushing syndrome can be found in any age, but usually occurs between 30 and 50 years of age.

Pathophysiology

Causes of hypercortisolism often involve excessive circulating ACTH, which may result from a variety of pathophysiologic alterations. Dysregulation of hypothalamic or anterior pituitary hormones may lead to increased levels of ACTH. Autonomous, ectopic ACTH secretion by a tumor outside the pituitary, usually a malignant tumor, and frequently an oat cell carcinoma of the lung, also may cause the development of Cushing syndrome.

Elevated levels of ACTH account for approximately 75% to 80% of all cases of Cushing syndrome. Autonomous secretion of cortisol by an adrenal neoplasm, which may be either benign or malignant, accounts for approximately 10% of the cases of hypercorticoadrenalism.

Whatever the cause, two observations consistently apply to individuals with Cushing syndrome: (1) they do not have diurnal or circadian secretion patterns of ACTH and cortisol, and (2) they do not increase ACTH and cortisol secretion in response to a stressor. In individuals with ACTH-stimulated hypercorticoadrenalism, secretion of both cortisol and adrenal androgens is increased. Hormone-secreting tumors of the adrenal cortex, however, generally only secrete cortisol. When the secretion of cortisol by the tumor exceeds normal cortisol levels, symptoms of hypercortisolism develop.

The elevated cortisol levels suppress CRH and ACTH secretion by the hypothalamus and anterior pituitary, respectively, because normal feedback mechanisms still function. The low circulating levels of ACTH cause atrophy of the remaining normal portions of the adrenal cortex. This atrophy is not considered irreversible if the hypercortisolism is resolved, although recovery of cortisol-secreting activity of such cells may take several months.

Clinical Manifestations

Most of the clinical signs and symptoms of Cushing syndrome are caused by hypercortisolism (see Chapter 9 and Table 18-9). Weight gain is the most common feature and results from the accumulation of adipose tissue in the trunk, facial, and cervical areas. These characteristic patterns of fat deposition have been described as "truncal obesity," "moon face," and "buffalo hump" (Figs. 18-14 and 18-15). Transient weight gain from sodium and water retention may be present because of the mineralocorticoid effects of cortisol, exhibited when cortisol is present in high levels.

Glucose intolerance occurs because of cortisol-induced insulin resistance and increased gluconeogenesis by the liver. Overt diabetes mellitus develops in approximately 20% of individuals with hypercortisolism. Polyuria, which is sometimes seen in hypercortisolism, is a manifestation of hyperglycemia and resultant glycosuria.

Protein wasting is commonly observed in hypercortisolism and is caused by the catabolic effects of cortisol on peripheral tissues. Muscle wasting, especially obvious in the muscles of the extremities, leads to muscle weakness. In bone, loss of the protein matrix leads to osteoporosis, with pathologic fractures, vertebral compression fractures, bone and back pain, kyphosis, and reduced height. Bone disease may contribute to hypercalsuria and resulting renal stones, which are experienced by approximately 20% of individuals with disease. Loss of collagen also leads to thin, weakened integumentary tissues through which capillaries are more visible and which are easily stretched by adipose deposits. Together, these changes account for the characteristic purple striae most frequently observed in the trunk area. Loss of collagenous support around small vessels makes them susceptible to rupture, leading to easy bruising, even with minor trauma. Thin, atrophic skin is also easily damaged, leading to skin breaks and ulcerations.

Hyperpigmentation in Cushing syndrome is associated with very high serum levels of ACTH. The precise hormonal basis for this hyperpigmentation is still undetermined; however, current speculation focuses on the melanotropic activity of ACTH (Franco-Saenz, 1986). The pigmentation involves the mucous membranes, hair, and skin, all of which acquire a characteristic brownish or bronze color.

Cortisol has a permissive effect on the actions of the catecholamines. With elevated cortisol levels, vascular sensitivity to catecholamines is significantly increased, leading to vasoconstriction and hypertension. Elevated blood pressure occurs in most individuals with Cushing syndrome. Chronically elevated cortisol levels also cause

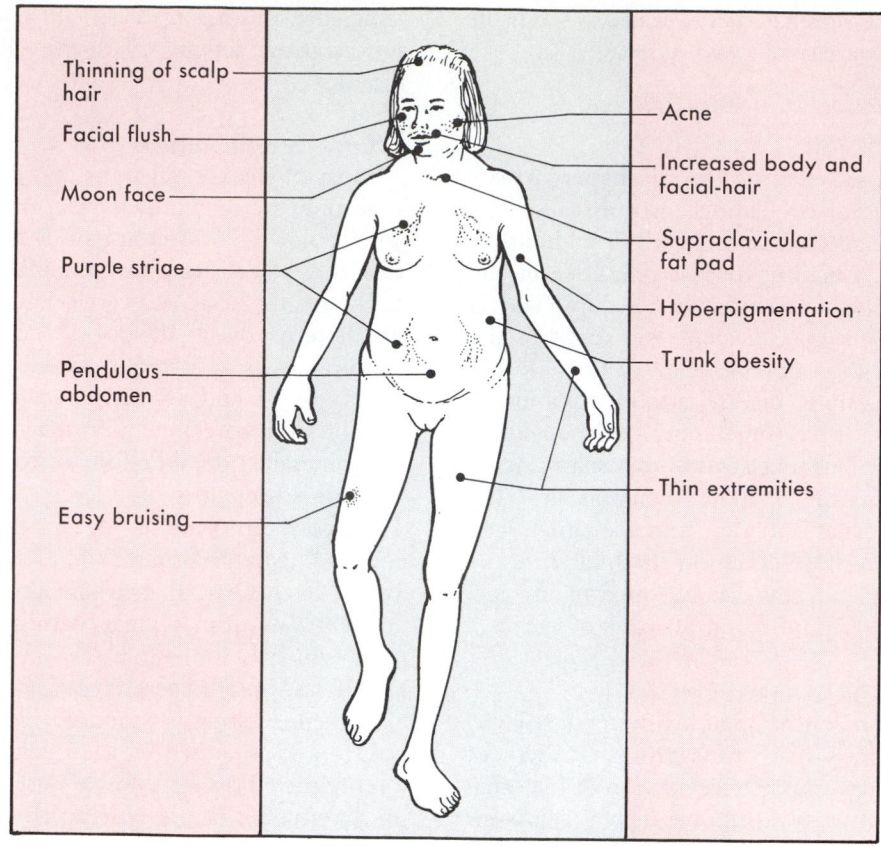

FIG. 18-14. Symptoms of Cushing disease.

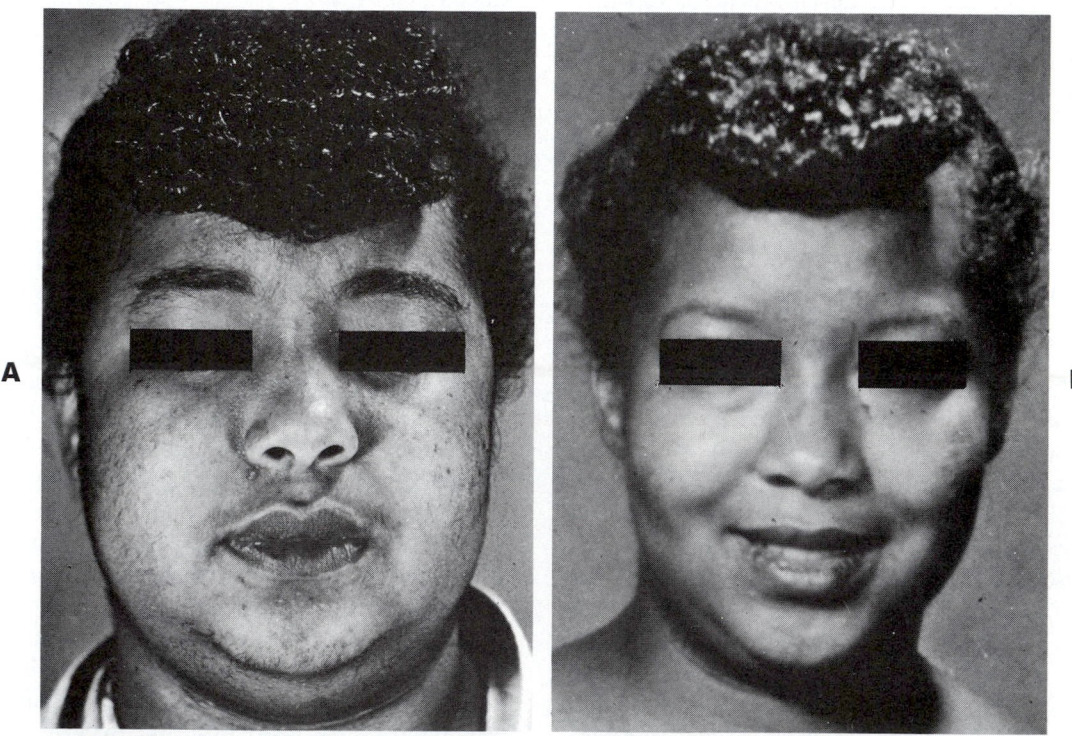

FIG. 18-15. Cushing syndrome. **A,** Preoperatively. **B,** Six months postoperatively. (From Thibodeau, 1987.)

suppression of the immune system, so that individuals with Cushing syndrome have an increased susceptibility to infections.

Approximately 50% of individuals with Cushing syndrome experience alterations in their mental status. These may range from irritability and depression to severe psychiatric disturbances such as schizophrenia. The effects of glucocorticoids on mood are complex and are just beginning to be examined (Majewska, 1986).

Females may experience symptoms of increased adrenal androgen levels, increased hair growth (especially facial hair), acne, and oligoamenorrhea. Rarely do androgen levels become high enough to cause changes of the voice, recession of the hairline, and clitoral hypertrophy unless an adrenal carcinoma is involved. Routine laboratory examinations may reveal hyperglycemia, glycosuria, hypokalemia, and metabolic alkalosis.

Evaluation and Treatment

A variety of laboratory tests must be used to diagnose Cushing syndrome. These include urinary free cortisol (17-hydroxycorticosterol) greater than 100 μg/24 hours, plasma cortisol obtained late in the evening greater than 20 μ/dl, and cortisol excretion rate greater than 20 μ/g creatinine. If laboratory tests are positive, a dexamethasone suppression test may be used to confirm the diagnosis and determine the cause.

Without treatment, approximately 50% of individuals with Cushing syndrome die within 5 years of onset. Major causes of death are overwhelming infection, suicide, complications from generalized arteriosclerosis, and hypertensive disease. Treatment is specific for the cause of hypercorticoadrenalism and includes medication, radiation, and surgery. Therefore differentiation among pituitary, adrenal, and ectopic causes of the hypercortisolism is essential for effective treatment.

Hyperaldosteronism

Hyperaldosteronism is characterized by excessive aldosterone secretion by the adrenal glands. The excessive secretion can result from a primary adrenal disorder, such as an aldosterone secreting adenoma, or from excessive stimulation of the normal adrenal cortex by substances such as angiotensin, ACTH, or elevated potassium. Hyperaldosteronism may be primary or secondary. **Primary hyperaldosteronism** refers to an excessive secretion of aldosterone caused by an abnormality of the adrenal cortex. **Secondary hyperaldosteronism** involves excessive aldosterone secretion from an extra-adrenal stimulus, most frequently angiotensin.

Primary hyperaldosteronism (Conn disease, primary aldosteronism) presents a clinical picture of hypertension, hypokalemia, renal potassium wasting, and neuromuscular manifestations (Young & Klee, 1988). The most common cause of primary aldosteronism is the benign, single adrenal adenoma (80% to 90% of cases), followed by multiple tumors or idiopathic hyperplasia of the adrenals (10% to 15% of cases). Adrenal carcinomas and unknown causes account for the remainder of cases. The incidence of primary hyperaldosteronism is not known; but estimated to be 1% to 7% of all hypertensives (Conn, 1967; Tan, 1986a).

Because aldosterone secretion is normally stimulated by the renin-angiotensin system, secondary hyperaldosteronism can be expected to result from sustained elevated renin release and activation of angiotensin. (Factors that affect renin and aldosterone secretion are summarized in Table 18-15.) Increased renin-angiotensin secretion occurs in a variety of situations. In general, these include decreased circulating blood volume (e.g., in dehydration, shock, or hypoalbuminemia) and decreased delivery of blood to the kidneys (e.g., renal artery stenosis, heart failure, or hepatic cirrhosis). In many of these instances, the activation of the renin-angiotensin system and subsequent aldosterone secretion may be seen as compensatory, although in some instances (e.g., congestive heart failure), the increased circulating volume may further worsen the condition.

Increased estrogen levels associated with pregnancy and use of oral contraceptives also increase renin-

TABLE 18-15 Physiologic factors affecting renin and aldosterone secretion

Factors	Renin secretion	Aldosterone secretion
Age	Highest in infants; lowest in the aged	Highest in infants
Menstrual cycle	Highest in luteal phase (see Chapter 19)	Highest in luteal phase
Sodium intake	Increased by salt restriction Decreased by salt loading	Increased by salt restriction Decreased by salt loading
Potassium status	Increased by K^+ depletion	Decreased by K^+ depletion
Posture	Increased with erect posture	Increased with erect posture
Sympathetic nervous stimulation	Increased by catecholamines	Increased through renin secretion
Time of sampling	Highest before noon; lowest in evening	Diurnal rhythm (as for ACTH)

angiotensin levels, apparently by stimulating renin substrate production by the liver. These pregnancy-induced changes may, however, represent adaptation to pregnancy and are therefore not representative pathophysiologic alterations.

Other causes of secondary hyperaldosteronism are Bartter syndrome, in which the underlying disorder is a renal tubular defect leading to hypokalemia, and renin-secreting tumors of the kidney. Such tumors, however, cause secondary hyperaldosteronism. (Renal disorders are discussed in Chapter 33.)

Pathophysiology

In primary hyperaldosteronism, pathophysiologic alterations are caused by excessive aldosterone secretion and the fluid and electrolyte imbalances that ensue. Hyperaldosteronism promotes increased sodium reabsorption with corresponding hypervolemia (see Chapter 3). The extracellular fluid volume overload and suppression

of normal feedback mechanisms of renin secretion are characteristic of primary disorders.

Edema usually does not occur with primary aldosteronism, possibly because of the renal tubular "escape" phenomenon that is activated in chronic hyperaldosteronism. The escape phenomenon changes or resets the rate of sodium excretion and prevents more severe sodium retention. The escape phenomenon operates in the proximal tubules and causes additional sodium to pass to the distal tubules, where the sodium is, to some extent, reabsorbed in exchange for potassium. This mechanism, while protecting from excessive sodium reabsorption and edema, increases urinary losses of potassium (Fig. 18-16).

In secondary hyperaldosteronism the effect of increased extracellular volume on renin secretion may vary. If renin secretion is being stimulated by variables other than pressure-initiated cellular changes at the juxtaglomerular apparatus (see Chapter 32), then increased

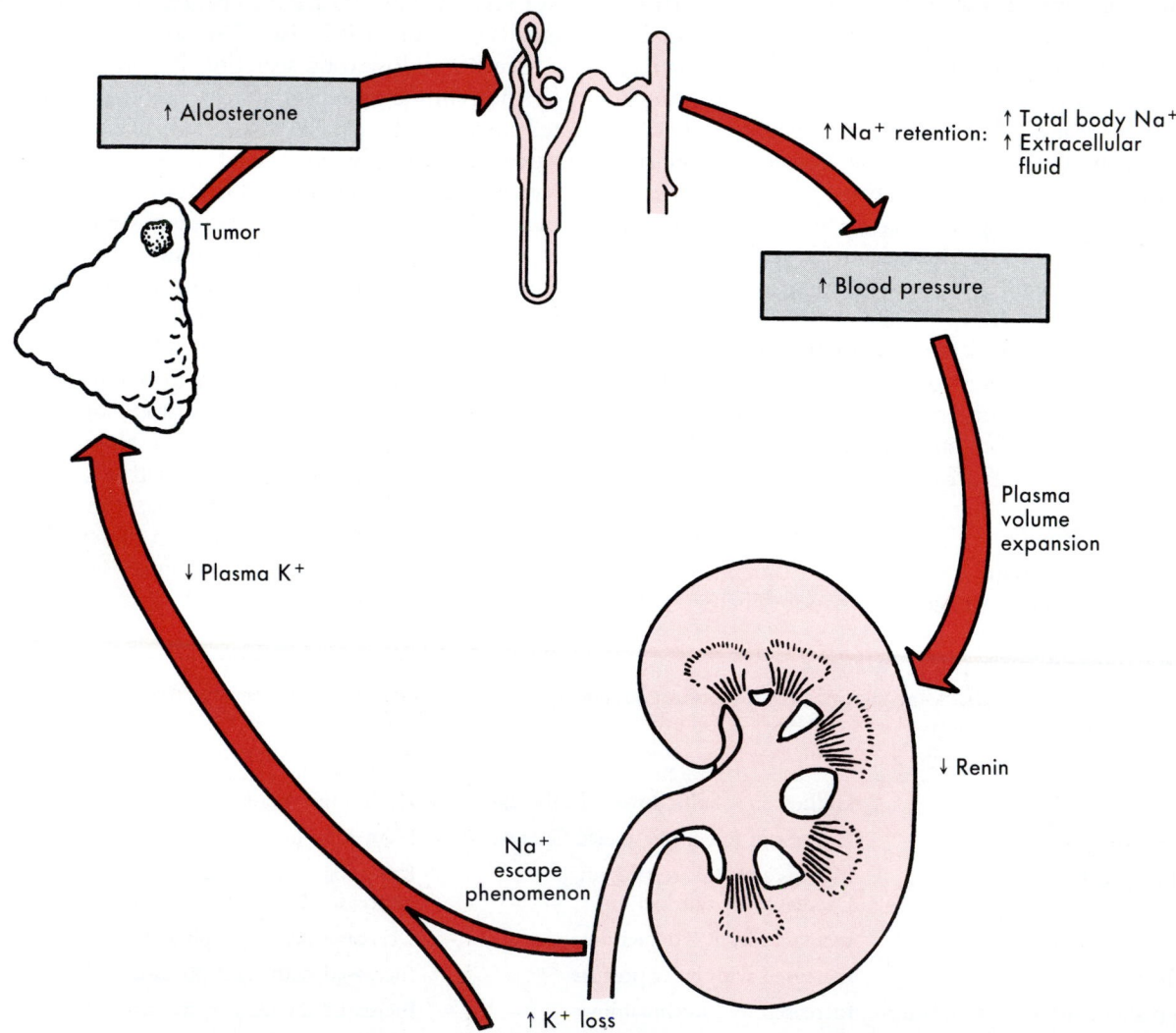

FIG. 18-16. Pathophysiology of mineralcorticoid excess syndromes in primary hyperaldosteronism.

circulating blood volume may not decrease renin secretion through feedback mechanisms. This process occurs, for instance, in states of increased estrogen levels.

In Bartter syndrome, a state of hypokalemia develops because of defective renal tubular reabsorptive mechanisms. The hypokalemic state may induce the formation of prostaglandins (especially PGE_2) by the renal cells, which stimulates renin and hence aldosterone secretion. The stimulatory effect on aldosterone secretion is offset somewhat by the aldosterone-suppressing effects of hypokalemia.

Potassium secretion is also promoted by aldosterone, so that with excessive circulating levels of aldosterone, hypokalemia occurs (see Chapter 3). In hyperaldosteronism, hypokalemic alkalosis, changes in myocardial conduction, and skeletal muscle alterations may be seen, particularly with severe potassium depletion (i.e., the renal tubules may become insensitive to ADH, thus promoting excessive loss of free water). In this situation, hypernatremia may also occur because water is not able to follow the sodium that is reabsorbed.

Clinical Manifestations

Hypertension and hypokalemia are the hallmarks of hyperaldosteronism. Hypertension may result from increased intravascular volume, from altered sodium concentrations in vessel walls, or from a state of aldosterone-mediated vasoconstriction, although this requires very high levels of aldosterone. If hypertension is sustained, the chronic effects of elevated arterial pressure become evident. These effects include left ventricular hypertrophy and progressive arteriosclerosis. Because of the increased arterial pressure, renin secretion is typically suppressed, although it may be increased in secondary aldosteronism.

Aldosterone-stimulated potassium loss can be substantial. Serum potassium levels of less than 3.0 mEq/L result in the typical manifestations of hypokalemia: hypokalemic alkalosis due to the movement of potassium from the intercellular to extracellular space in exchange for hydrogen ions as well as renal loss of hydrogen ions to facilitate sodium reabsorption (see Chapter 3). Individuals with hypokalemic alkalosis may experience (1) tetany and paresthesia caused by an alkalosis-induced lowering of ionized calcium levels, (2) skeletal muscle weakness that can be so severe as to mimic flaccid paralysis, (3) cardiovascular alterations, including depressed T waves and ST segment, appearance of U waves on the electrocardiogram, and ventricular ectopy, which may or may not be associated with syncope, and (4) loss of urine-concentrating mechanisms leading to polyuria or nocturia.

Evaluation and Treatment

A variety of clinical and laboratory measurements are useful in the assessment of hyperaldosteronism. These include blood pressure, serum and urinary electrolyte levels, serum and urinary levels of aldosterone and renin, and aldosterone suppression testing. Blood pressure is elevated; serum sodium may be normal or elevated; and serum potassium is depressed, while urinary potassium is elevated (i.e., > 30 mmol/day). Serum aldosterone, as measured by radioimmunoassay is usually greater than 20 ng/dl. Plasma renin activity is generally less than 1 ng/ml/hour for individuals with primary aldosteronism. Serum aldosterone and plasma renin activity must both be measured under controlled situations and after careful dietary regulation of sodium and potassium intake (see Table 18-15). Aldosterone-suppression testing is commonly accomplished with florinef. Imaging techniques, such as CT scans or nuclear magnetic resonance (NMR), may be used to localize an aldosterone-secreting adenoma.

Treatment includes management of hypertension and hypokalemia, as well as correction of any underlying causal abnormalities. If an aldosterone-secreting adenoma is present, it must be surgically removed.

Hypersecretion of Adrenal Androgens and Estrogens

Hypersecretion of adrenal androgens and estrogens may be caused by adrenal tumors, either adenomas or carcinomas. The clinical syndrome that results depends on the hormone secreted, the sex of the individual, and the ages at which the hypersecretion was initiated. Hypersecretion of estrogens causes **feminization,** the development of female sex characteristics. Hypersecretion of androgens causes **virilization,** the development of male sex characteristics (Fig. 18-17).

The effects of an estrogen-secreting tumor are most evident in males and results in gynecomastia (98% of cases), testicular atrophy, and decreased libido. In female children, such tumors may lead to early development of secondary sex characteristics. An androgen-secreting tumor indicates changes more easily observed in females, including excessive hair growth, clitoral enlargement, deepening of the voice, amenorrhea, acne, and breast atrophy. In children, virilizing tumors promote precocious sexual development and bone aging. Treatment of androgen-secreting tumors usually involves surgical excision.

Hypocortical Functioning

Hypofunction of the adrenal cortex may affect glucocorticoid or mineralocorticoid secretion or a combination of both. The hypofunction may result either from a deficiency of adrenal-stimulating substances (i.e., ACTH) or from a primary deficiency of the gland to secrete cortisol, aldosterone, or both.

Hypocortisolism (low levels of cortisol secretion) develops either because of inadequate stimulation of the adrenal glands by ACTH or because of a primary inabil-

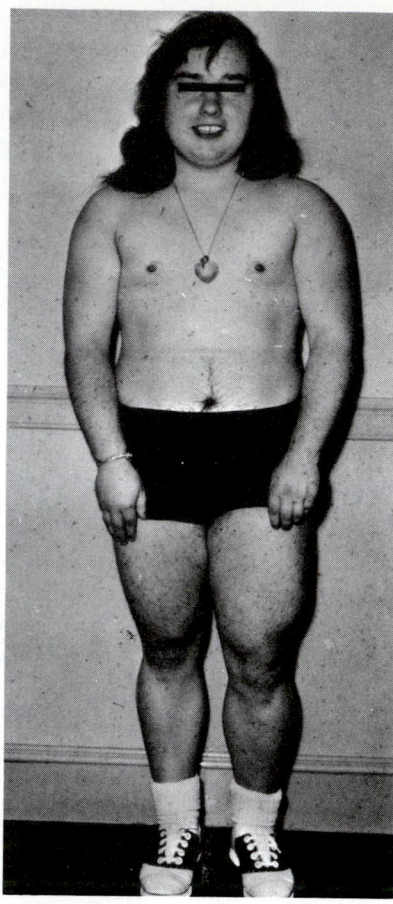

FIG. 18-17. Virilization of a young girl by a virilizing tumor of the adrenal cortex. The tumor secretes excess androgens, thereby producing masculinizing adrenogenital syndrome. (From Thibodeau, 1987.)

ity of the adrenals to produce and secrete the adrenal cortical hormones. In some syndromes, however, there is partial dysfunction of the adrenal cortex so that only synthesis of aldosterone or the adrenal androgens is affected.

Primary adrenal insufficiency is termed **Addison disease.** Addison disease is a relatively rare disease, occurring most often in adults ages 30 to 60, although it may appear at any time throughout the life span. Addison disease, caused by autoimmune mechanisms, is more common in females. Addison disease from tuberculosis affects both sexes equally.

Pathophysiology

Addison disease is characterized by elevated serum ACTH levels wth inadequate corticosteroid synthesis and output. The most common causes are idiopathic organ-specific autoimmune disease and tuberculosis of the adrenal gland. Other causes include familial adrenal insufficiency, amyloidosis, metastatic destruction of the adrenal glands, and adrenal hemorrhage. Before clinical

manifestations of hypocortisolism are evident, more than 90% of total adrenocortical tissue must be destroyed.

Idiopathic Addison Disease   **Idiopathic Addison disease (organ-specific autoimmune adrenalitis),** which causes adrenal atrophy and hypofunction, is generally recognized as an organ-specific autoimmune disease. (Autoimmunity is discussed in Chapter 8.) Autoantibodies are present in 50% to 70% of individuals with idiopathic Addison disease, and this percentage increases in younger persons and in those with other autoimmune diseases. The autoantibodies appear to be specific for the cells of the zona fasciculata. Apparently, a genetic defect in immune surveillance mechanisms causes a deficiency of immune suppressor cells. This deficiency allows the proliferation of immunocytes directed against specific antigens within the adrenocortical cells (Franco-Saenz, 1986).

Idiopathic Addison disease is frequently associated with other autoimmune diseases, especially Hashimoto thyroiditis, pernicious anemia, and idiopathic hypoparathyroidism. In these cases, Addison disease may be inherited as an autosomal recessive trait (Kaffe et al., 1975). (Mechanisms of inheritance are described in Chapter 4.)

The adrenal glands in idiopathic Addison disease are smaller than normal and may be misshapen. Microscopically, gland atrophy is evident throughout the cortex, although the medulla appears intact. Extensive diffuse cortical lymphocytic infiltrate supports the immune component of the disease process.

Secondary hypocortisolism   **Secondary hypocortisolism** is characterized by low-to-absent ACTH levels, which cause inadequate adrenal stimulation, adrenal atrophy, and ultimately decreased corticosteroidogenesis. The exogenous administration of glycocorticoids for nonendocrine disease results in this form of hypocortisolism. Cortisol-producing endocrine tumors also cause secondary hypocortisolism. In these cases, increased glucocorticoid levels suppress ACTH production through normal feedback mechanisms. With decreased ACTH levels, corticosteroid synthesis by the adrenal gland is suppressed. This mechanism is ineffective in reducing corticosteroid levels, however, because the alteration in cortisol secretion lies outside the regulation of the normal feedback loop. Pituitary hypofunction, as occurs in postpartum pituitary infarction (Sheehan syndrome) and panhypopituitarism, hypophysectomy, or isolated ACTH deficiency causes inadequate ACTH production and secretion and absence of pituitary responsiveness to normal feedback mechanisms. In all instances of low ACTH levels, adrenal atrophy occurs, and endogenous adrenal steroidogenesis is depressed.

In the United States and Europe, tuberculosis (TB) is a rare cause of Addison disease. In Japan, however, TB

TABLE 18-16 Clinical manifestations and pathophysiologic mechanisms of Addison disease

Clinical manifestation	Pathyphysiologic mechanism
Weakness and easy fatiguability that worsens as the day progresses, seen especially after exposure to stressors	Not known, may be related to hypoglycemia, decreased metabolism of proteins
Gastrointestinal disturbances: anorexia, nausea, vomiting, diarrhea, abdominal pain	Not known
Hypoglycemia, manifested by fatigue, mental confusion, apathy, psychosis	Absence of cortisol leads to decreased gluconeogenesis, decreased glycogen storage by liver, decreased metabolism of proteins, increased insulin sensitivity
Hyperpigmentation (only seen in cases of Addison disease with increased ACTH)	Increased secretion of ACTH is accompanied by increased secretion of beta-lipotropin and melanocyte-stimulating hormone; both hormones induce pigment changes in epithelial cells
Vitiligo, white patchy areas of depigmented skin	Autoimmune destruction of melanocytes
Hypotension	Decreased blood volume due to hypoaldosteronism causing increased renal sodium losses
Addisonian crisis: severe hypotension and vascular collapse	Combined effects of hypocortisolism, hypoaldosteronism, extracellular volume depletion, and some precipitating stressor (such as infection, vomiting, diarrhea)

continues to account for most cases. Once the adrenals are attacked by TB, the destructive process is irreversible and leads to progressive loss of the gland. Amyloidosis, another rare cause of Addison disease, also destroys the tissue of the adrenal cortex. Adrenoleukodystrophy and adrenomyeloneuropathy are two rare types of familial adrenal deficiency that lead to symptoms of hypocortisolism.

Clinical manifestations of secondary hypocortisolism are similar to those of Addison disease. One difference is that with the typically low levels of ACTH seen in secondary hypocortisolism, hyperpigmentation does not usually occur. Second, the renin-angiotensin system is usually normal in these individuals; therefore aldosterone and potassium levels also tend to be normal.

Clinical Manifestations

The symptoms of Addison disease are primarily a result of hypocortisolism and hypoaldosteronism. Decreased adrenal androgen secretion is usually not clinically obvious in males because the adrenals are not a major source of male androgens. Females may experience a loss of some secondary sex characteristics, such as pubic and axillary hair, normally maintained by the adrenal androgens. The symptoms of Addison disease are summarized in Table 18-16.

Evaluation and Treatment

Serum and urine levels of cortisol, aldosterone, and 17-ketosteroids are all depressed with hypocortisolism.

ACTH levels may be increased if there is adrenocortical insufficiency. Because of dehydration, blood urea nitrogen levels and hematocrit levels are increased. Serum glucose is low. Eosinophil and lymphocyte counts are frequently elevated. Hyperkalemia may cause mild alkalosis (see Chapter 3). The ACTH stimulation test may be used to evaluate adrenal cortical function. This is achieved by administering ACTH and monitoring the adrenal steroid levels.

The treatment of Addison disease involves glucocorticoid and possibly mineralocorticoid replacement therapy, together with dietary modifications. All individuals with hypocortisolism require daily chronic glucocorticoid replacement therapy. In the event of acute stressors, additional cortisol must be administered to approximate the amount of cortisol that might be expected to be secreted if normal adrenal function was present (approximately 100 to 300 μ/day).

The individual's diet should include at least 150 mEq of sodium per day, with sodium intake increased in the event of excessive sweating or diarrhea. Treatment must also include correction of any underlying disorders such as tuberculosis.

Disorders of the Adrenal Medulla
Adrenal Medulla Hypofunction

No known physiologic alterations are associated with hypofunction of the adrenal medulla. Bilateral adrenalectomy, for example, is followed by a rapid decrease in urinary excretion of epinephrine, but that of norepinephrine remains relatively stable. Pathophysiologic alterations are instead associated with hyperfunctioning of the adrenal medulla.

Adrenal Medulla Hyperfunction

The most prominent cause of adrenal medulla hypersecretion is pheochromocytoma. A **pheochromocytoma** is a catecholamine-producing tumor, usually derived from the adrenal medullary cells (Fig. 18-18). Fewer than 10% of these tumors metastasize; if they do, they are usually found in the lungs, liver, bones, or para-aortic lymph glands. Most pheochromocytomas produce norepinephrine, although large tumors secrete both epinephrine and norepinephrine (DeQuattro, Myers, & Campese, 1989).

The true incidence of pheochromocytoma in the general population is not known. One tenth of one percent of the hypertensive population have a pheochromocytoma (Braunwald et al., 1987). The tumors are most common in people in their 40s and 50s, with males and females equally affected.

Pathophysiology

Pheochromocytomas cause excessive production of catecholamines due to autonomous functioning of the

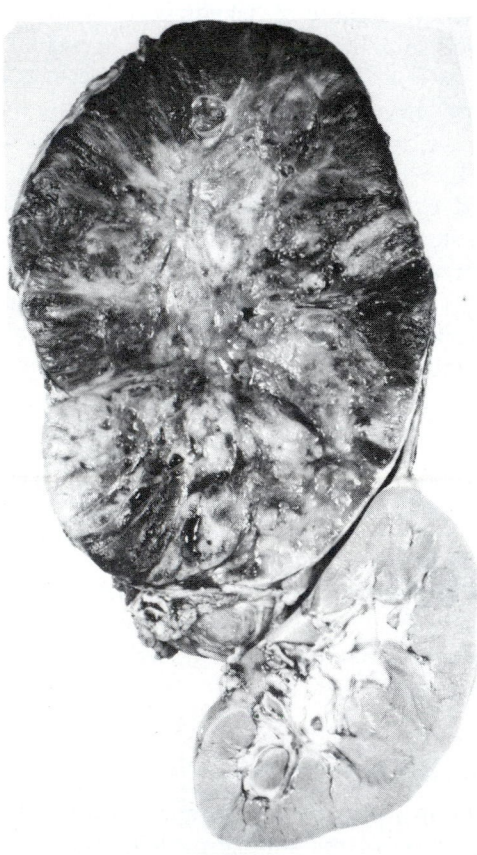

FIG. 18-18. Large pheochromocytoma replacing entire adrenal gland and displacing kidney. (From Rosai, 1989.)

tumor. Other causes of elevated levels of catecholamines include defects in the normal inhibition of tyrosine hydroxylate or defects in the control mechanisms responsible for the regulation of catecholamine synthesis and release. Approximately 5% of people with pheochromocytomas have no symptoms, apparently because the tumor is nonfunctioning. Such tumors can, however, release catecholamines, especially in response to a stressor.

Clinical Manifestations

The clinical manifestations of a pheochromocytoma are related to the chronic effects of catecholamine secretion and include persistent hypertension associated with flushing, diaphoresis, tachycardia, and palpitations. Hypertension is a result of increased peripheral vascular resistance and may be sustained or paroxsysmal. Headaches appear because of sudden changes in catecholamine levels in the blood, affecting cerebral blood flow. Hypermetabolism may be related to increased thyroid hormone levels resulting from stimulation of the thyroid gland by the catecholamines. Glucose intolerance may occur because of catecholamine-induced inhibition of insulin release by the pancreas. Complaints of warmth, heat intolerance, and weight loss are common despite a normal-to-increased appetite. Other symptoms of catecholamine excess include excessive sweating, palpitations and tachycardia, and gastrointestinal alterations, especially constipation.

An acute episode of hypertension related to hypersecretion of catecholamines may follow specific events. Exercise, excessive ingestion of tyrosine-containing foods (aged cheese, red wine, beer, yogurt), ingestion of caffeine-containing foods, external pressure on the tumor, and induction of anesthesia can all increase secretion of catecholamines by the tumor.

These tumors tend to be extremely vascular and can rupture. Such an event can cause massive and potentially fatal hemorrhage. Rupture of a pheochromocytoma is characterized by a sudden unexplained decrease in blood pressure, sudden severe abdominal pain, and a rigid abdomen.

Evaluation and Treatment

A diagnosis of pheochromocytoma is made when increased catecholamine production is demonstrated in the blood or urine. Individuals with this disorder can have total catecholamines greater than 250 μ/day. After elevation of urinary or plasma catecholamines is documented, the site of the tumor is determined by using radiographic techniques and surgical exploration of the abdomen. Because of the possibility of metastasis, whole-body scanning may be done.

The usual treatment of pheochromocytoma is surgical excision of the tumor. Medical therapy is used to stabilize blood pressure prior to surgery. Drugs used include alpha-adrenergic blocking agents and, possibly later, beta-adrenergic blocking agents (DeQuattro et al, 1989).

SUMMARY REVIEW

Mechanisms of Hormonal Pathology

1 Abnormalities in endocrine function may be caused by hypersecretion or hyposecretion of hormones, causing alterations in normal hormone levels.
2 Endocrine abnormalities may also be caused by alterations in receptor function through a variety of mechanisms: (1) a decrease in number of receptors, (2) receptor insensitivity to the hormone, (3) antibodies against specific receptors, and (4) general receptor dysfunction.
3 Abnormally high levels of circulating hormones are sometimes due to hormone release from tissues outside the endocrine system (ectopic foci), which may not respond to normal feedback mechanisms, in which case they are said to function autonomously.

Alterations of the Hypothalamic-Pituitary System

1 Dysfunction in the release of hypothalamic hormones is probably related to interruption of the connection between the hypothalamus and pituitary, the infundibular stem.
2 Disorders of the posterior pituitary include syndrome of inappropriate ADH secretion (SIADH) and diabetes insipidus. SIADH is characterized by abnormally high ADH secretion; diabetes insipidus is characterized by abnormally low ADH secretion.
3 In SIADH, high ADH levels interfere with renal function, leading to hyponatremia and hypoosmolality. SIADH is associated with certain forms of cancer, apparently because of ectopic secretion of ADH by tumor cells.
4 Diabetes insipidus may be neurogenic, caused by insufficient amounts of ADH, or nephrogenic, caused by an inadequate response to ADH. Its principal clinical features are polyuria and polydipsia.
5 Hypopituitarism is dysfunction of the anterior pituitary that causes failure of hormonal functions. Symptoms may be mild to severe.
6 The most common cause of hypopituitarism is pituitary infarction, in which an initiating event leads to circulatory collapse and compensatory vasospasm. Pregnant and postpartum women are most at risk for pituitary infarction.
7 Hyperpituitarism is caused by pituitary adenomas. These are usually benign, slow-growing tumors that arise from cells of the anterior pituitary.
8 Expansion of a pituitary adenoma causes both neurologic and secretory effects. Pressure from the expanding tumor causes hyposecretion of cells, dysfunction of the optic chiasma (leading to visual disturbances), and dysfunction of the hypothalamus and some cranial nerves.
9 Hypersecretion of GH causes acromegaly, in which GH secretion becomes high and unpredictable. Pituitary adenoma is the most common cause of acromegaly.
10 Prolonged, abnormally high levels of GH lead to proliferation in body and connective tissue and in the cytoplasmic matrix. Renal, thyroid, and reproductive dysfunction develop slowly, together with a change in body proportions.

Alterations of Thyroid Function

1 Hyperthyroidism is a general condition in which TH levels cause greater-than-normal physiologic responses. The condition can be caused by a variety of specific diseases, each of which has its own pathophysiology and course of treatment.
2 In general, hyperthyroidism has a range of endocrine, reproductive, gastrointestinal, integumentary, and ocular manifestations. These are caused by increased circulating levels of TH and by stimulation of the sympathetic division of the autonomic nervous system.
3 Graves disease, the most common form of hyperthyroidism, is probably caused by an autoimmune mechanism that overrides normal mechanisms for control of TH secretion.
4 Manifestations of Graves disease can include symptoms of hyperthyroidism, diffuse thyroid enlargement, disorders of the skin, and effects on the extremities.
5 Effects on the extremities cause pretibial myxedema, a condition characterized by subcutaneous swelling of the legs and, occasionally, the hands.
6 Ocular manifestations of Graves disease are caused by hyperactivity of the sympathetic division of the autonomic nervous system and by unknown mechanisms that cause infiltrative changes.
7 Toxic nodular goiter and toxic multinodular goiter occur when TH-regulating mechanisms and abnormal hypertrophy of the thyroid gland cause hyperthyroidism.
8 Toxic nodular goiters are follicular cell adenomas that produce symptoms similar to those of Graves disease.
9 Toxic multinodular goiter is caused by independently functioning follicular cells diffused throughout the thyroid gland.
10 Thyrotoxic crisis is a severe form of hyperthyroidism that is often associated with physiologic or psychologic stress. Without treatment, death occurs quickly.
11 Hypothyroidism is caused by deficient production of TH by the thyroid gland. The condition may be primary or secondary.
12 Hypothyroid conditions include a variety of specific disease processes. Hypothyroidism can also be caused by hypothalamic-pituitary dysfunction in which TRH and TSH is not produced in sufficient amounts.
13 Hypothyroidism affects all body systems. Symptoms depend on the degree of TH deficiency. Common manifestations include decreased energy metabolism and heat production.
14 Myxedema is the characteristic sign of hypothyroidism. Myxedema is caused by alterations in connective tissue with water-binding proteins. The excess water leads to edema and thickened mucous membranes.

15 Acute thyroiditis, a form of hypothyroidism, is caused by a bacterial infection.

16 Subacute thyroiditis, a form of hypothyroidism, is a self-limiting nonbacterial inflammation of the thyroid gland. The inflammatory process damages follicular cells, causing leakage of T_3 and T_4. Hyperthyroidism is then followed by transient hypothyroidism, which is corrected by cellular repair and a return to normal levels in the thyroid.

17 Autoimmune thyroiditis is associated with infiltration or fibrosis of the thyroid, circulating thyroid antibodies, and gradual loss of thyroid function. Autoimmune thyroiditis occurs in those individuals with genetic susceptibility to an autoimmune mechanism that causes thyroid damage and eventual hypothyroidism.

18 Myxedema coma is a severe form of hypothyroidism, which may be life threatening without emergency medical treatment.

19 Thyroid carcinoma is a relatively rare cancer. The most consistent causal risk factor associated with thyroid carcinoma is exposure to ionizing radiation, especially in childhood.

Alterations of Parathyroid Function

1 Hyperparathyroidism, which may be primary, secondary, or tertiary, is characterized by greater than normal secretion of PTH.

2 Primary hyperparathyroidism is caused by an interruption of the normal mechanisms that regulate calcium and PTH levels. Manifestations include chronic hypercalcemia, increased bone resorption, and hypercalcuria.

3 Secondary hyperparathyroidism is a compensatory response to hypocalcemia and often occurs with chronic renal failure.

4 Tertiary hyperparathyroidism is associated with hyperplasia of the parathyroid glands and a loss of the regulatory mechanism that governs PTH and calcium levels.

5 Hypoparathyroidism, defined by abnormally low PTH levels, is caused by thyroid surgery or by hereditary mechanisms.

6 The lack of circulating PTH in hypoparathyroidism causes depressed serum calcium levels, increased serum phosphate levels, decreased bone resorption, and eventual hypocalcuria.

Dysfunction of the Endocrine Pancreas: Diabetes Mellitus

1 Diabetes mellitus is a complex syndrome that causes a number of physiologic changes, some of which are metabolic processes and others of which are vascular.

2 A diagnosis of diabetes mellitus is based on elevated plasma glucose concentrations. Classic signs and symptoms are often present as well.

3 The two types of diabetes mellitus are type I and type II, also called insulin-dependent diabetes mellitus (IDDM) and non-insulin-dependent diabetes mellitus (NIDDM).

4 Type I diabetes mellitus is characterized by a lack of insulin and a relative excess of glucagon, which causes improper metabolism of fat, protein, and carbohydrates.

5 Type I diabetes mellitus is most commonly diagnosed among whites under 30 years of age.

6 In type I diabetes mellitus, beta cells are destroyed, and islet cell antibodies (ICA) appear. The function of these antibodies is unknown, and they tend to disappear with time.

7 Type I diabetes mellitus currently seems to be caused by a gradual process of autoimmune destruction in genetically susceptible individuals.

8 In type I diabetes mellitus, decreased use of glucose causes glucose accumulation in the blood and subsequent loss in the urine. This in turn causes polyuria and polydipsia resulting from osmotic diuresis.

9 Ketoacidosis, caused by increased levels of circulating ketones without the inhibiting effects of insulin; increased levels of circulating fatty acids; and weight loss are all manifestations of type I diabetes mellitus.

10 Type II diabetes mellitus is probably caused by genetic susceptibility that is triggered by environmental factors. The most compelling environmental risk factor is obesity.

11 In the obese, insulin has a diminished ability to influence glucose uptake and metabolism.

12 In type II diabetes, hyalinization of the islets, fatty atrophy of the pancreas and liver, and vascular sclerosis (causing ischemia) are generally present.

13 Some insulin production continues in type II diabetes mellitus, but the weight and number of beta cells decrease.

14 Because the ratio of alpha cells to beta cells may be normal in the individual with type II diabetes, hypotheses suggest that the disease is caused by dysfunctional levels of both insulin and glucagon.

15 Acute complications of diabetes mellitus include hypoglycemia, diabetic ketoacidosis, hyperosmolar hyperglycemic nonketotic coma (HHNK), and the Somogyi effect.

16 Hypoglycemia is a lowered blood glucose level, which may be related to exogenous, endogenous, or functional causes.

17 Symptoms of hypoglycemia are caused by an adrenergic reaction, which occurs when the neuron receives inadequate amounts of carbohydrates to metabolize, and cellular malnutrition, which causes further neurologic symptoms.

18 Diabetic ketoacidosis develops when there is an absolute or relative deficiency of insulin and an increase in stress with accompanying hormonal shifts in insulin antagonists.

19 Hyperosmolar hyperglycemic nonketotic coma (HHNK) is pathophysiologically similar to diabetic ketoacidosis, although levels of free fatty acids are lower in HHNK and lack of ketosis indicates that some level of insulin is present.

20 The Somogyi effect is a combination of hypoglycemia and ketosis. It is most common in those with type I diabetes mellitus and in children.

21 Chronic sequelae of diabetes mellitus include diabetic neuropathies, microvascular disease (e.g., retinopathy, nephrology), macrovascular disease (e.g., coronary

heart disease, stroke, and peripheral vascular disease), and infection.

22 Diabetic neuropathies may be caused by vascular or metabolic mechanisms or a combination of both.

23 In diabetic neuropathy, axonal and Schwann cell degeneration and metabolic aberrations are related to abnormalities in motor nerve conduction velocity, electromyography, and sensory perception.

24 Microangiopathy is caused by thickening of the capillary basement membrane and eventual decreased tissue perfusion affecting the microcirculation.

25 Diabetic retinopathy is caused by retinal ischemia related to microvascular occlusion associated with diabetes mellitus.

26 Diabetic neuropathy is related to glomerular enlargement and glomerular basement membrane thickening, which in turn cause diffuse intercapillary glomerulosclerosis.

27 Macrovascular disease associated with diabetes mellitus is probably related to the proliferation of fibrous plaques in the arterial wall and to elevated levels of various lipids.

28 Incidence of coronary heart disease, peripheral vascular disease, and stroke are greater in diabetics than in nondiabetics.

29 Diabetics are at risk for a variety of infections.

30 Infection may be related to sensory impairment and resulting injury, hypoxia, increased proliferation of pathogens in elevated concentrations of glucose, decreased blood supply associated with vascular damage, and impaired white cell function.

Alterations of Adrenal Function

1 Disorders of the adrenal cortex are related to hyperfunction or hypofunction. No known disorders are associated with hypofunction of the adrenal medulla, but medullary hyperfunction causes clinically defined syndromes.

2 Cortical hyperfunction, or hypercortisolism, causes Cushing syndrome, which may or may not involve the pituitary gland, and Cushing disease, which is hypercortisolism with pituitary involvement.

3 Cushing syndrome may be caused by excessive circulating ACTH related to CRH secretion, a pituitary adenoma, autonomous secretion by a tumor outside the pituitary, or autonomous secretion by an adrenal neoplasm and its metastases.

4 Individuals with Cushing disease lose diurnal and circadian patterns of ACTH and cortisol secretion, and they lack the ability to increase secretion of these hormones in response to a stressor. Individuals experience weight gain, glucose intolerance, protein wasting, bone disease, hyperpigmentation, and immune suppression.

5 Excessive aldosterone secretion causes hyperaldosteronism, which may be primary or secondary. Primary hyperaldosteronism is caused by an abnormality of the adrenal cortex. Secondary hyperaldosteronism involves an extra-adrenal stimulus, often angiotensin.

6 Primary hyperaldosteronism is usually caused by an adrenal adenoma or carcinoma. The condition is characterized by hypertension, hypokalemia, renal potassium wasting, and neuromuscular manifestations.

7 Secondary hyperaldosterone secretion is related to a variety of conditions associated wtih elevated renin release and activation of angiotensin. These include decreased circulating blood volume and decreased renal blood supply, elevated estrogen levels, Bartter syndrome, and renin-secreting tumors.

8 Hyperaldosteronism promotes increased sodium reabsorption, corresponding hypervolemia, increased extracellular volume (which is variable), and hypokalemia related to renal reabsorption of sodium.

9 Hypersecretion of adrenal androgens and estrogens causes adrenal tumors, either adenomas or carcinomas. Hypersecretion of estrogens causes feminization, the development of female sex characteristics. Hypersecretion of androgens causes virilization, the development of male sex characteristics.

10 Hypofunction of the adrenal cortex can affect glucocorticoid or mineralocorticoid secretion, or both. Hypofunction can be caused by a deficiency of adrenal-stimulating substance or by a primary deficiency in the gland itself.

11 Hypocortisolism, or low levels of cortisol, is caused by inadequate adrenal stimulation by ACTH or by primary cortisol hyposecretion. Primary adrenal insufficiency is termed Addison disease.

12 Addison disease is characterized by elevated ACTH levels with inadequate corticosteroid synthesis and output.

13 Causes of Addison disease include idiopathic autoimmune disease, tuberculosis of the adrenal gland, familial adrenal insufficiency, amyloidosis, metastatic destruction of the adrenal glands, and adrenal hemorrhage.

14 Secondary hypercortisolism is characterized by low to absent ACTH levels, leading to inadequate adrenal stimulation, adrenal atrophy, and decreased corticosteroidogenesis. The most common cause is exogenous administration of glucocorticoids.

15 Manifestations of Addison disease are related to hypocortisolism and hypoaldosteronism. Symptoms include weakness, fatiguability, hypoglycemia and related metabolic problems, lowered response to stressors, vitiligo, and manifestations of hypovolemia and hyperkalemia.

16 Hyperfunction of the adrenal medulla is usually caused by a pheochromocytoma, a catecholamine-producing tumor. Symptoms of catecholamine excess are related to their sympathetic nervous system effects and include hypertension, palpitations, tachycardia, glucose intolerance, excessive sweating, and constipation.

KEY TERMS

Acromegaly, 602

Acute thyroiditis, 608

Addison disease (primary adrenal insufficiency), 634

Autoimmune thyroiditis (Hashimoto disease, chronic lymphocyte thyroiditis), 608

Cushing disease (pituitary-dependent hypercortisolism), 629

Cushing syndrome (chronic hypercortisolism), 629

Dawn phenomenon, 623

Diabetes insipidus, 598

Diabetes mellitus, 612

Diabetic ketoacidosis (diabetic coma), 619

Diabetic neuropathy, 624

Feminization, 633

Gestational diabetes, 618

Giantism, 602

Graves disease, 604

Hyperaldosteronism

Hypercortisolism, 629

Hyperosmolar hyperglycemic nonketotic coma (HHNK; insulin shock, insulin reaction), 622

Hyperparathyroidism, 609

Hyperpituitarism, 599

Hyperthyroidism, 603

Hypocortisolism, 633

Hypoglycemia, 618

Hypoparathyroidism, 611

Hypopituitarism, 599

Hypothyroidism, 606

Idiopathic Addison disease (organ-specific autoimmune adrenalitis), 634

Islet cell antibodies (ICA), 612

Myxedema, 607

Myxedema coma, 608

Panhypopituitarism, 599

Pheochromocytoma, 636

Pituitary adenoma, 600

Pretibial myxedema (Graves dermopathy), 605

Primary hyperaldosteronism (Conn disease, primary aldosteronism), 631

Primary hyperparathyroidism, 609

Secondary hyperaldosteronism, 631

Secondary hypercortisolism, 634

Secondary hyperparathyroidism, 609

Somogyi effect, 624

Subacute thyroiditis, 608

Syndrome of inappropriate ADH secretion (SIADH), 597

Tertiary hyperparathyroidism, 610

Thyrotoxic crisis (thyroid storm), 605

Toxic nodular goiter, 605

Type I diabetes mellitus (insulin-dependent diabetes mellitus [IDDM]), 612

Type II diabetes mellitus (non-insulin-dependent diabetes mellitus [NIDDM]), 612

Virilization, 633

REFERENCES

Abbasi, A. A. (1981). Diabetes: Diagnostic and therapeutic significance of taste impairment. *Geriatrics, 36*(12), 3-78.

Ahren, B. (1986). Thyroid neuroendocrinology: Neural regulation of thyroid hormone secretion. *Endocrine Reveiws, 7*(2), 149-155.

American Cancer Society. (1988). *Cancer facts & figures 1988.* New York: Author.

American Diabetes Association. (1979). Policy statement, 1979. *Diabetes Care, 2,* 1-3.

Arky, R. A. (1983). Nutritional management of the diabetic. In M. Ellenberg & H. Rifkin (Eds.), *Diabetes mellitus theory and practice* (3rd ed.). New York: Medical Examination Publishing.

Barnes, D. M. (1986, June). Steroids may influence changes in mood. *Science, 232,* 1344-1345.

Bautter, F. C., & Schwartz, W. B. (1967). The syndrome of inappropriate secretion of antidiuretic hormone. *American Journal of Medicine, 42,* 790-806.

Bernstein, R. (1981). *Diabetes: The glucograph method for normalizing blood sugar.* New York: Crown.

Borsey, D. P., Fraser, D. M., Gray, R. S., Elton, R. A., Smith A. F., & Clarke B. F. (1982). Glycosylated hemoglobin and its temporal relationship to plasma glucose in non-insulin dependent (type 2) diabetes mellitus. *Metabolism Clinical and Experimental 31*(4), 362-365.

Brashear, H. R., & Raney, R. B. (1986). *Shand's handbook of orthopaedic surgery* (10th ed.). St. Louis: C. V. Mosby.

Braunwald, E., Isselbacher, K. J., Petersdorf, R. G., Wilson, J., Martin, J. B., & Fauci, A. S. (1987). *Harrison's principles of internal medicine* (11th ed.). New York: McGraw-Hill.

Brodoff, B. N., & Bleicher, S. J. (Eds.). (1982). *Diabetes mellitus and Obesity.* Baltimore: Williams & Wilkins.

Brown, B. L., Walker S. W., & Tomlinson, S., (1985). Calcium calmodulin and hormone secretion. *Clinical Endocrinology, 23*(2), 201-218.

Burchfield, S. R. (1979, December). The stress response: A new perspective. *Psychomotor Medicine, 41*(8), 661-670.

Burkholder, P. M. (Ed.). (1974). *Atlas of human glomerular pathology.* Hagerston, MD: Harper & Row.

Burry, M., & Martens, L. (1980, February). ADH and its inappropriate secretion. *Canadian Nurse,* 41-43.

Camargo, C. A., & Kolb, K. O. (1988). Endocrine disorders. In S. A. Schroeder, M. A. Krupp, & L. W. Tierney (Eds.), *Current medical diagnosis and treatment.* Norwalk, CT: Langer.

Campbell, P. J., Bolli, G. B., Cryer, P. E., & Gerich, J. E. (1985). Pathogenesis of the dawn phenomenon in patients with insulin-dependent diabetes mellitus. Accelerated glucose production and impaired glucose utilization due to nocturnal surges in growth hormone secretion. *New England Journal of Medicine, 312,* 1473-1479.

Cecil, R. L., Wyngaarden, J. B., & Smith, L. H. (1988). *Cecil's textbook of medicine* (8th ed.). Philadelphia: W. B. Saunders.

Cobb, W. E. (1984). Management of neurogenic DI. In S. Reichlin (Ed.), *The neurohypophysis.* New York: Plenum Medical Book Co.

Coleman, P. (1979). ADH: Physiology and pathophysiology—A review. *Journal of Neurosurgical Nursing, 11*(4), 199-204.

Colwell, J. A., Nair, R. M., Halusoka, P. V., Rogers, C., Whetsell A., & Sagel, J. (1979). Platelet adhesion and aggregation in diabetes mellitus. *Metabolism Clinical and Experimental 28*(4), 394-400.

Conn, J. W. (1967). Diagnosis of normokalemic primary aldosteronism: A new form of primary aldosteronism. *Science, 158,* 525-526.

Cryer, P. E. (1980). Physiology and pathophysiology of the human sympatho-adrenal neuroendocrine system. *New England Journal of Medicine, 303*(8), 436-444.

Culpepper, R. M., Heber, S. C., & Andreoli, T. E. (1985). The posterior pituitary and water metabolism. In J. D. Wilson & D. W. Foster (Eds.), *Williams textbook of endocrinology* (9th ed.). Philadelphia: W. B. Saunders.

Daughaday, W. H. (1982). Pathophysiology of acromegaly. In J. Givens (Ed.), *Hormone-secreting pituitary tumors.* Chicago: Year Book Medical Publishers, Inc.

DeQuattro, V., Myers, M., Campese, V. M. (1989). Pheochromocytoma: Diagnosis and therapy. In L. J. DeGroot (Ed.), *Endocrinology* (2nd ed.). Philadelphia: W. B. Saunders.

Donald, R. A. (1984). *Endocrine disorders: A guide to diagnosis.* New York: Marcel Dekker, Inc.

Ellenberg, M., & Rifkin, H. (Eds.). (1983). *Diabetes mellitus, theory and practice* (3rd ed.). New York: Medical Exam.

Ezrin, C. (1979). *Systemic endocrinology.* Hagerstown, MD: Harper & Row.

Ezrin, C., Horvath, C., Kaufman, B., Kovacs, K., & Weiss, M. (1980). *Pituitary disease.* Boca Raton, FL: CRC Press.

Farid, N. R., & Stenszky, V. (1988). Graves' disease. In N. Fand (Ed.), *Immunogenetics of endocrine disorders.* New York: Alan R. Liss, Inc.

Fein, F. S., & Schever, J. (1983). Heart disease in diabetes. In M. Ellenberg & H. Rifkin (Eds.), *Diabetes mellitus theory and practice* (3rd ed.). New York: Medical Examination Publishing.

Felig, P., Baxter, J. D., Broadus, A. E., & Frohman, L. A. (1987). *Endocrinology and metabolism* (2nd ed.). New York: McGraw-Hill.

Fitzgerald, M. G., & Kilveat, A. (1985). The endocrine system—Diabetes. In J. C. Brocklehurst (Ed.), *Textbook of geriatric medicine and gerontology.* London: Churchill Livingstone.

Flavin, K., & Haire-Joshu, D., (1986). The pharmacologic repertoire . . . Drugs for diabetes. *American Journal of Nursing, 86*(11), 1244-1251.

Franco, L. A. (1982, October). Syndrome of inappropriate secretion of antidiuretic hormone. *Journal of Neurosurgical Nursing, 14*(5).

Franco-Saenz, R. (1986). Diseases of the adrenal cortex. In P. J. Mulrow (Ed.), *The adrenal gland.* New York: Elsevier.

Friedman, E. A., & L'Esperance, F. A. (Eds.). (1981). *Diabetic renal-retinal syndrome.* New York: Grune & Stratton.

Frohlich, E. D. (1984). *Pathophysiology: Altered regulatory mechanisms in disease* (3rd ed.). Philadelphia: Lippincott.

Gamble, D. R., Taylor, K. W., & Cumming, H. (1973). Coxsackie viruses and diabetes mellitus. *British Medical Journal, 4,* 260-262.

Ganda, O. P. (1980). Pathogenesis of macrovascular disease in the human diabetic. *Diabetes, 29,* 931-942.

Genazzani, A. R., Thijsser, J. H., & Siteri, P. K. (1980). *Adrenal androgens,* New York: Raven Press.

Gerich, J. E. (1983). Somatostatin and analogues. In M. Ellenberg & H. Rifkin (Eds.), *Diabetes mellitus theory and practice* (3rd ed.). New York: Medical Examination Publishing.

Givens, J. R. (1982). *Hormone-secreting pituitary tumors.* Chicago: Year Book Publishers, Inc.

Gomez-Pan, A., & Rodrigquez-Arnao, M. (1983). Somatosin and GH-releasing factor and synthesis, location, metabolism, and function. *Clinical Endocrinology and Metabolism, 12*(3), 469-508.

Goto, Y., Horivchi, A., & Kyuya, K. (Eds.). (1982). *Diabetic neuropathy.* Amsterdam: Exerpta Medica.

Haire-Joshu, D., Flavin, K., & Cutter, W. (1986). Contrasting type I and type II diabetes. *American Journal of Nursing, 86*(11), 1240-1243.

Halder, J. B., Beard, J. C., & Porte, D. (1984). Islet function and stress hyperglycemia: Plasma glucose and epinephrine interaction. *American Journal of Physiology, 247*(E), 47-51.

Hays, R. M., & Leine, S. D. (1981). Pathophysiology of water metabolism. In B. Brenner & F. Rector (Eds.), *The kidney.* Philadelphia: Saunders Publishing.

Henry, H. L. (1987). The complications of diabetes mellitus. *Journal of the National Medical Association, 79*(6), 677-680.

Hersey, R. M. & Distefano, V. (1979). Control of phenyletahnolamine N-methyl transferase by glucocorticoids in cultured bovine adrenal medullary cells. *Journal of Pharmacology and Experimental Therapeutics, 209,* 147-152.

Hollenbeck, C. B. (1987). Effect of variation in diet on lipoprotein metabolism in patients with diabetes mellitus. *Diabetes Metabolic Review, 3*(3), 669-689.

Huff, T. A. (1981). Exercise planning of insulin-dependent diabetics. *Consultant, 21,* 71-72.

Imera, H. (Ed.). (1985). *The pituitary gland: Comprehensive endocrinology.* New York: Raven Press.

Jaffe, R. B. (Ed.). (1981). *Prolactin.* New York: Elsevier.

Jaffe, R. B. (1984). Stress and health. *Annual Review of Public Health, 5,* 319-341.

Jubiz, W. (1985). *Endocrinology* (2nd ed.). New York: McGraw-Hill.

Kaffe, S., Pettigrow, C. S., Cahill, L. T., Perlman, D., Moloshok, R. E., Hirschhorn, K., & Papageorgiou, P. S. (1975). Variable cell-mediated immune defects in a family with *candida* endocrinopathy syndrome. *Clinical and Experimental Immunology, 20,* 397-408.

Khachadurian, A. K. (1982). Diabetics: New systems for classification and diagnosis. *Geriatrics, 37*(1), 111-115.

Kreisberg, R. A. (1983). Diabetic ketoacidosis, alcoholic ketosis, lactic acidosis, and hyporeninemic hypoaldosteronism. In M. Ellenberg & H. Rifkin (Eds.), *Diabetes mellitus theory and practice* (3rd ed.). New York: Medical Examination Publishing.

Kubo, W. M., & Grant, M. M. (1978). The syndrome of inappropriate secretion of antidiuretic hormone. *Heart & Lung, 7*(3), 469-476.

L'Esperance, A., & James, A. (1980). *Diabetic retinopathy: Clinical evaluation and management.* St. Louis: C. V. Mosby.

L'Esperance, A., & James, A. (1983). The eye and diabetes mellitus. In M. Ellenberg & H. Rifkin (Eds.), *Diabetes mellitus theory and practice,* (3rd ed.). New York: Medical Examination Publishing.

Labhart, A. (1986). *Clinical endocrinology: Theory and Practice.* Berlin: Springer-Verlag.

Laron, Z., & Galatzer, A. (1982). *Psychological aspects of diabetes in children and adolescents.* Basel: Karger.

Lefebvre, P. J., & Luyckx, A. S. (1983). Hypoglycemia. In M. Ellenberg & H. Rifkin (Eds.), *Diabetes mellitus theory and practice* (3rd ed.). New York: Medical Examination Publishing.

Levin, M. E., & O'Neal, L. W. (1983). Peripheral vascular disease. In M. Ellenberg & H. Rifkin (Eds.), *Diabetes mellitus theory and practice,* (3rd ed.). New York: Medical Examination Publishing.

Lewis, M. E., & O'Neal, L. W. (Eds.). (1983). *The diabetic foot* (3rd ed.). St. Louis: C. V. Mosby.

Little, H. L. (1980). Preventing progressive diabetic retinopathy. In E. A. Friedman & F. A. L'Esperance (Eds.), *Diabetic renal-retinal syndrome.* New York: Grune & Stratton, pp. 171-183.

Little, H. L. Jack, R. L., Patz, A., & Forsham, P. H. (1983). *Diabetic retinopathy.* New York: Thieme-Stratton, Inc.

Majewska, M. D. (1986). Steroid hormone metabolites are barbituate-like modulators of the GABA receptor. *Science, 232,* 1004.

Mann, J. I., Pyorala., K., & Teuscher, A. (Eds.). (1983). *Diabetes in epidemiological perspective.* New York: Churchill Livingstone.

Martin, C. (1985). *Endocrine physiology.* New York: Oxford University Press.

Matz, R. (1983). Coma in the nonketotic diabetic. In M. Ellenberg & H. Rifkin (Eds.), *Diabetes mellitus theory and practice* (3rd ed.). New York: Medical Examination Publishing.

Melnik, J. & Potter, J. L. (1982). Variance in capillary and venous glucose levels during a glucose tolerance test. *American Journal of Medical Technology, 48*(6), 543-545.

Moses, A., & Notman, D. D. (1982). Diabetes insipidus and syndrome of inappropriate antidiuretic hormone secretion (SIADH). In G. J. Stollerman (Ed.), *Advances in internal medicine* (vol. 27). Year Book Medical Publishers, pp. 73-100.

Moskowitz, J. (Ed.). (1981). *Diabetes and atherosclerosis connection.* New York: Juvenile Diabetes Foundation.

Munck, A., Guyre, P. M., & Holbrook, N. J. (1984). Physiological functions of glucocorticoids in stress and their relation to pharmocological actions. *Endocrine Review, 5*(1), 25-42.

National Diabetes Data Group. (1979). Classification and diagnosis of diabetes mellitus and other categories of glucose intolerance. *Diabetes, 28,* 1039-1057.

Neville, A. M., & O'Hare, M. J. (1982). *The human adrenal cortex.* Berlin: Springer-Verlag.

Nikolics, K. Mason, A. J., Szony, E., Ramachandran, J., & Seebury P. H. (1985). A prolactin-inhibiting factor within the precursor for human gonadotropin-releasing hormone. *Nature, 316*(6028), 511-517.

Olefsky, J. (1983). Insulin antagonists and resistance. In M.

Ellenberg & H. Rifkin (Eds.), *Diabetes mellitus theory and practice* (3rd ed.). New York: Medical Examination Publishing.

Osterby, R. (1983). Basement membrane morphology in diabetes mellitus. In M. Ellenberg & H. Rifkin (Eds.), *Diabetes mellitus theory and practice* (3rd ed.). New York: Medical Examination Publishing.

Phipps, W. J., Long, B. C., & Woods, N. F. (1987). *Medical surgical nursing: Concepts and clinical practice* (3rd ed.). St. Louis: C. V. Mosby.

Pickup, J. C., Keen, H., Parsons, J. A., Alterti, K. G. M. M., & Rowe, H. J. (1979). Continuous subcutaneous insulin infusion: Improved blood glucose and intermediary metabolite control in diabetics. *Lancet, 1,* 1255-1258.

Pietri, A., Dunn, F. L., & Raskin, P. (1980). The effect of improved diabetic control on plasma lipid and lipoprotein levels: A comparison of conventional therapy and continuous insulin infusion. *Diabetes, 29,* 1001-1005.

Podolsky, S. (Ed.). (1980). *Clinical diabetes: Modern management.* New York: Appleton-Century-Crofts.

Porte, D, & Woods, S. C. (1983). Neural regulation of islet hormones and its role in energy balance and stress hyperglycemia. In M. Ellenberg & H. Rifkin (Eds.), *Diabetes mellitus theory and practice* (3rd ed.). New York: Medical Examination Publishing.

Pyke, D. A. (1979). Diabetes: The genetic connection. *Diabetologia, 17,* 333-343.

Rabin, D., & McKenna, T. J. (1982). *Clinical endocrinology and metabolism: Principles and practice.* New York: Grune & Stratton.

Rapp, J. P. (1986). Adrenal steroid biosynthesis and metabolism. In P. J. Mulrow (Ed.), *The adrenal gland.* New York: Elsevier.

Rayfield, E. J., Ault, M. J., Keusch, G. T., Brothers, M. J., Nechemias, C., & Smith, H. (1982). Infection and diabetes: The case for glucose control. *American Journal of Medicine, 72*(3), 439-450.

Reichlin, S. (Ed.). (1984). *The neurohypophysis.* New York: Plenum Medical Book Co.

Rosai, J. (1981). *Ackerman's surgical pathology* (6th ed.). St. Louis: C. V. Mosby.

Rose, R. M. (1980, August). Endocrine responses to stressful psychological events: Advances in psychoneuroendocrinology. *Psychiatric Clinics of North America, 3*(2), 251-275

Ross, H., Bernstein, G., & Rifkin, H. (1983). Relationship of metabolic control of diabetes mellitus to long-term complications. In M. Ellenberg & H. Rifkin (Eds.), *Diabetes mellitus theory and practice* (3rd ed.). New York: Medical Examination Publishing.

Schade, D. S., & Eaton, R. R. (1978). Pathophysiology of diabetes mellitus. *Medical Clinical of North America, 62*(4), 695-771.

Sheehan, H. L., & Davis, J. C. (1982). *Postpartum hypopituitarism.* Springfield, IL: Charles C. Thomas Publisher.

Sheehan, H. L., & Stanfield, J. P. (1961). The pathogenesis and postpartum necrosis of the anterior lobe of the pituitary gland. *Acta Endocrinol (Copenh), 37,* 479-510.

Smith, J. (1981). Nursing mangement of diabetes insipidus. *Journal of Neurological Nursing, 13*(6), 313-317.

Streeten, D. H. P., Anderson, G. H., Dalakos, T. G., & Seeley, D. (1984). Normal and abnormal function of the hypothalamic-pituitary-adrenocortical system in man. *Endocrine Review, 5*(1), 371-384.

Tan, S. Y. (1986a). Diseases of hyper- and hypomineralocorticoid production. In P. J. Mulrow (Ed.), *The adrenal gland.* New York: Elsevier.

Tan, S. Y. (1986b). Control of adrenal secretion of mineralocorticoids. In P. J. Mulrow (Ed.), *The adrenal gland.* New York: Elsevier.

Thibodeau, G. A. (1987). *Anatomy and physiology.* St. Louis: Times Mirror/Mosby.

Vorherr, H., Massry, S., Fallet, R., Kaplan, L., & Kleeman, C. R. (1970). Antidiuretic principle in tuberculous lung tissue of a patient with pulmonary tuberculosis and gyponatremia. *Annals of Internal Medicine, 72,* 383-387.

Waldhausl, W.K. (Ed.). (1980). *Diabetes 1979.* Amsterdam: Excerpta Medica.

West, K. M. (1978). *Epidemiology of diabetes and its vascular lesions.* New York: Elsevier.

Williams, R. H. (Ed.) (1981). *Textbook of endocrinology* (6th ed.). Philadelphia: W. B. Saunders.

Wilson, J. D., & Foster, D. W. (1985). *Williams textbook of endocrinology* (7th ed.). Philadelphia: W. B. Saunders.

Wollesein, F., Anderson, T., & Karle, A. (1982). Size reduction of extracellular pituitary tumors during bromocriptine treatment. *Annals of Internal Medicine, 96,* 281-286.

World Health Organization. (1980). WHO expert committee on diabetes mellitus, second report. *Technical Report Series, 646.*

Yao, Y. (1981). Current review of thyroid function tests. *Hospital Practice, 16*(9), 149-164.

Young, W., & Klee, G. (Eds.). (1988). Diagnostic evaluation of endocrine disorders. *Endocrine and Metabolic Clinics of North America, 17*(2).

Zimmet, P. (1983). Epidemiology of diabetes mellitus. In M. Ellenberg & H. Rifkin (Eds.), *Diabetes mellitus theory and practice* (3rd ed.). New York: Medical Examination Publishing.

Zimmet, P., Kirk, R., Sujeanston, S., Whitehouse, S., & Taylor, R. (1982). Diabetes in pacific populations: genetic and environmental interactions. In J. S. Melish, J. Hanna, & S. Baba (Eds.), *Genetic environmental interaction in diabetes mellitus.* Amsterdam: Exerpta Medica, pp. 9-17.

Zoneraich, S. (Ed.). (1978). *Diabetes and the heart.* Springfield, Illinois: Charles C. Thomas.

UNIT VII

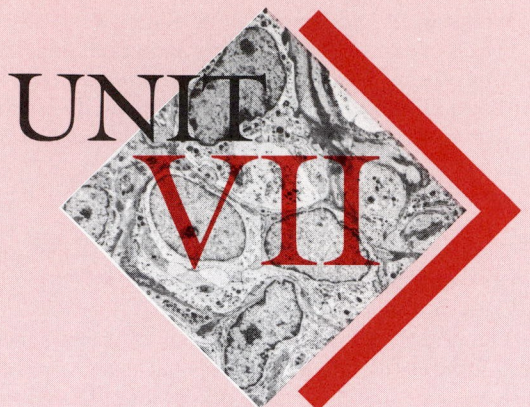

The Reproductive System

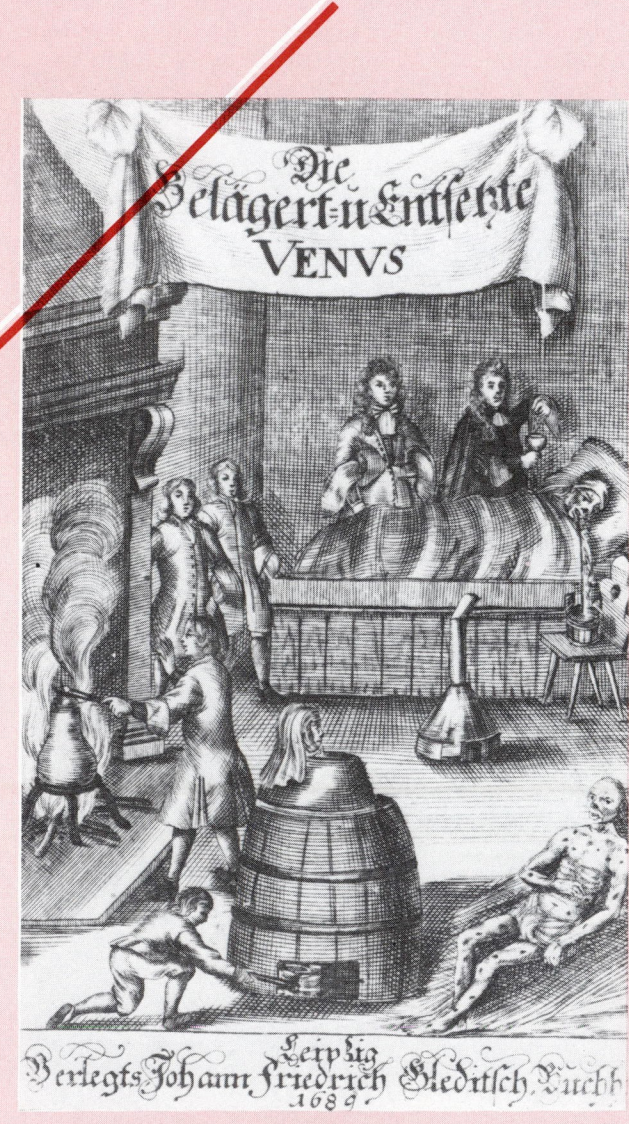

Interior scene showing people involved in various methods of syphilis treatment, including mercury fumigation. A victim in the last stages is in the foreground. (From Blankaart, S.: Die belagertund entsetzte Venus, Leipzig, 1689. Courtesy National Library of Medicine.)

MOST recorded history about the female and male reproductive systems has focused on issues of fertility, the female reproductive cycle, and venereal diseases. In ancient times the female reproductive cycle and birth were viewed as divine mysteries. As civilizations evolved reproduction and birth were sometimes viewed as dirty or sinful. This perspective was slow to change, even with the development of modern medicine. The idea that health problems peculiar to women deserved separate attention was not conceived before the middle of the nineteenth century. The first women's hospital in the United States was opened in 1855 by a physician in New York City.

In 1809 in Kentucky the first ovariotomy was performed. Physicians thought that removal of the ovaries might be a successful treatment for "female hysteria." Between 1846 and 1849 Dr. Marion Sims developed expertise in the surgical correction of vesicovaginal fistula by performing 30 operations on a female slave. Also in 1846 practitioners began to associate postpartum infections with the lack of hand washing. In 1871 the first hysterectomy was performed in the United States, and between 1878 and 1882, Poro and Saenger improved techniques of cesarean section, thereby establishing it as a routine procedure. Today the routine performance of cesarean section is receiving intense scrutiny.

Control of fertility was not available until the early 1900s, except through methods developed by lay healers and midwives. Spermatozoa had been known about since the seventeenth century, and the ovum was described in early 1800. Medically the first means of fertility control was the intrauterine device, first described in 1909 by Richard Richter. It was not until the 1930s that physicians knew enough about the menstrual cycle to predict the timing of ovulation and fertilization. This knowledge led to development of the rhythm method of birth control, which was proposed independently by Ogino in Japan and Knaus in Austria. Penile protectors were known to the ancient Egyptians, and the first description of the condom was written in 1854, primarily for protection against syphilis. By the middle of the eighteenth century sheaths of animal intestine were widely sold in France and England for safety and for prevention of conception.

Knowledge about the specific hormones involved in male and female reproductive function has increased dramatically since the development of techniques to isolate hormones and their derivatives. One of the first sex hormones to be isolated was progesterone; it was discovered by G. W. Corner and W. M. Allen in 1929. This was followed by the isolation of estrogen. This knowledge, together with information regarding the events of the menstrual cycle, led to the development of female birth control pills, which were introduced in the United States in the 1950s. Information about central nervous system control of the reproductive cycle became available in the 1960s with the isolation of follicle-stimulating hormone and luteinizing hormone. These hormones were initially thought to affect only the female reproductive cycle, but in the 1970s they were found to affect the male reproductive system as well.

Testosterone was first isolated in 1935, although evidence for male sex hormones was described in 1849 when testes were transplanted into castrated male chicks and the secondary characteristics of roosters appeared. The most recently discovered reproductive hormone is inhibin, a hormone that influences sperm production.

The recorded history of venereal diseases begins in the fifteenth century. The first major epidemic of syphilis occurred among sailors returning to the Old World on Columbus's first voyage. The disease spread to Spanish soldiers who were fighting for the king of Naples and then to the French troops of Charles VIII, after which it became known as the "French disease." Girolamo Francastoro of Verona (1483-1553), a poet, physician, geologist, classicist, and pathologist, wrote *Syphilis sive Morbus Gallicus* (1530), in which he named the French disease syphilis and noted its sexual means of spread. Jean Fernel (1497-1588), a physician trained in Paris, was the first to suggest that gonorrhea and syphilis were quite separate illnesses that merely shared a common mode of transmission. Syphilis was treated with mercury or guaiac. In the sixteenth century gonorrhea and syphilis became very common. Fear of these two venereal diseases prompted the closing of communal baths. This was a great loss, as adequate water for bathing was not generally available.

Not until the 1970s, as medical practitioners realized the complexity of sexually transmitted conditions, did thinking about venereal diseases undergo a major shift. Health care workers and policymakers became increasingly aware of the great number of infections spread from person to person during sexual contact. This new understanding caused the term *sexually transmitted diseases* to replace *venereal diseases* gradually.

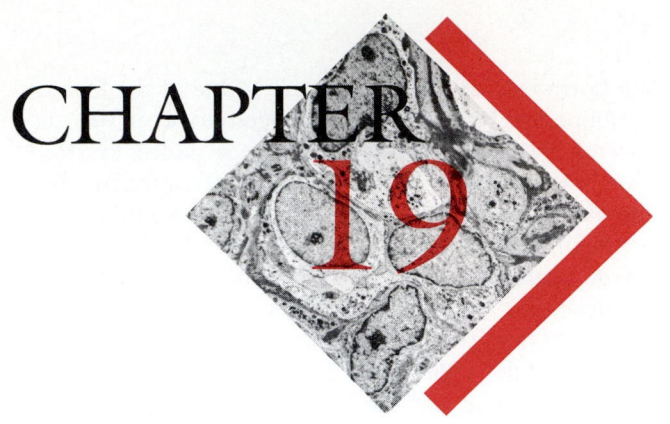

CHAPTER 19

Structure and Function of the Reproductive Systems

D. Patricia Gray
Sue E. Huether

Development of the reproductive systems, 646
    Sexual differentiation in utero, 646
    Puberty, 649
The female reproductive system, 650
    External genitalia, 650
    Internal genitalia, 650
      Vagina, 650
      Uterus, 651
      Fallopian tubes, 653
      Ovaries, 654
    Female sex hormones, 655
      Estrogens, 655
      Progesterone, 656
      Androgens, 657
    The menstrual cycle, 657
      Phases of the menstrual cycle, 657
      Hormonal controls, 659
      Ovarian cycle, 659
      Uterine phases, 660
      Vaginal response, 660
      Body temperature, 660
The male reproductive system, 660
    External genitalia, 660
      Testes, 660
      Epididymis, 662
      Scrotum, 662
      Penis, 663
    Internal genitalia, 663
      Spermatogenesis, 664
      Male sex hormones, 665
Structure and function of the breast, 666
    The female breast, 666
    The male breast, 668
Tests of reproductive function, 668
    Infection and cancer tests, 668
    Fertility tests, 670
Aging and reproductive function, 671
    Aging and the female reproductive system, 671
    Aging and the male reproductive system, 672

The male and female reproductive systems have several anatomic and physiologic features in common. Most obvious is their major function, reproduction, through which a 23-chromosome female gamete, the **ovum,** and a 23-chromosome male gamete, the **spermatozoan** (**sperm** cell) unite to form a 46-chromosome zygote that is capable of developing into a new individual. The male reproductive system produces the sperm and delivers them to the female reproductive tract. The female reproductive system produces the ovum and, if it is fertilized, can nurture and protect it while it develops and expel it at birth. These functions are determined not only by anatomic structures but also by complex hormonal, neurologic, and psychogenic factors.

DEVELOPMENT OF THE REPRODUCTIVE SYSTEMS

The structure and function of both male and female reproductive systems depend on steroid hormones called **sex hormones.** Hormonal effects on the reproductive systems begin well before birth and continue for life.

Sexual Differentiation in Utero

During embryonic development the most important sex hormone is the primary male sex hormone, **testosterone.** Until the eighth week of gestation, the initial reproductive structures of male and female embryos are homologous (the same), consisting of one pair of primary sex organs, or **gonads,** and two pairs of ducts, the mesonephric ducts (Wolffian ducts) and the paramesonephric ducts (mullerian ducts) (Fig. 19-1). Both pairs of ducts empty into an opening called the urogenital sinus.

UNDIFFERENTIATED

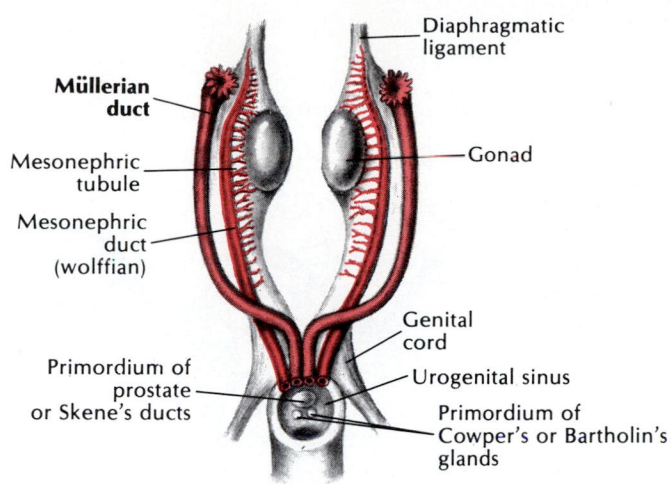

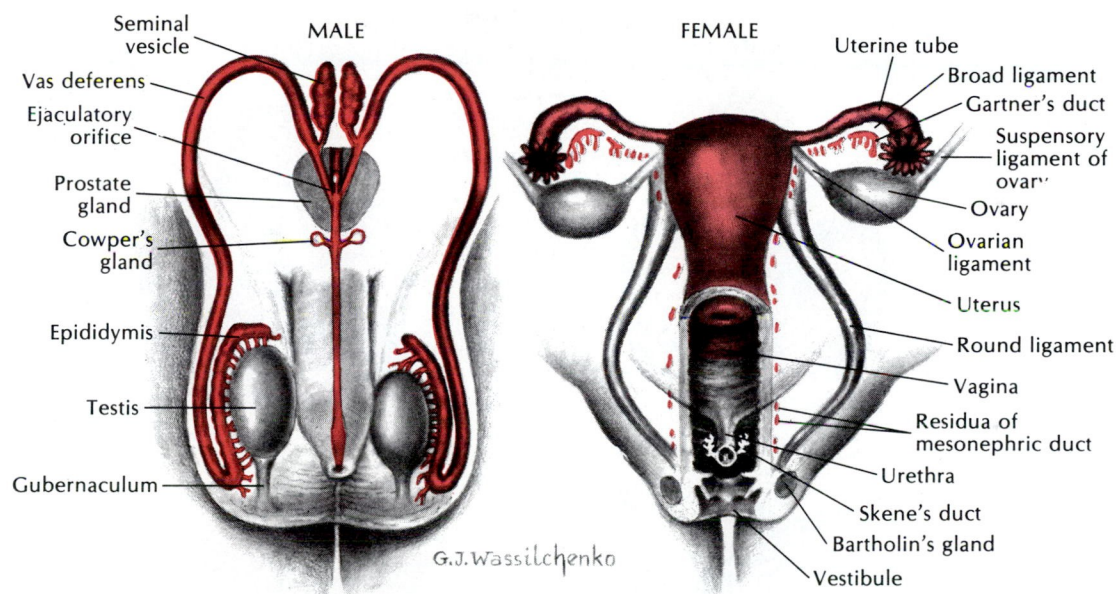

FIG. 19-1. Embryonic and fetal development of the internal genitalia. (From Bobak, Jensen, & Zular, 1989.)

At about 8 weeks' gestation, the gonads of genetically male embryos begin to produce testosterone. Under the influence of testosterone, the male gonads develop into the two testes, which produce sperm. The paramesonephric ducts degenerate, and the mesonephric ducts develop into the vas deferens, the two tubes that will carry sperm from the testes to the urethra.

In female embryos the gonads do not produce testosterone. Lack of testosterone causes the two female gonads to develop into ovaries, which will produce ova. In females the mesonephric ducts deteriorate, and the lower ends of the paramesonephric ducts join to become the uterus. The upper portions of the paramesonephric ducts develop into the fallopian (uterine) tubes. These two ducts will carry ova from the ovaries to the uterus.

Like the internal reproductive structures the external structures develop from homologous embryonic tissues. During the first 8 weeks of gestation both male and female embryos develop an elevated structure called the genital tubercle. Fig. 19-2 shows how the undifferentiated genital tubercle develops into the external reproductive organs of male or female. In male embryos testosterone causes the genital tubercle to form the male external genitalia. Absence of testosterone causes development of the external female genitalia. By 9 months' gestation the internal and external genital structures are all present, and the male gonads (the testes) have descended into the scrotum.

UNDIFFERENTIATED

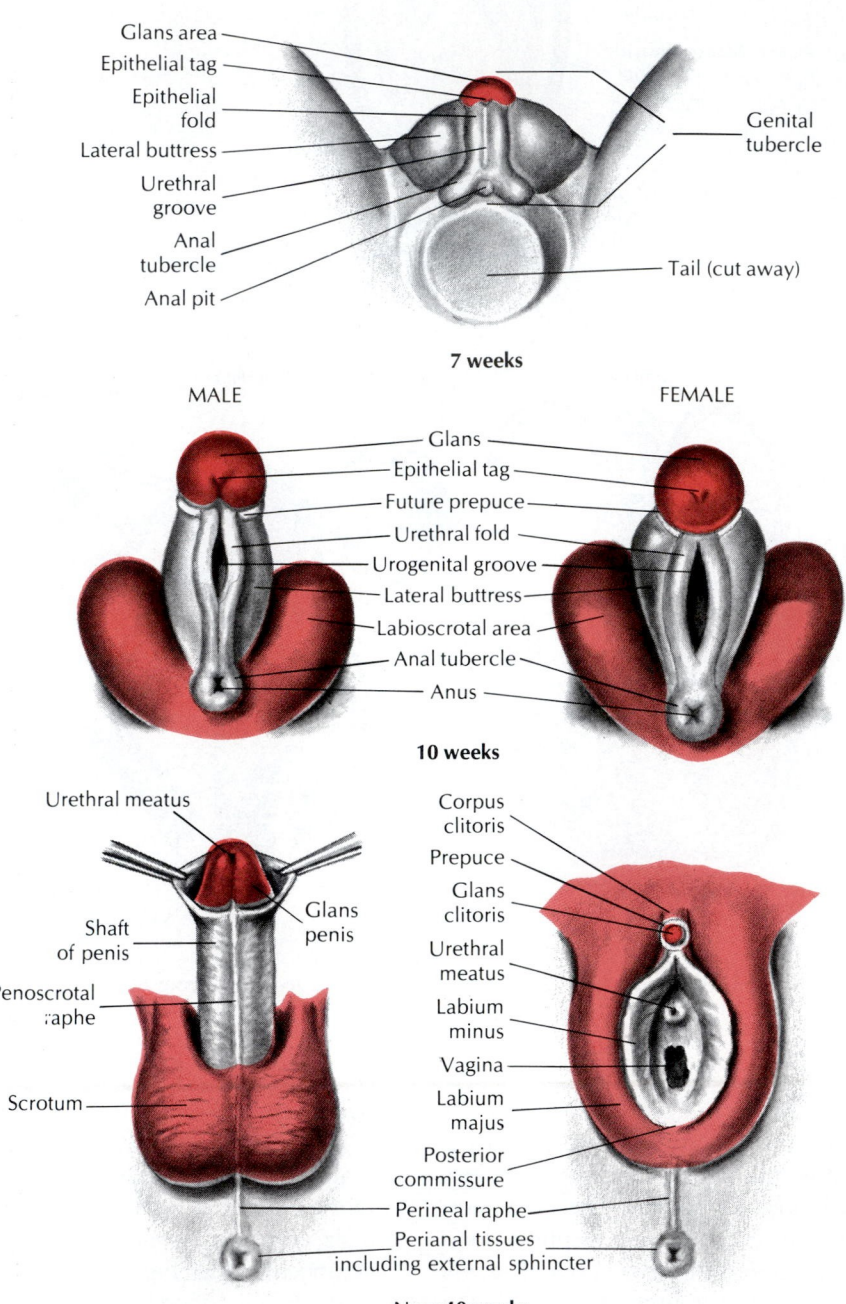

Glans area
Epithelial tag
Epithelial fold
Lateral buttress
Urethral groove
Anal tubercle
Anal pit

Genital tubercle

Tail (cut away)

7 weeks

MALE   FEMALE

Glans
Epithelial tag
Future prepuce
Urethral fold
Urogenital groove
Lateral buttress
Labioscrotal area
Anal tubercle
Anus

10 weeks

Urethral meatus

Glans penis

Shaft of penis

Penoscrotal raphe

Scrotum

Corpus clitoris
Prepuce
Glans clitoris
Urethral meatus
Labium minus
Vagina
Labium majus
Posterior commissure
Perineal raphe
Perianal tissues including external sphincter

Near 40 weeks

FIG. 19-2. Embryonic and fetal development of the external genitalia. (From Bobak, Jensen, & Zular, 1989.)

Puberty

From fetal life through childhood the testes secrete low levels of testosterone, and the ovaries secrete low levels of the primary female sex hormone, **estrogen.** Between the ages of 9 and 12 the gonads begin to produce more of the sex hormones. This triggers sexual maturation, or puberty. In girls puberty begins at about age 10. In boys it begins later, at about age 11. Puberty lasts 2 or 3 years and is complete when the individual is capable of reproduction. *Puberty* is not the same as adolescence. Puberty refers solely to sexual maturation; *adolescence* refers to all aspects of development that occur between the ages of 11 and 19.

Hormonal stimulation of the reproductive systems involves the central nervous systems, the endocrine system, and the gonads themselves. As can be seen in Fig. 19-3 specific structures involved are the hypothalamus, the anterior pituitary, and the gonads (ovaries and tes-

tes). At the time of puberty the hypothalamus of the brain begins to produce greater amounts of **gonadotropin-releasing hormone** (GnRH). Increased levels of GnRH stimulate the anterior pituitary to increase its production of the **gonadotropins: luteinizing hormone** (LH) and **follicle-stimulating hormone** (FSH). The gonadotropins then stimulate the gonads to produce more of the sex hormones. (The sex hormones are discussed in sections on the female and male systems.)

Increased sex hormone production causes the genitalia to grow into their adult proportions. It also stimulates the development of male and female secondary sex characteristics (beard, voice changes, breast development, and pubic and axillary hair). The most important hormonal effects occur in the gonads, however. In males the testes begin to produce mature sperm that are capable of fertilizing an ovum. Male puberty is complete with the first ejaculation that contains mature sperm. In

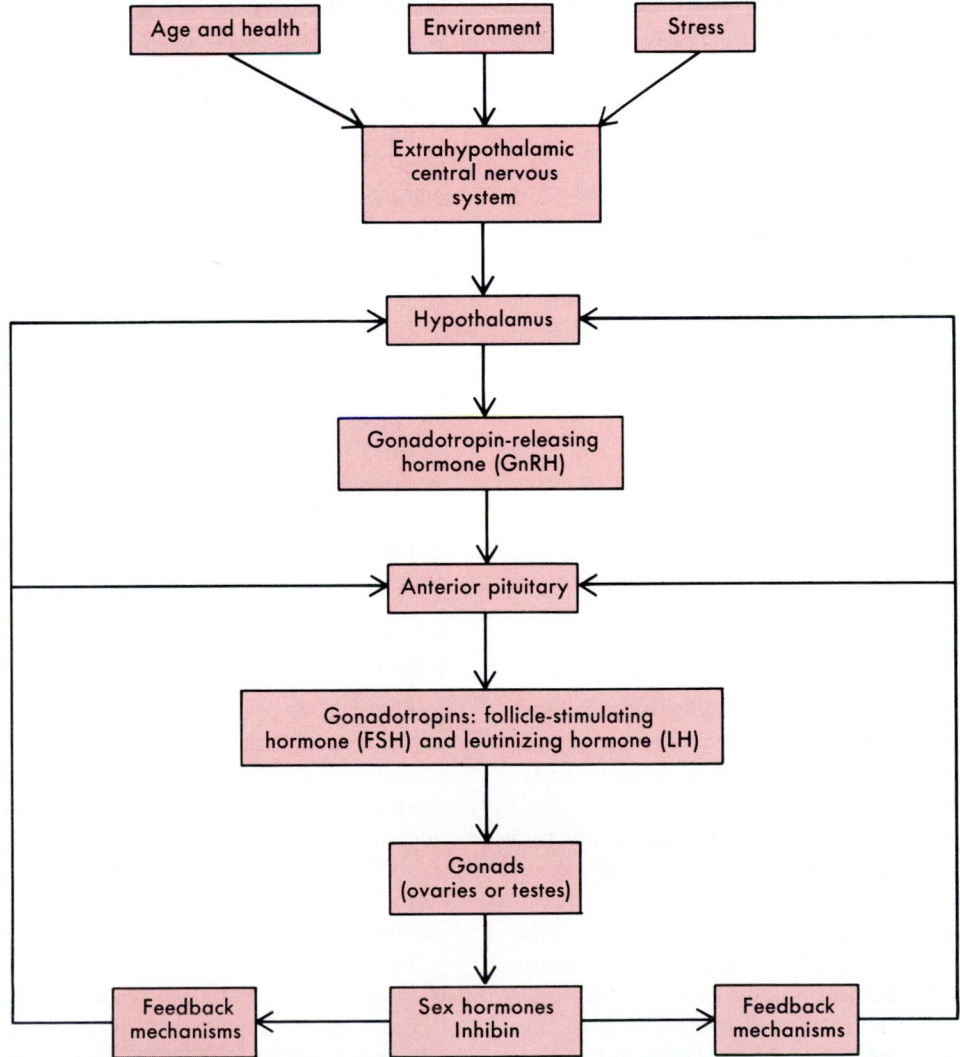

FIG. 19-3. Hormonal stimulation of the gonads: The hypothalamic-pituitary-gonadal axis.

Secondary Sex Characteristics That Develop at Puberty

Female	Male
Growth of long bones; widening of pelvis	Growth of long bones; widening of shoulders
Increase of subcutaneous fat, particularly at hips, thighs	Decrease of subcutaneous fat and increase of muscle mass
Growth of pubic and axillary hair	Growth of pubic and axillary hair
Activation of sebaceous and sweat glands in skin	Activation of sebaceous and sweat glands in skin
Some change of voice	Deepening of voice
Development of breasts	Growth of facial hair

---

females the ovaries begin to release mature ova. Female puberty is complete at the time of the first menstrual period.

THE FEMALE REPRODUCTIVE SYSTEM

In females the most important reproductive organs, or genitalia, are internal. They are the ovaries, fallopian tubes, uterus, and vagina. These organs are essential to reproduction. The external genitalia have accessory functions. They protect body openings and play an important role in sexual functioning.

External Genitalia

Fig. 19-4 shows the external female genitalia, which are known collectively as the **vulva,** or pudendum. The **mons pubis** (veneris) is a fatty layer of tissue over the pubic symphysis (joint of the pubic bones). During puberty the mons pubis becomes covered with pubic hair, and its sebaceous and sweat glands become more active. Estrogen causes fat to be deposited under the skin, giving the mons pubis a moundlike shape. This cushion of tissue protects the pubic symphysis during sexual intercourse.

The **labia majora** (singular, **labium majus**) are two folds of skin that arise at the mons pubis and extend back to the fourchette, forming a cleft. Like the mons pubis the labia majora undergo changes at puberty: the amount of fatty tissue increases, pubic hair grows on the lateral surfaces, and sebaceous glands on the hairless medial surfaces begin to secrete lubricants. The labia majora protect the inner structures of the vulva and are homologous to the male scrotum (Fig. 19-1).

Within the labia majora lie two smaller, thinner folds of skin, the **labia minora** (singular, **labium minus**). The labia minora are hairless, pink, and moist and are well supplied with nerves, blood vessels, and sebaceous glands. These glands secrete lubricating fluid having a distinct odor. During sexual arousal the labia minora become swollen with blood.

The **clitoris** is a richly innervated, erectile organ that lies anterior to the labia minora. It is a small, cylindrical structure having a glans that is visible and a shaft that lies beneath the skin (Fig. 19-4). The clitoris is homologous to the male penis. Like the penis the clitoris is a major site of sexual stimulation and orgasm. With sexual arousal erectile tissues in the clitoris fill with blood, causing it to enlarge somewhat.

The area protected by the labia minora is called the **vestibule.** The vestibule contains the external opening of the vagina, which is called the **introitus** or vaginal orifice. The introitus may be covered by a thin, perforated membrane called the hymen. The vestibule also contains the opening of the urethra, or **urinary meatus** (orifice). These structures are lubricated by two pairs of glands: Skene glands and Bartholin glands. The ducts of **Skene glands** (also called the lesser vestibular or paraurethral glands) open on both sides of the urinary meatus. The ducts of **Bartholin glands** (greater vestibular glands; vulvovaginal glands) open on either side of the introitus. In response to sexual stimulation Bartholin glands secrete mucus that lubricates the inner labial surfaces. Skene glands help to lubricate the urinary meatus.

The vulva is a common site of infection, particularly sexually transmitted infection. Its moist, warm surfaces provide an ideal growth medium for microorganisms of all kinds, which may ascend to internal structures through the urethra, vagina, or glandular ducts. Pubic lice may infest the hair of the mons pubis and labia majora, and the entire perineal area is susceptible to skin irritation and dermatologic disorders. (Skin disorders are described in Chapter 41.)

Internal Genitalia
Vagina

The **vagina** is an elastic, fibromuscular canal, 9 to 10 cm in length, that extends up and back from the introitus to the lower portion of the uterus. As Fig. 19-5 shows, it lies between the urethra (and part of the bladder) and the rectum. Mucosal secretions from the upper genital organs, menstrual fluids, and products of conception leave the body through the vagina, which also receives the penis during coitus.

The vaginal wall is composed of four layers. Its lining is a mucous membrane of squamous epithelial cells. (Types of epithelium are described and illustrated in Chapter 1, Table 1-3.) This layer thickens and thins in response to hormones, particularly estrogen. The

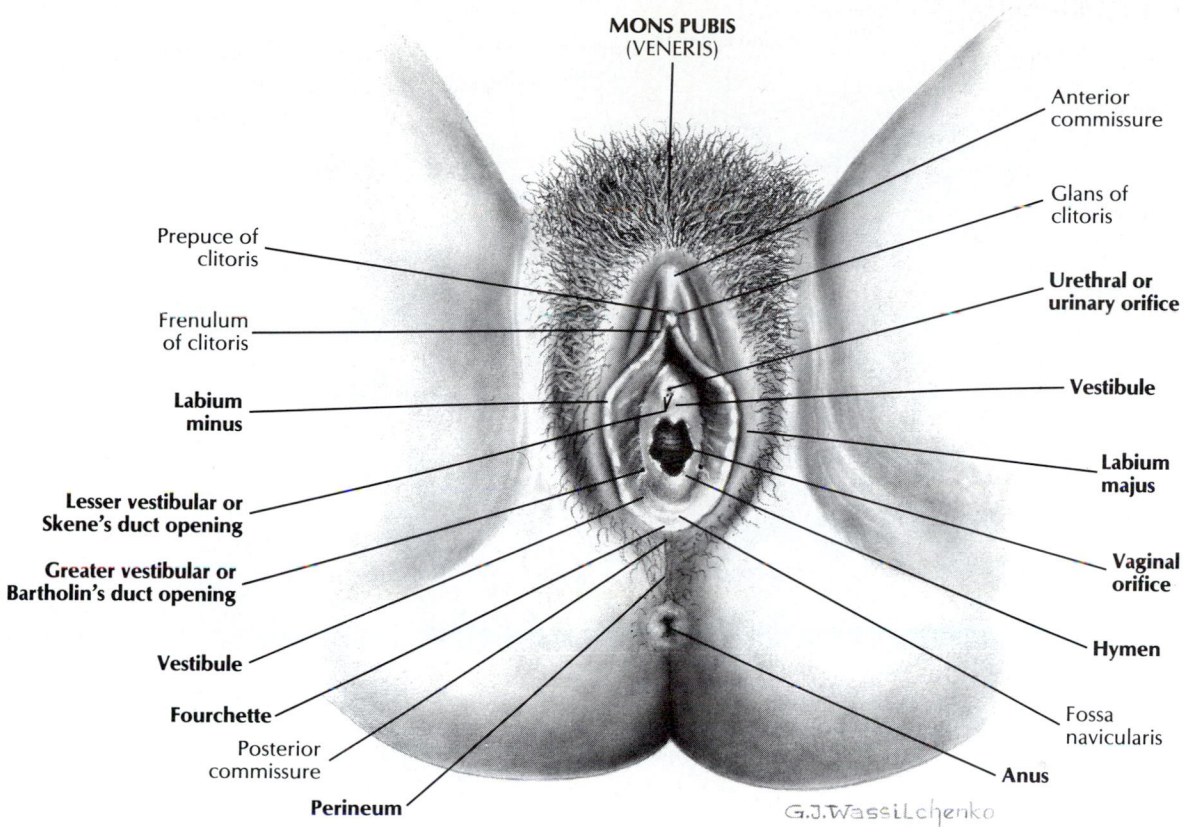

FIG. 19-4. External female genitalia. (From Bobak, Jensen, & Zular, 1989.)

squamous epithelial membrane is continuous with the membrane that covers the lower part of the uterus. In women of reproductive age the mucosal layer is arranged in transverse wrinkles, or folds, called **rugae** (singular, **ruga**). The rugae permit the mucosal layer to stretch during coitus and childbirth. The second layer consists of fibrous connective tissue containing numerous blood and lymphatic vessels. Smooth muscle comprises the third layer. The outermost layer consists of connective tissue and a rich network of blood vessels.

The upper part of the vagina surrounds the cervix, the lower end of the uterus (Fig. 19-5). The pouchlike space around the cervix is called the **fornix** of the vagina. The posterior fornix is "deeper" than the anterior fornix because of the angle at which the cervix meets the vaginal canal. In most women this angle is about 90 degrees.

Its elasticity and relatively sparse nerve supply enhance the vagina's function as the birth canal. During sexual arousal the vaginal wall becomes engorged with blood, like the labia minora and clitoris. Engorgement pushes some fluid to the surface of the mucosa, enhancing lubrication. The vaginal wall does not contain mucus-secreting glands; rather, secretions drain into the vagina from the uterus or enter from the vestibule.

Two factors help to defend the vagina from infection,

particularly during the reproductive years. They are (1) an acid-base balance that discourages the proliferation of most pathogenic bacteria and (2) thickness of the vaginal epithelium. Before puberty vaginal pH is about 7.0 (neutral), and the vaginal epithelium is thin. At puberty the pH becomes more acidic (4.0 to 5.0), and the squamous epithelial lining thickens. These changes are maintained until menopause (cessation of menstruation), at which time the pH rises again to more alkaline levels, and the epithelium thins out. Therefore, protection from infection is greatest during the years when a woman is most likely to be sexually active. Between puberty and menopause, vulnerability to infection varies somewhat with cyclical changes in pH and epithelial thickness. Both defenses are greatest when estrogen levels are high and the vagina contains a normal population of *Lactobacillus acidophilus,* a harmless resident bacterium that helps to maintain pH at acidic levels. Any condition that causes vaginal pH to rise, such as low estrogen levels or destruction of *L. acidophilus* by antibiotics, lowers vaginal defenses against infection.

Uterus

The **uterus** is a hollow, pear-shaped organ whose lower end opens into the vagina. The functions of the uterus are to anchor and protect a fertilized ovum, pro-

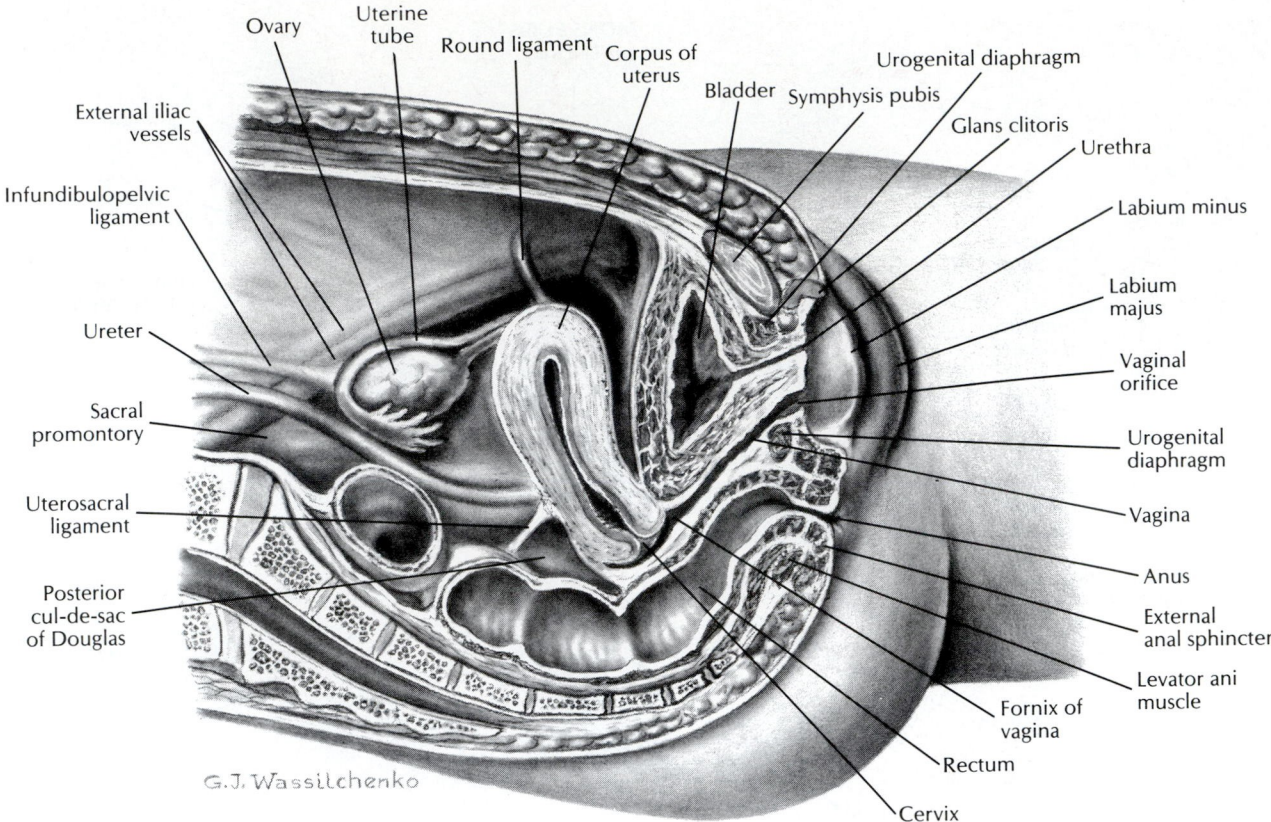

External iliac vessels

Infundibulopelvic ligament

Ureter

Sacral promontory

Uterosacral ligament

Posterior cul-de-sac of Douglas

Ovary

Uterine tube

Round ligament

Corpus of uterus

Bladder

Symphysis pubis

Urogenital diaphragm

Glans clitoris

Urethra

Labium minus

Labium majus

Vaginal orifice

Urogenital diaphragm

Vagina

Anus

External anal sphincter

Levator ani muscle

Fornix of vagina

Rectum

Cervix

G.J. Wassilchenko

FIG. 19-5. Internal female genitalia and other pelvic organs; midsagittal view, with woman lying supine. (From Bobak, Jensen, & Zular, 1989.)

vide an optimal environment while it develops, and push the fetus out at birth.

At puberty the uterus attains its adult size and proportions and descends from the abdomen to the lower pelvis, between the bladder and the rectum (Fig. 19-5). The uterus of a mature, nonpregnant female is approximately 9 cm long and 6.5 cm wide, with muscular walls 3.5 cm thick. It is held loosely in position by ligaments, peritoneal tissue folds, and pressure of adjacent organs, especially the urinary bladder, sigmoid colon, and rectum. In most women the uterus is anteverted: that is, it is tipped forward so that it rests on the urinary bladder. But it may be retroverted, or tipped backward. Various degrees of retroversion are normal (Fig. 19-6).

Fig. 19-7 shows a cross section of the uterus. The uterus has two major parts: the body, or **corpus,** and the cervix. The top of the corpus, above the insertion of the fallopian tubes, is called the **fundus.** The diameter of the uterine cavity is widest at the fundus and narrowest at the **isthmus,** which is the narrowed part of the corpus just above the cervix. The **cervix,** or "neck of the uterus," extends from the isthmus to the vagina. The passageway between the cervix's upper opening (the internal os) and its lower opening (the external os) is

called the **endocervical canal.** The entire uterus, like the upper vagina, is innervated exclusively by motor and sensory fibers of the autonomic nervous system.

The uterine wall is composed of three layers: the perimetrium, the myometrium, and the endometrium (Fig. 19-7). The **perimetrium,** or parietal peritoneum, is the outer serous membrane that covers the uterus. The **myometrium** is the thick, muscular middle layer. The myometrium is thickest at the fundus, apparently to facilitate birth. The **endometrium,** or uterine lining, is composed of a functional layer (superficial compact layer and spongy middle layer) and a basal layer. The functional layer of the endometrium is responsive to sex hormones. Between puberty and menopause this layer proliferates and sloughs off monthly. The basal layer, which is attached to the myometrium, regenerates the functional layer after the sloughing off (menstruation).

The endocervical canal does not have an endometrial layer. Rather, it is lined with columnar epithelial cells (Chapter 1, Table 1-3). The endocervical lining is continuous with that of the outer cervix and vagina, but it is not made up of the same type of epithelial cells. The point at which the columnar epithelium of the cervix meets the squamous epithelium of the vagina is called

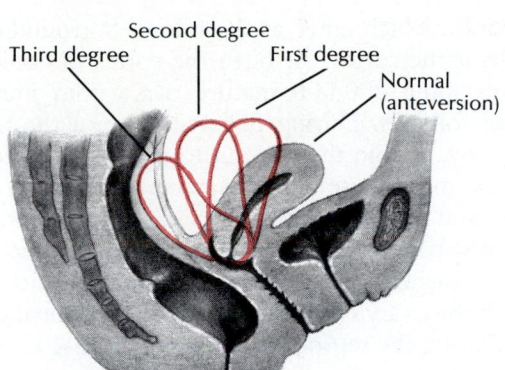

FIG. 19-6. The three degrees of uterine retroversion. (From Bobak, Jensen, & Zular, 1989.)

the transformation zone, or the **squamous-columnar junction** (Fig. 19-7). The transformation zone is the usual site of cervical carcinoma in situ.

The cervix acts as a mechanical barrier to infectious microorganisms that may be present in the vagina. The external cervical os is a very small opening that contains thick, sticky mucus (the mucous "plug") during most of the menstrual cycle and all of pregnancy. In addition the downward flow of cervical secretions moves microor-

ganisms away from the cervix and uterus. In women of reproductive age the pH of these secretions is inhospitable to most bacteria. Furthermore, mucosal secretions contain enzymes and antibodies (mostly immunoglobulin A) of the secretory immune system. (The secretory immune system is discussed in Chapter 6.) These defenses do not always prevent infection, even if they are intact. Besides infection, uterine pathophysiology includes displacement of the uterus within the pelvis, benign growths of the uterine wall, and cancer.

Fallopian Tubes

The two **fallopian tubes** (oviducts, uterine tubes) enter the uterus bilaterally just beneath the fundus (Fig. 19-7). Their function is to conduct the ova from the spaces around the ovaries to the uterus. From the uterus the fallopian tubes curve up and over the two ovaries. Each tube is 8 to 12 cm long and about 1 cm in diameter, except at its ovarian end, which flares out like the bell of a trumpet. This widened end, called the **infundibulum,** is fringed or fimbriated. The **fimbriae** (fringes) move, creating a current that draws the ovum into the infundibulum. Once it has entered the fallopian tube cilia and peristalsis (muscle contractions) keep the ovum moving toward the uterus.

The ampulla of the fallopian tube is the usual site of

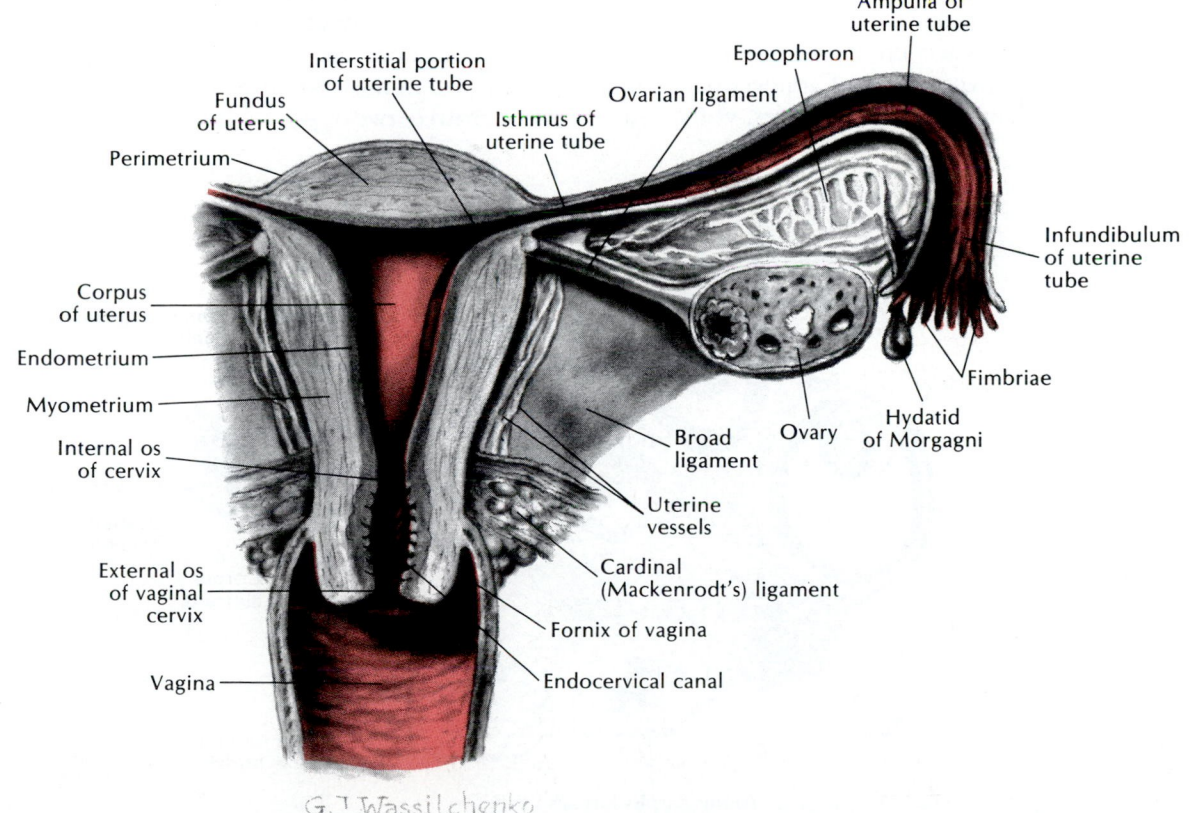

FIG. 19-7. Cross section of uterus, fallopian tube, and ovary. (From Bobak, Jensen, & Zular, 1989.)

fertilization (Fig. 19-7). Sperm released into the vagina travel upward through the endocervical canal and uterine cavity and enter the fallopian tubes. If an ovum is present in either tube fertilization can occur. Whether or not it encounters sperm, the ovum continues to travel through the fallopian tube to the uterus. If fertilized the ovum (now called a blastocyst) implants itself in the endometrial layer of the uterine wall. If not fertilized the ovum breaks down and leaves the uterus with menstrual fluids.

Disorders that affect the fallopian tubes can block the path of both sperm and ovum and cause infertility. Such disorders include congenital malformations, infection, and inflammation.

Ovaries

The **ovaries,** the female gonads, are the primary female reproductive organs. They have two main functions: secretion of female sex hormones and development and release of female gametes, or ova.

The almond-shaped ovaries are located on both sides of the uterus and are suspended and supported by the mesovarian portions of the broad ligament, ovarian ligaments, and suspensory ligaments (Fig. 19-7). The ovaries are smaller than their male homologues, the testes. In women of reproductive age each ovary is 3 to 5 cm long, 2.5 cm wide, and 2 cm thick and weighs 4 to 8. Size and weight vary somewhat from phase to phase of the menstrual cycle (see p. 657).

Fig. 19-8 shows a cross section of an ovary. The central part, or medulla, is composed of connective tissue and contains a large number of small arteries, veins, and

lymphatics, which enter at the hilum. Surrounding the medulla is the cortex. At birth the cortex of each ovary contains some 200,000 mature ova within immature **ovarian follicles.** During puberty some of the follicles and the ova within them begin to mature. Between puberty and menopause the ovarian cortex always contains follicles and ova in various stages of development. Once every menstrual cycle (about every 28 days) one of the follicles reaches maturation and discharges its ovum through the ovary's outer covering, the germinal epithelium. During the reproductive years 300 to 400 ovarian follicles mature completely and release an ovum, an event termed **ovulation.** The rest either fail to develop at all or degenerate without maturing completely.

Having ejected a mature ovum, the follicle develops into another structure, the **corpus luteum** (Fig. 19-8). The immediate fate of the corpus luteum depends on whether or not the ejected ovum is fertilized. If fertilization occurs the corpus luteum enlarges and begins to secrete hormones that maintain and support pregnancy. If fertilization does not occur the corpus luteum secretes these hormones for a few days and then degenerates while another follicle matures and releases its ovum. The **ovarian cycle**—the process of follicular maturation, ovulation, corpus luteum development, and corpus luteum degeneration—is continuous from puberty to menopause, except during pregnancy. At menopause this process ceases, and the ovaries may shrink to the point that they cannot be felt upon palpation.

Sex hormones are secreted by four types of cells present within the ovarian cortex: cells of the stroma, or tissue matrix; two types of cells in the ovarian follicle,

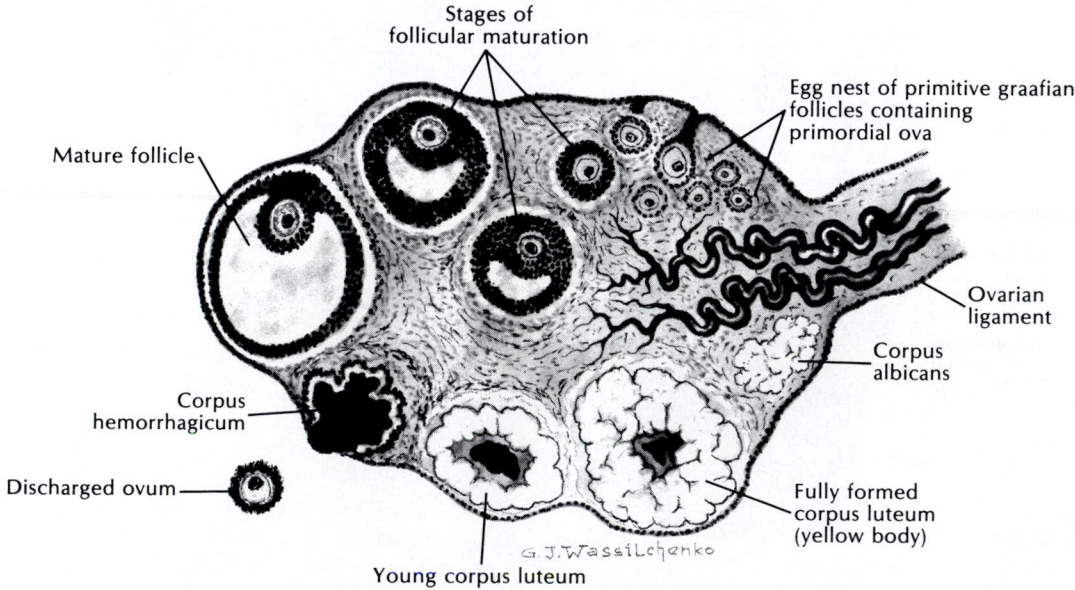

FIG. 19-8. Cross section of ovary during reproductive years. (From Bobak, Jensen, & Zular, 1989.)

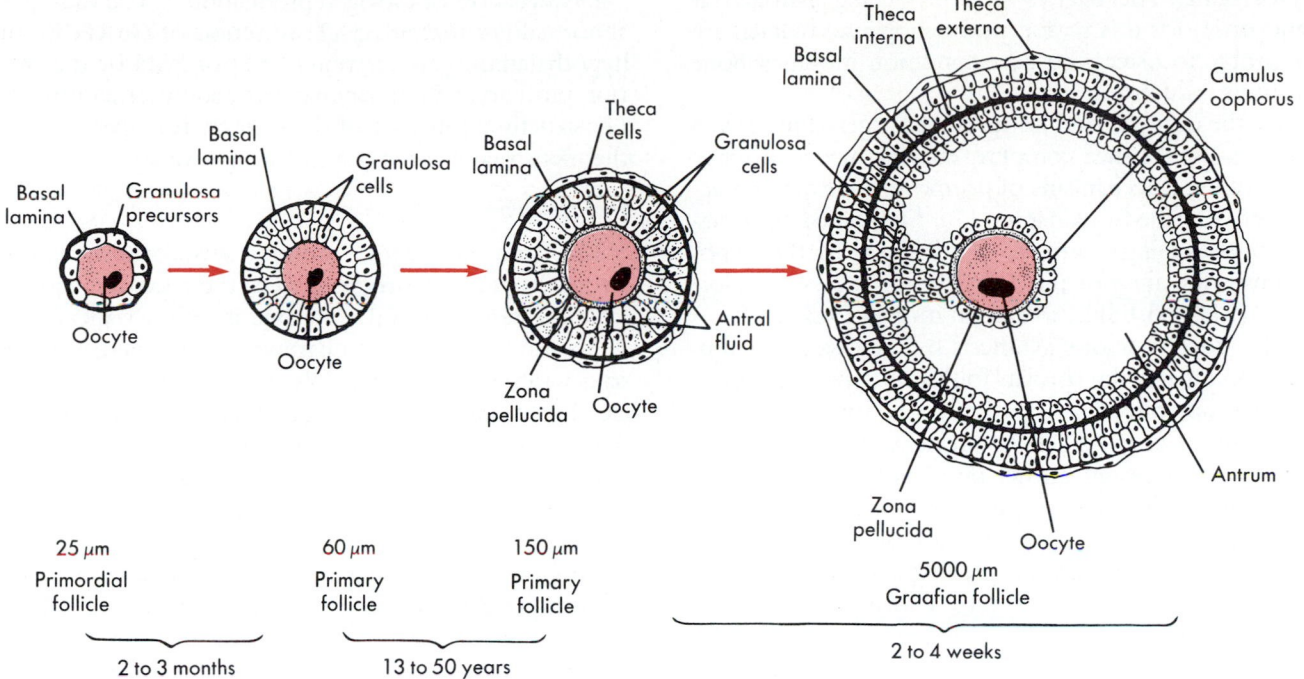

FIG. 19-9. The development of an ovarian follicle (not to scale). The Graafian follicle has more layers of granulosa and theca cells than shown here. (From Berne & Levy, 1988.)

granulosa cells and **theca cells;** and cells of the corpus luteum (Fig. 19-9). These cells all contain receptors for the gonadotropins (LH and FSH) or for the sex hormones, which are discussed in the next section.

Because ovarian function is regulated by hormones any disorder that disrupts hormone secretion or reception by target cells can cause ovarian dysfunction and infertility. Ovarian pathology can also be caused by benign or malignant growths, cysts, infection, or inflammation.

Female Sex Hormones

The sex hormones are all steroid hormones: that is, they are synthesized from cholesterol (Chapter 17). Most of the sex hormones, both male and female, are present in adults of both sexes all the time. The female body contains low levels of testosterone, for example, and the male body contains low levels of estrogen. The effects of the sex hormones depend on their amount and concentration in the blood.

Steroid hormones produced by the ovaries maintain female characteristics throughout life. During fetal development, infancy, and childhood, sex hormone production is low. At puberty hormone production surges, causing sexual maturation and development of secondary sex characteristics. From puberty to menopause the sex hormones control the ovarian-menstrual cycle, pregnancy, and lactation. The dominant female sex hormones are estrogen and progesterone. These two hormones are not produced steadily. Rather their production surges and diminishes monthly, creating the ovarian-menstrual cycle. The androgens, which are actually male sex hormones, also have important functions in females. The female body normally produces small amounts of androgens and other male sex hormones.

Estrogens

Estrogen is a generic term for any of three similar hormones: estradiol, estrone, and estriol. **Estradiol** is the most potent and plentiful of the three. The main site of estrogen production is the ovaries (ovarian follicle and corpus luteum), but limited amounts of estrogen are secreted by the cortices of the adrenal glands and the placenta during pregnancy. Androgens are converted to estrogen in peripheral adipose tissue; this process is the major source of estrogen in postmenopausal women and in men.

Estrogen has numerous biological effects, many of which involve interactions with other hormones. Estrogen is needed for maturation of reproductive organs, development of secondary sex characteristics, closure of long bones after the pubertal growth spurt, regulation of the ovarian-menstrual cycle, endometrial regeneration following menstruation, endometrial maintenance during pregnancy, and lactation. Estrogen also has metabolic effects on the bones, liver, blood vessels, blood, central nervous system, kidneys, and skin. During the reproductive years estrogen helps to maintain the density of bone. The ovaries stop producing estrogen at menopause; for this reason postmenopausal women are susceptible to osteoporosis, a condition in which bone density is reduced.

Like the other steroid hormones estrogens are derived from cholesterol in a complex, enzyme-mediated series of reactions. (Mechanisms of hormone synthesis and action are described in Chapter 17.) Stimulated by gonadotropin-releasing hormone (GnRH) from the hypothalamus, the anterior pituitary gland secretes gonadotropins (LH and FSH), as shown in Fig. 19-3.

LH induces estradiol synthesis by the corpus luteum. It also stimulates the ovarian follicle to synthesize estradiol, but not directly. Apparently LH stimulates theca cells of the ovarian follicle to produce androgens. (Androgens are discussed further on p. 666 and in the section on male reproductive function.) Some of these androgens are converted to estradiol by the theca cells themselves; others diffuse into the granulosa cells, where they are converted (aromatozed) to estradiol (Droegemueller et al., 1987). Conversion within the granulosa cells is made possible by FSH (Fig. 19-10).

Disturbances of estrogen production can be caused by abnormalities that affect (1) secretion of GnRH by the hypothalamus, (2) secretion of LH or FSH by the anterior pituitary, (3) hormonal feedback mechanisms, or (4) structural integrity of the ovaries. Estrogen's role in the menstrual cycle is described on p. 659.

Progesterone

LH from the anterior pituitary stimulates the corpus luteum to secrete **progesterone,** the second major female sex hormone. Progesterone is an early product in the enzymatic conversion pathway of estrogen. With estrogen progesterone controls the ovarian-menstrual cycle. Large amounts of progesterone are secreted while the corpus luteum is active, for about 9 days after ovulation. Small amounts of progesterone are secreted by the adrenal cortices. Adrenal secretion is not cyclical, however.

Progesterone secreted by the corpus luteum stimulates the thickened endometrium to become more complex in preparation for implantation of a blastocyte. If conception and implantation do occur the corpus lu-

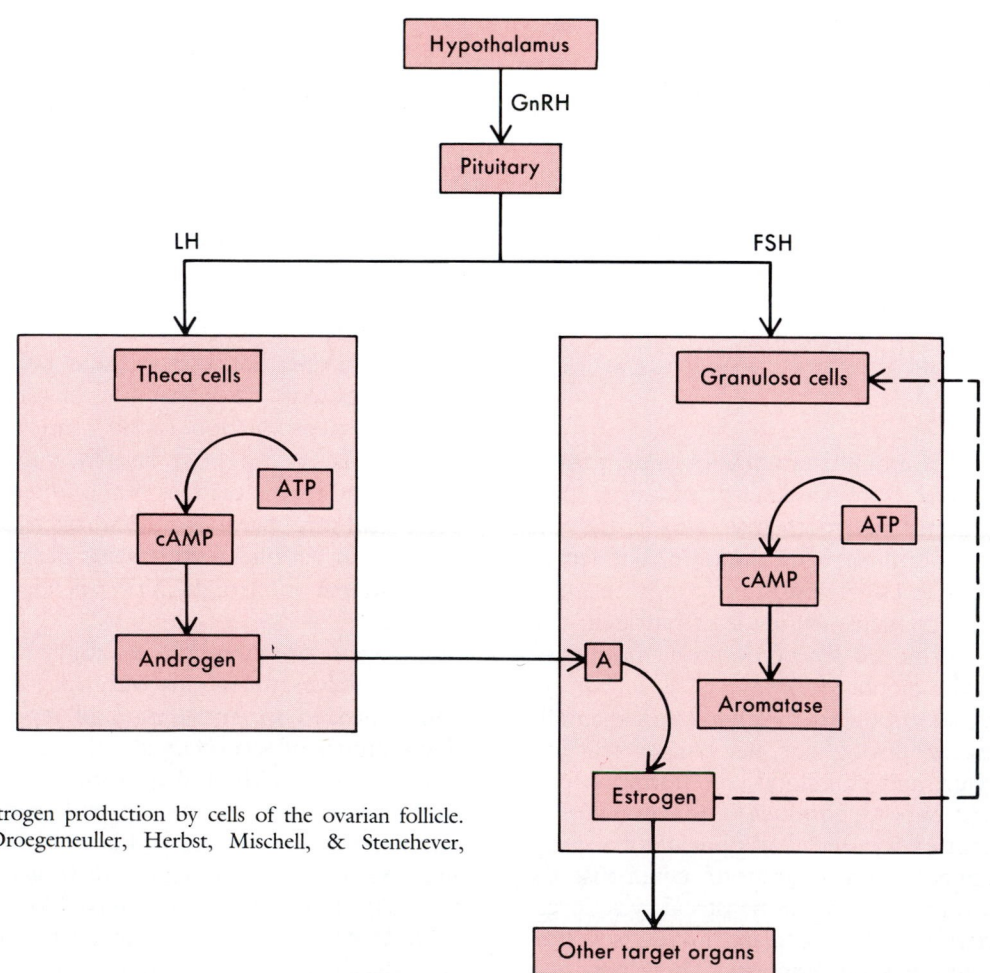

FIG. 19-10. Estrogen production by cells of the ovarian follicle. (Adapted from Droegemueller, Herbst, Mischell, & Stenehever, 1987.)

TABLE 19-1 Complementary and opposing effects of estrogen and progesterone

Structure	Effect of estrogen	Effect of progesterone
Vaginal mucosa	Proliferation of squamous epithelium; increase in glycogen content of cells; layering (cornification) of cells	Thinning of squamous epithelium; decornification
Cervical mucosa	Production of abundant fluid secretions that favor survival and enhance motility of sperm	Production of thick, sticky secretions that tend to "plug" the cervical os
Smooth muscle of uterus and fallopian tubes	Increased motility and ciliary action	Decreased motility and ciliary action; relaxes myometrium
Endometrium	Stimulation of growth; increase in number of receptors for progesterone	Activation of glands and blood vessels; accumulation of glucogen and enzymes
Breasts	Promotion of effects of prolactin (hormone that stimulates milk production)	Inhibition of effects of prolactin

teum persists and secretes progesterone (and estrogen) throughout pregnancy.

Progesterone is sometimes called "the hormone of pregnancy." During pregnancy it is produced not only by the corpus luteum but also by the placenta. Its effects in pregnancy include (1) maintenance of the thickened endometrium; (2) relaxation of smooth muscle in the myometrium, which prevents premature contractions and helps the uterus to expand; (3) thickening of the myometrium, which prepares it for the muscular work of labor; and (4) prevention of lactation until the fetus is born. Progesterone and estrogen have some opposing and complementary effects, which are summarized in Table 19-1.

Androgens

Although **androgens** are primarily male sex hormones, small amounts of them are produced in the ovaries and adrenal cortices of females. Some androgens are precursors of female sex hormones, notably estrogen and androstenedione. At puberty androgens contribute to the skeletal growth spurt and cause growth of pubic and axillary hair. The androgens also activate sebaceous glands, accounting for some cases of acne during puberty.

The Menstrual Cycle

Besides pregnancy the obvious manifestation of female reproductive functioning is menstrual bleeding (the menses), which starts with the **menarche** (first menstruation) and ends with **menopause.** In the United States the average age of first menstruation is 12.5 years, with a range from 9 to 17 years. Menarche appears to be related to body weight, especially percentage of body fat (ratio of fat to lean tissue), which may trigger a change in the metabolic rate and lead to hormonal changes associated with ovulation. At first cycles may vary in length from 10 to 60 days. As adolescence proceeds regular patterns of menstruation and ovulation are established. The average menstrual cycle takes 28.3 days, with a range from 26 to 34 days. During adulthood the cycles of most women gradually become shorter. The mean cycle for women of 40 is 27 days. Then about 3 years before menopause the mean cycle lengthens to 33 days (Droegemueller et al., 1987).

Phases of the Menstrual Cycle

The menstrual cycle consists of three phases of one event. The event is ovulation: the release of an ovum from a mature ovarian follicle. The three phases are the follicular/proliferative phase, the luteal/secretory phase, and menstruation (Fig. 19-11).

During **menstruation** the functional layer of the endometrium disintegrates and is discharged through the vagina. Menstruation is followed by the **follicular/proliferative phase.** This phase is named for two simultaneous processes: maturation of an ovarian follicle and proliferation of the endometrium (Fig. 19-7). During the follicular/proliferative phase the anterior pituitary gland secretes FSH, which causes an ovarian follicle to develop. While the follicle is developing, its granulosa cells secrete estrogen, and the estrogen causes cells of the endometrium to proliferate. By the time the ovarian follicle is mature the endometrial lining is restored. At this point ovulation occurs.

Ovulation marks the beginning of the **luteal/secretory phase** of the menstrual cycle. The ovarian follicle begins its transformation into a corpus luteum (Fig. 19-8), hence the name *luteal phase.* LH from the anterior pituitary stimulates the corpus luteum to secrete progesterone, which, in turn, initiates the secretory phase of endometrial development. Glands and

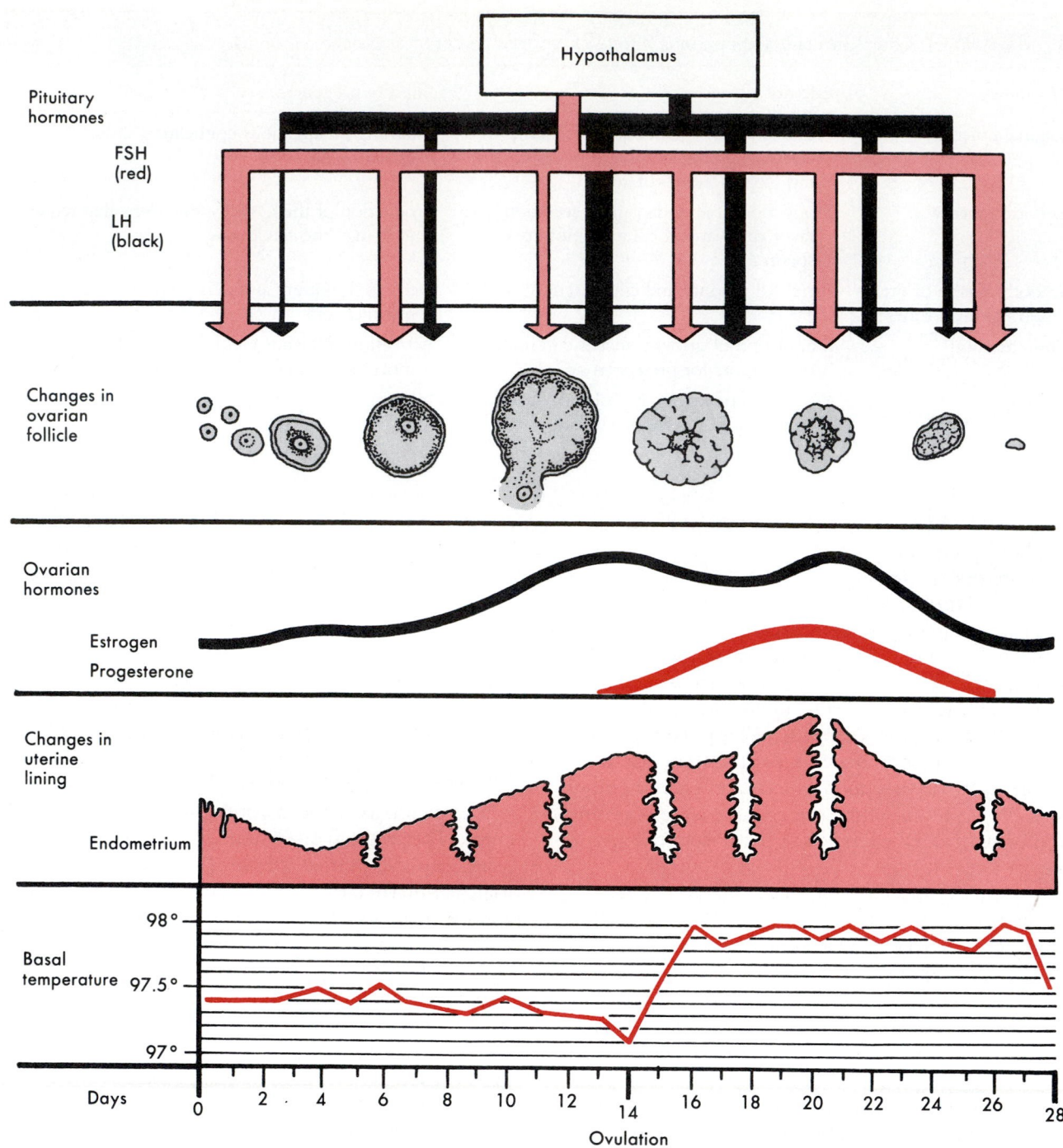

FIG. 19-11. The menstrual cycle. (Adapted from Bobak, Jensen, & Zular, 1989.)

blood vessels in the endometrium branch and curl throughout the functional layer, and the glands begin to secrete a thin, glycogen-containing fluid, hence the name *secretory phase*. If conception should occur, the nutrient-laden endometrium is ready for implantation. If conception and implantation do not occur the corpus luteum degenerates and ceases its production of progesterone and estrogen (which it has been producing in lesser amounts). Without progesterone or estrogen to maintain it the endometrium enters the ischemic ("blood-starved") phase and disintegrates. Then menstruation occurs, marking the beginning of another cycle.

Ovarian cycles appear to have a minimum length of 25 to 26 days: the ovarian follicle requires 12.5 days to develop, and the luteal phase appears fixed at 14 days. Menstrual blood flow lasts from 3 to 5 days, with approximately 2 ounces of blood lost each cycle. Environ-

TABLE 19-2 Hormonal feedback mechanisms in the menstrual cycle

Phase of cycle and ovarian hormone levels	Feedback to hypothalamus and anterior pituitary	Resultant GnRH, FSH, and LH levels	Ovarian and menstrual events
Early follicular phase: estrogen levels low; no progesterone secreted	Negative and inhibitory	All low	Ovarian follicle develops; endometrium proliferates
Late follicular phase: estrogen levels high; no progesterone secreted	Positive and stimulatory	All surge; LH dominates	Process of ovulation begins; endometrial proliferation complete
Ovulatory phase: estrogen levels dip; progesterone levels begin to rise	Negative and inhibitory	All fall sharply	Corpus luteum begins to develop; endometrium enters secretory phase
Early luteal phase: estrogen and progesterone levels high; progesterone dominates	Negative and inhibitory	All continue to decline, but gradually	Corpus luteum fully developed; endometrium ready for implantation
Late luteal phase: estrogen and progesterone levels fall sharply	Negative and inhibitory; feedback lessens slightly	All rise slightly	Corpus luteum regresses; endometrium breaks down; menstruation begins
Menstrual phase: estrogen levels low; no progesterone secreted	Negative and inhibitory	All low	More ovarian follicles begin to develop; functional layer of endometrium is shed

mental factors (e.g., severe emotional stress, illness, malnutrition, and seasonal variation) may affect the length of the menstrual cycle.

Hormonal Controls

Hormonal control of the menstrual cycle depends upon complex interactions among the hypothalamus, the anterior pituitary, and the ovaries. Gonadotropin-releasing hormone (GnRH) is secreted by the hypothalamus into the hypophyseal portal system and travels to the anterior pituitary, where it stimulates the secretion of LH and FSH. FSH and LH are released from the anterior pituitary in pulses that correspond to the secretion of GnRH.

Blood levels of estrogen and progesterone exert a feedback effect on the anterior pituitary, thereby determining how much FSH and LH is secreted (Table 19-2). FSH and LH secretion are not completely parallel: that is, FSH and LH are not secreted simultaneously in equal amounts throughout the menstrual cycle. Nonparallel secretion is due to cyclic changes in feedback mechanisms. During the early follicular phase low levels of estrogen inhibit the FSH-secreting cells of the anterior pituitary. In addition the developing ovarian follicle secretes **inhibin,** a protein hormone that inhibits both GnRH and FSH secretion. As the ovarian follicle grows it produces more and more estrogen. In the late follicular phase estrogen levels begin to rise, stimulating a

surge of FSH and LH secretion from the anterior pituitary. The midcycle surge of LH causes ovulation. Rising estrogen and progesterone levels during the luteal phase may have some inhibitory effect on the anterior pituitary, thereby inhibiting LH and FSH secretion. Just before the onset of menstruation FSH and LH levels begin to increase slightly, probably because of declining estrogen and progesterone levels.

Ovarian Cycle

To grow and mature ovarian follicles require FSH, LH, and estradiol. At the end of a cycle in which pregnancy does not occur FSH and LH levels increase slightly (Fig. 19-11). At this time or 5 or 6 ovarian follicles begin to mature. It is not understood why these particular follicles respond to the increase in FSH and LH. As the follicles mature granulosa cells multiply, increasing the secretion of estradiol. At this time one follicle becomes dominant, and the others atrophy. It is not clear why one follicle becomes dominant, but it may be because this follicle has more FSH receptors, or better blood supply, or greater ability to convert androgens to estradiol. The dominant follicle begins to secrete progressively larger amounts of estradiol, which exerts a positive-feedback effect, causing the LH surge. Ovulation generally occurs an average of 16 hours after the LH surge, with a range of 8 to 40 hours. Mechanisms controlling follicular rupture and release of the ovum may include contraction of smooth muscle cells of the follicle, forcing the ovum out; the actions of proteolytic enzymes; or the actions of prostaglandins, especially prostaglandin $F_2\alpha$ (Hadley, 1984).

The LH surge also transforms the granulosa cells of the ovulatory follicle into the corpus luteum. The corpus luteum secretes both estrogen and progesterone in amounts that depend, in part, on adequate development of the follicle before ovulation. If pregnancy does not occur the corpus luteum persists for 14 days, then regresses and eventually disappears.

Uterine Phases

Uterine phases of the menstrual cycle—the proliferative phase, the secretory phase, and menstruation—involve the cyclic changes that occur in the endometrium. During the midfollicular phase increasing levels of estrogen contribute to endometrial repair and proliferation, thus increasing endometrial thickness. Once ovulation occurs and serum progesterone levels rise the endometrial tissue develops secretory characteristics. If implantation of a fertilized ovum does not take place endometrial tissue begins to break down approximately 11 days after ovulation. The period of breakdown is sometimes called the ischemic phase (Fig. 19-11). Sloughing of tissue (menstrual bleeding) begins about 14 days after ovulation.

Cervical mucus also undergoes cyclic changes. During the proliferative phase the cervical mucus is thin and watery. With the preovulatory surge of LH and estradiol the mucus becomes thicker and more elastic. Increasing progesterone levels apparently contribute to the development of tiny channels in the mucus of the cervical os, providing access for sperm. Changes in the consistency of cervical mucus can be used to identify fertile intervals.

Vaginal Response

The vaginal endothelium also responds to the cyclic hormonal changes of the menstrual cycle. Under the influence of estrogen cells of the vaginal epithelium grow maximally during the follicular/proliferative phase. After ovulation layers of keratinized cells overgrow the basal epithelium, a process known as **cornification.** Near the end of the luteal phase leukocytes invade vaginal epithelium, removing the outer layers in a process termed **decornification.**

Body Temperature

Basal body temperature (BBT) undergoes characteristic biphasic changes during menstrual cycles in which ovulation occurs. During the follicular phase the BBT fluctuates around 98° F (37° C). During the luteal phase the average temperature increases by 0.4° to 1.0° F (0.2° to 0.5° C). At the end of the luteal phase, 1 to 3 days before the onset of menstruation, BBT declines to follicular-phase levels. The shift in temperature is related to ovulation, corpus luteum formation, and increased serum progesterone levels. Progesterone probably acts on the thermoregulatory center of the hypothalamus to increase body temperature. Changes in BBT are used to document ovulatory cycles, but they are not good predictors of the exact time of ovulation (Mishell & Davajan, 1986).

THE MALE REPRODUCTIVE SYSTEM

In males, the external genitalia perform the major functions of reproduction, which are to produce sperm and deliver them to the female reproductive tract. Sperm are produced in the male gonads, the testes, and delivered to the female vagina by the penis. The internal male genitalia have a more accessory function. They consist of conducting tubes and fluid-producing glands, all of which aid in the transport of sperm from the testes to the urethral opening of the penis. The male reproductive and urinary structures are shown in Fig. 19-12.

External Genitalia

Testes

In males the testes are the essential organs of reproduction. Like the ovaries the testes have two functions: (1) production of gametes (in this case, sperm) and (2) production of sex hormones (in this case, androgens and testosterone). The testes are suspended outside the pelvic cavity because sperm production requires an environment that is 2 or 3 degrees cooler than body temperature.

During embryonic and fetal life the testes develop within the abdomen (Fig. 19-1). Then, about 3 months before birth, the testes start to descend toward the developing scrotum. About 1 month before birth they enter twin passageways called **inguinal canals.** The inguinal canals are vaginal processes created by outpouchings of the peritoneum (lining of the abdominal cavity). The descent of a testis is shown in Fig. 19-13. Each testis moves down outside the peritoneum until it is suspended in the scrotal sac by its supply lines: the ducts, blood vessels, lymphatic vessels, and nerves of the **spermatic cord.** When descent is complete the abdominal end of each vaginal process closes up and the inguinal canal disappears. If peritoneal closure at the site of the inguinal canal is incomplete or weak, an inguinal hernia may occur later in life. Failure of the testes to descend through the inguinal canal is known as cryptorchidism. The scrotal end of each vaginal process becomes the outer covering of the testis, the **tunica vaginalis.** A hy-

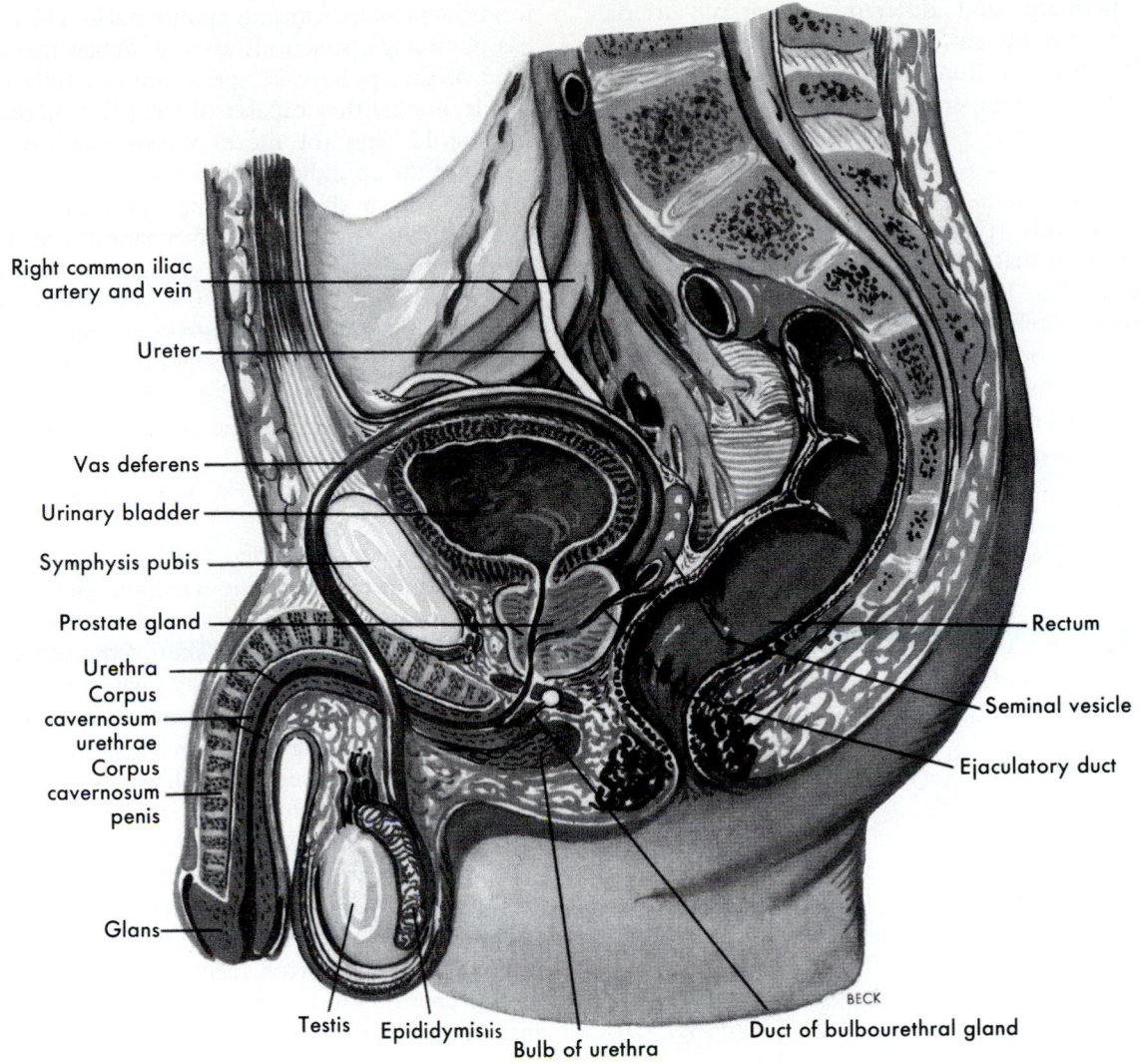

Right common iliac
artery and vein

Ureter

Vas deferens

Urinary bladder

Symphysis pubis

Prostate gland

Urethra
Corpus
cavernosum
urethrae
Corpus
cavernosum
penis

Glans

Rectum

Seminal vesicle

Ejaculatory duct

BECK

Testis   Epididymisiis   Duct of bulbourethral gland
                 Bulb of urethra

FIG. 19-12. Sagittal section of the male penis showing the location of the reproductive organs. (From Thibodeau, 1987.)

drocele is the accumulation of fluid within the tunica vaginalis.

Fig. 19-14 shows a sagittal section of a mature testis. The testis of an adult male is 4 to 5 cm long, 2.5 to 3.0 cm wide; it weighs approximately 32 g. The testis is almost entirely surrounded by an outer covering, the tunica vaginalis, and an inner covering, the **tunica albuginea.** Inward extensions of the tunica albuginea form septa that separate the testis into about 250 compartments, or lobules, each of which contains several tortuously coiled ducts called **seminiferous tubules** (Fig. 19-14). Sperm are produced within the seminiferous tubules. (Sperm production, termed **spermatogenesis,** is described on p. 664.) Tissue surrounding the seminiferous tubules contains blood and lymphatic vessels, fibroblastic support cells, macrophages, mast cells, and Ley-

dig cells. **Leydig cells,** which occur in clusters and account for about 12% of testicular volume, produce androgens, chiefly testosterone. Abnormal dilation of the veins in the testes is referred to as varicocele. Inflammation of the testes is known as orchitis and is a complication of the mumps virus.

The two ends of each seminiferous tubule join and leave the lobule through a short, straight section called the **tubulus rectus.** Sperm travel from the seminiferous tubules into these straight sections, which lead to the central portion of the testis, the **rete testis.** From the rete testis sperm move through the **efferent tubules** to the epididymis, where they mature.

The testes are innervated by adrenergic fibers, whose sole function apparently is to regulate blood flow to the Leydig cells. The testes receive arterial blood from the internal spermatic and differential arteries. Arterial blood flows over the surface of the testes before entering the parenchyma (functional tissues). Surface flow cools the blood to temperatures that promote spermatogenesis.

Epididymis

The **epididymis** (plural, *epididymides*) is a comma-shaped structure that curves over the posterior portion of each testis (Fig. 19-14). It consists of a single, coiled duct, approximately 5 m in length, whose structural function is to conduct sperm from the efferent tubules to the vas deferens. The duct can become inflamed from infection by microorganisms that ascend the urethra or

from the prostate, causing epididymitis. The epididymis has physiologic functions as well. When they enter the head of the epididymis, sperm are not fully mature or motile, nor are they capable of fertilizing an ovum. During the 12 days (or more) sperm takes to travel the length of the epididymis, they receive nutrients and testosterone from the epididymal epithelium, and some biochemical or physiologic mechanism enhances their capacity for fertilization.

The tail of the epididymis is continuous with the **vas deferens,** the duct that transports sperm toward the urethra. After traveling the length of the epididymis, sperm are stored in the epididymal tail and vas deferens. The vas deferens enters the pelvic cavity through the spermatic cord.

Scrotum

The testes, epididymides, and spermatic cord are enclosed and protected by the scrotum. The **scrotum** is a skin-covered, fibromuscular sac that is homologous to the female labia majora. The skin of the scrotum is thin and has rugae (wrinkles or folds), which enable it to enlarge or relax away from the body. At puberty the scrotal skin darkens, develops active sebaceous glands, and becomes sparsely covered with hair. Just under the skin lies a layer of connective tissue (fascia) and smooth muscle, the **tunica dartos.** The tunica dartos also forms a septum that separates the two testes. Exposure to cold temperatures causes the tunica dartos to contract, pulling the testes close to the warm body. In warm temperatures the tunica dartos relaxes, suspending the testes away from body heat. These mechanisms promote optimal temperatures for spermatogenesis.

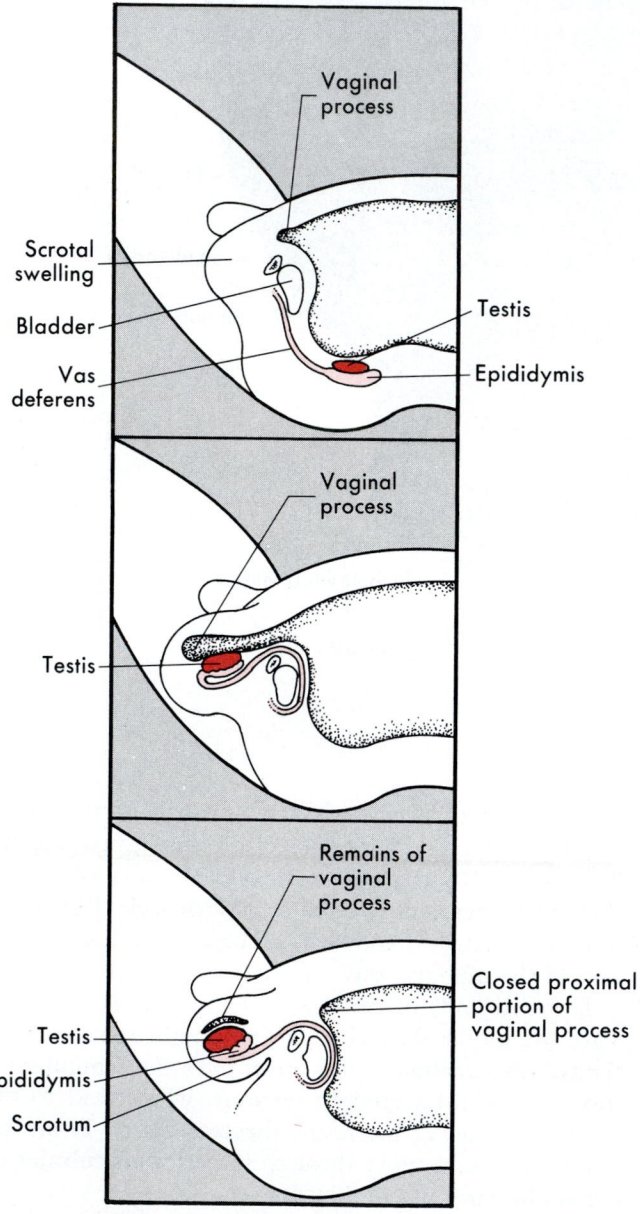

FIG. 19-13. Descent of a testis. The testes descend from the abdominal cavity to the scrotum during the last 3 months of fetal development.

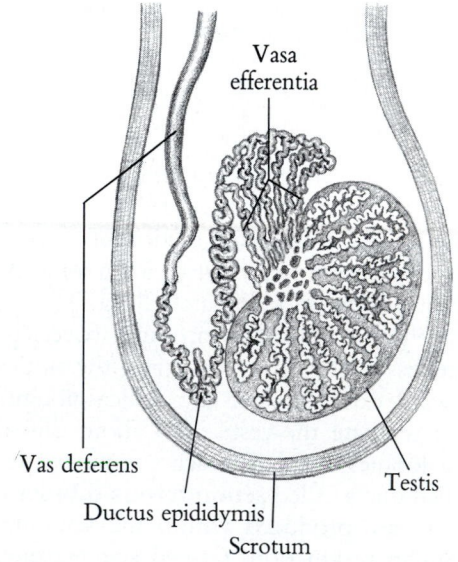

FIG. 19-14. Sagittal section of a mature testis. (From Seidel, Ball, Dains, & Benedict, 1987.)

Penis

The **penis** has two main functions: delivery of sperm to the female vagina and elimination of urine. (Urine formation and excretion are the subjects of Chapter 32.) Embryonically the penis is homologous to the female clitoris.

Fig. 19-12 shows a sagittal section of the adult penis and its anatomic relation to other urogenital structures. Externally the penis consists of a shaft with a tip, the **glans,** which contains the opening of the urethra. Balanitis is an inflammation of the glans. The skin of the glans folds over the tip of the penis, forming the prepuce, or **foreskin.** Soon after birth the foreskin may be removed in a surgical procedure termed circumcision. If the prepuce or opening of the foreskin is too small to slide over the glans, the condition is known as phimosis. The skin of the penis is continuous with that of the groin, scrotum, and inner thighs. It is hairless, movable, and darker than surrounding skin.

Internally the penis consists of the urethra and three compartments: two **corpora cavernosa** and a **corpus spongiosum** (Fig. 19-15). The **urethra** passes through the corpus spongiosum and ends at a sagittal slit in the glans. The three compartments are separated by fascia and, like the testis, enclosed by a tunica albuginea.

Penetration of the female vagina is made possible by the **erectile reflex,** a process in which erectile tissues within the corpora cavernosa and corpus spongiosum become engorged with blood. The erectile tissues consist of vascular spaces, or chambers, which are supplied with blood by arterioles (small arteries). Most of the time the arterioles are constricted, so that not much blood flows through the erectile tissues. Sexual stimulation, however, causes the arterioles to dilate and fill with blood. Their rapid expansion fills the erectile tissues, causing an erection. Erection apparently is maintained by compression or constriction of veins that drain the corpora cavernosa and corpus spongiosum. When sexual stimulation ceases or orgasm and ejaculation occur, these veins open up, blood flows out of the arterioles, and the penis becomes flaccid (soft and pendulous).

Erection is under the control of the autonomic nervous system but can be stimulated or inhibited by central nervous system input. Stimulation of mechanoreceptors of the penis, particularly of the glans, causes parasympathetic nerves of the autonomic nervous system to relax smooth muscle in the walls of penile arterioles. At the same time the effects of sympathetic nerves, which normally cause arteriolar smooth muscle to constrict, are inhibited.

Erections occur throughout life, from infancy through old age, but ejaculation does not occur until sperm production begins at puberty. Growth of the penis and scrotal contents continues well past puberty, however, and may not be complete until the late teens or early 20s.

Internal Genitalia

Fig. 19-12 shows the anatomy of the internal genitalia and their relation to other pelvic organs. The internal genitalia consist of ducts and glands. The ducts—the two vas deferens, the ejaculatory duct, and the ure-

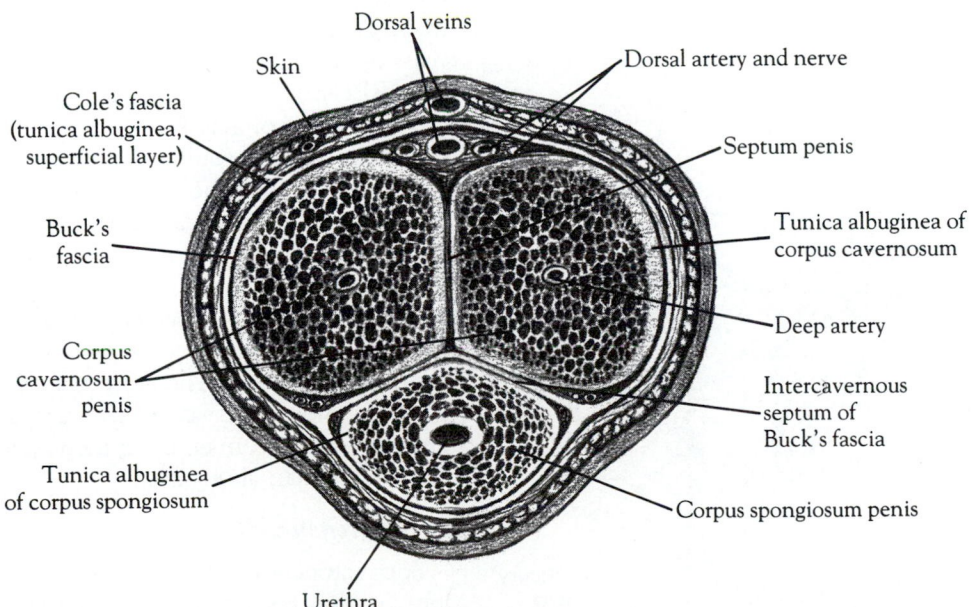

FIG. 19-15. Cross section of the penis. (From Thompson, McFarland, Hirsch, Tucker, & Bowers, 1989.)

thra—conduct sperm and glandular secretions from the testes to the urethral opening of the penis. The glands—the prostate gland, two seminal vesicles, and two Cowper (or bulbourethral) glands—secrete fluids that serve as a vehicle for sperm transport and create an alkaline, nutritious medium that promotes sperm motility and survival. Together, the sperm and the glandular fluids compose **semen.**

Sperm leave the epididymides and travel rapidly through the internal ducts in a process called **emission.** Emission occurs just seconds before ejaculation, at the moment when sexual arousal peaks. Emission always leads to ejaculation.

Emission occurs as smooth muscle in the walls of the epididymides and vas deferens begins to contract rhyth-

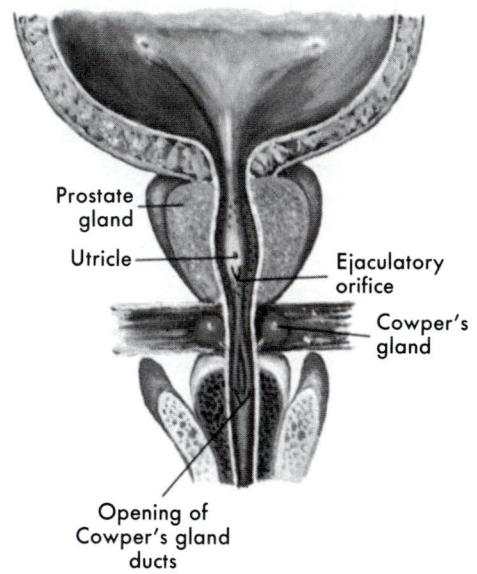

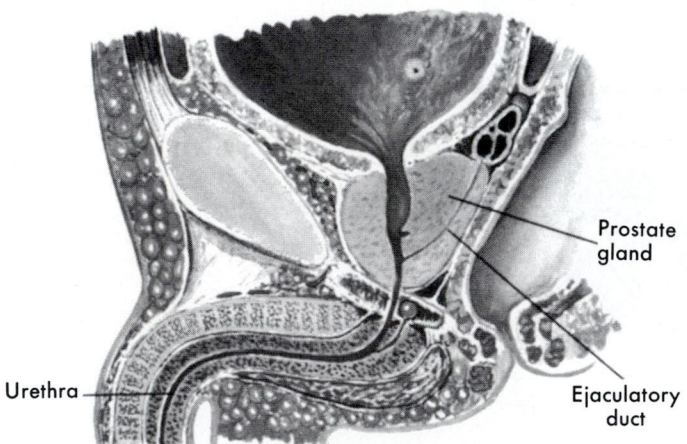

FIG. 19-16. Anatomy of the prostate gland and seminal vesicles. (From Seidel, Ball, Dains, & Benedict, 1987.)

mically, pushing sperm and epididymal secretions through the vas deferens. Each vas deferens is a firm, elastic, fibromuscular tube that begins at the tail of the epididymis, enters the pelvic cavity within the spermatic cord, loops up and over the bladder, and ends in the prostate gland (Figs. 19-12 and 19-16). Sperm are moved along by peristaltic contractions of smooth muscle in the walls of the vas deferens.

As sperm leave the ampulla (wide portion) of the vas deferens, the seminal vesicles secrete a nutritive, glucose-rich fluid into the ejaculate (semen). The **seminal vesicles** are a pair of glands, each about 4 cm long, that lie behind the urinary bladder and in front of the rectum. The ducts of the seminal vesicles join the ampulla of the vas deferens to become the **ejaculatory duct,** which contracts rhythmically during emission and ejaculation. As can be seen in Figs. 19-12 and 19-16 the ejaculatory duct joins the urethra; where both pass through the prostate gland. During emission and ejaculation a sphincter (muscle surrounding a duct) closes, preventing urine from entering the prostatic urethra.

The **prostate gland** is composed of alveoli and ducts embedded in fibromuscular tissue. It is about the size of a walnut and weighs approximately 20 g. While semen moves through the prostatic portion of the urethra the prostate gland contracts rhythmically and secretes prostatic fluid into the mixture. Prostatic fluid is a thin, milky substance with an alkaline pH that helps sperm to survive in the acid environment of the female reproductive tract. In addition substances in seminal and prostatic fluids help to mobilize sperm after ejaculation. Prostatitis is an inflammation of the prostate often caused by infecting microorganisms from the urinary tract. Enlargement of the prostate is common after 50 years of age and is known as benign prostatic hypertrophy (BPH).

The last pair of glands to add fluid to the ejaculate are **Cowper's glands** (bulbourethral glands), whose ducts secrete mucus into the urethra near the base of the penis. Ejaculation occurs as semen reaches the base of the penis and muscles there begin the rhythmic contractions that push semen out. Normally a man ejaculates between 2 and 5 ml of semen containing 75 million to 400 million sperm. About 98% of the ejaculate consists of glandular fluids. Therefore the ejaculate of a man who has undergone vasectomy (surgical procedure that prevents sperm from entering the vas deferens) is not reduced by much: about 2%.

Spermatogenesis

Spermatogenesis begins at puberty and continues for life. In this respect spermatogenesis differs markedly from oogenesis (production of primordial ova), which occurs during fetal life only.

Spermatogenesis takes place within the seminiferous

A

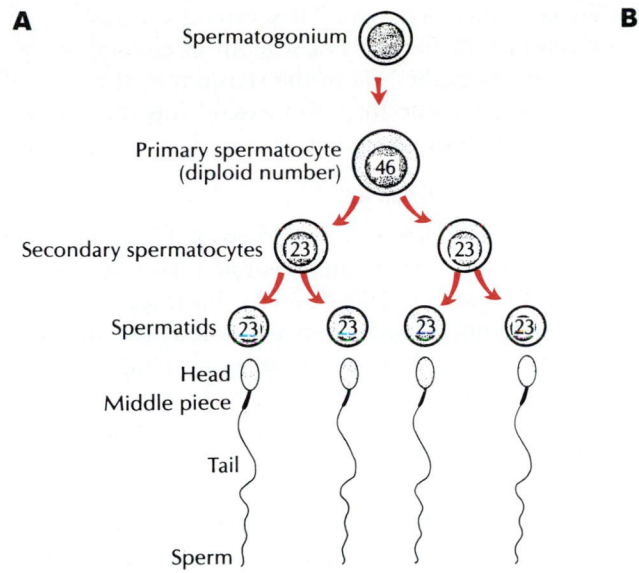

B

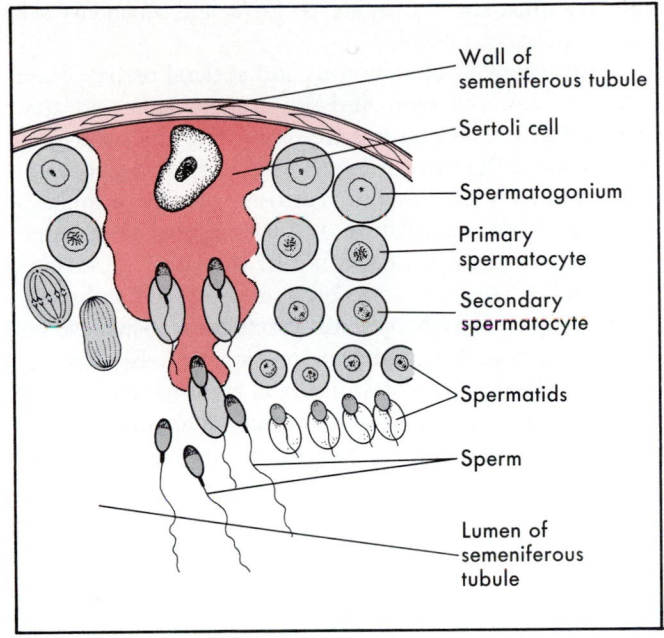

FIG. 19-17. Spermatogenesis. **A**, Cell division; **B**, sperm developing within seminiferous tubule. (From Bobak, Jensen, & Zular, 1989.)

tubules of the testes (Fig. 19-14). The basement membrane of each seminiferous tubule is lined with diploid (46-chromosome) germ cells called **spermatogonia** (singular, *spermatogonium*). These cells undergo continuous mitotic division. (Mitotic division, in which a cell divides into two identical cells, is described in Chapter 1.) Some of the spermatogonia move away from the basement membrane and mature, becoming **primary spermatocytes** (Fig. 19-17). The primary spermatocytes undergo meiosis, a type of cell division that results in two haploid (23-chromosome) cells called **secondary spermatocytes.** (Meiosis is described and illustrated in Chapter 4.) The two secondary spermatocytes then undergo meiosis, resulting in four **spermatids.** It is the spermatids that differentiate into spermatozoa, or sperm, each of which contains 23 chromosomes (Fig. 19-18).

The development of spermatids into sperm depends on the presence of **Sertoli cells** (sustentacular cells, nurse cells) within the seminiferous tubules. The spermatids attach themselves to Sertoli cells, from which they receive the nutrients and the hormonal signals they need to develop into sperm.

The process of spermatogenesis, from mitotic division of a spermatogonium to maturation of the spermatids, takes about 72 days. Mature sperm migrate from the seminiferous tubules to the epididymides, where their capacity for fertilization continues to develop. Though they are completely mature by the time they are ejaculated the sperm do not become motile (capable of movement) until they are activated by biochemicals in semen and in the female reproductive tract.

Male Sex Hormones

The male sex hormones are androgens. Testosterone, the primary male sex hormone, is an androgen. Testosterone and other androgens are produced mainly by Leydig cells of the testes, but they are also produced by the adrenal glands. In males sex hormone production is relatively constant and does not occur in a cyclical pattern, as it does in females.

The androgens have a number of physiologic actions related to the growth and development of male tissues and organs. The androgens are responsible for the fetal differentiation and development of the male urogenital system and have some effects on the fetal brain. After birth the Leydig cells become quiescent until activated by the gonadotropins during puberty. At puberty an-

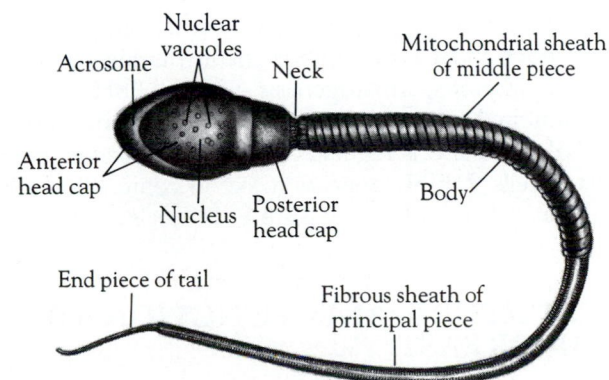

FIG. 19-18. Mature sperm cell (spermatozoon). (From Thompson, McFarland, Hirsch, Tucker, & Bowers, 1989.)

drogens cause the sex organs to grow and secondary sex characteristics to develop.

Testosterone affects nervous and skeletal tissues, bone marrow, skin and hair, and sex organs. It has an anabolic effect on skeletal muscle tissue, thereby contributing to the difference in body weight and composition between males and females. Testosterone also stimulates growth of the musculature and cartilage of the larynx, causing a permanent deepening of the voice. Testosterone directly stimulates the bone marrow and indirectly stimulates renal erythropoietin production to achieve increased hemoglobin and hematocrit levels. Because sebaceous gland activity is stimulated by testosterone acne may develop. Hair becomes coarser in texture, and facial, axillary, and pubic hair grows in male patterns. Later in life testosterone causes baldness in genetically susceptible individuals. Testosterone is required for spermatogenesis and for secretion of fluid by the prostate gland, seminal vesicles, and Cowper glands. Testosterone is also associated with an increase in libido (sex drive). Other, less well understood effects of testosterone include alterations in fatty acid and cholesterol metabolism.

The regulation of androgen production and spermatogenesis is achieved by a complex feedback system involving the extrahypothalamic central nervous system, the hypothalamus, the anterior pituitary, the testes, and the androgen-sensitive end organs. These relationships, which are essentially the same in females, are summarized in Fig. 19-3. Extrahypothalamic influences include such variables as physiologic and psychological stress. These factors may inhibit or augment hypothalamic activity. Gonadotropic-releasing hormone (GnRH) secretion by the hypothalamus is stimulated by norepinephrine and inhibited by both serotonin and dopamine. GnRH is transported by portal flow to the median eminence of the pituitary gland, where it stimulates the secretion of luteinizing hormone (LH) and follicle-stimulating hormone (FSH). LH and FSH, which are named for their effects in the female reproductive system, have important effects on the male system as well. LH acts on the Leydig cells to stimulate testosterone secretion; both FSH and LH are important in the initiation and maintenance of spermatogenesis. LH and FSH secretion are inhibited by testosterone, other androgens, and estradiol. FSH also is regulated by inhibin secreted by the Sertoli cells. Inhibin appears to act in conjunction with the gonadal steroids to regulate FSH levels.

STRUCTURE AND FUNCTION OF THE BREAST

The **breasts** are modified sebaceous glands that lie on the ventral surface of the thorax, within the superficial fascia of the chest wall. They extend vertically from the second rib to the sixth or seventh intercostal space, and laterally from the side of the sternum to the midaxillary line. Breast tissue may also extend into the axilla; this tissue is known as the tail of Spence.

The Female Breast

The female breast is composed of 15 to 20 pyramid-shaped lobes which are separated and supported by Cooper ligaments (Fig. 19-19). Each lobe contains 20 to 40 lobules (alveoli), which subdivide further into many functional units called **acini** (singular, *acinus*). Each acinus is lined with a layer of epithelial cells capable of secreting milk and a layer of subepithelial cells capable of contracting to squeeze milk from the acinus. The acini empty into a network of lobular collecting ducts, which empty into interlobular collecting and ejecting ducts. These ducts reach the skin through openings (pores) in the nipple. The lobes and lobules are surrounded and separated by muscle strands and fatty connective tissue. The amount of fatty connective tissue varies from individual to individual, depending on weight and genetic and endocrine factors, and contributes to the diversity of breast size and shape.

An extensive capillary network surrounds the acini and is supplied by the internal and lateral thoracic arteries and the intercostal arteries. Venous return follows arterial supply, with relatively rapid emptying into the superior vena cava. The breasts receive sensory innervation from branches of the second and sixth intercostal nerves and the cervical plexus. This accounts for the fact that breast pain may be referred to the chest, back, scapula, medial arm, and neck. Lymphatic drainage of the breast occurs largely through axillary nodes, but approximately 25% occurs through transpectoral and internal mammary routes (Fig. 19-20).

The **nipple** is a pigmented, cylindrical structure that is usually located at the fourth or fifth intercostal space. It is approximately 10 to 12 mm in height when erect. On its surface lie multiple openings, one from each lobe. The **areola** is the pigmented, circular area around the nipple. It may be from 15 to 60 mm in diameter. A number of sebaceous glands, the **glands of Montgomery,** are located within the areola and aid in lubrication of the nipple during lactation. The nipple and areola contain smooth muscles, which receive motor innervation from the sympathetic nervous system. Sexual stimulation and exposure to cold cause the nipple to become erect.

The fetal and early postnatal development of breast tissue does not depend on hormones, although fetal breast tissue does become progressively responsive to hormonal stimulation. During childhood breast growth is latent, and growth of the nipple and areola keeps pace with body surface growth. (Male breast development

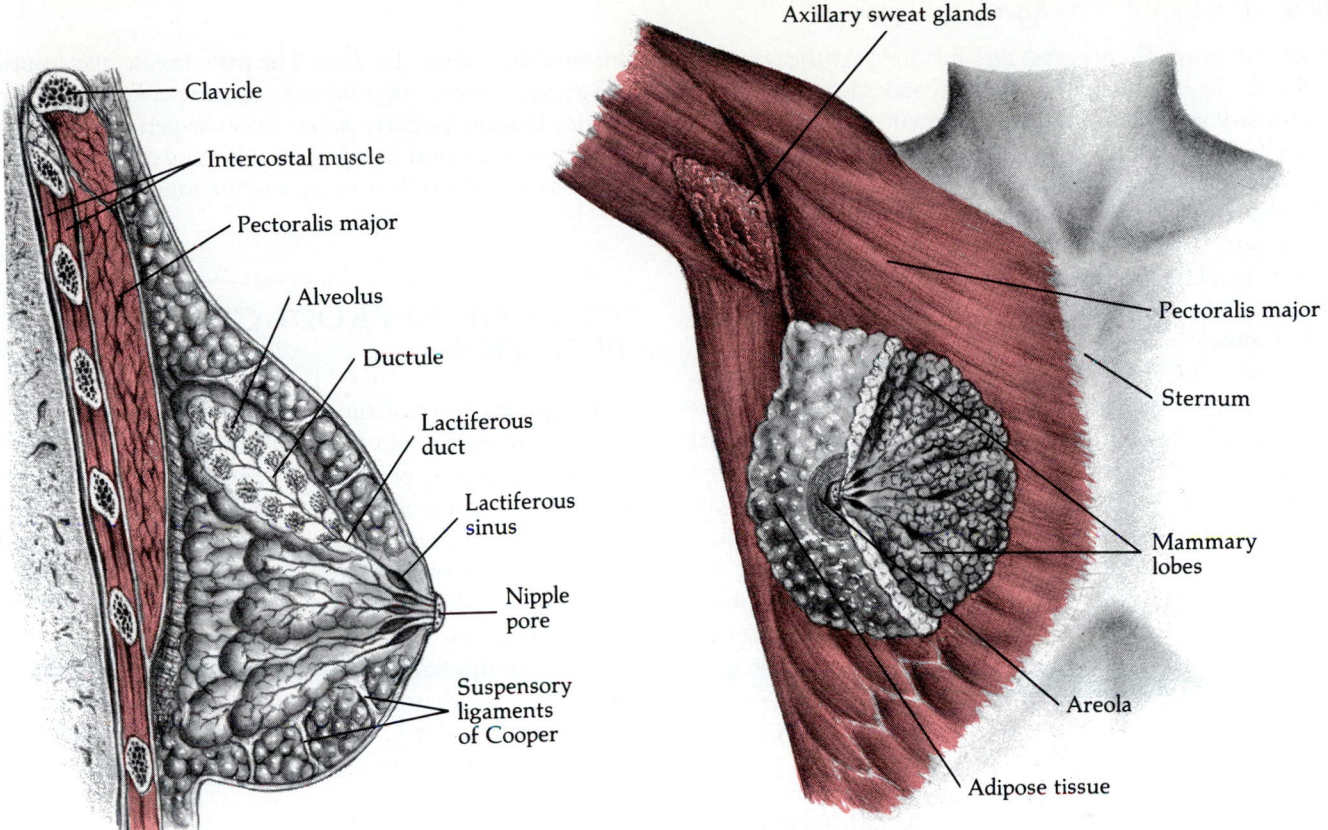

FIG. 19-19. The female breast. (From Thompson, McFarland, Hirsch, Tucker, & Bowers, 1989.)

Clavicle

Intercostal muscle

Pectoralis major

Alveolus

Ductule

Lactiferous duct

Lactiferous sinus

Nipple pore

Suspensory ligaments of Cooper

Axillary sweat glands

Pectoralis major

Sternum

Mammary lobes

Areola

Adipose tissue

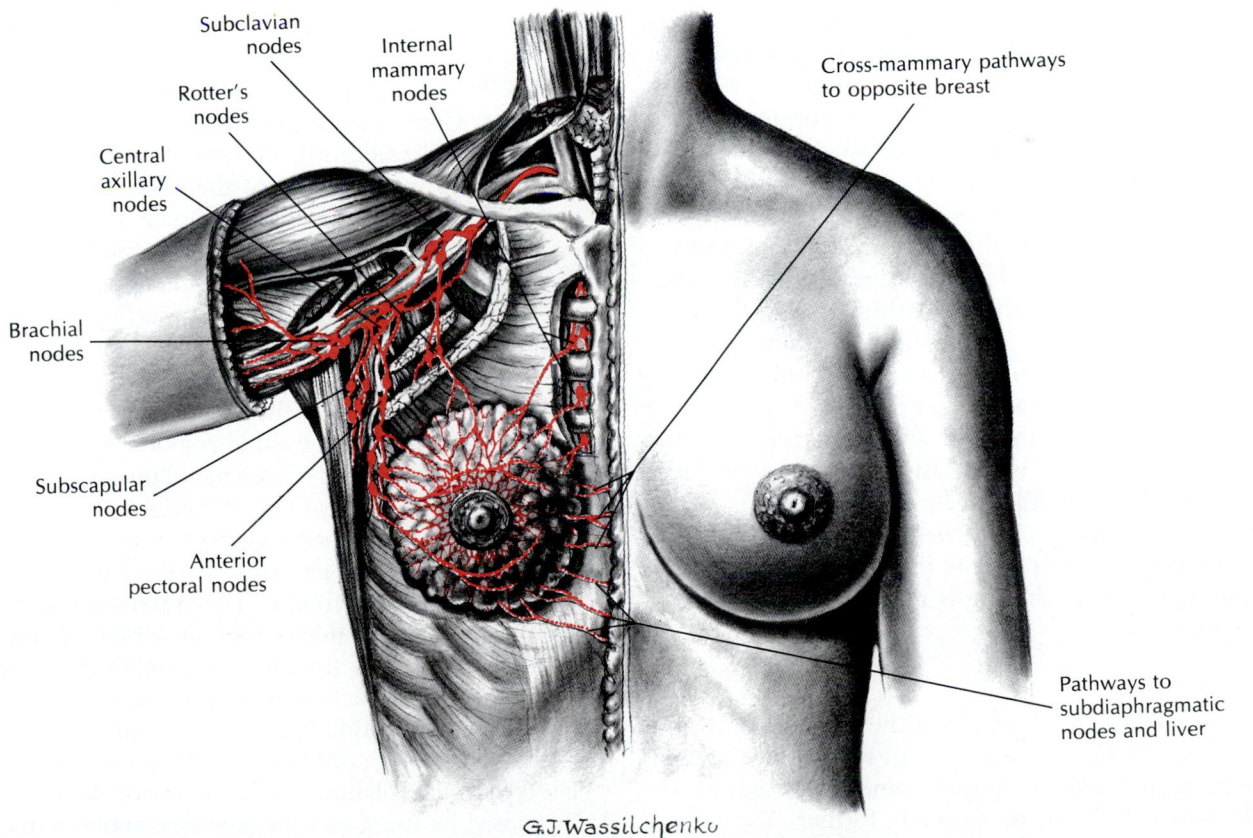

Subclavian nodes

Internal mammary nodes

Rotter's nodes

Central axillary nodes

Brachial nodes

Subscapular nodes

Anterior pectoral nodes

Cross-mammary pathways to opposite breast

Pathways to subdiaphragmatic nodes and liver

G.J.Wassilchenko

FIG. 19-20. Lymphatic drainage of the female breast. (From Bobak, Jensen, & Zular, 1989.)

does not normally progress any further.) At the onset of puberty in the female estrogen secretion stimulates mammary growth. Breast development, or **thelarche,** is usually the first sign of puberty in the female. Full differentiation and development of breast tissue are mediated by a variety of hormones, including estrogen, progesterone, prolactin, growth hormone, thyroid hormone, insulin, and cortisol. Estrogen promotes development of the lobular ducts; progesterone stimulates development of cells lining the acini.

During the reproductive years the breast undergoes cyclic changes in response to changes in the levels of estrogen and progesterone associated with the menstrual cycle. During the follicular/proliferative phase of the menstrual cycle high estradiol levels increase the vascularity of breast tissue and stimulate proliferation of ductal and acinar tissue. This effect is sustained into the luteal/secretory phase of the cycle. During this phase progesterone levels increase and contribute to the breast changes induced by estradiol. Specific effects of progesterone include dilatation of the ducts and conversion of the acinar cells into secretory cells. Most women experience premenstrual breast fullness, tenderness, and increased breast nodularity. Breast volume may increase as much as 10 to 30 ml. Because the length of the menstrual cycle does not allow for complete regression of new cell growth, breast growth continues at a slow rate until approximately age 35. Because of the cyclic changes that occur in breast tissue, breast examination should be conducted at the conclusion of or a few days following the menstrual cycle, when hormonal effects are minimal and breasts are at their smallest.

The function of the female breast is primarily to provide a source of nourishment for the newborn. Physiologically breast milk is the most appropriate nourishment for newborns. Not only does its composition change over time to meet the changing digestive capabilities and nutritional requirements of the infant, but breast milk also contains specific immunoglobulins, especially IgA, and nonspecific antimicrobial factors, such as lysosomes and lactoferrin, which protect the infant against infection. During lactation high prolactin levels interfere with hypothalamic-pituitary hormones that stimulate ovulation. This mechanism suppresses the menstrual cycle and prevents ovulation. In many parts of the world breast feeding is the major means of contraception.

The Male Breast

Until puberty development of the male breast is similar to that of the female breast. In the absence of sufficiently high levels of estrogen and progesterone the male breast does not develop any further. The normal male breast consists of a small, underdeveloped nipple; some fatty and fibrous tissue; and a few ductlike struc-

tures in the subareolar area. The male breast may appear enlarged in obese men because of accumulation of fatty tissue. During puberty some males experience gynecomastia, a condition in which the breasts enlarge temporarily as a result of hormonal fluctuations.

TESTS OF REPRODUCTIVE FUNCTION

Diagnostic tests of the male and female reproductive systems are performed to determine the cause of infertility, to detect the presence of cancerous lesions, or to identify the presence of sexually transmitted diseases. (Alterations of the reproductive systems are discussed in Chapter 20; sexually transmitted diseases are discussed in Chapter 21.) Procedures include laboratory tests, such as cultures, smears, stains, biopsies, serologic testing, and hormonal assays. Radiographic procedures are performed to identify abnormal growths or structures. Direct observation of reproductive organs is completed by laparoscopy or culdoscopy.

Infection and Cancer Tests

Smears, stains, cultures, and serologic testing are commonly used to detect infectious diseases. Smears are prepared by spreading a thick layer of specimen material on a glass slide. The specimen may be evaluated microscopically as a wet mount, dried, or stained with different dyes. Gram staining is a technique that allows the differential identification of two categories of bacteria according to the tendency of the microorganism to absorb different components of the stain selectively.

A **culture** is the growth of microorganism in a nutrient medium selectively prepared to support the growth of particular microorganisms that are obtained from body secretions or tissues. Both bacteria and viruses, such as cytomegalovirus, can be cultured.

Serological testing identifies whether an antigen-antibody reaction has occurred in response to an infectious microorganism. Several different techniques can be used to identify the formation of antigen-antibody complexes. With immunofluorescent testing fluorescein-labeled antibodies react with specific antigen, such as the spirochetes of syphilis. The fluorescent pattern of the reaction can be microscopically observed under ultraviolet light. The flocculation (agglutination) test is the precipitation of clumped cells caused by the reaction of antigen with homologous antiserum. The Venereal Disease Research Laboratory (VDRL) test for syphilis is a type of flocculation test. Certain viral diseases can be diagnosed by using specific serologic antibody markers, for example, the diagnosis of hepatitis A and hepatitis B viruses. Radioimmune assay (RIA) and enzyme-linked

TABLE 19-3 Diagnosis of sexually transmitted diseases

Test	Description	Normal value
Serologic test for syphilis	Detection of antibodies to *Treponema pallidum*	Negative or nonreactive
VDRL	Venereal Disease Research Laboratory	Nonspecific
RPR	Rapid plasma reagin	More specific
FTA	Fluorescent treponemal antibody absorption test	More specific
Gonorrhea culture	Culture of cervix in women and urethra in men to detect *Neisseria gonorrhoeae*	Negative
Chlamydia smear	Culture of cervix in women and urethra in men to detect polymorphonuclear leukocytes	Negative
ELISA (enzyme-linked immuno-absorbent assay)	Detects the presence of antibodies to human immuno-deficiency virus (HIV), an AIDS test	Nonreactive
IFA (indirect fluorescent antibody)	A more specific test for HIV	Nonreactive
WB (Western blot)	A more specific test for HIV	Nonreactive
TORCH test	Detects elevations of IgA or IgM caused by toxoplasma, rubella, cytomegalovirus, syphilis, and herpes simplex in mother and newborn infant; herpes requires more specific testing when result is positive	No elevation in antibodies
Cytomegalovirus (herpes virus 5)	Can be grown in cell culture with samples from urine, cervix, semen, saliva, blood	No growth

immunoabsorbent assay (ELISA) are more specific tests used to document viral infections. A summary of tests used for the diagnosis of sexually transmitted diseases is presented in Table 19-3.

Tissue biopsy is the surgical resection of a tissue specimen from a suspect site. The biopsy provides cells and tissues to identify infectious processes; to differentiate benign from malignant conditions, and primary from metastatic lesions. In the reproductive tract tissue may be obtained from the vagina, cervix (by cone or brush biopsy), endometrium of the uterus (by curettage), ovary, testes, prostate, or penis.

Needle biopsy is a technique of aspirating small amounts of tissue by positioning a needle in the tissue and applying negative pressure by pulling back on the plunger of the attached syringe as the needle is moved back and forth at the biopsy site. There is relatively less discomfort with this procedure than with a tissue biopsy that requires opening the surface of the skin to localize the tissue site. Normal findings indicate no abnormal cells or tissues on histologic examination.

The **Papanicolaou smear** is a procedure commonly used for the cytologic examination of the female reproductive tract. Cells from body tissues and fluids (from the vagina or cervix) are stained and examined for the number and types of cells and abnormalities in their morphology. Specimens may also be obtained from the mouth, nipple discharge, or amniotic, pleural, or spinal fluid aspirations. The Papanicolaou smear is particularly useful for diagnosis of premalignant, malignant, atypical, and inflammatory cells.

Evaluations of the breast are commonly performed to detect tumors. Mammography, thermography, and biopsy are specific examination techniques. **Mammography** is a low-dose radiographic examination used to identify nonpalpable (less than 1 cm) or unrecognized lesions. Breast cancer can be detected by radiography 2 to 3 years before its clinical presentation, providing an excellent prognosis for cure. The American Cancer Society (1988) recommends a baseline mammogram of all women at age 35 to 40 years, annual or biannual mammogram between 40 and 49 years, and yearly mammogram after age 50.

Thermography is a method of measuring patterns of temperature distribution by using an infrared camera for photography. The pictorial representation of the normal breast has an even distribution of temperature patterns. When there is increased or decreased blood supply, these areas are represented as hot spots (black areas) or cold spots (white areas) on a thermogram. Infection, tumor, and fibrocystic disease are associated with hot spots, making the test nonspecific. False negatives are also possible because not all breast cancers are associated with increased blood supply. However, since the test is easy and inexpensive it may be used for screening and followed by other diagnostic procedures.

TABLE 19-4 Tests and normal values of reproductive function

Test	Description	Normal value
Semen analysis	Determines normal number, motility, and structure of sperm cells	Volume = 2-6 million Number = 20-200 million/ml Motility = 60%-80% motile Morphology = 70%-90% normal shape
Antisperm antibody	Detects antibodies to sperm	No sperm agglutins present
Basal body temperature	Determines whether ovulation has occurred	Decrease in basal body temperature before ovulation followed by a rise in temperature at the time of ovulation
Cervical mucus	Evaluates presence of ovulation from estrogenic effects at ovulation; mucus may also be examined for pH, glucose, or proteins or cultured for presence of infection	Fern pattern appears when cervical mucus dries on a clean slide; mucus is clear, watery, and elastic (spinnbarkeit) with no inflammatory cells
Postcoital cervical mucus (Sims-Hunher test)	Tests ability of sperm to penetrate and maintain motility in cervical mucus 2-4 hours after coitus	6-20 motile sperm in each high power field; previous sperm analysis normal
Endometrial biopsy	Determines whether ovulation has occurred by obtaining endometrial tissue on day 27 or 28 of menstrual cycle	Finding is "secretory-type" endometrium if ovulation has occurred
Hysterosalpingogram	Assessment of uterus and fallopian tubes for obstructions using transuterine injection of contrast material and radiography	No obstruction evident
Uterotubal insufflation (Rubin test)	Assesses patency of fallopian tubes using transuterine tubal insufflation with carbon dioxide and pressure measurement	Pressures <180-200 mm Hg, no obstruction; pressures >200 mm Hg indicate tubal obstruction; repeated studies differentiate obstruction from tubal spasm
Laparoscopy (pelvic endoscopy)	Visualization of reproductive organs using a laparoscope inserted within the pelvic cavity through the abdomen to assess structure or determine presence of adhesions, endometriosis, tumors, or infection	Normal structure and position of organs
Culdoscopy	Visualization of pelvic organs using a culdoscope inserted through incision in the cul-de-sac	Normal structure and position of organs
Dilation and curettage (D & C)	Biopsy of uterine endometrium for diagnosis of endometrial hyperplasia	No abnormal tissue
Papanicolaou test	Stained smear of specimen obtained from the cervix, vagina, nipple; used for identification of abnormal cells	No atypical, premalignant, or malignant cells present

Fertility Tests

Tests of reproductive function are performed most commonly when infertility exists. Both the male and female partner are examined and several diagnostic evaluations may be completed. The types of tests and their normal values are summarized in Tables 19-4 and 19-5. The male must have normal numbers, amounts, structure, and motility of sperm with no obstruction along the reproductive tract. Tests for females determine whether (1) the reproductive tract (cervix, uterus, fallopian tubes) is adequately patent to allow for passage of ovum and sperm, (2) ovulation occurs normally, (3) the endometrium is responding normally to hormones, and (4) no tumors or infections are present. Hormonal assays evaluate the adequacy of pituitary function and target organ response. The position and size of organs or the presence of tumors can be detected by direct observation procedures using a laparoscope or by radiographic studies, such as plain films, computerized scans, or tomography.

TABLE 19-5 Serum hormone values

Hormone	Value
Serum progesterone	Normal = >10 ng/dl <10 ng/ml = inadequate luteal function <3 ng/ml suggests anovulation
Serum-free testosterone	Normal = 9-30 ng/dl Low values suggest abnormality of hypothalamic-pituitary-gonadal axis with male hypogonadism
Serum testosterone	Normal = 300-1200 ng/dl Low values in male hypogonadism
Serum estradiol	Normal = 3-40 ng/dl Low values in hypogonadism caused by either ovarian disease or hypothalamic-pituitary disease
Serum prolactin	Normal = 0-23 mg/ml Elevations associated with hypogonadism caused by hypothalamic-pituitary dysfunction
Serum FSH and LH	FSH = <22 IU/L LH = 4-24 IU/L High values in males indicate primary testicular disease; low values in males indicate hypogonadism caused by hypothalamic-pituitary dysfunction

AGING AND REPRODUCTIVE FUNCTION

Aging and the Female Reproductive System

Menopause is a normal developmental event that is universally experienced by middle-aged women. The average age at which menopause occurs is 50 to 51 years and does not appear to be affected by age at menarche, childbearing, weight, socioeconomic factors, or race. Because life expectancy has increased significantly women can now expect to spend one third of their lives after their last menstrual period.

The physiologic changes of menopause are primarily caused by declining ovarian function and a resulting decrease in ovarian hormone secretion. During the 5 to 10 years preceding menopause approximately 90% of women note extreme variability in the frequency of menstruation and in the quality of menstrual flow. This transitional interval begins with the onset of changes in ovarian function, including decreased frequency of ovulation, reduced estrogen production by the ovaries, and, finally, menopause. Primordial follicles are present in the ovaries, but they apparently resist gonadotropin stimulation. It is not clear exactly what mechanisms cause this resistance.

Hormonal findings during the years surrounding menopause include significantly elevated FSH and LH levels and maintenance of pulsatile secretion by the pituitary. In the ovary, however, the follicle and corpus luteum no longer develop and thus do not secrete estradiol and progesterone. Therefore, serum levels of both these hormones decline. The stroma of the ovaries does continue to secrete androstenedione, which is converted peripherally to estrone (a form of estrogen). The conversion takes place in adipose tissue; therefore, obese women tend to have higher serum levels of estrone. The physiologic role of estrone is not clearly understood, but increased estrone levels (unopposed by progesterone) are associated with an increased incidence of endometrial cancer. This may account for the higher incidence of endometrial cancer in obese women.

As ovarian function diminishes breast tissue begins to become involuted. Two phases of involution have been described: (1) the premenopausal phase and (2) the menopausal phase. The premenopausal phase occurs between 35 and 45 years of age. During this phase there is a moderate decrease in mammary tissue. During the menopausal phase glandular breast tissue is significantly reduced, and there is some increase of fat deposits and connective tissue. These changes contribute to the reduction in size and firmness of breast tissue.

Several systemic changes are associated with declining ovarian function. They include changes in vasomotor tone, urogenital structures, bone density, and artery walls. The severity of these changes may depend on such variables as the rate at which tissue levels of estradiol decline. Vasomotor changes can cause a hot flash, or **vasomotor flush.** This event is characterized by a rise in skin temperature, dilation of peripheral blood vessels, changes of electrical resistance in the skin, and transient increase in heart rate. Vasomotor flush usually occurs in the face and neck initially and may progress to the chest.

The flush may be accompanied by dizziness, nausea, headaches, palpitations, diaphoresis (sweating), or night sweats. Vasomotor flushes vary in intensity and in duration, lasting from 1 to 4 minutes. Approximately 75% to 85% of all menopausal women experience vasomotor flushes. Most have symptoms for more than 1 year, and 25% have symptoms for more than 5 years. Vasomotor flushes apparently are triggered by estrogen withdrawal rather than estrogen lack. They can also be triggered by emotional stress, excitement, fear, or anxiety. The exact causal mechanisms are not known.

The urogenital tract undergoes a number of changes. The ovaries begin to decrease in size around the age of 30 years, and shrinkage accelerates after the age of 60. During the years surrounding menopause the uterus atrophies and decreases in size. The vagina shortens and narrows. The vaginal pH, usually maintained at 4.0 to 6.0 as a result of estrogen stimulation, rises to between 6.5 and 8.0 and contributes to a higher incidence of vaginitis. The cervix atrophies, and the cervical os decreases in size. The vaginal epithelium also atrophies; this atrophy can cause vaginal irritation, burning, itching (pruritus), white discharge (leukorrhea), painful intercourse (dyspareunia), and vaginal bleeding. The labia majora and minora become less prominent, and some pubic hair is lost. Urethral tone declines, as does muscle tone throughout the pelvic area. Urinary frequency or urgency, urinary tract infections, and incontinence are thought to be associated with menopausal changes because these symptoms diminish with estrogen therapy (Droegemueller et al., 1987).

Loss of bone mass is also associated with menopause. Bone mass reaches a peak in the early 30s and then begins to decline. The decline amounts to 1% to 2% per year after menopause. Insufficient bone mass leads to increased brittleness and porosity of bone (osteoporosis), predisposing some women to pathologic bone fractures, usually after the age of 60. It is not understood how diminished estrogen production causes loss of bone mass. Bone loss appears to be prevented by estrogen therapy, however, and can be minimized with weight-bearing exercise. Smoking doubles a woman's risk for the development of osteoporosis, as does intake of more than two alcoholic drinks per day. Calcium intake in childhood and adolescence determines peak bone mass in adulthood. Those with greater bone mass are less likely to develop osteoporosis after menopause (Riggs & Melton, 1986). Increased calcium intake during the postmenopausal years does *not* appear to prevent osteoporosis.

Premenopausal women have significantly lower risk of developing coronary heart disease than do age-matched men, but immediately after menopause, women are at increased risk of coronary disease. This increase is significant after the age of 55 (Gordon et al., 1978). Levels of serum cholesterol and triglycerides increase after menopause, whether the menopause is spontaneous or surgically induced, increasing the risk of coronary disease (Mischnell, 1987).

The assumption that menopause is a distressing and depressing time is prevalent, but systematic investigations have failed to identify a psychological syndrome associated with menopause (Voda, 1984). It may be that responses to the physiologic changes of menopause are influenced by other life changes that tend to occur in the 50s. During these years a woman may be coping with increased responsibility for aging parents, loss of parents, changes in the dependent status of children, daily care of grandchildren, or illness of significant others.

Aging and the Male Reproductive System

Males maintain reproductive capacity longer than females, despite the popular perception that men over the age of 50 are somehow sexually impaired (Masters & Johnson, 1981). There is no known discrete event, comparable to menopause, that characterizes aging of the male reproductive system. Changes do occur, however, in male sexual behavior and in testicular structure and function, including hormonal secretion and spermatogenesis.

Components of male sexual behavior include both sexual drive and erectile/ejaculatory capacity. **Libido,** or sexual drive, is a complex phenomenon that requires a baseline hormonal milieu but is influenced significantly by health status and environmental, social, and psychological factors. Aging causes specific physical changes that influence erectile and ejaculatory capabilities. Alterations in sexual response include the need for longer stimulation to achieve full erection, slower and less forceful ejaculation, with less pelvic muscle involvement; decreased vasocongestive response; and longer refractory period (time during which erection and ejaculation are not possible, up to 24 hours in some males (Schneider, 1979).

The testes undergo several age-related structural changes including decreased weight, atrophy, and softening. Degenerative changes in the seminiferous tubules may include thickening of the basement membrane; increase in lumen size; germ cell (spermatogonium) arrest and a decrease in spermatogenic activity; and collapse of tubules, followed by complete obstruction caused by sclerosis and fibrosis (Schneider, 1979). Areas of mild to severe degenerative change may be interspersed with areas having intact tubules. These morphologic changes may result from atherosclerosis (arterial clogging) in the testicular vascular bed (Mastroianni & Paulsen, 1986). Alterations of the seminiferous tubules do not appear to diminish sperm counts (Swerdloff & Heber, 1982), but they do reduce fertility because a greater percentage of the sperm lack motility or have structural abnormalities (Schneider, 1979).

Aging probably causes changes in the production of male sex hormones and responsiveness of target tissues. Hormone synthesis by the testes, testicular responsiveness to the gonadotropins (FSH and LH), and pituitary secretion of these gonadotropins are altered. Most studies of testosterone levels in aging men show that their serum testosterone levels are lower than levels in younger men (Brenner, Vitiello, & Primz, 1983; Royer et al., 1984; Vermeulen, Rubens, & Verdonck, 1972).

The reduced levels of testosterone may be related to alterations in the Leydig cells, the testosterone producers of the testes. The number of Leydig cells decreases as age increases, perhaps because of atherosclerotic changes in arteries that supply blood to the testes (Kaler & Neaves, 1978). Even if testosterone levels are not decreased older men may have less unbound testosterone in their blood, decreasing the amount of unbound hormone available to stimulate target tissues (Vermeulen et al., 1972). Decreased testosterone levels have several effects, including functional deterioration of the accessory sex organs (the prostate gland, seminal vesicles, epididymis, and ductus deferens); loss of muscle mass, strength, and endurance (Valenta & Elias, 1983); and, in many men, decrease in libido. This last effect may also be caused by alterations in other variables that affect libido.

Serum levels of the gonadotropins, particularly FSH, increase with age. The change in gonadotropin secretion may result from primary testicular failure or from some hypothalamic-pituitary disregulation of the gonadotropins (Swerdloff & Heber, 1982).

Androgen replacement therapy is problematic because androgens have adverse systemic effects. Androgens are associated with coronary atherosclerosis, exacerbations of benign prostatic hypertrophy, and induction of prostatic carcinoma (Mastroianni & Paulsen, 1986).

SUMMARY REVIEW

Development of the Reproductive System

1 Differentiation of female and male genitalia begins in the eighth week of embryonic development, when the gonads of genetically male embryos begin to secrete male sex hormones, primarily testosterone. Until that time, the primitive reproductive organs of males and females are homologous (the same).

2 The structure and function of both male and female reproductive systems are controlled by the hypothalamic-pituitary-ovarian axis, a set of complex neurologic and hormonal interactions that accelerate at puberty, causing sexual maturation and making reproduction possible.

3 Extrahypothalamic factors cause the hypothalamus to secrete gonadotropin-releasing hormone (GnRH), which stimulates the anterior pituitary to secrete gonadotropins—follicle-stimulating hormone (FSH) and luteinizing hormone (LH)—which stimulate the gonads (ovaries or testes) to secrete female or male sex hormones.

4 Production of primitive female gametes (ova) occurs solely during fetal life. From puberty to menopause one female gamete matures per menstrual cycle. Production of the male gametes (sperm) begins at puberty; after that, millions are produced daily, normally for life.

The Female Reproductive System

1 The function of the reproductive system is to produce mature ova and, when they are fertilized, to protect and nourish them through embryonic and fetal life and expel them at birth.

2 The external female genitalia are the mons pubis, labia majora, labia minora, clitoris, vestibule (urinary and vaginal openings), Bartholin glands, and Skene glands.

3 The internal female genitalia are the vagina, uterus, fallopian tubes, and ovaries. Though all of these organs are needed for reproduction, the ovaries are the most essential because they produce the female gametes and female sex hormones.

4 The vagina is a fibromuscular canal that receives the penis during sexual intercourse and is the exit route for menstrual fluids and products of conception. The vagina leads from the introitus (its external opening) to the cervical portion of the uterus.

5 The uterus is the hollow, muscular organ in which a fertilized ovum develops until birth. The uterine walls have three layers: the endometrium (lining), myometrium (muscular layer), and perimetrium (outer covering, which is continuous with the pelvic peritoneum). The endometrium proliferates (thickens) and sloughs off in response to cyclical changes in levels of female sex hormones. The cervix is the narrow, lower portion of the uterus that opens into the vagina.

6 The two fallopian tubes extend from the uterus to the ovaries. Their function is to conduct ova from the spaces around the ovaries to the uterus. Fertilization normally occurs in the fallopian tubes.

7 From puberty to menopause, the ovaries are the site of (a) ovum maturation and release and (b) production of female sex hormones (estrogen and progesterone) and androgens. The female sex hormones are involved in sexual differentiation and development, the menstrual cycle, pregnancy, and lactation. Though they are primarily male sex hormones, androgens in females contribute to the prepubertal growth spurt, pubic and axillary hair growth, and activation of sebaceous glands.

8 Estrogen (primarily estradiol) is produced by cells in the developing ovarian follicle (structure that encloses the ovum). Progesterone is produced by cells of the corpus luteum, the structure that develops from the ruptured ovarian follicle after ovulation (ovum release). Androgens are produced within the ovarian follicle, adrenal glands, and adipose tissue.

9 The average menstrual cycle takes 28.3 days and consists of four phases, which are named for ovarian and endometrial changes: the follicular/proliferative phase, ovulation, the luteal/secretory phase, and menstruation.

10 Ovarian events of the menstrual cycle are controlled by gonadotropins. High FSH levels stimulate follicle and ovum maturation (follicular phase); then a surge of LH causes ovulation, which is followed by development of the corpus luteum (luteal phase).

11 Uterine (endometrial) events of the menstrual cycle are caused by ovarian hormones. During the follicular phase of the ovarian cycle estrogen produced by the follicle causes the endometrium to proliferate (proliferative phase). During the luteal phase estrogen maintains the thickened endometrium while progesterone causes it to develop blood vessels and secretory glands (secretory phase). As the corpus luteum degenerates production of both hormones drops sharply, and the "starved" endometrium degenerates and sloughs off, causing menstruation.

12 Cyclical changes in hormone levels also cause thinning and thickening of the vaginal epithelium, thinning and thickening of cervical secretions, and changes in basal body temperature.

The Male Reproductive System

1 The function of the male reproductive system is to produce male gametes (sperm) and deliver them to the female reproductive tract.

2 The external male genitalia are the testes, epididymides, scrotum, and penis. The internal genitalia are the vas deferens, ejaculatory duct, prostatic and membraneous sections of the urethra, seminal vesicles, prostate gland, and Cowper glands.

3 The testes (male gonads) are paired glands suspended within the scrotum. The testes have two functions: spermatogenesis (sperm production) and production of male sex hormones (androgens, chiefly testosterone).

4 The epididymis is a long, coiled tube arranged in a comma-shaped compartment that curves over the top and rear of the testis. The epididymis receives sperm from the testis and stores them while they develop further. Sperm travel the length of the epididymis and then are ejaculated into the vas deferens.

5 The scrotum is a skin-covered, fibromuscular sac that encloses the testes and epididymides, which are suspended within the scrotum by the spermatic cord. The scrotum keeps these organs at optimal temperatures for sperm survival (about 3 degrees lower than body temperature) by contracting in cold environments and relaxing in warm environments.

6 The penis is a cylindrical organ consisting of three longitudinal compartments (two corpora cavernosa and one corpus spongiosum) and the urethra. The urethra runs through the corpus spongiosum. The corpora cavernosa and corpus spongiosum consist of erectile tissue. Externally the penis consists of a shaft and a tip, which is called the glans. The glans contains sebaceous glands and the opening of the urethra. It is covered by a flap of skin (the foreskin), which may be removed in a procedure called circumcision.

7 The penis has two functions: delivery of sperm to the female vagina and elimination of urine. Semen (sperm and glandular secretions) and urine both leave the penis through the urethra, but these two fluids are never in the urethra at the same time.

8 Sexual intercourse is made possible by the erectile reflex, in which tactile or psychogenic stimulation of the parasympathetic nerves causes arterioles in the corpora cavernosa and corpus spongiosum to dilate and fill with blood, causing the penis to enlarge and become firm.

9 Emission, which occurs at the peak of sexual arousal, is the movement of semen from the epididymides to the penis. Ejaculation, which is a continuation of emission, is the pulsatile ejection of semen from the penis. Both emission and ejaculation involve rhythmic contractions of smooth muscle within the internal glands and ducts.

10 Spermatogenesis is a continuous process because spermatogonia, the primitive male gametes, undergo continuous mitosis within the seminiferous tubules of the testes. Some of the spermatogonia develop into primary spermatocytes, which divide meiotically into secondary spermatocytes, then spermatids. The spermatids develop into sperm with the help of nutrients and hormonal signals from Sertoli cells.

11 Production of the male sex hormones is controlled (like production of the female sex hormones) by the hypothalamic-pituitary-gonadal axis and by complex feedback mechanisms. However, the male hormones are produced steadily rather than cyclically.

Structure and Function of the Breast

1 Until puberty the female and male breasts are similar, consisting of a small, underdeveloped nipple, some fatty and fibrous tissue, and a few ductlike structures under the areola. At puberty, however, a variety of hormones (estrogen, progesterone, prolactin, growth hormone, insulin, and cortisol) cause the female breast to develop into a system of glands and ducts that is capable of producing and ejecting milk.

2 The basic functional unit of the female breast is the lobe, a system of ducts that branches from the nipple to milk-producing units called lobules. The lobules contain acini, which are convoluted spaces lined with epithelial cells that secrete milk and subepithelial cells that contract, moving the milk into the system of ducts that leads to the nipple.

3 Each breast contains 15 to 20 lobes, which are separated and supported by Cooper ligaments.

4 Milk production occurs in response to prolactin, a hormone that is secreted after delivery of the fetus. Milk ejection is under the control of oxytocin, another hormone of pregnancy and parturition. Milk production continues in response to sucking.

5 During the reproductive years breast tissue undergoes cyclic changes in response to hormonal changes of the menstrual cycle.

Tests of Reproductive Function

1 Diagnostic tests are performed to evaluate fertility or presence of tumors, infection, or sexually transmitted diseases.

2 Smears, stains, cultures, and serological tests are used to diagnose infections. These tests specifically identify microorganisms or types of infections.

3 Tissue biopsy can be performed by resection or needle aspiration. Specimen analysis permits identification of abnormal cells.

4 The Papanicolaou smear is a cytologic examination of cells taken from body fluids and tissues. Although cells can be obtained from many sites, the smear is most commonly used for diagnosis of cervical carcinoma.

5 Mammography is a low-dose radiographic examination of the breast for cancer detection.

6 Thermography measures patterns of temperature variation. The test is useful for identifying sites of infection or tumor growth, which frequently have an increased blood supply and show as "hot spots."

7 Evaluation of fertility includes reproductive hormone assays and assessment of structural alterations, normal ovulation, adequate sperm motility and count, and absence of infection.

Aging and Reproductive Function

1 In females the reproductive years end with menopause, which occurs at the average age of 51. At menopause the menstrual cycle ceases and levels of sex hormones fall.

2 Reduced levels of female sex hormones cause all the reproductive organs to atrophy. In addition the vaginal epithelium thins, and glandular secretions diminish and become more alkaline.

3 Nonreproductive effects of reduced estrogen levels include increased risk of osteoporosis and coronary artery disease.

4 Male reproductive function diminishes with age, but it does not cease in healthy men.

5 The testes atrophy and produce less testosterone, and some seminiferous tubules may degenerate and become fibrotic. These changes affect sex drive (libido) and sperm morphology. Though sperm count remains normal, the semen tends to contain more defective and nonmotile sperm.

6 The erectile reflex is somewhat diminished and occurs more slowly as age advances.

7 Reduced testosterone levels cause some loss of function in the internal genitalia and enlargement (hypertrophy) of the prostate gland.

KEY TERMS

Acinus of breast, 666

Androgen, 657

Areola, 666

Bartholin gland (greater vestibular gland), 650

Breast, 666

Cervix, 652

Clitoris, 650

Cornification, 660

Corpus cavernosum, 663

Corpus luteum, 654

Corpus spongiosum, 663

Corpus of uterus (body of uterus), 652

Cowper gland (bulbourethral gland), 664

Culture, 668

Decornification, 660

Efferent tubules, 661

Ejaculatory duct, 664

Emission, 664

Endocervical canal, 652

Endometrium, 652

Epididymis, 662

Erectile reflex, 663

Estradiol, 655

Estrogen, 655

Fallopian tube (oviduct, uterine tube), 653

Fimbriae, 653

Follicle-stimulating hormone (FSH), 649

Follicular/proliferative phase, 657

Foreskin (prepuce), 663

Fornix, 651

Fundus of uterus, 652

Glands of Montgomery, 666

Glans, 663

Gonad, 646

Gonadotropin, 649

Gonadotropin-releasing hormone (GnRH), 649

Granulosa cell, 655

Infundibulum, 653

Inguinal canal, 660

Inhibin, 659

Introitus, 650

Isthmus, 652

Labia majora, 650

Labia minora, 650

Leydig cell, 661

Libido, 672

Luteal/secretory phase, 657

Luteinizing hormone (LH), 649

Mammography, 669

Menarche, 657

Menopause, 657

Menstrual cycle, 657

Menstruation (menses), 657

Mons pubis, 650

Myometrium, 652

Needle biopsy, 669

Nipple, 666

Ovarian cycle, 654

Ovarian follicle, 654

Ovary, 654

Ovulation, 654

Ovum, 646

Papanicolaou smear, 669

Penis, 663

Perimetrium (peritonium), 652

Primary spermatocyte, 665

Progesterone, 656

Prostate gland, 664

Rete testis, 661

Ruga, 651

Scrotum, 662

Secondary spermatocyte, 665

Semen, 664

Seminal vesicle, 664

Seminiferous tubule, 661

Serological test, 668

Sertoli cell (sustentacular cell, nurse cell), 665

Sex hormone, 646

Skene gland (lesser vestibular gland), 650

Sperm (spermatozoa), 646

Spermatic cord, 660

Spermatid, 665

Spermatogenesis, 661

Spermatogonium, 665

Squamous-columnar junction, 653

Testis, 660

Testosterone, 646

Theca cell, 655

Thelarche, 668

Thermography, 669

Tissue biopsy, 669

Tubulus rectus, 661

Tunica albuginea, 661

Tunica dartos, 662

Tunica vaginalis, 660

Urethra, 663

Urinary meatus, 650

Uterus, 651

Vagina, 650

Vas deferens (ductus deferens), 662

Vasomotor flush, 671

Vestibule, 650

Vulva, 650

REFERENCES

American Cancer Society. (1988). *Cancer facts and figures 1988*. New York: Author.

Bobak, I. M., Jensen, M. D., & Zular, M. K. (1989). *Maternity and gynecologic care: The nurse and the family* (4th ed.). St. Louis: C. V. Mosby.

Brenner, W. J., Vitiello, M. V., & Primz, P. N. (1983). A loss of circadian rhythmicity in blood testosterone levels with aging in normal men. *Journal of Clinical Endocrine Metabolism, 56,* 1278-1281.

Droegemeuller, W. D., Herbst, A. L., Mischell, D. R., & Stenehever, M. A. (1987). *Comprehensive gynecology*. St. Louis: C. V. Mosby.

Gordon, T., Castelli, W. P., Hjortland, M. C., & McNamara, P. M. (1978). Menopause and coronary heart disease: The Framingham study. *Annals of Internal Medicine, 89,* 157-161.

Hadley, M. E. (1984). *Endocrinology*. Englewood Cliffs, N.J.: Prentice Hall.

Kaler, R., & Neaves, A. (1978). Attrition of the human leydig cell population with advancing age. *Anatomical Records, 192,* 513-518.

Masters, W. H., & Johnson, V. E. (1981). Sex and the aging process. *Journal of the American Gerontological Society, 29,* 385-390.

Mastroianni, L., & Paulsen, C. A. (1986). *Aging, reproduction and the climacteric*. New York: Plenum Press.

Mischell, D. R., & Davajan, B. (1986). *Infertility, contraception, and reproductive history*. Oradell, N.J.: Medical Economics Books.

Riggs, B. L., & Melton, L. J. (1986). Involutional osteoporosis. *New England Journal of Medicine, 314*(26), 1676-1686.

Royer, G. L., Seckman, C. E., Schwartz, J. H., Bennett, K. P., & Hendrix, J. W. (1984). Relationship between age and levels of total, free, and bound testosterone in healthy subjects. *Current Therapeutic Research, 35,* 345-353.

Schneider, E. L. (1979). *The aging reproductive system*. New York: Raven Press.

Seidel, H. M., Ball, J. W., Dains, J. E., & Benedict, G. W. (1987). *Mosby's guide to physical examination*. St. Louis: C. V. Mosby.

Swerdloff, R. S., & Heber, D. (1982). Effects of aging on male reproductive function. In S. G. Korenman (Ed.), *Endocrine aspects of aging*. New York: Elsevier.

Thibodeau, G. A. (1987). *Anatomy and physiology*. St. Louis: Times Mirror/Mosby College Publications.

Thompson, J. M., McFarland, G., Hirsch, J., Tucker, S., & Bowers, A. (1989). *Mosby's manual of clinical nursing* (2nd ed.). St. Louis: C. V. Mosby.

Valenta, L. H., & Elias, A. N. (1983). Pituitary-gonadal function in the aging male: The male climacteric. *Geriatrics, 38*(12), 67-72.

Vander, A. J., Sherman, J. H., & Luciano, D. S. (1980). *Human physiology: The mechanisms of body functions* (3rd ed.). New York: McGraw-Hill.

Vermeulen, A., Rubens, R., & Verdonck, L. (1972). Testosterone secretion and metabolism in male senescence. *Journal of Clinical Endocrine Metabolism, 34,* 730-735.

Voda, A. (1984). Menopause research in nursing practice. *Annual Review of Nursing Research,* (4), 55-75.

CHAPTER 20

Alterations of the Reproductive Systems

D. Patricia Gray
Sue E. Huether

Alterations of sexual maturation, 678
  Delayed puberty, 678
  Precocious puberty, 678
Disorders of the female reproductive system, 680
  Hormonal and menstrual alterations, 680
    Primary dysmenorrhea, 680
      Pathophysiology, 680
      Clinical manifestations, 680
      Evaluation and treatment, 680
    Primary amenorrhea, 680
      Pathophysiology, 680
      Clinical manifestations, 681
      Evaluation and treatment, 681
    Secondary amenorrhea, 681
      Pathophysiology, 681
      Clinical manifestations, 681
      Evaluation and treatment, 681
    Dysfunctional uterine bleeding, 682
      Pathophysiology, 682
      Clinical manifestations, 683
      Evaluation and treatment, 683
    Polycystic ovarian syndrome, 683
      Pathophysiology, 683
      Clinical manifestations, 683
      Evaluation and treatment, 683
    Premenstrual syndrome, 683
      Clinical manifestations, 683
      Evaluation and treatment, 684
  Infection and inflammation, 684
    Pelvic inflammatory disease, 685
      Pathophysiology, 685
      Clinical manifestations, 685
      Evaluation and treatment, 686
    Vaginitis, 686
    Cervicitis, 687
    Vulvitis, 687
    Bartholinitis, 687
  Pelvic relaxation disorders, 687
  Benign growths and proliferative conditions, 690
    Benign ovarian cysts, 690
    Endometrial polyps, 690
    Leiomyomas, 691

      Pathophysiology, 691
      Clinical manifestations, 691
      Evaluation and treatment, 691
    Endometriosis, 691
      Pathophysiology, 692
      Clinical manifestations, 692
      Evaluation and treatment, 692
  Cancer, 693
    Cervical cancer, 693
      Pathogenesis, 693
      Clinical manifestations, 695
      Evaluation and treatment, 696
    Vaginal cancer, 696
    Endometrial cancer, 696
    Ovarian cancer, 697
      Pathogenesis, 697
      Clinical manifestations, 697
      Evaluation and treatment, 698
Disorders of the male reproductive system, 699
  Disorders of the urethra, 699
    Urethritis, 699
    Urethral strictures, 699
  Disorders of the penis, 699
    Phimosis and paraphimosis, 699
    Peyronie disease, 699
    Priapism, 700
    Balanitis, 700
    Penile cancer, 700
  Disorders of the scrotum, testis, and epididymis, 701
    Disorders of the scrotum, 701
    Cryptorchidism, 702
    Torsion of the testis, 703
    Orchitis, 703
      Pathophysiology, 703
      Clinical manifestations, 703
      Evaluation and treatment, 703
    Cancer of the testis, 704
      Pathogenesis, 704
      Clinical manifestations, 704
      Evaluation and treatment, 704
    Impairment of sperm production and quality, 705
    Epididymitis, 706

Pathophysiology, 706
Clinical manifestations, 706
Evaluation and treatment, 707
Disorders of the prostate gland, 707
Benign prostatic hyperplasia, 707
Prostatitis, 707
Bacterial prostatitis, 708
Nonbacterial prostatitis, 709
Cancer of the prostate, 709
Pathogenesis, 709
Clinical manifestations, 709
Evaluation and treatment, 710
Sexual dysfunction, 710
Pathophysiology, 710
Evaluation and treatment, 711
Disorders of the breast, 711
Disorders of the female breast, 711
Galactorrhea, 711
Pathophysiology, 711
Clinical manifestations, 712
Evaluation and treatment, 712
Fibrocystic disease, 712
Pathophysiology, 713
Clinical manifestations, 713
Evaluation and treatment, 713
Breast cancer, 715
Reproductive factors, 715
Hormonal factors, 715
Environmental factors, 715
Familial factors, 715
Pathogenesis, 715
Clinical manifestations, 717
Evaluation and treatment, 717
Disorders of the male breast, 717
Gynecomastia, 717
Pathophysiology, 718
Evaluation and treatment, 719
Carcinoma, 719

ALTERATIONS OF SEXUAL MATURATION

A variety of congenital and endocrine disorders can disrupt the timing of puberty, or sexual maturation. These disorders may cause puberty to occur too late (delayed puberty) or too early (precocious puberty). Both types of disorders involve the inappropriate onset of sex hormone production by the gonads.

Delayed Puberty

The first sign of puberty in girls is thelarche, or breast development. Thelarche should begin by the time a girl is 13. In boys the first sign is enlargement of testes and thinning of the scrotal skin; this should happen by age 14. In **delayed puberty** these secondary sex characteristics show no sign of appearing in a girl of 13 or a boy of 14.

In 90% of cases the delayed puberty is a constitutional delay; that is, hormonal levels are normal and the hypothalamic-pituitary-ovarian axis is intact, but maturation is happening slowly. Constitutional delay is much more common in boys than in girls.

The other 5% of cases are caused by some disruption of the hypothalamic-pituitary-gonadal axis or to a systemic disease. The disruption can consist of deficient secretion of gonadotropin-releasing hormone (GnRH) by the hypothalamus, deficient gonadotropin secretion by the pituitary, or gonadal disorders. Treatment of pathophysiologic delayed puberty depends on the cause. Insufficient sex hormone secretion can be corrected by hormone replacement therapy.

Constitutional delay seldom requires treatment, unless the delayed puberty is causing psychosocial problems. The well-being of a boy with constitutional delay sometimes is improved by a short course of testosterone replacement, which will accelerate development.

Precocious Puberty

Precocious puberty is the onset of sexual maturation before the age of 8 in females and 9 in males. Girls are more often affected, sometimes in infancy, and the precocious puberty is usually idiopathic. Boys are affected less often, and the cause is more likely to be organic pathology.

Precocious puberty occurs in three forms: isosexual, heterosexual, and incomplete. **Isosexual precocious puberty** is premature development of appropriate characteristics for the child's sex. In true isosexual precocious puberty the hypothalamic-pituitary-ovarian axis is working normally but prematurely. In pseudoprecocious puberty the sex hormones are being produced by some mechanism other than stimulation by the gonadotropins.

Heterosexual precocious puberty causes the child to develop some secondary sex characteristics of the opposite sex. This condition is usually evident at birth and is rare in older children.

Incomplete precocious puberty is the partial development of appropriate secondary sex characteristics. A girl with incomplete precocious puberty might undergo thelarche only or adrenarche (growth of pubic hair) only. Premature thelarche is seen in girls between 6 months and 2 years of age. It does not progress to complete puberty (ovulation and menstruation). Premature adrenarche tends to occur between the ages of 5 and 8. This condition can progress to complete precocious puberty.

All forms of precocious puberty are treated by identifying and removing the underlying cause or administering appropriate hormones. In many cases precocious puberty can be reversed. The most common form, idiopathic isosexual precocity, is difficult to treat. Besides

Causes of Delayed Puberty

I. Deficiency of GnRH secretion by hypothalamus
- A. Genetic
  1. Familial
  2. Kallman syndrome
  3. Lawrence Moon-Biedel syndrome
  4. Prader-Willi syndrome
- B. Acquired
  1. Infections
     a. Encephalitis
     b. Granuloma
  2. Neoplasms
     a. Hypothalamus
     b. Pineal region

II. Deficiency of gonadotropic secretion by pituitary
- A. Genetic
  1. Panhypopituitarism
  2. Isolated gonadotropin deficiency
  3. Fertile eunuch (normal FSH, low LH)
- B. Acquired
  1. Infections
  2. Neoplasms
  3. After trauma

III. Gonadal disorders
- A. Genetic
  1. Turner syndrome (45, X or structural X abnormalities or mosaicism)
  2. Kleinfelter syndrome (47, XXY)
  3. Noonan syndrome
  4. Syndromes of complete androgen insensitivity (no pubic hair)
  5. Del Castillo syndrome (Sertoli cells only)
  6. Pure gonadal dysgenesis
  7. Myotonic dystrophy
- B. Acquired
  1. Infections
     a. Gonorrhea (male)
     b. Virus (usually mumps)
     c. Tuberculosis (male)
  2. Radiotherapy or chemotherapy
  3. Mechanical causes
     a. After torsion
     b. After surgery

IV. Adrenal and gonadal steroid enzyme deficiencies

V. Chronic systemic diseases
- A. Congenital heart disease
- B. Chronic pulmonary disease
- C. Inflammatory bowel disease
- D. Chronic renal failure and renal tubular acidosis
- E. Hypothyroidism
- F. Poorly controlled diabetes mellitus
- G. Sickle cell anemia
- H. Collagen-vascular disease
- I. Anorexia nervosa

From Hoekelman, Blatman, Friedman, Nelson, & Seidel, 1987.

Causes of Isosexual Precocious Puberty

I. True puberty (with gonadotropin secretion)
- A. Idiopathic (constitutional predisposition)
- B. CNS abnormalities
  1. Congenital anomalies (hydrocephalus)
  2. Tumors (hypothalamic, pineal, other)
  3. Hamartoma
  4. Postinflammatory condition
  5. Trauma
  6. Syndromes
     a. McCune-Albright (polyostotic fibrous dysplasia)
     b. Neurofibromatosis
     c. Tuberous sclerosis
- C. Hypothyroidism (severe)
- D. Ectopic gonadotropin-secreting tumors (chorioepithelioma, hepatoblastoma, teratoma)

II. Pseudopuberty
- A. Exogenous sex steroids
- B. Gonadal tumors
  1. Ovarian
  2. Testicular

From Hoekelman, Blatman, Friedman, Nelson, & Seidel, 1987.

Causes of Heterosexual Precocious Puberty

I. Female
- A. Congenital adrenal hyperplasia
- B. Androgen-secreting tumors
  1. Adrenal
  2. Ovarian
  3. Teratoma

II. Male
- A. Estrogen-producing tumors
  1. Adrenal
  2. Teratoma
- B. Exogenous estrogens

From: Hoekelman, Blatman, Friedman, Nelson, & Seidel, 1987.

the premature development of secondary sex characteristics, it can cause long bones to stop growing before the child has reached normal height.

DISORDERS OF THE FEMALE REPRODUCTIVE SYSTEM

Hormonal and Menstrual Alterations

Primary Dysmenorrhea

Primary dysmenorrhea is painful menstruation not associated with pelvic disease. The incidence varies, ranging from 30% to 50% among menstruating women (Rosenwaks & Jones, 1980). Dysmenorrhea usually begins with the onset of ovulation or within the first year after menarche.

Pathophysiology

Several factors may be associated with dysmenorrhea but the exact causal relationships are not clear. One prevalent theory implicates prostaglandin synthesis during the late luteal phase of the menstrual cycle. Concentrations of prostaglandins PGE_2 and $PGF_{2\alpha}$ were measured in menstrual blood and endometrial tissue and found to be increased in dysmenorrheic women (Pickles, Hall, & Best, 1965). This suggests that primary dysmenorrhea is mediated by prostaglandins. Prostaglandins increase myometrial contractions and constrict endometrial blood vessels, causing ischemia, endometrial bleeding, and pain.

Prostaglandins are also known to produce headache, diarrhea, and vomiting, which are secondary manifestations of dysmenorrhea. The relief of menstrual pain with prostaglandin-inhibiting drugs provides additional support to the theory that prostaglandins are a cause of dysmenorrhea.

Women who are anovulatory because they use oral contraceptives do not have primary dysmenorrhea. In these women the progesterone and estrogen in the pill may mediate the release of prostaglandins or increase the sensitivity of myometrial nerves to these substances.

Clinical Manifestations

The chief symptom of dysmenorrhea is pelvic pain associated with the onset of menses. The pain frequently radiates into the groin and may be accompanied by backache, anorexia, vomiting, diarrhea, syncope, and headache. The symptoms may last from a few hours to 2 days.

Evaluation and Treatment

Primary dysmenorrhea must be differentiated from secondary dysmenorrhea caused by disorders such as endometriosis, endometrial polyps, inflammatory disease, or cervical stenosis. A thorough medical history and pelvic examination are completed to exclude pelvic pathology.

Primary dysmenorrhea can be relieved with oral contraceptives, which decrease endometrial proliferation. Prostaglandin inhibitors are effective in 75% to 80% of cases. Local application of heat is a commonly used comfort measure.

Primary Amenorrhea

Amenorrhea means lack of menstruation. **Primary amenorrhea** is the failure of menarche and the absence of menstruation beyond the age of 16. In most cases girls with primary amenorrhea do not develop secondary sex characteristics. The etiology of primary amenorrhea includes a diverse group of abnormalities, such as congenital defects of gonadotropin production (Prader-Willi, Kallmann, and Laurence-Moon-Biedl syndromes); genetic disorders (Turner syndrome); congenital central nervous system defects, such as hydrocephalus; congenital anatomic malformations of the reproductive system (e.g., absence of vagina or uterus); and acquired central nervous system (CNS) lesions, including trauma, infection, and tumors.

Pathophysiology

In some of the congenital syndromes that cause primary amenorrhea the hypothalamic-pituitary-ovarian axis is dysfunctional. The hypothalamus is unable to synthesize GnRH, so the pituitary fails to secrete leutinizing hormone (LH) and follicle-stimulating hormone (FSH). Therefore, the ovary does not receive the hormonal signals that normally initiate the ovarian and endometrial changes of the menstrual cycle, and ovulation and menstruation do not occur. Because the ovarian hormones are absent, secondary sex characteristics do not develop.

Some anatomic defects of the central nervous system, whether congenital or acquired, impinge on the hypothalamic-pituitary unit so as to interfere with or interrupt the secretion of GnRH or FSH and LH. Examples of such defects include hydrocephalus, craniopharyngiomas, and other space-occupying lesions of the central nervous system. Again the target organ, the ovary, does not receive the necessary signals, and ovulation and menstruation do not occur. In some cases these lesions develop between the onset and conclusion of puberty. Therefore skeletal growth may occur and secondary sex characteristics may develop, but sexual maturation is interrupted before menarche, which normally concludes puberty.

Anatomic defects of the genitalia are also associated with primary amenorrhea. They include congenital absence of the vagina and uterus and congenital uterine hypoplasia (infantile uterus). Females without a uterus or vagina usually have normal ovarian function. Therefore, skeletal growth occurs, and secondary sex characteristics develop in the proper sequence, but menstruation does not occur. In cases of uterine hypoplasia the uterus does not respond to hormonal stimulation during puberty.

Several genetic disorders are associated with primary amenorrhea. These include gonadal dysgenesis (Turner syndrome); testicular feminizing syndrome (male pseudohermaphroditism); and poly-X, or superfemale syndrome. With the chromosomal abnormalities of Turner syndrome (XO) the ovaries lack gametes, and ovarian failure is complete. Without primitive gametes and follicles follicular development and estrogen secretion cannot occur. Lack of estrogen accounts for failure of secondary sex characteristic development, amenorrhea, and high levels of circulating FSH and LH. In male pseudohermaphroditism the individual is male genetically but female morphologically. The individual does not develop male genitalia because androgen receptors are absent in undifferentiated target organs. The gonads are found either in the abdomen or in the inguinal canal, and they produce both androgens and estrogens. Because target tissues lack androgen receptors but have estrogen receptors, most individuals with male pseudohermaphroditism acquire female external genitalia and female secondary sex characteristics. With the exception of a small vagina internal female genitalia are absent, accounting for amenorrhea and infertility.

Clinical Manifestations

The major clinical manifestation of primary amenorrhea is the absence of the menses. The etiology of the amenorrhea determines whether secondary sex characteristics and height are affected.

Evaluation and Treatment

Diagnosis of primary amenorrhea is based on history and physical examination. If ovarian steroid hormone levels are low, the individual has the appearance of an immature female. Physical examination may reveal structural or physiologic alterations. Laboratory studies may be required to document abnormal levels of gonadotropins and ovarian hormones. Diagnostic imaging is used to document structural abnormalities.

Treatment involves correction of any underlying disorders and hormone replacement therapy to induce the development of secondary sex characteristics. Surgical alteration of the genitals may be undertaken to correct structural abnormalities. Hormonal manipulation or embryo transplantation may make pregnancy possible for women with primary amenorrhea.

Secondary Amenorrhea

Secondary amenorrhea is the occurrence of menstruation three or fewer times per year in women who have previously menstruated. A wide variety of disorders and physiologic conditions are associated with secondary amenorrhea. Besides disease secondary amenorrhea can be triggered by dramatic weight loss, whether the loss results from malnutrition or excessive exercise. Secondary amenorrhea is normal during early adolescence, pregnancy, and lactation and when approaching menopause.

Pathophysiology

The pathophysiology of secondary amenorrhea is summarized in Fig. 20-1. In women with normal ovarian steroid hormone levels secondary amenorrhea is caused by structural abnormalities or removal of the uterus. In women with elevated ovarian steroid hormone levels inhibited ovulation leads to amenorrhea. An excess of ovarian hormones apparently disrupts feedback relationships between the various hormones of the hypothalamic-pituitary-ovarian axis, preventing ovulation. Depressed ovarian hormone levels, which are associated with a variety of clinical disorders, also cause amenorrhea by preventing ovulation. Lack of ovulation, termed **anovulation,** may result from increased levels of prolactin, decreased levels of gonadotropins, irregular secretion of gonadotropins, or abnormally low levels of central nervous system neurotransmitters. Any of these variables alters the feedback effects that the ovarian hormones have on the hypothalamus and pituitary.

Hyperprolactinemia (overproduction of prolactin by the pituitary) may have short-loop feedback effects that lead to decreased secretion of GnRH by the hypothalamus. The result is a loss of pulsatile LH secretion and an overall reduction in LH levels. Anovulation and secondary amenorrhea may result. In the ovary elevated prolactin levels appear to inhibit the secretion of progesterone by the granulosa cells of the follicle. This leads to anovulation caused by follicular atresia. These abnormalities may act singly or in combination to cause other alterations in the menstrual cycle.

Clinical Manifestations

The major manifestation of secondary amenorrhea is the absence of menses. Infertility, vasomotor flushes, vaginal atrophy, acne, and **hirsutism** (abnormal hairiness) may also be present, depending on the underlying cause of the amenorrhea.

Evaluation and Treatment

Diagnosis of secondary amenorrhea involves the identification of underlying hormonal or anatomic alterations. A woman with secondary amenorrhea and normal secondary sex characteristics should have a complete history and physical examination, thyroid function test, and 2-hour postprandial blood glucose analysis. Pregnancy is ruled out before any further endocrine workup

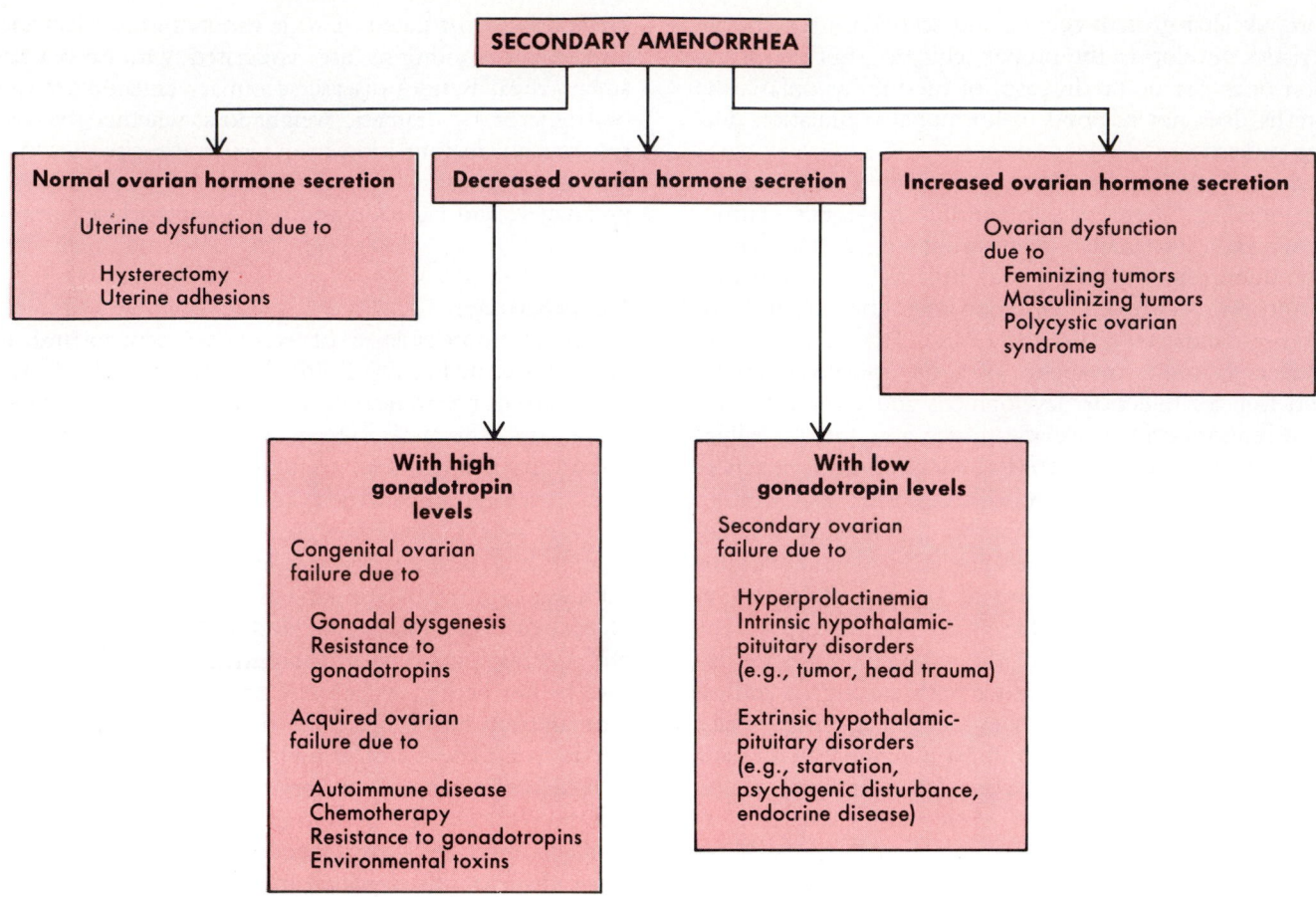

FIG. 20-1. Disorders that cause secondary amenorrhea.

is undertaken. Depending on the cause of the amenorrhea, treatment may involve hormone replacement therapy (e.g., estrogens, thyroid hormone, glucocorticoids, clomiphene citrate, gonadotropins, bromocriptine) or a corrective procedure, such as surgical removal of pituitary tumors.

Dysfunctional Uterine Bleeding

Dysfunctional uterine bleeding is abnormal uterine bleeding *resulting from a disturbance of the menstrual cycle.* It is not associated with other causes of abnormal uterine bleeding, such as tumor, infection, or systemic disease.

Pathophysiology

Dysfunctional uterine bleeding may be associated with either ovulatory or anovulatory menstrual cycles. In anovulatory cycles, which occur most often in women over 40 years of age, abnormal bleeding results from low levels of both estrogen and progesterone or from high levels of estrogen with low levels of progesterone. Low levels of both estrogen and progesterone cause the endometrium to become hypoplastic (thin and

underdeveloped) and to bleed with any downward fluctuation of estrogen levels. High estrogen levels, combined with low progesterone levels, cause the endometrium to become hyperplastic (to overproliferate). When a portion of the overproliferating endometrium outgrows its blood supply, tissue breakdown, sloughing, and bleeding occur. Because this process is ongoing throughout the endometrium, bleeding occurs at different sites and at different times. Bleeding caused by endometrial hyperplasia may be persistent and profuse.

In ovulatory cycles dysfunctional uterine bleeding may be regular or irregular. Excessive blood loss can occur during the menstrual phase of a normal-length cycle. This pattern of dysfunctional bleeding is most common in women over 30 who have had two or more children. Irregular dysfunctional uterine bleeding can result from luteal phase defects in which the corpus luteum degenerates prematurely. In this pattern of dysfunctional bleeding menstrual flow is normal but occurs too often. Conversely if corpus luteum degeneration is prolonged, the progesterone effect persists into the next cycle, and irregular bleeding occurs.

Clinical Manifestations

Dysfunctional uterine bleeding is characterized by irregular or heavy bleeding or both. Dysfunctional bleeding may also involve the passage of large clots, which often indicate excessive blood loss. It is difficult to estimate the severity of blood loss in otherwise healthy women because such women do not become anemic until blood loss exceeds 1.6 L over a short interval. Iron stores are usually depleted (Smith, 1985).

Evaluation and Treatment

Dysfunctional uterine bleeding is diagnosed after other organic conditions that could cause abnormal bleeding are ruled out. An endometrial biopsy or dilation and curettage (D & C) is performed before medical therapy is initiated. The clinician may prescribe an antifibrolytic agent, oral contraceptive, prostaglandin synthetase inhibitor, ovulation stimulator, or danazol. Because long-term drug therapy is inadvisable, women over 40 years of age who do not wish to extend their childbearing years may be advised to have a hysterectomy.

Polycystic Ovarian Syndrome

Polycystic ovarian syndrome (PCO) includes a variety of symptoms and physiologic abnormalities. In women with PCO nothing is intrinsically wrong with the ovary. Rather the ovary is affected by the production of excessive amounts of androgens and conversion of these androgens to estrogen in the peripheral tissues. This hormonal imbalance prevents ovulation. There is no proven cause of PCO, but possible ones include heredity, catecholamine abnormalities, obesity, and psychologic stress.

Pathophysiology

The biochemical basis of PCO is complex. The most common biochemical abnormality is inappropriate gonadotropin secretion. Levels of FSH are typically low or below normal, and the midcycle peak is absent. Levels of LH are elevated, and LH does not surge correctly at midcycle. The persistent LH elevation causes both adrenal and ovarian androgen secretion to increase. The androgen is converted to estrogen in peripheral tissues. Thus PCO is characterized by excessive production of both androgen and estrogen.

In about 50% of cases, the ovaries are enlarged, sometimes to two or three times their normal size, and may have numerous small cysts beneath a thickened surface. Because estrogen promotes endometrial proliferation, women with PCO are at risk for endometrial polyps and endometrial cancer.

Clinical Manifestations

Clinical manifestations of PCO usually appear during adolescence or young adulthood. They include increasingly light menstrual bleeding and periods of amenorrhea or total cessation of the menses. Because women with PCO do not ovulate, they are infertile. Excessive androgen levels usually cause hirsutism and acne. Approximately 15% of women with PCO are obese.

Evaluation and Treatment

Diagnosis of PCO is based on evidence of androgen excess, chronic anovulation, and inappropriate gonadotropin secretion. Treatment of PCO includes progesterone therapy to oppose estrogen's effects and medication to stimulate ovulation. Most often, chlomiphene citrate, an antiestrogen, is used, with resultant fall in estrogen, rise in FSH, then ovulation. Corticosteroids, oral contraceptives, and/or spironolactone may be given to suppress androgen production, particularly if hirsutism is present. Wedge resection of the ovary, a surgical procedure, can also decrease hirsutism and improve fertility, but the effects of this procedure are transient. Approximately 40% of women with PCO can become pregnant with the proper medical management.

Premenstrual Syndrome

Premenstrual syndrome (PMS) is the cyclic recurrence (in the luteal phase of the menstrual cycle) of physical, psychologic, or behavioral changes distressing enough to impair interpersonal relationships or interfere with usual activities (Reid, 1985). The prevalence of PMS is difficult to determine. It has been estimated that 5% to 10% of menstruating women have severe to disabling premenstrual symptoms, and 30% to 40% have moderately distressing symptoms. A predisposition to PMS runs in families: 70% of PMS mothers have PMS daughters; 63% of non-PMS mothers have symptom-free daughters (Reid, 1985).

The etiology of PMS is unknown, but it is thought to involve cyclic fluctuations of ovarian hormone levels or fluctuations of endogenous opiate peptides and serum glucose levels. The pathophysiology of PMS is unclear at present.

Clinical Manifestations

The clinical manifestations of PMS have been categorized according to four patterns based on the time of onset and duration of symptoms (Fig. 20-2). Most women with PMS experience patterns A and B, in which symptoms occur during the luteal phase of the menstrual cycle (see Chapter 19). Pattern C is characterized by PMS symptoms at the time of ovulation and again during the luteal phase. Most severe is pattern D, in which PMS is absent only 1 week per month.

The most common manifestations of PMS are abdominal bloating, breast tenderness and swelling, and constipation. Abdominal bloating and breast swelling are apparently caused by local fluid shifts, since total

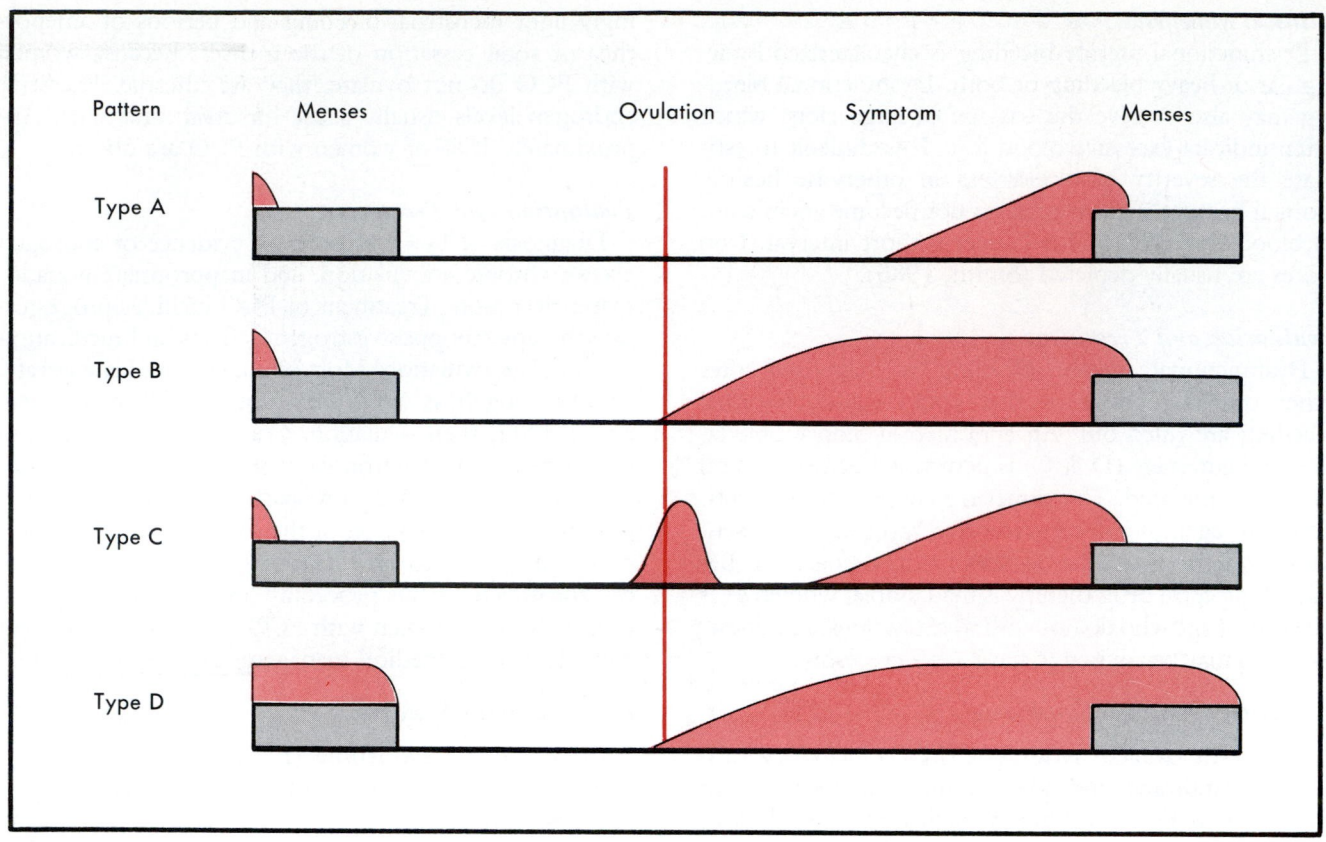

FIG. 20-2. Types of premenstrual syndrome (PMS) based on timing and duration of symptoms.

body weight does not generally change. Symptoms include an increase in appetite, fatigue, depression, and emotional lability. As the cycle progresses toward menstruation, anxiety and tension increase and may lead to physical unrest and irritability. In the final days of the cycle, tension, restlessness, inability to concentrate, and insomnia become extreme. Most women with PMS experience relief only after the second or third day of menstruation.

Evaluation and Treatment

Diagnosis of PMS is based on health history and symptoms. Research criteria for the diagnosis of PMS are presented in Table 20-1.

The current treatment for PMS is to relieve symptoms. Teaching the individual about the nature of the syndrome, counseling, stress-reduction techniques, and treatment of coexisting disorders are all recommended. Dietary changes, such as reduction of caffeine, alcohol, and sugar consumption and a switch from three large meals to several small meals each day, are sometimes beneficial. The effectiveness of these changes has not been proved, however. Drugs frequently prescribed include progesterone, vitamins, analgesics, antidepressants, magnesium, and tranquilizers. The efficacy of pro-

gesterone in the treatment of PMS has not been documented. Vitamin therapy, especially with megadoses, is not beneficial and may cause vitamin toxicity. Because the edema associated with PMS is a result of local fluid shifts rather than fluid retention, diuretics are not recommended (Reid, 1985). The effectiveness of narcotic antagonists and α-$_2$-adrenergic antagonists is currently being evaluated. Oophrectomy (ovary removal) may be considered in severe cases, but only for women who (1) do not wish to maintain fertility and (2) have experienced relief from symptoms after 3 months of pharmacologic suppression of ovulation and menstruation.

Infection and Inflammation

Infections of the genital tract may result from exogenous or endogenous microorganisms. Exogenous pathogens are most frequently sexually transmitted (see Chapter 21). Endogenous causes of infection include microorganisms that are normally resident in the vagina, bowel, or vulva. Infection occurs if these microorganisms migrate to a new location or overproliferate or if the immune system and other defense mechanisms are impaired.

A number of skin disorders can affect the vulva. They include reactive dermatitis, contact dermatitis, psoriasis,

TABLE 20-1 Research diagnostic criteria for PMS

Scale	Diagnostic criteria
A	Individual reports at least five of the following sets of symptoms for a definite diagnosis and four for a probable diagnosis during the current episode. Individual says she feels: 1. Irritable, hostile, angry, short-fused 2. Tense, restless, jittery, upset, high-strung, unable to relax 3. Less efficient than usual, fatigued 4. Dysphoric; experiences marked spontaneous, emotional lability, crying 5. Uncoordinated, clumsy, accident-prone 6. Distracted, confused, forgetful, unable to concentrate and exercise good judgment 7. A desire to change her eating habits (e.g., has cravings, overeats)
B	Overall disturbance is so severe that at least one of the following is true: 1. Individual experiences seriously impaired social interactions (e.g., with family, friends, co-workers) 2. Patient sought or was referred for medical help or took medication (especially tranquilizers and/or diuretics) at least once during a premenstrual episode
C	Premenstrual dysphoric symptoms have occurred for at least the 6 preceding menstrual cycles
D	Symptoms occur only during the premenstrual period, with relief soon after onset of menstruation

Adapted from Steiner, Haskett, Osmun, & Caroll, 1980.

and impetigo. (For a discussion of skin disorders, see Chapter 41.) Most infectious disorders that affect the vulva and vagina are sexually transmitted, however. These disorders are described in Chapter 21.

Pelvic Inflammatory Disease

Pelvic inflammatory disease (PID) is an acute inflammatory process caused by infection (Fig. 20-3). PID may involve any organ of the upper genital tract—the uterus, fallopian tubes, or ovaries—and, in its most severe form, the entire peritoneal cavity. (Infection of the fallopian tubes is termed **salpingitis** [Fig. 20-4]; infection of the ovaries is called **oophritis.**) Most cases of PID are caused by sexually transmitted microorganisms that migrate from the vagina to the uterus, fallopian tubes, and ovaries.

Pathophysiology

The development of upper genital infections is mediated by a number of defense mechanisms that are usually very effective in preventing PID (see Chapter 19). Virulence of the organism, size of the inoculum, and defense status of the individual all determine whether or not an infectious process results.

Clinical Manifestations

The clinical manifestations of PID vary from sudden, severe abdominal pain with fever to no symptoms at all.

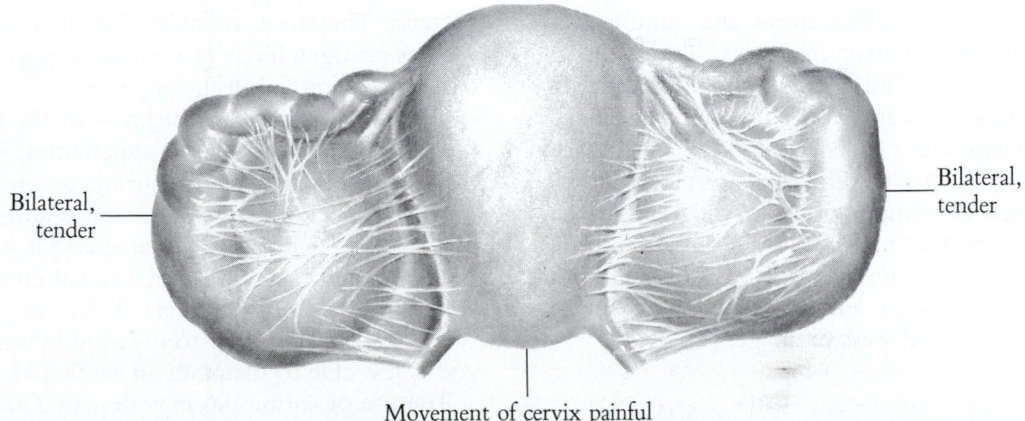

Bilateral, tender

Bilateral, tender

Movement of cervix painful

FIG. 20-3. Pelvic inflammatory disease. (From Seidel, Ball, Dains, & Benedict, 1987.)

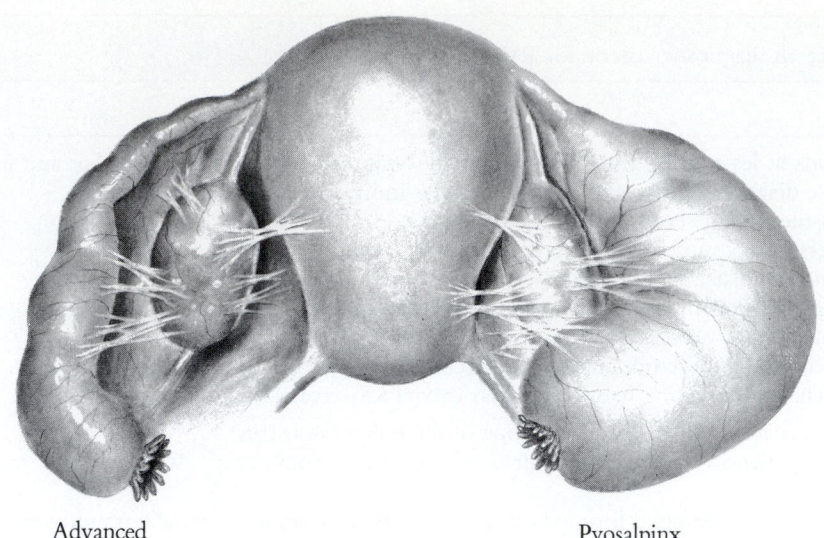

Advanced   Pyosalpinx

FIG. 20-4. Salpingitis. (From Seidel, Ball, Dains, & Benedict, 1987.)

A lower genital infection, such as vaginitis, may be present for some time before PID develops. The first sign of the ascending infection may be the onset of low bilateral abdominal pain, most often characterized as dull and gradual in onset. If the PID is caused by *Neisseria gonorrhoeae* (a sexually transmitted bacterium), the pain is often associated with menstrual bleeding. The pain of PID may worsen with intercourse. Other manifestations of PID include dysuria (difficult or painful urination) and vaginal discharge.

PID can lead to serious complications, including infertility. Infection that involves the entire peritoneal cavity can cause ileus (paralysis of the bowel). The mortality rate associated with PID is 8% to 9% of cases. Most deaths resulting from PID are caused by septic shock (cardiovascular shock brought on by infection of the blood; see Chapter 29).

Evaluation and Treatment

PID is difficult to diagnose on the basis of symptoms alone. Laparoscopy or culdocentesis and cultures may be necessary for a definitive diagnosis. Treatment involves rest, avoidance of intercourse, and administration of antibiotics. Common antibiotics used include penicillin G or ampicillin with probenecid followed by tetracycline or doxycycline plus cefoxitin. It it not known which antibiotics or combinations are most effective in preventing long-term complications, such as infertility. From 25% to 40% of women require hospitalization for IV administration of antibiotics, pelvic drainage, peritoneal lavage, and abscess drainage.

Vaginitis

Vaginitis is infection of the vagina. The major causes of vaginitis are sexually transmitted pathogens (see

Chapter 21) and *Candida albicans.* The incidence of sexually transmitted vaginitis is highest in young women. Susceptibility to vaginitis increases after menopause, however, because defense mechanisms mediated by ovarian hormones are somewhat compromised.

The development of vaginal infection is related to alterations in normal defense mechanisms of the vagina, particularly the vaginal pH and histologic characteristics of the vaginal epithelium. The pH of the vagina varies according to age and reproductive status, estrogen levels, and specific area of the vagina. Prior to puberty the vaginal pH is neutral. After puberty the pH falls to between 4.0 and 5.0. Variations in pH are associated with cyclic changes in estrogen levels: pH is lowest during the luteal phase of the menstrual cycle (between ovulation and the beginning of menstruation). After menopause pH rises to neutral or even alkaline values. Vaginal pH is lowest near the cervix. Vaginal pH is an important regulator of bacterial growth: pH of about 4.1 to 4.9 will not support the growth of most pathogenic bacteria. Therefore, variables that alter the vaginal pH, such as estrogen levels or even douching, can contribute to the onset of an infectious process.

The composition and thickness of the vaginal epithelium also determine defense capabilities. The thick vaginal epithelium that forms during pregnancy offers the most resistance to bacterial invasion and is best able to maintain an acidic pH. Premenarchal and postmenopausal females have the thin vaginal epithelium associated with low estrogen levels. A thin vaginal epithelium is a less effective barrier to invasion by infectious agents and is less able to maintain an acidic pH.

The use of antibiotics may destroy *Lactobacillus acidophilus,* an anaerobic, gram-positive rod normally found in the vagina that helps to maintain an acidic pH. In its absence alkalinity increases and vaginal infection may occur. Such infections are often caused by an overgrowth of organisms, such as *C. albicans,* that are normally found in the vagina.

Vaginitis is characterized by **leukorrhea,** a whitish, sticky discharge. The composition and copiousness of the discharge vary, depending on the cause of infection. Diagnosis is based on history, physical examination, and culture and examination of the discharge. Treatment involves developing and maintaining an acidic pH, relieving symptoms (usually pruritus), and administering antibiotics to eradicate the infectious organism.

Cervicitis

Cervicitis is an inflammation of the cervix. **Mucopurulent cervicitis,** formerly called acute cervicitis, is usually caused by a sexually transmitted pathogen or fungus, such as *C. albicans*. Infection causes the cervix to become red and edematous. A mucopurulent (mucus- and pus-containing) exudate drains from the external cervical os, and the individual may report vague pelvic pain. The infectious organisms are cultured or identified by immunoassay. Definitive diagnosis is followed by oral antibiotic therapy.

Chronic cervicitis is persistent infection and inflammation of the cervix. Long-term inflammation can result in scarring or metaplasia. If local or systemic antibiotics do not eradicate the infection, cautery or cryotherapy may be tried.

Vulvitis

Inflammation of the vulva is termed **vulvitis.** Acute vulvitis is an inflammation of the skin (dermatitis) of the vulva and often of the perianal area. Vulvitis can be caused by contact with soaps, detergents, lotions, hygienic sprays, or perfumed toilet paper or to nonabsorbent or tight-fitting clothes. Vulvitis is also caused by vaginal infections (e.g., candidiasis) that spread to the labia, where they cause inflammation and edema. Other skin diseases, such as tinea cruris, psoriasis, and inflammation of the apocrine (sweat) glands can involve the vulva (see Chapter 41).

Avoidance of irritants; wearing of loose, cotton clothing; and antibiotics are usually effective cures for acute vulvitis. Chronic vulvitis is usually treated with fluorinated hydrocortisone. Biopsy specimens of persistent lesions are examined for the presence of malignancy.

Bartholinitis

Bartholinitis, or Bartholin cyst, is an inflammation of one or both of the ducts that lead from the introitus (vaginal opening) to Bartholin glands (Fig. 20-5). The usual causes of bartholinitis are microorganisms that infect the lower female reproductive tract, such as streptococci, staphylococci, and sexually transmitted patho-

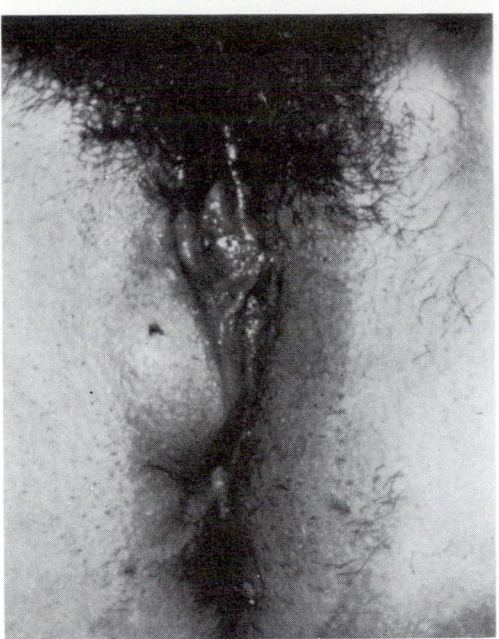

FIG. 20-5. Inflammation of Bartholin glands. (From Gardner & Kaufman, 1969.)

gens. Acute bartholinitis is usually preceded by an infection, such as cervicitis, vaginitis, or urethritis.

Infection or trauma causes inflammatory changes that narrow the distal portion of the duct, leading to obstruction and stasis of glandular secretions. The obstruction, or cyst, varies from 1 to 8 cm in diameter and is located in the posterolateral portion of the vulva. The cyst is usually reddened and painful, and pus may be visible at the opening of the duct. The individual may have symptoms of the initiating infection, fever, and malaise.

Most Bartholin cysts are asymptomatic and require no treatment. Chronic bartholinitis is characterized by the presence of a small cyst that is slightly tender but otherwise is asymptomatic. Symptoms occur if an exacerbation of infection causes an abscess to form in the gland itself.

Diagnosis of bartholinitis is based on the clinical manifestations and the identification of infectious microorganisms. Antibiotics are given to treat infection, and pain is relieved with analgesics and warm sitz baths. If an abscess forms, it is surgically drained.

Pelvic Relaxation Disorders

The bladder, urethra, and rectum are supported by the endopelvic fascia and the perineal muscles. This muscular and fascial tissue loses tone and strength with aging and may fail to maintain the pelvic organs in the proper position. Progressive relaxation of the pelvic support structures may cause uterine displacement. Uterine displacement can also result if trauma, such as

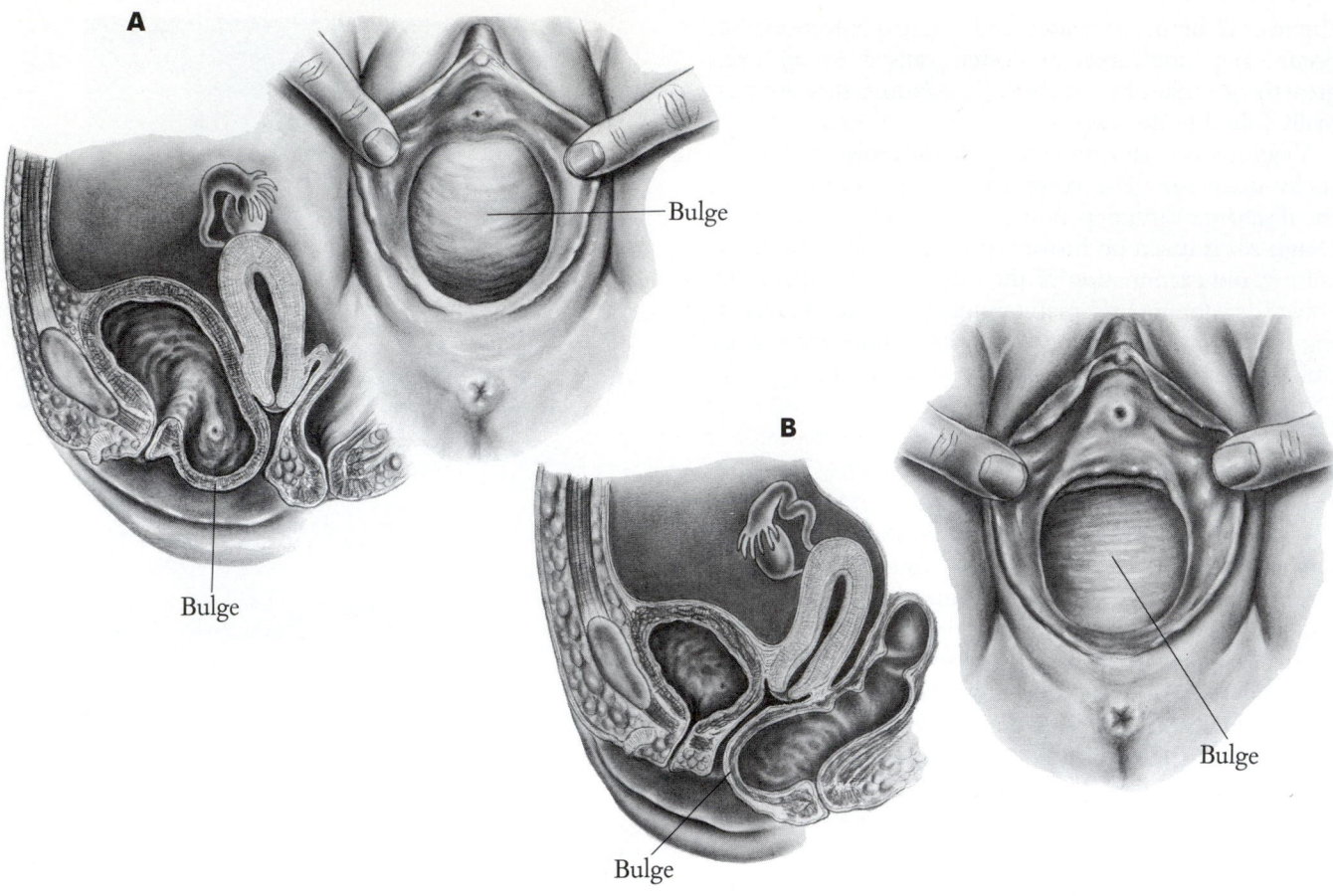

FIG. 20-6. **A,** Cystocele, **B,** Rectocele. (From Seidel, Ball, Dains, & Benedict, 1987.)

TABLE 20-2 Cystocele, urethrocele, and rectocele

Condition	Etiology	Symptoms	Treatment
Cystocele	Laceration, stretching, or weakening of supporting fascial tissue; usually caused by prolonged labor, multiple births, or birth of a large baby	Urinary frequency, urgency, and occasional incontinence Difficulty in complete emptying of the bladder Low backache Symptoms become problematic pre- or postmenopausally	Depending on age of woman and severity of the condition, includes: Isometric exercise to strengthen the pubococcygeal muscle Oral or topical estrogen to improve tone and vascularity of fascial support Pessary, a removable device that holds the bladder in position Surgical correction
Urethrocele	Pressure of fetal head on urethra and attachments beneath the symphysis pubis	Asymptomatic, unless it occurs in conjunction with cystocele	Isometric exercises (see Cystocele)
Rectocele	Trauma to the fascia and levator muscles; usually caused by childbirth	Constipation or feeling of rectal fullness Difficult defecation Pressure and sensation of fullness in the vagina	Isometric exercises Diet counseling to prevent constipation Stool softeners or laxatives Surgery

childbirth or pelvic surgery, damages or weakens the supporting structures. Pelvic relaxation is progressive. Malpositioning of the bladder, urethra, or rectum (and hence the uterus) may occur many years after an initial injury to the supporting structure.

Fig. 20-6 shows vaginal prolapse caused by cystocele, rectocele, and enterocele. **Cystocele** is descent of the bladder and the anterior vaginal wall into the vaginal canal. In severe cases the bladder and anterior vaginal wall bulge outside the introitus. A cystocele may cause the woman to lose urine when she laughs, sneezes, coughs, or does anything that strains the abdominal muscles. Cystocele is usually accompanied by **urethrocele,** or sagging of the urethra. Urethrocele is usually caused by the shearing effect of the fetal head on the urethra dur-

ing childbirth. A **rectocele** is the bulging of the rectum and posterior vaginal wall into the vaginal canal. If this condition is severe, defecation is difficult and can only be accomplished by applying manual pressure to the posterior vaginal wall. An enterocele is herniation of the rectouterine pouch into the rectovaginal septum (between the rectum and posterior vaginal wall). It is usually associated with other pelvic relaxation disorders such as uterine prolapse, cystocele, and rectocele. Table 20-2 summarizes the etiology, symptoms, and treatment of cystocele, urethrocele, and rectocele.

Uterine prolapse is descent of the cervix or entire uterus into the vaginal canal (Fig. 20-7). In severe cases the uterus falls completely through the vagina and protrudes from the introitus. First-degree uterine prolapse

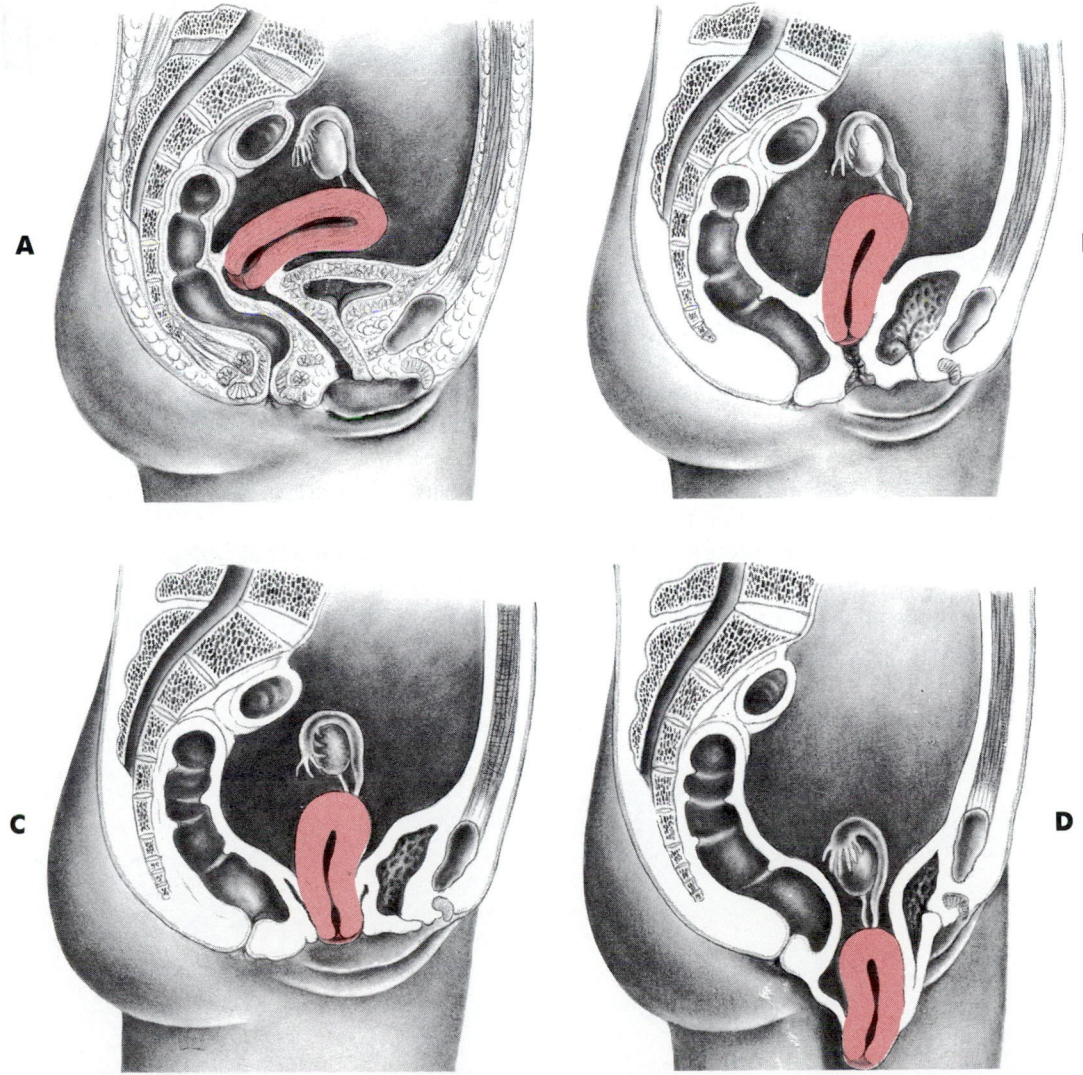

FIG. 20-7. Degrees of uterine prolapse. **A,** Normal uterus. **B,** First-degree prolapse: descent within the vagina. **C,** Second-degree prolapse: the cervix protrudes through the introitus. **D,** Third-degree prolapse: the vagina is completely everted. (From Seidel, Ball, Dains, & Benedict, 1987.)

is not treated unless it causes discomfort. Second- and third-degree prolapse cause feelings of fullness, heaviness, and collapse through the vagina. Symptoms of other pelvic relaxation disorders may also be present. Treatment in these cases is the insertion of a **pessary,** which is a removable mechanical device that holds the uterus in position. The pelvic fascia may be strengthened by a course of estrogen therapy, particularly if the woman is past menopause. Surgical repair is the treatment of last resort.

Benign Growths and Proliferative Conditions
Benign Ovarian Cysts

Benign cysts of the ovary may occur at any time during the life span but are most common between puberty and menopause (Fig. 20-8). Two common causes of benign ovarian enlargement in ovulating women are follicular cysts and corpus luteum cysts. These cysts are called functional cysts because they are caused by pathologic variations of normal physiologic events. Follicular and corpus luteum cysts are unilateral. They are typically 5 to 6 cm in diameter but can grow as large as 8 to 10 cm.

A **follicular cyst** develops from a dominant ovarian follicle that does not release its ovum but remains active or from a degenerating follicle whose fluid is not reabsorbed. Most follicular cysts are not symptomatic, require no treatment, and either regress or rupture spontaneously within 60 days. A large follicular cyst may cause low back pain, painful intercourse (dyspareunia), chronic lower abdominal pain, and menstrual irregularities.

A **corpus luteum cyst** develops if a mature corpus luteum persists abnormally and continues to secrete progesterone. The cyst consists of blood and/or fluid that accumulates in the cavity of the corpus luteum. Corpus luteum cysts are less common than follicular cysts, but luteal cysts typically cause more symptoms, particularly if they rupture. Manifestations include dull pelvic pain and amenorrhea or delayed menstruation, followed by irregular or heavier-than-normal bleeding. Rupture can cause massive bleeding and require immediate surgery. Corpus luteum cysts usually regress spontaneously, however, within 2 months in nonpregnant women.

Endometrial Polyps

Endometrial polyps are overgrowths of endometrial tissue. These polyps usually arise from the uterine fundus and vary tremendously in size. They develop most often in women between the ages of 40 and 49 but have been found in individuals from 12 to 81 years of age. The etiology of endometrial polyps is unknown. Since they are commonly seen during the years preceding menopause, hormonal alterations may be involved. During these years estrogen levels are higher than progesterone levels throughout the menstrual cycle, an imbalance that contributes to endometrial hyperplasia in general. The hormonal environment that supports endometrial hyperplasia may also facilitate the development of uterine polyps.

An endometrial polyp consists of stromal tissue covered by a layer of columnar epithelial cells. Approximately one third of these polyps is composed of mature, functional endometrial tissue that responds to hormonal fluctuations. The other two thirds are composed of immature endometrium that does not respond to hormonal changes. Fewer than 1% of endometrial polyps are thought to become malignant.

Most endometrial polyps do not produce signs or symptoms. Clinical manifestations that do occur consist of abdominal bleeding, spotting between periods, or excessive menstrual bleeding. Asymptomatic polyps are found on D & C or hysterectomy performed for other reasons.

Suspected endometrial polyps are diagnosed by D & C. Treatment involves surgical removal of the polyp. The base of the polyp must be scraped during D & C. If this is not possible, hysterectomy is recommended.

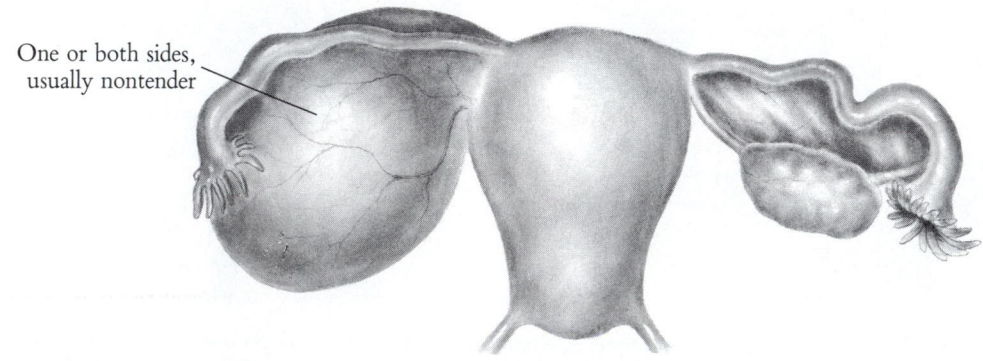

One or both sides, usually nontender

FIG. 20-8. Ovarian cyst. (From Seidel, Ball, Dains, & Benedict, 1987.)

Leiomyomas

Leiomyomas, commonly called uterine fibroids, are benign tumors that develop from smooth muscle cells in the myometrium. Leiomyomas are the most common benign tumors of the uterus. One fifth of all women over the age of 35 years have a uterine leiomyoma. The incidence of leiomyomas in black and oriental females is two to five times higher than that in white females. Uterine leiomyomas are not seen prior to menarche, and those that develop during the reproductive years generally decrease in size after menopause.

The etiology of uterine leiomyomas is unknown, although their size appears to be related to hormonal fluctuations. Tumors in pregnant women and those taking oral contraceptives often enlarge rapidly. These tumors decrease in size on withdrawal of the oral contraceptive or termination of the pregnancy.

Pathophysiology

Most leiomyomas occur in multiples in the fundus of the uterus, although they may occur singly and throughout the uterus. Leiomyomas are classified as subserous, submucous, or intramural, according to their location within the various layers of the uterine wall (Fig. 20-9). Uterine leiomyomas are usually firm and surrounded by a pseudocapsule composed of com-

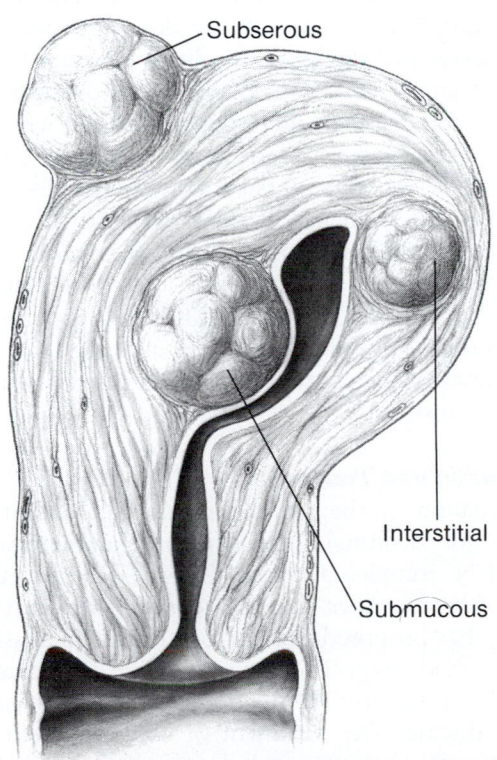

FIG. 20-9. Uterine section showing whorl-like appearance and locations of leiomyomas, which are also called uterine fibroids. (From Droegemueller, Herbst, Mischell, & Stenehever, 1987.)

pressed but otherwise normal uterine myometrium. Degenerative changes may occur when the leiomyoma outgrows its blood supply; therefore, degeneration is more common in larger tumors.

Clinical Manifestations

The major clinical manifestations of leiomyomas are abnormal uterine bleeding, pain, and symptoms related to pressure on nearby structures. The leiomyoma tends to make the uterine cavity larger, thereby increasing the endometrial surface area. This increase may account for the increased menstrual bleeding that is associated with leiomyomas. Pain is not an early symptom but tends to occur with the devascularization of larger leiomyomas. It is also associated with blood vessel compression that limits blood supply to adjacent structures. Symptoms of abdominal pressure are slow to develop, apparently because the tumor is relatively slow-growing, enabling adjacent structures to adapt to pressure. Pressure on the bladder may contribute to urinary frequency, urgency, and dysuria. Pressure on the ureter may cause it to become distended "upstream" from the pressure point; rectosigmoid pressure may lead to constipation. A sensation of abdominal or genital heaviness may be felt with larger tumors.

Evaluation and Treatment

Uterine leiomyomas are diagnosed by physical examination. The bimanual examination reveals irregular, nontender nodularity of the uterus. Treatment depends upon the symptoms, tumor size, age, reproductive status, and overall health of the individual. Oral contraceptives are usually discontinued, and the individual is examined at regular intervals to make sure the leiomyomas are not growing rapidly. Myomectomy may be undertaken, especially in women who wish to preserve fertility. Hysterectomy is recommended for women who have severe symptoms or who have an extremely large leiomyoma.

Endometriosis

Endometriosis is the presence of functioning endometrial tissue or implants outside the uterus. Like normal endometrial tissue, the ectopic (out-of-place) endometrium responds to the hormonal fluctuations of the menstrual cycle.

The incidence of endometriosis is difficult to determine, particularly in asymptomatic fertile women and adolescents. Up to 50% of women evaluated for pelvic pain, infertility, or a pelvic mass are diagnosed as having endometriosis.

The etiology of endometriosis is not known, but several theories have been proposed. In 1927 J. A. Sampson proposed that endometriosis is caused by the implantation of endometrial cells during **retrograde men-**

struation, in which menstrual fluids move through the fallopian tubes and empty into the pelvic cavity. It is now known that retrograde menstruation occurs in almost all women; however, not all women develop endometriosis.

Another theory is that women with endometriosis have a slightly depressed cytotoxic T cell response to endometrial cells or some other defect of the immune response. These alterations may cause the body to tolerate ectopic implantation of endometrial cells. Researchers have also proposed that endometrial cells spread through the lymphatic system or that multipotential cells in the epithelial coverings of reproductive organs are stimulated somehow to develop into endometrial cells. A genetic predisposition to endometriosis has been documented. Studies show that incidence and severity of disease are greatest among women with female relatives who also have endometriosis.

Pathophysiology

Endometrial implants can occur throughout the body. The most common sites of implantation are the ovaries, uterine ligaments, rectovaginal septum, and pelvic peritoneum (Fig. 20-10). Other sites of implantation are the sigmoid colon, small intestine, rectum, appendix, bladder, uterus, vulva, vagina, cervix, lymph nodes, extremities, pleural cavity, lungs, laparotomy scars, and hernial sacs.

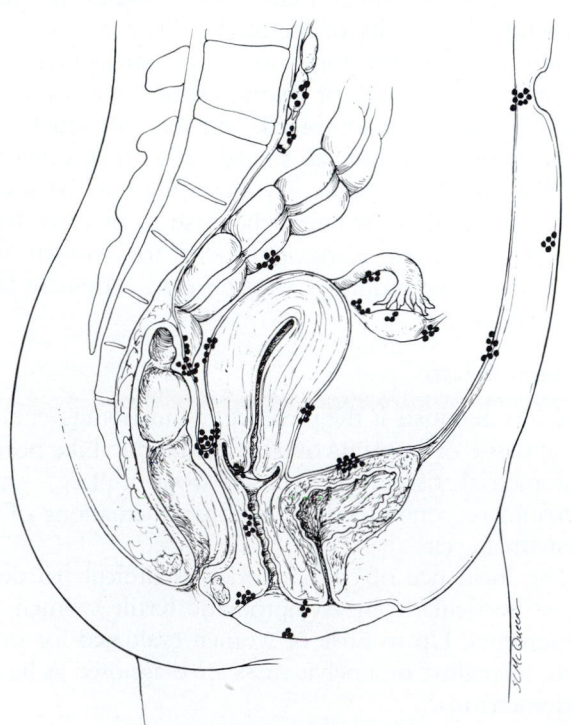

FIG. 20-10. Pelvic sites of endometrial implantation. Endometrial cells may enter the pelvic cavity during retrograde menstruation. (From Droegemeuller, Herbst, Mischell, & Stenehever, 1987.)

Cyclic changes depend on the blood supply of the implants. Given that blood supply is sufficient, the ectopic endometrium proliferates, breaks down, and bleeds in conjunction with the normal menstrual cycle. The bleeding causes inflammation and pain in surrounding tissues. The inflammation may lead to fibrosis, scarring, and adhesions.

Clinical Manifestations

The clinical manifestations of endometriosis include infertility; abnormal vaginal bleeding, dysmenorrhea, dyschezia (pain on defecation); constipation; dyspareunia (pain on intercourse); and, if implants are located within the pelvis, asymptomatic pelvic mass having irregular, movable nodules and a fixed, retroverted uterus. Most symptoms of endometriosis can be explained by the proliferation, breakdown, and bleeding of the ectopic endometrial tissue, with subsequent formation of adhesions. In many instances, however, the degree of endometriosis is not related to the frequency or severity of symptoms. Dysmenorrhea, for example, does not appear to be related to the degree of endometriosis. With involvement of the rectovaginal septum or the uterosacral ligaments, dyspareunia develops. Dyschezia occurs with bleeding of ectopic endometrium in the rectosigmoid musculature and subsequent fibrosis.

Approximately 30% to 40% of individuals with endometriosis are infertile. The link between endometriosis and infertility is not clear, but it does not appear to involve severity of disease. Infertility may result from mechanical interference with ovulation or ovum transport through the fallopian tube, but mechanical interference is an unlikely cause of infertility in women with mild endometriosis. Another possible cause is phagocytosis of sperm by macrophages in the reproductive tract. It is known that endometriosis causes macrophages in the peritoneal fluid to become more aggressive phagocytes ("eater cells"; see Chapter 7). These macrophages have been found in the fallopian tubes and may account for some cases of infertility, especially in women with mild endometriosis.

Evaluation and Treatment

Evaluation of the pelvis through laparoscopy is required for definitive diagnosis of endometriosis and should be completed before therapy is begun. On the basis of the extent of the disease, the American Fertility Society has proposed that endometriosis be classified as stage I, mild; stage II, moderate; stage III, severe; and stage IV, extensive. All treatment is based on the stage of the disease. The treatment of mild endometriosis is controversial and may include use of danazol, laparoscopic removal of endometrial implants, or both. Moderate endometriosis usually is treated surgically; surgery may include removal of all abdominal implants, resection of the uterosacral ligaments, uterine suspension, and, if dysmenorrhea is a problem, presacral neurectomy. If severe endometriosis is present, ablative or reconstructive surgery may be performed. If the woman's family is complete and moderate to severe disease is present, a complete abdominal hysterectomy may be performed.

Cancer

Malignant tumors of the female reproductive system are common. Endometrial carcinoma accounts for 7% of all cancers in women; ovarian tumors, 5%; cervical tumors, 6%; and other malignant tumors, 1% to 3% (American Cancer Society, 1989; Knapp, 1986). The malignant neoplasms of the female reproductive tract account for about 1 of 6 diagnosed cancers and 1 of 10 cancer deaths in women in the United States (Knapp, 1986).

Cervical Cancer

Cervical cancer affects 1 of every 63 newborn females in the United States. Women who are 40 to 49 years of age are most frequently affected. However, the number of new cases of cervical cancer occurring in women under 35 years of age has increased from 9% to nearly 25% of the total (Elliott et al., 1989). In addition, the increase in incidence has been the result of an unusual histologic type that is likely to metastasize more frequently in young women today compared with a couple of decades ago (Elliott et al., 1989). Young age at first coitus, large number of sex partners, infection with certain sexually transmitted viruses, and frequent intercourse with men whose previous partners have had cervical cancer are all associated with increased risk of developing cervical cancer. Of these risk factors it appears that young age at first coitus is the most important predictor. Recently researchers have documented an association between cervical cancer and cigarette smoking or exposure to "sidestream" smoke (Layde, 1989; Slattry et al., 1989).

Oral contraceptives are apparently a risk factor for carcinoma in situ and invasive cancer of the cervix. A recent study by Beral and coworkers showed that pill users had an excess incidence of genital cancers of 37 per 100,000 women-years, primarily carcinoma in situ (Beral, Hannaford, & Clifford, 1988). Incidence rates of cervical cancer increased steadily with increasing duration of pill use. Beral found that women who had used the pill for more than 10 years had more than four times the incidence of cervical cancer of those who had never used it.

Pathogenesis

There are several theories concerning the cause of cervical cell transformation. Most involve more than one mechanism. For example, the herpes simplex virus may initiate a multistage process leading to epithelial neoplasia, but additional unidentified factors probably are required for epithelial neoplasia to progress to invasive carcinoma (carcinoma that invades tissues beneath the epithelial layer).

A second group of theories proposes sperm as the causative agent. Semen may contain mutant sperm, whose mutant DNA may be incorporated into a cervical epithelial cell genome, leading to cellular neoplasia. It has also been suggested that exposure of cervical cells to particular concentrations of amino acids found in sperm heads, especially high levels of protamine, may cause cellular alterations that predispose cervical cells to neoplastic changes. In animals the exposure of cervical cells to chemical carcinogens has resulted in neoplastic changes; however, this development has not been demonstrated in humans.

The progressive changes of cervical cells are classified as (1) cervical intraepithelial neoplasia, (2) cervical carcinoma in situ, and (3) invasive carcinoma. **Cervical intraepithelial neoplasia** (CIN), commonly called cervical dysplasia, is replacement of some epithelial cells by atypical, neoplastic cells. CIN is graded as mild (CIN 1), moderate (CIN 2), or severe (CIN 3), depending on the depth of epithelial involvement (Fig. 20-11).

In **cervical carcinoma in situ** all or most of the cervical epithelium shows cellular features of carcinoma, but underlying tissue is not affected. Women with CIN 1 and 2 are not at risk for development of carcinoma in situ, but the incidence of progression is not known, and there are no reliable predictors to indicate which cases of CIN 1 and 2 will spontaneously regress and which will progress to carcinoma in situ.

Carcinoma in situ is most likely to develop in the squamous-columnar junction—the so-called transformation zone—where the columnar epithelium of the cervical lining meets the squamous epithelium of the outer cervix and vagina (Fig. 20-12). In this zone columnar epithelium is constantly being replaced by squamous epithelium in a process known as metaplasia. Metaplasia is pronounced during fetal and neonatal life, in early adolescence, and during a first pregnancy. Metaplasia seems to be stimulated by the difference in pH between the endocervical canal, where pH is 8.5, and the vagina, where pH is 4 to 6.8. Because metaplastic cells are at increased risk of incorporating foreign or abnormal genetic material, neoplastic changes are most common in the transformation zone.

The spontaneous regression of carcinoma in situ is extremely rare. Carcinoma in situ is generally a precursor of invasive carcinoma of the cervix. A number of factors, including tumor type, contribute to the rate at which carcinoma in situ becomes invasive. Invasive carcinoma of the cervix consists of direct invasion into adjacent tis-

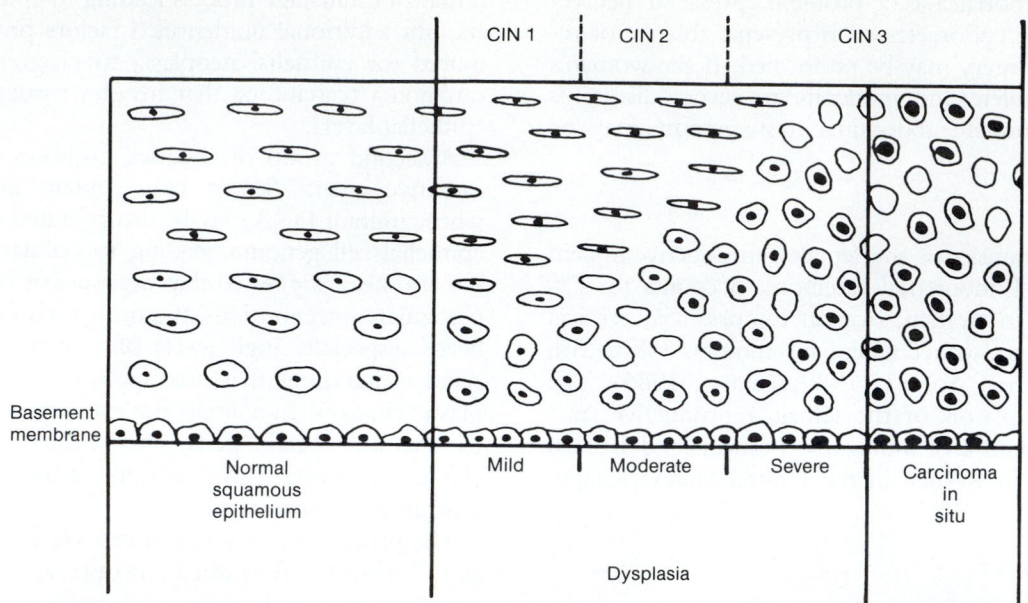

FIG. 20-11. Diagram of cervical endothelium showing progressive degrees of cervical intraepithelial neoplasia (CIN). (From Droegemeuller, Herbst, Mischell, & Stenehever, 1987.)

TABLE 20-3 FIGO* staging of carcinoma of the cervix

Stage		Characteristics
I		Carcinoma is strictly confined to cervix (extension to corpus disregarded)
	IA	Preclinical carcinoma
	IA1	Minimal microscopically evident stromal invasion
	IA2	Microscopic lesions no more than 5 mm depth measured from base of epithelium, either surface or glandular, from which it originates, and horizontal spread not to exceed 7 mm
	IB	All other cases of stage I; occult cancer is marked "occ"
II		Carcinoma extends beyond cervix but has not extended to pelvic wall; it involves vagina, but not as far as lower third
	IIA	No obvious parametrial involvement
	IIB	Obvious parametrial involvement
III		Carcinoma has extended to pelvic wall; rectal examination reveals no cancer-free space between tumor and pelvic wall; tumor involves lower third of vagina; all cases with hydronephrosis or nonfunctioning kidney are included, unless they are known to have another cause
	IIIA	No extension to pelvic wall, but involvement of lower third of vagina
	IIIB	Extension to pelvic wall or hydronephrosis or nonfunctioning kidney caused by tumor
IV		Carcinoma has extended beyond true pelvis or has clinically involved mucosa of bladder or rectum
	IVA	Spread of growth to adjacent pelvic organs
	IVB	Spread to distant organs

From Droegemeuller, Herbst, Mischell, & Stenehever, 1987.
*The International Federation of Gynecologists and Obstetricians.

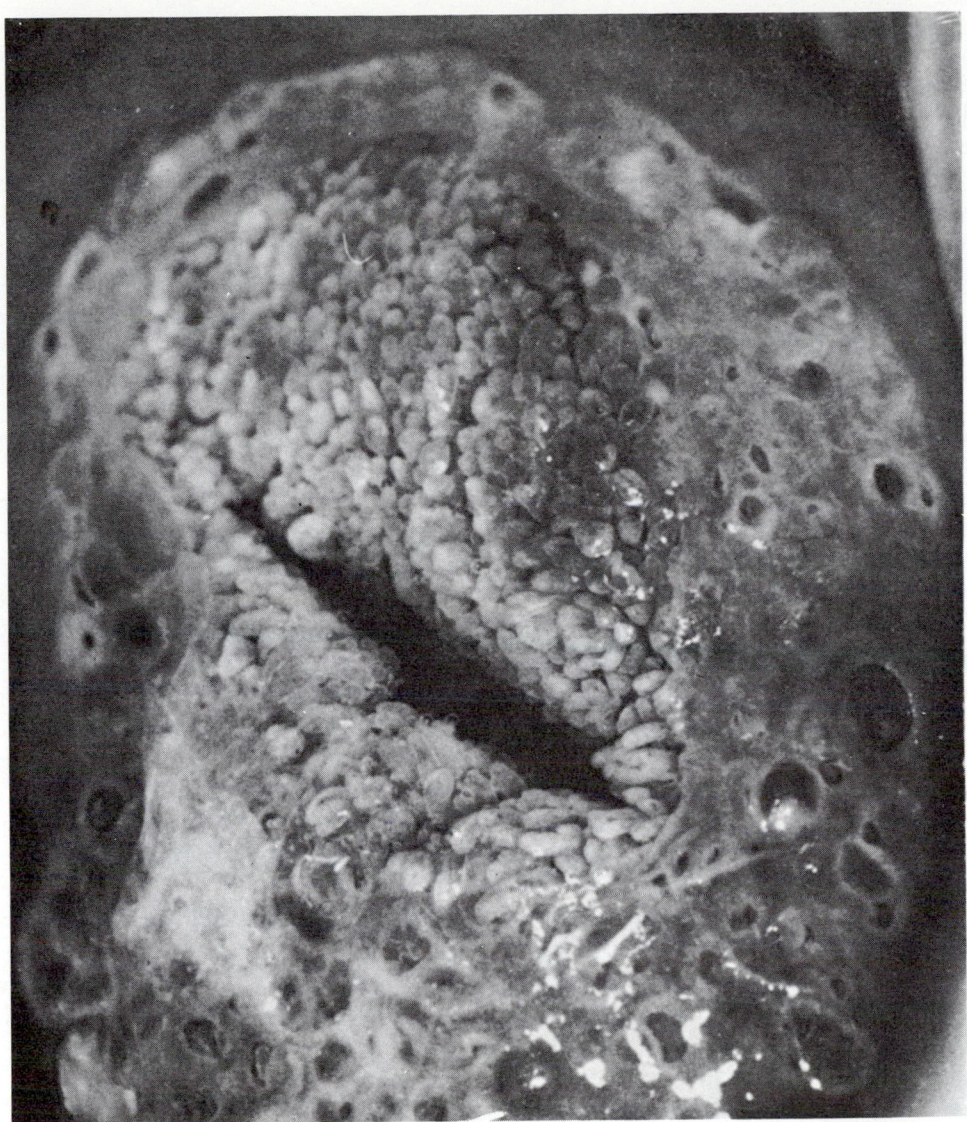

FIG. 20-12. Typical transformation zone, where the columnar (grapelike) epithelium is replaced by metaplastic epithelium. At its outer edge, the metaplastic epithelium adjoins the squamous epithelium, which extends into the vagina. (From Coppleson, Pixley, & Reed, 1971, and Droegemueller, Herbst, Mischell, & Stenehever, 1987.)

sues and metastasis (spread of cancer cells) through the lymphatics. Adjacent tissues most often involved are the ureters and structures of the lateral pelvic wall, the vaginal stroma and epithelium, and the lower uterine segment and myometrium. The internal, external, and common iliac lymph nodes and the obturator nodes are common sites of lymphatic involvement. A staging system for carcinoma of the cervix is set forth in Table 20-3.

Clinical Manifestations

Because cervical neoplasms are asymptomatic, regular cytologic screening (Papanicolaou smear) is necessary. Early signs of cervical cancer can include abnormally long menstrual periods, slight but constant watery discharge, and spotting after physical exertion, intercourse, or travel (del Regato, Spjut, & Cox, 1985). Bleeding and discharge are likely to be disregarded by premenopausal women, who mistake these signs for variations of normal processes. Postmenopausal women are more likely to seek medical attention if these signs appear. Some women feel a dull lower back ache preceding menstrual periods. Signs of advanced disease include vaginal bleeding, yellow vaginal discharge, and pain that extends from the lower back through the hip and into the thigh. Urinary symptoms are variable and may result from inflammation or tumor invasion. Signs of late disease include weight loss and anemia.

Evaluation and Treatment

Cervical cytology is most accurate if cells obtained by endocervical swabbing and ectocervical scraping are examined. Self-collected specimens from vaginal irrigations provide very little information regarding cervical pathology. Cervical biopsy and endocervical curettage are required, and histologic confirmation of the tumor and colposcopy are extremely useful in identifying sites that should be biopsied. The transformation zone moves higher into the cervix as age increases, making biopsy more difficult. If invasive carcinoma is found, lymphangiography, computed tomography (CT) scan, ultrasonography, or radioimmunodetection methods are used to assess lymphatic involvement.

The treatment depends on the degree of neoplastic change, the size and location of the lesion, and the extent of metastatic spread. For CIN 1 and 2 and carcinoma in situ, a cervical conization may be performed. The amount of tissue removed depends on the location of the lesion. Cryotherapy, electrocautery, and carbon dioxide laser surgery may also be used to eradicate neoplastic endothelium. None of these measures affects fertility or childbearing. If fertility is not desired, a hysterectomy may be performed.

For invasive cervical carcinoma treatment depends on the stage of the tumor (see Table 20-3). Surgical intervention may include a hysterectomy, pelvic lymphadenectomy, and pelvic exoneration. Radiation therapy is used most frequently in cases of small cell cancer with lymphatic involvement. External radiation is usually combined with use of one or two intracavity implants. Multidrug chemotherapy regimens have also been used. Approximately 50% of individuals with invasive cervical carcinoma have a recurrence within the first year, and 75% have a recurrence within 2 years. However, the recurrence rate is only 5% 5 years after the first occurrence.

Vaginal Cancer

Cancer of the vagina is the rarest of the female genital cancers. It is found predominantly in women 70 years of age and older. Over 90% of women with vaginal cancer have squamous cell carcinoma, although melanomas, sarcomas, and adenocarcinomas are also seen. (Types of tumors are described in Chapter 10.)

Exposure to nonsteroidal estrogens in utero, exposure to herpes simplex virus or papillomavirus, chronic irritation from use of a pessary, and ionizing radiation received as treatment for uterine or cervical cancer have all been implicated as causes of malignant transformation in the vagina. It has been estimated that 100,000 to 160,000 women were exposed in utero to such nonsteroidal estrogens as diethylstilbestrol (DES), dienestrol, or hexestrol from 1960 to 1970. Apparently exposure to such hormones during the first 3 months of gestation

inhibits the normal replacement of columnar epithelium by squamous epithelium in the vagina of the fetus. The columnar epithelium, which is not normally found in the vagina, may then undergo malignant transformation. Not all women exposed to DES in utero develop neoplastic changes in the vagina, however. Between 0.14 and 1.4 cases of vaginal cancer develop per 1000 women at risk. Nineteen is the average age at which clear cell carcinoma develops as a result of DES exposure.

Like cervical neoplasms, vaginal cancers are classified as intraepithelial neoplasia (dysplasia), carcinoma in situ, or invasive carcinoma. The lesion is usually not invasive, and it most frequently occurs in the upper third of the vagina.

Vaginal cancer is generally asymptomatic. Therefore, regular pelvic examinations, particularly for those exposed to DES in utero, are extremely important. Clinical manifestations that do occur include abnormal vaginal bleeding or discharge and urinary symptoms. Pain is a symptom of advanced disease.

Biopsy techniques confirm the tumor type and determine its size, location, and extent. Treatment depends on these findings and on the age of the individual. Vaginal dysplasia or carcinoma in situ is excised by using standard surgical techniques, cryotherapy, or laser surgery. Topical 5-fluorouracil (5-FU) may also be used. If the lesion is invasive, surgery may include hysterectomy, vaginectomy, and pelvic bilateral inguinal lymphadenectomy. Radiation and chemotherapy may follow surgery. Approximately 40% of individuals with invasive vaginal cancer develop recurrent cancer, which is usually confined to the pelvic area.

Endometrial Cancer

The incidence of endometrial cancer has increased since the 1960s. Approximately 1 of every 45 newborn females will develop invasive cancer of the endometrium during their lifetime. It most frequently affects women between the ages of 50 and 64, with the average and most frequently affected age being 61 years.

Although the etiology of endometrial cancer is not clear, a number of risk factors have been identified. They include overnutrition, particularly excessive carbohydrate and fat intake; decreased glucose tolerance; hypertension; nulliparity; early menarche; habitual abortion; and indicators of hyperestrogenism, such as dysfunctional uterine bleeding, anovulation, and prolonged amenorrhea. Postmenopausal women who have endometrial hyperplasia secondary to estrogen replacement therapy or to estrogens produced by a feminizing ovarian tumor are particularly at risk for the development of endometrial carcinoma. Overall, exposure to estrogen without progesterone is associated with 1.4 times the risk of endometrial cancer (Persson et al., 1989). Certain types of estrogen are associated with a higher risk: for more than 3 years estradiol compounds or conjugated estrogens alone had double to triple the risk. These findings strongly suggest that progesterone decreases the risk of endometrial cancer and should be used in conjunction with estrogen (i.e., hormone replacement therapy instead of estrogen replacement therapy) (Persson et al., 1989). Autosomal dominant inheritance may increase susceptibility to endometrial cancer, perhaps through an HLA phenotype. The incidence of endometrial carcinoma is low among Japanese women and high among those of Jewish descent. It is not known whether susceptibility is based on race or reflects life-style and dietary patterns. Women with a history of endometrial polyps or leiomyomas are also at increased risk.

Approximately 95% of endometrial cancers are adenocarcinomas. About three fourths are local lesions. Abnormal vaginal bleeding is the only clinical manifestation of endometrial cancer. The bleeding is caused by disruption of the endometrial surface by neoplastic processes.

Screening methods for the early detection of endometrial cancer are as effective as those for cervical cancer. Direct cytologic sampling of the endometrium is required for diagnosis. This may be accomplished by endometrial biopsy or fractional curettage that includes biopsies of all sectors of the uterus. Hysteroscopy and hysterography may also be used to examine the endometrium, but these methods may result in uterine perforation or enhancement of tumor cell migration if disease is advanced. Evaluation for metastasis includes routine blood work, metabolic studies, chest x-ray films, intravenous pyelography (IVP), barium enema, ultrasonography, and lymphangiography.

Treatment is based on the extent of the disease and includes surgical removal of the obvious tumor and radiation for control of residual microscopic disease. Surgical interventions may include curettage for carcinoma in situ, total abdominal hysterectomy with bilateral salpingo-oophrectomy, and lymphadenectomy. Chemotherapy may also be used. Progesterone may benefit individuals with advanced or recurrent disease. Multidrug protocols are currently under investigation because the results of single-drug therapy for endometrial cancer have been disappointing.

Ovarian Cancer

Cancer of the ovaries is the sixth most frequent cancer in women. The ovary is the site of a greater histologic variety of tumors than any other organ in the body. Ovarian cancer accounts for 5% of all female cancer deaths and causes more deaths than any other cancer of the female reproductive system (American Cancer Society, 1989). The incidence of ovarian cancer is highest in industrialized countries. In the United States white women are at greatest risk for the development of ovarian cancer; the risk for Japanese, Chinese, Hispanic, and black women is 19% to 42% lower.

Pathogenesis

The etiology of ovarian cancer is unknown at present. The risk of disease is greatest for women who have not borne children, have borne few children, are married but have never been pregnant, have undergone estrogen replacement therapy after menopause, smoke, or have been exposed to asbestos and talc. Dietary factors, such as caffeine, alcohol, iodine, and fat intake have been explored, but the results are inconclusive. Ovarian cancer does not appear to occur in family groups; this suggests that genetic susceptibility is not a risk factor. The risk of ovarian cancer is slightly decreased in women who use oral contraceptives for many years. Exposure to mumps virus and early exposure (before 12 years of age) to measles and rubella also appear to have some protective effect.

There are two major types of ovarian cancer: epithelial ovarian neoplasms and germ cell neoplasms. Ninety percent of ovarian malignancies are epithelial ovarian neoplasms, which usually develop from the surface epithelium of the ovary. Epithelial ovarian tumors may be serous, mucinous, endometrial, Brenner, or clear cell tumors. These tumors are classified as (1) benign, (2) borderline malignant, or (3) frankly malignant. The malignant forms are collectively classed as ovarian adenocarcinomas, which account for 90% of all ovarian malignancies. Of the ovarian adenocarcinomas 40% to 50% are serous epithelial malignancies, which usually involve both ovaries and tend to be bulky. Serous tumors generally affect women from 50 to 55 years of age and are extremely rare in prepubertal girls. The 5-year survival rate is 25% to 30%.

Germ cell tumors are derived from the primitive germ cells (gametes) of the embryonic gonad and may be either malignant or benign. The benign cystic teratoma accounts for 10% to 20% of all ovarian tumors. If the germ cell tumor is malignant, it tends to be a highly aggressive and rapidly growing tumor with a poor prognosis. Malignant germ cell tumors tend to affect women under the age of 30 years.

Clinical Manifestations

The intrapelvic location of the ovaries and the range of tumor activity (from slow to rapid and relentless growth) cause diverse signs and symptoms. Ovarian cancer is generally considered a silent disease, meaning that by the time the individual experiences symptoms and seeks treatment, the disease has spread beyond the primary site.

The most obvious symptoms are pain and abdominal

TABLE 20-4 FIGO* staging of carcinoma of the ovary

Stage		Characteristics
I		Growth limited to the ovaries
	IA	Growth limited to one ovary; no ascites
		i. No tumor on the external surface; capsule intact (90% 5-year survival, with treatment)
		ii. Tumor present on the external surface, or capsule(s) ruptured, or both
	IB	Growth limited to both ovaries; no ascites
		i. No tumor on the external surface; capsule intact
		ii. Tumor present on the external surface, or capsule(s) ruptured, or both
	IC	Tumor either Stage IA or Stage IB, with ascites present or with positive peritoneal washings
II		Growth involving one or both ovaries with pelvic extension
	IIA	Extension and/or metastases to the uterus and/or tubes
	IIB	Extension to other pelvic tissues
	IIC	Tumor either Stage IIA or Stage IIB, but with ascites present or with positive peritoneal washings
III		Growth involving one or both ovaries with intraperitoneal metastases outside the pelvis, or positive retroperitoneal nodes, or both. Tumor limited to the true pelvis with histologically proven malignant extension to small bowel or omentum
IV		Growth involving one or both ovaries with distant metastases. If pleural effusion is present, there must be positive cytology to allot a case to Stage IV. Parenchymal liver metastases indicate Stage IV
Special category		Unexplored cases that are thought to be ovarian carcinoma

From Droegemeuller, Herbst, Mischell, & Stenehever, 1987.
*The International Federation of Gynecologists and Obstetricians.

swelling that arises from the primary ovarian mass, epigastricomental plaques, or ascites. Gastrointestinal manifestations may include dyspepsia, vomiting, and alterations in bowel habits caused by the mechanical obstruction by the tumor. Abnormal vaginal bleeding may occur if the postmenopausal endometrium is stimulated by a hormone-secreting tumor. The tumor may also cause ulcerations through the vaginal wall that result in bleeding.

Systemic manifestations of nonmetastatic malignant disease include connective tissue inflammation (dermatomyositis), abnormal pigmentation (acanthosis nigricans), and subacute cerebellar degeneration. Tumor obstruction of vascular channels can cause venous and, occasionally, arterial thrombosis. Alterations in coagulability also occur, contributing to clot formation. Metastasis frequently causes pleural effusion.

Evaluation and Treatment

Because ovarian cancer has no early symptoms and there are no effective screening techniques to detect it, disease is usually advanced by the time treatment is sought. Diagnosis is made after ultrasound, CT scan, magnetic resonance imaging (MRI), or other imaging techniques that enable clinicians to localize the tumor mass. Staging of disease requires exploratory surgery. The International Federation of Gynecologists and Obstetricians (FIGO) staging system is described in Table 20-4. Other preoperative studies may be used to determine the extent of metastasis. These include an upper gastrointestinal series, barium enema, intravenous pyelogram, mammography, and lymphography.

The initial approach to treatment is surgery, which is performed to determine the stage of disease and remove as much of the tumor as possible. Radiation therapy may follow if the tumor is less than 2.0 cm in size and is confined to the abdominopelvic area without involvement of the kidneys or liver. Radiation therapy may be administered externally, intraperitoneally, or in both ways. The success of chemotherapy depends on whether the tumor is a discrete mass, the extent of disease, and whether there has been prior exposure to chemotherapeutic agents. Alkylating agents are given alone or in combination with antimetabolites. Chemotherapy can reduce tumor size, but it does not reduce mortality.

The mortality rate associated with ovarian cancer has not changed significantly over the past 20 years, mostly because disease is already advanced at the time of diagnosis. Five-year mortality rates for epithelial neoplasms range from 30% for women with early disease (stage IA) to 96% for women with advanced disease (stage IV) (diSaia & Creasman, 1989).

DISORDERS OF THE MALE REPRODUCTIVE SYSTEM

Disorders of the Urethra

Urethritis and urethral strictures are common disorders of the male urethra. Urethral carcinoma occurs in males over 60, but it is an extremely rare form of cancer.

Urethritis

Urethritis is an inflammatory process that is usually, but not always, caused by a sexually transmitted microorganism. Biologic agents associated with infectious urethritis in males include *Neisseria gonorrhoeae* and *Chlamydia trachomatis,* and, less commonly, *Ureaplasma urealyticum.* Infectious urethritis caused by *N. gonorrhoeae* is often called gonococcal urethritis (GU); that caused by other microorganisms is called nongonococcal urethritis (NGU). (Sexually transmitted urethritis is described in Chapter 21.) Nonsexual transmission of urethritis can result from urologic procedures, insertion of foreign bodies into the urethra, anatomic abnormalities, or trauma.

Noninfectious urethritis is rare and is associated with the ingestion of wood or ethyl alcohol or turpentine. It is also seen with Reiter syndrome, which involves a number of mucocutaneous lesions.

Symptoms of urethritis include a burning sensation upon urinating, frequency, and urgency. The individual may notice a purulent discharge from the urethra. Treatment consists of appropriate antibiotic therapy for infectious urethritis and avoidance of future exposure or mechanical irritation.

Urethral Strictures

A **urethral stricture** is a narrowing of the urethra caused by scarring. The scars may be congenital or may result from trauma (e.g., injury or urologic instrumentation) or untreated or severe urethral infections.

The clinical manifestations of urethral structure are caused by bladder outlet obstruction. Symptoms include urinary frequency and hesitancy, diminished force and caliber of the urinary stream, dribbling after voiding, and nocturia.

Urethral stricture is diagnosed on the basis of history, physical examination, and cytoscopy. Treatment is usually surgical and may involve urethral dilation, urethrotomy, or a variety of open surgical techniques. The choice of surgical intervention depends on the age of the individual and the severity of the problem.

Disorders of the Penis

Phimosis and Paraphimosis

Phimosis and paraphimosis are both disorders in which the foreskin (prepuce) is "too tight" to be moved easily over the glans penis. **Phimosis** is a condition in which the foreskin cannot be retracted back over the glans, whereas **paraphimosis** is the opposite: the foreskin is retracted and cannot be moved forward (reduced) to cover the glans (Fig. 20-13). Both conditions can cause penile pathology.

Because phimosis prevents adequate cleansing of the glans and the underside of the foreskin, it can lead to infection and is a risk factor for penile cancer. Severe constriction of the foreskin causes urinary obstruction, which can be fatal in infants. Congenital phimosis is treated by gently stretching the foreskin so that it can be retracted. If this is not effective, circumcision is performed. Acquired phimosis is often caused by fibrosis following infection and inflammation beneath the foreskin. Circumcision is performed after the infection has been eradicated.

Paraphimosis, in which the foreskin is retracted, can constrict the penis, causing edema of the glans. If edema is such that the foreskin cannot be reduced manually, surgery must be performed to prevent necrosis of the glans caused by constricted blood vessels. Severe paraphimosis is a surgical emergency.

Peyronie Disease

Peyronie disease is a fibrotic condition that causes lateral curvature of the penis during erection (Fig. 20-14). The problem usually affects middle-aged men and is associated with painful erection and painful intercourse or impotence. A dense, fibrous plaque is usually palpable on the dorsum of the penile shaft. Peyronie disease is associated with Dupuytren contracture (a flex-

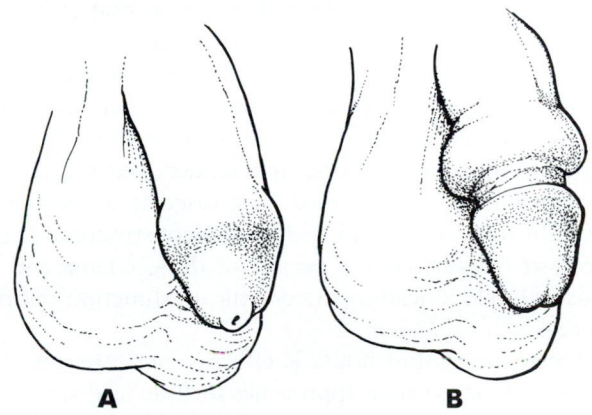

FIG. 20-13. **A,** Phimosis: the foreskin has a pinpoint opening that is not large enough to permit retraction over the glans, **B,** Paraphimosis: the foreskin is retracted over the glans but cannot be reduced to its normal position. Here it has formed a constricting band around the penis. (From Phipps, Long, & Woods, 1987.)

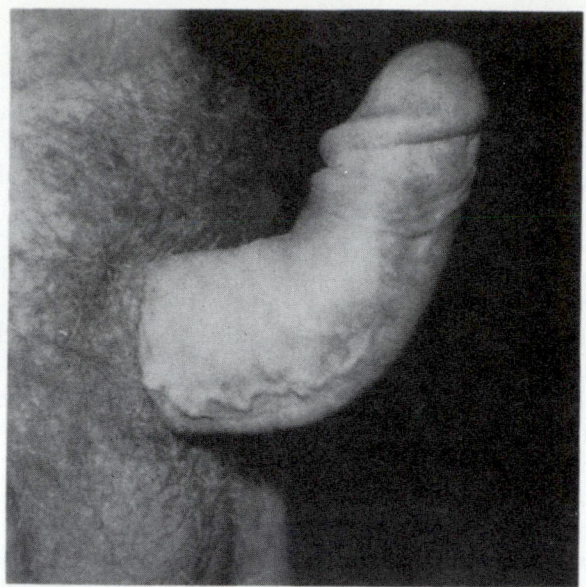

FIG. 20-14. Peyronie disease. (Courtesy Patrick C. Walsh MD. The Johns Hopkins University School of Medicine, Baltimore.) (From Seidel, Ball, Dains, & Benedict, 1987.)

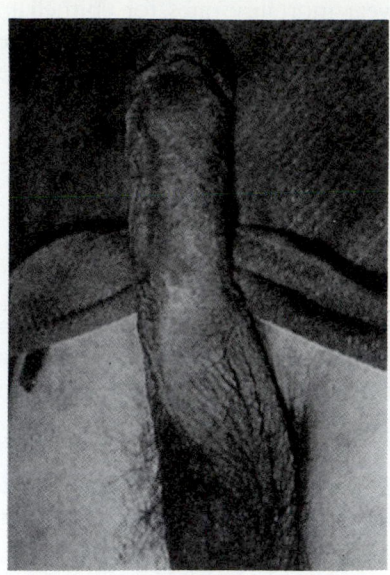

FIG. 20-15. Priaprism. (From Lloyd-Davies, Gow, & Davies, 1983.)

ion deformity of the fingers or toes caused by shortening or fibrosis of the palmar or plantar fascia), diabetes, and the tendency to develop keloids.

There is no definitive treatment for Peyronie disease. Spontaneous remissions occur up to 50% of the time. Pharmacologic therapies that may be beneficial include administration of vitamin E, cortisone, or para-aminobenzoic acid. Radiotherapy can relieve pain. Surgical resection of the fibrous plaque followed by grafting has been successful (Wild, Devine, & Horton, 1979).

Priapism

Priapism is prolonged penile erection that is usually painful and is not associated with sexual arousal (Fig. 20-15). Priapism can be idiopathic or associated with spinal cord trauma, sickle cell disease, leukemia, or pelvic tumors. The two corpora cavernosa within the erect penis are filled with blood and tender, but the corpus spongiosum is not engorged. The vascular congestion is thought to be associated with venous obstruction. If the erection remains over a period of days, edema and fibrosis develop, leading to erectile dysfunction (impotence).

Treatment within hours is effective and prevents impotence. Conservative approaches include iced saline enemas, ketamine administration, and spinal anesthesia. Needle aspiration of blood from the corpus through the dorsal glans is often effective and is followed by catheterization and pressure dressings to maintain decompression. More aggressive surgical treatments include

the creation of vascular shunts to maintain blood flow. Erectile dysfunction results in up to 50% of cases.

Balanitis

Balanitis is an inflammation of the glans penis (Fig. 20-16). It usually occurs in uncircumcised males, often in cases of phimosis. The accumulation under the foreskin of glandular secretions (smegma), sloughed epithelial cells, and *Mycobacterium smegmatis* can irritate the glans directly or lead to infection. Skin disorders (e.g., psoriasis, lichen planus, eczema) and candidiasis must be differentiated from inflammation resulting from poor hygienic practices. Antibiotics are used to treat infection. Circumcision can prevent recurrences.

Penile Cancer

Carcinoma in situ of the penis (erythroplasia of Queyrat; Bowen disease) is a red, smooth, well-defined lesion of the glans penis and, less commonly, of the foreskin. Microscopic examination of a tissue biopsy differentiates carcinoma in situ from chronic balanitis. Treatment consists of local excision. Radiation therapy and local application of 5-fluorouracil have also been successful.

Invasive carcinoma of the penis usually occurs in men between 60 and 70 years of age, but it can occur in younger men. Invasive carcinoma represents less than 1% of malignancies among males. This cancer tends to occur in uncircumcised individuals, probably because of chronic irritation by smegma or the presence of phimosis. The incidence of penile carcinoma is highest in

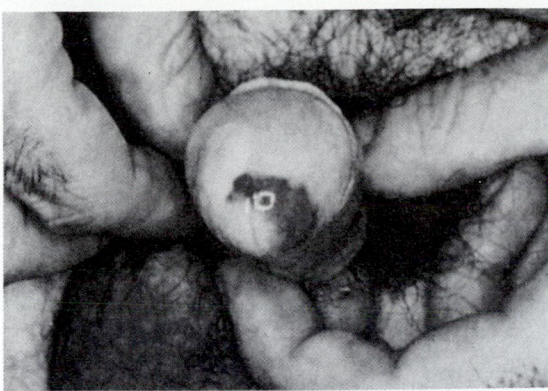

FIG. 20-16. Balanitis (From Lloyd-Davies, Gow, & Davies, 1983.)

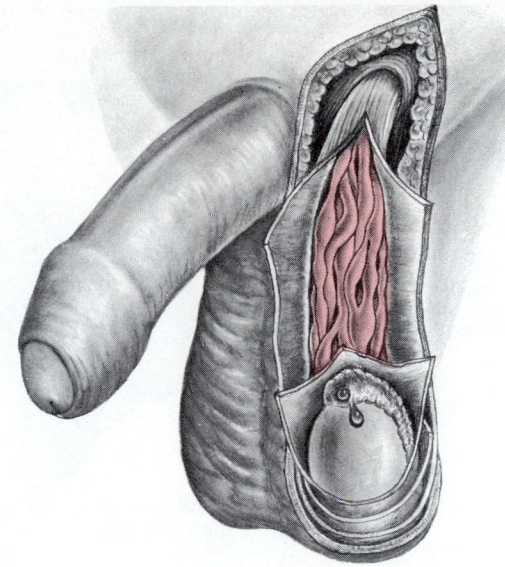

FIG. 20-17. Varicocele: dilatation of veins within the spermatic cord. (From Seidel, Ball, Dains, & Benedict, 1987.)

countries where circumcision is uncommon (Schell-hammer & Grabstald, 1986). Despite this circumstantial evidence, the exact etiology of invasive penile carcinoma is unknown.

The carcinoma usually begins as a small, fat ulcerative or papillary lesion on the glans or foreskin that grows to involve the entire penile shaft. Extensive lesions are associated with metastases and a poor prognosis. These lesions are not as painful as the amount of tissue involvement would seem to indicate. The regional femoral and iliac nodes are common metastatic sites. Rarely the urethra and bladder are involved. Weight loss, fatigue, and malaise accompany chronic suppurative lesions. Untreated, progressive disease causes death within 2 years.

The specific diagnosis is made by biopsy after examination to document the location, size, and fixation of the lesion and the absence or presence of regional adenopathy. Distant metastases are uncommon. Classifications of carcinoma of the penis are presented in Table 20-5.

Treatment usually involves partial or total penectomy (surgical resection). If the glans and distal shaft are the primary site, the penis is amputated, leaving a 2-cm margin proximal to the tumor. Inguinal lymph nodes also are removed if metastasis to these structures is

known or suspected. Radical surgery—excision of the penis, dorsal lymphatics, and inguinal lymph nodes—is seldom performed today (del Regato et al., 1985). More advanced tumors, with erosion of the scrotum or groin nodes, may require radical resection, however. Small superficial lesions can be treated with radiation therapy, which is most effective in young men. The 5-year survival for stages I and II is 65% to 95%.

Disorders of the Scrotum, Testis, and Epididymis
Disorders of the Scrotum

Varicocele, hydrocele, and spermatocele are common intrascrotal disorders. A **varicocele** is an abnormal dilatation of a vein within the spermatic cord (Fig. 20-17). The majority occur on the left side, probably because the left spermatic cord is longer than the right. Varicocele occurs in 10% to 15% of males and is seen most frequently after puberty.

The cause of varicocele is incompetent or congenitally absent valves in the spermatic veins. The valves that normally prevent backflow are absent or do not close adequately, permitting blood to pool in the veins rather than flow into the venous system. Varicocele decreases blood flow through the testis. This interferes with spermatogenesis and is a cause of infertility. If infertility is a problem, treatment consists of ligation of the spermatic vein. If varicocele is mild and fertility is not an issue, a scrotal support is usually sufficient to relieve symptoms of scrotal heaviness or "dragging."

A **hydrocele** is a collection of fluid within the tunica vaginalis (Fig. 20-18). It is the most common cause of

TABLE 20-5 Classifications of carcinoma of the penis	
Stage	**Definition**
I	Tumor limited to the glans or foreskin
II	Tumor extends to shaft of penis
III	Inguinal lymph nodes involved but operable
IV	Inguinal nodes inoperable or distant metastasis has occurred

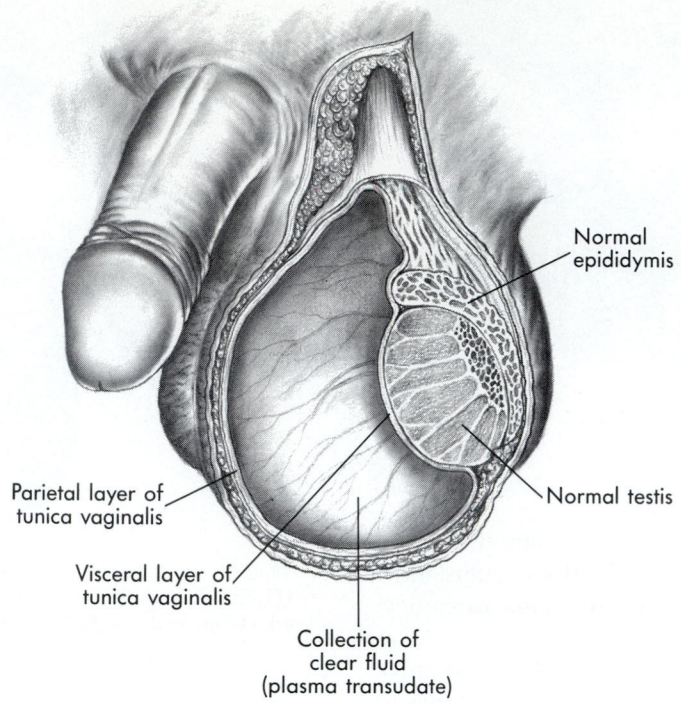

Normal
epididymis

Normal testis

Parietal layer of
tunica vaginalis

Visceral layer of
tunica vaginalis

Collection of
clear fluid
(plasma transudate)

FIG. 20-18. Hydrocele: accumulation of clear fluid between the visceral and parietal layers of the tunica vaginalis.

scrotal swelling. Hydroceles in infants are congenital malformations that frequently resolve spontaneously by 1 year of age. Hydroceles in adults may be caused by an imbalance between the secreting and absorptive capacities of scrotal tissues. Hydroceles range in size from slightly larger than the testes to the size of a grapefruit or larger.

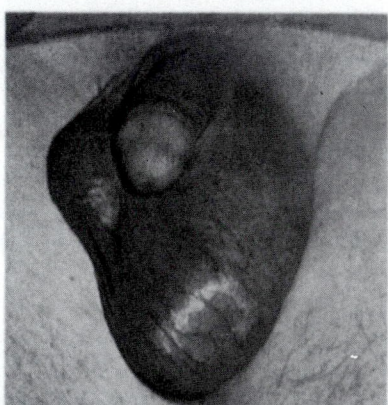

FIG. 20-19. Spermatocele: retention cyst of the head of the epididymis or of an aberrant tubule or tubules of the rete testis. The spermatocele lies outside the tunica vaginalis; therefore, on palpation it can be readily distinguished and separated from the testis. (From Lloyd-Davies, Gow, & Davies, 1983.)

The exact mechanism of idiopathic hydrocele is unknown. Secondary hydrocele may result from trauma or infection of the testis or epididymis. Treatment for uncomplicated hydrocele is aspiration of the fluid and injection of a sclerosing drug into the scrotal sac. The goal of treatment is to remove the hydrocele and prevent recurrence by causing sclerosis of the tunica vaginalis. Treatment for recurrent hydroceles is excision of the tunica vaginalis.

A **spermatocele** is a cyst of the testis or epididymis that is filled with milky fluid that contains sperm (Fig. 20-19). Spermatoceles that cause pain or discomfort are excised. Usually, however, spermatoceles are asymptomatic or produce mild discomfort that is relieved by scrotal support.

Cryptorchidism

Cryptorchidism is a condition in which one or both testes fail to descend into the scrotum. It is the most common congenital condition involving the testes. Approximately 1% to 3% of all full-term males and 20% of all premature males have undescended testes at birth. The testes may remain in the abdomen, or descent may be arrested in the inguinal canal or the puboscrotal junction. In approximately 80% of infants with cryptorchidism, the testes descend into the scrotum by 1 year of age.

Cryptorchidism may result from a developmental delay, a defect of the testis, or some mechanical factor that prevents descent through the inguinal canal. Mechanical possibilities include a short spermatic cord, fibrous bands or adhesions in the normal path of the testes, or a narrowed inguinal canal. Endocrine disorders, such as Klinefelter syndrome, are also associated with cryptorchidism.

Untreated cryptorchidism is associated with a lowered sperm count and, therefore, impaired fertility. Impaired spermatogenesis is caused by higher temperatures within the abdomen. Cryptorchidism does not prevent puberty or maintenance of secondary sex characteristics if the testis is otherwise normal. Undescended testes are susceptible to neoplastic processes: the risk of testicular cancer is 35 to 50 times greater for men with cryptorchidism or a history of cryptorchidism than for the general male population.

Physical examination reveals the absence of one or both testes in the scrotum. Ultrasonography or a CAT scan can help clinicians to locate a testis that has migrated intraabdominally. Treatment often begins with administration of human chorionic gonadotropin (HGC), a hormone that may initiate descent, making surgery unnecessary. If hormonal therapy is not successful, the testis is located and moved surgically. To preserve fertility, surgical correction of cryptorchidism should be attempted when the child is about 2 years of age. Undescended testis must be treated before age 6 to reduce the risk of neoplastic disease.

Torsion of the Testis

Torsion of the testis is a condition in which the testis rotates on its vascular pedicle, interrupting its blood supply. This event tends to occur in childhood and adolescence, with highest incidence at the time of puberty. Onset may be spontaneous or follow physical exertion or trauma. Torsion twists the arteries and veins in the spermatic cord, reducing or stopping circulation to the testis. Vascular engorgement and ischemia develop, causing scrotal swelling. These manifestations are not relieved by rest or scrotal support. Tortion of the testis is a surgical emergency. If the torsion cannot be reduced manually, surgery must be performed within 6 hours after the onset of symptoms to prevent testicular atrophy or abscess and preserve fertility. Surgery includes untwisting the spermatic cord and anchoring both testicles in correct position within the scrotum to prevent recurrences.

Orchitis

Orchitis is an acute infection of the testes (Fig. 20-20). This condition is rare because the testes have a rich blood supply, which helps them to resist infection. Infectious organisms may reach the testes through the

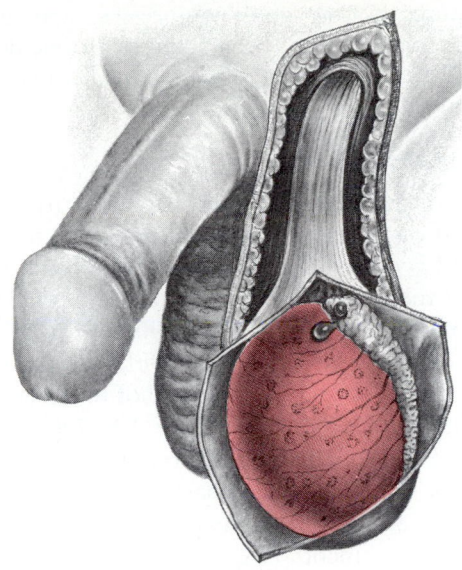

FIG. 20-20. Orchitis. (From Seidel, Ball, Dains, & Benedict, 1987.)

blood, through the lymphatics, or, most commonly, by ascent through the urethra, vas deferens, and epididymis. Most cases of orchitis are actually cases of epididymo-orchitis.

Pathophysiology

The usual causes of orchitis are bacteria: *Escherichia coli, Klebsiella pneumoniae,* Streptococci, Staphylococci, and *Pseudomonas aeruginosa.* Bacterial invasion of the testes is almost always secondary to infection of the epididymides or urinary tract or instrumental procedures, such as catheterization. Rarely acute orchitis is secondary to a systemic disease, such as diphtheria, influenza, typhoid fever, syphilis, scarlet fever, malaria, infectious mononucleosis, or mumps. Orchitis occurs in approximately 18% of mumps cases and usually occurs in adults.

Clinical Manifestations

Clinical manifestations of orchitis include high fever and sudden pain in the involved testis. The pain often radiates to the inguinal canal. Systemic manifestations include nausea, vomiting, and chills. The infected testis is swollen, tense, and tender, and the scrotum may be red and swollen. Complications of orchitis include abscess formation, acute hydrocele, and atrophy and infertility caused by fibrosis and destruction of the tubule system.

Evaluation and Treatment

Diagnosis of orchitis is based on physical examination. Antibiotics are given to treat infection. Supportive therapies include bed rest, scrotal support, elevation of the scrotum, hot or cold compresses, and analgesic agents for relief of pain. If an acute hydrocele develops, it is aspirated. Testicular abscess usually requires orchiectomy (removal of the testis).

Cancer of the Testis

Cancer of the testis is rare in most age groups, but it is the most common malignancy in males 25 to 35 years of age and is one of the leading causes of cancer deaths in men in their twenties and thirties. The estimated incidence of testicular cancer was 5700 new cases in 1989 (American Cancer Society, 1989) with an estimated 350 cancer deaths. The annual incidence of testicular tumors consistently ranges from 2 to 3 per 100,000 men (Garnick et al., 1986). The 5-year survival rate for all types of testicular cancer is approximately 85%, although men with large tumors and those who do not respond to standard management have a much poorer prognosis (Ellis & Sikora, 1987). Testicular tumors occur more frequently in the right testis than the left and are bilateral in only 2% of cases (Fig. 20-21).

Pathogenesis

Most testicular cancers are germ cell tumors: that is, they arise from the male gametes. Germ cell tumors include seminomas, embryonal carcinomas, teratomas, and choriosarcomas. Of these tumors seminomas are the least and choriosarcomas are the most aggressive. Testicular tumors can also arise from specialized cells of the gonadal stroma. These tumors, which are named for

their cellular origins, are the Leydig cell, Sertoli cell, granulosa cell, and theca cell tumors.

The etiology of testicular neoplasms is unknown. Because young men are affected most frequently, it is thought that high levels of androgens may contribute to tumorigenesis. A genetic predisposition is suggested by the fact that the incidence is higher among brothers, identical twins, and other close male relatives. Genetic predisposition is supported further by statistics showing that the disease is relatively rare among black Africans, black Americans, Asians, and native New Zealanders. Cryptorchidism is statistically associated with the development of testicular cancer. Apparently the undescended testis has a developmental defect or undergoes gradual involution and degeneration over time, which may contribute to neoplastic changes. A history of trauma or infection also is associated with the development of testicular neoplasms, but it may be that coexisting testicular tumors are discovered by "accident" in men who undergo examination because of trauma or infections.

Clinical Manifestations

Testicular enlargement, with or without pain, is usually the first sign of testicular cancer. Pain, if present, is frequently described as a dull ache. The testicular mass is usually discovered by the individual or by his sexual partner. A hydrocele is present in about 5% to 25% of all cases of testicular cancer. Approximately 10% to 20% of individuals already have metastases at the time of initial diagnosis. Lumbar pain may also be present and is usually caused by retroperitoneal node metastasis. Signs of metastasis to the lungs include cough, dyspnea, and bloody sputum (hemoptysis). Supraclavicular node involvement may cause difficulty swallowing (dysphagia) and neck swelling. Alterations in vision or mental status, papilledema, and seizures may be experienced with metastasis to the central nervous system.

Evaluation and Treatment

Evaluation begins with careful physical examination, including palpation of the scrotal contents with the individual in the erect and supine positions. Signs of testicular cancer include abnormal consistency, induration, nodularity, or irregularity of the testis. Translumination may be helpful in identifying scrotal contents. The abdomen and lymph nodes are palpated to seek evidence of metastasis. Tumor type is identified after orchiectomy. Testicular biopsy is not recommended because it may cause dissemination of the tumor and increase the risk of local recurrence. Chest x-ray films, lymphangiograms, intravenous pyelograms, abdominal ultrasound or CT scan, and measurement of serum markers (α-fetoprotein and β-subunit gonadotropin) are used in clinical staging of disease. Besides surgery treatment involves ra-

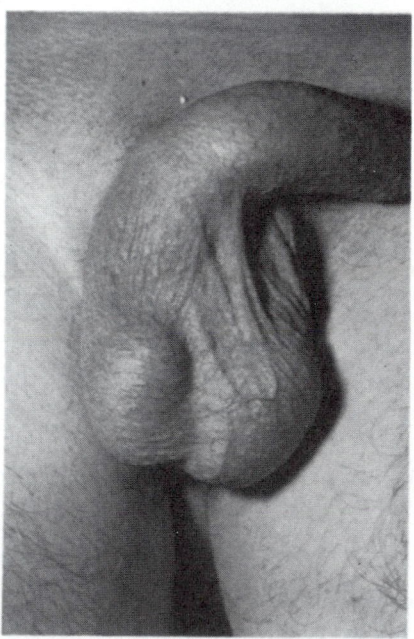

FIG. 20-21. Testicular tumor. (From 400 Self-assessment picture tests, 1984.)

TABLE 20-6 Testicular tumors of germ cell origin

Cell types	Occurrence	Metastatic pattern	Prognosis/remission rate
SINGLE-CELL TUMORS			
Seminoma (germinoma)	30%-40% of all germ cell tumors	Rarely to retroperitoneal lymph nodes	Excellent; tumor usually remains localized and is responsive to radiation
Embryonal carcinoma	15%-20% of all germ cell tumors	Earlier to regional lymphatics, also lung, liver, bone, gestrointestinal tract	Good; complete remission rate of 75%
Teratoma	Less than 10% of all germ cell tumors	Through lymphatics and bloodstream; affects same organ systems as embryonal type	Fair; complete remission rate of 45%
Choriocarcinoma	2% of all germ cell tumors	Earliest and widest, initially through bloodstream	Poor; early metastasis; complete remission rate of 40%
MIXED TUMORS			
Teratocarcinoma	30%-40% of all germ cell tumors	Mixed pattern; depends on cell types	Variable; worst prognosis of the cell types
Teratocarcinoma with seminoma			
Embryonal cancer with seminoma			
Teratoma with seminoma			
Any combination with choriocarcinoma			

From Mostofi & Sobin, 1977.

diation and chemotherapy singly or in combination. A number of factors influence the prognosis (Table 20-6). They include histology of the tumor, α-fetoprotein and HCG levels, and tumor volume. The serum markers are useful for detecting metastases and assessing responses to therapy. The presence of any masses or nodes greater than 2 cm in diameter indicates a poor prognosis.

Impairment of Sperm Production and Quality

Spermatogenesis requires adequate secretion of FSH and LH by the pituitary and sufficient secretion of testosterone by the testes. Inadequate secretion of gonadotropins may be caused by hypothyroidism, hyperadrenocortisolism, hyperprolactinemia, or hypogonadotropic hypogonadism. In these situations gonadotropin levels are low because of feedback inhibition or idiopathic hyposecretion. In the absence of adequate gonadotropin levels the Leydig cells are not stimulated to secrete testosterone, and sperm maturation is not promoted in the Sertoli cells. Spermatogenesis depends not only on appropriate stimulation by the gonadotropins, but also on an appropriate response by the testes. Defects in testicular response to the gonadotropins result

in decreased secretion of testosterone and, as a result of normal feedback mechanisms, high levels of circulating gonadotropins. In the absence of adequate testosterone levels spermatogenesis is impaired.

Impaired spermatogenesis can also be caused by testicular trauma, infection, or atrophy of the testes from any cause. Other conditions associated with impaired spermatogenesis include systemic illness involving high fever, ingestion of various drugs, exposure to environmental toxins, and cryptorchidism.

Fertility is adversely affected if spermatogenesis is normal but the sperm are chromosomally or morphologically abnormal or are produced in insufficient quantities. Chromosomal abnormalities are caused by genetic factors and by external variables, such as exposure to radiation or toxic substances. A sperm count of 20 million sperm per milliliter of semen has been suggested as the minimum concentration required for fertility. Average fertile men have 50 to 100 million sperm per milliliter.

Sperm motility is another important variable affecting fertility. Mobility appears to be affected by the sperm's chemical environment, that is, the characteristics of semen (Table 20-7). Prostatic dysfunction, excessive se-

TABLE 20-7 Volume and characteristics of semen			
	Normal semen quality	Marginal semen quality	Abnormal semen quality
Semen volume (ml)	1-5*	1-2	<1
Sperm count ($\times 10^6$ ml [million/ml])	10-250*	10-20	<10
Sperm motility (% motility)	50	40-50	<40
Mean swimming speed (μm/sec)	25	20-25	<20

From Overstreet & Katz, 1987.

*Values that exceed the upper range of normal may result in classification of semen as marginal or abnormal.

men viscosity, presence of drugs or toxins in the semen, and presence of antisperm antibodies are associated with impaired sperm motility. Approximately 17% of infertile males have antisperm antibodies in their semen. Antisperm antibodies may develop as a result of trauma to or obstruction of the reproductive organs or genetic defect in self-recognition or may be stimulated by cross-reactive microbial antigens present in urinary tract infections. Antisperm antibodies may be (1) cytotoxic antibodies, which attack sperm and reduce their number in the semen, or (2) sperm-immobilizing antibodies, which impair sperm motility and reduce their ability to transverse the endocervical canal.

Treatment for impaired spermatogenesis involves correction of any underlying disorders and avoidance of radiation or toxins. Androgens, human gonadotropins, and antiestrogens (such as clomiphene citrate or tamoxifen eitrate) may enhance spermatogenesis. Semen can be modified to improve sperm motility. If conception is desired, the semen is obtained by masturbation, after which it can be diluted, concentrated, or washed to re-

move antisperm antibodies. These alterations are followed by artificial insemination.

Epididymitis

Epididymitis, or inflammation of the epididymis, generally occurs in sexually active young males and is rare before puberty (Fig. 20-22). In young men the usual cause is a sexually transmitted microorganism, such as *Neisseria gonorrhoeae* or *Chlamydia trachomatis*. *N. gonorrhoeae* accounts for between 20% and 50% of cases of epididymitis in males under the age of 35. Enterobacteriaceae (intestinal bacteria) and *P. aeruginosa* also cause epididymitis. Rarely epididymitis occurs after strenuous lifting or straining, or after scrotal trauma. In older men chronic bacterial prostatitis or some structural pathology is the most frequent cause of epididymitis.

Pathophysiology

The pathogenic microorganism usually reaches the epididymis by ascending the vasa deferentia from an already infected urethra or bladder. The presence of bacteria initiates the inflammatory response, causing symptoms of bacterial epididymitis. Epididymitis caused by heavy lifting or straining results from reflux of urine from the bladder into the vas deferens and epididymis. Urine is extremely irritating to the epididymis and initiates an inflammatory response called chemical epididymitis.

Clinical Manifestations

Pain is the main symptom of epididymitis. Scrotal or inguinal pain is caused by inflammation of the epididymis and surrounding tissues. The pain is usually acute and severe. Flank pain may occur if, as the urethra passes over the spermatic cord, edematous swelling of the cord obstructs the urethra. The individual may have a history of urinary symptoms, especially if a urinary tract infection is the source of the bacteria affecting the epididymis. The scrotum on the involved side is red and edematous as a result of inflammatory changes. The tail

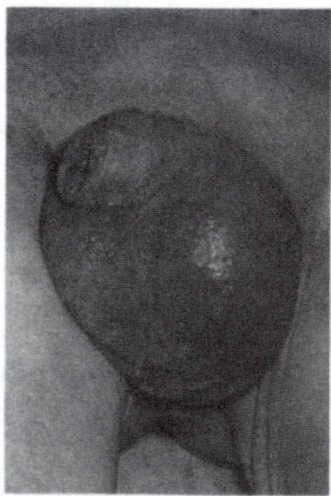

FIG. 20-22. Epididymitis. (From Lloyd-Davis, Gow, & Davies, 1983.)

of the epididymis near the lower pole of the testis usually swells first, then swelling ascends to the head of the epididymis. The spermatic cord may also be swollen and tender.

Complications of epididymitis include abscess formation, infarction of the testis, recurrent infection, and infertility. Infarction is probably caused by thrombosis (obstruction by blood clots) of the prostatic vessels secondary to severe inflammation. Recurrent epididymitis may result from inadequate initial treatment or failure to identify or treat predisposing factors. Chronic epididymitis can cause scarring of the epididymal endothelium. Once scarring has occurred, treatment with antibiotics is ineffective because adequate antibiotic levels cannot be achieved within the epididymis.

Evaluation and Treatment

A history of recent urinary tract infection or urethral discharge suggests the diagnosis of epididymitis. The relief of pain when the inflamed testis and epididymis are elevated (Phren sign) is also diagnostic. Definitive diagnosis is based on culture or Gram stain of a urethral swab. Epididymal aspiration may be necessary to obtain a specimen, especially if the individual has been taking antibiotics and has sterile urine.

Treatment includes antibiotic therapy for the infection itself and various measures to provide symptomatic relief. Bed rest and scrotal elevation are recommended until the scrotum is no longer tender. Scrotal elevation facilitates maximal lymphatic and venous drainage. Abscess formation is rare with antibiotic therapy. If an abscess occurs and persists, it is drained surgically. The individual's sexual partner should be treated with antibiotics if the causative microorganism is a sexually transmitted pathogen.

Disorders of the Prostate Gland
Benign Prostatic Hyperplasia

Benign prostatic hyperplasia (BPH), also called benign prostatic hypertrophy, is the enlargement of the prostate gland (Fig. 20-23). This condition becomes problematic as prostatic tissue compresses the urethra, where it passes through the prostate. About half of all men over the age of 65 have some prostatic enlargement. Although BPH is common, its etiology remains obscure. Most speculations regarding the pathogenesis of BPH involve endocrine changes associated with aging. Excessive dihydroxytestosterone accumulation in the prostate, estrogen stimulation, and action by a local growth hormone all have been proposed as causes of BPH (Heible & Caine, 1986).

The prostate enlarges as nodules form and grow (nodular hyperplasia) and glandular cells enlarge (hypertrophy). As nodular hyperplasia and cellular hypertrophy progress, tissues that surround the prostatic urethra

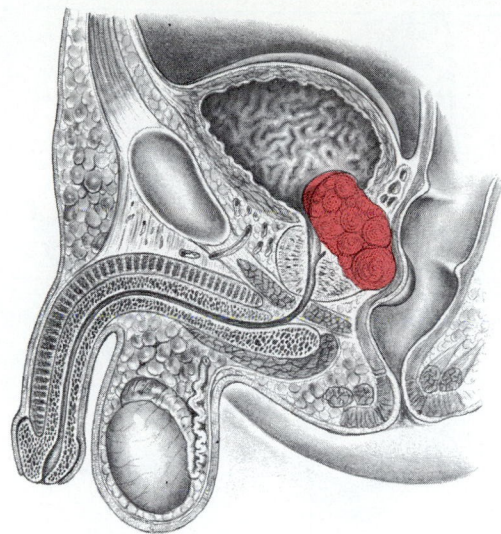

FIG. 20-23. Benign prostatic hypertrophy. (From Seidel, Ball, Dains, & Benedict, 1987.)

compress it, causing bladder outflow obstruction.

During the early stages of urethral obstruction, the detrusor muscle hypertrophies to help the bladder force urine out against increasing resistance. Symptoms include the urge to urinate frequently, some delay in starting urination, and decreased force of the urinary stream. As the obstruction progresses, often over a period of several years, the bladder is unable to empty all of the urine. Increasing volumes of urine are retained until urine retention is chronic. The volume of urine retained may be great enough to produce uncontrolled "overflow incontinence" with any increase in intraabdominal pressure. At this stage the force of the urinary stream is significantly reduced, and it takes much more time to initiate and complete voiding.

Progressive bladder distention causes sacculations or diverticular outpouchings of the bladder wall. The ureters may be obstructed where they pass through the hypertrophied detrusor muscle. Hydroureter, hydronephrosis, and bladder or kidney infection then develop.

There is no way to reverse progressive BPH, but the hyperplasia is not always progressive. The hyperplastic tissue may be removed surgically to prevent the serious consequences of urethral obstruction. A permanent indwelling catheter is inserted if the individual cannot tolerate surgery. Drugs are used to treat secondary infections.

Prostatitis

Prostatitis is an inflammation of the prostate. Some degree of prostatic inflammation is present in 4% to 36% of the male population. This percentage increases to 50% in older males. Inflammation is usually limited to a few of the gland's excretory ducts (Fig. 20-24).

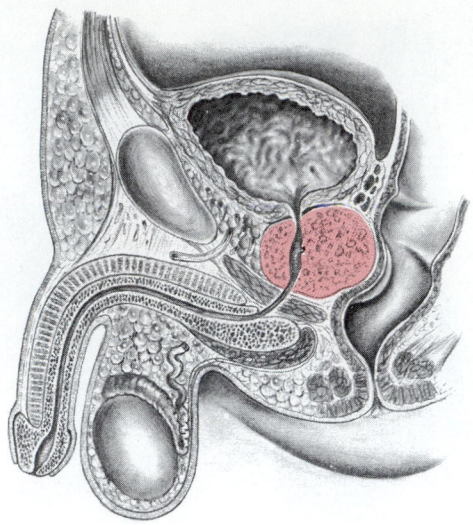

FIG. 20-24. Prostatitis. (From Seidel, Ball, Dains, & Benedict, 1987.)

Prostatitis is characterized as (1) acute bacterial prostatitis, (2) chronic bacterial prostatitis, or (3) nonbacterial prostatitis. **Prostatodynia** (pain in the prostate) is sometimes considered a form of prostatitis. Men with prostatodynia have the same clinical manifestations as those with nonbacterial prostatitis, but physical and laboratory examinations do not reveal prostatic pathology. Prostatodynia may not be caused by a pathologic condition of the prostate but rather by spasms in the genitourinary tract or tension in the muscles of the pelvic floor.

A number of defense mechanisms normally protect the lower urogenital tract from infection. Mechanical defenses include urethral length, micturition (urination), and ejaculation. Structural malformations and instrumentation of the genitourinary tract may weaken these defense mechanisms. Chemical defenses include antimicrobial substances in the prostatic fluid. The most important of these is a zinc-containing polypeptide known as prostatic antibacterial factor.

Bacterial Prostatitis

Acute bacterial prostatitis is an ascending infection of the urinary tract that tends to occur in men between the ages of 30 and 50 but is also associated with BPH in older men. Coliform bacteria, particularly *Escherichia coli* and *Streptococcus faecalis,* are common causes of acute bacterial prostatis. *Aeruginosa, Staphylococcus,* and *Salmonella* are other causes. Infection stimulates an inflammatory response in which the prostate becomes enlarged, tender, and firm. The onset of prostatis may be acute and unrelated to previous illnesses, or it may follow catheterization or cystocopy.

Clinical manifestations of acute bacterial prostatitis are those of urinary tract infection. Symptoms include dysuria and urinary frequency, which result from bacterial contamination and inflammation of the bladder. Lower abdominal and suprapubic discomfort is another symptom of bladder infection. The individual may also have symptoms of lower urinary tract obstruction, such as slow, small urinary stream, inability to empty the bladder, and nocturia (need to urinate frequently during the night). Acute inflammatory prostatic edema can compress the urethra, causing urinary obstruction. Systemic signs of infection include sudden onset of a high fever (up to 40° C [104° F]), fatigue, arthralgia, and myalgia. Prostatic pain may occur, especially when the individual is in an upright position, because the pelvic floor muscles tighten with standing and compression of the prostate gland occurs. Some individuals experience painful ejaculation and rectal pain. Palpation reveals an extremely tender and enlarged prostate.

Because acute bacterial prostatitis is usually associated with a bladder infection caused by the same microorganism, urine cultures reveal its identity. Prostatic massage may express enough secretions from the urethra for direct bacterial examination, but massage increases the risk that the infection will ascend to adjacent structures or enter the bloodstream.

Long-term, broad-spectrum-antibiotic therapy (up to 6 weeks) may be required to resolve the infection and control its spread. In severe cases the individual is hospitalized and treated with an aminoglyoside, such as gentamicin sulfate, kanamycin sulfate, or tobramycin sulfate. Pain relievers, antipyretics, bed rest, and adequate hydration are also therapeutic.

Chronic bacterial prostatitis is characterized by recurrent urinary tract infections and persistence of pathogenic bacteria. This form of prostatitis is the most common recurrent urinary tract infection in men. Symptoms are similar to those of an acute bladder infection: frequency, urgency, dysuria, perineal discomfort, low back pain, myalgia, and arthralgia. The prostate may be only slightly enlarged, but fibrosis can cause it to be firm and irregular in shape.

Definitive diagnosis requires bacteriologic localization by culture of sequentially collected urine specimens (initially voided urine and midstream urine) and expressed prostatic secretions (Pfau, 1986). In individuals with chronic bacterial prostatitis the pH of the prostatic secretions becomes increasingly alkaline and zinc levels and specific gravity decrease. The prostatic fluid also contains high levels of antigen-specific immunoglobulin A (IgA).

Treatment of chronic bacterial prostatitis is difficult, mainly because damage caused by chronic inflammation blocks passage of antibiotics into prostatic tissues. Therefore, therapeutic levels are hard to achieve. The usual treatment is a 6-week course of trimethoprim-sulfamethoxazole. Kanamycin sulfate or tobramycin sulfate is used to eradicate gram-negative microorganisms or *Aeruginosa*. Newer drugs, such as doxycycline hyclate and minocycline are selectively useful.

Nonbacterial Prostatitis

Nonbacterial prostatitis consists of prostatic inflammation without evidence of bacterial infection. The etiology of nonbacterial prostatitis is not clear. Microbiologic, urodynamic, and psychologic factors have been studied, but results are inconclusive.

Men with nonbacterial prostatitis may complain of pain or a dull ache that is continuous or spasmodic in the suprapubic, infrapubic, scrotal, penile, or inguinal area. Other symptoms are pain on ejaculation and urinary symptoms, such as frequency of urination. The prostate gland generally feels normal upon palpation.

Digital examination of the prostate, bacterial cultures of the urogenital tract, microscopic examination of expressed prostatic fluid, urethroscopy, and urodynamic studies are used to verify the diagnosis of nonbacterial prostatitis. Nonbacterial prostatitis is diagnosed when all bacterial causes are excluded.

There is no generally accepted treatment for nonbacterial prostatitis. Some clinicians prescribe a 1- to 3-week course of antibiotics for both affected individuals and sexual partners. This approach sometimes reduces symptoms. Symptoms can be relieved by hot sitz baths, bed rest, anticholinergics, and anti-inflammatory drugs.

Cancer of the Prostate

Cancer of the prostate accounts for approximately 10% of all cancer deaths in men in the United States; only lung and colorectal cancer account for more. Prostatic cancer usually occurs in men after the age of 50, and incidence increases with advancing age.

Prostatic cancer is more common in North America and Northern Europe and is relatively rare in Eastern Europe and the Far East. Migration from low-incidence to high-incidence areas increases the risk of developing this cancer, indicating that an environmental risk factor is involved. In the United States, the incidence and mortality among blacks are approximately 50% higher than those among whites.

The etiology of prostatic cancer is poorly understood. The five possible etiologies studied thus far are genetic predisposition, endogenous hormones, environmental factors, sexually transmitted infectious pathogens, and impaired immunologic competence. Evidence from most of these studies is inconclusive or conflicting.

Pathogenesis

More than 95% of prostatic neoplasms are adenocarcinomas, and most occur in the periphery of the pros-

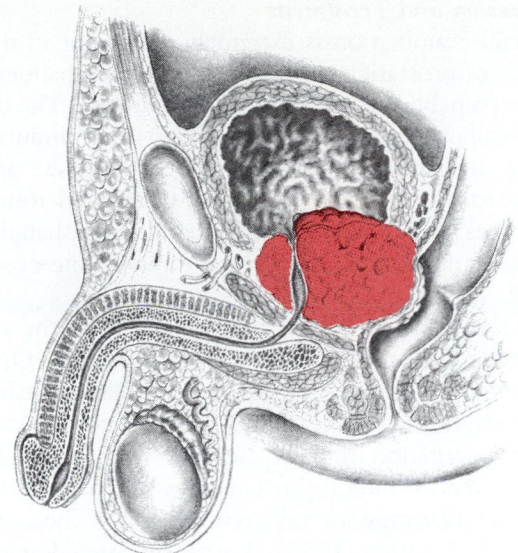

FIG. 20-25. Carcinoma of prostate. (From Seidel, Ball, Dains, & Benedict, 1987.)

tate. Several histologic grading systems have been developed on the basis of the glandular pattern, the degree of differentiation (anaplasia) of the cancer cells, or both. The biologic aggressiveness of the neoplasm appears to be related to the degree of differentiation rather than the size of the tumor.

Prostatic cancer is thought to metastasize by local extension and through lymphatic and blood vessels. The most frequent sites of distant metastasis are the lymph nodes, bones, lungs, liver, and adrenals. The pelvis, lumbar spine, femur, thoracic spine, and ribs are the most common sites of bone metastasis. Local extension is usually posterior, although late in the disease the tumor may invade the rectum or encroach on the prostatic urethra and cause bladder outlet obstruction (Fig. 20-25).

Clinical Manifestations

Prostatic cancer often causes no symptoms until it is far advanced. The first manifestations of disease are those of bladder outlet obstruction: slow urinary stream, hesitancy, incomplete emptying, frequency, nocturia, and dysuria. Unlike the symptoms of obstruction caused by BPH, the symptoms of obstruction caused by prostatic cancer are progressive and do not remit. Local extension of prostatic cancer can obstruct the upper urinary tract ureters as well. If rectal obstruction occurs, the individual may experience a large bowel obstruction or difficulty in defecation. Symptoms of late disease include bone pain at sites of bone metastasis, edema of the lower extremities, enlargement of lymph nodes, liver enlargement, pathologic bone fractures, and mental confusion associated with brain metastases.

Evaluation and Treatment

Rectal examination is extremely important in the diagnosis of prostatic cancer; however, abnormalities may not be palpable in the early stages of disease. The tumor is typically palpated as an area of extreme induration. Biopsy and microscopic examination of tissue are required to establish the diagnosis. Computed tomography scans, bone scans, arteriography, lymphangiography, and ultrasound can be used to assess the extent of spread.

Treatment of prostatic cancer depends on the age of the individual and the stage of the neoplasm. Options include no treatment, hormonal manipulation (estrogen administration), orchiectomy, adrenalectomy, chemotherapy, radiation therapy, surgery (radical prostatectomy, extended radical prostatectomy, or pelvic exteneration), cryotherapy, or any combination of these (Culp, Fallon, & Loening, 1985). Treatments aimed at relieving symptoms of urinary obstruction, bladder outlet obstruction, colon obstruction, and spinal cord compression may be undertaken. Pain, especially that of bony metastases, may be relieved by narcotics.

Sexual Dysfunction

In males the normal sexual response involves three processes: erection, emission, and ejaculation. **Sexual dysfunction** is the impairment of any or all of these processes. Impairment can be caused by a number of physiologic, psychologic, and emotional factors.

Until the late 1970s most cases of male sexual dysfunction were thought to be psychogenic. Recent studies of this problem indicate that, in men over 40 years of age, organic factors are involved in more than 50% of cases. The causes of organic sexual dysfunction include (1) vascular, endocrine, and neurologic disorders; (2) chronic disease, including renal failure and diabetes mellitus; (3) penile diseases and penile trauma; and (4) iatrogenic factors, such as surgery and pharmacologic therapies. Most of these disorders cause erectile dysfunction.

Pathophysiology

Vascular disorders can prevent erection. Some arterial diseases diminish or interrupt circulation to the penis. This prevents engorgement of erectile tissues in the corpora cavernosa and corpus spongiosum. Rarely excessive venous drainage of the corpora cavernosa prevents erection.

Endocrine disorders that reduce testosterone production affect sexual function and libido. The reduction may be caused by inadequate secretion of the gonadotropins caused by pituitary dysfunction or hyperprolactinemia. Feminizing tumors and estrogen therapy reduce relative levels of testosterone. Testicular atrophy from any cause also decreases testosterone levels and contributes to sexual dysfunction.

Neurologic disorders can interfere with the important sympathetic, parasympathetic, and central nervous system mechanisms required for erection, emission, and ejaculation. They include spinal cord injury or tumor, multiple sclerosis, and disorders that cause peripheral neuropathies, for example, diabetes mellitus and chronic renal failure. Spinal cord injuries or tumors can alter one or more components of the sexual response, depending on the location of the lesion. For example, in most men with upper motor neuron lesions, reflexogenic erection is possible, but emission and ejaculation (i.e., orgasm) are not possible. Lesions affecting the lower motor neurons usually prevent erection. In approximately 40% of such cases emission and ejaculation are prevented.

Many chronic diseases are associated with sexual dysfunction. In some conditions the sexual dysfunction has a specific physiologic cause. Diabetes mellitus, for example, causes both peripheral vascular and neurologic pathology that can lead to erectile dysfunction. In other chronic conditions sexual dysfunction is associated with low energy levels and loss of libido. The pathophysiologic mechanisms responsible for such changes are not known.

Priapism causes fibrosis of trabeculae (erectile tissues) within the corpora cavernosa, making erection difficult. The penile curvature caused by Peyronie disease does not make erection impossible but may make it extremely painful and intercourse impossible. Penile trauma can damage the erectile tissue, disrupt the posterior urethra, and disrupt the pudendal arteries or nerves.

Iatrogenic factors, including drugs and surgery, have a significant impact on erectile function. The following surgical procedures all carry the risk of erectile dysfunction: radical pelvic surgery; radical prostatectomy; transurethral, suprapubic, or simple retropubic prostatectomy; and aortoiliac surgery. Erectile dysfunction is caused by the severing of small nerve branches that are essential for erection (Silber, 1984). Aortoiliac surgery, retroperitoneal lymphadenectomy, and sympathectomy cause the loss of ejaculation capacity in some individuals.

A few pharmacologic agents enhance the sexual response, but most have the opposite effect (Table 20-8). Men who are taking antihypertensives, antidepressants, antihistamines, antispasmodics, sedatives or tranquilizers, barbiturates, diuretics, sex hormone preparations, narcotics, or psychoactive drugs may experience some degree of sexual dysfunction. Ethyl alcohol also has a negative effect on sexual function. Drug-induced sexual dysfunction consists of decreased desire, decreased erectile ability, or decreased ejaculatory ability. A number of pharmacologic agents also diminish the quality or quantity of sperm.

TABLE 20-8 Examples of pharmacologic agents associated with male sexual dysfunction

Drug	Decreased desire	Decreased erectile ability	Decreased ejaculatory ability	Decreased sperm quality
Spironolactone	Common	4%-30%	None	None
Propranolol	1%-4%	Up to 28%	None	None
Methyldopa	7%-14%	2%-80%	7%-19%	None
Guanethidine	29%	4%-100%	2%-100%	None
Estrogens	Common	Common	Common	Common
Methadone	6%-38%	6%-50%	5%-88%	Common
Disulfiram	None	10%-12%	None	None
Digoxin	36%	36%	None	None
Cyclophosphamide	Common	Common	None	Common

Data from Drugs that cause sexual dysfunction, 1983, and Wein & Van Arsdalen, 1988.

Evaluation and Treatment

Evaluation of sexual dysfunction includes a physical examination, with particular attention to the genitalia, prostate, and nervous system, and basic laboratory tests to identify the presence of endocrinopathies or other underlying disorders that can cause the dysfunction. If no physiologic cause is found and the condition does not improve with psychotherapy, the man is referred for further investigation of organic causes. Psychologic evaluation is indicated for younger men with a sudden onset of sexual dysfunction or men of any age who are able to achieve but not maintain an erection.

Sophisticated diagnostic techniques can be used to assess penile blood flow, erectile tissue anatomy, nervous system function, and occurrence of erection and/or emission during sleep (nocturnal emission). Penile blood flow is measured by Doppler techniques and penile arteriography. Corpus cavernosography, in which contrast material is injected into the corpora cavernosa, provides information about the anatomy of the erectile tissue of the penis. Neuropathic causes of sexual dysfunction are evaluated by measuring the speed of the bulbocavernous reflex. Nocturnal penile tumescence monitoring measures the frequency of nocturnal erections. Depending on the equipment used, this information may be correlated to rapid-eye-movement (REM) or non-REM sleep.

Treatments for organic sexual dysfunction include both medical and surgical interventions. Nonsurgical interventions include correction of underlying disorders, particularly drug-induced dysfunction and endocrinopathy-related (e.g., reduced testosterone associated with chronic renal failure) dysfunction. Vasodilators and cessation of smoking can benefit individuals with vasculogenic erectile dysfunction. Surgical interventions include penile implants, penile revascularization, and correction of other anatomic defects contributing to sexual dysfunction.

DISORDERS OF THE BREAST

Disorders of the Female Breast
Galactorrhea

Galactorrhea (inappropriate lactation) is the persistent and sometimes excessive secretion of a milky fluid from the breasts of a woman who is not pregnant or nursing an infant. Galactorrhea, which can also occur in men, may involve one or both breasts and is not associated with breast cancer.

The incidence of galactorrhea is difficult to estimate because of differences among definitions of the condition, examination techniques, and populations of women who have been studied. Prevalence has been documented as 0.1% to 32% of all women.

Pathophysiology

Galactorrhea is not a breast disorder per se. Rather it is a manifestation of pathophysiologic processes elsewhere in the body. These processes are chiefly hormone imbalances caused by hypothalamic-pituitary disturbances, pituitary tumors, or neurologic damage. Exogenous causes include drugs, estrogen (e.g., in oral contraceptives), and manipulation of the nipples.

The most common cause of galactorrhea is **nonpuerperal hyperprolactinemia,** or excessive amounts of prolactin in the blood not related to pregnancy or childbirth. Prolactin is a pituitary hormone that stimulates milk production. Elevated prolactin levels are found in 49% to 77% of cases of galactorrhea. Nonpuerperal hyperprolactinemia can be caused by any factor that (1) stimulates or overstimulates the prolactin-secreting units of the pituitary gland; (2) interferes with production of **prolactin-inhibiting factor** (PIF), a neurotransmitter (probably dopamine) that inhibits prolactin secretion; or (3) interferes with pituitary receptors for PIF. A variety of exogenous agents and disorders can trigger one of these three mechanisms, thereby causing hyperprolactinemia.

Several drugs can cause nonpuerperal hyperprolactinemia. They include the phenothiazines, reserpine, and methyldopa; exogenous estrogens, particularly in oral contraceptives; morphine; and the tricyclic antidepressants.

Hypothyroidism causes increased secretion of hypothalamic thyroid-releasing hormone (TRH), which stimulates prolactin release from the pituitary. Hypothyroidism also is associated with reduced metabolic clearance of prolactin, which prolongs its effects.

Many types of pituitary tumors cause hyperprolactinemia. Approximately 20% of cases of galactorrhea are caused by a prolactin-secreting pituitary adenoma or prolactinoma. Prolactinomas cause hyperprolactinemia by secreting prolactin, decreasing production of PIF, or putting pressure on the pituitary stalk such that delivery of PIF to the anterior pituitary is prevented. Growth-hormone-secreting pituitary tumors may cause galactorrhea through the intrinsic lactogenic effect that growth hormone appears to have on mammary tissue. Prolactin-secreting lung and kidney tumors also cause hyperprolactinemia.

Chronic stress may cause hyperprolactinemia by inhibiting PIF release. Cervical spinal injuries, head trauma, encephalitis, meningitis, herpes zoster, or thoracotomy scars may stimulate the afferent portion of the suckling-reflex arc, which is carried in the second to sixth thoracic nerves. The suckling reflex increases prolactin secretion.

Galactorrhea can be induced by persistent and repeated sucking or squeezing of the nipples and has been documented in women who manipulate their breasts and nipples daily (Haagensen, 1986). Monthly examination of the breasts for nipple discharge is usually not associated with the development of galactorrhea.

Clinical Manifestations

Inappropriate lactation is manifested by the appearance of a milky breast secretion, usually from both breasts. Most women with galactorrhea have some menstrual abnormality. In fact, the most common complaint for which evaluation is sought is infertility, not galactorrhea.

If a hypothalamic or pituitary process is involved, the individual may report central nervous system symptoms. These include intractable headache, visual field abnormalities, and abnormal temperature, thirst, or appetite.

Evaluation and Treatment

The evaluation of galactorrhea includes a variety of diagnostic tests. Breast secretions are examined for fat globulets and neoplastic cells to verify their source. Serum prolactin levels are measured. Because such variables as eating, sleeping, stress, and breast examinations all increase prolactin levels, at least two positive results are needed for diagnosis of hyperprolactinemia. Prolactin levels greater than 25 to 30 ng/ml (by radioimmunoassay) are considered elevated. Those in the range of 75 to 100 ng/ml are considered to be caused by a pituitary tumor until proved otherwise. Serum T_4 and TSH levels are measured to rule out hypothyroidism, and LH and FSH levels are obtained if the individual is amenorrheic. CT scans MRI evaluations, and carotid angiography may assist in the localization of adenomas.

Treatment for galactorrhea consists of identification and treatment of the cause. Medical and surgical therapies may be involved. If a pituitary microadenoma is found, it may be surgically removed, particularly if there has been progressive tumor growth, loss of visual field or acuity, cranial nerve dysfunction, increased intracranial pressure, cerebrospinal fluid leak or obstruction, or infertility. A microadenoma may be treated medically with bromocriptine (Parlodel). This drug controls the tumor, but does not cure it, and must be taken indefinitely. A pituitary macroadenoma is usually treated medically because surgical and radiologic therapies seldom succeed.

Fibrocystic Disease

A great many terms have been used to describe benign breast lesions of epithelial origin. **Fibrocystic disease** (physiologic nodularity) is perhaps most descriptive of the clinical manifestations: palpable lumps in the breast that fluctuate with the menstrual cycle and may become progressively worse until menopause. *Fibrocystic disease* is not, however, an accurate term for the wide range of breast lesions it has been used to describe. Microcysts, macrocysts, adenosis, apocrine change, fibrosis, fibroadenomas, and ductal hyperplasia are all termed *fibrocystic disease*. This is unfortunate for two reasons. First, physiologic nodularity is present in approximately 50% of all menstruating women, and at least some of these pathophysiologic changes are seen in up to 90% of all women. It is probably a misnomer to term so widespread a process a "disease" (Hutter, 1985; Love, Gellman, & Silen, 1982). Second, some of the lesions called fibrocystic disease are associated with an increased risk of breast cancer, particularly when such variables as age and family history are considered. Having all these epithelial processes grouped together under one name generates significant confusion regarding potential outcomes, particularly the development of breast cancer.

A. Microscopic features normally seen in the breasts of women. They do not form a palpable tumor and are not predisposing factors for carcinoma.
  1. Blunt ducts.
  2. Microcysts: cysts less than 3 mm in diameter that evolve from blunt ducts.
  3. Apocrine gland epithelium.
B. Microscopic lesions frequently seen in the breasts of modern women, but not often enough to be regarded as normal components of breast tissue. They do not form a palpable tumor and are not predisposing factors for carcinoma.
  4. Adenosis: When very extensive, it may form a palpable tumor and therefore constitute a separate category.
  5. Papillomatosis.
C. Clinically evident lesions that often form a palpable tumor but are not predisposing factors for carcinoma.
  6. Fibrous disease.
  7. Solitary intraductal papilloma in a subareolar terminal duct.
D. A microscopic lesion that does not form a palpable tumor but is a predisposing factor for carcinoma.
  8. Lobular neoplasia (misnamed lobular carcinoma in situ).
E. Clinically evident breast lesions that form a palpable tumor and are predisposing factors for carcinoma.
  9. Multiple intraductal papilloma. A number of ducts, usually peripheral, are involved.
  10. Gross cysts that are 3 mm and more in diameter and are visible to the naked eye. When they reach 10 mm in diameter, they are usually palpable.

Adapted from Haagensen, 1986.
*Also called chronic cystic mastitis, cystic mastitis, mammary dysplasia, and, in Sweden, fibroadenomatosis.

On the basis of a study of 3303 women and at least a 15-year follow-up, Dupont and Page (1985) devised a three-category classification system for benign breast lesions and a risk index for the development of breast cancer. The three classifications are (1) lesions with no proliferative activity (nonproliferative lesions), including mild hyperplasia, microcysts, epithelium-related calcification, and fibroadenomas; (2) proliferative lesion without atypia, including moderate to florid hyperplasia,

TABLE 20-9 Relative risk of breast cancer in women with proliferative breast disease

Lesion	Risk
Proliferative lesion without atypia	
Age 46-55	1.1
Without calcifications	1.5
Without family history	1.5
Age greater than 55	1.7
Age 20-45	1.8
With calcifications	1.9
With family history	2.1
Atypical hyperplasia	
Without family history	3.5
Without calcifications	4.0
With calcifications	6.5
With family history	8.9
Overall risk, all women	1.5

From Dupont, & Page, 1985.

papillomas, ductal involvement with atypical lobular hyperplasia, and sclerosing adenosis; and (3) atypical hyperplasia, including the so-called borderline lesion (a lesion with some of the morphologic characteristics of carcinoma in situ). The risk index for classifications 2 and 3 is shown in Table 20-9.

Pathophysiology
The histologic changes associated with fibrocystic breast disease appear to be responses to hormonal stimulation; however, the exact causative mechanisms are not known at present. The hormone involved appears to be estrogen, but it is not known whether estrogen level alone or the estrogen-to-progesterone ratio is more important. Histologic changes may result from inappropriate responses by breast tissue to hormones rather than inappropriate hormone levels.

Clinical Manifestations
Pain or tenderness is the most common complaint associated with fibrocystic disease. Discomfort increases as menstruation approaches. Pain, fluctuation in lesion size, and presence of multiple lesions distinguish benign fibrocystic lesions from carcinoma.

Evaluation and Treatment
Breast biopsy is used to make a definitive diagnosis and assess an individual's risk for the development of

TABLE 20-10 Benign breast disorders

Benign breast disease	Period of greatest risk	Pathophysiology	Clinical manifestations of lesion	Treatment
Fibroadenoma	Puberty, early adulthood, rare after menopause	Unknown, but thought to be associated with exposure to increased estrogen levels	Painless, firm, solitary, well-circumscribed mobile mass; usually in upper outer quadrant of breast	Surgical excision of mass
Mammary duct ectasia (comedomastitis)	Menopausal, postmenopause, during lactation and nursing	Subareolar ducts become dilated and fill with cellular debris, initiating inflammatory reaction, rupture of ducts may occur	Blood-stained, sticky, thick spontaneous, multiple-duct discharge; ductal rupture creates palpable mass; burning pain swelling of areolar area may occur	Condition usually resolves 7-10 days after onset with or without antibiotic therapy
Solitary intraductal papilloma	Age 40-50	Unknown	Lesion is slow-growing, cauliflowerlike, and extends length of involved duct, nipple discharge from one or two ductal openings may be watery, serous, serosanguinous or sanguinous	Surgical excision of involved duct
Multiple papilloma	Age 35-40	Unknown	Similar to solitary intraductal papilloma, except that discharge is from multiple ductal openings	Depends on extent of involvement; if lesion is small, excision of that breast segment; total mastectomy if disease is widespread
Fat necrosis	Age 14-80, average age 50	Breast trauma, including silicone injections and breast biopsy, cause hemorrhage and induration, leading to formation of a palpable mass	Unilateral, fairly immobile breast mass, located close to the surface, mass is usually tender and painful	Mass may be reabsorbed spontaneously; biopsy, excision may be required if no resorption occurs

breast cancer. Mammography may be helpful, but the very dense breast tissue frequently seen in young women can make interpretation extremely difficult. Sonography can be used to differentiate a solid mass from a cystic (fluid-filled) mass.

Treatment consists largely of relieving symptoms. The individual can minimize breast pain by wearing a brassiere that provides good support. Cystic pain is reduced by draining the cysts under local anesthesia. Many women find that the elimination or reduction of caffeine in their diet reduces both the pain and the nodularity.

Danazol, a synthetic androgen, has been used to treat individuals with severe pain caused by proliferative breast disease. Danazol is thought to minimize the hormonal fluctuations to which breast tissue is exposed (Krupp, Chatton, & Tierney, 1986).

Benign breast tumors include fibroadenomas, mammary ductectasia, solitary intraductal papilloma, multiple papilloma, and fat necrosis. These benign conditions are summarized in Table 20-10.

Breast Cancer

Breast cancer incidence is second only to that of lung cancer in women. Breast cancer afflicts approximately 1 in every 10 women (American Cancer Society, 1989). It is the second most frequent cause of cancer death in both black and white women, killing approximately 43,000 women each year (American Cancer Society, 1989). Generally incidence is much higher among North American and Northern European women than among South American and Asian women. The risk of breast cancer increases as age advances, reaching a peak in women aged 45 to 64. After age 64 incidence increases slightly but less sharply (Ernster, 1984). Breast cancer is the leading cause of death in women between 40 and 44 years of age. The risk factors and possible etiologies of breast cancer can be classified as reproductive, hormonal, environmental, and familial.

Reproductive Factors

A woman's age when her first child is born affects her risk for developing breast cancer (American Cancer Society, 1989). The younger she is, the lower the risk. Pregnancies that do not proceed to term apparently have no protective effect. Women who have never given birth are at greater risk than those who have. The duration of a woman's reproductive life also affects her risk of developing breast cancer. Late menarche and early menopause (i.e., a short reproductive life) reduce risk.

Hormonal Factors

The link between breast cancer and hormones is based on three factors that affect risk: (1) the protective effect of an early first pregnancy; (2) the protective effect of removal of the ovaries and pituitary gland; and (3) the increased risk associated with early menarche, late menopause, and nulliparity. Oral contraceptive use and estrogen replacement therapy may be risk factors for breast cancer. Study results to date are conflicting and inconclusive.

Environmental Factors

High doses of ionizing radiation are associated with an increased risk of breast cancer, especially if exposure occurs during adolescence or pregnancy. These are periods when breast cells are proliferating rapidly.

A high-fat diet may increase the risk of breast cancer. The incidence of breast cancer is significantly higher in populations with high fat intake than in those with low fat intake. Breast cancer is rare in Japan, but not in Japanese immigrants in the United States who adopt Western eating habits. In 1980 a group of 89,538 registered nurses in the United States participated in a study to measure individual fat consumption and incidence of breast cancer (Willett, Stampfer, Colditz et al., 1987). Although the study period was limited (4 years), results

suggested that total fat intake or consumption of specific types of fat among women did not increase the risk of breast cancer.

Several studies have shown some correlation between breast cancer and alcohol ingestion (Graham, 1987). A higher risk of breast cancer is associated with even moderate drinking. According to one study as few as three drinks per week can increase a woman's risk of developing breast cancer by about 30% (Willett, Rosner, & Speizer, 1987). If the average woman's risk of developing breast cancer is 1 in 10, or 10%, drinking alcohol increases the risk to 13%. It does not matter whether the alcohol consumed is beer, wine, or hard liquor (Schatzkin et al., 1987).

The mechanisms by which alcohol increases the risk of breast cancer are unknown. Alcohol may hinder the liver's ability to rid the body of cancer-causing agents, impair the body's immune system, or make breast tissue more susceptible to cancer cells. It is not known whether decreasing or stopping alcohol consumption in midlife lessens the risk of breast cancer.

Familial Factors

A history of breast cancer in first-degree relatives (mother or sister) increases a woman's risk two to three times. Risk increases even more if two first-degree relatives are involved, especially if the disease occurred before menopause and was bilateral. In some families breast cancer occurs at an earlier age and the frequency of bilateral tumors is greater.

Pathogenesis

Table 20-11 lists the different types of breast carcinomas and summarizes their major characteristics. Most breast cancers arise from the ductal epithelium. Tumors of the infiltrating ductal type do not grow to a large size, but they metastasize early. This type accounts for 70% of breast cancers.

Metastatic spread of malignant cells occurs through the lymph vessels and the lymph nodes. The breast has three major pathways of lymphatic drainage: the axillary, internal mammary, and transpectoral routes. The axillary pathway is the usual route of metastatic spread. The lateral part of the mammary gland is drained into the anterior axillary or interpectoral node (Rotter node). Carcinoma of the breast metastasizes to the axillary nodes by embolization. That is, a small mass of cells, called a cancer embolus, breaks off from the tumor and enters the lymphatic system. When the cancer embolus reaches a lymph node, it may remain and enlarge the node or travel to a nearby or distant node. The embolus may bypass some of the axillary nodes and lodge in a node in the infraclavicular or supraclavicular area. About 60% of carcinomas of the breast occur in the upper outer quadrant because most of the glandular tissue

TABLE 20-11 Types of breast carcinomas and major distinguishing features

Histologic type	Distinguishing features
CARCINOMA OF MAMMARY DUCTS	
Papillary	Well-delineated cystic masses in multiple areas. Hemorrhage often present. Majority appear in 40-60 age group. Often involves skin.
Intraductal (comedo)	Often accompanied by evidence of infection. Well-circumscribed tumors within the duct, well-differentiated tumor cells. Rarely ulcerates the skin.
Infiltrating carcinoma	
Ductal	Fibrous, firm, glistening, gray-tan mass with chalky streaks, mixture of patterns. Infrequent, slow-growing, causes discharge from the nipple.
Mucinous	Usually large, >3 cm in diameter, circumscribed and encapsulated, glistening appearance, varies in color. Two types: pure and mixed. Pure tumor is surrounded by mucin. Infrequent; found in the lateral half of the breast.
Medullary	Encapsulated and grows to be very large (7-8 cm in diameter). Commonly infiltrates lymphoid tissue. Occurs after age 50.
Tubular	Well-differentiated with orderly tubules in center (stroma) of mass. Associated with the noninfiltrating ductal carcinoma. Occurs in women about 50 years of age. Nodal metastasis infrequent.
Adenoid cystic	Very rare. Well-circumscribed, painless mass arising from the nipple and areola.
Metaplastic	Involves cartilage or bone, mixed tumors or osteogenic sarcomas.
Squamous cell	Frequent in blacks. Originates in ductal epithelium.
CARCINOMA OF MAMMARY LOBULES	
Lobular carcinoma in situ	Found in individuals with fibrocystic disease. Localized to upper breast quadrants. Risk of 10%-35% becoming invasive. Occurs frequently in mid-40s. Infiltrating variety occurs in early 50s.
Infiltrating lobular	Infiltrates from duct. Firm mass with chalk streaks.
Paget disease	Eczema of the nipple that extends to the areola. Cancer usually found underneath the nipple. Poorly circumscribed. Large Paget cells arise from the duct and directly invade nipple. History of scaly, red rash spreading from the nipple. Lesion palpable beneath the nipple, often bilateral. Occurs in middle age.
Inflammatory carcinomas	Not a histologic type. Fairly diffuse within the breast tissue; diffuse edema of the overlying skin. Extremely undifferentiated, very rare, most metastasize to axilla.
Sarcoma of the breast	
Cytosarcoma phyllodes	Usually large (>17 cm in diameter). Mostly localized, but can rupture through the skin. Rarely metastasizes to lymph nodes. History of painless nodule present for years before it forms a large mass. Ulceration and bleeding of skin often present. Occurs in wide age range (13-77 years).
Fibrosarcoma	Well-circumscribed, firm, and usually do not involve the skin or nipple. Well-differentiated to extremely undifferentiated. Arise from connective tissue; are extremely rare (e.g., liposarcoma, angiosarcoma).

of the breast is there (Fig. 20-26). The lymphatic spread of cancer to the opposite breast, to lymph nodes in the base of the neck, and to the abdominal cavity is caused by obstruction of the normal lymphatic pathways or destruction of lymphatic vessels by surgery or radiotherapy. The less common inner-quadrant tumors may spread to mediastinal nodes or Rotter nodes, which are located between the pectoral muscles. Internal mammary chain nodes are frequent sites of metastasis.

Metastases from the vertebral veins can involve the vertebrae, pelvic bones, ribs, and skull. The lungs, kidneys, liver, adrenal glands, ovaries, and pituitary gland are also sites of metastasis.

Approximately one third of breast cancers are hormone-dependent and regress in response to surgical removal of the ovaries. Estrogens are of primary significance in maintaining some breast cancer growths. Not all breast tumors, however, are estrogen-receptor- (ER-)

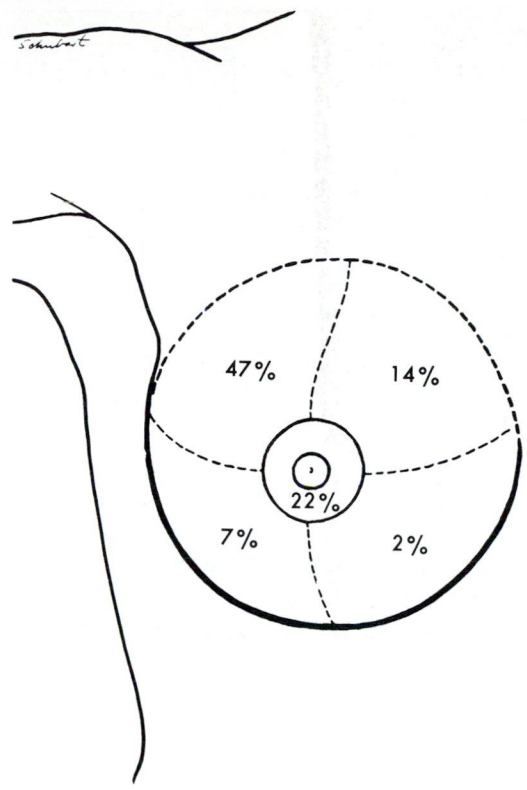

FIG. 20-26. Distribution of carcinomas in different areas of the breast. (From del Regato, Spjut, & Cox, 1985.)

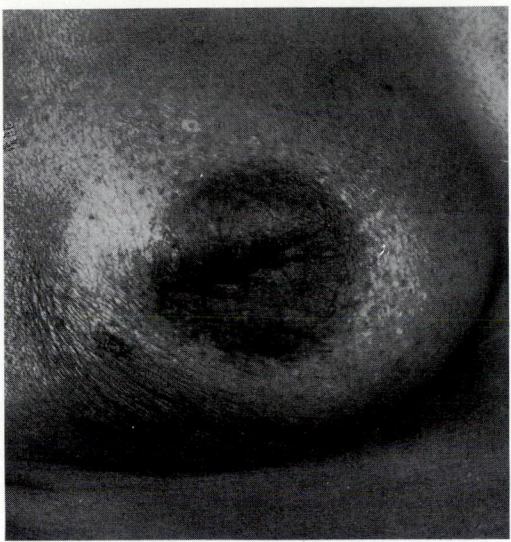

FIG. 20-27. Retraction of nipple caused by carcinoma. (From del Regato, Spjut, & Cox, 1985.)

positive. Whether the estrogen receptor is initially present in all tumor types and is lost as the tumor matures or whether ER-positive and ER-negative tumors represent different types is not clear at present.

Clinical Manifestations

The first sign of breast cancer is usually a painless lump. Lumps caused by breast tumors do not have any classic characteristics. Other presenting signs include palpable nodes in the axilla; retraction of tissue (dimpling) (Fig. 20-27) or bone pain due to metastasis to the vertebrae. Table 20-12 summarizes the clinical manifestations of breast cancers. Manifestations vary according to the type of tumor and stage of disease.

Evaluation and Treatment

Mammography, thermography, and biopsy are generally utilized in evaluating breast cancer. Biopsy is the definitive diagnostic test.

Treatment is based on the extent or stage of the cancer (Table 20-13). The extent of the tumor at the primary site, the presence and extent of lymph node metastasis, and the presence of distant metastases are all evaluated to determine the stage of disease.

Surgery, radiation, and chemotherapy may be used to treat breast cancer. The extent of the surgery depends on the tumor's histology, predictability, and stage and the individual's age and medical and psychologic history. Beginning with the most conservative, the surgical procedures commonly used are (1) tylectomy or lumpectomy, in which the tumor and a small amount of surrounding tissue are removed; (2) quadrant excision, in which a quadrant of the breast is removed; (3) partial mastectomy, in which a larger amount of tissue is removed; (4) total or simple mastectomy, in which the tumor and all breast tissue are removed (the nipple may or may not be removed); (5) modified radical mastectomy, in which the breast, pectoralis minor, and axillary contents are removed; and (6) radical mastectomy, in which the breast, axillary contents, and pectoralis major and minor are removed. Radiation therapy is infrequently used except to prevent metastasis of a small tumor (<2 cm) that has been surgically excised. Chemotherapy is most successful as an adjunct to surgery in premenopausal women with hormone-dependent tumors. It is also used in individuals with advanced disease. Endocrine therapy (androgens, estrogens, progesterones, and steroids) may be used to prolong survival time and appears most effective in women with ER-positive tumors. ER-negative tumors are unlikely to respond to hormonal therapy.

Disorders of the Male Breast
Gynecomastia

Gynecomastia is the overdevelopment of breast tissue in a male. Gynecomastia accounts for approximately 85% of all masses that develop in the male breast and affects 32% to 40% of the male population. If only one

TABLE 20-12 Clinical manifestations of breast cancer

Clinical manifestation	Pathophysiology
Local pain	Local obstruction caused by the tumor
Dimpling of the skin	Can occur with invasion of the dermal lymphatics because of retraction of Cooper ligament, or involvement of the pectoralis fascia
Nipple retraction	Shortening of the mammary ducts
Skin retraction	Involvement of the suspensory ligaments
Edema	Local inflammation or lymphatic obstruction
Nipple/areolar eczema	Paget disease
Pitting of the skin (similar to the surface of an orange [*peau d'orange*])	Obstruction of the subcutaneous lymphatics, resulting in the accumulation of fluid
Reddened skin, local tenderness, and warmth	Inflammation
Dilated blood vessels	Obstruction of venous return by a fast-growing tumor; obstruction dilates superficial veins
Nipple discharge in a non-lactating woman	Spontaneous and intermittent discharge caused by tumor obstruction
Ulceration	Tumor necrosis
Hemorrhage	Erosion of blood vessels
Edema of the arm	Obstruction of lymphatic drainage in the axilla
Chest pain	Metastasis to the lung

Adapted from Griffiths, Murray, & Russo, 1984.

breast is involved, it is typically the left. Incidence is greatest among adolescents and men over 50.

Gynecomastia results from hormonal alterations, which may be idiopathic or caused by systemic disorders, drugs, or neoplasms. Gynecomastia usually involves an imbalance of the estrogen/testosterone ratio. The normal estrogen/testosterone ratio can be altered in one of two ways. First, estrogen levels may be excessively high, although testosterone levels are normal. This is the case in drug-induced and tumor-induced cases of hyperestrogenism. Second, testosterone levels may be extremely low, although estrogen levels are normal, as is the case in hypergonadism. Gynecomastia can also be caused by alterations in breast-tissue responsiveness to hormonal stimulation. Breast tissue may have increased responsiveness to estrogen or decreased responsiveness to androgen. Alterations of responsiveness may cause many cases of idiopathic gynecomastia.

Besides puberty and aging, estrogen-testosterone imbalances are associated with hypogonadism, Klinefelter syndrome, and testicular neoplasms. Hormone-induced gynecomastia is usually bilateral. Pubertal gynecomastia is a self-limiting phenomenon that usually disappears within 4 to 6 months. Senescent gynecomastia usually regresses spontaneously within 6 to 12 months.

Systemic disorders associated with gynecomastia include cirrhosis of the liver, infectious hepatitis, chronic renal failure, chronic obstructive lung disease, hyperthyroidism, tuberculosis, and chronic malnutrition. It may be that these disorders ultimately alter the estrogen/testosterone ratio, initiating the gynecomastia.

Gynecomastia is frequently seen in males receiving estrogen therapy, either in preparation for a sex-change operation or for prostatic carcinoma. Other drugs that can cause gynecomastia include digitalis, cimetidine, spironolactone, reserpine, thiazide, isoniazid, ergotamine, tricyclic antidepressants, amphetamines, vincristine, and busulfan. Gynecomastia is usually unilateral in these instances.

Malignancies of the testes, adrenals, or liver can cause gynecomastia if they alter the estrogen/testosterone ratio. Pituitary adenomas and lung cancer are also associated with gynecomastia.

Pathophysiology

The enlargement consists of hyperplastic stroma and ductal tissue. Hyperplasia results in a firm, palpable mass, at least 2 cm in diameter and located beneath the areola.

TABLE 20-13	Staging and TMN classification of breast cancer

Stage	TNM Classification
Stage 1	T_1 (tumor 2 cm or less)
	N_0 (no palpable axillary nodes)
	M_0 (no evident metastasis)
Stage 2	T_0 (no palpable tumor)
	T_1 (tumor 2 cm or less)
	T_2 (tumor less than 5 cm)
	N_1 (palpable axillary nodes with histologic evidence of breast malignancy)
Stage 3	T_3 (tumor more than 5 cm; may be fixed to muscle or fascia)
	N_1 or N_2 (fixed nodes)
	M_0
Stage 4	T_4 (tumor any size with fixation to chest wall or skin; presence of edema, including *peau d'orange;* ulceration; skin nodules; inflammatory carcinoma)
	N_3 (supraclavicular or intraclavicular nodes or arm edema)
	M_1 (distant metastasis present or suspected)

From Phipps, Long, & Woods, 1987.

Evaluation and Treatment

The diagnosis of gynecomastia is based on physical examination. Identification and treatment of the cause are likely to be followed by resolution of the gynecomastia. The man should be taught to perform breast self-examination and is examined at 6- and 12-month intervals if the gynecomastia persists.

Carcinoma

Breast cancer in males accounts for 0.2% of all male cancers and 1% of all breast cancers. Breast cancer in men is seen most commonly after the age of 60, with the peak incidence between 60 and 69 years. It has, however, been reported in males as young as 6 and in adolescents. Possible risk factors include gynecomastia, radiation of the chest wall, and family history of breast cancer. The relationship between these factors and risk of disease is not clearly defined at present.

Male breast tumors frequently resemble carcinoma of the breast in women. Estrogen receptors have been found in up to 84% of biopsied specimens from men (deVita, Hellman, & Rosenberg, 1985). The malignant male breast lesion is usually a unilateral solid mass located near the nipple. Because the nipple is commonly involved, crusting and nipple discharge are typical clini-

cal manifestations. Other findings include skin retraction, ulceration of the skin over the tumor, and axillary node involvement. Patterns of metastasis are similar to those in females.

The diagnosis of cancer is confirmed by biopsy. Because of delays in seeking treatment male breast cancer tends to be advanced at the time of diagnosis and therefore to have a poor prognosis. Treatment protocols are similar to those for female breast cancer, but endocrine therapy is used more frequently for males because a higher percentage of male tumors are hormone-dependent. Orchiectomy is performed to treat metastatic disease.

SUMMARY REVIEW

Alterations of Sexual Maturation

1 Sexual maturation, or puberty, should begin in girls between the ages of 8 and 13, and in boys between the ages of 9 and 14. Delayed puberty is the onset of sexual maturation after these ages; precocious puberty is onset before these ages.

2 Alterations of sexual maturation can be idiopathic or caused by a disease or congenital anomaly. In most cases of delayed puberty the hypothalamic-pituitary-gonad axis is intact, but the surge of activity that stimulates puberty is delayed. This situation is common in boys. Precocious puberty, which is more common in girls, can also be caused by mistiming of the stimulatory surge in a child whose hypothalamic-pituitary-ovarian system is otherwise normal.

3 Precocious puberty can be isosexual (sex-appropriate), heterosexual (not sex-appropriate), or partial (development of one secondary sex characteristic only).

Disorders of the Female Reproductive System

1 The female reproductive system can be altered by hormonal imbalances, infectious microorganisms, inflammation, structural abnormalities, and benign or malignant proliferative conditions.

2 Menstrual disorders usually involve some disruption of the hypothalamic-pituitary-ovarian axis and subsequent alteration of hormone production, reception by target organs, or feedback mechanisms.

3 Primary dysmenorrhea is painful menstruation not associated with pelvic disease. Its cause is not known for certain, but primary dysmenorrhea probably results from excessive synthesis of prostaglandins, which cause the myometrium to contract and constrict blood verssels, resulting in ischemic pain.

4 Primary amenorrhea is the continued absence of menarche and menstrual function after 16 years of age. Usually secondary characteristics fail to develop.

5 Primary amenorrhea may be caused by decreased or absent secretion of GnRH, FSH, or LH; ovarian resistance to FSH or LH; anatomic defects, such as congen-

ital absence of the uterus; or genetic disorders, including Turner syndrome.

6　Secondary amenorrhea is the occurrence of menstruation three or fewer times per year in women who have previously menstruated. Secondary amenorrhea is associated with anovulation.

7　Secondary amenorrhea can be physiologic (e.g., during adolscence, premenopause, during pregnancy) or pathophysiologic. This condition develops if the uterus is removed or if levels of regulatory hormones are altered so as to inhibit ovulation.

8　Dysfunctional uterine bleeding is heavy or irregular bleeding caused by a disturbance of the menstrual cycle.

9　Polycystic ovarian syndrome (PCO) is a condition in which excessive androgen production is triggered by inappropriate secretion of gonadotropins. Depressed FSH and elevated LH levels perpetuate adrenal and ovarian secretion of androgens, which are converted to estrogen in peripheral tissues. This hormonal imbalance prevents ovulation and causes enlargement and cyst formation in the ovaries, excessive endometrial proliferation in the uterus, and, occasionally, hirsutism.

10　Premenstrual syndrome (PMS) is the cyclic recurrence of physical, psychological, or behavioral changes distressing enough to disrupt normal activities or interpersonal relationships. Physical symptoms include abdominal bloating, breast tenderness and swelling, and constipation. The usual psychological symptoms are irritability and emotional lability.

11　Infection and inflammation of the female genitalia can result from microorganisms from the environment or overproliferation of microorganisms that normally populate the genital tract.

12　Pelvic inflammatory disease (PID) is an acute ascending infection of the upper genital tract. Its usual cause is a sexually transmitted pathogen.

13　Vaginitis, or vaginal infection, is usually caused by sexually transmitted pathogens or to *Candida albicans,* which causes candidiasis. Susceptibility to infection is highest when estrogen levels are lowest (e.g., before puberty, after menopause, and during the luteal phase of the menstrual cycle). Risk factors associated with low estrogen levels are alkaline pH, relatively thin epithelium, and decreased populations of lactobacilli.

14　Cervicitis, which is infection of the cervix, can be acute (mucopurulent cervicitis) or chronic. Its most common cause is a sexually transmitted pathogen.

15　Vulvitis is an inflammation of the skin of the vulva. It can be caused by chemical irritants, allergens, skin disorders, irritation from tight-fitting clothing, or spread of vaginal infections, such as candidiasis.

16　Bartholinitis, also called Bartholin cyst, is an infection of the ducts that lead from the Bartholin glands to the surface of the vulva. Infection blocks the glands, preventing the outflow of glandular secretions.

17　The pelvic relaxation disorders—uterine displacement, uterine prolapse, cystocele, rectocele, and urethrocele—are caused by the relaxation of muscles and fascial supports, usually with age or after childbirth or other trauma.

18　Benign growths and proliferative conditions of the female reproductive tract tend to affect the ovaries (benign ovarian cysts) or uterine tissues (endometrial polyps, leiomyomas, and endometriosis).

19　Benign ovarian cysts develop from mature ovarian follicles that do not release their ova (follicular cysts) or from a corpus luteum that persists abnormally instead of degenerating (corpus luteum cyst).

20　Endometrial polyps consist of overgrowths of endometrial tissue. Though their etiology is unknown, these polyps are associated with high estrogen levels, which promote endometrial proliferation. Some of the polyps wax and wane with estrogen levels during the menstrual cycle.

21　Leiomyomas, also called uterine fibroids, are tumors arising from the muscle layer of the uterus, the myometrium. Their etiology is unknown, but, like endometrial polyps, they tend to grow when estrogen levels are high.

22　Endometriosis is the presence of functional endometrial tissue (i.e., tissue that responds to hormonal stimulation) at sites outside the uterus. Endometriosis causes an inflammatory reaction at the site of implantation and is a cause of infertility.

23　Most cancers of the female genitalia involve the uterus (particularly the cervix) and the ovaries. Cancer of the vagina is rare.

24　Risk factors for cervical cancer are young age at first coitus, multiple sexual partners, exposure to sexually transmitted viral infection, long-term use of oral contraceptives, and exposure to cigarette smoke. Incidence is greatest among women in their 40s; however, it is increasing in younger women.

25　Cervical cancer arises from the cervical epithelium. The progressively serious neoplastic alterations are (a) cervical intraepithelial neoplasia (cervical dysplasia), cervical carcinoma in situ, and invasive cervical carcinoma.

26　Risk factors for cancer of the vagina are exposure in utero to nonsteroidal estrogens (e.g., DES), exposure to sexually transmitted viral infection, radiation therapy for other genital cancers, and chronic irritation from use of a pessary. Incidence is greatest in women over 70.

27　Most vaginal cancers are not invasive. Like cervical cancers, they arise from the epithelium and are identified as intraepithelial neoplasia (dysplasia), carcinoma in situ, or invasive carcinoma.

28　Risk factors for endometrial cancer include overnutrition, decreased glucose tolerance, high blood pressure, lack of childbearing (nulliparity), early menarche, habitual abortion, family history of the disease, history of endometrial polyps or leiomyomas, and hyperestrogenism (abnormally high estrogen levels). Incidence of endometrial cancer is greatest among women in their 50s and early 60s.

29　Risk factors for ovarian cancer include residence in an industrialized country, white race, nulliparity or low parity, estrogen replacement therapy after menopause, exposure to cigarette smoke, and exposure to asbestos or talc. Ovarian cancer causes more deaths than any other genital cancer in women.

30 Ovarian tumors can arise from the ovarian epithelium or from the female germ cells (developing ova). Epithelial neoplasms account for 90% of all ovarian malignancies.

Disorders of the Male Reproductive System

1 Disorders of the urethra include urethritis (infection of the urethra) and urethral strictures (narrowing or obstruction of the urethral lumen caused by scarring).

2 Most cases of urethritis result from sexually transmitted pathogens. Infectious urethritis can also be caused by urologic instrumentation, foreign bodies inserted into the urethra, trauma, or an anatomic abnormality. Noninfectious urethritis can be caused by drinking a toxic fluid (wood or ethyl alcohol, turpentine) and by Reiter syndrome.

3 Urethritis causes urinary symptoms (dysuria), including a burning sensation during urination, frequency, and urgency.

4 The scarring that causes urethral stricture can be caused by trauma or by severe untreated urethritis.

5 Manifestations of urethral stricture include those of bladder outlet obstruction: urinary frequency and hesitancy, diminished force and caliber of the urinary stream, dribbling after voiding, and nocturia.

6 Phimosis and paraphimosis are penile disorders involving the foreskin (prepuce). In phimosis the foreskin cannot be retracted over the glans. In paraphimosis the foreskin is retracted and cannot be reduced (returned in its normal anatomic position over the glans). Phimosis prevents cleansing and is a risk factor for penile cancer. Paraphimosis can constrict the penile blood vessels, preventing circulation to the glans.

7 Peyronie disease consists of fibrosis, usually affecting one of the corpora cavernosa, which causes penile curvature during erection. Fibrosis prevents engorgement on the affected side, causing a lateral curvature that can prevent intercourse.

8 Priapism is a prolonged, painful erection that is not stimulated by sexual arousal. The corpora cavernosa (but not the corpus spongiosum) fill with blood that does not drain out, probably because of venous obstruction. Priapism is associated with spinal cord trauma, sickle cell disease, leukemia, and pelvic tumors. It can also be idiopathic.

9 Balanitis is an inflammation of the glans penis. It is associated with phimosis, inadequate cleansing under the foreskin, skin disorders, and pathogens (e.g., *Candida albicans*).

10 Cancer of the penis is rare and tends to occur in uncircumcised men and men with phimosis. Penile carcinoma in situ tends to involve the glans; invasive carcinoma of the penis involves the shaft as well.

11 A varicocele is an abnormal dilation of the veins within the spermatic cord caused by either congenital absence of valves in the internal spermatic vein or acquired valvular incompetence.

12 A hydrocele is a collection of fluid between the testicular and scrotal layers of the tunica vaginalis. Hydroceles can be idiopathic or caused by trauma or infection of the testes.

13 A spermatocele is a cyst of the testis or epididymis that is filled with fluid and sperm.

14 Cryptorchidism is a congenital condition in which one or both testes fail to descend into the scrotum. It may be caused by a developmental delay of descent, presence of a defective testicle, or some mechanical factor preventing descent, such as a short spermatic cord or a narrowed inguinal canal. Uncorrected cryptorchidism is associated with infertility and significantly increased risk of testicular cancer.

15 Testicular torsion is the rotation of a testis, which twists blood vessels in the spermatic cord. This interrupts blood supply to the testis, resulting in edema and, if not corrected within 6 hours, necrosis and atrophy of testicular tissues.

16 Orchitis is an acute infection of the testes. Pathogenic organisms may reach the testes through the blood or the lymphatics; most commonly, they reach the testes by ascending through the vas deferens and epididymis. Complications of orchitis include hydrocele and abscess formation.

17 Testicular cancer is the most common malignancy in males from 25 to 35 years of age. Although its etiology is unknown, high androgen levels, genetic predisposition, and history of cryptorchidism, trauma, or infection may contribute to tumorigenesis. Most testicular neoplasms are germ cell tumors.

18 Spermatogenesis (sperm production by the testes) can be impaired by disruptions of the hypothalamic-pituitary-testicular axis that reduce testosterone secretion and by testicular trauma, infection, or atrophy from any cause. Sperm production is also impaired by neoplastic disease, cryptorchidism, or any factor (e.g., circulatory impairment, wearing of tight clothing) that causes testicular temperature to rise.

19 Sperm quality is impaired by chromosomal abnormalities resulting from genetic factors, irradiation, or toxins. Sperm motility can be impaired by unfavorable constituents or characteristics of semen. Reductions in quality, motility, or number (per milliliter of semen) all impair fertility.

20 Epididymitis, an inflammation of the epididymis, is usually caused by a sexually transmitted pathogen that ascends through the vasa deferentia from an already infected urethra or bladder.

21 Benign prostatic hyperplasia (BPH), also called benign prostatic hypertrophy, is the enlargement of the prostate gland. This condition becomes symptomatic as the enlarging prostate compresses the urethra, causing symptoms of bladder outlet obstruction and urine retention.

22 Bacterial prostatitis is an infection of the prostate. Acute bacterial prostatitis causes an inflammatory response in which the prostate becomes enlarged, tender, and firm. Infection may spread to the bladder. Chronic

bacterial prostatitis is recurrent prostatic infection that eventually causes fibrosis.

23 Nonbacterial prostatitis is prostatic inflammation without evidence of bacterial infection.

24 Prostate cancer is the third leading cause of cancer deaths in men (after lung and colorectal cancer). Possible etiologies involve genetic predisposition, environmental factors, sexually transmitted pathogens, and impaired immune function. Incidence is greatest among Northern European and North American men (particularly blacks) over 50.

25 Most cancers of the prostate are adenocarcinomas that develop at the periphery of the gland. Because there are no early symptoms, disease is often advanced at the time of diagnosis.

26 Sexual dysfunction in males can be caused by any physical or psychologic factor that impairs erection, emission, or ejaculation.

27 Vascular disorders can prevent initiation or maintenance of an erection; endocrine disorders that reduce testosterone levels can decrease libido; neurologic disorders can interfere with erection, emission, and ejaculation; chronic diseases can cause physiologic or psychologic dysfunction; priapism and Peyronie disease can impair erectile function; and surgical procedures and many drugs can disrupt processes necessary for sexual function.

Disorders of the Breast

1 Most disorders of the breast are disorders of the mammary gland, that is, the female breast.

2 Galactorrhea, or inappropriate lactation, is the persistent secretion of a milky substance by the breasts of a woman who is not in the postpartum state or nursing an infant. Its most common cause is nonpuerperal hyperprolactinemia, a rise in serum prolactin levels that is not associated with pregnancy and childbirth.

3 *Fibrocystic breast disease* is a catch-all term used to describe a variety of benign epithelial breast lesions, including microcysts, macrocysts, adenosis, apocrine gland change, fibroadenomas, and ductal hyperplasia. Many of these lesions are risk factors for breast cancer, and most appear to represent a response of breast tissue to estrogen stimulation.

4 The lesions of fibrocystic disease are nodular, are multiple, and become tender and large as menstruation approaches. They are palpable and may worsen until menopause. Physiologic nodularity is present in about 50% of menstruating women.

5 Other benign breast lesions are fibroadenomas, mammary duct ectasia (an inflammatory condition), intraductal papillomas, and fat necrosis.

6 Breast cancer is the second most common form of cancer in women and second to lung cancer as the most frequent cause of cancer death.

7 The major risk factors for breast cancer are environmental factors, such as a high-fat diet; reproductive factors, such as nulliparity; and familial factors, such as a family history of breast cancer.

8 Approximately one third of breast cancers are hormone-dependent, or estrogen-receptor-positive. Treatment protocols are often based on whether the tumor is estrogen-receptor-positive or -negative.

9 Most breast cancers arise from the ductal epithelium and then may metastasize to the lymphatics, opposite breast, abdominal cavity, lungs, bones, kidneys, liver, adrenal glands, ovaries, and pituitary glands.

10 The first clinical manifestation of breast cancer is usually a small, painless lump in the breast. Other manifestations include palpable lymph nodes in the axilla, dimpling of the skin, nipple and skin retraction, nipple discharge, ulcerations, reddened skin, and bone pain associated with bony metastases.

11 Gynecomastia is the overdevelopment (hyperplasia) of breast tissue in a male. It presents as a firm, palpable mass at least 2 cm in diameter and is located in the subareolar area.

12 Gynecomastia affects 32% to 40% of the male population. Incidence is greatest among adolescents and men over 50.

13 Gynecomastia is caused by hormonal or breast tissue alterations that cause estrogen to dominate. These alterations can result from systemic disorders, drugs, neoplasms, or idiopathic causes.

14 Breast cancer is relatively uncommon in males, but it has a poor prognosis because men tend to delay seeking treatment until the disease is advanced. Incidence is greatest in men in their sixties.

15 Most breast cancers in men are estrogen-receptor-positive.

KEY TERMS

Acute bacterial prostatitis, 708

Amenorrhea, 680

Anovulation, 681

Balanitis, 700

Bartholinitis (Bartholin cyst), 687

Benign prostatic hyperplasia (BPH); benign prostatic hypertrophy, 707

Cervical carcinoma in situ, 693

Cervical intraepithelial neoplasm (CIN); cervical dysplasia, 693

Cervicitis, 687

Chronic bacterial prostatitis, 708

Corpus luteum cyst, 690

Cryptorchidism, 702

Cystocele, 689

Delayed puberty, 678

Dysfunctional uterine bleeding, 682

Endometrial polyp, 690

Endometriosis, 691

Epididymitis, 706

Fibrocystic disease (physiologic nodularity), 712

Follicular cyst, 690

Galactorrhea, 711

Gynecomastia, 717

Heterosexual precocious puberty, 678

Hirsutism, 681

Hydrocele, 701

Hyperprolactinemia, 681

Incomplete precocious puberty, 678

Invasive carcinoma of the cervix, 693

Isosexual precocious puberty, 678

Leiomyoma (uterine fibroid), 691

Leukorrhea, 687

Mucopurulent cervicitis, 687

Nonbacterial prostatitis, 708

Nonpuerperal hyperprolactinemia, 711

Oophritis, 685

Orchitis, 703

Paraphimosis, 699

Pelvic inflammatory disease (PID), 685

Pessary, 690

Peyronie disease, 699

Phimosis, 699

Polycystic ovarian syndrome (PCO), 683

Precocious puberty, 678

Premenstrual syndrome (PMS), 683

Priapism, 700

Primary amenorrhea, 680

Primary dysmenorrhea, 680

Prolactin-inhibiting factor, 712

Prostatitis, 707

Prostatodynia, 708

Retrocele, 689

Retrograde menstruation, 691

Secondary amenorrhea, 681

Salpingitis, 685

Sexual dysfunction, 710

Spermatocele, 702

Torsion of the testis, 703

Urethral stricture, 699

Urethritis, 699

Urethrocele, 689

Uterine prolapse, 689

Vaginitis, 686

Varicocele, 701

Vulvitis, 687

REFERENCES

American Cancer Society. (1989). *Cancer statistics. Ca—A Cancer: Journal for Clinicians, 39*(1).

Beral, V., Hannaford, P., & Clifford, K. (1988). Oral contraceptive use and malignancies of the genital tract. *Lancet, 2,* 1331-1335.

Coppleson, M., Pixley, E., & Reed, B. (1971). *Colposcopy: A scientific approach to the cervix in health and disease.* Springfield, Ill.: Charles C Thomas.

Culp, D., Fallon, B., & Loening, A. H. (1985). *Surgical urology.* Chicago: Year Book Medical.

del Regato, J. A., Spjut, H. J., & Cox, J. D. (1985). *Ackerman and del Regato's cancer: Diagnosis, treatment, and prognosis* (6th ed.). St. Louis: C. V. Mosby

deVita, V. T., Hellman, S., & Rosenberg, S. A. (1985). *Cancer principles and practice of oncology* (2 ed.). Philadelphia: Lippincott.

diSaia, P. J., & Creasman, W. T. (1989). *Clinical gynecologic oncology* (3 ed.). St. Louis: C. V. Mosby.

Droegemueller, W. D., Herbst, A. L., Mischell, D. R., & Stenehever, M. A. (1987). *Comprehensive gynecology.* St. Louis: C. V. Mosby.

Drugs that cause sexual dysfunction. (1983). *Medical Letter, 25* (641), 73-76.

Dupont, W., & Page, D. (1985). Risk factors for breast cancer in women with proliferative breast disease. *New England Journal of Medicine, 312*(2), 146-151.

Elliott, P. M., Tattersall, M. H. N., Coppelson, M., Russell, P., Wong, F., Coates, A. S., Solomon, H. J., Bannatyne, P. M., Atkinson, K. H., & Murray, J. C. (1989). Changing character of cervical cancer in young women. *British Medical Journal, 298,* 288-290.

Ellis, M., & Sikora, K. (1987, January). The current management of testicular cancer. *British Journal of Urology, 59*(1), 2-9.

Ernster, V. L. (1984). Risk factors for benign and malignant breast disease. In E. B. Gold (Ed.), *The changing risk of disease in women: An epidemiologic appproach.* Lexington, Mass.: Collamore Press.

400 Self-assessment picture tests in clinical medicine. (1984.) London: Wolfe Medical Publications, Ltd.

Gardner, H. L., & Kaufman, R. H. (1969). *Benign diseases of the vulva and vagina.* St. Louis: C. V. Mosby.

Garnick, M. B., Scully, R. E., Weber, E. T., & Krane, J. R. (1986). Cancer of the testis. In *Cancer Manual.* Boston: American Cancer Society.

Graham, B. J. (1987). Extramural programs of the Fogarty International Center. *National Institutes of Health Psychologist, 30*(5), 160, 249, 251-253. 160.

Griffiths, M. J., Murray, K. H., & Russo, P. C. (1984). *Oncology nursing: Pathophysiology, assessment, and intervention.* New York: Macmillan.

Haagensen, C. D. (1986). *Diseases of the breast.* Philadelphia: W. B. Saunders.

Heible, J. P., & Caine, M. (1986, October). Etiology of benign prostatic hyperplasia and approaches to its pharmacological management. *Federation Proceedings, 45*(11), 2601-2603.

Hoekelman, R. A., Blatman, S., Friedman, S. B., Nelson, N. M., & Seidel, H. M. (1987) *Primary pediatric care.*St. Louis: C. V. Mosby.

Hutter, R. V. P. (1985). Goodbye to fibrocystic disease. *New England Journal of Medicine, 312*(3), 179-181.

Kissane, J. M. (Ed.). (1985). *Anderson's pathology* (8th ed.). St. Louis: C.V. Mosby.

Knapp, R. C. (1986). Cancer of the female genital tract. In *Cancer Manual.* Boston: American Cancer Society.

Kritzler, R. K., Plotnick, L. P., & Migeon, C. J. (1987). Sexual development alterations. In R. A. Hoekelman et al. (Eds.), *Primary pediatric care.* St. Louis: C. V. Mosby.

Krupp, M., Chatton, M., & Tierney, L. (1986). *Current medical diagnosis and treatment, 1986.* Los Altos, Calif.: Lange Medical.

Layde, P. M. (1989). Smoking and cervical cancer: Cause or coincidence? *Journal of the American Medical Association, 261,* 1631-1633.

Lloyd-Davies, R. W., Gow, J. G., & Davies, D. R. (1983). Color atlas of urology. London: Wolfe Medical Publications, Ltd.

Love, S. M., Gellman, R. S., & Silen, W. (1982). Fibrocystic "disease" of the breast—a non-disease? *New England Journal of Medicine, 307,* 1010-1014.

Mostofi, F. K., & Sobin, L. H. (1977). Histologic typing of testicular tumors. In *International histological classification of tumors, 16.* Geneva: World Health Organization.

Overstreet, J. W., & Katz, D. F. (1987). Semen analysis. *Urologic Clinics of North America, 14*(3), 441-449.

Persson, I., Adami, O., Bergkvist, L., Lindgren, A., Petterson, B., Hoover, R., & Schairer, C. (1989). Endometrial cancer after treatment with oestrogens alone or in conjunction with progesterones: Results of a prospective study. *British Medical Journal, 298,* 147-151.

Pfau, A. (1986). Prostatis. *Urologic Clinics of North America, 13*(4), 695-714.

Phipps, W. P., Long, B. C., & Woods, N. F. (1987). *Medical-surgical nursing: Concepts and clinical practice.* St. Louis: C. V. Mosby.

Pickles, V. R., Hall, W. S., & Best, F. A. (1965). Prostaglandins in endometrium and menstrual fluid from normal and dysmenorrheic subjects. *British Journal of Obstetrics and Gynecology, 72,* 185.

Reid, R. (1985). *Premenstrual syndrome: Current problems in obstetrics, gynecology, and fertility* (Vol. VIII, No. 2). Chicago: Year Book Medical.

Rosenwaks, Z., & Jones, G. S. (1980). Menstrual pain: Its origin and pathogenesis. *Journal of Reproductive Medicine, 25,* 207-221.

Sampson, J. A. (1927). Peritoneal endometriosis due to the menstrual dissemination of endometrial tissue into the peritoneal cavity. *American Journal of Obstetrics & Gynecology, 14,* 422.

Schatzkin, A., Jones, D. Y., Hoover, R. N., Taylor, P. R., Brinton, L. A., Ziegler, R. G., Harvey, E. B., Carter, C. L., Licitra, L. M., Dufour, M. C., & Larson, D. B. (1987). Alcohol consumption and breast cancer in the epidemiologic follow-up study of the first national health and nutrition examination survey. *New England Journal of Medicine, 19*(316), 1169-1173.

Schellhammer, P. F., & Grabstald, H. (1986). Tumors of the penis. In P. C. Walsh, R. F. Gittes, A. D. Perlmutter, & T. A. Stanley (Eds.), *Campbell's urology* (5th ed.). Philadelphia: W. B. Saunders.

Seidel, H., Ball, J., Dains, J., & Benedict, G. W. (1987). *Mosby's guide to physical examination.* St. Louis: C. V. Mosby.

Silber, S. J. (1984). *Reproductive microsurgery in male and female.* Baltimore: Williams & Wilkins.

Slattry, M. L., Robinson, L. M., Schuman, K. L., French, T. K., Abbot, T. M., Overall, J. C., & Gardner, J. M. (1989). Cigarette smoking and exposure to passive smoke as risk factors for cervial cancer. *Journal of the American Medical Association, 261*(11), 1593-1589.

Smith, S. D. (1985). Dysfunctional uterine bleeding. *British Journal of Hospital Medicine, 34*(6).

Steiner, M., Haskett, R. F., Osmun, J. N., & Carroll, B. J. (1980). Treatment of premenstrual tension with lithium carbonate: A pilot study. *Acta Psychiatrica Scandinavica, 61*(2), 96-102.

Wein, A. J., & Van Arsdalen, K. N. (1988). Drug-induced male sexual dysfunction. *Urologic Clinics of North America, 15*(1), 23-31.

Whaley, L. F., & Wong, D. L. (1987). *Nursing care of infants and children* (3 ed.). St. Louis: C. V. Mosby.

Wild, R. M., Devine, C. J., & Horton, C. E. (1979). Dermal graft repair of Peyronie's disease: Survey of 50 patients. *Journal of Urology, 121,* 47.

Willett, W. G., Rosner, B. A., & Speizer, F. E. (1987). Moderate alcohol consumption and the risk of breast cancer. *New England Journal of Medicine, 316,* 1174-1180.

Willett, W. G., Stampfer, M. J., Colditz, G. A., Rosner, B. A., Hennekens, C. J., & Speizer, F. E. (1987). Dietary fat and the risk of breast cancer. *New England Journal of Medicine, 316,* 22.

CHAPTER 21

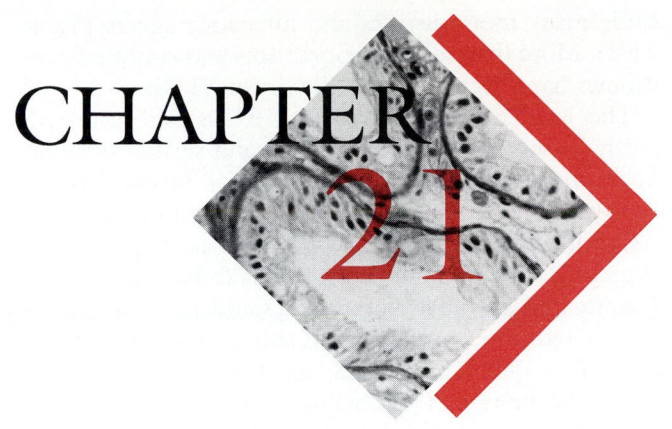

Sexually Transmitted Diseases

Deborah L. Greener

Sexually transmitted urogenital infections, 727
  Bacterial infections, 727
    Gonorrhea, 727
      Pathophysiology, 727
      Clinical manifestations, 728
      Evaluation and treatment, 729
    Syphilis, 729
      Pathophysiology, 730
      Clinical manifestations, 731
        Primary stage, 731
        Secondary stage, 731
        Latent and tertiary stages, 732
        Congenital syphilis, 732
      Evaluation and treatment, 732
    Chancroid, 734
      Pathophysiology, 734
      Clinical manifestations, 735
      Evaluation and treatment, 735
    Granuloma inguinale, 735
      Pathophysiology, 735
      Clinical manifestations, 735
      Evaluation and treatment, 735
    Gardnerella vaginalis, 735
      Pathophysiology, 736
      Clinical manifestations, 736
      Evaluation and treatment, 736
  Chlamydial infections, 736
    Urogenital infections, 736
      Pathophysiology, 736
      Clinical manifestations, 737
      Evaluation and treatment, 738
    Lymphogranuloma venereum, 738
      Pathophysiology, 738
      Clinical manifestations, 738
      Evaluation and treatment, 739
  Viral infections, 739
    Genital herpes, 739
      Pathophysiology, 740
      Clinical manifestations, 740
      Evaluation and treatment, 741

Condylomata acuminata, 741
      Pathophysiology, 741
      Clinical manifestations, 741
      Evaluation and treatment, 741
    Molluscum contagiosum, 742
  Parasitic infections, 743
    Trichomoniasis, 743
      Pathophysiology, 743
      Clinical manifestations, 743
      Evaluation and treatment, 743
    Scabies, 743
      Pathophysiology, 744
      Clinical manifestations, 744
      Evaluation and treatment, 744
    Pediculosis pubis, 745
      Pathophysiology, 745
      Clinical manifestations, 745
      Evaluation and treatment, 745
Sexually transmitted infections of other body systems, 745
  Gastrointestinal infections, 745
    Shigellosis and Campylobacter enteritis, 745
      Pathophysiology, 745
      Clinical manifestations, 746
      Evaluation and treatment, 746
    Giardiasis and amebiasis, 746
      Pathophysiology, 746
      Clinical manifestations, 746
      Evaluation and treatment, 746
    Hepatitis B, 746
      Pathophysiology, 747
      Clinical manifestations, 747
      Evaluation and treatment, 747
  Systemic diseases, 747
    Acquired immune deficiency syndrome, 747
    Cytomegalovirus infection, 747
      Pathophysiology, 747
      Clinical manifestations, 747
      Evaluation and treatment, 748

Throughout recorded history humans have been threatened by infectious diseases. Even into this century epidemics of diphtheria, smallpox, tuberculosis, typhoid, and other catastrophic infections could decimate entire communities almost overnight. Today, however, many of these diseases are virtually unknown, or at least under control, in the United States. Unfortunately, despite medical advances, improved living standards, and better nutrition, new epidemics are now considered major public health problems, and some pose lethal threats to individuals and communities. These epidemics are the venereal, or sexually transmitted, diseases (STDs).

Until quite recently the label venereal was applied to a very limited number of diseases caused by bacterial agents: gonorrhea, syphilis, chancroid, lymphogranuloma vereneum, and granuloma inguinale (Cates & Holmes, 1986). Today through increased diagnostic capabilities and extensive epidemiologic investigations into modes of transmission, the list has expanded to include many more diseases and infectious agents (Table 21-1). More than 20 microorganisms and countless syndromes have been added to the list of STDs.

The incidence of the "newer" STDs has increased, partly because of changes in social and sexual behavior. Such changes include earlier onset of sexual activity, later marriage, and rising divorce rates, all of which increase the number of sexual partners and exposure to sexually transmitted infections (Cates & Holmes, 1986). Despite changes in sexual mores, standards, and behaviors in recent years, STDs are still associated with sin and immorality. This stigma, and the fear of it, can affect health behaviors and help-seeking behaviors.

Education about safe sexual practices may be the most important nursing intervention for individuals who are undergoing treatment for STDs. Nurses and other health professionals are challenged to (1) teach individuals how to avoid contracting and transmitting a STD; (2) convince individuals to seek medical treatment at the

TABLE 21-1 Currently recognized sexually transmitted infections

Causal microorganism	Disease
BACTERIA	
Campylobacter	Campylobacter enteritis
Calymmatobacterium granulomatis	Granuloma inguinale
Chlamydia trachomatis	Urogenital infections; lymphogranuloma venereum
Gardnerella vaginalis	Nonspecific vaginitis (bacterial vaginosis)
Haemophilus ducreyi	Chancroid
Mycoplasma	Mycoplasmosis
Neisseria gonorrhoeae	Gonorrhea
Shigella	Shigellosis
Treponema pallidum	Syphilis
VIRUSES	
Cytometalovirus	Cytomegalic inclusion disease
Hepatitis B virus (HBV)	Hepatitis
Herpes simplex virus (HSV)	Genital herpes
Human immunodeficiency virus (HIV)	Acquired immune deficiency syndrome (AIDS)
Human papillomavirus	Condylomata acuminata
Molluscum contagiosum virus	Molluscum contagiosum
PROTOZOA	
Entamoeba histolitica	Amebiasis; amebic dysentery
Giardia lamblia	Giardiasis
Trichomonas vaginalis	Trichomoniasis
ECTOPARASITES	
Phthirus pubis	Pediculosis pubis
Sarcoptes scabtiei	Scabies
FUNGUS	
Candida albicans	Candidiasis

first sign of disease; (3) convince individuals to comply with medical treatment; and (4) help individuals to take control of their sexual health. Information about safe sexual practices, from the proper use of condoms to "safe sex" guidelines, can be obtained from numerous sources (e.g., Hatcher et al., 1988; Parra, Weisner, & Drotman, 1984). Helping individuals take control of their sexual health is perhaps the most difficult and most pressing challenge, because an individual who is unwilling to take responsibility for his or her sexual health will not choose health-promoting sexual practices, seek medical help, or comply with treatment.

Not all of the sexually transmitted diseases are reportable; that is, the Centers for Disease Control (CDC) do not require health care providers to report the cases they diagnose. This makes estimating the incidence of many common STDs difficult. Another difficulty that skews epidemiologic data, even for the reportable diseases, is the fact that most reports of diagnoses are made by public health clinics. Private physicians often do not report STDs. Therefore, many of the demographic data about STDs give the impression that these diseases exist primarily among the poor urban clients of STD clinics, although, in fact, STDs are prevalent today among all socioeconomic groups.

SEXUALLY TRANSMITTED UROGENITAL INFECTIONS

Bacterial Infections
Gonorrhea

Gonorrhea is caused by **gonococci** (singular, *gonococcus*), which are microorganisms of the species *Neisseria gonorrhoeae*. Gonococci were first identified by Neisser in stained smears of vaginal, urethral, and conjunctival exudate in 1879. Gonorrhea can be local or systemic, uncomplicated or complicated. Uncomplicated gonorrhea is gonococcal infection that is limited to the site of original infection, causes minimal symptoms, and, once treated, rarely has sequelae (Handsfield, 1984). Gonococcal urethritis in men is a typical uncomplicated gonococcal infection. Unfortunately gonorrhea can result in complications, particularly in those who delay treatment or have minimal access to medical care. Such complications include pelvic inflammatory disease (PID) in women, involving cervicitis, endometritis, salpingitis, tubal abscesses, infertility, or ectopic pregnancy; and disseminated gonococcal infections, which affect the skin, the joints, and the heart.

Gonorrhea is the most commonly reported communicable disease in the United States. In 1987, 780,905 cases (not including military cases) were reported (CDC, 1987a). Because most private physicians do not report gonorrhea, actual prevalence and morbidity may exceed reported figures by 30% to 200% (Lossick, 1985). Researchers estimate that the inclusion of unreported cases would bring the total to over 2 million cases per year (Hatcher et al., 1988).

About one half of the reported cases of gonorrhea occur in men, most of whom are between 20 and 24 years of age. Sexually active women between 15 and 19 are also at high risk for gonorrhea. Other demographic risk factors include nonwhite race, low socioeconomic status, urban residence, early onset of sexual activity, single marital status, male homosexuality, and previous gonorrhea (Handsfield, 1984).

Transmission of gonococcal infection generally requires contact of epithelial surfaces, such as occurs during sexual intercourse. If one partner is infected, the risk that the other will contract the disease is between 36% and 92% for females and 40% and 90% for males (Spagna, 1985). Gonorrhea can also be transmitted by a pregnant women to her fetus. The infection passes from mother to child across the amniotic membranes, by direct inoculation with a fetal scalp electrode during labor monitoring, during passage through the birth canal, or through mother-infant contact following birth. **Fomites** (contaminated objects) are rarely involved in the transmission of *N. gonorrhoeae,* primarily because the gonococcus requires a rich medium (such as bodily fluids) and an environment high in carbon dioxide (5% to 10%) for growth.

Pathophysiology

Humans are the only natural hosts for *N. gonorrhoeae,* which is an aerobic, non-spore-forming, oxidase-positive, gram-negative coccal (round) microorganism that usually appears in pairs (diplococci) with the adjacent sites slightly flattened. Hairlike filaments, called pili, appear to help the microorganisms attach themselves to host cells: the epithelial cells of mucous membranes. Columnar, transitional, and stratified squamous epithelial cells are most frequently infected. First the microorganisms become attached to the plasma membranes (cell walls) of these cells, then they invade the cells and begin to damage the mucosa. Generally a quick leukocytic (inflammatory) response and exudation at the site of infection occur.

In females the endocervical canal (inner portion of the cervix) is the usual site of original gonococcal infection, although urethral colonization is also common, as is the infection of Skene and Bartholin glands. Several factors can facilitate ascent of gonococci into the uterus and the fallopian tubes, where they cause pelvic inflammatory disease. Among these factors are menstruation, presence of an intrauterine contraceptive device, orgasm, and attachment of the gonococci to sperm, which transport the pathogens to the upper genital tract (McGee, 1984). In the fallopian tubes progressive mucosal and submucosal invasion and sloughing of normal, ciliated tubal epithelium are accompanied by marked inflammatory response, causing the fallopian tubes to fill with exudate. In males the gonococci typically infect the urethra. Infection of the epididymis and other complications in men are rare (Handsfield, 1984).

Disseminated gonococcal infection (DGI) is the spread of infection through the bloodstream. Gonococci may enter the bloodstream from the urogenital tract, the rectum, or the pharynx. In women most cases of DGI occur close to the menstrual period or during pregnancy (Mills & Brooks, 1984).

Clinical Manifestations

The incubation period for urethral gonococcal infection in men is usually 2 to 5 days but may be up to 3 weeks. About 60% of those infected suddenly experience marked dysuria (painful or difficult urination), and a profuse, mucopurulent discharge spontaneously appears at the urethral meatus. Some individuals have little discharge, however, and some may have no symptoms at all. Most cases of untreated gonococcal urethritis resolve spontaneously after several weeks, and more than 95% of individuals are asymptomatic by 6 months after infection (Pelouze, 1941).

In females the incubation period varies, but those who develop symptoms generally do so within 10 days of exposure. Symptoms may not appear until after the next menstrual period, when pelvic inflammatory disease begins (McGee, 1984). The clinical manifestations of uncomplicated gonorrhea in women may be slight or very severe; they include a vaginal discharge that is often yellowish, dysuria, bleeding or spotting between menstrual periods, and heavy menses. Physical examination may reveal cervical friability and erythema (redness) and purulent or mucopurulent discharge from the os. There may be a discharge from the Skene or Bartholin glands if these sites are involved (Fig. 21-1). If pelvic inflammatory disease develops, the onset of symptoms may be very rapid and include chills, fever, nausea, vomiting, and lower abdominal pain that worsens with coughing, sneezing, or intercourse. Abdominal palpation often reveals bilateral lower quadrant tenderness and rebound tenderness resulting from peritoneal irritation caused by tubal exudate. Marked tenderness of the internal genitalia is frequently noted during pelvic examination. Enlargements or masses may also be palpable in the upper genital tract.

Gonococcal infection of the anus and rectum is found in 35% to 50% of women who are diagnosed with urogenital gonorrhea. Anorectal infection probably is caused by the spread of infected exudate from the cervix and vagina, since few such individuals report having had anogenital sexual contact. Among homosexual men the infection results from rectal intercourse.

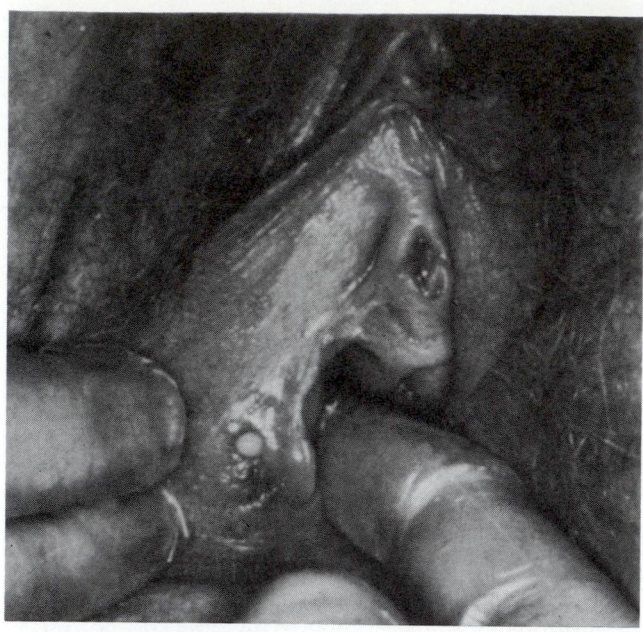

FIG. 21-1. Gonorrhea that has caused bartholinitis with purulent exudate. (From Handsfield, 1984.)

Symptoms of anorectal gonorrhea range from mild anal pruritus (itching), mucopurulent rectal discharge, and slight rectal bleeding, to severe rectal pain, tenesmus (painful and ineffectual straining at stool), and constipation. Physical examination may reveal anal erythema and discharge and evidence of mucosal damage to the anus and rectum, such as friability, edema, and purulent exudate. The frequency of such signs and symptoms is not well known.

Gonococcal infection can be transmitted to the pharynx by orogenital sexual contact, particularly fellatio. Pharyngeal infection occurs in 3% to 25% of cases of gonorrhea, primarily in heterosexual women and homosexual men. Most of these infections are asymptomatic, but acute pharyngitis or tonsillitis with lymphadenopathy and fever may occasionally occur.

Disseminated gonococcal infection is usually associated with systemic manifestations of infections such as fever, shaking, chills, anorexia, and malaise. Tissue-specific manifestations of DGI include skin lesions, tenosynovitis (inflammation of a tendon sheath), and arthritis (inflammation of a joint). The skin lesions are commonly seen near the joints of the fingers and toes. These erythematous macules are 1 to 5 mm in diameter and often develop into pustular, bleeding, or necrotic lesions, but they only appear early in the course of the illness. Tenosynovitis usually affects one or more joints of the hands and feet. The arthritis of DGI is most commonly a migratory polyarthralgia, although occasionally a septic arthritis occurs in the knee, elbow, ankle, or hand. Residual joint deformity is possible. Rarely DGI is associated with endocarditis (cardiac inflammation) or meningitis.

Gonococcal infection of the newborn is usually manifested as an eye infection **(ophthalmia neonatorum).** Onset generally occurs 1 to 12 days after birth, with a mean of 4 to 6 days. Affected newborns are usually born to mothers who have had prolonged ruptured membranes. In these cases immediate treatment with a topical antibiotic or chemical eyedrop (e.g., silver nitrate) is not effective, because the infection is already established. Established infection causes bilateral corneal ulceration, with a profuse yellow or gray purulent exudate, and is followed by necrosis, scarring, and compromised vision. Signs of systemic disease are seldom apparent.

Evaluation and Treatment

Clinical signs and symptoms are not sufficient for the differential diagnosis of gonococcal infections. Microscopic evaluation of Gram-stained slides of clinical specimens are deemed positive for *N. gonorrhoeae* if gramnegative diplococci with typical "kidney bean" morphology are seen inside polymorphonuclear leukocytes. Such a finding is considered adequate for the diagnosis of gonococcal urethritis in a symptomatic male. For screening purposes or diagnosis of pharyngeal or anorectal gonorrhea, cultures are recommended. For females the Gram stain technique is less accurate and reliable and is replaced with a single culture of endocervical secretions. Since the pharynx or anus and rectum are rarely the only sites of infection for females, routine cultures of these sites are optional.

The many different strains of *N. gonorrhoeae* vary with respect to pathogenicity, virulence, and susceptibility to antibiotics. In 1976 researchers identified a penicillinase-producing strain of the microorganism (PPNG). By 1986 this strain accounted for 2% of all reported gononorrheal infections in the United States (CDC, 1987b). The ability of PPNG to inactivate penicillin has made penicillin useless in individuals infected with this strain of gonococcus. Other antibiotics, including tetracycline and spectinomycin hydrochloride, are ineffective against other new strains of *N. gonorrhoeae.*

The Centers for Disease Control (CDC) recommend drug regimens for the treatment of uncomplicated gonorrhea, gonococcal pelvic inflammatory disease, DGI, and gonorrhea in newborns (CDC, 1985). After clinical and laboratory evaluation women and heterosexual men known to have been exposed to gonorrhea within the past 30 days or thought to have gonorrhea are evaluated and treated with a regimen that covers both gonococcal and chlamydial infections. (*Chlamydia* will be discussed in a later section.) Because homosexual men are less likely to have chlamydial infections, they are treated for gonorrhea only. The treatment of choice for non-PPNG infections is a single dose of oral ampicillin or amoxicillin and probenecid. The single-dose regimen is preferred because it eliminates compliance problems, is accepted well by individuals, and can be followed with a 7-day course of tetracycline or doxycycline (or erythromycin in pregnancy) to eliminate any coexisting chlamydial infection. A single dose of intramuscular ceftriaxone or procaine penicillin and oral probenecid can also be followed by tetracycline, doxycycline, or erythromycin, but this regimen is painful and carries an increased risk of anaphylaxis. It may be best for homosexual men, however, because these drugs are highly effective against anorectal gonorrhea. In cases of penicillin allergy or proven or highly suspected infection with PPNG, the CDC recommends the use of intramuscular spectinomycin or ceftriaxone, but followed by tetracycline or doxycycline (unless the individual is a male homosexual).

Sexual partners are also assessed and treated according to these protocols, and sexual contact is avoided by all until treatment is completed. Condoms are strongly recommended to prevent future infection.

Syphilis

Syphilis, a disease having local and systemic manifestations, has been well known throughout history. Many famous figures from biblical and Roman times, the royal families of the Old World, and the United States were thought or known to have had syphilis (Brandt, 1987). In the early half of the 1900s, it was estimated that the prevalence of syphilis in the United States was between 5% and 25% (Sparling, 1984).

There were 35,147 new cases of syphilis (excluding military cases) reported in the United States during 1987 (CDC, 1987a). This number brought the total of all known cases to 86,545, a 32% increase over the total in 1986. In some locations the annual incidence of syphilis rose 70% to 74% between 1984 and 1987 (CDC, 1988).

The incidence of syphilis is down in homosexual and bisexual males, probably because of changes in sexual practices brought about by AIDS. Incidence is up, however, among heterosexual men and women, particularly those between 20 and 24 years of age. The rise in incidence may be caused by an increase of cocaine-related prostitution (where sex is bartered for drugs) or the increased use of spectinomycin to treat PPNG. Unlike other drugs used to treat gonorrhea, spectinomycin is ineffective against syphilis. The recent increase in cases may also be the result of less vigilant case finding and screening and reduced government spending for syphilis-related programs (CDC, 1988). The increased incidence of syphilis is a grave public health concern, not only because of the morbidity and mortality involved in late-stage syphilis and congenital syphilis, but also because the open sores of primary syphilis are sites of entry for human immune deficiency virus, the cause of acquired immunodeficiency syndrome (AIDS).

Pathophysiology

Treponema pallidum, the cause of syphilis, is an anaerobic bacterium. The *treponemes* (individual microorganisms) look like corkscrews, with regular, tight spirals and a rotary motion (Fig. 21-2). *T. pallidum* has never been cultured in vitro.

The bacterium is present in exudate from the moist mucosal or cutaneous lesions of early syphilis and is transmitted through macroscopically invisible abrasions produced during sexual intercourse. Approximately one third of individuals who have sexual intercourse with a partner who has early-stage syphilis develop the disease (Musher, 1984). Syphilis becomes a systemic disease shortly after infection and can be transmitted from a pregnant women to her fetus as early as the ninth week of gestation. The risk of transmission to the fetus gradually declines with each subsequent pregnancy; therefore, a mother who has had several children with severe congenital syphilis may go on to bear a healthy child. After about 8 years, even without treatment, the mother's infection is not transmitted to her fetus (Sparling, 1984).

The course of untreated syphilis consists of four stages: primary, secondary, latent, and tertiary. **Primary syphilis** begins at the site of bacterial invasion. There *T. pallidum* multiplies in the epithelium, producing a granulomatous tissue reaction called **chancre.** Some microorganisms drain with lymph into adjacent lymph nodes. Within the nodes and at the site of the chancre, the cell-mediated and humoral immune responses are stimulated.

Secondary syphilis is systemic. During this stage blood-borne bacteria spread to all major organ systems. The secondary stage is followed by a period during which the immune system is able to suppress the infection. Skin lesions disappear during this period, which is called **latent syphilis.** Medical history and serologic

studies show that syphilis is present, but the individual has no clinical manifestations. Transmission is possible during the secondary and early latent stages.

Tertiary syphilis is the most severe stage, involving significant morbidity and mortality. The pathogenesis of syphilitic manifestations at this stage remains unclear. The destructive skin, bone, and soft tissue lesions (called **gummas**) of tertiary syphilis are probably caused by a severe hypersensitivity reaction to the microorganism. Within the cardiovascular system infection with *T. pallidum* may cause aneurysms, heart valve insufficiencies, and heart failure. Within the central nervous system

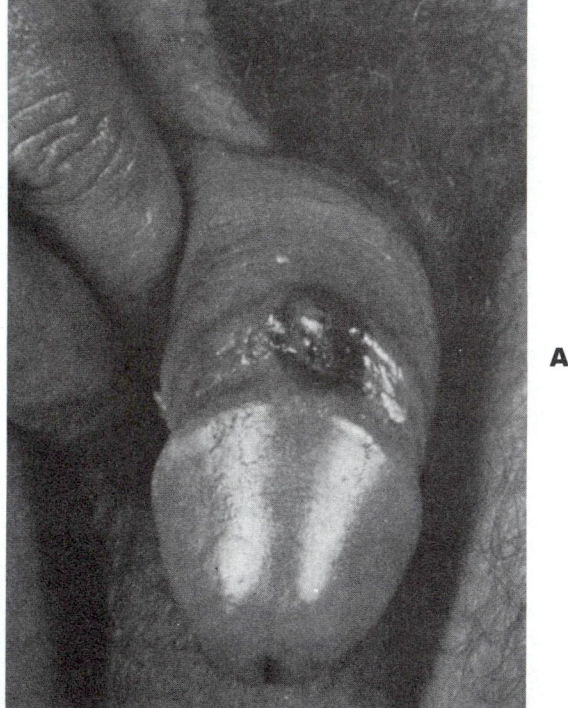

A

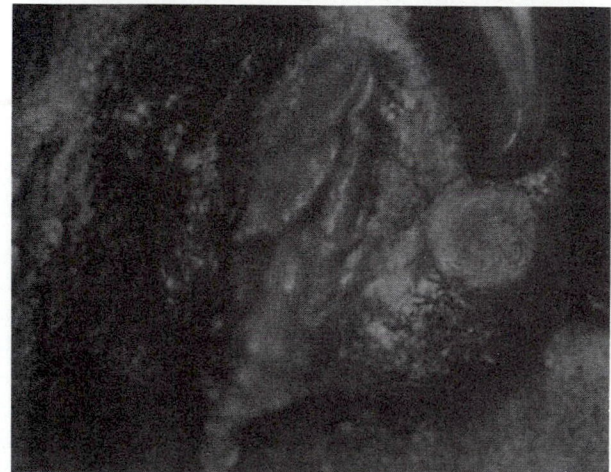

B

FIG. 21-3. Primary syphilis. **A,** Chancre of the penis, **B,** Chancre of the vulva. (From Wehrle & Top, 1981.)

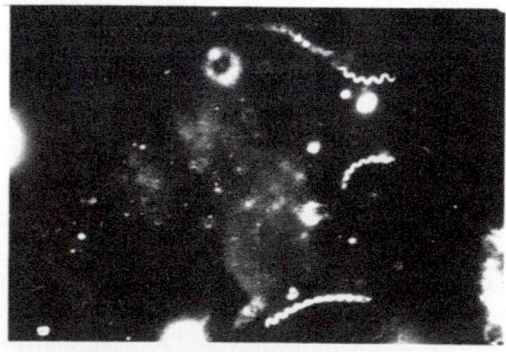

FIG. 21-2. Syphilis. *Treponema pallidum* as seen with dark-field microscope. (From Habif, 1985.)

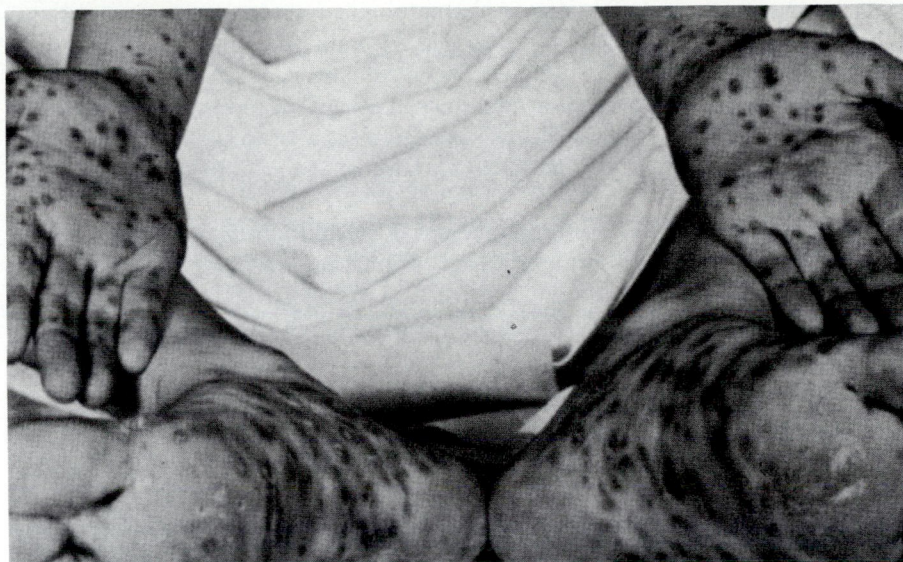

FIG. 21-4. Secondary syphilis. Papulosquamous lesions of an infant with secondary syphilis. (From Wehrle & Top, 1981.)

(CNS) the presence of *T. pallidum* in cerebrospinal fluid may cause the manifestations of **neurosyphilis** (Sparling, 1984).

Congenital syphilis is characterized by vasculitis, necrosis, fibrosis, and distribution of *T. pallidum* throughout the tissues. Dental malformations and extensive, destructive bone lesions are also found in the affected infant. Pathophysiology depends on gestational age at the time of infection. The placenta itself may be infected, causing it to become pale and diffusely fibrotic.

Clinical Manifestations

Primary Stage In adults the incubation period of syphilis ranges from 12 days to 12 weeks after exposure and averages 3 weeks. At the site of treponemal entry a sore, or "hard chancre," develops. Typically the chancre is an eroded, painless, firm, and indurated (hard) ulcer that may be from a few millimeters to 2 centimeters in diameter. Chancres are accompanied by firm, enlarged, and nontender regional lymph nodes. Fig. 21-3 shows typical chancres of the penis and vulva. Syphilitic chancres are not always typical, however. Secondary infection can cause chancres to become necrotic and painful, and lesions on the fingers may be dry, scaly, and papular or moist and vegetative. If left untreated, the chancre of primary syphilis heals in 2 to 8 weeks and then spontaneously disappears, usually without leaving a scar.

Secondary Stage Clinical manifestations of secondary syphilis may overlap with those of the primary stage or may not appear for several weeks. Generally about 6 weeks after the appearance of the chancre the individual develops cutaneous (skin) lesions of any type, from macular to pustular. These lesions are usually widespread, bilateral, and almost always present on the palms and soles (Fig. 21-4). Some moist papules may become elevated and bumpy, or vegetative; these are known as **condylomata lata.** The condylomata lata are usually whitish and flattened and appear most frequently in women, in the labial folds and on the skin of the groin and inner thighs (Fig. 21-5). Men and women may also develop these highly infectious lesions in the anal area.

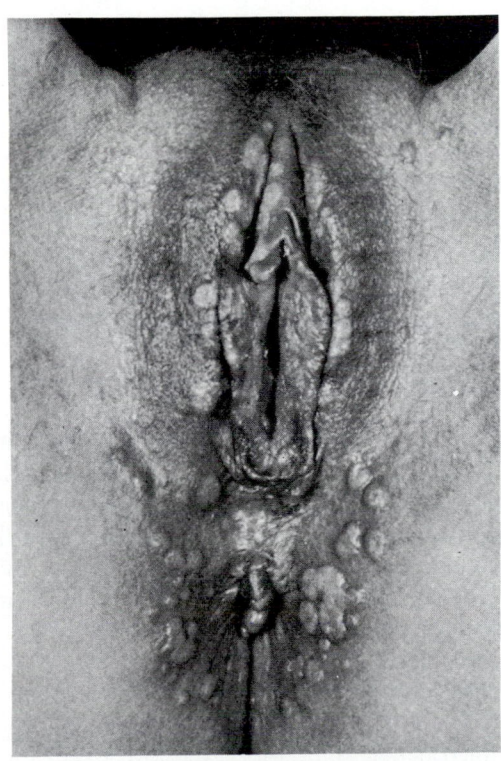

FIG. 21-5. Secondary syphilis. Condylomata lata of the vulva. (From Wehrle & Top, 1981.)

Mild to severe systemic signs and symptoms, such as malaise, fever, sore throat, headache, hoarseness, anorexia, and joint pain, may occur with secondary syphilis. Lymphadenopathy, pruritus, and alopecia are commonly present. Some individuals develop anemia, leukocytosis, increased sedimentation rate, hepatitis, transitory proteinuria, arthritis, electrocardiographic abnormalities, and CNS symptoms. Whether treatment is given or not, the cutaneous lesions generally heal in 2 to 10 weeks, but relapses may occur for several years (Knox & Rudolph, 1984; Para & Baird, 1985).

Latent and Tertiary Stages The asymptomatic, latent stage of syphilis may be as long as the life of the individual or as short as 1 year. The clinical manifestations of tertiary syphilis may then appear. These include gummas, cardiovascular lesions, and neurosyphilis. Because antibiotics can cure syphilis, manifestations of tertiary syphilis are quite rare.

Congenital Syphilis Congenital syphilis is usually divided into two clinical syndromes: early (manifested in the first 2 years of life) and late (manifested later, often near puberty). Newborns with congenital syphilis are often premature and show evidence of intrauterine growth retardation, hepatosplenomegaly, nasal discharge, varied cutaneous lesions, osteochondritis, anemia, leukocytosis or leukopenia, thrombocytopenia, nephrotic syndrome, varying degrees of CNS involvement, retinal inflammation, and glaucoma (Murphy & Patamasucon, 1984). The late clinical manifestations of classic congenital syphilis correspond to those of tertiary syphilis in the adult and are now rare.

Evaluation and Treatment

Because *T. pallidum* cannot be cultured in vitro, definitive diagnosis of early syphilis depends upon dark-field microscopy of a specimen taken from the chancre. The examination is repeated on 2 successive days if the result is initially negative (Knox & Rudolph, 1984). Genital ulcers are sometimes difficult to diagnose; an algorithm outlining an approach to the diagnosis of the individual presenting with a genital ulcer is given in Fig. 21-6.

Serologic tests for primary syphilis provide indirect evidence of infection. The VDRL antigen or rapid plasmin reagin (RPR) test yields a positive result in over half of infected individuals; the more sensitive fluorescent treponemal antibody absorption (FTA-ABS) test has a positive result in approximately three fourths of infected individuals (Knox & Rudolph, 1984). However, the VDRL, RPR, and FTA-ABS tests can also have false-positive results under numerous conditions (see the box on p. 734) Another *T. pallidum*-specific test is the microhemagglutination assay (MHA-TP) for antibodies to the microorganism.

Numerous dermatologic disorders can mimic the skin lesions of secondary syphilis, making differential diagnosis difficult. Again laboratory confirmation is important; dark-field microscopy of scrapings from the condylomata lata or other skin lesions reveals the treponemes. Serologic tests are almost always strongly positive in this stage.

During the latent stage individuals continue to have serologic evidence of untreated disease, but it is difficult to obtain confirmation through dark-field microscopy. Examination of cerebrospinal fluid may confirm that the treponemes are present and the insidious onset of neurosyphilis has begun.

Treatment for all stages of syphilis is parenteral injection of benzathine penicillin G. If the individual has had signs of disease for less than 1 year, a single dose is appropriate. If signs have been present for more than 1 year, the treatment is three weekly injections. This therapy is also appropriate in pregnancy. Individuals who are allergic to penicillin receive tetracycline, or if pregnant, erythromycin (CDC, 1985). Because treatment failures do occur, all individuals should have follow-up evaluation. Sexual partners are also examined and treated, and the use of condoms is recommended.

Definitive diagnosis of congenital syphilis is made by microscopic identification of *T. pallidum* in material from skin lesions or nasal discharge. Probable diagnosis is assumed on the basis of a rising or persistently reactive FTA-ABS value and clinical manifestations. In all cases of maternal syphilis the goal is to treat the mother in order to prevent congenital syphilis. Maternal treatment with penicillin before delivery usually prevents congenital syphilis. If the infant requires treatment, penicillin is the drug of choice, since allergy does not pose a problem in the neonatal period. Such infants are then followed with serologic tests for syphilis at 3, 6, and 12 months. Nearly all of the tests become nonreactive (negative) by the time the infant is 6 months of age (Murphy & Patamasucon, 1984).

Chancroid

Chancroid, or soft chancre, is an acute infectious disease that was first differentiated from syphilis in 1852. It is caused by the bacterium *Haemophilus ducreyi*.

Chancroid is most common in men (more than 90% of reported cases), particularly those who are not circumcised. Chancroid lesions in women tend to be asymptomatic and internal (in the vagina and cervix); this may account for the low incidence of reported cases among women. There is no evidence that chancroid is transmitted from mother to fetus, either before or during delivery.

Chancroid is rare in the United States; however, recent outbreaks have occurred in high-risk groups, par-

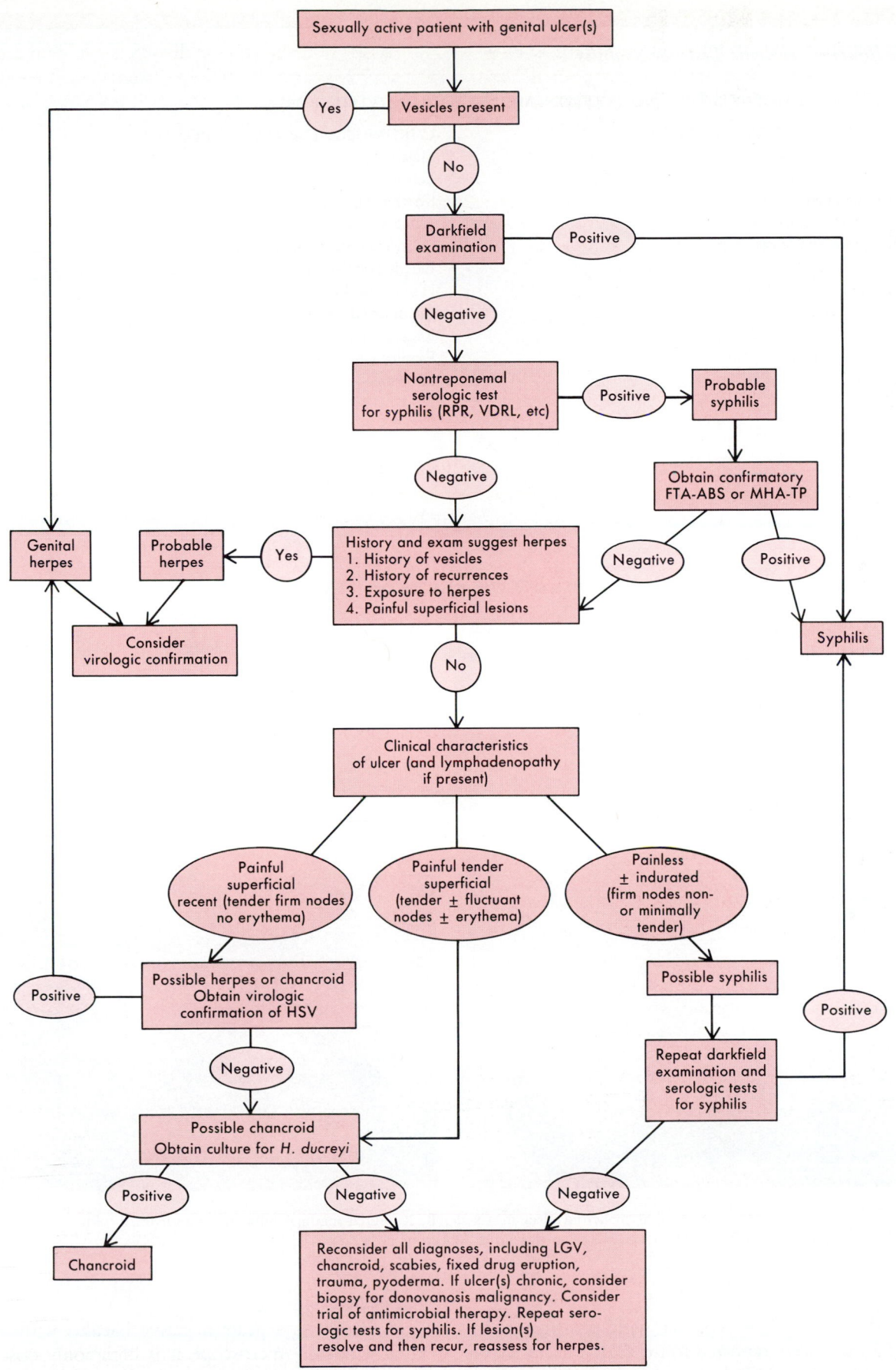

FIG. 21-6. Algorithm outlining an approach to the diagnosis of an individual who presents with a genital ulceration. (From Kraus, 1984.)

REASONS FOR FALSE-POSITIVE, NONTREPONEMAL REACTIONS (VDRL, RPR):

TRANSIENT REACTIONS (<6 MONTHS)

Technical error (low titer)
Smallpox vaccination
Mycoplasma pneumonia
Enterovirus infections
Infectious mononucleosis
Pregnancy
Narcotic abuse
Advanced tuberculosis
Scarlet fever
Viral and atypical pneumonia
Brucellosis
Ratbite fever
Leptospirosis
Measles
Mumps
Lymphogranuloma venecreum
Malaria
Trypanosomiasis
Varicella

CHRONIC REACTIONS (>6 MONTHS)

Malaria
Leprosy
Systemic lupus erythematosus
Narcotic abuse
Other connective tissue diseases
Elderly population
Hashimoto thyroiditis
Rheumatoid arthritis
Reticuloendothelial malignancy
Familial false-positives
Idiopathic

REASONS FOR FALSE-POSITIVE, *TREPONEMA*-SPECIFIC REACTIONS (FTA-ABS)

Technical error
Inefficient sorbents
Healthy individuals without syphilis
Genital herpes simplex
Pregnancy
Lupus erythematosus (skin only or systemic)
Alcoholic cirrhosis
Scleroderma
Mixed connective tissue disease

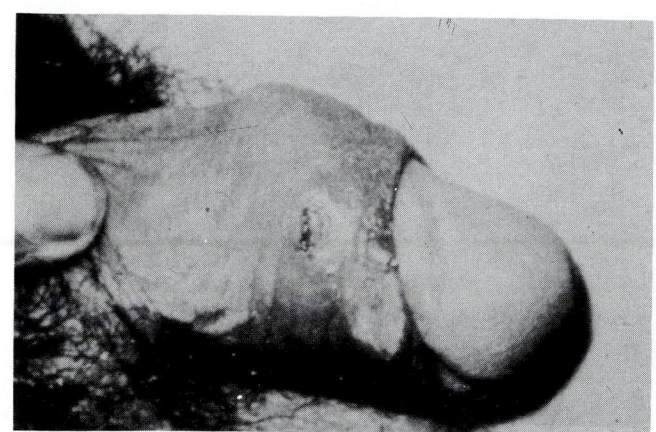
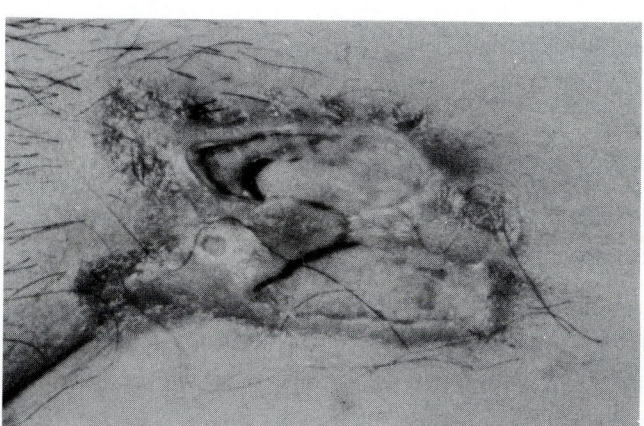

FIG. 21-7. A, Typical chancroid ulcer in a male, **B,** Ruptured inguinal bubo in an individual with chancroid from STD. (**A** and **B** from Ronald & Albritton, 1984.)

ticularly those who have contact with prostitutes. In 1984, 665 cases were reported to the CDC (exclusive of military cases). In 1987 the number had increased to 4995 (CDC, 1987a).

Pathophysiology

H. ducreyi is a gram-negative bacillus with rounded ends. Under a microscope it is commonly observed in small clusters along strands of mucus. Transmission occurs through intimate contact with infected lesions or mucosal surfaces. Like other pathogens *H. ducreyi* does not easily penetrate intact skin or mucous membranes. Therefore, it is thought that these surfaces must be abraded or traumatized to permit entry of the organism (Ronald & Albritton, 1984). Chancroid lesions are usually found on the internal surface of the foreskin or its point of attachment to the penis (the frenulum) in men, and on the labia, clitoris, or fourchette in women. Initially the papule enlarges, then erodes into a soft, circumscribed ulcer containing a superficial exudate. Beneath the ulcer is a lesion characterized by edema, endothelial proliferation, and a base of granulation tissue that is full of lymphocytes and plasma cells. Adjacent lymph nodes are acutely inflamed and full of polymorphonuclear leukocytes and necrotic cells (Para & Baird, 1985).

Clinical Manifestations

Chancroid has an incubation period of 1 to 14 days, after which the primary lesion appears. This lesion is inflamed and painful. It erodes to an irregular ulcer that is 3 to 20 mm in diameter (Fig. 21-7). Occasionally more than one lesion is present. Lymphadenopathy is usually unilateral, and an inguinal **bubo** (fluid-filled lymph node lesion) develops 7 to 10 days after the initial chancre in about 25% of individuals, primarily men (Para & Baird, 1985). The bubo may fill with exudate and rupture spontaneously.

Evaluation and Treatment

Chancroid is easily confused with other types of genital ulcers, particularly those of syphilis, genital herpes, and granuloma inguinale (Fig. 21-7). Microscopic analysis of a Gram-stained smear from the chancroid helps to identify the microorganism. Definitive diagnosis depends on recovery of *H. ducreyi* from cultured specimens. All individuals with ulcers are tested for syphilis. At present there are no serologic tests specific for *H. ducreyi*.

The CDC (1985) recommends that chancroid be treated with a 1-week regimen of oral erythromycin or a single, intramuscular injection of ceftriaxone. Sexual partners are treated simultaneously. Buboes and inflamed nodes are not excised and drained, because these procedures would delay healing. Rather, fluctuant (fluid-filled) lymph nodes or buboes are generallly aspirated through adjacent, healthy skin. The use of condoms is recommended to prevent future infections.

Granuloma Inguinale

Granuloma inguinale is a chronic, progressively destructive bacterial infection caused by the microorganism *Calymmatobacterium granulomatis,* formerly known as *Donovania granulomatis.* The infection is also known by other names, the most common of which is *donovanosis.*

Granuloma inguinale is among the most prevalent sexually transmitted diseases in some parts of the world, particularly India and Papau New Guinea. Granuloma inguinale is rare in the United States. Only 22 cases were reported to the CDC during 1987, a drop from 64 cases in 1986 (CDC, 1987a). Although it is sexually transmissible, granuloma inguinale is only mildly contagious. Repeated exposure is necessary to cause disease.

Pathophysiology

C. granulomatis is a gram-negative, nonmotile, nonsporing, encapsulated rod. After exposure the bacteria survive and multiply within vacuoles inside the macrophages, called **Donovan bodies.** (Macrophages are phagocytes of inflammation; see Chapter 7.) The initial lesion is an indurated nodule. Single lesions often coalesce with nearby lesions or form new lesions by autoinoculation of nearby skin surfaces. The progression from the initial nodule to a large, granulomatous heaped ulcer occurs slowly. Secondary infection may occur, increasing tissue damage and residual scarring. The disease may spread to the bones, joints, and liver .

Clinical Manifestations

The incubation period of granuloma inguinale is between 8 and 80 days. The first signs of disease are the indurated nodules, which are sharply defined and usually painless. They bleed easily; contain abundant, red, beefy-looking granulation tissue; and enlarge slowly. Subcutaneous inguinal involvement may mimic the buboes of other STDs. In the male lesions usually occur on the foreskin or glans of the penis; in the female labial lesions are most common (Hart, 1984).

Evaluation and Treatment

Although the clinical manifestations of this disease are important for diagnosis, confirmation involves microscopic examination in which Donovan bodies are seen in a smear or biopsy specimen. Cultures and serologic tests for granuloma inguinale are not available (Para & Baird, 1985).

Many antibiotics have been used successfully against *C. granulomatis.* They include tetracycline, streptomycin, chloramphenicol, gentamicin, and trimethoprim with sulfamethoxasole. If an antibiotic is effective, the lesions begin to heal within 7 days. Treatment is continued for 21 days or until all lesions are healed. Relapses can occur, so prolonged follow-up is necessary, as is treatment of sexual partners (Hart, 1984; Hatcher et al., 1988; Para & Baird, 1985).

Gardnerella Vaginalis

Gardnerella vaginalis (initially called *Haemophilus vaginalis,* then *Corynebacterium vaginale*) contributes to the clinical syndrome of nonspecific vaginitis known as **bacterial vaginosis.** Epidemiologic studies of *Gardnerella-*

associated bacterial vaginosis are scarce, and the evidence for sexual transmission is circumstantial. Although 50% or more of sexually active women may be infected with *G. vaginalis* at any time, only a small percentage of these infections cause symptoms. Active disease occurs almost exclusively in sexually active women. There may be a correlation between *G. vaginalis*-associated infection and race, promiscuity, marital stability, previous pregnancy, other sexually transmitted infections, and presence of an intrauterine device (Piot & Vanderheyden, 1984). Although most male sexual partners of infected women harbor the microorganism in their urethra, *G. vaginalis* does not cause disease in males.

Pathophysiology

G. vaginalis is a nonmotile, gram-negative or gram-variable rod. Its exact role in the development of bacterial vaginosis is unclear, primarily because *G. vaginalis* is part of the normal flora of the vagina. Apparently the microorganism acts in concert with anaerobic bacteria to produce some of the clinical manifestations of vaginitis. These anaerobic bacteria, probably bacteroides and peptococci, produce various aromatic amines, including abundant amounts of foul-smelling putrescine and cadaverine. These amines raise the pH of vaginal secretions, thus further promoting the growth of *G. vaginalis*. *G. vaginalis* adheres readily to vaginal epithelial cells and mucosal surfaces but is not invasive and produces a minimal inflammatory response. The microorganism is not associated with ascending infections or pelvic inflammatory disease (Piot & Vanderheyden, 1984; Remington & Swartz, 1983).

Clinical Manifestations

Bacterial vaginosis associated with *G. vaginalis* is characterized by a thin, gray, homogenous and malodorous discharge, which adheres to the vaginal walls but is often copious enough to drain into the vulva. Occasionally the discharge is bubbly or frothy. Usually the vaginal pH is 5.0 to 5.5 and there are no signs of vaginal or cervical inflammation. Individuals often complain of a strong, fishy vaginal odor, particularly after intercourse. Odor is caused by the release of aromatic amines following bacterial contact with alkaline semen.

Evaluation and Treatment

Diagnosis is made by microscopic analysis of a wet mount (a specimen of vaginal secretions placed on a slide and mixed with normal saline). The wet mount shows "clue cells," which are considered to be almost pathognomonic for *Gardnerella*-associated bacterial vaginosis. The clue cells are vaginal epithelial cells that are covered with bacteria and look as if pepper has been shaken on them. Few leukocytes are visible on the wet mount, and lactobacilli are also absent. If a drop of potassium hydroxide (KOH) solution is added to vaginal secretions, a characteristic foul, fishy odor is immediately released. Cultures are rarely required or performed.

The most effective and commonly used treatment for *Gardnerella*-associated bacterial vaginosis is a week-long course of metronidazole (Flagyl). Ampicillin is the drug of choice in pregnancy, but it is often less effective than metronidazole. Sulfa preparations, either oral or topical, are ineffective in the treatment of *Gardnerella*-associated infection. Some clinicians routinely treat sexual partners; others treat partners only if infection recurs after at least one successful course of treatment. The use of condoms helps to prevent future infections.

Chlamydial Infections
Urogenital Infections

Chlamydia trachomatis is a sexually transmitted urogenital pathogen responsible for many clinical manifestations in both men and women. Transmission from mother to fetus can result in substantial newborn morbidity.

Infection with *C. trachomatis* is not a reportable disease in the United States, is often not microbiologically confirmed, and may often be asymptomatic. Therefore, it is difficult to assess the incidence of infections in men or women. Local prevalence studies lead to estimates that over 800,000 cases of symptomatic chlamydial urethritis occur annually in men. The incidence of chlamydial cervicitis in women is thought to be about the same (Stamm & Holmes, 1984). These estimates suggest that *C. trachomatis* infections are the most prevalent STDs in the United States.

Evidence of chlamydial infection is rare in the sexually inexperienced. It is most common among heterosexuals under the age of 30. Pregnancy and use of oral contraceptives are associated with chlamydial infection in women, probably as a result of the hormone-induced increase in cervical ectopy, which exposes more columnar epithelial cells to the microorganism. The incidence of *Chlamydia* infection in pregnancy is between 2% and 30%, and the estimated rate of transmission from infected mother to neonate ranges from 23% to 70% (Heggie et al., 1981; Harrison & Alexander, 1984; Marecki, 1988). Like gonorrhea *Chlamydia* infection is transmitted from mother to infant during passage through the infected birth canal.

Pathophysiology

C. trachomatis is an obligate, gram-negative, intracellular parasite that is similar to a bacterium but lacks the ability to reproduce independently. Like viruses *Chlamydia* can only reproduce within host cells. *Chlamydia* organisms are always pathogens; they are not part of the normal flora of the urogenital tract, despite

TABLE 21-2 Similarity of clinical syndromes caused by *C. trachomatis* and *N. gonorrhoeae*

| Site of infection | Clinical syndrome | |
	N. gonorrhoeae	*C. trachomatis*
MEN		
Urethra	Urethritis	Nongonococcal urethritis; postgonococcal urethritis
Epididymis	Epididymitis	Epididymitis
Rectum	Proctitis	Proctitis
Conjunctiva	Conjunctivitis	Conjunctivitis
Systemic	Disseminated gonococcal	Reiter syndrome
WOMEN		
Urethra	Acute urethral syndrome	Acute urethral syndrome
Bartholin gland	Bartholinitis	Bartholinitis
Cervix	Cervicitis	Cervicitis; cervical dysplasia
Fallopian tube	Salpingitis	Salpingitis
Conjunctiva	Conjunctivitis	Conjunctivitis
Liver capsule	Perihepatitis	Perihepatitis
Systemic	Disseminated gonococcal infection	Arthritis-dermatitis syndrome

Adapted from Stamm & Holmes, 1984.

the fact that infection is often asymptomatic. There are numerous different serotypes, or strains, of *C. trachomatis*. Some cause urogenital infection, some ocular trachoma, and others lymphogranuloma venereum, which is discussed in the next section.

The strains of *C. trachomatis* that cause urogenital infection apparently require squamous-columnar and columnar epithelial cells as hosts. After gaining entry, they undergo a unique growth cycle that eventually results in death of the host cell. The disease process and clinical manifestations of infection are probably caused by both pathogen-mediated tissue damage and the inflammatory response. *C. trachomatis* infects and disrupts epithelial tissues but does not seem to invade or destroy deeper tissues or organs. Urogenital chlamydial infections may have a fairly self-limited acute course, which is followed by a chronic, low-grade, persistent infection that lasts for years (Schachter, 1984).

In newborns several sites may be inoculated with *Chlamydia* during passage through the infected maternal cervix. These include the eye, nasopharynx, rectum, and vagina. The infant may also aspirate infected secretions with its first breath.

Clinical Manifestations

Asymptomatic chlamydial infection is very common. Urogenital infections caused by *Chlamydia* closely parallel those caused by gonorrhea. Both microorganisms infect superficial genital tract tissues, such as mucosa of

the urethra and cervix, and both can invade the epididymides, fallopian tubes, and hepatic capsule. Table 21-2 lists the pathophysiologic similarities of chlamydial and gonococcal infections.

Chlamydial infection accounts for 35% to 50% of cases of nongonococcal urethritis (NGU) in men. Clinically urethritis caused by gonorrhea and chlamydia cannot be differentiated, since both have a 7- to 21-day incubation period and individuals with either infection present with dysuria and a whitish urethral discharge. Chlamydial urethritis is generally milder and more likely to be asymptomatic, however. Gram-stained smears of the urethral discharge reveal numerous polymorphonuclear leukocytes, which indicate ongoing inflammation. Chlamydial epididymitis can accompany chlamydial urethritis and is characterized by fever and a unilaterally painful, swollen scrotum. Chlamydial infection also causes proctitis (rectal inflammation) in homosexual men and occasionally in heterosexual women and is linked to the practice of passive anal intercourse. Chlamydial proctitis is generally mild, although it may, like gonorrheal proctitis, cause rectal bleeding, mucous discharge, and diarrhea. Reiter syndrome (urethritis, conjunctivitis, arthritis, and characteristic mucocutaneous lesions) is also associated with untreated chlamydial infections of the urogenital tract.

In young, sexually active women, *C. trachomatis* is a cause of **acute urethral syndrome** (dysuria, urinary frequency, and presence of sterile pus in the urine). *C. tra-*

chomatis also causes asymptomatic urethral infection in women. Chlamydial infection of Bartholin glands can cause purulent discharge and formation of a Bartholin cyst. Women with chlamydial cervicitis may be asymptomatic or may have a yellow mucopurulent discharge from the os and a hypertrophic, edematous, and friable area of cervical ectopy. The woman may also report intermenstrual or postcoital spotting. Although ectopy alone is not indicative of pathology, a raised, erythematous, raw, and friable ectopy is abnormal and strongly suggestive of chlamydial cervicitis. Chlamydial cervicitis is also often associated with cytologic atypia suggestive of cervical dysplasia (Stamm & Holmes, 1984) and is a leading cause of pelvic inflammatory disease.

The most common clinical manifestations of chlamydial infections in the newborn are conjunctivitis and pneumonia. Chlamydial conjunctivitis begins between 5 and 14 days after delivery, when the infant's eyes begin to water. This discharge may become purulent, and both eyes become red and swollen. Scarring of the conjunctivae may result, but this infection does not cause blindness, as does the ophthalmia neonatorium caused by *N. gonorrhoeae*. *C. trachomatis* accounts for 20% to 60% of all cases of pneumonia in infants up to 6 months of age (Maurice, 1983). The pneumonia is mild or severe and may accompany the conjunctivitis. Infants with chlamydial pneumonia present at 3 to 11 weeks of age with staccato coughing spells, nasal congestion, dyspnea, and minimal fever. Other signs include otitis media, tachypnea, wheezing, bronchospasm, crepitant inspiratory rales, and apneic spells.

Evaluation and Treatment

Methods for diagnosing chlamydial infections include tissue culture techniques, direct chlamydia enzyme immunoassay, and fluorescein-labeled monoclonal antibody tests, such as Microtrak. The last two techniques are the least expensive and time consuming. Papanicolaou smears may suggest the presence of chlamydial cervicitis, but they cannot confirm the diagnosis. Cultures for *N. gonorrhoeae* must also be performed, because chlamydial infection and gonorrhea frequently coexist and have similar clinical manifestations.

Treatment for urogenital infections with *C. trachomatis* include a week of tetracycline or doxycycline for men and nonpregnant women and erythromycin for pregnant women and newborns (CDC, 1985). Sexual partners should be identified, examined, and treated, and all individuals should avoid sex until the chlamydial infection is cured. Condoms should be used to prevent future infections.

Lymphogranuloma Venereum

C. trachomatis can also cause a chronic sexually transmitted disease known as **lymphogranuloma venereum** (LGV), which is often confused with other STDs, particularly syphilis, genital herpes, and chancroid (see Fig. 21-7). LGV is uncommon in the United States: during 1987 only 303 cases were reported to the CDC (1987a). In contrast, LGV is endemic in many other areas, including Africa, India, Southeast Asia, South America, and the Caribbean. Like other STDs it is more common in urban areas, among those with multiple sexual partners, and in men.

Pathophysiology

The strain of *C. trachomatis* that causes LGV probably penetrates skin and mucous membranes through tiny abrasions. LGV begins as a skin lesion and spreads to lymphatic tissue, where it causes marked inflammation, necrosis, buboes, abscesses of inguinal lymph nodes, and infection of surrounding tissues. Healing occurs by fibrosis after several weeks or months and results in scarring, which damages the lymph nodes and disrupts nodal function. Affected nodes become chronically swollen, hardened, and enlarged. *C. trachomatis* also spreads systematically through the bloodstream and can enter the CNS (Perine & Osoba, 1984).

Clinical Manifestations

The primary lesion of LGV appears after an incubation period of 3 to 12 days or more. The lesion is most commonly a herpetiform (multivesicular) ulcer, but it can take various forms. The ulcer generally is asymptomatic and inconspicuous and heals rapidly, leaving no scar. In men the lesion is most commonly found on the penis or scrotum; in women it is found on the vaginal wall, cervix, or labia. Other signs of primary LGV include a large, tender lymphatic nodule or bubo, urethritis, and cervicitis.

The secondary stage of untreated LGV in men is characterized by inflammation and swelling of the lymph nodes. At first the inguinal bubo is a firm, somewhat painful mass. As the bubo gradually enlarges it becomes very painful, thereby restricting mobility, and takes on a deep blue color (Fig. 21-8). This color change signals impending rupture of the bubo through the skin. Thick yellow pus may drain from the site for weeks or months. Healing is very slow and results in scar formation. Systemic manifestations of secondary LGV can include meningitis, pneumonitis, and other major infections. In some cases the bubo does not rupture but rather involutes and becomes firm. Bubo formation is most common in men. In women the inguinal lymph nodes are involved in fewer than one third of cases.

Anorectal LGV may be caused by direct inoculation during anal intercourse, or it may be a chronic or late manifestation of lymphatic spread from the inguinal area. The vast majority of individuals with anorectal

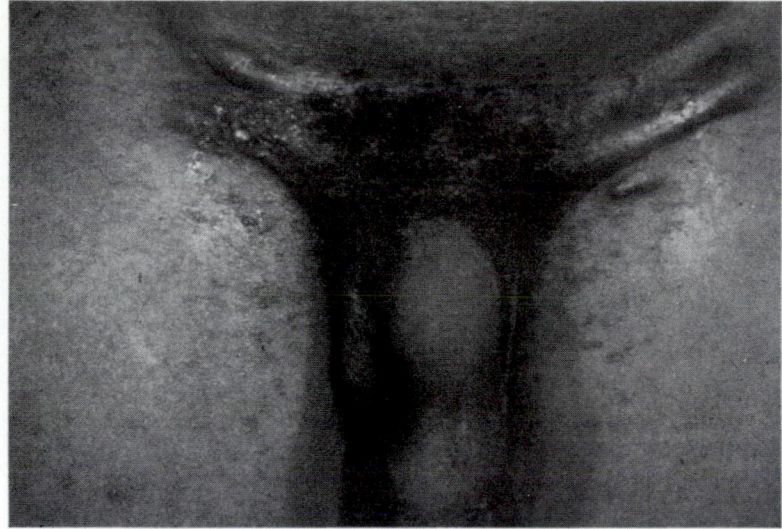

FIG. 21-8. Lymphogranuloma venereum. Bilateral inguinal buboes that discharge purulent material. (From Habif, 1985.)

LGV are women and homosexual men. Clinical symptoms include multiple ulcerations of the rectal mucosa, chronic inflammation, mucopurulent rectal discharge, and rectovaginal fistulas in women. Individuals may have fever, rectal pain, and tenesmus. Rectal strictures, perirectal abscesses, and anal fissures may develop and are the cause of most of the severe morbidity associated with LGV.

Evaluation and Treatment

Clinical manifestations and laboratory tests are used to diagnose LGV. Tests include the LGV complement-fixation tests, isolation of the microorganism in tissue culture, and monoclonal antibody tests. LGV is treated with a 2-week course of tetracycline. Sex partners should also be treated (CDC, 1985).

Viral Infections
Genital Herpes

Genital herpes, which causes blisterlike lesions, is the most common infectious genital ulceration in the United States. In fact, genital infection with the herpes simplex virus (HSV) is an epidemic in the United States. Genital herpes can be caused by either of the two serotypes of HSV, type 1 (HSV-1) or type 2 (HSV-2). Although infections caused by the serotypes are clinically indistinguishable, serologic studies show that over 80% of initial and 98% of recurrent genital HSV infections are caused by HSV-2 (Para & Baird, 1985).

Though national statistics for genital herpes are not available, primary HSV infections are estimated by various sources to affect 200,000 to 300,000 persons each year. Recurrent HSV infections are even more common: estimated at up to 20 million episodes yearly

(Hatcher et al., 1988). Individuals with genital herpes infections are usually well-educated, single men and women in their midtwenties. Most do not have other STDs, such as gonorrhea (Corey, 1984).

HSV-2 infections are usually transmitted through close contact with a person who is shedding the virus in a secretion or from a peripheral lesion or mucosal surface. Exposure to HSV-1 is almost universal. Most children are exposed to HSV-1 within the first 18 months of life. They contract an oral infection that is often asymptomatic but may cause a typical "cold sore" or stomatitis, with mild fever and vesicles on the gums and oral mucosa. Some time after exposure the virus enters neural cells and remains latent for the lifetime of the host. Initial infection with HSV-2 follows the onset of sexual activity. After the primary infection HSV-2 becomes latent. Latent HSV-1 and HSV-2 both can be reactivated and cause symptoms to recur. Although about 80% of the population harbors latent oral HSV-1, very few experience recurrent disease. HSV-1 or HSV-2 may reactivate in response to some nonspecific stimulus, such as fever, exposure to sunshine, or stress. The mechanisms of HSV latency and reactivation are not fully understood (Rapp, 1984).

Orogenital sexual contact has been implicated in the transmission of HSV: HSV-1 is found in an increasing number of genital lesions, and HSV-2 is found in oral lesions. Fomites (contaminated objects, such as washcloths and bathtubs) may also play a role in transmission, since the virus can live on wet surfaces for several hours (Para & Baird, 1985; Rapp, 1984).

Genital herpes causes extensive perinatal morbidity and mortality. HSV infection can be transmitted to the fetus in utero (across the placenta) and during passage

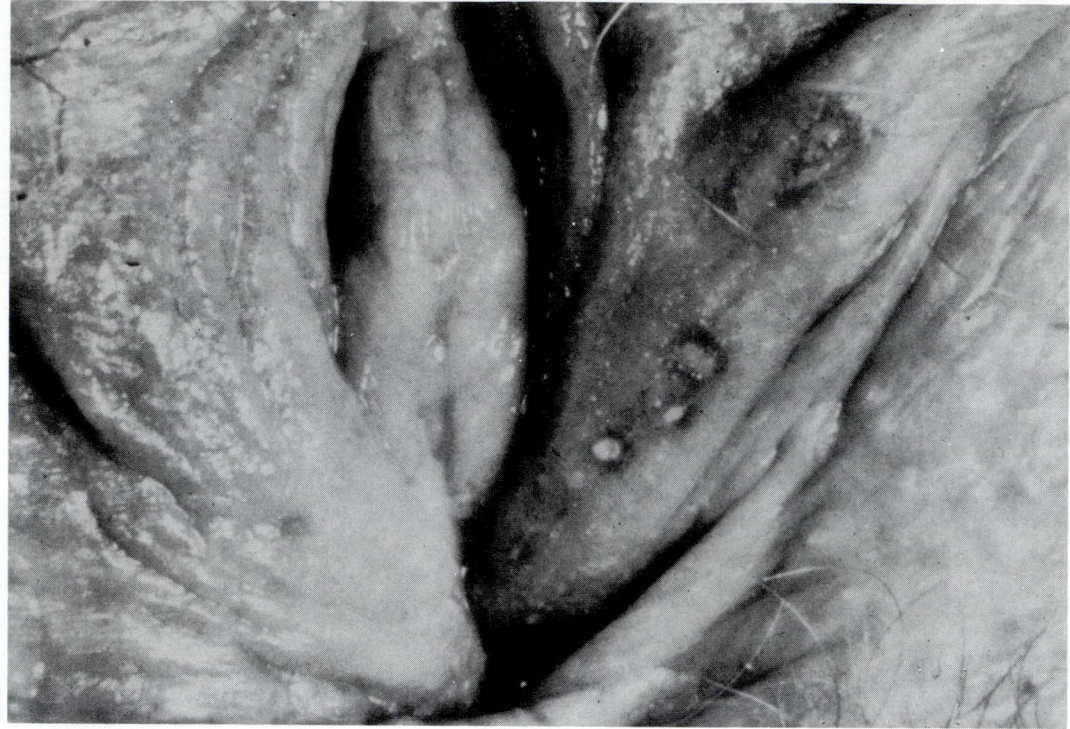

FIG. 21-9. Recurrent herpes genitalis. Ulcers are noted following rupture of vesicles. (From Kaufman & Faro, 1985.)

through an infected birth canal. HSV infection in utero can cause spontaneous abortion or premature delivery (Corey, 1984). The risk of neonatal infection is highest for infants born to women who are culture-positive at the time of delivery, have a primary HSV infection, and experience ruptured membranes more than 6 hours prior to delivery (American Academy of Pediatrics Committee on the Fetus and Newborn, 1980). Fortunately the rate of mother-infant transmission is very low. Transmission of HSV infection in utero occurs in about 0.1% to 1% of all pregnancies (Bolognese, Adlinger, & Roberts, 1981), and the incidence of transmission during delivery is as low as 1 in 20,000 births.

Pathophysiology

Infection by HSV is generally fatal to the cell. Within 1 to 2 hours of inoculation extensive damage to host chromosomes has occurred. Soon inclusion bodies develop in the host nucleus, and the virus begins replication. After oral infection the latent virus resides in the trigeminal ganglion; after genital infections it resides in the dorsal sacral nerve roots.

The genital lesions caused by HSV-1 and HSV-2 are indistinguishable to the naked eye. Multiple, small, 1-mm to 2-mm vesicular or ulcerated lesions develop on the labia minora, fourchette, or penis (Fig. 21-9). These lesions may also appear on the cervix, buttocks, and

thighs and are generally painful and pruritic. The small vesicles may coalesce into larger ulcers, which tend to become secondarily infected. These wet lesions actively shed virus for about 10 to 14 days, after which they gradually heal by crusting and reepithelialization.

Clinical Manifestations

A wide range of clinical manifestations are caused by HSV infection. Primary genital infection is generally more severe than recurrent infection, but both can be asymptomatic. In a person with HSV antibodies from previous "cold sores" the clinical course of the first genital herpes infection is generally shorter and milder and is termed an initial rather than a primary infection.

Fig. 21-10 illustrates the clinical course of primary genital herpes. Besides the genital lesions, local clinical manifestations can include inguinal lymphadenopathy, urethral and vaginal discharge, and dysuria. Systemic manifestations can include fever, headache, photophobia, and malaise. Viremia, meningitis, and urinary retention are possible complications.

Recurrent genital infection develops after about 55% of primary infections with HSV-1 and 88% of primary genital infections with HSV-2 (Corey et al., 1983). Recurrent episodes are generally less severe and of shorter duration than the primary infection. Pain and viral shedding may only last 4 to 5 days, and the lesions dry and

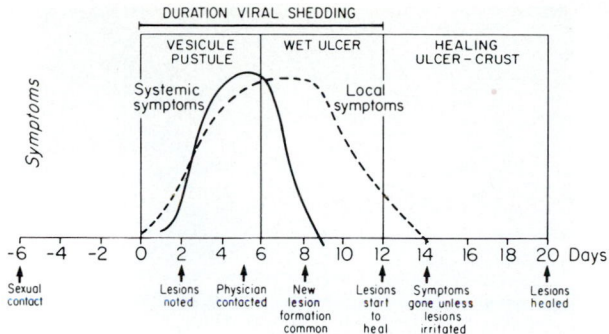

FIG. 21-10. Clinical course of primary genital herpes. (From Corey, 1984.)

heal in about 10 days. Before each outbreak some individuals experience a prodromal syndrome manifested by itching, tingling, or aching at the site where the lesions subsequently appear. Some individuals have outbreaks several times each year; others never experience a recurrence. Transmission is possible during latent periods: HSV can be shed from the saliva, cervix, and semen of asymptomatic individuals (Adam et al., 1979).

Symptomatic HSV infection of the newborn may occur any time in the first month of life. Manifestations range from a local infection of the eyes, skin, or mucous membranes to a severe, disseminated infection with CNS involvement. About 70% of affected infants present with skin lesions. CNS involvement includes seizures and is associated with a mortality rate of over 50% and extensive neurologic sequelae in survivors.

Evaluation and Treatment

Genital HSV infection is suspected if typical genital lesions are present. A presumptive diagnosis of HSV-associated infection is supported by the identification in a Papanicolaou smear of multinucleated giant cells with intranuclear inclusions. Definitive diagnosis is made after viral tissue culture. HSV-1 and HSV-2 are distinguished by fluorescent antibody, neutralization, or other serologic techniques.

There is currently no curative treatment for HSV infection, but the antiviral drug acyclovir can reduce symptoms and suppress recurrent outbreaks. Although condoms offer some protection, individuals with HSV should refrain from all sexual contact in areas of lesions and understand that an undetermined risk of transmission exists even during asymptomatic periods (Hatcher et al., 1988).

Condylomata Acuminata

Condylomata acuminata, or genital warts, are caused by species of the human papillomavirus (HPV). These lesions also have been called gonorrheal warts, venereal warts, and condylomata. Condylomata acuminata

were once confused with the lesions of secondary syphilis (condylomata lata) and later were thought to be caused by gonorrhea.

Condylomata acuminata are often found in conjunction with other STDs. Although it is not a reportable STD in the United States, condylomata acuminata is common: over 3 million cases are diagnosed yearly (Hatcher et al., 1988). HPV infection is associated with multiple sexual partners and early onset of sexual activity and is most common among men and women aged 16 to 25. Genital warts are quite contagious: approximately 60% of exposed sexual partners develop the disease after an incubation period of 2 to 3 months. HPV has also been implicated in the development of cervical dysplasia. The infection can be passed from mother to fetus during passage through an infected birth canal.

Pathophysiology

Papillomaviruses are not well studied because they cannot yet be grown in cell cultures; an additional problem is that very few virus particles are present in each wart. It is known, however, that epithelial cells infected by HPV undergo transformation, proliferate, and form a warty growth. Susceptibility is greatest in immunosuppressed individuals, pregnant women, and diabetics.

Transmission occurs by contact with infected epithelium. Local trauma or friction during intercourse may cause tiny abrasions that permit HPV to enter. Excoriation of epithelial surfaces caused by other infections, such as vulvovaginitis, may promote entry of HPV through small fissures or abrasions (Oriel, 1984).

Clinical Manifestations

Condylomata acuminata are soft, skin-colored, whitish pink to reddish brown, discrete, growths. They may occur singly or in clusters and may be broad-based or pedunculated, feathery, or smooth (Fig. 21-11). Sometimes the warts enlarge to form cauliflowerlike masses on the male frenulum, glans, foreskin, urinary meatus, shaft, scrotum, and/or anus and on the female labia, clitoris, perineum, vagina, and/or anus (Fig. 21-12). Although the lesions are usually not painful, they may cause dyspareunia (painful intercourse) and may be friable and bleed easily. Some individuals complain of pruritus. Cervical lesions are generally flattened and may not be seen easily without colposcopy (Camisa, 1985).

Laryngeal papillomas can occur in infants whose mothers had genital warts at the time of delivery. Clinical manifestations of laryngeal warts include stridor, hoarseness, abnormal cry, cough, and respiratory distress (Camisa, 1985).

Evaluation and Treatment

Generally diagnosis of condylomata acuminata is made on the basis of clinical manifestations. Koilocyto-

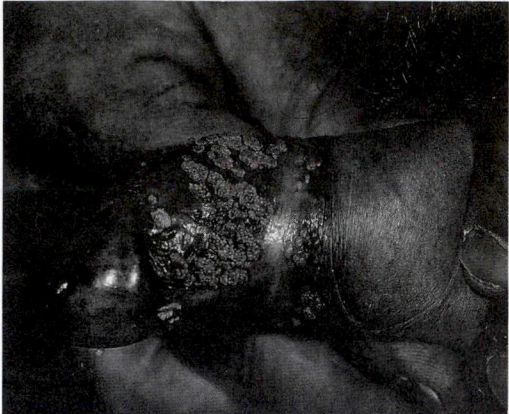

FIG. 21-11. Condylomata acuminata. Multiple, small warts under the foreskin, the type of moist area where autoinoculations tend to occur. (From Habif, 1985.)

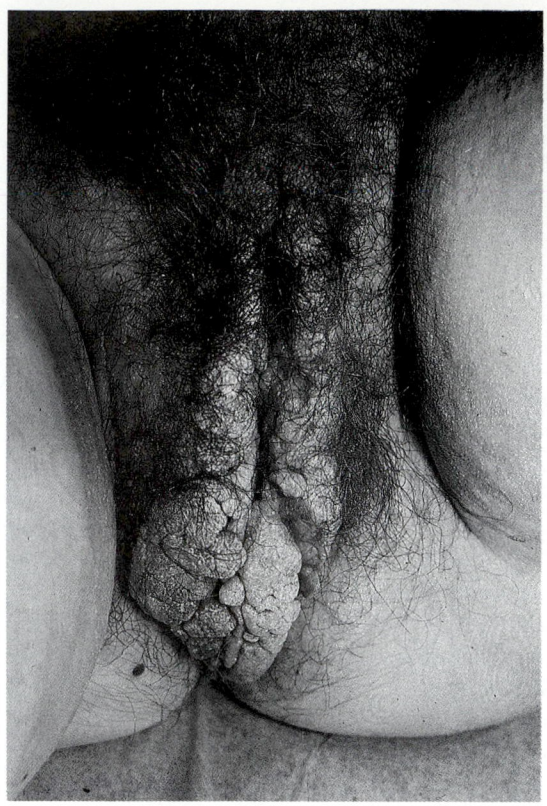

FIG. 21-12. Condylomata acuminata. Massive, cauliflower-like inoculation of warts on the vulva. (From Habif, 1985.)

sis (typical cellular changes of HPV infection) seen on the Papanicolaou smear aid in the diagnosis of cervical HPV infection. Pointy, fleshy pink lesions caused by HPV must be differentiated from condylomata lata (the whitish-gray, flat lesions) of secondary syphilis. Because HPV infection often accompanies other STDs, gonorrhea culture, chlamydia culture, serology test for syphilis, and wet mount for other vaginal microorganisms should also be performed. HPV infection is also associated with the development of squamous cell carcinoma; therefore, all atypical or persistent lesions should have biopsy examination (CDC, 1985). Some clinicians recommend that Papanicolaou smears be repeated every 6 months for women with a history of HPV infection.

Treatments for genital warts include application of topical agents, such as podophyllin, trichloroacetic acid, and 5-fluorouracil cream; cryosugery, CO$_2$ laser surgery, electrosurgery, and surgical excision. Podophyllin is quite toxic and must be used with extreme care; it should never be used in pregnancy. Surgery and CO$_2$ laser surgery require local or regional anesthesia, but these therapies are precise and sterile and cause minimal bleeding (Bourcier & Seidler, 1987; CDC, 1985). Surgical excision is the treatment for laryngeal warts in infants.

Molluscum Contagiosum

Molluscum contagiosum is a benign viral infection of the skin in children and adults. It adults it tends to occur on the genitals and to be transmitted by sexual contact.

Molluscum contagiosum occurs throughout the world and is a very common childhood disease in Papua New Guinea and Fiji. It is much less common in the United States, where incidence is highest among young adults. The childhood disease is transmitted by skin-to-skin contact and fomites (swimming pools, towels, gym equipment) and affects the face, trunk, and limbs. Adult disease is more commonly sexually transmitted and affects the lower abdomen, genitals, and perianal area (Brown, 1984).

The molluscum contagiosum virus is taken into epithelial cells by phagocytosis and replicates within the cytoplasm, where it produces cytoplasmic inclusions (**molluscous bodies**) and cellular hyperplasia. The underlying skin usually is not affected (Lambert & Yoder, 1985).

After an incubation period of 2 to 7 weeks white or flesh-colored, round or oval, dome-shaped papules appear. The surface has a characteristic central umbilication, from which a thick, creamy core material can be expressed (Fig. 21-13). Generally the lesions are not painful or pruritic unless secondarily infected. The papules may last several months or several years and spread by autoinoculation.

The appearance of the lesions is generally all that is needed to make the diagnosis, although direct microscopic examination of stained material from the core of the papule reveals molluscous bodies within the swollen and rounded epithelial cells. Treatment consists of cryo-

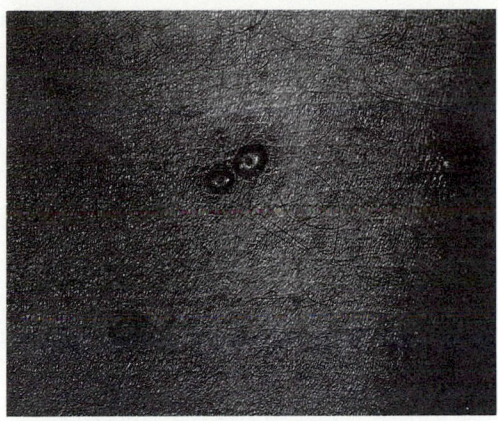

FIG. 21-13. Papules typical of molluscum contagiosum. (From Habif, 1985.)

therapy or use of topical irritants, such as podophyllin or silver nitrate (Brown, 1984).

Parasitic Infections
Trichomoniasis

Originally discovered in 1836, *Trichomonas vaginalis* was at first thought to be a harmless commensal microorganism. *T. vaginalis* is now known to be one of the most common causes of sexually transmitted lower genital tract infection.

Because **trichomoniasis** (infection by *T. vaginalis*) is not a reportable disease, its prevalence can only be estimated. Between 2.5 and 3 million American women are infected with trichomoniasis every year, and *T. vaginalis* accounts for one out of four cases of infectious vaginitis (Droegemueller et al., 1987). Trichomoniasis is usually found in both sexual partners and often coexists with gonorrhea. Although sexual transmission is clearly the most common means of disease spread, transmission through fomites is theoretically possible. To cause infection the fomite would have to introduce an inoculum of about 10,000 microorganisms directly into the vagina (Rein & Holmes, 1983).

Pathophysiology

T. vaginalis is an anaerobic, unicellular, flagellated, parasitic protozoan that adheres to and damages squamous epithelial cells. Because this protozoan selectively affects squamous epithelium, vaginal and urethral tissue are often infected, as are Skene and Bartholin glands. The endocervical canal is not affected because it is lined with columnar epithelium. In men the urethra is the most common site of infection, although the protozoa, called **trichomonads,** also can infect the epididymis and (rarely) the prostate. Zinc, which has potent antibacterial properties, is found in high concentrations in the prostate. Hence many trichomonads are cleared

from the male urethra during ejaculation. This action makes urethral trichomoniasis a fairly self-limiting infection in men. Most infections of the male urethra clear up within 2 weeks.

Trichomoniasis is most common in women of reproductive age, and it is primarily an infection of the vagina. *T. vaginalis* can induce a marked inflammatory response in the vagina, causing a copious discharge that contains large numbers of polymorphonuclear neutrophils. Trichomonads adhere to, but do not invade, the squamous epithelial cells.

Clinical Manifestations

Manifestations of vaginal trichomoniasis range from none to severe, with some women reporting an increase in distressing symptoms immediately after menses. Vaginal discharge and internal pruritus are the most common complaints. Dyspareunia and dysuria are also fairly common. Secretions are usually copious, sometimes frothy or bubbly, and gray-green. The vaginal walls may appear erythematous and sore. Rarely small, punctate red marks, the so-called strawberry spots, are visible. Vaginal pH is usually greater than 5.0.

Most men with trichomoniasis remain asymptomatic. Possible clinical manifestations include scant intermittent discharge, slight pruritus, and mild dysuria.

Evaluation and Treatment

History and symptoms are inadequate for diagnosis of trichomoniasis. Microscopic confirmation of the presence of the trichomonads in vaginal secretions or urine provides a definitive diagnosis. In a fresh wet mount preparation that has been warmed slightly, the epithelial cells have relatively clean and sharp edges, the ratio of polymorphonuclear leukocytes to epithelial cells exceeds 1:1, and the trichomonads are visible. The ovoid microorganism is slightly larger than a polymorphonuclear leukocyte and has one rounded, flagellated end and one slightly pointed, flagellated end. The flagella give the trichomonads their characteristic twisting motility. In an acidic environment, such as urine, the trichomonads assume a "balled-up" or spherical shape and become less motile.

The treatment of choice for trichomoniasis is a single dose of metronidazole (Flagyl). The single-dose therapy is effective, has few side effects, and obviates the need for individual compliance with longer regimens. Sexual partners, even if asymptomatic, are also treated and examined for coexisting STDs. Metronidazole is contraindicated in pregnancy, during which topical clotrimazole is the treatment of choice (CDC, 1985).

Scabies

Scabies is a rather benign, common parasitic infection that can be spread by skin-to-skin and sexual contact. Discovered by Bonomo in 1687, it is considered to be the first human disease with a known cause (Orkin & Maibach, 1984).

Scabies has a worldwide distribution and accounts for approximately 2% to 3% of visits to dermatologists in the United States (Shaw & Juranek, 1976). Traditionally the disease was attributed to conditions of poverty, overcrowding, uncleanliness, and sexual promiscuity. Today it is recognized that scabies occurs in individuals with good personal hygiene and is not limited to any social class. Outbreaks of scabies occur every 30 years or so and last about 15 years. The most recent outbreak in the United States began in 1971 and subsided in the 1980s (Fitzpatrick, Polano, & Suurmond, 1983).

Transmission of scabies requires close skin-to-skin contact, which typically occurs within families or between sexual partners. Transmission through fomites is possible but not likely (Lambert & Yoder, 1985).

Pathophysiology

The adult female itch mite, *Sarcoptes scabiei,* is 0.3 to 0.4 mm long and has a life span of about 30 days. Once deposited on human skin, it burrows through the horny layer of the stratum granulosum. Within hours of burrowing the female begins laying two to three large eggs per day, each of which progresses through larval and nymphal stages to become an adult itch mite in about

10 days. The most common places for scabies to burrow are on the hands (between the fingers) and on the flexor surfaces of the wrists and the extensor surfaces of the elbows. Genital burrowing occurs on the penis and buttocks and in the crease of skin where the buttock meets the thigh (Orkin & Maibach, 1984). Fig. 21-14 shows the typical sites of scabies burrows.

Clinical Manifestations

The classic symptom of scabies is intense pruritus, which may be pronounced at night. The typical burrow of the *S. scabiei* is a short, wavy line (Fig. 21-15). There may be small, erythematous, excoriated larval papules near the burrows. Secondary infections are common and are caused by scratching. In some individuals a hypersensitivity reaction occurs 1 or more months after the infestation and causes multiple reddish-brown, pruritic nodules to develop on the covered portions of the body, most commonly the upper thighs, buttocks, male genitalia, and axillary regions. These nodules may persist for more than a year, despite treatment with a scabicide.

Evaluation and Treatment

Although the diagnosis is often made on clinical grounds, microscopic identification of the mite or its eggs, larvae, or feces is recommended because the symptoms of scabies can imitate those of many other dermatologic conditions. Superficial scrapings from a recently developed, unexcoriated papule or burrow can easily be observed under the microscope; the addition of potassium hydroxide allows easier visualization of the mite.

Treatment consists of topical application of lindane 1% cream or lotion (Kwell, Gammexane, Scabene). Close household and sexual contacts should also be treated. For very young children and pregnant or lactating women crotamiton 10% cream (Eurax) or sulfur 6% in petrolatum is substituted. To prevent reinfestation clothing and bed linen should be machine washed and dried at high temperatures (CDC, 1985; Orkin & Maibach, 1984).

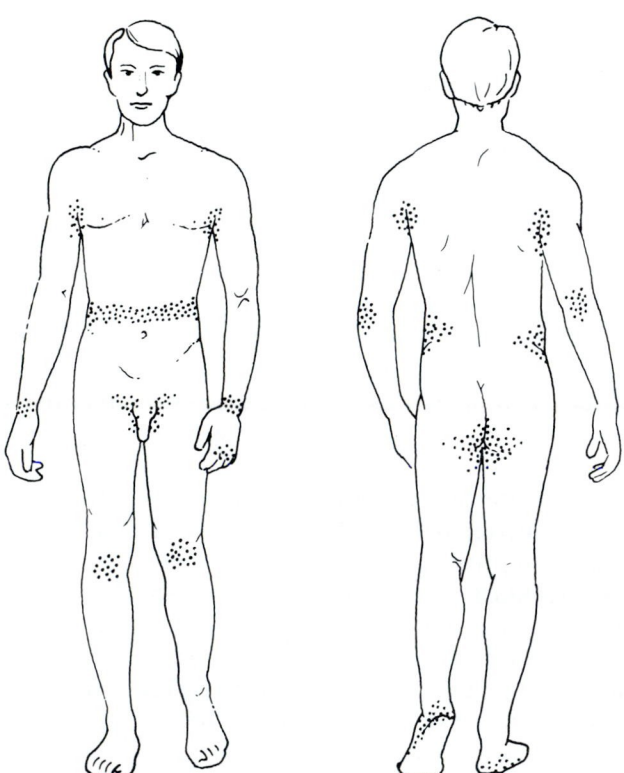

FIG. 21-14. Scabies. Typical distribution of lesions. (From Habif, 1985.)

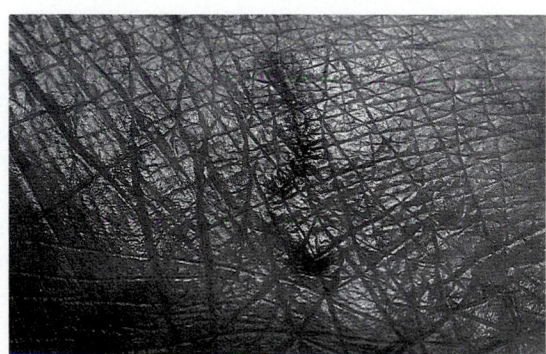

FIG. 21-15. Scabies. An S-shaped burrow with a tiny vesicle at one end. (From Habif, 1985.)

Pediculosis Pubis

Phthirus pubis, the crab louse, is one of three species of lice that infest humans. *P. pubis* is commonly transmitted sexually and causes **pediculosis pubis,** or "crabs."

The prevalence of pubic lice infestation is difficult to estimate. Pediculosis pubis is common among individuals being treated for other STDs. Statistics show that incidence is somewhat higher in women than in men (Hatcher et al., 1988) and that the disease is most common in single persons aged 15 to 25 (Billstein, 1984). *P. pubis* is transmitted primarily by intimate sexual contact, although fomites (toilet seats and beds) do play a role in some cases.

Pathophysiology

The crab louse has a five-stage life cycle: an egg (or nit) stage, three nymphal stages, and an adult stage, all of which occur in the host. The nits of crab lice are found "glued" to hairs; they are oval, 0.8 by 0.3 mm, and whitish and hatch in 5 to 10 days (Fig. 21-16). In the adult stage pubic lice are grayish, are approximately 1 mm in length, and have a segmented body and claws particularly designed for clinging to pubic hairs. Dependent on blood for nutrition, the lice bite into the skin to obtain food.

Clinical Manifestations

Symptoms range from mild pruritus to severe, intolerable itching, depending on the individual's sensitivity to louse bites. Allergic sensitization occurs in about 5 days, when itching, erythema, and inflammation may worsen. Excessive scratching may lead to secondary infection.

Evaluation and Treatment

The individual's history usually reveals a recent exposure and the typical symptoms of infestation. Since both the lice and nits are visible to the naked eye, a thorough clinical examination permits definitive diagnosis. Pediculosis pubis is treated with lindane 1% lotion, cream, or shampoo (by prescription) or by pyrethin and piperonyl butoxide (Rid, Triple X, or A-200 Pyrinate, available without a prescription). Sexual contacts and any other intimate household contacts should also be examined and treated, and clothing and bed linen should be machine washed and dried at high temperatures (Billstein, 1984).

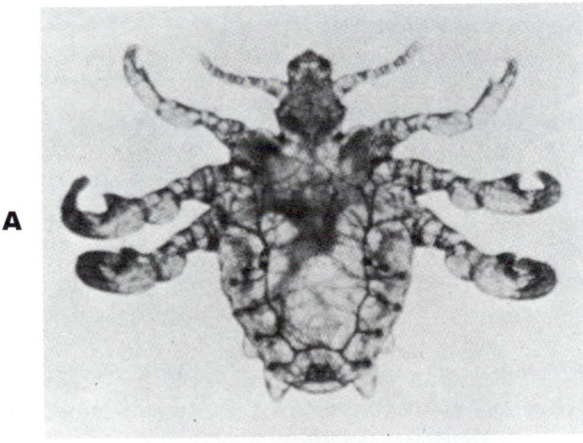

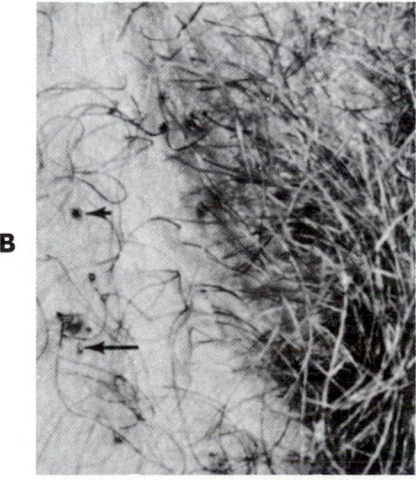

FIG. 21-16. A, Pubic louse, **B,** Crab lice and nits of pediculosis pubis (arrows). (**A** from Billistein, 1984; **B** from Droegemeuller, Herbst, Mischell, & Stenehever, 1987.)

SEXUALLY TRANSMITTED INFECTIONS OF OTHER BODY SYSTEMS

Gastrointestinal Infections

Shigellosis and Campylobacter Enteritis

A variety of enteric bacterial pathogens are now recognized as sexually transmitted, particularly among homosexual men. The bacteria most frequently implicated in the so-called gay bowel syndrome are species of *Shigella* and *Campylobacter*. *Shigella* infection, termed **shigellosis,** is transmitted by contact with infected feces. Very few microorganisms are needed to cause infection. Anal-oral spread occurs very easily through household contact and anal-oral sexual practices. *Campylobacter jejuni,* which causes **campylobacter enteritis,** is primarily an animal pathogen but may also be transmitted among humans through anal-oral sexual practices. Again very few microorganisms are necessary for inoculation and infection.

Pathophysiology

Shigella are nonmotile, gram-negative rods that are related to *Escherichia coli.* They invade and kill intestinal epithelial cells, thereby inducing a marked inflammatory response and diarrhea. *Campylobacter* are highly motile, curved, gram-negative rods that also invade and kill intestinal cells and cause bloody, inflammatory exudate and diarrhea.

Clinical Manifestations

Either microorganism may cause a mild, self-limited gastroenteritis or severe dysentery. After a 24- to 48-hour incubation period shigellosis begins with fever, abdominal distress, and diarrhea. It may resolve completely or progress to dysentery with severe cramping, abdominal pain, tenesmus, and bloody mucoid discharge from the rectum. Campylobacter enteritis typically begins, after a 1- to 7-day incubation period, with sudden fever and abdominal pain followed by diarrhea. Malaise, anorexia, headache, arthralgia, and myalgia are common (Caldwell, 1985).

Evaluation and Treatment

Clinical manifestations and cultures of fresh stool samples are used to diagnose shigellosis. Culturing *Campylobacter* is expensive; therefore, microscopic analysis of a Gram-stained smear of rectal exudate may be used as a diagnostic aid.

Treatment for mild illness includes correction of fluid and electrolyte imbalance. Antidiarrheals are avoided because they may delay clearance of the microorganism. Because *Shigella* and *Campylobacter* are both highly contagious, antibiotic treatment may be advisable even for mild cases. The usual treatment for shigellosis is 1 week of trimethoprim and sulfamethoxazole. Erythromycin is used to treat campylobacter enteritis (Caldwell, 1985; CDC, 1985). Sexual partners are examined and treated, and individuals are instructed to avoid oral-anal contact until the infection is cured.

Giardiasis and Amebiasis

Two enteric protozoa that are sexually transmitted, primarily among homosexual men, are *Giardia lamblia,* the cause of **giardiasis,** and *Entamoeba histolytica,* the cause of **amebiasis.** Among homosexual men the prevalence of these two infections is between 30% and 40% (Quinn & Holmes, 1984). Although the principal route of transmission is contaminated drinking water, giardiasis and amebiasis are also transmitted by anal-oral or genital-anal contact.

Pathophysiology

G. lamblia and *E. histolytica* are both parasites having two forms, cysts and **traphozoites** (uncysted protozoa). The cysts are the infective form because they can survive in moist environments outside the host. Giardiasis commonly begins with ingestion of a small number of *G. lamblia* cysts. Once in the upper small bowel each cyst becomes a traphozoite, which multiplies and attaches to

the bowel mucosa. Enzyme deficiencies, inflammation, and immunologic damage then apparently occur, resulting in intestinal malabsorption. Amebiasis begins similarly: the ingested cysts pass to the small or large bowel, where each returns to the traphozoite state, multiplies quickly, and begins to invade the mucosa through cytotoxic activity. Mucosal invasion results in the development of ulcers and an inflammatory response (Guerrant & Ravdin, 1984). Individuals infected with *E. histolytica* may excrete up to 45 million cysts per day.

Clinical Manifestations

Giardiasis begins with sudden, explosive diarrhea; distention; and flatulence. Upper gastrointestinal symptoms are also prominent and may include epigastric pain; vomiting; foul, sulfuric burping; and nausea. After the acute illness, which usually lasts several days, milder symptoms may persist for months, with evidence of malabsorption and weight loss. Amebiasis is often asymptomatic. Symptoms that do occur range from mild diarrhea to severe dysentery. Amebiasis may spread from the intestine to other organs, such as the liver.

Evaluation and Treatment

Diagnosis of both entities is usually made by history and microscopic examination of fresh stool specimens for either trophozoites or cysts. Small bowel biopsy may aid in the diagnosis of giardiasis; rectal biopsy may aid in the diagnosis of amebiasis. Serologic testing is useful in the differential diagnosis of symptomatic individuals with amebiasis. Metronidazole (Flagyl) is the usual treatment for both conditions (Quinn & Holmes, 1984).

Hepatitis B

Hepatitis is a liver infection that can be caused by three types of viruses: hepatitis A, hepatitis B, and hepatitis non-A, non-B. All cause a syndrome of acute, icteric (jaundice-producing) liver inflammation. Of the three types, the **hepatitis B virus** (HBV) is known to be sexually transmitted. (Hepatitis A, like most other predominantly enteric infections, may occasionally be sexually transmitted.) Additional information about hepatitis is found in Chapter 36.

The prevalence of HBV infection varies dramatically worldwide. In Southeast Asia and Africa 60% to 80% of the population may harbor serologic evidence of past or current infection. In the United States approximately 5% to 20% of the general population have evidence of HBV infection. Seropositivity generally increases with age. At risk for HBV infection are those with low socioeconomic status, blacks, Indochinese refugees, health care workers, and male homosexuals. In groups of male homosexuals the seropositivity rates may be as high as 80%. Other groups at risk are intravenous drug users, institutionalized mentally retarded persons, hemodialysis patients, and heterosexual partners of HBV carriers (Lemon, 1984).

Transmission of HBV can occur through needle puncture, blood transfusion, cuts or abrasions in the skin, and absorption by mucosal surfaces. Direct contact with infected body fluids, such as tears, cerebrospinal fluid, synovial fluid, gastric juices, pleural fluid, semen, and urine may pass the infection. Fomites can also transmit hepatitis: HBV can survive on inanimate objects for up to 1 week (Klein, 1988).

Perinatal transmission of HBV is relatively common. Neonates whose mothers are infectious have a 70% to 90% chance of becoming infected with HBV during labor or delivery and a 90% chance of becoming chronic carriers. HBV can be found in maternal vaginal secretions, blood, amniotic fluid, saliva, and breast milk (Klein, 1988).

Pathophysiology

After exposure HBV passes through the bloodstream to the liver, where it infects liver cells and multiplies. The infection is usually self-limiting, with most patients mounting an effective immune response. About 6% to 10% of infected individuals are unable to eradicate the virus and become chronic carriers of HBV.

Clinical Manifestations

Most HBV infections are clinically inapparent and result in solid and permanent immunity. Symptoms of hepatitis usually develop only after a certain HBV antigen has been circulating in the blood for 3 to 6 weeks. About 15% to 20% of individuals develop a prodromal syndrome that is similar to serum sickness. This syndrome is characterized by an erythematous rash, urticaria, polyarthralgias, and arthritis. Symptoms of infection may also include lassitude, anorexia, nausea, vomiting, headache, fever, dark urine, jaundice, and moderate liver enlargement with tenderness. Long-term sequelae include chronic persistent and chronic active hepatitis, cirrhosis, hepatocellular carcinoma, hepatic failure, and death. In neonates who contract HBV the disease may be manifested in many ways, from mild illness to a severe, fulminant infection with a mortality rate of 75%.

Evaluation and Treatment

HBV infection is clinically indistinguishable from other types of hepatitis. Diagnosis can only be made through serologic testing.

No specific therapy exists for HBV infection in adults. Treatment consists of supportive care and relief of symptoms. Vaccination is urged for members of high-risk groups.

The infant who is born to a mother with infectious HBV is given HBV immune globulin and Hepatavax-B

vaccine within 12 hours of birth. The HBV vaccine is administered again at 1 and 6 months, provided that serologic tests show that a chronic carrier state has not developed (CDC, 1985).

Systemic Diseases
Acquired Immune Deficiency Syndrome

Epidemiology, modes of transmission, pathophysiology, clinical manifestations, and evaluation and treatment of acquired immunodeficiency syndrome (AIDS) are discussed in detail in Chapter 8.

Cytomegalovirus Infection

Cytomegalovirus (CMV) is a sexually transmissible herpes virus. It is associated with a number of clinical syndromes in newborns, otherwise healthy adults, and immunosuppressed individuals.

CMV infection causes no specific genital disease, but its incidence is high in individuals being treated for other STDs. CMV infection is prevalent worldwide, especially in developing countries and lower socioeconomic groups. The virus is found in semen, cervical secretions, urine, blood, saliva, breast milk, and stool, and transmission is associated with close (although not always genital) interpersonal contact or direct transfer of cells or body fluids (Lang, 1984). It is more common in homosexual men and in young women with multiple sexual partners. Perinatal transmission of CMV may occur across the placenta, by contamination with infected secretions during passage through the birth canal, or during breastfeeding. Approximately 1% of infants born in the United States are infected with CMV (Lang, 1984).

Pathophysiology

After CMV infects a human cell it may replicate and destroy the infected cell or become incorporated into the host cell's DNA. Local CMV infections can persist despite the presence of large quantities of systemic antibody to CMV. Cell-mediated immunity seems to have a particular role in protecting against CMV infections. Depression of CMV-specific cell-mediated immunity has been noted in otherwise normal hosts with CMV infection. This may be caused by injury of T cells or macrophages by the cytomegalovirus (Lang, 1984).

Clinical Manifestations

In healthy individuals CMV infection can cause a number of mild subclinical or nonspecific illnesses, including mononucleosis, pneumonitis, hemolytic anemia, and thrombocytopenia purpura. In contrast, a CMV infection in an immunocompromised individual, such as a transplant recipient or an individual with AIDS, can cause a devastating, life-threatening illness.

Most babies born with CMV infection are asymptomatic. It is estimated that between 10% and 20% of these infants with silent CMV infection ultimately show signs of sensorineural deafness, or developmental delay, or both (Hanshaw et al., 1976). In classic congenital CMV infection the infant is small, with microcephaly, hepatosplenomegaly, chorioretinitis, jaundice, and purpura. The long-term effects are unknown but may include permanent CNS and developmental sequelae.

Evaluation and Treatment

The most definitive diagnostic test for CMV is isolation of the virus, usually through growth in human fibroblast cell culture. Several methods for measuring antibodies to CMV are available, including complement fixation (CF) tests and indirect immunofluorescent antibody (IFA) tests. These methods are frequently used in clinical situations.

Experimental antiviral drugs may prove helpful in the treatment of severe CMV infection, and preliminary studies to develop a vaccine appear promising. However, no treatment is indicated in most cases of CMV infection.

SUMMARY REVIEW

Sexually Transmitted Urogenital Infections

1 Gonorrhea is a communicable disease that can be local or systemic and is usually transmitted sexually. Complications, such as pelvic inflammatory disease in women and disseminated infections, spread through the bloodstream to the skin, joints, and heart.

2 Gonorrhea passed to the fetus from the mother is usually manifest as an eye infection and develops 1 to 12 days after birth.

3 Penicillin is the drug of choice for treatment of gonorrheal infections.

4 Syphilis is a sexually transmitted disease that becomes systemic shortly after infection. The four stages of the disease are: (a) primary syphilis with a chancre at the site of infection, (b) secondary syphilis with systemic spread to all body systems, (c) latent syphilis with minimal symptoms or the development of skin lesions, and (d) tertiary syphilis, the most severe stage, with destruction of bone, skin, and soft tissues.

5 Congenital syphilis contributes to prematurity of the newborn with bone marrow depression, CNS involvement, renal failure, and eye disorders. Late clinical manifestations are those of tertiary syphilis and are rare.

6 Serologic testing is used to diagnose syphilis, and penicillin is the drug of choice.

7 Chancroid is a soft genital chancre most common among uncircumcised men. The lesion appears 1 to 14 days after exposure and is painful and inflamed. The infected person and sexual partner are treated with erythromycin.

8 Granuloma inguinale (donovanosis) is rare in the United States. The bacteria are gram-negative and survive within macrophages. Localized nodules coalesce to form granulomas and ulcers on the penis in men and labia in women. Antibiotics provide effective treatment.

9 Bacterial vaginitis (*Gardnerella vaginalis*) is caused by anaerobic bacteria that produce aromatic amines that raise the pH of the vagina, promoting further bacterial growth with an inflammatory response and a fishy smelling odor. "Clue cells" are found on the wet mount. Flagyl provides effective treatment.

10 Infections of *Chlamydia trachomatis* are probably the most common STD in the United States. Cervicitis associated with pregnancy and use of oral contraceptives is common in women, and urethritis is common in men. *C. trachomatis* localizes to epithelial tissue and can spread throughout the urogenital system. Microorganisms may also pass from the mother to the eyes and respiratory tract of the infant during birth. Tetracycline or doxycycline is used for treatment in men and nonpregnant women, and erythromycin in infants and pregnant women.

11 Lymphogranuloma venereum is a chronic STD that is uncommon in the United States. The lesion begins as a skin infection and spreads to the lymph tissue, causing inflammation, necrosis, buboes, and abscesses of the inguinal lymph nodes. Primary lesions appear on the penis and scrotum in men, and on the cervix, vaginal wall, and labia in women. Secondary lesions involve inflammation and swelling of the lymph nodes with formation of large blue buboes that rupture and form draining ulcerative lesions. Tetracycline provides effective treatment.

12 Genital herpes is the most common genital ulceration in the United States and is caused by either type 1 (HSV-1) or type 2 (HSV-2) herpes virus. HSV-1 often presents as a "cold sore" of the oral mucosa and HSV-2 is commonly a genital lesion. Lesions initially appear as groups of vesicles that progress to ulceration with pain, lymphadenopathy, and fever. HSV passed from mother to fetus can cause spontaneous abortion or prematurity. Acyclovir reduces symptoms but does not cure the disease.

13 Condylomata acuminata (genital warts) is associated with multiple sexual partners and is highly contagious. The velvety cauliflowerlike lesions occur in the genital and anal areas, vagina, and cervix and are painless. They can be transmitted to the infant at birth. Surgical excision with laser or cryosurgery is most effective.

14 Trichomoniasis (*T. vaginalis*) is a common cause of genital infection, vaginitis in women, and urethritis. Both partners are usually infected. Women usually have a copious gray-green discharge with pruritus. Men are usually asymptomatic. Metronidazole is the treatment for both partners.

15 Scabies is a common parasitic infection that can be spread by skin-to-skin contact and sexual contact. The scabies mite burrows through the skin, depositing two or three large eggs per day. Intense pruritis is the most

pronounced clinical manifestation. Treatment consists of topical application of lindane 1% cream or lotion.

16 Pediculosis pubis (crabs) is commonly transmitted sexually and is caused by the crab louse, *Phthirus pubis*. The lice bite into the skin for nutrition. Symptoms include mild and severe pruritus. Treatment consists of lindane 1% cream, lotion, or shampoo, or pryethrins and piperonyl butoxide.

Sexually Transmitted Infections of Other Body Systems

1 A variety of enteric bacterial pathogens are now recognized as sexually transmitted, particularly among homosexual men. The infections include shigellosis, campylobacter enteritis, giardiasis, amebiasis, and hepatitis B.

2 Shigellosis is transmitted by contact with infected feces. Campylobacter enteritis can be transmitted through anal-oral sexual practices.

3 Giardiasis and amebiasis are primarily transmitted through contaminated drinking water but are also transmitted by anal-oral and genital-anal contact.

4 Transmission of hepatitis B virus (HBV) can occur through needle puncture, blood transfusion, cuts in the skin, and contact with infected body fluids.

5 Perinatal transmission of HBV is relatively common.

6 Systemic diseases known to be sexually transmitted include AIDS (see Chapter 8) and cytomegalovirus infection.

7 Cytomegalovirus (CMV) is a sexually transmissible herpesvirus. The infection causes no specific genital disease, but its incidence is high in individuals being treated for other STDs. The virus is found in semen, cervical secretions, urine, blood, saliva, breast milk, and stool.

8 CMV infection is more common in homosexual men and in young women with multiple sexual partners.

9 CMV infection can cause mononucleosis, pneumonitis, hemolytic anemia, and thrombocytopenia purpura. A CMV infection in an immunosuppressed individual can cause a life-threatening illness. No treatment is indicated in most cases of CMV infection.

KEY TERMS

Acute urethral syndrome, 737

Amebiasis, 746

Bacterial vaginosis, 735

Bubo, 735

Campylobacter enteritis, 745

Chancre, 730

Chancroid, 733

Condylomata acuminata, 741

Condylomata lata, 731

Cytomegalovirus (CMV), 747

Disseminated gonococcal infection (DGI), 728

Donovan body, 735

Fomite, 727

Genital herpes, 739

Giardiasis, 746

Gonococcus, 727

Gonorrhea, 727

Granuloma inguinale, 735

Gumma, 730

Hepatitis B virus (HBV), 746

Latent syphilis, 730

Lymphogranuloma venereum (LGV), 738

Molluscous body, 742

Molluscum contagiosum, 742

Neurosyphilis, 731

Ophthalmia neonatorum, 729

Pediculosis pubis, 745

Primary syphilis, 730

Scabies, 743

Secondary syphilis, 730

Shigellosis, 745

Syphilis, 729

Tertiary syphilis, 730

Traphozoite, 746

Trichomonad, 743

Trichomoniasis, 743

REFERENCES

Adam, E., Kaurman, R. H., Mirkovic, R. R., & Melnick, J. L. (1979). Persistence of virus shedding in asymptomatic women after recovery from herpes genitalis. *Obstetrics & Gynecology, 54,* 171-173.

American Academy of Pediatrics Committee on the Fetus and Newborn. (1980). Perinatal herpes simplex virus infection. *Pediatric Infectious Diseases, 1,* 253-255.

Billstein, S. (1984). Human lice. In K. K. Holmes, P. A. Mardh, P. F. Sparling, & P. J. Weisner (Eds.), *Sexually transmitted diseases* (pp. 513-516). New York: McGraw-Hill.

Bolognese, R. J., Adlinger, R., & Roberts, N. (1981). Prenatal care in the prevention of infection. *Clinics in Perinatology, 8,* 605-637.

Bourcier, K. M., & Seidler, A. J. (1987). Chlamydia and condlyomata acuminata: An update for the nurse practitioner. *Journal of Obstetric, Gynecologic, and Neonatal Nursing, 16*(1), 17-22.

Brant, A. M. (1987). *No magic bullet: A social history of venereal disease in the United States since 1180, expanded edition.* New York: Oxford University Press.

Brown, S. T. (1984). Molluscum contagiosum. In K. K. Holmes, P. A. Mardh, P. F. Sparling, & P. J. Weisner

(Eds.), *Sexually transmitted diseases* (pp. 507-512). New York: McGraw-Hill.

Caldwell, J. H. (1985). The "gay bowel" syndrome. In V. A. Spagna & R. B. Prior (Eds.), *Sexually transmitted disease: A clinical syndrome approach* (pp. 255-274). New York: Marcel Dekker.

Camisa, C. (1985). Condyloma acuminatum and other human papillomavirus-induced diseases. In V. A. Spagna & R. B. Prior (Eds.), *Sexually transmitted disease: A clinical syndrome* (pp. 309-332). New York: Marcel Dekker.

Cates, W., & Holmes, K. K. (1986). Sexually transmitted diseases. In J. M. Last, J. Chin, J. E. Fielding, A. L. Frank, J. C. Lashof, & R. B. Wallace (Eds.), *Maxcy-Rosenau public health and preventive medicine* (12th ed.) (pp. 257-295). East Norwalk, Conn.: Appleton-Century-Crofts.

Centers for Disease Control. (1985). 1985 STD treatment guidelines. *Morbidity and Mortality Weekly, 34*(4s), 137-139.

Centers for Disease Control. (1987a). Summary of notifiable diseases—United States 1987. *Morbidity and Mortality Weekly, 36*(54).

Centers for Disease Control. (1987b). Penicillinase-producing *Neisseria gonorrhoeae*—United States 1986. *Morbidity and Mortality Weekly, 36*(34), 585-593.

Centers for Disease Control. (1988). Continuing increase in infectious syphilis—United States. *Morbidity and Mortality Weekly, 37*(3), pp. 35-38.

Corey, L. (1984). Genital herpes. In K. K. Holmes, P. A. Mardh, P. F. Sparling, & P. J. Weisner (Eds.), *Sexually transmitted diseases* (pp. 449-473). New York: McGraw-Hill.

Corey, L., Adams, H. G., Brown, Z. A., & Holmes, K. K. (1983). Genital herpes simplex infections: Clinical manifestations, course, and complications. *Annals of Internal Medicine, 98,* 958-972.

Droegemueller, W. D., Herbst, A. L., Mischell, D. R., & Stenehever, M. A. (1987). *Comprehensive gynecology.* St. Louis: C. V. Mosby.

Fitzpatrick, T. B., Polano, M. K., & Suurmond, D. (1983). *Color atlas and synopsis of clinical dermatology.* New York: McGraw-Hill.

Guerrant, R. L., & Ravdin, J. I. (1984). *Giardia lamblia* and *Entamoeba histolytica.* In K. K. Holmes, P. A. Mardh, P. F. Sparling, & P. J. Weisner (Eds.), *Sexually transmitted diseases* (pp. 537-556). New York: McGraw-Hill.

Habif, T. P. (1985). *Clinical dermatology: A color guide to diagnosis and therapy.* St. Louis: C. V. Mosby.

Handsfield, H. H. (1984). Gonorrhea and uncomplicated gonococcal infection. In K. K. Holmes, P. A. Mardh, P. F. Sparling, & P. J. Weisner (Eds.), *Sexually transmitted diseases* (pp. 205-219). New York: McGraw-Hill.

Hanshaw, J. B., Scheiner, A. P., Moxley, A. W., Goev, L., Abel, V., & Scheiner, B. (1976). School failure and deafness after "silent" congenital cytomegalovirus infection. *New England Journal of Medicine, 295,* 468-470.

Harrison, H. R., & Alexander, E. R. (1984). *Chlamydia trachomatis* infections of the infant. In K. K. Holmes, P. A. Mardh, P. F. Sparling, & P. J. Weisner (Eds.), *Sexually transmitted diseases* (pp. 270-280). New York: McGraw-Hill.

Hart, G. (1984). Donovanosis. In K. K. Holmes, P. A.

Mardh, P. F. Sparling, & P. J. Weisner (Eds.), *Sexually transmitted diseases* (pp. 393-396). New York: McGraw-Hill.

Hatcher, R. A., Guest, F., Stewart, F., Stewart, G. K., Trussell, J., Bowen, S. C., & Cates, W. (1988). *Contraceptive technology 1988-1989* (14th revised ed.). Atlanta, Ga.: Irvington.

Heggie, A. D., Lamicao, C. G., Stuart, L. A., & Gyves, M. T. (1981). *Chlamydia trachomatis* infections in mothers and infants. *American Journal of Diseases of Children, 135* (6), 507-511.

Holmes, K. K. (1984). Cystitis/urethritis. In K. K. Holmes, P. A. Mardh, P. F. Sparling, & P. J. Weisner (Eds.), *Sexually transmitted diseases.* New York: McGraw-Hill.

Kaufman, R. N., & Faro, S. (1985). Herpes genitalis: Clinical features and treatment. *Clinical Obstetrics & Gynecology, 28,* 156.

Klein, M. B. (1988). Hepatitis B virus: Perinatal management. *Journal of Perinatal and Neonatal Nursing, 1*(4), 12-23.

Knox, J. M., & Rudolph, A. H. (1984). Acquired infectious syphilis. In K. K. Holmes, P. A. Mardh, P. F. Sparling, & P. J. Weisner (Eds.), *Sexually transmitted diseases* (pp. 305-312). New York: McGraw-Hill.

Kraus, S. J. (1984). Genital ulcer adenopathy syndrome. In K. K. Holmes, P. A. Mardh, P. F. Sparling, & P. J. Weisner (Eds.), *Sexually transmitted diseases.* New York: McGraw-Hill.

Lambert, D. R., & Yoder, F. W. (1985). Ectoparasites and molluscum contagiosum. In V. A. Spagna, & R. B. Prior (Eds.), *Sexually transmitted diseases: A clinical syndrome approach* (pp. 333-356). New York: Marcel Dekker.

Lang, D. J. (1984). Cytomegalovirus infections. In K. K. Holmes, P. A. Mardh, P. F. Sparling, & P. J. Weisner (Eds.), *Sexually transmitted diseases* (pp. 474-478). New York: McGraw-Hill.

Lemon, S. M. (1984). Viral hepatitis. In K. K. Holmes, P. A. Mardh, P. F. Sparling, & P. J. Weisner (Eds.), *Sexually transmitted diseases* (pp. 479-495). New York: McGraw-Hill.

Lossick, J. G. (1985). Epidemiology of sexually transmitted diseases. In V. A. Spagna & R. B. Prior (Eds.), *Sexually transmitted diseases: A clinical syndrome approach* (pp. 21-62). New York: Marcel Dekker.

Marecki, M. A. (1988). *Chlamydia trachomatis:* A developing perinatal problem. *Journal of Perinatal & Neonatal Nursing, 1*(4), 1-11.

Maurice, J. (1983). Ubiquitous parasites: Chlamydia infections now commonest sexually transmitted disease. *International Health, 3,* 19-20.

McGee, Z. A. (1984). Gonococcal pelvic inflammatory disease. In K. K. Holmes, P. A. Mardh, P. F. Sparling, & P. J. Weisner (Eds.), *Sexually transmitted diseases* (pp. 220-228). New York: McGraw-Hill.

Mills, J., & Brooks, G. F. (1984). Disseminated gonococcal infection. In K. K. Holmes, P. A. Mardh, P. F. Sparling, & P. J. Weisner (Eds.), *Sexually transmitted diseases* (pp. 229-237). New York: McGraw-Hill.

Murphy, F. K., & Patamasucon, P. (1984). Congenital syphilis. In K. K. Holmes, P. A. Mardh, P. F. Sparling, & P. J.

Weisner (Eds.), *Sexually transmitted diseases* (pp. 352-373). New York: McGraw-Hill.

Musher, D. M. (1984). Biology of *Treponemia pallidum*. In K. K. Holmes, P. A. Mardh, P. F. Sparling, & P. J. Weisner (Eds.), *Sexually transmitted diseases* (pp. 291-297). New York: McGraw-Hill.

Oriel, J. D. (1984). Genital warts. In K. K. Holmes, P. A. Mardh, P. F. Sparling, & P. J. Weisner (Eds.), *Sexually transmitted diseases* (pp. 496-506). New York: McGraw-Hill.

Orkin, M., & Maibach, H. I. (1984). Scabies. In K. K. Holmes, P. A. Mardh, P. F. Sparling, & P. J. Weisner (Eds.), *Sexually transmitted diseases* (pp. 517-524). New York: McGraw-Hill.

Para, M. F., & Baird, I. M. (1985). Genital ulcer syndromes. In V. A. Spagna, & R. B. Prior (Eds.), *Sexually transmitted diseases: A clinical syndrome approach* (pp. 161-186). New York: Marcel Dekker.

Parra, W. C., Weisner, P. J., & Drotman, D. P. (1984). Patient counseling. In K. K. Holmes, P. A. Mardh, P. F. Sparling, & P. J. Weisner (Eds.), *Sexually transmitted diseases* (pp. 953-964). New York: McGraw-Hill.

Pelouze, P. S. (1941). *Gonorrhea in the male and female*. Philadelphia: Saunders.

Perine, P. L., & Osoba, A. O. (1984). Lymphogranuloma vereneum. In K. K. Holmes, P. A. Mardh, P. F. Sparling, & P. J. Weisner (Eds.), *Sexually transmitted diseases* (pp. 281-290). New York: McGraw-Hill.

Piot, P., & Vanderheyden, J. (1984). *Gardnerella vaginalis* and nonspecific vaginitis. In K. K. Holmes, P. A. Mardh, P. F. Sparling, & P. J. Weisner (Eds.), *Sexually transmitted diseases* (pp. 421-426). New York: McGraw-Hill.

Quinn, T. C., & Holmes, K. K. (1984). Proctitis proctocolitis, and enteritis in homosexual men. In K. K. Holmes, P. A. Mardh, P. F. Sparling, & P. J. Weisner (Eds.), *Sexually transmitted diseases* (pp. 672-690). New York: McGraw-Hill.

Rapp, F. (1984). Herpes simplex viruses. In K. K. Holmes, P. A. Mardh, P. F. Sparling, & P. J. Weisner (Eds.), *Sexually transmitted diseases* (pp. 438-448). New York: McGraw-Hill.

Rein, M. R., & Holmes, K. K. (1983). "Nonspecific vaginitis," vulvovaginal candidiasis, and trichomoniasis: Clinical features, diagnosis, and management. In J. Remington & M. N. Swartz (Eds.), *Current clinical topics in infectious diseases* (pp. 281-315). New York: McGraw-Hill.

Remington, J., & Swartz, M. N. (Eds.). (1983). *Current clinical topics in infectious diseases*. New York: McGraw-Hill.

Ronald, A. R., & Albritton, W. L. (1984). Chancroid and *Haemophilus ducreyi*. In K. K. Holmes, P. A. Mardh, P. F. Sparling, & P. J. Weisner (Eds.), *Sexually transmitted diseases* (pp. 385-392). New York: McGraw-Hill.

Schachter, J. (1984). Biology of *Chlamydia trachomatis*. In K. K. Holmes, P. A. Mardh, P. F. Sparling, & P. J. Weisner (Eds.), *Sexually transmitted diseases* (pp. 243-257). New York: McGraw-Hill.

Shaw, P., & Juranek, D. (1976). Recent trends in scabies in the United States. *Journal of Infectious Disease, 134,* 414-416.

Spagna, V. A. (1985). Urethritis syndromes. In V. A. Spagna & R. B. Prior (Eds.), *Sexually transmitted diseases: A clinical syndrome approach* (pp. 63-88). New York: Marcel Dekker.

Sparling, P. F. (1984). Natural history of syphilis. In K. K. Holmes, P. A. Mardh, P. F. Sparling, & P. J. Weisner (Eds.), *Sexually transmitted diseases* (pp. 298-304). New York: McGraw-Hill.

Stamm, W. E., & Holmes, K. K. (1984). *Chlamydia trachomatis* infections of the adult. In K. K. Holmes, P. A. Mardh, P. F. Sparling, & P. J. Weisner (Eds.), *Sexually transmitted diseases* (pp. 258-269). New York: McGraw-Hill.

Wehrle, P. F., & Top, F. H. (1981). *Communicable and infectious diseases* (9th ed.). St. Louis: C. V. Mosby.

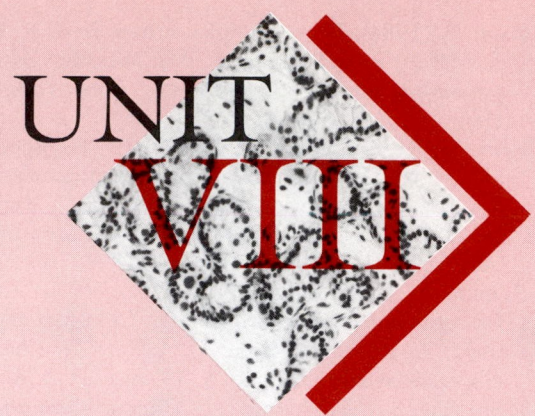

UNIT
VIII

The Hematologic System

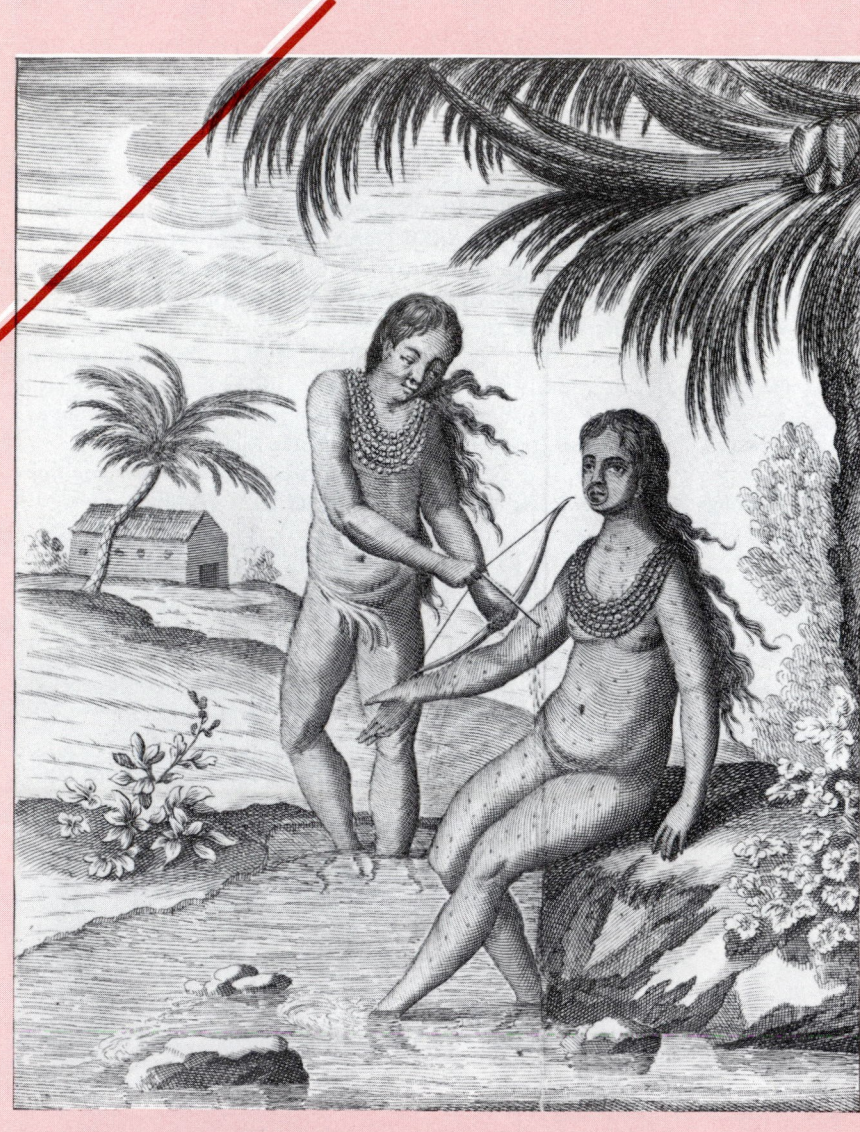

A female Indian sits on the bank of a stream, being bled with a bow and arrow by a male Indian. Many puncture points can be seen on her body. (From Wafer, L.: A new voyage and description of the Isthmus of America, London, 1699, Courtesy National Library of Medicine.)

THE idea that blood is a life force has intrigued people since ancient times. Healers in primitive cultures apparently recognized that without blood life ceased. Depictions of blood in relation to the heart are found in ancient drawings made in Paleolithic times (Breuil & Obermaier, 1935). The ancient Greeks also referred to the life-giving role of blood. In Greek mythology, Aesculapius, the son of Apollo and god of medicine, was given Gargon's blood from the goddess of wisdom, Athena. Aesculapius supposedly used this blood to raise the dead (Hart, 1980).

Early writing, painting, and sculpture refer to blood-related diseases. Expert paleopathologic analyses reveal that anemia is illustrated in certain Roman paintings and Greek vases showing women with varying degrees of pallor. Archaeological surveys of Egyptian mummies also reveal that blood diseases were indeed ancient maladies.

Anthony van Leeuwenhoek (1632-1723), a janitor from Holland, is given credit for the first description of erythrocytes (red blood cells). A rudimentary microscope enabled examination and measurement of the red corpuscles. Although van Leeuwenhoek may have seen the white blood cells, it was William Hewson (1739-1774) who first described them. Hewson is often called the "father of hematology."

Leukemia was simultaneously discovered by Rudolph Virchow in Berlin (leukamie) and by John Bennett in Edinburgh in 1845 (Wintrobe, 1980). Both investigators used autopsy findings to report their patient's symptoms and two important features: an enlarged spleen and a peculiar appearance of the blood with changes in both color and consistency. The question that was pursued for many years was why the colorless corpuscles were almost as numerous as the red corpuscles. Virchow made an important distinction that leukemia could be subdivided into two forms: one characterized by swelling of the spleen (splenic leukemia) and the other by swelling of the lymph nodes (lymphatic leukemia). Each form had its own dominant type of corpuscle. Although still observed, this distinction was further qualified in 1870 by Ernst Neumann, who suggested that in splenic leukemia the marrow, rather than the spleen, is the source of the excess corpuscles. This observation lead to the term *myeloid,* or marrow derived. The classifications of leukemia started in 1889 when A. Epstein introduced the term *acute.*

The first case of Hodgkin disease was reported by Thomas Hodgkin of Gay's Hospital in London in 1832. He had seven patients who were admitted to the hospital shortly before they died. They all had enlarged lymph nodes and some had an enlarged spleen. Hodgkin's observations were apparently ignored, because the condition was rediscovered in 1856 by Samuel Wilks, also of Gay's Hospital (Wintrobe, 1980). Later, when Wilks discovered that Hodgkin had already described the condition, he bestowed the name of Hodgkin's disease and gave a more complete account of the condition.

Paul Ehrlich's (1854-1915) development of a triacid stain, one of the most significant advances for hematology, enabled researchers to distinguish the cell's nucleus, cytoplasm, and other details. Leukocytes were discovered after the red corpuscles, probably because they are fewer in number and colorless, thus easily overlooked (Wintrobe, 1980). With Paul Ehrlich's discovery of the triacid stain (1877) and the improved microscope, he was the first to differentiate various types of white cells in the blood. Ehrlich's discovery dramatically changed the course of hematology (Wintrobe, 1980). Until that time, study of the blood was done with unstained, fresh material from the living animal. Ehrlich's techniques allowed fixation and, consequently, death of the cells— which for almost 50 years was the focus of attention rather than living cells. Ehrlich termed the many varieties of leukocytic granules "specific," meaning that each type of leukocyte had its own unique and specific cell constituents. He noted the process of degranulation in abscesses and specific conditions would elicit specific leukocytotic responses. For example, he observed eosinophilia with bronchial asthma, acute and chronic dermatitides, and malignant tumors (Wintrobe, 1980).

The modern era of hematology commenced in the 1920s, with the investigations of George Whipple, George Minot, and William Castle. These investigators promoted understanding of the pathogenesis of pernicious anemia and the role of certain foods, particularly liver, in promoting production of hemoglobin, the oxygen-carrying molecules of the blood (Wintrobe, 1980). It was during this time that hematology evolved into a quantitative science based on intricate observation and measurement. Methods of blood examination were developed, for example, measurement of the percentage of red cells in the blood (the hematocrit).

The study of leukocytes in terms of their numbers and function, kinetics, and biochemical behavior followed the study of anemia. The quantitative measurements of marrow compartments of neutrophils and their precursors were accomplished in 1958 using radioactive iron. Once neutrophil production became measurable, the humoral mechanisms of granulopoietic regulation were started.

By 1960, the shape and structure of the hemoglobin molecule were defined by the x-ray studies of Max Perutz. Since then, hematologists have made great progress in learning about abnormal hemoglobin disorders, anemias, the function of platelets and the process of coagulation, the white blood cell and its role in immunity, and effective treatments for many blood disorders.

CHAPTER 22

Structure and Function of the Hematologic System

Kathryn L. McCance
Pamela F. Cipriano

Components of the hematologic system, 755
  Composition of the blood, 755
    Plasma and plasma proteins, 755
    Cellular components of the blood, 757
        Erythrocytes, 757
        Leukocytes, 758
          Granulocytes, 758
          Agranulocytes, 760
        Platelets, 760
  Lymphoid organs, 760
    Spleen, 760
    Lymph nodes, 761
  The mononuclear phagocyte system (MPS), 761
Development of blood cells, 763
  Hematopoiesis, 763
    Stem cell system, 763
    Bone marrow, 764
  Development of erythrocytes, 764
    Hemoglobin synthesis, 765
    Nutritional requirements for erythropoiesis, 766
    Iron cycle, 767
    Regulation of erythropoiesis, 769
    Normal destruction of senescent erythrocytes, 769
  Development of leukocytes, 770
  Development of platelets, 771
Mechanisms of hemostasis, 771
  Function of platelets, 771
  Function of clotting factors, 772
  Control of hemostatic mechanisms, 773
  Retraction and lysis of blood clots, 776
Clinical evaluation of the hematologic system, 776
  Tests of bone marrow function, 776
  Blood tests, 777
Aging and the hematologic system, 780

COMPONENTS OF THE HEMATOLOGIC SYSTEM

Composition of the Blood

Blood consists of a variety of formed elements (cells and proteins) that circulate in the cardiovascular system suspended in plasma, which is about 90% water and 10% dissolved substances (solutes). All of these elements comprise blood volume, which in adults amounts to about 6 quarts (5.5 L). Approximately 45% to 50% of blood volume consists of formed elements, and the remainder is plasma. The continuous movement of blood keeps the formed elements dispersed throughout the plasma, where they are available to carry out their chief functions: (1) delivery of substances needed for cellular metabolism in the tissues and (2) defense against invading microorganisms and injury.

Plasma and Plasma Proteins

In adults, plasma accounts for 55% to 60% of blood volume. **Plasma** is a complex aqueous liquid containing a number of organic and inorganic elements Table 22-1). The concentration of these elements varies depending on diet, metabolic demand, hormones, and vitamins. Plasma differs from serum in that **serum** is plasma that has been altered in the laboratory so as to remove fibrinogen (a clotting factor) or some other element that is unwanted or unneeded in the sample.

In circulating plasma, the dominant elements by weight are the plasma proteins, which comprise about 7% of the total plasma weight. The **plasma proteins** vary in structure and function but can be classified into three major groups: the **albumins, globulins,** and **clotting factors.** The albumins are the most numerous, followed by the various globulins (immunoglobulins or

TABLE 22-1 Organic and inorganic components of arterial plasma

Constituent	Amount/concentration	Major functions
Water	93% of plasma weight	Medium for carrying all other constituents
Electrolytes	Total <1% of plasma weight	Kept H_2O in extracellular compartment; act as buffers; function in membrane excitability
Na^+	142 mEq/L (142 mM)	
K^+	4 mEq/L (4 mM)	
CA^{++}	5 mEq/L (2.5 mM)	
Mg^{++}	3 mEq/L (1.5 mM)	
CL^-	103 mEq/L (103 mM)	
HCO_3^-	27 mEq/L (27 mM)	
Phosphate (mostly HPO_4^{2-})	2 mEq/L (1 mM)	
SO_4^{2-}	1 mEq/L (0.5 mM)	
Proteins	7.3 g/dl (2.5 mM)	Provide colloid osmotic pressure of plasma; act as buffers; bind other plasma constituents (lipids, hormones, vitamins, metals, etc.); clotting factors; enzymes; enzyme precursors; antibodies (immune globulins); hormones
Albumins	4.5 g/dl	
Globulins	2.5 g/dl	
Fibrinogen	0.3 g/dl	
Gases		
CO_2 content	22-20 mmol/L plasma	By-product of oxygenation, most CO_2 content is from HCO_3 and acts as a buffer
O_2	Pao_2 80 torr or greater (arterial); Pvo_2 30-40 torr (venous)	Oxygenation
N_2	0.9 ml/dl	By-product of protein catabolism
Nutrients		Provide nutrition and substances for tissue repair
Glucose and other carbohydrates	100 mg/dl (5.6 mM)	
Total amino acids	40 mg/dl (2 mM)	
Total lipids	500 mg/dl (7.5 mM)	
Cholesterol	150-250 mg/dl (4-7 mM)	
Individual vitamins	0.0001-2.5 mg/dl	
Individual trace elements	0.001-0.3 mg/dl	
Waste products		
Urea (BUN)	7-18 mg/dl (5.7 mM)	End product of protein catabolism
Creatinine	1 mg/dl (0.09 mM)	End product from energy metabolism
Uric acid	5 mg/dl (0.3 mM)	End product of protein metabolism
Bilirubin	0.2-1.2 mg/dl (0.003-0.018 mM)	End product of red blood cell destruction
Individual hormones	0.000001-0.05 mg/dl	Functions specific to target tissue

From Vander, Sherman & Luciano, 1980.

gamma globulins), and the clotting factors, chiefly fibrinogen. The plasma proteins are synthesized in the liver with the exception of the immunoglobulins, which are synthesized by lymphocytes in the lymph nodes and other lymphoid tissues (see Chapter 6 and p. 760).

Albumin is present at a concentration of about 4 g/dl and is essential for regulating the passage of water and solutes through the capillaries. Since albumin molecules are large and do not diffuse freely through the vascular endothelium, they provide the critical colloid osmotic or oncotic pressure that regulates the passage of water and solutes through the microcirculation (arterioles, capillaries, and venules) (Berne & Levy, 1988) (see Chapters 1 and 3). Water and solute particles diffuse out of the arterial portions of the capillaries because blood pressure is greater in arterial than in venous blood vessels (see Chapter 29). Water and solutes move from tissue cells into the venous portions of the capillaries, where the pressures are reversed, oncotic pressure being greater than intravascular pressure. Albumin also serves as a carrier molecule for both normal components of blood and exogenous agents, such as drugs.

TABLE 22-2 Cellular components of the blood

Cell	Structural characteristics	Normal amounts in circulating blood	Function	Life span
Erythrocyte (red blood cell)	Nonnucleated cytoplasmic disk containing hemoglobin	4.2-6.2 million/mm³	Gas transport to and from tissue cells and lungs	80-120 days
Leukocyte (white blood cell)	Nucleated cell	5000-10,000/mm³	Bodily defense mechanisms	See below
Lymphocyte	Mononuclear immunocyte	25% to 33% of leukocyte count (leukocyte differential)	Humoral and cell-mediated immunity (see Chapter 6)	Days or years depending on type
Monocyte and macrophage	Large mononuclear phagocyte	3% to 7% of leukocyte differential	Phagocytosis; mononuclear phagocyte system	Months or years
Eosinophil	Segmented polymorphonuclear granulocyte	1% to 4% of leukocyte differential	Phagocytosis, antibody-mediated defense against parasites, allergic reactions, associated with Hodgkin disease, recovery phase of infection	Unknown
Neutrophil	Segmented polymorphonuclear granulocyte	57% to 67% of leukocyte differential	Phagocytosis, particularly during early phase of inflammation	4 days
Basophil	Segmented polymorphonuclear granulocyte	0% to 0.75% of leukocyte differential	Unknown, but associated with allergic reactions and mechanical irritation	Unknown
Platelet	Irregularly shaped cytoplasmic fragment (not a cell)	140,000 to 340,000/mm³	Hemostasis following vascular injury; normal coagulation and clot formation/retraction	8 to 11 days

The immunoglobulins, or antibodies, are synthesized by mature lymphocytes called plasma cells in the lymphoid organs, chiefly lymph nodes. The immunoglobulins include IgA, IgG, IgM, IgD, and IgE. Most of them are critical for defense against infectious microorganisms. (Lymphocyte and antibody function is described in Chapter 6.)

The third important class of plasma proteins is the clotting factors, which stop bleeding from damaged blood vessels. Fibrinogen is the most plentiful of the clotting factors and is the precursor of the fibrin clot (see p. 772). Other plasma proteins include complement proteins, a group of proteins involved in the immune response, a variety of enzymes and their inhibitors, and specific carriers of such elements as iron and copper. The plasma lipids, triglycerides, phospholipids, cholesterol, and fatty acids are carried through the blood as complexes with plasma proteins; they are known as **lipoproteins** (see Chapters 1 and 27).

The electrolytes (electrically charged solutes) of the plasma maintain the osmolarity and pH of blood within a physiologic range (see Table 22-1). (Electrolytes are described in Chapters 1 and 3.)

Cellular Components of the Blood

The cellular elements of the blood are broadly classified as **erythrocytes** (red blood cells), **leukocytes** (white blood cells), and **platelets** (thrombocytes). The components of the blood are listed in Table 22-2.

Erythrocytes

In 1628 Robert Burton described blood as a "hot, temperate red humor whose office is to nourish the whole body, to give it strength and color being dispersed by the veins through every part of it" (Babior & Stossel, 1984). A few years later, with the invention of the microscope, researchers learned that erythrocytes give blood its red color.

Erythrocytes are the most abundant cells of the blood, occupying about 48% of the blood volume in men and about 42% in women. Erythrocytes are primarily responsible for tissue oxygenation. Their shape, size, and structure reflect their unique function as deliverers of gases throughout the body. The erythrocyte's cytoplasm consists of a solution containing protein (mostly **hemoglobin [Hb]**, which carries the gases) and electrolytes, which regulate diffusion through the cell's plasma membrane. The mature erythrocyte lacks the cytoplasmic organelles—a nucleus, mitochondria, and ribosomes—that would enable it to divide or carry out metabolic functions. Therefore it cannot synthesize protein or carry out oxidative reactions. Because it cannot undergo mitotic division, it lives out its life span (about 120 days) in the circulation, dies, and is replaced by a new erythrocyte.

The erythrocyte's size and shape are ideally suited to its function as a gas carrier. It is a small disk with two unique properties: (1) **biconcavity** and (2) **reversible deformability** (Fig. 22-1). The flattened, biconcave shape provides a surface area/volume ratio that is optimal for gas diffusion into and out of the cell. Reversible deformity enables the erythrocyte to alter its shape to squeeze through the microcirculation and then return to normal. During its 120-day life span, the erythrocyte, which is 8 μm in diameter, must repeatedly circulate through splenic sinusoids (see p. 760) and capillaries that are only 2 μm in diameter. To do this, the erythrocyte assumes the torpedo like conformation.

Several hypotheses attempt to explain how the erythrocyte's resting biconcave shape is maintained. Sakagami, Minari, and Orii (1965) proposed that the convex portion of the cell's plasma membrane may have a higher concentration of cholesterol than the concave portion and that the cholesterol molecules may serve as a wedge, bending the membrane into the biconcave shape. (See Chapter 1 for a discussion of plasma membrane structure.) Other investigators have suggested that biconcavity is maintained by the interaction of elastic or electrical forces, surface tension, and colloid osmotic pressure (Lopez, Duck, & Hung, 1968). Whatever the mechanism, maintenance of erythrocyte shape apparently depends on both internal and external factors.

Leukocytes

Leukocytes are white blood cells that defend the body against organisms that cause infection and remove debris, including dead or injured host cells of all kinds (Fig. 22-2). The leukocytes act primarily in the tissues but are transported in the circulation. They are fewer in number than erythrocytes; the average adult has approximately 5000 to 10000 leukocytes/mm³ of blood.

Leukocytes are classified according to structure as either **granulocytes** or **agranulocytes** and according to function as either **phagocytes** or **immunocytes.** The granulocytes, which include neutrophils, basophils, and eosinophils, are all phagocytes. (Phagocytic action is described in Chapter 7.) Of the agranulocytes, the monocytes and macrophages are phagocytes, whereas the lymphocytes are immunocytes (cells that create immunity; see Chapter 6).

Granulocytes The granulocytes are so called because of the many membrane-bounded granules in their cytoplasm. The granules contain enzymes capable of killing microorganisms and catabolizing debris ingested by the process of phagocytosis. The granules also contain pow-

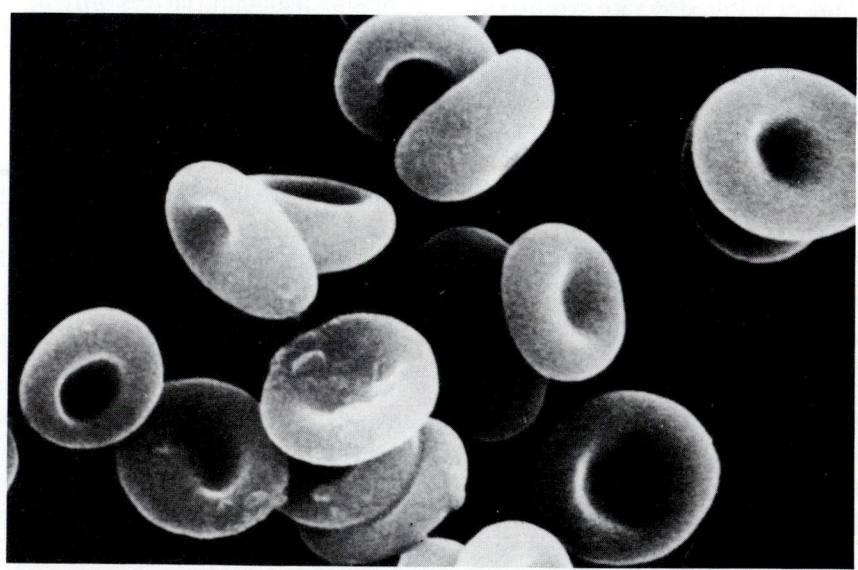

FIG. 22-1. Scanning electron micrograph of mature erythrocytes (×3000). (From Thibodeau, 1987.)

erful biochemical mediators with a variety of inflammatory and immune functions. These mediators, along with the digestive enzymes, are released from some granulocytes in response to specific stimuli and from all granulocytes as they reach the end of their natural life span and die. The biochemical mediators have various vascular and intercellular effects, and the enzymes participate in the breakdown of free-floating debris from sites of infection or injury.

Granulocytes are capable of ameboid movement, by which they migrate through vessel walls and then to sites where their action is needed. Migration through vessel walls, called diapedesis, and movement through the tissues, which occurs in response to chemotactic factors, are described and illustrated in Chapter 7.

The **neutrophil** (polymorphonuclear neutrophil, or PMN) is the most numerous and best understood of the granulocytes (Fig. 22-3). Neutrophils comprise about 55% of the total leukocyte count in adults. The cytoplasm of neutrophils contains small lysosomal granules and a central nucleus with two to five distinct lobes. Immature neutrophils are called bands or stabs. Mature neutrophils are called segmented neutrophils because of the characteristic appearance of their nucleus.

Neutrophils are the chief phagocytes of early inflammation. Soon after bacterial invasion or tissue injury, neutrophils migrate out of the capillaries and into the inflamed site, where they ingest and destroy microorganisms and debris, then die in a day or two. The dissolution of dead neutrophils releases digestive enzymes

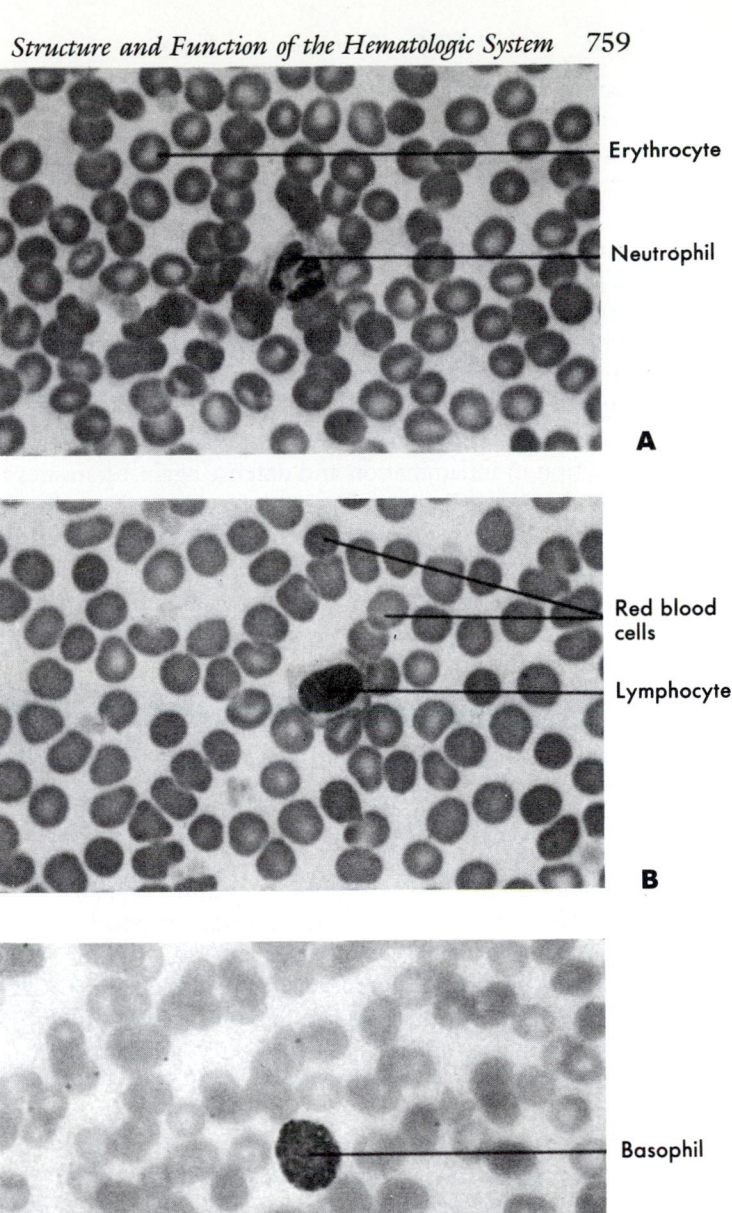

A — Erythrocyte, Neutrophil

B — Red blood cells, Lymphocyte

C — Basophil

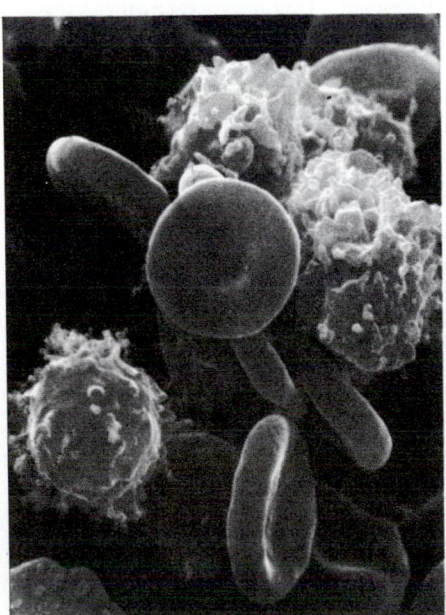

FIG. 22-2. Blood cells. Leukocytes are spherical and have irregular surfaces with numerous extending pili. Erythrocytes are flattened spheres with a depressed center. (From Raven & Johnson, 1989.)

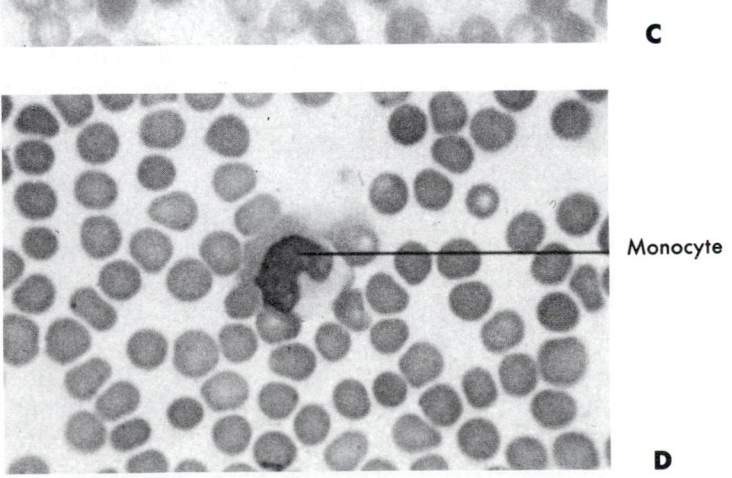

D — Monocyte

FIG. 22-3. Some leukocytes in human blood smear: (*a*) neutrophil, (*b*) lymphocyte, (*c*) basophil, (*d*) monocyte. (From Thibodeau, 1987.)

from their cytoplasmic granules. These enzymes dissolve cellular debris and prepare the site for healing. (This final function, called debridement, is described in Chapter 7.)

Eosinophils, which have large, coarse granules, comprise only 1% to 4% of the normal leukocyte count in adults. Like neutrophils, eosinophils are capable of ameboid movement and phagocytosis. Unlike neutrophils, which ingest cellular debris, eosinophils ingest antigen-antibody complexes and are induced by IgE-mediated hypersensitivity reactions to attack parasites. Eosinophils also help to control inflammatory processes. (Their function in inflammation and defense against parasites is described in Chapter 7.) High eosinophil counts in atopic (allergy-prone) individuals experiencing type I allergic reactions, such as asthma or allergic rhinitis, have led researchers to think that eosinophils participate in hypersensitivity reactions to allergens besides parasites (see Chapter 8).

Basophils, which make up less than 1% of the leukocytes, are structurally similar to the mast cells found throughout extravascular tissue. Like the mast cells, whose role in stimulating the inflammatory response is described in Chapter 7, the basophils have cytoplasmic granules that contain vasoactive amines (histamine, bradykinin, and serotonin) and an anticoagulant (heparin). The precise function of basophils is poorly understood.

Agranulocytes The agranulocytes—monocytes, macrophages, and lymphocytes—differ from the granulocytes in that they do not contain lysosomal granules in their cytoplasm. The lymphocytes do not contain *any* enzyme-filled digestive vacuoles, and the digestive vacuoles of the monocytes and macrophages are larger and fewer than those of the granulocytes.

The **monocytes** and **macrophages** make up the **mononuclear phagocyte system (MPS),** formerly called the reticuloendothelial system (RES). (The MPS is described on p. 761.) Both monocytes and macrophages participate in the immune and inflammatory response, being powerful phagocytes. They also ingest dead or defective host cells, particularly blood cells.

Monocytes are immature macrophages. After monocytes are formed and released by the bone marrow, they enter the bloodstream and circulate for about 36 hours while maturing into macrophages. Some of the circulating macrophages migrate out of the vessels in response to infection or inflammation anywhere in the body. Other macrophages migrate to fixed sites in lymphoid tissues of the liver, spleen, lymph nodes, peritoneum, or gastrointestinal tract where they are active for months or years.

Lymphocytes, which comprise approximately 36% of the total leukocyte count, are the primary cells of the immune response. Most lymphocytes are located in lymphoid tissues; only a small percent circulate in the blood. There are many types of lymphocytes, the most important of which are T cells, B cells, and mature B cells (plasma cells). The life span of the lymphocyte can be days, months, or years, depending on its type and subtype. (Lymphocyte function and dysfunction are described in detail in Unit 3.)

Platelets

Platelets are not cells, but disk-shaped cytoplasmic fragments. Platelets are essential for blood coagulation and control of bleeding. They lack a nucleus; therefore they have no DNA and are incapable of mitotic division. They do, however, contain cytoplasmic granules capable of releasing biochemical mediators when stimulated to do so by injury to a blood vessel.

There are about 150,000 to 400,000 platelets/mm^3 of circulating blood. An additional one third of the body's available platelets are in a reserve pool in the spleen. A platelet lives approximately 10 days, after which time it dies and is removed by macrophages of the MPS, mostly in the spleen.

Lymphoid Organs

The lymphoid organs, some of which are merely aggregations of lymphoid tissue, are classified as primary or secondary. The **primary lymphoid organs** are the thymus and the bone marrow. The **secondary lymphoid organs** consist of the spleen, lymph nodes, tonsils, and Peyer's patches of the small intestine (see Fig. 6-4). All of the lymphoid organs link the hematologic and immune systems in that they are sites of residence, proliferation, differentiation, or function of lymphocytes and mononuclear phagocytes (monocytes and macrophages). (The liver, which also has hematologic functions, is primarily a digestive organ and is described in Chapter 35.)

Spleen

The **spleen** is the largest of the secondary lymphoid organs. It is a site of fetal hematopoiesis, its mononuclear phagocytes filter and cleanse the blood, its lymphocytes mount an immune response to blood-borne microorganisms, and it serves as a blood reservoir (see Chapter 24).

The spleen is a concave, encapsulated organ that weighs about 150 g and is about the size of a fist (see Chapter 6; Fig. 6-4). It is located in the upper abdominal cavity, curved around a portion of the stomach. Strands of connective tissue (trabeculae) extend throughout the spleen from the splenic capsule, dividing the spleen into compartments. The compartments contain masses of lymphoid tissue called splenic pulp. The spleen is interlaced with many blood vessels, some of which are capable of distending to store blood.

Blood that circulates through the spleen comes from the splenic artery, which branches from the descending aorta and reenters the circulatory system through the splenic vein, which feeds into the portal vein. The portion of arterial blood that enters the spleen first encounters the white splenic pulp, which consists of masses of lymphoid tissue containing lymphocytes and macrophages. The white pulp forms clumps around the splenic arterioles and is the chief site of immune and phagocytic function within the spleen. Here blood-borne antigens encounter lymphocytes, initiating the immune response (see Chapter 6).

Some of the blood that enters the terminal capillaries of the spleen continues through the microcirculation and enters highly distensible storage areas called venous sinuses. Most of the blood, however, oozes through the extremely permeable capillary walls into the principal site of splenic filtration, the red pulp. Here the resident macrophages of the MPS phagocytose old, damaged, or dead blood cells of all kinds (but chiefly erythrocytes), microorganisms, and particles of debris. Hemoglobin from phagocytosed erythrocytes is catabolized, and heme (iron) is stored in the cytoplasm of the macrophages or released back into the blood plasma (see p. 767 and Fig. 22-8). The macrophages can also remove certain particulate inclusions from erythrocytes without harming the cells themselves. Blood that filters through the red pulp also finds its way into the venous sinuses and hence into the portal circulation.

The venous sinuses (and the red pulp) are capable of storing more than 300 ml of blood. Passive dilation of the venous sinuses enables the spleen to increase its storage capacity as needed by the body. Sudden reductions in blood pressure cause the sympathetic nervous system to stimulate constriction of the sinuses. Constriction, which can expel as much as 200 ml of blood into the venous circulation, helps to restore blood volume or pressure in the circulation and can also increase the hematocrit by as much as 4% (Guyton, 1987).

The spleen is not necessary for life or for adequate hematologic function. Splenic absence from any cause, however, whether it be atrophy, traumatic injury, or removal because of disease, has several effects that indicate its function. For example, leukocytosis (high levels of circulating leukocytes) often occurs after splenectomy. This suggests that the spleen exerts some control over the rate of proliferation of leukocyte stem cells in the bone marrow or their release into the bloodstream. Splenic absence is also associated with decreased levels of iron in the circulation, reflecting the spleen's role in the iron cycle (see p. 767). Immune function decreases in the absence of the spleen. Antibody production in response to small doses of soluble (i.e., blood-borne) antigen diminishes. Finally, the splenic function of removing old and defective blood cells seems to be confirmed by the fact that the blood of individuals lacking spleens contains more morphologically defective blood cells than normal.

Lymph Nodes

Structurally, **lymph nodes** are part of the lymphatic system. Thousands of them are clustered around the lymphatic veins, the vessels that collect interstitial fluid from the tissues and transport it, as lymph, back into the circulatory system near the heart. Functionally, however, lymph nodes are part of the hematologic and immune systems because they are the site of development or activity of large numbers of lymphocytes, monocytes, and macrophages. As the lymph filters through the bean-shaped lymph nodes clustered in the inguinal, axillary, and cervical regions of the body, it is cleansed of foreign particles and microorganisms by the monocytes and macrophages. The microorganisms in lymph stimulate the resident lymphocytes to develop into antibody-producing plasma cells (see Chapter 6). Lymphocytes, monocytes, and macrophages proliferate in the lymph nodes and are released into the lymphatic stream. During an infection, the rate of proliferation of macrophages within the nodes is so great that the nodes enlarge and become tender.

Each lymph node is enclosed in a fibrous capsule (Fig. 22-4). Strands of connective tissue (trabeculae) extend inward from the capsule, dividing the node into several compartments. Reticular fibers that extend between the trabeculae divide the compartments into smaller sections. The reticular fibers trap and store large numbers of lymphocytes, monocytes, and macrophages. The node is composed of an outer cortex area and an inner medullary area. Within the cortex of each node are germinal centers, or separate masses of lymphoid tissue. Lymph enters the node through several afferent lymphatic vessels, filters through the sinuses in the node, and leaves by way of efferent lymphatic vessels. Lymph flows slowly through the nodes, which facilitates the phagocytosis of foreign substances within the node and prevents them from reentering the bloodstream.

The Mononuclear Phagocyte System (MPS)

The MPS consists of a line of cells originating in the bone marrow, being transported by the bloodstream, and localizing in the tissues (Lasser, 1983). It is composed of monoblasts, promonocytes, and monocytes in bone marrow, monocytes in peripheral blood, and macrophages in tissue (Lasser, 1983; Robbins, Cotran, & Kumar, 1984). Table 22-3 lists the various names given to macrophages localized in specific tissues.

The cells of the MPS ingest and destroy (by phagocytosis) unwanted materials in the blood and in organs. During inflammation, they engulf and digest foreign protein particles, microorganisms, debris from dead or

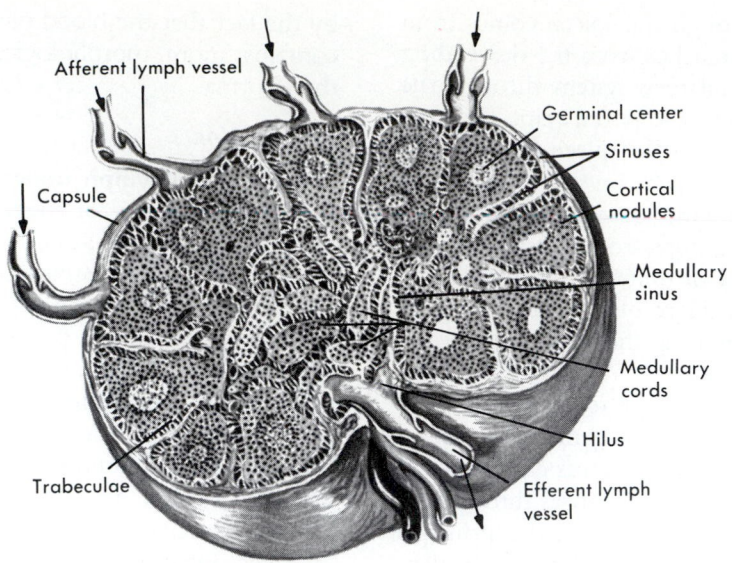

FIG. 22-4. Cross-section of lymph node. Several afferent valved lymphatics bring lymph to node. Efferent lymphatics leave node at the hilus. Blood vessels enter and leave at the hilus. (From Thibodeau, 1987.)

TABLE 22-3 Mononuclear phagocyte system (reticuloendothelial system)

Name of cell	Location
Committed stem cells*	Bone marrow
Monoblasts	Bone marrow
Promonoblasts	Bone marrow
Monocytes	Bone marrow and peripheral blood
Macrophages	Tissue
Kupffer cells (inflammatory macrophages)	Liver
Alveolar macrophages	Lung
Histiocytes	Connective tissue
Macrophages	Bone marrow
Fixed and free macrophages	Spleen and lymph nodes
Pleural and peritoneal macrophages	Serous cavities
Microglial cells	Nervous system
Osteoclasts	Bone
Langerhan's cells	Skin
Dendritic cells	Lymphoid tissue

*Development of blood cells from stem cells in the marrow is described on p. 763, and illustrated in Fig. 22-5.
From Robbins, Cotran, & Kumar, 1984.

injured cells, defective or injured erythrocytes, and dead neutrophils (see Fig. 7-15). The MPS (mostly in the liver and spleen) also is the main line of defense against bacteria in the bloodstream. In addition, the MPS cleanses the blood by removing old, injured, or dead erythrocytes, leukocytes, platelets, coagulation products, antigen-antibody complexes, and macromolecules, such as lipids and carbohydrates synthesized by the body as the result of faulty metabolism (as in storage diseases). Macrophages also play a role in blood coagulation, wound healing, tissue remodeling, and the control of blood production.

Monocytes and macrophages secrete a substance called colony-stimulating factor (CSF), which is necessary for the formation and growth of colonies of granulocytes and macrophages in the bone marrow (Burgess & Metcalf, 1980; Fitchen, Foon, & Cline, 1981; Metcalf, Johnson, & Burgess, 1980). Prostaglandin E, which is also secreted by macrophages, inhibits colony-forming cells, particularly those committed to monocytic differentiation (Williams, 1979). Macrophages may indirectly regulate erythrocyte differentiation because they have been reported to produce a substance **(erythropoietin)** that stimulates erythrocyte production in bone marrow (Peschle et al., 1976; Rich & Kubanek, 1982).

The origin and turnover of all the tissue macrophages named in Table 22-3 are not precisely known. It seems clear that once monocytes leave the circulation, they do not return. In the tissues, monocytes differentiate into macrophages without dividing. They can survive many months or perhaps even years (Shand & Bell, 1972). Under normal circumstances, macrophages show little evidence of mitotic division, but under certain stimulating conditions some may proliferate (Lasser, 1983). For example, alveolar macrophages and, to some degree, liver macrophages (Kupffer cells) may arise from local proliferation (Diesselhoff-den Dulk, Crofton, & Van Furth, 1979). Most of the macrophages that migrate to sites of inflammation develop from circulating monocytes (Robbins et al., 1984).

DEVELOPMENT OF BLOOD CELLS

Hematopoiesis

Blood cell production, termed **hematopoiesis,** occurs in the liver and spleen of the fetus, but after birth it normally occurs only in bone marrow (see Chapter 28). Blood cell production in bone marrow is known as medullary hematopoiesis. It is still a mystery why hematopoiesis is restricted to bone marrow after birth. Two explanations are possible: (1) some factor that enhances blood cell development is only present in marrow or (2) some factor that inhibits development is present in organs other than marrow. To date, neither factor has been identified (Wintrobe et al., 1981).

Hematopoiesis is a two-stage process that involves mitotic division, or **proliferation,** and maturation, or **differentiation.** Each type of blood cell has parent cells, called **stem cells,** that undergo mitosis when they receive specific biochemical signals indicating that populations of circulating blood cells have diminished to a certain point. The stem cells continue to proliferate until the requisite number of mature daughter cells has entered the circulation. The stem cells of lymphocytes and possibly monocytes are stimulated to proliferate and differentiate by other mechanisms, particularly activation of the immune response, but they, too, originate in bone marrow.

Certain blood cells proliferate and differentiate simultaneously for a period. Proliferation usually ceases after a number of doubling divisions, but differentiation continues. Erythrocytes and neutrophils are usually mature before entering the blood. Monocytes and other leukocytes are not. They enter the bloodstream and continue to mature as they travel to the spleen, peritoneal cavity, and lung.

Hematopoiesis continues throughout life to replace blood cells that grow old and die, are killed by disease, or are lost through bleeding. Medullary hematopoiesis increases in response to proliferative disease, hemorrhage, hemolytic anemia (in which erythrocytes are destroyed), chronic infection, idiopathic thrombocy-topenic purpura (bleeding caused by platelet insufficiency, see Chapter 28), and other disorders that deplete blood cells. In general, long-term stimuli, such as chronic diseases, cause a greater increase in hematopoiesis than acute conditions, such as hemorrhage. Abnormal proliferation of erythrocytes occurs in polycythemia vera, a myeloproliferative disease.

Medullary hematopoiesis can be accelerated by any or all of three mechanisms: (1) conversion of yellow bone marrow, which does not produce blood cells, to red marrow, which does; (2) faster differentiation of daughter cells; and presumably (3) faster proliferation of stem cells. Marrow conversion is stimulated by erythropoietin, the hormone that stimulates erythrocyte production (Maniatis, Tavassoli, & Crosby, 1971). Another possible stimulus to conversion is increase in body temperature (Wintrobe et al., 1981).

In adults, extramedullary hematopoiesis—blood cell production in tissues other than bone marrow—is usually a sign of disease. Extramedullary production of one or more types occurs in disease states that affect erythrocytes (e.g., pernicious anemia, sickle cell anemia, thalassemia, hemolytic disease of the newborn [erythroblastosis fetalis], hereditary spherocytosis), and leukocytes (certain leukemias). Extramedullary hematopoiesis of apparently normal blood cells has also been reported to occur in the spleen and liver and, less frequently, in lymph nodes, adrenal glands, cartilage, adipose tissue, intrathoracic areas, and kidneys (Wintrobe et al., 1981).

Stem Cell System

The processes by which blood cells develop from a common ancestor, or stem cell, are known collectively as the **stem cell system.** This system is a hierarchy in which the earliest, most primitive ancestor is the **totipotential hematopoietic stem cell (THSC)** (Fig. 22-5). Because these cells have the potential to develop into many types of blood cells, they are also called multipotential stem cells. One pathway of development leads to various lymphoid tissues, where T and B lymphocytes mature. The other pathway leads to myeloid tissue—the bone marrow. The stem cell of the myeloid pathway is called the pluripotential myeloid stem cell (MPSC), or simply the **pluripotential stem cell.** The pluripotential stem cell triggers differentiation of (1) neutrophils and monocytes, (2) eosinophils, (3) erythrocytes, and (4) platelets (Fig. 22-5).

The exact mechanisms governing stem cell proliferation and differentiation are not all known. Apparently, humoral factors (hormones, such as erythropoietin, thrombopoietin, or granulopoietin) stimulate stem cells to divide in response to either reduced amounts of hematopoietic (blood-cell-producing) bone marrow or an increased need for mature blood cells in the circulation.

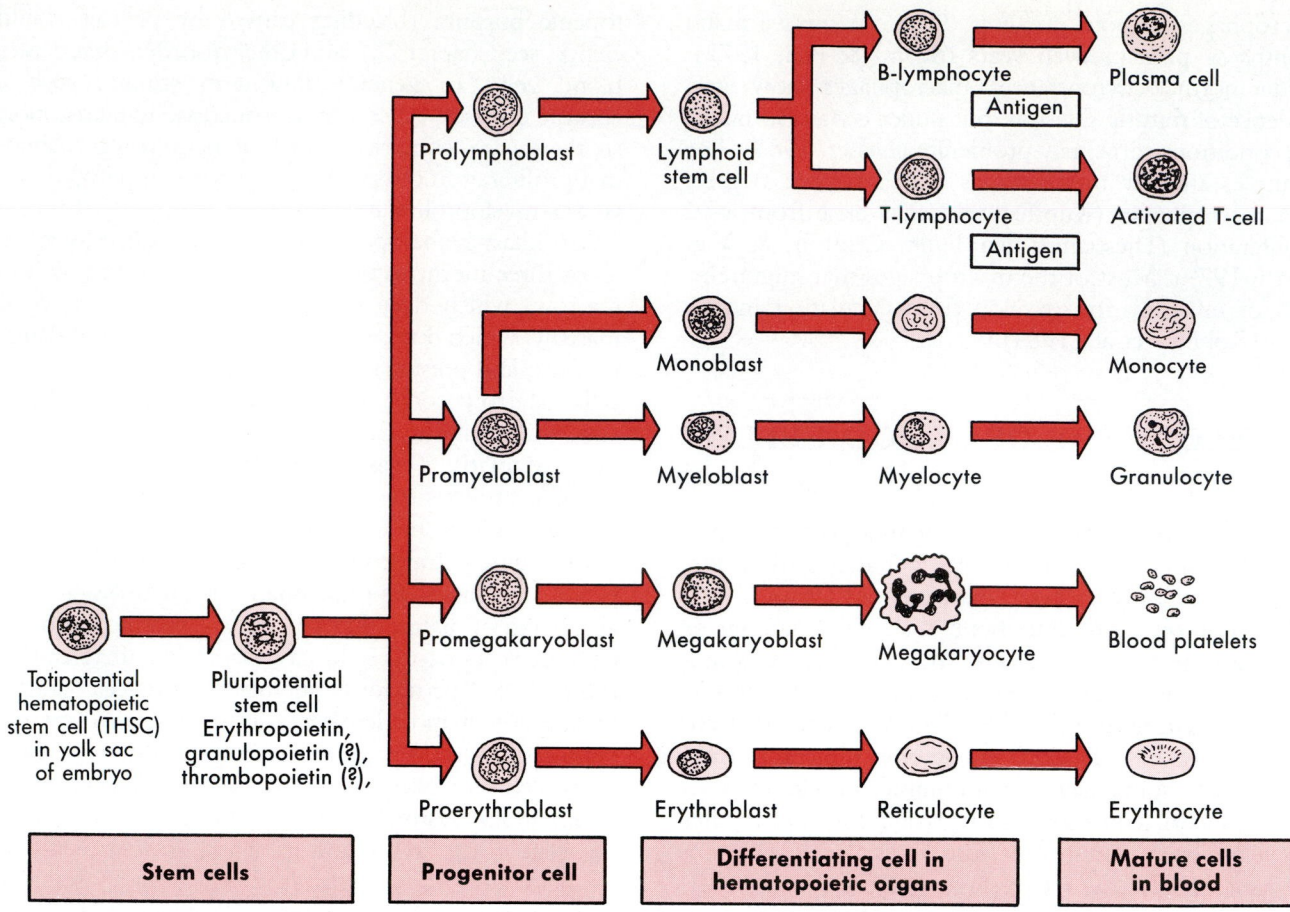

FIG. 22-5. Probable pathways of blood cell differentiation, from the totipotential hematopoietic stem cell to mature blood cells or platelets. (Adapted from Purtilo, 1978.)

Bone Marrow

Bone marrow, also called myeloid tissue (*myelos* = marrow), is confined to the cavities of bone. Bone marrow consists of blood vessels, nerves, mononuclear phagocytes, stem cells, blood cells in various stages of differentiation, and fatty tissue. Adults have two kinds of bone marrow: red, or active (hematopoietic), marrow and yellow, or inactive, marrow. The large quantities of fat in inactive marrow make it yellow. Not all bones contain active marrow. In adults there is active marrow in the pelvic bones (34%), vertebrae (28%), cranium and mandible (13%), sternum and ribs (10%), and extreme proximal portions of the humerus and femur (4% to 8%) (Russell et al., 1966). Inactive marrow predominates in cavities of other bones. (Bones are discussed further in Chapter 38.)

Stem cells in hematopoietic marrow receive the oxygen and nutrients they need for mitosis and maturation from the primary or nutrient arteries of the bones. Branches of these arteries terminate in a capillary net-

work that coalesces into large venous sinuses, which eventually drain into a central vein. Hematopoietic marrow and fat fill the spaces surrounding the network of venous sinuses. Some mechanism of transport enables the newly produced blood cells to traverse narrow openings in venous sinus walls and thus enter the circulation. It is not known whether the movement of the new blood cells forces an opening or whether certain sites open in response to the presence of the newly formed cells. Normally, cells do not enter the circulation until they have differentiated to a certain extent, but premature release is known to occur in certain diseases.

Development of Erythrocytes

For almost 100 years, it was believed that erythrocytes developed from lymphocytes that were transformed in the spleen. It was not until the 1850s that the bone marrow was accepted as the site of **erythropoiesis** (Wintrobe et al., 1981). It is now known that erythrocytes are derived from precursor cells called **erythro-**

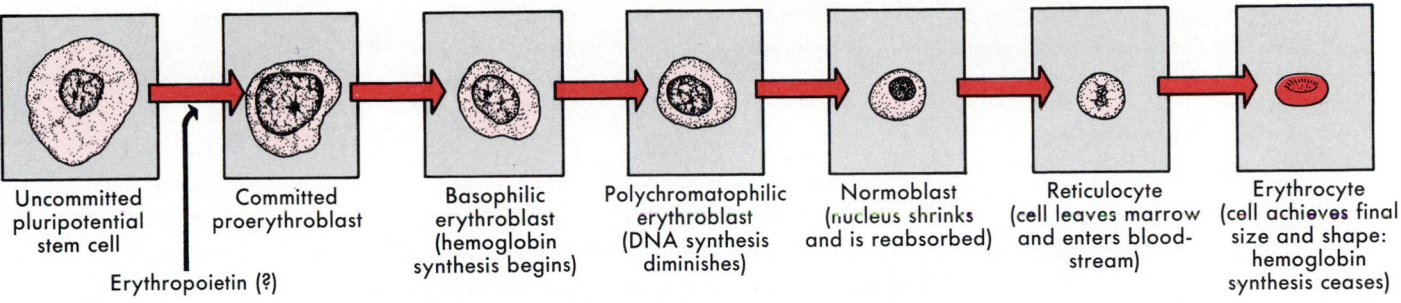

| Uncommitted pluripotential stem cell | Committed proerythroblast | Basophilic erythroblast (hemoglobin synthesis begins) | Polychromatophilic erythroblast (DNA synthesis diminishes) | Normoblast (nucleus shrinks and is reabsorbed) | Reticulocyte (cell leaves marrow and enters blood-stream) | Erythrocyte (cell achieves final size and shape: hemoglobin synthesis ceases) |

Erythropoietin (?)

FIG. 22-6. Erythrocyte differentiation from large, nucleated stem cell to small, nonnucleated erythrocyte.

blasts (see Fig. 22-6). Normal erythroblasts are also called **normoblasts,** whereas abnormal ones are called **megaloblasts.**

Erythrocyte development is shown in detail in Fig. 22-6. The proerythroblast (pronormoblast) possesses a huge nucleus, is rich in ribosomes, and can synthesize protein. Research suggests that the hormone erythropoietin stimulates uncommitted stem cells to differentiate into proerythroblasts (Wintrobe et al., 1981). Whether hemoglobin has been synthesized at this stage is controversial. Hemoglobin is, however, readily apparent and increases in quantity as nuclear size shrinks throughout the basophilic and polychromatophilic stages. The orthochromatic erythroblast (normoblast) is the smallest of the nucleated erythrocyte precursors. Once the nucleus is lost, the cell that remains is called a **reticulocyte.** Although it lacks a nucleus, the reticulocyte contains polyribosomes (for globin synthesis) and mitochondria (for oxidative metabolism and heme synthesis). The reticulocyte matures to an erythrocyte within 24 to 48 hours. During this period, mitochondria and ribosomes disappear, and the cell becomes smaller and more disklike. With these final changes, the erythrocyte loses its capacity for hemoglobin synthesis and oxidative metabolism.

Reticulocytes remain in the marrow approximately 1 day and are then released into the venous sinuses before maturation is complete. Reticulocytes continue to mature in the bloodstream and may travel to the spleen for several days of additional maturation. The normal reticulocyte count is 1% of the total red blood cell count. Approximately 1% of the body's circulating erythrocyte mass normally is generated every 24 hours. Therefore the reticulocyte count is a useful clinical index of erythropoietic activity and will indicate whether or not new red cells are being produced. The concept "erythron" has been used to describe all the tissues that produce erythrocytes and their precursors. Thus included in this term are stem cells, all stages of developing erythrocytes, and mature red blood cells.

Hemoglobin Synthesis

Hemoglobin, the oxygen-carrying protein of the erythrocyte, comprises about 90% of the cell's dry weight. The cytoplasm of a single erythrocyte can contain as much as 300 hemoglobin molecules. Hemoglobin enables the blood to transport 100 times more oxygen than could be transported dissolved in plasma alone. Hemoglobin is not one but a family of molecules whose members differ slightly in primary structure. Nonetheless, each member is composed of two pairs of polypeptide chains (the **globins**) and four colorful complexes of iron plus protoporphyrin (the **hemes**) (Fig. 22-7).

Hemoglobin synthesis is precisely coordinated by mechanisms not completely understood. Three requisites for hemoglobin synthesis are (1) formation of protoporphyrin, (2) availability of iron (heme), and (3) generation of the proteinaceous globin. Several genes dictate the synthesis of globin in maturing human eryth-

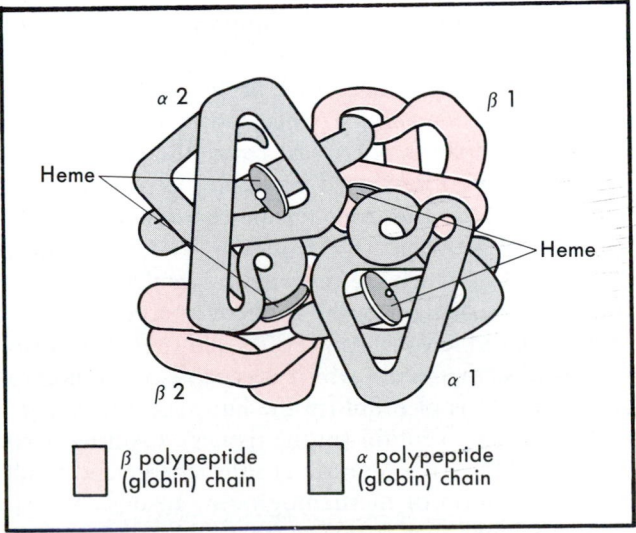

FIG. 22-7. Molecular structure of hemoglobin. Molecule is spherical tetramer weighing approximately 64,500 daltons. It contains a pair of α and a pair of β polypeptide chains and several heme groups.

TABLE 22-4 Structure of normal hemoglobin molecules

Type of hemoglobin (Hb)	Identity of polypeptide chain	Significance
Hb A	$\alpha_2\beta_2$	92% of adult Hb
Hb A$_{1c}$	α_2 (β-NH-glucose)	5% of adult Hb; increased in diabetes (see Chapter 19)
Hb A$_2$	$\alpha_2\delta_2$	2% of adult Hb; increased in β-thalassemia (see Chapter 23)
Hb F	$\alpha_2\gamma_2$	Major fetal Hb from the third through ninth month of gestation; promotes oxygen transfer across platelets; increase in β-thalassemia
Hb Gower I	ϵ_4 or $\zeta_2\epsilon_2$	Present in early embryo; function unknown
Hb Gower 2	$\alpha_2\epsilon_2$	Present in early embryo; function unknown
Hb Portland	$\zeta_2\gamma_2$	Present in early embryo; function unknown

Adapted from Bunn, 1977.

roblasts, each gene resulting in the formation of a structurally different polypeptide chain (alpha, beta, gamma, delta, epsilon, or zeta). Each polypeptide chain contains approximately 150 amino acids and is arranged in the knotted-sausage configuration shown in Fig. 22-7. The chains assemble to form a tetrahedron containing two pairs of identical chains. Hemoglobin A, the most common type of hemoglobin in adults, is composed of two alpha and two beta polypeptide chains. Seven different types of hemoglobin have been identified in healthy human blood at all stages, from fetal life to adulthood—testimony to the heterogeneity of the molecule (Table 22-4). The timing of synthesis and relative amount of each type of hemoglobin is determined by complex developmental processes.

Heme is a large, flat, iron-protoporphyrin disk that is capable of carrying one molecule of oxygen (O_2). Recall that hemoglobin contains four heme groups, thus it is capable of carrying four oxygen molecules. Through a series of complex biochemical reactions, protoporphyrin, a complex four-ringed molecule, is produced and abounds with ferrous iron. The biochemical reactions of heme synthesis include condensation, oxidation, and reduction, all of which are powered by catalytic enzymes. It is crucial that the iron be correctly charged. Presence of the reduced ferrous iron (Fe_2^{++}) allows the formation of normal hemoglobin, which is capable of binding oxygen where it is plentiful (in the lungs) and releasing it where it is less plentiful (in the tissues). Oxidized ferric iron (Fe_3^{+++}) carries an extra positive charge and results in the formation of **methemoglobin,** an unstable type of hemoglobin that is not capable of binding oxygen. An excess of ferric iron occurs in the presence of certain drugs and chemicals, such as nitrates and sulfonamides.

Hemoglobin that is carrying oxygen is called **oxyhe-moglobin.** If all four oxygen-binding sites on the oxyhemoglobin's hemes are occupied by oxygen, the molecule is said to be saturated. Oxyhemoglobin that has released its oxygen or is not bound to oxygen for some other reason is called reduced hemoglobin, or **deoxyhemoglobin.**

Nutritional Requirements for Erythropoiesis

Normal development of erythrocytes and synthesis of hemoglobin depend on an optimal biochemical milieu and adequate supplies of the necessary building blocks, including protein, vitamins, and minerals (Table 22-5). If these components are lacking, it is usually the result of a nutritional deficiency or a metabolic imbalance in which other organs or tissues use up a disproportionate share of these nutrients or are unable to absorb the needed nutrients (Wintrobe et al., 1981). If abnormal distribution of nutrients is prolonged, erythrocyte production slows, and anemia (insufficient numbers of functional erythrocytes) may result (see Chapter 23).

Protein is an important structural component of the erythrocyte's plasma membrane, contributing to its strength, flexibility, and elasticity. Amino acid chains form hemoglobin. Without proteins and amino acids, erythrocyte production decreases, and the life span of cells that are produced may be shortened because of structural defects (Delmonte, Aschkenasy, & Eyquem, 1964). One of the most important proteins is **intrinsic factor (IF),** a glycoprotein necessary for gastrointestinal absorption of vitamin B$_{12}$. Lack of vitamin B$_{12}$ causes pernicious anemia. IF is secreted by the parietal cells in the gastric mucosa and facilitates vitamin B$_{12}$ uptake at its absorptive site, the ileum.

Erythropoiesis cannot proceed in the absence of vitamins, especially B$_{12}$, folate (folic acid), B$_6$, riboflavin,

TABLE 22-5 Nutritional requirements for erythropoiesis

Nutrient	Role in erythropoiesis	Consequence of deficiency
Protein (amino acids)	Structural component of plasma membrane	Decreased strength, elasticity, and flexibility of membrane, hemolytic anemia
	Synthesis of hemoglobin	Decreased erythropoiesis and life span of erythrocytes
Cobalamin (vitamin B_{12})	Synthesis of DNA, maturation of erythrocytes, facilitator of folate metabolism	Macrocytic (megaloblastic) anemia
Folate (folic acid)	Synthesis of DNA and RNA, maturation of erythrocytes	Macrocytic (megaloblastic) anemia
Vitamin B_6 (pyridoxine)	Heme synthesis	Hypochromic, microcytic anemia
Vitamin B_2 (riboflavin)	Oxidative reactions	Normochromic, normocytic anemia
Vitamin C (ascorbic acid)	Iron metabolism, acts as a reducing agent to maintain iron in its ferrous (Fe^{++}) form	Normochromic, normocytic anemia
Pantothenic acid	Heme synthesis	Unknown*
Niacin	None, but needed for respiration in mature erythrocytes	Unknown
Vitamin E	Heme synthesis (?); protection against oxidative damage in mature erythrocytes	Hemolytic anemia with increased cell membrane fragility
Iron	Hemoglobin synthesis	Iron deficiency anemia
Copper	Required for optimal mobilization of iron from tissues to plasma	Hypochromic microcytic anemia

*Although pantothenic acid is important for optimal synthesis of heme, experimentally induced deficiency *failed* to produce anemia or other hematopoietic disturbances (Wintrobe, 1981).

pantothenic acid, niacin, ascorbic acid, and vitamin E. Vitamin B_{12} is a large molecule; therefore it requires assistance from IF to penetrate the gastrointestinal mucosa. Once absorbed, vitamin B_{12} is stored in the liver and used as needed in erythropoiesis.

Folate is the second most important vitamin for erythrocyte production and maturation. Folate is necessary for deoxyribonucleic acid (DNA) synthesis, being a component of three of the four DNA bases (thymine, adenine, and guanine). Folate is also needed for ribonucleic acid (RNA) synthesis. Intrinsic factor is not required for folate absorption, which occurs principally in the upper small intestine. Folate is stored in and circulates through the liver. Folate deficiency is more common than vitamin B_{12} deficiency and occurs more rapidly. Folate stores can be depleted within a few months, whereas vitamin B_{12} depletion can take years. Folate supplements are prescribed for pregnant women because pregnancy increases the demand for folate and deficiency can cause anemia.

Iron Cycle

About 67% of total body iron is bound to heme in erythrocytes and muscle cells, and about 30% is stored bound to ferritin or hemosiderin mononuclear phagocytes (i.e., macrophages) and hepatic parenchymal cells. The remaining 3% (less than 1 mg) is lost daily in urine, sweat, bile, and epithelial cells shed from the gut. Iron not lost is continuously recycled as shown in Fig. 22-8. Recycling is made possible by **transferrin,** a glycoprotein synthesized primarily by the liver but also by tissue macrophages, submaxillary and mammary glands, and ovaries or testes.

Dietary iron is absorbed primarily in the duodenum and proximal jejunum. Some of it passes into the bloodstream and the rest is sequestered in intestinal epithelial cells as ferritin. This iron is lost when epithelial cells are sloughed off in the intestinal lumen. Iron that is released to the bloodstream is picked up by transferrin, which is the body's major iron-transport molecule. Iron for hemoglobin production is delivered to erythroblasts in erythropoietic bone marrow. Under normal conditions, only one third of the iron-binding sites on transferrin molecules are occupied.

It is postulated that iron is transferred from transferrin to erythroblasts in the marrow as follows: (1) the transferrin-iron complex binds to a receptor on the erythroblast's plasma membrane; (2) the complex moves

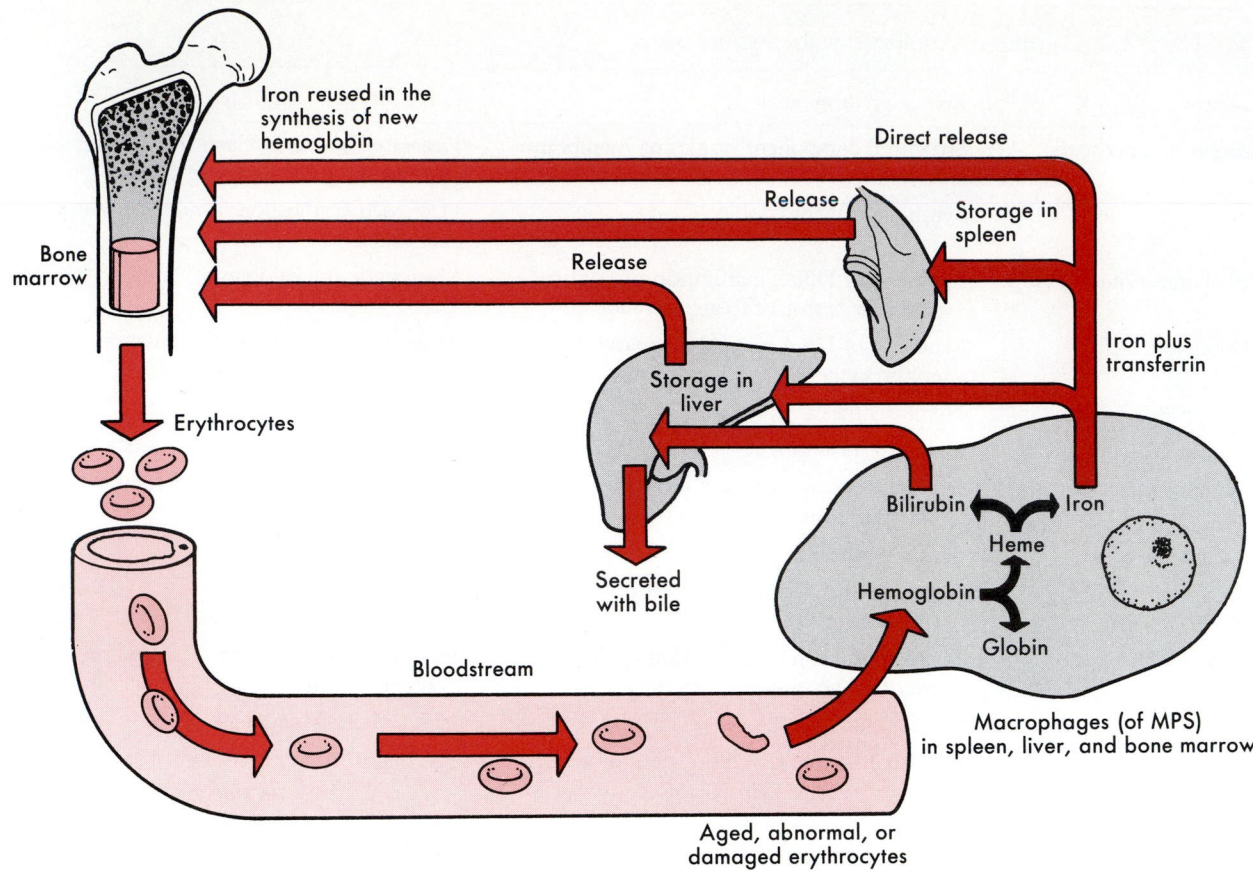

FIG. 22-8. Iron cycle. Iron *(Fe)* released from gastrointestinal epithelial cells circulates in bloodstream associated with its plasma carrier, transferrin. It is delivered to erythroblasts in bone marrow, where most of it is incorporated into hemoglobin. Mature erythrocytes circulate for approximately 120 days, after which they become senescent and are removed by MPS. Macrophages of MPS (mostly in spleen) break down ingested erythrocytes and return iron to bloodstream directly or after storing it as ferritin or hemosiderin.

into the cell, possibly by active transport; (3) iron is released (dissociated) from transferrin; and (4) the dissociated transferrin is returned to the bloodstream (see Fig. 22-8) (Wintrobe et al., 1981). Another source of iron for erythropoiesis is the iron stored by ferritin and hemosiderin in the cytoplasm of mononuclear phagocytes (macrophages) resident in the marrow. Once the iron is released into the marrow and incorporated into the erythroblast's mitochondria, the enzyme heme synthetase inserts ferrous iron into protoporphyrin to form heme. Heme is then bound to globin to form hemoglobin. Iron not used in erythropoiesis is stored temporarily as ferritin or hemosiderin and later excreted.

After mature erythrocytes have circulated for 120 days, they are removed from the bloodstream by macrophages of the MPS—chiefly in the spleen. Within the phagolyssomes (digestive vacuole) of the macrophage, the erythrocyte is catabolized and the iron in hemoglobin is oxidized, forming Fe_3^{+++} (methemoglobin). The

heme and globin of methemoglobin dissociate easily, and globin may be reduced to its component amino acids. The iron released by methemoglobin dissociation is stored in the macrophage's cytoplasm as ferritin or hemosiderin or released into the bloodstream, where it is free to bind again to transferrin (see Fig. 22-8). A minute amount of iron is stored in muscle cells by the heme-containing protein myoglobin. Unavailable stores of iron are present in cytochromes, catalases, and peroxidase enzymes.

Iron balance is achieved through mechanisms controlling its absorption rather than its excretion. Regulation of iron transport across the plasma membrane of gastrointestinal epithelial cells is related to the cell's iron content and the overall rate of erythropoiesis. If the body's iron stores are low or the demand for erythropoiesis is increased, iron passes rapidly through the epithelial cell and into the plasma, probably by mechanisms of active transport. (Transport mechanisms are described in Chapter 1.) If body stores are high and erythropoiesis is not increased, iron crosses the epithelial cell's plasma membrane passively and is stored there bound to ferritin. Excretion of iron occurs when the epithelial cells of the intestinal mucosa slough off.

Regulation of Erythropoiesis

In healthy humans the total volume of circulating erythrocytes remains surprisingly constant. The feedback mechanism that maintains an optimal population of erythrocytes is mediated by erythropoietin. Erythropoietin induces the selective proliferation and differentiation of proerythroblasts (see Fig. 22-5). Its earliest effects are to stimulate RNA synthesis, following either binding to receptors on the erythroblast's plasma membrane or entrance into the cell. Hemoglobin synthesis begins hours after initial stimulation by erythropoietin.

Erythropoietin is secreted by the kidney in response to tissue hypoxia (insufficient oxygen in tissue cells) (Fig. 22-9). Erythropoietin causes a compensatory increase in erythrocyte production if the oxygen content of blood decreases because of anemia, high altitude, or pulmonary disease. The receptors that detect hypoxia are postulated to be within the kidney because production of erythropoietin is known to increase after renal artery constriction, which reduces oxygen supply to renal cells (Fisher & Langston, 1967; Fisher, Samuels, & Langston, 1967). Unlike the peripheral chemoreceptors of the carotid body and aortic arch that send messengers to the brain to increase respiration in individuals with hypoxia, receptors in the kidney are on cells that synthesize and secrete erythropoietin. Thus the body responds to reduced oxygenation of blood in two ways: (1) by increasing intake of oxygen through increased respiration and (2) by increasing the oxygen-carrying capacity of the blood through increased erythropoiesis. Erythropoietin not only stimulates proliferation of committed stem cells in the marrow but also accelerates maturation of existing erythroblasts. This activity results in expansion of the erythron, including erythropoietic marrow. Erythron enlargement restores tissue oxygen levels. A negative-feedback mechanism is thought to monitor erythropoietin activity (Anagnostou, Fried, & Kurtzman, 1981; Fried & Marley, 1985).

Normal Destruction of Senescent Erythrocytes

Although mature erythrocytes lack nuclei, mitochondria, and endoplasmic reticulum, they do have cytoplasmic enzymes capable of glycolysis (anaerobic glucose metabolism) and production of small quantities of ATP. The ATP provides the energy necessary to keep the cell alive and its plasma membrane pliable (see Fig. 22-1, *B*). Metabolic processes diminish as the erythrocyte ages. Consequently, less ATP is available to maintain the functions essential for life. The senescent red cell be-

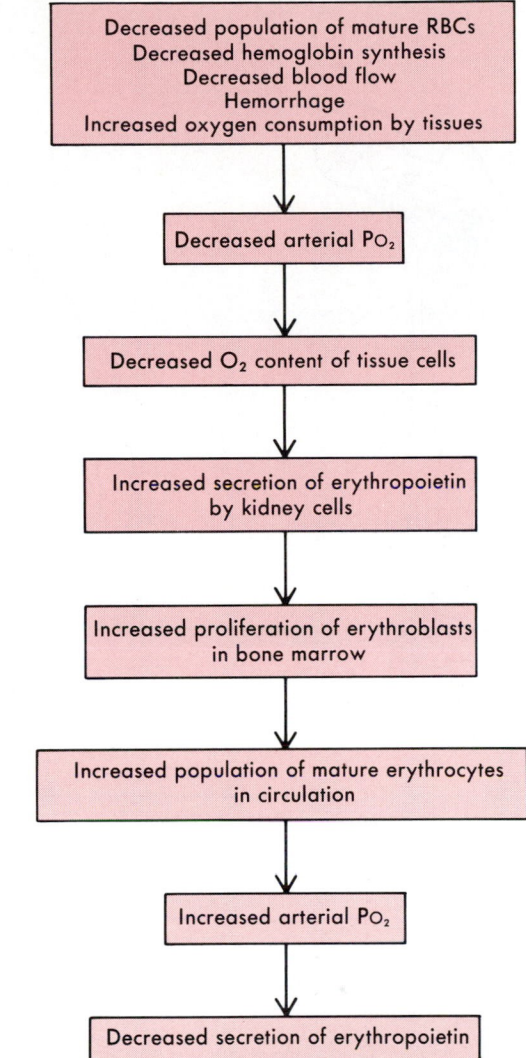

Decreased arterial oxygen levels stimulate production of erythropoietin, which in turn stimulates red cell production and expansion of the erythron. The increase in red cells frequently corrects the problem of low oxygen levels (hypoxia). This restoration to normal oxygen levels alerts the kidney to stop producing erythropoietin (negative feedback). Further erythrocyte production is not needed.

FIG. 22-9. Role of erythropoietin in regulation of erythropoiesis Po2, and partial pressure of oxygen in the blood (see Chapter 29).

comes increasingly fragile and loses its property of reversible deformability. Its membrane is therefore susceptible to rupture during passage through narrowed regions of the microcirculation.

Aged red cells are selectively sequestered and destroyed by macrophages of the MPS, primarily in the spleen. If the spleen is dysfunctional or absent, macrophages in the liver (Kupffer's cells) take over. The signal that identifies an erythrocyte as senescent and ready for disposal by the MPS is not known for certain. Alterations in the erythrocyte's plasma membrane, including

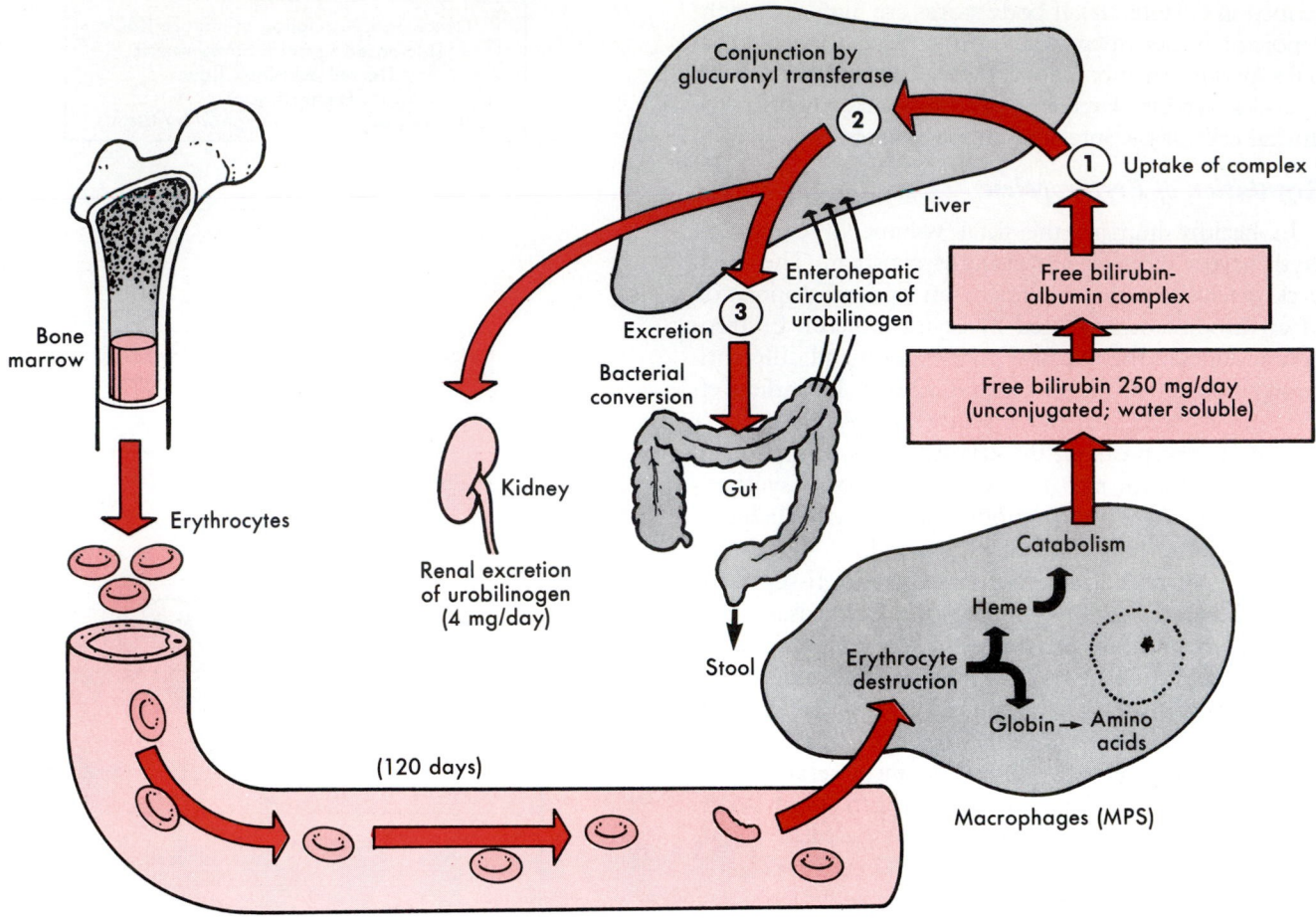

FIG. 22-10. Metabolism of bilirubin released by heme breakdown.

altered ionic and osmotic gradients across it and a decrease in its electrical charge, and an increase in methemoglobin within the erythrocyte all accompany cellular aging. These factors may contribute to sluggish erythrocyte movement through the spleen and other lymphoid tissues, increasing opportunities for phagocytosis by resident macrophages.

Phagocytosis of the erythrocyte is followed by its digestion by proteolytic and lipolytic enzymes within the phagolysosome of the macrophage. Globin is broken down into amino acids, and iron is recycled (Fig. 22-8). Porphyrin is reduced to bilirubin, which is transported to the liver, conjugated, and finally excreted in the bile as glucuronide (Fig. 22-10). Approximately 6 g of hemoglobin is catabolized daily, producing 200 mg of bilirubin. (Liver function is described in Chapter 35.) Bacteria in the intestinal lumen transform conjugated bilirubin into urobilinogen. A small portion of this urobilinogen is reabsorbed, either to be metabolized further by the liver or excreted by the kidney into the urine. Most of the urobilinogen is excreted in feces.

Conditions causing accelerated erythrocyte destruc-

tion increase the load of bilirubin for hepatic clearance, leading to increased serum levels of unconjugated bilirubin and increased urinary excretion of urobilinogen. Gallstones (cholelithiasis) can result from a chronically elevated rate of bilirubin excretion.

Development of Leukocytes

All of the leukocytes arise from stem cells in the bone marrow (their pathways of differentiation are shown in Fig. 22-5). The granulocytes (neutrophils, eosinophils, and basophils) normally mature fully in the marrow and then are released into the bloodstream. The agranulocytes (monocytes and lymphocytes), however, are released into the bloodstream before they undergo their final phase of maturation. The monocytes mature into macrophages within a day or two of release, and the lymphocytes travel to lymphoid tissues, where they are stimulated to differentiate into T cells or B cells (see Chapter 6).

The bone marrow exhibits selective retention of immature granulocytes. It is theorized that a humoral factor, sometimes referred to as granulocyte releasing factor or leukocytosis-inducing factor, causes an increase in release of granulocytes. The mechanism that controls selective retention is poorly understood. **Granulopoietin,** a plasma glycoprotein that stimulates granulopoiesis (proliferation of granulocytes), has been discovered that may be responsible for regulation of granulocyte levels in the circulation (Vick, 1984).

Maintenance of optimal levels of granulocytes and monocytes in the blood depends on the availability of pluripotential stem cells in the marrow, induction of these into committed stem cells, and timely release of new cells from the marrow. The marrow contains a reserve pool that can be rapidly mobilized in response to the body's needs. Once cells are released from the marrow, they join the marginating pool or the circulating pool. The cells in the marginating pool lie along the capillary walls and can move into tissues and mucous membranes. Cells from the circulating pool join the marginating pool to replace the cells that have migrated out of the capillaries. Leukocyte production increases in response to infection, to the presence of steroids, and to reduction or depletion of reserves in the marrow. It is also associated with strenuous exercise, convulsive seizures, heat, intense radiation, paroxysmal tachycardias, pain, nausea and vomiting, and anxiety (Wintrobe, 1986).

Normally, some leukocytes are lost in saliva, urine, the lungs, liver, spleen, and gastrointestinal tract. Most exist in the body from days to years, depending on type (see Table 22-2).

Development of Platelets

Platelets (thrombocytes) develop from megakaryocytes by a unique process of proliferation termed endomitosis (see Fig. 22-5). In endomitosis the megakaryocyte undergoes the nuclear phase of cellular division (mitosis) but fails to undergo the cytoplasmic phase (cytokinesis) (see Chapter 1). Without cytokinesis, the cell does not divide into two daughter cells. Rather, the megakaryocyte expands to accommodate the doubling of its DNA (nuclear) content, and breaks up into fragments known as platelets.

An optimal number of platelets and committed platelet precursors (megakaryoblasts) in the bone marrow are maintained in part by the action of **thrombopoietin,** a platelet-stimulating factor that binds to plasma membranes of pluripotential stem cells in the bone marrow, causing them to become committed megakaryoblasts. Thrombopoietin also stimulates committed cells at further stages of differentiation to differentiate faster. Processes of megakaryocyte development, endomitosis, and platelet release are all speeded up (Harker, 1984).

Approximately 4 days after thrombopoietin enters the bone marrow, platelets are released into the bloodstream (Fischbach & Fogdall, 1981). They circulate for 10 days before they begin to lose their capacity to carry out biochemical reactions. The initial alteration of function is possibly due to proteolytic enzymes present at sites of chronic vascular inflammation. (See Chapter 7 for a discussion of biochemicals involved in inflammation.) Senescent platelets are phagocytosed by neutrophils and monocytes if they are circulating freely or by neutrophils and macrophages if they are part of a clot, or thrombus. Senescent platelets may also be removed by tissue macrophages of the MPS in the liver or spleen.

MECHANISMS OF HEMOSTASIS

Hemostasis means arrest of bleeding. Mechanisms of hemostasis maintain a relatively steady state of blood volume, pressure, and flow through injured blood vessels. Hemostasis following vascular damage and bleeding involves a complex sequence of events: (1) vasoconstriction (vasospasm), (2) formation of a platelet plug, (3) activation of the coagulation (or clotting) cascade, and (4) formation of a blood clot. All four of these events are necessary for hemostasis and all four involve platelets or clotting factors or both in some way.

Function of Platelets

Mechanisms of platelet participation include adherence of platelets to injured vessel walls; platelet degranulation, which releases biochemical mediators; and platelet aggregation into clumps, or plugs. Normally, platelets circulate freely, suspended in plasma, and do not adhere to endothelial cells that line the vessels. When a vessel is damaged, however, collagen-containing subendothelial tissue is exposed. Collagen attracts platelets out of the plasma within 15 to 20 seconds after injury. The platelets adhere rapidly to this "foreign" surface, after which they undergo dynamic changes in shape, develop protrusions (pseudopods) and degranulate, releasing a variety of potent biochemicals (Fig. 22-11).

Several factors affect platelet adherence to exposed subendothelial tissues. The platelets must contain sufficient concentrations of calcium to change shape, aggregate, degranulate, and activate arachidonic pathways. Evidence suggests that calcium within platelets activates degranulation. Erythrocytes apparently increase the rate of platelet adherence by facilitating migration of circulating platelets toward vascular surfaces and by liberating ADP, which enables platelets to stick to exposed collagen.

Two of the biochemical mediators released by adhered platelets have immediate effects on smooth muscle in the vascular endothelium. These mediators, serotonin and histamine, cause an immediate temporary constriction of the injured vessel. Vasoconstriction reduces

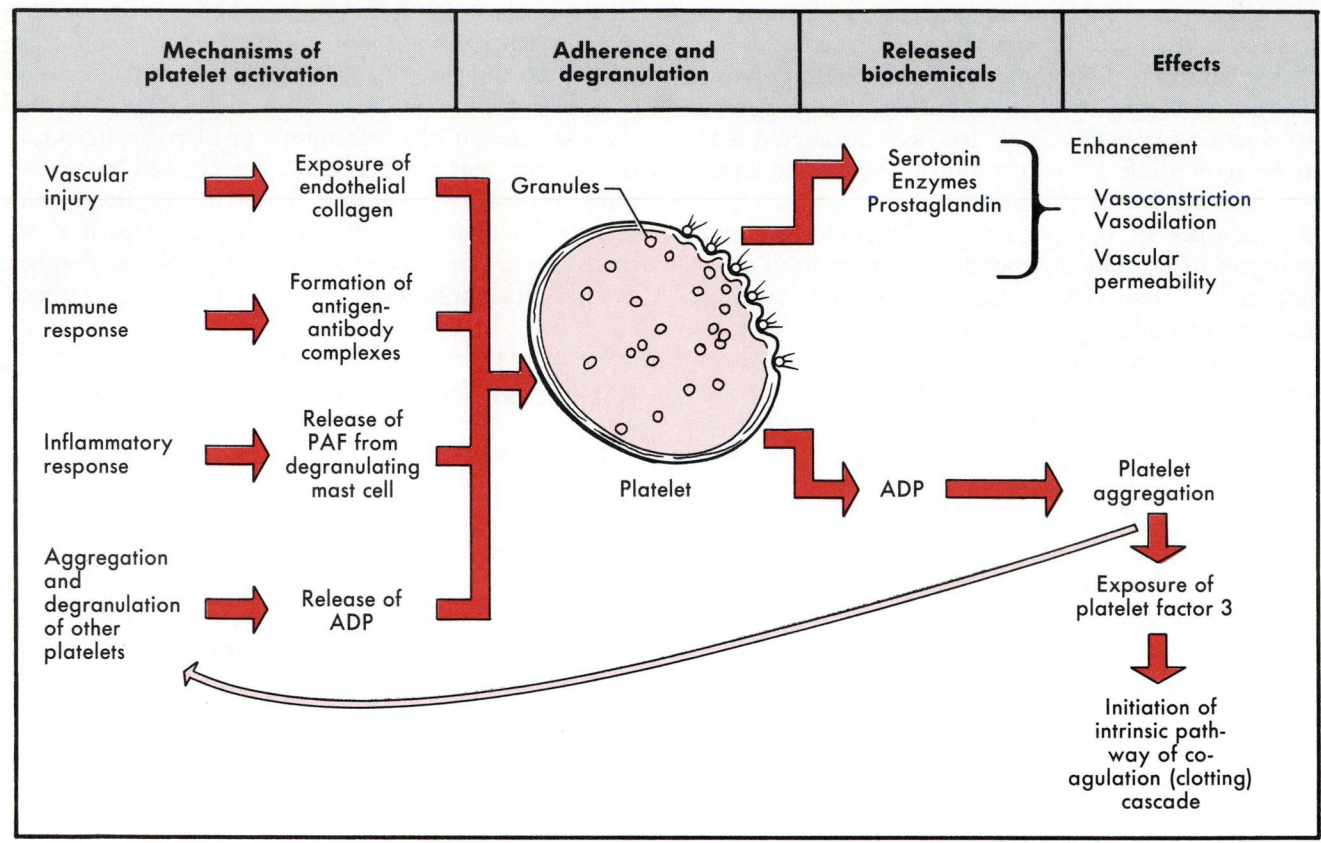

FIG. 22-11. Platelet degranulation. PAF, Platelet-activating factor.

blood flow and thereby diminishes bleeding. (Vasoconstriction is also produced by local reflexes of the nervous system.) Vasodilation soon follows, permitting the inflammatory response to proceed. (The inflammatory response is necessary for healing; see Chapter 7.)

Other biochemical mediators released by degranulation (also called the platelet-release reaction) either promote or inhibit platelet activity and the eventual process of clot formation (see Fig. 7-8). ADP promotes the adherence and subsequent degranulation of nearby platelets by causing their plasma membranes to become ruffly and sticky. The new activated platelets also adhere to the exposed collagen, causing a platelet plug to seal the injured endothelium. If the effects of ADP were not counteracted and laminar flow was not sufficient, platelet aggregation could continue indefinitely. This eventuality is prevented by two mutually antagonistic prostaglandin derivatives, thromboxane A_2 (TxA_2) and prostacyclin$_2$ (PGI_2). TxA_2 is synthesized and released by degranulating platelets. It causes vasoconstriction and promotes the degranulation of other platelets, which then release more ADP. PGI_2 is synthesized and released by uninjured endothelial cells in vessel walls. PGI_2 is a thromboxane antagonist: it inhibits the effects of

TxA_2 by promoting vasodilation and inhibiting platelet degranulation. The net effect of TxA_2 and PGI_2 is to permit platelet aggregation to proceed at the site of injury while preventing adherence to normal vascular endothelium (Fischbach & Fogdall, 1981). Heparin-neutralizing factor (platelet factor 4), which is also released by degranulating platelets, enhances clot formation at the site of injury.

If blood vessel injury is minor, hemostasis is achieved temporarily by the platelet plug, which usually forms within 3 to 5 minutes of injury. Platelet plugs seal the many minute ruptures that occur daily in the microcirculation, particularly in capillaries. In the absence of sufficient numbers of platelets, numerous small hemorrhagic areas called purpuras develop under the skin and throughout the tissues (see Chapters 24 and 25). The plug becomes stable during the process of clot formation.

Function of Clotting Factors

Clot formation is the third major event of hemostasis, following vasoconstriction and formation of the platelet plug. A **blood clot** is a meshwork of protein strands that stabilizes the platelet plug and traps other cells,

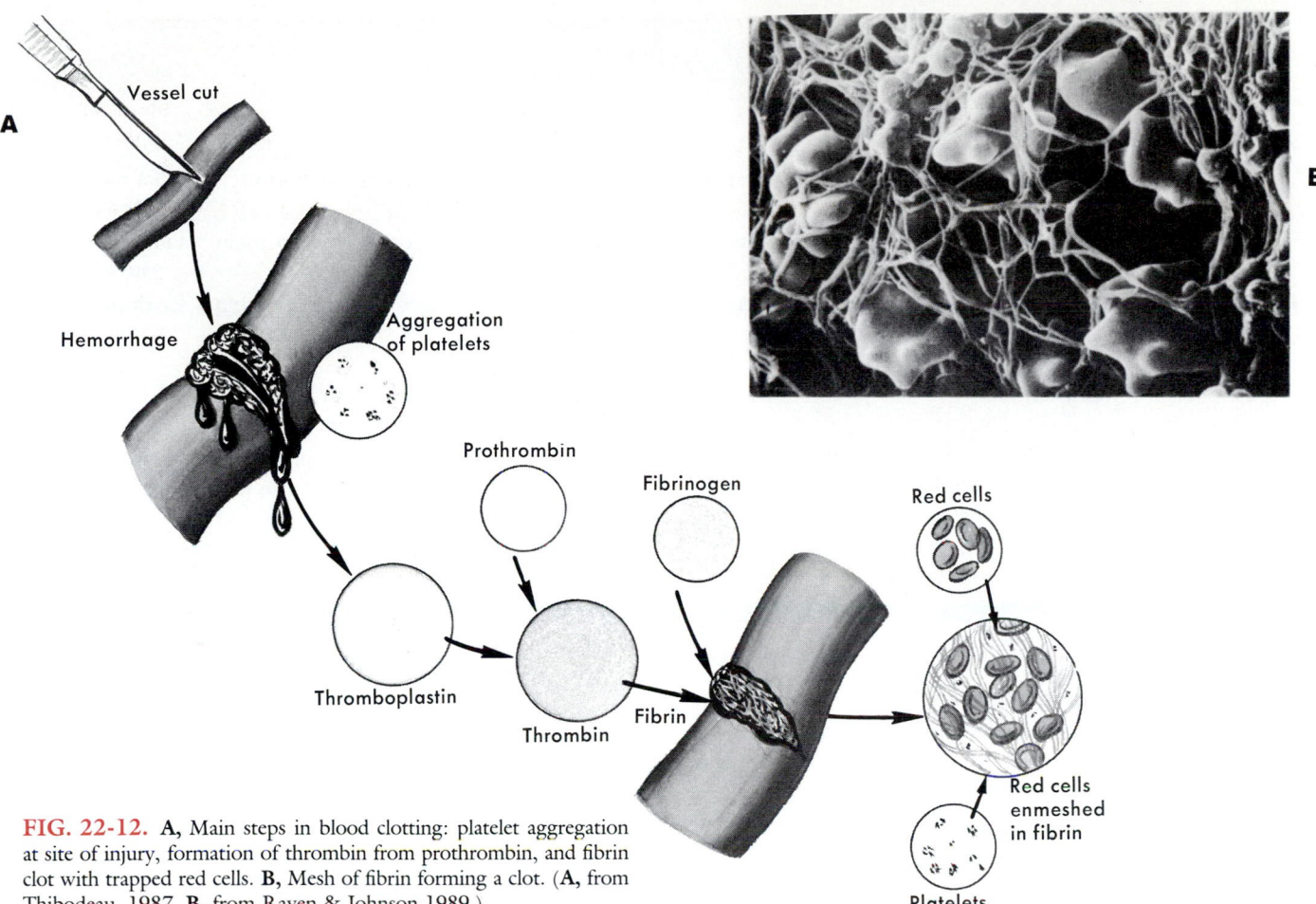

FIG. 22-12. A, Main steps in blood clotting: platelet aggregation at site of injury, formation of thrombin from prothrombin, and fibrin clot with trapped red cells. **B,** Mesh of fibrin forming a clot. (**A,** from Thibodeau, 1987. **B,** from Raven & Johnson 1989.)

such as erythrocytes, phagocytes, and microorganisms (Fig. 22-12). The strands are made of fibrin. Unlike platelets, which are formed elements of the blood, fibrin is not normally present in the circulation. Rather, it is the end product of the **coagulation cascade,** a series of enzymatic reactions among the clotting factors (Fig. 22-13). During the coagulation cascade, clotting factors in the blood are activated and transformed, in turn, until fibrin is produced. (Characteristics of the clotting factors are listed in Table 22-6.) In effect, soluble clotting factors become insoluble fibrin.

The coagulation cascade is initiated through two mechanisms. The intrinsic pathway is activated when Hageman factor (factor XII) in plasma comes into contact with subendothelial substances exposed by vascular injury. The extrinsic pathway is activated when tissue thromboplastin, a substance released by damaged endothelial cells, comes into contact with one of the clotting factors, serum prothrombin conversion factor (factor VII). Both pathways lead to a final common pathway when each has activated factor X (Stuart-Prower factor). The common pathway proceeds to clot formation.

Control of Hemostatic Mechanisms

Despite the continual presence of clotting factors and platelets in the circulation, blood normally remains fluid. Two properties of normal vascular endothelium prevent clotting. The first is the smooth texture of the endothelial lining, which prevents adherence of platelets. The second is the negative charge of protein in the endothelial cells, which repels some negatively charged platelets and clotting factors. Damage to the vascular endothelium destroys both of these properties, enabling platelets to adhere and initiating the intrinsic pathway of coagulation.

Once activated, the processes of coagulation are controlled by anticoagulants, some of which are products of the coagulation cascade itself. For example, once a clot has formed, its fibrin strands will absorb 85% to 90% of the thrombin subsequently produced at the site. The remaining thrombin is inactivated rapidly by antithrombin III, another plasma protein. Other anticoagulants, most notably heparin, are produced and secreted locally by tissue mast cells and basophils that have been activated by the injury (see Chapter 7). Heparin not only

TABLE 22-6 Clotting factors

International nomenclature	Synonyms	Substance	Source	Enzymatic function	Pathway of activation
I	Fibrinogen	Plasma protein	Liver	Precursor of fibrin	Final common pathway
II	Prothrombin	Plasma protein	Liver	Precursor of thrombin	Final common pathway
III	Tissue thromboplastin Tissue factor Thrombokinase	Lipoprotein and phospholipid	Released from damaged tissues	Activates prothrombin	Extrinsic pathway
IV	Calcium ion	Ion in plasma	Diet and bones	Activates prothrombin and fibrin formation	All
V	Labile factor Proaccelerin accelerator globulin (AcG) Thrombogen	Plasma protein	Liver	Accelerates conversion of prothrombin to thrombin	Final common pathway
VI	Obsolete; same as V				
VII	Serum prothrombin conversion factor Proconvertin Stable factor	Plasma protein	Liver	Accelerates conversion of prothrombin to thrombin; part of enzyme complex	Extrinsic pathway
VIII	Antihemophilic globulin (AGH) Antihemophilic factor (AHF) Thromboplastinogen Platelet cofactor 1	Plasma protein (three subunits)	Large molecular weight Subunit by endothelium	Associated with platelet factor 3 and Christmas factor (IX), activates prothrombin (II)	Intrinsic pathway
IX	Plasma thromboplastin component (PTC) Christmas factor Antihemophilic factor B Autoprothrombin II Platelet cofactor 2	Plasma protein	Liver	Associated with platelet factors 3 and 6; activates prothrombin	Intrinsic pathway
X	Stuart-Prower factor Stuart factor Autoprothrombin III	Plasma protein	Liver and plasma	Activated by Hageman factor	Extrinsic and intrinsic pathway
XI	Plasma thromboplastin antecedent (PTA) Antihemophilic factor C	Plasma protein	Possibly liver	Activated by Hageman factor; accelerates thrombin formation; substrate for activator enzymatic complex	Intrinsic pathway
XII	Hageman factor Contact factor Glass factor Antihemophilic factor D	Plasma protein	Liver and plasma	Involved in first step of activation of intrinsic pathway; activates XI	Intrinsic pathway
XIII	Fibrin stabilizing factor (FSF) Fibrinase Fibrinoligase Laki-Lorand factor (LLF) Plasma transglutaminase	Plasma protein	Present in plasma and platelets Liver	Produces stronger fibrin clot; stabilizes clot formation	Common

TABLE 22-6 Clotting factors—cont'd

International nomenclature	Synonyms	Substance	Source	Enzymatic function	Pathway of activation
High-molecular weight kininogen	HMWK Fitzgerald factor Williams factor Fluajeac factor Reid factor Washington factor	α globulin	Tissues	Activates contraction of clot	Intrinsic kinin cascade
Prekallikrein	Fletcher factor	γ-globulin	Tissues	Activates contraction of clot	Intrinsic kinin cascade

NOTE: The factors are numbered in the order of their discovery. Numerals do not denote their sequence of activation in the coagulation cascade.

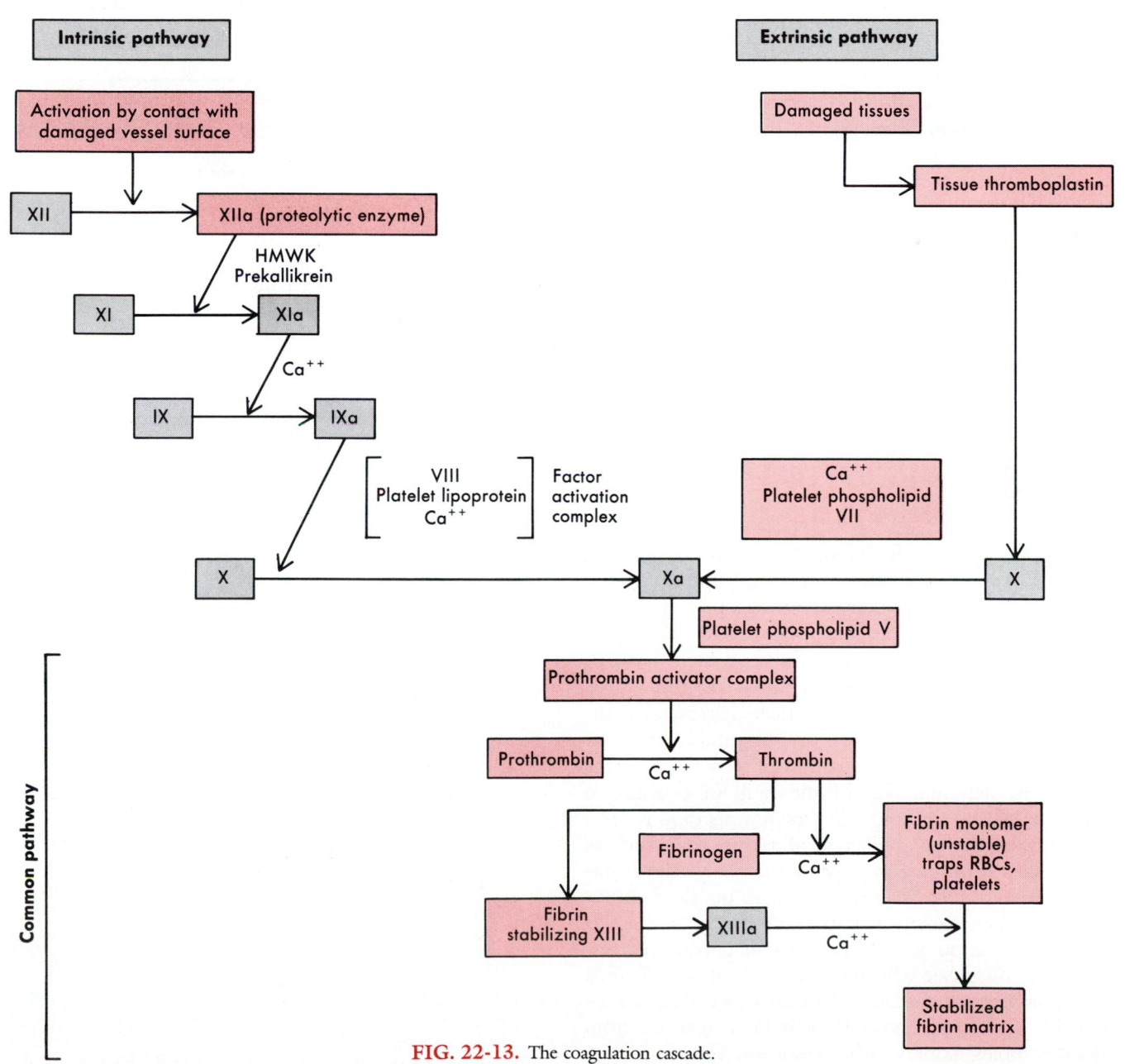

FIG. 22-13. The coagulation cascade.

halts the coagulation cascade but also enhances throm-bin absorption by fibrin in the clot.

Retraction and Lysis of Blood Clots

After a clot is formed, it retracts, or "solidifies." Clot retraction is the final stage of hemostasis. Fibrin strands shorten, becoming denser and stronger. This helps to approximate the edges of the injured vessel wall and seal the site of injury. Retraction is facilitated by the large numbers of platelets trapped within the fibrin mesh-work. The platelets, which contain actomyosin-like con-tractile protein, contract and "pull" the fibrin threads closer together while releasing a factor that stabilizes the fibrin. Contraction expels protein-free serum from the fibrin meshwork. This process usually begins within a few minutes after a clot has formed, and most of the se-rum is expressed within 30 to 60 minutes (Guyton, 1981).

Lysis (breakdown) of blood clots is carried out by the **fibrinolytic system** (Fig. 22-14). Lysis is mediated by plasmin (fibrinolysin), a proteolytic enzyme that is acti-vated by substances present during coagulation and in-flammation, such as factor XII, thrombin, and lysosomal enzymes. Plasmin splits fibrin and fibrinogen into **fibrin degradation products (FDP),** which dissolve the clot. The fibrinolytic system removes clotted blood from tis-sues and dissolves small clots (thrombi) in blood vessels. A balance between amounts of thrombin and plasmin in the circulation maintain normal coagulation and lysis.

CLINICAL EVALUATION OF THE HEMATOLOGIC SYSTEM

Tests of Bone Marrow Function

In tests of marrow function, or hematopoiesis, small amounts of myeloid tissue are removed from the bone cavity and examined under a microscope. Cells con-tained in the marrow specimen are assessed with respect to (1) relative numbers of stem cells and their develop-ing daughter cells and (2) morphologic structure.

Bone marrow aspiration, in which marrow is with-drawn using a hollow needle, provides information on gross cellular structure, estimation of iron stores in re-ticulocytes, determination of the ratio of erythrocyte precursor cells to myeloid cells (the normal ratio is 3:3), and the presence or absence of abnormal cells, such as tumor cells. A marrow aspirate that is richly cellular im-plies normal or increased hematopoiesis but does not in-dicate whether marrow activity is effective.

Bone aspiration is an important diagnostic test for several anemias (see Chapter 23) and is also performed to diagnose suspected acute leukemia (see Chapters 24 and 25). (Chronic leukemias can be diagnosed from blood samples alone.) Other disorders requiring mar-row aspiration for assessment include platelet disorders

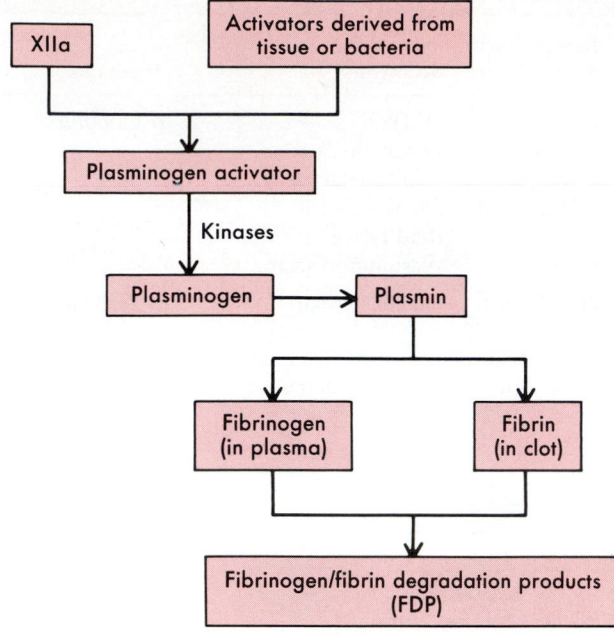

FIG. 22-14. The fibrinolytic system.

(to determine whether platelet counts are increased, de-creased, or normal; see Chapter 24) and immunoglobu-lin disorders (to gauge populations of plasma cells and lymphocytes; see Chapter 8).

Bone marrow biopsy, a surgical procedure in which a "slice" of marrow is removed, is performed if aspiration is not diagnostic, tumors are suspected (tumors are more easily detected in biopsy sections), marrow is fi-brotic, or populations of more than one type of blood cell are reduced. Because marrow aspiration disturbs

TABLE 22-7 Differential cell counts in bone marrow with age

Developing cells in marrow	Birth	1 mo-1 yr	1-4 yr	4-12 yr	Adult
Erythrocytic series	14	8	19	21	20
Lymphocytic series	14	47	22	18	17
Eosinophilic series	3	3	6	3	3
Neutrophilic series	60	33	50	52	57
Myeloid-erythroid ratio	4:3	4:0	1:3	2:5	1:3

NOTE: Values are percentages of cell types counted during examination of a marrow specimen containing approximately 400 nucleated cells.

marrow structure, only general cellularity (numbers of constituent cells) of the marrow can be gauged. Biopsy specimens provide the most reliable and specific information about marrow cellularity. Marrow biopsy is, however, usually more painful and expensive than marrow aspiration. Therefore biopsy is not performed unless insufficient information is obtained from aspiration.

A direct measure of iron stores can only be obtained from liver or marrow biopsy specimens. The bone marrow technique is preferred, not only because it is safer than liver biopsy but also because the red cell is the immediate source of plasma iron destined for erythrocyte production.

Examination of biopsy specimens and aspirate routinely includes a differential cell count (Table 22-7). The differential cell count involves examining approximately 400 nucleated cells under oil-immersion magnification and counting populations of different stem cells. The relative number of each type of stem cell is expressed as a percentage of 400.

Blood Tests

Blood tests provide information about the absolute and relative numbers of blood cells in a specimen of blood, as well as various structural and functional characteristics of the cells. Deviations from normal can reflect disease, physiologic states (e.g., pregnancy, infancy, old age), injury, or dysfunction in almost any part of the body. Blood tests that reflect chiefly hematologic disorders are listed in Table 22-8.

TABLE 22-8 Blood tests for hematologic disorders

Cell type and test	Property evaluated by test	Possible hematologic cause of abnormal findings
Erythrocyte		
Red cell count	Number (in millions) of erythrocytes/μL of blood	Altered erythropoiesis, anemias, hemorrhage, Hodgkin disease, leukemia
Mean corpuscular volume	Size of erythrocytes	Anemias, thalassemias
Mean corpuscular hemoglobin (MCH)	Amount of hemoglobin in each erythrocyte (by weight)	Anemias, hemoglobinopathy
Mean corpuscular hemoglobin concentration (MCHC)	Concentration of hemoglobin in each erythrocyte (percentage of erythrocyte occupied by hemoglobin)	Anemias, hereditary spherocytosis
Hemoglobin determination	Amount of hemoglobin/(by weight)/dl of blood	Anemias
Hematocrit determination	Percentage of a given volume of blood that is occupied by erthrocytes	Hemorrhage, polycythemia, erythrocytosis, anemias, leukemia
Reticulocyte count	Number of reticulocytes/μL of blood (also expressed as percentage of reticulocytes in total red cell count)	Hyperactive or hypoactive bone marrow function
Erythrocyte osmotic fragility test	Cellular shape (biconcavity), structure of plasma membrane	Anemias, hemolytic disease due to ABO or Rh incompatibility, Hodgkin disease, polycythemia vera, thalassemia major
Hemoglobin electrophoresis	Relative percentage of different types of hemoglobin in erythrocytes	Sickle cell disease, sickle cell trait, hemoglobin C disease, hemoglobin C trait, thalassemias
Sickle cell test	Presence of hemoglobin S in erythrocytes	Sickle cell trait, sickle cell anemia
Glucose-6-phosphate dehydrogenase (G-6-PD) deficiency test	Deficiency of G-6-PD in erythrocytes	Hemolytic anemia
Hemoglobin metabolism		
Serum ferritin determination	Depletion of body iron (potential deficiency of heme synthesis)	Iron deficiency anemias

From Byrne, C.J., et al. (1986). *Laboratory tests: Implications for nursing care*, Menlo Park, CA: Addison-Wesley.
NOTE: See Fig. 22-13 and Table 22-6 for information about clotting factors and their sequence of activation in the coagulation cascade.

Continued.

TABLE 22-8 Blood tests for hematologic disorders—cont'd

Cell type and test	Property evaluated by test	Possible hematologic cause of abnormal findings
Total iron-binding capacity (TICB)	Amount of iron in serum plus amount of transferrin available in serum(μg/dl)	Hemorrhage, iron deficiency anemia, hemochromatosis, hemosiderosis, iron overload, anemias, thalassemia
Transferrin saturation	Percentage of transferrin that is saturated with iron	Acute hemorrhage, hemochromatosis, hemosiderosis, sideroblastic anemia, iron deficiency anemia, iron overload, thalassemia
Porphyrin analysis (protoporphyrin analysis)	Concentration of protoporphyrin in erythrocytes (μg/dl); an indicator of iron-deficient erythropoiesis	Megaloblastic anemia, congenital erythropoietic porphyria
Direct antiglobulin test (DAT)	Antibody binding to erythrocytes	Hemolytic disease of the newborn, autoimmune hemolytic anemia, drug-induced hemolytic anemia, transfusion reaction
Antibody screen (indirect Coomb's test)	Detection of antibodies to erythrocyte antigens (other than the ABO antigens)	Same as for DAT
Leukocytes: differential white cell count (Absolute number of a type of leukocyte/μL of blood)	See below	See below
Neutrophil count	Neutrophils/μL	Myeloproliferative disorders, hematopoietic disorders, hemolysis
Lymphocyte count	Lymphocytes/μL	Infectious lymphocytosis, infectious mononucleosis, hematopoietic disorders, anemias, leukemia, lymphosarcoma, Hodgkin disease
Plasma cell count	Plasma cells/μL	Infectious mononucleosis, lymphocytosis, plasma cell leukemia
Monocyte count	Monocytes/μL	Hodgkin disease, infectious mononucleosis, monocytic leukemia, nonHodgkin lymphoma, polycythemia vera
Eosinophil count	Eosinophils/μL	Hematopoietic disorders
Basophil count	Basophils/μL	Chronic myelogenous leukemia, hemolytic anemias, Hodgkin disease, polycythemia vera
Platelets and clotting factors		
Platelet count	Number of circulating platelets (in thousands)/μL of blood	Anemias, multiple myeloma, myelofibrosis, polycythemia vera, leukemia, disseminated intravascular coagulation (DIC), hemolytic disease of the newborn, idiopathic thrombocytopenic purpura, transfusion reaction, lymphoproliferative disorders
Bleeding time	Duration of bleeding following a standardized superficial puncture wound of the skin, integrity of the platelet plug, measured in minutes following puncture	Leukemia, anemias, DIC, fibrinolytic activity, purpuras, hemorrhagic disease of the newborn, infectious mononucleosis, multiple myeloma, clotting factor deficiencies, thrombasthenia, thrombocytopathia, von Willibrand disease

TABLE 22-8 Blood tests for hematologic disorders—cont'd

Cell type and test	Property evaluated by test	Possible hematologic cause of abnormal findings
Clot retraction test	Platelet number and function, fibrinogen quantity and use, measured in hours required for expression of serum from a clot incubated in a test tube	Acute leukemia, aplastic anemia, factor XIII deficiency, increased fibronolytic activity, Hodgkin disease, hyperfibrinogenemia or hypofibrinogenemia, idiopathic thrombocytopenia purpura, multiple myeloma, polycythemia vera, secondary thrombocytopenia, thrombasthenia
Platelet adhesion studies	Ability of platelets to adhere to foreign surfaces	Anemia, macroglobulinemia, Barnard-Soulier syndrome, multiple myeloma, myeloid metaplasia, plasma cell dyscrasias, thrombasthenia, thrombocytopathy, von Willebrand disease
Platelet aggregation tests	Ability of platelets to adhere to one another	Afibrinogenemia, Barnard-Soulier syndrome, thrombosthenia, hemorrhagic thrombocythemia, myeloid metaplasia, plasma cell dyscrasias, platelet release defects, polycythemia vera, preleukemia, sideroblastic anemia, von Willebrand disease, Waldenstrom macroglobulinemia, hypercoagulability
Whole blood clotting time (Lee-White coagulation time)	Overall ability of blood to clot, as measured in minutes in a test tube	Afibrogenemia, clotting factor deficiencies, excessive fibrinolysis, hemorrhagic disease of the newborn, hypofibrinogenemia, hypoprothrombinemia, leukemia
Circulating anticoagulants (IgG antibodies that inhibit coagulation)	Presence of antibodies that neutralize clotting factors and inhibit coagulation, as indicated by prolonged clotting time, prothrombin time, or partial thromboplastin time	Afibrinogenemia, presence of fibrin-fibrinogen degradation products, macroglobulinemia, multiple myeloma, DIC, plasma cell dyscrasias
Partial thromboplastin time (PTT)	Effectiveness of clotting factors (except factor VII and VIII), effectiveness of intrinsic pathway of coagulation cascade, as measured by a test tube (in seconds)	Presence of circulating anticoagulants, DIC, clotting factor deficiencies, excessive fibrinolysis, hemorrhagic disease of the newborn, hypofibrinogenemia and afibrinogenemia, prothrombin deficiency, von Willebrand disease, acute hemorrhage
Prothrombin time	Effectiveness of activity of prothrombin, fibrinogen, and factors V, VII, and X: effectiveness of vitamin K–dependent coagulation factors of the extrinsic and common pathways of the coagulation cascade as measured in a test tube in seconds)	Hypofibrinogenemia, dysfibrinogenemia, and afibrinogenemia; presence of circulating anticoagulants; DIC; deficiency of factors V, VII, or X; presence of fibrin degradation products, increased fibrinolytic activity, hemolytic jaundice, hemorrhagic disease of the newborn; acute leukemia, polycythemia vera, prothrombin deficiency, multiple myeloma
Thrombin time	Quantity and activity of fibrinogen as measured in a test tube (in seconds)	Hypofibrinogenemia, dysfibrinogenemia, and afibrinogenemia; presence of circulating anticoagulants; hemorrhagic disease of the newborn, polycythemia vera; increase in fibrinogen-fibrin degradation products; increased fibrinolytic activity

Continued.

TABLE 22-8 Blood tests for hematologic disorders—cont'd

Cell type and test	Property evaluated by test	Possible hematologic cause of abnormal findings
Fibrinogen assay	Amount of fibrinogen available for fibrin formation	Acute leukemia, congenital hypofibrinogenemia or afibrinogenemia, DIC, increased fibrinolytic activity, severe hemorrhage
Fibrin-fibrinogen degradation products (fibrin-fibrinogen split products)	Fibrinogenic activity as measured by levels of fibrin-fibrinogen degradation products (in μg/ml of blood)	Transfusion reactions, DIC, internal hemorrhage in the newborn, deep vein thrombosis, pulmonary embolism

From Byrne, C.J., et al. (1986). Laboratory tests: Implications for nursing care, Menlo Park, CA: Addison-Wesley.
NOTE: See Fig. 22-13 and Table 22-6 for information about clotting factors and their sequence of activation in the coagulation cascade.

AGING AND THE HEMATOLOGIC SYSTEM

Blood composition changes little with age. Although anemia is frequent in the elderly population, it is usually a result of other conditions. Erythrocyte life span is normal in the elderly, although a delay in erythrocyte replenishment may occur after bleeding, probably because of iron depletion. Total serum iron, total iron-binding capacity, and intestinal iron absorption are all decreased in the elderly (Bothwell & Finch, 1962). The plasma membranes of erythrocytes become increasingly fragile because they contain fewer and fewer proteins and membrane-associated enzymes (Kadlubowski, 1978; Kadlubowski & Agutter, 1977). Increased fragility causes portions of the membrane to be lost, presumably because of physical trauma inflicted during circulation.

Although aging does not appear to alter numbers of lymphocytes, their function does decrease with age (see Chapters 6 and 7). The most significant changes are with cellular immunity with some decline in T cell function. The humoral immune system has a decreased ability to respond to antigenic challenge (Siskind, 1987).

No changes in platelet numbers or structure have been observed in the elderly, yet evidence shows that platelet adhesiveness probably increases (Adams & Mayet, 1966). There is disagreement about whether hemostasis and coagulation are altered with age. Although fibrinogen levels tend to be increased in the elderly, evidence about hypercoagulability is inconclusive.

SUMMARY REVIEW

Components of the Hematologic System

1 Blood consists of a variety of formed elements; about 90% water and 10% solutes. In adults the total blood volume is about 5.5 L.

2 Plasma, a complex aqueous liquid, contains three major groups of plasma proteins: (1) albumins, (2) globulins, and (3) clotting factors.

3 The cellular elements of blood are the erythrocytes, leukocytes, and platelets.

4 Erythrocytes are the most abundant cells of the blood, occupying about 48% of the blood volume in men and about 42% in women. Erythrocytes are responsible for tissue oxygenation.

5 Leukocytes are fewer in number than erythrocytes and comprise about 5000 to 10,000 cells/mm³ of blood. Leukocytes defend the body against infection and remove dead or injured host cells.

6 Leukocytes are classified as either granulocytes (neutrophils, basophils, and eosinophils) or agranulocytes (monocytes, macrophages, and lymphocytes).

7 Platelets are not cells, but disk-shaped cytoplasmic fragments. Platelets are essential for blood coagulation and control of bleeding.

8 The lymphoid organs are classified as primary (thymus and bone marrow) or secondary (spleen, lymph nodes, tonsils, and Peyer's patches of the small intestine).

9 The lymphoid organs are sites of residence, proliferation, differentiation, or function of lymphocytes and mononuclear phagocytes.

10 The spleen is the largest of the secondary lymphoid organs and functions as the site of fetal hematopoiesis, filters and cleanses the blood, and is a reservoir for lymphocytes and other blood cells.

11 The lymph nodes are the site of development or activity of large numbers of lymphocytes, monocytes, and macrophages.

12 The mononuclear phagocyte system (MPS), previously called the reticuloendothelial system (RES), is composed of monoblasts, promonocytes, and monocytes in bone marrow, monocytes in peripheral blood, and macrophages in tissue.

13 The MPS is the main line of defense against bacteria in the bloodstream and cleanses the blood by removing old, injured, or dead blood cells; antigen-antibody complexes; and macromolecules.

Development of Blood Cells

1 Hematopoiesis, or blood cell production, occurs in the liver and spleen of the fetus and in the bone marrow after birth.

2 Hematopoiesis involves two stages: (1) proliferation and (2) differentiation, or maturation. Each type of blood cell has parent cells called stem cells.

3 Hematopoiesis continues throughout life to replace blood cells that grow old and die, are killed by disease, or are lost through bleeding.

4 Bone marrow consists of blood vessels, nerves, mononuclear phagocytes, stem cells, blood cells in various stages of differentiation, and fatty tissue.

5 Hemoglobin, the oxygen-carrying protein of the erythrocyte, enables the blood to transport 100 times more oxygen than could be transported dissolved in plasma alone.

6 Erythropoiesis depends on the presence of vitamins (especially vitamin B_{12} folate, B_6, riboflavin, pantothenic acid, niacin, ascorbic acid, and vitamin E).

7 Regulation of erythropoiesis is mediated by erythropoietin. Erythropoietin is secreted by the kidneys in response to tissue hypoxia and causes a compensatory increase in erythrocyte production if the oxygen content of the blood decreases because of anemia, high altitude, or pulmonary disease.

8 Maintenance of optimal levels of granulocytes and monocytes in the blood depends on the availability of pluripotential stem cells in the marrow, induction of these into committed stem cells, and timely release of new cells from the marrow.

9 The mechanism that controls retention of granulocytes is poorly understood. Granulopoietin, a plasma glycoprotein, has been discovered and may be responsible for regulation of granulocyte levels in the circulation.

10 Platelets develop from megakaryocytes by a process called endomitosis. In endomitosis, the megakaryocytes undergo mitosis but not cytokinesis, thus the cell does not divide into two daughter cells.

11 The number of platelets in the bone marrow is maintained, in part, by the action of thrombopoietin.

Mechanisms of Hemostasis

1 Hemostasis, or arrest of bleeding, involves (1) vasoconstriction (vasospasm), (2) formation of a platelet plug, (3) activation of the clotting cascade, and (4) formation of a blood clot.

2 Two properties of normal vascular endothelium prevent clotting: (1) the smooth texture of the endothelial lining that prevents adherence of platelets and (2) the negative charge of protein in the endothelial cells that repels some negatively charged platelets and clotting factors.

3 Lysis of blood clots is the function of the fibrinolytic system. Plasmin, a proteolytic enzyme, splits fibrin and fibrinogen into fibrin degradation products that dissolve the clot.

Tests of the Hematologic System

1 Tests of bone marrow function include bone marrow aspiration and bone marrow biopsy.

Aging and the Hematologic System

1 Blood composition changes little with age. A delay in erythrocyte replenishment may occur after bleeding, presumably because of iron deficiency.

2 Lymphocyte function appears to decrease with age. Particularly affected is a decrease in cellular immunity.

3 Platelet adhesiveness probably increases with age.

KEY TERMS

Agranulocyte, 758

Albumin, 755

Basophil, 760

Biconcavity, 758

Blood clot, 772

Bone marrow (myeloid tissue), 764

Clotting factor, 755

Coagulation cascade, 773

Deoxyhemoglobin (reduced hemoglobin), 766

Differentiation (maturation), 763

Eosinophil, 760

Erythroblast, 764

Erythrocyte (red blood cell [RBC], corpuscle), 757

Erythropoiesis, 764

Erythropoietin, 762

Fibrin degradation product (FDP), 776

Fibrinolytic system, 776

Globin, 765

Globulin (immunoglobulin, antibody), 755

Granulocyte, 758

Granulopoietin, 771

Hematopoiesis, 763

Heme, 765

Hemoglobin (Hb), 758

Hemostasis, 771

Immunocyte, 758

Intrinsic factor (IF), 766

Leukocyte (white blood cell), 757

Lipoprotein, 757

Lymph node, 761

Lymphocyte, 760

Macrophage, 760

Megaloblast, 765

Methemoglobin, 766

Monocyte, 760

Mononuclear phagocyte system (MPS) (reticuloendothelial system[RES]), 760

Neutrophil, 759

Normoblast, 765

Oxyhemoglobin, 766

Phagocyte, 758

Plasma, 755

Plasma protein, 755

Platelet (thrombocyte), 757

Pluripotential stem cell (pluripotential myeloid stem cell [PMSC]), 763

Primary lymphoid organ, 760

Proliferation (mitotic division), 763

Reticulocyte, 765

Reversible deformability, 758

Secondary lymphoid organ, 760

Serum, 755

Spleen, 760

Stem cell, 763

Stem cell system, 763

Totipotential hematopoietic stem cell (THSC) (multipotential stem cell), 763

Thrombopoietin, 771

Transferrin, 767

REFERENCES

Adams, E. B., & Meyet, F. G. (1966). Hypochromic anaemia in chronic infections. *South African Medical Journal, 40,* 738-740.

Anagnostou, F. W., & Kurtzman, N. A. (1981). Hematologic consequences of renal failure. In B. M. Brenner & D. C. Rector (Eds.), *The kidney* (2nd ed.). Philadelphia: W. B. Saunders.

Babior, B. M., & Stossel, T. P. (1984). *Hematology: A pathophysiological approach.* New York: Churchill-Livingstone.

Berne, R. M., & Levy, M. N. (1988). *Physiology* (2nd ed.). St. Louis: C. V. Mosby.

Bothwell, T. H., & Finch, C. A. (1962). *Iron metabolism.* Boston: Little, Brown & Co.

Breuil, J., & Obermaier, H. (1935). *The case of altumira at santillana del mar* (Madrid, Spain, Tip. de Archivos, Plate XIX). In M. W. Wintrobe (Ed.), (1980). *Blood, pure and eloquent: A story of discovery, of people, and of ideas.* New York: McGraw-Hill.

Bunn, H. F, (1977. Hemoglobin I structure and function. In W. S. Beck (Ed.). *Hematology* (2nd ed.). Cambridge, MA: MIT Press.

Burgess, A. W., & Metcalf, D. (1980). The nature and action of granulocyte-macrophage colony stimulating factors. *Blood, 56,* 947.

Byrne, C. J., et al. (1986). *Laboratory tests: Implications for nursing care.* Menlo Park, CA: Addison-Wesley.

Cook, J. D. (1982). Clinical evaluation of iron deficiency. *Seminars in Hematology, 19*(1), 6-18.

Cunningham, A. S. (1975). Eosinophil counts: Age and sex differences. *Journal of Pediatrics, 87,* 426.

Dallman, P. R. (1981, June). Iron deficiency: Diagnosis and treatment. *The Western Journal of Medicine, 134,* 496-505.

DeGabriele, G., & Penington, D. G. (1967). Physiology of the regulation of platelet production. *British Journal of Haematology, 13,* 202.

Delmonte, L., Aschkenasy, A., & Eyquem, A. (1964). Studies of the hemolytic nature of protein deficiency anemia in the rat. *Blood, 24,* 49.

Diesselhoff-den Dulk, M. M. C., Crofton, R. W., & Van Furth, R. (1979). Origin and kinetics of Kupffer cells during an acute inflammatory response. *Immunology, 37,* 7.

Donohue, D. M., Gabrio, B. W., & Finch, C. A. (1958). Quantitative measurements of hemopoietic cells of the marrow. *Journal of Clinical Investigation, 37,* 1564-1567.

Fischbach, D., & Fogdall, R. (1981). *Coagulation, the essentials.* Baltimore: Williams & Wilkins.

Fishback, F. (1984). *A manual of laboratory diagnostic tests* (2nd ed.). Philadelphia: J. B. Lippincott.

Fisher, J. W. & Langston, J. W. (1967). The influence of hypoxemia and cobalt on erythropoietin production in the isolated perfused dog kidney. *Blood, 29,* 114.

Fisher, J. W., Samuels, A. I., & Langston, J. W. (1967). Effects of angiotensin and renal artery constriction on erythropoietin production. *Journal of Pharmacological and Experimental Therapeutics, 157*(3), 618.

Fitchen, J. H., Foon, K. A., & Cline, M. J. (1981). The antigenic characteristics of hematopoietic stem cells. *New England Journal of Medicine, 305,* 17.

Flynn, K. T. (1978, November-December). Iron deficiency among the elderly. *Nurse Practitioner, 3*(6), 20-24.

Fried, W., & Morley, C. (1985, March). Update on erythropoietin. *International Journal of Artificial Organs, 8*(2), 79-82.

Guyton, A. C. (1981). *Textbook of medical physiology* (6th ed.). Philadelphia: W. B. Saunders.

Guyton, A. C. (1987). *Human physiology and mechanisms of disease* (4th ed.). Philadelphia: W. B. Saunders.

Harker, L. A. (1984). Platelet survival time: Its measurement and use. In T. H. Spaet (Ed.), *Progress in hemostasis and thrombosis* (vol. 7) pp. 321-340. New York: Grune & Stratton.

Hart, G. (1980). Ancient diseases of the blood. In M. W. Wintrobe (Ed.), *Blood pure and eloquent: A story of discovery, of people, and of ideas.* New York: McGraw-Hill.

Kadlubowski, M. (1978). The effect of in vivo aging of the human erythrocyte on the protein of the plasma membrane. A characterization. *International Journal of Biochemistry, 9*(2), 67-78.

Kadlubowski, M., & Agutter, P. S. (1977). Changes in the activities of some membrane associated enzymes during in vivo aging of the normal human erythrocyte. *British Journal of Haematology, 37*(1), 111-125.

Kinlough-Rathbone, R., Packham, M., & Mustard, F. (1983, November/December). Vessel injury, platelet adherence, and platelet survival. *Arteriosclerosis, 3*(6), 529-546.

Kruckeberg, W. C., et al. (Eds.). (1984). Erythrocyte membranes: Recent clinical and experimental advances. *Progress in Clinical and Biological Research, 159.*

Lasser, A. (1983). The mononuclear phagocyte system: A review. *Human Pathology, 24,* 108.

Lewis, R., McReynolds, L., & Penman S. (1977). Coordinate regulation of protein synthesis and messenger RNA content during growth arrest of suspension Chinese hamster ovary cells. *Journal of Cellular Physiology, 90*(3) 485-502.

Lopez, L., Duck, I. M., & Hung, W. A. (1968). On the shape of the erythrocyte. *Biophysical Journal, 8,* 1228.

MacKinney, A. A., Jr. (1978). Effect of aging on the peripheral blood lymphocyte count. *Journal of Gerontology, 33,* 213.

Maniatis, A., Tavassoli, M., & Crosby, W. H. (1971). Factors affecting the conversion of yellow to red marrow. *Blood, 37,* 581.

Metcalf, D., Johnson, G. R., & Burgess, A. W. (1980). Direct stimulation by purified GM-CSF of the proliferation of multipotential and erythroid precursor cells. *Blood, 55,* 138.

Nathan, C. F., et al. (1980). The macrophage as an effector cell. *New England Journal of Medicine, 303,* 622.

Nemerson, Y. (1983, May-June). Regulation of the initiation of coagulation by factor VII. *Haemostasis, 13*(3), 150-155.

Packham, M., & Mustard, J. F. (1978). Platelet adhesion. In T. H. Spaet (Ed.), *Progress in hemostasis and thrombosis* (vol. 4) (pp. 211-267). New York: Grune & Stratton.

Peschle, C., Marone, G., Genovese A., Rappaport, I. A., & Condorelli, M. (1976). Increased erythropoietin production in anephric rats with hyperplasia of the reticuloendothelial system induced by colloidal carbon or zymosan. *Blood, 47,* 325.

Price, G. B., & McCullough, E. A. (1978). Cell surfaces and the regulation of hematopoiesis. *Seminars in Hematology, 15,* 283.

Prydz, H. (1983, May-June). The role of factor VII in the intrinsic pathway: A brief review. *Haemostasis, 13*(3), 156-160.

Purtilo, D. T. (1978). *A survey of human diseases.* Menlo Park, CA: Addison-Wesley.

Raven, P.H., & Johnson, G. B. (1989). *Biology.* (2nd ed.). St. Louis: Times Mirror/Mosby.

Rich, I. N., & Kubanek, B. (1982). Release of erythropoietin from macrophages mediated by phagocytons of crystalline silica. *Journal of Reticulo-endothelial Science, 31,* 17.

Robbins, S., Cotran, R. S., & Kumar, V. (1984). *Pathologic basis of disease* (3rd ed.). Philadelphia: W. B. Saunders.

Russell, W. J., Yoshinaga, H., Shigetoshi, A., & Mizuno, M. (1966). Active bone marrow distribution in the adult. *British Journal of Radiology, 39,* 735.

Sakagami, T., Minari, D., & Orii, T. (1965). Interaction of individual phospholipids between rat plasma and erythrocytes in vitro. *Biochimica et Biophysica Acta, 98,* 356-364.

Schumacher, H. R., Garvin, D. F., & Triplett, D. A. (1984). *Introduction to laboratory hematology and hematopathology.* New York: Alan R. Liss.

Shand, F. L., & Bell, E. B. (1972). Studies on the distribution of macrophages derived from rat bone marrow cells in xenogenic radiation chimaeras. *Immunology, 22,* 549.

Siskind, G.W. (1987). Aging and the immune system. In H. R. Warner, R. N. Butler, R. L. Sprott, & E. L. Schneider, (eds) *Modern biological theories of aging.* New York: Raven Press.

Thibodeau, G. A. (1987). *Anatomy and physiology.* St. Louis: Times Mirror/Mosby.

Vander, A. J., Sherman, J. H., & Luchiano, D. S. (1980). *Human physiology: The mechanisms of body function.*

Vick, R. L. (1984). *Contemporary medical physiology.* Menlo Park, CA: Addison-Wesley.

Williams, N. (1979). Preferential inhibitions of murine macrophage colony formation by prostaglandin E. *Blood, 53,* 1089.

Williams, W., Beutler, E., Erslev, A., & Lichtman, M. (1983). *Hematology* (3rd ed.). New York: McGraw-Hill.

Wintrobe, M. M. (1986). *Hematology, the blossoming of a science: A story of inspiration and effort.* Philadelphia: Lea & Febiger.

Wintrobe, M. M., Lee, G. R., Boggs, D. R., Bithell, T. C., Foerster, J., Athens J. W., & Lukens J. N. (1981). *Clinical hematology* (8th ed.). Philadelphia: Lea & Febiger.

Wintrobe, M. M. (Ed.). (1980). *Blood pure and eloquent: A story of discovery, of people, and of ideas.* New York: McGraw-Hill.

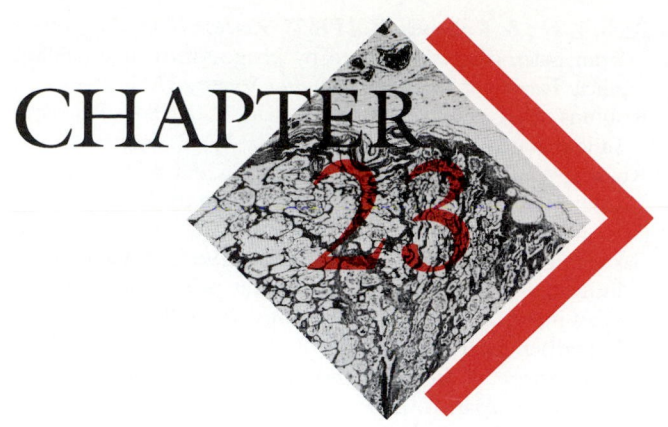

CHAPTER 23

Alterations of Erythrocyte Function

Pamela D. Parker-Cohen
Kathryn L. McCance

Anemia, 784
    Classification of anemias, 784
    Clinical manifestations of anemias, 785
    Macrocytic-normochromic anemias, 788
      Pernicious anemia, 788
        Pathophysiology, 788
        Clinical manifestations, 788
        Evaluation and treatment, 789
      Folate deficiency anemias, 789
    Microcytic-hypochromic anemias, 789
      Iron deficiency anemia, 789
        Pathophysiology, 789
        Clinical manifestations, 790
        Evaluation and treatment, 790
      Sideroblastic anemia, 790
        Pathophysiology, 790
        Clinical manifestations, 791
        Evaluation and treatment, 791
    Normocytic-normochromic anemias, 791
      Aplastic anemia, 791
        Pathophysiology, 791
        Clinical manifestations, 791
        Evaluation and treatment, 791
      Posthemorrhagic anemia, 792
      Hemolytic anemia, 792
        Pathophysiology, 792
        Clinical manifestations, 792
        Evaluation and treatment, 793
      Anemia of chronic disease, 794
        Pathophysiology, 795
        Clinical manifestations, 795
        Evaluation and treatment, 795
    Myeloproliferative red cell disorders (polycythemia vera), 796
      Pathophysiology, 796
      Clinical manifestations, 797
      Evaluation and treatment, 797

Alterations of erythrocyte function involve either insufficient or excessive numbers of erythrocytes in the circulation or normal numbers of cells with abnormal components. Anemias are conditions in which there are too few erythrocytes or an insufficient volume of erythrocytes in the blood. Polycythemias are conditions in which erythrocyte numbers or volume are excessive. Each of these two conditions has many causes, which is why each has so many names. Anemia and polycythemia are not diseases per se, but rather they are pathophysiologic manifestations of a variety of disease states.

ANEMIA

Strictly speaking, **anemia** is a reduction in the total number of circulating erythrocytes or a decrease in the quality or quantity of hemoglobin. Anemic conditions are usually a result of (1) impaired erythrocyte production, (2) blood loss, (3) increased erythrocyte destruction, or (4) a combination of the three.

Classification of Anemias

Anemias are classified in many ways, and no one system of classification is best or most clear. The most common classification of anemias is based on cellular morphology or structure. Descriptions of anemias based on erythrocyte morphology refer to the cell's size and hemoglobin content. Because all anemias can be described with respect to these two cellular features, the morphologic classification is widely used (Table 23-1). Terms that refer to cellular size end with "cytic," whereas terms that describe hemoglobin content end with "chromic." An erythrocyte can be **macrocytic** (abnormally large) or **microcytic** (abnormally small); **hy-**

TABLE 23-1 Morphologic classification of anemias

Morphology and cause of reduced oxygen-carrying capacity of the blood	Name and mechanism of anemic condition	Primary cause of associated disorder
Macrocytic-normochromic anemia: large, abnormally shaped erythrocytes but normal hemoglobin concentrations	Pernicious anemia: lack of vitamin B_{12} (cobalamin) for erythropoiesis; abnormal DNA and RNA synthesis in the erythroblast; premature cell death	Congenital or acquired deficiency of intrinsic factor (IF); genetic disorder of DNA synthesis
	Folate-deficiency anemia: lack of folate for erythropoiesis; premature cell death	Dietary folate deficiency
Microcytic hypochromic anemia: small, abnormally shaped erythrocytes and reduced hemoglobin concentration	Iron-deficiency anemia: lack of iron for hemoglobin production; insufficient hemoglobin	Chronic blood loss; dietary iron deficiency, disruption of iron metabolism or iron cycle (see Chapter 22)
	Sideroblastic anemia: dysfunctional iron uptake by erythroblasts and defective porphyrin and heme synthesis	Congenital dysfunction of iron metabolism in erythroblasts, acquired dysfunction of iron metabolism as a result of drugs or toxins
	Thalassemia: impaired synthesis of α or β chain of hemoglobin A; phagocytosis of abnormal erythroblasts in the marrow (see Chapter 27)	Congenital genetic defect of globin synthesis
Normocytic-normochromic anemia: destruction or depletion of normal erythroblasts or mature erythrocytes	Aplasic anemia: insufficient erythropoiesis	Depressed stem cell proliferation resulting in bone marrow aplasia
	Posthemorrhagic anemia: blood loss	Acute or chronic hemorrhage that stimulates increased erythropoiesis, which eventually depletes body iron
	Hemolytic anemia: premature destruction (lysis) of mature erythrocytes in the circulation	Any condition that increases fragility of erythrocytes
	Sickle cell anemia: abnormal hemoglobin synthesis, abnormal cell shape with susceptibility to damage, lysis, and phagocytosis	Congenital dysfunction of hemoglobin synthesis
	Anemia of chronic disease: abnormally increased demand for new erythrocytes	Chronic infection or inflammation; malignancy

perchromic (containing an unusually high concentration of hemoglobin within its cytoplasm) or **hypochromic** (containing an abnormally low concentration of hemoglobin). For comparison, cells of normal size are termed **normocytic,** and cells with normal amounts of hemoglobin are termed **normochromic.** In some anemias, the erythrocytes take on various sizes (**anisocytosis**) or they have various shapes (**poikilocytosis**) (Fig. 23-1).

Clinical Manifestations of Anemias

The number and severity of symptoms caused by anemia depend on the body's ability to compensate for the reduced oxygen-carrying capacity of the blood. If the anemia is mild and its onset is gradual, compensation may be so successful that the individual is asymptomatic except during periods of physical exertion. Although anemia may manifest itself in many organs and systems, compensation generally involves the cardiovascular, respiratory, and hematologic systems. Hematologic findings in various anemias are listed in Table 23-2.

A reduction in the number of circulating erythrocytes, such as seen after hemorrhage, affects the consistency and volume of the blood. To compensate for reduced blood volume, fluids from the interstitium move into the blood vessels, and plasma volume expands. Al-

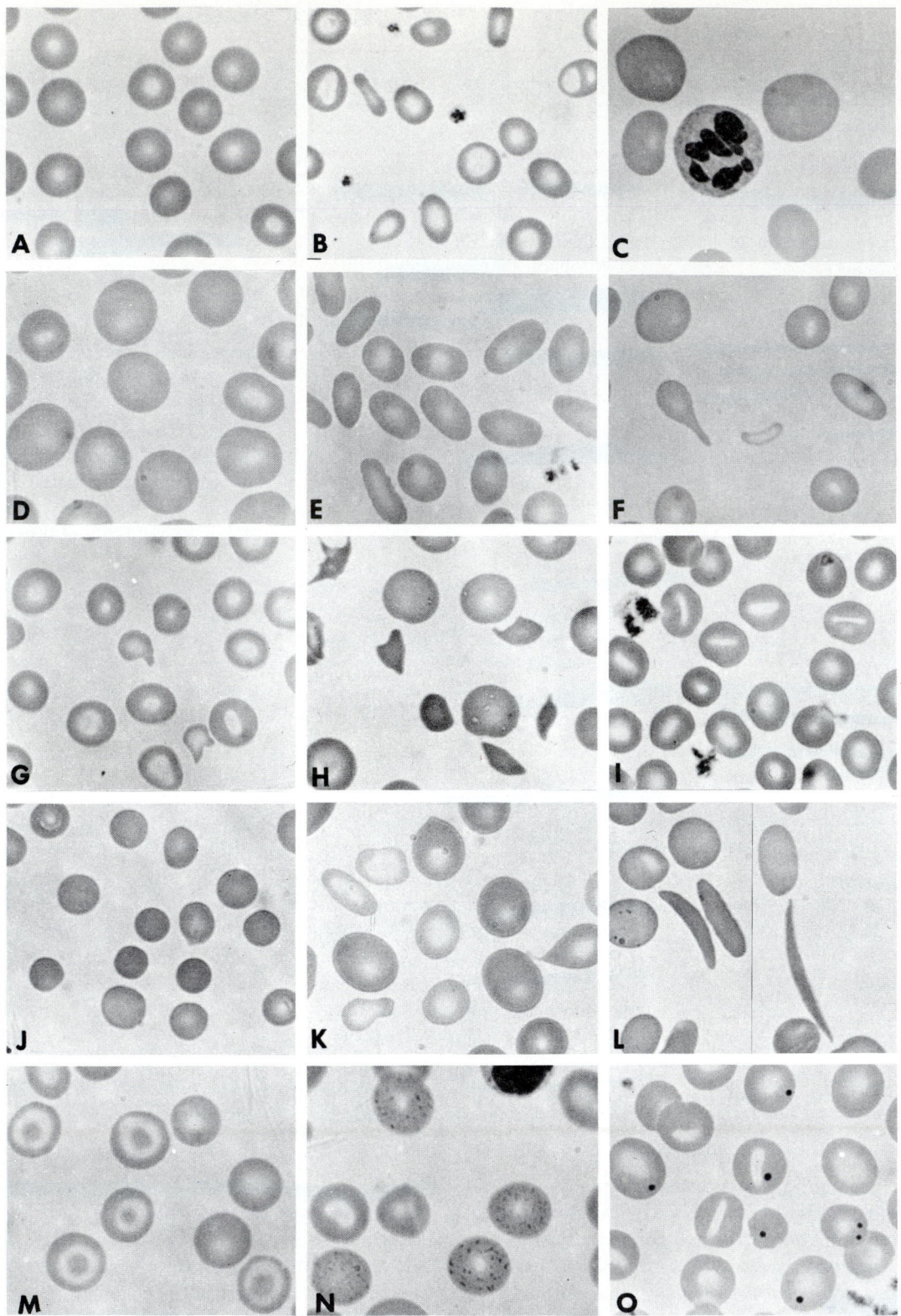

FIG. 23-1. Appearance of red blood cells in various disorders. **A,** Normal blood smear. **B,** Hypochromic microcytic anemia (iron deficiency). **C,** Macrocytic anemia (pernicious anemia). **D,** Macrocytic anemia in pregnancy. **E,** Hereditary elliptocytosis. **F,** Myelofibrosis (teardrop). **G,** Hemolytic anemia associated with prosthetic heart valve. **H,** Microangiopathic anemia. **I,** Stromatocytes. **J,** Spherocytes (hereditary spherocytosis). **K,** Sideroblastic anemia; note the double population of red blood cells. **L,** Sickle cell anemia. **M,** Target cells (after splenectomy). **N,** Basophil strippling in case of unexplained anemia. **O,** Howell-Jolly bodies (after splenectomy). (From Wintrobe et al., 1981.)

TABLE 23-2 Laboratory findings for various anemias

Test	Pernicious anemia	Folate deficiency anemia	Iron deficiency anemia	Sideroblastic anemia	Aplastic anemia	Posthemorrhagic anemia	Hemolytic anemia	Anemia of chronic disease
Hemoglobin	Low	Low	Low	Low	Low/ normal	Normal/low	Low	Low
Hematocrit	Low	Low	Low	Low	Low/ normal	Normal/low	Low	Low
Reticulocyte count	Low	Low	Normal or slightly high or low	Normal or slightly high	Low	Increased	High	Normal
Mean corpuscular volume	High	High	Low	Low	Normal or slightly high	Slightly low	Normal or high	Normal or low
Plasma iron	High	High	Low	High	High	Normal	Normal or high	Low
Total iron-binding capacity	Normal	Normal	High	Normal	Normal	Normal	Normal	Low
Ferritin	High	High	Low	High	Normal	Normal	Normal	Normal
Serum B_{12}	Low	Normal	Normal	Normal	Normal	Normal	Normal	Normal
Folate	Normal	Low	Normal	Normal	Normal	Normal	Normal	Normal
Bilirubin	Slightly high	Slightly high	Normal	High	Normal	Normal	Slightly high	Normal
Free erythrocyte protoporphyrin	Normal	Normal	High	Increased or normal	High	Normal	Normal	Normal or slightly high
Transferrin	Slightly high	Slightly high	Low	High	Normal	Normal	Normal	Slightly low

though this compensatory mechanism maintains adequate blood volume, it decreases the viscosity (thickness) of the blood. The "diluted" blood flows faster and more turbulently than normal blood. Increased blood flow within the heart can cause ventricular dysfunction, cardiac dilation, and heart valve insufficiency. Some cardiovascular manifestations of anemia are due to hypoxia, which causes arterioles, capillaries, and venules to dilate, speeding blood flow even further. As venous return to the heart increases, the heart must pump harder and faster to prevent cardiopulmonary congestion. All of these mechanisms of cardiovascular compensation can cause congestive heart failure. (Mechanisms of congestive heart failure are described in Chapter 27.)

Tissue hypoxia has other effects on the heart and lungs. The rate and depth of breathing increase in an attempt to make more oxygen available to the remaining erythrocytes. Cardiac output increases to handle the increased venous return and speed the remaining oxygen-carrying erythrocytes to and from hypoxic tissue cells. Hemoglobin in the erythrocytes releases its oxygen more readily than usual at the tissue level. (Mechanisms of oxygen transport and release by hemoglobin are described in Chapter 29.)

If anemia is severe enough to overcome the usual compensatory mechanisms, the individual will experience shortness of breath (dyspnea), a rapid pounding heartbeat, dizziness, and fatigue, even at rest.

When anemia is severe or sudden in onset, peripheral blood vessels constrict so as to direct available blood flow chiefly to the vital organs. A number of systemic symptoms result from this lifesaving maneuver. Decreased blood flow is sensed by the kidneys and in an effort to improve kidney perfusion, the renal renin-angiotensin response is activated, resulting in salt and water retention. The skin, mucous membranes, lips, nailbeds, and conjunctivae become pale as a result of reduced hemoglobin concentration; or yellowish as a result of the presence of products of red blood cell breakdown (**hemolysis**). Decreased oxygen delivery to the skin results in impaired healing and loss of elasticity, as well as thinning and early graying of the hair. If the anemia is due to vitamin B_{12} deficiency, the nervous system is affected. Myelin degeneration may occur with loss of nerve fibers in the spinal cord. Paresthesias (numbness), gait disturbances, extreme weakness, spasticity, and reflex abnormalities can result. Decreased oxygen supply to the gastrointestinal tract often produces abdominal pain, nausea, vomiting, and anorexia. Low-grade fever (less than 101° F) occurs in some anemic individuals and may be the result of leukocyte pyrogens being released from ischemic tissues.

Therapeutic intervention for any anemic condition calls for treatment of the underlying disorder and palliation of symptoms. Therapies for anemia include transfusions, dietary corrections, and administration of supplemental vitamins or iron.

Macrocytic-Normochromic Anemias

The **macrocytic anemias,** also termed megaloblastic anemias, are characterized by unusually large stem cells (megaloblasts) in the marrow that mature into unusually large erythrocytes (macrocytes) in the circulation. Megaloblastic stem cells are larger at all maturational stages than normal stem cells (normoblasts). In addition, the nucleus of the megaloblast is disproportionately small in relation to the size of the cell. As the cell matures and begins to synthesize hemoglobin, chromatin in the nucleus fails to clump normally. Hemoglobin content is normal, however. The macrocytic anemias are morphologically classified as macrocytic-normochromic anemias (see Table 23-1).

Defective DNA synthesis, usually caused by deficiences of vitamin B_{12} or folate, produces a pattern of ineffective erythropoiesis in the macrocytic anemias. The cause of these anemias is premature cell death with reduced numbers of mature erythrocytes as a result of ineffective erythropoiesis.

It is unknown why a deficiency of cobalamin or folate causes ineffective erythropoiesis and premature cell death. Suggested mechanisms include a delay in nuclear maturation and an imbalance in the normal distribution of ribonucleic acid (RNA) and deoxyribonucleic acid (DNA) (Wintrobe et al., 1981). Nuclear functions or DNA replication and cell division are blocked or delayed. RNA and protein synthesis, both cytoplasmic functions, proceed normally. The imbalance in the RNA/DNA ratio causes derangement of cell growth.

Pernicious Anemia

Pernicious anemia, the most common type of megaloblastic anemia, is a chronic condition caused by malabsorption of vitamin B_{12} (Fig. 23-1, *C*). The term per-

nicious means highly injurious or destructive and reflects the fact that this condition was once fatal. Pernicious anemia is most common in late adult life and rare in individuals younger than 30, except in the congenital type that usually occurs before 2 years of age. Pernicious anemia is most common among Scandinavian, English, and Irish peoples. In Great Britain and Scandinavia, women are more commonly affected than men. In the United States, both sexes appear to be equally affected.

Pathophysiology

The underlying disorder in pernicious anemia is defective gastric secretion of intrinsic factor (IF), which is necessary for absorption of vitamin B_{12}. Vitamin B_{12} is in turn necessary for nuclear maturation and DNA synthesis in red blood cells. Pernicious anemias can be due to a congenital deficiency of IF alone or to adult-onset atrophy of the gastric mucosa that causes deficiencies of all gastric secretions including IF. Partial or complete surgical excision of the stomach (gastrectomy) will also produce a deficiency of IF.

The specific cause of the gastric atrophy that results in IF deficiency in adult-onset pernicious anemia is unknown. A genetic predisposition is probable, but because of the late age of onset certain precipitating environmental agents are thought to interact with the genetic defect. Evidence suggests that the congenital type of pernicious anemia is an autosomal recessive trait (Sullivan, 1970). Because the risk of developing pernicious anemia is greatest in individuals whose family members have had the disorder, some inherited mechanism is postulated. Siblings of affected persons are at highest risk.

Conditions associated with development of pernicious anemia include immunologic aberrations, chronic gastritis, and gastrectomy. Autoantibodies against parietal cells, IF, and thyroid tissues have been found in the serum of individuals with pernicious anemia. Chronic fundal gastritis destroys glandular structures and diminishes gastric secretion of IF, hydrochloric acid, and pepsin. Impaired vitamin B_{12} absorption parallels the progress of gastric atrophy.

Pernicious anemia affects both erythrocyte and leukocyte precursors in the marrow. Platelet precursors are less affected. The number and size of all developing erythroid cells increase, and enormous leukocytes with large and unusual shaped nuclei are found. Hematopoietic alterations vary depending on the degree of cobalamin deficiency and metabolic causes leading to the anemia.

Clinical Manifestations

Pernicious anemia develops slowly. By the time it is diagnosed, it is usually severe. Vague early symptoms often are ignored by the individual, including infections, mood swings, and gastrointestinal, cardiac, or kidney ailments. When the hemoglobin has decreased significantly (7 to 8 g/dl), the individual experiences the classic symptoms of anemia: weakness, fatigue, paresthesias of feet and fingers, sore tongue, loss of appetite, abdominal pain, weight loss, and difficulty walking.

Evaluation and Treatment

Evaluation is based on blood tests (see Table 23-2), bone marrow aspiration, clinical manifestations, and the Schilling test. In the Schilling test cobalamin absorption is measured indirectly by administering radioactive cobalamin and measuring its excretion in the urine.

Untreated pernicious anemia is fatal, usually because of heart failure. Death occurs after a course of remissions and exacerbations lasting from 1 to 3 years. Since the advent in 1926 of replacement therapy with vitamin B$_{12}$, mortality has decreased significantly. Today, death caused by pernicious anemia is rare, and relapses are caused primarily by the individual's noncompliance with therapy.

Treatment for pernicious anemia and other anemias caused by cobalamin deficiency is the administration of cobalamin. Cyanocobalamin or hydroxocobalamin are administered intramuscularly or subcutaneously approximately once a month (weekly until the deficiency is corrected). Oral preparations are poorly absorbed. The effectiveness of cobalamin replacement therapy is manifested by a rising reticulocyte count. Within 5 to 6 weeks, blood counts can return to normal. Pernicious anemia cannot be cured, so maintenance therapy must continue for life. Blood transfusions are given if the individual shows signs of circulatory collapse, heart failure, or severe angina pectoris.

Folate Deficiency Anemias

Folate (folic acid) is a vitamin essential to erythrocyte production and maturation. Folate is necessary for DNA synthesis, being a component of three of the four DNA bases (that is, thymine, adenine, and guanine). Folic acid is also required for RNA synthesis. Absorption of folate occurs primarily in the upper small intestine and does not depend on IF. Folate circulates through and is stored in the liver. Deficiency of folate is more common than cobalamin deficiency, especially in alcoholics and other chronically malnourished individuals. Folate stores are depleted more rapidly than cobalamin stores. Without proper dietary intake of folate, megaloblastic anemia will develop.

Clinical manifestations are similar to those of pernicious anemia, except for the lack of neurologic symptoms associated with folate deficiency. Evaluation is based on blood tests, measurement of serum folate levels, and clinical manifestations.

Treatment of folate deficiency anemia requires administration of oral folate preparations daily. One mg per day is sufficient for most individuals, although alcoholics may require 5 mg. Alcohol interferes with folate metabolism in the liver and results in profound depletion of folate stores (Wintrobe et al., 1981). Prophylactic doses of 0.1 to 0.4 mg/day are sometimes given in pregnancy. Parenteral administration of folic acid can relieve acute symptoms within 48 hours. Blood transfusions are given to treat severe cardiac or respiratory distress.

Microcytic-Hypochromic Anemias

The microcytic-hypochromic anemias are characterized by erythrocytes that are abnormally small and contain abnormally reduced amounts of hemoglobin (Fig. 23-1, *B*). Hypochromia occurs even in cells of normal size.

Microcytic-hypochromic anemia can result from a variety of conditions that are due to (1) disorders of iron metabolism, (2) disorders of porphyrin and heme synthesis, or (3) disorders of globin synthesis. Specific disorders include iron deficiency anemia, sideroblastic anemia, and thalassemia.

Iron Deficiency Anemia

There are several interesting historic tales about iron deficiency anemia (Wintrobe et al., 1981). The Greek mythologic character, Iphiclus, supposedly drank iron rust dissolved in wine and thereby was cured of impotence. From the sixteenth through the early nineteenth centuries, adolescent girls suffered a malady called chlorosis ("green sickness") that caused a greenish pallor associated with palpitations, breathlessness, ankle edema, thrombophlebitis, and diffuse gastrointestinal complaints. Around 1830, scientists defined chlorosis as a disease of the blood characterized by anemia and lack of iron. Pierre Blaud became famous by successfully treating affected individuals with a combination of ferrous sulfate and potassium carbonate (Haden, 1938). Between 1890 and 1920, the incidence of chlorosis decreased dramatically, not because of iron therapy but because women stopped wearing tight-fitting corsets. Apparently, tight-fitting garments compressed the liver and other abdominal organs or induced reflux of stomach contents, causing blood loss resulting from esophageal inflammation. Women who wore corsets may also have had restricted dietary intake in the pursuit of the fashionably small waist.

Pathophysiology

Bleeding is the usual cause of **iron deficiency anemia,** although inadequate dietary intake is also a problem in impoverished populations. A daily blood loss of 2 to 4 ml/day is sufficient to cause this anemia (Wintrobe et al., 1981). In men gastrointestinal bleeding is most common and may be due to gastric or duodenal ulcers, hiatal hernia, esophageal varices, cirrhosis, hemorrhoids, ulcerative colitis, or carcinoma. In women menorrhagia (profuse menstruation) and pregnancy are reasons for primary iron deficiency anemia. Other causes in both sexes are (1) use of medications that cause gastrointestinal bleeding; (2) surgical procedures that decrease stomach acidity, intestinal transit time, and absorption; (3) insufficient dietary intake of iron; and (4) eating disorders such as pica, the craving and eating of nonnutritional substances. Iron deficiency is common in children less than 2 years of age because of greatly increased iron requirements associated with growth.

Iron deficiency anemia develops slowly through three overlapping stages. In stage I, the body's iron stores for erythropoiesis are depleted. At this stage, erythropoiesis remains normal as does the hemoglobin content of the maturing erythrocytes. In stage II, however, not enough iron is transported to the marrow, and iron-deficient erythropoiesis begins. Stage III begins when the small, hemoblobin-deficient cells enter the circulation in sufficient numbers, replacing normal erythrocytes that have grown old and have been removed from the circulation. The development of iron deficiency anemia occurs in stage III and is associated with depleted transport of iron stores and diminished hemoglobin production.

Clinical Manifestations

The onset of symptoms is gradual, and individuals usually do not seek medical attention until hemoglobin levels drop to a certain point (about 7 to 8 g/dl). Fatigue, weakness, and shortness of breath are common symptoms (see p. 785). Pale ear lobes, palms, and conjunctivae are common signs.

Structurally or functionally altered epithelial tissue is often found in individuals with iron deficiency anemia. The nails become brittle, thin, and "spoon-shaped" or concave as a result of impaired capillary circulation. The tongue may be sore, with redness and burning caused by atrophy of the papillae. These changes can be reversed after 1 to 2 weeks of iron replacement. Changes also occur in the epithelium at the corners of the mouth, causing soreness and dryness. This defect is called angular stomatitis. Difficulty swallowing is often associated with a "web" of mucous and inflammatory cells at the juncture between the hypopharynx and esophagus. These lesions may become malignant. The pathophysiology of the epithelial changes is unclear.

Since iron is a component of compounds other than hemoglobin (e.g., cytochromes, myoglobin, catalase), deficiencies probably alter several tissue enzymes. Deficient iron enzymes may cause many of the clinical manifestations. Individuals with iron deficiency anemia also exhibit gastritis, neuromuscular changes, irritability, headache, numbness, tingling, and vasomotor disturbances. The pathogenesis of neurologic symptoms is unknown but may be caused by hypoxia in already compromised cerebral vessels. Gait disturbances are rare. Mental confusion, memory loss, and disorientation are frequently associated with anemia in the elderly and may be overlooked as "normal" changes caused by aging.

Evaluation and Treatment

Evaluation is based on clinical manifestations and laboratory tests (see Table 23-2). Iron stores are measured directly, by bone marrow biopsy, or indirectly, by tests that measure serum ferritin, transferrin saturation, or total iron-binding capacity. A sensitive indicator of heme synthesis is the amount of free erythrocyte protoporphyrin (FEP) within erythrocytes.

The first step in treatment of iron deficiency anemia is to find and eliminate, or rule out, sources of blood loss. Without this strategy, any pharmacologic therapy will simply be palliative. Iron replacement is very effective in the treatment of iron deficiency anemia. In fact, the most conclusive evidence for the diagnosis of iron deficiency anemia is an increase in hemoglobin of 1 to 2 g/dl after iron therapy is initiated. Iron preparations can be administered orally, intramuscularly, or intravenously. Oral administration of ferrous sulfate, gluconate, or fumarate that provides about 200 mg of elemental iron daily is effective. Side effects of oral iron preparations include a change in stool color to green or black. Iron frequently produces loose stools but constipation is occasionally seen. Once iron therapy has been instituted, individuals often show a rapid decrease in fatigue, lethargy, and other symptoms. Two thirds of the hemoglobin deficit is generally corrected within the first month of therapy, regardless of the severity of the anemia (Dallman, 1981). Therapy is usually continued for 6 to 12 months after bleeding has been contained. For menstruating women, daily therapy may be needed until menopause. An increase in reticulocyte count is a good measure of response to iron therapy.

Sideroblastic Anemia

Sideroblastic anemia is a microcytic-hypochromic anemia resulting from abnormal erythropoiesis. The chief defect is the sequestration of iron complexes in the mitochondria of erythroblasts, transforming the erythroblasts into **sideroblasts** (Fig. 23-1, K).

Pathophysiology

The inherited form of sideroblastic anemia may be due to a recessive X-linked trait. This condition, however, is rare. Idiopathic sideroblastic anemia is less rare and usually affects elderly persons. The idiopathic form can "convert" to acute myeloblastic leukemia. Secondary sideroblastic anemia is caused by drugs or toxins, such as ethanol, isoniazid, chloramphenicol, phenylbutazone, antineoplastic medications, and lead.

Anemia occurs when hemoglobin levels in the circulation fall as a result of interruption of the iron cycle by iron sequestration in sideroblasts. Formation of small, hypochromic erythrocytes of various sizes and shapes (anisocytosis and poikilocytosis) occurs, and destruction of defective erythroblasts by phagocytes residing in the marrow is seen. Low hemoglobin levels stimulate erythropoiesis, which causes the marrow to become grossly hyperplastic and perpetuates the anemia.

Clinical Manifestations

In addition to the cardiovascular and respiratory manifestations common to all anemias (see p. 785), sideroblastic anemia causes mild-to-moderate enlargement of the liver (hepatomegaly) and spleen (splenomegaly) and, occasionally, abnormal skin pigmentation (bronze-tinted) related to iron overload. Other epithelial manifestations and all neurologic manifestations are absent.

Evaluation and Treatment

At first, sideroblastic anemia may be mistaken for deficiency of stem cells in the marrow (**hypoplastic anemia**) or iron deficiency anemia. (Laboratory findings are listed in Table 23-2.) Bone marrow examination establishes the diagnosis of sideroblastic anemia. The marrow is packed with erythrocyte stem cells, and mononuclear phagocytes in the marrow are loaded with iron in the form of hemosiderin. Presence of sideroblasts, the erythrocyte precursors with a necklace-like ring of iron granules around the nucleus, confirms the diagnosis of sideroblastic anemia.

Treatment and management of sideroblastic anemia is straightforward. If the anemia results from a drug or noxious substance, the offending treatment is discontinued or the substance is avoided. Pyridoxine therapy is sometimes beneficial. *Iron is not given.* Blood transfusions are limited to prevent hemochromatosis (an accumulation of iron in tissues), which would result in cellular damage. The course and prognosis of sideroblastic anemia are variable. Death may occur because of infection, bone marrow failure, liver failure, or cardiac dysrhythmias.

Normocytic-Normochromic Anemias

Normocytic-normochromic anemias are anemias in which erythrocytes are relatively normal in size and hemoglobin content but insufficient in number. The normocytic-normochromic anemias do not share any common cause, pathologic mechanism, or morphologic characteristics. These anemias are less common than the macrocytic-normochromic and microcytic-hypochromic anemias. Five distinct anemic conditions—aplastic anemia, posthemorrhagic anemia, hemolytic anemia, anemia of chronic disease, and sickle cell anemia—exemplify the diversity of the normocytic-normochromic classification.

Aplastic Anemia

Aplastic anemia is due to **bone marrow hypoplasia or aplasia,** conditions in which hematopoietic marrow or erythrocyte stem cells are underdeveloped, defective, or absent. Many disease processes interfere temporarily or permanently with the viability of the pluripotential stem cell. Reduction in numbers of pluripotential stem cells or their ability to become committed stem cells causes reduced hematopoiesis. If all the cell lines are affected, all cellular components of circulating blood are reduced. A life-threatening condition known as **pancytopenia** results. If only the erythrocyte stem cells are affected, the condition in the marrow is termed **pure red cell aplasia** and in the circulation is called aplastic anemia.

Pathophysiology

Pure red cell aplasia has many possible causes: infiltrative disorders of the bone marrow (myelofibrosis, leukemia, myeloma, or carcinoma); autoimmune diseases; renal failure; splenic dysfunction; cobalamin or folate deficiency; infection; and exposure to radiation, drugs, and toxins.

The exact mechanism that halts erythropoiesis is not known, but two theories have been proposed. The first, called the seed or stem cell-deficiency theory, proposes that a common stem cell population is irreversibly altered, rendering it incapable of proliferation and differentiation. The second theory, the microenvironmental deficiency theory, proposes that the stem cell environment (i.e., the marrow) is altered so as to inhibit erythropoiesis (Wintrobe et al., 1981).

If the erythrocyte stem cells or the marrow is unable to recover from the insult within months, bone marrow aplasia leads to death from anemia, infection, or hemorrhage. If the insult is mild, causing bone marrow hypoplasia, anemia is less severe and the individual may live for years.

Clinical Manifestations

Aplastic anemia causes the classic cardiovascular and respiratory manifestations of anemia. If the stem cells of platelets and leukocytes also are damaged or deficient, anemia is accompanied by platelet deficiency (thrombocytopenia), which results in hemorrhage into the tissues and leukocyte deficiency (leukopenia), and infection.

Evaluation and Treatment

Bone marrow biopsy is necessary to determine whether the anemia is due to pure red cell aplasia or hypoplasia (see Table 23-2).

The most important aspect of treatment for aplastic

anemia is to treat the underlying disorder or prevent further exposure to the causal agent. Hemoglobin levels can be improved temporarily with blood transfusions. Definitive treatment is marrow transplant or pharmacologic stimulation of the marrow function. Hemorrhage or infection is treated as needed. Splenectomy is considered if transfused erythrocytes are being destroyed in the spleen.

Posthemorrhagic Anemia

Posthemorrhagic anemia is a normocytic-normochromic anemia caused by sudden blood loss in an individual with normal iron stores. Hemorrhage may be obvious (after surgery or before trauma) or occult, such as that caused by malignancy or gastrointestinal disorders. Minor prolonged hemorrhage does not result in classic posthemorrhagic anemia, but rather in iron deficiency anemia—a microcytic-hypochromic anemia (see p. 789).

Within 24 hours of blood loss, the body begins to replace lost plasma and blood cells. Water and electrolytes from tissues and interstitial spaces are mobilized to expand plasma volume and accelerate hematopoiesis. Clinical manifestations of anemia are likely to be obscured by the cardiovascular manifestations of acute hemorrhage. Severe shock, lactic acidosis, and death can occur if blood loss exceeds 40% to 50% of plasma volume.

Treatment entails restoring blood volume by intravenous administration of saline, dextran, albumin, or plasma. For large blood losses, transfusion of fresh whole blood is the treatment of choice. The anemia itself does not require specific therapy unless it is associated with iron, folate, or cobalamin deficiency. A normal erythrocyte count is usually evident in 4 to 6 weeks, but hemoglobin restoration can take 6 to 8 weeks.

Hemolytic Anemia

Premature, accelerated destruction of erythrocytes is a clinical manifestation of many diseases. In **hemolytic anemias,** however, premature red cell destruction is the predominant pathogenic event (Fig. 23-1, *G*). Erythropoiesis is normal; the cause of the decreased hemoglobin in the blood is an abnormally short erythrocyte life span, as many as 100 days shorter than normal. Erythropoiesis accelerates to compensate for hemolysis, but production cannot keep up with destruction.

Pathophysiology

Hemolytic anemias may be acquired or hereditary. Acquired hemolytic anemias are generally caused by extrinsic (extracellular) defects, such as infection, systemic disease, drugs or toxins, liver disease, kidney disease, or abnormal immune responses. Hereditary forms are due to intrinsic (cellular) abnormalities, typically of the erythrocyte's plasma membrane or cytoplasmic contents (enzymes of hemoglobin). Congenital hemolytic ane-

mias are present at birth and may or may not be inherited. Causes of acquired and inherited hemolytic anemias are listed in Table 23-3.

Hemolysis occurs within blood vessels or in lymphoid tissues that filter the blood. Hemolysis that occurs within the vessels tends to be caused by chemicals (drugs or toxins), antibodies, or erythrocyte fragility. Hemolysis within lymphoid tissues is mostly due to phagocytosis by macrophages of the mononuclear phagocyte system (MPS).

Autoimmune hemolytic anemias, all of which are acquired forms, consist of warm antibody disease, cold antibody disease, and drug-induced anemia. Hemolysis occurs within blood vessels. **Warm antibody disease** is mediated by immunoglobulin (IgG antibody) that is specific for erythrocyte antigens and binds to the surface of the erythrocyte at normal body temperature (37° C). The antibody can activate the complement cascade, resulting in intravascular destruction of the erythrocyte. Chronic anemia caused by warm antibody disease is frequently observed in association with other diseases, including chronic lymphocytic leukemia, lymphoid tumors, and systemic lupus erythematosus.

Cold antibody disease is mediated by a different immunoglobulin (IgM) specific for erythrocyte antigens. The IgM binds to erythrocytes only at colder temperatures (below 31° C), which may occur in the fingers and toes during cold weather. Agglutination of IgM-bound erythrocytes in the extremities produces pain and tissue destruction. In addition, when the antibody-coated cells are warmed on reentering the general circulation, the antibody may dissociate from the erythrocyte. If it does not, hemolysis of the cell may occur. Thus, cold antibody disease is more a problem of vascular obstruction than hemolysis. Cold antibody disease is often a complication of infectious mononucleosis, **mycoplasma pneumoniae** infections, and lymphoid malignancies.

Drug-induced immune hemolytic anemia can be due to either of two mechanisms. One stems from an immune reaction against a drug, resulting in the formation of antigen-antibody (drug-antibody) complexes that adhere to the surfaces of erythrocytes. Alternately, a drug, or a metabolite of a drug, may bind directly to the surface of the erythrocyte, forming a neoantigen that attracts antibodies. Both mechanisms result in the activation of the complement cascade and hemolysis.

Clinical Manifestations

The presence and severity of signs and symptoms of hemolytic anemia depend on the degree of hemolysis and the success of compensatory erythropoiesis. The spleen enlarges as it removes more and more dead or defective erythrocytes from the circulation. Jaundice (icterus) occurs if heme breakdown exceeds the liver's ability to conjugate and excrete bilirubin.

TABLE 23-3 Causes of hemolytic anemias

Type of hemolytic disorder	Primary cause or associated disorder	Mechanisms of erythrocyte destruction
Acquired forms		
Immune system—mediated hemolysis	Transfusion reaction Hemolytic disease of the newborn (see Chapter 25) Autoimmune hemolytic anemia (see text)	Antibody-mediated erythrocytes by enzymes of the complement system (see Chapter 7)
Traumatic hemolysis	Presence of prosthetic heart valves Structural abnormalities of the heart Hemolytic uremic syndrome Disseminated intravascular coagulation Hemodialysis	Physical destruction of erythrocytes by "mechanical" means (trauma)
Infectious hemolysis	Bacterial infection (clostridia, cholera, typhoid fever) Protozoal infection (malaria, toxoplasmosis)	Infection of erythrocytes
Toxic (chemical) hemolysis	Exposure to toxic chemical agents Hemodialysis or uremia Venoms	Chemical injury of erythrocytes (see Chapter 2)
Physical hemolysis	Burns Radiation	Heat or radiation injury (see Chapter 2)
Hypophosphatemic hemolysis	Hypophosphatemia (phosphate deficiency in plasma; see Chapter 3)	Diminished cellular production of substances required for erythrocyte life and function
Hereditary forms		
Structural defects	Plasma membrane defects	Fragility of the erythrocyte
Enzyme deficiencies	Deficiency of glycolytic enzymes Deficiency of metabolic enzymes (i.e., glucose-6-phosphate dehydrogenase deficiency)	Diminished cellular function
Defects of globin synthesis or structure	Sickle cell anemia	Increased membrane fragility and deformation during sickle crises
	Thalassemia	Defective hemoglobin structure and function
	Miscellaneous hemoglobin defects	Defective hemoglobin structure and function

From Wintrobe, et al., 1981.

Acute conditions—aplastic, hemolytic, or megaloblastic crises—frequently develop if other diseases, particularly viral infections, are also present. Crises are associated with further declines in levels of hemoglobin in the peripheral blood and occasionally bone marrow hypoplasia or aplasia.

In severe hemolytic anemia, the bones become deformed as a result of expansion of hematopoietic bone marrow, and pathologic fractures often occur. Cardiovascular and respiratory manifestations vary with the degree of anemia.

Evaluation and Treatment

Evaluation is based on clinical manifestations, bone marrow studies, and blood tests (Table 23-2). Abnormally increased numbers of erythrocyte stem cells are found in the marrow, a finding termed erythroid hyperplasia. Acceleration of erythropoiesis causes large numbers of fragile and immature erythrocytes (stem cells and reticulocytes) to be released prematurely into the circulation. These cells are seen in blood smears.

Acquired hemolytic anemias can be treated by removing the cause or treating the underlying disorder. Acute, fulminating hemolytic anemia (hemolytic crisis) is treated with fluid and electrolyte replacement to prevent shock and renal damage from clogging the kidney tubules by red cell debris. Transfusions of blood products are sometimes given. Splenectomy is performed if the spleen is the major site of hemolysis and splenomegaly is significant.

Steroids are often used to treat autoimmune hemolytic anemias. Folate is given for chronic hemolytic disease because long-term erythrocyte turnover increases folate requirements.

Anemia of Chronic Disease

Anemia of chronic disease is a mild-to-moderate anemia associated with chronic infections, chronic non-infectious inflammatory diseases, and malignancies. The anemia develops after 1 to 2 months of active disease. The severity of anemia is related to that of the underlying disorder and may be an asymptomatic or coincidental clinical finding. Morphologically, anemia of chronic disease is usually normocytic-normochromic, but it may also be normocytic-hypochromic or microcytic-hypochromic. Anemia of chronic disease is commonly associated with rheumatoid arthritis, systemic lupus erythematosus (and other autoimmune collagen disorders), Hodgkin disease, colitis, and regional enteritis. The exact incidence of anemia of chronic disease is unknown. Because it is associated with so many pathologic conditions, it is probably second only to iron deficiency anemia in overall incidence.

normocytic–normochromic

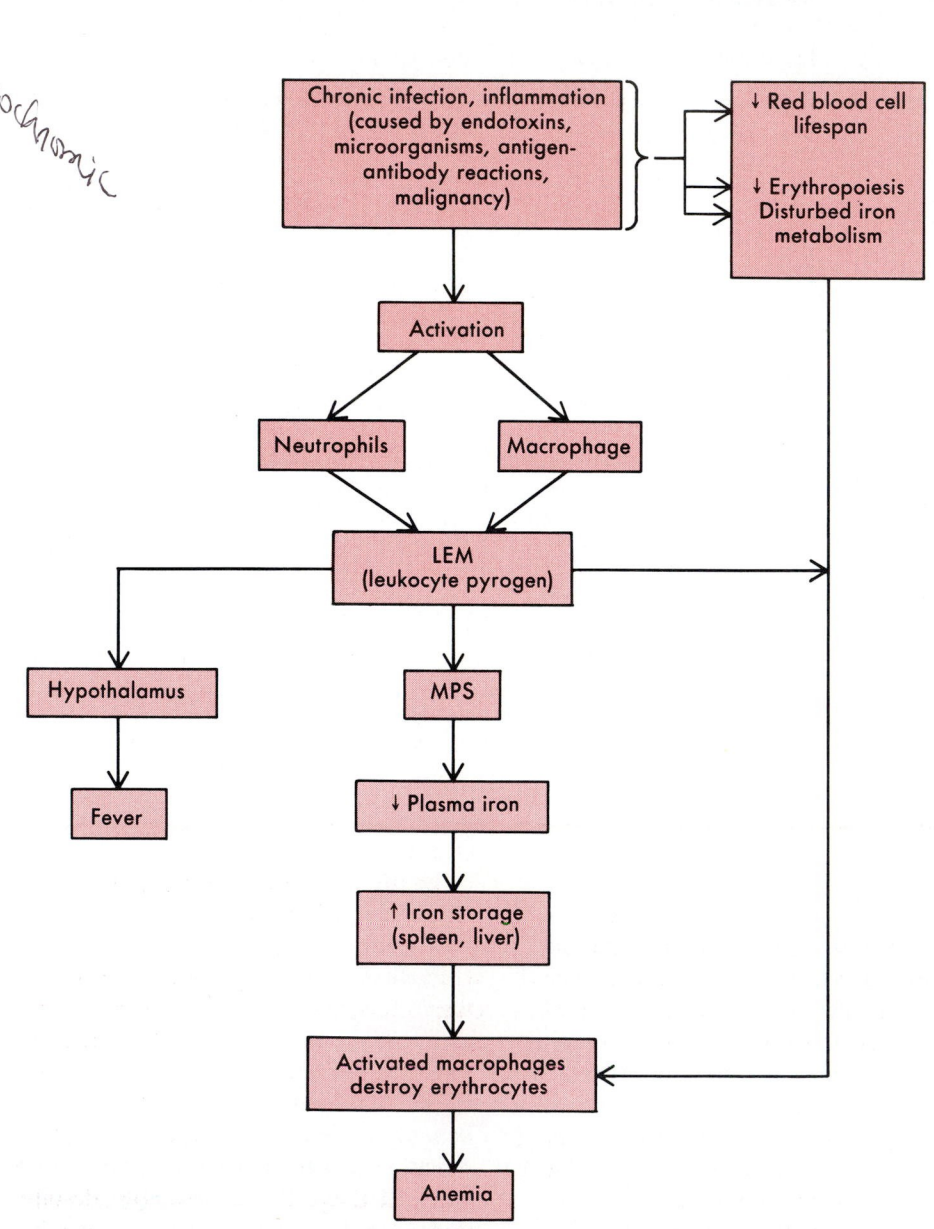

FIG. 23-2. Anemia of chronic disease and LEM. (*MPS*, Mononuclear phagocyte system).

Pathophysiology

Three pathogenic mechanisms cause anemia of chronic disease: (1) decreased erythrocyte life span, (2) failure of mechanisms of compensatory erythropoiesis, and (3) disturbances of the iron cycle.

An extrinsic factor may accelerate erythrocyte destruction in anemia of chronic disease. Several attempts have been made to identify an extrinsic hemolytic factor in individuals with anemia associated with cancer. Researchers have suggested four possibilities: (1) hemolytic agents (hemolipins) are released from the tumor (Sheets et al., 1954); (2) erythrocytes are destroyed by entering the tumor (Price & Greenfield, 1958); (3) the tumor stimulates the immune system to produce antibodies against erythrocyte antigens; and (4) erythrocytes are destroyed by macrophages activated by the disease (Atkinson & Frank, 1974). Anemia associated with chronic infection is thought to be due to the hemolytic action of bacterial toxins.

The erythropoietic defect in anemia of chronic disease apparently is a failure to *increase* erythropoiesis in response to hemolysis. Erythropoiesis does not accelerate, but rather continues at the normal rate. This failure may be due to substances released from phagocytes, which tend to be numerous when inflammation or infection is present in the body. These substances, known collectively as **leukocyte endogenous mediator (LEM),** or leukocyte pyrogen, are released by neutrophils and macrophages (Kampschmidt, 1978; Kampschmidt & Upchurch, 1980). Research indicates that LEM causes an abrupt drop in plasma iron levels (Fig. 23-2). With long-term secretion of LEM, iron content apparently continues to decrease in plasma and increase in the spleen and liver.

LEM apparently interferes with the iron cycle (Fig. 23-3). Research suggests that the cycle is disrupted at the point where iron released from macrophages of the MPS is returned to plasma (VanSnick, Markowetz, & Masson, 1977; Wintrobe et al., 1981). If this hypothesis is correct, LEM may consist of **lactoferrin,** an iron-binding protein normally present in neutrophils and body secretions. Lactoferrin is nearly identical to transferrin, the protein that normally transports iron by binding it in plasma and carrying it to the marrow for erythropoiesis. Lactoferrin has an iron-binding capacity 260 times that of transferrin, however. When lactoferrin is present in the plasma, as occurs with increased levels of neutrophils in the blood, it competes with transferrin for the available iron molecules and wins. Iron that is bound to lactoferrin instead of transferrin is removed by the MPS instead of traveling to the marrow. Normally, lactoferrin in mucosal secretions prevents iron overload by preventing gastrointestinal absorption of iron. Its presence in plasma is apparently due to increased levels of neutrophils in the blood caused by chronic inflammation, infection, or malignancy.

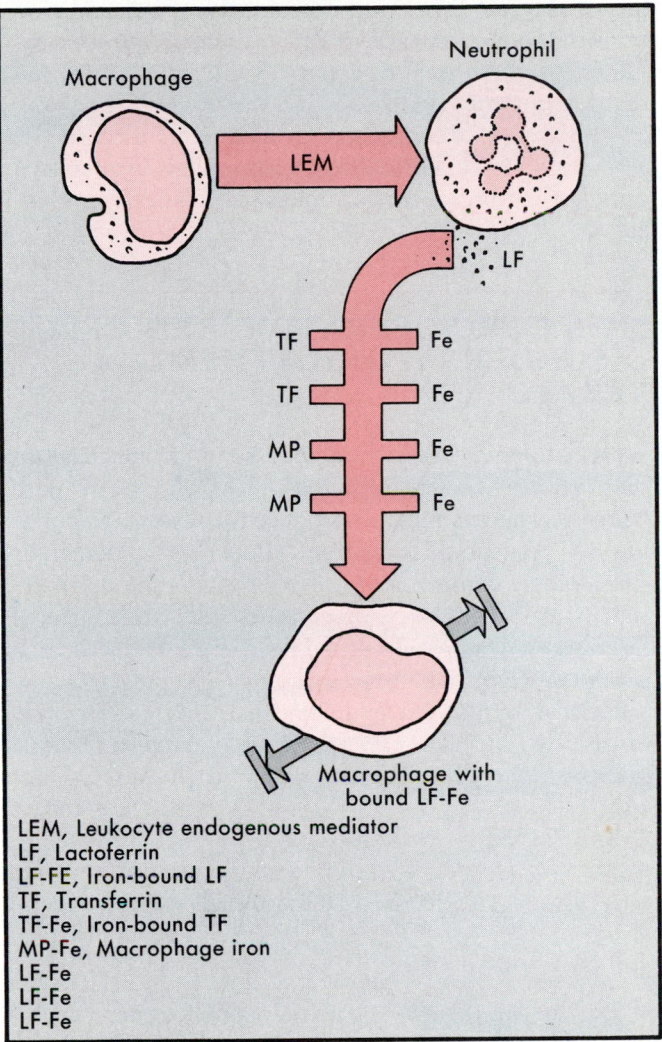

LEM, Leukocyte endogenous mediator
LF, Lactoferrin
LF-FE, Iron-bound LF
TF, Transferrin
TF-Fe, Iron-bound TF
MP-Fe, Macrophage iron
LF-Fe
LF-Fe
LF-Fe

FIG. 23-3. Iron binding in anemia of chronic disease. Defective iron metabolism in anemia of chronic disease results from (1) release of LEM by macrophages; (2) LEM stimulates neutrophils to release lactoferrin from secondary storage granules; (3) lactoferrin binds to iron, preventing iron reuse in normal pathways; and (4) lactoferrin-iron complex is engulfed by macrophage and cannot be returned to plasma. (Adapted from Schumacher, Garvn, & Triplett, 1984).

Clinical Manifestations

Anemia of chronic disease has fewer and milder clinical manifestations than most other anemias. Manifestations depend on the degree of anemia. As a rule, disability caused by chronic disease limits physical activity, so that hemoglobin levels are adequate. If hemoglobin levels drop significantly, however, the clinical manifestations of iron deficiency anemia appear (see p. 790).

Evaluation and Treatment

The significant finding in anemia of chronic disease is iron deficiency in the marrow despite normal or increased iron stores elsewhere in the body. (Blood test findings are listed in Table 23-2.) Individuals with anemia of chronic disease but no evidence of inflammation or infection are screened for the presence of neoplasms.

Anemia of chronic disease does not respond to iron replacement therapy because iron is unable to reach the bone marrow. The mainstay of treatment, therefore, is alleviation of the underlying disorder. The anemia itself does not require treatment unless it becomes symptomatic.

MYELOPROLIFERATIVE RED CELL DISORDERS (POLYCYTHEMIA VERA)

Hematologic dysfunction may result from an overproduction of cells, as well as a deficiency. One or more marrow elements may be produced in excess, responding to exogenous (radiation, drugs) or endogenous (physiologic compensatory response, immune disorder) signals. An overabundance of white cells results in leukemia (see Chapters 24 and 25). An excess of red cells produces a group of disorders classified as polycythemia.

Polycythemia vera is an unusual myeloproliferative disease that causes **erythrocytosis**—excessively large numbers of erythrocytes in the blood. It was first de-

scribed in 1892 by a French physician, M. H. Vaquez. In the early 1900s, William Osler undertook an extensive investigation of the disease. Not much more was learned about polycythemia vera until the 1960s, at which time researchers began to investigate a link between polycythemias of all kinds and neoplasia affecting stem cells.

Pathophysiology

Polycythemia vera is due to excessive proliferation of erythrocyte precursors in the marrow. The fact that it typically is accompanied by increases of circulating platelets and granulocytes suggests that polycythemia vera is caused by an abnormality of the pluripotential stem cell. Controversy exists as to whether polycythemia vera should be classified as a leukemia (see Chapter 24) or a problem of marrow hyperplasia (i.e., myeloproliferative disorder).

There are three types of polycythemia: primary, secondary, and familial (Table 23-4). The primary form of polycythemia vera is relatively rare and tends to occur in men between the ages of 40 and 60. It is more common in whites, particularly Jews of European ancestry, than in blacks. The cause of polycythemia is unknown. Secondary polycythemia is the more commonly seen form

TABLE 23-4 Types of polycythemia

Type of polycythemia	Mechanism of increased erythropoiesis	Cause or associated disorder
Primary polycythemia (polycythemia vera)	Excessive proliferation of erythroid precursors in marrow; increased sensitivity of pluripotential stem cell to erythropoietin	Unknown
Secondary polycythemia	Physiologic increase in erythropoietin secretion by the kidneys in response to underlying systemic disorder	Tissue hypoxia caused by cardiopulmonary disorders (chronic obstruction pulmonary disease, congestive heart failure), decreased barometric pressure, cardiovascular malformations causing mixing of arterial and venous blood, methemoglobinemia, carboxyhemoglobinemia, smoking, obesity
	"Nonphysiologic"* increase in erythropoietin secretion	Renal disorders, cerebellar hemangioblastomas, hepatoma (liver tumor), ovarian carcinoma, uterine leiomyoma, pheochromocytoma, adrenocortical hypersecretion
Familial polycythemia	Genetically induced increase in erythroid precursors of the marrow Abnormal Hb with increased oxygen affinity Decreased 2, 3-DPG Increased sensitivity of stem cells to erythropoietin Increased erythropoietin in secretion	Genetic defect

*Nonphysiologic means that there is no obvious physiologic explanation for hypersecretion of erythropoietin.

of the disorder. It is an essentially physiologic response to hypoxia. Therefore it is not uncommon to find an increased red cell count in individuals living at high altitudes (10,000 feet) and in smokers and individuals with congestive heart failure and chronic obstructive pulmonary disease.

Erythrocytosis causes blood volume and blood viscosity to increase because of an increased erythrocyte count. The liver and spleen become increasingly congested with erythrocytes as viscosity causes blood flow to slow. Eventually, the thick, sticky, slow-flowing blood becomes an ideal environment for clotting and acidosis. If thrombi obstruct vessels, tissue or organ infarction (blood deprivation) results.

Clinical Manifestations

The clinical manifestations of polycythemia vera are caused by increased blood volume and viscosity and clogging of microcirculatory blood vessels. They include (1) plethora (ruddy, red color of the face, hands, feet, ears, and mucous membranes), (2) engorgement of retinal and sublingual veins, (3) splenomegaly, and (4) hepatomegaly. Symptoms include headache, a feeling of fullness in the head, dizziness, weakness, elevated blood pressure, itching, sweating, weight loss, epigastric distress, fatigue on exertion, backache, and visual disturbances. The eyes may be bloodshot, and intense pruritus (itching) after bathing may be so troublesome that the individual avoids bathing with warm water. The cause of the pruritus is unknown and the symptoms do not respond to antihistamines.

Clinical manifestations of vascular disease may predominate, including angina pectoris, calf pain associated with walking induced vasospasm (intermittent claudication), thrombotic disease, and cerebral insufficiency. Thrombosis of gastric vessels can cause ulcers and mesenteric pain. Respiratory infections are common, as is hoarseness. Some individuals with polycythemia vera tend to bleed, especially from the gastrointestinal and genitourinary tracts. Microvascular clots interfere with normal coagulation mechanisms and a disseminated intravascular coagulation-like syndrome can occur.

Evaluation and Treatment

Blood and laboratory findings establish the diagnosis. Diagnosis is characterized by an absolute increase in red blood cells and in the total blood volume, although it is not unusual to also have increases in white blood cells and platelets. A bone marrow examination may be done; however it is incapable of definitively establishing the diagnosis. Treatment for polycythemia vera consists of reducing erythrocytosis and blood volume, controlling symptoms, and preventing thrombosis. Erythrocytosis and blood volume are reduced by phlebotomy, a procedure in which a vein is opened and blood is re-

moved. Three hundred to 500 ml may be removed two to three times per week until hematocrit drops sufficiently. After that, phlebotomy may be done every 3 to 4 months. Smokers should be urged to quit and patients with congestive heart failure and chronic obstructive pulmonary disease require appropriate pharmaceutical intervention.

Radioactive phosphorus is sometimes given orally or intravenously to suppress erythropoiesis. Unfortunately, a side effect of this therapy can be the general suppression of hematopoiesis, resulting in anemia, leukopenia, or thrombocytopenia. Radioactive phosphorus is not given at frequent intervals—as many as 18 months may elapse between treatments. Myelosuppressive drugs (marrow suppressants) are also used, but their effects can be more unpleasant than the disease.

Without proper treatment, 50% of individuals with polycythemia vera die within 18 months of the onset of initial symptoms. The major cause of death is thrombosis or hemorrhage. Although polycythemia vera is a chronic disorder, appropriate therapy results in remissions and prevention of significant morbidity and mortality.

SUMMARY REVIEW

Anemia

1 Anemia is generally defined as a reduction in the number or volume of circulating red cells or an alteration in hemoglobin.

2 Anemias can be classified according to erythrocyte size or concentration of hemoglobin, cause of low blood count, or according to the kinetics of why constant and adequate numbers of mature erythrocytes are not maintained in the circulation.

3 Clinical manifestations of anemia can be found in all organs and tissues throughout the body. Decreased oxygen delivery to tissues can cause fatigue, dyspnea, syncope, angina, compensatory tachycardia, and organ dysfunction.

4 Macrocytic/megaloblastic anemias are most commonly caused by deficiency of vitamin B_{12}. Pernicious anemia can be fatal unless vitamin B_{12} replacement is given.

5 Microcytic-hypochromic anemias are characterized by abnormally small red cells with insufficient hemoglobin content. The most common cause is iron deficiency.

6 Iron deficiency anemia usually develops slowly, with gradual insidious onset of symptoms. Fatigue, weakness, dyspnea, alteration of various epithelial tissues, and vague neuromuscular complaints result.

7 Iron deficiency anemia is usually a result of blood loss or poor nutritional intake. Once the source of blood loss is defined and corrected, iron replacement therapy can be initiated. Elevated reticulocyte count is a good index of response to iron therapy.

8 Sideroblastic anemia results from impaired iron metabolism and abnormal sequestration of iron. Treatment varies depending on the cause.

9 Normocytic-normochromic anemias are characterized by insufficient numbers of normal erythrocytes. Included in this category are aplastic, posthemorrhagic, and hemolytic anemia, and anemia of chronic disease.

10 In aplastic anemia erythrocyte stem cells are underdeveloped, defective, or absent. Unless the cause is determined, bone marrow aplasia will result in death.

11 Sudden blood loss after hemorrhage results in a normocytic-normochromic anemia. Restoration of blood volume by plasma expanders or transfusions may diminish subjective symptoms of anemia. Hemoglobin restoration may take 6 to 8 weeks.

12 Premature destruction of erythrocytes (hemolytic anemia) may be acquired or hereditary. Of the acquired forms, autoimmune reaction and drug-induced hemolysis are the most common.

13 Failure of erythropoiesis in anemia of chronic disease may result in release of leukocyte endogenous mediator (LEM) by phagocytic cells. LEM has been shown to cause abrupt decreases in plasma iron levels and interferes with the normal iron cycle.

Myeloproliferative Red Cell Disorders (Polycythemia Vera)

1 Polycythemia vera is characterized by excessive proliferation of erythrocyte precursors in the bone marrow. Signs and symptoms result directly from increased blood volume and viscosity. Therapeutic phlebotomy to remove excessive blood volume and use of radioactive phosphorus have been helpful in decreasing the excessive red cell pool.

KEY TERMS

Anemia, 784

Anemia of chronic disease, 794

Anisocytosis, 785

Aplastic anemia, 791

Autoimmune hemolytic anemia, 792

Bone marrow aplasia, 791

Bone marrow hypoplasia, 791

Cold antibody disease, 792

Drug-induced immune hemolytic anemia, 792

Erythrocytosis, 796

Hemolysis, 788

Hemolytic anemia, 792

Hyperchromic erythrocyte, 784

Hypochromic erythrocyte, 784

Hypoplastic anemia, 791

Iron deficiency anemia, 789

Lactoferrin, 795

Leukocyte endogenous mediator (LEM), 795

Macrocytic anemia (megaloblastic anemia), 788

Macrocytic erythrocyte, 784

Microcytic erythrocyte, 784

Mycoplasma pneumoniae, 792

Normochromic erythrocyte, 785

Normocytic erythrocyte, 785

Pancytopenia, 791

Pernicious anemia, 788

Poikilocytosis, 791

Polycythemia vera, 796

Posthemorrhagic anemia, 792

Pure red cell aplasia, 791

Sideroblast, 790

Sideroblastic anemia, 790

Warm antibody disease, 792

REFERENCES

Adamson, J. W. (1968). Erythropoietin in the polycythemias. *Annals of the New York Academy of Sciences, 149,* 560.

Adamson, J. W. (1968). The erythropoietin/hematocrit relationship in normal and polycythemic man: Implications of marrow regulation. *Blood, 32,* 597.

Atkinson, J. P., & Frank, M. M. (1974). The effect of bacillus Calmette-Guerin-induced macrophage activation on the in vivo clearance of sensitized erythrocytes. *Journal of Clinical Investigation, 53,* 1742.

Ballas, S. K. (1978, July-August). Disorders of the red cell membrane: A reclassification of hemolytic anemias. *The American Journal of the Medical Sciences, 276*(1), 4f.

Birgens, H. S. (1984). The biological significance of lactoferrin in haematology. *Scandinavian Journal of Haemotology, 33,* 225-230.

Brewer, G. J. (Ed.). (1984). Progress in clinical and biological research. *Proceedings of the Sixth Ann Arbor Conference, 165,* 198. New York: Alan R. Liss, Inc.

Cartwright, G. E. (1966). The anemia of chronic disorders. *Seminars in Hematology, 3,* 351.

Dallman, P. R. (1981). Anemia of prematurity. *Annual Review of Medicine, 32,* 143-160.

Delmonte, L., Aschkenasy, A., & Eyquem, A. (1964). Studies on the hemolytic nature of protein deficiency anemia in the rat. *Blood, 24,* 49.

Editorial Staff. (1983). Pale blood, thin blood. *Emergency Medicine, 15*(21), 26-47.

Fisher, J. W., & Langston, J. W. (1967). The influence of hypoxemia and cobalt on erythropoietin production in the isolated perfused dog kidney. *Blood, 29,* 114.

Fisher, J. W., Samuels, A. I., & Langston, J. W. (1967). Effects of angiotensin and renal artery constriction on erythropoietin production. *Journal of Pharmacology and Experimental Therapeutics, 157,* 618.

Fitch, C. D. (1968). The red cell in the vitamin E deficient monkey. *American Journal of Clinical Nutrition, 21,* 51.

Fitch, C. D. (1972). The hematopoietic system in vitamin E-deficient animals. *Annals of the New York Academy of Sciences, 203,* 172.

Freedman, M. L. (1982, May). Anemias in the elderly: Physiologic or pathologic? *Hospital Practice, 17*(5), 121-136.

Goodman, S. R., Shiffer, K., Coleman, D. B., & Whitfield, C. F. (1984). Erythrocyte membrane skeletal protein: A brief review. In G. J. Brewer (Ed.), *The red cell. Proceedings of the 6th Ann Arbor Conference (pp. 415-439).* New York: Alan R. Liss,

Guyton, A. C. (1982). *Human physiology and mechanisms of disease* (3rd ed.). Philadelphia: W. B. Saunders.

Haden, R. L. (1938). Historical aspects of iron therapy in anemia. *JAMA, 111,* 1059.

Hansen, N. E. (1983). The anemia of chronic disorders: A bag of unresolved questions. *Scandinavian Journal of Haematology, 31,* 397-402.

Horadam, V. W., & Hutton, J. J. (1983, January). Anemia of chronic disease: Basic concepts and management. *Geriatrics, 38*(1), 51-58.

Kampschmidt, R. F. (1978). Leukocytic endogenous mediator. *Journal of the Reticuloendothelial Society, 23,* 287.

Kampschmidt, M. S., & Upchurch, H. F. (1980, August). Neutrophil release after infection of endotoxin or leukocytic endogenous mediator into rats. *Journal of the Reticuloendothelial Society, 28*(2), 191-201.

Klein, H. (1983). *Polycythemia: Theory and management.* Springfield, IL: Charles C Thomas.

Krantz, S. B. (1968). Response of polycythemia vera marrow to erythropoietin in vitro. *Journal of Laboratory and Clinical Medicine, 71,* 999.

LaCelle, P. L. (1970). Alteration of membrane deformabilities in hemolytic anemias. *Seminars in Hematology, 7,* 355-371.

Mohandas, N., Wyatt, J., Mel, S. F., Rossi, M. E., & Shohet, S. B. (1982). Lipid translocation across the human erythrocyte membrane: Regulatory factors. *Journal of Biological Chemistry, 257*(11), 6537.

Murphy, J. R. (1962). Erythrocyte metabolism I. V. equilibrium of cholesteral-4-C^{14} between erythrocytes and variously tested sera. *Journal of Laboratory and Clinical Medicine, 60,* 571-578.

Prasad, A. S. (1984). Zinc deficiencies in sickle cell disease: The red cell. In G. J. Brewer (Ed.): *Proceedings of the Sixth Ann Arbor Conference on Progress in Clinical and Biological Research, 165,* 49-58. New York: Alan R. Liss, Inc.

Price, V. E., & Greenfield, R. E. (1958). Anemia in cancer. In J. P. Greenstein & A. Haddow (Eds.), *Advances in cancer research* (Vol. 5). New York: Academic Press.

Sakagami, T., Minari, D., & Orii, T. (1965). Interaction of individual phospholipids between rat plasma and erythrocytes in vitro. *Biochimica et Biophysica Acta, 98,* 356-364.

Schumacher, H. R., Garvn, D. F., & Triplett, D. A. (1984). *Introduction to laboratory hematology and hematopathology.* New York: Alan R. Liss.

Sheets, R. F., Hamilton, H. E., DeGowin, E. L., & Janney, C. D. (1954). Spontaneous and x-ray induced hemolysis in malignancy. *Journal of Clinical Investigations, 33,* 179.

Steinberg, M. H., & Drieling, B. J. (1983). Microcytosis: Its significance and evaluation. *JAMA, 249*(1), 85-87.

Stolhman, F., Jr. (1972). Aplastic anemia. *Blood, 40,* 282.

Sullivan, L. W. (1970). Vitamin B_{12} metabolism and megaloblastic anemia. *Seminars in Hematology, 7*(6).

Tosteson, D. C. (1967). Electrolyte composition and transport in red blood cells. *Federal Proceedings, 26,* 1805-1812.

VanNeer, G., & OgdenKamp, J. A. F. (1982). Transbilayer movement of various phosphatidylcholine species in intact human erythrocytes. *Journal of Cellular Biochemistry, 19,* 193.

VanSnick, J. L., Markowetz, B., & Masson, P. L. (1977). The involvement of lactoferrin in the hyposideremia of acute inflammation. *Journal of Experimental Medicine, 146,* 817.

West, J. B. (Ed.). (1985). *Best and Taylor's physiological basis of medical practice* (11th ed.). Baltimore: Williams & Wilkins.

Windson, C. W. O., & Collins, J. L. (1967). Anemia and hiatus hernia. *Thorax, 22,* 73.

Wintrobe, M. M., Lee, G. R., Boggs, D. R., Bithell, T. C., Foerster, J., Athens, J. W., & Lukens, J. N. (1981). *Clinical hematology* (8th ed.). Philadelphia: Lea & Febiger.

Witts, L. F. (1969). *Hypochromic anemia.* Philadephia: F. A. Davis.

Young, N. S., Humphries, K., & Levin, A. S. (Eds.) (1984). Aplastic anemia: Stem cell biology and advances in treatment. In *Progress in clinical and biological research* (vol. 148). New York: Alan R. Liss.

CHAPTER 24

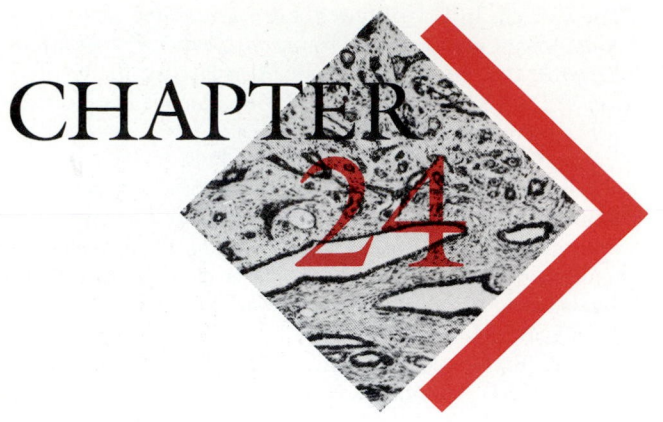

Alterations of Leukocyte, Lymphoid, and Hemostatic Function

Pamela F. Cipriano
Kathryn L. McCance

Alterations of leukocyte function, 800
  Quantitative alterations of leukocytes, 801
   Granulocytes and monocytes, 801
   Lymphocytes, 802
  Infectious mononucleosis, 802
  Leukemias, 803
   Acute leukemias, 803
    Pathogenesis, 804
    Clinical manifestations, 804
    Evaluation and treatment, 804
   Chronic leukemias, 805
  Multiple myeloma, 809
   Pathophysiology, 810
   Clinical manifestations, 810
   Evaluation and treatment, 810
Alterations in lymphoid function, 810
  Lymphadenopathy, 810
  Malignant lymphomas, 811
   Hodgkin disease, 811
    Pathogenesis, 811
    Clinical manifestations, 813
    Evaluation and treatment, 814
   Non-Hodgkin lymphoma, 814
    Pathogenesis, 814
    Clinical manifestations, 814
    Evaluation and treatment, 815
   Burkitt lymphoma, 815
   Conditions that mimic lymphomas, 816
Alterations of splenic function, 816
  Splenomegaly, 816
  Hypersplenism, 816
Alterations of platelets and coagulation, 816
  Disorders of platelets, 817
   Thrombocytopenia, 817
   Thrombocytosis, 818
  Alterations of platelet function, 818
  Disorders of coagulation, 818
   Vitamin K deficiency, 819
   Liver disease, 819
   Disseminated intravascular coagulation (DIC), 819
   Thromboembolic disease, 821

ALTERATIONS OF LEUKOCYTE FUNCTION

Leukocyte function is affected if too many or too few cells are present in the blood or if the cells that are present are structurally or functionally defective. The presence of too many or too few cells, the so-called quantitative disorders, can be the result of bone marrow dysfunction or premature destruction of cells in the circulation. Many quantitative alterations, however, originate in the circulation or lymphoid organs in response to invasion by infectious microorganisms.

Most qualitative disorders consist of disruptions of leukocyte function in mechanisms of self-defense. The phagocytic cells (granulocytes, monocytes, and macrophages) may lose their capacity to function as effective phagocytes. The lymphocytes may lose their capacity to respond to antigens. (Disruptions of inflammatory and immune processes caused by leukocyte disorders are described in Chapter 8.) Other leukocyte alterations are not primarily immune or inflammatory defects, but rather are hematologic defects. These disorders include infectious mononucleosis, and cancers of the blood—leukemia and multiple myeloma.

Quantitative Alterations of Leukocytes

Quantitative alterations are increases and decreases in numbers of leukocytes in the blood. **Leukocytosis** is a condition in which the leukocyte count is higher than normal; **leukopenia** is a condition in which the count is lower than normal. Usually leukocytosis or leukopenia affects a specific type of leukocyte.

Leukocytosis and leukopenia can result from a variety of bodily conditions and alterations. Leukocytosis is a normal protective response to physiologic stressors, such as invading microorganisms, strenuous exercise, emotional changes, temperature changes, anesthesia, surgery, pregnancy, and some drugs, hormones, and toxins. It is also caused by pathologic conditions, such as malignancies and hematologic disorders. Unlike leukocytosis, leukopenia is never beneficial. As the leukocyte count falls below 1000 per cubic millimeter, the individual is at risk for infection. With counts below 500 per cubic millimeter, the risk for very serious life-threatening infections is high. Leukopenia can be caused by radiation, anaphylactic shock, systemic lupus erythymatosus, and certain chemotherapeutic agents.

Granulocytes and monocytes

Increased levels of circulating granulocytes (neutrophils, eosinophils, and basophils) and monocytes are chiefly a physiologic response to infection, but can also be stimulated by diseases that increase stem cell proliferation in the bone marrow. Decreases occur when infectious processes "use up" the circulating granulocytes and monocytes, drawing them out of the circulation and into infected tissues faster than they can be replaced. Decreases can also be caused by disorders that suppress marrow function.

Granulocytosis begins with the release of blood cells that have been stored in the venous sinuses of the marrow. Because the neutrophil is the most numerous of the granulocytes, the term granulocytosis is often used to describe **neutrophilia** (see Table 22-2). Neutrophilia is prevalent in the early stages of infection or inflammation. Release of stored neutrophils from the marrow causes immediate neutrophilia because twenty to forty times more neutrophils are stored than are present in circulating blood. Emptying of the venous sinuses stimulates granulopoiesis to replenish stores in the marrow.

If infection is severe, neutrophils migrate out of the circulation faster than they can be replaced. (Mechanisms of granulocyte migration from blood vessels to sites of infection or inflammation are described in Chapter 7.) When the demand for neutrophils exceeds the supply in the circulation, the marrow begins to release immature neutrophils (and other leukocytes) into the blood. Premature release of the immature cells is responsible for the phenomenon that hematologists call the shift to the left. The **shift to the left** refers to the microscopic detection of disproportionate numbers of immature leukocytes in smears of peripheral blood. The term can be understood if one visualizes cellular differentiation and maturation as occurring from left to right, as is shown in Chapter 22, Fig. 22-5. (The shift to the left is sometimes called a leukomoid reaction because it is similar to morphologic findings in blood smears of individuals with leukemia.) As infection or inflammation diminish and granulopoiesis replenishes circulating granulocytes, a **shift to the right,** or back to normal, occurs.

An increase in eosinophils, termed **eosinophilia**, can be caused by (1) parasitic invasion, (2) intake of toxic foreign particles, (3) presence of blood clots, or (4) presence of allergens. The most common cause of eosinophilia is invasion of the body by parasites. Eosinophils are attracted out of the circulation in great numbers, after which they migrate to sites of infestation and degranulate powerful enzymes onto the parasites. (This process is described and illustrated in Chapter 7.) The second most common cause of eosinophilia is inhalation or oral ingestion of toxic foreign particles. Eosinophils migrate into the respiratory or gastrointestinal mucosa, where they phagocytose (ingest) and thereby detoxify the foreign particles. The third cause of eosinophilia, presence of blood clots, stimulates eosinophils to migrate into the clots and release profibrinolysin, an enzyme that dissolves fibrin. The fourth cause of eosinophilia is allergic reactions. Eosinophils collect at sites of antigen-antibody (allergen-immunoglobulin) binding in tissues, where they phagocytose the antigen-antibody complexes. (Antigen-antibody binding is described in Chapter 6.) This mechanism of eosinophilia is not clearly understood.

Basophilia occurs during the healing phase of inflammation, during which coagulation and clotting need to be inhibited. Basophils release heparin, an anticoagulant that inhibits the hemostatic functions of platelets and coagulation factors (see Chapter 22).

Monocytosis occurs during the late or recuperative phase of infection. As infection subsides, monocytes (which mature into macrophages) enter the inflammatory site to phagocytose surviving microorganisms and debris (see Chapter 7). Monocytosis is a manifestation of long-lasting or chronic infections, particularly granulomatous diseases, such as tuberculosis and sarcoidosis.

A decrease in numbers of circulating granulocytes and monocytes can be caused by prolonged, overwhelming infections, anaphylactic shock, systemic lupus erythematosus, radiation, or chemotherapy. **Neutropenia** may result from ineffective or defective neutrophil production, such as occurs in hypoplastic or aplastic anemia, starvation, and cancers in which normal stem cells in bone marrow are replaced by malignant cells.

If neutrophils are absent and the entire granulocyte count is extremely low, a very serious condition called **granulocytopenia,** or **agranulocytosis,** results. The usual cause is interference with hematopoiesis in the bone marrow or increased cell destruction in the circulation. Chemotherapeutic agents commonly used in the treatment of hematologic and other malignancies cause bone marrow suppression. Such drugs as analgesics, antibiotics, and antihistamines rarely cause neutropenia or granulocytopenia. Clinical manifestations of granulocytopenia include infection (particularly of the respiratory system), general malaise, septicemia, fever, tachycardia, and ulcers in the mouth and colon. If untreated, sepsis caused by granulocytopenia will result with death in 3 to 6 days.

Lymphocytes

Quantitative alterations of lymphocytes occur when lymphocytes are activated by antigenic stimuli, usually microorganisms (see Chapter 6). A **lymphocytosis** occurs in infectious mononucleosis, infectious hepatitis, toxoplasmosis, measles, mumps, varicella, some allergic reactions, drug sensitivities, pertussis, lymphocyte leukemia, lymphomas, and some chronic infections, such as tuberculosis.

Lymphocytopenia occurs with acute infections and many diseases, such as heart failure, pneumonia, active tuberculosis, carcinomas, lymphomas, some immunologic deficiency syndromes, and in some individuals with no apparent disease (Wintrobe et al., 1981). The lymphocytopenia associated with heart failure and possibly other acute illnesses may be caused by elevated plasma cortisol levels; however, mechanisms in other conditions are poorly understood. Other substances (including chemotherapeutic agents and exogenous adrenal steroid, as well as irradiation) can cause **lymphopenia.**

Infectious Mononucleosis

Infectious mononucleosis is an acute infection of B lymphocytes (B cells) by the Epstein-Barr virus, a type of herpes virus. Infectious mononucleosis usually affects young adults between the ages of fifteen and twenty-five. It has been called "kissing disease" because the virus is transmitted in oropharyngeal secretions. Infectious mononucleosis does not develop in many individuals who are infected with the Epstein-Barr virus because their immune systems neutralize the virus and kill the infected B cells before infection becomes widespread. This produces a carrier who can transmit the virus to others during a time period of 1 to 18 months.

Active infectious mononucleosis begins with widespread invasion of B cells by the virus. (Mechanisms of cellular viral invasion are described in Chapter 2.) Unaf-

fected B cells produce antibodies against the virus, and T lymphocytes (T cells) assist the B cell response to attack the virus directly (see Chapter 6). The proliferation of clones of B and T cells and removal of dead and damaged leukocytes are largely responsible for the swelling of lymphoid tissues (lymph nodes, spleen, tonsils, and occasionally, liver). Sore throat and fever, two of the earliest manifestations of infectious mononucleosis, are caused by inflammation at the site of viral entry (and initial infection), the mouth and throat.

The incubation period for infectious mononucleosis is approximately 30 to 50 days. Mild symptoms, such as headache, malaise, and fatigue, appear during the first 3 to 5 days, with symptoms varying in severity for the next 7 to 20 days. The majority of cases include fever with temperature elevation lasting 7 to 10 days, sore throat, and enlargement and tenderness of the cervical lymph nodes. Sore throat is the most common symptom. It appears in the first week and is usually accompanied by hyperplasia of the pharyngeal lymphoid tissue with inflammation and edema, as well as exudative tonsillitis.

Lymph node enlargement is the predominant clinical manifestation of infectious mononucleosis. Enlargement occurs gradually, most commonly in the anterior and posterior cervical chains, and generalized lymph node enlargement may also develop. Splenomegaly occurs in about one half of affected individuals.

On rare occasions, other manifestations may occur, including hepatitis, erythematous maculopapular rash on the trunk and extremities, and edema around the eyes. Neurologic involvement can include aseptic meningitis, encephalitis, blurred vision, coma, acute cerebellar syndrome, and Guillain-Barré syndrome (inflammation of the nerves).

Infectious mononucleosis is usually self-limiting, and recovery occurs in a few weeks. Treatment consists of rest and alleviation of symptoms with analgesics. Rarely, however, infection with Epstein-Barr virus results in fatal infectious mononucleosis or malignant lymphoma. (Epstein-Barr virus also causes Burkitt lymphoma; see p. 815.) This outcome is probably the result of a genetic immune deficiency syndrome in which the individual's B cells are unable to produce antibodies to the Epstein-Barr virus (Purtilo, 1978).

Laboratory findings include an increase in relative and absolute lymphocyte and monocyte counts, with 10% to 20% atypical forms. In early phases of infectious mononucleosis, this is caused by an increase in both B and T cells. Atypical T cells predominate later. The atypical lymphocytes are large, with oval, horseshoe-shaped, or indented nuclei and vacuolated, spongy cytoplasm, similar to that of basophils. During the first week of infection, the leukocyte count may be normal or slightly low, secondary to mild neutropenia. After the first week, the leukocyte count (predominantly lymphocytes and monocytes) rises to 10,000 to 20,000 per microliter and persists at this level from 4 to 8 weeks. Platelet counts are low (less than 140,000 per cubic millimeter).

Serologic tests are necessary to diagnose infection by Epstein-Barr virus. A Monospot agglutination test is performed to show the presence of heterophilic antibodies associated with infection by Epstein-Barr virus. (Heterophilic antibodies are a heterogeneous group of antibodies that are agglutins against sheep red blood cells.) Specificity can be increased by differential agglutination tests. Other serologic tests that detect antibodies specific for the virus are used in children.

Leukemias

Leukemia is a disease of the blood-forming organs. Primary tumors are found predominantly in the bone marrow, but are also found in lymphoid tissues (liver, spleen, and lymph nodes) and other organs. The common pathologic feature of all forms of leukemia is an uncontrolled proliferation of leukocytes. This lack of control causes normal bone marrow to be replaced by immature and undifferentiated leukocytes or "blast cells." Abnormal, immature leukocytes then circulate in the blood and infiltrate the liver, spleen, lymph nodes, and other sites throughout the body.

Much controversy has surrounded the classification and pathogenesis of leukemia. Perhaps the first description of a "leukemic" individual was by Velpean in 1827 (Gunz, 1980). His patient, a florist and seller of lemonade, age 63 years, "who had abandoned himself to the abuse of spiritous liquor and of women, without, however, becoming syphilitic," became ill in 1825. This patient had great swelling of the abdomen, fever, weakness, and symptoms related to urinary stones. On autopsy, he was found to have a very large liver and spleen, and blood and pus resembling the color of yeast and red wine (Gunz, 1980). Not until 1945, however, did the physiologist Bennet and pathologist Virchow separately describe leukemia. Virchow coined the term "white blood" (weissus blut) and later the term "leukemia." He is largely credited with discoveries that have led to current knowledge of the pathology of leukemia.

Since Virchow's time, the classification of leukemia has become increasingly complex. All leukemias can be designated as (1) lymphocytic, (2) myelocytic or myelogenous, or (3) monocytic. Classification systems for the leukemias vary from scientist to scientist, from clinician to clinician, and, therefore, from text to text. Part of this confusion is because of the great variability in the maturity of leukemic cells. Compounding the problem is the difficulty of separating some **lymphomas** (tumors of the lymph nodes, spleen, and liver) from leukemias whose cells have remarkably identical phenotypes. In addition to this chaos, accurate survival and mortality data have been most difficult to disentangle when records use different classification types.

One common method of classification distinguishes acute and chronic forms. With this method, the term **acute leukemia** refers to undifferentiated or poorly differentiated blast cells characterized by a rapidly fatal course (approximately 2 to 4 months) when left untreated. The acute leukemias are divided into two major types: (1) **acute nonlymphoblastic leukemia (ANLL)** or **acute myelogenous leukemia (AML)**, and (2) **acute lymphoblastic leukemia (ALL).** Chemotherapy and bone marrow transplants have significantly increased the survival time for individuals with acute leukemia. In **chronic leukemia** the leukemic cell is well differentiated, and cell types are more easily identified. Chronic leukemias permit longer survival even when untreated. Two principal types of chronic leukemia are (1) **chronic granulocytic leukemia (CGL)** or **chronic myelocytic leukemia (CML)** and (2) **chronic lymphocytic leukemia (CLL).**

Leukemia occurs with varying frequencies at different ages and is more frequent in older people (about 27,300 cases/year) than in younger people (2200 cases/year) (American Cancer Society, 1989). Acute lymphoblastic leukemia is the most common type in children and accounts for more than two-thirds of all cases. Acute nonlymphoblastic leukemia (about 8000 cases/year) and chronic lymphocytic leukemia (about 9600 cases/year) are the most common types in adults (American Cancer Society, 1988). The sites of highest overall incidence are the United States, Canada, Sweden, and New Zealand.

Acute Leukemias

For all types of acute leukemia, the mortality rate for the United States is about 7 per 100,000 individuals. North America and the Scandanavian countries have the highest mortality; Eastern European countries, Asia (except Japan), and Central America have the lowest mortality. The higher mortality in Japan is the result of the atomic bombs. Black Americans have consistently shown a lower mortality than whites.

The incidence in males is greater than in females in all age groups. Recent data have revealed a reduction in mortality from ALL at all ages, except among male children ages 10 to 14, and have revealed increases in mortality from ANLL, especially in the older age groups. The decrease in mortality for ALL appears to be the result of chemotherapy. The reasons for the increase in mortality from ANLL are not clear. One possibility is that because chemotherapeutic agents are capable of producing cancerous transformation of the bone marrow, such transformation leads to the development of ANLL (Selvin et al., 1983).

Pathogenesis

Leukemias are considered clonal disorders, in that a single cell undergoes transformation and leukemic cells then proliferate. An interesting paradox is that leukemic cells apparently divide more *slowly* and take longer to synthesize DNA than other blood precursors. Acute leukemia therefore is not caused by rapid cellular proliferation, but is instead caused by the blocking of blood cell precursors. Leukemic cells do accumulate relentlessly in most affected individuals, and they compete with normal cellular proliferation. Thus, acute leukemia has also been termed an accumulation disorder, as well as a proliferation disorder.

Although the exact cause of leukemia is unknown, it is clear that causal risk factors acting together with a genetic predisposition can alter nuclear DNA. The leukemic cell is then unable to mature and respond to normal regulatory mechanisms. Abnormal chromosomes are reported in 40% to 50% of patients with acute leukemia, and certain chromosomes are repeatedly more involved than others. It thus appears that a mutation in a single cell gives rise to some leukemias.

Although the genetic mechanism remains unknown, a high incidence of acute leukemias and CLL is reported in certain families. Hereditary abnormalities are also associated with an increased incidence of leukemia. Down syndrome, Fanconi aplastic anemia, Bloom syndrome, ataxia telangiectasia, trisomy 13 (Patau syndrome), Wiskott-Aldrich syndrome, and congenital X-linked agamaglobulinemia.

Acquired disorders that progress to acute leukemia include CGL, polycythemia vera, myelofibrosis, Hodgkin disease, multiple myeloma, ovarian cancer, CLL, and sideroblastic anemia. Large doses of ionizing radiation are associated with an increased incidence in myelogenous leukemia. Viruses are known to cause leukemia in certain animals, but have not yet been proved to cause leukemia in human beings. Drugs that cause bone marrow depression (e.g., chloramphenicol, phenylbutazone) can also predispose an individual to leukemia. Cancer chemotherapeutic agents that cause bone marrow depression can thus be a contributing factor in the development of leukemia.

In some cases, the development of leukemia occurs in the most primitive blood precursors—pluripotential stem cells—that give rise to all other blood cells (Fig. 24-1). The leukemia blasts, or precursor cells, literally "crowd out" the marrow and cause cellular proliferation of the other cell lines to cease. Normal granulocytic-monocytic, lymphocytic, erythrocytic, and megakaryocytic stem cells cease to function, causing **pancytopenia** (a reduction in all cellular components of the blood). Transformation also may occur specifically in the granulocyte-monocyte series and not in the erythrocyte series. Much research in acute leukemia has concerned the depression of granulopoietic precursors and the subsequent granulocytopenia. Granulocytes fail to proliferate if cultured in vitro with leukemic cells. The process created in vitro is termed **leukemia-associated inhibitory activity (LIA).** LIA is produced by lymphoidlike cells from patients with ANLL, ALL, acute erythroleukemia (AEL), CGL, and acute transformation of CGL. Individuals in remission exhibit LIA, but the process is usually not detectable because of an inhibitor produced by rapid sedimenting of bone marrow cells (Broxmeyer et al., 1977). During remission, leukemic granulopoietic precursors are thus resistant to LIA.

Clinical Manifestations

The clinical manifestations of all the varieties of acute leukemia are generally similar. (Mechanisms associated with common manifestations are summarized in Table 24-1.) Signs and symptoms related to bone marrow depression include fatigue caused by anemia, bleeding resulting from **thrombocytopenia** (reduced numbers of circulating platelets), and fever caused by infection. Bleeding can occur in skin, gums, mucous membranes, and gastrointestinal and genitourinary tracts. Signs of bleeding include discoloration visible through the skin, oozing from the gums, and hematuria (blood in the urine).

Acute leukemia in children is abrupt, resembling an infection. Sites of infection include gums, throat, respiratory tract, lower colon, urinary tract, and skin. Common organisms include the gram-negative bacilli *Escherichia coli, Pseudomonas aeruginosa,* and *Klebsiella pneumonia* and some gram-positive organisms, particularly *Staphylococcus aureus.* Fever is an early sign. Chills and tissue infiltration are common.

Anorexia is associated with weight loss, diminished sensitivity to sour and sweet tastes, wasting away of muscle, and difficulty swallowing. Liver, spleen, and lymph node enlargement are more common in ALL than in ANLL. Splenomegaly and hepatomegaly usually occur together. The leukemic individual often experiences abdominal pain and tenderness and breast tenderness.

Headache, vomiting, and papilledema are associated with central nervous system involvement. Facial nerve involvement causes facial palsy. Blurred vision, auditory disturbances, and meningeal irritation can occur if leukemic cells infiltrate the cerebral or spinal meninges. Because chemotherapeutic agents do not pass the blood-brain barrier, leukemia cells can grow easily. Intracranial hemorrhage and compression can also occur.

Evaluation and Treatment

Because leukemia is frequently confused with other conditions, early detection is difficult. Persistent symptoms need intensive medical investigation. The diagno-

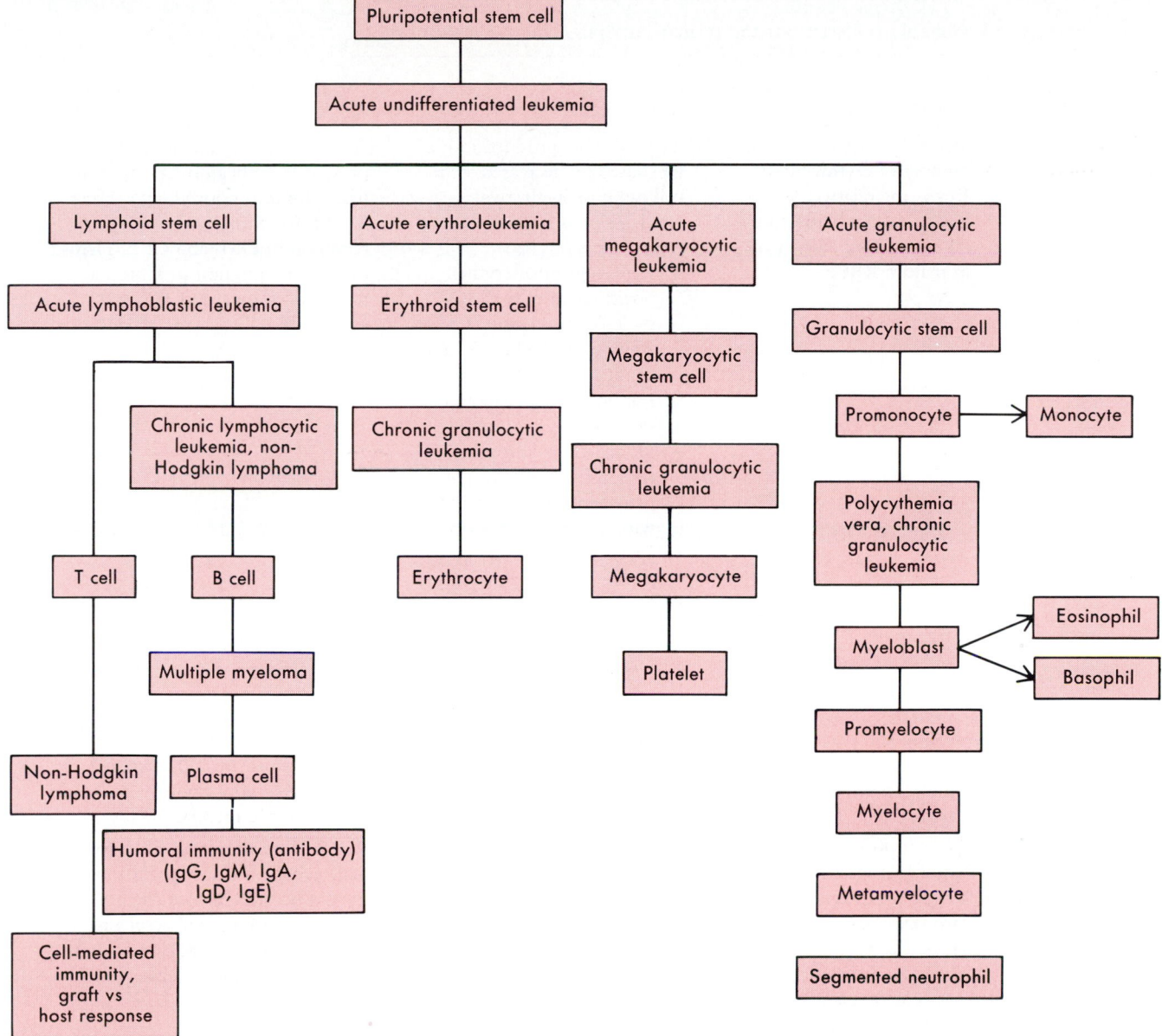

FIG. 24-1. Differentiation pathways of blood-forming cells and reported sites of block resulting in cell-specific leukemias.

sis is made through blood tests and examination of bone marrow.

Chemotherapy is the treatment of choice for leukemia. Drugs are used singly or in combination. Supportive measures include blood transfusions, antibiotics, and allopurinol for preventing production of uric acid.

Acute leukemias are associated with a 20% to 50% long-term survival (American Cancer Society, 1988). Recent improvements have been made in survival of individuals with ALL. In children, ALL remissions are obtained in 85% to 98% of cases, but 50% of children die in the first 5 years. Remissions for adult ALL occur

in about 78% of all cases. ANLL still demonstrates poor survival rates.

Chronic Leukemias

The two main types of chronic leukemia are (1) granulocytic (CGL) and (2) lymphocytic (CLL). Unlike cells in acute leukemia, chronic leukemic cells are well differentiated and can be readily identified. Individuals with chronic leukemia have a longer life expectancy, usually of several years from the time of diagnosis.

The chronic leukemias have a presentation and progression different from the acute leukemias. Chronic

TABLE 24-1 Clinical manifestations and related pathophysiology in leukemia

Clinical manifestations	Laboratory abnormalities	Cause	Comments
Anemia	Either a decrease or normal number of erythroblasts. Key is the relative *proportion* of erythroblasts to total count. Decreased iron in mature RBC.	Decreased RBC production may be caused by decreased stem cell input or ineffective erythropoeisis or is both. Proposed reasons are: 1. Replacement of erythropoeitic stem cells (ESCs) by leukemic clone 2. Inhibition of ESCs by leukemic cells 3. Inhibition of pluripotent stem cell 4. Decreased erythropoeitin responsiveness from impaired interaction of ESCs with T-lymphocytes (in leukemia there is an increase in T-lymphocytes) 5. Hemorrhage 6. Splenic pooling of RBC 7. Drug therapy Marrow crowding is probably not a major cause.	In acute leukemia, anemia is usually present from beginning, often the first symptom noticed, and severe. Mild form without symptoms is common in CGL and CLL. Hemorrhage is common in acute forms, occasional in CGL, but rare in CLL.
Bleeding	Decreased and possibly abnormal platelets.	Reduction in megakaryocytes leading to thrombocytopenia.	Bleeding occurs more commonly in acute than in chronic leukemia. Bleeding is more frequent and serious in the presence of fever.
Disseminated intravascular coagulation (DIC)	Abnormal promyelocytes; hypofibrinogenemia; prolonged prothrombin, thrombin, and reptilase times; elevated fibrin degranulation products; and decreased levels of factor V, fibrinogen, and platelets.	Abnormal promyelocytic granules are known to have procoagulant activity and can be reversed by low-dose heparin. DIC will worsen pre-existing thrombocytopenia by using platelets.	AML patients almost always have hemorrhage. Prior heparinization should be done before chemotherapy because DIC will accelerate from the increased release of granules from destroyed cells.
Infection	Infection is likely with granulocyte levels below 500/mm^3.	Infections are caused by acquired organisms during and after hospitalization and are not merely normal endogenous flora. The rapid overturn of squamous epithelial cells in the alimentary and respiratory tracts encourages organisms to colonize. Granulocytopenic patients have an impaired inflammatory response. Immunodeficiency is secondary to chemotherapy and the disease process.	Major causes of infection are medical personnel, food, and water. Aseptic techniques are absolutely essential for preventing infection. Usually, a combination of antibiotic agents is used.

TABLE 24-1 Clinical manifestations and related pathophysiology in leukemia—cont'd

Clinical manifestations	Laboratory abnormalities	Cause	Comments
Anorexia	Decreased 24-hour urinary creatinine excretion.	Loss of appetite is part of the cachexic syndrome (see p. 306). Condition can be attributed to pain, depression, chemotherapy, radiotherapy, some unknown circulating inhibitor, and alterations in taste.	Causes of anorexia are poorly understood. Severe alterations in taste; highly seasoned foods seem bland, aggravate condition. Patients with liver involvement often detest red meat. Some patients have good appetites in the morning, but become satiated later.
Bone pain	Frequently no radiographic evidence of bone problems.	Result of bone infiltration by leukemic cells or intramedullary infarction.	If combination drug regimens are ineffective, radiotherapy is used.
Elevated uric acid	Normal excretion of uric acid is 300 to 500 mg daily. The leukemic patient can excrete 50 times more. Uric acid precipitates (urates) are commonly found in the proximal collecting tubules and pelvices of the kidney. Oliguria and concentrated urine are sometimes found.	Uric acid is a normal by-product of protein catabolism. Nucleic acid catabolism is accelerated in the leukemic patient. Uric acid precipitation occurs at an acidic, or low, pH. Urate precipitation in the leukemic patient is increased from dehydration caused by anorexia or fever and drug therapy.	Hyperuricemia is present in both acute leukemia and CGL. Kidney pathology can be prevented by ensuring increased urine flow, increasing urine pH by administering sodium bicarbonate, or decreasing acid production through allopurinol, which inhibits the enzyme xanthine oxidase.
Liver, spleen, and lymph node enlargement	Biopsy is abnormal for liver and spleen.	Leukemic cell infiltration causes splenic, hepatic, and lymph node enlargement. Lymph nodes also undergo leukemic proliferation as in CLL.	
Fluid and electrolyte alterations (Na, K, Ca)	Hypernatremia and hypokalemia are common. Hyperkalemia can also be present. Hypercalcemia, although common in other cancers, is rare in leukemia.	Hypernatremia is caused by dehydration or diabetes insipidus. Inappropriate secretion of antidiuretic hormone can spontaneously occur after drug treatment. Hyponatremia can follow drug therapy. Hypokalemia, frequently seen in AML and ALL, may follow drug therapy. Hyperkalemia is seen as a result of cell catabolism and antileukemic therapy. Calcium metabolism may be altered because of parathormone, prostaglandins, or an osteolytic factor causing calcium release from bone.	

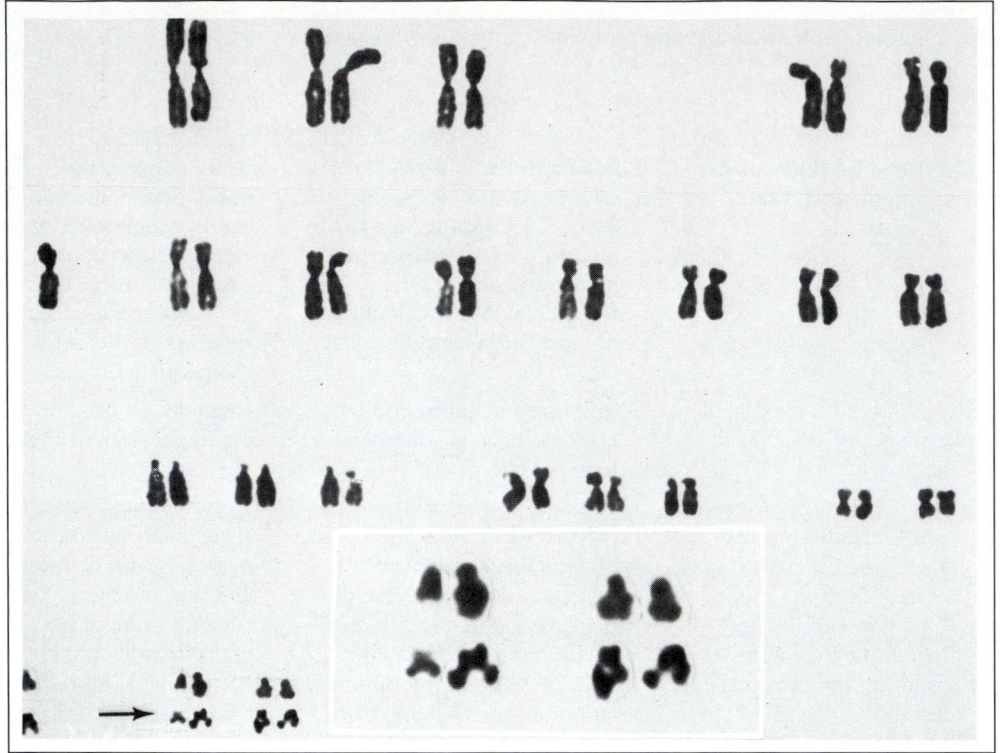

FIG. 24-2. Philadelphia chromosome. Metaphase spread of marrow cell in chronic myelocytic leukemia. Ph[1] chromosome is G21 (arrow and enlarged inset). It is recognized by partial deletion of long arm. (Courtesy Dr. A. K. Sinha, Houston, Texas. From del Regato, Spjut, & Cox, 1985.)

leukemia advances slowly and surreptitiously, without warning. Symptoms—when they do appear—include extreme fatigue, weight loss, night sweats, and low-grade fever.

The incidence of CGL is about 1 per 100,000 people, with most cases occurring in those between 30 and 50 years of age. CGL is also classified as one of the myeloproliferative disorders, along with polycythemia vera, primary thrombocytosis, and idiopathic myelofibrosis (invasion of bone marrow by fibrous tissue).

The presence of the Philadelphia chromosome (a shortened arm on chromosome 22) is diagnostic of CGL (Fig. 24-2). Identifying the Philadelphia chromosome allows the clinician to follow the transformation process. Transformation is identified in erythroid, megakaryocytic, and macrophage cell lines. The chromosome appears not to be genetically transmitted, but to occur because of mitotic error. Evidence thus indicates that CGL has a clonal origin. The malignant transformation arises from pluripotential stem cells or lymphoid stem cells (see Fig. 24-1). Structural cellular abnormalities are not readily identified in CGL. Absent or low levels of the enzyme neutrophil alkaline phosphatase, with subse-

quent decreased phagocytic capabilities, do, however, indicate that cells fail to differentiate normally.

Although the Philadelphia chromosome is present in erythrocytes, monocytes, and megakaryocytes, erythrocytes and platelets are produced and function relatively normally. The acute effects of CGL resemble those of acute leukemia, but with more prominent and painful splenomegaly. Liver function is rarely altered despite enlargement, and lymphadenopathy is generally found only in the acute phase of the disease. Hyperuricemia is invariably present and produces gouty arthritis. Infections, fever, and weight loss are common findings in patients with CGL.

CLL predominantly involves malignant transformation of B cells, although T cell CLL occurs less commonly. The major pathophysiologic deficit in CLL of B cells is their failure to mature into plasma cells that synthesize immunoglobulin (antibody; see Chapter 6). A possible mechanism responsible for CLL of B cells is a deficiency of normal helper T cells with an increase in suppressor T cells. Together, the T cell abnormalities might account for the impaired differentiation of B cells in CLL.

Suppression of humoral immunity caused by reduction in normally functioning B cells is the most significant effect of CLL. Individuals are at risk for both infections commonly combated by B cell-produced immunoglobulins and for the development of autoimmune diseases that result in secondary cancers. Anemia, thrombocytopenia, and neutropenia are typically present with overt CLL (see Table 24-1). Invasion of most organs is uncommon, but infiltration does occur in lymph nodes, liver, spleen, and salivary glands. Central nervous system involvement is rare. Elevated levels of the enzyme lactic dehydrogenase (LDH) and hyperuricemia are common, whereas hypercalcemia is rarely evident.

Multiple Myeloma

Multiple myeloma is a neoplasm of B cells (immature plasma cells) and mature plasma cells. (These lymphocytes are described in Chapter 6.) It is characterized by multiple malignant tumor masses of plasma cells scattered throughout the skeletal system and sometimes in soft tissue. The reported incidence of multiple myeloma has doubled in the past two decades, possibly because of more sensitive testing used for diagnosis (McPhedron, Heath, & Garcia, 1972; Wintrobe et al., 1981). The incidence of multiple myeloma is three times greater than all other malignant tumors of bone combined. It has an annual incidence rate of about 10,000 cases in the United States (Schnipper, Wagner, & McCaffrey, 1986). Malignant myeloma has been reported in all races, but the incidence rate in blacks (2 to 4 per 100,000) is at least twice that in whites (1 to 2 per 100,000) (McPhedran et al., 1972; Young, Percy, & Asire, 1981). It is rare before the age of 40 and then occurs increasingly with age, reaching a peak during the seventh decade. The neoplasm is also more common in men than women.

The exact cause of multiple myeloma remains uncertain, but a few clues have been gleaned from studies of animals and clinical observations of human disease. Genetic factors are suggested as a possible cause because tumors occur in specific strains of mice and in human siblings and other near relatives. Chronic stimulation of the mononuclear phagocyte system by chemicals, bacteria, and viral agents has also been suggested as a possible cause. This suggestion is supported by the increased frequency of plasma cell neoplasms in individuals with long-standing chronic infections, such as tuberculosis, osteomyelitis, and pneumonitis, and by the effects of chemical injections in mice (Robbins, Cotran, & Kumar, 1984).

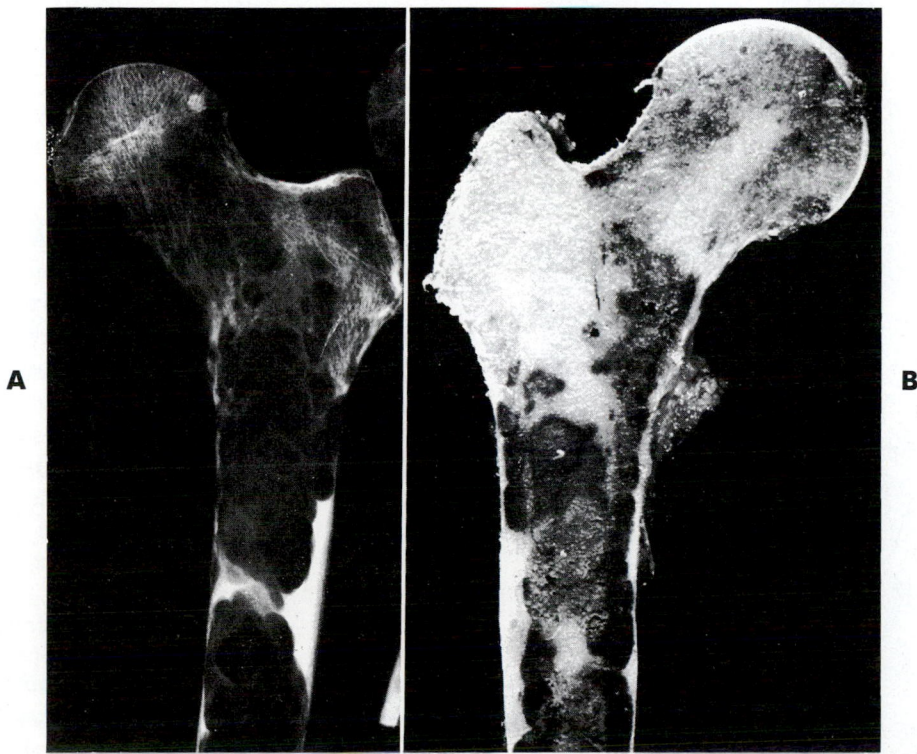

FIG. 24-3. Multiple (plasma cell) myeloma. **A,** Roentgenogram of femur showing extensive bone destruction caused by tumor. Note absence of reactive bone formation. **B,** Gross specimen from same individual; myelomatous sections appear as dark granular sections (From Kissane, 1985.)

Pathophysiology

Malignant plasma cells arise from one clone of B cells that produce abnormally large amounts of one class of immunoglobulin (usually IgG, occasionally IgA, and rarely IgM, IgD, or IgE). Blood levels of the immunoglobulin, called the **M component**, are elevated, and immunoglobulin fragments are present in the urine. **Bence Jones proteins** are present in the urine and the M components in the blood of 60% to 80% of all individuals with multiple myeloma (Solomon, 1981).

Multiple myeloma becomes evident as diffuse destructive bone lesions (Fig. 24-3). The bones most commonly affected are the vertebrae (66%), ribs (44%), skull (41%), pelvis, (28%), femur (24%), clavicle (10%), and scapula (10%) (Robbins et al., 1984). The lesions progressively destroy the cortical bone. (Bone structures are described in Chapter 38.)

Clinical Manifestations

Clinical manifestations are the result of (1) infiltration and destruction of organs, particularly bone, by the neoplastic plasma cells and (2) an M component consisting of an excess of immunoglobulins with altered physio-logic properties and immune function. Infiltration of bones by malignant plasma cells causes pain and pathologic fractures. Hypercalcemia resulting from bone resorption can cause neurologic disturbances, such as confusion, lethargy, and weakness and can contribute to renal disease.

A major clinical manifestation is recurrent infections resulting from suppression of the humoral (antibody-mediated) immune response. Cell-mediated immune function (i.e., T cell function) is relatively normal (Robbins et al., 1984). Humoral immune function is thought to be suppressed by unknown factors secreted from malignant plasma cells. These factors activate macrophages that inhibit maturation of B cells into plasma cells that would be capable of producing immunoglobulins normally (Ullrich & Zolla-Pazner, 1982; Wintrobe et al., 1981). Renal disease, a complication of multiple myeloma, is thought to be the result of Bence Jones proteinuria. The excreted Bence Jones proteins may be toxic to the tubular epithelial cells of the kidney (Defonzo et al., 1978).

Evaluation and Treatment

Diagnosis of multiple myeloma is made by radiographic and laboratory studies and biopsy of a lesion. Chemotherapy is used for treatment. Individuals with mutiple bony lesions, if untreated, rarely survive for more than 6 to 12 months. With chemotherapy, survival is still only 2 to 3 years.

ALTERATIONS IN LYMPHOID FUNCTION

Lymphadenopathy

Normally, lymph nodes are not palpable or only barely palpable. Nodes are generally classified as tender or nontender, and movable or fixed. **Lymphadenopathy** is characterized by enlarged lymph nodes (Fig. 24-4). Localized lymphadenopathy usually indicates drainage of an inflammatory lesion. Generalized lymphadenopathy occurs less frequently as a result of infection and is, therefore, usually associated with a malignant or nonmalignant disease. Lymphadenopathy reflects significant diseases more often in adults than in children.

Enlargement of the lymph node is often caused by an increase in size and number of the germinal centers within the node caused by proliferation of lymphocytes or monocytes (immature macrophages). Enlargement may also be caused by invasion of the node by malignant cells or cells not normally present within the node. Palpable nodes, however, do not always indicate serious disease and may only indicate a reaction to minor trauma or infection of a specific structure. The location and size of the enlarged node are important factors in

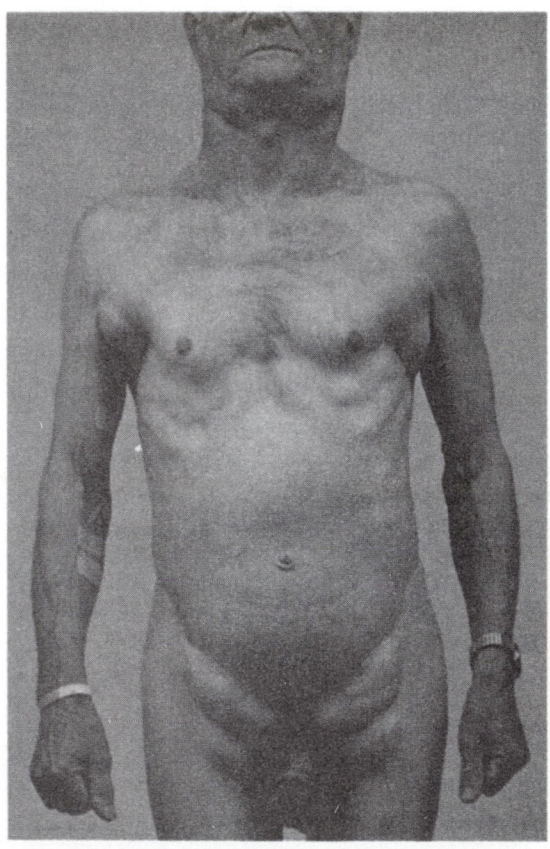

FIG. 24-4. Individual with lymphocyte leukemia with extreme but symmetrical lymphadenopathy. (Courtesy Dr. A. R. Kagan, Los Angeles. From del Regato, Spjut, & Cox, 1985.)

diagnosing the cause of the lymphadenopathy, as are the individual's age, sex, and geographic location. Generalized lymphadenopathy occurs with non-Hodgkin lymphomas, chronic lymphocytic leukemia, histiocytoses, and disorders that produce lymphocytosis. In general, lymphadenopathy results from four types of conditions: (1) neoplastic disease, (2) immunologic or inflammatory conditions, (3) endocrine disorders, or (4) lipid storage diseases. Diseases of unknown cause, including autoimmune diseases and reactions to drugs, may also lead to generalized lymphadenopathy.

Malignant Lymphomas

Lymphomas are tumors of primary lymphoid tissue (thymus and bone marrow) or secondary tissue (lymph nodes, spleen, tonsils, and intestinal lymphoid tissue). Most lymphomas are neoplasms of secondary lymphoid tissue and involve mostly lymph nodes and/or spleen. Malignant lymphoid cells are sometimes found in circulating blood, indicating bone marrow involvement. The major subdivisions of malignant lymphomas are **Hodgkin disease** and **non-Hodgkin lymphoma.** Bone marrow involvement occurs more often in non-Hodgkin lymphoma than in Hodgkin disease.

Histopathologic classifications for Hodgkin disease have grown and changed since the first attempt by Ewing in 1928 to the present widely used Rye classification (Table 24-2). Undoubtedly, more changes will ensue. Non-Hodgkin lymphoma also has several classifications. Rappaport's widely used classification distinguishes two major histopathologic patterns: nodular and diffuse (Table 24-3). The diffuse pattern does not show the cell aggregates that are evident in the nodular pattern.

These two patterns in non-Hodgkin lymphoma illustrate two different pathologic states. The nodular (and diffuse, well-differentiated lymphocytic) pattern involves nodal and extranodal sites. Initially, the disease is slow-growing with few symptoms. After a time, rapid growth

can cause the disease to become diffuse. With the diffuse pattern, disease is rapidly growing with early extranodal invasion.

Incidence rates differ with respect to age, sex, geographic locations, and socioeconomic class. The incidence rate of Hodgkin disease is about 2.6 per 100,000 in men and 2.2 per 100,000 in women (Skarin et al., 1986). The incidence rate of non-Hodgkin lymphoma in men is about 5.0 per 100,000 and 3.4 per 100,000 in women (Skarin et al., 1986). Both diseases occur more frequently in men than in women. Hodgkin disease peaks at two different ages, one between 15 and 35 years (the majority of cases) and the other at about age 50 years. Non-Hodgkin lymphoma is a disease of the middle years, usually over the age of 40. The Netherlands, Denmark, and the United States have the highest incidence of Hodgkin disease; Japan and Australia have the lowest rates. High socioeconomic status is also associated with the disease.

Hodgkin Disease

Pathogenesis
Distinctive abnormal chromosomes are present in multiple cells from the lymph nodes of an individual with Hodgkin disease. Hodgkin disease is therefore a

TABLE 24-2 Major classifications of Hodgkin disease

Rye (1966) and Rosenberg (1966)	Lukes, Butler, Hicks (1966)	Jackson & Parker (1944)
Lymphocytic predominant	Nodular or diffuse lymphocytic/ histiocytic	Paragranuloma
Nodular sclerosis	Nodular sclerosis	None
Mixed cellularity	Mixed	Granuloma
Lymphocytic depletion	Diffuse fibrosis or reticular	Sarcoma

TABLE 24-3 Classification of non-Hodgkin lymphoma

New terminology (Rappaport, 1966)	Old terminology (Gall & Mallory, 1944)
LOW GRADE	
Lymphocyte well differentiated, nodular or diffuse	Giant follicular lymphoma (Brill-Symmer)
Nodular, poorly differentiated, lymphocytic	None
Nodular mixed lymphocytic-histiocytic	None
INTERMEDIATE GRADE	
Nodular histiocytic	Lymphosarcoma
Diffuse poorly differentiated lymphocytic	None
Diffuse mixed lymphocytic-histiocytic	None
Diffuse histiocytic	None
HIGH GRADE	
Diffuse histiocytic	Reticulum cell sarcoma
Lymphoblastic	None
Diffuse undifferentiated (Burkitt/non-Burkitt)	None

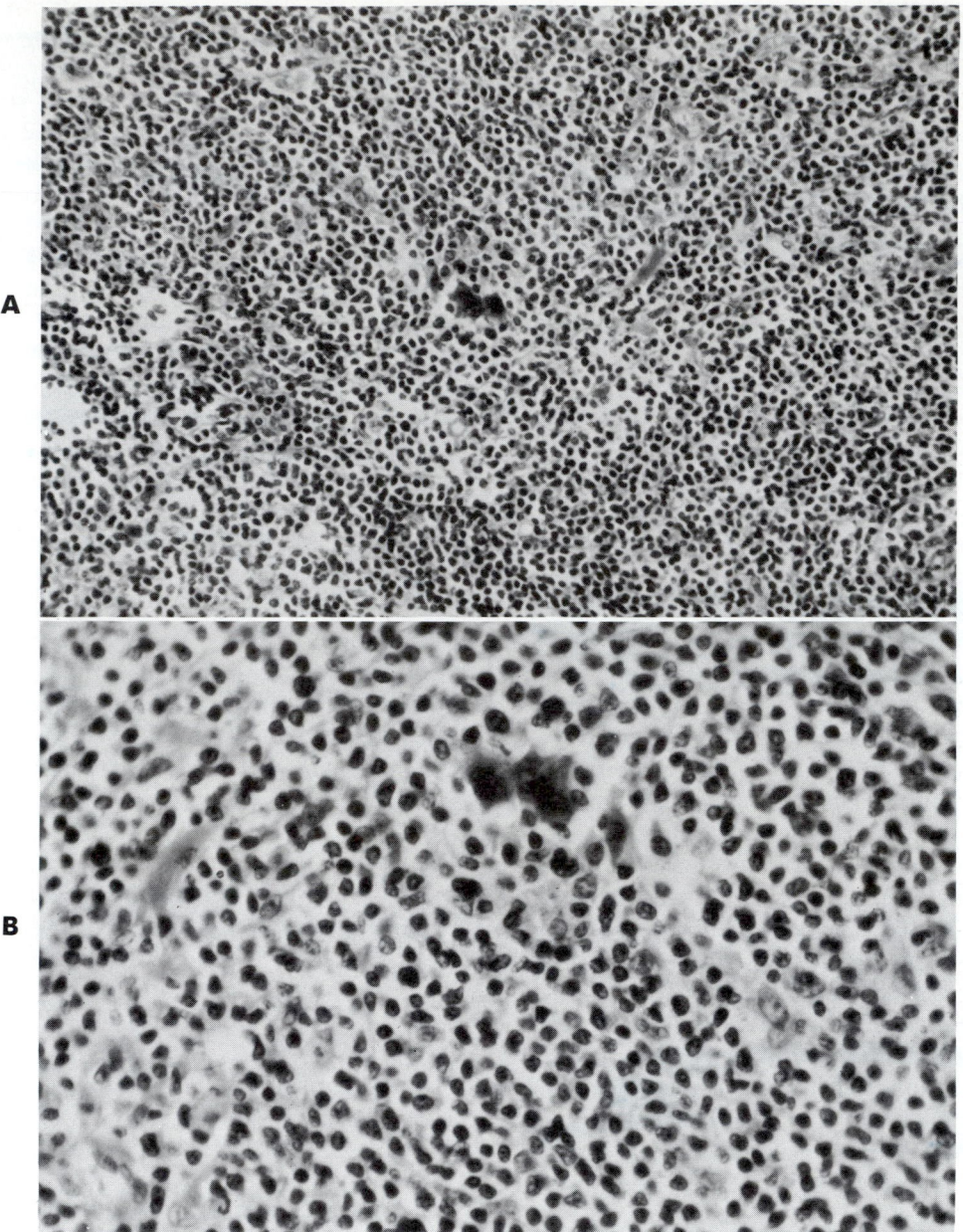

FIG. 24-5. Lymph node. **A,** Hodgkin disease, lymphocytic predominance type (125×). **B,** Note large darker cell. Sternberg-Reed cell, characteristic of Hodgkin disease with lymphocytic predominance (250×). (From Kissane, 1985.)

clonal disorder. The classically abnormal cell is the Sternberg-Reed cell, which is large and often confused with giant cells found in tuberculosis (Fig. 24-5). Sternberg-Reed cells are polyploid with large nuclei and are derived from the monocyte-macrophage series.

Cancerous transformation occurs from a particular site in the lymph node. With continuing growth, the entire node becomes replaced, with zones of necrosis obscuring the normal nodular pattern.

Current evidence indicates that an inhibitor in the se-

rum and spleen of individuals with Hodgkin disease selectively binds to T cells and interferes with their function. Another reported mechanism is suppressor activity by monocytes. Individuals in sustained long remission after total lymphoid radiation continue to exhibit deficient cell-mediated immunity, which is associated with a T-lymphocytopenia and a B-lymphocytosis (Kaplan, 1980). Impaired cell-mediated immunity causes delayed responsiveness to natural antigens (hypersensitivity) and delayed homograft rejection.

Two theories are proposed for the mechanism of spread of Hodgkin disease: (1) the contiguity theory and (2) the susceptibility theory. The contiguity theory suggests that Hodgkin disease spreads by the movement of existing tumor cells through lymphatic routes. This theory is based on the notion that spread occurs through immediate connections between pairs of lymph node chains connected by one or more lymphatic channels. Thus transmission is orderly, from one chain to another.

The susceptibility theory suggests that Hodgkin disease is a disorder of the whole lymphatic system, involving certain susceptible multiple sites of origin. Thus the spread occurs because of a traveling causative agent rather than spread of pre-existing tumor cells. This theory also suggests that Hodgkin cells may travel to different lymph nodes through the bloodstream, much as normal lymphocytes do. Because Hodgkin disease is currently more accepted as a clonal disorder and contiguous lymph nodes have been described, the contiguity theory is better supported.

Clusters of cases in high schools and certain geographic locations suggest that transmissible agents, such as a virus, might be involved in the pathogenesis of Hodgkin disease. The isolation of herpes virus in individuals with Hodgkin disease (i.e., the presence of Sternberg-Reed cells in lymph nodes of individuals with infectious mononucleosis) further substantiate the viral theory. Higher-than-normal antibody titers to the Epstein-Barr virus are also reported in individuals with Hodgkin disease. Some familial clustering of Hodgkin disease suggests an unknown genetic mechanism.

Clinical Manifestations

An enlarged painless mass, lump, or swelling, most commonly in the neck, is frequently an initial sign of Hodgkin disease (Fig. 24-6). Fever, especially in the evening for several days, may occur intermittently. Older persons more readily experience weakness, malaise, weight loss, and anemia. Back and neck pain with hyperreflexia can be present in both Hodgkin disease and non-Hodgkin lymphoma, suggesting epidural involvement. Alcohol ingestion is often followed by pain and discomfort in a state of lymphadenopathy.

The cervical, axillary, inguinal, and retroperitoneal lymph nodes are most commonly affected in Hodgkin disease, whereas the mesenteric epitrochlear, bronchial, and popliteal nodes are rarely involved (Fig. 24-7). Local symptoms are produced by lymphadenopathy, usually caused by pressure or obstruction. Extremity in-

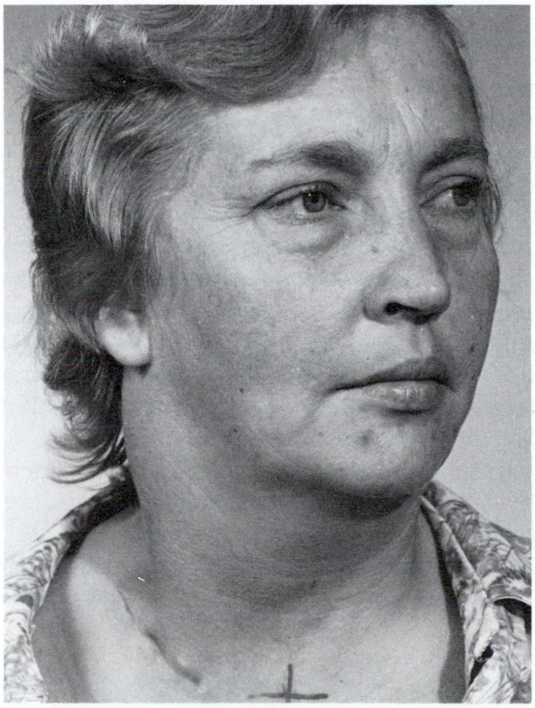

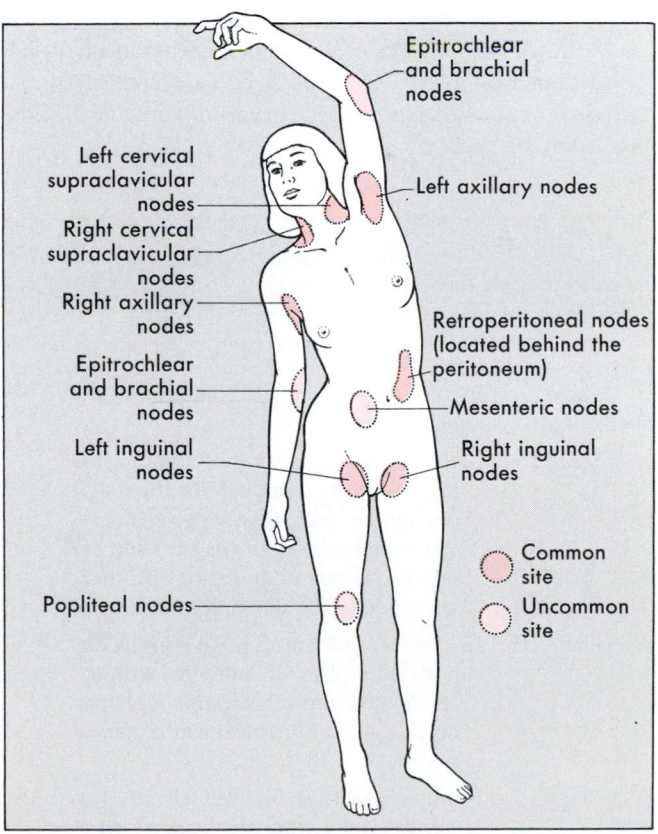

FIG. 24-6. Typical enlarged cervical lymph node in the neck of a 35-year-old woman with Hodgkin disease. (From del Regato, Spjut, & Cox, 1985.)

FIG. 24-7. Common and uncommon involved lymph nodes sites for Hodgkin disease.

volvement can manifest itself by pain, nerve irritation, and obliteration of the pulse.

Although Hodgkin disease rarely arises in the lung, mediastinal, and hilar node, adenopathy can cause secondary involvement of the trachea, bronchi, pleura, or lungs. Determination that pulmonary involvement is because of Hodgkin disease is complicated by infections that can occur together with Hodgkin disease in the same lung. Retroperitoneal nodes can involve vertebral bodies and nerves and can cause displacement of ureters. In the spinal cord, involvement is more common in the dorsal and lumbar regions than in the cervical region. Although infrequent, skin manifestations can include psoriasis and eczematoid lesions, causing itching and scratching.

Pericardial involvement can occur by direct invasion from mediastinal lymph nodes. This involvement can cause pericardial friction rub, pericardial effusion, and engorgement of neck veins. The gastrointestinal tract and urinary tract are rarely sites of involvement. Anemia is frequently found in individuals with a low serum iron and iron-binding capacity. Hemolytic anemia is rare. Other laboratory findings include elevated sedimentation rate, leukocytosis, and eosinophilia. With advanced stages of Hodgkin disease, leukopenia occurs.

Splenic involvement in Hodgkin disease depends on histopathologic type (see Table 24-2). The spleen is involved in 60% of cases of mixed-cellularity and lymphocyte depletion types. Only 34% of cases reveal splenic involvement with lymphocyte predominance and nodular sclerosis types.

TABLE 24-4 Stanford clinical staging classification in Hodgkin disease

Stage	Extent of involvement
Stage I	Involvement of a single lymph node site or lymphatic region
Stage II	Involvement of two or more lymph node regions on the same side of the diaphragm or single involvement of an extralymphatic organ (or site) and one or more lymph node regions on the same side of the diaphragm
Stage III	Involvement of lymph node regions on both sides of the diaphragm, with local involvement of an extralymphatic organ (or site), involvement of the spleen, or both
Stage IV	Multiple or diffuse involvement of one or more extralymphatic organs or tissue, with or without associated lymph node involvement

---

Mixed-cellularity and lymphocyte depletion patterns are usually widespread at time of diagnosis. In the lymphocyte depletion type of Hodgkin, an abundance of Sternberg-Reed cells with few lymphocytes is evident. This type has a higher incidence of spleen, liver, and bone marrow involvement. (Initially, the lymphocytic predominance pattern tends to involve a single peripheral node or chain of nodes.) At diagnosis, nodular sclerosing Hodgkin disease can include groups of nodes in the cervical regions as well as mediastinal involvement. (Clinical staging classification is presented in Table 24-4.)

Evaluation and Treatment

Because of the variability in symptoms, early definitive detection may be difficult. Asymptomatic lymphadenopathy can progress undetected for several years. Careful evaluation, including chest x-ray films, lymphangiography, and biopsy, should be carried out for individuals with fever of unknown origin and peripheral lymphadenopathy. Biopsy establishes the diagnosis for both Hodgkin disease and non-Hodgkin lymphoma. Both are treated with radiotherapy and chemotherapy (Fig. 24-8). Localized gastrointestinal lymphoma is occasionally cured by surgery.

With proper treatment, cure of stage I or II Hodgkin disease is relatively assured. Stage III has a 75% long-term cure rate, and stage IV about 60%. Individuals treated with chemotherapy who relapse in less than 2 years have poor prognoses.

Non-Hodgkin Lymphoma

Pathogenesis

The cause of lymph node enlargement and cancerous transformation in non-Hodgkin lymphoma is unknown. The diffuse form is characterized by more systemic symptoms (see Table 24-3).

Immunosuppressed persons have greater incidence of non-Hodgkin lymphoma, suggesting an immune mechanism. In contrast to Hodgkin disease, T cell function is minimally affected. B-cell abnormalities, such as impaired and decreased antibody production, are more common in non-Hodgkin lymphoma than in Hodgkin disease. Disorders of mononuclear phagocytes, particular macrophages fixed in tissues, occur more often in individuals with non-Hodgkin lymphoma. A greater-than-expected incidence of non-Hodgkin lymphoma is reported in individuals with ataxia-telangiectasia, Wiskott-Aldrich syndrome, and Chediak-Higashi syndrome.

Clinical Manifestations

The cervical, axillary, inguinal, and femoral chains are the most frequent sites of lymph node enlargement. Generally, the swelling is painless and the nodes have enlarged and transformed over a period of months or

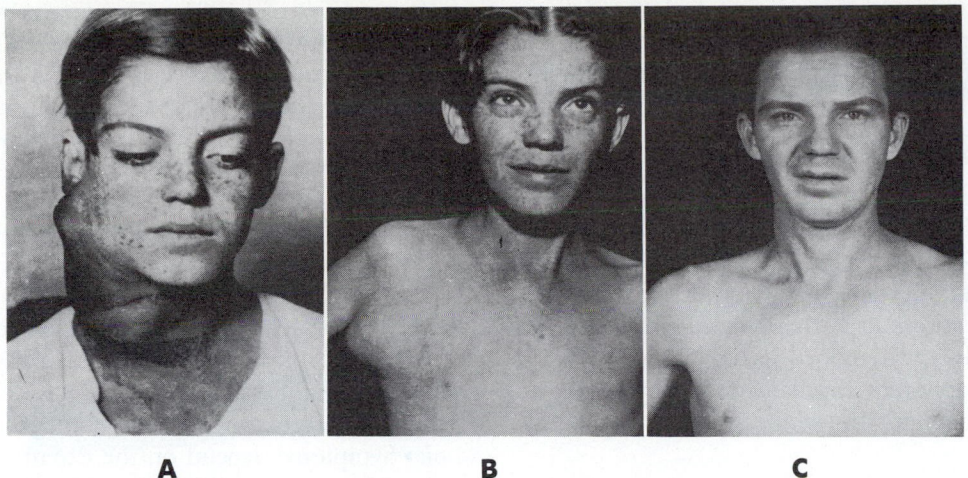

FIG. 24-8. A, Young boy with extensive cervical Hodgkin disease. **B,** Appearance several years later, when axillary manifestation developed. **C,** Appearance 23 years after initial treatment with radiation. (From del Regato, Spjut, & Cox, 1985.)

years. Extranodal sites of involvement are the nasopharynx, gastrointestinal tract, bone, thyroid, testes, and soft tissue. Some individuals have retroperitoneal and abdominal masses with symptoms of abdominal fullness, back pain, ascites (fluid in the peritoneal cavity), and leg swelling. Several sites of involvement for non-Hodgkin lymphoma are not common for Hodgkin disease. These sites include Waldeyer's ring (lymphoid tissue that encircles the tonsils), stomach, small and large bowel, mesenteric lymph nodes, thyroid, skin, pancreas, kidney, and central nervous system. With diffuse non-Hodgkin lymphoma, symptoms are variable and generally involve more systemic findings.

Initially, the blood count at diagnosis for non-Hodgkin lymphoma is normal. Blood abnormalities are not seen until the disease is advanced, although the bone marrow is involved earlier than in Hodgkin disease. Pancytopenia, when present, indicates hypersplenism or extensive replacement of bone marrow by lymphoma.

Evaluation and Treatment

Individuals with non-Hodgkin lymphoma can survive for long periods. Survival with nodular lymphoma ranges up to 15 years. Individuals with diffuse disease generally do not survive as long. Recently, however, 30% of those who were treated with aggressive chemotherapy and who entered complete remission demonstrated a 3-year disease-free interval. These data suggest a possible cure.

Burkitt Lymphoma

Burkitt lymphoma is a tumor with unique clinical and epidemiologic features. It occurs in children from Eastern Central Africa and New Guinea and primarily involves the jaw and facial bones (Fig. 24-9). The Epstein-Barr virus is associated with Burkitt lymphoma in African children. The virus is found in nasopharyngeal secretions (Borden, Steeves, & Hogan, 1983).

The American type of Burkitt lymphoma usually involves the abdomen and is characterized by extensive marrow replacement. The cancerous cell is a B cell that

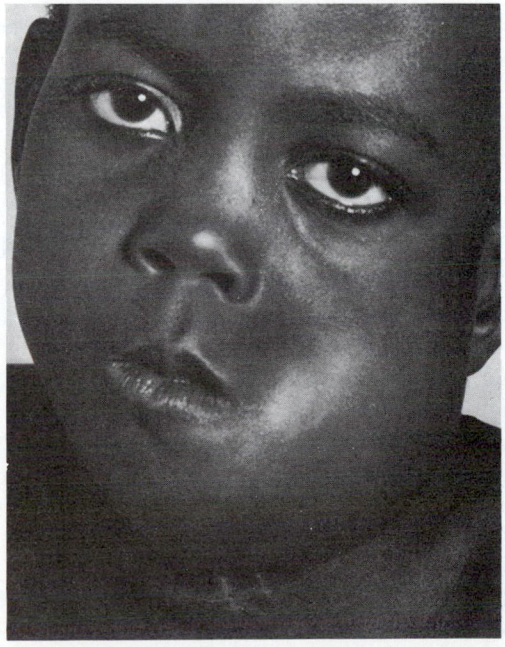

FIG. 24-9. Burkitt lymphoma involving the jaw in young African boy. (Courtesy Dr. J. N. P. Davies, Albany, NY. From del Regato, Spjut, & Cox, 1985.)

undergoes cancerous transformation and progression. The African variety has been successfully treated with radiotherapy and cyclophosphamide. The American type is more resistant to treatment.

Conditions that Mimic Lymphomas

Certain other clinical conditions mimic the malignant lymphomas. These conditions include tuberculosis, syphilis, systemic lupus erythematosus, lung cancer, and bone cancer. An important distinction between lymphomas and other conditions is that lymphomas usually involve localized lymphadenopathy. Infectious precursors of malignant lymphomas are characterized by more generalized lymphadenopathy with systemic signs and symptoms.

ALTERATIONS OF SPLENIC FUNCTION

Most alterations of splenic function, particularly those caused by **splenomegaly** (splenic enlargement) result from disorders elsewhere in the body. Sometimes, however, primary physiologic or anatomic alterations do occur. Primary anatomic alterations include splenic rupture (usually caused by trauma), tumors, cysts, and vascular anomalies, particularly infarction (blockage) or aneurysm (a sac or outpouching in a vessel wall). **Hypersplenism** (hyperactivity of the spleen) is the most common primary physiologic alteration.

Splenomegaly

Splenic enlargement can be caused by proliferation of lymphocytes or macrophages of the white pulp, invasion of neoplastic cells, or chronic congestion with blood. These mechanisms of splenomegaly have several different causes. Proliferation of lymphocytes is caused by infection and is almost always associated with lymphadenopathy. Proliferation of macrophages, on the other hand, is usually the result of a blood disorder, such as hemolytic anemia, in which macrophages increase in number so as to phagocytose the defective or dead erythrocytes. Infiltration of neoplastic cells causes splenomegaly resulting from tumor growth. Congestive splenomegaly, or congestion with blood, is caused by hypertension in the portal vein (the vein that receives blood from the spleen), causing blood to leave the spleen more slowly and with more turbulence than it enters. Other causes of splenomegaly include metabolic-infiltrative disorders and splenic abnormalities.

Infiltrative splenomegaly is caused by engorgement of macrophages within the spleen. These macrophages contain indigestible materials associated with specific rare diseases, such as Gaucher disease, Niemann-Pick disease, amyloidosis, diabetic lipemia, and gargoylism

(Wintrobe et al., 1981). The spleen may also develop cysts that cause enlargement. Cysts are benign tumors.

The spleen is usually not palpable in the adult. Splenomegaly without lymphadenopathy is associated with such conditions as hemolytic anemia and portal hypertension. Splenomegaly with lympadenopathy is very common and is likely to be associated with any condition involving inflammation or infection.

Hypersplenism

Hypersplenism is a primary or secondary syndrome of accelerated splenic function, particularly the function of blood cell filtration and removal. Hypersplenism is therefore associated with splenomegaly and pancytopenia. Symptoms depend on the extent of the pancytopenia. Neutropenia causes frequent bacterial infections, whereas thrombocytopenia (platelet counts less than 50,000 per cubic millimeter) cause easy bruising and hemorrhage from mucous membranes of the gastrointestinal and genitourinary tracts or from cerebral blood vessels.

Treatment for hypersplenism is splenectomy, which is performed if granulocytopenia (granulocyte count less than 5,000 cells per cubic millimeter) or thrombocytopenia are severe. Improvement after splenectomy is fairly rapid and dramatic. Long-term effects of splenectomy are not entirely beneficial, however, and include leukocytosis, decreased levels of serum iron, and slight decreases in immune function.

ALTERATIONS OF PLATELETS AND COAGULATION

Alterations of platelets and coagulation all affect hemostasis, either by preventing hemostasis or by causing hemostasis to occur when it is not needed. (Hemostasis is described in Chapter 22.) Platelet and coagulation disorders can prevent hemostasis to varying degrees, causing (or failing to cause) internal or external hemorrhage. Diffuse internal hemorrhage that is visible through the skin causes a discoloration identified as a **purpura.** Purpuric disorders occur when there are not enough normal platelets to plug damaged vessels or prevent leakage from the many minute tears that occur daily in normal capillaries. Coagulation disorders tend to result in more serious bleeding and are usually caused by a deficiency of one or several clotting factors. Hemorrhagic manifestations of deficient platelet and coagulative function are defined in Table 24-5.

Disorders in which coagulation proceeds unnecessarily tend to result from vascular abnormalities that stimulate clotting. These disorders are known collectively as thromboembolic disease.

TABLE 24-5 Manifestations of bleeding disorders

Manifestation	Mechanism	Appearance and characteristics	Primary hematologic disturbance	
			Platelet	Coagulation
Purpura	Hemorrhage into tissues	Reddish brown discoloration visible through skin	X	
Petechia	Hemorrhage from a damaged capillary	Tiny red or brownish purple dot on skin or mucous membrane. Develops in dependent areas having high venous pressure; tends to occur in groups and in association with ecchymosis	X	
Ecchymosis	Seepage of blood through walls of various small vessels	Red or brownish purple patch on skin or mucous membrane, larger than petechia. Develops because of seepage rather than vessel damage		X
		Small, superficial (cutaneous) ecchymosis	X	
		Large, subcutaneous ecchymosis		X
Hematoma	Hemorrhage from damaged blood vessel	Large, spreading collection of blood in deeper tissues		X
Bruise	Effusion of blood from superficial vessels damaged by blunt impact without laceration of the skin.	Bluish purple area that may be raised (swollen) and tender; changes color as hemoglobin is broken down by phagocytes	X	X
Hemarthrosis	Hemorrhage into a synovial joint	Impaired mobility of the joint		X
Persistent bleeding from superficial injury	Hemorrhage of blood vessels damaged by superficial trauma	Bleeding immediately after injury Delayed bleeding	X	X

Disorders of Platelets

Quantitative or qualitative abnormalities of platelets can interrupt normal blood coagulation and prevent hemostasis. The quantitative abnormalities are **thrombocytopenia,** a decrease in the number of circulating platelets, and **thrombocytosis,** an increase in the number of platelets. Qualitative disorders affect the structure or function of individual platelets and can coexist with the quantitative disorders. Qualitative disorders usually prevent platelet adherence and aggregation, preventing formation of a platelet plug.

Thrombocytopenia

Thrombocytopenia is defined as a platelet count below 100,000 platelets per cubic millimeter of blood. A count of 50,000 or less increases the potential for hemorrhage associated with minor trauma. Spontaneous bleeding can occur with counts between 20,000 and 10,000, resulting in petechiae, ecchymoses, larger purpuric spots, or frank bleeding from mucous membranes. Severe bleeding results if the count is below 10,000 and can be fatal if it occurs in the gastrointestinal tract, respiratory system, or central nervous system.

Three mechanisms can cause thrombocytopenia: (1) defective platelet production in bone marrow, (2) disordered platelet distribution, and (3) accelerated platelet destruction. Defective platelet production occurs if too few platelet stem cells proliferate or if their maturation is defective. Reduced proliferation of stem cells is usually caused by drugs or malignancies that suppress or replace normal stem cells in the bone marrow. (Stem cell development is described in Chapter 22; see Fig. 22-5.)

Disordered platelet distribution is associated with splenomegaly, in which disproportionate numbers of platelets (as much as 80% of the total) are sequestered in the spleen. Platelets adhere to reticular cells of the red pulp and sinus endothelial cells of the spleen, thus any condition that causes splenomegaly can also cause thrombocytopenia (Wintrobe et al., 1981). Splenic sequestration of platelets is usually not sufficient to cause hemorrhage.

Accelerated platelet destruction or consumption (utilization) is the most common cause of thrombocytopenia. Accelerated destruction can be caused by antibody-mediated injury or to nonimmunologic causes, such as injury resulting from infectious processes. Thrombocytopenia caused by increased consumption occurs in disseminated intravascular coagulation (DIC; see p. 819), and thrombotic thrombocytopenic purpura (TTP). TTP is a disorder that affects young adults and is characterized by hemolytic anemia, thrombocytopenia, viral disease, neurologic changes, and fever (see Chapter 25).

Thrombocytopenia may be idiopathic or secondary, and acute or chronic. Idiopathic thrombocytopenic purpura (ITP) is thought to be an autoimmune disorder. (Children and young adults are most commonly affected with acute ITP, which is described in Chapter 25.) Chronic ITP sometimes occurs in women between 20 and 40 years of age. The pathogenic mechanism in all types of thrombocytopenic purpura is destruction of platelets by the host's immune system.

Secondary thrombocytopenia is caused by conditions associated with drug hypersensitivities that produce antibodies, viral and bacterial infections, and some autoimmune conditions. Viruses produce thrombocytopenia by (1) involving the megakaryocyte and inhibiting platelet production, (2) destroying circulating platelets, or (3) forming viral antigen-antibody complexes. Bacterial infections may increase consumption of platelets in the setting of septicemia associated with DIC.

Thrombocytosis

Thrombocytosis is defined as a platelet count greater than 400,000 per cubic millimeter of blood. Thrombocytosis may be primary or secondary and is usually asymptomatic until the count exceeds 1 million/mm^3. At that point, intravascular clot formation (thrombosis), hemorrhage, or other abnormalities can occur.

Transient thrombocytosis is a normal, physiologic response to stress, infection, trauma, exercise, and ovulation. Abnormal thrombocytosis is caused by accelerated platelet production in the bone marrow.

Primary thrombocytosis (also called hemorrhagic thrombocythemia) is a myeloproliferative disorder in which megakaryocytes in the marrow overproliferate. It is associated with other myeloproliferative disorders, such as chronic nonlymphoblastic leukemia, polycythemia vera, and myelofibrosis (replacement of hematopoietic bone marrow with fibrous tissue). Clinical manifestations of primary thrombocytosis typically include thrombosis of peripheral blood vessels

(particularly in the digits) or, in severe episodes, thrombosis of hepatic, mesenteric, or pulmonary vessels. The other clinical hallmarks are splenomegaly and easy bruising.

Bleeding time may be prolonged or normal. If the course is benign, treatment is not necessary. In those with thrombotic and hemorrhagic complications, the goal of therapy is to lower the platelet count by use of chemotherapy agents or phlebotomy. Splenectomy is usually contraindicated because it causes a transient rise in the platelet count.

Secondary thrombocytosis occurs after splenectomy because platelets that normally would be stored in the spleen remain in circulating blood. The increase in platelets may be gradual, so that thrombocytosis does not occur for up to 3 weeks following splenectomy. Other forms of secondary thrombocytosis (reactive thrombocytosis) usually consist of a moderate rise in the platelet count that resolves with treatment of the underlying condition, such as rheumatoid arthritis and cancers. Secondary thrombocytosis can also be caused by the accelerated thrombopoiesis that commonly accompanies accelerated erythropoiesis. This form of secondary thrombocytosis may be seen in conjunction with hemolytic anemias and some polycythemias, or as compensatory thrombocytosis following thrombocytopenia.

Alterations of Platelet Function

Alterations of platelet adherence (or adhesion) and aggregation can result in prolonged bleeding times despite a normal platelet count. These disorders of platelet function may be inherited or acquired. Inherited disorders of platelet function are grouped as (1) disorders in which platelet function is the only abnormality, (2) disorders in which abnormal platelet function is associated with mild to moderate thrombocytopenia, and (3) disorders in which abnormal platelet function is only one of a number of manifestations of an inherited systemic disorder (Wintrobe et al., 1981).

Acquired disorders of platelet function result in membrane abnormalities, intracellular abnormalities, deficiencies in cellular contents, or defects in thromboxane synthesis. These disorders of platelet function are commonly caused by drugs, such as anti-inflammatory agents, antimicrobials, antidepressants, and adrenergic blocking agents. Drugs interrupt and inhibit the synthesis of thromboxane A$_2$, as well as alter normal platelet adherence to endothelium. Uremia and a variety of other disorders that affect the hematopoietic system can also result in acquired disorders of platelet function.

Disorders of Coagulation

Disorders of coagulation are usually caused by defects or deficiencies of one or more of the clotting factors. (The characteristics of normal function of the clotting factors are described in Chapter 22.) Qualitative or quantitative abnormalities of clotting factors prevent the enzymatic reactions by which these factors are normally transformed from circulating plasma proteins to a stable fibrin clot (see Fig. 22-12).

Some clotting factor defects are inherited and usually involve a single factor. Two of the most common inherited disorders, the hemophilias and Von Willebrand disease, are caused by deficiencies of clotting factors (see Chapter 25). Other coagulation defects are acquired and tend to result from deficient synthesis of clotting factors by the liver. Liver disease is one cause of acquired coagulation deficiency. Another is a dietary deficiency of vitamin K, which is necessary for normal synthesis of the clotting factors.

Other coagulation disorders that are not caused by quantitative or qualitative clotting factor defects, are attributed to pathologic conditions that trigger coagulation inappropriately, engaging the clotting factors and causing detrimental clotting within blood vessels. For example, any cardiovascular abnormality that alters normal blood flow by speeding it up, slowing it down, or obstructing it can create conditions in which coagulation proceeds within the vessels. This is a cause of **thromboembolic disease,** in which blood clots obstruct blood vessels. Coagulation is also stimulated by the presence of tissue thromboplastin, which is released by damaged or dead tissues. Therefore, any condition in which tissue decay or damage releases a great deal of tissue thromboplastin, such as occurs in complications of pregnancy, including death of the fetus and placental decay within the mother, can cause widespread and possibly fetal intravascular coagulation. Another cause of detrimental coagulation processes is vasculitis, or inflammation of the blood vessels. Damage to inflamed vessels causes platelet activation, which in turn activates the coagulation cascade. In extensive or prolonged vasculitis, blood clot formation can overcome mechanisms that normally control clot formation and breakdown, leading to clogging of the vessels. In each of these acquired conditions, normal hemostatic function proves detrimental to the body by consuming coagulation factors excessively or by overwhelming normal control of clot formation and breakdown (fibrinolysis).

Vitamin K Deficiency

Vitamin K, a fat-soluble vitamin, is necessary for synthesis of normal prothrombin and clotting factors II, VII, IX, and X. Vitamin K is usually taken into the body in green, leafy vegetables. Resident intestinal bacteria also are a source of vitamin K. Deficiencies occur because of insufficient dietary intake, the absence of bile salts necessary for vitamin K absorption, intestinal malabsorption syndromes, and oral antibiotics that kill resident intestinal bacteria. Bleeding caused by vitamin K

deficiency resembles that of other coagulation defects and may be moderate to fatal. Laboratory tests reveal an elevated prothrombin time.

Parenteral administration of vitamin K and transfusion of fresh frozen plasma are appropriate ways to replace vitamin K as well as factors II, VII, IX, and X. Resolution of the condition that caused vitamin K deficiency is also necessary. Neonates are deficient in vitamin K because of the immaturity of their livers and lack of normal intestinal flora, so some clinicians administer vitamin K routinely at birth to eliminate the risk of hemorrhagic disease of the newborn.

Liver Disease

A pattern of hemostatic derangements is seen with advanced liver disease that disrupts synthesis of clotting factors and is frequently associated with thrombocytopenia resulting from portal hypertension and congestive splenomegaly. Consequent bleeding is gastrointestinal and is usually associated with a local lesion. Generalized, recurrent ecchymoses and epistaxis can also occur. Treatment is administration of vitamin K and replacement of plasma and blood volume as indicated.

Disseminated Intravascular Coagulation (DIC)

Disseminated intravascular coagulation (DIC) is a complex syndrome resulting from a variety of chemical conditions in which clotting occurs throughout the vascular system. Intravascular clotting is followed by active bleeding because of (1) consumption of coagulation factors and platelets and (2) diffuse fibrinolysis. DIC is rare, life threatening, and usually associated with another critical illness. It is commonly associated with circulatory shock, sepsis, acute hemolysis resulting from incompatible transfusion, and anaphylactic shock. Infection, tissue trauma, obstetric complications, neoplasms, and vascular and hematopoietic disorders can initiate DIC. Venomous snake bites also cause DIC and are one of the common causes associated with the syndrome.

The pathophysiology of DIC is shown in Fig. 24-10. DIC is initiated when tissue thromboplastin is liberated by tissue destruction, thereby activating the extrinsic pathway of coagulation, or when endothelial damage activates the intrinsic pathway. Widespread coagulation consumes clotting factors and platelets, such that activation of the fibrinolytic system ensues, causing diffuse fibrinolysis. Fibrin degradation products (FDP) combine with the fibrin monomer, preventing the laying down of fibrin threads and inhibiting platelet aggregation. Normal compensatory processes may become impaired so as to create a self-perpetuating "vicious cycle." The outcome is determined by the interplay between the various pathologic processes and compensatory mechanisms (i.e., fibrin deposition vs. fibrinolysis; depletion vs. repletion of clotting factors and platelets; production vs.

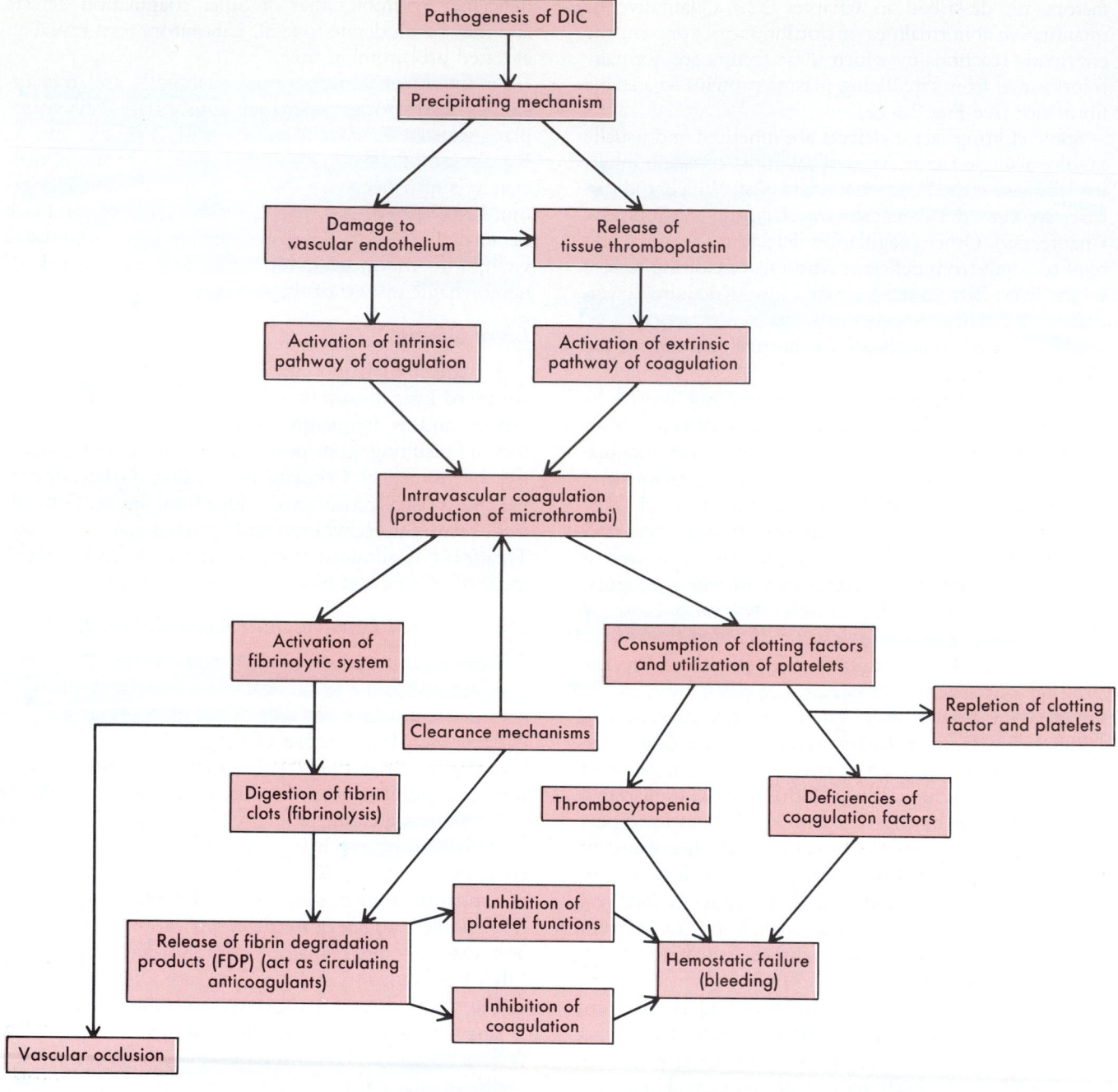

FIG. 24-10. Pathogenesis and cyclic nature of DIC. The coagulation cascade is activated if sufficient amounts of specific substances are released into the blood. If the linings of the blood vessels are damaged, the substance released by the injured endothelium initiates the intrinsic pathway for coagulation (see Chapter 22). If tissues anywhere in the body are dead, their decay releases tissue thromboplastin into the blood, initiating the extrinsic pathway of coagulation. (Adapted from Wintrobe, M. M. et al., 1981.)

clearance of fibrin, FDP, and other products of coagulation) (Wintrobe et al., 1981). Because clotting factors and platelets are deficient or prevented from functioning, a cycle of bleeding, clotting, and fibrinolysis perpetuates itself.

The onset of DIC can be either acute, as is seen in such obstetric emergencies as placenta previa or retained placenta, or gradual, as is common with malignant processes. Bleeding from numerous sites becomes the predominant problem. Oozing or frank bleeding occurs from mucous membranes, deep tissue, injured tissues, sites of venipuncture or injection, and every natural orifice. Petechiae and ecchymoses are common. Though major organ dysfunction is sometimes caused by underlying disorders, DIC is often the cause, particularly of pulmonary, renal, hepatic, and central nervous system dysfunction. The mechanism of injury is vascular obstruction by microthrombi that occlude small vessels.

Laboratory tests reveal accelerated clotting. Fibrinogen levels and platelet count are decreased. Treatment is directed toward correction of the underlying cause and may necessitate administration of many different drugs. Plasma factors are replaced by administration of fresh frozen plasma and cryoprecipitate (factor VIII). Platelets and erythrocytes are given if the condition is severe.

The role of heparin in treating DIC remains controversial. Heparin is known to inhibit the coagulation process by preventing tissue thromboplastin from activating the extrinsic pathway, thereby retarding the consumption of coagulation factors and deposition of fibrin. Though this may help to break the cycle of DIC, it does nothing to stop bleeding that is already occurring.

Thromboembolic Disease

Abnormal clots may occur occasionally within the vascular system. If the clot is stationary or adheres to the vessel wall, it is called a **thrombus** Fig. 24-11). A thrombus may block blood flow within a vessel that supplies nutrients to tissue critical to survival, such as the heart, brain, or lungs. It is not completely known why the endothelial lining of these vessels changes, but many causes are under investigation.

An intravascular clot that floats within the blood is called an **embolus.** The mobile embolus will travel within the bloodstream until it comes to rest in a very small vessel, where it usually blocks circulation to distal structures. This has dangerous effects in vessels that supply vital organs.

The term **triad of Virchow** refers to the three factors that can cause thrombus formation: (1) loss of integrity of the vessel wall, (2) abnormalities of blood flow, and (3) alterations in the blood constituents. The vessel wall can be injured, for example, by atherosclerosis (plaque deposits on arterial walls). Atherosclerosis initiates platelet adhesion, aggregation, and formation of a thrombus that resembles a platelet plug. It is not known why atherosclerosis causes arterial thrombosis. Venous thrombosis is apparently caused by alterations of the integrity and tone of the veins by extrinsic factors.

Several abnormalities of blood flow can cause thrombus formation. In arterial vessels, thrombosis occurs in conditions of rapid flow. Changes that create turbulence or change the rate of blood flow promote thrombus enlargement that can ultimately occlude the vessel. In veins, slow blood flow contributes to thrombosis, which becomes more severe with further slowing or stagnation. The slower the flow, the greater the quantity of activated clotting factors that remain in close proximity in the vessels. This is the mechanism by which thrombosis occurs in conditions of venous stasis.

Quantitative or qualitative alterations of blood constituents (chiefly clotting factors and platelets) also contribute to thrombosis. Thrombocytopenia, thrombocytosis, elevated levels of clotting factors, deficiencies of antithrombin III, and reduced fibrinolytic activity can all increase the risk or presence of thromboembolism. Increased viscosity of the blood and increased platelet activity also can lead to thrombus formation.

Numerous clinical conditions (pulmonary embolus, deep vein thrombosis, cerebral vascular accident [stroke], myocardial infarction, mesenteric thrombosis) are associated with thromboembolic disease. Whether or not episodes of thromboembolism are life threatening depends on the site of vessel occlusion. Therapy consists of removal or breakdown of the clot and supportive measures.

Anticoagulant therapy is effective in treating or preventing venous thrombosis; it is not useful in treating or preventing arterial thrombosis. Parenteral heparin is the major anticoagulant used to treat thromboembolism. Oral coumarin drugs are also widely used, particularly for outpatients.

More aggressive therapy may be indicated for such conditions as pulmonary embolism, coronary thrombo-

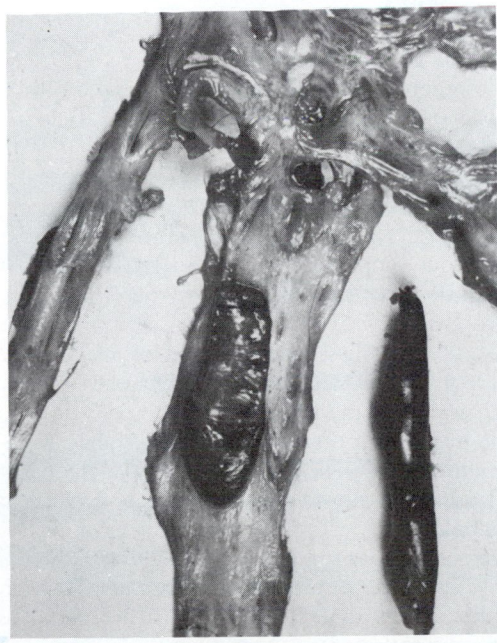

FIG. 24-11. Thrombus arising in valve pocket at upper end of superficial femoral vein. Postmortem clot on the right is shown for comparison. (From McLachlin & Paterson JC: Some basic observations on venous thrombosis and pulmonary embolism. Surg Gynecol Obstet **93**:1-8, 1951; by permission of Surgery, Gynecology, & Obstetrics.)

sis, or thrombophlebitis. Streptokinase and urokinase activate the fibrinolytic system, and are administered to accelerate the lysis of known thrombus. Thrombolytic therapy has limited uses and is prescribed with a high degree of caution because it can cause hemorrhagic complications.

SUMMARY REVIEW

Alterations of Leukocyte Function

1 Quantitative alterations of leukocytes (too many or too few) can be caused by bone marrow dysfunction or premature destruction of cells in the circulation.

2 Many quantitative changes in leukocytes occur in response to invasion by microorganisms.

3 Leukocytosis is a condition in which the leukocyte count is higher than normal and is usually a response to stress and invasion of microorganisms.

4 Leukopenia is a condition in which the leukocyte count is lower than normal and is caused by pathologic conditions, such as malignancies and hematologic disorders.

5 Granulocytosis (particularly as a result of neutrophilia) occurs in response to infection.

6 When the demand for neutrophils exceeds the supply in the circulation, the marrow releases immature cells, causing a shift to the left.

7 Eosinophilia results most commonly from parasitic invasion and ingestion or inhalation of toxic foreign particles.

8 Basophilia occurs in the healing phase of inflammation during which coagulation and clotting need to be inhibited and are accomplished through the release of heparin.

9 Monocytosis occurs during the late or recuperative phase of infection when macrophages (mature monocytes) phagocytose surviving microorganisms and debris.

10 Granulocytopenia, a condition resulting in a decrease in neutrophils, can be a life-threatening condition if sepsis occurs; it is often caused by chemotherapeutic agents, severe infection, and radiation.

11 The common pathologic feature of all forms of leukemia is an uncontrolled proliferation of leukocytes.

12 All leukemias can be designated as (1) lymphocytic, (2) myelocytic or myelogenous, or (3) monocytic. The acute leukemias are divided into two major types: (1) acute nonlymphoblastic leukemia (ANLL) or acute myelogenous leukemia (AML), and (2) acute lymphoblastic leukemia (ALL).

13 The two principal types of chronic leukemia are (1) chronic granulocytic leukemia (CGL) or chronic myelocytic leukemia (CML), and (2) chronic lymphocytic leukemias (CLL).

14 Although the exact cause of leukemia is unknown, it is considered a clonal disorder. A high incidence of acute leukemias and CLL is reported in certain families, suggesting a genetic predisposition.

15 In leukemia, blasts (precursor cells) "crowd out" the marrow and cause cellular proliferation of the other cell lines to cease.

16 The major clinical manifestations of leukemia include fatigue caused by anemia, bleeding caused by thrombocytopenia, fever secondary to infection, anorexia, and weight loss.

17 Chemotherapy is the treatment of choice for leukemia. Acute leukemias are associated with a 20% to 50% long-term survival. Chronic leukemias are associated with a longer life expectancy.

18 Chronic leukemias progress differently than acute leukemias, advancing slowly and unknowingly, without warning.

19 Multiple myeloma is a neoplasm of B cells (immature plasma cells) and mature plasma cells. It is characterized by multiple malignant tumor masses of plasma cells scattered throughout the skeletal system and sometimes in soft tissue.

20 The exact cause of multiple myeloma is unknown, but genetic factors and chronic stimulation of the mononuclear phagocyte system by bacteria, viral agents, and chemicals has been suggested.

21 The major clinical manifestations for multiple myeloma include recurrent infections caused by suppression of the humoral immune response and renal disease as a result of Bence Jones proteinuria.

22 Chemotherapy is the treatment for multiple myeloma. However, survival is still only two to three years with chemotherapy.

Alterations of Lymphoid Function

1 The number of lymphocytes is decreased (lymphocytopenia) in most acute infections and in some immune deficiency syndromes.

2 Lymphocytosis occurs in viral infections, infectious mononucleosis and infectious hepatitis, in particular, leukemia, lymphomas, and some chronic infections.

3 Infectious mononucleosis is an acute infection of B-lymphocytes by the Epstein-Barr virus (EBV) (a type of herpes virus).

4 Two of the earliest manifestations of infectious mononucleosis are sore throat and fever caused by inflammation at the site of viral entry.

5 The majority of cases of EBV include fever with temperature elevation lasting 7 to 10 days, sore throat, and enlargement and tenderness of the cervical lymph nodes.

6 Lymphomas are tumors of primary lymphoid tissue (thymus and bone marrow) or secondary tissue (lymph nodes, spleen, tonsils, and intestinal lymphoid tissue). The two major types of malignant lymphomas are (1) Hodgkin disease and (2) non-Hodgkin disease.

7 Distinctive abnormal chromosomes are present in multiple cells of the lymph nodes of an individual with

Hodgkin disease. The abnormal cell is called the Sternberg-Reed cell.

8 A virus might be involved in the pathogenesis of Hodgkin disease. Some familial clustering suggests an unknown genetic mechanism.

9 An enlarged, painless mass or swelling, most commonly in the neck, is an initial sign of Hodgkin disease. Local symptoms are produced by lymphadenopathy, usually caused by pressure or obstruction.

10 Treatment of Hodgkin disease includes radiotherapy and chemotherapy. A cure is possible regardless of stage of Hodgkin disease; however, individuals treated with chemotherapy and who relapse in less than 2 years have a poor prognosis.

11 The cause of lymph node enlargement and cancerous transformation in non-Hodgkin lymphoma is unknown. Immunosuppressed persons have greater incidence of non-Hodgkin lymphoma, suggesting an immune mechanism.

12 Generally, with non-Hodgkin lymphoma, the swelling of lymph nodes is painless and the nodes have enlarged and transformed over a period of months or years.

13 Individuals with non-Hodgkin lymphoma can survive for long periods. Treatment is with chemotherapy.

14 Burkitt lymphoma involves the jaw and facial bones and occurs in children from east-central Africa and New Guinea.

15 Splenomegaly (enlargement of the spleen) is a secondary effect to other disorders in the body.

16 Splenomegaly results from (1) proliferation of lymphocytes or macrophages of the white pulp, (2) invasion of neoplastic cells, or (3) chronic congestion with blood.

17 Hypersplenism is associated with splenomegaly and pancytopenia.

Alterations of Platelet Function and Coagulation

1 Thrombocytopenia is characterized by a platelet count below 100,000 platelets per cubic millimeter of blood; a count below 50,000 increases the potential for hemorrhage associated with minor trauma.

2 Three mechanisms cause thrombocytopenia: (1) defective platelet production in bone marrow, (2) disordered platelet distribution, and (3) accelerated platelet destruction.

3 Thrombocytopenia is commonly associated with autoimmune diseases and viral infections; bacterial sepsis with DIC also results in thrombocytopenia.

4 Thrombocytosis is characterized by a platelet count greater than 400,000 platelets per cubic millimeter of blood and is symptomatic when the count exceeds one million when risk for intravascular clotting (thrombosis) is high.

5 Thrombocytosis is caused by accelerated platelet production in the bone marrow.

6 Alterations in normal platelet adherence or aggregation prevents platelet plug formation and may result in prolonged bleeding times.

7 Platelet dysfunction results from changes in the cellular contents and integrity.

8 Disorders of coagulation are usually caused by defects or deficiencies of one or more of the clotting factors.

9 Pathologic conditions can trigger coagulation, inappropriately using up the clotting factors causing detrimental clotting within blood vessels.

10 Coagulation is impaired when there is a deficiency of vitamin K because of insufficient production of prothrombin and clotting factors II, VII, IX, and X.

11 Liver disease accounts for a pattern of hemostatic derangement caused by a disruption of the synthesis of clotting factors.

12 Disseminated intravascular coagulation (DIC) is a complex syndrome resulting from a variety of chemical conditions that cause clotting through the vascular system.

13 DIC is characterized by a cycle of intravascular clotting followed by active bleeding because of the consumption of coagulation factors, platelets, and diffuse fibrinolysis.

14 Thromboembolic disease results from a fixed (thrombus) or moving (embolism) clot that blocks flow within a vessel, denying nutrients to tissues distal to the occlusion; death can result when clots are located in the heart, brain, or lungs.

15 The term *Triad of Virchow* refers to three factors that can cause thrombus formation: (1) loss of integrity of the vessel wall, (2) abnormalities of blood flow, and (3) alterations in the blood constituents.

KEY TERMS

Acute leukemia, 803

Acute lymphoblastic leukemia (ALL), 803

Acute nonlymphoblastic leukemia (ANLL) (acute myelogenous leukemia), 803

Agranulocytosis, 802

Basophilia, 801

Bence Jones protein, 810

Burkitt lymphoma, 815

Chronic granulocytic leukemia (CGL) (chronic myelocytic leukemia), 803

Chronic leukemia, 803

Chronic lymphocytic leukemia (CLL), 803

Disseminated intravascular coagulation (DIC), 819

Embolus, 821

Eosinophilia, 801

Granulocytosis, 801

Granulocytopenia, 802

Hodgkin disease, 811

Hypersplenism, 816

Infectious mononucleosis, 802

Leukemia, 803

Leukemia-associated inhibitory activity (LIA), 804

Leukocytosis, 801

Leukopenia, 801

Lymphadenopathy, 810

Lymphocytopenia, 802

Lymphocytosis, 802

Lymphoma, 803

Lymphopenia, 802

M component, 810

Monocytosis, 801

Multiple myeloma, 809

Neutropenia, 801

Neutrophilia, 801

Non-Hodgkin disease, 811

Pancytopenia, 804

Primary thrombocytosis (hemorrhagic thrombocythemia), 818

Purpura, 816

Secondary thrombocytosis, 818

Shift to the left (leukemoid reaction), 801

Shift to the right, 801

Splenomegaly, 816

Thrombocytopenia, 804

Thrombocytosis, 817

Thromboembolic disease, 819

Thrombus, 821

Triad of Virchow, 821

REFERENCES

American Cancer Society. (1988). *Cancer facts & figures 1988.* New York: American Cancer Society

American Cancer Society. (1989). Cancer statistics. *Ca-A Cancer: Journal for Clinicians, 39*(1).

Borden, E. C., Steeves, R. A., & Hogan, J. F. (1983). Infectious carcinogenesis: Viruses and human neoplasia. In S. B. Kahn, R. R. Lone, C. Sherman, & R. Chakravorty (Eds.), *Concepts in cancer medicine.* New York: Grune & Stratton.

Broxmeyer, H. E., Mendelsohn, N., Moore, M., & Alcolm, A. S. (1977). Abnormal granulocyte feedback regulation of colony forming and colony stimulating activity—Producing cells from patients with chronic myelogenous leukemia. *Leukemia Research, 1,* 3.

Defonzo, R., Cooke, C. R., Wright, J. R., & Humphrey, R. L. (1978). Renal function in patients with multiple myeloma. *Medicine, 57,* 151.

DelRegato, J. A., Spjut, H. J., & Cox, J. D. (1985).*Cancer: Diagnosis, treatment, and prognosis* (6th ed.). St. Louis: C. V. Mosby.

Fundenberg, H. J., Stiles, D. P., Caldwell, J. L., & Wells, J. V. (1978). *Basic and clinical immunology* (2nd ed.). Los Altos, CA: Lange Medical Publishers.

Gall, E. A. & Mallory, T. B. (1942). Malignant lymphoma—a clinico-pathologic survey of 618 cases. *American Journal of Pathology, 18,* 381-429.

Gunz, F. W. (1980). The dread leukemias and the lymphomas: Their nature and their prospects. In M. M. Wintrope (Ed.), *Blood, pure and eloquent: A story of discovery, of people, and of ideas.* New York: McGraw-Hill.

Guyton, A. C. (1981). *Textbook of medical physiology* (6th ed.). Philadelphia: W. B. Saunders.

Hirschaut, Y. et al. (1973). Epstein-Barr virus antibodies in American and African Burkitt's lymphoma. *Lancet, 2,* 144.

Isselbacher, K., Adams, R., Braunwald, E., Petersdorf, R., & Wilson, J. (Eds.). (1980). *Harrison's principles of internal medicine* (9th ed.). New York: McGraw-Hill Co.

Jackson, H. Jr. & Parker F. Jr. (1944). Hodgkin's disease, II. Pathology, *New England J Med 231:*35-44.

Kaplan, H. S. (1980). *Hodgkin's disease* (2nd ed.). Cambridge, MA: Harvard University Press.

King, Fenoglio, & Lefkowitch (1983). *General pathology: Principles and Dynamics.* Philadelphia: Lea & Febiger.

Lukes, R. J. & Butler, J. J. (1966). The pathology and nomenclature of Hodgkin's disease, *Cancer Research 26,* 1063-1081.

McLachlin, J. & Paterson, J. C. (1951). Some basic observations on venous thrombi and pulmonary embolism, *Surgery, Gynecology and Obstetrics, 93,* 1-8.

McPhedran, P., Heath, C. W., & Garcia, J. (1972). Multiple myeloma incidence in metropolitan Atlanta, Georgia: Racial and seasonal variations. *Blood, 39,* 866.

Purtilo, D. T. (1978). *A survey of human diseases.* Menlo Park, CA: Addison-Wesley.

Rappapart H. (1966). Tumors of the hematopoietic system. In *Atlas of tumor pathology.* Section III. Facile 8. Washington D.C.: Armed Forces/Institutes of Pathology.

Robbins, S., Cotran, R. S., & Kumar, V. (1984). *Pathophysiologic basis for disease* (3rd ed.). Philadelphia: W. B. Saunders.

Rosenberg, S. A. (1966). Report of the committee on the staging of Hodgkin's disease. *Cancer Research 26,* 1310.

Schnipper, L. E., Wagner, H., & McCaffrey, R. P. (1986). Multiple myeloma and plasma cell dyscrasias. In *Cancer Manual.* Boston, MA: American Cancer Society.

Selvin, S., Levin, L. I., Merrill, D. W., & Winkelstein, W., Jr. (1983). Selected epidemiologic observations of cell-specific leukemia mortality in the U. S. *American Journal of Epidemiology, 117*(2), 140-152.

Skarin, A. T., Canellos, G. P., Maych, P. M., & Nieman, R. S. (1986). Lymphoma. In *Cancer Manual.* Boston, MA: American Cancer Society.

Solomon, A. (1981). Bence Jones proteins: Malignant or benign. *New England Journal or Medicine, 306,* 605.

Ullrich, S., & Zolla-Pazner, S. (1982). Immunoregulatory circuits in myeloma. *Clinical Hematology, 11,* 87.

Wintrobe, M. M., Lee, G. R., Boggs, D. R., Bithell, T. C., Foerster, J., Athens, J. W., & Lukens, J. N. (1981). *Clinical hematology* (8th ed.). Philadelphia: Lea & Febiger.

Wolach, B., Baehner, R., & Boxer, L. (1982). Clinical and laboratory approach to management of neutrophil dysfunction. *Israel Journal of Medical Science* (Review), *18*(9), 897-911.

Young, J. L., Jr., Percy, C. L., & Asire, A. J. (1981). Surveillance, epidemiology, and end results: Incidence and mortality data, 1973-77. *NCI Monograph, 57,* 1-1082.

CHAPTER 25

Alterations in Hematologic Function in Children

Margaret Andrews
Kathleen Hardin Mooney

Fetal and neonatal hematopoiesis, 826
Postnatal changes in the blood, 826
   Erythrocytes, 829
   Leukocytes and platelets, 829
Disorders of erythrocytes, 829
   Acquired disorders, 830
    Iron deficiency anemia, 830
     Pathophysiology, 831
     Clinical manifestations, 831
     Evaluation and treatment, 831
    Hemolytic disease in the newborn (HDN), 831
     Pathophysiology, 832
     Clinical manifestations, 832
     Evaluation and treatment, 834
    Anemia of infectious disease, 834
   Inherited disorders, 834
    Glucose-6-phosphate dehydrogenase (G-6-PD)
     deficiency, 834
     Pathophysiology, 834
     Clinical manifestations, 835
     Evaluation and treatment, 835
    Hereditary spherocytosis, 835
     Pathophysiology, 835
     Clinical manifestations, 836
     Evaluation and treatment, 836
    Sickle cell disease, 836
     Pathophysiology, 836
     Clinical manifestations, 839
     Evaluation and treatment, 840
    The thalassemias, 841
     Pathophysiology, 841
     Clinical manifestations, 841
     Evaluation and treatment, 842
Disorders of coagulation and platelets, 842
   Inherited hemorrhagic disease, 842
    The hemophilias, 842
     Types of hemophilia, 842
     Pathophysiology, 844
     Clinical manifestations, 844
     Evaluation and treatment, 844
   Antibody-mediated hemorrhagic disease, 845
    Idiopathic thrombocytopenic purpura, 845
     Pathophysiology, 845
     Clinical manifestations, 845
     Evaluation and treatment, 845
    Transient neonatal thrombocytopenias, 846
    Autoimmune vascular purpura, 846
Leukemias and lymphomas, 847
   Leukemia, 847
    Types of leukemia, 847
     Pathogenesis, 848
     Clinical manifestations, 849
     Evaluation and treatment, 850
   Lymphomas, 851
    Non-Hodgkin lymphoma, 851
     Pathogenesis, 851
     Clinical manifestations, 851
     Evaluation and treatment, 852
    Hodgkin disease, 852

In this chapter a brief explanation of fetal and neonatal hematopoiesis and postnatal changes in blood is presented as a foundation for understanding the pathophysiology of specific blood disorders in childhood. Among the diseases that affect erythrocytes are: acquired disorders, such as iron deficiency anemia, hemolytic disease of the newborn (HDN), and anemia of infectious disease; and inherited disorders, such as glucose-6-phosphate dehydrogenase deficiency (G-6-PD), hereditary spherocytosis, sickle cell disease, and the thalassemias. Disorders of coagulation and platelets include inherited hemorrhagic diseases, such as the hemophilias, and antibody-mediated hemorrhagic diseases, which include idiopathic thrombocytopenic purpura (ITP), transient neonatal thrombocytopenias, and autoimmune vascular purpuras. Finally, leukocyte disorders, such as leukemia and the lymphomas (both non-Hodgkin lymphoma and Hodgkin disease) are discussed.

FETAL AND NEONATAL HEMATOPOIESIS

As the developing embryo becomes too large for oxygenation of tissues by simple diffusion, the production of erythrocytes begins within the vessels of the yolk sac. Shortly after 2 weeks' gestation, circulating erythrocytes play a major role in delivering oxygen to the tissues. At approximately the eighth week of gestation, the site of erythrocyte production shifts from the vessels to the liver sinusoids, and the production of leukocytes and platelets begins in the liver and spleen. Erythropoiesis in the liver and, to a lesser extent in the spleen and lymph nodes, reaches a peak at approximately 4 months. Hepatic blood formation declines steadily thereafter, but does not disappear entirely during the remainder of gestation. By the fifth month of gestation, hematopoiesis begins to occur in the bone marrow and increases rapidly until hematopoietic (red) marrow fills the entire bone marrow space. By the time of delivery, the marrow is the only significant site of hematopoiesis.

In neonates and young infants, hematopoietic marrow progressively fills the bony cavities of the entire axial skeleton (skull, vertebrae, ribs, and sternum), the long bones of the limbs, and many intramenbranous bones. (These structures are described in Chapter 38.) Fatty (yellow) marrow gradually replaces hematopoietic marrow in some bones. During childhood, hematopoietic tissue retreats centrally to the vertebrae, ribs, sternum, pelvis, scapulae, skull, and proximal ends of the femur and humerus.

In diseases characterized by hemolysis, erythrocyte production can increase as many as eight times normal because erythropoietin causes hematopoietic marrow to increase in volume. Initially, hematopoietic marrow expands from the ends of the long bones toward the middle of the shafts, replacing fatty marrow. Next, blood cell production begins to occur outside the marrow cavities, especially in the liver and spleen. Extramedullary hematopoiesis is more likely to occur in children than in adults because the bony cavities of children are already filled with red marrow (Fig. 25-1). This is why he-

molytic disease causes especially pronounced enlargement of the spleen and liver in children.

The erythrocytes undergo striking changes during gestation, particularly during the first two trimesters, during which they nearly double in numbers and in hemoglobin content. A proportionate increase in hematocrit also occurs. By the end of gestation, the erythrocyte count has more than tripled, but the size of each erythrocyte has decreased.

A biochemically distinct type of hemoglobin is synthesized during fetal life. The three **embryonic hemoglobins** (Gower 1, Gower 2, and Portland) and the **fetal hemoglobin (Hb F)** are composed of two alpha and two gamma chains of polypeptides, whereas the adult hemoglobins (Hb A and Hb A_2) are composed of two alpha and two beta chains. (The structure of an adult hemoglobin molecule is illustrated in Chapter 22, Fig. 22-7, and types of hemoglobin are defined in Table 22-3.) Some unknown regulatory mechanism promotes gamma chain synthesis and inhibits beta and delta chain synthesis in utero. This results in production of embryonic or fetal hemoglobin. After birth, gamma chain synthesis is inhibited, while beta and delta chain synthesis are facilitated, resulting in production of adult hemoglobins.

Fetal hemoglobin has greater affinity for oxygen than adult hemoglobin because it interacts less readily with an enzyme (2,3-diphosphoglycerate, or 2,3-DPG) that inhibits hemoglobin-oxygen binding. The decreased inhibitory effects of 2,3-DPG enable fetal blood to transport oxygen despite the relative lack of oxygen in the uterine environment. The increased affinity for oxygen enables fetal hemoglobin to bind with maternal oxygen in the placental circulation.

During the first trimester, nearly all of the hemoglobin in the fetus is embryonic, but some Hb A can be detected. Therefore, it is possible to identify as early as 16 to 20 weeks gestation some disorders of adult hemoglobin, such as sickle cell anemia and thalassemia major. In the 6-month-old fetus, Hb F constitutes 90% of the total. This percentage then begins to decline. At birth, neonatal hemoglobin consists of 70% Hb F, 29% Hb A, and 1% Hb A_2. Between 6 and 12 months of age, normal adult hemoglobin percentages are established (see Chapter 22).

POSTNATAL CHANGES IN THE BLOOD

Blood cell counts tend to rise above adult levels at birth, then decline gradually throughout childhood. Table 25-1 lists normal ranges during infancy and childhood. The immediate rise in values is the result of accel-

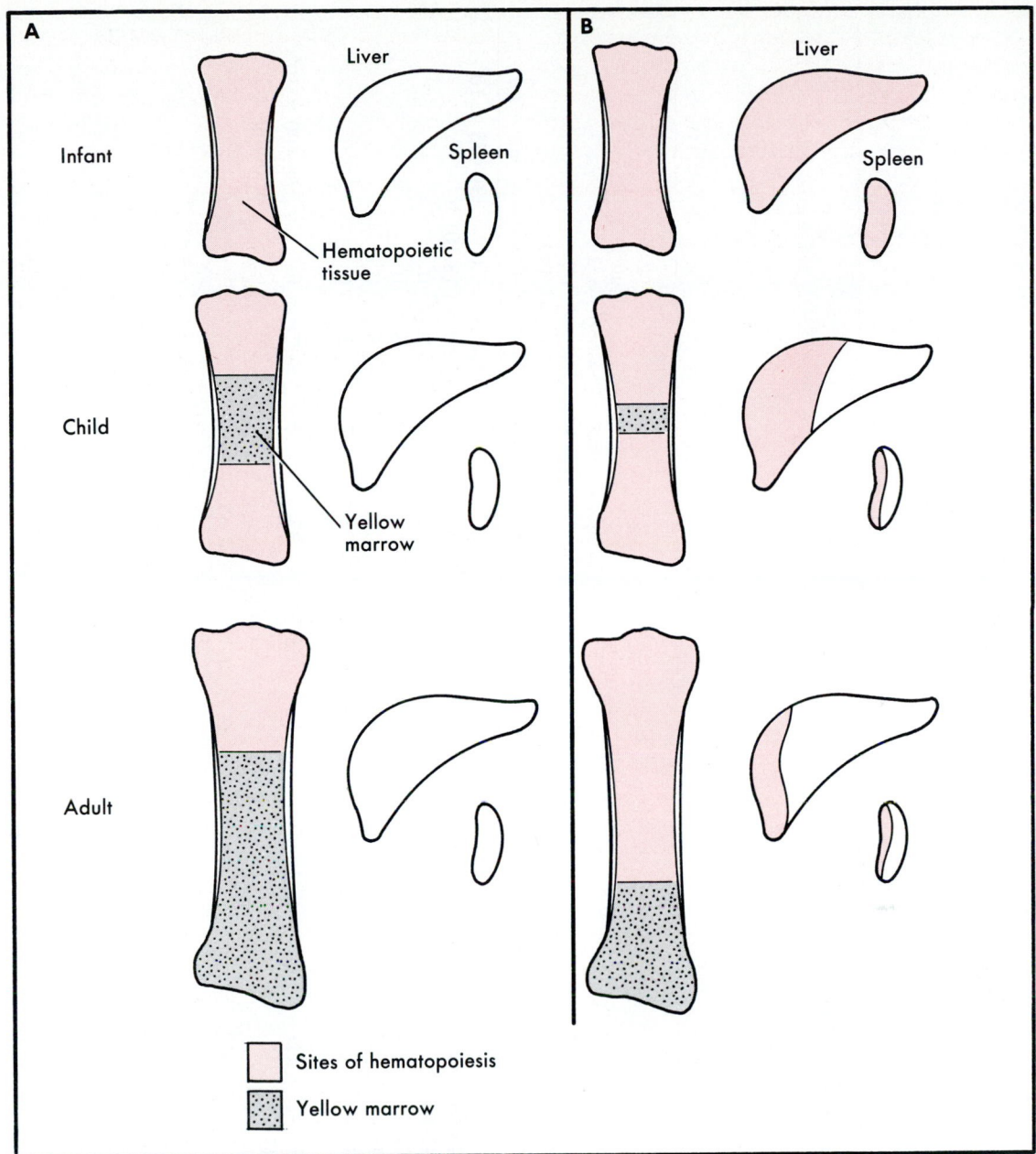

FIG. 25-1. Sites of hematopoiesis in health and illness. With normal maturation, red marrow is partly replaced by yellow marrow in the shafts of the long bones. In adults, red marrow is largely restricted to the proximal ends of the femur and humerus. In response to hemolysis, red marrow replaces yellow marrow in the long bones. In infants, whose long bones are already filled with red marrow, additional hematopoiesis takes place in the liver and spleen. In children and adults, red marrow can replace yellow marrow in response to hemolysis, necessitating less hematopoiesis in the liver and spleen.

erated hematopoiesis during fetal life, increased numbers of cells that result from the trauma of birth, and cutting of the umbilical cord. These events surrounding the birth are also accompanied by a shift to the "left," i.e., the presence of large numbers of immature erythrocytes and leukocytes (particularly granulocytes) in peripheral blood (see Chapter 24). The shift to the left disappears as the child develops, usually within the first

2 to 3 months of life. Other unique postnatal characteristics, particularly of lymphocytes, may be caused by exogenous factors, such as viral infections.

Average blood volume in the full-term neonate is 85 ml/kg body weight. The premature infant has a slightly larger average blood volume of 90 ml/kg of body weight, with the mean increasing to 150 mg/kg, during the first few days after birth. In both full-term and pre-

TABLE 25-1 Hematologic values during infancy and childhood

Age	Hemoglobin (gM/dL) Mean	Range	Hematocrit (%) Mean	Range	Reticulocytes (%) Mean	Leukocytes (WBC/mM³) Mean	Range	Neutrophils (%) Mean	Range	Lymphocytes (%) Mean*	Eosinophils (%) Mean	Monocytes (%) Mean	Nucleated red cells (100 WBC)	Platelets (/mm³)
Cord blood	16.8	13.7-20.1	55	45-65	5.0	18,000	(9-30,000)	61	(40-80)	31	2	6	7.0	$84\text{-}478 \times 10^3$
2 wk	16.5	13.0-20.0	50	42-66	1.0	12,000	(5-21,000)	40		48	3	9	(3-10)	
3 mo	12.0	9.5-14.5	36	31-41	1.0	12,000	(6-18,000)	30		63	2	5	0	
6 mo-6 yr	12.0	10.5-14.0	37	33-42	1.0	10,000	(6-15,000)	45		48	2	5	0	
7-12 yr	13.0	11.0-16.0	38	34-40	1.0	8000	(4500-13,500)	55		38	2	5	0	
Adult														
Female	14	12.0-16.0	42	37-47	1.6	7500	(5-10,000)	55	(35-70)	35	3	7	0	$150\text{-}400 \times 10^6$
Male	16	14.0-18.0	47	42-52										$150\text{-}400 \times 10^6$

Adapted from Behrman & Vaughan, 1983.
*Relatively wide range.

Polycythemia — ↑ (above normal) in # of RBC

mature infants, blood volume decreases during the first few months. Thereafter, the average blood volume is 75 to 77 ml/kg, which is similar to that of older children and adults.

Erythrocytes

The hypoxic intrauterine environment stimulates erythropoietin production in the fetus. This accelerates fetal erythropoiesis, producing polycythemia of the newborn. After birth, the oxygen from the lungs saturates arterial blood, and the amount of oxygen delivered to the tissues increases. In response to the change from a placental to a pulmonary oxygen supply during the first few days of life, levels of erythropoietin and the rate of blood cell formation decrease. The very active rate of fetal erythropoiesis is reflected by the large numbers of immature erythrocytes (reticulocytes) in the peripheral blood of full-term neonates. After birth, the number of reticulocytes decreases about 50% every 12 hours, so that it is rare to find an elevated reticulocyte count after the first week of life. A decrease in extramedullary hematopoiesis also occurs at this time. In the peripheral blood, the erythrocyte count drops for 6 to 8 weeks after birth. During this period of rapid growth, the rate of erythrocyte destruction is greater than that in later childhood and adulthood. In full-term infants, normal erythrocyte life span is 60 to 80 days; in premature infants, it may be as short as 20 to 30 days; and in children and adolescents it is the same as that in adults— 120 days. (Mechanisms of hemolysis are described in Chapter 22.)

In the premature infant, the postnatal fall in hemoglobin and hematocrit is more marked than in the full-term infant. In the pre-school and school-age child, there is a gradual rise in hemoglobin, hematocrit, and red cell count. Values in males and females first begin to diverge in adolescence. In the female, the gradual hemoglobin increase continues into early puberty, at which time it stabilizes. In the male, the hemoglobin increase keeps pace with growth and maturation and eventually surpasses that of the female. This higher value in the mature male is related to androgen secretion.

Metabolic processes within the erythrocytes of neonates differ significantly from those of erythrocytes in the normal adult. The relatively young population of erythrocytes in the newborn consumes greater quantities of glucose than do erythrocytes in adults. This phenomenon is related to enzymatic activity. Several enzymes that regulate glucose consumption are increased in the erythrocytes of neonates, with a subsequent increase in the rate of glycolysis.

Leukocytes and Platelets

The lymphocytes of children tend to have more cytoplasm and less compact nuclear chromatin than the lymphocytes of adults. The significance of these differences is unknown. One possible explanation is that children tend to have more frequent viral infections, which are associated with atypical lymphocytes. Even minor infections, in which the child fails to exhibit clinical manifestations of illness and administration of immunizations, may result in lymphocyte changes (Mauer, 1969).

The lymphocyte count is high at birth and continues to rise in some healthy infants during the first year of life. Then a steady decline occurs throughout childhood and adolescence, until lower adult values are reached. It is unknown whether these developmental variations are physiologic or are a pathologic response to frequent viral infections and immunizations in children.

At birth, the neutrophil count is very high and rises during the early days of life (Manroe et al., 1979). After 2 weeks, neutrophil counts fall to within or below normal adult ranges. By approximately 4 years of age, the neutrophil count is the same as that of an adult. White children have slightly higher counts than black children (Caramihai et al., 1975).

Eosinophil count is high in the first year of life and is higher in children than in teenagers or adults (Cunningham, 1975). Monocyte counts are high in the first year of life and then decrease to adult levels. No relationship between age and basophil count has been found.

Platelet counts in full-term neonates are comparable to platelet counts in adults, and remain so throughout infancy and childhood (Albin et al., 1961). Controversy exists as to whether premature infants are usually thrombocytopenic.

DISORDERS OF ERYTHROCYTES

Anemia is the most common blood disorder in children. Like the anemias of adulthood, the anemias of childhood are caused by ineffective erythropoiesis or premature destruction of erythrocytes. The most common cause of insufficient erythropoiesis is iron deficiency, which may result from insufficient dietary intake or chronic loss of iron caused by bleeding. The hemolytic anemias of childhood may be divided into two large categories. The first consists of disorders that result from premature destruction caused by intrinsic abnormalities of the erythrocytes, whereas the second consists of disorders that result from damaging extra-erythrocytic factors. The hemolytic anemias tend to be inherited (because of a genetic anomaly), congenital (acquired or manifested before birth), or both.

The most dramatic form of acquired congenital hemolytic anemia is **hemolytic disease of the newborn (HDN)**, also termed **erythroblastosis fetalis**. HDN is an isoimmune disease in which maternal and fetal blood are antigenically incompatible, causing the mother's im-

TABLE 25-2 Anemias of childhood

Cause	Anemic condition
DEFICIENT ERYTHROPOIESIS OR HEMOGLOBIN SYNTHESIS	
Decreased stem cell population in marrow (congenital or acquired pure red cell aplasia)	Normocytic-normochromic anemia
Decreased erythropoiesis despite normal stem cell population in marrow (infection, inflammation, cancer, chronic renal disease, congenital dyserythropoeisis)	Normocytic-normochromic anemia
Deficiency of a factor or nutrient needed for erythropoiesis	
Cobalamin (vitamin B_{12}), folate	Megaloblastic anemia
Iron	Microcytic-hypochromic anemia
INCREASED OR PREMATURE HEMOLYSIS	
Isoimmune disease (maternal-fetal Rh, ABO, or minor blood group incompatibility)	Hemolytic disease of the newborn (HDN)
Autoimmune disease (idiopathic autoimmune hemolytic anemia, symptomatic systemic lupus erythematosus, lymphoma, drug-induced autoimmune processes)	Autoimmune hemolytic anemia
Inherited defects of plasma membrane structure (spherocytosis, elliptocytosis, stomatocytosis) or cellular size, or both (pyknocytosis)	Hemolytic anemia
Infection (bacterial sepsis; congenital syphilis, malaria, cytomegalovirus infection, rubella, toxoplasmosis, disseminated herpes)	Hemolytic anemia
Intrinsic and inherited enzymatic defects (deficiencies of glucose-6-phosphate dehydrogenase [G-6-PD], pyruvate kinase, 5'-nucleotidase, glucose phosphate isomerase)	Hemolytic anemia
Inherited defects of hemoglobin synthesis	Sickle cell anemia Thalassemia
Disseminated intravascular coagulation (see Chapter 24)	Hemoytic anemia
Galactosemia	Hemolytic anemia
Prolonged or recurrent respiratory or metabolic acidosis	Hemolytic anemia
Blood vessel disorders (cavernous hemangioma, large vessel thrombus, renal artery stenosis, severe coarctation of the aorta) (see Chapter 28)	Hemolytic anemia

mune system to produce antibodies against fetal erythrocytes. Fetal erythrocytes that have been attacked by (i.e., bound to) maternal antibodies are recognized as foreign or defective by the fetal mononuclear phagocyte system and are removed from the circulation by phagocytosis, usually in the fetal spleen. (For a complete discussion on HDN see p. 831.) Other acquired hemolytic anemias—some of which begin in utero—include those caused by infections or the presence of toxic chemicals.

The inherited forms of hemolytic anemia result from intrinsic defects of the child's erythrocytes, any of which can lead to erythrocyte removal by the mononuclear phagocyte system. Structural defects include abnormal cellular size or shape and abnormalities of plasma membrane structure (spherocytosis). Intracellular defects include enzyme deficiencies, the most common of which is **glucose-6-phosphate dehydrogenase (G-6-PD) deficiency,** and defects of hemoglobin synthesis, which are manifested as **sickle cell disease** or **thalassemia,** depending on which component of hemoglobin is defective. These and other causes of childhood anemia, some more common than others, are listed in Table 25-2.

Acquired Disorders
Iron Deficiency Anemia

Iron deficiency anemia is the most frequent blood disorder of infancy and childhood, with the highest incidence occurring between 6 months and 2 years of age. Incidence is not related to sex or race, but socioeconomic factors are important because they affect nutrition. Iron deficiency anemia is a common disorder in children because of their extremely high need for normal growth to occur.

Between 4 years of age and the onset of puberty, dietary iron deficiency is uncommon. During adolescence, however, it is relatively common, especially in menstruating females. Rapid growth, together with the average teenager's dietary habits, cause iron depletion to occur readily. (Mechanisms of iron depletion are described in Chapter 22.)

Pathophysiology

While inadequate intake of iron is the most common cause of iron deficiency anemia during the first few years of life and during adolescence, blood loss is the most frequent cause in childhood. Chronic iron deficiency anemia from occult ("hidden") blood loss may be caused by a gastrointestinal lesion, parasitic infestation, or hemorrhagic disease. As many as one third of infants with severe iron deficiency anemia have chronic intestinal blood loss induced by exposure to a heat-labile protein in cow's milk. Such exposure causes an inflammatory gastrointestinal reaction that damages the mucosa and results in diffuse hemorrhage.

The amount of iron available for hemoglobin synthesis in the infant depends on iron stores present at birth, rate of growth, the amount of dietary iron absorbed, and physiologic or pathologic loss of iron. During the period of inactive erythropoiesis immediately after birth, iron from erythrocytes that die at the end of their normal life span is stored in bone marrow and liver tissue, as hemosiderin. This creates an iron reserve that can be used in lieu of dietary intake. The greatest stores are present 4 to 8 weeks after birth. Until erythropoiesis resumes, these iron stores are mobilized. In the premature infant, resumption of erythropoiesis depletes iron stores within 6 to 12 weeks; in the full-term infant, depletion takes longer—about 16 to 20 weeks. Once iron stores have been used, the infant depends on dietary iron.

The amount of dietary iron available for erythropoiesis depends on which foods are consumed. Iron-fortified cereals, green and yellow vegetables, fruits, and milk are common in the average 6-month-old infant's diet, and provide iron in the amount of 0.9 to 1.5 mg/kg per day, amounts that satisfy the normal average daily requirement. Iron fortified formulas are commercially available and are being used with increasing frequency.

Clinical Manifestations

The symptoms of mild anemia—lethargy and lassitude—are not usually present or not detectable in infants and young children, who are unable to describe these symptoms. Therefore, parents usually do not notice any change in the child's behavior or appearance until moderate anemia has developed. General irritability, decreased activity tolerance, weakness, and lack of interest in play are nonspecific indications of anemia. In mild to moderate iron deficiency anemia (Hb 6 to 10

gm/dl), compensatory mechanisms of tissue oxygenation, such as increased amounts of 2,3-DPG within erythrocytes and a shift of the oxyhemoglobin dissociation curve, may be so effective that few clinical manifestations are apparent. When the hemoglobin determination falls below 5.0 gm/dl, however, pallor, anorexia, tachycardia, and systolic murmurs may occur.

Splenomegaly is evident in 10% to 15% of children with iron deficiency anemia and, if the condition is long-standing, the sutures of the skull may be widened. Chronic anemia may also result in decreased physical growth and developmental delays. Some children exhibit pica, a behavior in which nonfood substances are eaten. Because children with iron deficiency anemia may be obese, underweight, or normal weight, other manifestations of undernutrition must be identified.

Iron deficiency anemia may have effects on neurologic and intellectual function. Some research findings indicate that low iron in the blood affects attention span, alertness, and learning ability, even when anemia is not severe (Pollit & Leibel, 1976).

Evaluation and Treatment

Evaluation and treatment of iron deficiency anemia in children is similar to that in adults (see Chapter 23). Oral administration of simple ferrous salts is usually satisfactory, but additional vitamin C may be needed to promote absorption because vitamin C must be present in adequate amounts. Supplementary trace metals or other vitamins are not necessary. If malabsorption is the cause of the anemia (or if oral administration has not been successful), iron dextran (Inferon) is given intravenously. Iron therapy continues for 4 to 6 weeks after erythrocyte indices have returned to normal.

Dietary modification is required to prevent recurrences of iron deficiency anemia. The child's intake of iron-rich foods is increased, and the intake of cow's milk may be restricted with the exact amount depending on the child's age (from 1 pint to 32 ozs). Limiting milk intake makes the child hungrier for other, iron-rich foods and prevents gastrointestinal blood loss in children whose anemia is aggravated or caused by inflammatory reactions to proteins in cow's milk.

Hemolytic Disease in the Newborn (HDN)

HDN can only occur if antigens on fetal erythrocytes differ from antigens on maternal erythrocytes. The antigenic properties of erythrocytes are determined genetically: they may be type A, B, or O, and may or may not include Rh antigen D. Erythrocytes that express Rh antigen D are Rh-positive; those that do not are Rh-negative. Maternal-fetal incompatibility exists if mother and fetus differ in ABO blood type or if the fetus is Rh-positive and the mother is Rh-negative. (The antigenic properties of erythrocytes are described in Chapter 6.)

ABO incompatibility exists in about 20% to 25% of all pregnancies, but only one in ten cases of ABO incompatibility results in HDN. Rh incompatibility occurs in less than 10% of pregnancies and rarely causes HDN in the first incompatible fetus. Even after five or more pregnancies, only 5% have babies with hemolytic disease. Usually, erythrocytes from the first incompatible fetus cause the mother's immune system to produce antibodies that affect the fetuses of subsequent incompatible pregnancies. Only one in three cases of HDN is due to Rh incompatibility; most cases are caused by ABO incompatibility.

Pathophysiology

Given that the mother and fetus have antigenically incompatible erythrocytes, HDN will result if (1) the mother's blood contains preformed antibodies against fetal erythrocytes or produces them upon exposure to fetal erythrocytes, (2) sufficient amounts of antibody (usually IgG) cross the placenta and enter fetal blood, and (3) IgG binds with sufficient numbers of fetal erythrocytes to cause widespread antibody-mediated hemolysis or splenic removal. (Antibody-mediated cellular destruction is described in Chapter 6.)

Maternal antibodies may be formed against type B erythrocytes if the mother is type A, or against type A if the mother is type B. Usually, however, the mother is type O and the fetus is A or B. ABO incompatibility can cause HDN even if fetal erythrocytes do not escape into the maternal circulation during pregnancy. This is because the blood of most adults already contains anti-A or anti-B antibodies, which are produced upon exposure to certain foods or infection by gram-negative bacteria. (There are not anti-O antibodies because type O erythrocytes are not antigenic.) Therefore, IgG against type A or B erythrocytes is usually preformed in maternal blood and can enter the fetal circulation throughout the first incompatible pregnancy.

Anti-Rh antibodies, on the other hand, are *only* formed in response to the presence of incompatible (Rh-positive) erythrocytes in the blood of an Rh-negative mother. Sources of exposure include fetal blood that is mixed with the mother's blood at the time of delivery, transfused blood, and, rarely, previous sensitization of the mother by her own mother's incompatible blood.

The first Rh-incompatible pregnancy usually presents no difficulties because very few fetal erythrocytes cross the placental barrier during gestation. When the placenta detaches at birth, however, a large number of fetal erythrocytes usually enters the mother's bloodstream. If the mother is Rh-negative and the fetus is Rh-positive, the mother produces anti-Rh antibodies. The capacity of the mother's immune system to produce anti-Rh antibodies depends on many factors, including her genetic capacity to make antibodies against the Rh antigen D, the amount of fetal-to-maternal bleeding, and the occurrence of any bleeding earlier in the pregnancy. Anti-Rh antibodies persist in the bloodstream for a very long time, and if the next offspring is Rh-positive, the mother's anti-Rh antibodies can enter the fetus's bloodstream and destroy the erythrocytes. Antibodies against Rh antigen D are of the IgG class and easily cross the placenta.

IgG-coated fetal erythrocytes are destroyed extravascularly, primarily by mononuclear phagocytoses in the spleen. As hemolysis proceeds, the fetus becomes anemic. Erythropoiesis accelerates, particularly in the liver and spleen, and immature nucleated cells (erythroblasts) are released into the bloodstream. (This phenomenon is responsible for the other name of HDN, the erythroblastosis fetalis). The degree of anemia depends on the length of time the antibody has been in the fetal circulation, antibody concentration, and the ability of the fetus to compensate for increased hemolysis. Unconjugated (indirect) bilirubin, which is formed during catabolism (breakdown) of hemoglobin, is transported across the placental barrier into the maternal circulation and is excreted by the mother. **Hyperbilirubinemia** occurs in the neonate after birth because excretion of lipid-soluble unconjugated bilirubin through the placenta is no longer possible.

The pathophysiologic effects of HDN are more severe in Rh incompatibility than in ABO incompatibility. ABO incompatibility may resolve after birth without life-threatening complications. Maternal-fetal incompatibility in which a mother with type O blood has a child with type A or B blood is usually so mild that it does not require treatment.

Rh incompatibility is more likely than ABO incompatibility to cause severe or even life-threatening anemia, death in utero, or damage to the central nervous system. Severe anemia alone can cause death resulting from cardiovascular complications (see Chapter 23). Extensive hemolysis also results in increased levels of unconjugated bilirubin in the neonate's circulation. If bilirubin levels exceed the liver's ability to conjugate and excrete bilirubin, some of it is deposited in the brain, causing cellular damage and eventually, if the neonate does not receive exchange transfusions, death.

Fetuses that do not survive anemia in utero are usually stillborn with gross edema in the entire body, a condition called **hydrops fetalis.** Death can occur as early as 17 weeks' gestation and result in spontaneous abortion.

Clinical Manifestations

A wide spectrum of hemolytic disease occurs in affected infants born to sensitized mothers. Neonates with mild HDN may appear healthy or slightly pale, with slight enlargement of the liver or spleen. Pronounced pallor, splenomegaly, and hepatomegaly indicate severe anemia, which predisposes the neonate to cardiovascular failure and shock.

Because the maternal antibodies remain in the neonate's circulatory system after birth, erythrocyte destruction can continue. This causes hyperbilirubinemia and a jaundiced appearance (**icterus neonatorum**) shortly after birth. Without replacement transfusions, in which the child receives Rh-negative erythrocytes, the bilirubin is deposited in the brain, a condition termed **kernicterus.** Kernicterus produces cerebral damage and usually

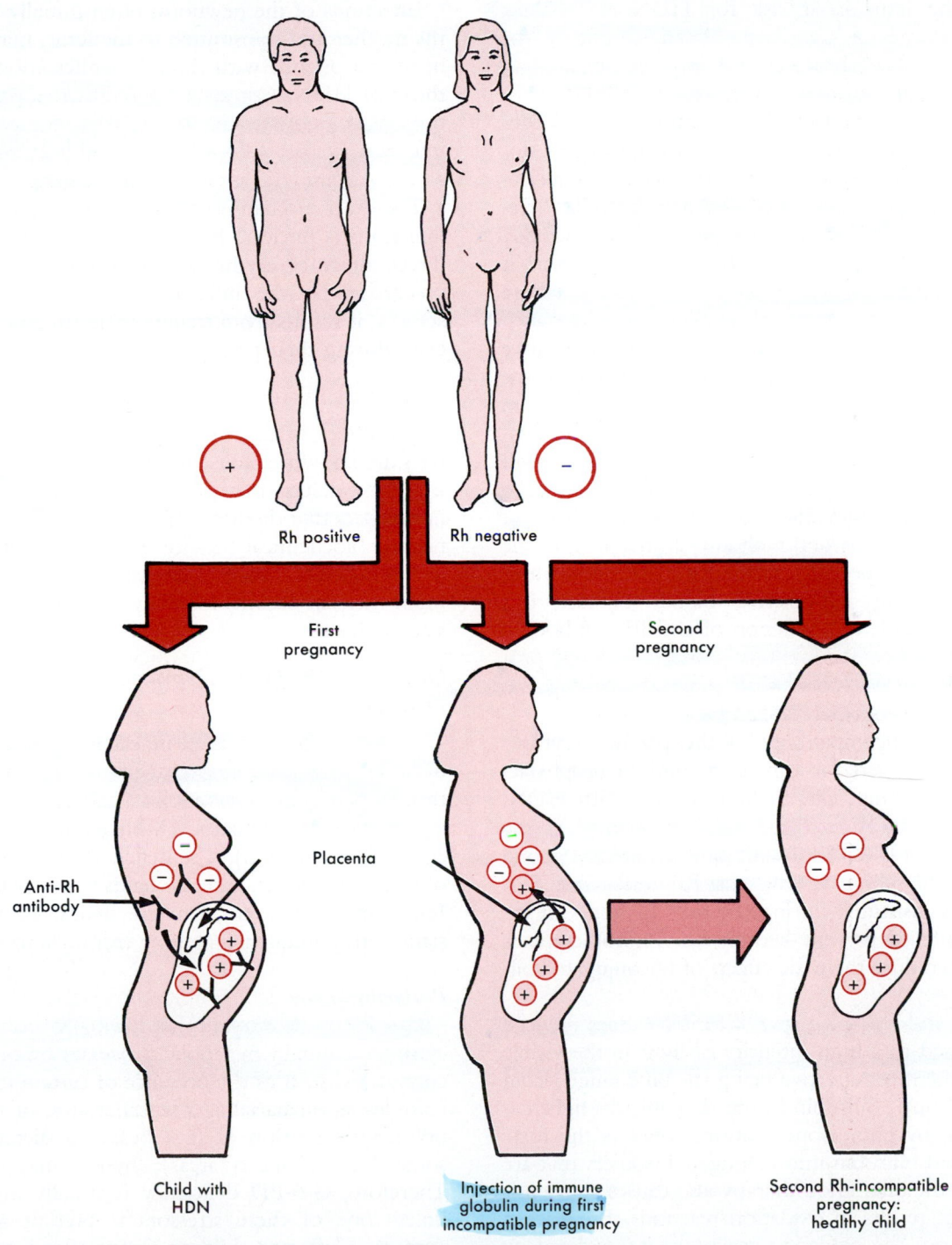

FIG. 25-2. Occurrence and prevention of HDN caused by Rh incompatibility.

causes death (**icterus gravis neonatorum**). Infants that do not die may have mental retardation, cerebal palsy, or high-frequency deafness.

Evaluation and Treatment

Routine evaluation of fetuses at risk for HDN (i.e., fetuses resulting from Rh- or ABO-incompatible matings) includes the Coombs test. The indirect Coombs test measures antibody in the mother's circulation and indicates the fetus is at risk for HDN. The direct Coombs test measures antibody already bound to the surfaces of fetal erythrocytes and is primarily used to confirm the diagnosis of antibody-mediated HDN.

The key to treatment of HDN resulting from Rh-incompatibility lies in prevention. One of the success stories of immunology has been the spectacular results obtained through the use of Rh-immune globulin (frequently called RhoGam), a preparation of antibody against Rh antigen D. If an Rh-negative woman is given Rh-immune globulin within 72 hours of exposure to Rh-positive erythrocytes, she will not produce antibody against the D antigen, and the next Rh-positive baby will be protected (see Fig. 25-2). Apparently, the injected antibodies remain in the mother's bloodstream long enough to prevent her immune system from producing its own anti-Rh antibodies, but not long enough to affect subsequent offspring. The mother must be given Rh-immune globulin injections after the birth of each Rh-positive baby and with any abortion. Also, the mother must be especially careful not to receive a transfusion containing Rh-positive blood, because this would also stimulate production of anti-Rh antibodies. In many hospitals, Rh-immune globulin is given prophylactically at 28 weeks to all pregnant Rh-negative women with Rh-positive husbands.

If antigenic incompatiblity of the parents' erythrocytes is not discovered in time to administer prophylactic immune globulin and a child is born with HDN, treatment consists of exchange transfusions in which the neonate's blood is replaced with new Rh-positive blood that is not contaminated with anti-Rh antibodies. This treatment is instituted during the first 24 hours of extrauterine life to prevent kernicterus. Phototherapy is also used to reduce the toxic effects of unconjugated bilirubin.

Jaundice and indirect hyperbilirubinemia are reduced when exposed to a high intensity of light in the visible spectrum, the most effective being the blue range (from 420 to 470 nm). Bilirubin in the skin absorbs light energy which, by photoisomerization, converts the toxic unconjugated bilirubin into conjugated isomers that are excreted in the bile. Phototherapy also causes autosensitization that results in oxidation reactions. Breakdown products from the oxidation reactions are excreted by the liver and kidney without need for conjugation. The therapeutic effect of phototherapy depends upon the light energy emitted in the effective wave lengths, the distance between the infant and the light source, and the amount of skin exposed; the rate of hemolysis and the infant's ability to excrete bilirubin are also factors in determining the effectiveness of phototherapy in lowering serum bilirubin levels.

Anemia of Infectious Disease

Infections of the newborn, often initially acquired by the mother and transmitted to the fetus, may result in a hemolytic anemia with clinical manifestations similar to those of HDN. Congenital syphilis, toxoplasmosis, cytomegalic inclusion disease, rubella, coxsackie virus B infection, herpes virus infection, and bacterial sepsis can all cause hemolytic anemia in the neonate.

The exact mechanism of anemia caused by congenital infections is unclear. In some instances, it is related to direct injury of erythrocyte membranes or erythrocyte precursors by the infectious organism. In other instances, it results from traumatic destruction of erythrocytes during their passage through inflamed capillaries.

Inherited Disorders

A number of inherited and intrinsic erythrocyte defects are known to cause increased hemolysis (Table 25-2). These defects may be associated with enzymatic abnormalities that disrupt metabolic processes and prevent normal biochemical balance within the cell, alterations of hemoglobin structure or synthesis, or plasma membrane defects accompanied by changes in erythrocyte size or shape.

Glucose-6-Phosphate Dehydrogenase (G-6-PD) Deficiency

G-6-PD deficiency is an inherited, X-linked, recessive disorder, most fully expressed in homozygous males, although partial expression (and a carrier state) is possible in heterozygous females. (X-linked inheritance is discussed in Chapter 5). The deficiency is present in 10% of black Americans, and also tends to occur in Sephardic Jews, Greeks, Iranians, Chinese, Filipinos, and Indonesians with a frequency ranging from 5% to 40%.

Pathophysiology

G-6-PD is an enzyme that normally enables erythrocytes to maintain metabolic processes despite injurious conditions, such as the presence of certain drugs (sulfonamides, antimalarial agents, salicylates, or naphthaquinolones); ingestion of fava beans (a dietary staple in some Mediterranean areas); hypoxemia; or acidosis. Therefore, G-6-PD deficiency is usually asymptomatic unless one of these stressors is present. Erythrocyte damage in affected children begins after intense or prolonged exposure to one of these injurious substances or conditions, and ceases when they are removed. In black American males, the G-6-PD defect becomes more pronounced as the erythrocyte ages; in other populations, the defect is profound even in young erythrocytes. By ingesting a substance with oxidant properties, such as a salicylate (aspirin), a pregnant woman may precipitate an episode of hemolysis in a fetus with G-6-PD deficiency.

In the absence of G-6-PD, oxidative stressors damage hemoglobin and erythrocyte's plasma membrane, and possibly interfere with the activities of other enzymes within the cell. Hemoglobin is oxidized progressively to methemoglobin, sulfhemoglobin, and denatured globin-glutathione complexes. Eventually, exposure to oxidating substances results in the precipitation of insoluble hemoglobin inclusions, called Heinz bodies, within the cell. Plasma damage and the presence of Heinz bodies cause hemolysis, chiefly in the spleen.

Clinical Manifestations

In Oriental and Mediterranean infants, G-6-PD deficiency is likely to be associated with icterus neonatorum. The most common clinical manifestation of G-6-PD deficiency is acute hemolytic anemia, usually following infections or the ingestion of certain oxidative drugs. The fava bean produces a severe hemolytic reaction called "favism" in infants with G-6-PD deficiency.

Hemolytic episodes are characterized by pallor, icterus, dark urine, back pain, and, in severe cases, shock, cardiovascular collapse, and death. Between hemolytic episodes, anemia is absent and erythrocyte survival is normal.

Evaluation and Treatment

Direct or indirect demonstration of reduced G-6-PD activity in erythrocytes is required for evaluation. Satis-factory screening tests are based on discoloration of methylene blue and on reduction of methemoglobin. Immediately after a hemolytic episode, reticulocytes and young erythrocytes predominate. Because young erythrocytes have significantly higher enzyme activity than older cells, testing should be done a few weeks after a crisis, so that a low level of enzyme activity can be demonstrated. The disorder can be suspected when G-6-PD activity is within the low normal range in the presence of a high reticulocyte count. G-6-PD can also be detected by electrophoretic analysis.

Prevention of hemolysis is the most important therapeutic measure. Males belonging to high-risk groups (Greeks, Southern Italians, Sephardic Jews, Filipinos, Chinese, Blacks, and Thais) should be tested for the defect before being given drugs known to be oxidant. When hemolysis has occurred, supportive treatment may include blood transfusions and oral iron therapy. Spontaneous recovery generally follows treatment.

Hereditary Spherocytosis

Hereditary spherocytosis, also known as congenital hemolytic anemia or congenital acholuric jaundice, is the most common of the hemolytic disorders in which there is no abnormality of hemoglobin.

Pathophysiology

Transmitted as an autosomal dominant trait, hereditary spherocytosis is presumed to represent new mutations in about 25% of cases. The defect is believed to be caused by an undefined abnormality of proteins or spectrins of the erythrocyte membrane. Affected cells are unduly permeable to sodium and acquire a particular characteristic structure (Fig. 25-3). An increased concentration of intracellular sodium is believed to lead to increased use of ATP to drive the so-called cation pump.

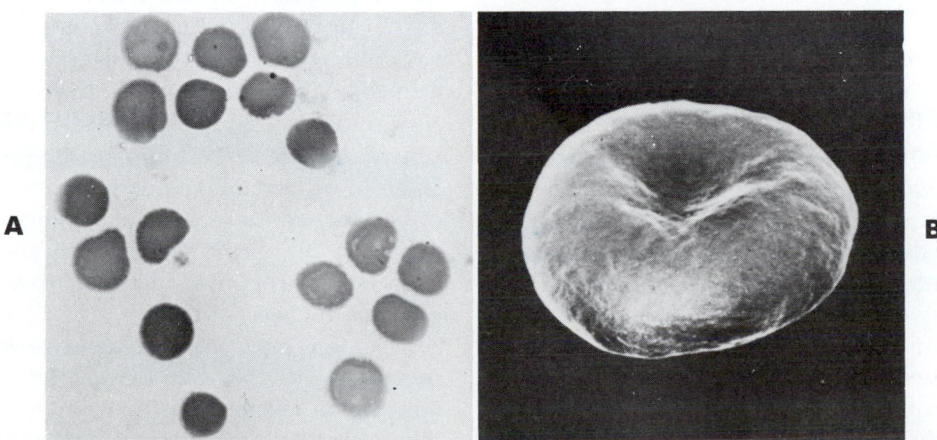

FIG. 25-3. The microspherocyte. **A,** Blood smear from patient with hereditary spherocytosis. (Wright's stain.) **B,** Scanning electron microscope photograph. (Courtesy Dr. M. Bessis. From Miale, 1982.)

Early aging and destruction of erythrocytes are believed to result from metabolic overwork and loss of erythrocyte membrane (Bellingham & Prankerd, 1975; Valentine, 1977).

Circulation of blood to the spleen creates a metabolic environment that is stressful to the spherocyte cell, and repeated passages through this stressful environment results in their sequestration and destruction. The spherocyte is relatively rigid and passes with difficulty through the small openings between the splenic cords and sinuses. Thus, the spleen is intimately involved in the hemolytic process.

Clinical Manifestations

With onset in the neonatal period or in early infancy, anemia and hyperbilirubinemia are severe enough to require phototherapy or exchange transfusions. During infancy and childhood, severity of the anemia varies widely, but tends to be similar within families. Slight jaundice is usually present. Moderate expansion of the marrow cavity of the skull may occur because of compensatory mechanisms to overproduce cells. After infancy, the spleen is almost always enlarged. Although gallstones have been reported to occur as early as 4 to 5 years of age, they usually do not develop until late childhood or early adolescence. If the spleen is not surgically removed, gallstones will form in approximately one half of cases. Aplastic crises are the most serious complication occurring during childhood (Behrman & Vaughan, 1983).

Evaluation and Treatment

The family history, blood smear, and studies of osmotic fragility and autohemolysis are important to evaluate. Surgical removal of the spleen invariably produces a clinical cure and should be performed when the child is 5 to 6 years of age or older.

Sickle Cell Disease

Sickle cell disease is a group of disorders characterized by the presence of an abnormal form of hemoglobin— hemoglobin S (Hb S) within the erythrocytes. Hb S is formed by a genetic mutation in which one amino acid (valine) replaces another (glutamic acid) (Fig. 25-4). Hb S, the so-called sickle hemoglobin, reacts to deoxygenation and dehydration by solidifying and stretching the erythrocyte into an elongated sickle shape. This change has a variety of pathologic consequences, including hemolytic anemia.

Sickle cell disease is an inherited, autosomal recessive disorder that is expressed as sickle cell anemia, sickle cell–thalassemia disease or sickle cell–hemoglobin C disease, depending on mode of inheritance (Table 25-3). (See Chapter 4 for a discussion of genetic inheritance of disease.) Sickle cell anemia, a homozygous form, is the most severe. Sickle cell–thalassemia and sickle cell–Hb C disease are heterozygous forms in which the child simultaneously inherits another type of abnormal hemoglobin from one parent. Sickle cell trait, in which the child inherits Hb S from one parent and normal hemoglobin (Hb A) from the other, is a heterozygous carrier state that rarely has clinical manifestations. Because the child has more than 50% Hb S, clinical manifestations occur only with extreme stress. All forms of sickle cell disease are life-long conditions and have no known cure.

Sickle cell disease tends to occur in people with origins in equatorial countries, particularly central Africa, the Near East, the Mediterranean area, and parts of India. In the United States, sickle cell disease is most common in blacks, with a reported incidence ranging from 1:400 to 1:500 live births within the black population. In the general population, the risk of two black parents having a child with sickle cell anemia is 0.7%. Sickle cell hemoglobin C disease is less common (1 in 800 births), and sickle cell–thalassemia occurs in 1 in 1700 births.

Sickle cell trait occurs in 7% to 13% of the black American population, whereas its incidence among East African blacks may be as high as 45%. The sickle cell trait may provide protection against lethal forms of malaria. This would be a genetic advantage to carriers residing in endemic regions for malaria (Mediterranean and African zones) but is of no advantage to carriers living in the United States.

Pathophysiology

Though the precise mechanisms of sickling is not clearly understood, Hb S that is not bound with oxygen forms aggregates of semisolid gel that become stacked within the erythrocyte, stretching it into an elongated crescent (Figs. 25-5 and 25-6). It is widely theorized that sickling occurs in deoxygenated blood as a consequence of stress. Sickled erythrocytes are stiff and cannot change shape as easily as normal cells when they pass through the microcirculation. (The reversible deformability of erythrocytes is described in Chapter 22.) As a result, sickled erythrocytes tend to plug the blood vessels, causing vascular occlusion, pain, and organ infarction. Sickled cells undergo hemolysis in the spleen or become sequestered there, causing blood pooling and infarction of splenic vessels. The anemia that follows triggers erythropoiesis in the marrow and, in extreme cases, in the liver.

Sickling is not usually permanent; most sickled erythrocytes regain a normal shape after reoxygenation and rehydration. Some cells, however, do become irreversibly sickled despite treatment. Irreversible sickling is not caused by irreversible hemoglobin changes, but rather by irreversible plasma membrane damage caused by sickling. The precise nature of the permanent membrane

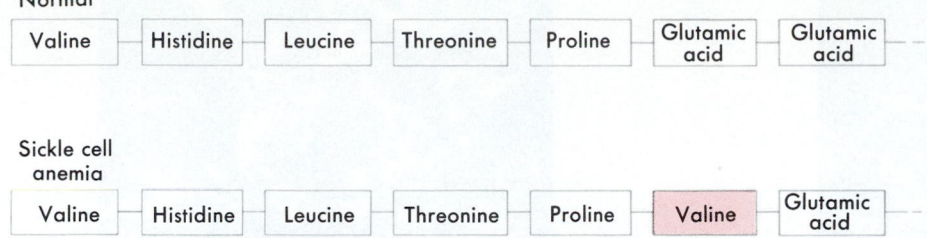

First seven amino acids in normal and sickle cell hemoglobin

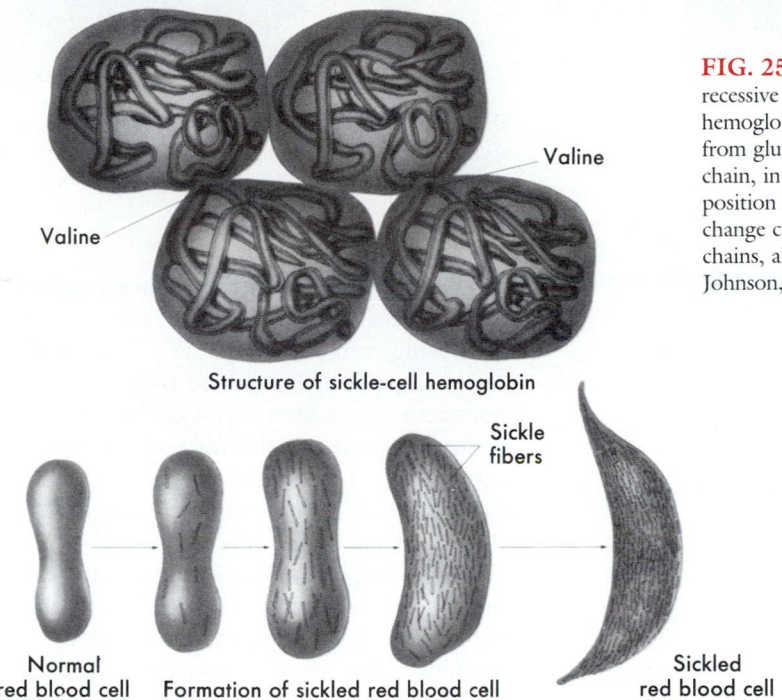

Structure of sickle-cell hemoglobin

FIG. 25-4. Sickle cell hemoglobin is produced by a recessive allele of the gene encoding the beta chain of hemoglobin. It represents a single amino acid change from glutamic acid to valine at the sixth position in the chain, in the folded beta chain molecule the sixth position contacts the alpha chain, and the amino acid change causes the hemoglobins to aggregate into long chains, altering the shape of the cell. (From Raven & Johnson, 1989.)

TABLE 25-3 Inheritance of sickle cell disease

Hemoglobin inherited from first parent	Hemoglobin inherited from second parent	Form of sickle cell disease in child
Hb S (an abnormal hemoglobin)	Hb S	Sickle cell anemia: homozygous inheritance in which the child's hemoglobin is mostly Hb S, with the remainder Hb F (fetal hemoglobin)
Hb S	Defective or insufficient alpha or beta chains of Hb A (alpha- or beta-thalassemia)	Sickle cell—thalassemia disease (heterozygous inheritance of Hb S and alpha-or beta-thalassemia
Hb S	Hb C or D (both abnormal hemoglobins)	Sickle cell—hemoglobin C (or D) disease (heterozygous inheritance of hemoglobin S and either C or D)
Hb S	Normal hemoglobins (mostly Hb A)	Sickle cell trait, the carrier state (heterozygous inheritance of Hb S and normal hemoglobin)

NOTE: See Chapter 22 for a description of normal fetal and adult hemoglobins.

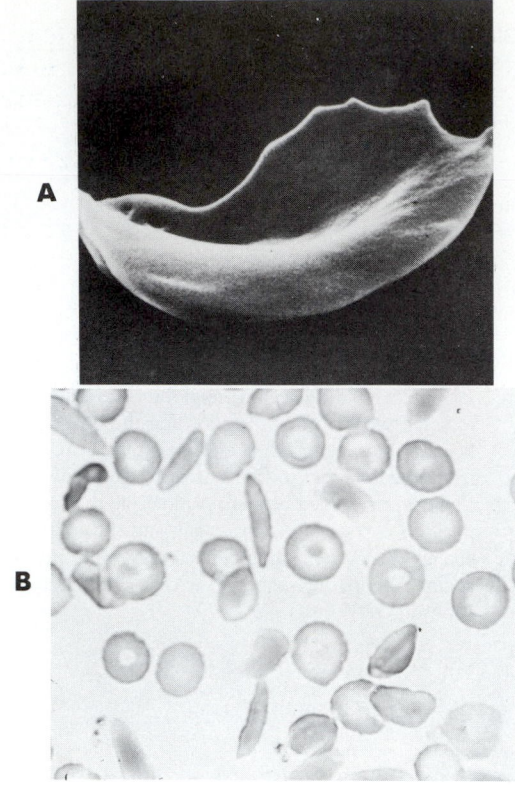

FIG. 25-5. **A,** A sickled cell. **B,** Peripheral blood smear in sickle cell anemia. (Courtesy Dr. M. Bessis. From Miale, 1982.)

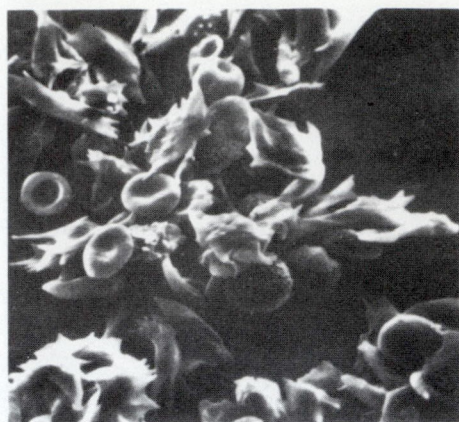

FIG. 25-6. Scanning electron micrograph of normal and sickle-shaped red blood cells. The irregularly shaped cells are the sickle cells; the circular cells are the normal blood cells. (From Raven, 1989.)

The level of Po_2 in the microcirculation also affects sickling because hemoglobin releases whatever oxygen it is carrying to tissues. Thus Po_2 is normally lower in the microcirculation. The added reduction in Po_2 caused by persistent hypoxemia—caused by stressors—eventually results in sickling in the microcirculation of all cells that contain Hb S in that site (not throughout the body). Sickling within the microcirculation decreases blood flow as sickled cells clog the vessels. Slow blood flow promotes hypoxemia and perpetuates sickling. Finally, decreased blood pH decreases hemoglobin's affinity for oxygen. As less oxygen is taken up by hemoglobin in the lungs, Po_2 drops, promoting sickling further.

Increased osmolality of the plasma (increased concentration of solutes; see Chapter 1) draws water out of the erythrocytes. This promotes sickling by raising the relative Hb S content in erythrocytes. Decreased plasma volume, which occurs in states of dehydration, causes the blood to become viscous (thick and sticky). Increased viscosity of the blood is the final common pathway leading to many pathologic effects of sickle cell disease. Viscous blood flows slowly and promotes vascular obstruction by increasing opportunities for sickling while decreasing opportunities for reoxygenation in the lungs. This is an example of positive feedback in a vicious cycle of events.

Once sickling begins, it tends to perpetuate itself until Po_2 returns to normal, then it ceases spontaneously. The extent, severity, and clinical manifestations of sickling depend to a great extent on the percentage of hemoglobin that is Hb S. That is why homozygous inheritance of Hb S produces the severest form of sickle cell disease, sickle cell anemia. Heterozygous inheritance of sickle cell disease results in less sickling because the individual's erythrocytes contain other forms of abnormal hemoglobin that, though defective, do not participate in

injury is not known, but it is known that, while in the sickled state, the plasma membrane loses some of its capacity for active transport, permitting an influx of calcium ions. (Membrane transport and the effects of calcium influx are described in Unit I.) In individuals with sickle cell anemia, in which the erythrocytes contain a high percentage of Hb S (75% to 95%), up to 30% of the erythrocytes can become irreversibly sickled. Occasionally, irreversible sickling occurs in sickle cell disease, but never in the carrier state (sickle cell trait).

Sickling is an occasional, intermittent phenomenon that can be triggered or sustained by one or more of the following stressors: decreased oxygen tension (Po_2) of the blood (i.e., hypoxemia), increased hydrogen ion concentration in the blood (decreased pH), increased plasma osmolality, and decreased plasma volume. The same decrease in Po_2 will cause the most sickling in individuals with sickle cell anemia (high concentrations of Hb S), the second most in children with sickle cell–thalassemia, the third most in those with sickle cell–hemoglobin C disease, and the least or none in those with sickle cell trait. The duration of the Po_2 disease is also important, as sickling tends to occur only after the inciting stimulus has been present for some time.

sickling to any great degree. Heterozygous inheritance (sickle cell trait) in which abnormal hemoglobin is inherited from one parent and normal hemoglobins from the other, rarely results in sickling because normal fetal hemoglobin (Hb F) and adult hemoglobin (Hb A) do not participate in sickling at all. Anemia persists because fetal hemoglobin does not live 120 days.

Clinical Manifestations

When sickling occurs, the general manifestations of hemolytic anemia—pallor, fatigue, jaundice, and irritability—are sometimes accompanied by acute manifestations called crises. Extensive sickling can precipitate four types of crises: (1) vasoocclusive (or thrombotic) crisis, (2) aplastic crisis, (3) sequestration crisis, or,

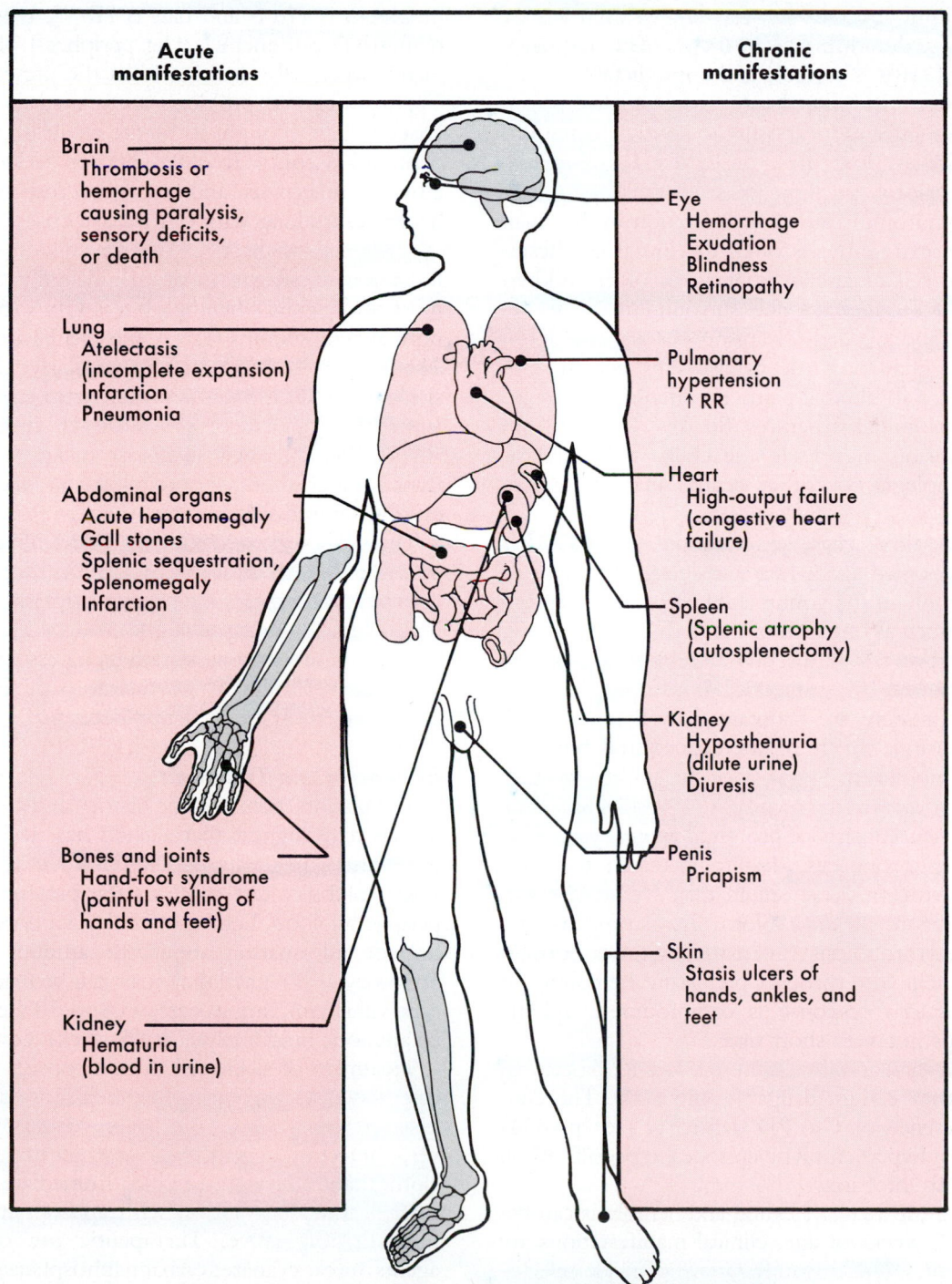

Acute manifestations

Brain
  Thrombosis or hemorrhage causing paralysis, sensory deficits, or death

Lung
  Atelectasis (incomplete expansion)
  Infarction
  Pneumonia

Abdominal organs
  Acute hepatomegaly
  Gall stones
  Splenic sequestration, Splenomegaly
  Infarction

Bones and joints
  Hand-foot syndrome (painful swelling of hands and feet)

Kidney
  Hematuria (blood in urine)

Chronic manifestations

Eye
  Hemorrhage
  Exudation
  Blindness
  Retinopathy

Pulmonary hypertension
  ↑ RR

Heart
  High-output failure (congestive heart failure)

Spleen
  (Splenic atrophy (autosplenectomy)

Kidney
  Hyposthenuria (dilute urine)
  Diuresis

Penis
  Priapism

Skin
  Stasis ulcers of hands, ankles, and feet

FIG. 25-7. Clinical manifestations of sickle cell disease.

rarely, (4) hyperhemolytic crisis. Sites of specific dysfunction are shown in Fig. 25-7.

Vasoocclusive crisis begins with sickling in the microcirculation. As blood flow is obstructed by tangled masses of rigid, sickled cells, some degree of vasospasm occurs, and a "log-jam" effect brings all blood flow through the vessel to a halt. Unless the process is reversed, thrombosis and infarction (death caused by lack of oxygen) of local tissue follows. Vasoocclusive crisis is extremely painful and may last for days or even weeks, with an average duration of 4 to 6 days. The frequency of this type of crisis is variable and unpredictable.

Vasoocclusive crises may develop spontaneously or be precipitated by infection, exposure to cold, dehydration, low Po_2, acidosis (low pH), or localized hypoxemia. Symmetric, painful swelling of the hands and feet (hand-foot syndrome) caused by infarction in the small vessels of the extremities is often the initial manifestation of sickle cell disease in infancy. In older children and adults the large joints and surrounding tissue become painful and swollen. Priapism (persistent erection of the penis) may occur if penile veins become obstructed. Severe abdominal pains are often caused by infarction in abdominal structures. Strokes resulting from cerebral occlusion may leave the child with paralysis (usually hemiplegia) or other central nervous system deficits.

In **sequestration crisis,** large amounts of blood become acutely pooled in the liver and spleen. This type of crisis is seen only in the young child. Because the spleen can hold as much as one fifth of the body's blood supply at one time, up to 50% mortality rate has been reported with death caused by cardiovascular collapse. If blood volume and pressure are maintained by hydration and blood transfusion, much of the sequestered blood is eventually remobilized. Removal of the spleen (splenectomy) is the treatment for recurrent sequestration crises.

Aplastic crisis consists of profound anemia caused by diminished erythropoiesis, despite increased need for new erythrocytes. In sickle cell anemia, erythrocyte survival is only 10 to 20 days. Normally, a compensatory increase in erythropoiesis (five to eight times normal) replaces the cells lost through premature hemolysis. If this compensatory response is compromised, aplastic crisis develops in a very short time.

Hyperhemolytic crisis is unusual, but may occur in association with certain drugs or infections. The concomitant presence of G-6-PD deficiency (see p. 834) contributes to hyperhemolytic episodes, especially when combined with infections.

Although intravascular sickling and hemolysis can begin by 6 to 8 weeks of age, clinical manifestations are not yet present. Clinical manifestations of sickle cell disease do not usually appear until the infant is at least six months old, at which time the postnatal decrease in Hb F causes concentrations of Hb S to rise.

Infection is the most frequent cause of death because of sickle cell disease. Sepsis and meningitis develop in as many as 10% of children with sickle cell anemia during the first 5 years of life, with a mortality rate of 25%. Survival time is unpredictable, but averages in the twenties.

Sickle cell–Hb C disease, in which about half the hemoglobin is Hb S and half is Hb C, is usually milder than sickle cell anemia. The peripheral blood contains many target cells resulting from the presence of Hb C. The main clinical problems are related to vasoocclusive crises and are thought to be the result of higher hematocrit and viscosity. In older children, sickle cell retinopathy, renal necrosis, and aseptic necrosis of the femoral heads occur along with obstructive crises.

Sickle cell–thalassemia has the mildest clinical manifestations of all the sickle cell diseases. Even though most of the child's hemoglobin is Hb S (60% to 90%), normal hemoglobins (Hb A and Hb F) are also present. The normal hemoglobins, particularly Hb F, inhibit sickling. In addition, the erythrocytes tend to be small (microcytic) and to contain relatively little hemoglobin (hypochromic). Their small size makes them less likely than normal sized cells to clog the microcirculation, even when in a sickled state.

The sickle cell trait does not affect life expectancy or interfere with daily activities. Yet on rare occasions, *severe* hypoxia caused by shock, vigorous exercising at high altitudes, flying at high altitudes in unpressurized aircraft, or undergoing anesthesia is associated with vasoocclusive episodes in individuals with sickle cell trait. These cells form an ivy shape instead of a sickle shape.

Evaluation and Treatment

The parents' hematologic history and clinical manifestations may suggest that a child has sickle cell disease, but hematologic tests are necessary for diagnosis. If the sickle solubility test confirms the presence of Hb S in peripheral blood, hemoglobin electrophoresis is done to provide information about the amount of Hb S in erythrocytes. Prenatal diagnosis can be made after chorionic villus sampling as early as 8 to 10 weeks' gestation or amniotic fluid analysis at 15 weeks' gestation.

Treatment of sickle cell disease consists of supportive care aimed at preventing consequences of anemia and avoiding crises. Crises can be prevented by avoiding fever, infection, acidosis, dehydration, constricting clothes, and exposure to cold. Immediate correction of acidosis and dehydration with appropriate intravenous fluids is imperative. Therapeutic use of antisickling agents (urea, cyanate, carbamylphosphate) is still in the experimental stages. Acetaminophen is preferable to salicylates for antipyretic therapy in order to avoid increased acidosis. Immunization against influenzae and pneumococcis should be seriously considered. Blood transfusion can be very effective, but must be weighed against the risks of hepatitis, hemosiderosis, and splenic overload. Oral maintenance therapy with folic acid and/or iron is needed to meet the increased demands of chronic hemolytic anemia. Splenectomy may be performed if sequestration crises recur.

Genetic counseling and psychological support are important for the child and family. Genetic counseling enables individuals with sickle cell disease or trait to make informed decisions about perpetuating this genetic disorder to their offspring, since there is a 25% chance with each pregnancy that a child born to two parents with sickle cell trait will have sickle cell disease.

The Thalassemias

The **alpha-** and **beta-thalassemias** are inherited, autosomal recessive disorders that cause an impaired *rate* of synthesis of one of the two chains—alpha or beta—of adult hemoglobin (Hb A). The disorder was named "thalassemia," which is derived from the Greek word for "sea," because it was initially defined in persons with origins near the Mediterranean Sea. Beta-thalassemia, in which synthesis of the beta globin chain is slowed or defective, is prevalent among Greeks, Italians, and some Arabs and Sephardic Jews. Alpha-thalassemia, in which the alpha chain is affected, is most common among Chinese, Vietnamese, Cambodians, and Laotians. Both alpha- and beta-thalassemia are common among American blacks.

Alpha- and beta-thalassemia can be major or minor, depending on (1) how many of the genes that control alpha or beta chain synthesis are defective and (2) whether the defects are inherited homozygously (thalassemia major) or heterozygously (thalassemia minor). Pathophysiologic effects range from mild microcytosis to death in utero, depending on the number of defective genes and mode of inheritance. The anemic manifestation of thalassemia is microcytic-hypochromic hemolytic anemia.

Pathophysiology

Normally, two genes control beta chain synthesis and four genes control alpha chain synthesis. The number of genetic defects in the controlling genes determines the severity of the disorder. As in sickle cell disease, the hemoglobin abnormality usually consists of the substitution of a single amino acid for another. Other molecular abnormalities that cause thalassemia are two amino acid substitutions, amino acid deletions or fusions, and synthesis of elongated chains.

The fundamental defect in beta-thalassemia is the uncoupling of alpha and beta chain synthesis. Beta chain production is depressesed—moderately in the heterozygous form, **beta-thalassemia minor,** and severely in the homozygous form, **beta-thalassemia major** (also called Cooley anemia). Depression of beta chain synthesis results in erythrocytes having a reduced amount of hemoglobin and accumulations of free alpha chains. The free alpha chains are unstable and easily precipitate in the cell. Most erythroblasts that contain precipitates are destroyed by mononuclear phagocytes in the marrow, resulting in ineffective erythropoiesis and anemia. Some of the precipitate-carrying cells do mature and enter the bloodstream but they are destroyed prematurely in the spleen, resulting in mild hemolytic anemia.

There are four forms of alpha-thalassemia: (1) **alpha trait** (the carrier state), in which a single alpha-chain-forming gene is defective; (2) **alpha-thalassemia minor,** in which two genes are defective; (3) **hemoglobin H disease,** in which three genes are defective; and (4) **alpha-thalassemia major,** a fatal condition in which all four alpha-forming genes are defective. Death is inevitable because alpha chains are absent and oxygen cannot be released to the tissues.

Beta-thalassemia occurs more commonly than alpha-thalassemia. Occasionally, synthesis of gamma or delta polypeptide chains is defective, resulting in gamma- or delta-thalassemia. (Hemoglobin chains are described in Chapter 22.)

Clinical Manifestations

Beta-thalassemia minor causes mild to moderate microcytic-hypochromic anemia, mild splenomegaly, bronze coloring of the skin, and hyperplasia of the bone marrow. The degree of reticulocytosis depends on the severity of the anemia, resulting in skeletal changes. Hemolysis of immature (and therefore fragile) erythrocytes may cause a slight elevation in serum iron and indirect bilirubin levels. Individuals with beta-thalassemia minor are usually asymptomatic.

Individuals with beta-thalassemia major may become quite ill. Anemia is severe and results in a signficant cardiovascular burden, with high-output congestive heart failure. In the past, death resulted from cardiac failure. Today, blood transfusions can increase life span by a decade or two, and death is usually caused by hemochromatosis (from transfusions). (Hemosiderosis and hematochromatosis are described in Chapter 23.) Liver enlargement occurs as a result of progressive hemosiderosis, whereas enlargement of the spleen is caused by extramedullary hemopoiesis and increased destruction of red blood cells. Growth and maturation are retarded, and a characteristic deformity (chipmunk deformity) develops on the face, caused by expansion of bones to accommodate hyperplastic marrow.

Individuals who inherit the mildest form of alpha-thalassemia, the alpha trait, are usually asymptomatic, having at most, mild microcytosis. Alpha-thalassemia minor has clinical manifestations that are virtually identical to those of beta-thalassemia minor: mild microcytic-hypochromic reticulocytosis, bone marrow hyperplasia, increased serum iron concentrations, and moderate splenomegaly.

Signs and symptoms of alpha thalassemia are similar to those of beta-thalassemia major, but milder. Moderate microcytic-hypochromic anemia, enlargement of the liver and spleen, and bone marrow hyperplasia are evident.

Alpha-thalassemia major causes hydrops fetalis and fulminant intrauterine congestive heart failure. The fetus has a grossly enlarged heart and liver, in addition to edema and massive ascites. Diagnosis is usually made post mortem. Prenatal screening for this disorder can be done using chorionic villus sampling. These cells can be analyzed and a DNA genetic map can be constructed and evaluated for the abnormalities characteristic of hydrops fetalis.

Both alpha- and beta-thalassemia major are life-threatening. Children with thalassemia major are generally weak, fail to thrive, show poor development, and experience cardiovascular compromise with high output failure secondary to anemia. Untreated, they will die by 5 to 6 years of age.

Evaluation and Treatment

Evaluation of thalassemia is based on familial disease history, clinical manifestations, and blood tests. Peripheral blood smears showing microcytosis, and hemoglobin electrophoresis that demonstrates diminished amounts of alpha or beta chains, are used to make the diagnosis. Analysis of fetal DNA from withdrawn amniotic fluid is used as a screening test to detect hydrops fetalis (alpha-thalassemia major).

Individuals who are "silent" carriers or have thalassemia minor generally have few if any symptoms and require no specific treatment. Therapies to support and prolong life are necessary, however, for thalassemia major. There is no cure for either condition.

At present, thalassemia major is treated with the following:
1. Blood transfusions, which can return hemoglobin and hematocrit to normal, thus alleviating the anemia-induced cardiac failure. Iron overload and hemochromatosis are complications of transfusion therapy.
2. Iron chelation therapy in combination with hypertransfusion (transfusion to a hematocrit of 35 to correct all manifestations of thalassemia). This therapy is currently under investigation. If it is

proved effective, what once was a fatal disease may in the future be merely an expensive nuisance.
3. Splenectomy, which can reduce the need for transfusions by eliminating a site of hemolysis, thus prolonging erythrocyte survival.
4. Neocyte transfusion, in which young erythrocytes (neocytes) in a unit of blood are separated by centrifugation from old erythrocytes (gerocytes). Neocytes may last longer in the circulation and thus reduce the problem of hemolysis and premature cell destruction. This therapy is being investigated.

For both asymptomatic carriers and those with the disease, prenatal diagnosis and genetic counseling may be the most important therapeutic measures that can be offered.

DISORDERS OF COAGULATION AND PLATELETS

Inherited Hemorrhagic Disease

The Hemophilias

Awareness of a serious bleeding disorder in males was documented nearly 2000 years ago in the Babylonian Talmud, which exempted from the rite of circumcision those boys having male relatives prone to excessive bleeding. In 1803, the first description of this disorder appeared in the medical literature, where it was noted to be X-linked in nature and associated with joint bleeding and crippling.

Table 25-4 lists the coagulation factors that are associated with clinical bleeding. Until 1952, the term "hemophilia" was reserved for deficiency of factor VIII (antihemophilic factor). Since that time two additional coagulation proteins, factor IX (plasma thromboplastin component [PTC]) and factor XI (plasma thromboplastin antecedent [PTA]), have been identified and their deficiency associated with similar clinical manifestations. Congenital deficiencies of these three plasma clotting factors—VIII, IX, and XI—account for 90% to 95% of the hemorrhagic bleeding disorders collectively called hemophilia. (Table 25-5 lists coagulation disorders in children.)

Types of Hemophilia

Hemophilia A (classic hemophilia) is caused by factor VIII deficiency. It is the most common of the hemophilias. Inherited as an X-linked recessive disorder affecting males and transmitted by females, its estimated incidence rate is 1 per 10,000 male births.

Hemophilia B (Christmas disease), caused by factor IX deficiency, is also transmitted as an X-linked recessive trait and is clinically indistinguishable from factor VIII

TABLE 25-4 Phase, factor, and disease name for coagulation disorders in children

Phase/factor	Synonyms
PHASE I DISORDERS	
Factor VIII deficiencies	Classic hemophilia; hemophilia A; antihemophilic factor (AHF) deficiency
Factor IX deficiency	Christmas disease; hemophilia B
Factor XI deficiency	Plasma thromboplastin antecedent (PTA) deficiency; hemophilia C
Factor XII deficiency	Hageman factor deficiency
von Willbrand disease	Vascular hemophilia
PHASE II DISORDERS	
Congenital deficiency of factors II, V, & VII	Hemorrhagic disease of the newborn; parahemophilia, Owren disease (factor V)
PHASE III DISORDERS	
Congenital afibrinogenemia	Congenital fibrinogen deficiency
Congenital dysfibrinogenemia	Congenital fibrinogen deficiency
Factor XIII deficiency	Fibrin-stabilizing factor deficiency

deficiency. Approximately 15% of cases of hemophilia are caused by factor IX.

Hemophilia A and B occur with varying degrees of clinical severity, depending on concentrations of clotting factor VIII or IX in the blood. Severe hemophilia (concentration of clotting factors less than 1% of normal) is associated with spontaneous bleeding. In moderate hemophilia (1% to 5% of normal), bleeding usually occurs only after trauma; and in the mild form (5% to 35% of normal), bleeding occurs only after severe trauma or surgery. The severity of hemophilia is similar in all affected members of a family.

Hemophilia C (factor XI deficiency) occurs as an autosomal recessive disease and occurs equally in males

TABLE 25-5 Coagulation disorders in children

Factor/deficient	Genetics	Frequency in population (per 10^6)	Disorder
I (fibrinogen)	AR	0.1	Afibrinogenemia, hypofibrinogenemia
II (prothrombin)	AR	0.1	Hypoprothrombinemia
III (thromboplastin)			
IV (Ca^{++})			
V	AR	0.1	Parahemophilia, factor V deficiency
VII	AR	0.1	Factor VII deficiency
VIII (AHP)	X-R	30-40	Hemophilia A, classic hemophilia; von Willibrand disease
IX (PTC)	X-R	3-4	Hemophilia B, Christmas disease
X	AR	0.1	Factor X deficiency
XI (PTA)	AR	1	Hemophilia C, PTA deficiency
XII	AR	0.1	Hageman trait
XIII	AR	0.1	Factor XIII deficiency

Adapted from Kelly, 1983.
AR, autosomal recessive; X-R, sex-linked recessive.

and females. Bleeding is usually less severe than in hemophilia A or B.

Von Willebrand disease is an inherited autosomal dominant trait with variable clinical manifestations and hematologic findings. The factor VIII deficiency differs from that of hemophilia A in mode of inheritance and response to treatment. In hemophilia A, the deficiency is inherited as an X-linked recessive trait, whereas in von Willebrand disease it is inherited as an autosomal dominant trait. The most important difference, however, is manifested by the responses to the infusion of plasma. In von Willebrand disease, infusion of plasma causes factor VIII activity to increase for several days because infusion of factor VIII temporarily induces endogenous synthesis of factor VIII.

Pathophysiology

As discussed in Chapter 22, the blood is in dynamic equilibrium between fluidity and coagulation. This balance must be maintained to assure that exsanguination does not follow minor injury or that clotting does not occur spontaneously. The complex process by which this balance is maintained involves local reaction of the blood vessels, a variety of activities by platelets, and the interactions of specific coagulation factors that circulate in the blood. The primary barrier against hemorrhage is the vascular endothelium. When small blood vessels are traumatized, active vasoconstriction and local tissue pressure control minute areas of bleeding without mobilization of the coagulation mechanism, but the action of platelets is essential for maintaining small blood vessels and supporting endothelial stability. Defects caused by abnormalities of the blood vessels result in small intracutaneous hemorrhages and petechiae. Defects of platelets and the soluble coagulation proteins result in serious bleeding disorders, with dramatic and urgent clinical manifestations.

In the classic schema of coagulation, three phases are identified. In phase I, a hypothetical substance, called thromboplastin, is formed by the interaction of plasma, platelets, and tissue fluid. Both intrinsic and extrinsic mechanisms are also responsible during this phase. The intrinsic mechanism involves the successive enzymatic conversion of the inactive forms of factors XII, XI, and IX. Activated factor IX interacts with factor VIII, platelet factor 3, and calcium to activate factor X. Once factor X is activated, it interacts with factor V to generate prothrombinase, an enzyme responsible for converting prothrombin to thrombin. The extrinsic mechanism involves the conversion of inactive factor VII to its active state by thromboplastin, a substance derived from tissue fluid. In the extrinsic system, active factor VIII directly activates factor X (see p. 772).

In phase II, prothrombin is converted to thrombin in the presence of thromboplastin and calcium. This phase requires factors II and V, active factor V, and calcium.

Finally, in phase III, thrombin is converted by soluble fibrinogen into the fibrin clot. Thrombin splits four small peptides from the fibrinogen molecule and uncovers reactive sites in the fibrin monomer. These monomers polymerize, both side-to-side and end-to-end, to form fibrin. Factor VIII promotes cross-linking between fibrin strands to form a stable three-dimensional clot. Other systems, such as the Kallikrein and fibrinolytic systems, interact with the coagulation mechanisms and are discussed in Chapter 7.

Table 25-4 summarizes the types of coagulation disorders according to the phase of coagulation affected. Not all of the disorders are discussed in this chapter because some are extremely rare (congenital dysfibrinogenemias), whereas others have no clinical significance (e.g., Hegeman factor deficiency, a condition in which profound laboratory deficiency of factor XII has absolutely no clinical effects on the child).

Clinical Manifestations

While abnormal bleeding may occur in the newborn period, particularly after circumcision, spontaneous bleeding due to hemophilia is infrequent during the first year of life. Although there is no transfer of maternal clotting factor to the fetus, many boys with hemophilia are circumcised without excessive bleeding. Normal hemostasis is achieved in these infants because clotting is activated through the extrinsic coagulation cascade, which does not involve factors VII, IX, or XI.

During the first year, spontaneous bleeding is often minimal, but hematoma formation may result from injections and from firm holding (such as under the arms). Easy bruising and/or hemarthrosis (bleeding into joints) occurs with ambulation. By age 3 to 4 years, 90% of children with hemophilia have had episodes of persistent bleeding from relatively minor traumatic lacerations (e.g., to the lip or tongue). This is usually the first clinical manifestation of hemophilia. Hemorrhage into the elbows, knees, and ankles causes pain, limits joint movement, and predisposes the child to degenerative joint changes. Spontaneous hematuria and epistaxis are troublesome but minor complications.

Recurrent bleeding, both spontaneous and after minor trauma, is a life-long problem. Many individuals experience phases or cycles of spontaneous bleeding episodes. Mechanisms that cause this phenomenon are unknown. Intracranial hemorrhage and bleeding into the neck constitute life-threatening emergencies.

Evaluation and Treatment

Although laboratory tests are of primary value in the evaluation of hemorrhagic disorders, the history and physical assessment should also be given careful consideration. The three phases of coagulation can be individually assessed by simple, reliable tests. In any hemorrhagic condition, the adequacy of phase III should be determined first. Unless adequate fibrinogen is present, the blood is incapable of coagulation, and other laboratory tests requiring formation of a visible clot will be invalid. Phase III can be evaluated by the **thrombin time,** the time required for plasma to clot after the addition of bovine thrombin. Fibrinogen can be measured by chemical or immunologic methods.

Phase II is assessed by the **prothrombin time,** the time required for plasma to clot after the addition of thromboplastin and calcium. If phase III is intact, a prolonged prothrombin time indicates a deficiency involving factors II, V, VII, or X, alone or in combination. Specific assays for each of the factors is available.

Phase I, the most complex part of coagulation, can be evaluated by several tests. The **activated partial thromboplastin time (PTT)** is the time required for clotting of plasma that has been activated by incubation with Koalin when calcium and platelets, or partial thromboplastin, are added. PTT assesses the adequacy of factors XII, XI, IX, and VII. The **prothrombin consumption time** is a standard prothrombin test of serum instead of plasma. Because prothrombin is used up during coagulation, the serum normally contains little prothrombin and the serum prothrombin time is prolonged. Deficiencies of the phase I factors are associated with poor use of prothrombin. If the serum and plasma prothrombin times are similar, deficiency of a phase I factor is likely. The **thromboplastin generation** test is the most sensitive of all phase I tests. The test can precisely identify deficiencies of factors VIII and IX. If the PTT, prothrombin consumption, or thromboplastin generation test results are abnormal, the way in which they can be corrected identifies the specific deficiency.

For superficial and minor injuries, local pressure and/or topical application of hemostatic agents may be useful. Quick-frozen plasma (cryoprecipitate) containing the missing clotting factor may be administered to promote hemostasis and as a prophylactic measure.

The prognosis for children with hemophilia is far more promising now than in the past. Programs of comprehensive care and home treatment have improved the quality of life for hemophiliacs and enhanced their general physical capabilities.

Antibody-mediated Hemorrhagic Disease

The antibody-mediated hemorrhagic diseases are a group of disorders caused by the immune response. Antibody-mediated destruction of platelets or antibody-mediated inflammatory reactions to allergens damage blood vessels and cause seepage into tissues. The thrombocytopenic purpuras may be intrinsic, or idiopathic, or may be transient phenomena transmitted from mother to fetus. The inflammatory, or "allergic" purpuras occur in response to allergens in the blood. All of these disorders first appear during infancy or childhood.

Idiopathic Thrombocytopenic Purpura

Acute **idiopathic thrombocytopenic purpura (ITP),** is the most common of the thrombocytopenic purpuras of childhood. ITP, a so-called autoimmune or primary thrombocytopenic purpura, is a disorder of platelet consumption in which antiplatelet antibodies bind to the plasma membranes of platelets, causing platelet sequestration and destruction by mononuclear phagocytes in the spleen and other lymphoid tissues at a rate that exceeds the ability of the bone marrow to produce them.

Pathophysiology

Platelets have several tissue-specific antigens on their plasma markers that may be targets for antiplatelet antibody. In approximately 70% of cases of ITP, there is an antecedent viral disease (such as rubella, rubeola, or viral respiratory infection), thus suggesting that viral sensitization has occurred. The interval between infection and onset of purpura averages 2 weeks. By analogy with purpura seen in adults, an immune mechanism has been identified as the basis for ITP. High levels of IgG have been found bound to platelets and may represent immune complexes on the platelet surface (Karpatkin, 1981; Lightsey & Koenig, 1979; Simons, Main, & Yarsh, 1975; Weiss, 1975).

Clinical Manifestations

One to four weeks after a viral infection, bruising and a generalized petechial rash often occurs with acute onset. Asymmetrical bleeding is typical and is found most frequently covering the legs. Hemorrhage bullae of the gums, lips, and other mucous membranes may be prominent. Epistaxis (nose bleeding) may be severe and difficult to control. Except for the signs of bleeding, the child appears well. The acute phase of the disease associated with spontaneous hemorrhages lasts 1 to 2 weeks, but thrombocytopenia often persists even longer. Although its incidence is less than 1%, intracranial hemorrhage is the most serious complication of ITP. In some cases, the onset is more gradual and clinical manifestations consist of moderate bruising and a few petechiae.

Evaluation and Treatment

Upon examination of the blood, the platelet count is reduced and the few platelets observed on a smear are large in size, reflecting increased bone marrow production. The tourniquet test and tests of bleeding time and clot reaction give abnormal results. Bone marrow aspiration reveals normal or increased megakaryocytes and normal erythrocytes and granulocytes.

Even without treatment, ITP has an excellent prognosis. Three fourths of children recover completely within

3 months. After the initial acute phase, spontaneous clinical manifestations subside. By 9 to 12 months after onset, about 90% of affected children have regained normal platelet counts.

Because of the short life-span of platelets (10 days), fresh blood or platelets are of no value or of transient benefit, but are indicated when life-threatening hemorrhage occurs. For 20% of cases, corticosteroid therapy reduces the severity and shortens the duration of the initial phase by suppressing the immune attack on platelets. Bacterial infections should be treated with antibiotics. Parents should be instructed to protect the child from falls or other trauma that might result in bleeding. Splenectomy should be reserved for chronic cases that fail to respond to nonsurgical intervention.

Transient Neonatal Thrombocytopenias

Antibody-mediated thrombocytopenic purpura occurs in neonates in either autoimmune or isoimmune form. Both forms are characterized by the immunologic destruction of platelets by antibodies (IgG) against tissue-specific antigens expressed by the platelets (i.e., platelet-specific antigens).

Transient neonatal thrombocytopenia was first noted in the early 1950s when it was observed that mothers with ITP frequently delivered infants who were transiently thrombocytopenic. Neonatal thrombocytopenia was observed in approximately 50% of infants at risk and lasted an average of 1 month. As platelet counts returned to normal, there was a concomitant drop in the level of maternal antiplatelet antibody on the child's platelets. The particular platelet-specific antigens that are the targets of antiplatelets have not yet been identified, but do not appear to be among known platelet-specific antigens. The prognosis is generally favorable, but several fetal complications do occur. Perinatal intracranial hemorrhage, for example, occurs in approximately 6% to 17% of affected infants born by vaginal delivery.

Isoimmune thrombocytopenic purpura (IITP) is less common, occurring in approximately 1 in 5000 births. IITP is suspected in thrombocytopenic infants of mothers with normal platelet counts and no history of purpura. The disorder is caused by the production of a maternal antibody against a fetal platelet-specific antigen inherited from the father and not shared by the mother. Approximately 50% of IITP cases are associated with the presence of the PlA1 antigen on neonatal and paternal platelets, but not on maternal platelets.

It is not known why IITP occurs in only half of the neonates genetically at risk for IITP. Because 98% of the population is PlA1 positive, approximately 1 in 50 pregnancies would be expected to show maternal-fetal incompatibility, but the incidence of IITP is 100 times

less. IITP does not develop in neonates born to some mothers with high antiplatelet antibody levels.

The diagnosis of IITP is confirmed by detection in the maternal serum of antibody that reacts with platelets from the infant and father, but not with platelets from the mother. IITP has an approximately 75% to 85% chance of recurrence in subsequent pregnancies. Purpura usually develops in the affected infant shortly after delivery, and intracranial, renal, and gastrointestinal hemorrhages are possible. Mortality rates from intracranial hemorrhage have been estimated at 10% to 15%.

Most of the life-threatening clinical manifestations of both transient neonatal thrombocytopenia and IITP can be avoided through delivery by cesarean section. If the mother has antiplatelet disease, however, surgery can result in hemorrhage and serious maternal morbidity. Maternal mortality resulting from ATP during pregnancy is low (less than 5%): the principal maternal risk is bleeding from surgical incisions during cesarean section. This poses a problem for the obstetrician. The incidence of transient thrombocytopenia in infants born to mothers with ATP is about 50%. If all deliveries were performed by cesarean section, half the mothers would undergo cesarean section unnecessarily. Conversely, if all deliveries were vaginal, then half the infants—those with thrombocytopenia—would be at risk for intracranial bleeding. A considerable amount of research has focused on methods of predicting whether or not the fetus is thrombocytopenic, so that the route of delivery can be chosen to minimize the risks for both mother and child. No satisfactory method has been found, despite reports from many laboratories that fetal platelet counts correlate closely with levels of antiplatelet antibody on maternal platelets or in the maternal circulation. Equally unreliable are predictions of neonatal thrombocytopenia based on immunosuppression with corticosteroids. Research continues in such areas as the identification of specific subclasses of antiplatelet antibodies.

Autoimmune Vascular Purpura

Autoimmune vascular purpura, also called allergic purpura, is caused by antibody-mediated injury of blood vessel walls, typically the arterioles and capillaries. The inflammatory reaction is to foreign proteins or chemicals in the blood (microorganisms, drugs, or other chemicals).

Autoimmune vascular purpura is usually seen in children, with the incidence decreasing in adolescents and adults and occurring only rarely in the elderly. The average age at onset is 5 years, with a slightly higher proportion of males affected. Purpura occurs as vessel integrity is disrupted by inflammatory processes, causing effusion of serosanguinous exudate to perivascular tissues.

Clinical manifestations may vary and include headache, anorexia, fever, abdominal pain, arthralgias, and skin lesions (urticaria and erythema). The lesions are usually located symmetrically on the proximal portions of the extremities, particularly on the legs and buttocks, and may be accompanied by itching or paresthesias (Wintrobe et al., 1981). Abdominal pain results from hemorrhage into the bowel, which may lead to colic, nausea, and vomiting. These symptoms may precede the appearance of skin lesions. The pain is usually midabdominal, but may radiate to other parts of the abdomen. Constipation may occur.

Some forms of autoimmune vascular purpura may produce joint pain and tenderness. Periarticular swelling and edema of the hands and feet are common, but hemarthrosis does not occur. These symptoms may precede the onset of symptoms associated with abdominal pain and purpura. Subacute glomerulonephritis occurs in some cases, but is usually reversible.

The characteristic skin lesions (purpura and cutaneous manifestations of allergy), accompanied by a history of joint and abdominal pain, are clues for diagnosis. Laboratory tests often reveal no major abnormalities. Attacks may last several weeks and may recur at odd intervals and with changing manifestations with each episode. Treatment, if necessary, is the alleviation of symptoms.

LEUKEMIA AND LYMPHOMA

Leukemia is the most common malignancy of children less than 15 years of age. The lymphomas of childhood are the third most common malignant neoplasm of children in the United States. (See Chapter 24 for a discussion of leukemia in adults.)

Leukemia

Of the varieties of childhood leukemia, 80% to 85% of leukemias in children are acute lymphoblastic leukemia (ALL) or acute undifferentiated leukemia (AUL). The remaining 15% to 20% are acute nonlymphoblastic leukemias (ANLL) (which include myeloblastic, promyelocytic, monocytic, myelomonoblastic) and the very rare red blood cell leukemia, erythroleukemia. Leukemia accounts for 25% of cases of cancer in black children and 34% of cases of cancer in white children. A total of 2200 new cases are diagnosed each year in the United States (American Cancer Society, 1988). Of those 2200 children, 1700 are diagnosed with ALL. Both a juvenile and an adult form of chronic granulocytic leukemia (CGL) in children develop, but this condition is uncommon and accounts for only 2% of all leukemias in childhood. Chronic lymphocytic leukemia (CLL) is virtually nonexistent in children.

The peak incidence for childhood ALL is between 2 and 6 years of age. Although this peak is very evident in white children in the United States, it is not observed in black children. The reason for this difference is unknown, but it may be related to genetic susceptibility or to exposure to the environmental influences that might play a role in leukemia. Furthermore, acute leukemia is nearly twice as common in white children than in nonwhite children (4.2/100,000 vs. 2.4/100,000, respectively). For a white child, the risk of acute leukemia developing before the age of ten is 1/2,800 (Pendergrass, 1985). Childhood ALL is also more common in boys than in girls (1.3:1.0). The reason for this difference is again unknown, although sex hormones may play a role in the leukemia process.

Types of Leukemia

A number of different classifications are used for the leukemias. First, acute leukemia is differentiated from chronic leukemia. Second, the cell line determines whether lymphoid cells or myeloid cells are involved. In acute leukemia, this separates ALL from ANLL and vice versa. Then, within each of these categories, further subdivisions have been developed. (See Chapter 24 for a discussion of leukemias that occur in adults.)

Two additional classifications of ALL, morphologic and immunologic, have proved clinically useful because they have prognostic value. Although a number of different morphologic classifications have been developed, the accepted system was developed by a cooperative effort of French, American, and British scientists and is known as the FAB system (Bennett et al., 1981). This classification system divides lymphoblasts into three categories—L_1, L_2, and L_3—on the basis of histologic appearance of the abnormal lymphoblast. Approximately 85% of ALL is of the L_1 subtype; less than 15% is L_2 and is more common in adults with ALL, and the L_3 subtype is very rare and seen in less than 1% of children with ALL.

The immunologic classification of ALL is currently evolving as advances are made in immunologic techniques (Greaves et al., 1981). Because of the new techniques, distinguishing between lymphoblastic and nonlymphoblastic leukemia is much easier than in the past, when the degree of immaturity of the cell had sometimes made such distinction difficult. In addition, immunologic classifications have assisted clinicians in determining the degree of aggressive therapy needed.

Immunologic classification has been based on identification of various surface markers. Five categories of ALL have been identified. These are (1) T cell acute lymphoblastic, characterized by the presence of abnormal T lymphoblasts (20% of ALL); (2) B cell acute lymphoblastic, characterized by the presence of abnormal B lymphoblasts (5% of ALL); (3) pre-B cell acute lymphoblastic, characterized by the presence of pre-B lymphoblasts (20% of ALL); (4) unclassified acute lymphoblastic, also known as "null cell" meaning neither T nor B lymphoblasts are identified (15% of ALL); and (5) common acute lymphoblastic, characterized by the presence of a specific antigen known as the common acute lymphoblastic leukemia antigen or CALLA (39% of ALL). The identification of the CALLA is important because this type of ALL has a more favorable prognosis.

As more progress is made in immunologic classifications, these categories will be revised. As recently as 1980, only three categories were recognized; currently consideration of a sixth category (a pre-T cell leukemia) is under way. Health care providers should therefore view these categories as a developing system for classifying ALL. Unlike ALL, current studies of cell surface markers on ANLL cells have not proved helpful.

Pathogenesis

The exact cause of childhood leukemia is unclear. Investigations have focused on genetic susceptibility, environmental factors, and viral infections. (Theories on carcinogenesis are discussed in Chapter 11.) Observations of a familial tendency and links with a number of inherited disorders have implicated genetic factors in the origin of leukemia. For example, if ALL develops in one identical twin, the other twin is at very high risk for development of the disease—particularly during the first year after diagnosis of the leukemic twin. Miller (1963) found the risk of development of leukemia in the co-twin to be 1 in 4. After approximately 7 years, the risk to the unaffected twin returns to the same risk as that of the general population. Some evidence suggests that multiple cases of leukemia occur in families. The incidence of leukemia in siblings of leukemic children is reported to be between 1:720 and 1:1000, which represents a fourfold risk over that of the general population (Miller, 1967).

Inherited diseases that predispose a child to leukemia (both ALL and ANLL) include Down syndrome (1:74 before the age of 10), Fanconi anemia (1:12 before the age of 21), Bloom syndrome (1:8 before the age of 26), and ataxia telangiectasia (1:8 before the age of 25) (Pendergrass, 1985). Leukemia has also been associated with known genetic diseases, such as congenital agammaglobulinemia. ANLL in children is sometimes associated with loss or deletions of chromosome 7 (Grier & Weinstein, 1985). ANLL can develop from preexisting myeloproliferative disorders that are also preleukemia syndromes. When these disorders progress to ANLL, an insidious pattern of leukemic dysfunction is usually revealed.

Most research on environmental factors as etiologic agents has centered on exposure to ionizing radiation. Atomic bomb survivors have been shown to have an increased risk for leukemia. The degree of risk depends on the distance from the hypocenter. The peak incidence period is 4 to 8 years after exposure to the radiation. Whereas ANLL most often develops in adults who are exposed to radiation, ALL is more likely to develop in children. The therapeutic use of x-rays for thymic enlargement in children has also been linked to subsequent development of ALL in children (Murray, Heckel, & Hempelmann, 1959). Some doubt remains concerning the relative risk of prenatal exposure to radiation. A study conducted by the National Academy of Sciences (1980), however, found that radiation exposure during the prenatal period was associated with a marked risk of development of a variety of pediatric cancers. During the first trimester the risk was five fold; the risk dropped to 1.5 times the normal rate during the second and third trimesters. Leukemia accounted for approximately one half of the subsequent cancers.

Although chemicals such as benzene have been associated with the development of ANLL in adults, no evidence suggests a similar chemical or drug association in childhood leukemia. Leukemia (primarily ANLL) has been reported as a secondary malignancy (development of a second cancer after the first) in children treated for Hodgkin disease and Wilms tumor, although such cases are rare. In most cases, the children received both chemotherapy (alkylating agents or dactinomycin) and radiation therapy for the primary cancer, perhaps accounting for the subsequent development of another cancer.

Leukemic "clusters" representing a greater number of leukemia cases occurring in a particular geographic location have raised speculation about environmental factors of infectious patterns of transmission. Careful followup, however, has failed to document the abnormal clustering. Explanations for this phenomenon are therefore statistical artifact and coincidence.

Current interest focuses on the role viruses may play in the development of leukemia. Viruses clearly have been known to cause leukemia in a number of animals, including cats, fowl, and mice. Although a similar relationship has not been clearly established between viruses and human leukemia, progress is being made. Scientists have recently linked a retrovirus with an unusual form of adult T cell lymphoblastic leukemia-lymphoma (Reitz et al., 1984). The difficulty in understanding the role of viruses in the case of leukemia in human beings is primarily one of technology and the state of knowledge of viral activity.

Evidence suggests that the virus genetically alters the cell it invades. The expression of the defect remains dormant until a second event, such as radiation or some other unknown factor, activates it. The two events together then lead to cancerous transformation. Should this discovery be confirmed, it would demonstrate a link between genetic changes and an environmentally acquired agent. Further work is required to demonstrate a relationship between viruses and the development of childhood leukemias. Although this initial discovery explains only a few cases of leukemia, it will contribute to an understanding of the role of viruses in other forms of leukemia, including the leukemias of childhood.

Gibson and colleagues (1968) have reported findings that also indicate the interaction of multiple factors in the cause of childhood leukemia. They investigated risk factors in children in whom leukemia developed between the ages of one and four years. They found that children exposed to four specific factors had a 4.64 times greater risk for development of leukemia than children who did not experience similar exposures. The four factors are (1) radiation of the mother before conception, (2) prenatal radiation of the child, (3) maternal history of miscarriages, and (4) early viral illness in the child. These, along with other evidence, strongly suggest that childhood leukemia is likely to be the result of a multiple interaction between hereditary or genetic predisposition and environmental influences (Fernbach, 1984).

Clinical Manifestations

Few variations appear in the presenting symptoms of the various cell types of acute leukemia. The onset may be abrupt or insidious, but the most common symptoms reflect the consequence of bone marrow failure resulting in decreased red blood cells, platelets, and changes in white blood cells. Pallor, fatigue, petechiae, purpura, bleeding, and fever are generally present. Approximately 45% of children have a hemoglobin below 7 gm/ml; in contrast to adults, children seem to demonstrate fewer symptoms. If acute blood loss occurs, however, characteristic symptoms of tachycardia, air hunger, restlessness, and thirst may be present. Epistaxis is frequently seen if the child has severe thrombocytopenia. Three-fourths of children with ALL have platelet counts below 100,000/mm^3 at diagnosis, and 28% have a platelet count below 20,000/mm^3. Half of all children newly diagnosed with ANLL have platelet counts below 50,000/mm^3. Disseminated intravascular coagulation occurs more commonly with ANLL, particularly with promyelocytic leukemia. The granules in the leukemic promyelocytes may then indicate thromboplastin activity.

Fever is usually present as a result of two causes: (1) infection associated with the decrease in functional neutrophils and (2) hypermetabolism associated with the ongoing rapid growth and destruction of leukemic cells. In most children with ALL, the total white blood count is less than 10,000/mm^3, and in ANLL most have white cell counts below 50,000/mm^3. In a few children, how-

ever, the peripheral white blood count can go well above 100,000/mm^3. White counts greater than 200,000/mm^3 can cause leukostasis, an intravascular clumping of cells that causes infarction and hemorrhage, usually in the brain and lung.

Renal failure as a result of hyperuremia (high uric acid levels) can be associated with ALL, particularly at diagnosis or during active treatment. Cell breakdown results as a natural process in the presence of a high white blood cell count and/or as a result of cellular breakdown caused by chemotherapy. Uric acid levels rise as an end-product of purine metabolism from cellular destruction. Because the major excretory pathway is through the kidney, urates can precipitate in renal tubules or ureters and can lead to oliguria and acute renal failure. Renal failure is preventable if uric acid levels are monitored and treatment is aimed at optimal hydration, alkalinization of urine to assist with the excretion of soluble urates, and blockage of further uric acid formation by administration of the drug allopurinol.

Extramedullary invasion with leukemic cells can occur in nearly all body tissue. Most children with ALL have some extramedullary involvement at diagnosis. Leukemic invasion of tissue other than bone marrow is thought to represent metastatic infiltration. Hepatosplenomegaly and lymphadenopathy, resulting from extramedullary hematopoiesis, occur in nearly one half of children with ALL, but is less common in children with ANLL.

The central nervous system (CNS) is a common site of infiltration of extramedullary leukemias, although fewer than 10% of children with ALL have CNS involvement at diagnosis. CNS infiltration manifests itself later in the course of the disease. As successful chemotherapy prolongs the time of remission, the incidence of CNS involvement has increased. The most common symptoms of CNS involvement relate to increased intracranial pressure, causing early morning headaches, nausea, vomiting, irritability, and lethargy. Prophylactic CNS treatment is therefore necessary, since systemic treatment with chemotherapy does not cross the blood-brain barrier.

Gonad involvement with testicular and ovarian infiltration has been demonstrated in postmortem examination in 57% and 35% of children, respectively. Clinical detection of gonad involvement is much less frequent (5% to 30% in boys and approximately 17% in girls) (Fernbach, 1984). The incidence of testicular involvement, like CNS involvement, has increased with lengthened duration of remission. Prophylactic treatment has not been successful, however, and is currently not recommended.

Leukemic infiltration into bones and joints is frequent in children. Reports of bone or joint pain actually lead to the diagnosis of leukemia in some children. In most children, bone pain is characterized as migratory, vague, and without areas of swelling or inflammation. If joint pain is the primary symptom and some swelling is associated with the pain, however, misdiagnoses of rheumatoid arthritis or rheumatic fever have occurred.

Other organs reported to be sites of leukemic invasion include the kidneys, heart, lungs, thymus, eyes, skin, and the gastrointestinal tract. Of these, kidneys, lungs, and the gastrointestinal tract are the most frequently reported sites. Skin involvement is more common in ANLL than ALL.

Evaluation and Treatment

Although examination of the blood raises the suspicion of leukemia to the clinician, a bone marrow aspiration is required to establish the diagnosis. The **blast cell** is the hallmark of acute leukemia. The blast cell is a relatively undifferentiated cell characterized by diffusely distributed nuclear chromatin, with one or more nucleoli and basophilic cytoplasm. Normal children have less than 5% blast cells in the bone marrow and none in the peripheral blood. In ALL, the bone marrow is often replaced by 80% to 100% blast cells, with a reduction in normal developing red blood cells and granulocytes. The marrow is considered hypercellular and composed of a homogenous population of cells. Occasionally, however, the marrow appears hypocellular, making the diagnosis difficult to differentiate from aplastic anemia. When this occurs, bone marrow biopsy or biopsy of extramedullary sites is necessary to confirm the diagnosis.

Combination chemotherapy, with or without radiation therapy to localize sites, such as the CNS, is the treatment of choice for acute leukemia. In ALL, identification of various risk groups has led to the development of different intensities of drug protocols. Thus, treatment is tailored specifically for a particular risk group. (Table 25-6 outlines the various prognostic factors for ALL that are considered in determining the degree of risk).

TABLE 25-6 Prognostic factors in ALL

Prognostic factors	Better prognosis	Worse prognosis
*Age		
<2 years or >10 years		X
2-7 years	X	
*Sex		
Male		X
Female	X	
*Initial white blood count		
$>50{,}000/mm^3$		X
$<10{,}000/mm^3$	X	
Race		
Black		X
White	X	
Morphology		
L_2 or L_3		X
L_1	X	
Immunology		
T or B cell ALL		X
Unclassified or common ALL	X	
Leukemic involvement		
Mediastinal mass		X
Central nervous system involvement at diagnosis		X
Splenic enlargement		X

*The three most reliable prognostic factors. Initial prognostic factors become less effective predictors with increasing length of remission. Age and sex are not significant after 15 months of continuous remission and white blood count after 24 months of continuous remission.

Most ALL treatment programs have four distinct phases: (1) induction of remission, (2) preventive therapy for the CNS, (3) consolidation, and (4) maintenance. In remission induction, the goal is the child's remission (i.e., no clinical evidence of disease and a normal bone marrow biopsy). Ninety-five percent of children with ALL achieve initial remission. Prophylatic CNS treatment has included both chemotherapy and radiation in the past, but evidence has increasingly shown that this therapy, while effective in preventing CNS leukemia, adversely affects neurologic and intellectual function. A marked incidence of learning disabilities has been identified in children previously treated to prevent CNS disease. New, less toxic treatment protocols are now being studied to deal with this problem. Once remission is achieved and CNS preventive treatment completed, additional maintenance chemotherapy is required for remission to continue. The optimal duration of maintenance therapy is not well defined, but it usually continues for 2½ to 3 years. During maintenance therapy, intermittent "pulses" of additional drugs may be given to "consolidate" the therapeutic process. Periods of intensified therapy are thought to minimize the development of drug resistance.

ALL is a curable disease. This prognosis is indeed a dramatic reversal of the outlook for a child diagnosed with this disease 30 years ago, when ALL was uniformly fatal, the average survival time being only 2 to 3 months. Today, with prompt and appropriate treatment, more than 60% of children with ALL are in continuous and complete remission 5 years after initial diagnosis. Most of these children are then considered cured (Poplack, 1985).

Lymphomas

Non-Hodgkin lymphoma (NHL) and Hodgkin disease comprise approximately 10% of all childhood cancer. Either group of diseases is rare before the age of 5, and the relative incidence increases throughout childhood. Non-Hodgkin lymphoma is 1.5 times more common than Hodgkin disease in children. Boys are more likely to be diagnosed with a malignant lymphoma than are girls, and high-risk groups have been identified. At particular risk are children with inherited or acquired immunodeficiency syndromes. These children have been found to have increased rates of lymphoreticular cancers that range between 100 and 10,000 times the rate of normal children. The cancers are most commonly non-Hodgkin lymphomas (Link, 1985). Children who are artifically immune suppressed after organ transplantation, especially if cyclosporine is the immunosuppresive agent, are also at increased risk for lymphomas.

Non-Hodgkin Lymphoma

The classification of non-Hodgkin lymphoma has been confusing because of the heterogeneity of this group of diseases. Generally, most classification systems divide non-Hodgkin lymphoma into two categories, nodular or diffuse, on the basis of cellular pattern. Whereas one half of all adults with non-Hodgkin lymphoma have a nodular form of the disease, children rarely demonstrate this pattern. Nodular disease represents a less aggressive form of lymphoma. Almost without exception, childhood non-Hodgkin lymphoma becomes evident as a diffuse disease and can be further subdivided into three groups: (1) histocytic, (2) lymphoblastic, and (3) undifferentiated (Burkitt or non-Burkitt lymphoma).

An area of intensive study concerns the apparent biologic similarities of non-Hodgkin lymphoma and ALL in children. These two diseases are cytologically identical, and the distinction between them, histologically, has been made by the degree of infiltration in the blood and bone marrow. The more bone marrow involvement and less nodal and organ infiltration disease present, the more likely the disease is to be classified as ALL. Childhood non-Hodgkin lymphoma also is much more like ALL in its clinical manifestations and much less like Hodgkin disease or adult non-Hodgkin lymphoma.

Like ALL, immunophenotyping is an important part of the classification of childhood non-Hodgkin lymphoma. Almost 45% of the disease in children originate from T cells; an equal number originate from B cells. The remaining group, representing less than 10% of childhood non-Hodgkin lymphomas is classified as non-T, non-B. This distribution is quite different from that found in ALL, where 80% of children have neither T nor B cell origins (unclassified ALL and common ALL).

Pathogenesis

The origin of non-Hodgkin lymphoma (NHL) in childhood is still elusive. While defective host immunity is implicated in most children in whom non-Hodgkin lymphoma develops, an immune deficit cannot be identified. Viral etiology is suggested, but the role in development of human lymphoma is still unclear. The strongest correlation exists between the Epstein-Barr virus and African Burkitt lymphoma. The relationship between the Epstein-Barr virus infection in Burkitt lymphoma outside Africa is weak, however, even though the tumor is histopathologically and clinically indistinguishable. Chronic immunostimulation has also been suggested as a factor in the development of lymphomas because these diseases are seen more frequently when chronic persistent antigenic stimulation occurs from infection, such as malaria or intestinal parasites. Genetic susceptibility may also play a role in the process of malignant transformation. This hypothesis is based on the observation of chromosomal rearrangement in the malignant cells of non-Hodgkin lymphoma.

Clinical Manifestations

In children, non-Hodgkin lymphoma has been found to arise from any lymphoid tissue. Signs and symptoms are therefore specific for the site involved. Some children have such widespread involvement that no original site can be determined. Because childhood non-Hodgkin lymphoma is a rapidly progressive disease, symptoms are generally only present a few weeks before diagnosis is made. Rapidly enlarging lymphoid tissue and painless lymphadenopathy are very common in about one third of children with abdominal sites of involvement, usually representing a gastrointestinal origin for the disease. Symptoms often include abdominal pain and vomiting, but a palpable mass is not always present. Most children with abdominal symptoms have diffuse, undifferentiated lymphomas (Burkitt or non-Burkitt) of B cell origin. If the tumor recurs, it appears again in the abdomen before distant spread.

The other frequent site of childhood non-Hodgkin lymphoma is the chest region. An anterior mediastinal mass, with or without pleural effusion, is often present. If the mass is large enough, respiratory compromise, tracheal compression, and superior vena cava syndrome may arise, constituting a medical emergency. Children with anterior mediastinal involvement are often male adolescents and usually have diffuse lymphoblastic lymphoma of T cell origin. This form of diffuse lymphoblastic lymphoma often evolves into extensive bone marrow involvement and is considered to be an overt leukemic phase, therefore referred to as leukemic transformation. CNS involvement and testicular infiltration often then occur.

The bone marrow is less common than other primary

sites, whereas CNS involvement is common. A relatively small number (10% to 20%) of children with non-Hodgkin lymphoma have lymphoid tissue involvement of the head and neck (Waldeyer's ring, nasopharyngeal and sinuses). Signs and symptoms include tonsillitis, sinusitis, and a painless nasopharaynx mass. In African Burkitt lymphoma, involvement of facial bones is common, although this occurs infrequently in non-African cases.

Evaluation and Treatment

Diagnosis is made by observing the pathologic changes in biopsy material, usually from excised lymph nodes. Other sites of biopsy include the tonsils, bone marrow, spleen, liver, bowel, or skin. Advances in understanding the disease and progress in treatment strategies have meant that most children with non-Hodgkin lymphoma are cured of the disease. Optimal treatment is still being developed, but combination chemotherapy, with or without radiation therapy for prevention of CNS involvement, is currently being used successfully. Treatment programs are based on the same four phases for ALL: (1) induction of remission, (2) therapy for the CNS, (3) consolidation, and (4) maintenance. Radiation therapy may be combined with chemotherapy in treatment of lymphomatous masses because lymphoma cells are easily destroyed by radiation.

Children with advanced undifferentiated lymphoma of the abdomen have the poorest prognoses. Although more than 90% of these children can achieve remission, most experience subsequent relapses. Even in the presence of advanced lymphoblastic lymphoma, however, 60% to 80% of children can be cured. Children with localized disease in more easily treated sites are very likely to be cured with prompt and appropriate treatment. Approximately one third of non-Hodgkin lymphoma in children falls into this category.

Hodgkin Disease

Although the etiologic agent for Hodgkin disease, a lymphoma, has not been identified in children, an infectious mode of transmission has been implicated. Major interest currently concerns viral activity, particularly in light of the association between the Epstein-Barr virus and African Burkitt lymphoma. Many individuals with Hodgkin disease have high Epstein-Barr virus titers. At this time, however, the evidence is not sufficient to link an Epstein-Barr virus infection to Hodgkin disease.

The interest in a viral cause of Hodgkin disease has been supported by epidemiologic studies (Gutensohn & Cole, 1981; Gutensohn & Shapiro, 1982). Childhood factors that might influence the time of exposure to an infectious agent were studied. A striking similarity between the epidemiology of Hodgkin disease in children and the prevaccine era of poliomyelitis gives support to the theory that Hodgkin disease may be the rare consequence of a common infection. Gutensohn (1982) has suggested that the pathogenesis of Hodgkin disease in children may be different from that of adults.

Genetic susceptibility has also been suggested. Observations show that siblings have a sevenfold increase in risk, particularly siblings of the same sex. In general, Hodgkin disease is more common in males—in childhood, 60% of all cases occur in males.

Hodgkin disease is rare in childhood. The disease is rarely seen in children less than 2 years of age, and few cases are observed before the age of 5. A gradual rise in incidence occurs through the age of 11, with a marked increase through adolescence that continues into the thirties. The annual incidence of Hodgkin disease in the United States is 4:1,000,000 in children less than 15 years of age.

Painless adenopathy in the lower cervical chain, with or without fever, is the most common symptom in children. Extranodal primary sites of Hodgkin disease are rare. Initial symptoms consist of anorexia, malaise, and lassitude. Intermittent fever is present in 30% of children, and weight loss may also accompany these symptoms. Treatment and prognosis for children are the same as for adults (see Chapter 24).

SUMMARY REVIEW

Disorders of Erythrocytes

1 Iron deficiency anemia is the most frequent blood disorder of infancy and childhood; the highest incidence occurs at 6 months and 2 years of age.

2 Hemolytic disease of the newborn (HDN) results from incompatibility between the maternal and the fetal blood, which may involve differences in Rh factors or blood type (ABO). Maternal antibodies enter the fetal circulation and cause hemolysis of fetal erythrocytes. Because the immature liver is unable to conjugate and excrete the excess bilirubin resulting from the hemolysis, icterus neonatorum and/or kernicterus can develop. Kernicterus may also result from other causes that result in increased breakdown of red blood cells or decreased liver output of enzymes.

3 Infections of the newborn, often acquired by the mother and transmitted to the infant, may result in hemolytic anemia.

4 Glucose-6-phosphate dehydrogenase (G-6-PD) deficiency is an inherited enzyme deficiency in erythrocytes that results in a disruption of a common pathway of glycolysis, shortening erythrocyte life span to a pathologic state.

5 Hereditary spherocytosis is the most common of the hereditary hemolytic states in which there is no abnormality of hemoglobin. The basic defect is an undefined abnormality of the proteins or spectrins of the erythro-

cyte membrane in which affected cells are unduly permeable to sodium and acquire a characteristic structure.

6 Sickle cell disease is a genetically determined defect of hemoglobin synthesis, inherited by an autosomal recessive transmission and causing a change in the shape of a red blood cell to decreased oxygen or hydration. It is most common among blacks and those of Mediterranean descent.

7 The thalassemias are a heterogenous group of hereditary hypochromic anemias of varying severity. Basic genetic defects include abnormalities of messenger-RNA processing or deletion of genetic materials, resulting in a decrease in the chains for hemoglobin.

Disorders of Coagulation and Platelets

1 Hemophilia is a condition characterized by impairment of the coagulation of blood or subsequent tendency to bleed. The classic disease is hereditary and limited to males, being transmitted through the female to the second generation. Many similar conditions attributable to the absence of different clotting factors from the blood are now recognized.

2 Von Willebrand disease is a dominantly inherited disease characterized by a vascular abnormality that produces a prolongation of bleeding time and by decreased levels of clotting factor VIII. The platelets in von Willebrand disease have decreased adhesiveness resulting from absence of the plasma factor.

3 The acquired antibody-mediated hemorrhagic diseases include idiopathic thrombocytopenia purpura (ITP), transient neonatal thrombocytopenia, and autoimmune vascular purpura.

4 ITP, the most common of the childhood thrombocytopenic purpuras, is a disorder of platelet consumption in which antiplatelet antibodies bind to the plasma membranes of platelets. This results in platelet sequestration and destruction by mononuclear phagocytes at a rate that exceeds the ability of the bone marrow to produce them.

5 Transient neonatal thrombocytopenia is an antibody-mediated disorder that occurs in either autoimmune or isoimmune form.

6 The autoimmune vascular purpuras (allergic purpuras) are caused by the body's responses to allergens in the blood.

Leukemia and Lymphoma

1 The childhood leukemias include, in order of their rate of incidence, acute lymphoblastic, acute nonlymphoblastic, and the very rare chronic granulocytic leukemia.

2 Although the cause of childhood leukemia is not known, it is probably the result of multiple interactions between hereditary or genetic predisposition and environmental influences.

3 Acute lymphoblastic leukemia is a potentially curable disease with more than 60% of cases cured.

4 The lymphomas of childhood are non-Hodgkin lymphoma and Hodgkin disease.

5 The origin of non-Hodgkin lymphoma is unknown.

Factors that have been implicated include defective host immunity, a viral agent, chronic immunostimulation, and genetic predisposition.

6 Non-Hodgkin lymphoma has a favorable prognosis, with a 60% to 80% rate of cure.

7 Hodgkin disease is thought to be caused by a yet unidentified etiologic agent.

8 Hodgkin disease is a readily curable disease with survival statistics similar to those of adults.

KEY TERMS

Activated partial thromboplastic time (PTT), 845

Alpha-thalassemia major, 841

Alpha-thalassemia minor, 841

Alpha trait, 841

Aplastic crisis, 840

Autoimmune vascular purpura (allergic purpura), 846

Beta-thalassemia major (Cooley anemia), 841

Beta-thalassemia minor, 841

Blast cell, 850

Embryonic hemoglobin, 826

Fetal hemoglobin (Hb F), 826

Glucose-6-phosphate dehydrogenase (G-6-PD) deficiency, 830

Hemoglobin H disease, 841

Hemoglobin S (Hb S), 836

Hemolytic disease in the newborn (HDN) (erythroblastosis fetalis), 829

Hemophilia A (classic hemophilia), 842

Hemophilia B (Christmas disease), 842

Hemophilia C (factor XI deficiency), 843

Hereditary spherocytosis, 835

Hydrops fetalis, 832

Hyperbilirubinemia, 832

Hyperhemolytic crisis, 840

Icterus gravis neonatorum, 834

Icterus neonatorum (neonatal jaundice), 833

Idiopathic thrombocytopenic purpura (ITP) (immune, or primary thrombocytopenic purpura), 845

Isoimmune thrombocytopenic purpura (IITP), 846

Kernicterus, 833

Prothrombin consumption time, 845

Prothrombin time, 845

Sequestration crisis, 840

Sickle cell anemia, 836

Sickle cell disease, 830

Sickle cell–Hb C disease, 836

Sickle cell–thalassemia, 836

Sickle cell trait, 836

Thalassemia, 830

Thrombin time, 845

Thromboplastin generation, 845

Transient neonatal thrombocytopenia, 846

Vasoocclusive crisis (thrombotic crisis), 840

von Willebrand disease, 844

REFERENCES

Abramson, H. F., Bertles, J. F., & Wethers, D. L. (Eds.). (1973). *Sickle cell disease: Diagnosis, management, education, and research.* St. Louis: C. V. Mosby.

Albin, A. R., Kushner, J. H., Murphy, A., & Zippin, C. (1961). Platelet enumeration in the neonatal period. *Pediatrics, 28,* 822.

American Cancer Society. (1988). *Cancer facts & figures 1988.* New York: American Cancer Society.

Behrman, R. E., & Vaughn, V. C. (1983). *Nelson textbook of pediatrics* (12th ed.). Philadelphia: W. B. Saunders.

Bellingham, A. J., & Prankerd, S. F. (1975). Hereditary spherocytosis. *Clinical Haematology, 4,* 139-142.

Bennett, J., Catovsky, D., Daniel, M., Flandrin, G., Galton, D. A. G., Gralnick, H. R., Sultan, C., & The French-American-British (FAB) Cooperative Group. (1981). French-American-British (FAB) cooperative group: The morphological classification of acute lymphoblastic leukaemia-Concordance among observers and clinical correlations. *British Journal of Haematology, 47,* 553-561.

Berenson, A. S. (Ed.). (1980). *Control of communicable diseases in man* (13th ed.). Washington, DC: The American Public Health Association.

Bevers, E. M. et al. (1985). Development of procoagulant binding sites on the platelet surface. *Advances in Experimental Medicine & Biology, 192,* 359-371.

Capel, P. et al. (1986). Factor VIII inhibitor in mild hemophilia. *British Journal of Haematology, 62*(4), 786-787.

Caramihai, E., Karayaclin, G., Aballi, A. J., & Lanzkowsky, P. (1975). Leukocyte count differences in healthy white and black children. *Journal of Pediatrics, 86,* 252.

Castle, V. et al. (1986). Frequency and mechanism of neonatal thrombocytopenia. *Journal of Pediatrics, 108,* 749-755.

Cunningham, A. S. (1975). Eosinophil counts—Age and sex differences. *Journal of Pediatrics, 87,* 426.

Ekert, H. (Ed.). (1982). *Clinical pediatric haematology and oncology.* Boston: Blackwell Scientific Publications.

Ellis, V. et al. (1985). Mechanism of inhibition of platelet coagulant activity. *Advances in Experimental Medicine & Biology, 192,* 373-387.

Embury, S. H. (1986). The clinical pathophysiology of sickle cell disease. *Annual Review of Medicine, 37,* 361-376.

Fernbach, D. (1984). Natural history of acute leukemia. In W. Sutow, D. Fernbach, & T. Vietti (Eds.), *Clinical pediatric oncology* (3rd ed.). St. Louis: C. V. Mosby.

Gibson, R. W., Bross, I., Graham, S., Lilienfield, A. M., Schu-man, L. M., Levin, M. L., & Dowd, J. E. (1968). Leukemia in children exposed to multiple risk factors. *New England Journal of Medicine, 279,* 906.

Gilchrist, G., & Evans, R. (1985). Contemporary issues in pediatric Hodgkin's disease. *Pediatric Clinics of North America, 32,* 721-734.

Greaves, M., Janossy, G., Peto, J., & Humphrey, K. (1981). Immunological defined subclasses of acute lymphoblastic leukemia in children: Their relationship to presentation features and prognosis. *British Journal of Haematology, 48,* 179-197.

Greer, I. A. et al. (1986). Endothelial stimulation by DDAVP in von Willebrand's disease and haemophilia. *Haemostasis, 16*(1), 15-19.

Grier, H., & Weinstein, H. (1985). Acute nonlymphocytic leukemia. *Pediatric Clinics of North America, 32,* 653-668.

Gutensohn, N. (1982). Social class and age at diagnosis of Hodgkin's disease: New epidemiologic evidence for the "two-disease hypothesis." *Cancer Treatment Report, 66,* 689-695.

Gutensohn, N., & Cole, P. (1981). Childhood social environment and Hodgkin's disease. *New England Journal of Medicine, 304,* 135-140.

Gutensohn, N., & Shapiro, D. (1982). Social class risk factors among children with Hodgkin's disease. *Internal Journal of Cancer, 30,* 433-435.

Karpatkin, S. (1981). Autoimmune thrombocytopenic purpura. *Blood, 56,* 329-333.

Kelley, V. S. (1983). *Practice of Pediatrics* (vol. 5). New York: Harper & Row.

Lanzkowsky, P. (1980). *Pediatric hematology-Oncology.* New York: McGraw-Hill.

Lanzkowsky, P., & Shende, A. (1983). Leukemias. In P. Lanzkowsky (Ed.), *Pediatric oncology.* New York: McGraw-Hill.

Lefrere, J. J. et al. (1986). Six cases of hereditary spherocytosis revealed by human parovirus infection. *British Journal of Haemotology, 62*(2), 653-658.

Li, F., & Bader, J. (1981). Epidemiology of cancer in childhood. In D. Nathan & F. Oski (Eds.), *Hematology in infancy and childhood* (vol. 21). Philadelphia: W. B. Saunders.

Lightsey, A. L., & Koenig, H. M. (1979). Platelet associated immunoglobulin G in childhood idiopathic thrombocytopenic purpura. *Journal of Pediatrics, 94,* 20-22.

Link, M. (1985). Non-Hodgkin's lymphoma in children. *Pediatric Clinics of North America, 32,* 699-720.

Magrath, I. (1982). Malignant lymphomas. In A. Levine (Ed.), *Cancer in the young.* New York: Masson Publishing.

Manroe, B. L., Weinberg, A. G., Rosenfeld, C. R., & Browne, R. (1979). The neonatal blood count in health and disease. Reference values for neutrophilic cells. *Journal of Pediatrics, 95,* 89-98.

Mauer, A. M. (1969). *Pediatric hematology.* New York: McGraw-Hill.

Miale, J. B. *Laboratory medicine: hematoloy* (6th ed.). St. Louis: C. V. Mosby.

Miller, C. H. (1986). Concurrence of von Willebrand's disease and hemophilia A: Implications for carrier detection and prevalence. *American Journal of Medical Genetics, 24*(1), 83-94.

Miller, D. R., Pearson, H. A., Baehner, R. L. & McMillan, C.

W. (Eds.). (1990). *Blood disorders of infancy and childhood* (6th ed.) St. Louis: C. V. Mosby.

Miller, R. (1967). Persons with exceptionally high risk of leukemia. *Cancer Research, 27,* 2420.

Miller, R. W. (1963). Down's syndrome (mongolism), other congenital malformations, and cancers among the siblings of leukemic children. *New England Journal of Medicine, 268*(8), 393-401.

Murray, R., Heckel, P., & Hempelmann, L. (1959). Leukemia in children exposed to ionizing radiation. *New England Journal of Medicine, 261,* 585-589.

Nathan, D. G., & Oski, F. A. (1981). *Hematology of infancy and childhood.* Philadelphia: W. B. Saunders.

National Academy of Sciences. (1980). *Biological effects of atomic radiation.* Washington, DC: National Research Council.

Oski, F. A., & Naiman, J. L. (1982). *Hematologic problems in the newborn* (3rd ed.). Philadelphia: W. B. Saunders.

Pendergrass, T. (1985). Epidemiology of ALL. *Seminars in Oncology, 12*(2), 80-91.

Pollit, E., & Leibel, R. L. (1976). Iron deficiency and behavior. *Journal of Pediatrics, 88,* 372-376.

Poplack, D. (1985). Acute lymphoblastic leukemia in childhood. *Pediatric Clinics of North America, 32,* 669-697.

Rao, A. K. et al. (1986). Congenital disorders of platelet function. *Seminars in Hematology, 23*(2), 102-118.

Raven, P. H., & Johnson, G. B. (1989). *Biology* (2nd ed.). St. Louis: Times Mirror/Mosby.

Reitz, M., Jr., Robert-Guroff, M., Kalyanaraman, V., Sarngadharan, M. G., Sarin, P., Popovic, M., & Gallo, R. C. (1984). A retrovirus associated with human adult T-cell leukemia-lymphoma. In I. Magrath, G. O'Conor, & B. Ramot (Eds.), *Pathogenesis of leukemia and lymphomas: Environmental influences.* New York: Raven Press.

Robinson, L. A., Brown, A. L., & Underwood, T. (1978, November-December). Iron therapy. Helps and hazards. *Pediatric Nursing, 4*(6), 9-14.

Rote, N. S. (1982). Pathophysiology of Rh isoimmunization. *Clinical Obstetrics and Gynecology, 25,* 243-254.

Rudolph, A. M. (Ed.). (1982). *Pediatrics* (17th ed.). Norwalk, CT: Appleton-Century-Crofts.

Schwartz, E. (1980). *Hemoglobinopathies in children.* Littletown, MA: PSG Publishing.

Simons, S. M., Main, C. A., & Yarsh, H. M. (1975). Idiopatyhic thrombocytopenic purpura in children. *Journal of Pediatrics, 293,* 531-535.

Steuber, P. (1984). Chronic myelogenous leukemia and other myeloproliferative disorders. In W. Sutow, D. Fernbach, & T. Vietti (Eds.), *Clinical pediatric oncology* (3rd ed.). St. Louis: C. V. Mosby.

Valentine, W. N. (1977). The molecular lesion of hereditary spherocytosis: A continuing enigma. *Blood, 49,* 241-245.

Vander, A. J., Sherman, J. H., & Luciano, D. S. (1980). *Human physiology: The mechanism of body fucntion.* New York: McGraw-Hill.

Volkl, K. P. (1986). The estimation of the platelet survival time from a biological point of view. *Thrombosis Research, 42*(1), 109-112.

Weinstein, H., & Link, M. (1979). Non-Hodgkin's lymphoma in childhood. *Clinical Hematology, 8,* 699-716.

Weiss, H. J. (1975). Platelet physiology and abnormalities of platelet function. *Journal of Medicine, 293,* 531-535.

Whaley, L. F. & Wong, D. L. (1983). *Nursing care of infants and children* (2nd ed.). St. Louis: C. V. Mosby.

Williams, W. J., Beutler, E., Elsleu, A. J., & Lichtman, M. A. (1983). *Hematology* (3rd ed.). New York: McGraw-Hill.

Wintrobe, M. M., Lee, G. R., Boggs, D. R., Bithell, T. C., Foerster, J., Athens, J. W., & Lukens, J. N. (1981). *Clinical hematology* (8th ed.). Philadelphia: Lea & Febiger.

Ziegler, J. L. (1981). Burkitt's lymphoma. *New England Journal of Medicine, 305,* 733-745.

UNIT
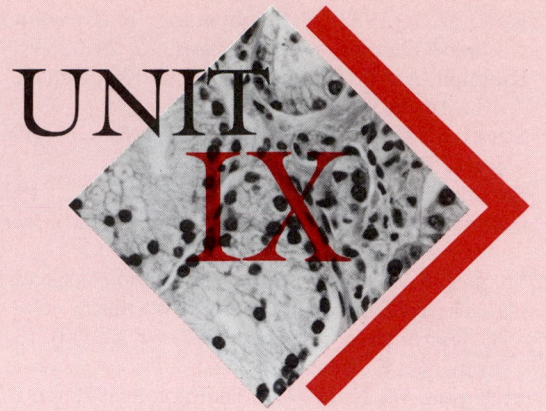
IX

The Cardiovascular and Lymphatic System

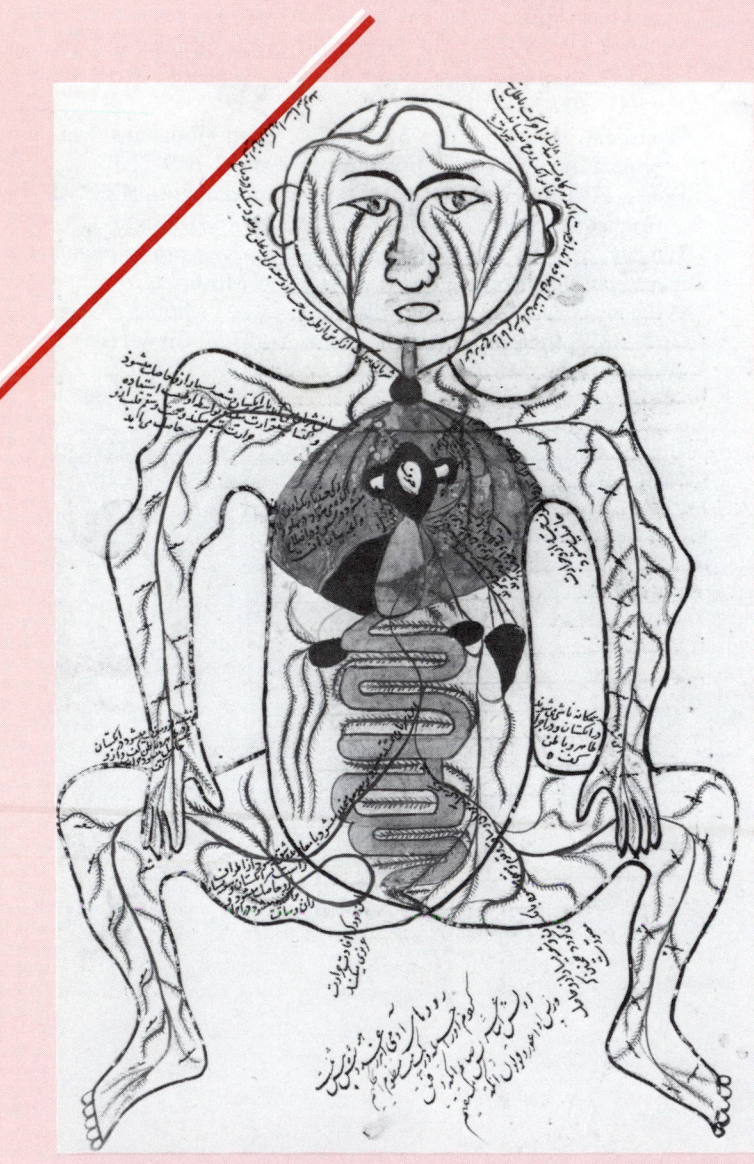

Human figure showing arterial system. (From Mansur ibn Muhammad ibn Ahmad ibn Yusuf ibn Faqih Ilyas: *Tashrih al-badan*. Courtesy National Library of Medicine.)

THE role of the heart was questioned by ancient societies. For example, the Egyptians attributed breathing to the heart, whereas the ancient Chinese connected the action of the heart to the pulse. The *Nei Ching,* a collection of Chinese medical writings, reported that all the blood was under the control of the heart and that the heart was the seat of happiness. The Greeks thought of the heart as the region in the body in which thinking originated.

The works of the renowned Greek physician, Galen (ca AD 129 to 200), survived for nearly 1500 years as the "unimpeachable authority on medicine." Galen thought blood was produced in the liver, where it received "natural spirit" and from which it was pulled to the periphery of the body by some attractive force. When he first looked at the heart in the second century AD, Galen noted that the sides of the heart did not contract simultaneously, as he thought a pump should. Galen concluded that blood was displaced from the right to the left chambers of the heart through tiny pores in the membrane that separated the chambers. He believed that the arterial and venous circulatory systems were joined by these pores.

Galen's theories finally collapsed when William Harvey (1578-1657), an Englishman, published his studies on circulation. Harvey's writings were based on dissection of cadavers and physiologic experiments performed on animals. He showed that the heart pumped blood continuously and that the veins returned the blood to the heart. Observing that both ventricles of the heart contracted and expanded together, Harvey concluded that there was no pressure difference between these chambers to drive blood through the thick membrane that separated them. He also noted that when the heart was removed from an animal, it continued to contract and expand like a muscle. This demonstrated that the heart was an independent pump and not just an organ that sucked in blood. Harvey's achievement became the foundation of modern cardiovascular physiology.

Thomas Wharton (1614-1673) described the distinguishing characteristics of the lymphatic glands. He denied the old and persistent idea that the brain was a gland that secreted mucus, yet he continued to believe that tears came from the brain. He recognized that there were ductless glands (now called endocrine glands), whose secretions entered the blood, and ductile glands, whose secretions were discharged into cavities (exocrine glands). In 1661, Niels Steensen made the distinction between the exocrine glands and the lymph nodes. He also disproved the idea that tears originated in the brain.

In 1733, more than 100 years after Harvey's work was published, Stephan Hales (1677-1761), a clergyman, made the first blood pressure measurements. He inserted a hollow tube into the neck artery of a horse and was surprised to see the blood rise 9 feet in a glass column. In the middle of the nineteenth century, Harry Goldblatt, R. Tigerstedt, P. G. Bergman, and others first showed that blood pressure could be affected by a substance thought to be from the kidney. A little later, intensive studies by several researchers, including G. W. Pickering, M. Prinzmetal, I. Page, and D. vanSlyke, revealed the existence of a complex enzymatic hormonal mechanism of blood pressure regulation involving the adrenal glands, kidneys, and nervous system.

In the early twentieth century a Dutch physicist, Willem Einthoven, invented the string galvanometer, an instrument to measure electric circuits. This instrument was the forerunner of the electrocardiogram. By the end of World War I, the string galvanometer and its applications had been developed by Englishman Thomas Lewis, establishing the science of electrocardiography.

In 1929, Weiner Forssmann, a young intern in a German hospital, worked out a technique for emergency injection of drugs directly into the heart. While looking into a mirror and standing behind a fluoroscopic screen, he threaded a thin catheter into his own arm vein, through the venous channels, and into his heart. Dangerous as the procedure was, it had been performed 15 years earlier by three other researchers without the aid of x-rays. Forssmann, along with A. Cournand and D. W. Richards, Jr., received the Nobel Prize in 1956 for developing the procedure of intracardiac catheterization.

Until midcentury, surgical repair of congenital heart defects and malarrangements of the large blood vessels were performed entirely by feel, since the heart could not be stopped during surgery. In 1939, Robert Gross reported the first successful cure of a congenital heart anomaly. After 19 years of experimentation, John Gibbon, his wife, and others developed a heart-lung machine that could take over the pumping function of the heart during surgery. This advancement enabled Gibbon to repair a heart defect under direct visualization in 1953.

In 1967, in South Africa, Christiaan Barnard performed the first heart transplantation in a human being. But by 1977 the procedure was practically abandoned because there were virtually no long-term survivors of heart transplantation. The problem was, and still is, rejection of the transplanted heart by the recipient's immune system.

In 1958, T. Akusu and Wilhelm Kolff, and later Michael DeBakey, experimented with mechanical devices to support or replace diseased hearts for short periods in animals. In 1969, Denton Cooley and his colleagues used an artificial heart to keep a patient alive for 2½ days to await the transplantation of a living heart. In 1982, a total artificial heart developed at the University of Utah was implanted in Dr. Barney Clark. Dr. Clark was the first person to live with an artificial heart that was implanted as a permanent replacement of his own heart. He died of circulatory collapse because of multisystem failure in March of 1983.

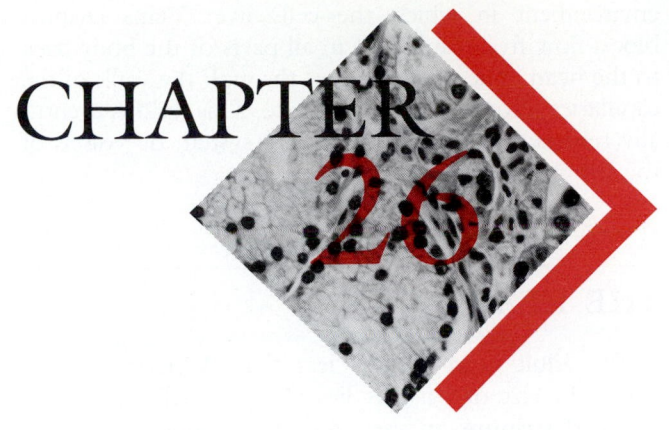

Structure and Function of the Cardiovascular and Lymphatic Systems

Kathryn L. McCance
Stephanie J. Richardson

The circulatory system, 860
The heart, 860
  Structures that direct circulation through the heart, 860
    The heart wall, 860
    Chambers of the heart, 862
    Fibrous skeleton of the heart, 863
    Valves of the heart, 864
    The great vessels, 864
    Blood flow during the cardiac cycle, 864
    Normal intracardiac pressures, 865
  Structures that support cardiac metabolism: the coronary vessels, 866
    Coronary arteries, 866
    Collateral arteries, 868
    Coronary capillaries, 868
    Coronary veins and lymphatic vessels, 868
  Structures that control heart action, 868
    The conduction system, 869
      Cardiac excitation, 870
      Propagation of cardiac action potentials, 871
        The normal electrocardiogram, 872
        Automaticity, 873
        Rhythmicity, 873
    Cardiac innervation, 873
      Sympathetic and parasympathetic nerves, 873
      Adrenergic receptor function, 873
    Myocardial cells, 874
      Actin, myosin, and the troponin-tropomyosin complex, 875
      Myocardial metabolism, 876
    Myocardial contraction and relaxation, 876
      The crossbridge theory, 877
      Calcium and excitation-contraction coupling, 878
      Myocardial relaxation, 878

Factors affecting cardiac performance, 879
  Frank-Starling law of the heart, 879
  Laplace's law, 880
  Preload, 881
  Afterload, 881
  Heart rate, 881
    Cardiovascular control centers in the brain, 881
    Neural reflexes, 882
    Hormones and biochemicals, 882
  Myocardial contractility, 882
  Factors determining cardiac output, 883
  The suction-pump theory of heart action, 883
The systemic circulation, 886
  Structure of blood vessels, 886
    Arterial vessels, 886
    Veins, 889
  Factors affecting blood flow, 890
    Pressure and resistance, 890
    Neural control of total peripheral resistance, 892
      Baroreceptors, 893
      Arterial chemoreceptors, 894
      Velocity, 894
      Laminar versus turbulent flow, 894
    Vascular compliance, 895
  Regulation of blood pressure, 895
    Arterial pressure, 895
      Effects of cardiac output, 896
      Effects of total peripheral resistance, 896
      Effect of hyperemia, 896
      Effects of hormones, 896
      The systemic renin-angiotensin system, 896
    Venous pressure, 897
  Regulation of the coronary circulation, 897

Autoregulation, 898
Autonomic regulation, 898
The lymphatic system, 898
Tests of cardiovascular function, 901
    Noninvasive assessment of function, 901
        Sensorium of the individual, 901
        Mucous membrane color, 901
        Manually palpated pulse, 901
        Auscultation of heart sounds, 901
        Cardiography, 902
        Pulse tracing, 904
        Doppler studies, 904
        Stress testing, 905
        Chest x-ray examinations, 905
    Invasive assessment of cardiac function, 905
        X-ray films with barium, 905
        Nuclear imaging with radiolabeled pharmaceuticals, 905
        Arterioventricular bundle electrocardiography, 905
        Cardiac catheterization, 906
        Coronary angiography, 907
    Combined indicators of cardiac function, 907
Aging and the cardiovascular system, 907
    Resting cardiac performance, 907
    Exercise cardiac performance, 908

THE CIRCULATORY SYSTEM

The function of the circulatory system is quite simple: to deliver oxygen, nutrients, and other substances to all of the body's cells and to remove the waste products of cellular metabolism. Delivery and removal are achieved by a wonderfully complex array of tubing—the blood vessels—connected to a pump—the heart. The heart pumps blood continuously through the blood vessels with cooperation from other systems, particularly the nervous and endocrine systems, which are intrinsic regulators of the heart and blood vessels. Nutrients and oxygen are supplied by the digestive and respiratory systems; gaseous wastes of cellular metabolism are blown off by the lungs; and other wastes are removed by the kidneys.

The heart pumps blood through two separate circulatory systems, one to the lungs and one to all other parts of the body. Structures on the right side of the heart, or **right heart,** pump blood through the lungs. (This system, termed the **pulmonary circulation,** is described in Chapter 29.) The left side of the heart, or **left heart,** sends blood throughout the **systemic circulation,** which supplies all of the body except the lungs (Fig. 26-1). These two systems are serially connected; thus the output of one becomes the input of the other.

Arteries carry blood flow from the heart to all parts of the body, where they branch into even smaller vessels until they become a fine meshwork of capillaries. Capillaries allow the closest contact and exchange between the blood and the interstitial space, or interstitium—the environment in which the cells live. Veins channel blood flow from capillaries in all parts of the body back to the heart. The plasma passes through the walls of the capillaries into the interstitial space. This fluid is eventually returned to the cardiovascular system by vessels of the lymphatic system.

THE HEART

The adult heart weighs less than 1 pound and is about the size of a fist. It lies obliquely (diagonally) in the **mediastinum,** an area above the diaphragm and between the lungs.

Heart structures can be described with respect to three general categories of function: (1) structural support of heart tissues and circulation of pulmonary and systemic blood through the heart; (2) maintenance of heart cells; and (3) stimulation and control of heart action. Included in the first category are the heart wall and fibrous skeleton, which enclose and support the heart and divide it into four heart chambers: the valves that direct flow through the chambers, and the great vessels that conduct blood to and from the heart. The second category comprises vessels of the coronary circulation—the arteries and veins that serve the metabolic needs of all the *heart's* cells, particularly its muscle cells. Also included in the second category are the lymphatic vessels of the heart. The third category of structures, those responsible for heart action, consists of the nerves and specialized muscle cells that direct the rhythmic contraction and relaxation of the heart muscles, which propel blood throughout the pulmonary and systemic circulatory systems.

Structures that Direct Circulation Through the Heart
The Heart Wall

The heart wall has three layers—the pericardium, myocardium, and endocardium. The **pericardium** is a double-walled membranous sac that encloses the heart (Fig. 26-2). The pericardium has several functions. It (1) prevents displacement of the heart during gravitational acceleration or deceleration, (2) is a physical barrier that protects the heart against infection and inflammation from the lungs and pleural space, and (3) contains pain receptors and mechanoreceptors that can elicit reflex changes in blood pressure and heart rate. The outer layer of the pericardium, the **parietal pericardium,** is composed of a surface layer of mesothelium over a thin layer of connective tissue. The **visceral pericardium,** or epicardium, is the inner layer of the pericardium. At one point, the visceral pericardium folds back and becomes continuous with parietal pericardium,

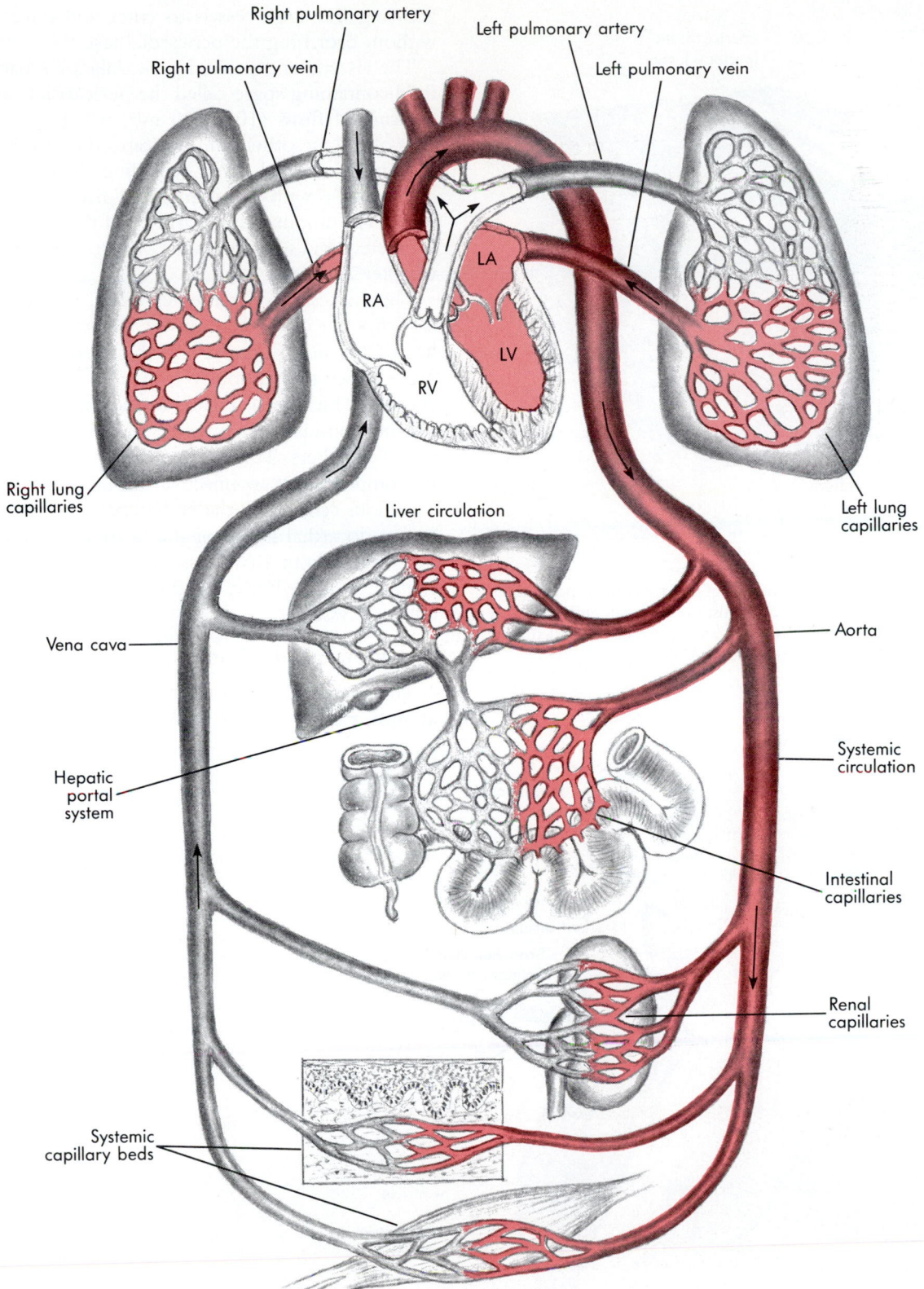

FIG. 26-1. Diagram showing serially connected pulmonary and systemic circulatory systems. Right heart chambers propel unoxygenated blood through pulmonary circulation, while left heart propels oxygenated blood through systemic circulation.

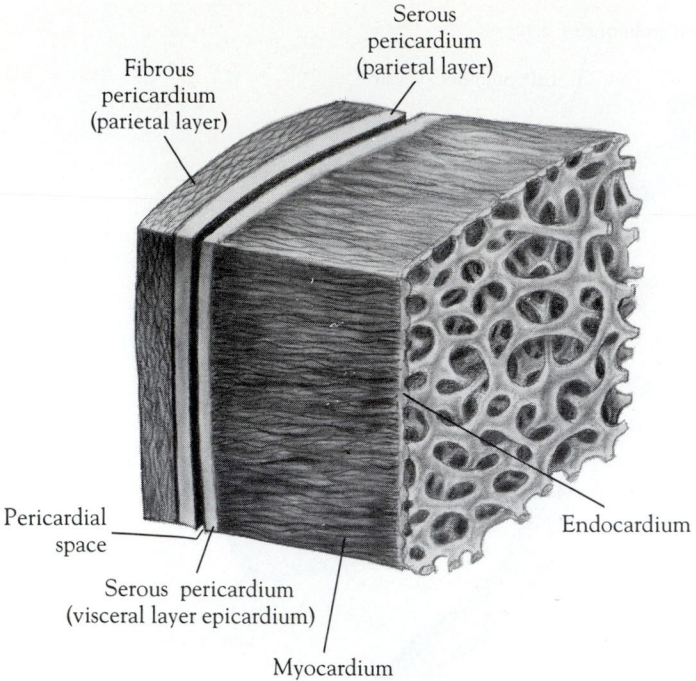

FIG. 26-2. Section through wall of heart, showing pericardium (outer sac), myocardium (cardiac muscle), and endocardium (inner lining). Heart wall encloses chambers (atria and ventricle) of left heart and right heart. (From Thompson et al., 1989.)

allowing the large vessels to enter and leave the heart without breaching the pericardial layers.

The visceral and parietal pericardia are separated by a fluid-containing space called the **pericardial cavity.** The **pericardial fluid** (10 to 30 ml), which is secreted by cells of the mesothelium, lubricates the membranes that line the pericardial cavity, enabling them to slide over one another with a minimum of friction as the heart beats. The amount and character of the pericardial fluid is altered by inflammation of the pericardium (see Chapter 27).

The thickest layer of the heart wall, the **myocardium,** is composed of cardiac muscle and is anchored to the heart's fibrous skeleton. The thickness of the myocardium varies tremendously from one heart chamber to another. Thickness is related to the amount of resistance the muscle must overcome to pump blood from the different chambers. The internal lining of the myocardium is composed of connective tissue and a layer of squamous cells called the **endocardium** (see Fig. 26-2). The endocardial lining of the heart is continuous with the endothelium that lines all the arteries, veins, and capillaries of the body, creating a continuous, closed circulatory system.

Chambers of the Heart

The heart has four chambers, the **right atrium, left atrium, right ventricle,** and **left ventricle.** (Blood flow

FIG. 26-3. Structures that direct blood flow through the heart. *Arrows* indicate path of blood flow through chambers, valves, and major vessels. (From Thibodeau, 1987.)

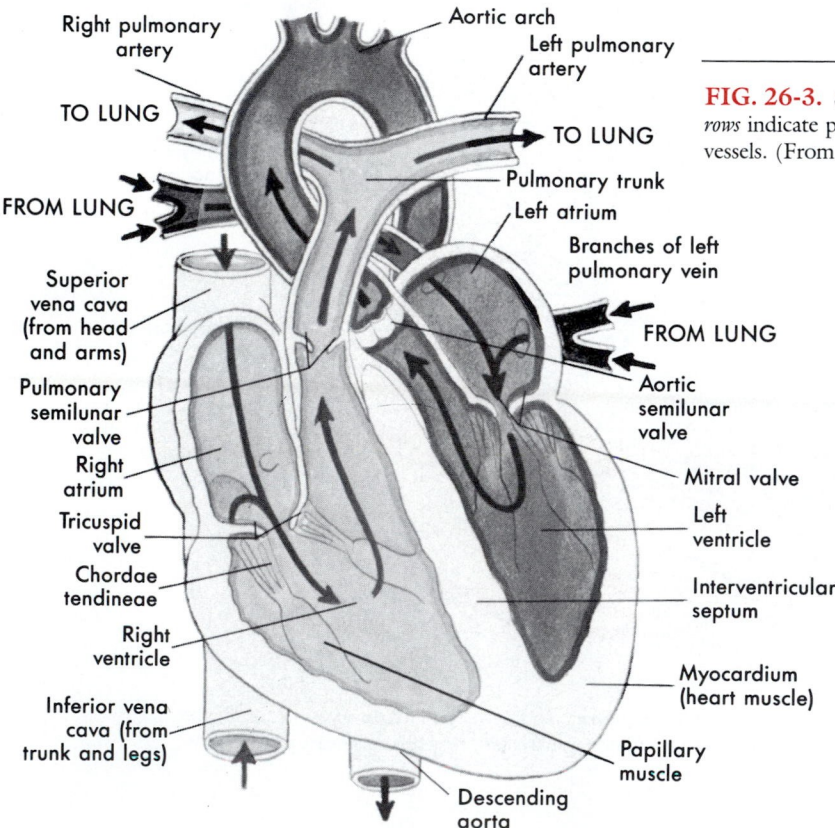

through these chambers is illustrated in Fig. 26-3.) The atria are smaller than the ventricles and have thinner walls. The wall of the right atrium is about 2 mm thick, and that of the left atrium is about 3 to 5 mm thick. The ventricles have a thicker myocardial layer and comprise much of the bulk of the heart. The wall of the right ventricle is about 3 to 5 mm thick and that of the left ventricle, the most muscular chamber, is about 13 to 15 mm (Underhill et al., 1989).

The myocardial thickness of each cardiac chamber depends on the amount of pressure or resistance it must overcome to eject blood. The two atria have the thinnest walls because they are low-pressure chambers that serve as storage units and conduits for blood that is emptied into the ventricles. Normally, there is little resistance to flow from the atria to the ventricles. The ventricles, on the other hand, must propel blood all the way through the pulmonary or systemic circulation. The ventricular myocardium must also be strong enough to pump against pressures in the pulmonary or systemic vessels. Pressure is greatest in the systemic circulation, which is driven by the left ventricle. This explains why the left ventricle's myocardium is several times thicker than that of the right ventricle, which sends blood through the low-pressure pulmonary circulation.

The shapes of the right and left ventricles also differ according to their function. The right ventricle is shaped like a crescent, or triangle, enabling its bellows-like action, which efficiently ejects large volumes of blood through a very small valve into the low-pressure pulmonary system (Rushmer, 1976). The left ventricle is larger and bullet shaped. Its shape and thick myocardium help it to eject blood through a relatively large valve opening into the high-pressure systemic circulation.

The ventricles are structurally more complex than the atria. Each ventricle contains muscle fibers that divide it roughly into an **inflow tract,** which receives blood from the atrium, and an **outflow tract,** which sends blood to the circulation (see Fig. 26-3).

Normally, blood does not flow between the chambers of the right side of the heart and the chambers of the left side of the heart. The adult right and left sides of heart are separated by an intact septal membrane. The atria are separated by the interatrial septum, and the ventricles by the interventricular septum. The interventricular septum is an extension of the fibrous skeleton of the heart. Indentations of the endocardium form valves that separate the atria from the ventricles and the ventricles from the aorta and pulmonary arteries.

Fibrous Skeleton of the Heart

Four rings of dense fibrous connective tissue provide a firm anchorage for the attachments of the atrial and ventricular musculature, as well as the valvular tissue. The fibrous rings are adjacent and form a central, fi-

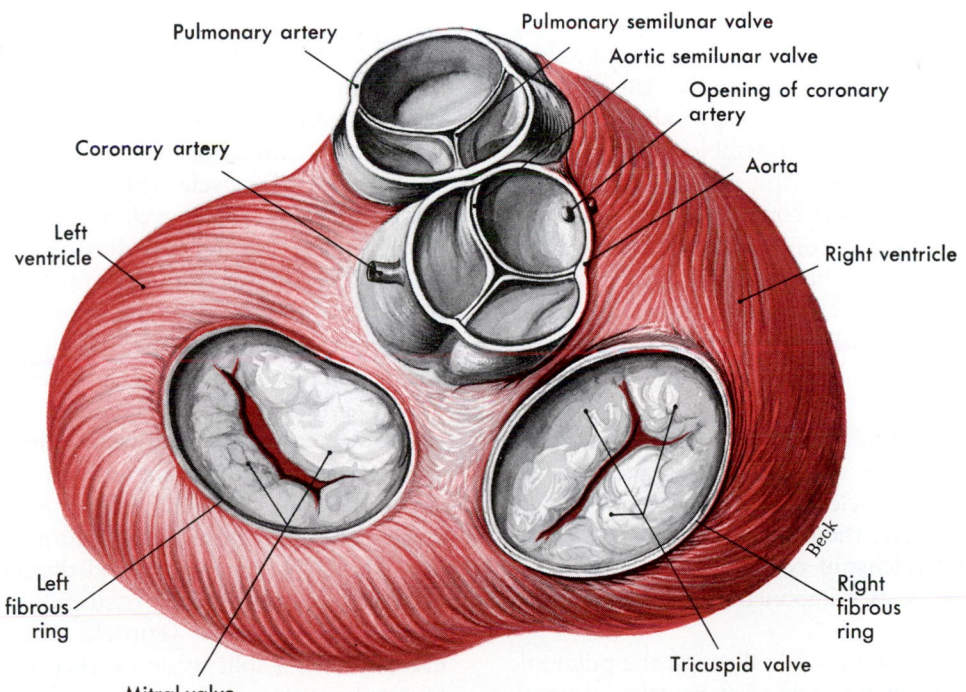

FIG. 26-4. Fibrous skeleton and valves of heart. Fibrous rings serve as attachments for all of the heart's valves. Two atrioventricular valves, mitral and tricuspid, separate atria from ventricles, while pulmonic and aortic semilunar valves separate ventricles from their receiving vessels, pulmonary artery, and aorta, respectively. (From Thibodeau, 1987.)

brous supporting structure collectively termed the an-nuli fibrosi cordis. The fibrous rings serve as attachments for the four heart valves (Fig. 26-4).

Valves of the Heart

One-way blood flow through the heart is ensured by the four heart valves. During ventricular relaxation the two **atrioventricular valves** open and blood flows from the higher pressure atria to the relaxed ventricles. With increasing ventricular pressure these valves close and prevent backflow into the atria as the ventricles contract. The **semilunar valves** of the heart open when intraventricular pressure exceeds aortic and pulmonary pressures and blood flows out of the ventricles and into the pulmonary and systemic circulations. After ventricular contraction and ejection, intraventricular pressure falls and the **pulmonic** and **aortic semilunar valves** close, preventing backflow into the right and left ventricle (see Figs. 26-3 and 26-4).

The openings of the heart valves are guarded by flaps of tissue called leaflets or cusps. The cusps of the atrioventricular valves are attached to the papillary muscles by the **chordae tendineae** (see Fig. 26-3). The **papillary muscles** are extensions of the myocardium that pull the cusps together and downward at the onset of ventricular contraction, thus preventing their backward expulsion into the atria. (See p. 865 for a description of pressure changes and valvular function.)

The right atrioventricular valve is called the **tricuspid valve** because it has three cusps. The tricuspid opening (orifice) has the largest diameter of all the heart valves. The three cusps are unequal in size. The left atrioventricular valve is a bicuspid (two-cusp) valve called the **mitral valve.** The mitral valve resembles a cone-shaped funnel that extends into the cusps, which are connected by a fibrous tissue called the commissure. The anterior cusp of the mitral valve is continuous with supporting tissues of the aortic semilunar valve cusps and the left coronary valve cusps. (The coronary circulation is described on p. 866). Thus, damage to this continuous tissue can alter function of both the aortic and mitral valves.

The tricuspid and mitral valves function as a unit because the atrium, fibrous rings, valvular tissue, chordae tendineae, papillary muscles, and ventricular walls are connected. Collectively, these six structures are known as the **mitral and tricuspid complex.** Damage to any one of the complex's six components can alter function significantly.

Blood leaves the right ventricle through the pulmonic semilunar valve, and it leaves the left ventricle through the aortic semilunar valve (see Figs. 26-3 and 26-4). Both the pulmonic and aortic semilunar valves have three cup-shaped cusps that arise from the fibrous skeleton. The pulmonic cusps are slightly thinner than the aortic cusps. The lower edges of each cusp are suspended from the root of the pulmonary artery or aorta, with the upper valve edges freely projecting into the vessel lumen. When the ventricles contract, the cusps behave like one-way swinging doors. The force of the blood propels the cusps outward against the vessel wall. When the ventricles relax, blood fills the cusps and causes their free edges to meet in the middle of the vessel, closing the valve and preventing any backflow.

The Great Vessels

Blood moves in and out of the heart through several large vessels (see Fig. 26-3). The right heart receives venous blood from the systemic circulation through the **superior** and **inferior venae cavae.** These vessels enter the right atrium. Blood leaves the right ventricle and enters the pulmonary circulation through the **pulmonary artery.** The pulmonary artery divides into **right** and **left pulmonary arteries** to transport unoxygenated blood from the right heart to the right and left lungs. The pulmonary arteries branch further into the pulmonary capillary bed, where oxygen and carbon dioxide exchange occurs.

The four **pulmonary veins,** two from the right lung and two from the left lung, carry oxygenated blood from the lungs to the left side of the heart. The oxygenated blood moves through the left atrium and ventricle and out into the **aorta,** which delivers it to systemic vessels that supply the body.

Blood Flow during the Cardiac Cycle

The pumping action of the heart consists of contraction and relaxation of the myocardial layer of the heart wall. Each contraction, and the relaxation that follows it, is one **cardiac cycle.** (Blood flow through the heart during a single cardiac cycle is illustrated in Fig. 26-5.) During relaxation, termed **diastole,** blood fills the ventricles. The contraction that follows, termed **systole,** propels the blood out of the ventricles and into the circulation. Contraction of the left ventricle is slightly earlier than contraction of the right ventricle.

During diastole, blood from the veins of the systemic circulation enters the thin-walled right atrium from the superior vena cava and the inferior vena cava (see Figs. 26-3 and 26-5). Venous blood from the coronary circulation enters the right atrium through the coronary sinus. The right atrium fills and distends, pushing open the right atrioventricular (tricuspid) valve. This permits blood to fill the right ventricle. The same sequence of events occurs a split second earlier in the left heart. The four pulmonary veins, two from the right lung and two from the left lung, carry blood from the pulmonary circulation to the left atrium. As the left atrium fills, it pushes the cusps of the mitral valve open, and blood flows into the left ventricle. Filling of the right and left

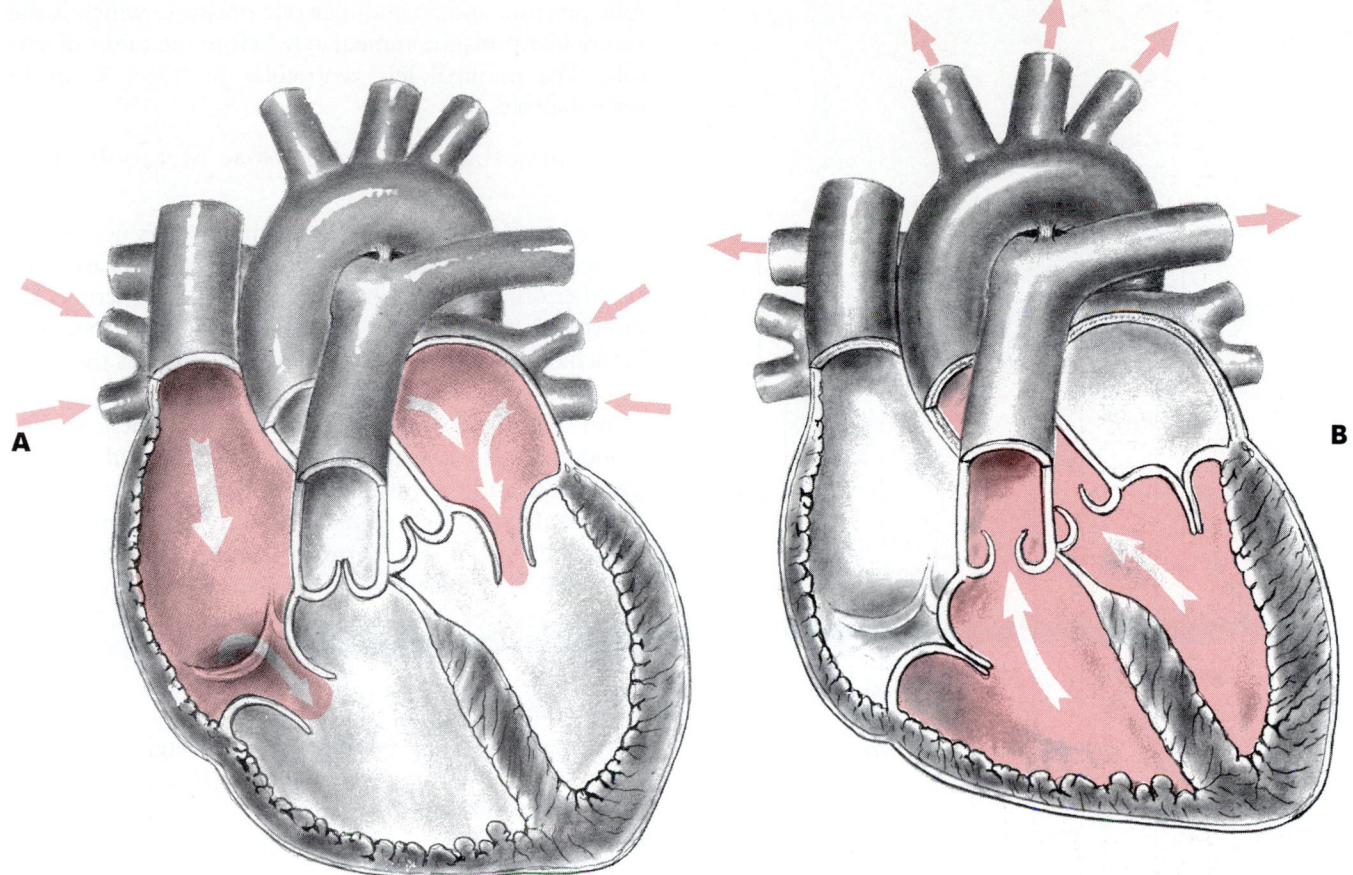

FIG. 26-5. Blood flow through the heart during a single cardiac cycle. **A,** During diastole, blood flows into atria, atrioventricular valves are pushed open, and blood begins to fill ventricles. Atrial systole (center) squeezes any blood remaining in atria out into ventricles. **B,** During ventricular systole *(right),* ventricles contract, pushing blood out through semilunar valves into pulmonary artery (right ventricle) and aorta (left ventricle).

sides of the heart occur during one period of diastole.

Four phases of the cardiac cycle can be identified on initiation of ventricular myocardial contraction (Fig. 26-6).

Phase 1: Systole begins with "isovolumic contraction," the first detectable rise in left ventricular pressure. Contraction pushes the atrioventricular valves shut. Their cusps bulge backward but are prevented from opening back into the atria by their anchors, the chordae tendineae (see Fig. 26-3).

Phase 2: When left ventricular pressure reaches that of the aorta, the aortic valve opens and ventricular ejection occurs. Intraventricular pressure and ventricular volume decrease rapidly.

Phase 3: With left ventricular relaxation and ventricular pressure decreases, the aortic valve closes and "isovolumic relaxation" occurs.

Phase 4: When sufficient decreases exist in left ventricular pressure, the mitral valve opens and ventricular filling from the atrium occurs.

The ventricle fills rapidly in early diastole and again in late diastole when the atrium contracts. As blood is pushed through the inflow and outflow tracts of the ventricles, it flows around the **crista supraventricularis**—the muscle that separates the inflow from the outflow tracts—and is mixed by passing through the strands of the **trabeculae carneae.** Expulsion of blood from the ventricles marks the end of one cardiac cycle.

Normal Intracardiac Pressures

Normal intracardiac pressures are shown in Table 26-1 and Fig. 26-7. Atrial pressure curves are composed of the **a wave,** which is generated by atrial contraction, and the **v wave,** which is an early diastolic peak caused by filling of the atrium from the peripheral veins. The **x descent** follows the a wave and the **y descent** follows the v wave. A small deflection, the **c wave,** occurs after the a wave in early systole and may represent bulging of the tricuspid valve into the left atrium during early systole. Ventricular pressures are illustrated by a peak sys-

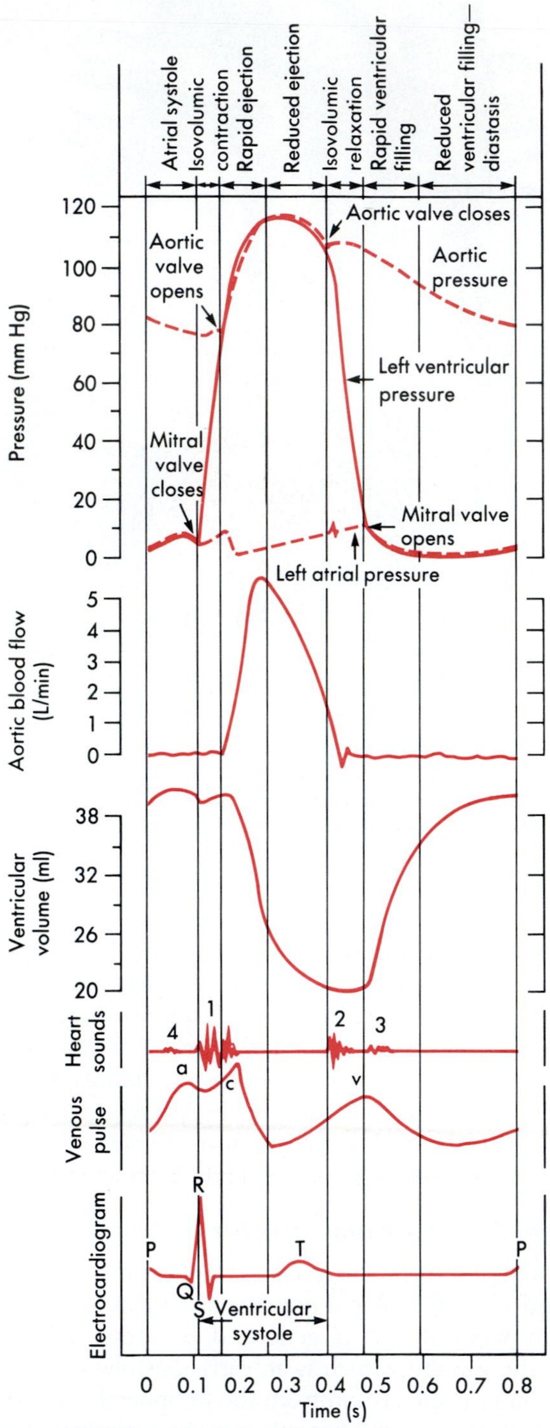

FIG. 26-6. Schematic at top shows four major phases of cardiac cycle. Left atrial, aortic, and left ventricular pressure pulses correlated in time with aortic flow, ventricular volume, heart sounds, venous pulse, and electrocardiogram for a complete cardiac cycle in the dog. (From Berne & Levy, 1988a.)

tolic pressure and an end-diastolic pressure, which is the ventricular pressure immediately before the onset of systole. The minimal left ventricular pressure occurs in early diastole.

Structures that Support Cardiac Metabolism: The Coronary Vessels

The blood within the heart chambers does not supply oxygen and other nutrients to the cells of the heart. Like all other organs, including the lungs, heart structures are nourished by vessels of the systemic circulation. The branch of the systemic circulation that supplies the heart is termed the **coronary circulation.** The coronary circulation consists of **coronary arteries,** which receive blood through openings in the aorta called the **coronary ostia,** and the **cardiac veins,** which empty into the right atrium through another ostium, the opening of a large vein called the **coronary sinus** (see Fig. 26-3). (Regulation of the coronary circulation, which is similar to regulation of flow through systemic and pulmonary vessels, is described elsewhere.)

Coronary Arteries

The major coronary arteries are the **right coronary artery** and the **left coronary artery** (Fig. 26-8). These arteries traverse the epicardium and branch several times. The pattern of branching through the visceral pericardium differs from heart to heart. The branches enter the myocardium and endocardium and branch further to become arterioles, then capillaries.

The left coronary artery arises from a single ostium (opening) behind the left cusp of the aortic semilunar valve. This artery ranges from a few millimeters to a few centimeters in length. It passes between the left atrial appendage and the pulmonary artery and generally divides into two branches, the left anterior descending artery and the circumflex artery. Other branches of the left main coronary artery are distributed diagonally across the free wall of the left ventricle.

TABLE 26-1 Normal intracardiac pressures

	Mean (mm Hg)	Range (mm Hg)
Right atrium	4	0-8
Right ventricle		
Systolic	24	15-28
End-diastolic	4	0-8
Left atrium	7	4-12
Left ventricle		
Systolic	130	90-140
End-diastolic	7	4-12

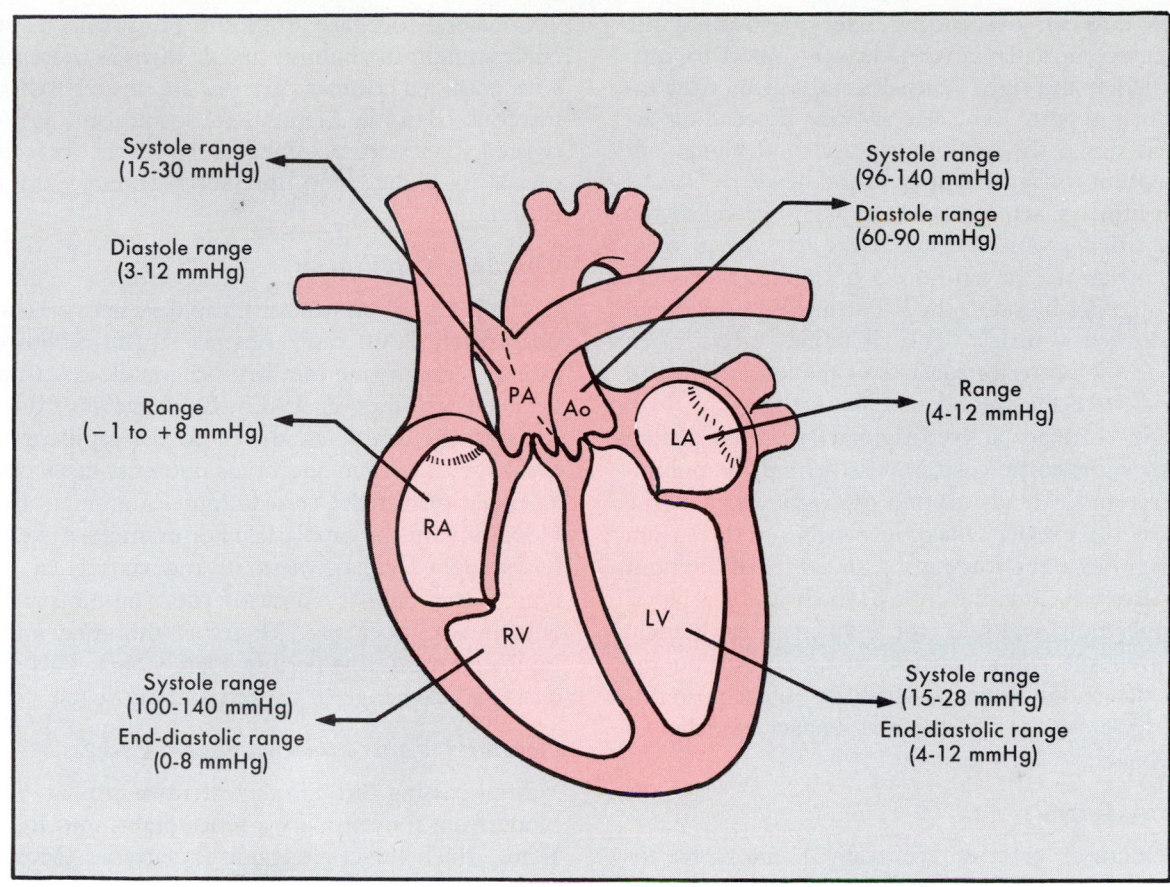

FIG. 26-7. Normal intracardiac pressures. *RA,* Right atrium; *LA,* left atrium; *RV,* right ventricle; *LV,* left ventricle; *PA,* pulmonary artery; *AO,* aorta.

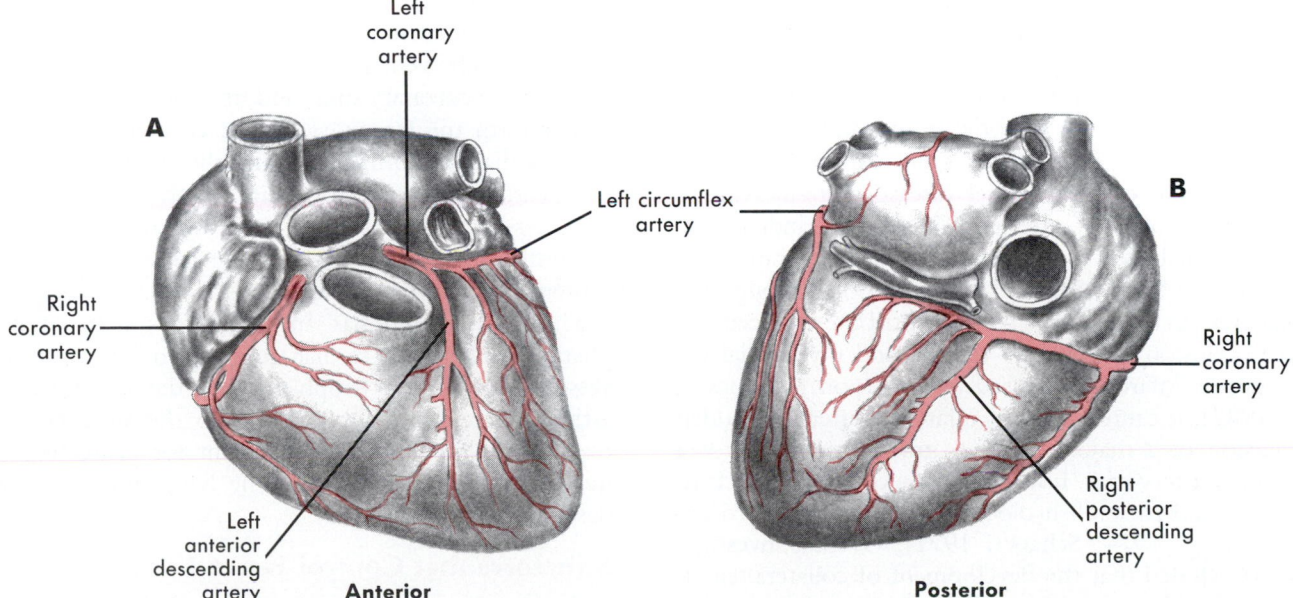

FIG. 26-8. A, Blood vessels of anterior surface of heart. **B,** Blood vessels of posterior surface of heart. (From Thelan, Davie, and Urden, 1990.)

The **left anterior descending artery,** also called the anterior interventricular artery, delivers blood to portions of the left and right ventricles and much of the interventricular septum. The left anterior descending artery travels down the anterior surface of the interventricular septum toward the apex of the heart.

The **circumflex artery** travels in a groove called the **coronary sulcus,** which separates the left atrium from the left ventricle, to the left border of the heart (see Fig. 26-8). It supplies blood to the left atrium and the lateral wall of the left ventricle. The circumflex artery often branches to the posterior surfaces of the left atrium and left ventricle (see Fig. 26-8).

The right coronary artery originates from an ostium behind the right aortic cusp, travels behind the pulmonary artery, and extends around the right heart to the heart's posterior surface, where it branches to the atrium and the ventricle. The three major branches of the right coronary artery include the conus, which supplies blood to the upper right ventricle; the right marginal branch, which travels the right ventricle to the apex; and the posterior descending branch, which lies in the posterior interventricular sulcus and supplies smaller branches to both ventricles.

Collateral Arteries

The **collateral arteries** are really connections, or anastomoses, between two branches of the same coronary artery or connections of branches of the right coronary artery with branches of the left. They are particularly common within the interventricular and interatrial septa, at the apex of the heart, over the anterior surface of the right ventricle, and around the sinus node (Thomas et al., 1982). The epicardium contains more collateral vessels than the endocardium.

The functional importance of the collateral circulation is debated: does it protect the heart or does it represent more severe ischemia? In some studies individuals with good collateral arteries had a significantly higher prevalence of two- or three-vessel disease than individuals with poor collateral arteries. These same individuals, however, had a lower prevalence of acute myocardial infarction and heart failure (Hansen, 1989). Although the collateral circulation apparently contributes to recovery after occlusion of coronary arteries and myocardial tissue death (infarction) caused by occlusion (Thomas et al., 1982), it cannot prevent infarction after the sudden occlusion of a major vessel. A gradual occlusion of a coronary artery may, however, cause collateral vessels to develop and reestablish blood flow to the deprived tissue (Gregg, 1974; Schaper, 1971). Overall, investigators concluded that the development of collateral circulation provides some protection against the myocardial effects of coronary occlusion (Hansen, 1989; Kirk & Jennings, 1985).

Collateral coronary arteries in normal hearts are generally straight or slightly curved, whereas those in hearts with occluded coronary arteries are severely twisted and tortuous (Baroldi, Manteo, & Scomozoni, 1956). The twisted shapes are possibly caused by the wear and tear caused by higher blood pressures generated by the occlusion.

Coronary Capillaries

The heart has an extensive capillary network, with approximately 3300 capillaries per square millimeter (ca/mm^2) or about one capillary per muscle cell (muscle fiber) (Underhill et al., 1982). Blood travels from the arteries to the arterioles, then into the capillaries, where exchange of oxygen and other nutrients takes place.

Alterations of the cardiac muscles dramatically affect blood flow in the capillaries. For example, in ventricular hypertrophy (enlargement of the ventricular myocardium), the capillary network does not expand along with muscle fiber size. Therefore the same number of capillaries must now perfuse a larger area. This results in decreased exchange of oxygen and nutrients.

Coronary Veins and Lymphatic Vessels

After passing through the extensive capillary network, blood from the coronary arteries drains into the cardiac veins, which travel alongside the arteries. Most of the venous drainage of the heart occurs through veins in the visceral pericardium.

The cardiac veins feed into the **great cardiac vein** and then into the enlarged vessel cavity called the coronary sinus. The coronary sinus is located on the posterior surface of the heart, between the atria and ventricles, in the coronary sulcus. Venous coronary blood empties into the right atrium from the coronary sinus. Blood from the left ventricular walls is generally drained through the coronary sinus and its tributaries, which together form the largest system of coronary veins. The great cardiac vein primarily drains the anterior surface of the heart. The **posterior vein of the left ventricle** branches from the coronary sinus and accompanies the circumflex artery. This vein is the largest vein on the posterior surface of the heart.

The myocardium has an extensive system of lymphatic vessels. With cardiac contraction, the lymphatic vessels drain fluid to lymph nodes in the anterior mediastinum that eventually empty into the superior vena cava. The lymphatics are important for protecting the myocardium against injury. (The lymphatic vessels are described on p. 898.)

Structures that Control Heart Action

Continuous, rhythmic repetition of the cardiac cycle (systole and diastole) depends on the continuous, rhythmic transmission of electrical impulses, termed **cardiac**

action potentials, through the myocardium. (Action potentials are described in Chapters 1 and 3.) As an electrical impulse passes from cell to cell (fiber to fiber) in the myocardium, it stimulates the fibers to shorten. Shortening causes muscular contraction, or systole. After the action potential passes, the fibers relax and return to their resting length, causing diastole. The muscle fibers of the myocardium are uniquely joined so that action potentials pass from cell to cell very rapidly and efficiently. Therefore an action potential generated in one part of the myocardium passes almost simultaneously through all its contiguous fibers, causing rapid contraction.

The myocardium differs from other muscle tissues in that it contains its own **conduction system**—specialized cells that enable it to generate and transmit action potentials without stimulation from the nervous system. These cells are concentrated at certain sites in the myocardium called **nodes.** Although the heart is innervated by the autonomic nervous system (both sympathetic and parasympathetic fibers), neural impulses are not needed to maintain the cardiac cycle. Rather the cardiac cycle is stimulated by the nodes of specialized cells and "fine tuned" as needed by the autonomic fibers. The sympathetic and parasympathetic nerves have different effects on the speed of the cardiac cycle (**heart rate,** or beats per minute) and on the diameter of the coronary vessels (see Fig. 26-12).

Other factors that influence heart action are substances delivered to the myocardium in coronary blood. Nutrients and oxygen are needed for cellular survival and normal function, whereas hormones and biochemicals affect the strength and duration of myocardial contraction and the degree and duration of myocardial relaxation. Normal or appropriate function depends on the availability of these substances, which is why coronary artery disease can seriously disrupt heart function.

The Conduction System

Normally electrical impulses arise in the **sinoatrial node** (SA node, sinus node), which is often called the pacemaker of the heart. The SA node is located at the junction of the right atrium and superior vena cava, just above the tricuspid valve (Fig. 26-9). The SA node lies only a millimeter or less beneath the visceral pericardium, making it vulnerable to injury and disease, especially pericardial inflammation (James, 1962). The SA node is nourished by the sinus node artery, which passes through the center of the node. There are numerous autonomic nerve endings within the node. The SA node's

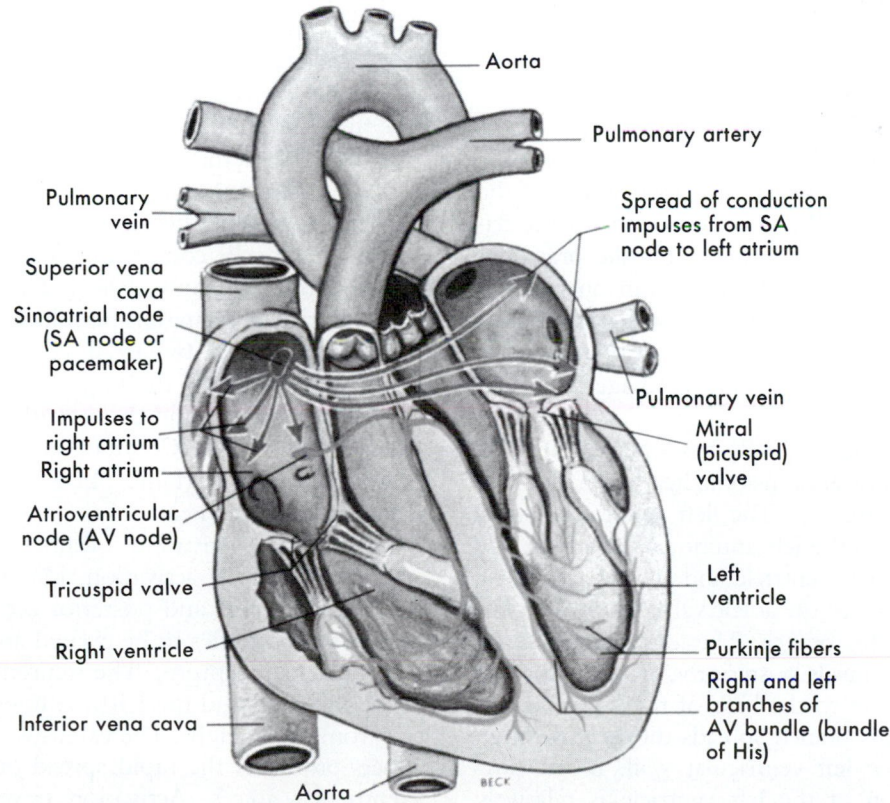

FIG. 26-9. Excitation and conduction system of heart. Arrows indicate stimulatory impulse from sinoatrial node as it travels through myocardium of both atria and stimulates conduction through ventricle. (From Thibodeau, 1987.)

P cells, so called because they are pale and primitive appearing, are assumed to be the site of impulse formation (DeHaan, 1965; Harary, 1962).

In the resting adult the SA node generates about 75 action potentials per minute. Each action potential travels rapidly from cell to cell and through special pathways in the atrial myocardium, causing both atria to contract. Atrial contraction begins systole. Ventricular contraction is delayed because the fibrous skeleton of the heart interrupts cell-to-cell transmission of the electrical impulses. Transmission of the action potential from the atrial to the ventricular myocardium occurs through fibers of the conduction system. The action potential travels first to the **atrioventricular node** (AV node), then to the **bundle of His** (atrioventricular bundle, common bundle), and finally through the **bundle branches** of the interventricular septum to Purkinje fibers in the heart wall (see Fig. 26-9).

The AV node is well situated for mediating conduction between the atria and ventricles. It is located in the right atrial wall above the tricuspid valve and anterior to the ostium of the coronary sinus. There is much variation from one heart to another in the size and length of the AV node fibers. Generally the AV node is thicker and shorter and has fewer P cells than the SA node. Behind the AV node are numerous autonomic ganglia, presumably vagal (parasympathetic) (James, 1968). (The nervous systems are described in Chapter 12.) These ganglia may serve as receptors for the vagus nerve and cause slowing of the cardiac cycle.

Conducting fibers from the AV node converge to form the bundle of His. The bundle of His, which is triangular in shape, lies within the posterior border of the interventricular septum. The two lower ends of the triangle give rise to the right and left bundle branches. The **right bundle branch** (RBB) is thin and travels without much branching to the right ventricular apex. Because of its thinness and relative lack of branches, the RBB is susceptible to interruption by damage to the endocardium.

The **left bundle branch** (LBB) arises perpendicularly from the bundle of His and, in some hearts, divides into two branches, or fascicles. The left anterior bundle branch (LABB) passes the left anterior papillary muscle and the base of the left ventricle and crosses the aortic outflow tract. Damage to the aortic valve or the left ventricle can interrupt this branch. The left posterior bundle branch (LPBB) travels posteriorly, crossing the left ventricular inflow tract to the base of the left posterior papillary muscle. This branch spreads diffusely through the posterior inferior left ventricular wall. Blood flow through this portion of the left ventricle is relatively nonturbulent, so the LPBB is somewhat protected from injury caused by wear and tear.

Because the LBB divides and crosses the ventricles to the anterior and posterior papillary muscles, action potentials reach the left ventricle before they reach the right ventricle. Therefore the left ventricle contracts slightly ahead of the right.

The **Purkinje fibers** are the terminal branches of the right and left bundle branches. They extend from the ventricular apices to the fibrous rings and penetrate the heart wall to the outer myocardium. P cells are also found among the Purkinje fibers.

Because impulses from the SA node arrive at the AV node extremely quickly, investigators have proposed that these nodes are connected by internodal pathways. In 1916, Bachmann first described a pathway between the right atrium and the left atrium. Although controversy exists as to whether this pathway, termed **Bachmann's bundle,** is made up of conducting fibers, the bundle is well developed and has been extensively demonstrated in autopsy dissections. Purkinje fibers also have been found in Bachmann's bundle (James et al., 1985). Two other pathways, the middle internodal pathway and the posterior internodal pathway, apparently connect the SA node and the AV node (Berne & Levy, 1988; Katz, 1977; Soderstrom, 1948; Thorel, 1909; Wenckebach, 1908).

Cardiac Excitation

From the SA node, the impulse that begins systole spreads throughout the right atrium at a conduction velocity of about 1 m/sec. Bachmann's bundle conducts the impulse from the SA node to the left atrium, and the three internodal pathways conduct the impulse from the SA node to the AV node.

The action potential is delayed in the region of the AV node, possibly because of electrophysiologic differences in the cells comprising the AV region (Berne & Levy, 1988; Halpenny, 1982). The delay between atrial and ventricular excitation permits an additional boost to ventricular filling by atrial contraction (atrial kick). From the AV node, the impulse travels from the atrioventricular bundle and through the bundle branches to the Purkinje fibers. Conduction velocities in the atrioventricular and Purkinje fibers are 2 to 4 m/sec, the most rapid in the heart.

Ventricular activation occurs sequentially in three phases: (1) septal activation, (2) apical activation, and (3) basal (upper) and posterior activation. The first areas of the ventricles to be excited are portions of the interventricular septum. The septum is activated from both the RBB and the LBB, although the impulse travels from left to right. The extensive network of Purkinje fibers promotes the rapid spread of the impulse to the ventricular apices. Activation traverses the heart wall from the inside outward (from the endocardium to the epicardium; see Fig. 26-2). The basal and posterior portions of the ventricles are the last to be activated. Deactivation, which begins diastole, occurs in the opposite direction, spreading from the outside inward (epicardium to endocardium). All areas of the ventricle recover at about the same time.

Propagation of Cardiac Action Potentials

Electrical activation of the muscle cells, termed **depolarization,** is caused by the movement of electrically charged solutes (ions) across cardiac cell membranes. Deactivation, called **repolarization,** occurs the same way. (Movement of ions across cell membranes is described in Chapter 1; electrical activation of muscle cells is described in Chapter 38.)

Movement of ions into and out of the cell creates an electrical (voltage) difference across the cell membrane called the membrane potential. The resting membrane potential of myocardial cells is -80 to -90 millivolts (mV), whereas that of SA and AV node cells is -60 mV. During depolarization, the inside of the cell becomes less negatively charged. In cardiac cells the difference between resting membrane potential (in millivolts) and the decreased negative charge caused by depolarizaton is termed the **cardiac action potential.** Table 26-2 summarizes the intracellular and extracellular ionic concentrations of cardiac muscle. The various phases of the cardiac action potential are related to changes in the permeability of the cell membrane, primarily to sodium and potassium. Threshold is the point at which the cell membrane's selective permeability to sodium and potassium is temporarily disrupted, leading to depolarization.

Normal myocardial cell depolarization and repolarization occur in four phases (Fig. 26-10). Phase 0 consists of depolarization. This phase lasts from 1 to 2 milliseconds (msec) and represents rapid sodium entry into the cell. Phase 1 is early repolarization, in which calcium slowly enters the cell. Phase 2, also called the **plateau,** is a continuation of repolarization, with slow entry of calcium and sodium into the cell. Potassium is moved out of the cell during phase 3, with a return to resting membrane potential in phase 4. This time between action potentials corresponds to diastole. If the resting mem-

brane potential becomes more negative, for example with a decrease in extracellular potassium concentration (hypokalemia), it is termed **hyperpolarization.**

The phases of depolarization and repolarization occur somewhat differently in the SA and AV node cells, a difference that enables these cells to generate cardiac action potentials independently. Although the cells of the Purkinje fibers, atria, and ventricles begin with a negative resting membrane potential and proceed to a rapid upstroke, or depolarization (phase 0), a rapid early repolarization (phase 1), a plateau (phase 2), and a rapid later repolarization (phase 3), cells of the SA and AV nodes begin with a less negative resting membrane potential, proceed to a slow upstroke (phase 0) and usually lack a plateau (phase 2) (see Fig. 26-10, *B*). The fast inward current, mediated by sodium ions flowing through "fast channels" in the cell membrane, causes the rapid upstroke of the action potential in Purkinje fibers, atria, and ventricles (see Fig. 26-10, *A*). The slow inward current, mediated by calcium and sodium ions flowing through "slow channels" of the cell membrane, is re-

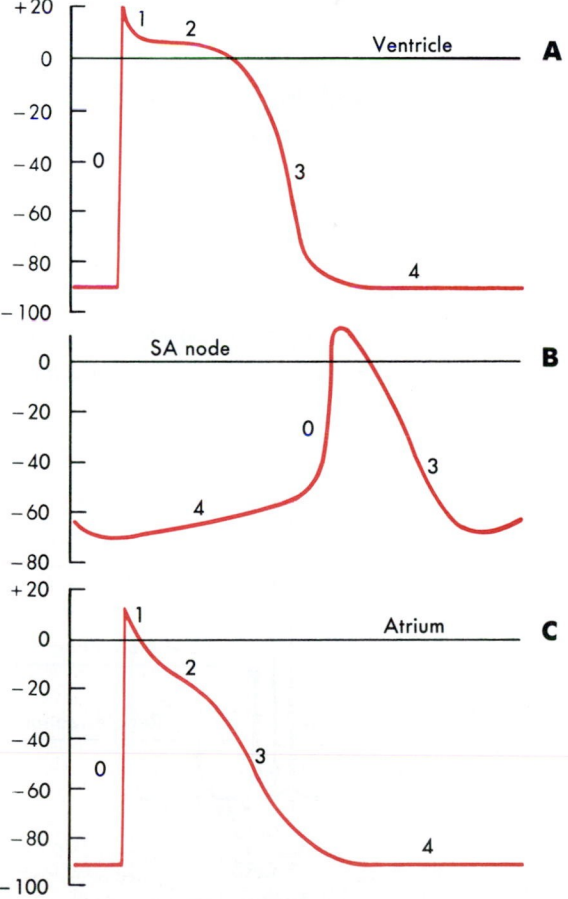

FIG. 26-10. Cardiac action potentials. **A,** SA node; **B,** atrium; and **C,** sweep velocity in **B** is one half that in **A** or **C.** (From Berne & Levy, 1988a.)

TABLE 26-2 Intracellular and extracellular ion concentrations in the myocardium		

Ion	Intracellular concentration	Extracellular concentration
Sodium (Na$^+$)	15 mM	145 mM
Potassium (K$^+$)	150 mM	4 mM
Chloride (Cl$^-$)	5 mM	120 mM
Calcium (Ca^{++})	10^{-7} M	2 mM

NOTE: mM, millimoles per kilogram; M, moles.

sponsible for the action potential of the SA node and the AV node. Hence, drugs that block calcium have profound effects on the slow inward current and can alter heart rate (Wu, 1984). Slow channel-blocking drugs, such as verapamil, are used to treat a variety of cardiovascular disorders.

A **refractory period,** during which no new cardiac action potential can be initiated by a stimulus, follows depolarization. This period, called the effective or absolute refractory period, corresponds to the time needed for the reopening of channels that permit sodium and calcium influx (phase 0 through half of phase 3). A relative refractory period occurs near the end of repolarization, following the effective refractory period. During

this time the membrane can be depolarized again but only by a greater-than-normal stimulus. Abnormal refractory periods as a result of disease can cause abnormal heart rhythms or dysrhythmias (see Chapter 27).

The Normal Electrocardiogram The genesis of the normal electrocardiogram is from electrical activity recorded by skin electrodes, that is, the sum of all the cardiac action potentials (Fig. 26-11). The **P wave** represents atrial depolarization. The **PR interval** is a measure of time from the onset of atrial activation to the onset of ventricular activation; it normally ranges from 0.12 to 0.20 seconds. The PR interval represents the time necessary to travel from the sinus node through the atrium, AV node, and His-Purkinje system to activate ventricular

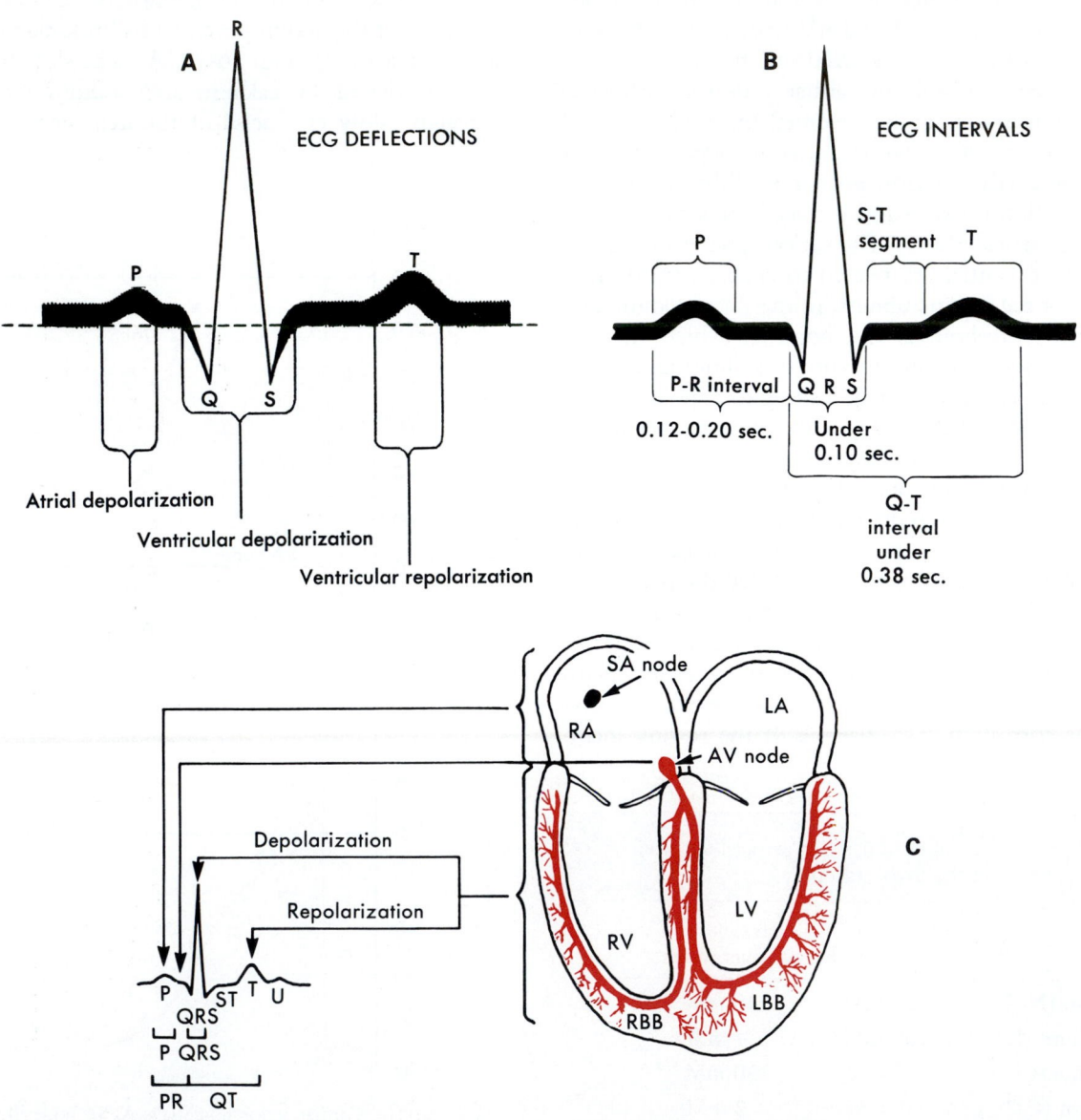

FIG. 26-11. A, Normal ECG. Depolarization and repolarization. **B,** ECG intervals between P, QRS, and T waves. **C,** Schematic representation of ECG and its relationship to cardiac electrical activity. (From Thibodeau, 1987.)

myocardial cells. The **QRS complex** represents the sum of all ventricular muscle cell depolarizations. The configuration and amplitude of the QRS complex vary considerably among individuals. The duration is normally between 0.06 and 0.10 second. During the **ST interval** the entire ventricular myocardium is depolarized. The **QT interval** is sometimes called the "electrical systole" of the ventricles. Its duration is about 0.4 second, but it varies inversely with the heart rate.

Automaticity **Automaticity,** or the property of generating spontaneous depolarization to threshold, enables the SA and AV nodes to generate cardiac action potentials without any stimulus. Cells capable of spontaneous depolarization are called **automatic cells.** The automatic cells of the cardiac conduction system can stimulate the heart to beat even when the heart is removed from the body. Spontaneous depolarization is possible in automatic cells because the membrane potential does not "rest" during phase 4. Instead, it slowly creeps toward threshold during the diastolic phase of the cardiac cycle. Because threshold is approached during diastole, phase 4 in automatic cells is called **diastolic depolarization.** The electrical impulse normally begins in the SA node because its cells depolarize more rapidly than other automatic cells.

Rhythmicity **Rhythmicity** is the regular generation of an action potential by the heart's conduction system. The SA node sets the pace, which is why it is called the natural pacemaker of the heart. The SA node depolarizes spontaneously 60 to 100 times a minute. If the SA node is damaged, the AV node will become the heart's pacemaker at a rate of about 40 to 60 spontaneous depolarizations per minute. Eventually, however, conduction cells in the atria usually take over from the AV node. Purkinje fibers are capable of spontaneous depolarization, but at a rate of only 30 to 40 beats/min.

Cardiac Innervation

Although the heart's nodes and conduction system generate cardiac action potentials independently, the autonomic nervous system influences the *rate* of impulse generation (firing), depolarization, and repolarization of the myocardium and the strength of atrial and ventricular contraction. Autonomic neural transmission produces changes in the heart and circulatory system faster than metabolic or humoral agents (Fig. 26-12). Speed is important, for example, in stimulating the heart to increase its pumping action during times of stress or fear, the so-called fight or flight response. Although increased delivery of oxygen, glucose, hormones, and other blood-borne factors sustains increased cardiac activity, the rapid initiation of increased activity depends on the sympathetic and parasympathetic fibers of the autonomic nervous system. (The autonomic nervous system is described and illustrated in Chapter 12.)

Sympathetic and Parasympathetic Nerves

Sympathetic nerve fibers innervate all parts of the atria and ventricles. Parasympathetic fibers from the vagus nerve innervate these structures plus the SA and AV nodes. Strong vagal stimulation can block cardiac action potentials transmitted from the atria. Sympathetic nerves can also shorten the conduction time through the AV node and increase the rhythmicity of the AV pacemaker fibers.

Efferent sympathetic fibers originate in the thoracic spinal cord and branch into the superior middle and inferior cardiac nerves. The efferent parasympathetic fibers originate in the medulla oblongata and travel by way of the vagus nerves to join the sympathetic nerves in the **cardiac plexus,** a neural junction located at the root of the aorta, in front of the trachea.

Ventricular function is regulated primarily by the sympathetic nervous system through the release of the neurotransmitter, norepinephrine. Heart rate is controlled primarily by the parasympathetic system through release of acetylcholine. In the heart, receptors for these neurotransmitters are found in the myocardium and in the coronary vessels.

Adrenergic Receptor Function

Sympathetic neural stimulation of the myocardium and coronary vessels depends on the presence of adrenergic receptors, which bind specifically with neurotransmitters of the sympathetic nervous system. (Receptor physiology is discussed in Chapter 1.) The effects of sympathetic stimulation depend on (1) whether α- or β-adrenergic receptors are most plentiful on cells of the effector tissue and (2) whether the neurotransmitter is norepinephrine or epinephrine.

Overall, cardiovascular structures have more β than α receptors; therefore effects mediated by the β receptors predominate. β_1 receptors are found mostly in the heart, specifically the conduction system (AV and SA nodes, Purkinje fibers) and the atrial and ventricular myocardium. Norepinephrine binding with β_1 receptors increases the rate of impulse generation (firing) and conduction and also the strength of myocardial contraction during systole. These effects enable the heart to pump more blood. At the same time, epinephrine binds with β_2 receptors, which are most plentiful in the coronary arterioles. This causes the coronary arterioles to dilate, supplying the hard-working myocardium with more oxygen and nutrients (see Table 12-6).

α-adrenergic receptors are also present in the coronary vessels, but in fewer numbers than the β receptors. Norepinephrine binding with α_1 receptors in the coronary arteries causes vasoconstriction. The α_2 receptors are located mostly on the sympathetic ganglia and nerve terminals. The effect of norepinephrine on the α_2 receptors is to inhibit release of more norepinephrine, which promotes vasodilation.

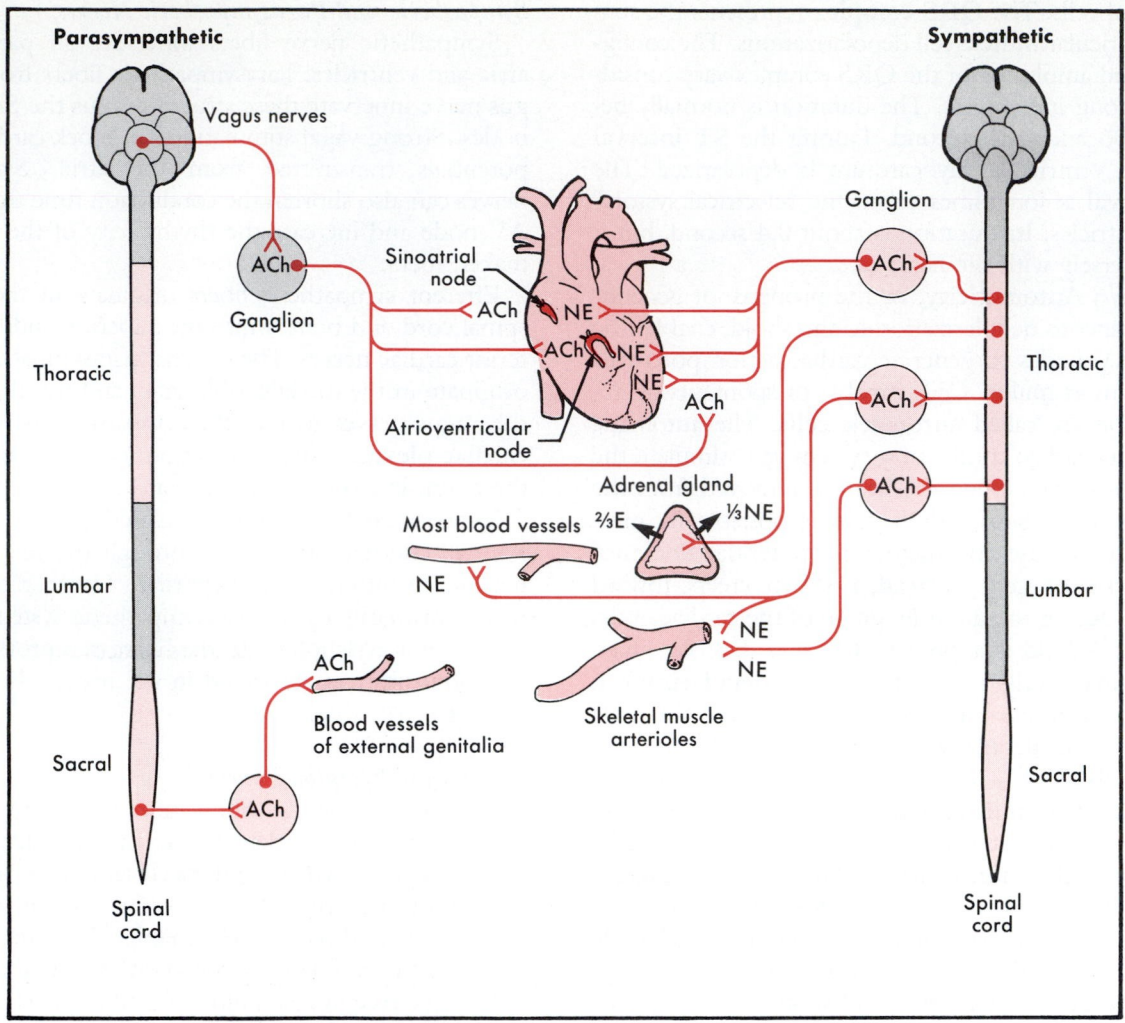

FIG. 26-12. Autonomic innervation of cardiovascular system. *ACh* Acetylcholine; *NE* norepinephrine; *E* epinephrine; *SA* sinoatrial node; *AV* atrioventricular node.

Epinephrine stimulates all four types of receptors (β_1, β_2, α_1, α_2) strongly; whereas norepinephrine stimulates α_1, α_2, and β_1 receptors and certain β_2 receptors weakly or not at all. Thus both epinephrine and norepinephrine stimulate the heart (β_1) and constrict certain blood vessels (α_1), but only epinephrine dilates certain blood vessels (β_2) (Vick, 1984).

Myocardial Cells

The cells of cardiac muscle (the myocardium) and of muscle that makes voluntary movement possible (skeletal muscle) are nearly identical in structure, function, and microscopic appearance. (The properties of skeletal muscle are described in detail in Chapter 38.) Both types of muscle tissue are composed of long, narrow cells, called fibers, which contain basically the same

structures: bundles of longitudinally arranged myofibrils; a nucleus (cardiac muscle) or many nuclei (skeletal muscle); mitochondria; an internal membrane system (the sarcoplasmic reticulum); cytoplasm (sarcoplasm); and a plasma membrane (the sarcolemma), which encloses the cell. Cardiac and skeletal muscle cells also have an "external" membrane system made up of transverse tubules (t-tubules) formed by invaginations of the sarcolemma. The sarcoplasmic reticulum forms a network of channels that surrounds the muscle fiber.

The microscopic appearance of cardiac and skeletal muscle is somewhat similar as well (see Chapter 1, Table 1-5). Because the myofibrils in both types of fibers are made up of alternating light and dark bands of protein, the fibers appear striped, or striated. The dark and light bands of the myofibrils comprise longitudinal repeating units called sarcomeres. The length of the sarcomeres, normally between 1.6 to 2.2 μm, is very important because it determines the limits of myocardial stretch at the end of diastole and subsequently the force of contraction during systole.

Cardiac muscle differs from skeletal muscle in several respects that reflect heart function. Cardiac cells are arranged in branching networks throughout the myocardium, whereas skeletal muscle cells tend to be arranged in parallel throughout the length of the muscle. Cardiac fibers have only one nucleus, whereas skeletal muscle cells have many nuclei. Other differences enable cardiac fibers to (1) transmit action potentials quickly from cell to cell, (2) maintain high levels of energy synthesis, and (3) gain access to more ions, particularly sodium and potassium, in the extracellular environment.

Rapid transmission of electrical impulses from cardiac fiber to cardiac fiber is possible because the network of fibers is connected at specialized intercellular junctions called intercalated disks (see the illustration in Chapter 1, Table 1-5). **Intercalated disks** are thickened portions of the sarcolemma that enable electrical impulses to spread quickly in a continuous cell-to-cell (syncytial) fashion. The intercalated disks contain two junctions: desmosomes, which attach one cell to another; and gap junctions, which allow the electrical impulse to spread from cell to cell (see Chapter 1). Together, these junctions provide a low-resistance pathway for impulse propagation.

Unlike skeletal muscle, the heart cannot rest and is in constant need of energy compounds, such as adenosine triphosphate (ATP). Therefore the cytoplasm surrounding the bundles of myofibrils in each cardiac muscle cell contains a superabundance of mitochondria (25% of the cellular volume). Cardiac muscle cells have more mitochondria than skeletal muscle cells. The large number of mitochondria provide the necessary respiratory enzymes for aerobic metabolism and supply quantities of ATP sufficient for the constant action of the myocardium. (The role of mitochondria in cellular energy production is described in Chapter 1.)

The third major difference between cardiac and skeletal muscle cells has to do with the transverse tubule (t-tubule) system. Cardiac fibers contain more t-tubules than skeletal muscle fibers. This feature gives each myofibril in the myocardium ready access to molecules it needs for the continuous transmission of action potentials, a process that involves transport of sodium and potassium through the walls of the t-tubules. (The mechanisms by which sodium and potassium transport cause transmission of cardiac action potentials are described in Chapters 1 and 38.)

Because the t-tubule system is continuous with the extracellular space and the interstitial fluid, it facilitates the rapid transmission of the electrical impulses from the surface of the sarcolemma to the myofibrils inside the fiber. This activates all the myofibrils of one fiber simultaneously. The sarcoplasmic reticulum is located around the myofibrils. When an action potential is transmitted through the t-tubules, it induces the sarcoplasmic reticulum to release its stored calcium, which activates the contractile proteins, actin and myosin.

Actin, Myosin, and the Troponin-Tropomyosin Complex

The thick filaments of **myosin** constitute the central dark band called the **anistropic** or **A bands** (Fig. 26-13). The myosin molecule resembles a golf club with two large bulbous heads protruding from one end of a straight shaft (Fig. 26-14). The bilobed heads contain an actin-binding site and a site of ATPase activity. A thick filament is composed of about 200 myosin molecules bundled together with the heads of the molecules (called crossbridges) facing outward (Fig. 26-14). The actin molecules are part of the thin filaments (Fig. 26-15). The light bands are called **isotropic** or **I bands** (see Fig. 26-13). The thin filaments of actin appear light and

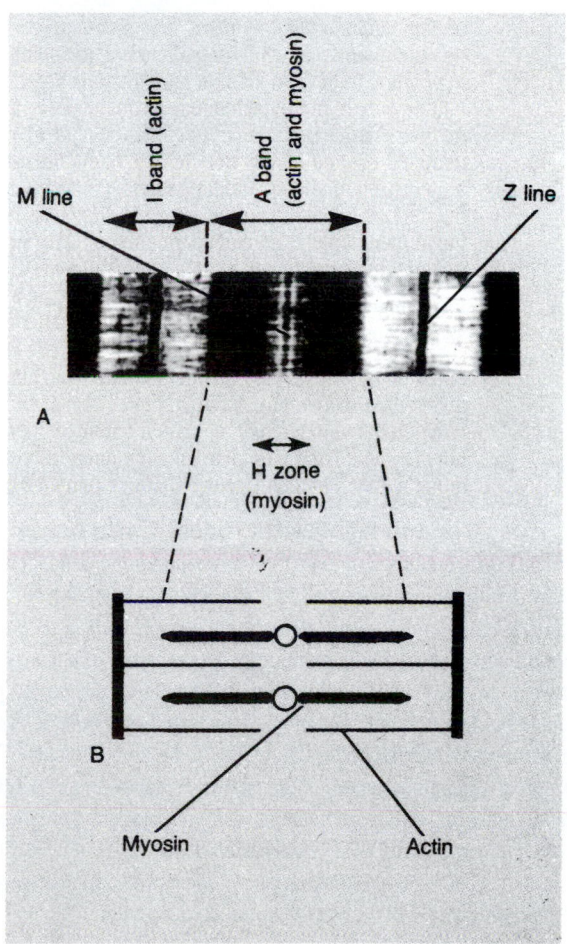

FIG. 26-13. A, Electron photomicrograph of sarcomere. **B,** Schematic of location and interaction of actin and myosin. (From Andreoli, Carpenter, Plum, & Smith, 1986.)

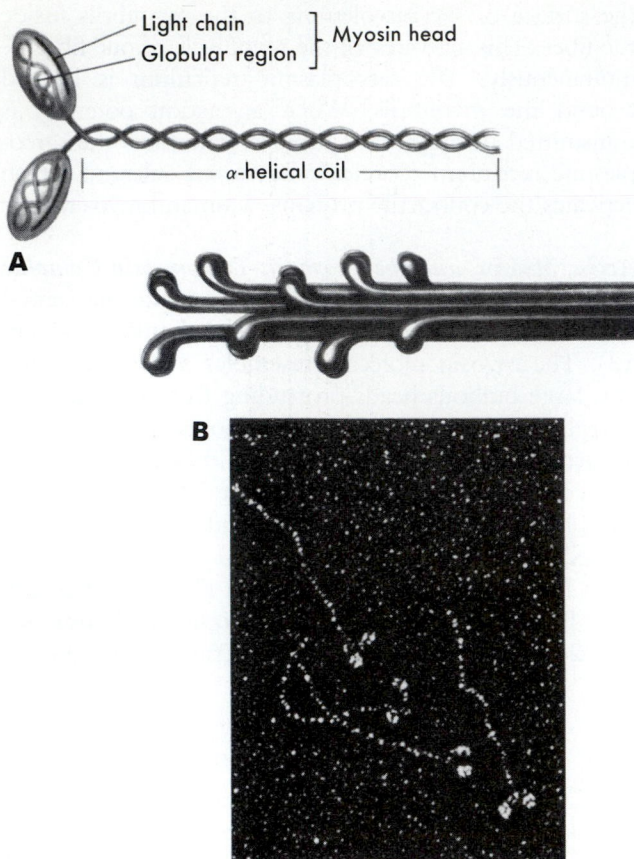

FIG. 26-14. Structure of myosin. **A,** Each myosin molecule is a coil of two chains wrapped around one another. At the end of each chain is a globular region, much like a golf club, called the "head." **B,** Myosin molecules are usually combined into filaments, which are stalks of myosin from which the heads protrude at regular intervals. (From Raven, & Johnson, 1986.)

extend from the Z line. The dense fibrous **Z line** crosses the center of each I band. A sarcomere is the area from one dark Z line to an adjacent Z line with a length that varies from 1.6 to 2.2 μm. In the center of a sarcomere is the H zone, a somewhat less dense region. A thin, dark **M line** travels the center of the H zone. A single tropomyosin molecule (a relaxing protein) lies alongside seven actin molecules. Troponin, another relaxing protein, associates with the tropomyosin molecule forming the **troponin-tropomyosin complex** (Fig. 26-16). The troponin complex, itself, has three components. **Troponin T** aids in the binding of the troponin complex to actin and tropomyosin; **troponin I** inhibits the ATPase of actomyosin; and **troponin C** contains binding sites for the calcium ions involved in contraction.

Myocardial Metabolism

Cardiac muscle, like other muscle tissue in the body, depends on the constant production of ATP for energy.

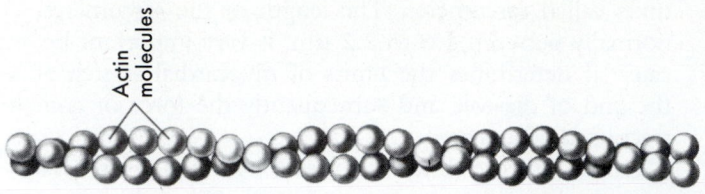

FIG. 26-15. Actin filament. (From Raven & Johnson, 1986.)

ATP is produced within the mitochondria mainly from glucose, fatty acids, and lactate. If the myocardium is inadequately perfused because of coronary artery disease, anaerobic metabolism becomes an essential source of energy (see Chapter 1). The energy produced by metabolic processes is used for muscle contraction and relaxation, electrical excitation, membrane transport, and synthesis of large molecules. Normally, the amount of ATP produced supplies sufficient energy to pump blood systemically.

Cardiac work is often expressed in terms of **myocardial oxygen consumption** (MVO_2). Because oxidative metabolism is the main process of cardiac energy generation, the rate of MVO_2 correlates closely with total cardiac energy requirements. MVO_2 is determined by three major and three minor factors. The three major determinants of MVO_2 include (1) the amount of wall stress during systole, which can be estimated by measuring the systolic blood pressure; (2) duration of systolic wall tension, which is measured indirectly by the heart rate; and (3) the contractile state of the myocardium. No clinical measurement for the contractile state exists. The three determinants of MVO_2 include the normal resting metabolism, energy for activating contraction, and myocardial fiber shortening (Cohn, 1985).

The oxygen supply to the myocardium is delivered exclusively by the coronary arteries. Approximately 70% to 75% of the oxygen from the coronary arteries is used immediately by cardiac muscle, leaving little oxygen in reserve. Therefore increased energy needs can only be met by increases of heart rate, which speeds blood flow through the coronary circulation. Oxygen content of the blood cannot be increased under normal atmospheric conditions, nor can the amount of oxygen extracted from the blood be appreciably increased from the resting level (see Chapter 29).

Myocardial Contraction and Relaxation

Myocardial contractility can be defined as a change in developed tension at a given resting fiber length. In functional terms, contractility is the ability of the heart muscle to shorten (Berne & Levy, 1988). The molecular basis of myocardial contraction is the sliding of the thin filaments of actin over thick filaments of myosin, called the **crossbridge theory of muscle contraction.** Anatomically, contraction occurs when the sarcomere short-

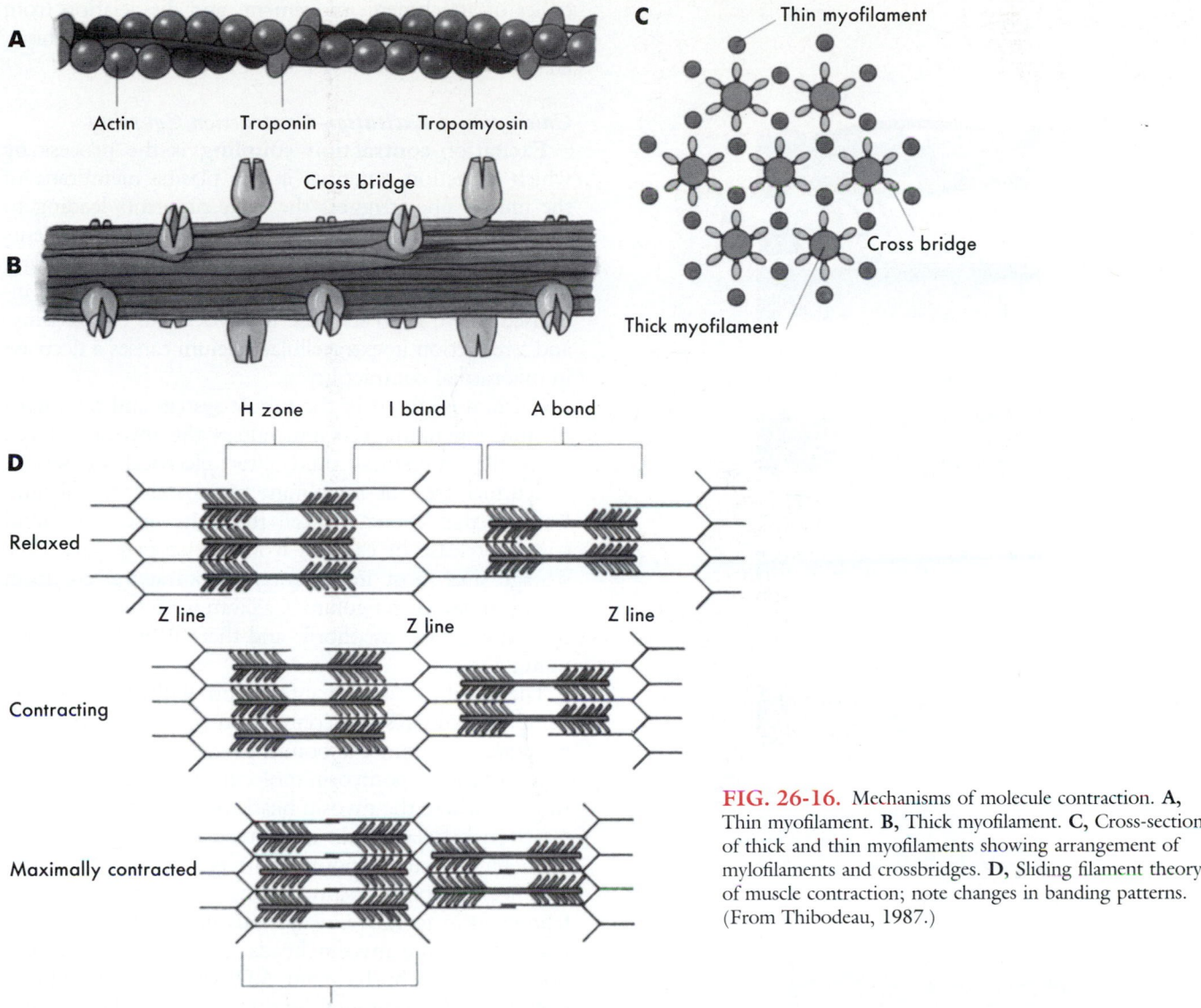

FIG. 26-16. Mechanisms of molecule contraction. **A,** Thin myofilament. **B,** Thick myofilament. **C,** Cross-section of thick and thin myofilaments showing arrangement of mylofilaments and crossbridges. **D,** Sliding filament theory of muscle contraction; note changes in banding patterns. (From Thibodeau, 1987.)

ens with adjacent Z lines moving closer together (Fig. 26-17). The width of the A band, which contains the thick myosin filaments, is unchanged. The movement comes from the long sets of filaments. The degree of shortening of the muscle fibers depends on how much the thin filaments overlap the thick filaments. Maximal contraction occurs when the sarcomere length is 2.2 μm. At 2.2 μm, the number of crossbridge attachments between actin and myosin is maximal.

The Crossbridge Theory

The globular head-end of the myosin contains a binding site for actin and a separate enzymatic site that catalyzes the breakdown of ATP to ADP and inorganic phosphate (Fig. 26-17). This reaction releases the chemical energy stored in ATP. Magnesium is required for the binding of ATP to the myosin site. The splitting of

ATP occurs on the myosin molecule before it attaches to actin, but the ADP and inorganic phosphate released remain bound to the active site on myosin. The chemical energy released is transferred to myosin (m), producing a high-energy form of myosin (M) (Vander, Sherman, & Luciano, 1980):

$$m \cdot ATP \rightarrow M \cdot ADP + P_i$$

The binding of this high-energy form of myosin to actin through a crossbridge releases the energy stored in myosin (e.g., ADP and P_i), producing the force necessary for movement of the crossbridge. With the attachment of actin to myosin at the crossbridge, the myosin head molecule undergoes a position change exerting traction on the rest of the myosin bridge, causing the thin filaments to slide past the thick filaments (see Fig. 26-17). During contraction, each crossbridge undergoes

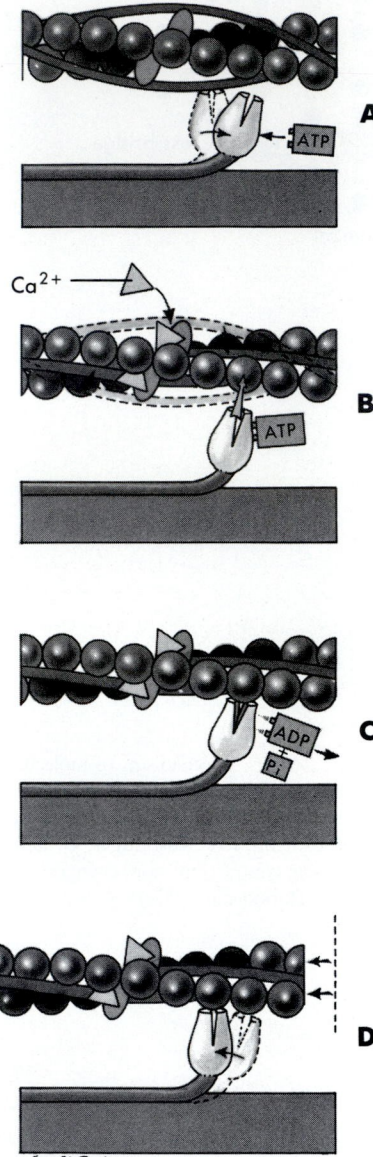

FIG. 26-17. Crossbridge theory of muscle contraction (or sliding filament theory). Crossbridges of single myosin fiber are thought to point at 60° angles at six actin filaments. Crossbridges bond to actin filaments and slide them toward center of sarcomere. Sequence of events in muscular contraction: **A,** in preparation for contraction, ATP bonding of myosin head causes conversion to high-energy form of myosin; **B,** Ca⁺⁺ is released from the sarcoplasmic reticulum and is bound to troponin-tropomyosin complex, changing its conformation so that troponin no longer holds tropomyosin in a blocking position between actin and myosin; **C,** as tropomyosin is pulled out of position, myosin head makes contact with actin molecule (bonding process displaces high-energy phosphate group [ADP + Pi]) from myosin head; **D,** loss of energy causes myosin to contract back to its original position, exerting traction on the rest of the myosin bridge, causing thin filaments to slide past the thick filaments. (From Thibodeau, 1987.)

cycles of attachment, movement, and dissociation from the thin filaments. It is estimated that each cycle shortens the muscle by about 1% (Cohn, 1985).

Calcium and Excitation-Contraction Coupling

Excitation-contraction coupling is the process by which an action potential in the plasma membrane of the muscle fiber triggers the cycle of events leading to crossbridge activity and contraction. This cycle of events and contraction depends on the availability of calcium. When the extracellular calcium concentration is increased, there is an increase in myocardial contractility, and a reduction in extracellular calcium causes a decrease in myocardial contractility.

Calcium is stored in the tubule system and the sarcoplasmic reticulum. Calcium enters the myocardial cell from the interstitial fluid after electrical excitation, which increases the membrane permeability to calcium. Calcium that enters the cell from the interstitial fluid triggers release of calcium from the storage sites. The storage sites most important for contraction are from the sarcoplasmic reticulum. Calcium from these sites diffuses toward the myofibrils and there it binds with troponin.

The calcium and its interaction with the troponin complex facilitates the contraction process. In the resting state, troponin I is bound to actin and the configuration of the tropomyosin molecule is such that it covers the sites where the myosin heads bind to actin. Thus interaction between actin and myosin is prevented. Calcium binding to troponin inhibits troponin C (which enhances troponin I-actin binding). This, in turn, causes tropomyosin to move away, thus uncovering the binding sites on the myosin heads. Myosin and actin can now form crossbridges and ATP can be dephosphorylated to ADP. Sliding of the thick and thin filaments can now occur and the muscle contracts.

Myocardial Relaxation

Adequate relaxation is just as vital to optimal cardiac function as contraction. Studies have shown that various heart diseases affect relaxation long before they result in inadequate contraction (Brutsaert, Rademakers, & Sys, 1984). Calcium also facilitates relaxation. After contraction, free calcium ions are actively pumped out of the cell back into the interstitial fluid or reaccumulated in the sarcoplasmic reticulum and stored. Troponin releases its bound calcium. The tropomyosin complex blocks the active sites on the actin molecule preventing crossbridges with the myosin heads. Each tropomyosin molecule is held in this blocking position by a molecule of troponin. Troponin is bound to both tropomyosin and actin (Figs. 26-16, *A* and 26-17).

Adequate relaxation is just as vital to optimal cardiac function as contraction. Studies have shown that various heart diseases affect relaxation long before they result in inadequate contraction (Brutsaert et al., 1984). Relaxation, or inhibition of contraction, is made possible by the so-called relaxing proteins in the myofibrils, troponin, and tropomyosin. The release of calcium also facilitates relaxation.

Factors Affecting Cardiac Performance

Four factors affect cardiac performance directly: (1) preload, (2) afterload, (3) heart rate, and (4) myocardial contractility. **Preload** (pressure generated at the end of diastole) and **afterload** (resistance to ejection during systole) depend on both the heart and the vascular system. Heart rate and contractility are characteristics of the cardiac tissue, per se, and are influenced by neural and humoral mechanisms (Fig. 26-18). To understand the role of these factors in cardiac performance, it is first necessary to understand two physical laws that explain the mechanisms of heart action: the Frank-Starling law of the heart and Laplace's law.

Frank-Starling Law of the Heart

Cardiac muscle, like other muscle, increases its strength of contraction when it is stretched. This relationship was described in 1914 by a British physiologist, Ernest Starling, who based his studies on the ear-

lier work of a German physiologist, Otto Frank. In 1914, Starling wrote that "the output of any heart can be varied within wide limits by alterations of the venous inflow, and that within these limits it varies directly as the venous inflow. So long as the functional condition of the heart remains constant, the amount put out at each beat depends directly on the diastolic filling" (Fye, 1983).

The **Frank-Starling law of the heart,** or the length-tension relationship of cardiac muscle, relates resting sarcomere length, expressed as the volume of blood in the heart at the end of diastole, or **end-diastolic volume,** to tension generation, described as development of left ventricular pressure. Thus there is a direct relationship between the volume of blood in the heart at the end of diastole (the length of its muscle fibers) and the force of contraction during the next systole. Although the change in pressure is related to volume of the ventricle and, consequently, to the length of the ventricular muscle fibers, it is common to use preload (i.e., filling pressure) as an index of ventricular volume. The length-tension mechanism is the major mechanism by which the normal right and left ventricles maintain equal minute outputs even though their stroke outputs may vary considerably during normal respiration (Schlant, Sonnenblick, & Gorlin, 1986). For example,

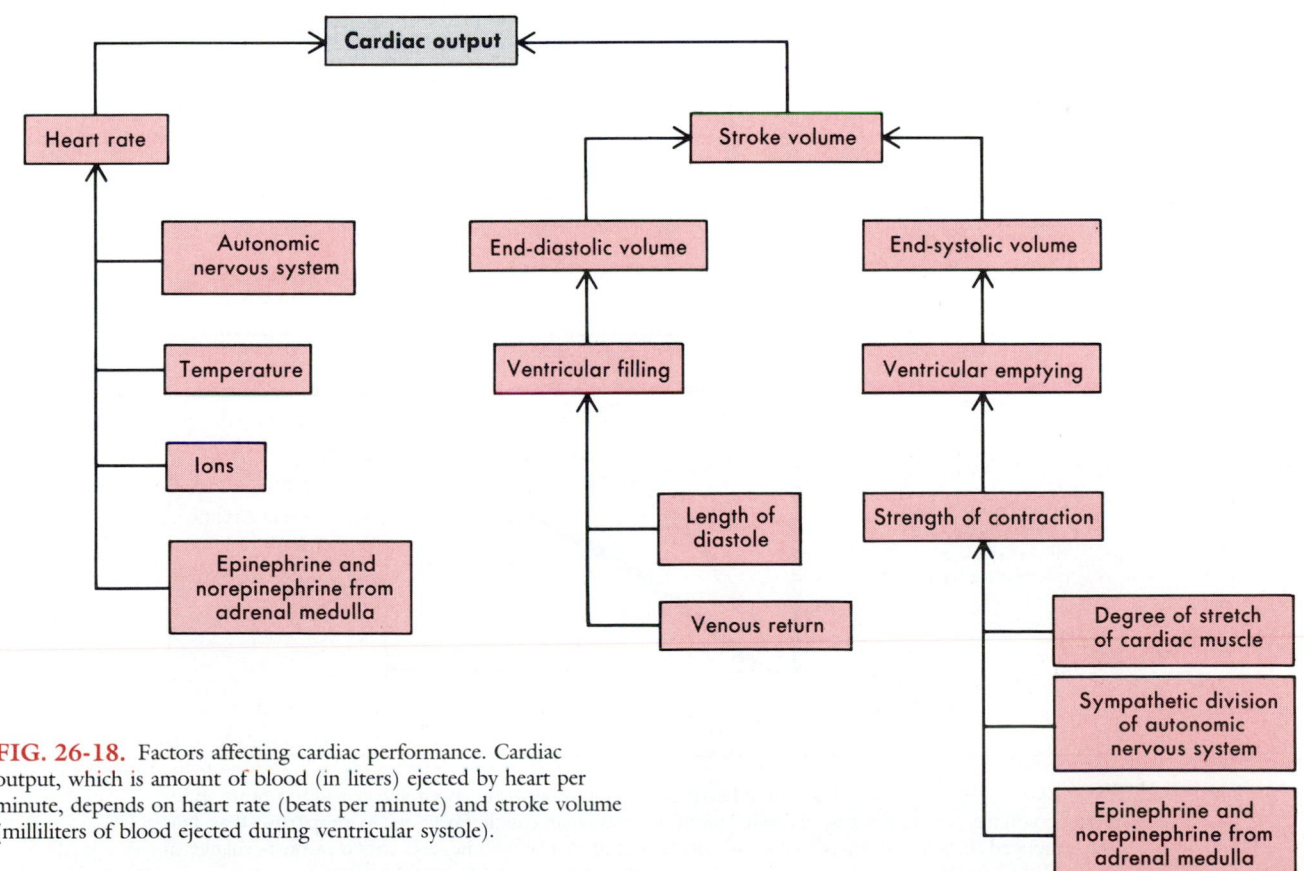

FIG. 26-18. Factors affecting cardiac performance. Cardiac output, which is amount of blood (in liters) ejected by heart per minute, depends on heart rate (beats per minute) and stroke volume (milliliters of blood ejected during ventricular systole).

changes in volume occur when an individual assumes a reclining position after being in a standing position; the volume of blood returning to the heart temporarily increases. The right ventricle stretches to accommodate this increase in volume and, thereby, increases its force of contraction. A larger stroke volume (i.e., the amount of blood ejected per beat) is pumped to the lungs, generating higher pressures. Pulmonary vascular pressure increases causing a rise in the left ventricular filling pressure or preload. Left ventricular volume and pressure increases. The left ventricle pumps a larger stroke volume and arterial vascular pressure rises (Bond, 1982).

The mechanical function of the heart is characterized by a number of length-tension curves (Fig. 26-19). Factors that increase contractility (i.e., positive inotropic), such as sympathetic nerve stimulation, cause the heart to operate on a higher length-tension curve (curve A). A higher tension or increase in ventricular stroke volume is generated without a necessary change in left ventricular end-diastolic volume or fiber length. Heart failure (curve C) is characterized by a lower length-tension curve (Chapter 27). The failing or dilated heart may not be able to use the Frank-Starling law of the heart because their fibers are lengthened maximally already. The failing heart is unable to respond significantly to increased filling or stretch with a greater force (Schlant et al., 1986). Thus at the same left ventricular end-diastolic volume as curves A and B, the force of contraction of stroke volume is decreased. The relationship between stretch and contraction can be compared to that of a rubber band. To a certain point, the more the rubber band is stretched, the farther it will fly when one end is released. Beyond that point, however, the rubber band will break.

The crossbridge theory partially accounts for the length-tension mechanism of cardiac muscle. According to the Frank-Starling law, the longer the initial resting length of the cardiac muscle fiber (optimal length is between 2.2 µm and 2.4 µm), the greater the strength of contraction. At 2.2 µm there is an optimal number of active crossbridges between actin and myosin. If the fibers are stretched beyond 2.2 µm to 2.4 µm, the force of contraction decreases because actin and myosin become partially disengaged, disrupting many of the crossbridges. Excessive stretching, to about 3.65 µm, causes actin and myosin to become completely disengaged and causes developed tension (force of contraction) to drop to zero. Heart failure occurs when it takes higher and higher filling pressures to accomplish normal contractile force.

Laplace's Law

Laplace's law demonstrates the relationship between wall thickness, pressure, and wall tension. Wall tension is related directly to the product of intraventricular pressure and internal radius, and inversely to the wall thickness. Wall tension can be calculated by Laplace's equation:

$$T = \frac{p \times r}{\mu}$$

where T = wall tension, p = intraventricular pressure, r = internal radius of the sphere, and µm = wall thickness. In other words, the amount of tension generated in the wall of the ventricle (or any chamber or vessel) to produce a given intraventricular pressure depends on the size (radius and wall thickness) of the ventricle.

The law of Laplace is useful for understanding aneu-

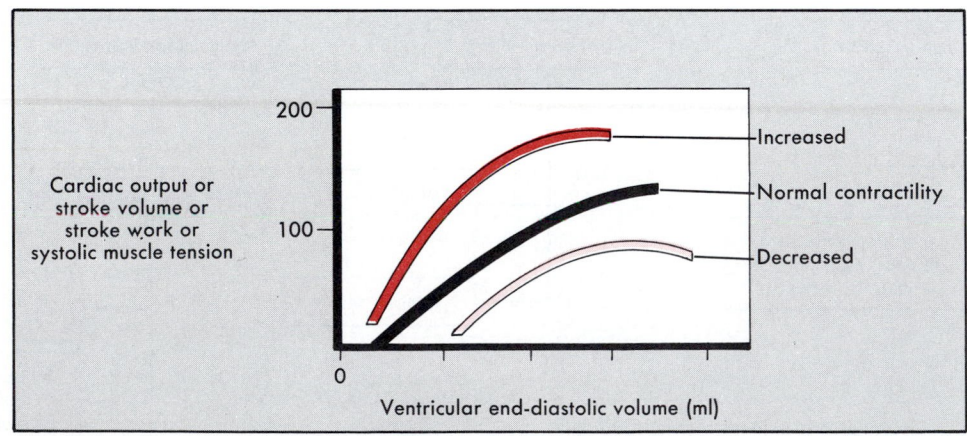

FIG. 26-19. Frank-Starling law of the heart. Relationship between length and tension in heart. End-diastolic volume determines end-diastolic length of ventricular muscle fibers and is proportional to tension generated during systole, as well as to cardiac output, stroke volume, and stroke work. A change in myocardial contractility causes the heart to perform on a different length-tension curve.

rysm formation, distensibility in blood vessels, and the effects of ventricular dilation on myocardial contraction. Dilation is an important factor in heart failure (see Chapter 27). With a dilated ventricle there is a need for the myocardial fibers in the wall to develop greater tension to produce a given pressure within the ventricle. The disadvantage of dilation is that the increased force, or tension, in the myocardial fibers required to develop a given pressure inside a dilated ventricle results in a decrease in the *rate* of fiber shortening, thereby decreasing the ability of the ventricle to eject blood (Schlant et al., 1986).

Preload

Left ventricular preload is the pressure generated in the left ventricle at the end of diastole, or left ventricular **end-diastolic pressure.** Preload is determined by end-diastolic volume. According to the Frank-Starling law, the end-diastolic volume stretches the cardiac muscle fibers, which in turn develop tension, or force, for contraction. Within a physiologic range of muscle stretching (2.2 μm to 2.4 μm), an increase in preload increases cardiac output (volume of blood pumped per minute; see Fig. 26-18). In monitoring preload the clinician measures indexes of left ventricular end-diastolic pressure. Pressure changes are important because increased left ventricular filling pressures "back up" into the pulmonary circulation, where they force plasma out through vessel walls, causing fluid to accumulate in lung tissues. (This condition is called pulmonary edema; see Chapter 30). Treatment goals are to maintain an end-diastolic volume that will maintain or increase cardiac output.

Afterload

Left ventricular afterload is the resistance or impedance to ejection of blood from the left ventricle. It is the load the muscle must move after it starts to contract. Aortic systolic pressure is a good index of afterload. Low aortic pressures (decreased afterload) enable the heart to contract more rapidly, whereas high aortic pressures (increased afterload) slow contraction. Increased afterload, or high aortic pressures, causes higher work loads against which the heart must function and therefore the less blood it can eject and vice versa. Pressure in the ventricle must exceed aortic pressure before blood can be pumped out during systole. Afterload involves a force-velocity relationship; that is, the lighter the afterload, the faster the contraction, and the heavier the afterload, the slower the contraction.

In addition to influencing the speed of shortening, afterload is related to extent of shortening. Increases in aortic pressure, with a constant preload, result in decreased blood pumped by the left ventricle. Decreased aortic pressure allows the left ventricle to pump a larger volume.

Heart Rate

The average heart rate in normal adults is about 70 beats/min. The average heart rate is significantly greater in children. Heart rate diminishes by 10 to 20 beats/min during sleep and can accelerate to more than 100 beats/min during muscular activity or emotional excitement. In well-conditioned athletes at rest the heart rate is normally about 50 to 60 beats/min.

Neural factors, including neural reflexes, and hormonal and chemical factors influence the heart rate. Neural control is exerted by both the central and autonomic nervous systems. Hormonal factors include the catecholamines (norepinephrine and epinephrine), thyroid hormones, growth hormones, and pancreatic hormones. (Hormonal function is described in Unit 6.) Stimulation by the sympathetic nervous system increases the rhythmicity of the cardiac pacemaker (SA node), whereas the parasympathetic stimulation has an inhibiting effect.

Cardiovascular Control Centers in the Brain

The major **cardiovascular control center** is in the brain stem in the medulla. Other areas of central cardiovascular control are in the hypothalamus, the cerebral cortex, the thalamus, and complex networks of exciting or inhibiting interneurons (connecting neurons) throughout the brain. The hypothalamic centers regulate cardiovascular responses to changes in temperature; the cerebral cortex centers adjust cardiac reaction to a variety of emotional states; and the medullary control center regulates heart rate and blood pressure (see p. 895 for a discussion of blood pressure regulation). The medullary neurons are often classified as cardiac and vasomotor (vasoconstrictor or vasodilator) centers; yet, because these centers are not discrete anatomic areas and actually constitute diffuse networks of interneurons, it is preferable to call the entire area the cardiovascular control center (Vander et al., 1980).

The nerve fibers from the cardiovascular control center synapse with the autonomic neurons (see Chapter 12, Fig. 12-15 and Table 12-7). When the parasympathetic nerves to the heart are stimulated, the sympathetic nerves to the heart, arterioles, and veins are usually inhibited. The opposite is also true: when the sympathetic nerves are stimulated, the parasympathetic nerves are usually inhibited. Because parasympathetic excitation and simultaneous sympathetic inhibition generally depress cardiac function (e.g., decrease the heart rate), these interneurons are often referred to as the **cardioinhibitory center** (Little, 1985). Excitation occurs with parasympathetic inhibition and sympathetic stimulation, and these interneurons are collectively called the **cardioexcitatory center** (Little, 1985). Therefore heart rate can be slowed by two simultaneous events that begin in the cardiovascular control center: (1) inhibition of sympathetic stimulation of the SA node and (2) activation of parasympathetic stimulation of the SA node. Heart rate can be increased by activation of sympathetic nerves and inhibition of parasympathetic nerves.

The resting heart rate in healthy individuals is primarily under the control of parasympathetic stimulation. While the individual is at rest, parasympathetic effects from the vagus nerves override sympathetic effects in the SA node. Interruption of the vagus nerves causes significant tachycardia (abnormally fast heart rate) because the inhibitory parasympathetic influence is lost.

Neural Reflexes

Two important neural reflexes that affect heart rate and rhythm are the Bainbridge reflex and the baroreceptor reflex. The **Bainbridge reflex** causes heart rate to increase after intravenous infusions of blood or other fluid. The increased rate is thought to be due to a reflex mediated by volume receptors in the atria that are innervated by the vagus nerves. (Volume receptors are thought to respond to increased plasma volume.) The magnitude of the change in heart rate depends on the initial heart rate. If the initial rate is slow, intravenous infusion usually accelerates it, but if the initial rate is rapid, infusions will usually slow it down (Berne & Levy, 1988). Contractility is usually not affected by the Bainbridge reflex (Cohn, 1985).

The **baroreceptor reflex** is a more important facilitator of blood pressure changes, but it also facilitates heart rate changes. The baroreceptor reflex is mediated by tissue pressure receptors (pressoreceptors) in the aortic arch and carotid arteries. (Because the receptors respond to mechanical factors, they are also called aortic and carotid mechanoreceptors.) The pressoreceptors increase their rate of discharge when stretched by blood pressure elevations. Neural impulses are then transmitted over the glossopharyngeal nerve (ninth cranial nerve) from the carotid artery and through the vagus nerve from the aorta to the cardiovascular control centers in the medulla. These centers initiate an increase in parasympathetic activity and a decrease in sympathetic activity, causing blood vessels to dilate and heart rate to decrease. In the heart, the initial response is caused by a decrease in sympathetic stimulation, but most of the decrease in heart rate is probably due to increased parasympathetic activity. Responses to the baroreceptor reflex return the blood pressure to its previous level, which may or may not be normal. The higher the blood pressure, the greater the reflexive decrease in heart rate.

If blood pressure is decreased, the baroreceptor reflex accelerates heart rate and causes vessels to constrict. These responses raise blood pressure back toward normal (see p. 893 and the section about shock in Chapter 27). The pressoreceptors are more effective in compensating for a decrease in arterial blood pressure than a rise in pressure (Kirchheim, 1976).

Neural receptors in the lungs cause heart rate to increase during inspiration and decrease during expiration. The increase in heart rate during inspiration is caused by the stretching (activation) of vagal fibers in the lungs that cause heart rate to speed up by inhibiting the cardioinhibitory center of the medulla. Inhibition of this center allows unopposed sympathetic acceleration of heart rate.

Hormones and Biochemicals

Hormones and biochemicals affect the arteries arterioles, venules, capillaries, and, both directly and indirectly, contractility of the myocardium. The catecholamines (norepinephrine and epinephrine) and hormones affect both heart rate and myocardial contractility. Norepinephrine increases heart rate, enhances myocardial contractility, and constricts blood vessels. Epinephrine dilates vessels of the liver and skeletal muscle and also causes an increase in myocardial contractility. Some adrenocortical hormones, such as hydrocortisone, potentiate the effects of the catecholamines.

Thyroid hormones enhance sympathetic activity, promoting an increase in cardiac output. The exact mechanism by which this occurs is not known. A decrease in growth hormone, as well as thyroid and adrenal hormones, results in bradycardia (heart rate below 60 beats/min), reduced cardiac output, and low blood pressure (hypotension; see Chapter 27).

Myocardial Contractility

Stroke volume, or the volume of blood ejected during systole, depends on the *force* of contraction, which depends on myocardial contractility, or the degree of myocardial fiber shortening. Two major factors determine the force of contraction: (1) changes in the stretching of the ventricular myocardium caused by changes in ventricular volume (preload) and (2) alterations in the sympathetic activation of the ventricles. An increase in the flow of blood from the veins into the heart distends the ventricle by increasing preload. Greater preload increases the stroke volume and, subsequently, cardiac output. Increased output then causes increased venous return, atrial volume and pressure, and eventually end-diastolic volume and stroke volume.

Myocardial contractility is difficult to measure because measurement requires keeping preload, afterload, and heart rate constant. Only when these factors are held constant can changes in cardiac performance be attributed to changes in the inotropic (contractile) state of the myocardium itself (Cohn, 1985).

Factors affecting contractility are called **inotropic agents.** Positive inotropic agents increase the velocity of myocardial contraction (phase 0) and stroke volume. The positive inotropic agents are excess thyroid hormone, epinephrine, norepinephrine, dopamine or isoproterenol infusion, and calcium salt infusion. The negative inotropic agents decrease the velocity of myocardial contraction and the stroke volume. These agents include alcohol, procainamide, quinidine, and propranolol.

Myocardial contractility is also affected by oxygen and carbon dioxide levels (tensions) in the coronary blood. (Blood gases are discussed in Chapter 29.) Different degrees of arterial oxygen deficiency—termed hypoxemia—affect contractility differently. With severe hypoxemia (arterial oxygen saturation less than 50%) contractility is decreased. With less severe hypoxemia (saturation more than 50%) contractility is stimulated. Moderate degrees of hypoxemia may increase contractility by enhancing the myocardial response to circulating catecholamines (Berne & Levy, 1988).

Factors Determining Cardiac Output

Cardiac output is a measure of the amount of blood flow in liters per minute. Heart rate and stroke volume determine cardiac output. The volume to which the ventricle fills is determined by the ventricular filling pressure and the compliance of the ventricle. The filling pressure of the right ventricle is the **right atrial pressure** and the filling pressure of the left ventricle is the **left atrial pressure.** A summary of the major factors that determine cardiac output is presented in Fig. 26-20. (Also see heart rate and myocardial contractility [stroke volume], p. 882.)

The ventricle does not eject all of the blood it contains; the amount ejected is called the **ejection fraction,** or the stroke volume divided by the end-diastolic volume. The end-diastolic volume of the normal ventricle is about 70 to 80 ml/m^2, the normal ejection fraction of the resting heart is about 60% to 75% (Vick, 1984). The ejection fraction is increased by factors that increase contractility (e.g., sympathetic nervous system activity), decrease contractility (e.g. heart failure), increase afterload (e.g., arterial hypertension), or decrease afterload (e.g., decreased peripheral resistance) (Vick, 1984).

The Suction-Pump Theory of Heart Action

Researchers have recently proposed a new model of the heart's function (Robinson, Factor, & Sonnenblick, 1986) that challenges and supplements the Frank-Star-

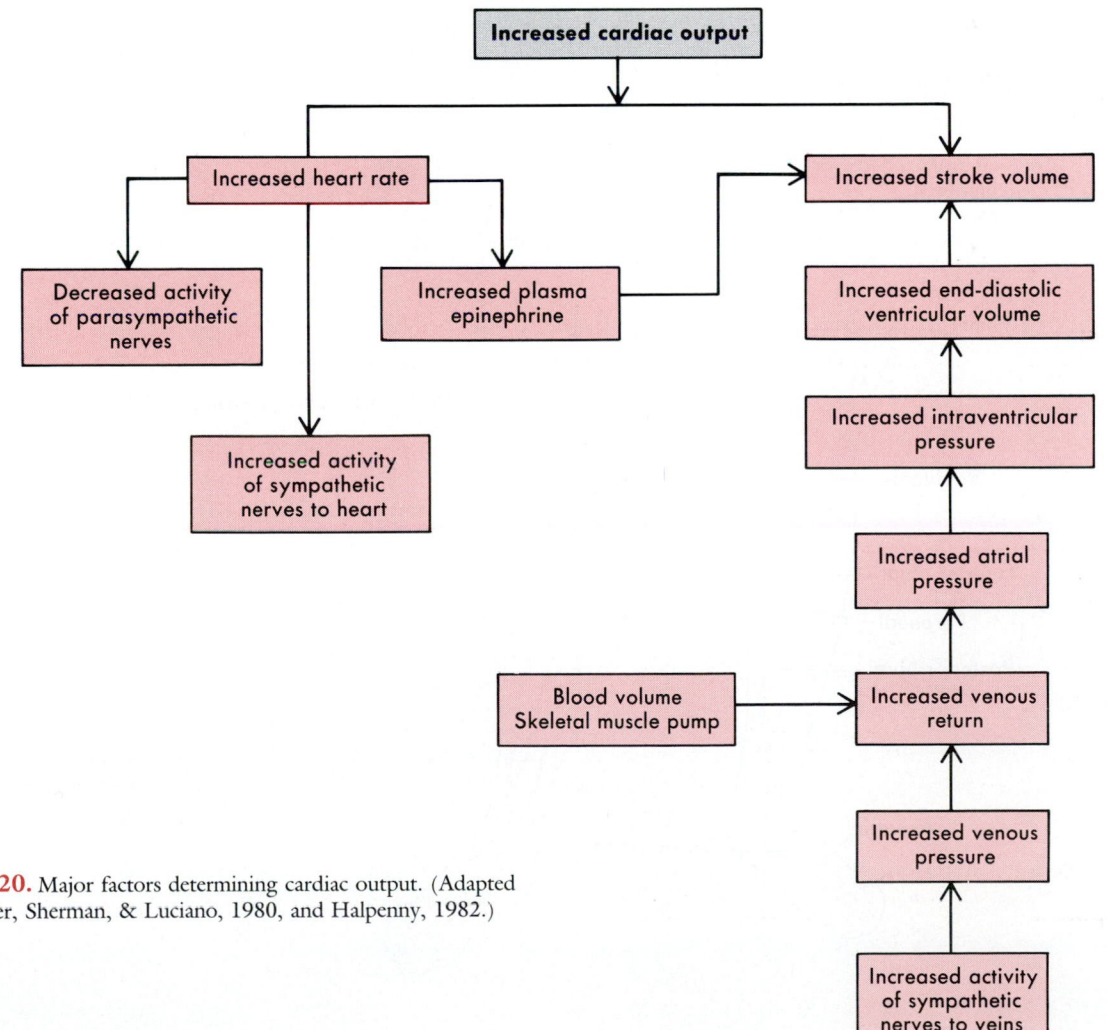

FIG. 26-20. Major factors determining cardiac output. (Adapted from Vander, Sherman, & Luciano, 1980, and Halpenny, 1982.)

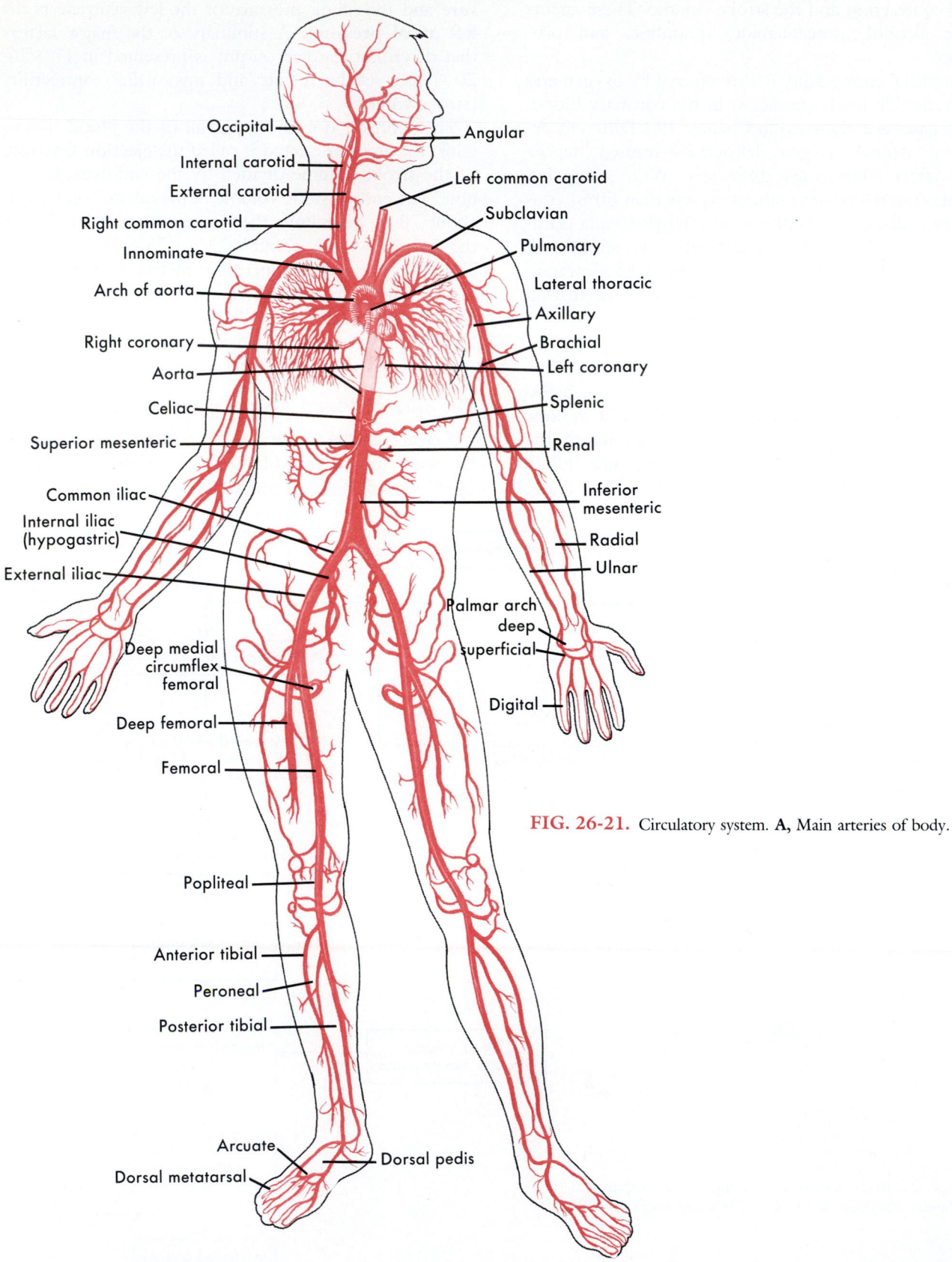

Occipital

Angular

Internal carotid

Left common carotid

External carotid

Right common carotid

Subclavian

Innominate

Pulmonary

Arch of aorta

Lateral thoracic

Right coronary

Axillary

Brachial

Aorta

Left coronary

Celiac

Splenic

Superior mesenteric

Renal

Common iliac

Inferior mesenteric

Internal iliac (hypogastric)

Radial

External iliac

Ulnar

Palmar arch deep

Deep medial circumflex femoral

superficial

Deep femoral

Digital

Femoral

Popliteal

Anterior tibial

Peroneal

Posterior tibial

Arcuate

Dorsal pedis

Dorsal metatarsal

FIG. 26-21. Circulatory system. **A,** Main arteries of body.

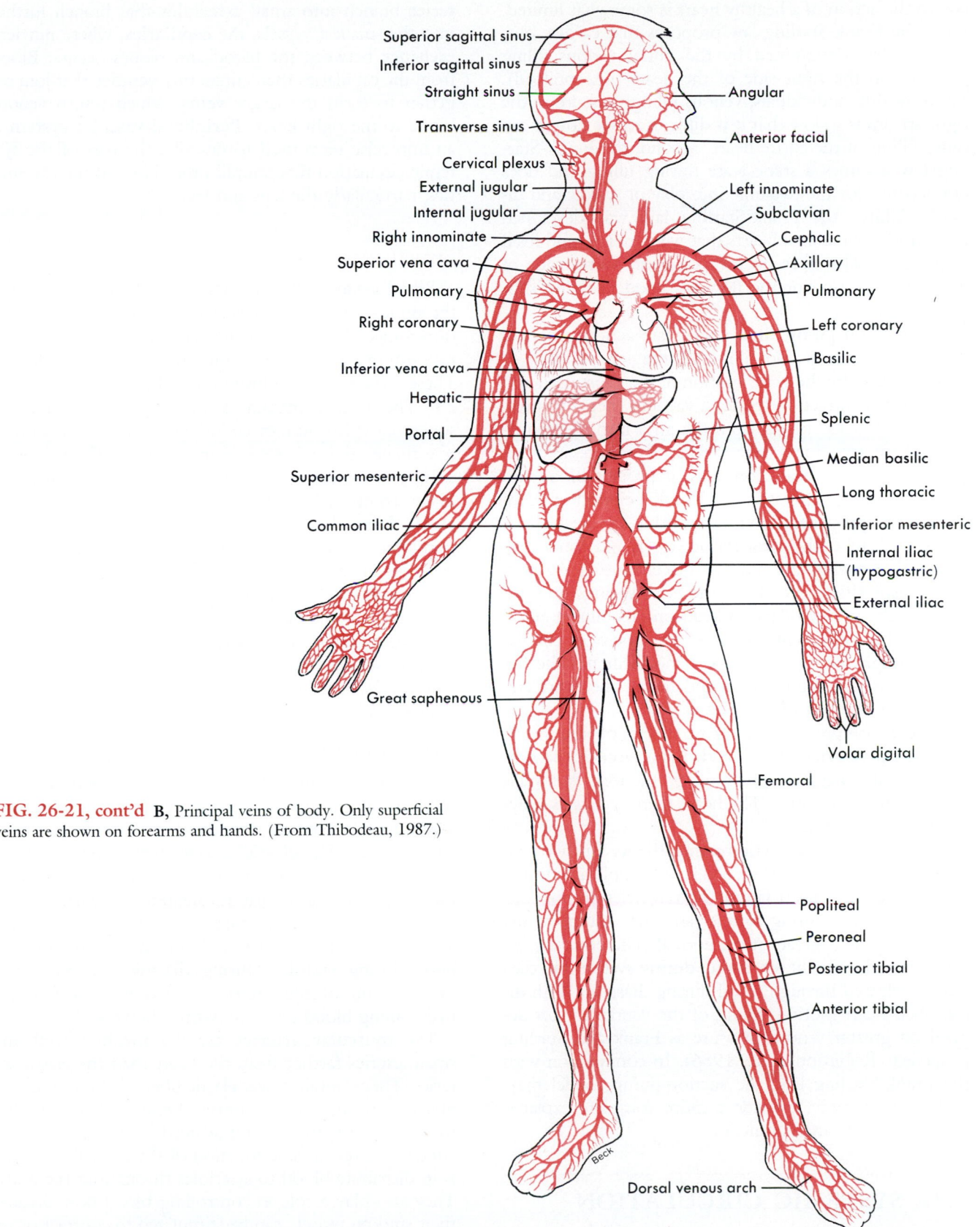

Superior sagittal sinus
Inferior sagittal sinus
Straight sinus
Transverse sinus
Cervical plexus
External jugular
Internal jugular
Right innominate
Superior vena cava
Pulmonary
Right coronary
Inferior vena cava
Hepatic
Portal
Superior mesenteric
Common iliac
Great saphenous

Angular
Anterior facial
Left innominate
Subclavian
Cephalic
Axillary
Pulmonary
Left coronary
Basilic
Splenic
Median basilic
Long thoracic
Inferior mesenteric
Internal iliac
(hypogastric)
External iliac
Volar digital
Femoral
Popliteal
Peroneal
Posterior tibial
Anterior tibial
Dorsal venous arch

Beck

FIG. 26-21, cont'd **B,** Principal veins of body. Only superficial veins are shown on forearms and hands. (From Thibodeau, 1987.)

ling law of the heart. Application of the Frank-Starling law to the action of a healthy heart is somewhat limited. First, the Frank-Starling law proposes that cardiac output is solely determined by the initial venous filling pressure on the right side of the heart (i.e., preload). Yet in healthy individuals, venous filling pressure in the right atrium is so low that it is difficult to see how it can cause filling of the entire heart. Second, the Frank-Starling law assumes a static state during filling and does not account for the dynamic interplay of systole and diastole. Third, the Frank-Starling law was developed from studies of animal hearts that were excised and fixed in position. Therefore no measurements were made of the heart's motion or the flow of blood in living subjects.

The **suction-pump theory** of heart action proposes that (1) expansion and filling of the left ventricle is caused in part by the gross motion of the heart itself and (2) systolic contraction creates a vacuum (negative pressure) that "sucks" blood from the atria into the ventricles. These two ideas take cardiac dynamics into account. When the heart contracts, it propels blood upward into the great vessels. As blood is ejected upward, the heart is propelled downward within the body. This reaction stretches the great elastic vessels and connective tissues that anchor the heart in place. During diastole, these elastic tissues recoil and the heart springs upward, meeting the inflow of blood head on (Robinson et al., 1986). This movement increases the velocity of circulation through the heart chambers and facilitates the filling process. Through stretch and recoil, the heart creates energy from its own motion.

Systole compresses the elastic fibers of the heart, which help ventricles to expand. Expansion of the ventricles creates negative pressure, or suction, that pulls blood in from the atria. The heart thereby acts as a dynamic suction pump.

Proponents of the suction-pump theory further propose that the Frank-Starling law is only applicable to the diseased heart. In heart failure the ventricles do not contract completely during systole, and the volume at the end of diastole is greater than normal. Therefore energy is not stored by tissue stretching during systole and cannot be released through recoil during diastole. With diminished heart motion, filling of the ventricles *does* depend on greater venous pressure as Frank and Starling proposed (Robinson et al., 1986). In conjunction with the Frank-Starling law, the suction-pump model may, with further study, provide a more complete explanation of normal cardiac function.

THE SYSTEMIC CIRCULATION

The arteries and veins of the systemic circulation are illustrated in Fig. 26-21. Blood from the left heart flows through the aorta and into the systemic arteries. The **arteries** branch into small **arterioles** that branch further into the smallest vessels, the **capillaries,** where nutrient exchange between the blood and tissues occurs. Blood from the capillaries then enters tiny **venules** that join together to form the larger **veins,** which return venous blood to the right heart. **Peripheral vascular system** is an imprecise term used to describe the part of the systemic circulation that supplies the skin and the extremities, particularly the legs and feet.

Structure of Blood Vessels

Blood vessel walls are composed of three layers: (1) the tunica intima (innermost or intimal layer), (2) the tunica medial (middle or medial layer), and (3) the tunica externa or adventitia (outermost or external layer). These structures are illustrated in Figs. 26-22 and 26-23. The **tunica intima** is composed of a layer of squamous epithelium or endothelium, a layer of connective tissue, and a basement membrane. (These cellular structures are described in Chapter 1). The **tunica media** is composed of smooth muscle fibers mixed with elastic fibers. The **tunica externa,** or adventitia, has a thin layer of connective tissue containing elastic and collagenous fibers that run lengthwise in the vessel. Blood vessel walls vary in thickness depending on the thickness or absence of one or more of these three layers. Cells of the larger vessels are nourished by the **vasa vasorum,** small vessels located in the tunica externa. The vasa vasorum arise from the blood vessel itself or from other vessels nearby.

Arterial Vessels

Arterial walls are composed of elastic connective tissue, fibrous connective tissue, and smooth muscle. There are two types of arteries: elastic arteries and muscular arteries. The **elastic arteries** have a very thick tunica media that contains more elastic fibers than smooth muscle fibers. Elastic arteries include the aorta and its major branches and the pulmonary trunk. Elasticity enables the vessel to stretch as blood is ejected from the heart during systole. During diastole, elasticity promotes recoil of the arteries, which is important for maintaining blood pressure within the vessels.

The **muscular arteries** are the medium-sized and small arteries farther from the heart than the elastic arteries. They contain fewer elastic fibers and more muscle fibers than the elastic arteries because, being farther from the heart, they have less need of the properties of stretch and recoil. The function of the muscular arteries is to distribute blood to arterioles throughout the body. They also play a role in controlling blood flow because their smooth muscle can be stimulated to contract or relax. Contraction narrows the vessel **lumen** (the internal cavity of the vessel), which diminishes flow through the

ARTERY VEIN

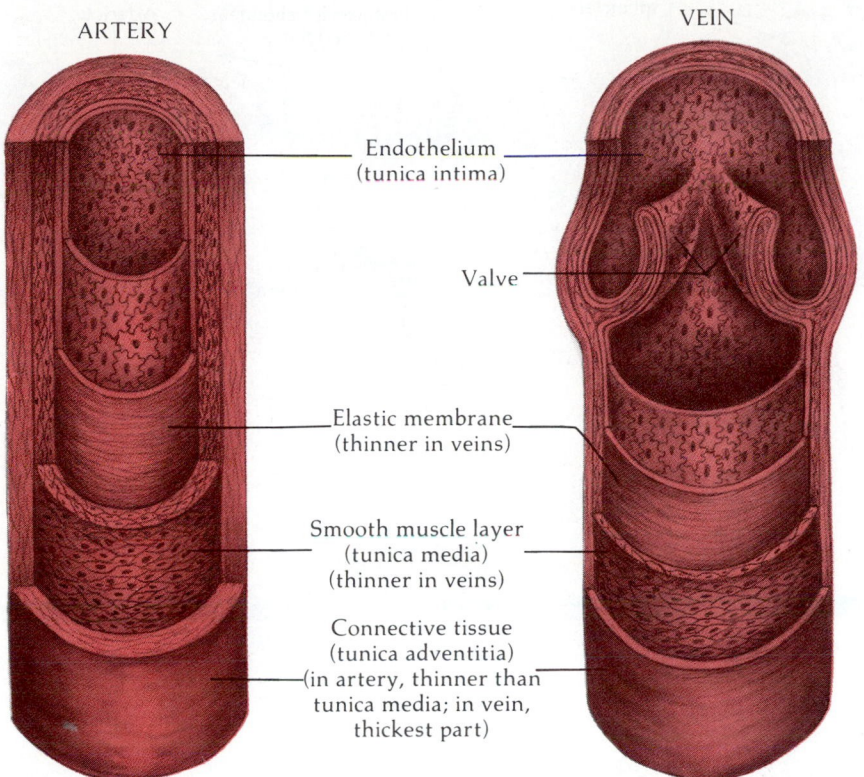

Endothelium
(tunica intima)

Valve

Elastic membrane
(thinner in veins)

Smooth muscle layer
(tunica media)
(thinner in veins)

Connective tissue
(tunica adventitia)
(in artery, thinner than
tunica media; in vein,
thickest part)

FIG. 26-22. Schematic drawings of artery and vein showing comparative thickness of three coats: outer coat (tunica adventitia), muscle coat (tunica media), and lining of endothelium (tunica intima). Note that muscle and outer coats are much thinner in veins than in arteries and that veins have valves. (From Thompson, 1987).

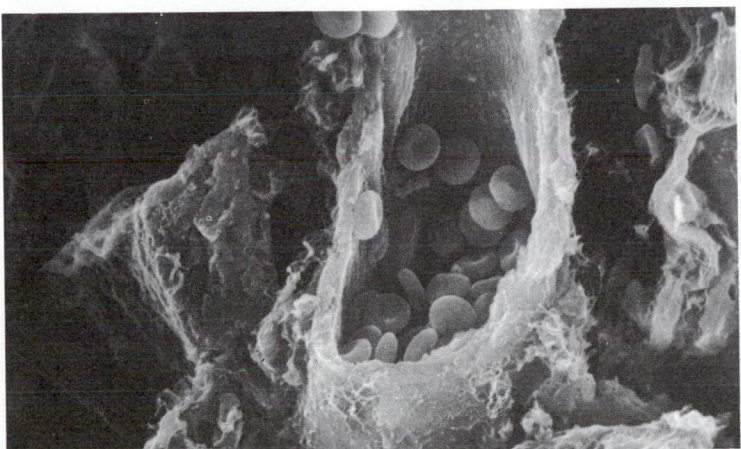

FIG. 26-23. This ruptured tube is a blood vessel. It is full of red blood cells, which move through these blood vessels transporting oxygen and carbon dioxide from one place to another in the body. (From Raven & Johnson, 1986.)

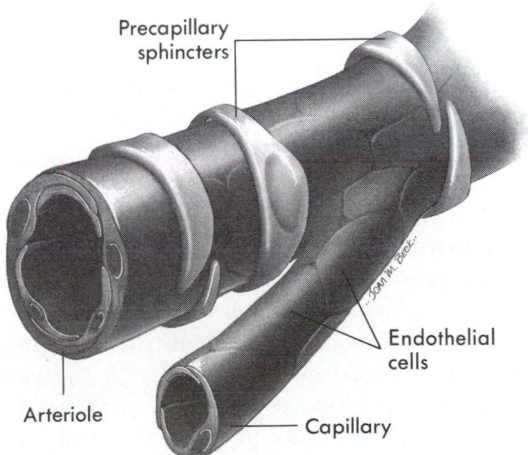

Precapillary
sphincters

Endothelial
cells

Arteriole

Capillary

FIG. 26-24. Walls of capillaries consist of only a single layer of epithelial cells. These thin, flattened cells permit rapid movement of substances between blood and interstitial fluid. Note thicker walls and presence of precapillary sphincters (smooth muscle cells) on arteriole. (From Thibodeau, 1987.)

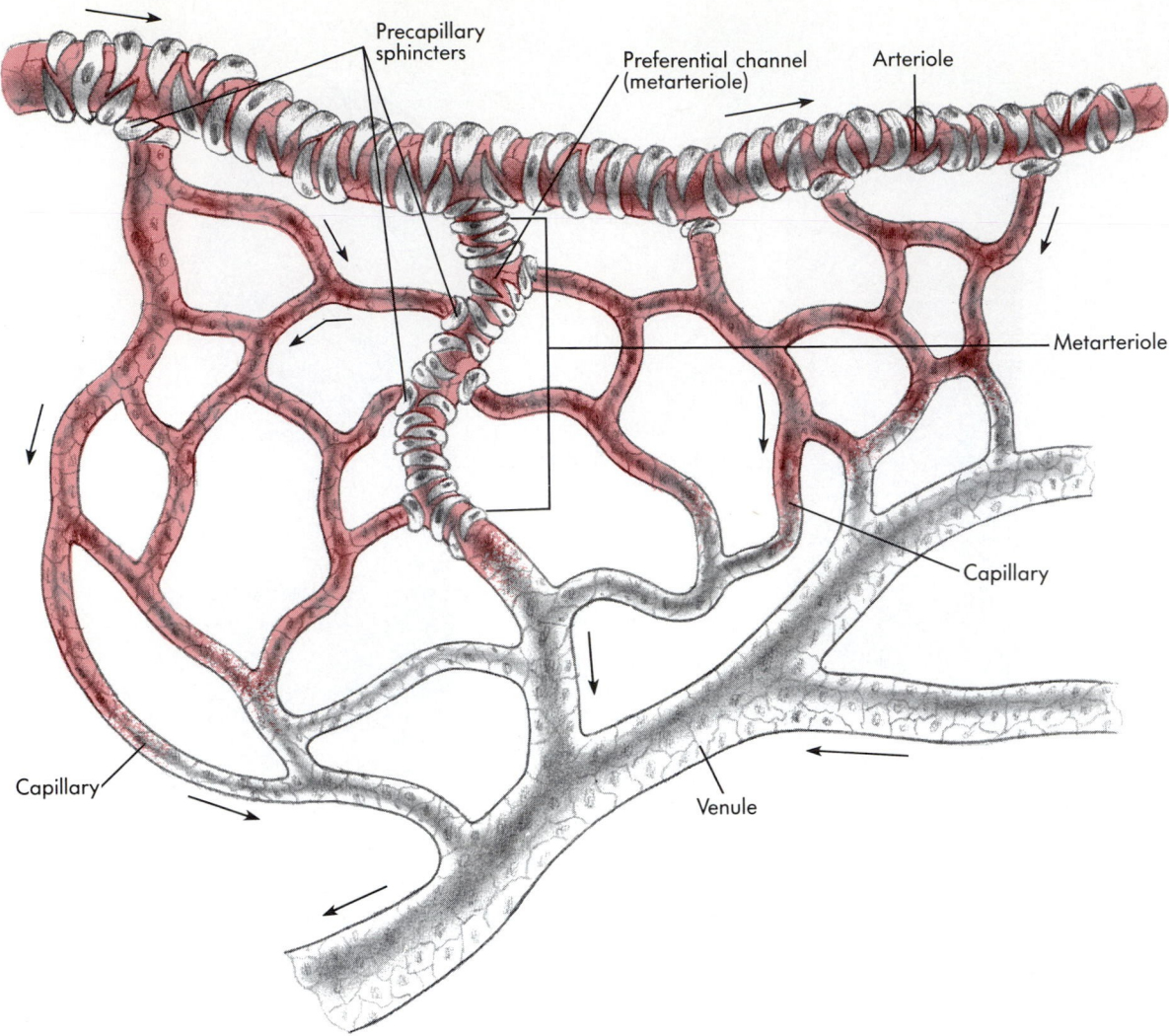

Precapillary
sphincters

Preferential channel
(metarteriole)

Arteriole

Metarteriole

Capillary

Capillary

Venule

FIG. 26-25. Capillary network. Blood enters network as arterial blood and exits as venous blood.

vessel. This condition is termed **vasoconstriction.** The smooth muscle layer can also be stimulated to relax, which permits more blood to flow through the vessel lumen. This state is called **vasodilation.**

An artery becomes an arteriole where the diameter of its lumen narrows to less than 0.5 mm. The arterioles are composed almost exclusively of smooth muscle, with little elastic tissue. Arterioles regulate the flow of blood into the capillaries by vasoconstriction, which retards the flow of blood into the capillaries, and vasodilation, which permits blood to enter the capillaries freely (Fig. 26-24). The thick smooth muscle layer of the arterioles is a major determinant of the resistance blood encounters as it flows through the systemic circulation.

The capillary network is composed of connective channels, or thoroughfares, called **metarterioles,** and "true" capillaries (Fig. 26-25). The capillaries branch from the metarterioles, which are the main channels connecting arterioles and venules. The metarteriole and capillary meet at a ring of smooth muscle called the **precapillary sphincter.** As the sphincters contract and relax, they regulate blood flow through the capillaries. Appropriately stimulated, the precapillary sphincters help to (1) maintain arterial pressure, (2) oppose the effects of gravity on blood flow in the arteries, and (3) regulate selective flow to vascular beds (Vick, 1984).

The capillary walls are very thin, making possible the rapid exchange of substrates, metabolites, and special products (such as hormones) between the blood and the interstitial fluid, from which they are taken up by the cells. The capillary wall consists of a single layer of endothelial cells surrounded by the thin basement membrane of the tunica intima. A single endothelial cell may form the entire vessel wall if the capillary has no tunica media or tunica externa. In some capillaries, the endothelial cells contain oval windows or pores termed **fenes-**

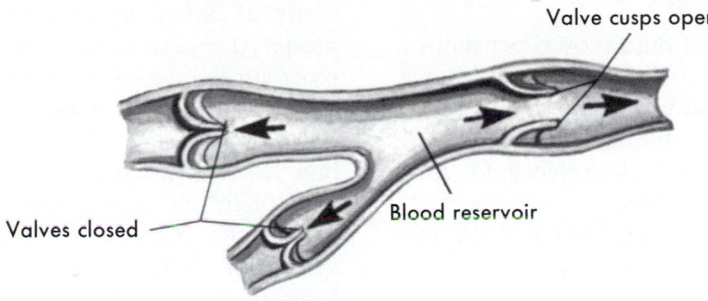

FIG. 26-26. Valves of vein. Pooled blood is moved toward heart as valves are forced open by pressure from volume of blood downstream. (From Thibodeau, 1987.)

trations. Fenestrations are generally covered by a thin diaphragm.

Substances pass between the capillary lumen and the interstitial fluid in several ways: (1) through junctions between endothelial cells, (2) through fenestrations in endothelial cells, (3) in vesicles moved by active transport across the endothelial cell membrane, or (4) by diffusion through the endothelial cell membrane. (Movement across cell membranes is described in Chapter 1.) A single capillary may be only 0.5 mm to 1 mm in length and 0.01 mm in diameter, but the capillaries are so numerous that their total surface area may be more than 600 m^2 (Spence & Mason, 1987).

Veins

The smallest venules closest to the capillaries have an inner lining, which is composed of the endothelium of the tunica intima and surrounded by some fibrous tissue. The largest venules, those farthest from the capillaries, are surrounded by a few smooth muscle fibers that comprise a thin tunica media.

Compared to arteries, veins are thin-walled, fibrous, and have a larger diameter (see Fig. 26-22). A given vein is larger than the artery that lies within the same sheath. Veins are more numerous than arteries. In veins the tunica externa has less elastic tissue than it does in the arteries. Therefore veins do not recoil after distention as quickly as arteries. Like arteries, veins receive nourishment from the tiny vasa vasorum. Some veins, most commonly in the lower limbs, contain valves that regulate the one-way flow of blood toward the heart (Fig. 26-26). These valves are folds of the tunica intima and resemble the semilunar valves of the heart. Backflow in veins of the legs is stopped as the flaps of the valves fill with blood and block the vessel. The position of the valves also facilitates blood flow in the proper direction during venous compression. When a person stands up, contraction of the skeletal muscles of the legs compresses the deep veins of the legs and assists the flow of blood toward the heart. This important mechanism of venous return is called the **muscle pump** (Fig. 26-27).

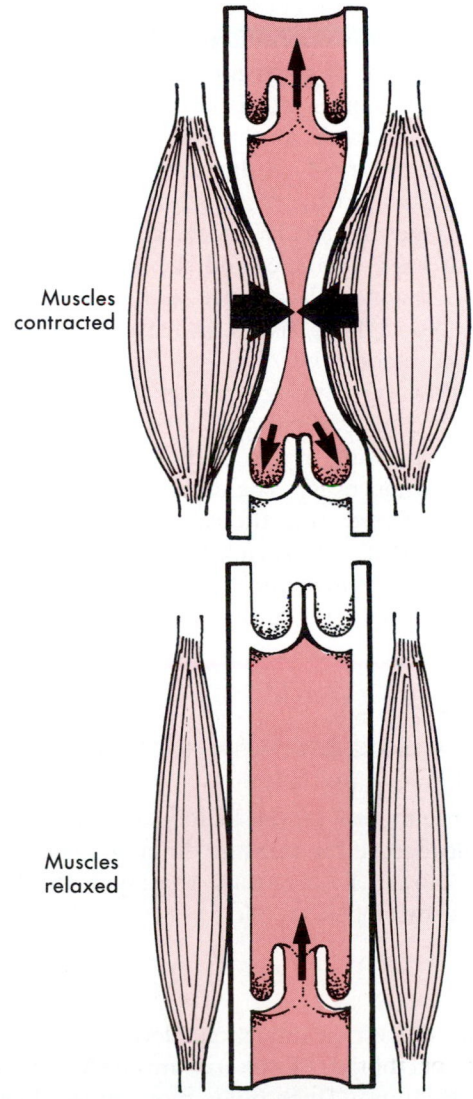

FIG. 26-27. Muscle pump.

Factors Affecting Blood Flow

Blood flow is the amount of fluid moved per unit of time and is usually expressed as liters or milliliters per minute (ml/min) or cubic centimeters per second (cm³/sec). Blood flow is regulated by the same physical properties that govern the movement of simple fluids in a closed, rigid system. These properties include pressure, resistance, velocity, turbulent versus laminar flow, and compliance.

Pressure and Resistance

Blood flow is determined primarily by two factors, pressure and resistance. **Pressure** in a liquid system is the force exerted on the liquid per unit area. Pressure is expressed as dynes per square centimeter (dyn/cm²) mm Hg, or torr. Blood flow depends partly on the difference between pressures in the arterial and venous vessels supplying the organ. Fluid moves from the arterial "side" of the capillaries, a region of greater pressure, to the venous side, a region of lesser pressure.

Resistance is the opposition to force. In the cardiovascular system most opposition to blood flow is provided by the diameter and length of the blood vessels themselves. Therefore most of the changes in blood flow through an organ are due to changes in the vascular resistance within the organ. The major mechanisms causing changes in vascular resistance are an increase or decrease in vessel diameter and the opening or closing of vascular channels. Resistance in a vessel is inversely related to blood flow; that is, increased resistance leads to decreased blood flow.

Blood flow (Q) through a vessel can be calculated from measurements of pressure at the inflow end of the vessel (P_1), pressure at the outflow end of the vessel (P_2), and resistance (R). The difference between P_1 and P_2 is often referred to as the change in pressure and is expressed as δP. The following formula, which expresses **Poiseuille's law,** shows the relationship between blood flow, pressure, and resistance:

$$Q = \frac{\delta P}{R}$$

where Q = blood flow, δP = the pressure difference (P_1-P_2), and R = resistance.

Resistance to flow cannot be measured directly, but it can be calculated if the pressure difference and flow volumes are known. To determine resistance, the equation for flow is rearranged as follows:

$$R = \frac{\delta P}{Q}$$

Another factor that influences blood flow is the consistency of the blood. Flow varies inversely with the viscosity of the fluid. Thick fluids move more slowly and cause greater resistance to flow than thin fluids. The viscosity of blood depends on its red cell content. The greater the percentage of red cells in the blood, the more viscous the blood. This relationship is expressed as the hematocrit, the ratio of the volume of red blood cells to the volume of whole blood (see Chapter 22). A high hematocrit reduces flow through the blood vessels, particularly the microcirculation (arterioles, capillaries, and venules). Conditions in which the hematocrit is elevated, for example, dehydration, cyanotic congenital heart disease (see Chapter 28), or polycythemia (see Chapter 23), can lead to increased cardiac work as a result of increased vascular resistance.

The viscosity of blood also increases if blood flow becomes very slow or stagnates. This condition is called **anomalous viscosity.** Anomalous viscosity is generally not significant unless cardiac output is low (Little, 1985). When cardiac output is reduced, as in shock, venous flow may be slowed to the point that anomalous viscosity develops. (Shock is described in Chapter 27.)

Poiseuille's formula for resistance to fluid flow through a tube takes into account the length of the tube, the viscosity of the fluid, and the radius of the tube's lumen. According to Poiseuille's formula, resistance (R) is proportional to a constant $8/\pi$, the viscosity of the blood (η), and the length of the vessel (l), *and is inversely proportional to the fourth power of the lumen's radius* (r_4) (Berne & Levy, 1988). Thus

$$R = \frac{8\eta l}{\pi r_4}$$

Because this equation was derived using straight, rigid tubes with steady, streamlined flow, it cannot be applied directly to the vascular system. Nevertheless, it is a useful model of vascular resistance.

The most important factor determining resistance *in a single vessel* is the caliber of the vessel's lumen, expressed in Poiseuille' formula as its radius and in Fig. 26-28 as its diameter. Small changes in the lumen's radius lead to large changes in vascular resistance. Because vessel length is relatively constant, length is not as important as lumen size in determining flow through a single vessel.

Generally, resistance to flow is greater in longer tubes because resistance increases with length. That resistance increases with increased length is demonstrated by comparing flow of the same amount of blood under the same pressure through vessels arranged in different configurations. Blood flowing through the distributing arteries, beginning with branches off the aorta and ending at arterioles in the capillary bed, encounters more resistance than blood flowing through the capillary bed itself, where flow is distributed among many short, tiny branches arranged in parallel. This is because the distributing arteries comprise a long system of tubes connected in series (end to end), whereas the arterioles and capil-

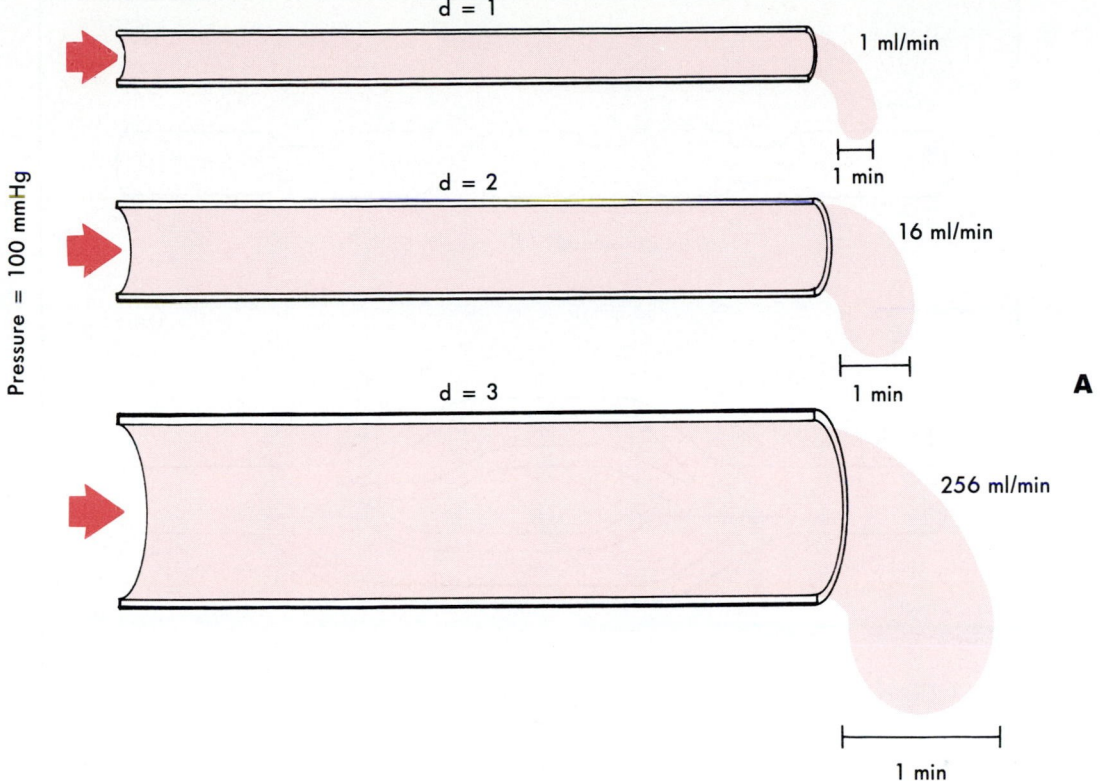

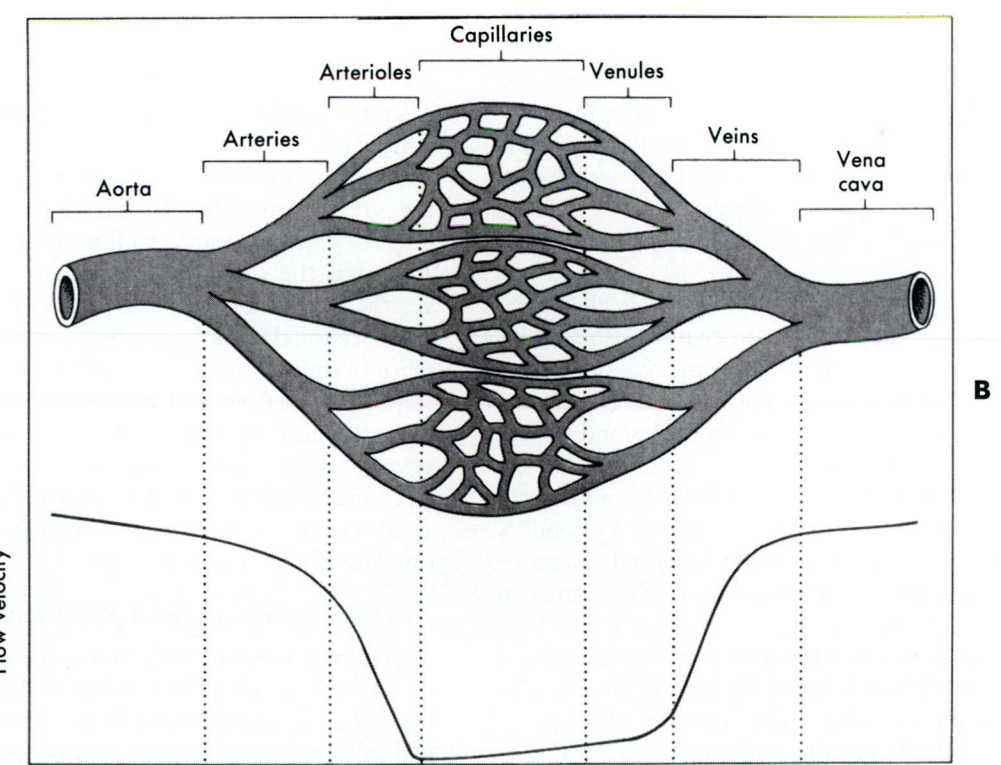

FIG. 26-28. **A,** Effect of lumen diameter on flow through vessel. **B,** Effect of vessel diameter on resistance and flow velocity. The narrower a tube, the greater the resistance it presents to liquid flowing through it. The resistance is inversely proportional to the fourth power of the radius of the tube. (**B** from Raven & Johnson, 1986.)

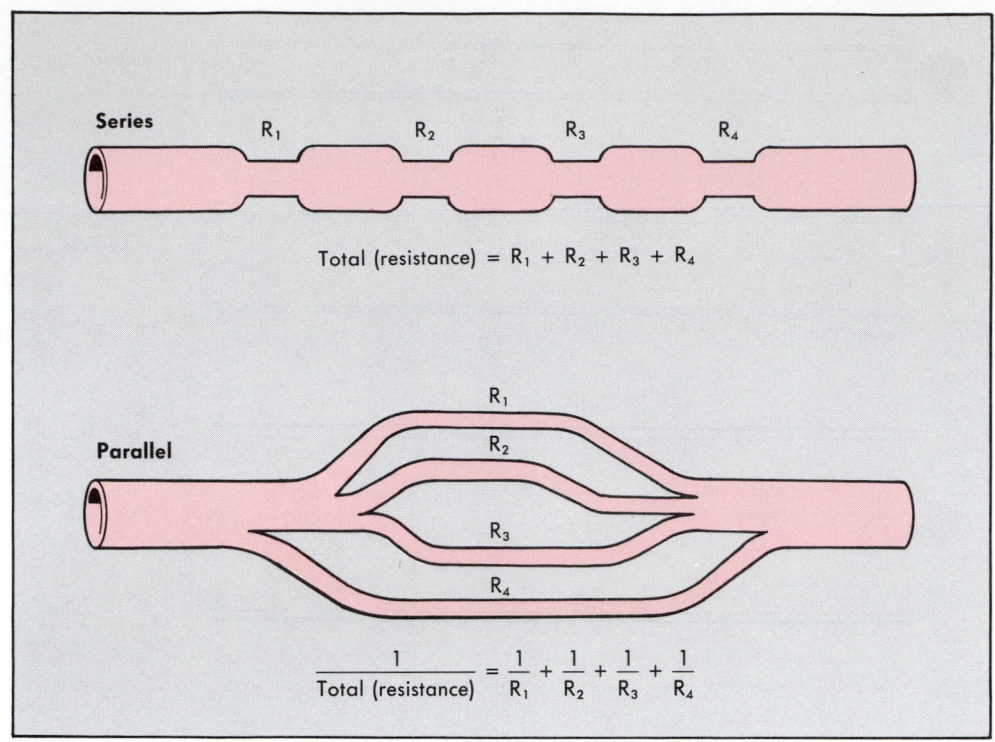

FIG. 26-29. Resistance in blood vessels arranged in series or parallel. *R*, Resistance in an individual vessel.

laries comprise a short system of many vessels arranged in parallel (side by side) (Fig. 26-29). Although the arterioles are arranged in series with the distributing arteries and the capillaries, they are arranged in parallel with other arterioles. Similarly, the capillaries are in series with the metarterioles, but they are in parallel with other capillaries.

Resistance to flow through a system of vessels, or **total resistance,** depends not only on characteristics of individual vessels but also on whether the vessels are arranged in series or in parallel. Total resistance is calculated differently for vessels arranged in series and in parallel (see Fig. 26-29). For vessels arranged in series, total resistance equals the sum obtained by adding all the individual resistances calculated using Poiseuille's formula. For vessels arranged in parallel, total resistance equals the sum of the reciprocals *(I/R)* of the individual resistances.

Total resistance is related to the total cross-sectional area of a system of vessels in parallel and to the number of vessels in parallel that make up the total cross-sectional area. The larger the total cross-sectional area, as in the capillary system, the lower the resistance. However, if a cross-sectional area is made up of a very large number of parallel vessels, the overall resistance will be greater than it would be if the cross-sectional area were made up of only two or three parallel vessels. Therefore, resistance is greater in smaller vessels than in larger vessels. The total cross-sectional area of the arteriolar system is greater than that of the arterial system, yet the greater number of arterioles arranged in parallel leads to great resistance to flow in the arteriolar system. Although the capillary system has a larger number of vessels in parallel than the arteriolar system, the total cross-sectional area is greater, resulting in lower resistance overall through the capillary system. The relationship between flow and cross-sectional area has physiologic significance. Despite the narrow diameter of each vessel (which normally increases resistance), total resistance in any capillary bed is relatively low. This, plus the slow velocity of flow in each vessel, promotes optimal capillary-tissue exchange.

Neural Control of Total Peripheral Resistance

Total resistance in the systemic circulation, sometimes called total peripheral resistance, is determined primarily by change in the diameter of the arterioles. Reflex control of total cardiac output and peripheral resistance includes (1) sympathetic stimulation of heart, arterioles, and veins; and (2) parasympathetic stimulation of the heart only.

The autonomic nervous system is monitored by the

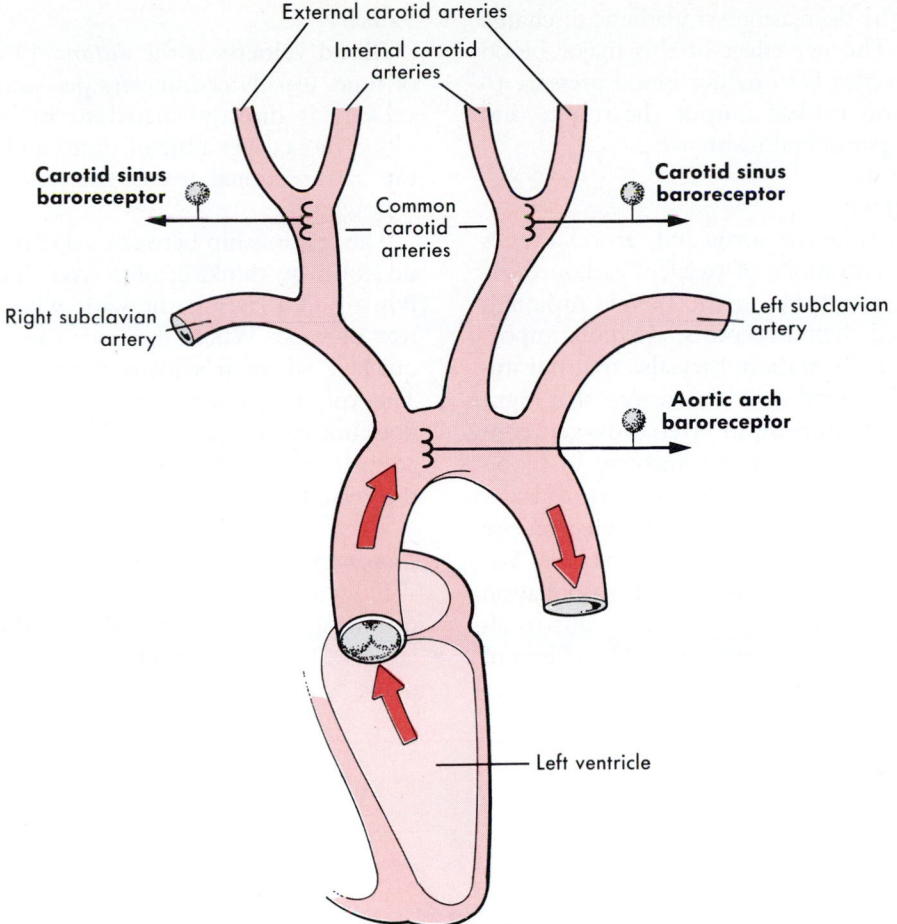

FIG. 26-30. Location of arterial baroreceptors.

cardiovascular control center in the brain (see p. 881). The hypothalamic centers regulate vascular (and cardiac) responses to changes in temperature. When the body's core temperature exceeds normal, the hypothalamus reflex initiates dilation of arterioles and veins in the skin. This causes shunting of blood to the skin, where heat is lost from sweating, radiation, conduction, or convection. When body core temperature decreases below normal, surface vessels constrict, shunting blood to the vital organs. Vasoconstriction is regulated by an area of the brain stem that maintains a constant (tonic) output of norepinephrine from sympathetic fibers in the peripheral arterioles. This tonic activity is essential for maintenance of blood pressure.

During exercise and stress, the sympathetic fibers that stimulate vasodilation of skeletal muscle arterioles are thought to be under the direct control of the cerebral cortex and hypothalamus, and *not* the medullary centers (Vander et al., 1980). Information about pressure and resistance is sensed by neural receptors (baroreceptors

and chemoreceptors) in arterial walls and delivered to the medullary centers.

Baroreceptors

Major stretch receptors are located in the aorta and in the carotid sinus (Fig. 26-30). These baroreceptors respond to changes in smooth muscle fiber length by altering their rate of discharge. (Technically, they are mechanoreceptors but are usually called baroreceptors or pressoreceptors.) The baroreceptors supply sensory information to the cardiovascular center that regulates blood pressure. The rate of firing of the baroreceptors increases and decreases with changes in blood pressure. An increase in arterial pressure increases the rate of firing of both the carotid sinus and aortic arch baroreceptors. These impulses travel up the afferent nerves to the medulla and (1) slow heart rate by decreasing sympathetic discharge and increasing parasympathetic discharge, (2) decrease myocardial contractility by inhibiting sympathetic discharge, and (3) decrease arteriolar and venous dilation by decreasing sympathetic discharge to smooth muscle. The net effect of this major blood pressure-regulating reflex is to reduce blood pressure to normal by decreasing cardiac output (heart rate and stroke volume) and peripheral resistance.

Arterial Chemoreceptors

Specialized areas within the aortic and carotid arteries are sensitive to concentrations of oxygen, carbon dioxide, and hydrogen ions (pH) in the blood. Although these receptors, called chemoreceptors, are more important for the control of respiration, they also transmit impulses to the medullary cardiovascular centers that regulate blood pressure. A decrease in arterial oxygen concentration or pH causes a reflexive increase in blood pressure, whereas an increase in carbon dioxide causes a decrease in blood pressure. Blood pressure changes are carried out by smooth muscle layers in the vessels. Vasoconstriction raises blood pressure and vasodilation lowers it. The major chemoreceptive reflex is due to alterations in arterial oxygen concentration. The effects of altered pH or carbon dioxide levels are minor.

Velocity

Blood velocity is the *distance* blood travels in a unit of time, usually centimeters per second (cm/sec). Blood velocity is directly related to blood flow (*amount* of blood moved per unit of time) and inversely related to the cross-sectional area of the vessel in which the blood is flowing.

The relationship between velocity and flow can be understood by thinking of a river. The volume of water flowing in a river is the same whether the river is narrow or wide. Where the river narrows, the water flows quickly; where it widens out the water flows slowly. The volume of water moving between the riverbanks does not change. In the body, as blood moves from the aorta to the capillaries, the total cross-sectional area of the vessels increases and velocity of flow decreases.

Laminar versus Turbulent Flow

Flow through any tubular system is either laminar or turbulent. Normally, blood flow through the vessels is laminar. In **laminar flow**, concentric layers of molecules move "straight ahead." Each concentric layer flows at a

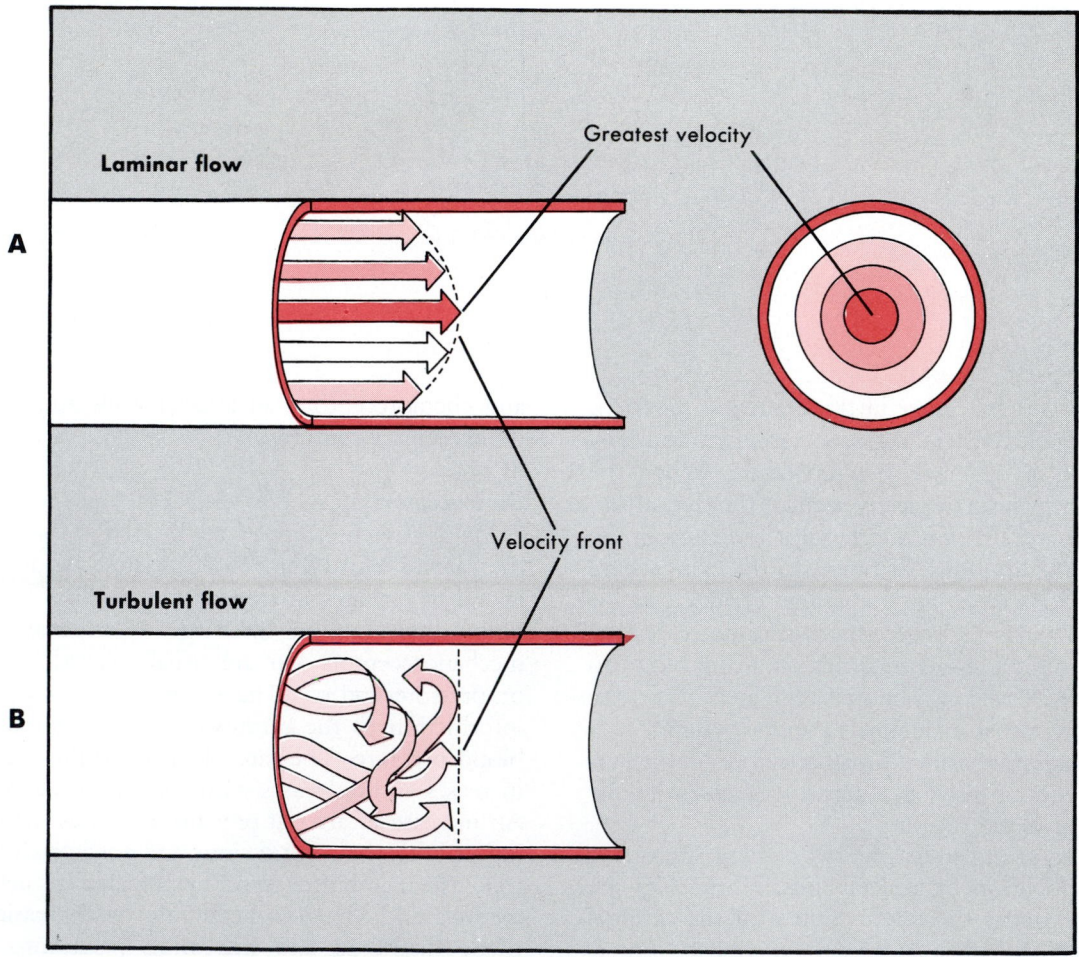

FIG. 26-31. Laminar and turbulent blood flow. **A,** Laminar flow, with the center stream having greatest velocity. **B,** Turbulent flow, with whorls.

different velocity (Fig. 26-31). The cohesive attraction between the fluid and the vessel wall prevents the molecules of blood that are in contact with the wall from moving. The next thin layer of blood is able to slide slowly past the stationary layer, and so on until, at the center, the blood velocity is greatest. The centermost concentric layer of fluid is not slowed by friction against the vessel wall. Large vessels have room for a large center layer; therefore they have less resistance to flow and greater flow and velocity than smaller vessels.

Where flow is obstructed, or the vessel turns, or blood flows over rough surfaces, it becomes turbulent. **Turbulent flow** consists of whorls or eddy currents and is noisy, causing a murmur to be heard on auscultation. Resistance increases with turbulence.

Vascular Compliance

Vascular compliance is the increase in volume a vessel is able to accommodate for a given increase in pressure. Compliance depends on the ratio of elastic fibers to muscle fibers in the vessel wall. The elastic arteries are more compliant than the muscular arteries, and the veins are more compliant than either type of artery because they serve as storage areas for the circulatory system.

Compliance determines a vessel's response to pressure changes. For example, with a very small increase in pressure, a large volume of blood can be accommodated by the venous system. In the less compliant arterial system, where smaller volumes and higher pressures are normal, small variations in pressure cause little or no change in the volume of blood within the arterial vessels.

Stiffness is the opposite of compliance. Several conditions and disorders can cause stiffness. The most common is arteriosclerosis (see Chapter 27). Arteriosclerosis increases the rigidity or stiffness of arterial walls, which in turn increases peak arterial pressure at a given volume of blood.

Regulation of Blood Pressure
Arterial Pressure

Arterial pressure is constantly regulated to maintain tissue **perfusion,** or blood supply to the capillary beds, during a wide range of physiologic conditions. These conditions include changes in body position, muscular activity, and circulating blood volume. The **mean arterial pressure,** which is the average pressure in the arteries throughout the cardiac cycle, depends on the elastic properties of the arterial walls and the volume of blood in the arterial system. Thus the mean arterial pressure is determined by (1) total peripheral resistance and (2) cardiac output. The major factors and relationships that regulate arterial blood pressure are summarized in Fig. 26-32.

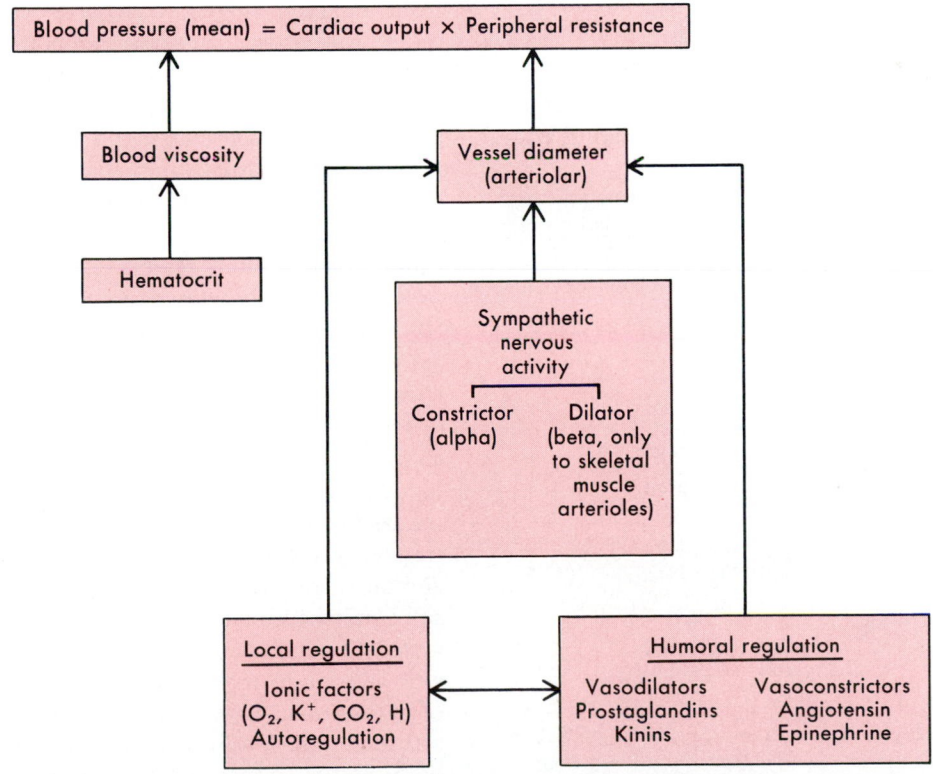

FIG. 26-32. Factors regulating blood pressure.

Effects of Cardiac Output

The cardiac output (minute volume) of the heart can be changed by alterations in heart rate, stroke volume (volume of blood ejected during each ventricular contraction), or both. An increase in cardiac output without a decrease in peripheral resistance will cause both arterial volume and mean blood pressure to increase. The higher arterial pressure increases blood flow through the arterioles. On the other hand, a decrease in the cardiac output causes an immediate drop in mean arterial blood pressure and arteriolar flow (Table 26-3).

Effects of Total Peripheral Resistance

Total peripheral resistance is primarily determined by a change in the diameter of the arterioles: arteriolar constriction raises mean arterial pressure by preventing the free flow of blood into the capillaries. Dilation has the opposite effect. Reflex control of vasoconstriction and vasodilation is mediated by the sympathetic nervous system.

Effect of Hyperemia

When metabolic activity is increased in the heart, skeletal muscle, and other muscular organs, it causes an increase in blood flow termed **hyperemia.** For example, the blood flow to exercising skeletal muscle increases in proportion to the activity of the muscle. This condition, known as active (exercise) hyperemia, is the result of arteriolar dilation and autoregulation of blood flow within the active organ.

Effects of Hormones

Many hormones cause contraction or relaxation of arteriolar smooth muscle. By constricting or dilating arterioles in specific vascular beds, hormones can (1) increase the blood supply to vital organs requiring more flow in times of stress, (2) redistribute blood volume during hemorrhage or shock, and (3) regulate heat loss.

Epinephrine, the hormone released from the adrenal medulla, causes vasoconstriction in most vascular beds (exceptions are the liver and skeletal muscles). However, the effects of norepinephrine (from the sympathetic nervous system and adrenal medulla) are quantitatively more vasoconstrictive than the effects of epinephrine.

The Systemic Renin-Angiotensin System

Renin is an enzyme synthesized and secreted by the juxtaglomerular cells of the kidney. To date, however, renin has also been found in the adrenal cortex, in the salivary gland, in the prolactin-producing and leutinizing hormone-producing cells of the pituitary, in arterial smooth muscle cells in the vascular endothelial cell, in the brain, and in the myocardium (Re, 1987). Factors that control renin release include (1) a drop in blood pressure (e.g., the renal artery); (2) a decrease in the amount of sodium delivered to the kidney (although recent evidence indicates a role for chloride in regulating renin secretion) (Re, 1987); (3) β-adrenergic stimuli stimulate renin release, whereas β-adrenergic inhibitors decrease renin release; (4) angiotensin II reduces renin release; and (5) low potassium concentrations in plasma stimulate renin release.

Once in the circulation, renin splits off a polypeptide from angiotensinogen to generate **angiotensin I.** Angiotensin I appears to be physiologically inactive (Re, 1987). Angiotensin I, however, is converted by an enzyme (kininase II) to **angiotensin II.** Angiotensin II is a powerful vasoconstrictor and also stimulates the secretion of **aldosterone** from the adrenal gland (Fig. 26-33; also see Fig. 17-5). Aldosterone causes reabsorption of sodium in the kidneys. In addition, angiotensin II causes some sodium retention in the kidneys and suppresses renin secretion from the juxtaglomerular cells (Re, 1987; Re et al., 1978). In some tissues, angiotensin II is converted to angiotensin III, which is also biologically active.

The kidney-based renin-angiotensin system serves as an important regulatory loop. For example, decreases in blood pressure or sodium delivery to the kidneys (macula densa), as might occur after hemorrhage or extracellular volume deficits (dehydration), stimulates secretion of renin, which acts in the blood on angiotensinogen to form angiotensin I. Angiotensin I is converted to angiotensin II and restores blood pressure, as well as sodium retention caused by increased secretion of aldosterone. Overall the renin-angiotensin system is activated after volume depletion or hypotension, or both, and is suppressed after volume repletion and hypertension.

TABLE 26-3 Factors that affect mean arterial pressure and capillary flow

	Mean arterial pressure	Capillary flow
Peripheral resistance*		
Increased	Increased	Decreased
Decreased	Decreased	Increased
Heart rate†		
Increased	Increased	Increased
Decreased	Decreased	Decreased
Stroke volume‡		
Increased	Increased	Increased
Decreased	Decreased	Decreased

From Little RC: *Physiology of the heart and circulation,* ed 3, Chicago, 1985, Year Book.
*Cardiac output maintained constant.
†Peripheral resistance and stroke volume constant.
‡Peripheral resistance and heart rate constant.

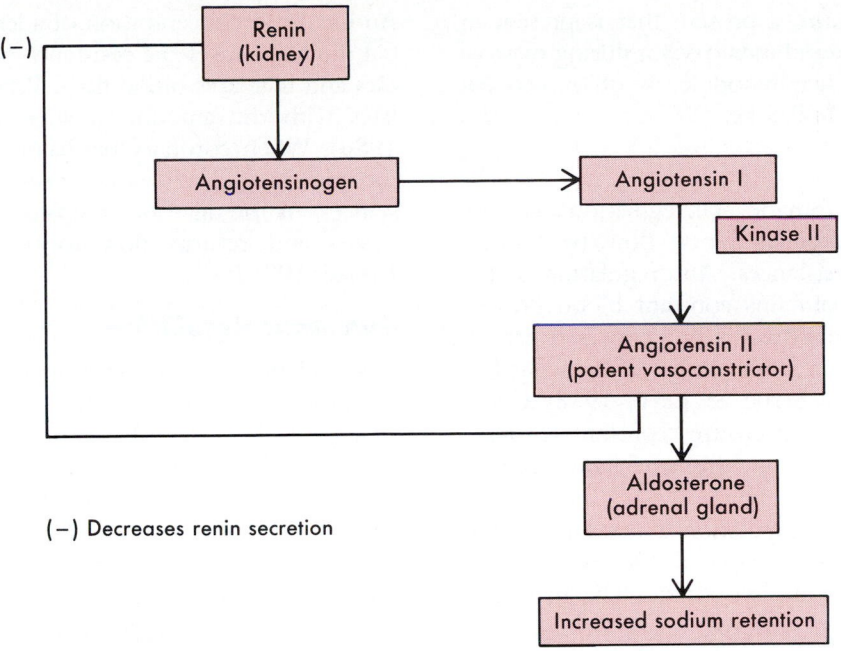

FIG. 26-33. Renin-angiotensin system.

Venous Pressure

The main determinants of venous blood pressure are (1) the volume of fluid within the veins and (2) the compliance (distensibility) of the vessel walls. Veins have much thinner walls than arteries and are more distensible than arteries. The venous system accommodates approximately 60% of the total blood volume at any given moment, with a venous pressure averaging less than 10 mm Hg. Conversely, the arteries accommodate about 15% of the total blood volume, with an average arterial pressure (blood pressure) of about 100 mm Hg (Vander et al., 1980).

The sympathetic nervous system regulates venous blood pressure by controlling compliance. The walls of the veins are highly innervated by sympathetic fibers that, when stimulated, cause venous smooth muscle to contract. This increases muscle tone (i.e., prevents distention) rather than causing vasoconstriction, as occurs in arterial vessels. The effect of increased muscle tone is to stiffen the wall of the vein, which reduces distensibility and increases blood pressure. The increased venous pressure forces more blood through the veins and into the right heart.

Two other mechanisms that increase venous pressure and venous return to the heart are (1) the skeletal muscle pump and (2) the respiratory pump. During skeletal muscle contraction, the veins within the muscles are partially compressed, causing a decrease in venous capacity and increased return to the heart. The respiratory pump acts during inspiration, when the veins of the ab-

domen are partially compressed by the downward movement of the diaphragm. Increased abdominal pressure moves blood toward the heart.

Regulation of the Coronary Circulation

Flow of blood (F) in the coronary circulation, as in vascular beds, is directly proportional to the perfusion pressure (P) and inversely proportional to the vascular resistance (R) of the bed ($F = P/R$). **Coronary perfusion pressure** is the difference between pressure in the aorta and pressure in the coronary vessels of the right atrium. Aortic pressure is the driving pressure that perfuses vessels of the myocardium. Mechanisms of vasodilation and vasoconstriction normally maintain coronary blood flow despite stresses imposed by the constant contraction and relaxation of the heart muscle and despite shifts (within a physiologic range) of coronary perfusion pressure.

Several anatomic factors influence coronary blood flow. Because of their location, the aortic valve cusps obstruct coronary blood flow by pushing against the openings of the coronary arteries during systole. Also during systole, the coronary arteries are compressed by ventricular contraction. These anatomic factors have a **systolic compressive effect,** which is particularly evident in the subendocardial layers of the left ventricular wall and can greatly decrease coronary blood flow. Therefore most coronary blood flow in the left ventricle occurs during diastole. During the period of systolic compression, when flow is slowed or stopped, oxygen is supplied by **myoglobulin,** a protein that is present in heart muscle. This protein binds oxygen during diastole and then releases it when blood levels of oxygen fall during systole (Sparks & Rooke, 1987).

Autoregulation

Autoregulation (automatic self-regulation) enables individual vessels to regulate blood flow by altering their own arteriolar resistances. Autoregulation in the coronary circulation maintains constant blood flow at perfusion pressures (mean arterial pressure) between 60 and 180 mm Hg, provided that other influencing factors are held constant (Berne & Levy, 1988; Cohn, 1985). Thus autoregulation ensures constant coronary blood flow despite shifts in the perfusion pressure within the stated range.

The mechanism of autoregulation is not known, but two explanations have been proposed: the myogenic hypothesis and the metabolic hypothesis. The myogenic hypothesis proposes that autoregulation originates in vascular smooth muscle, presumably of the arterioles, as a response to an increase in arterial pressure. According to the myogenic hypothesis of autoregulation, smooth muscle stretches in response to an increase in perfusion pressure. The stretching eventually stimulates contraction of the smooth muscles, which increases vascular resistance. Initially, coronary blood flow increases with the abrupt distention of the blood vessels. The return of more normal flow follows constriction of the arterioles. This mechanism also works in the opposite direction; that is, vasodilation is stimulated by decreased arterial pressure (Sparks & Rooke, 1987).

The myogenic hypothesis illustrates the law of Laplace (tension = pressure × radius). Increased coronary perfusion pressure increases the pressure against the vessel wall, and the stretch increases the vessel's radius, resulting in an increase in wall tension. The increase in tension stimulates constriction of the vessel to a radius less than the original radius, so that the product of pressure (increased) times radius (decreased) is restored to normal.

The metabolic hypothesis of autoregulation, which is better documented, proposes that autoregulation of coronary vessels originates in the myocardium. The stimulus is a drop in coronary perfusion pressure or an increase in the metabolic needs of the myocardium (e.g., because of strenuous exercise). The metabolic hypothesis proposes that with an increased myocardial oxygen requirement, myocardial cells release substances that promote vasodilation. The best known of these substances is adenosine, a potent vasodilator released in response to a decrease in myocardial oxygenation. Low coronary blood flow, hypoxemia, or increased metabolic activity of the heart can all increase the heart muscle's need for oxygen (Berne, 1980; Berne & Levy, 1988).

An increased concentration of adenosine in the interstitial fluid decreases the resistance of the coronary arterioles and increases blood flow. Perfusion strongly correlates with the amount of adenosine released (Berne, 1980). When coronary perfusion pressure is increased, the increased flow washes out the vasodilatory substances. As the dilators are washed out, vasoconstriction occurs and returns flow toward normal (Sparks & Rooke, 1987).

Autonomic Regulation

Stimulation of the sympathetic nerves to the heart causes a marked increase in coronary blood flow, even though it also causes vasoconstriction of the coronary vessels. Why? The increase in coronary flow is due to acceleration of heart rate and enhancement of myocardial contractility (more forceful systole). Although the longer, forceful myocardial contraction and the tachycardia (heart rate greater than 100 beats/min) tend to restrict coronary flow, the increase in myocardial metabolism tends to counteract these factors by dilating the coronary arterioles (Berne & Levy, 1988). Therefore the net effect of sympathetic stimulation is to increase coronary blood flow.

Although the coronary vessels themselves contain sympathetic (α- and β-adrenergic) and parasympathetic neural receptors, coronary blood flow is regulated locally through metabolic autoregulation. Metabolic autoregulation overrides neurogenic influences (Berne & Levy, 1988; Schlant et al., 1986).

THE LYMPHATIC SYSTEM

The lymphatic system is a special vascular system that picks up excess tissue fluid and returns it to the bloodstream. Normally, fluid is forced out of the blood at the arterial end of the capillary bed and is reabsorbed into the bloodstream at the venous end. Yet not all of this interstitial fluid returns to the blood at the venous end; capillary outflow exceeds venous reabsorption by about 3L/day. Thus some fluid lags behind in the interstitium. To maintain sufficient blood volume in the cardiovascular system, this fluid must eventually rejoin the bloodstream. Returning interstitial fluid to the bloodstream is the function of the lymphatic system.

The lymphatic system consists of lymphatic vessels and the lymph nodes (Fig. 26-34). (Lymph nodes are described in Chapter 8). It is a pumpless system in which a series of valves ensure one-way flow of the excess interstitial fluid (now called lymph) toward the heart. The lymphatic capillaries are closed at the ends as shown in Fig. 26-35.

Lymph consists primarily of water and small amounts of dissolved proteins, mostly albumin, that are too large

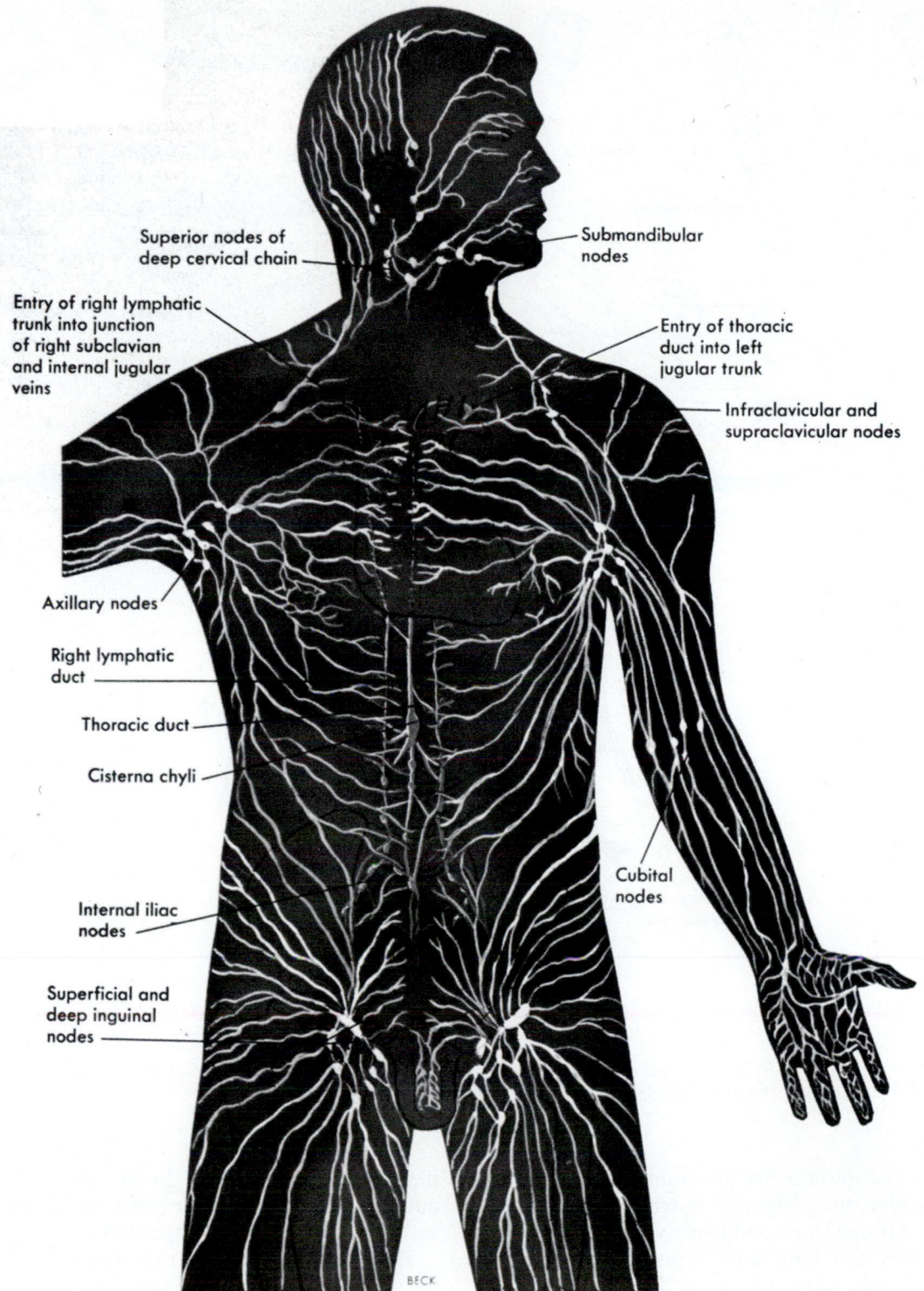

FIG. 26-34. Schematic representation of lymphatic vessels, larger lymphatic trunks, and lymph nodes. (From Thibodeau, 1987.)

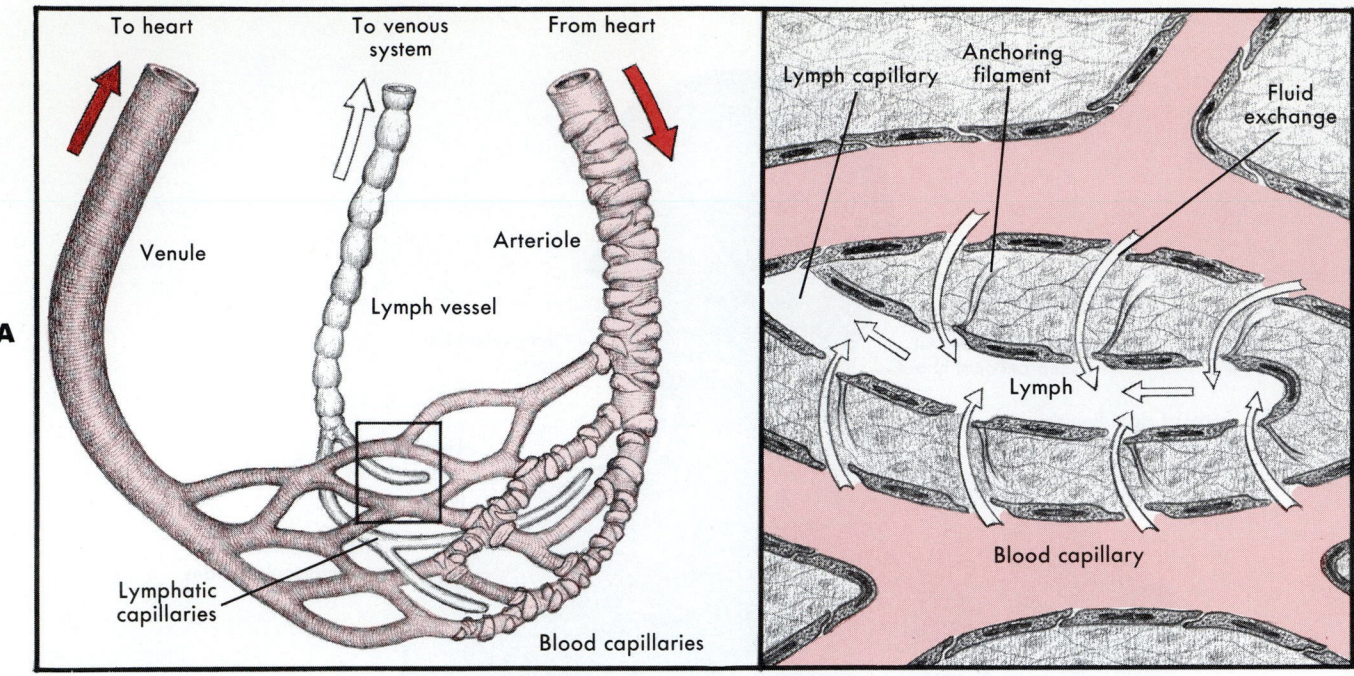

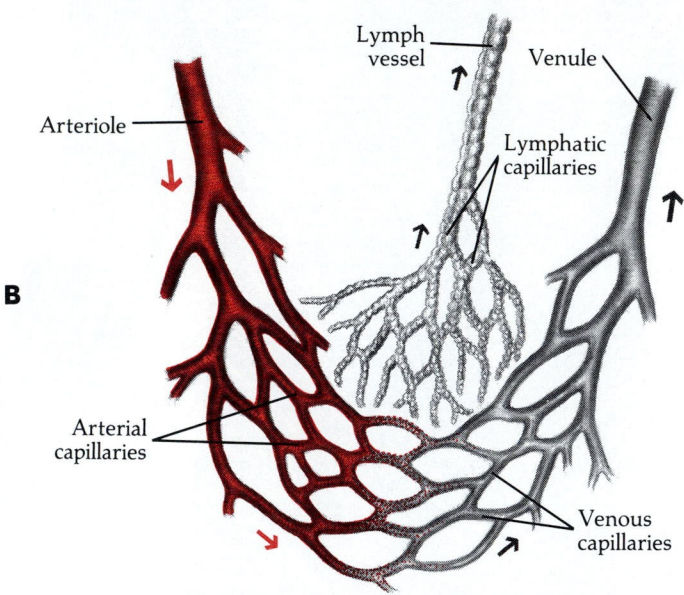

FIG. 26-35. **A,** Schematic representation of lymphatic capillaries. **B,** Anatomic components of microcirculation. (From Thompson, 1989.)

to be reabsorbed into the less permeable blood capillaries. Once within the lymphatic system, lymph travels successively through larger and larger vessels called **lymphatic venules** and **lymphatic veins.** The lymphatic vessels run in the same sheaths with the arteries and veins and eventually drain into one of two large ducts in the thorax, the right lymphatic duct and the thoracic duct. The **right lymphatic duct** drains lymph from the right arm and the right side of the head and thorax, whereas the larger **thoracic duct** receives lymph from

the rest of the body (Fig. 26-34). The right lymphatic duct and the thoracic duct drain lymph into the right and left subclavian vein, respectively.

The lymphatic veins are thin walled like the veins of the cardiovascular system. In the larger lymphatic veins, endothelial flaps form valves similar to those in the circulatory veins (see Fig. 26-26). The valves permit lymph to flow in only one direction because lymphatic vessels are compressed intermittently by contraction of skeletal muscles, pulsatile expansion of an artery in the same sheath, and contraction of the smooth muscles in the walls of the lymphatic vessel (Vick, 1984).

As lymph is transported toward the heart, it is filtered through thousands of bean-shaped lymph nodes clustered along the lymphatic vessels (see Fig. 26-34). Lymph enters the node through several **afferent lymphatic vessels,** filters through the sinuses in the node, and leaves by way of **efferent lymphatic vessels.** Lymph flows slowly through the node, which facilitates the phagocytosis of foreign substances within the node and prevents them from reentering the bloodstream. (Phagocytosis is described in Chapter 7.)

TESTS OF CARDIOVASCULAR FUNCTION

Historically, cardiac function was first measured by subjective means and by simple objective observations that included the individual's sensorium, mucous membrane color, and a manually palpated pulse. Currently, there are many sophisticated ways to measure heart function, ranging from no-risk, noninvasive electrocardiography to relatively high-risk, invasive cardiac catheterization.

Noninvasive Assessment of Function
Sensorium of the Individual

Often, the first observation indicating an impairment of cardiac function is a decreased level of consciousness. Should the pumping ability of the heart decrease for whatever reason, the amount and pressure of blood ejected from the heart will decrease. Consequently, the amount and pressure of blood that reaches all body tissues will be insufficient to supply oxygen and nutrients to cells and remove waste products.

Perhaps no other system is more sensitive to a decrease in oxygen and nutrient supply (particularly of glucose) than the central nervous system. A decrease in cardiac pumping ability, if sufficiently severe, will almost immediately be followed by a decrease in neural efficiency, which includes impairment of mentation and such simple motor functions as conjugate gaze, enunciation, and pupillary reflexes (see Chapters 12 and 13).

Mucous Membrane Color

Provided that lung, blood, and vessel structure and function are normal, a darkening or bluing of the mucous membranes, called cyanosis, signifies decreased cardiac function. Mucous membrane color is a reflection of hemoglobin saturation in the capillary blood (see Chapters 22 and 29). Well-oxygenated (well-saturated) hemoglobin takes on a bright red color, whereas poorly oxygenated hemoglobin is dark red or purple. These colors are best observed in the mucous membranes (for

example, the conjunctivae, gums, nail beds, and genitalia), where the capillary network is dense and the epithelium is thin.

Cardiac function indirectly affects the affinity of hemoglobin for oxygen. If blood is delivered at a decreased rate to the capillary beds, two changes occur. First, hemoglobin will come in contact with tissues for an extended time, allowing more oxygen to diffuse into the tissues. The capillary blood will darken, as will mucous membranes. Second, a decrease in the amount of oxygen delivered per minute to the tissues will result in a metabolic acidosis, as cells switch from aerobic to anaerobic metabolism and produce lactic acid. Interstitial pH and capillary blood pH will drop. Acidosis causes more oxygen to dissociate from hemoglobin and diffuse out of the capillaries (see Chapter 29). Capillary blood in mucous membranes will darken further.

Manually Palpated Pulse

If cardiac function is impaired, the pulse will be affected. When palpated, changes in the radial, femoral, and carotid pulses offer information regarding heart rate, regularity of heart rhythm, the length and strength of ventricular systole, and peripheral artery patency. A decrease in cardiac function may be detected as a decrease in pulsatile strength. A bilateral comparison of pulses may reveal decreased pulsatile flow unilaterally, in which case arterial narrowing or occlusion would be suspected.

Irregular heartbeats (dysrhythmias) may be reflected in changes in pulse rhythmicity and pulse pressure per beat. Turbulent blood flow caused by valve or septal disease may be reflected in the carotid pulses and felt as a "thrill." A pulsatile thrill elsewhere may indicate the presence of a fistula, or opening, between an artery and a nearby vein.

Auscultation of Heart Sounds

Auscultation (auditory examination) of the heart is done with a stethoscope placed over the valve, chamber, or great vessel being examined. Different sounds are normally heard over different heart structures during systole and diastole. The dominant sounds are made by the four heart valves as they close. The first sound, S_1, is made by atrioventricular valve closure. The second, S_2, is made by closure of the aortic and pulmonic semilunar valves. The first two heart sounds provide information about heart rate, heart rhythm, and the length of ventricular systole.

Abnormal heart sounds indicate abnormalities of the heart valves or chamber walls. In healthy adults, only S_1 and S_2 can be heard. Abnormalities of these sounds or detection of the third and fourth heart sounds (S_3 and S_4) indicates disease. The mechanisms causing the normal heart sounds are listed in Table 26-4. Causes of ab-

TABLE 26-4 Normal heart sounds

Sound	Event in cardiac style	Cause of sound	Comments
First sound (S_1)	Beginning of ventricular systole	Closure of atrioventricular valves, particularly mitral valve	With S_2, the loudest heart sound normally heard
Second sound (S_2)	End of ventricular systole	Closure of semilunar valves, particularly aortic valves	With S_1, the loudest heart sound normally heard
Third sound (S_3)	Early ventricular diastole (filling)	Vibration of ventricular walls as blood rushes in	Normally heard only in children and young adults
Fourth sound (S_4)	Atrial systole during late ventricular diastole (filling)	Uncertain, but thought to be the result of a sudden change in filling rate (i.e., shudder of the left ventricle)	Rarely heard in the normal heart

normal heart sounds, or **adventitious sounds,** are listed in Table 26-5.

Cardiography

Electrocardiography, typically the 12-lead electrocardiogram (ECG), gives information about heart rate and rhythm, the effects of electrolytes or drugs on the heart, and the electrical orientation of the cardiac muscle. An ECG gives no direct information about the contractile state or mechanical performance of the heart.

Einthoven's triangle places the heart in the center of a triangle, with angles placed at the right shoulder, left shoulder, and the pubic area. Body fluids conduct electrical potential differences that can be detected by bipolar or unipolar electrical leads placed on the skin. Einthoven's triangle gives a triaxial (three-axis) reference for the detection of cardiac electrical potentials.

Serial 12-lead ECGs are of primary importance in establishing the presence of myocardial infarction. This examination has become part of the routine hospital admission assessment, even when the admitting diagnosis is not cardiac in nature, because it establishes baseline information about the electrical function of the heart. Also, recent ECGs can be compared to ECGs obtained from the same individual in the past. Changes in the ECG over time assist in determining the cause, amount, or nature of changes in cardiac anatomy and physiology over time. Fig. 26-11 depicts a normal ECG.

In conjunction with a 12-lead ECG, a vectorcardiogram can assist to (1) precisely locate the site of a myocardial infarction, (2) diagnose conduction defects, and (3) diagnose chamber hypertrophy. Commonly, five electrodes are placed over the precordium, one electrode is placed on the left leg, and one is placed on the back of the neck. Recorded in conjunction with the ECG, the electrodes of the vectorcardiogram provide a series of dots over time that represent the vector of the heart in microseconds.

TABLE 26-5 Abnormal heart sounds

Sound	Cause of sound	Typical underlying abnormality
Accentuated S_1	Forceful closure of mitral valve	Rapid heart rate resulting from exercise, anemia, or hyperthyroidism Mitral valve stenosis (narrowing)
Diminished S_1	Premature partial closure of the mitral valve before systole, so that systole causes only the completion of closure	Prolonged diastole resulting from blockage in conduction system that slows impulse conduction to or within the atrioventricular node
	Failure of the mitral valve to close completely	Mitral valve incompetence (regurgitation)

TABLE 26-5   Abnormal heart sounds—cont'd

Sound	Cause of sound	Typical underlying abnormality
Accentuated S_2	Forceful closure of the aortic or pulmonic semilunar valve, which closes late and must close quickly	Prolonged systole resulting from high blood pressure in the systemic or pulmonary circulation; systole is slightly prolonged so as to force all the blood out against high pressure
	Valvular stiffness, which increases the impact of closure	Aortic valve syphilis
Diminshed S_2	Gentle closure of aortic semilunar valve	Low blood pressure in the systemic arteries, which reduces pressure that pushes valve leaflets shut
	Gentle closure of aortic semilunar valve caused by incomplete opening	Aortic stenosis
Split heart sounds (S_1 and S_2)	Delayed closure of various heart valves, usually caused by late right ventricular systole	Normal increase in venous return to the right heart with inspiration Conduction defects involving the right or left bundle branches Defect of the interatrial septum that raises pressures in the right heart Pulmonic semilunar valve stenosis, which causes delayed closure
Gallop sounds S_3 (in adults)	Possibly the "thud" of blood hitting noncompliant ventricular walls at the start of ventricular filling	Myocardial damage that stiffens muscle and prevents relaxation during systole
S_4 (in children)	Ejection of blood into overfilled ventricle during atrial systole	Incomplete emptying of ventricle during systole of preceding cardiac cycle, causing overfilling and overdistention during next cycle; causes include myocardial damage or disease, aortic stenosis, high blood pressure, fluid overload (see Chapter 3)
Murmurs	Turbulent blood flow at high blood pressure	Irregularity, constriction, or dilation of any structure that blood flows through, such as valvular stenosis or incompetence, perforation of interatrial or interventricular septum
		Increased rate of flow (blood flow) through normal structures (e.g., during pregnancy)
Rub	Friction within the pericardium, usually caused by disruption of the pericardial fluid; loss of fluid causes the visceral and parietal pericardium to rub against one another	Surgery, infection, inflammation, or adhesion that damages the parietal or visceral pericardium
Click	Sudden, abnormal movement of an aortic or pulmonic semilunar valve leaflet	Valve prolapse, in which valve leaflets open backward as well as forward; usually resulting from increased in valve opening (anulus)
Snap	Opening of stenotic (stiff) atrioventricular valve (mitral or tricuspid)	Atrioventricular valve stenosis
Hum	Vibration of heart walls or vessel walls caused by movement usually during turbulent blood flow at low pressure	Irregularity of any structure that blood flows through; normal in jugular veins of children

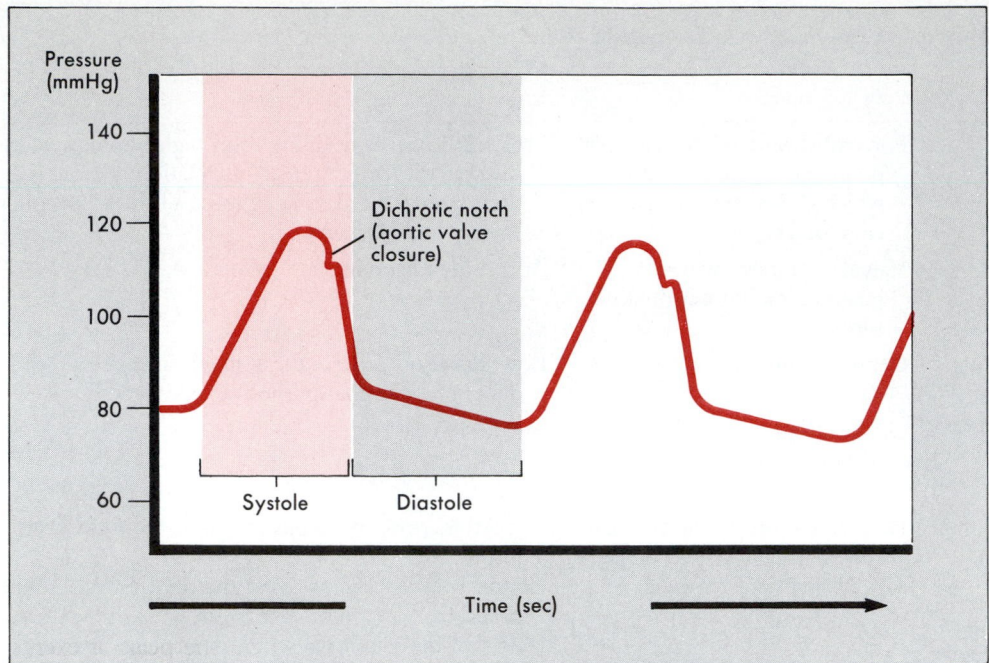

FIG. 26-36. Arterial pulse waveforms.

Pulse Tracing

The pulsation described by the flow of blood through an artery during the cardiac cycle can be drawn as a waveform plotting pressure against time (Fig. 26-36). The waveform can be obtained noninvasively by placing a transducer on the skin over the carotid artery, while the individual's head is turned slightly away from the transducer. In conjunction with phonocardiography and an ECG, the arterial pulse tracing gives a reference for the phonocardiograph and assists in the timing of the events of the cardiac cycle.

Like an arterial pulse tracing, a venous pulse tracing gives a reference for the phonocardiograph and assists in the timing of the cardiac cycle. A venous pulse tracing is obtained by placing a transducer over the jugular vein at the supraclavicular area near the manubrium. A waveform is produced that reflects pressures in the vein over time during the cardiac cycle.

Vibrations at the apex of the heart during the cardiac cycle are recorded by placing a transducer at the point of maximal impulse. An apexcardiogram is used to assist in the timing of the cardiac cycle and is made along with a phonocardiogram and an ECG.

A phonocardiogram is made by placing microphones over the precordium. An ECG is recorded simultaneously as a reference point. By recording the sounds made during the cardiac cycle, the phonocardiogram can assist to time the events and length of diastole and systole. Abnormal sounds can also be examined more closely for timing, characteristics, and sources of those sounds.

An echocardiogram is an ultrasonic examination. The skin is first prepared by applying a lubricating agent (usually cooking oil), and a piezoelectric crystal is placed against the chest. Ultrasonic sound waves are then generated and directed into the cardiac structures that reflect the waves at different angles and lengths according to structure and density. The crystal picks up these deflected waves and passes them through a transducer, which transforms the waves into electrical impulses. The impulses are displayed on an oscilloscope and are viewed with a simultaneously recorded ECG.

Like an ECG, an echocardiogram is recorded continuously over time so that changes in the heart during the cardiac cycle (such as valve position, chamber size, and myocardial wall position) can be examined. Information about cardiac anatomy and function, including stroke volume and cardiac output, is gained.

Doppler Studies

A Doppler study is made by using a hand-held microphone placed on the skin over a lubricating gel. The microphone amplifies and can record sounds made by blood flowing in peripheral vessels. The Doppler microphone is placed over the vessel to be studied, and sounds related to obstructions to flow, vessel wall mobility, and heart murmurs are transmitted through the gel to the microphone. The microphone amplifies sound waves so that they are audible to the human ear.

Stress Testing

Cardiac activity during exercise is examined during a stress test. Stress testing elicits signs and symptoms of heart disease and coronary artery disease that may not appear at rest. A 12-lead ECG, blood pressure measurement, and bipolar ECG strip-recording are done before the study and at regular intervals during and after the study. Cardiac stress from exercise is induced by having the individual walk on a treadmill. Other, less frequently used forms of exercise include stair climbing (the Master's double two-step) and bicycle ergometry. The individual exercises until the maximal heart rate for sex and age is reached or until other subjective or objective indicators of cardiac dysfunction or distress appear. Subjective indicators include chest pain, extreme fatigue, extreme dyspnea, leg pain, or the individual's request to stop the test. Objective criteria are ST segment elevation or depression, SA node or atrial dysrhythmias, atrioventricular node dysrhythmias, ventricular dysrhythmias, elevated or decreased blood pressure, signs of cerebral hypoxia, and signs of circulatory insufficiency.

A stress test is also useful in determining the rate or progress of recovery from a myocardial infarction or cardiac surgery. When a differential diagnosis for chest pain has been difficult to determine, stress testing may help distinguish coronary artery insufficiency from other causes of pain. There is some risk associated with stress testing. The mortality rate is about 1 per 10,000, and the morbidity rate is approximately 24 per 10,000 (Rochmis & Blackburn, 1971).

Chest X-ray Examinations

In a chest x-ray examination, the size and contour of the heart and related structures are visualized. A chest x-ray examination is a routine part of a cardiac examination. The most commonly obtained views are anteriorposterior and lateral, with the individual upright and the lungs fully expanded.

Invasive Assessment of Cardiac Function

Invasive studies generally carry a greater risk to the individual than noninvasive studies, with the possible exception of stress testing. Ingestion of substances is considered invasive.

X-ray Films with Barium

The cardiac silhouette obtained with routine radiographic studies of the chest can be enhanced by ingestion of barium. The contrast medium causes the esophagus to appear as white on the x-ray film, creating a bright background against which the heart is more distinctly outlined. X-ray films are taken using four different axes.

Nuclear Imaging with Radiolabeled Pharmaceuticals

Technetium pyrophosphate (^{99m}TcPYP) is injected intravenously into a resting individual during a hot spot imaging examination. Two hours after injection, the distribution pattern of the radioactive solution is recorded by nuclear scan. During the 2-hour delay, the injected material will have been taken up by infarcted areas of the myocardium, particularly 1 to 3 days after the onset of symptoms. This study is not definitive during the first 12 hours after an infarct.

Hot spot imaging is used when (1) there is a conflicting history for myocardial infarction, (2) there are equivocal ECG abnormalities, or (3) an individual's cardiac enzymes have been elevated because of surgery or trauma. Such small amounts of the injected material are used in this examination that the risks associated with radioactive substances are not an issue.

Thallium is the radioactive substance injected intravenously during a perfusion imaging examination. During stress testing and at the peak of exercise, thallium is injected intravenously. After a 1- or 2-minute delay, the distribution of thallium within the myocardium is determined by nuclear scan, and again after a period of rest. Thallium typically is not taken up by areas of ischemic or infarcted myocardium, creating "cold spots." Cold spots disappear at rest if the ischemia is reversible and remain at rest if infarction has occurred. Perfusion imaging is useful to differentiate a myocardial infarction from reversible angina (cardiac pain) in the presence of conflicting or equivocal enzymatic and historical data. Risks associated with perfusion imaging are the same as for stress testing. No risk attributable to the small quantity of injected material has been documented.

Atrioventricular Bundle Electrocardiography

Two electrode-tipped catheters are inserted percutaneously into the femoral vein, floated up the inferior vena cava, and positioned in or near the right atrium during atrioventricular bundle (His bundle) electrocardiography. The first electrode is quadripolar and is lodged against the right atrial wall. Two poles of this electrode record the difference in electrical potential between two points, and the other two poles are a pacing electrode and a ground (that allow for pacing of the right atrium). The second electrode is bipolar and is placed across the tricuspid valve, at the location of the bundle of His, and records the electrical potentials across the bundle. These recordings across the bundle divide the P-R interval into two segments: (1) the atrial-His interval (AHI), and (2) the His-ventricular interval. The atrial-His interval is the interval from the onset of atrial electrical activity to the arrival of the impulse at the bundle of His. The His-ventricular interval is the interval between the passage of the impulse through the His bundle and the passage of the impulse through the ventricular conduction system and muscle.

His bundle electrocardiography can detect secondary sites of impulse generation (ectopic foci), as well as accessory pathways of conduction. Other conduction defects and the effects of drugs on conduction can also be illuminated. Risks related to this procedure can be grave and include dysrhythmias, death, vessel or heart perforation, clot or plaque embolization, and kidney failure.

Cardiac Catheterization

One or both sides of the heart can be examined using cardiac catheterization. This procedure requires the use of fluoroscopy and strict sterile techniques and takes place in a specially equipped catheterization laboratory. Local anesthesia is given, and a catheter is introduced percutaneously into the vasculature and passed caudally into the atrium and ventricle. For a right-heart catheterization, the catheter is placed in the brachial or femoral vein. The femoral artery is commonly used for a left-heart study. Once the catheter has been guided into the atrium, pressures are recorded, blood samples are obtained to examine oxygen content, and a contrast medium is injected to visualize chamber function and valve patency. The catheter is then passed into the ventricles and the sequence repeated.

Cardiac catheterization provides a means to visualize the chambers of the heart continuously, although for a short time. A great deal of information can be obtained about heart structure and function. Pressures in each chamber and across heart valves can be precisely measured, along with timing of events in the cardiac cycle.

TABLE 26-6 Indicators of cardiac function

Indicator	Definition*	Common cause of abnormality
Heart rate (HR)	Number of heartbeats (cardiac cycles) per minute Normal adult value: 70 beats/min	Dysrhythmia
Cardiac output (CO)	Amount of blood (in liters) moved by the heart in 1 minute Normal range: 4-8 L/min	Decrease indicates heart failure
Cardiac index (CI)	Relationship between cardiac output and body surface area (BSA, in square meters) Normal range: 2.8-4.2 L/min/m²	Disturbance of perfusion pressure
Stroke volume (SV)	Amount of blood (in milliliters) ejected by the left ventricle during systole; i.e., per beat Normal range: 60-100 ml/beat	Disturbance of contractility
Stroke volume index (SVI)	Relationship between stroke volume and body surface area Normal range: 33-47 ml/beat/m²	Decrease indicates possible decrease of myocardial contractility (force of systole); heart failure
Oxygen consumption index (VO₂I)	Amount of oxygen (VO₂ in milliliters) consumed per minute in relation to body surface area	Decrease indicates decrease in coronary blood flow
Stroke work index (SWI)	Amount of work (expressed as done) by the left or right ventricle per systole per square meter of body surface area Normal value: 35 gmM	Decreases within specific ranges indicate cardiogenic or hypovolemic shock (see Chapter 27)
Systemic mean arterial pressure (MAP)	Mean blood pressure (in millimeters of mercury) in the systemic arteries Normal range: 70-100 mm Hg	Hypertension or hypotension
Pulmonary vascular resistance (PVR)	Relationship between cardiac output, preload, and afterload, expressed as units of force of resistance per second per centimeter of water Normal value: less than 250 dyn/sec/cm⁻⁵	Congestive heart failure
Systemic vascular resistance (SVR)	Same definition as for PVR Normal range: 770-1500 dyn/sec/cm⁻⁵	Hypertension or hypotension

*Values given are for adults at rest.

Of particular value is the ability to compare the oxygen content of blood in each heart chamber.

Risks for this procedure have decreased over time and mortality rates range from 0.1% to 0.3% (Abrams, 1983). Morbidity rates, including serious and relatively minor complications, ranged from 3.1% to 10.1% in 1968 (Braunwald, 1968), but are quoted currently as less than 0.5% (Silverman & Neeld, 1984). One of the most serious complications of cardiac catheterization is the development of dysrhythmias. Death is usually caused by cardiac arrest after ventricular fibrillation.

Coronary Angiography

Fluoroscopic visualization of the coronary arteries and left heart structures using contrast dye is called coronary angiography or arteriography. Like cardiac catheterization, this study takes place in a catheterization laboratory using local anesthesia and a sterile field. A catheter is threaded into the left ventricle through the femoral artery. A ventriculogram is generally performed first. Contrast dye is injected into the apex of the ventricle and the next few cardiac cycles are visualized and filmed. The contrast dye used is 66% diatrizoate meglumine and 10% diatrizoate sodium, an iodine preparation that is not tolerated by individuals who are allergic to iodine. Like cardiac catheterization, coronary angiography is used to gain information about the structure and function of the ventricle and related valves.

After the ventriculogram, catheters are introduced individually into the ostia of the coronary arteries. When the catheter is in position, 5 to 10 ml of contrast dye is mechanically and rapidly injected into the artery, and the results are visualized and filmed. Dye injection is repeated with the individual tilted at various angles to afford views of the artery other than the anterior-posterior view. The catheter is then either moved to the next artery to be studied or withdrawn to conclude the study. Pressures in the left side of the heart are usually obtained, but blood samples are not. The right side of the heart is not studied.

The risks of this procedure are similar to those of cardiac catheterization, but with exceptions. Because the blood supply to the cardiac muscle is briefly interrupted when dye is introduced into the coronary arteries, angina (chest pain) caused by ischemia (lack of perfusion) is much more common. Coronary artery spasms can also occur. Interrupted flow also causes decreased heart rate (bradycardia, as well as some tachydysrhythmias), hypotension, and ST segment depression. The administration of nitroglycerin sublingually or directly into the coronary artery can dilate the artery sufficiently to alleviate ischemic complications. Persistent bradycardia is corrected by having the individual cough to stimulate the heart rate or, in severe cases, by the administration of atropine. Bradycardia is such a common complication

that a temporary pacer is often introduced into the right ventricle through the femoral vein at the beginning of coronary angiography. Heparin is given to avoid thrombus formation. The effects of heparin may be reversed after the procedure by using protamine.

Combined Indicators of Cardiac Function

Cardiac function can be evaluated using indicators calculated from pressures and flow rates in the heart and vessels. Table 26-6 defines the indicators most frequently used in the clinical setting.

AGING AND THE CARDIOVASCULAR SYSTEM

Cardiovascular disease is the most common cause of hospitalization and death in the elderly population in Western society. The most common cardiovascular pathologic condition is coronary atherosclerosis. It is difficult to describe normal physiologic changes in cardiac function with aging because many pathologic changes are usually present as well. Studies of the effect of age on cardiovascular function must be rigorous in their distinction between persons who are free of disease and those who have disease that may only be evident during stress testing. To obtain an understanding of the effects of age on cardiovascular functioning it is, therefore, necessary to consider cardiac performance at rest and during exercise.

Resting Cardiac Performance

For many years it has been believed that advanced age is associated with a progressive decline in resting cardiovascular function. The physiologic changes were reported to involve most of the major determinants of cardiac performance: heart rate, cardiac output, blood volume, filling rate, filling volume, afterload, and blood pressure. However, recent studies are challenging these findings.

The Baltimore Longitudinal Study on Aging (BLSA) was conducted in a group of 61 participants, ranging from 26 to 79 years of age, who were free of heart disease (Rodeheffer et al., 1984). The volunteers were active but not conditioned athletes. Subjects were studied in the upright position at rest and during progressive bicycle exercise to exhaustion. In contrast to previous studies, there were no age-related changes in cardiac output. Resting heart rate has been reported to be unchanged with age (Strandell, 1964), but there was a trend toward lower heart rates in the BLSA subjects. Resting stroke volume has previously been reported to be decreased or unchanged with age (Julius et al., 1967; Strandell, 1964), but there was a slight age-related increase in stroke volume at rest in the BLSA population.

TABLE 26-7 Resting cardiac function in the elderly: a comparison of new and old data

Determinant	Previous studies	Baltimore Longitudinal Study
Cardiac output	Decreased	No change
Heart rate	No change	Slight decrease
Stroke volume	Decreased or unchanged	Slight increase
Ejection fraction	Unchanged	Unchanged
Afterload (systolic blood pressure)	Increased	Increased
End-diastolic volume	Unchanged	Unchanged
End-systolic volume	Unchanged	Unchanged
Contraction	Increased	Increased because of prolonged relaxation

Thus, the lack of any change in cardiac output in the BLSA subjects is possibly related to the slight decrease in heart rate and slight increase in stroke volume. Table 26-7 summarizes both the findings of the BLSA study and previous findings of resting cardiac function in the elderly.

In summary, resting healthy/fit subjects show no age-related changes in cardiac output or heart rate, and a small increase in stroke volume. No age-related changes were noted in cardiac volume and the ejection fraction; however, there may be an increase in the resting vascular components of left ventricular afterload with increasing age. There is also evidence of an age-related prolonged and delayed left ventricular relaxation in humans and in animal models (Rodeheffer & Gerstenblith, 1985).

Exercise Cardiac Performance

Stress testing is used to uncover changes in functional capacity that are not apparent at rest. Previous studies have reported an age-related decrease in maximal oxygen consumption (Julius et al., 1967; Robinson et al., 1973). Recent studies have shown that this decline in maximal oxygen consumption can be altered but not completely eliminated in elderly athletes. The decline in maximal oxygen consumption is present when statistically correcting for changes in lean body mass. The decrease in maximal oxygen consumption may be due to decreased cardiac function, decreased pulmonary gas exchange capacity, and altered distribution of peripheral blood flow (Gerstenblith, Lakatta, & Weisfeldt, 1976). Previous studies have also reported a decrease in car-

diac output with exercise in elderly individuals (Gerstenblith et al., 1976; Julius et al., 1967), but there was no age-related decrease in cardiac output in the BLSA study, even at high levels of exercise. The components of cardiac output, however, showed significant age-related alterations. As reported by others, there was a decrease in heart rate as a function of age. Exercise stroke volume, however, increased significantly and to such an extent that the elderly were able to maintain a cardiac output comparable to that of young subjects who had lower heart rates.

Examination of the ventricular volumes in the BLSA participants provided important information for understanding mechanisms by which young people and older people are able to maintain the same cardiac output. The end-diastolic volume (preload) remained at resting levels in young subjects at high levels of exercise, whereas end-systolic volume decreased significantly. In elderly subjects the end-diastolic volume increased at low levels of exercise and continued to increase progressively at higher levels of exercise. End-systolic volumes in elderly subjects also increased with exercise, although less significantly. The implications of these findings are that young people maintain cardiac output by achieving a high heart rate and *healthy* older individuals maintain cardiac output by dilating the ventricle and using the Frank-Starling mechanism to increase stroke volume (Rodeheffer & Gerstenblith, 1985).

Contrary to other studies, the BLSA found no age-related increase with exercise for systolic blood pressure and systemic vascular resistance. Ejection fraction in the BLSA subjects decreased with age at high levels of exercise but rarely fell below resting baseline.

In summary, previous investigators have stated that a decrease in exercise cardiac output is characteristic of adult aging. The BLSA challenges these findings and reports that cardiac output is preserved in fit elderly subjects; the findings in the BLSA stand in contrast to other studies.

Unlike previous studies, the BLSA subjects were not physically deconditioned and were free of clinically detectable ischemic heart disease. These two factors probably explain why they had preserved cardiac function, even at vigorous levels of exercise (Rodeheffer & Gerstenblith, 1985).

SUMMARY REVIEW

The Circulatory System

1 The circulatory system is the body's transport system. It delivers oxygen, nutrients, metabolites, hormones, neurochemicals, proteins, and blood cells through the body and carries metabolic wastes to the kidneys and lungs for excretion.

2 The circulatory system consists of the heart and blood vessels and is made up of two separate, serially connected systems: the pulmonary circulation and the systemic circulation.

3 The pulmonary circulation is driven by the right side of the heart. The function of the pulmonary circulation is to deliver blood to the lungs for oxygenation.

4 The systemic circulation is driven by the left side of the heart, and its function is to move oxygenated blood throughout the body.

5 The lymphatic vessels collect fluids from the interstitium and return the fluids to the circulatory system.

The Heart

1 The heart consists of four chambers (two atria and two ventricles), four valves (two atrioventricular valves and two semilunar valves), a muscular wall, a fibrous skeleton, a conduction sytem, nerve fibers, systemic vessels (the coronary circulation), and openings where the great vessels enter the atria and ventricles.

2 The heart wall, which encloses the heart and divides it into chambers, is made up of three layers: the pericardium (outer layer), the myocardium (muscular layer), and the endocardium (inner lining).

3 The myocardial layer of the two atria, which receive blood entering the heart, is thinner than the myocardial layer of the ventricles, which have to be stronger to squeeze blood out of the heart.

4 The right and left sides of the heart are separated by portions of the heart wall called the interatrial septum and the interventricular septum.

5 Unoxygenated (venous) blood from the systemic circulation enters the right atrium through the superior and inferior venae cavae. From the atrium the blood passes through the right atrioventricular (tricuspid) valve into the right ventricle. In the ventricle the blood flows from the inflow tract to the outflow tract and then through the pulmonic semilunar valve (pulmonary valve) into the pulmonary artery, which delivers it to the lungs for oxygenation.

6 Oxygenated blood from the lungs enters the left atrium through the four pulmonary valves (two from the left lung and two from the right lung). From the left atrium, the blood passes through the left atrioventricular valve (mitral valve) into the left ventricle. In the ventricle the blood flows from the inflow tract to the outflow tract and then through the aortic semilunar valve (aortic valve) into the aorta, which delivers it to systemic arteries of the entire body.

7 The heart valves ensure the one-way flow of blood from atrium to ventricle and from ventricle to artery.

8 Oxygenated blood enters the coronary arteries through an opening in the aorta, and unoxygenated blood from the coronary veins enters the right atrium through the coronary sinus.

9 The pumping action of the heart consists of two phases: diastole, during which the myocardium relaxes and the chambers fill with blood, and systole, during which the myocardium contracts, forcing blood out of the ventricles. A cardiac cycle consists of one systolic contraction and the diastolic relaxation that follows it. Each cardiac cycle comprises one "heartbeat."

10 The conduction system of the heart generates and transmits electrical impulses (cardiac action potentials) that stimulate systolic contractions. The autonomic nerves (sympathetic and parasympathetic fibers) can adjust heart rate and systolic force, but they do not stimulate the heart to beat.

11 The normal electrocardiogram is the sum of all action potentials. The P wave represents atrial depolarization; the QRS complex is the sum of all ventricular cell depolarizations. The ST interval occurs when the entire ventricular myocardium is depolarized.

12 Cardiac action potentials are generated by the sinoatrial node at the rate of about 75 impulses per minute. The impulses can travel through the conduction system of the heart, stimulating myocardial contraction as they go.

13 Cells of the cardiac conduction system possess the properties of automaticity and rhythmicity. Automatic cells return to threshold and depolarize rhythmically without outside stimulus. The cells of the sinoatrial node depolarize faster than other automatic cells, making it the natural pacemaker of the heart. If the sinoatrial node is disabled, the next fastest pacemaker, the atrioventricular node, takes over.

14 Each cardiac action potential travels from the sinoatrial node to the atrioventricular node to the bundle of His (atrioventricular bundle) through the bundle branches and finally to the Purkinje fibers. There the impulse is stopped. It is prevented from reversing its path by the refractory period of cells that have just been polarized. The refractory period ensures that diastole (relaxation) will occur, thereby completing the cardiac cycle.

15 Adrenergic receptor number, type, and function govern autonomic (sympathetic) regulation of heart rate, contractile force, and the dilation or constriction of coronary arteries. The presence of specific receptors (α-1, α-2; β-1, β-2) in the myocardium and coronary vessels determines the effects of the neurotransmitters norepinephrine and epinephrine.

16 Unique features that distinguish myocardial cells from skeletal cells enable myocardial cells to transmit action potentials faster (through intercalated disks), synthesize more ATP (because of a large number of mitochondria), and have readier access to ions in the interstitium (because of an abundance of transverse tubules). These combined differences enable the myocardium to work constantly, which skeletal muscle is not required to do.

17 Crossbridges between actin and myosin enable contraction. Calcium and its interaction with the troponin complex facilitates the contraction process. With troponin release of calcium, myocardial relaxation begins.

18 Cardiac performance is affected by preload, afterload, heart rate, and myocardial contractility.

19 Preload, or pressure generated in the ventricles at the end of diastole, depends on the amount of blood in the ventricle. Afterload is the resistance to ejection of the

blood from the ventricle. Afterload depends on pressure in the aorta.

20 Heart rate is determined by the sinoatrial node and by components of the autonomic nervous system, including cardiovascular control centers in the brain, neuroreceptors in the atria and aorta, hormones, and catecholamines (epinephrine and norepinephrine).

21 Contractility is the potential for myocardial fiber shortening during systole. It is determined by the amount of stretch during diastole (i.e., preload) and by sympathetic stimulation of the ventricles.

22 The Frank-Starling law of the heart states that the myocardial stretch determines the force of myocardial contraction (the greater the stretch, the stronger the contraction).

23 Laplace's law states that the amount of contractile force generated within a chamber depends on the radius of the chamber and the thickness of its wall (the smaller the radius the thicker the wall, the greater the force of contraction).

24 The suction-pump theory of heart action adds movement to the list of factors that influence cardiac performance. The physical laws of stretch and recoil, action and reaction, and behavior within a vacuum can all be applied to the function of a beating heart.

The Systemic Circulation

1 Blood flows from the left ventricle into the aorta and from the aorta into arteries that eventually branch into arterioles and capillaries, the smallest of the arterial vessels. Oxygen, nutrients, and other substances needed for cellular metabolism pass from the capillaries into the interstitium, where they are available for uptake by the cells. Capillaries also absorb products of cellular metabolism from the interstitium.

2 Venules, the smallest veins, receive capillary blood. From the venules, the venous blood flows into larger and larger veins until it reaches the venae cavae, through which it enters the right atrium.

3 Vessel walls consists of three layers: the tunica intima (inner layer), the tunica media (middle layer), and the tunica externa (the outer layer).

4 Layers of the vessel wall differ in thickness and composition from vessel to vessel, depending on the vessel's size and location within the circulatory system. In general, the tunica media of arteries close to the heart contains a greater proportion of elastic fibers because these arteries must be able to distend during systole and recoil during diastole. Distributing arteries farther from the heart contain a greater proportion of smooth muscle fibers because these arteries must be able to constrict and dilate to control blood pressure and volume within specific capillary beds.

5 Blood flow into the capillary beds is controlled by the contraction and relaxation of smooth muscle bands (precapillary sphincters) at junctions between metarterioles and capillaries.

6 Blood flow through the veins is assisted by the contraction of skeletal muscles (the muscle pump), and backflow in the lower body is prevented by one-way valves, particularly in the deep veins of the legs.

7 Blood flow is affected by blood pressure, resistance to flow within the vessels; blood consistency (which affects velocity); anatomic features that may cause turbulent or laminar flow; and compliance (distensibility) of the vessels.

8 Poiseuille's law describes the relationship of blood flow, pressure, and resistance as the difference between pressure at the inflow end of the vessel and pressure at the outflow end divided by resistance within the vessel.

9 According to Poiseuille's formula, resistance depends on the vessel's length and radius and on the viscosity of the blood. The greater the vessel's length and the blood's viscosity and the narrower the radius of the vessel's lumen, the greater the resistance within the vessel.

10 Total peripheral resistance, or the resistance to flow within the entire systemic circulatory system, depends on the combined lengths and radii of all the vessels within the system and on whether the vessels are arranged in series (greater resistance) or in parallel (lesser resistance).

11 Poiseuille's law and Poiseuille's formula are based on physical laws governing the behavior of fluids in a straight tube. In the body blood flow is also influenced by neural stimulation (of vasoconstriction or vasodilation) and by autonomic features that cause turbulence within the vascular lumen (e.g., protrusions from the vessel wall, twists and turns, bifurcations).

12 Arterial blood pressure is influenced and regulated by factors that affect cardiac output (heart rate and stroke volume), total resistance within the system, and blood volume.

13 Venous blood pressure is infuenced by blood volume within the venous system and compliance of the venous walls.

14 Blood flow through the coronary circulation is governed not only by the same principles as flow through other vascular beds but also by adaptations dictated by cardiac dynamics. First, blood flows into the coronary arteries during diastole rather than systole because, during systole, the cusps of the aortic semilunar valve block the openings of the coronary arteries. Second, systolic contraction inhibits coronary artery flow by compressing the coronary arteries.

15 Autoregulation enables the coronary vessels to maintain optimal perfusion pressure despite systolic effects, and myoglobulin in heart muscle stores oxygen for use during the systolic phase of the cardiac cycle.

The Lymphatic System

1 The vessels of the lymphatic system run in the same sheaths with the arteries and veins.

2 Lymph (interstitial fluid) is absorbed by lymphatic venules in the capillary beds and travels through ever larger lymphatic veins until it is emptied through the right or left thoracic duct into the right or left subclavian vein.

3 As lymph travels toward the thoracic ducts, it is filtered

by thousands of lymph nodes clustered around the lymphatic veins. The lymph nodes are sites of immune function.

Tests of Cardiovascular Function

1 Observable signs of cardiovascular disease include a decreased level of consciousness (caused by insufficient perfusion of brain tissue) and cyanosis, particularly mucous membrane color (caused by insufficient perfusion of vascular beds of the skin).
2 Palpable signs of cardiovascular disease include abnormal pulses of the radial, femoral, and carotid arteries.
3 Abnormal heart sounds, which are detected by auscultation with a stethoscope or by phonocardiography, are auditory signs of cardiovascular disease.
4 Stress tests elicit clinical manifestations of cardiovascular disease that might not be present at rest.
5 Noninvasive diagnostic tests include electrocardiography (ECG) and Holter monitoring, which detect disturbances of impulse generation or conduction; pulse tracings and Doppler studies, which detect abnormalities of blood flow; phonocardiograhy; ultrasound (echocardiography), which detects the structural and functional abnormalities over time; and chest x-ray films, which detect cardiac enlargement and structural abnormalities.
6 Invasive diagnostic tests involve intravenous injection of radiolabeled substances (barium x-rays, nuclear imaging) or the introduction of a catheter that is threaded through the vascular system to the heart (atrioventricular bundle ECG, cardiac catheterization, coronary angiography).
7 Cardiac catheterization is used to measure the oxygen content and pressure of blood in the heart's chambers and to inject contrast media for x-ray examination of the size and shape of the chambers and valves. Injection of contrast medium in the coronary arteries (coronary angiography), on the other hand, permits visualization of the coronary circulation and every tissue perfused by the coronary arteries.

Aging and the Cardiovascular System

1 Much controversy exists regarding the effects of normal aging on the cardiovascular system. Separating the physiologic from the pathologic alterations is difficult because of the presence of arteriosclerosis in the majority of the elderly population.
2 Recent studies have documented no change in cardiac output, a slight decrease in heart rate, and a slight increase in stroke volume in healthy (lack of ischemic heart disease) elderly persons at rest. Also no changes were noted at rest in ejection fraction. A slight increase in afterload (e.g., as systolic blood pressure) and prolonged left ventricular relaxation were noted.
3 With exercise, the healthy elderly subjects demonstrated a decrease in maximum oxygen consumption and no age-related changes in cardiac output but did demonstrate significant decreases in heart rate and increases in stroke volume. Thus the healthy elderly subjects main-

tained a normal cardiac output during exercise by dilating the ventricle and using the Frank-Starling mechanism to increase stroke volume.
4 Contrary to previous studies, recent studies have found no age-related increase with exercise for systolic blood pressure and systemic vascular resistance.

KEY TERMS

A band, 875

Adventitious sound, 902

Afferent lymphatic vessel, 901

Afterload, 879

Aldosterone, 896

Angiotensin I, 896

Angiotensin II, 896

Anistropic, 875

Anomalous viscosity, 890

Aorta, 864

Aortic semilunar valve (aortic valve), 864

Arteriole, 886

Artery, 886

Atrioventricular node (AV node), 870

Atrioventricular valve, 864

Automatic cell, 873

Automaticity, 873

Autoregulation, 898

a wave, 865

Bachmann's bundle, 870

Bainbridge reflex, 882

Baroreceptor reflex, 882

Blood flow, 890

Blood velocity, 894

Bundle branch, 870

Bundle of His (atrioventricular bundle, common bundle), 870

Capillary, 886

Cardiac action potential, 868

Cardiac cycle, 864

Cardiac output, 883

Cardiac plexus, 873

Cardiac vein, 866

Cardioexcitatory center, 881

Cardioinhibitory center, 881

Cardiovascular control center, 881

Chordae tendineae, 864

Circumflex artery, 868

Collateral artery (collateral circulation), 868

Conduction system, 869

Coronary artery, 866

Coronary circulation, 866

Coronary ostium, 866

Coronary perfusion pressure, 897

Coronary sinus, 866

Coronary sulcus, 868

Crista supraventricularis, 865

Crossbridge theory of muscle contraction, 876

c wave, 865

Depolarization, 871

Diastole, 864

Diastolic depolarization, 873

Efferent lymphatic vessel, 901

Ejection fraction, 883

Elastic artery, 886

End-diastolic pressure, 880

End-diastolic volume, 879

Endocardium, 862

Excitation-contraction coupling, 878

Fenestration, 888

Frank-Starling law of the heart, 879

Great cardiac vein, 868

Heart rate, 869

Hyperemia, 896

Hyperpolarization, 871

I band, 875

Inferior vena cava, 864

Inflow tract, 863

Inotropic agent, 882

Intercalated disk, 875

Isotropic, 875

Laminar flow, 894

Laplace's law, 880

Left anterior descending artery (anterior interventricular artery), 868

Left atrial pressure, 883

Left atrium, 862

Left bundle branch (LBB), 870

Left coronary artery, 866

Left heart, 860

Left pulmonary artery, 864

Left ventricle, 862

Lumen, 886

Lymph, 898

Lymphatic vein, 900

Lymphatic venule, 900

Mean arterial pressure, 895

Mediastinum, 860

M line, 876

Metarteriole, 888

Mitral and tricuspid complex, 864

Mitral valve (left atrioventricular valve, bicuspid valve), 864

Muscle pump, 889

Muscular artery, 886

Myocardial contractility, 876

Myocardial oxygen consumption (MVO_2), 876

Myocardium, 862

Myoglobulin, 898

Myosin, 875

Node, 869

Outflow tract, 863

Papillary muscle, 864

Parietal pericardium, 860

P cell, 870

Perfusion, 895

Pericardium, 860

Pericardial cavity, 862

Pericardial fluid, 862

Peripheral vascular system, 886

Plateau, 871

Poiseuille's formula, 890

Poiseuille's law, 890

Posterior vein of the left ventricle, 868

Precapillary sphincter, 888

Preload, 879

Pressure, 890

PR interval, 872

Pulmonary circulation, 860

Pulmonary artery, 864

Pulmonary vein, 864

Pulmonic semilunar valve (pulmonary valve), 864

Purkinje fiber, 870

P wave, 872

QRS complex, 873

QT interval, 873

Refractory period, 872

Renin, 896

Repolarization, 871

Resistance , 890

Rhythmicity, 873

Right atrial pressure, 883

Right atrium, 862

Right bundle branch (RBB), 870

Right coronary artery, 866

Right heart, 860

Right lymphatic duct, 900

Right pulmonary artery, 864

Right ventricle, 862

Semilunar valve, 864

Sinoatrial node (SA node, sinus node), 869

ST interval, 873

Stroke volume, 882

Suction-pump theory, 886

Superior vena cava, 864

Systemic circulation, 860

Systole, 864

Systolic compressive effect, 897

Thoracic duct, 900

Total resistance, 892

Trabeculae carneae, 865

Tricuspid valve (right atrioventricular valve), 864

Troponin C, 876

Troponin I, 876

Troponin T, 876

Troponin-tropomyosin complex, 876

Tunica externa (adventitial layer), 886

Tunica intima (intimal layer), 886

Tunica media (medial layer), 886

Turbulent flow, 895

Vasa vasorum, 886

Vascular compliance, 895

Vasoconstriction, 888

Vasodilation, 888

Vein, 886

Venule, 886

Visceral pericardium, 860

v wave, 865

X descent, 865

y descent, 865

Z line, 876

REFERENCES

Abrams, H. L. (1983). Complications of coronary arteriography (Chapter 23, pp. 503-518). In H. L. Abrams (Ed.), *Angiography: Vascular and interventional radiology* (3rd ed.). Boston: Little, Brown.

Ahlquist, R. P. (1948). A study of the adenotropic receptors. *American Journal of Physiology, 153,* 586.

Anderson, K. E., & Hogestatt, E. D. (1984). On the mechanism of action of calcium antagonists. *Acta Medica Scandinavian Supplementum, 681,* 12-24.

Andreoli, T. E., Carpenter, C.C.J., Plus, F., & Smith, L. H.

(1986). *Cecil essentials of medicine.* Philadelphia: W. B. Saunders.

Bachmann, G. (1916). The inter-auricular time interval. *American Journal of Physiology, 41,* 309.

Baroldi, G., Manteo, O., & Scomozoni, G. (1956). The collaterals of the coronary arteries in normal and pathologic heart. *Circulatory Research, 4,* 223.

Berne, R. M. (1980). The role of adenosine in the regulation of coronary blood flow. *Circulation Research, 47,* 807.

Berne, R. M., & Levy, M. N. (1988a). *Pathophysiology* (2nd ed.). St. Louis: C. V. Mosby.

Berne, R. M., & Levy, M. N. (Eds.). (1988b). *Physiology* (pp. 597-599) St. Louis: C. V. Mosby.

Bond, E. (1982). Physiology of the heart. In S. L. Underhill, S. L. Woods, E. S. Sivarajan, & C. J. Halpenny (Eds.), *Cardiac nursing.* Philadelphia: J. B. Lippincott.

Braunwald, E. (1968). Cooperative study on cardiac catheterization. *Circulation, 37,* (Suppl. 3).

Brutsaert, D. L., Rademakers, F. E., & Sys, S. U. (1984). Triple control of relaxation: Implications in cardiac disease. *Circulation, 69,* 190-196.

Burt, J. J., & Jackson, R. (1965). The effects of physical exercise on the coronary collateral circulation of dogs. *Journal of Sports Medicine, 5,* 203-206.

Burton, A. C. (1972). *Physiology and biophysics of the circulation: An introductory text* (2nd ed.). Chicago: Yearbook.

Carmeliet, E., & Vereecke, J. (1979). Electrogenesis of the action potential and automaticity. In R. M. Berne (Ed.), *Handbook of physiology. Vol. 1: The heart. Section 2: The cardiovascular system (pp.269-334).* Bethesda, MD: American Physiological Society.

Cobb, F. R., Ruby, R. L., & Fariss, B. L. (1968). Effects of exercise on acute coronary occlusion in dogs with prior partial occlusion [Abstract]. *Circulation, 37 & 38.*

Cohn, P. F. (1985). *Diagnosis and therapy of coronary heart disease* (2nd ed.). Boston: Nijhoff.

DeHaan, R. L. (1965). Development of pacemaker tissue in the embryonic heart. *Annals of the New York Academy of Sciences, 127,* 7.

Eckstein, R. W. (1957). Effect of exercise and coronary artery narrowing on coronary collateral circulation. *Circulatory Research, 5,* 230-235.

Fisch, C. (1982). Electrolytes and the heart. In J. W. Hurst et al. (Eds.), *Heart: Arteries and veins* (5th ed.) (p. 1599) New York: McGraw-Hill.

Fye, W. B. (1983). Ernest Henry Starling: His law and its growing signficance in the practice of medicine. *Circulation, 68*(5), 1145-1148.

Gerstenblith, G., Lakatta, E. G., & Weisfeldt, M. L. (1976). Age changes in myocardial function and exercise response. *Progressive Cardiovascular Disease, 19,* 1-21.

Gregg, D. E. (1974). The natural history of collateral development. *Circulation Research, 35,* 355.

Haber, E., & Wrenn, S. (1976). Problems in identification of the beta-adrenergic receptor. *Physiological Review, 56,* 317.

Halpenny, C. J. (1982). Cardiac electrophysiology. In S. L. Underhill, S. L. Woods, E. S. Sivarajan, & C. J. Halpenny (Eds.), *Cardiac nursing* (p. 36). Philadelphia: J. B. Lippincott.

Halpenny, C. J. (1982). Regulation of cardiac output and

blood pressure. In S. L. Underhill, S. L. Woods, E. S. Sivarajan, & C. J. Halpenny (Eds.), *Cardiac nursing*. Philadelphia: J. B. Lippincott.

Halpenny, C. J. (1982). Systemic and pulmonary circulations. In S. L. Underhill, S. L. Woods, E. S. Sivarajan, & C. J. Halpenny (Eds.), *Cardiac nursing*. Philadelphia: J. B. Lippincott.

Halpenny, C.J. (1982). Regulation of cardiac output and blood pressure. In S. L. Underhill, S. L. Woods, E. S. Sivarajan, & C. J. Halpenny [Eds.], *Cardiac nursing*. Philadelphia: J. B. Lippincott.)

Hansen, J. F. (1989). Coronary collateral circulation: Clinical significance and influence on survival in patients with coronary artery occlusion. *American Heart Journal, 117,* 290-295.

Harary, I. (1962). Heart cells in vitro. *Scientific American, 206,* 141.

Heath, G. W., Hagberg, J. M., Ehsani, A. A., & Holloszy, J. O. (1981). A physiological comparison of young and older endurance athletes. *Journal of Applied Physiology, 51,* 634-640.

His, W., Jr. (1893). Die thatigkeit des embryonaten herzens und deren bedeutung fur die lehre von der hersbewegung beim erwachsenen. *Arbeiten Mod Klinische, 14.*

James, T. N. (1962). Pericarditis and the sinus nodes. *Archives of Internal Medicine, 110,* 305.

James, T. N. (1967). Cardiac innervation: Anatomic and pharmacologic relations. *Bulletin of the New York Academy of Medicine, 43,* 1041.

James, T. N. (1968). The coronary circulation and conduction system in acute myocardial infarction. *Progressive Cardiovascular Disease, 10,* 410.

James, T. N., Sherf, L., Schlat, R. C., & Silverman, M. E. (1985). Anatomy of the heart. In J. W. Hurst & C. Rackley (Eds.), *The heart: Arteries and veins* (6th ed.). New York: McGraw-Hill.

Julius, S., Antoon, A., Whitlock, L. S., & Conway, J. (1967). Influence of age on the hemodynamic response to exercise. *Circulation, 36,* 222-230.

Katz, A. M. (1977). Physiology of the heart (pp.1-24). New York: Raven Press.

Keith, A., & Flack, M. (1907). The form and nature of the muscular connections between the primary divisions of the vertebrate heart. *Journal of Anatomy and Physiology, 41,* 172.

Kirchheim, H. R. (1976). Systemic arterial baroreceptor reflexes. *Physiological Review, 56*(1), 110-176.

Kirk, E. S., & Jennings, R. B. (1985). Pathophysiology of myocardial ischemia. In J. W. Hurst & C. Rackley (Eds.), *The heart: Arteries and veins* (6th ed.). New York: McGraw-Hill.

Little, R. C. (1985). *Physiology of the heart and circulation* (3rd ed.). Chicago: Year Book.

Raven, R. H. & Johnson, G. B. (1986). *Biology* St. Louis: Times Mirror/Mosby College Publications.

Re, R. N. (1987). The renin-angiotensin systems. In E. D. Frohlich (Ed.), *Essential hypertension. Medical Clinics of North America, 71*(5).

Re, R., Novelline, R., Escourrou, M. T., Atnansouhs, C., Burton, J., & Aarber, E. (1978). Inhibition of angiotensin-converting enzyme for diagnosis of renal artery stenosis. *New England Journal of Medicine, 298*(11), 582-586.

Roach, M. R., & Burton, A. C. (1959). The effect of age on the elasticity of human iliac arteries. *Canadian Journal of Biochemistry, 37,* 557.

Robinson, S., Dill, D. B., Ross, J. C., Robinson, R. D., Wagner, J. A., & Tzankoff, S. P. (1973). Training and physiological aging in man. *Federation Proceedings, 32,* 1628-1634.

Robinson, T. F., Factor, S. M., & Sonnenblick, E. H. (1986, June). The heart as a suction pump. *Scientific American, 254*(6), 84-91.

Rochmis, P., & Blackburn, H. (1971, August 23). Exercise tests: A survey of procedures, safety, and litigation experience in approximately 170,000 tests. *JAMA, 217,* 1061-1066.

Rodeheffer, R. J., & Gerstenblith, G. (1985). Effect of age on cardiovascular function. In H. A. Johnson (Ed.), *Relations between normal aging and disease*. New York: Raven Press.

Rodeheffer, R. J., Gerstenblith, G., Becker, L. C., Fleg, J. L., Weisfeldt, M. L., & Lakatta, E. G. (1984). With exercise cardiac output is maintained with advancing age in healthy human subjects: Cardiac dilatation and increased stroke volume compensate for a diminished heart rate. *Circulation, 69,* 203-213.

Rushmer, R. F. (1976). *Cardiovascular dynamics*. Philadelphia: W. B. Saunders.

Schaper, W. (1971). *The collateral circulation of the heart*. New York: American Elsevier.

Schlant, R. C., Sonnenblick, E. H., & Gorlin, R. (1982) Normal physiology of the cardiovascular system. In J. W. Hurst, R. B. Logue, C. E. Rackley, R. C. Schlant, E. H. Sonnenblick, A. G. Wallace, & N. K. Wenger (Eds.), *The heart* (5th ed.). New York: McGraw-Hill.

Shepard, J. T., & VanLouttle, P. M. (1979). *The human cardiovascular system: Facts and concepts* (pp. 107-193). New York: Raven Press.

Silverman, B. D., & Neeld, J. B., Jr. (1984). Evaluation of the cardiac patient for noncardiac surgery. *Journal of the Medical Association of Georgia, 73*(5), 315-318.

Soderstrom, M. (1948). Myocardial infarction and mival thrombosis in the atria of the heart. *Acta Medica Scandinavian Supplementum, 132*(217), 114.

Sparks, H. V., & Rooke, T. W. (1987). *Essentials of cardiovascular physiology*. Minneapolis: University of Minnesota Press.

Spence, A. P., & Mason, E. B. (1987). *Human anatomy and physiology* (3rd ed.). Menlo Park, CA: Benjamin/Cummings.

Starling, E. H. (1918). *The Linacre lecture on the law of the heart*. London: Longmans, Green & Co.

Strandell, T. (1964). Circulation studies on healthy old men. *Acta Medica Scandinavian Supplementum 175 (414),* 1-14.

Thomas, J. L., Dickstein, R. A., Parker, F. B., Jr., Potts, J. L., Poirer, R. A., et al. (1982). Prognostic significance of the development of left bundle conduction defects following aortic valve replacement. *Journal of Thoracic and Cardiovascular Surgery, 84*(3), 382-386.

Thorel, C. (1909). Vorlarifig mittelung uber eine beson dere muskel ver bindung zwischen der cava superior und dem hisschen bundel. *Munich Med Wochenschrift, 56,* 2159.

Thibodeau, G. A. (1987). *Anatomy and Physiology*. St. Louis: Times Mirror/Mosby.

Thompson, J. M., et al. (1989). *Mosby's manual of clinical nursing* (2nd ed.). St. Louis: C.V. Mosby.

Underhill, S. L., Woods, S. L., Sivarajan, E. S., & Halpenny, C. J. (Eds.). (1982). *Cardiac nursing*. Philadelphia: J. B. Lippincott.

Vander, A. J., Sherman, J. H., & Luciano, D. S. (1980). *Human physiology: The mechanisms of body function* (3rd ed.). New York: McGraw-Hill.

Vander, A., Sherman, J.H., & Luciano, D. S. (1980). *Human physiology* [3rd ed.]. New York: McGraw-Hill.

Vick, R. L. (1984). *Contemporary medical physiology*. Menlo Park, CA: Addison-Wesley.

Wenckebach, K. F. (1908). Bietrage zur kenntnis der mengchlichen hertztatigkeit. *Archives of Anatomy and Physiology, 3*, 53.

Wu, D. (1984). What is the role of calcium antagonists for ventricular tachycardia. *International Journal of Cardiology, 5*, 543-547.

CHAPTER 27

Alterations of Cardiovascular Function

Pamela D. Parker-Cohen
Stephanie J. Richardson
Sandra Haak

Diseases of the arteries and veins, 917
  Arteriosclerosis, 917
  Atherosclerosis, 917
    Pathophysiology, 919
    Clinical manifestations, 919
    Evaluation and treatment, 920
  Hypertension, 920
    Risk factors for primary hypertension, 920
    Pathophysiology, 921
      Primary hypertension, 921
      Secondary hypertension, 923
      Isolated systolic hypertension, 923
      Complicated hypertension, 923
    Clinical manifestations, 925
    Evaluation and treatment, 926
  Orthostatic (Postural) hypotension, 926
  Aneurysm, 927
  Thrombus formation, 930
  Embolism, 930
    Thromboembolism, 930
    Air embolism, 931
    Amniotic fluid embolism, 931
    Bacterial embolism, 931
    Fat embolism, 931
    Foreign matter, 931
  Peripheral arterial disease, 931
    Thromboangiitis obliterans (Buerger disease), 931
    Raynaud's phenomenon and disease, 932
  Diseases of the veins, 932
    Varicose veins and chronic venous insufficiency, 932
    Thrombus formation in veins, 933
    Superior vena cava syndrome, 933
  Coronary artery disease, myocardial ischemia, and
      myocardial infarction, 934
    Development of coronary artery disease, 934
      Hyperlipidemia, 934
      Hypertension, 936
      Cigarette smoking, 936

      Diabetes mellitus, 936
      Genetic predisposition, 936
      Obesity, 936
      Sedentary life-style, 936
      Hormone therapy, 937
      Alcohol, 937
      Women and coronary artery disease, 937
      Type A personality, 937
    Myocardial ischemia, 938
      Pathophysiology, 938
      Clinical manifestations, 939
      Evaluation and treatment, 940
    Myocardial infarction, 942
      Pathophysiology, 942
        Cellular injury, 942
        Cellular death, 943
        Structural and functional changes, 943
        Repair, 944
      Clinical manifestations, 944
      Evaluation and treatment, 945
      Complications, 946
Disorders of the heart wall, 947
  Disorders of the pericardium, 947
    Acute pericarditis, 947
    Pericardial effusion, 948
    Constrictive pericarditis, 949
  Disorders of the myocardium: the cardiomyopathies, 951
    Congestive cardiomyopathy, 951
    Hypertrophic cardiomyopathy, 953
    Restrictive cardiomyopathies, 953
  Disorders of the endocardium, 953
    Valvular dysfunction, 953
      Stenosis, 954
        Aortic stenosis, 954
        Mitral stenosis, 955
      Regurgitation, 956
        Aortic regurgitation, 956
        Mitral regurgitation, 957

Tricuspid regurgitation, 957
Mitral valve prolapse syndrome (MVPS), 957
Acute rheumatic fever and rheumatic heart disease, 958
Pathophysiology, 958
Clinical manifestations, 959
Carditis, 959
Polyarthritis, 959
Chorea, 959
Erythema marginatum, 959
Evaluation and treatment, 959
Infective endocarditis, 960
Pathophysiology, 960
Clinical manifestations, 962
Evaluation and treatment, 962
Manifestations of heart disease, 963
Dysrhythmias, 963
Heart failure, 963
Mechanisms of heart failure, 963
Altered contractility, 963
Altered ratio of oxygen supply and demand, 969
Types of heart failure, 969
Right heart failure (cor pulmonale), 969
Left heart failure (congestive heart failure), 971
Low-output failure, 975
High-output failure, 975
Shock, 976
Types of shock, 976
Cardiogenic shock, 976
Hypovolemic shock, 977
Neurogenic shock, 977
Anaphylactic shock, 979
Septic shock, 980
Impairment of cellular metabolism, 981

Impairment of oxygen use, 981
Impairment of glucose use, 983
Treatment for shock, 984

DISEASES OF THE ARTERIES AND VEINS

Arteriosclerosis

Arteriosclerosis is a chronic disease of the arterial system characterized by abnormal thickening and hardening of the vessel walls. In arteriosclerosis, the tunica intima undergoes a series of changes that decrease the artery's ability to change lumen size. Smooth muscle cells and collagen fibers migrate into the tunica intima, causing it to stiffen and thicken. This process gradually narrows the arterial lumen (Fig. 27-1). Changes in lipid, cholesterol, and phospholipid metabolism within the tunica intima also contribute to arteriosclerosis. Although these structural changes may be part of the normal aging process, they can cause or worsen pathophysiologic conditions such as high blood pressure, insufficient perfusion of tissues, or weakening and outpouching of arterial walls.

Atherosclerosis

Atherosclerosis is a form of arteriosclerosis in which the thickening and hardening of the vessel walls is caused by soft deposits of intraarterial fat and fibrin that harden over time. Atherosclerosis is not a single disease

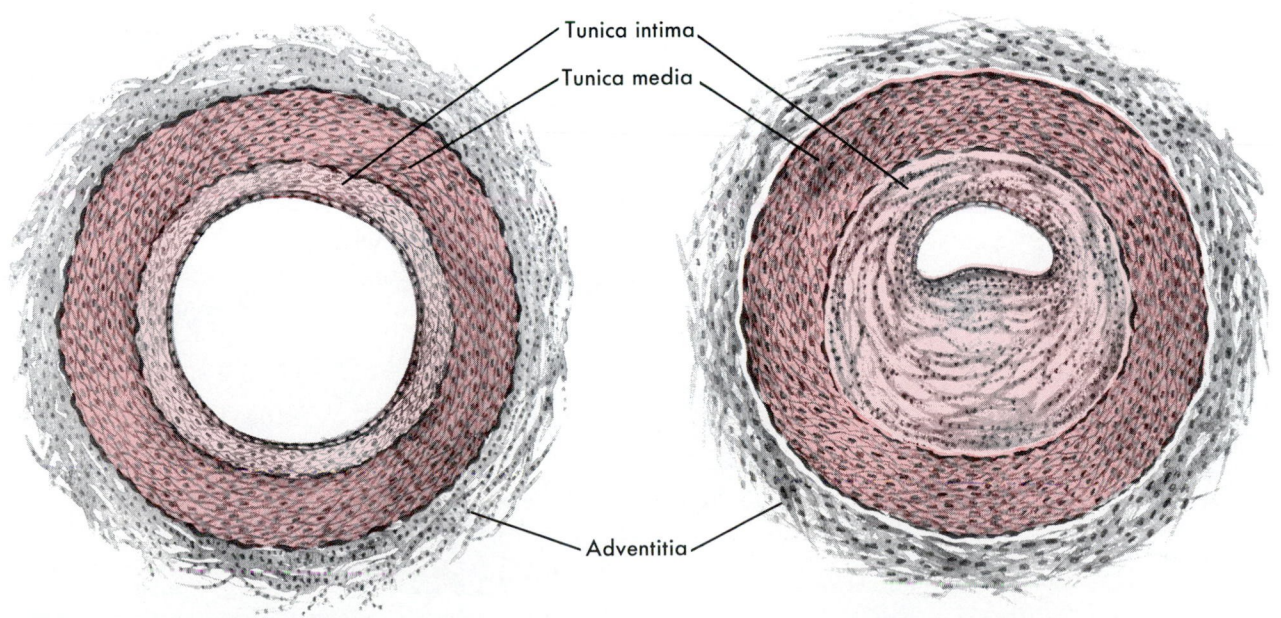

Tunica intima

Tunica media

Adventitia

Normal artery   Diseased (occluded) artery

FIG. 27-1. Arteriosclerosis. Cross-section of a normal artery and an artery altered by disease.

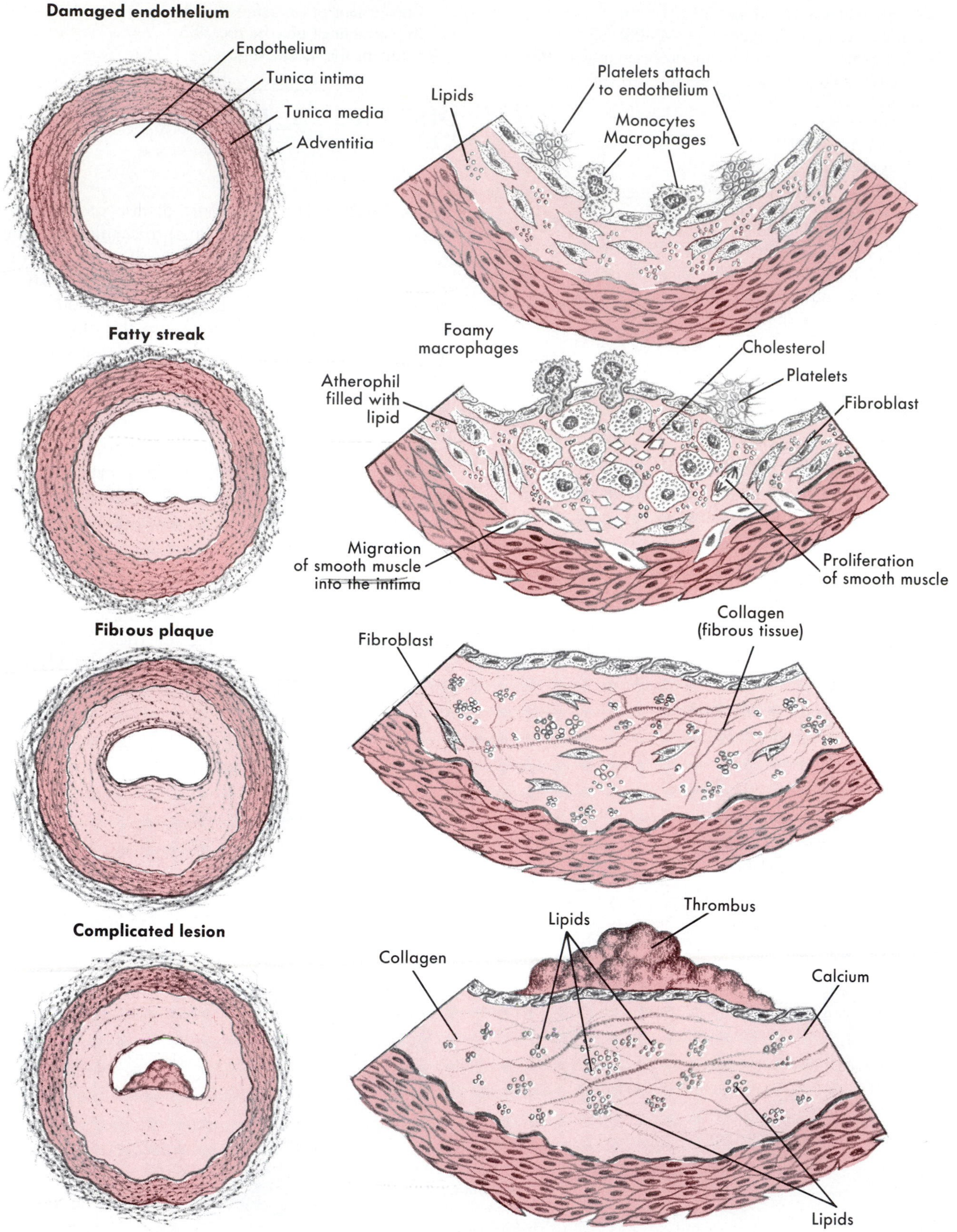

Damaged endothelium

Endothelium
Tunica intima
Tunica media
Adventitia

Lipids
Platelets attach
to endothelium
Monocytes
Macrophages

Fatty streak

Foamy
macrophages
Cholesterol
Platelets
Atherophil
filled with
lipid
Fibroblast
Migration
of smooth muscle
into the intima
Proliferation
of smooth muscle

Fibrous plaque

Collagen
(fibrous tissue)
Fibroblast

Complicated lesion

Thrombus
Lipids
Collagen
Calcium
Lipids

FIG. 27-2. Progression of atherosclerosis.

entity. It can take several forms, depending on the anatomic location, the age, genetic and physiologic status, and the risk factors to which each individual may have been exposed. (Atherosclerosis of the coronary arteries is described on p. 934; that of the cerebral arteries in Chapter 15.)

Pathophysiology

It has long been recognized that lipid deposition is an early event in atherogenesis and occurs when influx and deposition of cholesterol into the arterial wall exceeds efflux (Angelin, Eriksson, & Andersson, 1987). The lesions of atherosclerosis occur primarily within the tunica intima (innermost layer) and include the fatty streak, fibrous plaque, and the advanced or complicated lesion. The **fatty streak,** the earliest atherosclerotic lesion, is a flat, yellow, lipid-filled smooth muscle cell that causes no obstruction of the affected vessel. Fatty streaks are commonly present in the aorta of an affected individual by the age of 10 years and in the coronary arteries by the age of 15 years, regardless of race, sex, or environmental factors (Robbins, Cotran, & Kumar, 1984). These lesions are thought to be reversible.

Fibrous plaque is the characteristic lesion of advancing atherosclerosis and is rarely found in people under the age of 25 years. It consists of lipid-laden smooth muscle cells surrounded by collagen, elastic fibers, and a mucoprotein matrix. The lesion is white and elevated and protrudes into the lumen of the artery (Fig. 27-2). The growing mass fixes to the inner wall of the tunica intima and may invade the muscular tunica media. Fibrous plaques are thought to develop from fatty streaks in which cellular proliferation, lipid accumulation, and connective tissue formation occur. The core of the fibrous plaque may consist of lipids and debris resulting from cellular necrosis caused by insufficient blood supply. If the lesion progresses sufficiently, it can occlude the arterial lumen. This is most likely to occur at arterial bifurcations, curves, or regions in which the arteries taper.

Complicated or advanced lesions occur if the fibrous plaques are altered over time by hemorrhage, calcification, cellular necrosis, and mural thrombosis (occlusion by blood clots throughout the intimal layer). The intimal surface may disintegrate or ulcerate as the lipid-laden lesion enlarges and hardens. This rigid complex structure is often the cause of vascular occlusion.

Atherosclerotic lesions generally cause no symptoms until 60% or more of the tissue's blood supply is occluded. If plaque formation occurs slowly, collateral arteries may develop to supply tissue.

Several hypotheses have been proposed to explain the pathogenesis (atherogenesis) and progression of atherosclerosis, but there is disagreement about which is correct. Atherogenesis and atherosclerosis probably occur as a result of several of the hypotheses described in Table 27-1.

Clinical Manifestations

Atherosclerosis may have many different manifestations, again depending on the vessel involved, site of the lesion, and the age, genetic makeup, and physiologic

---

TABLE 27-1 Hypotheses of atherogenesis

Hypothesis	Mechanism of atherogenesis
Response to injury	Arterial endothelium is injured by altered hemodynamic forces (hypertension), harmful chemicals (nicotine, catecholamines), bacterial infection, hyperlipidemia, or mechanical trauma. Endothelial membrane is disrupted, permeability is altered, and platelets, lipids, and smooth muscle aggregate on the intimal layer.
Monoclonal hypothesis	Phenotypically identical smooth muscle cells are transformed into benign neoplasms by viruses or chemicals
Dipogenic hypothesis	Elevated levels of low-density lipoproteins (LDL), decreased levels of high-density lipoproteins (HDL) result in migration and accumulation of LDLs and cholesterol in the tunica intima and tunica media.
Clonal senescence	Aging interferes with immune function in the tunica intima and tunica media, and smooth muscle cell replication continues unchecked, allowing muscle cells and lipids to accumulate.
Thrombogenic hypothesis	Repeated deposition of blood elements (fibrin, platelets, etc.) on the endothelium result in formation of microthrombi. Old deposits degenerate as new material continues to accumulate and platelets release a factor that stimulates smooth muscle proliferation (Rokitansky, 1852).
Lipid infiltration	Circulating lipids enter arterial endothelium and accumulate around the smooth muscle. Endothelial permeability is adversely affected, allowing continued lipid filtration (Virchow, 1862).

status of the individual. High blood pressure ensues if atherosclerosis elevates systemic vascular resistance. Cerebral or myocardial ischemia is a life-threatening manifestation of atherosclerosis in vessels of the brain or heart.

Evaluation and Treatment

In evaluating individuals for the presence of atherosclerosis, the complete health history and physical examination, including laboratory data, are considered. Judicious use of x-ray films, electrocardiography, ultrasonography, nuclear scanning, and angiography may be necessary to identify affected vessels, particularly coronary vessels.

Dietary modification is always the first treatment for atherosclerosis. Fat intake should be reduced to 30% of daily calorie consumption, with no more than 10% saturated fats. Daily cholesterol intake must be reduced to 250 to 300 mg.

The NIH Consensus Development Conference has recommended target blood cholesterol levels of 200 mg/dl for individuals over 30 years of age and about 180 mg/dl for those under 30 years of age (Assmann, 1987). Drugs that decrease lipidemia are only prescribed if serum lipoproteins are not reduced by a reasonable trial of dietary modification or if lipid levels are dangerously elevated in an individual who will require a considerable period of time for significant dietary change and weight reduction.

Hypertension

Hypertension is consistent elevation of systemic arterial blood pressure. Adults are diagnosed as having hypertension when the average of two or more diastolic blood pressure measurements made on at least two consecutive clinical visits is 90 mm Hg or higher, or when the average of systolic blood pressure measurements made on two or more consecutive visits is greater than 140 mm Hg (Joint National Committee, 1985).

Hypertension is caused by increases in cardiac output, total peripheral resistance, or both. (The many factors affecting cardiac output and peripheral resistance are described in Chapter 26. See Figs. 26-10 and 26-31.) Cardiac output is increased by any condition that increases heart rate or stroke volume, whereas peripheral resistance is increased by any factor that increases blood viscosity or reduces vessel diameter, particularly arteriolar diameter.

Individuals with hypertensive disease may have combined systolic and diastolic hypertension or isolated systolic hypertension. Most cases of combined systolic and diastolic hypertension have no known cause and are therefore diagnosed as **primary hypertension.** Primary hypertension, also called essential or idiopathic hypertension, affects 89% to 95% of hypertensive individuals

(Berglund, Andersson, & Wilhemsen, 1976; Danielson & Dammstrom, 1981; Ferguson, 1975; Gifford, 1969; Joint National Committee, 1985; Kaplan, 1982; Rudnick et al., 1977). **Secondary hypertension** is caused by altered hemodynamics associated with a primary disease, such as arteriosclerosis. Although many diseases can cause secondary hypertension, this form of hypertension accounts for only 5% to 10% of cases. **Isolated systolic hypertension** is elevated systolic blood pressure accompanied by normal diastolic blood pressure (below 90 mm Hg). Isolated systolic hypertension is a manifestation of increased cardiac output, or rigidity of the aorta, or both.

Risk Factors for Primary Hypertension

Risk factors for primary hypertension include (1) family history of hypertension, (2) advancing age, (3) male gender, (4) black race, (5) obesity, (6) high sodium intake, (7) glucose intolerance (diabetes mellitus), (8) changeable (labile) blood pressure or borderline hypertension, (9) cigarette smoking, and (10) heavy alcohol consumption (Page, 1987; Sadler, 1984). These risk factors are associated with many other cardiovascular disorders as well. The chance of developing hypertension increases geometrically, rather than additively, with each additional risk factor.

Estimates of the prevalence of hypertension in the United States (Haynes, Eaker, & Feinleib, 1984) indicate that the prevalence rate of hypertension per 100 adults is lowest for white women (15.7) and highest for black women (28.6). The prevalence rate for white men (18.5) is lower than that for black men (27.8) (Roberts & Maurer, 1977). Among whites, the incidence of hypertension in men is higher than in women (Advance Data, 1976; Roberts & Maurer, 1977).

Obesity alone is not a significant risk factor for hypertension (Johnson et al., 1975; Katz et al., 1980). Obesity is, however, frequently associated with hypertension, hyperlipidemia, and glucose intolerance. Therefore, many obese individuals are at significant risk for cardiovascular morbidity and mortality (Keys et al., 1972a).

Although populations with high dietary sodium intake have long been shown to have a high incidence of hypertension, recent studies indicate that low dietary potassium and calcium intake are also risk factors (Genest et al., 1983; McCarron et al., 1984; Roberts & Maurer, 1977).

The nicotine in cigarette smoke is a vasoconstrictor that can elevate both systolic and diastolic blood pressure acutely (Aronow et al., 1974; Cryer et al., 1976). In habitual smokers, an individual cigarette may not raise blood pressure, yet habitual smoking is associated with a high incidence of severe hypertension and with death resulting from hypertension (Doll & Peto, 1976; Isles et al., 1979). The incidence of hypertension is higher among heavy drinkers of alcohol (more than three drinks per day) than among abstainers, but moderate drinkers (two to four drinks per week) appear to have lower blood pressures, as well as lower cardiovascular mortality, than either abstainers or heavy drinkers (Harburg et al., 1980; Hennekens et al., 1979; Klatsky, Friedman, & Siebelbaum, 1981).

Pathophysiology

Chronic hypertension damages the walls of systemic blood vessels. Prolonged vasoconstriction and high pressures within these vessels, particularly the arteries and arterioles, stimulates the vessels to thicken and strengthen to withstand the stress. Arterial smooth muscle undergoes hypertrophy (cellular enlargement) and hyperplasia (cellular proliferation). Eventually, the tunica intima and tunica media undergo fibromuscular thickening sufficient to narrow their lumina. At this point, regardless of stimuli that cause vasoconstriction, the vessels are permanently narrowed.

Hypertensive injury of vessel walls also stimulates the biochemical mediators of inflammation to increase the permeability of the vascular endothelium. As permeability increases, sodium, calcium, water, plasma proteins, and other blood-borne (humoral) substances enter vessel walls, causing further thickening and, in the case of calcium, increases responsiveness to stimuli that cause smooth muscle contraction (i.e., vasoconstriction).

In the coronary vessels, hypertension causes or aggravates other conditions, such as atherosclerosis, that diminish vessel caliber. Therefore, hypertension combined with coronary artery disease increases the risk of coronary artery occlusion and infarction of myocardial tissue.

Primary Hypertension

Despite research by numerous investigators, the exact pathogenesis of primary hypertension has not been established. In view of the multiple, interdependent factors involved in normal blood pressure regulation, it seems likely that no single cause or defect will be identified.

Several hypotheses have been proposed to explain the onset of primary hypertension in individuals at risk. They include (1) increases in blood volume, (2) inappropriate autoregulation, (3) overstimulation of sympathetic neural fibers in the heart and vessels, (4) water and sodium retention by the kidneys, and (5) hormonal inhibition of sodium-potassium transport across cell walls in the kidneys and blood vessels. Any or all of these mechanisms may be at work, but researchers disagree about which is dominant during pathogenesis of primary hypertension.

Fig. 27-3 illustrates the hemodynamic hypothesis of onset. This hypothesis, which is closely related to all but the neural hypothesis, attributes the onset of hypertension to fluid overload. According to the hemodynamic hypothesis, early primary hypertension consists of a series of cardiovascular adjustments to an increase in

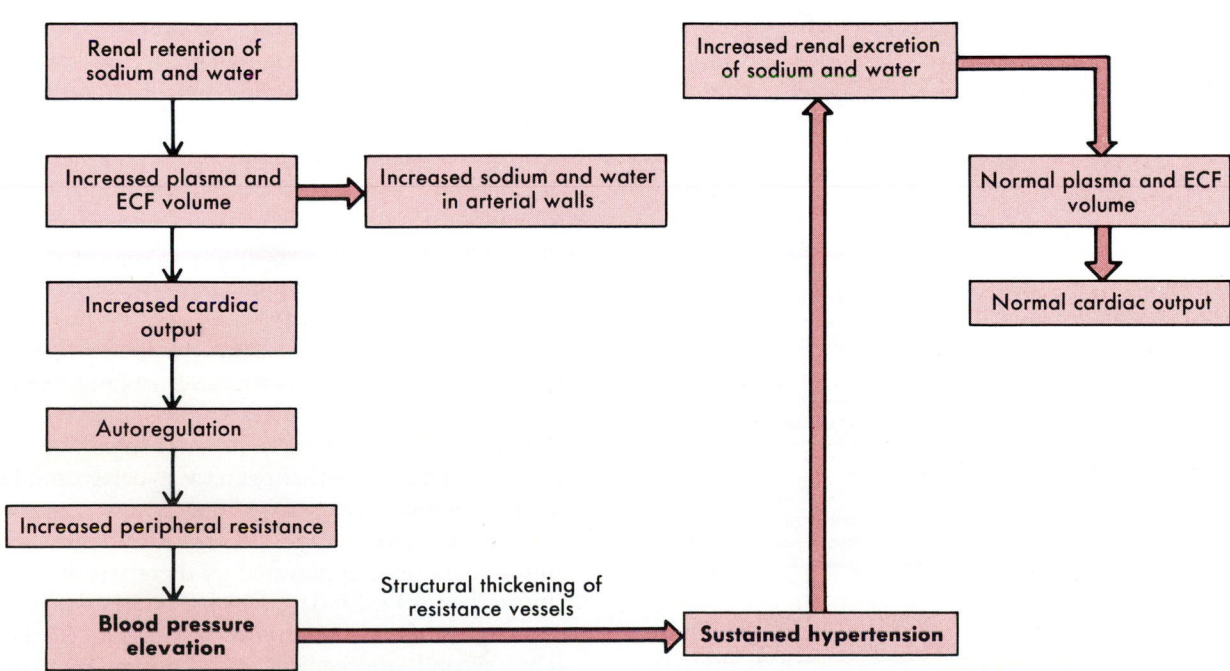

FIG. 27-3. Hemodynamic events of early primary hypertension *(thin arrows)* and established primary hypertension *(thick arrows)*. *ECF,* Extracellular fluid volume.

blood volume. First, cardiac output increases to handle the increased volume of blood circulating through the heart. As the systemic arteries sense the volume increase, their autoregulatory mechanisms try to slow things down by causing vasoconstriction. Because blood volume remains high, the increase in total peripheral resistance caused by vasoconstriction leads to hypertension. At this point, hypertension has not damaged the vessels and, if blood volume is reduced, cardiac output and vascular smooth muscle tone will return to normal.

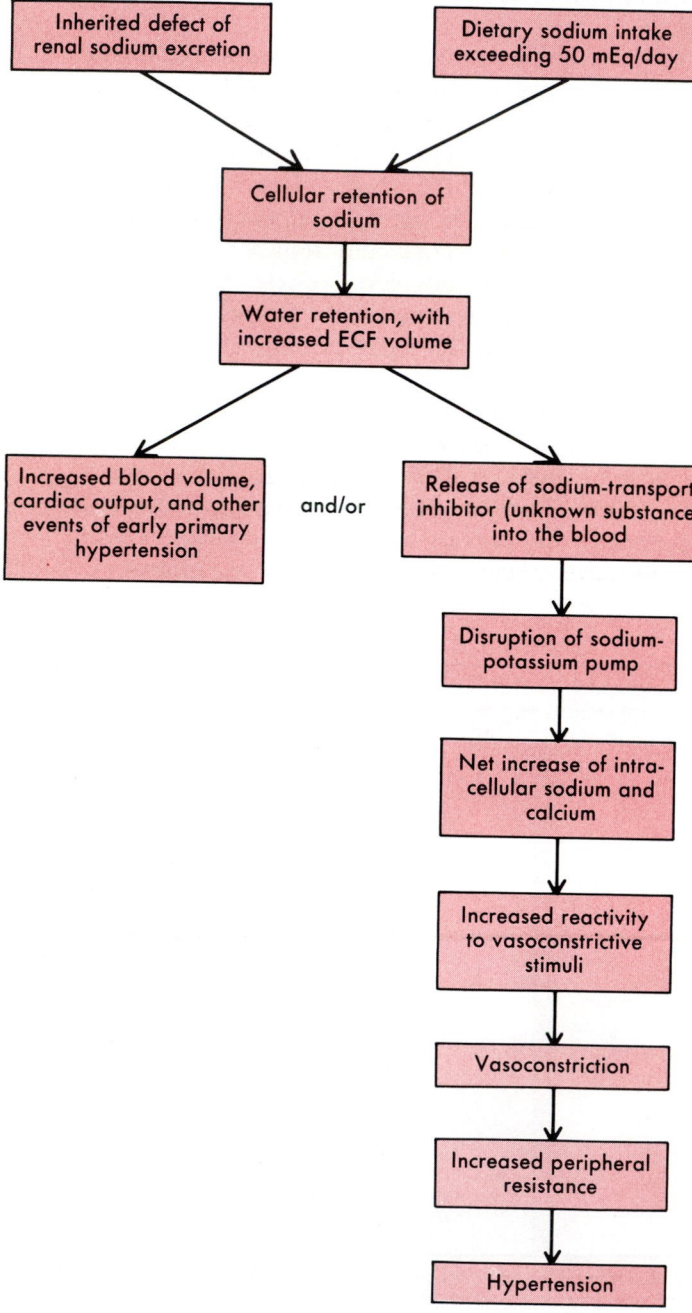

FIG. 27-4. Two related mechanisms of sodium-induced primary hypertension.

In individuals in whom persistent primary hypertension develops, however, cardiac output returns to normal but vascular smooth muscle tone does not, so peripheral resistance remains high. At this point, hypertension becomes established and vascular damage begins. This simple hypothesis leaves unexplained many mechanisms that might be involved. Unknown is the amount of increase in extracellular fluid and cardiac output that must occur before hypertension results (Page, 1987). Chronic hypervolemia and significant increases in cardiac output have not been found in individuals with essential hypertension or renovascular hypertension (Page, 1987).

Autoregulation in the cardiovascular system chiefly involves the intrinsic capability of the arterioles in the vascular beds to regulate the flow of blood according to the quantity of blood available, the concentration of metabolites carried in the blood, and the metabolic needs of surrounding tissues. The autoregulatory hypothesis proposes that, although primary hypertension begins with increased cardiac output (see Fig. 27-3), it is *maintained* by an alteration of vascular autoregulation. Normally, autoregulatory mechanisms adjust arterial and arteriolar vasoconstriction and vasodilation as needed to maintain normal, or baseline, blood pressure. According to the autoregulatory hypothesis, the defect consists of the failure of autoregulatory mechanisms to return vascular tone to normal after cardiac output and blood volume have returned toward baseline (because of water and sodium excretion by the kidneys). Hypertension is established as the new baseline, and autoregulation subsequently functions to maintain it.

The third hypothesis about the onset of primary hypertension is that neurally stimulated vasoconstriction is the initiating event. According to this hypothesis, the cardiovascular control centers in the brain overstimulate the sympathetic branch of the autonomic nervous system, causing vasoconstriction. Overstimulation could also be caused by some abnormality of α-adrenergic receptor function, or an oversupply of receptors for the neurotransmitter that stimulates vasoconstriction. Because the sympathetic nervous system innervates both the heart and the vessels, sympathetic overstimulation increases cardiac output, as well as peripheral resistance.

Researchers have proposed two mechanisms by which sodium retention can initiate primary hypertension (see Fig. 27-4). The first is that primary hypertension begins with an inherited defect of sodium excretion in the kidneys (Kaplan, 1982; Page, 1987). The defect in renal sodium excretion is aggravated by dietary sodium intake of more than 50 mEq/day, which initiates the hemodynamic events of early hypertension (see Fig. 27-3).

The second mechanism of sodium retention is thought to be an interruption of the sodium-potassium pump, which normally governs the transport of sodium and potassium across cell membranes (see Chapters 1 and 3). In individuals with this defect, a humoral factor (a hormone) is thought to inhibit sodium excretion from cells. The factor or factors have not been discovered. Elevated levels of the humoral sodium-transport inhibitor not only cause intracellular sodium to accumulate, but seem to also cause increases of intracellular calcium. Because intracellular calcium promotes smooth muscle contractility, the presence of extra calcium in vascular smooth muscle cells increases vascular reactivity. This vascular reactivity produces vasoconstriction with increased peripheral resistance and leads to the final outcome of hypertension. The cellular events related to sodium-induced hypertension are summarized in Fig. 27-4.

Secondary Hypertension

Secondary hypertension is caused by a systemic disease process that raises peripheral vascular resistance or cardiac output. If the cause is identified and removed before permanent structural changes occur, blood pressure will return to normal. Table 27-2 summarizes the pathogenesis of major forms of secondary hypertension.

Isolated Systolic Hypertension

Elevations of systolic pressure alone are usually caused by increases in cardiac output, or total peripheral vascular resistance, or both. Isolated systolic hypertension caused by increased cardiac output can be secondary to dysfunction of the aortic semilunar valve (aortic valve insufficiency), any abnormal opening between heart chambers (arterioventricular fistula, patent ductus arteriosus; see Chapter 28), thyrotoxic crisis (thyroid storm), Paget disease of the bone, and beriberi. Rigidity of the aorta is the chief vascular cause of isolated systolic hypertension.

Isolated systolic hypertension is most common in the elderly. Rigidity of the aorta is caused by arteriosclerosis, which increases total peripheral vascular resistance. Changes associated with aging alter the aortic valve so that increased cardiac output is needed to maintain blood flow into the systemic circulation.

Complicated Hypertension

Complicated hypertension is sustained primary hypertension that has pathologic effects besides hemodynamic alterations and fluid and electrolyte imbalances. Complicated hypertension commonly compromises the structure and function of the vessels themselves, the heart, aorta, kidneys, eyes, brain, and lower extremities. The two major mechanisms of tissue damage are ischemia and edema. Ischemia deprives tissues of the oxygen and nutrients they need for survival and function. Leakage of fluids into the interstitial space, and even hemorrhage, is caused by high pressures in the vessels. The heart is particularly susceptible to injury because while high cardiac output is stimulating myocardial hypertrophy, vasoconstriction is diminishing blood flow through the coronary arteries. The pathophysiology of complicated hypertension is summarized in Table 27-3.

Cardiovascular complications include left ventricular hypertrophy, angina pectoris, congestive heart failure (left heart failure), coronary artery disease, myocardial infarction, and sudden death. Vascular complications include the formation, dissection, and rupture of aneurysms (outpouchings in vessel walls); intermittent claudication; and gangrene resulting from vessel occlusion. Possible renal complications are parenchymal damage, nephrosclerosis, renal arteriosclerosis, and renal insufficiency or failure.

Changes in the vascular beds can be estimated by viewing the arterioles of the retina. Complications specific to the retina include retinal vascular sclerosis, exudation, and hemorrhage. Cerebrovascular complications

---

TABLE 27-2 Pathogenesis of major forms of secondary hypertension by cause

Primary disease	Pathogenesis of hypertension
RENAL DISORDERS	
Renal parenchymal disease	Disturbances in filtration and reabsorption of serum sodium, potassium, and calcium initiate the hemodynamics of early hypertension
Renovascular disease	Impaired blood flow and renal ischemia invoke the compensatory renin-angiotensin-aldosterone mechanism in an effort to raise the renal perfusion pressure
Renin-producing tumors	Elevated blood renin levels invoke elevations in angiotensin and aldosterone, which cause blood pressure to rise
Renal failure	Disturbances in filtration and reabsorption of serum sodium, potassium, and calcium initiate the hemodynamics of early hypertension
Primary sodium retention	Disturbance in filtration and/or reabsorption of serum sodium initiates the hemodynamics of early hypertension

Continued.

TABLE 27-2 Pathologies of major forms of secondary hypertention by cause—cont'd

Primary disease	Pathogenesis of hypertension
ENDOCRINE DISORDERS	
Acromegaly	Excess human growth hormone causes increased peripheral resistance
Hypothyroidism	Mucopolysaccharide deposits in vascular tissue increase resistance
Hypercalcemia	Calcium ion directly affects vascular tonicity. Elevated serum calcium levels increase vascular tone and peripheral resistance
Hyperthyroidism	Increased inotropic effect on the heart elevates systolic pressure. Diastolic pressure decreases as a result of decreased peripheral resistance
Adrenal disorders Cortical disturbances, Cushing syndrome	Glucocorticoids facilitate sodium and water retention, initiating the hemodynamics of early hypertension
Primary aldosteronism	Excess aldosterone promotes sodium retention and initiation of the hemodynamics of early hypertension
Congenital adrenal hyperplasia	Excess production of adrenal cortical hormones promotes sodium and water retention
Medullary disturbance: pheochromocytoma	Excess catecholamines raise vascular tone and increase peripheral resistance
Extraadrenal chromaffin tumors	Excess catecholamines raise vascular tone and increase peripheral resistance
VASCULAR DISORDERS	
Coarctation of the aorta	Decreased blood flow in distal areas initiates maximum peripheral resistance as an autoregulatory effort to adjust perfusion pressure
Arteriosclerosis	Loss of elasticity in vessel walls results in increased peripheral resistance
PREGNANCY-INDUCED HYPERTENSION	Pathogenesis unclear
NEUROLOGIC DISORDERS	
Elevated intracranial pressure (brain tumor, encephalitis, respiratory acidosis of pulmonary or CNS origin)	Higher systemic blood pressure required to maintain adequate cerebral perfusion
Quadriplegia, acute porphyria, familial dysautonomia, lead poisoning, Guillian-Barré syndrome,	Interface with neural control of blood pressure initiates increased systemic blood pressure
ACUTE STRESS	
Surgery, psychogenic hyperventilation, hypoglycemia, burns, pancreatitis, alcohol withdrawal, sickle-cell crisis, resuscitation, increased intravascular volume	Acute stress precipitates release of catecholamines and glucocorticoids
DRUGS AND OTHER SUBSTANCES	
Oral contraceptives and estrogen	Unknown; possibly caused by sodium retention, plasma retention, weight gain, changes in levels and actions of renin, angiotensin, aldosterone
Corticosteroids	Same as for Cushing disease
Sympathetic stimulants, appetite suppressants, antihistamines	Raises vascular tone and increases vascular resistance
Licorice	Contains glycerrhizic acid, a mineralocorticoid causing salt and water retention
Monamine inhibitorsoxidase	Hypertension may develop in an individual who routinely takes MAO inhibitor with ingestion of a food containing tyramine

TABLE 27-3 Pathologic effects of sustained, complicated primary hypertension

Site of injury	Mechanism of injury	Potential pathologic effect
Heart		
Myocardium	Increased workload combined with diminished blood flow through coronary arteries	Left ventricular hypertrophy, myocardial ischemia, congestive heart failure
Coronary arteries	Accelerated atherosclerosis (coronary artery disease)	Myocardial ischemia, myocardial infarction, sudden death
Kidneys	Renin and aldosterone secretion stimulated by reduced blood flow	Retention of sodium and water, leading to increased blood volume and perpetuation of hypertension
	Reduced oxygen supply	Tissue damage that compromises filtration
	High pressures in renal arterioles	Nephrosclerosis leading to renal failure
Brain	Reduced blood flow and oxygen supply; weakened vessel walls	Transient ischemic attacks, cerebral thrombosis, aneurysm, hemorrhage
Eyes (retinas)	Reduced blood flow	Retinal vascular sclerosis
	High arteriolar pressure	Exudation, hemorrhage
Aorta	Weakened vessel wall	Dissecting aneurysm (see p. 929)
Arterial vessels of lower extremities	Reduced blood flow and high pressures in arterioles	Intermittent claudication, gangrene

are similar to those of other arterial beds and include transient ischemia, stroke, cerebral thrombosis, aneurysm, and hemorrhage.

Malignant hypertension (rapidly progressive hypertension in which diastolic pressure is usually above 140 mm Hg) can cause encephalopathy, a profound cerebral edema that disrupts cerebral function and causes loss of consciousness. Encephalopathy occurs because high arterial pressure renders the cerebral arterioles incapable of regulating blood flow to the cerebral capillary beds. Capillary permeability is increased by high hydrostatic pressures in the capillaries and vascular fluid exudes into the interstitial space. If blood pressure is not reduced, cerebral edema and cerebral dysfunction increase until death occurs. Organ damage resulting from malignant hypertension is life-threatening. Besides encephalopathy, malignant hypertension can cause papilledema, cardiac failure, uremia, retinopathy, encephalopathy, and cerebrovascular accident.

Clinical Manifestations

The early stages of hypertension have no clinical manifestations other than elevated blood pressure. Most important, there are no signs and symptoms to cause the individual to seek health care. Some hypertensive individuals never have signs, symptoms, or complications, whereas others become very ill, in which case hypertension can be a cause of death. Others have anatomic and physiologic damage caused by past hypertensive disease, despite current blood pressures within normal ranges.

The chance of developing primary hypertension increases with age, over and above the natural rise in blood pressure associated with aging. In individuals at risk for primary hypertension, the factors leading to development of hypertension accumulate during the first two or three decades of life. Although hypertension is usually thought to be an adult health problem, it is important to remember that hypertension does occur in children and is being diagnosed with increasing frequency (Lieberman, 1982; Loggie, 1979). Usually, however, increased peripheral resistance and early hypertension develop in the second, third, and fourth decades of life. If elevated blood pressure is not detected and treated, it becomes established and may begin to accelerate atherosclerosis when the individual is 30 to 50 years of age. This sets the stage for the complications of hypertension that begin to appear during the fourth, fifth, and sixth decades of life.

Most of the clinical manifestations of hypertensive disease are caused by complications that damage organs and tissues outside the vascular system. Besides elevated blood pressure, the signs and symptoms, therefore, tend to be specific for the organs or tissues affected. Evidence of heart disease, renal insufficiency, central nervous system dysfunction, impaired vision, impaired mobility, vascular occlusion, or edema can all be caused by sus-

TABLE 27-4 Classification of hypertension by category of severity and recommended followup

Blood pressure (mm Hg)	Category of severity	Recommended followup
DIASTOLIC		
Below 85	Normal blood pressure	Recheck within 2 years
85-89	High normal blood pressure	Recheck within 1 year
90-104	Mild hypertension	Prompt confirmation (2 months or less)
105-114	Moderate hypertension	Prompt care (2 weeks or less)
Above 115	Severe hypertension	Immediate care (1 week or less)
Above 120 (organ damage present)	Malignant hypertension	Emergency care (24 hours or less)
SYSTOLIC (diastolic below 90 mm Hg)		
Below 140	Normal blood pressure	Recheck within 2 years
140-159	Boderline isolated systolic hypertension	Prompt confirmation (2 months or less)
Above 160	Isolated systolic hypertension	Prompt confirmation (2 months or less)
Above 200	Isolated systolic hypertension	Prompt care (2 weeks or less)

From Joint National Committee. The 1984 report of the Joint National Committee on detection, evaluation, and treatment of high blood pressure, 1985, © The Nurse Practitioner; Houston, 1986.

tained hypertension. (See appropriate chapters for specific clinical manifestations of organ dysfunction.)

Evaluation and Treatment

Diagnostic tests for suspected hypertension include repeated blood pressure measurements, complete blood count, urinalysis, biochemical blood profile (plasma glucose, potassium, creatinine, cholesterol, and triglycerides), and an electrocardiogram. Individuals who have elevated blood pressure are assumed to have primary hypertension unless their history, physical examination, or initial diagnostic screening indicates secondary hypertension.

Treatment of primary hypertension depends on its severity. Table 27-4 lists blood pressure levels and categories of severity used as guidelines for treatment.

Hypertension is usually managed with both pharmacologic and nonpharmacologic methods. Four groups of drugs are used to manage hypertension: (1) diuretics, (2) angiotensin inhibitors, (3) vascular smooth muscle relaxants, and (4) adrenergic blockers. Diuretics reduce blood pressure initially by facilitating renal excretion of sodium and water, thereby reducing blood volume and cardiac output. Subsequently, the cardiovascular system adjusts to restore cardiac output, but reduced blood pressure is maintained because peripheral resistance is lower. Angiotensin inhibitors reduce blood pressure by preventing the renin-angiotensin mechanism from acting upon the vascular smooth muscle, adrenal cortex, kidney, and brainstem. Captopril, for example, acts by inhibiting the enzyme that converts inactive angiotensin I to the active form, angiotensin II. With less active angiotensin II in the blood, blood pressure decreases. Vas-

cular smooth muscle relaxants lower blood pressure by blocking calcium influx to smooth muscle cells. This decreases vascular reactivity and promotes vasodilation. Adrenergic blockers interfere with the transmission of the neurohumoral facilitators (e.g., norepinephrine) of vasoconstriction and cardiac stimulation. These agents bind with adrenergic receptors, preventing receptor binding with neurohumoral stimulators of increased cardiac output and vasoconstriction.

Sometimes treatment consists of reducing or eliminating risk factors. Lifestyle modification can control hypertension and enhance the effects of drug treatment. The usual dietary recommendations are to restrict sodium intake to 2 gm/day, to increase potassium intake, to restrict saturated fat intake, and to adjust calorie intake as required to maintain optimum weight. An exercise program that promotes endurance and relaxation is usually recommended. Physical training increases stroke volume, which has the effect of lowering heart rate and hence systolic blood pressure. Relaxation is expected to reduce levels of circulating catecholamines, which have the effect of reducing vascular tone and blood pressure. Individuals are counseled to stop smoking cigarettes to eliminate vasoconstrictor effects of nicotine.

Orthostatic (Postural) Hypotension

The term **orthostatic (postural) hypotension** means a drop in both systolic and diastolic arterial blood pressure on standing. When a normal individual stands up, the resultant gravitational changes on the circulation are compensated for by several mechanisms that include reflex arteriolar and venous constriction, increased heart rate, and mechanical factors, such as the closure of valves in the venous system, pumping of the leg muscles, and a decrease in intrathoracic pressure (Hurst et al., 1986). The normally increased sympathetic activity during upright posture is mediated through stretch receptors (baroreceptors) in the carotid sinus and the aortic arch (see Chapter 26). Their reflex response to shifts in volume caused by postural changes leads to a prompt increase in heart rate and constriction of the systemic arterioles. Thus, despite a marked fall in cardiac output, arterial blood pressure is maintained.

Orthostatic hypotension is often accompanied by dizziness, blurring or loss of vision, and syncope or fainting. Fainting is caused by insufficient vasomotor compensation and reduction of blood flow through the brain. The normal or compensatory vasoconstrictor response to standing is thus replaced by a marked vasodilation and blood pooling in the muscle vasculature, as well as in the splanchnic and renal beds.

Orthostatic hypotension may be acute and temporary or chronic. **Acute orthostatic hypotension,** or temporary type, is caused when the normal regulatory mechanisms are sluggish. This delay may be the result of (1) anatomic variation, (2) altered body chemistry, (3) drug action (e.g., antihypertensives and antidepressants), (4) prolonged immobility caused by illness, (5) starvation, (6) physical exhaustion, (7) any condition that produces volume depletion (e.g., massive diuresis, potassium or sodium depletion), and (8) venous pooling (e.g., pregnancy, extensive varicosities of the lower extremities). The elderly are susceptible to this type of orthostatic hypotension in which postural reflexes are apparently slowed as part of the aging process. However, this is not a universal finding in the elderly.

The two forms of **chronic orthostatic hypotension** are (1) secondary to a specific disease and (2) idiopathic or primary. The diseases that cause secondary orthostatic hypotension are endocrine disorders (e.g., adrenal insufficiency, diabetes mellitus), metabolic disorders (e.g., porphyria), or diseases of the central or peripheral nervous system (e.g., intracranial tumors, cerebral infarcts, Wernicke's encephalopathy, and peripheral neuropathies).

Idiopathic, or primary, orthostatic hypotension is the term for the group in which there is no known initial cause (Silber, 1987). However, there is controversy about this group. Some define the disorder as a separate entity, whereas others suggest it is a part of a generalized degenerative central nervous system disease. Idiopathic orthostatic hypertension affects men more often than women and usually occurs between the ages of 40 and 70. In addition to cardiovascular symptoms, impotence and bowel and bladder dysfunction are often found in this type.

No curative treatment is available for idiopathic orthostatic hypertension. In the secondary form, syncope

---

Treatments for Orthostatic Hypotension

MECHANICAL MEASURES
Elevate head of bed
Lower body compression suit
Slow motion and calf muscle-flexing on arising
Elastic stockings

VOLUME EXPANSION
High-salt diet
Fluorohydrocortisone

DRUGS
Sympathomimetics
Vasoconstrictors
β-Receptor blockers
α_2-Receptor agonists
Prostaglandin synthesis inhibitors
Antiserotonergics
Monoamine oxidase inhibitors and tryamine
Vasopressin

---

will cease when the underlying disorder is corrected (Silber, 1987). Several treatments can help acute and chronic orthostatic hypotension.

Aneurysm

An **aneurysm** is a localized dilatation or outpouching of a vessel wall or cardiac chamber. The law of Laplace can provide an understanding of the hemodynamics of an aneurysm (Fig. 27-5). (The law of Laplace is discussed in detail in Chapter 26). Presumably, formation of an aneurysm occurs when intraventricular tension stretches the noncontracting infarcted muscle (Braunwald, 1988). The stretching produces infarct expansion, a weak and thin layer of necrotic muscle, and fibrous tissue that bulges with each systole. With time, the aneurysm becomes more fibrotic, but continues to bulge with each systole, thus acting as a "reservoir" for some of the stroke volume.

The aorta is particularly susceptible to aneurysm formation because of constant stress on the vessel wall and the absence of penetrating vasa vasorum in the adventitial layer. Three fourths of all aneurysms occur in the abdominal aorta (Fig. 27-6). Atherosclerosis is the most common cause of aneurysms because plaque formation erodes the vessel wall. Arteriosclerosis and hypertension are found in more than half of all individuals with aneurysms. Syphilis and other infections can also cause aortic aneurysms.

True aneurysms involve all three layers of the arterial wall and are best described as a weakening of the vessel wall. Most are fusiform and circumferential (Fig. 27-7). **False aneurysms** and **saccular aneurysms** are usually

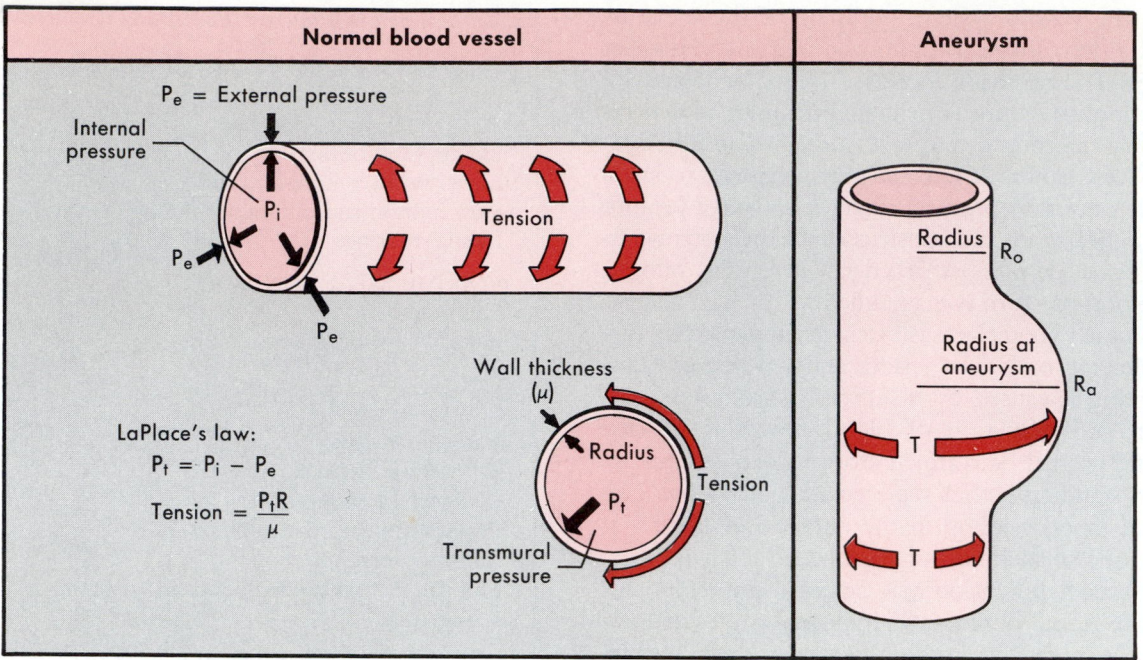

FIG. 27-5. Pressure-tension and wall thickness relations in blood vessels (Laplace's law). (From Kissane, 1985).

FIG. 27-6. Infrarenal atherosclerotic aneurysm of abdominal aorta. **A,** Origins of celiac axis and superior mesenteric artery, as well as the right and left renal arteries, are above aneurysm. Aortic bifurcation and common iliac arteries are below. **B,** Opened atherosclerotic aneurysm of distal abdominal aorta demonstrates laminated fibrin thrombus *(dark material)* in aneurysm. Renal arteries are at top of photograph, and aortic bifurcation with severely atherosclerotic and aneurysmal common iliac arteries is at bottom. (From Kissane, 1985.)

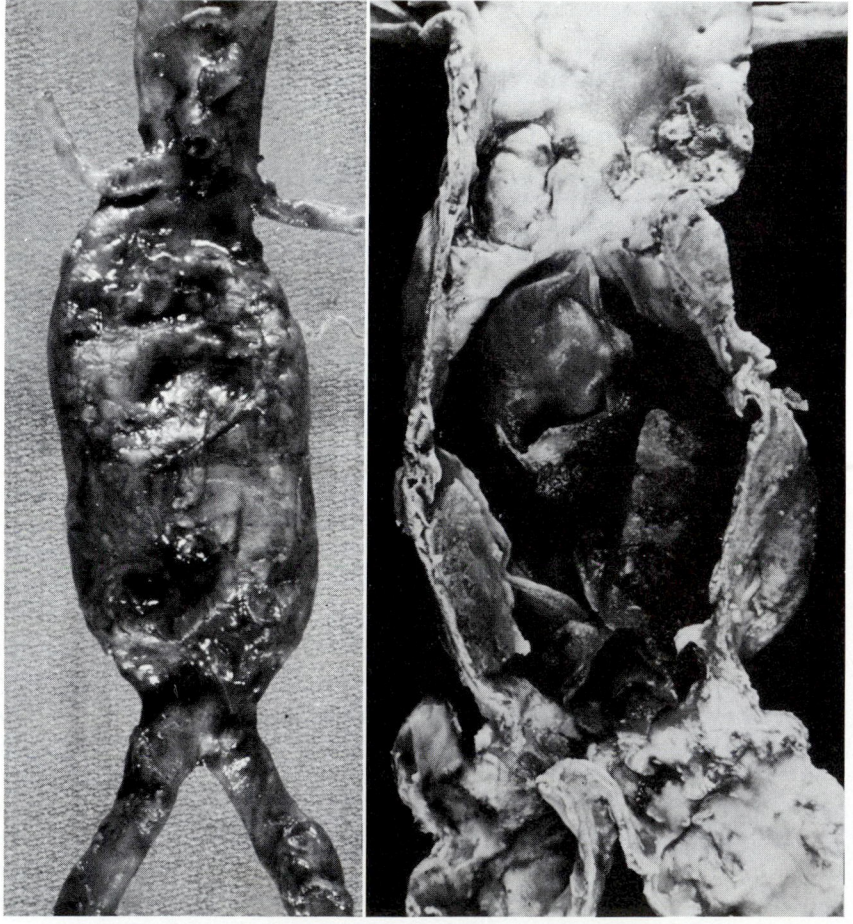

A   B

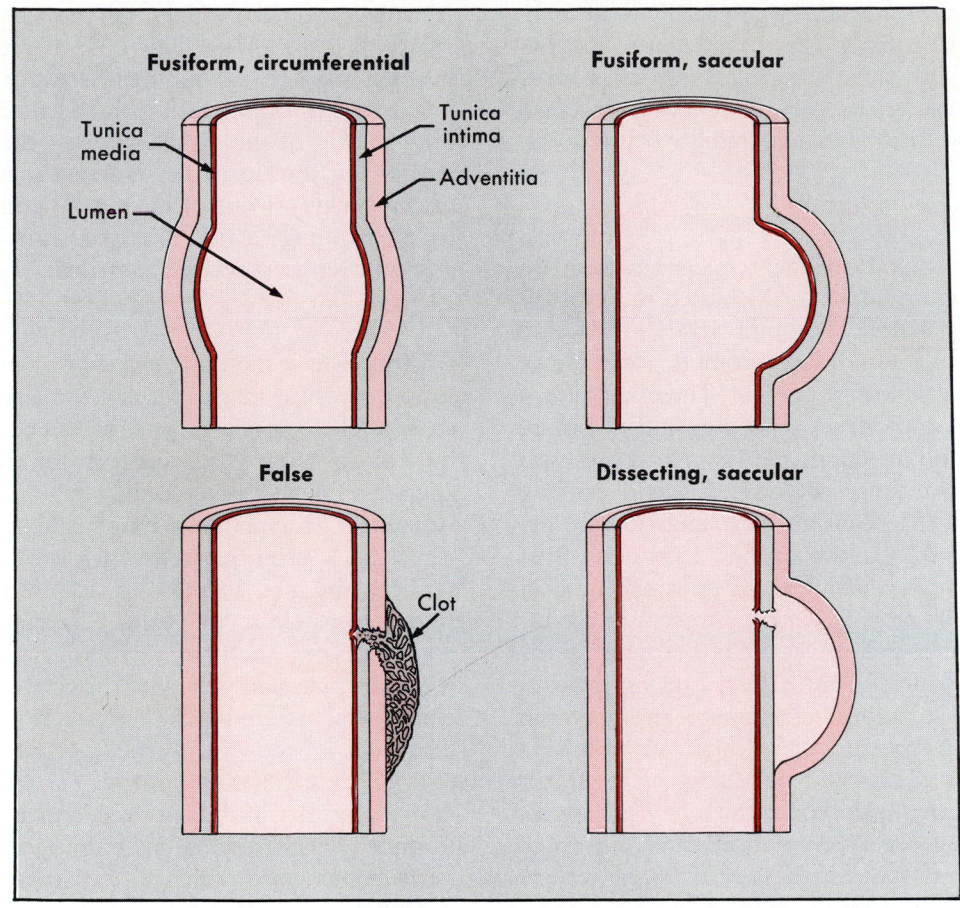

FIG. 27-7. Longitudinal sections showing types of aneurysms. The fusiform circumferential and fusiform saccular aneurysms are true aneurysms, caused by weakening of the vessel wall. False and saccular aneurysms involve a break in the vessel wall, usually caused by trauma.

the result of trauma. These aneurysms are caused by a dissection of the layers of the arterial wall, so that blood is contained at the point of aneurysm by the adventitial layer (dissecting saccular aneurysm) or by a clot (false aneurysm).

Clinical manifestations of aneurysm include a variety of symptoms. Aortic aneurysms can be very painful. Symptoms of dysphagia (difficulty swallowing) and dyspnea (breathlessness) are caused by the pressure of a large volume of blood on surrounding organs. An aneurysm that impairs flow to an extremity causes symptoms of ischemia. Cerebral aneurysms, which frequently occur in the circle of Willis, are associated with signs and symptoms of increased intracranial pressure. Signs and symptoms of stroke occur when cerebral aneurysms leak. (Cerebral aneurysms are described in Chapter 15.)

Treatment of aneurysms is nearly always surgical. Saccular aneurysms are repaired more easily than fusiform and circumferential aneurysms. If the weakness or separation of vascular layers spreads, the aneurysm becomes a **dissecting aneurysm** (Fig. 27-8). Dissecting aneurysms and leaking aneurysms require emergency treat-

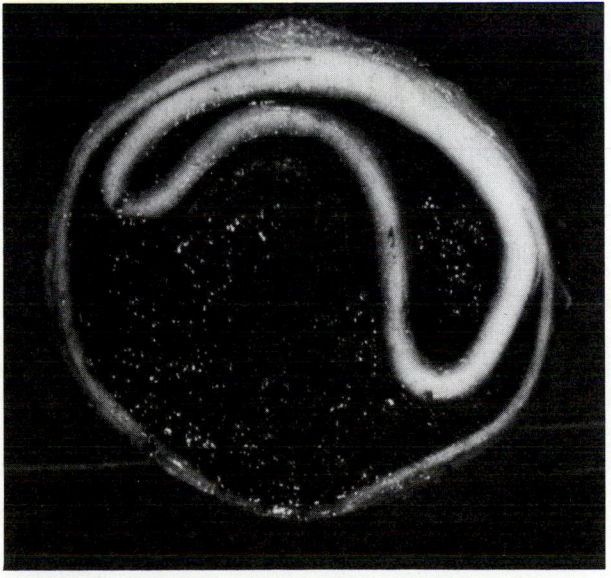

FIG. 27-8. Cross-section of the aorta with dissecting aneurysm showing true aortic lumen *(above and right)* compressed by dissecting column of blood that separates media and creates false lumen. (From Kissane, 1985.)

ment. Leaking cerebral aneurysms, especially those associated with vascular spasms as a compensatory mechanism, are treated with clot-stabilizing drugs and a number of clinical measures designed to reduce intracranial pressure and induce hemodynamic stability before surgical intervention.

Thrombus Formation

A **thrombus** is a blood clot that remains attached to a vessel wall (see Figure 24-11). A detached thrombus is called **thromboembolus.** Thrombi tend to develop wherever intravascular conditions promote activation of the coagulation, or clotting, cascade. These conditions include intimal irritation, roughening, inflammation, traumatic injury, and infection, and low blood pressures or obstructions that cause blood stasis and pooling within the vessels. (Mechanisms of coagulation are described in Chapter 22.) In the arteries, activation of the coagulation cascade is usually caused by roughening of the tunica intima by atherosclerosis. Invasion of the tunica intima by an infectious agent also roughens the normally smooth lining of the artery, causing platelets to adhere readily. Anatomic changes of an artery can stimulate thrombus formation, particularly if the change results in a pooling of arterial blood. This can occur, for example, in blood that is pooled within an aneurysm. In the veins, thrombus formation is more often associated with inflammation (phlebitis), a condition termed thrombophlebitis. Thrombi also form on heart valves altered by calcification or bacterial vegetation. Valvular thrombi are most commonly associated with inflammation of the endocardium (endocarditis) and rheumatic heart disease.

Shock (circulatory failure), particularly shock resulting from septicemia, can activate the intrinsic and extrinsic pathways of coagulation. The impaired cellular metabolism that occurs with all types of shock activates the extrinsic pathway of coagulation, whereas blood stasis caused by very low blood pressures activates the intrinsic pathway (see Chapter 22). Thrombus formation may be confined to one area or may progress to diffuse coagulopathy, such as disseminated intravascular coagulation (see Chapter 24).

A thrombus poses two potential threats to the circulation. First, the thrombus may grow large enough to occlude the artery, causing ischemia in tissue supplied by the artery. Second, the thrombus may dislodge, becoming a thromboembolus that travels through the arterial system until it occludes flow into a distal vascular bed.

Pharmacologic treatment includes the administration of heparin and warfarin derivatives that interfere with the clotting cascade by accelerating the activity of antithrombin III, thereby slowing or stopping thrombus growth, and by the intravenous or intraarterial administration of streptokinase, which dissolves the thrombus.

A balloon-tipped catheter can be used to remove or compress a thrombus. This type of catheter is inserted into the vessel containing the thrombus at a point proximal to the thrombus and is threaded past the thrombus until the tip of the catheter is past the thrombus. The balloon on the tip of the catheter is then inflated and drawn backward out of the vessel, pulling out the clot by a "dredging" action. Various combinations of drug and catheter therapies are sometimes used concurrently.

Embolism

Embolism is the obstruction of a vessel by an **embolus**—a bolus of matter that is circulating in the bloodstream. The embolus may consist of a dislodged thrombus; an air bubble; an aggregate of amniotic fluid; an aggregate of fat, bacteria, or cancer cells; or a foreign substance. An embolus travels in the bloodstream until it reaches a vessel through which it cannot fit. No matter how tiny it is, an embolus will eventually lodge in a systemic or pulmonary vessel. The source of the embolus determines whether the embolus will lodge in a vessel of the pulmonary or systemic circulation. Pulmonary emboli originate on the venous side (mostly from the deep veins of the legs) of the systemic circulation or in the right heart; systemic emboli (or arterial) most commonly originate in the left heart and are associated with thrombi after myocardial infarction, valvular disease, left heart failure, endocarditis, and dysrrythmias.

Embolism causes ischemia or infarction in tissues distal to the obstruction. A limb that is ischemic because of arterial occlusion is characterized by an almost waxy whiteness of the skin because the vasculature is devoid of erythrocytes, and by numbness and pain resulting from neural ischemia.

Embolism of a central organ causes organic dysfunction and pain. For example, pulmonary artery embolism causes chest pain and dyspnea; renal artery embolism causes abdominal pain and oliguria; and mesenteric artery embolism causes abdominal pain and a paralytic, ischemic bowel. Infarction and subsequent necrosis of a central organ is life-threatening, not only because of organ dysfunction but also because of sepsis. Necrotic tissue is a rich medium for the growth of bacteria from the lungs, bowel, and, occasionally, the bladder. Necrosis of the bladder, in particular, can quickly lead to peritonitis or septicemia.

Embolism of a coronary or cerebral artery is an immediate threat to life if the embolus severely obstructs a major vessel. Occlusion of a coronary artery will cause a myocardial infarction (see p. 934), whereas occlusion of a cerebral artery will cause a stroke (see Chapter 15).

Thromboembolism

Thromboembolism is a vascular obstruction by a dislodged thrombus. The most common source of arterial thromboemboli is the heart. Mitral or aortic valvular disease, especially that associated with abnormal heart rhythms (atrial fibrillation and flutter), causes thrombus formation on roughened vascular surfaces and in atrial blood as a result of stasis. More than half of these thromboemboli lodge in the lower extremities (in the femoral and popliteal arteries). Others lodge in the coronary arteries and the cerebral vasculature.

Air Embolism

Room air that enters the circulation through intravenous lines is probably the most common cause of air embolism. Room air is about 70% nitrogen. Although nitrogen dissolves quickly in blood, large amounts of air cannot be dissolved rapidly enough to prevent the displacement of blood in the arterioles and capillary beds. Ischemia and necrosis occur when air totally blocks a vessel.

Air can also be introduced into the bloodstream if trauma to the chest causes air from the lungs to enter the vascular space. For example, gunshot wounds and puncture wounds of the thorax sometimes introduce air emboli. Treatment for air embolism is supportive, once the connection between the source of air and the vascular system has been eliminated.

Amniotic Fluid Embolism

The great intraabdominal pressures generated during labor and delivery may force amniotic fluid into the bloodstream of the mother through the highly vascular uterine wall. Amniotic fluid not only displaces blood, reducing oxygen, nutrient, and waste exchange, but it also introduces antigens, cells, and protein aggregates that trigger inflammation, coagulation, and the immune response within the bloodstream. Capillary beds are usually affected by amniotic fluid emboli, especially the capillary beds of the lungs and kidneys. Treatment is supportive and may include dialysis, particularly after a cesarean section or hysterectomy.

Bacterial Embolism

Isolated bacteria in the bloodstream do not cause embolism, but aggregates of bacteria may be large enough to do so. The most common cause of bacterial embolism is subacute bacterial endocarditis, during which clumps of vegetation are dislodged from infected cardiac valves and ejected into the pulmonary or systemic circulation. A less common cause is erosion of an artery or vein by bacteria at a source of infection, such as an abscess. Treatment for bacterial embolism includes bed rest, supplemental oxygen, and antibiotics to eradicate the source of infection.

Fat Embolism

Trauma to the long bones is associated with fat embolism, particularly in the lungs. Two mechanisms have been proposed to account for the generation of fat em-

boli after skeletal trauma. The first is that trauma to the bones initiates defective fat metabolism, causing globules of fat to form in the blood. Platelets adhere to these globules until the conglomerate is large enough to lodge in a capillary bed. The second possible explanation is that globules of fat are released from fatty bone marrow exposed by fracture. Again, platelets adhere to the fat globules and embolism occurs.

Treatment for fat embolism consists of prompt immobilization of fractures and supportive measures that include administration of supplemental oxygen and steroids. Steroid administration may decrease the inflammation that occurs with vascular occlusion. Inflammation in the pulmonary bed is especially dangerous because it can cause adult respiratory distress syndrome (see Chapter 30). Intravenous administration of glucose is thought to prevent inappropriate fat metabolism.

Foreign Matter

Foreign matter can enter the bloodstream during trauma or through an intravenous or intraarterial line. If the bolus of foreign matter is relatively large, it is usually removed surgically. Small particles, such as drug precipitates, small glass shards, or fibers from linen are sometimes introduced unintentionally into a vessel through intravenous injections or manipulation of monitoring lines. Once in the blood, these small particles initiate the coagulation cascade. The thromboemboli that form around the particles are large enough to occlude a vessel and result in ischemia. Treatment is aimed at preventing thrombus formation around the particle, dissolution of the particle, and supportive measures to alleviate ischemia.

Peripheral Arterial Disease
Thromboangiitis Obliterans (Buerger Disease)

Thromboangiitis obliterans (Buerger disease), which tends to occur in young men who are heavy cigarette smokers, is an inflammatory disease of the peripheral arteries. The inflammatory lesions are accompanied by thrombi and sometimes by vasospasm of arterial segments. Inflammation, thrombus formation, and vasospasm can eventually occlude and obliterate (render physiologically useless) portions of small and medium-sized arteries in the feet and sometimes in the hands. Typically affected are the digital, tibial, and plantar arteries of the feet and the digital, palmar, and ulnar arteries of the hands. The disease is sometimes associated with inflammation of adjacent veins and nerves. The pathogenesis of thromboangiitis obliterans is not known.

The chief symptom of thromboangiitis obliterans is pain and tenderness of the affected part. Clinical manifestations are caused by sluggish blood flow and include rubor (redness and shininess of the skin), which is caused by dilated capillaries under the skin, and cyanosis, which is caused by blood that remains in the capillaries after its oxygen has diffused into the interstitium. Chronic ischemia causes the nails to become thickened and malformed. In advanced disease, ischemia resulting from vessel obliteration can cause gangrene.

The most important part of treatment is cessation of cigarette smoking. All other measures are aimed at improving circulation to the foot or hand. Vasodilators are prescribed to alleviate vasospasm, and exercises are taught that use gravity to improve blood flow. If vasospasm persists, sympathectomy may be performed. Gangrene necessitates amputation.

Raynaud Phenomenon and Disease

Raynaud phenomenon and **Raynaud disease** are both characterized by attacks of vasospasm in the small arteries and arterioles of the fingers and, less commonly, the toes. Though the clinical manifestations of the phenomenon and the disease are the same, their etiologies differ.

Raynaud phenomenon is secondary to systemic diseases, particularly collagen vascular disease (scleroderma), pulmonary hypertension, thoracic outlet syndrome, myxedema trauma, serum sickness (see Chapter 8), or long-term exposure to environmental conditions, such as cold or vibrating machinery in the workplace. (The effects of segmental vibration are described in Chapter 2.) Raynaud disease, though, is a primary vasospastic disorder of unknown origin. Raynaud disease tends to affect young women and to consist of vasospastic attacks triggered by brief exposure to cold or by emotional stress. Genetic predisposition may play a role in its development.

The clinical manifestations of the vasospastic attacks of either disorder are changes in skin color and sensation caused by ischemia. Vasospasm occurs with varying frequency and severity, and causes pallor, numbness, and the sensation of cold in the digits. Attacks tend to be bilateral, and manifestations usually begin at the tips of the digits and progress to the proximal phalanges. Sluggish blood flow resulting from ischemia may cause the skin to appear cyanotic. Rubor follows as vasospasm ends and the capillaries become engorged with oxygenated blood. Rubor is often accompanied by throbbing and paresthesias. Skin color returns to normal after the attack, but frequent, prolonged attacks interfere with cellular metabolism, causing the skin of the fingertips to thicken and the nails to become brittle. In severe, chronic Raynaud phenomenon or disease, ischemia can eventuallly cause ulceration and gangrene. This outcome is rare, however.

Treatment for Raynaud phenomenon consists of removing the stimulus or treating the primary disease process. Attacks of vasospasm can sometimes be alleviated at their onset by an exercise in which the arms are swung forward and backward. This maneuver increases hydrostatic pressure (and perfusion pressure) in the arteries by means of centrifugal force.

Treatment of Raynaud disease is limited to prevention or alleviation of vasospasm itself, because no underlying disorder has been identified. Stimuli that trigger attacks (e.g., cold and emotional stress) are avoided, and cigarette smoking is stopped to eliminate the vasoconstricting effects of nicotine. Exercises that build centrifugal force in the extremities are also helpful in the early stages of vasospasm. If attacks of vasospasm become frequent or prolonged, vasodilators (e.g., the antihypertensive drugs Dibenamine or Roniacal) and Rauwolfia alkaloids such as Reserpine, are administered. Sympathectomy, which is not always effective, is the next line of treatment. If ischemia leads to ulceration and gangrene, amputation is necessary. Calcium blockers may also be tried to decrease vasospasm caused by vascular reactivity from calcium influx.

Diseases of the Veins
Varicose Veins and Chronic Venous Insufficiency

A **varicose vein** is a vein in which blood has pooled. Varicose veins, typically the saphenous veins of the legs, are distended, tortuous, and palpable. Varicose veins are caused by (1) trauma to the saphenous veins that damages one or more valves or (2) gradual venous distention caused by a combination of standing for long periods, which diminishes the action of the muscle pump, and the action of gravity on blood within the legs.

Veins are thin-walled, highly distensible vessels. Normally, valves prevent backflow and pooling of blood. If a valve is damaged, permitting backflow, a section of the vein is subjected to the pressure exerted by a larger volume of blood under the influence of gravity. The vein swells as it becomes engorged and surrounding tissue becomes edematous because increased hydrostatic pressure pushes plasma through the stretched vessel wall.

Valvular incompetence is also caused by venous distention that develops over time in individuals who habitually stand for long periods of time, wear constricting garments, or cross the legs at the knees. Distention progresses until the pressure in the vein damages venous valves, rendering the valves incompetent. Damaged valves are unable to maintain normal venous pressure, which causes hydrostatic pressure in the vein to increase. As the vein distends further, it becomes tortuous, and edema develops in the extremity.

Varicose veins and valvular incompetence can progress to **chronic venous insufficiency** (CVI). CVI is inadequate venous return over a long period of time. It causes pathologic changes as a result of ischemia in the vasculature, skin, and supporting tissues. CVI is marked by chronic pooling of blood in the veins of the lower extremities and leads to hyperpigmentation of the skin over the feet and ankles. Edema of the feet and ankles becomes marked and may progress proximally to the knees.

Circulation to the extremities becomes so sluggish that the metabolic demands of the cells for oxygen, nutrients, and waste removal are barely met. Any trauma or pressure can, therefore, lower the oxygen supply to injurious levels by further reducing blood flow into the area. Cell death occurs and necrotic tissue develops into **venous stasis ulcers.** Persistent ulceration develops because the high metabolic demands of healing tissue, particularly an increased need for oxygen, cannot be met by the existing circulation. Venous stasis ulcers are susceptible to infection because poor circulation impairs the delivery of the cells and biochemicals of the immune and inflammatory responses. (The role of inflammation in processes of healing are described in Chapter 7.)

Treatment of varicose veins and chronic venous insufficiency begins conservatively. The individual wears antiembolism stockings and avoids standing and other factors, such as constrictive clothing, that contribute to venous stasis. If conservative treatment is ineffective or if thrombi develop in the varicose veins, stasis ulcers develop and saphenous vein stripping is performed.

Thrombus Formation in Veins

The process of thrombus formation in the veins is the same as that of thrombus formation in the arteries. Venous thrombi are more common than arterial thrombi, however, because flow and pressure are lower in the veins than in the arteries (Fig. 27-9). With aging, in particular, the deep veins in the lower extremities become susceptible to thrombus formation, particularly with long-term bedrest or the wearing of constrictive clothing.

The inflammatory response triggered by the clotting cascade causes extreme tenderness, swelling, and redness in the area of thrombus formation. Deep venous thrombi rarely detach and cause embolism. Thrombi that form in superficial veins are almost always caused by trauma to the venous intima.

The clinical manifestations of venous occlusion differ markedly from those of arterial occlusion. With venous occlusion, the skin is discolored rather than pale (ranging from an angry red to deep blue-purple), edema is prominent, and pain is most marked at the site of occlusion, though extreme edema can render all the skin of the limb quite tender. Neuralgia develops if the edema causes soft tissues to compress local nerves.

Superior Vena Cava Syndrome

Superior vena cava syndrome (SCVS) is a progressive occlusion of the superior vena cava (SVC) that leads to venous distention in the upper extremities and

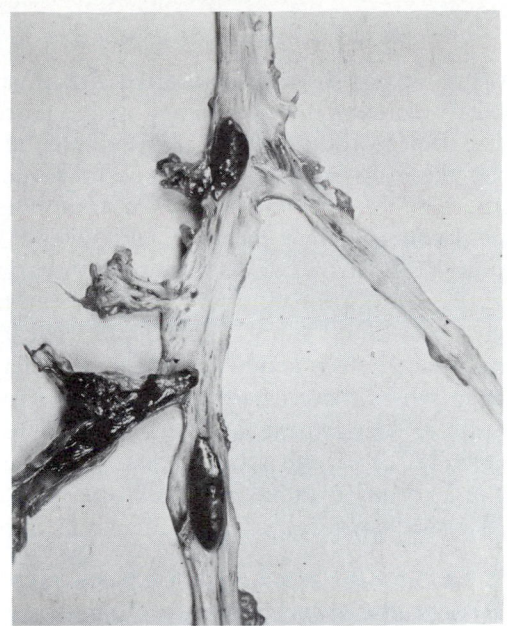

FIG. 27-9. Multiple venous thrombi. (From Rosai, 1981.)

head. The leading cause of SCVS is bronchogenic cancer (75% of cases), followed by lymphomas (15%), and metastasis of other cancers (7%). The right main stem bronchus abuts the SVC so that cancers occurring in this bronchus may press upon the SVC. The SVC is also a relatively low-pressure vessel that lies in the closed thoracic compartment; therefore, tissue expansion within the thoracic compartment can easily compress the SVC. Finally, the SVC is surrounded by lymph nodes and lymph chains that commonly become involved in thoracic cancers and compress the SVC during tumor growth. Because onset of SVCS is slow, collateral venous drainage to the azygous vein usually has time to develop.

Clinical manifestations of SVCS include edema and venous distension in the upper extremities and face, including the ocular beds. Cerebral and central nervous system edema may cause headache, visual disturbance, and impaired consciousness. The skin of the face and arms is purple and taut, and capillary refill time is prolonged. Respiratory distress may be present because of edema of bronchial structures or to compression of the bronchus by a carcinoma.

Treatment of SVCS is usually delayed for 24 hours to determine its cause. Because of its slow onset and the development of collateral venous drainage, SVCS is generally not a vascular emergency, but rather is an oncologic emergency. Treatment consists of radiotherapy and the administration of diuretics, steroids, and anticoagulants, as necessary (Varricchio, 1985).

Coronary Artery Disease, Myocardial Ischemia, and Myocardial Infarction

Coronary artery disease, myocardial ischemia, and myocardial infarction form a pathophysiologic continuum that impairs the pumping ability of the heart by depriving the heart muscle of blood-borne oxygen and nutrients. The earliest lesions of the continuum are those of **coronary artery disease**—virtually any vascular disorder that narrows or occludes the coronary arteries (Fig. 27-10). Coronary artery disease can diminish the myocardial blood supply until deprivation impairs myocardial metabolism enough to cause **ischemia,** a local state in which the cells are temporarily deprived of blood supply. They remain alive but are unable to function normally. Persistent ischemia or the complete occlusion of a coronary artery causes **infarction,** or death, of the deprived myocardial tissue. Infarction comprises the often-fatal event known as the "heart attack."

Development of Coronary Artery Disease

In the United States, coronary artery disease is responsible for nearly 50% of all deaths and one third of deaths of persons between 35 and 65 years of age (Hancock, 1986). In the 1960s, researchers began to identify risk factors that contribute to the onset and escalation of coronary artery disease. The factors were classified as either modifiable or nonmodifiable. The nonmodifiable risk factors refer to variables that cannot be altered by persons wishing to decrease their risk of cardiovascular disease. These include advanced age, male gender (until age 60), black or oriental race, genetic predisposition (which many consider modifiable if genetic risk means hypertension and hyperlipidemia, which are treatable), and diabetes mellitus type I. The modifiable risk factors include hyperlipidemia (high levels of circulating lipoproteins), hypertension, cigarette smoking, diabetes mellitus type II, obesity, sedentary life-style, psychoso-

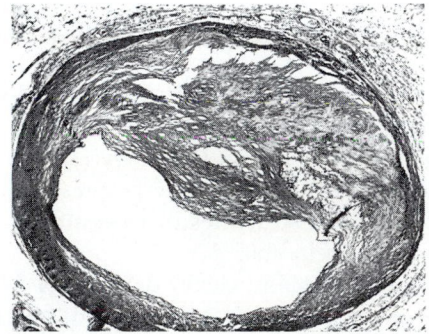

FIG. 27-10. Narrowed lumen of small branch of anterior descending coronary artery caused by atherosclerosis. Note thick fibrous and atheromatous plaque on one side, greatly reduced lumen, and reduced media. This woman died of a myocardial infarction. (From Kissane, 1985.)

cial factors (e.g., stress), hormone therapy, and heavy alcohol consumption. The role that some of the modifiable risk factors play in precipitating or exacerbating cardiovascular disease is controversial. Hyperlipidemia (e.g., hypercholesterolemia), hypertension, and cigarette smoking have, however, been identified objectively as most predictive of CAD (Criqui, 1986).

Hyperlipidemia

The strong link between coronary artery disease and elevated plasma lipoprotein concentrations is well documented by many authors (Assmann, 1987; Goldstein & Brown, 1985; Kottke, 1986; Ross & Glomset, 1976; Schaefer & Levy 1985). The term *lipoprotein* refers to lipids, phospholipids, cholesterol, and triglycerides bound to carrier proteins. Lipids (cholesterol in particular) are required by most cells for the manufacture and repair of plasma membranes. Cholesterol is also a necessary component for the manufacture of such essential substances as bile acids and steroid hormones. Although cholesterol can easily be obtained from dietary fat intake, most body cells are also able to manufacture cholesterol.

The cycle of lipid metabolism is quite complex. Dietary fat is packaged into particles known as **chylomicrons** in the small intestine. Chylomicrons are required for absorption of fat and function by transporting exogenous lipid from the intestine to the liver and peripheral cells. Chylomicrons are the least dense of the lipoproteins, and primarily contain triglyceride. Some of the triglyceride may be removed and either stored by adipose tissue or used by muscle as an energy source. The chylomicron remnants, comprised mainly of cholesterol, are taken up by the liver. A series of chemical reactions in the liver result in the production of several lipoproteins that vary in density and function. These include very low-density lipoproteins (VLDL), primarily triglyceride and protein; low-density lipoproteins (LDL), mostly cholesterol and protein; and high-density Lipoproteins (HDL), mainly phospholipids and protein. Investigators suggest that high levels of VLDL and LDL are directly related to increased risk of atherosclerosis of the coronary arteries because of their fat content. HDLs, on the other hand, are thought to prevent or delay atherogenesis and thus are thought to be protective. This may be because of their lower fat content or their possible role in carrying lipids away from body tissues to the liver for degradation; that is, "reverse" cholesterol transport (Assmann, 1987; Goldstein & Brown, 1985).

Hyperlipidemia may develop in individuals because of high dietary fat intake, systemic disease (pancreatitis, diabetes mellitus, hypothyroidism, nephrosis, systemis lupus erythematosus), and genetic defects (familial dyslipoproteinemias). The most convincing evidence that hy-

TABLE 27-5 Familial dyslipoproteinemias

Name	Laboratory findings	Clinical features	Therapy
Type I; exogenous hyperlipidemia; fat-induced hypertriglyceridemia	Cholesterol normal Triglycerides increased 3 times Chylomicrons increased	Abdominal pain Hepatosplenomegaly Skin and retinal lipid deposits Usual onset: childhood	Low fat diet
Type IIa; hypercholesterolemia	Triglycerides normal LDL increased Cholesterol increased	Premature vascular disease Xanthomas of tendons and bony prominences Common Onset: all ages	Low saturated fat and cholesterol diet Cholestyramine[1] Colestipol[2] Nicotinic acid[3] Neomycin[4] Intestinal bypass
Type IIb; combined hyperlipidemia; carbohydrate-induced hypertriglyceridemia	LDL, VLDL increased Cholesterol increased Triglycerides increased	Same as IIa	Same as IIa; *plus* carbohydrate restriction Clofibrate[5] Gemfibrozil[6]
Type III; dysbetalipoproteinemia	IDL or chylomicron remnants increased Cholesterol increased Triglycerides increased	Premature vascular disease Xanthomas of tendons and bony prominences Uncommon Onset: adulthood	Weight control Low carbohydrate, saturated fat, and cholesterol diet Alcohol restriction Clofibrate Gemfibrozil Nicotinic acid Estrogens[7] Intestinal bypass
Type IV; endogenous hyperlipidemia; carbohydrate-induced hypertriglyceridemia	Glucose intolerance Hyperuricemia Cholesterol normal or increased VLDL increased Triglycerides increased	Premature vascular disease Skin lipid deposits Obesity Hepatomegaly Common onset: adulthood	Weight control Low carbohydrate diet Alcohol restriction Clofibrate Nicotinic acid Intestinal bypass
Type V; mixed hyperlipidemia; carbohydrate and fat-induced hypertriglyceridemia	Glucose intolerance Hyperuricemia Chylomicrons increased VLDL increased LDL increased Cholesterol increased Triglycerides increased 3 times	Abdominal pain Hepatospenomegaly Skin lipid deposits Retinal lipid deposits Onset: childhood	Weight control Low carbohydrate and fat diet Clofibrate Nicotinic acid Progesterone[8] Intestinal bypass

[1]Cholestyramine (Questram): anion exchange resin; binds bile acids; enhances cholesterol excretion.
[2]Colestipol (Colistid): same as cholestyramine.
[3]Nicotinic acid (niacin): decreases release of free fatty acids from adipose tissue; increases lipogenesis in liver; decreases glucagon release; most effective for Type V disorder.
[4]Neomycin: experimental medication; questionable mode of action; decreases LDLs
[5]Clofibrate (Atromid S): decreases release of free fatty acids from adipose tissue; decreases hepatic secretion of VLDL and increased catabolism of VLDL.
[6]Gemfibrozil (Lopid): similar to clofibrate, but increases HDLs more.
[7]Estrogens: decrease IDL levels in type III disorders; experimental.
[8]Progesterone: decreases plasma triglycerides in type V disorders; experimental.

perlipidemia is an important risk factor in the development of atherosclerosis is seen in cases of familial hypercholesterolemia. Individuals who are homozygous for this disorder rarely reach the age of 20; most die of severe atherosclerosis in their teens. Myocardial infarctions have been documented in children as young as 3 to 5 years old in whom this familial disorder occurs (Assmann, 1987). Causes of the familial dyslipoproteinemias includes abnormalities of lipid-metabolizing enzymes and abnormal cellular lipid receptors (see Table 27-5) (Goldstein & Brown, 1985)

Hypertension

Elevated blood pressure may precipitate or exacerbate the atherosclerotic process by causing trauma to the arterial walls. A vicious cycle results as atherogenic plaques stiffen and narrow arterial walls, increasing peripheral resistance and myocardial workload. Escalating hypertension and cardiac muscle hypertrophy result.

Cigarette Smoking

Studies indicate that 30% of the annual mortality from coronary artery disease is traceable to cigarette smoking (Hancock, 1986). The mechanism by which smoking increases atherosclerosis is uncertain. Nicotine stimulates the release of catecholamines (epinephrine and norepinephrine), which increase heart rate and peripheral vascular constriction. As a result, blood pressure increases, as does cardiac workload and oxygen demand. Elevated catecholamines also stimulate release of free fatty acids. In one study, men and women who smoked more than 15 cigarettes per day were found to have lower HDL levels and higher LDL, cholesterol, and triglyceride levels (Brischetto et al., 1983). Cigarette smoking may also increase platelet adhesiveness, thereby increasing the risk of clot formation within the arteries. Furthermore, the carbon monoxide in cigarette smoke reduces the oxygen content of arterial blood. Hypoxemia (insufficient oxygen in arterial blood) may promote atherosclerosis by decreasing the availability of oxygen to the vessel walls and increasing vessel wall permeability. The cadmium in cigarette smoke may be related to elevations in blood pressure. One hypothesis suggests that tobacco tars are atherogenic because they cause proliferation of arterial monoclonal smooth muscle cells (Hancock, 1986). The risk of coronary artery disease increases with heavy smoking and decreases when smoking is stopped. After smoking is discontinued, the risks associated with coronary artery disease may decrease as much as 50% in one year (Braunwald, 1988).

Diabetes Mellitus

Diabetes mellitus is often associated with increased lipid levels, obesity, and hypertension. Glucose intolerance doubles the occurrence of coronary disease in men and may quadruple the incidence in women (Hurst et al., 1986). Control of hyperglycemia alone, however, does not eliminate the coronary risk. The pathophysiologic link to atherosclerosis is unclear, but multifactorial risk reduction is implied (see Chapter 5).

Genetic Predisposition

A very strong family predisposition to early coronary heart disease occurs in about 5% of the general population of families, however, these coronary-prone families account for more than 50% of cases of coronary disease occurring before the age of 55 (Williams, 1984). Serum cholesterol level is one of the most predictive risk factors for coronary heart disease (CHD) (Hjermann et al., 1981; Kannel et al., 1979). It is the cholesterol risk factor that clinicians most often refer to as the genetic contribution to CAD (McCance, 1983). Coronary disease usually develops by age 45 in men who have familial hypercholesterolemia (Williams, 1984).

A phenomenon called "tracking" exists in children, whereby the level of serum cholesterol at school age is predictive of the level 4 years later. This suggests an inborn genetic control of cholesterol over time (Schrott et al., 1979). The Framingham Offspring Study (Kannel et al., 1979), as well as twin studies (Feinleib & Garrison, 1979), indicate the cholesterol subfractions, LDL, HDL, and VLDL reveal familial associations and heritability similar to those of total cholesterol levels. Familial hypercholesterolemia (type IIa) has the greatest predictive power in characterizing genetic disorders leading to early CAD.

Hypertension also plays a significant role in about one fourth of coronary-prone families. Estimates of heritability for blood pressure indicate that about 50% of the population variability for blood pressure could be attributed to genetic factors (Williams, 1984).

Obesity

Obesity is not an independent factor. Obesity does affect the risk profile by predisposing individuals to hypertension, hyperlipidemias, and impaired glucose tolerance. Studies have consistently reported a decrease in HDL levels associated with obesity (Criqui, 1986). As obesity progresses, the heart increases in size, resulting in increased oxygen consumption and increased work load.

Sedentary Life-style

The concept that a sedentary life-style predisposes to coronary artery disease and that physical exercise may prevent its development is quite popular. The popularity, however, exceeds the supporting scientific evidence (Blair & Oberman, 1987; Lavie & Savage, 1987). Physical exercise may reduce blood pressure, decrease the urge to smoke and eat, improve carbohydrate metabolism, and improve psychologic outlook. (Increased fibrinolysis with decreased blood clotting has been noted in individuals who exercise regularly [Estok & Rudy, 1986]). In addition, persons who are habitually physically active tend to have higher plasma HDL levels than do sedentary individuals (Crique, 1986). There is no evidence that exercise increases development of coronary collateral vessels or results in regression of atheromatous plaques. However, physical activity does increase heart volume and mass, increases cardiac capillary vascularity, and decreases heart rate—all of which may protect from the effects of ischemic damage (Hurst et al., 1986). Studies on sudden death in joggers and runners over the age of 30 reveal coronary atherosclerosis is most often the cause (Estok & Rudy, 1986; Scragg et al., 1987; Thompson et al., 1979).

Hormone Therapy

Mortality from coronary artery disease has been reportedly reduced in women who receive estrogen replacement postmenopause (Criqui, 1986). It is thus interesting to note that estrogens do not reduce the incidence of coronary artery disease in men. Moreover, use of estrogen-containing oral contraceptives in premenopausal women may increase the risk of myocardial infarction (Hurst et al., 1986). The mechanism involved is enhanced thrombosis rather than accelerated atherogenesis. Presumably, contraceptives effect the coagulation profile, i.e., high platelet counts, short thromboplastin time, elevation of various clotting factors, increased platelet adhesiveness, lowered levels of antithrombin III (complexes with thrombin, a reduction promotes thrombosis), and decreased clearance of activated clotting factors (Braunwald, 1988). Oral contraceptives have been associated with increases in body weight, blood pressure, and triglyceride levels while decreasing glucose tolerance and HDL concentrations. Women who smoke may be at an even greater risk for untoward effects of estrogen therapy (Braunwald, 1988). Further research is needed to elucidate the relationship of estrogens and coronary artery disease.

The reason for the male-female differential in susceptibility to coronary artery disease is not understood. Although initial studies lauded estrogen as the reason women under the age of 50 experienced lower incidence of CAD, the previous paragraph disputes this claim. Perhaps androgen levels are responsible. Postmenopausal women experience increased effects from circulating androgens as a result of decreased estrogen opposition. It is possible that male-linked hormones may also be correlated significantly with increased coronary risk.

Alcohol

Moderate alcohol intake (less than three drinks per day) has been associated with increased HDL levels (Hopkins & Williams, 1986). Regardless, the apparent protective nature of alcohol may be more likely the consequence of multiple advantageous characteristics, such as low blood pressure, healthy genetic endowment, and so forth (Shaper, Phillips, Pocock, & Walker, 1987). Alcohol is known to increase body weight, triglyceride levels and systolic blood pressure and may impair left ventricular function. Some studies have demonstrated a direct cardiotoxic effect of excessive alcohol on myocardial tissue, resulting in collagen accumulation, diminished nucleic acid pools, and loss of membrane transport systems (Hurst et al., 1986). Further research is needed to clarify this issue.

Women and Coronary Artery Disease

There is concern that women will lose their survival advantage over men as they enter the work force in increasing numbers. This concern has its basis in the unsubstantiated assumption that men live fewer years than women because they work outside the home (Haynes et al., 1984). If working women smoke, drink alcohol to excess, indulge in fatty foods, and develop hypertension or diabetes mellitus, their risk of coronary artery disease will increase in comparison to nonworking women who do not so indulge (Detre, 1984). Premenopausal women, however, may still have a selective survival advantage when compared to men in the same age group, possibly because of hormonal effects.

Although high-density-lipoprotein (HDL) cholesterol levels are inversely related to the risk of cardiovascular disease in both men and women, the risk posed by high levels of low-density-lipoprotein (LDL) cholesterol is not as dramatic or clear-cut in women as it is in men (Crouse, 1989). Data from two large studies suggest that low HDL levels are riskier for women than high LDL levels (Crouse, 1989). The study of women and cardiovascular disease needs direct investigation and not just extrapolation from studies of men.

Type A Personality

Beginning in the 1950s, Friedman and Rosenman (1974) and other investigators argued compellingly that persons with the type A personality are at higher risk for the development of coronary disease. Many epidemiologic studies support that view; however, crucial support came from two other types of studies—a prospective study and a number of angiographic studies (Dimsdale, 1988).

The well-known prospective study was the Western Collaborative Group Study (WCGS), which followed 3154 healthy men for 8½ years. Data demonstrated three significant findings: (1) that persons with type A behavior had about twice the chance of acquiring coronary artery disease, (2) that the increased risk associated with type A behavior was not dependent on other known risk factors, and (3) that type A behavior was a predictor of subsequent reinfarction (Jenkins, Zyzanski,

& Rosenman, 1976). Three separate research groups found that persons with type A behavior had more extensive coronary artery disease at the time of coronary angiography (Blumenthal et al., 1978; Frank et al., 1978; Jenkins et al., 1976).

As a result of these studies, a review panel recognized type A behavior as a risk factor for coronary artery disease in 1981 (The Review Panel on Coronary-prone Behavior and Coronary Heart Disease, 1981). Since the early 1980s, however, a large number of contradictory findings have been reported regarding the risk status of type A behavior (Dimsdale, 1988). For example, Ragland and Brand (1988) found that subsequent coronary mortality in patients who had experienced a first coronary event was surprisingly lower among type A than among type B persons (an opposite type of behavior). Thus, type A behavior became a protective factor!

Recent studies now fail to demonstrate an association between type A behavior and the extent of coronary artery disease (Dimsdale, 1988). Nonetheless, type A behavior continues to appear, suggesting validity to the type A concept. One of the problems to keep in mind is how the type A behavior is described. Perhaps there is a better, tighter, more predictive description of the type A behavior. For example, suppressed hostility has been described as a more predictive core of the "coronary-prone personality" (MacDougall et al., 1985). Emotional stresses are known to precipitate an acute myocardial infarction (Braunwald, 1988). Rahe et al. (1974) noted a significant increase in stressful life events in individuals who subsequently experienced myocardial infarction or sudden death. Increased coronary risk has been correlated with certain behavior traits, specifically those of the so-called type A personality. Individuals with the type A personality are described as hard-driving, aggressive, compulsive, domineering, and deadline conscious (Rose, 1987).

Myocardial Ischemia

Pathophysiology

The coronary arteries normally supply blood flow sufficient to meet the demands of the myocardium as it labors under varying work loads. Oxygen extraction from these vessels occurs with maximal efficiency. If efficient exchange does not meet myocardial oxygen needs, healthy coronary arteries are able to dilate to increase the flow of oxygenated blood to the myocardium. A variety of pathologic mechanisms can interfere with blood flow through the coronary arteries, giving rise to myocardial ischemia. Narrowing of a major coronary artery by more than 50% impairs blood flow sufficiently to hamper cellular metabolism under conditions of increased myocardial demand (Fig. 27-10).

The most common cause of myocardial ischemia is atherosclerosis. Plaque formation within the arterial system often results in occlusion of vessel lumina, depriving the myocardium of oxygen and nutrients. Thrombus formation in the coronary arteries may result from ulceration of atherosclerotic plaques. The growing mass of plaque, platelets, fibrin, and cellular debris can eventually narrow the lumen enough to impede blood flow (see Fig. 27-2). Platelet aggregations are known to release the prostaglandin thromboxane A_2, a potent vasoconstrictor capable of causing spasm of the coronary arteries. Thromboxane A_2 also promotes platelet aggregation, resulting in a vicious positive feedback cycle of vasoconstriction and platelet buildup in the vessel walls.

Myocardial ischemia develops if coronary blood flow or the oxygen content of coronary blood is not sufficient to meet the metabolic demands of myocardial cells. Imbalances between blood supply and myocardial demand can result from a number of conditions. Supply is reduced by (1) hemodynamic factors, such as increased resistance in coronary vessels, hypotension, or decreased blood volume (e.g., due to hemorrhage); (2) cardiac factors, such as decreases of diastolic filling time, increases in heart rate, or valvular incompetence; (3) hematologic factors, such as the oxygen content of the blood; or (4) systemic disorders that reduce blood flow or the availability of oxygen (e.g., shock). Myocardial ischemia is usually caused by increased resistance in coronary vessels, but because the myocardium has little tolerance for hypoxia, it is particularly vulnerable (along with brain tissue) to the hypoxemia caused by respiratory disease (e.g., chronic obstructive pulmonary disease), anemia, or erythrocyte disorders that interfere with oxygen binding (see Chapters 23 and 30).

Demand is increased by (1) high systolic blood pressure; (2) increased ventricular volume; (3) increased thickness of the myocardium (e.g., left ventricular hypertrophy caused by increased systemic resistance, such as occurs with aortic valve stenosis and hypertension); (4) increased heart rate resulting from exercise, stress, hyperthyroidism, anemia, or hyperviscosity of the blood (e.g., polycythemia); or (5) conditions that heighten the myocardium's contractile response. Ischemia occurs if demand exceeds supply. For example, in an individual with coronary artery disease, supply may be adequate for myocardial function while the individual is at rest, provided respiratory and erythrocyte function are normal. Any factor that increases demand, such as strenuous exercise, or decreases supply, such as the development of anemia or respiratory disease, places the individual at risk for an episode of myocardial ischemia.

Myocardial cells become ischemic within 10 seconds of coronary occlusion. After several minutes, the heart cells lose the ability to contract, thus hampering pump function and depriving the myocardium of a glucose

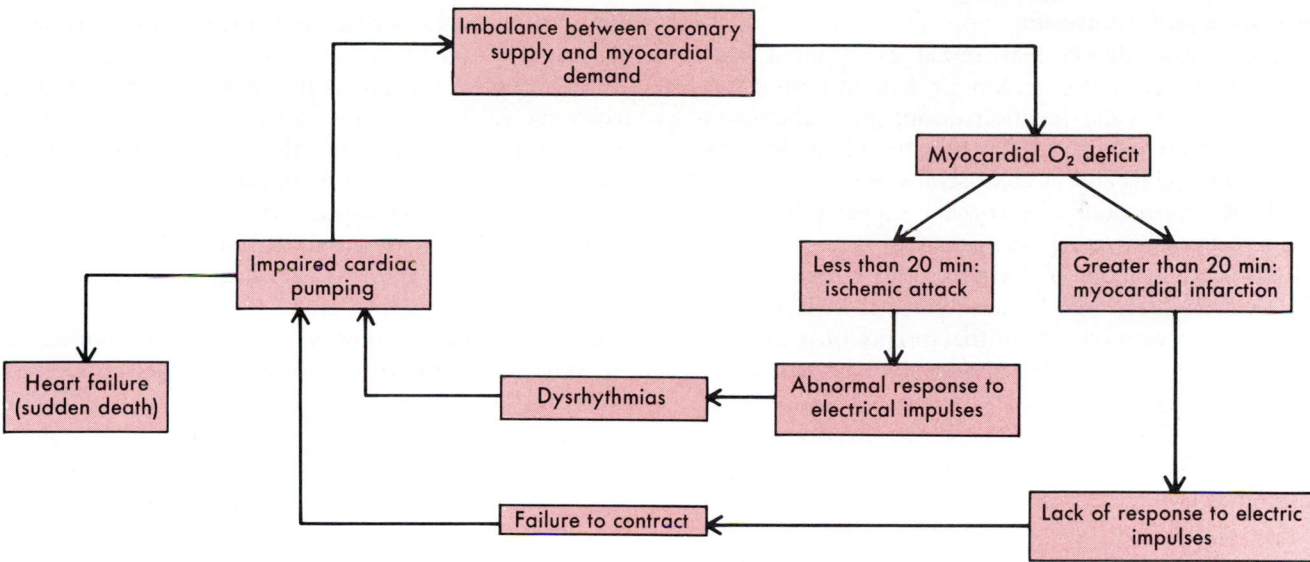

FIG. 27-11. Cycle of ischemic events.

source necessary for aerobic metabolism. Anaerobic processes take over, and lactic acid accumulates. Cardiac cells remain viable for approximately 20 minutes under ischemic conditions. If blood flow is restored, aerobic metabolism resumes, contractility is restored, and cellular repair begins. If the coronary arteries cannot compensate for lack of oxygen, myocardial infarction occurs (Fig. 27-11).

Clinical Manifestations

Angina pectoris is chest pain caused by myocardial ischemia. The discomfort is transient, lasting approximately 3 to 5 minutes. If blood flow is restored, no permanent change or damage results. The effects of temporary ischemia are reversible.

Angina pectoris is typically experienced as substernal chest discomfort, ranging from a sensation of heaviness or pressure to moderately severe pain. Individuals often describe the sensation by clenching a fist over their left chest. Discomfort may radiate to the neck, lower jaw, left arm, and left shoulder. It may occasionally radiate to the back or down the right arm. Discomfort is commonly mistaken for indigestion. The pain is presumably caused by the buildup of lactic acid or abnormal stretching of the ischemic myocardium that irritates myocardial nerve fibers. These afferent sympathetic fibers enter the spinal cord from levels C3 to T4, accounting for the variety of locations and radiation pattern of anginal pain. Pallor, diaphoresis, and dyspnea may be associated with the pain.

There are three types of angina: stable angina, unstable angina, and Prinzmetal angina. **Stable angina** (classic, exertional angina) is caused by luminal narrow-ing and hardening of the arterial walls, so that the affected vessels cannot dilate in response to increased myocardial demand associated with physical exertion or emotional stress. The discomfort of stable angina is generally predictable. It is brought on by known stimuli and causes the same type of sensation with each ischemic attack. Stable angina is usually relieved by rest and nitrates; if unrelieved by either treatment, the individual may be progressing toward an infarction.

Unstable angina (preinfarction angina, acute coronary insufficiency, crescendo angina) may indicate advanced ischemic heart disease. Unstable angina can seldom be predicted. The onset and course of pain differs with each attack, and attacks tend to increase in frequency and duration with time, often occurring at rest. Ischemia is often caused by a combination of vasospasm and atherosclerotic lesions that cause inadequate oxygen supply at rest. Unstable angina is a manifestation of ischemia that may signify impending infarction.

Prinzmetal angina (variant angina) is chest pain due to transmural ischemia of the myocardium (ischemia that involves the entire thickness of the myocardial layer). It occurs unpredictably and almost exclusively at rest. The underlying pathology is vasospasm of one or more of the major coronary arteries, with or without associated atherosclerosis. Variant angina frequently occurs at night, during rapid-eye-movement sleep. It may have a cyclical pattern of occurrence. The cause of vasospasm is postulated to be (1) hyperactivity of the sympathetic nervous system, (2) an increase in calcium flux within arterial smooth muscle, or (3) impaired production or release of prostaglandin I_2 or thromboxane A_2 (Oats et al., 1987; Vanhoutte & Houston, 1985).

Evaluation and Treatment

Physical examination may reveal extra, rapid heart sounds (left ventricular gallop or S₃), indicating impaired left ventricular function during the ischemic attack. The presence of xanthelasmas (small fat deposits) around the eyelids and/or arcus senilis of the eyes (a yellow lipid ring around the cornea) suggests hyperlipidemia and possible atherosclerosis.

Electrocardiography is a critical tool for the diagnosis of myocardial ischemia. Because many individuals have normal electrocardiograms in the absence of pain, diagnosis requires that electrocardiography be performed during an attack of angina. Transient ST segment depression and T wave inversion are characteristic signs of subendocardial ischemia. ST elevation, indicative of transmural ischemia, is seen in individuals with Prinzmetal's angina (Fig. 27-12). The electrocardiogram can also give some indication of which coronary artery is involved. Exercise stress testing is useful in differentiating angina from other types of chest pain, as well as detecting ischemic changes that occur in the absence of anginal pain.

Radioisotope imaging with thallium-201 is another technique used to diagnose coronary artery disease. Active transport mechanisms (the Na-K-ATPase system) cause thallium to enter myocardial cells. An area of myocardial infarction appears as a region of diminished activity or no activity (a "cold spot"). Defects that are absent at rest, but can be induced by exercise, represent ischemia.

Coronary angiography is useful in determining the anatomic extent of coronary artery disease. Though the procedure is expensive and carries some risk, it is considered essential in the diagnostic evaluation of angina.

The primary aim of therapy for myocardial ischemia and angina is to reduce myocardial oxygen consumption by altering its various determinants in a favorable way. The factors most amenable to pharmacologic manipulation are blood pressure, heart rate, contractility, and left ventricular volume.

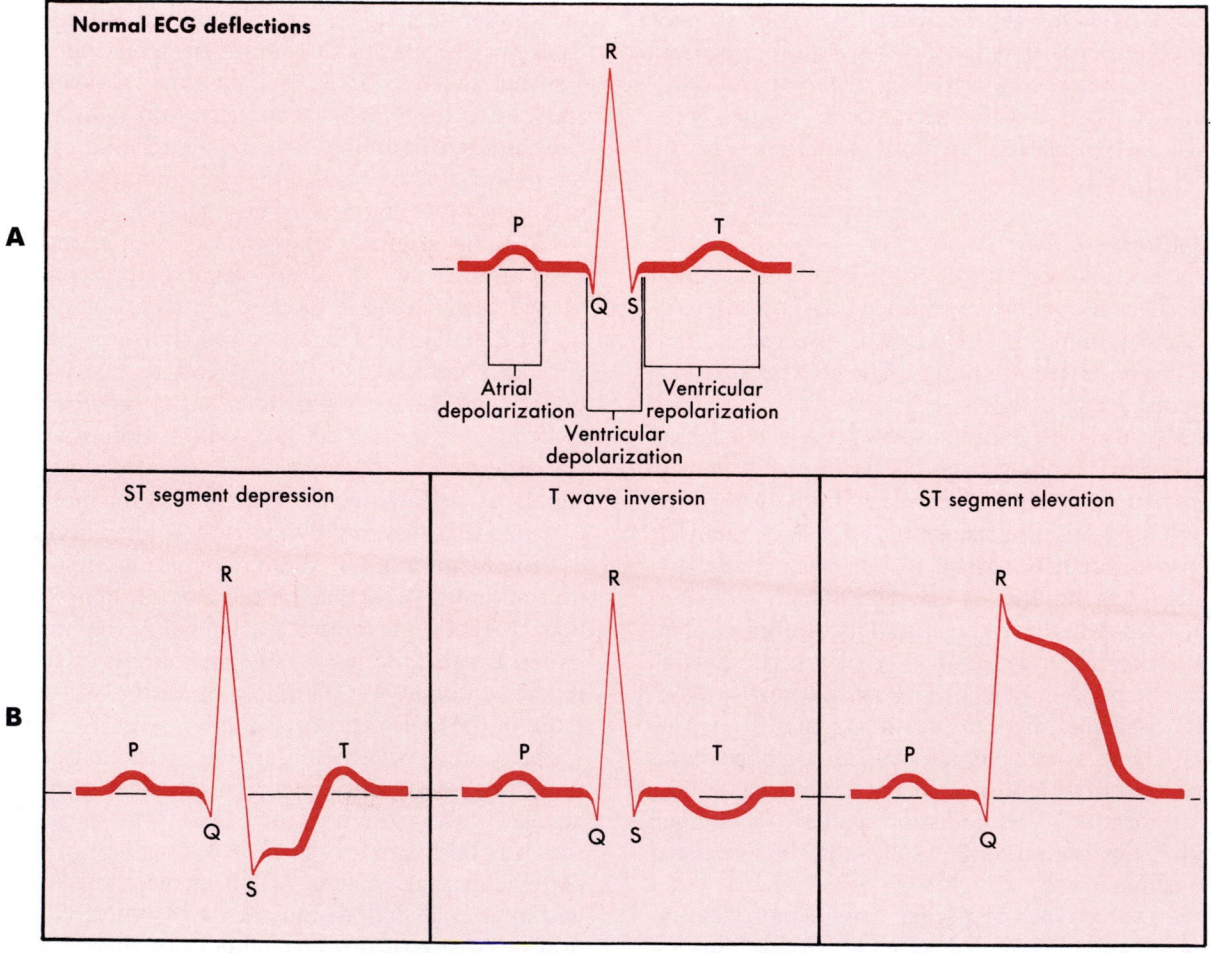

FIG. 27-12. **A,** Normal ECG. **B,** Electrocardiographic alterations associated with ischemia.

Nitrates are often the first drug of choice because they increase oxygen supply and reduce demand. Nitrates cause peripheral veins and, to a lesser extent, peripheral arteries to dilate. Dilation reduces both peripheral vascular resistance and venous return to the heart (preload) and thereby reduces left ventricular filling pressure and left ventricular volume. Reduced filling pressure and volume decrease workload (myocardial demand). Nitrates also improve coronary blood flow by reducing coronary artery spasm and thereby increase myocardial blood supply. These drugs cannot enhance vasodilation in coronary vessels altered by atherosclerosis or arteriosclerosis, because these disorders impair the vessels' ability to change lumen size.

β-Adrenergic blocking agents have had great impact on therapy for ischemic heart disease in the past 20 years. By blocking β receptors, these medications can increase oxygen supply and reduce myocardial demand. β blockers diminish catecholamine-induced elevations of heart rate, myocardial contractility, and blood pressure. Coronary blood flow also can be augmented by β blockade. Reduction in heart rate provides additional diastolic filling time for coronary perfusion, leading to enhanced oxygen delivery to the heart.

Calcium plays a key role in the electrical excitation of cardiac cells and in mechanical contraction of the myocardial and vascular smooth muscle cells (see Chapter 26). By blocking the influx of calcium into myocardial cells and vascular smooth muscle cells, the pacemaker activity of the sinoatrial node and conduction properties of the atrioventricular node can be modified. The three calcium channel blockers available in the United States are verapamil, nifedipine, and diltiazem. Combination of nitrates, β blockers, and calcium antagonists may provide dramatic relief from clinical manifestations of ischemic heart disease and make more invasive interventions unnecessary. The effects of these drugs are summarized in Table 27-6.

Experimental evidence linking platelet aggregation with decreased coronary blood flow has led to the use of antiplatelet agents for individuals with ischemic heart disease. Effective antiplatelet agents include aspirin, sulfinpyrazone, dipyridamole, or combinations of these drugs.

Percutaneous transluminal coronary angioplasty (PTCA) is a procedure whereby stenotic (narrowed) coronary vessels are dilated with a balloon dilatation catheter. The lesion most suitable for angioplasty is one that is discrete, concentric, located in a proximal portion of the vessel, noncalcified, and less than 10 mm in size (Hutter, Pasaoglu, & Williams, 1985). PTCA is generally used to treat single-vessel disease, but can be effective with multiple-vessel disease or stenosis of a coronary artery or a venous bypass graft.

Ischemic heart disease can be surgically treated by a coronary artery bypass graft. A saphenous vein from the thigh is most commonly used to bypass the obstructed coronary artery. A more recent technique, using the left internal mammary artery (LIMA) rather than the saphenous vein, has shown promise for significant improvement in long-term graft patency. One of the most common indications for bypass surgery is incapacitating angina in an individual who has good left ventricular function and technically operable coronary arteries, but who

TABLE 27-6 Effects of antianginal agents on myocardial supply and demand

	Nitrates	Beta blockers	Calcium antagonists
DEMAND			
Wall tension	Decrease	Increase	Increase or no apparent effect
Systolic blood pressure	Decrease	Decrease	Decrease
Ventricular volume	Decrease	Increase	Decrease or no apparent effect
Heart rate	Increase	Decrease	Increase, decrease, or no apparent effect
Contractility	No apparent effect	Decrease	Decrease
SUPPLY			
Coronary blood flow	Increase	Increase or no apparent effect	Increase
Coronary vascular resistance	Decrease	Increase or no apparent effec	Decrease
Coronary spasm	Decrease	Increase or no apparent effect	Decrease
Diastolic perfusion time	Decrease	Increase	Decrease, increase, or no apparent effect
Collateral blood flow	Increase	No apparent effect	Decrease

From: Kafka, Meltzer, & Frishman, 1985.

has not responded to medical therapy (Hutter et al., 1985). Although surgery has been shown to relieve angina, it does not halt the progress of atherosclerosis or prolong life. A successful coronary artery bypass graft can, however, diminish the probability of lethal insult to the coronary tissues.

Myocardial Infarction

Acute myocardial infarction can be considered the endpoint of the coronary artery disease-myocardial ischemia continuum. Prolonged, unrelieved ischemia that interrupts the blood supply to the myocardium will result in an acute coronary event. Unlike the temporary ischemia that causes angina and reversible cellular injury, the prolonged ischemia that causes infarction leads to irreversible hypoxia and cellular death (Fig. 27-13).

The precipitating cause of irreversible hypoxia is controversial. If myocardial infarction is on a continuum with the ischemic attacks of angina, then hypoxia could be the result of long-term obstruction by atherosclerotic plaques, hemorrhage into a plaque, embolism caused by thrombi or atheromatous material, or coronary spasm. Thrombus formation resulting from abnormal platelet aggregation seems to be the most likely cause of eventual arterial occlusion, but researchers cannot agree on what makes platelets *begin* to collect on arterial walls. One explanation is that if platelets were to aggregate in a normal coronary artery with healthy endothelium, the smooth muscles of the vessel walls would respond to platelet-released substances by relaxing. This reflex relaxation would prevent significant luminal occlusion, allowing the initial aggregate of debris to be washed away from the vessel wall. On the other hand, if the vascular endothelium were absent or damaged, platelets would adhere, and the response of the vessel to platelet products and thrombin would be to contract, obstructing blood flow (Vanhoutte & Houston, 1985). Though vasoconstriction in response to platelet aggregation has been noted under some experimental conditions, platelet aggregation is not universally accepted as the precursor of coronary artery obstruction. Such substances as serotonin, thromboxane A_2, adenosine diphosphate (ADP), adenosine triphosphate (ATP), platelet-activating factor (PAF), and platelet-activated growth factor may be responsible for the coronary occlusion seen in serious coronary artery disease.

Pathophysiology

Cellular Injury Cardiac cells can withstand ischemic conditions for about 20 minutes before cellular death

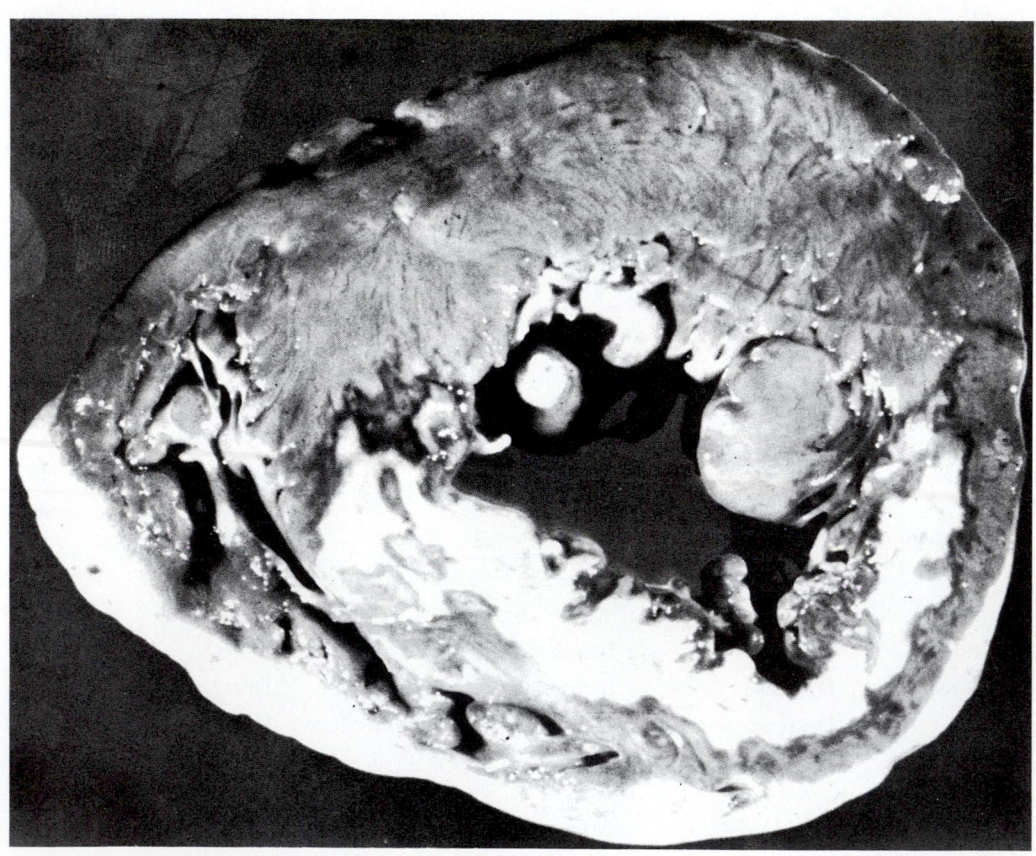

FIG. 27-13. Recent infarct of myocardium of left ventricle. (From Kissane, 1985.)

takes place. After only 30 to 60 seconds of hypoxia, electrocardiographic changes are visible. Yet even if cells are metabolically altered and nonfunctional, they can remain viable if blood flow returns within 20 minutes (Braunwald & Sobel, 1988).

After 8 to 10 seconds of decreased blood flow, the affected myocardium becomes cyanotic and cooler. Myocardial oxygen reserves are used very quickly (within about 8 seconds) after complete cessation of coronary flow. Glycogen stores decrease as anaerobic metabolism begins. Unfortunately, glycolysis can only supply 65% to 70% of the total myocardial energy requirement and produces much less ATP than aerobic processes. Hydrogen ions and lactic acid accumulate. Because myocardial tissues have poor buffering capabilities and myocardial cells are very sensitive to low cellular pH, accumulation of these products further compromises the myocardium. Acidosis may make the myocardium more vulnerable to the damaging effects of lysosomal enzymes, and may suppress impulse conduction and contractile function, thereby leading to heart failure.

Oxygen deprivation is also accompanied by electrolyte disturbances, specifically loss of potassium, calcium, and magnesium from cells. Myocardial cells deprived of necessary oxygen and nutrients lose contractility, thereby diminishing the pumping ability of the heart. Normally, the myocardium takes up varying quantities of catecholamines (epinephrine and norepinephrine). Significant arterial occlusion causes the myocardial cells to release catecholamines, predisposing the individual to serious imbalances of sympathetic and parasympathetic function, irregular heart beats (dysrhythmia), and heart failure. Catecholamines mediate the release of glycogen, glucose, and stored fat from body cells. Therefore,

plasma concentrations of free fatty acids and glycerol rise within 1 hour after onset of acute myocardial infarction. Excessive levels of free fatty acids can have a harmful detergent effect on cell membranes. Norepinephrine elevates blood sugar levels through stimulation of liver and skeletal muscle cells. It also suppresses pancreatic β-cell activity, which reduces insulin secretion and elevates blood glucose further. Not surprisingly, hyperglycemia is noted approximately 72 hours after an acute myocardial infarction.

Cellular Death After about 20 minutes of myocardial ischemia, irreversible hypoxic injury causes cellular death and tissue necrosis. (Types of necrosis are described in Chapter 2.) Necrosis of myocardial tissue results in the release of certain intracellular enzymes through the damaged cell membranes into the interstitial spaces. The lymphatics pick up the enzymes and transport them into the bloodstream, where they can be detected by serologic tests.

Structural and Functional Changes Myocardial infarction results in both structural and functional changes of cardiac tissues. Table 27-7 outlines the tissue changes that may follow myocardial infarction. Gross tissue changes may not become apparent for several hours, despite almost immediate onset (within 30 to 60 seconds) of ECG changes. Ischemic tissues around the area of necrosis may not be irreversibly damaged at the onset of myocardial infarction. Researchers are seeking ways to salvage these tissues and reduce the size of the infarction.

The severity of functional impairment depends on the size of the lesion and the site of infarction. Functional changes can include (1) decreased cardiac contractility

---

TABLE 27-7 Tissue changes after myocardial infarction

Time after myocardial infarction	Tissue changes	Stage of healing process
6-12 hours	No gross changes; subcellular cyanosis with decreased temperature	Not begun
18-24 hours	Pale to grey-brown; slight pallor	Inflammatory response; intercellular enzyme release
2-4 days	Visible necrosis: yellow-brown in center and hyperemic around edges	Proteolytic enzymes remove debris; catecholamines, lipolysis, and glycogenolysis elevate plasma glucose and increase free fatty acids to assist depleted myocardium recovery from anaerobic state
4-10 days	Area soft, with fatty changes in center, regions of hemorrhage in infarcted area	Debris cleared; collagen matrix laid down
10-14 days	Weak, fibrotic scar tissue with beginning revascularization	Healing continues, but area very mushy, vulnerable to stress
6 weeks	Scarring usually complete	Tough inelastic scar replaces necrotic myocardium

NOTE: Processes of tissue healing are described and illustrated in Chapter 7.

with abnormal wall motion, (2) altered left ventricular compliance, (3) decreased stroke volume, (4) decreased ejection fraction, (5) increased left ventricular end-diastolic pressure, and (6) sinoatrial node malfunction. Life-threatening dysrhythmias and heart failure often follow myocardial infarction.

Repair Myocardial infarction causes a severe inflammatory response that ends with wound repair (see Chapter 7). Repair consists of degradation of damaged cells, proliferation of fibroblasts, and synthesis of scar tissue. Many cell types, hormones, and nutrient substrates must be available for optimal healing to proceed. Within 24 hours, leukocytes infiltrate the necrotic area, and proteolytic enzymes from scavenger neutrophils degrade necrotic tissue. A pseudodiabetic state often develops as catecholamines released from damaged cells stimulate release of glucose and free fatty acids. By the second week, insulin secretion increases to mobilize glucose from the repair processes. The collagen matrix that is deposited is initially weak, mushy, and vulnerable to reinjury. Unfortunately it is at this time in the recovery period (10 to 14 days after infarction) that individuals feel more like increasing activities and may stress the newly formed scar tissue. After 6 weeks, the necrotic area is completely replaced by scar tissue, which is strong but is unable to contract and relax like healthy myocardial tissue.

Clinical Manifestations

The first symptom of acute myocardial infarction is usually sudden, severe chest pain. The pain is similar to angina pectoris but is more severe and persistent and is not relieved by nitrates. Radiation to the neck, jaw, back, shoulder, or left arm is common. Infarction often stimulates a sensation of unrelenting indigestion. Nausea and vomiting may occur because of reflex stimulation of vomiting centers by pain fibers. Vasovagal reflexes from the area of the infarcted myocardium may also affect the gastrointestinal tract. Catecholamine release results in sympathetic stimulation, producing diaphoresis and peripheral vasoconstriction that cause the skin to become cool and clammy. Fever may develop in the first 24 hours and persist for a week because of inflammatory activity within the myocardium.

A variety of cardiovascular changes may be found on physical examination. With an acute myocardial infarction, blood pressure may initially decrease. The drop in blood pressure reflexively activates the sympathetic nervous system to compensate and then causes a temporary increase in heart rate and blood pressure. Abnormal extra heart sounds (S_3, S_4) reflect left ventricular dysfunction. Inflammation can cause pericardial friction rub, along with a variety of cardiac murmurs.

Laboratory data reveal leukocytosis and elevated sedimentation rate, both of which indicate inflammation.

TABLE 27-8 Normal Values for SGOT and LDH_1 (CK-MD)*

Enzyme/isoenzyme	Value
SGOT	8 to 33 units/ml
	8 to 55 Units
LDH_1	17% to 27% (activity)

*CK-MD is not normally detectable in the serum; failure to detect this isoenzyme excludes the diagnosis of myocardial infarction, provided blood samples are drawn on admission and at 8-hour intervals for the next 24 hours.

Blood sugar is usually elevated, and glucose tolerance may remain abnormal for several weeks.

A transient rise in plasma enzyme levels can confirm the occurrence of myocardial infarction and indicate its severity. The enzymes released by myocardial cells include creatine phosphokinase (CK), lactic dehydrogenase (LDH), and, to a lesser extent, serum glutamic oxaloacetic transaminase (SGOT; also known as aspartate aminotransferase, or AST). These enzymes exist in several different active molecular forms called isoenzymes, which are present in different amounts within particular tissues. If serologic tests show abnormally high levels of isoenzymes associated with cardiac tissue (CK-MB, LDH-1), acute myocardial infarction has probably occurred. Of the three isoenzymes, CK-MB is most specific for myocardial infarction, although its level may also rise in individuals with certain other conditions (such as muscular dystrophy, hypothermia, chronic obstructive pulmonary disease associated with left heart failure and pulmonary embolism, extensive third-degree burns, or small bowel infarction). Elevation of CK-MB, LDH-1, and SGOT will be noted at characteristic times (Table 27-8). The amount of CK elevation may be correlated with severity of infarction. The higher the serum concentration of CK-MB, the more extensive the tissue damage that has occurred. Blood is drawn for enzyme determinations as soon as possible after the onset of symptoms, and serial enzyme levels are assessed for several days. Three consecutive days of negative enzyme elevations rule out myocardial infarction.

Myocardial infarction can occur in various regions of the heart wall and may be described as anterior, inferior, posterior, lateral, subendocardial, endocardial, subepicardial, epicardial, intramural, or transmural, depending on the anatomic location and extent of tissue damage from infarction. (For descriptions of these locations see Chapter 26.) Twelve-lead ECGs help to localize the affected area through identification of Q waves and changes in ST segments and T waves (Fig. 27-14). The infarcted myocardium is surrounded by a zone of hy-

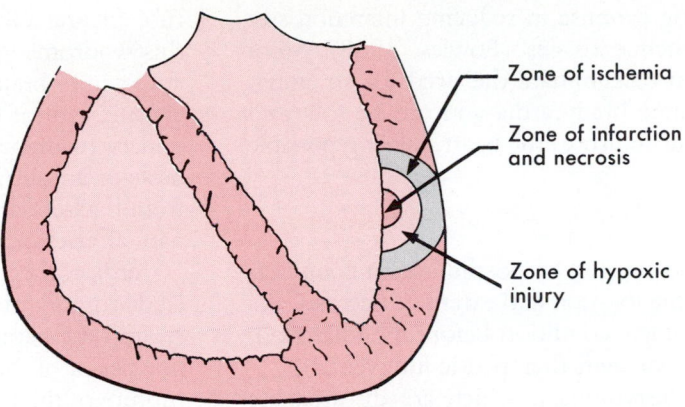

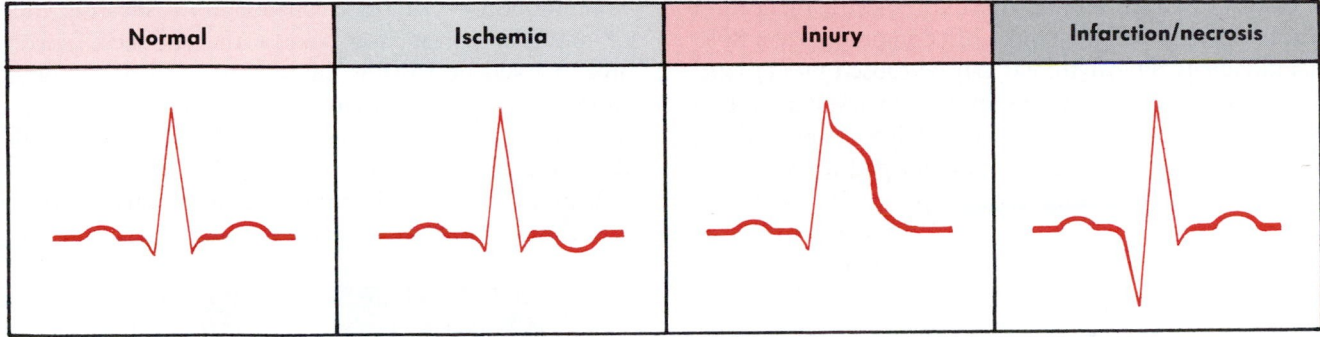

FIG. 27-14. Electrocardiographic alterations associated with the three zones of myocardial infarction.

poxic injury, which may progress to necrosis or return to normal. Infarcted tissue results in the inscription of a Q wave on the ECG. Adjacent to the zone of hypoxic injury is a zone of reversible ischemia. Ischemic and injured myocardial tissue causes ST and T wave changes. As the myocardium heals, the ST segment and T waves gradually return to normal, but abnormal Q waves generally persist.

Radionucleotide imaging with thallium-201 can provide a diagnostic picture in individuals with acute or healed myocardial infarction. Technetium-99m pyrophosphate is also taken up by areas of myocardial infarction, which appear as "hot spots." Unfortunately, the area of infarction must be large enough to visualize the hot spot, and the scan may remain positive for many months after infarction.

Evaluation and Treatment

The diagnosis of acute myocardial infarction is made on the basis of ECG, serial enzyme alterations, radionucleotide imaging, and physical examination (see Clinical Manifestations). Acute myocardial infarction requires immediate admission to a hospital with a coronary care unit, if possible. Continuous close monitoring of cardiac rhythms and enzymatic changes is especially important. The first 24 hours after onset of symptoms is the time of highest risk for sudden death. In complicated cases, in-

vasive monitoring techniques (such as arterial, central venous pressure, and Swan-Ganz lines) may be required. Intracoronary artery infusion of streptokinase (during coronary angiography), which dissolves blood clots and causes vasodilation, can relieve myocardial infarction caused by intracoronary thrombi. The treatment must be performed within 3 to 4 hours after the onset of infarction, and can reestablish blood flow in approximately 3 minutes.

Bed rest, followed by gradual return to activities of daily living, reduces the myocardial oxygen demands of the compromised heart. Pain relief is of utmost importance. If sublingual nitroglycerin is ineffective, small, carefully titrated doses of morphine sulfate (4 mg to 6 mg) may be given for sedation and vasodilation. Supplemental oxygen (2 to 4 L/min) is administered to increase arterial oxygen content and deliver more oxygen to the ischemic myocardium. Dietary measures are aimed at preventing nausea and vomiting, and consumption of sodium, saturated fats, sugar, and caffeine is limited.

Besides pain relief, pharmacologic intervention is used to limit infarction size, reduce vasoconstriction, prevent thrombus formation, and augment repair. Emergent utilization of PTCA, thrombolytic therapy (streptokinase, urokinase, tissue plasminogen activators), and judicious use of β blockers are among the techniques showing promise in reducing infarction size and salvaging ischemic tissues (Fowles, 1988). Stool softeners are given to eliminate the need for straining, which can precipitate bradycardia and can be followed by increased venous return to the heart, causing possible cardiac overload.

Complications

The number and severity of postinfarction complications depends on the location and extent of necrosis, the individual's physiologic condition before the infarction, and the availability of swift therapeutic intervention.

Dysrhythmias (arrythmias), which are disturbances of cardiac rhythm, are the most common complication of acute myocardial infarction, affecting more than 80% of individuals. Dysrhythmias can be caused by (1) ischemia, (2) hypoxia, (3) autonomic nervous system imbalances, (4) lactic acidosis, (5) electrolyte abnormalities, (6) alterations of impulse conduction pathways or conduction defects, (7) drug toxicity, or (8) hemodynamic abnormalities. Dysrhythmias may originate from the atria, ventricles, nodal regions, or conduction tissues. The seriousness of dysrhythmias depends on the hemodynamic consequences. There is no ventricular contraction in ventricular fibrillation, consequently no cardiac output. Atrial fibrillation, however, does not affect ventricular contraction and can thus be tolerated by most individuals. (Dysrhythmias are described on p. 963.)

Acute myocardial infarction is usually accompanied by some degree of left ventricular failure (congestive heart failure), which is characterized by pulmonary congestion, reduced myocardial contractility, and abnormal heart wall motion (see p. 963). Anterior infarction is associated with more severe congestive heart failure than is inferior infarction (Hancock, 1982). Mortality from acute myocardial infarction is directly related to the reduction in stroke volume caused by the infarcted ventricle. If cardiac output is insufficient to maintain normal arterial pressure and to perfuse the kidneys and other organs adequately, cardiogenic shock develops. Cardiogenic shock characteristically develops if 40% or more of the left ventricular myocardium is infarcted. (Cardiogenic shock is discussed on p. 976.)

Inflammation of the pericardium (pericarditis) is a frequent complication of acute myocardial infarction. Pericardial friction rubs are often noted 2 to 3 days post infarction, associated with anterior chest pain that worsens with respiratory effort. Specific treatment is not required, but corticosteroids dramatically relieve symptoms.

Dressler's post infarction syndrome, which is essentially a delayed form of acute pericarditis, can occur from 1 week to several months after acute myocardial infarction. Though poorly understood, the syndrome is thought to be an immunologic (antigen-antibody) response to the necrotic myocardium. Pain, fever, friction rub, pleural effusion, and arthralgias may accompany this syndrome. Steroids may alleviate symptoms.

Organic brain syndrome may occur in acute or chronic form if blood flow to the brain is impaired secondary to myocardial infarction. Transient ischemic attacks or an outright cerebrovascular accident may result from thromboemboli that have broken loose from coronary arteries or cardiac valves.

Cardiac complications of myocardial infarction include rupture of heart structures. Necrosis of tissue in or around the papillary muscles can cause rupture of these muscles or of the chordae tendineae. Factors that lead to rupture of the free wall of the infarcted ventricle include thinning of the wall, poor collateral flow, shearing effect of muscular contraction against the stiffened necrotic area, marked necrosis at the terminal end of the blood supply, and aging of the myocardium with laceration of the myocardial microstructure (Pasternak, Braunwald, & Sobel, 1988).

Rupture of the wall of the infarcted ventricle may be

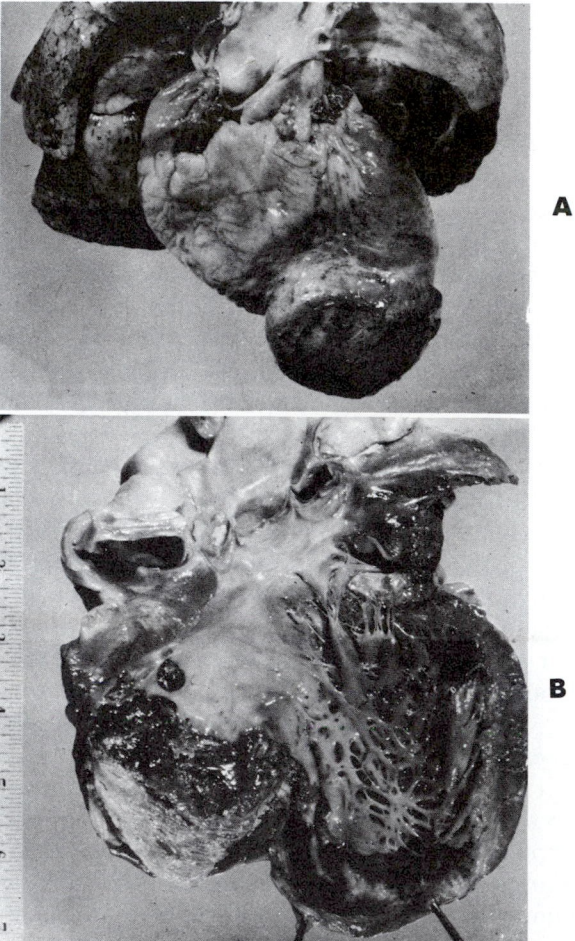

FIG. 27-15. Aneurysm of left ventricle, a result of myocardial infarct. **A,** External view. **B,** Interior view. On right, between forceps, is thin fibrotic wall. On left, aneurysm sac is filled with thrombus. (From Kissane, 1985.)

a consequence of aneurysm formation (Fig. 27-15). According to the law of Laplace, with decreased muscle mass at the infarcted site, the wall is weakened and tension stretches the noncontracting infarcted heart muscle, thus producing infarct expansion or aneurysm formation (see aneurysm, p. 927). Decreased muscle mass causes an increase in the radius of the ventricle and, because the radius is directly proportional to pressure and tension, both increase with time. The wall of the aneurysm becomes more fibrotic but continues to bulge with systole. The bulge results in impaired pump function. Although rare, rupture may occur when the tension becomes too great. Death in individuals with a left ventricular aneurysm is presumably related to ventricular tachyarrhythmias and not to ventricular rupture (Pasternak et al., 1988). Left ventricular aneurysm is a late complication of myocardial infarction, occurring months or years after the acute event.

Infarctions around septal structures that separate the heart chambers can lead to septal rupture. Ruptures are associated with audible, harsh cardiac murmurs, increased left ventricular end-diastolic pressure, and decreased systemic blood pressure.

Systemic thromboembolism is commonly found during postmortem examinations of individuals who have died of myocardial infarction. Thromboemboli may disseminate from debris and clots that collect inside dilated aneurysmal sacs, or from the infarcted endocardium. Pulmonary emboli are especially common, as are deep venous thrombi of the legs. Early mobilization and prophylactic anticoagulation therapy should reduce the incidence of this complication.

Sudden death resulting from cardiac arrest is often caused by dysrhythmias, particularly ventricular fibrillation. Other dysrhythmias may be equally lethal. Widespread knowledge of cardiopulmonary resuscitation has increased the probability of survival during the first few hours after cardiac insult. Immediate intervention and careful monitoring have also reduced mortality and have improved chances for long-term survival. However, several factors contribute to the risk of death during acute infarction or reduce the chances of long-term survival, despite the best possible treatment. They are (1) age greater than 65 years, (2) previous angina pectoris, (3) hypotension or cardiogenic shock, (4) acute systolic hypertension at the time of admission, (5) diabetes mellitus, (6) dysrhythmias or conduction defects, and (7) previous myocardial infarction (Pasternak et al., 1988).

DISORDERS OF THE HEART WALL

Disorders of the Pericardium

Pericardial disease is often a localized manifestation of another disorder, such as infection (bacterial, viral, fungal, rickettsial, or parasitic); trauma or surgery; neoplasm; or a metabolic, immunologic, or vascular disorder (uremia, rheumatoid arthritis, systemic lupus erythematosis, periarteritis nodosa). The pericardial response to injury from these diverse causes may consist of acute pericarditis, pericardial effusion, or constrictive pericarditis.

Acute Pericarditis

Though frequently idiopathic, **acute pericarditis** (acute inflammation of the pericardium) is also commonly caused by infection, connective tissue disease, or radiation therapy (Fig. 27-16). The pericardial membranes become inflamed and roughened, and an exudate may develop.

Symptoms include sudden onset of severe chest pain that worsens with respiratory movements. Although the pain may radiate to the back, it is generally felt in the anterior chest and may initially be confused with the pain of acute myocardial infarction. Individuals with acute pericarditis may also report dysphagia, restlessness, irritability, anxiety, weakness, and malaise.

Physical examination often reveals low-grade fever and sinus tachycardia. Friction rub, a short, scratchy, grating sensation similar to the sound of sandpaper,

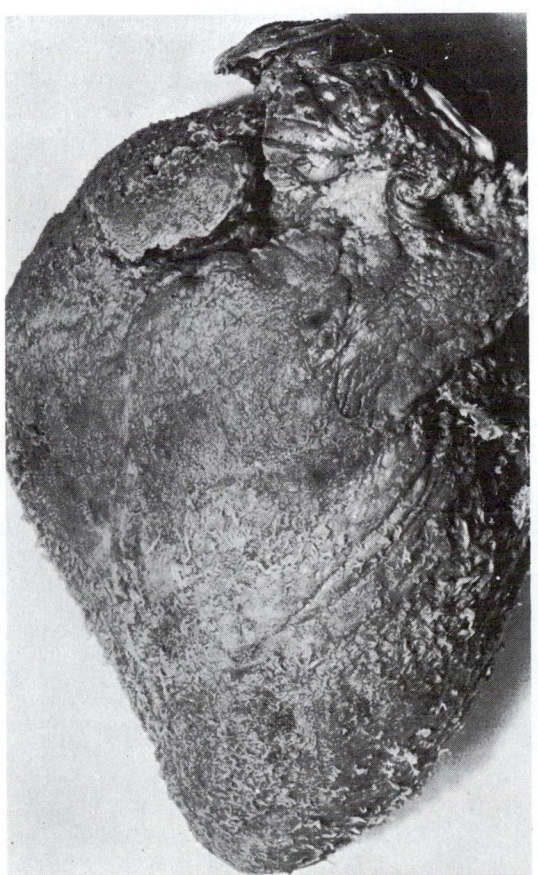

FIG. 27-16. Acute pericarditis. Note shaggy coat of fibers covering surface of heart. (From Anderson & Scotti, 1980.)

may be heard at the cardiac apex and left sternal border and is pathognomonic for pericarditis. The rub is caused by the roughened pericardial membranes rubbing against each other. Friction rubs are not always present, and may be intermittently heard and transient. Electrocardiographic changes may reflect inflammatory processes through diffuse ST segment elevation without Q waves.

Treatment for uncomplicated acute pericarditis consists of relieving symptoms. Analgesics are given to relieve pain, but doses are limited to avoid excessive respiratory depression in individuals who are already limiting respiratory effort because of pain. Salicylates and nonsteroidal antiinflammatory drugs will reduce inflammation. Corticosteroids may diminish symptoms, but rebound pain may occur after the steroids are discontinued. Rest is helpful during episodes of acute pain. Exploration of the underlying cause is important. If pericardial effusion develops, aspiration of the excessive fluid may be necessary. Acute pericarditis is usually self-limiting but may occasionally progress to chronic constrictive pericarditis.

Pericardial Effusion

Pericardial effusion—the accumulation of fluid in the pericardial cavity—can occur in all forms of pericarditis. The fluid may be a transudate, such as the serous effusion that develops with congestive heart failure, overhydration, or hypoproteinemia. More often, however, the fluid is an exudate, which reflects pericardial injury and inflammation (Fig. 27-17). (Types of exudate are described in Chapter 7.) If the fluid is serosanguinous, the underlying cause is likely to be tuberculosis, neoplasm, uremia, or radiation. Idiopathic serosanguinous (etiology unknown) effusion is possible, however. Effusions of frank blood are generally related to aneurysms, trauma, or coagulation defects. If chyle leaks from the thoracic duct, it may enter the pericardium and lead to cholesterol pericarditis.

Pericardial effusion, even in large amounts, is not necessarily clinically significant, except that it indicates an underlying disorder. The important consideration is whether the fluid is under sufficient pressure to cause cardiac compression, which is a serious condition known as **tamponade.** If an effusion develops gradually, the pericardium can stretch to accommodate large quantities of fluid without compressing the heart. If the fluid accumulates rapidly, however, even a small amount (50 to 100 ml) may cause serious tamponade. The danger is that pressure exerted by the pericardial fluid will eventually equal diastolic pressure within the heart chambers. The first structures to be affected by tamponade are the right atrium and ventricle, where diastolic pressures are normally lowest. Compression by pericardial fluid interferes with right atrial filling during diastole, resulting in increased venous pressure, systemic venous congestion, and signs and symptoms of right heart failure (distention of the jugular veins, edema, and hepatomegaly). Decreased atrial filling leads to decreased ventricular filling, decreased stroke volume, and reduced cardiac output. Life-threatening circulatory collapse may occur.

The most significant clinical finding is pulsus paradoxus, in which arterial blood pressure during expiration exceeds arterial pressure during inspiration by more than 10 mm Hg. Pulsus paradoxus indicates tamponade. This clinical finding reflects impairment of diastolic filling of the left ventricle plus reduction of blood volume within all four cardiac chambers. Presence of a large pericardial effusion or tamponade magnifies the normally insignificant effect of inspiration on intracardiac flow and volume.

Other clinical manifestations of pericardial effusion are distant or muffled heart sounds, poorly palpable apical pulse, dyspnea on exertion, and dull chest pain. A chest x-ray film may reveal a "water-bottle" configuration of the cardiac silhouette. An echocardiogram can detect an effusion as small as 20 ml.

Treatment of pericardial effusion or tamponade generally consists of pericardiocentesis (aspiration of excessive pericardial fluid). Pericardiocentesis is both diagnostic and therapeutic: the fluid is analyzed to identify the cause of the effusion and its removal alone may bring dramatic relief from symptoms. Persistent pain may be treated with analgesics, antiinflammatory medications, or steroids. Surgery may be required if the underlying cause of tamponade is trauma or aneurysm.

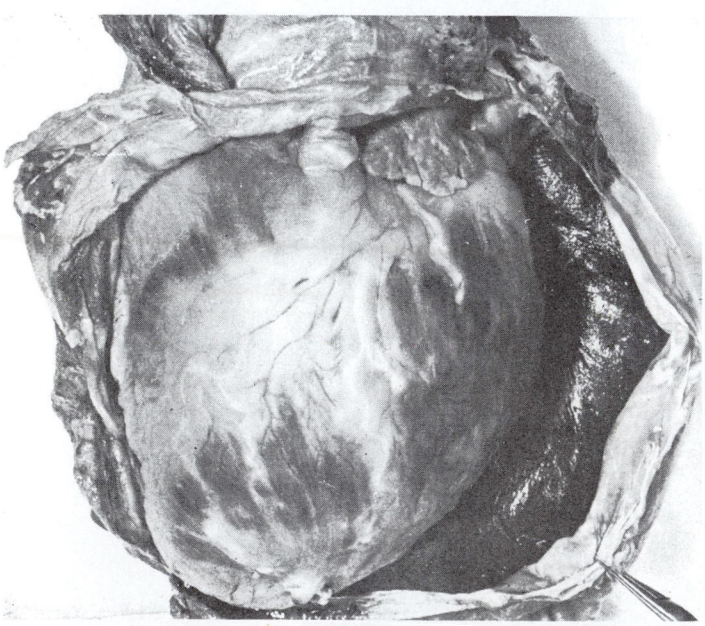

FIG. 27-17. Exudate of blood in the pericardial sac from rupture of aneurysm. (From Anderson, & Scotti, 1980.)

Individuals with acute pericarditis secondary to certain underlying conditions may have pericardial effusion. This manifestation is common in (1) individuals with uremia who are in need of dialysis and have fluid overload and left ventricular failure; (2) individuals who have lymphoma or breast cancer or who are receiving radiation therapy; (3) individuals who are taking such drugs as procainamide and minoxidil; and (4) individuals who have undergone surgery that involved an incision of the heart wall. If an effusion is neoplasm induced, chemotherapeutic agents may be injected into the pericardial space. Tetracycline may also be injected into the pericardium to induce pericardial sclerosis and prevent further fluid accumulation (Hancock, 1985).

Constrictive Pericarditis

Constrictive pericarditis (chronic pericarditis) was synonymous with tuberculosis years ago (Fig. 27-18). Currently in the United States, this form of pericardial disease is either idiopathic or associated with radiation exposure, rheumatoid arthritis, uremia, or coronary artery bypass graft. In constrictive pericarditis, fibrous scarring with occasional calcification of the pericardium causes the visceral and parietal pericardial layers to adhere, obliterating the pericardial cavity. The fibrotic lesions encase the heart in a rigid shell. Like tamponade, constrictive pericarditis compresses the heart and eventually reduces cardiac output. Unlike tamponade, however, constrictive pericarditis always develops gradually.

Because the onset of constrictive pericarditis is gradual, clinical manifestations seldom include pulsus paradoxus. Symptoms tend to be exercise intolerance, dyspnea on exertion, fatigue, and anorexia. Clinical assessment reveals weight loss, edema, distention of the jugular vein, and hepatic congestion. Restricted ventricular filling may cause a pericardial knock (early diastolic sound).

Electrocardiographic findings include T wave inversions and atrial fibrillation. An echocardiogram may suggest evidence of nonspecific pericardial thickening. Computed tomography is best able to detect constrictive processes (Hancock, 1985). Chest x-ray films frequently reveal prominent pulmonary vessels and calcification of the pericardium.

Initial treatment for constrictive pericarditis is pharmacologic and dietary. Digitalis glycosides, diuretics, and sodium restriction are often prescribed. If these modalities are successful, surgical excision of the restrictive pericardium is indicated. Removal of the pericardium (pericardectomy) results in no noticable cardiac impair-

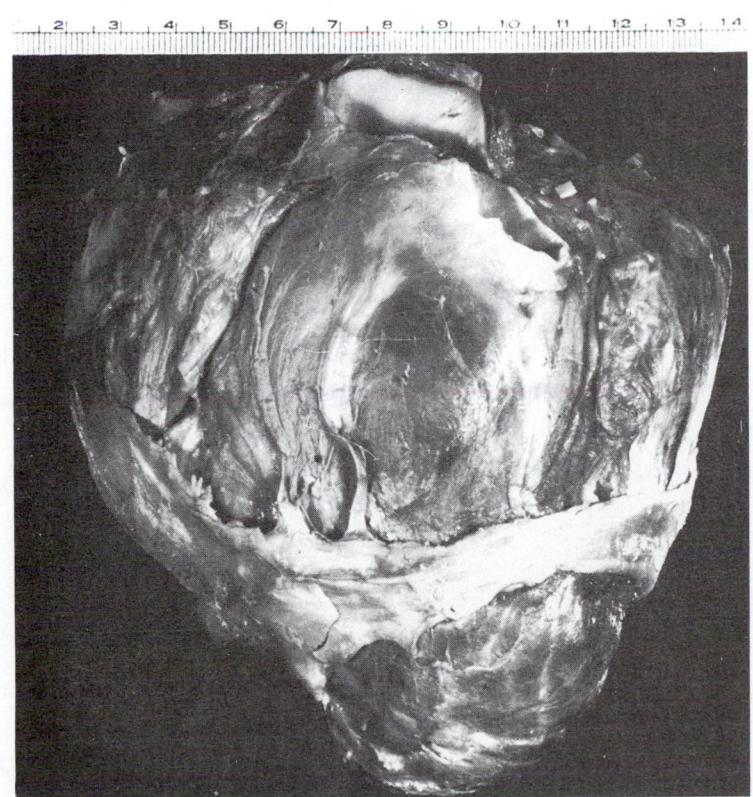

FIG. 27-18. Constrictive pericarditis. Note band of calcified tissue that constricts heart. (From Kissane, 1985.)

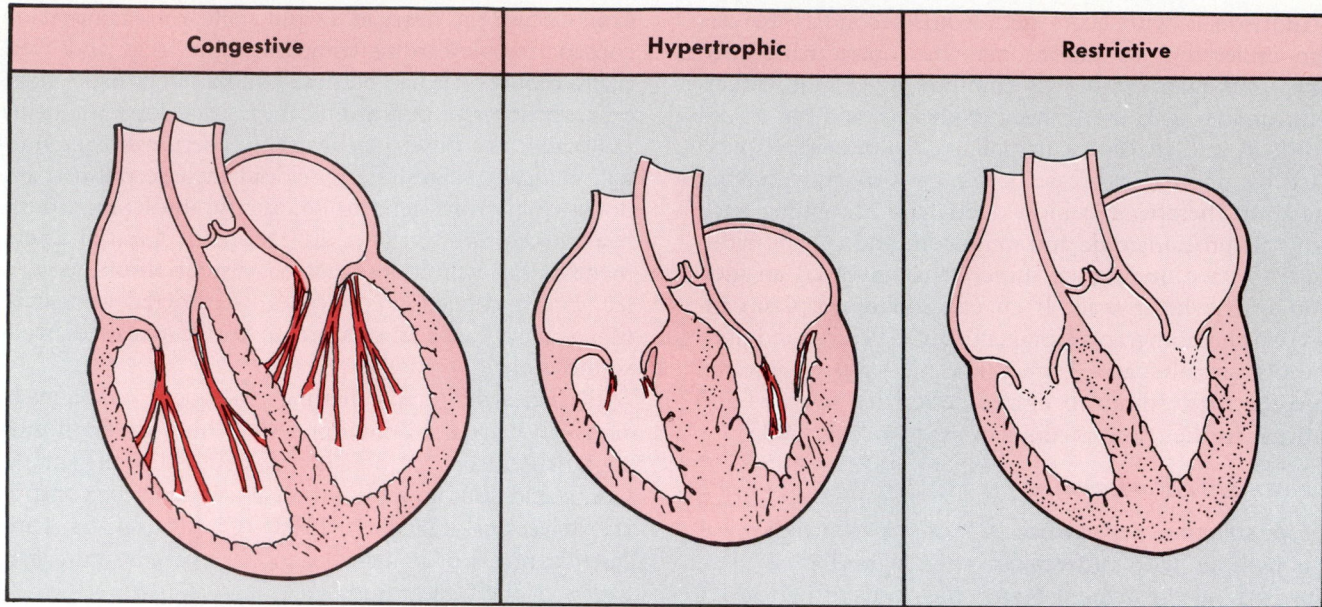

FIG. 27-19. Morphologic characteristics of the cardiomyopathies. Congestive, or dilated, cardiomyopathy *(left)* causes biventricular dilation. Hypertrophic cardiomyopathy *(center)* causes marked interventricular septal hypertrophy and contortion of the left ventricle. Restrictive cardiomyopathy *(right)* results in a decrease of ventricular compliance, usually from infiltration of the myocardium by deposits of hemosiderin (hemosiderosis), amyloid (amyloidosis), or glycogen (glycogen storage disease).

TABLE 27-9 Effects of cardiomyopathies on circulation through the heart

Effect	Type of cardiomyopathy		
	Congestive	Hypertrophic	Restrictive
Hemodynamic			
Cardiac output	Decreased	Normal	Normal or decreased
Stroke volume	Decreased	Normal or Increased	Decreased
Ventricular filling pressure	Increased	Normal Increased	Increased
Ejection fraction	Decreased	Increased	Normal or Decreased
Inflow resistance	Normal	Increased	Increased
Outflow tract obstruction	None	Increased	None
Formation of intracardiac thrombi	Increased	None	Increased
STRUCTURAL OR FUNCTIONAL			
Chamber size	Increased	Normal or Decreased	Decreased
Myocardial mass	Increased	Increased	Normal or Increased
Endocardial thickness	Normal or Increased	Increased	Increased
Contractility	Decreased	Increased or Decreased	Normal or Decreased
Mitral valve competence	Decreased	Decreased	Decreased

Data from DeSanctis, 1985; Hurst et al., 1984.

ment. For individuals with severe restrictive disease, pericardectomy may prevent untimely death from heart failure.

Disorders of the Myocardium: the Cardiomyopathies

The **cardiomyopathies** are a diverse group of diseases that primarily affect the myocardium itself and are not secondary to the usual cardiovascular disorders, such as coronary artery disease, hypertension, or valvular dysfunction. They may, however, be secondary to infectious disease, exposure to toxins, systemic connective tissue disease, infiltrative and proliferative disorders, or nutritional deficiencies. Despite this large number of possible causes, most cases of cardiomyopathy are idiopathic; that is, their cause is unknown. The cardiomyopathies are categorized as congestive, hypertrophic, or restrictive, depending on their physiologic effects on the heart (Fig. 27-19 and Table 27-9).

Congestive Cardiomyopathy

Congestive cardiomyopathy (dilated cardiomyopathy) is characterized by ventricular dilatation and grossly impaired systolic function, leading to congestive heart failure (Fig. 27-20). The basic problem is diminished myocardial contractility, which is reflected in diminished systolic performance of the heart. Congestive cardiomyopathy causes decreased ejection fractions, increased end-diastolic and residual volumes, decreased ventricular stroke volume, and biventricular failure.

About one half of the cases of congestive cardiomyopathy are idiopathic, and the remainder result from some known disease process. Serious myocardial damage can result from certain drugs used in cancer chemo-

therapy, especially doxorubicin and daunorubicin. Cardiotoxicity increases with dosage, and the severity of the toxic reaction is directly related to the cumulative dose. It is not known whether ischemia related to coronary artery disease can cause congestive cardiomyopathy. Recurrent and extensive myocardial infarction can, however, cause the same outcome as congestive cardiomyopathy; that is, left heart failure. Congestive cardiomyopathies occur most often in black men between 40 and 60 years of age.

A disproportionate number of individuals with idiopathic congestive cardiomyopathy are alcoholics. Evidently, alcohol depresses cardiac function and causes histologic changes in the myocardium. Disagreement exists, however, as to whether alcohol alone is a cause of cardiomyopathy in otherwise healthy individuals (Sereny et al., 1983). Alcohol abuse is frequently complicated by malnutrition, which may contribute to cardiomyopathy. In the 1960s, an epidemic of congestive cardiomyopathy in beer drinkers living in the midwestern United States and Canada was ascribed to toxicity from cobalt additives in beer (Sullivan, Egan, & George, 1969).

Peripartum cardiomyopathy is another idiopathic form of congestive cardiomyopathy. The cardiomyopathy usually develops in the first 3 to 4 months after completion of a pregnancy, after the period of maximum physiologic stress is thought to have ended. A few cases have resulted from acute myocardial inflammation (myocarditis).

A third group of congestive cardiomyopathies may be the late consequences of previous viral, bacterial, or parasitic infections or an autoimmune process. Endocardial biopsies have revealed a significant number of these

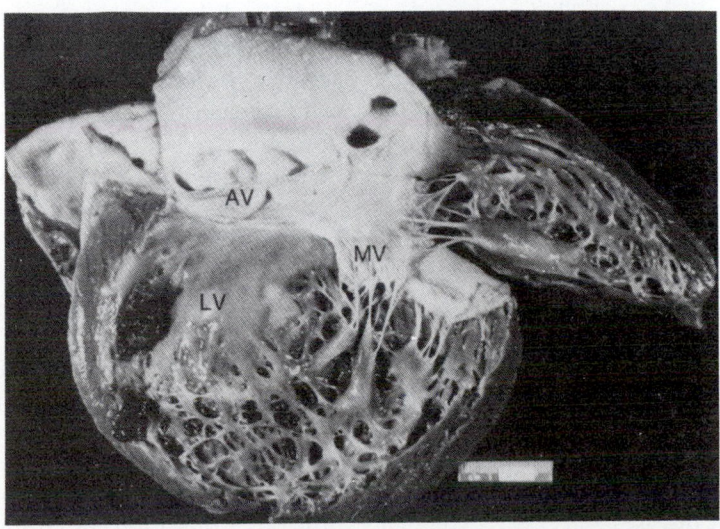

FIG. 27-20. Heart with idiopathic congestive cardiomyopathy. Opened left ventricle, *LV,* has dilated configuration. Aortic valves, *AV,* and mitral valves, *MV,* are normal. (From Kaye & Rose, 1983.)

TABLE 27-10 Pathophysiologic effects of the cardiomyopathies

| Pathophysiology | Type of cardiomyopathy | | |
	Congestive	Restrictive	Hypertrophic
Major symptoms	Fatigue, weakness, palpitations	Dyspnea, angina pectoris, fatigue, dizziness (syncope), palpitations	Dyspnea, fatigue
Cardiomegaly	Moderate to marked	Mild to moderate	Mild
Hypertrophy	Left ventricular myocardium	Left ventricular myocardium and interventricular septum	Left ventricular myocardium
Alterations of chamber volume	Volume increased	Volume decreased, particularly in left ventricle	Volume normal to decreased
Alterations of chamber compliance	Compliance increased	Compliance decreased, particularly in left ventricle	Compliance decreased, particularly in left ventricle
Alterations of systolic function (myocardial contractility)	Contractility decreased in left ventricle	Contractility increased or vigorous	None
Valvular incompetence	Atrioventricular valves, particularly mitral	Mitral valve	Atrioventricular valve
Conduction defects	Intraventricular	Nonspecific	Atrioventricular
Dysrhythmias	Sinoatrial tachycardia; atrial and ventricular dysrhythmias	Atrial and ventricular dysrhythmias	Tachyarrhythmias
Thromboembolism	Systemic or pulmonary	Systemic or pulmonary	Systemic or pulmonary
Associated conditions	Alcoholism, pregnancy, infection, nutritional deficiency, exposed to toxins	Possible inherited defect of muscle growth and development	Infiltrative disease
Eventual cardiovascular event	Congestive left heart failure	Congestive heart failure	Congestive right heart failure

cases also involve active myocarditis. The implications of these findings remain unclear. (Pathophysiologic effects of the cardiomyopathies are summarized in Table 27-10.)

The most common symptoms of congestive cardiomyopathy are dyspnea and fatigue. Pulmonary congestion is expected, but acute pulmonary edema is not. Palpitations are common, and associated dysrhythmias may cause dizziness (syncope). Systemic and pulmonary emboli are common complications. Chest pain may be present, but it is unlike anginal pain.

In the presence of congestive heart failure, blood pressure is often elevated. Extra heart sounds and cardiac murmurs may be present as well. Congestive cardiomyopathy may be difficult to distinguish from acute myocarditis, valvular heart disease, coronary artery disease, and hypertensive heart disease.

Treatment for congestive cardiomyopathy consists of salt restriction and the prescription of digitalis glyco-sides and diuretics. Anticoagulants are given to prevent pulmonary and systemic embolism. Bed rest for extended periods can be used to reduce the workload of the weakened heart. Corticosteroids and immunosuppressants can benefit individuals with documented inflammatory disease, and vasodilators are administered to combat congestion. Venous dilation reduces preload by promoting peripheral venous pooling, thereby decreasing central blood volume and alleviating pulmonary congestion. Arterial dilation reduces afterload and aortic impedance, making it easier for the failing left ventricle to eject blood. Combinations of these drugs have been effective in improving symptoms, although there is no indication that they prolong life.

The prognosis is poor. About 50% of individuals with congestive cardiomyopathy die within 2 years of the onset of symptoms (Ahumada, 1987). Sudden death from congestive failure or dysrhythmias is most common.

Hypertrophic Cardiomyopathy

This form of cardiomyopathy is also known as asymmetric septal hypertrophy, muscular subaortic stenosis, and idiopathic hypertrophic subaortic stenosis. The name *hypertrophic* is preferrable, however, because the cardiac changes are not always obstructive and the hypertrophy is not always subaortic or asymmetric (Robbins et al., 1984). An autosomal dominant inheritance has been linked to this disorder (Chung, 1987). Although its origin is unknown, the basic abnormality appears to reside in the contractile elements of the heart muscle. The hallmark of **hypertrophic cardiomyopathy** is disproportionate thickening of the interventricular septum (Fig. 27-21). There is disorganization of the septal muscle cells and greater hypertrophy of the ventricular septum than of the ventricular chambers. Thus the heart may actually appear to be of normal size. Thickening of the septum results in a hyperdynamic state, with subsequent increased myocardial contractility and ejection fraction (Orie & Liedtke, 1986). However, diastolic relaxation is impaired and ventricular compliance is decreased (increased stiffness). If the septum is asymmetrically enlarged, it may actually obstruct left ventricular outflow and result in decreased cardiac output. Under these circumstances, any condition or medication that increases contractility will also increase the degree of obstruction. For example, nitroglycerine aggravates obstruction by increasing the heart rate, decreasing chamber size, and decreasing blood pressure (afterload) (DeSanctis, 1984).

Major clinical manifestations of hypertrophic cardiomyopathy are angina, syncope, palpitations, and congestive heart failure. Myocardial infarction can occur if the hypertrophied myocardium outgrows its blood supply. Dysrhythmias are common, and extra heart sounds and murmurs are not unusual. Electrocardiography reveals left ventricular hypertrophy and dysrhythmias, if any are present. Echocardiograms may prove helpful in recognizing and assessing the severity of this disorder.

Beta-blockers, such as propanolol, are favored for initial therapy because they may decrease left ventricular stiffness and reduce the heart rate enough to permit a longer time for ventricular filling. Calcium antagonists may or may not be beneficial. Surgical resection of the hypertrophic tissue may be done to relieve symptoms in individuals who do not respond to pharmacologic therapy. Although the course and prognosis of hypertrophic cardiomyopathy vary, long-term survival is expected.

Restrictive Cardiomyopathies

Restrictive cardiomyopathy is usually caused by an infiltrative disease of the myocardium, such as amyloidosis, hemochromatosis, or glycogen storage disease. The myocardium becomes rigid and noncompliant, impeding ventricular filling and raising filling pressures during diastole. The overall clinical and hemodynamic picture mimics that of constrictive pericarditis.

The most common clinical manifestation of restrictive cardiomyopathy is congestive heart failure, particularly right heart failure. Cardiomegaly and dysrhythmias are common. In most cases, there is no therapy for restrictive cardiomyopathy other than treating the underlying disease process. Death occurs as a result of congestive failure or dysrhythmias.

Disorders of the Endocardium
Valvular Dysfunction

Disorders of the endocardium, the innermost lining of the heart wall, all damage the heart valves, which are made up of endocardial tissue. Endocardial damage can be either congenital or acquired. The acquired forms cause inflammatory, ischemic, traumatic, degenerative, or infectious alterations of valvular structure and function.

The usual cause of acquired valvular dysfunction is inflammation of the endocardium secondary to acute rheumatic fever or infectious endocarditis (see pp. 958-960). Structural alterations of the heart valves lead to stenosis, incompetence, or both.

In **valvular stenosis,** the valve orifice is constricted and narrowed, impeding the forward flow of blood and increasing the workload of the cardiac chamber "in front" of the diseased valve (Fig. 27-22). Pressure (intraventricular or atrial) increases in the chamber to overcome resistance to flow through the valve. Increased pressure causes the myocardium to work harder, causing myocardial hypertrophy. In **valvular regurgitation** (also called insufficiency or incompetence), the valve

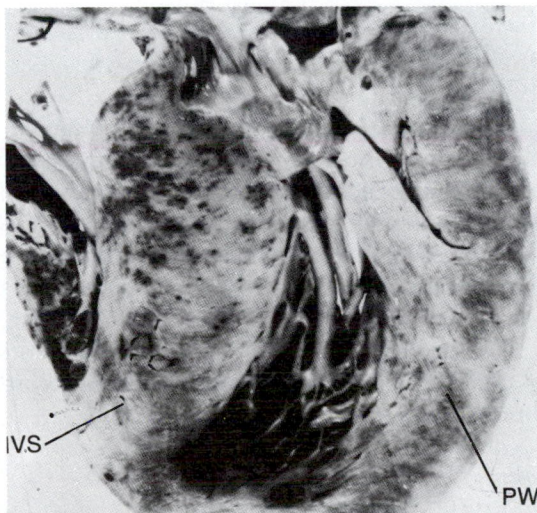

FIG. 27-21. Heart with hypertrophic cardiomyopathy. Interventricular septum, *IVS,* is thicker than posterior wall, *PW.* (From Bulkley, 1979.)

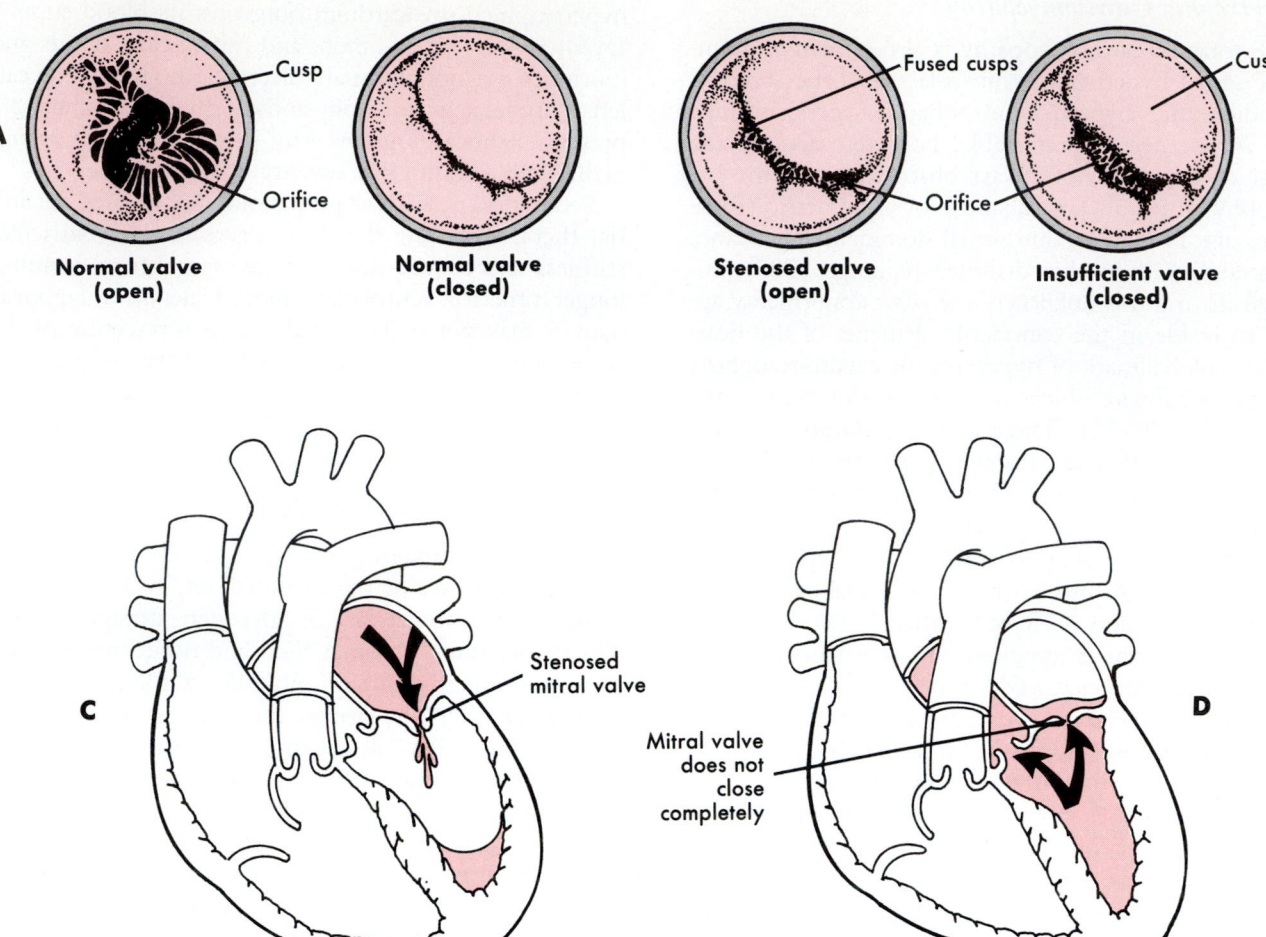

FIG. 27-22. Valvular stenosis and regurgitation. **A,** Normal position of the valve leaflets, or cusps, when the valve is open and closed. **B,** Open position of a stenosed valve *(left)* and open position of a closed regurgitant valve *(right)*. **C,** Hemodynamic effect of mitral stenosis. The stenosed valve is unable to open sufficiently during left atrial systole, inhibiting left ventricular filling. **D,** Hemodynamic effect of mitral regurgitation. The mitral valve does not close completely during left ventricular systole, permitting blood to reenter the left atrium.

leaflets, or cusps, fail to shut completely, permitting blood flow to continue even when the valve is supposed to be closed (see Fig. 27-21). During systole, some blood leaks back into the atrial chamber "upstream." Valvular regurgitation increases the volume of blood the heart must pump and increases the workload of both atrium and ventricle. Valvular incompetence causes cardiomegaly. Increased volume leads to chamber dilatation, and increased workload leads to hypertrophy. Although all four heart valves may be affected, those of the left heart (mitral and aortic semilunar valves) are far more commonly affected that those of the right heart (tricuspid and pulmonic semilunar valves).

Valvular dysfunction stimulates chamber dilatation and myocardial hypertrophy, both of which are compensatory mechanisms intended to increase the pump-

ing capability of the heart. Eventually, myocardial contractility is diminished, the ejection fraction is reduced, diastolic pressure increases, and the ventricles fail from overwork. Depending on the severity of the valvular dysfunction and the capacity of the heart to compensate, valvular alterations cause a range of symptoms and some degree of incapacitation (Table 27-11). Valvular dysfunction is treated with cardiac glycosides, diuretics, dietary salt restriction, and antibiotics until prosthetic valve replacement becomes necessary.

Stenosis

Aortic Stenosis **Aortic stenosis** has three common etiologies (1) inflammatory damage caused by rheumatic heart disease, (2) congenital malformation (see Chapter 3), and (3) degeneration resulting from calcification (see

TABLE 27-11 Clinical manifestations of valvular stenosis and regurgitation

Manifestation	Aortic stenosis	Mitral stenosis	Aortic regurgitation	Mitral regurgitation	Tricuspid regurgitation
Cardiovascular outcome*	Left ventricular failure	Right ventricular failure	Congestive left heart failure	Left heart failure	Right heart failure
General symptoms	Fatigue	Fatigue, weakness		Fatigue, weakness	Peripheral edema (with heart failure)
Respiratory effects	Dyspnea on exertion	Dyspnea on exertion, orthopnea, paroxysmal nocturnal dyspnea, predisposition to respiratory infections, hemoptysis, pulmonary hypertension, and edema	Dyspnea with effort	Dyspnea; occasional hemoptysis	Dyspnea
Central nervous system effects	Syncope, especially on exertion	Neural deficits only associated with emboli (e.g. hemiparesis)	Syncope	None	None
Gastrointestinal effects	None	Ascites; hepatic angina with hepatomegaly	None	None	Ascites, hepatomegaly (with heart failure)
Pain	Angina pectoris	Chest pain	Chest pain (anginal)	None	Palpitations
Heart rate rhythm	Bradycardia, dysrhythmias (with heart failure)	Palpitations (atrial fibrillation)	Palpitations, water-hammer pulse	Palpitations	Atrial fibrillations
Heart sounds	Systolic murmur	Diastolic murmur, accentuated first heart sound, opening snap	Diastolic and systolic murmurs	Murmur throughout systole	Murmur throughout systole
Most common cause	Congenital rheumatic fever	Rheumatic fever	Bacterial endocarditis	Rheumatic fever	Congenital

*Untreated disease.
Data from Lewis & Collier, 1983; Swanton, 1984; Cheng, 1986.

Chapter 2) (Cheitlin, Buckley, & Ramachandran, 1985). The orifice of the aortic semilunar valve narrows, causing diminished blood flow from the left ventricle into the aorta (see Fig. 27-22). Outflow obstruction increases pressure within the left ventricle as it tries to eject blood through the narrowed opening.

Aortic stenosis tends to develop gradually. Clinical manifestations include decreased stroke volume, reduced systolic blood pressure, and narrowed pulse pressure (difference between systolic and diastolic pressure). Heart rate is often slow, and pulses are faint. Resistance to flow gives rise to a crescendo-decrescendo systolic heart murmur. Left ventricular hypertrophy develops to compensate for the increased work load. Eventually, hypertrophy increases myocardial oxygen demand, which the coronary arteries may not be able to supply. If this

occurs, ischemia may cause attacks of angina. Untreated aortic stenosis can lead to dysrhythmias, myocardial infarction, and heart failure. Most symptoms of aortic stenosis are due to diminished stroke volume, which results in diminished tissue perfusion.

Mitral Stenosis **Mitral stenosis** impairs the flow of blood from the left atrium to the left ventricle. Mitral stenosis is most commonly caused by acute rheumatic fever or bacterial endocarditis, although uncommonly it can be congenital. Narrowing of the orifice occurs as inflammatory lesions in the valvular leaflets heal (Fig. 27-23). Scarring causes the leaflets to become fibrous and fused, and the chordae tendinea to become shortened.

Clinical manifestations depend on the size of the valvular orifice. As in aortic stenosis, impedance to blood flow results in incomplete emptying of the left atrium

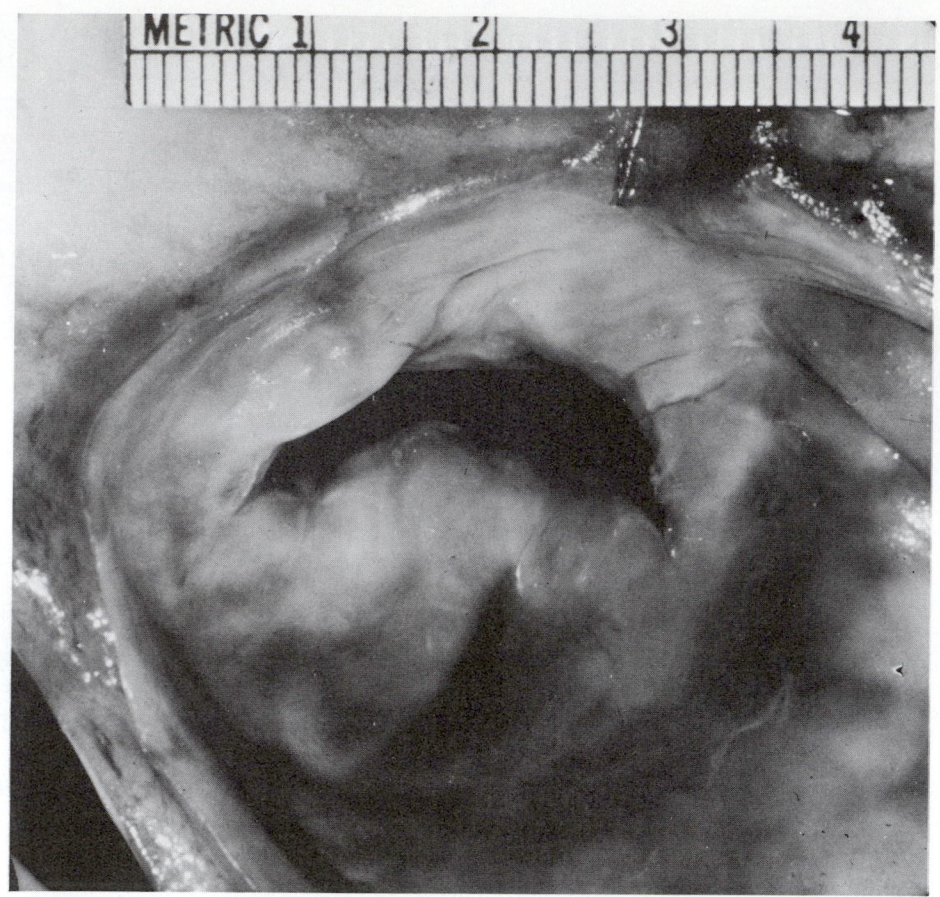

FIG. 27-23. Mitral stenosis with classic "fishmouth" orifice. (From Kissane, 1985.)

and elevated atrial pressure, as the chamber tries to force blood through the stenotic valve. Continued increases in left atrial volume and pressure cause chamber dilatation and hypertrophy. The risk of developing atrial dysrhythmias (especially fibrillation) and dysrhythmia-induced thrombi is high. As mitral stenosis progresses, symptoms of decreased cardiac output occur, especially during exertion. Continued elevation of left atrial pressure and volume causes pressure to rise in the pulmonary circulation. The outcome of untreated chronic mitral stenosis is pulmonary hypertension, edema, and right ventricular failure.

Atrial enlargement is demonstrated by chest x-ray films and electrocardiography. Blood flow through the stenotic valve gives rise to a rumbling decrescendo diastolic murmur. The first heart sound (S_1) is often accentuated and somewhat delayed because of increased left atrial pressure. Other signs and symptoms are generally those of pulmonary congestion and right heart failure.

Regurgitation

Aortic regurgitation **Aortic regurgitation** is caused by an acute or chronic lesion of rheumatic fever, bacterial endocarditis, syphilis, hypertension, connective tissue disorders (e.g., Marfan syndrome), or atherosclerosis. The hemodynamic repercussions depend on the size of the "leak." During systole, blood is ejected from the left ventricle into the aorta. If the aortic semilunar valve is affected, some of the ejected blood flows back into the left ventricle. Volume overload occurs in the ventricle because it receives blood from the left atrium during diastole and blood from the aorta during systole. Over time, the end-diastolic volume of the left ventricle increases, and myocardial fibers stretch to accommodate the extra fluid. Compensatory dilatation permits the left ventricle to increase its stroke volume and maintain cardiac output. Ventricular dilation and hypertrophy eventually cease to compensate for aortic incompetence, and heart failure develops.

Clinical manifestations include widened pulse pressure resulting from increased stroke volume and backflow. Turbulence across the aortic valve during diastole produces a characteristic murmur. Large stroke volume and rapid runoff of blood from the aorta result in prominent carotid pulsations and throbbing peripheral pulses (water-hammer pulse). Other symptoms are usually associated with heart failure that occurs when the ventricle can no longer enlarge. Dysrhythmias and endocarditis are common complications of aortic regurgitation.

Mitral Regurgitation **Mitral regurgitation,** unlike mitral stenosis, has a variety of etiologies. The most common are mitral valve prolapse and rheumatic heart disease. Other causes include infective endocarditis, coronary artery disease, connective tissue diseases (Marfan syndrome), and congestive cardiomyopathy. Mitral regurgitation permits backflow of blood from the left ventricle into the left atrium during ventricular systole, giving rise to a loud pansystolic (throughout systole) murmur that radiates into the back and axilla. The left ventricle becomes dilated and hypertrophied to maintain adequate cardiac output, despite increased volume from the left atrium. The volume of backflow reentering the left atrium gradually increases, causing atrial dilatation. As the left atrium enlarges, the valve structures stretch and become deformed, leading to further backflow. As mitral valve regurgitation progresses, left ventricular function may become impaired to the point of failure. Eventually, increased atrial pressure also causes pulmonary hypertension and failure of the right ventricle. Mitral incompetence is usually well-tolerated—often for years—until ventricular failure occurs. Most clinical manifestations are caused by heart failure.

Tricuspid Regurgitation **Tricuspid regurgitation** is more common than tricuspid stenosis and is usually associated with failure and dilatation of the right ventricle secondary to high blood pressure in the pulmonary circulation or right ventricle. Rheumatic heart disease and infective endocarditis are less common causes. Tricuspid valve incompetence leads to volume overload in the right ventricle, increased systemic venous blood pressure, and right heart failure. Pulmonic semilunar valve dysfunction can have the same consequences as tricuspid valve dysfunction.

Mitral Valve Prolapse Syndrome (MVPS)

Mitral valve prolapse syndrome is a condition in which the anterior and posterior cusps of the mitral valve billow upward (prolapse) into the atrium during systole (Fig. 27-24). The cusps are enlarged, thickened, and scalloped, possibly secondary to collagenous abnormalities, and the chordae tendineae may be elongated, permitting the valve cusps to stretch upward. Mitral regurgitation occurs if blood leaks back into the atrium through the ballooning valve.

Mitral valve prolapse is relatively common, occurring in 2.5% to 5% of the population of the United States (Lavie & Savage, 1987). It tends to be most prevalent in young women. Recent studies suggest an autosomal dominant inheritance pattern. Because mitral valve prolapse is often associated with other inherited connective tissue disorders (Marfan's syndrome, Ehlers-Danlos syndrome, osteogenesis imperfecta), it may result from a genetic or environmental disruption of valvular develop-

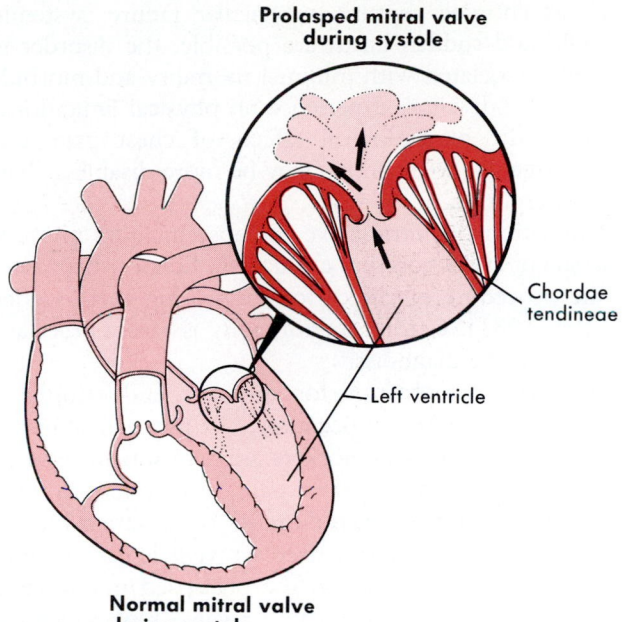

FIG. 27-24. Mitral valve prolapse. Normal mitral valve *(left)* and prolapsed mitral valve *(inset)*. Prolapse permits the valve leaflets to billow back into the atrium during left ventricular systole. The billowing causes the leaflets to part slightly, permitting regurgitation into the atrium.

ment during the fifth or sixth week of gestation (Come, 1981). There also may be a relationship between symptomatic mitral valve prolapse and hyperthyroidism.

Many cases of mitral valve prolapse are completely asymptomatic. Cardiac auscultation on routine physical examination may reveal a regurgitant murmur or midsystolic click in an otherwise healthy individual, or echocardiography may demonstrate the condition in the absence of auscultatory findings. Symptomatic mitral valve prolapse can cause palpitations related to dysrhythmias, tachycardia, light-headedness, syncope, fatigue (especially in the morning), lethargy, weakness, dyspnea, chest tightness, hyperventilation, anxiety, depression, panic attacks, and atypical chest pain (Cornell, 1985). Many symptoms are vague and puzzling and are unrelated to the degree of prolapse. Mitral valve prolapse was once considered a psychiatric malady. Recent research has suggested that individuals with mitral valve prolapse have an autonomic dysfunction in which inordinate quantities of catecholamines are produced, with or without adrenergic stimulation (Cornell, 1985). This finding could explain why mitral valve prolapse causes such a variety of subjective complaints.

Its high incidence rate suggests that mitral valve prolapse may be a normal variant rather than a pathologic entity. It is not clear whether mitral valve prolapse causes serious complications. Although severe sequelae, such as chordae rupture, ventricular failure, systemic emboli, and sudden death are possible, the disorder is actually associated with minimal mortality and morbidity. Most individuals experience no physical limitations. In fact, the psychological effects of chest pain and knowledge of the diagnosis may be more disabling than the disease itself.

Evaluation of mitral valve prolapse includes physical assessment and laboratory evaluation. Echocardiography is the procedure of choice for diagnosing the disorder (Come, 1981). Cardiac angiography is rarely necessary to confirm the diagnosis.

Antibiotic prophylaxis for infective endocarditis is given before invasive procedures, but physical activities are not restricted. Beta blockers are occasionally used to alleviate syncope, severe chest pain, or palpitations. Hypovolemia (resulting from diuretics or donating blood) is avoided because it can decrease ventricular volume, thereby increasing stress on the prolapsed mitral valve (Hunt, 1985). Surgical repair or valve replacement is rarely required.

Acute Rheumatic Fever and Rheumatic Heart Disease

Rheumatic fever is a diffuse, inflammatory disease caused by a delayed immune response to infection by the group A β-hemolytic streptococcus. In its acute form, rheumatic fever is a febrile illness characterized by inflammation of the joints, skin, nervous system, and heart. If untreated, rheumatic fever can cause the scarring and deformity of cardiac structures that compromise **rheumatic heart disease.**

The incidence of acute rheumatic fever has dramatically declined in the United States during the past 25 years because of medical and socioeconomic improvements (Markowitz & Gerber, 1987). Because crowding or poor hygiene are environmental risk factors for acute rheumatic fever, the disease continues to be a major cause of death and disability for underprivileged populations.

The acute disease occurs most frequently in children between the ages of 5 and 15 years. Only 3% of those in whom pharyngeal streptococcal infection develops will acquire acute rheumatic fever. Because the β-hemolytic streptococcus infection must persist for some time to cause acute rheumatic fever, appropriate antibiotic therapy given within the first 9 days of infection will usually prevent rheumatic fever (Stollerman, 1975). Initiation of antibiotic therapy 2 weeks after the start of streptococcal infection does not prevent rheumatic fever in susceptible indiviudals (Fitzmaurice, 1980).

The incidence of rheumatic fever tends to run in families, lending support to the concept of genetic predisposition (Zabriskie & Friedman, 1983), perhaps involving an abnormal immune response to antigens expressed by the bacterial membrane. Individuals who have experienced one attack of acute rheumatic fever are more susceptible than the general population to recurrent attacks.

Pathophysiology

Acute rheumatic fever can develop *only* as a sequel to pharyngeal infection by group A β-hemolytic streptococcus. Streptococcal skin infections do not progress to acute rheumatic fever, although both skin and pharyngeal infections can cause acute glomerulonephritis (Macek, 1983). Acute rheumatic fever probably affects the heart, joints, central nervous system, and skin through an abnormal humoral and cell-mediated response to group A streptococcal cell membrane antigens. These antigens can bind to receptors on heart, muscle, and brain cells. They also have an affinity for membrane receptors within synovial joints, where they trigger an autoimmune response.

Diffuse, proliferative, and exudative inflammatory lesions develop in the connective tissues, especially in the heart, joints, and skin. The inflammation may subside before treatment, leaving behind damage to the heart valves and increasing the individual's susceptibility to recurrent acute rheumatic fever following any subsequent streptococcal infections. Repeated attacks of acute rheumatic fever cause chronic proliferative changes in the previously mentioned organs as a result of scarring, granulomas, and thromboses.

Approximately 10% of cases of rheumatic fever develop rheumatic heart disease (Cheng, 1986). Rheumatic heart disease begins as **carditis,** or inflammation of the heart. Even mild cases of rheumatic fever can cause carditis in all three layers of the heart wall (endocardium, myocardium, and pericardium; see Chapter 26, Figure 26-2). The primary lesion usually involves the endocardium, which lines the heart chambers and includes the heart valves. Endocardial inflammation causes swelling of the valve leaflets, with secondary erosion along the lines of leaflet contact. Small, beadlike clumps of vegetation containing platelets and fibrin are deposited on eroded valvular tissue and on the chordae tendineae (Fig. 27-25). (The chordae tendineae anchor the valve leaflets; see Chapter 26, Figure 26-3.) These lesions can become progressively adherent. Scarring and shortening of the involved structures occur over time. The valves lose their elasticity and the leaflets may adhere to each other.

If inflammation penetrates the myocardium, localized fibrin deposits develop that are surrounded by areas of necrosis. These fibrinoid necrotic deposits are called Aschoff bodies. Pericardial inflammation is usually characterized by serofibrinous effusion within the pericardial cavity. Cardiomegaly and congestive heart failure may occur during episodes of untreated acute or recurrent

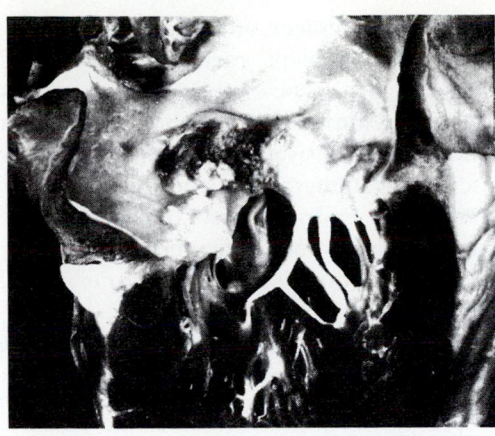

FIG. 27-25. Mitral stenosis. Mitral leaflets are thickened and fused and have clumps of vegetation containing platelets and fibrin. (From Kissane, 1985.)

rheumatic fever. Conduction defects and atrial fibrillation are frequently associated with rheumatic heart disease.

Clinical Manifestations

Many of the common clinical manifestations of acute rheumatic fever—fever, lymphadenopathy, arthralgia, nausea, vomiting, epistaxis, abdominal pain, and tachycardia—are associated with other disorders as well and are by no means diagnostic of the disease. The major specific manifestations of acute rheumatic fever are carditis, acute migratory polyarthritis, chorea, and erythema marginatum, which may occur singly or in combination after a latent period of 1 to 5 weeks after streptococcal infection of the pharynx.

Carditis The earliest cardiac manifestation of acute rheumatic fever may be a previously undetected murmur caused by mitral or aortic semilunar valve dysfunction. Chest pain is caused by pericardial inflammation. Pericardial effusion produces an audible friction rub. Extra heart sounds, heart block (see p. 966), atrial fibrillation, and a prolonged PR interval are frequently associated with chronic rheumatic heart disease.

Polyarthritis The classic presenting manifestation of acute rheumatic fever is acute migratory polyarthritis (inflammation of more than one joint). Although all of the synovial joints may be involved, the large joints of the extremities are most frequently affected. Two or more joints are usually involved simultaneously or in succession. Exudative synovitis causes heat, redness, swelling, severe pain, and tenderness, but no permanent disability. Palpable subcutaneous nodes often develop over bony prominences and along extensor tendons. They do not interfere with joint function and often go unnoticed.

Chorea Sydenham chorea, or St. Vitus dance, is a disorder of the central nervous system characterized by sudden, aimless, irregular, involuntary movements. (Chorea is described in Chapter 14.) It is more common in girls than in boys and may occur several months after the streptococcal infection. The chorea is self-limiting. It runs its course within weeks or months and has no permanent neural sequelae (Hurst et al., 1986).

Erythema Marginatum Erythema marginatum is a distinctive truncal rash that often accompanies acute rheumatic fever. It consists of nonpruritic, pink, erythematous macules that never occur on the face or hands. The rash is transitory and may change in appearance within minutes or hours. Heat (e.g., bathing) darkens the rash. The macules may fade in the center and be mistaken for ringworm.

Evaluation and Treatment

When correlated with physical assessment findings, laboratory values lend significant support to the diagnosis of acute rheumatic fever. A positive throat culture for group A β-hemolytic streptococci can be an important finding when associated with certain physical signs. However, cultures may be negative when the rheumatic attack begins. Documented recent scarlet fever is another potentially strong diagnostic aid to acute rheumatic fever, but diagnosis of scarlet fever may depend on a positive throat culture and may be difficult to distinguish from other disorders associated with a similar rash. A high or rising antistreptolysin O antibody titer (ASO) is a more accurate means of diagnosing the presence of a streptococcal infection. Most strains of group A β-hemolytic streptococcus produce a hemolytic factor called streptolysin O. Antibodies against this hemolytic factor increase as the individual's immune system fights the disease. ASO titers greater than 250 Todd units in adults and 333 Todd units in children are considered elevated. Several other antibody tests are sensitive prognosticators of streptococcal infection. These include antideoxyribonucleotidase (anti-DNase B), antihyaluronidase, and antistreptozyme (ASTZ).

Elevated white blood cell count, erythrocyte sedimentation rate, and C-reactive protein indicate inflammation. All three are usually increased at the time cardiac or joint symptoms begin to appear. They are more useful in identifying an acute inflammatory process and suggesting prognosis than in diagnosing acute rheumatic fever. The levels of these tests will decrease as the inflammatory process resolves.

In 1944, the Jones criteria were established to assist in the diagnosis of acute rheumatic fever. The criteria have been modified several times by the American Heart Association, most recently in 1966. No single laboratory test, sign, or symptom is pathognomonic of acute rheumatic fever, but certain combinations of criteria indicate that acute disease is probably present.

Therapy for acute rheumatic fever is aimed at eradicating the streptococcal infection. This is accomplished by a 10-day regimen of oral penicillin or erythromycin administration. Salicylates are used as antiinflammatory agents for both rheumatic carditis and arthritis. Serious carditis may require that cardiac glycosides, corticosteroids, diuretics, and bed rest be added to the regimen. Surgical repair of damaged valves may be necessary in cases of chronic recurrent rheumatic fever/carditis. Active disease is considered resolved when (1) the murmur has disappeared or cardiac status becomes stable, (2) major manifestations are no longer present, (3) the individual is afebrile, and (4) the erythrocyte sedimentation rate is normal or stabilized. This may take anywhere from 1 to 6 months (Macek, 1983).

Research suggests that a rheumatic recurrence will develop in approximately 50% of children with known rheumatic fever if they have another hemolytic streptococcal infection. Recurrence rates range from 25% for children under 13 years of age to 1.3% for individuals over 18. To prevent recurrence of acute rheumatic fever, continuous prophylactic antibiotic therapy is necessary.

Infective Endocarditis

Infective endocarditis is a general term used to describe inflammation of the endocardium—especially the cardiac valves. Causal agents include bacteria, viruses, fungi, rickettsiae, and parasites, but bacterial infection, particularly by streptococci or staphylococci, is most common. Infective carditis was once a lethal disease, but morbidity and mortality diminished significantly with the advent of antibiotics and improved diagnostic techniques.

Risk factors for infective carditis include acquired valvular heart disease (especially mitral valve prolapse) and implantation of prosthetic heart valves. Congenital lesions associated with highly turbulent flow, such as ventricular septal defect, are also risk factors. (Congenital lesions are discussed in Chapter 28.) Other risk factors include a previous attack of infective endocarditis, male gender, intravenous drug abuse, long-term indwelling catheterization (e.g., for pressure monitoring, hyperalimentation, or hemodialysis), and recent cardiac surgery.

Pathophysiology

The pathogenesis of infective endocarditis is a complex process that requires at least three critical elements (Fig. 27-26). First, the endocardium (e.g., heart valve) must be "prepared," usually by endothelial damage, for microorganism colonization. Second, blood-borne microorganisms must adhere to the damaged endocardial surface. Third, the adherent microorganisms must proliferate and promote the propagation of infective endocardial vegetation (Sullam, Drake, & Sande, 1985).

The first critical element, endocardial damage, exposes the endothelial basement membrane. The basement membrane contains a type of collagen that attracts platelets and thereby stimulates thrombus formation on the membrane. Platelet activation and thrombus formation can cause an inflammatory reaction termed **nonbacterial thrombotic endocarditis.** Infective endocarditis cannot develop unless microorganisms gain access to the bloodstream. Microorganisms may enter the bloodstream as a result of minor procedures, such as dental cleaning or bladder catheterization, or they may spread from uncomplicated upper respiratory or skin infections. Any time pathogens gain access to the bloodstream, the potential for endocardial infection exists. Bacteremia and adherence comprise the second critical element. Adherence of microorganisms to the endocardial surface is facilitated by the coexistence of nonbacterial thrombotic endocarditis. It should be noted, however, that bacteremia can cause infective endocarditis even on healthy, intact endocardium (Sullam et al., 1985). The third critical element, bacterial proliferation and vegetation formation, is also promoted by coexistant nonbacterial thrombotic endocarditis.

Not all microorganisms are capable of colonization. This capability, which determines the microorganism's pathogenicity, depends on the organism's ability to survive interactions with circulating serum complement, antibodies, and platelets aggregated on the endocardial surface. Complement, antibodies, and platelets may serve as effective inhibitors to bacterial colonization.

In addition to circumventing the host's defense mechanisms, the circulating microorganisms must adhere to the endocardial surface in order to initiate endocardial infection. Studies suggest that bacteria are able to synthesize extracellular polysaccharides, such as dextran or fibronectin, which promote stickiness on endocardial surfaces (Gould et al., 1975).

Once the endocardial surface is colonized, formation of infected vegetation proceeds by a series of complex steps (Fig. 27-27). Within 3 to 6 hours after infection, microbial replication occurs and bacterial colonies form within aggregates of fibrin and platelets. Within 24 hours, infected vegetation has increased in size, with colonies of microorganisms sandwiched between layers of fibrin and platelets. Bacteria may accelerate fibrin formation by activating the clotting cascade in some as yet undetermined manner (Sullam et al., 1985). As the growing bacterial colonies become progressively enmeshed in the tight fibrin network, which contains few phagocytic cells, they become less and less susceptible to the host's mechanisms of self-defense (Archer, 1977). Although endocardial tissue is constantly bathed in antibody-containing blood and is surrounded by scavenging monocytes and polymorphonuclear leukocytes, bacterial colonies are inaccessible to host defenses because they

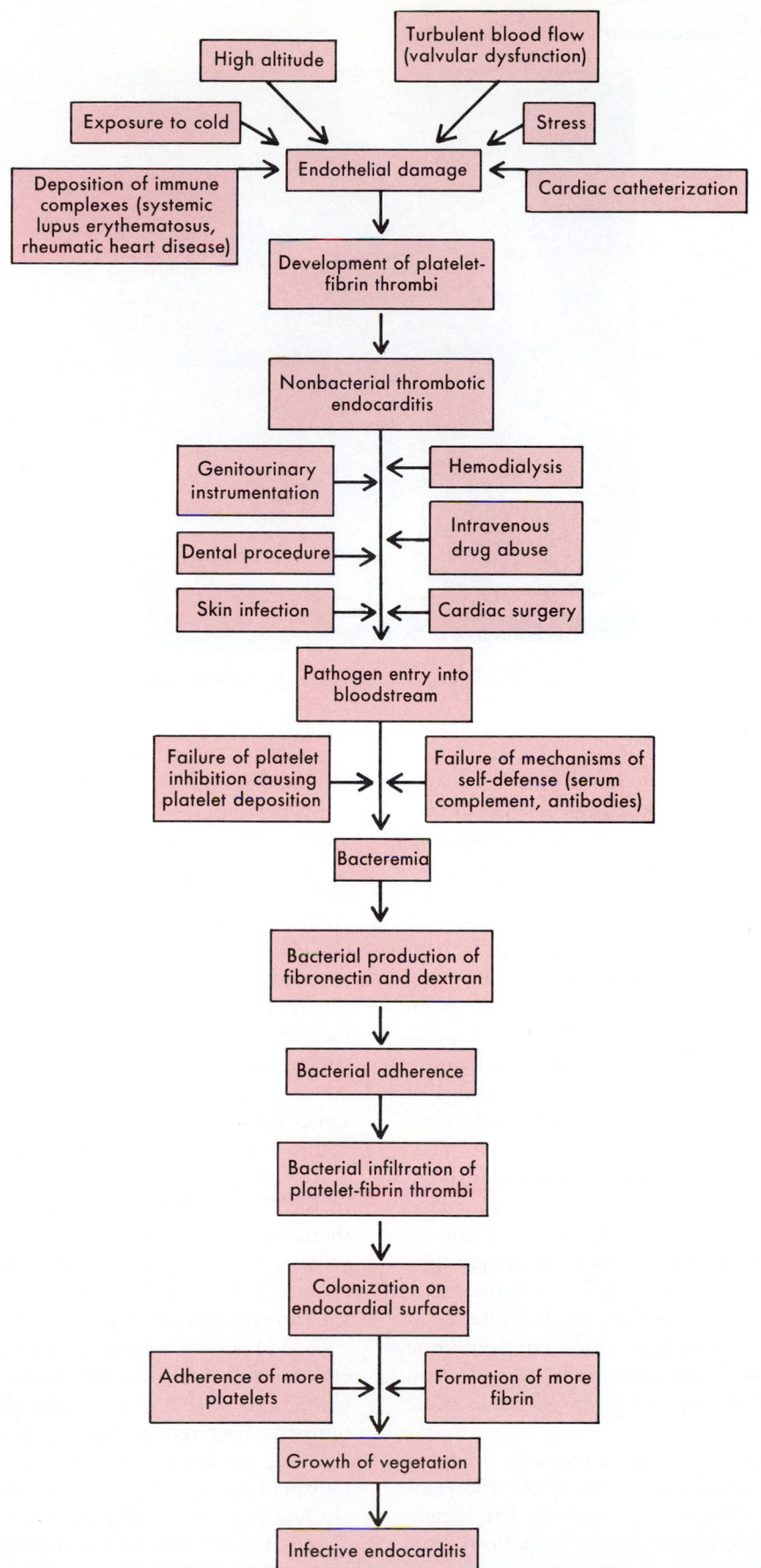

FIG. 27-26. Pathogenesis of infective endocarditis.

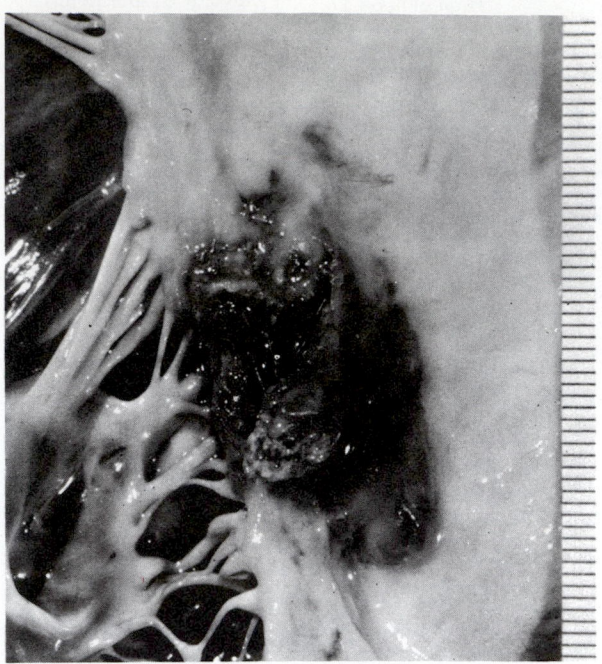

FIG. 27-27. Bacterial endocarditis of mitral valve. Lesion in combination with old rheumatic valvulitis. (From Kissane, 1985.)

are embedded in the protective fibrin clots (Donabedian, 1985). The lesions can form anywhere on the endocardium, but usually occur on the endocardial surfaces of heart valves and surrounding structures.

Clinical Manifestations

Infective endocarditis may be acute, subacute, or naggingly chronic. It causes varying degrees of valvular dysfunction and may be associated with manifestations involving any number of organ systems (lungs, eyes, kidneys, bones, joints, central nervous system), making diagnosis exceedingly difficult. The "classic" findings of fever, cardiac murmur, and petechial lesions of the skin, conjunctiva, and oral mucosa, are not always present.

Signs and symptoms of infective endocarditis are caused by infection and inflammation, systemic spread of microemboli, and immune complex deposition in various organs. A history of fever, anorexia, weight loss, back pain, and night sweats; a new or significantly changed cardiac murmur; petechiae; positive blood cultures; elevated erythrocyte sedimentation rate; and urine abnormalities make the diagnosis quite clear. Sudden onset of severely debilitating symptoms indicates acute disease.

If infective endocarditis extends farther into the heart wall and invades the conduction system, electrocardiography may reveal prolonged PR interval, left bundle branch block, or complete heart block (see p. 966). Emboli may travel to the coronary arteries and cause an acute myocardial infarction.

Evaluation and Treatment

Echocardiography is useful for diagnosing infective endocarditis and predicting the prognosis, especially in cases in which blood cultures are negative. If peripheral emboli are suspected, organ scans can be performed to confirm their presence. Antimicrobial therapy is generally given for 4 to 6 weeks, beginning with intravenous and ending with oral administration. In some cases, two different antibiotics are given simultaneously to eliminate the offending microorganism and prevent the development of drug resistance. Penicillin and streptomycin are commonly used to treat infective endocarditis. Other drugs may be necessary to treat congestive heart failure secondary to valvular dysfunction.

Recurrent infective endocarditis or severe impairment of the heart valves may require implantation of prosthetic valves. Unfortunately, the presence of an artificial valve is itself a significant risk factor for infective endocarditis. Valve failure and valve-induced embolization are known sequelae of prosthetic valve placement.

Individuals who are known to be at risk for infective endocarditis can avoid the disease by taking antibiotics before and after any procedure that carries the risk of transient bacteremia. Such procedures include dental cleaning, genitourinary instrumentation, and open cardiovascular surgery. The Committee on Rheumatic Fever and Infective Endocarditis of the Council on Cardiovascular Disease in the Young periodically updates its recommendations concerning prevention of infective endocarditis for individuals at risk.

MANIFESTATIONS OF HEART DISEASE

Dysrhythmias

A dysrhythmia, or arrhythmia, is a disturbance of heart rhythm. Normal heart rhythms are generated by the sinoatrial node (SA node) and travel through the heart's conduction system, causing the atrial and ventricular myocardium to contract and relax at a regular rate that is appropriate to maintain circulation at various levels of physical activity (see Chapter 26). Dysrhythmias range in severity from occasional "missed" or rapid beats to serious disturbances that impair the pumping ability of the heart, contributing to heart failure and death. Dysrhythmias can be caused by either an abnormal rate of impulse generation (see Table 27-12) by the SA node or other pacemaker, or the abnormal conduction of impulses (see Table 27-13) through the heart's conduction system, including the myocardial cells themselves.

Heart Failure

Heart failure is the inability of the heart to supply the body and heart muscle itself with adequate circulatory volume and pressure. Failure encompasses a large number of causes and a spectrum of clinical manifestations. Heart failure is occasionally defined as reduced stroke volume with adequate venous return. This definition does not, however, apply to heart failure in which venous return is excessive or cardiac output is high. The causes of heart failure include elevated systemic and pulmonic vascular resistance, myocardial infarction, infection, anemia, and beriberi. These and other causes of heart failure usually involve alterations of (1) contractility, (2) preload, (3) afterload, and (4) the ratio of oxygen supply to oxygen demand. (These factors are described in Chapter 26.)

Mechanisms of Heart Failure

Altered Contractility

According to Starling's law of the heart, contractility is optimal within a certain range of myocardial cell lengths. Within this range, the more the myocardium is stretched, the harder it contracts. This increases the force of systole and the amount of blood that is ejected with each ventricular contraction. In other words, an increase of diastolic stretch results in a larger systolic ejection force and a larger stroke volume.

As the sarcomeres of the muscle cell microfilaments are stretched to the upper limits of their length, two

---

TABLE 27-12 Disorders of impulse formation

Type	ECG	Effect	Pathophysiology	Treatment
Sinus bradycardia	P rate 60 or less PRI normal QRS for each P	Increased preload Decreased mean arterial pressure	Hyperkalemia: slows depolarization Vagal hyperactivity: unknown Digoxin toxicity common Late hypoxia: lack of ATP	If hypotensive, treat cause and support Follow with sympathomimetics, cardiotonics and pacer
Simple sinus tachycardial	P rate 100-150 PRI normal QRS for each P	Decreased filling times Decreased mean arterial pressure Increased myocardial demand	Catecholamines: rise in resting potential, calcium influx Fever: unknown Early failure and lung disease: hypoxic cell metabolism Hypercalcemia	Oxygen, bedrest Calcium blockers Vagolytics
Premature atrial contractions or beats*	Early P waves, that may have changed morphology PRI normal QRS for each P	Occasional decreased filling time and mean arterial pressure	Electrolyte disturbances: decrease all phases Hypoxia and elevated preload: cell membrane disturbances Hypercalcemia	Treat underlying cause Digoxin

*Most common in adults.
†Life-threatening in adults.

Continued.

TABLE 27-12 Disorders of impulse formation—cont'd

Type	ECG	Effect	Pathophysiology	Treatment
Sinus arrhythmia	Rate varies P-P regularly irregular, short with inspiration, long with exhalation PRI normal QRS for each P	Variable filling times Variable mean arterial pressures Variable oxygen demand	Unknown Common in young and young adults	None
Atria tachycardia (includes premature atrial tachycardia if onset is abrupt)	P rate 151-250 P morphology may differ from sinus P PRI normal P:QRS ratio variable	Decreased filling time Decreased mean arterial pressure Increased myocardial demand	Same as PACs: leads to increased atrial automaticity, atrial reentry Age: unknown Digoxin toxicity: many	Control ventricular rate Digoxin, calcium blockers, vagus stimulation Pace to override
Atrial flutter*	P rate 251-300, morphology may vary from sinus P PRI usually not observable P:QRS ratio variable	Decreased filling time Decreased mean arterial pressure	Same as atrial tachycardia Aging	Same as atrial tachycardia Synchronous cardioversion
Atrial fibrillation*	P rate >300 and usually not observable No PRI QRS rate variable and rhythm irregular	Same as atrial flutter	Same as atrial tachycardia Aging	Same as atrial tachycardia
Idiojunctional rhythm	P absent or independent QRS normal, rate 41-59, regular	Decreased cardiac output from loss of atrial contribution to ventricular preload Decreased mean atrial pressure as a result of bradycardia	Atrial and sinus bradycardia, or standstill, or block	Same as sinus bradycardia
Junctional bradycardia	P absent or independent QRS normal, rate 40 or less	Same as idiojunctional rhythm	Same as idiojunctional rhythm Vagal hyperactivity	Same as sinus bradycardia
Premature junctional contractions beats	Early beats without P waves QRS morphology normal	Decreased cardiac output from loss of atrial contribution to ventricular preload for that beat	Hyperkalemia (6-5.4 mEq/L) Hypercalcemia, hypoxia, and elevated preload (see PACs)	Same as PAC
Accelerated junctional rhythm	P absent or independent QRS morphology normal, rate 60-99	Decreased cardiac output from loss of atrial contribution to ventricular preload	Same as PJCs	Same as PAC

TABLE 27-12 Disorders of impulse formation—cont'd

Type	ECG	Effect	Pathophysiology	Treatment
Junctional tachy-cardia	P absent or independent QRS morphology normal, rate 100 or more	Decreased cardiac output from loss of atrial contribution to ventricular preload Increased myocardial demand because of tachycardia	Same as PJCs	Same as PAC
Idioventricular rhythm†	P absent or independent QRS >0.11 and rate 20-39	Same as idiojunctional rhythm	Sinus, atrial, and junctional bradycardia, standstill, or block	Same as sinus bradycardia
Ventricular bradycardia†	P absent or independent QRS > 0.11 and rate 60-21	Same as idiojunctional rhythm	Same as indiojunctional rhythm	Same as sinus bradycardia
Agonal rhythm/electromechanical dissociation†	P absent or independent QRS >0.11 and rate 20 or less	Absent or barely present cardiac output and pulse Not compatible with life	Depolarization and contraction not coupled: electrical activity present with little or no mechanical activity Usually due to profound hypoxia	Vigorous pharmacology aimed at restoring rate and force Usually ineffective May attempt to pace
Ventricular standstill or asystole†	P absent or independent QRS absent	No cardiac output Not compatible with life	Profound ischemia, infact: hyperkalemia, acidosis	Same as agonal rhythm, including electrical defibrillation
Premature ventricular contraction or depolarizations*	Early beats with P waves QRS occasionally opposite in deflection from usual QRS	Same as premature junctional contractions	Same as PJCs, including aging and induction of anesthesia Impulse originates in cell outside normal conduction system and spreads through intercalated discs	Pharmacology to change thresholds, refractory periods, reduce myocardial demand increase supply, Removal of cause
Accelerated ventricular rhythm	P absent or independent QRS >0.11 and rate 41-99	Same as accelerated junctional rhythm	Same as PVCs	Same as PVCs
Ventricular tachycardia†	P absent or independent QRS >0.11 and rate 100 or more	Same as junctional tachycardia	Same as PVCs	Same as PVCs, including electrical cardioversion
Ventricular fibrillation†	P absent QRS >300 and usually not observable	Same as ventricular standstill	Same as PVCs Rapid infusion of potassium	Same as PVCs including electrical defibrillation

TABLE 27-13 Disorders of impulse conduction

Type	ECG	Effect	Pathophysiology	Treatment
Sinus block	Occasionally absent P, with loss of QRS for that beat	Occasional decrease in cardiac output Increase in preload for the following beat	Local hypoxia, scarring of intraatrial conduction pathways, electrolyte imbalances Increased atrial preload	Conservative Usually do not progress in severity Pharmacologic treatment includes vagolytics, sympathomimetics, pacing
First-degree block*	PRI >.2	None	Same as sinus block Hyperkalemia (>7 mEq/L) Hypokalemia (>3.5 mEq/L) Formation of myocardial abscesses in endocarditis	Conservative Discovery and correction of cause
Second-degree block, Mobitz I, or Wenckeback*	Progressive prolongation of PRI until one QRS is dropped Pattern of prolongation resumes	Same as sinus block	Hypokalemia (>3.5 mEq/L) Faulty cell metabolism in A-V node Severity increases as heart rate increases Supports theory that A-V node is fatiguing Digoxin toxicity, betablockade CAD, MI, hypoxia, increased preload, valvular surgery and disease, diabetes	Same as sinus block
Second-degree block or Mobitz II	Same as sinus block	Same as sinus block	Hypokameia (>3.5 mEq/L) Faulty cell metabolism below A-V node Antiarrhythmics, cyclic antidepressants CAD, MI, hypoxia, increased preload, valvular surgery and disease, diabetes	More aggressively than Mobitz I, since can progress to type III Pacemaker after pharmacologic treatment
Third-degree block†	P waves present and independent of QRS No observed relationship between P and QRS Always A-V dissociation	Same as idiojunctional rhythm	Hypokalemia (>3.5 mEq/L) Faulty cell metabolism low in Bundle of His MI, especially inferior wall, as nodal artery interrupted, and results in ischemia of A-V node	Pharmacologic until pacemaker inserted Temporary pacing if caused by inferior MI, as ischemia usually resolves
Atrioventricular dissociation	P waves present and independent of QRS, but not always because of block (an example is ventricular tachycardia) A-V dissociation not always third-degree block	Decreased cardiac output from loss of atrial contribution to ventricular preload Variable effect on myocardial demand, depending on ventricular rate	May result from third-degree block or accelerated junctional or ventricular rhythm, or be caused by sinus, atrial, and junctional bradycardias	Treat according to cause Pacemaker or reducing rate of A-V or ventricular discharge, or increasing rate of sinus or A-V node discharge

*Most common in adults.
†Life-threatening in adults.

TABLE 27-13 Disorders of impulse conduction—cont'd

Type	ECG	Effect	Pathophysiology	Treatment
Ventricular block	QRS >.11 R-S-R' in V1, V2, V5, V6	None	Faulty cell metabolism in right and left bundle branches RBBB more common than LBBB because of dual blood supply to left bundle branch CHR, MR, especially anterior MI, because of infarct of fascicles Left anterior hemiblock more common than left posterior hemiblock, since posterior fascicles have dual blood supply	Isolated RBBB or LBBB or hemiblock not treated If acute and/or associated with acute anterior MI, treated with permanent pacer and vigorous pharmacology
Aberrant conduction	QRS >0.11	None, unless ventricular rate abnormalities present	Conduction of impulse through intercalated disks, since conduction system transiently blocked because of hypoxia, electrolyte imbalances, digoxin toxicity, excessively rapid rates of discharge	Correct underlying cause
Preexcitation syndromes (Wolf-Parkinson-White and Lown-Ganog-Levine)	P present with QRS for each P PRI >0.12 and QRS >0.11 because of presence of delta wave in PRI	None	Congenital presence of accessory pathways (Bundle of Kent and Fiber of Mahaim) that conduct very rapidly and bypass the A-V node, causing early ventricular depolarization in relation to atrial depolarization Prone (unknown why) to tachycardias and atrial fibrillation that can result in very rapid ventricular rates	Aimed at lining-up refractory periods of accessory pathway and A-V node to prevent reentry May slow rate with pharmacology May surgically cut pathways

things happen: not only do a large number of crossbridges have an opportunity to form, but more room is created within the cell to allow for the sliding of the microfilaments upon contraction. (The crossbridge theory and the Frank-Starling law of the heart are discussed in Chapter 25.) At a cell length of less than 0.5 μm, the microfilaments are overlapped so completely that there is little room for them to slide when the crossbridges are moved (Fig. 27-28). At 0.5 μm, the sarcomere is already nearly as short as it can get and still contract. At lengths less than 0.5 μm, the actin filaments themselves may have begun to overlap. Because actin filaments cannot form crossbridges with each other (i.e., they require the thick filaments of myosin), contractile force is lim-

ited. Clinically, 0.5 μm is the minimal length at which the myocardium contracts satisfactorily. Therefore, low blood volume resulting from hemorrhage, for example, can reduce contraction even in the absence of cardiac disease because the nearly empty ventricle is not stretched sufficiently to contract with much force.

At cell lengths greater than 2.2 μm, the amount of contact the filaments have with each other begins to be reduced. Contractile force progressively degenerates as length increases (see Fig. 27-28). The fewer the number of crossbridges, the less force will be generated, even though the stretched microfilaments have adequate room to move within the sarcomere. At 2.2 μm or more, the force of systole is reduced, causing the heart

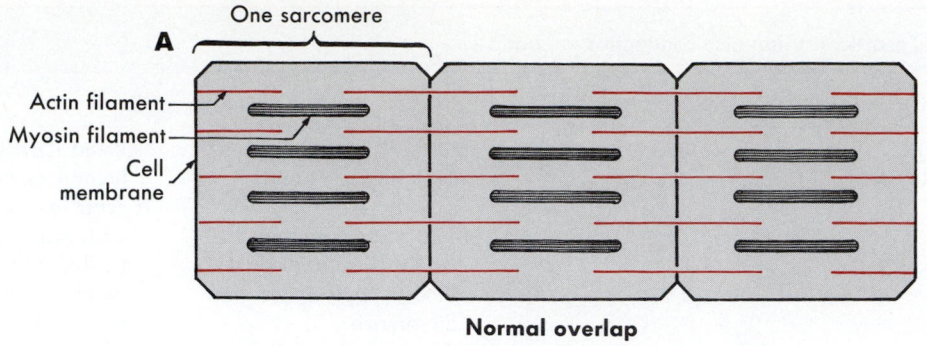

Normal overlap

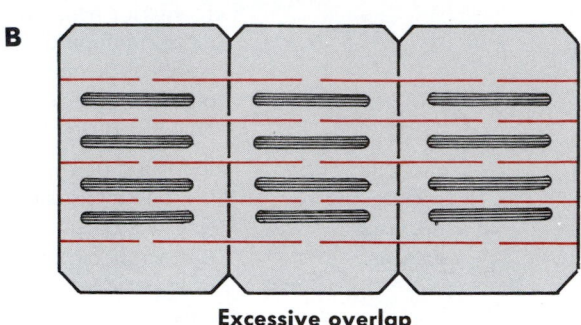

Excessive overlap

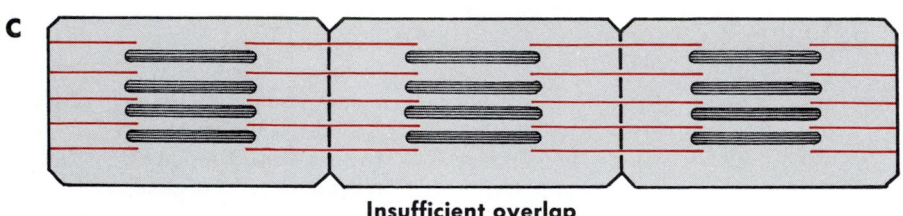

Insufficient overlap

FIG. 27-28. Effects of sarcomere overlap on myocardial contractility. **A,** The position of myocardial sarcomeres at lengths from 0.5 to 2.2 μm. **B,** The position of myocardial sarcomeres at a length of less than 0.5 μm. Overlap is excessive, and contractility is diminished. **C,** The position of myocardial sarcomeres at a length greater than 2.3 μm. Overlap is insufficient, and contractility is diminished.

chamber to supply inadequate blood volume and pressure to the body, even though the chamber is very full and stretched. Consequently, blood pressure drops. If the chamber empties poorly but venous return remains normal, the chamber will "overfill" during diastole. Overfilling increases stretch further, which weakens systole more. This forms a positive feedback loop that can lead to chamber failure.

Preload determines the amount of stretch, usually exerted by blood volume, that occurs before systole. Preload in the right heart depends on venous return to the heart from the systemic circulation. Preload in the left heart depends on venous return from the pulmonary system. Preload is also increased by outflow impedance from any chamber, even when venous return is not increased. If the chamber cannot empty fully, the end-di-

astolic volume increases, and myocardial stretch increases. Idiopathic hypertrophic subaortic stenosis and aortic stenosis increase left ventricular preload, whereas pulmonary stenosis increases right ventricular preload. Prolapse of the aortic semilunar valve enables blood to enter the ventricle during diastole from both the left atrium and the aorta. This increases the end-diastolic volume and increases stretch in the left ventricle. If the mitral valve is prolapsed, blood reenters the left atrium from the left ventricle during systole and from the pulmonary vasculature during diastole. Blood volume and pressures in the left atrium become very high prior to atrial systole, and atrial stretch occurs.

If preload stretches the sarcomere beyond 2.2 μm, contractile force diminishes, ejection is reduced, and the cardiac chamber contains more blood than usual at the

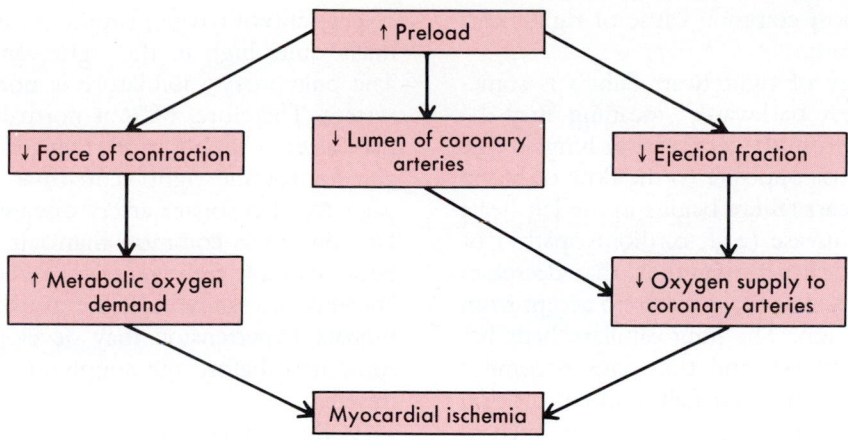

FIG. 27-29. The effect of elevated preload on myocardial oxygen supply and demand.

end of systole. Because there is no reduction in the amount of blood entering the chamber during diastole, the chamber is "overfilled" during diastole, preload climbs, and the systolic ejection fraction diminishes further.

Increases of preload also increase myocardial oxygen consumption by necessitating a greater force of contraction to accompish systole. The increased force of cardiac contraction is accompanied by increased metabolic demand in the myocardium, and more oxygen is required to support myocardial metabolism (Fig. 27-29). Unfortunately, elevated preload can also decrease the amount of oxygen available to the myocardium by two mechanisms. First, increased myocardial stretch decreases myocardial capillary perfusion by mechanically narrowing coronary capillary lumina. Second, if preload increases beyond the ventricle's ability to empty, the coronary artery blood supply will drop as the ejection fraction decreases. Increases of metabolic demand in the face of coronary capillary lumen narrowing and decreased blood flow to the coronary arteries will cause the overworked and overstretched myocardium to become hypoxic.

Afterload is the force or pressure against which a cardiac chamber must eject blood during systole. Increased afterload can be caused by and equated with mechanical outflow impedance, as in subaortic and aortic stenosis. Subaortic and aortic stenosis will, through impeding outflow of blood, eventually cause decreased left ventricular emptying, which will lead to elevated left ventricular preload. More commonly, increased afterload is equated with increased systemic vascular resistance (SVR) or pulmonary vascular resistance (PVR), such as occurs in systemic or pulmonary hypertension. To maintain cardiac output, the left ventricle must eject the same amount of blood over the same amount of time into an area of higher resistance. Therefore, the ventricular myocardium must use greater force during ejection

and consume more oxygen with each contraction. In order to maintain blood pressure, the heart rate and stroke volume must rise. To increase stroke volume, the ventricle must contract with more force than usual and raise the ejection fraction. The ventricular myocardium will also require more oxygen as the force of contraction increases.

Altered Ratio of Oxygen Supply and Demand

The myocardial need for oxygen is affected by a number of factors—among them heart rate, force of contraction, and metabolic rate. The myocardial oxygen supply is affected by the patency or lumen size of the coronary arteries, oxygen content of the blood, and the oxygen content of ambient air.

Because both oxygen supply and oxygen demand are always in states of flux, they are thought of as a ratio. The optimum ratio of supply to demand is 1:0 or greater. When the ratio falls below 1.0 (i.e., demand exceeds supply), the myocardium suffers grave consequences. Two of the most common and devastating sequelae to a ratio of less than 1 are myocardial infarction and impaired myocardial contractility. A decrease in the ratio can precipitate, exacerbate, or follow heart failure.

Types of Heart Failure

The four major types of heart failure are (1) right heart failure, (2) left heart failure, (3) low-output failure, and (4) high-output failure.

Right Heart Failure (Cor Pulmonale)

Right heart failure (cor pulmonale) is rarely caused by excessive systemic venous return. However, high venous return to a right heart that is on the verge of failing as a result of myocarditis or other diseases can be forced "over the line" into frank failure. Right heart failure more commonly results from pulmonary disease and elevated PVR. The most common cause of right heart failure is left heart failure.

The pathophysiology of right heart failure is sometimes said to "progress backward," meaning that the disease process moves from the left heart or lungs to the right atrium, contrary or opposite to the flow of blood (Fig. 27-30). Right heart failure begins in the left heart because of left heart disease (e.g., cardiomyopathy) or an event, such as myocardial infarction, that decreases the amount of blood the left heart is able to accept from the pulmonary circulation. The lung capillary beds become engorged with blood, and the lungs become a high-pressure system. Right heart failure can also begin in the lungs as a result of disease or an event, such as pulmonary embolism, that alters the alveolocapillary membrane (the blood-air interface in the lungs). Elevated pressures across affected capillary beds are transferred to the pulmonary arteries, and PVR is increased. Whether it is caused by left heart disease or lung disease, elevated PVR promotes right heart failure because the right ventricle must work harder to maintain its systolic ejection fraction; therefore, more oxygen is required and consumed with each contraction.

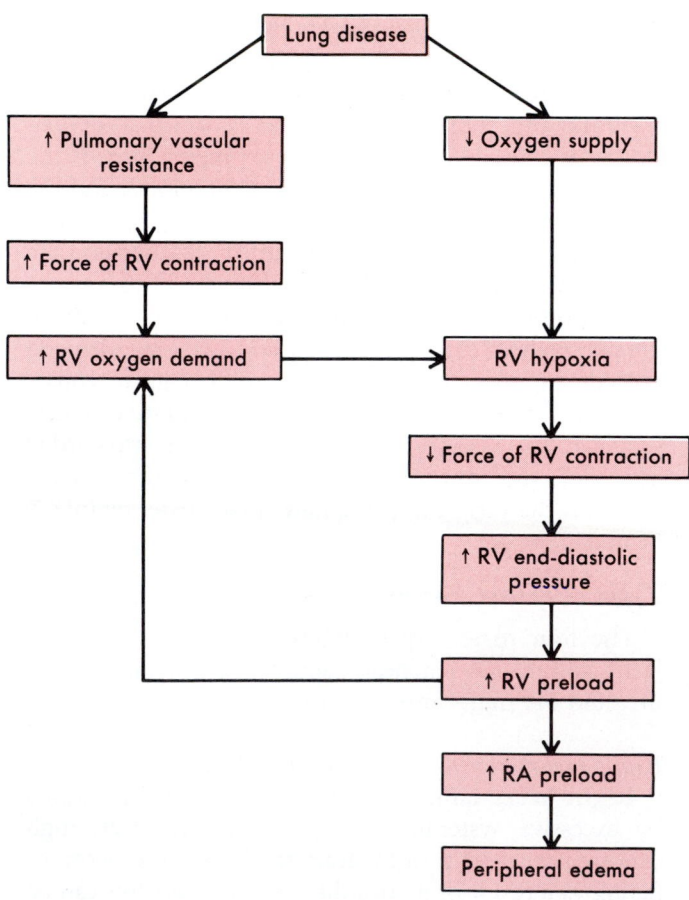

FIG. 27-30. Right heart failure (cor pulmonale) caused by lung disease. *RV,* Right ventricular; *RA,* right atrial.

The ratio of oxygen supply to oxygen demand is normally quite high in the right ventricular myocardium. The pulmonary vasculature is normally a low-pressure system. Therefore, PVR is normally low, and the coronary arteries supply more than enough blood and oxygen for routine right ventricular activity. Even in the presence of coronary artery disease, right ventricular infarction is less common than left ventricular infarction because of low right ventricular demand. Unless coexistent lung disease reduces the availability of oxygen, pulmonary hypertension may develop and exist for quite some time before the supply-demand ratio is compromised.

As the supply-demand ratio falls, the right ventricle loses its ability to maintain a normal ejection fraction and empties less completely with each beat. In addition, if rising PVR makes ejection of a normal volume of blood more and more difficult for the right ventricle, right ventricular end-diastolic pressure (RVEDP) will rise.

Increases of RVEDP and volume cause increases of right ventricular preload, which stretch the right ventricle. Within the optimum range of stretch, the right ventricle increases its force of contraction as the myofibrils lenghten. The increased force of contraction increases the amount of oxygen required with each systole. This lowers the supply-demand ratio further and contributes to ventricular weakening as myocardial metabolism becomes anaerobic. Preload continues to increase, and the ventricle continues to weaken.

The high RVEDP causes right atrial preload to rise because the right atrium begins to have trouble emptying fully into the engorged right ventricle. The right atrium stretches, and its contractility and oxygen consumption increase until it, too, begins to fail.

Blood volume and pressure rise in the vena cavae as the right atrial preload increases because blood cannot empty from the cavae into the engorged right atrium. Elevated blood volumes and pressures are transmitted backwards from the vena cavae through the veins, venules, and capillaries of the systemic circulation. Elevated central venous pressure (CVP) occurs early in right heart failure. In the absence of central venous pressure monitoring, distention of the jugular vein is used as an indicator of elevated right atrial and ventricular end-diastolic pressures. As pressures in the capillaries rise, hydrostatic pressure exceeds interstitial pressure, and fluid leaks out of the capillaries, causing peripheral edema. Peripheral edema progresses to anasarca (generalized, massive edema) and abdominal organ distension, especially of the liver and spleen.

Treatment for right heart failure begins with treatment of underlying left heart failure (see p. 975), or pulmonary disease. The goal is to reduce pulmonary hypertension and increase arterial oxygen content. Diuretics, in conjuction with restricted water and sodium intake, are used to reduce venous blood volume (preload). Myocardial contractility is enhanced with digoxin or other cardiotonic medications. Bed rest reduces myocardial oxygen demand and promotes diuresis by increasing renal perfusion.

Left Heart Failure (Congestive Heart Failure)

Left heart failure, commonly called congestive heart failure, is really left ventricular failure. Myocardial infarction resulting from coronary artery disease is a very common cause of left heart failure that can be thought of as intrinsic to the myocardium (Castaner et al., 1984). Causes extrinsic to the myocardium are systemic hypertension, and aortic stenosis and regurgitation.

In left heart failure resulting from systemic hypertension or elevated SVR, the progression of events is similar to that of right heart failure (Fig. 27-31). Elevated SVR increases myocardial oxygen demand until contractile force is decreased. As the ejection fraction falls, left ventricular end-diastolic pressure (LVEDP) rises, as does ventricular preload. The left ventricle stretches, works harder, and requires more oxygen. When the increased demand for oxygen is not met, contractile force decreases further.

The rise in LVEDP makes it difficult for the left atrium to empty fully into the engorged left ventricle, and the ejection fraction of the left atrium decreases. Preload in the left atrium then rises, the atrium fails, and blood pressure and volume rise in the pulmonary veins.

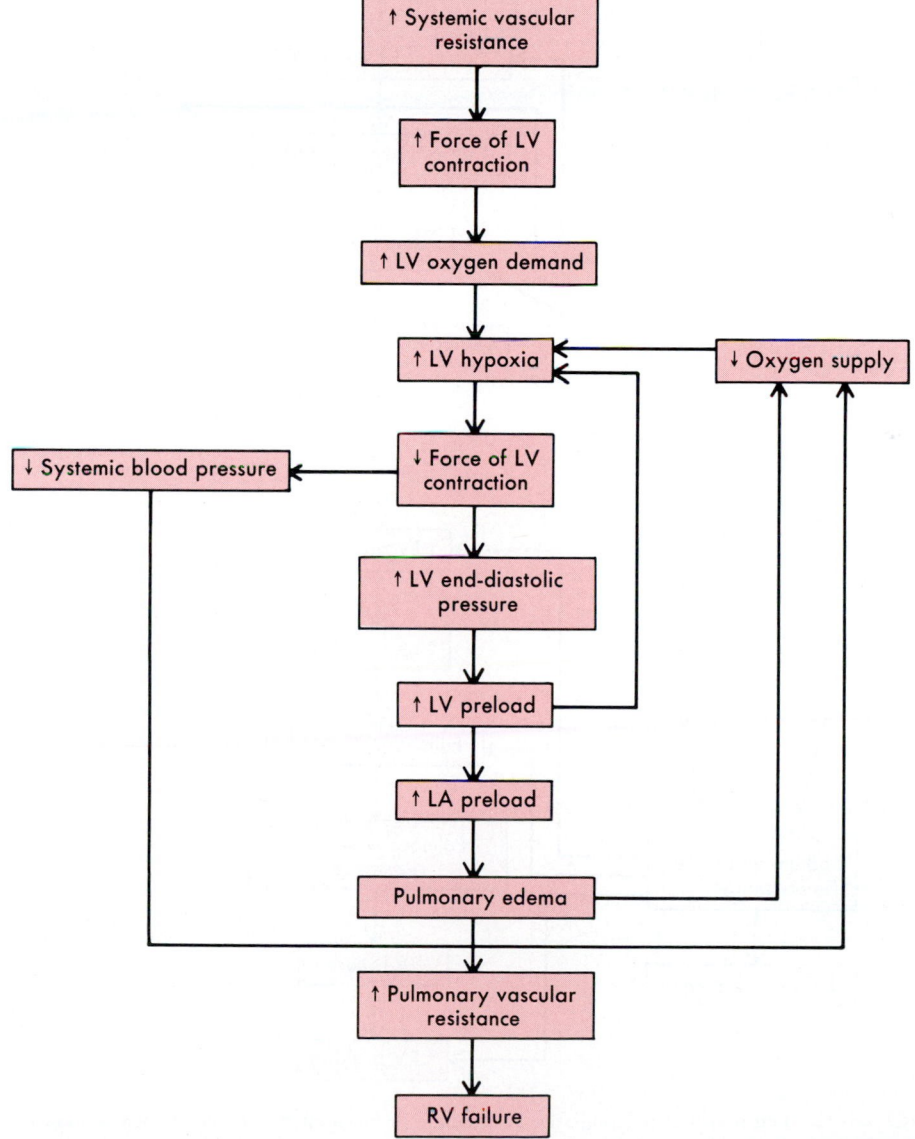

FIG. 27-31. Left heart failure resulting from systemic hypertension. Left heart failure leads to right heart failure. *LV,* Left ventricular; *LA,* left atrial; *RV,* right ventricular.

Elevated pressure and volume are transmitted from the pulmonary veins to the pulmonary capillary beds, where increased hydrostatic pressure drives fluid into the low-pressure air sacs (alveoli; see Chapter 30). The alveoli fill with plasma, and pulmonary edema results.

When the lungs become fluid-filled, gas exchange is impaired, and the failing left ventricle is faced with a decrease in oxygen supply. This further impairs ventricular metabolism and contractility. Pressures increase in the lungs, and pressures in the systemic circulation fail.

PVR will rise if the pulmonary edema is not treated or if the left heart failure persists. Elevated PVR causes right ventricular failure (see Fig. 27-32). **Biventricular heart failure** is failure of both ventricles.

Systemic blood pressure falls because of decreased contractile force and decreased ejection fraction of the left ventricle (Fig. 27-32). This triggers receptors in the glomerular apparatus of the kidneys to release renin. Renin converts angiotensinogen (produced in the liver and circulating in the blood) to angiotensin. Angiotensin stimulates release of aldosterone by the adrenal cortex. Under the influence of aldosterone, renal tubular reabsorption of sodium increases. As sodium and water is reabsorbed, plasma volume increases.

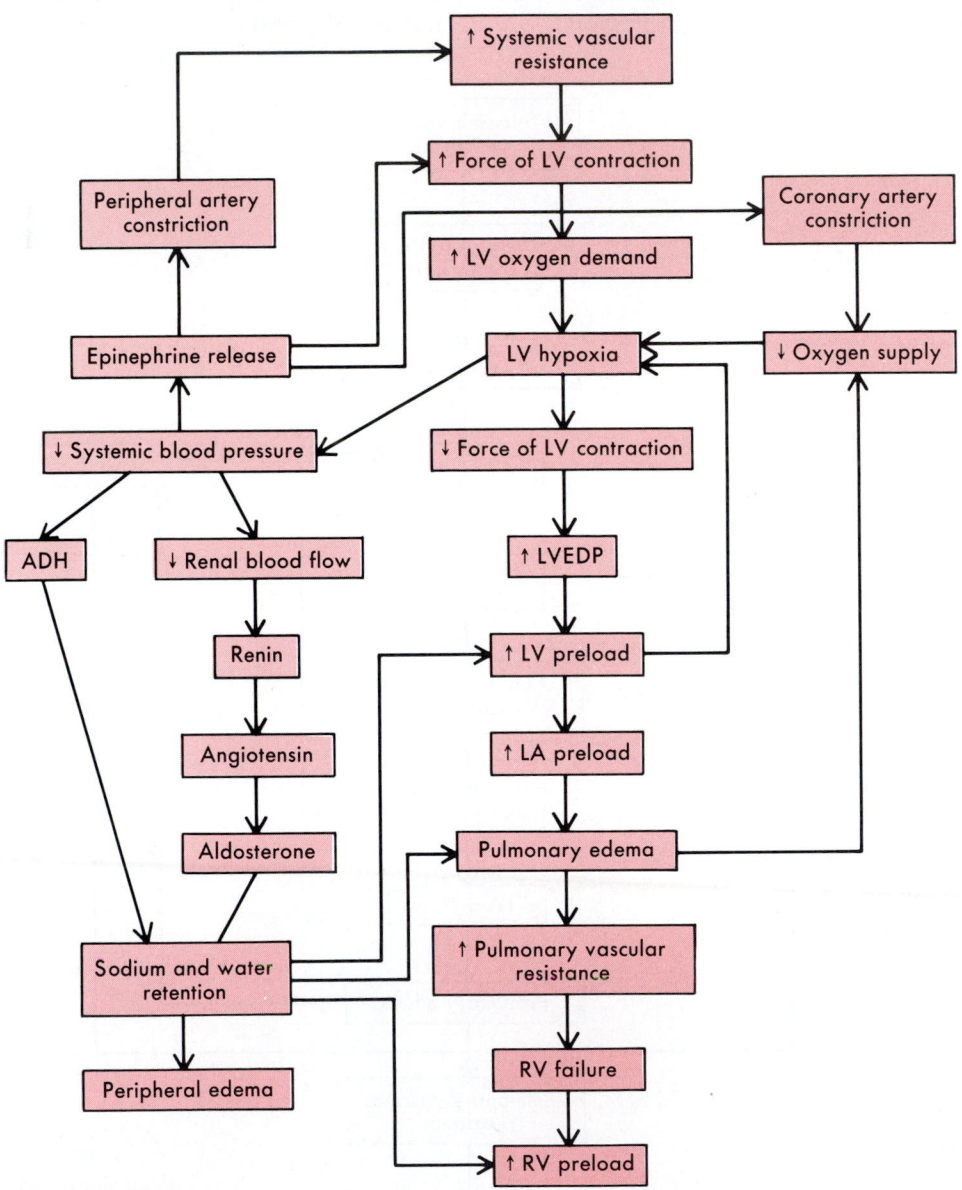

FIG. 27-32. Left heart failure (congestive heart failure) from elevated systemic vascular resistance. Left heart failure leads to right heart failure. Systemic vascular resistance and preload are exacerbated by renal and adrenal mechanisms. *LV,* Left ventricular; *LVEDP,* left ventricular end-diastolic pressure; *LA,* left atrial; *ADH,* antidiuretic hormone.

The extent to which renin and angiotensin contribute to congestive heart failure varies. Cody, Covit, Schaer, and Laragh (1984) demonstrated that occupation of receptor sites for angiotensin II in individuals with heart failure range from low (with low SVR) to quite high (with high SVR). This has implications for treatment aimed at manipulation of vascular resistance.

The fall in systemic blood pressure is also detected by various baroreceptors (Sleight, 1984). Through neuronal pathways, baroreceptors stimulate the hypothalamus to cause the symptom of thirst. The hypothalamus also causes the posterior pituitary to release antidiuretic hormone (ADH). ADH increases the renal tubular permeability to water. This causes water reabsorption to increase, and plasma volume increases further.

Increased plasma volume increases right ventricular preload. High preload will exacerbate right ventricular failure if that chamber has begun to be affected by elevated PVR. If right ventricular function is intact, a greater volume of blood will be delivered to the pulmonary vasculature. If pulmonary edema has not already developed, it will soon do so, causing an increase in PVR and a decrease in oxygen diffusion into the pulmonary capillaries. The right ventricle will fail if the PVR rises high enough and/or if the atrial oxygen content falls low enough to affect right ventricular contractility.

As blood pressure drops, sympathetic activity is stimulated, causing the release of epinephrine and norepinephrine (Sleight, 1984). These neurotransmitters are cardiotonic; that is, they increase the action of the myo-cardium. This lowers the supply-demand ratio further while contributing to decreased left ventricular contractility.

Epinephrine also constricts arterioles, reducing their radii. Arteriolar constriction increases SVR directly, and may decrease blood flow to the coronary arteries. An increased SVR contributes to failure by increasing oxygen demand, whereas a narrowing of the coronary arteries' radii decreases the oxygen supply.

If left heart failure is caused by ventricular infarction, contractility is not decreased by an elevated SVR, but rather by the loss of functional myofibrils (Fig. 27-33). In this case, heart failure begins with a drop in contractility, which leads to decreased blood pressure and increased left ventricular preload. Left heart failure resulting from infarction will eventually cause the same array of manifestations as failure resulting from elevated SVR. Risk factors for left heart failure as a result of myocardial infarction include triple-vessel coronary artery disease (Castaner et al., 1984), left bundle branch block with coronary artery disease (Hamby et al., 1983), diabetes mellitus (Jaffe et al., 1984), and early atrioventricular node block with anterior myocardial infarction (Sclarovsky et al., 1984).

In the elderly, ventricular diastolic stiffness can lead to pulmonary circulatory congestion without a concomitant decrease in left ventricular ejection fraction (Luchi et al., 1982). Aortic stenosis and aortic insufficiency, which are rather common in individuals over the age of

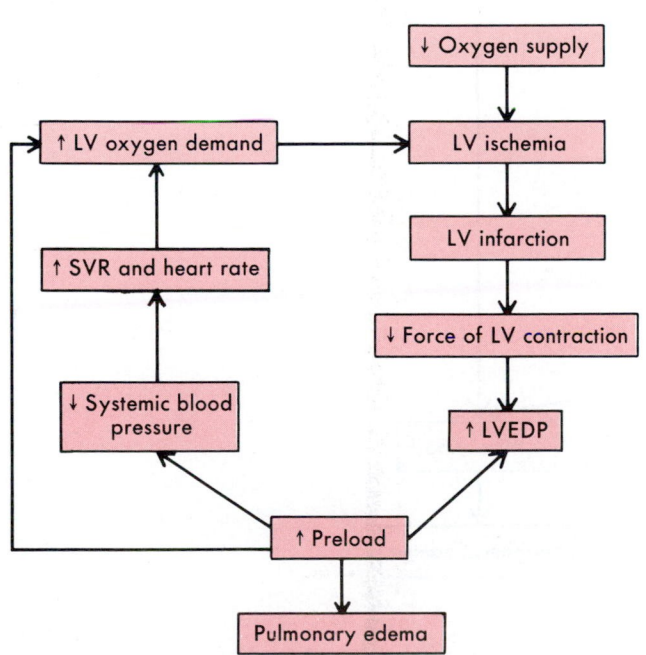

FIG. 27-33. Left heart failure from left ventricular myocardial infarction. *SVR,* Systemic vascular resistance. (See Fig. 27-32 for key to abbreviations.)

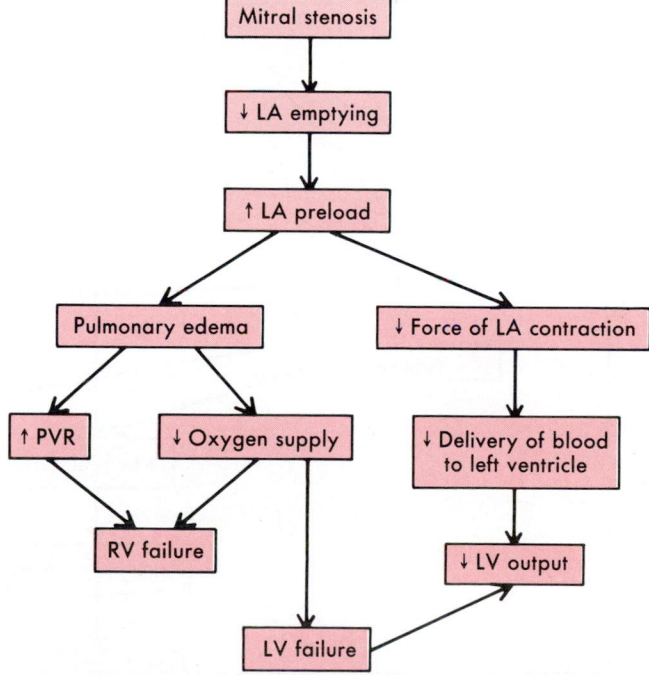

FIG. 27-34. Left atrial failure caused by mitral stenosis. *LA,* Left atrial; *PVR,* pulmonary vascular resistance; *LV,* left ventricular.

75 years, elevate left ventricular preload to the point where the left ventricle becomes relatively stiff and noncompliant. Elevated pressures are transmitted to the pulmonary vasculature and lead to pulmonary edema and other manifestations of left heart failure, despite the fact that left ventricular systole remains normal.

The pathogenesis of left atrial failure caused by mitral stenosis is shown in Fig. 27-34. Left atrial failure progresses to the right ventricle without a drop in cardiac output. If the valvular stenosis is severe, however, cardiac output will diminish because of a drop in the volume of blood delivered to the ventricle during diastole.

The earliest clinical manifestation of left ventricular failure is a rise in LVEDP, which corresponds to a rise in the pulmonary capillary wedge pressure as measured by a Swan-Ganz catheter. Because compensatory mechanisms enable the body to maintain systemic blood pressure for a while, a drop in blood pressure is usually not the first sign of left ventricular failure. Cardiac output may drop quite early, however. Decreased cardiac output is accompanied by a rise in the SVR. Pulmonary edema, which is manifested by frothy sputum, dyspnea, falling oxygen content of the blood, and white fields visible on lung x-ray films, is a later sign of left ventricular failure.

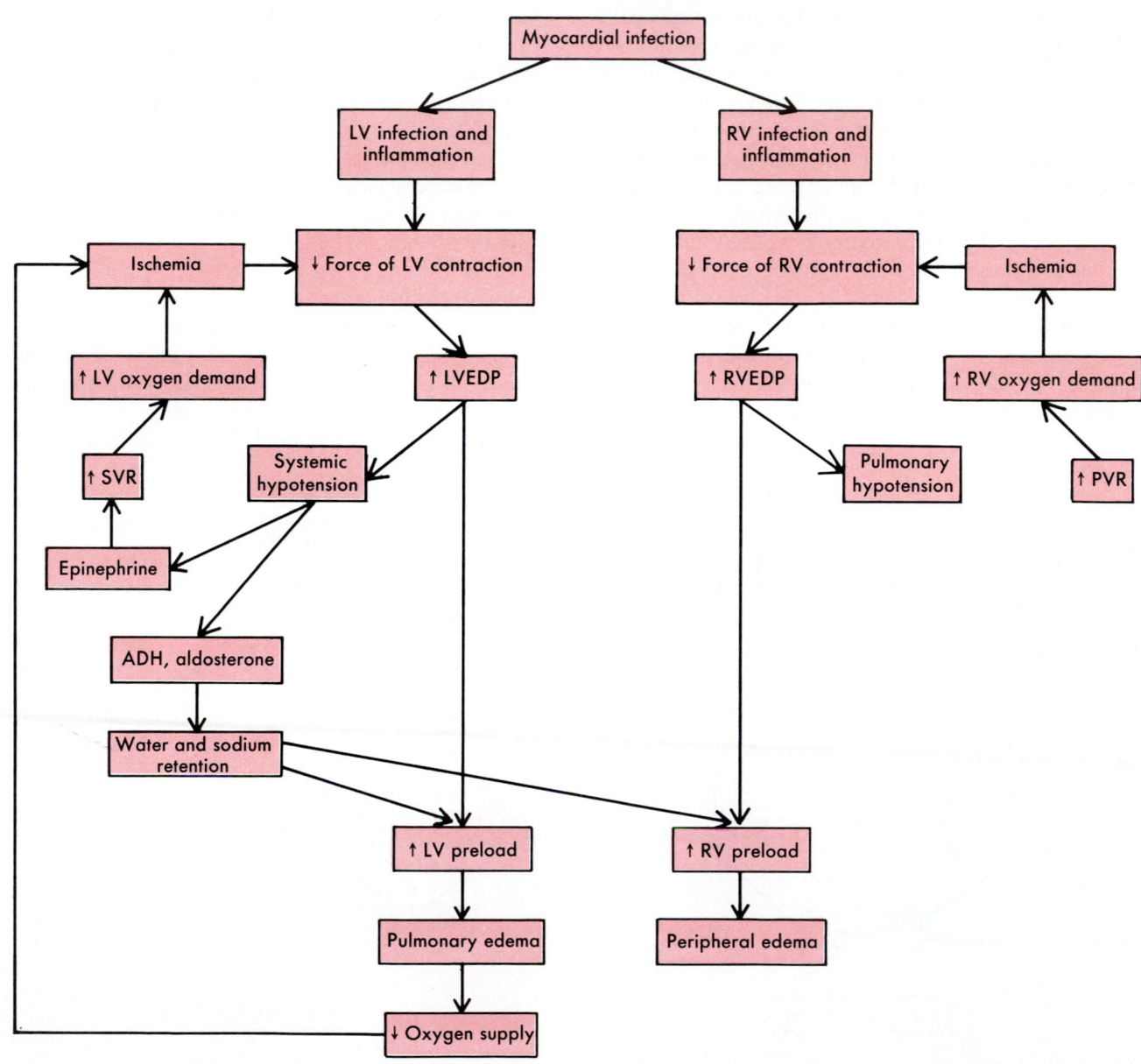

FIG. 27-35. Low-output failure. *EDP,* End-diastolic pressure. (See legends to preceding figures for key to other abbreviations.)

Treatment of left heart failure is aimed at the underlying cause. Valvular dysfunction may require surgery. Elevated SVR is treated with vasodilators, such as nitroprusside and nitroglycerine. Vasodilators can also improve coronary artery perfusion. However, the **hypotension** associated with left ventricular failure is usually treated with a cardiotonic antihypotensive, such as dopamine or dobutamine, especially if vasodilators are also being given to treat elevated SVR. At low doses, dopamine also increases renal perfusion.

Oxygen is administered continuously to increase the supply of oxygen to the myocardium, and diuretics are given to decrease pulmonary edema and blood volume. Sodium and fluid intake are restricted. Bed rest can reduce oxygen consumption further.

Morphine sulfate is often used to treat left ventricular failure accompanied by pulmonary edema, because morphine dilates the pulmonary and systemic vessels enough to decrease pulmonary and systemic capillary hydrostatic pressure. Morphine sulfate is also an analgesic and an opiate. These properties help to improve the emotional state of the individual and may limit the cerebrally mediated release of epinephrine.

The intra-aortic balloon pump (IABP) is sometimes used to treat left heart failure. The IABP is a counter-pulsation device that sits in the aorta and decreases afterload, decreases preload, increases coronary artery perfusion, and increases mean systemic arterial blood pressure. However, the IABP has not been shown to change the mortality rate of left heart failure, which is 60% to 80% despite treatment.

Low-Output Failure

Low-output failure is biventricular. Common causes of low-output failure are cardiomyopathies and myocardial infection (myocarditis). The pathophysiology of low-output failure, like that of failure caused by myocardial infarction, begins with a loss of contractility and a drop in cardiac output (Fig. 27-35). Because myocardial disease renders the myocardium unable to contract more forcefully no matter what the stimulus, low-output failure may be unresponsive to treatments aimed at elevating preload (Howard, Puri, & Paidipaty, 1984), to cardiotonic drugs, or to sympathetic stimulation.

High-Output Failure

High-output failure is the inability of the heart to adequately supply the body with blood-borne nutrients, despite adequate blood volume and normal or elevated myocardial contractility. In high-output failure, the

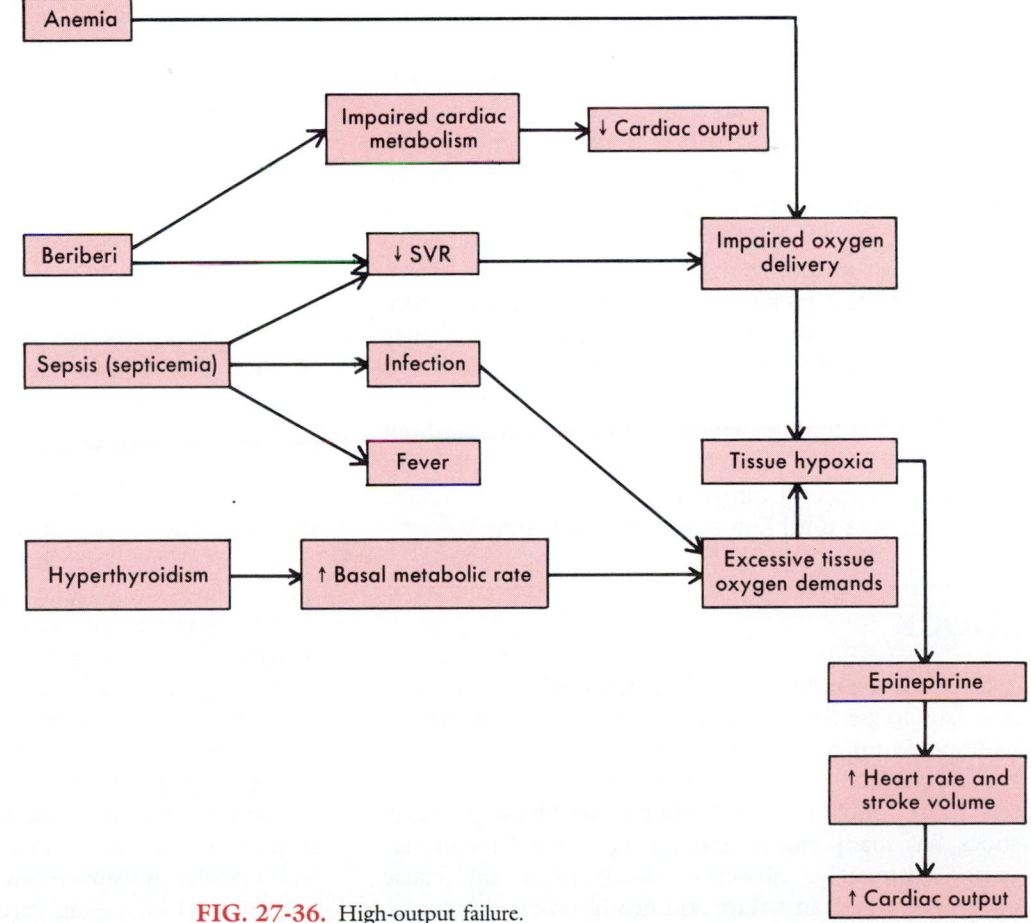

FIG. 27-36. High-output failure.

heart increases its output, but the body's metabolic needs are still not met. Common causes of high-output failure are anemia, septicemia, hyperthyroidism, and beriberi (Fig. 27-36).

Anemia decreases the oxygen-carrying capacity of the blood (see Chapter 23). Metabolic acidosis occurs as the body's cells switch to anaerobic metabolism (see Chapter 3). In response to metabolic acidosis, heart rate and stroke volume increase in an attempt to circulate blood faster. If anemia is severe, however, even maximum cardiac output will not supply the cells with enough oxygen for metabolism.

In septicemia, disturbed metabolism, bacterial toxins, and the inflammatory process cause systemic vasodilation and fever. Faced with a lowered SVR and an elevated metabolic rate, cardiac output increases to maintain blood pressure and prevent metabolic acidosis. In overwhelming septicemia, however, the heart may not be able to raise its output enough to compensate for vasodilation. Body tissues will show signs of inadequate blood supply despite a very high cardiac output.

Hyperthyroidism accelerates cellular metabolism through the actions of elevated levels of thyroxine from the thyroid gland. This may occur chronically (e.g., thyrotoxicosis) or acutely, (e.g., thyroid storm). As the body's demand for oxygen threatens to cause metabolic acidosis, cardiac output increases. If blood levels of thyroxine are high and the metabolic response to thyroxine is quite vigorous, even an abnormally elevated cardiac output may be inadequate.

In the United States, beriberi (thiamine deficiency) is usually caused by malnutrition secondary to chronic alcoholism. Beriberi actually causes a mixed type of heart failure. Thiamine deficiency impairs cellular metabolism in all tissues, including the myocardium. In the heart, impaired cardiac metabolism leads to insufficient contractile strength. In blood vessels, thiamine deficiency leads mainly to peripheral vasodilation, which decreases SVR. Heart failure ensues as decreased SVR triggers increased cardiac output, which the impaired myocardium is unable to deliver. The strain of demands for increased output in the face of impaired metabolism may deplete cardiac reserves until low-output failure begins.

SHOCK

Shock is a condition in which the cardiovascular system fails to perfuse the tissues adequately, resulting in widespread impairment of cellular metabolism. Because tissue perfusion can be disrupted by any factor that alters heart function, blood volume, or blood pressure, shock has many causes and various clinical manifestations. Ultimately, however, shock from any cause progresses to organ failure and death, unless compensa-

tory mechanisms reverse the process or clinical intervention succeeds. Untreated severe shock overwhelms the body's compensatory mechanisms through positive feedback loops that initiate and maintain a downward physiologic spiral.

Because the body is made up of many cells, which may function or malfunction at different stages of metabolic impairment, shock causes many diverse signs and symptoms. Subjective complaints are usually nonspecific, and may not be particularly helpful to the clinician who is attempting diagnosis and treatment. The individual may report feeling sick, weak, cold, hot, nauseated, dizzy, confused, afraid, thirsty, and short of breath. Observable and measurable signs and symptoms are often conflicting in nature. Blood pressure, cardiac output, and urinary output are usually—but not always—decreased. Respiratory rate is usually increased. Variable indicators of shock include alterations of heart rate, core body temperature, skin temperature, systemic vascular resistance, and skin color. Dyspnea, diaphoresis, and altered sensorium may be obvious.

Types of Shock

Shock can be classified by cause, by principal pathophysiologic process, or by clinical manifestations. Classification by cause is perhaps the most useful because it suggests the principal pathophysiologic process and focuses on the underlying disorder, which must be treated to prevent the irreversible impairment of cellular metabolism. Shock is classifed by cause as cardiogenic (caused by heart failure), hypovolemic (caused by insufficient intravascular fluid volume), neurogenic (caused by neural alterations of vascular smooth muscle tone), anaphylactic (caused by immunologic processes), or septic (caused by infection). Each type of shock involves numerous clinical manifestations that are also characteristic of many other conditions, making diagnosis difficult. In addition, the body's many compensatory mechanisms can mask, for a time, many definitive signs of shock.

Cardiogenic Shock

Cardiogenic shock results from heart failure from any cause. Most cases of cardiogenic shock follow myocardial infarction, but shock can also follow congestive heart failure, myocardial ischemia, myocardial or pericardial infections, and heart failure resulting from drug toxicity. The pathophysiology of cardiogenic shock is shown in Fig. 27-37. As cardiac output decreases, renal and hypothalamic adaptive responses maintain or increase blood volume. Blood pressure is maintained through vasoconstriction in response to catecholamine release from the adrenals. Catecholamines also increase contractility and heart rate. Increases in blood volume and vascular resistance succeed in normalizing blood pressure and increasing cardiac performance, but at the

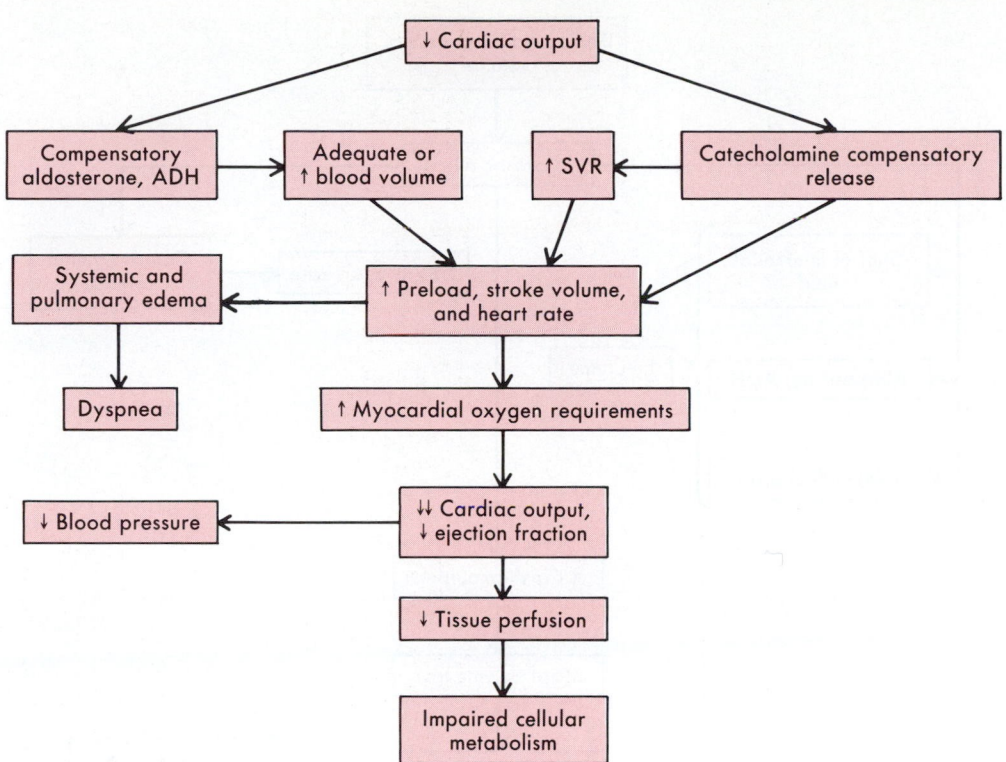

FIG. 27-37. Cardiogenic shock. Shock becomes life threatening when compensatory mechanisms (colored labels) cause increased myocardial oxygen requirements.

cost of increasing myocardial demands for oxygen and nutrients. Increasing myocardial requirements further strain the already failing heart, which can no longer pump an adequate volume of blood with sufficient force to perfuse the tissues. The direct effect of decreased tissue perfusion is impaired cellular metabolism. (Normal cellular metabolism is discussed in Chapter 1.)

The clinical manifestations of cardiogenic shock are caused by widespread impairment of cellular metabolism. They include impaired mentation, elevated preload in the systemic and pulmonary vasculature, systemic and pulmonary edema, dusky skin color, low blood pressure, oliguria, ileus, and dyspnea. Elevated preloads and low cardiac output are manifestations of heart failure (Howard et al., 1984).

Hypovolemic Shock

Hypovolemic shock is caused by loss of whole blood (hemorrhage), plasma (burns), or interstitial fluid (diaphoresis, diabetes mellitus, diabetes insipidus, emesis, or diuresis) in large amounts. Loss of whole blood or plasma causes hypovolemia directly. Loss of interstitial fluid causes it indirectly by promoting diffusion of plasma from the intravascular to the extravascular space. Hypovolemic shock begins to develop when intravascular volume has decreased by about 15%.

Hypovolemia is offset initially by compensatory mechanisms (Fig. 27-38). Heart rate and SVR increase as a result of catecholamine release by the adrenals. This boosts both cardiac output and tissue perfusion pressures. Compelled by a drop in capillary hydrostatic pressures, interstitial fluid moves into the vascular compartment. The liver and spleen add to blood volume by disgorging stored red blood cells and plasma. In the kidneys, renin (through several intermediaries) stimulates aldosterone release and the retention of sodium (and hence water), whereas ADH from the posterior pituitary gland increases water retention.

These compensatory mechanisms are finite, however. If the initial fluid or blood loss is great, or if loss continues, compensation fails, resulting in decreased tissue perfusion. As in cardiogenic shock, nutrient delivery to the cells is impaired, and cellular metabolism fails.

The clinical manifestations of hypovolemic shock include high SVR, poor skin turgor, thirst, oliguria, low systemic and pulmonary preloads, and rapid heart rates. The differences between the signs and symptoms of hypovolemic shock and those of cardiogenic shock are mainly because of differences in fluid volume and cardiac muscle health (Howard et al., 1984).

Neurogenic Shock

Neurogenic shock is sometimes called vasogenic shock. Both terms refer to a widespread and massive va-

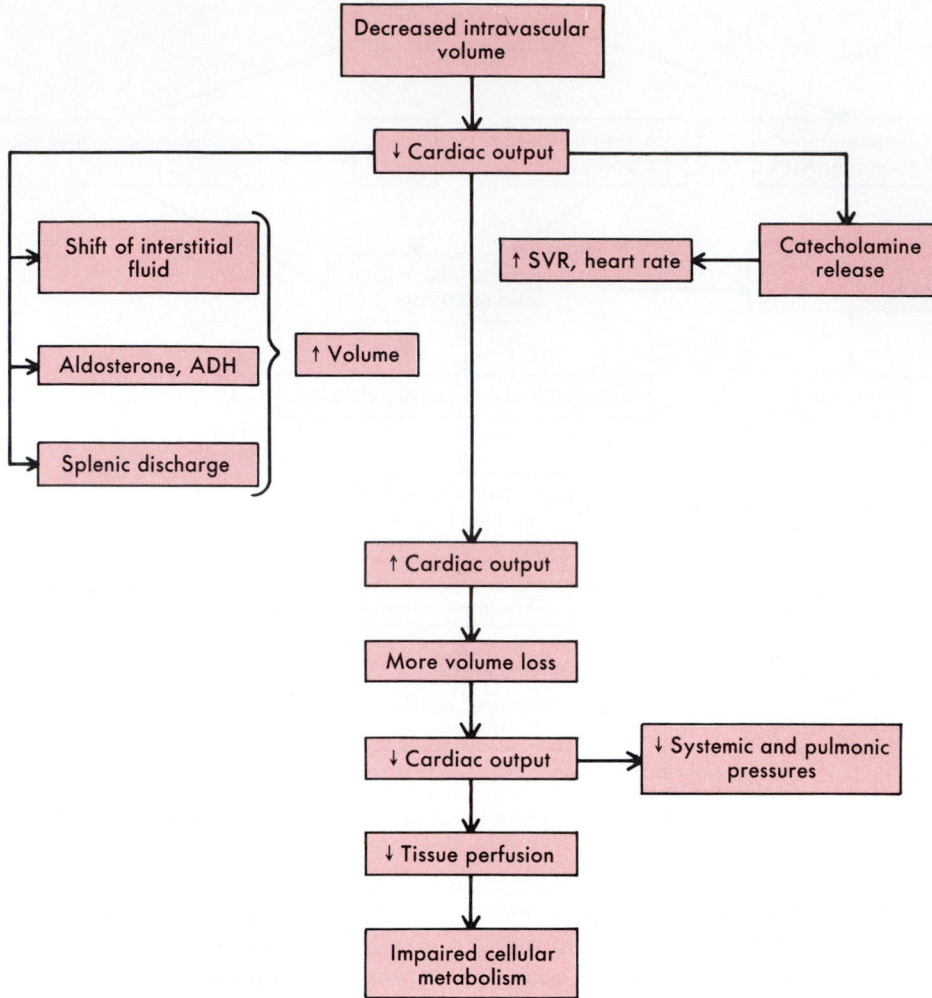

FIG. 27-38. Hypovolemic shock. This type of shock becomes life threatening when compensatory mechanisms (colored labels) are overwhelmed by continued loss of intravascular volume.

sodilation that results from an imbalance between parasympathetic and sympathetic stimulation of vascular smooth muscle (see Chapter 26). Occasionally, parasympathetic overstimulation or sympathetic understimulation persists, causing vasodilation for an extended period of time. Extreme, persistent vasodilation leads to neurogenic shock (Fig. 27-39). Neurogenic shock creates "relative hypovolemia." Blood volume has not changed, but the amount of space containing the blood has increased, so that SVR drops drastically. With a decreased SVR, pressure in the vessels is inadequate to drive nutrients across capillary membranes, and nutrient delivery to the cells is impaired. As with other types of shock, this leads to impaired cellular metabolism.

Neurogenic shock can be caused by any factor that stimulates parasympathetic or inhibits sympathetic stimulation of vascular smooth muscle. (Parasympathetic stimulation automatically inhibits sympathetic activity,

and vice versa; see Chapter 26.) Normally, sympathetic stimulation maintains muscle tone. If sympathetic stimulation is interrupted or inhibited, vasodilation occurs. Therefore, trauma to the spinal cord or medulla, conditions that interrupt the supply of oxygen to the medulla, or conditions that deprive the medulla of glucose (e.g., insulin reactions) can all cause neurogenic shock by interrupting sympathetic activity. Depressive drugs, anesthetic agents, and severe emotional stress and pain are other causes of neurogenic shock.

The clinical hallmark of neurogenic shock is a very low SVR, along with other indicators of excessive parasympathetic activity. Bradycardia is the most obvious manifestation, especially in the early stages. Bradycardia may cease when compensatory mechanisms, particularly an increase in sympathetic system activity, have been initiated. The ejection fraction remains high, indicating a healthy myocardium, whereas central venous pressure drops as the veins dilate. Neurogenic shock causes fainting if blood pressure decreases to the point that cerebral metabolism is not sufficient to support consciousness. Most episodes of fainting are *not* shock, however; for such episodes to progress to shock is rare. By allowing the blood pressure to equalize from head to toe as the individual becomes prone, fainting can actually prevent shock.

Anaphylactic Shock

Anaphylactic shock is the outcome of a widespread hypersensitivity reaction known as anaphylaxis. The basic physiologic alteration in anaphylactic shock is the same as that of neurogenic shock; that is, vasodilaton, **peripheral pooling,** and relative hypovolemia, leading to decreased tissue perfusion and impaired cellular metabolism (Fig. 27-40). Anaphylactic shock is often more severe than other types of normovolemic shock because the hypersensitivity reaction that triggers vasodilation has other pathophysiologic effects that rapidly involve the entire body.

Anaphylactic shock begins as an allergic reaction—an immune and inflammatory response—to an allergen. (An allergen is an antigen to which an individual is hy-

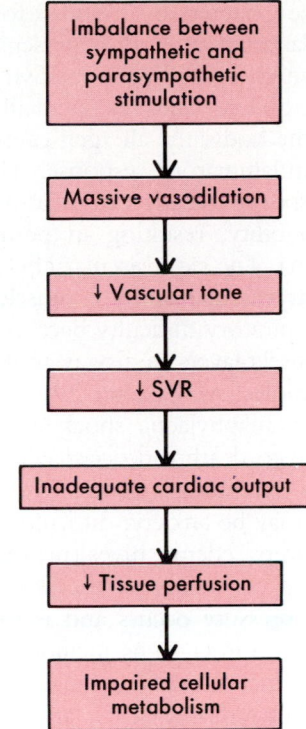

FIG. 27-39. Neurogenic shock.

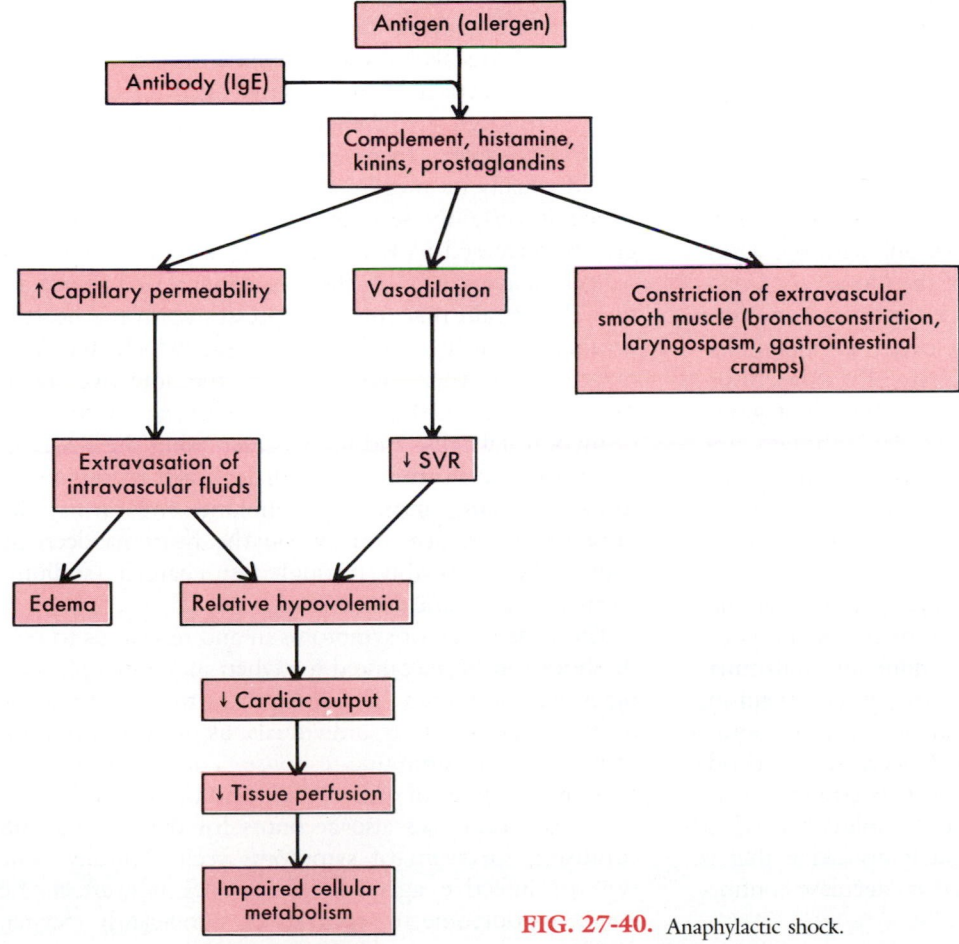

FIG. 27-40. Anaphylactic shock.

persensitive; see Chapters 6, 7, and 8 for discussion of immunity, inflammation, and hypersensitivity.) Some allergens known to cause hypersensitivity reactions are insect venoms, pollens, shellfish, penicillin, and animal sera. Once in the body, the allergen causes an extensive immune and inflammatory response. The vascular effects of this response include vasodilation and increased vascular permeability, resulting in peripheral pooling and tissue edema. The extravascular effects include constriction of extravascular smooth muscle. Constriction often causes respiratory difficulty because it tends to affect smooth muscle layers in airway walls (e.g., the larynx and bronchioles; see Chapter 29).

The onset of anaphylactic shock is usually sudden, and progression to death can occur within minutes unless emergency treatment is given. The first manifestations of shock may be anxiety, difficulty breathing, gastrointestinal cramps, edema, hives (urticaria), and sensations of burning or itching of the skin. A precipitous drop in blood pressure occurs and is followed by impaired mentation. Other signs include decreased SVR, with high or normal cardiac output, and oliguria. Treatment begins with removal of the antigen (if possible). Epinephrine is administered to cause vasoconstriction and reverse airway constriction. Volume expanders (such as lactated Ringer's solution) are given intravenously to reverse the relative hypovolemia, and antihistamines and steroids are given to stop the inflammatory reaction.

Septic Shock

Septic shock is complex and presents the most confusing and rapidly changing clinical manifestations of all the types of shock. **Septic shock** begins with the development of septicemia (infection of the blood; see Chapter 2). Septicemia, which may exist for quite some time before shock develops, tends to occur in individuals who are debilitated or are being treated for other disorders. The infectious agent is most commonly a gramnegative bacteria, such as *Escherichia coli,* although viral septicemia sometimes occurs. The pathophysiologic processes leading to shock are similar, at first, to those of anaphylactic shock (Fig. 27-41), but differ in three ways.

First, septicemia triggers an immune and inflammatory response that causes vasodilation, peripheral pooling, and decreased SVR. If the immune and inflammatory responses cannot eradicate the microorganism, these responses are perpetuated and vasodilation continues. The sustained decrease in SVR decreases afterload, making it easier for the heart to eject its contents. Cardiac output may increase dramatically unless it is offset by myocardial depressant factor, a lymphokine that is believed to act directly on the heart to decrease contractility (Demeules, 1984).

Second, the infective agent itself is affecting the metabolism of all tissues. All tissue may be invaded and affected by the infecting agent, which is circulating freely in the bloodstream. If bacteria are responsible for the septicemia, an increase in the release of bacterial endotoxins is seen. Bacterial endotoxins cause direct cellular damage and trigger the release of lysosomal enzymes from the ruptured cells. If the infecting agent is viral, an increase in the number of host cells damaged in the course of viral reproduction is seen. These infected tissues will not be able to metabolize efficiently, nor will they be able to perform their functions well.

Third, the fever that accompanies septicemia increases the basal metabolic rate (BMR) of nearly all body tissues. Fever is probably initiated and maintained by the hypothalamus, in response to the release from leukocytes of endogenous pyrogen, a lymphokine. Fever increases the metabolic oxygen requirements of peripheral tissues. Because of the greatly decreased SVR, however, less oxygen is reaching the cells, even though cardiac output is increased. Cellular metabolism becomes anaerobic, which is a less energy-efficient form of metabolism. Lactic acidosis is a hallmark of septic shock (Howard et al., 1984).

In septic shock, cellular metabolism is impaired through three pathways: (1) through a relative hypovolemia, resulting from the decreased SVR caused by vasoactive chemicals of the inflammatory response; (2) through the action of the infective agent on all tissues; and (3) through the increased oxygen needs of all tissue caused by fever. Increased oxygen needs of tissues would usually be met by an increase in cardiac output, which is certainly seen in early shock. However, the greatly decreased SVR of septic shock prevents effective oxygen delivery even in the face of increased pump action. The strain that this cycle presses upon the heart is profound: cardiac output increases, which increases myocardial oxygen requirements; the infective agent may be acting on the heart, decreasing the effectiveness of myocardial cells; and fever is increasing the BMR of the heart, which raises myocardial oxygen requirements further. Finally, another lymphokine, myocardial depressant factor, acts directly on the heart to decrease contractility, probably through fast channel (sodium) mechanisms (Demeules, 1984).

The wide range of symptoms in and responses to septic shock can be accounted for when individual physiologies are considered. The strength of the inflammatory response varies among individuals, as does the strength of each person's immune response. The involvement of a varying number of cells, tissues, and organs as the septic shock progresses also accounts for the varying and confusing spectrum of symptoms seen clinically. The type of infective agent involved does not affect the course or outcome of septic shock significantly (Siegel, 1983).

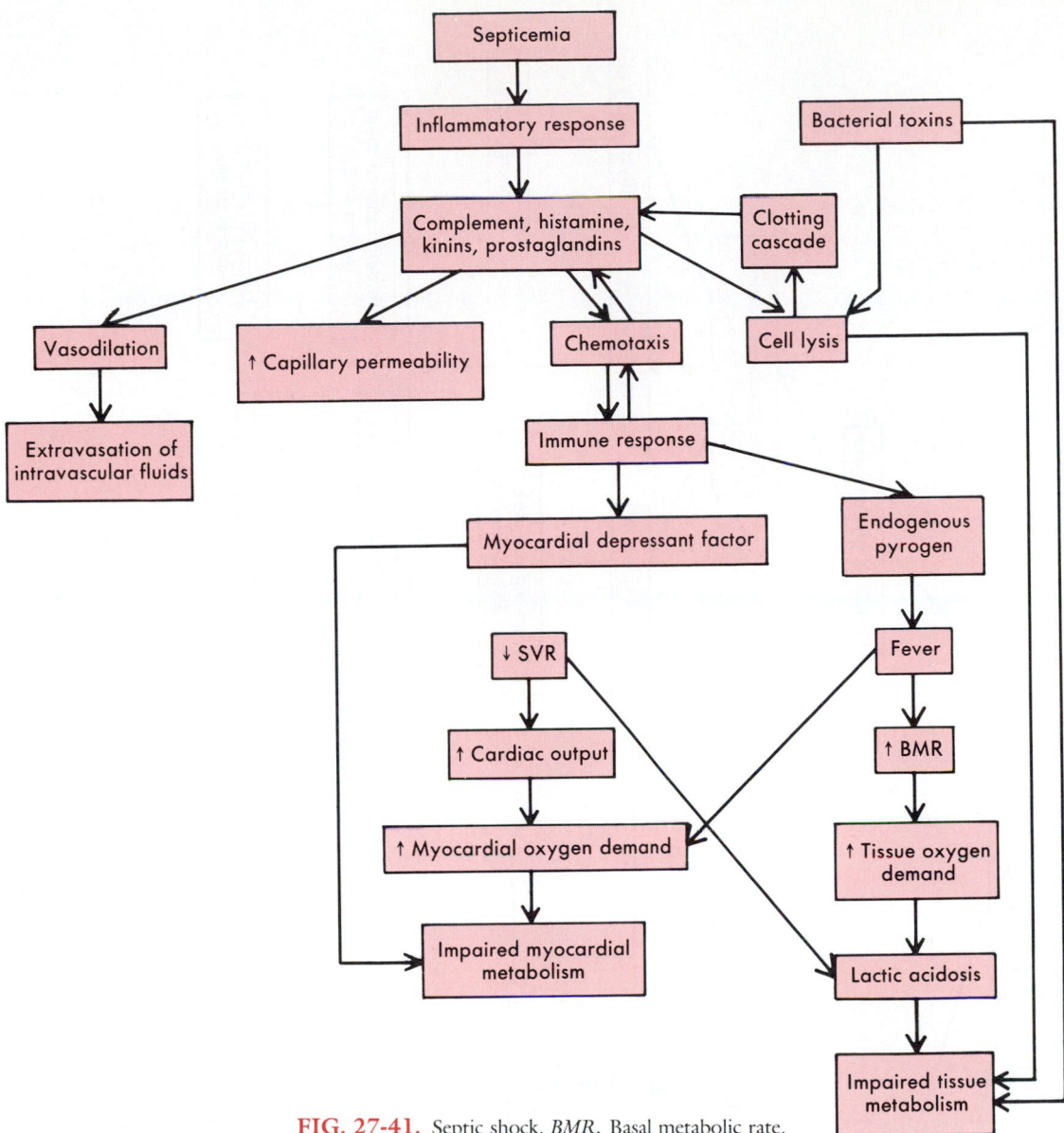

FIG. 27-41. Septic shock. *BMR,* Basal metabolic rate.

Toxic shock syndrome, which is most common in menstruating women, is a form of septic shock with a similar set of clinical manifestations. Toxic shock syndrome is characterized by extremely low blood pressure, high fever, cerebral manifestations (confusion, syncope, headache), and skin rash. In toxic shock, bacterial toxins, usually those of *Staphylococcus aureus*, may migrate from the site of infection (e.g., the vagina) into the blood, triggering a widespread inflammatory response that leads to peripheral vasodilation, impaired cellular metabolism, and septic shock.

Impairment of Cellular Metabolism

The final common pathway in all types of shock is impairment of cellular metabolism, which is a complex concept in itself. Fig. 27-42 illustrates the pathophysiology of shock at the cellular level.

Impairment of Oxygen Use

In all types of shock, the cell either is not receiving an adequate amount of oxygen or is unable to use oxygen (see Fig. 27-42). In cardiogenic shock, cardiac output is too low to deliver adequate oxygen to the cell. In hypovolemic shock, oxygen delivery is impaired by inadequate numbers of red cells or inadequate volume of intravascular fluid. In neurogenic, anaphylactic, and septic shock, SVR is too low and perfusion pressure in the capillaries is inadequate to drive oxygen across cell membranes. In septic shock, hypoxia is made worse by fever, which increases the cell's oxygen consumption

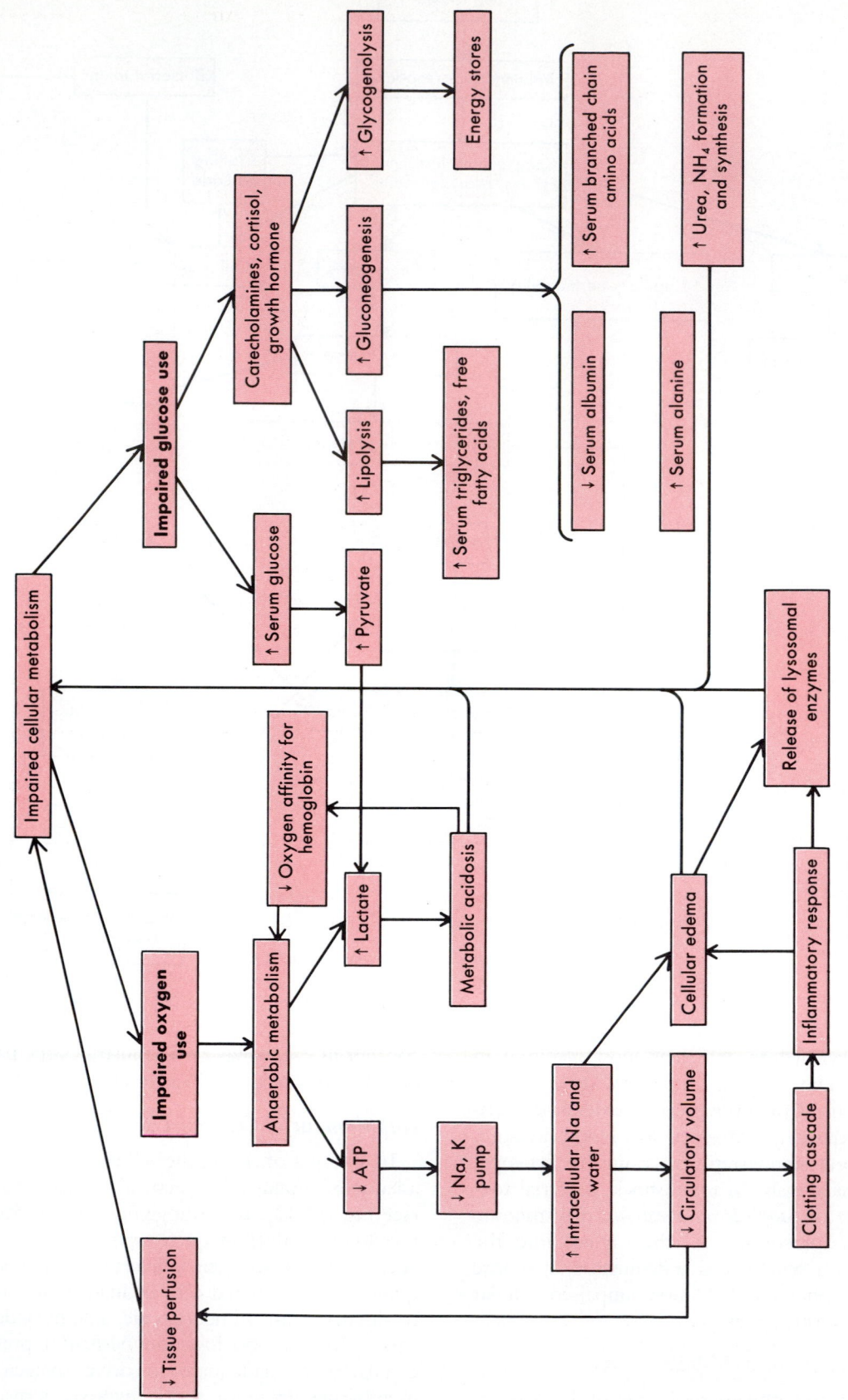

FIG. 27-42. Impairment of cellular metabolism by shock.

rate, and by bacterial disruption of cells' metabolism, which impairs the cells' ability to use oxygen.

Without oxygen, the cell shifts from aerobic to anaerobic metabolism. Anaerobic metabolism is a less efficient method of extracting energy from carbon bonds, and the cell will begin to use its stores of adenosine triphosphate (ATP) faster than stores can be replaced. Without ATP, the cell loses its ability to maintain an electrochemical gradient across its selectively permeable membrane. Specifically, the cell cannot operate the sodium-potassium pump. Sodium and chloride accumulate inside the cell, and potassium exits. Cells of the nervous system and myocardium are profoundly and immediately affected. The resting potentials of these cells are reduced, and action potentials decrease in amplitude. Myocardial depressant factor also decreases the contractility of the heart. A variety of clinical manifestations of impaired central nervous system and myocardial function result.

As sodium moves into the cell, water follows. Throughout the body, the water drawn from the interstitium into the cells is "replaced" by water that is, in turn, drawn out of the vascular space. This decreases circulatory volume. Within the cells, water causes cellular edema that disrupts cellular membranes, releasing lysosomal enzymes that injure the cells internally and leak into the interstitium.

Three positive feedback loops now begin that further impair oxygen use: (1) activation of the clotting cascade, (2) decreased circulatory volume, and (3) lysosomal enzyme release. First, enzymatic processes are disrupted by the change in the normal ionic and osmotic levels in the cell, as are those processes governed by the physical laws of diffusion. Diffusion of nutrients and wastes into and out of the cell takes longer, and cellular metabolism is further altered. At the same time, diffusion across capillary membranes occurs more slowly as blood flow in the capillary beds becomes sluggish. Sluggish capillary flow decreases tissue perfusion further and activates the clotting cascade (see Chapter 22). The clotting cascade activates the inflammatory response and also accounts for common complications of shock, such as acute tubular necrosis, adult respiratory distress syndrome, and disseminated intravascular coagulation.

Decreased circulatory volume causes the second positive feedback loop and magnifies decreased tissue perfusion in all types of shock. Decreased intravascular volume causes decreased cardiac output in septic shock and further decreases cardiac output in cardiogenic shock. In individuals with anaphylactic, neurogenic, or septic shock and an already dilated vasculature, hypotension worsens as a result of decreased circulatory volume.

The third positive feedback loop involves the release of lysosomal enzymes. Lysosomal enzymes not only injure the cell that released them, but also injure adjacent cells. By damaging the mechanisms of surrounding cells, lysosomal enzymes extend areas of impaired metabolism and cellular injury.

In addition to decreasing ATP stores, anaerobic metabolism affects the pH of the cell and metabolic acidosis develops (Siegel, 1983). A compensatory mechanism is initiated that enables cardiac and skeletal muscles to use lactic acid as a fuel source, but only for a limited time.

The decreasing pH of the cell that is functioning anaerobically has serious consequences. Enzymes necessary for cellular function dissociate under acid conditions. Enzyme dissociation stops cell function, repair, and division. As lactic acid is released systemically, blood pH drops, reducing the oxygen-carrying capacity of the blood (see Chapter 2). Therefore, less oxygen is delivered to the cells. Further acidosis triggers the release of more lysosomal enzymes because the low pH disrupts lysosomal membrane integrity.

Impairment of Glucose Use

Impaired glucose use can be caused by either impaired glucose delivery or impaired glucose uptake by the cells (see Fig. 27-42). The reasons for inadequate glucose delivery are the same as those enumerated for inadequate oxygen delivery. Additionally, in septic and anaphylactic shock, glucose metabolism may be increased or disrupted because of fever or bacteria, and glucose uptake can be prevented by the presence of vasoactive toxins, endotoxins, histamine, and kinins.

Some of the compensatory mechanisms activated by shock contribute to decreased glucose uptake by the cells. High serum levels of cortisol, growth hormone, and catecholamines account for hyperglycemia and insulin resistance, tachycardia, increased SVR, and increased cardiac contractility. Cells shift to glycogenolysis, gluconeogenesis, and lypolysis to generate fuel for survival (see Chapter 1). Except in the liver, kidneys, and muscles, the body's cells have extremely limited stores of glycogen. In fact, total body stores can only fuel the metabolism for about 10 hours. The depletion of fat and glycogen stores is not itself a cause of organ failure, but the energy costs of glycogenolysis and lypolysis are considerable and contribute to the cells' failure.

The depletion of protein is, however, a cause of organ failure. When gluconeogenesis causes proteins to be used for fuel, these proteins are no longer available to maintain cellular structure, function, repair, and replication. The breakdown of protein occurs in starvation states, hyperdynamic metabolic states, and septic shock. The breakdown of protein into amino acids that occurs with septicemia is called septic autocannibalism (Siegel, 1983). Under anaerobic metabolism, protein breakdown liberates alanine, which is converted to pyruvate. In sepsis, pyruvic acid is changed into lactic acid, and a positive feedback loop is formed.

As proteins are broken down anaerobically, ammonia and urea are produced. Ammonia is toxic to living cells. Uremia develops and uric acid further disrupts cellular metabolism.

Proteins are broken down preferentially. Serum albumin and other plasma proteins are consumed for fuel first. Serum protein consumption decreases capillary osmotic pressure and contributes to the development of interstitial edema, creating another positive feedback loop that decreases circulatory volume. In septic shock, plasma protein breakdown includes breakdown of immunoglobulins (Siegel, 1983), thereby impairing immune system function when it is most needed.

Muscle wasting caused by protein breakdown weakens skeletal and cardial muscle. Skeletal muscle wasting impairs the muscles that facilitate breathing. Muscle wasting therefore alters the actions of both heart and lungs. The delivery of oxygen and glucose to the cells is directly reduced, as is the removal of waste products, forming another positive feedback loop.

A final outcome of impaired cellular metabolism is the buildup of metabolic end-products in the cell and interstitial spaces. Waste products are toxic to the cells and further disrupt cellular function and membrane integrity. In septic shock, for example, a deficiency in cellular metabolism and the build up of toxins may precede and cause decreased tissue perfusion.

Treatment for Shock

The first treatment for shock is to discover and correct or remove the underlying cause. Though this seems a simple tenet, it is one that is not always remembered. Thus, treatment for cardiogenic shock begins with treatment of heart failure or at least enhancement of cardiac output. If hypovolemia is the cause of shock, hemorrhage and other causes of fluid loss must be stopped. In neurogenic shock, as a result of spinal cord trauma, stabilization of the spine and surrounding tissue is a beginning, and pain can usually be decreased to a level at which neurally mediated decreases of SVR cease. The initial treatment for anaphylactic shock is to remove or neutralize the antigen. Treatment for septic shock begins with eradication of the infective agent, usually with antibiotics.

After the underlying cause or condition is corrected as far as possible, treatment is supportive. Intravenous fluid is administered to expand intravascular volume, except in cardiogenic shock, which requires diuresis to reduce preload. Supplemental oxygen is always given. Cardiotonic drugs are given early in cardiogenic shock, and later in other forms of shock. Once positive feedback loops are established, intervention is difficult.

SUMMARY REVIEW

Diseases of the Arteries and Veins

1 Arteriosclerosis is a thickening and hardening of the arteries, involving the intimal layer and leading to hypertension. It seems to be a part of the normal aging process, but is a disease state when occurring to the point of symptom development.

2 Arteriosclerosis raises the systolic pressure by decreasing arterial distensibility and lumen diameter. With arteriosclerotic changes in the artery causing narrowing and decreased elasticity, diastolic blood pressure will be elevated.

3 Hypertension is the elevation of systemic arterial blood pressure resulting from increases in cardiac output or total peripheral resistance or both.

4 Hypertension can be primary, without a known cause, or secondary, caused by a primary disease.

5 The risk factors for hypertension include a positive family history, male gender, advancing age, black race, obesity, high sodium intake, diabetes mellitus, labile blood pressure, cigarette smoking, and heavy alcohol consumption.

6 The pathophysiology of hypertension includes damage and inflammation of the vessel walls that stimulates the vessels to thicken, harden, and become narrow. Narrowing causes vasoconstriction and increases the permeability of the vessel walls leading to the influx of sodium, calcium, water, plasma proteins, and other substances. Calcium further increases smooth muscle contraction.

7 The exact cause of primary hypertension is unknown, although several hypotheses are proposed, including increases in blood volume, inappropriate autoregulation, an increase in sympathetic stimulation, water and sodium retention by the kidneys, and inhibition of the sodium-potassium active pump.

8 Clinical manifestations of hypertension result from damage of organs and tissues outside the vascular system. These include heart disease, renal disease, central nervous system problems, and musculoskeletal dysfunction.

9 Hypertension is managed with both pharmacologic and nonpharmacologic methods, for example, dietary alterations.

10 Orthostatic hypotension is a drop in blood pressure that occurs on standing. The compensatory vasoconstriction response to standing is altered by a marked vasodilation and blood pooling in the muscle vasculature.

11 Orthostatic hypotension may be acute or chronic. The acute form is caused by a delay in the normal regulatory mechanisms. The chronic forms are secondary to a specific disease or are idiopathic in nature.

12 The clinical manifestations of orthostatic hypotension include fainting and may involve cardiovascular symptoms, as well as impotence and bowel and bladder dysfunction.

13 An aneurysm is a localized dilatation of a vessel wall, to which the aorta is particularly susceptible.

14 A thrombus is a clot that remains attached to a vascular wall. Arteriosclerosis can generate thrombus formation through roughening of the intima that activates the clotting cascade. Thrombus formation may be discrete or diffuse.

15 An embolus is a mobile aggregate of a variety of substances that occludes the vasculature. Sources of emboli include clots, air, amniotic fluid, bacteria, fat, and foreign matter.

16 The most common cause of arterial thrombotic emboli is the heart, as a result of mitral and aortic valvular disease and atrial fibrillation, followed by myxomas. Organs affected include the lower extremities, the brain, and the heart.

17 Emboli to the central organs cause tissue death in lungs, kidneys, and mesentery.

18 The generation of air emboli requires a connection between the vascular compartment and a source of air. These emboli cause ischemia and necrosis when a vessel is totally blocked.

19 Amniotic fluid may be forced into the bloodstream and generate an embolus during the labor and delivery of pregnancy.

20 Aggregates of bacteria in the vasculature may be large enough to form an embolus.

21 Fat emboli are caused mainly by trauma to the long bones, through either defective fat metabolism following trauma or through the release of fat globules from bone marrow exposed by fracture.

22 The introduction of foreign matter into the vasculature can occur with trauma and can also occur in a hospital setting in which intravenous and intraarterial lines are being used.

23 Vasospastic disorders include Raynaud disease, involving arterioles of the extremities; Prinzmetal angina, involving coronary arteries; and Buerger disease, involving arteries of the hands and feet.

24 Diabetic lesions of the arteries may be caused by a defect in glycoprotein metabolism that involves the capillary basement membranes in kidneys, retinas, and extremities.

25 Varicosities are areas of veins in which blood has pooled, usually in the saphenous veins. Varicosities may be caused by damaged valves as a result of trauma to the valve, or by chronic venous distention involving gravity and venous constriction.

26 Chronic venous insufficiency is inadequate venous return over a long period of time that causes pathologic ischemic changes in the vasculature, skin, and supporting tissues.

27 Venous stasis ulcers follow the development of chronic venous insufficiency and probably develop as a result of the borderline metabolic state of the cells in the affected extremities.

28 The pathophysiology of thrombus formation in the veins is the same as for thrombus formation in the arteries. Because of the triggering of the inflammatory response at the site of formation, deep vein thrombi are characterized by tenderness, swelling, and redness.

29 Superior vena cava syndrome is a progressive occlusion of the superior vena cava that leads to venous distention in the upper extremities and head. Because this syndrome is usually caused by bronchogenic cancer, it is generally not a vascular emergency, but is an oncologic emergency.

Coronary Artery Disease, Myocardial Ischemia, Myocardial Infarction

1 Coronary artery disease (CAD) is any disorder that narrows or occludes the coronary arteries. Many risk factors contribute to the onset and escalation of CAD, including: hyperlipidemia (primarily hypercholesterolemia), smoking, hypertension, male gender, diabetes mellitus, advancing age, obesity, sedentary lifestyle, psychosocial factors, hormone therapy, and heavy consumption of alcohol.

2 The three risk factors most predictive of CAD are hypercholesterolemia, cigarette smoking, and hypertension.

3 Ischemic heart disease is most commonly the result of coronary artery disease and the resultant decrease in myocardial blood supply.

4 Angina pectoris is chest pain caused by myocardial ischemia.

5 Therapeutic interventions for CAD include use of vasodilators and medications to reduce cardiac workload (e.g., beta blockers), as well as surgical procedures.

6 Myocardial infarction is caused by prolonged, unrelieved ischemia that interrupts blood supply to the myocardium. After about 20 minutes of myocardial ischemia, irreversible hypoxic injury causes cellular death and tissue necrosis.

7 A transient rise in plasma enzyme levels may diagnose the occurrence of myocardial infarction and indicate its severity. Elevations of the isoenzymes creatine phosphokinase (CK-MB) and lactic dehydrogenase (LDH-1) are the isoenzymes most predictive of a myocardial infarction.

8 Treatment of a myocardial infarction includes bed rest, pain relief, and drug interventions to limit infarct size, prevent thrombus formation, and augment repair. Dysrhythmias are the most common complication of acute myocardial infarction.

Disorders of the Heart Wall

1 Inflammation of the pericardium, pericarditis, may result from innumerable sources (infection, drug therapy, tumors). Pericarditis presents with symptoms that are physically troublesome, but in and of themselves are not life-threatening.

2 Fluid may collect within the pericardial sac (pericardial effusion). Cardiac function may be severely impaired if the accumulation of fluid occurs rapidly and involves a large volume.

3 Cardiomyopathies are a diverse group of primary myocardial disorders that are poorly understood. The cardiomyopathies are categorized as congestive (dilated), restrictive (rigid and noncompliant), and hypertrophic

(asymmetric). Size of the cardiac muscle walls and chambers may increase or decrease, depending on the type of cardiomyopathy, thereby altering contractile activity.

4 Hemodynamic integrity of the cardiovascular system depends to a great extent on properly functioning cardiac valves. Congenital or acquired disorders that result in stenosis or incompetence or both can structurally alter the valves.

5 Characteristic heart sounds, cardiac murmurs, and systemic complaints assist in determination of which valve is abnormal. If severely compromised function exists, a prosthetic heart valve may be surgically implanted to replace the faulty one.

6 Mitral valve prolapse (MVP) is a common finding, especially in young women. Although not grossly abnormal, the mitral valve leaflets do not position themselves properly during systole. MVP may be a completely asymptomatic condition or could result in severe subjective symptoms. Afflicted valves may be at greater risk for developing infective endocarditis.

7 Rheumatic fever is an inflammatory disease that results from a delayed immune response to a streptococcal infection. The disorder usually resolves without sequelae if treated early.

8 Severe or untreated cases of rheumatic fever may progress to rheumatic heart disease, a potentially disabling cardiovascular disorder.

9 Infective endocarditis is a general term for inflammation of the endocardium, especially the cardiac valves. A wide range of conditions predispose the development of this disorder. In the mildest cases, valvular function may be slightly impaired by vegetations that collect on the valve leaflets. If left unchecked, severe valve abnormalities, chronic bacteremia, and systemic emboli may occur as vegetations break off the valve surface and travel through the bloodstream. Antibiotic therapy can limit the extension of this disease.

Manifestations of Heart Disease

1 A dysrhythmia (arrhythmia) is a disturbance of heart rhythm. Dysrhythmias range in severity from occasional missed beats or rapid beats to disturbances that impair myocardial contractility and are life-threatening.

2 Dysrhythmias can occur because of an abnormal rate of impulse generation or the abnormal conduction of impulses.

3 Heart failure is an inability of the heart to supply the metabolism with adequate circulatory volume and pressure.

4 The supply:demand oxygen ratio is one of the major components of heart failure. A decrease in the ratio can precipitate, exacerbate, or follow heart failure.

5 The most common cause of right heart failure is left heart failure, followed by pulmonary disease with an elevated pulmonary vascular resistance.

6 Since the right ventricle normally has a high oxygen supply:demand ratio, and the pulmonary vasculature is normally low, right ventricular infarction is rare, and

left ventricular failure or pulmonary disease may be present for quite some time before the right ventricle begins to fail.

7 As oxygen supply:demand ratio falls and pulmonary vascular resistance increases, right ventricular preload increases, and the right heart begins to fail.

8 Symptoms of right heart failure arise in the systemic venous system because of elevated venous pressures and volumes.

9 The most common causes of left ventricular failure are myocardial infarction, systemic hypertension, and valvular incompetence or stenosis.

10 The pathophysiology of left heart failure resembles that of right heart failure.

11 Biventricular failure is failure of the right and left ventricles.

12 A decrease in left ventricular output triggers sodium and water retention through renal, adrenal, and posterior pituitary hormone actions. This increases vascular volume and preload, and contributes to additional failure.

13 Epinephrine and norepinephrine release is triggered by a lowered ventricular output. These neurotransmitters increased oxygen demand through cardiotonic and vascular resistance increases.

14 Left ventricular failure in the aged does not necessarily include a reduction in left ventricular ejection force.

15 The earliest clinical indicator of left heart failure is a rise in the left ventricular end-diastolic pressure or pulmonary capillary wedge pressure.

16 Low-output failure is (1) biventricular, (2) commonly caused by cardiomyopathies and myocarditis, and (3) usually refractory to treatment.

17 High-output failure is the inability of the heart to adequately supply the metabolism with blood, despite adequate blood volume and a normal myocardial contractility. Common causes are anemia, sepsis, hyperthyroidism, and beriberi.

Shock

1 Shock is a widespread impairment of cellular metabolism involving positive feedback loops that places the individual on a downward physiologic spiral leading to multiple organ failure.

2 Types of shock are cardiogenic, hypovolemic, neurogenic, anaphylactic, and septic.

3 Cardiogenic shock is due to heart failure and is characterized by a decrease in cardiac output and impaired cellular metabolism.

4 Hypovolemic shock is caused by loss of blood or fluid in large amounts. The use of compensatory mechanisms may be vigorous, but tissue perfusion ultimately decreases and results in impaired cellular metabolism.

5 Neurogenic shock results from massive vasodilation, causing a relative hypovolemia, even though cardiac output may be high, and results in impaired cellular metabolism.

6 Anaphylactic shock is caused by physiologic recognition of a foreign substance. The inflammatory response

is triggered and a massive vasodilation with fluid shift into the interstitium follows. The relative hypovolemia leads to impaired cellular metabolism.

7 Septic shock begins with impaired cellular metabolism caused by uncontrolled septicemia. The infecting agent triggers the inflammatory and immune responses, and cellular metabolism is impaired further by (1) the resulting hypovolemia, (2) the actions of the agent on target tissue, and (3) fever.

8 Oxygen use in impaired cellular metabolism is affected—cells switch from aerobic to anerobic metabolism. Energy stores drop and cellular mechanisms relative to membrane permeability, action potentials, and lysosyme release fail.

9 Anaerobic metabolism results in activation of the inflammatory response, decreased circulatory volume, and decreasing pH.

10 Impaired cellular metabolism results in cellular inability to use glucose because of impaired glucose delivery or impaired glucose intake, resulting in a shift of glycogenolysis, gluconeogenesis, and lipolysis for fuel generation.

11 Glycogenolysis is affected for up to 10 hours. Gluconeogenesis results in the use of proteins necessary for structure, function, repair, and replication that leads to more impaired cellular metabolism. Lipolysis is ineffective because of a lack of transport serum proteins and malfunction of the Kreb's cycle.

12 Gluconeogenesis contributes to lactic acid, uric acid and ammonia build-up, interstitial edema, and impairement of the immune system, as well as general muscle weakness leading to decreased respiratory function and cardiac output.

KEY TERMS

Acute orthostatic hypotension, 927

Acute pericarditis, 947

Anaphylactic shock, 979

Aneurysm, 927

Angina pectoris, 939

Aortic regurgitation (aortic insufficiency, aortic incompetence), 956

Aortic stenosis, 954

Arteriosclerosis, 917

Atherosclerosis, 917

Biventricular heart failure, 972

Cardiogenic shock, 976

Cardiomyopathy, 951

Carditis, 958

Chronic orthostatic hypotension, 927

Chronic venous insufficiency (CVI), 932

Chylomicron, 934

Complicated hypertension, 923

Congestive cardiomyopathy (dilated cardiomyopathy), 951

Constrictive pericarditis, 949

Coronary artery disease, 934

Dissecting aneurysm, 929

Dysrhythmia (arrhythmia), 946

Embolism, 930

Embolus, 930

False aneurysm, 927

Fatty streak, 919

Fibrous plaque, 919

Heart failure, 963

High-output failure, 975

Hypertension, 920

Hypertrophic cardiomyopathy, 953

Hypotension, 975

Hypovolemic shock, 977

Infarction, 934

Infective endocarditis, 960

Ischemia, 934

Isolated systolic hypertension, 920

Left heart failure (left ventricular failure, congestive heart failure), 971

Low-ouput failure, 975

Malignant hypertension, 925

Mitral regurgitation (mitral insufficiency, mitral incompetence), 957

Mitral stenosis, 955

Mitral valve prolapse syndrome, 957

Neurogenic shock (vasogenic shock), 977

Nonbacterial thrombotic endocarditis, 960

Orthostatic (postural) hypotension, 926

Pericardial effusion, 948

Peripheral pooling, 979

Primary hypertension (essential hypertension, idiopathic hypertension), 920

Prinzmetal angina, 939

Raynaud disease, 932

Raynaud phenomenon, 932

Restrictive cardiomyopathy, 953

Rheumatic fever, 958

Rheumatic heart disease, 958

Right heart failure (cor pulmonale), 969

Saccular aneurysm, 927

Secondary hypertension, 920

Septic shock, 980

Shock, 976

Stable angina, 939

Superior vena cava syndrome (SVCS), 933

Tamponade, 948

Thromboangiitis obliterans (Buerger disease), 931

Thromboembolus, 930

Thromboembolism, 930

Thrombus, 930

Toxic shock syndrome, 981

Tricuspid regurgitation (tricuspid insufficiency, tricuspid incompetence), 957

True aneurysm, 927

Unstable angina, 939

Valvular regurgitation (valvular insufficiency, valvular incompetence), 953

Valvular stenosis, 953

Varicose vein, 932

Venous stasis ulcers, 933

REFERENCES

Advance Data. (1976). *Vital and Health Statistics* (October), *1*.

Ahumada, G. G. (Ed.). (1987). *Cardiovascular pathophysiology.* New York: Oxford University Press.

Alonzo, A. A., Simon, A. B., & Feinlit, M. (1975). Prodromata of myocardial infarction and sudden death. *Circulation, 52,* 1056.

Anderson, W. A. D., & Scotti, T. M. (1980). *Synopsis of pathology* (10th ed.). St. Louis: C. V. Mosby.

Angelin, B., Eriksson, M., & Andersson, O. (1987). Studies of human macrophage lipoprotein uptake: Relation to atherosclerosis. *Acta Medica Scandinavica* [Supplement], *715,* 45-49.

Archer, G. L. (1977). Experimental endocarditis. In R. J. Duma (Ed.), *Infections of prosthetic heart valves and vascular grafts. Prevention, diagnosis, and treatment.* Baltimore: University Park Press, pp. 43-57.

Aronow, W. S., Goldsmith, J. R., Kern, J. C., & Johnson, L. L. (1974). Effect of smoking on cardiovascular hemodynamics. *Archives of Environmental Health, 28,* 331-332.

Assmann, G. (1987). Lipoproteins and apolipoproteins in the prediction of coronary artery disease. *Acta Medica Scandinavica* [Supplement], *715,* 67-77.

Berglund, G., Andersson, O., & Wilhemsen, L. (1976). Prevalence of primary and secondary hypertension: Studies in a random sample population. *British Medical Journal, 2,* 554-556.

Blair, S. N., & Oberman, A. (1987). Epidemiologic analysis of coronary heart disease and exercise. *Cardiology Clinics, 5*(2), 217-283.

Blumenthal, J. A., Williams, R. G. J., Kong, Y., Schanberg, S. M., & Thompson, L. W. (1978). Type A behavior pattern and coronary atherosclerosis. *Circulation, 58,* 634-639.

Braunwald, E. (Ed.). (1988). *Heart disease: A textbook of cardiovascular medicine* (3rd ed.). Philadelphia: W. B. Saunders.

Braunwald, E., & Sobel, B. E. (1988). Coronary blood flow and myocardial ischemia. In E. Braunwald (Ed.), *Heart disease: A textbook of cardiovascular medicine.* Philadelphia: W. B. Saunders.

Brischetto, C. S., Connor, W. E., Connor, S. L., & Matarazzo, J. D. (1983). Plasma lipid and lipoprotein profiles of cigarette smokers from randomly selected families: enhancement of hyperlipidemia and depression of high density lipoprotein. *American Journal of Cardiology, 52,* 675.

Bulkley, B. H. (1979), Advances in cardiac pathology. In J. W. Hurst (Ed.), *The heart: Update I.* McGraw-Hill.

Castaner, A., Betriu, A., Sanz, G., Pare, J. C., Coll, S., Soler, J., Roig, E., & Navarro-Lopez, F. (1984). Natural history of severe left ventricular hypertrophy after myocardial infarction. *Chest, 85*(6), 744-750.

Cheitlin, R., Buckley, D. I., & Ramachandran, J. (1985). The role of extracellular calcium in corticotropin-stimulated steroidogenesis. *Journal of Biological Chemistry, 260*(9), 5323-5327.

Cheng, T. O. (1986). *The international textbook of cardiology.* New York: Pergamon Press.

Chung, E. K. (1987). *Cardiovascular diseases, quick reference to.* Baltimore: Williams & Wilkins.

Cody, R. J., Covit, A. B., Schaer, G. L., & Laragh, J. H. (1984). Estimation of angiotension II receptor activity in chronic congestive heart failure. *American Heart Journal, 108*(1), 81-89.

Come, P. C. (1981). Mitral valve prolapse: clinical features, laboratory abnormalities, complications, and prognosis. *Journal of Family Practice, 12*(3), 431-446.

Cornell, L. V. (1985). Mitral valve prolapse syndrome: etiology and symptomatology. *Nurse Practitioner* (April), 25-34.

Criqui, M. H. (1986). Epidemiology of atherosclerosis: an updated overview. *American Journal of Cardiology, 57*(5), 18C-23C.

Crouse, J. R., III. (1989, February). Gender, lipoproteins, diet, and cardiovascular risk. *Lancet, 1,* 318-320.

Cryer, P. E., Haymond, M. W., Santigo, J. V., & Shah, S. D. (1976). Norepinephrine and epinephrine release and adrenergic mediation of smoking-associated hemodynamic and metabolic events. *New England Journal of Medicine, 295,* 573-577.

Danielson, M., & Dammstrom, B. G. (1981). The prevalence of secondary and curable hypertension. *Acta Medica Scandinavica, 209,* 451-455.

Demeules, J. E. (1984). A physiologic explanation for cardiac deterioration in septic shock. *Journal of Surgical Research, 36*(6), 553-562.

DeSanctis, R. W. (1984). Cardiomyopathies. *Scientific American Medicine Index, 8.*

Detre, K. M. (1984). Hypertension in women—a review. In E. G. Gold (Ed.), *The changing risk of disease in women: an epidemiologic approach.* Lexington, MA: D. C. Heath Co.

Dimsdale, J. E. (1988). A perspective on type A behavior and coronary disease. *New England Journal of Medicine, 318*(2), 110-112.

Doll, R., & Peto, R. (1976). Mortality in relation to smoking: 20 years observations on male British doctors. *British Medical Journal, 2,* 1525-1536.

Donabedian, H. (1985). Human mononuclear cells exposed

to staphylococci rapidly produce an inhibitor of neutrophil chemotaxis. *Journal of Infectious Disease, 152*(1), 24-32.

Estok, P. J., & Rudy, E. B. (1986). Jogging: cardiovascular benefits and risks. *Nurse Practitioner, 11*(5), 21-28.

Feinleib, M., & Garrison, R. J. (1979). The contribution of family studies to the partitioning of population variation of blood pressure. In C. F. Sing, M. Skolnick, & A. R. Liss (Eds.), *Genetic analysis of common diseases: application to predictive factors in coronary disease.* New York: Alan R. Liss, p. 653.

Ferguson, R. K. (1975). Cost and yield of the hypertensive evaluation. *Annals of Internal Medicine, 82,* 761-765.

Fitzmaurice, J. B. (1980). *Rheumatic heart disease and mitral valve disease.* New York: Appleton-Century-Crofts.

Fowles, R. E. (1988). Acute myocardial infarction. The primary care physician as gatekeeper. *Postgraduate Medicine, 84*(7), 89-111.

Frank, K. A., Heller, S. S., Kornfield, D. S., Sporn, A. A., & Weiss, M. B. (1978). Type A behavior pattern and coronary angiographic findings. *Journal of the American Medical Association, 240,* 761-763.

Friedman, M., & Rosenman, R. H. (1974). *Type A behavior and your heart.* New York: Knopf.

Genest, J., Kuchel, O., Hamet, P., & Cantin, M. (1983). *Hypertension: physiopathology and treatment* (2nd ed.). New York: McGraw-Hill.

Gifford, R. W., Jr. (1969). Evaluation of the hypertensive patient with emphasis on detecting curable causes. *Milbank Memorial Fund Quarterly, 47,* 170-212.

Goldstein, J. L., & Brown, M. S. (1985). Familial hypercholesterolemia. A genetic receptor disease. *Hospital Practice, 20*(11), 35-46.

Gould, K., Ramirez-Ronda, C. J., Holmes, R. K., & Stanford, J. P. (1975). Adherence of bacteria to heart valves in vitro. *Journal of Clinical Investigation, 56,* 1364-1370.

Hamby, J. I., Weissman, R. H., Prakash, M. N., & Hoffman, I. (1983). Left bundle branch block: a predictor of poor left ventricular function in CAD. *American Heart Journal, 106*(3), 471-477.

Hancock, E. W. (1982). Ischemic heart disease: Acute myocardial infarction. *Scientific American Medicine Index, 5.*

Hancock, E. W. (1985). Diseases of the pericardium. *Scientific American Medicine Index, 8.*

Hancock, E. W. (1986). Coronary artery disease—Epidemiology and prevention. *Scientific American Medicine Index* (January), *9*(1).

Hancock, E. W. (1986). Coronary artery disease—epidemiology and prevention. *Scientific American Medicine Index* (January), *9*(1). *Health, 70,* 813-820.

Haynes, S., Eaker, E. D., & Feinleib, M. (1984). The effects of employment, family, and job stress on coronary heart disease patterns in women. In E. B. Gold (Ed.), *The changing risk of disease in women: An epidemiological approach.* Lexington, MA: D. C. Heath and Company.

Hennekens, C. H., Willett, W., Rosner, B., Cole, D. S., & Mayrent, S. L. (1979). Effects of beer, wine, and liquor on coronary deaths. *Journal of the American Medical Association, 242,* 1973-1974.

Hjermann, I., Velve Byrek, K., Holm, I., & Leren, P. (1981). Effect of diet and smoking intervention on the incidence of cardiac heart disease: report from the Oslo study group of a randomized trial of healthy men. *Lancet, 2*(8259)m, 1303-1310.

Hopkins, P. N., & Williams, R. R. (1986). Identification and relative weight of cardiovascular risk factors. *Cardiology Clinics, 4*(1), 3-31.

Houston, M. (1986). Hypertensive emergencies and urgencies: pathophysiology and clinical aspects. *American Heart Journal III* (1), 205-210.

Howard, M., Puri, V. K., & Paidipaty, B. B. (1984). The effects of fluid resuscitation in the critically ill patient. *Heart & Lung, 13*(6), 649-654.

Hunt, A. H. (1985). Mitral valve prolapse. Physical assessment, complications, and management. *Nurse Practitioner,* April, 15-21.

Hurst, J. W., Logue, R. B., Rackley, C. E., Schlant, R. B., Sonnenblick, E. H., Wallace, A. G., & Wenger, N. K. (Eds.). (1986). *The heart, arteries, and veins* (6th ed.). New York: McGraw-Hill.

Hutter, R. A., Pasaoglu, I., & Williams, B. T. (1985). The incidence and management of coronary ostial stenosis. *Journal of Cardiovascular Surgery, 26*(6), 581-584.

Isles, C., Brown, J. J., Cumming, A. M., Lever,. A. F., MacAreavey, D., Robertson, J. J., Hawthorne, V. M., Steward, G. M., Robertson, J. W., & Wapshaw, J. (1979). Excess smoking in malignant phase hypertension. *British Medical Journal, 1,* 579-581.

Jaffe, A. S., Spandaro, J. J., Schechtman, K., Roberts, R., Gettman, E. M., & Sobel, B. E. (1984). Incidence of congestive heart failure after MI of modest extent in patients with DM. *American Heart Journal, 108*(1), 31-37.

Jenkins, C. D., Zyzanski, S. J., & Rosenman, R. H. (1976). Risk of new myocardial infarction in middle-aged men with manifest coronary heart disease. *Circulation, 53,* 342-347.

Johnson, A. L., Cornoni, J. C., Cassel, J. C., Tyroler, H. A., Heyden, S., & Hames, C. G. (1975). Influence of race, sex, and weight on blood pressure behavior in young adults. *American Journal of Cardiology, 35,* 523-530.

Joint National Committee. (1985). The 1984 report of the Joint National Committee on detection, evaluation, and treatment of high blood pressure. *Nurse Practitioner, 10*(7), 9-10, 13-14, 19-20, 23-26, 31-32, 34.

Kannel, W. B., Feinleib, M., McNamara, P. M., Garrison, J. R., & Castelli, W. P. (1979). An investigation of coronary heart disease in families. The Framingham offspring study. *American Journal of Epidemiology, 110,* 281.

Kafka, K. R.,

Kaplan, N. M. (1982). *Clinical hypertension* (3rd ed.). Baltimore: Williams & Wilkins.

Katz, S. H., Hediger, M. L., Schall, J. I., Bowers, E. J., Barker, W. F., Aurand, S., Eveleth, P. B., Gruskin, A. B., & Parks, J. S. (1980). Blood pressure growth and maturation from childhood through adolescence. *Hypertension* [Supplement I], *2,* 155-169.

Kafka, K. R., Meltzer, A. H., & Frishman, W. H. (1985). Antianginal agents part I: Ischemic heart disease and the role of nitrates. *Hospital Formulary 20*(1), 1144-1153.

Kaye, D., & Rose, L. F. (1983), *Fundamentals of internal medicine.* St. Louis: C. V. Mosby.

Keys, A., Aravanis, C., Blackburn, H., van Buchem, F. S. P., Buzina, R., Djordjevic, B. S., Fidanza, F., Karvanen, M. et al. (1972a). Coronary heart disease: Overweight and obesity as risk factors. *Annals of Internal Medicine, 77,* 15-27.

Kissane, J.M. Ed., (1985), *Anderson's Pathology,* 8th ed, St. Louis: C. V. Mosby.

Klatsky, A. L., Friedman, G. D., & Siebelbaum, A. B. (1981). Alcohol and mortality. A ten year Kaiser-Permanente experience. *Annals of Internal Medicine, 95*(2), 139-145.

Kottke, B. A. (1986). Lipid markers for atherosclerosis. *American Journal of Cardiology, 57*(5), 11C-15C.

Lavie, D., & Savage, D. (1987). Prevalence and clinical features of mitral valve prolapse. *American Heart Journal, 113*(5), 1281-1290.

Lieberman, E. (1982). Hypertension in childhood and adolescence. In N. M. Kaplan (Ed.), *Clinical hypertension* (3rd ed.). Baltimore: William & Wilkins.

Loggie, J. M. H. (1979). Identification and management of juvenile hypertension. *Postgraduate Medicine, 65*(5), 103-107, 110-112.

Luchi, R. J., Snow, E., Luchi, J. M., Nelson, C. S., & Pircher, F. J. (1982). Left ventricular function in hospitalized geriatric patients. *Journal of the American Geriatric Society, 30*(11), 700-705.

MacDougall, J. M., Dembroski, T. M., Dimsdale, J. B., & Hackett, T. P. (1985). Components of type A, hostility, and anger in further relationships to angiographic findings. *Health Psychology, 4,* 137-150.

Macek, L. (1983). Acute rheumatic fever. *Nurse Practitioner,* 17-19.

Markowitz, M., & Gerber, M. A. (1987). Rheumatic fever: Recent outbreaks of an old disease. *Connecticut Medicine, 51*(4), 229-233.

Massachusetts Nurses Association. (1980). Hypertension: a disease of impaired regulation of blood pressure. *Massachusetts Nurse, Special Edition, Revised,* p. 5, Table 1.

Massachusetts Nurses Association (1986). Hypertension: a disease of impaired regulation of blood pressure. *Massachusetts Nurse, Special Edition, Revised*p. 5, Table 1.

McCance, K. L. (1983). Genetics: Implications for preventative nursing practice. *Journal of Advanced Nursing, 8,* 359-364.

McCarron, D. A., Morris, C. D., Henry, H. J., & Stanton, J. L. (1984). Blood pressure and nutrient intake in the United States. *Science, 224,* 1392-1398.

Oates, J. A., Fitzgerald, G. A., Branch, R. A., Jackson, E. K., Knapp, H. R., & Roberts, I. J. (1987). Clinical implications of prostaglandin and thromboxane A_2 formation. *New England Journal of Medicine, 319*(11), 689-698.

Orie, J. E., & Liedtke, A. J. (1986). Cardiomyopathy. *Postgraduate Medicine, 79*(5), 83-91, 95-106.

Page, I. H. (1987). *Hypotension mechanisms.* New York: Grune & Stratton.

Pasternak, R. C., Braunwald, E., & Sobel, B. E. (1988) Acute myocardial infarction. In E. Baumwald (Ed.), *Heart disease: A textbook of cardiovascular medicine* (3rd ed.). Philadelphia: W. B. Saunders.

Ragland, D. R., & Brand, R. J. (1988). Type A behavior and mortality from coronary heart disease. *New England Journal of Medicine, 318,* 5-9.

Rahe, R. H., Romo, M., Bennett, L., & Sietonen, P. (1974). Recent life changes, myocardial infarction, and abrupt coronary death. *Arch Intero Med, 133,* 221.

Robbins, S. L., Cotran, R. S., & Kumar, V. (1984). *Pathologic basis disease.* Philadelphia: W. B. Saunders.

Roberts, J., & Maurer, K. (1977). Blood pressure levels of persons 6-74 years. United States, 1971-1974. *Vital and Health Statistics, Series 11*(203). DHEW Publication No.

Rosai, J. (1981). *Ackerman's surgical pathology* (6th ed.). St. Louis: C. V. Mosby.

Rose, M. I. (1987). Type A behavior pattern: a concept revisited. *Canadian Medical Association Journal, 136*(4), 345-350.

Ross, R., & Glomset, J. A. (1976). The pathogenesis of atherosclerosis, Part I. *New England Journal of Medicine, 295*(7), 369-374.

Rudnick, K. V., Sackett, D. L., Hirst, S., & Holmes, C. (1977). Hypertension in a family practice. *Canadian Medical Association Journal, 117*(5), 492-497.

Sadler, D. (1984). *Nursing for cardiovascular health.* Norwalk, CT: Appleton-Century-Crofts.

Schaefer, E. J., & Levy, R. I. (1985). Pathogenesis and management of lipoprotein disorders. *New England Journal of Medicine, 312*(29), 1300-1309.

Schrott, H. G., Bucker, K. A., Clarke, W. R., & Lauer, R. M. (1979). The Muscatine hyperlipidemia family study program. In C. F. Sing & M. Skolnick (Eds.), *Genetic analysis of common diseases: Application to preventive factors in coronary disease.* New York: Alan R. Liss, p. 629.

Sclarovsky, S., Strasberg, B., Hirshberg, A., Arditi, A., Lewin, R. J., & Agman, J. (1984). Advanced early and late atrioventricular block in acute inferior wall MI. *American Heart Journal, 108*(1), 19-24.

Scragg, R., Stewart, A., Jackson, R., & Beaglehole, R. (1987). Alcohol and exercise in myocardial infarction and sudden coronary death in men and women. *American Journal of Epidemiology, 126*(1), 77-85.

Sereny, G., Lane, F., Knandelwal, B., & Saraswhat, S. (1983). Chronic alcoholism and myocardial disease. *Drug and Alcohol Dependence, 12,* 303-313.

Shaper, A. G., Phillips, A. N., Pocock, S. J., & Walker, M. (1987). Alcohol and ischaemic heart disease in middle aged British men. *British Medical Journal, 294,* 733-737.

Siegel, J. H. (1983). Cardiorespiratory manifestations of metabolic failure in sepsis and multiple organ failure syndrome. *Surgical Clinics of North America, 63*(2), 379-399.

Silber, E. N. (1987). *Heart disease* (2nd ed.). New York: MacMillan.

Sleight, P. (1984). Hemodynamics in hypertension and heart failure. *American Journal of Medicine, 76*(58), 3-13.

Sobel, B. E. (1972, February). Biochemical and morphologic changes in infarcting myocardium. *Hospital Practice,* 59-71.

Stollerman, G. J. (1975). *Rheumatic fever and streptococcal infection.* New York: Grune & Stratton.

Sullam, P. M., Drake, T. A., & Sande, M. A. (1985, June). Pathogenesis of endocarditis. *The American Journal of Medicine* [Supplement], *78*(6B), 110-115.

Sullivan, J. F., Egan, J. D., & George, R. P. (1969). A distinctive cardiomyopathy occurring in Omaha, Nebraska: Clinical aspects. *Annals of the New York Academy of Science, 156,* 526.

The Review Panel on Coronary Prone Behavior and Coronary Heart Disease. (1981). Coronary prone behavior and coronary heart disease: a critical review. *Circulation, 63,* 1199-1215.

Thompson, P. D., Stern, M. P., Williams, P., Duncan, K., Haskell, W. L., & Wood, P. D. (1979). Death during jogging or running: A study of 18 cases. *Journal of the American Medical Association, 242,* 1265.

Vanhoutte, P. M., & Houston, D. S. (1985). Platelets, endothelium, and vasospasm. *Circulation, 72*(4), 728-734.

von Rokitansky, C. (1852). *A manual of physiological anatomy* (vol 4). London: Sydenham Society p. 204.

Varricchio, C. (1985). Clinical management of superior vena cava syndrome. *Heart & Lung, 14*(4), 411-416.

Williams, R. R. (1984). Understanding genetic and environmental risk factors in susceptible persons. *Western Journal of Medicine, 141*(6), 799-806.

Zabriskie, J. B., & Friedman, J. E. (1983). The role of heart binding antibodies in rheumatic fever. *Advances in Experimental Medicine and Biology, 161,* 457-470.

Virchow, R. (1862). Phlogose und thrombose in geyfassytem. *Gesammelte abhandlungen zur wissen chaftlichen medizin.* Berlin: Max Hirsch.

CHAPTER 28

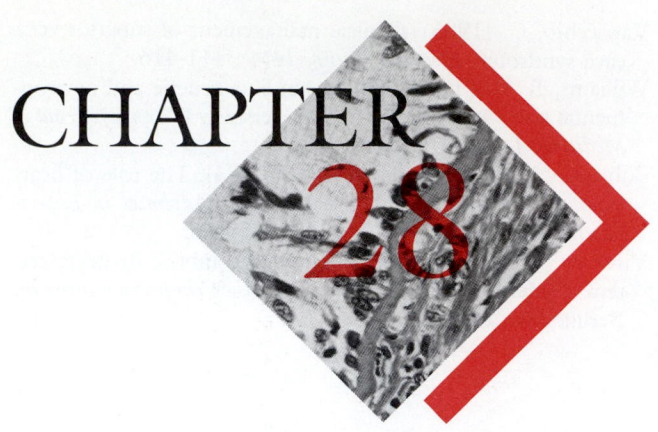

Alterations of Cardiovascular Function in Children

Sharon L. Sims

Development of the cardiovascular system, 993
   Development of the heart, 993
   Development of the circulation, 994
   Changes in circulation at birth, 995
Congenital heart defects, 996
   Restriction of ventricular outflow, 999
      Pulmonary stenosis, 1000
         Pathophysiology, 1000
         Clinical manifestations, 1000
         Evaluation and treatment, 1001
      Coarctation of the aorta, 1001
         Pathophysiology, 1001
            Postductal coarctation, 1001
            Preductal coarctation, 1002
         Clinical manifestations, 1002
         Evaluation and treatment, 1002
   Acyanotic heart defects with increased pulmonary blood
      flow, 1003
      Ventricular septal defect, 1003
         Pathophysiology, 1003
         Clinical manifestations, 1004
         Evaluation and treatment, 1005
      Patent ductus arteriosus, 1005
         Pathophysiology, 1005
         Clinical manifestations, 1005
         Evaluation and treatment, 1006
      Atrial septal defect, 1006
         Pathophysiology, 1006
         Clinical manifestations, 1007
         Evaluation and treatment, 1007
   Cyanotic heart defects with increased pulmonary blood
      flow, 1007
      Persistent truncus arteriosus, 1007
         Pathophysiology, 1007
         Clinical manifestations, 1008
         Evaluation and treatment, 1008
      Complete transposition of the great vessels, 1009
         Pathophysiology, 1009

         Clinical manifestations, 1010
         Evaluation and treatment, 1010
      Total anomalous pulmonary venous connection, 1010
         Pathophysiology, 1010
         Clinical manifestations, 1011
         Evaluation and treatment, 1012
   Cyanotic heart defects with decreased pulmonary blood
      flow, 1012
      Tetralogy of Fallot, 1012
         Pathophysiology, 1012
         Clinical manifestations, 1013
         Evaluation and treatment, 1014
      Tricuspid atresia, 1014
         Pathophysiology, 1014
         Clinical manifestations, 1015
         Evaluation and treatment, 1015
Acquired cardiovascular disorders, 1015
   Congestive heart failure, 1015
   Rheumatic heart disease, 1017
   Primary hypertension, 1017
   Course of the disease, 1018
   Pathophysiology, 1018

Cardiovascular disorders in children can be classified as congenital or acquired. Though this is an oversimplification in some ways, it does facilitate discussion. Certainly the most dramatic and most highly documented cardiovascular disorders in children are the congenital defects. The acquired cardiovascular disorders of childhood are less studied and less well documented. They include heart failure (congestive heart failure), rheumatic heart disease, and hypertension.

DEVELOPMENT OF THE CARDIOVASCULAR SYSTEM

In order to understand the pathophysiology of congenital heart defects, it is first necessary to have a clear idea of how the heart develops, the fetal circulation, and what changes occur in the circulation after birth. Heart defects can often be traced to disturbances in these events.

Development of the Heart

The heart arises from the mesenchyme and begins its development as an enlarged blood vessel with a large lumen and a muscular wall (Fig. 28-1, *A*). During the fifth week of gestation, the midsection of this tube be-

gins to grow faster than its ends. This causes the tube to bulge and twist (Fig. 28-1, *B* and *C*) until both ends of the tube come together and fuse (Fig. 28-1, *B* to *D*). The part of the tube at the cranial end of the embryo is the **truncus arteriosus,** which divides longitudinally into the pulmonary artery and aorta. The part of the tube at the caudal end of the embryo becomes the superior and inferior vena cavae.

On the inside of the developing heart, other changes occur that result in the eventual formation of the four chambers. These changes are illustrated in Fig. 28-2. The development of the cardiac septa, which eventually divide the four chambers, is an intricate process. If the parts of the septa do not develop or fuse properly, several types of defects may occur, among them abnormal openings between chambers, formation of a single

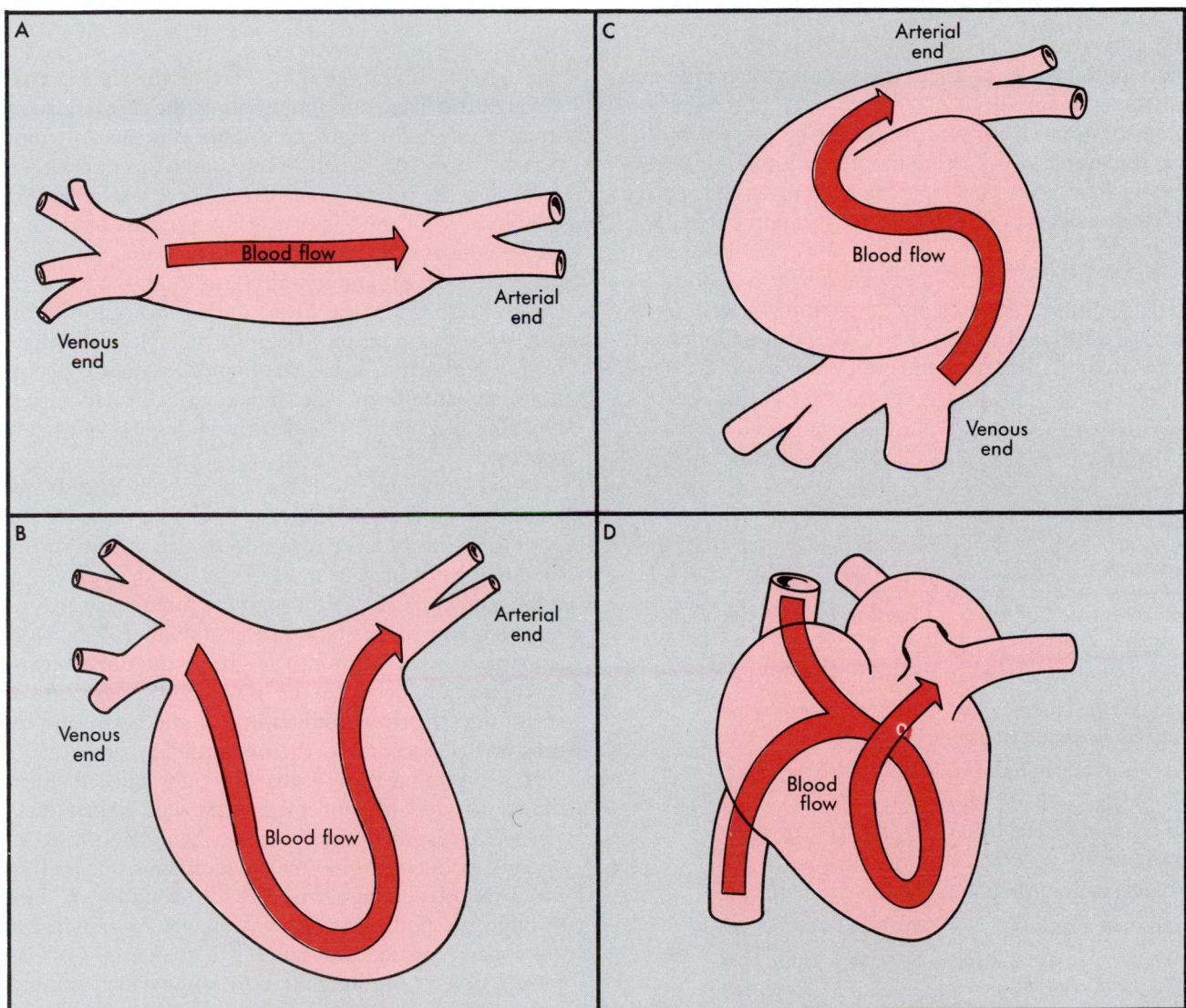

FIG. 28-1. Embryologic development of the heart. The earliest heart structure, **A,** consists of a muscular tube with a large lumen. About the fifth week of gestation, **B,** the tube bulges and, **C,** twists until, **D,** the ends come together and fuse.

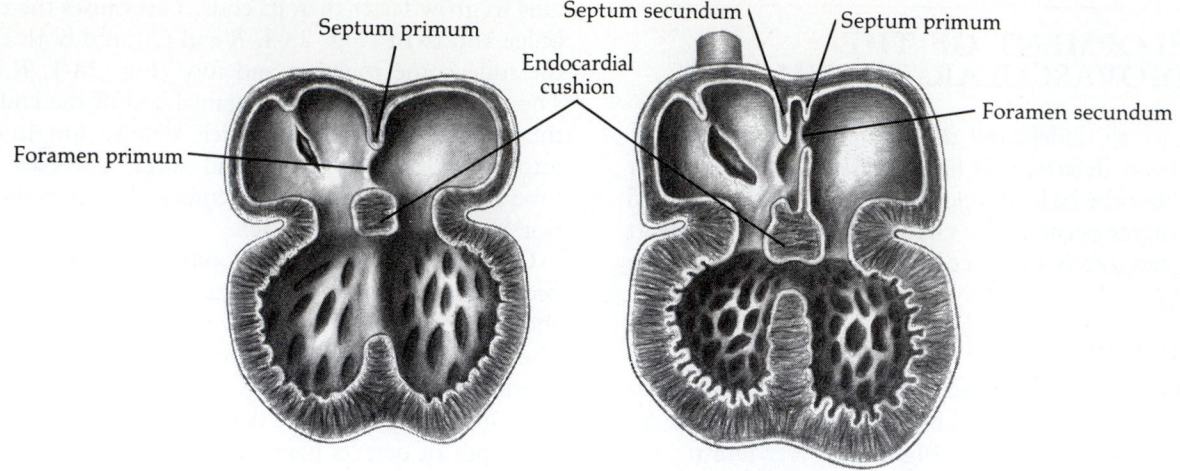

Septum primum | Septum secundum | Septum primum

Endocardial cushion

Foramen primum

Foramen secundum

FIG. 28-2. Development of the cardiac septa. (From Thompson et al., 1989.)

atrium or ventricle, or a lack of septa between atria and ventricles. If development of the septa proceeds normally, the four-chambered heart will be present by the sixth or seventh week of gestation. Examples of crucial times in fetal heart development with regard to specific defects described in this chapter are listed in Table 28-1.

Development of the Circulation

The anatomic features and direction of fetal blood flow are illustrated in Fig. 28-3. Blood for the fetus is oxygenated in the placenta and returns to the fetus

TABLE 28-1 Critical times in fetal heart development related to specific defects

Defect	Critical time in gestation
Transposition of the great vessels	Third to fourth week
Patent ductus arteriosus	Third to eighth week
Anomalous pulmonary venous connection	Third to eighth week
Tricuspid or mitral atresia	Third to sixth week
Ventricular septal defect (muscular)	Fourth to sixth week
Coarctation of the aorta	Fourth week on
Truncus arteriosus	Sixth to seventh week
Ventricular septal defect (membranous)	Sixth to seventh week
Persistent foramen ovale	Eighth week on

From Keith, Roe, & Vlad, 1978.

through the umbilical vein. Part of this blood passes through the liver, but about half of the flow is diverted from the liver through the **ductus venosus** (a connection between the hepatic vessels and the inferior vena cava) into the inferior vena cava, where it is mixed with the blood from the lower extremities. This blood flows into the heart through the **foramen ovale** (the opening between the right and left atria), through the left ventricle, and into the aorta. From there it flows to the head and upper extremities. Because this blood is mainly from the placenta, it has the highest oxygen concentration, or saturation. The brain and coronary arteries therefore receive the blood with the highest oxygen saturation.

Blood returning from the upper body (head, neck, and arms) collects in the superior vena cava. A small portion of this blood passes into the left atrium through the foramen ovale, but most of the blood flows into the right ventricle and out through the pulmonary artery. A small amount of this blood enters the lungs. The largest amount, however, flows through the **ductus arteriosus** (a connection between the pulmonary artery and the aorta) into the descending aorta, to the body, and then back to the placenta via the two umbilical arteries.

It is important to note that the right and left sides of the fetal heart are connected in parallel, rather than in series. That is, they work side by side as almost separate systems, connected only by the foramen ovale and ductus arteriosus. Therefore, the distribution of blood through the body depends on vascular resistance. Fetal pulmonary vascular resistance is high because of vasoconstriction in the lungs due to low oxygen saturation (this phenomenon is sometimes called hypoxic vasoconstriction). Oxygen saturation is low because no gas exchange is taking place in the fetus's uninflated lungs. On the other hand, fetal systemic resistance is low because

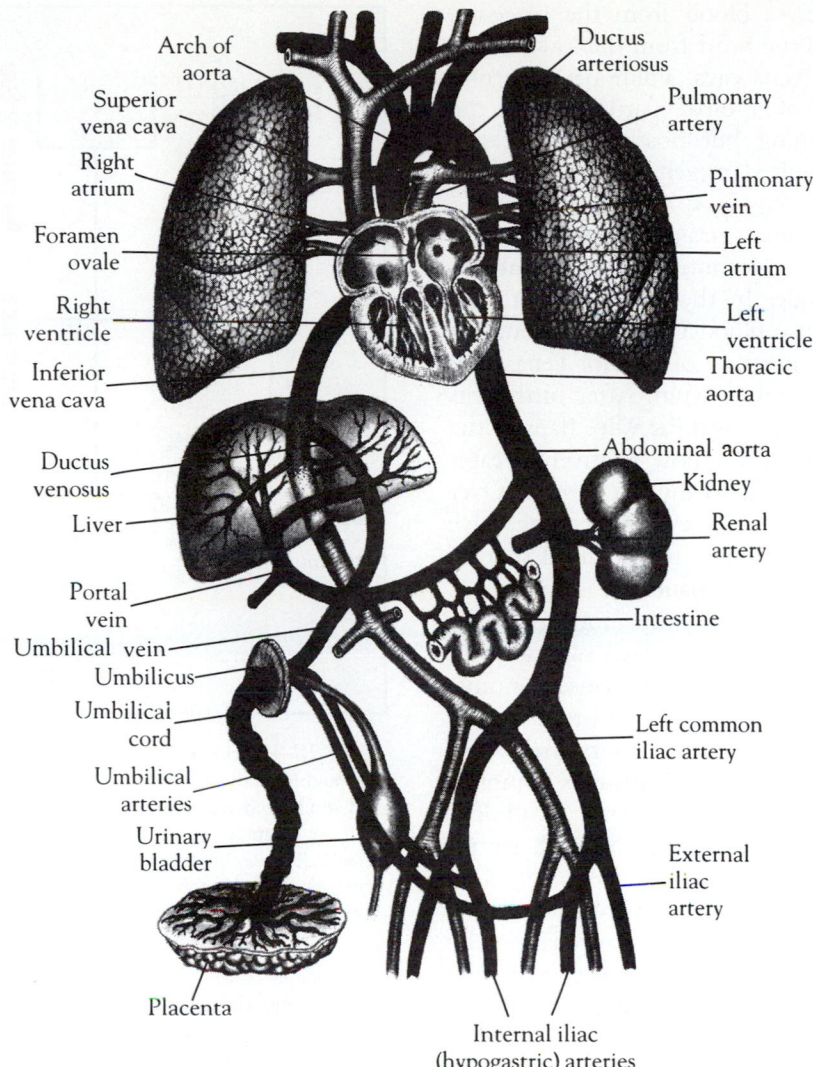

FIG. 28-3. Fetal circulation. Circulation of the fetus reflects the fact that oxygenation of fetal blood does not take place in the lungs, but rather in the placenta. Therefore, the pulmonary circulatory system is essentially "bypassed." Instead of traveling from the right heart to the lungs, as occurs after birth, most blood entering the right heart passes through the ductus arteriosus and into the systemic circulation. (From Thompson et al., 1985).

the large-volume placenta is a low-resistance organ. High resistance impedes blood flow and low resistance encourages it. Because of this, very little blood flows into the high-resistance lungs, and most of the blood flows into the low-resistance systemic circulation. High pulmonary resistance diverts most of the blood flow into the pulmonary artery, through the ductus arteriosus, and into the aorta, thereby equalizing the pressure in those two vessels. Because resistance determines the flow, when pressure is equal, the blood returns to the low-resistance placenta.

Changes in Circulation at Birth

At birth, a series of circulatory changes occur, some sudden and some gradual, that affect blood flow dra-

matically. The most important change taking place in the circulation at birth is the shift of gas exchange from the placenta to the lungs. In addition, changes in pressure and volume of blood flowing through the heart's chambers functionally close the ductus arteriosus, ductus venosus, and foramen ovale. A decrease of pulmonary vascular resistance and an increase of systemic vascular resistance leads to changes in the size and shape of the heart's chambers. The most immediate changes are due to the severing of the umbilical cord. This removes the low-resistance placenta from the neonate's circulation and causes an immediate increase in systemic vascular resistance, to about twice that prior to birth. The absence of the placenta also causes a decrease in blood flow through the inferior vena cava because the ductus venosus no longer receives blood from the placenta. Only blood returning to the heart from the lower body now enters the inferior vena cava. Pulmonary vascular resistance falls suddenly after birth, partly because the lungs expand with breathing, but mostly because exposure to blood with a higher oxygen saturation dilates the pulmonary vessels.

Increased pulmonary venous return and decreased inferior vena caval return cause immediate functional closure of the foramen ovale. In the fetus, the foramen ovale is held open because blood is pushed through it by the relatively greater pressure of inferior vena caval (systemic) return to the right atrium. After birth, this pressure difference is reversed, and the valve flaps of the foramen ovale are closed by the now relatively greater pressure of pulmonary return to the left atrium. Over the course of several months, or even years, the valve flaps of the foramen ovale adhere to the atrial septum and the foramen ovale closes permanently.

The ductus arteriosus closes a little more gradually than the foramen ovale. Increased oxygen saturation in the systemic arterial blood is thought to cause the muscular wall of the ductus arteriosus to constrict, which occludes the opening within 15 to 18 hours after birth. Permanent closure of the ductus arteriosus is complete within about 10 to 21 days after birth (Rudolph, 1974). Low arterial oxygen saturation at birth stimulates the ductus arteriosus to remain open.

Another change that occurs in the first week of life is the closure of the ductus venosus. The mechanism by which this happens is unclear, but closure is usually complete within 7 days of birth. Blood flow through the ductus venosus falls instantly when the umbilical cord is cut, because the umbilical veins no longer bring placental blood to it.

Other more gradual changes combine to decrease pulmonary vascular resistance during the 6 to 8 weeks after birth. The inner medial linings of the small pulmonary arterioles thin out in response to decreased pulmonary arterial pressure. The resulting larger diameters of these vessels cause a decrease in pulmonary resistance. As the lungs grow, so does the pulmonary arterial bed, which further decreases resistance to flow. Finally, increased oxygen saturation causes vasodilation in the pulmonary bed.

The high pulmonary vascular resistance during fetal life affects the anatomy of the ventricles in a significant way. Before birth, high pressure in the pulmonary circulation causes high pressure in the right ventricle. The right ventricle is subject to high afterload, which causes the right ventricular myocardium to become as thick and strong as the left. In addition, the fetal right ventricle is heavier than the left ventricle. After birth, when the pulmonary vascular resistance decreases, the right ventricular myocardium begins to thin out. By 1 month

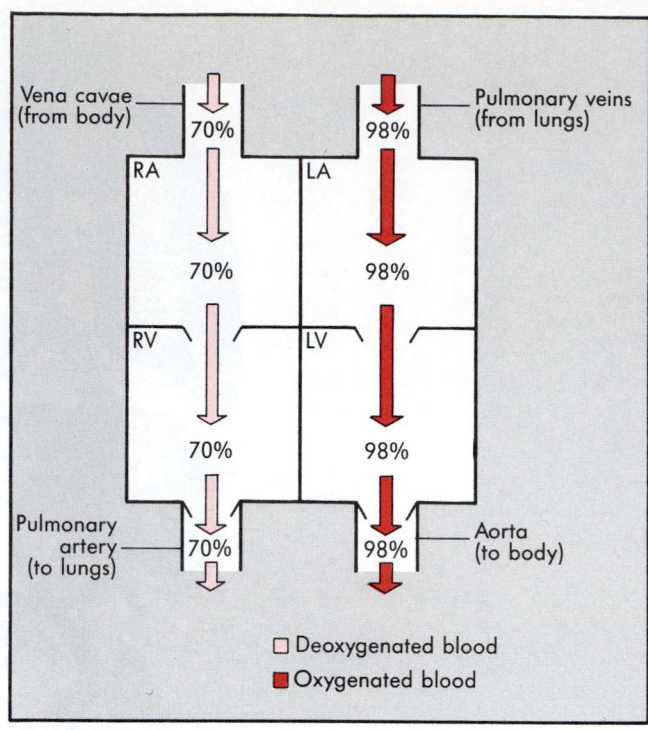

FIG. 28-4. Schematic representation of normal oxygen saturation (%) and hemodynamics in the neonatal heart and great vessels. This and similar schematics throughout the chapter are extremely simplified; see Chapter 26, Figure 26-5 for correct placement of the great vessels. *RA,* Right atrium; *LA,* left atrium; *RV,* right ventricle. Percentages equal the percentage of hemoglobin (per unit of blood) that is bound with oxygen molecules, or saturated.

of age, the neonate's ventricles are approximately equal in weight. As systemic resistance rises, the left ventricular myocardium becomes thicker than the right, and the ventricles begin to assume the relative size and shape of maturity (Moller & Neal, 1981). Fig. 28-4 represents normal hemodynamics and oxygen saturation in the neonatal heart.

CONGENITAL HEART DEFECTS

Statistics on the incidence of congenital heart defects have been kept with some consistency since the late 1930s. These figures have been shown to vary widely from medical center to medical center, however, and they depend on criteria used for diagnosis, thoroughness of follow-up, the child's age, and autopsy findings. Reviews of such data for the past 20 years indicate that the overall incidence of congenital heart defects is 1% to 2% of all live births (Keith, Rowe, & Vlad, 1978; Moller & Neal, 1981). Other sources estimate the overall incidence of congenital heart defects at 8 in 1000 live births (Guzzetta & Dossey, 1984; Smith, 1983). Stillbirths and spontaneous abortions are generally excluded

TABLE 28-2 Environmental factors and associated congenital heart defects

Cause	Type of congenital heart defect
Infection	
Intrauterine	Patent ductus arteriosus (PDA), pulmonary stenosis, coarctation of aorta
Systemic viral	PDA, pulmonary stenosis, coarctation of aorta
Rubella	PDA, pulmonary stenosis, coarctation of aorta
Coxsackie B	Endocardial fibroelastosis
Radiation	Specific cardiovascular effect not known
Metabolic disorders	
Diabetes	Ventricular septal defect (VSD), cardiomegaly, transposition of the great vessels
Phenylketonuria (PKU)	Coarctation of aorta, PDA
Hypercalcemia	Supravalvular aortic stenosis, pulmonic stenosis; aortic hyperplasia
Drugs	
Thalidomide	No specific lesion
Dextroamphetamine	One case of reported transposition
Peripheral conditions	
Increased maternal age	VSD, tetralogy of Fallot (relationship unclear)
Antepartal bleeding	Various defects (relationship unclear)
Prematurity	PDA, VSD
High altitude	PDA, atrial septal defect (increased incidence)

From Doyle & Rutkowski, 1970.

from these estimates because the incidence of heart defects is much higher in this group.

Though their incidence is significant, the morbidity and mortality rates for congenital heart defects are more significant. It is currently estimated that most deaths due to congenital heart defects occur in the first year of life (35%) and that over one third of all children with such defects will eventually die of congenital heart disease (Moller & Neal, 1981).

Several environmental and genetic risk factors are associated with the incidence of various types of congenital heart defects. Among the environmental factors are maternal conditions, such as intrauterine viral infection (especially rubella), diabetes mellitus, phenylketonuria, maternal alcoholism, maternal hypercalcemia, drugs (e.g., thalidomide, lithium, dilantin, and dextroamphetamine), and complications of increased maternal age, antepartal bleeding, and prematurity. These risk factors and associated heart defects are summarized in Table 28-2.

Genetic factors have also been implicated in the incidence of congenital heart defects, though the mechanism of causation is often unknown. Family studies have shown that the incidence of congenital heart defects in siblings of affected children is three to four times higher than in the general population (Doyle & Rutkowski, 1970). Chromosomal aberrations account for about 6% of all congenital heart defects (Doyle & Rutkowski, 1970). Down syndrome, trisomy 13-15 syndrome, Turner syndrome, and cri du chat syndrome have all been associated with a relatively high incidence of heart defects. (Genetic inheritance is discussed in Chapter 4.) These syndromes and their associated defects are summarized in Table 28-3. Other disorders associated with congenital heart defects are presented in Table 28-4. Only a small percentage of congenital heart defects are clearly linked solely to genetic or to environmental factors. The cause of most defects is probably multifactorial.

Congenital heart defects can be described with respect to anatomic abnormality, hemodynamic abnormality, or the status of tissue oxgenation. Possible anatomic defects include valvular abnormalities; abnormal openings in the septa, including persistence of the foramen ovale; continued patency of the ductus arteriosus; and malformation or abnormal placement of the great vessels. The hemodynamic alterations caused by these anatomic defects consist of (1) increases or decreases of blood flow through the pulmonary or systemic circulatory systems and (2) the mixing of pulmonary and systemic blood through an abnormal communication that permits flow between the two circulatory systems. The movement of

TABLE 28-3 Genetic factors and congenital heart defects

Chromosomal aberrations or syndrome	Incidence of defects	Type of defect
Trisomy 13-15	80%	Ventricular septal defect (VSD), atrial septal defect (ASD), patent ductus arteriosus (PDA), anomalous pulmonary venous connection, bicuspid aorta, overriding aorta
Trisomy 18	90%	VSD, PDA, patent foramen ovale, bicuspid aorta, dextrocardia
Down syndrome	12%-44%	Endocardial cushion defects, VSD, PDA, ASD, transposition of great vessels, tetralogy of Fallot, persistent truncus arteriosus, coarctation of aorta, endocardial fibroelastosis
Cri-du-chat syndrome	20%	PDA, mixed defects
Turner syndrome	20%-40%	Coarctation of aorta, pulmonary stenosis, subaortic and aortic stenosis, PDA, septal defects

From Doyle & Rutkowsky, 1970.

TABLE 28-4 Disorders coexistent with congenital heart defects

Disorder	Associated cardiovascular defect
Connective tissue disorders	
Marfan syndrome	Aortic or mitral regurgitation, aortic aneurysm
Hurler syndrome	Pseudoatherosclerosis
Hunter syndrome	Pseudoatherosclerosis, hypertension
Osteogenesis imperfecta	Incompetent aortic valve
Complex syndromes	
Kartagener syndrome	Dextrocardia
Holt-Oram syndrome	Atrial septal defect (ASD), ventricular septal defect (VSD)
Ellis–van Creveld syndrome	Defect or absence of atrial septum
Laurence-Moon-Biedl syndrome	Tetralogy of Fallot, single ventricle, transposition of aorta
Inborn errors of metabolism	
Pompe disease	Cardiomegaly, congestive heart failure
Homocuptinuria	Thromboembolic episodes, pulmonic and aortic regurgitation
Phakomatosis	
Neurofibromatosis (von Recklinghausen disease)	Hypertension, pheochromocytoma
von Hippel-Lindau disease	Hypertension, pheochromocytoma
Sturge-Weber-Dimitri disease	VASC, anomalies of carotid and meningeal arteries
Vascular malformations	
Osler-Weber-Rendu disease (hereditary hemorrhagic telangiectasia)	Atrioventricular fistula, telangiectasia
Milroy disease (lymphedema)	Hypoplasia of lymphatic vessels

From Doyle & Rutkowski, 1970.

TABLE 28-5 Classification of congenital heart defects		
Pulmonary blood flow	**Shunt direction**	**Specific defects**
ACYANOTIC		
Normal pulmonary flow	None	Pulmonary stenosis; pulmonary valvular dysplasia; peripheral pulmonary arterial stenosis; obstruction to left ventricular outflow (coarctation of aorta, interruption of aortic arch, vascular aortic stenosis, systemic hypertension); endocardial fibroelastosis; myocarditis
Increased pulmonary flow	Left to right	Ventricular septal defect (VSD); patent ductus arteriosus; corrected transposition of the great vessels with VSD; aortico-pulmonary septal defect; aortic origin of pulmonary artery; atrial shunts (endocardial cushion defect, atrial septal defect)
Decreased pulmonary* flow	Usually none	Cor triatriatum; parachute mitral valve; supravalvular stenosing ring; pulmonary vein stenosis
CYANOTIC		
Increased pulmonary flow	Either direction	Admixture lesions; persistent truncus arteriosus; transposition of great vessels; single ventricle; tricuspid atresia; total anomalous pulmonary venous connection (TAPVC) without obstruction
Decreased pulmonary flow	Right to left	Ventricular septal communications (tetralogy of Fallot and variants); mixed lesions (e.g., single ventricle with pulmonary stenosis); atrial septal communications (pulmonary valve atresia, tricuspid valve atresia, Ebstein anomaly, tricuspid insufficiency)
Increased pulmonary venous markings	Left to right	TAPVC with obstruction

Adapted from Moller & Neal, 1981.
*Decreased pulmonary flow causes a characteristic x-ray finding called pulmonary venous markings. The pulmonary veins become distended, which makes them more visible on x-ray films.

blood between the normally separate pulmonary and systemic circulations is termed a **shunt.** Movement from the pulmonary to the systemic circulation (i.e., from the right heart to the left heart) is called a **right-to-left shunt.** Movement from the systemic to the pulmonary circulation (from the left heart to the right heart) is a **left-to-right shunt.** Shunt direction depends on relative pressures and resistances (see Chapter 26), and can be obligatory or dependent. In an obligatory shunt, pressure gradients determine the direction of blood flow through an opening, whereas in a dependent shunt, vascular resistance or ventricular compliance determines the direction of flow.

The status of tissue oxygenation is gauged by the presence or absence of cyanosis. **Cyanosis** is a bluish discoloration of the skin. It is a sign that the tissues are not receiving enough oxygen, a condition known as hypoxia. (See Chapter 29 for more discussion about cyanosis and hypoxia. Hypoxic injury to cells is described in Chapter 2.) Hypoxia may be the result of any disorder that prevents oxygen from reaching the body's cells. Ischemia, for example, is hypoxia from lack of blood

flow. Congenital heart defects that cause hypoxia, and therefore cyanosis, usually involve a right-to-left shunt, which directs blood flow away from the lungs, or **stenosis** (restrictive narrowing) of structures in the right heart, which restricts outflow to the lungs. Such defects are commonly called **cyanotic defects.** Congenital defects that do not cause cyanosis, or **acyanotic defects,** usually involve a left-to-right shunt, which directs blood toward the lungs, or no shunt at all. For the sake of convenience, congenital heart defects can be categorized according to (1) whether or not they cause cyanosis, (2) whether they increase or decrease blood flow into the pulmonary circulation, and (3) shunt direction. Table 28-5 categorizes the congenital heart defects based on these three characteristics (Moller & Neal, 1981). Many, but not all, of these defects are described in this chapter.

Restriction of Ventricular Outflow

Acyanotic defects with normal pulmonary blood flow are those that cause right ventricular outflow obstruction, such as pulmonary stenosis, and those that cause left ventricular outflow obstruction, such as coarctation of the aorta.

Pulmonary Stenosis

Right ventricular outflow can be obstructed by any anatomic abnormality that affects the pulmonic semilunar valve, also called the pulmonary valve. The pulmonic valve is located between the right ventricle and the pulmonary artery. **Pulmonary stenosis** is the narrowing of the valvular opening, either by partial fusing or abnormal thickening of the valve leaflets. Sometimes the annulus, or muscular ring around the valve, is severely narrowed, a variation of pulmonic stenosis termed **pulmonary atresia.** Narrowing can also occur on the arterial side of the valve (**supravalvular stenosis**) or on the ventricular side (**infundibular stenosis**). Pulmonic stenosis accounts for 5% to 8% of all congenital heart defects (Park, 1988).

Pathophysiology

Whatever the anatomic features in a given child, their effect is to create an opening too small for normal outflow during systole (Fig. 28-5, *A*). Less blood can pass through the pulmonary valve under normal systolic pressure, and some of it remains in the right ventricle, causing increased afterload (see Chapter 26). Essentially, valvular stenosis causes the whole system to "back up," which further increases pressures in the right ventricle. The smaller the valve opening, the harder it will be for the right ventricle to maintain output. To do so, the right ventricular myocardium undergoes hypertrophy. If the outflow obstruction is very severe, blood backs up in the right atrium, causing dilation and hypertrophy, and leads to the reopening of the foramen ovale. Higher pressures in the right atrium can create a right-to-left shunt across the foramen ovale. Children with this condition will also develop cyanosis, since the blood shunting from right to left is deoxygenated (Fig. 28-5, *B*). Related conditions with similar cardiac effects are stenosis of the peripheral pulmonary arteries and dysplasia of the pulmonary valve.

Clinical Manifestations

In **mild to moderate** cases of right ventricular outflow obstruction, the right ventricle and atrium remain almost normal in size, and the foramen ovale does not reopen, so that shunting and cyanosis do not occur. The child looks healthy and may be asymptomatic. Growth and development usually are normal. A systolic murmur is heard because blood flow through the narrowed valve is turbulent. The electrocardiogram (ECG) is likely to be normal or indicates some right ventricular hypertrophy. X-ray films show a normal-sized heart and normal pulmonary vessels.

In **severe** cases of right ventricular outflow obstruction, decreased growth and development, cyanosis, dys-

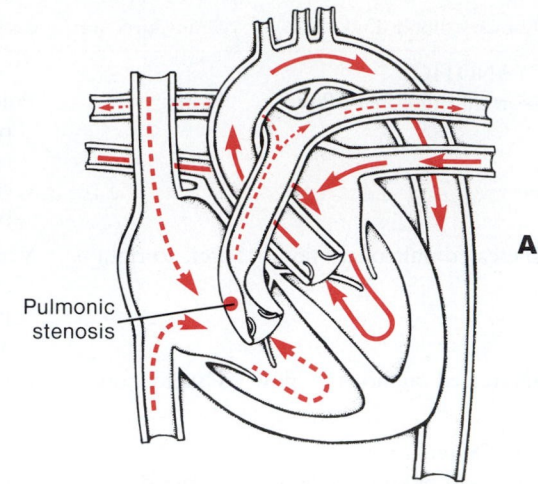

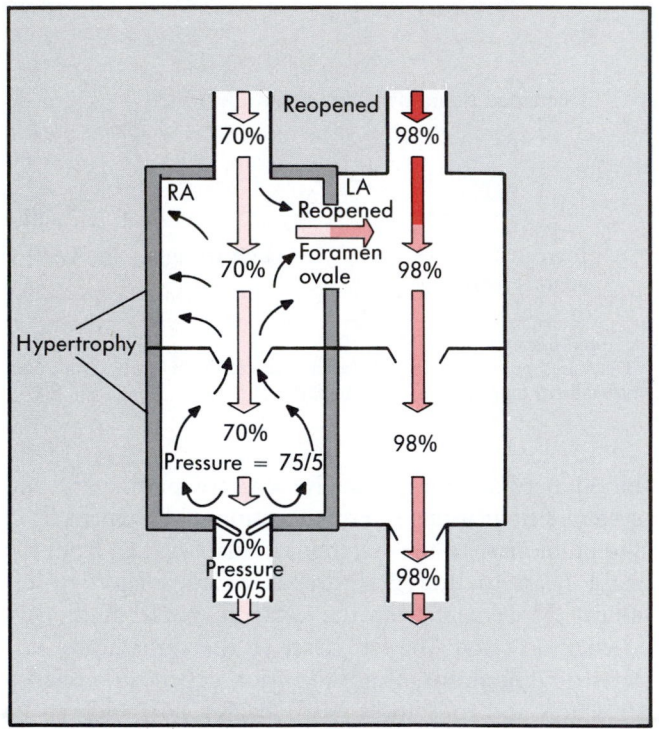

FIG. 28-5. A, Obstruction of right ventricular outflow due to pulmonary stenosis. Pressure on the ventricular side of the pulmonic semilunar valve (pulmonary valve) is much greater than that on the pulmonary arterial side. This difference disrupts the normal pressure gradient across the valve. Pulmonary stenosis increases ventricular afterload by decreasing blood flow through the valve *(dashed arrows),* which causes ventricular hypertrophy. **B,** The backup of ventricular afterload into the right atrium reopens the foramen ovale. Venous blood then flows from the area of higher pressure (the right atrium) to the area of lower pressure (the left atrium) causing a right-to-left shunt. Cyanosis occurs if enough venous blood shunts from right to left to reduce oxygen saturation in the systemic circulation by 3% to 5%. (From Whaley & Wong, 1987.)

pnea, and breathlessness caused by congestive heart failure may be evident. The systolic murmur is louder than in a mild case, and the ECG indicates hypertrophy of the right ventricle and, perhaps, of the right atrium.

Evaluation and Treatment

Besides electrocardiography and chest x-ray films, diagnostic procedures include cardiac catheterization, angiocardiography, and echocardiogram. The treatment of pulmonary stenosis consists of pulmonary valvotomy, in which fused pulmonary valve leaflets are freed from one another or the narrow opening is widened.

Coarctation of the Aorta

Pathophysiology

Obstruction of outflow from the left ventricle often is the result of a localized malformation of the aorta that narrows its lumen sufficiently to impede blood flow. This congenital defect, termed **coarctation of the aorta,** may occur anywhere between the origin of the aortic arch and bifurcation of the aorta in the lower abdomen. Coarctation is most common (98% of cases) in the aortic arch, just below the origin of the left subclavian artery (Vaughn, McKay, & Berhman, 1985). Narrowing may occur before, at, or after the opening of the ductus arteriosus.

The location of the coarctation determines its hemodynamic consequences. When the narrowing is distal to the opening of the ductus arteriosus, and the ductus is closed, it is called **postductal coarctation** (Fig. 28-6). When the narrowing is proximal to the ductus arteriosus, it is called a **preductal coarctation.**

Postductal Coarctation Closure of the ductus arteriosus, which occurs 10 to 21 days after birth, proceeds from its pulmonary to its aortic end. While the aortic end of the ductus arteriosus is open, blood can flow around the coarctation through the orifice of the ductus arteriosus. As the opening of the ductus arteriosus closes, the degree of obstruction increases. Systolic pressure rises in the ascending aorta and the left ventricle and falls in the descending aorta beyond the coarctation (Fig. 28-7). Because the vessels branching off the ascending aorta (the subclavian arteries) supply the head and upper extremities, systolic blood pressure in these parts of the body will be elevated, and because the descending aorta ultimately supplies the lower extremities, systolic blood pressure in the legs will be depressed. The classic clinical manifestations of postductal coarctation are decreased or absent pulses in the femoral arteries and lower extremities, sometimes accompanied by mottled skin or cyanosis of the lower extremities and epistaxis (nosebleeds).

The likelihood of congestive left heart failure depends on the severity and location of the coarctation and the age of the child. In the first month of life, the ventricles have a limited ability to compensate for the higher afterload that occurs with coarctation. As a consequence of

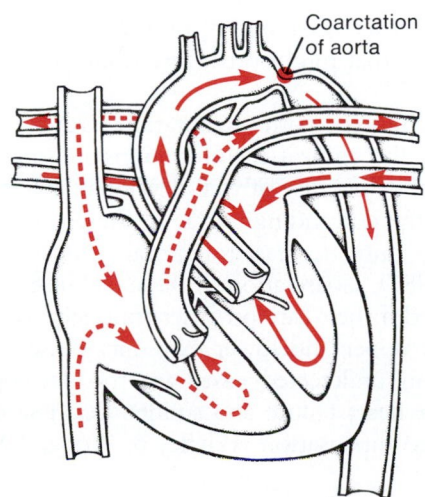

FIG. 28-6. Coarctation of the aorta. Postductal coarctation occurs distal to ("after") the insertion of the closed ductus arteriosus into the aortic arch. Preductal coarctation occurs proximal to ("before") insertion of the patent ductus arteriosus. The coarctation consists of a flap of tissue that protrudes from the tunica media of the aortic wall. (From Whaley & Wong, 1987.)

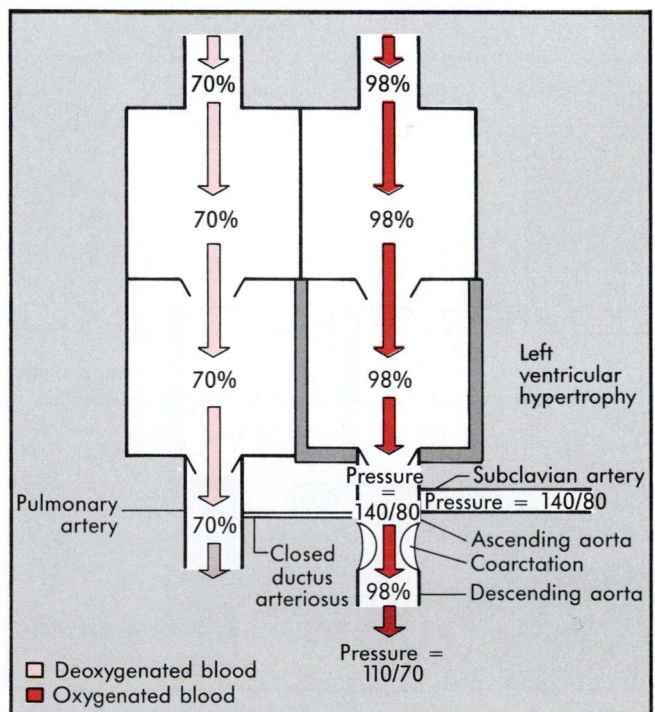

FIG. 28-7. Hemodynamics of postductal coarctation of the aorta. Blood pressure increases in the ascending aorta and subclavian artery and decreases in the descending aorta. These pressure changes eventually occur in the parts of the systemic circulation served by arteries that branch from the aorta before and after the coarctation.

the increased afterload, the left ventricle and atrium enlarge. To bypass the coarctation, collateral circulation develops around the obstruction. Small arteries bypass the coarctation by branching from the subclavian arteries and joining the intercostal arteries that branch from the descending aorta. This bypass around the coarctation supplies more oxygenated blood to the lower extremities. The collateral vessels become enlarged and kinked, and leave telltale "notches" that are visible on x-ray films where they pass over the ribs.

Preductal Coarctation   Preductal coarctation of the aorta (infantile coarctation), occurs proximal to the opening of the ductus arteriosus (see Fig. 28-6). Preductal coarctation is often associated with other congenital defects, particularly continued patency of the ductus arteriosus and openings in the interventricular septum.

A shunt is created if the ductus remains patent. The direction of the shunt depends first on the difference in blood pressure between the aorta and pulmonary artery. If there is no difference in pressure between these vessels, the direction of the shunt is determined by differences in total pulmonary and systemic resistance. For example, if pulmonary vascular resistance is higher than systemic resistance (as it is in the neonate before pulmo-

nary vascular resistance falls), blood flow through the patent ductus arteriosus will be from right to left. The right ventricle acts as a systemic pump, sending unoxygenated blood through the ductus into the descending aorta below the coarctation. When this occurs, the classic difference between pulses in the upper and lower extremities disappears.

If the blood pressure is greater in the aorta than in the pulmonary artery, blood flow through the ductus will be left to right, toward the lungs (Fig. 28-8). This can cause more than the normal amount of blood to be sent to the lungs. As the increased pulmonary blood volume reaches the left heart, it puts a strain on the left atrium and ventricle, often leading to congestive heart failure. The left heart has two sources of afterload: increased volume from the pulmonary circulation and obstruction to outflow caused by coarctation of the aorta. Both cause left ventricular hypertrophy.

Clinical Manifestations

The most important clinical manifestation of coarctation of the aorta is congestive heart failure (see p. 1015). Its onset and associated problems depend on how soon after birth the neonate's pulmonary vascular resistance decreases and the ductus arteriosus closes, the location and degree of coarctation, and whether the neonate has associated cardiac defects.

Usually the first manifestations of coarctation of the aorta are manifestations of congestive heart failure (see p. 1015 and Chapter 27). Once heart failure has developed, cyanosis occurs in the whole body, not just in the lower extremities. Fine crackles can be heard in the lungs. If the heart failure is advanced, insufficient cardiac output causes decreased blood pressures in both the upper and lower extremities, obliterating the difference in pressures that might otherwise result from the coarctation.

Most children with coarctation are symptomatic. However, the clinical manifestations in some children may be subtle because of well-developed collateral circulation to the descending aorta. In these cases, the child may have only decreased femoral pulses (Whaley & Wong, 1987). Coarctation in these children would only be detected if their care provider routinely compares the quality of upper and lower extremity pulses. The risks inherent in undetected cases are the development of congestive heart failure and sudden death secondary to cardiac decompensation (Whaley & Wong, 1987).

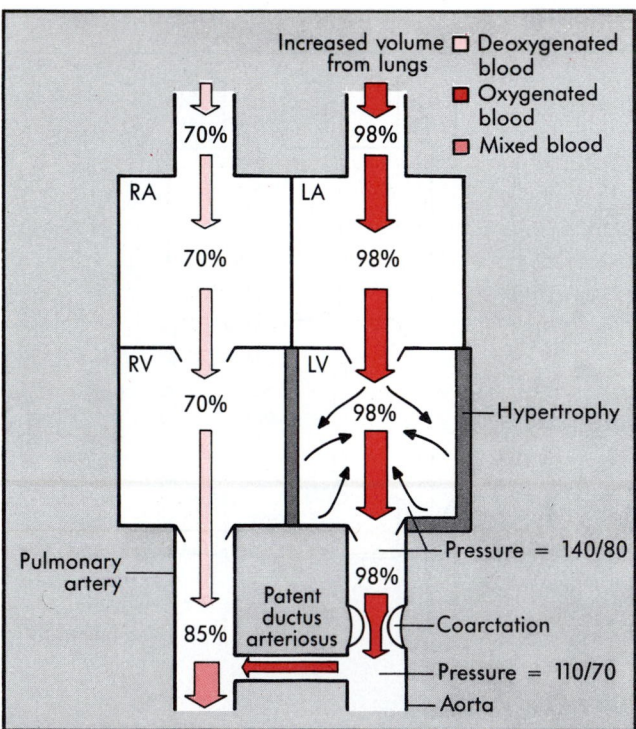

FIG. 28-8. Hemodynamics of preductal coarctation of the aorta with a patent ductus arteriosus. The left-to-right shunt through the ductus arteriosus increases the volume of blood in the pulmonary circulation. Afterload (indicated by dashed arrows) is increased in the left heart by (1) increased return from the lungs and (2) decreased ventricular outflow due to the coarctation. The outcome is left heart failure (congestive heart failure).

Evaluation and Treatment

Chest x-ray examinations reveal an enlarged heart with left atrial and ventricular hypertrophy. Cardiac catherization may be performed to measure pressures in the heart's chambers, the pulmonary artery, and the aorta. Oxygen saturation of blood within these structures is measured to determine the direction of the shunt. Angiocardiography may also be performed to visualize the aorta, the location of the coarctation, and any associated malformations of the interventricular septum, and aortic valve.

The first step in treatment of coarctation is to stabilize the child's vital signs and treat the congestive heart failure. High concentrations of supplemental oxygen are avoided because the ductus arteriosus (unlike other vessels) responds to oxygen by constricting, which worsens the effects of the coarctation. Diuretics are given to decrease fluid overload and edema, and prostaglandins may be given to dilate the ductus arteriosus.

Resection of the coarctation is the classic surgical treatment for localized postductal coarctation. Surgery is performed when the congestive heart failure is under control or when the child's aorta has grown to near-maximum size, between the ages of 4 and 8 years (Arciniegas, 1985; Smith, 1983). Preductal coarctation requires resection of a larger portion of the aorta, closure of the ductus arteriosus, and closure of interventricular septal openings, which are commonly associated with preductal coarctations. Bypass grafts and subclavian flap aortoplasty are examples of other surgical techniques used to correct coarctations.

Acyanotic Heart Defects with Increased Pulmonary Blood Flow

Acyanotic heart defects with increased pulmonary blood flow results in a left-to-right shunt. Some of the most common conditions in this category are ventricular septal defects, patent ductus arteriosus, and atrial septal defects. Other such defects, which will not be discussed here, are endocardial cushion defect and systemic arteriovenous fistulous connection.

Ventricular Septal Defect

A **ventricular septal defect (VSD)** is a hole in the interventricular septum. As an isolated (single) defect, VSD occurs at a rate of 1.3 to 2.4 per 1000 live births (Keith et al., 1978) and as 20% to 30% of all congenital heart defects (Guzzetta & Dossey, 1984; Smith, 1983). VSDs occur in conjunction with other heart defects in about 50% of children who have congenital heart disease.

Pathophysiology

The interventricular septum is formed by the fusion of several tissues: the right and left bulbar ridges, the endocardial cushions, the muscular septum, and the aorticopulmonary system (Fig. 28-2). Fusion is usually complete by the seventh week of gestation. A VSD can occur if any of these tissues fail to fuse with any of the others, creating an opening almost anywhere between the left and right ventricles (Fig. 28-9). The size of the

opening, which can vary widely, determines the amount of blood that is shunted through it. The position of the opening can also vary, but its size affects hemodynamics more than its location does.

If the VSD is very small, the flow of blood through the opening may be minimal and often causes no symptoms. Small VSDs often close spontaneously and require no treatment. The controlling factor in shunt direction through a small VSD is the pressure difference between the right and left ventricles. Normally, pressure is greater in the left ventricle, causing blood to shunt from left to right through the VSD (see Fig. 28-9, *B*). If the pressure is greater in the right ventricle than in the left, blood will shunt from right to left through the VSD.

Hemodynamics are quite different if the VSD is large (see Fig. 28-9, *C*). With a large VSD, the blood flows through the opening unimpeded, leading to equal pressure in both ventricles. Since there is no pressure gradient to produce a shunt, the difference between pulmonary and systemic vascular resistance becomes the determinant of shunt direction through a large VSD. Because systemic resistance is usually higher than pulmonary resistance, blood flows from the left (the area of greatest resistance) to the right (the area of lowest resistance).

When a large amount of blood shunts from left to right through a VSD, it has nowhere to go except into the lungs through the pulmonary artery and then back to the left side of the heart, where it creates serious strain. To compensate for volume overload, the left ventricle enlarges. Enlargement (hypertrophy) reduces compliance and increases contractility. For a time, the larger ventricle pumps more effectively. Eventually, however, the heart can no longer handle the increased volume, and heart failure ensues.

The pulmonary vascular bed also undergoes changes due to the increased volume it receives. In an attempt to maintain normal blood volume, the vessels undergo changes that increase their resistance to flow. The smooth muscle layer in the arteriolar walls increases and extends further than normal into the metarterioles. Proliferation of the intimal layer also occurs. The effect of these changes is to decrease the diameter of the vessels, which increases their resistance to blood flow. This protective mechanism of pulmonary hypertension succeeds at first, because it helps to decrease the volume of blood flowing into the lungs. Eventually, however, the changes become permanent, and pulmonary vascular resistance continues to rise. In some cases, it eventually exceeds systemic vascular resistance, causing the shunt through the VSD to reverse directions. At this point, deoxygenated blood is forced into the systemic circulation, and cyanosis occurs. This phenomenon, known as **Eisenmenger syndrome,** is a late and usually fatal complication of a VSD.

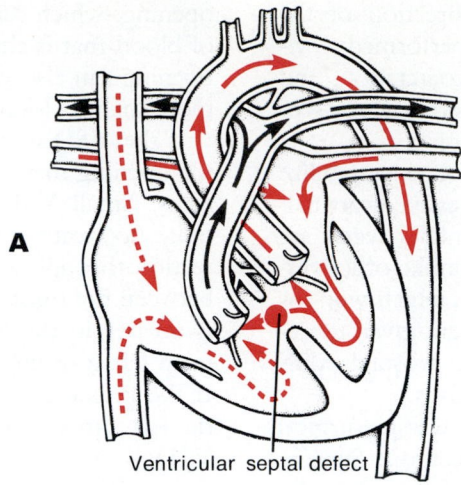

Ventricular septal defect

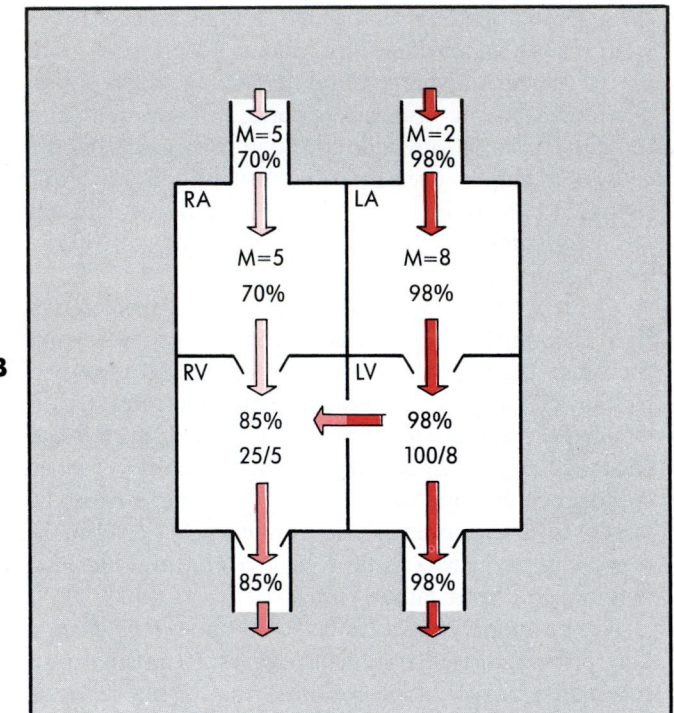

B

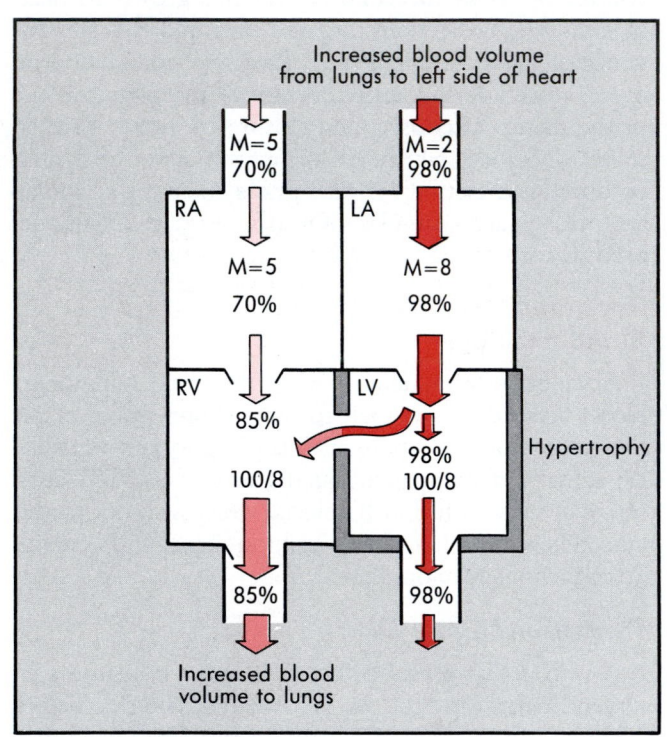

C

FIG. 28-9. **A,** Ventricular septal defect (VSD) with left-to-right shunt. **B,** Hemodynamics of a small VSD with left-to-right shunt. Mean (M) indicates mean of pressure; systolic/diastolic pressures are in mm Hg; and percentages indicate oxygen saturation. **C,** Hemodynamics of a large VSD with left-to-right shunt. Like the shunting that occurs in preductal coarctation of the aorta, the shunting pictured here causes left ventricular overload and hypertrophy. (From Whaley & Wong, 1987.)

Clinical Manifestations

Neonates with small VSDs are usually acyanotic and have no symptoms. Those with large VSDs have obvious manifestations. The murmur is usually heard shortly after birth, and is a harsh, loud, systolic murmur heard at the left lower sternal border and radiating to the pericardium (Whaley & Wong, 1987). The loudness of the murmur is not directly correlated with the size of the VSD; rather, the smaller the opening, the louder the murmur. This is because there is a greater pressure gradient across a small VSD, which creates greater turbulence of blood flow through the opening. The more turbulent the flow, the louder the murmur. Congestive heart failure develops when the infant is 4 to 12 weeks of age (Keith et al., 1978). Cyanosis is due to low cardiac output caused by heart failure and not to the VSD itself. Cyanosis does not result directly from a left-to-right shunt. Only in the case of Eisenmener syndrome, in which the shunt is reversed, does the VSD itself cause cyanosis.

Evaluation and Treatment

Diagnosis of a VSD is made on the basis of chest x-ray films, ECGs, cardiac catheterization, angiography, or echocardiogram. Chest x-ray films will show cardiac enlargement and pronounced or intensified pulmonary vascular markings, which indicate vascular adaptations to pulmonary hypertension. The ECG is usually normal if the VSD is small, but may indicate biventricular hypertrophy if the VSD is large and congestive heart failure is well established. Cardiac catheterization is used to measure pressures and oxygen levels in the chambers and great vessels. If the VSD is large, pressures will be equal or nearly equal in both ventricles and in the aorta at systemic levels. If the shunt is left to right, oxygen saturation will be higher in the right ventricle than in the right atrium. (Normally they are the same.) The difference indicates that oxygenated blood from the left ventricle has entered the right ventricle through the VSD. Angiography is performed to visualize and locate the VSD and to determine whether any other defects are present.

If the child is asymptomatic or has a small VSD, treatment may not be required. Fifty percent of VSDs close spontaneously or shrink to an insignificant size within 5 years of birth (Arciniegas, 1985). Infants who have congestive heart failure are treated with digoxin and diuretics until surgery can be performed. Though the surgical closure is sometimes performed on an infant, many surgeons prefer to wait until the child is 1 to 3 years old, provided that the VSD is asymptomatic. Waiting until the heart is larger lowers the risks of surgery. The surgery must, however, be done before increases in pulmonary vascular resistance become permanent. In some cases, the pulmonary artery is banded, or artificially constricted, before the VSD is closed. This decreases the left-to-right shunt and protects the pulmonary vasculature from overload. Permanent repair is made with a synthetic patch over the VSD. Because the conduction system of the heart runs through the ventricular septum, surgical manipulation carries some risk of heart block.

Patent Ductus Arteriosus

The aortic arch system develops between the fifth and sixth weeks of gestation. Six pairs of arches branch off the truncus arteriosus and connect with the dorsal aorta. Eventually, most of these arches develop into arteries, such as the right and left pulmonary arteries, and lose their connection to the aorta. The sixth arch on the left side, however, retains an attachment to the aorta and becomes the ductus arteriosus. Its function is to shunt blood away from the fetal lungs and into the systemic circulation. Normally, the ductus arteriosus becomes functionally closed shortly after birth and anatomically by constriction and fibrosis within 10 to 21 days after birth. Sometimes closure does not occur and the ductus arteriosus remains open, or patent. This condition is termed **patent ductus arteriosus** (PDA).

Estimates of incidence vary. PDA occurs in isolation or with other defects in approximately 10% of children with congenital heart defects (Moller & Neal, 1981). The incidence of PDA is greater in females than in males, and it is greater in premature infants than in full-term infants.

Pathophysiology

The pathogenesis of PDA is not known. Because it is not known precisely what causes the ductus arteriosus to close, it is difficult to pinpoint what might cause it to remain open.

The PDA may be long and narrow or short and wide. At the short extreme, it consists of only a "window" between the aorta and pulmonary artery. Its hemodynamic effects depend on the size of its lumen and, as always, the relative resistance in the pulmonary and systemic circulations (Keith et al., 1978) (Fig. 28-10, *A*). In general, as pulmonary resistance decreases and systemic resistance increases at birth, blood flow through the PDA reverses, becoming left to right. This shunts oxygenated blood into the pulmonary circulation. The hemodynamic effect of a left-to-right shunt is to increase pulmonary blood flow (Fig. 28-10, *B*). The hemodynamic effects of a PDA are similar to those of a VSD, and so are the possible complications: pulmonary hypertension and congestive heart failure. Subacute bacterial endocarditis is also seen as a complication of PDA. These complications are most common in premature infants who also have respiratory distress syndrome (see Chapter 31).

Clinical Manifestations

Full-term infants do not exhibit clinical manifestations of PDA at birth. No murmur is heard at birth because the systemic and pulmonary vascular resistances are still approximately equal, which prevents shunting of blood through the PDA. As the pulmonary and systemic resistances approach mature values—between 2 and 6 weeks after birth—left-to-right shunting begins. With its onset, a murmur is heard. The murmur begins as a systolic murmur, but both systolic and diastolic components of the typical "machinery" murmur are evident by the end of the first year. This occurs because the shunting begins to take place during both phases of the cardiac cycle (Fink, 1985). If the left ventricle does not accommodate the increased load of blood returning from the lungs, the infant may develop congestive heart failure (see p. 1015).

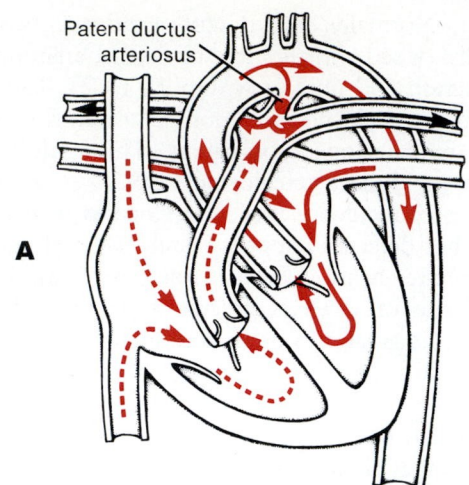

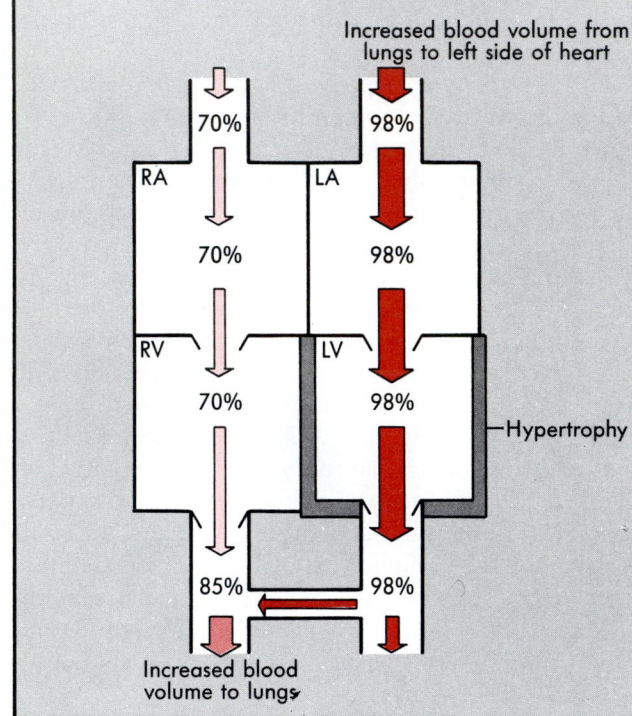

FIG. 28-10. **A,** Patent ductus arteriosus with left-to-right shunt. **B,** Changes in oxygen saturation, left ventricular volume, and the myocardium due to left-to-right shunt through a patent ductus arteriosus. (From Whaley & Wong, 1987.)

Evaluation and Treatment

Chest x-rays usually reveal cardiomegaly and intensified pulmonary vascular markings. Cardiac catheterization and angiography may be performed to determine the size and location of the PDA. These procedures are used if the child has congestive heart failure or pulmonary hypertension, or if the diagnosis cannot be made on the basis of the characteristic murmur.

Digoxin and diuretics are given if the infant has congestive heart failure. Drug therapy is followed by ligation of the PDA. Ligation has a mortality rate of less than 1%, even in premature infants (Tyson, 1975). The procedure does not require cardiopulmonary bypass or incisions into the heart itself. The ductus arteriosus is simply ligated with a suture and allowed to fibrose. In older children, the ductus may be ligated and oversewn (Arciniegas, 1985). In critically ill infants, medical closure is attempted through the use of prostaglandin inhibitors, such as indomethacin (Whaley & Wong, 1987).

Atrial Septal Defect

An **atrial septal defect** (ASD) is an abnormal opening in the interatrial septum (Fig. 28-11, *A*). ASDs account for about 8% of congenital heart defects. The interatrial septum develops during the fourth to sixth weeks of gestation, from a series of tissue walls (septum primum and septum secundum) that are laid down and resorbed (see Fig. 28-2). The fetal atrial septum contains one opening, the foramen ovale, which is covered by a flap of tissue on the left side creating a one-way valve from right to left. During fetal life, blood flows through the foramen ovale from right to left, shunting blood away from the pulmonary circulation into the systemic circulation (see Fig. 28-3). Normal development of the atrial septum involves a delicate balance between the laying down of tissue and its reabsorption.

Pathophysiology

The hemodynamics of ASDs are similar to those of VSDs. The size of the ASD determines the direction of blood flow through the opening. If the opening is small, the normal pressure difference between the right and left atria is maintained; that is, pressure is greater on the left side. This gradient causes blood to shunt from left to right through the ASD. If the opening is large, however, pressures in the atria are equalized and shunt direction is determined by relative resistance in the ventricles. In this respect, the hemodynamics of ASDs differ somewhat from the hemodynamics of VSDs. Shunt direction through a large VSD is determined by relative resistance in the pulmonary and systemic circulation, because these circuits receive ventricular outflow. Because atrial outflow is received by the ventricles, relative ventricular resistance is the crucial factor determining shunt direction through a large ASD.

Resistance to blood flow from the atria to the ventricles is determined by ventricular compliance. Ventricular compliance, or elasticity, depends on the thickness of the ventricular walls: the thicker the myocardium, the less compliant it is (see Chapter 26). At birth, the walls of both ventricles are about equal in thickness, so they are equally compliant, and no blood flows through the ASD. As the infant grows, the left ventricular wall thickens and the right ventricular wall thins. Compli-

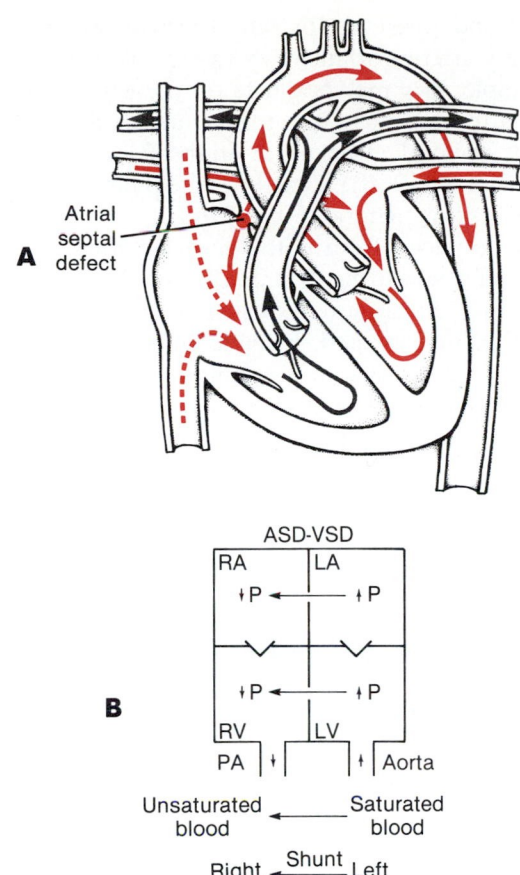

FIG. 28-11. A, Atrial septal defect. **B,** Hemodynamics of atrial septal defect with left-to-right shunt. (From Whaley & Wong, 1987.)

ance decreases on the left and increases on the right, causing blood to flow through the ASD from left to right (see Fig. 28-11, *B*).

Clinical Manifestations

Because the shunt through a simple ASD is from left to right, cyanosis does not occur. Most neonates and infants with isolated ASDs are asymptomatic until changes in myocardial thickness affect compliance. Therefore the defect may go undetected until the child is of preschool age. Only about 2% of children with ASDs develop congestive heart failure (Moller & Neal, 1981). (Manifestations of congestive heart failure are described on p. 1015.) Children with congestive heart failure due to ASDs are prone to develop respiratory infections, such as pneumonia. The soft murmur associated with ASD is usually heard at the 2nd intercostal space and is caused by the increased flow of blood across the pulmonic semilunar valve. The second heart sound may have a fixed, wide split because the right ventricle is always overloaded, which causes continuous

delayed closure of the pulmonic valve. (In the normal heart, delayed closure is only detected on inspiration.)

Evaluation and Treatment

Chest x-ray films of symptomatic children reveal an enlarged heart and increased pulmonary vascular markings. ECGs often indicate an enlarged right ventricle and, in about one half of cases, an enlarged right atrium (Moller & Neal, 1981). Cardiac catheterization may not be performed unless the cause of the congestive heart failure is undetermined. Because oxygenated blood enters the right atrium, oxygen saturation in the right heart is greater than normal. Pressures will be equal in both atria if the ASD is large.

Congestive heart failure must be stabilized before surgery can be performed. Stabilization includes administration of digoxin and diuretics, sometimes for several months. If the pharmacologic treatment is effective, respiratory infections will decrease, and the child will be able to eat and grow more normally while awaiting surgery. If the child is too stressed to eat, gastrostomy feedings become part of the medical management. Surgery consists of patching the ASD with a synthetic graft or simply stitching it shut. Though surgery has been performed on very young infants, the preferred approach is to wait until the child is older and risk decreases. There is also the possibility that the defect will close spontaneously.

Cyanotic Heart Defects with Increased Pulmonary Blood Flow
Persistent Truncus Arteriosus

Persistent truncus arteriosus (PTA) is the failure of the large embryonic artery, the truncus arteriosus, to divide into the pulmonary artery and the aorta. Instead, the truncus arteriosus persists and, through a single valve, empties both ventricles, which communicate through a large VSD at the top of the interventricular septum (Fig. 28-12, *A*). This single valve takes the place of the aortic and pulmonic valves. PTA causes the combined output of the ventricles to flow into both the systemic and pulmonary circulations. PTA is fairly rare. One estimate of incidence is 1 in 11,600 live births (Keith et al., 1978). The defect is reported to account for between 0.7% and 2.2% of all congenital heart defects (Guzzetta & Dossey, 1984).

Pathophysiology

The truncus arteriosus normally divides into the aorta and pulmonary trunk through the development of a spiral septum, which also closes the upper part of the interventricular septum. Any interruption of this process of division results in a large, single artery (the truncus arteriosus), which overrides a VSD.

The truncus arteriosus usually lies over both ventricles

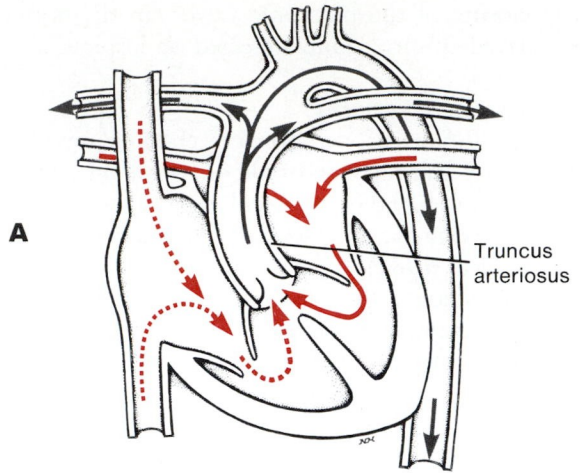

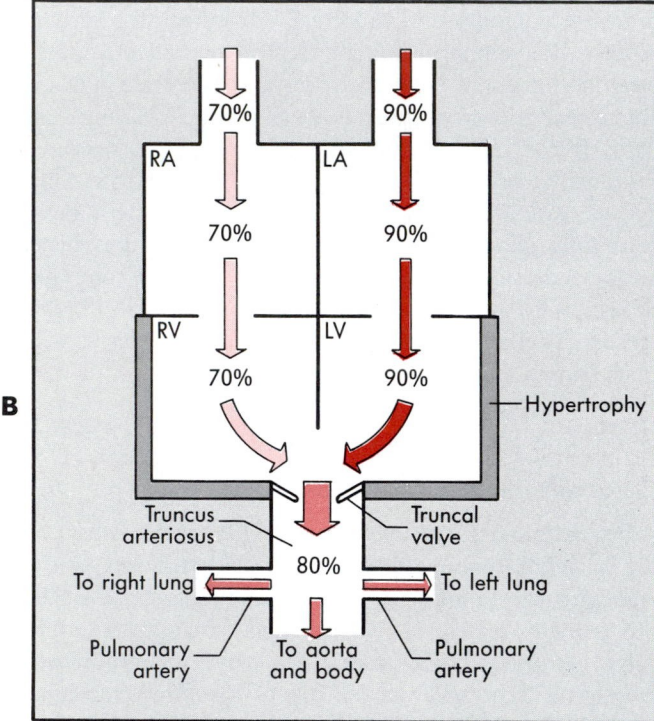

FIG. 28-12. **A,** Persistent truncus arteriosus. The truncus arteriosus fails to divide into the pulmonary artery and aorta, and the interventricular septum fails to close at the top. Blood from both ventricles mixes in the truncus arteriosus and then enters the pulmonary and systemic circuits. **B,** Alterations of hemodynamics and oxygen saturation by persistent truncus arteriosus. (From Whaley & Wong, 1987.)

and all blood flowing from both chambers enters through the truncal valve. A mixture of oxygenated and deoxygenated blood is thus pumped to the lungs and to the body (see Fig. 28-12, *B*). Because the VSD is usually high on the septal wall, just below the truncal valve, the mitral valve adjoins the truncal valve. Occasionally, the tricuspid valve is part of this complex as well. (Normally, all of the valves are part of the heart's fibrous skeleton; see Chapter 26). The truncal valve is often

stenosed and thickened or has defective leaflets. The pulmonary arteries originate in various abnormal sites. For example, they may originate on the left side of the truncus arteriosus, just above the truncal valve; on the posterior side of the truncus; or on the sides of the truncus (see Fig. 28-12, *B*). Sometimes the pulmonary arteries are absent or stenotic (Fink, 1985).

All of the blood from both ventricles flows into the truncus, after which the volume of flow that enters the aorta and pulmonary arteries depends on the difference between pulmonary and systemic resistance. In most cases, blood pressures in the pulmonary arteries and aorta are equal, so that relative total systemic and pulmonary resistances determine which system will receive the greatest amount of blood. The hemodynamic pattern is basically that of a VSD. If, however, the ductus arteriosus is stenosed, a natural pulmonary artery banding occurs that limits blood flow to the lungs. If pulmonary vascular resistance is high and blood flow to the lungs is low, less oxygenated blood returns to the left heart, and cyanosis is increased. If pulmonary vascular resistance falls, cyanosis decreases because more blood flows to the lungs.

Clinical Manifestations

Congestive heart failure is a common manifestation of persistent truncus arteriosus, and the child may fail to thrive from an early age. Fine crackles in the lungs are common. Cyanosis is present in varying degrees. It usually is mild in the neonate, but increases with age. The degree of cyanosis depends on the amount of blood flowing to the lungs. Usually, PTA causes an increase in pulmonary blood flow, so cyanosis is mild. If, however, blood flow to the lungs is significantly restricted over time, the child will develop polycythemia (overproliferation of red blood cells), plethora (reddened skin due to excessive blood volume), and clubbing of the fingers, as well as bluish lips and mucous membranes. Like a large VSD, PTA can increase pulmonary vascular resistance to the point of causing Eisenmenger syndrome (see p. 1003). Cyanosis then becomes chronic.

PTA causes a wide pulse pressure (a greater-than-average difference between systolic and diastolic blood pressures). Systolic pressure is increased because the output of *both* ventricles enters the truncus arteriosus with each systolic contraction. Diastolic pressure is lower than usual because blood is diverted from the aorta (systemic circulation) into the pulmonary arteries (pulmonary circulation) during the diastolic phase of the cardiac cycle.

Evaluation and Treatment

Chest x-ray films reveal cardiac enlargement that includes both ventricles and increased pulmonary vascular markings, which indicate increased pulmonary blood flow. ECGs indicate ventricular hypertrophy. Cardiac catheterization usually detects equal pressures in the right and left ventricles and aorta and very slight differences in oxygen saturation between the aorta and pulmonary arteries (Moller & Neal, 1981). Angiography is the most useful diagnostic technique because it enables the clinician to visualize the PTA, hypertrophied ventricles, and location and size of the pulmonary arteries (Keith et al., 1978).

Treatment of PTA is surgical. The pulmonary artery is disconnected from the truncus, and the VSD is closed so that blood will flow from the left ventricle into the truncus and then into the aorta. Next, a connection is created between the right ventricle and the pulmonary artery. A conduit graft with a valve is inserted between the right ventricle on one end and the pulmonary artery on the other. The success of this procedure depends on the status of the child's pulmonary vascular resistance. Mortality is 39% if pulmonary vascular resistance is high and 14% if it is low (Arciniegas, 1985). Untreated PTA is fatal, usually within the first few months of life.

Complete Transposition of the Great Vessels

Complete transposition of the great vessels is a defect in which the aorta and pulmonary arteries are completely switched; that is, the aorta arises from the right ventricle, and the pulmonary artery arises from the left ventricle. Complete transposition of the great vessels accounts for 8% to 9% of congenital heart disorders. Various studies have shown that the incidence of this condition is 1 in 4000 to 4500 live births (Keith et al., 1978). Males are affected twice as often as females, and maternal diabetes is a risk factor. Until an effective treatment was developed in the 1960s, transposition of the great vessels was fatal in 95% of cases. By the early 1980s, the mortality rate had dropped to less than 10% (Guzzetta & Dossey, 1984).

Pathophysiology

It is not known precisely which embryologic events lead to transposition, but researchers have proposed that the fault lies in the development of conal tissue in the fibrous skeleton of the heart (Moller & Neal, 1981). The conus is a segment of muscle that separates the atrioventricular (tricuspid and mitral) valves from the semilunar (aortic and pulmonic) valves. (The fibrous skeleton and heart valves are described and illustrated in Chapter 26; see Figure 26-4.) Normally, this conus grows more on the left side, under the pulmonic valve. This pushes the pulmonic valve anteriorly and to the left of the aortic valve. Some researchers believe that in transposition of the great vessels, nearly the opposite occurs; that is, the conus beneath the aortic valve grows more, pushing the aortic valve until it is anterior (forward) and superior to the pulmonic valve. This causes the aorta to rise anteriorly and to the right of the pulmonary artery (Fink, 1985; Keith et al., 1978). The in-

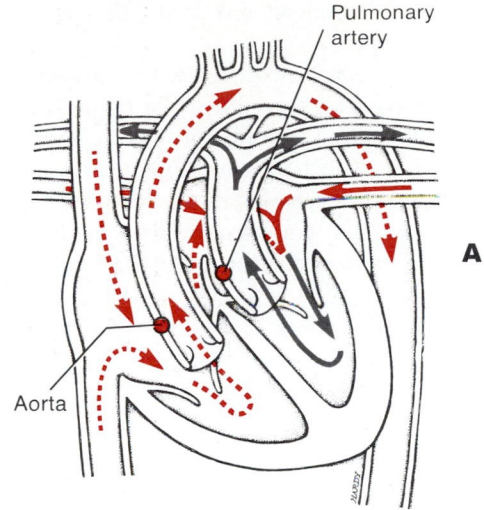

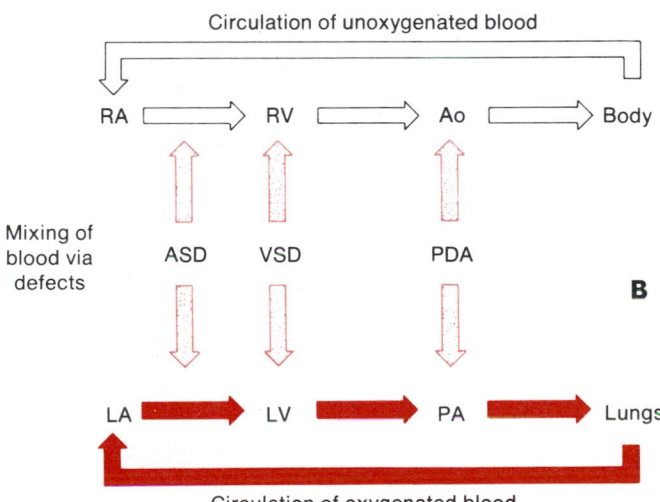

FIG. 28-13. **A,** Complete transposition of the great vessels with an intact interventricular septum. The aorta arises from the right ventricle and the pulmonary artery from the left. **B,** Oxygen saturation in the two parallel circuits. (From Whaley & Wong, 1987.)

terventricular septum is intact in about 60% of cases of transposition; a VSD is present in the remaining 40%. Pulmonary stenosis is associated with the transposition in about 4% to 6% of children with intact septums and in 28% to 31% of children with VSDs (Keith et al., 1978). The discussion that follows is limited to the pathophysiology of complete transposition with an intact interventricular septum.

The outstanding feature of complete transposition is that it creates two closed systems: blood from the pulmonary circulation does not enter the systemic circulation, and vice versa (Fig. 28-13). This, of course, is not conducive to life, because unoxygenated blood circulates continuously through the systemic circulation, and oxygenated blood circulates repeatedly through the pulmonary circulation.

Two factors allow neonates with complete transposition to survive long enough to be treated. First, blood from the two closed systems can mix through the ductus arteriosus for a short time following birth if pulmonary vascular resistance remains high. Some mixing may also occur through the foramen ovale. (If the child has a VSD, mixing will occur through that opening as well.)

Clinical Manifestations

The degree of mixing permitted by fetal structures determines the type and severity of clinical manifestations. The neonate with complete transposition and an intact ventricular septum will develop cyanosis within 24 hours of birth. Cyanosis may be mild shortly after and worsen during the first day due to functional closure of the ductus arteriosus. Breathing is not effective because the oxygen taken in by the lungs never reaches the systemic circulation. Low oxygen levels in the blood (hypoxemia) cause metabolic acidosis, tachycardia, and tachypnea.

The first heart sound is normal and the second sound may be heard as a single sound, even though both the aortic and pulmonic valves are functioning. The single sound (S_2) may occur because transposition places the aortic valve closer to the chest wall than the pulmonic valve. A systolic murmur is heard in about 50% of cases, even if no other lesion, such as a VSD, is present. The murmur is fairly nonspecific, and varies in loudness.

Evaluation and Treatment

On chest x-ray films the heart is seen to have a characteristic shape—like an egg on its side—and pulmonary vascular markings are increased. The heart may be enlarged if the infant is a few weeks old and has a VSD. ECG findings in the neonate are usually normal; that is, they indicate a right-axis deviation and some right ventricular hypertrophy. These findings reflect the initially larger and heavier right ventricle of the neonate. In the normal infant, however, the ECG pattern changes, reverting to an axis more to the left. In the infant with transposition, the axis remains to the right (Keith et al., 1978).

The neonate's response to supplemental oxygen indicates whether cyanosis is the result of pulmonary disease or transposition of the great vessels. If the infant has pulmonary problems, inhalation of supplemental oxygen increases arterial oxygen saturation. Arterial oxygen saturation remains unchanged in an infant with transposition.

Cardiac catheterization and angiography are usually performed on an emergency basis if transposition is suspected, in order to (1) confirm the diagnosis, (2) check for other lesions, such as VSD or pulmonary stenosis,

and (3) enlarge the foramen ovale to increase mixing of the circulations, a procedure termed balloon septostomy. Prior to the septostomy, catheterization is used to measure the percentage of desaturated blood in the peripheral system, to measure pressure in the right ventricle, and to confirm that the aorta and pulmonary artery are transposed (Fink, 1985).

Within 1 year of birth, a Mustard procedure is usually performed to correct complete transposition of the great vessels. The atrial septum is removed and replaced with a baffle (a chutelike arrangement that reroutes blood flow) made of pericardium or synthetic material. Oxygenated blood from the pulmonary veins is rerouted from the left atrium into the right ventricle, from which it is pumped out into the systemic circulation through the aorta. Unoxygenated blood is rerouted from the right atrium into the left ventricle, from which it is pumped to the lungs through the pulmonary artery. After the Mustard procedure, the great vessels remain transposed, but circulation through the chambers has been altered so that blood will flow into the correct circuit. In other words, the pump is altered to conform to the transposition. Because the Mustard procedure was developed less than 30 years ago, it is not known whether the right ventricle can sustain systemic pressures over a lifetime without failing (Arciniegas, 1985). Right ventricular failure could limit survival. Although the Mustard procedure and similar procedures are used to treat most children with transposition of the great vessels, arterial switching is sometimes performed. Current opinion is that arterial switching works best if the transposition is accompanied by a VSD (Arciniegas, 1985).

Total Anomalous Pulmonary Venous Connection

Total anomalous pulmonary venous connection (TAPVC), also called total anomalous pulmonary venous return, is a condition in which blood from the pulmonary circulation enters the right atrium instead of the left. Several developmental defects can cause TAPVC, which is thought to account for 1% of all congenital cardiac defects (Smith, 1983).

Pathophysiology

During about the third week of fetal life, the lung buds begin to develop a venous drainage system. This system consists of indirect connections to embryonic vessels—the umbilical vitelline veins (veins that return blood from the yolk sac to the heart of the embryo) and the cardinal veins—through the splanchnic plexus. At the same time, another embryonic vessel, the common pulmonary vein, grows out of the common atrium of the embryo. There is no direct connnection between the lungs and the common pulmonary vein at this time. As the common pulmonary vein grows from the atrium toward the lung buds, the cardinal and umbilical vitelline veins lose their connection with the splanchnic plexus, which develops into the four pulmonary veins that will eventually enter the left atrium. The common pulmonary vein continues to grow into these veins, establishing a direct connection between the lungs and the pulmonary vein. Ultimately, the common pulmonary vein is reabsorbed, leaving the four pulmonary veins that enter the heart at the left atrium. If the common pulmonary vein fails to develop fully from the left atrium, the earlier connections between the cardinal and umbilical vitelline veins may persist and cause a TAPVC.

TAPVCs can take various forms, depending on the vascular abnormality that causes pulmonary venous return to the right atrium. The four common forms are (1) drainage of the pulmonary veins into the superior vena cava and right atrium through the right anterior cardinal vein; (2) drainage into the right atrium through the coronary sinus through a remnant of the left anterior cardinal vein; (3) attachment of the four pulmonary veins directly to the right (instead of the left) atrium; or (4) drainage into the right atrium from the common pulmonary vein through the portal system into the inferior vena cava and right atrium. This particular connection is due to persistence of a remnant of the umbilical vitelline veins (Fink, 1985). Atrial septal defects accompany all forms of TAPVC, and pulmonary venous obstruction accompanies most forms. Obstruction is most common with the fourth form, however.

Pulmonary venous obstruction limits the return of oxygenated blood to the heart. The obstruction may be caused by external compression of the venous channel where it passes through the diaphragm, stenosis at the junction of the pulmonary venous channel and portal vein, or narrowing of the channel at any point along the route to the inferior vena cava. The blood that cannot pass the obstruction exerts pressure backward into the pulmonary capillary bed, causing pulmonary hypertension. As hydrostatic pressure rises in the pulmonary capillaries, plasma extravasates into the lung tissues, causing pulmonary edema. Obstruction also increases pulmonary vascular resistance, which in turn inhibits blood flow to the lungs from the right ventricle.

Oxygenated blood that enters the right atrium from the lungs mixes with unoxygenated blood returning from the body through the vena cavae. After that, the blood can flow (1) into the right ventricle and back to the lungs to be oxygenated or (2) through the ASD into the left atrium, the left ventricle, and out to the body. Ventricular compliance is a major determinant of the path the blood will take. Because pulmonary vascular resistance does not fall to normal levels in infants with TAPVC, the right ventricular wall does not thin out and become more compliant as it should. Lack of right ventricular compliance limits the amount of blood that

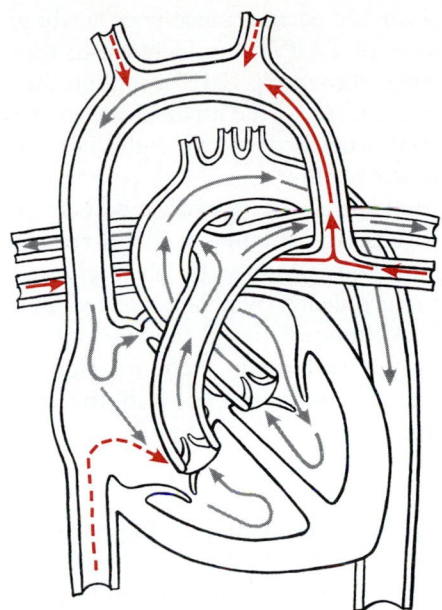

FIG. 28-14. Hemodynamics of total anomalous venous connection (TAPVC). In the form of TAPVC represented here, the pulmonary veins enter the left anomalous vertical vein instead of the left atrium. From the left anomalous vertical vein, the mixed blood from the lungs flows into the superior vena cava through an innominate vein (literally, a "vein with out a name"). Oxygen saturation within the four heart chambers, the pulmonary artery, and the aorta is the same. Blood pressure in the right heart exceeds that in the left heart because the right heart is receiving blood from both the pulmonary and systemic circulatory systems. (Abnormal vessels are shaded.) (From Whaley & Wong, 1987.)

will flow from the right atrium into the right ventricle and out to the lungs. Therefore, much of the mixed blood in the right atrium shunts through the ASD into the left ventricle. This hemodynamic pattern causes mixed blood to be pumped throughout the systemic circulation (Fig. 28-14).

Clinical Manifestations

Because TAPVC causes a mixture of oxygenated and deoxygenated blood to enter the systemic circulation, cyanosis is the predominant clinical manifestation. The degree of cyanosis ultimately depends on pulmonary blood flow; that is, pulmonary vascular resistance. The higher the resistance, the lower the flow; and the lower the flow, the greater the cyanosis. The cyanosis may worsen with feeding, elimination, or any strain that increases intrathoracic pressure by causing exhalation against a closed glottis (Valsalva maneuver). Pressure on the pulmonary venous channel further decreases the amount of oxygenated blood that flows to the right atrium.

Tachypnea and dyspnea are other early signs of TAPVC. These respiratory manifestations, which are due to pulmonary edema, cause poor feeding. The respiratory signs of TAPVC are identical to those of congestive heart failure (see p. 1015), though their underlying cause is different. If the infant survives long enough, the increased workload of the right heart may cause congestive heart failure.

Heart sounds may be normal and there may be no murmur because the amount of blood returning to the right atrium is often limited by obstruction. (Murmurs are due to turbulence, which is created by high volumes.) The volume of blood flowing out of the right ventricle is not increased; therefore right ventricular ejection time is not increased, and the second heart sound is normal.

Evaluation and Treatment

ECGs indicate right ventricular hypertrophy. Chest x-ray films reveal a normal-sized heart with increased pulmonary venous markings and a prominent pulmonary trunk. Pulmonary edema is apparent in the lung fields. Cardiac catheterization and angiography are the most useful diagnostic procedures. Catheterization reveals that oxygen saturation is equally low in all chambers of the heart, the aorta, and the pulmonary artery. Normally, the oxygen saturation of blood in the aorta is about 97%. In an infant with TAPVC, aortic oxygen may range from 20% to 70% (Fink, 1985; Moller & Neal, 1981). Catheterization also indicates pulmonary hypertension. TAPVC often causes pulmonary arterial pressure to exceed systemic arterial pressure. Pressures in the right atrium and ventricle may also be higher than normal. Angiography reveals the route of the anomalous pulmonary venous blood flow and right-to-left atrial shunting through the ASD.

If not treated surgically, most infants with TAPVC and pulmonary venous obstruction will die within months of birth. Surgical treatment consists of attaching the common pulmonary vein to the left atrium and tying off the anomalous connecting vein. The atrial septal defect is usually closed at this time. The likelihood of postoperative mortality depends on the infant's condition prior to surgery; for example, degree of pulmonary hypertension, nutritional status, condition of the lungs, presence or absence of obstruction, and the size of the left atrium.

Cyanotic Heart Defects with Decreased Pulmonary Blood Flow

Malformations of the chambers or valves of the right heart can cause cyanosis by reducing the volume of blood that flows to the lungs to be oxygenated. Several congenital heart defects restrict pulmonary blood flow. They include endocardial fibroelastosis of the right ventricle, in which ventricular hypertrophy and endocardial fibrosis reduce flow by reducing ventricular compliance;

Ebstein anomaly, in which the tricuspid valve is malformed; tricuspid atresia, in which the tricuspid opening is abnormally narrow; and **tetralogy of Fallot,** which consists of four defects involving the valves, the aorta, the interventricular septum, and the right ventricular myocardium. Tetralogy of Fallot and pulmonary atresia are useful examples of right heart defects that cause cyanosis by restricting pulmonary blood flow.

Tetralogy of Fallot

Tetralogy of Fallot, a syndrome of four defects, is the most common of the cyanotic heart defects and accounts for approximately 10% of all congenital heart defects. Tetralogy of Fallot has been associated with Down syndrome, first-trimester rubella, and Noonan syndrome (male Turner syndrome, in which stature and overall appearance are altered because the gonads fail to develop). The risk for recurrence of tetralogy of Fallot in a family with an affected child is about 3% (Keith et al., 1978).

Pathophysiology

The anatomic features of tetralogy of Fallot are (1) a ventricular septal defect, which is high on the septum and usually large, (2) an overriding aorta, which straddles the VSD, (3) pulmonary stenosis, usually due to hypertrophy of the arterial infundibulum (funnel-shaped opening at the entrance of the pulmonary artery), and (4) right ventricular hypertrophy (Fig. 28-15, *A*). Right ventricular hypertrophy develops because afterload is increased by the obstruction of flow from the right ventricle.

Tetralogy of Fallot develops during two phases of embryologic growth: (1) during the division of the truncus arteriosus by the spiral septum in the third or fourth week of gestation and (2) during the division of the ventricles between the fourth and eighth weeks of gestation (see Fig. 28-2). Normally, as these events progress, the truncal septum fuses with the bulbar ridges and, in turn, with the endocardial cushions. The membranous portion of the interventricular septum grows upward to meet the endocardial cushions and, ultimately, all of these tissues come together to complete the interventricular septum.

The embryologic error that causes tetralogy of Fallot is not known for certain, but two theories have been proposed (Fink, 1985). The first is that the truncus arteriosus divides unevenly, resulting in great vessels of unequal size. Because of this asymmetry, the part of the spiral septum that normally fuses with the atrioventricular septa is not where it should be, causing a VSD. Concomitantly, pulmonary stenosis develops because there is a larger than normal amount of tissue in the infundibulum of the right ventricle. (This infundibulum is on the ventricular side of the pulmonic valve.) The sec-

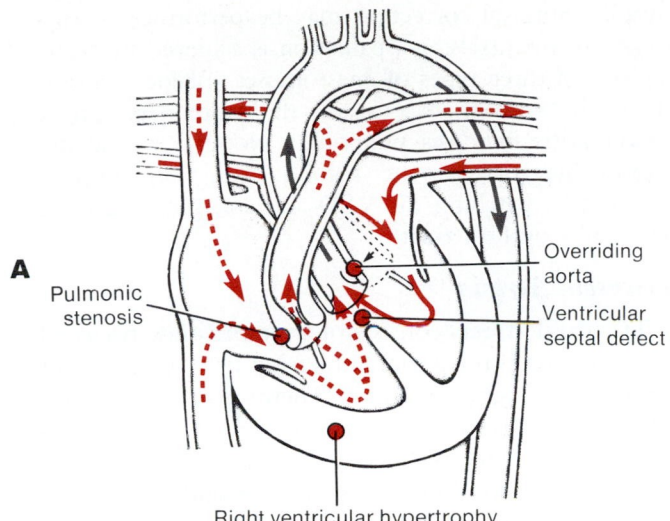

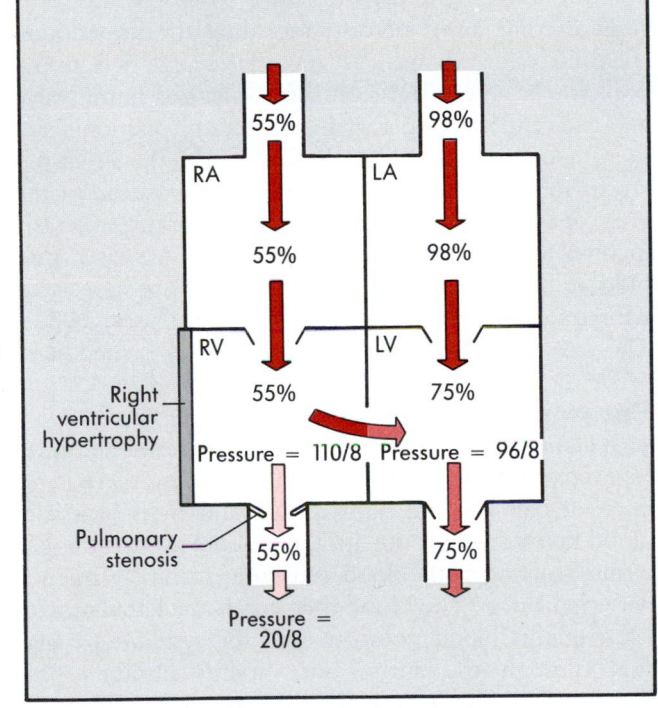

FIG. 28-15. **A**, Anatomic defects in tetralogy of Fallot. **B**, Hemodynamics of tetralogy of Fallot with right-to-left shunt. (**A** from Whaley & Wong, 1987.)

The pathophysiology associated with tetralogy of Fallot varies widely, depending primarily on the degree of pulmonary stenosis, but also on the size of the VSD and the pulmonary and systemic resistance to flow. Because the VSD is usually large, pressures may be equal in the right and left ventricles. Therefore the major determinant of shunt direction through the VSD is the difference between pulmonary and systemic vascular resistance. If pulmonary vascular resistance is higher than systemic resistance, the shunt is from right to left. If systemic resistance is higher than pulmonary resistance, the shunt is from left to right. Because many factors can alter the balance between pulmonary and systemic resistance, shunt direction is not necessarily constant (see Fig. 28-15, *B*).

Stenosis decreases blood flow to the lungs and, consequently, the amount of oxygenated blood that returns to the left heart. If blood also shunts from right to left through the VSD, deoxygenated blood mixes with the small amount of relatively oxygenated blood returning from the lungs. The result is low oxygen saturation (hypoxemia) in the systemic circulation. The body attempts to compensate for hypoxemia by producing more red cells (thereby causing polycythemia) and by increasing blood flow to the lungs through collateral bronchial vessels.

Clinical Manifestations

As long as the ductus arteriosus remains open, the neonate's pulmonary blood flow may be adequate. As the ductus closes, however, cyanosis becomes apparent. Many factors can affect the degree of cyanosis, especially those which change the balance between systemic and pulmonary resistance. For example, a hot environment causes peripheral vessels to dilate, thereby lowering systemic vascular resistance and shifting more unoxygenated blood through the VSD into the aorta. (This increases cyanosis.) Physical exertion (e.g., playing or eating) also lowers systemic resistance as blood travels to the muscles. Chronic cyanosis causes clubbing of the fingers and toes (see Chapter 30).

A common manifestation of tetralogy of Fallot is the sudden onset of dyspnea, cyanosis, and restlessness, sometimes called a hypoxic spell or a "tet spell." These spells generally occur in the morning or early evening and in the summer, often with crying and exertion. No one knows for sure what causes these episodes, but it is theorized that the right ventricular outflow tract goes into spasm or the systemic resistance drops suddenly (Moller & Neal, 1981; Perloff et al., 1983). In either case, the relative or actual increase in pulmonary vascular resistance increases the right to left shunt and the cyanosis. Other signs associated with these episodes, such as loss of consciousness and seizures, are the result of hypoxia (lack of tissue oxygenation).

ond theory proposes that infundibular overgrowth in the right ventricle is the major developmental anomaly. The extra tissue restricts the blood flow through the pulmonary artery, causing the artery to be smaller than normal at birth. Concomitantly, the aorta is subjected to greater-than-normal blood flow during fetal life, causing it to be larger than normal at birth. In addition, infundibular overgrowth in the right ventricle prevents normal closure of the ventricular septum, causing the VSD.

Squatting is a spontaneous compensatory mechanism used by older children to alleviate hypoxic spells. Squatting and its variants increase systemic resistance while decreasing backflow to the heart from the inferior vena cava. The decrease of systemic return makes relatively more oxygenated blood available to the body. The increase of systemic resistance also reverses the shunt through the VSD to a left-to-right shunt, which has the effect of increasing pulmonary blood flow. Through both of these mechanisms, squatting decreases cyanosis temporarily. Infants do not squat, but may assume a knee-chest position, which accomplishes the same thing. Infants and children also experience slow growth and failure to thrive. Infants often have difficulty with feeding because the exertion required increases hypoxia.

Congestive heart failure is not usually a manifestation of tetralogy, because blood can exit from the right heart through the overriding aorta. This prevents afterload from building in the right heart, despite pulmonary stenosis.

Polycythemia can lead to iron-deficiency anemia if the child's iron intake does not keep pace with the increased production of red blood cells (see Chapter 23). Polycythemia may also cause thromboembolism by making the blood more viscous, which slows flow and promotes clotting. The brain is particularly vulnerable to thromboembolism in children with tetralogy of Fallot.

The typical heart murmur of tetralogy is a pulmonary systolic ejection murmur caused by the obstruction in the outflow tract, which creates turbulence during systole. The smaller the obstruction, the louder the murmur. This explains why the murmur often disappears during a hypoxic spell, when obstruction increases. The second heart sound seems to be single, but in fact it is not. The pulmonary component is very soft and delayed and is usually not heard, although it is present. The enlarged right ventricle may cause the left side of the chest to be more prominent, and a "heave" may also be felt.

Evaluation and Treatment

The ECG indicates right ventricular hypertrophy. Chest x-ray examination reveals that the heart is shaped like a boot and that pulmonary vascular markings are decreased. Measurements made during cardiac catheterization demonstrate normal systemic pressure in the right ventricle, decreased pressure in the right ventricular outflow tract, and low oxygen saturation in the aorta. Angiograms enable the clinician to see the size and position of the VSD, the stenotic pulmonary infundibulum or valve, the smaller-than-normal pulmonary artery, and the overriding aorta.

Children who are not treated surgically have a life expectancy of about 12 years (Keith et al., 1978). Pulmonary stenosis tends to progress with age. Surgical treatment has been available since the mid-1940s, and the age at which surgery is performed has decreased

steadily. Surgical correction may be performed in two stages. In the first stage, palliation is achieved by creating one of three types of anastomoses (Blalock-Taussig shunt) between the aorta and the pulmonary artery. Anastomosis increases pulmonary blood flow and decreases hypoxia. In the second step, correction is achieved by patching the VSD and enlarging the right ventricular outflow tract.

Tricuspid Atresia

Tricuspid atresia consists of an imperforate tricuspid valve, resulting in no communication between the right atrium and right ventricle. There may be a small "dimple" on the floor of the right atrium, but there is no opening (Roberts, 1987). This defect accounts for 2% to 3% of congenital heart defects and is the third most common cyanotic heart defect (Adams & Emmanouilides, 1983; Arciniegas, 1985). Tricuspid atresia is really a complex of defects, including the imperforate tricuspid valve, as well as an atrial septal defect, hypoplastic or absent right ventricle, enlarged mitral valve and left ventricle, and varying degrees of pulmonic stenosis (Arciniegas, 1985; Roberts, 1987). Tricuspid atresia may also be associated with transposition of the great vessels. The most common type of tricuspid atresia involves a hypoplastic right atrium with decreased pulmonary blood flow and a VSD, and is not associated with transposition (Adams & Emmanouilides, 1983). The pathophysiology of this type will be presented here.

Pathophysiology

Systemic blood returns through the superior and inferior vena cavae to the right atrium. Because there is no opening between the right atrium and right ventricle, blood flows through the atrial septal defect into the left atrium, mixing with blood returning from the pulmonary circulation. The blood then enters the left ventricle. Most of this blood goes out into the systemic circulation through the aorta, but varying amounts pass through the VSD into the hypoplastic right atrium and then out through the pulmonary valve to the lungs. Pulmonary circulation depends on the presence of a VSD, which in turn assumes a right ventricle of some size is present. If the right ventricle is absent, the pulmonary valve is usually imperforate as well. If this is the case, a PDA is necessary to ensure that some blood flows into the pulmonary circulation (Adams & Emmanouilides, 1983).

As is the case with tetralogy of Fallot, pulmonary circulation also depends on the relationship between pulmonary and systemic vascular resistance. As long as pulmonary resistance is lower than systemic resistance, blood will flow through the VSD from left to right, feeding the pulmonary circulation. If pulmonary resistance rises above systemic resistance, blood will not reach the pulmonary circulation through the VSD.

Clinical Manifestations

Central cyanosis in some degree is a common manifestation in tricuspid atresia. As with tetralogy of Fallot, these children also experience exertional dyspnea and squatting. Long-term effects of hypoxia are polycythemia and clubbing. These children may also display hypoxic "spells," like the tet spells (Adams & Emmanouilides, 1983) (see p. 1013). It is not coincidental that the clinical manifestations of tricuspid atresia (type 1-b) described here are so similar to the clinical manifestations of tetralogy. Although the anatomic features are somewhat different, the hemodynamic effects are the same.

The ECG in tricuspid atresia reveals right atrial and left ventricular hypertrophy, and left axis deviation. There is a single first heart sound because there is no tricuspid valve to make a sound on closing. The second sound may also be single because of the presence of pulmonic stenosis. The murmur heard with tricuspid atresia may have several components depending on the anatomic features of each case. Pulmonic stenosis produces a systolic murmur, the loudness of which depends on the degree of stenosis. A severely stenotic valve will produce a soft murmur because very little blood flows through the valve. A less stenotic valve will produce a louder murmur from more blood flow. The VSD also causes a murmur that is systolic; the larger the VSD, the softer and shorter the murmur is likely to be.

Evaluation and Treatment

Although cardiac catheterization and angiocardiography are still frequently done to ascertain the anatomic and hemodynamic features of tricuspid atresia, echocardiography and magnetic resonance imaging are gaining popularity in the evaluation of this and most other congenital heart defects (Roberts, 1987). These techniques are noninvasive and can provide information about anatomy and some information about hemodynamic characteristics.

Surgical treatment of tricuspid atresia consists of maximizing systemic and pulmonary blood flow and increasing pulmonary blood flow (Arciniegas, 1985). The Fontan procedure, developed in the early 1970s, establishes a more normal circulation by creating a four-chambered, four-valve heart and eliminates systemic-pulmonary mixing (Arciniegas, 1985; Roberts, 1987).

ACQUIRED CARDIOVASCULAR DISORDERS

Acquired heart diseases in children include congestive heart failure, rheumatic heart disease, and essential or primary hypertension. (Rheumatic heart disease is discussed in Chapter 27; as are adult forms of heart failure and primary hypertension.)

Congestive Heart Failure

Congestive heart failure (CHF) is a common complication of many congenital heart defects. The effect of congestive heart failure is the same in all age groups: the heart is unable to maintain sufficient output to meet the body's metabolic needs. The most common causes of CHF in infancy are pressure and volume overloads secondary to congenital disease. (Table 28-6 lists the congenital heart defects that cause CHF, by age.) Ninety percent of children who develop CHF do so within 12 months of birth (Guzzetta & Dossey, 1984), often by the age of 6 months (Park, 1988).

In general, the pathophysiologic mechanisms of CHF in infants and children are very similar to those in adults. The same compensatory mechanisms are activated in the face of inadequate cardiac output. A decrease in blood pressure stimulates stretch receptors and baroreceptors in the aorta and carotid arteries, which in turn stimulate the sympathetic nervous system. With the release of catecholamines and the stimulation of β receptors, heart rate and the force of myocardial contraction increase. Venous smooth muscle tone also increases, which increases return of venous blood to the heart. Sympathetic stimulation also decreases blood flow to the kidneys, skin, spleen, and extremities, so that maximum flow to the brain, heart, and lungs can be maintained. Decreased blood flow to the kidneys causes the release of renin, angiotensin, and aldosterone. This cycle results in retention of sodium and fluid by the kidneys, which in turn increases volume in the circulatory system.

The myocardium hypertrophies in CHF, which increases ventricular pressure. The myocardium fibers also stretch to accommodate the increased volume. This increases contractility and hence the force of ventricular contraction. Both hypertrophy and increased stretch eventually fail to maintain cardiac output as CHF progresses. A review of the Frank-Starling law of the heart is useful for an understanding of the cycle of compensation and decompensation that occurs in CHF. (The Frank-Starling law is described in Chapter 26.)

Despite its different causes, CHF in infants is not generally differentiated as right or left ventricular failure. Usually, both ventricles are involved by the time signs and symptoms are apparent (Mott, Fazekas, & James, 1985; Smith, 1983).

Congestive heart failure in infants is manifested as poor feeding and sucking (leading to failure to thrive), diaphoresis (increased perspiration), breathlessness (dyspnea), and irritability. Most of the symptoms of congestive heart failure are due to low cardiac output and venous congestion (see Chapter 27). The body tries to compensate for low output by increasing the pulse rate until the infant has tachycardia even at rest. Any increase in exertion, such as eating, will have the same effect. Blood flow to all peripheral organs, including the

TABLE 28-6 Congenital heart defects causing congestive heart failure

Age	Congenital heart defect
Time of birth	Hypoplastic left heart syndrome Volume overload due to tricuspid regurgitation Arterial venous fistula
Birth to 1 week	Hypoplastic left heart syndrome Aortic atresia Transposition of the great vessels Coarctation of the aorta Total anomalous pulmonary venous connection (TAPVC) with obstruction Patent ductus arteriosus (PDA) in premature infants
First 4 weeks	Coarctation of the aorta TAPVC Large left-to-right shunt due to ventricular septal defect (VSD), PDA in premature infants Tricuspid atresia All previously mentioned defects
4-6 weeks	Transposition of the great vessels Large left-to-right shunt due to endocardial cushion defect
6 weeks to 6 months	VSD
6 months	Endocardial fibroelastosis Persistent truncus arteriosus with large left-to-right shunt

Data from Keith, Rowe, & Vlad, 1978; Park 1988.

skin, diminishes to conserve flow to the brain and heart. This causes peripheral hypotension, cool extremities, and muscular flaccidity. Decreased flow to the skin decreases elimination of body heat through radiation, and the body compensates by increasing perspiration. (Mechanisms of temperature regulation are described in Chapter 13.)

The failing heart eventually causes venous congestion throughout the body, resulting in hepatomegaly, edema, and dyspnea. Edema may appear in the periorbital area early in congestive heart failure and progress to peripheral edema later in the course of the condition. Dyspnea occurs when the hydrostatic pressure in the pulmonary veins exceeds that in the surrounding tissue, enabling fluid to leak out into the lung tissue. Edema decreases lung compliance, in effect creating a stiff lung and increasing the work of breathing. (Dyspnea and pulmonary edema are defined in Chapter 30.) Cyanosis is sometimes a sign of congestive heart failure in children, but other skin changes, such as pallor or mottling, are more common.

Dyspnea on exertion is manifested in infants as difficulty with feeding. When the infant tries to suck and swallow, breathing is interrupted, and the child becomes exhausted. Poor feeding, coupled with failure to thrive, is one of the primary indicators of CHF in infants. The child's growth is slowed, and parents report

that it can take 45 to 60 minutes for the infant to finish 1 to 2 ounces of formula.

The infant's respiratory rate may be greater than 40 breaths per minute. In severe CHF, tachypnea may be accompanied by retractions, grunting, nasal flaring, wheezing, coughing, and rales (Smith, 1983).

Hepatomegaly (enlargement of the liver) is typically due to systemic venous congestion caused by right ventricular failure. In infants, the normal liver is sharp-edged and palpable 1 to 2 cm below the costal margin. In the infant with CHF, the liver has a dull, rounded edge that is felt more than 3 cm below the costal margin, and may be tender (Guzzetta & Dossy, 1984; Keith et al., 1978).

Although peripheral edema is a common finding in adults with CHF, it is unusual in infants and young children. Periorbital tissue may be the only site of obvious edema in infants. Another manifestation in adults, distention of the jugular veins, is seldom apparent in infants becaue of their relatively short necks. Fluid retention in infants is usually manifested by a weight gain without any increase in calorie intake.

A chest x-ray examination is performed to ascertain the presence of cardiomegaly (a reflection of hypertrophy). An ECG is also performed to determine the presence of arrhythmias and as an indirect indicator of heart size. Plotting the child's growth (height, weight, and head circumference) is an important method of assessing failure to thrive. A thorough physical examination reveals the extent of tachycardia, tachypnea, dyspnea, diaphoresis, edema, and hepatomegaly.

Treatment is aimed at decreasing cardiac workload and increasing the efficiency of the heart (Moller & Neal, 1981). Digitalis and diuretics are prescribed for these same reasons. Other treatments may include the administration of oxygen, sedation, gastrostomy feedings, and keeping the child in a semi-upright position. The semi-upright position causes fluid to pool in the lung bases, limiting areas of fluid reabsorption by lymphatic vessels in the lungs. This decreases the volume of blood that returns to the heart (Smith, 1983). Diuretics usually make salt and fluid restrictions unnecessary for infants (Guzzetta & Dossey, 1984; Park, 1988).

Rheumatic Heart Disease

The incidence of rheumatic fever and rheumatic heart disease has a wide geographic variation. In many Third World countries, it remains a common, virulent disease with early cardiac sequelae and a much-shortened lifespan. In the United States, this disease has decreased markedly in the last 50 to 60 years. In the late 1920s, it was estimated that rheumatic heart disease accounted for 40% of all heart disease, but by the 1950s, this estimate was only 23% (Keith et al., 1978). One estimate of incidence of rheumatic heart disease in the 1970s was 2 cases per 1000 children, with an equal number contracting rheumatic fever without cardiac complications (Keith et al., 1978). In recent years, there has been a dramatic increase in the incidence of rheumatic fever in some regions of the United States, such as the Intermountain West, Ohio, Texas, and Hawaii (Ruttenberg, 1986; Kaplan, 1988). The incidence figures for the nation as a whole remain very low. Nonetheless, rheumatic fever remains the leading cause of acquired heart disease in children.

The usual age of onset is between 5 and 10 years, though some cases occur before the age of 5. Demographic characteristics, such as race and sex, are not strongly related to the incidence of rheumatic fever (Keith et al., 1978). The possibility of a genetic predisposition has been discussed but not proven (Vaughn et al., 1985).

The initiating cause of rheumatic fever is infection by group A β-hemolytic streptococcus. The streptococcal infection usually preceeds the onset of rheumatic fever by several days. It has been suggested that rheumatic fever may be the result of a hypersensitivity reaction to some antigen in the streptococcus or its toxins. If this is so, rheumatic fever could be categorized as an autoimmune disease. Other theories of pathogenesis include actual infection of the cardiac valves with living bacteria in altered forms. (See Chapter 27 for a detailed discussion of rheumatic fever and its sequelae.)

Conditions Associated with Secondary Hypertension in Children

CARDIOVASCULAR
Coarctation of the aorta
Hypoplastic aorta
Abnormalities of renal artery
Renal vein thrombosis

RENAL
Hydronephrosis
Chronic glomerulonephritis
Chronic pydonephritis
Dysplastic kidney
Hydronephrosis
Polycystic kidneys
Renal trauma
Renal tumors
Medullary cystic disease
Post-transplantation

ADRENAL
Neuroblastoma
Cushings disease
Pheochromocytoma
Adrenogenital syndrome
Primary aldosteronism
Adrenal carcinoma

OTHER
Intracranial tumors
Chronic use of steroids
Excessive intake of licorice
Renal disease secondary to irradiation
Lead neuropathy

From Adams & Emmanouilides, 1983.

Primary Hypertension

In the past, most hypertension in children was thought to be secondary to other diseases, such as chronic glomerulonephritis or renal tumors, to name but two (see the box above). In the 1950s, this opinion began to change because autopsies done on young Korean War casualties revealed significant arterial disease, which is known to cause hypertension. It was discovered that many of these young men (and later, young casualties of the Vietnam War) had significant atherosclerosis in major blood vessels. The autopsies showed that even the late lesions of atherosclerosis, fibrous plaques, can be present by late adolesence (Berenson, 1980). Since then, autopsies on infants have revealed fatty streaks—the earliest lesions of atherosclerosis—in the intimal lining of blood vessels (Engle, 1981). Evidently, hypertension-causing arterial disease can begin extremely early in life.

The incidence of primary (or essential) hypertension in childhood is at present a controversial topic, partly because normal blood pressure values, a consistent definition, and diagnostic criteria are still being established (Berenson, 1980; Kotchen & Kotchen, 1983).

It is unclear whether the pathophysiologic mechanisms of primary hypertension in adults and children are the same, or even exactly what those mechanisms are. Primary hypertension is thought to result from a complex interaction of disturbances in sympathetic vascular smooth muscle tone, humoral agents (angiotensin, catecholamines), renal sodium excretion, and cardiac output. (See Chapter 26 for a full discussion of these mechanisms.) Ultimately, these factors impair the ability of the peripheral vascular bed to adjust its own resistance to meet tissue perfusion needs (Kotchen & Kotchen, 1983).

Course of the Disease

Pathophysiology

Hypertension is thought to result from a complex interaction of disturbances in sympathetic smooth muscle tone, humoral agents (angiotensin, catecholamines), re-

nal function, sodium balance, blood volume, vasopressor responses, and cardiac output. Ultimately, these factors alter the ability of the peripheral vascular bed to adjust its own resistance to meet tissue perfusion needs (Kotchen & Kotchen, 1983).

An increase in peripheral vascular resistance decreases the body's ability to perfuse its tissues at normal arterial pressures. Over a period of time, the increased pressures resulting from those changes cause permanent thickening of vessel walls, which in turn leads to further increases in resistance, setting up a vicious cycle, This cycle serves as another illustration of Poiseuille's equation in action, where thickening of vessel walls causes a decreased radius, which in turn results in increased resistance to flow (see Chapter 26).

Changes in cardiac output provide the other hemodynamic element in hypertension. The aorta is a distensible tube that is subjected to intermittent pressure increases with each systole. These pressure increases drive the blood through the arterial system to the capillaries and then back to the heart through the veins. The distensibility of the aorta determines how easily it can adjust to systemic pressure changes. If the walls of the

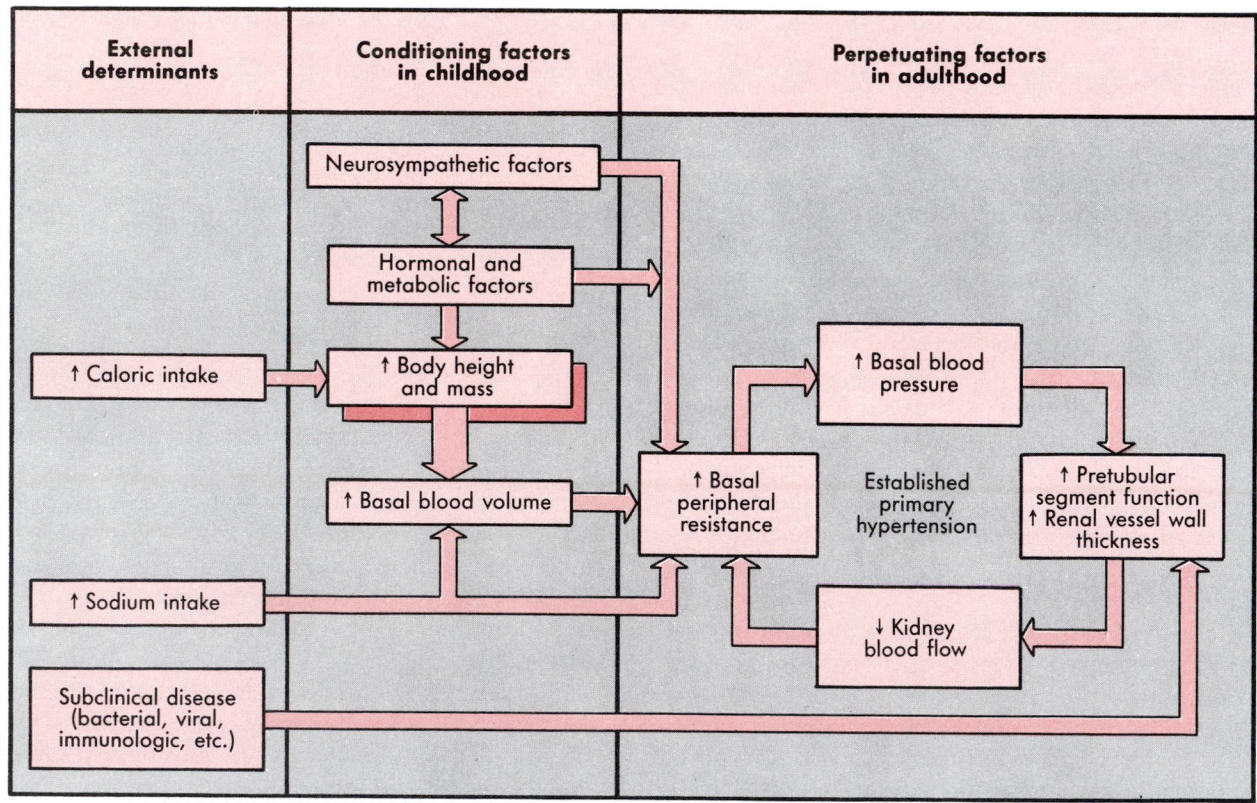

FIG. 28-16. Mechanisms believed to influence blood pressure in childhood. According to this model, a critical factor in the development of hypertension is obesity during childhood. Increased body mass, coupled with excessive sodium intake, can cause primary hypertension in children or set the stage for its development later in life. (Adapted from Voors & Berenson, 1981.)

aorta become less distensible (i.e., more rigid), greater systolic pressure will be generated within it, even if the volume remains the same.

Peripheral vascular resistance helps to determine diastolic pressure. Because increased resistance causes decreased flow, any increase in peripheral vascular resistance will result in decreased flow to the microcirculation from the arteries. This in essence creates a pressure backup and results in a smaller than usual decrease in blood pressure during diastole.

Risk factors (such as smoking, obesity, hypercholesteremia, diabetes mellitus, positive family history, poor fitness, and increased sodium intake) have been correlated with the development of hypertension in adults. In recent years, much research has been done to assess the importance and interrelatedness of these factors in the development of hypertension (and coronary artery disease) in children (Fig. 28-16).

Obesity has been identified as one of these factors. Approximately 50% to 60% of hypertensive children are obese. Obesity in the high school population as a whole is about 10% to 15%. For many hypertensive children, a weight loss of 15 pounds can cause a decrease in diastolic pressure of 15 mm Hg. Conversely, another study showed that weight gain was associated with the development of hypertension in a group of adolescents (Kotchen & Kotchen, 1983). Sodium intake is also a known correlate of hypertension. In industrialized nations with a high salt intake, the incidence of hypertension is greater than in those countries with low salt intake (Berenson, 1980). This correlation gains strength in those individuals with a family history of hypertension—there may undoubtedly be a genetic interaction as well.

Some differences in the development of hypertension in children are race related (Berenson et al., 1984). Black children generally develop a greater body mass than white children and also have a decreased ability to achieve sodium and water balance. (Imbalances of sodium and water are described in Chapter 3.) Increased body mass could increase blood volume and cardiac output, both of which can increase blood pressure (Berenson et al., 1984). In addition, if sodium intake is high, the decreased sodium-handling ability in blacks may contribute to the earlier onset of hypertension. The race-related risk factors differ slightly for white children. White children have a greater percentage of body fat for their weight (as opposed to greater body mass), more of a tendency toward obesity, faster heart rates, higher levels of blood sugar, and higher renin and dopamine-β-hydroxylase levels than black children. These findings suggest that hypertension in black children is associated with body mass and renal mechanisms, whereas hypertension in white children is associated with obesity and neurohumoral factors (Berenson et al., 1984).

High cholesterol levels may also be a significant risk factor for hypertension in children because high cholesterol levels are associated with atherosclerosis. Several studies in different areas of the United States show that 5% to 9% of school-age children tested have serum cholesterol levels of 220 mg/dl or more (Engle, 1981). Though it is hard to say with certainty that all of those children are at risk for atherosclerosis, it is known that the incidence of hypercholesteremia is much greater in children with a family history of heart disease and hypercholesteremia than in children with no such history (Croft, et al., 1988).

Smoking doubles the risk of hypertension and other cardiovascular diseases at any age. The number of children who smoke seems to be increasing. It is estimated that approximately 40% of both black and white adolescents are smoking by high school age (Berensen et al., 1984).

The interrelationships among these risk factors are currently being studied in children. The precise relevance of each is not yet known. It seems logical to assume that the more factors that are present, the greater the risk of hypertension will be. What remains to be seen is how assessment of these factors can be used to identify and treat children at risk for hypertension and the later development of cardiovascular disease.

Diagnosis of primary hypertension in children is difficult because (1) the early stages of primary hypertension (which children are likely to have) are asymptomatic, and (2) normal blood pressures vary from child to child and change continuously as the child grows. It is not surprising that "normal" blood pressure in children is still being debated. Longitudinal studies in which blood pressure was measured under controlled conditions in children of various races and economic backgrounds indicated that normal systolic and diastolic values are considerably lower than was previously thought (Berenson, 1980; Kotchen & Kotchen, 1983). Currently, normal values are usually computed by age, but research indicates that height and weight (body mass) are more important than age in determining normal blood pressure in children (Berenson, 1980). (In Fig. 28-17, blood pressures are plotted by age, weight, and height.)

Blood pressure tends to remain at about the same percentile as the child grows older. A child who is consistently at the 95th percentile may well be at risk for adult hypertension and cardiovascular disease. Some clinicians base their treatment of childhood hypertension on this belief, and prescribe antihypertensive medications for children whose blood pressures are above the 90th or 95th percentile. The preventive efficacy of antihypertensive therapy during childhood is debated among researchers and clinicians, some of whom prefer to emphasize the control or elimination of risk factors.

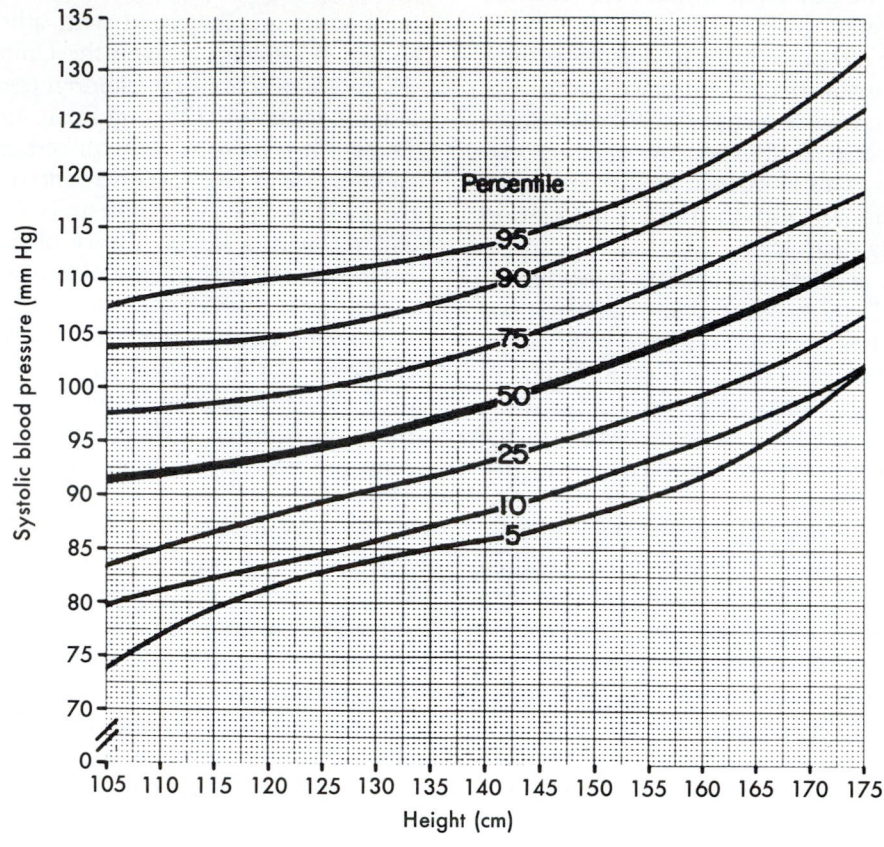

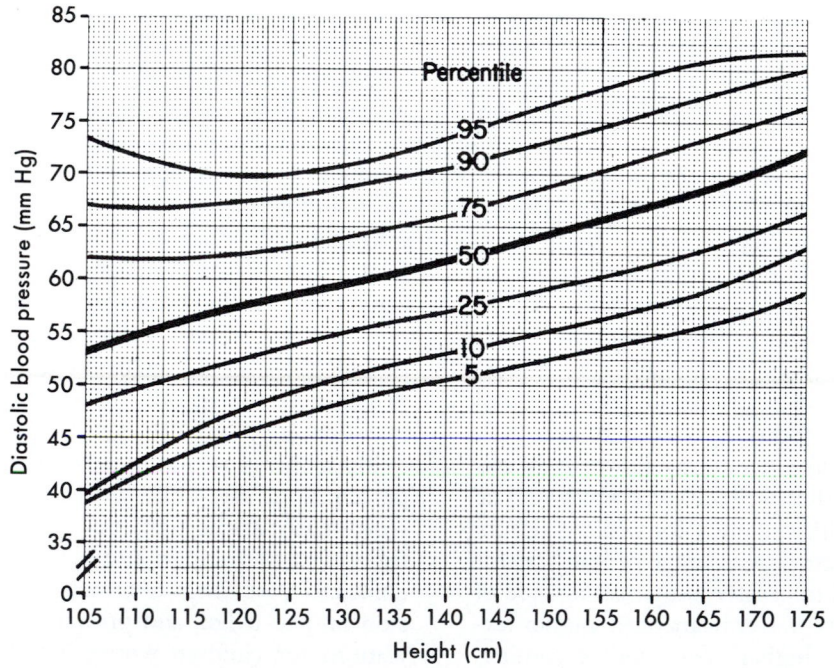

FIG. 28-17. Systolic and diastolic blood pressures by weight. The heavy lines indicate 50th percentile, or the midpoint in distribution of blood pressure values. Children who are above the 90th percentile for their age are hypertensive. (From Berenson, 1980.)

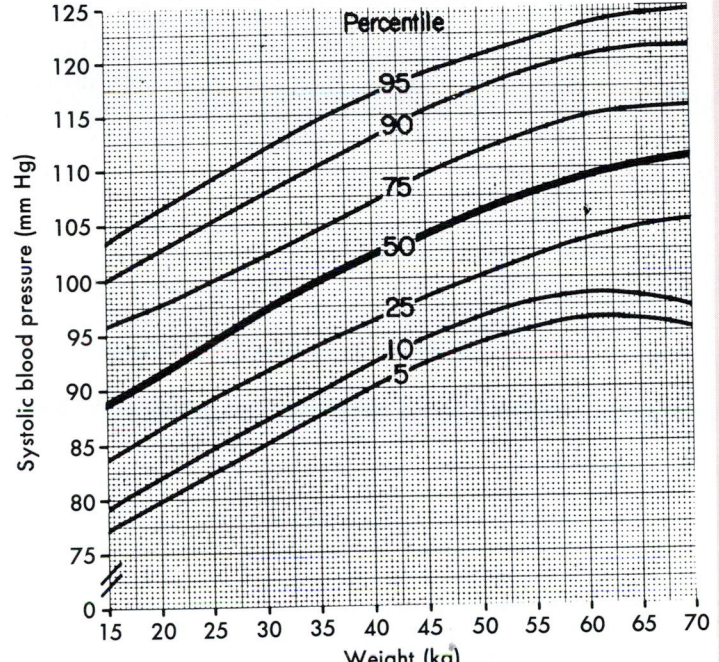

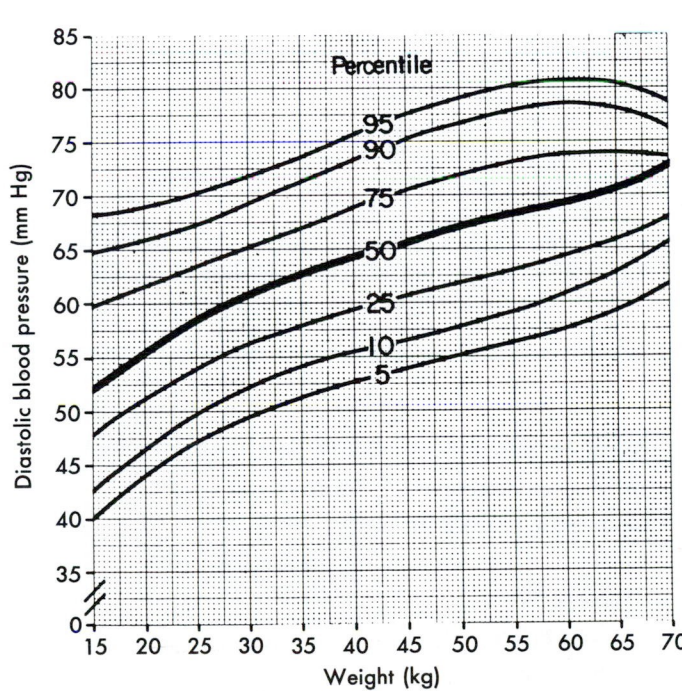

FIG. 28-17, **cont'd.** For legend see opposite page.

SUMMARY REVIEW

Development of the Cardiovascular System

1 The heart arises from the mesenchyme and begins as an enlarged blood vessel with a large lumen and a muscular wall. By about the eighth week of gestation, all of the structures of the fetal heart and vascular system are present.

2 Fetal blood is oxygenated in the placenta and returned to the fetus through the umbilical vein.

3 In the fetus, the pulmonary and systemic circulatory systems are connected by the foramen ovale, an opening between the atria; by the ductus arteriosus, a fetal vessel that joins the pulmonary artery to the aorta; and by the ductus venosus, a fetal vessel that connects the inferior vena cava to the umbilical vein.

4 Fetal blood flow depends on resistance for its distribution through the body. Resistance in the pulmonary circulation is higher than resistance in the systemic circulation, so myocardial thickness is about the same in the right heart and the left heart.

5 After birth, systemic resistance rises and pulmonary resistance falls.

6 Pulmonary vascular resistance drops suddenly at birth because the lungs expand and the pulmonary vessels dilate. It continues to decrease gradually over the first 6 to 8 weeks after birth. Decreased resistance causes the right myocardium to thin out.

7 Systemic vascular resistance increases markedly at birth because severance of the umbilical cord removes the low resistance placenta from the systemic circulation. Increased systemic resistance causes the right myocardium to thicken.

8 Changes in resistance cause the fetal connections between the pulmonary and systemic circulatory systems to disappear. The foramen ovale closes functionally at birth and anatomically several months later; the ductus arteriosus closes functionally 15 to 18 hours after birth and anatomically within 10 to 21 days; and the ductus venosus closes within 1 week after birth.

Congenital Heart Defects

1 Most congenital cardiovascular defects have begun to develop by the eighth week of gestation, and most have many causes, both environmental and genetic.

2 Environmental risk factors associated with the incidence of congenital heart defects typically are maternal conditions. Among these are viral infections, diabetes, drug intake, and advanced maternal age.

3 Genetic factors associated with congenital heart defects include but are not limited to Down syndrome, trisomy 13-16, trisomy 18, cri-du-chat syndrome, and Turner syndrome.

4 Classification of congenital heart defects is based on (a) whether they cause blood flow to the lungs to increase, decrease, or remain normal and (b) whether they cause cyanosis.

5 Cyanosis, a bluish discoloration of the skin, indicates

that the tissues are not receiving adequate oxygenated blood. Cyanosis can be caused by defects that (a) restrict blood flow into the pulmonary circulation, (b) overload the pulmonary circulation, causing pulmonary hypertension, pulmonary edema, and respiratory difficulty, or (c) cause large amounts of unoxygenated blood to shunt from the pulmonary to the systemic circulation.

6 Congenital defects that maintain or create direct communication between the pulmonary and systemic circulatory systems cause blood to shunt from one system to another, mixing oxygenated and unoxygenated blood and increasing blood volume and pressure on the receiving side of the shunt.

7 The direction of shunting through an abnormal communication depends on differences in pressure and resistance between the two systems. Flow is always from an area of high pressure to an area of low pressure.

8 Obstruction of ventricular outflow is commonly due to pulmonary stenosis (right ventricle) or coarctation of the aorta (left ventricle).

9 Despite obstruction, ventricular outflow remains normal because of compensatory ventricular hypertrophy stimulated by increased afterload and, in postductal coarctation of the aorta, development of collateral circulation around the coarctation.

10 Congestive heart failure can develop as a result of right ventricular obstruction if afterload backs up into the pulmonary circulation. Congestive heart failure can result from left ventricular obstruction in preductal coarctation of the aorta in which left-to-right shunting through the patent ductus arteriosus greatly increases blood flow into the pulmonary circulation.

11 Acyanotic congenital defects that increase pulmonary blood flow consist of abnormal openings (ventricular septal defect, patent ductus arteriosus, or atrial septal defect) that permit blood to shunt from left (systemic circulation) to right (pulmonary circulation). Cyanosis does not occur because the left-to-right shunt does not interfere with the flow of oxygenated blood through the systemic circulation.

12 If the abnormal communication between the left and right circuits is large, volume and pressure overload in the pulmonary circulation leads to congestive heart failure.

13 Cyanotic congenital defects that increase pulmonary blood flow are due to abnormal development of the great vessels. These defects include persistent truncus arteriosus, complete transposition of the great vessels, and total anomalous pulmonary venous connection.

14 In persistent truncus arteriosus, the truncus arteriosus fails to divide longitudinally into the aorta and pulmonary artery. All of the blood from both ventricles enters the truncus, so that mixed blood is delivered to both circulatory systems, causing cyanosis and failure to thrive.

15 In complete transposition of the great vessels, the circulatory systems are not connected serially or through a shunt, so that oxygenated blood remains permanently in the pulmonary circulation and unoxygenated blood remains permanently in the systemic circulation. Life is possible while the ductus arteriosus remains patent; after that, surgical intervention is mandatory.

16 Total anomalous pulmonary venous connection is caused by the persistence of the fetal common pulmonary artery and the lack of pulmonary venous return to the left atrium. All blood from the pulmonary and systemic circulations enters the right atrium. Mixed blood enters the left atrium through an atrial septal defect, then flows into the systemic circulation and causes cyanosis. Obstruction in the common pulmonary vein causes pressure to back up into the lungs, leading to congestive heart failure.

17 In cyanotic heart defects that decrease pulmonary blood flow (tetralogy of Fallot, tricuspid atresia), myocardial hypertrophy cannot compensate for restricted right ventricular outflow. Flow to the lungs decreases, and cyanosis is due to an insufficient volume of oxygenated blood.

18 Treatment for all congenital defects is surgical correction of the anomaly and management of cyanosis and congestive heart failure.

Acquired Cardiovascular Disorders

1 The most common acquired cardiovascular disorders of childhood are congestive heart failure, rheumatic heart disease, and hypertension.

2 Congestive heart failure is usually the result of congenital heart defects that increase blood volume and pressure in the pulmonary circulation. Clinical manifestations are almost the same as the manifestations of congestive heart failure in adults. Unique manifestations in children include failure to thrive and periorbital edema.

3 Rheumatic heart disease, like rheumatic heart disease in adults, begins with acute pharyngeal infection by a group A β-hemolytic streptococcus that leads to valvular dysfunction.

4 Primary hypertension in children is the same as that in adults, except that it is more likely to be in its early, asymptomatic stage.

KEY TERMS

Acyanotic defect, 999

Atrial septal defect (ASD), 1006

Coarctation of the aorta, 1001

Complete transposition of the great vessels, 1009

Cyanosis, 999

Cyanotic defect, 999

Ductus arteriosus, 994

Ductus venosus, 994

Eisenmenger syndrome, 1003

Foramen ovale, 994

Infundibular stenosis, 1000

Left-to-right shunt, 999

Patent ductus arteriosus (PDA), 1005

Persistent truncus arteriosus (PTA), 1007

Postductal coarctation, 1001

Preductal coarctation (infantile coarctation), 1001

Pulmonary atresia, 1000

Pulmonary stenosis, 1000

Right-to-left shunt, 999

Shunt, 999

Stenosis, 999

Supravalvular stenosis, 1000

Tetralogy of Fallot, 1012

Total anomalous pulmonary venous connection (TAPVC), 1010

Tricuspid atresia , 1014

Truncus arteriosus, 993

Ventricular septal defect (VSD), 1003

REFERENCES

Adams, F. H., & Emmanouilides, G. C. (Eds.). (1983). *Moss' heart disease in infants, children, and adolescents* (3rd ed.). Baltimore: Williams & Wilkins.

Arciniegas, E. (Ed.). (1985). *Pediatric cardiovascular surgery*. Chicago: Year Book Medical Publishers.

Berenson, G. S. (1980). *Cardiovascular risk factors in children*. New York: Oxford University Press.

Berenson, G. S., Webber, L. S., Srinivasan, S. R., Cresanta, J. L., Frank, G. C., & Farris, R. P. (1984). Black-white contrasts as determinants of cardiovascular risk in childhood: Precursors of coronary artery and primary hypertensive diseases. *American Heart Journal, 108,* 3.

Croft J. B., Cresanta, J. L., Webber, L.S., Srinivasan, S. R., Freedman, D. S., Burke, G. L., Berenson, G. S. (1988). Cardiovascular risk in parents of children with extreme lipoprotein cholesterol levels: the Bogalusa Heart Study. *Southern Medical Journal, 81*(3), 341-349, 353.

Doyle, E. F., & Rutkowski, M. (1970). Etiology of congenital heart disease. *Cardiovascular Clinics, 2,* 2.

Engle, M. E. (Ed.). (1981). *Pediatric cardiovascular disease*. Philadelphia: F. A. Davis.

Fink, B. W. (1985). *Congenital heart disease* (2nd ed.). Chicago: Year Book Medical Publishers.

Ganong, W. F. (1975). *Review of medical physiology*. Los Altos, CA: Lange Medical Publications.

Giboney, G. S. (1983). Ventricular septal defect. *Heart and Lung, 12,* 3.

Gow, B. S. (1980). Circulatory correlates: Vascular impedance, resistance and capacity. In D. F. Bohr, A. P. Somlyo, & H. V. Sparks, Jr. (Eds.), *Handbook of physiology, Section 2: The cardiovascualr system*. Bethesda, MD: American Physiological Society.

Graham, G., & Rossi, E. (Eds.). (1980). *Heart disease in infants and children*. Chicago: Year Book Medical Publications.

Guyton, A. C. (1986). *Textbook of medical physiology* (7th ed.). Philadelphia: W. B. Saunders.

Guzzetta, C., & Dossey, B. M. (Eds.). (1984). *Cardiovascular nursing: Bodymind tapestry*. St. Louis: C. V. Mosby.

Hedges, J. R. (1983). Preload and afterload revisited. *Journal of Emergency Nursing, 9,* 5.

Kaplan, E. L. (1988). A comeback for rheumatic fever? *Patient Care, 22*(5), 80-84.

Keith, J. D., Rowe, R. D., & Vlad, P. (Eds.). (1978). *Heart disease in infancy and childhood* (3rd ed.). New York: MacMillan.

Kotchen, T. A., & Kotchen, J. M. (Eds.). (1983). *Clinical approaches to high blood pressure in the young*. Boston: John Wright·PSG Inc.

Langley, L. L., Telford, I. R., & Christensen, J. B. (1974). *Dynamic anatomy and physiology*. New York: McGraw-Hill.

Levine, H. E. (Ed.). (1976). *Clinical cardiovascular physiology*. New York: Grune & Stratton.

Moller, J. H., & Neal, W. A. (1981). *Heart disease in infancy*. New York: Appleton-Century-Crofts.

Mott, W. R., Fazekas, N. F., & James, S. R. (1985). *Nursing care of children and families*. Menlo Park, CA: Addison-Wesley.

Park, M. K. (1988). *Pediatric cardiology for practitioners* (2nd ed.). Chicago: Year Book Medical Publishers.

Perloff, J. K., Friedman, W. F., Laks, H., & Child, J. S. (1983). From cyanotic infant to a cyanotic adult—The odyssey of blue babies. *The Western Journal of Medicine, 139*(5), 673-687.

Roberts, W. C. (1987). *Adult congenital heart disease*. Philadelphia: F. A. Davis.

Ruch, T. L., & Patton, H. D. (1974). *Physiology and biophysics*. Philadelphia: W. B. Saunders.

Rudolph, A. M. (1974). *Congenital diseases of the heart: Clinical-physiologic considerations in diagnosis and management*. Chicago: Year Book Medical Publishers.

Rushmer, R. F. (1972). *Structure and function of the cardiovascular system*. Philladelphia: W. B. Saunders.

Ruttenberg, A. D. (1986). Acute rheumatic fever in the 1980s. *Pediatrician, 13*(4), 180-188.

Smith, J. B. (Ed.). (1983). *Pediatric critical care*. New York: John Wiley & Sons.

Thompson, J. M., McFarland, G. K., Hirsch, J. E., Tucker, S. M., & bowers, A. C. (1989). *Mosby's manual of clinical nursing* (2nd ed.). St. Louis: C. V. Mosby.

Tyson, K. R. T. (1975). Congenital heart disease in infants. *Ciba Clinical Symposia, 27,* 3.

Vaughn, V. C., McKay, R. J., & Behrman, R. E. (Eds.). (1985). *Nelson textbook of pediatrics* (12th ed.). Philadelphia: W. B. Saunders.

Voors, A. W., & Berenson, G. S. (1981). In G. Onesti & K. E. Kin (Eds.), *Phasic pressor mechanisms: Hypertension in the young and the old*. New York: Grune & Stratton.

West, J. B. (1985). *Best and Taylor's physiologic basis of medical practice* (11th ed.). Baltimore: Williams & Wilkins.

Whaley, L. F., & Wong, D. L. (1987). *Nursing care of infants and children* (3rd ed.). St. Louis: C. V. Mosby.

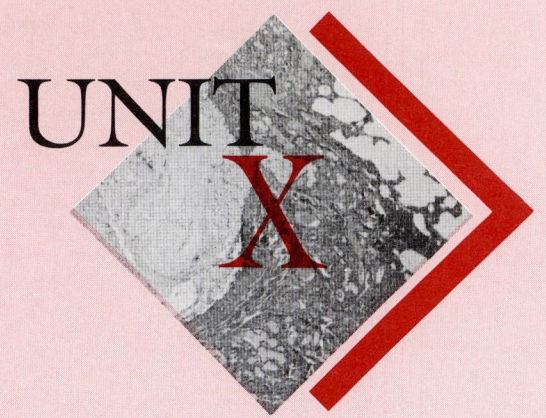

UNIT
X

The Pulmonary System

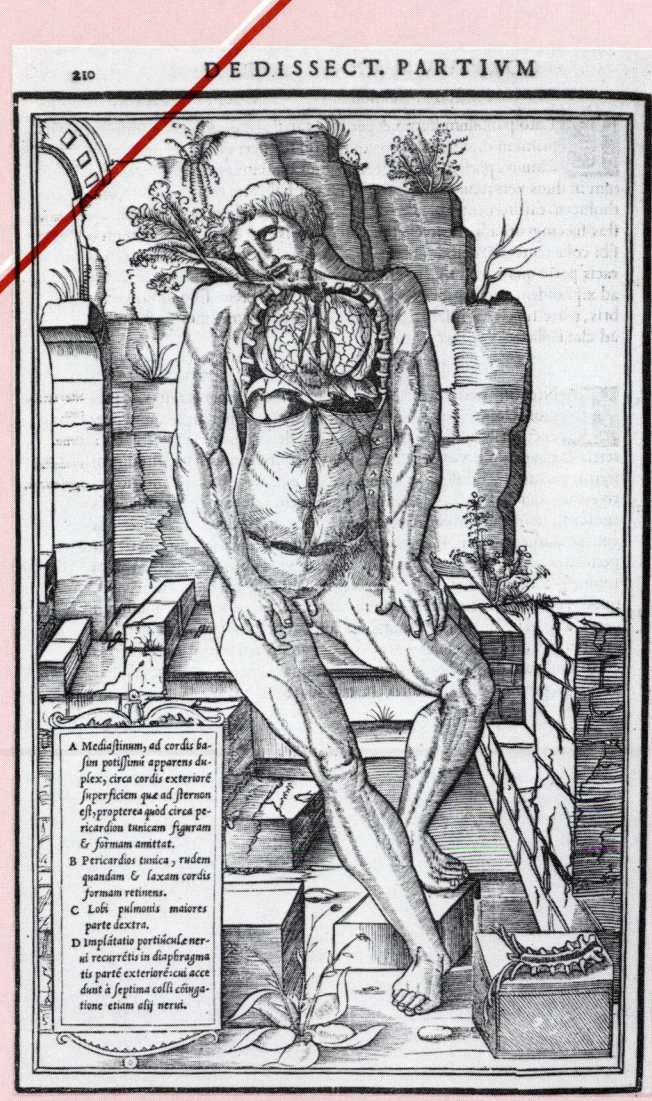

Respiratory system. Cadaver seated on ruin. Front view, with chest open to show lungs, diaphragm, etc. (From Estienne, C.: *De dissectione partium corporis humani,* Paris, 1545. Courtesy National Library of Medicine.)

THOUGH pulmonary disease has been documented as a significant problem since the time of Hippocrates, human understanding and knowledge of respiratory physiology, pathology, and therapy were extremely limited until the end of the nineteenth and beginning of the twentieth century. At the time of Hippocrates it was believed that the purpose of the lungs was to cool the heart. Early physicians thought air entered the heart directly through the lungs and pulmonary vein, bringing to the body "vital forces" responsible for life. An imbalance of these forces, or "humors," was felt to cause disease. In the second century A.D., asthma, the term then used to describe most respiratory diseases, was felt to be the result of excessive and thick secretions that dripped into the lung from the brain.

Leonardo DaVinci was the first to document that the airways of the lungs had no direct connection to the heart, and in the 1600s William Harvey accurately described the pulmonary circulation. Oxygen and carbon dioxide were not identified until the 1700s. In the 1800s the hemoglobin molecule was discovered, and Adolph Fick described the relationship of blood oxygen content, metabolism, and cardiac output. It was not until 1910 that the mechanism for the exchange of oxygen and carbon dioxide in the lung was established. Pulmonary mechanics and the principles of acid-base physiology were first understood in the early 1900s.

Misconceptions about the structure and function of the pulmonary system severely limited early attempts to treat respiratory disease. For example, during the time of the Romans, tuberculosis was treated with a special root that was dug up before dawn and wrapped in the wool of a sheep who had just given birth to a ewe lamb. The treatment recommended for tuberculosis in the first century A.D., rest and a good diet, remained essentially the same for centuries. It was not until the Middle Ages that tuberculosis was even considered to be contagious. By the 1800s contagion was feared to the extent that individuals with tuberculosis were sent to sanitoriums, where they were isolated from the general population. The tubercle bacillus was not identified by Robert Koch until 1890, and there was little change in treatment until 1944, when streptomycin was developed.

Within the last 100 years mortality and morbidity from pulmonary diseases have decreased dramatically, yet these diseases are a major cause of death and disability today. Such diseases as asthma, bronchitis, and emphysema are now better understood, but a definitive treatment for them has not yet been discovered. Others, particularly chronic obstructive pulmonary disease, lung cancer, and occupational diseases, are on the increase. Some respiratory diseases, such as respiratory distress syndrome, are "new" in that they occur in individuals whose treatments have enabled them to survive other disorders that proved fatal in the past. Today progress is being made toward (1) further understanding of the mechanisms of pulmonary disease, (2) early detection and treatment of disease, (3) development of new therapies, and (4) prevention of disease through public education, improvements in environmental and occupational safety standards, and air quality.

CHAPTER 29

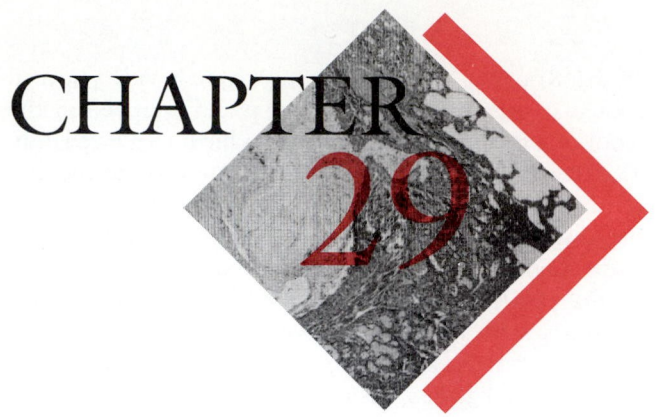

Structure and Function of the Pulmonary System

Marjorie Budd

Structures of the pulmonary system, 1026
    Conducting airways, 1026
    Gas-exchange airways, 1030
    Pulmonary and bronchial circulation, 1031
    Chest wall and pleura, 1034
Function of the pulmonary system, 1034
    Ventilation, 1034
        Measurement of gas pressure, 1034
        Measurement of lung volumes and capacities, 1036
        Mechanics of breathing, 1037
            Major and accessory muscles, 1037
            Alveolar surface tension, 1038
            Elastic properties of the lung and chest wall, 1038
            Airway resistance, 1039
            Work of breathing, 1040
    Neurochemical control of ventilation, 1040
        Lung receptors, 1041
        Chemoreceptors, 1042
    Control of the pulmonary circulation, 1042
    Gas transport, 1043
        Distribution of ventilation and perfusion, 1043
        Oxygen transport, 1044
            Diffusion across the alveolocapillary membrane, 1044
            Determinants of arterial oxygenation, 1045
            Oxyhemoglobin association and dissociation, 1046
        Carbon dioxide transport, 1047
Tests of pulmonary function, 1048
Aging and the pulmonary system, 1050

The pulmonary system consists of the lungs, airways, chest wall, and pulmonary circulation. Its primary function is the exchange of gases between the environmental air and the blood. There are three steps in this process: (1) ventilation, the movement of air into and out of the lungs; (2) diffusion, the movement of gases between air spaces in the lungs and the bloodstream; and (3) perfusion, the movement of blood into and out of the capillary beds of the lungs to body organs, and tissues. The first two functions are carried out by the pulmonary system and the third by the cardiovascular system (see Chapter 26). Normally the pulmonary system functions efficiently under a variety of conditions and with little energy expenditure.

STRUCTURES OF THE PULMONARY SYSTEM

The pulmonary system is made up of two lungs, their airways, and the blood vessels that serve them (Fig. 29-1) and the chest wall, or thoracic cage. The lungs are divided into lobes, three in the right lung (upper, middle, and lower) and two in the left lung (upper and lower). Each lobe is further divided into segments and lobules. The space between the lungs, which contains the heart, is called the mediastinum. A set of tubes, or conducting airways, delivers air to each section of the lung. The lung tissue that surrounds the airways supports them, preventing their distortion or collapse as gas moves in and out during ventilation.

The lungs are exposed to a variety of exogenous contaminants, yet the defense mechanisms of the respiratory system are such that contamination of lung tissue itself, particularly by infectious agents, is rare. Table 29-1 summarizes the mechanical barriers that protect the lungs. (Other mechanisms of self-defense are discussed in Chapters 6 and 7.)

Conducting Airways

The conducting airways are the portion of the pulmonary system that provides a passage for the movement of air into and out of the gas-exchange portions of the lung. They consist of upper and lower airways. The **nasopharynx** and **oropharynx** and related structures are often called the upper airway (Fig. 29-2). These structures are lined with a ciliated mucosa with a very rich vascular supply. The mucosal lining warms and humidifies inspired air and removes foreign particles from it as it passes into the lungs. During quiet breathing gas usually flows through the nose, nasopharynx, and oropharynx to the lower airways. The mouth and oropharynx are also used for ventilation when the nose is obstructed or when increased flow is required, for example, during exercise. Filtering and humidifying are not, however, as efficient with mouth breathing.

The **larynx** connects the upper and lower airways. The structure of the larynx consists of the endolarynx and its surrounding triangular-shaped bony and cartilaginous structures. The endolarynx is formed by two pairs of folds that form the false vocal cords (supraglottis) and the true vocal cords. The slit-shaped space between the true cords forms the glottis (Fig. 29-3). The vestibule is the space above the false vocal cords. The laryngeal box is formed of three large cartilages—the epiglottis, thyroid, and cricoid—and three smaller cartilages—the arytenoid, corniculate, and cuneiform—that are connected by ligaments. The supporting cartilages prevent collapse of the larynx during inspiration and swallowing. The internal laryngeal muscles control vocal cord length and tension, and the external laryngeal muscles move the larynx as a whole. Both sets of muscles are important to swallowing, respiration, and vocalization. The internal muscles contract during swallowing to prevent aspiration into the trachea and also contribute to voice pitch. The ciliated epithelium of the larynx warms, filters, and humidifies the air.

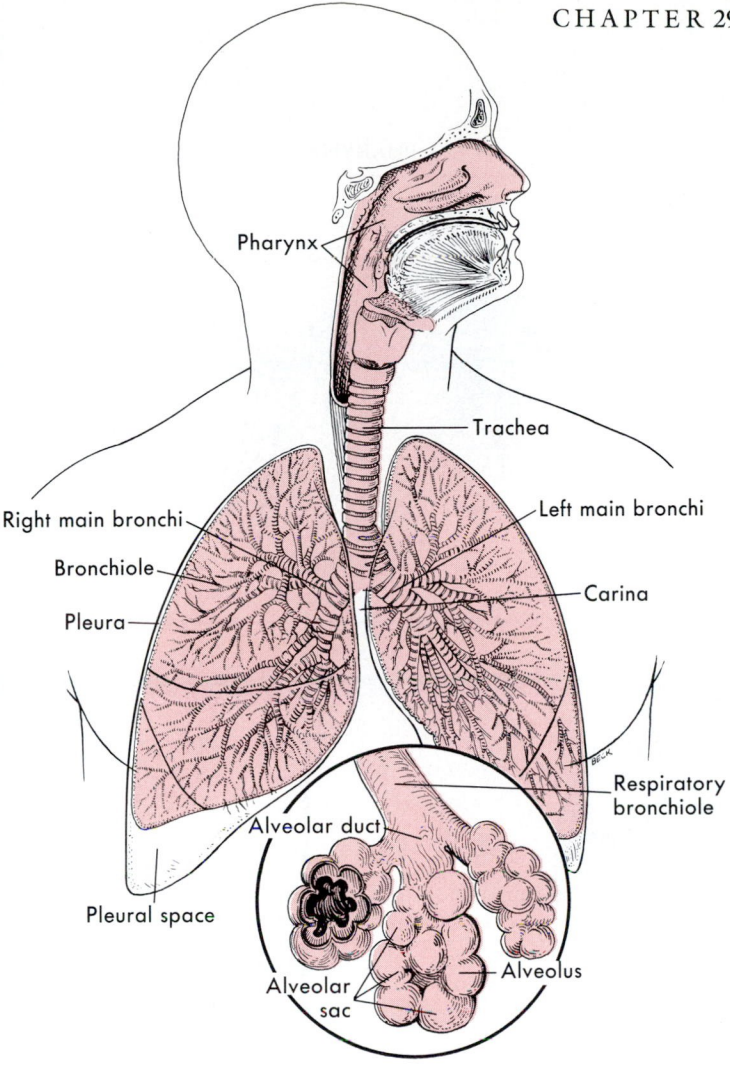

FIG. 29-1. Structures of the pulmonary system. The circle denotes the acinus, where oxygen and carbon dioxide are exchanged. (From Thibodeau, 1987.)

TABLE 29-1 Pulmonary defense mechanisms	
Structure or substance	**Mechanism of defense**
Upper respiratory tract mucosa	Maintains constant temperature and humidification of gas entering the lungs; traps and removes foreign particles, some bacteria, and noxious gases from inspired air
Nasal hairs and turbinates	Trap and remove foreign particles, some bacteria, and noxious gases from inspired air
Mucous blanket	Protects trachea and bronchi from injury; traps most foreign particles and bacteria that reach the lower airways
Cilia	Propel mucous blanket and entrapped particles toward the oropharynx, where they can be swallowed or expectorated
Alveolar macrophages	Ingest and removes bacteria and other foreign material from alveoli by phagocytosis (Chapters 6 and 7)
Irritant receptors in nares (nostrils)	Stimulation by chemical or mechanical irritants triggers sneeze reflex, which results in rapid removal of irritants from nasal passages
Irritant receptors in trachea and large airways	Stimulation by chemical or mechanical irritants triggers cough reflex, which results in removal of the irritant from the lower airways

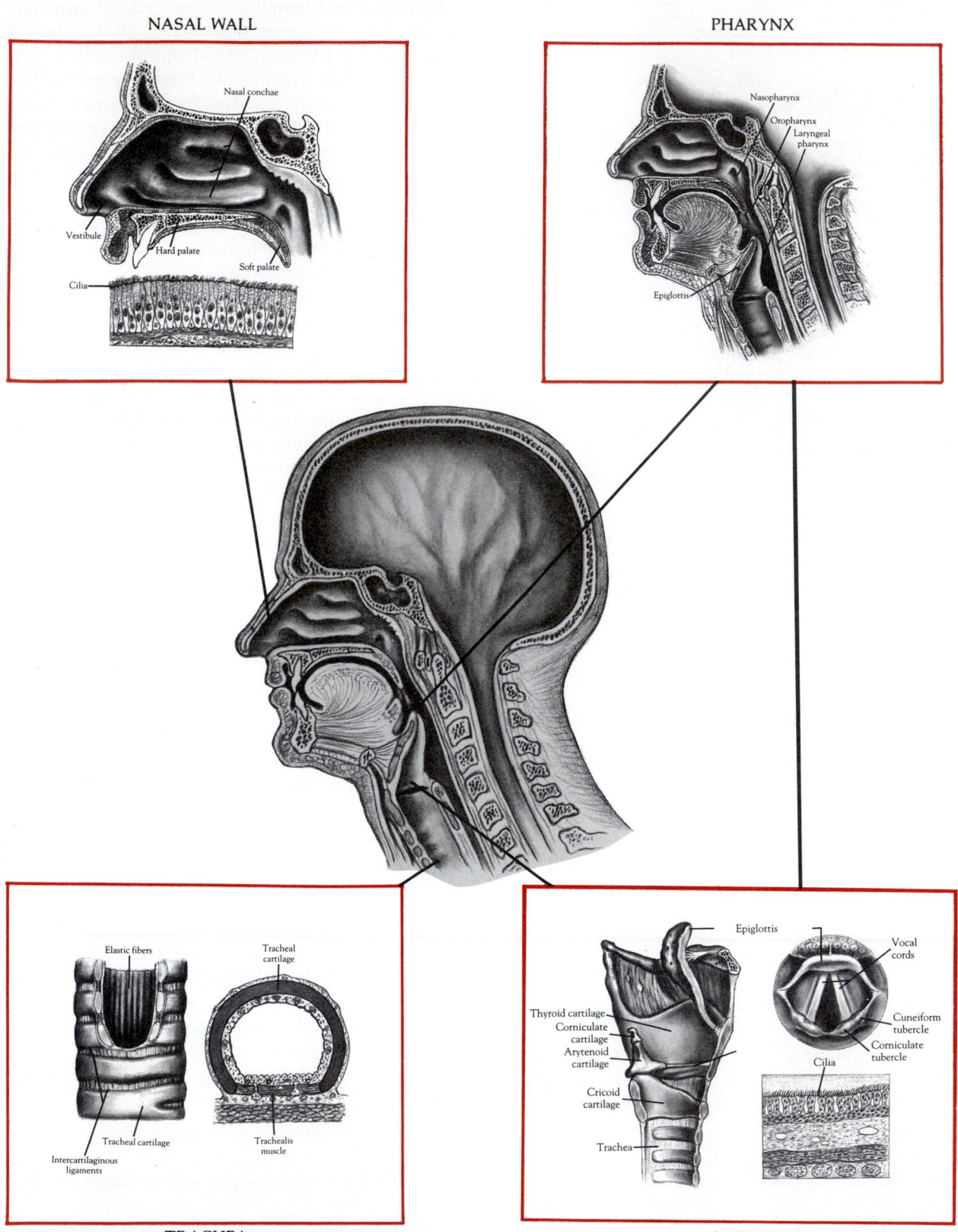

FIG. 29-2. Structures of the upper airway. (From Thompson et al., 1989.)

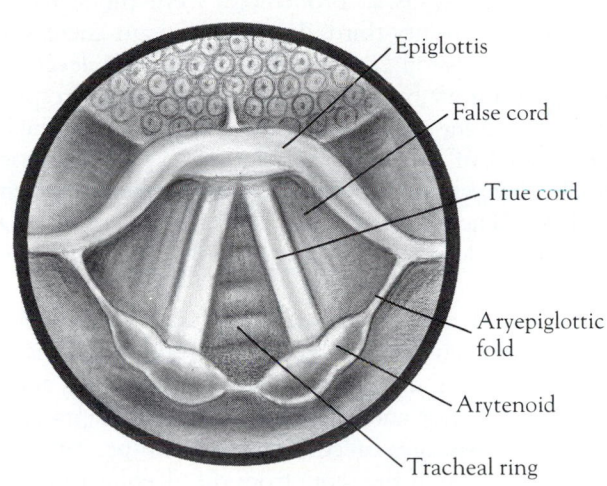

FIG. 29-3. Larynx in quiet respiration. (From Thompson et al., 1989).

The **trachea,** which is supported by U-shaped cartilage, connects the larynx to the **bronchi,** the conducting airways of the lungs. The trachea divides into the two main airways, or **bronchi,** at the **carina** (see Fig. 29-1). This area is very sensitive and when stimulated can cause coughing and airway narrowing. The right main bronchus extends from the trachea more vertically than the left main bronchus, so that aspirated fluids or foreign particles tend to enter the right lung rather than the left. The right and left main bronchi enter the lungs at the **hila,** or "roots" of the lungs, along with the pulmonary blood and lymphatic vessels. From the hila the main bronchi branch into lobar bronchi, then to segmental and subsegmental bronchi, and finally end at the sixteenth division in the smallest of the conducting airways, the terminal **bronchioles.**

The bronchial walls have three layers: an epithelial lining, a smooth muscle layer, and a connective tissue layer. In the large bronchi (to about the tenth division), the connective tissue layer contains cartilage. The epithelial lining of the bronchi contains single-celled exo-

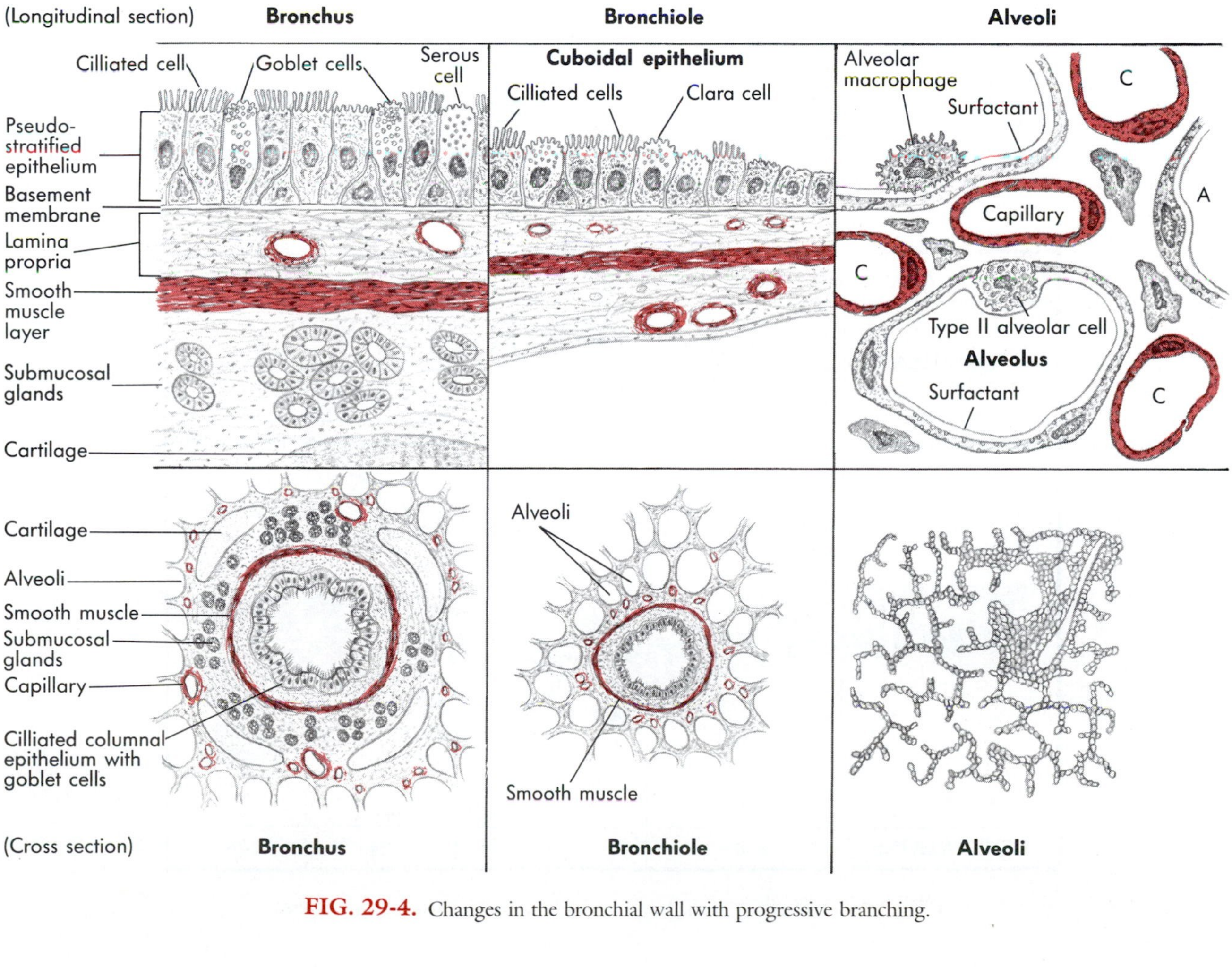

FIG. 29-4. Changes in the bronchial wall with progressive branching.

crine glands—the mucus-secreting **goblet cells**—and ciliated cells. High columnar pseudostratified epithelium lines the larger airways, changing to columnar cuboidal epithelium in the bronchioles (types of epithelium are illustrated in Chapter 1). The submucosal glands of the bronchial lining also produce mucus, contributing to the mucus blanket that covers the bronchial epithelium. The ciliated epithelial cells rhythmically beat this mucus blanket toward the trachea and pharynx, where it can be swallowed or expectorated by coughing. Foreign particles and microorganisms that are not expelled by mucociliary clearance and coughing are attacked by cellular components of the inflammatory response and antibodies of the secretory immune system (see Unit III). The biochemical mediators released early in inflammation also play a part in antibody-mediated hypersensitivity reactions, such as asthma, because they stimulate bronchial smooth muscles and blood vessels to constrict.

With branching the layers of epithelium that line the bronchi become thinner (Fig. 29-4). Mucus-producing glands are found only in the bronchi, and goblet cells are not found past the terminal bronchioles (seventeenth division). Ciliated cells are more sparse, and smooth muscle and connective tissue layers thin toward the terminal bronchioles.

Gas-Exchange Airways

The conducting airways terminate in gas-exchange airways, where oxygen (O_2) enters the blood and carbon dioxide (CO_2) is removed from it. The gas-exchange airways are made up of **respiratory bronchi-oles, alevolar ducts,** and **alveoli.** These structures together are sometimes called the **acinus** (Fig. 29-5), and all of them participate in gas exchange.

Because the walls of bronchioles from the sixteenth through the twenty-third divisions contain increasing numbers of alveoli, the bronchioles at this level are called respiratory bronchioles. The walls of the respiratory bronchioles are very thin, consisting of an epithelial layer devoid of cilia and goblet cells, very little smooth muscle fiber, and a very thin and elastic connective tissue layer. The respiratory bronchioles end in alveolar ducts, which lead to alveolar sacs made up of numerous alveoli.

The alveoli are the gas-exchange units of the lung, where oxygen enters the blood and carbon dioxide is removed. They are thin-walled, spherical structures about 3 mm in diameter and have shared walls, or septa (Fig. 29-6). Tiny passages called pores of Kohn permit some air to pass through the septa from the alveolus to alveolus, promoting collateral ventilation and even distribution of air among the alveoli. In cross sections alveoli appear similar to common sponges. The lungs contain approximately 25 million alveoli at birth and 300 million by adulthood. The alveoli of the lungs comprise a surface area of 70 to $100/m^2$, equivalent to that of a tennis court.

The alveolar septa consist of an epithelial layer and a thin, elastic basement membrane, but no muscle layer (Fig. 29-7). Two major types of epithelial cells appear in the alveolus. Type I alveolar cells provide structure, and type II alveolar cells secrete **surfactant,** a lipopro-

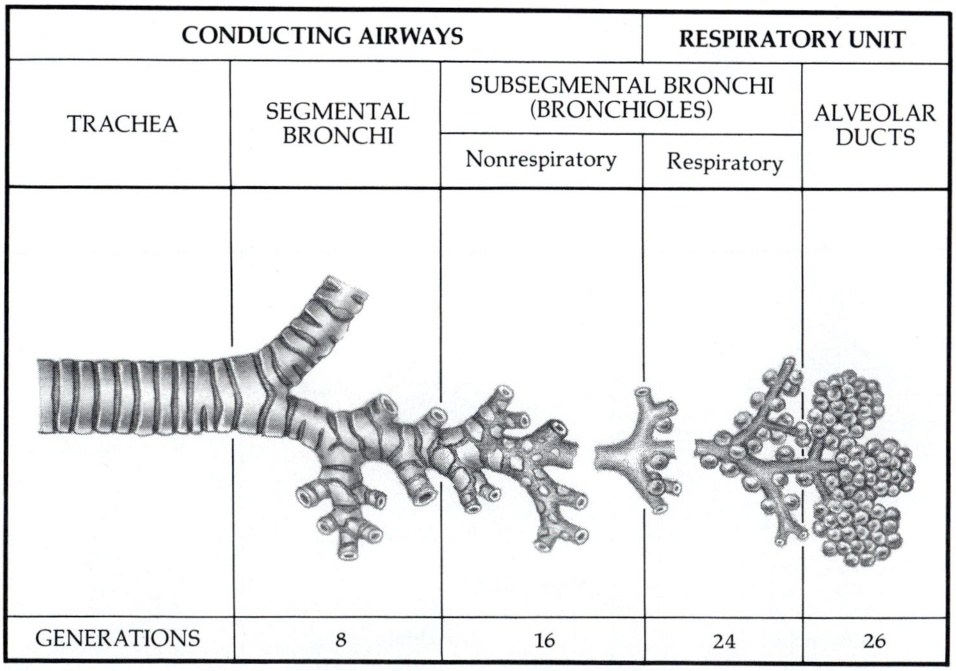

CONDUCTING AIRWAYS				RESPIRATORY UNIT
TRACHEA	SEGMENTAL BRONCHI	SUBSEGMENTAL BRONCHI (BRONCHIOLES)		ALVEOLAR DUCTS
		Nonrespiratory	Respiratory	
GENERATIONS	8	16	24	26

FIG. 29-5. Structures of the lower airway. (From Thompson et al., 1989.)

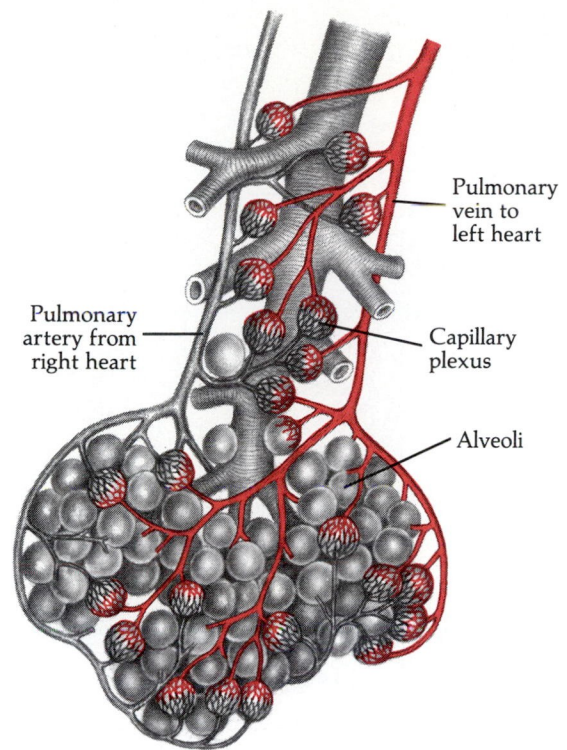

FIG. 29-6. Terminal respiratory units. (From Thompson et al., 1989.)

tein that coats the inner surface of the alveolus and facilitates its expansion during inspiration.

Like the bronchi, alveoli contain cellular components of inflammation and immunity, particularly the mononuclear phagocytes. The mononuclear phagocytes of the lungs are called alveolar macrophages. These cells ingest foreign material that reaches the alveolus and prepare it for removal via the lymphatics. (Phagocytosis and the mononuclear phagocyte system are described in Chapters 6 and 7.)

Pulmonary and Bronchial Circulation

The main function of the pulmonary circulation is to facilitate gas exchange. Its other functions are to deliver nutrients to lung tissues, act as a reservoir for the left ventricle, and serve as a filtering system that removes clots, air, and other debris from the circulation. The pulmonary circulation is illustrated in Fig. 29-8.

The pulmonary circulation has a lower pressure and resistance than the systemic circulation. Pulmonary arteries are exposed to about one fifth the pressure of the systemic circulation (mean pulmonary artery pressure is 18 mm Hg; mean aortic pressure is 90 mm Hg). The smooth muscle layer in normal pulmonary artery walls is much thinner than that in systemic vessel walls, and pulmonary arteries are more distensible than their systemic counterparts. (Systemic vessels are described in Chapter 26.)

Usually about one third of the pulmonary vessels are filled with blood (perfused) at any given time. Additional vessels become perfused when cardiac output increases. Therefore, increased delivery of blood to the lungs does not normally increase mean pulmonary artery pressure.

The pulmonary artery divides and enters the lung at the hilus with each main bronchus and branches with the bronchus at every division, so that every bronchus and bronchiole has an accompanying artery or arteriole.

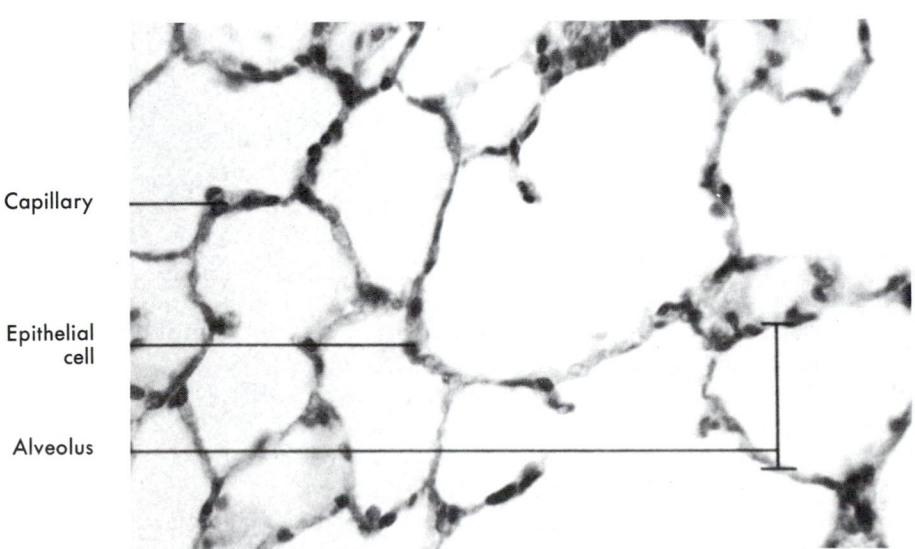

FIG. 29-7. Photomicrograph of lung, showing several alveoli. Note the proximity of the capillary to the alveolar wall (×140). (From Thibodeau, 1987.)

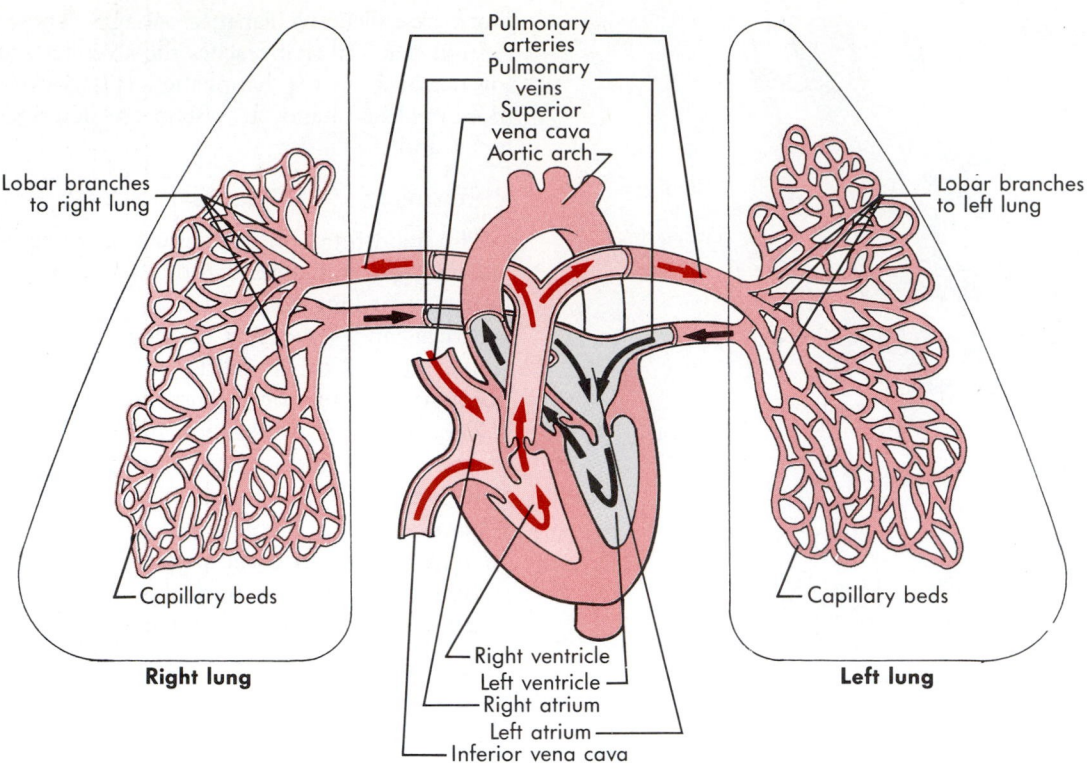

Lobar branches
to right lung

Pulmonary
arteries
Pulmonary
veins
Superior
vena cava
Aortic arch

Lobar branches
to left lung

Capillary beds

Capillary beds

Right lung

Left lung

Right ventricle
Left ventricle
Right atrium
Left atrium
Inferior vena cava

FIG. 29-8. The pulmonary circulation, illustrating the right and left pulmonary veins and arteries and the branching capillaries.

The arterioles, less than 1 mm in diameter, are thought to regulate blood flow through their respective capillary beds.

The arterioles divide at the terminal bronchiole to form a network of pulmonary capillaries around the acinus. The capillaries are an integral part of the alveolar septa. Capillary walls consist of an endothelial layer and a thin basement membrane, which often fuses with the basement membrane of the alveolar septum. This results in very little separation between blood in the capillary and gas in the alveolus.

The shared alveolar and capillary walls compose the **alveolocapillary membrane,** a very thin membrane made up of the alveolar epithelium, the alveolar basement membrane, an interstitial space, the capillary basement membrane, and the capillary endothelium (Fig. 29-9). Gas exchange occurs across the alveolocapillary membrane. With normal perfusion approximately 100 ml of blood in the pulmonary capillary bed is spread very thinly over 70 to 100 m^2 of alveolar surface area. This could be compared to spreading 100 ml of blood over a tennis court and covering it with a sheet of cellophane to separate it from the air. The alveolocapillary membrane efficiently exposes large quantities of blood

to gas in the alveoli. Any disorder that thickens the membrane impairs gas exchange.

Each pulmonary vein drains several pulmonary capillaries. Unlike the pulmonary arteries, which follow the branching bronchi, pulmonary veins are dispersed randomly throughout the lung, then leave the lung at the hila and enter the left atrium. They are similar to veins in the systemic circulation but have no valves.

The bronchial circulation is part of the systemic circulation. It supplies nutrients to the conducting airways, large pulmonary vessels, and membranes (pleura) that surround the lungs. The bronchial circulation is unique in that not all of its capillaries drain into its own venous system. Some of the bronchial capillaries empty into the pulmonary vein and contribute to the normal venous admixture (mixing of oxygenated and deoxygenated blood) or right-to-left shunt. It does not, however, participate in gas exchange.

Lung vasculature also includes deep and superficial lymphatic capillaries. The deep lymphatic capillaries begin at the level of the terminal bronchioles; there are no lymphatic structures in the acinus. Fluid and alveolar macrophages migrate from the alveoli to the terminal bronchioles, where they enter the lymphatic system. The

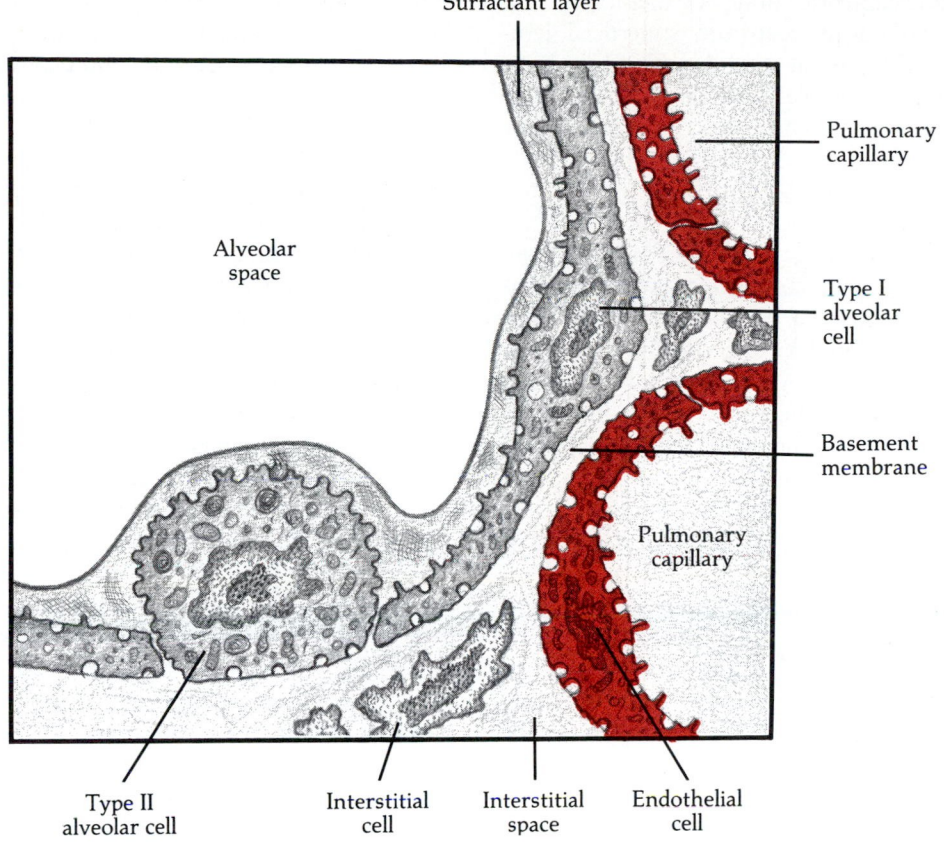

FIG. 29-9. Alveolar wall and space. (From Thompson et al., 1989.)

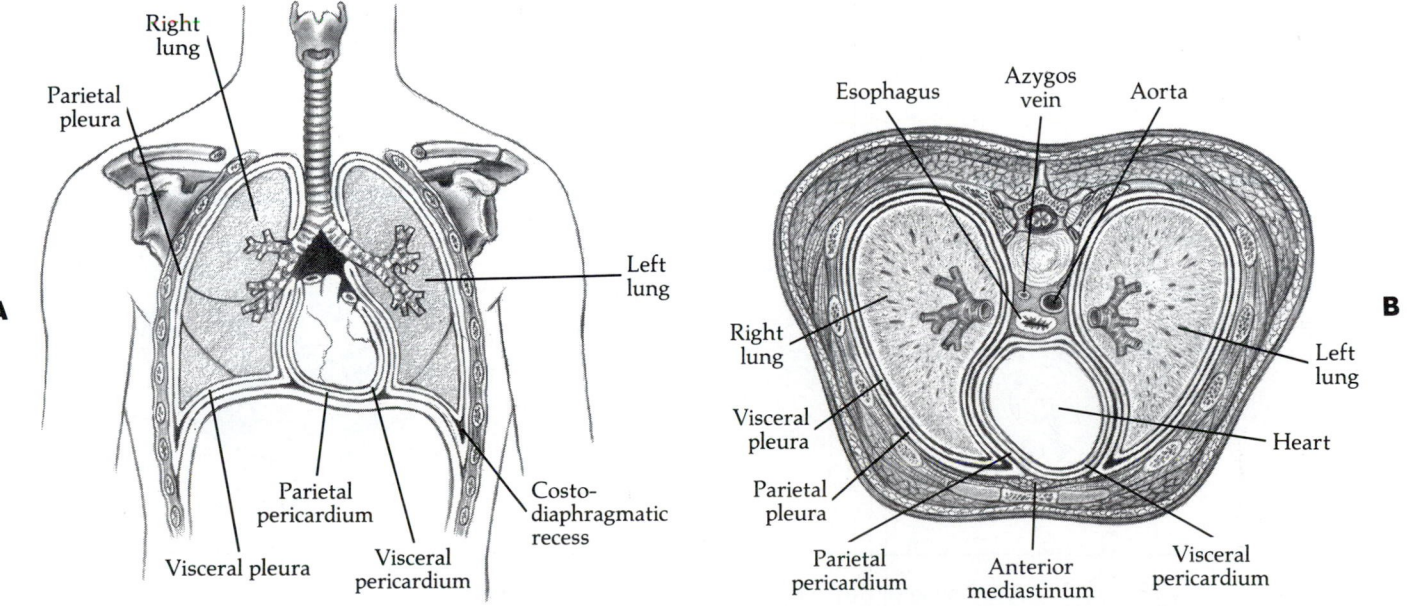

FIG. 29-10. Chest cavity and related structures. **A,** Anterior view; **B,** cross section. (From Thompson et al., 1989.)

superficial lymphatic capillaries drain the membrane that surrounds the lungs. Both deep and superficial lymphatic vessels leave the lung at the hilus. The lymphatic system plays an important role in keeping the lung free of fluid. (The lymphatic system is described in Chapter 26.)

Chest Wall and Pleura

The chest wall (thoracic cage) protects the lungs from injury, and its muscles, in conjunction with the diaphragm, perform the muscular work of breathing. The **thoracic cavity** is contained by the chest wall and encases the lungs (Fig. 29-10). A serous membrane called the **pleura** adheres firmly to the lungs. It then folds over itself and attaches firmly to the chest wall. The pleural membrane covering the lungs is the visceral pleura; that lining the thoracic cavity is the parietal pleura. The area between the two pleurae is called the **pleural space,** or pleural cavity. Normally only a thin layer of fluid secreted by the pleura (pleural fluid) fills the pleural space. This lubricates the pleural surfaces, allowing the two layers to slide over each other without separating. Pressure in the pleural space is usually negative or subatmospheric (-4 to -10 mm Hg).

FUNCTION OF THE PULMONARY SYSTEM

Ventilation

Ventilation is the mechanical movement of gas or air into and out of the lungs. Ventilation is often misnamed respiration, which is actually the exchange of oxygen and carbon dioxide during cellular metabolism. "Respiratory rate" is actually the ventilatory rate, or the number of times gas is inspired and expired per minute.

Measurement of Gas Pressure

A few physical characteristics of gas are important for an understanding of ventilation. A gas is made up of millions of molecules moving randomly. As they move they collide with each other and the wall of the space in which they are contained. These collisions exert pressure. If more molecules are present in the space, the pressure, or number of collisions, increases (Fig. 29-11). If the same number of gas molecules is contained in a small and a large container, the pressure is greater in the small container because more collisions occur in the smaller space. Increases in temperature increase the speed of the molecules, which increases the number of collisions. Therefore, pressure also increases at higher temperatures.

Barometric pressure (P_B) (atmospheric pressure) is the pressure exerted by gas molecules in air at specific altitudes. At sea level barometric pressure is 760 mm Hg. This number is the sum of the pressure exerted by each gas in the air at sea level. The portion of the total pressure exerted by any individual gas is its **partial pressure** (see Fig. 29-11). At sea level the air is made up of oxygen (20.9%), nitrogen (69.9%), and a few other trace gases. The partial pressure of oxygen is equal to the percentage of oxygen in the air (20.9) times the total pressure (760 mm Hg), or 159 mm Hg (760 × 0.209 = 158.84). (Symbols used in the measurement of gas pressures and pulmonary ventilation are defined in Table 29-2.)

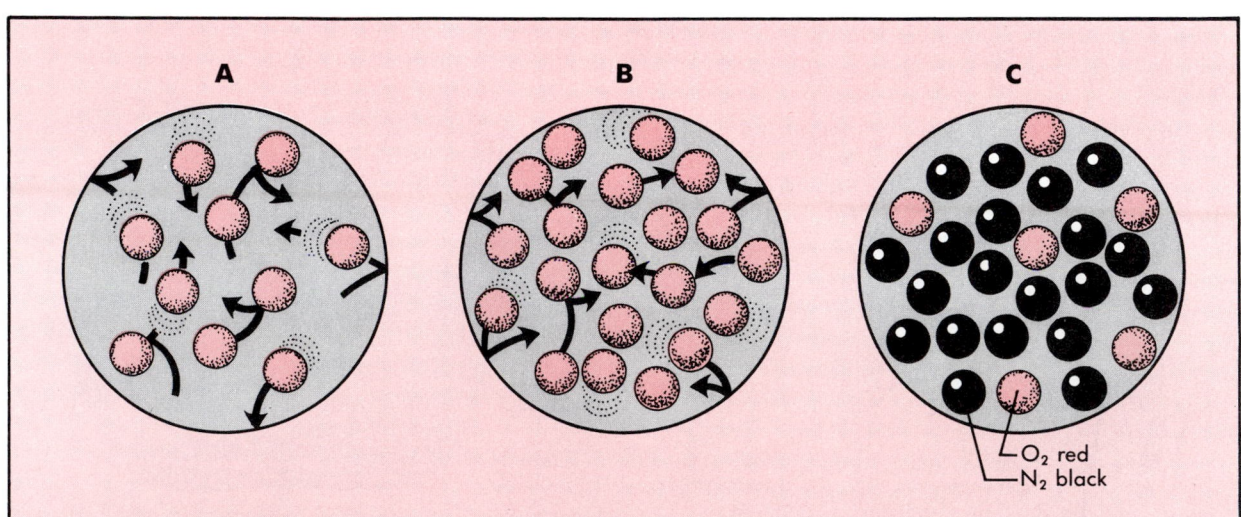

O_2 red
N_2 black

FIG. 29-11. Relationship between number of gas molecules and pressure exerted by the gas in an enclosed space. **A,** Theoretically 10 molecules of the same gas exert a total pressure of 10 within the space. **B,** If the number of molecules is increased to 20, total pressure is 20. **C,** If there are different gases in the space, each gas exerts a partial pressure: Here the partial pressure of nitrogen (N_2) is 18, that of oxygen (O_2) is 6, and total pressure is 24.

TABLE 29-2 Common pulmonary abbreviations

Symbol	Definition
V	Volume or amount of gas
Q	Perfusion or blood flow
P	Pressure (usually partial pressure) of a gas
S	Percentage of hemoglobin saturation with a gas (usually oxygen)
F	Fraction of gas, or gas flow (in a laboratory test)
C	Content or amount of gas
C_{TH}	Thoracic compliance
E	Expired gas
i	Inspired gas
A	Alveolar gas
a	Arterial blood
$\bar{v}$	Mixed venous or pulmonary artery blood
D	Dead space
Pa_{O_2}	Partial pressure of oxygen in arterial blood
PA_{O_2}	Partial pressure of oxygen in alveolar gas
Pa_{CO_2}	Partial pressure of carbon dioxide in arterial blood
$P\bar{v}_{O_2}$	Partial pressure of oxygen in mixed venous or pulmonary artery blood
$P(A-a)_{O_2}$	Difference between alevolar and arterial partial pressure of oxygen (A−a gradient)
P_B	Barometric or atmospheric pressure
Sa_{O_2}	Saturation of hemoglobin (in arterial blood) with oxygen
$S\bar{v}_{O_2}$	Saturation of hemoglobin (in mixed venous blood) with O_2
Ca_{O_2}	Content or amount (volume) of oxygen in arterial blood
$C\bar{v}_{O_2}$	Content of oxygen in mixed venous blood
$C(a-\bar{v})_{O_2}$	Oxygen content difference between arterial and mixed venous blood
$\dot{V}_A$	Alveolar ventilation
$\dot{V}_D$	Dead-space ventilation
$\dot{V}_E$	Minute volume
VC	Vital capacity
TV or V_T	Tidal volume or average breath
$\dot{Q}T$	Total perfusion or blood flow (cardiac output)
$\dot{V}/\dot{Q}$	Ratio of ventilation to perfusion
Fi_{O_2}	Fraction of inspired oxygen
FRC	Functional residual capacity
IC	Inspiratory capacity

NOTE: Subscripts identify the particular gas, volume, or pressure being discussed. A dot (·) means measurement over time, usually 1 minute.

The amount of water vapor contained in a gas mixture is determined by the temperature of the gas and is unrelated to barometric pressure. Gas that enters the lungs becomes saturated with water vapor (humidified) as it passes through the upper airway. At body temperature (37° C) water vapor exerts a pressure of 47 mm Hg. Because this is true regardless of total (barometric) pressure, the partial pressure of water vapor (always 47 mm Hg) must be subtracted from the barometric pressure before the partial pressure of other gases in the mixture can be determined. In saturated air at sea level, the partial pressure of oxygen is, therefore, $(760 - 47) \times 0.209 = 149$. All pressure and volume measurements made in pulmonary function laboratories specify the temperature and humidity of a gas at the time of measurement.

Many pressure measurements are stated as variations from barometric pressure, rather than percentages of it. On such scales barometric pressure is considered zero, and pressure varies up or down from zero. Physiologic pressure measurements that involve fluids, rather than gases, are measured as variations from barometric pressure. For example, a systolic blood pressure of 120 mm Hg indicates that systolic pressure is 120 mm Hg above barometric pressure.

Measurement of Lung Volumes and Capacities

Tidal volume (V_T or TV) is the amount of gas inspired and expired during normal breathing (Fig. 29-12). **Inspiratory reserve volume (IRV)** is the amount of gas that can be inspired in addition to tidal volume. **Expiratory reserve volume (ERV)** is the amount of gas that can be expired after a passive (relaxed) expiration. **Residual volume (RV)** is the volume of gas that cannot be expired and is always present in the lungs.

Total lung capacity (TLC) is the total gas volume in the lung when it is maximally inflated. It is made up of RV, ERV, TV, and IRV. **Vital capacity (VC)** is the maximum amount of gas that can be displaced (expired) from the lung. It includes IRV, TV, and ERV. **Functional residual capacity (FRC)** is the amount of gas remaining in the lung at the end of a passive expiration (RV and ERV). At this point the lungs are at rest, or in a state of mechanical equilibrium. **Inspiratory capacity**

(IC) is the amount of gas that can be inspired after a passive expiration (from FRC). It includes TV and IRV. The lung capacities are always the sum of two or more volumes. Norms for volumes and capacities are based on age, sex, and height and are referred to as predicted values. Changes from predicted or baseline values are taken into account in diagnosing and assessing respiratory disorders.

With each breath a portion of the tidal volume remains in the conducting airways. Because it does not reach the alveoli, this gas does not participate in gas exchange and is called wasted ventilation, or **dead-space ventilation ($\dot{V}_D$)**. Dead-space ventilation is usually 1 ml per pound of lean body weight, or 150 cc in an average-sized man (approximately one third of each breath). This normal dead space is called anatomic dead space. In some disease states a portion of the alveoli and respiratory bronchioles do not participate in gas exchange and, therefore, increase the amount of dead-space ventilation. The combination of this additional dead space and the anatomic dead space is called physiologic dead space.

Alveolar ventilation ($\dot{V}_A$) is that portion of the tidal volume that reaches the alveoli. Adequate alveolar ventilation is required for sufficient gas exchange. During expiration a portion of this alveolar gas remains in the conducting airways and moves back into the alveoli with the next inspiration.

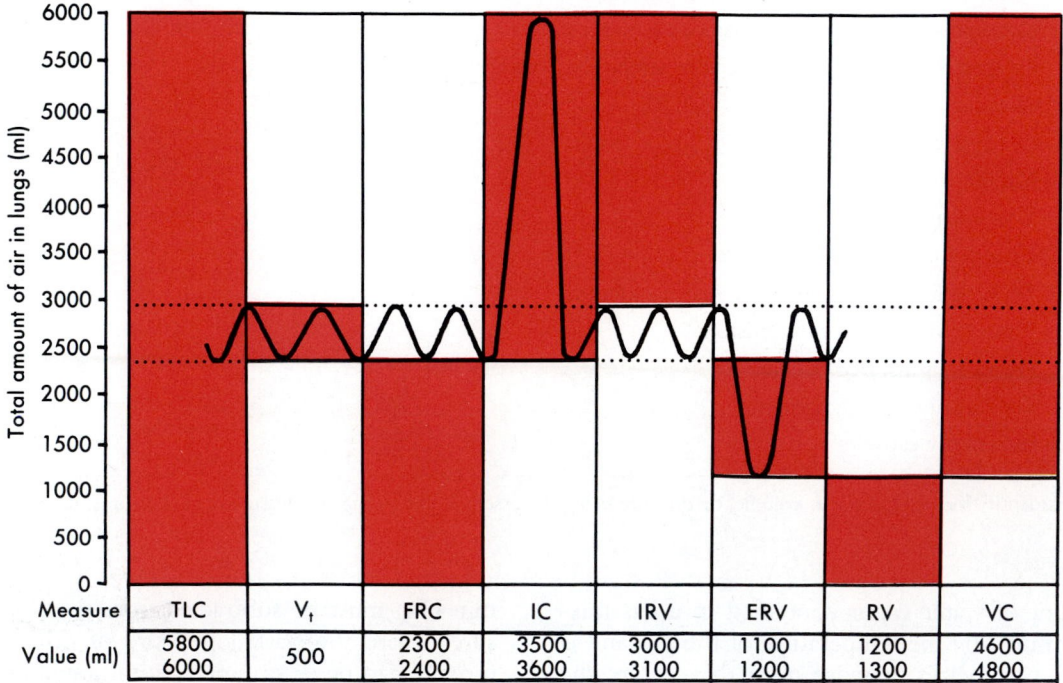

Measure	TLC	V_t	FRC	IC	IRV	ERV	RV	VC
Value (ml)	5800 6000	500	2300 2400	3500 3600	3000 3100	1100 1200	1200 1300	4600 4800

FIG. 29-12. Lung volume measurements. All values are approximately 25% lower in women. *TLC,* Total lung capacity; V_T, *tidal volume; FRC,* functional residual capacity; *IC,* inspiratory capacity; *IRV,* inspiratory reserve volume; *ERV,* expiratory reserve volume; *RV,* residual volume; *VC,* vital capacity. (From Thompson et al., 1989.)

Carbon dioxide (CO_2), the gaseous form of carbonic acid (H_2CO_3), is a product of cellular metabolism. The lung eliminates about 10,000 milliequivalents (mEq) of carbonic acid per day in the form of CO_2, which is produced at the rate of approximately 200 ml/min. Carbon dioxide elimination is necessary to maintain a normal arterial CO_2 (Pa_{CO_2}) of 40 mm Hg and normal acid-base balance (see Chapter 3 for a discussion of acid-base regulation).

The adequacy of alveolar ventilation *cannot* be determined by observation of ventilatory rate, pattern, or effort. If a health professional has a question about the adequacy of ventilation, an arterial blood gas analysis or its equivalent must be performed to measure Pa_{CO_2}.

Mechanics of Breathing

The mechanical aspects of inspiration and expiration are known collectively as the mechanics of breathing. The mechanics of breathing involve (1) major and accessory muscles of inspiration and expiration, (2) alveolar surface tension, (3) elastic properties of the lungs and chest wall, and (4) resistance to air flow through the conducting airways. Alterations in any of these properties increase the work of breathing, or the metabolic energy that must be expended to achieve adequate ventilation and oxygenation of the blood (see p. 1040).

Major and Accessory Muscles

The major muscles of inspiration are the diaphragm and the external intercostal muscles (muscles between the ribs) (Fig. 29-13). The diaphragm is a dome-shaped muscle that separates the abdominal and thoracic cavities. When the diaphragm contracts, it flattens downward, increasing the volume of the thoracic cavity, and creates a vacuum that draws gas into the lungs. Contraction of external intercostal muscles elevates the anterior portion of the ribs. This increases the volume of the thoracic cavity by increasing its front-to-back (anterior-posterior [A-P]) diameter. Although the external intercostals may contract during quiet breathing, inspiration at rest is usually assisted by the diaphragm alone.

The accessory muscles of inspiration are the sternocleidomastoid and scalene muscles. Like the external intercostals these muscles enlarge the thorax by increasing its A-P diameter. The accessory muscles of inspiration assist inspiration when minute volume (volume of air inspired and expired per minute) is very high, as during strenuous exercise or when the work of breathing is increased because of disease. The accessory muscles do not increase the volume of the thorax as efficiently as the diaphragm does.

There are no major muscles of expiration because normal, relaxed expiration is passive and requires no muscular effort. The accessory muscles of expiration, the abdominal and internal intercostal muscles, assist expiration when minute volume is high, when expiration exceeds FRC, or when airway obstruction is present. When the abdominal muscles contract intraabdominal pressure increases, pushing up the diaphragm and decreasing the volume of the thorax. The internal intercostal muscles pull down the anterior ribs, decreasing the A-P diameter of the thorax.

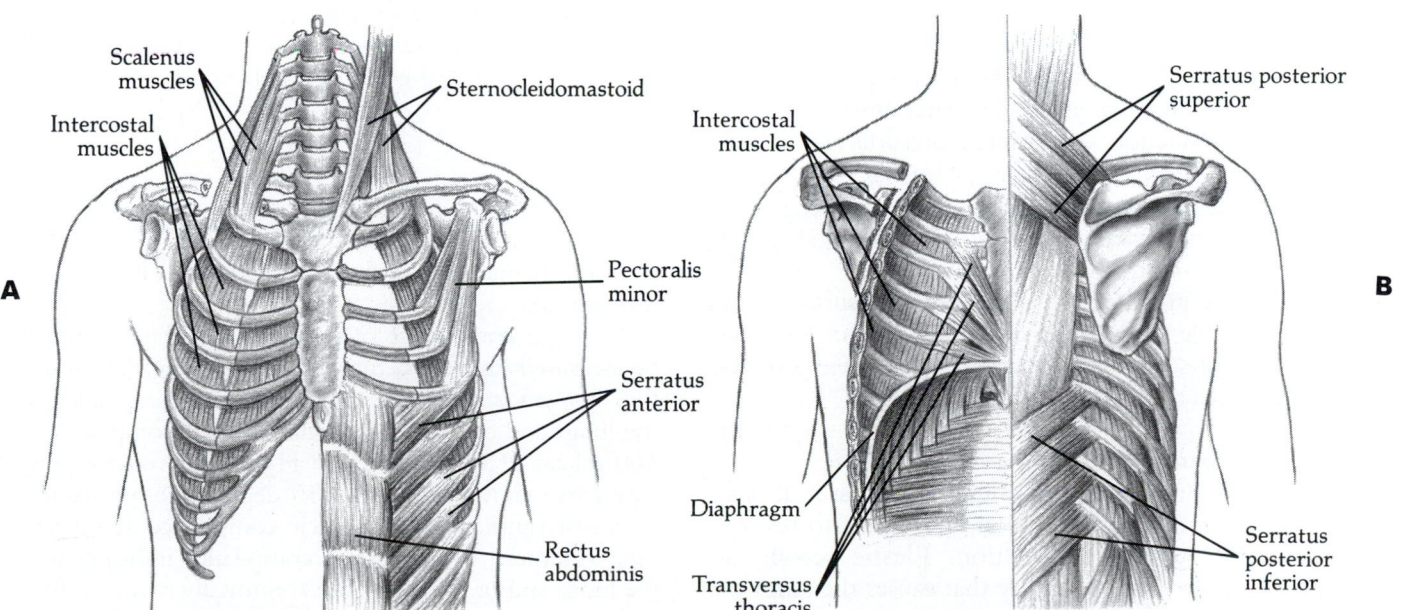

FIG. 29-13. Muscles of ventilation. **A,** Anterior view; **B,** posterior view. (From Thompson et al., 1989.)

Alveolar Surface Tension

Surface tension occurs at any gas-liquid interface. **Surface tension** is the tendency for liquid molecules that are exposed to air to adhere to one another, forming a sort of "skin." This phenomenon can be seen, for example, in a glass of liquid that is about to overflow or in the way liquids "bead" when splashed on a waterproof surface. In both examples, this behavior decreases the surface area exposed to the air.

Within a sphere, such as an alveolus, surface tension tends to make expansion difficult. According to the law of Laplace, the pressure (P) required to inflate a sphere is equal to two times the surface tension ($2T$) divided by the radius (r) of the sphere, or $P = (2T/r)$. As the radius of the sphere (or alveolus) becomes smaller, more and more pressure is required to inflate it. If the alveoli were lined with a waterlike fluid, taking breaths would be extremely difficult.

Alveolar ventilation, or distention, is made possible by surfactant, which lowers surface tension by coating the air-liquid interface in the alveoli. Surfactant, a lipoprotein produced by type II alveolar cells, has a detergentlike effect that separates the liquid molecules, thereby decreasing alveolar surface tension.

Surfactant lines the alveolar side of the alveolocapillary membrane and, in effect, reverses the law of Laplace. In the lung the relationship between surface tension and radius is opposite to that of the law of Laplace. As the radius of a surfactant-lined sphere (alveolus) grows smaller, the surface tension *decreases,* and as the radius grows larger, the surface tension *increases.* This occurs because the smaller radius causes surfactant molecules to crowd together, then repel one another strongly. A larger radius spreads them apart, decreasing their mutual repellence. Therefore, the alveoli are much easier to inflate at low lung volumes (i.e., after expiration) than at high volumes (i.e., after inspiration). If surfactant production is disrupted or surfactant is not produced in adequate quantities, alveolar surface tension increases and results in alveolar collapse, decreased lung expansion, increased work of breathing, and severe gas-exchange abnormalities.

The change in surface tension caused by surfactant is also responsible for keeping the alveoli free of fluid. In the absence of surfactant the surface tension tends to attract fluid into the alveoli.

Elastic Properties of the Lung and Chest Wall

The elastic properties of the lung and chest wall permit expansion during inspiration and return to resting volume (FRC) during expiration. **Elastic recoil,** or elastance, is the elastic property that causes the lungs to return to the resting state after expiration. Normal elastic recoil permits passive expiration, which is why there are no major muscles of expiration. Passive elastic recoil may be insufficient during labored breathing (high minute volume), in which case the accessory muscles of expiration are used. The accessory muscles are also used if disease compromises elastic recoil (e.g., in emphysema) or blocks the conducting airways.

Normal elastic recoil depends on an equilibrium between opposing forces of recoil in the lungs and chest wall. Under normal conditions the chest wall tends to recoil by expanding outward. This can be readily observed during open heart surgery. When the sternum is split to open the thoracic cavity, the chest wall moves outward laterally. The tendency of the chest wall to recoil by expanding is balanced by the tendency of the lungs to recoil or collapse around the hila. The tendency of the lungs to collapse can be demonstrated if the chest is opened without mechanically ventilating the lungs (for example, at postmortem examination). As the thorax is opened the lungs immediately collapse like inflated balloons that have been released. This reaction is due to elastic recoil and surface tension in the alveoli.

During inspiration the diaphragm and intercostal muscles contract, air flows into the lungs, and the chest wall expands. Inspiration continues until the tendency of the lungs to collapse is equal to the chest wall's tendency to expand. During expiration the muscles relax and the thorax decreases in volume until once again the tendency for the lungs to collapse is equal to the chest wall's tendency to expand (Fig. 29-14). Functional residual capacity is reached when, with no muscular effort, the recoil forces of the lungs and chest wall are equal. Pleural pressure is negative because of this balance of opposing forces.

Compliance is a measure of lung and chest wall distensibility. Compliance is determined by alveolar surface tension and the elastic recoil of the lung and chest wall and can be measured by using the formula

$$C = \frac{\Delta V}{\Delta P},$$

where C = compliance in liters/centimeter of water, ΔV = volume change (usually tidal volume), and ΔP = pressure change (airway or pleural pressure) in centimeters of water.

Although compliance of the lung and chest wall can be measured separately, the value used in the clinical setting is *thoracic compliance:* the combined compliance of the lungs and chest wall. Normal thoracic compliance is 100 ml/cm H_2O or 0.1 L/cm H_2O. The volume-pressure curve shown in Fig. 29-15 depicts the mechanical forces of ventilation or thoracic compliance at varying lung volumes. An increase in compliance indicates that the lungs and/or chest wall are abnormally easy to inflate and have lost some elastic recoil. A decrease indicates that the lungs and/or chest wall are abnormally stiff or difficult to inflate. Compliance is increased in emphy-

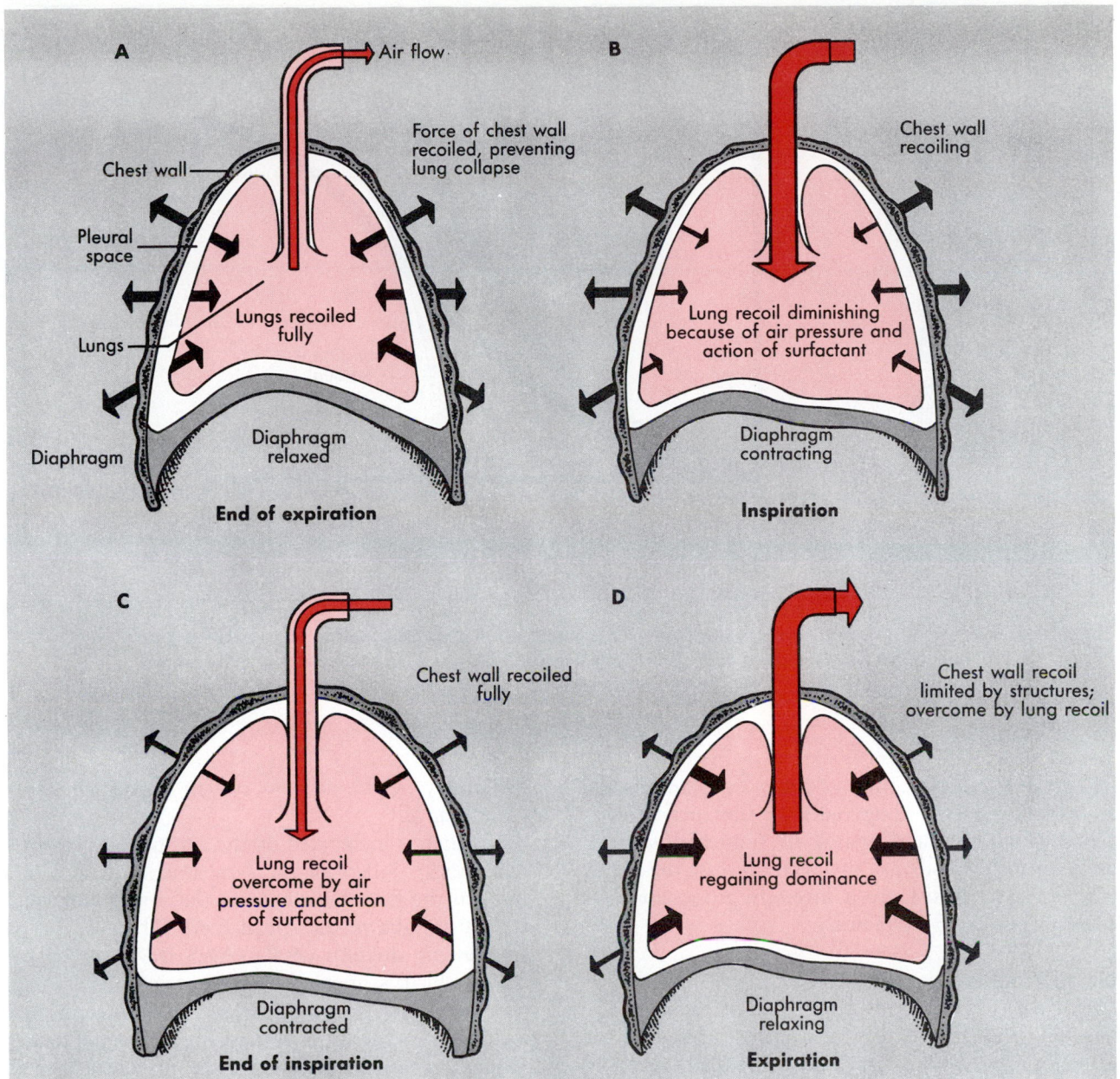

FIG. 29-14. Equilibrium between recoil tendencies of lungs (to move inward) and chest wall (to move outward) is reached at the end of each normal expiration **(A)** and inspiration **(C)**. **B,** During inspiration, the equilibrium is disrupted, with the chest wall's tendencies dominant. **D,** During expiration, the lung's recoil tendencies are dominant. (Thick arrows indicate dominant recoil forces.) Whichever recoil tendency is dominant, the lungs and chest wall move together because of negative pressures in the pleural space.

sema and decreased in adult respiratory distress syndrome, pneumonia, pulmonary edema, or fibrosis. (These disorders are described in Chapter 30.)

Airway Resistance

Airway resistance, which is similar to resistance to blood flow (described in Chapter 26), is determined by the length, radius, and cross-sectional area of the air-

ways and density, viscosity, and velocity of the gas (Poiseuille law). Resistance is computed by dividing change in pressure *(P)* by rate of flow *(F)*, or $R = P/F$ (Ohm's law). Airway resistance is normally very low. One half to two thirds of total airway resistance occurs in the nose. The next highest resistance is in the oropharynx and larynx. There is very little resistance in the conducting airways of the lungs because of their large cross-sec-

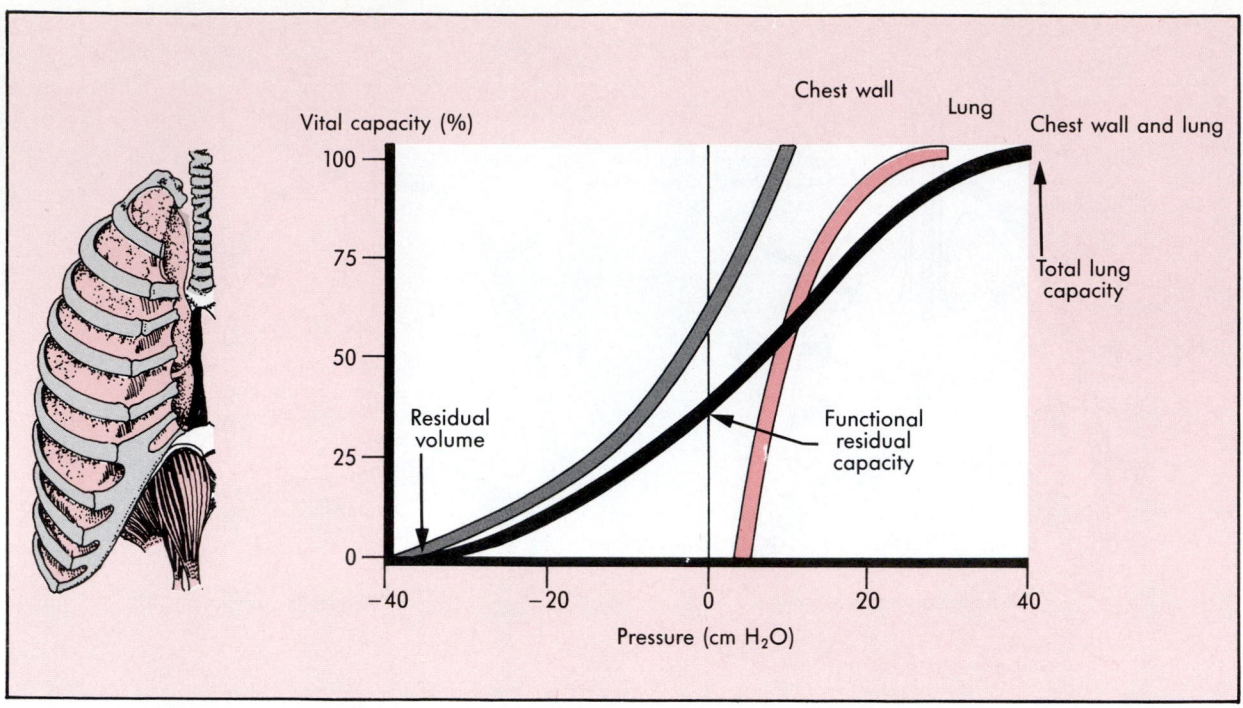

FIG. 29-15. Volume-pressure curve, or compliance curve, of the lungs and chest wall. Recoil pressures of the lungs and chest wall together *(solid line)* equal the sum of recoil pressures of each structure combined, or the thoracic compliance *(dotted lines)*.

tional area. The most common causes of increased airway resistance are swelling (edema), obstruction (i.e., mucous plugging), and spasm of bronchial smooth muscle (bronchospasm), all of which decrease the radius of the airways. (Resistance is inversely proportional to the fourth power of the radius.)

Work of Breathing

The work of breathing is determined by the muscular effort (and therefore oxygen and energy) required for ventilation. The work of breathing is normally very low but may increase considerably in diseases that disrupt the equilibrium between forces exerted by the lung and chest wall. More muscular effort is required when lung compliance is decreased (e.g., in pulmonary edema), chest wall compliance is decreased (e.g., in spinal deformity or obesity), or airways are obstructed by bronchospasm or mucous plugging (e.g., in asthma or bronchitis). An increase in the work of breathing can be life-threatening when oxygen delivery also is impaired (e.g., in anemia).

Neurochemical Control of Ventilation

Breathing is usually involuntary, although voluntary breathing is necessary for talking, singing, laughing, and deliberately holding one's breath, because homeostasis changes in ventilatory rate and volume are adjusted au-

tomatically by the nervous system to maintain normal gas exchange.

The lung is innervated by the autonomic nervous system (ANS). Fibers of the sympathetic division of the ANS in the lung branch from the upper thoracic and cervical ganglia of the spinal cord. Fibers of the parasympathetic division of the ANS travel in the vagus nerve, which is important in the regulation of ventilation. The respiratory centers in the brain stem control involuntary ventilation by transmitting impulses to the respiratory muscles, causing them to contract or relax (Fig. 29-16). (Structure and function of the autonomic nervous system are covered in detail in Chapter 12.) The pneumotaxic center in the upper pons functions to maintain rhythmic respirations. It stimulates the expiratory center, which then sends inhibitory signals to the inspiratory center. Inspiration ends and expiration begins. Strong stimuli from the pneumotaxic center result in shorter inspiration, and mild stimuli result in longer inspiration. The apneustic center sends stimuli to the inspiratory center and prolongs inspiration. The pneumotaxic center usually overrides the apneustic center.

Impulses are transmitted from **lung receptors** (receptors that respond to physical changes in the pulmonary system) and **chemoreceptors** (receptors that respond to changes in oxygen or carbon dioxide concentrations) through the sympathetic and parasympathetic divisions

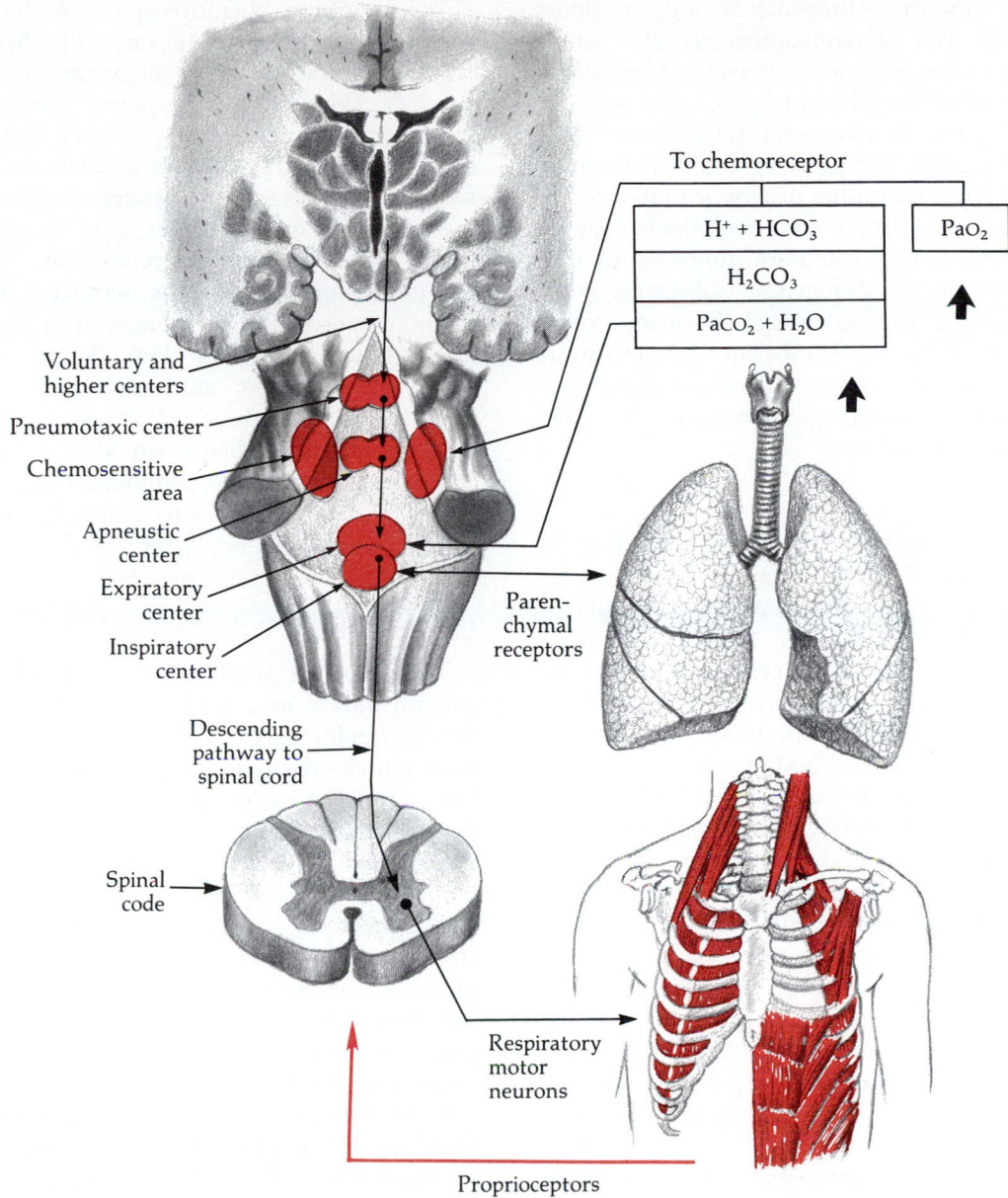

FIG. 29-16. Respiratory control system. (From Thompson et al., 1989.)

of the ANS and the respiratory centers in the brain stem.

Lung Receptors

Three types of lung receptors send impulses from the lungs to the respiratory centers: (1) irritant receptors, (2) stretch receptors, and (3) *j*-receptors. **Irritant receptors** are found in the epithelium of all conducting airways. They are sensitive to noxious aerosols (vapors), gases, and particulate matter (inhaled dusts, etc.), which cause them to initiate the cough reflex. When stimulated, irritant receptors cause bronchoconstriction and increased ventilatory rate. **Stretch receptors** are located

in the smooth muscles of airways and are sensitive to increases in the size or volume of the lungs. Stretch receptors decrease ventilatory rate and volume when stimulated, an occurrence sometimes referred to as the Hering-Breuer expiratory reflex. This reflex is not thought to play a major role in the regulation of ventilation in adults, though it may be important in infants. J-receptors are located near the capillaries in the alveolar septa. J-receptors are sensitive to decreases in alveolar size (e.g., in edema and fibrosis), which stimulate them to initiate rapid, shallow breathing.

The parasympathetic and sympathetic divisions of the ANS control airway caliber (interior diameter of the airway lumen) by stimulating bronchial smooth muscle to contract or relax. The parasympathetic receptors cause smooth muscle to contract, whereas sympathetic receptors cause it to relax. Bronchial smooth muscle tone depends on equilibrium, that is, equal stimulation of contraction and relaxation. The parasympathetic division of the ANS is the main controller of airway caliber under normal conditions. Constriction occurs if the irritant receptors in the airway epithelium are stimulated by irritants in inspired air, by endogenous substances (e.g., histamine, serotonin, prostaglandins), by many drugs, and by humoral substances. The balance between parasympathetic and sympathetic stimulation of the airway is important in many pathologic conditions, the most important of which is asthma.

Chemoreceptors

Chemoreceptors monitor the pH, $Paco_2$, and Pao_2 of arterial blood. **Central chemoreceptors** monitor arterial blood indirectly by sensing changes in the pH of cerebrospinal fluid (CSF). They are located in the myelencephalon, near the respiratory center, and are sensitive to hydrogen ion concentration in the CSF. (Chapter 3 describes the relationship between ions and the pH, or acid-base status, of body fluids.) The pH, or concentration of hydrogen ions in the CSF, reflects $Paco_2$ because unlike H^+ ions, carbon dioxide in arterial blood diffuses across the blood-brain barrier (the barrier separating blood from cells of the central nervous system) into the CSF until the partial pressure of carbon dioxide (Pco_2) is equal on both sides. Carbon dioxide that has entered the CSF combines with H_2O to form carbonic acid, which subsequently dissociates into hydrogen ions that are capable of stimulating the central chemoreceptors. In this way $Paco_2$ regulates ventilation through its impact on the pH (hydrogen ion content) of the CSF.

If alveolar ventilation is inadequate, $Paco_2$ increases. Carbon dioxide diffuses across the blood-brain barrier until Pco_2 in blood and CSF reaches equilibrium. As the central chemoreceptors sense the resulting decrease in pH (increase in hydrogen ion concentration) they stimulate the respiratory center to increase the depth and rate of ventilation. Increased ventilation causes the Pco_2 of arterial blood to decrease below that of the CSF, and carbon dioxide diffuses back out of the CSF, returning its pH to normal.

The central chemoreceptors are sensitive to very small changes in the pH of CSF (equivalent to a 1 to 2 mm Hg change in Pco_2) and are able to maintain a normal $Paco_2$ under many different conditions, including strenuous exercise. If inadequate ventilation, or hypoventilation, is long-term, for example, in chronic obstructive pulmonary disease, these receptors become insensitive to small changes in $Paco_2$ and become poor regulators of ventilation.

The **peripheral chemoreceptors** are located in aortic bodies, the aortic arch, and carotid bodies at the bifurcation of the carotids, near the baroreceptors (see Chapter 26). Although the peripheral chemoreceptors are sensitive to changes in $Paco_2$ and pH, they are primarily sensitive to oxygen levels in arterial blood (Pao_2). As Pao_2 and pH decrease, peripheral chemoreceptors, particularly in the carotid bodies, send signals to the respiratory center to increase ventilation. The peripheral chemoreceptors are not as sensitive as the central chemoreceptors. The Pao_2 must drop well below normal (to about 60 mm Hg) before the peripheral chemoreceptors have much influence on ventilation. If $Paco_2$ is elevated as well, however, ventilation increases much more than it would in response to either abnormality alone. The peripheral chemoreceptors become the major stimulus to ventilation when the central chemoreceptors are "reset" by chronic hypoventilation.

Control of the Pulmonary Circulation

The caliber of pulmonary artery lumina decreases as smooth muscle in arterial walls contracts. Contraction increases pulmonary artery pressure. Caliber increases as these muscles relax, decreasing blood pressure. Contraction (vasoconstriction) and relaxation (vasodilation) apparently occur in response to local humoral conditions, even though the pulmonary circulation is innervated by the ANS in the same manner as the systemic circulation.

The most important cause of pulmonary artery constriction is a low alveolar Po_2 (Pao_2). Vasoconstriction due to alveolar hypoxia, often termed **hypoxic vasoconstriction,** can affect only one portion of the lung (i.e., one lobe that is obstructed, decreasing its Pao_2) or the entire lung. If only one segment of the lung is involved, the arterioles to that segment constrict, shunting blood to other, well-ventilated portions of the lung. This reflex improves the lung's efficiency by better matching ventilation and perfusion. If hypoventilation affects all segments of the lung, however, pulmonary hypertension (elevated pulmonary artery pressure) can result. The pulmonary vasoconstriction caused by low alveolar Po_2 is reversible if the alveolar Po_2 is corrected. Chronic alveolar hypoxia can result in permanent pulmonary artery hypertension, which eventually leads to cor pulmonale and heart failure.

Acidosis also causes pulmonary artery constriction. If the acidosis is corrected, the vasoconstriction is reversed. (Respiratory acidosis and metabolic acidosis are described in Chapter 3.) It is important to note that an elevated $Paco_2$ without a drop in pH does not cause pulmonary artery constriction. Other biochemial factors that affect the caliber of vessels in pulmonary circulation are histamine, prostaglandins, serotonin, and bradykinin.

Gas Transport

Gas transport, the delivery of oxygen to the cells of the body and the removal of carbon dioxide, has four steps: (1) ventilation of the lungs, (2) diffusion of oxygen from the alveoli into the capillary blood, (3) perfusion of systemic capillaries with oxygenated blood, and (4) diffusion of oxygen from systemic capillaries into the cells. Steps in the transport of carbon dioxide occur in reverse order: (1) diffusion of carbon dixoide from the cells into the systemic capillaries, (2) perfusion of the pulmonary capillary bed by venous blood, (3) diffusion of carbon dioxide into the alveoli, and (4) removal of carbon dioxide from the lung by ventilation. If any step in gas transport is impaired by a respiratory or cardiovascular disorder, gas exchange at the cellular level is compromised.

Distribution of Ventilation and Perfusion

Effective gas exchange depends on an approximately even distribution of gas (ventilation) and blood (perfusion) in all portions of the lungs. Gas exchange would not be very efficient if the most of each inspired breath went to the right lung and most of the pulmonary blood flow went to the left lung.

The lungs are suspended from the hila in the thoracic cavity. When the individual is in an upright position (sitting or standing), gravity pulls the lungs down toward the diaphragm and compresses their lower portions or bases. As a result the alveoli in the upper portions, or apices, of the lungs contain a greater residual volume of gas than those in the lower portions. Because surface tension increases as the alveoli become larger, the larger alveoli in the upper portions of the lung are more difficult to inflate (less compliant) than the smaller alveoli in the lower portions of the lung. Therefore, during ventilation most of the tidal volume is distributed to the bases of the lungs, where compliance is greater.

The heart pumps against gravity to perfuse the pulmonary circulation. As blood is pumped into the lung apices, some blood pressure is dissipated in overcoming gravity. As a result blood pressure at the apices is lower than that at the bases. Because greater pressure causes greater perfusion, the bases of the lungs are better perfused than the apices (Fig. 29-17). Thus ventilation and perfusion are greatest in the same lung portions: the lower lobes.

Distribution of perfusion in the pulmonary circulation also is affected by alveolar pressure (gas pressure in the alveoli). The pulmonary capillary bed differs from the systemic capillary bed in that it is surrounded by gas-containing alveoli. If the gas pressure in the alveoli exceeds the blood pressure in the capillary, the capillary collapses and flow ceases. This is most likely to occur in portions of the lung where blood pressure is lowest and alveolar gas volume, and therefore pressure, is greatest: that is, the apex of the lung.

The lungs have been divided into three zones on the basis of the relationships among all the factors affecting pulmonary blood flow (West, Dollery, & Naimark, 1974). Alveolar pressure plus the forces of gravity, arterial blood pressure, and venous blood pressure affect the distribution of perfusion as shown in Fig. 29-18.

Zone I is that portion of the lung in which alveolar pressure exceeds pulmonary arterial and venous pressures. The capillary bed collapses, and normal blood

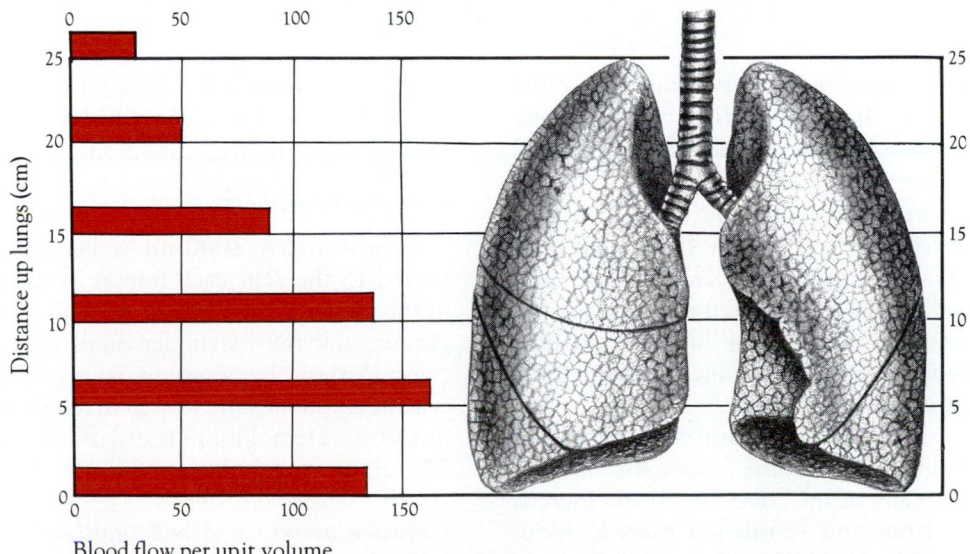

FIG. 29-17. Measurements of distribution of blood flow in lungs of individual sitting in an upright position. (From Thompson et al., 1989.)

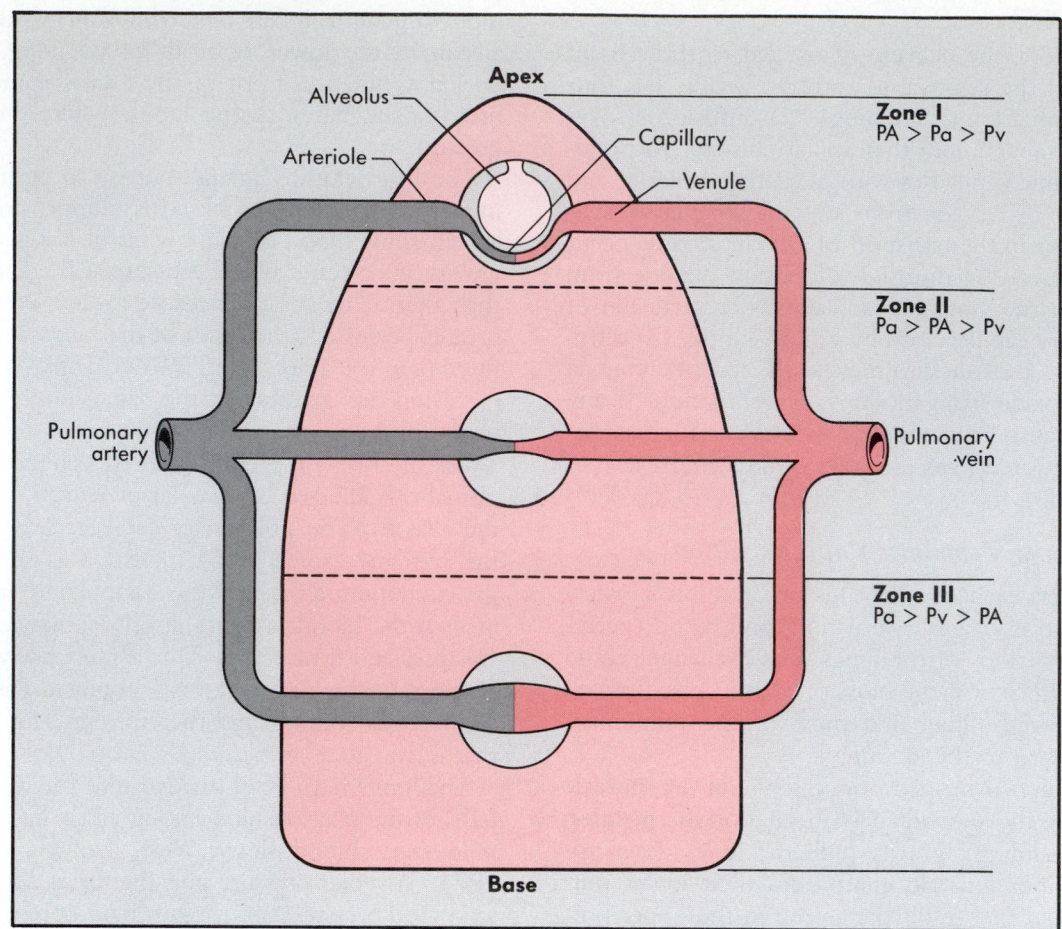

FIG. 29-18. Effects of gravity and alveolar pressure on pulmonary blood flow in the three lung zones. In zone I, alveolar pressure (P_A) is greater than arterial and venous pressure, and no blood flow occurs. In zone II, arterial pressure (P_a) exceeds alveolar pressure, but alveolar pressure exceeds venous pressure (P_v). Blood flow occurs in this zone, but alveolar pressure compresses the venules (venous ends of the capillaries). In zone III, both arterial and venous pressure are greater than alveolar pressure, and blood flow fluctuates, depending on the difference between arterial and venous pressure.

flow ceases. Normally zone I is a very small part of the lung at the apex. Zone II is the portion where alveolar pressure is greater than venous pressure but not arterial pressure. Blood flows through zone II, but it is impeded to a certain extent by alveolar pressure. Zone II is normally above the level of the left atrium. In zone III both arterial and venous pressures are greater than alveolar pressure and blood flow is not affected by alveolar pressure. Zone III is in the base of the lung. Blood flow through the pulmonary capillary bed increases in regular increments from the apex to the base.

Although both blood flow and ventilation are greater at the base of the lungs than at the apices, they are not perfectly matched in any of the zones. Perfusion exceeds ventilation in the bases and ventilation exceeds perfusion in the apices of the lung. The relationship between ventilation and perfusion is expresssed as a ratio called the **ventilation-perfusion ratio,** or $\dot{V}/\dot{Q}$ The normal

$\dot{V}/\dot{Q}$ ratio, sometimes called the $\dot{V}/\dot{Q}$ mismatch, is 0.8. This is the amount by which perfusion exceeds ventilation under normal conditions.

Oxygen Transport

Approximately 1000 ml (1 liter) of oxygen is transported to the cells each minute. Oxygen is transported in the blood in two forms. A small amount dissolves in plasma, and the remainder binds to hemoglobin molecules. Without hemoglobin oxygen would not reach the cells in amounts sufficient to maintain normal metabolic function. (Hemoglobin is discussed in detail in Chapter 22; cellular metabolism in Chapter 1.)

Diffusion across the Alveolocapillary Membrane

The alveolocapillary membrane is the ideal medium for oxygen diffusion because it has a large total surface area (70 to 100 m²) and is very thin (0.5 micrometer

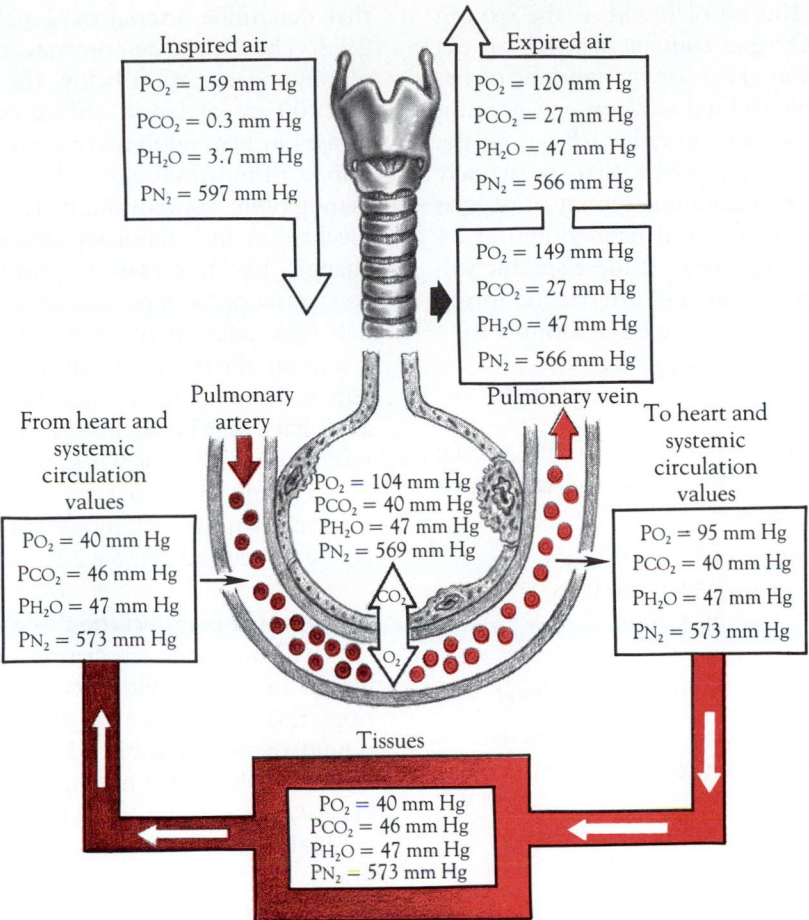

FIG. 29-19. Partial pressure of respiratory gases in normal respiration. (From Thompson et al., 1989.)

[µm]). In addition the concentration of oxygen molecules (PO_2) is much greater in alveolar gas than in capillary blood, a condition that promotes rapid diffusion down the concentration gradient from the alveolus into the capillary. The partial pressure of oxygen (oxygen tension) in mixed venous or pulmonary artery blood ($P-vO_2$) is about 40 mm Hg as it enters the capillary, and alveolar oxygen tension (PAO_2) is 100 mm Hg at sea level. Therefore, a pressure gradient of 60 mm Hg facilitates the diffusion of oxygen from the alveolus into the capillary.

Blood remains in the pulmonary capillary for about 0.75 sec, but only 0.25 sec is required for oxygen concentration to equilibrate (equalize) across the alveolocapillary membrane. Therefore, oxygen has ample time to diffuse into the blood, even during increased cardiac output, which speeds blood flow, shortening the time the blood remains in the capillary.

Determinants of Arterial Oxygenation

As oxygen diffuses across the alveolocapillary membrane, it dissolves in the plasma, where it exerts pressure (the partial pressure of oxygen in arterial blood, or PaO_2). As the PaO_2 rises, oxygen moves from the plasma into the red blood cells (erythrocytes) and binds with hemoglobin molecules. Oxygen continues to bind with hemoglobin until the hemoglobin binding sites are filled or saturated. Oxygen then continues to diffuse across the alveolocapillary membrane until the PaO_2 (oxygen dissolved in plasma) and PAO_2 equilibrate, eliminating the pressure gradient across the alveolocapillary membrane. At this point diffusion ceases (Fig. 29-19).

Normally about 20 ml of oxygen is transported per 100 ml of blood. Because oxygen is not very soluble in plasma, most of the oxygen molecules bind with hemoglobin. Plasma carries only about 0.3 ml of oxygen per 100 ml of blood (at sea level). Although the remaining 19.7 ml is carried by hemoglobin, it is the small amount of oxygen dissolved in plasma that is responsible for oxygen's partial pressure in the blood.

Although PaO_2 is important in that it provides the driving pressure that loads the hemoglobin with oxygen, it gives little information about the *amount* of oxygen carried in the blood. This amount, which is measured in milliliters per 100 ml of blood, is the oxygen content of the blood. Oxygen content depends on (1) hemoglobin concentration (Hb), or the amount of hemoglobin that is available to bind with oxygen per unit volume of blood; (2) oxygen saturation (So_2), or the percentage of available hemoglobin that is actually bound to oxygen; and (3) maximum amount of oxygen that can be transported per gram of hemoglobin (1.34 ml of O_2 per gram of hemoglobin). If these specific values are known, the oxygen content of arterial and mixed venous blood can be calculated. The basic formula is

$$O_2 \text{ content} = (1.34 \times Hb) \, So_2$$
$$Vol \% = ml/g \times g/\%.$$

If hemoglobin concentration (Hb) = 15 and arterial oxygen saturation (Sao_2) = 98%, then arterial oxygen content is computed as follows:

$$
\begin{aligned}
\text{Arterial } O_2 \text{ content} &= (1.34 \times Hb) \, Sao_2 \\
&= (1.34 \times 15) \, 0.96 \\
&= (20.1) \, 0.96 \\
&= 19.3. \\
\text{Normal} &= 19\text{-}20 \text{ ml/100 ml blood.}
\end{aligned}
$$

If Hb = 15 and mixed venous saturation ($S\text{-}vo_2$) = 75%, then mixed venous oxygen content is computed as follows:

$$
\begin{aligned}
\text{Mixed venous } O_2 \text{ content} &= (1.34 \times Hb) \, S\text{-}vo_2 \\
&= (1.34 \times 15) \, 0.75 \\
&= (20.1) \, 0.75 \\
&= 15.08. \\
\text{Normal} &= 15\text{-}16 \text{ ml/100 ml blood.}
\end{aligned}
$$

Because hemoblogin transports all but 0.3 ml of the 20 ml of oxygen carried per 100 ml of arterial blood, increases or decreases in hemoglobin concentration affect the oxygen content of the blood. The relationship between hemoglobin concentration and other values that determine arterial oxygenation is shown in Table 29-3. These data demonstrate that decreases in hemoglobin concentration below the normal value of 15 ml per 100 ml of blood reduce oxygen content, and increases in hemoglobin concentration may minimize the impact of impaired gas exchange. In fact, an increase in hemoglobin concentration is a major compensatory mechanism in pulmonary diseases that impair gas exchange. For this reason measurement of hemoglobin concentration is important in the assessment of individuals with pulmonary disease. If cardiovascular function is normal, the body's initial response to low oxygen content is to speed up cardiac output. In individuals who also have cardiovascular disease, this compensatory mechanism does not work, making increased hemoglobin concentration an even more important compensatory mechanism. (Hemoglobin structure and function are described in Chapter 22.)

Oxyhemoglobin Association and Dissociation

Oxyhemoglobin association is the binding of hemoglobin molecules with oxygen, or hemoglobin saturation, that takes place in the lungs, forming the compound **oxyhemoglobin (HbO_2)**. Oxyhemoglobin dissociation, also called hemoglobin desaturation, is the reverse process, by which oxygen is freed from hemoglobin at the cellular level. When plotted on a graph, conditions under which association and dissociation occur result in an S-shaped curve called the **oxyhemoglobin dissociation curve** (Fig. 29-20).

The association portion of the curve, sometimes called the arterial portion, is the horizontal or flat segment at the top of the graph, and the dissociation or venous portion is the vertical or steep segment at the lower left. The association portion of the curve tends to be flat because partial pressure changes between 60 and 100 mm Hg do not alter saturation significantly. The

---

TABLE 29-3 Effects of hemoglobin concentration on arterial oxygenation

Gas-exchange status	Hemoglobin concentration* (gm/100 ml)	Arterial oxygen content (ml/100 ml)	Arterial oxygen saturation (Sao_2) (%)	Oxygen partial pressure (Pao_2) (mm Hg)	Adjusted Sao_2† (%)	Adjusted Pao_2† (%)
Normal	15	19.98	98	90	None	None
Normal	11.5	15.38	98	90	75	40
Normal	7.5	10.13	98	90	50	26
Impaired	17	20.21	88	55	99	100
Impaired	15	17.86	88	55	None	None
Impaired	13	15.5	88	55	78	41

*Normal hemoglobin concentration is 15. Normal oxygen content is 19-20 ml/dl. Sao_2 and Pao_2 reflect gas-exchange status.
†Approximate values necessary to cause equivalent arterial oxygen content if hemoglobin concentrations were normal.

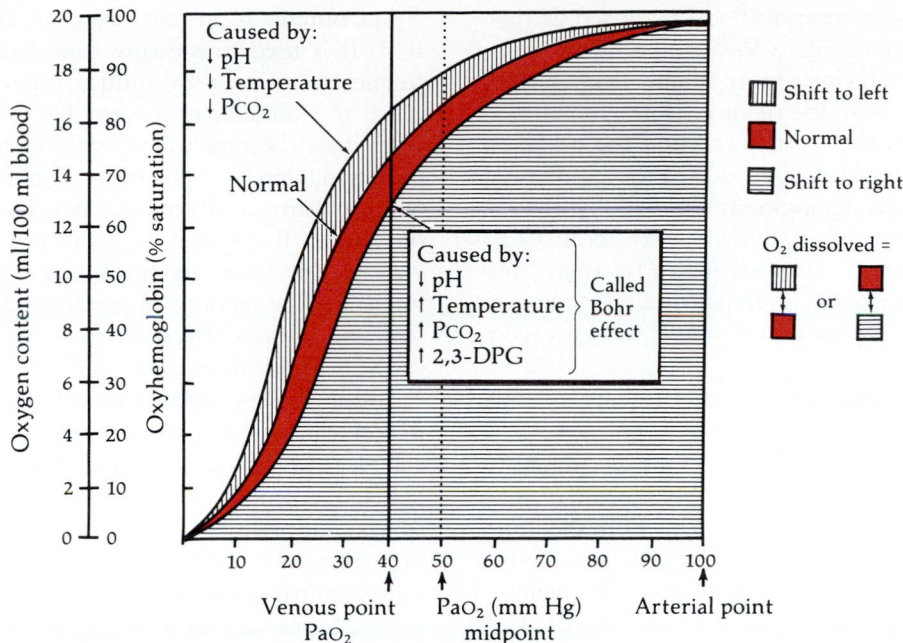

FIG. 29-20. Oxyhemoglobin dissociation curve with pH 7.4 and temperature 98.6° F (37° C). (From Thompson et al., 1989.)

wide range of partial pressures that results in adequate hemoglobin saturation enables people to exist at a variety of altitudes without significant effects on tissue oxygenation. For example, a P_{O_2} of 100 mm Hg at sea level results in 98% saturation. At an altitude of about 5000, where P_{O_2} is only 70 mm Hg, saturation is only 4% less than at sea level, or 94%. If the relationship between S_{O_2} and P_{O_2} were linear (1:1), life could not be sustained much above sea level: at a P_{O_2} of 70 mm Hg, saturation would be only be 70%, which is equivalent to normal *venous saturation*.

Oxyhemoglobin dissociation occurs readily once P_{O_2} drops below 60 mm Hg. The steepness of this portion of the curve enables oxygen to dissociate from hemoglobin and diffuse from the blood into tissue cells with little drop in the pressure gradient, ensuring that the cells will receive sufficient concentrations of oxygen molecules by diffusion.

Several factors can change the relationship between P_{O_2} and S_{O_2}, causing the oxyhemoglobin dissociation curve to shift to the right or left (see Fig. 29-20). A shift to the right depicts an increase in the ease with which oxyhemoglobin dissociates and oxygen moves into the cells. A shift to the left depicts hemoglobin's increased affinity for oxygen, which promotes association in the lungs and inhibits dissociation in the tissues.

The oxyhemoglobin dissociation curve is shifted to the right by acidosis (low pH), hypercapnia (increased Pa_{CO_2}), and hyperthermia (elevated temperature). The curve is shifted to the left by alkalosis (high pH), hypo-

capnia (decreased Pa_{CO_2}), hypothermia (low temperature), decreased 2,3-diphosphoglycerate in erythrocytes, and carbon monoxide (CO).

Carbon Dioxide Transport

About 200 ml of CO_2 is produced by the tissues per minute as a by-product of cellular metabolism. This CO_2 equilibrates with carbonic acid ($H_2O + CO_2 \rightleftharpoons H_2CO_3 \rightleftharpoons H^+ HCO_3^-$) and must be eliminated continuously in order to prevent acidosis. The elimination of carbon dioxide by the lungs plays an important role in the regulation of acid-base balance (see Chapter 3).

Carbon dioxide is carried in the blood in three ways: (1) dissolved in plasma (P_{CO_2}), (2) as bicarbonate, and (3) as carbamino compounds. As CO_2 diffuses out of the cells into the blood, it dissolves in the plasma. About 10% of the total CO_2 in venous and 5% of the CO_2 in arterial blood is carried dissolved in the plasma (P_{CO_2}). As CO_2 moves into the blood it diffuses into the red blood cells. Within the red cells carbon dioxide, with the help of the enzyme carbonic anhydrase, combines with water to form carbonic acid and then quickly dissociates into H^+ and HCO_3^-. As carbonic acid dissociates, the H^+ binds to hemoglobin, where it is buffered, and the HCO_3^- moves out of the red cell into the plasma. About 60% of the CO_2 in venous blood and 90% of the CO_2 in arterial blood are carried in the form of bicarbonate. The remainder combines with blood proteins, hemoglobin in particular, to form carbamino compounds. About 30% of the CO_2 in venous blood and 5% of the CO_2 in arterial blood is carried as carbamino compounds (see Fig. 3-9, Chapter 3).

Carbon dioxide is 20 times more soluble than O_2 and diffuses very quickly from the tissue cells into the blood. The amount of CO_2 that is able to enter the blood is enhanced by diffusion of oxygen out of the blood and into the cells. Reduced hemoglobin (hemoglobin that is dissociated from oxygen) is able to carry more CO_2 than hemoglobin that is saturated with O_2. Therefore, the drop in So_2 at the tissue level increases the ability of the blood to carry CO_2 back to the lung. This is called the **Haldane effect.**

The diffusion gradient for CO_2 in the lung is only about 6 mm Hg (venous Pco_2 = 46; alveolar Pco_2 = 40 mm Hg). Yet CO_2 is so soluble in the alveolocapillary membrane that the CO_2 in the blood quickly diffuses into the alveoli, where it is removed from the lung with each expiration. The diffusion of CO_2 out of the blood is also enhanced by oxygen binding with hemoglobin in the lung. As hemoglobin binds with O_2 the amount of CO_2 it can carry is decreased, a reversal of the Haldane effect called the **Bohr effect.** The CO_2 is released from the hemoglobin and diffuses into the alveolus. Diffusion of CO_2 in the lung is so efficient that diffusion defects that cause hypoxemia (low oxygen content of arterial blood) do not cause hypercapnia (excessive carbon dioxide in the blood).

TESTS OF PULMONARY FUNCTION

Several laboratory tests aid in the diagnosis and evaluation of pulmonary system abnormalities. Most of them are easy to perform and are performed in most hospitals and many clinics. They provide valuable information as to the possible cause of a respiratory abnormality and are also helpful in evaluating the progression or resolution of disease.

Spirometry is an important test of pulmonary function. It is used to measure forced expiration, which is frequently affected by diffuse pulmonary disease. Because the pulmonary system has remarkable reserves, disease may become well established before clinical manifestations appear. Spirometry enables clinicians to detect restrictive or obstructive deficits early in the course of disease. Restrictive lung diseases restrict the lung's volume: the lungs are unable to expand normally, diminishing the amount of gas that can be inspired. Obstructive diseases affect gas flow: air flow into and out of the lungs is obstructed.

Spirometry measures both volume and flow. The test is performed with a spirometer, which is a water-filled cylinder into which an inverted cylinder or bell has been inserted. A length of tubing runs from the inverted bell to a mouthpiece through which a person breathes during testing. The bell is attached to a pen that writes on calibrated paper rotating at a constant speed. As the person performs various breathing maneuvers, the inverted bell moves up and down, causing the pen to move on the calibrated paper. This produces a spirogram, which records the individual's ventilation in relation to time. (Values measured by spirometry are listed in Table 29-4.) Normal values depend on the individual's age, height, and sex (Table 29-3). Findings are usually considered normal if the individual's values are within 80% of normal for his or her age, sex, and height.

To ensure the accuracy of spirometry, the individual must be cooperative and perform the ventilatory maneuvers with maximal effort. Cooperation and effort of the individual are evaluated according to (1) the reproducibility of the spirogram and (2) the perceptions of the technicians administering the test.

Calculation of alveolar-arterial oxygen gradient, or A − a gradient $P(A-a)O_2$, and measurement of right-to-left shunt $(\dot{Q}s/\dot{Q}t)$ are sometimes used to determine the cause of a low Pao_2. These values, calculated

---

TABLE 29-4 Values measured by spirometry

Symbol	Ventilatory property measured
FVC	Forced vital capacity: maximum amount of gas that can be displaced from the lung during a forced expiration
FEV_1	Forced expiratory volume in 1 second: maximum amount of gas that can be displaced from the lung in 1 second
FEV_1/FVC	Percentage of forced vital capacity that is expired in 1 second, usually 80% of FVC
FEV_3	Forced expiratory volume in 3 seconds; maximum amount of gas that can be expired in 3 seconds
FEV_3/FVC	Percentage of FVC that is expired in 3 seconds; usually 95% of FVC
$FEF_{25-75\%}$	Forced expiratory flow rate during the middle 50% of expiration; is sometimes reported as maximum midexpiratory flow rate (MMFR)

from blood gas analysis of samples drawn while the person is breathing 100% oxygen, are often helpful in the management of severe acute respiratory failure.

Diffusing capacity is a measure of the rate of gas diffusion across the alveolocapillary membrane. Oxygen, or more commonly carbon monoxide, is used to measured diffusing capacity. The measurement is made by determining how much carbon dioxide is taken up by the blood and dividing this amount by the pressure gradient across the alveolocapillary membrane. Helium is often added to the gas mixture in order to obtain a simultaneous measurement of RV, FRC, and TLC. Individuals are asked to perform ventilatory maneuvers similar to those of spirometry. A decreased diffusing capacity can be the result of an abnormal ventilation/perfusion ratio or an actual diffusion defect. Diffusing capacity is decreased in individuals with emphysema.

Arterial blood gas analysis is commonly performed for individuals with suspected or diagnosed pulmonary disease. Direct analysis of the pH and gas concentrations in arterial blood provides valuable information about an individual's gas exchange and acid-base status. Acidosis (low pH), alkalosis (high pH), ventilatory alterations, and decreased Pa_{O_2} can only be diagnosed by arterial blood gas analysis. A blood gas report may be divided into an acid-base/ventilation portion and an oxygenation portion. (Normal values for arterial blood gases can be seen in Table 29-5.) (Acid-base alterations are described in Chapter 3.)

Signs and symptoms of most respiratory abnormalities first appear when the system is stressed during exercise. Therefore, if pulmonary disease is suspected, the individual is evaluated at rest and during exercise. During exercise the usual procedures are spirometry and withdrawal of arterial blood for gas analysis. The exercise usually consists of riding a stationary bicycle or walking on a treadmill. Exercise testing enables clinicians to detect early changes in respiratory function and begin treatment. Exercise tests are also used in planning and evaluating exercise and rehabilitation programs.

Chest radiograms are among the most common examinations of the pulmonary system. A few of the abnormalities detected in chest radiographs are air trapping in the alveoli and airways (e.g., in asthma or emphysema), consolidation of lung tissue (in pneumonia or pulmonary edema), cavities (abcesses or tuberculosis), and nodules (lung cancer). Often pulmonary abnormalities are detected in routine chest radiographs of asymptomatic individuals. A variety of radiographic techniques are available for the diagnosis and evaluation

---

TABLE 29-5 Normal ranges for arterial and mixed venous blood gases

Measurement	Arterial blood	Mixed venous blood*	Clinical notes
Acid-base status (pH)	7.35-7.45	7.33-7.43	Most important acid-base value; detects acidosis or alkalosis
Partial pressure of carbon dioxide (P_{CO_2})	35-45 mm Hg	41-57 mm Hg	Measures adequacy of ventilation and respiratory contribution to acid-base abnormality (respiratory acidosis)
Bicarbonate (HCO_3^-)	22-26 mEq/L	24-28 mEq/L	Measures metabolic contribution to acid-base abnormality (metabolic acidosis); calculated from pH and P_{CO_2}
Base excess (BE)	−2 - +2	0 - +4	Reflects deviation of bicarbonate concentration from normal
Partial pressure of oxygen (P_{O_2}) (sea level)	80-100 mm Hg	35-40 mm Hg	Indicates driving pressure that causes oxygen-hemoglobin binding; varies with age and barometric pressure
Saturation of hemoglobin with oxygen (S_{O_2})	96-98%	70-75%	Indicates abnormalities of oxyhemoglobin association and dissociation; may be measured directly or calculated from P_{O_2}, pH, and body temperature
Concentration of hemoglobin in the blood	15 g/100 ml	15 g/100 ml	Detects alterations of gas transport caused by anemia
Oxygen content of the blood	19-20 ml/100 ml	14-15 ml/100 ml	Detects hypoxemia

*Mixed venous (pulmonary artery) blood is analyzed for critically ill individuals and those undergoing cardiac catheterization (it is not practical to withdraw samples except from a pulmonary artery catheter). Mixed venous blood gas analysis, in conjunction with arterial analysis, provides important information about the adequacy of cardiac output and tissue oxygenation.

of respiratory disorders. It is important that radiographs be repeated under similar conditions and that such material as catheters and cables be removed from the individual's chest. This is not usually a problem if the individual can be examined in the radiology department but may pose difficulties if portable x-ray machines are used in the individual's room. The clinician assists the radiology technician in positioning the person and removing material or equipment from the person's chest.

AGING AND THE PULMONARY SYSTEM

Most knowledge about pulmonary structure and function is based on norms for the middle years. Less is known about structure and function in the very young (see Chapter 31) and the elderly, but a few normal physiologic (developmental and degenerative) changes are known to occur from birth to old age. An understanding of these changes is needed to provide appropriate care and to differentiate between normal alterations and disease. Normal alterations can be categorized as (1) structural changes, (2) mechanical changes, and (3) alterations in gas exchange.

During adulthood and as age advances the alveoli tend to enlarge, atrophy, and lose capillaries. This process diminishes alveolar surface area available for gas diffusion and decreases airway support provided by normal lung tissues. Mechanical changes involve elastic properties of the lungs and chest wall. Chest wall compliance decreases with age because the ribs become ossified (less flexible) and their joints become stiffer. As a result the chest wall loses some of its ability to expand. Lung changes occur in reverse order. Elastic recoil diminishes with advancing age, possibly because of loss of elastic fibers in the lung tissue. This leads to an increase in lung compliance. These mechanical changes in the lung and chest wall, along with structural changes in the alveoli, reduce ventilatory capacity in old age. Vital capacity decreases and residual volume increases; however, total lung capacity remains unchanged. This is probably a result of airway instability and collapse at lower lung volumes. These changes decrease ventilatory reserves and lead to decreased ventilation/perfusion ratios.

Alterations in gas exchange are reflected by blood gas analysis. With advancing age, pH or Pco_2 does not change much, even though it has been documented that the chemoreceptors become less sensitive to gas partial pressures with age. Po_2, however, does decline with age as a result of structural and mechanical changes, such as loss of alveolar surface area and increased ventilation-perfusion mismatch. The maximum Pao_2 in an elderly individual at sea level can be estimated by multiplying the person's age by 0.3 and subtracting the product

from 100. For example, an 80-year-old individual would have an estimated maximum Po_2 of 76 mm Hg (0.3 x 80 = 24; 100 - 24 = 76).

The decrease in Pao_2 and diminished ventilatory reserve in the elderly lead to a decrease in exercise tolerance. Changes in respiratory function can vary considerably from person to person, however. They are also affected by activity and fitness earlier in life. A very active, physically fit individual will, all else being equal, have fewer changes in function at any age than one who has been sedentary.

SUMMARY REVIEW

Structures of the Pulmonary System
1 The pulmonary system consists of the lungs, airways, chest wall, and pulmonary and bronchial circulation.
2 Air is inspired and expired through the conducting airways, which include the nasopharynx, oropharynx, trachea, bronchi, and bronchioles to the sixteenth division.
3 Gas exchange occurs in structures beyond the sixteenth division: the respiratory bronchioles, alveolar ducts, and the alveoli. Airways consist of the respiratory bronchioles, alveolar ducts, and alveoli. Together these structures compose the acinus.
4 The chief gas-exchange units of the lungs are the alveoli. The membrane that surrounds each alveolus and contains the pulmonary capillaries is called the alveolocapillary membrane.
5 The gas-exchange airways are served by the pulmonary circulation, a separate division of the circulatory system. The bronchi and other lung structures are served by a branch of the systemic circulation called the bronchial circulation.
6 The chest wall, which contains and protects the contents of the thoracic cavity, consists of the skin, ribs, and intercostal muscles, which lie between the ribs.
7 The chest wall is lined by a serous membrane called the parietal pleura; the lungs are encased in a separate membrane called the visceral pleura. The area where these two pleurae come into contact and slide over one another is called the pleural space.

Function of the Pulmonary System
1 The pulmonary system enables oxygen to diffuse into the blood and carbon dixoide to diffuse out of the blood.
2 Ventilation is the process by which air flows into and out of the gas-exchange airways.
3 Successful ventilation involves the mechanics of breathing: the interaction of forces and counterforces involving the muscles of inspiration and expiration, alveolar surface tension, elastic properties of the lungs and chest wall, and resistance to airflow.
4 The major muscle of inspiration is the diaphragm.

When the diaphragm contracts it moves downward in the thoracic cavity, creating a vacuum that causes air to flow into the lungs.

5 The alveoli produce surfactant, a lipoprotein that lines the alveoli. Surfactant reduces alveolar surface tension and permits the alveoli to expand as air flows in.

6 Compliance is the ability of the lungs and chest wall to expand during inspiration. Lung compliance is ensured by adequate production of surfactant, whereas chest wall expansion depends on flexibility.

7 Elastic recoil is the tendency of the lungs and chest wall to return to their resting state after inspiration. The elastic recoil forces of the lungs and chest wall are in opposition and pull upon each other, creating the normally negative pressure of the pleural space.

8 Most of the time ventilation is involuntary. It is controlled by the sympathetic and parasympathetic divisions of the autonomic nervous system, which adjust airway caliber (by causing bronchial smooth muscle to contract or relax) and control the rate and depth of ventilation.

9 Neuroreceptors in the lungs (lung receptors) monitor the mechanical aspects of ventilation. Irritant receptors sense the need to expel unwanted substances, stretch receptors sense lung volume (lung expansion), and J-receptors sense alveolar size.

10 Chemoreceptors in the circulatory system and brain stem sense the effectiveness of ventilation by monitoring the pH status of cerebrospinal fluid and the oxygen content (Po_2) of arterial blood.

11 The pulmonary circulation is innervated by the ANS, but vasodilation and vasoconstriction are controlled mainly by local and humoral factors, particularly arterial oxygenation and acid-base status.

12 Gas transport depends on ventilation of the alveoli, diffusion across the alveolocapillary membrane, perfusion of the pulmonary capillaries or circulation and systemic capillaries, and diffusion between systemic capillaries and tissue cells.

13 Efficient gas exchange depends on an even distribution of ventilation and perfusion within the lungs. Both ventilation and perfusion are greatest in the bases of the lungs because the alveoli in the bases are more compliant (their resting volume is low) and perfusion is greater in the bases as a result of gravity.

14 Almost all of the oxygen that diffuses into pulmonary capillary blood is transported by hemoglobin, a protein contained within red blood cells. The remainder of the oxygen is transported dissolved in plasma.

15 Oxygen enters the body by diffusing down the concentration gradient, from high concentrations in the alveoli to lower concentrations in the capillaries. Diffusion ceases when alveolar and capillary oxygen pressures equilibrate.

16 Oxygen is loaded onto hemoglobin by the driving pressure exerted by Pao_2 in the plasma. As pressure decreases at the tissue level, oxygen dissociates from hemoglobin and enters tissue cells by diffusion, again down the concentration gradient.

17 Carbon dioxide is more soluble in plasma than oxygen is. Therefore, carbon dioxide diffuses readily from tissue cells into plasma. Carbon dioxide returns to the lungs dissolved in plasma, as bicarbonate, or in carbamino compounds (e.g., bound to hemoglobin).

Tests of Pulmonary Function

1 Spirometry measures both volume and flow rate during forced expiration.

2 The alveolar-arterial oxygen gradient is used to evaluate the cause of hypoxia.

3 Diffusing capacity is a measure of the gas diffusion rate at the alveolocapillary membrane.

4 Arterial blood gas (ABG) analysis can be used to determine pH and oxygen and carbon dioxide concentrations.

5 Radiographic examination of the chest evaluates air trapping, consolidation, cavity formation, or presence of tumors.

Aging and the Pulmonary System

1 Aging affects the mechanical aspects of ventilation by decreasing chest wall compliance and elastic recoil of the lungs. Changes in these elastic properties reduce ventilatory reserve.

2 Aging causes the Pao_2 to decrease but does not affect the $Paco_2$.

KEY TERMS

Acinus, 1030

Alveolar duct, 1030

Alveolar ventilation ($\dot{V}_A$), 1036

Alveolocapillary membrane, 1032

Alveolus, 1032

Bohr effect, 1048

Bronchiole, 1029

Bronchus, 1029

Carina, 1029

Central chemoreceptor, 1042

Chemoreceptor, 1040

Chest radiogram, 1049

Compliance, 1038

Dead-space ventilation ($\dot{V}_D$), 1036

Diffusing capacity, 1049

Elastic recoil (elastance), 1038

Expiratory reserve volume (ERV), 1036

Functional residual capacity (FRC), 1036

Goblet cell, 1030

Haldane effect, 1048

Hilus, 1029

Hypoxic vasoconstriction, 1042

Inspiratory capacity (IC), 1036

Inspiratory reserve volume (IRV), 1036

Irritant receptor, 1041

J-receptor, 1041

Larynx, 1027

Lung receptor, 1040

Nasopharynx, 1027

Oropharynx, 1027

Oxyhemoglobin (HbO_2), 1046

Oxyhemoglobin dissociation curve, 1046

Partial pressure (tension) of a gas, 1034

Peripheral chemoreceptor, 1042

Pleura, 1034

Pleural space, 1034

Residual volume (RV), 1036

Respiratory bronchiole, 1030

Spirometry, 1048

Stretch receptor, 1041

Surface tension, 1038

Surfactant, 1030

Thoracic cavity, 1034

Tidal volume (TV), 1036

Total lung capacity (TLC), 1036

Trachea, 1029

Ventilation, 1034

Ventilation/perfusion ratio, or mismatch ($\dot{V}/\dot{Q}$), 1044

Vital capacity (VC), 1036

REFERENCES

Altose, M. D. (1979). The physiological basis of pulmonary function testing. CIBA, *Clinical Symposia, 31*(2), 1-39.

Bogartz, L. J. (1983). Control of respiration: A review and update. *Current Revue of Respiratory Theory, 8*(21), 167-172.

Brian, , & Ingles, . (1965). *A history of medicine.* : World Publishing Company.

Brigham, K. L., & Newman, J. H. (1979). The pulmonary circulation. *Basics of Respiratory Disease, 8*(1), 1-6.

Burton, J. (1982, November). Acid-base balance. *Critical Care Update, 9*(10), 23-25.

Burton, J. (1982, November). Arterial blood gases. *Critical Care Update, 9*(10), 23-25.

Burton, J. (1982, November). Compensation of acid-base disturbances. *Critical Care Update, 9*(11), 15-16.

Carrieri, V. K., Murdaugh, C., & Janson-Bjerklie, S. (1984, April). A framework for assessing pulmonary disease categories. *Focus on Critical Care, 11*(2), 10-24.

Cherniak, R. M. & Cherniak, L. (1982). *Respiration in health and disease* (3d ed.). Philadelphia: W. B. Saunders.

Clemmer, T. P. (1982). Oxygen transport. *International Anesthetic Clinics, 19*(3), 21-38.

Comroe, J. H. (1974). *Physiology of respiration* (2d ed.). Chicago: Yearbook Medical.

Crapo, R. O., Morris, A. H., & Gardner, R. M. (1981). Reference spirometric values using techniques and equipment that meet ATS recommendations. *American Review of Respiratory Diseases, 123,* 659-664.

Davenport, H. W. (1975). *The ABC of acid-base chemistry* (6th ed.). Chicago: University of Chicago Press.

Finch, C. A., & Lenfant, C. (1972). Oxygen transport in man. *New England Journal of Medicine, 286*(8), 407-415.

Fishman, A. P. (1980). *Pulmonary diseases and disorders.* New York: McGraw-Hill.

Freeman, E. (1985). The respiratory system. In J. C. Brocklehurst (Ed.), *Textbook of geriatric medicine and gerontology.* London: Churchill Livingstone.

Gray, H. (1977). *Gray's anatomy.* New York: Bounty Books.

Guyton, A. (1986). *Textbook of medical physiology* (7th ed.). Philadelphia: W. B. Saunders.

Hedemark, L. L. & Kronenberg, R. S. (1982, October). Chemical regulation of respiration: Normal variations and abnormal responses. *Chest, 82*(4), 488-494.

Janson-Bjerklie, S. (1983, November). Defense mechanisms: Protecting the healthy lung. *Heart & Lung, 12*(6), 643-649.

Keyes, J. L. (1976, March-April). Basic mechanisms involved in acid-base homeostasis. *Heart & Lung, 5*(2), 239-246.

Keyes, J. L. (1976, March-April). Blood gas analysis and the assessment of acid-base status. *Heart & Lung, 5*(2), 247-255.

Litrell, K. (1983, August). Arterial blood gas analysis: The matching game. *Focus on Critical Care, 10*(4), 49-51.

McFadden, E. R. (1977). Pulmonary functioning testing: Theory and practical applications. *Asthma and Allergy, 4*(1), 10-21.

Micca, R. (1983). The physiology and physics of ventilation: Mechanisms. *Current Reviews for Recovery Room Nurses, 5*(12), 99-104.

Micca, R. (1983). The physiology and physics of ventilation: Static lung volumes. *Current Reviews for Recovery Room Nurses, 5*(11), 91-96.

Murray, J. F. (1986). *The normal lung.* Philadelphia: W. B. Saunders.

Pavlin, E. G., & Hornbein, T. F. (1978, November). The control of breathing. *Basics of Respiratory Disease, 7*(2), 1-6.

Rochester, D. F. (1984, July). Respiratory muscle function in health. *Heart & Lung, 13*(4), 349-354.

Roussos, C. (1985, August). Function and fatigue of respiratory muscles. *Chest, 88*(2), 1245.

Shapiro, B. A., Harrison, R. A., & Walton, S. R. (1985). *Clinical application of blood gases* (4th ed.). Chicago: Yearbook Medical.

Singer, C. J., & Underwood, E. A. (1962). *A short history of medicine.* New York: Oxford University Press.

Thibodeau, G. A. (1987). *Anatomy and physiology.* St. Louis: C.V. Mosby Co.

Thompson, J. M., et al. (1989). *Mosby's manual of clinical nursing,* (2nd ed.) St. Louis: C.V. Mosby Co.

Weibel, E. R. (1983, April). How does lung structure affect gas exchange. *Chest, 83*(4), 657-665.

West, J. (1985). *Respiratory physiology—the essentials* (3rd ed.). Baltimore: Williams & Wilkins.

West, J. B., Dollery, C. T., & Naimark, A. (1974). Distribution of blood flow in isolated lung: Relation to vascular and alveolar pressures. *Journal of Applied Physiology, 19,* 713-724.

Woodson, R. D. (1977, March). O_2 transport; DPG and P50. *Basics of Respiratory Disease, 5*(4), 1-6.

CHAPTER 30

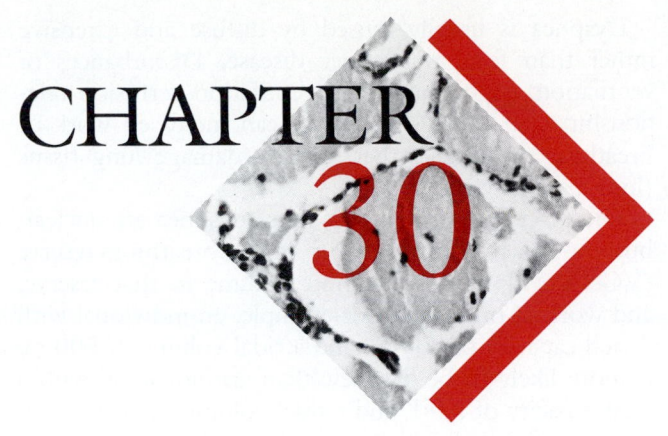

Alterations of Pulmonary Function

Marjorie Budd
Kathryn L. McCance

Clinical manifestations of pulmonary alterations, 1054
  Signs and symptoms of pulmonary disease, 1054
    Dyspnea, 1054
    Abnormal breathing patterns, 1055
    Hypoventilation/hyperventilation, 1055
    Cough, 1055
    Hemoptysis, 1055
    Cyanosis, 1056
    Pain, 1056
    Clubbing, 1056
    Abnormal sputum, 1057
  Conditions caused by pulmonary disease or injury, 1057
    Hypoxemia, 1057
    Pulmonary edema, 1058
    Aspiration, 1060
      Atelectasis, 1060
    Bronchiectasis, 1060
    Bronchiolitis, 1062
    Pleural abnormalities, 1062
      Pneumothorax, 1062
      Pleural effusion, 1063
      Empyema, 1064
      Pleurisy, 1064
    Abscess formation and cavitation, 1064
    Pulmonary fibrosis, 1065
    Chest wall restriction, 1065
    Flail chest, 1065
    Inhalation disorders, 1065
      Exposure to toxic gases, 1065
      Pneumoconiosis, 1066
      Allergic alveolitis, 1067
    Systemic disorders, 1067
Pulmonary disorders, 1067
  Acute respiratory failure, 1067
    Adult respiratory distress syndrome, 1067
      Pathophysiology, 1067
      Clinical manifestations, 1068
      Evaluation and treatment, 1068
    Postoperative respiratory failure, 1069

Obstructive pulmonary disease, 1069
  Asthma, 1069
    Types of asthma, 1069
    Pathophysiology, 1070
    Clinical manifestations, 1071
    Evaluation and treatment, 1071
  Chronic bronchitis, 1072
    Pathophysiology, 1072
    Clinical manifestations, 1073
    Evaluation and treatment, 1073
  Emphysema, 1074
    Pathophysiology, 1074
    Clinical manifestations, 1074
    Evaluation and treatment, 1076
Respiratory tract infections, 1076
  Pneumonia, 1076
    Pathophysiology, 1077
      Pneumococcal pneumonia, 1077
      Viral pneumonia, 1077
    Clinical manifestations, 1078
    Evaluation and treatment, 1078
  Tuberculosis, 1079
    Pathophysiology, 1079
    Clinical manifestations, 1079
    Evaluation and treatment, 1079
  Acute bronchitis, 1080
Pulmonary vascular disease, 1080
  Pulmonary embolism, 1080
    Pathophysiology, 1080
    Clinical manifestations, 1081
    Evaluation and treatment, 1081
  Pulmonary hypertension, 1082
    Pathophysiology, 1082
    Clinical manifestations, 1082
    Evaluation and treatment, 1082
  Cor pulmonale, 1082
    Pathophysiology, 1083
    Clinical manifestations, 1083
    Evaluation and treatment, 1083

Lip cancer, 1083
  Pathophysiology, 1083
  Clinical manifestations, 1084
  Evaluation and treatment, 1084
Laryngeal cancer, 1084
  Pathophysiology, 1085
  Clinical manifestations, 1085
  Evaluation and treatment, 1085
Lung cancer, 1085
  Types of lung cancer, 1086
    Squamous cell carcinoma, 1087
    Small cell carcinoma, 1087
    Adenocarcinoma, 1088
    Large cell carcinoma, 1088
  Pathogenesis, 1088
  Clinical manifestations, 1088
  Evaluation and treatment, 1088
  Other lung cancers, 1088
    Bronchial adenomas, 1088
    Mesotheliomas, 1090
  Staging of lung cancer, 1090

Pulmonary disease is often classified as acute or chronic, obstructive or restrictive, infectious or noninfectious, and is caused by lung or heart failure. Because skillful and knowledgeable clinical care plays a major role in decreasing respiratory mortality and morbidity, the nurse who has a clear understanding of the pathophysiology of common respiratory problems can greatly affect the outcome for each individual.

CLINICAL MANIFESTATIONS OF PULMONARY ALTERATIONS

Signs and Symptoms of Pulmonary Disease

Pulmonary disease is associated with many common signs and symptoms. The most common of these are cough and respiratory distress. Other manifestations include abnormal sputum, bluish discoloration of skin, coughing up of blood, chest pain, fever, and altered breathing patterns. The signs and symptoms present and their specific characteristics often help in identifying the underlying disorder.

Dyspnea

Dyspnea is the subjective sensation of breathlessness, shortness of breath, or respiratory distress. The individual has an abnormal awareness or preoccupation with breathing, and ventilation may be excessive in relation to physical exertion. Dyspnea is not synonymous with **tachypnea,** or increased ventilatory rate, as many individuals have tachypnea without any sensation of breathlessness.

Dyspnea is usually caused by diffuse and extensive rather than focal pulmonary disease. Disturbances of ventilation, gas exchange, or ventilation-perfusion relationships can cause dyspnea, as can increased work of breathing or diseases that severely damage lung tissue (lung parenchyma).

The exact mechanisms that cause dyspnea are unclear, but the major factors appear to be breathing reserve (VC-TV), closeness of minute volume to that reserve, and work of breathing. For example, an individual with a vital capacity of 800 ml and a tidal volume of 500 ml is more likely to be dyspneic than an individual with a vital capacity of 3.0 L and a tidal volume of 500 ml because the first individual's average breath is very close to the maximum possible breath. (These volumes and capacities are shown schematically in Chapter 29, Fig. 29-12.) Similarly an individual with compliance of 25 ml/cm H_2O and tidal volume of 500 ml is more likely to be dyspneic than an individual with a compliance of 80 ml/cm H_2O with the same tidal volume because the first individual has to work harder to inspire the same amount of air. Neurologic mechanisms may also contribute to dyspnea, particularly the irritant and J-receptors in the lung, which send impulses to the vagus nerve, and receptors in the respiratory muscles, particularly the diaphragm, which signal the central nervous system through the phrenic nerve.

The signs of dyspnea include flaring of the nostrils, use of accessory muscles of respiration, and retraction (pulling back) of the intercostal spaces. In dyspnea caused by parenchymal disease (e.g., pneumonia), retractions of tissue between the ribs (subcostal and intercostal retractions) are observed more frequently than supercostal retractions (retractions of tissues above the ribs), which predominate in upper-airway obstruction.

Dyspnea can occur transiently or in specific circumstances. Frequently the first episode occurs with exercise and is called dyspnea on exertion. Pulmonary congestion tends to cause dyspnea when the individual is lying down. This type is called **orthopnea** (positional dyspnea). Orthopnea is caused by the horizontal position, which redistributes body water, causes the abdominal contents to exert pressure on the diaphragm, or decreases the efficiency of the respiratory muscles. Orthopnea is generally relieved by sitting up or supporting the upper body on several pillows. Some individuals with left ventricular failure wake up at night gasping for air and have to sit up or stand to relieve the dyspnea. This type of positional dyspnea is termed paroxysmal nocturnal dypsnea (PND). PND results from fluid in the lungs caused by the redistribution of body water while the individual is recumbent. **Apnea** is the cessation of breathing.

Abnormal Breathing Patterns

Normal breathing (eupnea) is rhythmic and effortless. Ventilatory rate is 8 to 16 breaths per minute, and tidal volume ranges from 400 to 800 ml. A short expiratory pause occurs with each breath, and the individual takes an occasional deeper breath or sighs.

The rate, depth, regularity, and effort of breathing undergo characteristic alterations in response to physiologic and pathophysiologic conditions. Patterns of breathing automatically adjust to minimize the work of respiratory muscles. Strenuous exercise or metabolic acidosis induce **Kussmaul respiration** (hyperpnea). Kussmaul respiration is characterized by a slightly increased ventilatory rate; very large, effortless tidal volumes; and no expiratory pause.

Labored, or obstructed, breathing occurs if the airways are obstructed, as in chronic obstructive pulmonary disease. Obstructed breathing consists of slow ventilatory rate, large tidal volume, increased effort, and prolonged inspiration or expiration, depending on the site of obstruction. Audible wheezing (whistling sounds) or stridor (high-pitched sounds made during inspiration) is often present.

Restricted breathing is commonly caused by disorders, such as pulmonary fibrosis, that stiffen the lungs or chest wall and decrease compliance. Restricted breathing is characterized by small tidal volumes and rapid ventilatory rate (tachypnea), both of which minimize the work of breathing. Panting occurs with exercise. Shock and severe cerebral hypoxia (insufficient oxygen in the brain) contribute to gasping respirations that consist of irregular, quick inspirations with an expiratory pause.

Cheyne-Stokes respirations are characterized by alternating periods of deep and shallow breathing. Apnea lasting from 15 to 60 seconds is followed by ventilations that increase in volume until a peak is reached, after which ventilation (tidal volume) decreases again to apnea. Cheyne-Stokes respirations result from any condition that slows the blood flow to the brain stem, which, in turn, slows impulses sending information to the respiratory centers of the brain stem. Neurologic impairment above the brain stem is also a contributing factor.

Sighing respirations consist of irregular breathing characterized by frequent, deep sighing inspirations. Sighing respirations are caused by anxiety.

Hypoventilation/Hyperventilation

Hypoventilation is inadequate alveolar ventilation in relation to metabolic demands. It is always caused by alterations in pulmonary mechanics or in the neurologic control of breathing. When alveolar ventilation is normal, carbon dioxide is removed from the lungs at the same rate as it is produced by cellular metabolism. This maintains arterial and alveolar Pco_2 at normal levels (40 mm Hg). With hypoventilation CO_2 removal does not keep up with CO_2 production and $Paco_2$ rises, causing **hypercapnea** ($Paco_2$ greater than 44 mm Hg). (See Chapter 29, Table 29-2, for a definition of gas partial pressures and other pulmonary abbreviations.)

Hypoventilation is often overlooked until it is severe because breathing pattern and ventilatory rate may appear to be normal. Hypoventilation can only be determined by blood gas analysis (i.e., by measurement of the $Paco_2$ of arterial blood). Pronounced hypoventilation can cause somnolence or disorientation. Pao_2 may be reduced in those breathing room air.

Hyperventilation is alveolar ventilation that exceeds metabolic demands. The lungs remove CO_2 at a faster rate than it is produced by cellular metabolism, resulting in decreased $Paco_2$, or **hypocapnea** ($Paco_2$ less than 36 mm Hg). Like hypoventilation, hyperventilation can only be determined by arterial blood gas analysis. Hyperventilation commonly occurs with severe anxiety, acute head injury, and conditions that cause insufficient oxygenation of the blood.

Cough

A **cough** is a protective reflex that cleanses the lower airways by an explosive expiration. Inhaled particles, accumulated mucus, inflammation, or presence of a foreign body initiates the cough reflex by stimulating the irritant receptors in the airway. The cough consists of inspiration, closure of the glottis and vocal cords, contraction of the expiratory muscles, and reopening of the glottis, causing a sudden, forceful expiration that removes the offending matter. The effectiveness of the cough depends on the depth of the inspiration and the degree to which the airways narrow, increasing the velocity of expiratory gas flow.

A persistent cough indicates the presence of a disorder or disease. An acute nonproductive cough often indicates bronchitis or viral pneumonia. Aspiration of a foreign body or irritating fumes can cause a dry cough. A persistent dry cough is commonly caused by a tumor or congestion. A cough that produces purulent sputum usually indicates infection, whereas a cough that produces nonpurulent sputum is nonspecific and merely indicates irritation. It is important to remember that many individuals swallow their sputum, and a lack of expectorated sputum does not mean that a cough is nonproductive.

Hemoptysis

Hemoptysis is the coughing up of blood or bloody secretions. Hemoptysis is sometimes confused with hematemesis, which is the vomiting of blood. Blood that is coughed up is usually bright red, has an alkaline pH, and is mixed with frothy sputum, whereas blood that is vomited is dark, has an acidic pH, and is mixed with food particles.

Hemoptysis indicates a localized abnormality, usually infection or inflammation that damages the bronchi (bronchitis, bronchiectasis) or the lung parenchyma (tuberculosis, lung abscess). Other causes include cancer and pulmonary infarction. The amount and duration of bleeding (i.e., a sudden large amount versus a persistent slight amount) provide important clues about the source of the bleeding. Bronchoscopy is used to confirm the site of bleeding.

Cyanosis

Cyanosis is a bluish discoloration of the skin caused by increasing amounts of desaturated or reduced hemoglobin (which is bluish) in the blood. Cyanosis generally develops when 5 g of hemoglobin is desaturated, regardless of hemoglobin concentration. For example, if total hemoglobin concentration is 15 g/100 ml of blood, then 5 g/100 ml must be desaturated to cause cyanosis. If total Hb is 11 g/100 ml, 5 g/100 ml must still be desaturated for cyanosis to occur.

Cyanosis can result from decreased arterial oxygenation (low Pao_2), pulmonary or cardiac right-to-left shunts, or decreased cardiac output. A cold environment or anxiety can cause cyanosis because of peripheral vasoconstriction. Lack of cyanosis does not necessarily indicate that oxygenation is normal. Sometimes impaired cellular oxygenation is not accompanied by cyanosis. For example, severe anemia (inadequate hemoglobin concentration) and carbon monoxide poisoning (in which hemoglobin binds to carbon monoxide instead of to oxygen) can cause inadequate oxygenation of tissues without causing cyanosis. Individuals with polycythemia (an abnormal increase in numbers of red blood cells), on the other hand, may have cyanosis when oxygenation is adequate. Because polycythemia causes hemoglobin concentration to be greater than normal, 5 g/100 ml can be desturated, causing cyanosis, without having much effect on oxygenation. Therefore, the significance of cyanosis as a clinical finding must be interpreted in relation to the underlying pathophysiology. The ear lobes, nail beds, lips, and mucous membranes are good areas to observe for cyanosis because the capillaries in these areas are close to the surface.

Pain

Pain caused by pulmonary disorders originates in the pleurae, the lungs, or the chest wall. Pleural pain is the most common pain caused by pulmonary disease. Infection and inflammation of the parietal pleura cause pain when the pleura stretches during inspiration. The pain is usually localized to a portion of the chest wall, where a unique breath sound called a pleural friction rub can be heard over the painful area. Laughing or coughing makes pleural pain worse. Pleural pain is also common with pulmonary infarction (tissue death) caused by pulmonary embolism. In the case of infarction, the pain eminates from the area around the infarction.

Pulmonary pain is central chest pain that is pronounced after coughing and occurs in individuals with infection and inflammation of the trachea and/or bronchi (tracheitis or tracheobronchitis). Central chest pain has to be differentiated from cardiac pain (see Chapter 27). High blood pressure in the pulmonary circulation (pulmonary hypertension) can cause pain during exercise that is often mistaken for cardiac pain (angina pectoris).

Pain in the chest wall is muscle pain or rib pain (costochondritis). The common causes of chest wall pain are excessive coughing, which makes the muscles sore, and rib fractures. Chest wall pain often mimics pleural pain.

Clubbing

Clubbing is the selective bulbous enlargement of the end (distal segment) of a digit (finger or toe) (Fig. 30-1). Usually it is painless. Clubbing is commonly associated with diseases that interfere with oxygenation, such as lung cancer, bronchiectasis, cystic fibrosis, pulmonary fibrosis, lung abscess, emphysema, and congenital heart disease. Its pathogenesis is unknown.

Clubbing—early

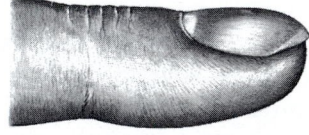

Clubbing—middle

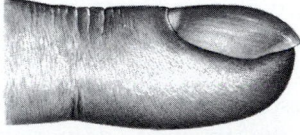

Clubbing—severe

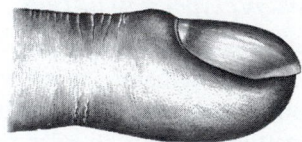

FIG. 30-1. Clubbing of fingers caused by chronic hypoxemia. (From Seidel, Ball, Dains, & Benedict, 1987.)

Abnormal Sputum

The color, consistency, odor, and amount of sputum vary with different pulmonary disorders. A distinctive color or odor may indicate infection by a specific microorganism. Changes in the amount and consistency of sputum provide information about progression of disease and effectiveness of therapy. The gross and microscopic appearances of sputum enable the clinician to identify cellular debris or microorganisms that aid in diagnosis and choice of therapy.

Conditions Caused by Pulmonary Disease or Injury

Hypoxemia

Hypoxemia, or reduced oxygenation of arterial blood (reduced Pa_{O_2}) is caused by respiratory alterations, whereas **hypoxia,** or reduced oxygenation of cells in tissues, may be caused by alterations of other systems as well. (Hypoxia can occur anywhere in the body; if it occurs in arterial blood, it is correctly called hypoxemia.) Although hypoxemia can lead to tissue hypoxia, tissue hypoxia can result from other abnormalities, such as low cardiac output or cyanide poisoning, that have no relation to alterations of pulmonary function.

There are five causes of hypoxemia: (1) decreased oxygen content (P_{O_2}) of inspired gas, (2) hypoventilation, (3) diffusion abnormalities, (4) abnormal ventilation/perfusion ratios, and (5) pulmonary right-to-left shunt (Table 30-1). The physiologic mechanisms for each cause of hypoxemia are different, and each requires different clinical management.

The P_{O_2} of arterial blood depends on the P_{O_2} of inspired gas (Pi_{O_2}). If the P_{O_2} of inspired gas is below normal, then less oxygen is available to diffuse into the blood. The most common cause of a decrease in inspired oxygen is the drop in atmospheric pressure that occurs at high altitudes. Pi_{O_2} drops proportionately with atmospheric pressure, resulting in a drop in Pa_{O_2}. Hypoxemia caused by high altitude is prevented by the use of supplemental oxygen.

Hypoventilation of the alveoli causes elevated Pa_{CO_2} (hypercapnea). If fresh, oxygen-rich gas is not delivered to the alveoli, the oxygen content of alveolar gas (PA_{O_2}) falls as Pa_{CO_2} rises. As PA_{O_2} falls less oxygen diffuses into the blood, causing hypoxemia. This type of hypoxemia can be completely corrected if alveolar ventilation is improved by increases in the rate and depth of breathing. Hypoventilation is a common cause of hypoxemia in unconscious persons and in individuals who have chronic obstructive pulmonary disease.

Diffusion of oxygen through the alveolocapillary membrane is impaired if the alveolocapillary membrane is thickened or the surface area available for diffusion is decreased. Abnormal thickness, such as that which occurs with edema (tissue swelling) and fibrosis (formation of fibrous lesions), increases the time required for diffusion across the alveolocapillary membrane. If diffusion is slowed enough, the P_{O_2} of alveolar gas and capillary blood does not have time to equilibrate during the fraction of a second that blood remains in the capillary. Destruction of alveoli, such as that which occurs in emphysema, decreases the surface area available for diffusion. Hypoxemia caused by impaired diffusion alone is rare, however, and hypercapnea is never produced by impaired diffusion because carbon dioxide diffuses so easily from capillary to alveolus that the individual with

---

TABLE 30-1 Causes of hypoxemia

Mechanism	Common clinical cause
Decrease in inspired oxygen	High altitude Low oxygen content of gas mixture Enclosed breathing space (suffocation)
Hypoventilation	Lack of neurologic stimulation of the respiratory center (oversedation, drug overdose, neurologic damage) Chronic obstructive pulmonary disease
Alveolocapillary diffusion abnormality	Emphysema Fibrosis Edema
Increased ventilation-perfusion mismatch	Asthma Chronic bronchitis Pneumonia
Shunting	Adult respiratory distress syndrome Respiratory distress syndrome of the newborn (hyaline membrane disease) Atelectasis

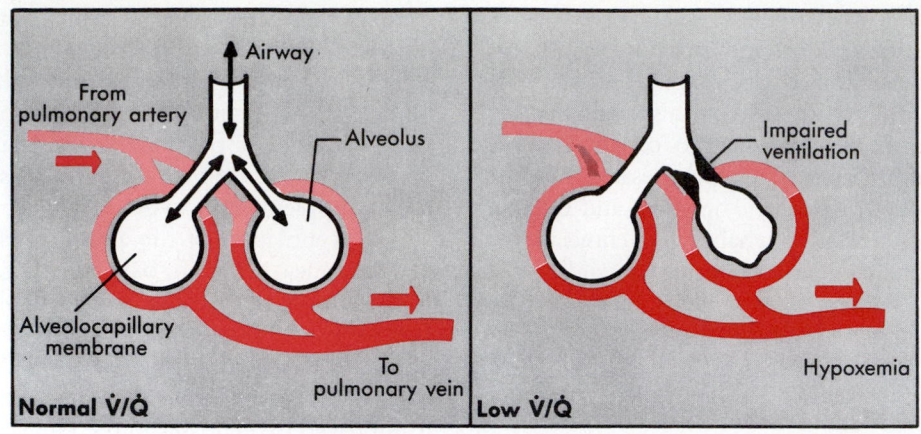

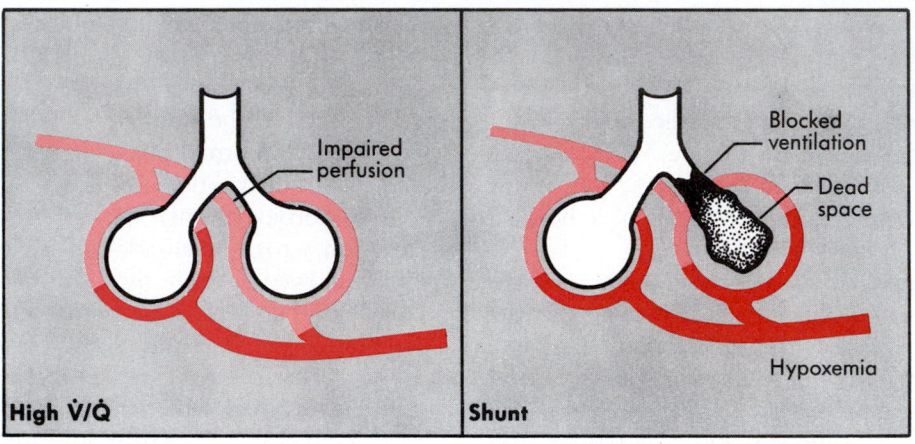

FIG. 30-2. Ventilation-perfusion abnormalities.

impaired diffusion would succumb from hypoxemia before hypercapnea could occur.

An abnormal ventilation/perfusion ratio ($\dot{V}/\dot{Q}$) is the most common cause of hypoxemia. (Normal $\dot{V}/\dot{Q}$ is 0.8; see Chapter 29.) Hypoxemia is caused by inadequate ventilation of well-perfused areas of the lung, poor perfusion of well-ventilated areas, or both (Fig. 30-2). Low $\dot{V}/\dot{Q}$, or poor ventilation of a well-perfused segment of the lung, might be caused by mucous plugging of a bronchus. The resulting low PA_{O_2} would lead to a low Pa_{O_2}, hypoxemia, and, when severe, to hypercapnea. Mismatching of this type is common in bronchitis and asthma.

High $\dot{V}/\dot{Q}$, or poor perfusion of a well-ventilated portion of the lung, may result from a pulmonary embolus that has impaired blood flow to a lung segment. In this case PA_{O_2} would be elevated because little blood could flow through the capillary bed to remove oxygen from the alveoli. Areas of high $\dot{V}/\dot{Q}$ are often termed **physiologic dead space.**

In pulmonary right-to-left shunt, blood passes through portions of the pulmonary capillary bed that receive no ventilation, either because the airway leading to the alveoli is completely obstructed or because the alveoli are collapsed or filled with fluid. Blood flows from the pulmonary artery and through the pulmonary capillary bed, enters the pulmonary vein, and passes into the systemic arterial circulation without unloading carbon dioxide and taking on oxygen. This decreases systemic Pa_{O_2} and results in hypoxemia. Pa_{CO_2} is usually not affected except by severe shunting.

The hypoxemia resulting from pulmonary shunting does not respond to increases in inspired oxygen concentration (supplemental oxygen) because a portion of the pulmonary capillary blood is never exposed to oxygen-rich alveolar gas. This makes hypoxemia produced by shunting very difficult to treat. Shunting is the cause of hypoxemia in adult respiratory distress syndrome and respiratory distress syndrome of the newborn. Hypoxemia from other causes can be corrected by administration of 100% oxygen.

Pulmonary Edema

Pulmonary edema is excess water in the lung. The normal lung contains very little water or fluid. It is kept dry by lymphatic drainage and a balance among capil-

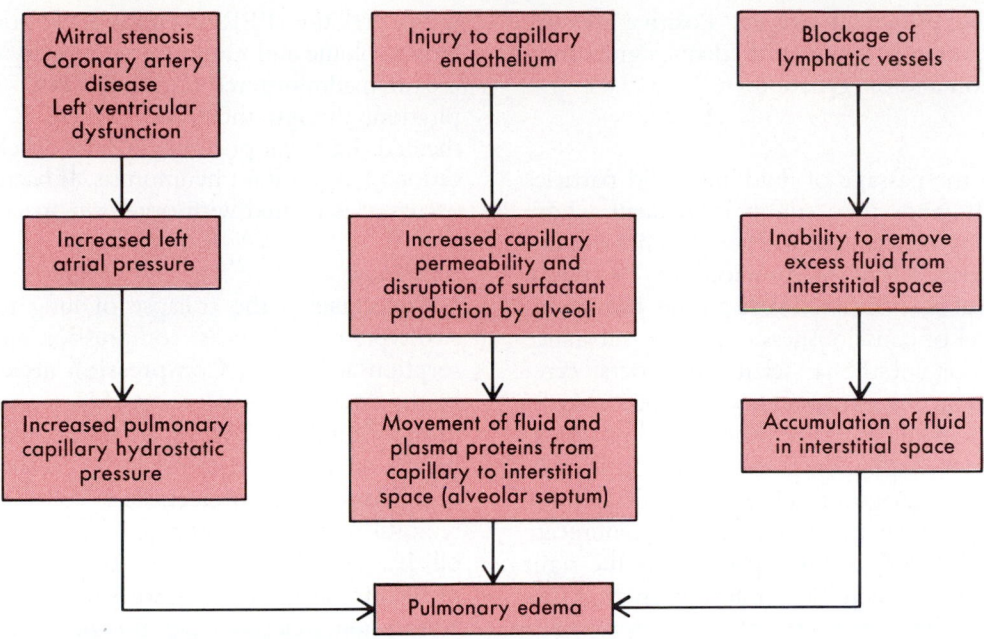

FIG. 30-3. Pathogenesis of pulmonary edema.

lary hydrostatic pressure, capillary oncotic pressure, and capillary permeability. (The mechanisms that determine this balance and water movement across the capillary membrane are described in Chapters 1 and 3.) Predisposing factors for pulmonary edema include heart disease, adult respiratory distress syndrome, and inhalation of toxic gases. The pathogenesis of pulmonary edema is shown in Fig. 30-3.

The most common cause of pulmonary edema is heart disease. When the left ventricle fails, filling pressures on the left side of the heart increase and cause a concomitant increase in pulmonary capillary hydrostatic pressure. When the hydrostatic pressure push exceeds oncotic pressure, which holds fluid in the capillary, fluid moves out into the interstitium, or interstitial space (the space within the alveolar septum between alveolus and capillary). Initially fluid is picked up by lymphatic vessels and removed from the lung. When the flow of fluid out of the capillaries exceeds the lymphatic system's ability to remove it, pulmonary edema develops.

Pulmonary edema usually begins to develop at a pulmonary capillary wedge pressure or left atrial pressure of 20 mm Hg. If the capillary oncotic pressure is decreased for any reason (such as anemia or decreased plasma proteins) pulmonary edema develops at a lower hydrostatic pressure. Individuals with chronically elevated hydrostatic pressure tend to develop pulmonary edema at higher left atrial pressures.

Another cause of pulmonary edema is capillary injury that increases capillary permeability. Capillary injury causes edema in cases of adult respiratory distress syndrome or inhalation of toxic gases, such as ammonia.

Capillary injury causes water and plasma proteins to leak out of the capillary and move into the interstitium. When plasma proteins move into the lung interstitium, they increase the lung's oncotic pressure, which is usually very low. As the lung's oncotic pressure begins to equal capillary oncotic pressure, water moves out of the capillary and into the lung. (This phenomenon is discussed in Chapter 3, Fig. 3-1.)

High altitude (over 7000 feet) sometimes causes a unique form of pulmonary edema (Hultgren, 1970). Although the exact mechanism of high-altitude pulmonary edema is not certain, edema may begin with nonuniform hypoxic vasoconstriction that occurs in the pulmonary vasculature because of hypoxemia. Vasoconstriction causes pulmonary artery pressure to rise, forcing water out of the capillaries.

Clinical manifestations of pulmonary edema include dyspnea, hypoxemia, and increased work of breathing. In severe edema pink frothy sputum is expectorated and P_{CO_2} rises.

The treatment of pulmonary edema depends on its cause. If the edema is caused by increased hydrostatic pressure, therapy is geared toward reducing blood pressure with diuretics, vasodilators, and drugs that improve the contraction of the heart muscle. If edema is the result of increased capillary permeability resulting from injury, the treatment is focused on removing the offending agent and increasing capillary oncotic pressure by adding plasma proteins (colloids) to the blood. Restoration of plasma proteins increases capillary oncotic pressure and draws water from the lung back into the blood vessels. Individuals with either type of pulmonary edema require supplemental oxygen. Positive-pressure mechanical ventilation is also used if edema significantly impairs ventilation and oxygenation.

Aspiration

Aspiration is the passage of fluid and solid particles into the lung. It tends to occur in individuals whose normal swallowing mechanism and cough reflex are impaired by a decreased level of consciousness or central nervous system abnormalities. Predisposing factors include altered level of consciousness caused by substance abuse, sedation, or anesthesia; seizure disorders; cerebrovascular accident; myasthenia gravis (a neuromuscular disorder); and Guillain-Barre syndrome (inflammation of the nerves). Aspiration is also common in children with tracheoesophageal fistula (a congenital abnormality in which the trachea and esophagus communicate (see Chapter 37). The right lung, particularly the right lower lobe, is more susceptible to aspiration than the left lung.

The effects of aspiration depend on the material aspirated. The aspiration of large food particles or gastric fluid with pH of less than 2.5 has serious consequences. Solid food particles can obstruct a bronchus, resulting in bronchial inflammation and collapse of airways distal to the obstruction. If the aspirated solid is not identified and removed by bronchoscopy, a chronic, local inflammation develops that may lead to recurrent infection and bronchiectasis (permanent dilatation of the bronchus). Once the pathologic process has progressed to bronchiectasis, surgical resection of the affected area is usually required.

Aspiration of acidic gastric fluid may cause severe pneumonitis (localized lung inflammation). Bronchial damage includes inflammation, loss of ciliary function, and bronchospasm. In the alveoli acidic fluid damages the alveolocapillary membrane. This allows plasma and blood cells to move from capillaries into the alveoli, resulting in hemorrhagic pneumonitis. Movement of serous exudate into the lung causes systemic hypovolemia and hypotension. The lung becomes stiff and noncompliant as surfactant production is disrupted, leading to further edema and collapse.

Preventive measures for individuals at risk are more effective than treatment of known aspiration. Surgical patients do not receive food or fluid for several hours preoperatively. Antacids are sometimes given to persons at risk in order to keep gastric pH above 2.5. Individuals who have difficulty swallowing are fed with extreme caution and positioned so as to minimize the likelihood of aspiration. Nasogastric tubes, which are often used to remove stomach contents, can also cause aspiration.

Mortality caused by aspiration-caused pneumonitis is greater than 50%. Treatment includes supplemental oxygen and mechanical ventilation with positive end-expiratory pressure (PEEP). Fluids are restricted to decrease blood volume and minimize pulmonary edema. Steroids are often administered during the first 72 hours after aspiration, though their effectiveness is not well documented. Bacterial pneumonia may develop as a complication of aspiration pneumonitis. If bacterial pneumonia occurs, it is treated with organism-specific antibiotics.

Atelectasis

Atelectasis is the collapse of lung tissue. There are two types of atelectasis: compression atelectasis and absorption atelectasis. **Compression atelectasis** is caused by the external pressure exerted by a tumor, fluid, or air in the pleural space or by an abdominal distension that presses on a portion of the lung, causing collapse of alveoli. **Absorption atelectasis** is collapse resulting from removal of air from obstructed or hypoventilated alveoli. If a bronchus is obstructed, atelectasis occurs as air in the alveoli is slowly absorbed into the bloodstream. Absorption atelectasis can also be caused by inhalation of concentrated oxygen or anesthetic agents, which are quickly absorbed into the bloodstream and can lead to collapse of alveoli in dependent portions of the lung, particularly when tidal volumes are small. Clinical manifestations of atelectasis are similar to those of pulmonary infection: dyspnea, cough, fever, and leukocytosis.

Atelectasis tends to occur postoperatively. Postoperative patients may have received supplemental oxygen or inhaled anesthetics, and they are usually in pain, breathe shallowly, are reluctant to change position, and produce viscous secretions that tend to pool in dependent portions of the lung. Prevention and treatment of postoperative atelectasis usually include deep breathing, frequent position changes, and early ambulation. Deep breathing is beneficial because it (1) promotes the ciliary clearance of secretions, (2) stabilizes the alveoli by redistributing surfactant, and (3) permits collateral ventilation of the alveoli, through pores of Kohn in the alveolar septa. The pores of Kohn, which open only during deep breathing, allow air to pass from well-ventilated alveoli to obstructed alveoli, minimizing their tendency to collapse and facilitating obstruction removal (Fig. 30-4).

Bronchiectasis

Bronchiectasis is persistent abnormal dilatation of the bronchi. It usually occurs in conjunction with other respiratory conditions and can be caused by obstruction of an airway with mucous plugs, atelectasis, aspiration of a foreign body, infection, cystic fibrosis, tuberculosis, congenital weakness of the bronchial wall, or impaired defense mechanisms. Bronchiectasis is frequently associated with inflammation of the bronchi (bronchitis) and has similar symptoms (see p. 1072).

Bronchial dilatation may be cylindrical, saccular, or

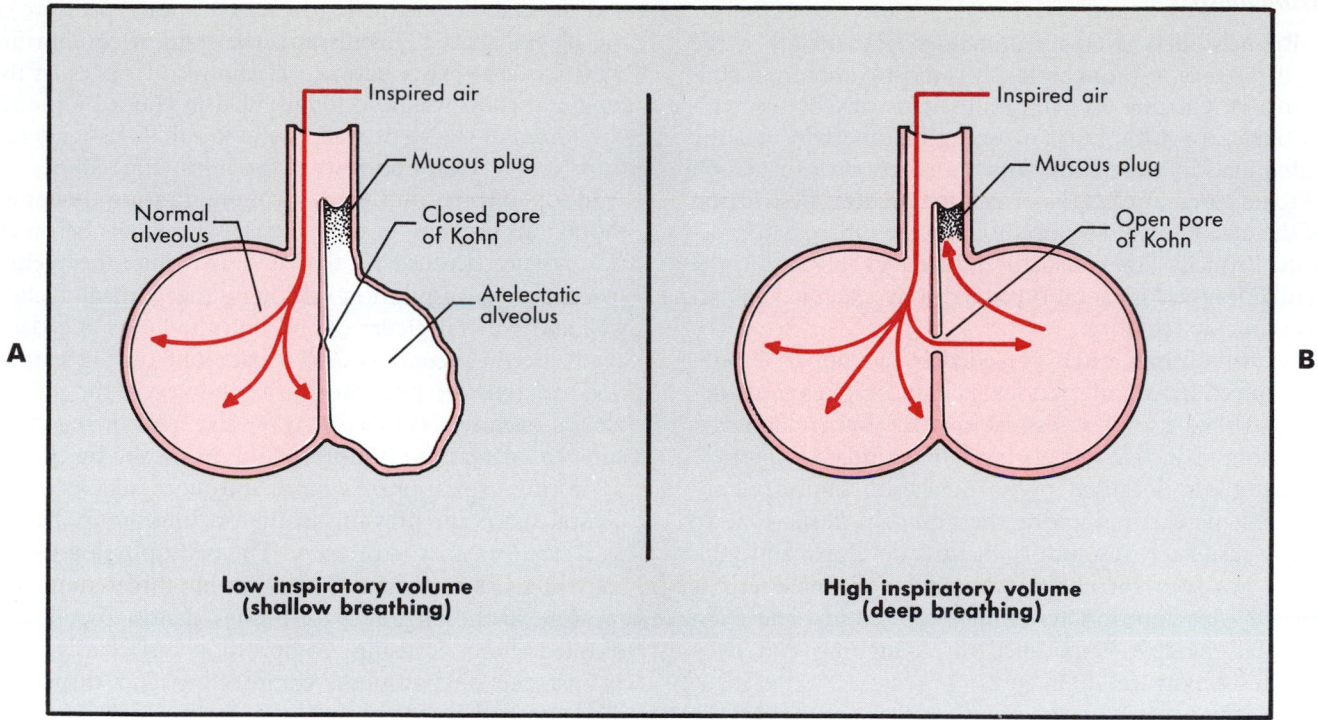

FIG. 30-4. A, Absorption atelectasis caused by lack of collateral ventilation through pores of Kohn;
B, restoration of collateral ventilation during deep breathing.

varicose (Fig. 30-5). In **cylindrical bronchiectasis** the airways are symmetrically dilatated. Cylindrical bronchiectasis is commonly seen after pneumonia and is reversible. In **saccular bronchiectasis** the bronchi become large and balloon like. In **varicose bronchiectasis** constrictions and dilatations deform the bronchi. In both varicose and saccular bronchiectasis the smaller bronchial divisions are plugged with secretions or obliterated by fibrosis. Large anastomoses (connections) develop between the bronchial and pulmonary blood vessels, in-

creasing blood flow through the bronchial circulation. These anastomoses are thought to cause the hemoptysis experienced by individuals with bronchiectasis. Airway damage leads to bronchospasm and copious production of purulent mucus. Ventilation-perfusion abnormalities develop and result in hypoxemia. In severe cases $Paco_2$ may also be elevated.

The symptoms of bronchiectasis may date back to a childhood illness or infection. The disease is commonly associated with recurrent lower respiratory tract infections and expectoration of voluminous amounts of purulent sputum (measured in cupfuls). If the individual is not receiving antibiotics the sputum has a foul odor. Hemoptysis and clubbing of the fingers are common. Pulmonary function studies show a decrease in vital capacity (VC) and in expiratory flow rates. Bronchiectasis is often associated with bronchitis and atelectasis. Hypoxemia eventually leads to cor pulmonale (see p. 1082).

The goals of treatment for bronchiectasis are removal of secretions and prevention of infection. Adequate hydration, percussion, and postural drainage are essential parts of therapy. Bronchodilators are administered to relieve spasms of bronchial smooth muscle, and appropriate antibiotics are given. Hemoptysis is monitored closely, and lung resection may be required to stop severe bleeding. If symptoms are severe and disease is confined to one lobe or area of the lung, surgical resection is sometimes the treatment of choice.

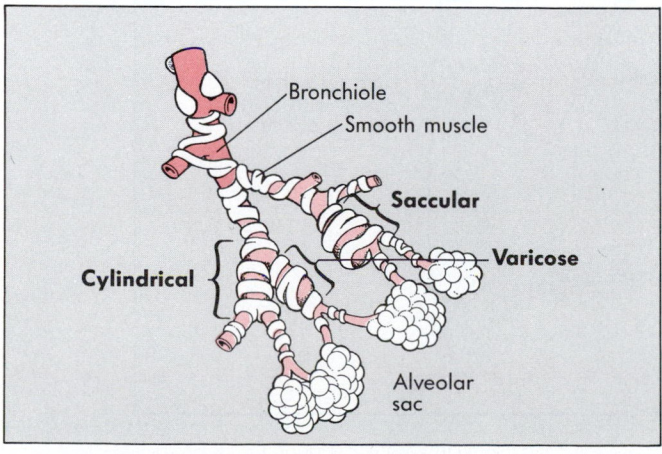

FIG. 30-5. Types of bronchiectasis.

Bronchiolitis

Bronchiolitis is an inflammatory obstruction of the small airways or bronchioles. It is most common in children (see Chapter 31). In adults it usually occurs with chronic bronchitis but can occur in otherwise healthy individuals in association with an infection or inhalation of toxic gases. Atelectasis or emphysematous destruction of the alveoli may develop distal to the inflammatory lesion. Bronchiolitis is usually diffuse. An increase in the ventilation/perfusion ratio results in hypoxemia and carbon dioxide retention.

Bronchiolitis is often preceded by an upper respiratory infection. Manifestations include a rapid ventilatory rate, marked use of accessory muscles, low-grade fever, dry nonproductive cough, and hyperinflated chest. If bronchiolitis is caused by an inhalation injury pulmonary edema occurs rapidly, then quickly clears. One to two weeks later, respiratory distress develops, and infiltrates are seen on chest radiographs. Bronchiolitis is treated with appropriate antibiotics, steroids, and chest physical therapy (humidified air, coughing and deep breathing, postural drainage).

Pleural Abnormalities

Pneumothorax

Pneumothorax is the presence of air or gas in the pleural space caused by a rupture in the visceral pleura (which surrounds the lungs) or the parietal pleura and chest wall (see Chapter 29). As air separates the visceral and parietal pleurae, it destroys the negative pressure of the pleural space. This disrupts the state of equilibrium that normally exists between elastic recoil forces of the lung and chest wall. No longer held in check by the recoil forces of the chest wall, the lung fulfills its tendency to recoil by collapsing toward the hilus (Fig. 30-6).

In **open pneumothorax** (communicating pneumothorax) air pressure in the pleural space equals barometric pressure because air that is drawn into the pleural space during inspiration (through the damaged chest wall and parietal pleura or through the lungs and damaged visceral pleura) is forced back out during expiration. In **tension pneumothorax,** however, the site of pleural rupture acts as a one-way valve, permitting air to enter on inspiration but preventing its escape by closing up during expiration. As more and more air enters the pleural space, air pressure in the pneumothorax begins to exceed barometric pressure. The pathophysiologic effects of tension pneumothorax are life-threatening. Air pressure in the pleural space pushes against the already recoiled lung, causing compression atelectasis, and against the mediastinum, compressing and displacing the heart and great vessels.

Spontaneous pneumothorax, which occurs unexpectedly in healthy individuals (usually men) between the ages of 20 and 40, is caused by the spontaneous rupture of blebs (blisterlike formations) on the visceral pleura. Bleb rupture tends to occur during sleep or rest. The ruptured bleb or blebs are usually located in the apices

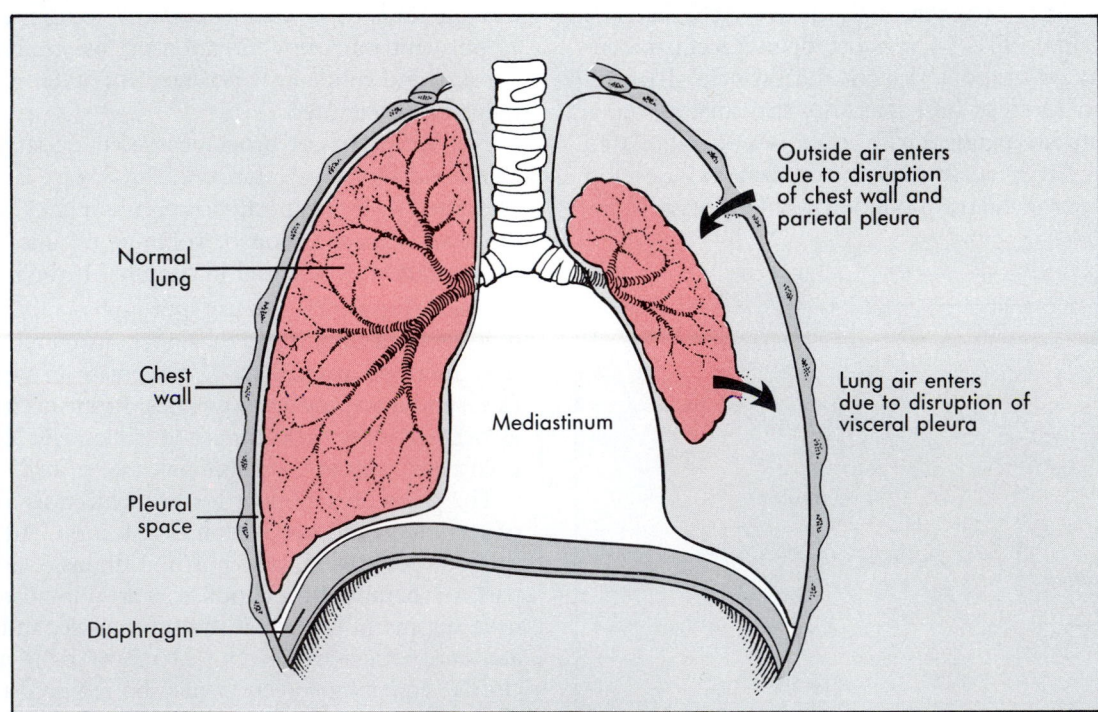

FIG. 30-6. Pneumothorax. Air in the pleural space causes the lung to collapse around the hilus and may push mediastinal contents (heart and great vessels) toward the other lung.

of the lungs. The cause of bleb formation is not known. Tension pneumothroax can develop with bleb rupture.

Clinical manifestations of spontaneous pneumothorax begin with sudden pleural pain, tachypnea, and possibly mild dyspnea. The manifestations depend on the size of the pneumothorax. If the pneumothorax is large or if there is a tension pneumothorax, it may push the mediastinum toward the unaffected lung, causing the chest to appear asymmetrical. Hypoxemia may develop. Lung collapse causes diminished breath sounds over the affected lung. Diagnosis is made with chest radiographs.

A secondary pneumothorax can be caused by chest trauma, such as a rib fracture that tears the pleura; rupture of a bleb or bulla (larger vesicle), as occurs in chronic obstructive pulmonary disease; or mechanical ventilation, particularly if it includes positive end-expiratory pressure (PEEP). Secondary pneumothorax is usually open.

The pathophysiology and clinical manifestations of secondary pneumothorax are similar to those of spontaneous pneumothorax. Occasionally air enters the mediastinum. Secondary pneumothorax (and other open pneumothoraces if large enough) is treated with a chest tube that is attached to a water-seal drainage system with suction. After the pneumothorax is evacuated and the pleural rupture is healed, the chest tube is clamped. If the pneumothorax does not reaccumulate, the chest tube is removed.

Tension pneumothorax, in which air in the pleural space cannot escape through the rupture, is a life-threatening emergency. As increasing positive pressure in the pleural space compresses lung tissue and thoracic blood vessels, venous return and cardiac output decrease. Clinical manifestations of tension pneumothorax include severe hypoxemia, dyspnea, and hypotension (low blood pressure), as well as the other signs and symptoms of pneumothorax. Deterioration occurs rapidly, and shock and bradycardia (reduced heart rate) may develop.

Tension pneumothorax requires immediate treatment. A chest tube is placed quickly, usually after physical examination alone. If a chest tube is not readily available, a large-bore needle is inserted into the pleural space to decompress it until a chest tube can be placed. An outward gush of air as the needle or chest tube is inserted confirms the presence of tension pneumothorax. The chest tube is connected to a water-seal drainage and suction until the damaged pleura is healed.

Pleural Effusion

Pleural effusion is the presence of fluid in the pleural space. The source of the fluid is usually blood vessels or lymphatic vessels lying beneath either pleura, but occasionally the source is an abscess or other lesion that drains into the pleural space. Because the pleura is a relatively permeable membrane fluids that accumulate in the lung can cross into the pleural space.

Like pneumothorax pleural effusion can cause compression atelectasis and displace mediastinal contents. Unlike pneumothroax, however, pleural effusion does not cause the lung to collapse as a result of elastic recoil. Because there is no communication between the pleural space and environmental air, pressure in the pleural space remains negative and atelectasis is caused solely by pressure exerted by the effusion.

The most common mechanism of pleural effusion is migration of fluids and other blood components through the walls of intact capillaries bordering the pleura. Pleural effusions that enter the pleural space from the intact blood vessels can be transudative or exudative. In **transudative effusion** the fluid, or transudate, is watery and diffuses out of the capillaries as a result of disorders that increase blood pressure or decrease capillary oncotic pressure. Examples are congestive heart failure, in which venous and left arterial pressures are increased, and liver or kidney disorders that diminish synthesis of plasma proteins, causing hypoproteinemia. Hypoproteinemia decreases capillary oncotic pressure, which promotes diffusion of water out of the capillaries. (This mechanism is discussed in Chapter 3.)

Exudative effusion is less watery and contains high concentrations of white blood cells and plasma proteins. Exudative effusion occurs in response to inflammation, infection, or malignancy and involves inflammatory processes that increase capillary permeability (see Chapter 7). When stimulated by biochemical mediators of inflammation, junctions in the capillary endothelium separate slightly, enabling leukocytes and plasma proteins to migrate out into affected tissues.

Other fluids occasionally accumulate in the pleural space. Overproduction of the serous fluid that enables the pleurae to slide over one another can cause pleural effusion. Rupture of a blood vessel or leakage of blood from an injured vessel causes a form of pleural effusion termed hemothorax.

Lymphatic blockage from any cause can result in drainage of the contents of lymphatic vessels into the pleural space. Lymphatic contents, which can include pus being drained from infectious lesions in the lungs or substances being transported from other areas of the body to the thoracic duct (which lies near the pleural space), sometimes drain to the pleural space. (Mechanisms of pleural effusion are summarized in Table 30-2.)

Small collections of fluid can normally be drained away by the lymphatics. Large effusions cause clinical manifestations related to their volume and the rate at which they accumulate in the pleural space. Dyspnea, compression atelectasis with impaired ventilation, and mediastinal shift occur with large effusions. Pleural pain

TABLE 30-2 Mechanisms of pleural effusion

Type of fluid/effusion	Source of accumulation	Primary or associated disorder
Transudate (hydrothorax)	Water fluid that diffuses out of capillaries beneath the pleurae (i.e., capillaries in lung or chest wall)	Cardiovascular disease that causes high blood pressure; liver or kidney disease that disrupts plasma protein production, causing hypyproteinemia (decreased oncotic pressure in the blood vessels)
Exudate	Fluid rich in proteins (leukocytes, plasma proteins of all kinds; see Chapter 34), that migrates out of the capillaries	Infection, inflammation, or malignancy of the pleurae that stimulates mast cells to release biochemical mediators that increase capillary permeability
Pus (empyema)	Detritus of infection (microorganisms, leukocytes, and cellular debris) dumped into the pleural space by blocked lymphatic vessels	Pulmonary infections, such as pneumonia; lung abscesses; infected wounds
Blood (hemothorax)	Hemorrhage into the pleural space	Traumatic injury, surgery, rupture, or malignancy that damages blood vessels
Chyle (chylothorax)	Chyle (milky fluid containing lymph and fat droplets) that is dumped by lymphatic vessels into the pleural space instead of passing from the gastrointestinal tract to the thoracic duct	Traumatic injury, infection, or disorder that disrupts lymphatic transport

NOTE:The principles of diffusion are described in Chapter 1; mechanisms that increase capillary permeability and cause exudation of cells and proteins are discussed in Chapter 7.

is present if the pleura is inflamed, and cardiovascular manifestations occur in large, rapid hemothorax. A pleural friction rub can be heard over areas of extensive effusion.

If the effusion is causing considerable impairment of pulmonary function, thoracentesis (needle aspiration) may be performed to drain the fluid from the pleural space. A pleural effusion can contain several liters of fluid.

Empyema

Empyema (infected pleural effusion), the presence of pus in the pleural space, is a complication of respiratory infection, usually pneumonia caused by *Staphylococcus aureus, Escherichia coli,* or *Klebsiella pneumoniae.* (*Staphylococcus* is responsible for more than 90% of empyemas in children.) Empyema is thought to develop when the pulmonary lymphatics become blocked, leading to an outpouring of contaminated lymphatic fluid into the pleural space.

Individuals with empyema have clinical manifestations of toxicity, including cyanosis, fever, tachycardia (rapid heart rate), cough, and pleural pain. Breath sounds are decreased directly over the empyema. Diagnosis is made by chest radiographs and thoracentesis, though positive cultures from fluids are obtained only about 50% of the time. Therefore, the offending micro-

organism is usually identified by its preponderance in a sputum culture.

The treatment for empyema is similar to that for pneumonia (see p. 1076). Antibiotics are given, and thoracentesis is performed to drain the pleural space. Chest tube placement and continuous drainage may also be required. In severe cases surgical debridement of the pleural space is performed to prevent reaccumulation.

Pleurisy

Pleurisy (pleuritis) is inflammation of the pleura. Pleurisy causes pleura to become reddened and covered with an exudate of lymph, fibrin, and cellular elements and may lead to pleural effusion. The most common signs and symptoms of pleurisy are chills, fever, and pain on inspiration. Often a pleural friction rub can be heard over the affected area. Pleurisy is frequently preceded by upper respiratory infection.

Abscess Formation and Cavitation

An **abscess** is a circumscribed area of suppuration and destruction of lung parenchyma. Abscess formation follows **consolidation** of lung tissue, in which inflammation causes alveoli to fill with fluid, pus, and microorganisms. Necrosis (death and decay) of consolidated tissue may progress proximally until it communicates with a bronchus. If this occurs, the abscess empties into the bronchus, leaving a cavity that has a radiographic appearance similar to that of a lesion of tuberculosis. **Cavitation** is the process of abscess emptying and cavity formation. The diagnosis is made by radiography.

Pneumonia caused by aspiration, Klebsiella, or Staphylococcus is the most common cause of abscess formation. Aspiration abscess is usually associated with alcohol abuse, seizure disorders, general anesthesia, and swallowing disorders. The clinical manifestations of abscess formation are similar to those of pneumonitis: fever, cough, chills, sputum production, and pleural pain. Abscess communication with a bronchus causes a severe cough, copious amounts of often foul-smelling sputum, and occasionally hemoptysis.

Treatment includes the administration of appropriate antibiotics and chest physiotherapy, chest percussion, and postural drainage. Sometimes bronchoscopy is performed to drain the abscess. Mortality is influenced by the severity of the primary disease that initially caused consolidation.

Pulmonary Fibrosis

Pulmonary fibrosis is an excessive amount of fibrous or connective tissue in the lung. It can be caused by healing (formation of scar tissue) after active disease (e.g., adult respiratory distress syndrome or tuberculosis) or by inhalation of harmful substances (such as coal dust or asbestos). When no cause for the development of fibrosis is known, it is called idiopathic pulmonary fibrosis.

Fibrosis causes a marked loss of lung compliance. The lung becomes stiff and difficult to ventilate, and the diffusing capacity of the alveolocapillary membrane may decrease, causing hypoxemia. Diffuse pulmonary fibrosis has a very poor prognosis.

Chest Wall Restriction

If the chest wall is deformed, immobilized, or made heavy by fat, the work of breathing is increased and ventilation may be compromised. The degree of ventilatory impairment depends on the severity of the chest wall abnormality. Grossly obese individuals are often dyspneic on exertion or when recumbent. Individuals with severe kyphoscoliosis (lateral bending and rotation of the spinal column, with distortion of the thoracic cage) often present with dyspnea on exertion that can progress to respiratory failure. Such individuals are also susceptible to lower respiratory tract infections. Both obesity and kyphoscoliosis are risk factors for respiratory disease in hospital patients admitted for other problems, particularly those who require surgery. Other musculoskeletal abnormalities that can impair ventilation are ankylosing spondylitis (rheumatoid arthritis of the spine; see Chapters 39 and 40) and pectus excavatum, or funnel chest (a deformity characterized by depression of the sternum).

Impairment of respiratory muscle function caused by neuromuscular disease can also restrict the chest wall and impair pulmonary function. Muscle weakness can result in hypoventilation, inability to remove secretions, and hypoxemia. The most common cause of hospital admission for individuals with such neuromuscular diseases as polio myelitis, muscular dystrophy, myasthenia gravis, and Guillain-Barre syndrome is respiratory difficulty. (See Unit V for a more complete discussion of these disorders.)

Flail Chest

Flail chest results from the fracture of several consecutive ribs in more than one place, or the fracture of the sternum plus several consecutive ribs. These multiple fractures result in instability of a portion of the chest wall, causing paradoxical movement of the chest with breathing. During inspiration the unstable portion of the chest wall moves inward, and during expiration it moves outward, impairing movement of gas in and out of the lungs (Fig. 30-7).

The clinical manifestations of flail chest are pain, dyspnea, unequal chest expansion, hypoventilation, and hypoxemia. Treatment is internal fixation by controlled mechanical ventilation until the chest wall has stabilized.

Inhalation Disorders

Exposure to Toxic Gases

Inhalation of gaseous irritants can cause significant respiratory dysfunction. Commonly encountered toxic gases include smoke, ammonia, hydrogen chloride, sulfur dioxide, chlorine, phosgene, and nitrogen dioxide. Inhalation of a toxic gas results in severe inflammation of the airways, alveolar and capillary damage, and pulmonary edema. (The cellular effects of toxic gases are described in Chapter 2.) Initial symptoms include burning of the eyes, nose, and throat; coughing; chest tightness; and dyspnea. Hypoxemia is common. Treatment includes supplemental oxygen, mechanical ventilation with PEEP, and support of the cardiovascular system. Steroids are sometimes used, though their effectiveness has not been well documented. Most individuals respond very quickly to therapy. Some, however, may improve initially and then deteriorate as a result of bronchiectasis or bronchiolitis (inflammation of the bronchioles).

Oxygen toxicity is an iatrogenic condition caused by prolonged exposure to high concentrations of supplemental oxygen (Deneke & Fanburg, 1980). The higher the oxygen concentration, the more likely the occurrence of toxicity. Oxygen toxicity damages the alveolocapillary membrane, disrupts surfactant production, causes alveolar edema, and decreases functional residual capacity. The mechanism of cellular injury is unclear. Toxicity is often undetected because it occurs in individ-

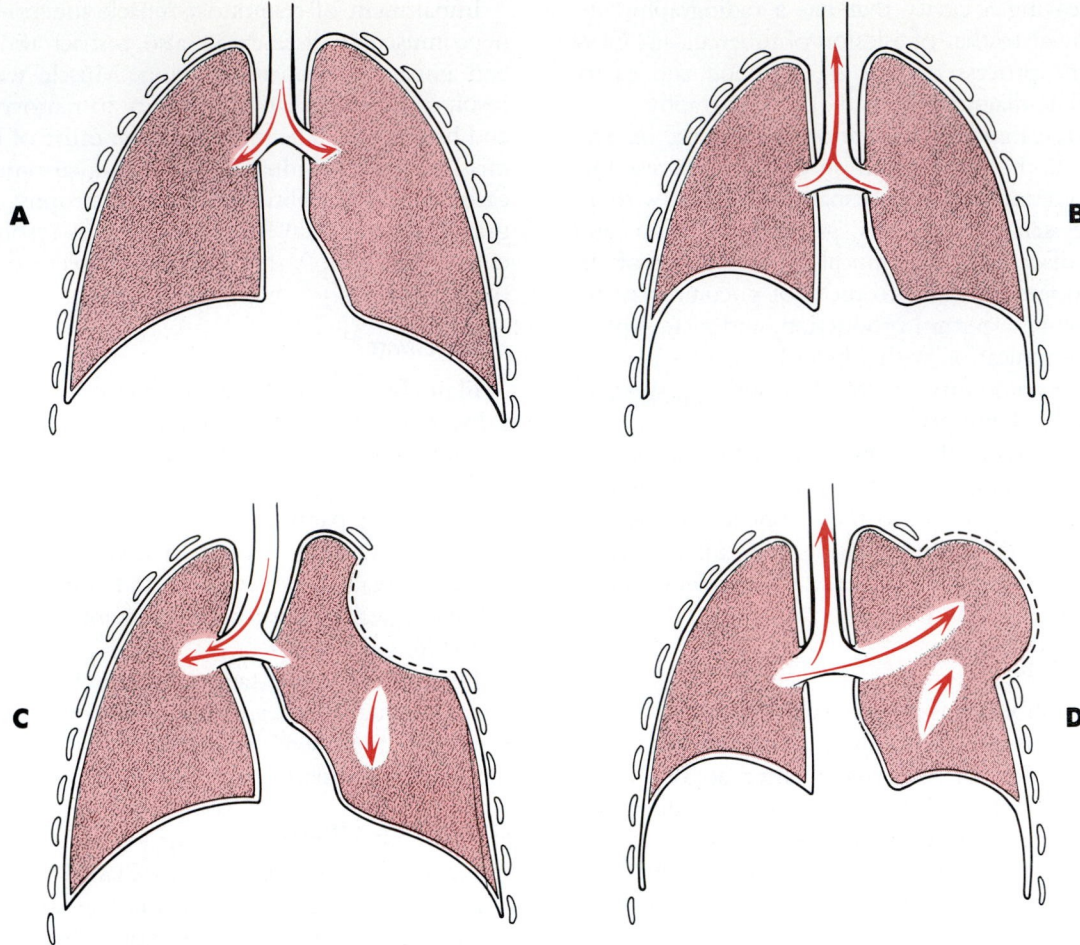

FIG. 30-7. Flail chest. The unstable chest wall causes paradoxical movement during inspiration and expiration. **A,** Normal inspiration; **B,** normal expiration; **C,** paradoximcal collapse of lung with inspiration; **D,** paradoxical expansion of lung with expression. (From Phipps, Long, & Woods, 1987.)

uals who already have acute respiratory failure. Clinical manifestations are indistinguishable from those of adult respiratory distress syndrome (see p. 1067). Treatment involves ventilatory support and reduction of inspired oxygen concentration to less than 60% as soon as possible.

Pneumoconiosis

Pneumoconiosis is caused by inhalation of dust particles, usually in the workplace. As in all cases of environmentally acquired lung disease, the individual's history of exposure is important in determining the diagnosis. Pneumoconiosis often occurs after years of exposure to the offending dust, and manifestations are often difficult to differentiate from those resulting from smoking.

The dusts of silica, asbestos, and coal are the most common causes of pneumoconiosis. Others include talc, fiberglass, clays, sillimanite, mica, slate, cement, cadmium, beryllium, tungsten, cobalt, aluminum, and iron.

No matter what the substance, the dust deposits are permanent. Treatment, therefore, is palliative and focuses on preventing further exposure and improving working conditions.

Silicosis, a type of pneumoconiosis resulting from silica dust deposits, produces fibrous nodules within the lung. Exposed individuals usually remain asymptomatic long after the nodules are visible on chest radiography. When they do appear, clinical manifestations include cough and dyspnea. Silicosis is also a predisposing factor for lower respiratory tract infection. There is no specific treatment for the disease, though corticosteroids may produce some improvement. Silica exposure occurs in mining and other industries involved with the extraction and processing of ores; preparation and use of sand; and manufacture of pipe, building, and roofing material.

Coal worker's pneumoconiosis, sometimes called coal miner's lung or black lung, is caused by coal dust deposits in the lung. Its mild form is asymptomatic, except for possible chronic bronchitis. Its advanced form consists of severe pulmonary fibrosis. Individuals usually present with a productive cough and wheezing. Symptoms are more severe with advanced disease and mimic those of chronic bronchitis (see p. 1072). Diagnosis is made by history of exposure and characteristic chest radiographs. There is no specific treatment for coal worker's pneumoconiosis. Individuals with the mild form of the disease usually do well. Those with more complicated forms often develop marked cardiopulmonary dysfunction.

Asbestos exposure affects not only factory workers but also individuals who live in areas of asbestos emission. Asbestos exposure can result in a type of pulmonary fibrosis called **asbestosis** or in tumor formation, depending on the amount of exposure. The most prominent clinical manifestations of fibrosis are dyspnea on exertion a nonproductive cough, hypoxemia, and decreased lung volume. Progressive disease may lead to respiratory failure and cardiac complications. Asbestos workers who smoke have a marked increase in risk for developing bronchogenic cancer (see p. 1085).

Allergic Alveolitis

Inhalation of organic dusts can result in an allergic inflammatory response called **allergic alveolitis,** hypersensitivity pneumonitis, or type II extrinsic asthma (see p. 00). Many allergens can cause this disorder, including grains, silage, bird droppings or feathers, wood dust (particularly redwood and maple), cork dust, animal pelts, coffee beans, fish meal, mushroom compost, and molds that grow on sugarcane, barley, and straw. The lung inflammation, or pneumonitis, occurs after repeated, prolonged exposure to the allergen.

Allergic alveolitis can be acute, subacute, or chronic. The acute form causes a fever, cough, and chills a few hours after exposure. In the subacute form coughing and dyspnea are common and sometimes necessitate hospital care. Recovery is complete if the offending agent can be avoided in the future. With continued exposure the disease becomes chronic and pulmonary fibrosis develops. (The mechanisms of hypersensitivity reactions are discussed in Chapter 8.)

Systemic Disorders

Several systemic diseases affect the airways, pleurae, or lung parenchyma, causing fibrosis, vasculitis, pulmonary hemorrhage, or granuloma formation. Clinical manifestations of lung involvement are usually nonspecific, and the diagnosis is based on involvement of other organs. There is usually no specific treatment, though corticosteroids are frequently used. Some of the systemic diseases affecting the lung are granulomatous disorders such as sarcoidosis, Wegener granulomatosis, lymphomatoid granulomatosis, and eosinophilic granuloma; connective tissue diseases such as rheumatoid disease, systemic lupus erythematosus, scleroderma, polymyositis or dermatomyositis, Sjogren syndrome, and polyarteritis nodosa; angioimmunoblastic or immunoblastic lymphadenopathy, a disease of the lymph nodes; cystic fibrosis (see Chapter 31); and Goodpasture syndrome, a renal disorder.

PULMONARY DISORDERS

Acute Respiratory Failure

Respiratory failure is defined as inadequate gas exchange, that is, hypoxemia, where $Pao_2 \leq 50$ mmHg and/or where $Paco_2 \geq 50$ mmHg with pH ≤ 7.25. Respiratory failure can result from direct injury to the lungs, airways, or chest wall or to another body system. It can occur in individuals who have an otherwise normal respiratory system or in those with underlying chronic pulmonary disease. Most pulmonary diseases can cause episodes of acute respiratory failure. Whatever the cause of acute respiratory failure, its pathophysiologic results and treatment are quite similar.

Adult Respiratory Distress Syndrome

Adult respiratory distress syndrome (ARDS) is charcterized by diffuse alveolocapillary injury. Identified within the last 20 years, the syndrome affects approximately 150,000 people per year and has a 50% mortality rate, despite therapy. It often affects young people who were previously in excellent health. Predisposing factors commonly associated with ARDS are shock, pneumonia, sepsis, trauma, aspiration, cardiopulmonary bypass surgery, pancreatitis, massive blood transfusions, drug overdose, pregnancy-induced hypertension, increased intracranial pressure, inhalation of smoke or noxious gases, fat emboli, high concentrations of supplemental oxygen, radiation therapy, and intravascular coagulation.

Pathophysiology

All disorders that result in ARDS acutely injure the alveolocapillary membrane and are associated with increased fluid in the lungs. The alveolocapillary damage can occur directly with the aspiration of highly acidic gastric contents or inhalation of toxic gases. Chemical damage can also occur indirectly from activation and aggregation of formed elements, such as neutrophils, with release of inflammatory mediators in response to diffuse pulmonary infection or septicemia.

Whether the damage is direct or indirect, the alveolocapillary membrane becomes more permeabile, causing fluid, plasma proteins, and blood cells to diffuse from the capillary bed into the pulmonary interstitium and al-

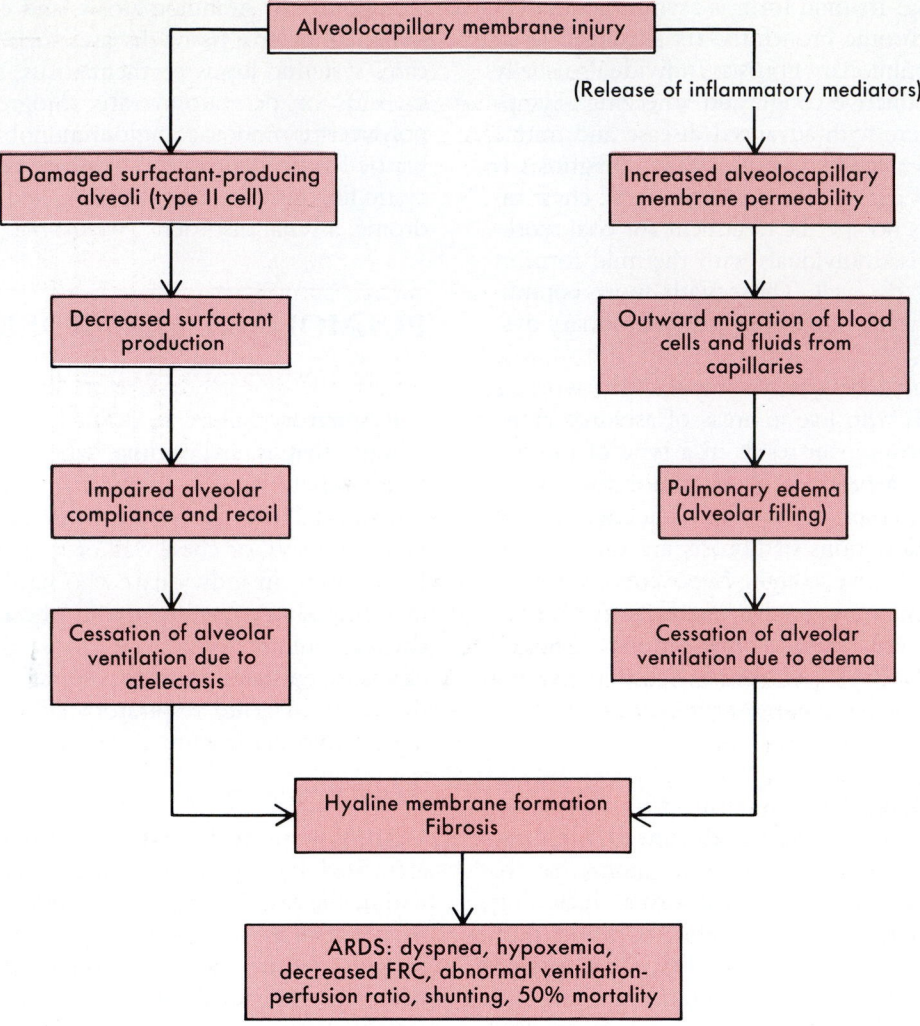

FIG. 30-8. Pathogenesis of adult respiratory distress syndrome (ARDS). FRC, functional residual capacity.

veoli, resulting in pulmonary edema. Surfactant is inactivated, and its production by the type II alveolar cells is impaired as alveoli and respiratory bronchioles fill with fluid or collapse. The lungs become less compliant or stiff with decreased ventilation of alveoli and shunting of pulmonary blood flow. Twenty-four to forty-eight hours after the acute, hemorrhagic phase of ARDS, hyaline membranes form, and fibrosis progressively obliterates the alveoli, respiratory bronchioles, and interstitium. This leads to a decrease in functional residual capacity, a marked decrease in lung compliance, decreased $\dot{V}/\dot{Q}$, and an increased right-to-left shunt (Fig. 30-8).

Clinical Manifestations

The classic signs and symptoms of ARDS are rapid, shallow breathing; respiratory alkalosis; marked dyspnea; decreased chest wall compliance; hypoxemia unresponsive to oxygen therapy; and diffuse alveolar infiltration seen on chest radiographs, without evidence of cardiac disease. Initially individuals hyperventilate, causing respiratory alkalosis. As the work of breathing increases, because of the decrease in compliance caused by alveolar filling and collapse, dyspnea and hypoxemia develop. Hypoxemia worsens despite oxygen therapy, and diffuse rales can be heard on auscultation. Metabolic acidosis develops from the increased work of breathing and hypoxemia, and fluffy infiltrates appear on chest radiographs. If ARDS is not reversed respiratory acidosis develops, and further hypoxemia results in hypotension, decreased cardiac output, metabolic acidosis, and death.

Evaluation and Treatment

Diagnosis is made on the basis of physical examination, analyses of blood gases, and radiologic examination. Initial physical examination may reveal fine rales and the chest film may be clear or show a few scattered infiltrates. With progressive respiratory involvement rales are heard throughout both lungs and radiographs show extensive bilateral infiltrates. Hypoxia cannot be corrected with oxygen.

Treatment is based on early detection, supportive therapy, and prevention of complications. Therapy involves fluid management, oxygen administration, mechanical ventilation with PEEP, steroid administration, and cardiac drugs, if needed.

Postoperative Respiratory Failure

Although usually not as severe as ARDS, postoperative respiratory failure can result in the same pathophysiology and clinical manifestations as ARDS. Smokers are at risk, particularly if they have preexisting lung disease. Limited cardiac reserve, chronic renal failure, chronic hepatic disease, and infection also increase the tendency to develop postoperative respiratory failure. Surgical procedures involving the thorax or abdomen carry the greatest risk.

The most common postoperative pulmonary problems are atelectasis, pneumonia, pulmonary edema, and pulmonary emboli. These problems usually result in reduced functional residual capacity, decreased compliance, and increased ventilation-perfusion mismatching. Individuals in whom ARDS develops have usually had a period of hypotension during surgery, and many have sepsis.

Prevention of postoperative respiratory failure includes frequent turning, deep breathing, and early ambulation in order to prevent atelectasis and accumulation of secretions. Humidification of inspired air can help loosen secretions. Incentive spirometry gives individuals immediate feedback about tidal volumes, which encourages them to breathe deeply (spirometry is described in Chapter 29). Supplemental oxygen is given for hypoxemia, and antibiotics are given as appropriate to treat infection. If respiratory failure develops the individual may require mechanical ventilation for a period of time. Treatment is then very similar to that for ARDS.

Obstructive Pulmonary Disease

Obstructive pulmonary disease is characterized by difficult expiration. Either more force (i.e., use of accessory muscles of expiration) is required to expire a given volume of air, or emptying of the lungs is slowed, or both. The most common obstructive diseases are asthma, chronic bronchitis, and emphysema. Because many individuals have both chronic bronchitis and emphysema, these diseases together are often called **chronic obstructive pulmonary disease (COPD).** Asthma is more acute and intermittent than COPD, even though it can be chronic (Fig. 30-9).

COPD is second only to heart disease as a cause of disability in adults less than 65 years of age. Over one third of all patients admitted to VA hospitals have evidence of COPD. The direct and indirect costs of the disease have been estimated at $2 billion. The primary cause of COPD is cigarette smoking. Air pollution and occupational exposure to noxious dusts and gases may also contribute to the development of obstructive pulmonary disease.

Asthma

Asthma is a condition involving episodic periods of **bronchospasm** (spasm, or prolonged contractions, of the bronchial smooth muscle). It is a complex disorder involving biochemical, autonomic, immunologic, infectious, endocrine, and psychological factors in varying degrees in different individuals. Most attacks of asthmatic bronchospasm are short-lived, with freedom from symptoms and complete recovery between episodes.

Asthma occurs in families, suggesting that a predisposition is transmitted genetically, although the mode of genetic transmission is unclear. Apparently environmental factors interact with inherited factors to cause attacks of bronchospasm. For example, asthma can develop when "predisposed" individuals are infected by viruses or exposed to allergens or pollutants. Other inciting factors, including psychological factors, remain to be identified. The severity of asthma attacks varies among individuals, over time, and with the degree of exposure to inciting factors. About half of all cases of asthma develop during childhood. Another third develop before the age of 40.

Because some individuals with asthma seem to have an exaggerated response to allergens and others apparently have none, a "nonallergenic" theory has been proposed to explain the cause of asthma. Proponents of this theory believe that bronchospasm is caused by an imbalance between the sympathetic and parasympathetic divisions of the autonomic nervous system (ANS). Because airway caliber is controlled by a balance between the sympathetic division, which causes dilatation, and the parasympathetic division, which causes constriction, parasympathetic domination would cause bronchospasm. It is not yet clear whether the imbalance results from a problem in central or local regulation of the ANS.

Types of Asthma

Asthma is described as extrinsic if it is triggered by allergens and intrinsic if it is not (Table 30-3). However, some recent studies indicate that both extrinsic and intrinsic asthma are related to serum IgE activity (Burrows et al., 1989). **Extrinsic asthma**, or allergic asthma, is classified as type I or type II, depending on the type of hypersensitivity reaction (allergic response) involved (see Chapter 8). Type I extrinsic asthma is the classic allergic asthma. It is common in children and young adults who are highly sensitive to commonly inhaled antigens, such as dust and pollen, and is often seasonal in nature. Children frequently outgrow this disease, and they tend to have sudden, brief, intermittent attacks that respond well to bronchodilators (see Chapter 29).

Type II extrinsic asthma (sometimes called allergic alveolitis) develops in adults under the age of 35 after long exposure to irritants. The attacks are more prolonged than those of type I extrinsic asthma and tend to be more inflammatory. Fever and infiltrates visible on chest radiographs often accompany bronchospasm. Individuals with type II extrinsic asthma commonly exhibit Arthus phenomenon, or reaction, a skin wheal that forms in response to intradermal injection of the causal antigen.

Intrinsic asthma has no known immunologic (antigenic) cause and no seasonal variation. It usually occurs in adults over the age of 35, many of whom are sensitive to aspirin and have nasal polyps. The attacks are often severe and do not respond well to sympathomimetic bronchodilators.

Asthma that occurs in otherwise normal individuals after moderate to severe exertion is called exercise-induced asthma. These attacks can usually be prevented by susceptible individual's using a bronchodilator before exercising.

Pathophysiology

The common factor in all types of asthma is hyperreactivity of the airways. The hyperreactivity is related to the interaction of an antigen with mast cell-bound IgE molecules that produce an immediate inflammatory response of bronchial smooth muscle spasm, edema formation, bronchial constriction, inflammation of mucous membranes, and production of thick, tenacious mucus (Fig. 30-10). The released mediators include histamine bradykinins, leukotrienes, prostaglandins, and thromboxane A_2. Mucus plugs the inflamed airways, causing obstruction and air trapping in the distal portions of the lung. These abnormalities lead to increased ventilation-perfusion mismatching, hypoxemia, and increased work of breathing. In a few individuals a second episode of bronchoconstriction occurs 6 to 10 hours later (the late response).

Airway obstruction increases resistance to airflow and decreases flow rates, including expiratory flow. Impaired expiration causes hyperinflation distal to obstructions,

FIG. 30-9. Airway obstruction caused by emphysema, chronic bronchitis, and asthma. **A,** Emphysema: enlargement and destruction of alveolar walls with loss of elasticity and trapping of air; **B,** chronic bronchitis: inflammation and thickening of mucous membrane with accumulation of mucus and pus leading to obstruction; **C,** bronchial asthma: Thick mucus, mucosal edema, and smooth muscle spasm causing obstruction of small airways.

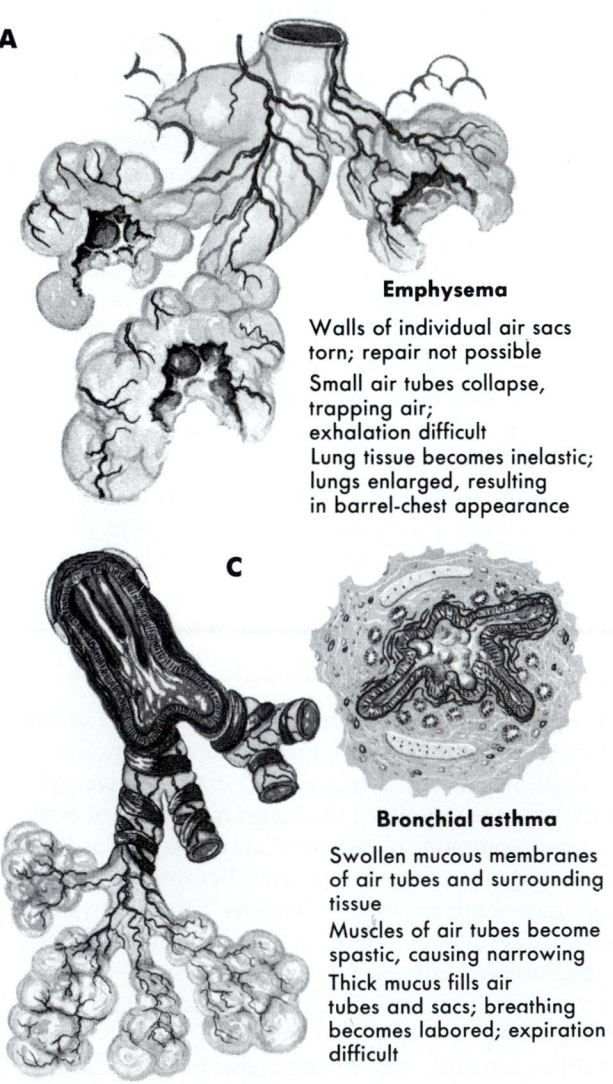

A

Emphysema

Walls of individual air sacs torn; repair not possible

Small air tubes collapse, trapping air; exhalation difficult

Lung tissue becomes inelastic; lungs enlarged, resulting in barrel-chest appearance

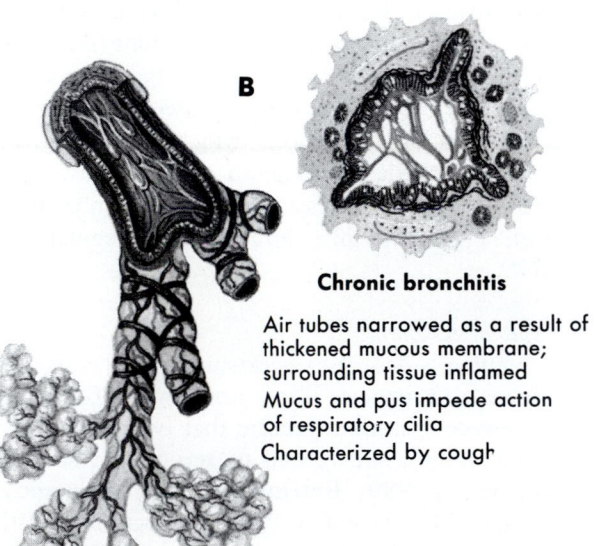

B

Chronic bronchitis

Air tubes narrowed as a result of thickened mucous membrane; surrounding tissue inflamed

Mucus and pus impede action of respiratory cilia

Characterized by cough

C

Bronchial asthma

Swollen mucous membranes of air tubes and surrounding tissue

Muscles of air tubes become spastic, causing narrowing

Thick mucus fills air tubes and sacs; breathing becomes labored; expiration difficult

TABLE 30-3 Comparison of extrinsic and intrinsic asthma

Characteristic	Extrinsic asthma	Intrinsic asthma
Age at onset	Under 35	Over 35
Allergies	Present	Absent
Skin tests	Positive	Negative
Bronchospasm	Intermittent	More continuous
Family history of allergies	Common	Uncommon

altered pulmonary mechanics, and increased work of breathing. Changes in resistance to airflow are not uniform throughout the lungs. Because of regional differences in airway resistance, the distribution of inspired air is uneven, with more air flowing to the less resistant portions.

Hyperventilation is eventually triggered by lung receptors' responding to increased lung volume and obstruction. Continued air trapping increases intrapleural and alveolar gas pressures and causes decreased perfusion of the alveoli. Increased alveolar gas pressure, decreased ventilation, and decreased perfusion lead to variable and uneven ventilation-perfusion relationships within different lung segments. The result is early hypoxemia without hypercapnea. Hypoxemia further increases hyperventilation through stimulation of the respiratory center, causing $Paco_2$ to fall and pH to rise (respiratory alkalosis). As the obstruction becomes more severe, however, and the number of alveoli being inadequately ventilated and perfused increases, a point at which CO_2 retention (hypercapnea) and respiratory acidosis develop is reached. Respiratory acidosis signals respiratory failure.

Clinical Manifestations

During full remission individuals are asymptomatic and pulmonary function tests are normal. During partial remission, there are no clinical symptoms but pulmonary function tests are abnormal. During attacks individuals are dyspneic and respiratory effort is marked. Breath sounds are decreased except for considerable wheezing. The severity of alterations in blood gases is difficult to evaluate by clinical signs alone, and arterial blood gas tensions should be measured.

At the beginning of an attack there are a sensation of chest constriction, inspiratory and expiratory wheezing, dyspnea, nonproductive coughing, prolonged expiration, tachycardia, and tachypnea. With severe attacks the accessory muscles of respiration are prominent. As the episode resolves coughing produces a thick, stringy mu-

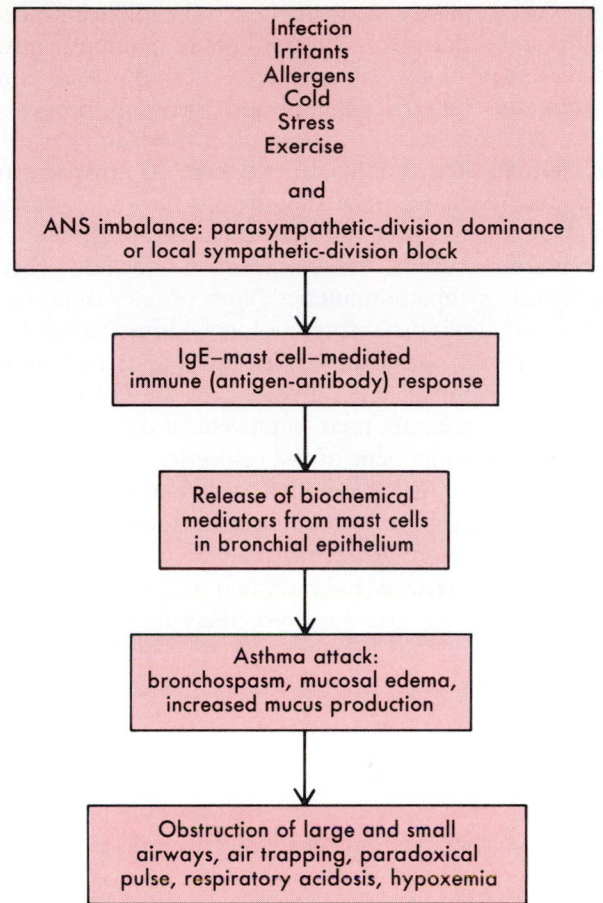

FIG. 30-10. Pathogenesis of asthma.

cus with casts of the small airways that can be seen microscopically.

Evaluation and Treatment

Spirometry reveals decreases in expiratory flow rate, forced expiratory volume (FEV_1), and forced vital capacity (FVC) (see Chapter 29). Functional residual capacity (FRC) and total lung capacity (TLC) are increased. Blood gas analysis reveals hypoxemia and respiratory alkalosis. There are no specific tests for the different types of asthma.

If bronchospasm is not reversed by usual measures the individual is considered to have severe bronchospasm, or **status asthmaticus.** With severe bronchospasm work of breathing can be 5 to 10 times normal. When air trapping is severe paradoxical pulse (manifested as a blood pressure drop of more than 10 mm Hg during inspiration) develops and pneumothorax is common. If status asthmaticus continues hypoxemia worsens, expiratory flows and volumes decrease further, and the individual begins to tire. Acidosis develops as arterial Pco_2 begins to rise. Asthma becomes life-threatening at this point if treatment does not reverse this process quickly. A silent chest (no audible air movement) and a P_{CO_2} over 70 mm Hg are ominous signs.

Treatment of an asthma attack is geared toward eliminating the causative agents and reversing bronchospasm and airway obstruction. Bronchodilators usually are administered, singly or in concert, to increase sympathetic ANS control of the airways through a variety of mechanisms. Often no other intervention is required. Commonly used bronchodilators include beta-adrenergic sympathomimetics (epinephrine, isoproterenol, isoetharine, metaproterenol, ephedrine, terbutaline, or salbutamol); anticholinergics (atropine); methylxanthines (theophylline). Corticosteroids are not bronchodilators, but they are used to prevent or decrease the inflammatory component of the response.

Chronic Bronchitis **Bronchitis** is inflammation of the bronchi caused by irritants (cigarette smoke, air pollutants) or infection. Bronchitis can be acute or chronic and is characterized by increased mucus production, mucosal swelling, and impaired ciliary function.

Pathophysiology

Chronic bronchitis is defined as hypersecretion of mucus and chronic productive cough that continues for at least 3 months of the year (usually the winter months) for at least 2 consecutive years. Incidence is increased in smokers (up to 20-fold) and even more so in workers exposed to air pollution. Repeated infections are common.

Inspired irritants not only increase mucus production but also increase the size and number of mucus glands and goblet cells in airway epithelium. The mucus produced is thicker and more tenacious than normal. Ciliary function is impaired, reducing mucus clearance further. The lung's defense mechanisms are therefore compromised, increasing susceptibility to pulmonary infection and injury. As infection and injury increase mucus production further, the bronchial walls become inflamed and thickened from edema and accumulation of inflammatory cells. (The pathogenesis of chronic bronchitis is shown in Fig. 30-11.)

Initially chronic bronchitis affects only the larger

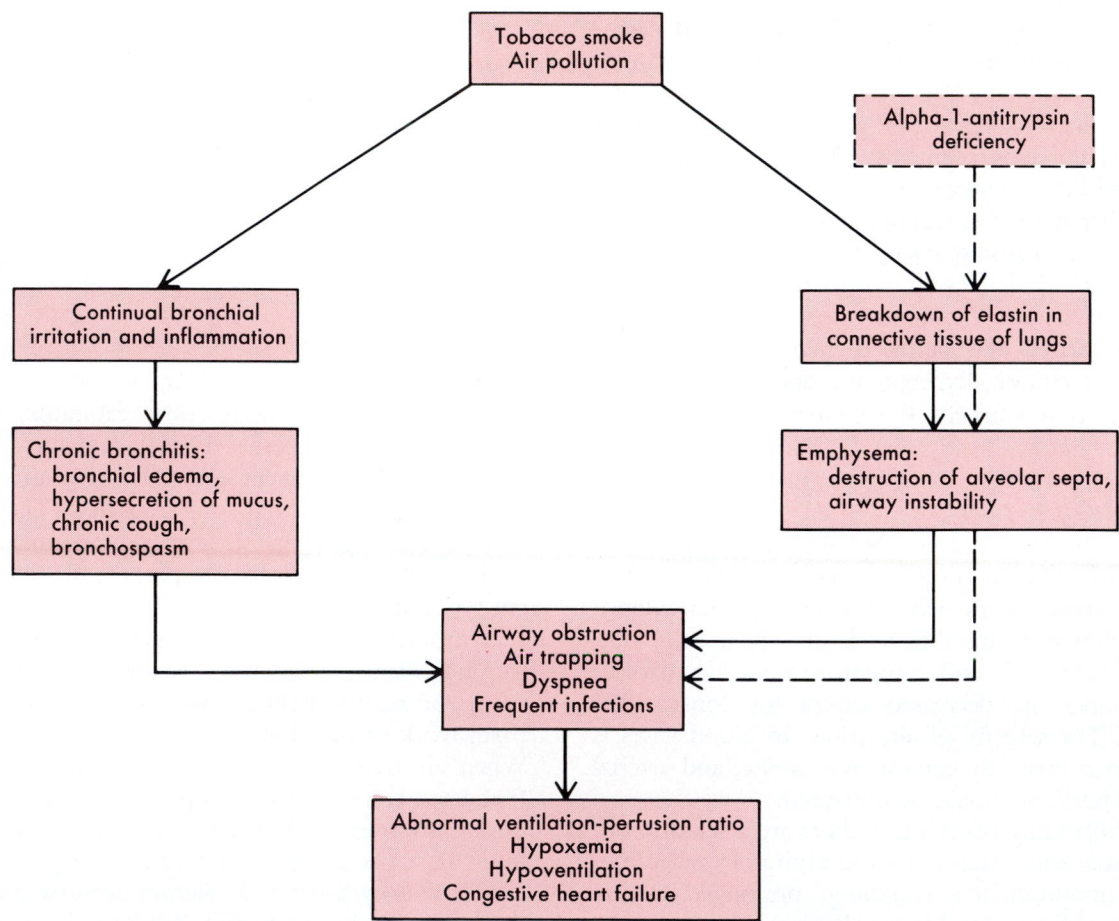

FIG. 30-11. Pathogenesis of chronic bronchitis and emphysema (chronic obstructive pulmonary disease [COPD]). (Dashed arrows indicate role of α_1-antitrypsin deficiency, if present.)

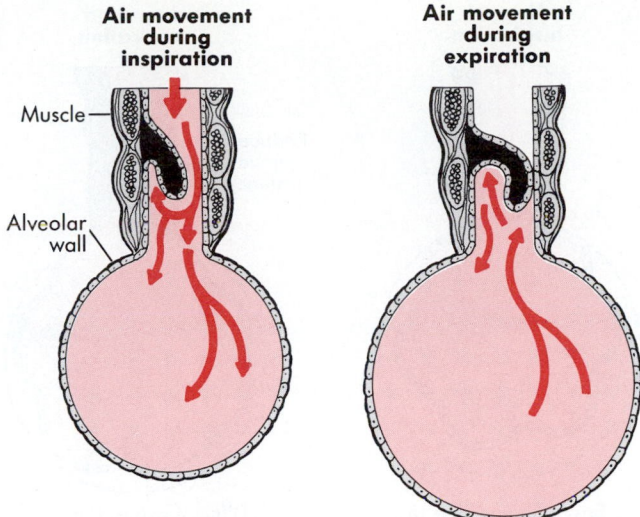

Air movement during inspiration

Air movement during expiration

Muscle

Alveolar wall

FIG. 30-12. Mechanisms of air trapping in COPD. Mucus plugs and narrowed airways cause air trapping and hyperinflation on expiration. During inspiration the airways enlarge, allowing gas to flow past the obstruction. During expiration the airways narrow and prevent gas flow. This mechanism of air trapping, known as "ball valving," occurs in asthma and chronic bronchitis.

TABLE 30-4 Clinical manifestations of chronic obstructive lung disease

Clinical manifestation	Bronchitis	Emphysema
Productive cough	Classic sign	Late in course
Dyspnea	Late in course	Common
Wheezing	Intermitten	Minimal
History of smoking	Common	Common
Barrel chest	Occasionally	Classic
Prolonged expiration	Always present	Always present
Cyanosis	Common	Uncommon
Chronic hypoventilation	Common	Late in course
Polycythemia	Common	Late in course
Cor pulmonale	Common	Late in course

bronchi, but eventually all airways are involved. The thick mucus and hypertrophied bronchial smooth muscle obstruct the airways and lead to closure, particularly during expiration, when the airways are narrowed (Fig. 30-12). The airways collapse early in expiration, trapping gas in the distal portions of the lung. Obstruction eventually leads to ventilation-perfusion mismatch, hypoventilation (increased Pa_{CO_2}), and hypoxemia.

Clinical Manifestations

The symptoms that lead individuals with chronic bronchitis to seek medical care include decreased exercise tolerance, wheezing, and shortness of breath. Individuals usually have a productive cough ("smoker's cough"), and evidence of airway obstruction (decreased FEV_1) is shown by spirometry. Hypoxemia may occur with exercise. As the disease progresses copious amounts of sputum are produced, accompanied by frequent pulmonary infections. Forced vital capacity and FEV_1 become markedly reduced, and FRC and residual volume (RV) are increased as airway obstruction and air trapping become more pronounced.

Airway obstruction results in decreased alveolar ventilation and increased Pa_{CO_2}. Marked hypoxemia leads to polycythemia (overproduction of erythrocytes) and cyanosis. If not reversed, hypoxemia leads to pulmonary hypertension and eventually results in cor pulmonale and congestive heart failure (see Chapter 27) and can lead to severe disability or death. (Table 30-4 lists the common clinical manifestations of chronic bronchitis.) Cyanosis and peripheral edema are responsible for the

slang term "blue bloater," an unfortunate description of individuals with advanced chronic bronchitis.

Evaluation and Treatment

Diagnosis is made on the basis of physical examination, chest radiograph, pulmonary function tests, and blood gas analyses; these tests reflect the progressive nature of the disease. The best "treatment" for chronic bronchitis is prevention, because pathologic changes are not reversible. By the time an individual seeks medical care for symptoms considerable airway damage is present. If the individual stops smoking disease progression can be halted. If smoking is stopped before symptoms occur the risk of chronic bronchitis drops considerably and eventually reaches that of nonsmokers.

Bronchodilators and expectorants are prescribed to increase airway caliber, improve secretion removal, and maximize gas exchange. Chest physiotherapy, including deep breathing (incentive spirometry or intermittent positive pressure breathing [IPPB], a type of mechanical ventilation); postural drainage; and percussion are also used to remove secretions and open airways. Teaching of individuals includes nutritional counseling, respiratory hygiene, recognition of the early signs of infection, and techniques that relieve dyspnea, such as pursed-lip breathing. Some individuals receive prophylactic antibiotic therapy, particularly during the winter months. Steroids are often used late in the course of the disease. Digitalis and diuretics are used to treat congestive heart failure.

Low-flow oxygen is administered with care to individuals with severe hypoxemia. Because of the chronic elevation of PaCO$_2$, the central chemoreceptors no longer act as the primary stimulus for breathing. (Chemoreceptors are described in Chapter 29). This role is taken over by the peripheral chemoreceptors, which are sensitive to changes in PaO$_2$. Peripheral chemoreceptors do not stimulate breathing if the PaO$_2$ is much over 60 mm Hg. Therefore, if oxygen therapy causes PaO$_2$ to exceed 60 mm Hg, the stimulus to breathe is lost, PaCO$_2$ rises, and apnea results. Oxygen is used only to keep PaO$_2$ above 50 mm Hg.

Emphysema

Emphysema is abnormal permanent enlargement of gas-exchange airways (acini) accompanied by destruction of alveolar walls (Snider et al., 1985). In emphysema obstruction results from changes in lung tissues, rather than mucus production and inflammation, as in chronic bronchitis. Difficult expiration in emphysema is caused by destruction of alveolar septa, partial airway collapse, and loss of elastic recoil. Some degree of emphysema is considered normal in old age. When it occurs earlier in life, however, it is usually secondary to chronic bronchitis and cigarette smoking.

Primary emphysema is commonly linked to an inherited deficiency of the enzyme α$_1$-antitrypsin. α$_1$-Antitrypsin is a major component of α$_1$ globulin, a plasma protein. Normally α$_1$-antitrypsin inhibits the action of many proteolytic enzymes (enzymes that break down proteins). Individuals who have α$_1$-antitrypsin deficiency (an autosomal recessive trait) have an increased likelihood of developing emphysema because proteolysis in lung tissues is not inhibited. Homozygous individuals have a 70 to 80% likelihood of developing lung disease. Heterozygous individuals also seem to have an increased risk. (Mechanisms of genetic inheritance are described in Chapter 4.) Persons with α$_1$-Antitrypsin deficiency who smoke are even more susceptible to emphysema than those with the deficiency alone (Janus, Philipps, & Carrell, 1985). A$_1$-Antitrypsin deficiency is suspected in individuals who develop emphysema before age 40 or in their early 40s and in nonsmokers who develop the disease. (The principles of risk-factor analysis are discussed in Chapter 5.)

Pathophysiology

Emphysema begins with destruction of alveolar septa, probably because of elastin breakdown within the septa. Septal destruction eliminates portions of the pulmonary capillary bed and increases the volume of air in the acinus. Expiration becomes difficult because loss of elastic recoil reduces the volume of air that can be expired passively. Hyperinflation of alveoli causes large air spaces (bullae) and subpleural air spaces (blebs) to develop. Septal destruction also affects airway caliber because the force that normal alveoli exert on bronchiolar walls is

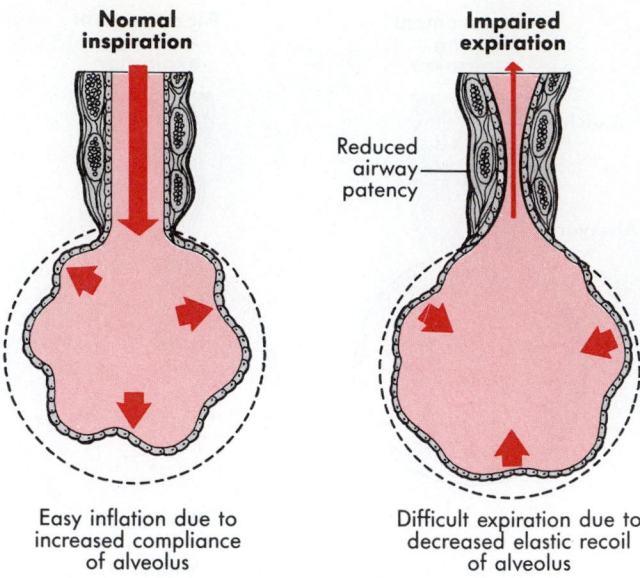

Normal inspiration   **Impaired expiration**

Reduced airway patency

Easy inflation due to increased compliance of alveolus

Difficult expiration due to decreased elastic recoil of alveolus

FIG. 30-13. Mechanisms of air trapping in emphysema. Damage or destroyed alveolar walls no longer support and hold open the airways, and alveoli lose their property of passive elastic recoil. Both of these factors contribute to collapse during expiration.

diminished. The combination of increased residual volume in the alveoli and diminished caliber of the bronchioles causes part of each inspiration to be trapped in the acinus (Fig. 30-13).

Emphysema can be centriacinar (centrilobular) or panacinar (panlobular), depending on site of involvement (Fig. 30-14). In **centriacinar emphysema** septal destruction occurs in the respiratory bronchioles and alveolar ducts, usually in the upper lobes of the lung. Inflammation develops in the bronchioles, but the alveolar sac (alveoli distal to respiratory bronchiole) remains intact. Smokers tend to develop centriacinar emphysema, and it tends to occur with chronic bronchitis. In **panacinar emphysema** the whole acinus is involved (Fig. 30-15). The damage is more randomly distributed and tends to involve the lower lobes of the lung. Panacinar emphysema occurs in the elderly and in patients with α$_1$-antitrypsin deficiency.

Clinical Manifestations

Individuals with emphysema usually present with dyspnea on exertion that later progresses to marked dyspnea, even at rest (see Table 30-4). There is no cough and very little sputum production. The individual is often thin, has tachypnea with prolonged expiration, and must use accessory muscles for ventilation. The anterior-posterior diameter of the chest is increased and has a hyperresonant sound with percussion. The individual often leans forward with arms extended and braced on knees when sitting.

Normal lungs

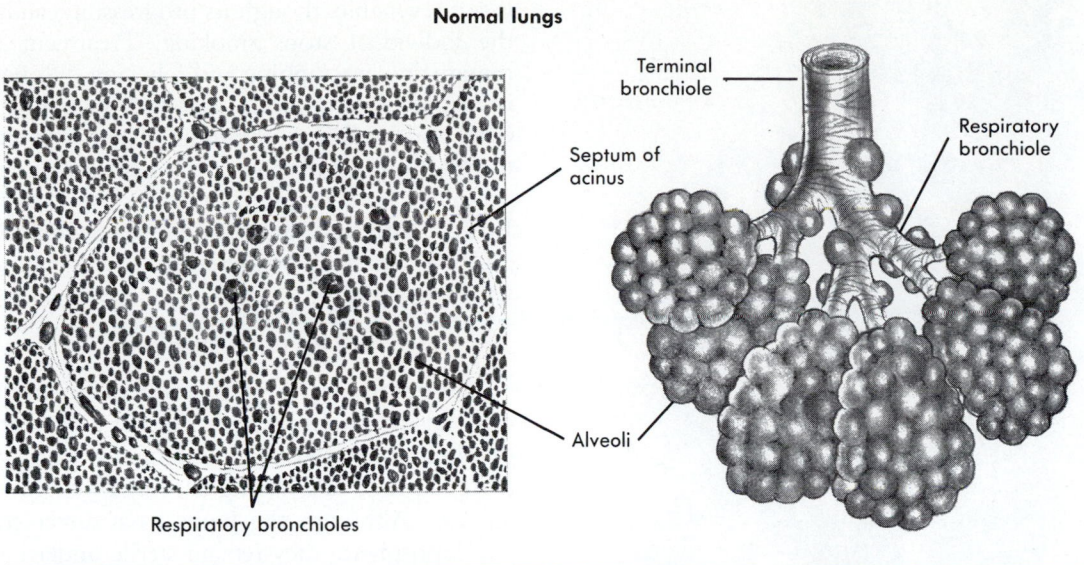

Centriacinar emphysema

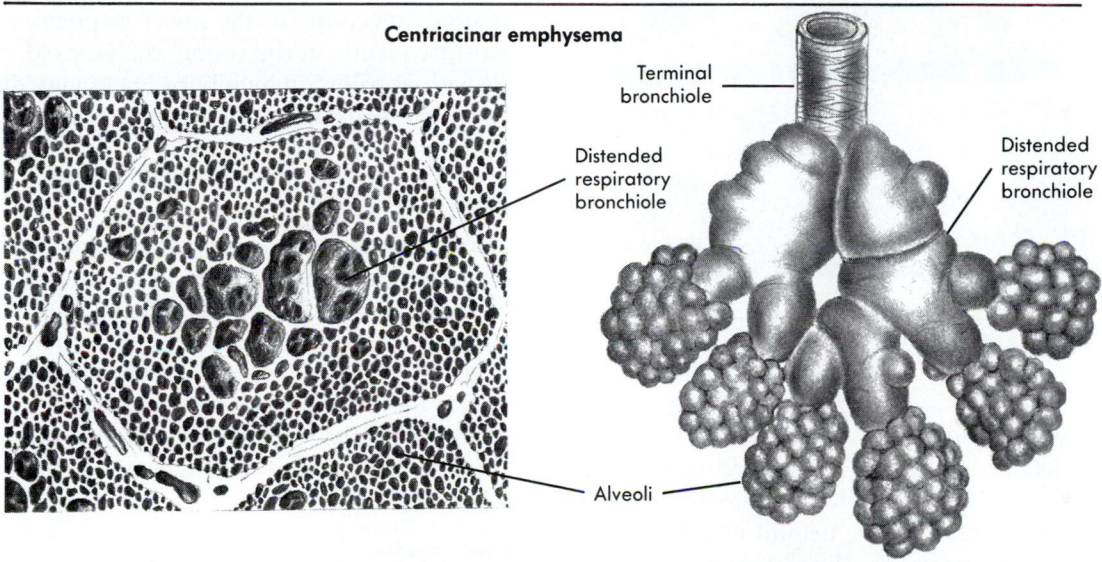

Panacinar emphysema

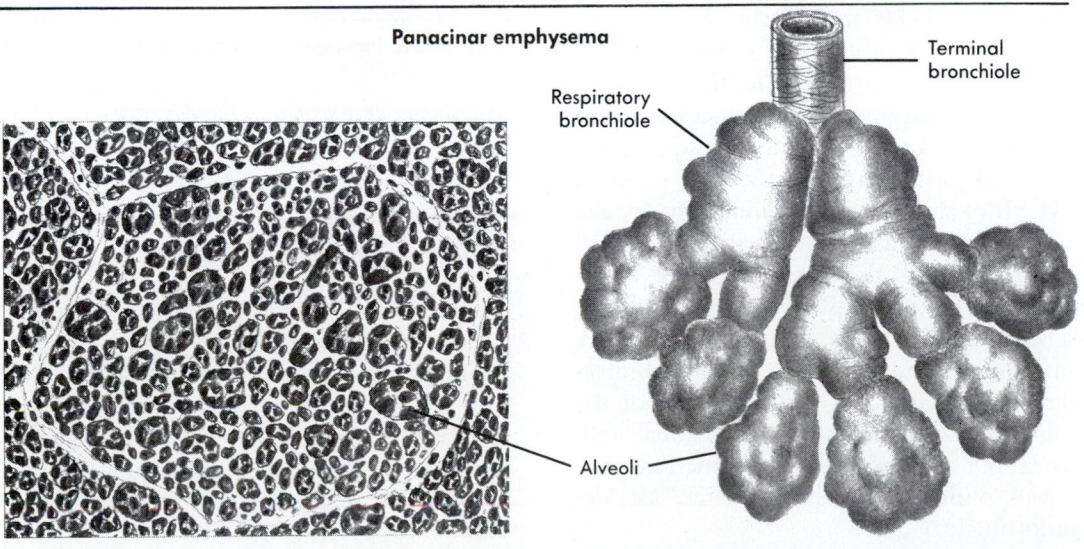

FIG. 30-14. Types of emphysema.

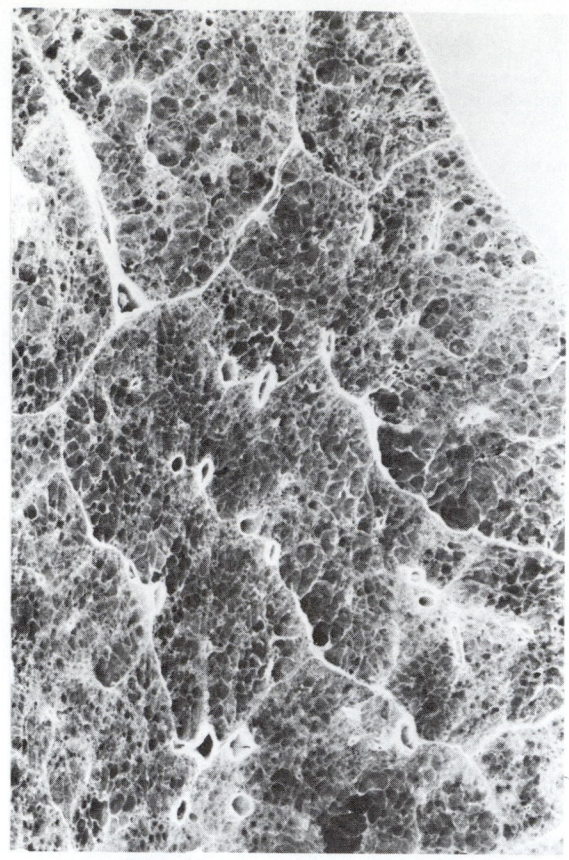

FIG. 30-15. Paracinar emphysema. Uniformly enlarged air spaces. (From Kissane, 1985.)

Evaluation and Treatment

The most definitive evidence for the presence of emphysema is obtained from the chest radiograph. Pulmonary function measurements are helpful in determining a prognosis. On radiographs the diaphragm appears flattened and the lung fields translucent. Marked and persistent overdistention of the lungs is suggestive of emphysema. Pulmonary function tests indicate obstruction to gas flow during expiration. Airway collapse and air trapping in distal portions of the lung lead to a decrease in forced vital capacity (FVC) and FEV_1 and an increase in FRC, RV, and TLC. Total lung capacity can increase to twice normal. Diffusing capacity is decreased because of destruction of the alveolocapillary membrane. Arterial blood gases are usually normal until late in the disease. The disease course is usually prolonged, with increasing dyspnea and intermittent bouts of infection that culminate in failure of the right side of the heart (cor pulmonale) and death. The individual with marked dyspnea but normal Pao_2 is sometimes described as a "pink puffer." Like "blue bloater," the description is unfortunate.

Treatment for emphysema is similar to that for chronic bronchitis. Like chronic bronchitis emphysema

is not reversible, though its progression can be slowed if the individual stops smoking. Treatment focuses on minimizing air trapping and relieving dyspnea. Dyspnea is relieved by relaxation exercises, reconditioning exercises, and breathing retraining. The individual is taught to maximize ventilation, avoid respiratory irritants, and stay away from people with upper respiratory infections. Because infection can prove life-threatening, prophylactic antibiotics may be prescribed, particularly during the winter months.

Respiratory Tract Infections

Respiratory tract infections are the most common cause of short-term disability in the United States. Most of these infections—the common cold, pharyngitis (sore throat), and laryngitis—involve only the upper airways. Although the lungs have direct contact with the atmosphere, they remain sterile under most circumstances. Infections of the lower respiratory tract occur most frequently in the young, the very old, or individuals with impaired immunity or underlying disease. In all cases the body's normal defense mechanisms are impaired.

Pneumonia

Pneumonia is an acute infection of the lung caused by bacteria or viruses. Over 1 million cases of pneumonia are diagnosed each year. Pneumonia primarily occurs during the winter months and is frequently associated with recent upper respiratory tract infection.

Many microorganisms can cause pneumonia. Most of them are carried in the oropharynx of normal individuals. The most common causal microorganisms are the following:

Gram-positive bacteria	Gram-negative bacteria	Nonbacterial organisms
Streptococcus pneumoniae	*Escherichia coli*	Pneumocystis carinii
Mycoplasma pneumoniae	*Pseudomonas aeruginosa*	Funguses
Klebsiella pneumoniae	Proteus species	Viruses
Staphylococcus aureus	Bacteroides species	
Streptococcus pyogenes	Haemophilus species	
	Legionella species	

Fungi are an uncommon cause of pneumonia, but fungal pneumonia can develop as a result of immunosuppression from microorganisms, such as *Candida, Mucor,* and *Aspergillus.* Fungi associated with histoplasmosis and coccidiomycosis can infect both normal and immunosuppressed individuals.

The microorganisms that cause "community-acquired" pneumonia usually differ in identity, virulence, and mortality from those that cause hospital-acquired, or nosocomial, pneumonia. The most common cause of community-acquired pneumonia is *Streptococcus pneumoniae*. This microorganism causes more than 70% of all diagnosed cases of pneumonia (community-acquired and nosocomial). *Mycoplasma pneumoniae* is the next most common cause of community-acquired pneumonia. Mortality from these two organisms is very low (less than 5%). *Staphylococcus aureus* and *Klebsiella pneumoniae* cause some community-acquired disease, usually in individuals with other health problems, such as COPD or alcoholism. *Staphylococcus aureus* and *Klebsiella pneumoniae*, can also cause secondary infection in individuals with a primary viral illness. Viral pneumonia is usually caused by influenza viruses.

Most nosocomial pneumonias are caused by gram-negative bacteria, commonly *Escherichia coli*, *Klebsiella pneumoniae*, and *Pseudomonas aeruginosa*, though *Staphylococcus aureus*, which is gram-positive, also causes pneumonia in some hospital patients. The gram-positive organisms result in more serious infection, with an average mortality rate of 50%. They are also more likely to result in lung necrosis, abscess, or empyema.

The *Legionella* species are widely distributed in water environments and are present in cooling systems, condensers, shower heads, and water reservoirs. Infections may occur in outbreaks, as with the 1976 incident at the American Legion Convention in Philadelphia, or more sporadically.

Pathophysiology

Pathogenic microorganisms can reach the lung by several routes. A common mode of transmission is inspiration. When an infected individual coughs, sneezes, or talks, microorganisms are released into the air in tiny droplets that can be inhaled by other people. Microorganisms can also be inspired with aerosols (nebulized gas) from contaminated respiratory therapy equipment. One of the few microorganisms transmitted via inhalation outside the hospital is influenza.

Another common pathway is aspiration of oropharyngeal secretions. Aspiration of small amounts is normal, particularly during sleep. The oropharynx is normally colonized by a variety of potential pathogens, mostly gram-positive bacteria. In illness or cases of poor dental hygiene the oropharynx is often colonized by gram-negative bacteria. Whether pneumonia develops depends on the virulence of microorganisms aspirated and the effectiveness of the individual's immune system.

Infection can also be spread via the circulation. *Staphylococcus* and gram-negative bacteria are the most common organisms transmitted by this route. The source is usually systemic infection, sepsis, or contaminated needles of intravenous drug abusers.

In healthy individuals pathogens that reach the lung are expelled or held in check by mechanisms of self-defense (see Chapters 6 and 7). The lungs' defense mechanisms—the cough reflex, mucociliary clearance, and phagocytosis by alveolar macrophages—are backed up by the body's immune system and various components of the inflammatory response, including the release of biochemical mediators by alveolar mast cells. In susceptible individuals the invading pathogen is not held in check but multiplies, releasing damaging toxins and stimulating full-scale inflammatory and immune responses, both of which have damaging side effects. The immune response (antigen-antibody reaction) and the endotoxins released by some microorganisms damage bronchial mucous membranes and alveolocapillary membranes. Inflammation and edema cause the acinus and terminal bronchioles to fill with infectious debris and exudate, leading to ventilation-perfusion abnormalities. If the pneumonia is caused by staphylococcus or gram-negative bacteria, necrosis of lung parenchyma may also occur.

Pneumococcal Pneumonia The pathogenesis of pneumococcal pneumonia is best understood (Fig. 30-16). *Streptococcus pneumoniae* organisms initiate the inflammatory response (see Chapter 7), and inflammatory exudate causes alveolar edema. Edema creates a medium for the multiplication of bacteria and aids in the spread of infection into adjacent portions of the lung. The involved lobe undergoes consolidation (solidification of the tissue caused by filling with exudate). There follows a stage of red hepatization in which alveoli fill with blood cells, fibrin, edematous fluid, and pneumococci, giving lung tissue a red appearance. This passes into the stage of gray hepatization, in which affected tissues become gray because of fibrin deposition over the pleural surfaces and the presence of fibrin and leukocytes (neutrophils) in the consolidated alveoli, where phagocytosis is rapidly taking place. With resolution increasing numbers of macrophages appear in the alveolar spaces, the neutrophils degenerate, and the fibrin threads and remaining bacteria are digested by macrophages and removed by lymphatic vessels. Usually infection is limited to one or two lobes.

Viral Pneumonia Viral pneumonia is usually mild and self-limiting but can set the stage for a secondary bacterial infection by providing an ideal environment for bacterial growth and by damaging ciliated epithelial cells, which normally prevent pathogens from reaching the lower airways. Viral pneumonia can be a primary infection or a complication of another viral illness (such as chickenpox or measles). The virus not only destroys the ciliated epithelial cells but also invades the goblet cells and bronchial mucus glands. Sloughing of destroyed bronchial epithelium occurs throughout the respiratory tract, preventing mucociliary clearance. Bronchial walls become edematous and infiltrated with leukocytes.

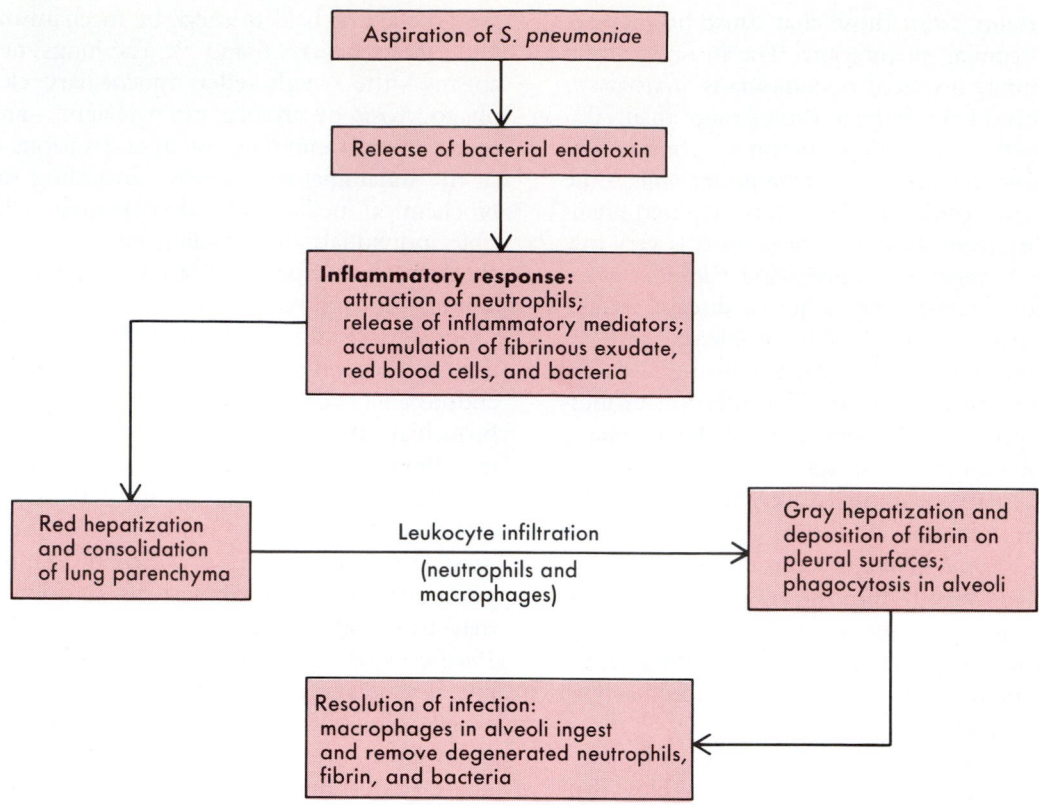

FIG. 30-16. Pathophysiologic course of bacterial pneumonia.

Clinical Manifestations

Most cases of pneumonia are preceded by an upper respiratory infection, which is frequently viral. Individuals then develop fever, chills, productive or dry cough, malaise, pleural pain, and sometimes dyspnea and hemoptysis.

The white blood count is usually elevated (greater than 10,000), though it may be low (less than 6,000) if the individual is debilitated. Chest radiographs reveal infiltrates that may involve a single lobe of the lung (**lobar pneumonia**) or may be more diffuse (**bronchopneumonia**).

Once the diagnosis of pneumonia has been made the pathogen is identified by means of sputum characteristics (gram stain, color, odor) and cultures or, if sputum is absent, blood cultures. Purulent sputum is expectorated by individuals with bacterial pneumonia, and the appearance and odor of the sputum aid in pathogen identification. For example, infection by *Streptococcus pneumoniae*, results in rusty-colored sputum, infection by *Staphylococcus aureus,* results in salmon-pink sputum, and infection by *Pseudomonas aerugenosa,* causes greenish sputum with a distinctive odor. Viral pneumonia and pneumonia caused by *Mycoplasma pneumoniae,* characteristically result in scanty sputum production. Because many pathogens are part of the normal flora in the

oropharynx the specimen may be contaminated with pathogens from oral secretions. Transtracheal aspiration is used to obtain an uncontaminated sputum specimen.

If sputum studies fail to identify the pathogen, pneumonia is assumed to be viral. Positive identification of the virus is often difficult. Blood cultures often help to identify the virus if systemic disease is present.

Evaluation and Treatment

Diagnosis is made on the basis of physical examination, cultures of blood, and cultures of respiratory secretions. Antibiotics are used to treat bacterial pneumonia. Selection of the appropriate antibiotic is based on the sputum culture and specific bacterial sensitivity. The individual's condition usually begins to improve 24 hours after antibiotic therapy is instituted. The duration of antibiotic therapy depends on the identity of the microorganism and the severity of the illness. The development of a complication, such as abscess or empyema, necessitates longer antibiotic therapy. Viral pneumonia is treated with supportive therapy alone, unless secondary bacterial infection is present.

Adequate hydration and good pulmonary hygiene (deep breathing, coughing, chest physiotherapy, etc.) are important aspects of treatment for all types of pneumonia. Mechanical ventilation and supplemental oxygen are provided as needed to maintain adequate gas exchange. Severe pneumonia may develop into ARDS, in which case PEEP is added to ventilatory support measures.

Tuberculosis

Tuberculosis, is an infection caused by *Mycobacterium tuberculosis,* an acid-fast bacillus that usually affects the lungs but may invade other body systems. Before the advent of specific antimicrobial therapy tuberculosis was an important cause of death and disability in North America. Now though it is still a considerable health problem in underdeveloped areas of the world, in North America it affects approximately 28,000 people each year. The risk of developing the disease is highest for the elderly, military personnel (because of their extensive travel), American Indians, and individuals with inadequate nutrition and crowded living conditions.

Pathophysiology

Like some types of pneumonia tuberculosis is transmitted from person to person in airborne droplets. Microorganisms lodge in the lung periphery, usually in the upper lobe. Once the bacilli are inspired into the lung, they multiply and cause nonspecific pneumonitis (lung inflammation). Some bacilli migrate through the lymphatics and become lodged in the lymph nodes, where they encounter lymphocytes and initiate the immune response.

Inflammation in the lung causes neutrophils to migrate to the area, then alveolar macrophages. These cells are phagocytes that engulf the bacilli and begin the process by which the body's defense mechanisms isolate the bacilli, preventing their spread. The neutrophils and macrophages seal off the colonies of bacilli, forming a granulomatous lesion called a tubercle (see Chapter 7). Infected tissues within the tubercle die, forming cheese-like material called caseation necrosis. (Necrosis is described in Chapter 2.) Collagenous scar tissue then grows around the tubercle, completing isolation of the bacilli. The immune response is complete after 10 days or so, preventing further multiplication of the bacilli.

Once the bacilli are isolated in tubercles and immunity develops tuberculosis may remain dormant for life. If the immune system is impaired, however, or if live bacilli escape into the bronchi, active disease occurs.

Clinical Manifestations

In many infected individuals tuberculosis is asymptomatic. In others symptoms develop so gradually that they are not noticed until the disease is advanced. Common clinical manifestations include fatigue, weight loss, lethargy, anorexia (loss of appetite), and a low-grade fever that usually occurs in the afternoon. (These are common signs and symptoms of all chronic infections.) A cough that produces purulent sputum develops slowly and becomes more frequent over several weeks or months. "Night sweats" and general anxiety are often present. Dyspnea, chest pain, and hemoptysis are uncommon findings.

Evaluation and Treatment

Tuberculosis is diagnosed by a positive tuberculin skin test, sputum culture, and chest radiographs. A positive tuberculin skin test indicates that an individual has been infected and has produced antibodies against the bacillus. By itself the positive skin test does not indicate the presence of active disease. It is important that the material used for skin testing be standardized in order to minimize the number of false-positive and false-negative results.

When active disease is present the tubercle bacillus can be cultured from the sputum and may be seen with an acid-fast stain. Chest radiographs of individuals with current or previous active disease demonstrate characteristic changes. Nodules, calcifications, cavities, or hilar enlargement (enlarged mediastinal lymph nodes) is commonly seen in the upper lobes. A positive skin test indicates the need for yearly chest radiographs to detect active disease.

Tuberculosis is graded as follows to aid in evaluation and determination of appropriate therapy (American Thoracic Society, 1981):

0 No TUBERCULOSIS, NO EXPOSURE, NO INFECTION
1 Exposure to tuberculosis, no infection
2 Tuberculosis infection, no disease
3 Tuberculosis, active disease
4 Tuberculosis, no active disease
5 Tuberculosis suspected

Tuberculosis poses a real treatment challenge because once an individual is infected, the tubercle bacilli can lie dormant in the host for life, causing active disease any time the immune system is impaired. Treatment consists of antibiotic therapy to contol active or dormant tuberculosis and prevent transmission. Today most new cases of active tuberculosis occur in previously infected individuals. Prophylactic treatment is, therefore, a major part of disease management.

The choice of drugs and the duration of treatment depend on the individual's health history, the likelihood of bacterial resistance to certain drugs, and the presence of active disease. Individuals whose tuberculin skin tests have converted from negative to positive are treated for 1 year. To prevent the emergence of drug-resistant strains two effective drugs are required: for example, isoniazid and rifampin or isoniazid and ethambutol.

Prophylaxis with isoniazid is frequently prescribed for individuals who have been exposed to active tuberculosis. If an exposed adult has a negative skin test, the test is repeated in 3 months. If it is still negative at that time no antibiotic therapy is necessary. Children and young adults with negative skin tests begin prophylactic isoniazid therapy, and a skin test is repeated in 3 months. If the skin test is still negative after 3 months medication is stopped. If the skin test is positive, therapy is continued for 1 year.

Individuals with active tuberculosis require antibiotic therapy to kill dormant bacilli, eliminate bacilli that may be resistant to one drug, and prevent reactivation of the disease at a later date. Tuberculosis acquired in the Far East or Asia is highly resistant to isoniazid. Therefore, Asian immigrants or travelers who have been exposed to tuberculosis in Asia are given three drugs. Daily medications are taken for 9 months. If the individual's cooperation is in question the drugs are administered biweekly by health care workers.

In the past individuals with active tuberculosis were isolated from the community and their families. Today individuals remain at home or, rarely, in the hospital, until sputum cultures show that the active bacilli have been eliminated. This usually takes a few weeks. After that isolation is unnecessary.

Acute Bronchitis

Acute bronchitis is acute infection or inflammation of the airways or bronchi. Acute bronchitis commonly follows a viral illness and is usually self-limiting. Many of the clinical manifestations are similar to those of pneumonia (i.e., fever, cough, chills, and malaise), but chest radiographs show no infiltrates. Individuals with viral bronchitis present with a nonproductive cough that frequently occurs in paroxysms and is aggravated by cold, dry, or dusty air. Chest pain often develops from the effort of coughing. Purulent sputum may be produced. Treatment consists of rest, aspirin, humidity, and a cough suppressant, such as codeine.

Individuals with bacterial bronchitis present with a productive cough, fever, and pain behind the sternum (breastbone) that is aggravated by coughing. It is rare in previously healthy adults except after viral infection but is common in patients with COPD. Bacterial bronchitis is treated with rest, aspirin, humidity, and antibiotics (usually a penicillinase resistant penicillin). If the cough is nonproductive cough suppressant is given, because a dry cough can cause bronchial irritation and damage. Acute bronchitis may lead to pneumonia.

Pulmonary Vascular Disease

Blood flow through the lungs can be disrupted by a number of disorders that result in occlusion of the vessels, an increase in pulmonary vascular resistance, or destruction of the vascular bed. The consequences of altered pulmonary blood flow may be of no functional significance or can result in severe and life-threatening changes in ventilation/perfusion ratios. Major disorders include pulmonary embolism, pulmonary hypertension, and cor pulmonale.

Pulmonary Embolism

Pulmonary embolism is occlusion of a portion of the pulmonary vascular bed by an embolus: a thrombus (blood clot), tissue fragment, lipids (fats), or air bubble. The most common emboli are thrombi dislodged from deep veins in the calf. They can also originate in the pelvis, particularly in pregnant women.

Risk factors for **pulmonary thromboembolism,** the obstruction of a pulmonary vessel by a thrombus, include many conditions and disorders that promote blood clotting (see Chapter 22). Clotting within the vessels is promoted by venous stasis (slowing or stagnation of blood flow through the veins), hypercoagulability (increased tendency of the blood to form clots), and injuries that cause bleeding. Venous stasis is usually caused by immobility associated with prolonged bed rest or sitting, obesity, and old age, but it can also be caused by pregnancy, congestive heart failure, sickle cell disease, and systemic lupus erythematosus. Hypercoagulability can result from coagulation disorders of the blood or oral contraceptive use. Clot formation also proceeds if vessel damage occurs, as in traumatic injury, surgery, or spontaneous rupture (e.g., cerebrovascular accident).

No matter what its source, a blood clot becomes an embolus when all or part of it breaks away from the site of formation and begins to travel in the bloodstream. (Thromboembolism is described further in Chapter 24.)

Pulmonary emboli are the most common cause of acute pulmonary disease in hospital patients. Approximately 200,000 people die of pulmonary embolism each year in the United States. Half die within 2 hours of embolization, which often is undetected and therefore untreated.

Pathophysiology

The impact or effect of the embolus depends on the extent of pulmonary blood flow obstruction, the size of the affected vessels, the nature of the embolus, and the secondary effects. Pulmonary emboli can occur as any of the following:

1. Massive occlusion, an embolus that occludes a major portion of the pulmonary circulation (i.e., main pulmonary artery embolus)
2. Embolus with infarction, an embolus that is large enough to cause infarction (death) of a portion of lung tissue
3. Embolus without infarction, an embolus that is not severe enough to cause permanent lung injury
4. Multiple pulmonary emboli, which may be chronic or recurrent

Depending on its pattern of occurrence and severity,

pulmonary embolism causes varying degrees of hypoxic vasoconstriction, pulmonary edema, atelectasis, stimulation of the vagus nerve, and release of neurohumoral substances such as histamine. The embolus may also cause systemic hypotension, decreased cardiac output, and pulmonary hypertension, which, when severe, results in acute right ventricular failure and death. The pathogenesis of pulmonary embolism due to a thrombus is summarized in Fig. 30-17.

If the embolus does not cause infarction, the clot is dissolved by the fibrinolytic system (see Chapter 24), and pulmonary function returns to normal. If pulmonary infarction occurs shrinking and scarring develop in the affected area of the lung. (Infarction, or cellular death caused by lack of blood supply, is described in detail in Chapter 27.)

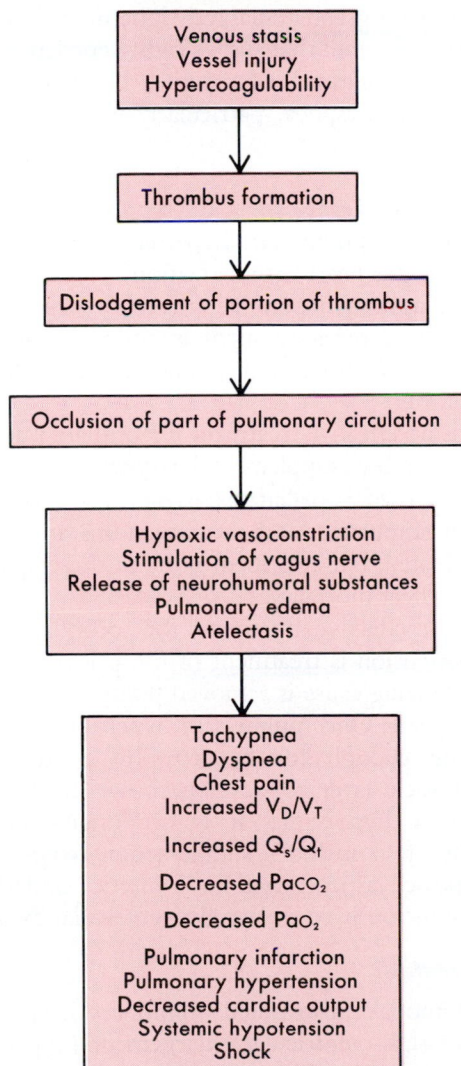

FIG. 30-17. Pathogenesis of pulmonary embolism caused by a thrombus (pulmonary thromboembolism).

Clinical Manifestations

In most cases the clinical manifestations of pulmonary embolism are nonspecific, so that evaluation of risk factors and predisposing factors is an important aspect of diagnosis. The characteristic signs of deep vein thrombosis, the most important predisposing factor, are leg swelling, duskiness, and a positive Homan sign (calf pain on palpation and dorsiflexion of the foot). Sometimes the thrombus is palpable, but quite often the legs appear normal or signs are masked by superficial thrombophlebitis.

The clinical manifestations of pulmonary embolism vary, depending on its type. Massive occlusion causes profound shock, hypotension, tachypnea, tachycardia, severe pulmonary hypertension, and chest pain. Once these manifestations occur death is imminent.

Manifestations of emboli that cause infarction are pleural pain, dyspnea, pleural friction rub, pleural effusion, hemoptysis, fever, and leukocytosis. On chest radiographs, the infarcted portion of the lung shows up as a nonspecific infiltrate in a classic wedge shape bordering the pleura. Pulmonary infarction is most likely in individuals with underlying pulmonary disease.

Pulmonary embolism without infarction is the most common type and is the most difficult to evaluate. The individual usually presents with tachypnea, tachycardia, dyspnea, and unexplained anxiety. Occasionally syncope (fainting) or pleural pain occurs. Recurrent pulmonary emboli occur in indviduals who have had a history of previous emboli. Recurrent emboli may not be detected until progressive incapacitation, precordial pain, anxiety, dyspnea, and right ventricular enlargement are exhibited.

Evaluation and Treatment

Routine chest radiographs and pulmonary function tests are not definitive tests for pulmonary embolism. Pulmonary embolism is suspected if arterial blood gas analyses demonstrate unexplained hypoxemia and hyperventilation. A perfusion scan, in which lungs are scanned after injection of a radioactive substance into the venous circulation, may indicate embolism.

The ideal treatment for pulmonary embolism is prevention through risk-factor analysis and elimination of predisposing factors for individuals at risk. (Risk factor analysis is described in Chapter 5.) Venous stasis in hospital patients is minimized by leg elevation, bed exercises, position changes, early postoperative ambulation, and pneumatic calf compression. Clot formation is also prevented by prophylactic low-dose anticoagulant therapy; less anticoagulant is required to prevent a clot than to treat one.

Anticoagulant therapy is the primary treatment for pulmonary embolism. Intravenous administration of heparin is begun immediately and is followed by oral doses of coumarin. If massive life-threatening embolism occurs, a fibrinolytic agent, such as streptokinase, is sometimes used. (Streptokinase is contraindicated for 10 days after surgery.)

Pulmonary Hypertension

Pulmonary hypertension is high blood pressure in the pulmonary arteries. Normally pulmonary artery pressure is lower than systemic artery pressure. Pulmonary hypertension is defined as a rise in pulmonary artery pressure (normally 15 to 18 mm Hg) of 5 to 10 mm Hg.

Primary pulmonary hypertension is very rare. It has no known cause, usually occurs in women between the ages of 20 and 40, and may be hereditary in some cases. Primary pulmonary hypertension has a very poor prognosis: most individuals die within 5 years of diagnosis.

Secondary pulmonary hypertension is more common. It can be secondary to any respiratory or cardiovascular disorder that (1) increases the volume or pressure of blood entering the pulmonary arteries or (2) narrows or obstructs the pulmonary arteries. The first cause overloads the pulmonary circulation from without; the second elevates blood pressure by increasing resistance to flow within the lungs.

Pathophysiology

In primary hypertension the small pulmonary arteries (arterioles) become narrow or obliterated as a result of hypertrophy (enlargement) of smooth muscle in the vessel walls and formation of fibrous lesions around the vessels. The mechanisms that cause these changes are not known. Vessel narrowing or obliteration increases resistance and causes the pulmonary hypertension. Pressures in the left ventricle, which receives blood from the lungs, remain normal, but high pressures generated in the lungs are transmitted to the right ventricle, which supplies the pulmonary arteries. Eventually the right ventricle fails. (Right ventricular disease resulting from pulmonary hypertension is termed **cor pulmonale.** Oxygenation is not severely affected, though mild hypoxia and cyanosis do occur. Death eventually results from cor pulmonale. (Mechanisms of heart failure are described in Chapter 27.)

There are four causes of secondary pulmonary hypertension. The first is elevated left ventricular filling pressures, such as occur with coronary artery disease and mitral valve disease. When pressures on the left side of the heart are elevated, the pulmonary artery pressure rises proportionally in order to maintain normal blood flow. The second cause of secondary pulmonary hypertension is increased blood flow through the pulmonary circulation (left-to-right shunts), as occurs with a ventricular septal defect or patent ductus arteriosus. (These congenital heart defects are discussed in Chapter 28.) The third cause is obliteration or obstruction of the pulmonary

vascular bed by a pulmonary embolus, and the fourth is vasoconstriction of the vascular bed. Vasoconstriction is usually caused by hypoxemia, acidosis, or both.

Secondary pulmonary hypertension can be reversed if the primary disorder is resolved. If hypertension persists hypertrophy occurs in the medial smooth muscle layer of the arterioles. The larger arteries stiffen, and hypertension progresses until pulmonary artery pressure equals systemic blood pressure. The result is ventricular hypertrophy and eventual cor pulmonale. The pathogenesis of heart failure caused by secondary pulmonary hypertension is shown in Fig. 30-18.

Clinical Manifestations

Pulmonary hypertension may not be detected until pulmonary artery pressure is equal to systemic blood pressure. The symptoms are often masked by primary pulmonary or cardiovascular disease. The first indication of pulmonary hypertension is often an abnormality seen on a chest radiograph (enlarged right heart border) or an electrocardiogram that shows right ventricular hypertrophy. Manifestations of fatigue, chest discomfort, tachypnea, and dyspnea, particularly with exercise, are common.

Evaluation and Treatment

Diagnosis of pulmonary hypertension can only be made with right heart catheterization. The diagnosis of primary pulmonary hypertension is made when all other causes of hypertension, such as mitral stenosis (see Chapter 27), COPD, and pulmonary embolus have been ruled out.

There is no effective treatment for primary pulmonary hypertension, but supplemental oxygen, digitalis, and diuretics are used as palliatives. α-Blockers, vasodilators, β-receptor stimulants, and prostaglandins are currently being evaluated, but at present none of these agents has proved to affect mortality.

The most effective treatment for secondary pulmonary hypertension is treatment of the primary disorder. If the underlying cause is removed pulmonary hypertension disappears. Once pulmonary hypertension has persisted long enough for hypertrophy of the medial smooth muscle layer to develop, however, as it does with chronic hypoxemia, it is no longer reversible. Treatment often includes supplemental oxygen to reverse hypoxic vasoconstriction. Diuretics and digitalis are used judiciously to treat right ventricular failure.

Cor Pulmonale

Cor pulmonale, also called pulmonary heart disease, consists of right ventricular enlargement (hypertrophy, dilatation, or both). It is secondary to pulmonary hypertension caused by disorders of the lungs or chest wall.

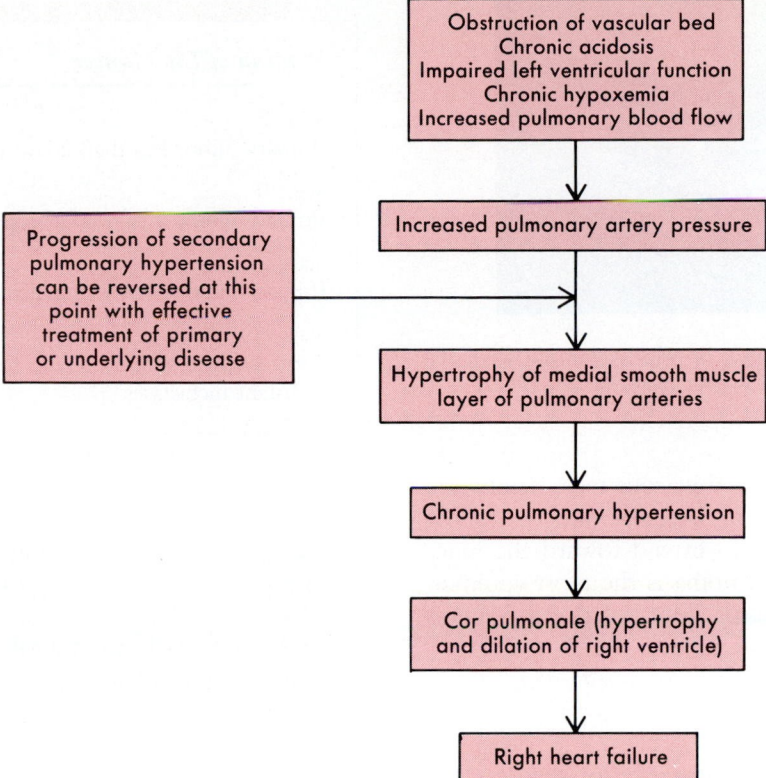

FIG. 30-18. Pathogenesis of pulmonary hypertension and cor pulmonale.

Pathophysiology

Cor pulmonale develops as pulmonary hypertension creates chronic pressure overload in the right ventricle similar to that created in the left ventricle by systemic hypertension. (Systemic hypertension is discussed in Chapter 27.) Pressure overload increases the work of the right ventricle and causes hypertrophy of the normally thin-walled heart muscle. Acute hypoxemia, such as might occur with pneumonia, can exaggerate pulmonary hypertension and dilate the ventricle as well. Right ventricular filling pressures are normal until failure occurs. The right ventricle usually fails when pulmonary artery pressure equals systemic blood pressure.

Clinical Manifestations

The clinical manifestations of cor pulmonale may be obscured by primary respiratory disease and only appear during exercise testing. The heart appears normal at rest, but with exercise cardiac output falls and the electrocardiogram shows right ventricular hypertrophy. Chest pain is common. The pulmonary component of the second heart sound, which represents closure of the pulmonic valve, may be accentuated, and a pulmonic valve murmur may also be present. Tricuspid valve murmur may accompany the development of right ventricular failure.

Evaluation and Treatment

Diagnosis is made on the basis of physical examination, radiologic examination, and electrocardiogram or echocardiography, or both. Physical examination findings are often similar to those of chronic lung disease with dyspnea and distended neck veins. The goal of treatment for cor pulmonale is to decrease the workload of the right ventricle by lowering pulmonary artery pressure. Treatment is the same as that for pulmonary hypertension, and its success depends on reversal of the underlying lung disease.

Lip Cancer

Cancer of the lip is more prevalent in men, with 3700 new cases per year accounting for about 1% of all cancers in men (American Cancer Society, 1989). Chronic exposure to sun, wind, and cold over a period of years results in dryness, chapping, hyperkeratosis, and predisposition to malignancy. The lower lip is the most common site.

Pathophysiology

The most common form of lower lip cancer is termed exophytic. The lesion usually develops in the outer part of the lip along the vermilion border. The lip becomes thickened and evolves to an ulcerated center with a

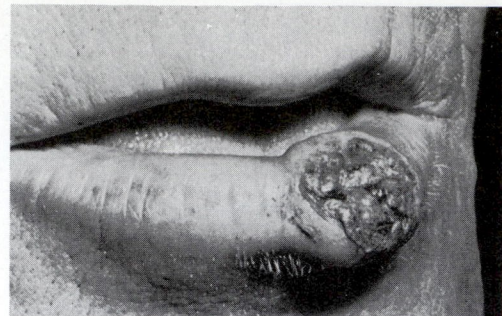

FIG. 30-19. Carcinoma of lower lip with central ulceration and raised, rolled borders. (From del Regato, Spjut, & Cox, 1985.)

Staging of Lip Cancer

Stage I
Primary tumor less than 2 cm; no palpable nodes

Stage II
Primary tumor 2 to 4 cm; no palpable nodes

Stage III
Primary tumor over 4 cm; metastatic lymph nodes

Stage IV
Large primary tumors; nodes fixed to mandible or distant metastases

---

raised border (Fig. 30-19). Verricous-type lesions are less common. They have an irregular surface, follow cracks in the lip, and tend to extend toward the inner surface. Squamous cell carcinoma is the most common cell type. Basal cell carcinoma does not develop unless there is extension beyond the mucous membrane or vermilion border of the lip.

Clinical Manifestations

Malignant lesions are often preceded by the development of a blister that evolves into a superficial ulceration. In some cases there is a history of recurrent scales that precede development of a bleeding ulceration. Metastases to the cervical lymph nodes have a low rate of occurrence (2% to 8%) and are more likely when the primary lesion is larger and exists for a longer period of time.

Evaluation and Treatment

Diagnosis is commonly made by clinical history and presentation of the lesion. Biopsy confirms the presence

of malignant cells. The staging for lip cancer is summarized in the box above. Surgical excision is effective for smaller lesions. Larger lesions that require extensive resection may be followed by subsequent cosmetic surgeries. Interstitial irradiation and radioactive implants have been proved effective for control of primary lesions (Pigneaux, Richard, & LaGarde, 1979). The prognosis for recovery is excellent and deaths are usually the result of inadequate treatment.

Laryngeal Cancer

Cancer of the larynx represents about 2 to 3% of all cancers in the United States. There are approximately 12,300 new cases per year, 10,000 of them in men (American Cancer Society, 1989). The risk of laryngeal cancer is increased by the amount of tobacco smoked; risk is further heightened with the combination of smoking and alcohol consumption. The highest incidence is in men between 50 and 75 years of age.

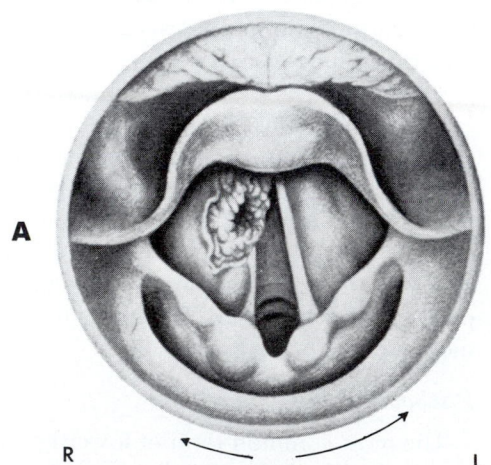
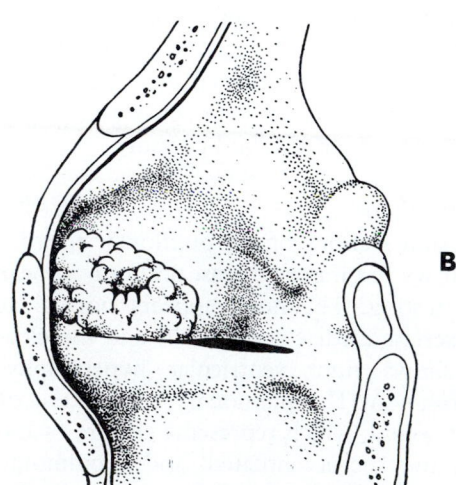

FIG. 30-20. **A,** Mirror view of carcinoma of right false cord partially hiding true cord; **B,** lateral view. (From del Regato, Spjut, & Cox, 1985.)

Pathophysiology

Carcinoma of the true vocal cords (glottis) is more common than that of the supraglottic structures (epiglottis, aryepiglottic folds, arytenoids, and false cords). Tumors of the subglottic area are rare. Squamous cell carcinoma is the most frequent cell type, although small cell carcinomas also occur (Fig. 30-20). Metastasis develops by spread to the draining lymph nodes, and distant metastasis, usually to the lung, is rare.

Clinical Manifestations

The presenting symptoms of laryngeal cancer include hoarseness, dyspnea, and cough. Progressive hoarseness is the most significant symptom and can result in voice loss. Dyspnea is rare in the case of supraglottic tumors but can be severe in subglottic tumors. Cough occurs less commonly and may follow swallowing. Laryngeal pain or a sore throat is likely to be present with supraglottic lesions.

Evaluation and Treatment

Evaluation of the larynx includes external inspection and palpation of the larynx and the lymph nodes of the neck. Indirect laryngoscopy provides a steroscopic view of the structure and movement of the larynx. A biopsy can also be obtained during this procedure. Direct laryngoscopy provides specific visualization of the tumor. Plain films of the larynx and computed tomography facilitate the identification of tumor boundaries and the degree of extension to surrounding tissue.

Radiation therapy has shown good results for early carcinoma of the vocal cords. Partial laryngectomies are the preferred treatment for small supraglottic and subglottic malignancies. Total laryngectomy is required when lesions are extensive and involve the cartilage.

Lung Cancer

Lung cancers (bronchogenic carcinomas) arise from the epithelium of the respiratory tract. As such the term *lung cancer* excludes other pulmonary tumors including sarcomas, lymphomas, blastomas, hematomas, and mesotheliomas. Lung cancer is an epidemic in the United States, with an estimated 155,000 new cases in 1989 (American Cancer Society, 1989) (see Box, 30-b). It is the most frequent cause of cancer death in the United States and, along with malignant melanoma, is the only major cancer type whose incidence is rapidly increasing (Gazdar & Linnoila, 1988). Although there has been some slowing of deaths caused by lung cancer in men, the increase among women has been extraordinarily high. The lung cancer death rate for women is now higher than that of any other cancer because of increased cigarette smoking by women (American Cancer Society, 1989). Deaths from lung cancer appear at ages 35 to 44 years; a sharp increase occurs between the ages

Important Trends for Lung Cancer

Incidence
An estimated 155,000 new cases in 1989: 101,000 in males and 54,000 in females.

Mortality
An estimated 142,000 deaths in 1989: 93,000 in males and 49,000 in females. The death rate for women is now higher than that of any other cancer.

Risk Factors
Heavy cigarette smoking (more than 20 cigarettes/day) is the number one risk factor. Passive smoking (exposure to someone else's cigarette smoke) increases the risk of lung cancer. Occupational risk factors include exposure to asbestos dust, arsenic, chromium, nickel, ionizing radiation, chloromethyl ethers, coal products, mustard gas, and vinyl chloride. Cigarette smoking and exposure to asbestos may have a synergistic effect on the production of lung cancer.

Warning Signs
A persistent cough, sputum streaked with blood, chest pain, recurring attacks of pneumonia or bronchitis.

Early Detection and Prevention
Lung cancer is very difficult to detect early. If a smoker quits at the time of early cellular changes, altered bronchial lining often returns to normal. Periodic chest x-ray films and sputum cytologic analysis can detect presymptomatic, early-stage lung cancers, particularly of the squamous cell type; however, no conclusive evidence of reduction in lung cancer mortality as a consequence of screening has been found.

Treatment
Surgery, radiation therapy, and chemotherapy are all used. Surgery is usually the treatment of choice, and with improved ventilation machinery and antibiotics, surgical complications are infrequent. Tumor spread requiring chemotherapy or radiation therapy is evident in about one third of all surgical lung cancer patients.

Survival
Only 13% of white and black patients live 5 or more years after diagnosis. Non−small cell carcinomas are considered separately from small cell carcinomas (see text). Rates have improved only sightly over a recent 10-year period.

From American Cancer Society. (1989). Cancer statistics 1989. *Ca—A Cancer Journal for Clinicians, 39(1)*.

of 45 and 55, and the incidence rate continues to rise through ages 65 to 74, after which it levels off and decreases among the very old.

The most common cause of lung cancer is cigarette smoking. Heavy smokers have about 25 times greater chance of developing lung cancer than nonsmokers. Cigarette smoke contains several organ-specific carcinogens, and smoking has been causally related to carcinogenesis at several sites, including the larynx, oral cavity, esophagus, and urinary bladder. Genetic predisposition to developing lung cancer, which is evident in analysis of pedigrees, also plays a role in its pathophysiology (see Chapter 5).

The cancer death rates for pipe and cigar users are about equal to those of cigarette smokers for cancer of the larynx, oral cavity, and esophagus. The incidence of lung cancer decreases among people who stop smoking, and it reaches a level almost as low as that of nonsmokers 15 years after smoking has stopped. Theories of carcinogenesis are discussed in Chapter 11.

Environmental or occupational risk factors *associated,* with lung cancer include benzopyrene and radon particles associated with uranium mining, radiation, and nuclear bombs. Others are polycyclic aromatic hydrocarbons and arsenicals, asbestos fibers, diesel exhauset, nitrogen mustard gases, nickel, silica, vinyl chloride, and chloromethyl methyl ether. Air pollution, coal, and iron mining are also considered risk factors (Matthews & Linniola, 1988).

Types of Lung Cancer

At least a dozen different cell types of tumors are included under the broad heading of lung cancer. The four major histologic types are squamous cell carcinoma, small cell carcinoma, large cell carcinoma, and adenocarcinoma (including broncholoalveolar cell carcinoma). However, for clinical and therapeutic reasons, lung cancers are frequently classified in small cell lung cancer (SCLC) and non-SCLC (NSCLC) subdivisions. Characteristics of these tumors, including evaluation

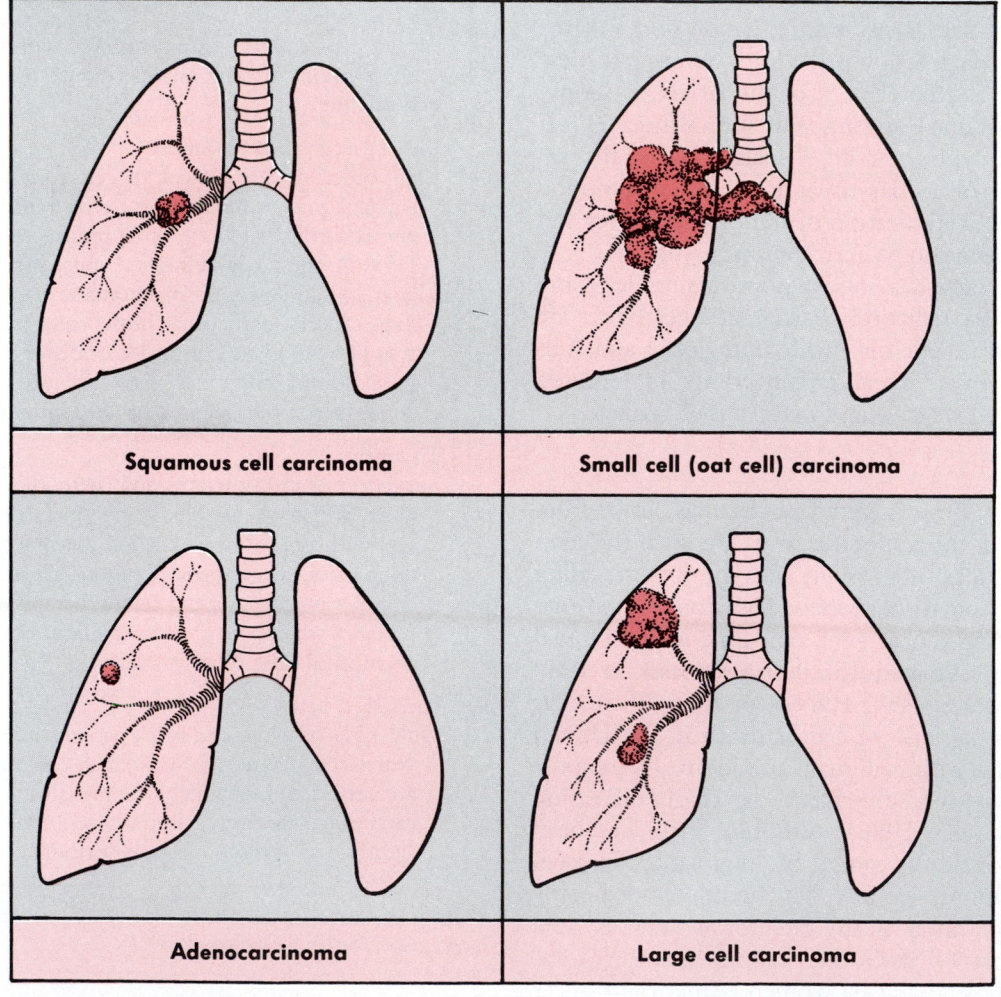

FIG. 30-21. Predominant sites of types of lung cancer. (Tumor characteristics are summarized in Table 30-5.)

and treatment, are listed in Table 30-5. Some controversy exists as to the most frequently encountered cell type of bronchogenic carcinoma. In the past squamous cell carcinoma was considered the most common type, but the incidence of adenocarcinoma is currently greater. Common sites of involvement for all four types of bronchogenic carcinoma are shown in Fig. 30-21. (Tumor biology is the subject of Chapter 10.)

Squamous Cell Carcinoma

Squamous cell carcinoma, accounts for about 30% of bronchogenic carcinomas, representing a sharp decline in incidence in the past two decades. These tumors are typically located near the hilus and project into bronchi (Fig. 30-22).

Because of the location in the central bronchi obstructive manifestations such as pneumonia and atelectasis are often associated with squamous cell carcinoma (see Fig. 30-22). These tumors can remain fairly well localized and tend not to metastasize until late in the course of the disease. The preferred treatment is surgical resection, although once metastasis has taken place, total surgical resection is most difficult and survival rates dramatically drop.

Small Cell Carcinoma

Small cell carcinomas, comprise between 20 and 25% of bronchogenic carcinomas. It is estimated that most of these tumors are central in origin (Fig. 30-21). Cell sizes range from 6 to 8 micrometers. When almost no cytoplasm is present (because of density of cells) and the cells are compressed into an ovid mass, the tumor is called **oat cell carcinoma.** This cell type has the strongest correlation with cigarette smoking. Because these tumors show a rapid rate of growth and tend to metastasize early and widely, small cell carcinomas have the worst prognosis. The most frequent survival time for small cell carcimona is between 9 and 10 months. Fewer than 5% of individuals are alive 2 years after diagnosis.

Small cell carcinoma is most often associated with ectopic hormone production, production of hormones by tumors of nonendocrine origin, or production of an inappropriate hormone by an endocrine gland. Neuroendocrine cells (NE cells) containing neurosecretory granules exist throughout the tracheobronchial tree (Matthews & Linnoila, 1988). Ectopic hormone production is important to the clinician because resulting signs and symptoms may be the first manifestation of the underlying cancer. Small cell carcinomas commonly produce

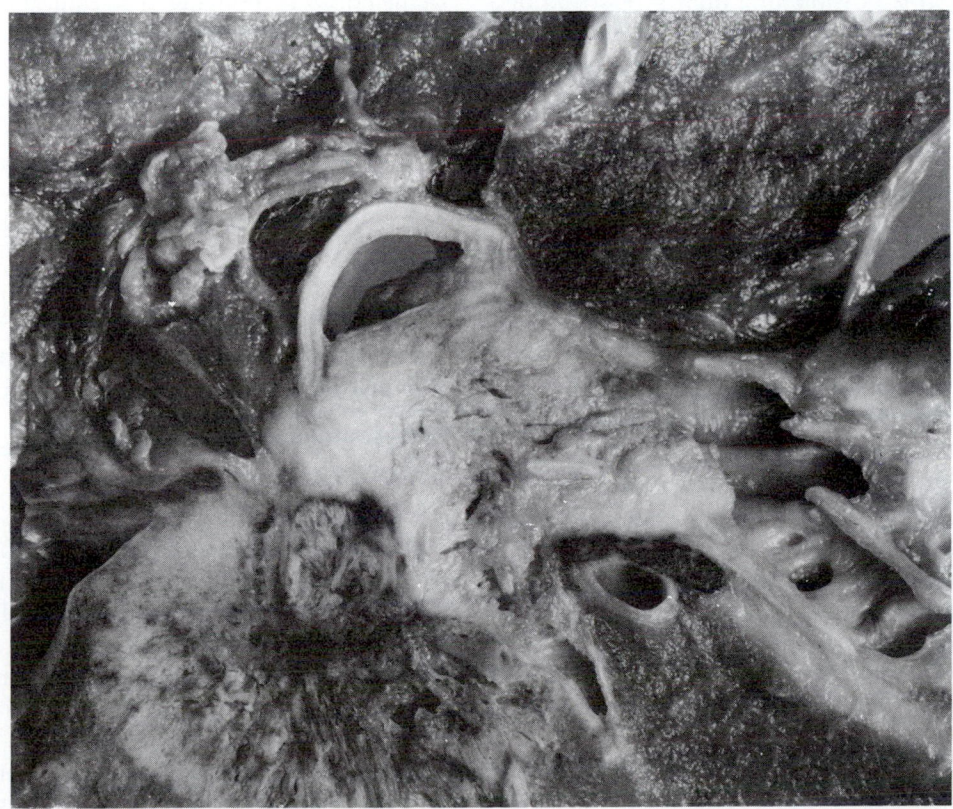

FIG. 30-22. Bronchogenic carcinoma extending into a major bronchial airway. Bronchogenic squamous cell carcinoma arising in major bronchus. Tumor disrupts bronchial wall and extends into surrounding tissue. Pneumonia can be seen at periphery. (From Rosai, 1981.)

gastrin-releasing peptide, calcitonin, arginine vaso-pressin, and adenocorticotrophin hormone (ACTH) (Matthews & Linnoila, 1988). As a result of ACTH secretion, lung cancer patients secrete large quantities of 17-hydroxy steriods and 17-ketosteriods, leading to the development of an atypical Cushing syndrome. Signs and symptoms related to this condition include muscular weakness, facial edema, hypokalemia, alkalosis, hyperglycemia, hypertension, and increased pigmentation.

Adenocarcinoma

Adenocarcinoma, (tumor arising from glands) of the lung comprises 30 to 35% of all bronchogenic carcinomas. The recent increase in incidence of adenocarcinoma has been ascribed to the increasing frequency of lung cancer in women, environmental and occupational carcinogens, and changes in the histologic criteria for diagnosis. These tumors, which are usually smaller than 4 cm, more commonly arise in the peripheral regions of the pulmonary parenchyma.

Included in the category of adenocarcinoma is bronchioloalveolar cell carcinoma. These tumors tend to arise from the terminal bronchioles and alveoli. They are slow-growing tumors with an unpredictable pattern of metastasis. This cell type has the weakest association with smoking.

Surgical resection is possible in a high proportion of cases, but because metastasis occurs early, the 5-year survival rate is less than 10%. Neither chemotherapy nor radiation therapy has, as yet, increased the survival rate.

Large Cell Carcinoma

Large cell carcinomas, constitute between 10 and 15% of bronchogenic carcinomas. This cell type has lost all evidence of differentiation and is therefore commonly referred to as **large cell anaplastic cancer.** Because large cell carcinomas show none of the histologic findings of squamous cell carcinoma or adenocarcinoma, this type is diagnosed by a process of exclusion. The cells are generally larger than leukocytes and contain large, darkly stained nuclei. These tumors commonly arise peripherally but are found centrally and can grow to distort the trachea and cause widening of the carina.

Once metastasis has occurred surgical therapy is limited to palliative procedures (comfort measures) designed to relieve obstructive pneumonitis or prevent recurrence of pleural effusion. Neither radiation therapy nor chemotherapy has been successful in increasing survival.

Pathogenesis

A number of investigators have stressed that at sites of segmental bronchial bifurcations airflow and mucus production are altered and bronchial epithelium become very susteptible to injury (Matthews & Linnoila, 1988). It is proposed that carcinogenic agents are likely to be deposited and absorbed in these areas. Saccomanno (1971) and others who studied uraniuim miners reported that metaplastic squamous cells were replaced in a progressive manner over time by dysplastic, in situ, and invasive neoplastic cells.

The single most important risk factor in lung cancer is tobacco smoke. The effects of smoking include structural, functional, malignant, and toxic changes. For example, there are specific central nervous system receptor sites for nicotine that produce an opiatelike state (Smoking & Health, 1979). Individuals with lung cancer demonstrate bronchial epithelial changes progressing from squamous cell alteration or metaplasia to carcinoma in situ. Histologic changes are evident with bronchitis and emphysema. Thickening of the bronchial epithelium, mucous gland hypertrophy, and alveolar cell rupture occur more frequently in smokers that nonsmokers. Cigarette smokers also have altered alveolar macrophage functions or phagocytosis, which may increase the risk of pulmonary infections.

Clinical Manifestations

Symptoms of early-stage, localized disease are nonspecific and are likely to be attributed by the individual to the effects of smoking. The clinical manifestations are ambiguous and insidious; they include coughing, sputum production, hemoptysis, pneumonia, airway obstruction, and pleural effusions. Table 30-5 summarizes the clinical manifestations according to tumor type. Important to remember is that by the time there are manifestations severe enough to motivate the individual to seek medical advice the disease is usually advanced (Jeff, Cortese, & Fontana, 1983).

Evaluation and Treatment

The specific means of diagnosis and treatment for each cell type of lung cancer are summarized in Table 30-5.

Other Lung Cancers
Bronchial Adenomas

Another broad category of lung neoplasm are **bronchial adenomas,** or tumors of glandular epithelium. Bronchial adenomas comprise about 1% to 5% of all bronchial tumors. Traditionally they are divided into carcinoid and salivary gland subcategories, although recent evidence suggests that they arise from different cellular precursors.

Carcinoid tumors tend to occur earlier in life than bronchogenic carcinoma; the average age at diagnosis is about 45 years. The tumors arise more commonly in the main or segmental bronchi, are easily visualized bronchoscopically, and are found on routine chest radio-

TABLE 30-5 Characteristics of lung cancers

Tumor type	Growth rate	Metastasis	Means of diagnosis	Clinical manifestations and treatment
Squamous cell carcinoma	Slow	Late; mostly to hilar lymph nodes	Biopsy, sputum analysis, bronchoscopy, electron microscopy, immunohistochemistry	Cough, sputum production, airway obstruction; treated surgically
Small cell (oat cell) carcinoma	Very rapid	Very early; to mediastinum or distally in lung	Radiography, sputum analysis, bronchoscopy, electron microscopy, immunohistochemistry, and clinical manifestations (cough, chest pain, dyspnea hemoptysis, localized wheezing)	Airway obstruction caused by pneumonitis, signs and symptoms of excessive hormone secretion; treated by chemotherapy and ionizing radiation to thorax and central nervous system
Adenocarcinoma	Moderate	Early	Radiography, fiber-optic bronchoscopy, electron microscopy	Pleural effusion; treated surgically
Large cell carcinoma	Rapid	Early and widespread	Sputum analysis, bronchoscopy, electron microscopy (by exclusion of other cell types)	Chest wall pain, pleural effusion, cough, sputum production, hemoptysis, airway obstruction caused by pneumonia (if airways involved); treated surgically

TABLE 30-6 TNM classification of lung cancer

Symbol	Definition
Primary tumors (T)	
T_o	No evidence of primary tumor
Tx	Presence of tumor proved by malignant cells in bronchopulmonary secretions but not visualized by x-ray or bronchoscopy
Tis	Carcinoma in situ
T_1	Tumor 3.0 cm or less in diameter, surrounded by lung or visceral pleura, no evidence of invasion proximal to a lobar bronchus at bronchoscopy
T_2	Tumor more than 3.0 cm in diameter, or a tumor of any size that invades the visceral pleura or has associated atelectasis or obstructive pneumonitis to the hilar regions
T_3	Tumor of any size with direct extension into an adjacent structure, such as chest wall, diaphragm, or mediastinum; or tumor demonstrated bronchoscopically to involve a main bronchus less than 2.0 cm to the carina; any tumor associated with atelectasis or obstructive pneumonitis of an entire lung or pleural effusion
Lymph node involvement (N)	
N_0	No demonstrable metastasis to regional lympho nodes
N_1	Metastasis to nodes in the peribronchial and/or ipsalateral hilar region
N_2	Metastasis to lymph nodes within the mediastinum
Metastasis (M)	
M_0	No distant metastasis
M_1	Distant metastasis, such as to scalene or contralateral hilar lymph nodes, brain, bones, lung, liver

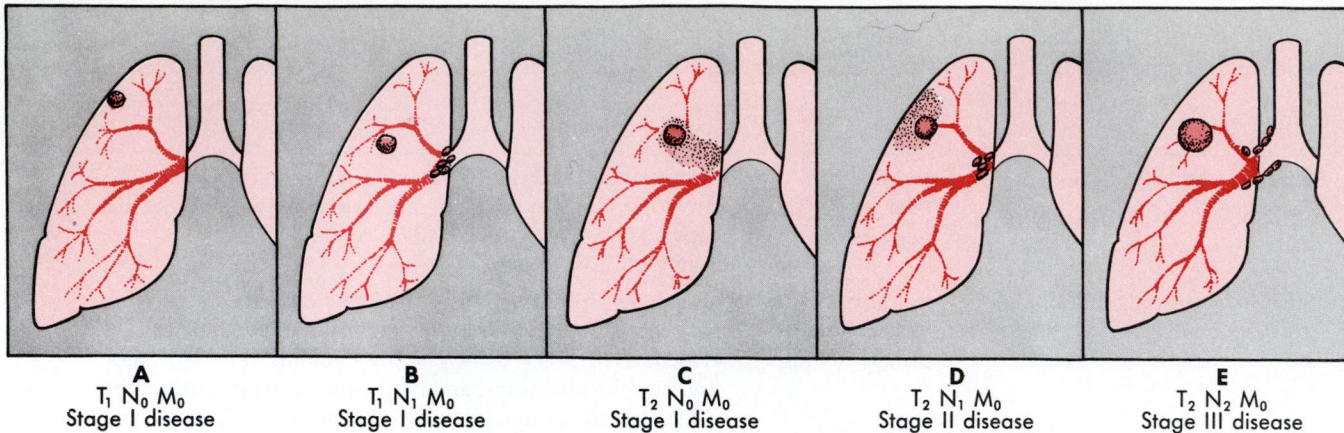

A
$T_1\ N_0\ M_0$
Stage I disease

B
$T_1\ N_1\ M_0$
Stage I disease

C
$T_2\ N_0\ M_0$
Stage I disease

D
$T_2\ N_1\ M_0$
Stage II disease

E
$T_2\ N_2\ M_0$
Stage III disease

FIG. 30-23. Staging of lung cancer by the TNM classification system. **A and B,** Stage I disease includes tumors classified at T_1, with or without matastasis to the lumph nodes in the ipsilateral hilar region. **C,** also included in Stage I are tumors classified as T_2, but having no nodal or distant metastases. **D,** Stage II disease includes those tumors classified as T_2, with metastasis only to the ipsilateral hilar lymph nodes. **E,** Stage III includes all tumors more extensive than T_2, or any tumor with metastasis to the lymph nodes in the mediastinum or with distant metastasis.

graphs. These tumors are slow-growing cancers, so that 50% of individuals with bronchial carcinoid tumors are asymptomatic. Local surgical resection is curative if metastasis has not occurred.

Salivary gland tumors comprise only about 10% of bronchial adenomas. There are three subgroups: adenocystic carcinoma, or culindroma; mucoepidermoid adenoma; and the extremely rare pleomorphic-type adenoma. Cylindromas predominately arise in the trachea or large airways. The tumor is highly malignant, as it metastasizes early, although distal pulmonary metastases are usually slow-growing. Thus it is not unusual for a patient to survive 10 to 15 years after diagnosis.

Mesotheliomas

Mesotheliomas, are benign or malignant sarcomas arising from the epithelium covering the serous membranes, most importantly from the pleura and peritoneum. Benign pleural mesotheliomas have a slow clinical onset and are usually asymptomatic but over a period of years can cause dyspnea. These tumors can grow to be very large and fill the entire pleural cavity. Mesotheliomas are more likely to be malignant than benign.

Recently of more concern is the reported excess incidence of malignant mesotheliomas in asbestos workers. Conflicting data exist about the incidence of asbestos-induced mesotheoliomas (Doll & Peto, 1981; Selikoff, Lilis, & Nicholson, 1979). These data have mostly been generated from populations exposed to asbestos in the workplace during the 1940s. A long latent interval between exposure to asbestos and appearance of mesothelioma occurs; onset of symptoms may take 20 to 30

years. Asbestos-induced mesotheliomas arise largely from the pleura, although a considerable number involve the peritoneum.

Staging of Lung Cancer

The histologic cell type and the stage of the disease are the major factors that influence choice of therapy for patients. The current accepted system for the staging of lung cancer is the **TNM classification,** (Table 30-6). This system is a code in which T denotes the extent of the primary tumor, N indicates the nodal involvement, and M describes the extent of metastasis. Staging of lung cancer is illustrated in Fig. 30-23.

SUMMARY REVIEW

Clinical Manifestations of Pulmonary Alterations

1 Dyspnea is the feeling of breathlessness that tends to occur if minute volume is close to breathing reserve and work of breathing.
2 Abnormal breathing patterns are adjustments made by the body to minimize the work of respiratory muscles, they include Kussmaul, obstructed, restricted, gasping, and Cheyne-Stokes respirations, and sighing.
3 Hypoventilation is decreased alveolar ventilation caused by airway obstruction, chest wall restriction, or altered neurologic control of breathing. Hypoventilation causes increased Pa_{CO_2}.
4 Hyperventilation is increased alveolar ventilation produced by anxiety, head injury, or severe hypoxemia. Hyperventilation causes decreased Pa_{CO_2}.

5 Coughing is a protective reflex that expels secretions and irritants from the lower airways.

6 Hemoptysis is expectoration of bloody mucus, which can be caused by bronchitis, tuberculosis, abscess, neoplasms, and other conditions that cause hemorrhage from damaged vessels.

7 Cyanosis is a bluish discoloration of the skin caused by desaturation of hemoglobin, polycythemia, or peripheral vasoconstriction.

8 Chest pain can result from inflamed pleurae, trachea, bronchi, or respiratory muscles.

9 Clubbing of the fingertips is associated with diseases that interfere with oxygenation of the tissues.

10 Hypoxemia is a reduced Pao_2 caused by (a) decreased oxygen content of inspired gas, (b) hypoventilation, (c) diffusion abnormality, (d) ventilation-perfusion mismatch, or (e) shunting.

11 Pulmonary edema is excess water in the lung caused by disturbances of capillary hydrostatic pressure, capillary oncotic pressure, or capillary permeability. A common cause is left heart failure that increases the hydrostatic pressure in the pulmonary circulation.

12 Atelectasis is the collapse of alveoli resulting from compression of lung tissue or absorption of gas from obstructed alveoli.

13 Bronchiectasis is abnormal dilatation of the bronchi secondary to another pulmonary disorder, usually infection or inflammation.

14 Pneumothorax is the accumulation of air in the pleural space. It can be caused by spontaneous rupture of weakened areas of a pleura or secondary to pleural damage caused by disease, trauma, or mechanical ventilation.

15 Pleural effusion is the accumulation of fluid in the pleural space, usually resulting from disorders that promote transudation or exudation from capillaries underlying the pleura, but occasionally from blockage or injury that causes lymphatic vessels to drain into the pleural space.

16 Empyema is the presence of pus in the pleural space (infected pleural effusion). The source of the pus is usually lymphatic drainage from sites of bacterial pneumonia.

17 Pleurisy is inflammation of the pleura.

18 Pulmonary fibrosis is an excessive amount of connective tissue in the lung. It diminishes lung compliance and may be idiopathic or disease caused.

19 Chest wall compliance is diminished by obesity and kyphoscoliosis, which compress the lungs, and by neuromuscular diseases that impair chest wall muscle function.

20 Flail chest results from rib or sternal fractures that disrupt the mechanics of breathing.

21 Inhalation of noxious gases or prolonged exposure to high concentrations of oxygen can damage the bronchial mucosa or alveolocapillary membrane and cause inflammation or acute respiratory failure.

22 Pneumoconiosis, which is caused by inhalation of dust particles in the workplace, can cause pulmonary fibrosis, susceptibility to lower airway infection, and tumor formation.

23 Allergic alveolitis is an allergic or hypersensitivity reaction to many allergens.

24 Bronchiolitis is the inflammatory obstruction of small airways. It is most common in children.

Pulmonary Disorders

1 Acute respiratory failure is caused by inadequate gas exchange or ventilation ($PaoO_2$ equal to or less than 50 mm Hg or Pao_2 equal to or greater than 50 mm Hg and pH equal to or less than 7.25).

2 Adult respiratory distress syndrome (ARDS) results from an acute, diffuse injury to the alveolocapillary membrane and decreased surfactant production, which increases membrane permeability, causes edema, and atelectasis.

3 Postoperative respiratory failure is most common in surgical patients who smoke or have chronic disease.

4 Obstructive pulmonary disease is characterized by airway obstruction that causes difficult expiration. Obstructive disease can be acute or chronic in nature and includes asthma, chronic bronchitis, and emphysema.

5 In asthma obstruction is caused by episodic attacks of bronchospasm, bronchial inflammation, mucosal edema, and increased mucus production.

6 Extrinsic asthma is caused by an immune response to allergens or other irritants and may be a type I (classic) or type II (delayed) hypersensitivity reaction.

7 Intrinsic asthma is not caused by allergens and occurs in adults over 35.

8 A local imbalance between the parasypathetic and sympathetic divisions of the autonomic nervous system is thought to facilitate bronchospasm in individuals with asthma.

9 Chronic bronchitis causes airway obstruction resulting from bronchial smooth muscle hypertrophy and production of thick, tenacious mucus.

10 In emphysema destruction of the alveolar septa and loss of passive elastic recoil lead to airway collapse and obstruct gas flow during expiration.

11 Emphysema, in which septal deterioration is caused by α_{-1}-antitrypsin deficiency or old age, tends to be panacinar.

12 Emphysema, in which septal deterioration results from smoking, tends to be centriacinar.

13 Chronic obstructive pulmonary disease (COPD) is the coexistence of chronic bronchitis and emphysema.

14 Upper respiratory tract infections, which are the most common cause of short-term disability in the United States, include rhinitis (the common cold), pharyngitis, and laryngitis.

15 Serious lower respiratory tract infections, which occur most frequently in the very old and individuals with impaired immunity or underlying disease, include pneumonia and tuberculosis.

16 Pneumococcal pneumonia is an acute lung infection resulting in an inflammatory response with four phases:

(a) consolidation, (b) red hepatization, (c) gray hepatization, and (d) resolution.

17 Viral pneumonia is an acute, self-limiting lung infection usually caused by the influenza virus.

18 Tuberculosis is a lung infection caused by *Myobacterium tuberculosis,* (tubercle bacillus).

19 In tuberculosis the inflammatory response proceeds to isolate colonies of bacilli by enclosing them in tubercles and surrounding the tubercles with scar tissue.

20 Bacilli may remain dormant within the tubercles for life or, if the immune system breaks down, cause recurrence of active disease.

21 Pulmonary vascular diseases are caused by embolism or hypertension in the pulmonary circulation.

22 Pulmonary embolism is occlusion of a portion of the pulmonary vascular bed by a thrombus (most common), tissue fragment, or air bubble. Depending on its size and location, the embolus can cause hypoxic vasoconstriction, pulmonary edema, atelectasis, pulmonary hypertension, shock, and even death.

23 Pulmonary hypertension (pulmonary artery pressure 5 to 10 mm Hg above normal) is caused by (a) elevated left ventricular pressure, (b) increased blood flow through the pulmonary circulation, (c) obliteration or obstruction of the vascular bed, or (d) active constriction of the vascular bed produced by hypoxemia or acidosis.

24 Cor pulmonale is right ventricular enlargment caused by chronic pulmonary hypertension. Cor pulmonale progresses to right ventricular failure if the pulmonary hypertension is not reversed.

25 Lip cancer is most common in men and represents about 1% of all cancers. In the most common cell type, squamous cell, metastasis is rare when lesions are diagnosed and treated early.

26 Laryngeal cancer occurs primarily in men and represents 2 to 3% of all cancers. Squamous cell carcinoma of the true vocal cords is most common and presents with a clinical symptom of progressive hoarseness.

27 Lung cancer, the most frequent cause of cancer death in the United States, is commonly caused by cigarette smoking.

28 Cancer cell types include squamous cell carcinoma, small cell (oat cell) carcinoma, adenocarcinoma, large cell carcinoma, bronchial adenoma, and mesothelima. Each type arises in a characteristic site or type of tissue, causes distinctive clinical manifestations, and differs in likelihood of metastasis and prognosis.

KEY TERMS

Abscess, 1064

Absorption atelectasis, 1060

Adenocarcimona, 1088

Adult respiratory distress syndrome (ARDS), 1067

Allergic alveolitis (hypersensitivity pneumonitis; type II extrinsic asthma), 1067

Apnea, 1054

Asbestosis, 1066

Aspiration, 1060

Asthma, 1069

Atelectasis, 1060

Bronchiectasis, 1060

Bronchial adenoma, 1088

Bronchiolitis, 1062

Bronchitis, 1072

Bronchopneumonia, 1078

Bronchospasm, 1069

Cavitation, 1065

Centriacinar (centrilobular) emphysema, 1074

Cheyne-Stokes respirations, 1055

Chronic obstructive pulmonary disease (COPD), 1069

Clubbing, 1056

Coal worker's pneumoconiosis (coal miner's lung), 1066

Compression atelectasis, 1060

Consolidation, 1064

Cor pulmonale, 1082

Cough, 1055

Cyanosis, 1056

Cylindrical bronchiectasis, 1061

Dyspnea, 1054

Emphysema, 1074

Empyema (infected pleural effusion), 1064

Extrinsic asthma, 1069

Exudative effusion, 1063

Flail chest, 1065

Hemoptysis, 1055

Hypercapnea, 1055

Hyperventilation, 1055

Hypocapnea, 1055

Hypoventilation, 1055

Hypoxemia, 1057

Hypoxia, 1057

Intrinsic asthma, 1069

Kussmaul respiration (hyperypnea), 1055

Large cell carcinoma (large cell anaplastic cancer), 1088

Lobar pneumonia, 1078

Mesothelioma, 1090

Oat cell carcinoma, 1087

Open pneumothorax (communicating pneumothorax), 1062

Orthopnea (positional dyspnea), 1054

Panacinar (panlobular) emphysema, 1074

Physiologic dead space, 1058

Pleural effusion, 1063

Pleurisy (pleuritis), 1064

Pneumoconiosis, 1066

Pneumonia, 1076

Pneumothorax, 1062

Pulmonary edema, 1058

Pulmonary embolism, 1080

Pulmonary fibrosis, 1065

Pulmonary hypertension, 1082

Pulmonary thromboembolism, 1080

Saccular bronchiectasis, 1061

Silicosis, 1066

Small cell carcimona, 1087

Squamous cell carcinoma, 1087

Status asthmaticus, 1071

Tachypnea, 1054

Tension pneumothorax, 1062

TNM classification, 1090

Transudative effusion, 1063

Tuberculosis, 1079

Varicose bronchiectasis, 1061

REFERENCES

Addington, W. W. (1979). Patient compliance: The most serious remaining problem in control of tuberculosis in the United States. *Chest* (Suppl.), *76*,(6), 741-743.

Alexander, J. C., Jr., & Wolfe, W. G. (1980, August). Lung abscess and emphysema of the thorax. *Surgical Clinics of North America, 60*,(4), 835-850.

American Cancer Society. (1989). Cancer statistics 1989. *Ca-A Cancer Journal for Clinicians, 39*,(1).

American Thoracic Society (ATS). (1981). Diagnostic standards and classification of tuberculosis and other myocobacterial diseases (14th ed.). *American Review of Respiratory Diseases, 123*, 343.

Anderson, R. W., & Arentzen, C. E. (1980, August). Carcinoma of the lung. *Surgical Clinics of North America, 60*,(4), 793-814.

Anderson, S. D., Silverman, H., Konig, P., & Godfrey, S. (1975). Exercise induced asthma. *British Journal of Diseases of the Chest, 69*,(1), 1-39.

Ayers, S. M. (1982). Mechanisms and consequences of pulmonary edema: Cardiac lung, shock lung, and principles of ventilatory therapy in adult respiratory distress syndrome. *American Heart Journal, 103*,(1), 97-112.

Barlow, P. B. (1976, September). Treatment of tuberculosis. *Basics of Respiratory Disease, 5*,(1), 1-6.

Becklacke, M. (1976). State-of-the-art: Asbestos related diseases of the lung and other organs: Their epidemiology and implications for clinical practice. *American Review of Respiratory Diseases, 114*, 187-227.

Bell, W. R., & Simon, T. L. (1982, February). Current status of pulmonary thromboembolic disease: Pathophysiology, diagnosis, prevention, and treatment. *American Heart Journal, 103*,(2), 239-262.

Bolman, R. M., & Wolfe, W. G. (1980, August). Bronchiectasis and bronchopulmonary sequestration. *Surgical Clinics of North America, 60*,(4), 867-881.

Bradley, R. B. (1987). Adult respiratory distress syndrome. *Focus on Critical Care, 14*,(5), 48-59.

Brandstetter, R. D. (1986). The adult respiratory distress syndrome-1986. *Heart & Lung, 15*,(2), 155-164.

Braun, S. R., doPico, G. A., Tsiatis, A., Horvaln, E., & Dickie, H. A. (1979). Farmer's lung disease: Long term clinical and physiologic outcome. *American Review of Respiratory Disease, 119*, 185-191.

Brigham, K. L., & Newman, J. H. (1979). The pulmonary circulation. *Basics of Respiratory Disease, 8*,(1), 1-6.

Burrows, B., Martinez, F. D., Halonen, M., Barbee, R. A., & Cline, M. G. (1989, February). Association of asthma with serum IgE levels and skin-test reactivity to allergens. *New England Journal of Medicine, 310*,(5), 271-277.

Carr, D. T. (1977, May). Bronchogenic carcinoma. *Basics of Respiratory Disease, 5*,(5), 1-6.

Cerrina, J., Denjean, A. Alexandre, G., Lockhart, A., & Puroux, P. (1981). Inhibition of exercise-induced asthma by a calcium antagonist, nifedipine. *American Review of Respiratory Diseases, 123*, 156-160.

Cherniack, R., & Cherniack, L. (1983). *Respiration in health and disease,* (3d ed.). Philadelphia: W. B. Saunders.

Colice, G. L. (1986). Pulmonary edema. *Clinical Geriatric Medicine, 2*,(2), 411-432.

Crapo, R. O. (1981, October). Smoke inhalation injuries. *Journal of the American Medical Association, 246*,(15), 1694-1698.

Crockcroft, D., & Dosman, J. (1981, September). Respiratory health risks in farmers. *Annals of Internal Medicine, 95*,(3), 380-382.

Dannenberg, A. M., Jr. (1982, March). Pathogenesis of pulmonary tuberculosis. *American Review of Respiratory Diseases,* Koch Centennial Supplement, *125*,(3), 25-29.

del Regato, J. A., Spjut, H. J., & Cox, J. D. (1985). *Ackerman and del Regato's Cancer* (6th ed.) St. Louis: C. V. Mosby.

Deneke, S. M., & Fanburg, B. L. (1980, July). Normobaric oxygen toxicity of the lung. *New England Journal of Medicine, 303*,(2), 76-86.

Doll, R., & Peto, R. (1981). *The causes of cancer: Qualitative estimates of avoidable risks of cancer in the U.S. today,*. New York: Oxford University Press.

Edelson, J. D., & Rebuck, A. S. (1985, February). The clinical assessment of severe asthma. *Archives of Internal Medicine, 145*,(2), 321-323.

Elliot, C. G., Miehock, R. J., Brown, R., & Ottesen, O. E. (1982, February/March). Heparin requirements in pulmonary embolism and venous thrombosis: A prospective study. *Journal of Clinical Pharmacology, 22*,(1,2), 102-109.

Fishman, A. P. (1976). Chronic cor pulmonale. *American Review of Respiratory Diseases,* (vol. 2) *114*, 775-794.

Fishman, A. P. (1979). *Pulmonary diseases and disorders,* (2nd vol.). New York: McGraw-Hill.

Fishman, A. P. (1982). *Pulmonary disease and disorders: Update 1,*. New York: McGraw-Hill.

Fuster, V., Guiliani, E. R., Brandenburg, R. O., Weidman,

W. H., & Edwards, W. D. (1981). The natural history of ideopathic pulmonary hypertension. *American Journal of Cardiology, 47,* 422. (Abstract)

Gazdar, A. F. & Linnoila, R. I. (1988). The pathology of lung cancer; changing concepts and newer diagnostic techniques. *Seminars in Oncology, 15,*(3), 215-225.

George, W. L., & Finegold, S. M. (1982, April). Bacterial infections of the lung. *Chest, 81,*(4), 502-507.

Glassroth, J., Robins, A. G., & Snider D. E. (1980, June). Tuberculosis in the 1980s. *New England Journal of Medicine, 302,*(26), 1441-1450.

Gold, W. M. (1976). Asthma. *Basics of RD Books, 4,*(3), 1-6.

Gosink, B., Friedman, P. J., & Liebew, A. (1973, April). Bronchiolitis obliterans. *American Journal of Roentgenology, 177,*(4), 816-832.

Guenter, C. A., & Welch, M. H. (Eds.). (1982). *Pulmonary medicine,* (2d ed.). Philadelphia: J. B. Lippincott.

Hartman, R. B. (1979). Pulmonary heart disease. *Postgraduate Medicine, 66,*(3), 58.

Heim, C. R. & Des Prez, R. M. (1986). Pulmonary embolism: A review. *Advances in Internal Medicine, 31,* 187-212.

Hirsh, J. (1987). Treatment of pulmonary embolism. *Annual Review of Medicine, 38,* 91-105.

Hodgkin, J. E., Balchum O. J., Kass, I., Glaser, E. M., Miller, W. F., Haas, A., Shaw, D. B., Kimbel, P., & Petty, T. L. (1975, June). Chronic obstructive airway diseases. *Journal of the American Medical Association, 232,*(12), 1243-1260.

Hogg, J. C. (1981). Bronchial mucosal premeability and its relationship to airway hyperactivity. *Journal of Allergy and Clinical Immunology, 67*(6), 421-425.

Holbrook, J. (1983). Cigarette smoking. In W. N. Rom (Ed.), *Environmental and occupational medicine,* (p. 788). Boston: Little, Brown.

Hopewell, P. C. (1972, March). Adult respiratory distress syndrome. *Basics of Respiratory Disease, 7*(4), 1-6.

Hultgren, H. N. (1970). High altitude pulmonary edema. *Advanced Cardiology, 5* 24-31.

Israel, H. L., & Atkinson, G. W. (1978, September). Sarcoidosis. *Basics of Respiratory Disease, 7*(1), 1-6.

Janus, E. D., Philipps, N. T., & Carrell, R. N. (1985). Smoking, lung function, and alpha-1-antitrypsin deficiency. *Lancet, 1*(8421), 152.

Jeff, J. R., Cortese, D. A., & Fontana, R. S. (1983). Lung cancer: Current concepts and prospects. *CA-A Cancer Journal for Clinicians, 33,* 74-86.

Johanson, W. G., Jr., & Harris, G. D. (1980, May). Aspiration pneumonia, anerobic infections, and lung abscess. *Medical Clinics of North America, 64*(3), 385-394.

Kanemoto, N., & Sasamoto, H. (1979, July). Pulmonary hemodynamics in primary pulmonary hypertension. *Japanese Heart Journal, 20*(4), 395-405.

Karnad, A., Alvarez, S., & Berk, S. L. (1985). Pneumonia caused by gram-negative bacilli. *American Journal of Medicine, 79*(1A), 61.

Kissane, J. M., (Ed.). (1985). *Anderson's Pathology,* (8th ed.). St. Louis: C. V. Mosby.

Leff, A. (1982, February). Pathogenesis of asthma. *Chest, 81*(2), 224-229.

Mariencheck, W. I. (1979). Continuing treatment of respiratory insufficiency. *Advances in Internal Medicine, 24* 359-384.

Matthay, R. A., & Balmes, J. R. (1982, February). Lung cancer: A persistent challenge. *Geriatrics, 37*(2), 109-131.

Matthews, M. J., & Linnoila, R. I. (1988). Pathology of lung cancer. An update. In J. D. Britan, H. M. Golomb, A. G. Little (Eds.), *Lung cancer: A comprehensive treatise,*. New York: Grune & Stratton.

McFadden, E. R., Jr. (1987). Exercise-induced asthma. Assessment of current etiologic concepts. *Chest,* (Suppl.), *91,* 1515-1575.

McKellar, P. P. (1985). Treatment of community acquired pneumonias. *American Journal of Medicine,* (Suppl.), *79*(2A), 25-31.

Michaelson, E. D. (1978, July-August). Oxygen therapy and delivery in obstructive pulmonary disease. *Heart & Lung, 7*(4), 627-634.

Middleton, E., Jr., Atkins, F. M., Fanning, M., & Georgitis, J. W. (1981, September). Cellular mechanisms in the pathogenesis and pathophysiology of asthma. *Medical Clinics of North America, 65*(5), 1013-1031.

Miller, W. C. (1981, October). Acute respiratory failure. *American Family Physician, 24*(4), 176-182.

Morgan, W. K. C. (1980, August). International conference on occupational diseases. *Chest,* (Suppl.), *78*(2), 359-414.

Morgan, W. K. C., Lapp, L., & Seaton, D. (1980). Respiratory disability in coal miners. *Journal of the American Medical Association, 243*(23), 2401-2404.

Morse, J. O. (1978). Alpha-antitrypsin deficiency. *New England Journal of Medicine, 299*(19), 1045-1048.

Murray, H. W., & Tuazon, C. (1980, May). Atypical pneumonias. *Medical Clinics of North America, 64*(3), 507-527.

Nadel, J. A. (1977, June). Autonomic control of airway smooth muscle and airway secretions. *American Review of Respiratory Diseases, 115*(6), 117-126.

National Heart, Lung, and Blood Institute (NHLBI), Division of Lung Diseases. (1979). *Extracorporeal support for respiratory insufficiency,*. Bethesda, Md.: National Institues of Health.

Osbern, L. N., & Crapo, R. O. (1981). Dung lung: A report of toxic exposure to liquid manure. *Annals of Internal Medicine, 95*(3), 312-314.

Phipps, W., Long, B., & Woods, N. (1987). *Medical-surgical nursing* (3rd ed.). St. Louis: C. V. Mosby.

Pigneaux, J., Richard, P. M., & LaGarde, C. (1979). The place of interstitial therapy using 192 iridium in the managent of carcinoma of the lip. *Cancer, 43,* 1073-1077.

Pohlson, E. C., McNamara, J. J., Char, C., Kurata, L. (1985, July). Lung abscess: A changing pattern of the disease. *American Journal of Surgery, 150*(1), 97.

Pontoppidan, H., Geffin G., & Lowen, S. E. (1972). Acute respiratory failure in the adult. *New England Journal of Medicine, 287*(15), 743-752.

Pontoppidan, H., Geffin, B., & Lowen, S. E. (1972). Acute respiratory failure in the adult. *New England Journal of Medicine, 287*(14), 690-698.

Reichman, R. C., & Dolin, R. (1980, May), Viral pneumonias. *Medical Clinics of North America, 64*(3), 491-506.

Reyes, M. P. (1980, May). The aerobic gram negative bacillary pneumonias. *Medical Clinics of North America, 64*(3), 363-383.

Rinaldo, J. E., & Rogers, R. M. (1982, April). Adult respiratory distress syndrome: Changing concepts of injury and repair. *New England Journal of Medicine, 306*(15), 900-909.

Roberts, R. C., & Moore, V. C. (1977, December). Immunopathogenesis of hypersensitivity pneumonitis. *American Review of Respiratory Disease, 116*(6), 1075-1090.

Rogers, R. M. K., & Juers, J. A. (1975). Physiologic considerations in the treatment of acute respiratory failure. *Basics of Respiratory Disease, 3*(4), 1-6.

Rom, W. K. N., Rom, N. W., Kanner, R. E., Renzetti, A. D., Shigeoka, J. W., Barkman, H. W., Nicols, M., Turner, W. A., Coleman, M., & Wright, W. E. (1981). Respiratory distress in Utah coal miners. *American Review of Respiratory Disease, 123,*(1), 372-377.

Rosai, J. (1981). *Ackerman's surgical pathology* (6th ed.). St. Louis: C. V. Mosby.

Roussos, C., & Macklem, P. T. (1982, September). The respiratory muscles. *New England Journal of Medicine, 307,*(13), 786-797.

Saccomanno, G., Archer, V. E., Auerbach, O., Kuschner, M., Saunders, R. P., & Klein, M. P. (1971). Histologic types of lung cancer among uranium miners. *Cancer, 27,* 515-523.

Sbarburo, J. A. (1980, May). Tuberculosis. *Medical Clinics of North America, 64,*(3), 417-431.

Seidel, H. M., Ball, J. W., Dains, J. E., & Benedict, G. W. (1987). *Physical examination.* St. Louis: C. V. Mosby.

Selikoff, I. J., Lilis, R., & Nicholson, W. J. (1979). Asbestos disease in United States shipyards. *Annual New York Academy of Science, 330,* 295-311.

Sheller, J. R. (1987). Asthma: Emerging concepts and potential therapies. *American Journal of Medical Science, 293,*(5), 298-308.

Smith, S. B. (1985, June). Exercise-induced asthma. *Postgraduate Medicine, 77,*(8), 42-50.

Smoking and Health. (1979). A report of the surgeon general. Rockville, Md.: U.S. Department of Health, Education, and Welfare (DHEW).

Snider, G. L. (1981, September). Pulmonary perspective: A pathogenesis of emphysema—twenty years of progress. *American Review of Respiratory Disease, 124,*(3), 321-324.

Snider, G. L., Kleinerman, J., Thurlbeck, W. M., & Bengali, Z. H. (1985). The definition of emphysema. Report of a national heart, lung, blood institute, division of lung diseases workshop. *American Review of Respiratory Diseases, 132,*(1), 182.

Stead, W. W., & Dutt, A. K. (1981, July). What's new in tuberculosis. *American Journal of Medicine, 71,* 1-4.

Stead, W. W., & Dutt, A. K. (1982, March). Chemotherapy for tuberculosis today. *American Review of Respiratory Disease, 125,*(3), 94-101.

Stokley, R. A. (1987). Alpha-1-antitrypsin and the pathogenesis of emphysema. *Lung, 165,*(2), 61-77.

Stratton, C. W. (1986). Bacterial pneumonias—an overview with emphasis on pathogenesis, diagnosis, and treatment. *Heart & Lung, 15,*(3), 226-244.

Tuazon, C. U. (1980, May). Gram-positive pneumonias. *Medical Clinics of North America, 64,*(3), 343-361.

Wagenvoort, C. A., & Wagenvoort, N. (1970, December). Primary pulmonary hypertension: A pathologic study of the lung vessels in 156 clinically diagnoses cases. *Circulation, 42,* 1163-1184.

Weisman, I. M., Rinaldo, J. E., & Rogers, R. M. (1982, November). Positive end-expiratory pressure in acute respiratory failure. *New England Journal of Medicine, 307,*(22), 1381-1384.

Weiss, E. B., & Faling, L. J. (1968, October). Clinical significance of $Paco_2$, during status asthma: The cross-over point. *Annals of Allergy, 26,*(10), 545-551.

West, J. B. (1985). *Pulmonary pathophysiology: The essentials,* (3d ed.). Baltimore, Md.: Williams & Wilkins.

Woolf, C. R., & Zamel, N. (1980, November). The respiratory effects of regular cigarette smoking on women. *Chest, 78,*(5), 707-713.

Ziskind, M., Jones, M., & Weill, H. (1975). State-of-the-art: Silicosis. *American Review of Respiratory Disease, 113*(5), 643-645.

CHAPTER 31

Alterations of Pulmonary Function in Children

Margaret M. Andrews

Structure and function of the pulmonary system in children, 1096
Pulmonary disorders, 1098
  Disorders of the upper airways, 1098
    Croup syndrome, 1098
      Pathophysiology, 1099
      Clinical manifestations, 1099
      Evaluation and treatment, 1099
    Types of croup,1100
      Acute epiglottitis, 1100
      Viral croup and acute laryngotracheobronchitis, 1100
    Sudden infant death syndrome (SIDS), 1100
  Disorders of the lower airways, 1101
    Asthma, 1101
      Pathophysiology, 1101
      Clinical manifestations, 1101
      Evaluation and treatment, 1101
    Infection, 1102
      Pneumonia, 1102
      Bronchitis, 1103
      Bronchiolitis, 1103
      Pathophysiology, 1103
        Clinical manifestations, 1103
        Evaluation and treatment, 1103
      Bronchiolitis obliterans, 1103
    Respiratory distress syndrome of the newborn, 1104
      Pathophysiology, 1104
      Clinical manifestations, 1106
      Evaluation and treatment, 1106
    Bronchopulmonary dysplasia, 1106
    Cystic fibrosis, 1106
      Pathophysiology, 1107
      Clinical manifestations, 1107
      Evaluation and treatment, 1107

STRUCTURE AND FUNCTION OF THE PULMONARY SYSTEM IN CHILDREN

There are a number of structural differences between mature and immature upper airways and lungs that influence the way in which children respond to respiratory disturbances. Children are less well equipped than adults to overcome pulmonary infections. Their airways are shorter and narrower from the trachea through the terminal bronchioles, so that a relatively small amount of mucus or mucosal edema can cause obstruction. The trachea bifurcates higher in infants than in adults (Fig. 31-1), the accessory muscles of respiration are not fully

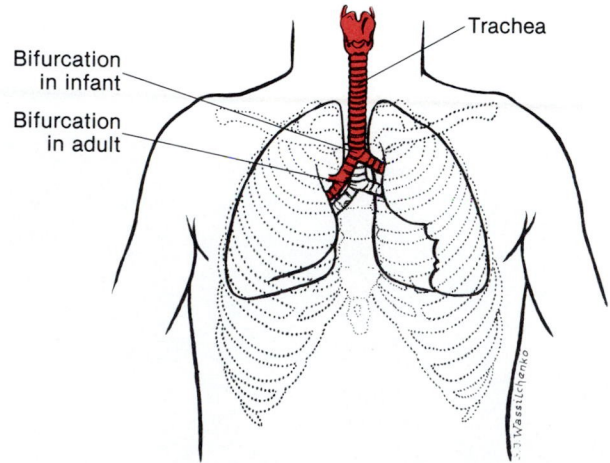

FIG. 31-1. Level of bifurcation of the trachea in infants and adults. (From Whaley & Wong, 1987.)

1096

developed in infants, and respiratory and coughing efforts are not as effective or sustained. The upper airway is narrow, and its caliber may be reduced further by hypertrophied tonsils and adenoids, or by posterior displacement of the tongue, which diminishes air flow.

All the conducting airways are present at birth and change only in size through adulthood. During the first 5 years of life, the respiratory tract grows longer, but the lumen remains narrow. Only after age 5 does lumen caliber increase. Infants do not have as many alveoli as older children and adults. There are only about 25 million alveoli at birth and they are less complex than alveoli in an adult. The lack of development and the reduced number of pores of Kuhn make collateral ventilation of alveoli less efficient than in adults. Until age 8,

alveoli and their vascular supply multiply until there are several hundred million (approximately 300,000,000). The alveoli then increase in size and complexity through puberty.

Surfactant production is thought to begin during the twenty-fourth week of gestation. Production continues to increase through term (fortieth week of gestation). At term, surfactant production is comparable to that of an adult and remains so throughout life. If an infant is born prematurely, however, surfactant production is frequently inadequate to maintain normal alveolar surface tension. Without surfactant, the alveoli do not inflate sufficiently. This leads to alveolar edema and collapse, resulting in respiratory distress syndrome of the newborn, or hyaline membrane disease (see p. 1104).

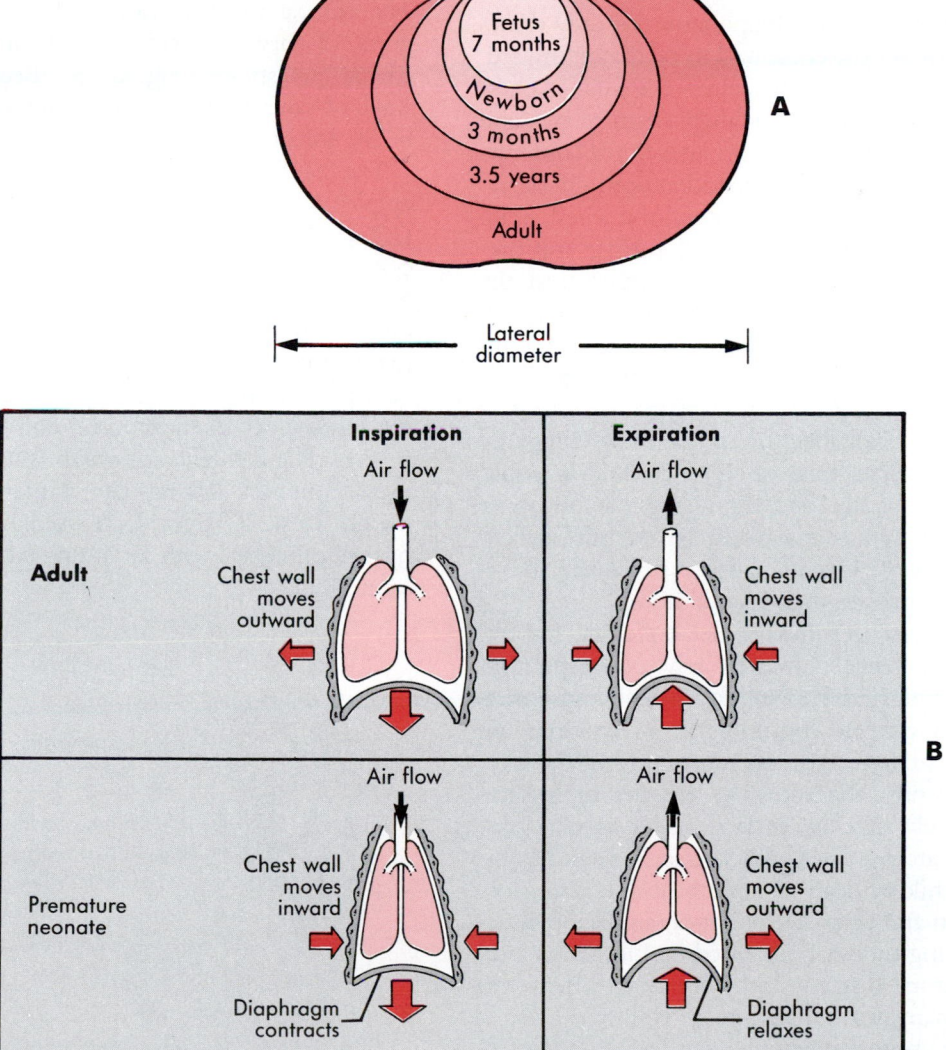

FIG. 31-2. **A**, Changes in chest wall shape and lung mechanics with age. **B**, Differences in lung mechanics due to differences in chest wall compliance (degree of rigidity) in premature neonates and adults. (Arrows indicate direction of airflow, chest wall movement, and diaphragm movement.)

At birth the chest wall is soft and compliant. Chest wall compliance decreases with bone and muscle development throughout childhood until adult compliance is approached at puberty. Compliance increases to adult values by around age 20.

The thoracic cage (chest wall) is less rigid in childhood as well and its contents are more easily displaced by the abdominal organs. This reduces its efficiency in assisting or preserving ventilation. Fig. 31-2 shows developmental differences in chest wall shape and rigidity.

Lung mechanics, or the interaction and equilibrium between compliance and elastic recoil, differ in adults and infants, as can be seen in Fig. 31-2, *B*. (Lung mechanics are described in Chapter 29.) The adult's wider and more rigid chest wall expands during inspiration because the vacuum created by downward movement of the diaphragm draws air inward. In the preterm infant, the chest wall is so flexible that the vacuum created by downward movement of the diaphragm not only draws in air, but also causes the chest wall to be drawn inward. Expiration relieves the force that drew the infant's chest wall inward, and it expands. The diaphragm relaxes and is pushed upward by pressure from abdominal contents. In adults, an equilibrium is reached between elastic recoil of the lungs and compliance of the chest wall, which keeps the lungs from collapsing further and prevents the relaxed diaphragm from pushing against the lungs. At the end of expiration, the adult's residual volume is 50% greater than the residual volume of the infant. (Lung volumes and capacities are defined in Chapter 29.)

The infant's tracheobronchial cartilaginous rings are also more flexible than those of an older child or adult. The rings collapse easily, and the lumina of the upper airways are not sufficiently wide to permit airflow around obstructions. Overall, airway resistance in infancy is 15 times greater than in adulthood.

Physiologic differences involve metabolic rate and immunologic competence. Children rely on respiratory function to a greater extent than do adults because metabolic rate and oxygen consumption in children are much higher. Children have less muscle glycogen in reserve. Consequently, the accessory muscles of inspiration tire relatively quickly, as lactic acidosis develops. The proportionately greater body surface area and respiratory rate of children lead to rapid heat and water loss during infection and fever. Dehydration and acidosis occur rapidly during times of decreased oral intake as a result of respiratory distress and vomiting, which frequently accompany acute infections in children.

Children are more susceptible than adults to infections of the respiratory tract because their immune systems are immature, they have not had time to develop immunity to most microorganisms, and they are frequently exposed to respiratory tract infections through contact with other children with similar immunologic incompetence. (The development of immunity is discussed in Chapter 6). The physiology of children and adults is otherwise the same. Within a few hours of birth, the infant achieves normal arterial pH, P_{CO_2}, and P_{O_2}. Gas exchange and chemoreceptor activity is not affected by immaturity of the respiratory system.

PULMONARY DISORDERS

Disorders of the Upper Airways

Croup Syndrome

Croup is a syndrome of clinical manifestations caused by infection of the upper airways. Croup is characterized by inspiratory stridor, hoarseness, and a resonant cough described as "barking," "brassy," or "croupy." The clinical manifestations are caused by varying degrees of laryngeal obstruction due to inflammatory edema and spasm (Fig. 31-3). Because the upper airways of young children are easily occluded, croup can be life threatening.

The conditions frequently referred to as croup include **epiglottitis, laryngitis,** and **laryngotracheobronchitis (LTB).** The actual incidence of these disorders is difficult to determine, but they comprise a significant number of respiratory illnesses in young children. In 85% of cases, croup is caused by a virus and affects children between 3 months and 5 years of age. Croup caused by bacteria (*Haemophilus influenzae* and *Corynebacterium diphtheriae*) occurs more rarely and in children aged 3 to 7 years. The incidence of croup is higher in males and is most common during the winter months. Approximately 15% of affected children have a strong family history of croup, with laryngitis tending to recur in the same child.

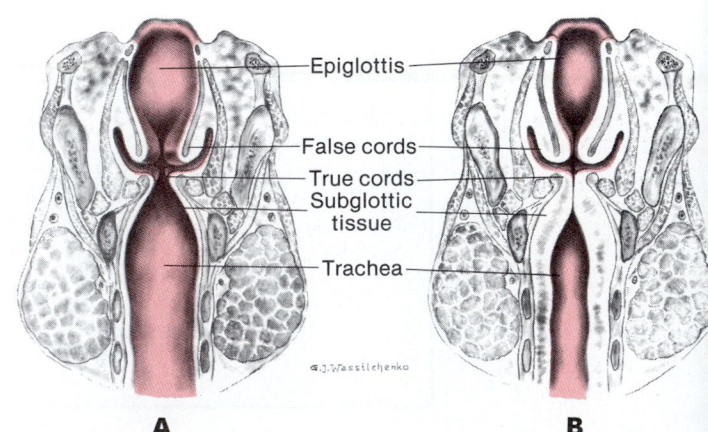

FIG. 31-3. **A,** Normal larynx. **B,** Narrowing and obstruction from edema of croup. (From Whaley & Wong, 1987.)

Pathophysiology

The anatomic differences between the larynx of the child and of the adult explain why croup is principally a disease of children. Not only are the diameter and surface area of the immature airway relatively smaller, but the mucous membrane is more loosely attached and more vascular. The glottis is small and is rapidly compromised by inflammatory edema and spasm, and the submucosa of the region contains many lymphoid cell aggregates that cause edema and dyspnea if they become inflamed. (Lymphoid tissues are described in Chapters 24 and 26.)

Children with viral croup may have a preceding infection of the upper respiratory passages (e.g., rhinitis or the common cold), which primarily involves the nasal mucosa. After 3 or 4 days, the infection spreads to the larynx, where the true vocal cords and subglottic structures become inflamed and edematous. In addition, spasms of smooth muscle in laryngeal walls contribute to the laryngeal obstruction.

In infections due to *H. influenzae,* the primary site of inflammation is the epiglottis. This is a serious, life-threatening condition, as the inflammatory edema can obstruct the airway. Inflammation may spread above and below the epiglottis to involve the trachea and bronchi. If this occurs, respiratory distress is more severe and the outcome of the disease is less favorable.

In croup caused by *C. diphtheriae,* inflammation and infection of the upper airways, including pharyngitis and rhinitis, precedes laryngeal inflammation. Diptheria causes the mucosa of the larynx to become coated with a fibrous exudate, occluding the airway. Fortunately, immunization against diphtheria has made this serious disease a rare occurrence in the United States today.

Regardless of the causal microorganism, certain endogenous factors are believed to predispose a child to croup. Evidence for this includes (1) the tendency for croup to recur in children who have had one episode and (2) the likelihood that the same virus will cause croup in susceptible children while causing a variety of other, milder illnesses in children who are not susceptible. An anatomically defective or abnormally immature larynx may be a predisposing factor for croup. Hypersensitivity to allergens has also been suggested as an endogenous predisposing factor (Gerbeaux, Couvreur, & Tournier, 1982; Phelan, Landau, & Olinsky, 1982).

Clinical Manifestations

The clinical manifestations of croup are mainly produced by obstruction of the larynx. Soon after the onset of cough and hoarseness, the child exhibits inspiratory stridor, a harsh, high crowing noise that is most distinct during inspiration. Unlike wheezing, inspiratory stridor originates high in the respiratory tract, usually in the trachea or larynx. It indicates obstruction and may be

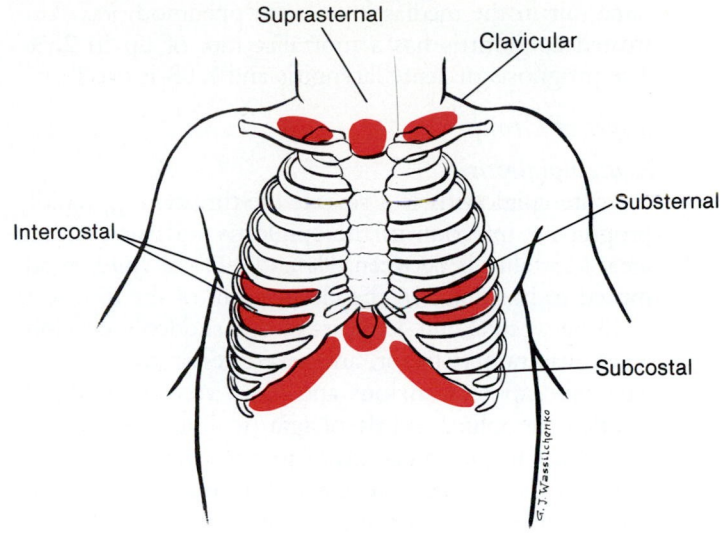

Location of retractions.

FIG. 31-4. Areas of chest muscle retraction.(From Whaley Wong, 1987.)

combined with cough, dyspnea, hoarseness, retractions of the chest wall with respiration, and tachypnea. The degree of nasal flaring, tracheal tugging, and retraction of the chest muscles depends on the degree of airway resistance (Fig. 31-4). The child becomes apprehensive and agitated as dyspnea and airway obstruction worsen. Cyanosis, pallor, weakness, rapid pulse, low tidal volumes, and stridor are all signs of hypoxemia. Death may occur from hypoventilation.

Most cases of croup progress only as far as stridor and slight dyspnea, and the child recovers from the acute crisis in a few hours. Complete recovery from croup often requires 24 to 48 hours.

Evaluation and Treatment

Diagnosis is made on the basis of physical examination and radiologic examination. Treatment for croup consists of (1) restricting the child's activity to avoid aggravating respiratory distress, (2) administering humidifier and oxygen (25% to 30%) to alleviate anxiety and reverse hypoxemia, (3) administering intravenous fluids to ensure adequate hydration, (4) instituting mechanical ventilation (intermittent positive-pressure breathing) with aerosol epinephrine to relieve obstruction, (5) administering antibiotics (if croup is bacterial in origin), and (6) tracheotomy or nasal intubation for laryngeal obstruction.

With the exception of epiglottitis, which is a localized and frequently fatal infection, the likelihood of death increases as the infection extends to involve a greater portion of the respiratory tract. Most deaths from croup are the result of laryngeal obstruction or the complications of tracheotomy, most commonly mediastinal emphysema (air in the mediastinum) and pneumothorax. Untreated epiglotittis has a mortality rate of up to 25%. The prognosis of acute laryngitis and LTB is excellent.

Types of Croup

Acute Epiglottitis

Acute epiglottitis is a severe, life-threatening, rapidly progressive infection of the epiglottis and surrounding area. Mortality is between 8% and 12% of children admitted to hospitals. In the classic form of the disease, a child between 2 and 12 years of age suddenly develops fever, inspiratory stridor, and severe respiratory distress. The child appears anxious and has a voice that sounds muffled. Drooling and dysphagia (inability to swallow) are common. Death can occur in a few hours. Nasotracheal intubation or tracheotomy is mandatory in instances of rapidly increasing obstruction. Examination of the throat may trigger laryngospasm and cause respiratory collapse. Pneumonia, cervical lymph node inflammation, otitis, and, rarely, meningitis or septic arthritis may occur during the course of epiglottitis.

Viral Croup and Acute Laryngotracheobronchitis

Viral croup and acute laryngotracheobronchitis are frequently caused by the same virus. Viral croup usually occurs in children between the ages of 6 months and 3 years. It follows an upper respiratory infection consisting of rhinorrhea, coryza (severe infection, with discharge, of the nasal mucosa), and fever. After 2 to 3 days, the child suddenly develops symptoms of croup, with inspiratory stridor and a harsh, barking cough. Difficulty in breathing makes the child apprehensive and restless. In viral croup, the obstruction is caused by inflammatory swelling of the subglottic tissues with impingement on the airway below the level of the glottis. Spasm of the vocal cords occurs with tracheobronchitis as the inflammatory process extends.

Acute laryngotracheobronchitis (LTB) (sometimes called acute laryngotracheitis) is the most common form of croup. Affected children have frequent recurrences between ages 3 and 6 years, after which airway growth decreases susceptibility. Symptoms characteristically appear worse at night. A considerable number of children with LTB require tracheotomy for the establishment of an adequate airway.

Complications occur in approximately 15% of children with viral croup or LTB. The most common complication is extension of the infection to other regions of the respiratory tract, such as the middle ear, terminal bronchioles, or pulmonary parenchyma.

Sudden Infant Death Syndrome (SIDS)

The greatest single cause of death among infants between 1 week and 1 year of age is **sudden infant death syndrome (SIDS),** also called crib death or cot death.

The syndrome refers to the sudden, unexpected death of any infant or young child in whom a postmortem examination fails to demonstrate a cause for death. The incidence is 2 to 3 per 1000 live births.

The highest incidence of SIDS is between 2 and 4 months of age; it almost always occurs during sleep, with higher frequencies during the winter months. SIDS is the leading cause of postneonatal death and claims 700 to 10,000 lives each year (Beckwith, 1970). Risk factors associated with SIDS include (1) poor, unmarried mothers, less than 20 years of age; (2) low birth weight; (3) preterm delivery; (4) multiple pregnancies; and (5) siblings who died of SIDS (Avery & Taeusch, 1984).

The cause of SIDS is unknown and no single factor is predictive of the sudden death. There is no treatment because the death is sudden and unexplained. Apnea is a common finding in infants with "near miss" SIDS, and these infants have survived with successful resuscitation. The apnea leads to manifestations of asphyxia, including pallor or cyanosis, bradycardia, gasping respiratory efforts, limpness, and unresponsiveness. Home monitoring of respiratory and cardiovascular functions have been successful for infant apnea. Research is continuing to find the cause and prevention of this mysterious syndrome.

SIDS occurs most often between 2 and 4 months of age, with fewer than 1% of deaths occurring during the first 2 months of life, and more than 90% of the deaths occurring within the first 6 months. SIDS is known to occur more frequently in males (60%), in siblings of SIDS victims (2 of 100 live births), in twins of SIDS victims (5 to 10 of 100 live births) (Spitzer & Fox, 1984), and in low birth weight or small for gestational age infants (Shannon & Kelly, 1982). SIDS is reportedly more frequent in families of low socioeconomic status and occurs often during the winter months when upper respiratory infections are most prevalent. SIDS occurs most often during sleep with 50% to 80% of deaths occurring between midnight and 6:00 AM (Aranda et al., 1983; Brooks, Cloutier, & Afshani, 1982; Nuttall, 1986; Shannon & Kelly, 1982).

Despite much medical controversy, evidence substantiates a relationship between SIDS, periodic apneic episodes, and sleep-related disorders, but the etiology remains unclear. In studies of infants who have almost succumbed, five abnormalities have been identified: hypoventilation, depressed ventilatory response to carbon dioxide, prolonged sleep apnea, frequent short apneic episodes, and excessive periodic breathing (Aranda et al., 1983; Ariagno, 1984; Shannon & Kelly, 1982; Nuttall, 1986; Steinschneider, Weinstein, & Diamond, 1982; Ward et al., 1986).

Although the procedure can be burdensome to parents, infants considered at risk are often placed on home apnea monitors during sleep until they are past the age of vulnerability and demonstrate normal lung functioning as evidenced by normal pneumatograms (Nuttall, 1986).

Disorders of the Lower Airways

Lung disease is the single major cause of death in the first year of life, accounting for 46% of deaths. Death is usually caused by lower airway obstruction by foreign bodies, inflammation, mucus, and edema. In addition, the child's poorly supported large airways may collapse during forced expiration, such as in crying, or as a result of disturbance of lung pressures caused by acceleration of expired gas past a partially occluded segment of the large bronchi.

Asthma

Asthma is characterized by mild to severe obstruction of air movement into and out of the lungs (see Chapter 29). Asthma is usually extrinsic or type I and is usually caused by an allergen. It is a leading chronic illness in childhood, affecting 5% to 10% of children to some degree. Prior to puberty, about twice as many boys as girls are affected. After puberty, the incidence of asthma is evenly divided between the sexes. About 80% to 90% of asthmatic children have their first symptoms before 4 or 5 years of age.

Pathophysiology

Edema of the bronchial mucosa, bronchospasm, and mucous plugging vary in severity depending on the age of the child, the size and anatomy of the airways, the type of irritant that precipitates obstruction, and the duration and severity of the asthma attack. The increased work of breathing caused by use of accessory muscles during an asthma attack increases oxygen consumption and cardiac output. This level of exertion is difficult for young children to maintain because of their small glycogen reserves and the likelihood that caloric intake is inadequate because of illness. Hyperventilation can be severe and prolonged and cause permanent anatomic changes (e.g., barrel chest, prominent sternum, and malformation of the ribs), particularly in young children with soft, developing rib cages.

The site and degree of obstruction may differ in a given child from one asthma attack to another. In most children, both larger and smaller airways are obstructed. Even when the bronchi at all levels are involved, the large and small airways can respond differently to inciting agents. Acute, relatively short-lived asthma attacks may chiefly involve the large bronchi. Obstruction of the small airways occurs more slowly. It follows that relief of obstruction occurs more rapidly in larger than in smaller airways. Chronic, partially irreversible small airway obstruction may occur in asymptomatic children with asthma.

The severity, location, and sites of obstruction by asthma are related to age. In general, the younger the child, the greater the risk of morbidity and mortality. Infants in particular are at an anatomic and physiologic disadvantage because of (1) their relatively small alveolocapillary surface area; (2) the increased resistance to airflow in their narrow airways; (3) the horizontal insertion angle of their diaphragm, which is mechanically disadvantageous and increases the work of breathing; and (4) the relatively large number of mucous glands per square centimeter of bronchial mucosa. The one anatomic advantage of infants is the relatively small amount of smooth muscle in their smaller airways, making bronchospasm less severe. In infants, mechanical obstruction from edema, mucus, and inflammatory cell infiltrates, which is slow to resolve, is a more important component of airway obstruction than bronchospasm, which can be reversed with drugs. This difference is reflected in the higher number of infants and very young children requiring hospitalization for control of asthma.

The effects of asthma also depend on the duration of attacks. In short attacks of acute asthma, bronchospasm and/or mucosal edema usually predominate, and obstruction from secretions is of secondary importance. Mucous secretions become a more important cause of obstruction if inflammation is intense and prolonged, such as in viral infections of the lung.

Clinical Manifestations

In typical cases, previously well infants or young children develop what seems to be a cold with rhinorrhea, which is rapidly followed by signs and symptoms of asthma. These include the high-pitched, wheezing sound heard mostly on expiration; cough, sometimes so severe as to induce gagging and vomiting; an anxious facial expression; irritability or restlessness; dyspnea; labored breathing; tachypnea; use of accessory muscles of respiration; nasal flaring; assumption of an upright posture, with raised shoulder, expanded upper chest, and arms extended behind to prop the upper torso; and, in severe attacks, cyanosis, pallor, and diaphoresis (sweating). Respiratory symptoms may be preceded by exposure to irritants, animals, molds or dusty areas, pollens, tobacco smoke, or cold air. Sometimes exercise precipitates an asthma attack (see Chapter 30) or the attack follows bronchitis or recurrent chest colds. Chronic asthma causes chest abnormalities, such as pectus excavatum (funnel chest), or barrel chest, an abnormal prominence of the ribs. Growth may be retarded, resulting in abnormally small stature or low weight, and puberty may be delayed.

Evaluation and Treatment

Diagnosis is determined on the basis of history, clinical manifestations, physical examination, and to a lesser extent, laboratory tests. Treatment for mild and moderate asthma consists of avoidance of contact with suspected allergens or irritants; hyposensitization therapy; promotion of liquification and expectoration of mucus through adequate hydration, administration of adrenergic aerosols, and postural drainage; administration of oral or aerosol bronchodilators; correction of metabolic acidosis; and administration of corticosteroids (prednisone) in severe acute and chronic asthma unresponsive to other measures. Between attacks, the child is encouraged to exercise, and prophylactic medication (theophylline or cromolyn sodium or adrenergic aerosol) may be prescribed.

Severe asthma or status asthmaticus (intractable asthma in which the child continues to have incapacitating dyspnea, cough, and obstruction of airways despite treatment) is a life-threatening emergency requiring admission to an intensive care unit. Emergency care includes administration of epinephrine, oxygen, corticosteriods, methylxanthines, sedatives (contraindicated in status asthmaticus), intravenous hydration, correction of acidosis, and administration of antibiotics.

Although there is a widespread notion that children usually "outgrow" their asthma in adolescence, half of them do not. Many children whose overt symptoms disappear continue to have persistent airway obstruction. The recurrence of overt asthma after years of freedom from symptoms is not unusual. Thus, asthma is often a life-long disorder with periodic exacerbations and remissions.

The likelihood of becoming asymptomatic is greater if the asthma is mild and the child is free from symptoms between attacks. Few deaths are caused by asthma. The 1% to 4% mortality reported in children is usually from associated factors rather than the asthma itself.

Infection

Children have approximately six to eight upper respiratory infections a year. The incidence of lower respiratory infections is approximately 50 infections per 1000 individuals each year for children less than 6 years of age. Most of these illnesses are pneumonia.

The etiology of lower airway infection depends on the infectious microorganism, the age of the child, immune function, seasonal and geographic variables, and environment. Microorganisms transmitted from the maternal genital tract during childbirth, particularly gram-negative bacteria, group B streptococci, and *Chlamydia trachomatis,* can cause pulmonary infections in infants up to 3 months of age. Later in infancy and during early childhood, viral rather than bacterial infections predominate. Respiratory syncytial virus and parainfluenza 3 virus infections are most common. Ninety percent of bacterial pneumonias in children are caused by *S. pneumoniae,* with the remainder caused by staphylococcus and *H. influenzae.* The incidence of *Mycoplasma pneumoniae*

infection peaks between the ages of 5 and 10 years, and as the incidence of all pneumonia decreases during adolescence, *M. pneumoniae* becomes the most common cause of bacterial pneumonia.

In infants and young children, viral infections tend to be more common during the winter and early spring, with other minor peaks in the fall. During influenza epidemics, pneumonia and croup may develop in infants and children of all ages.

Familial and environmental factors are associated with certain types of respiratory infection. For example, *M. pneumoniae* infections tend to occur with overcrowding and affect multiple members of a family. (Predisposing environmental and familial risk factors are described in Unit X.)

Pneumonia

Viral pneumonia causes varying degrees of illness in children. In severe cases the child may rapidly become dangerously ill with fever, respiratory distress, and circulatory failure. Death may occur in 1 to 3 days because of marked tissue necrosis. This pattern occurs primarily with adenovirus infection. The mildest cases of viral pneumonia occur in infants or young children, who develop a cough, fever, and tachypnea with mild systemic disturbance following a cold. There are few or no clinical signs of lung involvement, but radiographs reveal consolidation.

Bacterial pneumonia in children is usually lobar pneumonia caused by *Streptococcus pneumoniae* (90% of cases). It occurs at all ages but is most common in children aged 3 to 8 years during late winter and early spring, when respiratory infections are at their peak.

The classic clinical manifestations of a shaking chill followed by a high fever, cough, and chest pain may occur in older children with streptococcal pneumonia but are rarely observed in infants and young children, in whom the clinical picture is considerably more variable. A mild upper respiratory tract infection characterized by stuffy nose, irritability, and poor feeding usually precedes the onset of streptococcal pneumonia in infants. This mild illness of several days' duration ends with an abrupt onset of fever, restlessness, apprehension, and respiratory distress. The respiratory distress is manifested by grunting; flaring of the nostrils; retraction of the supraclavicular, intercostal, and subcostal areas; tachypnea; and tachycardia. Cyanosis is often apparent.

Clinical manifestations in children and adolescents are similar to those in adults. A brief, mild, upper respiratory infection is followed by the onset of a shaking chill, then fever. These manifestations are accompanied by drowsiness, intermittent periods of restlessness, tachypnea, a dry, hacking, unproductive cough, anxiety, and cyanosis around the mouth. Many children splint the affected side to minimize pleural pain and improve ventilation and may lie on their side with knees drawn up to the chest. Children with pneumonia may have pain referred to the abdomen. Abdominal distention may occur because of swallowed air or air ileus (intestinal blockage by gas) associated with the pneumonia.

S. pneumoniae is treated with penicillin. Supplemental oxygen is given for significant respiratory distress, and aspirin for high fever. With appropriate antibiotic therapy instituted early in the course of illness, the mortality rate from bacterial pneumonia is now less than 1%.

Bronchitis

Bronchitis in children tends to occur in association with a number of other conditions of the upper and lower airways. Bronchitis occurs most commonly following a respiratory illness, such as croup, pneumonia, or even a mild upper respiratory tract infection, and it is aggravated by dry environmental air (e.g., in homes with forced-air heating). When the dry, hacking cough is severe enough to interfere with eating or resting, demulcents such as lollipops or cough drops are quite effective. Recurring bronchitis in childhood may be a predisposing factor for later bronchial lesions that cause chronic obstruction (Boule et al., 1979).

Bronchiolitis

Bronchiolitis is a common disease of the lower respiratory tract in infants. Caused by inflammatory obstruction of the bronchioles it tends to occur during the first 2 years of life, with a peak incidence at approximately 6 months of age, particularly during the winter and spring. Bronchiolitis is a major reason for hospital admission of infants less than 1 year of age.

Respiratory syncytial virus causes over 50% of cases of bronchiolitis, but parainfluenza 3 virus, mycoplasma, some adenoviruses, and occasionally other viruses or bacteria cause acute bronchiolitis. Infection is usually transmitted to the infant from a family member with a minor respiratory illness.

Pathophysiology

Viral infection causes necrosis of the bronchial epithelium and destruction of ciliated epithelial cells, followed by infiltration with lymphocytes around the bronchioles. As the submucosa becomes edematous, cellular debris and fibrin form plugs within the bronchioles.

Edema of the bronchiolar wall, accumulation of mucus and cellular debris, and bronchospasm narrows many peripheral airways. Other airways become partially or completely occluded. Obstruction varies in degree and location. Atelectasis occurs in some areas of the lung and hyperinflation in others.

The mechanics of breathing are disrupted by bronchiolitis. Tidal volume is high and functional residual capacity is approximately twice normal. Compliance is decreased because the lungs are already highly inflated and because airway resistance within the lung is uneven and

increased. The decrease in compliance and the increase in airway resistance results in a substantial increase in the work of breathing.

Serious alterations in gas exchange occur because of airway obstruction and patchy atelectasis. Hypoxemia and hypercapnea develop due to ventilation-perfusion abnormalities (see Chapter 30), and hypercapnea is incresed further because the increased work of breathing causes hypoventilation. Although pH varies, metabolic acidosis occurs more frequently than respiratory alkalosis. The causes of metabolic acidosis is complex. Poor caloric and fluid intake and the administration of salicylate (aspirin) may contribute to ketoacidosis, and carbon dioxide retention can produce respiratory acidosis. (Acid-base disturbances are discussed in Chapter 3.)

Clinical Manifestations Older children and adults can tolerate bronchiolar edema better than infants and thus seldom develop the clinical manifestations of bronchiolitis. In infants and young children, bronchiolitis is characterized by difficulty in expiration, tachypnea, chest wall retractions, and cyanosis around the mouth. Severely affected infants appear anxious and distressed because of dyspnea. The thoracic cage is overexpanded, particularly in its anteroposterior diameter. The infant takes rapid, short breaths, and wheezing and rales are often heard on auscultation. With overexpansion of the lungs, the diaphragm is flattened, causing downward displacement of the liver and spleen. Abdominal distention results from air swallowing.

Evaluation and Treatment Diagnosis of bronchiolitis is made on the basis of physical examination (e.g., rhinitis, cough, and tachypnea), and radiologic examination. Humidification of inspired air is the traditional treatment for bronchiolitis in children. Cold, humidified oxygen relieves hypoxemia and possibly reduces the insensible water loss due to tachypnea. Placing the child in a croup tent with the head elevated at a 30- to 34-degree angle relieves dyspnea, cyanosis, anxiety, and restlessness.

Some children recover from bronchiolitis within 3 to 4 days, whereas others require a week or more. Recently, concern has been focused on the long-term complications of bronchiolitis. Lung development continues during the neonatal period, and the insults inflicted on developing lungs by viruses are as yet unknown. Long-term follow-up of infants who have had bronchiolitis reveals an increased incidence of asthma during childhood (Eisen, & Bacal, 1963). For example, a history of frequent bronchiolitis in infancy is more common in asthmatic children than in normal children.

Bronchiolitis Obliterans

In **bronchiolitis obliterans,** the bronchioles and some of the small bronchi are partially or completely obliterated by nodular masses containing granulomatous and fibrotic tissue. In adults, some cases can be related to chemical injury by nitrogen oxide or other toxic gases. Most cases in children are associated with pulmonary infections, such as influenza, adenoviral infection, or pertussis (whooping cough), or to measles. Cough, respiratory distress, and cyanosis occur initially, followed by a brief period of improvement. The progression of disease is then reflected by increasing dyspnea, cough, sputum production, and wheezing.

There is no specific treatment for bronchiolitis obliterans. Some children deteriorate rapidly and die within weeks, while others follow a more chronic course.

Respiratory Distress Syndrome of the Newborn

The names **respiratory distress syndrome of the newborn (RDS),** *idiopathic respiratory distress syndrome* (IRDS), and *hyaline membrane disease* (HMD) all refer to the severe lung disorder that is responsible for more neonatal deaths than any other condition. RDS affects 5% to 10% of premature infants, or 0.05% to 0.1% of all neonates. RDS or its complications are responsible for 30% to 50% of all neonatal deaths and up to 70% of deaths in premature infants.

The chief predisposing factor is premature birth, but several other factors are important. The condition is twice as common in males as in females. It frequently follows delivery by cesarean section, particularly if the procedure is done before labor has begun. Infants of diabetic mothers are five times more likely to develop RDS than infants of nondiabetic mothers, regardless of gestational age, sex, and mode of delivery. Asphyxia increases the possibility that a premature infant will develop RDS because acidosis (caused by hypoxemia) interferes with production of alveolar surfactant, increasing the likelihood of atelectasis. Other predisposing factors are hypo-or hypervolemia, maternal antepartum hemorrhage, and shock.

Pathophysiology

During the third trimester of gestation, the final unfolding of the alveolar septum takes place, an event that significantly increases the alveolocapillary surface area of the lungs. Because alveolar septal unfolding is incomplete in premature infants, they are born with many underdeveloped and uninflatable alveoli. In addition, pulmonary blood flow is limited by fetal atelectasis and incomplete vascular development, particularly of the alveolocapillary network. Because of increased pulmonary vascular resistance, most fetal blood is shunted from the lungs through the fetal cardiac structures, the ductus arteriosus and foramen ovale. (These structures are described in Chapter 28.)

At birth, the infant must initiate breathing and keep the previously fluid-filled lungs inflated with air. With the onset of ventilation a marked increase in pulmonary blood flow occurs because oxygen dilates the constricted pulmonary blood vessels. Pulmonary venous return is thus increased and, consequently, so is left ventricular output. In the normal neonate, ductal closure and the fall of pulmonary vascular resistance result in a fall of pulmonary arterial and right ventricular pressures. The major decline from the high fetal pressures to low adult pressures usually occurs within the first 2 to 3 days following birth but may be prolonged for 7 or more days (Behrman & Vaughan, 1983). At the same time, the volume of pulmonary capillary blood flow must increase approximately 10 times to provide adequate pulmonary perfusion and alter intracardiac pressure enough to close the ductus arteriosus and foramen ovale. Most full-term infants are successful in making these changes, but the premature infant with RDS is not.

The primary problem in RDS is atelectasis, which develops in premature infants as a result of three interrelated developmental factors: (1) small alveoli that are difficult to inflate; (2) a weak, compliant chest wall (see Fig. 31-2, *B*); and (3) insufficient production of pulmonary surfactant, which is needed to reduce surface tension and permit alveolar inflation. (The principles that govern alveolar inflation are described in Chapter 29.) These factors combined contribute to the greater respiratory effort required to expand the alveoli of premature infants and the greater end-expiratory pressure (functional residual capacity) required to prevent chest wall collapse. Incomplete initial inflation and small lung volume at end-inspiration both promote atelectasis.

Premature infants who do not have RDS have developed sufficient alveolar surface area to meet their metabolic needs and have produced and accumulated sufficient surfactant to permit alveolar inflation. Infants with RDS have not developed the ability to synthesize, store, and secrete surfactant onto the alveolocapillary membrane. Surfactant reaches the alveolar surface of the membrane at approximately 28 to 38 weeks of gestation, as demonstrated by its detection in amniotic fluid. This variation in ages at detection is evidence that the lung matures at different rates in different individuals. It also explains why some infants with a gestational age of <30 weeks do not acquire RDS, while other infants with greater gestational age may do so.

Without surfactant, each breath requires as much negative pressure as the initial lung expansion at birth. The infant uses more oxygen to sustain the work of breathing than is gained from ventilation. This leads to exhaustion and a decreased ability to maintain lung expansion. The result is widespread atelectasis, one of the characteristics of RDS.

In the absence of alveolar stability (normal functional residual capacity) and with progressive atelectasis, pulmonary vascular resistance is increased instead of decreased, as in normal lungs. This results in hypoperfusion of the lung and a decrease in effective pulmonary blood flow. Increased pulmonary vascular resistance causes a partial return to fetal circulation, with right-to-left shunting of blood through the ductus arteriosus and foramen ovale. Inadequate pulmonary perfusion and ventilation produce hypoxemia and hypercapnia. Because the thick muscular layer of the pulmonary arterioles is sensitive to diminished oxygen concentration and decreased blood pH, hypoxic vasoconstriction occurs. Hypoxic vasoconstriction contributes to further increases in pulmonary vascular resistance.

Capillary permeability increases, resulting in the leakage of plasma proteins into the interstitium, where clotting causes fibrin formation. Fibrin deposited in the alveolocapillary interstitium creates the hyaline appear-

ance seen upon histologic examination; hence the name hyaline membrane disease.

To make the situation more complex, prolonged hypoxemia activates anaerobic glycolysis, which produces increased amounts of lactic acid and promotes metabolic acidosis. Because the collapsed alveoli are unable to get rid of excess carbon dioxide, respiratory acidosis also develops. Lowered pH causes further vasoconstriction. With inadequate pulmonary circulation and alveolar perfusion, the oxygen content of the blood continues to decrease, pH falls, and materials needed for surfactant production are not circulated to the alveoli. The pathogenesis of RDS is summarized in Fig. 31-5.

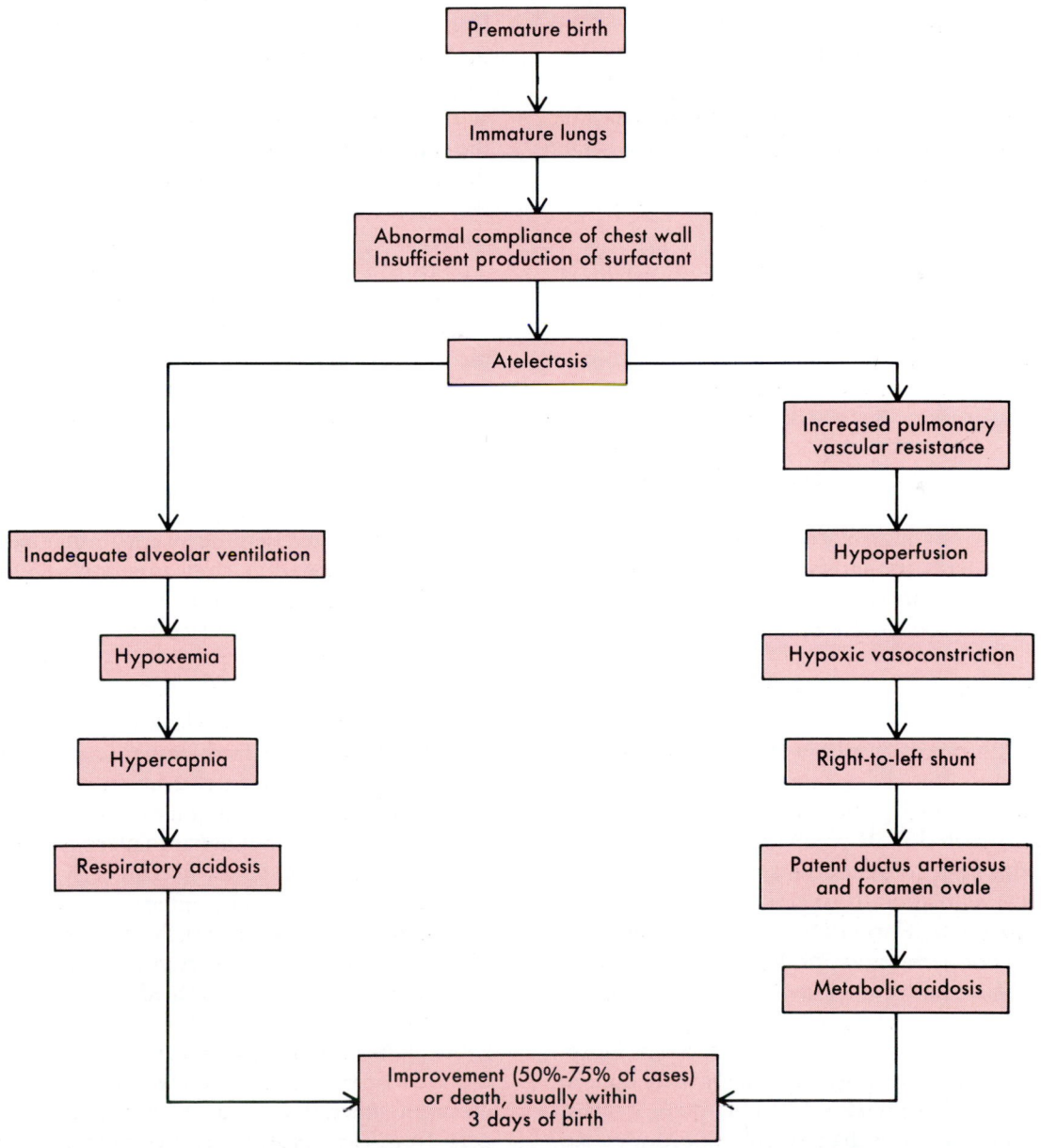

FIG. 31-5. Pathogenesis of respiratory distress syndrome of the newborn (RDS), also known as hyaline membrane disease.

Clinical Manifestations

Signs of RDS appear within minutes of birth. Some neonates require resuscitation at birth because of asphyxia or initial severe respiratory disease. Tachypnea (respiratory rate over 70 per minute), expiratory grunting or whining, intercostal and subcostal retractions, nasal flaring, duskiness of the skin, and low body temperature are the most striking clinical manifestations of RDS. The natural course is characterized by progressive hypoxemia and dyspnea. Blood pressure and body temperature fall. Fatigue, cyanosis, and pallor increase, and grunting decreases or disappears as the condition worsens. Apnea and irregular respirations occur as the infant tires. Edema of the extremities, ileus, and oliguria may also occur during the first 2 to 3 days of life. Signs of asphyxia as a result of apnea or partial respiratory failure indicate rapid progression of the disease. RDS can progress to death in severe cases, but in milder cases the clinical manifestations reach a peak within 3 days, after which time gradual improvement is seen. Death is rare after 3 days.

Evaluation and Treatment

Diagnosis is made on the basis of clinical manifestations, blood gas analysis, shunting, and chest radiographs. The course of RDS can be altered dramatically by supportive treatment that maintains adequate oxygenation, circulation, acid-base balance, and nutrition. Mechanical ventilation, often used successfully in managing RDS, can create such secondary problems as bronchopulmonary dysplasia, however. Approximately 50% to 70% of infants survive with treatment. Even in severe cases, recovery may be complete within 10 to 14 days. The long-term prognosis for normal pulmonary function in most infants is excellent. Neurologic deficits, however, occur in about 20% of neonates weighing less than 1500 g.

Bronchopulmonary Dysplasia

Bronchopulmonary dysplasia (BPD), also known as chronic or respiratory lung disease, is abnormal size, shape, or organization of the bronchopulmonary structures. It is associated with premature birth, RDS, and treatment with high concentrations of oxygen delivered by mechanical ventilation. (Oxygen toxicity is described in Chapter 29.) The relationship of these factors to the condition has not been assessed fully. Other theories implicate mechanical injury and patent ductus arteriosus as the cause of BPD.

The incidence of BPD is difficult to ascertain. Hospitals in which a relatively large number of premature infants survive RDS have reported BPD in 20% of infants whose birth weight is less than 1000 g (Northway, Rosan, & Porter, 1967).

The process of BPD is one of continuous injury and repair of lung tissue, causing delays in both lung and body growth. Pulmonary alterations include scarring and emphysema. Alveoli fail to multiply, and alveolar walls or capillaries become inflamed and may be destroyed. The pulmonary arteries have smaller lumina and thicker walls than is normal for the infant's age. Ciliated epithelium is lost, and mucous plugs and debris clog the airways. Ventilation/perfusion mismatch is severe, and the infant may develop an infection, cor pulmonale, and right heart failure (Behrman & Vaughan, 1983).

In its mildest form, BPD appears to be a prolonged phase of RDS. Episodes of atelectasis, hyperinflation, pneumothorax, and air in the interstitium are characteristic. The infant may seem to be improving but suddenly becomes apneic, or develops more severe respiratory distress and cyanosis. In many, a murmur is heard at 1 or 2 weeks of age, and a left-to-right shunt through the ductus arteriosus becomes evident. As resistance in the pulmonary vascular bed falls, blood flow through the ductus arteriosus increases, resulting in pulmonary edema and increased oxygen demands. (Patent ductus arteriosus is described in Chapter 28.) BPD can cause death within a few weeks or can continue for months or years. Either death or recovery is possible regardless of the length of disease.

Because the pathogenic mechanisms of BPD are not fully understood, treatment consists of supportive care. Regulation of the environmental temperature, monitoring of oxygen requirements, prevention of infection, and maintenance of nutritional status are essential aspects of care. Because fluid overload may be important in the etiology of BPD, close attention to hydration status and early surgical closure of the patent ductus arteriosus have been advocated (Rudolph, 1987).

Cystic Fibrosis

Cystic fibrosis (mucoidvicidosis) is an inherited disease of the exocrine glands resulting in the production of excessive, thick mucus that obstructs the gastrointestinal system and lungs. Although cystic fibrosis (CF) is a multiorgan disease, pulmonary failure is the most common cause of death. Cystic fibrosis is the most common fatal genetic disease and it affects about 1 out of every 2000 children. The disease is characterized by pancreatic enzyme deficiency, progressive obstructive infectious pulmonary disease, and elevated sodium chloride concentrations in the sweat. The incidence is highest in white children, although occurrence in any race is possible. Genetic transmission follows an autosomal recessive mode of inheritance (a child must inherit a defective gene from each parent). The cystic fibrosis gene is located in the middle of the long arm of chromosome 7

(Rommens, et al., 1989). Clinical manifestations are only present in homozygotes. About 2% to 5% of the white population are carriers. The biochemical defect of CF remains unknown.

Pathophysiology

CF is a generalized disease with complications that affect nearly every organ system. The exocrine, or mucus-producing, glands secrete an abnormally thick mucus that coagulates in the ducts of organs or the airways of the lung with obstruction and dilation that alters or destroys structure and function. Pancreatic function may be normal or completely altered. Loss of pancreatic function occurs with the obstruction of pancreatic ducts by thick mucus secretions that lead to dilation and fibrosis. Pancreatic exocrine function declines with a decrease in the production and secretion of pancreatic enzymes (lipase, amylase, trypsin), resulting in maldigestion and malabsorption. The islet tissues are usually involved with a decrease in insulin secretion and glucose intolerance.

Bronchiolar obstruction with thick mucus is the first stage of pulmonary involvement. The obstruction predisposes the lung to infection and with chronic inflammation there is hyperplasia of goblet cells with enlargement and destruction of airway walls causing bronchiectasis. The disease progresses from bronchiolitis to bronchitis, followed by bronchiectasis, pneumonia, peribronchial fibrosis, and to the formation of large cystic dilations that involve all bronchi. Alveolar involvement ensues with infection, atelectasis, and hemorrhagic pneumonia. Recurrent pneumothroax, hemoptysis, pulmonary hypertension, and cor pulmonale are serious and life-threatening complications of severe and diffuse pulmonary disease.

Alteration in hepatic function develops with obstruction and fibrosis. Multinodular biliary cirrhosis is accompanied by symptoms of portal hypertension and splenomegaly. Reproductive function is affected in females by dilated cervical mucus glands and there may be decreased fertility. The function of the vans deferens, epididymus, and seminal vesicles are usually abnormal in males, resulting in sterility. Sweat and salivary gland secretions have elevated sodium chloride concentrations as a result of abnormal reabsorption of chloride by the duct epithelium.

Clinical Manifestations

Children with CF may have few or numerous clinical manifestations. The eccrine sweat abnormality will appear as powdery white crystals on the forehead or hairline and tastes salty. The malabsorption associated with pancreatic insufficiency results in steatorrhea, a protuberent abdomen, and failure to gain weight. The child looks pale and the skin may have a transparent quality from diminished subcutaneous fat. Chronic cough and sputum production are symptomatic of lung involvement. There is labored ventilation resulting in hypoxia, clubbing of the fingers, and cyanosis.

The chronic pulmonary infection and malabsorption can lead to secondary manifestations of barrel chest, pectus carinatum, and kyphosis. Vitamin K deficiency related to malabsorption may lead to bleeding disorders, purpura, and ecchymoses. Some children have transient polyarticular or monoarticular arthritis of the large joints. Edema may be a function of hypoproteinemia from nutritional deficiency or from elevated venous pressures associated with right-sided congestive heart failure caused by cor pulmonale. Chronic rhinitis is common among children with CF. Although diffuse organ involvement can be characteristic of the complications of CF, the pulmonary disorders are the most common cause of morbidity and mortality.

Evaluation and Treatment

Recently, new genetic markers make it possible to diagnose CF prenatally and to detect carriers in over 70% of families with a history of CF (O'Connell et al., 1987). CF is traditionally diagnosed when a sweat test reveals a sodium chloride concentration greater than 60 mEq/L. The sweat test is performed when there is a family history of CF or when there are pulmonary or gastrointestinal symptoms consistent with the disease. The stool may be examined for increased fat and the absence of pancreatic enzymes.

Management of CF requires a multidisciplinary effort to relieve symptoms from generalized organ involvement and the social and financial burdens of the disease. The management plan includes judicious use of antibiotics to control pulmonary infection; aggressive pulmonary therapy with drugs to thin mucous secretions, humidified air, postural drainage, ventilator treatments, and oxygen; oral pancreatic enzyme replacement; nutrition and diet counseling; and psychological and social support of the child and family.

Cystic fibrosis was first described in 1936, and the natural history of the disease has changed from death in early childhood to a mean life expectancy of 18 years, primarily as a function of improved clinical management. There is a need to provide genetic counseling, in addition to educating the entire family about the nature of the disease with instruction in pulmonary and nutritional therapy. Once a couple has a child with CF, the risk for a subsequent child with CF is 1:4 (25%) and 2:4 (50%) will be carriers. The chance of a healthy sibling being a carrier is 2:3 (66%).

SUMMARY REVIEW

Structure and Function of the Pulmonary System in Children

1 The airways of infants and children are shorter and narrower from the trachea through the terminal bronchioles, thus making them more prone to obstruction than the airways of adults.

2 The accessory muscles of respiration are not fully developed in infants and children, making respiratory efforts and coughing less effective than those of adults.

3 Infants have fewer alveoli than older children and adults.

4 The immature chest wall is soft and compliant, contributing to inefficient mechanisms of breathing.

Pulmonary Disorders

1 Croup is a syndrome of clinical manifestations due to acute obstruction of the larynx caused by infection, aspiration of a foreign body, or allergy.

2 Acute epiglottitis is the most life-threatening type of croup. Acute laryngotracheobronchitis, which is less dangerous, is the most common type.

3 The severity of asthma in children depends on the child's age (because age determines the caliber of airway lumina), the child's hypersensitivity to the variant, and the duration of the asthma attack.

4 Children are less well-equipped than adults to sustain the work of breathing during asthma attacks.

5 Viral and bacterial pneumonia cause varying degrees of illness in children; symptoms range from mild respiratory distress to rapid death.

6 Bronchiolitis, the inflammatory obstruction of the bronchioles, is most common in infants and is usually caused by infection by a virus that would cause only mild illness in older children or adults.

7 In bronchiolitis obliterans, the bronchioles and some small bronchi are partially or completely obliterated by nodular masses containing granulomatous or fibrous tissue.

8 Respiratory distress syndrome (RDS) of the newborn usually occurs in premature infants who are born before surfactant production and alveolocapillary development are complete. Atelectasis and hypoventilation cause shunting, hypoxemia, and hypercapnea.

9 Bronchopulmonary dysplasia (BPD) is an iatrogenic abnormality of pulmonary and bronchial development in premature neonates. It is caused by administration of oxygen via positive pressure, which injures tissues and delays both lung and body growth. Alterations include scarring of the alveoli and emphysema.

10 Cystic fibrosis is an autosomal recessive genetic disease characterized by excessive secretion of thick, tenacious mucus and elevated sodium chloride concentrations in the sweat. Symptoms vary from minimal to multiorgan involvement with pancreatic insufficiency and malnutrition, and progressive obstructive lung disease, resulting in pulmonary failure and death.

KEY TERMS

Asthma, 1101

Bronchiolitis obliterans, 1103

Bronchopulmonary dysplasia (BPD) (chronic or respiratory lung disease), 1106

Croup, 1098

Cystic fibrosis (CF), 1106

Epiglottitis, 1098

Laryngitis, 1098

Laryngotracheobronchitis (LTB), 1098

Sudden infant death syndrome (SID), 1100

Respiratory distress syndrome of the newborn (RDS, idiopathic RDS, hyaline membrane disease), 1104

REFERENCES

Anderson, C. M., & Goodchild, M. C. (1976). *Cystic fibrosis: Manual of diagnosis and management.* London: Blackwell Scientific Publications.

Aranda, J. B., Trippenbach, T., Turmen, T., Lopes J. M. (1983). Apnea and control of breathing in newborn infants. In L. Stern (Ed.), *Diagnosis and management of respiratory disorders in the newborn* pp. 134-157. Reading, MA.: Addison-Wesley.

Ariagno, R. L. (1984). Evaluation and management of infantile apnea. *Pediatric Annals, 13,* 210-217.

Avery, G. B. (Ed.). (1987). *Neonatology: Pathophysiology and management of the newborn* (3rd ed.). Philadelphia: J. B. Lippincott.

Avery, M. E., & Teusch, H. W. (Eds.). (1984). *Snaffer's diseases of the newborn* (5th ed.). Philadelphia: W. B. Saunders.

Bakke, K., & Dougherty, J. (1981, March-April). Sudden infant death syndrome and infant apnea: Current questions, clinical management, and research dissections. *Issues in Comprehensive Pediatric Nursing, 5*(2), 77-88.

Beckwith, B. (1970). Observation on the pathologic anatomy of the SIDS. In A. B. Bergman, J. B. Beckwith, & C. G. Ray (Eds.), *Sudden infant death syndrome.* Seattle: University of Washington Press.

Behrman, R. E., & Vaughan, V. C. (1983). *Nelson textbook of pediatrics* (12th ed.). Philadelphia: W. B. Saunders.

Berry, C. L. (1981). *Pediatric pathology.* New York: Springer-Verlag.

Bierman, C. W., & Pearlman, D. S. (1987). *Allergic diseases of infancy, childhood, and adolescence* (2nd ed.). Philadelphia: W. B. Saunders.

Boule, M., Gaultier, C., Tournier, G., Allaire, Y., & Girard, F. (1979). Lung function in children with recurrent bronchitis. *Respirations, 38,* 127-129.

Brooks, L. J., Cloutier, M. M., & Afshani, E. (1982). Significance of roentgenographic abnormalities in children hospitalized for asthma. *Chest, 82*(3), 315-318.

Brown, E. R., Stark, A., Sosenko, I., Lawson, E. E., & Avery, M. E. (1982). Bronchopulmonary dysplasia: Possible relationship to pulmonary edema. *Journal of Pediatrics, 92,* 982.

Cerrina, J., Denjean, A., Alexandre, G., Lockhart, A., & Duroux, P. (1981). Inhibition of exercise-induced asthma by a calcium antagonist. *American Review of Respiratory Diseases, 123,* 156.

Crawford, L. V. (1977). *Pediatric allergy diseases.* Flushing, NY: Medical Examination Publishing, Co.

Eisen, A. H., & Bacal, H. L. (1963). The relationship of acute bronchiolitis to bronchial asthma: A 4 to 14-year follow-up. *Pediatrics, 31,* 859.

Felman, A. H. (1983). *The pediatric chest.* Springfield, IL: Charles C. Thomas Publisher.

Gerbeaux, J., Couvreur, J., & Tournier, G. (1982). *Pediatric respiratory disease* (2nd ed.). New York: Wiley.

Hogg, J. C. (1981). Bronchial permeability and its relationship to airway's hyperactivity. *Journal of Allergy and Clinical Immunology, 76,* 421.

Kelly, D. H., & Shannon, D. C. (1982). Sudden infant death syndrome and near-sudden infant death syndrome: A review of the literature 1964 to 1982. *Pediatric Clinics of North America, 29,* 1241-1261.

Kendig, E. L., & Chernick, V. (1983). *Disorders of the respiratory tract in children.* Philadelphia: W. B. Saunders, Co.

Klaustermeyer, W. B. (Ed.). (1983). *Practical allergy and immunology.* New York: Wiley.

Mangos, J. A., & Talamo, R. C. (Eds.). (1976). *Cystic fibrosis: Projections into the future.* New York: Stratton Intercontinental Medical Book Corporation.

Nadel, J. A. (1977). Autonomic control of airway smooth muscle and airway secretions. *American Review of Respiratory Diseases, 115,* 117.

Northway, W. H., Rosan, R. C., & Porter, D. Y. (1967). Pulmonary disease following respiratory therapy of hyaline membrane disease: Bronchopulmonary dysplasia. *New England Journal of Medicine, 276,* 357.

Nussbaum, E., & Galant, S. P. (Eds.). (1983). *Pediatric respiratory disorders.* San Francisco: Grune & Stratton.

Nuttall, P. (1986). Maternal and infant responses to home apnea monitoring (Doctoral dissertation). Salt Lake City: University of Utah.

O'Connell, D. M., Leppert, M., Park, A., Amos, J. A., Phillips, D. G., White, R., & Vande Woude, G. F. (1987). Three additional polymorphisms in the *met* gene and D758 locus: Use in prenatal diagnosis of cystic fibrosis. *The Journal of Pediatrics, III*(4), 490-495.

Phelan, P. D., Landau, L. I., & Olinsky, A. (1982). *Respiratory illness in children* (2nd ed.). Boston: Blackwell Scientific Publications.

Rommens, J. M., Iannuzzi, M. C., Kerem, B., et al. (1989). Identification of the cystic fibrosis gene: chromosome walking and jumping. *Science 245,* 1059.

Rudolph, A. M. (1987). *Pediatrics* (18th ed.). Norwalk, CT: Appleton & Lange.

Scarpelli, E. M. (1975). *Pulmonary physiology of the fetus, newborn, and child.* Philadelphia: Lea & Febiger.

Shannon, D. C., & Kelly, D. H. (1982). SIDS and near SIDS (Part I). *New England Journal of Medicine, 306*(16), 959-965.

Shannon, D. C., & Kelly, D. H. (1982). SIDS and near SIDS (Part II). *New England Journal of Medicine, 306*(17), 1022-1028.

Spitzer, A. R., & Fox, W. W. (1984). Sudden infant death syndrome: Guidelines for averting tragedy. *Post Grad Mel, 23*(7), 374-380.

Steinschneider, A., Weinstein, S. L., & Diamond, E. (1982). The sudden infant death syndrome and apnea/obstruction during neonatal sleep and feeding. *Pediatrics, 70,* 858-863.

Ward, L., Keens, T., Chan, L. S., Chipps, B., Carson, S., Deming, D., Krishna, V., MacDonald, H. M., Martin, G., Meredith, K. S., Merritt, T. A., Nickerson, B. G., Stoddard, R. A., & van der Hall, A. L. (1986). Sudden infant death syndrome in infant evaluated by apnea programs in California. *Pediatrics, 77*(840), 451-458.

Whaley, L. F., & Wong, D. L. (1987). *Nursing care of infants an) children* (3rd ed.). St. Louis: C. V. Mosby.

Wung, J. T., Koons, A. H., Driscoll, J. M., & James, S. (1979). Changing incidence of bronchopulmonary dysplasia. *Journal of Pediatrics, 95,* 845.

UNIT XI

The Renal and Urologic Systems

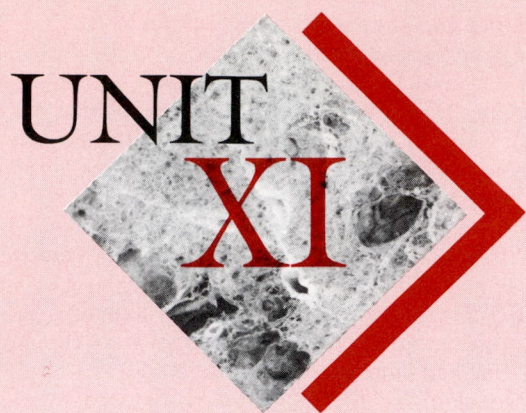

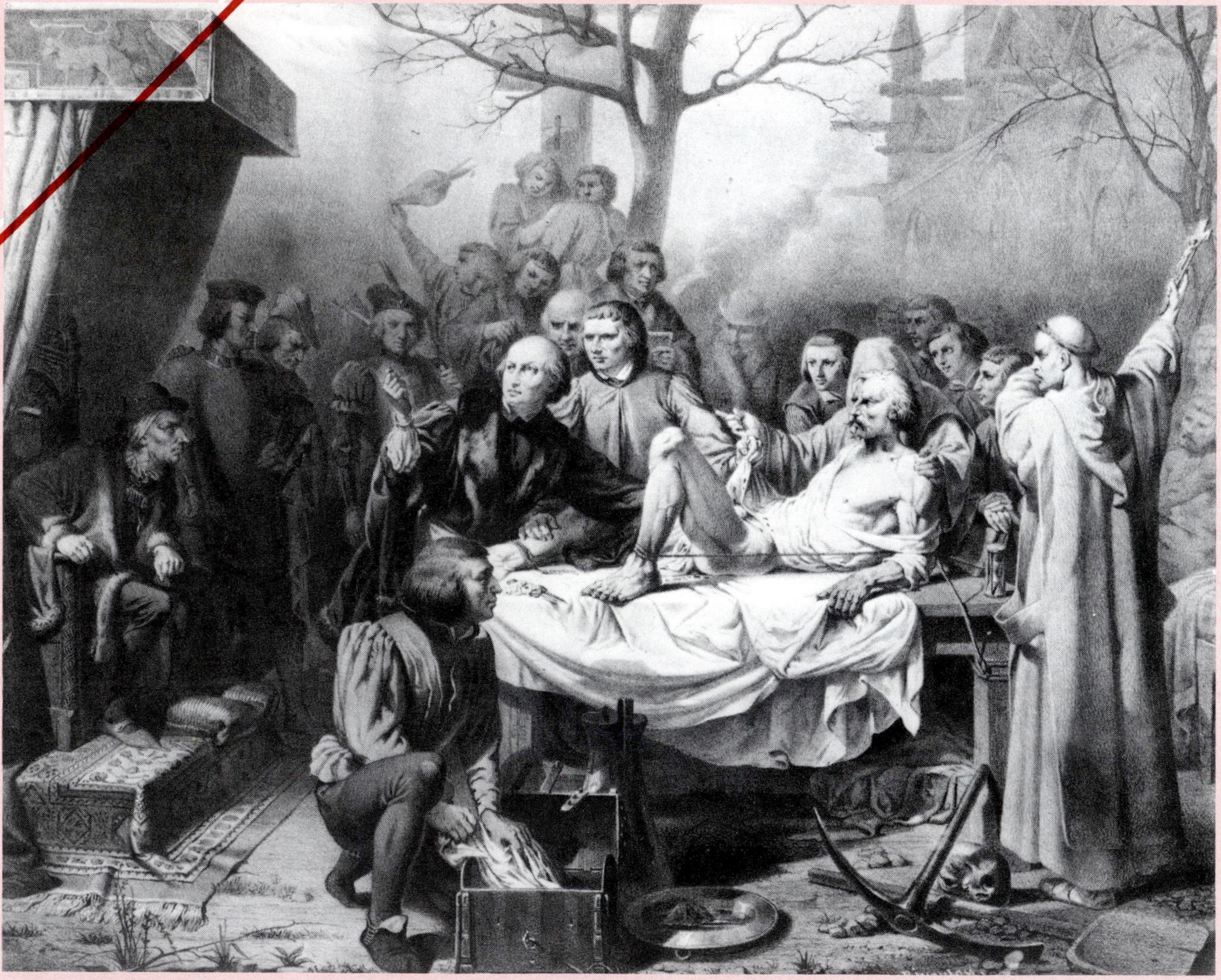

Premiere operation de la pierre. The earliest operation for removal of a urethral stone was performed in the presence of King Louis 11th. The surgeon is about to begin. Lithograph by Antoine Rivoulon, 1851. (Courtesy National Library of Medicine.)

HIPPOCRATES (400 BC) first wrote descriptions of the characteristics of urine as a basis for the appearance or progression of disease. Galen (130-200) dissected the kidney, ureters, and bladder in humans and animals and evolved a theory of how the kidneys "attract" waste products from the blood. After the prescientific era, Malpighi (1628-1694) made the greatest contribution to defining the anatomy of the kidney by using the microscope to describe the glomeruli (malpighian corpuscles). He described the glomeruli as glands but was unable to identify them as capillary tufts.

Bladder stones were removed during ancient and medieval times, but it was not until the invention of instruments that could be passed into the bladder for observation that modern urology was born. Cheselden (1688-1752), an expert anatomist from England, was especially adept in the removal of bladder stones (lithotomy), and it was reputed that he performed a lithotomy in less than 1 minute. In Germany, Nitze and Leiter invented the first practical cystoscope in 1879. In the 1920s, after Roentgen introduced x-rays, a technique was devised to adequately visualize the urologic tract.

Physicians before Richard Bright (1789-1858) had observed albuminuria (albumin in the urine), but Bright was the first to associate a coagulable urine with kidney disease and granular appearing kidneys. Lorenzo Bellini had previously described the tubules of the kidney, and William Bowman (1816-1892) described the microscopic anatomy of the kidney, including the spheric capsule still known as Bowman's capsule. From his understanding of the proximity of the glomerular blood flow to the fluid in Bowman's capsule he proposed a theory of the movement of water and salts to form urine. But this description, based on anatomy, was incomplete without physiologic experimentation.

Filtration as a function of hydrostatic pressure in the glomerular capillaries was described by Carl Ludwig in 1842, and tubular secretion was demonstrated by Rudolf Heidenhain (1834-1897). The processes of filtration, reabsorption, and secretion were then synthesized by Robert Cushny (1866-1926), thus completing a foundation for the advancement of modern renal physiology and a continued understanding of disease.

CHAPTER 32

Structure and Function of the Renal and Urologic Systems

Sue E. Huether

Structures of the renal system, 1112
  Structures of the kidney, 1112
    Nephron, 1113
    Blood vessels of the kidney, 1116
  Urinary structures, 1118
    Ureters, 1118
    Bladder and urethra, 1118
Renal blood fow, 1119
  Autoregulation, 1119
  Neural regulation, 1120
  Hormonal regulation, 1121
Kidney function, 1121
  Nephron function, 1121
    Glomerular filtration, 1122
      Filtration rate, 1124
      Tubular transport, 1124
        Proximal tubule, 1124
        Loop of Henle and distal tubule, 1125
      Glomerulotubular balance, 1126
  Concentration and dilution of urine, 1126
    Water, sodium, and chloride, 1126
    Urea, 1127
    Antidiuretic hormone (ADH), 1127
    Diuretics as a factor in urine flow, 1128
  Renal hormones, 1129
    Vitamin D, 1129
    Erythropoietin, 1129
    Natriuretic hormone, 1129
Tests of renal function, 1129
  The concept of clearance, 1129
    Clearance and glomerular filtration rate, 1129
    Clearance and renal blood flow, 1130
  Blood tests, 1130
    Plasma creatinine concentration, 1130
    Blood urea nitrogen, 1130
  Urinalysis, 1130
    Specific gravity, 1131
    Urine sediment, 1131
      Red blood cells, 1131
      Casts, 1131

      Crystals, 1131
      White blood cells, 1131
Aging and renal function, 1131

The primary function of the kidney is to maintain a stable internal environment for optimal cell and tissue metabolism. The kidneys accomplish these life-sustaining tasks by balancing solute outputs and water with inputs excreting metabolic waste products, conserving nutrients, and regulating acids and bases. The kidney also has an endocrine function and secretes the hormones renin, erythropoietin, and 1,25-dihydroxy vitamin D for regulation of blood pressure, erythrocyte production, and calcium metabolism, respectively. In times of severe fasting the kidney also can synthesize glucose from amino acids, performing the process of gluconeogenesis. The formation of urine is achieved through the process of filtration, reabsorption, and secretion by the glomeruli and tubules within the kidney.

Although the kidney controls the formation of urine and regulates fluid and electrolyte balance, other structures are involved in elimination. The bladder stores the urine that it receives from the kidney by way of the ureters. Urine is then removed from the body through the urethra.

STRUCTURES OF THE RENAL SYSTEM

Structures of the Kidney

The **kidneys** are paired organs located on the posterior abdominal wall outside the peritoneal cavity. They lie on either side of the vertebral column with their upper and lower poles extending from the twelfth thoracic

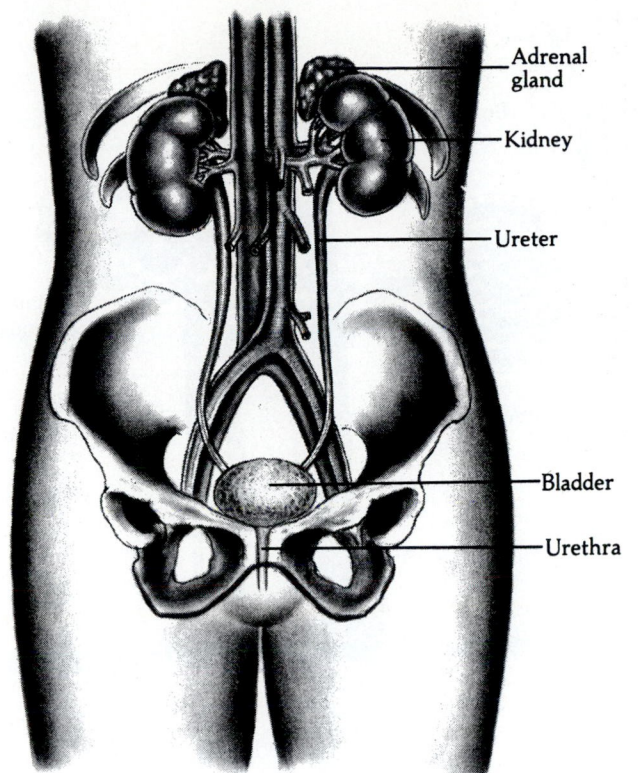

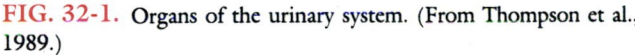

FIG. 32-1. Organs of the urinary system. (From Thompson et al., 1989.)

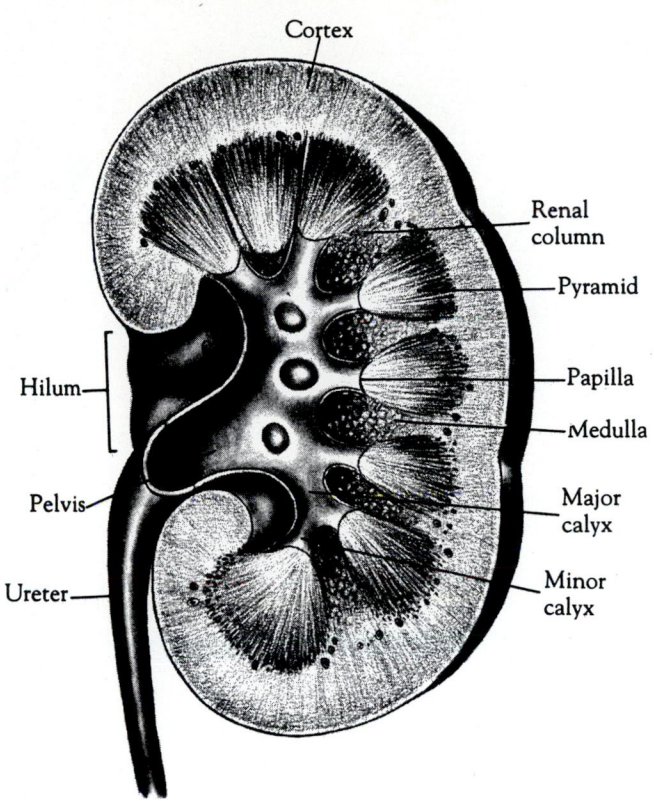

FIG. 32-2. Kidney structure. (From Thompson et al., 1989.)

to the third lumbar vertebrae (Fig. 32-1). Each kidney is approximately 11 cm long, 5 to 6 cm wide, and 3 to 4 cm thick. A tightly adhering capsule (the **renal capsule**) surrounds each kidney, and the kidney is then embedded in a mass of fat. The capsule and fatty layer are covered with a double layer of **renal fascia,** fibrous tissue that attaches the kidney to the posterior abdominal wall.

The cushion of fat and the position of the kidney between the abdominal organs and muscles of the back protect it from trauma. The right kidney is slightly lower than the left; it is displaced downward by the overlying liver. A medial indentation (the **hilus**) contains the entry and exit for the renal blood vessels, nerves, lymphatic vessels, and ureter.

The gross structure of the kidney can be identified when it is divided from top to bottom in a coronal plane (Fig. 32-2). The major components are the outer **renal cortex** and the inner **renal medulla.** The cortex contains all the glomeruli and portions of the tubules. The medulla consists of a series of wedges, called **renal pyramids,** with an outer zone close to the cortex and an inner zone. **Renal columns** extend from the cortex down between the renal pyramids. The apex of the pyramids project into a **minor calyx** (a cup-shaped cavity), which joins together to form a **major calyx.** The major

calyces join to form the **renal pelvis,** an extension of the upper end of the ureter.

Nephron

The **nephron** is the functional unit of the kidney. Approximately 1.2 million nephrons are contained in each kidney. The nephron is a tubular structure with subunits that include the glomerulus, proximal convoluted tubule, loop of Henle, distal convoluted tubule, and collecting duct, all of which contribute to the formation of final urine (Fig. 32-3). The different structures of the epithelial cells lining various segments of the tubule facilitate the special functions of secretion and reabsorption (Fig. 32-4).

The kidney has two kinds of nephrons: (1) **cortical nephrons,** which extend only partially into the medulla, and (2) **juxtamedullary nephrons,** which extend deep into the medulla and are important for the concentration of urine (Fig. 32-5). The **glomerulus** is a tuft of capillaries, the glomerular capillaries, that loop into a circular capsule, called **Bowman's capsule,** like fingers pushed into bread dough. **Mesangial cells** lie between the capillaries and hold them together. The space inside of Bowman's capsule is called **Bowman's space.**

The wall of the glomerular capillary serves as a filtra-

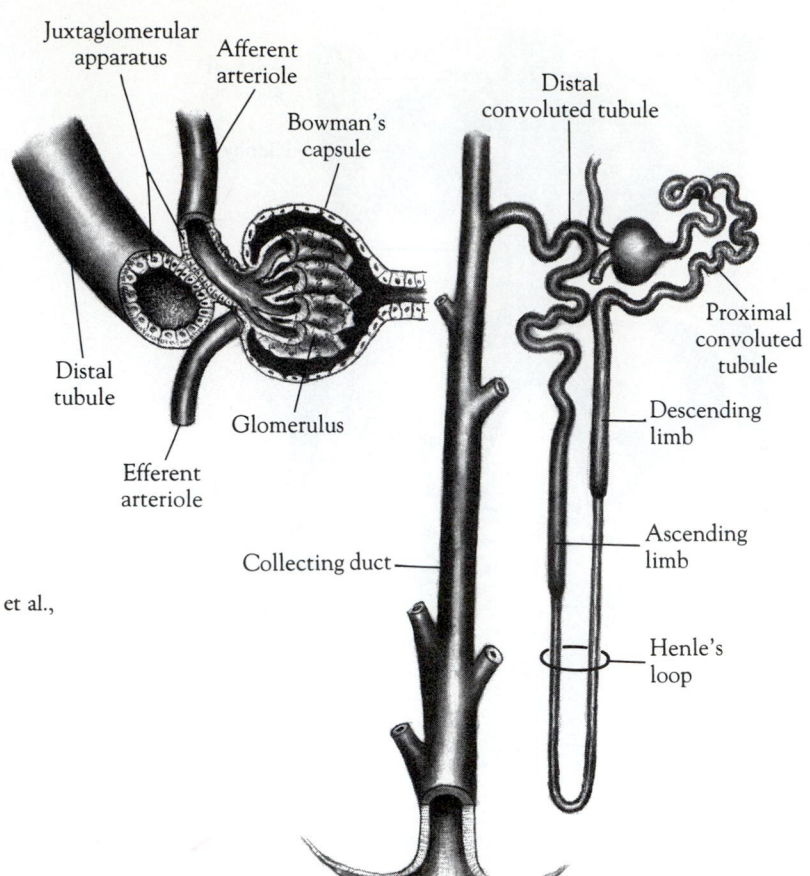

FIG. 32-3. Components of nephron. (From Thompson et al., 1989.).

tion membrane (the **glomerular filtration membrane**) and has three layers: (1) an inner capillary endothelium, (2) a middle basement membrane, and (3) an outer layer of capillary epithelium. Each layer has unique structural properties that allow all components of the blood to filter through, with the exception of blood cells and plasma proteins with a molecular weight greater than 70,000 (Figs. 32-6 and 32-7). The capillary endothelium is composed of cells in continuous contact with the basement membrane. It is perforated by many small openings or windows, called fenestrae. The middle basement membrane is a selectively permeable network of glycoproteins and mucopolysaccharides. The epithelium has specialized cells called **podocytes.** Footlike processes, or pedicles, radiate from the podocytes and adhere to the basement membrane. The pedicles of one podocyte interlock with the pedicles of adjacent podocytes, forming an elaborate network of intercellular clefts. These clefts are called **filtration slits** or slit membranes. The glomerular filtration membrane separates the blood of the glomerular capillaries from the fluid in Bowman's space. The glomerular filtrate passes through the three layers of the glomerular membrane and forms the primary urine.

The **proximal tubule** continues from Bowman's space and has an initial convoluted segment (pars convoluta) and then a straight segment (pars recta) that descends toward the medulla (see Fig. 32-3). The proximal tubular lumen consists of one layer of cuboidal cells. This is the only surface inside the nephron where the cells are covered with microvilli (a brush border). The microvilli create a brushlike surface that greatly expands the surface area of the tubule and enhances its reabsorptive function (Fig. 32-4). The proximal tubule joins the loop of Henle, a hairpin loop composed of thick and thin portions of a descending segment that goes into the medulla. The tube then loops and becomes the thickening ascending segment that extends toward the cortex. The thin segment is composed of thin squamous cells with no active transport function. The cells of the thick segment are cuboidal and actively transport several solutes.

The more numerous cortical nephrons have glomeruli originating close to the surface of the cortex or in the midcortex unlike the juxtamedullary nephrons, whose glomeruli are located deep in the cortex close to the medulla. The major structural difference between the glomeruli in the two types of nephrons is the length of the

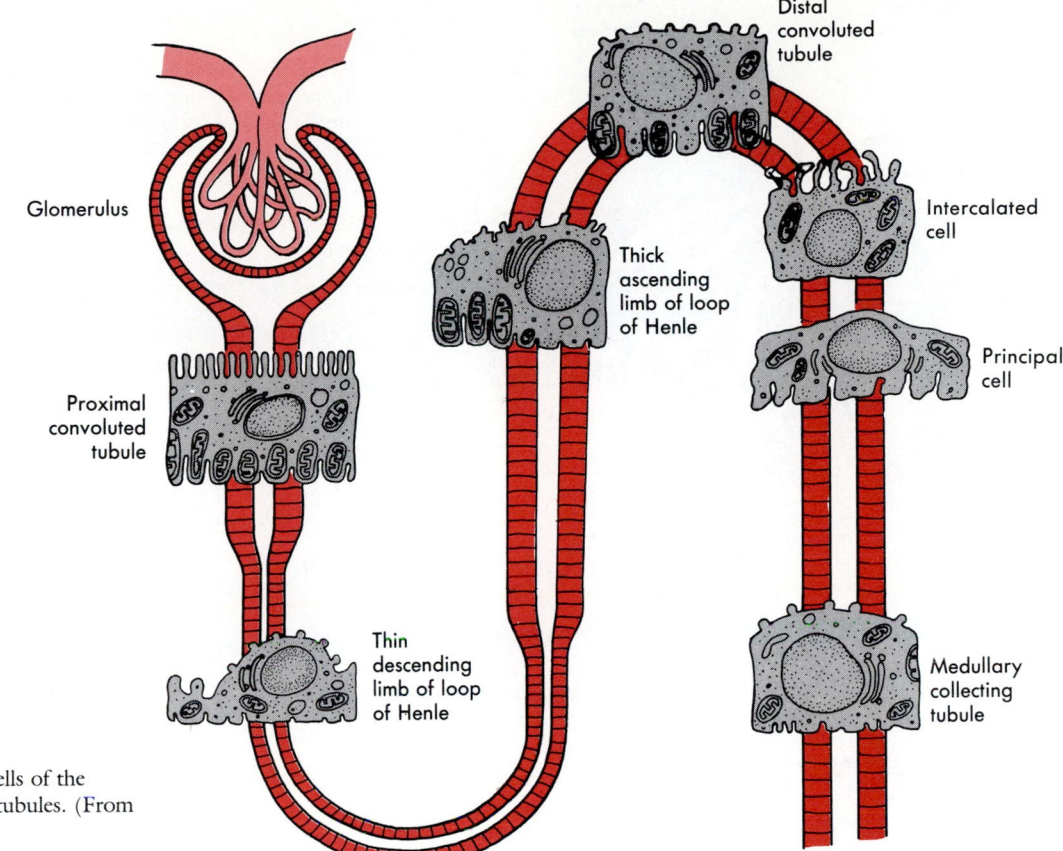

FIG. 32-4. The epithelial cells of the various segments of nephron tubules. (From Berne & Levy, 1988.)

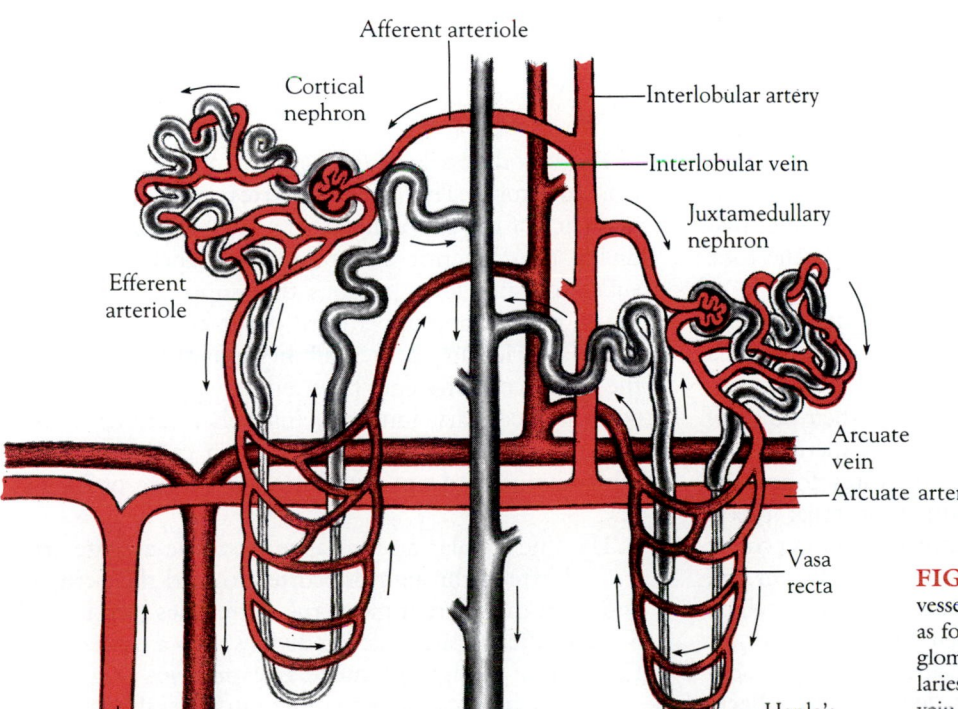

FIG. 32-5. The nephron unit with its blood vessels. Blood flows through nephron vessels as follows: interlobular artery afferent arteriole glomerulus efferent arteriole peritubular capillaries (around the tubules) venules interlobular vein. (From Thompson et al., 1989.).

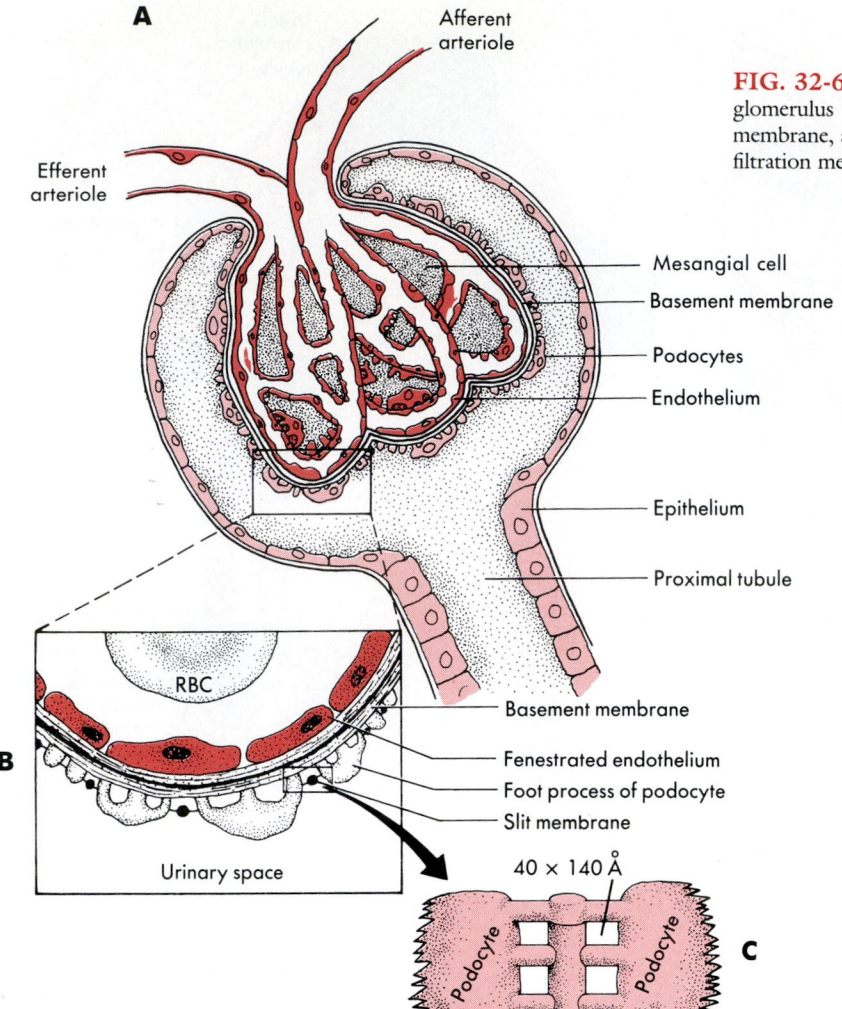

FIG. 32-6. Anatomy of the glomerulus. **A,** Cross section through glomerulus showing glomerular capillaries, endothelium, basement membrane, and podocytes of the epithelium. **B,** Expanded view of the filtration membrane. (From Berne & Levy, 1988).

loop of Henle. In cortical nephrons the loop is short and may not extend into the medulla. The loops of Henle for the juxtamedullary nephrons, however, may extend the whole length of the medulla (40 mm). Juxtamedullary nephrons represent about 12% of the total number of nephrons.

The transitional segment at the end of the ascending limb of the loop of Henle is known as the **macula densa.** Here the distal tubule passes between and contacts the afferent and efferent arterioles at their point of attachment to the macula densa's own glomerulus (see Fig. 32-3). The linkage of these structures forms the **juxtaglomerular apparatus.** Control of renal blood flow, glomerular filtration, and renin secretion occur at this site. Specialized cells in the walls of the afferent and efferent arterioles secrete the hormone renin, which contributes to the control of arterial blood pressure.

The **distal tubule** has straight and convoluted segments. It extends from the macula densa to the **collecting duct.** The collecting duct is a large tubule that descends down the cortex, through the renal pyramids of the inner and outer medulla, and into the minor calyx.

Blood Vessels of the Kidney

The blood vessels of the kidney closely parallel nephron structure. The **renal arteries** arise as the fifth branches of the abdominal aorta. At the renal hilus they divide into anterior and posterior branches and then subdivide into lobar arteries that supply blood to the lower, middle, and upper third of the kidney. The **interlobar arteries** are further subdivisions that travel down the renal columns and between the pyramids. At the cortical medullary junction, interlobar arteries branch into the **arcuate arteries,** which arch over the base of the pyramids and run parallel to the surface of the kidney.

The interlobular arteries arise from the arcuate arteries and extend through the cortex toward the periphery and form the afferent glomerular arterioles (see Fig. 32-5). The afferent arteriole subdivides into a fistlike structure of four to eight **glomerular capillaries** (Fig. 32-6). The glomerular capillaries empty into the efferent arteriole, which conveys blood to a second capillary bed, the peritubular capillaries. This is the only place in the body where an arteriole is positioned between two capillary

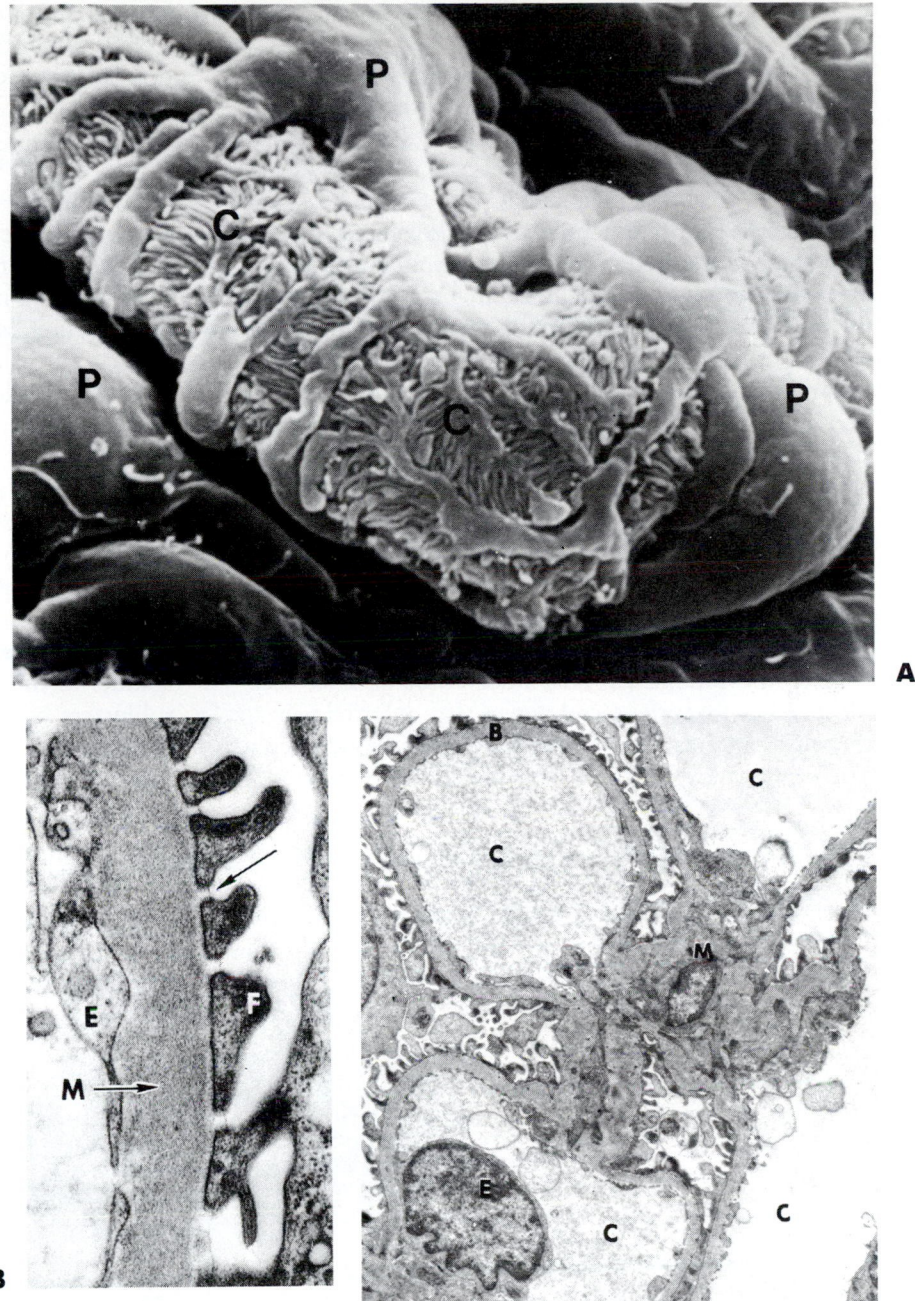

FIG. 32-7. A, Scanning electron micrograph of normal glomerular capillary *(C)* enclosed by podocytes *(P)* with primary processes and interdigitating foot processes. (×5200.) **B,** Glomerular capillary wall showing foot processes of endothelial podocytes *(F)* filtration slit membrane (arrow); basement membrane *(M)* and fenestrated endothelium *(E)*. (x40,000.) **C,** Portion of human glomerulus showing endothelial cell, E; mesangial cell, M; and capillaries *(C)*. Basement membrane (B) is somewhat thickened by hypertension. (×3600.) (From Kissane, 1985).

beds; this position is important for glomerular filtration.

The peritubular capillaries surround the convoluted portions of the proximal and distal tubules and the loop of Henle (see Fig. 32-5). The peritubular capillaries are adapted differently for the cortical and juxtamedullary nephrons. The peritubular capillaries surrounding the tubules of the cortical nephrons are similar to capillaries in other tissues. For the juxtamedullary nephrons, a network of capillaries called the **vasa recta** forms loops and closely follows the loops of Henle. The capillaries of the vasa recta are the only blood supply to the medulla. They influence the osmolar concentration of the medullary extracellular fluid, which is important to the formation of a concentrated urine. All capillaries then drain into the venous system. The renal veins follow the arterial path in a reverse direction and have the same names as the arteries. The lymphatic vessels tend also to follow the distribution of the blood vessels.

Urinary Structures
Ureters

The urine formed by the nephrons flows from the distal tubules and collecting ducts through the duct of Bellini, the **renal papillae** (projections of the ducts), and into the calyces and is collected in the renal pelvis (see Fig. 32-2). From the renal pelvis, urine is funneled into the **ureters.** Each adult ureter is approximately 30 cm long and is composed of long, intertwining muscle bundles. The lower ends of the ureters pass obliquely through the posterior aspect of the bladder wall. The close approximation of muscle cells permits the direct transmission of electrical stimulation, and the resulting peristaltic activity propels urine into the bladder. Peristaltic activity is affected by urine volume. When urine flow is slow, the contraction is segmented, with downward propulsion of urine. Increasing flow rates increase peristalsis. Peristalsis is maintained even when the ureter is denervated, so that ureters can be transplanted.

Sensory innervation for the upper part of the ureter arises from the tenth thoracic nerve roots, with referred pain to the umbilicus. The innervation of lower segments arises from the sacral nerves with referred pain to the vulva or penis. The ureters have a rich blood supply. The primary arteries come from the kidney with contri-butions from the lumbar and superior vesical artery. Contraction of the bladder during **micturition** (urination) compresses the lower end of the ureter, preventing reflux.

Bladder and Urethra

The **bladder** is a bag composed of a basket weave of smooth muscle fibers that forms the **detrusor muscle** and its smooth epithelial lining. The **trigone** is a smooth triangular area lying between the openings of the two ureters and the urethra (Fig. 32-8). The position of the bladder varies with age and sex. In infants and young children the bladder rises above the symphysis pubis, providing easy access for percutaneous aspiration. In adults it lies in the true pelvis, in front of the rectum and in front of the uterus in women. Inferiorly, the bladder sits on the prostate in men and on the anterior vagina in women. The bladder has a profuse blood supply, accounting for the bleeding that readily occurs with trauma, surgery, or inflammation.

The **urethra** extends from the inferior side of the bladder to the outside of the body. Two muscles called sphincters control excretion of urine from the bladder through the urethra. A ring of smooth muscle forms the **internal urethral sphincter** at the junction of the ure-

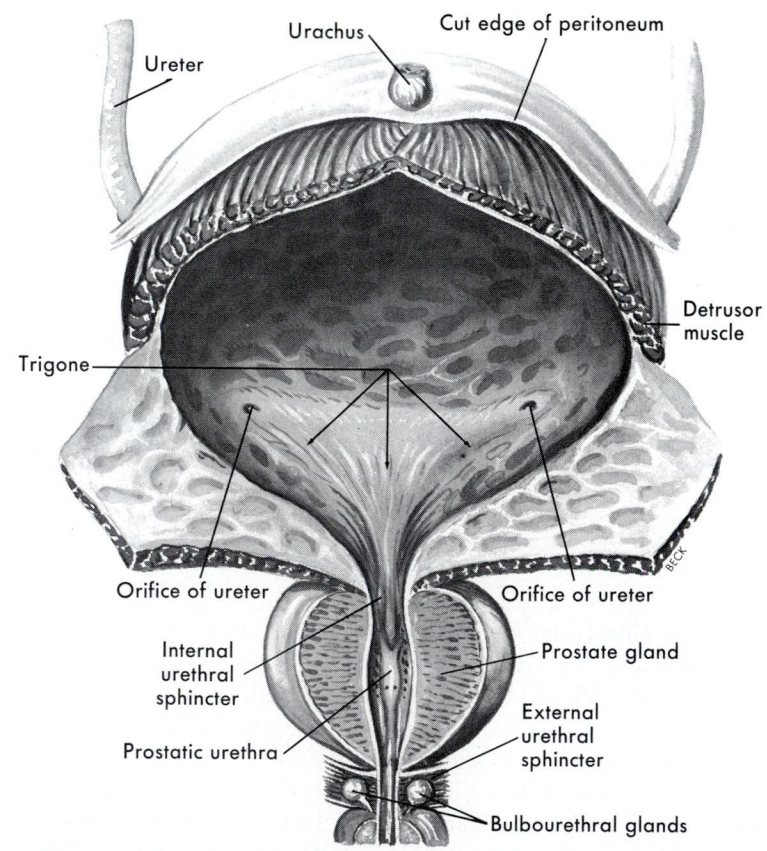

FIG. 32-8. The male urinary bladder cut to show the interior. (From Thibodeau, 1987.)

thra and bladder. The **external urethral sphincter** is composed of striated muscles and is under voluntary control. The entire urethra is lined with mucus-secreting glands. The female urethra is short (3 to 4 cm). The male urethra is long (18 to 20 cm) and has three segments: prostatic, membranous, and cavernous. The prostatic urethra is closest to the bladder. It passes through the prostate gland and contains the openings of the ejaculatory ducts. The membranous urethra is the segment that passes through the floor of the pelvis. The cavernous segment forms the remainder of the tube. The cavernous segment is surrounded by erectile tissue and contains the openings of the bulbourethral mucous glands.

The innervation of the bladder and internal urethral sphincter is supplied by parasympathetic fibers of the autonomic nervous system. They primarily pass with the arteries to and from the sacral levels of the spinal cord. Sensory fibers may extend as high as the T6 portion of the spinal cord. Motor fibers from the pudendal nerve supply the external urethral sphincter. The reflex arc required for micturition is stimulated by mechanoreceptors, which respond to stretching of tissue. The mechanoreceptors sense bladder fullness and send impulses to the sacral level of the cord with bladder filling. When the bladder accumulates 250 to 300 ml of urine, the bladder contracts, and the internal urethral sphincter relaxes through activation of the spinal reflex arc (known as the micturition reflex). At this time a person feels the urge to void. In older children and adults, the reflex can be inhibited or facilitated by impulses coming from the brain, resulting in voluntary control of micturition.

RENAL BLOOD FLOW

The kidneys are highly vascular organs and usually receive 1000 to 1200 ml of blood/min, or about 20% to 25% of the cardiac output. With a normal hematocrit of 45%, about 600 to 700 ml of blood flowing through the kidney per minute is plasma. From the renal plasma flow (RPF), 20% (about 120 to 140 ml/min) is filtered at the glomerulus and passes into Bowman's capsule. The filtration of the plasma per unit of time is known as the **glomerular filtration rate** (GFR), and the GFR is directly related to the perfusion pressure in the glomerular capillaries.

The remaining 80% (about 480 ml) of plasma flows through the efferent arterioles to the peritubular capillaries. The ratio of glomerular filtrate to renal plasma flow per minute (125/600 = 0.20) is called the filtration fraction. All but 1 to 2 ml of the glomerular filtrate is normally reabsorbed and returned to the circulation by the peritubular capillaries.

The GFR is directly related to renal blood flow

(RBF), which is regulated by intrinsic autoregulatory mechanisms, by neural regulation, and by hormonal regulation. In general, blood flow to any organ is determined by the arteriovenous pressure differences across the vascular bed. This relationship in the kidney is illustrated by the following formula:

Renal blood flow (RBF) =

$$\frac{\text{Mean arterial pressure (PA)} - \text{venous pressure (PV)}}{\text{Vascular resistance (R)}}$$

or

$$RBF = \frac{PA - PV}{R}$$

Autoregulation

In the kidney there is a local mechanism tending to keep the rate of blood flow and therefore the GFR fairly constant over a range of arterial pressures between 80 and 180 mm Hg (Fig. 32-9). This means that changes in afferent arteriolar resistance and arteriolar pressure occur in the same direction. Therefore RBF and GFR are relatively constant. This "constant" state is maintained by some intrinsic autoregulatory mechanism mediating the arteriolar resistance changes. The purpose of renal autoregulation is to prevent wide fluctuations in systemic arterial pressure from being transmitted to the glomerular capillaries. In this way, large fluctuations in GFR are prevented, and solute and water excretion is constantly maintained when arterial pressure changes.

One mechanism responsible for the autoregulatory response in the kidney is probably a myogenic mechanism. As arterial pressure declines, the stretch on the afferent arteriolar wall decreases and the arteriole relaxes, with an increase in renal blood flow; an increase in arteriolar pressure causes the arteriole to contract and de-

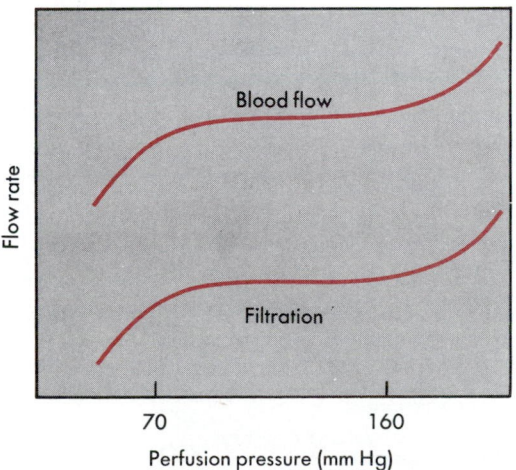

FIG. 32-9. Renal autoregulation. Blood flow and glomerular filtration rate are stabilized in the face of changes in perfusion pressure. (From Berne & Levy, 1988).

creases renal blood flow. Other mechanisms may operate to influence autoregulation, including changes in flow through the macula densa and the presence of metabolites (i.e., kinins and prostaglandins) (Brenner, Katz, & Ishikawa, 1986).

Neural Regulation

The blood vessels of the kidney are innervated by the autonomic nervous system through sympathetic fibers that cause vasoconstriction. The innervation of the kidney comes primarily from the celiac ganglion and greater splanchnic nerve (see Figure 12-23). Adrenergic fibers are mainly present and are generally distributed with the arteries and arterioles. The afferent and efferent arterioles are richly innervated, but nerves have not been observed in the glomerular capillaries.

The RBF is reflexly related to the systemic arterial pressure. When systemic arterial pressure decreases, increased renal sympathetic nerve activity is mediated re-

flexively through the carotid sinus and the baroreceptors of the aortic arch. This stimulates renal arteriolar vasoconstriction and decreases both RBF and GFR. Thus, RBF still changes when systemic arterial pressure is significantly reduced, although autoregulatory processes dampen the response. The decreased renal blood flow decreases the GFR and diminishes excretion of sodium and water, promoting an increase in blood volume and thus an increase in systemic pressure.

Exercise, body position, and hypoxia also influence RBF. Exercise and change of body position activate renal sympathetic neurons and cause mild vasoconstriction. Severe hypoxia stimulates the chemoreceptors of the carotid and aortic bodies and decreases RBF by means of sympathetic stimulation. Hemorrhage induces intense sympathetic stimulation and vasoconstriction and both glomerular filtration rate and blood flow are reduced.

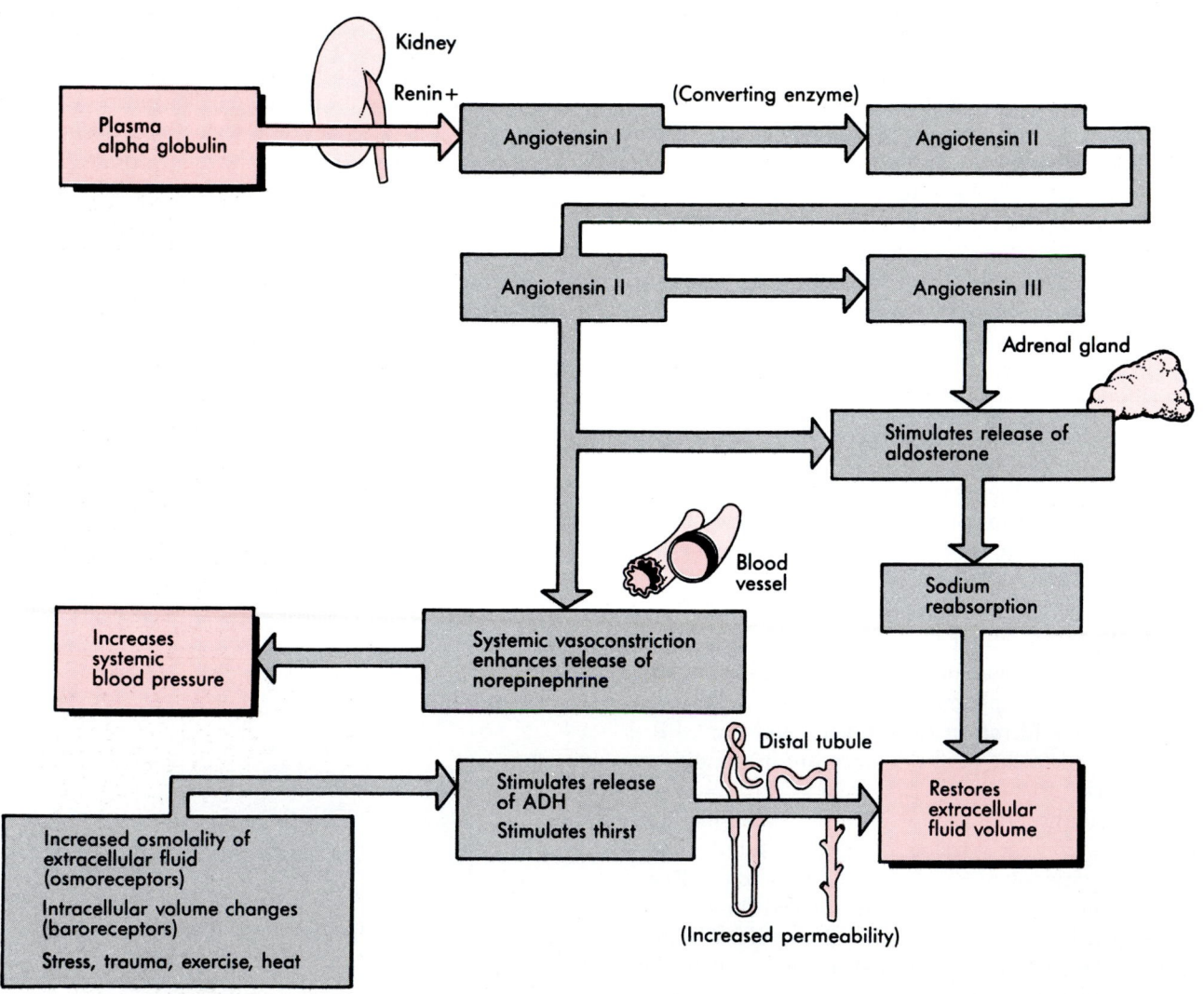

FIG. 32-10. Physiologic effects of renin-angiotensin system.

Hormonal Regulation

Hormonal factors can alter the resistance of the renal vasculature by stimulating vasodilation or vasoconstriction. A major hormonal regulator of renal blood flow is the **renin-angiotensin system,** which can increase systemic arterial pressure and change renal blood flow. Renin is an enzyme formed and stored in the cells of the arterioles of the juxtaglomerular apparatus (see Fig. 32-3). Several complex physiologic mechanisms stimulate the release of renin. These mechanisms are principally the following: decreased plasma sodium; decreased plasma potassium; decreased blood pressure in the afferent arterioles, which reduces stretch of the juxtaglomerular cells; and sympathetic nerve stimulation of β-adrenergic receptors on the juxtaglomerular cells (Re, 1987).

When renin is released, it cleaves an α-globulin (angiotensinogen) in the plasma to form angiotensin I, which is physiologically inactive. In the presence of a converting enzyme, angiotensin I is converted to angiotensin II and angiotensin III. Angiotensin II stimulates secretion of aldosterone by the adrenal cortex (see Chapter 17), is also a potent vasopressor, and inhibits renin release. Angiotensin III has less of an effect than angiotensin II. Numerous physiologic effects of the renin-angiotensin system serve the purpose of stabilizing systemic blood pressure and preserving the extracellular fluid volume during hypotension or hypovolemia, including sodium reabsorption, systemic vasoconstriction, sympathetic nerve stimulation, thirst stimulation, and drinking. (The effects are summarized in Fig. 32-10.)

Prostaglandins and kinins are other hormones that are formed in and act on the kidneys. The precise effect of locally produced prostaglandins is not clear, but different types of prostaglandins appear to have different actions. For example, prostaglandin E_2 in the kidney is a vasodilator.

KIDNEY FUNCTION

Nephron Function

The nephron is able to perform many functions simultaneously. It filters the plasma at the glomerulus and reabsorbs and secretes different substances at various parts of its tubular structure (Fig. 32-11). The function of the nephron is to form a filtrate of protein-free plasma. This process, known as **ultrafiltration,** occurs across the glomerular capillaries. The nephron then regulates the filtrate to maintain body fluid volume and electrolyte composition within narrow limits.

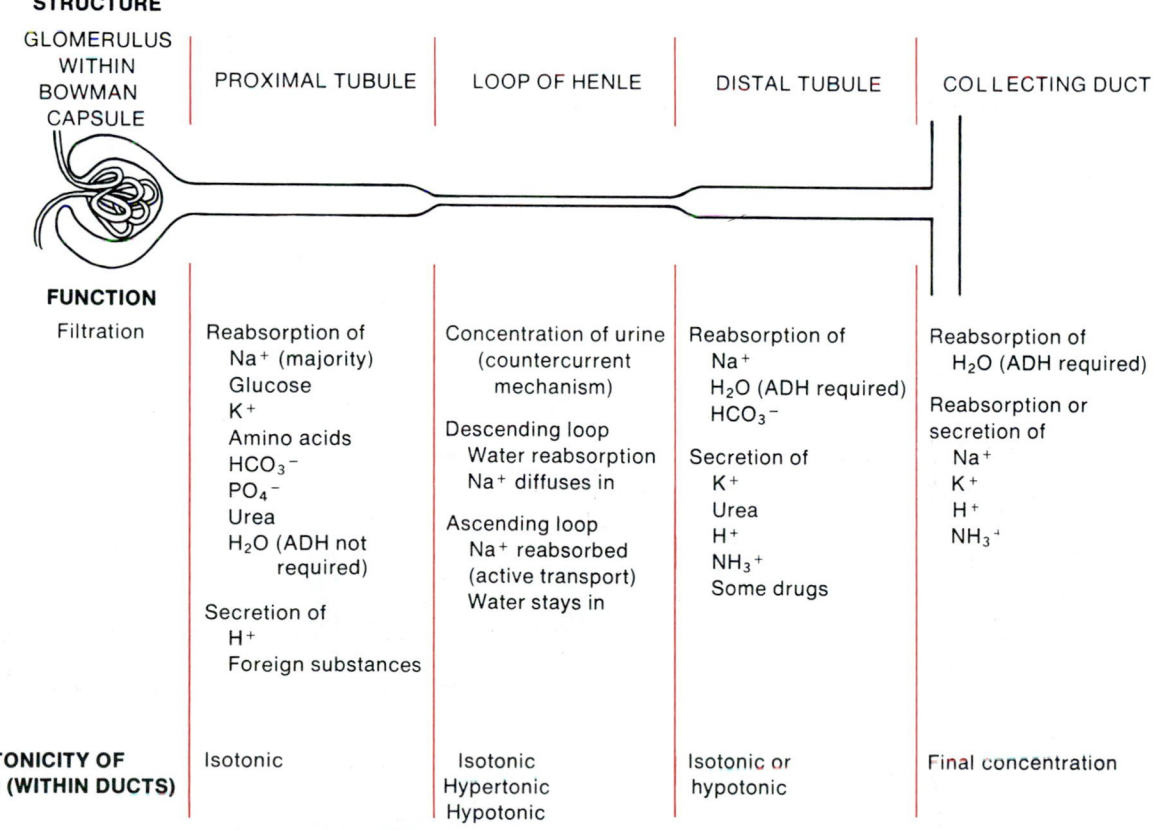

STRUCTURE				
GLOMERULUS WITHIN BOWMAN CAPSULE	PROXIMAL TUBULE	LOOP OF HENLE	DISTAL TUBULE	COLLECTING DUCT
FUNCTION				
Filtration	Reabsorption of Na⁺ (majority) Glucose K⁺ Amino acids HCO₃⁻ PO₄⁻ Urea H₂O (ADH not required) Secretion of H⁺ Foreign substances	Concentration of urine (countercurrent mechanism) Descending loop Water reabsorption Na⁺ diffuses in Ascending loop Na⁺ reabsorbed (active transport) Water stays in	Reabsorption of Na⁺ H₂O (ADH required) HCO₃⁻ Secretion of K⁺ Urea H⁺ NH₃⁺ Some drugs	Reabsorption of H₂O (ADH required) Reabsorption or secretion of Na⁺ K⁺ H⁺ NH₃⁺
TONICITY OF FLUID (WITHIN DUCTS)	Isotonic	Isotonic Hypertonic Hypotonic	Isotonic or hypotonic	Final concentration

FIG. 32-11. Major functions of nephron segments. (From Whaley & Wong, 1987).

Regulation of the filtrate occurs through two processes: tubular reabsorption and tubular secretion. **Tubular reabsorption** is the movement of fluids and solutes from the tubular lumen to the peritubular capillary plasma. Transfer of substances from the plasma of the peritubular capillary to the tubular lumen is **tubular secretion.** The transport mechanisms are both active and passive (processes defined in Chapter 3). The elimination of a substance in the final urine is known as **excretion** (Fig. 32-12).

Glomerular Filtration

The fluid filtered by the glomerular capillary filtration membrane is protein free but contains electrolytes such as sodium, chloride, and potassium and organic molecules such as creatinine, urea, and glucose in the same concentrations as in plasma. Like other capillary membranes, the glomerulus is freely permeable to water and relatively impermeable to large colloids such as plasma proteins. The size of the molecules and their electrical charge are important factors affecting the permeability

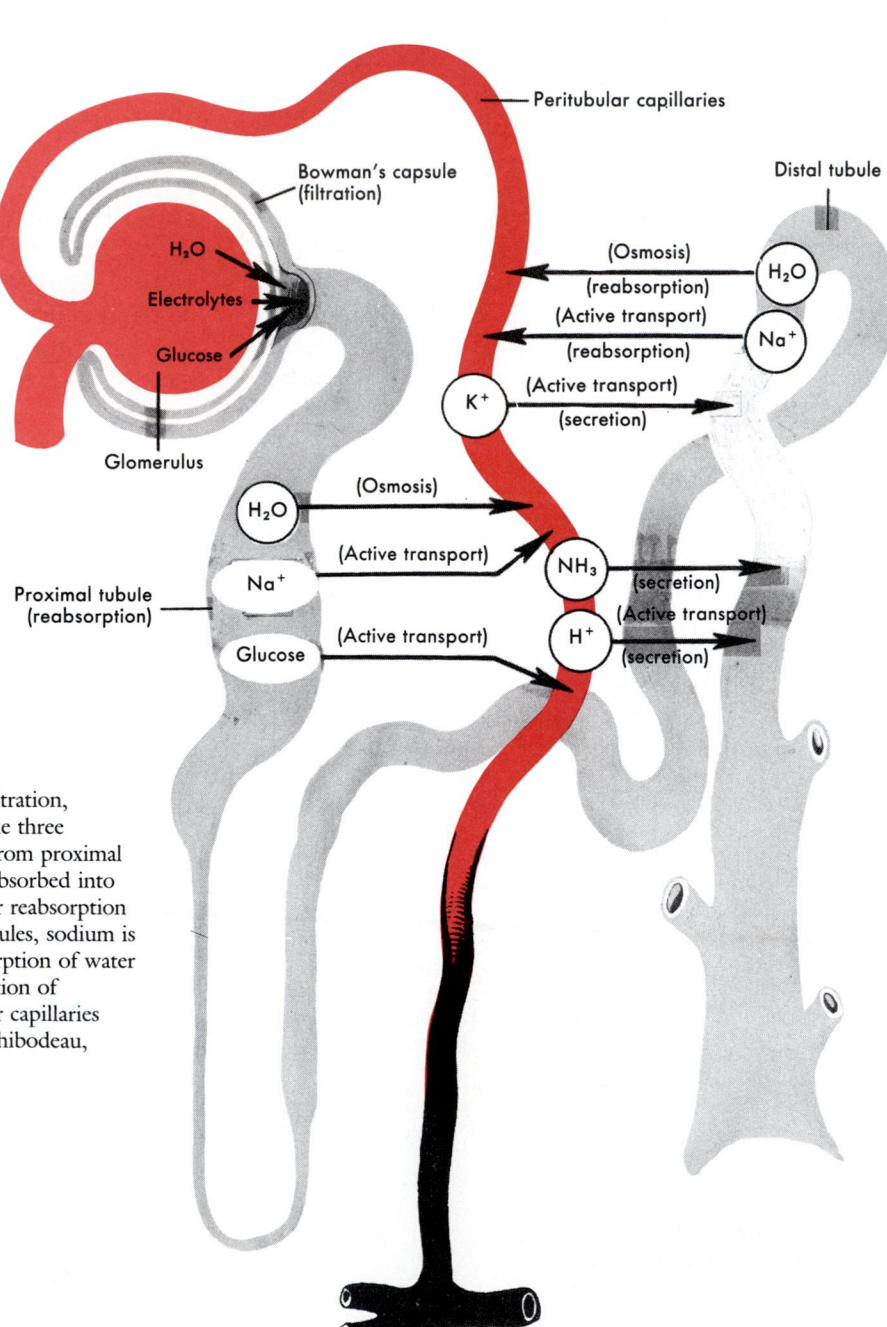

FIG. 32-12. Diagram showing glomerular filtration, tubular reabsorption, and tubular secretion—the three processes by which the kidneys excrete urine. From proximal convoluted tubules, sodium and glucose are reabsorbed into peritubular capillaries by active transport. Water reabsorption by osmosis follows. From distal convoluted tubules, sodium is reabsorbed by active transport. Osmotic reabsorption of water from them occurs when ADH is present. Secretion of ammonia and hydrogen occurs from peritubular capillaries into distal tubules by active transport. (From Thibodeau, 1987.)

of substances crossing the glomerulus. The small size of the filtration slits or pores in the membrane restricts the passage of proteins and other macromolecules. The negative charge along the filtration membrane further impedes the passage of negatively charged macromolecules (because like forces repel each other). Positively charged macromolecules therefore permeate the membrane more readily than neutrally charged particles.

Capillary pressure, as well as electrical charge, has an effect on glomerular filtration. The hydrostatic pressure within the capillary is the major force for inducing water and solutes across the filtration membrane and into Bowman's capsule. This pressure is determined indirectly by the efficiency of cardiac contraction and directly by the systemic arterial pressure and the resistances to blood flow in the afferent and efferent arterioles. Two forces oppose the filtration effects of the glomerular capillary hydrostatic pressure (P_{GC}): (1) the hydrostatic pressure in Bowman's space (P_{BC}) and (2) the effective oncotic pressure of the glomerular capillary blood (π_{GC}). (As explained in Chapter 3, hydrostatic presure is a pushing force in relation to water, and on-

cotic pressure is a pulling force.) Because the fluid in Bowman's space normally contains only minute amounts of protein, it does not normally have an oncotic influence on the plasma of the glomerular capillary (Fig. 32-13).

The combined effect of forces favoring and forces opposing filtration determines the filtration pressure. The **net filtration pressure** (NFP) is the sum of forces favoring and opposing filtration and is expressed by the following equation:

$$NFP = \underset{\substack{\text{Forces favoring} \\ \text{filtration}}}{[P_{GC} + \pi_{BC}]} - \underset{\substack{\text{Forces opposing} \\ \text{filtration}}}{[B_{BC} + \pi_{GC}]}$$

(The estimated values contributing to the forces of net filtration are presented in Table 32-1.)

As the protein-free fluid is filtered into Bowman's capsule, the plasma oncotic pressure rises, and the hydrostatic pressure falls. The increase in glomerular capillary oncotic pressure is great enough to reduce the net filtration pressure to zero at the efferent end of the cap-

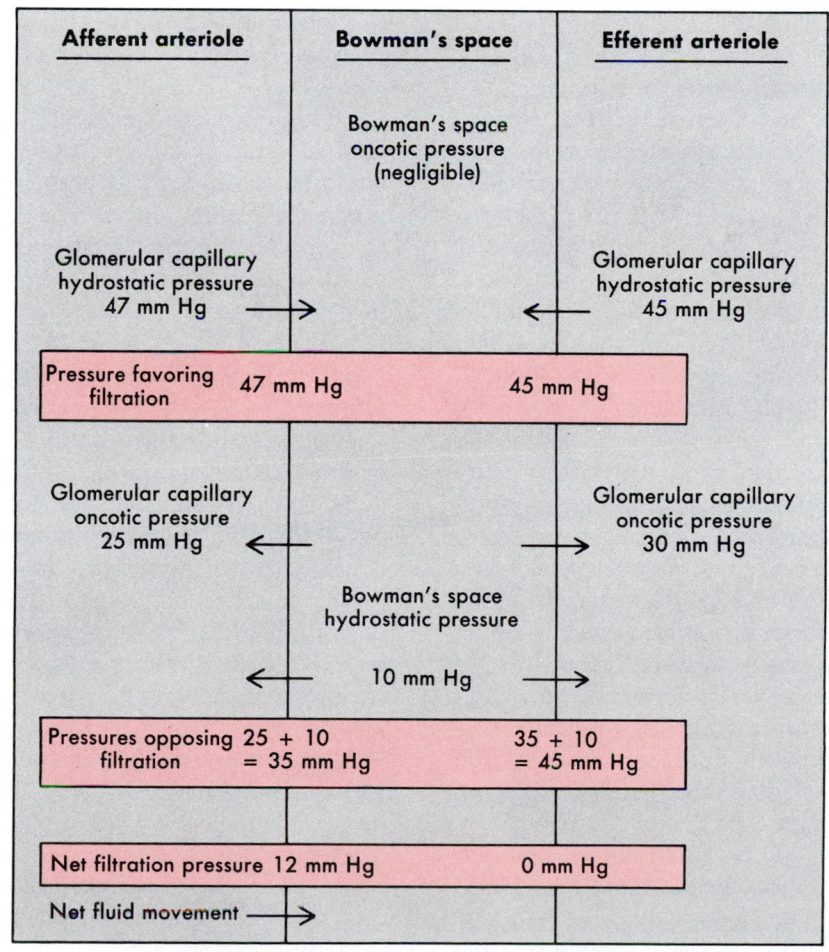

FIG. 32-13. Glomerular filtration pressures.

TABLE 32-1 Glomerular filtration pressures

| Forces | Pressures | Pressures (mm Hg) | |
		Beginning of capillary	End of capillary
Promoting filtration			
Glomerular capillary hydrostatic pressure	P_{GC}	47	45
Bowman's capsule oncotic pressure	π_{BC}	Negligible effect	
Opposing filtration			
Bowman's capsule hydrostatic pressure	P_{BC}	10	10
Glomerular capillary oncotic pressure	π_{GC}	25	35
Net filtration pressure		12	0

illary and to stop the filtration process effectively. The low hydrostatic pressure and increased oncotic pressure in the efferent arteriole are then transferred to the peritubular capillaries and facilitate reabsorption of fluid from the proximal tubules.

Filtration Rate

The total volume of fluid filtered by the glomeruli averages 180 L/day, or approximately 120 ml/min, a phenomenal amount considering the size of the kidneys. Because only 1 to 2 L of urine is excreted per day, 99% of the filtrate has been reabsorbed into the peritubular capillaries and returned to the blood. The factors determining the GFR are directly related to the pressures that favor or oppose filtration. Any changes in afferent or efferent arteriolar resistance will alter glomerular capillary hydrostatic pressure and GFR. Vasoconstriction of one or the other of these two arterioles will produce opposite effects on glomerular pressure. For example, if the afferent arteriole constricts, blood flow decreases with a corresponding drop in glomerular pressure. The GFR then decreases, and body fluids are conserved. On the other hand, constriction of the efferent arteriole increases the net filtration pressure, and the GFR rises. When both afferent and efferent arterioles constrict, little change occurs in filtration pressure, but renal blood flow is reduced.

Obstruction to the outflow of urine (caused by strictures, stones, or tumors along the urinary tract) can cause a retrograde increase in pressure at Bowman's capsule and a decrease in GFR. Excessive loss of protein-free fluid from vomiting, diarrhea, use of diuretics, or excessive sweating can increase glomerular capillary oncotic pressure and decrease the GFR. Renal disease can also cause changes in pressure relationships by altering capillary permeability and the surface area available for filtration (see Chapter 33).

Tubular Transport

By the end of the proximal tubule about 60% to 70% of filtered sodium and water and about 50% of urea have been reabsorbed, along with 90% or more of potassium, glucose, bicarbonate, calcium, phosphate, and uric acid. All this occurs by active transport. Chloride, water, and urea are reabsorbed passively but are linked to the active transport of sodium. Active transport in the renal tubules can be limited as the carrier molecules become saturated, a phenomenon known as **transport maximum** (Tm). Transport maximums exist for most substances actively transported by the tubular epithelium. The reabsorption of glucose is a significant example. Glucose is coupled to sodium transport and is almost completely reabsorbed in the proximal tubule. Like other actively transported substances, glucose has a maximal transport capacity, or renal threshold. This means that when the carrier molecules for glucose become saturated, the excess will be excreted in the urine. Normally, the plasma level and filtered glucose load are not high enough to saturate the carrier mechanism. When the plasma glucose reaches 180 mg/dl, however, as occurs in the individual with uncontrolled diabetes mellitus, the threshold for glucose is achieved. Any further increase in the plasma level causes loss of glucose in the urine.

Proximal Tubule Active reabsorption of sodium is the primary function of the proximal tubule. Water, most electrolytes, and organic substances are cotransported with sodium. The osmotic force generated by active sodium transport promotes the passive diffusion of water out of the tubular lumen and into the peritubular capillaries. Passive transport of water is further enhanced by the elevated oncotic pressure of the blood in the peritubular capillaries. The reabsorption of water leaves an increased concentration of urea within the tubular lumen, creating a gradient for its passive diffusion to the peritubular plasma.

As the positively charged sodium ions leave the tubular lumen, negatively charged chloride ions passively follow to maintain electroneutrality. Because the luminal membrane (the inside of the tubule) of the proximal tubular cell has a limited permeability to chloride, however, chloride reabsorption lags behind sodium.

Hydrogen ions are actively exchanged for sodium ions. The hydrogen ions (H+) then combine with bicarbonate (HCO_3^-). Bicarbonate is completely filtered at the glomerulus, and approximately 90% is reabsorbed in the proximal tubule. This process also occurs to a lesser extent in the ascending loop of Henle and the distal tubule.

In the tubular lumen hydrogen and bicarbonate ions form carbonic acid (H_2CO_3). The carbonic acid rapidly breaks down, or dissociates, to carbon dioxide (CO_2) and water (H_2O) in the presence of the enzyme carbonic anhydrase, which is in the luminal membrane. The CO_2 and H_2O then diffuse into the tubular cell, where carbonic anhydrase again catalyzes the CO_2 and H_2O to form HCO_3^- and H^+. The H_2CO_3 thus produces $H+$ and HCO_3^-. The $H+$ is secreted again, and HCO_3^- combines with sodium and is transported to the peritubular capillary blood.

Thus, because bicarbonate is not highly permeable at the peritubular capillary membrane, it is reabsorbed as $CO_2 + H_2O$, which are readily diffusable. One of the unusual aspects of this process is that the bicarbonate molecule filtered at the glomerulus is not the same molecule that is reabsorbed (because it dissociates) and the hydrogen ion secreted by the proximal tubule is not excreted in the urine. Bicarbonate is thus conserved, and the hydrogen is reabsorbed as water. Therefore these ions do not contribute to the urinary excretion of acid or the addition of acid to the blood (Fig. 32-14).

In addition to the proximal tubular secretion of hydrogen ions, secretory transport mechanisms exist for creatinine, other organic bases, and endogenous and exogenous organic acids including para-aminohippurate (PAH) and penicillin (Table 32-2). These secretory mechanisms are important for eliminating drugs and

TABLE 32-2 Substances transported by renal tubules	
Reabsorption	**Secretion**
Albumin	Choline
Ascorbate	Creatinine
Fructose	Histamine
Galactose	Methyl guanidine
Glutamate	Para-aminohippurate
Glucose	Penicillin
Phosphate	Steroid glucuronides
Sulfate	Thiamin
Xylose	

other exogenous chemical products from the body. Frequently, exogenous substances are conjugated with sulfate and glucuronic acid by the liver and then actively secreted by the renal tubules. This has important clinical implications because many drugs and their metabolites are eliminated from the body in this way. When the renal tubules are damaged, metabolic by-products and drugs may accumulate, causing toxic levels in the body.

Loop of Henle and Distal Tubule The filtrate entering and leaving the proximal tubule is essentially iso-osmotic with the plasma and has a concentration of about 285 mOsm. Although approximately 65% of salt and water are reabsorbed along the proximal tubule, they are reabsorbed in equal amounts, causing only minor changes in

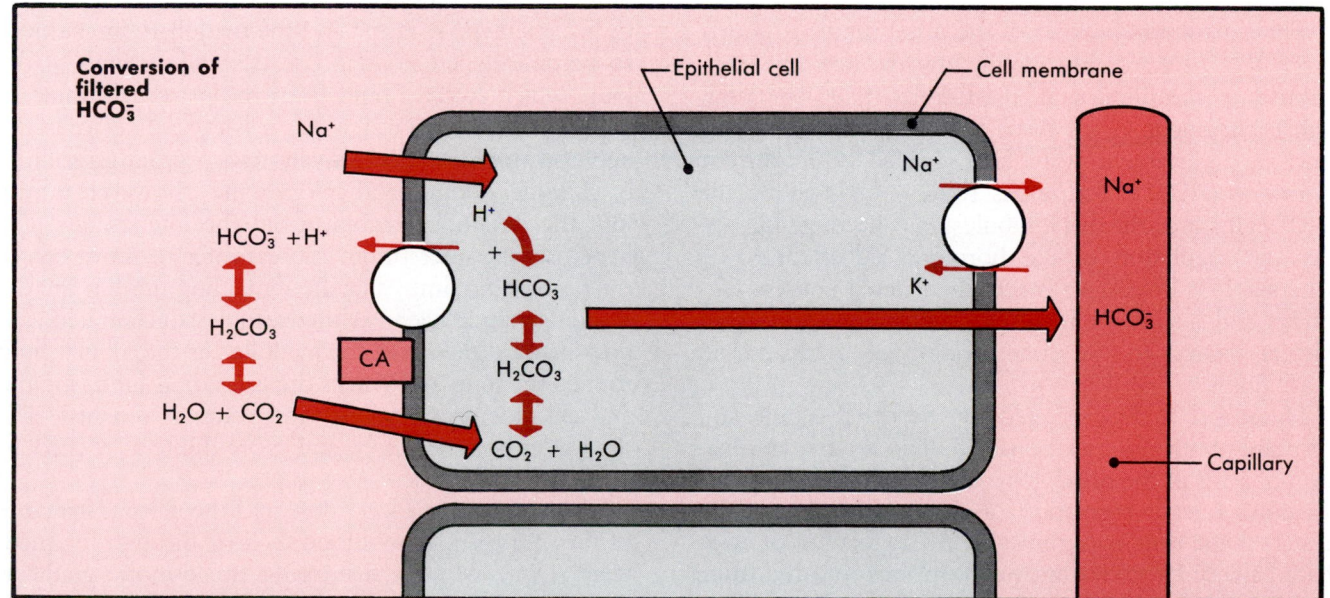

FIG. 32-14. Bicarbonate conservation. Filtered bicarbonate is reabsorbed by the tubular epithelium.

the osmotic and electrolyte concentrations of the fluid flowing into the loop of Henle. Therefore any concentration or dilution of urine occurs at more distal sites of the nephron, principally in the loop of Henle and collecting ducts.

These quantitative changes taking place in the loop of Henle are related to the length of the loop and its depth of penetration into the medulla. The structural features of the medullary hairpin loops provide the kidney with the ability to concentrate urine and conserve water for the body. The transition of the filtrate into urine is a function of the concentrating ability of the loops and final adjustments in urine compositon made by the distal tubule and collecting duct.

The primary function of the loop of Henle is to establish a hyperosmotic state within the medullary interstitial fluid. This is achieved by reabsorbing more solute than water into the interstitium. The fluid leaving the ascending limb of the loop is therefore hyposmotic, or more dilute than the fluid that entered. This dilution allows the distal tubule and collecting duct to make final adjustments in the concentration or dilution of the excreted urine according to body needs. The vasa recta act to maintain the high osmotic gradient established by the loop of Henle.

Different transport or permeability functions of the loop of Henle are important for dilution and concentration of urine. The thin, descending segment of the loop of Henle is highly permeable to water and moderately permeable to sodium, urea, and other solutes. The thin, ascending segment is more permeable to solutes and almost impermeable to water. The thick portion of the ascending segment is highly permeable to sodium, potassium, and chloride and significantly less permeable to water and urea.

The convoluted portion of the distal tubule is poorly permeable to water but readily absorbs ions and contributes to the dilution of the tubular fluid. The later, straight segment of the distal tubule and the collecting duct are permeable to water as controlled by antidiuretic hormone (ADH). Sodium is readily absorbed by the later segment of the distal tubule and collecting duct under the regulation of the hormone aldosterone (see Chapter 17). Potassium is actively secreted in these segments and is also controlled by aldosterone and other factors related to the concentration of potassium in body fluids.

Hydrogen is also secreted by the distal tubule and combines with nonbicarbonate buffers for the elimination of acids in the urine. (See Chapter 3 for further discussion of renal regulation of acid-base balance.) The distal tubule thus contributes to the regulation of acid-base balance by excreting hydrogen ions into the urine and by adding new bicarbonate to the plasma. The mechanism is similar to the conservation of bicarbonate

by the proximal tubule, except that the hydrogen ion is excreted in the urine. (The specific mechanisms of acid-base balance and acid excretion are described in Chapter 3.)

Glomerulotubular Balance

To regulate body fluid balance the kidney must not reabsorb or excrete too much water. Normally, 99% of the glomerular filtrate is reabsorbed. When the GFR decreases or increases, the renal tubules, primarily the proximal tubules, automatically adjust their rate of reabsorption of sodium and water to balance the change in GFR.

Concentration and Dilution of Urine

The production of a concentrated urine involves a **countercurrent exchange system,** in which a concentration gradient causes fluid to be exchanged across parallel pathways. In the nephron the fluid moves up and down the parallel sides of the hairpin loop of Henle in the medulla. The longer the loop, the greater the concentration gradient because the concentration gradient increases from the cortex to the tip of the medulla. The loops of Henle serve as multipliers of the concentration gradient, and the vasa recta acts as a countercurrent exchanger for maintaining the gradient.

Water, Sodium, and Chloride

The process is initiated in the thick ascending limb of the loop of Henle with the active transport of chloride and sodium out of the tubular lumen and into the medullary interstitium (Fig. 32-15). Because the lumen of the ascending limb is impermeable to water, water cannot follow the sodium-chloride transport. This lack of luminal permeability causes the ascending tubular fluid to become hypo-osmotic and the medullary interstitium to become hyperosmotic. The descending limb of the loop, which receives fluid from the proximal tubule, is highly permeable to water, but it is the only place in the nephron that does not actively transport either sodium or chloride. Sodium and chloride may, however, diffuse into the descending tubule from the interstitium. The hyperosmotic interstitium causes water to move out of the descending limb, and the remaining fluid in the descending tubule becomes increasingly concentrated as it flows toward the tip of the medulla. As the tubular fluid rounds the loop and enters the ascending limb, sodium and chloride are removed, and water is retained. The fluid then becomes more and more dilute as it encounters the distal tubule.

The slow rate of blood flow and the hairpin structure of the vasa recta allow blood to flow through the medullary tissue without disturbing the osmotic gradient. As blood flows into the descending limb of the vasa recta, it encounters the increasing osmotic concentration

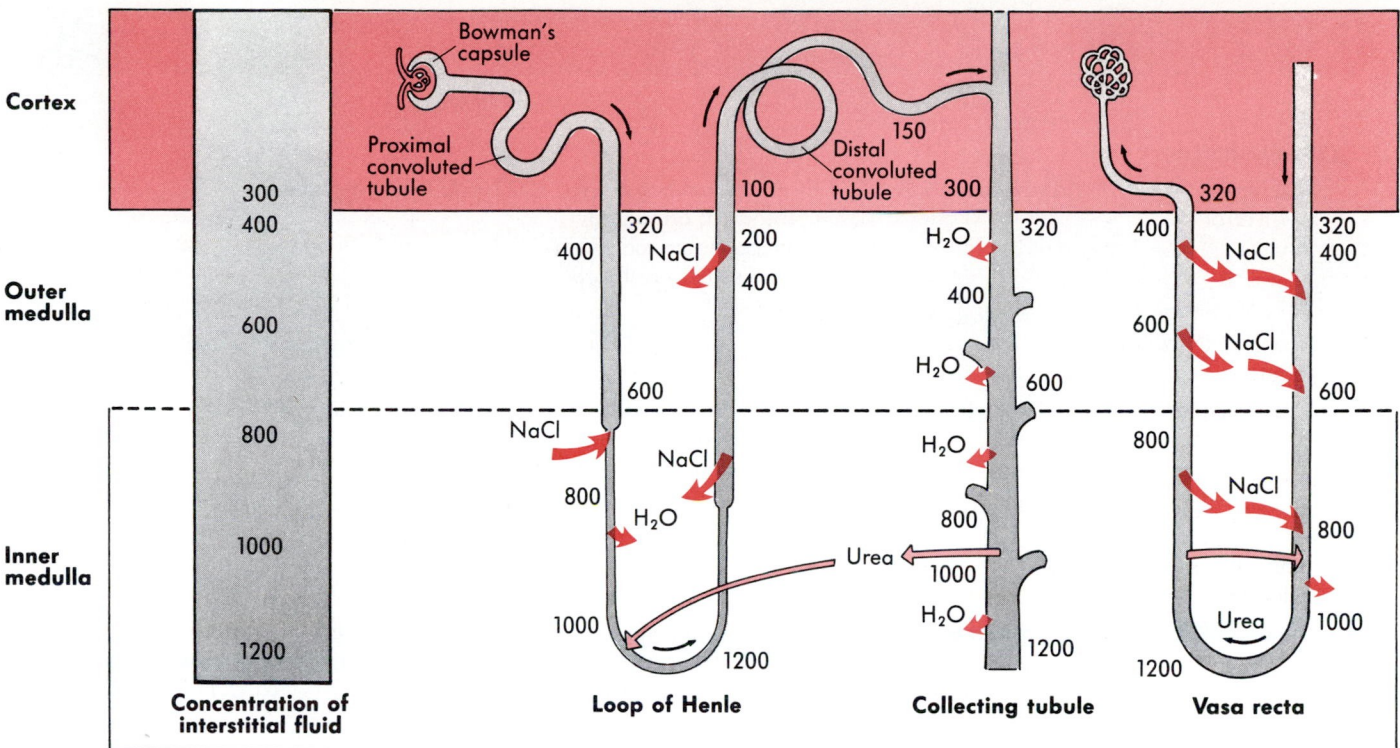

FIG. 32-15. Countercurrent mechanism for concentrating and diluting urine.

gradient of the medullary interstitium. Water moves out, and sodium and chloride diffuse into the descending vasa recta. The plasma becomes increasingly concentrated as it flows toward the tip of the medulla.

As the blood flow passes into the ascending limb and back toward the cortex, the surrounding interstitial fluid becomes comparatively more dilute. Water then moves back into the vasa recta, and sodium and chloride diffuse out. The net result is a preservation of the medullary osmotic gradient. If blood were to flow rapidly through the vasa recta, as occurs in some renal diseases, the medullary concentration gradient would be washed away, and the ability to concentrate urine and conserve water would be lost. The efficiency of water conservation is related to the length of the loops: the longer the loops, the greater the ability to concentrate the urine. Many desert animals have very long loops and can reabsorb water so efficiently that they rarely need to drink.

Urea

Urea is an end-product of protein metabolism and is the major constituent of urine along with water. The glomerulus freely filters urea, and tubular reabsorption of urea depends on urine flow rate with less reabsorption at higher flow rates. About 50% of urea is excreted in the urine and 50% is recycled within the kidney. The recycling of urea from the tubules and collecting ducts contributes to an osmotic gradient within the medulla and is necessary for the concentration and dilution of urine. Because urea is an end-product of protein metabolism, individuals with protein deprivation will not be able to maximally concentrate their urine.

Antidiuretic Hormone (ADH)

The distal tubule in the cortex receives the hypo-osmotic urine from the ascending limb of the loop of Henle. The concentration of the final urine is controlled by antidiuretic hormone (ADH). ADH increases water permeability in the last segment of the distal tubule and along the entire length of the collecting ducts, which pass through the inner and outer zones of the medulla.

In the presence of ADH, water reabsorption is high. Most of the water is reabsorbed in the medullary collecting ducts because of the high osmotic gradient in the medullary interstitium. The water diffuses into the ascending limb of the vasa recta and returns to the systemic circulation. The excreted urine can have a high osmotic concentration, up to 1400 mOsm. The volume is normally reduced to about 1% of what was filtered at the glomerulus.

ADH secretion is therefore one cause of **oliguria,** or diminished excretion of urine that is less than 400 ml/day or 30 ml/hr. Fluid imbalance may be related to the syndrome of inappropriate secretion of ADH, which is a cause of water excess (see Chapter 3).

TABLE 32-3 Action of diuretics

Diuretic	Site of action	Action	Side effects
Osmotic diuretic:			
Mannitol Glycerol Urea	Proximal tubule	Freely filtered but not re-absorbed; osmotically attacks water and diminishes sodium reabsorption	Hypokalemia, dehydration
Carboninic anhydrase inhibitors:			
Acetaxolamide	Proximal tubule	Inhibits carbonic anhydrase; blocks hydrogen ion secretion and reabsorption of sodium and bicarbonate	Hypokalemia, systemic acidosis, alkaline urine
Inhibitors of sodium/ chloride reabsorption:			
Thiazides	Between end of ascending loop and beginning of distal tubule	Blocks sodium and chloride reabsorption; mildly suppresses carbonic anhydrase	Hypokalemia, metabolic alkalosis
Furosemide Ethacrynic acid Bumetanide	Thick ascending limb of Henle's loop	Blocks active transport of chloride, sodium, and potassium	Hypokalemia, uric acid retention
	Cortical vasodilation	Increased rate of urine formation	Hypokalemia, uric acid retention
Aldosterone antagonists:			
Spironolactone	Distal tubule	Inhibits aldosterone, blocks sodium reabsorption, and results in potassium retention	Hyperkalemia, nausea, confusion, gynecomastia
Triamterene and amiloride	Distal tubule	Blocks sodium reabsorption and inhibits potassium excretion	Nausea, vomiting, headache, granulocytopenia, skin rash

In the absence of ADH, **water diuresis,** an increase in excretion of a highly dilute urine, takes place. The distal tubules and collecting ducts become impermeable to water. Water remains in the tubular lumen and is excreted as a dilute and large volume of urine. Because ADH has no effect on sodium reabsorption, it continues to be actively transported from the distal tubule. (The mechanism for the regulation of ADH and plasma osmolality is described in Chapter 3.)

Diuretics as a Factor in Urine Flow

A **diuretic** is any agent that enhances the flow of urine. Clinically, diuretics interfere with renal sodium reabsorption and reduce extracellular fluid volume. Di-

uretics are commonly used to treat hypertension and edema caused by heart failure, cirrhosis, and nephrotic syndrome.

Different diuretics affect different sites of tubular function and may produce side effects that alter acid-base and electrolyte balance. Therefore health professionals need to understand their indications for use, mechanisms of action, and toxic side effects. Diuretics are divided into four general categories: (1) osmotic diuretics, (2) carbonic anhydrase inhibitors (inhibitors of urinary acidification), (3) inhibitors of loop sodium or chloride transport, and (4) aldosterone antagonists. (The physiologic mechanism related to each category is summarized in Table 32-3.)

Renal Hormones

Certain hormones are either activated or synthesized by the kidney. These hormones have significant systemic effects and include the active form of vitamin D, erythropoietin, and natriuretic hormone.

Vitamin D

Vitamin D is a hormone that can be obtained in the diet or synthesized by the action of ultraviolet radiation on cholesterol in the skin. These forms of vitamin D_3 (cholecalciferol) are inactive and require two hydroxylations to establish a metabolically active form. The first step occurs in the liver with hydroxylation at the twenty-fifth carbon, and the second hydroxylation occurs at the first carbon position in the kidneys. The end product is l,25 dihydroxycholecalciferol, or more simply l,25 dihydroxy vitamin D_3 (1,25 OH_2D_3).

Vitamin D is necessary for the absorption of calcium and phosphate by the small intestine. The renal hydroxylation step is stimulated by parathyroid hormone. A decreased plasma calcium level (less than l0 mg/ldl) stimulates the secretion of parathyroid hormone. Parathyroid hormone then stimulates a sequence of events that help restore plasma calcium back toward normal:

Calcium mobilization from bone

Synthesis of l,25 dihydroxy vitamin D
↓
Absorption of calcium from the intestine
↓
Increased renal calcium reabsorption
↓
Decreased renal phosphate reabsorption.

Serum phosphate fluctuations also influence the renal hydroxylation of vitamin D. Decreased levels stimulate active 1,25 OH_2D_3 formation and increased levels inhibit formation. This results in compensatory changes in phosphate absorption from bone and the intestine. The clinical significance of the role of the kidney in calcium and phosphate metabolism is evident in renal disease. Patients with renal disease will have a deficiency of 1,25 OH_2D_3 and manifest symptoms of disturbed calcium and phosphate balance (Chapter 3).

Erythropoietin

Erythropoietin stimulates the bone marrow to produce red blood cells in response to tissue hypoxia. (Erythrocyte production is discussed in Chapter 22.) The stimulus for erythropoietin release is decreased oxygen delivery in the kidneys. The anemia of chronic renal failure, where kidney cells have become nonfunctional, may be related to the lack of this hormone.

Natriuretic Hormone

A substance called atrial natriuretic hormone (ANF) probably also contributes to the loss of sodium and water and the regulation of fluid balance (see Chapter 3). When ECF volume is expanded, ANF secretion is increased, sodium reabsorption is depressed, and increased amounts of sodium and water will be excreted in the urine. Natriuretic hormone is released from cardiocyte granules located in the atria of the heart in response to increased atrial stretch (Genest & Cantin, 1986).

TESTS OF RENAL FUNCTION

The Concept of Clearance

A number of specific renal functions can be measured by renal clearance. Renal clearance techniques determine how much of a substance can be cleared from the blood by the kidneys per given unit of time. The application of this principle permits an indirect measure of GFR, tubular secretion, tubular reabsorption, and renal blood flow.

Clearance and Glomerular Filtration Rate

The GFR provides the best estimate of functioning renal tissue. Loss or damage to nephrons leads to a corresponding decrease in GFR. The measurement of GFR requires use of a substance that has a stable plasma concentration, is freely filtered at the glomerulus, and is not secreted, reabsorbed, or metabolized by the tubules. Inulin (a fructose polysaccharide) is one substance that meets the criteria for measurement of GFR.

The kidney "clears" inulin from the plasma by filtering it at the glomerulus, reabsorbing nearly all of the fluid, and excreting the inulin left behind in the urine. The amount of inulin filtered is equal to the volume of plasma filtered (GFR) multiplied by the plasma concentration of inulin (P_{in}). The amount of inulin in the urine is equal to a volume of urine per unit of time ($\dot{V}$) (usually 24 hours) multiplied by the inulin concentration of urine (U_{in}). Because all the inulin filtered is excreted in the urine:

$$GFR \times P_{in} = U_{in} \times \dot{V}$$

GFR can be calculated by rearranging the formula:

$$GFR(ml/min) = \frac{U_{in} \times \dot{V}}{P_{in}}$$

The accurate determination of inulin clearance requires constant infusion to maintain a stable plasma level. This is time-consuming and inconvenient. Therefore the clearance of creatinine, a natural substance produced by muscle and released into the blood at a relatively constant rate, is commonly used clinically. It is freely filtered at the glomerulus, but a small amount is secreted by the renal tubules. Therefore creatinine clearance overestimates the GFR but within tolerable limits. Creatinine clearance provides a good measure of GFR because only one blood sample is required in addition to a 24 hour volume of urine. The GFR estimated by creatinine clearance is

$$GFR \times \frac{U_{cr}\dot{V}}{P_{cr}}$$

Similar calculations can be made for all solutes excreted in the urine per unit of time. Substances freely filtered at the glomerulus but with a clearance less than inulin or creatinine have been reabsorbed along the tubules. For example glucose is completely reabsorbed and has a clearance rate of nearly zero. Conversely, substances secreted by the tubules have a clearance rate greater than inulin or creatinine (i.e., greater than 1.0).

Clearance and Renal Blood Flow

The standard clearance formula can also be used to estimate renal plasma flow (RPF) and renal blood flow (RBF). The substance used for this evaluation is para-aminohippurate (PAH). Some PAH is filtered at the glomerulus, and most of the remainder is secreted into the tubules in one circulation through the kidney. If all of the PAH were removed from the plasma during a single pass through the kidney, then total renal plasma flow could be determined. Since the supporting and nonsecreting structures of the kidney receive 10% to 15% of renal blood flow, clearance of PAH (CPAH) only measures what is known as the **effective renal plasma flow** (ERPF), which is 85% to 90% of the true renal plasma flow:

$$ERBF = \frac{ERPF}{1 - Hematocrit} \quad (1.0 - .45)$$

The estimation of effective renal blood flow (ERBF) can then be calculated by considering the hematocrit in the formula:

$$ERPF = C_{PAH} = \frac{U_{PAH}\dot{V}}{B_{PAH}}$$

Blood Tests
Plasma Creatinine Concentration

A chronic decline in the GFR over weeks or months is reflected in the **plasma creatinine (P_{cr}) concentration** (normal value = 0.7 to 1.2 mg/dl). The P_{cr} concentration will have a stable value when the GFR is sta-

ble because creatinine has a constant rate of production as a product of muscle metabolism. The amount filtered is about equal to the amount excreted. When the GFR declines, the P_{cr} will rise proportionately. Thus the GFR and P_{cr} are inversely related. If the GFR were to decrease by 50%, the filtration and excretion of creatinine would be reduced by 50%, and creatinine would accumulate in plasma to twice the normal value. Therefore elevated P_{cr} values represent decreasing GFR. In the new steady state, however, the total amount of creatinine excreted in the urine would remain the same because of the proportionate decrease in GFR and increase in P_{cr}.

The application of this principle is simple and useful for monitoring progressive changes in renal function. The test is most valuable for monitoring the progress of chronic rather than acute renal disease because it takes 7 to 10 days for the plasma creatinine level to stabilize when GFR declines. Serial measures can be obtained over a long time and plotted as a curve of glomerular function. The P_{cr} also becomes elevated during trauma or breakdown of muscle tissue. In such instances the value is then not useful for estimating GFR.

Blood Urea Nitrogen

The concentration of urea nitrogen in the blood reflects glomerular filtration and urine-concentrating capacity. Because urea is filtered at the glomerulus, blood urea nitrogen (BUN) levels rise as glomerular filtration drops. Because urea is reabsorbed by the blood through the permeable tubules, the BUN rises in states of dehydration and acute and chronic renal failure when passage of fluid through the tubules is slowed. BUN also changes as a result of altered protein intake and protein catabolism. The normal range for BUN in the adult is 10 to 20 mg/dl of blood.

Urinalysis

Urinalysis is a noninvasive and relatively inexpensive diagnostic procedure. The best results are obtained from a fresh, clearly voided specimen, because decay permits changes in the composition of urine. Urinalysis includes evaluation of color, turbidity, protein, pH, specific gravity, sediment, and supernatant.

Urine normally has a clear light yellow color because of urochrome and other pigments. When formed substances (crystals, blood cells, or casts) are in the urine, it appears turbid. Protein in the urine creates marked foaming when shaken, and the foam will be yellow when the urine contains bile pigments.

Urine pH normally ranges between 5.0 and 6.5 but may vary from 4.5 to 8.0. Urine is more alkaline after eating and then declines before the next meal. Because sleep is accompanied by intermittent hypoventilation, a person will produce more acidic urine after awakening.

Specific Gravity

Specific gravity is an estimated measure of the solute concentration of the urine. Specific gravity of any solution is measured by comparing the weight of the solution compared to an equal volume of distilled water. Hence, specific gravity is not a true measure of the number or concentration of particles but it correlates well with osmolality and is a useful clinical tool. Specific gravity is usually measured with a hydrometer in a cylinder of urine; the normal value is 1.016 to 1.022.

The final urine osmolality is primarily a function of ADH, which controls water reabsorption in the collecting ducts. If the kidney is unable to concentrate or dilute urine, given a stimulus, the cause is usually a malfunction of the renal tubules or inappropriate ADH secretion by the posterior pituitary gland. The state of hydration also affects the urine specific gravity, so that hydration status should be evaluated before making a diagnosis. This determination is helpful for differentiating oliguria caused by intrinsic renal disease from hypovolemia as a result of dehydration.

Urine Sediment

The urine sediment is examined microscopically and may contain cells, casts, crystals, and bacteria. Epithelial cells may be seen in the microscopic field as they are shed naturally throughout the urinary tract.

Red Blood Cells

Normal urine contains few or no red blood cells. If large numbers of red cells are present, this is known as **hematuria** and the sediment may be red. An alkaline or hypotonic urine causes lysis of red cells, however, so that the cells will not be seen. Urine then will be positive for hemoglobin, and the specific gravity will be elevated. Hematuria can occur with the administration of anticoagulants and with several renal diseases.

Casts

Casts (accumulations of cellular precipitates) originate in the renal tubules, from which they take their shape. They are cylindric with distinct borders. All casts have a precipitated microprotein matrix and arise primarily from the ascending limb of the distal tubule. Red cell casts indicate bleeding into the tubules; white cell casts are associated with an inflammatory process. Epithelial cell casts indicate degeneration of the tubular lumen or necrosis of the renal tubules. The type of cast identified suggests the disease process occurring in the kidney.

Crystals

Numerous kinds of crystals can be observed in the urine. They may be composed of cystine, uric acid, calcium oxalate, or phosphate. They may not be initially observable, but as the urine cools, crystals will form.

Crystals tend to form in a concentrated acidic or alkaline urine. Generally, they are not clinically significant. Crystal formation is diagnostically significant, usually indicating inflammation, infection, or a metabolic disorder.

White Blood Cells

White blood cells (WBC) in the urine (a condition termed **pyuria**) are primarily indicative of urinary tract infection, particularly when bacteria are present. Glomerulonephritis and nephrotic syndrome may also demonstrate pyuria but usually in combination with proteinuria, red cells, and casts. The finding of white blood cell casts reflects a kidney infection, because these casts are not formed in the bladder or prostate. The presence of white cells in the urine should be followed by a culture for specific identification of bacteria and sensitivity of bacteria to antibiotics.

AGING AND RENAL FUNCTION

Throughout life the kidney responds to an increased work load by compensatory hypertrophy. This hypertrophy is marked in individuals who have donated a kidney for transplant or have lost functioning nephrons from trauma or disease. The glomeruli increase in diameter, and the tubules enlarge effectively to maintain the regulatory functions of the kidney. Hypertrophy occurs more rapidly and with a larger size increase in younger individuals and in those with high protein intake.

Changes in the kidneys occur throughout life, with a linear decrease in renal blood flow and GFR. With aging, the number of nephrons decreases. The primary mechanism appears to be a change in the renal vasculature and perfusion pattern, which leads to a reduction in numbers of nephrons. The rate of nephron loss accelerates between 40 and 80 years. By 75 years of age the nephron population will be reduced by 30% to 50%. Degenerative changes within nephrons also occur with aging. The glomerular capillaries atrophy with a reduction in the branching vessels. The glomeruli may then disappear completely. The arcuate and interlobular arteries become tortuous, contributing to ischemia. The loss of the glomerular tuft may cause a shunt between the afferent and efferent arterioles. Although loss of juxtaglomerular nephrons still allows the vasa recta to be perfused, the combination of events contributes to a decreasing ability to excrete a concentrated urine. Thus the specific gravity of the urine in older individuals tends to be on the low side of normal.

Tubular transport changes with aging. Glucose and bicarbonate are not as efficiently reabsorbed. Response to acid or base loads is delayed and prolonged. Sudden or large changes in pH or fluid load may lead to serious imbalances. Thus acute losses or chronic fluid deficits can lead to renal insufficiency in the elderly person. Administration of drugs eliminated by renal processes may require dose modifications and more astute observations for toxic side effects. The T_m for glucose reabsorption decreases with age, contributing to a greater amount of glucose in the urine. This is an important consideration when glycosuria is used for screening or monitoring the process of diabetes mellitus in the elderly. These changes occur independently of disease, however, indicating a normal process of aging. Previous or concurrent renal disease or urinary tract obstruction may amplify age-related changes in function.

SUMMARY REVIEW

Structures of the Renal System

1 The kidneys are paired structures lying bilaterally between the twelfth thoracic and third lumbar vertebrae.
2 The kidney is composed of an outer cortex and an inner medulla.
3 The calyces join to form the renal pelvis, which is continuous with the upper end of the ureter.
4 The nephron is the urine-forming unit of the kidney and is composed of the glomerulus, proximal tubule, hairpin loops of Henle, distal tubule, and collecting duct.
5 The glomerulus contains loops of capillaries. The capillary walls serve as a filtration membrane for the formation of the primary urine.
6 The proximal tubule is lined with microvilli to increase surface area and enhance reabsorption.
7 The hairpin loops of Henle transport solutes and water, contributing to the hypertonic state of the medulla.
8 The distal tubule adjusts acid-base balance by excreting acid into the urine and forming new bicarbonate ions.
9 The ureters extend from the renal pelvis to the posterior wall of the bladder. Urine flows through the ureters by means of peristaltic contraction of the ureteral muscles.
10 The bladder is a bag composed of the detrusor and trigone muscles and innervated by parasympathetic fibers. When accumulation of urine reaches 250 to 300 ml, mechanoreceptors, which respond to stretching of tissue, stimulate the micturition reflex.

Renal Blood Flow

1 Renal blood flows at about 1000 to 1200 ml/min, or 20% to 25% of the cardiac output.
2 Blood flow through the glomerular capillaries is maintained at a constant rate in spite of a wide range of arterial pressures.
3 The glomerular filtration rate (GFR) is the filtration of plasma per unit of time and is directly related to the perfusion pressure of renal blood flow.
4 Autoregulation of renal blood flow and neural regulation of vasoconstriction maintain a constant CFR.
5 Renin is an enzyme secreted from the juxtaglomerular apparatus and causes the generation of angiotensin, a potent vasoconstrictor. The renin-angiotensin system is thus a regulator of renal blood flow.

Kidney Function

1 The major function of the nephron is urine formation, which involves the processes of glomerular filtration, tubular reabsorption, and tubular secretion and excretion.
2 Glomerular filtration is favored by capillary hydrostatic pressure and opposed by oncotic pressure in the capillary and hydrostatic pressure in Bowman's capsule. The balance of favoring and opposing filtration forces is known as net filtration pressure (NFP).
3 The GFR is approximately 120 ml/min, and 99% of the filtrate is reabsorbed.
4 The proximal tubule reabsorbs about 60% to 70% of the filtered sodium and water and 90% of other electrolytes.
5 Since most molecules are reabsorbed by active transport, the carrier mechanism can become saturated at a point known as the transport maximum (T_m). Molecules not reabsorbed are excreted with the urine.
6 The distal tubules actively reabsorb sodium and secrete potassium and hydrogen for the regulation of electrolyte and acid-base balance.
7 The concentration of the final urine is a function of the level of antidiuretic hormone (ADH) that stimulates the distal tubules and collecting ducts to reabsorb water. The countercurrent exchange system of the long loops of Henle and their accompanying capillaries establishes a concentration gradient within the renal medulla to facilitate the reabsorption of water from the collecting duct.
8 The distal nephron regulates acid-base balance by excreting hydrogen ions and forming new bicarbonate.
9 The kidney secretes or activates a number of hormones that have systemic effects, including $1,25 \ OH_2D_3$, erythropoietin, and natriuretic hormone.

Tests of Renal Function

1 Tests that measure renal clearance indicate how much of a substance can be cleared from the blood by the kidneys per given amount of time.
2 Creatinine, a substance produced by muscle, is measured in both plasma and urine to calculate a commonly used clinical measurement of GFR.
3 Both the plasma creatinine concentration and the blood urea nitrogen (BUN) level indicate glomerular function. Plasma creatinine is measured to monitor progressive renal dysfunction; BUN is an indicator of hydration status.
4 Urinalysis involves evaluation of color, turbidity, protein, pH, specific gravity, sediment, and supernatant.
5 Presence of bacteria, red blood cells, white blood cells, casts, or crystals in the urine sediment may indicate a renal disorder.

Aging and Renal Function
1 As a person grows older, a decrease occurs in the number of nephrons. Both renal blood flow and GFR decline.
2 Tubular transport and reabsorption decrease with age. Response to acid-base changes and reabsorption of glucose is delayed. Drugs eliminated by the kidney can accumulate in the plasma, causing toxic reactions.

KEY TERMS

Arcuate artery, 1116

Bladder, 1118

Bowman's capsule, 1113

Bowman's space, 1113

Collecting duct, 1116

Cortical nephron, 1113

Countercurrent exchange system, 1126

Detrusor muscle, 1118

Distal tubule, 1116

Diuretic, 1128

Effective renal plasma flow, 1130

Excretion, 1122

External urethral sphincter, 1119

Filtration slit, 1114

Glomerular capillary, 1116

Glomerular filtration membrane, 1114

Glomerular filtration rate, 1119

Glomerulus, 1113

Hematuria, 1131

Hilus, 1113

Interlobar artery, 1116

Internal urethral sphincter, 1118

Juxtaglomerular apparatus, 1116

Juxtamedullary nephron, 1113

Kidney, 1112

Macula densa, 1116

Major calyx, 1113

Mesangial cell, 1113

Micturition, 1118

Minor calyx, 1113

Nephron, 1113

Net filtration pressure, 1123

Oliguria, 1127

Plasma creatinine (P_{cr}) concentration, 1130

Podocyte, 1114

Proximal tubule, 1114

Pyuria, 1131

Renal artery, 1116

Renal capsule, 1113

Renal column, 1113

Renal cortex, 1113

Renal fascia, 1113

Renal medulla, 1113

Renal papilla, 1118

Renal pelvis, 1113

Renal pyramids, 1113

Renin-angiotensin system, 1121

Transport maximum (Tm), 1124

Trigone, 1118

Tubular reabsorption, 1122

Tubular secretion, 1122

Ultrafiltration, 1121

Urea, 1127

Ureter, 1118

Urethra, 1118

Urinalysis, 1130

Vasa recta, 1117

Water diuresis, 1128

REFERENCES

Berg, M. B. & Green, N. (1973, March). Function of the thick ascending limb of Henle's loop. *American Journal of Physiology, 224,* 659-668.

Berne, R. M. & Levy, M. N. (Eds.). (1988). *Physiology* (2nd ed.). St. Louis: C. V. Mosby.

Brenner, B. M., Katz, R., & Ishikawa, I. (1986). The renal circulation. In B. M. Brenner & F. C. Rector (Eds.), *The kidney* (pp. 115-117). Philadelphia: W. B. Saunders.

Brezis, M., Rosen, S., & Epstein, F. H. (1986). Acute renal failure. In B. M. Brenner & F. C. Rector (Eds.), *The kidney* (3rd ed.) (p. 735-799). Philadelphia: W. B. Saunders.

Dretler, S., Watson, G., & Parrish, J. (1986). Laser fragmentation of ureteral calculi: Clinical experience. *Lasers in Surgery and Medicine, 6*(2) p.191.

Genest, J. & Cantin, M. (1986). Regulation of body fluid volume: The atrial naturiuretic factor. *News in Physiological Sciences, 1,* 3-5.

Hart, D. (Ed.). (1985). *French's index of differential diagnosis* (12th ed.). Briston: John Wright & Sons.

Kass, E. H (1978). Horatio at the orfice: The significance of bacteriuria. *Journal of Infectious Disease, 138,* 546-557.

Kissane, J. M. (Ed.). (1985). *Anderson's Pathology* (8th ed.). St. Louis: C. V. Mosby.

Krupp, M. A., Chatton, M. J., & Tierney, L. M. (1986). *Current medical diagnosis and treatment.* Los Altos, CA: Lange Medical Publications.

Marsh, D. J. (1983). *Renal physiology.* New York: Raven Press.

Re, R. N. (1987). The renin-angiotensin system. *Medical Clinics of North America, 71*(5), 877-895.

Rocha, A. S. & Kokko, J. P. (1981, April). Sodium chloride and water transport in the medullary thick ascending limb of Henle's loop in the rabbit kidney. *Pflugers Archiv European Journal of Physiology (Berlin), 390,* 30-37.

Rosenberg, S. J. & Williams, R. D. (1986). Photodynamic therapy of bladder carcinoma. *Urologic Clinics of North America, 13*(3), 435-444.

Schmidt, R. A. (1985). The urethral syndrome. *Urologic Clinics of North America, 12*(2), 349-354.

Spence, A. P. & Mason, E. B. (1983). *Human anatomy and physiology* (2nd ed.). Menlo Park, Ca: Addison-Wesley.

Sullivan, L. P. & Grantham, J. L. (1982). *Physiology of the kidney* (2nd ed.). Philadelphia: Lea & Febiger.

Thibodeau, G. A. (1987). *Anatomy and physiology.* St. Louis: Times Mirror/Mosby College Publications.

Thompson, J., et al. (1989). *Clinical nursing.* (2nd ed.). St. Louis: C. V. Mosby.

Vander, A. J. (1980). *Renal physiology* (2nd ed.). New York: McGraw-Hill.

Vick, R. L. (1984). *Contemporary medical physiology.* Menlo Park, Ca.: Addison-Wesley.

West, J. B. (Ed.). (1985). *Best and Taylors: The physiological basis of medical practice* (11th ed.). Baltimore: Williams & Wilkins.

Whaley, L. F. & Wong, D. L. (1987). *Nursing care of infants and children* (3rd ed.). St. Louis: C. V. Mosby.

CHAPTER 33

Alterations of Renal and Urinary Tract Function

Sue E. Huether

Urinary tract obstruction, 1136
  Consequences of obstruction, 1136
  Obstructive disorders, 1137
    Renal stones, 1137
      Pathophysiology, 1137
      Clinical manifestations, 1138
      Evaluation and treatment, 1138
    Neurogenic bladder, 1138
      Pathophysiology, 1138
      Clinical manifestations, 1139
      Evaluation and treatment, 1139
  Tumors, 1139
    Renal tumors, 1139
      Pathogenesis, 1139
      Clinical manifestations, 1139
      Evaluation and treatment, 1140
    Bladder tumors, 1140
      Pathogenesis, 1140
      Clinical manifestations, 1141
      Evaluation and treatment, 1141
Urinary tract infection, 1141
  Causes of urinary tract infection, 1141
  Types of urinary tract infection, 1141
    Cystitis, 1141
      Pathophysiology, 1141
      Clinical manifestations, 1141
      Evaluation and treatment, 1142
    "Nonbacterial" cystitis, 1142
    Acute pyelonephritis, 1142
      Pathophysiology, 1142
      Clinical manifestations, 1143
      Evaluation and treatment, 1143
    Chronic pyelonephritis, 1143
      Pathophysiology, 1143
      Clinical manifestations, 1143
      Evaluation and treatment, 1143

Glomerular disorders, 1144
  Glomerulonephritis, 1144
    Types of glomerulonephritis, 1145
      Acute glomerulonephritis, 1145
      Rapidly progressive glomerulonephritis, 1145
      Chronic glomerulonephritis, 1145
    Pathophysiology, 1145
    Clinical manifestations, 1148
    Evaluation and treatment, 1148
  Nephrotic syndrome, 1149
    Types of nephrotic syndrome, 1149
    Course of the disease, 1149
      Pathophysiology, 1149
      Clinical manifestations, 1150
      Evaluation and treatment, 1150
Renal failure, 1150
  Classification of renal dysfunction, 1150
  Types of renal failure, 1151
    Acute renal failure, 1151
      Pathophysiology, 1151
      Clinical manifestations, 1152
      Evaluation and treatment, 1153
    Chronic renal failure, 1153
      Pathophysiology, 1154
        Creatinine and urea clearance, 1154
        Sodium and water balance, 1155
        Potassium balance, 1155
        Acid-base balance, 1155
        Phosphate and calcium balance, 1155
      Clinical manifestations, 1156
      Evaluation and treatment, 1156
        Dietary management, 1156
        Sodium and fluids, 1156
        Potassium, 1156
        Caloric intake, 1156

Renal and urinary function can be affected by a variety of disorders. The most common type of urinary dysfunction is infection of the bladder. The urinary tract can also be obstructed by stones or tumors. Renal function can be impaired by disorders of the kidney itself or by many other systemic diseases. Because the kidney filters the blood, it is directly linked to every other organ system. Renal failure, whether acute or chronic, is therefore a life-threatening condition.

URINARY TRACT OBSTRUCTION

Urinary tract obstruction, or obstructive uropathy, is an interference with the flow of urine at any site along the urinary tract (Fig. 33-1). The obstruction causes stasis and accumulation of urine behind the obstruction that can lead to infection or damage to involved organs. Obstruction can be either congenital or acquired. (Congenital obstruction is discussed in Chapter 34.) Among the numerous causes of acquired obstruction are tumors, stones (calculi), and trauma. The obstruction can be within the urinary tract (as with renal calculi) or within the ureteral strictures. It can be caused by edema associated with infection or by tumors of the bladder or

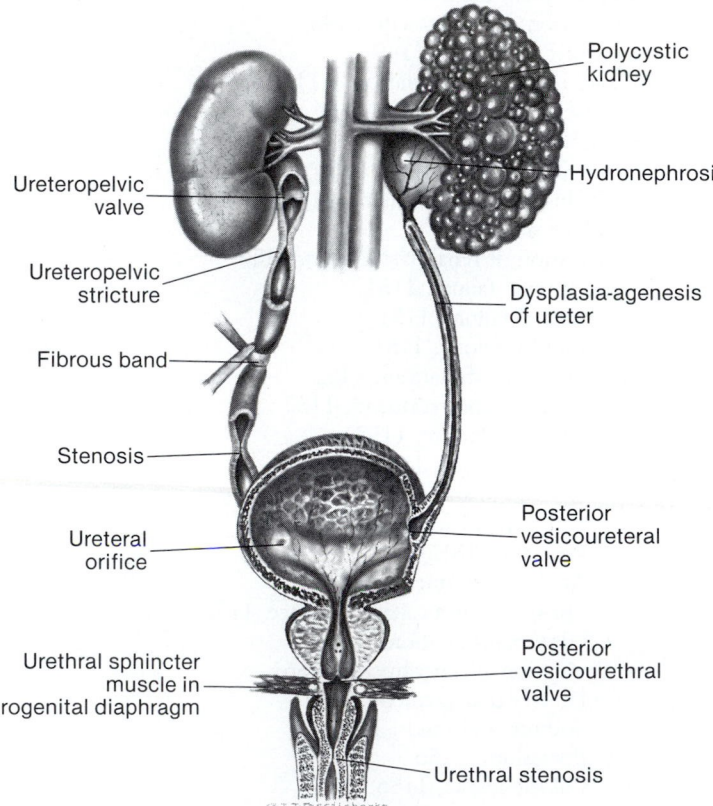

Major sites of urinary tract obstruction.

FIG. 33-1. Major sites of urinary tract obstruction. (From Whaley & Wong, 1987.)

urethra. Obstructions arising from outside the urinary tract can be related to pregnancy, benign prostatic hyperplasia or carcinoma, and inflammation of the gastrointestinal tract. Functional causes of obstruction are due to loss of ureteral peristaltic activity or bladder muscle function, which occur with vesicoureteral reflux (reflux of urine from the bladder into the ureter) or with neurogenic bladder. (Vesicoureteral reflux is discussed in Chapter 34.)

Urinary tract obstructions can develop acutely or evolve insidiously over weeks or months. Early recognition of obstruction is important to the prevention of infection and permanent loss of renal function. The pathophysiology of obstructive disorders can frequently be reversed by alleviating the obstruction.

Consequences of Obstruction

The pathophysiologic consequences of urinary tract obstruction are related to (1) location within the urinary tract, (2) unilateral or bilateral involvement, (3) partial or complete obstruction, (4) acute or chronic duration, and (5) the underlying cause. Whenever the flow of urine is obstructed, hydrostatic pressure increases, and structures behind the site of occlusion dilate. Obstructions lower in the urinary tract cause less severe pressure increases because more surface area is available for dilation.

Obstruction of the ureter causes **hydroureter** (accumulation of urine in the ureter). Retrograde increases in hydrostatic pressure involving the renal pelvis and calyces produce **hydronephrosis** (accumulation of urine in the renal collecting system). Acute, complete obstructions cause an increase in pressure that is transmitted to the proximal tubule and decreases glomerular filtration. If the obstruction is complete, the glomerular filtration rate (GFR) will decline to zero, with resulting renal failure. Partial obstructions generally do not cause a cessation of glomerular filtration (Wilson & Schrier, 1986). Complete unilateral obstruction may reduce the GFR to 30% of normal and is reflected by an increased plasma creatinine level (see Chapter 35).

Chronic partial obstruction causes compression of the kidney structures from accumulation of urine, with ischemic atrophy of the papilla and medulla. Although the kidneys will initially increase in size, progressive atrophy follows, with eventual loss of renal mass and smaller kidneys. The accompanying tubular damage decreases renal ability to conserve sodium and water and to excrete hydrogen ion and potassium. The resulting failure to concentrate the urine may produce excessive urine volumes even though the GFR has declined. Sodium and bicarbonate will be wasted with an increased risk of dehydration and metabolic acidosis.

The relief of urinary tract obstruction—in one or both kidneys—is usually followed by a variable period of diuresis (commonly called postobstructive diuresis) with losses of large amounts of urine. The diuresis is related to salt and water retention during the period of obstruction and a return to a normal GFR. The diuresis lasts for a few days, usually without symptoms of volume depletion such as postural hypotension or elevated BUN and plasma creatinine levels.

An uncommon result of obstruction relief is an excessive loss of sodium and water (greater than 10 L/day). These losses are particularly unusual when intake is matched with output. In such cases reducing fluid intake until output falls to normal is appropriate while monitoring for volume deficit. In some cases of chronic obstruction diuresis may not be significant after relief of obstruction because the GFR returns to normal slowly or not at all.

Complications of urinary tract obstruction include infection and renal failure. The type of complication depends on the site of obstruction. Obstructions below the bladder cause infection because the accumulated urine is an excellent medium for bacterial growth. Acute or chronic renal failure occurs with prolonged bilateral obstruction (see pp. 1151 to 1153). Acute renal failure can be prevented if the obstruction is relieved within 1 week. Chronic renal failure may be insidious.

Obstructive Disorders

Renal Stones

Calculi, or **renal stones** (nephrolithiasis), are a common cause of urinary tract obstruction in adults. Renal stones account for 1 of 1000 hospitalizations, with an incidence at autopsy of approximately 5%. A significant number of patients are treated in outpatient settings. About 1% of the U.S. population will have a renal stone at some time.

Three major kinds of renal stones are (1) calcium (75% to 80%); (2) struvite (15%); and (3) magnesium, ammonium, phosphate, and uric acid (7%). Cystine stones are relatively rare and account for less than 1% of all renal stones.

Pathophysiology

The formation of stones is complicated and not entirely understood. The factors that contribute to stone formation include high urinary concentration of stone-forming substances, urine pH, and facilitators and inhibitors of crystal growth. Various diseases, drugs, and diet can contribute to stone development, so each person will have to be reviewed carefully to establish the specific causes. Inhibitors of crystal aggregation are normally present in the urine. One theory of stone formation is a reduced excretion of these inhibitors in the urine (Fleisch, 1978).

The formation of a stone begins with a nucleus, or nidus. A **nidus** is a crystal that evolves in the presence of

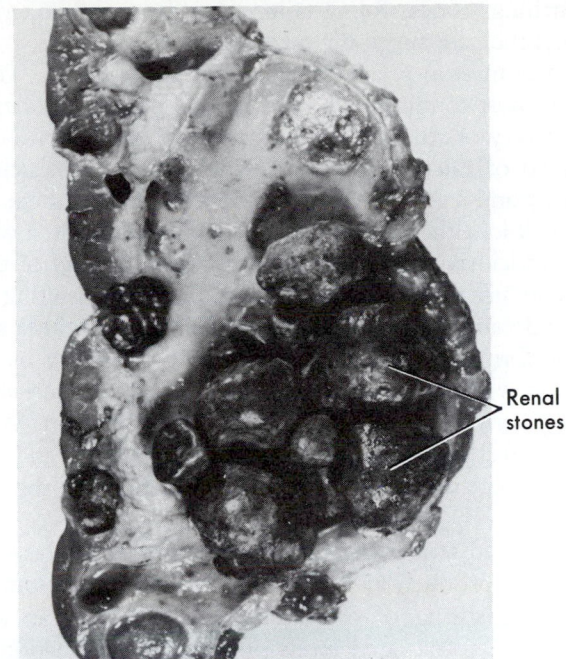

FIG. 33-2. Hydronephrosis with renal stones in renal pelvis and calyces. (From Kissane, 1985.)

stone-forming substances such as calcium oxalate, calcium phosphate, or struvite. After the nidus is formed, it may become trapped within the urinary tract. There it attracts other crystals and eventually grows into a stone. A high urinary saturation of stone-forming substances enhances crystal formation and stone growth (Fig. 33-2).

Some types of stones are aggregates of different substances. For example, people with high concentrations of uric acid will attract calcium oxalate crystals onto a uric acid nidus even though urinary calcium and oxalate levels are normal. An aggregate stone composed of these different substances will then form. The pH of the urine affects the solubility of many stone-forming substances. For instance, an alkaline urine decreases the solubility and enhances the crystallization of calcium carbonate and calcium phosphate. Keeping the urine more acidic increases the solubility of these substances and therefore helps to prevent supersaturation and stone formation. Uric acid tends to crystallize in an acidic urine, particularly when the pH remains below 5.5. Calcium oxalate and cystine stones will form independently of the urine pH.

Stones usually grow on the papillae or in the renal tubules, calyces, or renal pelvis. Stones may also form in the ureter or bladder. Many stones are less than 5 mm in diameter and are readily passed with the urine. Large stones are sometimes called **staghorn calculi,** as they grow in the pelvis and extend into the calyces to form branching stones. Renal failure may be a consequence, unless they are surgically removed.

Calcium stones are the most common stones. They occur most commonly in middle-aged men with a familial history of stone formation. Most of these stones are formed of calcium oxalate or an aggregate of calcium oxalate and calcium phosphate. About 80% of them are idiopathic, although they frequently are associated with hypercalciuria and hyperuricosuria (a high level of uric acid in urine). Prolonged immobilization resulting in bone demineralization can precipitate hypercalciuria and stone formation. Struvite stones are precipitated by infection with urea-splitting organisms (e.g., *Pseudomonas* and *Proteus*) and are more common in women. With such infections an alkaline urine is produced and the stones tend to form in the kidney or bladder and, although rarely, in the ureter.

Uric acid stones are caused by gout, an increase in uric acid production and hyperuricosuria. High-purine diets (consisting of meat, fish, and poultry) can also contribute to elevated levels of uric acid. Formation of uric acid stones is enhanced by a concentrated and acidic urine. Thus regional enteritis and ulcerative colitis can precipitate the formation of uric acid stones. Both of these diseases may cause fluid loss and a metabolic acidosis that develops from loss of bicarbonate (see Chapter 3). Patients with the rare hereditary disorder cystinuria develop cystine stones. In cystinuria an error in cystine metabolism causes decreased tubular reabsorption of cystine with an increased amount of this relatively insoluble substance in the urine.

Clinical Manifestations

Pain is the hallmark symptom of a renal stone. The location and severity vary with the site of occurrence. The presence of stones above the ureters is usually asymptomatic unless an infection or obstruction occurs. When a stone migrates into the ureter and obstructs the lumen, however, a colicky pain occurs as the rhythmic contractions of the ureter attempt to advance the stone. Distention and spasm of the ureter follow from the accumulation of urine behind the stone. The pain may be in the flank, at the costovertebral angle (between the last rib and the lumbar vertebrae), or it may radiate into the groin if the stone is lower in the ureter. The pain can be exquisitely severe, requiring narcotic analgesia for relief, and is frequently accompanied by nausea and vomiting. Gross or microscopic hematuria (blood in the urine) may be present.

Evaluation and Treatment

The diagnosis of renal stones requires a thorough medical and family history, diet history, previous history of urinary tract disease, and use of medications. Each of these factors may singularly or in combination contrib-

ute to stone formation. Both blood and urine tests should be performed to evaluate the presence of stone-forming substances. Urine pH and the presence of red or white blood cells should be evaluated. The GFR can be estimated by assessing the BUN and plasma creatinine (see Chapter 32). A plain (flat plate) film of the abdomen and an intravenous pyelogram will identify the presence of radiopaque stones and confirm the anatomic location.

The purpose of treatment is to prevent new stone formation and to reduce the size of stones that have already formed. Calcium stones reduce with difficulty, but struvite, uric acid, and cystine stones may dissolve with appropriate therapy. The principal components of treatment include (1) reducing the concentration of stone-forming substances by increasing the flow of urine with a high fluid intake or (2) decreasing the amount of the substance in the urine by decreasing dietary intake or endogenous production. The solubility of stone-forming substances can often be enhanced by altering the pH of the urine. Surgical removal may be required for large stones, obstruction, recurrent infections, or intractable pain. Smaller stones may pass spontaneously, or they can be extracted by instrumentation.

Extracorporeal shock-wave lithotripsy is a relatively noninvasive procedure that uses high energy shock waves to fragment stones for excretion in the urine (Walker, 1984). Lasers are also being used for the treatment of renal stones (Dretler, 1988). Immediate relief of obstruction caused by invading tumors can be obtained by placing ureteral catheters past the obstruction or by inserting a nephrostomy tube percutaneously into the renal pelvis. If the obstruction is not treatable, urinary diversion procedures may be required to prevent chronic infection.

Neurogenic Bladder

Neurogenic bladder is a functional urinary tract obstruction caused by an interruption of the nerve supply to the bladder. The neurologic disruption can occur in the central nervous system or at the level of the spinal cord.

Pathophysiology

The resulting bladder paralysis interferes with the normal flow of urine. This type of urinary dysfunction is related to the level of the neural lesion. Upper motor neuron lesions occur in the cortex or below the cortex but above the sacral level of the spinal cord. An upper motor neuron lesion causes loss of voluntary control of voiding. Lower motor neuron lesions affecting the bladder occur at the sacral level of the spinal cord and disrupt the sacral reflex arc. These lesions cause loss of both voluntary and involuntary control of urination. Some disease states or trauma may affect only the sen-

TABLE 33-1 Classification of neurogenic bladder

Type of neurogenic bladder	Cause	Neural lesion	Clinical manifestations	Treatment
Uninhibited (loss of cortical inhibition)	Lack of voluntary control in infancy, multiple sclerosis	Upper motor neuron	Smaller urine volume, frequency, urgency, incontinence, enuresis	
Reflex or automatic (reflex arc maintained below lesion with spontaneous voiding)	Spinal cord transsection, cord tumors, multiple sclerosis above level T_{12} of cord	Upper motor neuron	Involuntary voiding that may include incomplete emptying with retention and infection	Catheter or condom drainage; stimulation of reflex arc by stroking perineum, abdomen, or rectum
Autonomous (loss of cortical inhibition and interruption of spinal reflex arc)	Sacral cord trauma, tumors, herniated disk, abdominal surgery with transsection of pelvic parasympathetic nerves	Lower motor neuron	Overflow incontinence in which bladder does not empty spontaneously with stretch-fullness	Catheter, urinary diversion surgery
Motor paralysis (sensory functions intact)	Lesions at levels S_2, S_3, S_4; poliomyelitis, trauma; tumors	Lower motor neuron	Overflow incontinence caused by loss of bladder contraction	Manual, compression (Credé maneuver)
Sensory paralysis (motor functions intact)	Posterior lumbar nerve roots, diabetes mellitus, tabes dorsalis	Lower motor neuron	Dribbling, overflow incontinence; loss of sensation of bladder fullness	Bladder training to empty at regular intervals (i.e., every 3 hr)

sory or motor innervation of the bladder. (The types of neurogenic bladder are reviewed in Table 33-1.)

Clinical Manifestations

Infection with a neurogenic bladder may be associated with bladder distention and urine retention, placement of catheters, or the development of stones caused by bone resorption from physical immobility. Symptoms of infection in neurogenic bladder are often difficult to interpret because of disordered sensation and the presence of other neurologic disturbances. The condition may cause symptoms. Pain may not be experienced, but the individual may experience a burning sensation. The development of fever is frequently accompanied by chills and shivering, which aid in differentiating fever caused by other neurologic lesions.

Evaluation and Treatment

Sterile sampling of urine for bacterial analysis confirms the presence of bacteriuria. Antibiotic treatment for specific organisms is required.

Tumors
Renal Tumors

Renal adenomas (benign tumors) are uncommon. The tumors are encapsulated and are usually located near the cortex of the kidney. Because they can become malignant, they are usually surgically removed. **Renal cell carcinoma** is the most common renal neoplasm (85% of all renal neoplasms) and represents about 2% of cancer deaths. Renal cell carcinoma usually occurs in men between 50 and 60 years of age (Reiselbach & Garnick, 1982).

Pathogenesis

A moderate association has been identified between tobacco use and the incidence of renal cell carcinoma. Diethylstilbestrol and estrogen administration are linked to renal cell carcinoma in animals.

Renal cell carcinomas are classified according to cell type and extent of metastasis. Clear cell tumors present a better prognosis than granular cell tumors. Confinement within the renal capsule, together with treatment, is associated with a better survival rate. The tumors usually occur unilaterally and spread through the lymph nodes and blood vessels to the lungs, liver, lymph nodes, and bone (Fig. 33-3).

Clinical Manifestations

The classic clinical manifestations of renal cell carcinoma are flank pain, hematuria, palpable flank mass, and weight loss. Such signs and symptoms represent an

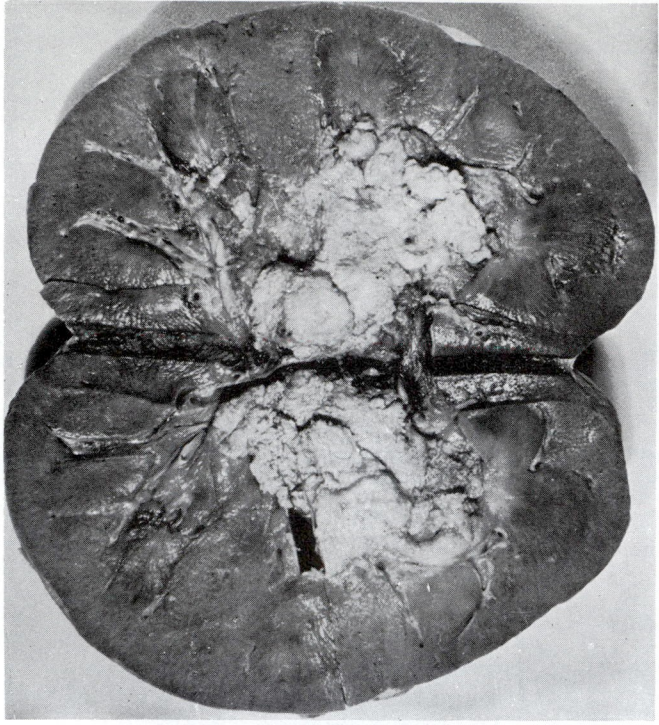

FIG. 33-3. Papillary carcinoma of renal pelvis. (From Kissane, 1985.)

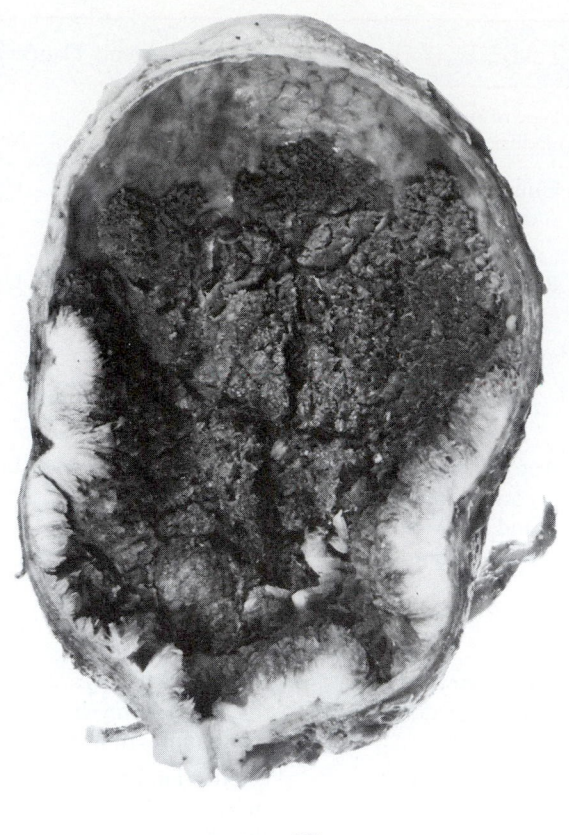

cm
0   1   2   3   4   5

FIG. 33-4. Cystectomy specimen. Multiple papillary tumors cover greater part of bladder wall. (From Kissane, 1985.)

advanced stage of disease, whereas earlier stages are often silent. Hematuria is the most common presenting symptom. The flank pain is usually dull and aching, and frequently associated with bleeding within the tumor. Tumor palpation is generally difficult but easier in thin people. Systemic manifestations include weight loss and fatigue; intermittent fever from tumor toxins; anemia from hematuria and lack of erythropoietin or polycythemia from secretion of erythropoietic factor; altered liver function with elevated serum alkaline phosphatase, prothrombin, and bilirubin; and hypertension from elevated renin levels. The most common sites of distant metastasis are the lung, liver, bone, thyroid, and central nervous system.

Evaluation and Treatment

Diagnosis is based on the clinical symptoms, plain x-ray films of the abdomen, intravenous pyelography, renal angiography, and computed tomography. (Staging of renal cell carcinoma is presented in Table 33-2). Treatment is usually surgical removal of the affected kidney (radical nephrectomy) with combined use of chemotherapeutic agents and, less effectively, hormonal agents (antiestrogen drugs). Radiation therapy may also be used. Survival is related to tumor grade, tumor cell type, and extent of metastasis.

Bladder Tumors

Bladder tumors represent about 2% of all malignant tumors. The development of bladder cancer is highest in men older than 60 years of age.

Pathogenesis

The risk of bladder cancer is greater for people who smoke, suggesting that smoking is a causative risk factor. The tumor is usually composed of transitional cells (the cells lining the bladder) and may or may not have a

---

TABLE 33-2 Staging of renal cell carcinoma

Stages	Metastasis
I	Tumor confined within kidney capsule
II	Invasion through renal capsule but within surrounding fascia
III	Involvement of regional lymph nodes, renal vein, or vena cava
IV	Distant metastases

TABLE 33-3 Staging of bladder carcinoma

Stages	Metastasis
O	Limited to mucosal involvement
A	Submucosal involvement
B	Involvement of the muscularis layer
C	Invasion of the perivesical fat
D_1	Spread to regional lymph nodes
D_2	Spread to distant sites, bone, and visceral organs

papillary growth pattern (a tuftlike lesion attached to a stalk) (Fig. 33-4). Nonpapillary tumors (representing 10% of bladder tumors) are not as common as papillary tumors, but they tend to be more invasive and have a poorer prognosis. Metastasis is usually to lymph nodes, liver, bones, and lungs. Staging for bladder carcinoma is presented in Table 33-3. Secondary bladder cancer develops by invasion of cancer from bordering organs, such as cervical carcinoma in women or prostatic carcinoma in men.

Clinical Manifestations

Bladder tumors may be asymptomatic or accompanied by hematuria. Advanced cancers are associated with pelvic pain and frequent urination.

Evaluation and Treatment

Diagnosis is made by cystoscopy (visual examination of the urinary tract through a cystoscope), cell studies, urograms (x-ray examinations), and transurethral biopsy. Treatment is related to the type and size of the lesion. Surgical resection is the treatment of choice because of the high propensity for bladder tumors to recur. Intravesicular (inside the bladder) chemotherapeutic agents have also been used with some success to prevent recurrence. Radiation therapy is not as effective, and candidates for radiation must be carefully selected based on tumor type. Photodynamic therapy, which involves photosensitizing agents and laser light to detect and kill cancer cells, is being clinically tested (Benson et al., 1983). Because of the risk of recurrence, cystoscopic evaluations are performed every 3 to 6 months after initial treatment.

URINARY TRACT INFECTION

Causes of Urinary Tract Infection

Urinary tract infections (UTIs) are usually caused by bacteria. Infections are diagnosed by culture of specific organisms with counts of 100,000 bacteria/ml of freshly voided urine. Bacterial contamination of the normally sterile urine usually occurs by retrograde movement of gram-negative bacilli (*Escherichia coli, Pseudomonas,* or *Proteus*) into the urethra and bladder. Gram-positive organisms (*Staphylococcus*), fungi, or tubercular bacillus are less common causes of infection. A UTI can occur anywhere along the urinary tract including the urethra, prostate, bladder, ureter, and kidney.

Several factors normally combine to protect against UTIs. Most bacteria are washed out of the urethra during micturition. The low pH and presence of urea in the urine provides a bactericidal effect. The ureterovesical junction closes during bladder contraction, preventing reflex of urine to the ureters and kidneys. Both the longer urethra and prostatic secretion decrease the risk of infection in men.

Types of Urinary Tract Infection
Cystitis

Cystitis is an inflammation of the bladder, the most common site of UTI. The morphologic appearance of the bladder through cystoscopy describes different types of cystitis. With mild inflammation the mucosa is hyperemic (red). More advanced cases may show diffuse hemorrhage (called hemorrhagic cystitis) or pus formation, suppurative exudate (called suppurative cystitis) on the epithelial surface of the bladder. Prolonged infection may lead to sloughing of the bladder mucosa with ulcer formation (termed ulcerative cystitis). The most severe infections may cause necrosis of the bladder wall (termed gangrenous cystitis). Generally, the infections are uncomplicated and resolve spontaneously.

Pathophysiology

The most common infecting organisms are *Escherichia coli, Klebsiella, Proteus, Pseudomonas,* and *Staphylococcus.* The disease may occur alone or in association with pyelonephritis or prostatitis. Cystitis is more common in women because of the shorter urethra, the closeness of the urethra to the anus, and the possibility of bacterial contamination from vaginal secretions. Introduction of bacteria and an environment that promotes bacterial growth are the common factors in cystitis. Sexually active and pregnant women, individuals with indwelling catheters, and persons with diabetes mellitus, neurogenic bladder, poor hygiene, and urinary tract obstruction are at greater risk for developing cystitis. Prostatitis and urethral obstruction from prostatic hypertrophy are predisposing factors to bacteriuria.

Clinical Manifestations

Many individuals with bacteriuria are asymptomatic. However, the clinical manifestations of cystitis usually include frequency, urgency, dysuria (painful urination), and suprapubic and low back pain. Hematuria, cloudy urine, and flank pain are more serious symptoms. About 10% of individuals with bacteriuria have no symptoms. Cystitis in the elderly may be asymptomatic (Kaye, 1980).

Evaluation and Treatment

Evaluation of the urine for bacteria is the most important diagnostic procedure. Risk factors, such as urinary tract obstruction, should be identified and treated. Evidence of bacteria from urine culture and sensitivity warrants treatment with an organism-specific antibiotic. A single large dose of antibiotic may be as effective as 3 to 10 days of treatment (Stamm and Turck, 1987). Twenty to 25% of women will have relapsing infection within 7 to 10 days, requiring prolonged antibiotic therapy (Hooten, Running, & Stamm, 1985). Follow-up urine cultures should be obtained 1 week after initiation of treatment and again at monthly intervals for 3 months. Clinical symptoms will frequently be relieved but bacteriuria may still be present. Repeated cultures should be obtained every 3 to 4 months until 1 year after treatment for evaluation of recurrent infection.

"Nonbacterial" Cystitis

A significant number of women will have symptoms of cystitis but a negative urine culture. This is more common in women 20 to 30 years of age and is called acute **urethral syndrome** or "irritable bladder" (O'Dowd et al., 1984). Its cause is obscure, but dysfunction of the external sphincter, vaginitis, urethritis, or inflammation of glands near the vagina and urethra are associated findings. Bacteria may develop in 60% of individuals up to 9 months after the initial symptoms. Symptoms are frequently relieved by a course of treatment with antibiotics, use of drugs that relax the external sphincter, or retraining of voiding habits.

A persistent and chronic form of "nonbacterial" cystitis occurring primarily in women is **interstitial cystitis.** The cause is not clearly known, but an autoimmune reaction may cause the inflammatory response. The inflammation is associated with a derangement of the bladder mucosa that makes it more susceptible to penetration by bacteria. Inflammation and fibrosis of the bladder wall are accompanied by the presence of hemorrhagic ulcers (Hunner's ulcers). Characteristic symptoms include bladder fullness, frequency, small urine volume, and lower abdominal pain. Response to treatment is generally good with fluid distention of the bladder followed by weekly instillations of dimethyl sulfoxide for up to 12 weeks.

Acute Pyelonephritis

Pyelonephritis is an infection of the renal pelvis and interstitium. The causative organism is usually bacterial but can be fungi or viruses. (Common causes of pyelonephritis are summarized in Table 33-4.) Urinary obstruction and reflux of urine from the bladder (vesicoureteral reflux) are the most common underlying risk factors. (See Chapter 34 for vesicoureteral reflux in children.) One or both kidneys may be involved. Most cases occur in women. The responsible organism is usually *E. coli, Proteus,* or *Pseudomonas.* The latter two organisms are more commonly associated with infections following urethral instrumentation or urinary tract surgery. These organisms also split urea to ammonia, making an alkaline urine that increases the risk of stone formation.

Pathophysiology

The infection is probably spread by ascending organisms along the ureters, but spread also may occur by way of the bloodstream. The inflammatory process is usually focal and irregular, primarily affecting the pelvis,

---

TABLE 33-4   Common causes of pyelonephritis

Predisposing factors	Pathologic mechanisms
Kidney stones	Obstruction and stasis of urine contributing to bacteriuria and hydronephrosis; irritation of epithelial lining with entrapment of bacteria
Vesicoureteral reflux	Chronic reflux of urine up the ureter and into kidney during micturition contributing to bacterial infection
Pregnancy	Dilation and relaxation of ureter with hydroureter and hydronephrosis; partly caused by obstruction from enlarged uterus and partly from ureteral relaxation caused by higher progesterone levels
Neurogenic bladder	Neurologic impairment interfering with normal bladder contraction with residual urine and ascending infection
Instrumentation	Introduction of organisms into urethra and bladder by catheters and endoscopes introduced into the urinary tract for diagnostic purposes
Female sexual trauma	Movement of organisms from the urethra into the bladder with infection and retrograde spread to kidney

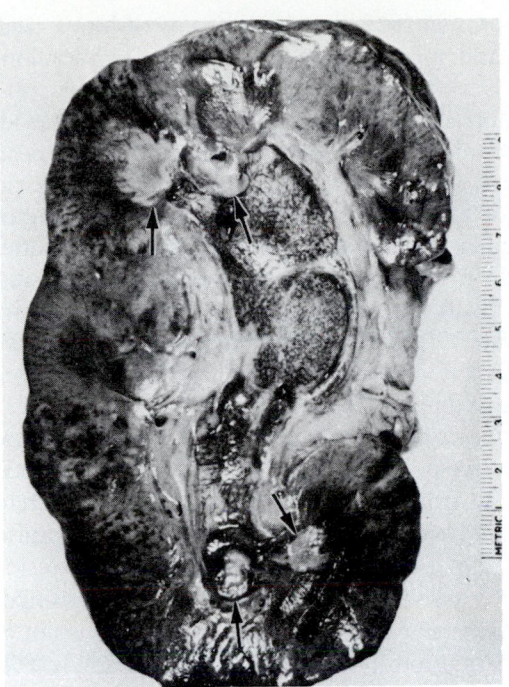

FIG. 33-5. Papillary necrosis resulting from acute pyelonephritis and obstruction. Note necrotic papillae *(arrows),* mottled patchy cortical infiltrate of acute pyelonephritis, and congested, dilated renal pelvis. (From Kissane, 1985.)

calyces, and medulla. The infection causes medullary infiltration of white blood cells with renal inflammation, renal edema, and purulent urine. In severe infections localized abscesses may form in the medulla and extend to the cortex. The tubules are primarily affected, but the glomeruli are usually spared. Necrosis of renal papillae can develop (Fig. 33-5). After the acute phase, healing occurs with deposition of scar tissue and atrophy of affected tubules. The number of bacteria decreases until the urine again becomes sterile.

Clinical Manifestations

The onset of symptoms is usually acute with fever, chills, flank or groin pain, frequency, dysuria, and costovertebral tenderness. Children and older adults may have nonspecific symptoms such as fever and malaise.

Evaluation and Treatment

Differentiating symptoms of cystitis from pyelonephritis may be difficult. The specific diagnosis is established by urine culture. The presence of antibody-coated bacteria is associated more closely with pyelonephritis (Ratner et al., 1981). White blood cell casts indicate pyelonephritis, but they are not always present in the urine.

Uncomplicated acute pyelonephritis responds well to 2 weeks of organism-specific antibiotic therapy. Follow-

up urine cultures are obtained at 1 and 4 weeks after treatment if symptoms recur. Antibiotic-resistant organisms or reinfection may occur in cases of urinary tract obstruction or reflux.

Chronic Pyelonephritis

Chronic pyelonephritis is a persistent or recurrent autoimmune infection of the kidney with inflammation and scarring of the kidney. The specific cause of chronic pyelonephritis is more difficult to determine, and controversy surrounds the criteria for constituting the diagnosis (Ronald & Simonsen, 1988). Recurrent infections from acute pyelonephritis may be associated with chronic pyelonephritis. The urine in chronic pyelonephritis may, however, contain only a few white cells and bacteria (Rubin, Tolkoff-Rubin, & Cotran, 1986). Generally, chronic pyelonephritis is more likely to occur in patients who have renal infections associated with some type of obstructive pathologic condition. This includes renal stones and vesicoureteral reflux.

Pathophysiology

Chronic urinary tract obstruction prevents elimination of bacteria in the normal flow of urine, resulting in progressive inflammation that causes fibrosis and scarring. The renal pelvis and calyces become dilated and blunted. Gradual destruction of the tubules occurs, with areas of atrophy or dilation and diffuse scarring. Impairment of function may affect urine-concentrating ability, with the excretion of a dilute urine, and can lead to chronic renal failure.

The lesions of chronic pyelonephritis are sometimes termed "chronic interstitial nephritis" because the inflammation and fibrosis are located in the interstitial spaces between the tubules. Chronic interstitial nephritis can occur from causes other than chronic pyelonephritis, including drug toxicity from analgesics such as phenacetin, aspirin, and acetaminophen; ischemia; irradiation; and immune complex diseases.

Clinical Manifestations

The early symptoms of chronic pyelonephritis are often minimal and may include hypertension. They may be similar to acute pyelonephritis with frequency, dysuria, and flank pain, although milder and more vague. Progression of the disease leads to renal failure.

Evaluation and Treatment

The urinalysis usually shows white blood cells and less commonly white blood cell casts. Bacteriuria may or may not be associated with the presenting symptoms. The diagnosis is commonly established by intravenous pyelogram and ultrasound, which reveals a small kidney with a characteristic "clubbing" of the affected calyces.

The choice of treatment is related to the underlying cause. When obstruction occurs, it must be relieved.

Appropriate antibiotic treatment is important and re-quires regular surveillance of the urine for bacterial growth. Antibiotics may be given in short courses when urine cultures are positive. Recurrent infection may re-quire prolonged antibiotic therapy.

GLOMERULAR DISORDERS

Immunologic mechanisms are primarily responsible for glomerular disease with the exception of hereditary disorders, nephritis associated with systemic diseases, and vascular pathologic conditions. Most information has been derived from animal studies and microscopic examination of renal biopsies.

The onset of glomerular disease may be sudden or in-sidious with hypertension, edema, and an elevated BUN. Some individuals are asymptomatic, so that dis-ease is detected through the presence of microscopic he-maturia from a routine urinalysis. The most definitive indication of glomerular disease is microscopic evalua-tion of tissue obtained by renal biopsy. The presence of clinical symptoms such as edema, hypertension, urinary changes, or systemic diseases associated with glomerular injury provides supporting evidence for the diagnosis.

Different types of glomerular disease may be associ-ated with patterns of urinary sediment. Urine in diseases associated with a **nephrotic sediment** have massive pro-teinuria, lipiduria, and microscopic or no hematuria. Urine in diseases associated with **nephritic sediment** is characterized by hematuria with red cell casts and vary-ing degrees of proteinuria, which is usually not severe. Severe glomerular disease is usually associated with dif-fuse lesions and may demonstrate oliguria, hyperten-sion, and renal failure. Focal lesions tend to produce less severe clinical symptoms. In some instances a combina-tion of hematuria may occur with excessive amounts of urine protein (as in renal symptoms of lupus erythema-tosus and membranous proliferative glomerulonephri-tis).

Reduced GFR during glomerular disease is evidenced by the plasma creatinine concentration or creatinine clearance (see Chapter 32). Glomerular damage causes a decrease in glomerular membrane surface area, glomeru-lar capillary blood flow, and driving hydrostatic pres-sure. In the presence of hypoalbuminemia plasma fluid tends to move to the interstitial spaces, contributing to decreased blood volume, decreased renal blood flow, and decreased glomerular capillary hydrostatic pressure with a decline in GFR.

Edema is commonly associated with nephrotic syn-drome (see p. 1149) or may be caused by salt and water retention from reduced GFR. Excessive fluid retention may cause systemic and pulmonary edema, requiring the use of diuretics or dialysis. The volume expansion that accompanies salt and water retention leads to hyperten-sion. Generally excessive renin production is not a cause of hypertension in glomerular diseases unless it is asso-ciated with ischemia, as in uremia (see p. 1150), or with profound hypovolemia.

Death occurs in 2% to 5% of all persons during acute glomerular disease. During the first few weeks, the ma-jor life-threatening problems are acute renal insuffi-ciency with fluid, electrolyte, and acid-base imbalances; acute hypertension that may cause hypertensive enceph-alopathy; circulatory failure; and pulmonary edema.

Glomerulonephritis

Glomerulonephritis is an inflammation of the glom-erulus that can be caused by a variety of factors includ-ing immunologic abnormalities, effects of drugs or tox-ins, vascular disorders, and systemic diseases. In some cases the exact cause of glomerular injury may be un-known. Immunologic alterations are most frequently re-

---

TABLE 33-5 Types of glomerular lesions

Lesion	Characteristics
Diffuse	Relatively uniform involvement of most or all glomeruli; most common form of glomerulo-nephritis
Focal	Changes in only some glomeruli while others are normal
Segmental-local	Changes in one part of the glomerulus with other parts unaffected
Mesangial	Deposits of immunoglobulins in the mesangial matrix
Membranous	Thickening of the glomerular capillary wall
Proliferative	An increase in the number of glomerular cells
Sclerotic	Glomerular scarring from previous glomerular injury
Crescentic	The accumulation of proliferating cells within Bowman's space making the appearance of a crescent

sponsible for glomerular injury (Wilson & Dixon, 1986). Glomerular disease is the most common cause of chronic and end-stage renal failure.

Types of Glomerulonephritis

The classification of glomerulonephritis is arbitrary and can be described according to cause, pathologic lesions, disease progression, or clinical presentation. (Types of glomerular lesions are reviewed in Table 33-5.)

Acute Glomerulonephritis

Acute glomerulonephritis is frequently associated with a poststreptococcal infection (acute poststreptococcal glomerulonephritis). The disease has an abrupt onset and usually occurs 7 to 10 days after a streptococcal infection of the throat or skin commonly in children (see Chapter 34). Sporadic occurrences have been observed following bacterial endocarditis, which may be associated with streptococcal or staphylococcal organisms, or after viral diseases such as varicella and hepatitis B.

The presenting symptoms are related to the preceding illness, and the manifestations of renal disease are variable. Acute onset of hematuria, red blood cell casts, proteinuria, decreased GFR, oliguria, edema, and hypertension are common. The edema of acute glomerulonephritis tends to be around the eyes but may involve dependent areas such as the feet and ankles. Occasionally, ascites or pleural effusions will develop. Immunofluorescent findings from renal biopsy indicate the presence of immune complex deposits in the glomerulus, with diffuse capillary endothelial cell proliferation (Fig. 33-6). The thickening of the glomerular membrane contributes to the decreased GFR. More severe renal disease is observed after a prolonged infection before antibiotic therapy. Specific antibiotic therapy is required. Most individuals, especially children, recover without loss of renal function or recurrence of the disease.

Rapidly Progressive Glomerulonephritis

Rapidly progressive glomerulonephritis (RPGN) is also known as subacute, crescentic, or extracapillary glomerulonephritis. The disease primarily affects adults in their 50s and 60s. RPGN may be idiopathic or associated with a number of proliferative glomerular diseases (with diffuse proliferation of extracapillary cells), such as poststreptococcal glomerulonephritis and Goodpasture syndrome.

Goodpasture syndrome is an example of RPGN. The disease is associated with antibody formation against both pulmonary capillary and glomerular basement membranes. The relationship between these two antibodies is unknown. Goodpasture syndrome is rare but occurs in men 20 to 30 years of age.

By the time RPGN is diagnosed, renal insufficiency is apparent. The disease is characterized by extensive proliferation of cells into Bowman's space with crescent formation. The cells become mixed with fibrin and form crescent-shaped deposits (Fig. 33-7). Typically, the glomerular injury is accompanied by a rapid decline in glomerular function progressing to renal failure in a few weeks or months (Leaf & Cotran, 1985). Hematuria is common and may or may not be accompanied by proteinuria, edema, or hypertension.

RPGN has a relatively poor prognosis. Prednisone alone or combined with immunosuppressant drugs such as cyclophosphamide or azathioprine has not been very effective. Pulsed methylprednisolone administration, which is given once a day for 3 to 5 days before prednisone therapy, is helpful in some cases. Anticoagulants, such as heparin or warfarin, may be of some benefit in reducing the fibrin component of crescent formation. Plasmapheresis (separation of the cells from the plasma) has been useful for removal of antibodies in Goodpasture syndrome and other causes of RPGN. Plasmapheresis is usually combined with prednisone and cyclophosphamide to suppress a rebound antibody production. Dialysis or transplantation is required when failure is irreversible.

Chronic Glomerulonephritis

Chronic glomerulonephritis includes a variety of glomerular diseases, each with a progressive course leading to chronic renal failure. Chronic glomerulonephritis may occur with no history of renal disease before the diagnosis, although several prior years of proteinuria and hematuria may have preceded the diagnosis. Various pathologic changes are evident in the glomerulus. Proliferation of mesangial cells (cells in connective tissue supporting the glomerular capillaries; see Figure 32-7, *B*) may be focal or diffuse with segmental fibrosis and glomerular deterioration. Secondary tubular dilation and atrophy may develop. The primary cause may be difficult to establish because advanced pathologic changes may obscure specific disease characteristics (Fig. 33-8).

Pathophysiology

Patterns of antigen-antibody complex deposition within the glomerular capillary filtration membrane have been established using light, electron, and immunofluorescent microscopy for different disease processes. The findings on light microscopy provide information about the distribution and extent of immune response injury (Table 33-6). Electron microscopy differentiates morphologic changes within the glomerular capillary wall. Staining with fluorescein identifies different antibodies and their configurations when viewed under ultraviolet (black) light with a microscope (Fig. 33-9).

Two types of immune mechanisms commonly con-

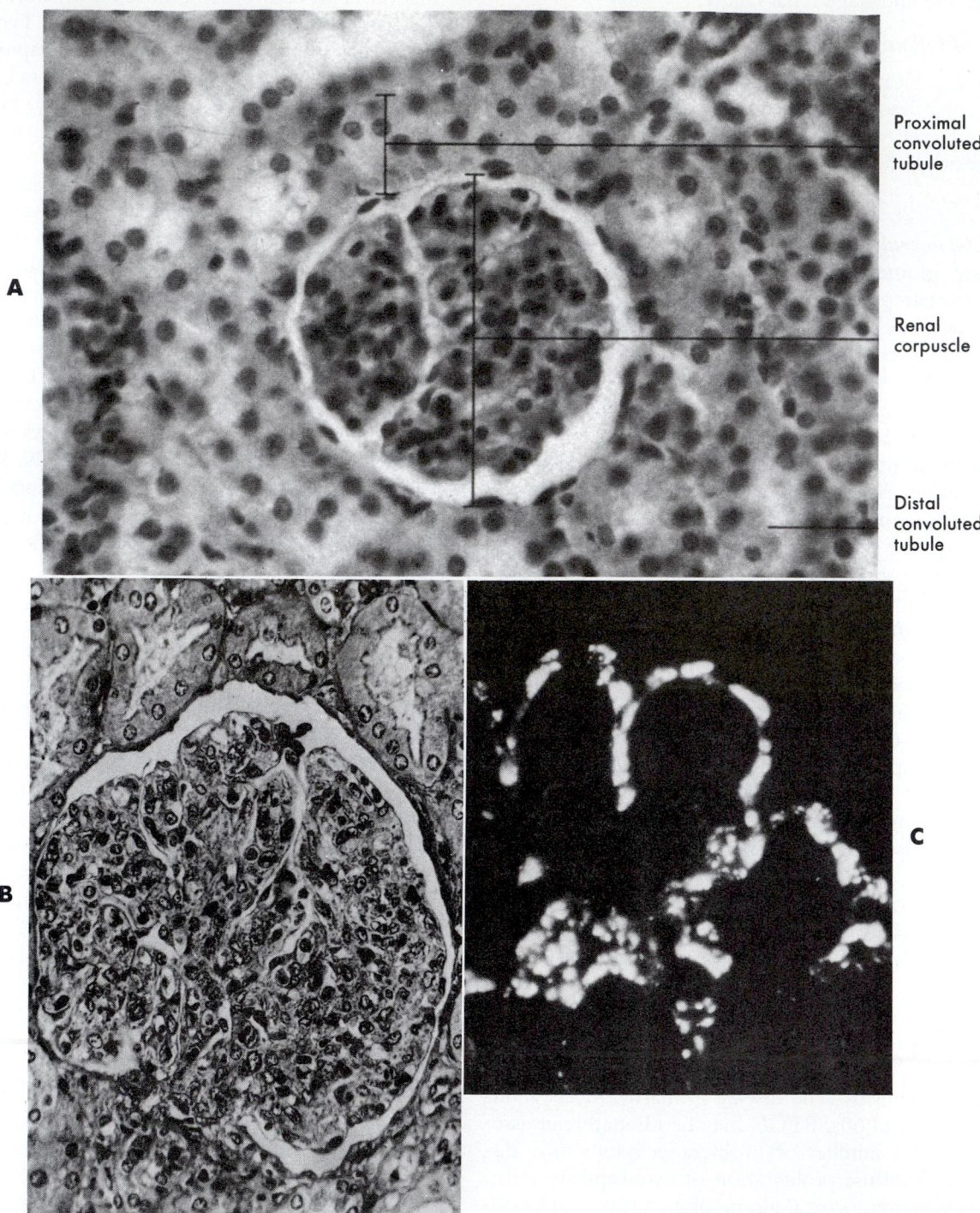

Proximal convoluted tubule

Renal corpuscle

Distal convoluted tubule

FIG. 33-6. A, Photomicrograph of kidney showing normal glomerulus surrounded by profiles of sectioned renal tubules. (×140.) **B,** Acute poststreptococcal glomerulonephritis. Swollen, hypercellular glomerular lobules with few open capillaries. (×250.) **C.** Acute poststreptococcal glomerulonephritis. "Humps" of immune complex stained with fluorescent antihuman complement (C3). (1000; courtesy Dr. Caude Cornwall, Syracuse, NY.). (**A** from Thibodeau, 1987; **B** and **C** from Kissane, 1987.)

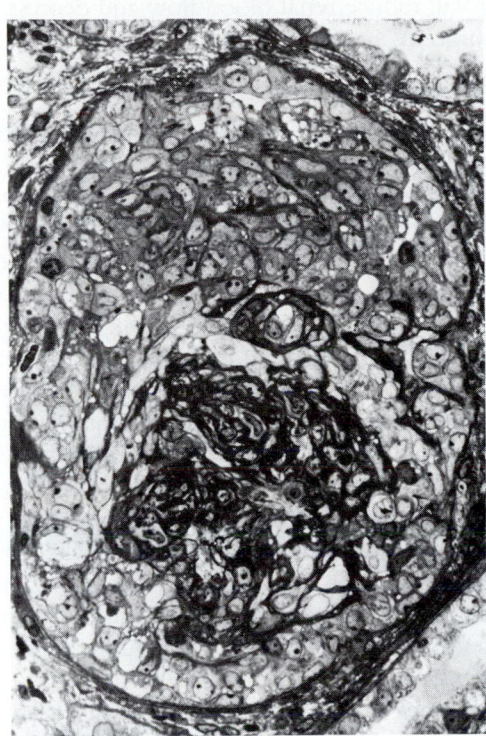

FIG. 33-7. Rapidly progressive glomerulonephritis, antiglomerular basement membrane type. Note crescent of epithelial cells encircling compressed glomerular tuft. (From Kissane, 1987.)

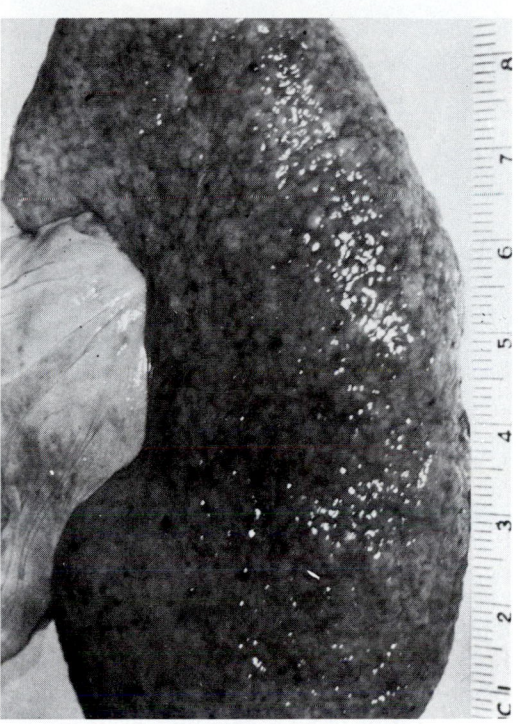

FIG. 33-8. End-stage chronic glomerulonephritis. Pebbly surface corresponds to surviving hypertrophied nephrons amid atrophy. (From Kissane, 1987.)

TABLE 33-6 Immunologic pathogenesis of glomerulonephritis

Glomerular injury	Mechanism
Soluble immune-complex glomerulonephritis (90%)	Formation of antibodies stimulated by the presence of endogenous or exogenous antigens results in circulating soluble antigen-antibody complexes, which are deposited in glomerular capillaries. Glomerular injury occurring with complement activation and release of immunologic substances that lyse cells and increase membrane permeability. Immune deposits with a microscopic appearance that fluoresce in a *granular pattern* when stained with fluorescene and viewed under ultraviolet light. Severity of glomerular injury related to the number of complexes formed.
Antiglomerular basement membrane glomerulonephritis (5%)	Antibodies are formed and act directly against the glomerular basement membrane; immune response that causes crescent formation and a *linear pattern* of immunofluorescence; generally associated with rapidly progressive renal failure such as Goodpasture syndrome.
Alternative complement pathway	A relatively obscure mechanism associated with low levels of complement and membranoproliferative glomerulonephritis.
Cell-mediated immunity	A delayed hypersensitivity response that damages the glomerulus. Actual cellular mechanism not clearly understood.

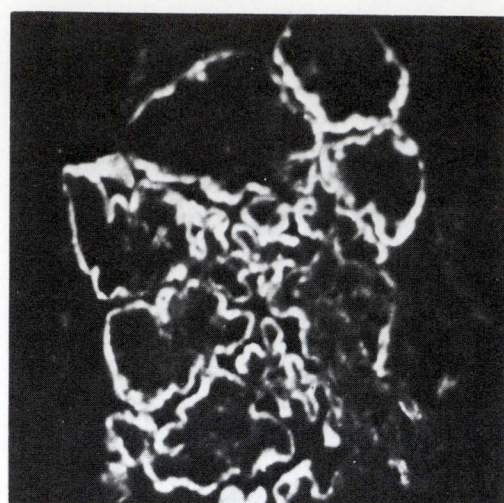

FIG. 33-9. Membranoproliferative glomerulonephritis, dense deposit type, stained with flurosecent antihuman complement (C3). (Courtesy Dr. Claude Cornwall, Syracuse, NY; from Kissane, 1987.)

tribute to glomerular injury: (1) deposition of circulating soluble antigen-antibody complexes and (2) formation of antibodies specific for the antiglomerular basement membrane (anti-GBM antibodies). The former is the most prevalent. Other immune mechanisms may also operate, but they have not been as clearly substantiated in humans. The severity of glomerular damage and renal insufficiency is related to the size, number, location (focal or diffuse), duration of exposure, and type of antigen-antibody complexes.

Glomerular damage generally occurs from activation of biochemical mediators of inflammation (complement, leukocytes, fibrin), which begins after the antibody or antigen-antibody complexes have localized in the glomerular capillary wall. Complement is deposited with the antibodies, followed by a sequence of metabolic events that initiate an attack on the glomerular membrane. Complement activation can serve as a chemotactic stimulus for attraction of neutrophils and monocytes. The neutrophils and monocytes further the inflammatory reaction by releasing lysosomal enzymes, which damage glomerular cell walls.

These processes alter membrane permeability and may cause loss of the negative electrical charge across the glomerular filtration membrane. Membrane damage can lead to platelet aggregation and degranulation, whereby platelets release vasoactive amines such as serotonin or histamine. These substances then increase glomerular permeability. Changes in membrane permeability and electrical charge permit the passage of protein molecules and/or red blood cells into the urine causing proteinuria and/or hematuria. The coagulation system may also be activated and lead to fibrin deposition in Bowman's

space, contributing to crescent formation (deposition of substance in Bowman's space). (Coagulation is discussed in Chapter 22.) Membrane proliferation and swelling will reduce renal blood flow and depress glomerular filtration.

Clinical Manifestations

Two major changes in the urine are distinctive of glomerulonephritis: (1) hematuria with red blood cell casts and (2) proteinuria exceeding 3 to 5 g/day, with albumin as the major protein. Several disorders may produce hematuria because bleeding can occur anywhere along the urinary tract. The characeristics of hematuria from red blood cells escaping through the glomerular membrane include a smoky brown-tinged urine, red blood cell casts, and an accompanying proteinuria. Bleeding from sites lower in the urinary tract may produce a pink- or red-colored urine. Glomerular bleeding provides prolonged contact with the acidic urine and transforms hemoglobin to methemoglobin, which has a brownish color and no blood clots. The immune-mediated inflammatory response with cellular infiltration decreases GFR, which leads to fluid retention. Salt and water are also reabsorbed, contributing to fluid volume expansion and hypertension. Additionally, the history and physical examination may reveal findings that differentiate glomerular disease from another source of urinary tract bleeding. Gross proteinuria is associated with nephrotic syndrome (see p. 1149); a decrease in urine output accompanies a decreased GFR.

Mild proteinuria and hematuria may occur during the early years of the disease. Blood pressure may be normal. After 10 or 20 years renal insufficiency will begin to develop, followed by nephrotic syndrome and an accelerated progression to end-stage renal failure. Symptom patterns will vary depending on the underlying cause. Steroids do not change the course of the disease, and dialysis or kidney transplantation may ultimately be necessary.

Evaluation and Treatment

The diagnosis of glomerular disease is confirmed by the progressive development of clinical manifestations and laboratory findings of abnormal urinalysis with proteinuria, red blood cells, white blood cells, and casts. In acute poststreptococcal glomerulonephritis, the streptococcal exoenzymes are elevated, such as antistreptolysin-O (ASO) and antistreptokinase (ASK). Serum complement is decreased. Creatinine clearance evaluates the extent of glomerular damage. Microscopic evaluation from renal biopsy provides a specific determination of renal injury.

The basic principles for treating glomerulonephritis are related to treating the primary disease, preventing or minimizing immune responses, and correcting accompa-

TABLE 33-7 Clinical manifestations of nephrotic syndrome

Manifestation	Contributing factors	Result
Proteinuria	Increased glomerular permeability, decreased proximal tubule reabsorption	Edema, increased susceptibility to infection from loss of immuno-globulins
Hypoalbuminemia	Increased urinary losses of protein	Edema
Edema	Hypoalbuminemia (decreased oncotic pressure, sodium and water retention, increased adolsterone and ADH secretion)	Soft, pitting, generalized edema
Hyperlipidemia	Decreased serum albumin; increased hepatic synthesis of very low-density lipoproteins, increased cholesterol, phospholipids, triglycerides	Increased athrogenesis
Lipiduria	Sloughing of tubular cells containing fat (oval fat bodies); free fat from hyperlipidemia	Fat droplets that may float in urine
Decreased vitamin D	The globulin, to which 25, vitamin D is attached for transport, passing through glomerulus and lost in the urine	Decreased absorption of calcium from gut

nying problems such as edema, hypertension, and hyperlipidemia. Specific treatment regimens are necessary for particular types of glomerulonephritis.

Antibiotic therapy is essential for management of underlying infections, which may be contributing to ongoing antigen-antibody responses. Several approaches have been instituted to control immune-mediated glomerular injury. Corticosteroids decrease antibody synthesis and suppress inflammatory responses. Different administrative protocols are implemented, including pulsed therapy (high doses once per day for 3 to 5 days) or more prolonged administration until clinical improvement is sustained.

Cytotoxic agents may be used cautiously because of their severe side effects. These drugs destroy lymphocytes or prevent their proliferation, and they are used more commonly when lupus erythematosus involves renal function. Immune complexes may be removed by removing the plasma and replacing it with fresh frozen plasma. Anticoagulants may be useful for controlling fibrin crescent formation in rapidly progressive glomerulonephritis.

Nephrotic Syndrome
Types of Nephrotic Syndrome

Nephrotic syndrome is simply defined as the excretion of 3.5 g or more of protein in the urine per day. This large amount of urine protein is characteristic of glomerular injury. A constellation of other clinical findings is usually associated with the proteinuria. These include hypoalbuminemia, edema, hyperlipidemia, and lipiduria (Table 33-7). Lipoid nephrosis and membranous glomerulonephritis are directly related to nephrotic syndrome, although these conditions can occur with other types of glomerular disease.

Secondary forms of nephrotic syndrome occur as a result of other organic pathologic processes. Systemic diseases often implicated in secondary nephrotic syndrome include diabetes mellitus, amyloidosis, systemic lupus erythematosus, and Henoch-Schonlein purpura. Nephrotic syndrome also is seen in association with certain drugs, infections, malignancies, and vascular disorders. When present as a secondary complication with renal diseases, nephrotic syndrome often signifies a more serious prognosis.

Course of the Disease
Pathophysiology

The pathophysiology of nephrotic syndrome is primarily related to loss of plasma proteins, particularly albumin and some immunoglobulins, across the injured glomerular filtration membrane. Disturbances in the glomerular basement membrane, which may be metabolic, biochemial, or physiochemical, lead to increased permeability to protein. Hypoalbuminemia is a consequence of the urinary loss of ablumin combined with a diminished synthesis of replacement albumin by the liver. Albumin is lost in the greatest quantity because of its high plasma concentration and low molecular weight.

Although synthesis of plasma proteins may be increased, the synthesis is insufficient to compensate for losses. Factors such as decreased dietary intake of protein from anorexia or malnutrition, or accompanying liver disease may contribute to lower levels of plasma albumin. Loss of immunoglobulins may increase susceptibility to infections.

Clinical Manifestations

Proteinuria is an excessive amount of protein in the urine (up to 10 g/24 hr). Urinary protein loss is related to increased glomerular permeability. Albumin is lost in greater amounts, although the smaller globulins also appear in the urine. Many of the clinical manifestations of nephrotic syndrome are related to loss of serum proteins (see Table 33-7).

Edema may be the first symptom noticed by the patient (see Chapter 3). Renal edema is usually associated with hypoalbuminemia and is soft, pitting, and in areas of low tissue pressure, such as the periorbital regions. According to Starling's law, hydrostatic pressure acts to force fluid into the interstitial space at the arterial end of the capillaries. The hydrostatic pressure is balanced by the oncotic pressure of the plasma proteins, which tends to draw the fluid back into the capillaries at the venous end (see Chapter 3). Plasma albumin concentration in nephrotic syndrome is often reduced to 20% of normal, with a considerable decrease in the plasma oncotic pressure. The threat of decreased plasma volume from the accumulation of fluid in the tissues stimulates compensatory mechanisms. Among these mechanisms are activation of the renin-angiotensin-aldosterone system and antidiuretic hormone, which together lead to excessive sodium and water retention. Increased lymph flow may allow some compensation. Edema in the interstitial space may facilitate lymph flow by elevating tissue pressure, facilitating the return of interstitial fluid into the plasma compartment.

Levels of all the plasma lipids (triglycerides, phospholipids, and cholesterol) are elevated, producing a hyperlipidemia. The inverse relationship between plasma albumin and plasma lipids indicates that hypoalbuminemia and the associated decrease in plasma oncotic pressure may play a causative role in hyperlipidemia. Hyperlipidemia is related to increased synthesis by the liver and decreased lipoprotein catabolism (Leaf & Cotran, 1985). **Lipiduria** is manifested by lipid casts or free fat droplets that leak across the glomerular capillary walls and into the urine. Tubular epithelial cells that reabsorb lipoprotein may also be shed and appear in the urine as "oval fat bodies."

Vitamin D deficiency may also be related to the proteinuria of nephrotic syndrome. The hormone 25-hydroxycholecalciferol is normally bound to a circulating globulin. If this is lost in the urine, there will be decreased absorption of intestinal calcium and hypocalcemia (see Chapter 3). Symptoms of vitamin D deficiency will develop, including low plasma levels of ionized calcium, secondary hyperparathyroidism, and osteomalacia.

Evaluation and Treatment

Nephrotic syndrome is diagnosed when the protein level in a 24-hour urine collection is greater than 3.5 g. Serum albumin decreases (to less than 3 g/dl), and serum cholesterol, phospholipids, and triglycerides increase. Fat bodies may be present in the urine.

Nephrotic syndrome is commonly treated with a high-protein diet, salt restriction, diuretics, and occasionally albumin replacement. Because the nephrotic state is primarily caused by protein depletion, dietary protein supplements (up to 100 g) are essential, unless renal failure has occurred. Diuretics may be used, particularly loop diuretics such as furosemide or ethacrynic acid, to control edema or hypertension. Care must be taken to observe for hypovolemia and hypokalemia or potassium toxicity in the presence of renal insufficiency. Aldactone may be combined with loop diuretics to suppress aldosterone activity and conserve potassium.

Because hyperlipidemia is associated with hypoalbuminemia, correction occurs when normal plasma albumin levels are reestablished. A low saturated-fat diet may be helpful in chronic nephrosis as a way of slowing down atherogenic processes. Drugs such as clofibrate are not safe to use when renal insufficiency exists. The underlying cause of nephrotic syndrome should be treated specifically if it is known.

RENAL FAILURE

Classification of Renal Dysfunction

The terms *renal insufficiency, renal failure, azotemia,* and *uremia* are all associated with decreasing renal function. Often, they are used synonymously, although with some distinctions. Generally, **renal insufficiency** refers to a decline in renal functions to about 25% of normal or a GFR of 25 to 30 ml/min. Levels of serum creatinine and urea will be mildly elevated. Renal failure often refers to significant loss of renal function. When less than 10% of renal function remains, this is termed **end-stage renal failure** (ESRF).

Renal failure may be acute and rapidly progressive, although the process may be reversible. Renal failure can also be chronic, progressing to ESRF over a period of months or years. **Uremia** is a syndrome of renal failure and includes elevated blood urea and creatinine levels accompanied by fatigue, anorexia, nausea, vomiting, pruritius, and neurologic changes. Azotemia and uremia are sometimes incorrectly used interchangeably. **Azotemia** means increased serum urea levels and frequently increased creatinine levels as well. Renal insufficiency or renal failure causes azotemia. Uremia represents the numerous consequences related to renal failure, including retention of toxic wastes, deficiency states, and electrolyte disorders. Both azotemia and uremia indicate an accumulation of nitrogenous waste products in the blood, a common characteristic that explains the overlap in definitions of terms (see p. 1156).

Types of Renal Failure
Acute Renal Failure

Acute renal failure is an abrupt reduction in renal function with elevation of BUN and plasma creatinine levels. Acute renal failure is usually associated with oliguria (urine output of less than 30 ml/hr or less than 400 ml of urine per day) although urine output may be normal or increased. Most types of acute renal failure are reversible if diagnosed and treated early. Acute renal failure is commonly classified as prerenal, intrarenal, or postrenal (Table 33-8).

Pathophysiology
Prerenal acute renal failure is caused by impaired renal blood flow. The GFR declines because of the decrease in filtration pressure. Poor perfusion can result from renal vasoconstriction, hypotension, hypovolemia, hemorrhage, or inadequate cardiac ouput. Acute prerenal failure may occur when chronic renal failure exists if

a sudden stress is imposed on already marginally functioning kidneys. Failure to restore blood volume or blood pressure may cause acute tubular necrosis or acute cortical necrosis.

Intrarenal acute renal failure may result from prerenal acute renal failure (e.g., acute tubular necrosis or cortical necrosis) or many other diseases, including acute glomerulonephritis, malignant hypertension, disseminated intravascular coagulation, and renal vasculitis. **Acute tubular necrosis** (ATN) is the most common cause of acute renal failure. ATN and acute renal failure are sometimes used interchangeably but they are not the same as acute renal failure that can occur without ATN. ATN is generally described as postischemic or nephrotoxic.

ATN caused by ischemia occurs most frequently after surgery (40% to 50% of cases), but ATN is also associated with sepsis or obstetric complications. A severe episode of hypotension often associated with hypovolemia is a significant contributing event. Nephrotoxic ATN can be produced by numerous antibiotics, but the aminoglycosides (particularly gentamicin) are the major culprits. The drugs tend to accumulate in the renal cortex and may not cause renal failure until after treatment is complete. Radiocontrast media (x-ray media) may also be nephrotoxic. Dehydration, advanced age, concurrent renal insufficiency, and diabetes mellitus tend to enhance nephrotoxicity from either agent. Other substances such as excessive myoglobin (oxygen-transporting substance in muscles), carbon tetrachloride, heavy metals (mercury, arsenic), or methoxyflurane

TABLE 33-8 Classifications of acute renal failure

Area of dysfunction	Possible causes
Prerenal	Hypovolemia
	Hemorrhagic blood loss (trauma, gastrointestinal bleeding, complications of childbirth)
	Loss of plasma volume (burns, peritonitis)
	Water and electrolyte losses (severe vomiting or diarrhea, intestinal obstruction, uncontrolled diabetes mellitus, inappropriate use of diuretics)
	Hypotension or hypoperfusion
	Septic shock
	Cardiac failure or shock
	Massive pulmonary embolism
	Stenosis or clamping of renal artery
Intrarenal	Acute tubular necrosis (postischemic or nephrotoxic)
	Glomerulopathies
	Malignant hypertension
	Coagulation defects
Postrenal	Obstructive uropathies (usually bilateral)
	Ureteral destruction (edema, tumors, stones)
	Bladder neck obstruction (enlarged prostate)

anethesia may promote renal failure. Necrosis caused by nephrotoxins is usually uniform and limited to the proximal tubules. Ischemic necrosis tends to be patchy and may be distributed along any part of the nephron.

Three pathophysiologic explanations have been proposed to account for the renal failure of ATN, but no single factor explains the condition adequately. The most classic explanation is the *tubular obstruction theory*. This theory suggests that necrosis of the tubules causes sloughing of cells, cast formation, or ischemic edema, resulting in tubular obstruction. Obstruction then causes a retrograde increase in pressure and reduces the GFR. Renal failure can occur within 24 hours. The theory does not always hold, however, since in some cases no cellular debris or casts can be observed in the urine.

The *back leak theory* suggests that glomerular filtration remains normal but that tubular reabsorption of filtrate is accelerated because of changes in permeability caused by ischemia. Most studies of renal function in ATN, however, indicate a decrease in glomerular filtration, and back leak may be only a minor aspect of acute failure.

Alterations in renal blood flow are considered by some authorities to be a major cause of decreased glomerular filtration. The exact mechanism is unknown, although afferent arteriolar constriction may be produced by an intrarenal release of angiotensin II or by a redistribution of blood flow from the cortex (where the glomeruli are located) to the medulla. Ischemia may also contribute to changes in glomerular permeability and decreased GFR.

Postrenal acute renal failure usually occurs with urinary tract obstruction that affects the kidneys bilaterally (e.g., bladder outlet obstruction, prostatic hypertrophy, or bilateral ureteral obstruction). A pattern of several hours of anuria with flank pain followed by polyuria is a characteristic finding. This type of renal failure can occur after diagnostic catheterization of the ureters, a procedure that may cause edema of the tubular lumen.

Clinical Manifestations

The clinical progression of acute renal failure with recovery of renal function occurs in three phases: oliguria, diuresis, and recovery. The initial phase of oliguria may begin within a day after a hypotensive event, although it may be delayed with exposure to nephrotoxic substances. Generally, the oliguria lasts for 1 to 2 weeks, but it may regress in several hours or extend for several weeks. Anuria (urine output less than 50 ml/day) is uncommon in ATN, but l0% to 20% of cases will have nonoliguric failure. The urine output may vary in volume, but the BUN and plasma creatinine concentratons will rise (plasma creatinine is inversely proportional to the GFR).

Other manifestations depend on the underlying cause of renal failure. Individuals who have experienced trauma or surgery, or those in a catabolic state may have more rapid elevations in BUN. They are prone to hyperkalemia and hyperphosphatemia from cellular breakdown. Fluid retention may cause edema. Symptoms of congestive heart failure develop in persons with cardiac disease. Nausea, vomiting, and fatigue accompany uremia and electrolyte imbalances. Wound healing will be delayed, and the risk of infection, particularly pneumonia, is greater. Nonoliguric renal failure generally has a better prognosis because of fewer complications. Oliguric patients may require maintenance dialysis to attenuate symptoms of renal failure.

As renal function improves, increase in urine volume (diuresis) is progressive. During the early diuretic phase, urea and creatinine excretion lag behind salt and water excretion. The lag occurs because tubular reabsorption may not recover as quickly as the GFR. Volume depletion may ensue with fluid losses of 3 to 4 L/day. Fluid and electrolyte balance must be carefully monitored and excessive urinary losses replaced.

Serial measurements of plasma creatinine provide an index of renal function during the recovery phase. Re-

---

TABLE 33-9   Differentiation of acute oliguric renal failure

	Urine volume	Urine specific gravity	Urine osmolality	Urine sodium	Bun/ plasma creatinine	FE$_{Na}$
Prerenal failure	<400 ml	1.16-1.020	>500 mOsm	<10 mEq/L	>15:1	<10% (also seen in acute glomerulonephritis)
Acute tubular necrosis	<400 ml	1.010-1.012	<400 mOsm	>30 mEq/L	<15:1	>10% (also seen in urinary tract obstruction and renal parenchymal disease)

turn to normal status may take from 3 to 12 months, and about 30% of individuals will not have full recovery of a normal GFR.

Evaluation and Treatment

The diagnosis of ATN is related to the cause of the disease. A history of surgery, trauma, or cardiovascular disorders is common. Exposure to nephrotoxins must also be considered. The diagnostic challenge is to differentiate prerenal acute renal failure from intrarenal acute renal failure. Urine composition provides helpful diagnostic clues to changes in tubular function. Urine osmolarity and specific gravity tend to be high in prerenal acute renal failure and are accompanied by low urinary sodium concentrations (Table 33-9). The ratios of the BUN to plasma creatinine concentration and fractional excretion of sodium (the ratio of filtered sodium to excreted sodium) are also helpful diagnostic indicators. The tests reflect renal tubular reabsorption ability. In prerenal failure tubular function is maintained and salt, water, and urea will be reabsorbed. With ATN, reabsorption and urinary concentration abilities are compromised. Other causes of renal failure may also exhibit similar clinical findings.

Prevention of acute renal failure is a major treatment factor. Maintenance of fluid volume before and after surgery or diagnostic procedures may significantly reduce acute renal failure precipitated by hypovolemia. Good hydration reduces the nephrotoxic risk of drugs, such as gentamicin or radiocontrast media, and sustains an adequate GFR. Mannitol has been used preoperatively in patients at high risk for developing acute renal failure (heart or aortic surgery) or during the oliguric phase of failure. Mannitol causes renal vasodilation with increased renal blood flow and glomerular filtration rate. The osmotic diuretic effect decreases sodium and water reabsorption and increases urine output. The net effect is a maintenance of renal blood flow and urine output with the prevention of accumulated tubular debris and obstruction. This drug is relatively safe but should be discontinued if the response is not immediate because it will disrupt the distribution of body fluids if not excreted.

The use of loop diuretics, furosemide and ethacrynic acid to treat acute renal failure is more controversial (Kjellstrand, Berkseth, & Klinkmann, 1988). These drugs increase renal blood flow and urine output but do not change the GFR. The therapeutic intent is to wash out cellular casts and relieve tubular obstruction. Whether these drugs alter the course of acute renal failure, however, has not been clearly established (Kjellstrand et al., 1988). In some instances a combination of diuretics may be successful.

The primary goal of therapy is to maintain the individual's life until renal function has been recovered.

Management principles directly related to physiologic alterations generally include (1) correcting fluid and electrolyte disturbances, (2) treating infections, and (3) maintaining nutrition. Fluid replacement must be carefuly calculated with consideration of urine losses, insensible losses (up to 1000 ml/day), and production of endogenous water by oxidation (450 ml/day). Overhydration of patients will dilute their plasma sodium concentration.

Hyperkalemia can be managed by restricting dietary sources of potassium or using cation-ion exchange resins, which may be administered orally or rectally. These resins exchange potassium for another cation, such as sodium in the bowel, and the potassium is then excreted attached to the resin. With tissue trauma or catabolic states large amounts of potassium may be liberated from cells. **Dialysis** (mechanical removal of water, electrolytes, and toxins from the blood) may be required, or potassium can temporarily be driven back into the cells by administering glucose and insulin or by infusing sodium bicarbonate. Glucose metabolism causes potassium to move to the intracellular fluid, and insulin infusions therefore can be effective in shifting potassium from the extracellular to intracellular space, along with the transport of glucose, within 30 minutes. (Glucose metabolism is discussed in Chapter 19.) Causing alkalemia with sodium bicarbonate also shifts potassium into cells in exchange for hydrogen ions.

Careful monitoring of the electrocardiogram for peaking T waves is essential for patients with hyperkalemia. Intravenous infusion of calcium is the most rapid method of treating cardiac effects of hyperkalemia. Calcium decreases the threshold potential and reduces the membrane excitability caused by hyperkalemia (see Chapter 3). Calcium should only be used in emergencies, however, because hypercalcemia may also cause cardiac arrest.

Azotemia is generally controlled and nutrition maintained with a low-protein, high-carbohydrate diet. Essential amino acid replacement, using products such as Nephramine, can be given orally or parenterally. Adequate carbohydrate intake slows protein catabolism and helps to prevent hyperkalemia. Because sepsis is a common serious complication of renal failure, observation for signs of infection and early treatment with antibiotics are necessary. Drug dosage levels may require adjustment if they are metabolized or excreted by the kidneys. Recovery may take up to 1 year.

Chronic Renal Failure

The kidney has many important regulatory functions including body fluid volume, solute concentration and dilution, acid-base balance, excretion of waste products, and secretion of hormones that regulate red blood cell production, blood pressure, and calcium metabolism.

Progressive loss of renal function (**chronic renal failure**), regardless of the cause, affects these vital processes with changes manifest throughout all organ systems. The kidneys, however, exhibit remarkable adaptive abilities, and symptomatic changes usually do not become apparent until the GFR declines to 25% of normal.

Pathophysiology

Two theories have been proposed to account for the adaptation to loss of renal function. One view suggests that the adaptive response depends on the particular location of kidney damage. For example, tubular interstitial diseases primarily damage the tubular or medullary parts of the nephron, producing problems such as renal tubular acidosis, salt wasting, and difficulty diluting or concentrating the urine. Conversely, when there is primarily vascular or glomerular damage, proteinuria, hematuria, and nephrotic syndrome are more prominent. This theory is useful for planning treatment in early stages of renal failure when symptomatic differences in renal disease may be distinct.

A second theory (the intact nephron hypothesis) proposes that loss of nephron mass with progressive kidney damage causes the remaining nephrons to sustain normal kidney function. These nephrons are capable of a compensatory expansion in their rates of reabsorption and secretion. They also can maintain a constant rate of excretion in the presence of a declining GFR. The increased work load is achieved primarily by hypertrophy of the remaining nephrons.

The intact nephron hypothesis explains adaptive changes in solute and water regulation that occur with advancing renal failure. Although the urine of an individual with chronic renal failure may contain abnormal amounts of protein and red and white blood cells or casts, the major end products of excretion will be similar to normally functioning kidneys until advanced stages of renal failure when there is a significant reduction of functioning nephrons.

Creatinine and Urea Clearance Creatinine is constantly released from muscle and excreted primarily by glomerular filtration with relatively no reabsorption or secretion. In a steady state the amount produced equals the amount filtered and excreted. If either the rate of production or the GFR changes, the plasma concentration of creatinine will change until the amount excreted again equals the amount produced. Therefore if the GFR falls, as in chronic renal failure, the plasma creatinine level will increase by a reciprocal amount to maintain a constant rate of excretion. Because no significant tubular adjustment occurs for creatinine (i.e., tubular secretion), the plasma levels will continue to rise as the GFR falls. This relationship allows the plasma creatinine concentration to serve as an index of changing glomerular function. (This relationship is represented in Fig. 33-10.)

The clearance of urea is similar, although urea is both filtered and reabsorbed and varies with the state of hydration and diet. Urea clearance, therefore, will be less than the GFR. If protein intake and metabolism are

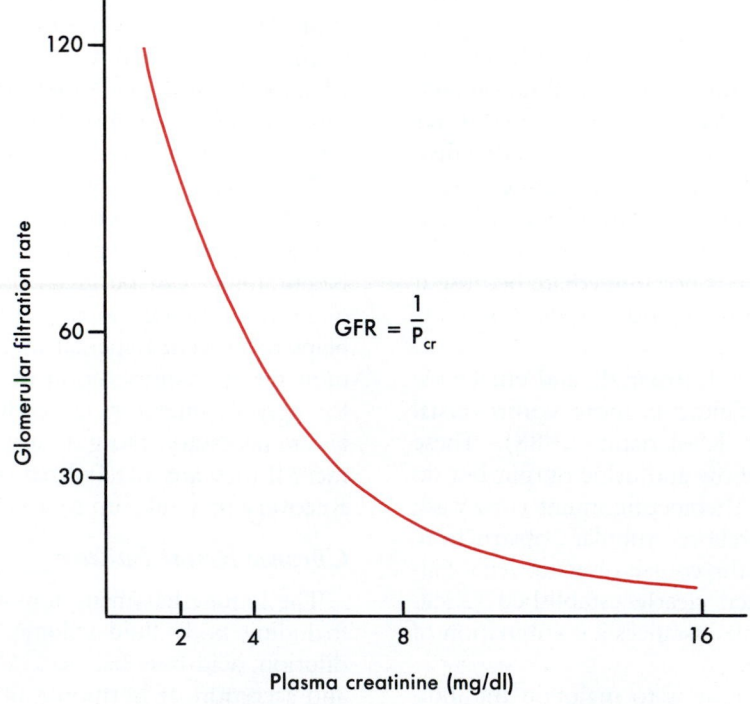

$$GFR = \frac{1}{P_{cr}}$$

FIG. 33-10. Plasma creatinine and glomerular filtration rate.

constant, however, plasma levels will increase as the GFR declines. Thus, no tubular adaptation modifies urea levels because urea is excreted primarily by glomerular filtration.

Sodium and Water Balance Levels of sodium must be regulated within narrow limits, because sodium is the major extracellular solute. In chronic renal failure the sodium load delivered to each remaining nephron will be greater than normal, so that the fractional excretion of sodium (the ratio of excreted to filtered sodium) must increase to maintain normal sodium balance. Increased excretion of sodium is accomplished by a decrease in the fractional reabsorption of sodium (ratio of reabsorbed to filtered sodium). Although the tubules will exhibit a compensatory increased reabsorption, a large obligatory loss remains. The exact regulatory mechanism, however, remains obscure.

Although the nephron is quite efficient at excreting sodium, it has difficulty conserving sodium when GFR falls to 25% (approximately 25 ml/min) of normal. At this GFR an obligatory loss of 20 to 40 mEq of sodium per day occurs. If dietary intake is less than this amount, sodium deficits and volume depletion will occur. These may be due to osmotic diuresis from loss of urea or to an inability to inhibit natriuretic hormone after a sudden decrease in sodium intake.

The regulation of water balance and osmolality is normally achieved by urinary concentration mediated by ADH. As GFR is reduced, ability to concentrate and dilute the urine diminishes. In earlier stages of renal failure this may be due to osmotic diuresis produced by increased fractional excretion of solutes by the remaining nephrons or to a decreased tubular response to ADH. Individual nephrons can maintain water balance until severe renal failure occurs and GFR declines to 15% to 20% of normal with extensive loss of nephron and tubular function. At this stage the urinary concentration becomes fixed and approaches that of the plasma at 285 mOsm/L with a specific gravity of about 1.010.

Potassium Balance Urinary excretion of potassium is primarily related to distal tubular secretion mediated by aldosterone and sodium-potassium ATPase (see Chapter 3). In renal failure there is increased tubular secretion that provides effective regulation until the onset of oliguria. Larger amounts of potassium are also lost through the bowel. Although nonoliguric patients can maintain potassium excretion with normal dietary intake, they are more prone to develop hyperkalemia with increased loading (i.e., use of salt substitutes). Use of potassium-sparing diuretics, such as spironolactone (Aldactone), or volume depletion may also precipitate elevated levels of serum potassium. With progression of disease to end-stage renal failure, total-body potassium can increase to life-threatening levels and will have to be controlled by dialysis.

Acid-Base Balance The intake of a normal diet produces 50 to 100 mEq of hydrogen per day. These ions are secreted from the renal tubules and excreted in the urine combined with phosphate and ammonia buffers (buffering is described in Chapter 3). During early stages of renal insufficiency, normal pH is maintained by an increased rate of acid excretion and bicarbonate reabsorption by individual nephrons. Metabolic acidosis begins to develop when the GFR falls by 30% to 40%, primarily because of decreased ammonia synthesis and decreased bicarbonate reabsorption. Phosphate buffers remain effective until late stages of chronic renal failure. When end-stage renal failure develops, serum bicarbonate levels will stabilize at 15 to 20 mEq/L, partly because the excess hydrogen is buffered by anions in bone. Individuals with end-stage renal failure develop metabolic acidosis, which may be severe enough to require dialysis.

Phosphate and Calcium Balance The metabolism of calcium and phosphate is mediated by parathyroid hormone (PTH) and vitamin D. Changes in acid-base balance also influence the status of calcium and phosphate (see Chapter 3). The major calcium and phosphate disorders associated with chronic renal failure are reduced renal phosphate excretion, decreased synthesis of 1,25 vitamin D, (the active form of vitamin D) and hypocalcemia, (Table 33-10).

In early chronic renal failure excreted phosphate levels decrease and the plasma phosphate concentration rises because of the fall in GFR. The elevated plasma phosphate binds calcium ($CaHPO_4$), causing hypocalcemia. The decreased calcium stimulates the secretion of PTH. The PTH causes release of calcium from bone and enhanced urinary excretion of phosphate. The adaptive effect is a secondary hyperparathyroidism with return of phosphate and calcium levels toward normal (see Chapter 18). With each incremental loss of GFR, however, the effectiveness of PTH in maintaining phosphate balance diminishes. Reducing the dietary intake of phosphate and providing calcium supplementation is helpful at this early stage of failure. When the GFR declines to 25% of normal, however, PTH is no longer effective in maintaining serum phosphate levels. The persistent decreased GFR and hyperparathyroidism causes progressive hyperphosphatemia, hypocalcemia, and dissolution of bone (e.g., osteitis fibrosa and osteomalacia).

Hypocalcemia and bone disease are accelerated by impaired synthesis of 1,25 vitamin D when loss of functioning nephrons is significant and GFR is less than 25% of normal. Lack of the active form of vitamin D reduces intestinal absorption of calcium and impairs the effectiveness of calcium and phosphate resorption from bone by PTH. The toxicity of uremia may also suppress vitamin D action in the gut. This depletion can be treated with vitamin D supplements, but larger than normal doses will be required. A negative calcium bal-

TABLE 33-10 Calcium and phosphate metabolism in chronic renal failure

Kidney	Plasma	Bone
Loss of nephron mass		
Decreased GFR		
Decreased phosphate excretion	Elevated phosphate	
	Formation of $CaPO_4$	
	Decreased ionized calcium	
Increased phosphate excretion (phosphaturia)	Increased PTH secretion (secondary hyperparathyroidism)	Release of calcium and phosphate
Increased calcium reabsorption and increased vitamin D formation (increased intestinal absorption of calcium)	Increased calcium	Osteitis fibrosa, osteomalacia, calcium deposits in soft tissue (occurs when kidney fails to respond to PTH secretion because of loss of renal mass and calcium and phosphate continue to be absorbed from bone)

ance also occurs when acidosis is present, which is common in chronic renal failure. Generally patients with advanced chronic renal failure will have high phosphate and low serum calcium concentrations. The secondary hyperparathyroidism, however, may cause calcium levels to approach normal, and in a small percentage of cases it may be elevated.

Clinical Manifestations

The clinical manifestations of chronic renal failure are often described using the term *uremia*. Uremia refers to a number of symptoms caused by decline in renal function with the accumulation of toxins in the plasma. The specific mechanisms contributing to toxic symptoms are unknown, although studies have shown that urea and creatinine are only minimally responsible. A combination of other end products of metabolism is associated with toxic symptoms and accompanies accumulations of urea and creatinine. Generally, the symptoms include anorexia, nausea, vomiting, diarrhea, weight loss, pruritus, edema, and neurologic changes (Table 33-11).

Evaluation and Treatment

Evaluation of chronic renal failure is based on the history and presenting signs and symptoms. Elevated serum creatinine concentrations and urea nitrogen are consistent with chronic renal failure. Ultrasound, intravenous pyelogram, or plain x-ray films will reveal small kidney size. Renal biopsy confirms the diagnosis.
Dietary Management The management of nutrition is essential for the person with chronic renal failure. Generally, nutritional management requires limiting the intake of some nutrients. Loss of renal function causes retention of end products of protein metabolism, and alterations in the ability to maintain fluid and electrolyte bal-

ance. Regulation of food and fluid intake may delay the need for dialysis. Diet therapy is planned according to individual needs by considering the type and severity of renal disease. The major objective is to maintain adequate nutrition while preventing the accumulation of metabolic waste products.
Sodium and Fluids Sodium requirements for individuals with renal failure may vary widely depending on the type of renal disease and use of diuretics. Glomerular disease tends to cause sodium retention, whereas tubulointerstitial diseases lead to sodium wasting. Sodium requirements can be evaluated by determining 24-hour urinary sodium levels. Usually sodium and fluids are restricted in patients with renal failure.

Fluid intake is usually limited to the amount of urine output, plus an additional amount for insensible water losses (500 to 1000 ml). Higher insensible losses occur with fever, excessive sweating, and elevations greater than 5000 feet.
Potassium Potassium is usually retained in chronic renal failure and requires dietary restriction. In the presence of anuria or oliguria, potassium is restricted to 0.5 mEq/kg of body weight/day (i.e., 50 meq or about 2 g/day). Many individuals with renal failure are able to maintain normal serum potassium levels if foods high in potassium are avoided.
Caloric Intake Adequate caloric intake is necessary to maintain ideal body weight. Calories are usually supplied in the form of fats and carbohydrates when protein intake is restricted. Individuals with chronic renal failure often have anorexia as a result of nausea, altered taste sensation, or psychologic depression, making it difficult to maintain an adequate caloric intake. A caloric intake of 35 kcal/kg of body weight/day usually spares tissue protein as a source of calories. Activity levels and

TABLE 33-11 Systemic effects of uremia

System	Manifestations	Mechanisms	Treatment
Skeletal	Osteitis fibrosa (bone inflammation with fibrous degeneration); bone demineralization (principally subperiosteal loss of cortical bone in the fibers, lateral ends of the clavicles, and lamina dura of the teeth); spontaneous fractures, bone pain; osteomalacia (rickets) with end-stage renal failure	Bone resorption associated with hyperparathyroidism, vitamin D deficiency, and demineralization; lowered calcium and raised phosphate levels	Control of hyperphosphatemia to reduce hyperparathyroidisms; administration of calcium and aluminum hydroxide antacids, which bind phosphate in the gut, together with a phosphate-restricted diet; vitamin D replacement; avoidance of magnesium antacids because of impaired magnesium excretion
Cardiopulmonary	Hypertension, pericarditis with fever, chest pain, and pericardial friction rub, pulmonary edema, Kussmaul's respirations	Extracellular volume expansion as cause of hypertension; hypersecretion of renin also associated with hypertension; fluid overload associated with pulmonary edema and acidosis leading to Kussmaul's respirations	Volume reduction with diuretics that are not potassium sparing (to avoid hyperkalemia); combination of propranolol, hydralazine, and minoxidil for those with high levels of renin; bilateral nephrectomy with dialysis or transplantation
Neurologic	Encephalopathy (fatigue, loss of attention, difficulty problem solving); peripheral neuropathy (pain and burning in the legs and feet, loss of vibration sense and deep tendon reflexes); loss of motor coordination, twitching, fasciculations, stupor, and coma with advanced uremia	Uremic toxins associated with end-stage renal disease	Dialysis
Hematologic	Anemia, usually normochromic normocytic; platelet disorders with prolonged bleeding times	Reduced erythropoietin secretion associated with loss of renal mass, leading to reduced red cell production in the bone marrow; uremic toxins associated with shortened red cell survival	Dialysis
Gastrointestinal	Anorexia, nausea, vomiting; mouth ulcers, stomatitis, urinous breath (uremic fetor), hiccups, peptic ulcers, gastrointestinal bleeding, and pancreatitis associated with end-stage renal failure	Retention of metabolic acids and other metabolic waste products	Protein-restricted diet for relief of nausea and vomiting
Integumentary	Abnormal pigmentation and pruritus	Retention of urochromes contributing to sallow, yellow color; high plasma calcium levels associated with pruritus	Dialysis with control of serum calcium levels
Immunologic	Increased risk of infection that can cause death	Suppression of cell-mediated immunity; reduction in number and function of lymphocytes, diminished phagocytosis	Routine dialysis
Reproductive	Sexual dysfunction: menorrhagia, amenorrhea, infertility, and decreased libido in women; decreased testosterone levels, infertility, and decreased libido in men	Probably related to dysfunction of ovaries and testes	No specific treatment

metabolic rate should also be considered when calculating caloric intake.

During dialysis, most water-soluble vitamins are lost into the dialysis bath, requiring replacement to maintain normal body requirements. Minerals, such as zinc and magnesium, may also be lost. Zinc replacement improves taste sensation and appetite.

When conservative management of chronic renal failure with diet, diuretics, and fluid restriction is no longer effective, dialysis or transplantation become necessary forms of treatment. Indications for initiating dialysis include uncontrollable hypertension, hyperkalemia, and signs of uremia, particularly neuropathies. When signs of neuropathy develop, dialysis should be initiated as soon as possible to prevent permanent damage.

SUMMARY REVIEW

Urinary Tract Obstruction
1 Obstruction can occur anywhere in the urinary tract and is usually caused by renal stones or tumors. The most serious complications are hydronephrosis, hydroureter, and infection caused by accumulation of urine behind the obstruction.
2 The most common kidney stone is formed from calcium and most often causes obstruction by lodging in the urethra.
3 Obstruction can be caused by a neural lesion that interrupts innervation of the bladder. The dysfunction is called a neurogenic bladder.
4 Renal cell carcinoma is the most common renal neoplasm. The larger neoplasms tend to metastasize to the lung, liver, and bone.
5 Bladder tumors are commonly composed of transitional cells with a papillary appearance and a high rate of recurrence.

Urinary Tract Infection
1 Urinary tract infections (UTIs) are usually caused by bacteria commonly from the retrograde movement of bacteria into the urethra and bladder.
2 Cystitis is an inflammation of the bladder commonly caused by bacteria, although types of "nonbacterial" cystitis may be caused by other conditions or by an autoimmune reaction.
3 Pyelonephritis is an acute or chronic inflammation of the renal pelvis that may cause abscess formation and scarring with an alteration in renal function. Pyelonephritis may be acute or chronic.

Glomerular Disorders
1 Glomerulonephritis is a group of related diseases of the glomerulus that can be caused by immune responses, toxins or drugs, vascular disorders, and other systemic diseases.
2 Acute glomerulonephritis commonly results from in-

flammatory damage to the glomerulus as a consequence of immune reactions following a streptococcal infection.
3 Rapidly progressive glomerulonephritis (RPGN) is associated with injury that results in proliferation of glomerular capillary endothelial cells and rapid loss of renal function.
4 Chronic glomerulonephritis is related to a variety of diseases that cause deterioration of the glomerulus and progressive loss of renal function.
5 Immune mechanisms in glomerulonephritis are the deposition of antigen-antibody complexes and the formation of antibodies specific for the glomerular basement membrane.
6 Nephrotic syndrome is the excretion of 3.5 g of protein in the urine per day. Its principal symptoms are hypoproteinuria, hyperlipidemia, and edema.
7 Nephrotic syndrome is caused by a loss of plasma proteins, principally albumin and some immunoglobulins, across the injured glomerular filtration membrane.

Renal Failure
1 Acute renal failure is classified as prerenal, intrarenal, or postrenal and is usually accompanied by oliguria with an elevated plasma BUN and plasma creatinine levels.
2 Prerenal acute renal failure is caused by decreased renal perfusion with a decreased GFR, ischemia, and tubular necrosis.
3 Intrarenal acute renal failure is associated with several systemic diseases but is commonly related to acute tubular necrosis (ATN).
4 Postrenal failure is associated with diseases that obstruct the flow of urine from the kidneys.
5 Chronic renal failure represents a progressive loss of renal function. Plasma creatinine levels gradually become elevated as GFR declines; sodium is lost in the urine; potassium is retained; acidosis develops; and calcium and phosphate metabolism is altered.

KEY TERMS

Acute glomerulonephritis, 1145

Acute renal failure, 1151

Acute tubular necrosis (ATN), 1151

Azotemia, 1151

Chronic glomerulonephritis, 1145

Chronic renal failure, 1154

Cystitis, 1141

End-stage renal failure, 1151

Dialysis, 1153

Glomerulonephritis, 1144

Goodpasture syndrome, 1145

Hydronephrosis, 1136

Hydroureter, 1136

Interstitial cystitis, 1142

Intrarenal acute renal failure, 1151

Lipiduria, 1150

Nephritic sediment, 1144

Nephrotic sediment, 1144

Nephrotic syndrome, 1149

Nidus, 1137

Neurogenic bladder, 1138

Postrenal acute renal failure, 1152

Prerenal acute renal failure, 1151

Pyelonephritis, 1142

Rapidly progressive glomerulonephritis, 1145

Renal adenoma, 1139

Renal cell carcinoma, 1139

Renal failure, 1150

Renal insufficiency, 1150

Renal stones (calculi, nephrolithiasis), 1137

Staghorn calculi, 1137

Uremia, 1150

Urethral syndrome ("irritable bladder"), 1142

Urinary tract infection, 1141

REFERENCES

Benson, R. C., Kinsey, J. H., Cortese, D. A., Farrow, G. M., & Utz, D. C. (1983). Treatment of transitional cell carcinoma of the bladder with hematoporphyrin derivative phototherapy. *Journal of Urology, 130,* 1090-1095.

Dretler, S. (1988). Laser lithotripsy: A review of 20 years of research and clinical applications. *Lasers in Surgery and Medicine, 8,* 341-356.

Fleisch, H. (1978). Inhibition and promotion of stone formation. *Kidney International, 13,* 361.

Hooten, T. M., Running, K., & Stamm, W. E. (1985). Single dose therapy for cystitis in women: A comparison of trimethoprim/sulfamethoxazole, amoxicillin, and clindicillin. *JAMA, 253,* 387.

Kaye, D. (1980). Urinary tract infection in the elderly. *Bulletin of the New York Academy of Medicine, 56,* 209.

Kjellstrand, C. M., Berkseth, R. O., & Klinkmann, H. (1988). Treatment of acute renal failure. In R. W. Schrier & C. W. Gottschalk (Eds.), *Diseases of the kidney* (4th ed.) (pp. 1510-1511). Boston: Little, Brown, & Co.

Kissane, J. M. (Ed.). (1985). *Anderson's Pathology* (8th ed.). St. Louis: C. V. Mosby.

Leaf, A. L. & Cotran, R. S. (1985). *Renal pathophysiology* (3rd ed.) p. 304. New York: Oxford University Press.

O'Dowd, T. C., Ribiero, C. D., Munro, J., West, R. R., Howells, C. H. L., & Davis, R. H. (1984). Urethral syndrome: A self-limiting illness. *British Medical Journal, 288,* 1349.

Ratner, J. J., Thomas, V. L., Sanford, B. A., & Forland, M. (1981). Bacteria-specific antibody in the urine of patients with acute pyeloneophritis and cystitis. *Journal of Infectious Diseases, 143,* 404.

Reiselbach, R. E. & Garnick, M. B. (Eds.). (1982). *Cancer and the kidney*. Philadelphia: Lea & Febiger.

Ronald, A. R. & Simonsen, N. (1988). Infections of the upper urinary tract. In R. W. Schrier & C. W. Gottschalk (Eds.), *Diseases of the kidney* (4th ed.) (p. 1084). Boston: Little, Brown, & Co.

Rubin, R. H., Tolkoff-Rubin, N. E., & Cotran, R. S. (1986). Urinary tract infection, pyelonephritis, and reflux nephropathy. In B. M. Brenner & R. C. Rector (Eds.), *The Kidney* (3rd ed.) (p. 1115). Philadelphia: W. B. Saunders.

Stamm W. E. & Turck, M. (1987). Urinary tract infection, pyelonephritis, and related conditions. In E. Braunwald, K. J. Isselbacher, R. G. Petersdorf, J. D., Wilson, J. B., Martin, & A. S., Fauli (Eds.), *Harrison's Principles of Internal Medicine*. (11th ed). (p. 1192). New York:McGraw Hill.

Thibodeau, G. A. (1987). *Anatomy and physiology*. St. Louis: C. V. Mosby.

Walker, P. L. (1984). Shock wave lithotripsy. *AORN Journal, 40,* 560.

Whaley, L. F. & Wong, D. L. (1987). *Nursing care of infants and children* (3rd ed.). St. Louis: C. V. Mosby.

Wilson, C. G. & Dixon, F. J. (1986). The renal response to immunological injury. In B. M. Brenner & F. C. Bector (Eds.), *The kidney* (3rd ed.). Philadelphia: W. B. Saunders.

Wilson, D. R. & Schrier, R. W. (1986). Obstructive nephropathy: Pathophysiology and management. In R. Sevier (Ed.), *Renal electrolyte disorders*. Boston: Little, Brown, & Co.

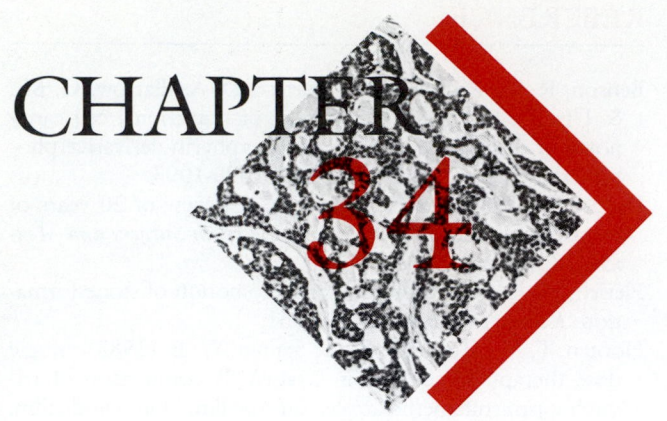

CHAPTER 34

Alterations of Renal and Urinary Tract Function in Children

Margaret M. Andrews
Kathleen Hardin Mooney

Structure and function of the renal system in children, 1160
    Development of the renal system, 1160
    Fluid and electrolyte balance in children, 1161
Alterations in renal function in children, 1161
    Structural abnormalities, 1161
        Hypospadias, 1162
        Epispadias, 1162
        Exstrophy of the bladder, 1163
        Renal agenesis, 1163
    Glomerular disorders, 1163
        Nephrotic syndrome, 1163
            Pathophysiology, 1163
            Clinical manifestations, 1164
            Evaluation and treatment, 1164
        Glomerulonephritis, 1164
        Hemolytic uremic syndrome, 1165
            Pathophysiology, 1166
            Clinical manifestations, 1166
            Evaluation and treatment, 1166
    Obstructive disorders, 1166
        Vesicoureteral reflux, 1166
            Pathophysiology, 1167
            Clinical manifestations, 1167
            Evaluation and treatment, 1167
        Wilms tumor, 1167
            Pathogenesis, 1167
            Clinical manifestations, 1167
            Evaluation and treatment, 1168
    Enuresis, 1168
        Types of enuresis, 1168
        Theories of enuresis, 1169

Some renal and urinary disorders occur in children as well as adults. In childhood, however, the kidney and genitourinary structures continue to develop, so that renal dysfunction may be associated with mechanisms and manifestations that are different from those in adults. In addition, some renal and urinary disorders are congenital. Many of these involve structural anomalies of the renal system.

STRUCTURE AND FUNCTION OF THE RENAL SYSTEM IN CHILDREN

Development of the Renal System

The embryonic kidneys develop as three sets of sequentially replaced organs, the pronephros, the mesonephros, and the metanephros (or the permanent kidney). The permanent kidneys are located in the pelvis, but their ascent to the abdomen begins by the seventh to ninth week of gestation. As the kidneys ascend, they rotate 90°. At birth, the kidneys occupy a large portion of the posterior abdominal wall, and the ureters are proportionately shorter than those of an adult. All the nephrons are present at birth, and their number does not increase as the kidney grows and matures. The kidney reaches adult size by adolescence and, because of maturation of the tubular system, increases in weight 10-fold from birth.

Urine formation and excretion begin by the third month of gestation, contributing to the amniotic fluid. In infancy, the bladder lies close to the abdominal wall, making urinary bladder aspiration for diagnostic pur-

TABLE 34-1 Average daily urine output in children	
Age	Output (ml/hr)
1 and 2 days	15-50
3-10 days	50-300
10 days to 2 mo	250-400
2 mo to 1 yr	400-500
1-3 yr	500-600
5-8 yr	700-1000
8-14 yr	700-1500

From Kempe, Silver, & O'Brien, 1982.

poses a relatively simple procedure. The bladder descends into the pelvis with growth, changing from a cylindric organ to the adult pyramidal shape. Although small amounts of urine are found in the bladder at birth, the newborn may not void for 12 to 24 hours. (The average daily urine output is shown in Table 34-1.)

Immediately at birth the renal blood flow and glomerular filtration rate (GFR) increase. These increases are caused by a decrease in vascular resistance and the need to perform excretory functions no longer performed by the placenta. Renal vascular resistance remains higher in newborns and infants, however, which may be attributed to increased levels of circulating renin. The resistance progressively declines during the first year of development with an increasing fraction of the cardiac output going to the kidney. The GFR continues to increase, becoming stable at 1 or 2 years but retaining 30% to 50% of adult levels until the end of the first year. Although glomerular filtration is important in removing nitrogenous and other wastes, the amount of urea to be removed is small.

Fluid and Electrolyte Balance in Children

Because the kidney develops from the center toward the periphery, renal distribution of blood flow during the newborn period is primarily to the renal medulla. The result is a preferential flow to the medullary nephrons, which have comparatively short loops at this stage of development. The combination of higher blood flow and shorter loops produces a more dilute urine, approximately 600 to 700 mOsm. The dilute urine is accentuated by a low rate of urea excretion because urea is necessary to establish the concentration gradient in the medulla. Urea excretion is low primarily because infants are in a high anabolic state and use their protein for growth.

Because of a high hydrogen ion concentration, limited ability to regulate the internal environment, and lowered osmotic pressure, the infant's renal system has a narrow chemical safety margin. The immaturity and smaller surface area of the tubules may also diminish the water reabsorption response to ADH. An immature tubular transport capacity means that the ability to excrete a potassium load, reabsorb bicarbonate, or buffer hydrogen with ammonia does not become efficient until about 2 years of age. Consequently, any disturbance, such as diarrhea, infection, fasting for diagnostic tests, or improper feeding, can rapidly lead to severe acidosis and fluid imbalance because the infant can rapidly develop overhydration, or edema.

After birth, the proportion of total body water to body weight does not change markedly. Considerable change occurs, however, in the location of that body water as the child matures (see Chapter 3). The percent of extracellular fluid volume of the newborn infant is nearly double that of the adult. Decrease in extracellular fluid volume occurs in two different periods of rapid growth, infancy and adolescence.

Not only does the infant have a greater content of extracellular fluid, but the fluid exchange rate also is greater. The adult takes in and excretes approximately 2000 ml of water daily, representing 5% of the total body fluid and 14% of the extracellular fluid. In contrast, the infant's daily exchange of 600 to 700 ml represents 290% of the total or nearly 50% of the extracellular volume, making control of dehydration and overhydration more difficult.

The composition of body fluids differs with age. The total electrolyte concentration in extracellular fluids is greater in the newborn than in the adult. The concentration of sodium, chloride, phosphates, and organic acids is also greater. The concentration of bicarbonate ions is lower in the infant than in the older child, with a mild acidosis evidenced by a lowered pH. These variations, combined with a lowered plasma protein level, cause a reduced oncotic pressure of the vascular compartment and favor accumulation of fluid in the tissue spaces and an increased GFR. In the healthy child, these differences remain for a few weeks or months. The premature infant and the normal newborn infant are usually in a state of well-compensated acidosis and potential edema.

ALTERATIONS IN RENAL FUNCTION IN CHILDREN

Structural Abnormalities

Variations from the normal anatomic structure of the urinary tract occur in 10% to 15% of the total population. The structural abnormalities range from minor, nonpathologic, or easily correctable anomalies to those that are incompatible with life. For example, the kidneys may fail to ascend from the pelvis to the abdomen, usually causing ectopic kidneys—an ectopic kidney usually functions normally. The kidneys may also fuse as they ascend, causing a **horseshoe kidney** that is U shaped. About one third of individuals with horseshoe kidneys are asymptomatic, and the most common problems are hydronephrosis, infection, and stone formation (Permutter, Retik, & Bauer, 1986). Collectively, structural anomalies of the renal system account for approximately 45% of cases of renal failure in children.

Some anomalies are obvious at birth, whereas others remain latent. Certain structural anomalies are commonly associated with urinary tract malformations (James, 1972). These include:

Low-set malformed ears
  Chromosomal disorders, especially trisomy 13 (Patau's syndrome) and trisomy 18
  Absent abdominal muscles
  Anomalies of the spinal cord and lower extremities
  Imperforate anus or genital deviation
  Wilms tumor
  Congenital ascities
  Cystic disease of the liver
  Positive family history of renal disease (hereditary nephritis or cystic disease)

Hypospadias

Hypospadias is a congenital condition in which the urethral meatus is located on the ventral or undersurface of the penis (Fig. 34-1). In more severe cases, it is located in the scrotum or perineum. This is the most common anomaly of the penis and occurs in about 1 in 300 infant boys. **Chordee** accompanies most cases of hypospadias. With chordee, a tough band of fibrous tissue replaces the normal tissue, causing the penis to bend or to "bow" ventrally (Fig. 34-2). Absence of the foreskin and cryptorchidism (undescended testicles, see Chapter 20) are associated with the anomaly.

Although hypospadias can have implications for sexual activity in the adult, the major problem for the hypospadic child is urination. The child must void sitting down until the problem is corrected surgically. Surgery is most effective at about 3 years of age when the penis has reached sufficient size. Psychologically, the preferred time to perform the correction comes before the child enters school and before he develops castration and mutilation anxiety.

Epispadias

Epispadias is a congenital condition with the urethral opening on the dorsal surface of the penis. The incidence of epispadias is about 1 in 30,000 infant boys. The urethral opening may be small and situated behind the glans, or a fissure may extend the entire length of the penis. This latter is associated with exstrophy of the bladder. Treatment is surgical, often requiring several operations over a prolonged time.

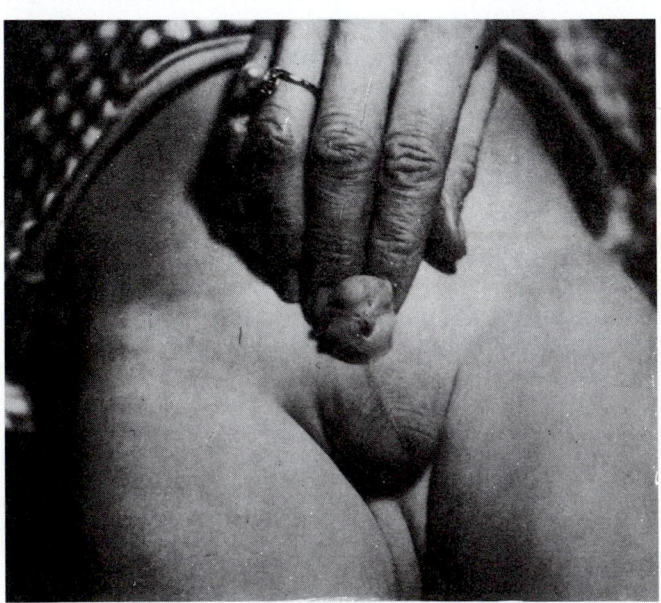

FIG. 34-1. Hypospadias. (Courtesy M. C. Gleason, M.D., San Diego, Calif.; from Ingalls & Salerno, 1979.)

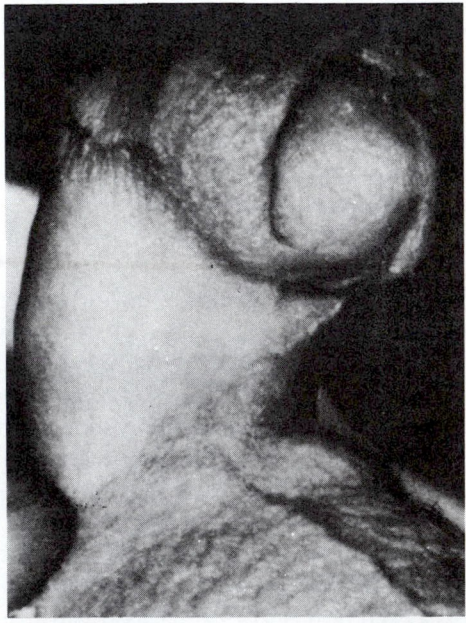

FIG. 34-2. Hypospadias with significant chordee. (From Shirkey, 1980.)

Exstrophy of the Bladder

Exstrophy of the bladder is an extensive congenital anomaly in which the lower urinary tract is exposed directly to the surface of the body (Fig. 34-3). The lining of the posterior portion of the bladder lining is exposed and appears bright red through a fissure in the abdominal wall. The incidence of exstrophy of the bladder is 1 in 40,000 live births. Between 100 and 200 children, mostly boys, are born with this defect each year.

Exstrophy of the bladder is caused by intrauterine failure of the abdominal wall and the mesoderm of the anterior bladder to fuse. The rectus muscles below the umbilicus are separated and the pubic rami (bony projections of the pubic bone) are not joined. The lack of bone fusion causes a waddling gait when the child walks. Urine seeps onto the abdominal wall from the ureters, causing a constant odor of urine and excoriation of the surrounding skin. Because the exposed bladder mucosa becomes hyperemic and edematous, it bleeds easily and is painful.

Surgical intervention is indicated between 6 months and 2 years of age. Objectives of management include preservation of renal function, attainment of urinary control, prevention of infection, reconstructive repair of the defect, and improvement of sexual function.

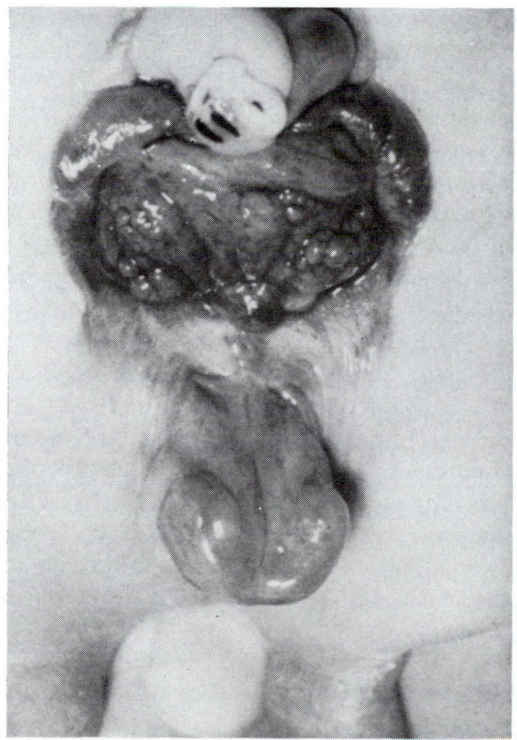

FIG. 34-3. Exstrophy of bladder. (Courtesy E. S. Tank, M.D., Division of Urology, University of Oregon Health Sciences Center, Portland, Ore.; from Whaley & Wong, 1987.)

Renal Agenesis

Renal agenesis (failure of a kidney to grow or develop) may be unilateral or bilateral, randomly occurring or clearly hereditary. The kidney is usually polycystic and dysplastic. The condition may occur as an isolated entity or as a problem associated with other unrelated disorders.

Unilateral renal agenesis occurs in about 1 of 1000 live births. The single kidney may be completely normal and without associated abnormalities, so that the child can expect a healthy and normal life. The normal solitary kidney grows because of compensatory hypertrophy after birth, and by the time the child is several years older, the volume of this kidney may approach twice the normal size.

In some instances, however, the single kidney is abnormally formed, and abnormalities are associated with its collecting system. Extrarenal congenital abnormalities are relatively more common with unilateral renal agenesis.

Bilateral renal agenesis (also called **Potter syndrome**) occurs in about 1 in 4000 live births, 75% being male. Bilateral renal agenesis results either from an abnormal development of the normal progression from pronephros to mesonephros to metanephros or from an isolated bilateral failure of development of the ureteral buds. The term *Potter syndrome* refers to the association with a specific group of facial anomalies (wide-set eyes, parrot-beak nose, low-set ears, and receding chin). Affected infants rarely live more than a few hours. Most die from respiratory distress caused by associated pulmonary hypoplasia rather than from renal failure. About 40% of affected infants are stillborn.

Glomerular Disorders

Nephrotic Syndrome

Nephrotic syndrome is a term used to describe a symptom complex characterized by proteinuria, hypoproteinemia, hyperlipidemia, and edema. Transient hematuria and/or hypertension may occur. Nephrotic syndrome is a clinical and biochemical state that may develop during the course of several different renal or systemic diseases. (The pathophysiology and common clinical manifestations of nephrotic syndrome in adults are described in Chapter 33.)

Pathophysiology

In children with nephrotic syndrome, the kidney is usually the only or principal organ involved. This condition is termed **primary nephrotic syndrome** and includes (1) the minimal change syndrome (also called idiopathic nephrotic syndrome, lipoid nephrosis, childhood nephrosis, and uncomplicated nephrosis), diffuse mesangial proliferation, and nephrotic syndrome with focal glomerulosclerosis, and (2) a group of disorders characterized by diffuse glomerular lesions, including membranoproliferative glomerulonephritis types I and II, membranous glomerulopathy, and idiopathic crescentic glomerulonephritis with antigen specific to the glomerular basement membrane.

Approximately 95% of nephrotic syndrome in children occurs in the absence of systemic or preexisting renal disease. Primary nephrotic syndrome is found predominantly in the preschool child with a peak incidence of onset between 2 and 3 years of age. It is rare after 8 years of age. Boys are affected more frequently than girls. No prevalent racial or geographic distributions are evident. The incidence is approximately 3 per 100,000 children per year.

Nephrotic syndrome may manifest itself during the first 6 months of life in infants with congenital syphilis. Nodular deposits on the glomerular basement membrane contain antigen-antibody complexes in which the antigen contains a component of the *Treponema pallidum* (the spirochete that causes syphilis). Antisyphilitic treatment results in complete recovery from the nephrotic syndrome and in resolution of the renal lesion.

Some nephrologists define nephrotic syndrome in infancy as a separate condition. This classification emphasizes its congenital origin and its association with congenital syphilis. **Infantile microcytic disease,** or Finnish-type congenital nephrotic syndrome, is an autosomal recessive condition that appears during the first year of life. The disease is chiefly characterized by early proteinuria and edema. Preeclampsia (toxemia of pregnancy), an enlarged placenta, and prematurity are other commonly associated features. No treatment is known to be effective, although some success has been reported with kidney transplantation. The disease is usually fatal within the first 2 years of life.

Clinical Manifestations

Onset of nephrotic syndrome is insidious with periorbital edema as the first sign (Fig. 34-4). The edema is most noticeable in the morning but subsides during the day as fluid shifts to the abdomen and lower extremities. Because toddlers have picky eating habits, parents are often pleased with the weight gain associated with edema. Parents become alerted to an abnormality when they notice diminished, "frothy," or "foamy" urine output and when edema becomes pronounced with ascites, respiratory difficulty from pleural effusion, and labial or scrotal swelling.

Edema of the intestinal mucosa may cause diarrhea, anorexia, and poor absorption. Edema often masks the malnutrition caused by malabsorption and protein loss. Because of protein deficiency, changes in the quality of hair indicates a malnourished state. Pallor, with shiny skin and prominent veins, is also common. Blood pressure is usually normal or slightly decreased. The child

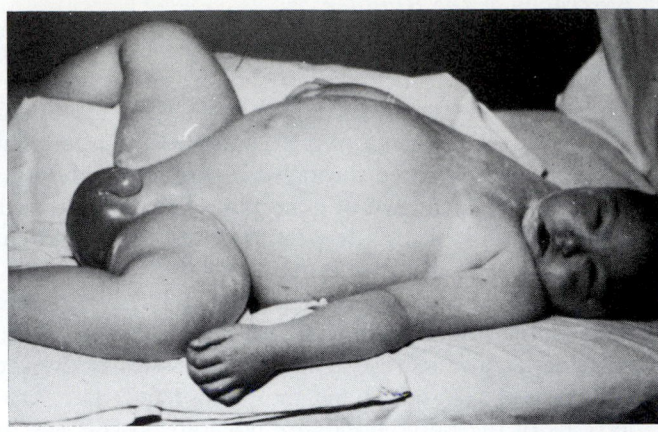

FIG. 34-4. Child with nephrotic syndrome. (From Shirkey, 1980.)

has an increased susceptibility to infection, especially pneumonia, peritonitis, cellulitis, and septicemia. Irritability, fatigue, and lethargy are common.

Evaluation and Treatment

The diagnosis of nephrotic syndrome is evident from the finding of proteinuria, hyperlipidemia, and lipiduria. Several different diagnostic tests, including kidney biopsy, may be required to determine whether the cause is an intrinsic renal disease or a consequence of systemic disease.

The goals of treatment are to reduce the excretion of protein and to maintain a protein-free urine. Prevention or treatment of infection, control of edema, establishment of a balanced nutritional state, and restoration of normal metabolic processes are also important in managing the disorder. Corticosteroids are the primary therapeutic agents, and children are often described according to their response to steroid therapy (Table 34-2). Basic management of nephrotic syndrome includes bed rest when edema is present; a low-sodium, high-protein diet; glucocorticosteroids (prednisone), diuretics (Lasix), and immunosuppressive agents (Cytoxan, Imuran); paracentesis (for ascites); and skin care.

Adults and children respond differently to management. Fifty-four percent of all children, as opposed to 21% of adults, have complete remission. Most children have minimal or no pathologic renal changes. The prognosis for ultimate recovery is quite good. Although relapses are common, most children can look forward to a healthy future.

Glomerulonephritis

Glomerulonephritis includes a number of renal disorders in which proliferation and inflammation of the glomerulus are secondary to an immune mechanism (Table 34-3). (The major glomerulopathies are de-

TABLE 34-2 Corticosteroid treatment in children with nephrotic syndrome

Response to corticosteroid	Incidence %	Outcomes
Steroid-sensitive	20-40	Single course of therapy, low recurrence rate
Steroid-dependent	60-80	Intermittent exacerbations with remissions over several years
Steroid-resistant	5-10	Resistance to steroids, eventual development of chronic renal failure

TABLE 34-3 Primary glomerulonephritis in children

Classification	Findings
Etiology	Poststreptococcal infection
	Related to other bacterial or viral infection
	Unknown
Immunologic mechanism	Antigen-antibody complex
	Anti-GMB disease
	No immunologic cause established
Histopathology	No lesion
	Diffuse, focal, or segmented
	Membranous, proliferative, or combination of types
	Lobular, exudative, necrotizing, and other types
	Chronic with glomerular proliferation
Clinical manifestations of disease	Acute glomerulonephritis
	Persistent (chronic) glomerulonephritis
	Idiopathic nephrotic syndrome

Adapted from James, 1972.

scribed in Chapter 33.) Chronic glomerulonephritis accounts for 53% of renal failure in children and is responsible for most patients requiring dialysis and kidney transplantation.

Acute glomerulonephritis (AGN) is the most common noninfectious renal disease in children. Whereas 95% of children can be expected to recover completely, a less favorable, 50% to 60% of adults can expect recovery. AGN occurs in children between 3 and 12 years, with a peak incidence at age 7 years. The 2:1 male/female ratio is unexplained. (The pathophysiology of acute glomerulonephritis is described in Chapter 33.)

Typically, a child is in good health until the onset of an upper respiratory or skin infection. One to 2 weeks later, mild proteinuria (less than l/G), hematuria, and periorbital edema appear. The urine is usually smoky brown or "cola" colored and the volume is reduced. The onset of symptoms in the child is abrupt and consists of flank or midabdominal pain, irritability, general malaise, and fever. Acute hypertension may cause headache, vomiting, somnolence, and other central nervous system manifestations including seizures. Cardiovascular symptoms are related to circulatory overload and are compounded by hypertension. These include dyspnea, tachypnea, and an enlarged, tender liver.

Improvement occurs within 2 to 3 weeks of onset although microscopic lesions remain for 2 months. Some children become oliguric and develop rapidly progressive glomerulonephritis, whereas others slowly progress to chronic glomerulonephritis. Prolonged proteinuria and abnormal GFR indicate an unfavorable prognosis.

AGN may be accompanied by a positive throat or skin culture for *Streptococcus*. The urine usually contains red blood cells and proteins. As a precautionary measure, penicillin is given in therapeutic doses for l0 to l4 days to eradicate residual *streptococci*. Because oliguria and hypertension are common, fluid, sodium, and potassium intake are restricted. Bed rest, antihypertensive medication, and diuretic agents are indicated during the acute phase.

Hemolytic Uremic Syndrome

Hemolytic uremic syndrome is an acute disorder characterized by hemolytic anemia originating in the microcirculation, acute renal failure, and thrombocytopenia. Although the cause remains unknown, evidence suggests that an abnormal host response to an infection triggers intravascular coagulation. (Normal hematologic function is discussed in Chapter 22.) An association between hemolytic uremic syndrome and both rickettsial and viral agents has been established, and the disease has been known to follow immunization with mumps and smallpox vaccines. Hemolytic uremic syndrome represents one of the most frequent causes of acute renal failure in children. The disease occurs in infants and children between the ages of 6 months and 3 years. When it occurs in adults, it is often associated with pregnancy and with use of oral contraceptives. Although the prognosis has improved dramatically in recent years, a l0% to 20% mortality rate has been reported.

Pathophysiology

In hemolytic uremic syndrome the endothelial lining of the glomerular arterioles becomes swollen and occluded with platelets and fibrin clots. Narrowed vessels damage erythrocytes, which become fragmented and assume a burrlike shape. These so-called burr cells are removed by the spleen, causing acute hemolytic anemia. Fibrinolysis, the process of dissolution of a clot, acts on precipitated fibrin, causing the fibrin-split products to appear in serum and urine. The platelet clustering within damaged vessels, combined with the damage and removal of platelets, produces thrombocytopenia.

Clinical Manifestations

A prodromal upper respiratory or gastrointestinal illness often precedes the onset of hemolytic uremic syndrome by 1 to 2 weeks. Pallor, bruising or purpura, irritability, and oliguria indicate the onset of the disease. Slight fever, anorexia, vomiting, and diarrhea, with the stool characteristically watery and blood stained, abdominal pain, mild jaundice, and circulatory overload are accompanying symptoms. Seizures and lethargy indicate CNS involvement. Renal failure is apparent within the first days of onset. The renal failure causes metabolic acidosis, azotemia, hyperkalemia, and often hypertension.

Evaluation and Treatment

Clinical evaluation includes history of preexisting illness, presenting symptoms, and urine and blood analysis. Management is supportive. When renal failure occurs, dialysis is indicated. Blood transfusions with packed red cells are needed to maintain reasonable hemoglobin levels.

Obstructive Disorders
Vesicoureteral Reflux

Vesicoureteral reflux is the retrograde flow of bladder urine into the ureters. Reflux allows infected urine from the bladder to be repeatedly swept up into the kidneys. The reflux perpetuates infection by preventing complete emptying of the bladder, as infected, refluxed urine drains back into the bladder at the end of each voiding. In addition, the reflux allows the maximal intravesical pressure to be transmitted to the renal calyces and pyramids (Fig. 34-5). The combination of reflux and infection is an important cause of pyelonephritis, especially in children less than 5 years of age.

Vesicoureteral reflux occurs more frequently in girls by a ratio of 10:1 and is uncommon in blacks. Its incidence is aproximately 1 in 1000 children, and siblings of those affected have a 25% chance of developing reflux. Although reflux is considered abnormal at any age, the shortness of the submucosal segment of the ureter during infancy and childhood renders the antireflux mechanism relatively inefficient and delicate. Thus reflux is seen commonly in association with infections during early childhood but rarely in older children and adults. (Among adults with urinary tract infections the incidence of reflux is approximately 5%.)

Reflux may be unilateral or bilateral, and it can be classified or graded for comparative purposes as follows:

Grade 1—Reflux into ureter only
Grade 2—Reflux up to the renal pelvis

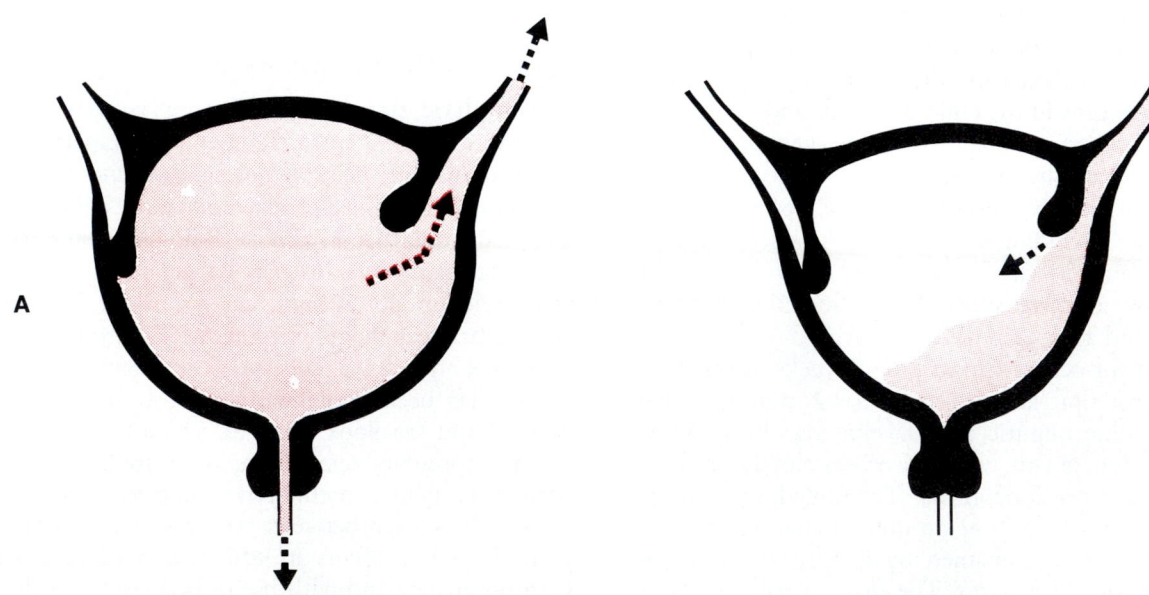

FIG. 34-5. Mechanisms of vesicoureteral reflux. **A,** During voiding, urine refluxes into ureter. **B,** After voiding, residual urine from ureter remains in bladder. (From Whaley & Wong, 1987.)

Grade 3—Ballooning of the pelvis and calyces
Grade 4—Tortuosity of the ureters and gross bal
looning

Pathophysiology

Primary reflux results from a congenitally abnormal or ectopic insertion of the ureter into the bladder. Occasionally, the condition is hereditary. Secondary reflux is of more serious importance and may be transient or persistent. It develops in association with infection, neurogenic bladder dysfunction, and other acquired disorders.

Clinical Manifestations

Children with reflux have recurrent urinary tract infection or unexplained fever, poor growth and development, irritability, and feeding problems. Both children and adults may have a family history of reflux or urinary tract infection, pain with voiding, and signs of urinary obstruction or neuropathy.

Evaluation and Treatment

In addition to the history of recurrent urinary tract infection and other symptoms, an intravenous pyelogram may be required for diagnosis. Most children with vesicoureteral reflux respond to nonoperative management which is aimed at prevention and treatment of infection. Spontaneous remission of reflux may occur in 30% to 60% of children less than 5 years of age. In cases of severe, persistent reflux, surgical intervention is indicated.

Wilms Tumor

Wilms tumor is an embryonal tumor of the kidney. Although the tumor was first described in 1814, it was named after Max Wilms, a German surgeon who wrote a detailed explanation of the tumor in 1899. At that time, Wilms proposed that the tumor was of embryonic origin and arose from undifferentiated mesoderm. Because it is an embryonal tumor of the kidney, Wilms tumor is also known by the histologic name of nephroblastoma.

The incidence of Wilms tumor remains constant in the United States with approximately 500 new cases identified each year. Because it is an embryonal tumor, most children are between 1 and 5 years of age when they are diagnosed. The peak incidence occurs between 1 and 3 years of age. Although generally limited in presentation, bilateral kidney involvement has been reported in up to 10% of children with this disease. Wilms tumor is the fifth most common childhood cancer and occurs in equal frequency among males and females. Wilms tumor constitutes slightly over 6% of cancer in white children and almost 8% of cancer in black children. It is less common than neuroblastoma in white

children but more common than neuroblastoma in black children.

Microscopically, Wilms tumor is composed of three cellular components (1) stromal, (2) epithelial, and (3) blastemal. This occurs because blastemal cells, which are primitive and undifferentiated, may have partially developed into epithelial or stromal tissue. With each of these three cellular components varying stages of differentiation may be evident.

Pathogenesis

Wilms tumor is thought to originate from the proliferation of the embryonic metanephric blastemal cells, primitive cells that normally differentiate into the renal tubules and glomeruli. Because normal renal development occurs during the eighth to thirty-fourth week of gestation, the mutation that causes the subsequent development of Wilms tumor should also occur between the eighth and thirty-fourth week of gestation (Belasco, Chatten, & D'Angio, 1984). The actual expression of Wilms tumor, however, may occur at birth or develop early in childhood.

Fifteen percent of children who have Wilms tumor also have a number of congenital anomalies, which suggests that the cancer is caused by an environmental agent that affects fetal development. The anomalies most commonly associated with Wilms tumor are aniridia (lack of an iris in the eye), hemihypertrophy (an asymmetry of the body), and genitourinary malformations (i.e., horseshoe kidneys, hypospadias, ureteral duplication, and polycystic kidneys) (Breslow & Beckwith, 1982). Children with both congenital anomalies and Wilms tumor are more likely to have bilateral disease.

Wilms tumor has both hereditary and nonhereditary origins. The hereditary form (accounting for only 1% to 2% of Wilms tumors) is transmitted as an autosomal dominant condition. Children with hereditary Wilms tumor are more likely to have bilateral or multifocal disease and congenital anomalies. The tumor usually is diagnosed at an earlier age than in those children seen with noninherited disease (Strong, 1976).

Clinical Manifestations

Most Wilms tumors are enlarging asymptomatic abdominal masses at the time of diagnosis. Many tumors are actually discovered by the child's parent, who feels or notices an abdominal swelling, usually while dressing or bathing the child. The child appears healthy and thriving. Other presenting complaints include vague abdominal pain (37%), hematuria (21%), and fever (23%) (Green, 1985). Hypertension may also be present. The reported frequency is quite variable, from 25% to as high as 63% in one report (Sukarochana, Tolentino, & Kiesewetter, 1972). Hypertension is probably caused by either encroachment by the tumor on the blood supply or secretion of renin by the tumor.

Wilms tumor may occur in any part of the kidney and varies greatly in size at the time of diagnosis. The tumor generally appears as a solitary tumor surrounded by a smooth, fibrous external capsule and may also contain cystic or hemorrhagic areas. A pseudocapsule generally separates the tumor from the renal parenchyma.

Evaluation and Treatment

On physical examination the tumor feels firm, nontender, and smooth. The mass is generally confined to one side of the abdomen. Should the tumor be palpable past the midline of the abdomen, it may be very large or may be arising from a horseshoe or ectopic kidney.

Diagnosis is based upon surgical biopsy. Additional laboratory and radiologic studies are used to evaluate the presence or absence of metastasis. The most common sites of metastasis are regional lymph nodes and the lungs. Metastases also occur in the liver, brain, and bone.

Several staging systems for Wilms tumor have been developed. The most widely accepted system was developed by the National Wilms Tumor Study Group (see Table 34-4). The system is based on surgical findings and the extent of disease at diagnosis (Farewell et al., 1981).

Surgical exploration and resection begins the treatment of Wilms tumor. The abdomen is explored to determine the extent of disease. In the case of bilateral disease, surgical intervention may include heminephrectomy of the least involved kidney and nephrectomy of the other. Wilms tumor is considered radiosensitive, and radiation therapy has been found to be most effective if begun within 1 to 3 days after surgery. Radiation therapy has not proven useful in stage I disease; it is used in stages II, III, and IV disease. Radiation therapy also is used for lung, nonresectable liver, brain, bone, and lymph node metastases should they be present.

The optimal protocol for chemotherapy is still under study for each stage of Wilms tumor. A combination of vincristine and actinomycin D currently appears to be more effective in stage I disease. Vincristine, actinomycin D, and doxorubicin hydrochloride (Adriamycin) are being tested in children with more advanced stages of disease. Cyclophosphamide also has shown some benefit.

Tremendous advances have been made in the treatment and cure of Wilms tumor. Before the 1930s, 90% of children died of Wilms tumor. Today, with modern treatment, the overall cure rate is greater than 90% for children with stage I through stage III disease. Prognosis is generally poor for children with metastases, although this is one of the few tumors for which lung metastases have been cured. Survival rates of 60% have

Stage	Tumor characteristics
Stage I	Tumor limited to the kidney, completely resected
Stage II	Tumor ascending beyond the kidney but appearing to be totally resected
Stage III	Residual nonhematogenous tumor confined to the abdomen
Stage IV	Hematogenous metastases
Stage V	Bilateral disease either at diagnosis or later

TABLE 34-4 Staging of Wilms tumor

NOTE: Staging system of the National Wilms' Tumor Study Group.

been reported for children with metastatic lung disease (Lanzkowsky, 1983).

A variety of factors affect the child's prognosis. These include tumor weight at diagnosis, the age of the child, lymph node invasion, and histologic category. The single most important prognostic factor, however, appears to be the histologic category.

Enuresis

Enuresis refers to the involuntary passage of urine by a child who is beyond the age when voluntary bladder control should have been acquired. Bladder control is accomplished by most children before the age of 4 years. However, 5 years of age is more accurate and widely accepted, being largely determined by cultural beliefs and practices of parents regarding toilet training. In 80% of children, enuresis occurs at night only and is then called **nocturnal enuresis.**

Types of Enuresis

Primary enuresis refers to a condition in which the child has never been continent. **Secondary enuresis,** or acquired enuresis, occurs when a child who has experienced a period of dryness of at least 3 to 6 months after toilet training becomes incontinent again. Secondary enuresis may be diurnal (daytime), nocturnal, or a combination of both. (Types of incontinence are defined in Table 34-5.)

The incidence of enuresis is difficult to determine because it is not a problem that parents readily share with others and because definitions vary according to cultural norms and family practices. Some families start toilet training before 1 year of age and expect continence by the age of 1 or 1 ½, whereas other families do not expect dryness earlier than 5 years. According to research data, the incidence of enuresis in children older than 5

TABLE 34-5 Classification of incontinence

Types of incontinence	Definition
Total incontinence	Inability to store any urine; indicates an anatomic or functional absence of urinary sphincters (e.g., epispadias or myelomeningocele) or a bypassing of urinary sphincters (e.g., vesicovaginal fistula)
Overflow incontinence	Frequent dribbling that relieves a constantly full bladder; occurs when urinary outlet is obstructed
Urge incontinence	Sudden and uncontrollable need to void that cannot be suppressed; suggests bladder irritation
Precipitate voiding	Voiding without a preceding urge to void; suggests neurologic origin
Stress incontinence	Uncontrollable voiding that occurs when intravesical pressure momentarily exceeds intravesical resistance, as in "giggle incontinence"
Paradox incontinence	Incontinence in spite of normal voiding; suggests an ectopic ureteral orifice outside the urinary sphincter mechanism (e.g., a girl who is constantly wet, yet voids normally)

years ranges from 15% to 26%. Boys are more enuretic than girls by a ratio of 3:2. Teenage enuresis is usually a continuation of childhood bedwetting. Sours (1978) reports that approximately 2% of men in the armed forces are enuretic.

Theories of Enuresis

Theories about the cause of enuresis abound. A combination of factors is likely to be responsible for enuresis. All or part of each one might be operating in a given child. Reasonable evaluation is to eliminate organic or physiologic causes for enuresis before exploring the psychologic ones.

Organic causes of enuresis account for 2% to 10% of cases. The causes include urinary tract infections; neurologic disturbances; congenital defects of the meatus, urethra, and bladder neck; and allergies. Disorders that increase the normal output of urine, such as diabetes mellitus and diabetes insipidus, or disorders that impair the concentrating ability of the kidney, such as chronic renal failure or sickle cell disease, must be considered in the evaluation of enuresis.

Enuresis in children is possibly caused by a maturational lag. Studies have demonstrated that the child with enuresis has a smaller functional bladder capacity than a nonenuretic child (Troup & Hodgson, 1971). A number of children show a general developmental delay along with elevated intravesical pressure and spikelike detrusor contractions during bladder filling. Enuresis may spontaneously disappear in these children as they get older.

Genetic factors as a cause of enuresis are speculative, but the condition does show a familial tendency (Koff, 1986). Bed-wetting does occur with high frequency among parents, siblings, and other near relatives of symptomatic children. These observations are further supported by a high concordance rate in enuretic monozygotic twins. Family studies indicate that the closer the relationship, the higher the incidence of enuresis.

A significant number of nocturnal enuretic episodes have been related to deep sleep. These children sleep more soundly than others. Many demonstrate increased frequency and magnitude of spontaneous bladder contractions during the non-rapid-eye-movement (non-NREM) stage of sleep preceding bed-wetting. Nocturnal enuresis occurs as the child moves from the deeper stages of non-REM sleep into the REM stage. Bed-wetting incidents are incorrectly associated with dreaming. Laboratory studies of sleep have demonstrated that very few incidents of bed-wetting occur when the child is dreaming (Kales & Kales, 1970). If the bed is not changed, however, the child may incorporate the feeling of wetness with the next REM dream cycle and may, therefore, incorrectly associate the enuresis with the dream. As the child develops, the deep sleep period, which is associated with a physiologic dysfunction of the reticular activating system, resolves, and the child "outgrows" the problem.

A variety of psychosocial theories have also been postulated as explanation of enuresis. Enuresis has been associated with temper tantrums, fear reactions, and excitability (Knopf, 1984).

Therapeutic management of enuresis includes conditioning devices, drug therapy (Tofranil), bladder training, withholding fluids, sleep interruption, and diet therapy. Psychotherapy and behavior modification are recommended when enuresis is associated with psychologic stress.

SUMMARY REVIEW

Structure and Function of the Renal System in Children

1 Because of high hydrogen ion concentration, limited ability to regulate the internal environment, and lowered osmotic pressure, children have a narrow chemical safety margin.

2 Any disturbance, such as diarrhea, infection, fasting, or feeding alterations can lead rapidly to severe acidosis and fluid imbalance.

3 The composition of body fluids differs with age, thus making children more vulnerable to pathophysiologic changes.

4 Because the kidney develops from the medulla to the cortex, blood flow to the medullary nephrons is limited in infancy, and infants thus have limited urine-concentrating capacity.

Alterations in Renal Function in Children

1 Congenital renal disorders affect 10% to 15% of the population. These disorders range in severity from minor, easily correctable anomalies, to those incompatible with life.

2 Hypospadias is a congenital condition in which the urethral meatus is located on the undersurface of the penis; epispadias is a congenital condition in which the urethral opening is located on the dorsal surface of the penis.

3 Exstrophy of the bladder is a congenital malformation in which the lower portion of the abdominal wall and anterior wall of the bladder are missing and the bladder is everted through the opening.

4 Renal agenesis is the failure of a kidney to grow or develop. (The condition may be unilateral or bilateral and may occur as an isolated entity or in association with other disorders.)

5 Nephrotic syndrome is a term used to describe a symptom complex characterized by proteinura, hypoproteinemia, hyperlipidemia, and edema. Metabolic, biochemical, or physiochemical disturbance in the glomerular basement membrane may lead to increased permeability to protein.

6 Glomerulonephritis is an inflammation of the glomeruli characterized by hematuria, edema, and hypertension. (The cause is unknown, but glomerulonephritis frequently follows other infections, especially those of the upper respiratory tract).

7 Hemolytic uremic syndrome is an acute disorder characterized by hemolytic anemia, acute renal failure, and thrombocytopenia.

Obstructive Disorders

1 Vesicoureteral reflux, which refers to the retrograde flow of bladder urine into the ureters, provides mechanisms for bladder infection in children whose ureters are shorter than those of adults.

2 Wilms tumor is an embryonal tumor of the kidney present at birth or evident by 5 years of age. The tumor can be successfully treated by surgery and radiation therapy.

Enuresis

1 Enuresis refers to the involuntary passage of urine.

2 The condition may occur during the daytime (diurnally) or during the night (nocturnally).

3 The disorder tends to occur during non-REM sleep and can have a variety of organic and psychologic causes.

KEY TERMS

Chordee, 1162

Enuresis, 1168

Epispadias, 1162

Exstrophy of the bladder, 1163

Hemolytic uremic syndrome, 1165

Horseshoe kidney, 1162

Hypospadias, 1162

Infantile microcytic disease, 1164

Nocturnal enuresis, 1168

Potter syndrome, 1163

Primary enuresis, 1168

Primary nephrotic syndrome, 1163

Renal agenesis, 1163

Secondary enuresis, 1168

Wilms tumor (nephroblastoma), 1167

REFERENCES

Belasco, J., Chatten, J., & D'Angio, G. (1984). Wilms' tumor. In W. Sutow, D. Fernbach, & T. Vietti (Eds.), *Clinical pediatric oncology* (3rd ed.). St. Louis: C. V. Mosby.

Breslow, N. E., & Beckwith, J. B. (1982). Epidemiological features of Wilms' tumor: Results of the national Wilms' tumor study. *Journal of the National Cancer Institute, 68,* 429-436.

Farewell, V. T., D'Angio, G. J., Breslow, N. E., & Norkool, P. (1981). Retrospective validation of a new staging system for Wilms' tumor. *Cancer Clinic Trials, 4,* 167-171.

Green, D. M. (1985). The diagnosis and management of Wilms' tumor. *Pediatric Clinics of North America, 32,* 735-754.

Ingalls, A. J., & Salerno, M. C. (1979.) *Maternal and child health nursing.* (4th ed.). St. Louis: C. V. Mosby.

James, J. A. (1972). *Renal disease in childhood* (2nd ed.) p. 84. St. Louis: C. V. Mosby.

Kales, A., & Kales, J. D. (1970, September). Evaluation, diagnosis, and treatment of clinical conditions related to sleep. *JAMA, 11,* 2229-2235.

Kempe, C.H., Silver, K. H., & O'Brien, D. (1982). *Current pediatric diagnosis and treatment.* Los Altos: Lange Medical Publishers.

Knopf, I. J. (1984). *Childhood psychopathology: A developmental approach* (2nd ed.). Englewood Cliffs, NJ: Prentice-Hall.

Koff, S. A. (1986). Enuresis [Chapter 54]. In P. C. Walsh, G. F. Ruben, A. D. Permutter, & T. A. Stanley (Eds.), *Campbell's urology* (vol. 2, 5th ed.). Philadelphia: W. B. Saunders.

Lanzkowsky, P. (1983). Wilms' tumor. In P. Lanzkowsky (Ed.), *Pediatric oncology.* New York: McGraw-Hill.

Permutter, A. D., Retik, A. B., & Bauer, S. B. (1986). Anomalies of the upper urinary tract [Chapter 38, p. 1165]. In P. C. Walsh, G. F. Ruben, A. D. Permutter, & T. A. Stanley (Eds.), *Campbell's urology* (vol. 2, 5th ed.). Philadelphia: W. B. Saunders.

Shirkey, H. C. (Ed.). (1980). *Pediatric therapy* (6th ed.). St. Louis: C. V. Mosby.

Sours, J. (1978). Enuresis. In B. Wolman (Ed.), *Handbook of treatment of mental disorders in childhood and adolescence* pp. 153-160. New Jersey: Prentice-Hall.

Strong, L. (1976). Genetic and teratogenic aspects of Wilms' tumor. In C. Pochedly & D. Miller (Eds.), *Wilms' tumor.* New York: John Wiley & Sons.

Sukarochana, K., Tolentino, W., & Kiesewetter, W. B. (1972). Wilms' tumor and hypertension. *Journal of Pediatric Surgery, 7,* 573-578.

Troup, C. W., & Hodgson, N. B. (1971, January). Nocturnal functional bladder capacity in enuretic children. *Journal of Urology, 105,* 129-136.

Whaley, L. F., & Wong, D. L. (1987). *Nursing care of infants and children* (3rd ed.). St. Louis: C. V. Mosby.

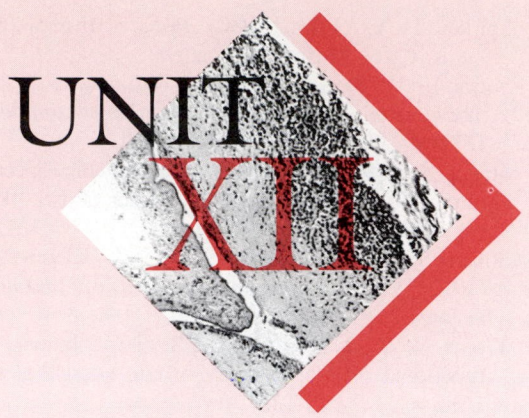

UNIT XI

The Digestive System

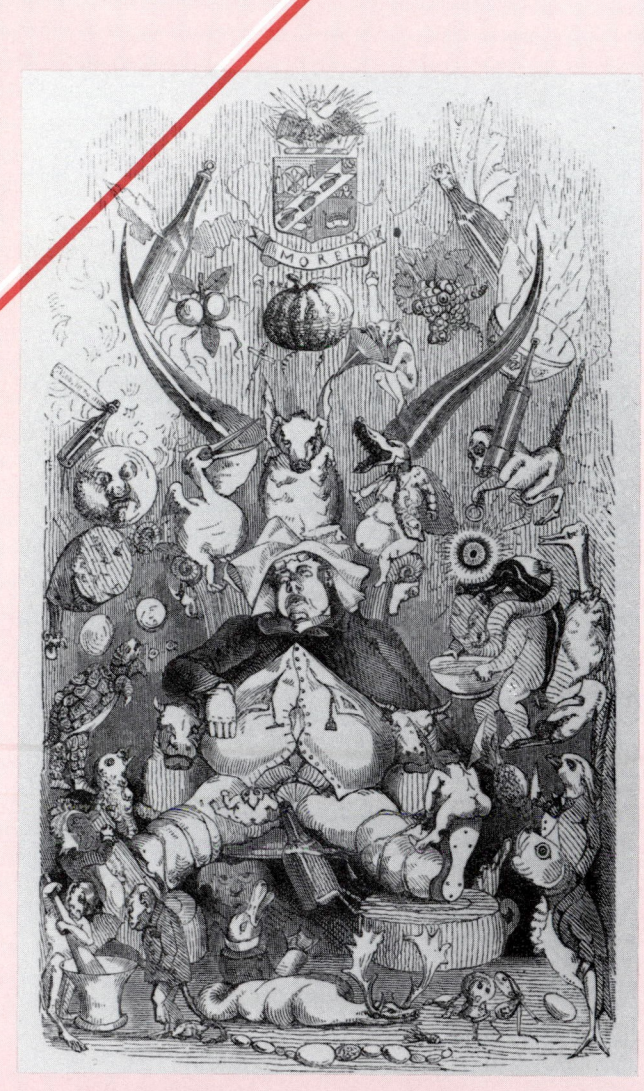

Overstuffed man dozes. He is plagued by visions (animals, food, bottles of wine, clyster, mortar and pestle, etc.) conjured up as a result of his overeating. (From Whiting, S,: Memoirs of a stomach, London, 1853. Courtesy National Library of Medicine.)

GASTROINTESTINAL disorders have been a source of human misery since ancient times. Hippocrates (460-370 BC) described clinical symptoms of dysentery, intestinal obstruction, and liver disease. Detailed descriptions of tumors and ulcers of the esophagus and stomach and hardening of the liver and ascites were made by Galen (131-201 AD). As one of the earliest physiologists, he offered ideas about processes of digestion and functions of the liver that provided the basis for his discussion of gastrointestinal diseases. Although his descriptions contained fundamental misconceptions, 1400 years passed before a Florentine physician, Antonius Benivenius (1507), accurately wrote about gastric ulcers, intestinal carcinoma, and gallstones on the basis of postmortem examinations.

By 1761 Morgangai had described the pathologic anatomy of gastritis, gastric and intestinal ulcers, and tumors and cirrhosis of the liver. The pathologic anatomy of gastrointestinal disease was advanced by Karl Rokitansky (1804-1878) from descriptions based on over 30,000 autopsies. Microscopic classifications of intestinal disease were first published by Rudolf Virchow in 1856.

Chemical processes of digestion were first introduced in the 1600s. Regner de Graaf (1641-1673) isolated pancreatic and salivary juices by creating parotid and pancreatic fistulas in a dog. Two hundred years later Claude Bernard (1813-1878) described the storage of sugar in the liver as glycogen and its release as glucose, as well as the digestive function of the pancreas. Pepsin was isolated in 1861, and the pancreatic enzyme trypsin was isolated in 1867. The first intestinal hormone, secretin, was identified in 1902, and the field of endocrinology began. Since that time more than two dozen intestinal hormones have been described. During World War II a Dutch physician observed that children with celiac sprue (gluten intolerance) who were deprived of bread had a great improvement in their symptoms. From this observation gluten was identified as the cause of celiac sprue. The virus-causing serum, hepatitis, was discovered by B. S. Blumberg in 1965; for this work he was awarded the Nobel Prize in 1976.

The functions of gastric juice were studied by the swallowing and retrieval of sponges from which the juice was squeezed. Swallowing linen bags or perforated metal tubes filled with food allowed analysis of gastric digestion. The presence of hydrochloric acid in gastric juice was established by an English physiologic chemist, William Prout, in 1824. An American frontier physician, William Beaumont (1785-1853), studied gastric function over many years by observing the gastric mucosa of a patient he treated who survived a gunshot wound in the abdomen. The wound healed, leaving a permanent gastric fistula, allowing Beaumont the opportunity to collect gastric secretions and study gastric activity under a variety of circumstances. He is credited as the father of American physiology and gastroenterology.

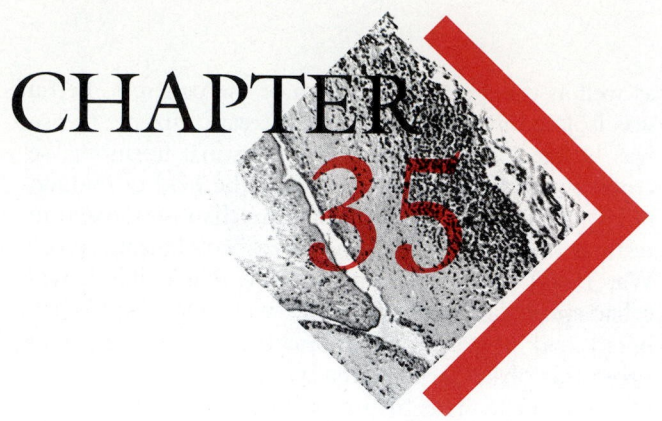

CHAPTER 35

Structure and Function of the Digestive System

Sue E. Huether

The gastrointestinal tract, 1175
  Mouth and esophagus, 1175
    Salivation, 1175
    Swallowing, 1176
  The stomach, 1177
    Gastric motility, 1178
    Gastric secretion, 1179
      Acid, 1180
      Pepsin secretion, 1181
      Mucus, 1181
    Phases of gastric secretion, 1181
      Cephalic phase, 1181
      Gastric phase, 1181
      Intestinal phase, 1182
  The small intestine, 1182
    Intestinal digestion and absorption, 1184
      Water and electrolytes, 1184
      Carbohydrates, 1186
      Proteins, 1187
      Fats, 1187
      Minerals and vitamins, 1188
    Intestinal motility, 1190
  The large intestine, 1190
  Intestinal bacteria, 1192
Accessory organs of digestion, 1193
  The liver, 1194
    Secretion of bile, 1195
    Metabolism of bilirubin, 1197
    Vascular and hematologic functions, 1198
    Metabolism of nutrients, 1198
      Fats, 1198
      Proteins, 1198
      Carbohydrates, 1198
    Metabolic detoxification, 1198
    Storage of minerals and vitamins, 1199
  The gallbladder, 1199
  The exocrine pancreas, 1200

Tests of digestive function, 1202
  The gastrointestinal tract, 1202
  The liver, 1202
  The gallbladder, 1203
  The exocrine pancreas, 1203
Aging and the gastrointestinal system, 1206

The digestive system breaks down ingested food, prepares it for uptake by the body's cells, and eliminates wastes. This system consists of the gastrointestinal tract, a long tube that extends from the mouth to the anus, and accessory organs of digestion: the liver, gallbladder, and exocrine pancreas.

Food breakdown begins in the mouth with chewing and continues in the stomach, where food is churned and mixed with acid, mucus, enzymes, and other secretions. From the stomach the fluid and partially digested food passes into the small intestine, where biochemicals and enzymes secreted by the liver and exocrine pancreas break it down into absorbable components of proteins, carbohydrates, and fats. These nutrients pass through the walls of the small intestine into blood vessels and lymphatics that carry them to the liver for storage or further processing.

Ingested substances and secretions that are not absorbed in the small intestine pass into the large intestine, where fluid continues to be absorbed. Fluid wastes travel to the kidneys and are eliminated in the urine. Solid wastes pass into the rectum and are eliminated from the body through the anus.

Except for chewing, swallowing, and defecation of solid wastes, the movements of the digestive system (gastrointestinal motility) are all controlled by hormones and the autonomic nervous system. As ingested substances move through the gastrointestinal tract, they trigger the release of hormones that stimulate or inhibit (1) the muscular contractions that mix and propel food from the esophagus to the anus and (2) the timely secretion of substances that aid in digestion. The autonomic innervation, both sympathetic and parasympathetic, is controlled by centers in the brain and by local stimuli that are mediated at plexuses (networks of nerve fibers) within the gastrointestinal walls.

THE GASTROINTESTINAL TRACT

The alimentary canal, or **gastrointestinal tract,** consists of the mouth, esophagus, stomach, small intestine, large intestine, rectum, and anus (Fig. 35-1). It carries out the following digestive processes:

1. Ingestion of food
2. Propulsion of food and wastes from the mouth to the anus
3. Mechanical breakdown of food particles
4. Chemical breakdown of food particles
5. Absorption of digested food
6. Elimination of waste products by defecation

Mouth and Esophagus

The **mouth** is a reservoir for the chewing and mixing of food with saliva. As food particles become smaller and move around in the mouth, the taste buds and olfactory nerves are continuously stimulated, adding to the satisfaction of eating. The tongue's surface contains thousands of chemoreceptors, or taste buds, which can distinguish salty, sour, bitter, and sweet tastes. Tastes and food odors help to initiate salivation and the secretion of gastric juice in the stomach.

Salivation

There are three pairs of **salivary glands,** the submandibular, sublingual, and parotid glands (Fig. 35-2). Together they secrete about 1 L of saliva per day. **Saliva** consists mostly of water that contains varying amounts of mucus, sodium, bicarbonate, chloride, potassium, and **salivary α-amylase** (ptyalin), an enzyme that initiates carbohydrate digestion in the mouth and stomach.

Both sympathetic and parasympathetic divisions of the autonomic nervous system control salivation. Because cholinergic parasympathetic fibers stimulate the salivary glands, atropine (an anticholinergic agent) inhibits salivation and makes the mouth dry. β-Adrenergic stimulation from sympathetic fibers also increases salivary secretion. The salivary glands, unlike other secretory glands of the gastrointestinal tract, are not regulated by hormones.

The composition of saliva depends on the rate of se-

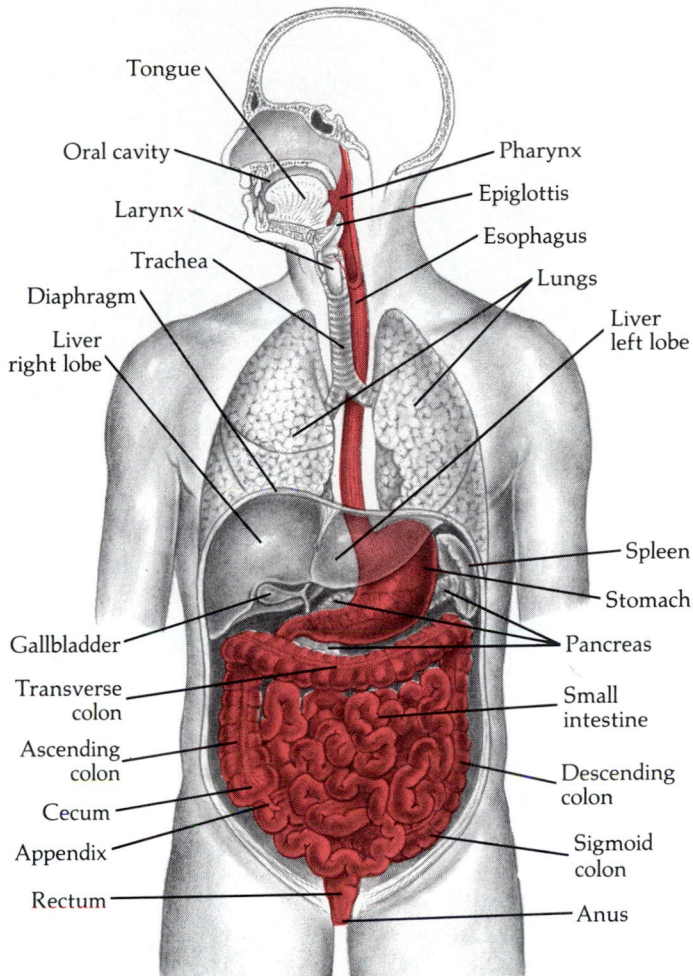

FIG. 35-1. Structure and function of the digestive system. Digestion begins in the mouth with chewing, which breaks down food mechanically and mixes it with saliva. Swallowing propels chewed food through the esophagus to the stomach, where acids and stomach motility liquefy it further. Next the liquefied food enters the small intestine, where secretions of the intestinal walls, liver, gallbladder, and pancreas digest it into absorbable nutrients. Nutrients are absorbed through intestinal walls, and unabsorbed wastes enter the large intestine (colon), where fluids are removed. Solid wastes then enter the rectum and leave the body through the anus. (From Thompson et al., 1989.)

cretion. At low rates of flow, such as those between meals, sodium, chloride, and bicarbonate are reabsorbed in the collecting ducts of the salivary glands, and the saliva contains fewer of these electrolytes (i.e., is more hypotonic). At higher flow rates, which are stimulated by food, reabsorption is decreased and there is more sodium, chloride, and bicarbonate in the saliva, making it hypertonic (Fig. 35-3). By this mechanism, sodium, chloride, and bicarbonate are recycled until they are released to help with digestion and absorption. Potassium secretion is fairly constant, independent of flow rate.

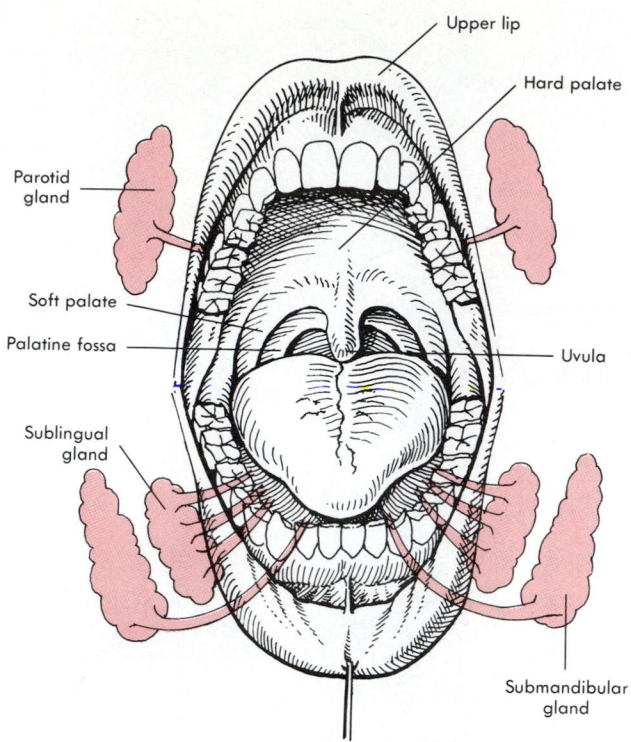

Upper lip

Hard palate

Parotid gland

Soft palate

Palatine fossa

Uvula

Sublingual gland

Submandibular gland

FIG. 35-2. Structures of the mouth. (From Phipps, Long, & Woods 1987.)

However, aldosterone can increase an exchange of sodium for potassium, increasing sodium conservation and potassium excretion. The bicarbonate concentration of saliva sustains a pH of about 7.4, which neutralizes bacterial acids and prevents tooth decay. Exogenous fluoride (e.g., fluoride in drinking water) is also secreted in the saliva, providing additional protection against tooth decay.

Swallowing

The **esophagus** is a hollow muscular tube that conducts substances from the oropharynx to the stomach (see Fig. 35-1). Swallowed food is moved to the stomach by **peristalsis,** the sequential contraction and relaxation of outer longitudinal and inner circular layers of muscles. The upper third of the esophagus contains striated muscle that is directly innervated by motor neurons. The lower two thirds contains smooth muscle that is innervated by preganglionic cholinergic fibers from the vagus nerve. The fibers are activated in a downward sequence. Peristalsis is stimulated when afferent fibers distributed along the length of the esophagus sense changes in wall tension caused by stretching as food passes. The greater the tension, the greater the intensity of esophageal contraction. Occasionally intense contractions cause pain similar to "heartburn" or angina.

Each end of the esophagus is opened and closed by a sphincter. The **upper esophageal sphincter** prevents

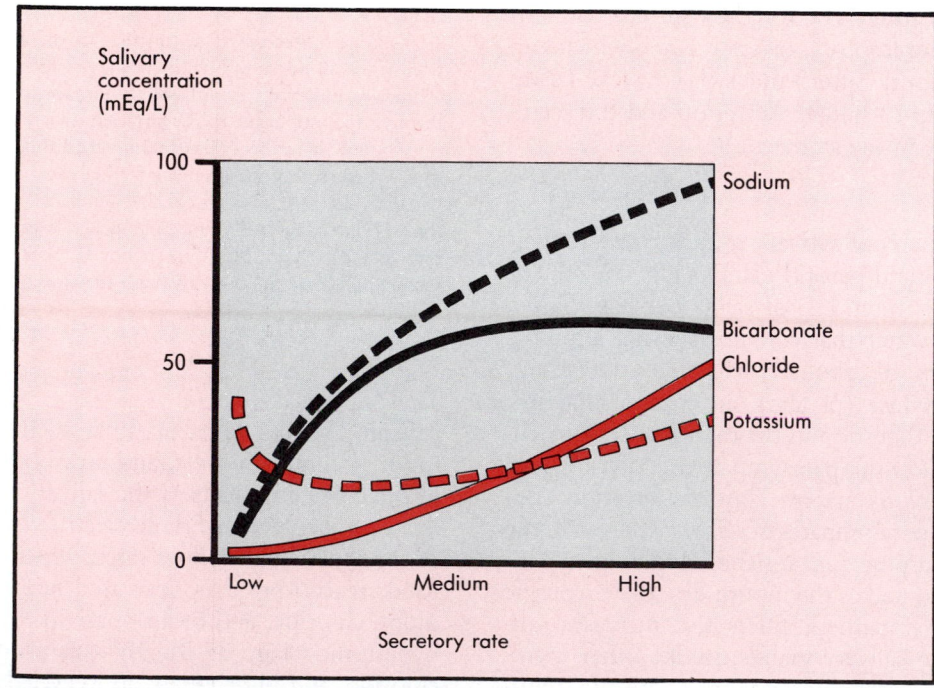

Salivary concentration (mEq/L)

Sodium

Bicarbonate

Chloride

Potassium

Low   Medium   High

Secretory rate

FIG. 35-3. Changes in concentration of sodium (Na^+), potassium (K^+), chloride (Cl^-), and bicarbonate (HCO_3^-) with increases in flow rate of saliva.

entry of air into the esophagus during respiration. The **lower esophageal sphincter** (cardiac sphincter) prevents regurgitation from the stomach. This is a necessary function because intra-abdominal pressure is greater than intrathoracic or atmospheric pressure.

Swallowing is a complex event mediated by the swallowing center, which is located in the reticular formation of the brain stem. Swallowing occurs in two phases, the oropharyngeal (voluntary) phase and the esophageal (involuntary) phase. During the **oropharyngeal phase** of swallowing, food is segmented into a bolus by the tongue and forced posteriorly toward the pharynx as the tongue pushes upward against the hard palate. The superior constrictor muscle of the pharynx contracts, preventing movement of food into the nasopharynx. At the same time, respiration is inhibited and the epiglottis slides downward to prevent the bolus from entering the trachea. The movements of the tongue and pharyngeal constrictors propel the food into the esophagus in a series of coordinated events taking less than 1 second (Christensen, 1987).

The **esophageal phase** of swallowing begins as the bolus of food enters the esophagus. The bolus is transported by peristalsis, the sequential waves of muscular contractions that travel down the esophagus and are preceded by receptive waves of relaxations. The wave of relaxation reduces resistance and allows food to pass, after which the wave of contraction pushes food farther along. The lower esophageal sphincter relaxes just before the arrival of a peristaltic wave. The sphincter muscles return to their resting tone after the bolus of food passes into the stomach. The esophageal phase of swallowing takes 5 to 10 seconds, with the bolus moving 2

to 6 cm/sec. Throughout swallowing the sphincters and esophagus work in concert with the peristaltic wave that moves food from the mouth to the stomach.

Peristalsis that immediately follows the oropharyngeal phase of swallowing is called **primary peristalsis.** If a bolus of food becomes stuck in the esophageal lumen, the distention of the esophageal wall stimulates **secondary peristalsis,** a wave of contraction and relaxation that is independent of voluntary swallowing. Secondary peristalsis is a response to stretch receptors that are stimulated by increased wall tension, causing an increase in impulses from the swallowing center of the brain.

When it is closed, the lower esophageal sphincter serves as a barrier between the stomach and esophagus. The muscle tone of the lower sphincter changes with neural and hormonal stimulation. Cholinergic vagal input and the digestive hormone gastrin increase sphincter tone. Nonadrenergic, noncholinergic vagal impulses relax the lower esophageal sphincter, as do the hormones progesterone, secretin, and glucagon. Relaxation during swallowing is mediated by the vagus.

The Stomach

The **stomach** is a hollow, muscular organ that stores food during eating, secretes digestive juices, mixes food with these juices, and propels partially digested food, called **chyme,** into the duodenum of the small intestine. The anatomy of the stomach is presented in Fig. 35-4. The stomach's major anatomic boundaries are the lower esophageal sphincter, where food passes through the **cardiac orifice** into the stomach; the greater and lesser curvatures; and the **pyloric sphincter,** which relaxes as food is propelled through the **pylorus** into the duode-

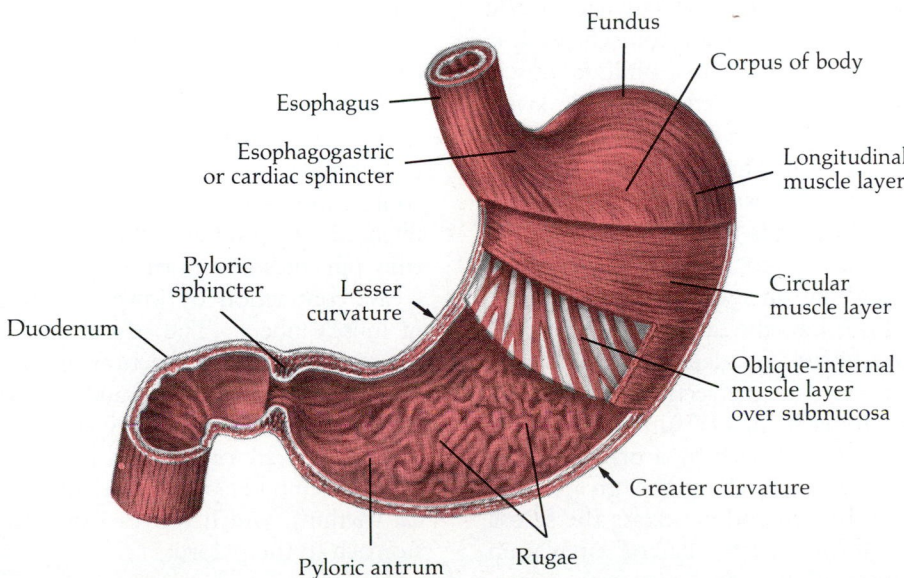

FIG. 35-4. Muscle layers and interior of the stomach. (From Thompson et al., 1989.)

Structural Layers of the Gastrointestinal Tract

Mucosa: a mucous membrane composed of three layers
  Epithelium
  Lamina propria: connective tissue containing blood vessels, lymph nodes, and glands
  Muscularis mucosa: thin layer of smooth muscle between mucosa and submucosa
Submucosa: connective tissue containing blood vessels, lymph channels, nerves, and glands (in some regions)
Tunica muscularis: layers of smooth muscle with a myenteric nerve plexus (Auerbach plexus) lying between them
  Oblique muscle layer (stomach only)
  Circular muscle layer
  Longitudinal muscle layer
Serosa or adventitia: a serous membrane covered with an outer layer of squamous epithelial cells

---

num. Functional areas of the stomach are the **fundus** (upper portion), **body** (middle portion), and **antrum** (lower portion).

The stomach wall consists of several layers: the **mucosa,** which lines the stomach cavity; the **muscularis mucosa,** a thin muscle layer separating the mucosa and submucosa; the **submucosa;** the **tunica muscularis,** or smooth muscle layer; and an outer, serous membrane, or **serosa** (see Fig. 35-4). With slight variation these layers form the walls of the entire gastrointestinal lumen, from the esophagus to the rectum.

The tunica muscularis consists of a circular muscle layer and a longitudinal layer. The stomach wall is unique in that it also contains a layer of oblique muscle between the submucosa and the circular muscle layer. The oblique muscle is prominent in the anterior and posterior walls of the stomach. The circular and longitudinal layers of muscle are thinnest in the fundus, where the stomach relaxes and expands to store food received from the esophagus. These layers become progressively thicker in the body and antrum, where food is mixed, churned, and pushed out into the duodenum. The mucosa of the stomach consists of glandular epithelium. This layer will be discussed in the section about secretory functions of the stomach (p. 1179).

Blood is supplied to the stomach by a branch of the celiac artery. Major arteries lie along the greater and lesser curvatures. They branch and penetrate the serosa and muscle layers to form a rich collateral circulation throughout the mucosa, submucosa, and tunica muscularis. The blood supply is so abundant that nearly all ar-

terial vessels must be occluded before ischemic changes occur in the stomach wall. The splenic vein drains the right side of the stomach, and the gastric vein drains the left side.

The stomach is innervated by sympathetic and parasympathetic divisions of the autonomic nervous system. Some of the autonomic fibers are extrinsic: that is, they originate outside the stomach and are controlled by nerve centers in the brain. Others are intrinsic: they originate within the stomach and also respond to local stimuli. Extrinsic sympathetic fibers reach the stomach through the celiac plexus (solar plexus), whereas extrinsic parasympathetic fibers enter through the gastric branch of the vagus nerve. Intrinsic nerves of the stomach and intestines are located solely within the gastrointestinal tract and are controlled by local and autonomic nervous system stimuli through the **enteric plexus,** three nerve plexuses located in different layers of the gastrointestinal walls. The **submucosal plexus** (Meissner plexus) is located in the muscularis mucosa, the **myenteric plexus** (Auerbach plexus) in the muscle layers (tunica muscularis), and the **subserosal plexus** just beneath the serosa.

Gastric Motility

In its resting state the stomach is small and contains about 50 ml of fluid. There is no wall tension, and the muscle layers in the fundus contract very little. Swallowing causes the fundus to relax (receptive relaxation) to receive a bolus of food from the esophagus. Relaxation is coordinated by efferent, nonadrenergic noncholinergic vagal fibers and is facilitated by **gastrin** and **cholecystokinin,** two polypeptide hormones secreted by the gastrointestinal mucosa. (The actions of digestive hormones are summarized in Table 35-1.) Food is stored in vertical or oblique layers as it arrives in the fundus, whereas fluids flow relatively quickly down to the antrum.

Gastric (stomach) motility increases with the initiation of peristaltic waves, which sweep over the body of the stomach toward the antrum. The rate of peristaltic contractions is approximately three per minute and is influenced by neural and hormonal activity. Gastrin, **motilin** (an intestinal hormone), and the vagus nerve increase contraction by lowering the threshold potential of muscle fibers. (The neural and biochemical mechanisms of muscle contraction are described in Chapter 12.) Sympathetic activity and **secretin** (another intestinal hormone) are inhibitory and raise the threshold potential. The rate of peristalsis is mediated by pacemaker cells that initiate a wave of depolarization (basic electrical rhythm), which moves from the upper part of the stomach to the pylorus.

The mixing and emptying of food from the stomach take several hours. Mixing occurs as food is propelled

TABLE 35-1 Hormones of the digestive system

Source	Hormone	Stimulus for secretion	Action
Mucosa of the stomach	Gastrin	Presence of partially digested proteins in the stomach	Stimulates gastric glands to secrete hydrochloric acid and pepsinogen
Mucosa of the small intestine	Motilin	Presence of acid and fat in the duodenum	Increases gastrointestinal motility
	Secretin	Presence of chyme (acid, partially digested proteins, and fats) in the duodenum	Stimulates pancreas to secrete alkaline pancreatic juice and liver to secrete bile; decreases gastrointestinal motility
	Cholecystokinin	Same as for secretin	Stimulates gallbladder to eject bile and pancreas to secrete alkaline fluid; decreases gastric motility
	Enterogastrone	Presence of fat in the duodenum	Inhibits gastric secretion and motility
	Entero-oxyntin	Presence of chyme in small intestine	Stimulates gastric glands to secrete hydrochloric acid

From Thibodeau, 1987.
NOTE: The digestive hormones are not secreted into the gastrointestinal lumen, but rather into the bloodstream, in which they travel to target tissues.

toward the antrum. As food approaches the pylorus the velocity of the peristaltic wave increases. The passage of the contractile wave over the gastric contents forces the contents back toward the body of the stomach. This action, which is known as **retropulsion,** effectively mixes food with digestive juices, and the oscillating motion breaks down large food particles. With each peristaltic wave, a small portion of the gastric contents (chyme) passes through the pylorus and into the duodenum. The pylorus is about 1.5 cm long and is always open about 2.0 mm. It opens wider during antral contraction. Normally there is no regurgitation from the duodenum into the antrum.

The rate of **gastic emptying** (movement of gastric contents into the duodenum) depends on the volume, osmotic pressure, and chemical composition of the gastric contents. Larger volumes of food increase gastric pressure, peristalsis, and rate of emptying. Solids, fats, and nonisotonic solutions delay gastric emptying. (Osmotic pressure and tonicity are described in Chapters 1 and 3.) Products of fat digestion, which are formed in the duodenum by the action of bile from the liver and enzymes from the pancreas, stimulate the secretion of cholecystokinin. This hormone inhibits gastric motility and decreases gastric emptying so that fats are not emptied into the duodenum at a rate that exceeds the rate of bile and enzyme secretion. Osmoreceptors in the wall of the duodenum are sensitive to the osmotic pressure of duodenal contents. The arrival of hypertonic or hypotonic gastric contents activates the osmoreceptors, which delay gastric emptying to facilitate formation of an iso-osmotic duodenal environment. The rate at which acid enters the duodenum also influences gastric emptying. Secretions from the pancreas, liver, and duodenal mucosa neutralize gastric acid in the duodenum. The rate of emptying is adjusted to the duodenum's ability to neutralize the incoming acidity (Berne & Levy, 1988).

Gastric Secretion

Stimulated by eating, the stomach secretes large volumes of gastric juices or gastric secretions. Specialized cells located throughout the gastric mucosa produce mucus, acid, enzymes, hormones, and intrinsic factor. (Intrinsic factor is necessary for the intestinal absorption of vitamin B_{12}.) The hormones are secreted into the blood and travel to target tissues in the bloodstream. The other gastric secretions are released directly into the stomach lumen. Different areas of the stomach mucosa secrete different substances with the exception of mucus, which is secreted by epithelial and mucous cells in all parts of the stomach. Mucus covers the entire mucosa, forming a protective barrier against acid and proteolytic enzymes, which otherwise would damage the gastric lining.

In the fundus and body of the stomach the **gastric glands** of the mucosa are the primary secretory units (Fig. 35-5). Several of these glands (three to seven) empty into a common duct known as the **gastric pit.** The **parietal cells** (oxyntic cells) within the glands se-

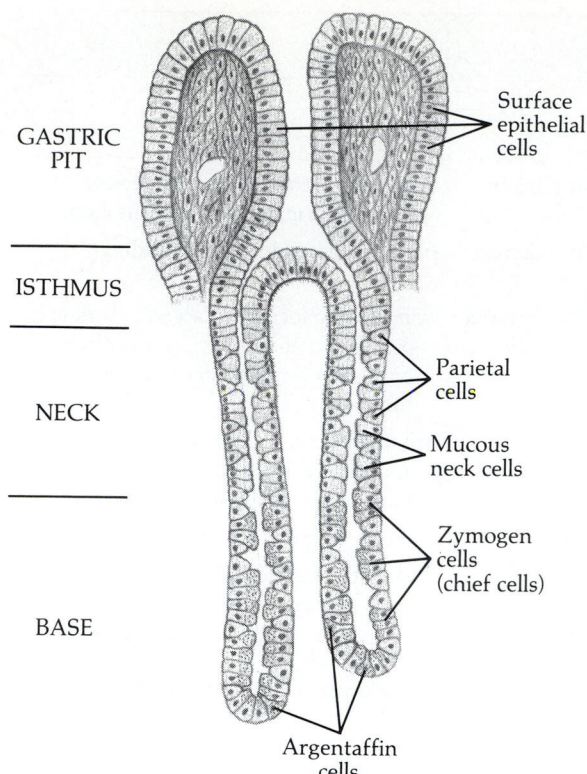

GASTRIC PIT

ISTHMUS

NECK

BASE

Surface epithelial cells

Parietal cells

Mucous neck cells

Zymogen cells (chief cells)

Argentaffin cells

FIG. 35-5. Gastric gland, which empties cellular secretions into a gastric pit. Secretions flow from the gastric pit into the lumen of the stomach. Surface epithelial cells have tight junctions and mucous coating. Parietal cells (oxyntic cells) secrete hydrochloric acid and intrinsic factor. Mucous neck cells secrete mucus. Chief cells (zymogen cells) secrete pepsinogen. Argentaffin cells secrete serotonin. (From Thompson et al., 1986.)

crete hydrochloric acid and intrinsic factor. The **chief cells** within the glands secrete **pepsinogen,** an enzyme precursor that is readily converted to **pepsin** (a proteolytic enzyme) in the gastric juice.

Like that of the secretions of salivary glands, the composition of gastric juice depends on volume and flow rate (Fig. 35-6). At low rates of secretion, hydrogen and chloride concentrations are low and sodium concentration is high. The reverse is true at high flow rates. Potassium remains relatively constant, but its concentration is greater in gastric juice than in plasma. The rate of secretion varies with the time of day. Generally the rate and volume of secretion are lowest in the morning and highest in the afternoon and evening. Loss of gastric juices through vomiting, drainage, or suction may decrease body stores of sodium and potassium.

Gastric secretion is inhibited by unpleasant odors and tastes and by rage, fear, or pain. These sensations and emotions cause a discharge of sympathetic impulses and inhibit parasympathetic impulses. Increased secretions may be associated with feelings of aggression or hostility and may contribute to some forms of gastric pathology.

Acid

The major functions of gastric acid are to dissolve food fibers, act as a bactericide against swallowed organisms, and convert pepsinogen to pepsin. The production of acid by the parietal cells requires the transport of hydrogen and chloride from the parietal cells to the stom-

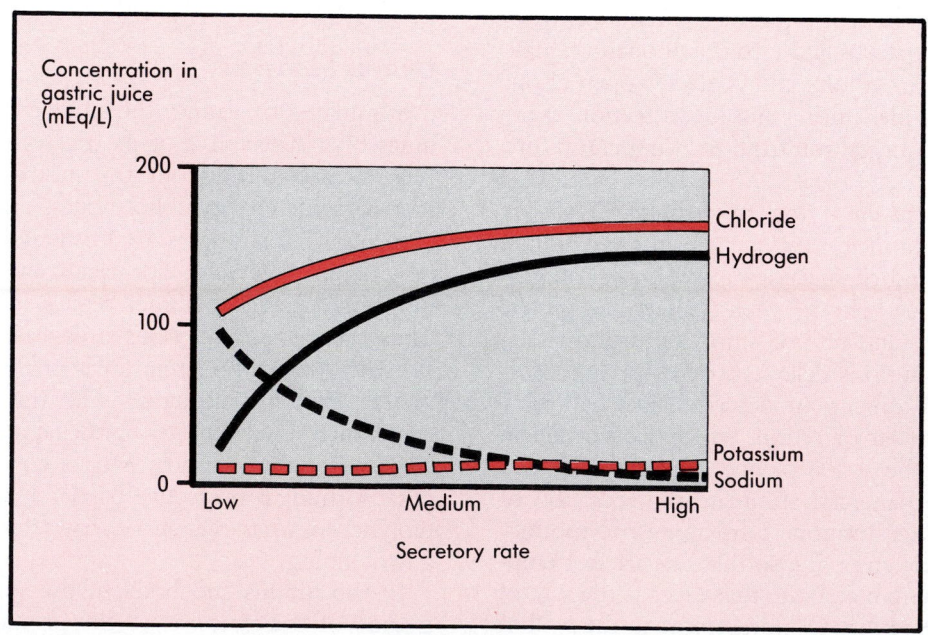

Concentration in gastric juice (mEq/L)

200

100

0

Chloride

Hydrogen

Potassium
Sodium

Low   Medium   High

Secretory rate

FIG. 35-6. Relationship between secretory rate and electrolyte composition of the gastric juice. Sodium (Na^+) concentration is lower in the gastric juice than in the plasma, whereas hydrogen (H^+), potassium (K^+), and chloride (Cl^-) concentrations are higher.

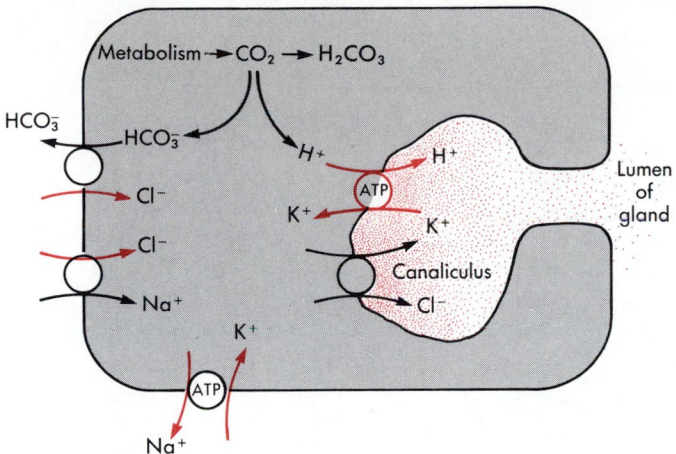

FIG. 35-7. One mechanism for secretion of hydrochloric acid. (From Berne & Levy., 1988.)

ach lumen. Acid is formed in the parietal cells primarily through the hydrolysis of water (Fig. 35-7). At a high rate of gastric secretion bicarbonate moves into the plasma, producing an "alkaline tide" in the venous blood, which may also result in a more alkaline urine (Davenport, 1982).

Acid secretion is stimulated by acetylcholine (a neurotransmitter), gastrin (a hormone), and histamine (a biochemical mediator). The vagus nerve releases acetylcholine and stimulates the secretion of gastrin, probably in response to histamine. Histamine is stored in enterochromaffin cells (mast cells; see Chapter 7) in the gastric mucosa. Histamine receptors in the gastric mucosa are H-2 receptors (unlike those in the bronchial mucosa, which are H-2 receptors). The drug cimetidine is an H-2 antagonist and is therefore effective in suppressing acid secretion in persons with ulcers. The regulation of histamine in the parietal cell area is not understood (Berne & Levy, 1988).

Pepsin Secretion

Acetylcholine, gastrin, and secretin stimulate the chief cells to release pepsinogen during eating. Gastrin indirectly stimulates pepsinogen secretion through a cholinergic reflex that it causes while stimulating acid secretion. Pepsinogen is quickly converted to pepsin in the acid gastric environment. Conversion to pepsin occurs at any pH below 5.0, but the optimum pH for pepsin activation is 2.0. Pepsin is a proteolytic enzyme: that is, it breaks down protein. Pepsin hydrolyzes peptide bonds at the anterior of protein molecules, thereby forming polypeptides. This action occurs in the stomach. Once chyme has entered the duodenum, the alkaline environment of the duodenum inactivates pepsin.

Mucus

The gastric mucosa is protected from the digestive actions of acid and pepsin by a coating of mucus called the **mucosal barrier.** The quality and quantity of mucus and the tight junctions between epithelial cells make gastric mucosa relatively impermeable to acid. Prostaglandins protect the mucosal barrier by stimulating the secretion of mucus and bicarbonate and by inhibiting secretion of acid. A break in the protective barrier may occur because of exposure to aspirin, ethanol, regurgitated bile, or ischemia. Breaks cause inflammation and ulceration.

Phases of Gastric Secretion

The secretion of gastric juice is influenced by numerous stimuli that together facilitate the process of digestion. The phases of gastric secretion are the cephalic phase, the gastric phase, and the intestinal phase (Fig. 35-8).

Cephalic Phase

The anticipatory and sensory experiences of smelling, seeing, tasting, chewing, and swallowing food contribute to the **cephalic phase** of secretion. Sensory experiences stimulate the secretion of acid, pepsinogens, and mucus in the body of the stomach and the release of gastrin from **G cells** (gastrin-secreting cells) in the antral region. The cephalic phase of gastric secretion is mediated by the vagus nerve via the myenteric plexus. Acetylcholine (ACh) is liberated and stimulates the parietal and chief cells to secrete acid and pepsinogen, respectively. The G cells in the antrum release gastrin into the bloodstream, through which it travels to the gastric glands and stimulates acid secretion. The secretion of gastric juice prior to the arrival of food in the stomach contributes to the desire for and enjoyment of food.

Insulin secretion by the endocrine pancreas, which is stimulated by hyperglycemia, is also a strong stimulus for gastric secretion. Acid secretion in response to insulin is mediated by the vagus through sensors located in the hypothalamus. These sensors respond to the decreased levels of serum glucose caused by insulin release. Maintenance of steady serum glucose levels suppresses the gastric response to insulin.

Gastric Phase

The **gastric phase** of secretion begins with the arrival of food in the stomach. The presence of food in the stomach is the most powerful stimulus of gastric secretion. Two major stimuli have a secretory effect: (1) distention of the stomach and (2) the presence of digested protein. Mechanoreceptors are activated as the stomach becomes distended with food, thereby stimulating secretions mediated by the vagus nerve. The enteric nerve plexus is also stimulated by distention and contributes

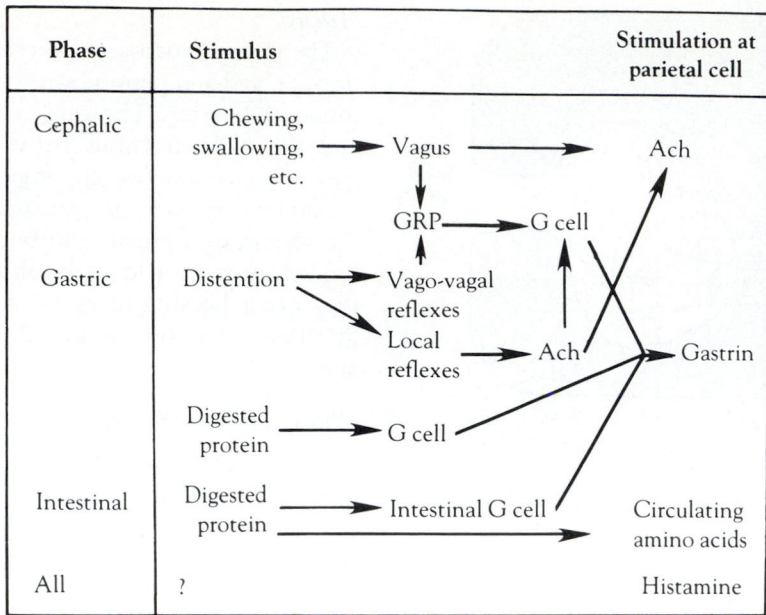

Phase	Stimulus		Stimulation at parietal cell
Cephalic	Chewing, swallowing, etc.	Vagus	Ach
		GRP → G cell	
Gastric	Distention	Vago-vagal reflexes	
		Local reflexes → Ach	Gastrin
	Digested protein	G cell	
Intestinal	Digested protein	Intestinal G cell	Circulating amino acids
All	?		Histamine

FIG. 35-8. The phases of gastric acid secretion. *GRP,* Gastrin-releasing peptide. (From Johnson, 1981.)

to gastric secretion through a local reflex. Because both neural reflexes are mediated by acetylcholine they can be blocked by atropine. As digestion proceeds products of protein breakdown come in contact with the pyloric mucosa and stimulate the release of gastrin from G cells in the antrum. Proteins activate the release of gastrin indirectly as well. Proteins in the stomach buffer the acid gastric juice and increase the gastric pH. The rise in pH promotes the secretion of gastrin because it cancels out the inhibitory effect of low pH on gastrin release in the antrum. Caffeine stimulates acid secretion, as does calcium.

Intestinal Phase

The movement of chyme from the stomach into the duodenum initiates the **intestinal phase** of gastric secretion. This phase represents a slowdown of the gastric secretory response and appears to be hormonally mediated. Apparently the presence of chyme in the small intestine causes a hormone called entero-oxyntin to be released into the bloodstream and travel to the gastric mucosa, where it causes the parietal cells to secrete acid. The intestinal absorption of some amino acids (products of protein breakdown) also stimulates gastric secretion. The intestinal phase of gastric secretion is limited by the fact that acidic chyme in the duodenum tends to inhibit both gastric acid secretion and gastric motility. Acid in the duodenum stimulates the release of hormones that inhibit acid secretion while stimulating pepsinogen secretion. One of these hormones, cholecystokinin-pancreozymin, inhibits gastrin-stimulated acid produc-

tion. There are probably other intestinal hormones that act synergistically to regulate gastric secretion.

The Small Intestine

The **small intestine** is about 5 meters long and is functionally divided into three segments: the **duodenum, jejunum,** and **ileum** (see Fig. 35-11). The duodenum begins at the pylorus and ends where it joins the jejunum at a suspensory ligament called the Treitz ligament. The end of the jejunum and beginning of the ileum are not distinguished by an anatomic marker. These structures are not grossly different, but the jejunum has a slightly larger lumen. The **ileocecal valve,** or sphincter, controls the flow of digested material from the ileum into the large intestine and prevents reflux into the small intestine.

The **peritoneum** is the serous membrane surrounding the organs of the abdomen and pelvic cavity. It is analogous to the pericardium and pleura that surround the heart and lungs, respectively. The peritoneum has two layers: the visceral peritoneum lies over the organs, and the parietal peritoneum lines the wall of the abdominal cavity. The space between these two layers is called the **peritoneal cavity.** This cavity normally contains just enough fluid to lubricate the two layers and prevent friction during organ movement. Inflammation of the peritoneum, called peritonitis, may occur with perforation of the large intestine or after abdominal surgery. As the inflammatory process resolves, adhesions may form and cause colonic obstruction.

The duodenum lies behind the peritoneum, or retroperitoneally, and is attached to the posterior abdominal wall. The ileum and jejunum are suspended in loose folds from the posterior abdominal wall by a peritoneal membrane called the **mesentery.** The mesentery facilitates intestinal motility and supports blood vessels, nerves, and lymphatics.

The arterial supply to the duodenum arises primarily from the gastroduodenal artery. The jejunum and ileum are supplied by branches of the superior mesenteric artery. The superior mesenteric vein joins the splenic vein and empties into the portal circulation to the liver. The regional lymph nodes and lymphatics drain into the thoracic duct. Both divisions of the autonomic nervous system innervate the small intestine. Secretion, motility, pain sensation, and intestinal reflexes (e.g., relaxation of the lower esophageal sphincter) are mediated by parasympathetic nerves. Sympathetic activity inhibits motil-

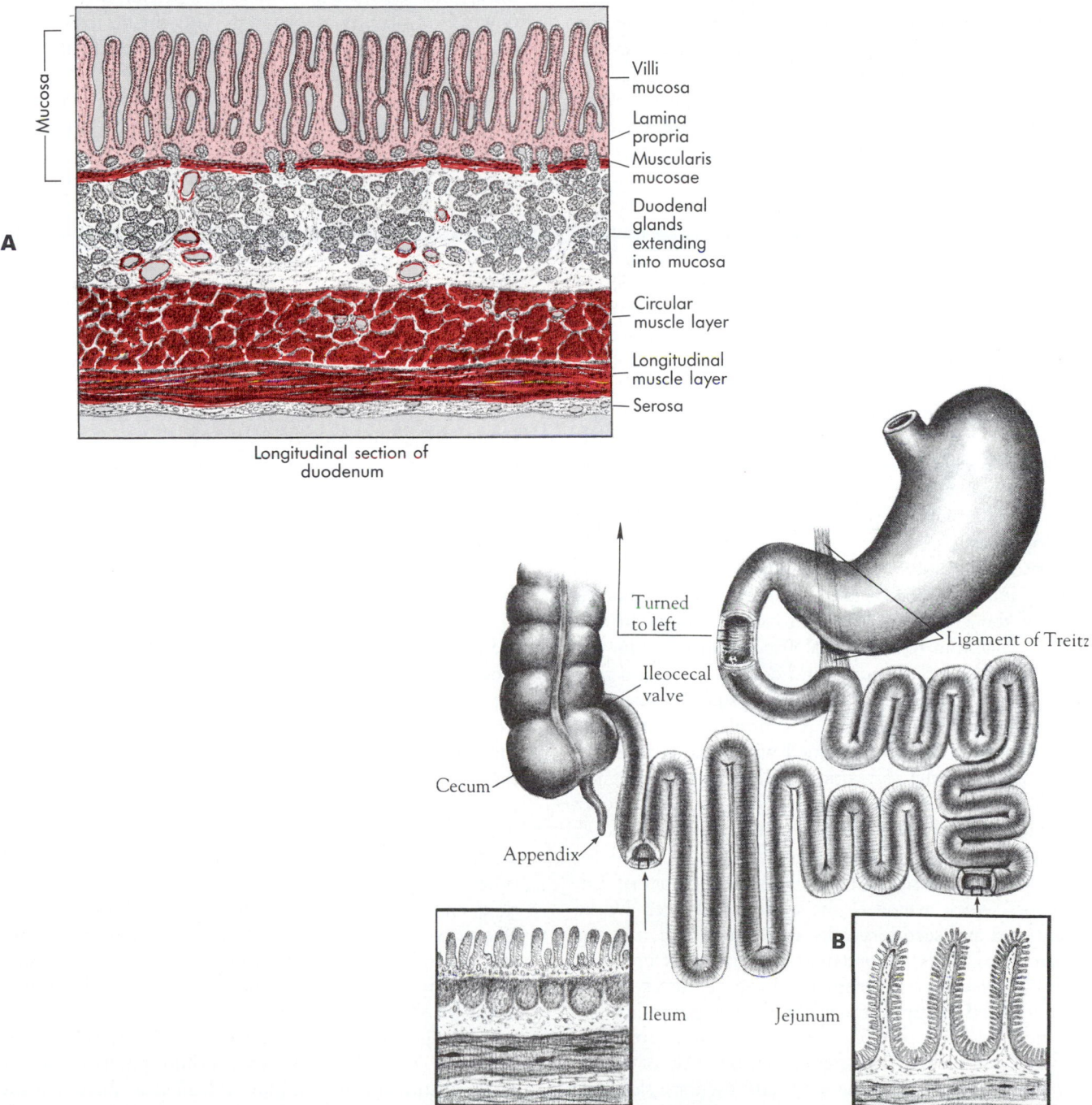

FIG. 35-9. The small intestine. (Adapted from Thompson et al., 1989.)

ity and produces vasoconstriction. Intrinsic motor innervation is mediated by the myenteric plexus (Auerbach plexuses) and the submucosal plexus (Meissner plexus).

The smooth muscles of the small intestine are arranged in two layers: a longitudinal outer layer and a thicker inner circular layer (Fig. 35-9, *A*). Mucosal folds (plica) within the small intestine slow the passage of food, thereby providing more time for digestion and absorption. The folds are most numerous and prominent in the jejunum and upper ileum (Fig. 35-9).

Absorption occurs through **villi,** which cover the mucosal folds and are the functional units of the intestine. (A single villus is shown in Fig. 35-9) Each villus secretes some of the enzymes necessary for digestion and absorbs nutrients. A villus is composed of absorptive columnar cells and mucus-secreting goblet cells of the mucosal epithelium. Near the surface columnar cells closely adhere to each other at sites called tight junctions. Water and electrolytes are absorbed through these intercellular spaces. The surface of each columnar epithelial cell contains tiny projections called **microvilli** (Fig. 35-9). Together the microvilli create a mucosal surface known as the **brush border.** The villi and microvilli greatly increase the surface area available for absorption. Coating the brush border is an "unstirred" layer of fluid that is important for the absorption of substances other than water and electrolytes. The **lamina propria** (a connective tissue layer of the mucous membrane) lies beneath the epithelial cells of the villi and contains lymphocytes; plasma cells, which produce immunoglobulins; and macrophages.

Central arterioles ascend within each villus and branch into a capillary array that extends around the base of the columnar cells and cascades down to the venules that lead to the portal circulation (see Fig. 35-9). The opposing ascending and descending blood flow provides a countercurrent exchange system for absorbed substances and blood gases. A central **lacteal,** or lymphatic channel, is also contained within each villus and is important for the absorption and transport of fat molecules. Contents of the lacteals flow to regional nodes and channels that eventually drain into the thoracic duct (Kvietys, Barrowman, & Granger, 1987).

Between the bases of the villi are the crypts of Lieberkuhn, which extend to the submucosal layer. Undifferentiated and secretory cells are located here. The undifferentiated cells are precursors of columnar epithelial cells. These cells arise from the base of the crypt and move toward the tip of the villus, maturing in shape and function as they progress. After becoming columnar cells and completing their migration to the tip of the villus, they function for a few days and then are sloughed into the intestinal lumen and digested. Sloughed epithelial cells are an important source of endogenous protein.

The entire epithelial population is replaced about every 4 to 7 days. Many factors can influence this process of cellular proliferation. Starvation, vitamin B_{12} deficiency, and cytotoxic drugs or irradiation suppress cell division and shorten the villi. The decreased absorption that results can cause diarrhea and malnutrition. Nutrient intake and intestinal resection stimulate cell production.

Intestinal Digestion and Absorption

The process of digestion is initiated in the stomach by the actions of hydrochloric acid and pepsin, which break down food fibers and proteins. The chyme that passes into the duodenum is a liquid that contains small particles of undigested food. Digestion is continued in the proximal portion of the small intestine by the action of pancreatic enzymes, intestinal enzymes, and bile salts. Here carbohydrates are broken down to monosaccharides and disaccharides; proteins are degraded further to amino acids and peptides; and fats are emulsified and reduced to fatty acids and monoglycerides (Fig. 35-10). These nutrients, along with water, vitamins, and electrolytes, are absorbed across the intestinal mucosa by active transport, diffusion, or facilitated diffusion. Products of carbohydrate and protein breakdown move into villus capillaries and then to the liver through the portal vein. Digested fats move into the lacteals and eventually reach the liver through the systemic circulation. Intestinal motility exposes nutrients to a large mucosal surface area by mixing chyme and moving it through the lumen. Different segments of the gastrointestinal tract absorb different nutrients. Sites of absorption are shown in Fig. 35-11.

Water and Electrolytes

The epithelial cell membranes of the small intestine are formed of lipids and therefore are hydrophobic, or tend to repel water. (The properties of cell membranes are described in Chapter 1.) Therefore, water and electrolytes are transported in both directions (toward the capillary blood or toward the intestinal lumen) through the tight junctions and intercellular spaces rather than across cell membranes. Water diffuses passively according to hydrostatic pressure and in relation to osmotic gradients established by the transport of sodium and other substances. Sodium passes through the tight junctions and is actively transported across cell membranes. The proximal part of the small intestine is more permeable to sodium than the distal part. Sodium is transported into the intestinal cells in exchange for hydrogen at the brush border, and chloride actively enters the cell in exchange for bicarbonate to maintain electroneutrality in the ileum. There is also a sodium pump at the basolateral membrane. Sodium and glucose share a common carrier mechanism, so that sodium absorption is enhanced by glucose transport (Fig. 35-12). Potassium

Action	Foodstuff	Enzymes/source	Site of action

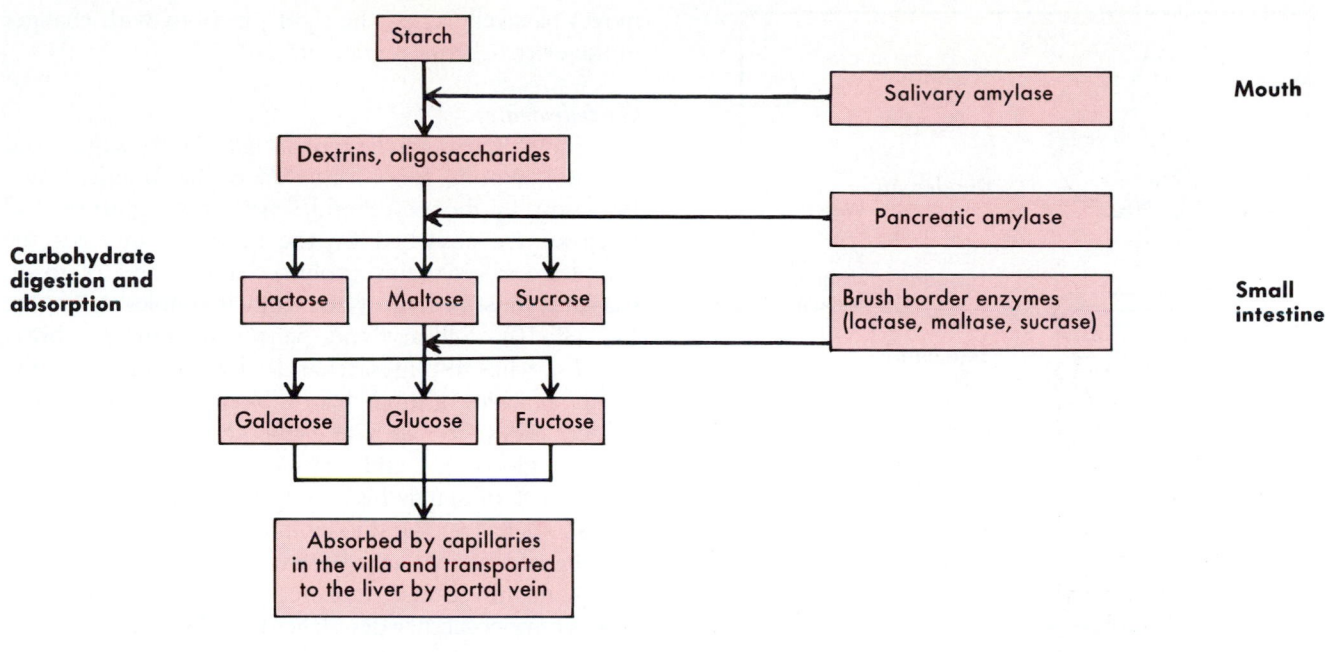

Carbohydrate digestion and absorption

Starch → (Salivary amylase, Mouth) → Dextrins, oligosaccharides → (Pancreatic amylase) → Lactose, Maltose, Sucrose → (Brush border enzymes (lactase, maltase, sucrase), Small intestine) → Galactose, Glucose, Fructose → Absorbed by capillaries in the villa and transported to the liver by portal vein

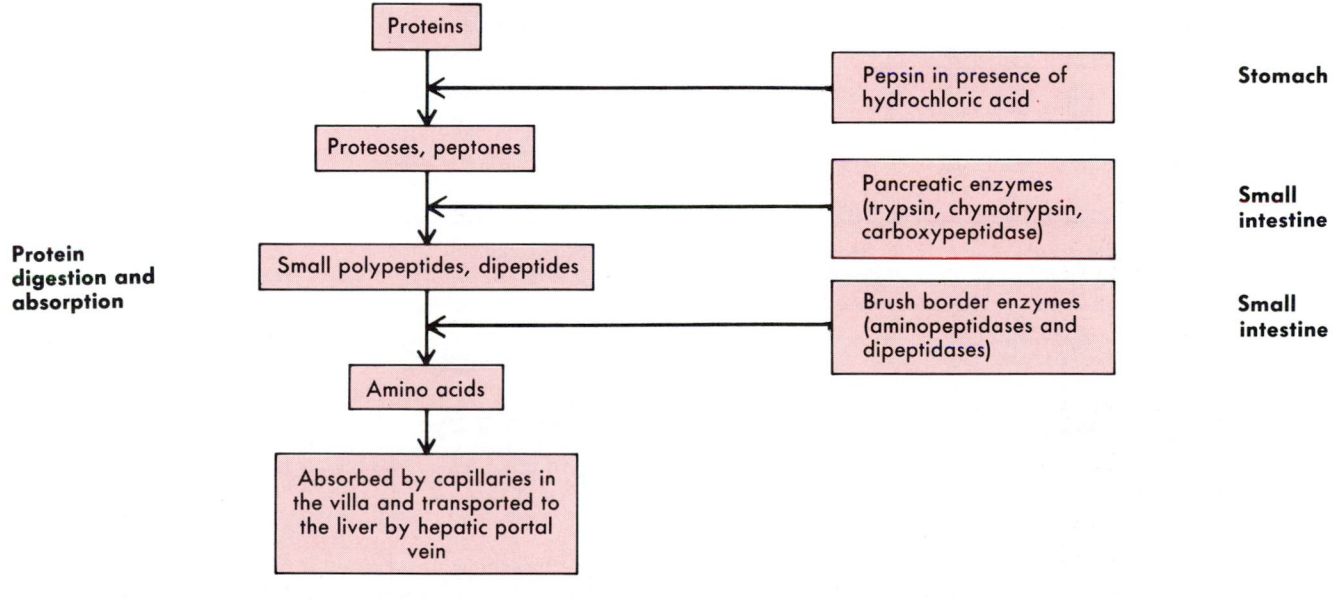

Protein digestion and absorption

Proteins → (Pepsin in presence of hydrochloric acid, Stomach) → Proteoses, peptones → (Pancreatic enzymes (trypsin, chymotrypsin, carboxypeptidase), Small intestine) → Small polypeptides, dipeptides → (Brush border enzymes (aminopeptidases and dipeptidases), Small intestine) → Amino acids → Absorbed by capillaries in the villa and transported to the liver by hepatic portal vein

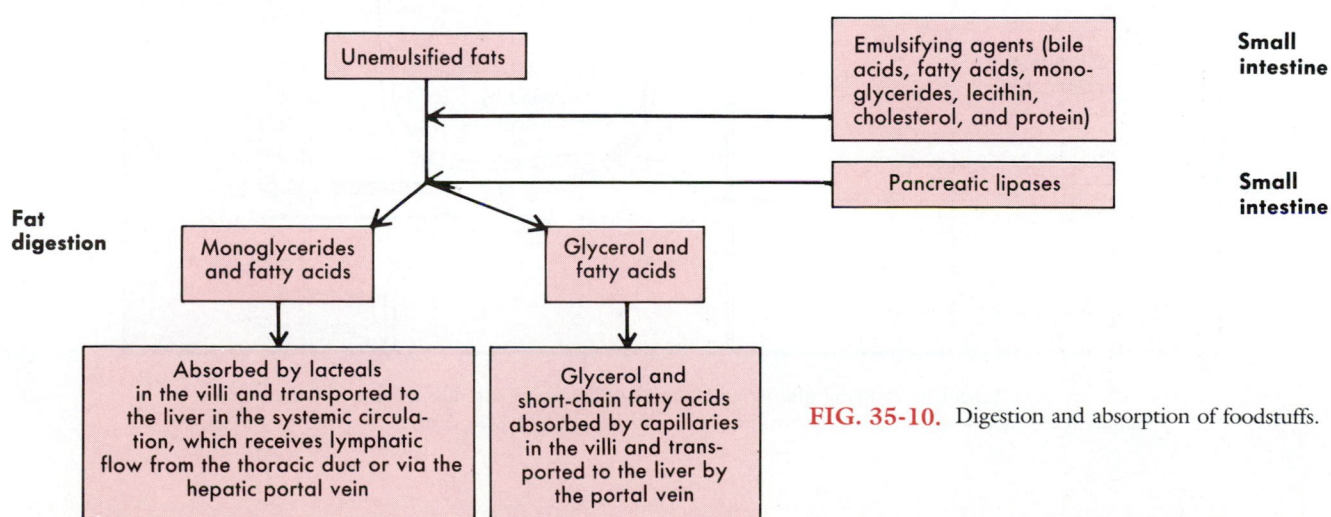

Fat digestion

Unemulsified fats → (Emulsifying agents (bile acids, fatty acids, monoglycerides, lecithin, cholesterol, and protein), Small intestine; Pancreatic lipases, Small intestine) → Monoglycerides and fatty acids → Absorbed by lacteals in the villi and transported to the liver in the systemic circulation, which receives lymphatic flow from the thoracic duct or via the hepatic portal vein; Glycerol and fatty acids → Glycerol and short-chain fatty acids absorbed by capillaries in the villi and transported to the liver by the portal vein

FIG. 35-10. Digestion and absorption of foodstuffs.

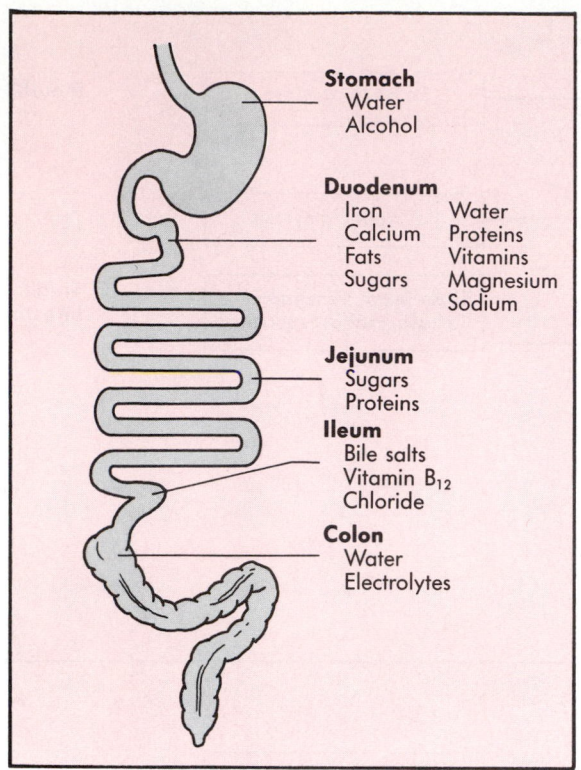

FIG. 35-11. Sites of absorption of major nutrients.

moves passively across the tight junctions with changes in the electrochemical gradient.

Carbohydrates

Carbohydrate (starch, table sugar, milk, sugar, and maltose) accounts for at least 50% of the American diet. Because only monosaccharides (galactose, glucose, and fructose) are absorbed by the intestinal mucosa, the complex carbohydrates (polysaccharides and oligosaccharides) must be hydrolyzed to their simplest form (see Fig. 35-10). Salivary and pancreatic amylases break down starches to oligosaccharides by splitting $\alpha_{-1,4}$-glycosidic linkages of long-chain molecules. The major oligosaccharides are sucrose (glucose-fructose), maltose (glucose-glucose), and lactose (glucose-galactose). About half of starch hydrolysis occurs in the stomach and about half in the duodenum. In the small intestine the oligosaccharides are hydrolyzed by brush-border enzymes, mainly sucrase, maltase, and lactase, to their respective monosaccharides (fructose, glucose, and galactose). The sugars then pass through the unstirred layer by diffusion. At the cell membrane glucose and galactose are actively transported with a sodium carrier and fructose is absorbed passively. Consequently glucose and galactose are absorbed more rapidly than fructose. Insulin is not required for the intestinal absorption of

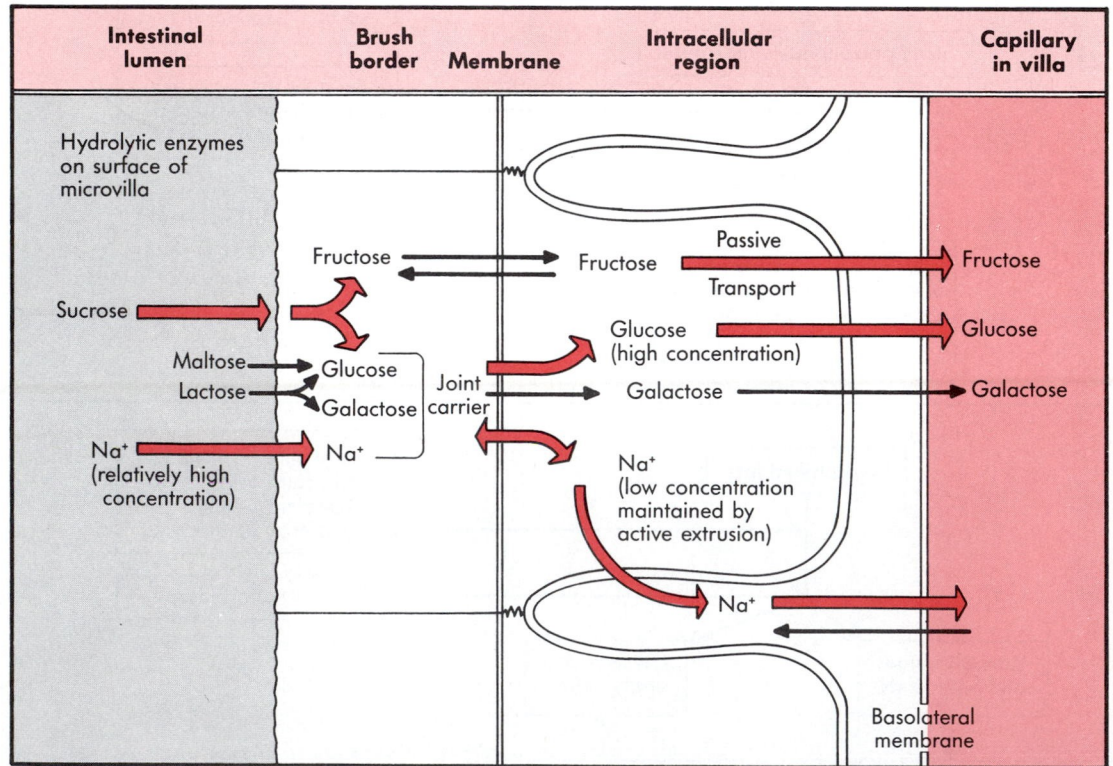

FIG. 35-12. Schematic showing glucose and sodium (Na^+) transport through the intestinal epithelium. Glucose and sodium are transported into the epithelial cell by a joint carrier.

carbohydrates. Fructose passes by diffusion into the bloodstream, and glucose and galactose enter by diffusion or active transport. The sugars are primarily absorbed in the duodenum and upper jejunum.

Proteins

Protein intake varies among different populations. Adults require 44 to 56 g of protein per day. About 20 to 30 g of protein is derived endogenously from shed epithelial cells and small amounts of plasma proteins. Most protein is absorbed; only 5% to 10% is eliminated in the stool.

Gastric digestion of protein by pepsin and acid is not essential. Major protein hydrolysis is accomplished in the small intestine by the pancreatic enzymes: trypsin, chymotrypsin, and carboxypeptidases (see Fig. 35-10). **Trypsin** and **chymotrypsin** hydrolyze the interior bonds of the large molecules, and the **carboxypeptidases** break away the end amino acids. Hydrolysis of proteins is also carried out by the brush-border enzymes and enzymes in the epithelial cytosol (intracellular fluid). The brush border enzymes hydrolyze the large oligopeptides (proteins composed of three to six amino acids) into smaller peptides, which can cross cell membranes. The cytosol then breaks them down to amino acids. Amino acids are actively transported by a carrier at the basal membrane. Protein absorption is directly linked to the active transport of sodium. There are three groups of free amino acids:

1. Neutral amino acids (methionine, glycine, phenylalanine, and tryptophan)
2. Basic amino acids (arginine, ornithine, lysine, and cystine)
3. Proline and hydroxyproline

Each group enters the circulation through a specific mechanism of transport. A small amount of protein may be taken into the cells by pinocytosis (Chapter 1).

Like the sugars, proteins are absorbed primarily in the proximal area of the small intestine. Protein absorption is impaired if inadequate amounts of proteolytic enzymes are secreted from the pancreas, as occurs with cystic fibrosis.

Fats

Approximately 90 to 100 g of fat is consumed daily by the average American. Fat is an important source of calories and is a primary structural component of cell membranes and organelles. Though triglycerides are the major dietary lipids, cholesterol, phospholipids, and fat-soluble vitamins also have nutritional importance. The digestion and absorption of fat occur in four phases: (1) emulsification and lipolysis, (2) micelle formation, (3) fat absorption, and (4) resynthesis of triglycerides and phospholipids.

The mechanical action of the stomach and small intes-

tine disperses the triglyceride droplets into small particles. **Emulsification** is the process by which emulsifying agents (fatty acids, monoglycerides, lecithin, cholesterol, protein, and bile salts) in the intestinal lumen cover the small fat particles and prevent them from reforming into fat droplets. Emulsified fat is then ready for **lipolysis** (lipid hydrolysis) by pancreatic lipase. Lipase breaks down triglycerides to diglycerides, monoglycerides, free fatty acids, and glycerol (see Fig. 35-10). The action of lipase requires the presence of colipase, a pancreatic enzyme that allows lipase to penetrate the triglyceride molecule.

The products of lipid hydrolysis must be made water soluble if they are to be absorbed efficiently from the intestinal lumen. This is accomplished by the formation of water-soluble molecules known as **micelles** (Fig. 35-13). Micelles are formed of bile salts, the products of fat hydrolysis, fat-soluble vitamins, and cholesterol. The

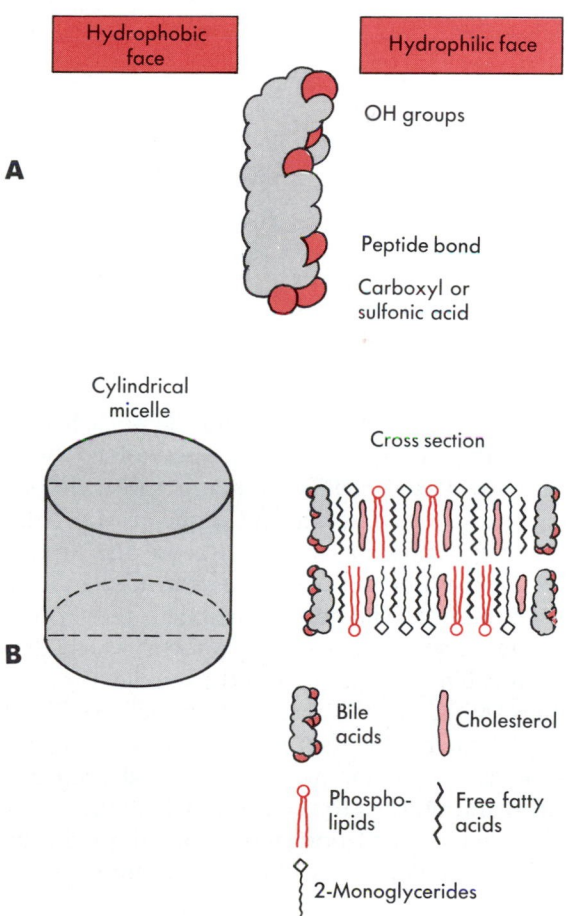

FIG. 35-13. Structure of bile acid and micelle. **A,** A bile acid molecule in solution. The molecule is amphipathic in that it has a hydrophilic face and a hydrophobic face. The amphipathic structure is key in the ability of the bile acids to emulsify lipids and form micelles. **B,** A model of the structure of a bile acid-lipid mixed micelle, an emulsified fat. (From Berne & Levy, 1988.)

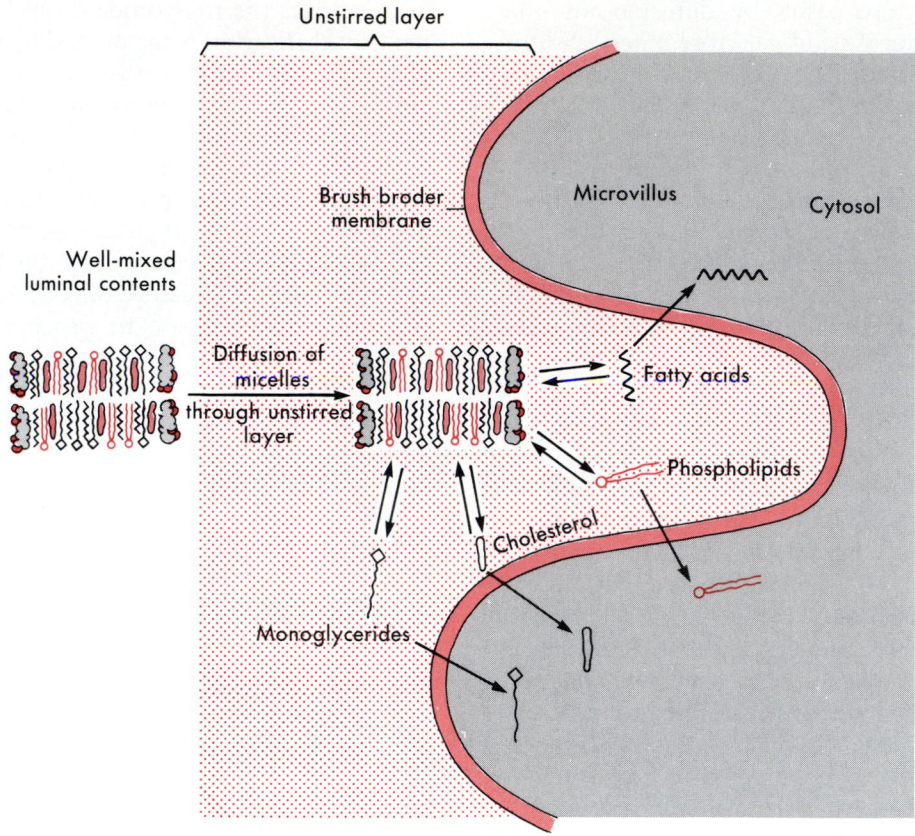

FIG. 35-14.   Lipid absorption in the small intestine. Micelles of bile salts and products of lipid digestion diffuse through the unstirred layer and among the microvilli. As digestive products are absorbed from free solution by epithelial cells of the villi, more digestive products dissociate from the micelles. (From Berne & Levy, 1988.)

fats form the core of the micelle and the polar bile salts form an outer shell, with the hydrophobic ("water-hating") side facing the interior and the hydrophilic ("water-loving") side facing the aqueous (waterlike) content of the intestinal lumen. Because the unstirred layer of the brush border is aqueous, the micelles readily diffuse through it. The micelles maintain the fat molecules in the dissolved or solubilized form, which allows them to move more rapidly from the micelle toward the absorbing surface of the intestinal epithelium. The fat products of the micelle then readily diffuse through the epithelial cell membrane, while the bile salts remain in the lumen and proceed to the ileum, where they are absorbed into the circulation and returned to the liver (Fig. 35-14). Almost all of the bile salts are recycled in this way.

When the fat products reach the inside of the epithelial cell, they are resynthesized into triglycerides and phospholipids. The triglycerides are covered with phospholipids, lipoproteins, and cholesterol to become particles called **chylomicrons.** The chylomicrons travel to the basolateral membrane of the columnar epithelial

cells, where they are extruded into the intercellular spaces of the villus. From here they enter the lacteals and lymphatic channels and, eventually, the systemic circulation.

Minerals and Vitamins

The recommended intake of calcium ranges from 1000 to 1500 mg/day. Between 500 and 600 mg is secreted or shed into the lumen with desquamated epithelial cells. Not all this calcium is absorbed. Daily absorption of calcium is about 600 mg. This amount increases with increased intake. When its concentration in the lumen is greater than 5 mM, calcium is absorbed by passive diffusion. At concentrations less than 5.0 mM calcium is transported actively across cell membranes, bound to a carrier protein. The carrier formation requires the presence of the active form of vitamin D (1,25-dihydroxy vitamin D). The calcium-protein complex moves into the epithelial cell, where the calcium binds to proteins or other substances. Then these complexes move through the basolateral membrane to the interstitial fluid by diffusion or active transport. Calcium is absorbed throughout the small intestine, but primarily in the ileum.

That calcium is absorbed more rapidly in children and pregnant or lactating women is evidence that increased demand results in increased uptake. Bile salts enhance calcium absorption indirectly by facilitating the absorption of vitamin D. Additionally bile salts promote the absorption of free fatty acids, which, at high concentrations, bind calcium and form soaps in the intestinal lumen. In older individuals calcium is absorbed less readily because of inadequate amounts of the active form of vitamin D.

The recommended intake of magnesium for adults is 300 to 350 mg/day. About 50% of it is absorbed by active transport or passive diffusion in the jejunum and ileum. Phosphate is also absorbed in the small intestine by passive diffusion and active transport.

The levels of iron in the body are regulated primarily by intestinal absorption and secretion. The average intake ranges from 15 to 30 mg/day. Of this amount menstruating women absorb 1.0 to 1.5 mg and men absorb 0.15 to 1.0 mg. Generally the amount of iron absorbed is equal to the amount required. Iron is absorbed more rapidly if a deficiency exists. The primary sources of iron are heme from hemoglobin and myoglobin from animal protein. This iron is rapidly absorbed by the epithelial cells of the duodenum and jejunum. Inorganic iron (e.g., iron in fruits, cereals, eggs, vegetables) is also readily absorbed. The presence of vitamin C reduces ferric iron to ferrous iron, which is the form more easily absorbed. Calcium phosphate and phosphoproteins (milk and antacids) in the intestinal lumen bind iron and reduce absorption. Tea also binds iron by forming iron tannate complexes.

Iron is primarily bound to the protein ferritin and to amino acid chelates in the cytosol of epithelial cells. Transport of iron across the basolateral membrane is determined by the amount of iron in the circulation. During hemorrhage, pregnancy, or growth, iron is actively transported from the epithelial cell to the plasma, where it is carried by the globulin protein transferrin (Chapter 22). When there is less need for iron, it remains in the cell and is carried into the lumen when the cell is sloughed from the end of the villus. The intestinal cells requires 3 days to increase their rate of iron absorption after hemorrhage. This is because the need for iron is perceived by the precursor cells in the crypts of Leiberkuhn and they take 3 days to mature and migrate to the tips of the villi, where they absorb more iron.

The absorption of vitamins is summarized in Table 35-2. Most of the water-soluble vitamins are absorbed by sodium-dependent active transport. Most vitamin B_{12} (cobalamin) is bound to intrinsic factor and absorbed in the terminal ileum, though a small amount of the vitamin is absorbed in its free (unbound) form. Because intrinsic factor is secreted by gastric cells of the stomach, gastric resection and gastric atrophy with achlorhydria diminish the secretion of intrinsic factor and hence the absorption of vitamin B_{12}. Lack of vitamin B_{12} prevents normal erythrocyte maturation and causes pernicious (macrocytic) anemia. (Anemias are discussed in Chapter 23.)

TABLE 35-2 Intestinal absorption of vitamins

Vitamin	Mechanisms of absorption	State of absorption
FAT-SOLUBLE VITAMINS		
A	Micelle formation with bile salts	Upper small intestine
D		
E		
K		
WATER-SOLUBLE VITAMINS		
B_1 (thiamine)	Active transport (sodium-dependent)	Duodenum and jejunum
B_2 (riboflavin)	Unknown	Duodenum and jejunum
Niacin (nicotinic acid)	Passive diusion	Jejunum
C (ascorbic acid)	Active transport (sodium-dependent)	Ileum
Folic acid	Active transport (sodium-dependent)	Jejunum
B_{12} (cobalamine)	Active transport (intrinsic-factor-dependent)	Terminal ileum
B_6 (pyridoxine, pyridoxamine, pyridoxal)	Passive diusion	Jejunum
Panthothenic acid	Passive diusion	Duodenum and jejunum
Biotin	Unknown	Unknown

Vitamin B_{12} is present in animal protein and is particularly abundant in liver and kidney. Gastric and pancreatic enzymes release vitamin B_{12} from food, after which the vitamin binds to intrinsic factor via an intermediary transport protein. The intrinsic factor-vitamin B_{12} complex then attaches to specific receptor sites on epithelial cells of the terminal ileum, where it is absorbed. After several hours the vitamin enters the plasma, attaches to the carrier protein transcobalamin, and is transported to tissues.

Intestinal Motility

The movements of the small intestine facilitate both digestion and absorption. Chyme coming from the stomach stimulates intestinal movements that mix in secretions from the liver, pancreas, and intestinal glands. A churning motion brings the luminal content into contact with the absorbing cells of the villi. Propulsive movements then advance the chyme toward the large intestine.

Intestinal motility is affected by two movements: haustral segmentation and peristalsis. **Haustral segmentation,** which occurs more frequently than peristalsis, consists of localized rhythmic contractions of the circular smooth muscles. The contractions occur at different rates in different parts of the small intestine. Frequency is greatest (12 per minute) in the upper small intestine and least (8 per minute) in the distal part of the ileum. Haustral segmentation divides and mixes the chyme, bringing it into contact with the absorbent mucosal surface. It also helps to propel the chyme toward the large intestine. The frequency of the haustral segmentation is regulated intrinsically by the frequency of the basic electrical rhythm (BER), which arises in the myenteric plexus of longitudinal smooth muscle. Although the basic rate of contraction is controlled intrinsically, the force of contraction can be enhanced by vagal stimulation (i.e., extrinsically).

Peristaltic movements involve short segments (about 10 cm) of longitudinal smooth muscle. The wave of contraction moves slowly (1 to 2 cm/sec) to allow time for digestion and absorption.

The intestinal villi move with contractions of the muscularis mucosa, a very thin layer of muscle that separates the mucosa and submucosa. Absorption is promoted by the swaying of villi in the luminal contents. Contractile activity also helps to empty the central lacteals, which contain products of fat digestion.

Neural reflexes along the length of the small intestine facilitate motility, digestion, and absorption. Through reflex action receptors in one part of the intestine transmit signals that influence the function of another part. The **ileogastric reflex** inhibits gastric motility when the ileum becomes distended. This prevents the continued movement of chyme into an already distended intestine.

The **intestinointestinal reflex** inhibits intestinal motility when one part of the intestine is overdistended. Both of these reflexes require extrinsic innervation. The **gastroileal reflex,** which is activated by an increase in gastric motility and secretion, stimulates an increase in ileal motility. This empties the ileum and prepares it to receive more chyme. The gastroileal reflex is probably regulated by the hormone gastrin.

During prolonged fasting or between meals, particularly overnight, slow waves sweep along the entire length of the intestinal tract from the stomach to terminal ileum. This is known as the interdigestive myoelectric complex, and it appears to propel residual gastric and intestinal contents into the colon.

The ileocecal valve (sphincter) marks the junction between the terminal ileum and the large intestine. This valve is intrinsically regulated and is normally closed. The arrival of peristaltic waves from the last few centimeters of the ileum causes the ileocecal valve to open, allowing a small amount of chyme to pass through. Distention of the upper large intestine causes the sphincter to constrict, preventing further distention or retrograde flow of intestinal contents.

The Large Intestine

The **large intestine** is about 1.5 m long and consists of the cecum, appendix, colon (ascending, transverse, descending, and sigmoid), rectum, and anal canal (Fig. 35-15). The **cecum** is a pouch that receives chyme from the ileum. Attached to the cecum is the **vermiform appendix,** an appendage having little or no physiologic function. From the cecum, chyme enters the **colon,** a four-part length of intestine that loops upward, traverses the abdominal cavity, and descends to the anal canal. The four parts of the colon are the **ascending colon, transverse colon, descending colon,** and **sigmoid colon.** Two sphincters control the flow of intestinal contents through the cecum and colon: the ileocecal valve, which admits chyme from the ileum to the cecum, and the **O'Beirne sphincter,** which controls the movement of wastes from the sigmoid colon into the rectum. A thick (2.5 to 3 cm) portion of smooth muscle surrounds the anal canal, forming the **internal anal sphincter.** Overlapping it distally is the striated muscle of the **external anal sphincter.**

In the cecum and colon the longitudinal muscle layer consists of three longitudinal bands called **teniae coli** (Fig. 35-15). The teniae coli are shorter than the colon, giving the colon its "gathered" appearance. The circular muscles of the colon separate the gathers into outpouchings called **haustra.** The haustra become more or less prominent with the contractions and relaxations of the circular muscles. The mucosal surface of the colon has rugae (folds), particularly between the haustra, and **Lieberkuhn crypts** but no villi. Columnar epithelial cells

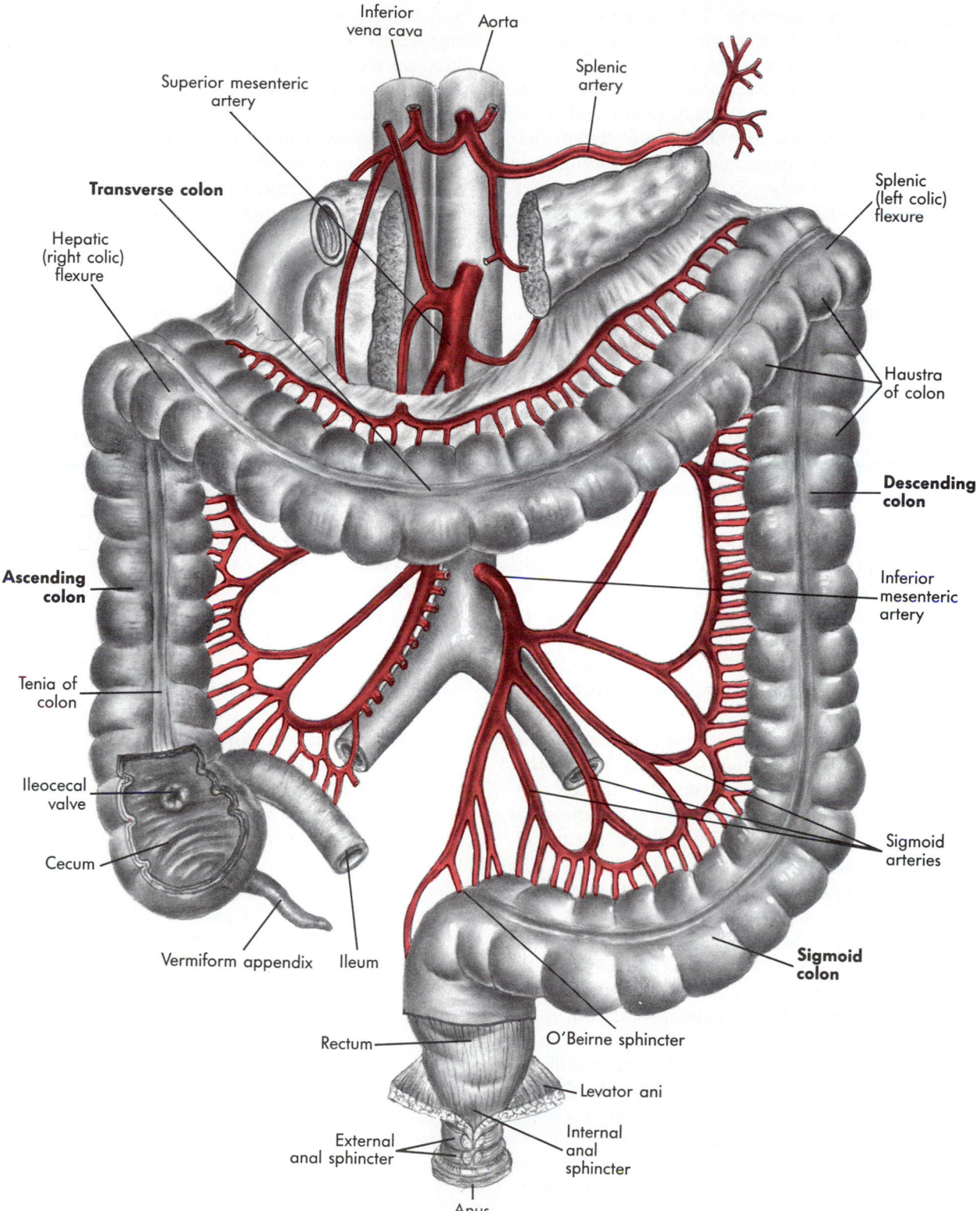

FIG. 35-15. Divisions of the large intestine. *Clockwise, from lower left:* the cecum, ascending colon, transverse colon, descending colon, sigmoid colon, rectum, and anal canal. Unlike the small intestine, the large intestine contains teniae coli, three bands of longitudinal muscle that are shorter than the intestinal wall. The teniae coli gather the large intestine lengthwise, forming outpouchings called haustra.

and mucus-secreting goblet cells form the mucosa throughout the large intestine. The columnar epithelium absorbs fluid and electrolytes, and the mucus-secreting cells lubricate the mucosa.

Intrinsic innervation in the colon is mediated by the myenteric plexus, which can regulate motor and secretory activity independently of the extrinsic system. Extrinsic parasympathetic innervation occurs through the vagus and extends from the cecum up to the first part of the transverse colon. Vagal stimulation increases rhythmic contraction of the proximal colon. Extrinsic parasympathetic fibers reach the distal colon via the pelvic nerves and can increase motility throughout the colon. The internal anal sphincter is usually in a state of contraction, and its reflex response is to relax when the rectum is distended. The intrinsic nerve plexuses provide the major innervation of the internal anal sphincter, which also receives sympathetic innervation to maintain contraction and parasympathetic innervation that facilitates relaxation when the rectum is full. The external anal sphincter is innervated by branches of the sacral division of the spinal cord. Sympathetic innervation of this sphincter arises from the celiac and superior mesenteric ganglia and the sphincter nerve. The external anal sphincter is paralyzed after destruction of the lower spinal cord, but the internal sphincter is not. Sympathetic activity in the entire large intestine modulates intestinal reflexes, conveys somatic sensation of fullness and pain, participates in the defecation reflex, and constricts blood vessels.

The primary type of colonic movement is segmental and is termed haustral shuttling, segmental propulsion, or multihaustral propulsion. The circular muscles contract and relax at different sites, shuttling the intestinal contents back and forth between the contracting and relaxing haustra, most commonly during fasting. The movements massage the intestinal contents, now called **fecal mass,** and facilitate the absorption of water. Propulsive movement occurs with the proximal-to-distal contraction of several haustral units. Peristaltic movements also occur and promote the emptying of the colon. The **gastrocolic reflex** initiates propulsion in the entire colon, usually during or immediately after eating, when chyme enters from the ileum. The gastrocolic reflex causes the fecal mass to pass rapidly into the sigmoid colon and rectum, stimulating defecation. Gastrin may participate in stimulating this reflex.

Approximately 500 to 700 ml of chyme flows from the ileum to the cecum per day. Most of the water is absorbed in the colon by diffusion and active transport. The electrochemical gradient established by sodium movement enhances the diffusion of serum potassium from the capillaries in the lumen. Aldosterone increases membrane permeability to sodium, thereby increasing both the diffusion of sodium into the cell and its active transport across the basolateral membrane to the interstitial fluid. (See Chapter 17 for a discussion of aldosterone secretion.) This increases the cell-to-lumen diffusion gradient for potassium. Potassium moves outward, and chloride is absorbed with sodium as the complementary anion. Chloride also enters the cell in exchange for bicarbonate. Sugars and amino acids are not absorbed by the colon, but some short-chain free fatty acids, which are produced by fermentation, are absorbed.

Absorption and epithelial transport occur in the cecum, ascending colon, transverse colon, and descending colon. By the time the fecal mass enters the sigmoid colon, the mass consists entirely of wastes and is called the feces. **Feces,** or excrement, consists of food residue, unabsorbed gastrointestinal secretions, shed epithelial cells, and bacteria.

The **rectum** receives feces from the sigmoid colon. The movement of feces into the sigmoid colon and rectum stimulates the **defecation reflex** (rectal reflex). Increased volume and pressure cause peristalsis in the sigmoid colon, forcing the feces into the normally empty rectum. This stretches the rectal wall and relaxes the tonically constricted internal anal sphincter, creating the urge to defecate. If the external anal sphincter is relaxed or paralyzed, defecation occurs. The defecation reflex can be overriden voluntarily by contraction of the external anal sphincter and muscles of the pelvic floor. The rectal wall gradually relaxes, reducing tension, and the urge to defecate passes. Retrograde contraction of the rectum may displace the feces out of the rectal vault until a more convenient time for evacuation. Pain or fear of pain associated with defecation, e. g., rectal fissures or hemorrhoids, can inhibit the defecation reflex. The defecation reflex is regulated by parasympathetic and cholinergic fibers. Voluntary inhibition or facilitation of defecation is mediated from cortical projections onto the medulla and down to sacral segments of the cord. Habit and diet affect the pattern of frequency.

Defecation is facilitated by squatting or sitting because these positions straighten the angle between the rectum and anal canal and increase the efficiency of straining (increasing intra-abdominal pressure). Intra-abdominal pressure is increased by initiating the Valsalva maneuver. This maneuver consists of inhaling and forcing the diaphram and chest muscles against the closed glottis. This increases both intrathoracic and intra-abdominal pressure, which is transmitted to the rectum.

Intestinal Bacteria

The type and number of bacteria vary greatly throughout the normal gastrointestinal tract. There is an increasing number of bacteria from the stomach to the distal colon. The stomach is relatively sterile because of the secretion of acid which kills injested pathogens or inhibits bacterial growth. Bile acid secretion, intestinal motility, and antibody production suppress bacterial growth in the duodenum, and in the duodenum and jejunum there is a low concentration of aerobes (10^{-1} to 10^{-4}/ml), primarily streptococci, lactobacilli, staphylococci, and enterobacteria. There are no anaerobes proximal to the ileum. The largest number of anaerobes are found distal to the ileocecal valve. They constitute about 95% of the fecal flora in the colon and contribute one third of the solid bulk of feces. Bacteriodes, clostridia, anaerobic lactobacilli, and coliforms are the most common microorganisms from the ileum to the cecum.

The intestinal tract is sterile at birth but becomes colonized with *Escherichia coli, Clostridium welchii,* and *Streptococcus* within a few hours. Within 3 to 4 weeks after birth the normal flora is established. The intestinal bacteria do not have major digestive or absorptive functions. They do play a role in the metabolism of bile salts, contributing to the intestinal reabsorption of bile and the elimination of toxic bile metabolites. Intestinal bacteria are also involved in the metabolism of estrogens and androgens, lipid metabolism, conversion of unabsorbed carbohydrates to absorbable organic acids, and metabolism of various nitrogenous substances and drugs.

Endogenous infections of the gastrointestinal tract occur by three major mechanisms: proliferation or overgrowth of bacteria, perforation of the intestine, and contamination of neighboring structures. Proliferation of bacteria occurs whenever there is obstruction to normal peristaltic flow of intestinal contents. The overpopulation of bacteria results in malabsorption of nutrients; bacterial utilization of folic acid and vitamin B_{12} may cause anemia. Ruptured appendix or external trauma can lead to perforation of the intestine, releasing bacteria into the peritoneum, and can lead to peritonitis or bacteremia. Movement of bacteria from the intestinal tract into the biliary tree can lead to colangitis (inflammation of the bile ducts). Colonization of the female urethra and bladder can result from fecal contamination caused by the close proximity of structures.

ACCESSORY ORGANS OF DIGESTION

The liver, gallbladder, and exocrine pancreas all secrete substances necessary for the digestion of chyme. These secretions are delivered to the duodenum through ducts (Fig. 35-16). The liver produces bile, which con-

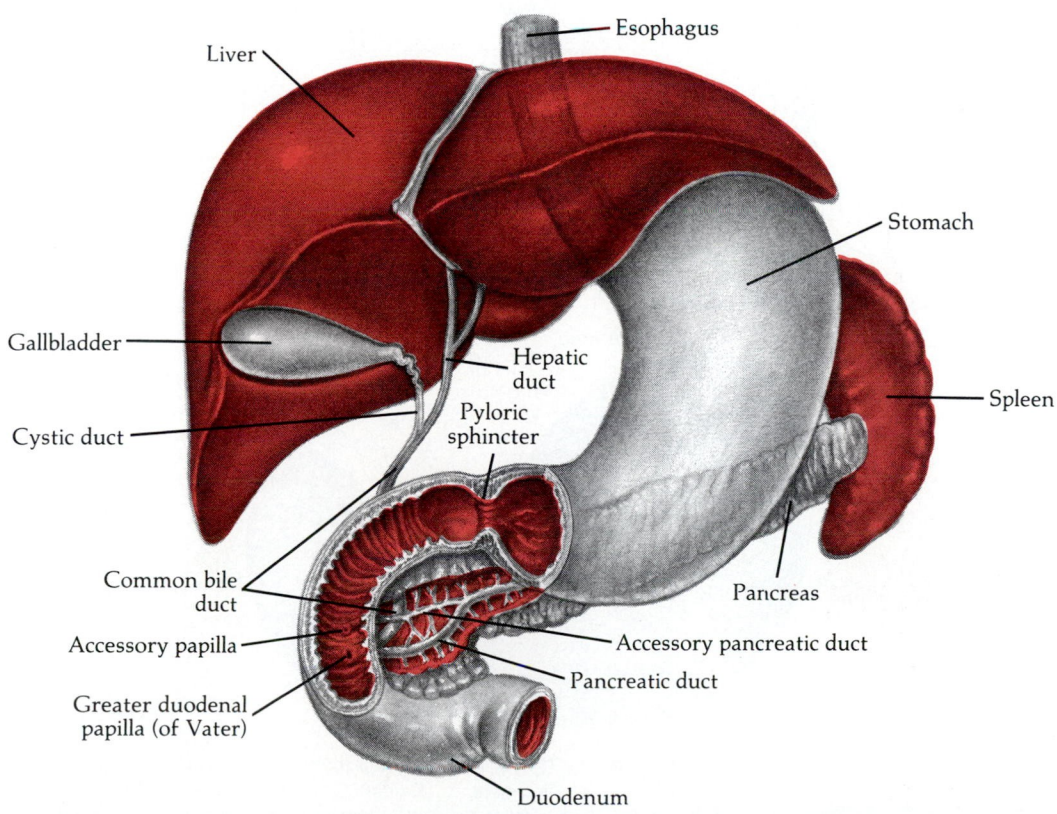

FIG. 35-16. Location of the liver, gallbladder, and exocrine pancreas, which are the accessory organs of digestion. (From Thompson et al., 1989.)

tains salts necessary for fat digestion and absorption. Between meals bile is stored in the gallbladder. The exocrine pancreas produces enzymes needed for the complete digestion of carbohydrates, proteins, and fats. The exocrine pancreas also produces an alkaline fluid that neutralizes chyme, creating a duodenal pH that supports enzymatic action.

The liver has many important functions besides bile secretion. It receives nutrients absorbed by the small intestine and metabolizes or synthesizes these nutrients into forms that can be absorbed by the body's cells. Having completed these processes, the liver releases the nutrients into the bloodstream or stores them for later use.

The Liver

The **liver,** which weighs 1200 to 1600 g, is the largest organ in the body. It is located under the right diaphragm and is divided into right and left lobes. The larger, right lobe is divided further into the caudate and quadrate lobes (Fig. 35-17). The falciform ligament separates the right and left lobes and attaches the liver to the anterior abdominal wall. A fibrous cord called the round ligament (ligamentum teres) extends along the free edge of the falciform ligament. The round ligament is the remnant of the umbilical vein and extends from the umbilicus to the inferior surface of the liver. The coronary ligament branches from the falciform ligament and extends over the superior surface of the right and left lobes, adhering the liver to the inferior surface of the diaphragm. The liver is covered by a fibroelastic capsule called **Glisson capsule.** Glisson capsule contains blood vessels, lymphatics, and nerves. When the liver is diseased or swollen, distention of the capsule causes pain and the lymphatics may ooze fluid into the peritoneal space.

The metabolic functions of the liver require a large amount of blood. The liver receives blood from both ar-

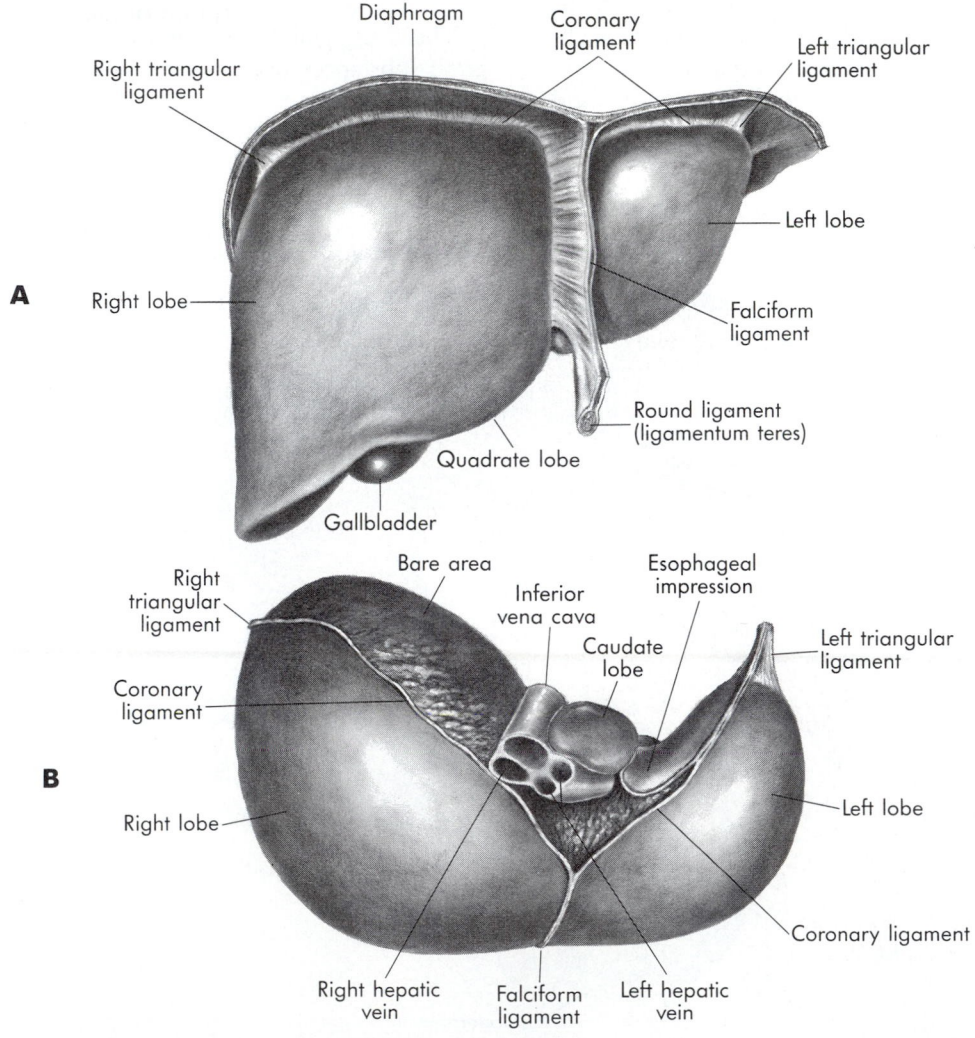

FIG. 35-17. Gross structure of the liver. **A,** Anterior view, showing supporting ligaments. **B,** Superior (diaphragmatic) surface of the liver.

terial and venous sources. The hepatic artery branches from the abdominal aorta and provides oxygenated blood at the rate of 400 to 500 ml/min (about 25% of the cardiac output). The hepatic portal vein, which receives deoxygenated blood from the inferior and superior mesenteric veins and the splenic vein, delivers about 1000 to 1200 ml/min to the liver. Portal venous blood constitutes 70% of the blood supply to the liver. This blood carries some oxygen and is rich in nutrients that have been absorbed from the digestive tract.

Within the liver lobes are multiple, smaller anatomic units called **liver lobules** (Fig. 35-18). The lobules are formed of cords or plates of **hepatocytes,** which are the functional cells of the liver. These cells are capable of regeneration; therefore, damaged or resected liver tissue can regrow. Small capillaries, or **sinusoids,** are located between the plates of hepatocytes. The sinusoids receive a mixture of venous and arterial blood from branches of the hepatic artery and portal vein. Blood from the sinusoids drains to a central vein in the middle of each liver lobule. Venous blood from all the lobules then flows into the hepatic vein, which empties into the inferior vena cava. Small channels known as **bile canaliculi** conduct bile, which is produced by the hepatocytes, outward to bile ducts and eventually drains into the **common bile duct** (Fig. 35-18). The common bile duct empties bile into the duodenum through an opening called the **major duodenal papilla.**

The sinusoids of the liver lobules are lined with highly permeable endothelium. This permeability enhances the transport of nutrients from the sinusoids into the hepatocytes, where they are metabolized. The sinusoids are also lined with phagocytic cells known as **Kupffer cells.** Kupffer cells are part of the mononuclear phagocyte system (Chapter 22). They remove foreign substances from the blood and trap bacteria. Between the endothelial lining of the sinusoid and the hepatocyte is the **Disse space** which drains interstitial fluid into the hepatic lymph system.

Secretion of Bile

The liver assists intestinal digestion by secreting 700 to 1200 ml of bile per day. **Bile** is an alkaline, bitter-tasting, yellowish green fluid that contains bile salts (conjugated bile acids), cholesterol, bilirubin (a pigment), electrolytes, and water. It is formed by hepatocytes and secreted into the canaliculi. **Bile salts,** which are conjugated bile acids, are required for the intestinal emulsification and absorption of fats. Having facilitated fat emulsification and absorption, most bile salts are actively absorbed in the terminal ileum and returned to the liver via the portal circulation for resecretion. The recycling of bile salts is termed the **enterohepatic circulation** (Fig. 35-19).

Bile has two fractional components: the acid-dependent fraction and the acid-independent fraction. Hepa-

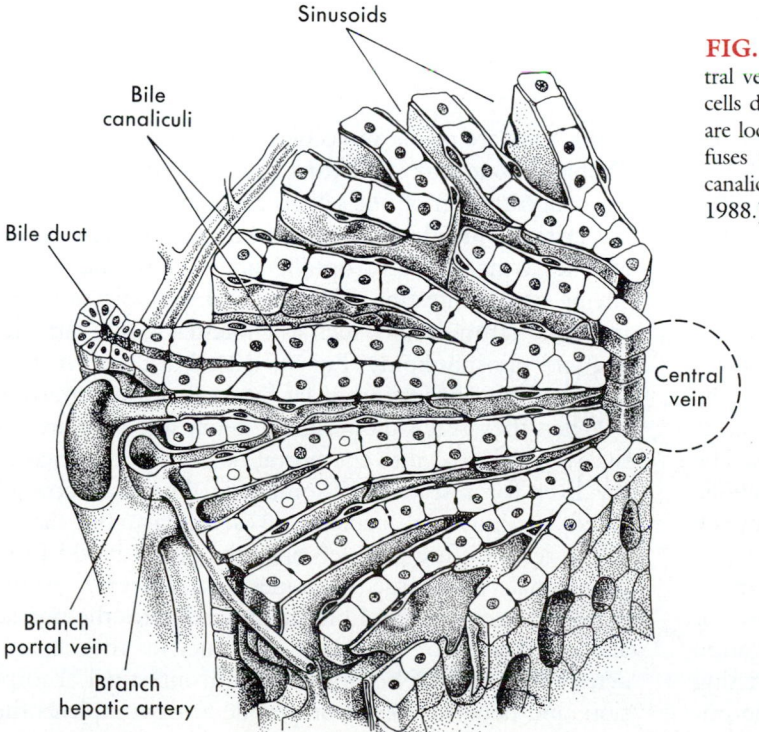

Sinusoids

Bile canaliculi

Bile duct

Branch portal vein

Branch hepatic artery

Central vein

FIG. 35-18. Diagrammatic representation of a liver lobule. A central vein is located in the center of the lobule with plates of hepatic cells disposed radially. Branches of the portal vein and hepatic artery are located on the periphery of the lobule, and blood from both perfuses the sinusoids. Peripherally located bile ducts drain the bile canaliculi that run between the hepatocytes. (From Berne & Levy, 1988.)

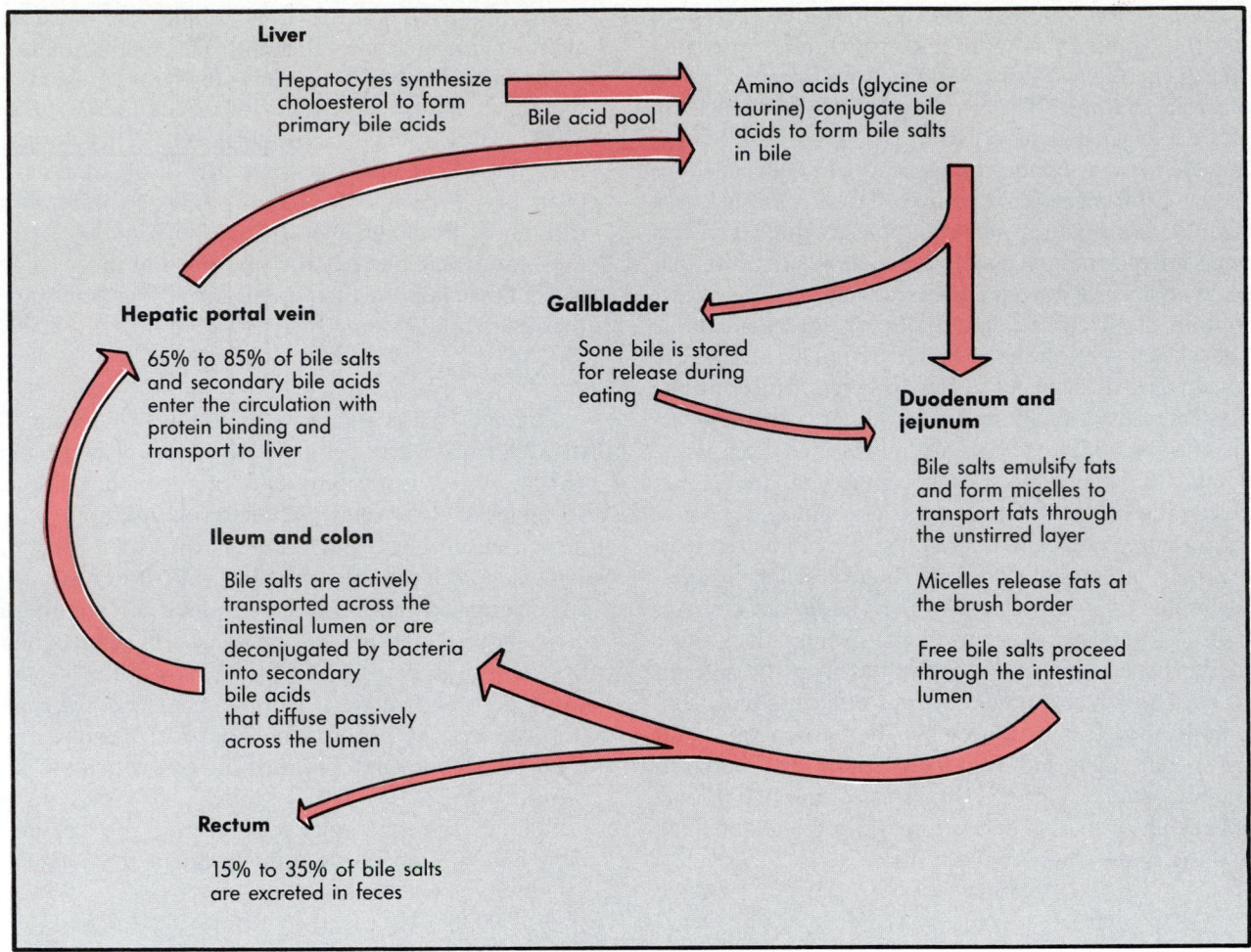

Liver

Hepatocytes synthesize choloesterol to form primary bile acids

Bile acid pool

Amino acids (glycine or taurine) conjugate bile acids to form bile salts in bile

Hepatic portal vein

65% to 85% of bile salts and secondary bile acids enter the circulation with protein binding and transport to liver

Gallbladder

Sone bile is stored for release during eating

Duodenum and jejunum

Bile salts emulsify fats and form micelles to transport fats through the unstirred layer

Micelles release fats at the brush border

Free bile salts proceed through the intestinal lumen

Ileum and colon

Bile salts are actively transported across the intestinal lumen or are deconjugated by bacteria into secondary bile acids that diffuse passively across the lumen

Rectum

15% to 35% of bile salts are excreted in feces

FIG. 35-19. The enterohepatic circulation of bile salts.

tocytes secrete the **bile acid-dependent fraction** of the bile. This fraction consists of bile acids, cholesterol, lecithin (a phospholipid), and bilirubin (a bile pigment). The **bile acid-dependent independent fraction** of the bile, which is secreted by the hepatocytes and epithelial cells of the bile canaliculi, is a bicarbonate-rich aqueous fluid that gives bile its alkaline pH.

Bile salts are conjugated in the liver from primary and secondary bile acids. The **primary bile acids** are cholic acid and chenodeoxycholic (chenic) acid. These acids are synthesized from cholesterol by the hepatocytes. The **secondary bile acids** are deoxycholic and lithocholic acid. These acids are formed in the small intestine by the action of intestinal bacteria, after which they are absorbed and flow to the liver (Fig. 35-19). Both forms of bile acids are conjugated with amino acids (glycine or taurine) in the liver to form bile salts. Conjugation makes the bile acids more water-soluble, thus restricting their diffusion from the duodenum and ileum. The primary and secondary bile acids together form the **bile acid pool.**

Bile salts are planar molecules: that is, they are hydrophobic on one end and hydrophilic on the other. When the concentration of bile salts is adequate or has reached the **critical micelle concentration,** the molecules form micelles with their hydrophilic side toward the watery chyme of the intestine and their hydrophobic side surrounding fat molecules such as cholesterol, free fatty acids, and phospholipids (Fig. 35-13). Micelle formation facilitates the absorption of fat by the intestinal mucosa.

When they reach the terminal ileum bile salts are actively transported into the portal blood and returned to the liver for resecretion. Some bile salts are deconjugated by intestinal bacteria to secondary bile acids. These acids diffuse passively into the portal blood from both small and large intestines. An increase in the plasma concentration of bile acids accelerates the uptake and resecretion of bile acids and salts by the hepatocytes. The cycle of hepatic secretion, intestinal absorption, and hepatic resecretion of bile acids completes the enterohepatic circulation.

Bile secretion is called **choleresis**. **A choleretic agent** is a substance that stimulates the liver to secrete bile. One strong stimulus is a high concentration of bile salts. Other choleretics include secretin, which increases the rate of bile flow by promoting the secretion of bicarbonate from canaliculi and other intrahepatic bile ducts; cholecystokinin; and vagal stimulation.

Metabolism of Bilirubin

Bilirubin is a by-product of destruction of aged red blood cells. It gives bile a greenish black color and produces the yellow tinge of jaundice. Aged red blood cells are taken up and destroyed by macrophages of the mononuclear phagocyte system (also called the reticuloendothelial system), primarily in the spleen and liver. (In the liver these macrophages are Kupffer cells.) Within these cells hemoglobin is separated into its component parts, heme and globin (Fig. 35-20). The globin component is further degraded into its constituent amino acids, which are recycled to form new protein. The heme moiety is converted to biliverdin by the enzymatic cleavage of iron. The iron attaches to transferrin in the plasma and can be stored in the liver or used by the bone marrow to make new red blood cells. The biliverdin is enzymatically converted to bilirubin in the macrophage of the mononuclear phagocytic system and

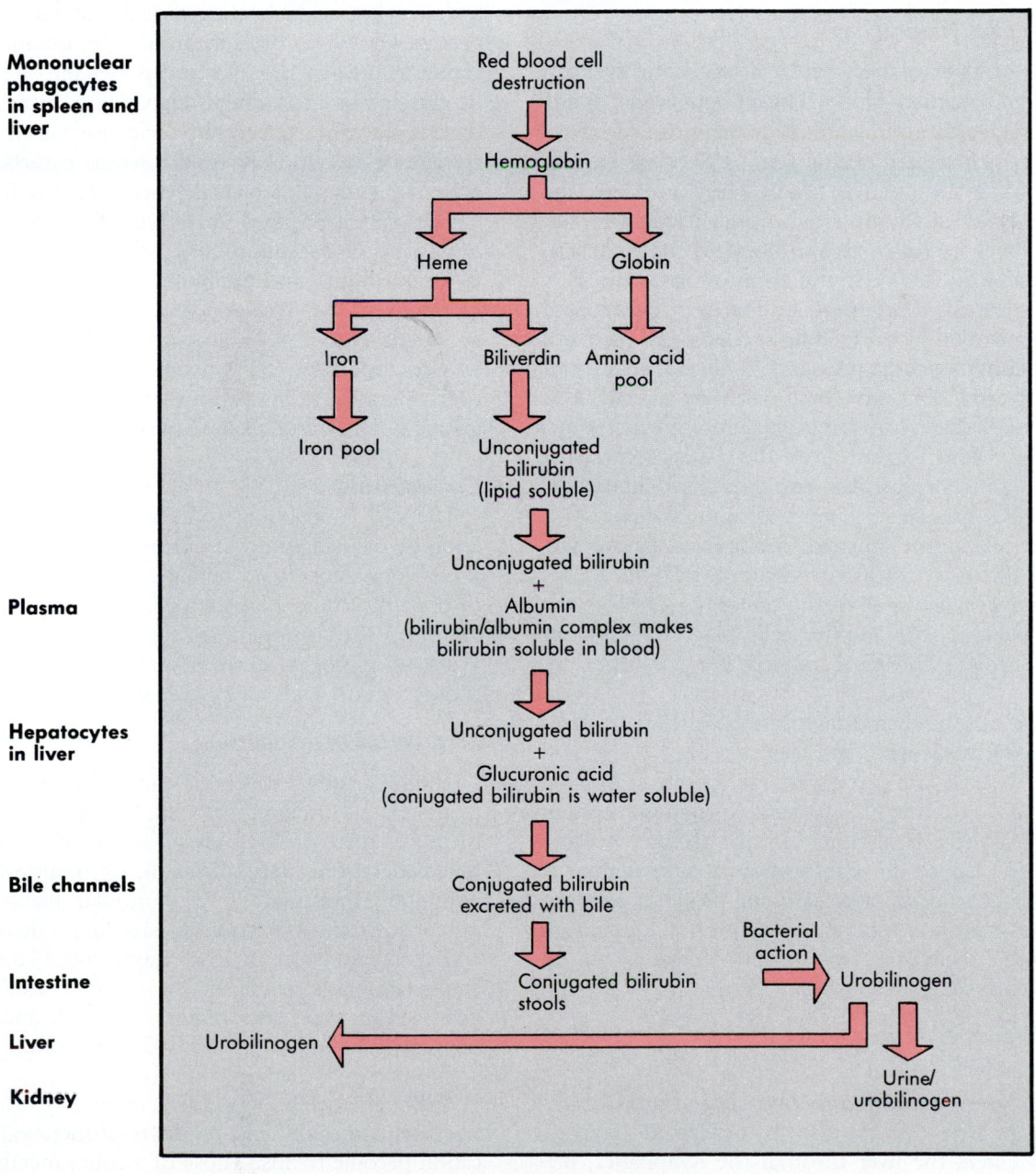

FIG. 35-20. Bilirubin metabolism.

then released into the plasma. In the plasma bilirubin binds to albumin and is known as **unconjugated bilirubin,** or free bilirubin, which is lipid-soluble.

In the liver unconjugated bilirubin moves from plasma in the sinusoids into the hepatocyte. Within hepatocytes it joins with glucuronic acid to form **conjugated bilirubin,** which is water-soluble. Conjugation transforms bilirubin from a lipid-soluble substance that can cross biologic membranes to a water-soluble substance that can be excreted in the bile. When conjugated bilirubin reaches the distal ileum and colon, it is deconjugated by bacteria and converted to **urobilinogen.** Most of the urobilinogen is then excreted in the urine, and a small amount is eliminated in feces.

Vascular and Hematologic Functions

Because of its extensive vascular network the liver can store a large volume of blood. The amount stored at any one time depends on pressure relationships in the arteries and veins. Increased central venous pressure, such as that caused by congestive heart failure, expands the venous capacity of the liver by several hundred milliliters. The liver can also release blood to maintain systemic circulatory volume in the event of hemorrhage.

Plasma proteins synthesized by the liver, particularly albumin, maintain blood volume and pressure by maintaining plasma oncotic pressure. Reduced concentrations of plasma proteins resulting from altered liver function or leakage of plasma proteins into interstitial spaces cause fluid to shift from the vascular compartment to the extravascular compartment (interstitial space). The consequence is reduced blood volume.

Kupffer cells in the sinusoids of the liver remove bacteria and foreign particles from the portal blood. Because the liver receives all of the venous blood from the gut and pancreas the Kupffer cells play an important role in destroying intestinal bacteria and preventing infections.

The liver also has hemostatic functions. It synthesizes prothrombin, fibrinogen, and factors I, II, VII, IX, and X, all of which are necessary for effective clotting (Chapter 22). Vitamin K, a fat-soluble vitamin, is essential for the synthesis of other clotting factors. Because bile salts are needed for reabsorption of fats, vitamin K absorption depends on adequate bile production in the liver. Impairment of vitamin K absorption diminishes production of clotting factors and increases risk of bleeding.

Metabolism of Nutrients

Fats

Fat is synthesized from carbohydrate and protein, primarily in the liver. Fat absorbed by lacteals in the intestinal villi enters the liver through the lymphatics, primarily as triglycerides. In the liver the triglycerides can be hydrolyzed to glycerol and free fatty acids and used to produce metabolic energy (ATP), or they can be released into the bloodstream as lipoproteins (lipids bound to proteins). Low-density lipoproteins have little protein and a lot of fat, and high-density lipoproteins have little fat and a lot of protein. The lipoproteins are carried by the blood to adipose cells for storage. The liver also synthesizes phospholipids and cholesterol, which are needed for the hepatic production of bile salts, steroid hormones, components of plasma membranes, and other special molecules.

Proteins

Within hepatocytes amino acids are converted to carbohydrates (ketoacids) by the removal of ammonia (NH_3), a process known as **deamination.** The ammonia is converted to urea by the liver and passes into the blood to be excreted by the kidneys. Depending on need, the ketoacids are converted to fatty acids for fat synthesis and storage or are oxidized by the Krebs tricarboxylic acid cycle (Chapter 1) to provide energy for the liver cells.

The plasma proteins, including albumins and globulins (with the exception of γ-globulin, which is formed in lymph nodes and lymphoid tissue), are synthesized by the liver. The liver also synthesizes several nonessential amino acids and serum enzymes, including aspartate aminotransferase (AST; previously SGOT), alanine aminotransferase (ALT; previously SGPT), lactate dehydrogenase (LDH), and alkaline phosphatase.

Carbohydrates

The liver contributes to the stability of blood glucose levels by releasing glucose during states of hypoglycemia (low blood sugar) and taking up glucose during states of hyperglycemia (high blood sugar) and storing it as glycogen (glyconeogenesis) or converting it to fat. When all glycogen stores have been used the liver can convert amino acids and glycerol to glucose.

Metabolic Detoxification

The liver alters exogenous and endogenous chemicals (e.g., drugs), foreign molecules, and hormones to make them less toxic or less biologically active. This process, called **metabolic detoxification,** or biotransformation, diminishes intestinal or renal tubular reabsorption of potentially toxic substances and facilitates their intestinal and renal excretion. In this way alcohol, barbiturates, amphetamines, steroids, and hormones (including estrogens, aldosterone, antidiuretic hormone, and testosterone) are metabolized or detoxified, preventing excessive accumulation and adverse effects.

Although metabolic detoxification is usually protective, sometimes the end products of metabolic detoxification become toxins. Those of alcohol metabolism, for example, are acetaldehyde and hydrogen. Excessive intake of alcohol over a prolonged period of time causes these end products to damage hepatocytes. Acetaldehyde damages cellular mitochondria, and the excess hydrogen promotes fat accumulation. This is how alcohol impairs the liver's ability to function.

Storage of Minerals and Vitamins

The liver stores certain vitamins and minerals in times of excessive intake and releases them in times of need. The liver can store vitamins B_{12} and D for several months and vitamin A for several years. Iron is stored in the liver as ferritin, an iron-protein complex, and is released as needed for red blood cell production.

The Gallbladder

The **gallbladder** is a saclike organ that lies on the inferior surface of the liver (Fig. 35-21). The primary function of the gallbladder is to store and concentrate bile between meals. During the interdigestive period bile flows from the liver through the right or left hepatic duct into the common hepatic duct and meets resistance at the closed **sphincter of Oddi,** which controls flow into the duodenum. Bile then flows to the **cystic duct** into the gallbladder, where it is concentrated and stored. The mucosa of the gallbladder wall readily absorbs water and electrolytes, leaving a high concentration of bile salts, bile pigments, and cholesterol. The gallbladder holds about 90 ml of bile.

Within 30 minutes after eating the gallbladder begins to contract and the sphincter of Oddi relaxes, forcing bile into the duodenum through the major duodenal papill. During the cephalic and gastric phases of digestion gallbladder contraction is mediated by cholinergic branches of the vagus nerve. Hormonal regulation of

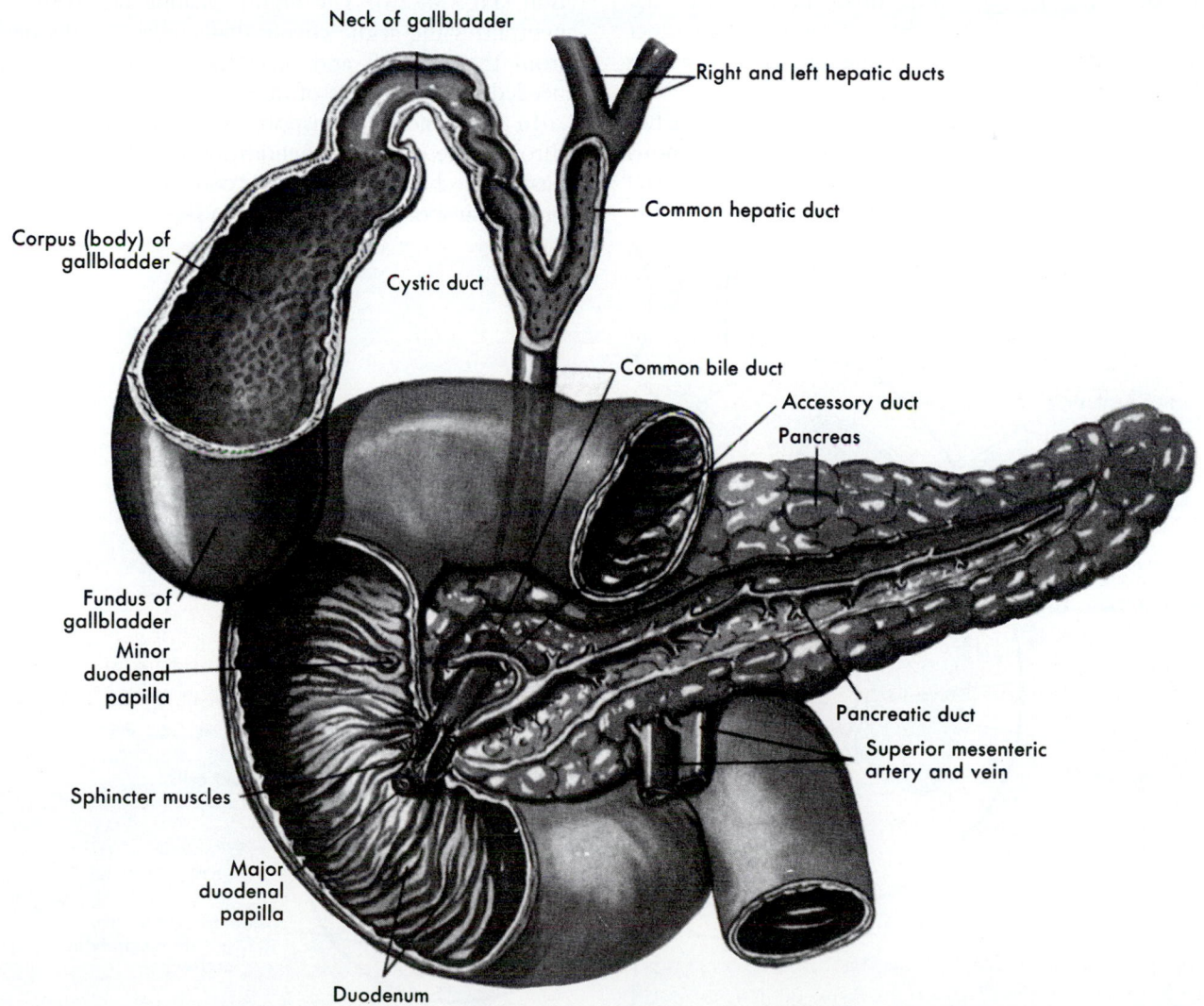

FIG. 35-21. The gallbladder and its divisions. Obstruction of either the hepatic or the common bile duct by stone or spasm prevents bile from being ejected into the duodenum. (From Thibodeau, 1987.)

gallbladder contraction is derived from the release of cholecystokinin and motilin secreted by the duodenal mucosa in the presence of fat (Way & Pellegrini, 1987).

The Exocrine Pancreas

The **pancreas** is approximately 20 cm long, with its head tucked into the curve of the duodenum and its tail touching the spleen. The body of the pancreas lies deep in the abdomen, behind the stomach (Fig. 35-21). The pancreas is unique in that it has both endocrine and exocrine functions. The endocrine pancreas secretes hormones, primarily insulin and glucagon.

The **exocrine pancreas** is composed of acini and networks of ducts that secrete enzymes and alkaline fluids with important digestive functions. The acinar cells are organized into spherical lobules around small secretory ducts (Fig. 35-22). Secretions drain into a system of ducts that leads to the **pancreatic duct** (Wirsung duct), which empties into the common bile duct at the **ampulla of Vater.** In some individuals an accessory duct (the duct of Santorini) branches off the pancreatic duct and drains directly into the duodenum at an opening called the minor duodenal papilla.

Arterial blood is supplied to the pancreas by branches of the celiac and superior mesenteric arteries. Venous blood leaves the head of the pancreas through the portal vein, with the body and tail being drained through the splenic vein. All hormonal pancreatic secretions also pass through the portal vein into the liver.

Pancreatic innervation arises from preganglionic parasympathetic fibers of the vagus nerve. The preganglionic fibers activate postganglionic fibers, which stimulate enzymatic and hormonal secretion. Sympathetic postganglionic fibers from the celiac and superior mesenteric plexuses innervate the blood vessels and cause vasoconstriction. Generally the sympathetic nerves inhibit pancreatic secretion and the parasympathetic nerves stimulate it.

The aqueous secretions of the exocrine pancreas are isotonic and contain potassium, sodium, bicarbonate, and chloride. Sodium and potassium concentrations are about equal to those in the plasma. The concentration of bicarbonate in pancreatic juice varies from 50 mEq/L at low secretory flow rates to 120 mEq/L at high flow rates. As bicarbonate secretion increases, chloride secretion decreases to maintain a constant anionic concentration (Fig. 35-23). The highly alkaline pancreatic juice neutralizes the acidic chyme that enters the duodenum from the stomach and provides the alkaline medium needed for the actions of digestive enzymes.

In the pancreas transport of water and electrolytes through the ductal epithelium involves both active and passive mechanisms. The most commonly proposed theory of transport is summarized in Fig. 35-24. The secre-

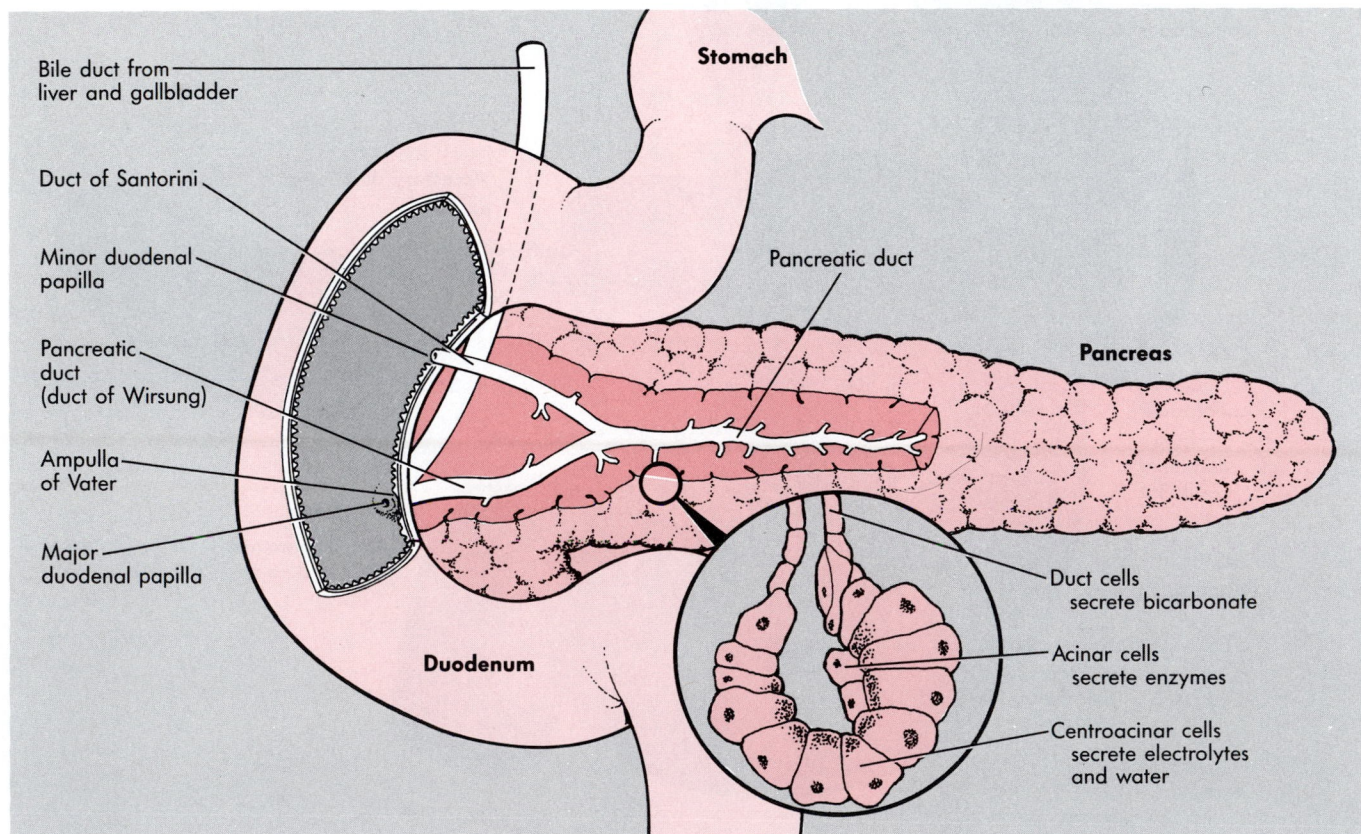

Bile duct from liver and gallbladder

Duct of Santorini

Minor duodenal papilla

Pancreatic duct (duct of Wirsung)

Ampulla of Vater

Major duodenal papilla

Stomach

Pancreatic duct

Pancreas

Duct cells secrete bicarbonate

Acinar cells secrete enzymes

Centroacinar cells secrete electrolytes and water

Duodenum

FIG. 35-22. Glands and ducts of the exocrine pancreas.

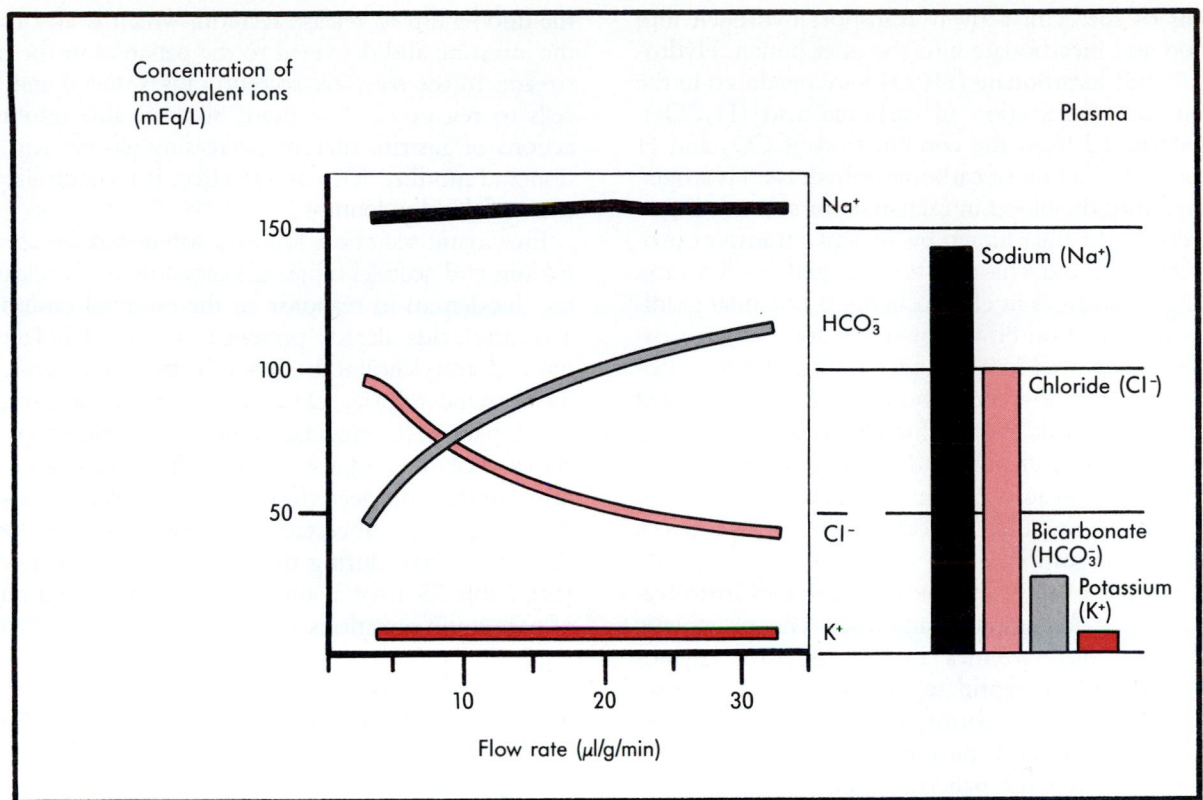

FIG. 35-23. Relationship between secretory rate and electrolyte composition of pancreatic juice in the rabbit. The concentrations of these electrolytes in plasma are shown for reference.

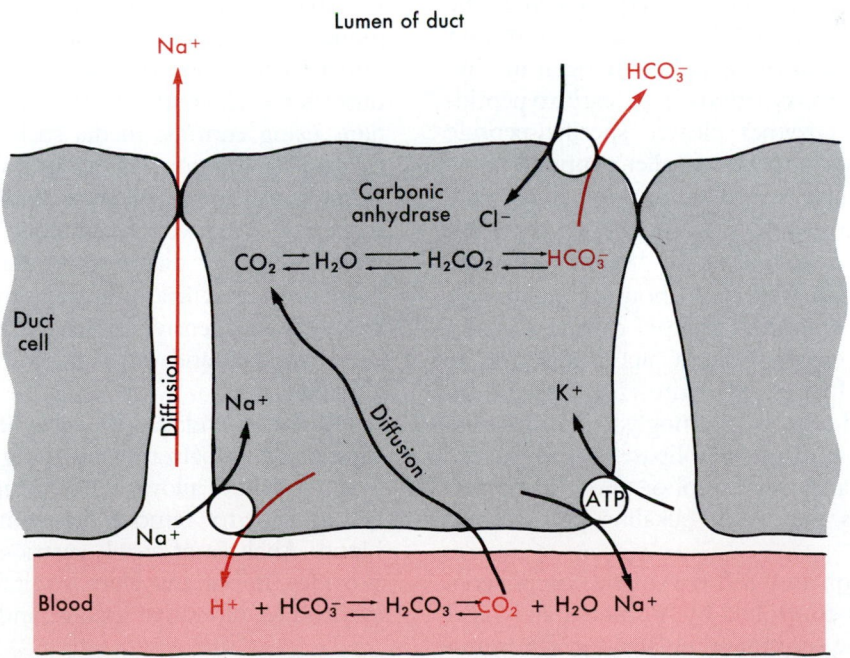

FIG. 35-24. A hypothetical mechanism for the secretion of bicarbonate (HCO.MDSD/3.MDSU/⁻) and sodium (Na⁺) by epithelial cells of the pancreatic duct. Acidification of the blood (driven by the Na⁺ gradient) is the primary mechanism driving bicarbonate transport. Na⁺ diffuses into the pancreatic duct through the intercellular junctions. (From Berne & Levy, 1988.)

tory cells of the acini actively transport hydrogen into the blood and bicarbonate into the duct lumen. Hydrogen (H^+) and bicarbonate (HCO_3^-) are produced in the cell from the dissociation of carbonic acid (H_2CO_3), which is formed from the combination of CO_2 and H_2O through the action of carbonic anhydrase. Hydrogen is secreted into the blood in exchange for sodium. Bicarbonate enters the duct lumen by an active transport process. Potassium and chloride are secreted by diffusion according to changes in electrochemical potential gradients. As the secretion flows down the duct, water is osmotically transported into the juice until it becomes iso-osmotic. At low flow rates bicarbonate is exchanged passively for chloride, but at higher flow rates there is less time for this exchange and bicarbonate concentration increases. Because eating stimulates the flow of pancreatic juice, the juice is most alkaline when it needs to be: during digestion.

The enzymes of the pancreas are capable of hydrolyzing proteins, carbohydrates, and fats. The proteolytic (protein-digesting) enzymes include **trypsin,** chymotrypsin, and carboxypeptidase. These enzymes are secreted in their inactive forms, that is, as trypsinogen, chymotrypsinogen, and procarboxypeptidase. This is necessary to protect the pancreas from the digestive effects of its own enzymes. For further protection the pancreas produces **trypsin inhibitor,** which prevents the activation of proteolytic enzymes while they are in the pancreas. Once in the duodenum the inactive forms (proenzymes) are activated by **enterokinase,** an enzyme secreted by the duodenal mucosa. Trypsinogen is the first proenzyme to be activated. Its conversion to trypsin stimulates the conversion of chymotrypsinogen to chymotrypsin and procarboxypeptidase to carboxypeptidase. Each of these enzymes cleaves specific peptide bonds to reduce polypeptides to smaller peptides.

Pancreatic α-amylase is secreted in active form. Like salivary amylase it participates in carbohydrate digestion by cleaving interior α-$_{1,4}$ glucosidic bonds. The optimum pH for α-amylase action is about 6.9, although enzymatic activity is supported at a pH of 4 to 11.

Several pancreatic enzymes digest fats. **Pancreatic lipase** (glycerol ester hydrolase) hydrolyzes triglycerides to one free fatty acid and two monoglycerides. Cholesterol ester hydrolase and phospholipase A and B produce free fatty acids and cholesterol or phosphate products. These enzymes require an alkaline pH ranging from 7 to 9.

Secretion of the aqueous and enzymatic components of pancreatic juice is controlled by hormonal and vagal stimuli. The hormone secretin stimulates the acinar and duct cells to secrete the bicarbonate-rich fluid that neutralize chyme and prepare it for enzymatic digestion. As chyme enters the duodenum its acidity (pH of 4.5 of less) stimulates the **S cells** (secretin-producing cells) of the duodenum to release secretin, which is absorbed by the intestine and delivered to the pancreas in the bloodstream. In the pancreas secretin causes ductal and acinar cells to release alkaline fluid. Secretin also inhibits the actions of gastrin, thereby decreasing gastric acid secretion and motility. The overall effect is to neutralize contents of the duodenum.

Enzymatic secretion follows, stimulated by cholecystokinin and acetylcholine. Cholecystokinin is released in the duodenum in response to the essential amino acids and fatty acids already present in chyme. Cholecystokinin and acetylcholine both act on the acinar cells, causing enzyme release. Once in the small intestine, activated pancreatic enzymes inhibit the release of more cholecystokinin and acetylcholine. This feedback mechanism inhibits the secretion of more pancreatic enzymes. Acetylcholine is liberated from pancreatic branches of the vagus nerve during the cephalic phase of digestion. (See Table 35-1 for a summary of hormonal stimulation of pancreatic secretions.)

TESTS OF DIGESTIVE FUNCTION

The Gastrointestinal Tract

Although important diagnostic information can be obtained from the history and presenting symptoms, numerous disease-specific tests must be performed to evaluate the structure and function of the gastrointestinal tract. A description of selected studies is presented in Tables 35-3 and 35-4. X-ray films and imaging techniques, including ultrasound and radionuclide and computed tomography (CT scanning), are common procedures for evaluating structure and function. Plain x-ray films using contrast media such as barium- or iodine-containing compounds can be used to outline the gastrointestinal lumen, biliary tree and pancreatic ducts, fistulas, and arteriovenous systems. CT scanning is particularly useful for diagnosis of pancreatic or hepatic tumors or cysts. Ultrasonic scanning is a safe, simple, and relatively inexpensive technique used to detect liver-related jaundice and intra-abdominal masses, particularly abscesses.

Fiberoptic endoscopy, using flexible endoscopes, allows direct visualization of the gastrointestinal tract. A biopsy channel allows tissue sampling, and suction can be applied to remove gastrointestinal secretions or blood. Analysis of stool, gastric secretions, and plasma provides important clues to infection, malabsorption syndromes, ulcerative lesions, and tumor growth.

The Liver

A variety of diagnostic tests can be performed to evaluate liver function (Table 35-5). Imaging techniques similar to those described for the gastrointestinal tract

TABLE 35-3 Selected studies of gastrointestinal structure

Test	Description	Application
Plain x-ray films	Use of high-energy electromagnetic radiation to evaluate tissue structure by radiopacity or radiolucency	Visualization of the position, size, and structure of abdominal contents
Air or barium contrast x-ray films	Introduction of radiopaque substances into the upper or lower gastrointestinal tract	Enhanced visualization of the contours, position, and size of the gastrointestinal tract to detect umbilical hernia, ulcers, diverticuli, congenital anomalies, polyps, tumors, strictures, obstructions
Endoscopy Esophagoscopy (esophagus) Gastroscopy (stomach) Duodenoscopy (duodenum) Colonoscopy (large intestine) Sigmoidoscopy (sigmoid colon)	Passage of rigid or flexible (fiberoptic) endoscope into the gastrointestinal tract for visualization of biopsy	Visualization or biopsy of inflamed hernias, polyps, ulcers, strictures, varices, tumors, sites of bleeding, mucosal or neoplastic lesions
Ultrasound	Use of piezoelectric crystal to generate sound waves that are reflected from tissue interfaces to provide an image	Imaging of abdominal organs (gallbladder, liver, pancreas, spleen), masses, stones, abscesses, structural abnormalities
Computed tomography (CT)	Use of a computer to integrate dierences in absorption of a large number of x-rays to produce a cross-sectional image, may be done with contrast agents	Imaging of gallbladder, liver, pancreas, spleen, cysts, hematomas, abscesses, stones, extrahepatic bile ducts, and portal vein
Magnetic resonance imaging (MRI)	Projection of dierences in magnetic properties of molecules within dierent cells and tissues, using the field of a large magnet	Same applications as CT scan; can also detect blood flow and vessel patency

are also useful to evaluate liver structure and function. Plasma chemistry findings are also altered with many liver diseases because of release of cytoplasmic enzymes into the circulation when there is damage to the hepatocyte. Of particular importance are elevations of aminotransferases and lactate dehydrogenate (LDH). Obstruction of bile canaliculi or ducts results in regurgitation of bile back into the hepatic sinusoids and into the circulation with elevation of bilirubin levels. Prothrombin times are often prolonged with both hepatitis and chronic liver disease. In severe disease other plasma proteins, such as albumin and globulins, may be diminished as a result of hepatocyte damage. Liver biopsies are often performed to evaluate the extent of liver involvement or degeneration with cirrhosis or hepatitis.

The Gallbladder

Evaluation of structural alterations in the gallbladder may be achieved by the use of different imaging techniques. Table 35-6 summarizes these techniques. Obstruction of the common ducts from stones, tumors, or inflammation prevents the flow of bile from the liver and gallbladder from reaching the gastrointestinal tract. Both the conjugated and total serum bilirubin values are elevated, urine urobilinogen is increased, stools are clay-colored, and jaundice develops. Fat absorption can be impaired and the prothrombin time prolonged if vitamin K is not absorbed. With inflammation of the gallbladder, the white cell count is elevated.

The Exocrine Pancreas

Tests of pancreatic function are summarized in Table 35-7. Evaluation of plasma and urinary amylase provides particularly significant measures of pancreatic function. Inflammation or obstruction of the pancreas results in an increase in serum amylase levels. Decreased renal absorption of amylase results in increased urine amylase levels. Increased stool fat can reflect pancreatic

TABLE 35-4 Selected tests of gastrointestinal function

Test	Normal findings	Clinical significance of abnormal findings
Stool studies	Resident microorganisms: clostridia, enterococci, pseudomonas, a few yeasts	Detection of *Salmonella typhi* (typhoid fever), *Shigella* (dysentery), *Vibrio cholerae* (cholera), *Yersinia* (enterocolitis), *Escherichia coli* (gastroenteritis), *Staphylococcus aureus* (food poisoning), *Clostridium botulinum* (food poisoning), *Clostridium perfringen* (food poisoning), *Aeromonas* (gastroenteritis)
	Fat: 2-6 g/24 hr	Steatorrhea (increased values) can result from intestinal malabsorption or pancreatic insufficiency
	Pus: none	Large amounts of pus are associated with chronic ulcerative colitis, abscesses, and anal-rectal fistula
	Occult blood: none (Ortho-Tolidin or Guaiac test)	Positive tests associated with bleeding
	Ova and parasites: none	Detection of *Entamoeba hystolytica* (amebiasis), *Giardia lamblia* (giardiasis), and worms
D-Xylose absorption	5-Hr urinary excretion: r4.5 g/L Peak blood level: >30 mg/dl	Dierentiation of pancreatic steatorrhea (normal D-xylose absorption) from intestinal steatorrhea (impaired D-xylose absorption)
Gastric acid stimulation	11-20 mEq/hr after stimulation	Detection of duodenal ulcers, Zollinger-Ellison syndrome (increased values), gastric atrophy, gastric carcinoma (decreased values)
Manometry (use of water-filled catheters connected to pressure transducers passed into the esophagus, stomach, colon, or rectum to evaluate contractility)	Values vary at dierent levels of the intestine	Inadequate swallowing, motility, sphincter function
Culture and sensitivity of duodenal contents	No pathogens	Detection of *Salmonella typhi* (typhoid fever)

TABLE 35-5 Common liver function tests

Test	Normal value	Interpretation
SERUM ENZYMES		
Alkaline phosphatase	13-39 U/ml	Increases with biliary obstruction and cholestatic hepatitis
Aspartate amino transferase (AST; previously SGOT)	5-40 U/ml	Increases with hepatocellular injury
Alanine amino transferase (ALT; previously SGPT)	5-35 U/ml	
LDH (lactate dehydrogenase)	200-500 U/ml	
5'-nucleotidase	2-11 U/ml	Increases with increase in alkaline phosphatase
BILIRUBIN METABOLISM Serum bilirubin		
Indirect (unconjugated)	<0.8 mg/dl	Increases with hemolysis (lysis of red blood cells)
Direct (conjugated)	0.2-0.4 mg/dl	Increases with hepatocellular injury or obstruction
Total	<1.0 mg/dl	Increase with biliary obstruction
Urine bilirubin	0	Decreases with biliary obstruction
Urine urobilinogen	0-4 mg/24 hr	Increases with hemolysis or shunting of portal blood flow
SERUM PROTEINS		
Albumin	3.5-5.5 gm/dl	Reduced with hepatocellular injury
Globulin	2.5-3.5 gm/dl	Increases with hepatitis
Total	6-7 gm/dl	
A/G ratio	1.5:1-2.5:1	Ratio reverses with chronic hepatitis or other chronic liver disease
Transferrin	250-300 mcg/dl	Liver damage with decreased values, iron deficiency with increased values
BLOOD CLOTTING FUNCTIONS		
Prothrombin time	11.5-14 sec or 90%-100% of control	Increases with chronic liver disease (cirrhosis) or vitamin K deficiency
Partial thromboplastin time	25-40 sec	Increases with severe liver disease or heparin therapy
BSP (bromsulphalein) excretion	<6% retention in 45 min	Increased retention with hepatocellular injury

---

TABLE 35-6 Diagnostic evaluation of the gallbladder

Test	Application
Plain film of the abdomen	Visualization of calcified gallstones
Oral cholecystogram (use of an oral contrast medium such as iodopanoic acid, which is excreted with bile and concentrated in the gallbladder for visualization by radiography; may be administered as a double dose)	Visualization of gallstones; evaluation of filling and emptying of gallbladder
Intravenous cholangiography (use of intravenous contrast agents for visualization of gallbladder and bile ducts)	Diagnosis of acute gallbladder inflammation (cholecystitis) or disease of bile ducts
Cholecystosonography (ultrasound imaging of gallbladder and bile ducts)	Preferred method for detecting gallstones; differentiation of hepatic disease from biliary obstruction; diagnosis of chronic cholecystitis
Cholescintigraphy (radioisotope imaging of gallbladder)	Diagnosis of cholecystitis in individuals allergic to iodine-containing contrast agents; diagnosis of cystic duct obstruction
Endoscopic retrograde cholangiography (instillation of contrast medium through cannulation of ampulla of Vater with a duodenoscope)	Differentiation of intra- or extrahepatic obstructive jaundice
Computed tomography (CT)	Diagnosis of biliary obstruction or malignancy when ultrasound is not successful

---

insufficiency caused by decreased lipase secretion when biliary function is normal.

AGING AND THE GASTROINTESTINAL SYSTEM

Age-related changes in gastrointestinal function begin to occur before age 50. Tooth enamel and dentin wear down, making the teeth vulnerable to cavities. Teeth are lost, frequently as a result of periodontal (gum) disease. Taste buds decline in number, and the sense of smell diminishes. Together these losses decrease the sense of taste. Salivary secretion decreases and contributes to dry mouth. In the very old these oral and sensory changes make eating less pleasurable and reduce appetite. Food may not be chewed or lubricated sufficiently, making swallowing difficult.

TABLE 35-7 Selected tests of pancreatic function

Test	Normal value	Clinical significance
Serum amylase	60-180 Somogyi units/ml	Elevated levels with pancreatic inflammation
Serum lipase	1.5 Somogyi units/ml	Elevated levels with pancreatic inflammation (may be elevated with other conditions; differentiates with amylase isoenzyme study)
Urine amylase	35-260 Somogyi units/hr	Elevated levels with pancreatic inflammaton
Secretin test	Volume r1.8 ml/kg/hr Bicarbonate concentration: >80 mEq/L Bicarbonate output: >10 mEq/L/30 sec	Decreased volume with pancreatic disease as secretin stimulates pancreatic secretion
Stool fat	2-5 g/25 hr Measures fatty acids	Decreased pancreatic lipase increases stool fat

Age also diminishes gastric motility and volume and acid content of gastric juice. These alterations cause hypochlorhydria (insufficient hydrochloric acid) and delayed gastric emptying, which are best managed with frequent and small meals. The villi of the small intestine become broader and shorter, perhaps because of a decrease in cell turnover. Intestinal absorption, motility, and blood flow decrease, impairing nutrient absorption. Carbohydrates, proteins, fats, minerals (including iron and calcium), and vitamins are absorbed more slowly and in lesser amounts. Interestingly intestinal absorption of drugs does not appear to decline (Brandt, 1984). Although constipation is often described as a condition of old age, it is probably caused by life-style factors rather than physiologic decline. Lifelong bowel habits, current diet, lack of fluid intake, and immobility are likely causes of constipation in the elderly.

The liver decreases in size and weight with advancing age, but liver function test results remain within normal ranges. Any alterations in liver function in older individuals are therefore signs of pathology. The pancreas undergoes structural changes, such as fibrosis, fatty acid deposits, and atrophy. Pancreatic secretion decreases, but there is usually no observable dysfunction. Aging does not cause apparent changes in the structure and function of the gallbladder and bile ducts.

SUMMARY REVIEW

The Gastrointestinal Tract

1 The major functions of the gastrointestinal tract are the mechanical and chemical breakdown of food and the absorption of digested nutrients.
2 The gastrointestinal tract is a hollow tube that extends from the mouth to the anus.
3 The walls of the gastrointestinal tract have several layers: mucosa, muscularis mucosae, submucosa, tunica muscularis (circular muscle and longitudinal muscle), and serosa.
4 The peritoneum is a double layer of membranous tissue. The visceral layer covers the abdominal organs, and the parietal layer extends along the abdominal wall.
5 Except for swallowing and defecation, which are controlled voluntarily, the functions of the gastrointestinal tract are controlled by extrinsic and intrinsic autonomic nerves and intestinal hormones.
6 Digestion begins in the mouth, with chewing and salivation. The digestive component of saliva is **α**-amylase, which initiates carbohydrate digestion.
7 The esophagus is a muscular tube that transports food from the mouth to the stomach. The tunica muscularis in the upper part of the esophagus is striated muscle and that in the lower part is smooth muscle.
8 Swallowing is controlled by the swallowing center in the reticular formation of the brain. The two phases of swallowing are the oropharyngeal phase (voluntary swallowing) and the esophageal phase (involuntary swallowing).
9 Food is propelled through the gastrointestinal tract by peristalsis: waves of sequential relaxations and contractions of the tunica muscularis.
10 The lower esophageal sphincter opens to admit swallowed food into the stomach, then closes to prevent regurgitation of food back into the esophagus.
11 The stomach is a baglike structure that secretes digestive juices, mixes and stores food, and propels partially digested food (chyme) into the duodenum.
12 The vagus nerve stimulates gastric (stomach) secretion and motility.
13 The hormones gastrin and motilin stimulate gastric emptying; the hormones secretin and cholecystokinin delay gastric emptying.
14 Mucus is secreted throughout the stomach and protects the stomach wall from acid and digestive enzymes.
15 Gastric glands in the fundus and body of the stomach secrete intrinsic factor, which is needed for vitamin B_{12} absorption, and hydrochloric acid, which dissolves food fibers, kills microorganisms, and activates the enzyme pepsin.
16 Chief cells in the stomach secrete pepsinogen, which is converted to pepsin in the acid environment created by hydrochloric acid.
17 Acid secretion is stimulated by the vagus nerve, gastrin, and histamine and inhibited by sympathetic stimulation and cholecystokinin.
18 The three phases of acid secretion by the stomach are the cephalic phase (anticipation and swallowing), the gastric phase (food in the stomach), and the intestinal phase (chyme in the intestine).
19 The small intestine is 5 m long and has three segments: the duodenum, jejunum, and ileum.
20 The duodenum receives chyme from the stomach through the pyloric valve. The presence of chyme stimulates the liver and gallbladder to deliver bile and the pancreas to deliver digestive enzymes. Bile and enzymes flow through an opening guarded by the sphincter of Oddi.
21 Bile is produced by the liver and is necessary for fat digestion and absorption. Bile's alkalinity helps to neutralize chyme, thereby creating a pH that enables the pancreatic enzymes to digest proteins, carbohydrates, and sugars.
22 Enzymes secreted by the small intestine (maltase, sucrose, and lactase), pancreatic enzymes, and bile salts act in the small intestine to digest proteins, carbohydrates, and fats.
23 Digested substances are absorbed across the intestinal wall then transported to the liver, where they are metabolized further.
24 The ileocecal valve connects the small and large intestines and prevents reflux into the small intestine.
25 Villi are small fingerlike projections that extend from

the small intestinal mucosa and increase its absorptive surface area.

26 Sugars, amino acids, and fats are primarily absorbed by the duodenum and jejunum; bile salts and vitamin B_{12} are absorbed by the ileum. Vitamin B_{12} absorption requires the presence of intrinsic factor.

27 Bile salts emulsify and hydrolyze fats and incorporate them into water-soluble micelles, which transport them through the unstirred layer to the brush border of the intestinal mucosa. The fat content of the micelles readily diffuses through the epithelium into lacteals (lymphatic ducts) in the villi. From there fats flow into lymphatics and into the systemic circulation, which delivers them to the liver.

28 Minerals and water-soluble vitamins are absorbed by both active and passive transport throughout the small intestine.

29 Peristaltic movements created by longitudinal muscles propel the chyme along the intestinal tract, while contractions of the circular muscles (haustral segmentation) mix the chyme.

30 The ileogastric reflex inhibits gastric motility when the ileum is distended.

31 The intestinointestinal reflex inhibits intestinal motility when one intestinal segment is overdistended.

32 The gastroileal reflex increases intestinal motility when gastric motility increases.

33 The large intestine consists of the cecum, appendix, colon (ascending, transverse, descending, and sigmoid), rectum, and anal canal.

34 The teniae coli are three bands of longitudinal muscle that extend the length of the colon.

35 Haustra are pouches of colon that are formed with alternating contraction and relaxation of the circular muscles.

36 The mucosa of the large intestine contains mucus-secreting cells and mucosal folds, but no villi.

37 The large intestine massages the fecal mass and absorbs water and electrolytes.

38 Distention of the ileum with chyme causes the gastrocolic reflex, or the mass propulsion of feces to the rectum.

39 Defecation is stimulated when the rectum is distended with feces. The conically contracted internal anal sphincter relaxes and, if the voluntarily regulated external sphincter relaxes, defecation occurs.

40 The largest number of intestinal bacteria are in the colon. They are anaerobes consisting of bacteriodes, clostridia, coliforms, and lactobacilli.

41 The intestinal tract is sterile at birth and becomes totally colonized within 3 to 4 weeks.

42 Endogenous infections of the gastrointestinal tract occur by excessive proliferation of bacteria, perforation of the intestine, or contamination from neighboring structures.

Accessory Organs of Digestion

1 The liver is the largest organ in the body. It has digestive, metabolic, hematologic, vascular, and immunologic functions.

2 The liver is divided into the right and left lobes and is supported by the falciform, round, and coronary ligaments.

3 Liver lobules consist of plates of hepatocytes, which are the functional cells of the liver.

4 The hepatocytes synthesize 700 to 1200 ml of bile per day and secrete it into the bile canaliculi, which are small channels between the hepatocytes. The bile canaliculi drain bile into the common bile duct and then into the duodenum through an opening called the major duodenal papilla. The sphincter of Oddi controls flow through the papilla.

5 Sinusoids are capillaries located between the plates of hepatocytes. Blood from the portal vein and hepatic artery flow through the sinusoids to a central vein in each lobule and then to the hepatic vein and inferior vena cava.

6 Kupffer cells, which are part of the mononuclear phagocyte system, line the sinusoids and destroy microorganisms in sinusoidal blood.

7 The primary bile acids are synthesized from cholesterol by the hepatocytes. The primary acids are then conjugated to form bile salts. The secondary bile acids are the product of bile salt deconjugation by bacteria in the intestinal lumen.

8 Most bile salts and acids are recycled. The absorption of bile salts and acids from the terminal ileum and their return to the liver are known as the enterohepatic circulation of bile.

9 Bilirubin is a pigment liberated by the lysis of aged red blood cells in the liver and spleen. Unconjugated bilirubin is fat-soluble and can cross cell membranes. Unconjugated bilirubin is converted to water-soluble, conjugated bilirubin by hepatocytes and is secreted with bile.

10 The gallbladder is a saclike organ located in the inferior surface of the liver. The gallbladder stores bile between meals and ejects it when chyme enters the duodenum.

11 Stimulated by cholecystokinin, the gallbladder contracts and forces bile through the cystic duct and into the common bile duct. The sphincter of Oddi relaxes, enabling bile to flow through the major duodenal papilla into the duodenum.

12 The pancreas is a gland located behind the stomach. The exocrine pancreas produces hormones (glucagon and insulin) which facilitate the formation and cellular update of glucose. The endocrine pancreas secretes an alkaline solution and the enzymes (trypsin, chymotrypsin, carboxypeptidase, α-amylase, and lipase) that digest proteins, carbohydrates, and fats.

13 Secretin stimulates pancreatic secretion of alkaline fluid, and cholecystokinin and acetylcholine stimulate secretion of enzymes. Pancreatic secretions originate in acini and ducts of the pancreas and empty into the duode-

num through the common bile duct or an accessory duct that opens directly into the duodenum.

Tests of the Digestive Function

1 Numerous diagnostic tests are performed to evaluate structure and function (digestion, secretion, and absorption) of the gastrointestinal tract. X-rays and scans are most commonly used to evaluate structure, in addition to direct observation by endoscopy. Gastric and stool analysis and blood studies provide important information about digestion, absorption, and secretion.

2 Plasma chemistries and imaging procedures are commonly used to diagnose alterations in liver function. Of particular importance are the enzymes LDH, AST, and GPT. Plasma bilirubin levels reflect alterations in bilirubin and bile metabolism, and prothrombin times are prolonged in hepatitis and chronic liver disease.

3 Obstructive diseases of the gallbladder are evident by elevated serum bilirubin, elevated urine urobilinogen, and increased stool fat. The serum leukocytes become elevated with inflammation of the gallbladder.

4 The most significant indicators of pancreatic dysfunction are serum amylase and stool fat. Both values are increased with diseases of the pancreas.

Aging and the Digestive System

1 Advancing age is often associated with the loss or wearing down of teeth, diminished senses of taste and smell, and diminished salivary secretions, all of which may make eating difficult and reduce appetite.

2 Aging reduces gastric motility and secretions, particularly of hydrochloric acid. These changes slow gastric digestion and emptying.

3 Intestinal motility and absorption of carbohydrates, proteins, fats, and minerals decrease with age.

KEY TERMS

α-Amylase (salivary, pancreatic), 1175

Ampulla of Vater, 1200

Antrum of stomach, 1178

Ascending colon, 1190

Bile, 1195

Bile acid-dependent fraction, 1196

Bile acid pool, 1196

Bile acid-independent fraction, 1196

Bile canaliculi, 1195

Bile salts, 1195

Bilirubin, 1197

Body of stomach, 1178

Brush border, 1184

Carboxypeptidase, 1187

Cardiac orifice, 1177

Cecum, 1190

Cephalic phase of secretion, 1181

Chief cell, 1180

Cholecystokinin, 1178

Choleresis, 1197

Choleretic agent, 1197

Chylomicron, 1188

Chyme, 1177

Chymotrypsin, 1187

Colon, 1190

Common bile duct, 1195

Conjugated bilirubin, 1198

Critical micelle concentration, 1196

Cystic duct, 1199

Deamination, 1198

Defecation reflex, 1192

Descending colon, 1190

Disse space, 1195

Duodenum, 1182

Emulsification, 1187

Enteric plexus, 1178

Enterohepatic circulation, 1195

Enterokinase, 1202

Esophageal phase of swallowing, 1177

Esophagus, 1176

Exocrine pancreas, 1200

External anal sphincter, 1190

Fecal mass, 1192

Feces, 1192

Fundus of stomach, 1178

Gallbladder, 1199

Gastric emptying, 1179

Gastric gland, 1179

Gastric phase of secretion, 1181

Gastric pit, 1179

Gastrin, 1178

Gastrocolic reflex, 1192

Gastroileal reflex, 1190

Gastrointestinal tract (alimentary canal), 1175

G cell, 1181

Glisson capsule, 1194

Haustral segmentation, 1190

Haustrum, 1190

Hepatocyte, 1195

Ileocecal valve (sphincter), 1182

Ileogastric reflex, 1190

Ileum, 1182

Internal anal sphincter, 1190

Intestinal phase of secretion, 1182

Intestinointestinal reflex, 1190

Jejunum, 1182

Kupffer cell, 1195

Lacteal, 1184

Lamina propria (basolateral membrane), 1184

Large intestine, 1190

Lieberkuhn crypts, 1190

Lipolysis, 1187

Liver, 1194

Liver lobule, 1195

Lower esophageal sphincter (cardiac sphincter), 1177

Major duodenal papilla, 1195

Mesentery, 1183

Metabolic detoxification (biotransformation), 1198

Micelle, 1187

Microvillus, 1184

Motilin, 1178

Mouth, 1175

Mucosa, 1178

Mucosal barrier, 1181

Muscularis mucosa, 1178

Myenteric plexus (Auerbach plexus), 1178

O'Beirne sphincter, 1190

Oropharyngeal phase of swallowing, 1177

Pancreas, 1200

Pancreatic α-amylase, 1202

Pancreatic duct (duct of Wirsung), 1200

Pancreatic lipase, 1202

Parietal cell (oxyntic cell), 1179

Pepsin, 1180

Pepsinogen, 1180

Peristalsis, 1176

Peritoneal cavity, 1182

Peritoneum, 1182

Primary bile acid, 1196

Primary peristalsis, 1177

Pyloric sphincter, 1177

Pylorus, 1177

Rectum, 1192

Retropulsion, 1179

Saliva, 1175

Salivary gland, 1175

S cell, 1202

Secretin, 1178

Secondary bile acid, 1196

Secondary peristalsis, 1177

Serosa, 1178

Sigmoid colon, 1190

Sinusoid, 1195

Small intestine, 1182

Sphincter of Oddi, 1199

Stomach, 1177

Submucosa, 1178

Submucosal plexus (Meissner plexus), 1178

Subserosal plexus, 1178

Swallowing, 1177

Teniae coli, 1190

Transverse colon, 1190

Trypsin, 1187

Trypsin inhibitor, 1202

Tunica muscularis, 1178

Unconjugated bilirubin, 1198

Upper esophageal sphincter, 1176

Urobilinogen, 1198

Vermiform appendix, 1190

Villus, 1184

REFERENCES

Berne, R. M., & Levy, M. N. (Eds.). (1988). *Physiology* (2d ed.). St. Louis: C. V. Mosby.

Brandt, L. J. (1984). *Gastrointestinal diseases of the elderly*. New York: Raven Press.

Christensen, J. (1987). Motor functions of the pharynx and esophagus. In L. R. Johnson (Ed.), *Physiology of the gastrointestinal tract* (vol. 7) (pp. 600-601). New York: Raven Press.

Davenport, H. W. (1982). *Physiology of the digestive tract* (8th ed.) (p. 119). Chicago: Yearbook Medical.

Johnson, L. R. (1981). *Gastrointestinal physiology* (2d ed.). St. Louis: C. V. Mosby.

Kvietys, P. R., Barrowman, J. A., & Granger, N. D. (1987). *Pathophysiology of the splanchnic circulation* (p. 5). Boca Raton, Fla.: CRC Press.

Phipps, W. J., Long, B. C., & Woods, W. F. (1987). *Medical surgical nursing: Concepts and clinical practice*. St. Louis: C. V. Mosby.

Sanford, P. A. (1982). *Digestive system physiology*. Baltimore: University Park Press.

Schlenker, E. D. (1984). *Nutrition in aging* (p. 76). St. Louis: C. V. Mosby.

Sernka, T., & Jacobson, E. (1983). *Gastrointestinal physiology*. Baltimore: Williams & Wilkins.

Thibodeau, G. A. (1987). *Anatomy and physiology*. St. Louis: Times Mirror/Mosby.

Thompson, J. M., McFarland, G. K., Hirsch, J. E., Tucker, S. M., & Bowers, A. C. (1989). *Mosby's manual of clinical nursing* (ed. 2). St. Louis: C. V. Mosby.

Way, L. W., & Pellegrini, C. A. (1987). *Surgery of the gallbladder and bile ducts* (p. 37). Philadelphia: W. B. Saunders.

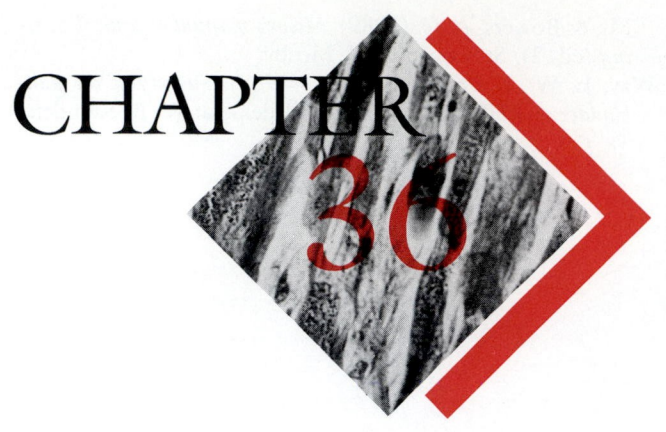

CHAPTER 36

Alterations of Digestive Function

Sue E. Huether
Kathryn L. McCance
Mary Suzanne Tarmina

Disorders of the gastrointestinal tract, 1213
  Clinical manifestations of gastrointestinal dysfunction,
    1214
  Anorexia, 1214
  Vomiting, 1214
  Constipation, 1214
    Pathophysiology, 1214
    Clinical manifestations, 1215
    Evaluation and treatment, 1215
  Diarrhea, 1215
    Pathophysiology, 1215
    Clinical manifestations, 1216
    Evaluation and treatment, 1216
  Abdominal pain, 1216
  Gastrointestinal bleeding, 1217
Disorders of motility, 1219
  Dysphagia, 1219
    Pathophysiology, 1219
    Clinical manifestations, 1219
    Evaluation and treatment, 1219
  Gastroesophageal reflux, 1219
    Pathophysiology, 1220
    Clinical manifestations, 1220
    Evaluation and treatment, 1220
  Hiatal hernia, 1220
    Pathophysiology, 1220
    Clinical manifestations, 1221
    Evaluation and treatment, 1221
  Pyloric obstruction, 1221
    Pathophysiology, 1221
    Clinical manifestations, 1221
    Evaluation and treatment, 1221
  Intestinal obstruction, 1223
    Pathophysiology, 1224
    Clinical manifestations, 1224
    Evaluation and treatment, 1224

Gastritis, 1224
Peptic ulcer disease, 1225
  Duodenal ulcers, 1226
    Pathophysiology, 1226
    Clinical manifestations, 1226
    Evaluation and treatment, 1226
  Gastric ulcers, 1226
    Pathophysiology, 1226
    Clinical manifestations, 1228
  Stress ulcers, 1228
  Surgical management of peptic ulcer disease, 1229
  Progastrectomy syndromes, 1229
    Dumping syndrome, 1229
    Alkaline reflux gastritis, 1230
    Afferent loop obstruction, 1230
    Diarrhea, 1230
    Weight loss, 1230
    Anemia, 1231
Malabsorption syndromes, 1231
  Pancreatic insufficiency, 1231
  Lactase deficiency, 1231
  Bile salt deficiency, 1231
  Ulcerative colitis, 1232
    Pathophysiology, 1232
    Clinical manifestations, 1232
    Evaluation and treatment, 1232
  Crohn disease, 1233
    Pathophysiology, 1233
    Clinical manifestations, 1234
    Evaluation and treatment, 1234
  Diverticulosis, 1234
    Pathophysiology, 1234
    Clinical manifestations, 1235
    Evaluation and treatment, 1235

Appendicitis, 1235
 Pathophysiology, 1235
 Clinical manifestations, 1235
 Evaluation and treatment, 1235
Vascular insufficiency, 1235
Disorders of nutrition, 1236
 Overnutrition, 1236
  Pathophysiology, 1236
  Evaluation and treatment, 1237
 Anorexia nervosa, 1237
 Bulimia, 1237
 Bulimarexia, 1238
 Starvation, 1238
Disorders of the accessory organs of digestion, 1238
 Clinical manifestations of liver disorders, 1238
  Portal hypertension, 1238
   Pathophysiology, 1239
   Clinical manifestations, 1240
   Evaluation and treatment, 1240
  Ascites, 1241
   Pathophysiology, 1241
   Clinical manifestations, 1241
   Evaluation and treatment, 1242
  Hepatic encephalopathy, 1242
   Pathophysiology, 1242
   Clinical manifestations, 1242
   Evaluation and treatment, 1242
  Jaundice, 1242
   Pathophysiology, 1242
   Clinical manifestations, 1243
   Evaluation and treatment, 1244
  Hepatorenal syndrome, 1244
   Pathophysiology, 1244
   Clinical manifestations, 1244
   Evaluation and treatment, 1245
 Disorders of the liver, 1245
  Viral hepatitis, 1245
   Types of hepatitis, 1245
    Hepatitis A, 1245
    Hepatitis B, 1246
    Hepatitis D, 1247
    Non-A, non-B hepatitis, 1247
   Pathophysiology, 1247
   Clinical manifestations, 1248
    Prodromal phase, 1248
    Icteric phase (Jaundice), 1248
    Recovery phase, 1248
   Evaluation and treatment, 1248
  Fulminant hepatitis, 1248
  Cirrhosis, 1248
  Alcoholic cirrhosis, 1249
   Pathophysiology, 1249
   Clinical manifestations, 1251
   Evaluation and treatment, 1251
  Biliary cirrhosis, 1252
   Primary biliary cirrhosis, 1252
   Secondary biliary cirrhosis, 1252
  Postnecrotic cirrhosis, 1252

Disorders of the gallbladder, 1253
 Cholelithiasis, 1253
  Pathophysiology, 1253
  Clinical manifestations, 1253
  Evaluation and treatment, 1253
 Cholecystitis, 1254
 Disorders of the pancreas, 1254
  Acute pancreatitis, 1254
   Pathophysiology, 1254
   Clinical manifestations, 1254
   Evaluation and treatment, 1254
  Chronic pancreatitis, 1255
Cancer of the digestive system, 1255
 Cancer of the gastrointestinal tract, 1255
  Cancer of the esophagus, 1255
   Pathogenesis, 1255
   Clinical manifestations, 1256
   Evaluation and treatment, 1256
  Cancer of the stomach, 1256
   Pathogenesis, 1256
   Clinical manifestations, 1256
   Evaluation and treatment, 1257
  Cancer of the colon and rectum, 1257
   Pathogenesis, 1257
   Clinical manifestations, 1257
   Evaluation and treatment, 1258
 Cancer of the accessory organs of digestion, 1259
  Cancer of the liver, 1259
   Pathogenesis, 1259
   Clinical manifestations, 1260
   Evaluation and treatment, 1260
  Cancer of the gallbladder, 1260
   Pathogenesis, 1260
   Clinical manifestations, 1260
   Evaluation and treatment, 1260
  Cancer of the pancreas, 1260
   Pathogenesis, 1261
   Clinical manifestations, 1261
   Evaluation and treatment, 1261

DISORDERS OF THE GASTROINTESTINAL TRACT

The gastrointestinal tract is a continuous, hollow organ that extends from the mouth to the anus. It includes the esophagus, stomach, small intestine (duodenum, jejunum, and ileum), large intestine (ascending, transverse, descending, and sigmoid colon), and rectum.

Disorders of the gastrointestinal tract disrupt one or more of its functions. Structural and neural abnormalities can slow, obstruct, or accelerate the movement of chyme at any level of the gastrointestinal tract. Inflammatory and ulcerative conditions of the gastrointestinal wall disrupt secretion, motility, and absorption. Many clinical manifestations of gastrointestinal tract disorders are nonspecific: that is, they can be caused by a variety of impairments. These manifestations are described in the next section.

Clinical Manifestations of Gastrointestinal Dysfunction

Anorexia

Anorexia is lack of a desire to eat despite physiologic stimuli that would normally produce hunger. Anorexia is a nonspecific symptom that is often associated with nausea, abdominal pain, and diarrhea. Disorders of other organ systems, including cancer, heart disease, and renal disease, are often accompanied by anorexia.

Vomiting

Vomiting is the forceful emptying of stomach and intestinal contents (chyme) through the mouth. Several types of stimuli initiate the vomiting reflex, including the presence of ipecac or copper salts in the duodenum; severe pain; distention of the stomach or duodenum; torsion or trauma affecting the ovaries, testes, uterus, bladder, or kidney; and activation of the chemoreceptor trigger zone in the medulla.

Nausea and retching usually precede vomiting. **Nausea** is a subjective experience that is associated with many different conditions. Specific neural pathways have not been identified with nausea. Hypersalivation and tachycardia are common associated symptoms. **Retching** begins with deep inspiration. The glottis closes, intrathoracic pressure falls, and the esophagus becomes distended. Simultaneously the abdominal muscles contract, creating a pressure gradient from abdomen to thorax. The lower esophageal sphincter and body of the stomach relax, but the duodenum and antrum of the stomach go into spasm. The reverse peristalsis and pressure gradient force chyme from the stomach and duodenum up into the esophagus. Since the upper esophageal sphincter is closed, chyme does not enter the mouth. As the abdominal muscles relax, the contents of the esophagus drop back into the stomach. This process may be repeated several times before vomiting occurs. A diffuse sympathetic discharge causes the tachycardia, tachypnea, and sweating that accompany retching and vomiting. The parasympathetic system mediates copious salivation, increased gastric motility, and relaxation of the upper and lower esophageal sphincters.

Vomiting usually follows retching. The duodenum and antrum of the stomach produce retrograde peristalsis, while the body of the stomach and esophagus relax. When the stomach is full of gastric contents, the diaphragm is forced high into the thoracic cavity by strong contractions of the abdominal muscles. The higher intrathoracic pressure forces the upper esophageal sphincter to open, and chyme is expelled from the mouth. Then the stomach relaxes and the upper part of the esophagus contracts, forcing the remaining chyme back into the stomach. The lower esophageal sphincter then closes. The cycle is repeated if there is a volume of chyme remaining in the stomach.

Spontaneous vomiting that is not preceded by nausea or retching is called **projectile vomiting**. Projectile vomiting is caused by direct stimulation of the vomiting center by neurologic lesions (e.g., tumors or aneurysms) involving the brain stem. The metabolic consequences of vomiting are fluid, electrolyte, and acid-base disturbances (see Chapter 3).

Constipation

Constipation is difficult or infrequent defecation. It is a common complaint caused by personal habits and a variety of disorders and drugs. Because patterns of bowel evacuation differ greatly among individuals, constipation must be individually defined. It usually means a decrease in the number of bowel movements per week, hard stools, and difficult evacuation. Normal bowel habits range from two or three evacuations per day to one per week.

Pathophysiology

Constipation can be caused by neurogenic disorders of the large intestine in which neural pathways are absent or degenerated. An example is Hirschsprung disease (congenital megacolon), the absence of ganglion cells in the myenteric plexus of the large intestine. Constipation is usually evident from birth, because the colon is incapable of the propulsive movements that move feces into the rectum (Chapter 37). Other disorders associated with constipation include acquired megacolon (enlarged or dilated colon), multiple sclerosis, spinal cord trauma, and cerebrovascular disease.

Many functional or mechanical conditions can cause constipation. Muscle weakness or pain caused by abdominal surgery can impair or inhibit defecation. Normally the abdominal muscles are used to create the intra-abdominal pressure required to evacuate the rectum. Weakness or pain can interfere with the generation of adequate intraabdominal pressure. Lesions of the anus, such as inflamed hemorrhoids, fissures, or fistulas, make defecation painful because of stretching. With the urge to defecate, the sphincter becomes hypertonic, and the stool is not eliminated.

A low-residue diet (the habitual consumption of highly refined foods) decreases the volume and number of stools and causes constipation. Increased consumption of cereals, fruits, and vegetables adds nonabsorbable fiber to the feces and is conducive to regular and easy evacuations.

A sedentary life-style and lack of regular exercise are frequent causes of constipation. Lack of access to toilet facilities and consistent suppression of the urge to empty the bowel are other causes. Depression often im-

Causes of Constipation

Megacolon (enlarged or dilated colon)
Abdominal muscle weakness
Painful anal lesions
Low-residue diet
Sedentary life-style
Delayed spontaneous defecation
Emotional depression
Selected drugs
   Opiates
   Anticholinergics
   Antacids (calcium carbonate, aluminum hydroxide)
Systemic diseases
   Hypothyroidism
   Diabetic neuropathy

pairs bowel evacuation, partly because depressed individuals tend to be sedentary and lack the motivation to eat healthfully. The problem is made worse if antidepressant drugs (e.g., anticholinergics) are used to treat the depression. Anticholinergics block parasympathetic impulses in the gastrointestinal tract, thereby impairing motility.

Excessive use of antacids containing calcium carbonate or aluminum hydroxide often results in constipation. Opiates, particularly codeine, tend to inhibit bowel motility.

Clinical Manifestations

Any change in bowel evacuation patterns may be significant. Changes such as less frequent defecation, smaller stool volume, difficulty in evacuating the rectum, or a feeling of bowel fullness and discomfort require investigation.

Evaluation and Treatment

The history and physical examination provide precise clues regarding the nature of constipation. Functional constipation, that is, constipation resulting from lifestyle or bowel habits, usually has a long history. Dysfunctional constipation is more likely to be sudden. Sudden-onset constipation can accompany the development of organic lesions and requires careful evaluation.

The individual's description of frequency, stool consistency, associated pain, and presence of blood is significant. Blood may be present as a result of bleeding hemorrhoids or a neoplastic lesion of the colon. Cramping abdominal pain may be symptomatic of partial bowel obstruction. In assessing frequency, it is important to discover whether evacuation was stimulated by enemas

or cathartics (laxatives). Palpation will reveal colonic distention, masses, and tenderness. Digital examination of the rectum is performed to assess sphincter tone and detect anal lesions. Proctosigmoidoscopy is used to visualize the lumen directly. A barium enema may be required if no lesions are directly visualized and symptoms continue after simple treatment.

The treatment for dysfunctional constipation is to manage the underlying lesion or disease. Management of functional constipation likewise depends on its cause. Treatment usually consists of bowel retraining, in which the individual establishes a satisfactory bowel evacuation routine without becoming preoccupied with bowel movements. The best time for defecation is during the period after a meal. The individual may also need to engage in moderate exercise, drink more fluids, and increase fiber intake. Bulk supplements (i.e., Metamucil or Konsyl), stool softeners, and laxative agents are useful for some individuals. Enemas can be used to establish bowel routine, but they should not be used habitually. Fluid instilled into the rectum causes distention, which stimulates propulsive movements and defecation. High colonic irrigations with large volumes of fluid should be avoided.

Diarrhea

Diarrhea is an increase in the frequency of defecation and the fluidity and volume of feces. Many factors determine stool volume and consistency, including water content of the colon and the presence of unabsorbed food, unabsorbable material, and intestinal secretions. Stool volume in the normal adult averages less than 200 g/day. Stool volume in children depends on age and size. An infant may pass up to 100 g/day. The adult intestine processes approximately 9 L of luminal content per day: 2 L is ingested, and the remaining 7 L consists of intestinal secretions. Of this volume, 99% of the fluid is absorbed: 90% (7 to 8 L) in the small intestine and 9% (1 to 2 L) in the colon. Normally, about 150 cc of water is excreted daily in the stool.

Pathophysiology

Diarrhea in which the volume of feces is increased is called large-volume diarrhea. Large-volume diarrhea generally is caused by excessive amounts of water or secretions or both in the intestines. Small-volume diarrhea, in which the volume of feces is not increased, usually results from excessive intestinal motility.

The three major mechanisms of diarrhea are osmotic, secretory, and motile. (Specific mechanisms of diarrhea in children are described in Chapter 37.)

In **osmotic diarrhea** the presence of a nonabsorbable substance in the intestine causes it to be drawn into the lumen by osmosis. The excess water is retained in the intestine and, along with the nonabsorbable substance, increases stool weight and volume. This causes large-volume diarrhea. **Lactase deficiency** is the most common cause of osmotic diarrhea. In this condition, the nonabsorbable substance is milk sugar, or lactose. The intestine does not produce enough lactase, the lactose-digesting enzyme. Lactose remains in the intestinal lumen because it is not digested and absorbed. Excessive ingestion of synthetic, nonabsorbable sugars (e.g., sorbitol) has a similar effect.

Secretory diarrhea is a form of large-volume diarrhea caused by excessive mucosal secretion of fluid and electrolytes. Primary stimuli of intestinal secretion are bacterial enterotoxins, particularly those released by cholera or strains of *Escherichia coli*. Secretory diarrhea can also be caused by neoplasms, such as gastrinoma or thyroid carcinoma. These tumors produce hormones that stimulate intestinal secretion.

Large-volume diarrhea can also result from excessive motility of the intestine. The cause is usually a lesion that impairs autonomic control of motility, such as diabetic neuropathy. Excessive motility decreases transit time, mucosal surface contact, and opportunities for fluid absorption. Therefore, a larger volume of stool reaches the rectum, producing urgency and frequency of elimination.

Small-volume diarrhea is usually caused by an inflammatory disorder of the intestine, such as ulcerative colitis or Crohn disease. Inflammation of the colon causes cramping pain, urgency, and frequency. Small-volume diarrhea can also be caused by fecal impaction, a severe form of constipation. In this case, the diarrhea consists of secretions (mucus and fluid) produced by the colon to lubricate the impacted feces and move it toward the anal canal. These secretions flow around the impaction and cause low-volume, secretory diarrhea.

Clinical Manifestations

Diarrhea can be acute or chronic, depending on its cause. Systemic effects of prolonged diarrhea are dehydration, electrolyte imbalance, and weight loss. Manifestations of acute bacterial or viral infection include fever, with or without cramping pain. Fever, cramping pain, and bloody stools accompany diarrhea caused by inflammatory bowel disease. Steatorrhea (fat in the stools) and diarrhea are common signs of malabsorption syndromes.

Evaluation and Treatment

A thorough history is taken to document the onset and frequency of diarrhea. Exposure to contaminated food or water is suspected if the individual has traveled in foreign countries or areas where drinking water might be contaminated. Iatrogenic diarrhea is suspected if the individual has undergone abdominal radiation therapy, intestinal resection, or treatment with selected drugs (e.g., antibiotics, diuretics, antihypertensives, or laxatives). Physical examination helps the clinician to identify underlying systemic disease. Stool culture, examination of stool specimens for blood, abdominal x-ray films, and intestinal biopsies provide more specific data.

Treatment for diarrhea includes restoration of fluid and electrolyte balance, management of distressing symptoms, and treatment of causal factors. In older adults and children, dehydration and electrolyte imbalance may be severe and require intravenous fluid therapy. Nutritional deficiencies need to be corrected in cases of chronic diarrhea or malabsorption. Substances that solidify stools decrease frequency and water content. Natural bran and commercial preparations of psyllium, such as Konsyl and Metamucil, are inexpensive and effective treatments for mild diarrhea. Opium alkaloids such as Lomotil suppress motility, relieve cramping, and reduce stool volume and frequency.

Abdominal Pain

Abdominal pain is the presenting symptom of a number of gastrointestinal diseases. (The physiology of pain is described in Chapter 13.) The causal mechanisms of abdominal pain are mechanical, inflammatory, or ischemic. Generally the abdominal organs are not sensitive to mechanical stimuli, such as cutting, tearing, or crushing. These organs are, however, sensitive to stretching and distention, which activate nerve endings in both hollow and solid structures. The onset of pain is associated with rapid distention; gradual distention causes little pain. Traction on the peritoneum caused by adhesions, distention of the common bile duct, or forceful peristalsis resulting from intestinal obstruction causes pain because of increased tension. Capsules that surround solid organs, such as the liver and gallbladder, contain pain fibers that are stimulated by stretching if these organs swell.

Biochemical mediators of the inflammatory response, such as histamine, bradykinin, and serotonin, stimulate organic nerve endings and produce abdominal pain. The edema and vascular congestion that accompany chemical, bacterial, or viral inflammation also cause painful stretching. Obstruction of blood flow from the distention of bowel obstruction or mesenteric vessel thrombosis produces the pain of ischemia and increased concentrations of tissue metabolites stimulate pain receptors.

Abdominal pain can be parietal (somatic), visceral, or referred. **Parietal pain** arises from the parietal peritoneum. This pain is more localized and intense than visceral pain, which arises from the organs themselves. Nerve fibers from the parietal peritoneum travel with peripheral nerves to the spinal cord, and the sensation of pain corresponds to skin dermatomes T_6 and L_1. Parietal pain lateralizes because, at any particular point, the parietal peritoneum is innervated from only one side of the nervous system.

Visceral pain arises from a stimulus acting on an abdominal organ. It is usually felt near the midline in the epigastrium (upper midabdomen), midabdomen, or lower abdomen. The pain is poorly localized and is dull rather than sharp. Its location is generally related to the corresponding skin dermatomes of the affected organ. Visceral pain is diffuse and vague because nerve endings in abdominal organs are sparse and multisegmented. Pain arising from the stomach, for example, is experienced as a sensation of fullness, cramping, or gnawing in the midepigastric area.

Referred pain is visceral pain felt at some distance from a diseased or affected organ. Referred pain is usually well localized and is felt in skin or deeper tissues that share a central afferent pathway with the affected organ. Generally referred pain develops as the intensity of a visceral pain stimulus increases. Intense gallbladder pain is, for example, referred to the back between the scapulae (shoulder blades). The pain may begin as a vague discomfort in the right epigastric region and then, as inflammation worsens, progress to a sharp, localized, referred pain between the shoulder blades.

Gastrointestinal Bleeding

Numerous disorders cause bleeding in the gastrointestinal tract. Upper **gastrointestinal bleeding,** which is defined as bleeding in the esophagus, stomach, or duodenum, is commonly caused by bleeding varices (varicose veins) in the esophagus or ulcers. Lower gastrointestinal bleeding, or bleeding from the jejunum, ileum, colon, or rectum, can be caused by polyps, inflammatory disease, cancer, or hemorrhoids. Acute, severe gastrointestinal bleeding is life-threatening. Mortality depends on the volume and rate of blood loss, associated disease, age, and effectiveness of treatment.

The signs of gastrointestinal bleeding are defined in Table 36-1. Acute blood loss is usually characterized by **hematemesis** (the presence of blood in the vomitus), **hematochezia** (frank bleeding from the rectum), or **melena** (dark, tarry stools). **Occult bleeding** is usually caused by slow, chronic blood loss that results in iron-deficiency anemia as iron stores in the bone marrow are slowly depleted. Physiologic response to gastrointestinal bleeding depends on the amount and rate of the loss (Fig. 36-1). Changes in blood pressure and heart rate are the best indicators of massive blood loss in the gastrointestinal tract. Blood losses of 1000 ml or more over a short period of time cause a decrease in cardiac output, a decrease in systolic and diastolic blood pressure,

TABLE 36-1 Presentations of gastrointestinal bleeding

Presentations	Definition
Acute bleeding	
Hematemesis	Bloody vomitus; either fresh, bright red blood or dark, grainy digested blood with "coffee grounds" appearance
Melena	Black, sticky, tarry, foul-smelling stools caused by digestion of blood in the gastrointestinal tract
Hematochezia	Fresh, bright red blood passed from the rectum
Occult bleeding	Trace amounts of blood in normal-appearing stools or gastric secretions; detectable only with a guaiac test

and an increase in pulse rate. With losses of 1000 ml or more, the heart rate is greater than 100 beats/min and systolic blood pressure is less than 100 mm Hg. During the early stages of blood volume depletion, the peripheral vascular compartment constricts to shunt blood to vital organs, including the brain (see Chapter 26). A sign that this is happening is postural hypotension, a drop in blood pressure, that occurs with a change from the recumbent position to a sitting or upright position. If blood loss continues, hypovolemic shock progresses. Diminished blood flow to the kidneys causes decreased urine output and may lead to oliguria (low urine output), tubular necrosis, and renal failure. Ultimately insufficient cerebral and coronary blood flow causes irreversible anoxia and death.

The accumulation of blood in the gastrointestinal tract is irritating and increases peristalsis, causing diarrhea. If bleeding is from the lower gastrointestinal tract, the diarrhea is frankly bloody. Bleeding from the upper gastrointestinal tract also can be rapid enough to produce bright red stools, but generally some digestion of the blood components will have occurred, producing melena. The digestion of blood proteins originating from massive upper gastrointestinal bleeding is reflected by an increase in blood urea nitrogen (BUN) levels (see Fig. 36-1).

The hematocrit and hemoglobin values are not the best indicators of acute gastrointestinal bleeding because plasma and red cell volume are lost proportionately. As the plasma volume is replaced, the hematocrit and hemoglobin values begin to reflect the extent of blood loss. The interpretation of these values is modified to ac-

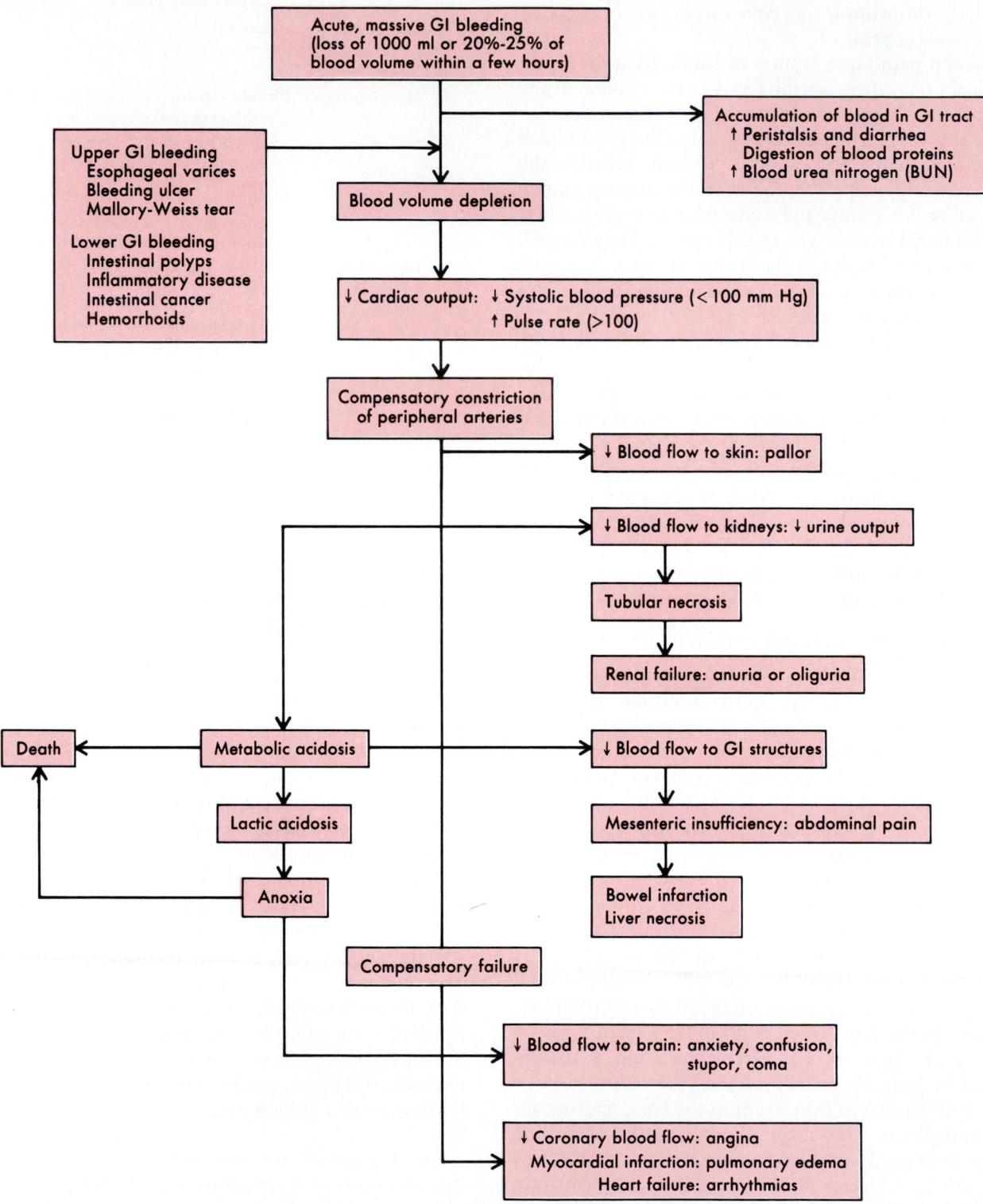

FIG. 36-1. Pathophysiology of gastrointestinal (GI) bleeding.

count for exogenous replacement of fluids and the hydration status of the tissues.

Disorders of Motility
Dysphagia
Pathophysiology

Dysphagia is difficulty swallowing. It can result from mechanical obstruction of the esophagus or a disorder that impairs esophageal motility. Mechanical obstructions can be intrinsic or extrinsic. Intrinsic obstructions originate in the wall of the esophageal lumen. Tumors, strictures, and diverticular herniations (outpouchings) are all causes of intrinsic mechanical obstruction. Extrinsic mechanical obstructions originate outside the esophageal lumen and narrow the esophagus by pressing inward on the esophageal wall. The most common cause of extrinsic mechanical obstruction is tumor.

Functional dysphagia is caused by neural or muscular disorders that interfere with voluntary swallowing or peristalsis (Merlo & Cohen, 1988). Disorders that affect the striated muscles of the upper esophagus interfere with the oropharyngeal (voluntary) phase of swallowing. Typical causes of functional dysphasia in the upper esophagus are dermatomyositis (a muscle disease) and neurologic impairments caused by cerebrovascular accidents or Parkinson disease.

Achalasia is a form of dysphagia that impairs (1) peristalsis of smooth muscle in the middle and lower portions of the esophagus and (2) lower esophageal sphincter (LES) functioning. Achalasia results from neural dysfunction, probably a decrease in the number of ganglion cells in the myenteric plexus and atrophy of smooth muscle cells or lesions along the vagus nerve. Disrupted innervation results in loss of neuromuscular coordination and muscle tone at the lower end of the esophagus. The three mechanisms that impair swallowing are decreased peristalsis of the middle esophagus, loss of tone in the lower esophageal sphincter, and decreased relaxation of the lower esophageal sphincter after swallowing. Food accumulates above the obstruction and distends the esophagus (Fig. 36-2). As hydrostatic pressure increases, food is slowly forced past the obstruction into the stomach.

Clinical Manifestations

Clinical manifestations of dysphagia vary according to the cause and location of the obstruction. Distention and spasm of the esophageal muscles during eating or drinking may cause a mild or severe stabbing pain at the level of obstruction. Discomfort occurring 2 to 4 seconds after swallowing is associated with upper esophageal obstruction. Discomfort occurring 10 to 15 seconds after swallowing is more common in obstructions of the lower esophagus. If the cause of obstruction is a growing tumor, dysphagia begins with difficulty swallowing solids and advances to difficulty swallowing semisolids and liquids (McCallum, 1987). If the cause is loss of motor function, dysphagia is experienced with both solids and liquids. Regurgitation of undigested food, unpleasant taste, vomiting, and weight loss are common manifestations of all types of dysphagia. Aspiration of esophageal contents can lead to pneumonia.

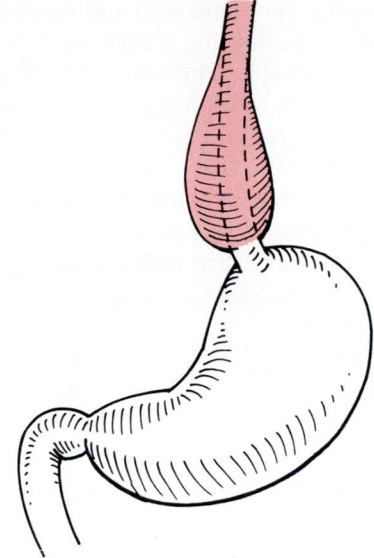

FIG. 36-2. Achalasia. Decreased muscle tone and peristaltic function prevent food from entering the stomach, causing esophageal distention. (From Phipps, Long, & Woods, 1987.)

Evaluation and Treatment

Knowledge of the patient's history and clinical manifestations contributes significantly to a diagnosis of dysphasia. A barium swallow is used to visualize the contours of the esophagus and identify structural defects. Manometry documents the duration and amplitude of abnormal pressure changes associated with obstruction or loss of neural regulation. Esophageal endoscopy is performed to examine the esophageal mucosa and obtain biopsy specimens.

The individual is taught to manage symptoms by eating slowly, eating small meals, taking fluid with meals, and sleeping with the head elevated to prevent regurgitation and aspiration. Anticholinergic drugs, such as dicyclomine (Bentyl), may alleviate achalasia. Definitive treatments include mechanical dilation of the esophageal sphincter and surgical separation of the lower esophageal muscles with a longitudinal incision (myotomy). Myotomy widens the passage into the stomach.

Gastroesophageal Reflux

Gastroesophageal reflux is the reflux of chyme from the stomach to the esophagus. The lower esophageal sphincter may relax spontaneously and transiently 1 to 2 hours after eating, permitting gastric contents to regurgitate into the esophagus. The acid is usually neutralized and cleared from the esophagus by peristaltic action within 1 to 3 minutes and sphincter tone is restored. Gastroesophageal reflux that does not cause symptoms is known as physiologic reflux. In some individuals, however, a combination of factors causes an inflammatory response to reflux called **reflux esophagitis.**

Pathophysiology

Normally the resting tone of the lower esophageal sphincter maintains a zone of high pressure that prevents gastroesophageal reflux. In individuals who develop reflux esophagitis, this pressure tends to be lower than normal (Behar, 1986). Vomiting, coughing, lifting, or bending can contribute to the development of reflux esophagitis. The severity of the esophagitis depends on the composition of the gastric contents and the length of time they are in contact with the esophageal mucosa. If the chyme is highly acidic or contains bile salts and pancreatic enzymes, reflux esophagitis can be severe. In individuals with weak esophageal peristalsis, refluxed chyme remains in the esophagus longer than usual. This increases the amount of time the esophageal mucosa is exposed to acids, bile, and enzymes. Finally delayed gastric emptying contributes to reflux esophagitis by (1) lengthening the period during which reflux is possible and (2) increasing the acid content of chyme. Disorders that delay emptying include gastric or duodenal ulcers, which can cause pyloric edema; strictures that narrow the pylorus; and hiatal hernia, which can weaken the lower esophageal sphincter.

Reflux esophagitis causes inflammatory responses in the esophageal wall, such as hyperemia, increased capillary permeability, edema, tissue fragility, and erosion. Fibrosis and thickening may develop.

Clinical Manifestations

The clinical manifestations of reflux esophagitis are heartburn and regurgitation of acidic chyme within an hour of eating. The symptoms worsen if the individual lies down or if intraabdominal pressure increases (e.g., as a result of coughing, vomiting, or straining at stool). Edema, fibrosis, esophageal spasm, or decreased esophageal motility may result in dysphagia. Alcohol or acid-containing foods, such as citrus fruits, can cause discomfort during swallowing.

Evaluation and Treatment

Diagnosis of reflux esophagitis is based on clinical manifestations and esophageal endoscopy, which reveals edema and erosion. A barium swallow is used to identify associated conditions, such as hiatal hernia, gastric ulcers, and abnormal contours of the esophageal lumen.

Antacids relieve symptoms by neutralizing gastric contents. Weight reduction and cessation of smoking also help to alleviate symptoms. Cimetidine (or another H_2 blocker) may be used to decrease nocturnal acid secretion; smooth muscle stimulants, such as bethanechol chloride (Urecholine) or metoclopramide (Reglan), can increase lower esophageal sphincter gastric motility and rate of gastric emptying. If other treatments fail, or if erosive esophagitis fails to heal, the lower esophageal sphincter may be narrowed surgically.

Hiatal Hernia

Pathophysiology

Hiatal hernia is the protrusion (herniation) of the upper part of the stomach through the diaphragm and

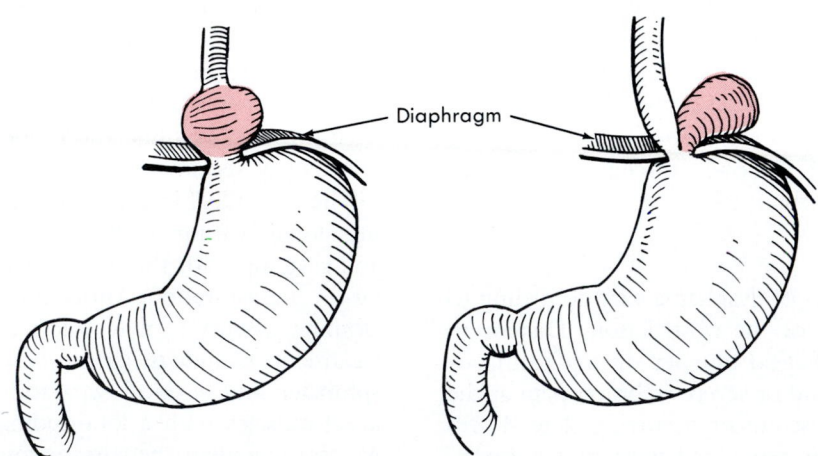

FIG. 36-3. Types of hiatal hernia. In sliding hiatal hernia the visceral peritoneum remains intact and restrains the size of the hernia. In paraesophageal hernia the membrane becomes thinned out or defective, allowing a true peritoneal sac to protrude into the posterior mediastinum, where negative intrathoracic pressure causes it to enlarge. (From Phipps, Long, & Woods, 1987.)

into the thorax. There are two types of hiatal hernia: (1) sliding (direct) hiatal hernia and (2) paraesophageal (rolling) hiatal hernia (Fig. 36-3). In **sliding hiatal hernia** the stomach slides or moves into the thoracic cavity through the esophageal hiatus, an opening in the diaphragm for the esophagus and vagus nerves. A congenitally short esophagus, trauma, or weakening of the diaphragmatic muscles at the gastroesophageal junction contributes to the hernia. While the individual is in the supine position, the lower esophagus and stomach are pulled into the thorax. Standing causes the stomach to "slide" back into the abdomen. Sliding hiatal hernia is exacerbated by factors that increase intra-abdominal pressure. Therefore, coughing, bending, tight clothing, ascites, or pregnancy accentuates the hernia. This type of hernia is associated with gastroesophageal reflux and esophagitis because the hernia diminishes the resting pressure of the lower esophageal sphincter. In pregnant women with sliding hiatal hernia, progesterone and estrogen may lower the resting pressure of the lower esophageal sphincter further.

Paraesophageal hiatal hernia (rolling hiatal hernia) is herniation of the greater curvature of the stomach through a secondary opening in the diaphragm (see Fig. 36-3). As the stomach protrudes through the opening into the thorax, it lies alongside the esophagus. The gastroesophageal junction remains below the diaphragm. With paraesophageal hernia, reflux is uncommon. The position of a portion of the stomach above the diaphragm, however, causes congestion of mucosal blood flow and can lead to gastritis and ulcer formation. A mechanical strangulation of the hernia is a major complication. Strangulation occludes blood vessels and causes vascular engorgement, edema, ischemia, and hemorrhage. Hiatal hernias of both types tend to occur in conjunction with several other diseases, including peptic ulcer, cholecystitis (gallbladder inflammation), cholelithiasis (gallstones), chronic pancreatitis, and diverticulosis.

Clinical Manifestations

Hiatal hernias are often asymptomatic. Generally a wide variety of symptoms develop later in life and are associated with other gastrointestinal disorders as well. Manifestations of the different types of hiatal hernia are difficult to distinguish and include gastroesophageal reflux, dysphasia, heartburn, and epigastric pain. Regurgitation and substernal discomfort after eating are common.

Evaluation and Treatment

Diagnostic procedures include barium x-rays and endoscopy. A chest x-ray film will often reveal the protrusion of the stomach into the thorax, indicating paraesophageal hiatal hernia.

Treatment for sliding hiatal hernia is usually conservative. The individual can diminish reflux by eating small, frequent meals and avoiding the recumbent position after eating. Abdominal supports or tight clothing are avoided, and weight control is recommended for obese individuals. Antacids alleviate reflux esophagitis. Anticholinergic drugs are contraindicated because they relax the lower esophageal sphincter and delay gastric emptying. Individuals who are uncomfortable at night benefit from sleeping in a semi-Fowler position. Surgery may be performed if medical management fails to control symptoms.

Pyloric Obstruction

Pathophysiology

Pyloric obstruction is the narrowing or blocking of the opening between the stomach and the duodenum. This condition can be congenital (see Chapter 37) or acquired. Acquired obstruction is caused by peptic ulcer disease or carcinoma near the pylorus. Duodenal ulcers are more likely than gastric ulcers to obstruct the pylorus. Ulceration causes obstruction resulting from inflammation, edema, spasm, fibrosis, or scarring. Tumors cause obstruction by growing into the pylorus.

Clinical Manifestations

Early in the course of pyloric obstruction the individual experiences vague epigastric fullness, which becomes more distressing after eating and later in the day. Nausea and epigastric pain may occur as the muscles of the stomach contract in attempts to force chyme past the obstruction. These symptoms disappear when the chyme finally moves into the duodenum. As obstruction progresses anorexia develops, sometimes accompanied by weight loss. Severe obstruction causes gastric distention and atony (lack of muscle tone and gastric motility). Gastric distention stimulates gastric secretion, which increases the feeling of fullness. Rolling or jarring of the abdomen produces a sloshing sound called the succussion splash. At this stage vomiting is a cardinal sign of obstruction. It is usually copious and occurs several hours after eating. The vomitus contains undigested food but no bile. Prolonged vomiting leads to dehydration, which is accompanied by a hypokalemic and hypochloremic metabolic alkalosis caused by loss of potassium and gastric acid. Because food does not enter the intestine, stools are infrequent and small. Prolonged pyloric obstruction causes malnutrition, dehydration, and extreme debilitation.

Evaluation and Treatment

Diagnosis is based on clinical manifestations, a history of ulcer disease, and examination of residual gastric contents. Endoscopy is performed if gastric carcinoma is the suspected cause of pyloric obstruction. Barium studies are contraindicated because the barium may harden and be retained in the stomach.

Obstructions resulting from ulceration often resolve with conservative management. A large-bore tube is used to aspirate stomach contents and relieve distention.

Then nasogastric suction is maintained for 2 to 3 days to decompress the stomach and restore normal motility. Gastric secretions that contribute to inflammation and edema can be suppressed with intravenous cimetidine. Fluids and electrolytes (saline and potassium) are given

---

TABLE 36-2 Common causes of intestinal obstruction

Cause	Pathophysiology
Hernia	Protrusion of the intestine through a weakness in the abdominal muscles or through the inguinal ring
Intussusception	Telescoping of one part of the intestine into another; this usually causes strangulation of the blood supply; more common in infants 10-15 months of age than in adults
Torsion (volvulus)	Twisting of the intestine on its mesenteric pedicle, with occlusion of the blood supply; often associated with fibrous adhesions; occurs most frequently in middle-aged and elderly men
Diverticulosis	Inflamed saccular herniations (diverticuli) of the mucosa and submucosa through the tunica muscularis of the colon; diverticuli are interspersed between thick, circular, fibrous bands; most common in obese individuals over 60 years of age
Tumor	Tumor growth into the intestinal lumen; adenocarcinoma of the colon and rectum is the most common tumoral obstruction; most common in individuals over 60 years of age
Paralytic (adynamic) ileus	Loss of peristaltic motor activity in the intestine; associated with abdominal surgery, peritonitis, hypokalemia, ischemic bowel, spinal trauma, or pneumonia

---

TABLE 36-3 Classification of intestinal obstruction

Criteria for classification	Definition
ONSET	
Acute	Sudden onset; often caused by torsion, intussusception, or herniation
Chronic	Protracted onset; more commonly from tumor growth or progressive formation of strictures
EXTENT OF OBSTRUCTION	
Partial	Incomplete obstruction of intestinal lumen
Complete	Complete obstruction of intestinal lumen
LOCATION OF OBSTRUCTING LESION	
Intrinsic	Obstruction develops within intestinal lumen; examples: luminal edema or hemorrhage, foreign bodies (gallstones), tumors, or intraluminal fibrosis
Extrinsic	Obstruction originates outside the intestine; examples: tumors, torsion, fibrosis, hernia, intussusception
EFFECTS ON INTESTINAL WALL	
Simple	Luminal obstruction without impairment of blood supply
Strangulated	Luminal obstruction with occlusion of blood supply
Closed Loop	Obstruction at each end of a segment of the intestine
CAUSAL FACTORS	
Mechanical	Blockage of the intestinal lumen by intrinsic or extrinsic lesions; usually treated surgically
Functional (paralytic ileus)	Paralysis of the intestinal musculature due to trauma, peritonitis, electrolyte imbalances, or spasmolytic agents; usually treated surgically

intravenously to effect rehydration and correct hypokalemia and alkalosis (see Chapter 3). Severely malnourished individuals may require parenteral hyperalimentation (intravenous nutrition). Surgery may be required to treat gastric carcinoma or persistent obstruction caused by fibrosis and scarring.

Intestinal Obstruction

Intestinal obstruction can be caused by any condition that prevents the normal flow of chyme through the intestinal lumen (Table 36-2). Criteria for classifying intestinal obstruction are summarized in Table 36-3.

Intestinal obstruction is classified by cause as simple or functional. Simple obstruction is mechanical blockage of the lumen by a lesion; functional obstruction is a failure of motility. Simple obstruction of the small intestine is the most common type of intestinal obstruction. Acute obstructions usually have mechanical causes, such as adhesions or hernias. Chronic or partial obstructions are more often associated with tumors or inflammatory disorders, particularly of the large intestine. Common causes of intestinal obstruction in children are presented in Chapter 37.

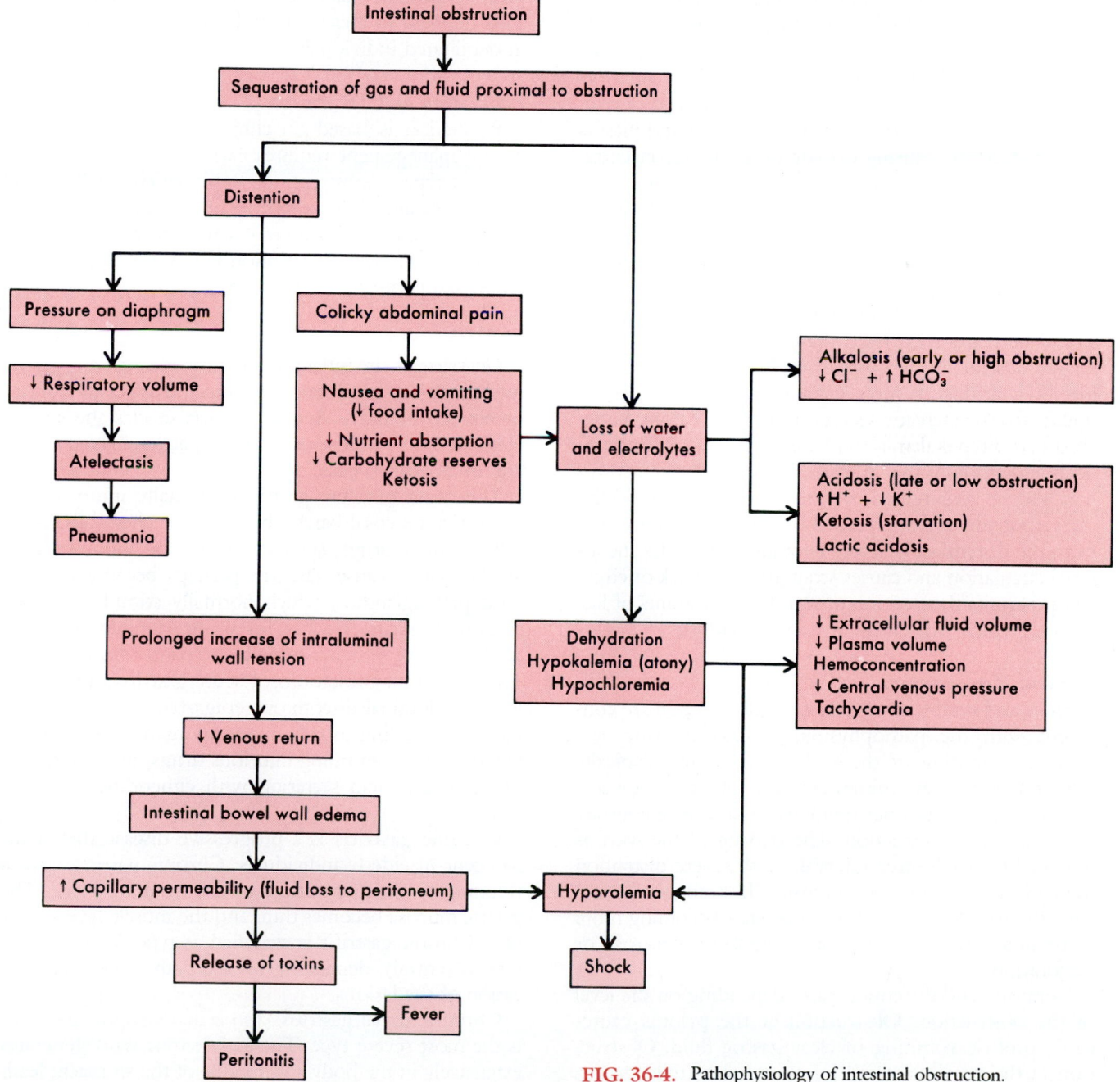

FIG. 36-4. Pathophysiology of intestinal obstruction.

Pathophysiology

The consequences of intestinal obstruction are related to its onset and location and the length of intestinal track proximal to the obstruction. The major pathophysiologic alterations are presented in Fig. 36-4. Usually the first symptoms of obstruction result from distention and the loss of fluids and electrolytes. Distention begins almost immediately, as gases and fluids accumulate proximal to the obstruction. The major source of gas is swallowed air, but some is contributed by bacterial fermentation. Distention decreases the intestine's ability to absorb water and electrolytes and increases the net secretion of these substances into the lumen. Within 24 hours up to 8 L of fluid and electrolytes enters the lumen in the form of saliva, gastric juice, bile, pancreatic juice, and intestinal secretions. Copious vomiting or sequestration of fluids in the intestinal lumen prevents their reabsorption and produces severe fluid and electrolyte disturbances. Extracellular fluid volume and plasma volume decrease, causing dehydration. Hemoconcentration (decreased plasma volume) elevates hematocrit, decreases central venous pressure, and causes tachycardia. Severe dehydration leads to hypovolemic shock.

If the obstruction is at the pylorus or high in the small intestine, metabolic alkalosis develops initially as a result of excessive loss of hydrogen ions that normally would be reabsorbed from the gastric juice. With prolonged obstruction or obstruction lower in the intestine, metabolic acidosis is more likely to occur because bicarbonate from pancreatic secretions and bile cannot be reabsorbed. Hypokalemia can be extreme, promoting acidosis and atony of the intestinal wall. Metabolic acidosis may also be accentuated by ketosis, the result of declining carbohydrate stores caused by starvation. If pressure from the distention is severe enough, it occludes the arterial circulation and causes strangulation. Lack of circulation permits the buildup of significant amounts of lactic acid, which worsen the metabolic acidosis.

Clinical Manifestations

Signs and symptoms of intestinal obstruction are consistent with the pathophysiology. Colicky pains followed by vomiting are the cardinal symptoms. Typically the pain occurs intermittently. Pain intensifies for seconds or minutes as a peristaltic wave of muscle contraction meets the obstruction. The passing of the wave is followed by a pain-free interval. With severe distention the pain may diminish in intensity. If strangulation occurs, the pain loses its colicky character, becoming more constant and severe as ischemia progresses to necrosis or perforation.

Vomiting and distention vary, depending on the level of the obstruction. Obstruction at the pylorus causes early, profuse vomiting of clear gastric fluid. Obstruction in the proximal small intestine causes mild disten-

tion and vomiting of bile-stained fluid. Obstruction lower in the intestine causes more pronounced distention because a greater length of intestine is proximal to the obstruction. In this cause vomiting may not occur or may occur later and contain fecal material. Partial obstruction can cause diarrhea or constipation, but complete obstruction usually causes constipation only. Complete obstruction increases the number of bowel sounds, which may be tinkly and accompanied by peristaltic rushes and crampy, abdominal pain. Signs of dehydration, hypovolemia, and metabolic acidosis may be observed as early as 24 hours after the occurrence of complete obstruction. Distention may be severe enough to push against the diaphragm and decrease lung volume. This can lead to atelectasis and pneumonia, particularly in debilitated individuals.

Evaluation and Treatment

Evaluation is based on clinical manifestations. Successful management requires early identification of the site and type of obstruction. Replacement of fluid and electrolytes and decompression of the lumen with gastric or intestinal suction are essential forms of therapy. Immediate surgical intervention is required for strangulation and complete obstruction.

Gastritis

Gastritis is an inflammatory disorder of the gastric mucosa. It can be acute or chronic and affect the fundus or antrum or both. **Acute gastritis** erodes the surface epithelium in a diffuse or localized pattern. The erosions are usually superficial.

The cause of acute gastritis is usually injury of the protective mucosal barrier by drugs or chemicals. Antiinflammatory drugs, such as aspirin and indomethacin, are known to cause gastritis, perhaps because they inhibit prostaglandins, which normally stimulate the secretion of mucus. Alcohol, histamine, digitalis, and metabolic disorders such as uremia are contributing factors. The clinical manifestations of acute gastritis can include vague abdominal discomfort, epigastric tenderness, and bleeding. Healing usually occurs spontaneously within a few days. Discontinuing injurious drugs, using antacids, or decreasing acid secretion with cimetidine facilitates healing.

Chronic gastritis is a progressive disease that tends to occur in elderly individuals. Chronic gastritis causes thinning and degeneration of the stomach wall. The gastric mucosa becomes thin, and the muscle layers atrophy. Chronic gastritis is classified as type A (fundal) or type B (antral), depending on the pathogenesis and location of the lesions.

Chronic fundal gastritis, also called atrophic gastritis, is the most severe type. The gastric mucosa degenerates extensively in the body and fundus of the stomach, lead-

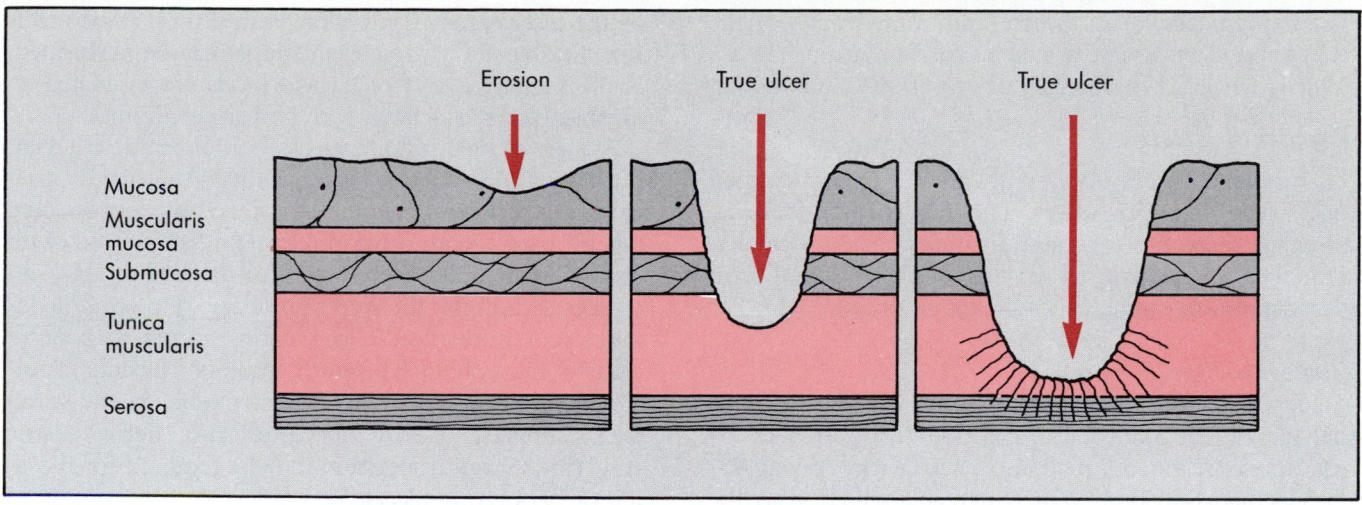

FIG. 36-5. Lesions caused by peptic ulcer disease.

ing to gastric atrophy. Loss of chief cells and parietal cells diminishes secretion of pepsinogen, hydrochloric acid, and intrinsic factor. Because acid secretion is insufficient, the feedback mechanism that normally inhibits gastrin secretion is impaired, causing elevated plasma levels of gastrin. Pernicious anemia develops because intrinsic factor is unavailable to facilitate vitamin B_{12} absorption.

A significant number of individuals with chronic fundal gastritis have antibodies to parietal cells, intrinsic factor, and gastric cells in their sera, suggesting that an autoimmune mechanism is involved in pathogenesis of the disease. The fact that chronic fundal gastritis occurs in association with other autoimmune diseases, such as diabetes, Addison disease, and thyroid disease, strengthens this association. Repeated mucosal injury caused by alcohol, aspirin, and other irritants exacerbates the gastritis. Chronic fundal gastritis is a risk factor for gastric carcinoma, particularly in individuals who develop pernicious anemia. Women develop fundal gastritis more frequently than men, and the incidence is higher in families with a history of pernicious anemia.

Chronic antral gastritis generally involves the antrum only. This type of chronic gastritis occurs about four times more frequently than fundal gastritis. It is not associated with decreased hydrochloric acid secretion, pernicious anemia, or presence of parietal cell antibodies. Antral gastritis causes mucosal inflammation, but mucosal atrophy is a rare finding. In approximately 10% of cases antibodies to gastrin-secreting cells are found in the serum. Chronic reflux of bile may contribute to the gastritis by persistently disrupting the mucosal barrier (Fig. 36-5).

Signs and symptoms of chronic gastritis often do not correlate with the severity of the disease. Gastroscopic examination may reveal a longstanding inflammatory process and gastric atrophy in an individual with no history of abdominal distress. Individuals may report vague symptoms, including anorexia, fullness, nausea, vomiting, and epigastric pain. Gastric bleeding may be the only clinical manifestation of gastritis.

Diagnosis of chronic gastritis is made by endoscopy and biopsy of the gastric mucosa. Failure to stimulate acid secretion confirms achlorhydria (diminished secretion of hydrochloric acid). The gastric secretions can also be evaluated for the presence of intrinsic factor. Symptoms can usually be managed with smaller meals; a soft, bland diet; and avoidance of alcohol and aspirin. Vitamin B_{12} is administered to correct pernicious anemia.

Peptic Ulcer Disease

A **peptic ulcer** is a break, or ulceration, in the protective mucosal lining of the lower esophagus, stomach, or upper small intestine. Such breaks expose submucosal areas to gastric secretions and autodigestion. Peptic ulcers can be acute or chronic, superficial or deep. Superficial ulcerations are called erosions because they erode the mucosa but do not penetrate the muscularis mucosa (Fig. 36-5). True ulcers extend through the muscularis mucosa and damage blood vessels, causing hemorrhage, or perforate the gastrointestinal wall.

Risk factors for peptic ulcer disease are smoking and habitual use of aspirin, alcohol, or antiinflammatory drugs. Some chronic diseases, such as emphysema, rheumatoid arthritis, and cirrhosis, are associated with the development of peptic ulcers. Infection of the gastric and duodenal mucosa with *Campylobacter pyloridis* also is proposed as a cause of peptic ulcers (Rathbone, Wyatt, & Heatley, 1986). Psychological stress may be a risk factor for peptic ulcer disease, although studies of life stress and ulcer disease are inconclusive (Feldman et al., 1986). The exact mechanism of causation is not known.

Duodenal Ulcers

Duodenal ulcers occur with greater frequency than other types of peptic ulcers. The incidence of duodenal ulcers is three times greater in males than in females. Duodenal ulcers tend to develop in the fifth and sixth decades and in individuals with type O blood.

Pathophysiology

Hypersecretion of acid is the primary cause of duodenal ulcers, but inadequate secretion of bicarbonate by the duodenal mucosa may also be a factor. Among the factors that contribute to increased acid secretion are the following:

1. A greater than usual number of parietal cells (acid-secreting cells) in the gastric mucosa
2. High serum gastrin levels that remain high longer than normal after eating and continue to stimulate secretion of acid
3. Failure of the feedback mechanism whereby acid in the gastric antrum inhibits gastrin release
4. Rapid gastric emptying, which overwhelms the buffering capacity of the bicarbonate-rich pancreatic secretions

All of these factors, singly or in combination, cause acid concentrations in the duodenum to penetrate the mucosal barrier and cause ulceration (Fig. 36-6).

Clinical Manifestations

The characteristic manifestation of a duodenal ulcer is chronic intermittent pain in the epigastric area. The pain begins 2 or 3 hours after eating, when the stomach is empty. It is not unusual for pain to occur in the middle of the night and disappear by morning. The pain results from sensorineural stimulation by acid, muscle spasm, or both. Pain is relieved rapidly by ingestion of food or antacids, creating a typical "pain-food-relief" pattern. Some individuals with duodenal ulcer may have no symptoms; the first manifestation may be hemorrhage or perforation.

Duodenal ulcers often heal spontaneously but recur within months. Exacerbations tend to develop in the spring and fall. Healing is accompanied by relief of pain. Constant, unremitting pain may be caused by complications, such as intestinal obstruction or perforation. Bleeding from duodenal ulcers causes hematemesis or melena.

Evaluation and Treatment

Several diagnostic approaches are used to differentiate duodenal ulcers from gastric ulcers or gastric carcinoma. Barium x-rays may show an anatomic deformity created by the ulcer crater. If the x-ray examination is inconclusive, flexible endoscopic evaluations may be performed. Radioimmune assays of gastrin levels are evaluated to identify ulcers associated with gastric carcinomas.

Management of duodenal ulcers is aimed at relieving the causes and effects of hyperacidity. Antacids neutralize gastric contents, elevate pH, inactivate pepsin, and relieve pain. Acid secretion can be suppressed with drugs (e.g., cimetidine) that block histamine (H_2) receptors and inhibit the secretion of acid. Omeprazole inhibits acid production. Ulcer-coating agents, such as sucralfate and colloidal bismuth, promote healing. Anticholinergic drugs may be used to inhibit gastric secretion, suppress gastric motility, and delay gastric emptying. Surgical resection may be required for bleeding or perforating ulcers.

Gastric Ulcers

Gastric ulcers are ulcers of the stomach. They occur about equally in males and females, usually after age 40, and are about one fourth as common as duodenal ulcers (Table 36-4).

Pathophysiology

Generally gastric ulcers develop in the antral region, adjacent to the acid-secreting mucosa of the body. The primary defect is an abnormality that increases the mucosal barrier's permeability to hydrogen ions. Gastric secretion may be normal or less than normal.

Chronic gastritis is often associated with development of gastric ulcers and may precipitate ulcer formation by limiting the mucosa's ability to secrete a protective layer of mucus (Fig. 36-7). Decreased mucosal synthesis of prostaglandin may be one factor causing decreased mucus secretion (Chailet, Gallo-Torres, & Bounameaux, 1985).

Other factors associated with gastric ulcer development include duodenal reflux of bile and use of ulcerogenic drugs (aspirin and indomethacin). Reflux of bile is caused by loss of tone at the pyloric sphincter. The pyloric sphincter may fail to respond to stimuli that normally increase resting tone, such as entry of acid, protein, and fat into the duodenum.

An increased concentration of bile salts disrupts the gastric mucosa; this disruption may decrease the electrical potential across the gastric mucosal membrane. The break damages the mucosal barrier by permitting hydrogen ions to diffuse into the mucosa, where they disrupt permeability and cellular structure. A vicious cycle can be established as the damaged mucosa liberates histamine, which stimulates the increase of acid and pepsinogen production, blood flow, and capillary permeability. The disrupted mucosa becomes edematous and loses plasma proteins. Destruction of small vessels causes bleeding.

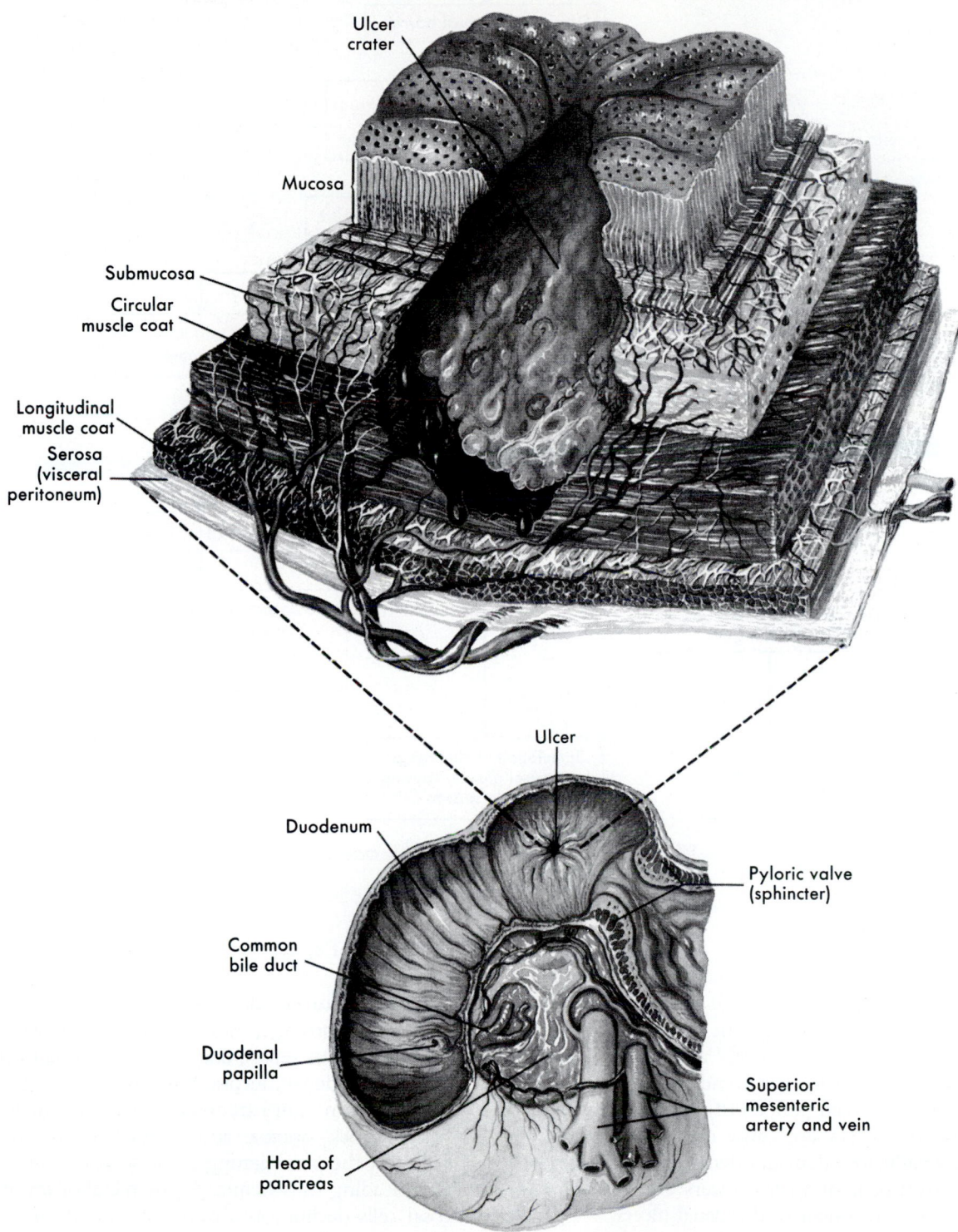

Ulcer crater

Mucosa

Submucosa

Circular muscle coat

Longitudinal muscle coat

Serosa (visceral peritoneum)

Ulcer

Duodenum

Common bile duct

Duodenal papilla

Head of pancreas

Pyloric valve (sphincter)

Superior mesenteric artery and vein

FIG. 36-6. Duodenal ulcer. The illustration depicts a deep ulceration in the duodenal wall extending as a crater through the entire mucosa and into the muscle layers. (From Thibodeau, 1987.)

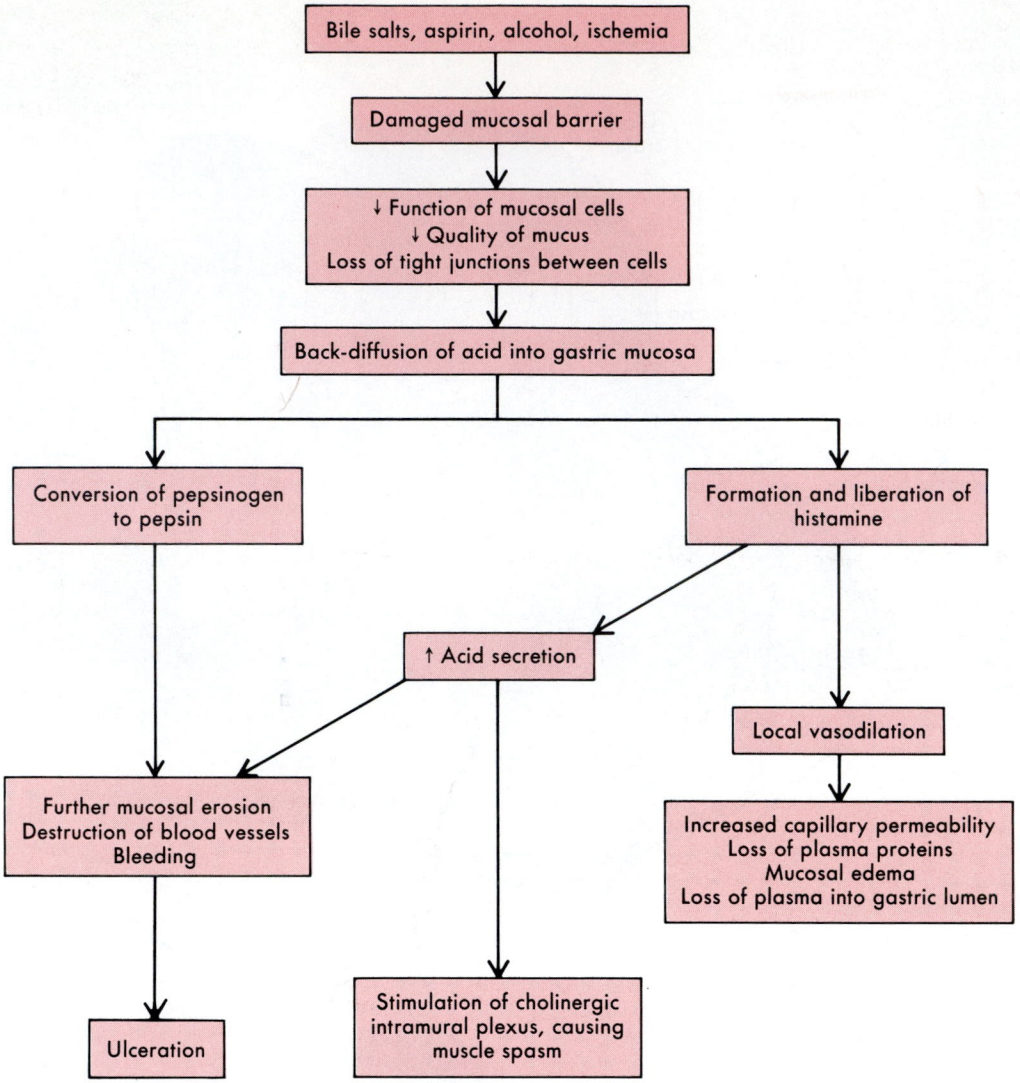

FIG. 36-7. Pathophysiology of gastric ulcer formation.

Clinical Manifestations

The clinical manifestations of gastric ulcers are similar to those of duodenal ulcers (Table 36-4). The pattern of "pain-food-relief" is common, but the pain of gastric ulcers may also occur immediately after eating. Another difference is that gastric ulcers tend to be chronic rather than alternate between periods of remission and exacerbation. Gastric ulcers also cause more anorexia, vomiting, and weight loss than duodenal ulcers. The evaluation and treatment of gastric ulcers are similar to the evaluation and treatment of duodenal ulcers.

Stress Ulcers

A **stress ulcer** is an acute form of peptic ulcer that tends to accompany severe illness, systemic trauma, or neural injury. Usually multiple sites of ulceration are distributed within the stomach or duodenum. There are two types of stress ulcers: ischemic ulcers and Cushing ulcers.

Ischemic ulcers develop within hours of an event, such as hemorrhage, multisystem trauma, severe burns, heart failure, or sepsis, that causes ischemia of the stomach and duodenal mucosa. Stress ulcers that develop as a result of burn injury are frequently called **Curling ulcer**.

The shock, anoxia, and sympathetic responses produced by the precipitating event decrease mucosal blood flow, leading to ischemia. As the metabolism of the mucosal cells declines as a result of lack of arterial blood, the mucosal lining degenerates. Acid diffuses back into the mucosa, causing inflammation, ulceration, hemorrhage, and necrosis. The ulcerative process is accelerated if bile or pancreatic enzymes are regurgitated from the duodenum.

Cushing ulcer is a stress ulcer associated with severe

TABLE 36-4 Characteristics of gastric and duodenal ulcers

Characteristics	Gastric ulcer	Duodenal ulcer
INCIDENCE		
Age at onset	50-70 years	20-50 years
Family history	Usually negative	Positive
Scx (prevalence)	Equal in women and men	Greater in men
Stress factors	Increased	Average
Ulcerogenic drugs	Normal use	Increased use
Cancer risk	Increased	Not increased
PATHOPHYSIOLOGY		
Parietal cell mass	Normal or decreased	Increased
Acid production	Normal or decreased	Increased
Serum gastrin	Increased	Normal
Serum pepsinogen	Normal	Increased
Associated gastritis	More common	Usually not present
CLINICAL MANIFESTATIONS		
Pain	Located in upper abdomen	Located in upper abdomen
	Intermittent	Intermittent
	Pain-antacid-relief pattern	Pain-antacid or food-relief pattern
	Food-pain pattern	Nocturnal pain common
Clinical course	Chronic ulcer without pattern of remission and exacerbation	Pattern of remissions and exacerbations for years

head trauma or brain surgery. This ulcer results from hypersecretion of acid caused by overstimulation of the vagal nuclei. Excessive acid damages the mucosal barrier, initiating the proccesses summarized in Fig. 36-7.

The primary clinical manifestation of stress ulcers is bleeding. Other symptoms may not be present. The bleeding may be slight or, if a small vessel is perforated, amount to hundreds of milliliters. Use of prophylactic antacids and suppression of vagal stimulation with anticholinergic drugs are effective forms of therapy. Stress ulcers seldom become chronic.

Surgical Management of Peptic Ulcer Disease

Advances in the medical treatment of peptic ulcer disease have reduced the number of cases requiring surgery to 10% to 15%. Despite this small percentage, clinicians care for a significant number of individuals who undergo upper gastrointestinal surgery and experience long-term complications.

The most common indications for ulcer surgery are recurrent or uncontrolled bleeding and perforation of the stomach or duodenum. The primary objectives of surgical treatment are to reduce stimuli for acid secretion, decrease the number of acid-secreting cells in the stomach, and correct complications of ulcer disease (Table 36-5).

Acute complications of gastrectomy or anastomosis, such as poor wound healing, abscess formation, or suture failure, are relatively uncommon except in the debilitated person. Chronic complications, however, occur more often and are likely to develop if a large portion of the stomach has been removed. These complications and their pathophysiologic mechanisms are described in the next section.

Progastrectomy Syndromes

Dumping Syndrome

Dumping syndrome is the rapid emptying of hypertonic chyme from the stomach into the small intestine 10 to 20 minutes after eating. It occurs with varying severity in 5% to 10% of individuals who have undergone partial gastrectomy or pyloroplasty. It is not common in individuals who have undergone a Billroth II anastomosis accompanied by vagotomy. Rapid gastric emptying and creation of a high osomotic gradient within the small intestine cause a sudden shift of fluid from the vascular compartment to the intestinal lumen. Plasma volume decreases, causing vasomotor responses, such as increased pulse rate, hypotension, weakness, pallor, sweating, and dizziness. Rapid distention of the intestine produces a feeling of epigastric fullness, cramping, nausea, vomiting, and diarrhea.

A less common form of dumping syndrome, termed

TABLE 36-5 Surgical management of peptic ulcer disease

Procedure	Definition	Purpose
Neural surgery		
Vagotomy	Severence of the vagus nerve	Eliminate neural stimulus of acid secretion
Selective vagotomy	Severence of vagal branches supplying acid-secreting (parietal) cells	Eliminate neural stimulus of acid secretion
Gastric surgery		
Pyloroplasty	Surgical widening or removal of obstruction of the pylorus	Facilitate gastric emptying
Antrectomy (partial gastrectomy)	Removal of the antrum	Eliminate hormonal stimulus of acid secretion; that is, the gastrin-secreting cells of the antral mucosa
Subtotal gastrectomy	Removal of most of the body and all of the antrum of the stomach	Remove acid-secreting and gastrin-secreting mucosa
Anastomosis (Billroth operation)	Reattachment of stomach to duodenum (Billroth I) or jejenum (Billroth II)	Restore continuity of the gastrointestinal tract after resection

late dumping syndrome, occurs 1 to 2 hours after eating. The symptoms include weakness, diaphoresis, and confusion, but they cannot be explained by rapid gastric emptying. After a high-carbohydrate meal, individuals who have undergone gastrectomy may develop hypoglycemia, which causes the symptoms. The hypoglycemia is caused by an increase in insulin secretion stimulated by the hyperglycemia that follows eating. Other hormonal responses may also participate in the development of hypoglycemia.

Most cases of dumping syndrome respond well to dietary management. Frequent small meals that are high in protein and low in carbohydrates relieve symptoms. Other measures include drinking fluids between meals instead of at mealtime and reclining on the left side after eating.

Alkaline Reflux Gastritis

Alkaline reflux gastritis is a stomach inflammation caused by reflux of bile and alkaline pancreatic secretions that contain proteolytic enzymes and disrupt the mucosal barrier. This form of gastritis occurs in 5% to 20% of individuals who have undergone gastrectomy or pyloroplasty. Clinical manifestations include nausea, bilious vomiting (vomiting in which the vomitus contains bile), and sustained epigastric pain that worsens after eating and is not relieved by antacids. Endoscopy reveals a hemorrhagic and friable gastric mucosa. Conservative management is often difficult because antacids do not consistently improve symptoms. Avoidance of use of aspirin and alcohol may decrease gastric irritation, and a low-fat diet may limit bile secretion. Surgical correction may ultimately be required.

Afferent Loop Obstruction

Afferent loop obstruction is an unusual problem that may occur after gastrojejunostomy (Billroth II; see Table 36-5). The problem is caused by volvulus, hernia, adhesion, or stenosis in the duodenal stump on the proximal side of the gastrojejunostomy. Partial obstruction causes bile and pancreatic secretions to accumulate and distend the loop. Obstruction also causes delayed emptying. The symptoms of afferent loop obstruction include intermittent severe pain and epigastric fullness after eating. Vomiting usually relieves symptoms. Conservative management consists of a low-fat diet. Surgical correction is required for complete obstruction.

Diarrhea

Diarrhea is one of the most common long-term alterations caused by gastric surgery. Diarrhea can accompany dumping syndrome or occur as a solitary symptom. Two forms of diarrhea can occur after gastrectomy. The first is the frequent, persistent elimination of liquid stool. The second is the intermittent, precipitous, and unpredictable elimination of a large volume of stool. Both types can be either mild or severe. Postgastrectomy diarrhea appears to be related to rapid gastric emptying, particularly after intake of large amounts of high-carbohydrate liquids, which increase the osmotic gradient and attract water into the intestinal lumen. Small, dry meals and anticholinergic drugs are effective control measures.

Weight Loss

Weight loss frequently follows gastric resection. Inadequate food intake is a common cause, as many individuals cannot tolerate carbohydrates or a normal-sized meal. Foods may be poorly absorbed because the stomach is less able to mix, churn, and break down food particles. Vomiting, diarrhea, and malabsorption of fats also contribute to weight loss.

Anemia

Anemia after gastrectomy results from iron, vitamin B_{12}, or folate deficiency. Iron malabsorption may be caused by decreased acid secretion. Acid changes iron from a trivalent to a divalent molecule, making it easier to absorb. Iron absorption is also compromised in individuals who have undergone a Billroth II procedure because the duodenum is no longer available to absorb iron.

Vitamin B_{12} deficiency may occur several years after gastrectomy. Contributing factors include loss of parietal cells, which secrete intrinsic factor. (Intrinsic factor facilitates absorption of vitamin B_{12}; see Chapter 35.) Vitamin B_{12} absorption is also compromised if gastric contents are not mixed adequately with pancreatic enzymes, as may occur after Billroth II anastomosis.

Folate deficiency is related to poor intake or malabsorption. Management of deficiencies consists of replacement of iron and folate with supplements. Vitamin B_{12} can be administered monthly by injection.

Malabsorption Syndromes

Malabsorption syndromes interfere with nutrient absorption in the small intestine. Historically malabsorption disorders have been classified as maldigestion or malabsorption. **Maldigestion** is failure of the chemical processes of digestion that take place in the intestinal lumen or at the brush border of the intestinal mucosa. **Malabsorption** is the failure of the intestinal mucosa to absorb (transport) the digested nutrients. Frequently maldigestion and malabsorption are interrelated or occur together, making classification difficult. Generally, however, maldigestion is caused by deficiencies of enzymes, such as pancreatic lipase or intestinal lactase, that are necessary for digestion. Inadequate secretion of bile salts and inadequate reabsorption of bile in the ileum also contribute to maldigestion. Malabsorption is the result of mucosal disruption caused by gastric or intestinal resection, vascular disorders, or intestinal disease.

Pancreatic Insufficiency

The pancreatic enzymes (lipase, amylase, trypsin, and chymotrypsin) are required for the digestion of proteins, carbohydrates, and fats. **Pancreatic insufficiency** is the deficient production of these enzymes by the pancreas. Causes of pancreatic insufficiency include chronic pancreatitis, pancreatic carcinoma, pancreatic resection, and cystic fibrosis. Significant damage to or loss of pancreatic tissue must occur before enzyme levels will decrease sufficiently to cause maldigestion. Although pancreatic insufficiency causes poor digestion of all nutrients, fat maldigestion is the chief problem. Salivary amylase and enzymes secreted by the intestinal brush border assist in carbohydrate and protein digestion, but these enzymes do not digest fats. Absence of pancreatic bicarbonate in the duodenum and jejunum causes an acidic pH that worsens maldigestion by preventing activation of pancreatic enzymes that are present. A large amount of fat in the stool (steatorrhea) is the most common sign of pancreatic insufficiency.

Lactase Deficiency

Deficiency of disaccharidase at the brush border of the small intestine is caused by a congenital defect in which a single enzyme, usually lactase, is lacking. **Lactase deficiency** inhibits the breakdown of lactose (milk sugar) into monosaccharides and therefore prevents lactose digestion and absorption across the intestinal wall. Lactase deficiency is most common in blacks. The deficiency usually does not develop until adulthood. Secondary (acquired) lactase deficiency can be caused by several diseases of the intestine, including gluten-sensitive enteropathy (see Chapter 37), enteritis, and bacterial overgrowth.

The undigested lactose remains in the intestine, where bacterial fermentation causes gases to form. Undigested lactose also increases the osmotic gradient in the intestine, causing irritation and osmotic diarrhea. Clinical manifestations of lactase deficiency are bloating, crampy pain, diarrhea, and flatulence. The disorder is diagnosed by a lactose-tolerance test. Avoiding milk and adhering to a lactose-free diet relieve symptoms.

Bile Salt Deficiency

Conjugated bile acids (bile salts) are necessary for the digestion and absorption of fats. Bile salts are conjugated in the bile that is secreted from the liver. When bile enters the duodenum, the bile salts aggregate with fatty acids and monoglycerides to form micelles. Micelle formation solubilizes fat molecules and allows them to pass through the unstirred layer at the brush border (see Chapter 35). A minimum concentration of bile salts, termed the critical micelle concentration, is required to allow micelles to form. Therefore, conditions that decrease the production or secretion of bile result in decreased micelle formation and fat malabsorption. These conditions include advanced liver disease, which decreases production of bile salts; obstruction of the common bile duct, which decreases flow of bile into the duodenum; intestinal stasis (lack of motility), which permits overgrowth of intestinal bacteria that deconjugate bile salts; and diseases of the ileum, which prevent the reabsorption and recycling of bile salts (enterohepatic circulation).

Clinical manifestations of bile salt deficiency are related to poor intestinal absorption of fat and fat-soluble vitamins (A, D, E, K). Increased fat in the stools (steatorrhea) leads to diarrhea and decreased plasma proteins. The loss of fat-soluble vitamins and their effects include the following:

1. Vitamin A deficiency results in night blindness
2. Vitamin D deficiency results in decreased calcium absorption with bone demineralization (osteoporosis), bone pain, and fractures
3. Vitamin K deficiency prolongs prothrombin time, leading to spontaneous development of purpura (bruising) and petechaie
4. Vitamin E deficiency has uncertain effects but may cause testicular atrophy and neurologic defects in children

The most effective treatment for fat-soluble vitamin deficiency is to increase medium-chain tryglycerides in the diet, for example, by using coconut oil for cooking. Vitamins A, D, and K are given parenterally.

Ulcerative Colitis

Ulcerative colitis is an inflammatory disease that causes ulceration of the colonic mucosa, usually in the rectum and sigmoid colon. The lesions appear in susceptible individuals between 20 and 40 years of age. Women are affected more frequently than men. Besides sex, risk factors include family history of disease and Jewish descent.

Although the etiology of ulcerative colitis is unknown, infectious, genetic, and immunologic factors are all suspected causes (Cello & Schneiderman, 1989). The hypothesis that inflammation is caused by infectious agents is not supported by consistent identification of specific viruses or bacteria in affected individuals. The familial tendency to develop ulcerative colitis and the occurrence of disease in identical twins support a genetic theory of causation. Perhaps most significant are immunologic factors associated with the disease. Anti-colon antibodies have been identified in the sera of individuals with ulcerative colitis. Lymphocytes (T cells) in individuals with ulcerative colitis may have cytotoxic effects on the epithelial cells of the colon. Furthermore, autoimmune disorders, such as systemic lupus erythematosus and erythema nodosum, often accompany ulcerative colitis.

Pathophysiology

The primary lesion of ulcerative colitis begins with inflammation at the base of the crypt of Lieberkuhn. The mucosa is hyperemic and may appear dark red and velvety (Fig. 36-8). Small erosions form and coalesce into ulcers. Abscess formation, necrosis, and ragged ulceration of the mucosa ensue. Edema and thickening of the muscularis mucosa may narrow the lumen of the involved colon. Mucosal destruction causes bleeding, cramping pain, and urge to defecate. Frequent diarrhea,

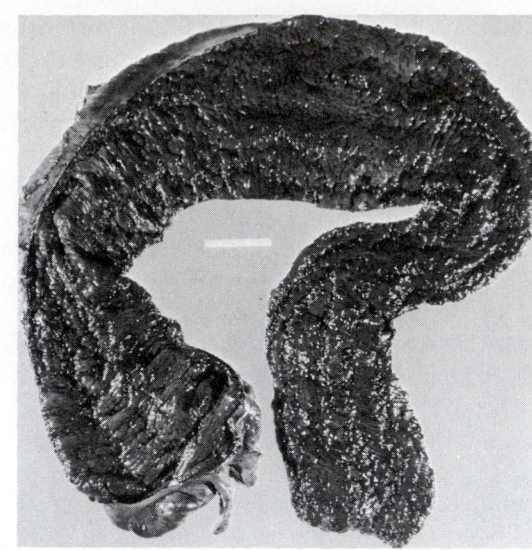

FIG. 36-8. Chronic ulcerative colitis. (From Kissane, 1985.)

with passage of small amounts of blood and purulent mucus, is common. Loss of the absorptive mucosal surface and decreased colonic transit time cause large volumes of watery diarrhea.

Clinical Manifestations

The course of ulcerative colitis consists of intermittent periods of remission and exacerbation. Clinical manifestations vary with the severity and extent of disease. Mild ulcerative colitis involves less mucosa, so that frequency of bowel movements, bleeding, and pain are minimal. Severe forms may involve the entire colon and are characterized by fever, elevated pulse rate, frequent diarrhea (10 to 20/day), obviously bloody stools, and continuous, crampy pain. Dehydration, weight loss, anemia, and fever result from fluid loss, bleeding, and inflammation. Complications include anal fissures, hemorrhoids, and pararectal abscess. Severe hemorrhage is rare, but chronic blood loss can precipitate hypotension and shock. Edema, strictures, or fibrosis can obstruct the colon. Perforation is an unusual but possible complication. The risk of colon cancer increases significantly after 10 years of ulcerative colitis.

Evaluation and Treatment

Diagnosis of ulcerative colitis is based on the medical history and clinical manifestations. Sigmoidoscopy reveals an inflamed and hemorrhagic mucosa. A barium enema and x-ray films may show loss of haustra, ulceration, and irregular mucosa. The laboratory data include low hemoglobin values, hypoalbuminemia, and low serum potassium levels. The symptoms of ulcerative colitis are very similar to those of Crohn disease, making differential diagnosis difficult.

TABLE 36-6 Features of ulcerative colitis and Crohn disease

Feature	Ulcerative colitis	Crohn disease
INCIDENCE		
Age at onset	Any age; 10-40 years most common	Any age; 10-30 years most common
Family history	Less common	More common
Sex (prevalence)	Greater in women	About equal in women and men
Cancer risk	Increased	Not increased
PATHOPHYSIOLOGY		
Location of lesions	Large intestine, no "skip" lesions	Large or small intestine, "skip" lesions common
Inflammation and ulceration	Mucosal layer involved	Entire intestinal wall involved
Granulomas	Rare	Common
Friable mucosa	Common	Less common
Anal and perianal fistulas and abscesses	Rare	Common
Narrowed lumen and possible obstruction	Rare	Common
CLINICAL MANIFESTATIONS		
Abdominal pain	Mild to severe	Mild to severe
Diarrhea	Common	Common
Bloody stools	Common	Less common
Abdominal mass	Rare	Common
Small intestinal malabsorption	Rare	Common
Steatorrhea	Rare	Common
Clinical course	Remissions and exacerbations	Remissions and exacerbations

Treatment depends on the severity of symptoms and the extent of mucosal involvement. The disease is often treated with sulfasalazine (a combination of a sulfa drug and aspirin). Steroids suppress the inflammatory response and help to alleviate the cramping pain. Broad-spectrum antibiotics may be prescribed if bacterial infection is suspected. Severe, unremitting disease can require hospital admission and administration of intravenous fluids. Extreme malnutrition may require intravenous hyperalimentation. Surgical resection of the colon or a colostomy may be performed if other forms of therapy are unsuccessful.

Crohn Disease

Crohn disease (granulomatous colitis or regional enteritis) is an inflammatory disorder that affects both the large and small intestines. In a small percentage of cases, Crohn disease is difficult to differentiate from ulcerative colitis (Table 36-6). The rectum is seldom involved, and the development of colon cancer is rare. Risk factors and theories of causation are the same as those for ulcerative colitis. Like ulcerative colitis, Crohn disease tends to run in families. Ten to twenty percent of affected individuals have a positive family history. Increased suppressor T cell activity and alterations in IgA production are the immunologic factors associated with Crohn disease. Psychologic stresses have been suggested as a cause of both inflammatory bowel diseases. Although stressful events may exacerbate illness, stress is probably not a cause of disease.

Pathophysiology

The inflammation process of Crohn disease begins in the intestinal submucosa and spreads inward and outward to involve the mucosa and serosa. The ascending and transverse colon is the most common site of the disease, but both the large and small intestine may be involved. The inflammation can affect some haustral segments but not others, creating a pattern called "skip lesions." One side of the intestinal wall may be affected and not the other.

The ulcerations of Crohn disease produce fissures that extend inflammation into lymphoid tissue. The typical lesion is a granuloma having projections of inflamed tissue surrounded by fibrous scarring. (Granulomas are described in Chapter 7.) Fistulas may form in the perianal area between loops of intestine or extend into the bladder.

Clinical Manifestations

Nonbloody diarrhea is the most common sign of Crohn disease. Other manifestations are related to the location and extent of intestinal involvement. Inflammation of the ileum, for example, causes tenderness in the lower right side of the abdomen. Weight loss and lower abdominal pain accompany Crohn disease. If the ileum is involved, the individual may be anemic as a result of malabsorption of vitamin B_{12}.

Evaluation and Treatment

The diagnosis and treatment of Crohn disease are similar to the diagnosis and treatment of ulcerative colitis. Surgical resection carries the risk of recurrence 10 to 15 years later (Speranza et al., 1986).

Diverticulosis

Diverticulosis is a disorder characterized by **diverticula,** which are herniations or saclike outpouchings of the mucosal layer of the colon through the muscle layers of the colon wall (Fig. 36-9). Diverticulosis is most common in the elderly, particularly those who live in developed countries where much of the diet consists of refined foods.

Pathophysiology

Although diverticula can occur anywhere in the gastrointestinal tract, the most frequent site is the sigmoid colon. The diverticula form at weak points in the colon wall, usually where arteries penetrate the tunica muscularis to nourish the mucosal layer. A common associated finding is thickening of the circular and longitudinal (teniae coli) muscles surrounding the diverticula. Hypertrophy and contraction of these muscles increase intraluminal pressure and degree of herniation. Habitual consumption of a low-residue diet reduces fecal bulk, thus reducing the diameter of the colon. According to the law of LaPlace (see Chapter 26), wall pressure increases as the diameter of a cylindrical structure decreases. Therefore, pressure within the narrow lumen can increase enough to rupture the diverticula. The resulting inflammatory response is known as **diverticulitis.** Diverticulitis can cause abscess formation or peritonitis.

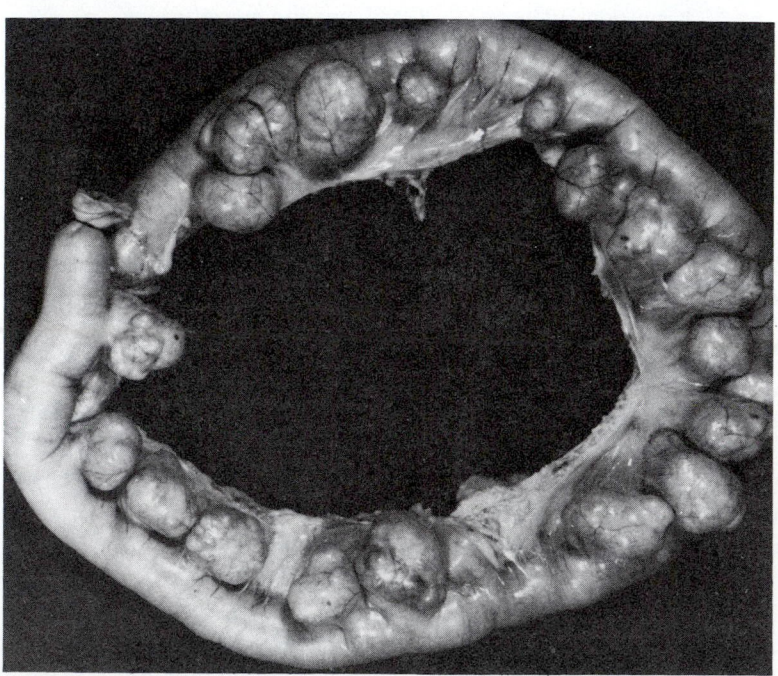

FIG. 36-9. Multiple diverticula in resected section of the colon. Weak spots in the muscle layers of the intestinal wall permitted the mucosa to bulge outward (herniate) into the pelvic cavity. (From Rosai, 1989.)

Clinical Manifestations

Symptoms of diverticulosis may be vague or absent. Cramping pain of the lower abdomen can accompany constriction of the hypertrophied colonic muscles. Diarrhea, constipation, distention, or flatulence may occur. If the diverticula become inflamed or abscesses form, the individual develops fever, leukocytosis (increased white blood cell count), and tenderness of the lower left quadrant. Severe complications, such as hemorrhage, peritonitis, bowel obstruction, and fistula formation, are rare.

Evaluation and Treatment

Diverticula are often discovered during diagnostic procedures performed for other problems. Sigmoidoscopy permits direct observation of the lesions. Barium enema reveals the muscle hypertrophy, but there is some risk that the barium will become trapped in the diverticula and form hard masses.

An increase of dietary fiber intake frequently relieves symptoms. Surgical resection may be required if there are severe complications.

Appendicitis

Appendicitis is an inflammation of the vermiform appendix, which is a projection from the apex of the cecum. It is the most common surgical emergency of the abdomen and affects 7% to 12% of the population. The most common occurrence is between 20 and 30 years of age, although it may develop at any age.

Pathophysiology

The exact mechanism of the cause of appendicitis is controversial. Obstruction of the lumen with stool, tumors, or foreign bodies with consequent bacterial infection is the most common theory. The obstructed lumen does not allow drainage of the appendix, and, as mucosal secretion continues, intraluminal pressure increases. The resultant increased pressure decreases mucosal blood flow and the appendix becomes hypoxic. The mucosa ulcerates, promoting bacterial invasion with further inflammation and edema. Inflammation may involve the distal or entire appendix. Gangrene develops from thrombosis of the luminal blood vessels, followed by perforation.

Clinical Manifestations

Epigastric or periumbilical pain is the typical symptom of an inflamed appendix. The pain may be vague at first, increasing in intensity over a period of 3 to 4 hours. It may subside and then recur with a shift of location to the right lower quadrant. Right lower quadrant pain is associated with extension of the inflammation to the surrounding tissues. Nausea, vomiting, and anorexia follow the onset of pain, and a low-grade fever is common. Diarrhea occurs in some individuals; others have a sensation of constipation. Perforation, peritonitis, and abscess formation are the most serious complications of appendicitis.

Evaluation and Treatment

In addition to clinical manifestations, the clinician can usually locate the painful site with one finger. Rebound tenderness is usually referred to the right lower quadrant. The white blood cell count ranges from 10,000 to 16,000 cells/mm³ with increased neutrophils. Plain films of the abdomen and computed tomography (CT) scans can assist in differentiating appendicitis from perforated ulcer or cholecystitis.

Appendectomy is the treatment for simple or perforated appendicitis. Surgery provides quick recovery for simple appendicitis. Recovery is more complicated in cases of perforation or abscess formation.

Vascular Insufficiency

The stomach and intestines are supplied by three branches of the abdominal aorta: the celiac axis and the superior and inferior mesenteric arteries. Atherosclerotic lesions, thrombi, and emboli can develop in these vessels, occluding blood flow and causing ischemia or necrosis in the gastrointestinal tract.

Chronic mesenteric insufficiency can develop secondary to congestive heart failure, acute myocardial infarction, hemorrhage, or any condition that decreases arterial blood flow. Elderly individuals with arteriosclerosis are particularly susceptible. Other causes of chronic occlusion of the mesenteric arteries are stenosis and thrombus formation. Chronic occlusion is often accompanied by formation of collateral circulation. The collateral vessels may be able to nourish the resting intestine. After eating, however, when the intestine requires more blood, the arterial supply may be insufficient. Ischemia develops, causing a cramping abdominal pain, called abdominal angina, after meals. Progressive vascular obstruction eventually causes continuous abdominal pain and necrosis of the intestinal tissue.

Acute occlusion of mesenteric blood flow results from dissecting aortic aneurysms or emboli. Embolic obstruction is associated with atrial fibrillation, mitral valve disease, and heart valve prostheses. The superior mesenteric artery has a more direct line of flow from the aorta; therefore, emboli enter it more readily than the inferior branch, causing ischemia and necrosis of the small intestine. Ischemia and necrosis alter membrane permeability. The damaged intestinal mucosa cannot produce enough mucus to protect itself from digestive enzymes (Kvietys, Barrowmand, & Granger, 1987). Mucosal dysfunction causes fluid to move from the blood vessels into the peritoneum. Fluid loss causes hypovolemia. As intestinal infarction progresses, shock, fever, bloody diarrhea, leukocytosis, and abdominal distention develop. Abdominal pain may be severe.

Colicky abdominal pain after eating is a cardinal symptom of chronic mesenteric insufficiency. Some individuals suffer significant weight loss because they stop eating to control the pain. Acute mesenteric insufficiency causes severe continuous pain, rigid abdomen, and bloody diarrhea. Manifestations of unrelieved acute obstruction are distended abdomen, loss of bowel sounds, shock, peritonitis, fever, and tachycardia.

Diagnosis of mesenteric artery occlusion is based on clinical manifestations, mesenteric artery angiography, and abdominal radiography. Frequently bruit can be heard over the occluded artery. After angiography a vasodilating agent may be injected into the vessels to improve the circulation. Surgery is required to remove necrotic tissue or repair sclerosed vessels. The mortality rate is high for individuals with acute occlusion and compromised cardiac output.

Disorders of Nutrition
Overnutrition

Overnutrition, or excessive caloric intake, is a major nutritional problem in the United States. It leads to **obesity** (excessive body fat), which is associated with the three leading causes of death: cardiovascular disease, cancer, and diabetes mellitus.

Obesity is classified by cause as either exogenous (resulting from an excess of ingested calories) or endogenous (resulting from inherent metabolic problems). Physiologically obesity can be classified according to the structure and distribution of the adipose tissue itself. Child-onset obesity is both hyperplastic (caused by a greater-than-normal number of fat cells) and hypertrophic (caused by a greater-than-normal size of fat cells). In children the adipose tissue is dispersed over the entire body, and few metabolic abnormalities exist. Adult-onset obesity is hypertrophic, the adipose tissue is centrally located, and metabolic abnormalities are more common.

A number of theories have been postulated to explain the physiology of obesity. The fat-cell theory proposes that individuals with hyperplastic fat (adipose) cells are overweight or obese because they have an excessive number of fat cells. The number of fat cells increases whenever a positive energy balance occurs (Faust et al., 1978).

The lipoprotein-lipase (LPL) theory involves biochemical mechanisms within the fat cells. Lipoprotein lipase is an enzyme synthesized by fat cells. It hydrolyzes triglycerides into glycerol and free fatty acids, which then enter the fat cells and are resterified into triglycerides. In other words, LPL promotes fat storage. According to theorists, obese individuals have elevated levels of LPL in their fat cells, and these levels rise even higher after weight reduction. The LPL works against the maintenance of reduced body weight and stimulates the fat cells to return to their hypertrophic size (Schwartz & Brunzell, 1981).

The lipostatic theory states that every individual has a biologic "set point" that maintains body weight. The set point is controlled by the ventromedial hypothalamus, which regulates an individual's appetite. Obese individuals are proposed to have a higher set point, which makes it difficult for them to maintain weight loss (Keesey, 1986).

Another theory of obesity is based on the thermogenesis of brown adipose tissue, the mitochondria-rich fat cells responsible for heat production. Individuals with a large number of subcutaneous brown fat cells release excess energy through heat production instead of converting the energy to fat stores. Obese people are believed to have very few brown fat cells compared to the average individual (Himms-Hagen, 1985; Miller, 1979).

The sodium-potassium-adenosine triphosphatase (ATPase) pump is believed to play a major role in the development of obesity. This enzyme pump transports sodium out of the cell and potassium into the cell and splits adenosine triphosphate, releasing energy. De Luise and colleagues (1980) discovered that obese people have an average of 22% fewer ATPase pumps than nonobese individuals. This lack could lead to less energy release and obesity.

The type II or non-insulin-dependent type of diabetes mellitus is often associated with obesity. Excessive food intake stimulates hyperinsulinemia. Through a negative-feedback mechanism, excessive insulin levels decrease the number of insulin receptor sites on adipose cells. The decrease of insulin receptor sites decreases the amount of glucose that can enter the cells. This promotes high blood levels of glucose. The excess glucose is stored as glycogen in the liver or as triglycerides in adipose cells, thereby enhancing hypertrophy and hyperplasia of fat cells in the already obese person. Weight reduction reverses this process.

Obesity probably has psychologic as well as physiologic causes (Wadden & Stunkard, 1985). One theory of psychologic causation proposes that obese people are directed more by external cues, such as the sight, smell, and taste of food, than by internal cues, such as hunger and satiety (Stunkard, 1980). Another psychologic theory is that eating creates the desire to eat more. Several studies have shown that some obese individuals eat more food after a snack or preload meal than nonobese individuals, who compensate for the preload meal by reducing food intake afterward.

Pathophysiology

Obese individuals are at risk for coronary artery disease resulting from hypercholesterolemia and hypertension. Obesity is also a risk factor for breast, cervical, endometrial, and liver cancer in women. Obese men are at greater risk for prostatic, colon, and rectal cancer (American Cancer Society, 1986). Pulmonary function can be compromised by a large amount of adipose tissue overlying the chest cage. Gas exchange, vital capacity, and expiratory volume all decrease, causing low arterial oxygen tension and high carbon dioxide tension. Sleep apnea can occur. Exercise intolerance and pain in the fingers and weight-bearing joints, particularly the knees, are common. Joint pain may be caused by premature erosion of cartilage (Bray, 1985).

Evaluation and Treatment

Obesity is evaluated by a number of methods including use of height and weight tables, body mass index (ratio of weight to height), skinfold thickness, hydrostatic weighing, measurement of oxygen intake, and bioelectric impedance analysis. If excess fat interferes with physiologic or psychological functioning, treatment may be initiated.

The treatment for obesity caused by excessive nutrient intake is a regimen of reduced nutrient intake and increased energy expenditure. Age at onset, laboratory data about metabolic function (e.g., glucose tolerance tests, serum triglyceride, and cholesterol analyses), and distribution of adipose tissue determine the weight-reduction goal. Individuals with adult-onset obesity can reduce the size of their adipose cells and achieve a standard weight. Those with child-onset obesity may never achieve a standard weight.

The goal of weight reduction is to return the adipose cells to normal size and correct any associated metabolic abnormalities. The diet-exercise regimen is tailored to the unique problems of each obese individual. Self-motivation and a support system are critical aspects of treatment. Additional treatments, such as psychotherapy, behavioral modification, medications, and surgery, are prescribed as needed.

Anorexia Nervosa

Many young adults and adolescents in the United States are affected by two complex and related eating disorders. **Anorexia nervosa** is a psychologic and physiologic syndrome characterized by bizarre eating habits, distorted body image, self-imposed starvation, very vigorous exercise, abuse of laxatives or diuretics, and voluntary vomiting. Persons with anorexia nervosa firmly deny that they have any eating problem. As the disease progresses, muscle and fat depletion give the individual a skeletonlike appearance. Amenorrhea and hirsutism (in females), impotence (in males), postural hypotension, edema, bradycardia, hypothermia, constipation, and sleep disturbances may ensue. The loss of 25% to 30% of ideal body weight can eventually lead to death

caused by starvation-induced cardiac failure.

Diagnosis of anorexia nervosa involves ruling out other causes of anorexia and malnutrition. The following findings confirm the diagnosis:

1. A fear of becoming obese despite progressive weight loss
2. A distorted body image; the perception that the body is fat when it is actually underweight
3. Body weight 15% less than normal for age and height because of refusal to eat
4. In females, absence of three consecutive menstrual periods

The treatment objectives for anorexia nervosa include reversing the compromised physical state, promoting positive self-image and interaction with family members, restoring developmental growth, and modifying food habits. Correction of nutritional status can require hospitalization. When the individual demonstrates the willingness to eat food for nourishment, dietary protein, carbohydrate, and fat are introduced in tolerable amounts. Psychotherapy begins as soon as the physical symptoms are stabilized and may continue for several years.

Bulimia

Bulimia is characterized by binging—the consumption of normal to large amounts of food, often several thousand calories at a time—followed by self-induced vomiting or purging of the intestines with laxatives. The group at risk is the same as that for anorexia nervosa, except that bulimia tends to occur in slightly older, less affluent women. About 50% of individuals with anorexia nervosa are bulimic as well (Halmi, 1987). Many young women stimulate vomiting inappropriately to control weight but are not classified as bulimic unless the pattern is obsessional or normal health or activity is interrupted. Diagnosis of bulimia is based on these findings:

1. Recurrent episodes of binge eating during which the individual fears not being able to stop
2. Self-induced vomiting, use of laxatives, or fasting to oppose the effect of binge eating
3. Two binge-eating episodes per week for at least 3 months

Although individuals with bulimia are afraid of gaining weight, their weight usually remains within normal range. Because of negative connotations associated with self-stimulated vomiting and purging, individuals who have bulimia binge and purge secretly. Bulimics may binge and purge as often as 20 times a day. Continual vomiting of acidic chyme can cause pitted teeth, pharyngeal and esophageal inflammation, and tracheoesophageal fistulas. Overuse of laxatives can cause rectal bleeding. Secret binging isolates the bulimic individual and leads to depression and anger that is turned inward. A vicious cycle of depression, overeating to try to feel better, vomiting and purging to maintain a normal weight, and returning depression perpetuates this eating disorder.

Because bulimics are usually older than individuals with anorexia nervosa and have usually separated from a family core, individual and/or group counseling is the treatment focus. Individuals with bulimia rarely have physical problems requiring hospital care.

Bulimarexia

Bulimarexia combines the major components of anorexia nervosa and bulimia. Individuals with bulimarexia binge and gorge with food, vomit and purge with laxatives, and starve themselves intermittently. Risk factors and treatment objectives for bulimarexia are the same as for anorexia nervosa.

Starvation

Short-term starvation and long-term starvation have different effects. Therapeutic short-term starvation is part of many weight-reduction programs because it causes an initial rapid weight loss that reinforces the individual's motivation to diet. Therapeutic long-term starvation is used in medically controlled environments to facilitate rapid weight loss in morbidly obese individuals. Pathologic long-term starvation can be caused by poverty; chronic diseases of the cardiovascular, pulmonary, hepatic, and digestive systems; malabsorption syndromes; and cancer.

Short-term starvation, or extended fasting, consists of several days of total dietary abstinence or deprivation. For 4 to 6 hours after the last meal, the body is in a well-fed state, and its energy requirements are supplied by glucose from recently ingested carbohydrates. Once all available energy has been absorbed from the intestine, glycogen in the liver is converted to glucose through **glycogenolysis,** the splitting of glycogen into glucose. This process peaks within 4 to 8 hours, and gluconeogenesis begins. **Gluconeogenesis** is the formation of glucose from noncarbohydrate molecules: lactate, pyruvate, amino acids, and the glycerol portion of fats. Like glycogenolysis, gluconeogenesis takes place within the liver. Both of these processes deplete stored nutrients and thus cannot meet the body's energy needs indefinitely. Proteins continue to be catabolized to a minimal degree, providing carbon for the synthesis of glucose.

Long-term starvation begins after several days of dietary abstinence and eventually causes death. The major characteristic of long-term starvation is a decreased dependence on gluconeogenesis and an increased use of ketone bodies (products of lipid and pyruvate metabolism) as a cellular energy source. During long-term starvation, depressed insulin and glucagon levels promote lipolysis in adipose tissue. Lipolysis liberates fatty acids, which supply energy to cardiac and skeletal muscle cells, and ketone bodies, which sustain brain tissue. Fatty acid or ketone body oxidation meets most of the energy needs of the cells. (Some glucose is still needed as fuel for brain tissue.) Once the supply of adipose tissue is depleted, proteolysis begins. The breakdown of muscle protein is the last process to supply energy for life. Death results from severe alterations in electrolyte balance and loss of renal, pulmonary, and cardiac function.

Adequate ingestion of appropriate nutrients is the obvious treatment for starvation. In medically induced starvation, the body is maintained in a ketotic state until the desired amount of adipose tissue has been lysed. Starvation imposed by chronic disease, long-term illness, or malabsorption is treated with enteral or parenteral nutrition.

DISORDERS OF THE ACCESSORY ORGANS OF DIGESTION

The accessory organs of digestion, the liver, gallbladder, and pancreas, secrete substances necessary for digestion and, in the case of the liver, carry out metabolic functions needed to maintain life. Inflammatory disease is a common cause of accessory organ dysfunction. Inflammation disrupts secretory function and prevents secretions from flowing into the duodenum. Lack of accessory organ secretions is a major cause of maldigestion and malabsorption in the small intestine. Other causes of accessory organ dysfunction are obstruction of ducts by aggregates in the secretions themselves (e.g., obstruction of bile flow by gallstones) or by tumors. (Cancers of the digestive tract are described at the end of the chapter.)

Clinical Manifestations of Liver Disorders

Of all the accessory organ disorders, acute or chronic liver disease leads to the most systemic, life-threatening complications. These complications include portal hypertension, ascites, hepatic encephalopathy, jaundice, and hepatorenal syndrome.

Portal Hypertension

Portal hypertension is abnormally high blood pressure in the portal venous system. Pressure in this system is normally 3 mm Hg; portal hypertension is a rise to at least 10 mm Hg. The portal veins carry blood from the gastrointestinal tract, pancreas, and spleen to the liver. In the liver the blood flows through the sinusoids and empties into the hepatic veins, which carry it into the inferior vena cava. The inferior vena cava delivers blood to the right atrium. The portal veins, sinusoids, and hepatic veins compose the portal venous system.

Pathophysiology

Portal hypertension is caused by disorders that obstruct or impede blood flow through any component of the portal venous system or vena cava. The obstruction can occur in the liver as a result of thrombosis, inflammation, or fibrosis of the sinusoids, as occurs in cirrhosis of the liver, viral hepatitis, or schistosomiasis (a parasitic infection). Portal outflow to the vena cava can be impeded by hepatic vein thrombosis or cardiac disorders, such as failure of the right side of the heart or constrictive pericarditis, that impair the pumping ability of the right heart. This causes blood to "back up" and increase pressure in the portal system. The most common

cause of portal hypertension is obstruction caused by cirrhosis of the liver (see p. 1248).

High pressure in the portal veins causes collateral vessels to open between the portal veins and the systemic veins, in which blood pressure is considerably lower (Fig. 36-10). This enables blood to bypass the obstructed portal vessels. The collateral veins develop in the esophagus, anterior abdominal wall, and rectum. High pressure and increased flow volume are transmitted through these veins from the portal to the system venous circulation.

Long-term portal hypertension causes several problems that are difficult to treat and can be fatal.

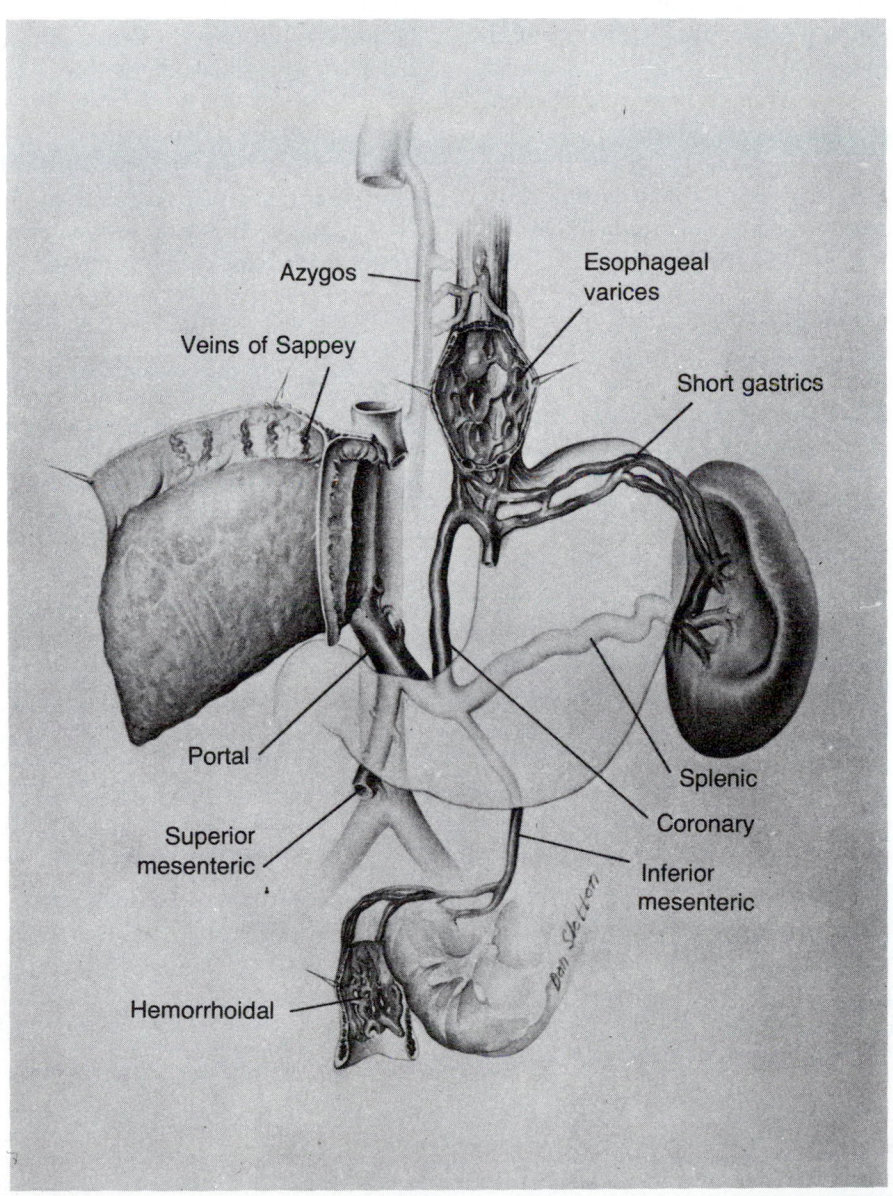

FIG. 36-10. Portal vein, its major tributaries, and the most important shunts (collateral veins) between the portal and caval systems. (From Kissane, 1985.)

1. **Varices** (distended, tortuous, collateral veins). Prolonged elevation of pressure in collateral veins causes their transformation into varices, particularly in the lower esophagus and stomach, but also in the rectum.
2. **Splenomegaly** (enlargement of the spleen) caused by increased pressure in the splenic vein, which branches from the portal vein.
3. **Ascites** (the accumulation of fluid in the peritoneal cavity, which is the space between the visceral peritoneum and the parietal peritoneum). Ascites is caused by increased pressure in the mesenteric tributaries of the portal vein. Hydrostatic pressure forces water out of these vessels and into the peritoneal cavity. (This process, termed transudative effusion, is described in Chapter 30.)
4. **Hepatic encephalopathy,** also called portal-systemic encephalopathy. This condition is characterized by central nervous system disturbances, particularly alterations of consciousness.

Blood that is shunted through collateral vessels to the systemic veins bypasses the liver, where toxins, hormones, and other harmful substances normally are removed. Hepatic encephalopathy results from the presence of these substances, particularly ammonia, in blood that reaches the brain.

Clinical Manifestations

The vomiting of blood from bleeding esophageal varices is the most common clinical manifestation of portal hypertension. Slow, chronic bleeding from varices causes anemia or melena. Usually the bleeding is from varices that have developed slowly over a period of years.

Rupture of esophageal varices causes hemorrhage and voluminous vomiting of dark-colored blood. The ruptured varices are usually painless. Rupture is caused by a combination of erosion by gastric acid and elevated venous pressure. The mortality rate of ruptured esophageal varices ranges from 30% to 60%. Recurrent bleeding of esophageal varices indicates a poor prognosis. Most individuals die within 1 year.

Evaluation and Treatment

Diagnosis of portal hypertension is often made at the time of variceal bleeding and confirmed by endoscopy and evaluation of portal venous pressure. Distended collateral veins may radiate over the abdomen, giving rise

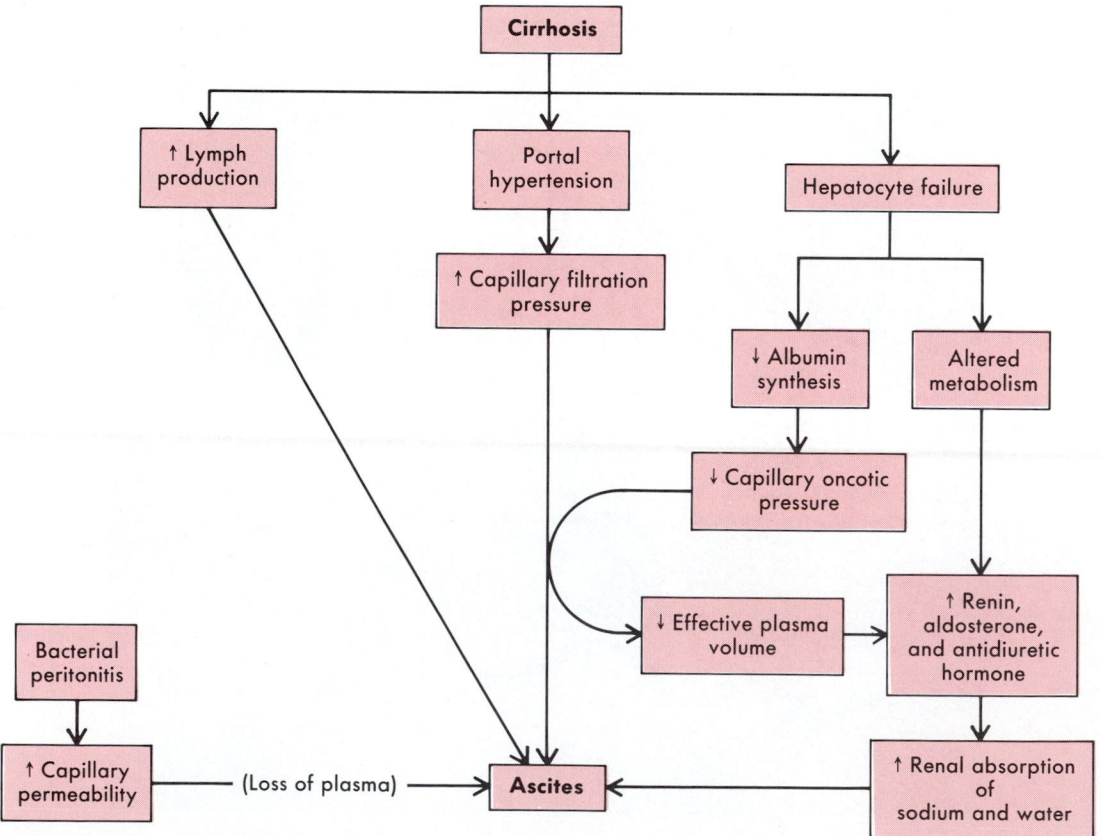

FIG. 36-11. Mechanisms of ascites caused by cirrhosis.

to the description caput medusae (Medusa's head). The individual usually has a history of jaundice, hepatitis, or alcoholism.

Emergency management of bleeding varices includes compression of the varices with an inflatable Seng-staken-Blakenmore tube, which is shaped like a cylindrical balloon with a bulb at the end. In some cases the varices are obliterated by injection of a sclerosing agent. Surgical construction of a portacaval shunt (anastomosis of the portal vein to the inferior vena cava) may decompress the varices, but this treatment can precipitate encephalopathy or liver failure resulting from reduced hepatic blood flow. There is no effective, definitive treatment for portal hypertension.

Ascites

Ascites is the accumulation of fluid in the peritoneal cavity. Ascites traps body fluid in a "third space" from which it cannot escape. The effect is to reduce the amount of fluid available for normal physiologic functions. Cirrhosis is the most common cause of ascites. Other diseases associated with ascites include heart failure, constrictive pericarditis, abdominal malignancies, nephrotic syndrome, and malnutrition. Twenty-five percent of individuals who develop ascites caused by cirrhosis die within 1 year. Continued heavy drinking is associated with this mortality rate.

Pathophysiology

Several factors contribute to the development of ascites. Portal hypertension and reduced serum albumin levels cause capillary hydrostatic pressure to exceed capillary osmotic pressure. This imbalance tends to push water into the peritoneal cavity. Portal hypertension also increases the production of hepatic lymph, which "weeps" into the peritoneal cavity.

In cases of cirrhosis both portal hypertension and decreased production of albumin by hepatocytes contribute to the ascites. Besides reducing albumin synthesis, deranged liver metabolism permits the accumulation of hormones that regulate sodium and water balance. Excessive amounts of aldosterone and antidiuretic hormone remain in the blood, stimulating the kidneys to retain sodium and water. High aldosterone levels can also be attributed to increased secretion mediated by excessive plasma renin activity. The increased plasma renin activity may develop because of decreased metabolic function of the liver, increased renal secretion stimulated by low blood flow, or both.

As ascites sequesters more and more bodily fluid, the kidneys respond by retaining sodium and water in amounts exceeding intake. Retention of sodium and water expands plasma volume, thereby accelerating portal hypertension and ascites formation.

Ascites can be complicated by bacterial peritonitis.

Peritonitis involves an inflammatory response that worsens ascites by increasing mesenteric capillary permeability. As plasma seeps out of the permeable mesenteric capillaries, it adds to the volume of ascitic fluid. Fig. 36-11 summarizes the mechanisms by which cirrhosis of the liver causes ascites.

Clinical Manifestations

The accumulation of ascitic fluid causes weight gain, abdominal distention, and increased abdominal girth (Fig. 36-12). Large volumes of fluid (10 to 20 L) displace the diaphragm and cause dyspnea by decreasing lung capacity. Respiratory rate increases, and the individual assumes a semi-Fowler position to relieve the dyspnea. Some peripheral edema is usually present. About 10% of individuals with ascites develop bacterial peritonitis, either spontaneously or as a result of paracentesis (needle aspiration of ascitic fluid). Peritonitis

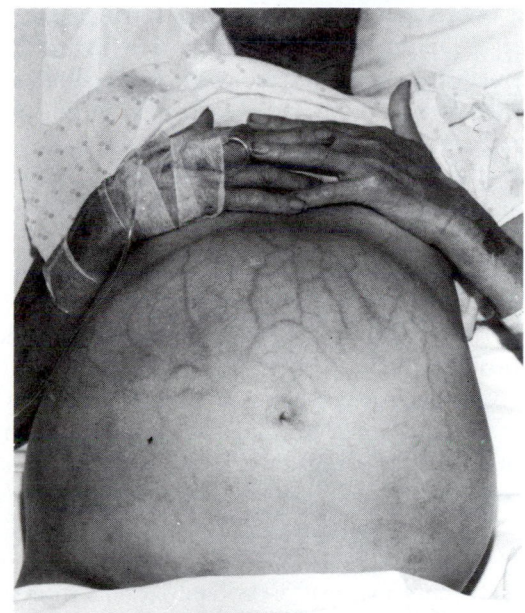

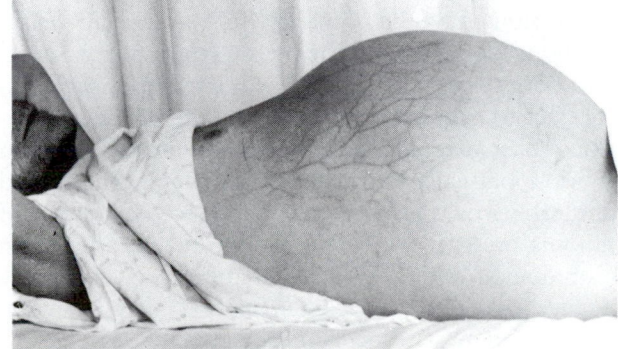

FIG. 36-12. Massive ascites in an individual with cirrhosis. Distended abdomen, dilated upper abdominal veins, and inverted umbilicus are classic manifestations. (From Prior, Silberstein, & Stang, 1981.)

causes fever, chills, abdominal pain, decreased bowel sounds, and cloudy ascitic fluid.

Evaluation and Treatment

Diagnosis of ascites is usually based on clinical manifestations and identification of liver disease. Paracentesis is used to aspirate ascitic fluid for bacterial culture, biochemical analysis, and microscopic examination. The goal of treatment is to relieve discomfort. If the restoration of liver function is possible (e.g., in ascites caused by viral hepatitis), the ascites diminishes spontaneously. In the meantime dietary salt restriction and potassium-sparing diuretics can reduce ascites. Strong diuretics, such as furosemide or ethacrynic acid, may be used. Serum electrolytes are monitored carefully because the individual is at risk for hyponatremia and hypokalemia.

Palliative measures include paracentesis to remove 1 or 2 L of ascitic fluid and relieve respiratory distress. This procedure can have serious complications, however. The removal of too much fluid relieves pressure on blood vessels and carries the risk of hypotension, shock, or death. Despite repeated paracentesis, ascitic fluid reaccumulates in individuals with irreversible disease, drawing more albumin and electrolytes out of the vascular compartment. Paracentesis is also likely to cause peritonitis. Individuals with ascites and portal hypertension have a poor prognosis.

Hepatic Encephalopathy

Hepatic encephalopathy (portal-systemic encephalopathy) is a complex neurologic syndrome characterized by impaired cerebral function, flapping tremor (asterixis), and electroencephalogram (EEG) changes. The syndrome may develop rapidly during acute fulminant hepatitis or slowly during the course of chronic liver disease.

Pathophysiology

Hepatic encephalopathy probably results from a combination of biochemical alterations that affect neurotransmission. Liver dysfunction and collateral vessels that shunt blood around the liver to the systemic circulation both permit toxins absorbed from the gastrointestinal tract to circulate freely to the brain. The most hazardous substances are end products of intestinal protein digestion, particularly ammonia. The digestion of blood from leaking or ruptured varices adds to the amount of ammonia present in systemic blood, as does the action of ammonia-forming bacteria in the colon. Ammonia that reaches the brain may alter cerebral energy metabolism or interfere with neurotransmitters.

Blood levels of ammonia do not account for all symptoms associated with hepatic encephalopathy. The accumulation of short-chain fatty acids, serotonin, tryptophan, and false neurotransmitters probably contrib-

utes to neural derangement. Infection, hemorrhage, electrolyte imbalance, sedatives, and analgesics can also precipitate stupor and coma in the presence of liver disease.

Clinical Manifestations

Subtle changes in personality, memory loss, irritability, lethargy, and sleep disturbances are common initial manifestations of hepatic encephalopathy. Symptoms can then progress to confusion, flapping tremor of the hands, stupor, convulsions, and coma. Coma is usually a sign of liver failure and ultimately results in death.

Evaluation and Treatment

Diagnosis of hepatic encephalopathy is based on a history of liver disease and clinical manifestations. Electroencephalography and blood chemistry tests provide supportive data.

Correction of fluid and electrolyte imbalances and withdrawal of depressant drugs metabolized by the liver are first steps in the treatment of hepatic encephalopathy. Reduction of blood ammonia levels is a major objective. This is accomplished by restricting dietary protein intake and eliminating intestinal bacteria. Neomycin is effective in sterilizing the bowel, but it can be nephrotoxic. Lactulose may be administered to prevent ammonia absorption in the colon. Lactulose passes unabsorbed into the large intestine, where bacteria hydrolyze it to a watery acid. The acid (1) converts ammonia to nonabsorbable ammonium and (2) produces diarrhea, which limits the amount of time feces are available for ammonia production by intestinal bacteria.

Jaundice

Jaundice, or icterus, is a yellow or greenish pigmentation of the skin caused by **hyperbilirubinemia** (plasma bilirubin concentrations above 1.2 mg/dl). Hyperbilirubinemia and jaundice can result from excessive hemolysis of red blood cells or disorders of the bile ducts or liver cells (Fig. 36-13). Jaundice in newborns is caused by impaired bilirubin uptake and conjugation (see Chapter 37).

Pathophysiology

Obstructive jaundice can result from extrahepatic or intrahepatic obstruction. Extrahepatic obstructive jaundice develops if the common bile duct is occluded by a gallstone or tumor. Because the bile duct is obstructed, bilirubin is conjugated by the hepatocytes but cannot flow into the duodenum. Therefore, it accumulates in the liver and enters the bloodstream, causing hyperbilirubinemia. Because conjugated bilirubin is water soluble, it appears in the urine. The stools may be light or clay-colored because they lack bile pigments. The stools also lack urobilinogen because bile is not available for conversion to urobilinogen.

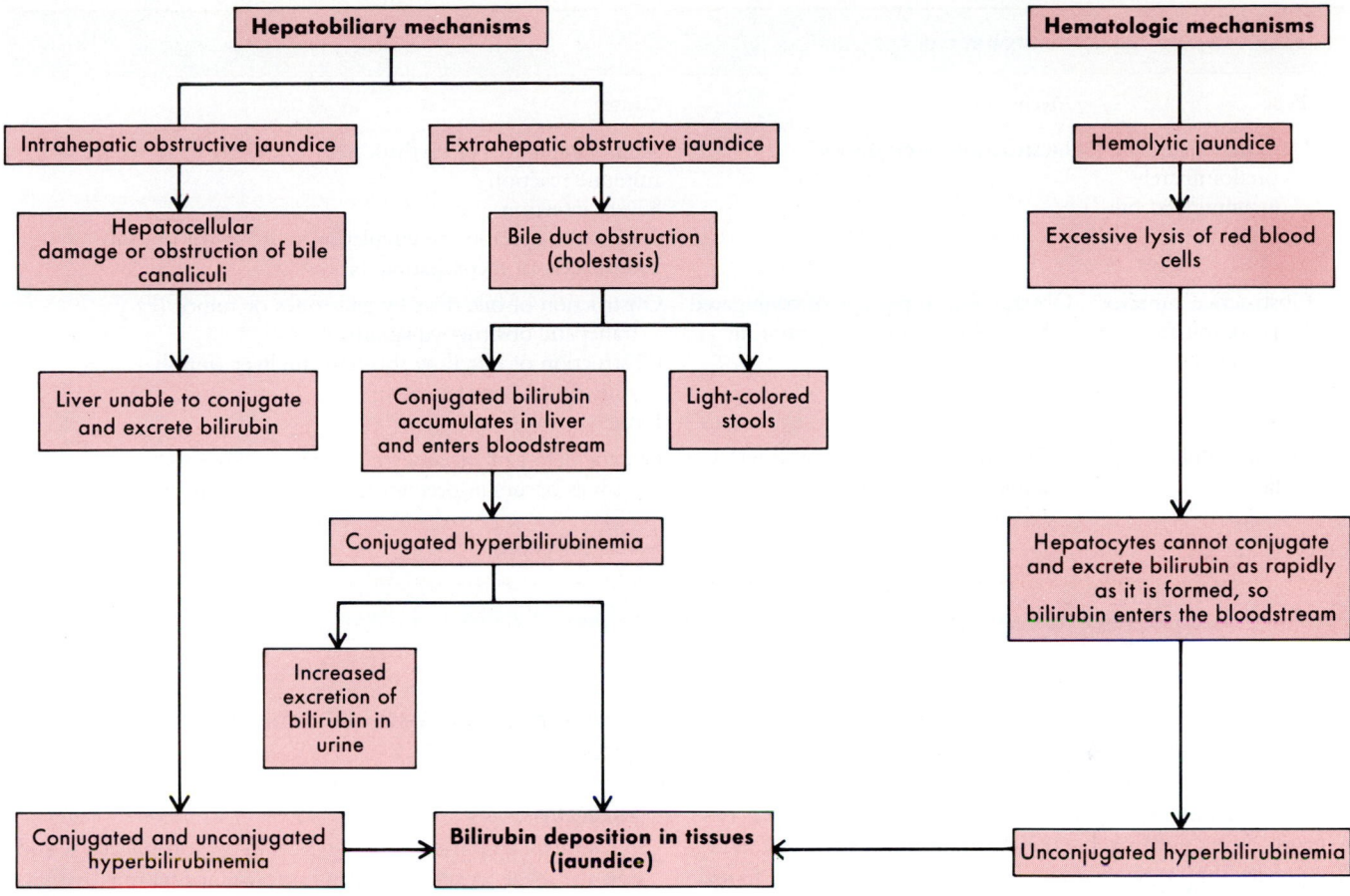

FIG. 36-13. Mechanisms of jaundice.

Intrahepatic obstructive jaundice involves disturbances in hepatocyte function and obstruction of bile canaliculi. The uptake, conjugation, and excretion of bilirubin are affected, because of elevated levels of both conjugated and unconjugated bilirubin. Hepatocellular damage increases plasma concentrations of unconjugated bilirubin. The major disorder, however, is obstruction of bile canaliculi, which diminishes flow of conjugated bilirubin into the common bile duct. In mild cases some of the bile canaliculi open. Consequently the amount of bilirubin in the intestinal tract may be only slightly decreased. The stools may appear normal or light-colored.

Excessive hemolysis (breakdown) of red blood cells can cause **hemolytic jaundice.** An increased amount of unconjugated bilirubin is formed through metabolism of the heme component of destroyed red blood cells. The extra amount of unconjugated bilirubin exceeds the conjugation ability of the liver, causing blood levels of unconjugated bilirubin to rise. Unconjugated bilirubinemia is the major cause of hemolytic jaundice. Because unconjugated bilirubin is not water soluble, it is not excreted in the urine. The reserve conjugation abil-

ity of the liver usually prevents long-term unconjugated hyperbilirubinemia greater than 4 to 5 mg/dl. Severe hemolytic crisis, such as that which occurs with sickle cell disease (see Chapter 25), is a cause of hemolytic jaundice. Hemolytic drugs can also cause jaundice. If unconjugated hyperbilirubinemia exceeds 5 mg/dl, both hemolytic and liver disorders are suspected.

Hyperbilirubinemia and jaundice can also be caused by metabolic defects that impair the uptake or conjugation of unconjugated bilirubin in the liver. Gilbert disease, for example, causes an elevation of unconjugated bilirubin in the plasma but no other symptoms of liver disease. Gilbert disease is probably caused by an inherited deficiency of glycuronyl transferase enzyme, which is required for the hepatic uptake of unconjugated bilirubin. The causes of jaundice are summarized in Table 36-7.

Clinical Manifestations

The clinical manifestations of jaundice vary and are related to the underlying pathology. Conjugated hyperbilirubinemia may cause the urine to darken several days prior to the onset of jaundice. The complete obstruction

TABLE 36-7 Three common types of jaundice

Type	Mechanism	Causes
Hemolytic jaundice (predominately unconjugated bilirubin	Destruction of erythrocytes	Membrane defect of erythrocytes Immune reaction Severe infection Toxic substances in the circulation (e.g., snake venom) Transfusion of incompatible blood
Obstructive jaundice (predominately conjugated bilirubin)	Obstruction of passage of conjugated bilirubin from liver to intestine	Obstruction of bile duct by gallstones or tumor (extrahepatic obstructive jaundice) Obstruction of bile flow through the liver (intrahepatic obstructive jaundice) Drugs
Hepatocellular jaundice	Failure of liver cells (hepatocytes) to conjugate bilirubin and of bilirubin to pass from liver to intestine	Genetic defect of hepatocyte (decreased enzymes), such as occurs in premature infants (see Chapter 37) Severe infections

of bile flow from the liver to the duodenum causes light-colored stools. With partial obstruction the stools are normal in color and bilirubin is present in the urine.

Fever, chills, and pain often accompany jaundice resulting from viral or bacterial inflammation of the liver (e.g., viral hepatitis). Manifestations of liver injury from any cause commonly include anorexia, malaise, and fatigue. Yellow discoloration may first occur in the sclera of the eye and then progress to the skin. Pruritus frequently accompanies jaundice because bilirubin accumulates in the skin.

Evaluation and Treatment

Laboratory evaluation of serum establishes whether plasma bilirubin is conjugated or unconjugated. Unconjugated bilirubinemia results from hemolysis or hereditary disorders of bilirubin metabolism. Elevations of conjugated bilirubin indicate liver injury or extrahepatic obstruction. The history and physical examination identify underlying disorders, such as alcoholism, exposure to hepatitis virus, or gallbladder disease. The treatment for jaundice consists of correcting the cause.

Hepatorenal Syndrome

Hepatorenal syndrome consists of advanced liver disease, functional renal failure, oliguria, sodium and water retention (with or without ascites and peripheral edema), hypotension, and peripheral vasodilation. Renal disorders associated with liver disease can have numerous causes, but hepatorenal syndrome is usually associated with portal hypertension and cirrhosis. The renal failure is not caused by primary renal disease or

other extrinsic factors, but rather by circulatory alterations.

Pathophysiology

Oliguric hepatic failure generally accompanies a sudden decrease in blood volume secondary to massive gastrointestinal bleeding or hypotension caused by failing liver function. Hypotension can also be caused by the excessive use of diuretics to treat ascites. The diuretics may decrease renal blood flow and glomerular filtration rate and cause oliguria. A significant number of individuals with advanced liver disease develop oliguria unrelated to any precipitating event. Liver failure is the apparent cause of functional renal failure in hepatorenal syndrome. Inappropriate constriction of renal arterioles is proposed as the causative mechanism. Intrarenal vasoconstriction may result from the selective effects of vasoactive substances that accumulate in the blood because of liver failure. The diseased liver fails to remove excessive angiotensin, vasopressin, prostaglandins, and catecholamines from the blood (Davidson & Dunn, 1987). These substances travel to the kidneys and cause vasoconstriction. Vasoconstriction may also be a compensatory response to portal hypotension and the pooling of blood in the splanchnic circulation. The exact reason for the vasoconstriction is unknown.

Clinical Manifestations

The onset of hepatorenal manifestations may be gradual or acute. Oliguria and complications of advanced liver disease, including jaundice, ascites, and gastrointestinal bleeding, are usually present. Systolic blood pressure is usually below 100 mm Hg. Nonspecific symptoms of hepatorenal syndrome include anorexia, weakness, and fatigue.

Evaluation and Treatment

Despite oliguria, serum potassium levels do not become dangerously elevated until the terminal stages of the hepatorenal syndrome. Blood urea increases, followed by an increase in creatinine concentration. Urine osmolality is increased, but urine sodium concentrations are below normal. Urine specific gravity is above 1.015.

The prognosis is usually poor and is related to liver function. Secondary problems, including fluid and electrolyte disorders, bleeding, infections, and encephalopathy, are vigorously treated.

Disorders of the Liver
Viral Hepatitis

Viral hepatitis is a relatively common systemic disease that primarily affects the liver. Three (or possibly four) strains of viruses cause different types of hepatitis: hepatitis A virus (HAV), hepatitis B virus (HBV), hepatitis D virus (HDV), and the non-A, non-B hepatitis

viruses. Hepatitis A used to be known as infectious hepatitis, and hepatitis B as serum hepatitis. The World Health Organization's nomenclature for hepatitis viruses and their corresponding antibodies is presented in Table 36-8. Characteristics of the different types are presented in Table 36-9.

Types of Hepatitis

Hepatitis A   The hepatitis A virus can be recovered from the feces, bile, and sera of infected individuals. The usual mode of transmission is the fecal-oral route (contaminated food or water), but the virus can also be spread by the transfusion of infected blood. Approximately 45% of adults in urban areas have HAV antibodies in their blood. The disease spreads readily in crowded, unsanitary conditions, usually through contaminated food or water. Person-to-person spread is more likely to occur in settings such as day care centers or institutions for the mentally retarded, where there is close contact between clients and caregivers (Hadler et al., 1982).

The incubation period (the time between exposure and onset of symptoms) for hepatitis A is 4 to 6 weeks (Fig. 36-14). Fecal shedding of the virus is greatest for

---

TABLE 36-8 Hepatitis viruses and antibodies

Virus, virus component, or antibody	Abbreviation
Hepatitis A virus	HAV
Hepatitis A virus antigen	HAAg
Antibody to HAV, immunoglobulin class not specified	Anti-HAV
Antibody to HAV, IgG class	Anti-HAV IgG
Antibody to HAV, IgM class	Anti-HAV IgM
Antibody to HAV, IgA class	Anti-HAV IgA
Hepatitis B virus	HBV
HBV surface antigen	HBsAg
HBV core antigen	HBcAg
HBV e antigen	HBeAg
Antibody to HBV surface antigen, immunoglobulin class not specified	Anti-HBs
Antibody to HBV core antigen, immunoglobulin class not specified	Anti-HBc
Antibody to HBV core antigen, IgG class	Anti-HBc IgG
Antibody to HBV core antigen, IgM class	Anti-HBc IgM
Antibody of HBV e antigen, immunoglobulin class not specified	Anti-HBe
HBV DNA-dependent DNA polymerase	HBV-DNA polymerase, HDNAP
Unidentified agents causing hepatitis non-A, non-B	HNANBV

TABLE 36-9 Characteristics of viral hepatitis

Characteristic	Hepatitis A	Hepatitis B	Non-A, Non-B
Size of virus	27 mm	42 mm	Unknown
Incubation period	30 days	60-180 days	35-60 days
Route of transmission	Fecal-oral, parenteral	Parenteral, sexual	Parenteral
Onset	Acute with fever	Insidious	Insidious
Carrier state	Negative	Positive	Positive
Severity	Mild	Severe; may be prolonged or chronic	Unknown
Age group affected	Children and young adults	Any	Any

10 to 14 days prior to the onset of symptoms and during the first week of symptoms. The disease is most contagious during this time. Antibodies to HAV (anti-HAV) develop about 4 weeks after infection. The serum IgM concentration increases initially and is followed by an increase of serum IgG. IgG levels remain elevated for several years following infection, creating immunity to the disease. (See Chapter 6 for a description of immune functions.)

Hepatitis B   Hepatitis B is transmitted through contact with infected blood, body fluids, or contaminated needles. Hepatitis B is also considered to be a sexually transmitted disease (see Chapter 21). People receiving hemodialysis, multiple blood transfusions, or immunosuppressive drugs have a greater risk of exposure or less resistance to HBV. Mother-infant transmission occurs if the mother becomes infected during the third trimester of pregnancy. Approximately 0.3% of adults in the

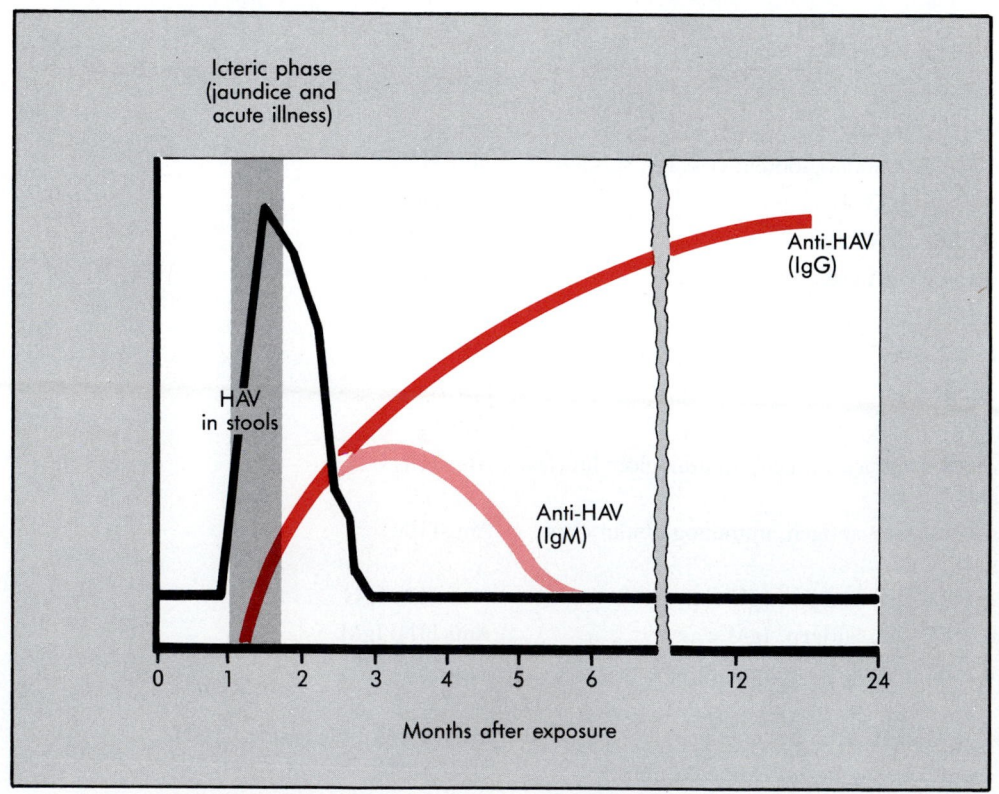

FIG. 36-14. Course of infection with the hepatitis A virus (HAV).

United States carry the HB$_s$Ag marker for active HBV (Gerety, 1985).

Three types of viral particles are involved in HBV infection. The larger (47 nm) Dane particle probably represents the intact HBV. The Dane particle has a double-layered outer coat and carries the hepatitis B surface antigen (HB$_s$Ag), which was originally called the Australian antigen. HB$_s$Ag can be identified in the serum by radioimmune assay. HBV has an incubation period of 6 to 8 weeks. The initial serologic change is a transient increase in IgM. Levels of IgG antibodies to HB$_s$Ag elevate more slowly and remain elevated for years (Fig. 36-15).

Hepatitis D The delta hepatitis virus (HDV) was identified in 1977 (Rizzetto et al., 1977). The delta virus depends on the hepatitis B virus for its replication because the coat of the delta virus consists of HB$_s$Ag molecules that are on the surface of the HBV virus. Parenteral drug users have a high incidence of HDV infection. HDV has been shown to suppress replication of hepatitis B virus (DeCock, Govindarajan, & Redeker, 1985). The clinical course of HDV is similar to that of hepatitis A and B, although it is sometimes more severe.

Non-A, Non-B Hepatitis When serologic tests for hepatitis A or hepatitis B are negative or other causes of viral liver disease are not identified, then non-A, non-B hepatitis is suspected. This type of viral hepatitis was originally diagnosed by exclusion in recipients of blood transfusions. The viruses involved have not been identified.

Pathophysiology

The pathologic lesions of hepatitis are similar to those caused by other viral infection. Hepatic cell necrosis, scarring, Kupffer cell hyperplasia, and infiltration by mononuclear phagocytes occur with varying severity. Regeneration of hepatic cells begins within 48 hours of injury. The inflammatory process can damage and obstruct bile canaliculi, leading to cholestasis and obstructive jaundice. In milder cases the liver parenchyma is not damaged. Damage tends to be most severe in cases of hepatitis B. Hepatitis B is also associated with acute fulminating hepatitis, a rare form of the disease that is characterized by massive hepatic necrosis. Acute fulminating hepatitis causes severe encephalopathy, which is manifested as confusion, stupor, and coma. Liver failure

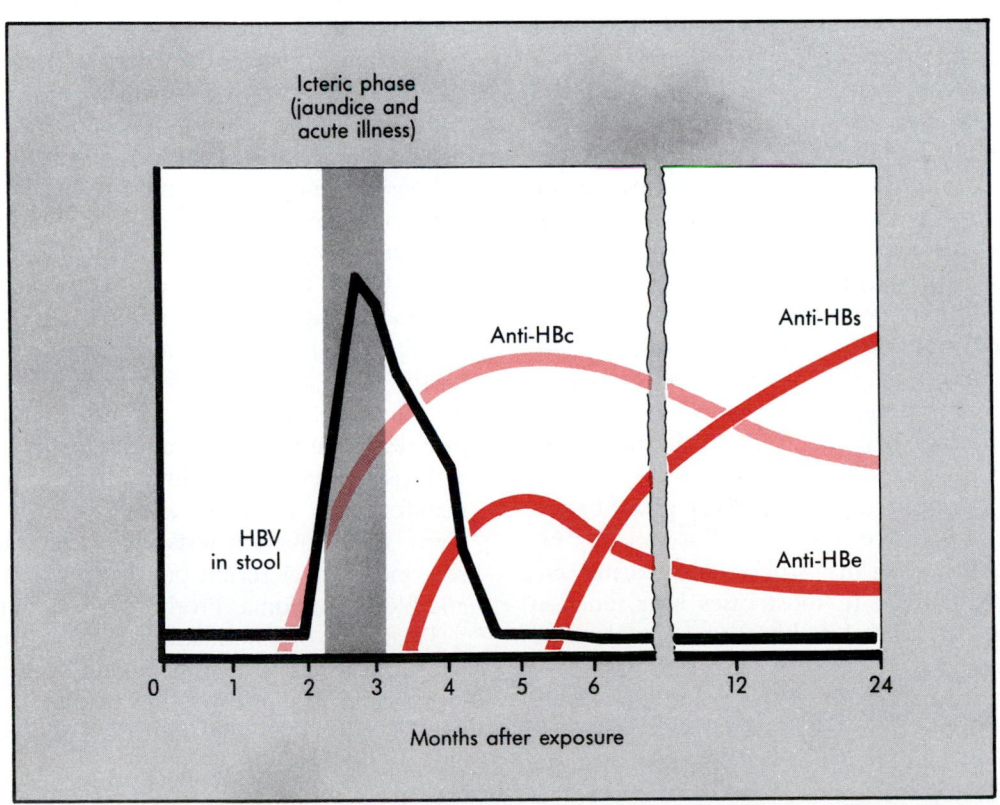

FIG. 36-15. Course of infection with the hepatitis B virus. (HBV). *HB$_s$Ag,* Hepatitis B surface antigen; *anti-HBs,* antibody to HB$_s$Ag; *HB$_e$Ag,* hepatitis Be antigen; *anti-HBe,* antibody to HB$_e$Ag; *anti-HB$_c$,* antibody to hepatitis B core antigen. The antibody to HB$_s$, (anti-HB$_s$,) is IgG, the immunoglobulin that creates immunity.

can occur, leading to intestinal bleeding, cardiorespiratory insufficiency, and renal failure. The mortality rate is high, but recovery can be complete.

Clinical Manifestations

The clinical manifestations of the different types of hepatitis are very similar. The spectrum of manifestations ranges from absence of symptoms to fulminating hepatitis, with rapid onset of liver failure and coma. Acute viral hepatitis causes abnormal liver function test results. The serum transaminase values, AST and ALT, are elevated, but their elevation may not be consistent with the extent of cellular damage. The clinical course of hepatitis usually consists of three phases: the prodromal, icteric, and recovery phases.

Prodromal Phase The **prodromal phase** of hepatitis begins about 2 weeks after exposure and ends with the appearance of jaundice. Fatigue, anorexia, malaise, nausea, vomiting, headache, hyperalgia, cough, and low-grade fever are prodromal symptoms that precede the onset of jaundice. Food odors often cause nausea, and changes in taste suppress the desire to smoke and drink alcohol. Right upper abdominal pain is common, and a weight loss of 2 to 4 kg is not unusual. The infection is highly transmissible during this phase.

Icteric Phase (Jaundice) The **icteric phase** begins about 1 to 2 weeks after the prodromal phase and lasts 2 to 6 weeks. Hepatocellular destruction and intrahepatic bile stasis cause jaundice (icterus). The urine may be dark and the stools clay-colored prior to the onset of jaundice. The icteric phase is the actual phase of illness. The liver is enlarged, smooth, and tender, and percussion over the liver causes pain. During the icteric phase gastrointestinal and respiratory symptoms subside, but fatigue and abdominal pain may persist or become more severe. Serum bilirubin levels range from 5 to 10 mg/dl, with both conjugated and unconjugated fractions increasing. The jaundice may last 2 to 6 weeks or longer. Mild and transient itching often accompanies jaundice. The prothrombin time may be prolonged in individuals with more serious forms of the disease.

Recovery Phase The posticteric or **recovery phase** begins with resolution of jaundice, about 6 to 8 weeks after exposure. Although the liver may still be enlarged and tender, symptoms diminish. In most cases liver function test results return to normal within 2 to 12 weeks after the onset of jaundice.

Chronic hepatitis may begin at this point and is associated with HBV infection. **Chronic active hepatitis** is the persistence of clinical manifestations and liver inflammation after acute hepatitis B. Liver function tests remain abnormal for longer than 6 months, and HB$_s$Ag persists.

Evaluation and Treatment

The most specific diagnostic test for viral hepatitis is serologic analysis for HB$_s$Ag, which is the marker for HBV. Diagnosis of type A hepatitis is based on the presence of anti-HAV. There is no specific serologic test for non-A, non-B hepatitis. Liver function tests can also indicate other viral liver diseases, drug toxicity, or alcoholic hepatitis.

There is no specific treatment for acute viral hepatitis. Physical activity may be restricted. A low-fat, high-carbohydrate diet is beneficial if bile flow is obstructed.

To prevent transmission of hepatitis A, hand washing and use of gloves for disposing of bed pans and fecal matter are imperative. There should be no direct contact with blood or body fluids of patients with hepatitis B or non-A, non-B hepatitis. The administration of immune globulin prior to exposure or early in the incubation period can prevent hepatitis A. Prophylactic immune globulin administered before exposure can also prevent hepatitis B. Prophylaxis is recommended for health care workers and others who are at risk for contact with infected body fluids.

Fulminant Hepatitis

Fulminant hepatitis is a clinical syndrome resulting in severe impairment or necrosis of liver cells and potential liver failure. The disorder may occur as a complication of non-A, non-B hepatitis or hepatitis B, particularly HBV infection compounded by infection with the delta virus. Toxic reactions to drugs and congenital metabolic disorders can also cause fulminant hepatitis.

Causative mechanisms of fulminant hepatic failure are poorly understood. Hepatocytes become edematous, and patchy areas of necrosis and inflammatory cell infiltrates disrupt the parenchyma. The death of hepatocytes may be caused by viral or immunologic damage.

Fulminant hepatitis usually develops 6 to 8 weeks after the initial symptoms of viral hepatitis or a metabolic liver disorder. Anorexia, vomiting, abdominal pain, and progressive jaundice are initial signs, followed by ascites and gastrointestinal bleeding. Hepatic encephalopathy is manifested as lethargy, altered motor functions, and coma. Liver function tests reveal elevations of both direct and indirect serum bilirubin, serum transaminases, and blood ammonia. Prothrombin time is prolonged.

Treatment of fulminant hepatitis is supportive. The hepatic necrosis is irreversible, and 60% to 90% of affected children die. Liver transplantation may be lifesaving. Survivors usually do not develop cirrhosis or chronic liver disease.

Cirrhosis

Cirrhosis is an irreversible inflammatory disease that disrupts liver structure and function. It is a leading

TABLE 36-10 Cirrhosis of the liver

Type and disease name	Causal mechanisms	Pathophysiology
Alcoholic cirrhosis, laennec cirrhosis, portal cirrhosis, fatty cirrhosis	Toxic effects of chronic, excessive alcohol intake; acetylaldehyde formed by alcohol metabolism damages hepatocytes	Fat accumulation, inflammation (alcoholic hepatitis), and derangement of the lobular architecture by necrosis and fibrosis (cirrhosis)
Biliary cirrhosis (intrahepatic or extrahepatic obstruction of bile flow)		
Primary biliary cirrhosis	Unknown; possibly an autoimmune mechanism	Inflammation and scarring of lobular bile ducts
Secondary biliary cirrhosis	Obstruction by neoplasms, strictures, or gallstones	Inflammation and scarring of bile ducts proximal to the obstruction
Postnecrotic cirrhosis	Viral hepatitis due to HAV or non-A non-B; drugs or other toxins; autoimmune destruction	Replacement of necrotic tissue with cirrhotic tissue, particularly fibrous, nodular scar tissue
Metabolic cirrhosis	Metabolic defects and storage disease, such as α-1-antitrypsin deficiency, glycogen storage disease, hemochromatosis, Wilson disease, glactosemia	Inflammation and scarring with specific morphologic changes related to etiology

cause of death in the United States. Cirrhosis is the disorganization of hepatic tissues caused by diffuse fibrosis and nodular regeneration. Nodules of regenerated tissue form between fibrous bands, giving the liver a cobbly appearance. The liver may be larger or smaller than normal, and usually it is firm or hard when palpated. A variety of disorders can cause cirrhosis. Therefore, it is often classified by etiology (Table 36-10). In many cases the cause of cirrhosis is unknown.

The precise cause of cellular injury depends on the type of cirrhosis, and the causes are not all clearly understood. Structural changes result from fibrosis, which is a consequence of inflammation. The parenchyma of the liver becomes distorted, and biliary channels may be altered or obstructed, producing jaundice. Obstruction caused by cirrhosis can cause portal hypertension. New vascular channels can form shunts, and blood from the portal vein bypasses the liver. These vascular changes compromise liver function further, and the process of regeneration is replaced by hypoxia, necrosis, atrophy, and, ultimately, liver failure.

Cirrhosis develops slowly over a period of years. Its severity and rate of progression depend on the cause. If toxins, such as alcohol, are involved, the rate of cell death and the severity of inflammation depend on the amount of toxin present (Orrego et al., 1987). Removal of the toxin slows the progression of liver damage and enhances the process of regeneration.

Alcoholic Cirrhosis

Deaths from alcohol-related liver disease have increased over the past decade. The incidence of alcoholic cirrhosis is greatest in middle-aged men. In the United States mortality resulting from cirrhosis is highest among nonwhites. Although alcoholic cirrhosis is the most prevalent of the different types of cirrhosis, the occurrence of cirrhosis among alcoholics is relatively low (about 25%). The amount and duration of alcohol consumption are positively related to the extent of liver damage. Abuse of any type of alcoholic beverage can cause cirrhosis. Malnutrition may add to the risk of cirrhosis in alcohol abusers.

Pathophysiology

Alcoholic cirrhosis is caused by the toxic effects of alcohol on the liver. The oxidative metabolism of alcohol occurs primarily in the liver. Alcohol is first transformed to acetylaldehyde. Excessive amounts of acetylaldehyde significantly alter hepatocyte function. Mitochondrial function is impaired, decreasing oxidation of fatty acid. Enzyme and protein synthesis may be depressed or altered, and hormone and ammonia degradation is diminished. Cellular damage initiates an inflammatory response. Inflammation and necrosis result in excessive collagen formation. (Collagen is the protein component of fibrous tissues.) Fibrosis and scarring alter the structure of the liver and obstruct biliary and vas-

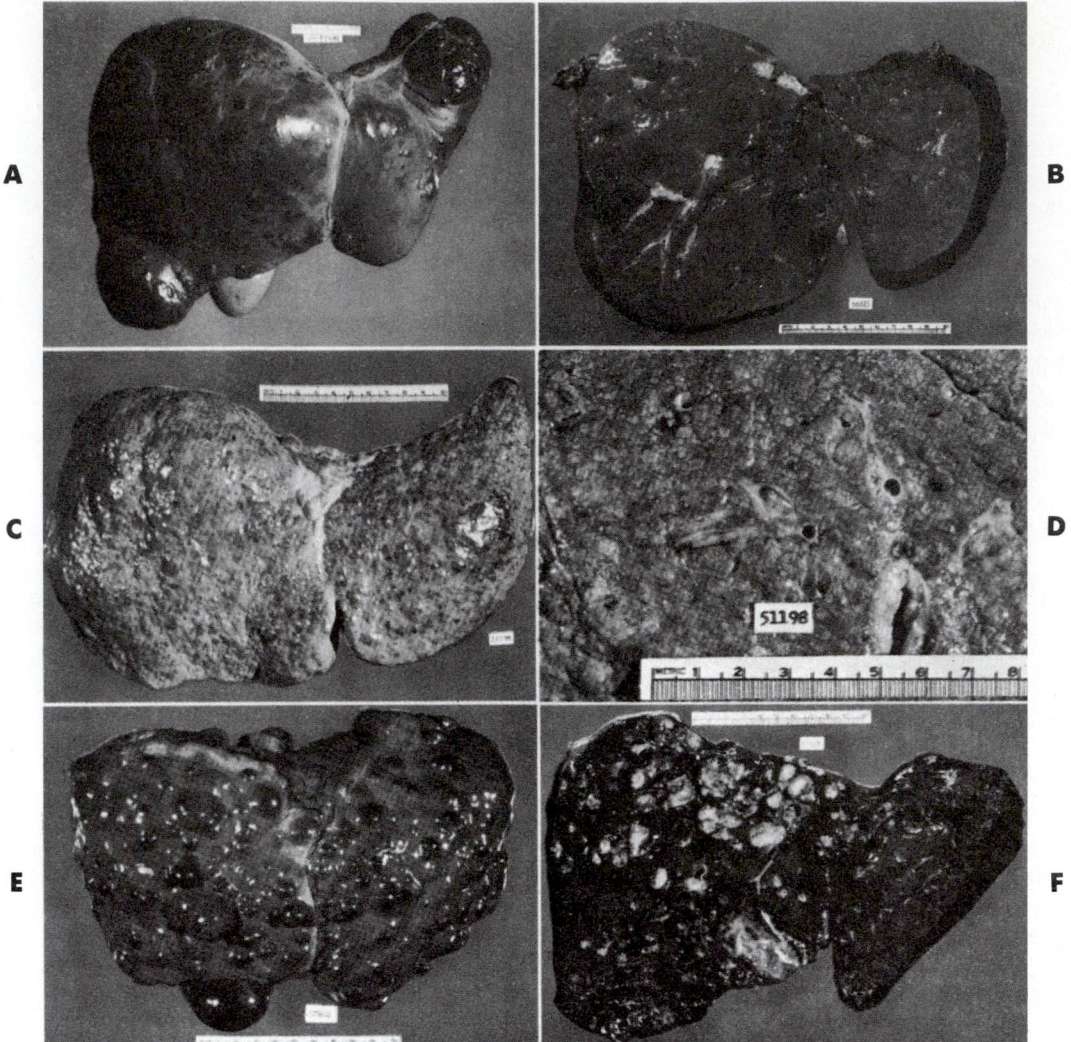

FIG. 36-16. Liver injury. **A,** Submassive hepatic necrosis from viral hepatitis, with bulging areas of residual liver and much shrinkage and collapse of left lobe. Individual lived 24 days after onset of clinical manifestations. **B,** Hypertrophic, firm, smooth alcoholic fatty liver. **C,** Eutrophic, hard, finely pseudolobular alcoholic cirrhosis in a 65-year-old man. **D,** Cut surface of alcoholic cirrhosis showing pseudolobular pattern. **E,** Atrophic, firm, megalonodular lupoid cirrhosis, quiescent in 20-year-old woman. **F,** Suppurative cholangitis with multiple abscesses resulting from carcinomatous obstruction of common duct. (From Kissane, 1985.)

cular channels. Examples of liver damage are shown in Fig. 36-16.

Alcoholic cirrhosis begins with fatty infiltration and cirrhosis. The relationship among these stages of alcoholic liver disease is not clear. Fatty infiltration can occur without subsequent hepatitis or cirrhosis. Fat deposition (deposition of tryglycerides) within the liver is primarily caused by increased lipogenesis and decreased fatty acid oxidation by hepatocytes. Lipids mobilized from adipose tissue or dietary fat intake may contribute to fat accumulation. Cessation of alcohol intake reverses the fatty accumulation.

The next stage, **alcoholic hepatitis,** is characterized by inflammation, degeneration, and necrosis of hepatocytes and infiltration of polymorphonuclear leukocytes and lymphocytes. The injured hepatocytes contain Mallory bodies (hyaline endoplasmic reticulum). The presence of Mallory bodies indicates the onset of fibrosis. The mechanism of hepatocyte injury is not clearly understood, but immunologic factors are suspected. Serum IgA is often elevated in individuals with alcoholic hepatitis, and liver antigens and antibodies have been identified in those with progressive alcoholic liver disease. The inflammation and necrosis caused by alcoholic hep-

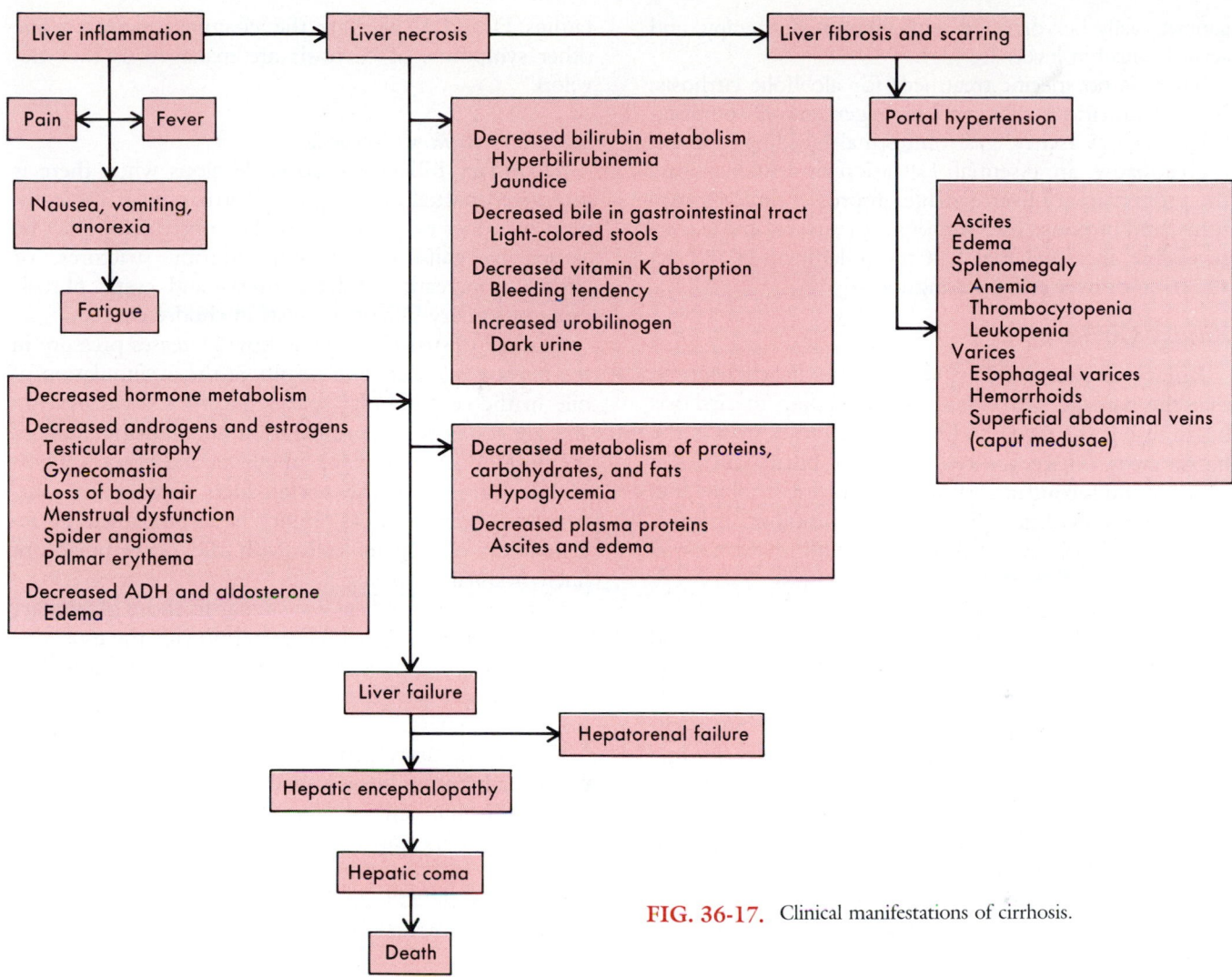

FIG. 36-17. Clinical manifestations of cirrhosis.

atitis stimulate the fibrosis characteristic of the cirrhotic stage of disease.

Clinical Manifestations

Fatty infiltration causes no specific symptoms or abnormal liver function test results. The liver is usually enlarged, however, and the individual has a history of continuous alcohol intake during the previous weeks or months. Anorexia, nausea, jaundice, and edema develop with advanced fatty infiltration or the onset of alcoholic hepatitis (Fig. 36-17).

The clinical manifestations of alcoholic hepatitis can be mild or severe. Nonspecific symptoms include fatigue, weight loss, and anorexia (Gine's et al., 1987). Manifestations of acute illness include nausea, anorexia, fever, abdominal pain, and jaundice. Cirrhosis causes hepatomegaly, splenomegaly, ascites, gastrointestinal hemorrhage, portal hypertension, hepatic encephalopathy, and esophageal varices. Anemia results from blood

loss, poor nutrition, and hypersplenism. The presence of numerous and severe manifestations increases the risk of death. The clinical features of alcoholic cirrhosis depend on the duration of the disease and the severity of liver damage.

Evaluation and Treatment

The diagnosis of alcoholic hepatitis is based on the individual's history and clinical manifestations. The results of liver function tests are abnormal, and serologic studies reveal elevated serum enzymes and bilirubin, decreased serum albumin, and prolonged prothrombin time.

Liver biopsy can confirm the diagnosis of cirrhosis, but biopsy is not necessary if clinical manifestations of cirrhosis are evident. Liver function test results are usually abnormal and reflect the severity of liver damage. In severe disease with a poor prognosis the serum albumin concentration is very low, prolonged prothrombin times cannot easily be corrected with vitamin K therapy, and serum bilirubin levels are high.

There is no specific treatment for alcoholic cirrhosis. Rest, a nutritious diet, and management of complications, such as ascites, gastrointestinal bleeding, and encephalopathy, are essential. Cessation of drinking slows the progression of liver damage, improves clinical symptoms, and prolongs life. Although the liver damage is irreversible, measures that halt the inflammation and destruction of liver cells prolong life.

Biliary Cirrhosis

Biliary cirrhosis differs from alcoholic cirrhosis in that the damage and inflammation leading to cirrhosis begin in bile canaliculi and bile ducts, rather than in the hepatocytes. There are two types of biliary cirrhosis: primary and secondary. Although both involve bile duct pathology, they differ with respect to etiology, risk factors, and mechanisms of obstruction and inflammation.

Primary Biliary Cirrhosis

Primary biliary cirrhosis causes inflammation and destruction of the intrahepatic bile ducts. Women are affected more commonly than men. Symptoms rarely develop before the age of 30 years. Primary biliary cirrhosis frequently accompanies collagen diseases, leading to speculation that autoimmune mechanisms initiate inflammation. The actual cause of the disease is unknown.

Primary biliary cirrhosis develops insidiously. It begins with inflammation, destruction, and fibrosis of the intrahepatic bile ducts. Nodular regeneration and cirrhosis follow. Portal hypertension develops during the later stages of the disease.

A significant number of individuals with primary biliary cirrhosis are asymptomatic. The earliest manifestations are pruritus, hyperbilirubinemia, jaundice, and light-colored stools. These symptoms are caused by intrahepatic obstruction of bile flow. Steatorrhea and fat-soluble vitamin deficiencies are present in some cases. Cirrhosis and symptoms of portal hypertension and encephalopathy ultimately develop. Life expectancy is about 5 to 10 years after onset of symptoms.

Serologic tests reveal elevated alkaline phosphatase levels and hyperlipidemia, with or without other clinical manifestations. Most individuals have a circulating IgG antimitochondrial antibody that is not found in other types of liver disease. Evaluation involves ruling out biliary obstruction caused by gallstones, tumor, or inflammation of the common bile duct (i.e., secondary biliary cirrhosis). Liver biopsy usually confirms the diagnosis of primary biliary cirrhosis.

No specific treatment is available. The distressing pruritus may be relieved by cholestyramine, which binds bile salts in the intestine. Intramuscular injections of vitamins D and K alleviate the vitamin deficiency. The other symptoms of cirrhosis are managed as they develop.

Secondary Biliary Cirrhosis

Secondary biliary cirrhosis develops when there is prolonged partial or complete obstruction of the common bile duct or its branches. The obstruction may be caused by gallstones, tumors, fibrotic strictures, or chronic pancreatitis. Biliary atresia and cystic fibrosis cause secondary biliary cirrhosis in children.

Chronic obstruction to bile flow increases pressure in the hepatic bile duct and results in the accumulation of bile in the centrilobular spaces. Necrotic areas develop and are followed by proliferation and inflammation of the portal ducts that result in edema and fibrosis. Pools of bile form when the portal ducts rupture into surrounding necrotic areas. Injury is accompanied by regeneration of hepatic cells with the development of finely nodular cirrhosis.

Clinical manifestations are similar to those of primary biliary cirrhosis, with jaundice and pruritis the most distressing. Right upper quadrant pain is common, and there may be a low-grade fever from bile duct inflammation (cholangitis).

Cholangiography provides the most definitive diagnosis. Laboratory tests usually reveal elevated conjugated bilirubin and alkaline phophatase levels. Aminotransferase increases if there is an accompanying cholangitis. Surgery or endoscopy relieves obstruction, prolongs survival, and diminishes or resolves symptoms. Continued obstruction leads to advanced cirrhosis and liver failure.

Postnecrotic Cirrhosis

Postnecrotic cirrhosis is a consequence of many types of chronic, severe liver disease. Twenty-five percent of individuals with non-A, non-B hepatitis progress to postnecrotic cirrhosis. Liver injury results from drugs or toxins; inherited metabolic disorders, such as Wilson disease; α1-antitrypsin deficiency; advanced alcoholic cirrhosis; or primary biliary cirrhosis that progresses to postnecrotic cirrhosis.

Clinical manifestations represent a progression of symptoms associated with an earlier stage of liver disease. Portal hypertension with ascites, bleeding varices, hypersplenism, and encephalopathy are the most prominent symptoms. As a consequence of progressive liver injury, broad and dense bands of fibrosis separate islands of liver cells, giving the liver a nodular appearance. The liver is small in size and distorted in shape.

Diagnosis is confirmed by needle biopsy, and treatment is directed toward relief of symptoms. Death usually occurs as a result of bleeding or encephalopathy.

Disorders of the Gallbladder

Obstruction and inflammation are the most common disorders of the gallbladder. Obstruction is caused by **gallstones,** which are aggregates of substances in the bile. The gallstones may remain in the gallbladder or be ejected, with bile, into the cystic duct. Gallstones that become lodged in the cystic duct obstruct the flow of bile into and out of the gallbladder and cause inflammation. Gallstone formation is termed **cholelithiasis.** Inflammation of the gallbladder or cystic duct is known as **cholecystitis.**

Cholelithiasis

Cholelithiasis is a prevalent disorder in developed countries, where incidence is 10% to 20%. The actual incidence is unknown because many individuals who have gallstones are asymptomatic. Gallstones are of two types: cholesterol and pigmented. Cholesterol stones are the most common. Risk factors include obesity, middle age, female gender, American Indian ancestry, and gallbladder, pancreatic, or ileal disease. Pigmented stones, which are common, occur later in life and are associated with cirrhosis.

Pathophysiology

Cholesterol gallstones form in bile that is supersaturated with cholesterol. Supersaturation sets the stage for cholesterol crystal formation, or the formation of "microstones." More crystals then aggregate on the microstones, which grow to form "macrostones." This process usually occurs in the gallbladder. The stones may lie "silent" or become lodged in the cystic or common duct, causing pain and cholecystitis. Gallstone formation may be such that the stones accumulate and fill the entire gallbladder (Fig. 36-18).

It is not known why the hepatocytes secrete bile that is supersaturated with cholesterol. Proposed mechanisms include (1) an enzymatic defect that affects the hepatocytes' synthesis of cholesterol; (2) diminished secretion of bile acids, which normally promote cholesterol solubility; (3) decreased resorption of bile salts from the ileum, which decrease the bile acid pool; and (4) some combination of these mechanisms. In obese individuals the mechanism appears to involve cholesterol synthesis, whereas in nonobese individuals, it appears to involve decreased secretion of bile acids.

Pigmented stones are created by cholesterol, calcium bilirubinate, or pigmented polymers. The formation of pigmented stones is associated with increased amounts of unconjugated bilirubin in bile. The unconjugated bilirubin precipitates in the gallbladder to form the stones.

Clinical Manifestations

Abdominal pain and jaundice are the cardinal manifestations of cholelithiasis. Vague symptoms include heartburn, flatulence, epigastric discomfort, and food intolerances, particularly to fats and cabbage. The pain, frequently called biliary colic, is caused by the lodging of one or more gallstones in the cystic or common duct. The pain can be intermittent or steady. It usually is located in the right upper quadrant and radiates to the midupper back. Jaundice indicates that the stone is located in the common bile duct. Abdominal tenderness and fever indicate cholecystitis.

Evaluation and Treatment

Diagnosis is based on the history, physical examination, and radiographic evaluation. An oral cholecystogram usually outlines the stones. Intravenous cholangiography is used to differentiate cholelithiasis from

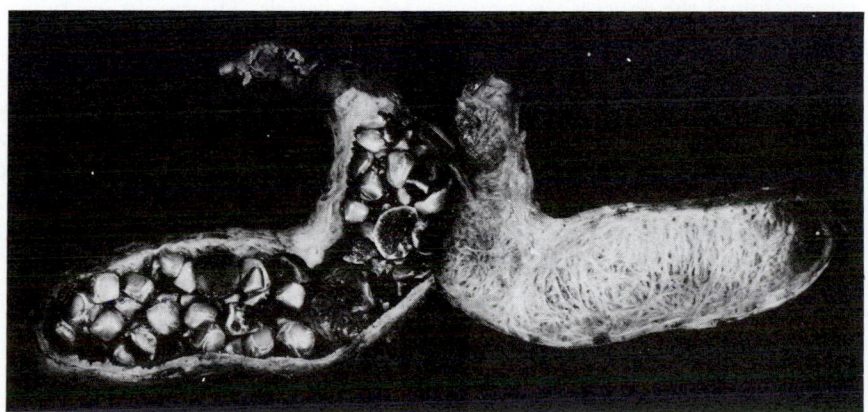

FIG. 36-18. Resected gallbladder containing mixed gallstones. (From Kissane, 1985.)

other causes of extrahepatic biliary obstruction if the cholecystogram is negative. Endoscopic or percutaneous cholangiography is also a diagnostic option.

Surgical removal is the traditional treatment for gallstones that cause obstruction or inflammation. An alternative treatment is the administration of drugs that dissolve the stones. For example, the bile acid chenodeoxycholic acid (CDCA) can completely or partially dissolve cholesterol gallstones. Ursodeoxycholic acid (UDCA), which is structurally similar to CDCA, is also effective, is less toxic to hepatocytes, and does not cause fatty diarrhea, as does CDCA.

Cholecystitis

Cholecystitis can be acute or chronic. Both forms are almost always caused by the lodging of a gallstone in the cystic duct. Obstruction causes the gallbladder to become distended and inflamed. The pain is similar to that caused by gallstones. Pressure against the distended wall of the gallbladder decreases blood flow. Ischemia, necrosis, and perforation of the gallbladder are possible. Fever, leukocytosis, rebound tenderness, and abdominal muscle guarding are common findings. Serum bilirubin and alkaline phosphatase levels may be elevated. Nevertheless the acute abdominal pain of cholecystitis must be differentiated from the pain caused by other disorders, such as pancreatitis, myocardial infarction, and acute pyelonephritis of the right kidney. Cholangiography or radioactive scan can confirm a diagnosis of cholecystitis.

Narcotics may be required to control pain, and antibiotics (e.g., gentamycin and clindomycin) are often prescribed to manage bacterial infection in severe cases. Persistent symptoms or development of chronic cholecystitis punctuated by recurrent, acute attacks usually requires gallbladder resection (cholecystectomy). If pancreatic abscesses develop, they are usually resected (Domschke, 1987).

Disorders of the Pancreas

Pancreatitis, or inflammation of the pancreas, is a relatively rare and potentially serious disorder. Incidence is about equal in men and women. The disease is most common during the fiftieth decade of life (Trapnell & Duncan, 1975). Pancreatitis can be acute or chronic. It is associated with several other clinical conditions, including alcoholism, obstructive biliary tract disease (particularly cholelithiasis), peptic ulcers, trauma, hyperlipidemia, and certain drugs (Ammann & Warshaw, 1985).

Acute Pancreatitis

Pathophysiology

Acute pancreatitis, also called acute hemorrhagic pancreatitis, is a severe pancreatic inflammation requiring hospital care. In many cases the precise pathogenic mechanism or sequence of events that triggers acute pancreatitis is unknown. Many causal factors are probably involved. The most common theory is that pancreatitis develops because of an injury or disruption of the pancreatic ducts or acini, which permits leakage of pancreatic enzymes into pancreatic tissue. The leaked enzymes become activated in the tissue, initiating autodigestion and acute pancreatitis. The exact mechanism of enzyme activation remains to be described (Steer, 1988), but activation is known to occur in the presence of bile. Bile reflux into the pancreas occurs if gallstones obstruct the common bile duct. The activated proteolases (trypsin, elastase, and lipases) break down tissue and cell membranes causing edema, vascular damage, hemorrhage, and necrosis (Nevalainen & Aho, 1987). (Fatty necrosis is described in Chapter 2.) Toxic enzymes also are released into the bloodstream and cause injury to vessels and other organs, such as the lungs and kidneys. These systemic effects are major causes of morbidity and mortality.

Clinical Manifestations

Epigastric or midabdominal pain is the cardinal symptom of acute pancreatitis. It can range from mild abdominal discomfort to severe, incapacitating pain. The pain may radiate to the back because of the retroperitoneal location of the pancreas. The pain is caused by edema, which distends the pancreatic ducts and capsule; chemical irritation and inflammation of the peritoneum; and irritation or obstruction of the biliary tract. Fever and leukocytosis accompany the inflammatory response.

Nausea and vomiting are common. These gastrointestinal symptoms are caused by hypermotility or paralytic ileus secondary to the pancreatitis or peritonitis.

Abdominal distention accompanies bowel hypermotility and the accumulation of fluids in the peritoneal cavity. Hypotension and shock occur frequently because plasma volume is lost as enzymes and kinins released into the circulation increase vascular permeability and dilate vessels. The results are hypovolemia, hypotension, and myocardial insufficiency. A small percentage of individuals develop tachypnea and hypoxemia secondary to pulmonary edema, atelectasis, or pleural effusions caused by circulating pancreatic enzymes. In severe cases hypovolemia decreases renal blood flow sufficiently to impair renal function. Tetany may develop as a result of deposition of calcium in areas of fat necrosis or as a decreased response to parahormone. Transient hyperglycemia can also occur if glucagon is released from damaged alpha cells in the pancreatic islets.

Evaluation and Treatment

Diagnosis of pancreatitis is based on clinical findings, identification of associated disorders, and laboratory studies. Elevated serum amylase is a characteristic diagnostic feature. The amylase level usually rises within 12 hours after the onset of symptoms and returns to normal within 3 to 5 days in most cases. Urine amylase and serum lipase are also elevated. The ratio of amylase clearance to creatinine clearance by the kidney can be diagnostic because, in cases of pancreatitis, amylase clearance increases significantly compared to creatinine clearance. Acute pancreatitis is difficult to diagnose because several other disorders can cause similar clinical and laboratory findings. These disorders include perforating duodenal ulcer, acute cholecystitis, small bowel obstruction, and kidney stones.

The goal of treatment for acute pancreatitis is to stop the process of autodigestion and prevent systemic complications. Narcotic medications may be needed to relieve pain. Demerol is used instead of morphine because it causes less spasm of the sphincter of Oddi than morphine. To decrease pancreatic secretions and "rest the gland," oral food and fluids are withheld and continuous gastric suction is instituted. Nasogastric suction may not be necessary with mild pancreatitis, but it helps to relieve pain and prevent paralytic ileus in individuals who are nauseated and vomiting. Parenteral fluids are given to restore blood volume and prevent hypotension and shock. Parenteral hyperalimentation may be required to reverse the catabolic state associated with severe pancreatitis. Drugs that decrease gastric acid production (e.g., cimetidine) can decrease stimulation of the pancreas by secretin. Severe, unremitting pancreatitis may require peritoneal lavage to remove toxic exudates or surgical drainage of the pancreas. The risk of mortality increases significantly with the development of pulmonary, cardiac, and renal complications.

Chronic Pancreatitis

Structural or functional impairment of the pancreas leads to **chronic pancreatitis.** Chronic alcohol abuse is the most common cause. Chronic pancreatitis causes continuous or intermittent abdominal pain, which usually intensifies after a meal. Individuals who require narcotic medications to relieve pain are at high risk for narcotic addiction. Occasionally manifestations of pancreatic enzyme deficiency, such as steatorrhea or a malabsorption syndrome, are present. To correct enzyme deficiencies and prevent malabsorption, oral enzyme replacements are taken before and during meals. Loss of islet cell function can cause insulin-dependent diabetes. Cessation of alcohol intake is essential for the management of chronic pancreatitis.

Pancreatic cysts are common lesions of chronic pancreatitis. The cysts are walled-off areas or pockets of pancreatic juice, necrotic debris, or blood within or adjacent to the pancreas. Surgical drainage or partial resection of the pancreas may be required to relieve pain and prevent cystic rupture.

CANCER OF THE DIGESTIVE SYSTEM

Cancer of the Gastrointestinal Tract

Cancer of the Esophagus

Carcinoma of the esophagus is a rare disease. The incidence in the United States and Europe is less than 1% of new cancers per year (American Cancer Society, 1989). The incidence in the United States is higher in blacks than in whites and peaks at about 60 years of age.

Dietary factors, particularly deficiencies of trace elements and vitamins, possibly influence carcinogenesis. Esophageal cancer is strongly associated with malnutrition caused by poor economic conditions, special dietary habits, or alcoholism (Dowlatshahi et al., 1984). Alcohol and tobacco use have long been established as risk factors for esophageal cancer. The risk of esophageal cancer increases with the amount of alcohol consumed. Alcohol abuse, in combination with dietary zinc deficiency, renders the esophageal mucosa susceptible to carcinogens. Although heavy cigarette smoking is known to increase the risk of esophageal cancer, esophageal cancer is found more frequently in pipe and cigar smokers than cigarette smokers.

Reflux esophagitis is associated with carcinomas of the esophagus, as is sliding hiatal hernia. Both of these conditions can cause erosive esophagitis and ulceration that can eventually lead to metaplasia and neoplastic changes.

Pathogenesis

Carcinoma of the esophagus is usually squamous cell carcinoma or, less commonly, adenocarcinoma. Adenocarcinomas of the esophagus are frequently secondary to infiltration by a gastric carcinoma or to the presence of Barrett's epithelium (columnar rather than squamous epithelium in the lower esophagus), which is associated with chronic gastroesophageal reflux. Carcinomas can occur at any level of the esophageal tract but are most common where the esophagus joins the stomach (the gastroesophageal junction).

The pathogenesis of esophageal carcinoma is facilitated by (1) alterations of esophageal structure and function that permit food and drink to remain in the esophagus for prolonged periods of time, (2) ulceration and metaplasia caused by esophageal reflux, and (3) chronic exposure to irritants, such as alcohol and tobacco, that cause neoplastic transformation (see Chapter 11). Chronic inadequate nutrition can impair both structure and function of the esophagus. Nutritional deprivation, particularly deficiencies of vitamin A and zinc, results in mucosal changes that make the esophageal mucosa vulnerable to neoplastic changes.

Clinical Manifestations

The two main manifestations of esophageal carcinoma are chest pain and dysphagia. The most common type of pain is heartburn (pyrosis). It is initiated by eating spicy or highly seasoned foods and by lying down. Dysphagia (pain on swallowing), another common symptom, is usually pressurelike and may radiate posteriorly between the scapulae. Odynophagia may be initiated by the swallowing of cold liquids. Spontaneous chest pain is more difficult to diagnose positively. Some individuals with esophageal cancer complain of a constant retrosternal pain that radiates to the back. Dysphagia usually progresses rapidly. It is mostly painless during the early stages of esophageal carcinoma.

Evaluation and Treatment

Individuals who present with dysphagia undergo endoscopy so that specimens can be obtained and examined for neoplastic change. Computed tomography (CT) studies of the thorax are also used for diagnosis. Esophageal cancer metastasizes rapidly and therefore has a poor prognosis. The lymphatic vessels of the esophagus are continuous with vital mediastinal structures and drain to the lymph nodes from the neck of the celiac axis, making it impossible to remove all the lymph nodes with the tumor. Removal of the primary lesion and the local lymph nodes can, however, benefit the individual with esophageal cancer. If the malignancy has not spread beyond these sites, cure is likely. If spread has occurred, however, an incomplete resection is of little benefit.

Cancer of the Stomach

Although the incidence of gastric cancer has declined in the United States, it still represents about 2% of all new cancer cases annually (American Cancer Society, 1989). In countries such as Japan, the British Isles, and Iceland, the incidence of stomach cancer has remained high consistently. The incidence rate in Japan is one of the highest in the world. Studies of Japanese immigrants to the United States show that offspring who are born and raised in the United States have an incidence rate comparable to that of Americans. These data illustrate the importance of environmental factors, such as diet, to carcinogenesis.

The most important environmental factors in the etiology of gastric cancer are (1) salt added to food; (2) food additives (e.g., nitrates) in pickled or salted foods (e.g., bacon); and (3) food factors found in water and vegetables, such as vitamin C (vitamin C is possibly a protective factor). Dietary salt enhances the conversion of nitrates to carcinogenic nitrosamines in the stomach. Salt is also caustic to the stomach and can cause chronic atrophic gastritis. Finally hypertonic salt solutions delay gastric emptying. Delayed emptying increases the time during which carcinogenic nitrosamines can exert their effects on the stomach mucosa.

The metabolism of nitrates and nitrites is very complex. Nitrates interact with amino acids in the stomach to form nitrosamines. The conversion of these carcinogenic nitrosamines is enhanced at a low pH by iodides and thiocyanotes. Nitrates are thought to be active only when converted to nitrites and to cause stomach cancer once atrophic gastritis has occurred.

The incidence of gastric cancer is greater in males than in females. Other nonenvironmental risk factors are a family history of gastric adenocarcinoma, blood type (blood group A), and pernicious anemia, which causes atrophy of the gastric mucosa in the same locations where gastric tumors arise.

Pathogenesis

Gastric cancer usually begins in the glands of the stomach mucosa. About 50% of all gastric cancers develop in the prepyloric antrum (Fig. 36-19). Atrophic gastritis and intestinal metaplasia are strongly linked to the development of gastric cancer. Insufficient acid secretion by the atrophic mucosa creates a relatively alkaline environment that permits bacteria to multiply and act on nitrates. The resulting increase in nitrosoamines damages the DNA of mucosal cells further, promoting metaplasia and neoplasia. Duodenal reflux may also contribute to intestinal metaplasia. The reflux contains caustic bile salts that destroy the mucosal barrier that normally protects the stomach.

Clinical Manifestations

The early stages of gastric cancer are generally asymptomatic or produce vague symptoms such as loss of appetite (especially for meat), malaise, and "indigestion." Later manifestations of gastric cancer include unex-

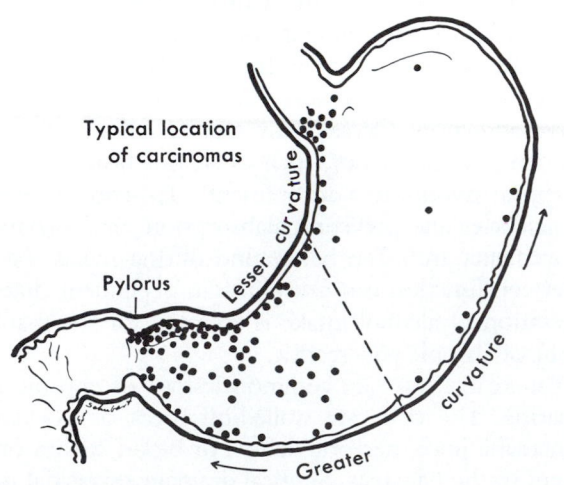

FIG. 36-19. Typical sites of stomach cancer. (From del Regato, Spjut, & Cox, 1985.)

plained weight loss, upper abdominal pain, vomiting, change in bowel habits, and anemia caused by persistent occult bleeding. The prognosis is poor because symptoms do not occur until the tumor has penetrated the muscle layers of the stomach, spread to surrounding tissues, and entered the draining lymph nodes and veins, causing distant metastases. Generally the first manifestations of carcinoma are caused by distant metastases.

Evaluation and Treatment

The choice of diagnostic tests depends on the clinical manifestations at the time of presentation. Most symptoms suggest a problem in the upper gastrointestinal tract, and the lesion is revealed by a barium x-ray film. Direct endoscopic visualization and biopsy usually establish the diagnosis. Another definitive technique is microscopic examination of exfoliated cells obtained by lavage during endoscopy.

Surgery is the usual treatment for gastric cancer. Staging is determined by pathologic findings following resection. Radiotherapy is generally unsuccessful, and immunotherapy is still experimental. Chemotherapy sometimes reduces the tumor. Individuals who respond well to chemotherapy generally live longer than those who do not.

Cancer of the Colon and Rectum

Cancer of the lower intestinal tract (colorectal cancer) is the second most frequent cause of cancer death in the United States, for both men and women. Colorectal cancer accounts for 10% to 15% of all cancer deaths (American Cancer Society, 1989). Cancer of the colon tends to occur in individuals over 50 years of age. It is rare in children. Worldwide the prevalence of colorectal cancer is highest in the United States and lowest in Japan, Finland, Puerto Rico, and Africa. Incidence is greatest in populations with high socioeconomic standards, possibly because of dietary habits.

Pathogenesis

Colorectal polyps are closely associated with development of cancer. A polyp, or papilloma, is a fingerlike projection arising from the mucosal epithelium. Most polyps are benign. The two major types of neoplastic polyps are: pedunculated (stalk), adenomatous polyps and sessile (papillary or villous) adenomas (Fig. 36-20). Once the adenoma traverses the muscularis mucosa, it becomes invasive and highly malignant. Adenomas can be detected early, however, and the submucosa may not be penetrated for several years. The larger the polyp, the greater the risk of colorectal cancer. Although lesions larger than 1.5 cm occur less frequently, they are more likely to be malignant than those smaller than 1.0 cm. For other conditions commonly confused with colorectal cancer see Table 36-11.

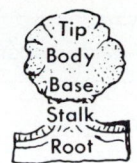

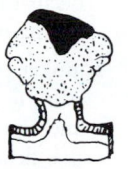 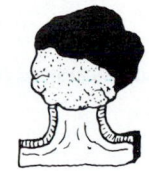

Focal atypia (cancer in situ)   Focal cancer (malignant adenoma)

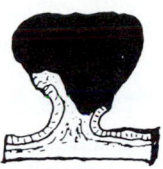 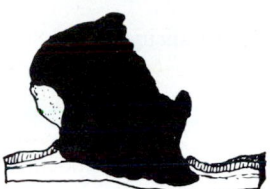

Focal cancer invading stalk with some "benign" polyp still in body

Invasive cancer containing piece of polyp

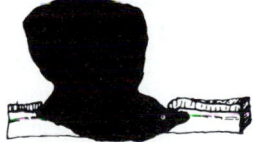 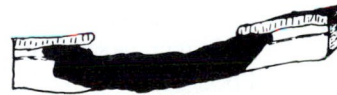

Polypoid invasive cancer without polyp remnant

Ulcerated invasive cancer without polyp remnant

FIG. 36-20. Development of cancer of the colon from adenomatous polyps. The tumor becomes invasive if it penetrates the muscularis mucosa and enters the submucosal layer. (From del Regato, Spjut, & Cox, 1985.)

Most colorectal cancers are moderately differentiated adenocarcinomas. These tumors have a long preinvasive phase, and when they invade they tend to grow slowly. Colorectal carcinoma starts in the glands of the mucosal lining. Because the lymphatic channels are located underneath the muscularis mucosa, the lesions must transverse this layer before metastasis can occur.

Clinical Manifestations

Tumors of the right (ascending) and left (descending) colon evolve into two distinct tumor types. On the right side the lesions are polypoid and extend along one wall of the cecum and ascending colon. Clinical manifestations include pain, palpable mass in the lower right

TABLE 36–11 Conditions commonly confused with colorectal cancer

Condition	Significant characteristics
Diverticulitis	Left-sided pain similar to that of appendicitis; tender lower left quadrant. Associated findings: nausea, vomiting, fever, obstruction, anorexia, and leukocytosis; mucosa is intact, and perforation peritonitis, and abscesses, occur more frequently than in cancer; protosigmoidoscopy and/or barium enema used to distinguish from cancer
Chronic ulcerative colitis	Younger people with chronic attacks of bloody diarrhea, crampy abdominal pain, fever, malnutrition, and dehydration; usually involves the left colon and rectum; endoscopy, barium enema, and biopsy performed for definitive diagnosis
Crohn disease (granulomatous colitis)	Generally involves the right colon; chronic diarrhea with abdominal cramps, fever, weight loss, and often a palpable abdominal mass; difficult at times to distinguish Crohn disease from ulcerative colitis; endoscopic examination and barium enema used to distinguish from cancer
Appendicitis	Vague abdominal symptoms, often with a tender or nontender mass in the lower right quadrant; associated symptoms: mild fever and leukycytosis; barium enema used to distinguish cancer of the cecum from appendiceal abscess
Thrombosed hemorrhoids	Examination shows a tender, swollen, bluish painful mass in the anus; patient will have a history of hemorroids

quadrant, anemia, and dark red or mahogany-colored blood mixed with the stool (Fig. 36-21). These large, bulky tumors become necrotic and ulcerated, contributing to persistent blood loss and anemia. Obstruction is unusual because the growth does not readily encircle the colon.

Tumors of the left or descending colon start as small, elevated buttonlike masses. This type grows circumferentially and spreads along the entire bowel wall, eventually ulcerating in the middle as the tumor penetrates the blood supply. Obstruction is frequent but occurs slowly. Manifestations include progressive abdominal distention, pain, vomiting, constipation, need for laxatives, cramps, and bright red blood on the surface of the stool.

Systematic lymphatic spread occurs along the aorta to the mesenteric and pancreatic lymph nodes. Liver metastasis follows invasion of the mesenteric veins (left colon) or superior veins (right colon), which drain into the portal circulation.

Rectal carcinomas are defined as tumors occurring up to 15 cm from the anal opening. Tumors of the rectum can spread through the rectal wall to nearby structures: the prostate in men and the vagina in women. Penetration occurs more readily in the lower third of the rectum because it has no serosal covering. Systemic and pulmonary metastases occur through the hemorrhoidal plexus, which drains into the vena cava.

Evaluation and Treatment

The staging of colorectal cancer involves preoperative testing and operative exploration. Preoperative testing begins with physical examination of the abdomen to detect liver enlargement and ascites and palpate appropriate lymph nodes. Elevations of carcinoembryonic antigen (CEA) are often detected in the sera of individuals with colorectal carcinoma. The amount of CEA in the serum is a function of the stage of the disease and the type of tumor. Operative staging consists of careful exploration during surgery and biopsy of possible metastases. The Duke classification for staging of colorectal cancer is as follows:

Stage A: cancer limited to the bowel wall

Stage B: cancer extending through the bowel wall

Stage C: nodal metastases regardless of extension into bowel wall

Stage D: distant metastases regardless of primary size

Treatment for cancer of the colon is always surgical. The location and amount of colon resected depend on the site of the cancer. Resection and anastomosis can be performed for cancer of the ascending, transverse, descending, or sigmoid colon and upper rectum. These surgeries are performed through abdominal incisions and natural defecation is preserved.

Growths in the lower portion of the rectum require removal of the entire rectum. The proximal end of the descending colon is brought out through a small inci-

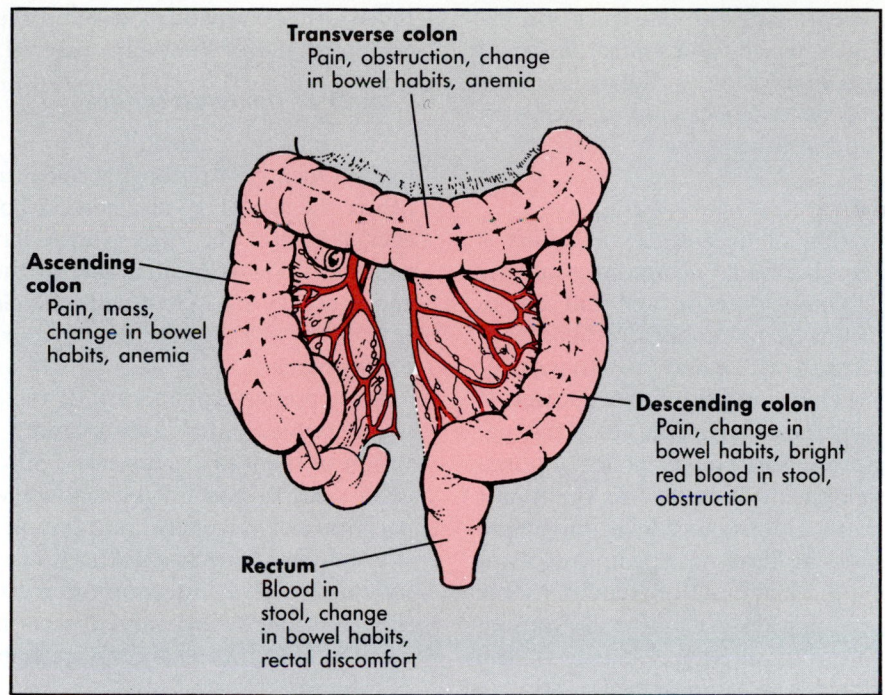

FIG. 36-21. Signs and symptoms of colorectal cancer by location of primary lesion. Clinical manifestations are listed in order of frequency for each region (lymphatics of colon also shown).

sion in the abdominal wall and becomes a permanent colostomy. Prognosis after surgery depends on the stage and location of the tumor.

Radiation therapy is often given before surgery in the hope that it will shrink the tumor, alter the malignant cells, or do both, so that these cells will not survive after surgery. Chemotherapy is used to treat metastatic disease and cases with a high risk of recurrence. Immunotherapy can boost the immune response.

Cancer of the Accessory Organs of Digestion
Cancer of the Liver

Cancer of the liver is usually caused by metastatic spread from a primary site elsewhere in the body. Primary liver cancer is relatively rare in the United States but is common in densely populated parts of the Far East, Southern Africa, China, and Greece. In the United States the incidence of primary liver cancer is higher in blacks than in whites (2 to 10 per 100,000 per annum). For reasons not understood, incidence is higher in males than in females. Primary liver cancer is rare before age 40 and most common during the sixth decade. Together, primary and secondary liver cancer account for 2% of all cancer deaths in the United States (American Cancer Society, 1989).

Risk factors for primary liver cancer include the following:

1. Exposure to mycotoxins. The most significant mycotoxins are the aflatoxins, particularly those pro-

duced by *Aspergillus flavus,* a mold found on spoiled corn, peanuts, and grain.
2. Chronic liver disease, especially cirrhosis.
3. Infection with hepatitis B virus (HBV), particularly in conjunction with cirrhosis. Hepatitis B virus acts either as a carcinogen or as a cocarcinogen in chronically infected hepatocytes.

Pathogenesis

Primary carcinomas of the liver are hepatocellular or cholangiocellular. **Hepatocellular carcinoma** (hepatocarcinoma) develops in the hepatocytes, whereas **cholangiocellular carcinoma** (cholangiocarcinoma) develops in the bile ducts. Hepatocellular carcinoma can be nodular (consisting of multiple, discrete nodules), massive (consisting of a large tumor mass having satellite nodules), or diffuse (consisting of very small nodules distributed throughout most of the liver). Hepatocellular carcinoma is the type of primary liver cancer that is closely associated with cirrhosis. Since carcinoma of the liver invades the hepatic and portal veins, it often spreads to the heart and lungs. Other sites of metastases are the brain, kidney, and spleen.

Cholangiocellular carcinomas occur less frequently than hepatocellular carcinomas. This type of primary liver cancer is most common in areas where liver fluke infestation is prevalent, such as Southeast China. The mechanism by which fluke infestation causes cholangiocellular carcinoma is unknown. Cholangiocellular carcinoma can occur anywhere along the bile duct and extend directly into the liver, usually as a solitary lesion. It is difficult to distinguish an invasion of cholangiocellular carcinoma from a metastatic adenocarcinoma except by neoplastic changes found in nearby ducts.

Clinical Manifestations

The clinical presentation of liver cancer in adults is characterized by vague abdominal symptoms, such as nausea and vomiting, fullness, pressure, and dull ache in the right hypochondrium. Manifestations of hepatocellular carcinoma can occur slowly or abruptly. In individuals with cirrhosis, deepening jaundice or abrupt lack of appetite is a sign of hepatocellular carcinoma. Obstruction by the tumor can cause sudden worsening of portal hypertension and development of ascites. As the tumor enlarges, it causes pain. Cholangiocellular carcinoma more commonly presents insidiously as pain, loss of appetite, weight loss, and gradual onset of jaundice. Some carcinomas of the liver rupture spontaneously, causing hemorrhage. Others are discovered accidentally during evaluation of a bone fracture or surgical exploration.

Evaluation and Treatment

There is no specific test for the diagnosis of liver cancer. The diagnosis is based on clinical manifestations, laboratory findings, radiologic examination, and exploratory laparotomy.

Levels of alkaline phosphatase, serum glutamic oxaloacetic transaminase (AST), and serum glutamic pyruvic transaminase (ALT) are commonly elevated in individuals with hepatocellular carcinoma. α-Fetoprotein is elevated (in excess of 400 ng/ml) in individuals with advanced hepatocellular carcinoma. Excessive levels of α-fetoprotein have been correlated with hepatitis B antigen, rapid tumor growth, and poor tumor differentiation. Erythrocytosis is secondary to erythropoietin production.

In individuals without cirrhosis liver scans can document filling defects. Computed tomography or ultrasonography is used to detect solid tumors, but neither can distinguish benign from malignant tumors. A liver biopsy can be diagnostic unless scattered nodules are missed by the examiner.

Surgical resection is possible only if the tumor is localized to a removable lobe of the liver. Tumors of the posterior segment of the right lobe are not resectable because this segment contains the right hepatic vein. Chemotherapeutic agents are administered systemically or locally. Radiation is not part of the treatment regimen because the dosages needed for effectiveness exceed the tolerance of liver tissue.

The overall median survival rate for individuals with liver cancer is only 3 to 4 months. Surgery is hazardous and is usually not undertaken if the individual has cirrhosis. Most individuals develop metastases after surgical resection, but long-term survival is possible.

Cancer of the Gallbladder

Cancer of the gallbladder is more common in women than in men by a ratio of about 3 to 1. It occurs rarely before the age of 40 and is most common between the ages of 50 and 60. Most gallbladder cancer is caused by metastasis. Primary carcinoma of the gallbladder is rare and is usually associated with cholelithiasis.

Pathogenesis

Most primary carcinomas of the gallbladder are adenocarcinomas. A few are squamous cell carcinomas. Invasion of the liver occurs early. Spreading occurs to the cystic and periportal lymph nodes with invasion of the pancreas and retroperitoneal lymph nodes. Direct invasion of the stomach and the duodenum can cause pyloric obstruction. Infection often accompanies cancer of the gallbladder. Generalized peritonitis, gangrene, perforation, and liver abscesses are potential complications of infection.

Clinical Manifestations

A typical presentation of carcinoma of the gallbladder is steady, upper-right-quadrant pain for a couple of months. Other manifestations include diarrhea, belching, weakness, loss of appetite, weight loss, and vomiting. Obstructive jaundice can occur if an enlarging tumor presses on the extrahepatic ducts.

Evaluation and Treatment

Early diagnosis of cancer of the gallbladder is not possible. Therefore, individuals with gallstones, especially older women, are evaluated carefully. Inflammatory disorders, such as cholangitis (bile duct inflammation) and peritonitis, often obscure an underlying malignancy. The most diagnostic procedure is the upper gastrointestinal barium study.

Complete surgical resection of the gallbladder is the only effective treatment. Because advanced malignancies cannot be resected, gallbladders containing stones are removed as a preventive measure. The prognosis of gallbladder cancer is extremely poor; most individuals die 1 year after surgery.

Cancer of the Pancreas

Pancreatic cancer now ranks fifth as a cause of cancer deaths in the United States. The incidence of pancreatic cancer rises steadily with age. Males are affected slightly more often than females, and blacks more often than whites. Pancreatic cancer accounts for about 25,000 deaths annually in the United States (American Cancer Society, 1989). The mortality rate is nearly 100%. The etiology of pancreatic cancer is not known, and with the exception of an association of risk with cigarette smoking, no external risk factors have been identified (American Cancer Society, 1988).

Pathogenesis

Cancer of the pancreas can arise from exocrine or endocrine cells. Most pancreatic tumors arise from exocrine cells in the ducts and are called ductal adenocarcinomas. Tumors arising in small ducts invade nearby glandular tissue, penetrate the covering of the pancreas, and extend into surrounding tissues.

Ductal adenocarcinomas can occur in the head, body, or tail of the pancreas. Tumors of the head quickly spread to obstruct the common bile duct and portal vein. These tumors can then infiltrate the superior mesenteric artery, the vena cava, and the aorta. Cancer cells that enter the blood vessels can form emboli. Tumors of the body and tail infiltrate the posterior abdominal wall. Lymphatic invasion occurs early and rapidly and involves local and regional lymph nodes. Venous invasion causes metastases to the liver. Tumor implants on the peritoneal surface can obstruct veins and promote development of ascites.

Ductal adenocarcinomas arising in the head of the pancreas cause biliary obstruction somewhat early in the disease. Individuals with such tumors survive slightly longer than those with cancer of the body and tail, presumably because they seek medical attention earlier.

Tumors of the endocrine pancreas are rare neoplasms of the islets of Langerhans known as "apudomas." The *apu* in *apudoma* is an acronym for *amine precursor uptake* and decarboxylation. The apudomas are so named because they contain neurosecretory granules. Endocrine neoplasms are fatal because they secrete abnormal amounts of hormones, such as insulin.

Clinical Manifestations

Cancer of the body and tail of the pancreas is generally asymptomatic until the tumor invades adjacent tissue. Frequently vague back pain is an initial symptom. Jaundice develops in most cases, usually caused by obstruction of the bile duct. Because it impairs enzyme secretion and flow to the duodenum, pancreatic cancer causes fat and protein malabsorption, resulting in weight loss. Distant metastases are found in the neck nodes, the lungs, and the brain. Most individuals die of hepatic failure, malnutrition, or systemic diseases.

Evaluation and Treatment

A laparotomy is often performed, particularly if jaundice is present. Ultrasonography and computed tomography may be needed to confirm the need for a laparotomy, especially in individuals without jaundice. Laparotomy is used to establish a definitive diagnosis, evaluate the extent of disease, and determine whether palliative bypass surgery (i.e., cholecystojejunostomy and gastrojejunostomy) is needed. Most individuals require palliative double bypass of the blocked bile ducts, as well as gastrojejunostomy to prevent duodenal obstruction.

Many surgeons recommend a total pancreatectomy because cancer of the pancreas seldom consists of a single lesion. Chemotherapy and radiation therapy are seldom beneficial, except as palliative measures. Because almost all pancreatic cancers are advanced at the time of diagnosis, staging has little relevance in determining treatment.

SUMMARY REVIEW

Disorders of the Gastrointestinal Tract

1 Anorexia (loss of appetite), vomiting, constipation, diarrhea, abdominal pain, and evidence of gastrointestinal bleeding are clinical manifestations of many disorders of the gastrointestinal tract.

2 Vomiting is the forceful emptying of the stomach effected by gastrointestinal contraction and reverse peristalsis of the esophagus. It is usually preceded by nausea and retching, with the exception of projectile vomiting, which is associated with direct stimulation of the vomiting center in the brain.

3 Constipation is frequently caused by unhealthy dietary and bowel habits combined with lack of exercise. Constipation can also result from a disorder that impairs intestinal motility or obstructs the intestinal lumen.

4 Diarrhea can be caused by excessive fluid drawn into the intestinal lumen by osmosis (osmotic diarrhea), excessive secretion of fluids by the intestinal mucosa (secretory diarrhea), or excessive gastrointestinal motility.

5 Abdominal pain is caused by stretching, inflammation, or ischemia (insufficient blood supply). Abdominal pain originates in the organs themselves (visceral pain) or in the peritoneum (parietal pain). Visceral pain is frequently referred to the back.

6 Obvious manifestations of gastrointestinal bleeding are hematemesis (vomiting of blood), melena (dark, tarry stools), and hematochezia (frank bleeding from the rectum). Occult bleeding can only be detected by testing stools or vomitus for presence of blood.

7 Dysphagia is difficulty in swallowing. It can be caused by a mechanical or functional obstruction of the esophagus. Functional obstruction is an impairment of esophageal motility.

8 Achalasia is a form of functional dysphagia caused by loss of esophageal innervation.

9 Gastroesophageal reflux is the regurgitation of chyme from the stomach into the esophagus. An inflammatory response (reflux esophagitis) ensues if the esophageal mucosa is repeatedly exposed to acids and enzymes in the regurgitated chyme.

10 Hiatal hernia is the protrusion of the upper part of the stomach through the hiatus (esophageal opening in the diaphragm) at the gastroesophageal junction. Hiatal hernia can be sliding or paraesophageal.

11 Pyloric obstruction is the narrowing or blockage of the pylorus, which is the opening between the stomach and the duodenum. It can be caused by a congenital defect, inflammation and scarring secondary to a gastric ulcer, or tumor growth.

12 Intestinal obstruction prevents the normal movement of chyme through the intestinal tract. It is usually mechanical, that is, caused by torsion, herniation, or tumor.

13 The most severe consequences of intestinal obstruction are fluid and electrolyte losses, hypovolemia, shock, intestinal necrosis, and perforation of the intestinal wall.

14 Gastritis is an acute or chronic inflammation of the gastric mucosa.

15 Regurgitation of bile, use of antiinflammatory drugs or alcohol, and some systemic diseases are associated with gastritis.

16 Chronic gastritis of the fundus and body is the most severe form of gastritis. It can result in gastric atrophy and decreased secretion of hydrochloric acid, pepsinogen, and intrinsic factor.

17 Chronic gastritis of the antrum, the most common type, is not usually associated with impaired secretion or gastric atrophy.

18 Appendicitis is the most common surgical emergency of the abdomen. Obstruction of the lumen leads to increased pressure, ischemia, and inflammation of the appendix. Inflammation may progress to gangrene, perforation, and peritonitis without surgical resection.

19 A peptic ulcer is a circumscribed area of mucosal inflammation and ulceration caused by excessive secretion of gastric acid, disruption of the protective mucosal barrier, or both.

20 There are three types of peptic ulcers: duodenal, gastric, and stress ulcers.

21 Duodenal ulcers, the most common peptic ulcers, are associated with increased numbers of parietal (acid-secreting) cells in the stomach, elevated gastrin levels, and rapid gastric emptying. Pain occurs when the stomach is empty and it is relieved with food or antacids. Duodenal ulcers tend to heal spontaneously and recur frequently.

22 Gastric ulcers develop near parietal cells, generally in the antrum, and tend to become chronic. Gastric secretions may be normal or decreased, and pain may occur after eating.

23 Ischemic stress ulcers develop suddenly after severe illness, systemic trauma, or neural injury. Ulceration follows mucosal damage caused by ischemia (decreased blood flow to the gastric mucosa).

24 Cushing ulcer is a stress ulcer caused by head trauma. Ulceration follows hypersecretion of hydrochloric acid caused by overstimulation of the vagal nuclei.

25 Postgastrectomy syndromes are long-term complications that follow gastrectomy, the resection of all or part of the stomach. The postgastrectomy syndromes include dumping syndrome, alkaline reflux gastritis, afferent loop obstruction, diarrhea, weight loss, and anemia.

26 Dumping syndrome is the rapid emptying of chyme into the small intestine. It causes an osmotic shift of fluid from the vascular compartment to the intestinal lumen, which decreases plasma volume.

27 Alkaline reflux gastritis is stomach inflammation caused by the reflux of bile and pancreatic secretions from the duodenum into the stomach. These substances disrupt the mucosal barrier and cause inflammation.

28 Afferent loop obstruction is an obstruction of the duodenal stump on the proximal side of a gastrojejunostomy. Biliary and pancreatic secretions accumulate in the stump, causing distention, intermittent pain, and vomiting.

29 Malabsorption syndromes result in impaired digestion or absorption of nutrients.

30 Pancreatic insufficiency causes malabsorption associated with impaired digestion. The pancreas does not produce sufficient amounts of the enzymes that digest protein, carbohydrates, and fats into components that can be absorbed by the intestine.

31 Deficient lactase production in the brush border of the small intestine inhibits the breakdown of lactose. This prevents lactose absorption and causes osmotic diarrhea.

32 Bile salt deficiency causes fat malabsorption and steatorrhea (fatty stools). Bile salt deficiency can result from inadequate secretion of bile, excessive bacterial deconjugation of bile, or impaired reabsorption of bile salts caused by ileal disease.

33 Ulcerative colitis is an inflammatory disease that causes ulceration, abscess formation, and necrosis of the colonic and rectal mucosa. Cramping pain, bleeding, frequent diarrhea, dehydration, and weight loss accompany severe forms of the disease. A course of frequent remissions and exacerbations is common.

34 Crohn disease is similar to ulcerative colitis, but it affects both the large and small intestines, and ulceration tends to involve all the layers of the lumen. "Skip lesion" fissures and granulomas are characteristic of Crohn disease. Abdominal tenderness, nonbloody diarrhea, and weight loss are the usual symptoms.

35 Diverticula are outpouchings of colonic mucosa through the muscle layers of the colon wall. Diverticulosis is the presence of these outpouchings; diverticulitis is inflammation of the diverticula.

36 Vascular insufficiency in the intestine is most often associated with occlusion or obstruction of the mesenteric vessels or insufficient arterial blood flow. The resulting ischemia and necrosis produce abdominal pain, fever, bloody diarrhea, hypovolemia, and shock.

37 Obesity can be classified as exogenous or endogenous, and adipose (fat) cells as hyperplastic or hypertrophic.

38 Susceptibility to obesity may involve an excessive num-

ber of fat cells, increased amounts of lipoprotein in fat cells, high biologic set point controlled by the hypothalamus, presence of relatively few brown (thermoregulating) fat cells, high blood glucose levels associated with type II diabetes, or decreased action of the ATPase pump.

39 Obesity increases the risk of developing coronary artery disease, cancer, and pulmonary disorders.

40 Anorexia nervosa, or self-imposed starvation, is a psychogenic disorder of adolescent and young women. It causes significant weight loss and developmental delays and can be fatal.

41 Bulimia, or binging and purging, involves eating normal or large amounts of food and then purging by inducing vomiting or abusing laxatives. Severe weight loss is rare, but frequent vomiting causes tooth decay, pharyngitis, and esophagitis.

42 Short-term starvation, or lack of dietary intake for 3 or 4 days, stimulates mobilization of stored glucose by two metabolic processes: glycogenolysis (splitting of glycogen into glucose) and gluconeogenesis (formation of glucose from noncarbohydrate molecules).

43 Long-term starvation triggers the breakdown of ketone bodies and fatty acids. Eventually proteolysis (protein breakdown) begins, and death ensues if nutrition is not restored.

Disorders of the Accessory Organs of Digestion

1 Portal hypertension, ascites, hepatic encephalopathy, jaundice, and hepatorenal syndrome are complications of many liver disorders.

2 Portal hypertension is an elevation of portal venous pressure to at least 10 mm Hg. It is caused by increased resistance to venous flow in the portal vein and its tributaries, including the sinusoids and hepatic vein.

3 Portal hypertension is the most serious complication of liver disease because it can cause potentially fatal complications, such as bleeding varices, ascites, and hepatic encephalopathy.

4 Ascites is the accumulation and sequestration of fluid in the peritoneal cavity, often as a result of portal hypertension and decreased concentrations of plasma proteins.

5 Hepatic encephalopathy (portal systemic encephalopathy) is impaired cerebral function caused by blood-borne toxins (particularly ammonia) not metabolized by the liver. Toxin-bearing blood may bypass the liver in collateral vessels opened as a result of portal hypertension, or diseased hepatocytes may be unable to carry out their metabolic functions.

6 Manifestations of hepatic encephalopathy range from confusion and asterixis (flapping tremor of the hands) to loss of consciousness, coma, and death.

7 Jaundice (icterus) is a yellow or greenish pigmentation of the skin or sclera of the eyes caused by increases in plasma bilirubin concentration (hyperbilirubinemia).

8 Obstructive jaundice is caused by obstructed bile canaliculi (intrahepatic obstructive jaundice) or obstructed bile ducts outside the liver (extrahepatic obstructive jaundice). Bilirubin accumulates proximal to sites of obstruction, enters the bloodstream, and is carried to the skin and deposited.

9 Hemolytic jaundice is caused by destruction of red blood cells at a rate that exceeds the liver's ability to metabolize unconjugated bilirubin.

10 Hepatorenal syndrome is functional kidney failure caused by advanced liver disease, particularly cirrhosis with portal hypertension. Renal failure is caused by a sudden decrease in blood flow to the kidneys, usually caused by massive gastrointestinal hemorrhage of liver failure. Its chief clinical manifestation is oliguria.

11 Viral hepatitis is an infection of the liver caused by a strain of the hepatitis virus: hepatitis A virus (HAV), hepatitis B virus (HBV), or non-A, non-B hepatitis. Though they differ with respect to modes of transmission and severity of acute illness, all cause hepatic cell necrosis, Kuppfer cell hyperplasia, and infiltration of liver tissue by mononuclear phagocytes. These changes obstruct bile flow and impair hepatocyte function.

12 The clinical manifestations of viral hepatitis depend on the stage of infection. Fever, malaise, anorexia, and liver enlargement and tenderness characterize the prodromal phase (stage 1). Jaundice and hyperbilirubinemia mark the icteric phase (stage 2). During the recovery phase (stage 3), symptoms resolve. Recovery takes several weeks.

13 Fulminant hepatitis is a complication of hepatitis B (with or without hepatitis D infection) or non-A, non-B hepatitis. It causes widespread hepatic necrosis and is often fatal.

14 Cirrhosis is an inflammatory disease of the liver that causes disorganization of lobular structure, fibrosis, and nodular regeneration. Cirrhosis can result from hepatitis or exposure to toxins, such as acetylaldehyde (a product of alcohol metabolism). The disease causes progressive irreversible liver damage, usually over a period of years.

15 Alcoholic cirrhosis impairs the hepatocytes' ability to oxidize fatty acids, synthesize enzymes and proteins, degrade hormones, and clear portal blood of ammonia and toxins. The inflammatory response includes excessive collagen formation, fibrosis, and scarring, which obstruct bile canaliculi and sinusoids. Bile obstruction causes jaundice. Vascular obstruction causes portal hypertension, shunting, and varices.

16 Primary biliary cirrhosis is the inflammatory destruction of intrahepatic bile ducts. Its cause is unknown.

17 Secondary biliary cirrhosis develops from prolonged obstruction of bile flow with increased pressure in the hepatic bile ducts that causes pooling of bile and necrosis of tissue. Relief of obstruction relieves symptoms of jaundice and pruritis. Continued obstruction causes cirrhosis and liver failure.

18 Postnecrotic cirrhosis is the consequence of many severe, chronic liver diseases. Fibrosis, atrophy, and nodular regeneration are characteristic of liver structure

with severely altered liver function and manifestations, including portal hypertension, ascites, bleeding varices, and encephalopathy.

19 Cholelithiasis (the formation of gallstones) is a common disorder of the gallbladder. Gallstones form in the bile as a result of the aggregation of cholesterol crystals (cholesterol stones) or precipitates of unconjugated bilirubin (pigmented stones). Gallstones that fill the gallbladder or obstruct the cystic or common bile duct cause abdominal pain and jaundice.

20 Cholecystitis is an inflammation of the gallbladder. It is usually associated with obstruction of the cystic duct by gallstones.

21 Acute pancreatitis (pancreatic inflammation) is a serious but relatively rare disorder. Some unknown factor injures the pancreatic ducts or acini. Injury permits leakage of digestive enzymes into pancreatic tissue, where they become activated and begin the process of autodigestion, inflammation, and destruction of tissues. Release of pancreatic enzymes into the bloodstream or abdominal cavity causes damage to other organs.

22 Chronic pancreatitis results from structural or functional impairment of the pancreas. It causes recurrent abdominal pain and digestive disorders.

Cancer of the Digestive System

1 Cancer of the esophagus is rare and tends to occur in people over 60 years of age. Alcohol and tobacco use, reflux esophagitis, and nutritional deficiencies are associated with esophageal carcinoma.

2 Dysphagia and chest pain are the primary manifestations of esophageal cancer. Early treatment of tumors that have not spread into the mediastinum or lymph nodes results in a good prognosis.

3 Gastric carcinoma is associated with high salt intake, food preservatives (nitrates and nitrites), and atrophic gastritis.

4 About 50% of all gastric cancers are located in the prepyloric antrum. Clinical manifestations (weight loss, upper abdominal pain, vomiting, hepatemesis, and anemia) develop only after the tumor has penetrated the wall of the stomach.

5 Cancer of the colon and rectum (colorectal cancer) is the second most common cause of cancer death in the United States. Preexisting polyps are highly associated with adenocarcinoma of the colon.

6 Tumors of the right (ascending) colon are usually large and bulky; tumors of the left (descending, sigmoid) colon develop as small, buttonlike masses. Manifestations of colon tumors include pain, bloody stools, and change in bowel habits.

7 Rectal carcinoma is located up to 15 cm from the opening of the anus. The tumor spreads transmurally to the vagina in women or prostate in men.

8 Metastatic invasion of the liver is more common than primary cancer of the liver.

9 Primary liver cancers are associated with chronic liver disease (cirrhosis and hepatitis B). Hepatocellular carcinomas arise from the hepatocytes, whereas cholangiocellular carcinomas arise from the bile ducts. Primary liver cancer spreads to the heart, lungs, brain, kidney, and spleen through the circulation.

10 Cancer of the gallbladder is relatively rare and tends to occur in women over 50. Adenocarcinoma is most common. Because clinical manifestations occur late in the disease, metastases to lymph channels have usually occurred by the time of diagnosis, and the prognosis is poor.

11 Cancer of the pancreas now ranks fifth as a cause of cancer deaths. The one known risk factor is heavy cigarette smoking. Most tumors are adenocarcinomas that arise in the exocrine cells of ducts in the head, body, or tail of the pancreas. Symptoms may not be evident until the tumor has spread to surrounding tissues. Treatment is palliative, and mortality is nearly 100%.

KEY TERMS

Achalasia, 1219

Acute gastritis, 1224

Acute pancreatitis (acute hemorrhagic pancreatitis), 1254

Afferent loop obstruction, 1230

Alcoholic cirrhosis, 1249

Alcoholic hepatitis, 1250

Anorexia, 1214

Alkaline reflux gastritis, 1230

Anorexia nervosa, 1237

Appendicitis, 1235

Ascites, 1240

Biliary cirrhosis, 1252

Bulimarexia, 1238

Bulimia, 1237

Cholangiocellular carcinoma (cholangiocarcinoma), 1259

Cholecystitis, 1253

Cholelithiasis (gallstone), 1253

Chronic active hepatitis, 1248

Chronic gastritis, 1224

Chronic pancreatitis, 1255

Cirrhosis, 1248

Constipation, 1214

Crohn disease, 1233

Curling ulcer, 1228

Cushing ulcer, 1228

Diarrhea, 1215

Diverticulitis, 1234

Diverticulosis, 1234

Dumping syndrome, 1229

Duodenal ulcer, 1226

Dysphagia, 1219

Fulminant hepatitis, 1248

Gallstone, 1253

Gastric ulcer, 1226

Gastritis, 1224

Gastroesophageal reflux, 1219

Gastrointestinal bleeding, 1217

Gluconeogenesis, 1238

Glycogenolysis, 1238

Hematemesis, 1217

Hematochezia, 1217

Hemolytic jaundice, 1243

Hepatic encephalopathy, 1240

Hepatocellular carcinoma (hepatocarcinoma), 1259

Hepatorenal syndrome, 1244

Hiatal hernia, 1220

Hyperbilirubinemia, 1242

Intestinal obstruction, 1223

Ischemic ulcer, 1228

Jaundice (icterus), 1242

Icteric phase of hepatitis, 1248

Lactase deficiency, 1216

Long-term starvation, 1238

Malabsorption, 1231

Maldigestion, 1231

Melena, 1217

Nausea, 1214

Obesity, 1236

Obstructive jaundice, 1242

Occult bleeding, 1217

Osmotic diarrhea, 1215

Overnutrition , 1236

Pancreatic insufficiency, 1231

Pancreatitis, 1254

Paraesophageal hiatal hernia, 1221

Parietal pain, 1216

Peptic ulcer, 1225

Portal hypertension, 1238

Postnecrotic cirrhosis, 1252

Primary biliary cirrhosis, 1252

Prodromal phase of hepatitis, 1248

Projectile vomiting, 1214

Pyloric obstruction, 1221

Recovery phase of hepatitis, 1248

Referred pain, 1217

Reflux esophagitis, 1220

Retching, 1214

Short-term starvation, 1238

Secondary biliary cirrhosis, 1252

Secretory diarrhea, 1216

Sliding hiatal hernia, 1221

Splenomegaly, 1240

Stress ulcer, 1228

Ulcerative colitis, 1232

Varices, 1240

Viral hepatitis, 1245

Visceral pain, 1217

Vomiting, 1214

REFERENCES

American Cancer Society. (1986). *Cancer facts and figures, 1986.* New York: American Cancer Society.

American Cancer Society. (1988). *Cancer facts and figures, 1988.* New York: American Cancer Society.

American Cancer Society. (1989). Cancer statistics. *Ca-A Cancer: Journal for Clinicians, 39,*(1).

Ammann, R., & Warshaw, A. L. (1985). Acute pancreatitis: Clinical aspects and medical and surgical management. In J. E. Berk (Ed.), *Bockus gastroenterology,* (4th ed.). (pp. 3993-4007), Philadelphia: W. B. Saunders.

Behar, J. (1986). The role of the lower esophageal sphincter in reflux prevention. *Journal of Clinical Gastroenterology, 8,*(1), 2-4.

Bray, G. A. (1985). The obese patient. In L. H. Smith (Ed.), *Major problems in internal medicine,* (Vol. 9). Philadelphia: W. B. Saunders.

Cello, J. P., & Schneiderman, D. L. (1989). Ulcerative colitis. In M. H. Sleisenger & J. S. Fortran (Eds.), *Gastrointestinal disease: Pathophysiology, diagnosis, and management,* (4th ed.) (pp. 1436-1438). Philadelphia: W. B. Saunders.

Chailet, N., Gallo-Torres, H. E., & Bounameaux, Y. (1985). Prostaglandins and the protection of the gastroduodenal mucosa in humans: A critical review. *Journal of Clinical Pharmacology, 25,* 564-582.

Davidson, E. W., & Dunn, M. S. (1987). Pathogenesis of hepatorenal syndrome. *Annual Review of Medicine, 38,* 361-372.

De Luise, M., Blackburn, G. L., & Flier, J. S. (1980). Reduced activity of the red cell sodium-potassium pump in human obesity. *New England Journal of Medicine, 303,* 1017.

DeCock, K. M., Govindarajan, S., & Redeker, A. G. (1985). Acute delta hepatitis without circulating HB_s,Ag. *Gut, 25,* 212-214.

del Regato, J. A., Spjut, H. J., & Cox, J. D. (1985). *Cancer: Diagnosis, treatment, and prognosis,* (6th ed.). St. Louis: C. V. Mosby.

Domschke, W. (1987). Medical and/or surgical treatment of severe pancreatitis. In H. G. Berger & M. Buchler (Eds.), *Acute pancreatitis,*. (pp. 295-302). New York: Springer-Verlag.

Dowlatshahi, K., Mehta, R. G., Levin, B., Gerny, W. L., Skinner, D. B., & Moon, R. C. (1984). Retinoic-acid-binding protein in normal and neoplastic human esophagus. *Cancer, 54,*(2), 308-311.

Faust, I. M., Johnson, P. R., Stern, J. S., & Hirsch, J. (1978). Diet-induced adipocyte number increases in adult rats: A new model for obesity. *American Journal of Physiology, 235,* E279-E286.

Feldman, M., Walker, P., Green, J. L., & Weingarden, K. (1986). Life events stress and psychosocial factors in men with peptic ulcer disease. A multidimensional case-controlled study. *Gastroenterology, 91,* 1370.

Gerety, R. J. (1985). *Hepatitis B,* (pp. 94, 121). Orlando: Academic Press.

Gine's, P., Ouintero, E., Arroyo, V., Teres, J., Bruguera, M., Rimola, A., Caballeri'a, J., Rodes, J., & Rozman, C. (1987). Compensated cirrhosis: Natural history and prognostic factors. *Hepatology, 7,*(1), 122-128.

Hadler, S. C., Erben, J. J., Francis, D. P., Webster, H. M., & Maynard, J. E. (1982). Risk factors for hepatitis A in day care centers. *Journal of Infectious Diseases, 145,* 255-261.

Halmi, K. A. (1987). Anorexia nervosa and bulimia. *Annual Review of Medicine, 38,* 373-380.

Himms-Hagen, J. (1985). Brown adipose tissue metabolism and thermogenesis. *Annual Review of Nutrition, 5,* 69-84.

Keesey, R. E. (1986). A set-point theory of obesity. In K. D. Brownell & J. P. Foreyt (Eds.), *Handbook of eating disorders.* New York: Basic Books, pp. 63-87.

Kissane, J. M. (Ed.). (1985). *Anderson's pathology,* (8th ed.). St. Louis: C. V. Mosby.

Kuhn, S. B., Love, R. R., Sherman, C., & Chakravorty, R. C. (1983). *Concepts in cancer medicine.* New York: Grune & Stratton.

Kvietys, P. R., Barrowmand, A., & Granger, N. D. (1987). *Pathophysiology of the splanchnic circulation,* (vol. 1) (p. 129). Boca Raton, Fla.: R. C. Press.

McCallum, R. W. (1987). The spectrum of esophageal motility disorders. *Hosppital Practice,* (December 15), *22,*(12), 71-83.

Merlo, A., & Cohen, S. (1988). Swallowing disorders. *Annul Review of Medicine, 39,* 17-28.

Miller, D. S. (1979). Theromogenesis and obesity. *Bibliotheca Nutritio et Dieta, 27,* 25-32.

Nevalainen, T. J., & Aho, H. J. (1987). Phospholipase A_2 in acute pancreatitis. In H. G. Berger & M. Buchler (Eds.), *Acute pancreatitis,* New York: Spinger-Verlag.

Orrego, H., Blake, J. E., Blendis, L. M., & Medline, A. (1987). Prognosis of alcoholic cirrhosis in the presence and absence of alcoholic hepatitis. *Gastroenterology, 92,* 208-214.

Phipps, W. J., Long, B. C., & Woods, W. F. (1987). *Medical surgical nursing: Concepts and clinical practice,* St. Louis: C. V. Mosby.

Prior, J.A., Silberstein, J.S., & Stang, J. M. (1981). Physical diagnosis: The history and examination of the patient (6th ed). St. Louis: C. V. Mosby.

Rathbone, B. J., Wyatt, J. I., & Heatley, R. V. (1986). *Campylobacter pyloridis-*A new factor in peptic ulcer disease. *Gut, 27,* 635-661.

Rizzetto, M., Carnese, M. G., Arico, S., Crivelli, O., Bonino, F., Trepo, C. G., & Verme, G. (1977). Immunofluorescence detection of a new antigen-antibody system (delta/antidelta) associated with hepatitis B virus in the liver and in the serum of HG_s,Ag carriers. *Gut, 18,* 997.

Rosai, J. (1989). *Ackerman's surgical pathology* (7th ed.). St. Louis: C. V. Mosby.

Schwartz, R. B., & Brunzell, J. D. (1981). Increase of adipose tissue lipoprotein lipase activity with weight loss. *Journal of Clinical Investigation, 67,* 1425.

Speranza, V., Simi, M., Leardi, S., & DelPapa, M. (1986). Recurrence of Crohn's disease after resection. *Journal of Clinical Gastroenterology, 8,* 640-646.

Steer, M. L. (1988). Pathogenesis of acute pancreatitis. *Annual Review of Medicine, 39,* 95-105.

Stunkard, A. J. (Ed.). (1980). *Obesity,* Philadelphia: W. B. Saunders.

Thibodeau, G. A. (1987). *Anatomy and physiology,* St. Louis: Times Mirror/Mosby College Publications.)

Trapnell, J. E., & Duncan, E. J. L. (1975). Patterns of incidence in acute pancreatits. *British Journal of Medicine,* (January), *2,* 179-183.

Wadden, T. A., & Stunkard, A. J. (1985). Social and psychological consequences of obesity. *Ann Intern Med, 103,* 1062-1067.

CHAPTER 37

Alterations of Digestive Function in Children

Margaret M. Andrews
Sue E. Huether

Disorders of the gastrointestinal tract, 1268
 Congenital impairment of motility, 1268
  Cleft lip and cleft palate, 1268
   Pathophysiology, 1268
    Cleft lip, 1268
    Cleft palate, 1268
   Clinical manifestations, 1268
   Evaluation and treatment, 1268
  Esophageal malformations, 1270
   Pathophysiology, 1270
   Clinical manifestations, 1270
   Evaluation and treatment, 1270
  Pyloric stenosis, 1271
   Pathophysiology, 1271
   Clinical manifestations, 1271
   Evaluation and treatment, 1271
  Malrotation, 1271
   Pathophysiology, 1271
   Clinical manifestations, 1271
   Evaluation and treatment, 1272
  Meconium ileus, 1272
   Pathophysiology, 1272
   Clinical manifestations, 1272
   Evaluation and treatment, 1272
  Obstructions of the duodenum, jejunum, and ileum, 1272
  Congenital Aganglionic Megacolon, 1273
   Pathophysiology, 1273
   Clinical manifestations, 1273
   Evaluation and treatment, 1273
  Anorectal malformations, 1273
 Acquired impairment of motility, 1274
  Intussusception, 1274
   Pathophysiology, 1274
   Clinical manifestations, 1275
   Evaluation and treatment, 1275
  Gastroesophageal reflux, 1275
   Pathophysiology, 1275

Clinical manifestations, 1275
   Evaluation and treatment, 1275
 Impairment of digestion, absorption, and nutrition, 1276
  Cystic fibrosis, 1276
   Pathophysiology, 1277
   Clinical manifestations, 1277
   Evaluation and treatment, 1277
  Gluten-sensitive enteropathy, 1277
   Pathophysiology, 1277
   Clinical manifestations, 1278
   Evaluation and treatment, 1278
    Protein energy malnutrition, 1279
   Pathophysiology, 1279
   Clinical manifestations, 1279
   Evaluation and treatment, 1279
  Failure to thrive, 1279
   Pathophysiology, 1279
   Clinical manifestations, 1280
   Evaluation and treatment, 1280
 Diarrhea, 1280
  Necrotizing enterocolitis, 1280
   Pathophysiology, 1280
   Clinical manifestations, 1281
   Evaluation and treatment, 1281
  Acute diarrhea in childhood, 1281
  Chronic diarrhea in children, 1281
   Chronic nonspecific diarrhea, 1281
   Primary lactose intolerance, 1281
Disorders of the liver, 1282
 Disorders of biliary metabolism and transport, 1282
  Physiologic jaundice of the newborn, 1282
   Pathophysiology, 1282
   Clinical manifestations, 1282
   Evaluation and treatment, 1282
  Biliary atresia, 1282
 Inflammatory disorders, 1282
  Hepatitis, 1282

       Hepatitis A, 1282

       Hepatitis B, 1283

       Non-A, non-B hepatitis, 1283

       Chronic hepatitis, 1283

     Cirrhosis, 1283

   Portal hypertension, 1283

     Types of portal hypertension, 1283

       Extrahepatic portal hypertension, 1283

       Intrahepatic portal hypertension, 1283

     Course of the disease, 1283

       Clinical manifestations, 1284

       Evaluation and treatment, 1284

   Metabolic disorders, 1284

     Galactosemia, 1284

       Pathophysiology, 1285

       Clinical manifestations, 1285

       Evaluation and treatment, 1285

     Fructosemia, 1285

       Pathophysiology, 1285

       Clinical manifestations, 1285

       Evaluation and treatment, 1285

     Wilson disease, 1285

       Pathophysiology, 1285

       Clinical manifestations, 1286

       Evaluation and treatment, 1286

DISORDERS OF THE GASTROINTESTINAL TRACT

Congenital Impairment of Motility

Cleft Lip and Cleft Palate

Cleft lip (harelip) and **cleft palate** are developmental anomalies of the first branchial arch (Fig. 37-1). These defects, which occur during embryonic development, vary in severity. Some are barely perceptible, while others are exceedingly handicapping functionally, cosmetically, and psychologically.

In whites the incidence of cleft lip or cleft palate ranges from 1 in 600 to 1 in 1250 births. The incidence of cleft lip, with or without cleft palate, is 1 in 1000 births, whereas the incidence of cleft palate alone is about 1 in 2500 births. Incidence is lower in black and higher in Japanese populations. Cleft lip, with or without cleft palate, is more frequent in females. Both anomalies can be unilateral or bilateral, partial or complete.

In most cases, cleft lip and cleft palate are caused by multiple factors, both genetic and nongenetic, each of which contributes only a minor developmental defect. (This phenomenon, called multifactorial inheritance, is discussed in Chapter 4.) Together, these factors reduce the amount of neural crest mesenchyme that migrates into the area that will develop into the face of the embryo. If the amount is sufficiently reduced, clefting occurs. The cleft can be part of a syndrome determined by single mutant genes or part of a chromosomal defect, usually trisomy 13. Rarely, the cleft is caused by a ter-

atogenic agent, such as an anticonvulsant drug (Mosher, 1986).

Pathophysiology

Cleft lip Cleft lip is caused by the incomplete fusion of the nasomedial or intermaxillary process during the second month of embryonic development. The deformity develops during a period of very rapid fetal growth. The cleft causes structures of the face and mouth to develop without the normal restraints of encircling lip muscles. A characteristic depression or flattening of the infant's midfacial contour may occur because normal antagonistic forces across the midline are absent, and growth of the involved facial segments is disturbed. The facial cleft may affect not only the lip but also the external nose, the nasal cartilages, the nasal septum, and the alveolar processes.

The cleft is usually just beneath the center of one nostril. The defect may occur bilaterally and may be symmetric or asymmetric. The cleft can range in severity from a slight indentation of the lip to a fissure that extends to the nostril, causing a sagging and flattening of the nose. The failure of lip fusion by 35 days of gestation may impair closure of the palatal shelves. The more complete the cleft lip, the greater the chance that teeth in the line of the cleft will be missing or malformed.

Cleft palate Cleft palate is often associated with cleft lip but may occur without it. The fissure may affect only the uvula and soft palate or may extend forward to the nostril and involve the hard palate and the maxillary alveolar ridge. It may be unilateral or bilateral, with the cleft occupying the midline posteriorly and as far forward as the alveolar process, where it deviates to the involved side. Clefts involving the palate only are usually but not necessarily in the midline. In some cases, the vomer and nasal septum are partly or completely undeveloped. When these facial bones are involved, the nasal cavity may freely communicate with the oral cavity.

Clinical Manifestations

Feeding the infant with cleft lip usually presents no difficulty if the cleft lip is simple and the palate intact. Nursing at breast or bottle depends on suction developed by pressing the nipple against the hard palate with the tongue. Closure of the lips is not necessary, but the tongue must work harder if the infant cannot purse its lips. A baby with cleft palate usually requires large, soft nipples with cross-cut openings. Breast feeding may be impossible for some infants. An orthodontic prosthesis for the roof of the mouth may facilitate sucking for some infants.

Evaluation and Treatment

Facial x-ray films confirm the extent of bone deformity. Soft tissue alterations are evaluated by history and physical examination.

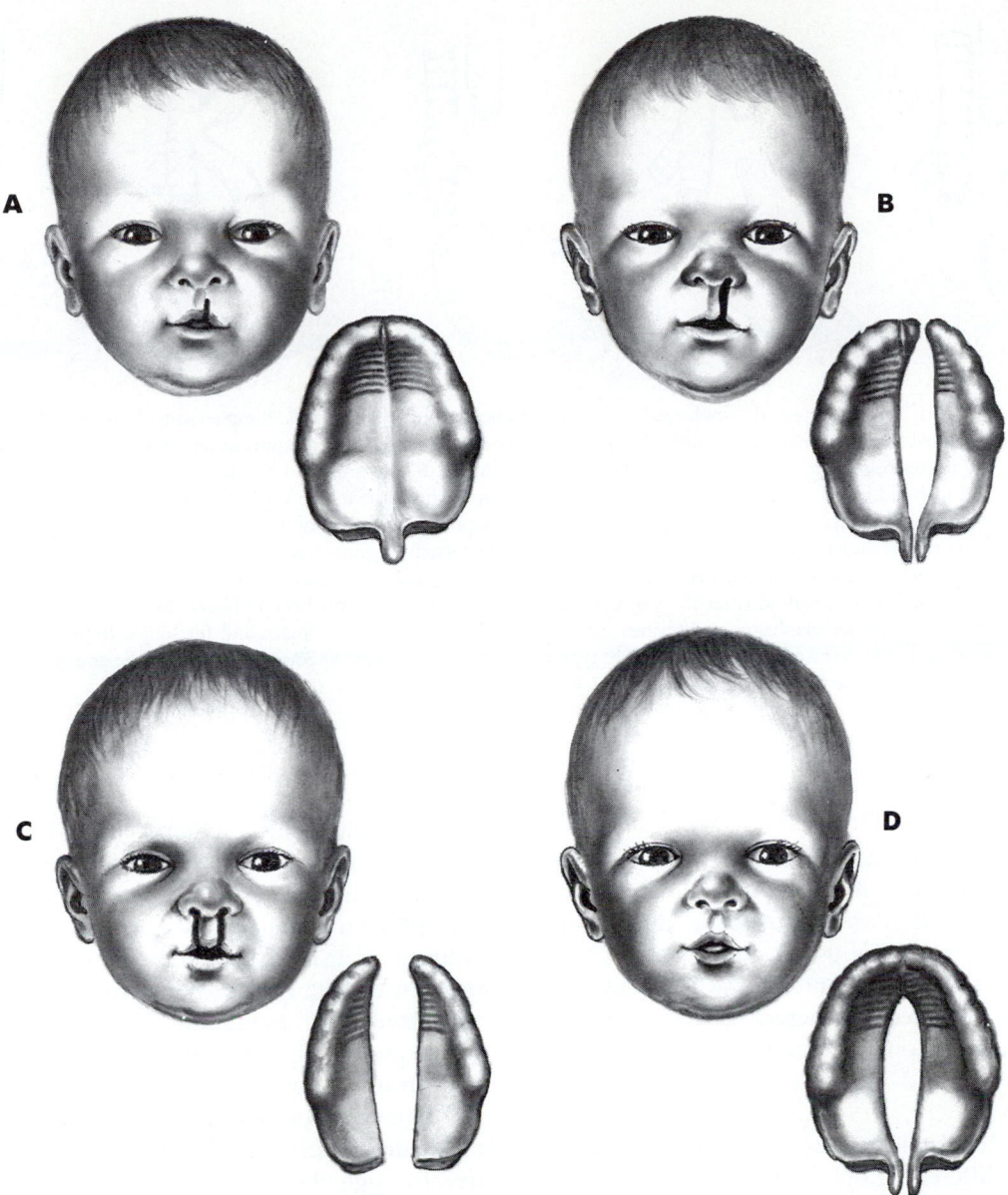

FIG. 37-1. Variations in clefts of the lip and palate. **A,** Notch in vermillion border. **B,** Unilateral cleft lip and palate. **C,** Bilateral cleft lip and cleft palate. **D,** Cleft palate. (From Whaley & Wong 1987).

The nature and extent of the cleft, the infant's condition, and the method of surgical correction proposed determine the course of treatment. Surgical correction is often planned in stages. The lip is united first. Although this can be done within a few weeks of birth, most surgeons prefer to wait until the infant is 2 to 3 months old to allow for sufficient growth to occur.

Repair of a cleft lip that is accompanied by bilateral cleft palate is technically more difficult, and so the procedure is often performed in two steps. The lip is repaired when the infant is a few weeks old. The palate is closed after the child is weaned from the nipple but before he or she has begun to talk, usually at about 18 months of age. The aim of surgery is to obtain an air-tight closure of the palatal cleft and to preserve the mobility and length of the soft palate. Even with early closure, the child may experience difficulty sealing off the nasopharynx from the buccal cavity during swallowing and while pronouncing certain consonants. Speech training and special attention by a prosthodontist and orthodontist are almost always required.

Both before and after surgery, children with cleft palate tend to suffer from repeated infections of the paranasal sinuses. Hypertrophy of tonsils and adenoids and otitis media are frequent accompaniments, and the child should be evaluated for hearing loss (Suslak & Desposito, 1988).

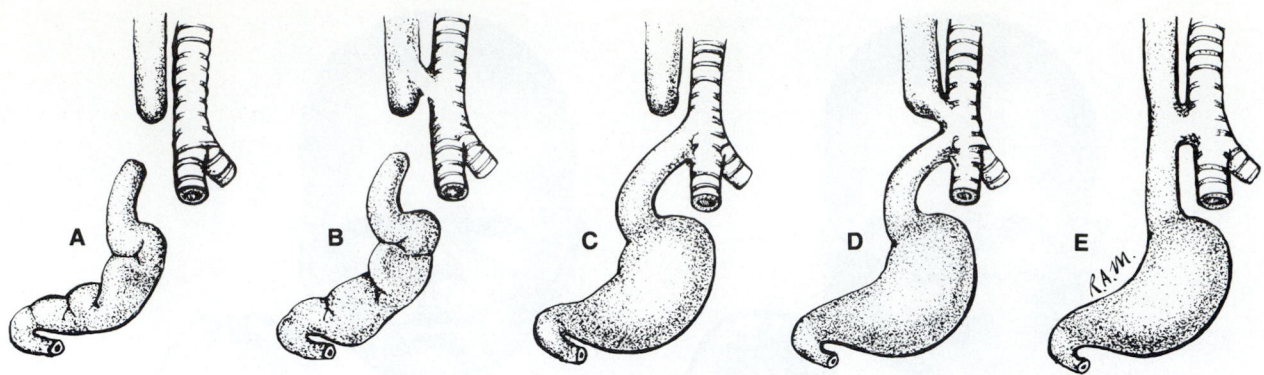

FIG. 37-2. Five types of esophageal atresia and tracheoesophageal fistula. **A,** Simple esophageal atresia. Proximal and distal esophagus end in blind pouches, and there is tracheal communication. Nothing enters the stomach; regurgitated food and fluid may enter the lungs. **B,** Proximal and distal esophageal segments end in blind pouches, and a fistula connects the proximal esophagus to the trachea. Nothing enters the stomach; food and fluid enter the lungs. **C,** Proximal esophagus ends in a blind pouch, and a fistula connects the trachea to the distal esophagus. Air enters the stomach; regurgitated gastric secretions enter the lungs through the fistula. **D,** Fistula connects both proximal and distal esophageal segments to the trachea. Air, food, and fluid enter the stomach and the lungs. **E,** Simple tracheoesophageal fistula between otherwise normal esophagus and trachea. Air, food, and fluid enter the stomach and the lungs. Between 95% and 90% of esophageal anomalies are type **C**; 6% to 8% are type **A**; 3% to 5% are type **E**; and less than 1% are type **B** or **D**. (From Whaley & Wong, 1987).

Esophageal Malformations

Congenital malformations of the esophagus occur in 1 of 3000 to 4500 live births. **Esophageal atresia** is a condition in which the esophagus ends in a blind pouch. Esophageal atresia is usually accompanied by a fistula between the esophagus and the trachea. This connection is called a **tracheoesophageal fistula** (TEF). Either defect can occur alone, however (Fig. 37-2).

Pathophysiology

The esophageal abnormalities are thought to arise from defective differentiation as the trachea separates from the esophagus during embryonic development. Defective growth of endodermal cells leads to atresia. Incomplete fusion of the lateral walls of the foregut leads to incomplete closure of the laryngeotracheal tube and fistula formation.

Clinical Manifestations

The blind end of the proximal esophagus has a capacity of only a few milliliters. As the infant with esophageal atresia swallows oral secretions, the pouch fills and overflows into the pharynx, resulting in drooling and occasionally in aspiration (see Fig. 37-2, *A* and *B*).

If a fistula connects the trachea with the distal esophagus, the abdomen fills with air and becomes distended. The distention may be great enough to interfere with breathing (see Fig. 37-2, *C* to *E*). If the fistula connects the proximal esophagus to the trachea, the first feeding after birth will be problematic (see Figure 37-2, *B* to *E*).

As the infant drinks, the blind end of the esophagus and the mouth fill with fluid. When the infant tries to take a breath, the fluid is aspirated into the lungs, which triggers protective cough and choke reflexes. Intermittent cyanosis may result. Plain water or glucose is recommended for the initial feeding to minimize the dangers associated with aspiration. If an abnormality of the esophagus is suspected, oral feedings are withheld until a diagnosis is confirmed.

Pulmonary complications are compounded by reflux of air and gastric secretions into the tracheobronchial tree through the fistula, causing severe chemical irritation. The upper lobe of the right lung is most commonly involved because of its proximity to the tracheoesophageal fistula. Infants with esophageal atresia but no fistula have scaphoid (boat-shaped), gasless abdomens. In fistula with atresia (Fig. 37-2, *B*), the usual symptoms are recurrent aspiration, pneumonia, and atelectasis that remains "silent" for days or even months.

In at least 30% of infants with esophageal defects, other congenital anomalies are present as well. Cardiovascular anomalies are the most common, but other digestive tract, urinary, vertebral, and central nervous system defects can accompany esophageal atresia and tracheoesophageal fistula.

Evaluation and Treatment

Esophageal atresia is usually diagnosed at birth when attempts to pass a catheter into the stomach fail. X-ray films will show the catheter coiled in the upper esophageal pouch. Barium x-ray examinations are used by some investigators (Beasley & Myers, 1988).

Treatment is surgical. Esophageal continuity is restored and the fistula is eliminated. Surgery is usually undertaken after birth, sometimes in stages. First, the tracheoesophageal fistula is ligated and a gastrostomy is created for feeding. Second, the two ends of the esophagus are joined. The child may continue to have problems with aspiration, gastroesophageal reflux, and esophagitis after surgical repair (Nakazato, Landing, & Wells, 1986). The overall survival rate for infants with esophageal defects is approximately 75%.

Pyloric Stenosis

Pyloric stenosis is an obstruction of the pyloric sphincter caused by hypertrophy of the sphincter muscle. Pyloric stenosis is one of the most common disorders of early infancy. It affects infants between the ages of 1 and 2 weeks or 3 and 4 months. The incidence of pyloric stenosis among males is approximately 5 in 1000, whereas that among females is only 1 in 1000. Whites are affected more frequently than blacks or orientals, and full-term infants are affected more frequently than premature infants. Increased gastrin secretion by the mother in the last trimester of pregnancy increases the likelihood of pyloric stenosis in the infant. The overproduction of gastric secretions in the infant may be due to stress-related factors in the mother.

Pathophysiology

The cause of the increased pyloric hypertrophy is unknown, but hereditary factors may be involved (Carter, 1961). Individual muscle fibers thicken, so that the whole pyloric sphincter becomes enlarged and inelastic. The mucosal lining of the pyloric opening is folded and narrowed by the encroaching muscle. Because of the extra peristaltic effort necessary to force the gastric contents through the narrow pylorus, the muscle layers of the stomach may become hypertrophied as well.

Clinical Manifestations

The clinical manifestations of pyloric stenosis usually evolve as follows. Between 2 and 3 weeks after birth, an infant that has fed well and gained weight begins to vomit without apparent reason. The vomiting gradually becomes more forceful. In some cases, stomach contents may shoot out 3 or 4 feet. Food is often regurgitated through the nose. The forceful, or projectile vomiting usually occurs immediately after eating, and the vomitus consists of the bulk of the feeding plus some food retained from previous feedings.

Prolonged retention of food in the stomach is a characteristic feature of pyloric stenosis. In healthy infants, the stomach empties within 2 to 3 hours after eating. In infants with pyloric stenosis, food is present after 4 hours unless vomiting has occurred. Constipation is the rule because not much food reaches the intestine.

In severe untreated cases, increased gastric peristalsis and vomiting lead to severe fluid and electrolyte imbalances, malnutrition, and weight loss that can be fatal within 4 to 6 weeks. Infants with pyloric stenosis are irritable because of hunger, and they may have esophageal discomfort caused by repeated vomiting.

Evaluation and Treatment

Diagnosis is based on the history of clinical manifestations and palpation of a pyloric mass. Occasionally, gastric peristalsis is observable over the abdomen. Contrast x-ray examinations confirm the diagnosis.

The standard treatment for hypertrophic pyloric stenosis is a pyloromyotomy, in which the muscles of the pylorus are split and separated. This procedure is almost uniformly successful.

Some infants respond to medical and nutritional management, which is based on the theory that the pylorus will open spontaneously by 6 to 8 months of age if nutrition can be maintained. To maintain nutrition, antispasmodic drugs are given to relax the pylorospasm, and the infant is refed after vomiting.

Malrotation

During the tenth week of embryonic development, the emerging ileum and cecum normally rotate, so that the cecum moves into the lower right quadrant of the abdomen and is fixed there by the mesentery. **Malrotation** is a condition in which rotation does not occur, and the colon remains in the upper right quadrant, where an abnormal membrane may press on and obstruct the duodenum. The obstructing band over the duodenum, called a **periduodenal band**, is one of the most significant findings in malrotation.

Pathophysiology

The small intestine lacks a normal posterior fixation in malrotation because it has only a rudimentary attachment near the origin of the superior mesenteric artery. Therefore the entire mass can twist when the mobile loops of intestine from the duodenojejunal junction to the middle of the transverse colon twist on themselves. The twisting is known as volvulus. Intestinal twisting around the rudimentary mesentery angulates and obstructs the intestinal lumen and partly or completely occludes the superior mesenteric artery, causing infarction and necrosis of the entire midgut.

Clinical Manifestations

Although most cases of malrotation-associated volvulus and infarction develop during the neonatal period, some develop during childhood or even adulthood. In infants the obstruction causes intermittent or persistent bile-stained vomiting after feedings. Abdominal distention is limited initially to the epigastrium because only the stomach and duodenum are dilated. The degree of distention depends on the pressure of swallowed air and the degree of obstruction caused by the volvulus. Dehydration and electrolyte imbalance may occur rapidly because large amounts of pancreatic juice, bile, and gastric secretions are lost through vomiting. Fever usually ensues. Scanty stools, diarrhea, and bloody stools are associated with progressive volvulus and infarction of the intestine in infants. Older children have minor abdominal complaints, such as nausea following meals, vomiting, or abdominal pain.

Evaluation and Treatment

Diagnosis of malrotation with volvulus and infarction is based on a review of the clinical manifestations. X-ray films of the abdomen show gas bubbles and distention proximal to the site of obstruction.

Treatment consists of opening the abdomen and reducing the volvulus manually. The surgeon takes the entire intestinal mass in hand and rotates it in a counterclockwise direction. In cases of malrotation without duodenal obstruction, operative survival is 80%. Operative survival is 40% to 50% in cases of malrotation complicated by obstruction caused by periduodenal bands or other intraabdominal anomalies.

Meconium Ileus

Meconium is a substance that fills the entire intestine before birth. It consists of intestinal gland secretions and some amniotic fluid. Normally, meconium is passed from the rectum during the first 12 to 72 hours after birth.

Meconium ileus is intestinal obstruction caused by thick, abnormal meconium that resists passage beyond the terminal ileum. The cause is usually a lack of digestive enzymes during fetal life. Most cases of meconium ileus are due to cystic fibrosis, but a few are not. In the cases *not* associated with cystic fibrosis, the cause usually is unknown. Partial aplasia of the pancreas is an associated factor, however, and one fifth of infants with meconium ileus are premature or have a history of maternal hydramnios (excessive amniotic fluid). After intestinal atresia and malrotation with volvulus, meconium ileus is the most common cause of small intestinal obstruction in newborns.

Pathophysiology

In infants with meconium ileus the terminal ileum is plugged with thick, viscous meconium. The viscosity of the meconium is due to the formation of an insoluble, calcium-glycoprotein compound in abnormal mucus. The segment of the ileum proximal to the obstruction is distended with liquid contents, and its walls may be hypertrophied. The segment distal to the obstruction is collapsed and filled with small pellets of pale-colored stool. Meconium in the obstructed segment has the consistency of thick syrup or glue. Peristalsis fails to propel this viscous material through the ileum, and so it becomes impacted. Volvulus, atresia, or perforation of the bowel sometimes accompanies meconium ileus.

Clinical Manifestations

Abdominal distention usually develops during the first few days after birth. The infant does not pass meconium and begins to vomit within hours or days of birth. Infants with cystic fibrosis may have signs of pulmonary involvement, such as tachypnea, intercostal retractions, and grunting respirations. The distended abdomen reveals patterns of dilated intestinal loops that feel dough-like when palpated. Some of the loops contain scattered, firm, movable masses. Despite hyperactive peristalsis, the rectal ampulla is empty.

Evaluation and Treatment

Radiologic examination is used to confirm the presence of meconium ileus. The sweat test, which is accurate in 90% of infants, is performed to detect or rule out cystic fibrosis. In approximately 50% of cases, an enema will evacuate the meconium. If this is not possible, the meconium is removed surgically.

Between 50% and 67% of infants with meconium ileus die of the disease. Mortality increases to 70% if obstruction is complicated by peritonitis. Of those with cystic fibrosis, more than one third die of pulmonary complications (Gryboski & Walker, 1983).

Obstructions of the Duodenum, Jejunum, and Ileum

Congenital obstruction of the duodenum can be due to intrinsic malformations or external pressure. Intrinsic duodenal obstruction is due to failure of canalization, which may be partial or complete. During embryonic development, the duodenal lumen does not become patent. The obstruction usually is located at or near the major duodenal papilla. Extrinsic obstructions can be caused by peritoneal bands that constrict the duodenum. This type of obstruction is associated with a partial failure of intestinal rotation and fixation during embryonic development. The duodenum can be obstructed by an annular pancreas, a defect in which the head of the pancreas surrounds part of the duodenum.

Congenital obstructions of the jejunum and ileum can be due to atresia, stenosis, meconium ileus, megacolon (Hirschsprung disease), intussusception, Meckel diverticulum, intestinal duplication, or strangulated hernia.

In **ileal** or **jejunal atresia**, the intestine ends blindly proximal and distal to an interruption in its continuity with or without a gap in the mesentery. Stenosis (narrowing of the lumen) causes dilation proximal to the obstruction and luminal collapse distal to it.

Congenital Aganglionic Megacolon

Congenital aganglionic megacolon (Hirschsprung disease) is a functional obstruction of the colon caused by inadequate motility. Congenital megacolon is the most common cause of colon obstruction; it accounts for about one third of all gastrointestinal obstructions in infants. The incidence is 1 in 5000 with a preponderance in males.

Pathophysiology

Congenital aganglionic megacolon is due to a malformation of the parasympathetic nervous system. It is characterized by absence of the intramural ganglion cells in the enteric nerve plexuses (Meissner and Auerbach plexuses). Lacking neural stimulation, the muscle layers of the colon wall fail to propel feces through the colon. In 80% of cases the aganglionic segment is limited to the rectal end of the sigmoid colon. In 3% of cases, the entire colon lacks ganglion cells. The abnormally innervated colon obstructs fecal movements, causing the proximal colon to become distended; hence the term megacolon (Fig. 37-3).

The ganglions normally develop between the muscle layers (tunica muscularis) in the submucosal area (muscularis mucosa) of the intestinal wall. In cases of congenital megacolon, large, nonmyelinated fibers develop in place of these ganglion cells. The segment of colon that lacks ganglion cells has a relatively normal lumen caliber and wall thickness. In the segment of the colon proximal to it, the lumen is dilated and the muscle hypertrophied. Therefore the abnormal portion of the colon appears to be normal, while the normal portion appears to be diseased.

The mechanism of propulsive failure is not entirely clear. Some investigators believe that the aganglionic segment simply fails to participate in normal peristalsis. Others suggest that tonic contraction of smooth muscle in the wall of the aganglionic colon narrows the lumen (Milla, 1988).

Clinical Manifestations

Constipation is the usual manifestation of congenital aganglionic megacolon. Diarrhea is the first sign, however, because only water can travel around the impacted feces.

Enterocolitis is a potentially serious complication of fecal impaction. Bowel dilation stretches and partly occludes the encircling blood and lymphatic vessels, causing edema, ischemia, infarction of the mucosa, and significant outflow of fluid into the bowel lumen. Copious, liquid stools result. Infarction and destruction of the mucosa enable enteric microorganisms to penetrate the

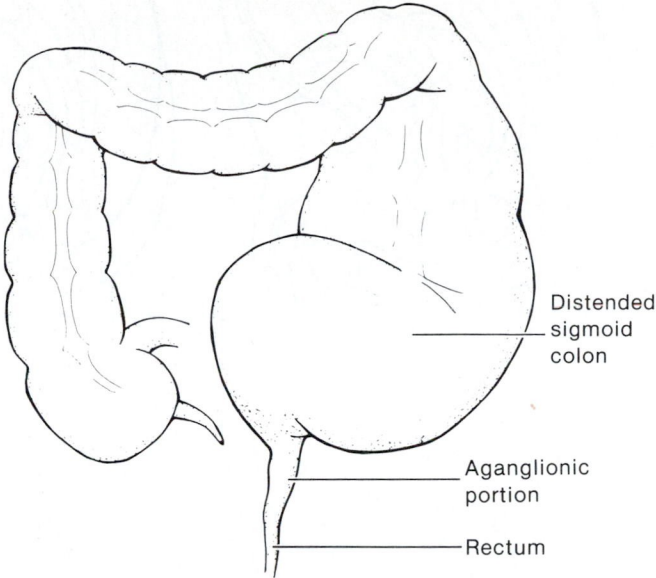

FIG. 37-3. Congenital aganglionic megacolon (Hirschsprung disease). (From Waley & Wong, 1989).

bowel wall. Frequently, gram-negative sepsis occurs, accompanied by fever and vomiting. Severe and rapid electrolyte changes may take place, causing collapse and rapid death.

Evaluation and Treatment

Biopsy findings reveal an absence of ganglion cells in the submucosa of the colon. X-ray films show dilated loops of colon and contrast films show aganglionic areas. The infant usually cannot expel the barium.

The involved segment is resected within the first few months of life. Alternatively, enemas are given until the lumen is clear, and then stool softeners are prescribed for life. The child is not treated for diarrhea.

After surgery, enterocolitis sometimes recurs. If the postoperative enterocolitis is allowed to persist, pseudopolyps may appear. Because these are essentially identical to the lesions of ulcerative colitis, they have malignant potential. Therefore a colectomy is indicated if pseudopolyps develop.

In general, the prognosis of congenital megacolon is satisfactory for children who undergo surgical treatment. Bowel training may be prolonged, but most children achieve bowel continence before puberty.

Anorectal Malformations

Several congenital malformations of anorectal structures can obstruct the passage of feces. The incidence of minor abnormalities is approximately 1 in 500, and that of major anomalies is approximately 1 in 5000.

Congenital anorectal malformations range from mild

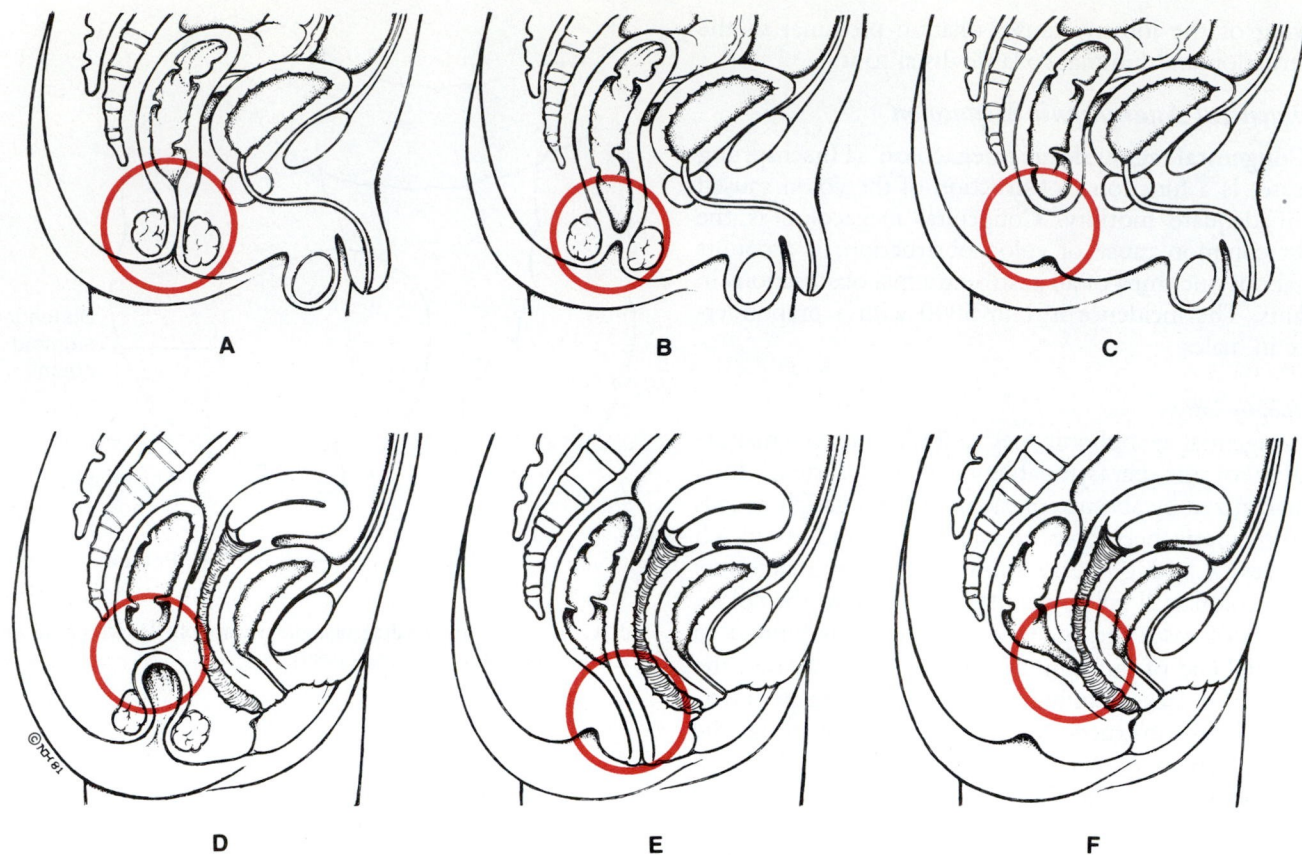

FIG. 37-4. Anorectal stenosis and imperforate anus. **A,** Congenital anal stenosis. **B,** Anal membrane atresia. **C,** Anal agenesis. **D,** Rectal atresia. **E,** Rectoperineal fistula. **F,** Rectovaginal fistula. (From Whaley & Wong, 1987).

anal stenosis, which is corrected by simple dilation, to complex deformities, such as anal or rectal agenesis, atresia, and fistula (Fig. 37-4). Deformities that cause complete obstruction are known collectively as **imperforate anus**.

About 40% of infants with anorectal malformations have other developmental anomalies as well. The most commonly associated major anomalies are congenital heart disease, renal abnormalities, esophageal atresia, and malformations of the spine.

Imperforate anus may not be obvious. It can be detected by gentle insertion of a rectal tube. X-ray films show dilations throughout the intestinal tract. Anal stenosis can be treated by dilations, but all other anorectal malformations require surgical correction. The overall mortality is about 10%. Children with a low (anal) anomaly usually achieve bowel continence, but those with a high (rectal) anomaly rarely do.

Acquired Impairment of Motility
Intussusception

The most frequent cause of acquired intestinal obstruction in infants is intussusception. **Intussusception**

is the telescoping or invagination of one portion of the intestine into another. Usually, the ileum invaginates the cecum and part of the ascending colon by collapsing through the ileocecal valve. Intussusception involving the ileum and colon (ileocolic intussusception) accounts for 80% to 90% of intestinal obstructions in infants and is two to three times more frequent in males than in females. Nearly 75% of intussusceptions occur before age 2; 70% occur before age 1. Intussusception is rare in infants less than 3 months of age and is infrequent after 36 months.

Pathophysiology

The proximal portion of the intestine, the intussusceptum, collapses into the distal portion, the intussuscepiens, in the direction of peristaltic flow (Fig. 37-5). As it does so, the intussusceptum drags its mesentery into the enveloping lumen. Initially, the mesentery is constricted, obstructing venous return. Compression of the mesenteric vessels between the two layers of intestinal wall and at the U-shaped angle at either end of the intussusceptum leads within hours to venous stasis, engorgement, edema, exudation, and further vascular

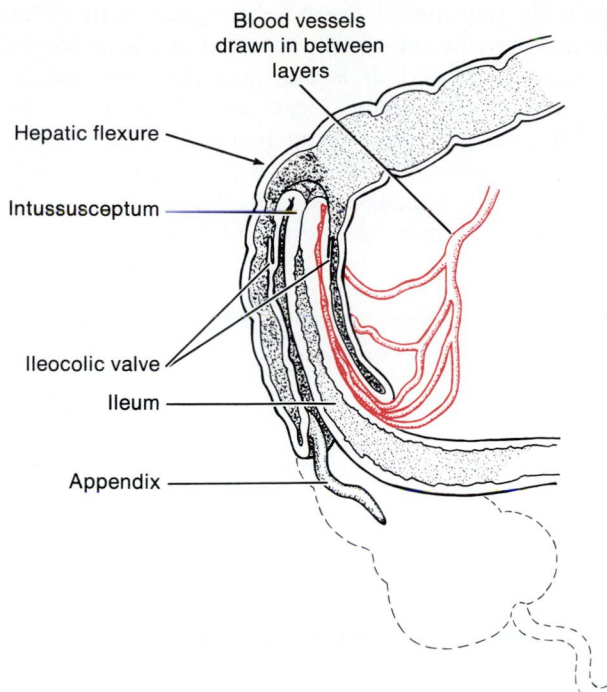

Blood vessels
drawn in between
layers

Hepatic flexure

Intussusceptum

Ileocolic valve

Ileum

Appendix

FIG. 37-5. Ileocolic intussusception. (From Whaley & Wong, 1987).

compression. Unless the intussusception is treated, gangrene ensues. The tension of the mesentery on the intussusceptum tends to arch the bowel in a curve having its center at the mesenteric root. Edema and compression obstruct the flow of chyme through the intestine.

Clinical Manifestations

Typically, intussusception occurs in thriving, previously healthy infants. The affected infant suddenly develops abdominal pain, becomes irritable (colicky), and draws up the knees. Vomiting occurs soon afterward. A single normal stool may be passed, evacuating the colon distal to the apex of the intussusception. After that, 60% of infants pass "currant jelly" stools, which appear dark and gelatinous because of their blood and mucus content. Most infants have a tender, sausage-shaped abdominal mass. Abdominal tenderness and distention develop as intestinal obstruction becomes more acute.

Evaluation and Treatment

Diagnosis of intussusception is based on clinical manifestations, onset of symptoms, and contrast x-rays. Reduction of the intussusception is an emergency procedure. Reduction is accomplished by hydrostatic pressure exerted by an enema given under fluoroscopic guidance or by surgery. Untreated intussusception in infants is nearly always fatal. Most infants will recover if the intussusception is reduced within 24 hours. The mortality rate rises rapidly after that time.

Gastroesophageal Reflux

Gastroesophageal reflux (GER) is the return of stomach contents into the esophagus because of relaxation or incompetence of the lower esophageal sphincter (see Chapter 36). In newborns, reflux is normal because neuromuscular control of the gastroesophageal sphincter is not fully developed. In a small percentage of infants, reflux persists and causes clinical manifestations.

Pathophysiology

The cause of gastroesophageal reflux in infants is unknown. Delayed maturation of the lower esophageal sphincter or impaired hormonal response mechanisms are possible causes. In addition, several factors besides pressure maintain lower esophageal sphincter integrity in children. These factors include location of the gastroesophageal junction in a high-pressure zone within the abdomen, mucosal gathering within the sphincter, and the angle at which the esophagus is inserted into the stomach. Reflux persists if any of these pressure-maintaining factors is altered. Irritation of the mucosa by acidic gastric contents results in deterioration of the esophageal epithelium and stimulation of the vomiting reflex.

Clinical Manifestations

The signs and symptoms of gastroesophageal reflux are caused by exposure of the esophageal epithelium to refluxed gastric contents. Eighty-five percent of affected infants vomit excessively during the first week of life, and all have symptoms by 6 weeks.

Vomiting may be forceful. Aspiration pneumonia develops in one third of infants with gastroesophageal reflux. In cases that persist into childhood, chronic cough, wheezing, and recurrent pneumonia are common. Because repeated vomiting leads to inadequate retention of nutrients, growth and weight gain are affected adversely. The major manifestation of esophagitis is bleeding from the esophagus. This causes hematemesis in some children. Approximately 25% suffer from iron deficiency anemia caused by frank or occult blood loss.

Evaluation and Treatment

The clinical manifestations are often adequate to confirm a diagnosis of gastroesophageal reflux. A barium swallow and esophageal pH monitoring with a probe are useful diagnostic procedures in complex cases.

Mild gastroesophageal reflux resolves without treatment. Upright positioning of the infant, particularly for the hour after a feeding, and the feeding of thickened foods, can prevent episodes of reflux. Symptoms diminish by age 2 because the child spends more time in an upright position and is eating solid foods. In severe, untreated cases, reflux may continue until the child is 4 years of age or older. If no improvement is seen within

6 weeks of diagnosis, a surgical procedure called fundal plication is performed.

Impairment of Digestion, Absorption, and Nutrition

Cystic Fibrosis

Cystic fibrosis (CF) of the pancreas, also called mucoviscidosis or fibrocystic disease of the pancreas, is a genetically transmitted disease that involves many organs and systems and usually causes death in childhood or young adulthood. It is the most frequent cause of chronic suppurative lung disease in children and is the most common life-threatening inherited disease in the white population. This section will focus on the deficiency of pancreatic enzymes. (Chapter 31 discusses the pulmonary consequences of cystic fibrosis.)

TABLE 37-1   Pathophysiology, clinical manifestations, and complications of cystic fibrosis

Organ involved	Secretory dysfunction	Clinical manifestations	Complications
Sweat glands	Elevated concentration of sodium and chloride in sweat	Hyponatremia; hypochloremia	Heat prostration; shock
Intestine			
Newborn	Viscid meconium	Meconium ileus with intestinal obstruction	Meconium peritonitis
Older child and adult	Inspissated (dried out) mucofecal masses (intestinal sludging)	Partial intestinal obstruction with severe cramping pains	Volvulus (obstruction), intussusception (prolapse)
Pancreas (enzyme deficiency)	Inspissation and precipitation of pancreatic secretions, causing obstruction of pancreatic ducts	Absence of pancreatic enzymes, causing malabsorption of food and fatty, bulky stools	Hypoproteinemia; iron deficiency anemia
		Decreased vitamin A, D, E, K absorption	Vitamin A, D, E, & K deficiency and rectal prolapse, and/or insulin deficiency, diabetes mellitus
Liver	Insulin deficiency; inspissation and precipitation of bile in biliary system	Glucose intolerance; focal bilary cirrhosis; shrunken, "hob-nail" liver	Portal hypertension with esophageal varices and hematemesis
Salivary glands	Inspissation and precepitation of secretions in small ducts of submaxillary and sublingual salivary glands	Mild patchy fibrosis of salivary glands	None
Paranasal structures	Viscid mucus	Retention of mucus; clouding seen on sinus roentgenograms	Mucopyoceles (pus accumulations) with nasal deformity or orbital cavity extension
Nose	Nasal polyps	Obstruction of nasal airflow	None
Lungs	Viscid mucus in bronchioles and bronchi	Obstruction of bronchioles causing bronchiolectasis, bronchiectasis, and chronic lung infection	Hemoptysis; pneumothorax; cor pulmonale; respiratory failure
Reproductive tract			
Male	Viscid genital tract secretions during embryologic development, causing failure of formation of normal vas deferens	Sterility	None
Female	Distention of endocervical epithelial cells with cytoplasmic mucin	Decreased fertility	Polypoid cervicitis (cervical inflammation) while taking oral contraceptives

From Rudolph & Hoffman, 1982.

Pathophysiology

Dysfunction of the exocrine glands, which secrete such substances as digestive enzymes, mucus, sweat, and tears onto internal and external body surfaces, is the predominant pathogenic mechanism in CF. The pathophysiologic triad that is the hallmark of CF includes (1) pancreatic enzyme deficiency, which causes maldigestion; (2) overproduction of mucus in the respiratory tract, which causes progressive, chronic, obstructive pulmonary disease; and (3) abnormally elevated sodium and chloride concentrations in sweat. Exocrine secretions tend to be abnormally thick and to precipitate in the glandular ducts, obstructing flow. Almost all clinical manifestations of CF are a result of overproduction of mucus and pancreatic enzyme deficiency. The full spectrum of involvement is evident from Table 37-1.

Pancreatic function may range from normal to completely ablated. Individuals with near-normal pancreatic function will have normal fat absorption, lower chloride values in sweat, and better pulmonary function. When pancreatic function is compromised, severe problems with maldigestion of proteins, carbohydrates, and fats occur because of insufficient secretion of pancreatic enzymes. Obstruction of the pancreatic ducts with thick mucus blocks the flow of pancreatic enzymes and causes degenerative and fibrotic changes in the pancreas.

Clinical Manifestations

Inadequate pancreatic secretions result in steatorrhea (fatty stools) and azotorrhea (excess nitrogen in stools). Maldigestion results in malnutrition. Children may have short stature, pitting edema, and anemia from untreated hypoproteinemia. Purpura and telangiectasia may develop from vitamin K deficiency related to fat malabsorption. Secondary biliary cirrhosis (see Chapter 36) may develop because of obstruction of the bile channels. Stomatitis (inflammation of the mucosa of the mouth) occurs with vitamin B_2 (riboflavin) deficiency.

Evaluation and Treatment

Seventy-two-hour stool fat measurements are used to determine the extent of pancreatic function. Stools may also be examined for absence of pancreatic enzymes, particularly trypsin and chymotrypsin. Pancreatic replacement enzymes are administered before or with meals.

Gluten-Sensitive Enteropathy

Gluten-sensitive enteropathy, formerly called celiac sprue or celiac disease, is the loss of mature villous epithelium caused by ingestion of gluten, the protein component of cereal grains. The gluten in wheat, rye, barley, and oats is toxic to the intestinal epithelial cells of genetically susceptible individuals (Auricchio, Greco, & Troncone, 1988).

Although it is known that the α-gliadin fraction of gluten induces the mucosal damage, the exact mechanism of injury is unknown. Elevations of gluten-specific serum IgG and IgA in individuals with gluten-sensitive enteropathy indicate that immunologic mechanisms are involved.

Pathophysiology

The mucosa of the upper small intestine appears shiny, cobble-stoned, and thin in children with gluten-sensitive enteropathy. The major pathophysiologic characteristics of the disease are atrophy of villi in the upper small intestine and malabsorption of most nutrients in the presence of cereal gluten (Fig. 37-6). The atrophy is caused by accelerated shedding of epithelial cells from the villi. To compensate for this loss, epithelial cell production increases, causing hypertrophy of the crypts of Leiberkuhn. Increased cell production is not sufficient to keep pace with cell loss, however. Inflammation and edema develop around the enlarged cysts. The villi shorten and atrophy, and their surface cells are not mature enough to sustain absorptive functions. The microvilli and brush border disappear, leaving patches of bald mucosa. The loss of mucosal surface area and brush border enzymes leads to severe malabsorption. The pathologic process is most pronounced in the duodenum and jejunum. The ileum may be spared.

Damage to the mucosa of the duodenum and jejunum have secondary effects that exacerbate malabsorption. The secretion of intestinal hormones, such as secretin and cholecystokinin-pancreozymin, may be diminished. Because these chemical messengers are scarce, secretion of pancreatic enzymes and expulsion of bile from the gallbladder decrease.

Destruction of mucosal cells causes inflammation. The inflamed mucosa secretes rather than absorbs water and electrolytes, leading to watery diarrhea. In addition, absorption that normally occurs by sodium-dependent, active transport or facilitated diffusion is impaired. Carbohydrates, amino acids, dipeptides, water-soluble vitamins, bile salts, and cations are not absorbed from the intestinal lumen. Potassium loss, which is more severe than sodium loss, leads to muscle weakness. Magnesium and calcium malabsorption can cause seizures or tetany. Unabsorbed fatty acids combine with calcium, and secondary hyperparathyroidism increases phosphorus excretion, resulting in bone reabsorption. Calcium is no longer available to bind oxalate in the intestine and is absorbed, which causes hyperoxaluria. Gallbladder function may be abnormal, and bile salt conjugation may be decreased.

Fat malabsorption in the jejunum is the major cause of steatorrhea (fatty stools). Malabsorption may be mild early in the disease. Fecal nitrogen is elevated because peptidase deficiencies impair protein absorption. Pan-

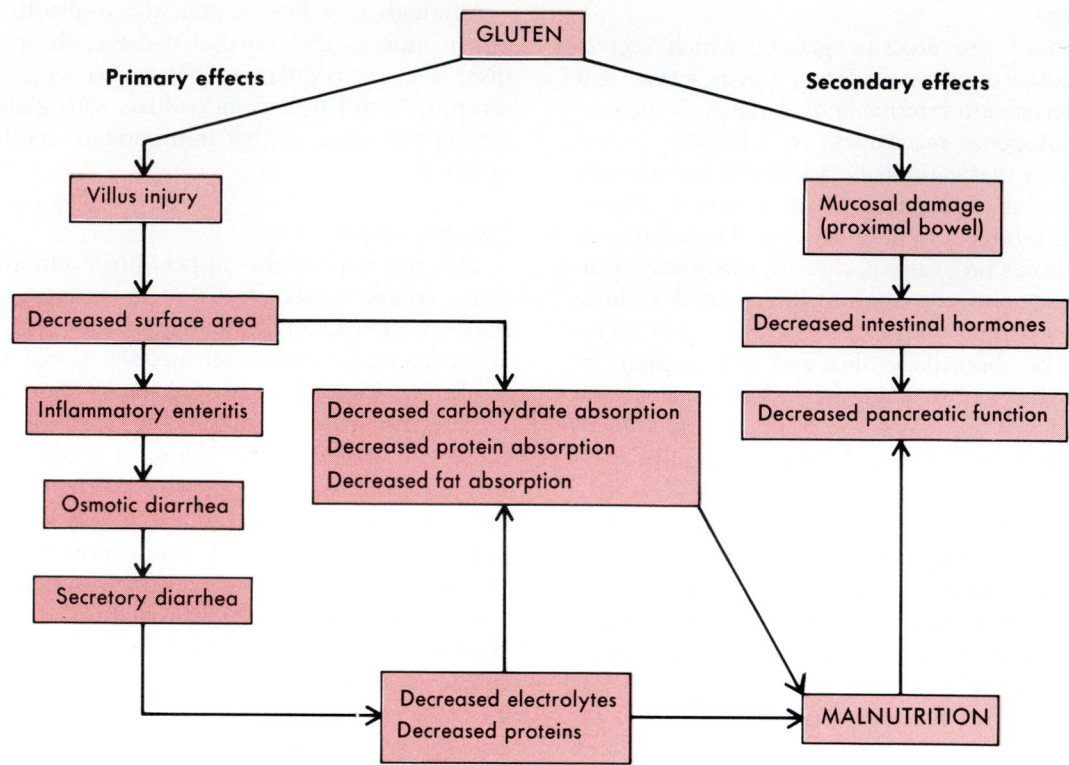

FIG. 37-6. Pathophysiology of gluten-sensitive enteropathy.

creatic function is decreased, not only because of decreased hormonal levels, but also because of malnutrition.

Deficiencies of fat-soluble vitamins are common in children with gluten-sensitive enteropathy. Vitamin K malabsorption leads to hypoprothrombinemia. In one third of cases, iron and folic acid malabsorption are manifested as cheilosis, anemia, and a smooth red tongue. Vitamin B$_{12}$ absorption is impaired in those with extensive ileal disease. Because the absorption of folate, iron, and myrodoxine is greatest in the proximal small intestine, deficiencies of these substances are common.

Clinical Manifestations

The onset of clinical manifestations of gluten-sensitive enteropathy depends on the age of the infant when gluten-containing substances are added to the diet. In 50% of affected children, onset occurs by 18 months of age, with latent intervals varying from months to years.

Diarrhea is an early sign in most infants. The stools are pale, bulky, greasy, and foul-smelling, and they may contain oil droplets. Three to five such movements occur daily. As early as 3 or 4 months of age, growth failure, anorexia, and constipation can begin. In older children, constipation is occasionally seen despite steatorrhea. Vomiting and abdominal pain are prominent in infants, but unusual in older children. Anorexia is prev-

alent. The classic physical manifestations of organic failure to thrive, such as abdominal protuberance, wasted buttocks and limbs, and hypotonia, occur in less than 50% of infants with gluten-sensitive enteropathy. Growth is usually diminished (Greco, Tozzi, & Mayer, 1987).

Manifestations of malabsorption, such as rickets, anemia, tetany, frank bleeding, or anemia, may be obvious. Some children urinate more at night. The tongue is smooth and red, and the child may bruise and bleed easily. Hypomagnesemia and hypocalcemia cause irritability, tremor, convulsions, tetany, bone pain, osteomalacia, and dental abnormalities. If vitamin D deficiency is prolonged, rickets and clubbing of the terminal phalanges are likely. Eighty-six percent of older children have fingerprint changes (ridge atrophy). Fingerprint changes are unusual before 5 years of age, and, if present, they resolve with treatment. In older children, delayed puberty and infertility may be a manifestation of otherwise subtle gluten-sensitive enteropathy.

An unusual complication of gluten-sensitive enteropathy in infancy is celiac crisis. Celiac crisis is characterized by severe diarrhea, dehydration, and hypoproteinemia as a result of malabsorption and protein loss.

Evaluation and Treatment

An intestinal biopsy is mandatory to detect mucosal changes caused by gluten-sensitive enteropathy. A wide variety of screening tests for malabsorption may also be useful. The best known tests are the serum D-xylose assay, which is used to assess upper intestinal surface area, and the quantitative, 72-hour, stool fat determination, which is used to detect steatorrhea. Steatorrhea is present in 80% of infants with gluten-sensitive enteropathy. Serum antibodies to gliaden may also be measured.

Treatment consists of the immediate and permanent institution of a diet free of cereal grains (wheat, rye, barley, oats, and malt). Lactose intolerance is presumed; therefore, lactose (milk sugar) is also excluded from the diet. Infants are routinely given vitamin D, iron, and folic acid supplements to treat deficiencies.

Approximately 25% of children suffer from recurrent relapses that interfere with growth. For most children, however, the long-term prognosis is excellent.

Protein Energy Malnutrition Kwashiorkor and marasmus are the two most common types of malnutrition in children. These disorders are known collectively as **protein energy malnutrition** (PEM). Both are states of long-term starvation (see Chapter 36). **Kwashiorkor** is a severe protein deficiency, while **marasmus** is a severe deficiency of all nutrients. Kwashiorkor is a widespread nutritional problem among children in developing countries and economically destitute populations. The disease usually occurs in infants or children from 1 to 4 years of age who have been weaned from breast milk to a high-starch, protein-deficient diet.

Marasmus, which means "to waste," can occur at any age, but it is common in children under 1 year of age. In marasmus, starvation is due to lack of protein and carbohydrates. In developing countries and impoverished populations, early weaning of breastfed infants to overdiluted commercial formulas is a risk factor for marasmus (Hegsted, 1976).

Protein energy malnutrition is also a complication of diseases, such as chronic fever, tuberculosis, malignancy, digestive and malabsorptive disorders, and psychogenic illness. Radiation therapy and chemotherapy can also contribute to protein energy malnutrition.

Pathophysiology

In cases of kwashiorkor the deficit dietary amino acids reduces protein synthesis in all tissues. Physical and mental growth are stunted permanently, and maintenance of minimal life processes is in jeopardy. The lack of sufficient plasma proteins, particularly albumin, causes systemic pressure changes that result in generalized edema. The volume of total body water and extracellular fluid increases, causing a substantial loss of potassium. The liver swells with stored fat because no hepatic proteins are synthesized to form and release lipoproteins. Kwashiorkor also causes malabsorption, reduced bone density, and impaired renal function. If

the condition is not reversed, the prognosis is very poor.

Because the intake of all dietary nutrients is reduced to a minimum in marasmus, metabolic processes, including liver function, are preserved, while growth is severely retarded. Caloric intake is too low to support protein synthesis for growth or the storage of fat. If more protein is needed than is ingested, muscle wasting occurs. Fat wasting and anemia are common and can be severe. The volume of total body water is high, extracellular fluid is somewhat increased, and potassium is depleted slightly. The serum lipoprotein level is high, but other serum values are normal or slightly reduced. Severe vitamin A deficiency commonly results in blindness.

Clinical Manifestations

Retarded physical, mental, and psychologic development; muscle wasting; diarrhea; and infection characterize marasmus. The presence of subcutaneous fat, hepatomegaly, and fatty liver distinguish kwashiorkor from marasmus. These manifestations are missing in marasmus because caloric intake is not sufficient to support fat synthesis and storage.

Evaluation and Treatment

Evaluation of PEM is based on nutritional history and clinical manifestations. The provision of deficient nutrients will resolve clinical symptoms in 4 to 6 weeks. Physical and mental retardation may not be reversible, however. Reversibility depends on the duration of PEM and the child's developmental status when the deficiency occurred.

Failure to Thrive

Failure to thrive (FTT) is the inadequate physical development of an infant or child. It is manifested as a deceleration in weight gain, a low weight height ratio, or a low weight/height/head circumference ratio. In the United States, FTT usually affects infants and young children. Failure to thrive is a nutritional disorder having organic or nonorganic causes. Nonorganic FTT is most common among psychosocially and economically deprived populations, whereas organic FTT occurs equally in all populations. The incidence of nonorganic FTT is greater than that of organic FTT (Cupoli, 1980).

Pathophysiology

Organic FTT has a pathophysiologic cause. Gastroesophageal reflux and pyloric stenosis, for example, cause nutrients to be lost through persistent vomiting. Gastroenteritis and infection by intestinal parasites cause nutrients to be lost through vomiting, diarrhea, and interference with mucosal absorption. Congenital anomalies or chronic diseases of major body systems can inhibit enzyme and hormone secretion, digestion, absorption, and the transport of nutrients to tissues. All of these factors reduce the availability of nutrients for maintenance and growth. Psychosocial problems can develop as a result of organic FTT. A chronic disease or congenital anomaly that causes weakness or reduced stature can create psychosocial and emotional problems for the child.

Nonorganic FTT is a syndrome with many psychosocial causes. The problem in nonorganic FTT is ineffective nurturing by primary caregivers. Infants and children are at risk for nonorganic FTT if their parents or primary caregivers are unable to provide nurturance. A variety of parental stressors may be involved, for example:
Lack of nurturance in the parents' own childhood
  Unwanted pregnancy
  Inability to bond with the infant because of health or other problems
  Postpartum depression
  Family crisis, such as a death or marital problems
  Stress caused by single parenthood or social isolation
  Mental, emotional, or physical illness

Clinical Manifestations

Clinical manifestations of organic FTT are retarded growth accompanied by manifestations of the underlying disease. Manifestations of nonorganic FTT are retarded growth plus reduced energy level, reduced responsiveness and interaction with the environment, social isolation, spasticity and rigidity when held or touched, inability to make eye contact or smile, refusal to eat, and rejection of foods. Weight loss and decelerated growth are accompanied by developmental retardation in many areas. Nonorganic FTT is a complex syndrome involving psychosocial, emotional, and parent-child problems that compound the pathophysiologic abnormalities (Chow et al., 1984).

Evaluation and Treatment

Failure to thrive is often complex and difficult to assess. The condition is suspected if a child falls below the third percentile on the growth curve. Organic FFT is manifested in infancy by weight, height, and head circumference measurements that are parallel to but below the normal ranges. If no genetic, endocrine, or other systemic disorder is identified, and if the physical and laboratory examination reveal no abnormalities other than delayed growth, an environmental cause is suspected.

Hospital admission is recommended if the diagnosis is unclear or the child is in nutritional or emotional jeopardy. Eating patterns, food preferences, caloric intake, and family interactions can be assessed during the hospital stay. If the cause is environmental, the hospitalized child with FTT usually begins to gain weight.

If an organic problem has been identified, management of FTT consists of treating the cause. Management of nonorganic FTT involves the immediate total care of the child and measures to address (1) the psychosocial and emotional problems of the caretakers, and (2) parent-child interactions. Counseling, parental modeling, and long-term family support are sometimes required.

Diarrhea

Diarrhea is a frequent gastrointestinal problem during infancy and early childhood. Severe diarrhea occurs between one and three times during the first 3 years of life. Most episodes are self-limiting and resolve within 72 hours.

The pathophysiologic mechanisms of diarrhea in children are similar to those described in Chapter 36 for adults. Prolonged diarrhea is more dangerous in children, however, because they have much smaller fluid reserves than adults. Therefore dehydration can develop rapidly if any disturbance increases fluid secretion into the gastrointestinal lumen (secretory diarrhea), draws fluid into the lumen by osmosis (osmotic diarrhea), or prevents fluid absorption in the intestine.

Infant diarrhea is of special concern because its cause may be a congenital or metabolic anomaly. Infants have low fluid reserves and relatively rapid peristalsis and metabolism. Therefore the danger of dehydration is great.

Common causes of acute diarrhea in infants include congenital aganglionic megacolon, infections, milk protein allergies, and necrotizing enterocolitis. Less common causes are adrenogenital syndrome, impaired chloride-bicarbonate exchange, congenital lactase deficiency, glucose-galactose malabsorption, and sucrase-isomaltase deficiency.

Infectious diarrhea in newborns is usually associated with nursery epidemics involving such pathogens as *Escherichea coli*, *Klebsiella*, staphylococci, salmonella, and *shigella*. Diarrhea caused by these agents has a rapid onset, and acidosis and shock can occur quickly. True milk protein allergy, which is uncommon, causes bloody, explosive stools after the introduction of milk into the diet.

Necrotizing Enterocolitis

Necrotizing enterocolitis is a potentially fatal condition that, if untreated, causes bowel necrosis or perforation. Its cause is unknown. The incidence reported in one study was 3 per 1000 live births and 30 per 1000 low-weight births (Pokorny, Garcia-Pratts, & Yvonne, 1986).

Pathophysiology

A number of factors can contribute to the development of necrotizing enterocolitis, including infections, immunologic injury, perinatal stress, and the effects of medications and feeding practices. Accumulation of gas in the mucosa and submucosa leads to ischemia and necrosis of intestinal segments.

Clinical Manifestations

Manifestations of necrotizing enterocolitis usually appear within 2 weeks of birth. They range from mild abdominal distention to bowel perforation, sepsis, and death. Abdominal pain, unstable temperature, bradycardia, and apnea are nonspecific signs. About 25% of affected infants have bloody stools, gastric retention, and abdominal distention. Premature infants often have more severe disease and other disorders, such as hyaline membrane disease (Barnard, Cotton, & Lutin, 1985).

Evaluation and Treatment

Diagnosis of necrotizing enterocolitis is based on clinical manifestations and plain films of the abdomen that show gas accumulation in the intestine. Treatments include cessation of feeding, gastric suction to decompress the intestines, fluid and electrolyte maintenance, and administration of antibiotics to control sepsis. Surgical resection is the treatment of choice for perforation (Cooper et al., 1988). Overall mortality is 20% to 40% (Walsh, Kleigman, & Fanaroff, 1988). Low-birth-weight infants are at greatest risk of death.

Causes of Chronic Diarrhea in Unwell Children with Retarded Growth

COMMON CAUSES
Cystic fibrosis
Gluten-sensitive enteropathy (celiac sprue)
Congenital aganglionic megacolon (Hirschsprung disease)
Short gut syndrome
Immune deficiency
Inflammatory bowel disease

LESS COMMON CAUSES
Acrodermatitis enteropathica
Bacterial overgrowth
Impaired chloride-bicarbonate exchange in the large intestine (familial chloride diarrhea)
Mild protein intolerance
Eosinophilic gastroenteritis
Intestinal lymphangiectasia
Isolated pancreatic enzyme deficiency
Radiation enteritis
Tropical sprue
Tumors (carcinoid, neural crest, gastrinoma, vipoma)
Poor nurturing by parents or primary caregivers

Acute Diarrhea in Childhood

Acute diarrhea in childhood is almost synonymous with acute viral or bacterial gastroenteritis. Viral gastroenteritis tends to be self-limiting. Bacterial gastroenteritis is treated with antibiotics if the causal pathogen can be identified. Other causes of acute diarrhea in the older child include antibiotic therapy, appendicitis, chemotherapy, inflammatory bowel disease, parasitic infestation, parenteral infections, and ingestion of toxic substances.

Chronic Diarrhea in Children

In adults, diarrhea is considered to be chronic if it lasts longer than 2 weeks. This definition does not apply to children, since children with acute gastroenteritis frequently remain mildly symptomatic for up to 4 weeks. In children, diarrhea that persists longer than 4 weeks is considered to be chronic.

Children with chronic diarrhea can be divided into two groups: (1) otherwise well children whose growth is normal and (2) ill children whose growth is retarded. Causes of chronic diarrhea in the first group include abnormal colonic motility, lactose intolerance, encopresis, parasitic infestation, and antibiotic use. Chronic diarrhea in the second group is usually due to a disease that impairs absorption.

Chronic Nonspecific Diarrhea

Chronic nonspecific diarrhea is a condition in which uncoordinated colonic motility causes forceful expulsion of feces. Apparently, the lower sigmoid colon remains in a tonically contracted state. Defecation occurs when pressure in the upper sigmoid colon and distal descending colon becomes great enough to force feces through the nonmotile, contracted segment.

In some instances, there is a family history of bowel complaints. As an infant, the child is likely to have experienced colic and diarrhea associated with teething and immunizations. In more than 90% of cases, chronic nonspecific diarrhea resolves by age 39 months. The cure frequently accompanies toilet training. Many children with chronic nonspecific diarrhea will develop irritable bowel syndrome (also called mucous colitis) as adults (Levine, 1987). Children with chronic nonspecific diarrhea usually do well with normal food and fluid intake. Special diets and medications are used with caution.

Primary Lactose Intolerance

Lactose intolerance, the inability to digest milk sugar, is due to inadequate production of lactase (see Chapter 36). Lactose intolerance is a common cause of diarrhea in children, particularly black children. The lactase deficiency causes osmotic diarrhea, in which fluids move by osmosis from the vascular compartment into the intestinal lumen. The diarrhea is accompanied by abdominal pain, bloating, and flatulence. These symptoms begin before the age of 7 in half of affected blacks. Treatment consists of reducing milk consumption. Some children can tolerate lactose in fermented forms, such as cheese and yogurt.

DISORDERS OF THE LIVER

Disorders of Biliary Metabolism and Transport
Physiologic Jaundice of the Newborn

Physiologic jaundice of the newborn is usually a transient, benign, icterus that occurs during the first week of life in otherwise healthy, full-term infants. It is caused by mild hyperbilirubinemia. Pathologic jaundice, on the other hand, is due to severe hyperbilirubinemia that persists and can cause brain damage. (Hyperbilirubinemia is described fully in Chapter 36.)

Pathophysiology

Physiologic jaundice results from the complex interaction of factors that cause (1) increased bilirubin production, (2) impaired hepatic uptake and excretion of bilirubin, and (3) reabsorption of bilirubin in the small intestine. Serum bilirubin values increase to 5 to 6 mg/dl by the second to fourth day after birth in full-term infants, and 10 to 15 mg/dl by the fifth to seventh day in premature infants.

Clinical Manifestations

Physiologic jaundice develops during the second or third day after birth. It usually subsides in 1 to 2 weeks in full-term infants and 2 to 4 weeks in premature infants. After this, increasing bilirubin values and persistent jaundice indicate pathologic hyperbilirubinemia. Bilirubin encephalopathy, which is due to the deposition of toxic, unconjugated bilirubin in brain cells, usually does not occur in healthy, full-term infants. Premature infants with respiratory distress, acidosis, or sepsis are at greater risk for encephalopathy. The mechanism by which bilirubin crosses the blood-brain barrier and precipitates into brain cells is not known (Stern & Brodersen, 1987).

Evaluation and Treatment

Laboratory tests are conducted to determine bilirubin levels. Both total and direct (conjugated) bilirubin levels are measured; the direct bilirubin should not exceed 1 mg/dl (Behrman & Vaughan, 1987). Other causes of jaundice must be eliminated to confirm physiologic jaundice. Treatment depends on the degree of hyperbilirubinemia. Physiologic jaundice is usually treated by phototherapy (ultraviolet light). Pathologic jaundice requires an exchange transfusion.

Biliary Atresia

Biliary atresia is a congenital malformation characterized by the absence or obstruction of intrahepatic or extrahepatic bile ducts. Extrahepatic ducts may end in a blind pouch. Intrahepatic ducts may be blocked by infection, metabolic disorders, anatomic malformations, or genetic defects (Fitzgerald, 1988). Extrahepatic biliary atresia may be caused by a virus (Glaser & Morecki, 1987).

The atresia or obstruction of the bile ducts leads to plugging, inflammation, and fibrosis of the bile canaliculi. Progressive obstruction may lead to biliary cirrhosis (see Chapter 36), portal hypertension, or liver failure.

Jaundice is the primary clinical manifestation of biliary atresia. Other signs are hepatomegaly and acholic (clay-colored) stools. Fat absorption is impaired for lack of bile salts, and the infant may fail to gain weight. Cirrhosis and liver failure can lead to death.

Diagnosis of biliary atresia is based on clinical manifestations and liver biopsy. Liver function test results are abnormal. Serum transaminase and alkaline phosphatase values are elevated, and conjugated serum bilirubin levels rise progressively.

Extrahepatic atresia can be relieved by surgical drainage and correction in about 10% of cases. Some infants benefit from the Kasai procedure, in which a hepatic duct remnant is anastomosed to the jejunum. This procedure has a 25% success rate. Liver transplantation is a possible alternative for children with atresia that cannot be corrected surgically (Alagille, 1987).

Inflammatory Disorders
Hepatitis

Hepatitis A, B, non-A, non-B, D (delta), and fulminant hepatitis affect children and adults. Hepatitis can also result from infection with other viruses, for example, herpesvirus, varicella, cytomegalovirus, rubella, coxsackie B, and Epstein-Barr virus. The pathophysiology of viral and fulminant hepatitis is described in Chapter 36.

Hepatitis A

About one third of the reported cases of hepatitis A occur in children (Francis et al., 1984). Incidence is highest among young children of nursery school age. Outbreaks tend to occur in day care centers with large numbers of children who are not toilet trained and staff members who practice poor handwashing techniques (Hadler & McFarland, 1986). Hepatitis A in children is usually mild and asymptomatic. When it does, clinical manifestations include nausea, vomiting, and diarrhea. Because jaundice is absent, infected children appear to have the "flu." Almost all children recover from hepatitis A without residual liver damage.

Hepatitis B

Infection with the hepatitis B virus (HBV) usually occurs among children in high-risk situations. Infants of mothers who are chronic HB$_s$Ag carriers, hemophiliacs who receive frequent blood transfusions, children who abuse parenteral drugs, and children who live in institutions for the mentally retarded are all at risk for HBV infection. Ninety percent of newborns infected by their mothers will develop chronic hepatitis and become carriers. Chronic hepatitis may develop because the infant's immune system is immature. Infected infants are at risk for cirrhosis and hepatocellular carcinoma (Balistreri, 1988). The most serious consequence of HBV infection is fulminant hepatitis, which occurs in 1% of cases. Hepatitis D infection depends on active infection with HBV. The addition of hepatitis D infection may increase the likelihood of chronicity or fulminant hepatitis.

Non-A, Non-B Hepatitis

Non-A, non-B hepatitis in children is primarily associated with blood transfusions. Children who receive frequent transfusions are at highest risk. Because there are no serologic markers for non-A, non-B hepatitis, other causes of acute hepatitis must be ruled out (Hay et al., 1987). Between 10% and 50% of affected children will develop chronic liver disease.

Chronic Hepatitis

Chronic hepatitis in adults is usually defined as liver disease lasting longer than 6 months. Chronic hepatitis in children is more difficult to define because the clinical manifestations of illness are milder than they are in adults. Hepatitis A, which is prevalent in childhood, neither persists nor progresses to chronic liver disease (Bortollotti et al., 1987). The cause of chronic hepatitis is unknown in most cases, but an autoimmune mechanism is suspected because inflammatory findings are commonly seen in biopsy specimens of the liver.

Manifestations of chronic hepatitis include malaise, anorexia, fever, gastrointestinal bleeding, hepatomegaly, edema, and transient joint pain. Serum transaminase and bilirubin levels are elevated and prothrombin time is prolonged. The diagnosis of chronic hepatitis is based on the clinical manifestations and liver biopsy. There is no effective therapy for chronic hepatitis B or chronic non-A, non-B hepatitis. Some success has been achieved with human alpha interferon (Hess et al., 1987), and young children respond to alternate-day treatment with steroids (Behrman, Vaughan, & Nelson, 1987).

Cirrhosis

Most forms of chronic liver diseases in children can progress to cirrhosis, but they seldom do so. Cirrhosis is the excessive formation of fibrous tissue in response to inflammation and tissue damage (see Chapter 36). The complications of cirrhosis in children are the same as those in adults: portal hypertension, the opening of collateral vessels between the portal and systemic veins, and varices. The cause of cirrhosis may influence its severity and course. Some types of cirrhosis can be stabilized if the cause is identified and treated early.

Portal Hypertension

Portal hypertension is a persistent increase in portal venous pressure (see Chapter 36). Because the portal system is relatively inaccessible, pressures in children are not often measured or are measured in unique ways. There are no standard values for portal pressure in children. In adults, however, portal hypertension is often defined as the presence of a pressure gradient of 10 to 15 cm H_2O between the portal and the systemic venous system.

There are two basic causes of portal hypertension in children: (1) increased resistance to blood flow within the portal system or (2) increased volume of portal blood flow. The second cause is quite rare in children and will not be discussed here. Increased resistance to flow can occur anywhere in the portal circulatory system. Portal hypertension can accompany cirrhosis, intraabdominal infections, portal vein thrombosis, congenital anomalies of the portal vein, and congenital hepatic fibrosis.

Types of Portal Hypertension

Extrahepatic Portal Hypertension

Extrahepatic (prehepatic) portal venous obstruction causes 50% to 70% of extrahepatic portal hypertension in children. In about two thirds of these children, no specific cause can be found (Behrman & Vaughan, 1987). Obstruction is almost always in the portal vein and is usually due to thrombosis. Portal vein thrombosis can occur as a complication of abdominal trauma, pancreatitis, abdominal infections, and some systemic disorders; however, these causes are rare. The liver is usually normal in cases of extrahepatic portal hypertension.

Intrahepatic Portal Hypertension

Cirrhosis is the primary cause of intrahepatic portal hypertension. In some cases of severe cirrhosis, the portal flow is thought to be reversed; whether this actually happens is controversial (Whitington, 1985). The most common finding is fibrosis, which increases resistance to portal blood flow by constricting and reducing the compliance of the hepatic sinusoids.

Course of the Disease

The important consequences of portal hypertension in children are the development of collateral circulation, with portal-systemic shunting; hypersplenism; and ascites. The pathophysiology of portal hypertension is described in Chapter 36.

Clinical Manifestations

The clinical manifestations of portal hypertension are (1) splenomegaly, (2) upper gastrointestinal bleeding, (3) ascites, and (4) hepatic encephalopathy. Splenomegaly is the most frequent sign of portal hypertension in children. The spleen may be firm or hard, depending on the duration of portal hypertension. Hematemesis, usually occurring some time after an episode of abdominal pain, is often associated with sudden pallor. Melena is observed, either at the time of hematemesis or soon afterward. In children, most episodes of gastrointestinal bleeding are due to the rupture of esophageal varices. Clotting abnormalities caused by altered liver function promote the bleeding. If plasma volume is increased, esophageal varices readily rupture during activities, such as coughing, that increase blood pressure. Acetylsalicylic acid (aspirin), which should not be administered to children, can trigger bleeding, but its exact mechanisms of action are not known. Severe bleeding episodes can cause hypovolemic shock and death. Symptoms of ascites include weight gain, protruding abdomen, and reduced tidal volumes if the ascites is severe.

Hepatic encephalopathy in children can be acute or chronic. Acute encephalopathy is characterized by major disorders of consciousness, which may progress to coma. Chronic, or minimal, encephalopathy is characterized by emotional or psychiatric disorders, decreased intellectual functioning, personality disorders caused by minimal brain dysfunction, and spatial disorientation.

Evaluation and Treatment

Assessment of portal hypertension in children must be thorough because the cause dictates the management. The objectives of the clinical investigation are to (1) locate the site of the venous block and (2) identify the disease responsible for the portal hypertension. Thorough physical examination, laboratory tests of liver function, imaging procedures, and biopsy may be included in the diagnostic evaluation (see Chapter 35). Severe liver disease is characterized by hypoalbuminemia, prolonged prothrombin times, hyperbilirubinemia, electrolyte imbalance, and hypoglycemia.

The outcome of portal hypertension depends almost entirely on its cause. Children with extrahepatic disease are expected to recover with little morbidity. For children with intrahepatic disease, the prognosis varies. For example, stable postnecrotic cirrhosis, complicated by variceal bleeding, has a much better prognosis than does cirrhosis with chronic acute liver disease and variceal bleeding. Postsinusoidal hypertension (high pressure

---

Clinical Management of Portal Hypertension in Children

POTENTIAL FOR GASTROINTESTINAL BLEEDING
Avoidance of aspirin-containing drugs
Surgical shunting

MASSIVE GASTROINTESTINAL HEMORRHAGE
Resuscitation
Arrest of hemorrhage
   Gastric cooling (debated)
   Vasopression
   Sengstaken-Blakemore tube (tamponade of esophageal varices)
   Blood transfusion
If bleeding stops, conservative therapy is continued, and shunt surgery is planned when indicated
If bleeding continues, emergency surgical transection of gastroesophageal varices is undertaken, to be followed by shunt procedure

ASCITES
Restriction of dietary sodium and fluid intake
Diuretics
Paracentesis (for diagnosis; exclusion of infection; relief of respiratory distress and painful, tense ascites; facilitation of physical or radiologic examination)

---

generated in the hepatic veins or vena cava) generally results in extreme morbidity and mortality. Encephalopathy has been reported in 22% to 29% of childern (Voorhes & Price, 1974).

Metabolic Disorders

Over 5000 genetically determined, metabolic pathways have been identified in liver tissue. The earliest possible identification of metabolic disorders is essential because (1) early treatment may prevent permanent damage to vital organs, such as the liver or brain; (2) precise genetic counseling may be possible with prenatal diagnosis; and (3) complications can be minimized, even if cure is not possible. Galactosemia, fructosemia, and Wilson disease are treatable metabolic disorders that have hepatic clinical manifestations.

Galactosemia

Galactosemia is a rare disorder caused by a deficiency of the enzyme galactose-1-phosphate uridyltransferase (a hepatic enzyme needed to convert galactose to glucose). This deficiency is inherited as a autosomal recessive trait. Because galactose cannot be incorporated into carbohydrate metabolism, it accumulates in all body tissues together with metabolites, which may be toxic. Galactosuria may occur after the ingestion of lactose.

Pathophysiology

A deficiency of galactose-1-phosphate uridyltransferase results in the accumulation of galactose-1-phosphate in body cells. These accumulations are most injurious in the liver, where they cause cirrhosis, and in the brain, where they cause mental retardation. Increasing accumulations cause severe and irreversible damage. Cataracts form because of increasing concentrations of galactitol resulting from uridyltransferase deficiency.

Clinical Manifestations

Signs of galactosemia appear in early infancy because milk (particularly breast milk) contains lactose. Some infants have mild failure to thrive and manifestations of cirrhosis that become evident at 2 to 6 months of age. Rarely are the early signs mental retardation, cataracts, or both.

Evaluation and Treatment

Diagnosis is based on a test for the presence of a reducing substance in the urine while the infant is receiving a formula containing lactose. Treatment consists of a galactose-free diet. Removal of dietary lactose causes rapid improvement in the infant's condition, including regression of jaundice, gastrointestial symptoms, bleeding, and other symptoms of cirrhosis. Most infants have no subsequent liver problems. Cataracts are stabilized and may regress slightly with treatment. Brain damage is irreversible. Long-term follow-up of adequately treated children shows that their mental development is often impaired. Children with galactose-1-phosphate uridyltransferase deficiency must continue a lactose-free diet for life.

Fructosemia

Fructosemia (hereditary fructose intolerance) is an inherited, autosomal recessive deficiency of the enzyme fructose-1-phosphate aldolase. If fructose is ingested, it has profound secondary effects on carbohydrate and nucleotide metabolism, particularly within the liver cells. Affected individuals develop an extreme aversion to fructose-containing foods.

Pathophysiology

Because of the fructose-1-phosphate aldolase deficiency, fructose-1-phosphate accumulates in hepatocytes. This accumulation is toxic in some children and results in severe, progressive liver disease. The accumulation of fructose-1-phosphate transiently inhibits the conversion of glycogen to glucose, causing severe hypoglycemia.

Clinical Manifestations

Signs of fructosemia include jaundice, vomiting, irritability, hepatomegaly, coagulation disorders, and convulsions that begin as soon as fructose is ingested. Onset occurs when breast milk is replaced by cow's milk, formula, or foods containing fructose, sucrose, or honey. In an older child, fructosemia may be seen as a feeding difficulty because ingestion of a fructose-containing food will cause anorexia and malaise. Older children and adults may develop manifestations when given intravenous fructose during an illness. Some children can tolerate a small amount of sucrose, but in most, sucrose ingestion provokes progressive liver damage, abdominal distention, and, ultimately, cirrhosis.

Evaluation and Treatment

A detailed dietary history is essential. The diagnosis is confirmed if low enzymatic activity is demonstrated in a liver or intestinal mucosal biopsy specimen.

Withdrawal of fructose from the diet causes vomiting to regress almost immediately, and other signs of liver disease improve within a few days. A fructose-free and sucrose-free diet must be maintained for life, and vitamin C supplements must be taken. If fructosemia causes acute liver failure, exchange transfusions, plasma and blood transfusions, and intravenous glucose may be required. With the institution of a fructose-free diet, the liver gradually decreases in size, and liver function tests return to normal. Fatty changes in liver tissue diminish but never disappear completely.

Wilson Disease

Wilson disease (hepatolenticular degeneration) is an autosomal recessive defect of copper metabolism that causes toxic amounts of copper to accumulate in the liver, brain, kidneys, and corneas. This defect in the uptake and excretion of copper by hepatocytes is an important cause of progressive liver disease in children and young adults. Wilson disease is very rare, with an incidence between 1 in 100,000 and 1 in 200,000 persons. Between 1 in 200 and 1 in 500 persons are carriers (Avery & First, 1986).

Pathophysiology

Two major abnormalities in copper metabolism have been identified: (1) diminished biliary excretion of copper and (2) impaired production of ceruloplasmin (a glycoprotein that transports copper in the blood). A positive copper balance is present from birth in children with Wilson disease, despite increased excretion of copper in the urine.

Early in the disease, intestinal absorption of copper is normal, as is hepatic clearance of albumin-bound, absorbed copper. As copper-binding proteins in the liver become saturated, hepatic uptake of copper diminishes. Decreased hepatic metabolism of copper causes elevated serum copper levels and biochemical and clinical evidence of liver damage caused by copper accumulation. In later stages of the disease, copper accumulates in extrahepatic tissues, including the eyes, brain, and kidneys.

Controversy exists over the pathogenesis of Wilson disease. One theory holds that the synthesis of the copper-binding protein, ceruloplasmin, may be deficient or abnormal; another suggests that biliary excretion of copper is impaired (Scheinberg & Sternlieb, 1984). When copper accumulating in liver cells (hepatocytes) reaches toxic levels, the liver cells die. Copper is released and accumulates in and damages other tissues.

When cerebral copper-binding proteins become saturated, a characteristic pattern of brain damage develops, particularly in the basal ganglia. Neural effects include intention tremor, unsteady gait, dystonia, and behavioral changes. Manifestations of renal tubular injury usually appear simultaneously. The uptake of copper by red blood cells is thought to cause hemolytic anemia, a condition sometimes seen early in the clinical course of Wilson disease.

Clinical Manifestations

The clinical manifestations of Wilson disease begin at about 4 years of age, the age by which control mechanisms responsible for copper homeostasis and biliary excretion should have matured. Some individuals, however, do not develop signs and symptoms until later in life.

The classic clinical presentation of Wilson disease is a triad of neuromuscular abnormalities, intention tremors, dysarthria (indistinct speech), and dystonia (disordered muscular tonicity); Kayser-Fleischer rings (accumulation of copper in the limbus of the cornea, causing a greenish yellow ring); cirrhosis associated with elevated serum copper; and low ceruloplasmin levels. Initial symptoms vary from malaise and abdominal pain to jaundice and changes in mental performance. The earliest signs of liver involvement include enlargement of the liver and spleen, jaundice, and anorexia. Edema and ascites may develop suddenly, or gastrointestinal hemorrhage may be the initial sign of the disease. Occasionally, Wilson disease begins with a hemolytic crisis caused by the toxic effects of copper on the red blood cells. Cirrhosis develops in all untreated cases. Copper deposition in the kidneys causes a proximal renal tubular defect that results in losses of glucose, amino acids, phosphate, and uric acid in the urine and renal tubular acidosis.

Evaluation and Treatment

Because Wilson disease is rare, it may not be diagnosed until clinical manifestations develop. Laboratory tests detect a serum ceruloplasmin concentration less than 30 mg/dl. Serum copper values may be normal or high and urine copper values are elevated. Liver biopsy is used to assess structural changes and measure copper concentrations.

Definitive treatment of Wilson disease is chelation therapy, the removal of excess copper from the tissues. Chelation is accomplished with d-penicillamine, an agent that incorporates copper into a complex that is readily eliminated in the urine. Children receiving penicillamine are given vitamin supplements, especially vitamin B_6. Copper intake is reduced by eliminating organ meats, nuts, legumes, shellfish, and chocolate from the diet. Physiotherapy may accelerate the recovery of gait and muscular coordination.

Children with untreated Wilson disease die from neural, hepatic, renal, or hematologic complications. The success of d-penicillamine therapy depends on early treatment and individual responsiveness. Therapy is seldom successful in children with chronic active liver disease, acute liver failure, or severe neuromuscular alterations.

SUMMARY REVIEW

Disorders of the Gastrointestinal Tract

1 Most alterations of digestive function in children are due to congenital obstructions of the intestinal tract; disorders of digestion, absorption, or nutrition; or liver disease.

2 Cleft lip (harelip) and cleft palate (failure of the bony palate to fuse in the midline) may occur separately or together. The fissure may affect the uvula, soft palate, hard palate, nostril, and maxillary alveolar ridge.

3 Esophageal atresia, a condition in which the esophagus ends in a blind pouch, may occur with or without tracheoesophageal fistula, or connection between the esophagus and the trachea. As the infant swallows oral secretions or ingests milk, the pouch fills, causing either drooling or aspiration into the lungs.

4 Pyloric stenosis, one of the most common disorders requiring surgery in early infancy, is an obstruction of the pyloric outlet caused by hypertrophy of circular muscles in the pyloric sphincter.

5 Malrotation of the intestine, with an obstructing band and volvulus (twisting of the bowel on itself), may partly or completely occlude the gastrointestinal tract and its blood vessels.

6 Meconium ileus is a condition in the newborn in which intestinal secretions and amniotic waste products produce a thick, tarry plug that obstructs the intestine. Cystic fibrosis is identified in 10% to 15% of infants with meconium ileus.

7 Duodenal, jejunal, and ileal obstructions can be due to

meconium ileus, atresia, congenital aganglionic mega-colon, and acquired obstructive disorders.

8 Congenital aganglionic megacolon (Hirschsprung disease) is caused by a malformation of the parasympathetic nervous system in a segment of the colon. It is characterized by the absence of nerves needed for stool propulsion.

9 Malformations of the anus and rectum range from mild congenital stenosis of the anus to complex deformities, all of which are classified as imperforate anus.

10 The most frequent cause of acquired intestinal obstruction in infants is intussusception, a condition in which one portion of the bowel telescopes, or invaginates, into another.

11 Gastroesophageal reflux is caused by the relaxation or incompetence of the lower esophageal sphincter. Infants are susceptible to reflux because mechanisms that prevent it are not fully mature, their diet consists of liquids, and they are seldom in an upright position.

12 Cystic fibrosis is an inherited exocrine gland abnormality that causes chronic suppurative lung disease and abnormalities in other organs that contain exocrine glands.

13 The pathophysiologic triad that is the hallmark of cystic fibrosis includes pancreatic enzyme deficiency (which causes maldigestion), overproduction of mucus in the respiratory tract, and abnormally elevated sodium and chloride concentrations in sweat. Affected individuals seldom survive beyond their 20s.

14 Gluten-sensitive enteropathy is a lifelong disease characterized by the loss of mature villous epithelium in the presence of a gluten-containing diet. It results in malabsorption and growth failure.

15 Protein energy malnutrition is a group of disorders resulting from a severe dietary deficiency of proteins, carbohydrates, or both. Starvation causes stunted mental and physical development.

16 Kwashiorkor is a severe protein deficiency that occurs in children who have stopped breast feeding and subsist on a high-carbohydrate diet. Marasmus is a deficiency of all dietary nutrients, including carbohydrates.

17 Failure to thrive is inadequate physical growth of a child. Organic failure to thrive is due to genetic, anatomic, or pathophysiologic factors that retard normal growth and development. Nonorganic failure to thrive is due to nutritional deficits associated with inadequate nurturing.

18 Diarrhea in infants and children can rapidly cause dehydration and electrolyte imbalances because fluid reserves are relatively small.

19 Necrotizing enterocolitis is a cause of diarrhea in newborns. It can be due to any gastrointestnal disturbance that causes gas to accumulate in the intestinal mucosa and submucosa, leading to ischemia, necrosis, and even perforation of the intestinal wall.

20 The most common cause of acute diarrhea in children is bacterial or viral enterocolitis (infection of the gastrointestinal tract).

21 Chronic diarrhea (diarrhea persisting longer than 4 weeks) can be caused by a wide variety of underlying conditions and frequently leads to growth failure and slow development.

Disorders of the Liver

1 Physiologic jaundice of the newborn is due to mild hyperbilirubinemia that subsides in a week or two. Pathologic jaundice is due to severe hyperbilirubinemia and can cause brain damage.

2 Biliary atresia is a congenital malformation of the bile ducts that obstructs bile flow. Atresia causes jaundice, cirrhosis, and liver failure if it is not corrected surgically.

3 Acute hepatitis has the same clinical course in children and adults, but children have milder cases of the disease. Hepatitis A is the most common form of childhood hepatitis.

4 Cirrhosis is rare in children, but it can develop from most forms of chronic liver disease.

5 Portal hypertension in children is usually due to extrahepatic obstruction. Thrombosis of the portal vein is the most common cause of portal hypertension in children, and splenomegaly is the most frequent sign.

6 The three most common metabolic disorders that cause liver damage in children are galactosemia, fructosemia, and Wilson disease. All three are inherited as genetic traits and permit the accumulation of toxins in the liver.

7 Galactosemia is due to a deficiency of the enzyme galactose-1-phosphate uridyltransferase. Galactose cannot be incorporated into carbohydrate metabolism, and salt accumulates in all body tissues, where it has toxic effects.

8 Fructosemia is due to a deficiency of the enzyme fructose-1-phosphate aldolase. Lack of this enzyme causes ingested fructose to disrupt carbohydrate and nucleotide metabolism.

9 Wilson disease causes defective copper uptake and metabolism. Unexcreted copper accumulates in the liver, brain, kidney, and corneal cells.

KEY TERMS

Biliary atresia, 1282

Cleft lip, 1268

Cleft palate, 1268

Chronic nonspecific diarrhea, 1281

Congenital aganglionic megacolon (Hirschsprung disease), 1273

Cystic fibrosis, 1276

Esophageal atresia, 1270

Failure to thrive (FTT), 1279

Fructosemia (hereditary fructose intolerance), 1285

Galactosemia, 1284

Gluten-sensitive enteropathy (celiac sprue), 1277

Ileal atresia, 1272

Imperforate anus, 1274

Infant diarrhea, 1280

Intussusception, 1274

Jejunal atresia, 1272

Kwashiorkor, 1279

Lactose intolerance, 1281

Malrotation, 1271

Marasmus, 1279

Meconium, 1272

Meconium ileus, 1272

Necrotizing enterocolitis, 1280

Nonorganic FTT, 1280

Organic FTT, 1279

Periduodenal band, 1271

Physiologic jaundice of the newborn, 1282

Protein energy malnutrition (PEM), 1279

Pyloric stenosis, 1271

Tracheoesophageal fistula (TEF), 1270

Wilson disease, 1285

REFERENCES

Alagille, D. (1987). Liver transplantation in children: Indications of cholestatic states. *Transplant Proceedings, XIX,* 3242-3248.

Auricchio, S., Greco, L., & Troncone, R. (1988). Gluten-sensitive enteropathy in childhood. *Pediatric Clinics of North America, 35*(1), 157-187.

Avery, M. E., & First, L. R. (1986). *Pediatric medicine* (p. 476). Baltimore: Williams & Wilkins.

Balistreri, W. F. (1988). Viral hepatitis. *Pediatric Clinics of North America, 35,* 375-407.

Barnard, J. A., Cotton, B. C., & Lutin, W. (1985). Necrotizing enterocolitis: Variables associated with severity of disease. *American Journal of Diseases of the Child, 139,* 375-377.

Beasley, S. W., & Meyers, W. A. (1988). The diagnosis of congenital tracheoesophageal fistula. *Journal of Pediatric Surgery, 23*(5), 415-417.

Behrman, R. E., & Vaughan, V. C. (1987). *Nelson textbook of pediatrics* (13th ed.). Philadelphia: W. B. Saunders.

Behrman, R. E., Vaughan, V. C., & Nelson, W. E. (1987). *Nelson textbook of pediatrics* (13th ed.). Philadelphia: W. B. Saunders.

Bortollotti, P., Cadrobbi, P., Armigliato, M., Rude, L., Rugge, M., & Realdi, G. (1987). Prognosis of chronic hepatitis B transmitted from HB$_s$Ag positive mother. *Archives of Disease in Childhood, 62,* 201-203.

Carter, C. O. (1961). The inheritance of congenital pyloric stenosis. *British Medical Bulletin, 17,* 251-254.

Chow, M. P., Durand, B. A., Feldman, M. N., & Mills, M. A. (1984). Failure to thrive. In M. P. Chow, B. Durand, M.

N. Feldman, & M. A. Mills (Eds.), *Handbook of pediatric primary care* (pp. 1185-1205). New York: Wiley & Sons.

Cooper, A., Ross, A. J., O'Neill, J. A., & Schnaufer, L. (1988). Resection with primary anastomosis for necrotizing enterocolitis: A contrasting view. *Journal of Pediatric Surgery, 23,* 64-68.

Cupoli, J. (1980). Failure to thrive. *Current Problems in Pediatrics, 10*:2-43.

Fitzgerald, J. F. (1988). Cholestatic disorders of infancy. *Pediatric Clinics of North America, 35,* 357-373.

Francis, D. P., Hadler, S. C., Prendergast, T. J., Peterson, E., Ginsberg, M. M., Loockbaugh, C., Holmes, J. R., & Maynard, J. E. (1984). Occurrence of hepatitis A, B, and non-A/non-B in the United States: CDC Sentinel County hepatitis study I. *American Journal of Medicine, 76,* 69-74.

Glaser, J. H., & Morecki, R. (1987). Retrovirus type 3 and neonatal cholestasis. *Seminars in Liver Disease, 7,* 100.

Greco, L., Tozzi A. E., & Mayer, M. (1987). Growth status of coeliac patients in the florid phase. *Italian Journal of Pediatrics, 13,* 161.

Gryboski, J., & Walker, A. (1983). *Gastrointestinal problems in the infant.* Philadelphia: W. B. Saunders.

Hadler, S. C., & McFarland, L. (1986). Hepatitis in day care centers. *Review of Infectious Diseases, 8,* 548-557.

Hay, C. R. M., Preston, F. E., Triger, D. R., Greaves, M., Underwood, J. C. E., & Westlake, L. (1987). Predictive markers of chronic liver disease in hemophilia. *Blood, 69,* 1595-1599.

Hegsted, D. M. (1976). Protein needs and possible modification of the American diet. *Journal of the American Dietetic Association, 68,* 317.

Hess, G., Gerlick, W., Gerken, G., Mann, M., Hutteroth, T. H., Meyer, Z. U. M., & Buschenfelde, K. H. (1987). The effect of recombinant alpha-interferon treatment on serum levels of hepatitis B virus-encoded proteins in man. *Hepatology, 7,* 704-708.

Kaye, D., & Rose, L. F. (1983). *Fundamentals of internal medicine.* St. Louis: C. V. Mosby.

Levine, J. J. (1987). Chronic nonspecific diarrhea. *Pediatric Annual, 10,* 822-829.

Milla, P. J. (1988). Gastrointestinal motility disorders in children. *Pediatric Clinics of North America, 35*(5), 311-330.

Mosher, M. S. (1986). Genetic counseling in cleft lip and palate. *Ear, Nose, and Throat Journal, 65,* 330-336.

Nakazato, Y., Landing, B. H., & Wells, T. R. (1986). Abnormal Auerbach plexus in the esophagus and stomach of patients with esophageal atresia and tracheoesophageal fistula. *Journal of Pediatric Surgery, 21,* 831-837.

Pokorny, W. J., Garcia-Pratts, J. A., & Yvonne, B. N. (1986). Necrotizing enterocolitis: Incidence, operative care, and outcome. *Journal of Pediatric Surgery, 21,* 1149-1154.

Rudolph, A. M., & Hoffman, J. I. E. (1982). *Pediatrics.* Norwalk NJ: Appleton-Century-Crofts.

Scheinberg, H. I., & Sternlieb, I. (1984). *Wilson's disease* (pp. 29-30). Philadelphia: W. B. Saunders.

Stern, L., & Brodersen, R. (1987). Kernicterus research and the basic sciences: A project for future development. *Pediatrics, 79,* 154-155.

Suslak, L., & Desposito, F. (1988). Infants with cleft lip/palate. *Pediatric Review, 9,* 331-334.

Voorhes, A. B., & Price, J. B. (1974). Extra-hepatic portal hypertension: Retrospective analysis of 127 cases and associated clinical implications. *Archives of Surgery, 108,* 138-144.

Walsh, M. C., Kleigman, R. M., & Fanaroff, A. A. (1988).

Necrotizing enterocolitis: A practitioner's perspective. *Pediatric Review, 9,* 219-226.

Whaley, L. F., & Wong, D. L. (1987). *Nursing care of infants and children* (3rd ed.). St. Louis: C. V. Mosby, p. 465.

Whitington, P. F. (1985). Portal hypertension in children. *Pediatric Annals, 14,* 494-499.

UNIT
XIII

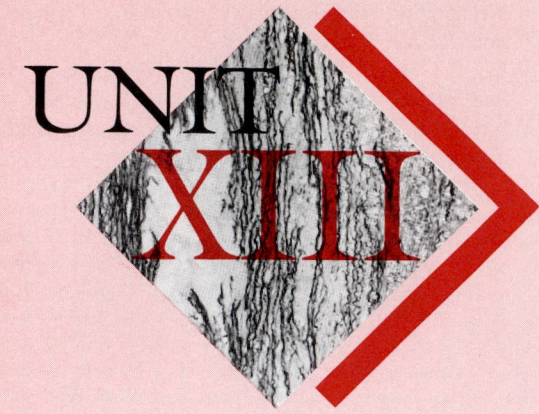

The Musculoskeletal System

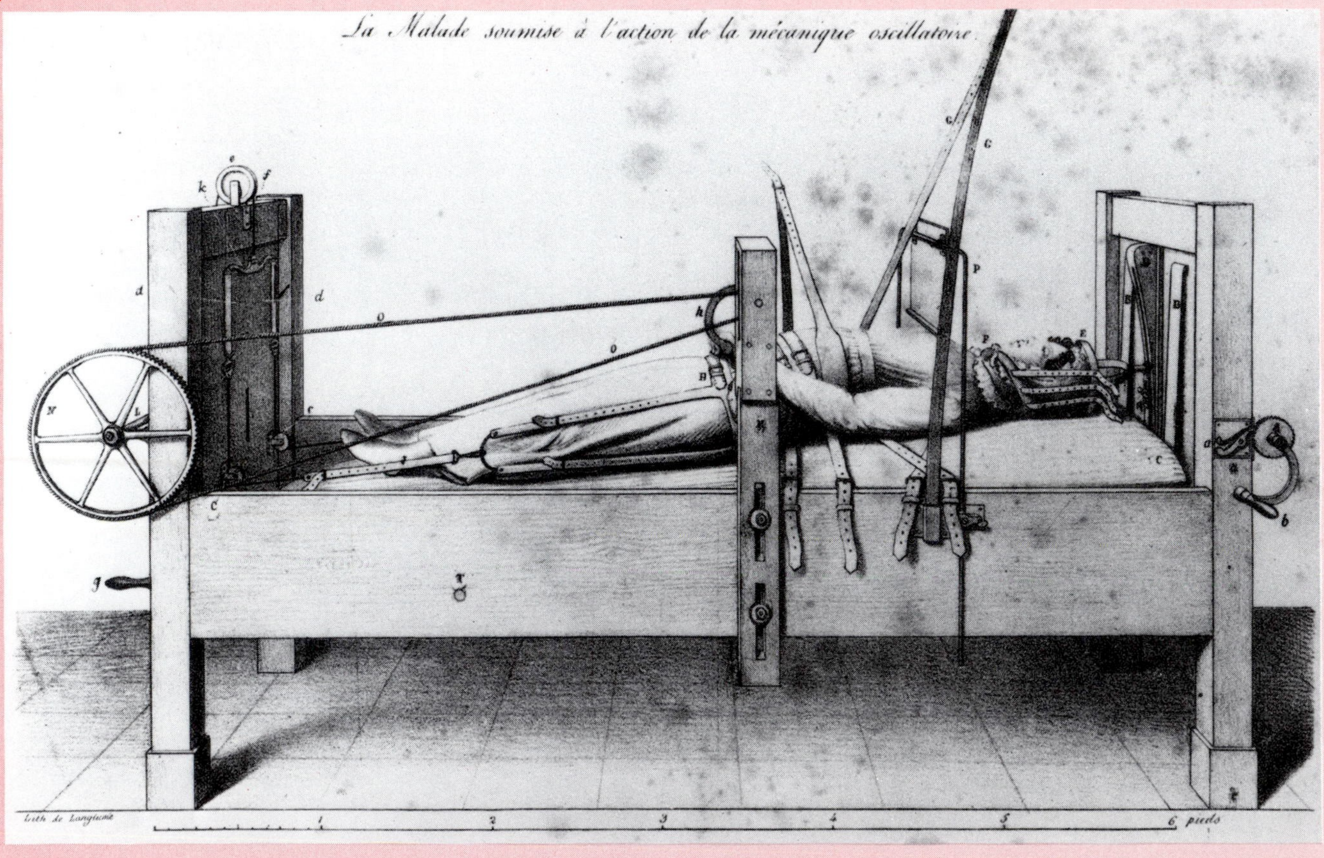

La Malade soumise à l'action de la mécanique oscillatoire.

Female patient strapped into an orthopedic bed. (From Jalade-Laford, G.: *Recherches pratiques sur les principales difformités du corps humain, Paris, 1827. Courtesy National Library of Medicine.*)

THE way an individual functions in daily life, moves about, or manipulates objects physically depends on the integrity of the musculoskeletal system. The musculoskeletal system is actually composed of two systems: (1) the skeleton proper, which is composed of bones and joints, and (2) skeletal muscles. Each of the systems contributes to mobility. The skeleton supports the body and provides leverage to the skeletal muscles so that movement of various parts of the body is possible. Movement of the various body parts is accomplished by contraction of the skeletal muscles and bending or rotation at the joints.

Alterations of the musculoskeletal system are among the oldest known diseases. Evidence of bone disease can be found in the earliest skeletal specimens of humans. The femur of Java man evidences a large, benign osteochondroma, a common bone tumor today. Evidence of a healed fracture is present in the ulna of a Neanderthal skeleton. Egyptian mummies from the Fifth Dynasty have been unearthed with fractured limbs bound in splints. Apparently fractures of the forearm and femur were fairly common during that time, probably as a result of constant warfare. Some fractures were healed, others not united, but usually some attempt had been made to immobilize the fracture. By the time Hippocrates (460-370 BC) wrote his books, *On Fractures* and *On Articulations,* the diagnosis and treatment of fractures had reached quite a level of sophistication. Closed fractures were differentially diagnosed from open fractures, and many types of fracture-dislocations of the clavicle, elbow, and hip were described. Along with bandages and splints, the books contained a carefully prescribed method of traction for reducing fractures. Maintaining a limb in its "natural" (anatomic) position during healing and early mobility after inflammation subsided were well-recognized fundamental principles of treatment. Both of these principles still underlie much of orthopedic treatment today.

The earliest evidence of joint disease (arthritides) is found in a fossil vertebrate (platycarpus) that lived about 100 million years ago. In the primitive species of humans, the earliest evidence of joint disease is found in the spine of the Ape man, who lived 2 million years ago. Joint disease can be traced further from the Ape man through the Java and Lansing men of 500,000 years ago to Egyptian mummies dating to 8000 BC. The prevalance of chronic joint disease can also be traced through the Roman civilization and is believed to be one of the reasons that Romans built extensive baths throughout their empire.

By far the most important description of muscle fibers was first made by Louis-Antoine Ranvier (1835-1922) over 100 years ago. In his study of animal muscle fibers he noted that "when electrically stimulated," red or dark muscle fibers fired less frequently and for longer duration than the rapid firing in white muscle. The white and dark meat of a holiday turkey also demonstrates this color difference. The fact that muscle fibers are not homogenous and differ on the basis of color has been further refined by modern histochemical techniques.

An understanding of the structure and function of normal skeletal muscle has been enhanced by the study of pathologic changes in muscle tissue. In 1861, the French neurologist Guillaume Benjamin Amand Duchenne introduced the skeletal muscle biopsy technique, similar to the technique still in use today. The report of this procedure sparked a lively debate in the nineteenth century press over the morality of studying living *human* tissue! Advances in the muscle and nerve biopsy technique, as well as biochemical electrical study, have immeasurably changed the understanding of skeletal muscle function.

CHAPTER
38

Structure and Function of the Musculoskeletal System

Katherine Hoare
Katharine M. Donohoe

Structure and function of bones, 1292
  Elements of bone tissue, 1293
  Bone cells, 1293
    Osteoblast, 1293
    Osteocyte, 1294
    Osteoclast, 1294
  Bone matrix, 1294
    Collagen fibers, 1294
    Proteoglycans, 1294
    Glycoproteins, 1294
  Bone minerals, 1295
  Types of bone tissue, 1295
  Characteristics of bone, 1296
  Maintenance of bone integrity, 1297
    Remodeling, 1297
    Repair, 1297
Structure and function of joints, 1298
  Fibrous joints, 1298
  Cartilaginous joints, 1298
  Synovial joints, 1298
    Structure of synovial joints, 1298
      Joint capsule, 1300
      Synovial membrane, 1300
      Joint cavity, 1300
      Synovial fluid, 1300
      Articular cartilage, 1301
    Movement of synovial joints, 1302
Structure and function of skeletal muscles, 1304
  Whole muscle, 1304
  Motor unit, 1306
    Sensory receptors, 1306
    Muscle fibers, 1306
    Myofibrils, 1310

    Muscle proteins, 1310
    Nonprotein constituents of muscle, 1311
  Components of muscle function, 1311
    Muscle contraction at the molecular level, 1311
    Muscle metabolism, 1312
    Muscle mechanics, 1313
    Types of muscle contraction, 1313
    Movement of muscle groups, 1314
Tests of musculoskeletal function, 1314
  Tests of bone function, 1314
  Tests of joint function, 1314
  Tests of muscular function, 1314
Aging and the musculoskeletal system, 1315
  Aging of bones, 1315
  Aging of joints, 1315
  Aging of muscles, 1315

STRUCTURE AND FUNCTION OF BONES

Bones give form to the body, support tissues, and permit movement by providing points of attachment for muscles. Many bones meet in movable joints that determine the type and extent of movement possible. Bones also protect many of the body's vital organs. For example, the bones of the skull, thorax, and pelvis are hard exterior shields that protect the brain, heart, lungs, and reproductive organs.

The marrow cavities within certain bones serve as sites of blood cell formation. In adults, blood cells originate exclusively in the marrow cavities of the skull, vertebrae, ribs, sternum, shoulders, and pelvis. Bones also have a crucial role in mineral homeostasis. They store minerals (i.e., calcium, phosphate, carbonate, magnesium) that are essential for the proper working of many delicate cellular mechanisms throughout the body. Through the action of certain cells within bone, the stored minerals can be mobilized and distributed as needed by the body.

Elements of Bone Tissue

Mature bone is a rigid connective tissue. Like other connective tissues, bone consists of cells, fibers, and a gelatinous material termed **ground substance.** Unlike other connective tissue, however, bone contains large amounts of crystallized minerals, mostly calcium, that give bone its rigidity. The structural elements of bone are summarized in Table 38-1.

Bone cells enable bone to grow, repair itself, and change shape. Even in mature bone, these cells continuously synthesize new bone tissue and resorb (dissolve or digest) old tissue. The fibers in bone are made of collagen, a protein that is synthesized and secreted by certain bone cells. The fibers give bone its tensile strength (the ability to hold itself together). Ground substance acts as a medium for the diffusion of nutrients, oxygen, metabolic wastes, biochemicals, and minerals between bone tissue and blood vessels.

Bone also contains blood vessels and nerves. Bone tissue is nourished by a network of capillaries, and major vessels serve the marrow cavities. The nerves in bone send messages to the central nervous system about stresses and pain stimuli that affect bone.

Bone formation begins during fetal life with the growth of cartilage—the precursor of bone tissue. In mature bone the formation of new tissue begins with the production of organic matrix by the bone cells. The organic components of bones' intercellular matrix, or **bone matrix,** consists of ground substances; collagen, which forms the fibers; and other proteins, which have several functions in bone formation and maintenance.

The next step in bone formation is **calcification,** the process of mineral deposition and crystallization. Minerals present in the matrix precipitate within and around the collagen fibers. A tight bond between the crystals and collagen fibers gives tensile and compressional strength (the ability to withstand pressure and weight bearing) to bone.

Bone Cells

Bone contains three types of cells: osteoblasts, osteocytes, and osteoclasts. **Osteoblasts** are the bone-forming cells. Their primary function is to lay down new bone. Once this function is complete, osteoblasts become osteocytes. **Osteocytes** are osteoblasts that have become "imprisoned" within the mineralized bone ma-

TABLE 38-1 Structural elements of bone

Structural element	Function
BONE CELLS	
Osteoblasts	Synthesize collagen and proteoglycans
Osteocytes	Maintain bone matrix
Osteoclasts	Resorb bone
BONE MATRIX	
Collagen fibers	Lend support and tensile strength
Proteoglycans	Control transport of ionized materials through matrix
Glycoproteins	
Sialoprotein	Promotes calcification
Osteocalcin	Inhibits calcium-phosphate precipitation; promotes bone resorption
Albumin	Transports essential elements to matrix; maintains osmotic pressure of bone fluid
Alphaglycoprotein	Promotes calcification
Minerals (elements)	
Calcium	Crystallizes to lend rigidity and compressive strength
Phosphate	Regulates vitamin D and thereby promotes mineralization

trix. They have an ill-defined role in maintaining the inorganic (mineral) and organic elements of bone matrix. **Osteoclasts** function primarily to resorb (remove) bone during processes of growth and repair.

Osteoblast

Osteoblasts are active near bone surfaces, where growth takes place. Osteoblasts usually form a single layer of cells on the surfaces of bone, where they synthesize and extrude **osteoid** (nonmineralized bone matrix). Osteoblasts also concentrate some of the plasma proteins found in bone matrix and may facilitate the deposition and exchange of calcium and other ions (Vaughan, 1981).

Osteoblasts have two functional states, an active state and a resting state. In its active state, the osteoblast synthesizes and secretes osteoid, mostly on the surfaces of young bone where osteoid is laid down in large areas. In its resting state the osteoblast (sometimes referred to as a lining cell) appears to be dormant. If appropriately stimulated, however, the resting osteoblast is believed capable of resuming activity.

Osteocyte

An osteocyte is an osteoblast that is trapped in osteoid as it hardens during calcification. As minerals enter the osteoid, each osteocyte is surrounded by a shell of mineralized bone matrix. The space within the hardened shell, termed a **lacuna,** contains the osteocyte surrounded by a thin layer of nonmineralized osteoid, somewhat like an egg yolk surrounded by egg white and a shell.

The function of osteocytes is still controversial, but several hypotheses have been proposed. Various researchers think that osteocytes play one or more of the following roles.

1. Maintenance of the bone matrix. Because osteocytes are located near capillaries and are in contact with nutrient-rich fluid in canaliculae, they may remove nutrients from these sources and concentrate them in the matrix. In addition, osteocytes may become reactivated as needed to synthesize and replace lost elements of the matrix (Resnick, 1981).

2. Maintenance of mineral homeostasis. In conjunction with osteoblasts and parathyroid hormone, osteocytes may facilitate the exchange of calcium and phosphorus between bone and tissue fluids, thereby maintaining optimal levels of calcium and other minerals in blood plasma (Albright & Brand, 1979).

3. Modification of bone matrix. Osteocytes may be able to release enzymes that dissolve the mineralized walls of the lacunae and prepare bone for remodeling (Wilson, 1983). (Remodeling is described on p. 1297.)

Osteoclast

The osteoclast is a multinucleated cell with a short life span that resorbs bone. The origin of the osteoclast is uncertain. One hypothesis is that osteoclasts arise from the fusion of osteoblasts, osteocytes, or both. Another hypothesis is that osteoclasts originate from mononuclear phagocytic cells (Hanaoka, 1979). (The mononuclear phagocyte system is discussed in Chapter 22.) The osteoclast is a large cell containing lysosomes (digestive vacuoles) filled with hydrolytic enzymes. Fine projections (microvilli) fan out from the cell's surface and terminate on bone surfaces that are being resorbed. Osteoclasts are found on the surface of bone in shallow, self-made excavations known as Howship's lacunae.

The exact mechanism by which an osteoclast resorbs bone is unclear. Some researchers believe that the osteoclast secretes acids that dissolve minerals in bone matrix, exposing collagen fibers and making them susceptible to digestion by other phagocytic cells. Others believe that the osteoclast carries out both of these functions, first dissolving the minerals and then ingesting the exposed matrix components. Whatever the mechanism, the osteoclast disappears once resorption is complete. Its disappearance has been attributed to mobility, degeneration, and reversion to its parent cell.

Bone Matrix

Bone matrix is made of the *extracellular* elements of bone tissue—collagen fibers, proteins, carbohydrate-protein complexes, ground substance, and minerals.

Collagen Fibers

Fibers comprise the bulk of bone matrix. The fibers are made of type I collagen, a protein synthesized and secreted by osteoblasts. Once secreted, the collagen molecules assemble into thin chains called alpha chains. The alpha chains combine in threes to form **fibrils.** The fibrils organize themselves into a staggered pattern in which each fibril overlaps its nearest neighbor by about one fourth of its length. Staggering and overlap create regular gaps into which mineral crystals are deposited. Approximately 50% to 90% of the crystallized minerals in bone are deposited in the gaps between staggered groups of fibrils (Urist, 1980; Wilson, 1983). After mineral deposition, the fibrils link together and twist to form a ropelike fiber. The fibers then join to form a framework that gives bone its tensile strength and enables it to bear weight.

Proteoglycans

Proteoglycans are proteins that strengthen bone by forming compression-resistant networks between the collagen fibrils. Proteoglycans also control the transport and distribution of ions (electrically charged particles), particularly calcium, through the bone matrix. Therefore proteoglycans may play a role in bone calcium deposition (calcification).

Glycoproteins

Glycoproteins are the carbohydrate-protein complexes of bone. Glycoproteins control the collagen interactions that lead to fibril formation. They may also play a role in calcification.

Bone matrix contains four glycoproteins: sialoprotein, osteocalcin, albumin, and alphaglycoprotein. **Sialoprotein** makes up about 8% of the noncollagenous matrix of bone. Sialoprotein binds easily with calcium, leading many researchers to believe that it plays a role in calcification (Vaughan, 1981).

Osteocalcin is also a calcium-binding protein but binds preferentially to calcium that has already crystallized. The physiologic role of osteocalcin has not yet been established, but it may inhibit calcium phosphate precipitation or play a part in bone resorption (Peck, 1984).

Bone albumin is identical to serum albumin (see Chapter 22). In calcified matrix, bone albumin is permanently fixed to bone mineral crystals and remains so until the bone is resorbed. The exact function of albumin in bone is unclear, but researchers believe it transports essential elements such as hormones, ions, and other metabolites to and from the bone cells and maintains the osmotic pressure of **bone fluid** (fluid surrounding mineral crystals and osteoblasts).

Alphaglycoprotein is thought to be synthesized in the liver, to be released into blood plasma, and to circulate to bone matrix, where it accumulates. Alphaglycoprotein's affinity for calcium is 40 times greater than that of albumin. Therefore it probably plays an important role in the calcification of growing bone. Alphaglycoprotein may also facilitate bone resorption by activating osteoclasts.

Bone Minerals

Mineralization is the final step in bone formation, following collagen synthesis and fiber formation. During mineralization, some unknown mechanism triggers calcium and phosphate precipitation and subsequent crystallization.

Table 38-2 lists the sequence in which calcium and phosphate form amorphous (fluid) calcium phosphate compounds that are converted, in stages, to solid hexagonal crystals of **hydroxyapatite (HAP).** As the calcium and phosphorus concentrations increase in the bone matrix, the first precipitate to form is dicalcium phosphate dihydrate (DCPD). Once DCPD precipitation begins, the remaining phases of bone crystal formation proceed spontaneously until insoluble HAP is produced (Urist, 1980). Approximately 80% to 90% of the HAP is incorporated into the collagen fibers (Urist, 1980),

whereas amorphous calcium phosphate is distributed throughout the bone matrix (Vaughan, 1981).

Types of Bone Tissue

Bone is made up of two types of bony (osseous) tissue: **compact bone** (cortical bone) and **spongy bone** (cancellous bone) (Fig. 38-1). Both types of bone tissue contain the same structural elements and, with a few exceptions, both compact and spongy tissue are present in every bone. The major difference between the two types of tissue is the organization of the elements.

Compact bone is highly organized, solid, and extremely strong. The basic structural unit in compact bone is the **haversian system** (Fig. 38-2). Each haversian system is made up of the following:

1. A central canal called the **haversian canal**
2. Concentric layers of bone matrix called **lamellae**
3. Tiny spaces (lacunae) between the lamellae
4. Bone cells (osteocytes) within the lacunae
5. Small channels or canals called **canaliculae**

Each haversian system is a separate cylindric entity that looks like a set of concentric rings. In the center of the haversian system is the haversian canal. The haversian canal runs through the long axis of bone and contains one or two blood vessels and nerve fibers. The blood vessels in the canal communicate with blood vessels in the periosteum (surface cover) and marrow cavity to transport nutrients and wastes to and from the osteo-

TABLE 38-2 Sequence of calcium and phosphate compound formation and crystallization

Formula	Name	Abbreviation
Ca(HPO$_4$)·2 H$_2$O	Dicalcium phosphate dihydrate	DCPD
Ca$_4$H(PO$_4$)$_3$	Octacalcium phosphate	OCP
Ca$_9$(PO$_4$)$_6$ (var.)	Amorphous calcium phosphate	ACP
Ca$_3$(PO$_4$)$_2$	Tricalcium phosphate	TCP
Ca$_5$(PO$_4$)$_3$OH	Hydroxyapatite	HAP

NOTE: Compounds are listed in the order in which precipitation and crystal formation occurs.

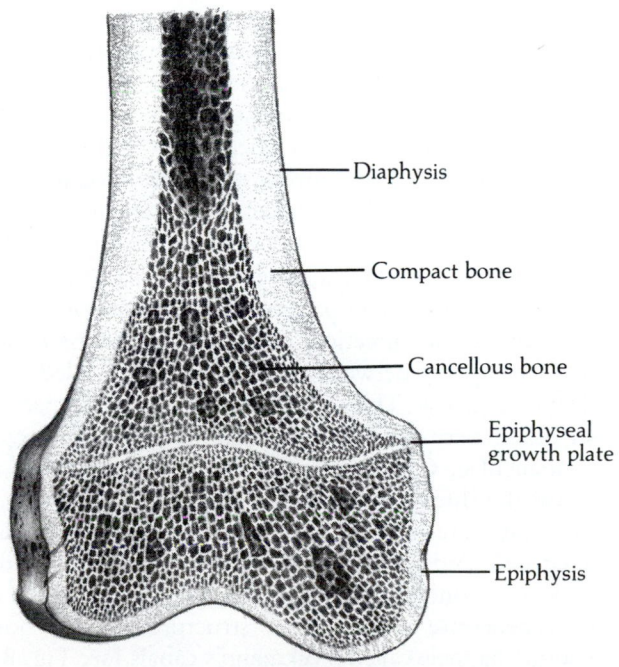

FIG. 38-1. Bone showing relationships of compact and cancellous bone, epiphysis, epiphyseal plate, and diaphysis. (From Thompson et al., 1989.)

Diaphysis

Compact bone

Cancellous bone

Epiphyseal growth plate

Epiphysis

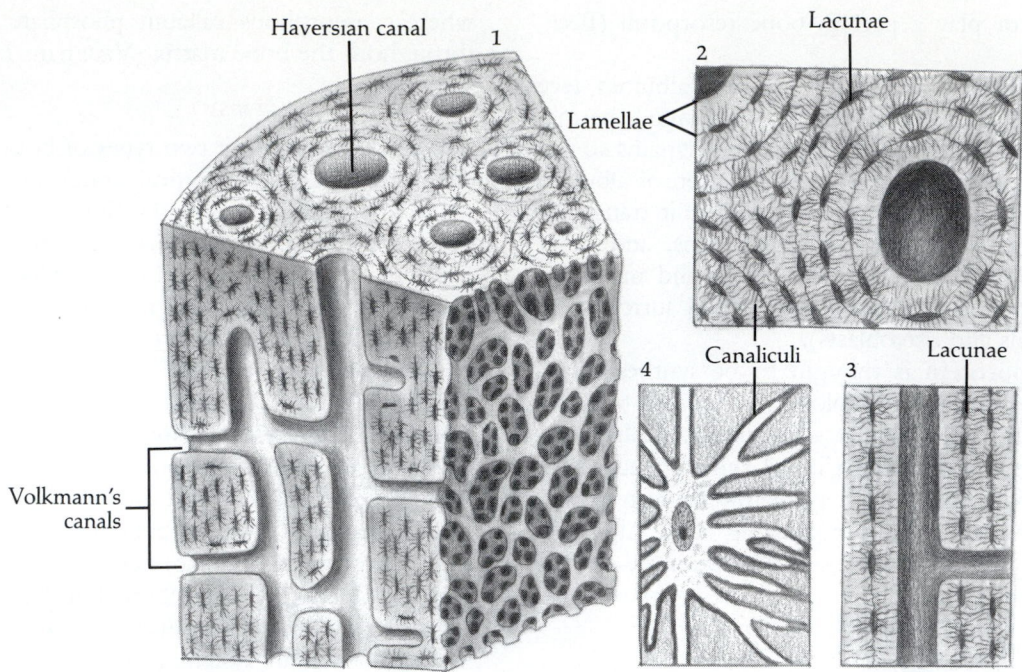

FIG. 38-2. *(1)* Three-demensional view of compact bone; *(2)* transverse section of compact bone depictng lamellae, lacunae, and canaliculi; *(3)* longitudinal section of bone with lacunae and canaliculi; *(4)* lacunae occupied by osteocyte. (From Thompson et al., 1989.)

cytes contained within the lacunae. Surrounding each haversian canal are the concentric lamellae. Between the lamellae are the lacunae, each of which contains one osteocyte. The lacunae are connected to each other and to the haversian canal by the caniculae, which run parallel to the horizontal axis of the bone. Each canaliculus encloses a small extension (cytoplasmic process) from the osteocyte contained in the lacuna.

Spongy bone is less complex and lacks haversian systems. In spongy bone the lamellae are not arranged in concentric layers but in plates or bars termed **trabeculae** that branch and unite with one another to form an irregular meshwork. The pattern of the meshwork is determined by the direction of stress on the particular bone. The spaces between the trabeculae are filled with red bone marrow. The osteocyte-containing lacunae are distributed between the trabeculae and interconnected by caniculae. Capillaries pass through the marrow to nourish the osteocytes.

All bones are covered with a double-layered connective tissue called the **periosteum.** The outer layer of the periosteum contains blood vessels and nerves, some of which penetrate to the inner structures of the bone through channels called Volkmann's canals (see Fig. 38-2). The inner layer of the periosteum is anchored to the bone by collagenous fibers (Sharpey's fibers) that penetrate the bone.

Characteristics of Bone

The human skeleton consists of 206 bones, which comprise the axial skeleton and the appendicular skeleton (Fig. 38-3). The **axial skeleton** consists of 80 bones that make up the skull, vertebral column, and thorax. The **appendicular skeleton** consists of 126 bones that make up the upper and lower extremities, the shoulder girdle (pectoral girdle), and the pelvic girdle (os coxae). The skeleton contributes about 14% of the weight of the adult body.

Bones can be classified by shape as long, flat, short (cubiodal), or irregular. **Long bones** are longer than they are wide and consist of a narrow tubular midportion **(diaphysis)** that merges into a broader neck **(metaphysis)** and a broad end **(epiphysis)** (see Fig. 38-1).

The diaphysis consists of thick, rigid compact bone (sometimes referred to as **cortex**) that is able to tolerate bending forces. Contained within the diaphysis is the elongated marrow (medullary) cavity. The marrow cavity of the diaphysis contains primarily fatty tissue, which is referred to as yellow marrow. The yellow marrow cavity of the diaphysis is continuous with marrow cavities in the spongy bone of the metaphysis and diaphysis. The marrow contained within the epiphysis is red because it contains primarily blood-forming tissue (see Chapter 22). A layer of connective tissue, **endosteum,** lines both types of marrow cavity.

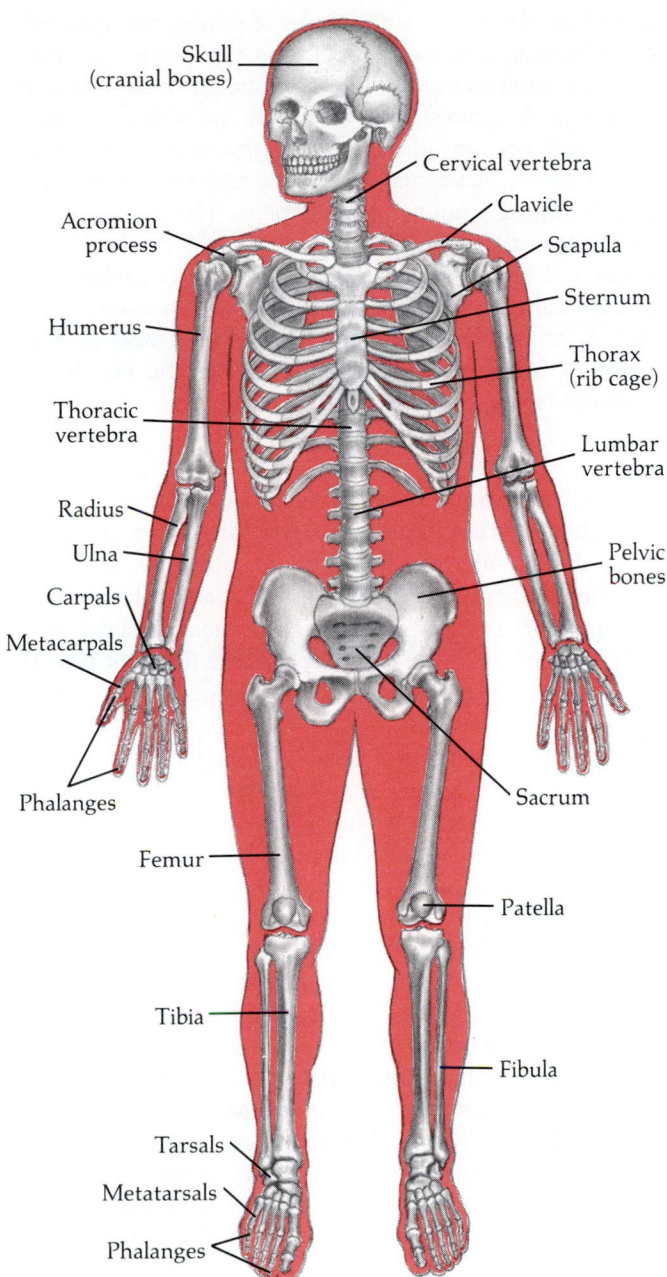

Skull
(cranial bones)

Acromion
process

Humerus

Thoracic
vertebra

Radius

Ulna

Carpals

Metacarpals

Phalanges

Femur

Tibia

Tarsals

Metatarsals

Phalanges

Cervical vertebra

Clavicle

Scapula

Sternum

Thorax
(rib cage)

Lumbar
vertebra

Pelvic
bones

Sacrum

Patella

Fibula

FIG. 38-3. Axial and appendicular skeleton. (From Thompson et al., 1989.)

The broadness of the epiphysis allows weight bearing to be distributed over a wide area. The epiphysis is made up of spongy bone covered by a very thin layer of compact bone. In a child the epiphysis is separated from the metaphysis by a cartilaginous growth plate, the **epiphyseal plate.** After puberty, the epiphyseal plate calcifies and the epiphysis and metaphysis merge. By adulthood, the line of demarcation between the epiphysis and metaphysis is undetectable.

In **flat bones,** two plates of compact bone are roughly parallel to each other. Between the compact-bone plates is a layer of spongy bone. **Short bones** (cuboidal bones) are often cuboidal in shape. They consist of spongy bone covered by a thin layer of compact bone.

Irregular bones have various shapes that include thin and thick segments. The thin part of an irregular bone consists of two plates of compact bone with spongy bone in between. The thick part consists of spongy bone surrounded by a layer of compact bone.

Maintenance of Bone Integrity
Remodeling

The internal structure of bone is maintained by **remodeling,** a three-phase process in which existing bone is resorbed and new bone is laid down to replace it. Remodeling is carried out by clusters of bone cells termed **basic multicellular units.** The basic multicellular units are made up of bone precursor cells that differentiate into osteoclasts and osteoblasts. Precursor cells are located on the free surfaces of bones and along the vascular channels (especially the marrow cavities).

In phase one of the remodeling cycle, a stimulus (e.g., hormone, drug, vitamin, physical stressor) activates the bone cell precursors in a localized area of bone to osteoclasts. In phase two, the osteoclasts form a "cutting cone," which gradually resorbs bone, leaving behind an elongated cavity termed a resorption cavity (Urist, 1980). The resorption cavity in compact bone follows the longitudinal axis of the haversian system; whereas the resorption cavity in spongy bone parallels the surface of the trabeculae.

Phase three is the laying down of new bone, termed secondary bone, by osteoblasts lining the walls of the resorption cavity. The osteoblasts "follow" the cutting cone, laying down new bone. Successive layers (lamellae) in compact bone are laid down, until the cavity is reduced to a narrow haversian canal around a blood vessel. In this way, old haversian systems are destroyed and new haversian systems are formed. New trabeculae are formed in spongy bone. The entire process of remodeling takes about 4 months.

Repair

The remodeling process can repair microscopic bone injuries, but gross injuries, such as fractures and surgical wounds (osteotomies), heal by the same stages as soft tissue injuries (see Chapter 7). In bone the stages of wound healing are as follows.

1. Hematoma formation. This occurs if vessels have been damaged, causing hemorrhage. Fibrin within the hematoma forms a meshwork, which is the initial framework for healing.
2. Procallus formation. Fibroblasts, capillary buds, and osteoblasts move into the wound to produce granulation tissue called **procallus.**

3. Callus formation. Osteoblasts in the procallus deposit disorganized cartilaginous clumps of primitive bone matrix termed woven bone, or **callus.**
4. Basic multicellular units replace the callus with lamellar bone or trabecular bone.
5. The periosteal and endosteal surfaces of the bone are remodeled to the size and shape of the bone before injury.

The speed with which bone heals depends on the severity of the bone disruption, the type and amount of bone tissue that needs to be replaced (spongy bone heals faster), blood supply to the site, presence of other disease, effects of aging, and effective treatment, including immobilization and the prevention of complications such as infection. In general, however, hematoma formation occurs within hours of fracture or surgery; formation of procallus by osteoblasts within days; callus formation within weeks; and replacement and contour modeling within years—up to 4 years in some cases.

STRUCTURE AND FUNCTION OF JOINTS

The site where two or more bones are attached is called a **joint,** or articulation. The primary function of joints is to provide stability and mobility to the skeleton. Whether a joint provides stability or mobility depends on its location and its structure. Generally, joints that stabilize the skeleton have a simpler structure than those that enable the skeleton to move. Most joints provide both stability and mobility to some degree (Fig. 38-4).

Joints are classified based on the degree of movement they permit or on the connecting tissues that hold them together. Based on movement, a joint is classified as a **synarthrosis** (immovable joint), an **amphiarthrosis** (slightly movable joint), or a **diarthrosis** (freely movable joint). On the basis of connective structures, joints are classified broadly as fibrous, cartilaginous, and synovial. Each of these three structural classifications can be subdivided according to the shape and contour of the articulating surfaces (ends) of the bones and the type of motion the joint permits.

Fibrous Joints

A joint in which bone is united directly to bone by fibrous connective tissue is called a **fibrous joint.** Generally, fibrous joints are synarthroses (immovable), but many fibrous joints allow some movement. The degree of movement depends on the distance between the bones and the flexibility of the fibrous connective tissue.

Fibrous joints are further subdivided into three types: sutures, syndesmoses, and gomphoses. A **suture** has a thin layer of dense fibrous tissue that binds together interlocking flat bones in the skulls of young children. Sutures form an extremely tight union that permits no motion. By adulthood, the fibrous tissue has been replaced by bone. A **syndesmosis** is a joint in which the two bony surfaces are united by a ligament or membrane. The fibers of ligaments are flexible and stretch, permitting a limited amount of movement. The paired bones of the lower arm (radius and ulna) and the lower leg (tibia and fibula) are syndesmotic joints. A **gomphosis** is a special type of fibrous joint in which a conical projection fits into a complementary socket and is held there by a ligament. The teeth held in the maxilla or mandible are gomphosis joints.

Cartilaginous Joints

Cartilaginous joints (amphiarthroses) are more movable than fibrous joints. A **cartilaginous joint** unites bone directly to bone by means of either fibrocartilage or hyaline cartilage (Fig. 38-4). The main difference between the two types of cartilage is their collagen content. Hyaline cartilage contains delicate fibers of type II collagen, whereas fibrocartilage has larger fibers of type I and type II collagen.

There are two types of cartilaginous joints—symphyses and synchondroses. A **symphysis** is a cartilaginous joint in which bones are united by a pad or disk of fibrocartilage. The articulating surfaces of the two bones are usually covered by a thin layer of hyaline cartilage and the thick pad of fibrocartilage acts as a shock absorber and stabilizer. Examples of symphyses are the symphysis pubis, which joins the two pubic bones, and the intervertebral discs, which join the bodies of the vertebrae. A **synchondrosis** is a joint in which hyaline cartilage, rather than fibrocartilage, connects the two bones. The joints between the ribs and the sternum are synchondroses. The hyaline cartilage of these joints is called costal cartilage (see Fig. 38-4). Slight movement at the synchondroses between the ribs and the sternum allows the chest to move outward and upward during breathing.

Synovial Joints
Structure of Synovial Joints

Synovial joints (diarthroses) are the most movable and the most complex joints in the body (Fig. 38-5). A synovial joint consists of:
1. A fibrous joint capsule (articular capsule)
2. A synovial membrane that lines the inner surface of the joint capsule
3. A joint cavity (synovial cavity), a space formed by the capsule
4. Synovial fluid, which fills the joint cavity and lubricates the joint surface
5. Articular cartilage, which covers and pads the articulating bony surfaces

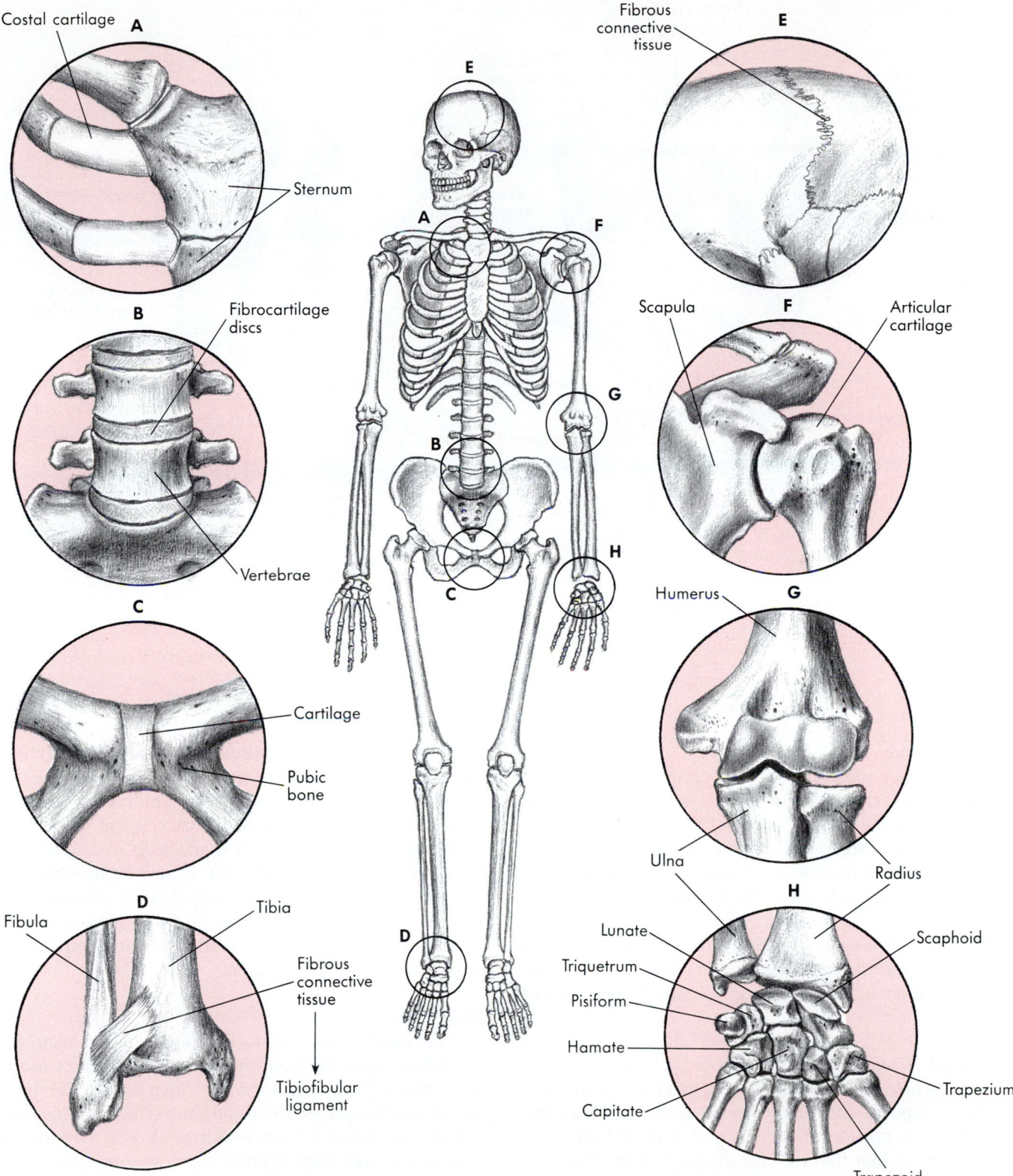

FIG. 38-4. Types of joints. Cartilaginous (amphiarthroidal) joints, which are slightly movable, include (**A**) a synchrondrosis that attaches ribs to costal cartilage; (**B**) a symphysis that connects vertebrae; and (**C**) the symphysis that connects the two pubic bones. Fibrous (synarthrodial) joints, which are immovable, include (**D**) the syndesmosis between the tibia and fibula, (**E**) sutures that connect the skull bones, and the gomophosis (not shown), which holds teeth in their sockets. The synovial joints include (**F**) the spheroid type at the shoulder, (**G**) the hinge type at the elbow, and (**H**) the gliding joints of the hand.

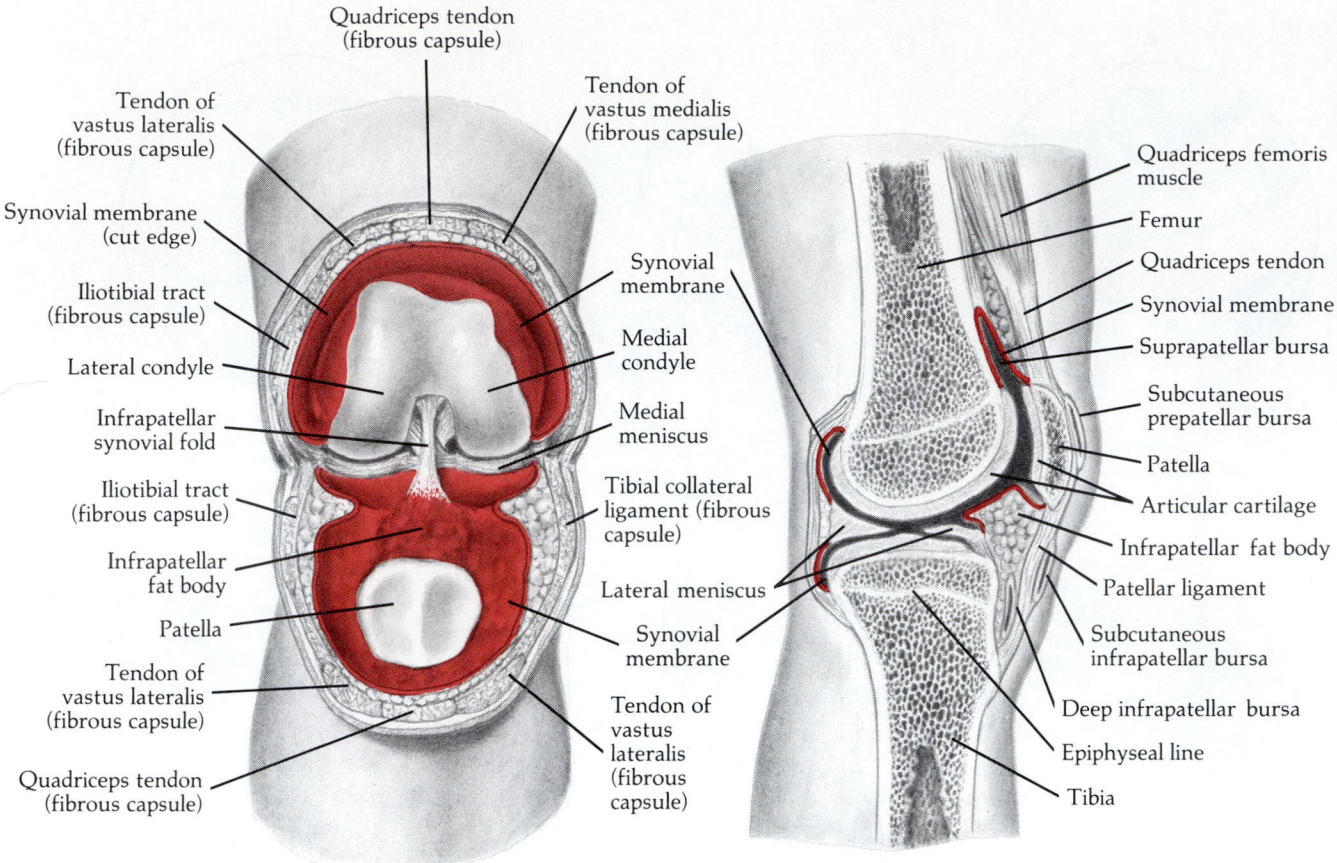

FIG. 38-5. Knee joint (synovial joint). (From Thompson et al., 1989.)

Joint Capsule

The fibrous **joint capsule** (articular capsule) is connective tissue that covers the ends of the bones where they meet in the joint. Sharpey's fibers firmly attach the proximal and distal capsule to the periosteum, and ligaments and tendons may also reinforce the capsule. The joint capsule is made up of parallel, interlacing bundles of dense, white fibrous tissue. It is richly supplied with nerves, blood vessels, and lymphatic vessels. The nerves in and around the joint capsule are sensitive to the rate and direction of motion, compression, tension, vibration, and pain.

Synovial Membrane

The **synovial membrane** (synovium) is the smooth, delicate inner lining of the joint capsule. It lines the nonarticular portion of the synovial joint and any ligaments or tendons that traverse the joint cavity. The synovial membrane is made up of two layers, a vascular layer called the **subintima** and a thin cellular layer called the **intima.** The vascular subintima merges with the fibrous joint capsule and is composed of loose fibrous connective tissue, elastin fibers, fat cells, fibroblasts, macrophages, and mast cells. The intima consists of

rows of synovial cells embedded in a fiber-free intercellular matrix. The intima contains two types of synovial cells, type A cells and type B cells. The **type A cells** ingest and remove (phagocytosis) bacteria and particles of debris in the joint cavity. (Phagocytosis is described in Chapter 7.) The **type B cells** secrete **hyaluronate,** a binding agent that gives synovial fluid its viscous quality. The synovial membrane is richly supplied with blood and lymphatic vessels; therefore it is capable of rapid repair and regeneration.

Joint Cavity

The **joint cavity** (synovial cavity) is an enclosed, fluid-filled space between the articulating surfaces of the two bones. This small cavity, often called the joint space, enables the two bones to move "against" one another. The synovial cavity is surrounded by the synovial membrane and filled with a clear, viscous, slick fluid called the synovial fluid.

Synovial Fluid

Synovial fluid is superfiltrated plasma from blood vessels in the synovial membrane. Synovial fluid lubricates the joint surfaces, nourishes the pad of the articu-

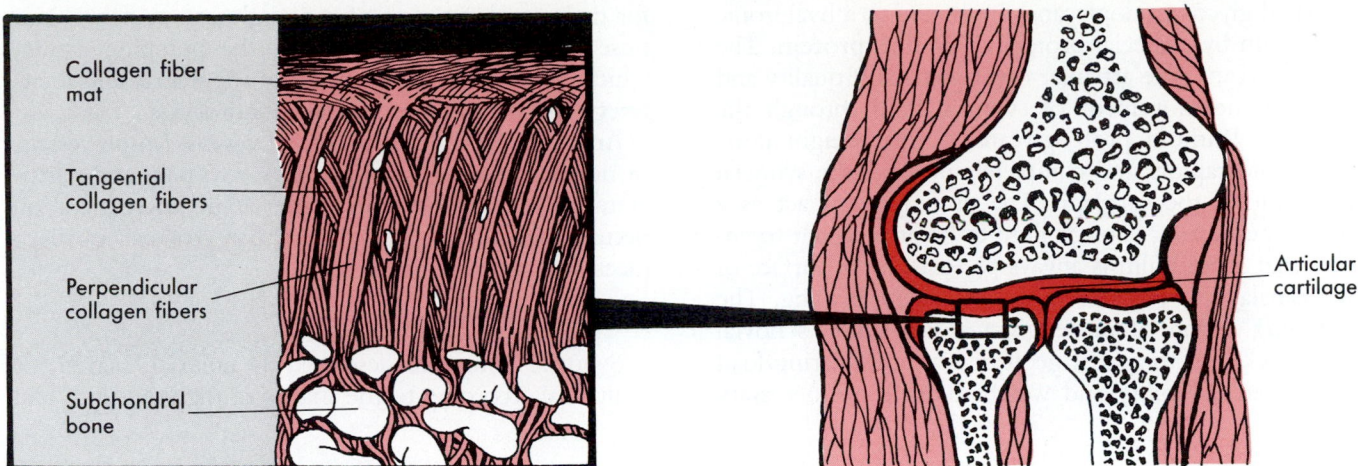

FIG. 38-6. Organization of collagen fibers in articular cartilage.

lar cartilage that covers the ends of the bones, and contains free-floating synovial cells and various leukocytes that phagocytose joint debris and microorganisms. Loss of synovial fluid leads to rapid deterioration of articular cartilage.

Articular Cartilage

Articular cartilage is a layer of hyaline cartilage that covers the end of each bone (see Fig. 38-5). It may be thick or thin, depending on the size of the joint, the fit of the two bone ends, and the amount of weight and shearing force the joint normally withstands. The function of articular cartilage is to reduce friction in the joint and to distribute the forces of weight bearing. Articular cartilage is composed of **chondrocytes** (cartilage cells) and an intercellular matrix made up of collagen, protein polysaccharides, and water. The intercellular matrix is produced by the chondrocytes. The chondrocytes synthesize and extrude collagen, which, like the collagen produced by bone cells, is distributed throughout the cartilage in a highly organized system of fibers. Collagen fibers in cartilage are made up of many fine fibrils that, like bone fibrils, are assembled in an orderly fashion that makes them resistant to physical, metabolic, or chemical breakdown. The main differences between bone collagen and cartilage collagen are the amino acid content of the alpha chains and the composition of the fibrils. Bone collagen fibrils are made up of two type I chains and one type II chain. Cartilage collagen fibrils are made up of three identical type II chains.

At the surface of articular cartilage (Figs. 38-6 and 38-7), the collagen fibers run parallel to the joint surface and are closely compacted into a dense, protective mat. (Loss of this dense, compacted configuration at the surface subjects the underlying fibers to splitting and thinning, in which case the cartilage is unable to tolerate weight bearing.) In the middle layer of the cartilage, the fibers are arranged tangential to the surface, which allows them to deform and absorb some of the force of weight bearing. In the bottom layer of the cartilage, the fibers are perpendicular to the joint surface and embedded in a calcified layer of cartilage called the **tidemark**. The tidemark anchors the collagen fibers to the underlying (subchondral) bone. Collagen fibers are important components of the cartilage matrix because they (1) anchor the cartilage securely to underlying bone, (2) provide a taut framework for the cartilage, (3) control the loss of fluid from the cartilage, and (4) prevent the escape of protein polysaccharides (proteoglycans) from the cartilage. The proteoglycans are macromolecules consisting of proteins, carbohydrates (**glycosaminoglycans**), and hyaluronic acid. The glycosaminoglycans (keratin sulfate and chondroitin sulfate) are attached to the **protein core,** and several protein cores (with their

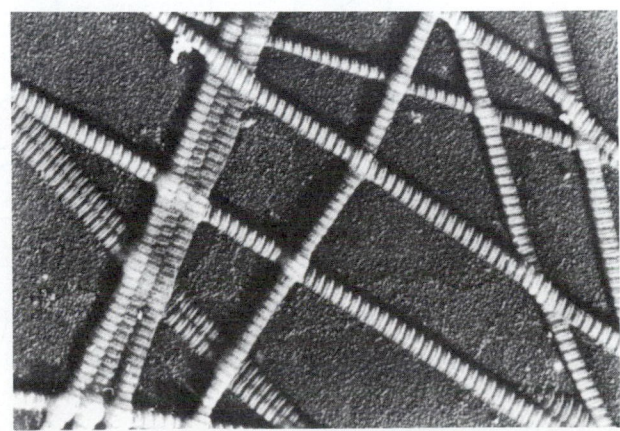

FIG. 38-7. Collagen fibers. Each fiber is composed of many collagen strands. (From Raven & Johnson, 1986.)

attached glycosaminoglycans) are bound to a hyaluronic acid chain by a special protein called **link protein.** The proteoglycans give articular cartilage its stiff quality and regulate the movement of synovial fluid through the cartilage. Without proteoglycans, normal weight bearing would rapidly and completely press all the synovial fluid out of the cartilage. The proteoglycans act as a pump, permitting enough fluid to be pressed out to ensure that a fluid film is always present on the surface of the cartilage, even after hours of weight bearing. The pumping action of proteoglycans also draws synovial fluid back into the cartilage after a weight-bearing load is released. Mobility and weight bearing are necessary for the pumping action of proteoglycans to occur. Nonuse of a joint quickly reduces the pumping action, which changes the composition of the matrix and interferes with the nutrition of the chondrocytes.

Articular cartilage has no blood vessels, lymph vessels, or nerves. Therefore it is insensitive to pain and regenerates slowly and minimally after injury. Regeneration occurs primarily at sites where the articular cartilage meets the synovial membrane.

Movement of Synovial Joints

Synovial joints are described as uniaxial, biaxial, or multiaxial according to the shapes of the bone ends and

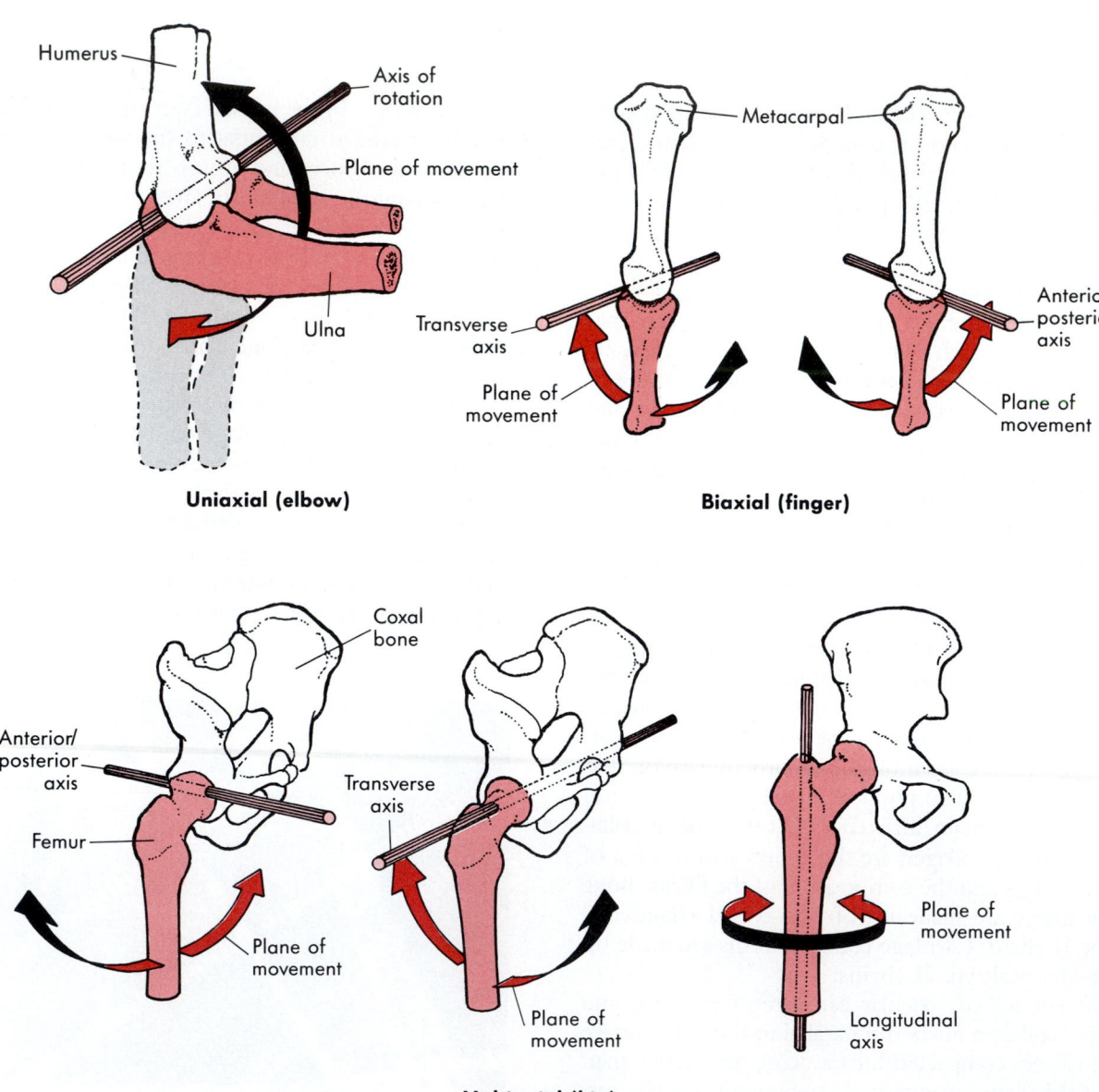

FIG. 38-8. Movements of synovial (diarthrodial) joints.

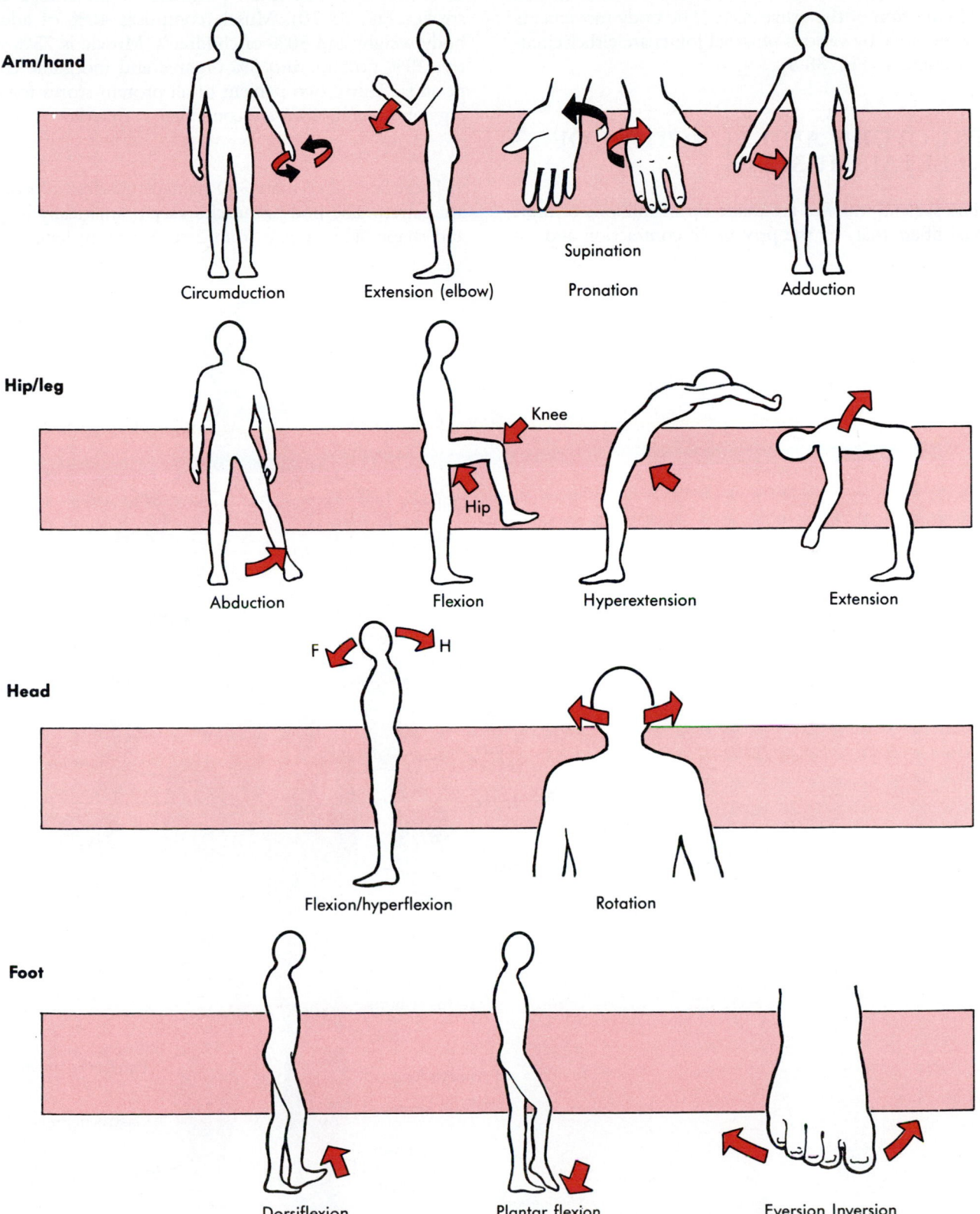

FIG. 38-9. Body movements provided by synovial (diarthrodial) joints.

the type of movement occurring at the joint (Fig. 38-8). Usually, one of the bones is stable and serves as an axis for the motion of the other bone. The body movements made possible by various synovial joints are either circular or angular (Fig. 38-9).

STRUCTURE AND FUNCTION OF SKELETAL MUSCLES

The skeletal muscles are made up of millions of individual fibers that, by the process of contraction and relaxation, do the work necessary to complete movements as varied as a ballerina's pirouette or an artist's deft stroke (Fig. 38-10). Muscle comprises 40% of adults' body weight and 50% of children's. Muscle is 75% water, 20% protein, and 5% organic and inorganic compounds. Thirty-two percent of all protein stores for energy and metabolism are contained in muscle.

Whole Muscle

There are more than 350 named muscles, almost all are paired. The body's muscles vary dramatically in size and shape. They range from 2 to 60 cm in length and

FIG. 38-10. Skeletal muscles of body. **A,** Anterior view.

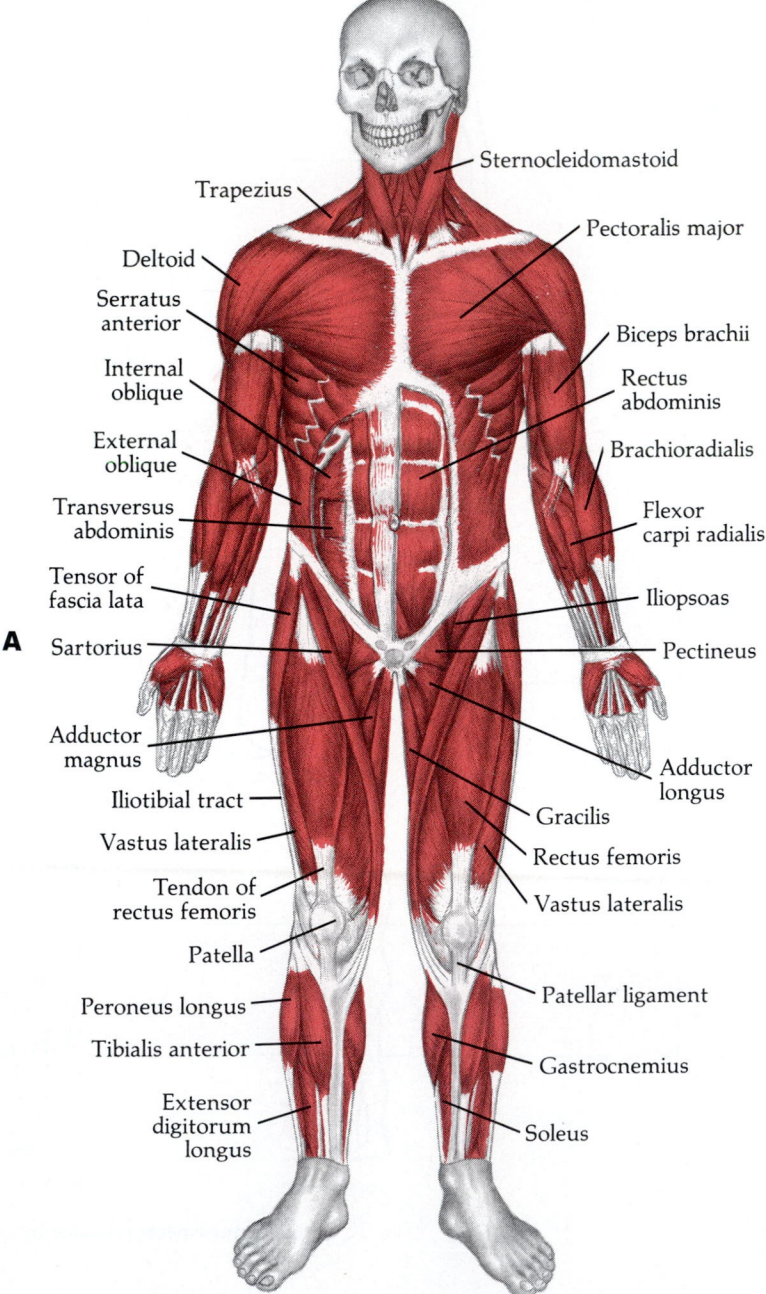

are shaped according to function. **Fusiform muscles** are elongated muscles shaped like straps and can run from one joint to another. **Pennate muscles** are broad, flat, and slightly fan shaped, with fibers running obliquely to the muscle's long axis. The multipennate deltoid muscle, which flexes and extends the arm, is a good example.

Each skeletal muscle is a separate organ, encased in a three-part connective tissue framework called **fascia.** The layers of connective tissue protect the muscle fibers, attach the muscle to bony prominences, and provide a structure for a network of nerve fibers, blood vessels, and lymphatic channels.

The outermost layer, the **epimysium,** is located on the surface of the muscle and tapers at each end to form the **tendon** (Fig. 38-11). Tendons allow a short muscle to exert power on a distant joint where a thick muscle would interfere with joint mobility. The next layer, the **perimysium,** further subdivides the muscle fibers into bundles of connective tissue, or **fascicles.** The **endomysium** surrounds the muscle fascicles, the smallest unit of muscle fibers visible without a microscope (Vick, 1984). The ligaments, tendons, and fascia are made up of connective tissue that also serves to buffer the limbs from the effects of sudden strains or changes in speed. The

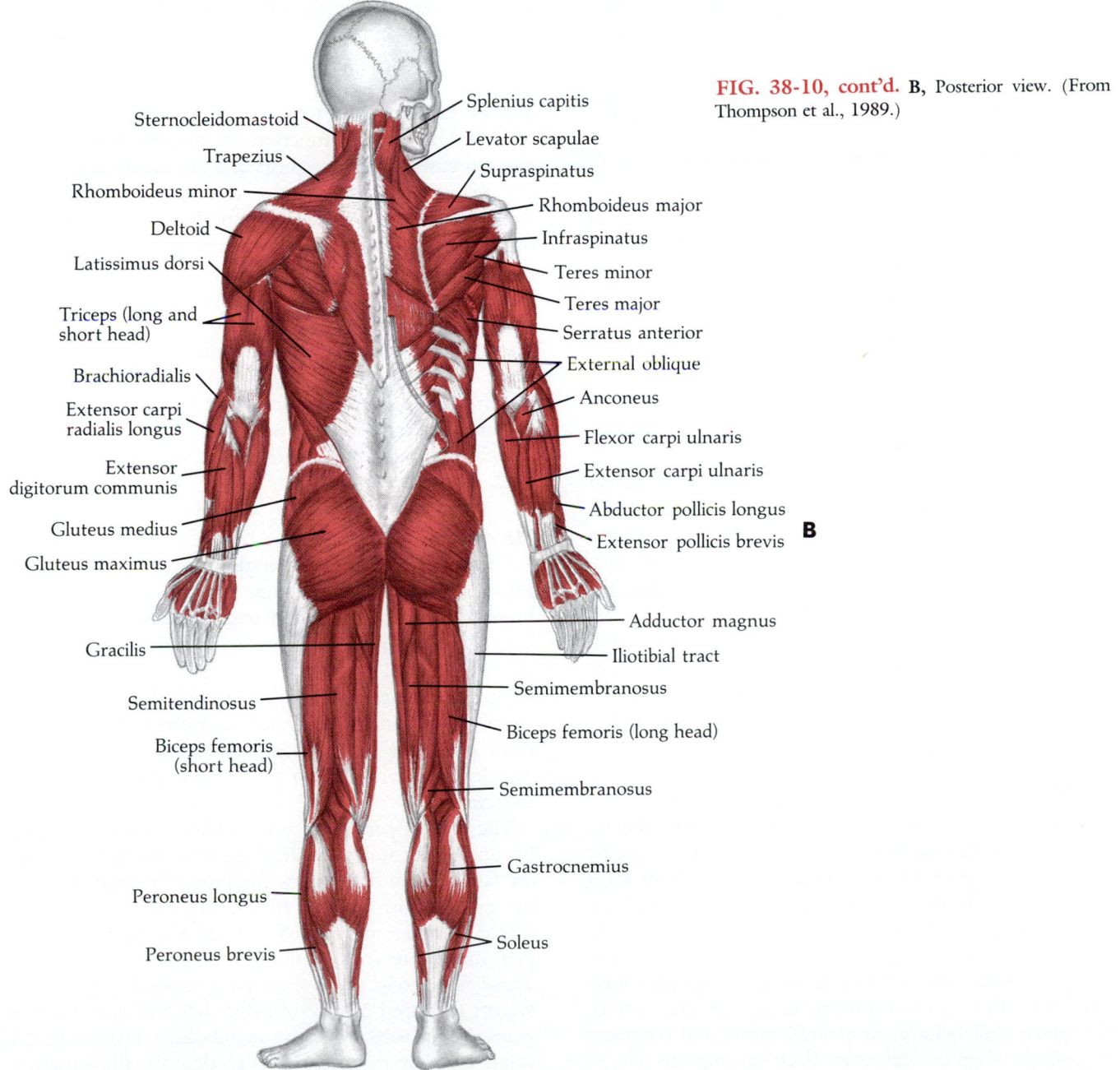

FIG. 38-10, cont'd. B, Posterior view. (From Thompson et al., 1989.)

Sternocleidomastoid
Trapezius
Rhomboideus minor
Deltoid
Latissimus dorsi
Triceps (long and short head)
Brachioradialis
Extensor carpi radialis longus
Extensor digitorum communis
Gluteus medius
Gluteus maximus
Gracilis
Semitendinosus
Biceps femoris (short head)
Peroneus longus
Peroneus brevis

Splenius capitis
Levator scapulae
Supraspinatus
Rhomboideus major
Infraspinatus
Teres minor
Teres major
Serratus anterior
External oblique
Anconeus
Flexor carpi ulnaris
Extensor carpi ulnaris
Abductor pollicis longus
Extensor pollicis brevis
Adductor magnus
Iliotibial tract
Semimembranosus
Biceps femoris (long head)
Semimembranosus
Gastrocnemius
Soleus

B

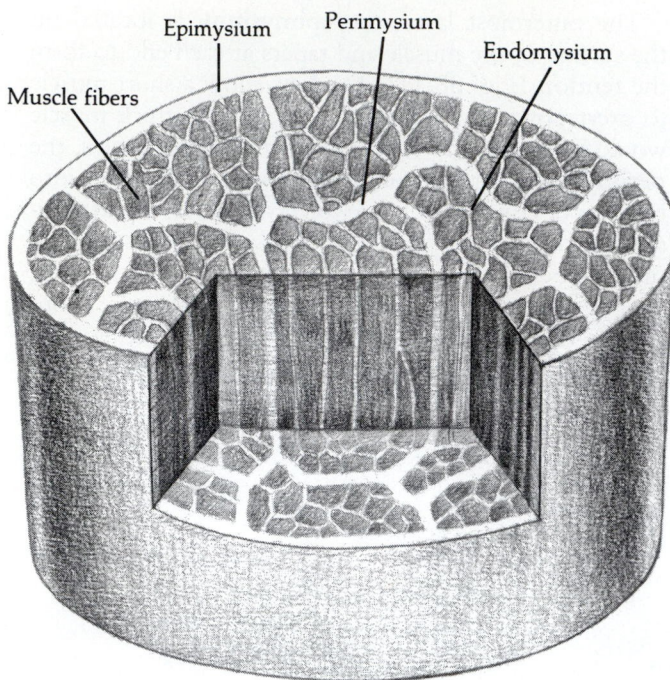

FIG. 38-11. Cross-section of skeletal muscle showing muscle fibers and their coverings. (From Thompson et al., 1989.)

rapid recovery necessary for strenuous exercise is supported by the elastic property of muscle and its connective tissue.

Skeletal muscle is described, almost interchangeably, as voluntary, striated, or extrafusal. "Voluntary" indicates that the muscle is controlled directly by the central nervous system. "Striated" describes the striated, or striped, pattern of skeletal muscle viewed under a light microscope. "Extrafusal" distinguishes the skeletal muscle fibers from other contractile fibers located within the sensory organs of the muscle.

Other components that are visible on gross inspection of the whole muscle include the motor and senory nerve fibers. These function together with the muscle, innervating portions of it and providing the electrical impulses needed for motor function.

Motor Unit

From the anterior horn cell of the spinal cord, the axons of motor nerves branch out to innervate a specific group of muscle fibers. Each anterior horn cell, its axon (part of lower motor neuron, see Chapter 12), and the muscle fibers innervated by it is called a **motor unit** (Fig. 38-12). The motor units are composed of lower motor neurons, which extend to skeletal muscles. Often termed the functional unit of the neuromuscular system, the motor unit behaves as a single entity and contracts as a whole when it receives an electrical impulse.

The whole muscle may be controlled by several motor nerve axons. These branch to innervate many motor units within the muscle. The whole muscle may then be made up of many motor units. The number of motor units per individual muscle varies greatly. In the calf, for example, one motor axon will innervate approximately 2000 muscle fibers, out of a total of 1,200,000 muscle fibers. This is a high innervation ratio of muscle fibers to axons, and it contrasts markedly with the low innervation ratio in the laryngeal muscles. There, two to three muscle fibers comprise each motor unit, and the innervation ratio can be of great functional significance. The greater the innervation ratio of a particular organ, the greater its endurance. Higher innervation ratios thus prevent fatigue, whereas lower innervation ratios allow for precision of movement (Goodgold & Epstein, 1977).

Sensory Receptors

Although muscles function as effector organs, they also contain sensory receptors and are involved in sending different signals to the central nervous system. Among these are the muscle spindles and Golgi tendon organs. **Spindles** are mechanoreceptors that lie parallel to muscle fibers and respond to muscle stretching. **Golgi tendon organs** are dendrites that terminate and branch to tendons near the neuromuscular junction. The muscle spindles, Golgi tendon organs, and free nerve endings provide a means of reporting changes in length, tension, velocity, and tone in the muscle. This system of afferent signals is responsible for the muscle stretch response and maintenance of normal muscle tone.

Muscle Fibers

Each **muscle fiber** is a single muscle cell. This long cell is cylindrical in structure surrounded by a membrane capable of excitation and impulse propagation. The muscle fiber contains bundles of **myofibrils,** the fiber's functional subunits, in a parallel arrangement along the longitudinal axis of the muscle (Fig. 38-13). At birth, the muscle fibers have completed development from precursor cells called **myoblasts.** All voluntary muscles are derived from the mesodermal layer of the embryo.

The type of peripheral nerve influences the muscle fiber and motor unit considerably. Whether motor nerves are fast or slow determines the type of muscle fibers in the motor unit. Type II fibers, also called white fast-motor fibers, are innervated by relatively large type II alpha motor neurons with fast conduction velocities. These fibers rely on a short-term anaerobic glycolytic system for rapid energy transfer; whereas type I fibers depend on aerobic oxidative metabolism. Histochemical stains are now routinely used to describe the structure

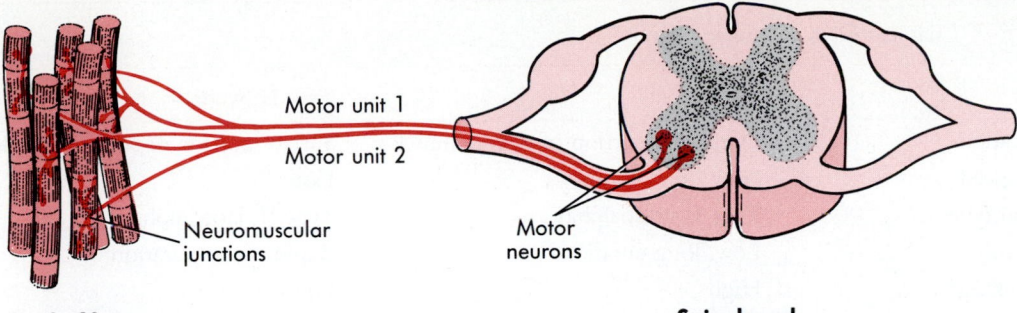

FIG. 38-12. Motor units of a muscle. Each motor unit consists of a motor neuron and all the muscle fibers (cells) supplied by the neuron.

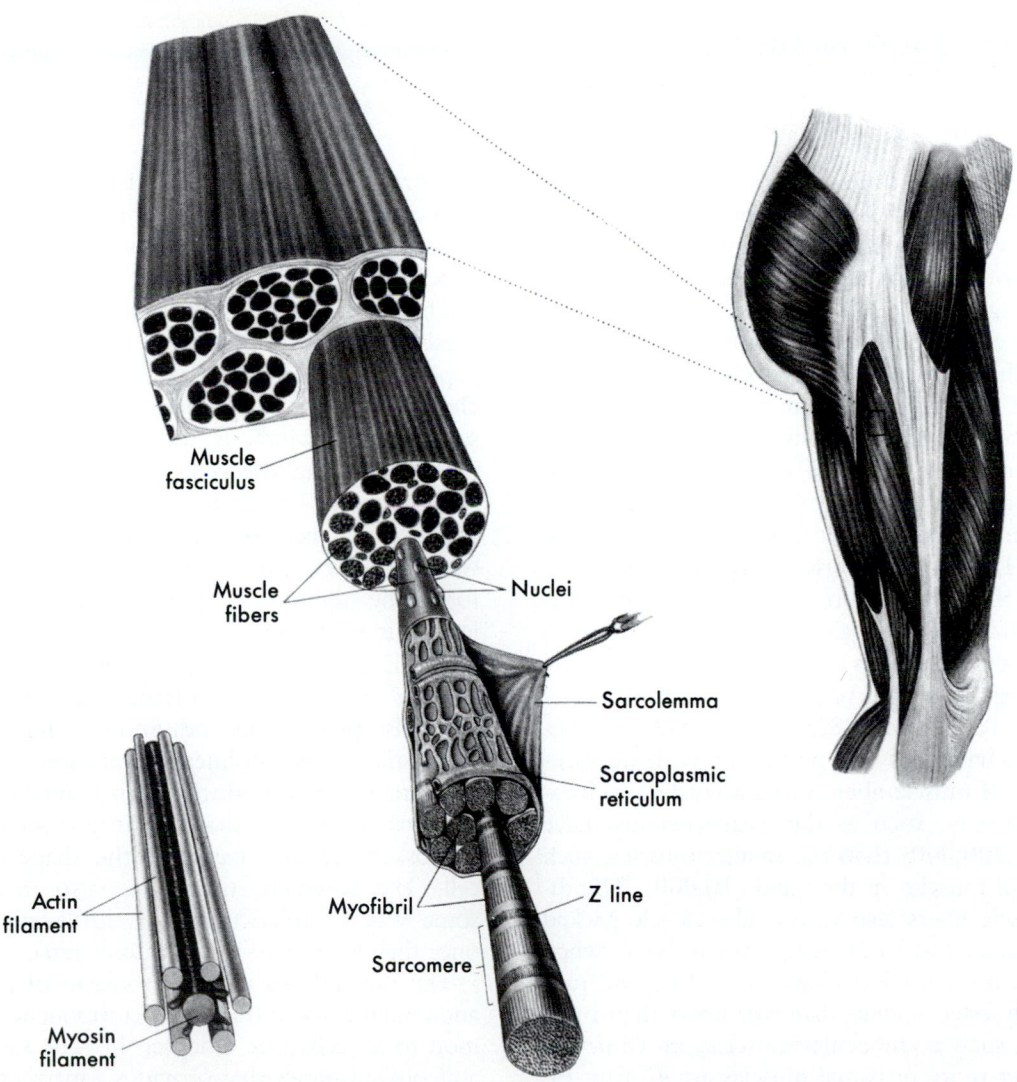

FIG. 38-13. Myofibrils of a skeletal muscle fiber (cell) and overall organization of skeletal muscle. (From Raven & Johnson, 1986.)

TABLE 38-3 Characteristics of muscle fibers

Characteristic	Type I (red)	Type II (white)
Anatomic location	Deep axial portion of surface muscle	Surface portion of surface muscle
Contraction speed	Slow	Fast
Motor neuron type	Type I, small alpha	Type II, large alpha
Firing frequently	Low, long duration	Rapid, short duration
Resistance to fatigue	High	Low
Myoglobin	High	Low
Capillary supply	Profuse	Intermediate to sparse
Metabolism	Oxidative	Glycolysis
Mitochondria	Many	Fewer
Enzymes	Lactate dehydrogenase, types 1-3	Lactate dehydrogenase types 4-5
Creatine kinase	Cardiac type	Fast, skeletal
Example (most muscles are mixed)	Greater proportion of slow-contracting fibers in soleus	Greater proportion of fast-contracting fibers in laryngeal and ocular muscles

From Ruch, T., & Patton, H. D. (Eds.). (1982). *Howell-Fulton's physiology and biophysics · IV · Excitable tissue and reflex control of muscle* (12th ed.). Philadelphia: W. B. Saunders.

of muscle fibers and contractile elements of muscle biopsy specimens. White muscle, or **type II fibers,** stains dark in the enzyme stain adenosine triphosphatase (AT-Pase) at a pH of 9.4. Red muscle, or **type I fibers,** appears lightly stained.

The overlap of muscle fibers that appears with staining gives the checkerboard appearance of muscle biopsy specimens and provides an equal distribution of fiber types throughout the muscle. This overlap also helps to compensate for muscle fiber loss and fatigue of individual motor units during activity. In spite of this, some muscles contain proportionally more of one fiber type than another. The postural muscles have more type I fibers, allowing them the high resistance to fatigue that is necessary to maintain the same position for extended periods. The ocular muscles have more type II muscle fibers, allowing them to respond rapidly to visual changes (Ruch & Patton, 1982). (Table 38-3 describes the specific characteristics of type I and type II fibers.)

The number of muscle fibers varies according to location. Large muscles, such as the gastrocnemius, have more fibers (1,200,000) than the smaller muscles, such as the lumbrical muscles in the hand (10,000). The diameter of muscle fibers also varies. The closely packed polygons are small (10 to 20 μm) until puberty, when they attain the normal adult diameter of 40 to 80 μm. Women usually have smaller diameter fibers than men. Small muscles, such as the ocular muscles, are 15 μm in diameter; larger more proximal muscles are 40 μm. Fiber size can have functional significance. Studies have shown that larger fiber diameter is associated with generation of greater forces. Fiber diameter can be increased by targeted exercise or occupational overuse, activities that cause hypertrophied muscle (Dubowitz & Brooke, 1973).

The major components of the muscle fiber include the muscle membrane, myofibrils, sarcotubular system, sarcoplasm, and mitochondria (see Fig. 38-13). The **muscle membrane** is a two-part membrane. It includes the **sarcolemma,** which is the plasma membrane of the muscle cell, and the cell's **basement membrane.** The sarcolemma is 7.5 nm thick and is capable of propagating electrical impulses. At the motor nerve endplate, where the nerve impulse is transmitted, the sarcolemma forms the highly convoluted synaptic cleft. The sarcolemma is made up of lipid molecules and protein systems. The protein systems perform special functions, such as transport of nutrients and protein synthesis. They also provide the sodium-potassium pump and include the cell's cholinergic receptor. The basement membrane is 50 nm thick and is composed primarily of proteins and polysaccharides. It also serves as the cell's microskeleton and maintains the shape of the muscle cell. The basement membrane also may function in some way to restrict further diffusion of electrolytes once they have crossed the sarcolemma.

The **sarcoplasm** is the cytoplasm of the muscle cell and contains the intracellular components that are common to all cells (see Chapter 1). The sarcoplasm is an aqueous substance that provides a matrix that surrounds the myofibrils. It contains numerous enzymes and proteins that are responsible for the cell's energy production, protein synthesis, and oxygen storage. The mitochondria houses enzyme systems for energy production, particularly those that regulate such processes as the citric acid cycle and adenosine triphosphate (ATP) formation. Many other structures are present in the sarcoplasm. The ribosomes are primarily composed of RNA and participate in the process of protein synthesis. The cell nucleus, satellite cells, glycogen granules, and lipid droplets are suspended in the sarcoplasmic matrix. Blood vessels, nerve endings, muscle spindles, and Golgi tendon organs are also directly located within this structure.

Unique to the muscle is the **sarcotubular system,** a network that includes the transverse tubules and the sarcoplasmic reticulum, which crosses the interior of the cell. The **sarcoplasmic reticulum** is made like the endoplasmic reticulum in other cells. In the muscle cells the sarcoplasmic reticulum is involved in calcium transport, which initiates muscle contraction at the **sarcomere,** a portion of the myofibril (see Fig. 38-13). The sarcoplasmic reticulum is composed of tubules that run parallel to the myofibrils. The longitudinal tubules are termed **sarcotubules.** The **transverse tubules,** which are closely associated with the sarcotubules, run across the sarco-

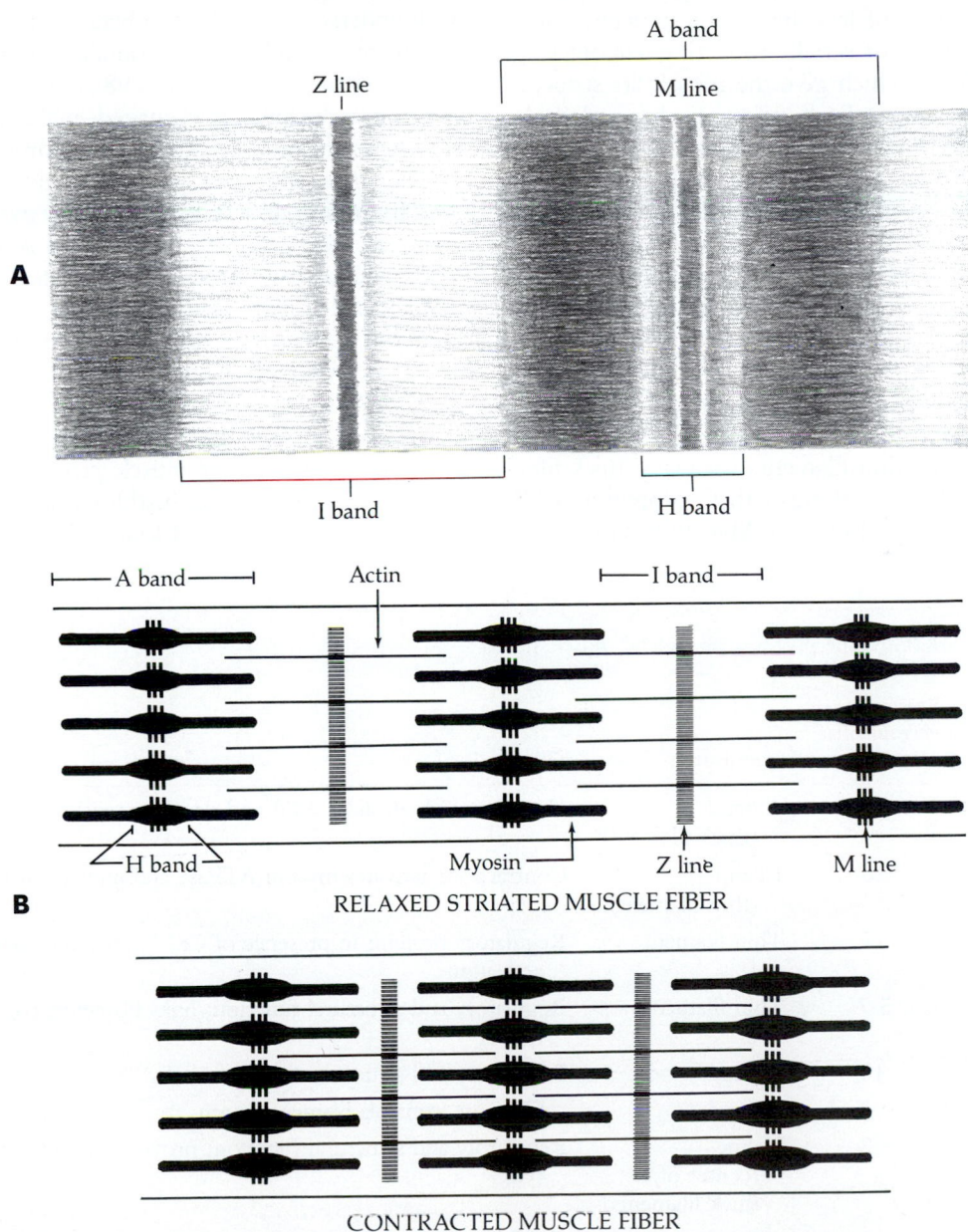

FIG. 38-14. **A,** Lines and bands in striated muscle. **B,** Relationships of bands, actin, myosin, and lines in relaxed and contracted muscle fibers. (From Thompson et al., 1989.)

plasm and communicate with the extracellular space. Together, the tubules of this membrane system allow for intracellular calcium uptake, regulation, and release during muscle contraction.

Myofibrils

The myofibrils are the functional units of muscle contraction. Each myofibril contains sarcomeres, which appear at intervals (see Fig. 38-13). The sarcomeres are composed of two contractile proteins, **actin** and **myosin.**

The myofibrils are the most abundant subcellular muscle component, equaling 85% to 90% of the total volume. On cross-section, they are irregular polygons with a mean diameter of less than a micrometer. Each myofibril is composed of serially repeating sarcomeres, separated by Z lines, which give the muscle its striped, cross-striated appearance. Each sarcomere has a dark A band and is flanked by two light I bands (Fig. 38-14). The A band is 1.5 to 1.6 μm long and contains the thick myosin filaments. Included in the A band is a lighter zone called the H band, and in the center of the H band is the dark M band, or M line. The I band, which contains actin, is divided at the midpoint of each sarcomere by the Z line. Its length varies with the start of muscle contraction.

Myofibrils are composed of myofilaments. Each myofilament is structured in a closely packed hexagonal arrangement, with two thin filaments for every thick filament. The thick filament, along with C protein and M line protein, is made up of myosin. Myosin has two subunits, heavy and light meromyosin, which resemble twisted golf club shafts. The thin filaments are twisted double strands, made up of actin, troponin, and tropomyosin (see Chapter 26 and Fig. 38-15).

Muscle Proteins

Eight proteins have been identified in the muscle fibrils. (Table 38-4 outlines their distribution, localization, and possible functional significance.) The contractile and regulatory functions of actin, myosin, and the troponin-tropomyosin complex (associated with actin) are the most commonly known. They also account for most of the protein found in the myofibril. The structural and regulatory processes of muscle proteins are less well understood. Alpha and beta actin are known to link the filaments. M protein contains the enzyme creatine kinase (Ruch & Patton, 1982). Creatine is released when muscle cells are damaged, making serum creatine an important test of pathologic conditions of muscles.

The most abundant proteins, actin and myosin, are also found in other cells, particularly motile cells such as platelets. The complete amino acid sequences of both actin and myosin have been identified. Noteworthy is the presence of the amino acid 3-methylhistidine, which is found only in the thin filament actin. Eighty-five to 90% of 3-methylhistidine is found in skeletal muscle. Because it is excreted unchanged (in the urine) after release from muscle and other tissue, 3-methylhistidine has been used to gauge muscle protein degradation. The amino acids lysine and histidine have been isolated in adult type II muscle and found absent in fetal, cardiac,

TABLE 38-4 Contractile proteins of skeletal muscle fibrils

Name	Percentage of myofibrillar protein	Localization	Function
Myosin	55	A band (thick filament)	Contraction; hydrolyzes ATP and develops tension
Actin	20	I band (thin filament)	Contraction; activates myosin ATPase and interacts with myosin
Troponin	7	Thin filament	Regulatory protein; in presence of Ca^{++}, promotes actin-myosin activation
Tropomyosin	5-7	Thin filament	Regulatory and structural function; links filaments, controls filament length
Alpha (α) actin	10	Z band	Regulatory and structural function; links
Beta (β) actin	2	Z band	filaments, controls filament length
M protein	<2	M line (center of thick filaments)	Regularoty and structural function; provides enzyme creatine kinase (CK)
C protein	2	A band (thick filaments)	Possible structural role

and type I muscle (Ruch & Patton, 1982). These amino acids, in addition to leucine, have been used to study protein synthesis by means of stable isotope infusion and muscle biopsy analysis.

Nonprotein Constituents of Muscle

Substances such as nitrogen, creatine, creatinine, phosphocreatine, purines, uric acid, and amino acids all serve in the complex process of muscle metabolism. Glycogen and its derivatives are present as energy sources.

Creatine and creatinine metabolism have been used to measure muscle mass. Plasma creatine is taken up by muscle and converted into the high-energy phosphate compound phosphocreatine by the enzyme creatine kinase. Creatinine is formed in muscle from creatine at a constant rate of 2%/day. (Tests for plasma creatine are discussed in Chapter 32). Creatine excretion is increased in muscle wasting, whereas creatinine excretion is reduced. This change reflects the reduction in total body creatine stores and loss of muscle mass.

Inorganic compounds, anions (phosphate and chloride), and cations (calcium, magnesium, sodium, and potassium) are important in the regulation of protein synthesis, muscle contraction, enzyme systems, and membrane stabilization. Total-body potassium (TBK), measured by the K^{40} method, has been used to measure muscle mass, also called lean body mass. Total-body potassium reflects changes in muscle mass seen during growth, malnutrition, and muscle wasting (Griggs et al., 1983).

Components of Muscle Function

The ultimate function of muscle is to accomplish work. Although variously expressed in such measures as foot-pounds or kilogram-meters, work usually refers to the amount of energy liberated or force exerted over a distance (work = force × distance). Muscles usually contract or tense while doing work. Muscle contraction occurs on the molecular level and leads to the observable phenomenon of muscle movement.

Muscle Contraction at the Molecular Level

Muscle contraction is a four-step process that includes (1) excitation, (2) coupling, (3) contraction, and (4) relaxation. The process involves the electrical properties of all cells and the movement of ions across the plasma membrane (see Chapter 1). The muscle fiber is an excitable tissue. At rest, an electric charge of −90 mV is continually maintained across the sarcolemma. This resting potential, generated by the separation of positive and negative charges on either side of the membrane, creates an electrochemical equilibrium caused by the selective permeability of the sarcolemma to electrolytes in the intracellular and extracellular fluids, particularly potassium and sodium.

Excitation, the first step of muscle contraction, begins with the spread of an action potential from the nerve terminal to the neuromuscular junction. The rapid depolarization of the membrane initiates an electrical impulse in the muscle fiber membrane called the **muscle fiber action potential.** As the action potential advances along the sarcolemmal membrane, it spreads to the transverse tubules. (The velocity of conduction is much slower in muscle fibers than in myelinated nerve fibers, only 3 to 5 m/sec compared to 54 to 90 m/sec in nerve fibers.)

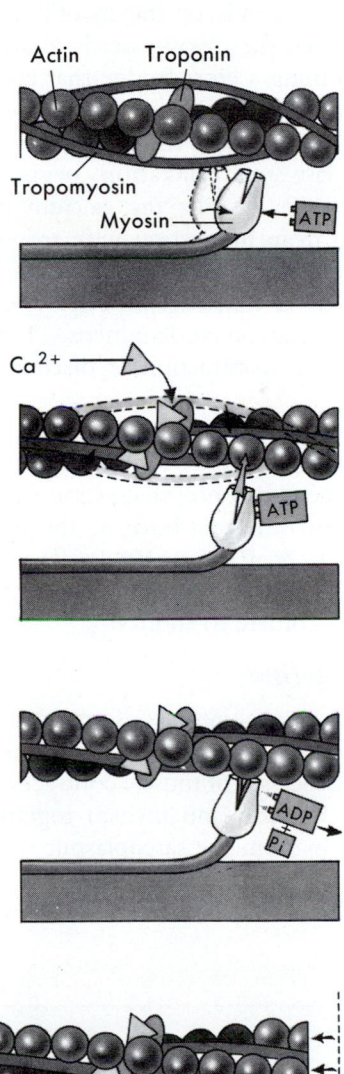

FIG. 38-15. Muscle contraction at the molecular level: the sliding filament theory. Muscle fiber shortens when thin filaments move past thick filaments toward centers of the sarcomeres and Z lines are drawn closer together. (From Thibodeau, 1987.)

The second stage, **coupling,** follows the depolarization of the transverse tubules. This stage consists of the migration of calcium ions, which are stored in the sarcoplasmic reticulum, to the myofilaments. Calcium affects troponin and tropomyosin, muscle proteins that bind with actin when the muscle is at rest. In the presence of calcium, however, both of these proteins are attracted to calcium ions, leaving the actin free to bind with myosin.

Contraction thus begins as the calcium ions combine with troponin, a reaction that overcomes the inhibitory function of the troponin-tropomyosin system. The thin filament, actin, then slides toward the thick filament, myosin. The two ends of the myofibril shorten after contraction when the myosin heads attach to the actin molecules, forming a cross-bridge that comprises an actin-myosin complex. ATP, located on the actin myosin complex, is released when the cross-bridges attach (Fig. 38-15). The last step, **relaxation,** begins as the sarcoplasmic reticulum absorbs the calcium molecules, removing them from interaction with troponin. Calcium is pumped back into the sarcoplasmic reticulum by means of an active transport process. The cross-bridges detach, and the sarcomere lengthens. (The cross-bridge theory of muscle contraction is discussed in Chapter 26.)

This is the **sliding filament theory** described in electron micrographs by A. F. Huxley in the 1950s, which is now the accepted conceptualization of the formation of the actin-myosin cross-bridges, the process of contraction (Ruch & Patton, 1982). The process is so named because the actin actually slides onto the myosin, causing the sarcomere to shorten.

Muscle Metabolism

Skeletal muscle requires a constant supply of ATP and phosphocreatine. These substances are necessary to fuel the complex processes of muscle contraction, driving the cross-bridges of actin and myosin together and transporting calcium from the sarcoplasmic reticulum to the myofibril.

In addition to muscle contraction, other internal processes of the muscular system require ATP. ATP is required for protein synthesis that replenishes muscle constituents and accommodates growth and repair. The rate of protein synthesis is related to hormone levels (particularly insulin), amino acid substrates, and overall nutritional status. At rest, the rate of ATP formation by oxidation of glucose or acetoacetate is sufficient to maintain internal processes, given normal nutritional status. During activity, the need for ATP increases almost 1000-fold (Edwards, 1984). The metabolic pathways for muscle activity in Table 38-5 show reactions to the immediate need for increased ATP caused by contraction. Activity lasting longer than 5 seconds expends the available stored ATP and phosphocreatine. Stored glycogen and blood glucose are converted anaerobically to sustain brief activity without increasing the demand for oxygen. Anaerobic glycolysis is much less efficient than aerobic glycolysis, using 6 to 8 times more glycogen to produce the same amount of ATP. With increased activity, such as intense exercise or with ischemia, an increase in lactic acid occurs because of the breakdown of glycogen, thus causing a shift in muscle pH (see Table 38-5). This short-term mechanism "buys time" by allowing ATP formation in spite of inadequate energy stores or oxygen supply. When the anaerobic threshold is reached and more oxygen is required, physiologic changes occur in addition to a rise in lactic acid. These include an increase in oxygen consumption, heart rate, respiratory rate, and muscle blood flow (McArdle, Katch, & Katch, 1986).

Strenuous exercise requires oxygen, which activates the aerobic glycogen pathway for ATP formation. During maximal exercise, free fatty-acid mobilization and the aerobic glycogen pathways provide ATP over an extended time. These pathways require oxygen both to maintain maximal activity and to return the muscle to the resting state. Maximal exercise increases oxygen uptake by 15 to 20 times over the resting state. When this system becomes exhausted or inadequate to respond to the need for ATP, fatigue and weakness finally force the muscle to reduce activity.

TABLE 38-5 Energy sources for muscular activity

Sources	Reactions
Short-term (anaerobic) sources	Adenosine triphosphate (ATP) → Adenosine diphosphate (ADP) + Inorganic phosphate (P_1) + Energy
	Phosphocreatine + ADP $\rightleftharpoons$ Creatine + ATP
	Glycogen/glucose + P_1 + ADP → Lactate + ATP
Long-term (aerobic) sources	Glycogen/glucose + ADP + P_1 + O_2 → H_2O + CO_2 + ATP
	Free fatty acids + ADP + P_1 + O_2 → H_2O + CO_2 + ATP

From Edwards, R. H. T. (1984). New techniques for studying human muscle function, metabolism, and fatigue. *Muscle and Nerve, 7*(8), 602.

The ability to sustain maximal muscular activity leads to the accumulation of oxygen debt. **Oxygen debt** is the amount of oxygen needed to oxidize the residual lactic acid, convert it back to glycogen, and replenish ATP and phosphocreatine stores (Honig, 1981). For example, after running at maximal speed for 10 seconds, the average person has consumed 1 L of oxygen. At rest, oxygen consumption for the same period is approximately 40 ml. As the person recovers, the measured oxygen debt is 4 L greater than the amount used during activity.

Measuring oxygen consumption as an indicator of energy expenditure is used to calculate the metabolic cost of activity in normal and diseased muscle. Indirect measures of energy expenditure include oxygen consumption, timed tests of activity, heart rate, and respiratory quotient (ratio of carbon dioxide to expired oxygen consumed). Energy expenditure is measured directly by the production of heat. Heat is released whenever work is accomplished, initially during muscle contraction and then during return to the resting state. Direct measures of energy expenditure require careful laboratory control and are not as useful as indirect measures for clinical studies (Ruch & Patton, 1982).

Another factor that changes energy requirements is muscle fiber type. Type II fibers rely on anaerobic glycolytic metabolism and fatigue readily. Type I fibers can resist fatigue for longer periods because of their capacity for oxidative metabolism.

Muscle Mechanics

Muscle contraction is not a process that can be viewed in isolation. Several factors determine how force is transmitted from the cross-bridges on individual muscle fibers to accomplish whole-muscle contraction. The first factor involves the motor unit. When a motor unit responds to a single nerve stimulus, it develops a phasic contraction, also called "twitch." Because the motor unit contracts in an "all or nothing" manner, the contraction that is generated by the stimulus will be a maximal contraction of the motor unit. The central nervous system smoothly grades the force generated by "recruiting" additional motor units and varying the discharge frequency of each active motor unit. This adding of motor units within the muscle is called **repetitive discharge.**

Recruitment and repetitive discharge of motor units allow the muscle to activate the number of motor units needed to generate the desired force. The total force developed is the sum of the force generated by each motor unit. As the strength, speed, and duration of stimuli increase, the summation of contractions reaches a critical frequency called **tetanus.** When tetanus is reached, no further increase in force can be achieved (Goodgold & Epstein, 1977).

Other variables, such as fiber type, innervation ratio,

muscle temperature, and muscle shape, influence the efficiency of muscular contraction. The two muscle fiber types differ in their responses to electrical activity. Tetanus and duration of phasic contractions, which take microseconds to accomplish, are achieved more rapidly in type II than in type I muscle fibers. Low innervation ratios promote control and coordination, whereas high ratios promote strength and endurance. For example, muscles with low innervation ratios, such as the laryngeal and ocular muscles, respond more rapidly than muscles with high innervation ratios to achieve fine control over movement. High innervation ratios, for example, in the calf, allow the muscle to sustain movement for prolonged periods or sustain the great forces needed for lifting. Muscle temperature also determines its degree of efficiency. Muscles work best at normal body temperature, 98.6° F (37° C). Muscle efficiency is also altered by the size of the load to be lifted and the shape of the muscle that carries the load. Heavier loads develop tension slowly. In some cases a load is necessary for the muscle to perform optimally. Muscles with a large cross-sectional area, such as the fan-shaped pennate muscles, develop greater contractile forces than smaller diameter muscles. The initial length of a muscle and the range of shortening that occur when the muscle contracts also determine the force it can generate. The long fusiform muscles have a greater range of shortening and can contract up to 57% of their resting length. A certain amount of elongation is necessary to generate sufficient tension and muscular force. The elongation that occurs during the swing of a golf club or tennis racket is an example of how stretch improves contractile force.

Types of Muscle Contraction

Two types of functional muscle contraction are isometric and isotonic. During **isometric contraction** (in Greek, *isos* = equal and *metron* = measure), the muscle maintains constant length as tension is increased. Isometric contraction occurs, for example, when the arm or leg is pushed against an immovable object. The muscle contracts, but the limb does not move. Isometric contraction is also called a static or holding contraction.

During **isotonic contraction** (in Greek, *isos* = equal and *tonus* = tension), the muscle maintains a constant tension as it moves. Isotonic contractions can be **eccentric** (lenghtening) or **concentric** (shortening). Positive work is accomplished during concentric contraction, and energy is released to exert force or lift a weight. Typical concentric contractions are stepping up on a stool or flexing the elbow during a pull-up. In contrast, during an eccentric contraction the muscle lengthens and absorbs energy. Negative work is accomplished on the muscle by the load. Examples include stepping down stairs, running downhill, or slowly lowering the forearm into the extended position from the flexed position during a pull-up (Basmajian, 1978). Eccentric contraction requires less energy to accomplish and has been said to result in the development of pain and stiffness after unaccustomed exercise.

Movement of Muscle Groups

Muscles do not act alone, but in groups, often under automatic control. When a muscle contracts and acts as a "prime mover," or **agonist,** its reciprocal muscle, or **antagonist,** relaxes. This is easily tested by holding the right arm in the horizontal position in front of the body, then bending the elbow while feeling the biceps in the front and the triceps in the back with the other hand. The biceps is firm, and the triceps is soft. As the arm is flexed, the muscles change. When the elbow is completely flexed, the biceps is soft and the triceps firm. Completing this movement causes the agonist and antagonist to change automatically; only the movement is commanded, not the alternate contraction and relaxation of the specific muscle groups.

In addition to the group action of muscles, other associated actions may be unheeded by the casual observer. During walking, as the foot leaves the ground, the paravertebral and gluteal muscles on the opposite sides of the body contract to maintain balance. One notices the loss of the associated muscle's action when paralysis offsets this process and decreases balance. Arm swing is another associated movement that can be reduced with a seemingly mild paralysis. Other associated movements include the involuntary movements of yawning and stretching. These same movements may be preserved when severe paralysis is present.

Muscles have a ligamentous action that prevents completing movements that would injure tissue. For example, the average person cannot relax the hamstrings sufficiently to touch the toes with the knees straight. This same muscle, if weakened by paralysis, can be damaged if forcibly stretched. Damage might occur, for example, in the supine position if hip flexion was forced while the knees were kept extended (Brunnstrom, 1979).

TESTS OF MUSCULOSKELETAL FUNCTION

Tests of Bone Function

Various diagnostic procedures are used to evaluate bone function, including gait analysis, serum calcium and phosphorus, x-ray films, angiography, and bone scanning. Roentgenograms visualize bone structure because bone absorbs x-ray beams better than soft tissue. Angiography is used to observe bone circulation. Bone scanning is the most frequently used procedure to evaluate bone function and can detect malignancy, trauma, necrosis, infection, metabolic bone disease, and osteoar-

thritis. The procedure for bone scanning involves the intravenous administration of radioactive isotopes (radionuclides) that have an affinity for bone tissue. The isotopes distribute in bone tissue and emit gamma rays. The spatial distribution of the rays is then visualized by a scanner or camera. Areas of bone that have prolific osteoblastic-osteoclastic activity (tumors, infection, fracture) concentrate greater amounts of isotopes than stable bone so these areas show a localized distribution of rays. Diffuse distribution of gamma rays is seen in metabolic bone disease.

Tests of Joint Function

Procedures used to diagnose joint function include arthrography, arthroscopy, magnetic resonance imaging, and synovial fluid analysis. Arthrography (the injection of dye into the joint) is particularly useful to diagnose tears in the fibrocartilage of the knee (meniscus) and the shoulder (rotator cuff). Arthroscopy is the direct visualization of a joint through an arthroscope.

Analysis of synovial fluid is an important diagnostic test because the composition of synovial fluid changes dramatically when the joint is injured or diseased. Analysis can reveal inflammatory, septic, and noninflammatory joint diseases. All of these disease conditions cause characteristic changes in the color, clarity, viscosity, and cellular elements of the fluid.

In normal synovial fluid, hyaluronate is joined to proteins. When the fluid is treated with dilute acid, several protein-hyaluronate complexes unite with each other to form a precipitate or clot. The characteristics of the clot, termed a **mucin clot,** provide a crude index of the amount and binding ability of the protein-hyaluronate complexes in the fluid. Normal joint fluid forms a tight, adherent clot, whereas the fluid in an inflamed joint will form a loose clot or a powder precipitate.

The presence of blood in the joint fluid (hemarthrosis) usually indicates joint trauma. Normally, blood in the synovial fluid does not coagulate well because the articular cartilage and synovial membrane release an enzyme that prevents the formation of a firm blood clot. Therefore the formation of a blood clot in the synovial fluid is indicative of a diseased joint.

Normal synovial fluid is sterile, so the presence of bacteria in the fluid is always indicative of disease. Cell fragments and fibrous tissue in the fluid are the result of inflammation or wear and tear on the articular surfaces.

Tests of Muscular Function

When the individual's history and physical examination reveal abnormalities, such as weakness, atrophy, muscle tenderness, cramps, and stiffness, specific tests of muscle function are in order. One of the most useful tests is the serum creatine kinase (CK) concentration. CK is found in large quantities in the muscle fibers, when these are diseased, CK leaks into the serum. Myoglobin is also detectable in the urine after acute muscle damage caused by crush injury, ischemic disorders, extreme exertion, and some inherited diseases.

Because the muscle membrane tissue is excitable and carries an electrical charge, its capacity to function can be assessed by electromyography. Using sensitive needle electrodes, the **electromyogram** (EMG) records the summation of action potentials of the muscle fibers in each motor unit. The EMG is often compared with the electrocardiogram (ECG), but the activity recorded on the EMG is on a much smaller scale. The amplitude of the ECG is measured in volts, the duration of impulse in seconds, and both are recorded as the heart rate (e.g., 80 volts per 60 seconds). On the EMG the amplitude is recorded in millivolts and the duration is measured in milliseconds, with a frequency of about 5 to 50 action potentials per second (Ruch & Patton, 1982). The motor unit potentials are measured to determine rate of firing, duration, and amplitude. Abnormalities in EMG and nerve conduction velocities help differentiate muscle diseases (myopathy) from peripheral nerve (neuropathy) and neuromuscular junction disorders. The muscle biopsy (using histologic, histochemical, and electron microscopic studies) is used to further define the presence of myopathic and neuropathic disorders. Many disorders can only be diagnosed by muscle biopsy (Golden, Powell & Jennings, 1985).

The forearm ischemic exercise test allows the clinician to determine the integrity of the glycolytic pathways and enzyme systems that function during intensive exercise. To perform this test, a catheter is placed in an antecubital vein and venous blood is collected for up to 20 minutes after intensive graded series of work loads at maximal grip strength. Any defect in the glycolytic pathway will be expressed by a lack of lactate production, such as is seen in McArdle disease. Mitochondrial disorders are associated with excessive lactate production at two levels of exercise. The absence of ammonia, usually proportional to the rise in lactate, is seen in myoadenylate deaminase deficiency.

Although manual muscle testing of strength and range of motion is still the most common way to detect changes, myometers are becoming increasingly popular. These hand-held devices measure strength of contraction in several muscle groups, the neck flexors, shoulder abductors, wrist extensors, hip flexors, knee extensors, and foot dorsiflexors.

AGING AND THE MUSCULOSKELETAL SYSTEM

Aging of Bones

Aging is accompanied by the loss of bone tissue. The haversian systems in compact bone undergo slow erosion, lacunae are enlarged, and canals nearest the marrow cavity become widened and the endosteal cortex converts to spongy bone. The endosteal surface gradually erodes until the rate of loss exceeds the rate of deposition on the subperiosteal surface. Newly forming haversian systems prematurely arrest and show incomplete closure. The end result is a thin and porous cortex. Bone erosion occurs first in the horizontal trabeculae of spongy bone, which considerably decreases the strength of the bone. Consolidation and erosion of the vertical trabeculae follow.

In both types of bone, the bone remodeling cycle takes longer to complete because the bone cells in the basic multicellular units are slower in their ability to resorb and deposit bone tissue. The rate of mineralization also slows down. The number of bone cells decreases because the bone marrow becomes fatty and is unable to provide an adequate supply of precursor cells. (Aging of bone marrow is discussed in Chapter 22.)

Aging of Joints

With increasing age, cartilage becomes more rigid, fragile, and susceptible to fibrillation. Loss of elasticity and resiliency is attributed to decreasing water content in the cartilage ground substance and decreasing concentrations of glycosaminoglycans (Wright, 1983).

Aging of Muscles

As the body ages, muscle bulk and strength decline. Studies of normal men show postpubertal increases in strength that peak in the third decade, coinciding with an increase in testosterone levels. Strength is maintained into the 50s, with a slow decline in dynamic and isometric strength evident after age 70. A corresponding loss is evident in the number of muscle fibers seen with age, particularly the type II fibers. Other observations include reduced RNA synthesis and loss of mitochondrial volume. In one study the loss of mitochondrial volume seen with aging was not associated with changes in energy production. Changes in RNA synthesis may be responsible for reduced protein synthesis, although the regenerative function of muscle tissue is reportedly normal in the aged (Mastaglia & Walton, 1982).

Several factors may explain these changes: change in activity level, reduced nerve supply to muscle, cardiovascular disease, and nutritional deficiencies. Reduced activity causes changes in strength and reduced fiber size owing to disuse. Although muscle fibers can regenerate into the seventh decade, nerve fibers cannot. Axonal regeneration and nerve terminal sprout are significantly reduced. Signs of neurogenic atrophy are quite common in the aged and may contribute significantly to the reduction in muscle size and strength.

One longitudinal study of energy expenditure reported that the "normal" elderly have reduced maximal oxygen uptake (Tzankoff & Norris, 1977). A follow-up study reanalyzed the group of individuals with the greatest reduction in oxygen uptake and found that they had died months later of cancer and cardiovascular disease (Tzankoff & Norris, 1978). The cachexia common among individuals with cancer produces muscle wasting and changes in muscle fiber volume similar to that seen in disuse atrophy. Reduced basal metabolic rate and lean body mass are also seen in the aged population. When the effects of aging are added to poor nutritional status, changes in basal metabolic rate and lean body mass are likely to be significant.

Because mobility is so important to the physiologic and psychologic health of the elderly, it would seem prudent to conduct an exhaustive search for treatable causes of muscle weakness and wasting before ascribing these changes to "old age." Given the normal muscle regenerative capabilities in this population, age should not be a deterrent to developing rehabilitation programs after muscle injury or illnesses that involve loss of muscular strength.

SUMMARY REVIEW

Structure and Function of Bones

1 Bones provide support and protection for the body's tissues and organs and are important sources of minerals and blood cells.

2 Bone formation begins with the production of an inorganic matrix by bone cells. Bone minerals crystallize in and around collagen fibers in the matrix giving bone its characteristic hardness and strength.

3 Bone tissue is continuously being resorbed and synthesized by basic multicellular units.

4 All bones in the body are made up of compact bone tissue and spongy bone tissue. Compact bone is highly organized into haversian systems that consist of concentric layers of crystallized matrix surrounding a central canal that contains blood vessels and nerves. Dispersed throughout the concentric layers of crystallized matrix are small spaces containing osteocytes. Smaller canals, called canaliculae, interconnect the osteocyte-containing spaces. The crystallized matrix in spongy bone is arranged in bars or plates. Spaces containing osteocytes are dispersed between the bars or plates and interconnected by canaliculae.

5 There are 206 bones in the body; these are divided into the axial skeleton and the appendicular skeleton. Bones are classified by shape as long, short, flat, or irregular. Long bones have a broad end (epiphysis), broad neck (metaphysis), and narrow midportion (diaphysis) that contains the medullary cavity.

6 Bone injuries are repaired in stages. Hematoma formation provides the fibrin framework for formation and organization of granulation tissue. The granulation tissue provides a cartilage model for the formation and crystallization of bone matrix.

Structure and Function of Joints

1 A joint is the site where two or more bones attach. Joints provide stability and mobility to the skeleton.

2 Joints are classified as synarthroses, amphiarthroses, or diarthroses depending on the degree of movement they allow. Joints are also classified by the type of connecting tissue holding them together. Fibrous joints are connected by dense fibrous tissue, ligaments, or membranes. Cartilaginous joints are connected by fibrocartilage of hyaline cartilage. Synovial joints are connected by a fibrous joint capsule. Within the capsule is a small fluid-filled space. The fluid in the space nourishes the articular cartilage that covers the ends of the bones meeting in the synovial joint.

3 Articular cartilage is a highly organized system of collagen fibers and proteoglycans. The fibers firmly anchor the cartilage to the bone and the proteoglycans control the loss of fluid from the cartilage.

Structure and Function of Muscle

1 Skeletal muscle is the largest organ in the body and is made up of millions of individual fibers.

2 Whole muscles vary in size (2 cm to 60 cm) and shape (fusiform and pennate). They are encased in a three-part connective tissue framework. The fundamental concept of muscle function is the motor unit, defined as all muscle fibers innervated by a single motor nerve.

3 Muscle fibers contain bundles of myofibrils arranged in parallel along the longitudinal axis and include the muscle membrane, myofibrils, sarcotubular system, aqueous sarcoplasm, and mitochondria. There are two types of muscle fibers, type I and type II, determined by motor nerve innervation.

4 Myofibrils and myofilaments contain the major muscle proteins, actin and myosin, which interact to form cross-bridges during muscle contraction. The nonprotein muscle constituents provide an energy source for contraction and regulate protein synthesis, enzyme systems, and membrane stabilization.

5 Muscle contraction includes excitation, coupling, contraction, and relaxation.

6 Muscle strength is graded by the "all or nothing" phenomenon and recruitment. Speed of contraction is affected by several factors: muscle fiber type, temperature, stretch, and weight of the load.

7 There are two types of muscle contraction, isometric and isotonic. Muscle shortening occurs during contraction but can also be seen during pathologic and physiologic contracture.

8 Skeletal muscle requires a constant supply of ATP and phosphocreatine to fuel muscle contraction and for growth and repair. ATP and phosphocreatine can be generated aerobically or anaerobically.

Tests of Musculoskeletal Function

1 Various diagnostic procedures are used to evaluate bone function including gait analysis, serum calcium and phosphorus, x-ray films, angiography, and bone scanning.

2 Procedures used to evaluate joint function include arthrography, arthroscopy, magnetic resonance imaging, and synovial fluid analysis.
3 Tests of muscular function include physical examination, serum creatine kinase, myoglobin, electromyogram, muscle biopsy, myometers, and the forearm ischemic exercise test.

Aging and the Musculoskeletal System
1 Muscle bulk and strength slowly decline although not to a pathologic degree. Age should not be a deterrent to developing an exercise program in the elderly.

KEY TERMS

Actin, 1310
Agonist, 1314
Alphaglycoprotein, 1295
Amphiarthrosis, 1298
Antagonist, 1314
Appendicular skeleton, 1296
Articular cartilage, 1301
Axial skeleton, 1296
Basement membrane, 1308
Basic multicellular unit, 1297
Bone albumin, 1295
Bone fluid, 1295
Bone matrix, 1293
Calcification, 1293
Callus (woven bone), 1298
Canaliculus, 1295
Cartilaginous joint, 1298
Chondrocyte, 1301
Compact bone (cortical or lamellar bone), 1295
Concentric contraction, 1313
Contraction, 1312
Coupling, 1312
Diaphysis, 1296
Diarthrosis, 1298
Eccentric contraction, 1313
Electromyogram, 1315
Endomysium, 1305
Epimysium, 1305
Endosteum, 1296
Epiphyseal plate (growth plate), 1297
Epiphysis, 1296
Excitation, 1311
Fascia, 1305
Fascicle, 1305
Fibril, 1294

Fibrous joint, 1298
Flat bone, 1297
Fusiform muscle, 1305
Glycoprotein, 1294
Glycosaminoglycans, 1301
Golgi tendon organ, 1306
Gomphosis, 1298
Ground substance, 1293
Haversian canal, 1295
Haversian system, 1295
Hyaluronate, 1300
Hydroxyapatite (HAP), 1295
Intima, 1300
Irregular bone, 1297
Isometric contraction, 1313
Isotonic contraction, 1313
Joint (articulation), 1298
Joint capsule (articular capsule), 1300
Joint cavity (synovial cavity, joint space), 1300
Lacuna, 1294
Lamella, 1295
Link protein, 1302
Long bone, 1296
Metaphysis, 1296
Motor unit, 1306
Mucin clot, 1314
Muscle fiber (muscle cell), 1306
Muscle fiber action potential, 1311
Muscle membrane, 1308
Myoblast, 1306
Myofibril, 1306
Myosin, 1310
Osteoblast, 1293
Osteocalcin, 1294
Osteoclast, 1293
Osteocyte, 1293
Osteoid, 1293
Oxygen debt, 1313
Pennate muscle, 1305
Perimysium, 1305
Periosteum, 1296
Procallus (granulation tissue), 1297
Protein core, 1301
Proteoglycans, 1294
Relaxation, 1312
Remodeling, 1297
Repetitive discharge, 1313

Sarcolemma, 1308

Sarcomere, 1309

Sarcoplasm, 1308

Sarcoplasmic reticulum, 1309

Sarcotubular system, 1309

Sarcotubule, 1309

Short bone (cuboidal bone), 1297

Sialoprotein, 1294

Skeletal muscle (voluntary, striated, or extrafusal muscle), 1306

Sliding filament theory, 1312

Spindle, 1306

Spongy bone (cancellous or trabecular bone), 1295

Subintima, 1300

Suture, 1298

Symphysis, 1298

Synarthrosis, 1298

Synchrondrosis, 1298

Syndesmosis, 1298

Synovial fluid, 1300

Synovial joint, 1298

Synovial membrane (synovium), 1300

Tendon, 1305

Tetanus, 1313

Tidemark, 1301

Trabecula, 1296

Transverse tubule, 1309

Type I fiber, 1308

Type II fiber, 1308

Type A synovial cell, 1300

Type B synovial cell, 1300

REFERENCES

Albright, J., & Brand, R. (1979). *The scientific basis of orthopedics*. New York: Appleton-Century-Crofts.

Basmajian, J. V. (1978). *Therapeutic exercise* (3rd ed.). Baltimore: Williams & Wilkins.

Brunnstrom, S. (1979). *Clinical kinesiology* (3rd ed.). Philadelphia: F. A. Davis.

Dubowitz, V., & Brooke, M. H. (Eds.). (1973). *Muscle biopsy: A modern approach*. Philadelphia: W. B. Saunders.

Edwards, R. H. T. (1984). New techniques for studying human muscle function, metabolism, and fatigue. *Muscle and Nerve, 7*(8), 599-609.

Golden, A., Powell, D. E., & Jennings, C. D. (1985). *Pathology: Understanding human disease* (2nd ed.). Baltimore: Williams & Wilkins.

Goodgold, J., & Epstein, A. (Eds.). (1977). *Electrodiagnosis of neuromuscular diseases* (2nd ed.). Baltimore: Williams & Wilkins.

Griggs, R. C., Forbes, G., Moxley, R. T., & Herr, B. E. (1983). The assessment of muscle mass in progressive neuromuscular disease. *Neurology, 33*(2), 158-165.

Hanaoka, H. (1979). The origin of the osteoclast. *Clinical Orthopedics and Related Research, 145,* 252.

Honig, C. (1981). *Modern cardiovascular physiology*. Boston: Little Brown & Company.

Mastaglia, F. L., & Walton, J. (Eds.). (1982). *Skeletal muscle pathology*. Edinburgh-London: Churchill-Livingstone.

McArdle, W. D., Katch, F. I., & Katch, V. L. (1986). *Exercise physiology: Energy, nutrition, and human performance* (2nd ed.). Philadelphia: Lea & Febiger.

Peck, W. (1984). *Bone and mineral research*. New York: Elsevier Sciences.

Raven, P. H., & Johnson, G. B. (1986). *Biology*. St. Louis: Mosby/Times Mirror.)

Resnick, D. (1981). Bone as living tissue. In D. Resnick & G. Niwayama (Eds.), *Diagnosis of bone and joint disorders*. Philadelphia: W. B. Saunders.

Ruch, T., & Patton, H. D. (Eds.). (1982). *Howell-Fulton's physiology and biophysics - IV - Excitable tissues and reflex control of muscle* (12th ed.). Philadelphia: W. B. Saunders.

Thompson, J. M., McFarland, G. K., Hirsch, J. E., Tucker, S. M., & Bowers, A. C. (1989). *Mosby's manual of clinical nursing* (2nd ed.). St. Louis: C. V. Mosby.

Tzankoff, S. P., & Norris, A. H. (1977). Effect of muscle mass decreases in age-related BMR changes. *Journal of Applied Physiology, 43,* 1001-1006.

Tzankoff, S. P., & Norris, A. H. (1978). Longitudinal changes in basal metabolism in man. *Journal of Applied Physiology, 45*(4), 536-539.

Urist, M. R. (Ed.). (1980). *Fundamental and clinical bone physiology*. Philadelphia: J. B. Lippincott.

Vaughan, J. (1981). *The physiology of bone* (3rd ed.). New York: Oxford University Press.

Vick, R. L. (1984). *Contemporary medical physiology*. Menlo Park, CA: Addison-Wesley.

Wilson, F. C. (1983). *The musculoskeletal system: Basic processes and disorders* (2nd ed.). Philadelphia: J. B. Lippincott.

Wright, V. (1983). *Bone and joint disease in the elderly*. New York: Churchill-Livingstone.

CHAPTER 39

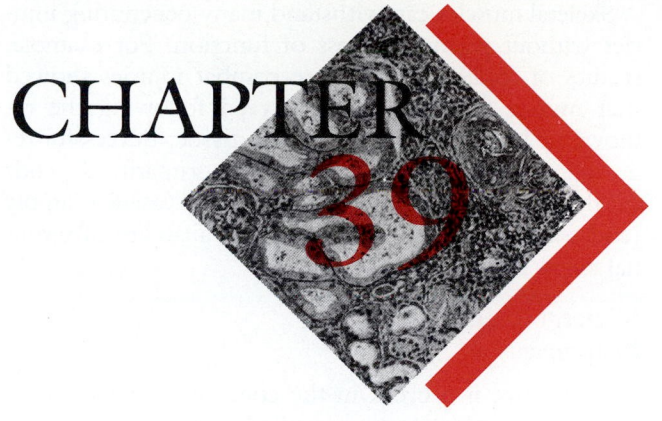

Alterations of Musculoskeletal Function

Katherine Hoare
Katharine M. Donohoe

Musculoskeletal injuries, 1320
  Skeletal trauma, 1320
    Fractures, 1320
      Classification of fractures, 1320
      Pathophysiology, 1322
      Clinical manifestations, 1322
      Evaluation and treatment, 1323
    Dislocation and subluxation, 1323
      Pathophysiology, 1324
      Clinical manifestations, 1324
      Evaluation and treatment, 1325
  Support structures, 1325
    Sprains and strains of tendons and ligaments, 1325
      Pathophysiology, 1325
      Clinical manifestations, 1325
      Evaluation and treatment, 1325
    Tendinitis and bursitis, 1326
      Pathophysiology, 1326
      Clinical manifestations, 1326
      Evaluation and treatment, 1326
    Muscle strains, 1326
    Myoglobinuria, 1327
      Pathophysiology, 1327
      Clinical manifestations, 1328
      Evaluation and treatment, 1328
Disorders of bones, 1328
  Metabolic bone diseases, 1328
    Osteoporosis, 1328
      Pathophysiology, 1329
      Clinical manifestations, 1329
      Evaluation and treatment, 1329
    Osteomalacia, 1330
      Pathophysiology, 1330
      Clinical manifestations, 1330
      Evaluation and treatment, 1330
    Paget disease, 1331
      Pathophysiology, 1331

Clinical manifestations, 1331
      Evaluation and treatment, 1332
  Infectious bone disease: osteomyelitis, 1332
    Pathophysiology, 1333
    Clinical manifestations, 1333
    Evaluation and treatment, 1334
  Bone tumors, 1334
    Incidence and etiology, 1335
    Patterns of bone destruction, 1335
    Types of tumors, 1335
      Osteogenic tumors: osteosarcoma, 1335
      Chondrogenic tumors: chondrosarcoma, 1337
      Collagenic tumors: fibrosarcoma, 1337
      Myelogenic tumors, 1338
        Giant cell tumor, 1338
        Myeloma, 1339
Disorders of the joints, 1339
  Noninflammatory joint disease, 1339
    Types of degenerative joint disease, 1340
    Course of degenerative joint disease, 1340
      Pathophysiology, 1340
      Clinical manifestations, 1341
      Evaluation and treatment, 1341
  Inflammatory joint disease, 1341
    Rheumatoid arthritis, 1342
      Pathophysiology, 1342
      Clinical manifestations, 1344
      Evaluation and treatment, 1345
    Ankylosing spondylitis, 1346
      Pathophysiology, 1346
      Clinical manifestations, 1347
      Evaluation and treatment, 1347
    Gout, 1347
      Pathophysiology, 1348
      Clinical manifestations, 1349
      Treatment, 1350

Disorders of skeletal muscle, 1350
    Secondary muscular dysfunction, 1351
        Contractures, 1351
        Stress-induced muscle tension, 1351
        Immobility, 1351
    Muscle membrane abnormalities, 1352
        Myotonia, 1352
        Periodic paralysis, 1352
    Metabolic muscle diseases, 1352
        Endocrine disorders, 1352
        Diseases of energy metabolism, 1353
            McArdle disease, 1353
            Acid maltase deficiency, 1353
            Myoadenylate deaminase deficiency, 1353
            Lipid deficiencies, 1354
    Inflammatory muscle diseases: myositis, 1354
        Viral, bacterial, and parasitic myositis, 1354
        Polymyositis and dermatomyositis, 1354
            Pathophysiology, 1354
            Clinical manifestations, 1354
            Evaluation and treatment, 1355
    Ocular myopathies, 1355
    Toxic myopathies, 1355
    Muscle tumors, 1356
        Rhabdomyoma, 1356
        Rhabdomyosarcoma, 1356
        Other tumors, 1356

MUSCULOSKELETAL INJURIES

Data accumulated by the National Center for Health Statistics reveal that each year, in the United States, an average of 1 out of 10 persons suffers an acute musculoskeletal injury, the most common being fracture, dislocation, sprain, and strain. Bone fracture is the most serious of these injuries.

Skeletal muscles can withstand many penetrating injuries without permanent loss of function. For example, studies of soldiers with severe combat injuries showed that muscle function was preserved following the removal of large portions of muscle tissue. Successful regeneration of skeletal muscle fibers primarily depends on the extent of injury, preservation of vascular supply (and source of nutrition), and the availability of terminal axons for reinnervation.

Skeletal Trauma
Fractures

A **fracture** is a break in the continuity of a bone. A break occurs when force is applied that exceeds the tensile or compressive strength of the bone. The incidence of fractures varies for individual bones according to age and sex. The highest incidence of fractures is in young males (between the ages of 15 and 24) and in the elderly (65 years of age and older). Fractures of healthy bones, particularly the tibia, clavicle, and lower humerus, tend to occur in the young and to be the result of trauma. Fractures of the hands and feet are usually caused by accidents in the workplace. The incidence of fractures of the upper femur, upper humerus, vertebrae, and pelvis is highest in the elderly and is associated with osteoporosis (see p. 1328).

Classification of Fractures

Fractures are classified as complete or incomplete and compound or simple (Fig. 39-1). In a **complete fracture,** the bone is broken all the way through, whereas in an **incomplete fracture,** the bone is damaged but is still in one piece. Complete or incomplete fractures can also be classified as **compound** (open) if the skin is broken

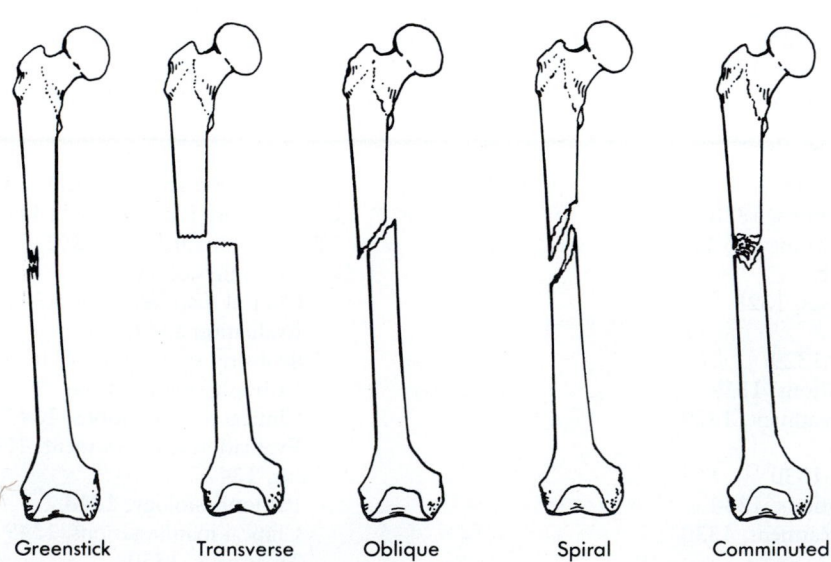

| Greenstick | Transverse | Oblique | Spiral | Comminuted |

FIG. 39-1. Five types of bone fracture. (From Phipps, Long, & Woods, 1987.)

or as **simple** (closed) if it is not. A fracture in which a bone breaks into two or more fragments is termed a **comminuted fracture.** Fractures are also classified according to the direction of the fracture line. A **linear fracture** runs parallel to the long axis of the bone. An **oblique fracture** occurs at a 45° angle (oblique angle) to the shaft of the bone. A **spiral fracture** encircles the bone, and a **transverse fracture** occurs straight across the bone.

Incomplete fractures tend to occur in the more flexible, growing bones of children. The three main types of incomplete fractures are greenstick, torus, and bowing fractures. A **greenstick fracture** perforates one cortex and splinters the spongy bone. The name is derived from the damage sustained by a young tree branch (a green stick) when it is bent sharply. The outer surface is disrupted, but the inner surface remains intact. Greenstick fractures typically occur in the proximal metaphysis or diaphysis of the tibia, radius, and ulna. In a **torus fracture,** the cortex buckles but does not break. Torus fractures are common in the metaphyses of persons with osteoporosis. **Bowing fractures** usually occur when longitudinal force is applied to bone. This type of fracture is common in children and usually involves the paired radius-ulna or the fibula-tibia. A complete dia-physeal fracture occurs in one of the bones of the pair, which disperses the stress sufficiently to prevent a complete fracture of the second bone, which bows. Bowing fractures resist correction (reduction) because the force necessary to reduce it must be equal to the force that bowed it. Treatment of bowing fractures is also difficult because the bowed bone interferes with reduction of the fractured bone. (Types of fractures are summarized in Table 39-1.)

Sometimes fractures are further classified by cause as pathologic, stress, or transchondral fractures. A **pathologic fracture** is a break at the site of a preexisting abnormality, usually by force that would not fracture a normal bone. Any disease process that weakens a bone (especially the cortex) predisposes the bone to pathologic fracture. Pathologic fractures are commonly associated with tumors, osteoporosis, infections, and metabolic bone disorders.

Stress fractures occur in normal or abnormal bone that is subjected to repeated stress, such as occurs during athletics. The stress is less than the stress that usually causes a fracture. Two types of stress fractures are recognized: fatigue fracture and insufficiency fracture. A **fatigue fracture** is caused by abnormal stress or torque applied to a bone with normal ability to deform and re-

TABLE 39-1 Types of fractures

Type	Definition
TYPICAL COMPLETE FRACTURES	
Closed (simple) fracture	Noncommunicating wound between bone and skin
Open (compound) fracture	Communicating wound between bone and skin
Comminuted fracture	Multiple bone fragments
Linear fracture	Fracture line parallel to long axis of bone
Oblique fracture	Fracture line at 45° angle to long axis of bone
Spiral fracture	Fracture line encircling bone
Transverse fracture	Fracture line perpendicular to long axis of bone
Impacted	Fracture fragments are pushed into each other
Pathologic	Fracture occurs at a point in the bone weakened by disease, for example with tumors or osteoporosis
Avulsion	A fragment of bone connected to a ligament breaks off from the main bone
Extracapsular	Fracture is close to the joint but remains outside the joint capsule
Intracapsular	Fracture is within the joint capsule
TYPICAL INCOMPLETE FRACTURES	
Greenstick fracture	Break on one cortex of bone with splintering of inner bone surface
Torus fracture	Buckling of cortex
Bowing fracture	Bending of the bone
Stress fracture	Microfracture
Transchondral fracture	Separation of cartilaginous joint surface (articular cartilage) from main shaft of bone

cover. Fatigue fractures usually occur in individuals (e.g., joggers, dancers, military recruits) who engage in a new or different activity that is both strenuous and repetitive. Because gains in muscle strength occur more rapidly than gains in bone strength, the newly developed muscles place exaggerated stress on the bones that are not ready for it. The imbalance between muscle and bone development causes microfractures to develop in the cortex. If the activity is controlled and increased gradually, new bone formation catches up to increased demands, and microfractures do not occur.

Insufficiency fractures are stress fractures that occur in bones lacking normal ability to deform and recover; normal weight bearing or activity fractures the bone. Rheumatoid arthritis, osteoporosis, Paget's disease, osteomalacia, rickets, hyperparathyroidism, and radiation therapy cause bone to lose its normal ability to deform and recover.

A **transchondral fracture** (also known as osteochondritis dissecans) consists of fragmentation and separation of a portion of the articular cartilage that covers the end of a bone at a joint. (Joint structures are defined in Chapter 38.) Single or multiple sites may be fractured, and the fragments may consist of cartilage alone or cartilage and bone. Typical sites of transchondral fracture are the head of the femur, the ankle, the knee cap, the elbow, and the wrist. Transchondral fractures are most prevalent in adolescents.

Pathophysiology

When a bone is broken, the periosteum and blood vessels in the cortex, marrow, and surrounding soft tissues are disrupted. Bleeding occurs from the damaged ends of the bone and from the neighboring soft tissue. A clot (hematoma) forms within the medullary canal, between the fractured ends of the bone, and beneath the periosteum. Bone tissue immediately adjacent to the fracture dies. This necrotic tissue (along with any debris in the fracture area) stimulates an intense inflammatory response characterized by vasodilation, exudation of plasma and leukocytes, and infiltration by inflammatory leukocytes and mast cells. Within 48 hours following the injury, vascular tissue invades the fracture area from surrounding soft tissue and the marrow cavity, and blood flow to the entire bone is increased. Bone-forming cells in the periosteum, endosteum, and marrow are activated to produce subperiosteal procallus along the outer surface of the shaft and over the broken ends of the bone (Fig. 39-2). Osteoblasts within the procallus synthesize collagen and matrix which becomes mineralized to form callus (woven bone). As the repair process continues, remodeling occurs, during which unnecessary callus is resorbed and trabeculae are formed along lines of stress (Fig. 39-3).

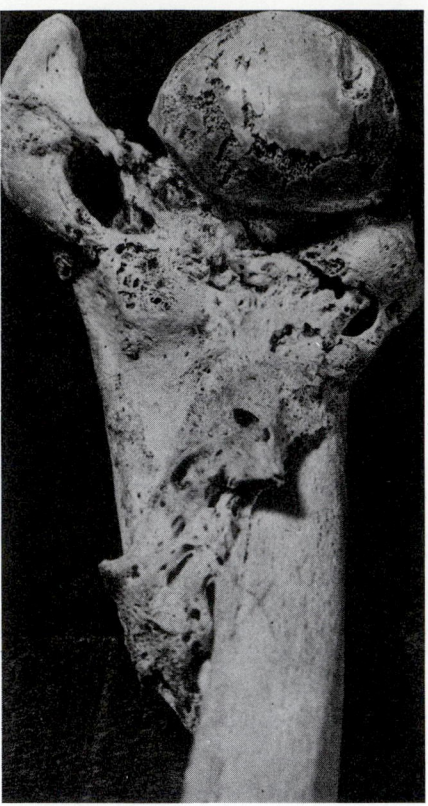

FIG. 39-2. Exuberant callus formation following fracture. (From Rosai, 1989.)

Clinical Manifestations

The clinical manifestations of a fracture vary according to the type of fracture, site of the fracture, and associated soft tissue injury. In general, the signs and symptoms of a fracture include unnatural alignment (deformity), swelling, muscle spasm, tenderness, pain, and impaired sensation. The position of the bone segments is determined by the pull of attached muscles, gravity, and the direction and magnitude of the force that caused the fracture. One or both segments may be rotated inward or outward on the bone's long axis (a condition termed rotation), misaligned at an angle (a condition termed angulation), or slide over the other segment (a condition termed overriding).

The immediate pain of a fracture is severe and usually caused by the trauma. Subsequent pain may be produced by muscle spasm, overriding of the fracture segments, or damage to adjacent soft tissues. Numbness is common and is caused by the pinching or severing of a nerve by the trauma or by bone fragments. Pathologic fractures usually cause angular deformity, painless swelling, or generalized bone pain. Pathologic fractures are not usually associated with trauma or trauma-related pain. Stress fractures are painful, not because of trauma,

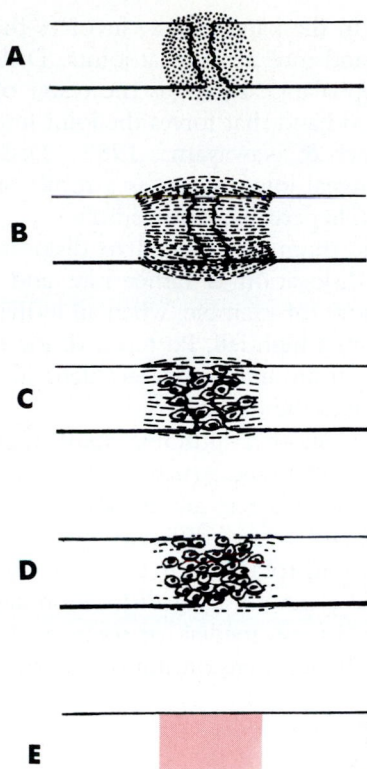

FIG. 39-3. Bone healing (schematic representation). **A,** Bleeding at broken ends of the bone with subsequent hematoma formation. **B,** Organization of hematoma into fibrous network. **C,** Invasion of osteoblasts, lengthening of collagen strands, and deposition of calcium. **D,** Callus formation: new bone is built up as osteoclasts destroy dead bone. **E,** Remodeling is accomplished as excess callus is reabsorbed and trabecular bone is laid down. (From Phipps, Long, & Woods, 1987.)

but because of accelerated remodeling. The pain occurs during activity and is usually relieved by rest. Stress fractures also cause local tenderness and soft tissue swelling. Transchondral fractures may be entirely asymptomatic or painful during movement. Range of motion in the joint is limited and movement may evoke audible clicking sounds (crepitus).

Evaluation and Treatment

Fracture treatment involves realigning the bone fragments close to their normal (anatomic) position (reduction) and holding the fragments in place (immobilization) so that bone union can occur. Several methods are available to reduce a fracture: closed manipulation, traction, and open reduction.

Most fractures can be reduced by closed manipulation: the skin is not opened (closed reduction); the bone is moved or manipulated into place. Closed manipulation is used when the contour of the bone is in fair alignment and can be maintained well with immobilization.

Traction is used to accomplish or maintain reduction. When bone fragments are displaced (not in their anatomic position), weights are used to apply firm, steady traction (pull) and countertraction to the long axis of the bone. Traction stretches and fatigues muscles that pull the bone fragments out of place, allowing the distal fragment to align with the proximal fragment. Traction can be applied to the skin (skin traction), directly to the involved bone, or distal to the involved bone (skeletal traction). Skin traction is used when only a few pounds of pulling force are needed to realign the fragments. A traction bow is applied to the skin with adhesive tape or elastic bandage and the weights are attached to the traction bow. In skeletal traction, a pin or wire is drilled through the bone and a traction bow and weights are attached to the pin or wire to apply tension and keep the wire or pin rigid.

Open reduction is a surgical procedure that exposes the fracture site; the fragments are brought into position under direct visualization. Some form of screw, plate, nail, or wire is usually used to maintain the reduction (fixation).

Splints and plaster casts are used to immobilize and hold a reduction in place. Improper immobilization of a fractured bone may result in nonunion or malunion. **Malunion** is the healing of a bone in a nonanatomic position. **Nonunion** is failure of the bone ends to grow together (Fig. 39-4). The gap between the broken ends of the bone fills with dense fibrous and fibrocartilaginous tissue instead of new bone. Occasionally, the fibrous tissue contains a fluid-filled space that resembles a joint and is termed a false joint, or pseudoarthrosis.

Dislocation and Subluxation

Dislocation and subluxation are usually caused by trauma. **Dislocation** is the temporary displacement of two bones in which the two bone surfaces lose contact entirely. If the contact between the two bone surfaces is only partially lost, the injury is called a **subluxation.**

Dislocation and subluxation are most common in persons under 20 years of age and are generally associated with fractures. Dislocation and subluxation may, however, be due to congenital or acquired disorders that cause (1) muscular imbalance, as occurs with congenital dislocation of the hip or neurologic disorders; (2) incongruities in the articulating surfaces of the bones, as occurs with rheumatoid arthritis (see p. 1342); or (3) joint instability.

The joints most often dislocated or subluxated are the joints of the shoulder, elbow, wrist, finger, hip, and knee. The shoulder joint most frequently injured is the glenohumeral joint. The glenohumeral joint is a rela-

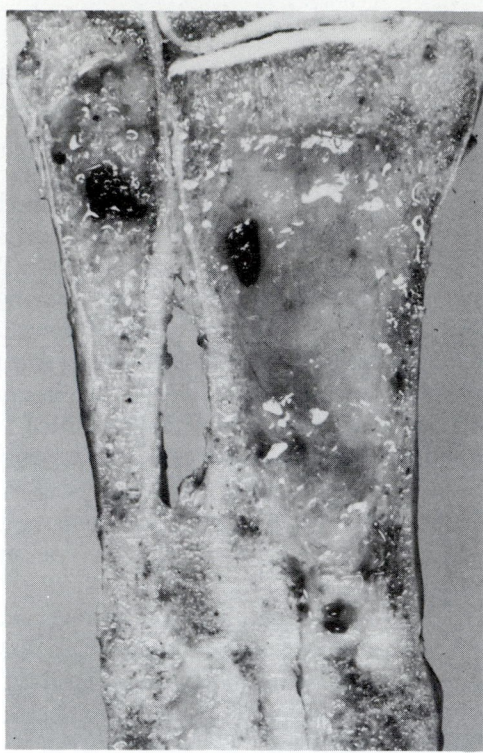

FIG. 39-4. Nonunion of old fracture of tibia and fibula in 53-year-old white man. Multiple fractures had occurred in 2 years previously and necessitated bone grafting. (From Rosai, 1989.)

tively unstable joint because the articular surface of the glenoid cavity is only one third as large as the surface of the humeral head. Physical trauma to the shoulder can cause anterior, posterior, superior, or inferior dislocation. Anterior dislocation is the most common and is usually associated with a compression fracture of the humeral head. Posterior dislocations usually occur spontaneously due to a general laxity in the ligaments that normally stabilize the joint. A superior dislocation is usually the result of an extreme forward and upward force on an adducted arm. An inferior displacement is frequently seen in persons with neurologic injuries of the brachial plexus and is believed to be caused by stretching of the supporting muscles or to joint effusion.

Traumatic dislocation of the elbow joint is common in the immature skeleton. In adults, an elbow dislocation is usually associated with a fracture of the ulna or head of the radius. Posterior dislocations occur when the individual falls on an outstretched hand with the arm in extension. Anterior dislocations are usually the result of a direct blow to the flexed elbow (Kelsey, 1982).

Traumatic dislocation of the wrist usually involves the distal ulna and carpal bones. Any one of the eight carpal bones can be dislocated following an injury. The most common cause is a fall on the hyperextended hand.

Dislocation in the hand usually involves the metacarpophalangeal and interphalangeal joints. Dislocation of the metacarpophalangeal joint is the result of a fall on the outstretched hand that forces the joint into hyperextension (Resnick & Nawayama, 1987). Dislocation of the interphalangeal joint occurs as a result of injury to the fingers in a hyperextended position.

Considerable trauma is needed to dislocate the hip. Anterior hip dislocation is rather rare and is due to forced abduction, for example, when an individual lands on the feet from a high fall. Posterior dislocation of the hip can occur in an automobile accident in which the flexed knee strikes the dashboard.

The knee is another unstable joint that depends heavily on the soft tissue structures around it for support. Because the knee is an unstable weight-bearing joint exposed to many different types of motion (flexion, extension, rotation), it is one of the most frequently injured joints. A knee dislocation can be anterior, posterior, lateral, medial, or rotatory. It is usually the result of a hyperextension injury that occurs during sports activities.

Pathophysiology

Dislocations and subluxations are often accompanied by fracture because stress is placed on areas of bone not usually subjected to stress. In addition, as the bone separates from the joint, it may bruise or tear adjacent nerves, blood vessels, ligaments, supporting structures, and soft tissue. Dislocation of the shoulder usually damages the shoulder capsule and the axillary nerve. Damage to the axillary nerve causes anesthesia in the sensory distribution of the nerve and paralysis of the deltoid muscle. Elbow dislocations are accompanied by torn periosteum and muscle. Bleeding from the damaged periosteum and muscle puts pressure on adjacent arteries that shuts off circulation to and from the forearm and hand. If the pressure is not promptly relieved, ischemic paralysis develops. Dislocations of the hand often result in permanent disability because of damage to the tendons and intricate mechanisms that allow smooth gliding in the joints. Avascular necrosis of the femoral head is a complication seen in hip dislocations. Knee dislocation usually tears both the collateral and cruciate ligaments.

Clinical Manifestations

The general signs and symptoms of dislocations or subluxations include pain, swelling, limitation of motion, and joint deformity. Pain may be due to effusion of inflammatory exudate into the joint or associated tendon and ligament injury. Joint deformity is usually caused by muscle contractions that exert pull on the dislocated or subluxated joint. Limitation of motion may be a result of effusion into the joint or the displacement of bones.

Tenderness and deformity are prominent in dislocations of the fingers. Unusual muscle pull and pain often result in abnormal posturing of the fingers; for example, the fingers or thumb may be abnormally flexed. A dislocated elbow is often held in a flexed position, and the joint resists active or passive movement. Pain is the key symptom of shoulder injuries. Attempts to lift the arm aggravate the pain. In most shoulder dislocations, the ability to elevate the arms is minimal and the individual supports the injured arm with the opposite hand. Pain and an abnormal gait or limp usually accompany traumatic dislocation of the hip. The pain is constant and severe and is often felt in the inguinal region or thigh. The thigh may assume a position of inward rotation, adduction, or flexion, and appears shortened. In a rare anterior dislocation, the limb is not shortened and the joint is fixed in abduction, outward rotation, and flexion.

Evaluation and Treatment

Evaluation of dislocations and subluxations is based on clinical manifestations and roentgenograms. Treatment consists of reduction immobilization for 2 to 6 weeks and exercise to maintain normal range of motion in the joint. Depending on the joint, healing is usually complete within months to years.

Support Structures
Sprains and Strains of Tendons and Ligaments

Tendon and ligament injuries can accompany fractures and dislocations. A tendon is fibrous connective tissue that attaches skeletal muscle to bone (see Chapter 38). A **ligament** is a band of fibrous connective tissue that connects bones where they meet at a joint. Tendons and ligaments support the bones and joints and either facilitate or limit motion. Tendons and ligaments can be torn, ruptured, or completely separated from bone at their points of attachment.

A tear in a tendon is commonly known as a **strain.** Major trauma can tear or rupture a tendon at any site in the body. Most frequently injured are the tendons of the hands and feet, the knee (patellar), the upper arm (biceps and triceps), the thigh (quadriceps), the ankle, and the heel (Achilles). Traumatic rupture of the biceps tendon is often due to lifting excessive weight with the arms. Rupture of the Achilles tendon occurs when body weight is forcefully applied to the foot when it is in plantar flexion. Spontaneous tendon ruptures can occur in individuals receiving local corticosteroid injections and persons with rheumatoid arthritis or systemic lupus erythematosus.

Ligament tears are commonly known as **sprains.** Ligament tears and ruptures can occur at any joint but are most common in the wrist, ankle, elbow, and knee joints. A complete separation of a tendon or ligament from its bony attachment site is known as an **avulsion.**

An avulsion is the result of abnormal stress on the ligament or tendon and is commonly seen in young athletes, especially sprinters, hurdlers, and runners.

Pathophysiology

When a tendon or ligament is torn, an inflammatory exudate develops between the torn ends. Later, granulation tissue containing macrophages, fibroblasts, and capillary buds grows inward from the surrounding soft tissue and cartilage to begin the repair process. Within four to five days after the injury, collagen formation begins. At first, collagen formation is random and disorganized. As the collagen fibers interweave and connect with preexisting tendon fibers, they become organized parallel to the lines of stress. Eventually vascular fibrous tissue fuses the new and surrounding tissues into a single mass. As reorganization takes place, the healing tendon or ligament separates from the surrounding soft tissue. Usually a healing tendon or ligament lacks sufficient strength to withstand strong pull for 4 to 5 weeks after the injury. If strong muscle pull does occur during this time, the tendon or ligament ends may separate again, which causes the tendon or ligament to heal in a lengthened shape with an excessive amount of scar tissue; this renders the tendon or ligament functionless.

Clinical Manifestations

Tendon and ligament injuries are painful and are usually accompanied by soft tissue swelling, changes in tendon or ligament contour, and dislocation/subluxation of bones. The pain is generally sharp and localized, and tenderness persists over the distribution of the tendon or ligament. Painful joint swelling can usually be seen in finger and elbow sprains. Flexion deformities of the fingers and thumb occur in injuries to the extensor tendons. Crepitus may accompany tendon injury in the wrist. Pain in the elbow may be accentuated by flexion, supination, and extension of the elbow or by extension of the wrist. Lifting small objects requires extension of the wrist and therefore aggravates the pain. Tendon injuries in the upper arm cause weakness when the individual tries to flex the forearm. Pain is often the key symptom of shoulder injuries. It may be referred to the deltoid muscle or extend down the arm. The pain is usually aggravated by attempts to lift the arms. Depending on the ligament or tendon involved, tendon and ligament injuries in the knee may produce pronounced mobility, lost lateral movement, instability when walking down stairs, semiflexion, crepitus, or an upward shift of the patella (De Gowin & De Gowin, 1981).

Evaluation and Treatment

Evaluation is based on clinical manifestations, stress radiography, or arthography. When possible, treatment consists of suturing the tendon or ligament ends in close approximation. If this is not possible because of the extent of damage, tendon or ligament grafting may be necessary.

Tendinitis and Bursitis

Trauma can also cause painful inflammation of tendons (tendinitis) and bursae (bursitis). Other causes of tendinitis include crystal deposits, postural misalignment, and hypermobility in a joint.

Bursae are small sacs lined with synovial membrane and filled with synovial fluid; they are located between tendons, muscles, and bony prominences. Their primary function is to separate and cushion these structures. Acute bursitis occurs primarily in the middle years and is caused by repeated trauma. Septic bursitis is caused by wound infection or bacterial infection of the skin overlying the bursae. The shoulder is the most common site of bursitis. Bursitis also frequently occurs in the hip, knee, elbow, and the toe with a bunion.

Pathophysiology

Fluid from inflammation accumulates in tendinitis, causing swelling of the tendon. The usual bursitis is an inflammation that is reactive to overuse or excessive pressure and decreases with rest, heat, and needle puncture. (Inflammation is discussed in Chapter 7.)

Clinical Manifestations

Clinical manifestations are usually localized to one side of the joint. Generally there is local tenderness and more pain with active motion than with passive motion. With tendonitis, the pain is localized over the involved tendon and movement in the affected joint is limited. The onset of pain may be gradual or sudden in bursitis, and movement in the joint is limited. Shoulder bursitis impairs arm abduction. Bursitis in the knee produces pain when climbing stairs, and crossing the legs is painful in bursitis of the hip. Signs of infectious bursitis include the presence of a puncture site, prior corticoster-

oid injection, severe inflammation, or an adjacent source of infection (McCune, 1989).

Evaluation and Treatment

Evaluation of tendinitis and bursitis is based on clinical manifestations and arthrography. Treatment includes immobilization of the joint with a sling, splint, or cast; systemic analgesics; ice or heat applications; or local injection of an anesthetic and corticosteroids to reduce inflammation. Physical therapy to prevent loss of function begins after acute inflammation subsides.

Muscle Strains

Mild injury such as **muscle strain** is usually seen after traumatic or sports injuries. Muscle strain is a general term for local muscle damage. It is often the result of sudden, forced motion causing the muscle to become stretched beyond normal capacity. Knife and gunshot wounds also cause traumatic rupture. Strains often involve the tendon as well. Muscles are ruptured more often than tendons in young people; the opposite is true in the older population. Muscle strain may be chronic when the muscle is repeatedly stretched beyond its usual capacity. There is evidence of tissue disruption with subsequent signs of muscle regeneration and connective tissue repair when a biopsy is performed. Hemorrhage into the surrounding tissue and signs of inflammation may also be present. Regardless of the cause of trauma, muscle cells are usually able to regenerate. Regeneration may take up to 6 weeks and the affected muscle should be protected during this time (Turek, 1984). (Degrees of acute muscle strain, together with their manifestations and treatment, are summarized in Table 39-2.)

A late complication of localized muscle injury is **myositis ossificans.** This condition is thought to be caused by scar tissue calcification and subsequent ossification. Examples include "rider's bone," in which the adductor muscle of the thigh of equestrians becomes calcified,

---

TABLE 39-2 Muscle strain

Type	Manifestations	Treatment
First degree (example: bench press in untrained athlete)	Muscle over-stretched, painful	Ice should be applied five or six times in the first 24-48 hours; complete rest for up to 2 weeks, followed by weight bearing 3 times per week and range of motion daily
Second degree (example: any muscle strain with bruising and pain)	Muscle intact with some tearing pain, mild bruising	Similar treatment for first-degree strains, with added mild analgesia; cryokinetics (a treatment system of alternating applications of heat and cold with progressive exercise)
Third degree (example: traumatic injury)	Due to tearing of fascia, muscle rupture palpable, bleeding present	Surgery to approximate ruptured edges; immobilization and rest for 6 weeks

and "drill bone," in which the same change is seen in the deltoid and pectoral muscles of fencers and infantry soldiers (Mastaglia & Walton, 1983).

Myoglobinuria

Myoglobinuria, also called rhabdomyolysis, can be a life-threatening complication of severe muscle trauma. Myoglobinuria is named for the principle manifestation of the condition, an excess of myoglobin, an intracellular muscle protein, in the urine. Muscle damage releases the myoglobin. The most severe form is often called crush syndrome. Less severe and more localized forms are called compartment syndromes (e.g., Volkmann's contracture in the forearm). Crush syndrome first gained notoriety in the reports of injuries seen following the London air raids in World War II. More recently it has been reported in individuals found unresponsive and immobile for long periods of time, usually after a drug overdose. Myoglobinuria can also be seen follow-ing viral infections, administration of certain anesthetic agents, strychnine poisoning, tetanus, heat stroke, electrolyte disturbances, and fractures. Excessive muscular activity has also been implicated in reports of myoglobinuria in athletes, such as long-distance runners, ice skaters, skiers, military recruits, and those subjected to fraternity hazing. Status epilepticus, electroconvulsive therapy, and high-voltage electrical shock are also associated with severe and sometimes fatal myoglobinuria.

Pathophysiology

The weight of a limp extremity can generate enough pressure to produce muscle ischemia (Fig. 39-5). This causes edema, rising compartment pressure, and tamponade that leads to muscle infarction and neural injury, and, finally, results in cell loss. Physical interruptions in the sarcolemmal membrane, called holes or delta lesions, suggest that the sarcolemmal membrane may be the route by which muscle constituents are released. (The

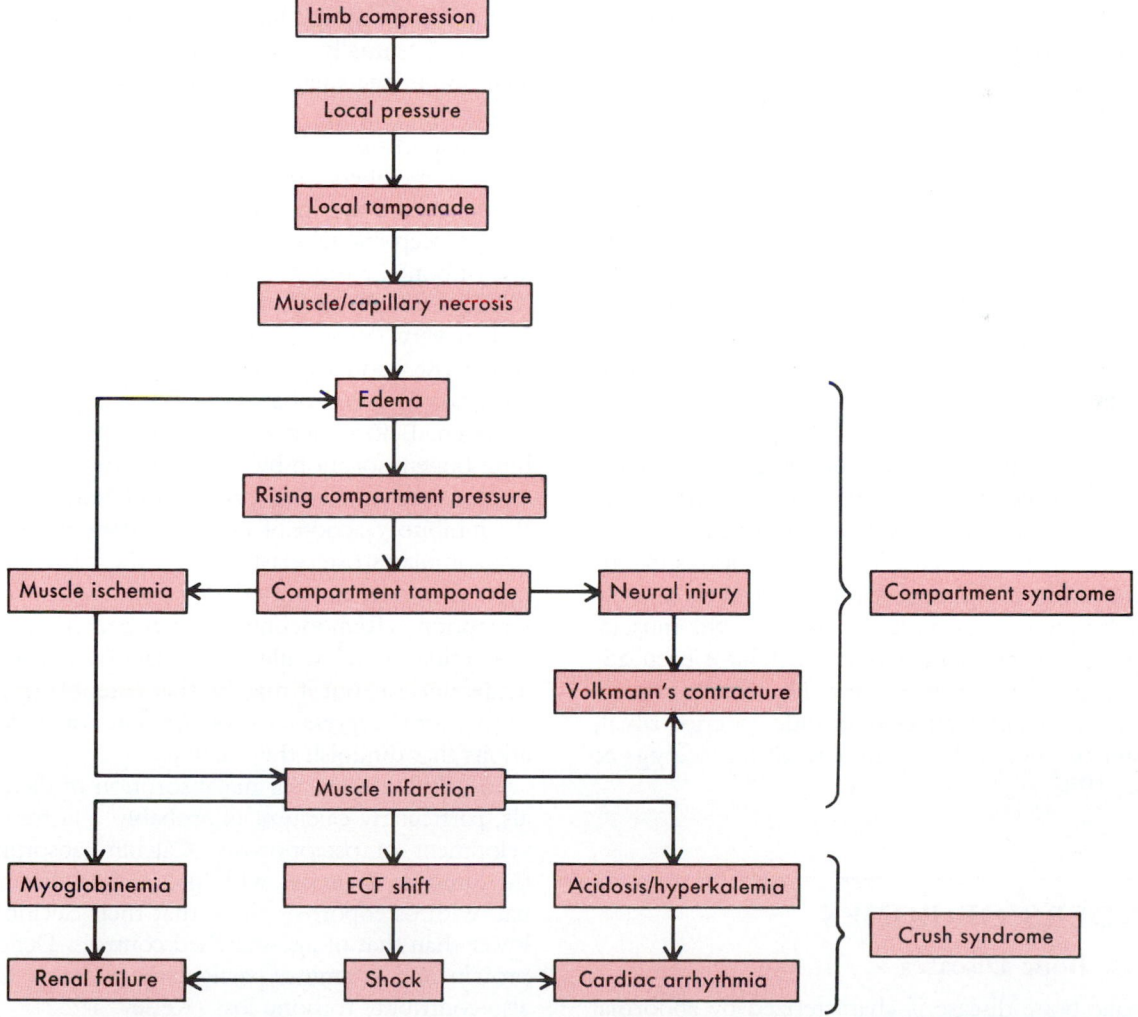

FIG. 39-5. Pathogenesis of compartment syndrome and crush syndrome due to prolonged muscle compression.

sarcolemmal membrane, the plasma membrane of the muscle cell, is described in Chapter 38.)

Clinical Manifestations

When myoglobin is released from the muscle fibers (cells) into the circulation, it can cause a visible, dark reddish brown pigmentation of the urine. The renal threshold for myoglobin is low, approximately 0.5 mg/100 ml urine, so that only 200 g of muscle need be damaged to cause visible changes in the urine. Along with the release of myoglobin, creatine kinase and other serum enzymes are released in massive quantities. The creatine kinase level is often 100 times greater than normal (5 to 25 U/ml for women and 5 to 35 U/ml for men). The efflux of proteins and enzymes also includes loss of potassium, phosphate, nucleotides, creatinine, and creatine. Serum hypocalcemia is seen early in the course of myoglobinuria and is followed by late hypercalcemia.

Evaluation and Treatment

Priorities in treatment of myoglobinuria include identifying and treating the underlying disorder and preventing life-threatening renal failure. Malignant hyperthermia and myoglobinuria caused by anesthetic agents can be treated by halting the anesthetic administration and infusing dantrolene sodium (Dantrium). Diluting the pigment using intravenous fluids and administration of mannitol, sodium bicarbonate, and furosemide (Lasix) to "flush" the kidney have been advocated to prevent renal failure. Other secondary problems include electrolyte imbalance, volume depletion, acidosis, hyperuricemia, hyperkalemia, and calcium imbalance. These need specific treatment. Short-term dialysis also may be necessary.

The compartment syndromes may require emergency treatment when blood flow to the affected extremity is compromised, producing a cycle of increased pressure, ischemia, and edema. When clinical evaluation is inconclusive, the rising compartment pressure can be directly measured by inserting a wick catheter into the muscle. Immediate fasciotomy and debridement have been advocated for pressures over 30 mm Hg. The compartments most frequently affected include anterior tibial, deep posterior tibial, volar, hand, and gluteal (Griggs & Donohoe, 1985).

DISORDERS OF BONES

Metabolic Bone Diseases

Metabolic bone disease is characterized by abnormal bone structure that is caused by altered or inadequate biochemical reactions. The altered or inadequate bio-

chemical reactions may be due to genetics, diet, or hormones.

Osteoporosis

Osteoporosis is a disease in which the density or mass of bone is reduced. The bone that remains is histologically and biochemically normal, but there is not enough of it to maintain skeletal integrity and mechanical support. The disease can be (1) generalized, involving major portions of the axial skeleton, or (2) regional, involving one segment of the appendicular skeleton. Both spongy and compact bone are lost, but spongy bone loss exceeds compact bone loss.

Osteoporosis is the most common metabolic disease. The incidence of fractures (a common complication of osteoporosis), indicates that osteoporosis occurs in women 2.5 times more frequently than in men (Urist, 1980). The incidence of osteoporosis also increases with age. Bone mass begins to decrease in both men and women at about age 40 and continues to decrease over the lifespan. It has been estimated that 50% of women over 45 years of age have significant decreases in bone density. Eventually, women may lose about one half and men about one quarter of their spongy bone (Kelsey, 1982).

Osteoporosis is most common in whites, probably because members of other races, particularly blacks, have denser bones to begin with. Whites are therefore more susceptible than other races to osteoporosis due to loss of bone density with age.

The etiology of generalized osteoporosis is diverse, and in very few cases is the cause certain. Postmenopausal osteoporosis, which occurs in middle-aged and older women, is probably caused by decreased levels of estrogen. Before menopause, higher estrogen levels inhibit bone resorption by decreasing the sensitivity of osteoclasts to circulating parathyroid hormone. Without the inhibitory action of estrogen, parathyroid hormone overstimulates osteoclasts within the basic multicellular units to initiate the remodeling cycle, which begins with resorption. (Remodeling is described in Chapter 38.) The etiology of senile (age-related) osteoporosis remains unclear, but it may be that osteoblasts and osteoclasts shrink, regress to a former state, or undergo alterations that diminish their activity.

Insufficient intake or malabsorption of dietary minerals, particularly calcium, is probably a factor in the development of osteoporosis. Calcium absorption from the intestine decreases with age, and studies of individuals with osteoporosis show that their calcium intake is lower than that of age-matched controls. Deficiencies of protein and vitamins, particularly vitamins C, and D, also contribute to bone loss (Kelsey, 1982).

A variety of hormonal imbalances may also contribute to osteoporosis. Skeletal homeostasis depends on a very narrow range of plasma calcium and phosphate concentrations, which are maintained by the endocrine system. Therefore, endocrine dysfunction can ultimately cause metabolic bone disease. The hormones most commonly associated with osteoporosis are parathyroid hormone (hyperparathyroidism), cortisol (Cushing syndrome), thyroid hormone (hyperthyroidism), and growth hormone (acromegaly). (Endocrine function is discussed in Unit VI.)

Iatrogenic osteoporosis sometimes develops temporarily in patients receiving large doses of heparin, perhaps because heparin promotes bone resorption by decreasing collagen synthesis or by increasing collagen breakdown. Osteoporosis caused by heparin therapy usually resolves when therapy ceases.

Regional osteoporosis—osteoporosis confined to a region or segment of the appendicular skeleton—usually has a known cause. Classic regional osteoporosis is associated with disuse or immoblization of a limb due to fractures, motor paralysis, or bone or joint inflammation. A negative calcium balance develops early and continues throughout the period of immobilization. After 8 weeks of immobilization, significant osteoporosis is present, although it may develop earlier in persons younger than 20 or older than 50 years. The pattern of bone loss may be uniform, spotty, or bandlike. Uniform bone loss usually occurs after long immobilization, for example, in quadriplegics or amputees. The bone loss initially appears in the appendicular skeleton or pelvis within 2 to 3 months following the paralysis. A uniform distribution of osteoporosis has also been observed in astronauts and in individuals treated with air suspension therapy as a result of weightlessness.

Pathophysiology

Whatever the cause, osteoporosis develops when the remodeling cycle—the process of bone resorption and bone formation—is disrupted. A complete remodeling cycle, consisting of basic multicellular unit activation (see Chapter 38), bone resorption, and bone formation, takes approximately 4 months in a normal, healthy adult. In an individual with osteoporosis, 2 years may be needed to complete one cycle. In normal bone, the frequency of multicellular unit activation, the rate of resorption, and the rate of new bone formation are relatively constant, so that replacement follows resorption immediately and the amount of bone replaced equals the amount of bone resorbed. In bones affected by osteoporosis, this equilibrium can be disrupted by (1) an increase in the number of basic multicellular units activated, (2) an increase in the frequency of basic multicellular unit activation, (3) an increase in the rate of resorption, (4) a delay in the rate of bone formation, or (5) a deficiency of cells in the multicellular unit. Any one of these changes causes a net decrease in total bone mass.

If the number of basic multicellular units increases, resorption occurs at more sites, or loci. Loci of resorption become so numerous that new bone is destroyed along with old bone, creating a state of "runaway" resorption. If a normal number of basic multicellular units is activated with abnormal frequency, the result is a net increase in the total amount of bone lost in a given period of time.

Another mechanism causing osteoporosis is an imbalance between the rate of resorption and the rate of new bone formation. Some hormones and drugs are thought to interfere with the relationship between osteoclast activity (bone resorption) and osteoblast (bone formation) activity. Anything that causes resorption to speed up or replacement to slow down causes resorption cavities to persist, weakening the bone.

Osteoporosis also occurs if the basic multicellular units fail to complete the three phases of the remodeling cycle. Failure occurs if there are inadequate numbers of osteoclasts and osteoblasts in bone tissue. Completion of the remodeling cycle requires delivery of a continuous supply of bone cell precursors from the marrow. Any interruption in the bone's vascular system will interfere with the delivery of osteoclast and osteoblast precursors to bone tissue.

Clinical Manifestations

The specific clinical manifestations of osteoporosis depend on the bones involved. The most common manifestations, however, are pain and bone deformity. Fractures are likely to occur because the trabeculae of spongy bone become thin and sparse, and compact bone becomes porous. As the bones lose volume, they become brittle and weak and may collapse or become misshapen. Vertebral collapse causes kyphosis (hunch back) and diminishes height. Fractures of the long bones (particularly the femur and humerus), the wrist, and the vertebrae are most common. Fracture of the neck of the femur—the so-called broken hip—tends to occur in elderly women with osteoporosis. Fatal complications of fractures include fat embolism, hemorrhage, and shock.

Evaluation and Treatment

Generally, osteoporosis is detected radiographically as increased radiolucency of bone. By the time abnormalities are detected by x-ray examination, approximately 30% of bone tissue has been lost. Other evaluation procedures include tests for levels of serum calcium, phosphorus, and alkaline phosphatase, and protein electrophoresis.

The goals of osteoporosis treatment are to slow down the rate of calcium and bone loss and to stop the disease before it progresses too far. Treatment includes increasing the dietary intake of calcium and vitamin D supplements to increase the intestinal absorption of calcium. Regular, moderate weight-bearing exercise can slow down the bone loss and, in some cases, reverse demineralization. Postmenopausal women are given estrogen in addition to exercise and dietary supplements of calcium and vitamin D.

The use of estrogen, however, is controversial. Studies have shown that estrogens decrease the rate of bone loss, but the long-term benefits and risks have been questioned. An increased risk of endometrial carcinoma is associated with estrogen therapy used to treat postmenopausal women with an intact uterus. Progesterone, however, seems to protect against the increased risk of endometrial cancer associated with estrogen use (Persson et al., 1989). The combined estrogen-progesterone regimen (hormone replacement therapy) will cause the woman to have cyclical uterine bleeding. A woman taking these hormones needs an annual gynecologic examination because of the associated side effects, including phlebitis and emboli.

Osteomalacia

Osteomalacia is a metabolic disease characterized by inadequate and delayed mineralization of osteoid in mature compact and spongy bone. In osteomalacia, the remodeling cycle proceeds normally through osteoid formation, but mineral calcification and deposition does not occur. Bone volume remains unchanged, but the replaced bone consists of soft osteoid instead of rigid bone. Rickets is similar to osteomalacia in pathogenesis, but it occurs in the growing bones of children, whereas osteomalacia occurs in adult bone. (Rickets is described in Chapter 40.)

Both osteomalacia and rickets are rare in the United States and western Europe but are significant health problems in Great Britian, Ethiopia, Pakistan, Iran, and India. In the United States, these diseases are prevalant in the elderly, in premature infants of very low birth weight, and in individuals adhering to rigid macrobiotic vegetarian diets.

Many factors contribute to the development of osteomalacia, but the most important is a deficiency of vitamin D. The major risk factors in vitamin D deficiency are diets deficient in vitamin D, decreased endogenous production of vitamin D, intestinal malabsorption of vitamin D, renal tubular diseases, and anticonvulsant therapy. Classic vitamin D deficiency is rare in the United States because of the addition of synthetic vitamin D to dairy products and bread.

Disorders of the small bowel, hepatobiliary system, and pancreas are common causes of vitamin D deficiency in the United States, however. In malabsorptive disease of the small bowel, vitamin D and calcium absorption are decreased, so that vitamin D is lost in feces. Liver disease interferes with the metabolism of vitamin D to its more active form, and diseases of the pancreas and biliary system cause a deficiency of bile salts, which are necessary for normal intestinal absorption of vitamin D.

The mechanism by which anticonvulsant drug therapy results in vitamin D deficiency is incompletely understood, but researchers think that the anticonvulsants phenobarbital and phenytoin interfere with calcium absorption in the intestine and with vitamin D metabolism in the liver.

Pathophysiology

Crystallization of minerals in osteoid requires adequate concentrations of calcium and phosphate. When the concentrations are too low, crystallization (and hence ossification) does not proceed normally.

Vitamin D deficiency disrupts mineralization because vitamin D normally regulates and enhances the absorption of calcium ions from the intestine. A lack of vitamin D causes the plasma calcium concentrations to fall. Low plasma calcium levels stimulate increased synthesis and secretion of parathyroid hormone. Although the increase in circulating parathyroid hormone raises the plasma calcium concentration, it also stimulates increased renal clearance of phosphate. When the concentration of phosphate in the bone falls below a critical level, mineralization cannot proceed normally.

Abnormalities occur in both spongy and compact bone. Trabeculae in spongy bone become thinner and fewer, while haversian systems in compact bone develop large channels and become irregular. Because osteoid continues to be produced but not mineralized, abnormal quantities of osteoid build up, coating the trabeculae and the linings of the haversian canals. Excessive osteoid can also accumulate in areas beneath the periosteum. The excess of osteoid leads to gross deformities of the long bones, spine, pelvis, and skull.

Clinical Manifestations

Osteomalacia causes varying degrees of diffuse skeletal pain and tenderness. Pain is noted particularly in the hips, and the individual may be hesitant to walk. Muscular weakness is common and may contribute to a waddling gait. Bone fractures and vertebral collapse occur with minimal trauma.

Evaluation and Treatment

Osteomalacia is evaluated on the basis of radiographic findings of radiolucent bands perpendicular to the surface of the bone. Other tests used to detect osteomalacia are plasma concentrations of calcium and phosphate, and tests of proximal tubular function in the kidney. Ultraviolet radiation therapy and dietary supplements of vitamin D and calcium are used to treat vitamin D deficiency.

Paget Disease

Paget disease (osteitis deformans) is a state of increased metabolic activity in bone. It is characterized by abnormal and excessive bone remodeling, both resorption and formation. Chronic accelerated remodeling eventually enlarges and softens the affected bones.

Paget disease can occur in any bone, but it most often affects the axial skeleton, especially the vertebrae, skull, sacrum, sternum, and pelvis. The femur is often affected in the appendicular skeleton. The disease process may occur in one or more bones without causing significant clinical manifestations.

Paget disease occurs with equal frequency in men and women over 40 years of age. Because it is often symptomless and can only be diagnosed by invasive procedures, few epidemiologic data are available. Autopsy data from England and Germany indicate that approximately 3% to 4% of the population over 40 years of age are afflicted with the disease. Survey data also indicate that the disease may be prevalent in Australia, Great Britain, certain areas of Europe, and the United States (Kelsey, 1982). Paget disease sometimes affects several members of the same family, leading to some speculation that it is inherited as an autosomal dominant trait.

The cause of Paget disease is unknown, but various researchers have suggested that it is the result of inflammatory processes, viral infection, benign or malignant bone tumors, vitamin D deficiency during childhood, mechanical stress to bone, autoimmune dysfunction, vascular disorders, or hormonal deficiencies. To date, however, little research has been done to support any of these hypotheses.

Pathophysiology

Paget disease begins with excessive resorption of spongy bone. The trabeculae diminish and bone marrow is replaced by extremely vascular fibrous tissue (Fig. 39-6).

The resorption phase of Paget disease is followed by the formation of abnormal new bone at an accelerated rate. The collagen fibers are disorganized, and glycoprotein levels in the matrix decrease. Mineralization may extend into the bone marrow. Bone formation is excessive around partially resorbed trabeculae, causing them to thicken and enlarge. Eventually, Paget disease progresses to an inactive phase, in which abnormal remodeling is minimal or absent.

Clinical Manifestations

In the skull, abnormal remodeling is first evident in the frontal or occipital regions; then it encroaches on the outer and inner surfaces of the entire skull. The skull thickens and assumes an asymmetric shape. Thickened segments of the skull may compress areas of the brain, producing altered mentality and dementia. Impingement of new bone on cranial nerves causes sensory abnormalities, impaired motor function, deafness, atrophy of the optic nerve, and obstruction of the lacrimal duct.

Extensive alterations of the facial bones are rare except in the jaw, where sclerosis and thickening of the maxilla and mandible displace teeth and produce malocclusion. In long bones, resorption begins in the subchondral regions of the epiphysis and extends into the metaphysis and diaphysis. Occasionally, Paget disease affects both ends of a tubular bone. In the femur, Paget

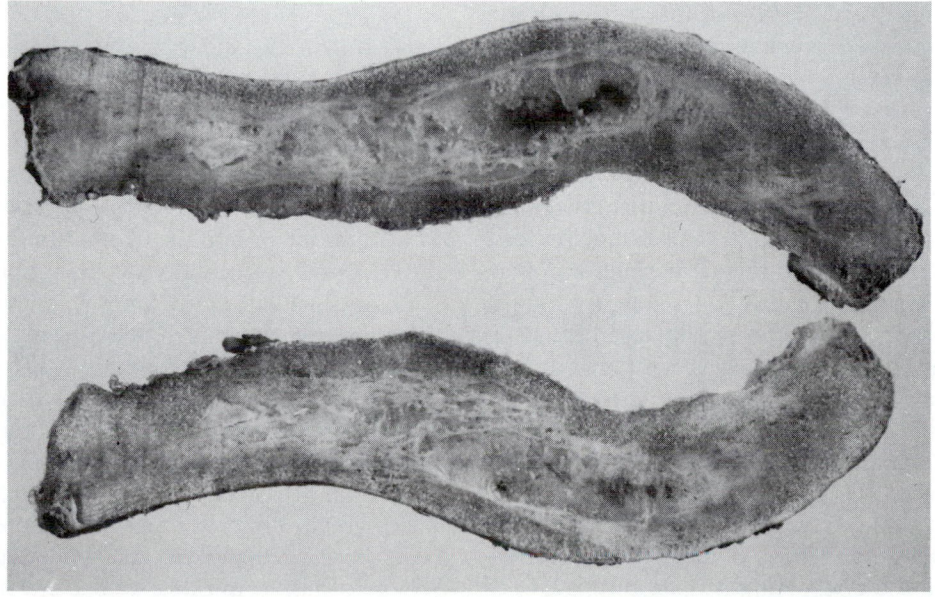

FIG. 39-6. Extensive Paget disease of clavicle of 60-year-old man. Note distortion and changes in cortex. (From Rosai, 1981.)

disease produces an exaggerated lateral curvature. In the tibia, anterior curvature is also exaggerated. Stress fractures are common in the lower extremities.

Clinical manifestations of Paget disease in the vertebral column depend on the level of involvement and are due to compression of adjacent structures. In the cervical spine, cord compression can lead to spastic quadriplegia.

Evaluation and Treatment

Evaluation of Paget disease is made on the basis of radiographic findings of irregular bone trabeculae with thickened and disorganized pattern. Early disease is detected by bone scanning that shows increased uptake of bone radionuclides.

Most individuals require no treatment because the disease is localized and does not cause symptoms. Treatment during active disease is for pain relief, prevention of deformity, or fracture. Corticosteroids, calcitonin, and cytotoxic drugs are sometimes used to slow down excessive resorption.

Infectious Bone Disease: Osteomyelitis

Infectious bone disease is expensive and difficult to treat and, often culminates in extensive physical disability. Several factors contribute to the difficulty in treating bone infection:

1. Bone contains multiple microscopic channels that are impermeable to the cells and biochemicals of the body's natural defenses. Once bacteria gain access to these channels, they are able to proliferate unimpeded.

2. The microcirculation of bone is highly vulnerable to damage and destruction by bacterial toxins. Vessel damage causes local thrombosis (blockage) of the small vessels, which leads to ischemic necrosis (death) of bone.

3. Bone cells have a limited capacity to replace bone destroyed by infections. Initially, osteoclasts are stimulated by infection to resorb bone, which opens up isolated bone channels so that cells of the inflammatory and immune systems can gain access to the infected bone. At the same time, however, resorption weakens the structural integrity of the bone. New bone formation usually lags behind resorption, and the Haversian systems in the new bone are incomplete.

Osteomyelitis is a bone infection caused by bacteria; however, fungi, parasites, and viruses can also cause bone infection (Fig. 39-7). It is further categorized according to the pathogen's mode of entry into bone tissue. **Exogenous osteomyelitis** is an infection that enters from outside the body, for example, through open fractures, penetrating wounds, or surgical procedures. In exogenous osteomyelitis, the infection spreads from

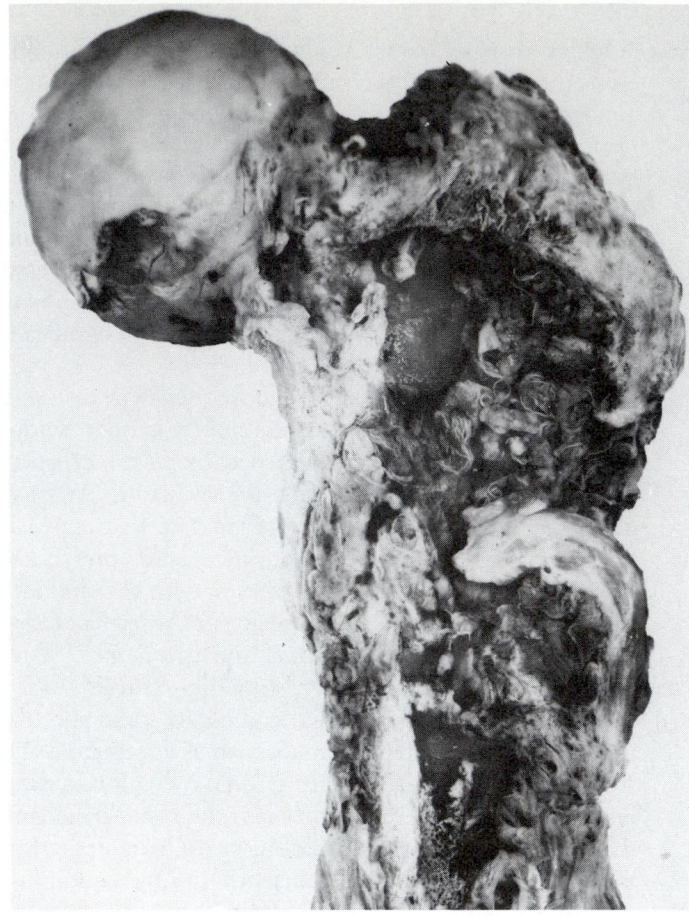

FIG. 39-7. Osteomyelitis of upper femur with massive bone destruction and reactive sclerosis. (Courtesy Dr. H. Rodriguez-Martinez, Mexico City, Mexico. From Rosai, 1981.)

soft tissues into adjacent bone. The other type of osteomyelitis, termed **hematogenous osteomyelitis,** is caused by pathogens carried in the blood from sites of infection elsewhere in the body. In hematogenous osteomyelitis, the bone infection spreads from bone outward to adjacent soft tissues. Hematogenous ostemylitis is commonly found in infants, children, and the elderly. (Osteomylitis in children is discussed in Chapter 40.) In infants, incidence rates among males and females are approximately equal. In children and older adults, however, males are most commonly affected.

Staphylococcus aureus is the usual cause of hematogenous osteomyelitis. Others include streptococcus B, *Haemophilus influenzae, Salmonella,* and gram-negative bacteria. Streptococcus B and *H. influenzae* tend to infect young children; *Salmonella* infection is associated with sickle cell anemia; and gram-negative infections are most common in older adults and individuals with impaired immunity.

Cutaneous, sinus, ear, and dental infections are the

primary sources of bacteria in hematogenous bone infections. Soft tissue infections, disorders of the gastrointestinal tract, infections of the genitourinary system, and respiratory infections are also important sources of bacterial contamination.

The vulnerability of specific bone depends on the anatomy of its vascular supply. In children, the long bones of the extremities (tibia, humerus, femur) are particularly susceptible to hematogenous infection. The bacteria pass through the bone's branching blood vessels until they reach the terminal capillaries on the metaphyseal side of the growth plate. In this area, the circulation is sluggish, creating an ideal site for bacterial growth and multiplication. The bacteria lodge in the small vascular channels, where they initiate inflammation.

In adults, hematogenous osteomyelitis is more common in the spine, pelvis, and the small bones. Microorganisms reach the vertebrae through arteries, veins, or lymphatic vessels. The spread of infection from pelvic organs to the vertebrae is well documented. Vaginal, uterine, ovarian, bladder, and intestinal infections can lead to iliac or sacral osteomyelitis.

Exogenous osteomyelitis can be caused by human bites or fist blows to the mouth. Superficial animal or human bites inoculate local soft tissue with bacteria that later spread to underlying bone. Deep bites can introduce microorganisms directly onto bone. The most common infecting organism in human bites is *S. aureus.* In animal bites, the most common infecting organism is *Pasteurella multocida,* which is part of the normal mouth flora of cats and dogs.

Direct contamination of bones with bacteria can also occur in open fractures or dislocations with an overlying skin wound. Intervertebral disk surgery and operative procedures involving implantation of large foreign objects, such as metallic plates or artificial joints, are associated with exogenous osteomyelitis. Local injections and venous punctures are significant causes of exogenous osteomyelitis. Exogenous osteomyelitis of the arm and hand bones tends to occur in drug abusers. *S. aureus* is the most common pathogen. In general, the chronically ill, diabetics, alcoholics, and those who are receiving large doses of steroids or immunosuppressive drugs are particularly susceptible to exogenous osteomyelitis.

Pathophysiology

Regardless of the source of the pathogen, the pathologic features of bone infection are similar to those in any other body tissue (see Chapters 6 and 7). First, the invading pathogen provokes an intense inflammatory response. Inflammation in bone is characterized by vascular engorgement, edema, leukocyte activity, and abscess formation. Once inflammation is initiated, the small terminal vessels thrombose, and exudate seals the bone's

canaliculi. Inflammatory exudate extends into the metaphysis and the marrow cavity and through small metaphyseal openings into the cortex. In children, exudate that reaches the outer surface of the cortex forms abscesses that lift the periosteum off underlying bone. Lifting of the periosteum disrupts blood vessels that enter bone through the periosteum, depriving underlying bone of its blood supply. Lifting of the periosteum also stimulates an intense osteoblastic response. Osteoblasts lay down new bone that can partially or completely surround the infected bone. This layer of new bone surrounding the infected bone is called an **involucrum.** Openings in the involucrum allow the exudate to escape into surrounding soft tissue and ultimately through the skin by way of sinuses.

In adults, this complication is rare because the periosteum is firmly attached to the cortex and resists displacement. Instead, infection disrupts and weakens the cortex, which predisposes the bone to pathologic fracture.

Clinical Manifestations

Clinical manifestations of osteomyelitis vary with the age of the individual, the site of involvement, the initiating event, the infecting organism, and whether the infection is acute, subacute, or chronic. Acute osteomyelitis causes aburpt onset of inflammation. If an acute infection is not completely eliminated, the disease may become subacute or chronic. In subacute osteomyelitis, signs and symptoms are usually vague. In the chronic stage, infection is indolent or silent between exacerbations. The microorganisms persist in small abscesses or fragments of necrotic bone and produce occasional flare-ups of acute osteomyelitis. The progression from acute to subacute or chronic osteomyelitis may be due to inadequate or inappropriate therapy or the development of drug-resistant microorganisms.

Acute hematogenous osteomyelitis in the child is usually manifested by a sudden onset of high fever, chills, nausea, and progressive pain at the site of bone involvement. Muscle spasm around the infected bone is common, and the child may refuse to move the affected limb. Tissues overlying the involved bone become edematous and warm due to the vascular changes and edema.

In the adult, hematogenous osteomyelitis has an insidious onset. The symptoms are usually vague and include fever, malaise, anorexia, and weight loss. Recent infection (urinary, respiratory, skin), or instrumentation (catheterization, cystoscopy, myleography, discography) usually precede onset of symptoms.

The primary symptom of acute osteomyelitis in the spine is back pain. The pain may be intermittent or constant, aggravated by motion, and throbbing at rest. It may radiate in a radicular distribution and is commonly accompanied by spinal tenderness and rigidity. Hip contracture occurs in the presence of soft tissue inflammation as a result of irritation of the psoas muscle.

The signs and symptoms of sacroiliac ("tailbone") osteomyelitis are generally severe and include local pain, tenderness, and a limp. The pain may radiate to the buttock or the abdomen.

Single or multiple abscesses (Brodie abscesses) characterize subacute or chronic osteomyelitis. Brodie abscesses are circumscribed lesions 1 to 4 cm in diameter, usually in the ends of long bones and surrounded by dense ossified bone matrix. The abscesses are thought to develop when the infectious microorganism has become less virulent or the individual's immune system is resisting the infection somewhat successfully.

In exogenous osteomyelitis, signs and symptoms of soft tissue infection predominate. Inflammatory exudate in the soft tissues disrupts muscles and supporting structures and forms abscesses. Low-grade fever, lymphadenopathy, local pain, and swelling usually occur within days of contamination by a puncture wound. Osteomyelitis in the hand causes exquisite tenderness over the course of tendon sheaths. The fingers are usually in a semiflexed, position and extension usually causes severe pain. Palmar swelling or symmetric swelling of the fingers may be present.

Evaluation and Treatment

Evaluation of osteomyelitis is done by radionuclide bone scanning and tomography. Tomography is a radiographic technique that produces an image of a slice through the bone rather than the whole bone. Treatment of osteomyelitis includes antibiotics and drainage of the inflammatory exudate. Tubes are placed into holes drilled into the cortex for continuous antibiotic irrigation and drainage. Chronic conditions may require surgical removal of the inflammatory exudate followed by continuous wound irrigation with antibiotic solutions in addition to systemic treatment with antibiotics.

Bone Tumors

Many different types of tumors involve the skeleton. The type is determined by the tissue from which the tumor is derived. Bone tumors may originate from bone cells, cartilage, fibrous tissue, marrow, or vascular tissue. Based on the tissue of origin, bone tumors are classified as osteogenic, chondrogenic, collagenic, and myelogenic. Each of the four types arises from one of the four stem cells that are ultimately derived from the primitive mesoderm (Fig. 39-8).

The mesoderm contributes the primitive fibroblast and reticulum cells. The fibroblast is the progenitor of the osteoblast, the chondroblast, and the fibroblast or fibrous connective tissue cell. Each cell synthesizes a specific type of intercellular ground substance, and the tumor derived from the cell is generally characterized by the type of ground substance produced by the cell. For example, osteogenic tumors usually contain cells which have the appearance of osteoblasts and produce an intercellular substance that can be recognized as osteoid. Chondrogenic tumors contain chondroblasts and produce an intercellular substance similar to chondroid (cartilage). Collagenic tumors contain fibrous tissue cells and produce an intercellular substance similar to the type of collagen found in fibrous connective tissue.

Besides being classified according to the tissue of origin, tumors are also classified as benign or malignant. The differences between malignant and nonmalignant bone tumors are nebulous, primarily because the criteria

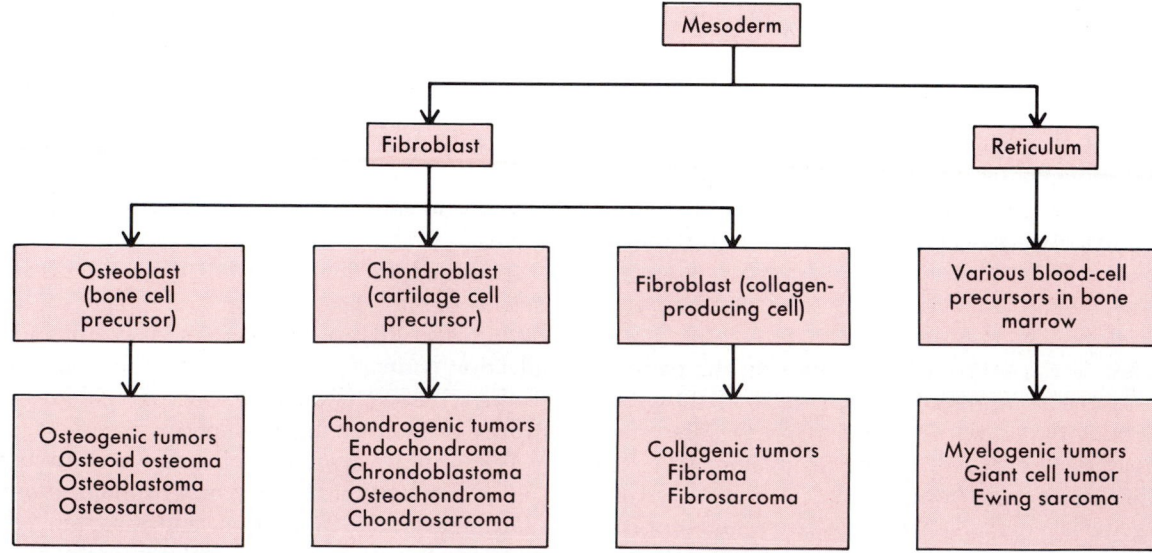

FIG. 39-8. Derivation of bone tumors.

used to differentiate them are vague (see Chapter 10). Generally, malignant bone tumors tend to be larger and more aggressive in their pattern of bone destruction, to invade surrounding tissue, and to initiate independent growth outside the site of origin (i.e., metastasize). Nonmalignant bone tumors, on the other hand, are less destructive to the host bone, tend to be limited to the anatomic confines of the host bone, and have a well-demarcated border. The criteria used to identify tumor cells as malignant are (1) an increased nuclear-cytoplasmic ratio, (2) an irregular nuclear border, (3) excess chromatin, (4) a prominent nucleolus, and (5) an increase in the number of cells undergoing mitosis. These criteria are sometimes confusing and misleading because many young, rapidly growing, normal cells and cells subjected to inflammation and change in their blood supply also exhibit many of these same characteristics (Aegerter & Kilpatrick, 1975). (Tumor characteristics in general are described in Chapter 10.)

Incidence and Etiology

The incidence rate of bone tumors varies with age. In children under the age of 15 years, the rate of bone tumors is relatively low, comprising approximately 3% of all malignancies. Adolescents have the highest incidence of bone tumors, and adults between the ages of 30 and 35 have the lowest incidence. After age 35, the incidence rate slowly increases until, at age 60, it equals the incidence rate in adolescents (Rubin, 1983).

The etiology of bone tumors is highly controversial. Part of the controversy stems from the lack of a common definition for tumor. In general, tumor refers to a new growth (neoplasia) or hyperplasia of cells. The new growth may be an excessive reparative proliferation of cells that ultimately mature. Thus, some tumors (or masses) may be the result of inflammation or trauma. Other tumors are the result of a spontaneous proliferation of cells which may or may not mature (differentiate), invade surrounding tissue, or metastasize.

Patterns of Bone Destruction

The general pathologic features of bone tumors include bone destruction, erosion or expansion of the cortex, and periosteal response to changes in underlying bone. The least amount of pathologic damage occurs with benign bone tumors, which push against neighboring tissue. Because they usually have a symmetrical, controlled growth pattern, benign bone tumors tend to compress and displace neighboring normal bone tissue, which weakens the bone's structure until it is incapable of withstanding the stress of ordinary use. Other tumors invade and destroy adjacent normal bone tissue. They do this by producing substances that promote resorption by changing osteoblasts into osteoclasts or by interfering with a bone's blood supply.

Lodwick (1983) identified three different patterns of bone destruction by bone tumors: (1) the geographic pattern, (2) the moth-eaten pattern, and (3) the permeative pattern of bone destruction. The **geographic pattern** of bone destruction is the least aggressive and is generally indicative of a slow-growing or benign tumor. Tumors associated with the geographic pattern have well-defined margins that can be easily separated from the surrounding normal bone. The margin may be smooth or irregular, but it is clearly demarcated by a short zone of transition between normal and abnormal bone tissue. A more aggressive pattern of bone destruction is the **moth-eaten pattern.** In this pattern, the tumorous lesion has a less-defined or demarcated margin that cannot be easily separated from normal bone. The moth-eaten pattern of bone destruction is characteristic of rapidly growing, malignant bone tumors. An aggressive, malignant tumor with rapid growth potential causes the **permeative pattern** of bone destruction. In this pattern, the margins of the tumor are poorly demarcated, and abnormal bone merges imperceptibly with surrounding normal bone tissue.

Tumors that erode the cortex of the bone usually stimulate a periosteal response, that is, new bone formation at the interface between the surface of the bone and the periosteum. Slow erosion of the cortex usually stimulates a uniform periosteal response. Additional layers of bone are added to the exterior surface of the bone so as to buttress the cortex. Eventually, the additional layers expand the bone's contour. Aggressive penetration of the cortex usually elevates the periosteum and stimulates erratic patterns of new bone formation. Examples of erratic patterns include concentric layers of new bone; a sunburst pattern, in which delicate rays of new bone radiate toward the periosteum from a single focus on the underlying surface; and rays of new bone that grow perpendicularly, creating a brush or bristle pattern.

Types of Tumors

An uncommonly large number of lesions are classified as bone tumors. Described here are the bone tumors most representative of the four derivative types (see Fig. 39-8): osteogenic, chondrogenic, and collagenic tumors.

Osteogenic Tumors: Osteosarcoma

Osteogenic tumors (bone-forming tumors) produce bone tissue. The tissue can have the appearance of callus, compact, or spongy bone (Mirra, 1980). The most common bone-forming tumor is the osteosarcoma.

Osteosarcoma is the most common of the primary bone tumors, accounting for 20% of them. Osteosarcoma occurs twice as frequently in males as in females, predominantly in adolescents and young adults. Sixty percent of osteosarcomas occur in the under-20 age group. A secondary peak incidence for osteosarcoma occurs in the 50 to 60 age group, primarily in individuals with a history of Paget disease (Fig. 39-9). Osteosarcoma may also develop as a complication of radiation therapy.

Osteosarcoma is a malignant bone-forming tumor. It is large, destructive, and most often found in bone marrow, and it has a moth-eaten pattern of bone destruction. The borders of the tumor are indistinct and merge into adjacent normal bone. Osteosarcomas always contain osteoid and callus, which is produced by anaplastic stromal cells. Anaplastic cells are atypical, abnormal cells not seen in normal developing bone; they are neither normal nor embryonal. The osteosarcoma may also contain chondroid (cartilage) and fibrinoid tissue. The osteoid is deposited as thick masses or "streamers" between the trabeculae of callus (Mirra, 1980). The streamers of osteoid infiltrate the normal compact bone, destroy it, and replace it with dense callus and masses of osteoid. Bone tissue produced by osteosarcomas never matures to compact bone.

Ninety percent of osteosarcomas are located in the metaphyses of long bones, especially the distal femur. The tumor typically breaks through the cortex, lifts the periosteum, and forms a soft tissue mass that is *not* cov-ered by a smooth shell of new bone. Lifting of the periosteum stimulates bizarre patterns of new bone formation called a periosteal reaction.

Osteosarcoma is rapidly fatal. The usual course of the disease is multiple pulmonary metastases and death within 2 years of diagnosis. Even with amputation and radiotherapy, the survival rate is rarely more than 5 years.

The most common initial symptoms are pain and swelling. Initially, the pain is slight and intermittent, but within a short time the pain increases in severity and duration. Serum alkaline phosphatase levels may also be elevated.

The location of the tumor dictates the extent of surgery. Amputation is the most satisfactory treatment of choice, however, in some cases the tumor and the tissue around it can be removed without amputation. Limb salvaging procedures have been made possible by advances in chemotherapy and endoprosthetics. Individuals must have achieved most of their bone growth to be candidates for these procedures. Following amputation, individuals are followed closely with chest roentgenograms and computed tomography. Pulmonary metastases are surgically resected, and chemotherapy is a common adjunctive therapy.

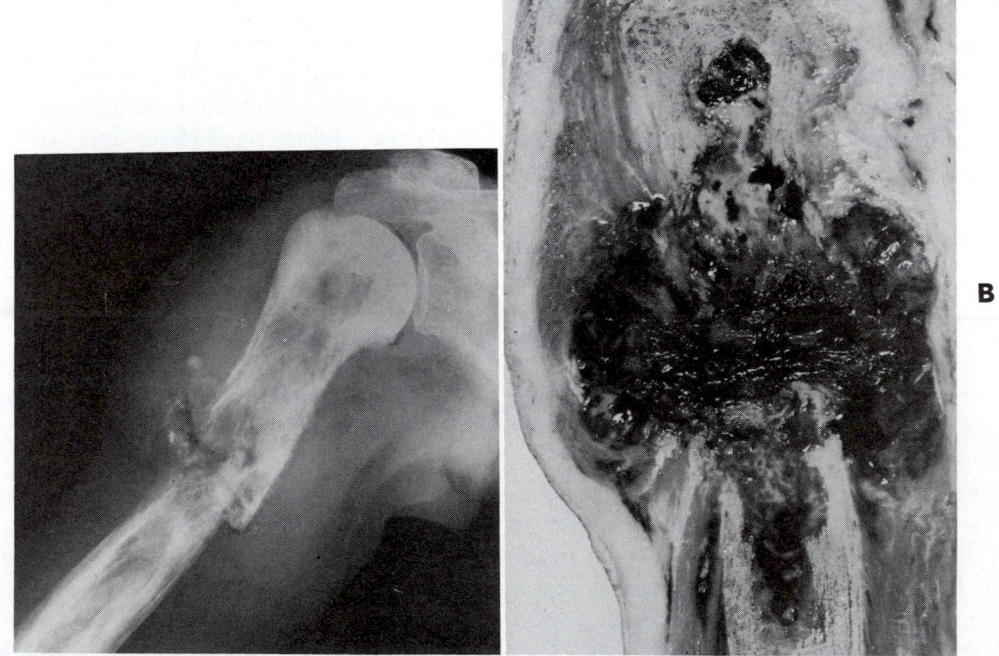

FIG. 39-9. A, Osteosarcoma of upper end of humerus associated with fracture and Paget disease. **B,** Point of fracture of humerous shown in **A** demonstrating extension of hemmorhagic neoplasm up shaft and out into soft tissues. Note porous, thickened cortical bone of Paget disease. (From Rosai, 1981.)

Chondrogenic Tumors: Chondrosarcoma

Chrondrogenic tumors (cartilage-forming tumors) produce cartilage or **chondroid,** a primitive cartilage or cartilagelike substance. The most common chrondrogenic tumor is chondrosarcoma.

Chondrosarcoma is a tumor of middle-aged and older adults. Most cases of primary chondrosarcoma are found in persons between 50 and 60 years of age. Secondary chondrosarcoma (a chondrosarcoma derived from an **endochondroma**) occurs most frequently in young adults between the ages of 20 to 30 years of age. The tumor is found more frequently in men than in women.

A chondrosarcoma is a large, ill-defined malignant tumor that infiltrates trabeculae in spongy bone. It occurs most often in the metaphysis or diaphysis of long bones, especially the femur, and in the bones of the pelvis (Fig. 39-10). The tumor contains large lobules of hyaline cartilage that are separated by bands of fibrous tissue and anaplastic cells. If located near the end of the bone, the tumor will infiltrate into the joint space. The tumor expands and enlarges the contour of the bone, causes extensive erosion of the cortex, and expands into the soft tissues.

Symptoms associated with the chondrosarcoma have an insidious onset. Local swelling and pain are the usual presenting symptoms. At first the pain is intermittent, then it gradually intensifies and becomes constant.

Surgical excision is generally regarded as the treatment of choice. Many surgically treated individuals demonstrate recurrences, however, so amputation is becoming one treatment of choice. Therefore, tumors located in the limbs have a better prognosis than, for example, pelvic lesions.

Collagenic Tumors: Fibrosarcoma

Collagenic tumors produce fibrous connective tissue. The most typical collagenic tumor is the fibrosarcoma (Fig. 39-11).

Fibrosarcomas represent 4% of the primary malignant bone tumors. The incidence of fibrosarcoma has a broad

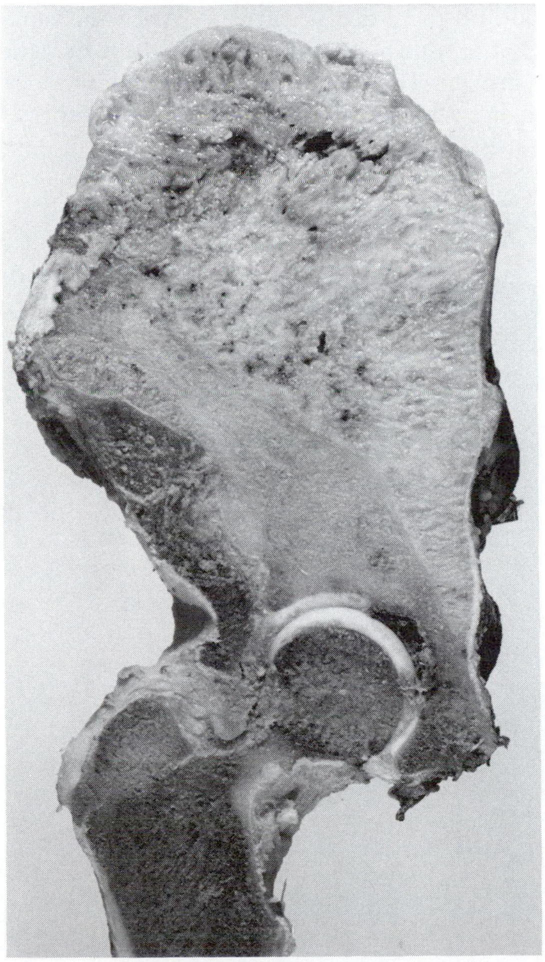

FIG. 39-10. Gross appearance of peripheral chondrosarcoma of pelvic bone. Huge tumor mass with heavy calcification protrudes into pelvis. (From Rosai, 1989.)

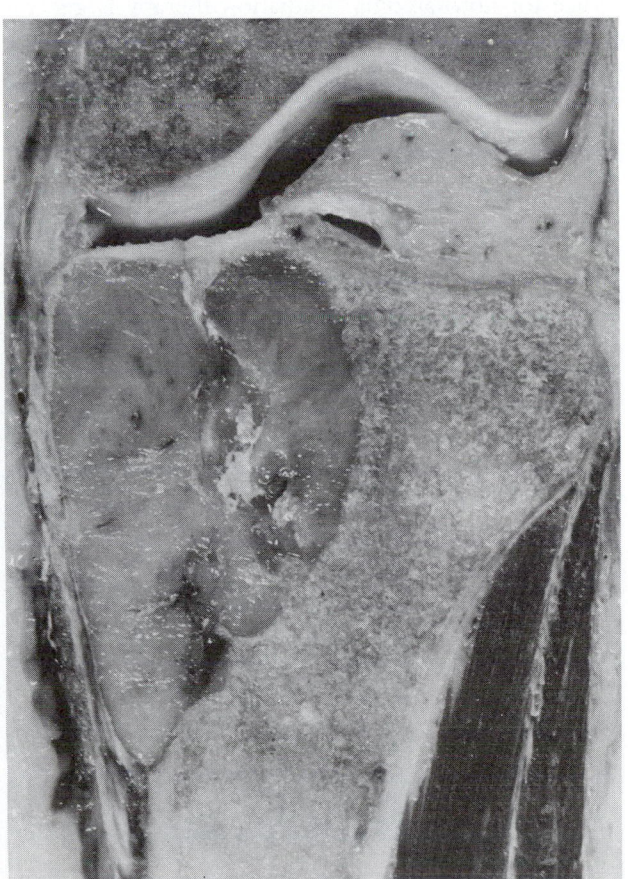

FIG. 39-11. Fibrosarcoma of tibia. Lesion produced osteolytic defect and was confused roentgenographically with giant cell tumor. (From Rosai, 1989.)

age distribution. It may occur in any age, but is most common in middle-aged adults between 40 and 50 years. The incidence is slightly greater in females. Fibrosarcoma may also be a secondary complication of radiation therapy, Paget disease, and long-standing osteomyelitis.

Fibrosarcoma is a solitary tumor that most frequently affects the metaphyseal region of the femur or tibia. The tumor is composed of a firm fibrous mass of tissue that contains collagen, malignant fibroblasts, and occasional osteoclastlike giant cells. Collagen fibers found within the tumor are quite thin.

The tumor begins in the marrow cavity of the bone and infiltrates the trabeculae. It demonstrates a permeative growth pattern, destroys the cortex, and extends into the soft tissue. Metastasis to the lung is common.

Symptoms associated with the tumor have an insidious onset, which delays diagnosis. Pain and swelling are the usual presenting symptoms and usually indicate that the tumor has broken through the cortex. Local tenderness, a palpable mass, and limitation of motion may also be present. A pathologic fracture in the affected bone is frequently the reason for seeking medical help.

Radical surgery and amputation are the treatments of choice for fibrosarcoma. Radiation therapy is generally considered ineffective treatment for this tumor.

Myelogenic Tumors

Myelogenic tumors originate from various bone marrow cells. Two types of myelogenic tumors are giant cell tumor and myeloma.

Giant Cell Tumor **Giant cell tumor** is the sixth most common of the primary bone tumors; it accounts for 4% of the bone tumors. Giant cell tumors have a wide age distribution; however, they are rare in persons younger than 10 years and older than 70 years. The majority of giant cell tumors are found in persons between 20 and 40 years of age. Unlike most other bone tumors, giant cell tumors affect females more frequently than males.

The giant cell tumor is a solitary, circumscribed tumor that causes extensive bone resorption because of its osteoclastic origin. The tumor is rich in osteoclastlike giant cells and anaplastic stromal cells. It may also contain osteoid, callus, and collagen. The giant cell tumor is located in the center of the epiphysis in the femur, tibia, or humerus (Fig. 39-12). The tumor has a slow relentless growth rate and is usually contained within the original contour of the affected bone. It may, however, extend into the articular cartilage. When the tumor extends, it is usually covered by periosteum or periosteal bone growth. The tumor may also extend into local soft tissue, but it has a low rate of metastasis to other organs or tissues.

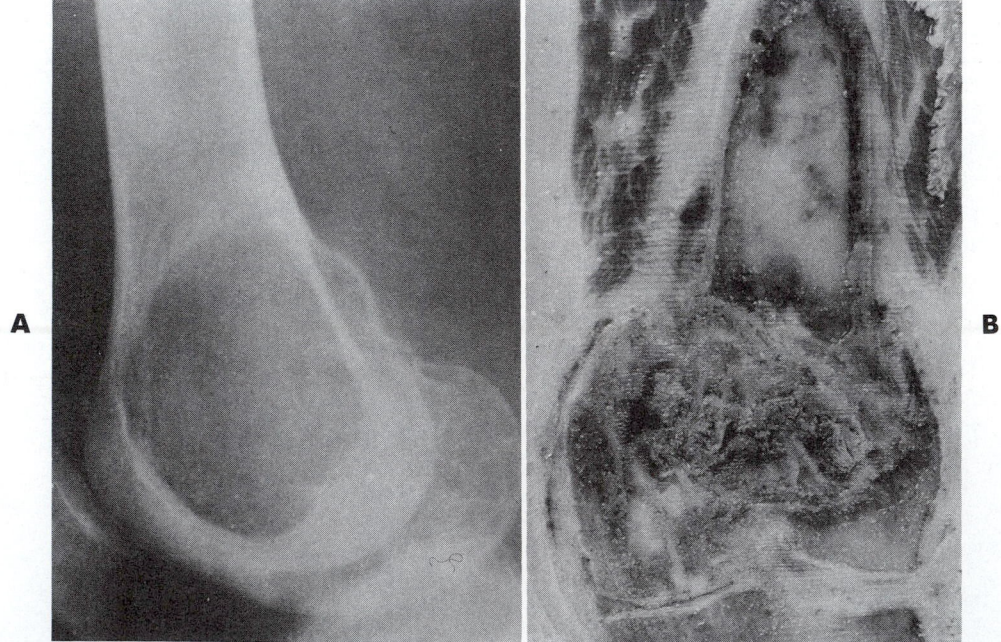

FIG. 39-12. **A,** Giant cell tumor of distant end of femur. Lesion was curetted and replaced with bone chips. **B,** Giant cell tumor shown in **A** recurred, necessitating amputation. Gross specimen demonstrates bone chips still in place, with tumor replacing femur. Review of original sections showed benign giant cell tumor, but recuts of curetted material demonstrated malignant stroma. (From Rosai, 1989.)

The most common symptoms associated with the giant cell tumor are pain, local swelling, and limitation of movement. Cryosurgery and resection of the tumor decrease recurrence and are more successful treatments than curettage and radiation. Depending on the extent of the tumor and its recurrence, amputation may be necessary.

Myeloma **Myeloma** is a neoplastic proliferation of immunocytes called plasma cells. The myeloma is the most common of the primary malignant tumors of the skeleton and accounts for 27% of bone tumors. The tumor may be solitary or multifocal (known as a multiple myeloma). Approximately 15% of the detected myelomas are multiple myelomas (see Chapter 24). The myeloma is common in persons over 40 years of age. Males are affected twice as frequently as females, and blacks have a higher incidence rate than whites.

Myelomas characteristically cause cortical and medullary bone lysis and infiltrate the bone marrow. The most common initiating symptom of myeloma is pain, which may be felt in a single bone or the entire skeleton. The usual sites of pain are the lower back, the upper spine, the pelvis, ribs, and sternum. The pain is initially aching, intermittent, and aggravated by weight bearing. As the disease progresses, the pain becomes severe and prolonged. It is common for the individual with myeloma to be treated for a slipped disk or arthritis before the correct diagnosis of myeloma is established. In addition to pain, the individual may also complain of weakness, fatigue, weight loss, and anorexia.

Myeloma has a poor prognosis, and the treatment is generally palliative. Pain is relieved with narcotics and special beds may be used to lessen pain and prevent pathologic fractures. Cord decompression may be necessary in persons with spinal myeloma. Radiotherapy and chemotherapy have very limited success.

DISORDERS OF THE JOINTS

The American Rheumatism Association recognizes thirteen groups of joint disease (arthropathies). Most of these disorders can be placed into two major categories: noninflammatory joint disease and inflammatory joint disease.

Noninflammatory Joint Disease

Noninflammatory joint disease is differentiated from inflammatory joint disease by: (1) the absence of synovial membrane inflammation; (2) the lack of systemic signs and symptoms; and (3) normal synovial fluid. **Degenerative joint disease** (osteoarthritis) is the most prevalent noninflammatory joint disease. Its chief pathologic feature is degeneration and loss of articular

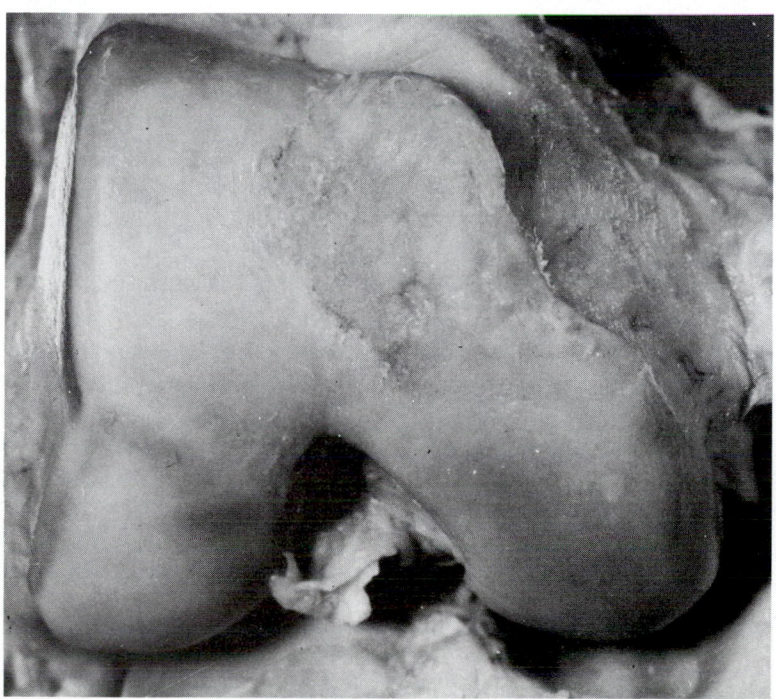

FIG. 39-13. Pronounced degenerative joint disease in 55-year-old man. Note degeneration and destruction of cartilage over wide area. (From Rosai, 1989.)

cartilage in synovial joints (Fig. 39-13). Degenerative joint disease tends to occur in men and women over 40 and becomes more common with increasing age. Although incidence rates are the same in men and women, women are more severely affected.

Types of Degenerative Joint Disease

Degenerative joint disease associated with known risk factors, such as joint stress, congenital abnormalities, or joint instability due to trauma, is referred to as **secondary degenerative joint disease. Primary degenerative joint disease** is not associated with known risk factors. Both primary and secondary degenerative joint disease have the same pathologic characteristics: (1) erosion of the articular cartilage, (2) sclerosis (thickening) of bone underneath the cartilage, and (3) formation of bone spurs or **osteophytes.** The two types differ in that primary disease tends to be generalized, whereas secondary disease involves only joints subjected to a particular risk factor.

Primary degenerative joint disease is the most common type of noninflammatory joint disease. The disease is generally distributed throughout the peripheral and central joints of the body and affects adult men more than women. The joints most characteristically affected are in the hand, wrist, neck (lower cervical spine), lower back (lumbar spine, sacroiliac), hip, knees, ankles, and feet. Though the etiology of primary degenerative joint disease is unknown, aging is the most important associated factor. With aging, the quality and quantity of the proteoglycans in cartilage decreases, rendering the cartilage more susceptible to breakdown. Evidence also suggests that primary disease may be inherited as an autosomal recessive trait (Resnick & Niwayama, 1987).

Secondary degenerative joint disease can be due to any condition that damages cartilage directly, subjects the joint surfaces or underlying bone to chronic, excessive, or abnormal forces, or causes instability in the joint. Specific risk factors include the following:

1. Trauma, particularly sprains, strains, joint dislocation, and fractures
2. Long-term mechanical stress associated with athletics, ballet dancing, or repetitive physical tasks
3. The presence of inflammation in joint structures, during which inflammatory cells release enzymes capable of digesting cartilage cells
4. Joint instability caused by damage to supporting structures, such as the joint capsule, ligaments, or tendons
5. Neurologic disorders (e.g., diabetic neuropathy, Charcot) in which pain and proprioceptive reflexes are diminished or lost, increasing the tendency for abnormal movement, positioning, or weight bearing
6. Congenital or acquired skeletal deformities

7. Hematologic or endocrine disorders, such as hemophilia, which causes chronic bleeding into the joints, or hyperparathyroidism, which causes bone to lose calcium
8. Drugs (e.g., colchicine, indomethacin, steroids) that stimulate the activity of collagen-digesting enzymes in the synovial membrane

All of these factors alter articular cartilage in some way and accelerate the rate of cartilage loss.

Course of Degenerative Joint Disease
Pathophysiology

The primary defect in primary and secondary degenerative joint disease is loss of articular cartilage. Early in the disease, the articular cartilage loses its glistening appearance. As the disease progresses, surface areas of the articular cartilage flake off, and deeper layers develop longitudinal fissures (fibrillation). The cartilage becomes thin and may be absent over some areas, leaving the underlying bone (subchondral bone) unprotected. Consequently, the unprotected subchondral bone becomes sclerotic (dense and hard). Cysts sometimes develop within the subchondral bone and communicate with the longitudinal fissures in the cartilage. Pressure builds in the cysts until the cystic contents are forced into the synovial cavity, breaking through the articular cartilage on the way. As the articular cartilage erodes, cartilage-coated osteophytes may grow outward from the underlying bone. These spurlike bony projections enlarge until small pieces, called "joint mice," break off into the synovial cavity. If osteophyte fragments irritate the synovial membrane, synovitis and joint effusion result.

Articular cartilage is probably lost through enzymatic breakdown of the cartilage matrix—the proteoglycans, glycosaminoglycans, and collagen. First, the enzymes break down the macromolecules of proteoglycans, glycosaminoglycans, and collagen into large, diffusable fragments. Then the fragments are taken up by the cartilage cells (chondrocytes) and digested by the cell's own lysosomal enzymes (Hall, Fitgerald, & Rosenblatt, 1983). (Processes of cellular uptake and lysosomal digestion are described in Chapter 1.)

It is not known for certain where cartilage-degrading enzymes come from or how they are activated, but researchers have proposed several hypotheses. Some of the enzymes may be present in latent form in the matrix or chondrocytes of the articular cartilage itself. Others might originate in the synovial membrane, blood plasma, or leukocytes that migrate into the synovial cavity. Possible mechanisms of enzyme activation include tissue injury, inflammation, or any other condition that causes excessive release of enzymes in the joint.

Enzymatic destruction of articular cartilage begins in the matrix, with destruction of proteoglycans and collagen fibers. Enzymes that affect proteoglycans do so by interfering with assembly of the proteoglycan subunit or the proteoglycan aggregate (see Chapter 38). Changes in the conformation of proteoglycans disrupts the pumping action that regulates movement of synovial fluid into and out of the cartilage. Without the regulatory action of the proteoglycan pump, cartilage imbibes too much fluid and becomes less able to withstand the stresses of weight bearing.

Enzymes that degrade collagen (i.e., collagenases) probably originate in the chondrocytes or in leukocytes. Collagen breakdown destroys the fibrils that give articular cartilage its tensile strength and exposes the chondrocytes to mechanical stress and enzyme attack. Thus a cycle of destruction begins that involves all the components of articular cartilage—proteoglycans, collagen fibers, and chrondrocytes.

Clinical Manifestations

Clinical manifestations of primary or secondary degenerative joint disease typically appear during the fifth or sixth decade of life, though asymptomatic, articular surface changes are common after age 40. Pain in one or more joints is the first symptom of a degenerative joint disease. Examination usually reveals general involvement of both peripheral and central joints. Peripheral joints most often involved are in the hands, wrists, knees, and feet. Central joints most often afflicted are in the lower cervical spine, lumbosacral spine, and hips.

Joint structures are capable of generating a limited number of signs and symptoms. The primary signs and symptoms of joint disease are pain, stiffness, enlargement or swelling, tenderness, limited range of motion, muscle wasting, instability, partial dislocation, and deformity.

Pain is the predominant symptom of degenerative joint disease. It is usually aggravated by weight bearing or use of the joint and relieved by resting the joint. Nocturnal pain is usually not relieved by rest and may be accompanied by paresthesias (numbness, tingling, or prickling) in the fingers. Sometimes pain is referred to another part of the body. For example, degenerative joint disease of the lumbosacral spine may mimic sciatica, causing severe pain in the back of the thigh along the course of the sciatic nerve. Degenerative joint disease in the lower cervical spine may cause brachial neuralgia (pain in the arm) aggravated by movement of the neck.

The actual mechanisms of joint pain are complex and poorly understood, but several explanations are possible. The pain could be due to articular distention and stretching of the fibrous joint capsule, which has an abundant nerve supply. Inflammation of the joint capsule also causes fibrous shrinking, so that movement of the joint in any direction causes painful stretching. Pain can also arise from the subchondral or periarticular bone.

The origin of joint stiffness is unknown. Joint stiffness is generally defined as difficulty in initiating joint movement, immobility, or a loss of range of motion. The stiffness usually occurs as joint movement begins, and it dissipates rapidly after a few minutes. Enlargement and bulging of joint contour, commonly described as swelling, may be due to bone enlargement or the proliferation of osteophytes around the margins of the joint. Swelling also occurs if inflammatory exudate or blood enters the joint cavity, thereby increasing the volume of synovial fluid. This condition, termed **joint effusion,** is caused by (1) the presence of osteophyte fragments in the synovial cavity, (2) drainage of cysts from diseased subchondral bone, or (3) acute trauma to joint structures, resulting in hemorrhage and inflammatory exudation into the synovial cavity.

Range of motion is limited to some degree, depending on the extent of cartilage degeneration. Frequently, joint motion is accompanied by sounds of crepitus, creaking, or grating. Hypermobility and subluxation of joints occurs in degenerative joint disease that is secondary to a neurologic disorder.

Evaluation and Treatment

Evaluation consists of clinical assessment and radiologic studies. Treatment is either conservative or surgical. Conservative treatment includes rest of the involved joint until inflammation subsides; range of motion to prevent joint capsule contraction; a cane, crutches, or walker to decrease weight bearing; and analgesic and antiinflammatory drug therapy to reduce swelling and pain. Surgery is used to improve joint movement, correct deformity or malalignment, or create a new joint with artificial implants.

Inflammatory Joint Disease

The second major type of joint disease is **inflammatory joint disease,** commonly termed arthritis. Inflammatory joint disease is characterized by inflammatory damage or destruction in the synovial membrane, articular cartilage, and by systemic signs of inflammation (fever, leukocytosis, malaise, anorexia, hyperfibrogenemia).

Inflammatory joint disease can be infectious or noninfectious. In infectious inflammatory joint disease, inflammation is caused by invasion of the joint by bacteria, mycoplasmas, viruses, fungi, or protozoa. These agents can invade the joint through a traumatic wound, surgical incision, or contaminated needle, or they can be delivered by the bloodstream from sites of infection elsewhere in the body, typically bones, heart valves, or blood vessels. In noninfectious inflammatory joint disease, which is the most common form, inflammation is due to immune reactions or the deposition of crystals of monosodium urate in and around the joint. Rheumatoid arthritis and ankylosing spondylitis are noninfectious inflammatory diseases caused by immune reactions; gout is a noninfectious inflammatory disease due to crystal deposition.

Rheumatoid Arthritis

Rheumatoid arthritis is an autoimmune disease that causes chronic inflammation of connective tissue, primarily in the joints. (Autoimmune disease is described in Chapter 8.) The first joint tissue to be affected is the synovial membrane, which lines the joint cavity (see Chapter 38, Fig. 38-5). Eventually, inflammation may spread to the articular cartilage, fibrous joint capsule, and surrounding ligaments and tendons, causing pain, joint deformity, and loss of function (Fig. 39-14). The joints most commonly afflicted are in the fingers, feet, wrists, elbows, ankles, and knees, but the shoulders, hips, and cervical spine may also be involved.

Rheumatoid arthritis affects 1% to 2% of adults and, like most autoimmune diseases, develops most often in women, with a female-to-male ratio of 3:1. Besides inflammation of the joints, rheumatoid arthritis can cause fever, malaise, rash, lymph node or spleen enlargement, and Reynaud phenomenon (transient lack of circulation to the fingertips and toes).

Despite intensive research, the etiology of rheumatoid arthritis remains obscure. Rheumatoid arthritis probably occurs in a genetically susceptible host because of an aberrant immune response to an unidentified antigen. Candidates for the precipitating antigen include three groups of infectious microorganisms: bacteria, mycoplasmas, and viruses (especially Epstein-Barr virus). With long-term or intensive exposure to the antigen, normal antibodies (immunoglobulins [Ig]) become autoantibodies—antibodies that attack host tissues (self-antigens). Because they are usually present in individuals with rheumatoid arthritis, the transformed antibodies are termed **rheumatoid factors (RFs).** The RFs usually consist of two classes of immunoglobulin-antibodies—antibodies for IgM and IgG—and, occasionally, IgA. Their main antigenic targets are portions of the immunoglobulin molecule. RFs bind with their target self-antigens in blood and synovial membrane, forming immune complexes (antigen-antibody complexes). (See Chapter 6 for a discussion about antigen-antibody binding in the immune response.)

Pathophysiology

Synovial inflammation (synovitis) occurs when immune complexes in blood and synovial tissue trigger the inflammatory response, chiefly by activating the plasma protein complement. (Complement activation by immune complexes is described in Chapter 7.) Complement activation stimulates kinin and prostaglandin release that increases the permeability of blood vessels in the synovial membranes and attacts leukocytes and lymphocytes to the synovial membrane.

Several types of leukocytes are attracted out of the circulation and to the synovial membrane. The phagocytes of inflammation (neutrophils and macrophages) ingest the immune complexes and, in the process of doing so, release powerful enzymes that degrade synovial tissue and articular cartilage. The immune system's B and T lymphocytes are also activated. The B lymphocytes are stimulated to produce more RFs, and the T lymphocytes produce enzymes that amplify and perpetuate the inflammatory response. Unlike the precipitating microorganism, which is killed off and removed from the

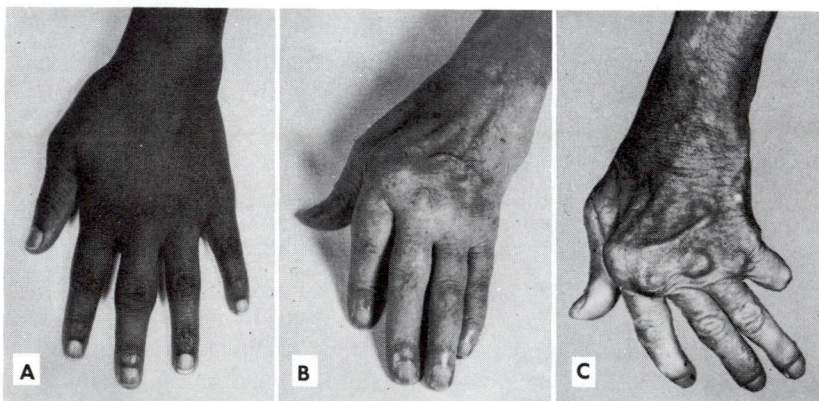

FIG. 39-14. Rheumatoid arthritis of the hand. **A,** Early stage. Note fusiform swelling of proximal interphalangeal joints, especially that of middle finger. **B,** Moderate involvement. Note swelling from chronic synovitis of metacarpophalangeal joints and early ulnar drift. **C,** Advanced stage. Note marked ulnar drift and subluxletion of metacarpophalangeal joints with extension of proximal interphalangeal joints and flexion of distal joints. Note also deformed position of thumb. Hand has wasted appearance. (From Raney and Brashear, 1971.)

body, the newly targeted self-antigens (immunoglobulin) are in relatively constant supply and can thus perpetuate inflammation and the formation of immune complexes indefinitely (Fig. 39-15).

Inflammatory and immune processes have several damaging effects on the synovial membrane (Fig. 39-

16). Along with the swelling caused by leukocyte infiltration, the synovial membrane undergoes hyperplastic thickening as its cells proliferate and enlarge abnormally. As synovial inflammation progresses to involve its blood vessels, small venules become occluded by hypertrophied endothelial cells, fibrin, platelets, and inflamma-

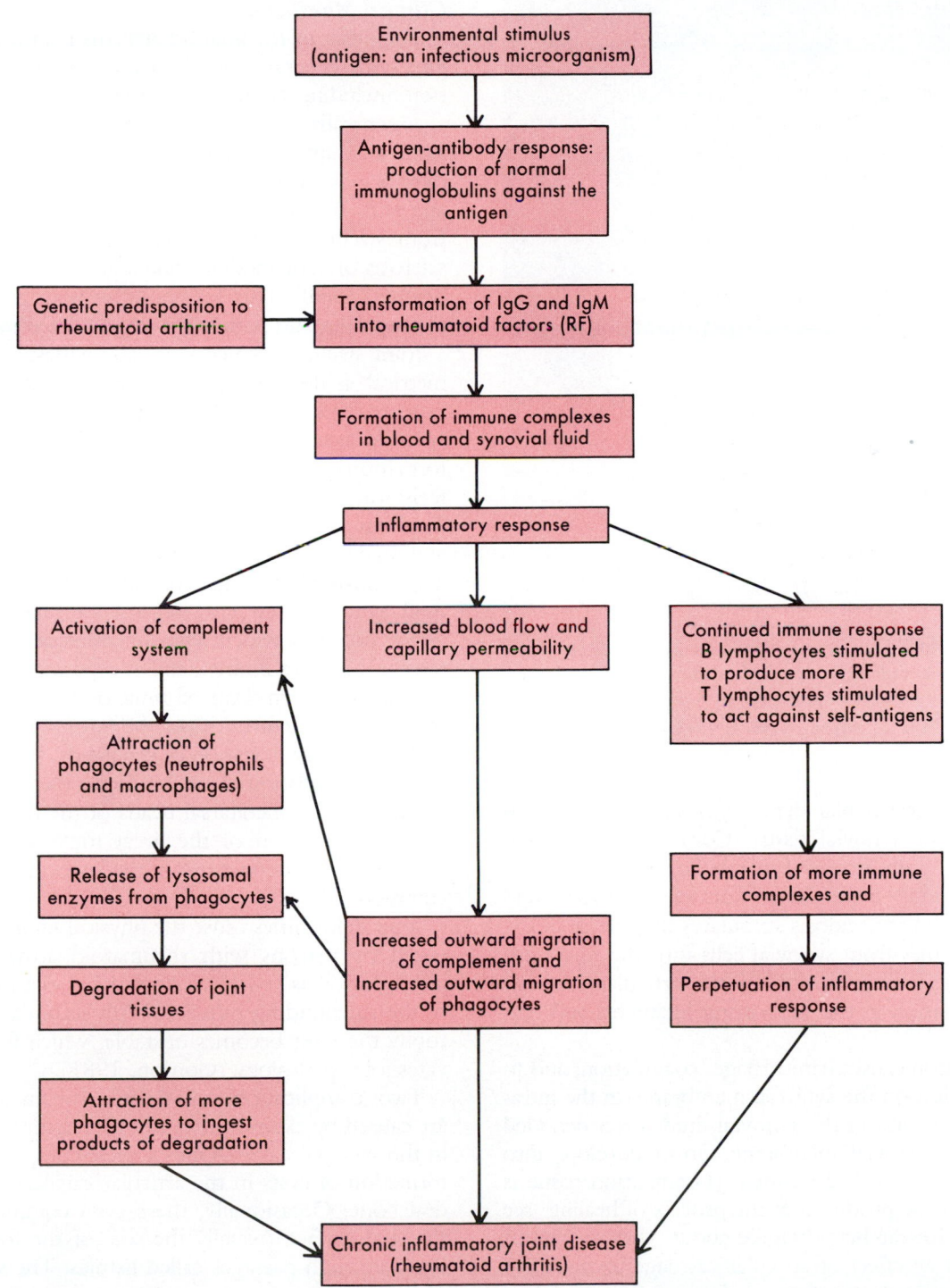

FIG. 39-15. Probable pathogenesis of rheumatoid arthritis.

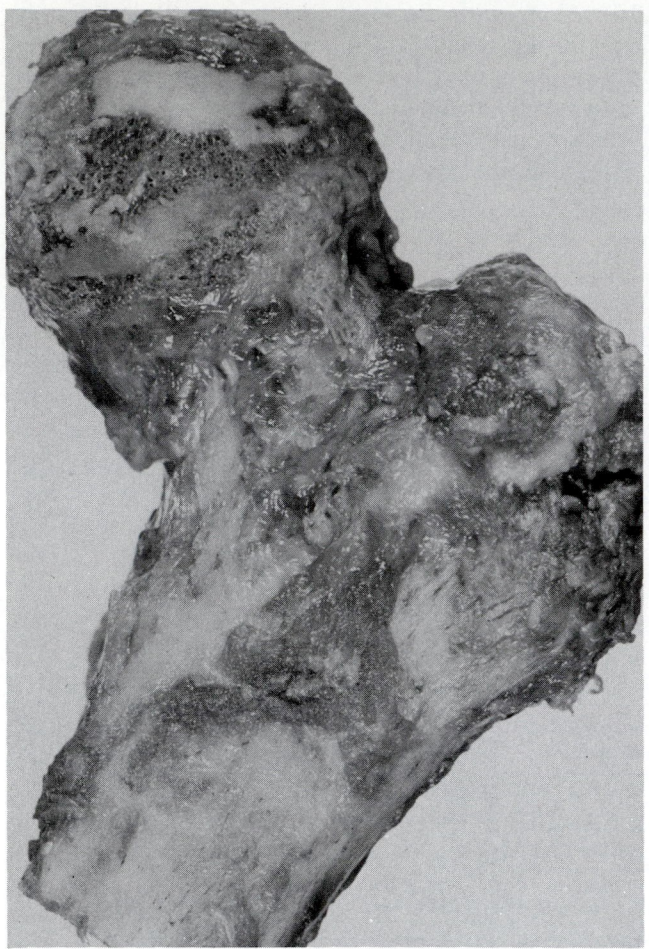

FIG. 39-16. Advanced rheumatoid arthritis involving femur. There is prominent proliferation of synovium and almost complete destruction of overlaying articular cartilage. (From Rosai, 1981.)

tory cells. These vascular derangements decrease vascular flow to the synovial tissue. Compromised circulation, coupled with increased metabolic needs due to hypertrophy and hyperplasia, causes hypoxia and metabolic acidosis. Acidosis stimulates the release of hydrolytic enzymes from synovial cells into the surrounding tissue, initiating erosion of the articular cartilage and inflammation in the supporting ligaments and tendons.

Inflammation causes hemorrhage, coagulation, and fibrin deposition on the synovial membrane, in the intracellular matrix, and in the synovial fluid. Over denuded areas of the synovial membrane, fibrin develops into granulation tissue called **pannus**. (Granulation tissue is the earliest tissue produced in the process of healing; see Chapter 7.) Researchers disagree about whether pannus is a cause or an effect of articular cartilage involvement in rheumatoid arthritis. Some believe that, as rheumatoid arthritis progresses, pannus extends from the synovial membrane into adjacent articular cartilage and destroys the cartilage. Other researchers think that pannus forms on articular cartilage after the cartilage has been destroyed by inflammation (Hall et al., 1983). In any case, pannus formation does not lead to synovial or articular regeneration but rather to formation of scar tissue that immobilizes the joint.

Clinical Manifestations

The onset of rheumatoid arthritis is insidious and begins with general systemic manifestations of inflammation, including fatigue, weakness, anorexia, weight loss, and generalized aching and stiffness. Local manifestations also appear gradually over a period of weeks or months. Typically, the joints become painful, tender, and stiff. Pain early in the disease is caused by pressure from swelling. Later in the disease pain is caused by sclerosis of subchondral bone and new bone formation. Stiffness usually lasts for about an hour after arising in the morning and is thought to be related to synovitis.

Joint swelling, which is usually widespread and symmetrical, is due to increasing amounts of inflammatory exudate (leukocytes, plasma, and plasma proteins) in the synovial membrane, hyperplasia of inflamed tissues, and formation of new bone. On palpation, the swollen joint feels warm and the synovial membrane feels "boggy." The skin over the joint may have a ruddy, cyanotic hue and may look thin and shiny.

An inflamed joint may lose some of its mobility. Even mild synovitis can lead to loss of range of motion, which becomes evident after inflammation subsides. Extension becomes limited, and is eventually lost if flexion contractures form. Loss of range of motion can progress to permanent deformities of the fingers, toes, and limbs, including ulnar deviation of the hands, boutonniere and swan-neck deformities of the finger joints, plantar subluxation of the metatarsal heads of the foot, and hallux valgus (angulation of the great toe toward the other toes). Flexion contractures of the knees and hips are also common.

Joint deformities cause the physical limitations experienced by persons with rheumatoid arthritis. Loss of joint motion is quickly followed by secondary atrophy of the surrounding muscles. With secondary muscle atrophy the joint becomes unstable, which further aggravates joint pathology (Gordon, 1981).

Two complications of chronic rheumatoid arthritis are caused by excessive amount of inflammatory exudate in the synovial cavity. One of these complications is the formation of cysts in the articular cartilage or subchondral bone. Occasionally, these cysts communicate with the skin surface (usually the sole of the foot) and can drain through passages called fistulas. The second complication is rupture of a cyst or of the synovial joint itself, usually due to strenuous physical activity that places excessive pressure on the joint. Rupture releases inflammatory exudate into adjacent tissues, thereby spreading inflammation.

Extrasynovial **rheumatoid nodules,** or swellings, are observed in areas of pressure or trauma in 20% of individuals with rheumatoid arthritis. Each nodule is an aggregate of inflammatory cells surrounding a central core of fibrinoid and cellular debris. T lymphocytes are the predominant leukocytes in the nodule. B lymphocytes, plasma cells, and phagocytes are found around the periphery. Nodules are most often found in subcutaneous tissue over the extensor surfaces of elbows and fingers. They may be movable or fixed to tendons or bone.

Rheumatoid nodules may also invade the skin, cardiac valves, pericardium, pleura, lung parenchyma, and spleen. These nodules are identical to those encountered in some individuals with rheumatic fever and are characterized by central tissue necrosis surrounded by proliferating connective tissue. Also noted are large numbers of lymphocytes and occassional plasma cells. The skin nodules appear in about 20% of those affected with rheumatoid arthritis, mostly involving the extensor surfaces of the arms and elbows. Less common sites are the scalp, back, hands, feet, buttocks, and knees (Fig. 39-17). Acute glaucoma may result with nodules forming on the sclera. Pulmonary involvement may result in diffuse pleuritis or multiple intraparenchymal nodules. Together, the occurrence of pulmonary nodules and pneumoconiosis (chronic inflammation of the lungs from inhalation of dust) creates the syndrome called **Caplan syndrome.** Diffuse pulmonary fibrosis may occur because of immunologically mediated immune complex deposition.

Rheumatoid nodules within the heart may cause valvular deformities, particularly of the aortic valve leaflets,

and pericarditis. Lymphadenopathy of the nodes close to the affected joints may develop. Rheumatoid nodules within the spleen result in splenomegaly. Involvement of blood vessels results in an acute necrotizing vasculitis, characteristic of that noted in other immunologic/inflammatory states. Thromboses of such involved vessels may give rise to myocardial infarctions, cerebrovascular occlusions, mesenteric infarction, kidney damage, and vascular insufficiency in the hands and fingers (Raynaud phenomenon). The vascular changes are primarily noted in individuals receiving steroid therapy, thus there is some concern that the therapy may play a role in initiating these lesions (Robbins, Cotran, & Kumar, 1984). Changes in skeletal muscle are often noted in the form of nonspecific atrophy secondary to joint dysfunction.

Evaluation and Treatment

Evaluation of rheumatoid arthritis is by clinical evaluation, roentgenography of the joint, and serologic tests for rheumatoid factor. The American Rheumatism Association lists eleven diagnostic criteria for rheumatoid arthritis (see box below). The presence of seven or more of the criteria is diagnostic of classic rheumatoid arthritis. Five criteria with joint signs or symptoms continuous for 6 weeks indicates definite rheumatoid arthritis. A diagnosis of probable rheumatid arthritis is made on the basis of three criteria with joint signs or symptoms continuous for 6 weeks.

Treatment is conservative or surgical. Conservative treatment includes rest of the inflamed joint and wholebody rest for several hours daily, use of hot and cold packs, physical therapy, antineoplastic medications, diet high in calories and vitamins, and antiinflammatory drugs taken orally or injected into the joint. Surgical

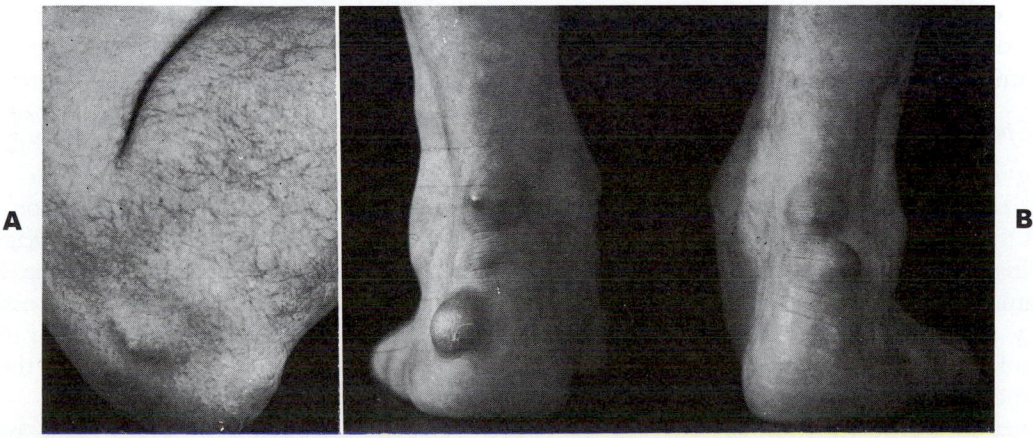

FIG. 39-17. Rheumatoid arthritis. **A,** Large subcutaneous nodule over olecranon process. **B,** Subcutaneous nodules of tendo achillis areas leaving typical morphologic features of nodule of rheumatoid arthritis. (Courtesy Dr. F. A. Chandler, Atlanta, GA. From Kissane, 1985.)

Eleven Diagnostic Criteria for Rheumatoid Arthritis

1. Morning stiffness
2. Motion pain or tenderness in at least one joint
3. Swelling (soft tissue or fluid) of at least one joint
4. Swelling of at least one other joint
5. Symmetrical joint swelling (same joint on each side of the body, excluding the terminal phalangeal joint
6. Subcutaneous nodules
7. X-ray changes (must include decalcified areas of at least one bone near joint margins, usually hands or wrist)
8. Positive rheumatoid factor
9. Poor mucin precipitate in synovial fluid
10. Characteristic histologic changes of synovium (chronic inflammatory infiltrate)
11. Characteristic histologic changes of nodules (granulomatous foci)

Classic rheumatoid arthritis: seven or more criteria observed

Definite rheumatoid arthritis: five criteria with joint signs or symptoms continuous for at least 6 weeks

Probably rheumatoid arthritis: three criteria with joint signs or symptoms continuous for at least 6 weeks

Possible rheumatoid arthritis: two criteria with joint signs or symptoms continuous for at least 6 weeks

Modified from: McDuffie, F. C. (1985). Rheumatoid factors A. Background. In A. S. Cohen (Ed.), *Laboratory diagnostic procedures in the rheumatic diseases.* (p. 103). Orlando, Florida: Grune & Stratton.

synovectomy may be done early in the disease to decrease inflammatory effusion and remove pannus. Surgery is used to correct deformity or mechanical deficiency in intermediate or late stages of the disease.

Ankylosing Spondylitis

Ankylosing spondylitis is a chronic, inflammatory joint disease characterized by stiffening and fusion (ankylosis) of the spine and sacroiliac joints. Like rheumatoid arthritis, ankylosing spondylitis is a systemic, immune inflammatory disease. Although inflammation is the primary pathologic process in both rheumatoid arthritis and ankylosing spondylitis, the two diseases differ in the primary site of inflammation and the end result. In rheumatoid arthritis, the primary site of inflammation is the synovial membrane resulting in the destruction and instability of synovial joints. In ankylosing spondylitis, the primary pathologic site is the **enthesis**—

the point at which ligaments, tendons, and the joint capsule are inserted into bone—and the end result is fibrosis, ossification, and fusion of the joint (Bywaters, 1980).

The incidence of ankylosing spondylitis is almost equal in men and women (McCarthy, 1985), but the disease tends to be more severe in men. In women, ankylosing spondylitis may affect the peripheral joints of the appendicular skeleton rather than the axial skeleton, progress less rapidly, and cause less dramatic spinal changes.

The prevalence of ankylosing spondylitis in the United States is approximately 0.5% to 1% among whites, 3% to 4% among blacks, and 18% to 50% among various tribes of American Indians (Kelley et al., 1985). Worldwide, however, the disease appears to be most prevalent in whites.

Primary ankylosing spondylitis usually develops in late adolescence and young adulthood, with peak incidence at about age 20. Secondary ankylosing spondylitis affects older age groups and is often associated with other inflammatory diseases (e.g., psoriatic arthropathy, inflammatory bowel disease, or Reiter syndrome).

The cause of ankylosing spondylitis is unknown, but the disease is strongly associated with the presence of histocompatiblity antigen HLA-B27 on the chromosomes of affected individuals, which suggests a genetic predisposition to the disease (Schlossteen et al., 1973). *Klebsiella* infection probably triggers or perpetuates the inflammatory response (Geczy et al., 1983; Kinsella, Fritzler, & McNeil; 1983; Sullivan, Pendergast, & Geczy, 1983).

Pathophysiology

Ankylosing spondylitis begins with inflammation of fibrocartilage in cartilaginous joints (see Chapter 38, Fig. 38-4). The fibrous tissue of the joint capsule, the cartilage that surrounds intervertebral discs, entheses, and periosteum are infiltrated by inflammatory cells. As inflammatory cells (chiefly macrophages) and lymphocytes infiltrate and erode bone and fibrocartilage in joint structures, repair begins to occur. Repair is the stage of the disease process that produces disability in individuals with ankylosing spondylitis. Repair of cartilaginous structures begins with the proliferation of fibroblasts. Fibroblasts synthesize and secrete collagen, which becomes organized into fibrous scar tissue. Eventually, the scar tissue undergoes calcification and ossification. With time, all the cartilaginous structures of the joint are replaced by ossified scar tissue, causing the joint to fuse, or lose flexibility.

Repair of eroded bone begins with osteoblast activation and proliferation. Osteoblasts lay down new bone (callus), which is remodeled and replaced by compact, lamellar bone. Bone repair changes the contour of the bone's surface because the new bone grows outward to form a new enthesis with the end of the eroded ligament. The new enthesis, which forms on top of the old one, is called **syndesmophyte.** As calcification of the spinal ligaments progresses, the vertebral bodies lose their concave anterior contour and appear square. The spine assumes the classic "bamboo spine" appearance of ankylosing spondylitis.

Clinical Manifestations

The most common signs and symptoms of early ankylosing spondylitis are low back pain and stiffness. Typically, the individual with primary disease develops low back pain during the early 20s. The pain is at first insidious but progressively becomes persistent. It is often worse after prolonged rest and is alleviated by physical activity. Eary morning stiffness usually accompanies the low back pain, and the individual typically has difficulty sitting up or twisting the spine. Forward flexion, rotation, and lateral flexion of the spine is restricted and painful. Early pain and resultant loss of motion are caused by the underlying inflammation and reflex muscle spasm rather than to soft tissue or bony fusion.

As the disease progresses, the normal convex curve of the lower spine (lumbar lordosis) diminishes, and concavity of the upper spine (kyphosis) increases. The individual becomes increasingly stooped. The thoracic spine becomes rounded, the head and neck are held forward on the shoulders, and the hips are flexed (Fig. 39-18).

Inflammation in the tendon insertions of the many costosternal and costovertebral muscles can cause "pleuritic" chest pain and restricted chest movement. The pain is usually worse on inspiration. Movement in the diaphragm is normal and full. Pressure on the anterior chest wall over the sternum, ribs, and costal cartilages may cause tenderness. Tenderness over the pelvic brim may cause discomfort at night and interfere with sleep because turning onto the iliac crests causes pain. Tenderness over the ischial tuberosities may make sitting on hard seats unbearable. Tenderness in the heels may contribute to a limp or the cautious placement of the feet during walking.

Evaluation and Treatment

Diagnosis of ankylosing spondylitis is made from the history and physical examination, roentgenograms, and serum analysis for the presence of the histocompatibility antigen HLA-B27. Treatment of individuals with ankylosing spondylitis consists of physical therapy to maintain skeletal mobility and prevent the natural progression of contractures. Prevention of deformity and maintenance of mobility require a continuous program of physical therapy. Exercises are performed several times a day to maintain chest expansion, full extension of the spine, and complete range of motion in the proximal joints.

Antiinflammatory and analgesic medications are prescribed to suppress some of the pain and stiffness and to facilitate exercise. The medications do not prevent disease progression, but they do provide relief from symptoms. Surgical procedures and radiotherapy are sometimes used to provide relief for individuals with end-stage disease or intolerable deformity.

Gout

Gout is a metabolic disorder that disrupts the body's control of uric acid production or excretion, causing high levels of uric acid in the blood (hyperuricemia) and in other body fluids, including synovial fluid. When the uric acid reaches a certain concentration in fluids, it crystallizes, forming insoluble precipitates that are deposited in connective tissues through the body. Crystallization in synovial fluid causes acute, painful inflammation of the joint, a condition known as **gouty arthritis.** With time, crystal deposition in subcutaneous tissues causes the formation of small, white nodules, or **tophi,** that are visible through the skin. Crystal aggregates deposited in the kidneys can form urate stones (renal stone) and lead to renal failure.

In classic gouty arthritis, inflammation of the joint is caused by the formation of monosodium urate crystals. Another condition, termed pseudogout, is due to the formation of calcium phosphate dehydrate crystals. The effect of either crystal is the same—the onset of an acute inflammatory response (see Chapter 7).

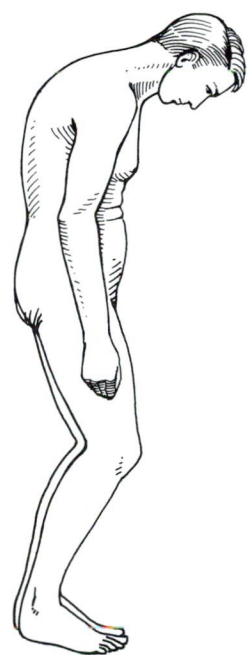

FIG. 39-18. Characteristic posture in advanced ankylosing spondylitis. (From Phipps, Long, & Woods, 1987.)

The number of people afflicted by gout is estimated at one-half million, almost all of them men. Approximately 95% of affected individuals have primary gout, in which hyperuricemia is due to an overproduction of uric acid. The exact biochemical defect in primary gout is unknown, but many researchers suspect inherited enzyme defects. The remaining 5% to 10% of those with gout have secondary gout, in which the hyperuricemia is the result of an acquired chronic disease or a drug that interferes with the normal balance between production and excretion of uric acid.

Both primary and secondary gout are most common in men over 40 years of age. Primary gout associated with specific enzyme defects has been diagnosed only in men. Secondary gout can afflict both men and women between the ages of 30 and 50, but gout seldom occurs in women until after menopause, probably because estrogen promotes excretion of uric acid.

Familial incidence of primary gout is reported in 18% to 50% of cases. Some studies suggest that gout is autosomal dominant; others that it is X-linked dominant. Gout may be a multifactorial inheritance disease (Kelley, 1972; Scott & Pollard, 1970). The fact that hyperuricemia is associated with obesity and with alcohol, drug, and purine (a protein) consumption indicates that environmental as well as genetic factors are important in the development of gout.

Secondary gout is due to drugs or disorders that promote hyperuricemia. Diuretics are the main class of drugs thought to cause secondary gout, particularly chlorothiazide, acetazolamide, ethacrynic acid, and furosemide. These diuretics decrease the renal tubular excretion of urate. Other causes of decreased uric acid excretion include chronic renal disease, hypertension, and starvation. Hyperuricemia from overproduction of uric acid can be due to myeloproliferative disorders of cancer, in which metabolic processes are speeded up (e.g., leukemia); hemolytic disorders, in which cellular breakdown is speeded up (e.g., hemolytic anemia); and genetic metabolic disorders in which hyperuricemia is just one of many clinical manifestations (e.g., Lesch-Nyhan syndrome).

Pathophysiology

The pathophysiology of gout is closely linked to (1) purine metabolism (or cellular metabolism of purines) and (2) kidney function. At the cellular level, purines are synthesized to purine nucleotides which are utilized in the synthesis of nucleic acids, adenosine triphosphate, cyclic AMP, and cyclic GMP. Uric acid is a breakdown product of purine nucleotides. Some individuals with gout have an accelerated rate of purine synthesis accompanied by an overproduction of uric acid. Even with restricted purine consumption, these individuals continue to overproduce uric acid. Other individuals breakdown

purine nucleotides at an accelerated rate that also results in an overproduction of uric acid. Overproduction of uric acid can also be the result of an increased turnover of nucleic acids, which is associated with an increased turnover of cells at other body sites. The increased turnover of nucleic acids leads to increased levels of uric acid with a compensatory increase in purine synthesis.

Kidney function is involved in the pathophysiology of gout because most uric acid is eliminated from the body through the kidneys. Urate (uric acid salt) is normally freely filtered at the glomerulus and undergoes both reabsorption and excretion within the renal tubules. In most individuals with primary gout, urate excretion by the kidneys is sluggish. The sluggish excretion may be the result of a decrease in glomerular filtration of urate or an acceleration in urate reabsorption (Emmerson, 1983). (Kidney function is described in Chapter 32).

The exact process by which crystals of monosodium urate are deposited in joints and induce gouty arthritis is unknown, but several mechanisms have been proposed based on observations that (1) monosodium urate precipitates at the periphery of the body, where lower body temperatures may reduce the solubility of monsodium urate; (2) decreases in albumin or glycosaminoglycan levels decrease urate solubility; (3) changes in ion concentration and decreases of pH enhance urate deposition; and (4) trauma promotes urate crystal precipitation (Kippin et al., 1974; Simpkin, 1973). The monosodium urate crystals may form in the synovial fluid or in the synovial membrane, cartilage, or other connective tissues in joints and elsewhere, such as in the heart, earlobes, and kidneys. Mechanical or metabolic changes probably cause release of the crystals from connective tissues into the synovial fluid.

Monosodium urate crystals are capable of both stimulating and perpetuating the inflammatory response (Fig. 39-19). The presence of the crystals triggers the acute inflammatory response, during which neutrophils are attracted out of the circulation and begin to phagocytose (ingest) the crystals. (Processes of acute inflammation and phagocytosis are described in Chapter 7.) Tissue damage begins to occur when the neutrophils release the contents of their digestive vacuoles (lysosomes). Lysosomal contents are released from neutrophils through one of three mechanisms: (1) dissolution of neutrophils that have died of "old age" (neutrophil life span is about 2 days), (2) leakage from neutrophils that have been injured by biochemical reactions with ingested urate crystals, or (3) rupture of neutrophils during attempts to ingest exceptionally large urate crystals.

The neutrophils' lysosomes contain substances that not only damage tissues, but also perpetuate inflammation. Most tissue damage in gouty arthritis is due to powerful lysosomal enzymes. Other lysosomal substances include the undigested urate crystals and bio-

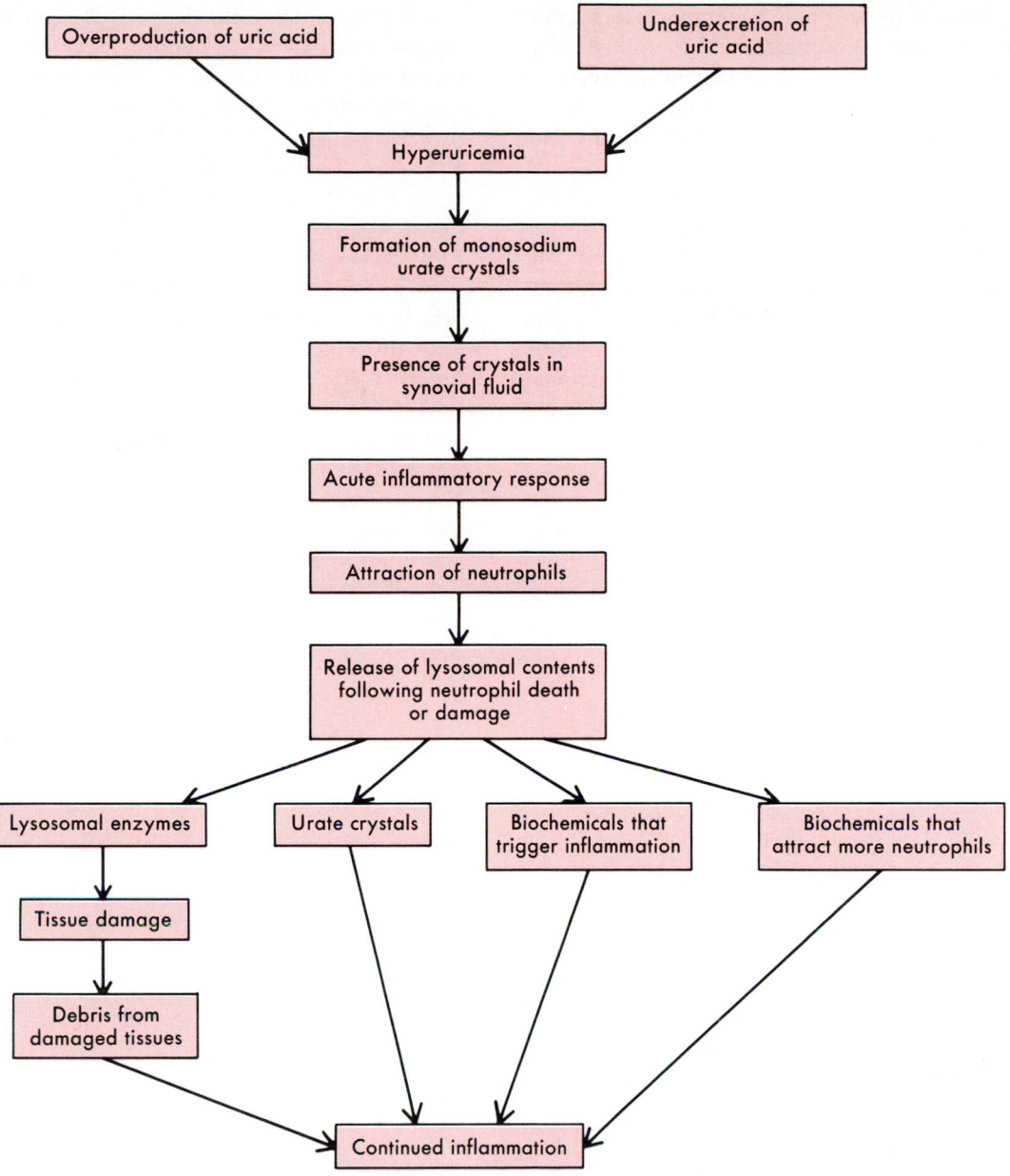

FIG. 39-19. Pathogenesis of acute gouty arthritis.

chemicals that attract more neutrophils to the site and trigger acute inflammation anew.

Clinical Manifestations

Gout is manifested by (1) an increase in serum urate concentration (uricemia), (2) recurrent attacks of monoarticular arthritis (inflammation of a single joint), (3) deposits of monosodium urate monohydrate (tophi) in and around the joints, (4) renal disease involving glomerular, tubular, and interstitial tissues and blood vessels, and (5) the formation of renal stones. These manifestations appear in three clinical stages: (1) asymp-

tomatic hyperuricemia, (2) acute gouty arthritis, and (3) chronic tophaceous gouty arthritis.

In asymptomatic hyperuricemia, the serum urate level is elevated, but arthritic symptoms, tophi, and renal stones are not present. Asymptomatic hyperuricemia may persist throughout life. Attacks of acute gouty arthritis and renal calculi develop with increased serum urate concentrations. Acute gouty arthritis tends to occur with sudden or sustained increases of hyperuricemia, but trauma, drugs, and alcohol can also trigger an acute attack.

Trauma is the most common aggravating factor. The

great toe is subject to chronic strain in walking and, subsequently, an acute gout attack may follow long walks. Trauma associated with occupations, such as truck driving, may also precipitate an attack.

Attacks of gouty arthritis occur abruptly, usually in a peripheral joint. The primary symptom is severe pain. Approximately 50% of the initial attacks occur in the great toe. The other 50% involve the heel, ankle, instep of the foot, knee, wrist, or elbow (Fig. 39-20). The pain is usually noticed at night. Within a few hours the affected joint becomes hot, red, and extremely tender and may be slightly swollen. Lymphangitis and systemic signs of inflammation (leukocytosis, fever, and elevated sedimentation rate) are occasionally present. Untreated, mild attacks usually subside in several hours but may persist for a day or two. Severe attacks may persist for several days or weeks. On recovery, the pain, swelling, and other symptoms resolve completely. The intervals between acute attacks of gouty arthritis are called intercritical periods. Some individuals never have a second attack. Others experience subsequent attacks 5 to 10 years after the first.

Tophaceous gout, the third and chronic stage of disease, can begin as early as 3 years or as late as 40 years after the initial attack of gouty arthritis. Progressive inability to excrete uric acid expands the urate pool until urate crystal deposits (tophis) appear in cartilage, synovial membranes, tendons, and soft tissue. The helix of the ear is the most common site of tophi, which are the

characteristic diagnostic lesions of chronic gout. Each tophus consists of a deposit of urate crystals, surrounded by a granuloma made up of mononuclear phagocytes (macrophages) that have developed into epithelial and giant cells. (Granuloma formation is described in and illustrated in Chapter 7.)

Tophaceous deposits produce irregular swellings of the fingers, hands, knees, and feet. Tophi commonly form lumps along the ulnar surface of the forearm, the tibial surface of the leg, the Achilles tendon, and olecranon bursae. Tophi may produce marked limitation of joint movement and eventually cause grotesque deformities of the hands and feet. Though the tophi themselves are painless, they often cause progressive stiffness and persistent aching of the affected joint. Tophi in the upper extremities may cause nerve compressions such as carpal tunnel syndrome. Tophi in the lower extremities may cause tarsal tunnel syndrome. They may also erode and drain through the skin.

Renal stones are 1000 times more prevalent in individuals with primary gout than in the general population (Wyngaarden & Kelley, 1976). The stones can be the size of a grain of sand or a piece of gravel, or can accumulate in massive deposits called staghorn calculi. They range in color from pale yellow to brown to reddish black, depending on their composition. Some stones consist of pure monosodium urate; others consist of calcium oxalate or calcium phosphate. Renal stones can form in the collecting tubules, pelvis, or ureters, causing obstruction, dilatation, and atrophy of the more proximal tubules and leading eventually to acute renal failure. Stones deposited directly in interstitial tissue initiate an inflammatory reaction that leads to chronic renal disease and progressive renal failure.

Treatment

The aims of gout treatment are to (1) terminate the acute gouty attack as promptly as possible, (2) prevent recurring attacks, (3) prevent or reverse complications associated with urate deposits in the joints and kidneys, and (4) prevent formation of kidney stones. Acute gouty arthritis is treated with antiinflammatory drugs. The drugs of choice are colchicine, indomethacin, and phenylbutazone. Hydrocortisone may be injected into the joint to relieve pain. Ice may also relieve some of the inflammation of the joint. Weight bearing on the involved joint is avoided until the acute attack subsides. The individual is put on a low purine diet and high fluid intake to increase urinary output. Antihyperuricemic drugs are given to reduce serum urate concentrations.

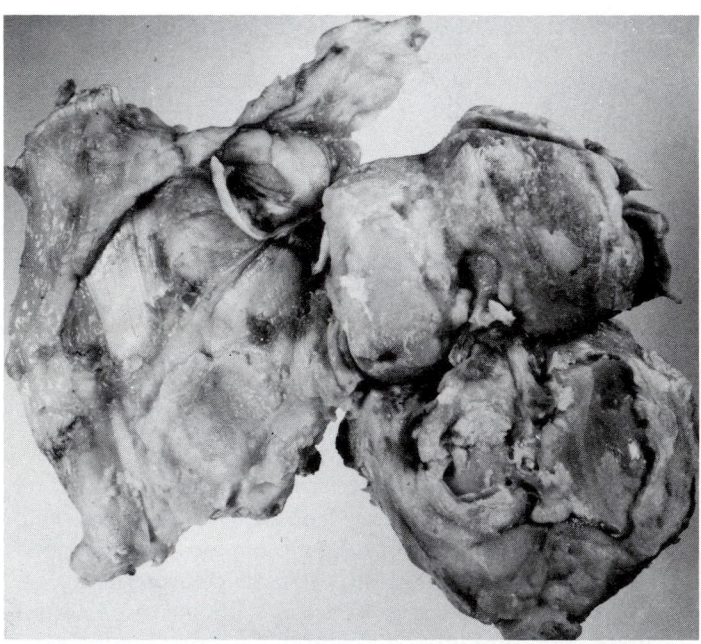

FIG. 39-20. Extensive involvement of knee joint and synovium by gout. In some areas, cartilage of condyles is completely missing and there is involvement of semilunar cartilages as well. Grayish white plaques represent deposits of uric acid crystals. The individual, an 83-year-old woman, had leg amputated because of arterial insufficiency, and finding of gout was unexpected. (From Rosai, 1981.)

DISORDERS OF SKELETAL MUSCLE

Muscle weakness and fatigue are common symptoms. In many cases, neural, traumatic, and psychogenic causes provide an adequate explanation for the failure to generate force (weakness) or sustain force (fatigue) seen in myopathies. Advances have been made in the understanding of the pathophysiologic mechanisms in some of the metabolic and inflammatory muscle diseases. The etiology of many of the myopathies, particularly the muscular dystrophies, remains obscure (see Chapter 40). The complex interaction between muscles and nerves affects muscular function as well. (Discussions of the disorders of neuromuscular transmission are found in Chapter 14; peripheral nerve and anterior horn cell diseases are in Chapters 15.) Only inherited and acquired disorders of skeletal muscles will be the focus here.

Secondary Muscular Dysfunction

Muscular symptoms arise from a variety of causes unrelated to the muscle itself. Secondary muscular phenomena (contracture, stress-related muscle tension, and immobility) are common disorders that influence muscular function.

Contractures

Several conditions cause the muscle fibers to shorten without contracting. This shortening, which is called a **contracture,** can be pathologic or physiologic. The physiologic contracture seen in primary muscle disease should be differentiated from the secondary contracture due to spasticity and paralysis. A physiologic muscle contracture occurs in the absence of a muscle action potential in the sarcolemma. Muscle shortening is explained on the basis of failure of the calcium pump in the presence of plentiful adenosine triphosphate (ATP). A physiologic contracture is seen in McArdle disease (muscle myophosphorylase deficiency) and malignant hyperthermia. The contracture is usually temporary if the underlying pathology is reversed.

A pathologic contracture is more commonly viewed as permanent muscle shortening due to muscle spasm or weakness. Heel cord (Achilles tendon) contractures are examples of pathologic contractures. They are associated with plentiful ATP and will occur in spite of a normal action potential. The most common form of contracture is seen in such conditions as muscular dystrophy (see Chapter 40) and central nervous system (CNS) injury. Rigor mortis causes terminal muscle shortening and contracture independent of action potential production. When ATP is depleted, the cross-bridges of myosin cannot be detached from the actin filaments (McComas, 1977).

Stress-Induced Muscle Tension

While not a uniformly recognized illness, abnormally increased muscle tension has been associated with chronic anxiety as well as a variety of stress-related muscular symptoms, including neck stiffness, back pain, and headache (Basmajian & Deluca, 1985). Abnormalities in the central nervous system, reticular activating system, and autonomic nervous system have been implicated. Although few studies have confirmed these complex interactions, the connection is intuitively plausible. For example, it is known that as an individual progressively relaxes, the amplitude of the kneejerk reflex diminishes (Feurstein, Labbe, & Kuczmierczyk, 1986). Conversely, individuals with absent reflexes are asked to increase tension by such maneuvers as clenching the teeth or handgrip. The underlying pathophysiology is thought to relate to the fact that as a muscle contracts, the muscle spindle is activated. This gamma-feedback system produces a series of impulses that are transmitted to the brain by the sensitive 1A afferent fibers. Unconscious tension is felt to increase the activity of the reticular-activating system as well. This influences increasing firing of the efferent loop of the gamma fibers producing further muscle contraction and increasing muscle tension. The connection with the autonomic nervous system that regulates increased blood flow to the muscle during sympathetic activity is thought to be related to increased muscle contraction tension.

In spite of the tentative nature of the pathophysiologic claims, various forms of treatment have been used to reduce the muscle tension associated with stress. Progressive relaxation training, yoga, meditation, and biofeedback are examples of stress-reduction therapies. **Biofeedback** uses an integrated electromyogram (EMG) to make recordings from the skin surface, as opposed to a needle EMG, which records electrical activity from a single muscle. The goal is to teach the individual to control tension that has been functioning maladaptively. It is particularly useful in individuals who have a connection between skeletal muscle tension and pain (Feurstein et al., 1986). **Progressive relaxation training** emphasizes the individual's ability to perceive the difference between tension and relaxation. This technique involves sequential tensing and relaxing of various muscle groups in a quiet, relaxing environment. The individual is taught to practice this routine daily, often with the use of audiotaped instructions. By teaching the individual to recognize excessive contraction of skeletal muscle, one hopes to enhance the ability to relax specific muscle groups to relieve tension and, thus, reduce CNS arousal as well as ANS arousal.

Immobility

The effects of muscular deconditioning associated with lack of physical activity may be apparent in a matter of days. The normal individual on bed rest loses muscle strength from baseline levels at a rate of 3% a day. Bed rest is also associated with cardiovascular, skeletal, and other organ system changes.

The term *disuse atrophy* has been used to describe the pathologic reduction in normal size of muscle fibers following prolonged inactivity due to bed rest, trauma (casting), or local nerve damage. Studies of experimental animals show a marked reduction in mitochondrial oxidative metabolism, leaving less energy available for muscle protein synthesis. This would explain the reduction in volume and number of myofibrils that has been demonstrated in studies on the effect of casting a fracture of one leg. These studies show that after 8 weeks, the casted limb demonstrates overall a 50% reduction in the number of muscle fibers, and the individual's maximum oxygen uptake is reduced. Some investigators report that, following knee injury, type I muscle fibers atrophy at a greater rate than type II fibers. Similar studies using the immobilized triceps report type II fiber atrophy (Vignos, 1983).

Measures to prevent atrophy include frequent forceful isometric muscle contractions and passive lengthening exercises. According to one report, when the muscle was encased in a cast in the stretched position, fiber atrophy was diminished (Mastaglia & Walton, 1983). If reuse is not restored within 1 year, regeneration of muscle fibers becomes impaired.

Muscle Membrane Abnormalities

Two defects of the muscle membrane (plasma membrane of the muscle fiber) have been linked to clinical syndromes: the hyperexcitable membrane seen in the myotonic disorders and the intermittently unresponsive membrane seen in the periodic paralyses. Although these are infrequent disorders, research into the pathologic processes has led to an improved understanding of the cell membrane.

Myotonia

Myotonia is both a physical and an electrical phenomenon. It is a delayed relaxation after such voluntary muscle contraction as grip, eye closure, or muscle percussion. The distinctive "dive bomber" noise, audible on needle EMG, is due to the prolonged depolarization of the muscle membrane. Because the depolarization is not terminated by neuromuscular blocking agents such as curare, the abnormality has been localized at the muscle membrane, outside the neuromuscular junction and sarcotubular system. (These structures are described in Chapter 38.)

In experimental animals, myotonia can be reproduced by removing extracellular chloride, thus reducing chloride conductance across the plasma membrane. The delicate balance in which sodium diffuses into the intracellular fluid, potassium diffuses out of the intracellular fluid, and chloride is in flux is thus interrupted. Because the normal diffusion processes (described in Chapter 3) stabilize the membrane, the shift in chloride ions is thought to increase membrane excitability. The chloride abnormality may explain the resting membrane hyperexcitability, but it does not explain the delayed relaxation present in myotonia and has not been detected in human myotonia.

Myotonia is seen in several disorders, myotonia congenita, paramyotonia congenita, myotonic muscular dystrophy, and some forms of periodic paralysis. Most are inherited disorders and are mild in symptomatology, with the exception of myotonic muscular dystrophy (see Chapter 40). Myotonia is treated by drugs that reduce muscle fiber excitability, such as procaine, procainamide, phenytoin, and quinine preparations. New treatments include acetazolamide, a carbonic anhydrase inhibitor, and verapamil, a calcium channel blocker.

Periodic Paralysis

During an attack of **periodic paralysis,** the muscle membrane is unresponsive to neutral stimuli, and the resting membrane potential is reduced from −90 to −45 millivolts. Periodic paralysis is triggered by exercise and any process or medication that increases serum potassium. The disorder is often inherited in an autosomal dominant pattern, although it can be seen in hyperthyroidism.

The paralysis, which leaves the individual flaccid and weak, does not affect the respiratory muscles. Many individuals have myotonia present on examination. In most cases the weakness is accompanied by a change in serum potassium, although in some individuals the change may be negligible. Cardiac dysrythmias have been present during attacks. Although the biochemical defect remains unknown, changes in the muscle membrane and sarcoplasmic reticulum have been described.

Hypokalemic periodic paralysis is triggered by high-carbohydrate meals, prolonged bed rest, or emotional stress. (The effects of potassium on the resting membrane potential is discussed in Chapter 3.) Glucose and insulin infusions and oral potassium loading are used as provocative tests; oral and intravenous potassium can relieve acute attacks. Treatment includes thiazides, diuretics, and a high-salt diet. Acetazolamide and a low-salt diet are useful for long-term therapy.

Metabolic Muscle Diseases

Disorders in muscle metabolism can be caused by endocrine abnormalities, or diseases of energy metabolism, such as glycogen storage disease, enzyme deficiencies, and abnormalities in lipid metabolism and mitochondrial function.

Endocrine Disorders

Often the systemic effects of hormonal imbalance overshadow the individual's muscular symptoms. For example, individuals with thyrotoxicosis may have signs of proximal weakness, paresis of the extraocular muscles (exophthalmic ophthalmoplegia), and, rarely, hypokalemic periodic paralysis. Hypothyroidism is often associated with an increase in muscle mass and strength. Common findings in hypothyroidism, myxedema, and delayed relaxation of the muscle stretch reflexes, can be confused with myotonia.

Thyroid hormone is believed to regulate muscle protein synthesis and electrolyte balance. Changes in muscle protein synthesis and electrolyte balance may, therefore, explain the changes in muscle mass and contractility seen in endocrine disorders. The muscular symptoms subside with appropriate treatment of the primary hormonal disorder.

Hyperparathyroidism also causes symptoms of muscular weakness and should be considered when the findings of proximal weakness, wasting, and fatigue, brisk reflexes, and bulbar symptoms predominate (Brooke, 1986).

Diseases of Energy Metabolism

The muscle relies on carbohydrates, such as glycogen and lipids (free fatty acids), for energy. When stored glycogen or lipids cannot be utilized due to a lack of the enzyme necessary to convert energy for contraction, the individual will experience cramps, fatigue, and exercise intolerance. Disorders of muscle metabolism can be self-limiting, such as is seen in McArdle disease and some lipid disorders, or cause widespread irreparable muscle destruction, as in acid maltase deficiency.

McArdle Disease

A severe metabolic defect in glycogen metabolism was first described in 1951 by B. McArdle, for whom the illness is named. Since then, three other deficiencies in glycotic enzymes have been described. **McArdle disease** was the first myopathy in which a single enzyme defect was identified. Although it is rare, over 110 cases have been reported from one clinic alone (Engel & Banker, 1986). Individuals with McArdle disease lack muscle phosphorylase, which is responsible for the breakdown of glycogen in muscle. Normally, after the body uses the short-term ATP and phosphocreatine stores, intramuscular lactic acid accumulates as glycogen is used (see Chapter 38). The individual with McArdle disease is not able to break down glycogen or produce lactic acid.

The lactic acid deficiency can be tested by nuclear magnetic resonance or the ischemic exercise test. On the nuclear magnetic resonance scan, lactic acid build-up appears as a change in the ratio of phosphocreatine to ATP and a decrease in muscle pH. The ischemic exercise test normally produces an exponential rise in the serum lactic acid, pyruvate, and ammonia levels following *intense* muscular work. For the individual with McArdle disease, however, there is no change in muscle pH in response to ischemic exercise.

The altered energy production manifests itself in exer-cise intolerance, fatigue, and painful muscle cramps. When exercise is carried to an extreme, painful muscle contracture and myoglobinuria develop. Some individuals describe a "second wind" phenomenon, in which exercise tolerance increases if they slow their pace once the initial sensation of fatigue commences. This may be caused by the use of free fatty acids as a secondary source of energy. As the disease progresses, some individuals have pronounced muscle weakness and wasting. Other organs are not involved, as the absence of phosphorylase is limited to muscle.

On muscle biopsy the muscle does not stain for myophosphorylase, and muscle cells demonstrate subsarcolemmal glycogen deposition and scattered necrotic fibers. Trials of glucose or fructose administration have been suggested to improve exercise tolerance, and a new high-fat, high-protein diet has received some support (Brooke, 1986). Generally, individuals with McArdle disease learn to adapt their daily routine to avoid muscle symptoms.

Acid Maltase Deficiency

Acid maltase deficiency is an uncommon glycogen storage disease associated with an accumulation of glycogen in the lysosomes of muscle cells and the cells of other tissues. The usual pathways of glycogen degradation are preserved. It appears that the absence of the enzyme acid maltase is responsible for the abnormality in glycogen metabolism, although the exact mechanism is unknown. It is an autosomal recessive disorder, with the gene located on the long arm of chromosome 17. Muscle biopsy shows vacuoles and glycogen deposition similar to the changes in McArdle disease, but the histochemical myophosphorylase reaction is normal.

The two forms of acid maltase deficiency are distinguished by the individual's age at onset. The infantile form is called **Pompe disease** and is recognized shortly after birth by hypotonia and an enlarged heart, tongue, and liver. Hypertrophy of these tissues is thought to be the result of glycogen deposition. The children die of cardiac or respiratory failure within a year of diagnosis. The adult variety becomes evident subacutely. The muscular symptoms resemble those of muscular dystrophy or polymyositis (see p. 1376). A distinguishing feature in adults may be the presence of severe respiratory muscle weakness (Brooke, 1986).

Myoadenylate Deaminase Deficiency

An enzyme deficiency that produces changes in skeletal muscle and is associated with exercise intolerance is **myoadenylate deaminase deficiency (MDD)**. Because of a lack of the enzyme myoadenylate deaminase, these individuals have a poor capacity for sustained energy production. Myoadenylate deaminase is the catalytic enzyme that forms phosphocreatine and ATP during exercise through a metabolic pathway that binds the purine and phosphate molecules that comprise ATP. Persons with MDD differ from those with McArdle disease in that, during the ischemic exercise test, lactate production is normal and ammonia production is absent. Ammonia is a by-product of the ATP and phosphocreatine synthesis. In muscle biopsies from affected individuals, cells fail to stain for the enzyme myoadenylate deaminase. The enzyme defect has been reported to be quite common, but in practice may be rarely recognized as a cause of exercise intolerance.

Lipid Deficiencies

Disorders of lipid metabolism are uncommon but account for severe changes in muscle metabolism. The lipid content of muscle cells consists of the free fatty acids, which are oxidized in the mitochondria. These acids require carnitine and the enzyme carnitine palmityl transferase (CPT) to transport metabolic by-products and energy to the myofibrils. Individuals with CPT deficiency have mild muscular symptoms but can experience bouts of renal failure caused by myoglobinuria. Individuals with a deficiency of carnitine alone have progressive muscle weakness and can experience sudden exacerbations.

Measuring the CPT and carnitine content in muscle aids in the diagnosis. Cells in the muscle biopsy will show vacuoles and lipid deposits. Treatments with riboflavin, medium-chain triglyceride, oral carnitine, and prednisone have been suggested (Brooke, 1977).

Inflammatory Muscle Diseases: Myositis
Viral, Bacterial, and Parasitic Myositis

Viral, bacterial, and parasitic infections of varying severity are known to produce inflammatory changes in skeletal muscle, a group of conditions collectively described by the term **myositis.** In the granulomatous diseases, tuberculosis and sarcoidosis, chronic inflammatory changes and granulomas are found in muscle as well as in other affected tissues. The parasitic infection trichinosis is said to affect up to 4% of the population. In trichinosis, *Trichinella* larvae reside in infected pork and, following ingestion, migrate to the intestinal mucosa and, from there, to the lymphatics. Symptoms include severe pain, rash, and muscle stiffness. Treatment includes administration of corticosteroids, prednisone, and the antiparasitic agent thiobendazole. Toxoplasmosis, a common parasitic infection, is also associated with a generalized polymyositis that responds rapidly to therapy.

In the tropics, more prevalent disorders include bacterial infections with *Staphylococcus aureus* and parasites such as cysticercus, the tape worm larva. Viral infections can be associated with an acute myositis. Muscle pain, tenderness, signs of inflammation, and creatine kinase elevation are common manifestations of viral myositis. The self-limiting symptoms of muscle aches and pains during a bout of influenza may actually be a subacute form of viral myopathy.

Polymyositis and Dermatomyositis

Polymyositis (generalized muscle inflammation) and **dermatomyositis** (polymyositis accompanied by skin lesions) are the most common inflammatory muscle diseases requiring chronic care. Prevalence rates are estimated to be up to 6 per 100,000.

Pathophysiology

Polymyositis and dermatomyositis are characterized by inflammation of connective tissue and muscle fibers that presumably causes the extensive necrosis and destruction of muscle fibers. The agent that causes the muscle inflammation has not been identified, but abnormalities in the immune system have been implicated. Experimental studies have not clarified whether the damage is produced by cell-mediated or humoral immune factors. There is growing support for the view that these two diseases should not be considered as a single autoimmune disease. Studies have shown that the inflammatory cells that surround the perimysial and perivascular sites are selectively enriched in Bcells and helper Tcells in dermatomyositis. (The immune response is discussed in Chapter 6.) Killer and natural killer T cells are rare. This suggests that a humoral immune mechanism may be an important factor.

The deposition of circulating immune complexes in the vascular endothelium is also present. This finding makes the presence of cell-mediated response difficult to exclude (Engel & Banker, 1986). There is less vascular involvement in polymyositis and a majority of the inflammatory cells, including B cells, T cells, and macrophages, surround the muscle fibers and fascicles. Immune complex deposits have not been located in the muscle fiber in polymyositis, but circulating antigen-antibody complexes were found in a majority of individuals (Brooke, 1986). Again, there is evidence for both cell-mediated and humoral immune responses.

Clinical Manifestations

The constellation of acute symptoms includes many of those seen in any inflammatory process: malaise, fever, muscle swelling, pain and tenderness, lethargy, and listlessness. Both illnesses are usually associated with a symmetric proximal muscle weakness and can be initially confused with other myopathies. They require a thorough evaluation to exclude other disorders. Clinical features common in both polymyositis and dermatomyositis are dysphagia, reduced esophageal motility, vasculitis, Raynaud phenomenon, cardiomyopathy, and interstitial pulmonary fibrosis. Some have other coexisting collagen vascular disorders, such as lupus and scleroderma.

The presence of skin rash, calcinosis, and eyelid edema most often suggests dermatomyositis. The skin rash is a purple (heliotrope) color and involves the eyelids, face, chest, and extensor surfaces of the extremities. Dermatomyositis is slightly more common in children and older adults, with an onset prior to age 15 and after age 50. The adult with dermatomyositis occasionally has underlying malignancies. Calcinosis, with calcium deposition in the subcutaneous tissue, can be a severe long-term complication of dermatomyositis.

Evaluation and Treatment

The muscle biopsy is striking in dermatomyositis, with most individuals showing inflammatory cells grouped around blood vessels and atrophy of cells in muscle fascile. This change, perifascicular atrophy, is absent in polymyositis. Creatine kinase and sedimentation rate are often acutely elevated in both disorders. EMG abnormalities include signs of muscle irritability and myopathic changes, usually large numbers of low-amplitude action potentials of brief duration. The EMG also shows a typical "myopathic" pattern, with short, low amplitude polyphasic potentials, as well as signs of marked muscle irritability.

Treatment primarily includes immunosuppressive drugs, although they are not always successful if uniformly applied. In one study, one third had functional disability after appropriate treatment for 4 years (Engel & Banker, 1986). Most clinicians choose corticosteroids initially, usually prednisone on a daily or alternating day schedule, tapering the dosage as the symptoms subside. Successful treatment with azathioprine, methotrexate, and cyclophosphamide has also been reported. All immunosuppressives have multiple side effects that require monitoring and frequent follow-up. Individuals with muscle weakness require careful physiotherapy to design a regular exercise program that prevents contractures and maximizes functional ability (Rowland, Clark, & Olarte, 1977).

Ocular Myopathies

Several rare muscle disorders cause particular severe ocular findings. One is **oculopharyngeal muscular dystrophy.** The age of onset for this autosomal dominant disorder is usually after age 40, with the symptoms of eyelid drooping (ptosis), ocular muscle weakness, difficulty swallowing (dysphagia), and weight loss. Occasionally, the individual will have mild proximal muscle weakness. Oculopharyngeal dystrophy is a mild, slowly progressive disorder. Findings are initially confined to ocular paresis and ptosis that spares the pupil. Later, the facial muscles may be involved. This disease is rare, but it appears to be clustered in two groups, Spanish-Amer-

icans in the southwestern United States and French-Canadians.

Diagnostic studies show only mild elevations in creatine kinase (CK) and a myopathic pattern on EMG. Muscle biopsy findings are generally similar to that of other individuals with dystrophic disorders, with the exception of intranuclear tubular filaments. These appear to be unique to this disease and may represent abnormal genetic material (Engel & Banker, 1986).

Ptosis and dysphagia are surgically correctable. Surgical elevation of the lids is recommended if visual acuity is impaired and lid crutches are helpful. The dysphagis seen in this disorder is often associated with a constriction of the circopharyngeus muscle, which, when released, permits a bolus of food to pass through the pharynx smoothly.

Chronic progressive external ophthalmoplegia (CPEO) is also characterized by ocular weakness. CPEO is known for the distinctive muscle biopsy finding of "ragged-red" fibers in 100% of cases. Mitochondrial abnormalities of the muscle fiber are an important feature of this disease. Whether or not a genetic defect causes these mitochondrial changes remains unclear (Engel & Banker, 1986). Individuals with CPEO have associated metabolic, cardiac, and neurologic deficits. Treatment of the lid weakness is the same as for oculopharyngeal muscular dystrophy.

Toxic Myopathies

The most common cause of **toxic myopathy** is alcohol abuse. Two clinical syndromes are prevalent: (1) an acute attack of muscle weakness, pain, and swelling after a binge; or (2) a more chronic, progressive proximal weakness in a drinker of long duration. The incidence of acute alcoholic myopathy has been estimated anywhere from 3% to 20% of individuals admitted with acute alcoholic withdrawal (Engel & Banker, 1986).

The pathologic abnormalities include necrosis of individual muscle fibers; whole segments can be found in the same stage of degeneration. Isolated, damaged fibers can be found next to undamaged fibers. Histochemistry of muscle biopsy specimens reveals patchy loss of oxidative enzymes in type I fibers. Electron microscopy reveals a marked accumulation of intracellular fluid and destruction of mitochondria (Engel & Banker, 1986). The mechanism by which alcohol affects the muscle fiber is uncertain, but direct toxic effect and nutritional deficiency have both received experimental support.

Acute alcoholic myopathy can range from benign cramps and pain resolving in a matter of hours, to severe weakness and markedly increased CK associated with myoglobinuria and renal failure. Individuals are prone to repeated attacks following recovery. The only treatment is abstinence from alcohol and improved nutrition. The individual with chronic alcoholic myopathy often has coexisting peripheral neuropathy that complicates the diagnosis.

Chemical agents have also been implicated in the development of myopathy. The drug chloroquine, an antimalarial and amebicial agent, in high doses has been associated with the development of generalized muscle weakness, particularly of the proximal muscles. Vacuoles and degeneration of muscle fibers, similar to that seen in glycogen storage disease, are present in muscle biopsies. These changes have been attributed to a molecular interaction between the drug and phospholipids in the cell with resultant accumulation on the lysosomes and impairment of the cell's digestive processes. Myopathy has also been caused by emetine (the major constituent of ipecac), vincristine, corticosteroids, and the toxic denatured rapeseed oil.

Rhabdomyolysis and myoglobinuria due to opioids (particularly heparin), clofibrate (hypolipidemic agent), the antifibrinolytic ε-amino capronate, and drugs that induce hypokalemia, such as amphotericin B, licorice, and azathioprine, have also been reported (Engle & Banker, 1986).

Repeated intramuscular injections have also been associated with changes in muscle fibers. Local necrosis of muscle fiber and elevated CK has been reported following intramuscular injections of cephalothin, lidocaine, diazepam, and digoxin; these effects were not produced with injections of saline. When drugs are injected over long periods of time, a chronic focal myopathy develops. Proliferation of connective tissue in both the muscle fiber and overlying skin and subcutaneous tissue has been reported. Over time, segments of the muscles, particularly the deltoid and quadriceps, are converted into fibrotic bands. These contractures have functional consequences. Contracture in the deltoid results in the arm becoming fixed in partial abduction. Pathophysiologic mechanisms for these changes include repeated needle trauma and infection, as well as nonphysiologic acidity and alkalinity of the injected material (Engel & Banker, 1986).

Muscle Tumors
Rhabdomyoma

Rhabdomyoma is a benign tumor of muscle, is extremely rare, and generally occurs in the tongue, neck muscles, larynx, uvula, nasal cavity, axilla, vulva, and heart. These tumors are usually treated by surgical excision and do not recur.

Rhabdomyosarcoma

Connective tissue sarcomas comprise 0.7% of all cancers; although they comprise 6.7% of all cancers in children under the age of 15 (DeVita, Hellman, & Rosenberg, 1985). (Muscle cancer in children is discussed in Chapter 40.) The malignant tumor of striated muscle is called rhabdomyosarcoma. The incidence of rhabdomy-

osarcoma ranges from 10% to 20% of all soft tissue cancers. Because of the relatively large size of muscles (40% of the total body weight, if tumor weight is related to body weight), rhabdomyosarcoma is the rarest of all tumors. This tumor is highly malignant because of rapid metastasis. The two age peaks in incidence statistics are 2 to 6 years and the early to late teens; although rhabdomyosarcoma can also be seen in adults and the elderly population. These tumors are located in the muscle tissue of the head, neck, and genitourinary tract in 75% of cases. The remainder are in the trunk and extremities.

There are three types of rhabdomyosarcoma differentiated on pathologic section: (1) pleomorphic, (2) embryonal, and (3) alveolar. The pleomorphic, or spindle cell, type is considered to be one of the most highly malignant tumors of the extremities seen in adulthood. Embryonal tumors are most frequently seen in childhood and appear to be shaped like a tadpole or tennis racket on biopsy. Alveolar type tumors appear latticelike and look like lung tissue alveoli.

The diagnosis of rhabdomyosarcoma is made by incisional biopsy and examination of the specimen by a pathologist. On electron microscopy, the tissue demonstrates myofilaments and Z-band material; computed tomography (CT) scan also helps define the tissue borders. Staging is based on pathologic grade of the tumor and is helpful in determining prognosis and treatment.

Treatment consists of a combination of surgical excision, radiation therapy, and systemic chemotherapy. Those individuals with only regional tumor growth, particularly tumors of the orbit and genitourinary tract, have been reported to have a 5 year survival of 76% (DeVita et al., 1985). Childhood rhabdomyosarcoma of any type with only regional involvement can be controlled in 60% of cases. Tumors of the trunk and extremities have a less favorable prognosis. Cure with distant metastasis is unlikely (DeVita et al., 1985).

Other Tumors

Metastatic deposits of tumors in muscles are rare in spite of the extensive vascular supply of skeletal muscles. It is suggested that local pH or metabolic changes prevent metastatic involvement from other tumors. When adjacent carcinomas do cause muscle damage, it is usually related to the compression of tissue and resultant muscle atrophy.

SUMMARY REVIEW

Musculoskeletal Injuries

1 One out of ten persons in the United States suffers an acute musculoskeletal injury each year.
2 The most serious musculoskeletal injury is a fracture. A bone can be completely or incompletely fractured. A

closed fracture leaves the skin intact. An open fracture has an overlying skin wound. The direction of the fracture line can be linear, oblique, spiral, or transverse. Greenstick, torus, and bowing fractures are examples of incomplete fractures that occur in children. Stress fractures occur in normal or abnormal bone that is subjected to repeated stress. Fatigue fractures occur in normal bone subjected to abnormal stress. Normal weight bearing can cause an insufficiency fracture in abnormal bone.

3 Dislocation is complete loss of contact between the surfaces of two bones. Subluxation is partial loss of contact between two bones. As a bone separates from a joint, it may damage adjacent nerves, blood vessels, ligaments, tendons, and muscle.

4 Tendon tears are called sprains and ligament tears are called strains. A complete separation of a tendon or ligament from its attachment is called an avulsion.

Disorders of Bones

1 Metabolic bone diseases are characterized by abnormal bone structure. In osteoporosis, the density or mass of bone is reduced because the bone remodeling cycle is disrupted. Osteomalacia is a metabolic bone disease characterized by inadequate bone mineralization. Excessive and abnormal bone remodeling occurs in Paget disease.

2 Osteomyelitis is a bone infection caused by bacteria. Bacteria can enter bone from outside the body (exogenous osteomyelitis) or from infection sites within the body (hematogenous osteomyelitis).

3 Bone tumors originate from bone cells, cartilage cells, fibrous tissue cells, or vascular marrow cells. Each cell produces a specific type of ground substance that is used to classify the tumor as osteogenic (bone cell), chondrogenic (cartilage cell), collagenic (fibrous tissue cell), or myelogenic (vascular marrow cell). Malignant bone tumors are large, aggressively destroy surrounding bone, invade surrounding tissue, and initiate independent growth outside the site of origin. Benign bone tumors are less destructive, limit their growth to the anatomic confines of the bone, and have a well-demarcated border.

Disorders of Joints

1 Noninflammatory joint disease is differentiated from inflammatory joint disease by the absence of synovial membrane inflammation, the absence of systemic signs and symptoms, and the presence of normal synovial fluid.

2 Degenerative joint disease is a noninflammatory joint disease characterized by the degeneration and loss of articular cartilage, sclerosis of underlying bone, and formation of bone spurs (osteophytes).

3 Rheumatoid arthritis is an inflammatory joint disease characterized by inflammatory destruction of the synovial membrane, articular cartilage, joint capsule, and surrounding ligaments and tendons. Rheumatoid nodules may also invade the skin, lung, spleen, and involve small and large arteries.

4 Ankylosing spondylitis is a chronic, inflammatory joint disease characterized by stiffening and fusion of the spine and sacroiliac joints.

5 Gout is a metabolic disorder associated with high levels of uric acid in the blood and body fluids. Uric acid crystallizes in the connective tissue of a joint where it initiates inflammatory destruction of the joint.

Disorders of Skeletal Muscle

1 A pathologic contracture is permanent muscle shortening due to muscle spasticity, as seen in CNS injury, or severe muscle weakness.

2 Stress-induced muscle tension is presumably caused by increased activity in the reticular activating system and gamma loop in the muscle fiber. The use of progressive relaxation training and biofeedback have been advocated to reduce muscle tension.

3 Atrophy of muscle fibers and overall diminished size of the muscle is seen following prolonged inactivity. Isometric contractions and passive lengthening exercises decrease atrophy to some degree in immobilized patients.

4 Hyperexcitable membranes cause the physical and electrical phenomenon, myotonia. The disorder is treated with drugs that reduce muscle fiber excitability. Periodic paralysis is caused by an unresponsive muscle membrane and is accompanied by changes in serum potassium. The biochemical defect is possibly related to changes in the muscle membrane and sarcoplasmic reticulum.

5 Metabolic muscle diseases are caused by endocrine disorders, glycogen storage disease, enzyme deficiencies, and abnormal lipid function. The muscle depends upon a complex system of carbohydrates and fats converted by enzymes to produce energy for the muscle cell. Abnormalities in these pathways can inhibit function or cause damage to the muscle fiber. These illnesses are rare, yet account for significant functional abnormalities.

6 Viral, bacterial, and parasitic infections of muscles produce the characteristic clinical and pathologic changes associated with inflammation. These are usually treatable and self-limiting disorders.

7 Polymyositis (generalized muscle inflammation) and dermatomyositis (polymyositis accompanied with skin lesions) are characterized by inflammation of connective tissue and muscle fibers, and muscle fiber necrosis. Cell-mediated and humoral immune factors have been implicated. Treatment with immunosuppressive agents is effective in many cases.

8 Oculopharyngeal muscular dystrophy differs from the more common muscular dystrophies in age of onset and affected musculature. It is a mild illness in which symptomatic therapy is often successful. Chronic, progressive external opthalnoplegia is characterized by multisystem deficits and ocular muscle weakness. Mitochondrial abnormality of the muscle fibers has been recognized.

9 The most common toxic myopathy is caused by alcohol abuse. Direct toxic effects of alcohol-producing necrosis

of muscle fibers and nutritional deficiency have been suggested. The only treatment is abstinence and improved nutrition. The toxic effects of many drugs on muscle fibers cause local trauma to the muscle fibers due to direct effects of the needle, secondary infection, and changes due to nonphysiologic acidity and alkalinity.

10 Sarcomas of muscle tissue are rare. Rhabdomyosarcoma has a uniformly poor prognosis due to an aggressive invasion and early, widespread dissemination. The usual treatment includes surgical excision, radiation therapy, and systemic chemotherapy.

KEY TERMS

Acid maltase deficiency, 1353

Ankylosing spondylitis, 1346

Avulsion, 1325

Biofeedback, 1351

Bowing fracture, 1321

Caplan syndrome, 1345

Chemical agents, 1356

Chondrogenic tumor (cartilage-forming tumor), 1337

Chondroid, 1337

Chondrosarcoma, 1337

Chronic progressive external ophthalmoplegia (CPEO), 1355

Collagenic tumor (collagen-forming tumor), 1337

Comminuted fracture, 1321

Complete fracture, 1320

Compound fracture (open fracture), 1320

Degenerative joint disease (osteoarthritis), 1339

Dermatomyositis, 1354

Dislocation, 1323

Endochondroma, 1337

Enthesis, 1346

Exogenous osteomyelitis, 1332

Fatigue fracture, 1321

Fibrosarcoma, 1338

Fracture, 1320

Geographic pattern, 1335

Giant cell tumor, 1338

Gout, 1347

Gouty arthritis, 1347

Greenstick fracture, 1321

Hematogenous osteomyelitis, 1332

Incomplete fracture, 1320

Inflammatory joint disease (arthritis), 1341

Insufficiency fracture, 1322

Involucrum, 1333

Ligament, 1325

Linear fracture, 1321

Malunion, 1323

McArdle disease, 1353

Motheaten pattern, 1335

Muscle strain, 1326

Myelogenic tumor, 1338

Myeloma, 1339

Myoadenylate deaminase deficiency (MDD), 1353

Myoglobulinuria, 1327

Myositis, 1354

Myositis ossificans, 1326

Myotonia, 1352

Noninflammatory joint disease, 1339

Nonunion, 1323

Oblique fracture, 1321

Oculopharyngeal muscular dystrophy, 1355

Osteogenic tumor (bone-forming tumor), 1335

Osteomalacia, 1330

Osteomyelitis, 1332

Osteophyte, 1340

Osteoporosis, 1328

Paget disease (osteitis deformans), 1331

Pannus, 1344

Pathological fracture, 1321

Periodic paralysis, 1352

Permeative pattern, 1335

Polymyositis, 1354

Pompe disease, 1353

Primary degenerative joint disease, 1340

Progressive relaxation training, 1351

Regional osteoporosis, 1329

Rheumatoid arthritis, 1342

Rheumatoid factor (RF), 1342

Rheumatoid nodule, 1345

Secondary degenerative joint disease, 1340

Simple fracture (closed fracture), 1321

Spiral fracture, 1321

Sprain, 1325

Strain, 1325

Stress fracture, 1321

Subluxation, 1323

Syndesmophyte, 1347

Tophaceous gout, 1350

Tophus, 1347

Torus fracture, 1321

Toxic myopathy, 1355

Transchondral fracture (osteochondritis dissecans), 1322

Transverse fracture, 1321

REFERENCES

Aegerter, E. E. & Kilpatrick, A., Jr. (1975). *Orthopedic diseases: Physiology, pathology, and radiology* (4th ed.). Philadelphia: W. B. Saunders.

Basmajian, J. V., & Deluca, C. J. (1985). *Muscle alive* (5th ed.). Baltimore: Williams & Wilkins.

Brooke, M. H. (1977). *A clinician's view of neuromuscular disease*. Baltimore: Williams & Wilkins.

Brooke, M. H. (1986). *A clinicians view of neuromuscular diseases* (2nd ed.). Baltimore: Williams and Wilkins.

Bywaters, E. G. (1980). Comparisons of the clinico-pathological aspects of ankylosing spondylitis, seropositive rheumatoid arthritis, and seronegative juvenile polyarthritis. *Scandinavian Journal of Rheumatology, 9,* 1-66.

DeGowin, E. L., & DeGowin, R. L. (1981). *Bedside diagnostic examination* (4th ed.). New York: Macmillan.

DeVita, V. T., Hellman, S., & Rosenberg, S. A. (1985). *Cancer: Principles and practice of oncology*. Philadelphia: J. B. Lippincott.

Emmerson, B. T. (1983). *Hyperuricemia and gout in clinical practice*. Boston: Adis Health Science Press.

Engel, A. G., & Banker, B. Q. (1986). *Myology*. New York: McGraw-Hill.

Feurstein, M., Labbe', E., & Kuczmierczyk, A. R. (1986). *Health psychology: A psychobiological perspective*. New York: Plenum.

Gecyz, A.F., Alexander, K., Bashir, H. V., Edmonds, J. P., Upfold, L., & Sullivan, J. (1983). HLA-B27, klebsiella and ankylosing spondylitis: Biological and chemical studies. *Immunological Review, 70,* 23-50.

Gordon, D. A. (1981). *Rheumatoid arthritis: Discussions in patient management*. New York: Medical Examination Publishing Company.

Griggs, R. G., & Donohoe, K. (1985). Emergency management of neuromuscular disease. *Handbook critical care neurology and neurosurgery*. New York: Praeger Press.

Hall, B. B., Fitgerald, R. H., Jr., & Rosenblatt, J. E. (1983). Anaerobic osteomylitis. *Journal of Bone and Joint Surgery, 65*(1), 30-35.

Kelley, W. N. (1972). Biochemistry of x-linked uric aciduria enzyme defect and its genetic variants. *Archives of Internal Medicine, 130,* 199-206.

Kelley, W., Harris, E., Ruddy, S., & Sledge, C. (1985). *Textbook of rheumatology*. Philadelphia: W. B. Saunders.

Kelsey, J. L. (1982). *Epidemiology of musculoskeletal disorders*. New York: Oxford University Press.

Kinsella, T. D., Fritzler, M. J., & McNeil, D. J. (1983). Ankylosing spondylitis, a disease in search of microbes. *Journal of Rheumatology, 10,* 2-4.

Kippin, I., Klineberg, J. R., Weinberger, A., & Wilcox, W. R. (1974). Factors affecting urate solubility in vitro. *Annals of Rheumatic Diseases, 33,* 313-317.

Kissane, J. M. (Ed.). (1985). *Anderson's Pathology* (8th ed.). St. Louis: C. V. Mosby.

Lodwick, G. S. (1983). Computeraided decision making slide. American Association of Physicist in Medicine, jointly sponsored by the Radiological Society of North America. Oak Brook, IL: The Soceity.

Mastaglia, F. L., & Walton, J. N. (1983). *Skeletal muscle pathology*. Churchill.

McArdle, B. (1951). Myopathy due to defect in muscle glycogen breakdown. *Clinical Sciencce, 10,* 13.

McCarthy, D. (1985). *Arthritis and allied conditions*. Philadelphia: Lea & Febiger.

McComas, A. J. (1977). *Neuromuscular function and disorders*. London: Butterworth.

McCune, W. J. (1989). *Monarticular arthritis*. In W. N. Kelley, E. D. Harris, S. Ruddy, & C. B. Sledge (Eds.), *Textbook of rheumatology* (3rd ed.). Philadelphia: W. B. Saunders.

Mirra, V. (1980). *Bone tumors: Diagnosis and treatment*. Philadelphia: J. B. Lippincott.

Persson, I., Adami, H., Bergkvist, L., Lindgren, A., Petterson, B., Hoover, R., & Schairer, C. (1989). Risk of endometrial cancer after treatment with estrogens alone or in conjunction with progestogens: Results of a prospective study. *British Medical Journal, 298,* 147-151.

Phipps, W. J., & Long, B. C., & Woods, W. F. (1987). *Medical surgical nursing: Concepts and clinical practice*. St. Louis: C. V. Mosby.

Raney, R., and Brashear, H: Shand's handbook of orthopaedic surgery, ed 8, St. Louis, 1971. The C.V. Mosby Co.

Resnick, D., & Niwayama, G. (1987). *Diagnosis of bone and joint disorders* (2nd ed.). Philadelphia: W. B. Saunders.

Robbins, S. L., Cotran, R. S., & Kumar, V. (1984). *Pathologic basis for disease*. Philadelphia: W. B. Saunders.

Rosai, J. (1989). *Ackerman's surgical pathology* (7th ed.). St. Louis: C. V. Mosby.

Rowland, L. P., Clark, C., & Olarte, M. (1977). Therapy for dermatomyositis and polymyositis. In R. G. Griggs & R. T. Moxley (Eds.), *Advances in neurology* (vol. 17). New York: Raven Press.

Rubin, P. (1983). *Clinical oncology: A multidisciplinary approach* (6th ed.). American Cancer Society.

Schlossteen, L., Terasaki, P. I., Bluestone, R., & Pearson, C. M. (1973). High association of HLA antigen W27 with ankylosing spondylitis. *New England Journal of Medicine, 288*(14), 704-706.

Scott, J. T., & Pollard, A. C. (1970). Uric acid excretion in relatives of patients with gout. *Annals of the Rheumatic Diseases, 29,* 397-400.

Simkin, P. A. (1973). Local concentration of urate in the pathogenesis of gout. *Lancet, 2,* 1295-1298.

Sullivan, J. S., Pendergast, S. D, & Geczy, A. F. (1983). The etiology of A.S. Does a plasmid trigger the disease in genetically susceptible individuals? *Human Immunology, 6,* 185-187.

Turek, S. L. (1984). *Orthopaedics: Principles and their application* (4th ed.). Philadelphia: J. B. Lippincott.

Urist, M. R. (Ed.). (1980). *Fundamentals and clinical bone physiology*. Philadelphia: J. B. Lippincott.

Vignos, P. L. (1983). Physical models of rehabilitation in neuromuscular disease. *Muscle and Nerve, 6,* 323-338.

Wyngaarden, J. B., & Kelley, W. N. (1976). *Gout and hyperuricemia*. New York: Grune and Stratton.

CHAPTER 40

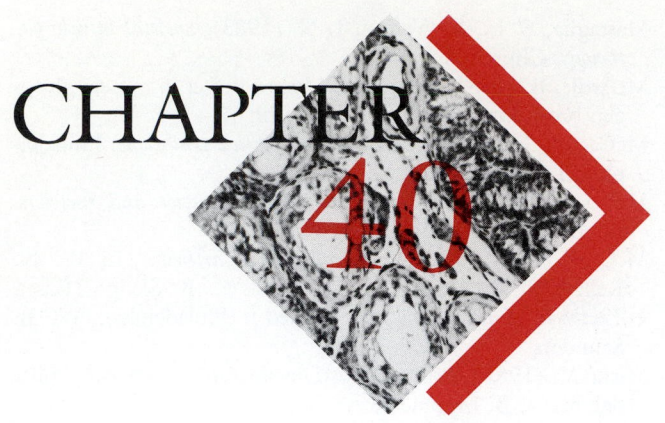

Alterations of Musculoskeletal Function in Children

Margaret M. Andrews
Kathleen Hardin Mooney

Musculoskeletal development in children, 1361
  Bone formation, 1361
  Bone growth, 1362
  Skeletal development, 1362
  Muscle growth, 1362
Musculoskeletal alterations in children, 1363
  Congenital defects, 1363
    Syndactyly, 1363
    Congenital dysplasia of the hip joint, 1363
      Pathophysiology, 1363
      Clinical manifestations, 1364
      Evaluation and treatment, 1364
    Talipes, 1364
      Pathophysiology, 1365
      Clinical manifestations, 1365
      Evaluation and treatment, 1365
    Congenital muscle disease, 1366
  Abnormal density or modeling of the skeleton, 1367
    Osteogenesis imperfecta, 1367
      Pathophysiology, 1367
      Clinical manifestations, 1367
      Evaluation and treatment, 1368
    Rickets, 1368
    Scoliosis, 1369
      Pathophysiology, 1369
      Clinical manifestations, 1370
      Evaluation and treatment, 1370
  Bone infection: osteomyelitis, 1370
    Pathophysiology, 1371
    Clinical manifestations, 1372
      Infants, 1372
      Children, 1372
      Adolescents and adults, 1372
    Evaluation and treatment, 1372
  Juvenile rheumatic arthritis, 1373
  Avascular diseases of the bone: osteochondrosis, 1373

Legg-Calvé-Perthes disease, 1374
  Pathophysiology, 1374
  Clinical manifestations, 1374
  Evaluation and treatment, 1375
Osgood-Schlatter disease, 1375
  Pathophysiology, 1375
  Clinical manifestations, 1375
  Evaluation and treatment, 1375
Muscular dystrophy, 1376
  Duchenne muscular dystrophy, 1376
    Pathophysiology, 1377
    Clinical manifestations, 1377
    Evaluation and treatment, 1378
  Becker muscular dystrophy, 1378
  Facioscapulohumeral muscular dystrophy, 1378
  Scapuloperoneal muscular dystrophy, 1379
  Limb girdle muscular dystrophy, 1379
  Myotonic muscular dystrophy, 1379
    Pathophysiology, 1379
    Clinical manifestations, 1380
    Evaluation and treatment, 1380
Musculoskeletal tumors in children, 1380
  Bone tumors, 1380
    Osteosarcoma, 1380
    Pathophysiology, 1381
    Clinical manifestations, 1381
    Evaluation and treatment, 1381
    Ewing sarcoma, 1382
    Pathophysiology, 1382
    Clinical manifestations, 1382
    Evaluation and treatment, 1382
    Fibroma, 1382
  Muscle tumors, 1382
    Pathophysiology, 1383
    Clinical manifestations, 1383
    Evaluation and treatment, 1384

MUSCULOSKELETAL DEVELOPMENT IN CHILDREN

Bone Formation

Bone formation, which begins at about the eighth week of gestation, involves two phases: (1) the delivery of bone cell precursors to sites of bone formation and (2) the aggregation of these cells at **primary centers of ossification,** where they mature and begin to secrete osteoid (see Chapter 38). Some of the bone cell precursors are present in fetal connective tissues, whereas others migrate in blood to sites of bone formation after blood vessels have grown into the tissue.

Cellular aggregation and maturation occur in two types of fetal tissue, depending on which bones are being formed. The cranium, facial bones, clavicles, and parts of the jaw bone arise from a fetal membrane termed the mesenchyme. Bones that develop on or within the mesenchyme grow by the process of **intramembranous formation.** As the mesenchyme becomes vascularized, the immature bone cells aggregate and mature into osteoblasts, which form the centers of ossification. Osteoblasts secrete osteoid, which surrounds them and quickly ossifies, forming the lacunae and canaliculae of compact bone. Spicules of bone radiate from the ossification centers to form the primary trabeculae characteristic of spongy bone. Later, some of the spongy bone is replaced by compact bone.

Endochondral formation is the development of new bone from cartilage. This process, by which the long bones of the appendicular skeleton develop, is more complex than intramembranous formation (Fig. 40-1). First, mesenchymal tissue forms a **cartilage model,** which defines the shape of the bone. The cartilage model is subsequently removed and replaced by bone. Endochondral bone formation begins in the outer layer of the cartilage model, which consists of a layer of dense connective tissue called **perichondrium.** The perichondrium contains cells that develop into osteoblasts, forming a collar of bone, termed the **periosteal collar,** around the cartilage model. Cartilage enclosed within the periosteal collar degenerates, and capillaries from outside the perichondrium invade the degenerating cartilage cells, carrying with them osteoblast precursors from the inner layer of the perichondrium and osteoclast precursors from the blood itself.

Endochondral bone formation begins at the primary center of ossification in the middle of the cartilage model and extends toward either end of the developing bone. At the same time, the periosteal collar thickens and becomes wider toward the epiphyses. By the end of gestation, **secondary centers of ossification,** the epiphyseal centers, begin to lay down bone at both ends of the cartilage model. Here, too, cartilage within the periosteal collar degenerates, and blood vessels grow inward, delivering bone cell precursors. Once the osteoblasts begin to secrete osteoid, ossification spreads from the secondary centers in all directions until all the cartilage within the model is replaced by bone.

Two regions of cartilage remain at the ends of long bones: (1) articular cartilage over the free ends of the bone and (2) the epiphyseal plate, a layer of cartilage between the diaphysis and epiphysis. (These structures

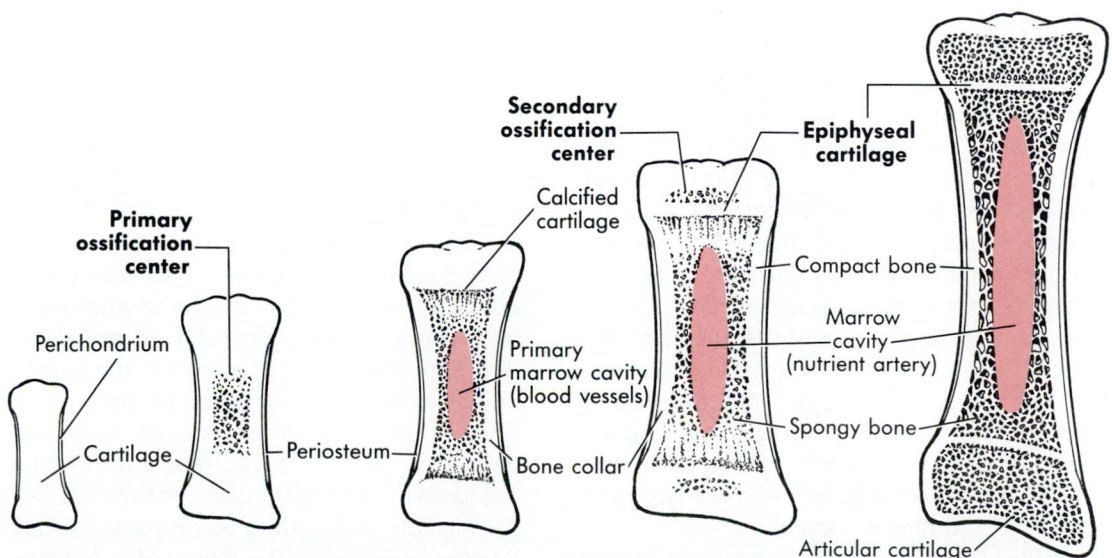

FIG. 40-1. Stages of endochondral bone formation and centers of ossification in long bone.

are described and illustrated in Chapter 38; see Figure 38-1.) The epiphyseal plate retains the ability to form and calcify new cartilage and deposit bone until the skeleton matures (at approximately 18 years of age).

Bone Growth

Until adult stature is reached, growth in the length of bone occurs at the epiphyseal plate through endochondral ossification. Cartilage cells in the proximal layer of the epiphyseal plate multiply and enlarge. As rapidly as new cartilage cells form, cartilage cells at the metaphyseal side of the plate are destroyed and replaced by bone.

In the shaft of new bone, where growth is relatively slow, the bone produced by accretion is compact and dense. The compact bone is thickest where it has to withstand the maximal stresses, which generally occur in the middle of the shaft.

More growth always takes place at one end of a long bone than at the other. The more active end is sometimes known as the "growing end" of the bone, and it is the end most likely to sustain a growth disturbance after injury. There are important differences in the rates of growth of individual bones. For example, the growing end of the femur lengthens twice as fast as the growing end of the tibia. The longitudinal growth rate of the extremities is greater at birth than at any other time. Longitudinal growth occurs by division of the cartilage cells on the epiphyseal side of the growth plate and by continued replacement of the calcified cartilage by bone on the metaphyseal side.

Growth in the diameter of bone occurs by deposition of new bone on an existing bone surface. Bone matrix is laid down by osteoblasts on the periosteal surface and subsequently becomes calcified. At the same time, bone resorption occurs on the endosteal surface. Endosteal resorption increases the diameter of the medullary cavity, which contains marrow and spongy bone.

Many factors affect the development, physiology, and rate of growth of the epiphyseal plate. Growth hormone has to be secreted by the pituitary gland at a constant rate to stimulate the growth plate consistently. Other known factors affecting growth include genetic makeup, nutrition, general health, and other hormones, such as thyroid hormone, adrenal and gonadal androgens, and estrogens. These factors influence both the rate of bone growth and the time of appearance of the secondary ossification centers. When the skeleton is mature, the epiphyseal plate is replaced by bone. This process, termed epiphyseal closure, unites the diaphysis and the epiphysis. Epiphyseal closure occurs earlier in females than males because of the accelerating influence of estrogens on cartilage growth and matrix formation.

Throughout life, bone is constantly being destroyed and reformed (see Chapter 38), but the process is at its maximum in children about 2½ years old. By young adulthood, bone turnover, or remodeling, occurs at a relatively low rate.

Skeletal Development

The axial skeleton changes shape with growth. (The axial skeleton and appendicular skeleton are described and illustrated in Chapter 38; see Fig. 38-3.) In a newborn the entire spine is concave anteriorly; the child's natural posture is "curled up." In the first 3 months of life, with the ability to control the head, the upper (cervical) spine begins to "arch," or become convex anteriorly. The normal arch in the lower (lumbar) spine begins to develop with sitting.

The appendicular skeleton (the extremities) grows faster during childhood than does the axial skeleton. The neonate has a relatively large head and long spine with disproportionately shorter limbs than an adult. By age 1, 50% of the total growth of the spine has occurred (Winter, 1977). Therefore failure of the spine to grow (e.g., spinal fusion) does not limit eventual height as much as the premature fusion of the growth plates of the lower extremities. In children with congenital curvature of the spine, growth tends to worsen the deformity rather than increase the length of the spine.

Besides getting longer, growing bones of the extremities undergo changes in rotation and alignment. In the newborn the femur is flexed forward up to 40 degrees, and the tibia is rotated inward. With growth, the femur assumes its normal alignment and tibial rotation disappears, usually at age 8. Bowlegs and knock-knees are normal at certain stages of growth. At birth, the neonate's legs are bowed because of stresses in utero. With growth, the knees gradually turn inward approximately 7 to 8 degrees, which is normal alignment in adults.

Muscle Growth

The composition and size of muscles varies with age. In the fetus muscle tissue contains a large amount of water and much intercellular matrix. After birth, both are reduced considerably as the muscle fibers (cells) enlarge by accumulating cytoplasm. Little information is available about the numbers of fibers in a given muscle at different ages, but the total mass of muscle in the body can be estimated from the amount of creatinine excreted in the urine because the conversion of creatine to creatinine takes place only in muscle (see Chapter 38). Between birth and maturity, the number of muscle nuclei in the body increases 14 times in boys and 10 times in girls. Muscle fibers reach their maximal size in girls at about the age of 10 and in boys by the age of 14. Growth in length occurs at the ends of muscles and the increase in length is accompanied by an increase in number of nuclei in the fibers. Muscle fibers increase in diameter as the fibrils become more numerous. The fibrils themselves do not increase in diameter. Connective tissue components of muscle grow where the tendon and muscle meet.

A potent stimulus to the growth of a muscle is the separation of its attachments as the skeleton grows. The length of a muscle fiber is the direct consequence of the range of movement it is called on to perform. The stimulus for the formation of a tendon is probably the pull of the muscle rudiment on undifferentiated connective tissue. The repair of a tendon from which a segment has been removed does not occur if the muscle is prevented from exercising tension on the damaged tendon. Replacement of muscle by tendon (tendinification) sometimes is the result of limitation of movement. If the normal opponents of a muscle are paralyzed, the muscle fails to grow properly, and it may be that the full development of a muscle is dependent on the progressive rise in the tension exerted on it by its antagonists.

Muscle growth during adolescence is a major factor in weight gain. Sex differences in muscle size and weight are minor in childhood, but become considerable with the onset of puberty.

In the infant muscle accounts for approximately 25% of total body weight compared with 40% in the adult. The muscles of the head, trunk, and upper limbs are relatively heavier in the infant because the lower extremities are poorly developed. In the adult, about 55% of muscle weight is accounted for by the lower limb muscles. The respiratory and facial muscles are well developed at birth so that the infant can perform the vital functions of breathing and sucking. Other muscle groups, such as the pelvic muscle, take several years to develop fully. Throughout life, the weight of the skeletal muscles can be increased by exercise. Less is known about the development of visceral and cardiac muscle. Visceral muscle fibers increase both in number and size, but the increase in fiber size is most important. Fiber enlargement alone can increase the bulk of visceral muscle by as many as eight times. Cardiac muscle also grows mainly by enlargement of existing fibers.

MUSCULOSKELETAL ALTERATIONS IN CHILDREN

Congenital Defects

Syndactyly

The most common congenital defect of the upper extremity is **syndactyly,** or webbing of the fingers (Fig. 40-2). Simple webbing involves the soft tissue envelope alone and is best released surgically when the child is 3 to 4 years of age. True syndactyly involves fusion of the bones and nails as well as the soft tissues, and may be associated with absence or anomaly of bony or neurovascular units. The primary goal in surgical correction

of these defects is to achieve maximal function and appearance. Ideally, corrective surgery is deferred until the child is 6 to 12 months of age and completed before the child enters school. **Vestigial tabs,** such as an extra digit, are best removed during the immediate neonatal period, however. Any neonate with a congenital anomaly of the upper extremity is examined for associated systemic anomalies, particularly of the heart and kidneys.

Congenital Dysplasia of the Hip Joint

Congenital hip dysplasia, or dislocation of the hip joint, is due to abnormal development of one or all of the components of the hip joint: the acetabulum (cup-shaped cavity in the pelvic girdle); the femoral head, which fits into the acetabulum; and the surrounding joint capsule and soft tissues.

The incidence of neonatal hip instability is about 1 in 60 live births. In most cases the hip stabilizes and becomes normal with time. Females are affected six to eight times more frequently than males. The left hip is affected three times more frequently than the right, perhaps because in utero the fetus's back is usually turned to the mother's left side, a position in which the lower left leg is pressed against the mother's lower spine. The pressure results in femoral adduction and possible anteversion, and the fetus is unable to move or kick the leg, preventing normal joint development.

The cause of congenital dysplasia of the hip is clearly multifactorial. There is a family history of congenital hip dysplasia in 20% to 30% of cases, which suggests genetic transmission of the disorder. Congenital hip dysplasia is also associated with first pregnancies (perhaps because of the mother's tight abdominal musculature), oligohydramnios (deficient volume of amniotic fluid), premature rupture of the amnion, spina bifida, breech presentation (up to 30%), and delivery by cesarean section. Maternal hormones have been reported to increase joint laxity, and studies have demonstrated changes in estrogen metabolism and excretion in infants with congenital hip dysplasia.

Environmental factors and local customs can exacerbate congenital hip instability. Neonatal hip dysplasia is common, for example, among the Lapps and American Indians, who swaddle their infants and secure them to cradle boards because this practice maintains the hips and adduction. Neonatal hip dysplasia is rare in Central Africa, Japan, China, and India where infants are carried with their hips flexed and abducted on the parent's hip or around the parent's back.

Pathophysiology

There are three main forms of congenital hip dysplasia: typical, fetal, and congenital dislocations. Typical dislocation, which takes place at or near the time of birth, is easily reduced in the newborn infant. Fetal dislocation, which occurs in utero usually early in fetal life, is characterized by displacement of the femoral head, a dysplastic (cartilaginous) acetabulum, and taut soft tissues. Fetal dislocation cannot be reduced by manipulation and requires early surgical treatment by open reduction and femoral shortening. Congenital dislocation of neuromuscular origin is associated with conditions involving contracture of the joint and with myelomeningocele.

Congenital hip dysplasia can be further classified according to severity. Most severe is a dislocated hip, in which the femoral head is completely displaced from the acetabulum (Fig. 40-3). In the dislocatable hip, the femoral head is in the acetabulum but can be totally displaced from the acetabulum by passive manipulation. In the subluxated hip, the femoral head is displaced laterally and proximally but not totally dislocated.

Clinical Manifestations

The neonate with congenital hip dysplasia usually

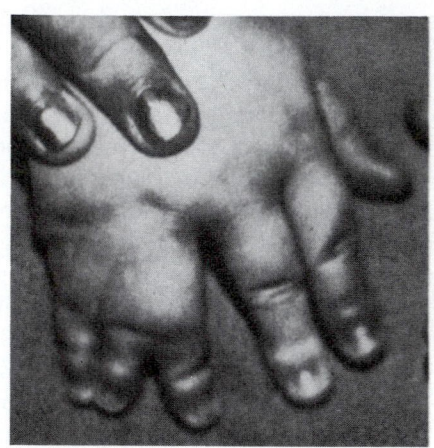

FIG. 40-2. Syndactyly.

does not exhibit abduction tightness or contracture. Therefore the diagnostic test at birth is demonstration of instability during physical examination. Signs of asymmetric skin folds, limited abduction, femoral shortening, and limited rotation may be present but are insufficient indications of dislocation.

Evaluation and Treatment

In the newborn period, the primary diagnostic tools are tests performed during the physical examination. In older infants and children radiographic examination is used to confirm the diagnosis.

Treatment depends on the age of the child and the duration of the hip dysplasia. The goal of treatment is to hold the legs in abduction until the joint capsule tightens. This can be accomplished with splints, braces, traction, or special casts. In a child whose dislocation of the hip has not been discovered until after 18 months of age, surgical intervention is often required.

Talipes

Talipes is a general term used to describe congenital deformities of the foot (Fig. 40-4). Talipes equinovarus (clubfoot) is the most common type, accounting for 95% of cases. Incidence of talipes is approximately 2 per 2000 live births. It is usually bilateral and affects males twice as often as females. Although the cause of talipes remains unkown, a neuromuscular cause has been implicated.

Pathophysiology

Arrested or abnormal embryonic development has been implicated in the development of talipes. The foot normally goes through a stage flexion and eversion during early development but gradually assumes a normal position by the seventh month. Arrested development during this early stage tends to result in a rigid defor-

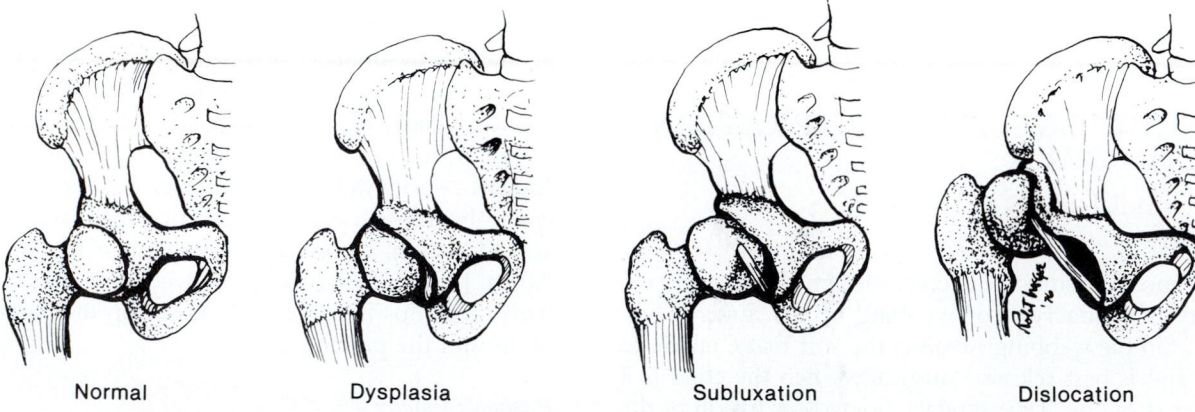

| Normal | Dysplasia | Subluxation | Dislocation |

FIG. 40-3. Configuration and relationship of structures in congenital hip deformities. (From Whaley & Wong, 1987.)

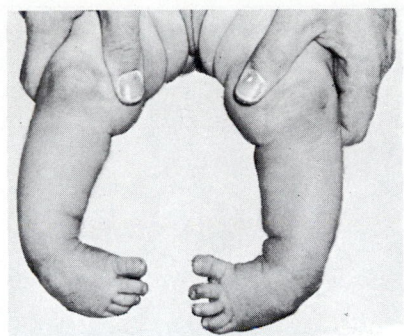

FIG. 40-4. Infant with bilateral congenital talipes equinovarus. (From Brashear & Raney, 1978.)

mity. The muscles on the posterior and medial aspect of the leg become unduly short, and the fibrous capsules (joint capsules) of all the deformed joints are thick and contracted on the concave side of the deformity. Soft tissue contractures become progressively resistant to correction, both in utero and after birth, and lead to secondary changes that involve the shape of the actively growing bones and the joints.

Clinical Manifestations

Talipes equinovarus, in which the heel and forefoot are inverted, the forefoot is adducted, and the entire foot is plantar flexed, is most severe. **Talipes calcaneovalgus** is characterized by eversion of the heel and forefoot, abduction of the forefoot, and dorsiflexion of the entire foot. (Terms that describe foot positions are defined in Table 40-1.)

Functional deformities of the feet as a result of in utero positioning frequently mimic talipes. These can be distinguished in that the functionally deformed foot can be easily brought to a neutral position and overcorrected. This is not possible when pathologic deformities are present.

Evaluation and Treatment

The deformity is readily observable and easily detected at birth. It must be differentiated, however, from other positional deformities that can be passively corrected or overcorrected. The true clubfoot is immobile.

Casting is usually required for initial correction of talipes. Tenotomies, muscle transplants, and arthrodeses (surgical fixation of joints) are necessary, in severe cases, when the child is older. Functional deformities are self-correcting and require no treatment at all.

Early treatment of talipes is critical and is started within the first hours after birth, when the joints of the foot are most flexible. Depending on the particular deformity, treatment for talipes may include:

1. Weekly application of a plaster cast (for about 6 weeks).

2. Denis Browne type of splint, in which the feet are strapped by adhesive tape and the affected foot is progressively turned to a normal position. The adhesive is changed weekly for about 12 weeks.
3. Denis Browne type of boot splint, which is worn day and night for 3 months, after which it is left off for increasingly longer periods until the child is walking.
4. Straight-last, outflare boots for day wear until age 3 years and occasionally the addition of an outside sole wedge.
5. Surgical treatment, the extent of which depends on the severity of the deformity.

If treatment is begun at birth, the foot may look relatively normal after 1 year. The lateral part of the foot will always have excess soft tissue, however, and the calf of that leg will be thinner. Because talipes tends to recur, orthopedic care is necessary throughout childhood. Approximately 10% of talipes are treated successfully without surgery.

Congenital Muscle Disease

Congenital muscle disorders, or myopathies, are rare and are generally mild. The possible congenital myopathies include congenital absence of muscles (failure of muscle cells to differentiate to a given region), congenital hypoplasia (local or generalized), congenital hyperplasia (local or generalized), faulty intrinsic development leading to disfigurement of fibers, and presenile abiotrophy (senescent polymyopathy).

Some persons are born without certain muscles. The muscles may be irrelevant in some instances or very important in others. The most commonly absent muscles are the pectoralis, trapezius, serratus anticus, and quadratus femoris. Congenital muscle absence is associated with other congenital abnormalities.

Many congenital deformities in children are a result of shortened muscles. Some conditions, such as myokymia and neuromyotonia, involve continuous muscle activity. Some true contracture states involve a contracted muscle's inability to relax because of a failure in the metabolic mechanism required for relaxation, such as in McArdle disease (see Chapter 39), in which there is a phosphorylase deficiency and a phosphofructokinase deficiency. Congenital myotonia (Thomsen disease) is a rare hereditary disease having two forms and is characterized by myotonia and muscular hypertrophy. Because no morphologic changes are evident in the muscles, an abnormality in the contracting mechanism must be the cause.

Because of new histologic technology in the past 25 years, a group of congenital polymyopathies that show an unusual pattern of central densification of sacroplasm (cores) has been described. This group of diseases in-

TABLE 40-1   Terms used to describe foot abnormalities

Term	Definition
POSITION	
Abduction	Lateral deviation away from the midline of the body
Adduction	Lateral deviation toward the midline of the body
Eversion	Twisting of the foot outward along its long axis
Inversion	Twisting of the foot inward on its long axis
Dorsiflexion	Bending of the foot upward and backward
Plantar flexion	Bending of the foot downward and forward
ABNORMALITY	
Talipes	Congenital abnormality of the foot (clubfoot)
Pes	Acquired deformity of the foot
Varus	Inversion and adduction of the heel and forefoot
Valgus	Eversion and abduction of the heel and forefoot
Equinus	Plantar flexion of the foot in which the heel is lower than the toes
Calcaneus	Dorsiflexion of the foot in which the heel is lower than the toes
Planus	Flattening of the medial longitudinal arch of the foot (flatfoot)
Cavus	Elevation of the medial longitudinal arch of the foot (high arch)
Equinovarus	Coexistent equinus and varus deformities
Calcaneovarus	Coexistent calcaneus and varus deformities
Equinovalgus	Coexistent equinus and valgus deformities
Calcaneovalgus	Coexistent calcaneus and valgus deformities

NOTE: The positions listed can all be achieved by voluntary movement of the normal foot; an abnormality exists if the foot is fixed in one or more of the positions while at rest.

volves a basic morphologic abnormality. Included in this category of congenital myopathies are central core disease, nemaline (rod-body) myopathy, mitochondrial (lipid storage) myopathy, and central myotubular myopathy.

Evidence first suggested that these myopathies are always manifested in infancy as delayed motor development with signs of hypotonia and weakness of the limbs, but now they have been shown to emerge later in life as well—up to middle age. Extremely slow progression characterizes these perhaps misnamed congenital myopathies.

Most diagnoses of congenital muscle disease that are made in childhood involve infants that are "floppy" at birth or show delays in reaching milestones for motor development. The muscle weakness does not fit the genetic pattern or progressive course of the muscular dystrophies (see p. 1376) or equal the distribution and severity seen in anterior horn cell disease. The distribution of weakness is usually greater in the limbs, particularly the quadriceps and elbow flexors, than in the bulbar musculature. Many disorders are not progressive and are associated with spinal deformities and hip dislocations.

Congenital muscle diseases are usually categorized by the striking abnormalities seen on muscle biopsy. Type I fiber predominance and fiber atrophy are also common features on muscle biopsy. Diagnosis is confirmed by histologic stain and phase and electron microscopy.

No specific treatment is yet available. Children require aggressive physiotherapy programs early in the course of the illness to prevent contractures and potentially improve strength. One study reported improvement in strength after a mild isometric exercise program in children with central core disease. In other respects the congenital myopathies require the same treatment programs followed for other individuals with neuromuscular disease. Cardiopulmonary failure is seen in myotubular myopathy and nemaline myopathy. These children should be closely monitored for any treatable complications, and families should be prepared for the difficult decision regarding ventilatory support that may ensue (Brooke, 1977).

A small number of cases are known to have been inherited in an autosomal dominant, autosomal recessive, or X-linked recessive pattern. Therefore genetic counseling, with documentation of a detailed pedigree and calculation of risk factors, is in order for young parents.

Abnormal Density or Modeling of the Skeleton
Osteogenesis Imperfecta

Osteogenesis imperfecta (brittle bone disease) is an inherited disorder of connective tissues that primarily affects bone. The disorder was first described in 1840 as a syndrome in newborns consisting of osteoporosis with fractures and skeletal deformities. The most severe form, **osteogenesis imperfecta congenita,** usually causes stillbirth or death soon after birth, although some neonates survive into childhood. Osteogenesis imperfecta congenita is obvious at birth because fractures and deformity have already occurred in utero. The less severe form, **osteogenesis imperfecta tarda,** usually becomes evident when the child begins to walk. Some children with this form experience numerous fractures in infancy and can be mistaken for battered children.

The incidence of the most common form, osteogenesis imperfecta, is about 1 in 40,000 live births. Inheritance is usually autosomal dominant but can be autosomal recessive. At least four syndromes have been identified that have various clinical manifestations and prognoses.

Pathophysiology

The major errors in osteogenesis imperfecta lie in the synthesis of collagen (Sykes, 1987). Very recent genetic studies have shown that the gene responsible for the encoding of collagen is "remarkably feeble," that is, easily mutates (Sykes, 1987). These mutations cause osteogenesis imperfecta. The large range of phenotypes are all mutants of the two collagen structural genes. (Genes are discussed in Chapter 4.) Abnormalities in collagen include: (1) an increase in collagen hydroxylysine residue in bones; (2) a decrease in hydroxylysino-norleucine in skin collagen; and (3) absence of alpha-2-polypeptide production in cultured skin fibroblasts (Zaleske, Doppelt, & Mankin, 1986).

A number of metabolic abnormalities have been reported. Some individuals have increased serum thyroxine levels suggesting hyperthyroidism. This is consistent with the findings of increased sweating, heat intolerance, increased body temperature, a resting tachycardia, and tachypnea. However, the hyperthyroid findings are not consistent in all individuals with osteogenesis imperfecta. Studies of leukocyte metabolism suggest an uncoupling of oxidative phosphorylation. Reports of alterations of platelet function with defects in adhesion and clot retraction also exist.

Clinical Manifestations

The classic clinical manifestations of osteogenesis imperfecta are bone fractures; osteoporosis; abnormally short, bowed, and deformed limbs; short stature; curvature of the spine; and bluish discoloration of the sclera (whites of the eyes) (Fig. 40-5). Four syndromes of clinical manifestations, designated type I through IV, have been identified. The most severe, types II and III, are osteogenesis imperfecta congenita. These two types are characterized by autosomal recessive inheritance and early onset of manifestations. Both can cause stillbirth or severe neonatal deformity and a short life expectancy. Less severe are types I and IV, which comprise osteogenesis imperfecta tarda. Types I and IV are slightly more common than types II and III. Types I and IV are inherited as autosomal dominant traits and vary in age of onset from birth to adulthood. Some children with type IV disease improve at puberty.

Evaluation and Treatment

Evaluation of osteogenesis imperfecta is based on clinical manifestations and serologic tests. Serum alkaline phosphatase is elevated in all forms of the disease.

For osteogenesis imperfecta congenita type II, no therapeutic intervention will be effective. For other types of osteogenesis imperfecta, careful positioning of the neonate on a firm mattress or pillows may prevent fractures. Beyond the neonatal period, various orthopedic measures are applied, such as prompt splinting of fractures and correction of deformities arising from the progressive bowing or bending of the skeleton. Although no clear benefit has been demonstrated, therapeutic regimens including supplements of calcium or fluoride, vitamin C, or magnesium oxide have been tried. Calcitron has been reported to increase the skeletal mass and decrease the frequency of fracture in some cases. Genetic counseling for affected families should aim at primary prevention (Behrman & Vaughan, 1983).

Rickets

Rickets is a disorder in which growing bone fails to become mineralized (ossified), resulting in "soft" bones and skeletal deformity. Incidence of rickets is greatest in children who receive insufficient dietary vitamin D, a mineral that is necessary for absorption and metabolism of calcium and phosphorus, the main minerals in bone. The pathophysiology of rickets is the same as that of osteomalacia, the "adult form" of rickets (see Chapter 39). The difference between osteomalacia and rickets is that in osteomalacia new bone formed during remodeling fails to ossify, whereas in rickets, new bone formed at the growing ends of bones fails to ossify.

The characteristic bone changes in rickets are identified in the epiphyseal plates (growth plates) before closure. The normal epiphyseal plate is a complex organized structure located at the ends of long bones between the epiphysis and metaphysis. The plate is organized into four distinct layers. The first layer, adjacent to the epiphysis, is composed of a few spherical cartilage

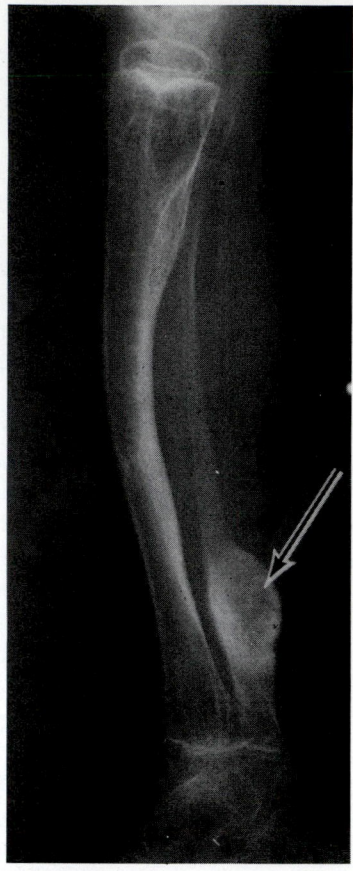

FIG. 40-5. Severely osteopenic and distorted tibia and fibula of child with osteogenesis imperfecta. Healing fracture shows abundant callus formation. (Courtesy Dr. James W. Debnam, Jr., Chesterfield, MS. From Kissane, 1985.)

cells (chondrocytes) randomly arranged in pairs. Their primary function is to store nutrients. The second layer is composed of flattened chondrocytes arranged longitudinally in parallel columns. The cells in this layer divide and produce cartilaginous matrix (see Chapter 38 for a description of bone formation). The third layer is composed of large spherical cells that participate in ossification of the cartilaginous matrix. The fourth layer is located within the metaphysis. This layer contains bars of collagen fibers that are partially or completely ossified. The bars are sheathed with osteoblasts that produce layers of osteoid.

In rickets the structure of the growth plate and metaphysis is disorganized. The first and second layers may not be significantly altered, but the third layer is grossly abnormal. There is a disorganized increase in the number of cells that decreases the length and width of the growth plate. In the fourth layer the cartilage bars are disorganized and decreased in size and number. In the metaphysis there is disorganized formation of lamellae and haversian systems.

Children with rickets are listless and irritable. They have profound hypotonia and muscle weakness and may be unable to walk without support. Abnormal parietal flattening and frontal bossing occur in the skull. The calvaria become soft and the sutures may widen. Cartilaginous attachments of the ribs become prominent, and the long bones of the extremities (tibia, femur, radius, and ulna) may be bowed. Growth is retarded, and fractures are common.

Scoliosis

Scoliosis is a lateral S-shaped or C-shaped curvature of the spinal column (Fig. 40-6). The milder form, **nonstructural scoliosis** (also termed postural scoliosis), does not involve permanent structural deformities of the spine and can be corrected by bending, exercises, or removal of an underlying disorder. **Structural scoliosis,** on the other hand, involves deformity or twisting of the vertebrae and, depending on the severity of the spinal curvature, compensatory changes in the bilateral symmetry positioning, and appearance of the hips, shoul-

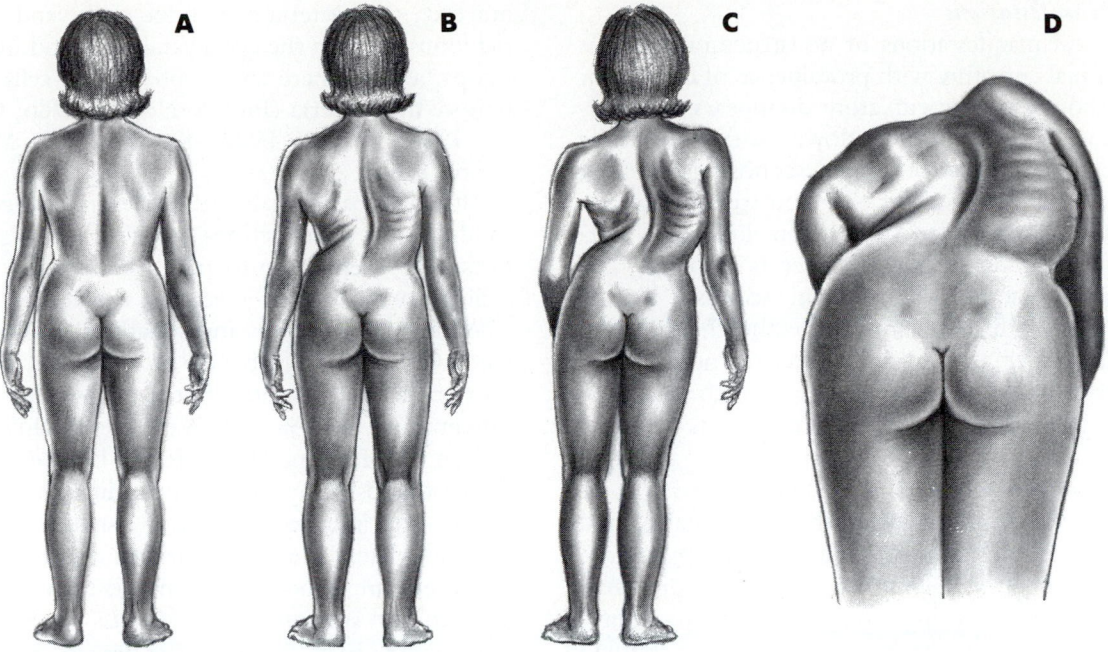

FIG. 40-6. Normal spinal alignment and abnormal spinal curvatures associated with scoliosis. **A,** Normal. **B,** Mild. **C,** Severe. **D,** Rotation and curvature of scoliosis. (From Thompson, et al., 1989.)

ders, and rib cage. In severe cases respiratory or digestive function is compromised because of compression or displacement of internal organs.

Structural scoliosis can be caused by a great variety of conditions. It can result from congenital skeletal abnormalities (15%), neuromuscular diseases (15%), trauma, extraspinal contractures, bone infections that involve the vertebrae, metabolic bone disorders (e.g., rickets, osteoporosis, osteogenesis imperfecta), joint disease, and tumors. Most cases of structural scoliosis, however, have no known cause, although genetic factors are suspected. Structural scoliosis with no known cause, termed **idiopathic scoliosis,** accounts for at least 65% of cases.

Idiopathic scoliosis is classified as infantile, juvenile, or adolescent, depending on the child's age at the time of onset. In infantile scoliosis spinal curvature develops during the first 3 years of life; in juvenile scoliosis, curvature develops between skeletal ages of 4 and 12 years in girls and 4 and 14 years in boys; and in adolescent scoliosis, it develops after the skeletal age of 12 years in girls and 14 years in boys. About 90% of children with adolescent idiopathic scoliosis are girls.

Pathophysiology

The earliest pathologic changes of idiopathic scoliosis occur in the soft tissues. The muscles, ligaments, and other soft tissues become shortened on the concave side of the curve long before bone deformities occur. With time, progressive deformities of the vertebral column and ribs develop. In growing children, lateral deviation of the spinal column ceases, and one-sided compression of the vertebral bodies on the concave side of the curve begins. Vertebral deformity occurs as asymmetric forces are applied to the epiphyseal center of the ossification by shortened and tight soft tissues on the concave side of the curve. The degree of compression and twisting varies according to the position of the vertebrae in the curve. The compressive force is greatest on the vertebrae in the apex of the concavity, so that the apical vertebrae become most deformed.

Deformity caused by idiopathic scoliosis increases quite rapidly during the growing years and then more slowly later in life. Although the rate of increase is greatest during adolescence, the total increase in curvature may be greatest during adult life. One reason is that it takes less force to bend the spine further once a curvature is established.

Gravity and increases of upper body weight during adulthood can apply sufficient force to increase the deformity. In addition, the muscles on the concave side have considerable mechanical advantage over those working around the curve on the convex side. All of these forces have cumulative effects on the spinal column through life. If the curve is greater than 35 to 40 degrees, particularly in the lumbar region where rib support is absent, the curve may continue to progress at about 1 degree per year throughout life (Riseborough & Herndon, 1975).

Clinical Manifestations

The clinical manifestations of nonstructural scoliosis are mild spinal curvature with prominence of one hip or rounded shoulders. The curvature disappears with forward flexion of the spine, lying down, or traction of the head. Treatment for nonstructural scoliosis is postural improvement and trunk exercises. Nonstructural scoliosis resulting from disorders such as spinal tumors is corrected when the underlying disorder is resolved. The clinical manifestations of structural scoliosis include asymmetry of hip height, shoulder height, shoulder and scapular (shoulder blade) prominence, rib prominence, and posterior humping of ribs or hips, which are visible when the child bends forward from the waist.

Evaluation and Treatment

Spinal curvature is usually visible or palpable, and muscles on one side of the lower back (the convex side) may be prominent or bulging. Most cases of idiopathic scoliosis are noticed during school screening programs. In girls the deformity may be noticed because clothing does not "hang" properly on the body. Diagnosis is made by x-ray examinations.

Treatment depends on the degree of lateral curvature. Traditional treatment is application of an upper body brace, the Milwaukee brace, which is worn 23 hours a day for months or years. Surgical fusion of the spine and insertion of a metal rod may be done if curvature exceeds 50 degrees and more conservative treatment has failed, particularly if the rib cage compresses the lungs or if other organs are affected by deformity of the spinal column.

The latest treatment for scoliosis is transcutaneous muscle stimulation, in which electrodes are placed on the skin of the back at night, and weak electrical impulses transmitted through the electrodes cause the muscles on the convex side of the curve to contract several times per minute. This treatment strengthens the muscles on the convex side of the curve and pulls the spine into alignment. Transcutaneous muscle stimulation has been used successfully as an alterative to the Milwaukee brace and apparently prevents progression of the curvature after treatment is stopped.

Bone Infection: Osteomyelitis

Osteomyelitis is an inflammation of the bone marrow. Occurring twice as often in males as females, acute osteomyelitis may affect infants and children of any age but occurs most frequently between 3 & 12 years of age (Behrman & Vaughan, 1983).

Bacteria enter the bone through the bloodstream and lodge in the medullary cavity where a rich phagocytic mechanism frequently prevents most of the bacteria from establishing an infectious state. In some cases, however, the bacteria may lodge at the end of the arterial loops beneath the epiphyseal plate and infection develops because there are no phagocytic cells present to remove the bacteria (Fink & Nelson, 1986; Gillespie et al., 1987; Hobbs, 1922; Karlin, 1987; Morrissy & Shore, 1986).

Although bacterial blood infections are common in children, not all infections result in osteomyelitis. Efforts have been made to better understand why some children with blood infections develop osteomyelitis whereas others do not. Investigations into the possible mechanism(s) responsible for osteomyelitis have focused on trauma, an associated factor in the development of osteomyelitis in 30% to 40% of cases in children (Dich, Nelson, & Haltalin, 1975). It has been experimentally shown that osteomyelitis can be induced with a subclinical bacterial infection by making a small crack in the epiphyseal plate. The same bacteria without the injury produce a rare, subclinical form of osteomyelitis that appears to heal spontaneously (Morrissy & Shore, 1986). Thus trauma may be one of the precursors or etiologic factors that allow the bacteria to settle in the bone or joint.

The organism responsible for osteomyelitis varies and is related to the age of the child (see box on p. 1370). Osteomyelitis in the newborn is caused primarily by *Staphylococcus aureus*. Group B streptococcus and *Escherichia coli* infections are responsible for some cases, especially those of multiple bone involvement and in high-risk infants (Carnsdale, 1987).

Causative microorganisms of osteomyelitis according to age

NEWBORNS
Staphylococcus aureus
Group B streptococcus
Gram-negative enteric rods

INFANTS
Staphylococcus aureus
Hemophilus influenzae

OLDER CHILDREN
Staphylococcus aureus
Pseudomonas
Salmonella
Neisseria gonorrhea

ADOLESCENTS AND ADULTS
Pseudomonas
Mycobacterium tuberculosis

S. aureus is the responsible organism in 60% to 90% of osteomyelitis in older children. Musculoskeletal infection caused by *Hemophilus influenzae* primarily occurs in children between the ages of 6 months and 4 years. At this stage of the child's immunity to the organism, a normal inhabitant of the upper respiratory tract is lowered because of the loss of passive immunity acquired from the mother at birth. Gram-negative microorganisms account for an increasing number of infections of the vertebrae (Abramovitz, Baston, & Yablon, 1986; Carnsdale, 1987; Ray & Bassett, 1985), whereas *Pseudomonas* infections are associated with heroin addiction (Chandrasekar & Narula, 1986).

Factors that predispose to the development of osteomyelitis include impetigo, furunculosis, infected lesions of varicella (chickenpox), infected burns, cerebral abscesses, immunization with bacillus Calmette-Guerin (BCG) vaccine, prolonged intravenous or central parenteral alimentation, drug addiction, and direct trauma to the area adjacent to the site of osteomyelitis (Arias et al., 1987; Behrman & Vaughan, 1983; Carnsdale, 1987; Fink & Nelson, 1986; Green, 1983; Gutman, 1985; Morrissy & Shore, 1986; Nelson & Lydiatt, 1987; Vizkelety, 1986; Wong & Wilhelmus, 1986).

Pathophysiology

Osteomyelitis usually begins as a bloody abscess in the metaphysis of the bone. The abscess ruptures under the periosteum and spreads along the bone shaft or into the bone marrow cavity if untreated. Infection rarely spreads down the medullary cavity of the bone but rather first gains entrance to the subperiosteal space in the metaphysis. This is the path of least resistance because the cortex of the bone in this area is porous or mazelike, and the inflammatory response blocks spread within the bone (Morrissy & Shore, 1986). Because of the accumulation of debris caused by the infection, the periosteum may separate and form a shell of new bone around the infected portion of the shaft. Because the periosteum is separated from an adequate blood supply, sections of the bone die with the pieces of dead bone, or **sequestrum** (see Fig. 40-7). The periosteum that maintains a blood supply generates new bone and is responsible for the appearance of the periosteal new bone, or **involucrum** (Fig. 40-7). The presence of the sequestra and involucrum indicate that the disease has progressed to subperiosteal abscess formation.

In cases where the infection in the metaphysis occurs near the joint, the accumulating pus (bacteria, white blood cells, and fluid) create increasing pressure that may cause a rupture into the joint cavity. If rupture into the joint occurs, the pus causes inflammation and a condition called **secondary suppurative arthritis** (Alderson et al., 1986). Osteomyelitis is most commonly

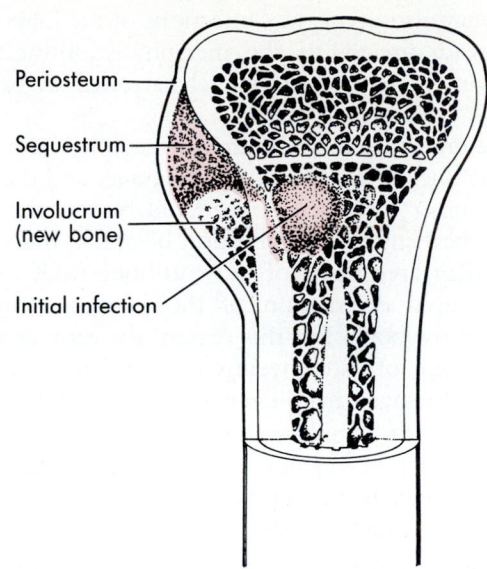

FIG. 40-7. Osteomyelitis in children. Infection starts in the metaphysis of the bone and easily spreads through the adjacent cortex. The inflammatory response decreases the infection's spread down the medullary cavity. In children the periosteum is easily elevated from the bone, allowing formation of a subperiosteal abscess. If allowed to continue, the infection can raise the periosteum from large segments of bone, depriving it of its blood supply and resulting in dead, infected bone called a *sequestrum*. Because the periosteum maintains a normal blood supply, it begins to produce new bone. If extensive, the new bone may surround parts of the dead bone and is called the *involucrum*.

caused by bacteria that reach the metaphysis through the bloodstream but may occur through secondary inoculation of microorganisms caused by trauma or contagious spread of infection from cellulitis in adjacent soft tissue.

Osteomyelitis in infants is frequently associated with septic arthritis because the infant's bone has blood vessels that perforate the growth plate. Because of the unique nature of blood supply to an infant's bones, osteomyelitis and septic arthritis frequently occur together. Normal anatomic variations in infants allow infection to spread directly to the epiphysis that causes both joint disease and permanent epiphyseal disease.

There are several reasons why children are susceptible to joint involvement. First, capillaries penetrate the epiphyseal plate and provide direct communication between the metaphysis of the bone and the joint cavity during the first month of life. Second, the capsules of the hip joints attach distally to the humerus. Because of these two structural differences during infancy, infections originating in the metaphysis of the bone, such as osteomyelitis, can spread rapidly to the joint cavity. The reverse may also occur, i.e., infections of the joint cavity may spread directly to the metaphysis of the bone. Bone growth may be completely arrested in extreme cases.

In the immature infant there is no epiphyseal plate or an ossific nucleus at the end of the bone, and the cartilage precursor of bone is penetrated by vascular channels. In these infants the infection begins in the vulnerable cartilage precursor of the end-bone itself that results in rapid destruction of the joint and arrested growth of the bone. For this reason, the early detection and treatment of osteomyelitis is crucial if the infant's joint is to be saved from later destruction. As the child matures and the epiphyseal plate forms, a temporary barrier is established against infection because the arterioles end beneath the epiphyseal plate (Morrissy & Shore, 1986; Trueta, 1959).

In children older than 2 years of age, the epiphyseal plate prevents the spread of a metaphyseal abscess into the epiphysis, and the cortex of the metaphysis is thicker. These anatomic differences increase the likelihood that the metaphyseal abscess will extend into the diaphysis and the blood supply of the bone will be disrupted. The periosteum is also more difficult to perforate in older children; this may lead to a larger subperiosteal abscess that could endanger the periosteal blood supply as well. This process commonly results in extensive sequestrum formation and chronic osteomyelitis (Morrissy & Shore, 1986).

Osteomyelitis is much less common after the epiphyses are closed, except in the vertebral body. Infection may develop in any part of a bone and abscesses spread slowly. Destruction of the cortex in a localized area may result in a pathologic fracture (Abramovitz et al., 1986; Ray & Bassett, 1985).

Spread of infection to contiguous joints is related to the child's age. Infection may spread to adjacent joints because the epiphyseal plate of the proximal femur is located within the hip joint capsule; the distal femur plate is partially located within the knee; and the proximal and distal humerus plates are partially located within the shoulder and elbow joints, respectively. There is a common blood supply for the metaphysis and the epiphysis in children younger than 2 years of age that crosses the epiphyseal plate. Infection may be carried through this common circulaton into the epiphysis and eventually involves the joint. An unossified epiphysis tends to be the site of initial infection more frequently than an ossified site; this common circulation ceases to exist in older children. After the epiphyses close, infection may extend directly from the metaphysis into the epiphyses and affect the joint. For this reason, osteomyelitis more commonly involves the joints in infants and adults rather that older children. However, epiphyseal separation may

occur in acute osteomyelitis in infants and children (Carnsdale, 1987; Morrissy & Shore, 1986).

Clinical Manifestations

The clinical manifestations of osteomyelitis are age dependent and are related to the differing vascular patterns found in the skeletal system at various ages. Three distinct groups may be identified: (1) infants younger than 1 year of age, (2) 1 year of age to puberty, and (3) after cessation of bone growth in adolescents and adults.

Infants

Osteomyelitis may be an acute illness characterized by fever and failure to move the affected limb (pseudoparalysis). Infantile osteomyelitis is characterized by permanent arrest in bone growth and involvement of multiple sites within the same bone or in multiple bones.

Children

Osteomyelitis is usually an abrupt illness in children between the ages of 1 year and puberty and is characterized by fever and systemic signs of toxicity. The illness is sometimes subacute with the child complaining of swelling, redness, tenderness, and slow movement of the affected bone or bones. Osteomyelitis during childhood most frequently affects the long bones but may also be found in the pelvis and small bones of the hands and feet. Clinical manifestations are usually accompanied by elevated white blood cell counts and elevated erythrocyte sedimentation rate counts. Evidence of infection using x-ray films may not be apparent until 10 to 14 days after the initial appearance of clinical manifestations and these manifestations, may be suppressed in the child receiving antibiotics for management of some other, nonrelated infection.

Adolescents and Adults

In addition to the sites previously mentioned, osteomyelitis in adolescents and adults may involve the vertebrae. Back pain, with a duration of several weeks, may be the only clinical complaint.

Evaluation and Treatment

White blood cell counts and erythrocyte sedimentation rate counts are sometimes elevated, but this is not a consistent finding. Monitoring of erythrocyte sedimentation rates is an indication of response to management. Blood cultures and aspiration of the soft tissue or bone, or both, should be obtained to identify the causative microorganism. Appropriate antibiotics should be prescribed after culture and sensitivity studies have been completed. A tuberculin test is also administered because *Mycobacterium tuberculosis* is sometimes the responsible microorganism. X-ray examinations of the affected area will reveal disease processes approximately 10 to 14 days after the appearance of clinical manifestations. Radionuclide imaging and bone scans are also useful.

Treatment includes administration of the appropriate antibiotic, drainage of infected bone, and symptomatic relief of pain and discomfort. Immobilization of the child is sometimes warranted.

Mortality is rare but serious sequelae may occur. The course of the disease and prognosis depend on the age of the child, the rapidity with which the diagnosis is established, the initiation of early treatment, and maintenance of the treatment for an adequate time. Dislocation of joints and bone growth arrest are the most serious complications of osteomyelitis (Bergdahl, Ekengren, & Eriksson, 1986; Behrman & Vaughan, 1987).

Juvenile Rheumatic Arthritis

The rheumatic diseases are a group of diverse conditions having in common the inflammation of connective tissues. They include rheumatoid arthritis, systemic lupus erythematosus, dermatomyositis, scleroderma, and polyarthritis. Incidence of these disorders in children is estimated in Table 40-2.

Juvenile rheumatoid arthritis (JRA) is the childhood form of rheumatoid arthritis (see Chapter 39). Like adult-onset rheumatoid arthritis, JRA is a syndrome that is often accompanied by systemic manifestations. About 5% of all cases of rheumatoid arthritis begin in childhood. An estimated quarter of a million children in the United States have JRA.

The basic pathophysiology of JRA is the same as that of adult rheumatoid arthritis. The clinical manifestations of JRA may differ, however, beginning with mode of onset. Unlike adult rheumatoid arthritis, which begins insidiously with systemic signs of inflammation and generalized aches, JRA has three distinct modes of onset: arthritis in fewer than five joints (oligoarthritis), arthritis in more than five joints (polyarthritis), and systemic disease. Onset is less gradual in JRA than in adult rheumatoid arthritis. JRA also differs from the adult form in the following respects (Cassidy, 1982):

1. Systemic disease is most common
2. The large joints are predominantly affected
3. Subluxation and ankylosis of the cervical spine is common
4. Joint pain is not as severe as the adult type
5. Chronic uveitis is common
6. Serologic tests often detect antinuclear antibody
7. Serologic tests seldom detect rheumatoid factor
8. Rheumatoid nodules are not limited to subcutaneous tissue but are found in the heart, lungs, eyes, and other organs.

Treatment for children with JRA is supportive but not curative. The aims of treatment are to control inflammation and other clinical manifestations of the disease and to minimize deformity.

Avascular Diseases of the Bone: Osteochondrosis

The avascular diseases of the bone, collectively termed **osteochondroses,** are due to insufficient blood supply to growing bones. Disturbances of blood supply to primary and secondary centers of ossification (see p. 1361) during periods of rapid bone growth result in a variety of skeletal abnormalities.

The cause of the osteochondroses remains obscure. In the past infection, nutritional deficiencies, and hormonal imbalances were blamed, but these causes have been largely disproven. Currently, vascular impairment and trauma, coupled with an underlying developmental or genetic predisposition, have been identified as probable causes of osteochrondroses. The most common osteochondroses involve the head of the femur femoral capital epiphysis, Legg Calvé-Perthes disease); the epiphyses

TABLE 40-2 Incidence of the connective tissue diseases in children

Disease	Annual rate/10^5	Sex ratio (F:M)	Race ratio (W:B)	Peak age group at risk (yr)	Childhood onset (%)
Rheumatoid arthritis	40	3:1	Equal	Increases with age (20-50)	5
Systemic lupus erythematosus	6	8:1	1:4	15-45	18
Dermatomyositis	0.8	2:1	1:3	45-65	20
Scleroderma	0.4	3:1	Equal	Increases with age (30-50)	3
Polyarteritis	0.2	1:3	Equal	Midadult	Rare

NOTE: F:M, Female to male; W:B = white to black.
From Cassidy, 1982.

of the vertebral bodies (Scheuermann disease); the proximal bones of the feet (tarsal navicular bones; Kohler bone disease); the shin bone (proximal tibial epiphysis; Blount disease); the anterior crest of the shin bone (tibial tuberosity; Osgood-Schlatter disease); and the heel bone (calcaneus). (These bones are illustrated in Chapter 38.)

The classic clinical course of the osteochondroses consists of three overlapping stages: (1) avascular necrosis, or death of newly formed bone or cartilage associated with diminished blood supply; (2) an acute inflammatory response in tissues adjacent to areas of necrosis; and (3) healing and repair. The first stage of osteochondrosis is characterized by extensive avascular necrosis without any evidence of adjacent tissue inflammation. A secondary defect at the subchondral interface frequently is associated with avascular necrosis of the spongy bone. Because the surface of the articular cartilage receives most of its nutrients from synovial fluid, it is not damaged by avascular necrosis. The deeper layers of the articular cartilage are adversely affected, however, because they depend on vascular support. Later, reabsorption of the spongy bone significantly alters the mechanical strength of the articular cartilage leading to transchondral fractures during joint stress.

In the second or intermediate stage of osteochondrosis, avascular necrosis causes reactive synovitis. Synovitis is often the cause of the first clinical manifestations—pain and muscle spasm. The extent of tissue damage and the outcome of osteochondrosis depend on how long the blood supply was diminished.

Most deformities become evident during the second or intermediate stage of osteochondrosis. Incongruity of the joint surfaces may occur if muscle spasms have resulted in contractures. Necrosis and articular damage are followed by processes of healing: ingrowth of new blood vessels and the appearance of primitive mesenchymal tissues that later differentiate into osteoblasts and contribute to the proliferation of reparative cells and new bone. Cysts in the articular cartilage and endochondral bone affect articular contour and congruity and future function and growth.

In the third or final stage of osteochondrosis, cysts disappear and bone and articular remodeling are completed. Foci of new bone grow outward and ultimately coalesce into remodeled bone tissue.

Osteochondroses have been reported in both primary and secondary ossification centers of all bone. The child is usually bothered by localized discomfort, a deformity, a limp, or an alteration of joint function.

Legg-Calvé-Perthes Disease

Legg-Calvé-Perthes disease, also called coxa plana, is one of the most common of the osteochondroses. This self-limited disease of the hip is produced by recurrent interruption of the blood supply to the femoral head. The ossification center first becomes necrotic and then is gradually replaced by live bone.

Legg-Calvé-Perthes disease is relatively common, usually occurring in children between the ages of 3 and 10 years, with a peak incidence at 6 years. It is more frequent in boys than in girls by a ratio of about 4:1. Incidence is 1 in 750 boys and 1 in 3700 girls. The condition is bilateral in about 12% of affected children.

The cause of decreased blood supply to the head of the femur is unknown. Several theories have been proposed, including thyroid deficiency, trauma, and infection. A plausible theory is that acute synovitis (infection of the synovial membrane) and increased hydrostatic pressure in the hip joint compress blood vessels that supply the femoral head.

Constitutional factors definitely play a role. Birth weight of children with Legg-Calvé-Perthes disease is much lower than that of unaffected children. Skeletal maturation is delayed in children with Legg-Calvé-Perthes disease, and affected children are between 2.5 and 7 cm shorter than unaffected children of the same age. Familial occurrence is common. The disease is rare in blacks and it is frequent in children of Japanese and Central European ancestry.

Pathophysiology

Legg-Calvé-Perthes disease runs its natural course in 2 to 5 years. In the incipient stage the soft tissues of the hip (synovial membrane and joint capsule) are swollen, edematous, and hyperemic, often with fluid present in the joint (Fig. 40-8). The joint space widens and the joint capsule bulges. The first stage lasts for only a few weeks. In the second, or active avascular necrotic stage, the entire or anterior half of the epiphysis of the femoral head is dead, and the metaphyseal bone at the junction of the femoral neck and capital epiphyseal plate is softened because of increased blood supply and decalcification. Soon granulation tissue (procallus) and blood vessels invade the dead bone. This stage lasts from several months to one year.

The third, or regenerative healing, stage ordinarily lasts 2 to 4 years. The dead femoral head is replaced by procallus and new bone is laid down. Collapse and flattening of the femoral head occurs, and the femoral neck becomes short and wide (see Fig. 40-8).

In the fourth, or residual, stage remodeling takes place, and the newly formed bone is organized into a live spongy bone. The restoration of the femoral head to a normal shape is more complete in younger than in older children. A complete return to normal is also more likely if only the anterior epiphysis was involved.

Clinical Manifestations

Injury or trauma precedes the onset of the clinical manifestations in approximately one third of children with Legg-Calvé-Perthes disease. Onset of symptoms is

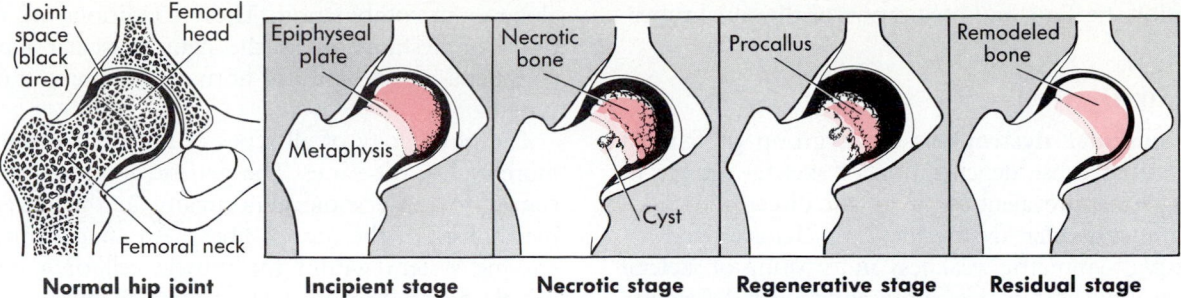

FIG. 40-8. Stages of Legg-Calvé-Perthes disease, a form of osteochondrosis.

insidious unless trauma aggravates the disease process. The child frequently complains of a limp and pain for several months. The pain usually is referred to the knee, inner thigh, and the groin, following the path of the obturator nerve. In some children, pain may be absent or minimal. If pain is present, it is usually aggravated by activity and relieved by rest.

The typical physical findings include spasm on rotation of the hip in extension, a limitation of internal rotation and abduction, and a hip flexion-abduction deformity. If the child is walking, an abnormal gait termed an **antalgic abductor lurch** is apparent. If the hip pain or limp has been present for a prolonged period, muscles of the hip and thigh atrophy.

Evaluation and Treatment

Diagnosis is confirmed by x-ray examination. The goals of treatment are to preserve normal congruity of the femoral head and acetabulum (hip socket) and maintain spasm-free and pain-free range of motion in the hip joint. In the past many children were treated successfully with bed rest or the use of braces to keep the affected limb off the ground, but a large percentage were left with distorted femoral heads. Current therapy allows the child to continue weight bearing but with the femur in an abducted position, so that the femoral head is held securely within the acetabulum. This decreases focal areas of increased load and minimizes distortion. Weight bearing in abduction is accomplished by Petrie casts (long leg casts with the legs held in abduction and medial rotation by a bar between the legs) or by braces that hold the legs in the same position. Surgical procedures can be used that keep the femoral head abducted in relation to the acetabulum.

Factors affecting the outcome of Legg-Calvé-Perthes disease are the age of the child, the extent of necrosis, and the stage of disease at the time treatment is begun. The outcome in 70% to 80% of appropriately treated children with Legg-Calvé-Perthes disease is satisfactory hip joint function.

Osgood-Schlatter Disease

Osgood-Schlatter disease consists of tendinitis of the anterior patellar tendon, within which the patella (kneecap) is embedded, and associated osteochondrosis of the tubercle of the tibia. Osgood-Schlatter disease occurs most frequently in preadolescents and adolescents who participate in sports. The incidence is higher in boys than in girls.

Pathophysiology

The severity of the lesion varies from mild tendinitis to a complete separation of the anterior extension of the tibial epiphysis, which is the part of the epiphysis that contributes to growth of the tibial tubercle. The underlying pathologic alterations also vary. The mildest form of Osgood-Schlatter disease causes ischemic (avascular) necrosis in the region of the bony tibial tubercle, with hypertrophic cartilage formation during the stages of repair. In more severe cases the abnormality involves a true epiphyseal separation of the tibial tubercle, with the characteristics of avascular necrosis described in the section on Legg-Calvé-Perthes disease.

Clinical Manifestations

The child complains of pain and swelling in the region of the patellar tendon and tibial tubercle, which becomes prominent and is tender to direct pressure. The pain is most severe after physical activity that involves vigorous quadriceps contraction or direct local trauma to the tibial tubercle area. Frequently, the child has complaints of sudden onset of acute discomfort referable to the affected region. Sudden onset of pain is caused by a pathologic fracture through an area of ischemic necrosis.

Evaluation and Treatment

Diagnosis is confirmed by x-ray examination. The goal of treatment for Osgood-Schlatter disease is to decrease the stress at the tubercle. Often a period of 4 to 8 weeks of restriction from strenuous physical activity, especially activities requiring deep knee bending, is sufficient. If relief from pain is not achieved, a cast is required to immobilize the knee, a situation that is particularly difficult if the condition is bilateral.

Gradual resumption of activity is permitted after 8 weeks, but return to unrestricted athletic participation requires an additional 8 weeks to allow for revascularization, healing, and ossification of the tibial tubercle.

Muscular Dystrophy

The **muscular dystrophies** are a group of familial disorders that cause degeneration of skeletal muscle fibers. The most prevalent of the muscle diseases in childhood, the muscular dystrophies are characterized by progressive, symmetric weakness and wasting of skeletal muscle groups, with increasing disability and deformity.

Classification of the muscular dystrophies is based on age of onset, rate of progression, distribution of muscular involvement, and inheritance patterns. The major types that are clinically and genetically distinct are the pseudohypertrophic (Duchenne), facioscapulohumeral, limb girdle, oculopharyngeal, and myotonic muscular dystrophies (Fig. 40-9). Because the clinical findings and genetic inheritance patterns are consistent for each type, some researchers believe that each involves a separate biochemical defect. The precise mechanisms, however, are still unknown. Current research points to defects in muscle fiber (cell) membrane as either a cause or result of an unknown biochemical abnormality. Genetic research has focused on identifying the locus for the abnormal genes. This will permit more accurate carrier detection and, eventually, description of the biochemcial aberration (Table 40-3 summarizes the types of muscular dystrophy.)

Muscle degeneration is characterized by biochemical, morphologic, or neurophysiologic changes that occur alone or in combination. These conditions are not the result of dysfunction of the neuromuscular junctions, peripheral nerves, anterior horn cells, or central nervous system.

The physiology of all types of muscular dystrophy is more or less the same. The genetic abnormality is presumed to cause some abnormality in the intracellular metabolism of the muscle fibers. An abnormality in an enzyme system within the muscle cell or a defect in muscle metabolism may result from inability to absorb or metabolize a substance vital to muscular function. A defect in creatine metabolism and a lowering of levels of intramuscular enzymes in the glycolytic system are involved.

The muscle cells have an increased number of nuclei that form chains and are moved centrally. The muscle cells also show necrosis and phagocytosis. Fragmentation and dissolution of myofilaments occur early. The muscle fibers may be swollen, indistinct, and homogenous, with disturbed striation. Some fibers may be hypertrophic and others atrophic. Muscle fibers are eventually replaced with fat (causing fatty infiltration) and connective tissues (causing fibrosis). The involved muscle fibers are randomly distributed, with no distinct pattern.

Duchenne Muscular Dystrophy

In 1868 the French neurologist G. B. A. Duchenne described a pseudohypertrophic muscular paralysis associated with large amounts of fat and connective tissue.

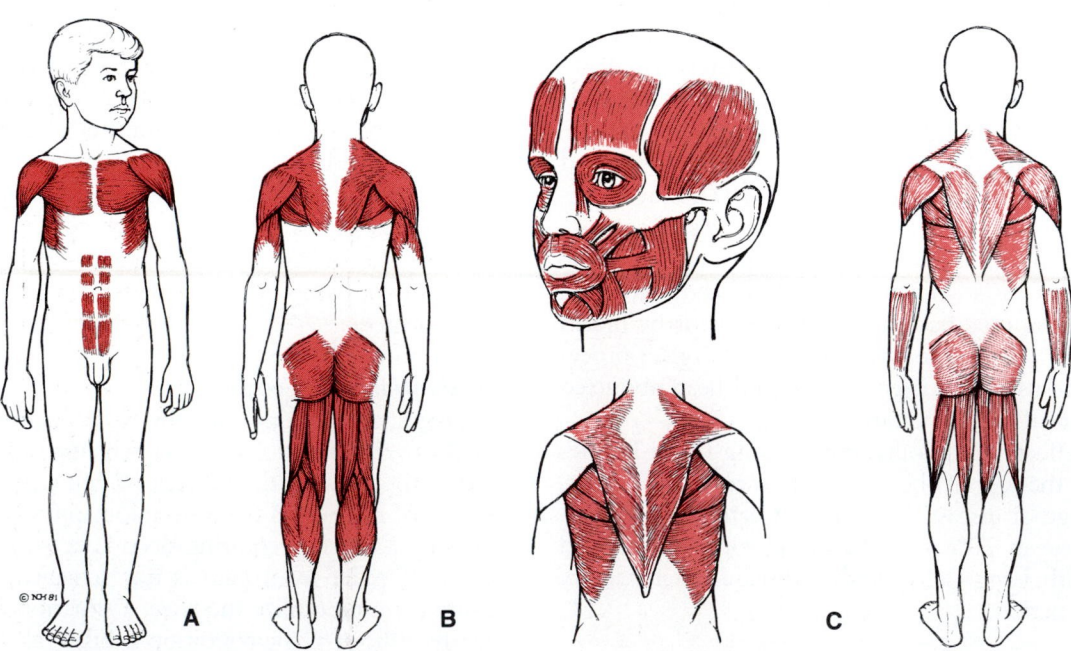

FIG. 40-9. Initial muscle groups involved in three types of muscular dystrophy. **A,** Pseudohypertrophic. **B,** Facioscapulohumeral. **C,** Limb girdle. (From Whaley & Wong, 1987.)

TABLE 40-3 Major muscular dystrophy syndromes

Disease	Mode of inheritance	Age at clinical onset	Usual distribution	Rate of progression	Mental retardation	Distinguished findings
Duchenne dystrophy (DMD)	X-linked recessive	About 3 years	Hips and shoulders, quadriceps femoris, gastrocenemius (pseudohypetrophy)	Rapid	Frequent	Elevated serum cnzymes (CPK, LDH, SGOT, aldolase)
Facioscapulo-humeral (FSH) dystrophy	Autodomal dominant	In first or second decade	Shoulder girdle, neck, face, pelvic girdle (late)	Moderate	Occasional	Several distinct muscle pathologies
Limb girdle (LG) dystrophy	Poorly defined or recessive	Variable	Pelvic and shoulder girdles	Variable	Variable	Collection of several diseases
Myotonic dystrophy (MyD)	Autosomal dominant	Variable—birth to fifth decade	Distal extensor muscle, eyelids, face, neck, hands, pharynx	Slow, related to age at clinical onset, faster with younger patients	Frequent	Percussion myotonia, cataracts, diabetic GTT despite increased insulin, testicular atrophy, decreased IgC

Adapted from Stanbury, 1983.

Today, this form of muscular dystrophy, called **Duchenne muscular dystrophy,** is the most common of the muscular dystrophies. Its incidence is approximately 1 in 3500 male births (Scott et al., 1988). Classic Duchenne muscular dystrophy occurs only in boys and has a history of X-linked inheritance in half of the cases.

Pathophysiology

The X-linked inherited type of Duchenne muscular dystrophy is thought to be due to a deletion of a segment of DNA (Scott et al., 1988). Other mechanisms causing Duchenne muscular dystrophy are unknown. Areas currently being investigated include: (1) a neurogenic basis, related primarily to abnormal motor neurons; (2) a vascular abnormality in which malformations or physiologic incompetence results in poor small-vessel perfusion, with or without abnormality in biogenic amine metabolism; and (3) an intrinsic abnormality within muscle fibers, possibly related to formation of inappropriate amounts of connective tissue, abnormality in enzyme metabolism, or structural defects (Swaiman & Wright, 1982).

Duchenne muscular dystrophy causes muscle bulk to diminish, and in later stages a predominant pink or yellowish pink replaces the dark red staining of normal muscle. Interstitial connective tissue and fat often replace muscle fibers.

Microscopic changes include a decrease in the number of fibers and necrosis of the fibers with associated phagocytosis. Overall, changes include increase of endomysial connective tissue and fat, loss of striations, and concomitant hyaline, granular, and fatty degeneration of fibers. Disorganization of tendinous insertions is associated with fat accumulation in these areas. Although fibers regenerate in the younger child, they are abnormal in many ways and become nonfunctional with time.

Clinical Manifestations

Duchenne muscular dystrophy is usually identified in children about 3 years of age when the parents notice slow motor development with progressive weakness and muscle wasting. Sitting, standing, and walking are delayed and the child is clumsy, falls frequently, and has difficulty climbing stairs.

Muscular weakness always begins in the pelvic girdle, causing a "waddling" gait. Hypertrophy of the calf muscles is apparent in 80% of cases. The method of rising from the floor by "climbing up the legs" (Gower sign) is characteristic and is due to weakness of the lumbar and gluteal muscles. The foot assumes a talipes equinovarus position (Fig. 40-4), and the child tends to walk on the toes because of weakness of the anterior tibial and peroneal muscles. Within 3 to 5 years, muscles of the shoulder girdle become involved. The deep tendon reflexes are usually depressed or absent. On rare occasions, a positive Babinski sign and other evidence of upper motor neuron lesions have been reported. Contractures and wasting of the muscles contribute to muscular atrophy and deformity of the skeleton.

Duchenne muscular dystrophy has serious complications. Pulmonary function is compromised greatly because of marked kyphoscoliosis ("humped" upper spine combined with scoliosis), which usually develops after the child is confined to a wheelchair. The incidence of cardiac involvement in Duchenne muscular dystrophy is as high as 95%. Chronic heart failure may occur in 50% of children. A moderate degree of mental retardation causes these children to have a mean IQ of about 80. Smooth muscle dysfunction may cause megacolon, volvulus, cramping pain, and malabsorption in the gastrointestinal tract.

Evaluation and Treatment

Diagnosis is confirmed by measurement of serum enzymes, electromyography (EMG), and muscle biopsy. The serum enzymes, especially creatine phosphokinase (CPK), are increased to more than 10 times normal, even during infancy and before the onset of weakness. Histologic changes in muscle include degeneration of muscle fibers, with variation in fiber size and central nuclei. Fat and connective tissue replace muscle fibers.

Although intrauterine diagnosis is not yet possible, elevated CPK levels at birth are diagnostic indicators of Duchenne muscular dystrophy. Identification of female carriers of the disease cannot be achieved with certainty, but serum CPK is elevated in 60% to 80% of carriers.

There is no effective treatment for Duchenne muscular dystrophy. Maintaining function in unaffected muscle groups for as long as possible is the primary goal. Although activity fosters maintenance of muscle function, strenuous exercise may hasten the breakdown of muscle fibers. Range of motion exercises, bracing, and surgical release of contracture deformities are used to maintain normal function for as long as possible. Genetic counseling is recommended. With X-linked inheritance, male siblings of an affected child have a 50% chance of being affected, and female siblings have a 50% chance of being carriers.

Progressive weakness leads to wheelchair confinement between the ages of 8 and 15 years, after which obesity or excessive thinness, kyphoscoliosis, and other complications of immobility develop. Death, usually resulting from respiratory or cardiac muscle weakness, occurs before age 20. Only 25% of children with Duchenne muscular dystrophy reach the age of 21.

Becker Muscular Dystrophy

Becker muscular dystrophy is often called "benign" Duchenne muscular dystrophy because it shares the X-linked inheritance pattern and similar clinical features. The two diseases are not found in the same pedigree, however, and are thought to involve different biochemical defects. Clinical symptoms often begin between the ages of 5 and 15. Children with Becker muscular dystrophy remain ambulatory into their teens and early 20s; in one study, the age at the time of disability and wheelchair use was 20 to 27 (Brooke, 1977). The incidence is one tenth that of Duchenne muscular dystrophy.

The pattern of muscle weakness for both dystrophies is almost identical, although calf hypertrophy and muscle cramps may precede clinical weakness as in Duchenne muscular dystrophy. Scoliosis and contractures are rare until the child with Becker muscular dystrophy is permanently wheelchair bound. The changes in creatine kinase levels and EMG and ECG readings are the same as those seen in Duchenne muscular dystrophy. Many individuals live well into middle age. Heart failure is infrequent but can be a cause of premature death and disability.

Maintaining ambulation and careful follow-up for evidence of cardiopulmonary complications are essential measures for long-term care. Children with Becker muscular dystrophy rarely show the mental changes seen in Duchenne dystrophy, and with appropriate vocational counseling and support may become exceedingly productive workers. The accurate diagnosis of Becker muscular dystrophy is important. If the affected individual marries and has children, all daughters will be carriers of this X-linked recessive disorder. Of course, genetic counseling should be offered to the mother, female siblings, offspring, and any maternal relatives (Brooke, 1977).

Facioscapulohumeral Muscular Dystrophy

Facioscapulohumeral muscular dystrophy is a mild form of progressive, autosomal dominant muscular dystrophy. Age at onset varies from early childhood to adult life, and the disease affects males and females equally. As the name implies, clinical manifestations begin with weakness and atrophy of facial and shoulder girdle (scapulohumeral) muscles. The illness progresses slowly. Inability to close the eyes completely may be noted from early childhood. The face is expressionless, and pouting of the lips makes whistling impossible. The first symptoms usually include drooping of the shoulders with difficulty in raising the arms above the head. Onset of weakness in the lower limbs often is delayed for 20 to 30 years, and pseudohypertrophy of muscles is rare. Contractures and skeletal deformities develop less frequently and are less prominent than in Duchenne muscular dystrophy.

Treatment includes supportive physiotherapy to prevent contractures and prolong ambulation. Lightweight plastic ankle-foot orthoses (AFO) for footdrop are extremely helpful. Surgery to stablize the shoulder is sometimes advised.

Some individuals with facioscapulohumeral muscular dystrophy improve with steroid therapy, particularly if the clinical picture includes rapidly progressive weakness. The disease may be arrested for prolonged periods; however, most individuals remain active and have a normal life expectancy. Vocational training and genetic counseling are important to provide them with the information necessary to plan their future.

Scapuloperoneal Muscular Dystrophy

Scapuloperoneal muscular dystrophy is considered a variant of facioscapulohumeral muscular dystrophy, but distal muscles in the lower extremity are involved early instead of the facial and shoulder muscle weakness that are the early signs in facioscapulohumeral dystrophy. Many seek initial treatment for troublesome footdrop and shoulder weakness. Analysis of inheritance patterns shows that the disease can be inherited both as an autosomal dominant trait or as an X-linked recessive trait.

The initial symptoms may resemble those of several other illnesses, including nemaline myopathy (a congenital muscle disease) and early hypertrophic peripheral neuropathy. A careful diagnostic evaluation therefore is in order. Other clinical findings include hypertrophy of the muscle that extends the toes, brought about by a futile attempt to overcome footdrop, and depressed or absent muscle stretch reflexes. Creatinine kinase is elevated two to 20 times normal; EMG readings reveal myopathy.

Treatment is directed toward treating symptoms and preserving ambulation and functional ability. Footdrop is easily treated with AFOs. Individuals with scapuloperoneal muscular dystrophy remain ambulatory for 40 or more years. Occasionally, walking may be hampered by paraspinal muscle contractures; in this case a wheelchair may assist the individual to cover long distances. The life span in this disorder is normal. Genetic counseling should be available to all persons (Brooke, 1977).

Limb Girdle Muscular Dystrophy

The diagnosis of **limb girdle muscular dystrophy** is considered when acute causes of proximal weakness are eliminated and the clinical findings and genetic pattern exclude Duchenne and facioscapulohumeral muscular dystrophy. The diagnosis is often determined by exclusion because few consistent clinical features make this type of muscular dystrophy unique. In fact, some researchers think that limb girdle dystrophy actually may be several separate diseases waiting for more sophisticated methods of evaluation to give them precise labels. Most individuals have a negative family history, making sporadic disease or an autosomal recessive pattern of inheritance likely. The prevalence rate for limb girdle muscular dystrophy is set at 20 per million.

The initial symptoms include shoulder and pelvic girdle weakness, which are usually noticed in the early 20s but can be seen as late as the 40s. The muscle weakness is often asymmetric and progresses at a much slower pace than in Duchenne muscular dystrophy. The biceps and deltoid muscles can be extremely atrophic and weak. Individuals can remain ambulatory for extended periods, often up to 20 years after initial diagnosis. When confined to wheelchairs, they show few of the severe effects of other dystrophies, such as contractures and scoliosis. Heart involvement and mental retardation also are rare.

The individual will have mild elevation in creatine kinase levels and a myopathic pattern on EMG. Muscle biopsy is often more characteristic, with fiber splitting and fibers that appear profusely "moth-eaten" and whorled. Treatment includes supportive measures to maintain ambulation and functional ability and frequent follow-up to eliminate secondary complications such as cardiopulmonary disease.

Myotonic Muscular Dystrophy

A multisystemic disorder, **myotonic muscular dystrophy** (MTD) is a common disease with a frequency ranging from 50 to 1200 per million, varying by geographic location. The myotonic muscular dystrophy gene has been identified on chromosome 19, a finding with implications for genetic counseling and for further understanding of biochemical defect.

Pathophysiology

The multisystemic nature of this disorder strongly suggests a defect of widespread involvement, potentially an abnormality of muscle cell membrane. Several studies have advanced this hypothesis. Electron microscopy shows a proliferation of transverse tubules coupled with an abnormal resting membrane potential. Researchers have identified the gene that governs the insulin receptors, and it is also located on chromosome 19. Because many indivdiuals with MTD show severe insulin resistance in skeletal muscle and abnormal insulin-mediated amino acid disposal after a glucose load, insulin studies are an exciting development. Individuals also show reduced protein synthesis; only 40% of normal or stable isotope studies. Because the mechanism of insulin uptake has such important effects on glucose use and protein synthesis in muscle, a defect in the insulin receptor and insulin action would have profound effects on muscle function and in particular may cause muscle wasting (Griggs & Rennie, 1983). Linking both the gene for myotonic muscular dystrophy and the gene for insulin uptake on chromosome 19 further substantiates the relationship between these phenomena.

Clinical Manifestations

The onset of the disease ranges from birth to the fifth decade. The peculiar attitudes of indifference seen in persons with myotonic muscular dystrophy make the onset of the disease and progression of symptoms difficult to qualify. Myotonic muscular dystrophy is typically more severe in the maternally transmitted neonatal and childhood forms than in adult forms.

The early clinical findings are the characteristic facial features and presence of myotonia (tonic muscle spasms). A common observation is that if the diagnosis of MTD is not made at first glance and handshake, the clinician misses it because of the myriad of individual complaints. Many are unrelated to the muscular system and individuals rarely complain of functional difficulties in spite of severe muscle weakness. The prominent temporal and masseter muscle wasting and severe neck flexor weakness gives rise to the terms "hatchet facies" and "swan-neck" deformity commonly applied to MTD. Myotonia usually affects the hands more than the eyelids, tongue, or facial muscles. As the disease progresses, weakness in the distal extremities is apparent, and footdrop is common. Weakness of the respiratory muscles and the pharyngeal and esophageal muscles is noted. In fact, abnormalities of all three types of muscles— smooth, skeletal, and cardiac—have been identified in pathologic analysis of sections from biopsies. Other organs are involved; defects in the lens, retina, brain, pancreas, testes, ovaries, skin, bone, gamma globulins, and red blood cells have been reported.

Mental retardation is often associated with neonatal MTD. A mean IQ of 66 was reported in one study (Brooke, 1977). Mental retardation is rarely seen in adolescence, adult-onset, and paternally transmitted disease.

Evaluation and Treatment

Diagnostic tests include the EMG, which shows myopathic findings and audible myotonia, the characteristic "dive bomber" noise heard when the needle is inserted. Creatine phosphokinase level is usually normal. Muscle biopsy shows type I fiber atrophy and type II fiber hypertrophy.

Cardiac abnormalities can be severe and can cause sudden death. Several studies have demonstrated that most individuals have abnormal His bundle conduction and prolonged P-R intervals. In one study all persons had abnormal His-ventricle intervals in spite of normal P-R intervals. Individuals who complain of syncope should be carefully evaluated for cardiac conduction abnormalities and potential pacemaker insertion.

Other systemic signs include bulbar weakness, with dysarthric nasal speech and swallowing difficulty. Many individuals aspirate and have reduced esophageal motility. If these problems are accompanied by weight loss and aspiration pneumonitis, they can be treated by insertion of a feeding tube. Abnormalities in endocrine function include insulin resistance, testicular atrophy, and infertility.

There is no treatment that alters the severe muscle wasting and weakness, yet treatment is available for many of the common symptoms. Drugs such as phenytoin and quinine can decrease functionally disabling myotonia. Cataract surgery can dramatically improve visual acuity. Hypersomnolence, in which individuals sleep more than 12 hours a day, can be treated with stimulants such as pemoline (Cylert) or methylphenidate (Ritalin). Braces and canes are prescribed when footdrop impedes ambulation.

Genetic counseling should be provided. Analysis of linkage to the ABO blood group has made prenatal prediction of an affected fetus possible in a small number of individuals. Genetic mapping studies have demonstrated that the blood groups ABO and Lutheran are on the same chromosome as myotonic dystrophy. If the patient secretes ABO blood group antigens in body secretions, analysis of the individual's family and spouse would permit prediction of the prenatal diagnosis of myotonic dystrophy.

Musculoskeletal Tumors in Children
Bone Tumors

Bone tumors are an uncommon form of cancer in childhood. The two main tumors are osteosarcoma and Ewing sarcoma. Children very rarely develop fibrosarcoma, chrondrosarcoma, or non-Hodgkin lymphoma of the bone.

Osteosarcoma

Osteosarcoma is the most common bone tumor during childhood and originates in bone-producing mesenchymal cells. Three fourths of cases occur between the age of 10 and 25 years—the majority are diagnosed between 15 and 19 years of age. Therefore it is predominantly a tumor that develops during the adolescent growth spurt. It is more common in males than females (1:6; 1:0), perhaps because males have longer growth periods and greater bone volume. The incidence of osteosarcoma before age 15 is the same for males and females.

The cause is unknown but it has been speculated that osteosarcoma may develop as a result of rapid local growth that increases the likelihood of mutation. Although controversial, there has been some evidence that these tumors occur more commonly in taller individuals, and it has also been well documented in animal studies that osteosarcoma is seen in giant dog breeds, such as Saint Bernards and Great Danes, but not in smaller dogs.

Osteosarcoma can be induced by ionizing radiation,

even with relatively low doses. This can be a tragic consequence of therapeutic radiation for other forms of cancer. The latent period after radiation exposure is 5 to 40 years, and it is estimated that 4% of all osteosarcomas occur in previously irradiated bone. Evidence for hereditary links have not been firmly established and no racial tendency is seen, although on rare occasions the tumor has been documented in multiple family members. There has also been a link to individuals with retinoblastoma (a hereditary eye tumor). In fact, osteosarcoma is more likely to occur if the individual has bilateral retinoblastoma, confirming a genetic transmission of the eye tumor rather than a spontaneous mutation in the genes. The link between retinoblastoma and subsequent osteosarcoma occurs whether or not radiation has been part of the treatment for retinoblastoma. Osteosarcoma has been associated with a few other medical syndromes. The most well-established association involves older individuals with Paget disease of the bone and is not seen during childhood.

There is no evidence that osteosarcoma can be caused by chemical carcinogens. In addition, there is no convincing evidence that there is a viral link. In the past, there has been some interest in investigating a viral link, since viruses have been shown to cause osteosarcoma in laboratory animals and C-type virus particles have been identified in human osteosarcoma growth in tissue culture. However, no DNA or RNA virus has been isolated.

Pathophysiology

Osteosarcoma occurs in the metaphysis of long bones. The majority of tumors arise in bones involved with the knee joint at the distal end of the femur or proximal end of the tibia. The ends of long bones are sites of most active epiphyseal growth. As a tumor of mesenchymal cells, osteosarcoma demonstrates production of osteoid cells.

Osteosarcoma is a bulky tumor that extends beyond the bone into a soft tissue mass. It may encircle the bone and destroy the trabeculae of the diseased bone. Osteosarcoma disseminates through the bloodstream, usually to the lung. Twenty-five percent of children diagnosed with osteosarcoma exhibit lung metastases at diagnosis. Other sites of metastatic spread include other bones and visceral organs.

Clinical Manifestations

The most common presenting complaint is pain. The pain can be intermittent at first, then continuing with increasing severity. There may be swelling and warmth and redness caused by the vascularity of the tumor. Symptoms may also include cough, dyspnea, and chest pain if lung metastasis is present. If a lower extremity is involved, a limp may be present and a pathologic frac-

ture may result if the disease is extensive. The child or family member may relate subsequent appearance of the tumor to a traumatic accident; however, osteosarcoma is not the result of trauma, but trauma may call attention to a preexisting tumor.

Initial evaluation includes x-ray examination that reveals osteosarcoma's characteristic osteoblastic and osteolytic changes. In addition, a laboratory study of blood serum alkaline phosphate levels may be performed because elevated levels may be due to osteoid production.

Evaluation and Treatment

Tissue biopsy will confirm the diagnosis, although needle biopsy is often sufficient to establish the diagnosis. At the present time, no standardized staging system exists for osteosarcoma.

Surgery and chemotherapy are the primary treatments for osteosarcoma; however, the tumor is resistant to radiation. Traditionally, surgery includes amputation at the joint above the involved bone; however, more recent limb salvage procedures have gained acceptance, and amputation may be avoided. The primary bone is removed and replaced with an internal prosthesis made of metal, cadaver bone, or bone graft. Certain requirements for eligibility for limb salvage surgery include a small tumor with minimal soft tissue involvement and linear bone growth that is nearly complete so that bone asymmetry will not develop as the uninvolved bone grows. The functional performance of the area salvaged must be considered because amputation and a prosthesis is sometimes more appropriate.

The efficacy of chemotherapy is still under investigation. Treatment with high-dose methotrexate and citrovorum "rescue" (as an antidote to the normal cell toxicity of the drug) has been the focus of many treatment approaches. Other drugs used in various combinations include doxorubicin bleomycin, cyclophosphamide, dactinomycin, and cisplatin. Some treatments used in conjunction with amputation or limb salvage advocate pretreatment with chemotherapy followed by surgery, in contrast to traditional treatments with surgery followed by chemotherapy. Immunotherapy with transfer factor and interferon have also been used but are not considered standard treatment.

A number of approaches have been used to treat pulmonary metastases. Because pulmonary metastases are generally solitary, focal lesions, thoracotomy with wedge resection has proven the most effective treatment. Investigators have searched for adjuvant treatment to prevent pulmonary metastases but to date nothing has proven useful.

Overall survival rates have been only 10% to 25% for osteosarcoma. However, more vigorous approaches for treatment have improved survival to above 50%.

Ewing Sarcoma

Ewing sarcoma is the second most common bone tumor during childhood. This tumor is named after James Ewing, who first saw it as a separate clinical diagnosis in 1921. Ewing sarcoma probably originates from cells within the bone marrow space and does not involve bone-forming cells. The most frequent period of diagnosis is between 5 and 15 years of age and is rare after 30. Like osteosarcoma, Ewing sarcoma is more common in males than females (1:6; 1:0) and the cause is also unknown. However, like osteosarcoma, there is a link with periods of rapid bone growth. Evidence for hereditary links has not been firmly established, however, Ewing sarcoma is very rare in blacks, both in the United States and Africa, perhaps indicating some genetic resistance.

Pathophysiology

Ewing sarcoma is most commonly located in the midshaft of long bones or in flat bones. The most frequent sites include the pelvis, femur, tibia, fibula, humerus, scapula, and ribs. An extremity is involved in the majority of cases, with the pelvis being the second most common site.

Arising from bone marrow, Ewing sarcoma can break through the cortex of the bone to form a soft tissue mass. Although the tumor does not form osteoid, it often contains areas of blood vessels and hemorrhage. Ewing sarcoma metastasizes to nearly every organ. Metastasis occurs early and is usually apparent at diagnosis or within 1 year. The most common sites are the lung, other bones, lymph nodes, bone marrow, liver, spleen, and central nervous system.

Clinical Manifestations

Like osteosarcoma, the most common complaint is pain that increases in severity. A soft tissue mass is often present. Additional symptoms may include fever, malaise, and anorexia. Both clinical and x-ray findings may mimic osteomyelitis. Additional radiographic and CT scans are used to evaluate the presence of metastatic disease.

Evaluation and Treatment

Needle biopsy is often sufficient to establish the diagnosis, but tissue biopsy will confirm the diagnosis. The primary treatment for Ewing sarcoma is radiation. Chemotherapy also plays an important role in the control of widespread disease. Surgery is effective if the tumor is resectable, and disfiguring surgery is avoided if possible. Amputation, however, may be considered in lower limb tumors of children less than 8 years of age because of the serious discrepancy in bone growth that results if the primary treatment used is radiation—growth is affected in the diseased bone whereas normal growth continues in the unaffected bone.

Treatment with high-dose (5500 to 5000 rad) radiation to the entire bone is used to control the primary tumor. Chemotherapy is generally administered before or concurrently with radiation. Agents used include vincristine, cyclophosphamide, doxorubicin, and dactinomycin (the last two agents are known to enhance the radiation effect). Intraarterial delivery of cisplatin also has been investigated.

Ewing sarcoma has had a dismal prognosis with 5-year survival rates no better than 5% to 10%. Combinations of aggressive radiation and chemotherapy have, however, improved the survival rate for localized disease to greater than 60%. The major predictor of prognosis appears to be the location of the primary tumor and whether metastases is present at diagnosis. The most favorable sites of involvement are the extremities; the worst prognosis involves tumors of the trunk, particularly the pelvis.

Fibroma

The **fibroma,** which is believed to be a defect in ossification rather than a true tumor, makes up approximately 50% of benign bone tumors. It is thought to begin as a fibrous, cystlike lesion, called a fibrous cortical defect, in children younger than 2 years of age. Most fibrous cortical defects resolve spontaneously or are obliterated by reparative ossification or remodeling. In some cases, however, the fibrous cortical defect persists and proliferates, becoming a fibroma. Fibromas are found primarily in children and adolescents. Ninety percent of these tumors occur in persons younger than 20 years of age.

The fibroma is a sharply demarcated tumor surrounded by a dense border of hardened bone. The tumor itself consists of fibrocytes arranged in whorled bundles, fibroblastic tissue, and osteoclast-like giant cells. As the tumor evolves, the fibrocytes imbibe lipids and assume a foamy appearance; thus they are known as foam cells. The tumor also contains extensive deposits of hemosiderin pigment. The tumor is characteristically located in the metaphyseal region of the bone and may cause a slight bulging of the cortex. The long axis of the tumor parallels the long axis of the bone.

The fibroma is usually asymptomatic and is found coincidentally. If the tumor is large enough, it may cause slight swelling or localized pain. An active adolescent may be first seen with a pathologic fracture.

The fibroma is generally not treated until is occupies more than 50% of the diameter of the bone or extends more than 3 to 4 cm into the cortex. When the tumor grows to this size, it is removed by curettage and the area is packed with bone chips.

Muscle Tumors

Soft tissue tumors in childhood are quite rare. The annual incidence is 8.4 per million for white children

TABLE 40-4 Classification of tumors by origin

Tissue	Tumor
Muscle	
Striated	Rhabdomyosarcoma
Smooth	Leiomyosarcoma
Adipose	Liposarcoma
Fibrous	Fibrosarcoma
Synovial mesothelium	Synovial sarcoma
Lymphatic structures	Lymphangiosarcoma
Blood vessels	Hemangiopericytoma
Nerve sheath	Neurogenic sarcoma

and 3.9 per million for black children. Soft tissue tumors originate from the primitive mesenchymal cells that normally give rise to muscle, tendons, blood vessels, lymphatic structures, fibrous and connective tissue, and bursa and fascia. Table 40-4 identifies the classification of soft tissue tumors depending on origin. All soft tissue tumors are characterized as highly aggressive tumors that invade surrounding structures and metastasize early.

Rhabdomyosarcoma (RMS) is the most common soft tissue sarcoma of childhood and accounts for over 50% of soft tissue tumors. RMS arises from embryonal rhabdomyoblasts that normally differentiate into mature striated muscle. The annual incidence of RMS is 4.4 per million in white children and 1.3 per million in black children. The five subclassifications of RMS are (1) embryonal (55%), (2) botryoid (7%), (3) alveolar (18%), (4) pleomorphic (2%), and (5) undifferentiated cell types I or II (5% each). The pleomorphic variety of rhabdomyosarcoma occurs in adults but is uncommon in children.

RMS can develop anywhere striated muscle is located. The primary locations and percentage range of incidence are (1) the head and neck (including the orbit), 61% to 36%; (2) the trunk, 33% to 8%; (3) the extremities, 24% to 14%; and (4) the genitourinary tract, 17% to 10%. Two age ranges (2 to 6 years of age and 15 to 19 years of age) are associated with RMS. Over two thirds of children with RMS are diagnosed by 10 years of age and RMS is slightly more common in males than females.

The cause of RMS is obscure. It can be induced in laboratory animals with viruses, chemical carcinogens, and heavy metal compounds. However, similar links have not been established in humans. On rare occasions, familial cases have been reported, sometimes associated with congenital malformations. RMS has also been reported to be a complication of neurofibromatosis and has been associated with breast cancer.

Pathophysiology

Rhabdomyosarcoma generally appears as a firm, fleshy, grayish-white mass. It sometimes exhibits variations, particularly with the botryoid subclassification that appears as a cystic polypoid mass. RMS has various appearances depending on the phase of differentiation of the rhabdomyoblast. The cells may be round or spindle shaped, racket or tadpole shaped, or multinucleated giant cells.

The **embryonal subclass of RMS** is the most common. The cells are generally round or spindle shaped because of their primitive stage. These tumors do not show striations and are consistent with the appearance of developing muscle in the 7- to 10-week-old fetus. Embryonal RMS is more common in younger children and is usually found in the head and neck region.

The **botryoides subclass of RMS** is very similar to the embryonal subclass. However, the gross appearance is often a bizarre polypoid, glistening, edematous "cluster of grapes" that is a mass of stroma and dilated blood vessels. Botryoides RMS is most common in young children and favors hollow viscera including the bladder, vagina, common bile duct, ear, nasopharnyx, and uterus.

The **alveolar subclass of RMS** is the most common type of RMS in adolescents. It generally involves an extremity or the perineal and perirectal areas. It appears as a firmer tumor than the embryonal and botryoides types. The tumor is composed of clusters of small, round rhabdomyoblasts and may have multinucleated giant cells. The alveolar subclass represents a higher degree of cellular differentiation than the embryonal or botryoides subtypes. The cell pattern is consistent with the hollow tube stage of normal muscle development seen in the 10- to 12-week-old fetus.

The **pleomorphic subclass of RMS** accounts for only 20% of pediatric RMS and is sometimes seen in adults during the third to fifth decade. It is composed of multinucleated giant cells and rackuet-shaped cells. The tumor cells appear as mature striated muscle that has become dedifferentiated.

The **undifferentiated cell types of RMS** are a relatively new subclass. They are similar in appearance to Ewing sarcoma (a bone tumor). They are most commonly found in the extremities.

RMS spreads by rapid local infiltration, as well as hematogenous and lymphatic routes. Hematogenous spread is thought to be the more common method of metastatic dissemination. At least 20% of children with RMS have metastatic disease at diagnosis. The preferred sites of metastases include the lungs, the lymph nodes, the bone marrow, the liver, the brain, and the bone.

Clinical Manifestations

The signs and symptoms of RMS depend on the anatomic location of the primary tumor and presence of

TABLE 40-5 Clinical manifestations of rhabdomyosarcoma

Location	Manifestation
HEAD AND NECK	
Orbit	Ptosis
	Exophthalmos
	Proptosis
Paranasal sinuses	Nasal obstruction
	Epistaxis
	Swelling
	Chronic sinusitis
Nasopharynx	Hypernasal speech
	Nasal discharge
	Visible polypoid mass
Oropharyngeal	Dysphagia
	Painful mastication
Middle ear	Chronic serous otitis media
	Discharge from affected ear
	Facial nerve palsy
	Conduction hearing loss
	Visible polypoid mass
EXTREMITIES	
All locations	Deep-seated, fixed palpable mass
RETROPERITO-NEAL	
All locations	Usually asymptomatic
	May have vague abdominal pain
	Bowel or genitourinary obstruction (late)
	Possible palpable mass
GENITOURINARY	
Vaginal	Abnormal vaginal bleeding
	Protruding polypoid mass
Prostate	Urinary tract obstruction
Bladder	Urinary retention
	Straining to void
	Hematuria
Paratesticular	Mass in scrotum that may or may not be painful

symptomatic metastases. The tumors are usually painless and early detection of RMS is facilitated by the presence of a palpable or visible mass. Deep-seated tumors cause functional impairment. The clinical manifestations of RMS are outlined in Table 40-5.

Evaluation and Treatment

Diagnostic studies during the pretreatment phase are used to determine the extent of the primary tumor and presence or absence of distant metastases. Specific diagnostic studies depend on the primary site, but a combination of radiographic, nuclear and CT scanning, and blood studies is used. Regional lymph nodes are assessed by lymphangiogram. Liver function, blood studies, and liver scans determine liver involvement, and bone scan determines the presence of bone metastases. Bone marrow aspiration may be used to determine bone marrow involvement. A lumbar puncture is performed to determine central nervous system involvement for tumors adjacent to the central nervous system. A biopsy of the primary tumor is necessary to confirm the diagnosis.

Staging of RMS is based on the classification system of the Intergroup Rhabdomyosarcoma Study, a national cooperative study group. Four stages are proposed based on the resectability of the tumor. About 15% of children have stage I disease (localized disease, completely resected); approximately 28% of children have stage II disease (grossly resected tumor with microscopic residual or regional disease that is totally resected); about 36% of children have stage III disease (gross residual disease); and approximately 20% of children have stage IV disease (metastatic disease present).

RMS is treated by a combination of surgery, radiation, and chemotherapy. Complete surgical resection provides the greatest assurance that cure can be achieved; however, cure occurs in only 16% of children. If surgical resection leads to serious disfigurement or functional disability (e.g., enucleation for orbital tumors or cystectomy for bladder tumors), chemotherapy and radiation will serve as the primary treatment and surgery will be avoided. However, if there is a high likelihood of local recurrence, as is the case for testicular and prostate tumors, radical orchiectomies and hemiscrotectomy will be used. For all tumors, except stage I disease, local radiation therapy is given. A variety of combination chemotherapy are used with RMS. Agents shown to be effective include vincristine, dactinomycin, and cyclophosphamide. Other drugs that have been used in combination are doxorubicin, VP-16, and cisplatin. Intrathecal chemotherapy is given to children whose tumor locations favor central nervous system spread.

The primary prognostic factor in RMS is the degree of residual disease that remains after surgical resection. Children with localized disease (stage I and II) have long-term survival rates reported at 70% to 80%. If widespread disease is present, long-term survival rates drop to 20%. Orbital tumors have an overall favorable prognosis, probably because of the lack of lymphatics in the area and early physical signs of disease.

SUMMARY REVIEW

Musculoskeletal Development in Children

1 Skeletal growth and development consist of two concurrent processes in healthy children: (1) the creation of new cells and tissues (growth), and (2) the consolidation of new tissues into a permanent form (maturation).

2 Ossification takes place in two centers in long bones: (1) the primary center or the diaphysis (the long, central portion of the bone), and (2) the secondary center or the epiphysis (the end portions of the bone).

3 Until adult stature is reached, age 17 for females and age 18 for males, growth in length of bones occurs at the epiphyseal plate through endochondrial ossification.

4 Fifty percent of the total growth of the spine has occurred by 1 year of age, and most children have achieved 50% of their adult height by 2 years of age.

5 The appendicular skeleton (extremities) grows faster during childhood than does the axial skeleton.

6 Muscle fibers reach their maximal size in females at 10 years of age and at 14 years of age in males.

Musculoskeletal Alterations in Children

1 The most common congenital defect of the upper extremities is syndactyly (webbing of the fingers).

2 Congenital hip dislocation is a serious and disabling condition in children.

3 Congenital muscle disorders (myopathies) include absence of muscles, hypoplasia, hyperplasia, and faulty intrinsic development.

4 Osteogenesis imperfecta (brittle bone disease) is an inherited disorder of collagen that primarily affects bones and results in serious fractures of many bones.

5 Rickets is a condition caused by deficiencies in vitamin D, calcium, and usually phosphorus, which is characterized by the failure of bones to become mineralized (ossified) and results in skeletal deformity.

6 Scoliosis is a lateral S-shaped or C-shaped curvature of the spinal column caused by congenital malformations of the spine, poliomyelitis, skeletal dysplasias, spastic paralysis, and unequal leg length.

7 Osteomyelitis is a local or generalized bacterial infection of bone and bone marrow. Bacteria is usually introduced by direct extension from a nearby infection, through the bloodstream, or by trauma.

8 Juvenile rheumatoid arthritis is an inflammatory joint disorder characterized by pain and swelling.

9 Avascular diseases of the bone are collectively referred to as osteochondroses and are caused by an insufficient blood supply to growing bones.

10 Legg-Calve-Perthes disease is one of the most common osteochondroses. This disorder is characterized by epiphyseal necrosis or degeneration of the head of the femur followed by regeneration or recalcification.

11 Osgood-Schlatter disease is characterized by inflammation or partial separation of the tibial tubercle caused by chronic irritation, usually as a result of overuse of the quadriceps muscles. The condition is primarily seen in muscular, athletic adolescent males.

12 The muscular dystrophies are a group of genetically transmitted diseases characterized by progressive atrophy of symmetric groups of skeletal muscles without evidence of involvement or degeneration of neural tissue. There is an insidious loss of strength in all forms of the disorder with increasing disability and deformity.

13 The two main types of childhood bone tumors are osteosarcoma and Ewing sarcoma.

14 Osteosarcoma, the most common childhood bone tumor, originates in bone-producing mesenchymal cells and is most often located in the distal end of the femur or proximal end of the tibia.

15 The majority of childhood osteosarcoma cases are diagnosed between 15 and 19 years of age and are most common in males.

16 Ewing sarcoma originates from cells within the bone marrow space and is most often located in the midshaft of long bones or in flat bones.

17 Ewing sarcoma is more common in males and is most frequently diagnosed between the ages of 5 and 15.

18 Pain is the usual presenting symptom for either osteosarcoma or Ewing sarcoma.

19 The primary treatments for osteosarcoma are surgery and chemotherapy. The primary treatment for Ewing sarcoma is radiation therapy; although surgery and chemotherapy may be added.

20 The most common type of childhood soft tissue tumor is rhabdomyosarcoma.

21 Rhabdomyosarcoma originates from embryonal rhabdomyoblasts that normally differentiate into mature striated muscle. There are five subtypes.

22 Clinical manifestations of rhabdomyosarcoma depend on the anatomic location; superficial tumors exhibit a painless palpable mass, whereas deep-seated tumors cause functional impairment.

23 Rhabdomyosarcoma is treated with a combination of surgery, radiation, and chemotherapy.

KEY TERMS

Alveolar subclass of RMS, 1383

Antalgic abductor lurch, 1375

Becker muscular dystrophy, 1378

Botryoides subclass of RMS, 1383

Cartilage model, 1361

Center of ossification, 1361

Congenital hip dysplasia, 1363

Duchenne muscular dystrophy, 1377

Embryonal subclass of RMS, 1383

Endochondral formation of bone, 1361

Ewing sarcoma, 1382

Facioscapulohumeral muscular dystrophy, 1378

Fibroma, 1382

Idiopathic scoliosis, 1369

Intramembranous formation of bone, 1361

Involucrum, 1371

Juvenile rheumatoid arthritis (JRA), 1373

Legg-Calvé-Perthes diseae, 1374

Limb girdle muscular dystrophy, 1379

Muscular dystrophy, 1376

Myotonic muscular dystrophy, 1379

Nonstructural scoliosis, 1369

Osgood-Schlatter disease, 1375

Osteochondrosis, 1373

Osteogenesis imperfecta (brittle bone disease), 1367

Osteogenesis imperfecta congenita, 1367

Osteogenesis imperfecta tarda, 1367

Osteomyelitis, 1370

Osteosarcoma, 1380

Perichondrium, 1361

Periosteal collar, 1361

Pleomorphic subclass of RMS, 1383

Primary center of ossification, 1361

Rhabdomyosarcoma (RMS), 1383

Rickets, 1368

Scapuloperoneal muscular dystrophy, 1379

Scoliosis, 1369

Secondary center of ossification, 1361

Secondary suppurative arthritis, 1371

Sequestra, 1371

Structural scoliosis, 1369

Syndactyly, 1363

Talipes (clubfoot), 1364

Talipes caleaneovalgus, 1365

Talipes equinovarus, 1365

Undifferentiated cell types of RMS, 1383

Vestigial tab, 1363

REFERENCES

Abramovitz, J. N., Baston, R. A., & Yablon, J. S. (1986). Vertebral osteomyelitis. The surgical management of neurologic complications. *Spine, 11*(5), 8-420.

Alderson, M., Speers, D., Emslie, K., & Nade, S. (1986). Acute haematogenous osteomyelitis and septic arthritis: A single disease. An hypothesis based upon the presence of transphyseal blood vessels. *Journal of Bone & Joint Surgery, 68*(2), 268-274.

Arias, F. G., Rodriguez, M., Hernandez, J. G., Gonzalvo, P., & Orense, M. (1987). Osteomyelitis deriving from BCG-vaccination. *Pediatric Radiology, 17*(2), 166-167.

Behrman, R. E., & Vaughan, V. C. (1983). *Nelson textbook of pediatrics* (12th ed.). Philadelphia: W. B. Saunders.

Bergdahl, S., Ekengren, K., & Eriksson, M. (1986). Neonatal hematogenous osteomyelitis: Risk factors for long-term sequelae. *Journal of Pediatric Orthopedics, 6*(2), 177-181.

Brashear, H. R., & Raney, R. B. (1978). *Shand's handbook of orthopedic surgery* (9th ed.). St. Louis: C. V. Mosby.

Brooke, M. H. (1977). *A clinician's view of neuromuscular diseases.* Baltimore: Williams & Wilkins.

Carnsdale, P. G., (1987). Osteomyelitis. In A. H. Crenshaw (Ed.), *Campbell's operative orthopaedics* (7th ed., vol. 1). St. Louis: C. V. Mosby.

Cassidy, J. T. (1982). *Textbook of pediatric rheumatology.* New York: John Wiley & Sons.

Chandrasekar, P. H., & Narula, A. P. (1986). Bone and joint infections in intravenous drug abusers. *Review of Infectious Diseases, 8*(6), 904-911.

Dich, V. Q., Nelson, J. D., & Haltalin, K. C. (1975). Osteomyelitis in infants and children. *American Journal of Diseases of Children, 129,* 1273-1276.

Fink, C. W., & Nelson, J. D. (1986). Septic arthritis and osteomyelitis in children. *Clinics in Rheumatic Diseases, 12*(2), 423-435

Gillespie, W. J., Haywood-Farmer, M., Fong, R., & Harding, S. M. (1987). Aspects of the microbe: Host relationship in staphylococcal hematogenous osteomyelitis. *Orthopedics, 10*(3), 475-480.

Green, N. E. (1983). Musculoskeletal infections in children. Part II. Primary subacute epiphyseal osteomyelitis. *Instructional Course Lectures, 32,* 37-40

Griggs, R. C., & Rennie, M. J. (1983). Muscle wasting in muscular dystrophy: Decreased protein synthesis or increased degradation? *Annals of Neurology, 13*(2), 125-132.

Gutman, L. T. (1985). Acute, subacute, and chronic osteomyelitis and pyogenic arthritis in children. *Current Problems in Pediatrics, 15*(12), 1-72.

Hobbs, R. (1922). *Treatment of puerperal infection by drainage.* Westland, MJ, London, xxvii, 16-32.

Karlin, J. M. (1987). Osteomyelitis in children. *Clinics in Podiatric Medicine and Surgery, 4*(1), 37-56.

Kissane, J. M. (Ed.). (1985). *Anderson's Pathology* (8th ed.). St. Louis: C. V. Mosby.

Morrissy, R. T., & Shore, S. L. (1986). Bone and joint sepsis. *Pediatric Clinics of North America, 33*(6), 1551-1564.

Nelson, L. W., & Lydiatt, D. D. (1987). Osteomyelitis of the head and neck. *Nebraska Medical Journal, 72*(5), 154-163.

Ray, M. J., & Basset, R. L. (1985). Pyogenic vertebral osteomyelitis. *Orthopedics, 8*(4), 504-506, 510, 512-513.

Riseborough, E. J., & Herndon, J. H. (1975). *Scoliosis and other deformities of the axial skeleton.* Boston: Little, Brown & Co.

Scott, M. O., Sylvester, J. E., Heiman-Patterson, T., Shi, Y. J., Fieles, W., Stedman, H., Burghes, A., Ray, P., Warton, R., & Fishbeck, K. H. (1988). Duchenne muscular dystrophy gene expression in normal and diseased human muscle. *Science, 239,* 1418-1420.

Swaiman, K. F., & Wright, F. S. (1982). *The practice of pediatic neurology.* St. Louis: C. V. Mosby.

Sykes, B. (1987). Molecular diagnostics: Genetics cracks bone disease. *Nature, 330,* 607-608.

Thompson, J. M. et al. (1989). *Mosby's manual of clinical nursing* (2nd ed.). St. Louis: C. V. Mosby.

Trueta, J. (1959). The three types of acute hematogenous osteomyelitis. *Journal of Bone and Joint Surgery, 41B,* 671-676.

Vizkelety, T. L. (1986). Partial destruction of the distal femoral epiphysis as a consequence of osteomyelitis: Regeneration after transplantation of a bone graft. *Journal of Pediatric Orthopedics, 5*(6), 731-733.

Whaley, L. F., & Wong, D. L. (1987). *Nursing care of infants and children* (3rd ed.). St. Louis: C. V. Mosby.

Winter, R. B. (1977). Scoliosis and spinal growth. *Orthopaedic Review, 6,* 17-20.

Wong, S. K., & Wilhelmus, K. R. (1986). Infantile maxillary osteomyelitis with cerebral abscess. *Journal of Pediatric Ophthalmology and Strabismus, 23*(3), 153-154.

Zaleske, D. J., Doppelt, S. H., & Mankin, H. J. (1986). Endocrine abnormalities of the immature skeleton. In W. W. Lovell & R. B. Winter (Eds.), *Pediatric orthopaedics* (2nd ed.). Philadelphia: J. B. Lippincott.

UNIT XIV

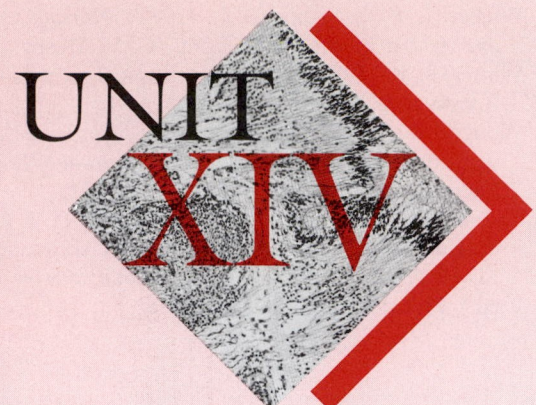

The Integumentary System

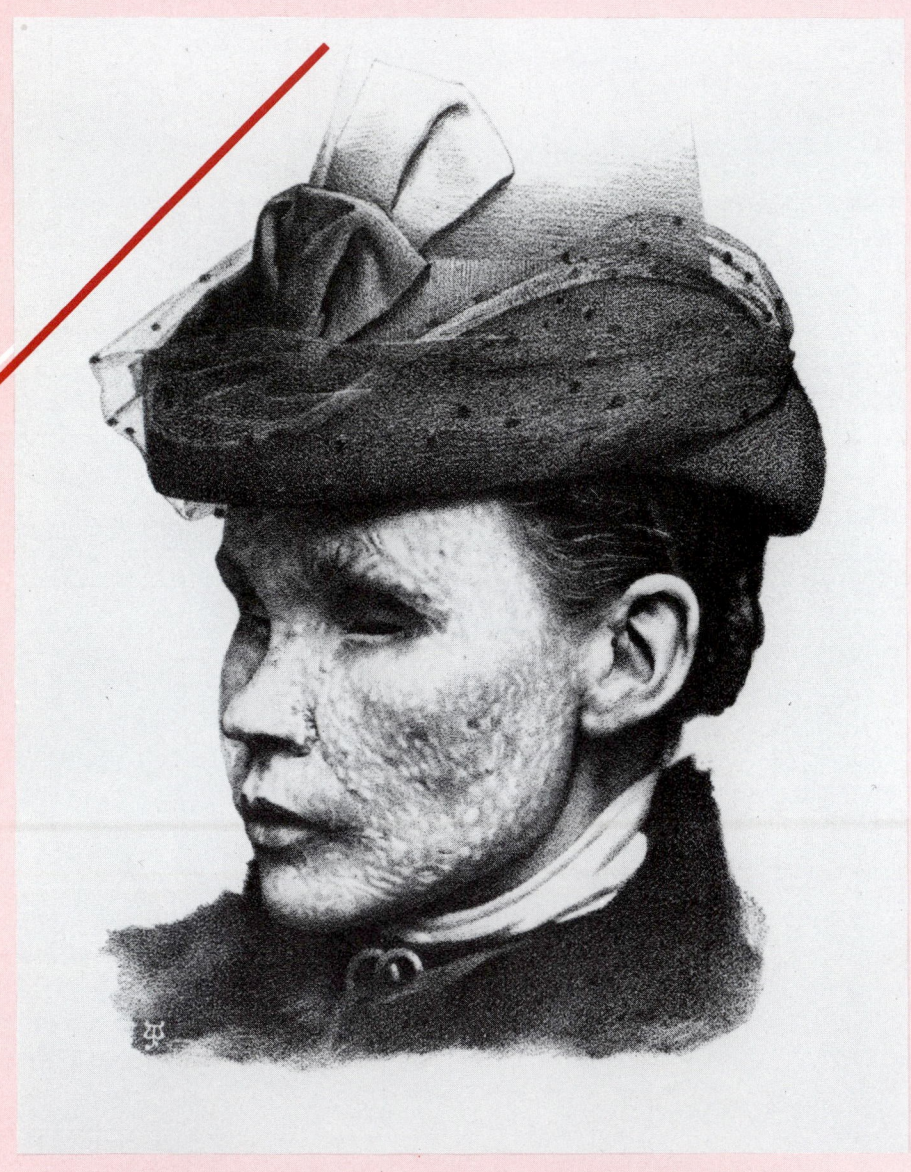

View of a blind woman, wearing hat and coat, her face pitted and scarred by smallpox. Note on caption: "The eyeballs were removed by Dr. Robertson on account of local pain and headache." (From Bramwell, B.: Atlas of clinical medicine, Edinburgh, 1892-96. Vol. I. Courtesy National Library of Medicine.)

SKIN diseases have been known since the early civilizations of the Egyptians, Greeks, Romans, and Arabs. In the time of Hippocrates, superficial ulcers were treated with warm baths, and the temperature of the water was important to prevent chilling and promote bleeding. Ulcers were then cleaned with vinegar, debrided, and covered with wool soaked in a herbal poultice including verdigris (copper acetate), flower of copper (copper oxide), molybdaina (lead oxide), alum, myrh, frankincense, gall nuts, vine flowers, and wool grease (Majno, 1975). Both the ancient Romans and Arabs used baths with both hot and cold water for treatment of some skin diseases. The Arabs developed theories of cleanliness in preventing skin diseases, particularly the bites of fleas, lice, and other insects. In the tenth century, Bagdad had more than 27,000 public baths. In second century BC China, "ulcer physicians" were designated to care for swollen ulcers, dripping ulcers, and ulcers caused by piercing instruments or fractures. Such wounds were treated with the five poisons, fortified with the five medicines, and tempered with the five flavors. Celcus, in AD 30, recommended sutures with women's hair to close small wounds and pins to close gaping wounds. He also advocated vinegar washes to avoid inflammation and loose closure for deep draining wounds. Leprosy, syphilis, smallpox, and skin tumors were evident in ancient times with epidemics of smallpox and bubonic plague affecting large populations. The major means of treatment were herbal applications, baths, and magical beliefs.

Early medical manuscripts from Britian (fifth to tenth century) indicate that the causes of skin diseases were unknown but often followed pestilence and trauma. Malnutrition, scabies, scurvy, and pellagra commonly occurred during and following wars, with lesions such as ulcers, eczema, impetigo, and erysipelas. Diseases such as psoriasis, scrofula (a tuberculous disease of lymph nodes and bones with draining abscesses), syphilis, and eczema were rampant during this period. Leprosy was associated with eating tainted or rotten meat and fish, and some leper hospitals of the time were noted for their treatment with fresh wholesome food. Scrofula was known as the "king's evil" because King Edward of Britian (1042 to 1066) believed the condition could be cured by the sovereign's touch. Elizabeth I practiced healing by touch; she knelt in prayer, laying her hands on the sores of her subjects (Huckbody, 1980). Hot herbal baths were often used for treatment. Fennel mint, yarrow, betony, and dill were most effective and are used in more sophisticated forms today. The recognition that pressure caused bedsores was first described by Paget in about 1855.

CHAPTER 41

Structure, Function, and Disorders of the Integument

Sue E. Huether
Melva Kravitz

Structure and function of the skin, 1391
  Layers of the skin, 1391
    Epidermis, 1391
    Dermis, 1392
  Hypodermis (subcutaneous layer), 1392
    Dermal appendages, 1392
    Blood supply and innervation, 1393
  Aging and skin integrity, 1393
  Tests of skin function, 1394
  Clinical manifestations of skin dysfunction, 1394
    Lesions, 1395
      Pressure ulcers, 1400
      Keloids, 1400
    Pruritus, 1401
Disorders of the skin, 1402
  Inflammatory disorders, 1402
    Allergic contact dermatitis, 1402
    Irritant contact dermatitis, 1402
    Atopic dermatitis, 1402
    Stasis dermatitis, 1403
    Seborrheic dermatitis, 1403
  Papulosquamous disorders, 1404
    Psoriasis, 1404
    Pityriasis rosea, 1405
    Lichen planus, 1405
    Acne vulgaris, 1406
    Acne rosacea, 1407
    Lupus erythematosus, 1408
      Discoid lupus erythematosus, 1408
      Systemic lupus erythematosus (SLE), 1409
  Vesiculobullous disorders, 1409
    Pemphigus, 1409
    Bullous pemphigoid, 1410
    Erythema multiforme, 1410
  Infections, 1411
    Bacterial infections, 1411

Folliculitis, 1411
    Furuncles and carbuncles, 1411
    Cellulitis, 1411
    Erysipelas, 1411
    Impetigo, 1411
  Viral infections, 1411
    Herpes simplex virus, 1411
    Herpes zoster and varicella, 1412
    Warts, 1413
  Fungal infections, 1414
    Tinea infections, 1414
    Candidiasis, 1414
Vascular disorders, 1415
  Cutaneous vasculitis, 1415
  Urticaria, 1415
  Scleroderma, 1416
Insect bites, 1416
  Ticks, 1416
  Mosquitoes and flies, 1416
Benign tumors, 1417
  Seborrheic keratosis, 1417
  Keratoacanthoma, 1417
  Actinic keratosis, 1418
  Nevi (moles), 1418
Cancer, 1418
  Basal cell carcinoma, 1419
  Squamous cell carcinoma, 1419
  Malignant melanoma, 1420
  Kaposi sarcoma, 1421
Thermal injury, 1423
  Burns, 1423
    Pathophysiology, 1423
      First-degree burns, 1423
      Second-degree burns, 1424
      Third-degree burns, 1425
    Clinical manifestations, 1426

Cardiovascular response to burn injury, 1427
Cellular response to burn injury, 1429
Evaporative water loss, 1431
Evaluation and treatment, 1431
Frostbite, 1431
Disorders of the hair, 1432
Alopecia, 1432
Male-pattern alopecia, 1432
Female-pattern alopecia, 1432
Alopecia areata, 1432
Hirsutism, 1433
Disorders of the nail, 1433
Paronychia, 1433
Onchyomycosis, 1433

STRUCTURE AND FUNCTION OF THE SKIN

The skin is the largest organ of the body. Combined with the accessory structures of hair, nails, and glands, it forms the **integumentary system.** The skin covers the entire body and accounts for approximately 20% of the body's weight. The primary function of the skin is to protect the body from the environment by serving as a

barrier against microorganisms, ultraviolet radiation, loss of body fluids, and the stress of mechanical forces. The skin also regulates body temperature within a very narrow range and is involved in the production of vitamin D. Touch and pressure receptors provide important protective functions and pleasurable sensations.

Layers of the Skin

The skin is formed of two major layers: (1) a superficial or outer layer of **epidermis** and (2) a deeper layer of **dermis** (the true skin) (Fig. 41-1 and Table 41-1). The subcutaneous tissue, or **hypodermis,** is an underlying layer of connective tissue. Each skin layer contains cells that represent progressive stages of skin cell differentiation as the skin grows.

Epidermis

The epidermis grows continually by shedding the superficial layer of **stratum corneum,** which is formed entirely of keratinocytes and melanocytes. These cells are named for the substances they produce. **Keratinocytes** produce **keratin,** a scleroprotein. Keratin is the main constituent of skin, hair, and nail cells. The thickness of the epidermis varies from 0.3 mm on the eyelids to 1.5

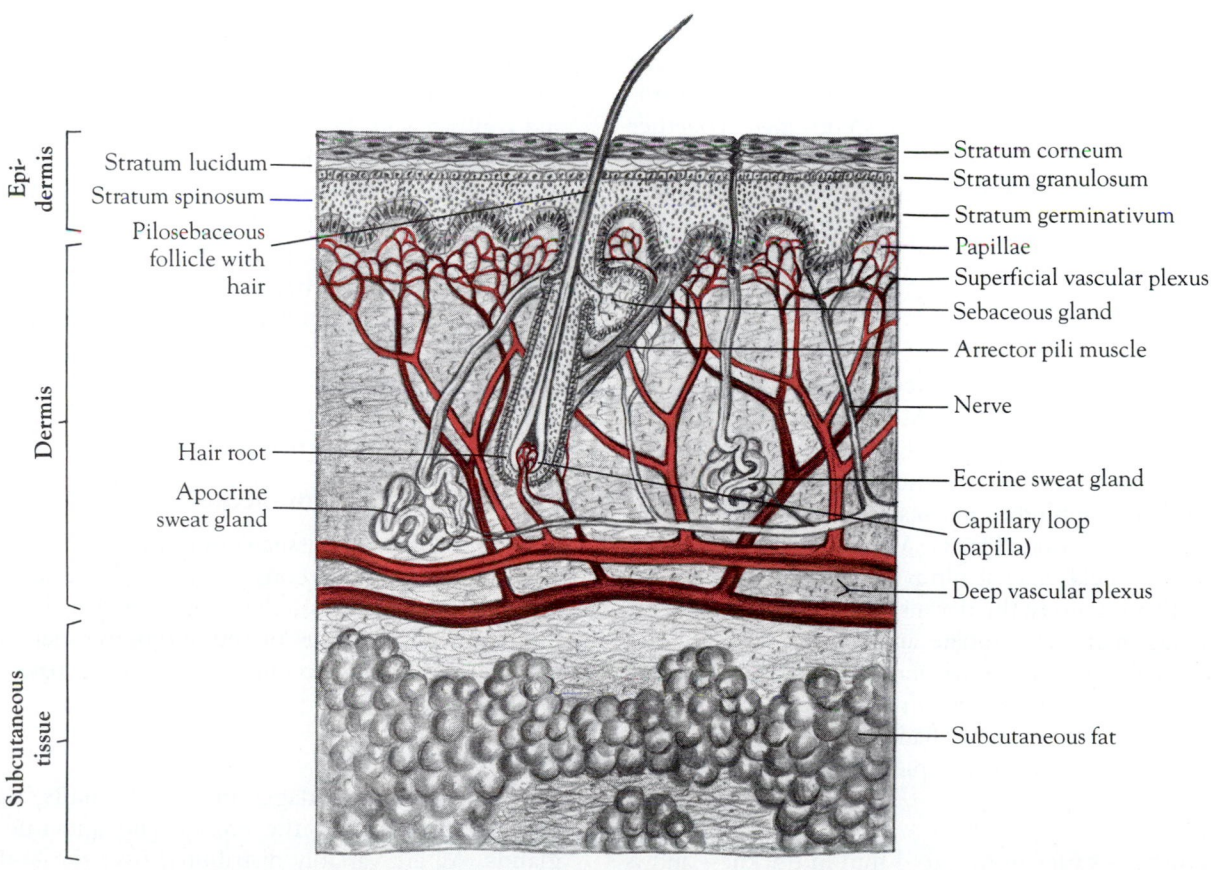

FIG. 41-1. Structure of the skin. (From Thompson et al., 1986.)

TABLE 41-1 Layers of the skin

Structure	Characteristics
Epidermis	The most important layer of the skin; normally very thin (0.12 mm) but can thicken and form corns or calluses in areas of constant pressure or friction
Stratum corneum	Dead keratinocytes that provide a tough covering over the body surface
Stratum lucidum	A clear layer of cells containing a substance called eleidin that is transformed into keratin as the cells differentiate into stratum corneum
Stratum granulosum	A layer of cells containing keratohyalin that gives a granular appearance
Stratum spinosum	A layer of cells on top of the basal cells that is polygonal shaped with spinous processes projecting between adjacent keratinocytes
Stratum germinativum	A basal cell layer closest to the basement membrane; keratinocytes divide and move upward to replace cells normally shed from the surface
Dermis	A 1-4 mm layer of irregular connective tissue composed of collagen and elastic and reticular fibers with a rich blood, lymphatic, and nerve supply; contains sensory receptors and special glands
Papillary layer	An irregular layer of collagen fibers containing capillary loops, sensory receptors, and a horizontal plexus of blood vessels
Reticular layer	A random array or reticulum of collagenous fibers that articulate (connect) with the hypodermis
Hypodermis	Subcutaneous tissue or superficial fascia of varying thickness that connects the overlying dermis to underlying muscle

mm on the palms of the hands and soles of the feet. New cells (keratinocytes) formed in the **basal layer** (stratum basale) move upward and differentiate, forming the **spinous layer** (stratum spinosum). Together they form the germinative layer (stratum germinativum). The cells enlarge and then become flattened, stacked, and cornified as they ascend to the skin surface. Cornification, or keratinization, prevents dehydration of deeper skin layers. The average turnover of the epidermis is about 30 days.

The epidermis has three different types of cells that facilitate its functional characteristics: (1) melanocytes, (2) Langerhans cells, and (3) Merkel cells. The **melanocytes** are usually located near the base of the epidermis. They synthesize and secrete the pigment melanin with exposure to sunlight in response to melanocyte-stimulating hormone (MSH). Melanin in the epidermis provides a shield against ultraviolet radiation. **Langerhans cells** migrate to the dermis from the bone marrow. The Langerhans cells initiate an immune response and provide defense against environmental antigens. **Merkel cells** are associated with touch receptors, and they function as slowly adapting mechanoreceptors when stimulated by deformation of the epidermis.

Dermis

The dermis varies from 1 to 4 mm in thickness and is composed of three types of fibrous connective tissue:
(1) collagen, (2) elastin and reticulin, and (3) a gel-like ground substance. The haphazard arrangement of connective tissue allows the skin to be mobile and stretch and contract with body movement. Hair follicles, sebaceous glands, sweat glands, blood vessels, lymphatic vessels, and nerves are contained in the dermis. The cone-like projections of the papillary dermis interface with the epidermis. The papillae provide texture to the surface of the skin by forming what are known as rete pegs.

The cells of the dermis include fibroblasts, mast cells, and macrophages. Fibroblasts secrete the connective tissue matrix. Mast cells release histamine and play a role in hypersensitivity reactions in the skin. Macrophages are phagocytic and participate in immune responses.

Hypodermis (Subcutaneous Layer)

The subcutaneous tissue contains the dermal appendages (nails, hair, sebaceous glands, and the eccrine and apocrine sweat glands), the supplying blood vessels of the dermis, and nerves of the autonomic nervous system. A layer of cushioning fat provides a base for the hypodermis.

Dermal Appendages

The **dermal appendages** include the **nails, hair, sebaceous glands,** and the eccrine and apocrine **sweat glands.** All are variably distributed over the body. The nails are protective keratinized plates that appear at the

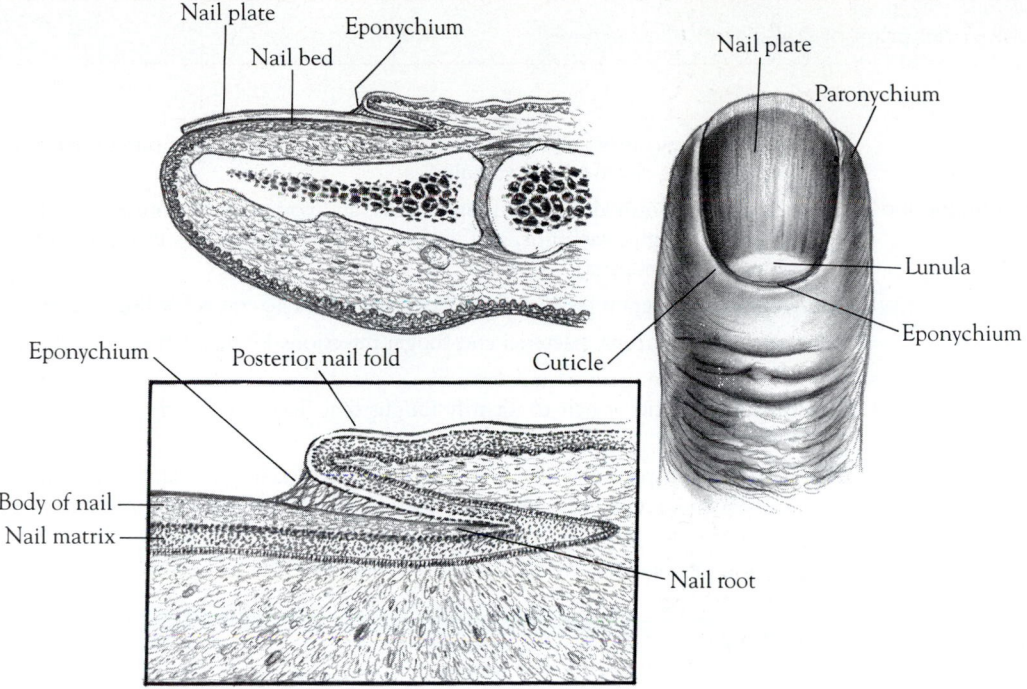

FIG. 41-2. Structures of the nail. (From Thompson et al., 1989.)

ends of fingers and toes. The nail is composed of four structural units: (1) the proximal nail fold, (2) the matrix from which the nail grows, (3) the hyponychiuam (the nail bed), and (3) the nail plate (Fig. 41-2). Nail growth is continuous throughout life at a rate of about 0 mm to 1 mm/day.

Hair follicles and sebaceous glands are integrated units (Fig. 41-1). Hair color, density, grain, and pattern of distribution have considerable variability and depend on age, sex, and race. Hair follicles arise from the matrix (or bulb) located deep in the dermis. They extend from the dermis at an angle and have an errector pili muscle attached near the mid-dermis that straightens the follicle when contracted causing the hair to stand up. Hair growth begins in the bulb, with cellular differentiation occurring as the hair progresses up the follicle. Hair is fully hardened, or cornified, by the time it emerges at the skin surface. Hair growth is cyclic with periods of growth and rest that vary over different body surfaces.

The **sebaceous glands** open onto the surface of the skin through a canal. They are found in greatest numbers on the face, chest, and back with modified glands on the eyelids, lips, nipple, glans penis, and prepuce. Sebaceous glands secrete sebum that is composed primarily of lipids. Growth of sebaceous glands is stimulated by testosterone, and their enlargement is one of the early signs of puberty.

The **eccrine sweat glands** are distributed over the body with the greatest numbers in the palms of the hands, soles of the feet, and forehead. These secretions are important in thermoregulation and cooling of the body through evaporation. The **apocrine sweat glands** are fewer in number and are located in the axillae, scalp, face, abdomen, and genital area.

Blood Supply and Innervation

The blood supply to the skin is limited to the **papillary capillaries,** or plexus, of the dermis. These capillary loops arise from a subpapillary plexus that is supplied by a deeper horizontal cutaneous arterial plexus. Branches from the deep plexus supply hair follicles and sweat glands. A subpapillary network of veins drains the capillary loops. There are arteriovenous anastomoses at the level of the dermis that facilitate the regulation of body temperature. Heat loss can be regulated by varying blood flow through the skin by opening and closing the arteriovenous anastomoses in conjunction with evaporative heat loss of sweat. The sympathetic nervous system regulates both vasoconstriction and vasodilation. There are only α-adrenergic receptors in the skin. The lymphatic vessels of the skin arise in the papillary dermis and drain into larger subcutaneous trunks, removing cells, proteins, and immunologic mediators.

Aging and Skin Integrity

Many of the age-associated changes in the skin are readily observable and appear over the body surface. Structurally, the skin becomes thinner, dryer, and wrin-

TABLE 41-2   Summary of skin diagnostic procedures

Test	Purpose
Skin biopsy	Differential diagnosis of cellular structure, i.e., benign growths vs carcinoma, chronic infections, blistering diseases, and vasculitis
Microscopic immunofluorescence	Identification of antibodies, immunoglobulins, and complement components for diseases such as pemphigus, vasculitis, and discoid lupus erythematosus using fluorescent light on slide-mounted biopsies.
Gram stain	Differentiation of gram-positive from gram-negative bacteria according to stain absorption
Culture	Identification of chronic bacterial and fungal infections by incubating skin specimens in culture media
Wood's lamp examination	Examination of skin or hair to identify fungus that fluoresces bright yellow-green under ultraviolet light
Patch and scratch tests	Application of suspected allergens to skin patch or scratch for evaluation of immune system responses to known allergens and evaluation of cell-mediated immune function (*Candida albicans,* skin fungus)
Skin scrapings	Application of potassium hydroxide (KOH) and low heat to skin scrapings on a glass slide to identify fungi
Side lighting	Indirect lighting of the skin using light to the side of the lesions to evaluate patterns of depression and elevation of skin lesions
Diascopy	Use of glass or clear plastic pressed on the skin to differentiate erythema caused by dilated capillaries (blanching) from extravasation of blood (no blanching)

kled with a change in pigmentation. The cellular alterations contributing to the changes include a flattening of the dermoepidermal border with a shortening and decrease in the number of capillary loops. There are fewer melanocytes with decreased protection against ultraviolet radiation. A significant decrease in the number of Langerhans cells decreases the skin's immune response with aging. The thickness of the dermis also decreases and accounts for the translucent, paper-thin quality of the skin. Loss of the rete pegs gives the skin a smooth, shiny appearance (Gilchrist, 1984).

The decreased vasculature probably contributes to the atrophy of eccrine, apocrine, and sebaceous glands that cause dry skin. Loss of elastin fibers is associated with wrinkling. The collagen fibers become less flexible and decrease the ability of the skin to stretch and regain shape. Decreased cell generation, blood supply, and depressed immune responses also delay wound healing in aging skin. Changes in hair color and distribution also occur. Greying is due to loss of melanocytes from hair bulbs, and thinning occurs from a gradual decline in the number of hair follicles and growth of finer hair.

The epidermal cells change shape, and the barrier function of the stratum corneum is reduced. There is increased permeability and decreased clearance of substances from the dermis. The accumulation of such substances is related to decreased vascularity and can cause

skin irritation. Temperature regulation is compromised in the elderly, and there is increased risk for both heat stroke and hypothermia. Loss of cutaneous vasomotion and subcutaneous fat and decreased eccrine sweat production are contributing factors. The pressure and touch receptors and free nerve endings all decrease in number and reduce sensory perception. In summary, many of the protective functions of the skin are decreased with aging.

Tests of Skin Function

Diagnostic evaluations of skin disorders can often be completed by the gathering of historical information and physical examination and observation of the distribution and characteristics of the presenting lesions. Additional diagnostic studies are summarized in Table 41-2.

Clinical Manifestations of Skin Dysfunction
Lesions

Lesions of the skin are readily observable and easily addressed for distribution and structure. The identification of the morphologic structure and appearance of the skin in combination with a health history is necessary to identify the underlying pathophysiology. Table 41-3 describes and illustrates the basic lesions of the skin. Special skin lesions are described in Table 41-4.

Text continued on p. 1400.

TABLE 41-3 Basic lesions of the skin

Type	Characteristics	Example
FLAT LESIONS		
Macule	A flat circumscribed lesion of any size differentiated from surrounding skin by color	Hyperpigmentation Erythema Telangiectasias Purpura
Patch	A flat, irregular lesion larger than 1 cm in diameter	Vitiligo
ELEVATED LESIONS		
Papule	Firm elevated lesions 1 cm or less in diameter from infiltration or hyperplasia of the dermis	Verruca (warts) Lichen planus Nevus
Plaque	Elevated lesions with a large surface area	Psoriasis Eczema

(Continued.)

TABLE 41-3 Basic lesions of the skin—cont'd

Type	Characteristics	Example	
Nodule	A palpable circumscribed lesion 1-2 cm in diameter located in the epidermis, dermis, or hypodermis; surface features may vary from smooth to ulcerated	Benign or malignant tumors Foreign body in flammation Calcium deposits	
Wheal	A dome or flat-topped elevated lesion with well-defined and often changing borders caused by edema of the dermis	Hives Angioedema	
Vesicle and bulla	A fluid-filled, thin-walled elevated lesion; a bulla is a vesicle greater than 0.5 cm in diameter	Herpes zoster Impetigo Pemphigus Second-degree burn	
Pustule	An elevated lesion containing an exudate of white blood cells that may be sterile or contaminated with bacteria	Acne Pustular psoriasis	

TABLE 41-3 Basic lesions of the skin—cont'd

Type	Characteristics	Example	
Scale	Accumulation of the stratum corneum from cellular retention or cellular overproduction	Psoriasis	
Crust	Accumulation of dried blood or serum; size may vary	Eczema Impetigo	
Lichenification	Thickening, toughening of the skin with accentuation of skin lines caused by scratching	Chronic dermatitis	
Cyst	An elevated, encapsulated mass of dermis or subcutaneous layers, solid or fluid filled	Sebaceous cyst	

(Continued.)

TABLE 41-3 Basic lesions of the skin—cont'd

Type	Characteristics	Example	
Tumor	A well-demarcated, elevated lesion greater than 2 cm in diameter	Fibroma Lipoma Melanoma Hemangioma	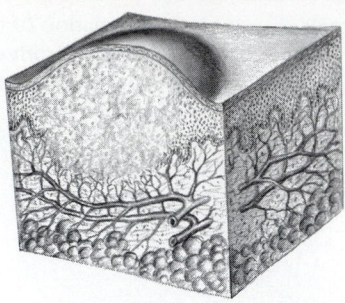
Scar	Thin or thick elevated fibrous tissue	Healed laceration, burn, or surgical incision	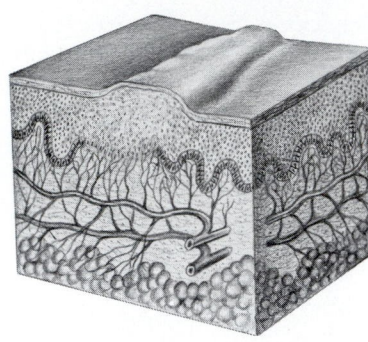

DEPRESSED LESIONS

Type	Characteristics	Example	
Atrophy	Thinning of the epidermis or dermis caused by a decrease in cell numbers of connective tissue	Thin facial skin of elderly Striae of pregnancy	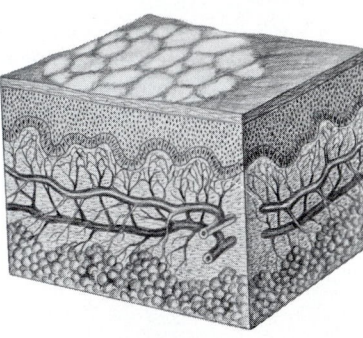
Ulcer	Loss of epidermis and dermis within a distinct border	Pressure sores Basal cell carcinoma	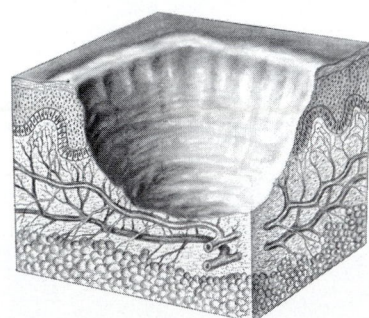

TABLE 41-3   Basic lesions of the skin—cont'd

Type	Characteristics	Example	
Excoriation	Loss of epidermis with exposed dermis	Scratches	
Fissure	Linear crack or break exposing dermis; small, deep, red	Athlete's foot Cheilosis	
Erosion	Depressed, moist, red break in epidermis; follows rupture of vesicle or bulla; larger than fissure	Chickenpox Diaper dermatitis	

TABLE 41-4   Special skin lesions

Type	Clinical manifestations
Comedone	A plug of sebaceous and keratin material lodged in the opening of a hair follicle; an open comedone has a dilated orifice (blackhead) and a closed comedone has a narrow opening (whitehead)
Burrow	A narrow, raised, irregular channel caused by a parasite
Petechiae	A circumscribed area of blood less than 0.5 cm in diameter
Purpura	A circumscribed area of blood greater than 0.5 cm in diameter
Telangiectasia	Dilated, superficial blood vessels

Pressure Ulcers

Pressure ulcers, or pressure sores, are the development of ischemic ulcers in normal skin as a result of pressure and shearing forces. The term decubitus ulcer refers to ulcers or pressure sores that develop from being in the recumbent position for a long time. The more general term of pressure sore or ulcer will be used here. Those at greatest risk are individuals who are immobilized, incontinent, or debilitated, particularly the elderly. The highest incidence occurs among individuals with a fractured neck of the femur (Versluysen, 1986).

Individuals with neurologic disorders, such as spinal cord injuries, dementia, or cerebrovascular disease, are particularly at risk, often as a result of loss of sensation rather than immobility. Chronic diseases accompanied by anemia, edema, renal failure, malnutrition, sepsis, and urinary or fecal incontinence increase the risk of pressure sores. The liability for developing a pressure sore is increased when individuals lie for hours on hard x-ray and operating tables or sit in wheelchairs or lie in bed for hours without changing position or relieving pressure. Use of coarse draw-sheets for turning and moving individuals in bed by dragging them about can cause shearing forces that lead to pressure sores.

Pressure sores usually develop over bony prominences. The sacrum, heels, ischia, and greater tronchanters are the most common sites. Continuous pressure on tissue between the bony prominence and a resistant outside surface distorts capillaries and occludes the blood supply. If the pressure is relieved within a few hours, a brief period of reactive hyperemia (redness) occurs with no lasting tissue damage. If the pressure continues unrelieved, the endothelial cells lining the capillaries become disrupted with platelet aggregation, forming microthrombi that block blood flow and cause anoxic necrosis of surrounding tissues. A layer of dead tissue forms that appears as a blister when there is superficial damage or a reddish blue discoloration when there is deeper tissue damage. Superficial sores are more common on the sacrum as a result of shearing or friction forces (forces parallel to the skin). Deep sores develop closer to the bone as a result of tissue distortion and vascular occlusion from pressure that is perpendicular to the tissue (over the heels, trochanter, and ischia).

The necrotic tissue initiates an inflammatory response with pain, fever, and leukocytosis. Although bacteria colonize the dead tissue, the infection is usually localized and self-limiting. Proteolytic enzymes from bacteria and macrophages dissolve necrotic tissues and cause a foul-smelling discharge that appears like, but is not, pus.

Pressure sores are often painful in individuals who do not have loss of sensation from spinal cord trauma or neuropathy. The presence of necrotic tissue produces an inflammatory response with hyperemia, fever, and increased white blood cell count. If the ulceration is large, toxicity and pain lead to loss of appetite, debility, and renal insufficiency. Individuals who are immunosuppressed or have diabetes mellitus may develop infection and inflammation of adjacent tissues (cellulitis) or septicemia.

The primary goal for those at risk for pressure ulcers is prevention. Pressure sores are not prevented by topical agents, such as benzoin, vitamin D ointment, zinc oxide, oils, or antibiotics. Turning every 2 hours or use of flotation devices and alternating pressure matresses are effective preventive techniques.

Superficial ulcers should be covered with flat, nonbulky dressings that cannot wrinkle and cause increased pressure or friction. Spontaneous healing will occur more quickly when the ulcer is kept moist with an occlusive dressing (Monk, Graham-Brown, & Sarkany, 1988). Antibiotics are seldom required. Antiseptics, such as hydrogen peroxide or iodine, are damaging to granulation tissue and should not be used. Successful healing requires continued adequate relief of pressure.

Large, deep pressure ulcers may require surgical debridement of necrotic tissue and opening of deep pockets for drainage. A variety of skin grafting techniques may be used for wound closure. The myocutaneous flap, a single unit of skin with its underlying muscle and vasculature, has been an effective treatment in large avascular areas over bony prominences.

Keloids

Keloids are sharply elevated, irregularly shaped, progressively enlarging scars caused by excessive amounts of collagen in the corneum during connective tissue repair. Seemingly inconsequential trauma may result in a keloidal reaction, particularly in blacks and Orientals. Burns incite this reaction more commonly than other types of injury.

Excessive or poorly aligned tension on a wound, introduction of foreign material into the skin, and certain types of trauma (such as burns) are all provocative factors. Those parts of the body at risk include shoulders, back, chin, ears, and lower legs. Most keloids appear within 1 year of trauma. Individuals 10 to 30 years of age develop lesions much more commonly than do children before puberty or older adults.

The fibrous tissue that accumulates in keloids is associated with increased cellularity and metabolic activity of fibroblasts. **Myofibroblasts,** cells with characteristics of both fibroblasts and smooth muscle cells, have been identified as the principal cell in keloids.

Type III collagen is increased with keloids. The swollen appearance of keloids is caused by an abundance of extracellular material. Collagenase activity in keloids has been found to be normal or increased, but the collagen may be protected from degradation by **proteoglycan,** a glycoprotein present in connective tissue that serves as a

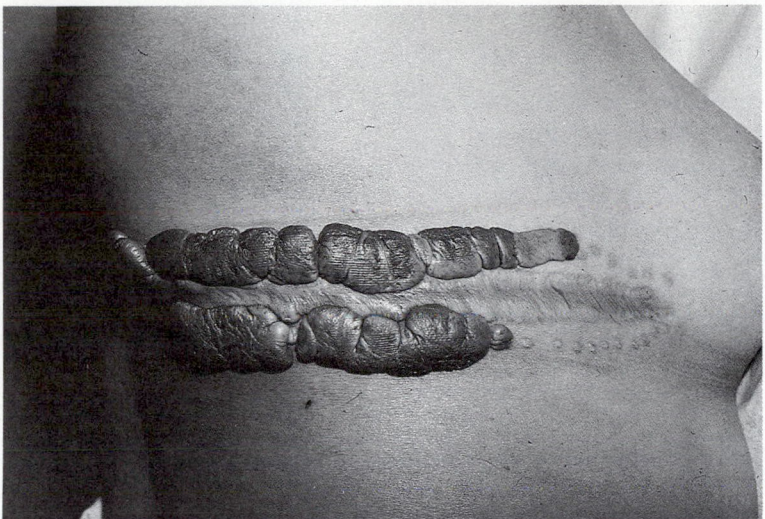

FIG. 41-3. Keloid formation. Mass of keloids arising from suture marks in a black individual. (From Habif, 1985.)

binding (cementing) material, and by specific inhibitors of proteolytic enzymes. A familial tendency for keloid formation has been found, with both autosomal recessive and autosomal dominant inheritance patterns being reported.

Keloids start as pink or red, firm, well-defined, rubbery plaques that persist for several months after trauma. Later, uncontrolled overgrowth causes extension beyond the site of the original wound and the tumor becomes smoother, irregularly shaped, hyperpigmented, harder, and more symptomatic. The tendency to send out **clawlike prolongations** is typical of keloids (Fig. 41-3).

Preventive measures such as the avoidance of unnecessary, elective surgeries are of paramount importance. When surgery is necessary for cosmetic reasons, early childhood is best. Scalpel surgery with strict aseptic technique and avoidance of wound tension should be imperative. Electrosurgery or chemosurgery should be avoided. Injection of corticosteroids into the lesion often brings excellent results and is the treatment of choice.

Pruritus

Pruritus, or itching, is a symptom associated with many primary skin disorders, such as eczema or lice infestations, or as a manifestation of systemic disease, such as chronic renal failure, cholestatic liver disease, thyroid disorders, iron deficiency, and opiate drugs. It may be localized or generalized and may move from one location to another.

The actual mechanisms causing pruritus are unknown. Multiple stimuli can produce itching including histamine, heat, and electrical stimulation with a fine probe. In experiments using cowage (a pruritogen or itch-causing substance), itching was most severe when applied at the junction of the dermis and epidermis (Shelley & Arthur, 1957). It is not known if the cowage stimulates the itching directly or induces histamine release. Antihistamines do not block this type of induced itching. Substance P, a neurotransmitter present throughout the nervous system, induces histamine release and wheal formation with itching when injected into the skin (Ebertz et al., 1987). Antihistamines and local anesthetics block substance P-induced itching.

Itching has also been linked to pain, since many stimuli that induce pain produce itching at lower intensities. Central nervous system mechanisms can also modulate itching and itching is less perceptible when the mind is concentrating on other things. How the central nervous system influences the itch sensation is unclear.

Chronic itching is an unpleasant sensation relieved by scratching, often severe enough to cause trauma to the skin, resulting in infection and scarring. Some individuals become so distraught with the constant irritation that they will apply heat with enough intensity and duration to produce burns.

Management of localized itching depends on the cause, and the primary condition must be treated. Symptomatic relief may be obtained from antihistamines, which also have a sedative effect. Minor tranquilizers, such as promethazine, may be effective for some causes of pruritus. Itching related to dry, rough skin (xerosis) can be managed with applications of emollients and increased environmental humidity. Topical steroids are immediately effective with some occurrences of pruritus; however, in some instances, pruritus is resistant to any type of therapy.

DISORDERS OF THE SKIN

Disruptions in skin integrity may be precipitated by trauma, abnormal cellular function, infection and inflammation, and systemic diseases. Many skin disorders are benign and self-limiting, whereas some are severe and life threatening.

Inflammatory Disorders

The most common inflammatory disorder of the skin is eczema (eczematous inflammation). **Eczema** is an inflammatory response of the skin caused by endogenous and exogenous agents and is often considered synonymous with dermatitis. Endogenous eczemas include atopic dermatitis and seborrheic dermatitis. Exogenous eczemas include irritant dermatitis and allergic contact dermatitis. Eczematous dermatitis is characterized by erythema, vesicles, scales, and itching. Edema, serous discharge, and crusting occur with continued irritation and scratching. In chronic eczema the skin becomes thickened, leathery, and hyperpigmented from recurrent irritation and scratching. The location of eczema is related to the underlying cause. Eczematous inflammations need to be differentiated from other rashes and dermatoses, particularly psoriasis.

Allergic Contact Dermatitis

Allergic contact dermatitis is a common form of cell-mediated or delayed hypersensitivity. (See Chapter 8 for different types of allergic responses.) A wide variety of allergens (e.g., microorganisms, chemicals, foreign proteins, drugs, metals) can form the sensitizing antigen. Contact with poison ivy is a common example (Fig. 41-4). As the allergen comes in contact with the skin, the allergen is bound to a carrier protein forming a sensitizing antigen. The Langerhans cells process the antigen and carry it to T cells that then become sensitized to the antigen.

Delayed hypersensitivity is characterized by the passing of several hours before an immunologic response is apparent. The T cells play an important role because they differentiate and secrete lymphokines that affect macrophage movement and aggregation, coagulation, and other inflammatory responses (see Chapter 2). Sensitization usually develops with first exposure to the antigen, and symptoms of dermatitis occur with reexposure.

The manifestations of allergic contact dermatitis include erythema and swelling with pruritic (itching) vesicular lesions in the areas of allergen contact. The pattern of distribution provides clues to the source of the antigen (i.e., hands exposed to chemical solutions or boundaries from rings and bracelets). Removal of the irritant is necessary for resolution of the inflammatory re-

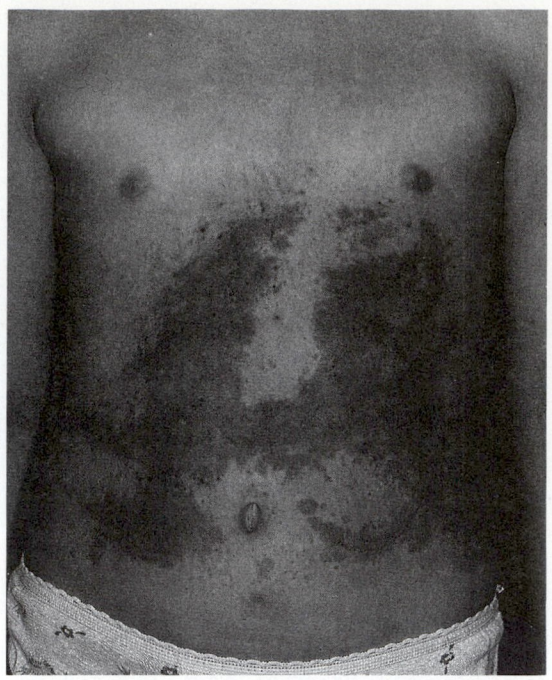

FIG. 41-4. Linear eruption caused by contact with poison ivy. Poison ivy dermatitis. Diffuse erythema with linear lesions. (From Habif, 1985.)

sponse and tissue repair. Topical or systemic steroids may be required for treatment, depending on the severity of the lesion.

Irritant Contact Dermatitis

Irritant contact dermatitis is a nonimmunologically mediated inflammation of the skin. Chemical irritation from acids or prolonged exposure to soaps and detergents are common causes (see box below). The skin lesions are similar in appearance to allergic contact dermatitis. Removing the source of irritation and use of topical agents provides effective treatment.

Atopic Dermatitis

Atopic dermatitis is a common disease affecting from 7 to 24 individuals per 1000 (Johnson, 1977). The prevalence is more common in infancy and childhood; however, some individuals are affected throughout life. A family history of asthma, allergic rhinitis, dry skin, and eczema accompany this disorder.

During infancy, the eczema is characterized by red, weeping, crusty lesions distributed over the face, neck, and buttocks (see Chapter 42). During adolescence and adulthood, the lesions are usually localized to the hands and feet and/or flexor surfaces (i.e., antecubital fossa and popliteal space) of the arms and legs. The erythema, scaling, and lichenification (thickened and leatherlike skin) are exacerbated by scratching as the lesions are

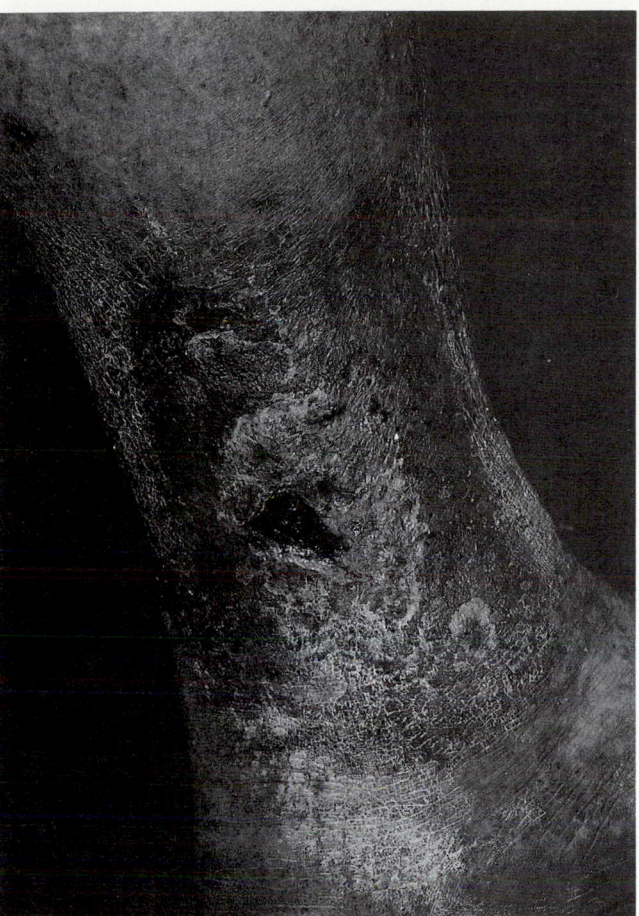

FIG. 41-5. Stasis dermatitis. The skin is diffusely red, thickened, and bound down by fibrosis. Ulceration occurs with the slightest trauma. (From Habif, 1985)

manifest by itching. The scratching increases susceptibility to infection from *Staphylococcus aureus* and predisposition of cutaneous dissemination of viruses, particularly herpes simplex and vaccinia. Affected individuals also have a higher incidence of cataracts. Although the cause of atopic dermatitis is unknown, depressed cell-mediated immunity, elevated IgE levels, and increased sensitivity to histamine are related factors (Stone, Muller, & Glech, 1973).

Management of atopic dermatitis includes avoidance of known irritants, good lubrication, and preservation of skin moisture. During the acute inflammatory stage, application of open wet compresses, using aluminum acetate solution (Burrow solution), soothes itching and cools and moistens the skin. Topical steroids in the lowest possible dosages may be used to treat the lesions. Relief of pruritus is difficult but oral antihistamines are occasionally prescribed. Affected individuals should avoid exposure to herpes simplex and vaccination with live virus.

Stasis Dermatitis

Stasis dermatitis usually occurs on the legs as a result of venous stasis and edema. The disorder is associated with varicosities, phlebitis, and vascular trauma. Initially there is erythema and pruritus with the development of scaling, petechiae, and hyperpigmentation. Progressive lesions become ulcerated, particularly around the ankles and tibia (Fig. 41-5).

Treatment includes elevating the legs as often as possible, not wearing tight clothes around the legs, and not standing for long periods. Acute inflammations are treated with antibiotics. Chronic lesions with ulceration are treated with wet dressings of Burrow solution or silver nitrate. Edema is controlled with external compression.

Seborrheic Dermatitis

Seborrheic dermatitis is a common chronic inflammation of the skin involving the scalp, eyebrows, eyelids, ear canals, nasolabial folds, axillae, chest, and back

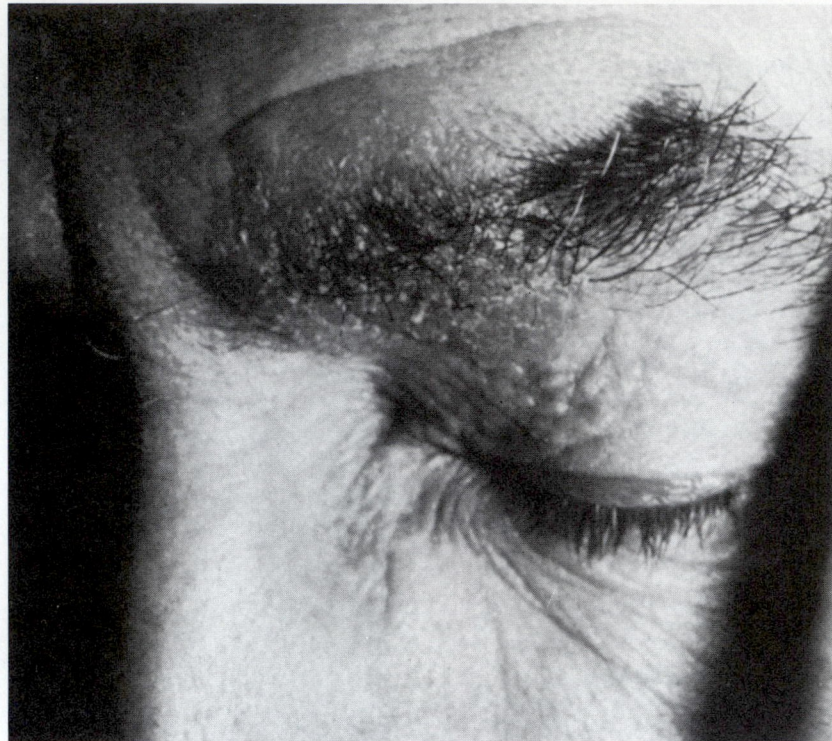

FIG. 41-6. Seborrheic dermatitis of eyebrow, a common site. (From Stewart, Danto, & Maddin, 1978.)

(Fig. 41-6). In infants, the occurrence is known as "cradle cap." The cause is unknown and the lesions appear from infancy to old age with periods of remission and exacerbation. The lesions appear as scaly, white or yellowish inflammatory plaques with mild pruritus. Mild cases are treated with shampoos containing sulfur, salicylic acid, or tar. Corticosteroid applications are useful for suppression of severe symptoms but should not be used for maintenance therapy.

Papulosquamous Disorders

Psoriasis, pityriasis rosea, and lichen planus are disorders characterized by inflammatory processes associated with papules, scales, plaques, and erythema. Collectively they are described as **papulosquamous disorders.**

Psoriasis

Psoriasis is a chronic relapsing proliferative skin disorder that can occur at any age and affects 1% to 2% of the population. The onset is generally established by 20 years of age. The cause of psoriasis is unknown, but genetic, immunologic, or biochemical alterations have been investigated (Dobson & Abele, 1985; Kragballe & Voorhees, 1985). A family history of psoriasis is often established, but the mode of inheritance is not clear (Fitzpatrick, et al., 1987).

Both the dermis and epidermis are thickened with cel-

lular proliferation and inflammation. The turnover time for shedding the epidermis is decreased from the normal 26 to 30 days to 3 to 4 days. There are increased numbers of germinative cells and an increase in transit time of cells through the dermis. The rapid cellular proliferation does not allow time for cell maturation and keratinization to occur. The cell proliferation contributes to a thickened epidermis and plaque formation. The loosely cohesive keratin gives the lesion a silvery appearance. There is frequently capillary dilation and increased vascularization to accommodate the increased cell metabolism. The increased vascularity causes erythema. The disease can be classified according to severity as mild, moderate, or severe depending on the size, distribution, and inflammation of the lesions. The progress of psoriasis is characterized by remissions and exacerbations. Arthritis develops in about 5% of individuals with psoriasis.

The typical psoriatic lesion is a well-demarcated, thick, silvery, scaly, erythematous plaque surrounded by normal skin (Fig. 41-7). Initial lesions usually develop insidiously as small erythematous papules that enlarge and coalesce into larger inflammatory lesions. The lesions are commonly located on the scalp, elbows, knees, and at sites of trauma. Lesions that develop in skin folds are smooth and have a deep red color. The scales are usually loosely adherent and may cause small bleeding points when removed.

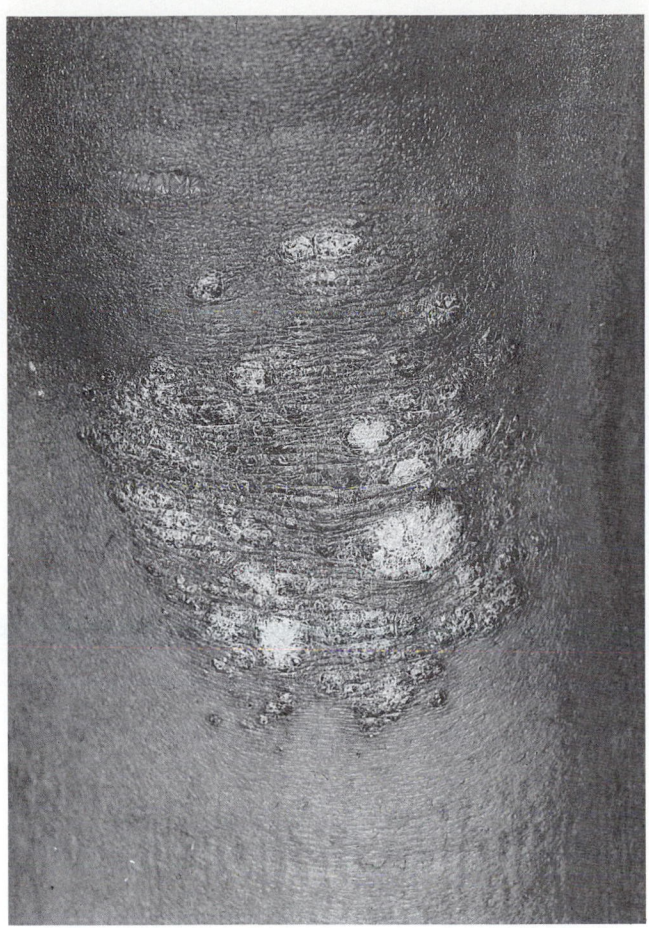

FIG. 41-7. Psoriasis. Typical oval plaque with well-defined borders and silvery scale. (From Habif, 1985.)

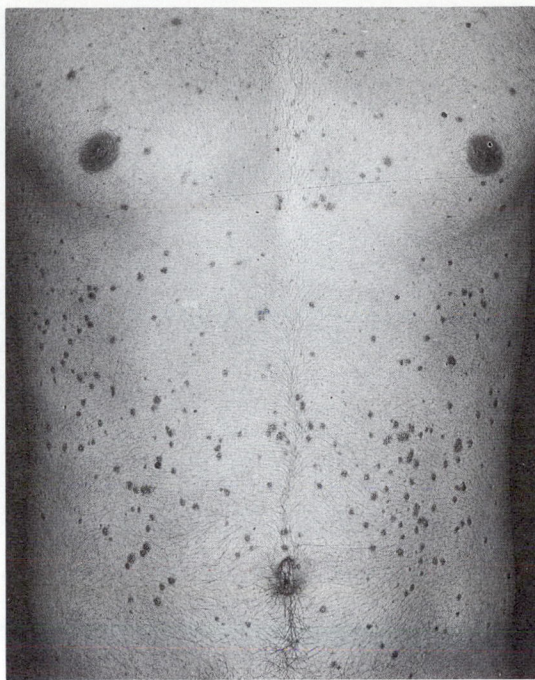

FIG. 41-8. Guttata psoriasis. Numerous uniformly small lesions may abruptly occur following streptococcal pharyngitis. (From Habif, 1985.)

Guttate psoriasis is the development of few to many small papules appearing suddenly on the trunk and extremities (Fig. 41-8). The lesions may appear a few weeks after a streptococcal respiratory infection and, in younger individuals, reflects a tendency to develop the disease. Guttate psoriasis may resolve spontaneously in weeks or months.

Treatment is related to reducing epidermal cell turnover. Mild lesions are usually treated with emollients, keratolytic agents, and corticosteroids. Moderate lesions may respond to ultraviolet light, tar preparations, or a combination of both. Severe disease may require hospitalization with a combination of topical agents and systemic corticosteroids and antimetabolites such as methotrexate. Lesions of the scalp, nails, and genitalia are treated with different lotions and shampoos.

Pityriasis Rosea

Pityriasis rosea is a self-limiting inflammatory disorder that occurs more frequently in young adults, usually during the winter months. The cause is unknown but is thought to be a virus (Ramsey & Hurley, 1985). It is more common during the colder months. Pityriasis rosea begins as a single lesion known as a **herald patch.** The patch is a circular, demarcated salmon-pink lesion about 3 to 4 cm in diameter and is usually located on the trunk. Early lesions are macular and papular. Secondary lesions develop within 14 to 21 days and extend over the trunk and upper part of the extremities (Fig. 41-9). Lesions are rarely located on the face. The lesions emerge as small erythematous papules that expand into characteristic oval lesions. There may be few or hundreds of lesions. The pattern of distribution follows the skin lines around the trunk and appears as a drooping pine tree. As scales flake off from the margin of the lesions, a "collarette" pattern is formed. Itching is the most common symptom. Occasionally headache, fatigue, or sore throat will precede the development of the lesions.

The diagnosis of pityriasis rosea is made by the clinical appearance of the lesion. It can be confused with secondary syphilis, psoriasis, or seborrheic dermatitis. The disorder is usually self-limiting and resolves in a few months with symptomatic treatment for pruritus. Ultraviolet light or systemic corticosteroids may be used to control itching. Sun exposure facilitates resolution of the lesions.

Lichen Planus

Lichen planus is a benign, inflammatory disorder of the skin and mucous membranes. The cause is unknown

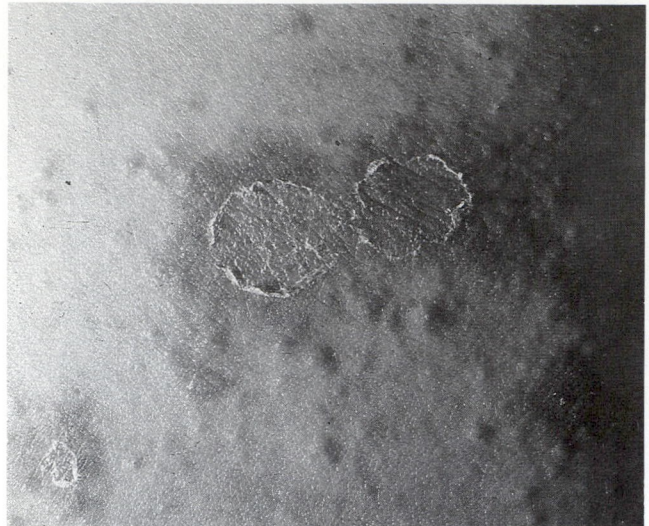

FIG. 41-9. Pityriasis rosea. A ring of tissuelike scale (collarette scale) remains attached within the border of the plaque. (From Habif, 1985.)

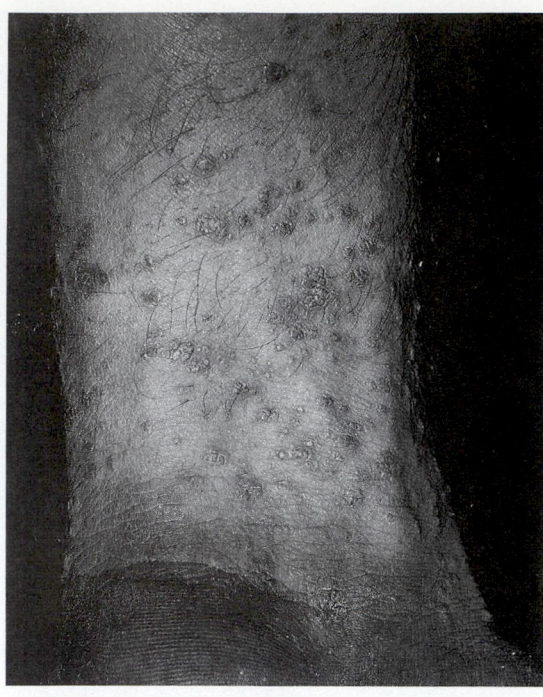

FIG. 41-10. Localized lichen planus. Early lesions are present on the flexor surface of the wrists, a common site for localized lichen planus. (From Habif, 1985.)

but some individuals develop lichenoid lesions after exposure to drugs or film processing chemicals. The age of onset is usually between 30 and 70 years. The disorder begins with nonscaling, violet-colored pruritic papules, 2 to 10 mm in size, usually located on the wrists, ankles, lower legs, and genitalia (Fig. 41-10). The papules are flat topped and have a polygonal shape often with a small central depression. New lesions are pale pink and evolve into a dark violet color. Persistent lesions may be thickened and red, forming hypertrophic lichen planus. The lesions often involve the oral mucous membranes appearing as lacy white rings that must be differentiated from leukoplakia or oral candidiasis. Fine white lines can be seen throughout the oral lesions on magnification. Mucous membrane lesions can also develop on the penis and vulvovaginal area. More commonly, oral lesions do not ulcerate, but localized or extensive painful ulcerations can occur. Chronic ulcerated lesions become malignant in 1% of individuals with the disease. Thinning and splitting of nails is common and part or all of the nail may be shed.

Pruritus is the most distressing symptom. The lesions are self-limiting and may last for months or years with an average duration of 12 to 18 months. Hyperpigmentation resulting from the inflammation is a common consequence of the lesion. About 20% of individuals will have a recurrence. Diagnosis is commonly made by the clinical appearance of the lesion. Antihistamines may be given for itching, and topical or systemic corticosteroids may be used to control inflammation. Mucous membrane lesions are treated with topical steroids or by injection into a single lesion.

Acne Vulgaris

Acne vulgaris is an inflammatory disorder of the pilosebaceous follicle (the sebaceous gland contiguous with a hair follicle). It occurs most commonly during adolescence and is slightly more prevalent in boys but may be more persistent in girls. Acne lesions may appear at age 9 or 10, with less active disease after adolescence. The primary lesions of acne are **comedones** (singular: comedo), pustules, papules, and nodules.

The precise cause of acne is unknown but several factors are associated with the development of the lesion. Studies have indicated that dietary factors do not promote acne. Individuals with acne generally have larger and more actively secreting sebaceous glands. An excessive production and accumulation of sebum appears directly related to androgenic hormones and the pathogenesis of acne. Testosterone is converted to dihydrotestosterone in the skin, which increases the size and productivity of the sebaceous glands. Estrogens decrease sebaceous secretion (Forstrom, 1980). Acne begins with sebum accumulation that obstructs the pilosebaceous unit. The mass of accumulated keratinous sebaceous material and bacteria within the pilosebaceous follicle (Fig. 41-11, A) causes inflammation when it is exposed to the dermis with rupture of a follicle. There are two types of acne, noninflammatory and inflammatory. In **noninflammatory acne,** the comedones are open

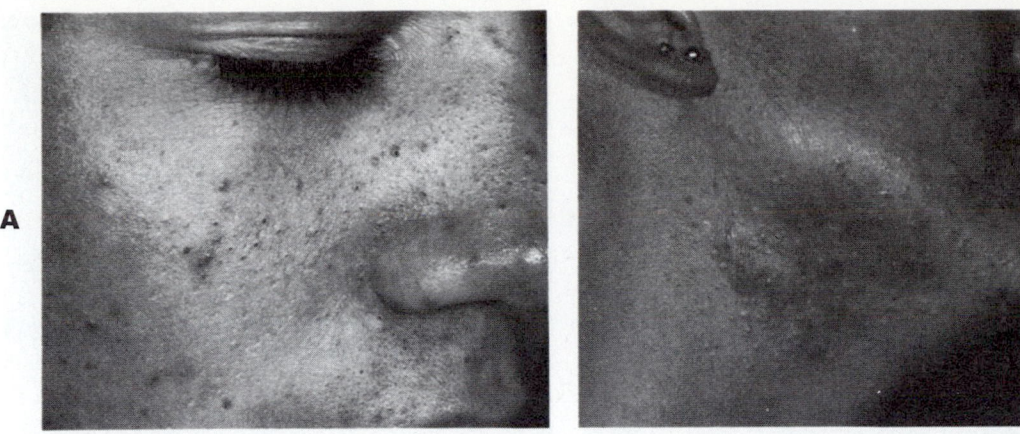

FIG. 41-11. A, Acne vulgaris (open and closed comedones). Comedones (blackheads) are occasionally inflamed. **B,** Acne vulgaris (erythematous papules and pustules). Pustular acne. Many pustules are present and several have become confluent on the chin area. (From Habif, 1985.)

(blackheads) and closed (whiteheads) with the accumulated material causing distention of the follicle and thinning of follicular canal walls. **Inflammatory acne** develops in closed comedones when the follicular wall ruptures expelling sebum into the surrounding dermis and initiating inflammation. Pustules form when the inflammation is close to the surface; papules and cystic nodules can develop when the inflammation is deeper, causing mild to severe scarring (Fig. 41-11, *B*).

Propionibacterium acnes is the major organism in the pilosebaceous follicle and it is very numerous in persons with acne. These bacteria produce substances that promote inflammation, including chemotactic factors and lipolytic and proteolytic enzymes. The hydrolytic action of the enzymes converts triglycerides into free fatty acids that stimulate inflammation and edema with breakdown of the follicle wall. Chemotactic substance may also be released with mediation of inflammation by attraction of polymorphonuclear leukocytes (Puhvel & Sakamoto, 1980).

The lesions of acne are most greatly distributed on the face, chest, and back. Both inflammatory and noninflammatory lesions are usually present. The lesions vary in size and may appear as pustules, nodules, or cysts. The greater the inflammatory response, the larger the lesion. Acne conglobata is a highly inflammatory form of acne with the formation of communicating cysts and abscesses beneath the skin. Remissions tend to occur during the summer, perhaps from more exposure to sunlight. Severe scarring may be treated with dermabrasion.

Treatment of acne is directed toward the pathogenesis of the lesion and there is no single effective treatment. Drugs, such as topical vitamin A and benzoyl peroxide, are comedolytic because they produce mild drying and peeling of the skin and facilitate a return of the normal sebum content of follicles. Benzoyl peroxide and an antibiotic (tetracycline, erythromycin, minocycline, or clindamyacin) are also effective for reducing the population of *Propionibacterium acnes*. Overactivity of sebaceous glands can be suppressed with estrogens, and oral contraceptives containing estrogens have been used to treat selected cases of acne in women. 13-cis-retinoic acid has been used for the successful treatment of nodular cystic acne but is contraindicated during pregnancy because of deforming effects on the fetus (Strauss, 1985). Prednisone or a single injection of a corticosteroid may be used for painful nodular cystic acne.

Acne Rosacea

Acne rosacea is an inflammation of the skin that develops in middle-aged adults. The disease is chronic with episodes of exacerbation. The most common lesions are erythema, papules, pustules, and telangiectasia. They occur in the middle third of the face, including the forehead, nose, cheeks, and chin (Fig. 41-12). The cause is unknown but the lesions are associated with chronic flushing and sensitivity to the sun. Hypertrophy of the sebaceous glands may be severe enough to produce an irreversible bulbous appearance of the nose, known as rhinophyma. Disorders of the eye frequently accompany rosacea, particularly conjunctivitis and more rarely, keratitis. Facial application of fluorinated topical steroids may precipitate rosacea-like lesions that are difficult to treat.

Hot drinks or alcohol should be taken cautiously as the heat and vasodilation accentuates erythema. Tetracycline is the drug of choice for treatment, and a low maintenance dose may be required after the most severe lesions are controlled. Surgical excision of excessive tissue may be required for rhinophyma.

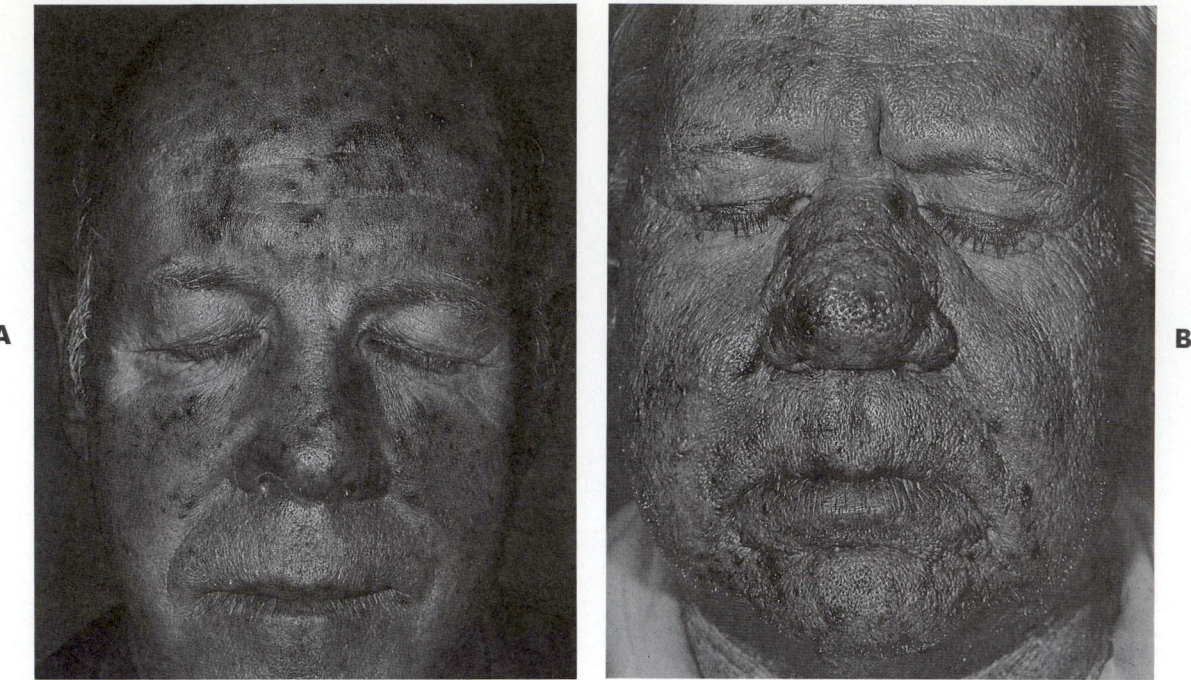

FIG. 41-12. **A,** Rosacea. Pustules and erythema occur on the forehead, cheeks, and nose. **B,** Rosacea and rhinophyma. Chronic rosacea of the nose has caused irreversible hypertrophy (rhinophyma). (From Habif, 1985.)

Lupus Erythematosus

Lupus erythematosus is an inflammatory disease that expresses cutaneous manifestations. Discoid, or cutaneous, lupus erythematosus (DLE) is limited to the skin and can lead to systemic lupus erythematosus. (Systemic lupus erythematosus [SLE], a diffuse, multisystem disease is discussed in Chapter 8.)

Discoid Lupus Erythematosus

Discoid lupus erythematosus (DLE) usually occurs in adults but any age can be affected. It is more common in women in their late 30s or early 40s. The lesions may be single or multiple and of various size. Often the lesions are located on light exposed areas of the skin and photosensitivity is common. The face is the most common site of lesion involvement with a characteristic butterfly distribution over the cheeks and bridge of the nose; however, the lesions may occur on any part of the body.

The cause is thought to be an altered immune response to an unknown antigen. DLE may be described as a subset of SLE, with cutaneous manifestations as the only symptom (Callen, 1986) (Fig. 41-13). On skin biopsy with immunofluorescent observation, there are lumpy deposits of immunoglobulins with IgM as the most common immunoglobulin. There are no deposits in normal skin.

The early lesion is asymmetric with a 1 to 2 cm raised red plaque with a brownish scale. The scale penetrates the hair follicle and leaves a carpet-tack appearance when removed. The lesions persist for months and then resolve spontaneously or atrophy. Healing progresses from the center of the lesion with a residual telangiectasia and scarring that is usually hypopigmented. Atrophy of the dermis and epidermis that results in a depressed scar can occur. Scalp lesions may lead to hair loss. Other symptoms of cutaneous lupus erythematosus include alopecia (hair loss), telangiectasias, urticaria, and Raynaud phenomenon. Scarring or atrophic alopecia is a common problem of DLE. Scaling and inflammation lead to destruction of hair follicles, followed by skin that is smooth and white with telangiectasias. Hair loss is random in distribution. Telangiectasias (prominent skin capillaries) are primarily distributed over the palms and fingers in association with erythema. Uritcaria of DLE may appear as typical hives but they usually stay localized, are not pruritic, and last for days. They probaby result from immune complex deposition rather than an allergic response. Raynaud phenomenon with a history of episodic vasospasm of the arterioles of the fingers and toes with stress or exposure to cold often precedes the onset of DLE by several years. Raynaud phenomenon is characterized by an initial stage of vasospasm that leads to white, numb, and cold digits followed by cyanosis and and then a reactive hyperemia as the vasospasm relaxes.

Diagnosis of DLE is made from the presenting symptoms, biopsy of skin lesions, and Wood tests. Individu-

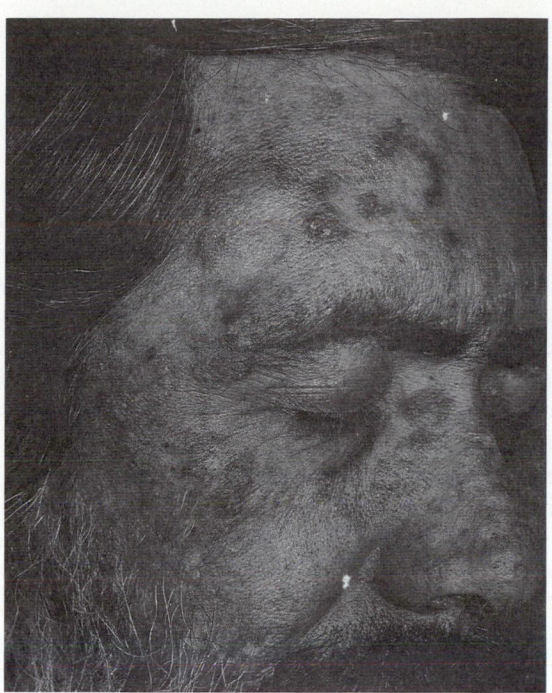

FIG. 41-13. Chronic cutaneous LE (discoid LE). Lesions that are several months old are hypopigmented and atropic. (From Habif, 1985.)

als with DLE should use sunscreen or limit direct exposure to the sun because this precipitates an exacerbation of lesions. Initial treatment with topical steroids relieves symptoms. Systemic therapy with antimalarial drugs (i.e., chloraquine sulfate) usually leads to clinical improvement within 1 to 3 months, but these medications must be used with caution to prevent serious side effects.

Systemic Lupus Erythematosus

Systemic lupus erythematosus (SLE) is a chronic inflammatory immune complex disorder that may affect the skin as well as other major body organs. The disease is more common in young women, although it can develop during early adolescence and later adulthood. It is rarely seen before 3 years of age. There is a strong genetic component with altered cellular immunity resulting in tissue inflammation and injury.

The most characteristic clinical manifestations are joint pain, fever, malaise, and diffuse facial erythema often with a butterfly pattern. Systemic manifestations can include oral ulcers, glomerulonephritis with hypertension and nephrotic syndrome, pleurisy, pericarditis, endocarditis, lymphadenopathy, and splenomegaly. The nervous system may be involved with polyneuropathy, seizures, and behavioral changes. Anemia and thrombocytopenia are frequently observed in individuals with SLE.

Diagnosis of SLE is based on clinical manifestations and histopathologic findings of low complement levels, the presence of antinuclear anbitodies, anti-DNA antibodies, and deposits of immunoglobulin and complement at the dermoepidermal junction.

Avoidance of sun and ultraviolet light is essential to prevent photosensitivity. Treatment of systemic manifestations depends on the degree and extent or organ system involvement. Antimalarials, salicylates, steroids, and immunosuppressive agents may be used. The disease can be controlled but is not curable.

Vesiculobulbous Disorders

Vesiculobullous skin disorders represent a group of diseases that have different causes and clinical courses but share a common characteristic of vesicle, or blister, formation. Two such diseases are pemphigus and erythema multiforme.

Pemphigus

Pemphigus is a chronic blister-forming disease of the skin and oral mucous membranes. There are several different types including pemphigus vulgaris, pemphigus foliaceus, and pemphigus erythematosus. The blisters form in the epidermis and occur more deeply in pemphigus vulgaris, with separation of the epidermis above the basal layer, and more superficially in pemphigus foliaceus and phemphigus erythematosus, with separation of the upper layer of epidermis. The disease is relatively rare and can occur in all age groups but is more prevalent between 40 and 50 years of age.

Pemphigus is an autoimmune disease caused by circulating IgG autoantibodies. Serum autoantibodies are formed that react with the intracellular cement or substance that holds the epidermal cells together. The antibody reaction is thought to cause the intraepidermal blister formation and acantholysis (loss of cohesion between epidermal cells) characteristics of pemphigus (Ahmed et al., 1980; Buschard, Dabelsteen, & Bretlau, 1981).

Pemphigus vulgaris is the most common form of the disease, with the epidermis separating above the basal layer with blister formation. It usually begins with the formation of a blister in the mouth or on the scalp. Within 6 months to 1 year, flaccid bullous lesions appear that rupture easily, leaving crusty denuded skin. The lesions spread to include the face, back, chest, umbilicus, and groin. Pressure on the blister may cause it to spread to adjacent skin (Nikolsky sign). Secondary infection of the open lesions is a potentially serious complication.

Pemphigus foliaceus and **pemphigus erythematosus** are less severe forms of the disease. Oral lesions are usually absent and erythema with crusting, scaling, and occasionally bullae develop and are more localized. Blisters that form are in the horizontal plane of the stratum corneum and rupture easily, forming crusts. Both forms of the disease can spread to become more generalized.

The diagnosis of pemphigus is made from the clinical manifestations and histologic examination of the skin. Immunofluorescence demonstrates the presence of antibodies at the site of blister formation. The clinical cause of the disease may range from rapidly fatal to relatively benign. The primary treatment for pemphigus is systemic corticosteroids usually in high doses during acute episodes or when there is widespread involvement. Immunosuppressive therapy may also be used and decreases the steroid dosage requirement. Newer methods of treatment and a clearer understanding of the pathogenesis have improved the prognosis.

Bullous Pemphigoid

Bullous pemphigoid is a more benign disease with the presence of serum and bound IgG and blistering of the subepidermal skin layer. It occurs more commonly after 60 years of age. The lesions of pemphigoid begin with localized erythema or as pruritic plaques that extend and become edematous. The plaques turn reddish purple by 2 to 3 weeks, with vesicles and bullae emerging on the surface (Fig. 41-14). The bulla do not extend with pressure. The blisters rupture within a week and heal rapidly.

Diagnosis is by skin biopsy and immunofluorescent examination. The presence of subepidermal blistering and eosinophils distinguishes pemphigoid from pemphigus. Treatment usually includes hydroxyzine (Atarax) for itching and prednisone with an immunosuppressive

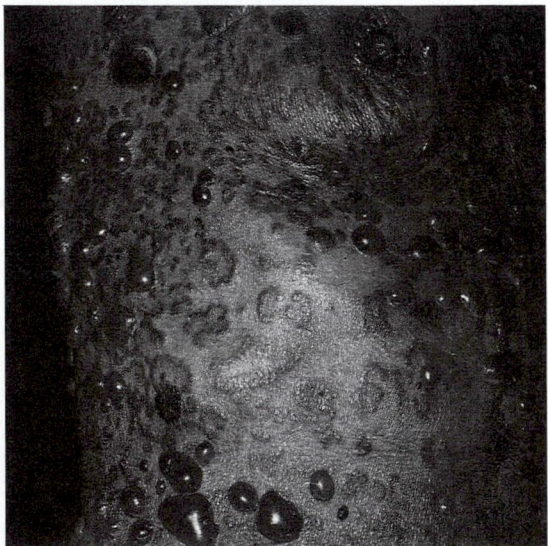

FIG. 41-14. Bullous pemphigoid. Generalized eruption with tense blisters arising from an edematous erythematous annular base. (From Habif, 1985.)

drug to control blistering. Individuals who respond to treatment with sulfapyridine or dapsone will not require prednisone.

Erythema Multiforme

Erythema multiforme is an acute, often recurrent, inflammatory disorder of the skin and mucous membranes, often associated with allergic or toxic reactions to drugs or microorganisms (i.e., *Mycoplasma pneumoniae* and herpes simplex). It can occur at any age but is more frequent between 20 and 40 years of age. Immune complex formation and deposition of C3, IgM, and fibrinogen around the superficial dermal blood vessels, basement membrane, and keratinocytes are found in most individuals with erythema multiforme. Edema develops in the superficial dermis leading to the formation of vesicles and bullae. The lesions vary in clinical presentation and may involve the skin or mucous membranes, or both. The characteristic "bull's-eye," or "target lesions," occur on the skin surface with a central erythematous region surrounded by concentric rings or alternating edema and inflammation. The lesions usually occur suddenly in groups over a period of 2 to 3 weeks. Urticarial plaques, 1 to 2 cm in diameter, can develop without the target lesion. A vesiculobullous form is characterized by mucous membrane lesions and erythematous plaques on the extensor surfaces of the extremities. Single or multiple vesicles or bullae may arise on a part of the plaque accompanied by pruritus and burning. The lesions heal within 3 to 4 weeks.

The most common form in children and young adults is **Stevens-Johnson syndrome** (severe bullous form), in which there are numerous erythematous bullous lesions on both the skin and mucous membranes. The cause is unknown but an immune mechanism is probably involved (White, 1985). Prodromal symptoms of fever, headache, malaise, sore throat, and cough develop in about one third of the cases. The bullous lesions form erosions and crusts when they rupture. The mouth, air passages, esophagus, urethra, and conjunctiva may be involved. Blindness can result from corneal ulcerations. Difficulty eating, breathing, and urinating may develop with severe manifestations. The disease can involve the kidneys and extend from the upper respiratory passages into the lungs. In rare instances, severe forms of the disease can be fatal.

Diagnosis is made by recognition of the target lesion or by skin biopsy if the target lesion is absent. Mild acute forms of the disease last 10 to 14 days. Mild forms of the disease, usually self-limiting, require no treatment. Any ongoing drug therapy should be reevaluated and underlying infections treated. Fluid and electrolyte balance should be monitored in severe forms of the disease and mucous membranes must be carefully managed with a bland diet, warm saline eyewashes, topical anesthetics, or corticosteroids to maintain comfort and prevent infection. Cutaneous blisters can be treated with wet compresses of Burrow solution. Ophthalmic, kidney, and lung involvement require special care. Resolution occurs in 8 to 10 days, usually without scarring. Mucosal lesions may take 6 weeks to heal.

Infections

Cutaneous infections are common forms of skin disease. The infections generally remain localized; however, serious complications can develop with systemic involvement. The type of skin infections include bacterial, viral, and fungal. Most infections tend to occur superficially; however, systemic signs and symptoms occasionally develop and rarely are life threatening. The normal flora of the skin consists of aerobes, yeast, and anerobes. These flora often provide protection against pathogens that cause skin infections, including *Staphylococcus* and *Streptococcus* (Singh, Marples, & Klingman, 1971).

Bacterial Infections

Most bacterial infections of the skin are caused by local invasion of pathogens. Coagulase-positive *S. aureus* and, less frequently, β-hemolytic streptococci are the common causative organisms.

Folliculitis

Folliculitis is a bacterial infection of the hair follicle. *Staphylococcus aureus* is the common causative organism. The infection develops from proliferation of the organism around the opening of the follicle with spread into the follicle. Inflammation is caused by the release of chemotactic factors and enzymes from the bacteria. The lesions appear as pustules with a surrounding area of erythema. They are most prominent on the scalp and extremities and rarely cause systemic symptoms. Prolonged skin moisture, skin trauma, and poor hygiene are associated contributing factors to the development of folliculitis. Cleaning with soap and water and topical application of antibiotics are effective forms of treatment.

Furuncles and Carbuncles

Furuncles, or "boils," are an inflammation of the hair follicles. They may develop from a preceding folliculitis with spread through the follicular wall into the surrounding dermis. The invading organism is usually *S. aureus*. The infecting strain may spread to the skin from the anterior nares. Any skin area with hair can be infected and one or several lesions may be present. The precipitating events are similar to folliculitis. The initial lesion is a deep, firm, red, painful nodule 1 to 5 cm in diameter. Within a few days, the initial erythematous nodules change to a large fluctuant and tender cystic nodule that may be accompanied by cellulitis. No systemic symptoms are present, and the lesion may drain large amounts of pus and necrotic tissue.

Carbuncles are a collection of infected hair follicles. The lesion occurs most frequently on the back of the neck, the upper back, and the lateral thighs. The lesion begins in the subcutaneous tissue and lower dermis as a firm mass that evolves into an erythematous, painful, swollen mass that drains through many openings. Abscesses may develop. Chills, fever, and malaise are systemic symptoms that can occur during the early stages of lesion development.

Furuncles and carbuncles are treated with warm compresses to provide comfort and promote localization and spontaneous drainage. Abscess formation requires incision and drainage, and recurrent infections are treated with systemic antibiotics.

Cellulitis

Cellulitis is an infection of the dermis and subcutaneous tissue usually caused by *Staphylococcus*. Cellulitis can occur as an extension of a skin wound, an ulcer, or from furuncles or carbuncles. The infected area is erythematous, swollen, and painful. The infection responds to systemic antibiotics, and Burrow soaks can be used to relieve pain.

Erysipelas

Erysipelas is an acute superficial infection of the skin most often caused by group A streptococci. The face, ears, and lower legs are common sites of involvement and the site of initial infection may not be identified. Chills, fever, and malaise precede the onset of lesions by 4 hours to 20 days. The initial lesions appear as firm, red spots that then enlarge and coalesce to form a clearly circumscribed, advancing bright red, hot lesion with a raised border. Vesicles may appear over the lesion and at the border. Itching, burning, and tenderness accompany the development of the lesion. Cold compresses provide symptomatic relief, and systemic antibiotics are required to arrest the infection.

Impetigo

Impetigo is a superficial lesion of the skin caused by coagulase-positive *Staphylococcus* and/or β-hemolytic streptococci. The disease occurs in adults but is more common in children (see Chapter 42).

Viral Infections

Herpes Simplex Virus

There are two types of **herpes simplex virus (HSV),** HSV-1 (type 1) and HSV-2 (type 2). A "cold sore" or "fever blister" is a type of HSV-1 infection and is the most common manifestation of the herpes simplex virus (Crumpacker, 1987). HSV-1 usually occurs in nongenital sites and causes infection of the cornea (herpes keratitis), mouth (gingivostomatitis), and labia (labialis). Genital infections are more commonly caused by HSV-2. The virus is spread by contact of the virus with the skin and there is a high risk of infection after sexual contact with infected individuals. After penetrating the skin, HSV is established in the sensory nerve ganglion innervating the primary site. Infection in one area does not protect the other areas from subsequent infection. The primary infection is asymptomatic and can only be determined by a rising antibody titer.

The incubation period ranges from 2 to 14 days, and clinical symptoms last from 1 to 3 weeks. An individual will then continue to shed the virus for 2 to 6 weeks. The virus remains dormant within sensory or autonomic nerve ganglia and can lead to recurrence of the disease. A number of factors stimulate recurrence, including sun exposure, fever, or stress, and lesions are usually located at or near the primary site. Since anti-HSV antibodies develop in response to infection, recurrence is also related to the titer or amount of antibodies present.

The lesions of HSV-1 appear as a rash or clusters of inflamed and painful vesicles within the mouth, over the tongue, or on the lips and around the nose (Fig. 41-15). Increased sensitivity, paresthesias, and mild burning may occur before onset of the lesion. The vesicles rupture forming a crust. Lesions may last for 2 to 6 weeks. Occasionally, there is an associated upper respiratory infection. Treatment is symptomatic and the lesions usually resolve within 2 weeks.

Genital herpes (HSV-2) may also occur in primary or recurrent forms and a large number of infections are sexually transmitted, usually within 3 to 14 days after exposure (see Chapter 21). The lesions begin as small vesicles that progress to ulceration within 3 to 4 days with pain, itching, and weeping. Treatment includes oral or topical administration of acyclovir, an antiviral drug that decreases new lesion formation and promotes healing.

Herpes Zoster and Varicella

Herpes zoster (shingles) and **varicella** (chickenpox) are caused by the same herpesvirus, varicella-zoster virus (VZV). Varicella occurs as a primary infection followed years later by herpes zoster. Chickenpox usually occurs in children (see Chapter 42).

Herpes zoster, or shingles, has initial symptoms of pain and paresthesia localized to the affected dermatome (the cutaneous area innervated by a single spinal nerve; see Chapter 12), followed by vesicular eruptions that follow along a facial, cervical, or thoracic lumbar dermatome (Fig. 41-16). Some individuals have vesicles scattered outside the area of the dermatome. Local symptoms are alleviated with compresses, calamine lotion, or baking soda. Antiviral drugs (vidarabine and

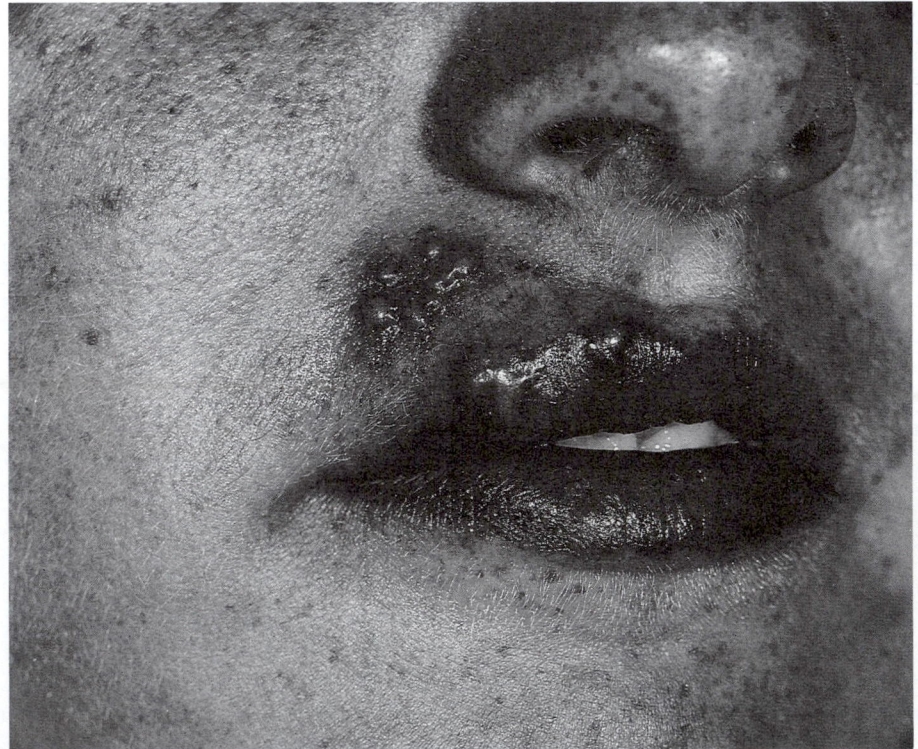

FIG. 41-15. Herpes simplex labialis. Typical presentation with tense vesicles appearing on the lips and extending onto the skin. (From Habif, 1985.)

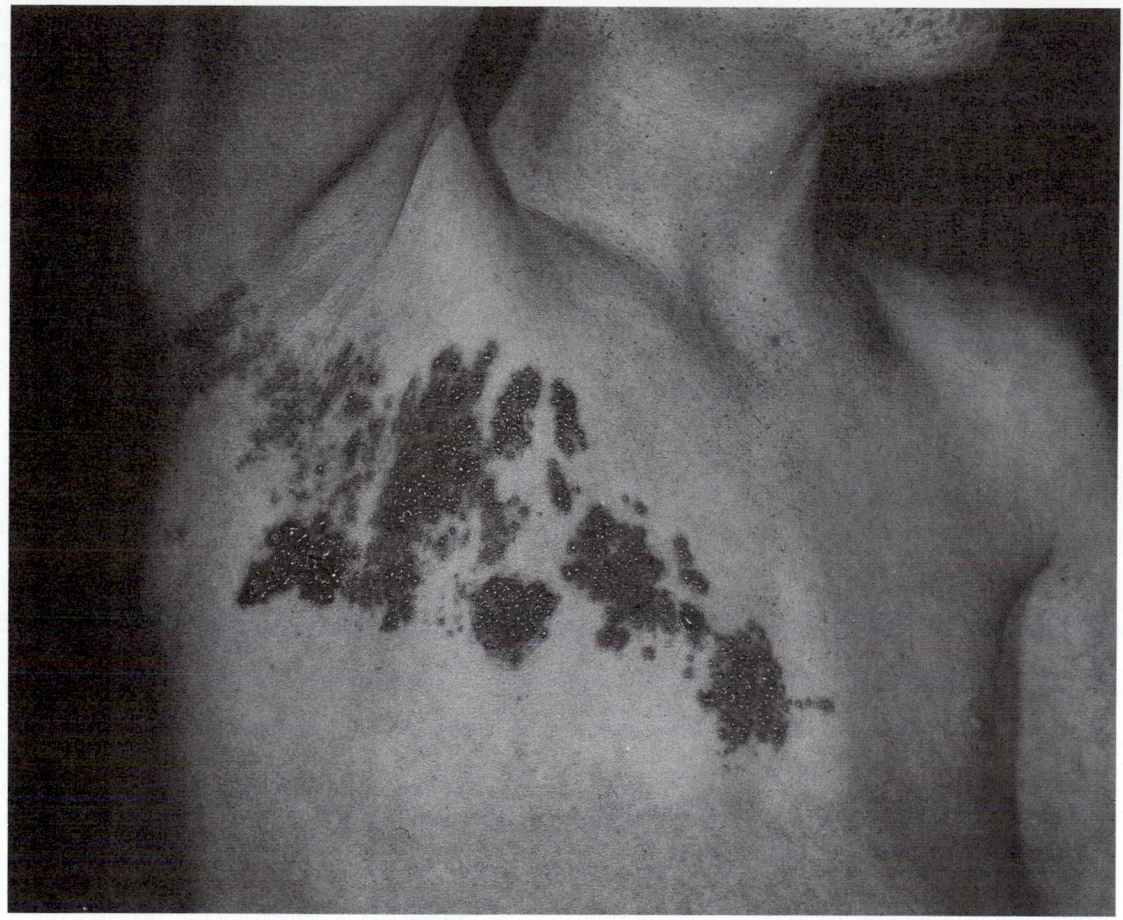

FIG. 41-16. Herpes zoster. Diffuse involvement of a dermatome in a 13-year-old boy. (From Habif, 1985.)

acyclovir) have provided useful treatment (Balfour, 1984; Whitely et al., 1982). About 20% of individuals experience postherpetic neuralgia (Ragozzino et al., 1982).

Warts

Warts (verrucae) are benign lesions of the skin caused by the human papillomavirus (HPV). There are many different types of HPV, and specific viruses are associated with specific kinds and locations of lesions. The lesions are round and elevated with a rough, grayish surface, and they can occur anywhere on the skin. Warts are transmitted by touch. Common warts (verucca vulgaris) occur most frequently in children and are usually on the fingers, although they may be located on any skin surface or mucous membrane. Warts vary in shape, size (flat, round, or fusiform), and location. Plantar warts are usually located at pressure points on the bottom of the feet (Fig. 41-17).

Condylomata accuminata (veneral warts) are cauliflower-like lesions that occur in moist areas, along the

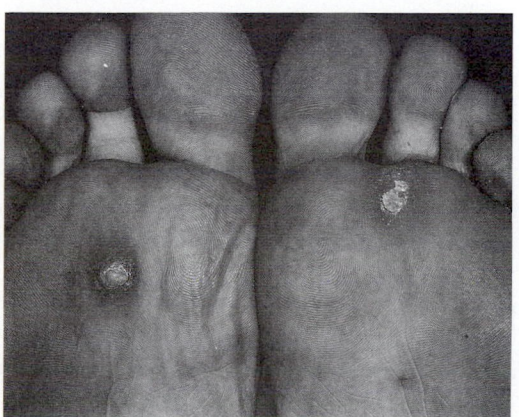

FIG. 41-17. Verruca plantaris. Corns (clavi) on the plantar surface are frequently mistaken for warts. (From Habif, 1985.)

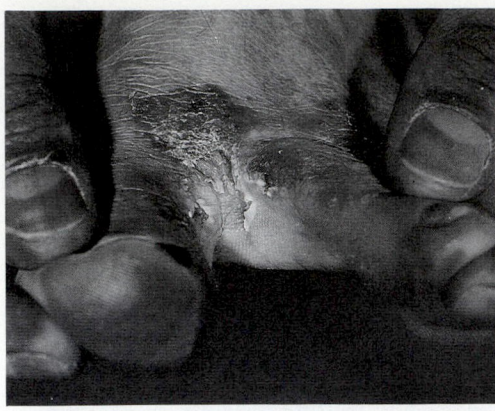

FIG. 41-18. Tinea pedis (toe web infection). The toe web space contains macerated scale. Inflammation has extended from the web area onto the dorsum of the foot. (From Habif, 1985.)

glans of the penis, vulva, and anus (see Chapter 21). Epidermodysplasia verruciformis is a rare condition and is associated with warts all over the body.

Diagnosis of warts is by visualization. Treatment considers age of the individual and size and location of the lesion. Warts can be removed by freezing with liquid nitrogen, electrocautery, vaporization with lasers, application of keratolytics, or application of irritants and corrosives, such as salicylic acid, formaldehyde, or saturated solution of potassium iodide. Many warts resolve spontaneously.

Fungal Infections

The fungi causing superficial skin infections are called dermatophytes and they thrive on keratin (stratum corneum, hair, and nails). Fungal disorders are known as mycoses; when caused by dermatophytes, the mycoses are termed tinea (dermatophytosis or ringworm). **Tinea pedis** is a chronic, superficial fungal infection of the skin of the foot common in adults (Fig. 41-18). In prepubertal children most scaling disorders of the toes and feet are eczema. **Tinea corporis** (ringworm) and **tinea capitis** (a fungal infection of the scalp) are much more common in children than adults. (See Chapter 42 for a discussion of fungal infections in children.)

Tinea Infections

Tinea infections are fungal infections of the skin and are classified according to their location on the body. The most common sites are summarized in Table 41-5. These infestations are common in children (see Chapter 42). Tinea is diagnosed by culture, microscopic examination of skin scrapings prepared with potassium hydroxide wet mount, or by observation of the skin with an ultraviolet light (Wood's lamp). Cultures establish the particular type of fungus and are necessary for hair and nail infections. Fungi have characteristic spores and filaments known as **hyphae** that are more prominent when prepared in potassium hydroxide. The spores fluoresce blue-green when exposed to ultraviolet light. Treatment is related to the type of fungi and includes both topical and systemic antifungal medication.

Candidiasis

Candidiasis is caused by the yeastlike fungus *Candida albicans* and can normally be found on mucous membranes, the skin, in the gastrointestinal tract, and in the vagina. *C. albicans* can, under certain circumstances, change from a commensal organism to a pathogen, particularly when the immune system is depressed. Among those factors that predispose to infection are (1) local

---

TABLE 41-5 Common sites of tinea infections

Site	Clinical manifestations
Tinea capitis (scalp)	Scaly, pruritic scalp with bald areas; hair breaks easily
Tinea corporis (skin areas, excluding scalp, face, hands, feet, groin)	Circular, clearly circumscribed, mildly erythematous scaly patches with a slightly elevated ringlike border; some forms are dry and macular and other forms are moist and vesicular
Tinea cruris (groin, also known as "jock itch")	Small erythematous and scaling of vesicular patches with a well-defined border that spread over the inner and upper surfaces of the thighs; occurs with heat and high humidity
Tinea pedis (foot, also known as "athlete's foot")	Occurs between the toes and may spread to the soles of feet, nails, and skin of toes; slight scaling, macerated painful skin, occasionally with fissures and vesiculation
Tinea manus (hand)	Dry, scaly, erythematous lesions, or moist vesicular lesions that begin with clusters of intensely itching, clear vesicles; often associated with fungal infection of the feet
Tinea unguium or onychomycosis (nails)	A superficial or deep inflammation of the nail that develops yellow-brown accumulations of brittle keratin over all or portions of the nail.

TABLE 41-6 Sites of candidiasis

	Risk factors	Clinical manifestations	Treatment
Vagina (vulvovaginitis)	Heat, moisture, occlusive clothing Pregnancy Systemic antibiotic therapy Diabetes mellitus	Vaginal itching; white, watery, or creamy discharge Red and swollen vaginal and labial membranes with erosions Lesions may spread to anus and groin	Miconazole cream Clotrimazole tablets or cream Nystatin tablets Ketoconazole cream Loose cotton clothing
Penis (balanitis)	Uncircumcised Sexual intercourse with infected female	Pinpoint red, tender papules and pustules on glans and shaft of penis	Any of creams listed above Topical steroids for severe inflammation
Mouth	Diabetes mellitus Immunosuppressive therapy Inhaled steroids	Red, swollen, painful tongue and oral mucous membranes Localized erosions and plaques appear with chronic infection	Nystatin oral suspension Myclex troches Ketoconazole

environment of moisture, warmth, maceration, and/or occlusion; (2) the systemic administration of antibiotics; (3) pregnancy; (4) diabetes mellitus; (5) Cushing disease; (6) debilitated states; (7) infants less than 6 months of age, as a result of decreased immune reactivity; (8) immunosuppressed persons; and (9) certain neoplastic diseases of the blood and monocyte/macrophage system. The resident bacteria on the skin, mainly cocci, inhibit proliferation of *C. albicans*. Cell-mediated immunity plays a major role in the defense against monilial infections. *C. albicans* can activate the complement system by the alternative pathway and include small abscesses. Candidiasis affects only the outer layers of mucous membranes and skin and occurs in the mouth, vagina, uncircumcised penis, and large skin folds. Table 41-6 lists the differentiation of different sites of candidiasis.

The initial lesion is a thin-walled pustule that extends under the stratum corneum with an inflammatory base that may burn or itch. The accumulation of inflammatory cells and scale produce a whitish yellow curdlike substance over the infected area. The lesion ceases to spread when reaching dry skin.

Vascular Disorders

Vascular abnormalities are commonly associated with skin diseases, or they may be present as congenital vascular malformations (see Chapter 42), or as vascular responses to local or systemic vasoactive substances. Blood vessels may increase in number, dilate, constrict, or become obliterated by disease processes.

Cutaneous Vasculitis

Vasculitis (angiitis) is an inflammation of the blood vessels. The initiating site of inflammation may be the blood, the vessel wall, or the adjacent tissue. Small vessels are usually affected. Immune complexes, which initiate an uncontrolled inflammatory response, are often the cause of damage, and the lesions are often polymorphic.

Cutaneous vasculitis develops from the deposit of immune complexes in small blood vessels as a toxic response to drugs (phenothiazines, barbiturates, and sulfonamides) or allergens, or as a response to streptococcal or viral infection. The precise mechanism is not known, but the deposit of immune complex activates complement, which is chemotactic for polymorphonuclear leukocytes. The cutaneous form usually resolves in a few weeks and is treated with steroids.

The disorder is also known as allergic vasculitis and occurs primarily in adults. A systemic form (cutaneous systemic vasculitis) can involve other organs including the kidneys, lungs, and gastrointestinal tract. The extremities are the chief sites, primarily the lower legs and feet. The lesions appear as palpable purpura (from the leakage of blood from damaged vessels) and progress to hemorrhagic bullae with necrosis and ulceration from occlusion of the vessel. Lesions appear in clusters and remain from 1 to 4 weeks. Recurrences are common. Biopsy may reveal the presence of complement or immunoglobins in the vessel walls.

Identifying and removing the antigen (chemical, drug, or source of infection) is the first step of treatment. Prednisone may be used when symptoms are severe.

Urticaria

Urticarial lesions are most commonly associated with type one hypersensitivity reactions to drugs (penicillin, aspirin), certain foods (strawberries, shellfish), systemic diseases (intestinal parasites, lupus erythematosus), or physical agents (heat or cold) (see Chapter 8). The lesions are mediated by histamine release, which causes the endothelial cells of skin blood vessels to contract. The leak of fluid from the vessel appears as wheals, welts, or hives and may be few or many and distributed over the entire body. Most lesions resolve spontaneously within 24 hours, but new lesions may appear. All possible causes should be removed. Antihistamines usually reduce hives and provide relief of itching. Corticosteroids may be required for treatment of severe attacks.

Scleroderma

Scleroderma means sclerosis of the skin and the cause is unknown. The disease is more prominent in women. Scleroderma may affect the visceral organs or remain localized to the skin. Systemic scleroderma involves the connective tissues of many organs, including the kidney, gastrointestinal tract, and lungs. Only a few organs are involved in some individuals. The cutaneous lesions are most often on the face and hands, the neck, and upper chest. However, the entire skin can be involved.

The disease is characterized by massive deposits of collagen with fibrosis, accompanied by inflammatory reactions, vascular changes in the capillary network with a decrease in the number of capillary loops, and dilation of the remaining capillaries (Theirs & Dobson, 1986). Fibrosis occurs in the papillary and reticular dermis and in the subcutaneous tissue and deep fascia. Autoimmunity and an immune reaction to a toxic substance are both possible initiating mechanisms of the disease, and autoantibodies are often recovered from the skin and serum of individuals with scleroderma.

The skin is hard, hypopigmented, taut, shiny, and tightly connected to the underlying tissue. The tightness of the facial skin projects an immobile masklike appearance, and the mouth may not open completely. The nose may assume a beaklike appearance. The hands are shiny and sometimes red and edematous. The fingers become tapered and flexed, often with depressed scars and loss of fingertips from atrophy. Raynaud phenomenon with episodic arteriolar vasoconstriction of the fingers contributes to ulcer formation. The nails may be shed (Fig. 41-19). Calcium deposits develop in the subcutaneous tissue and erupt through the skin. Progression to body organs may occur, and death is caused by subsequent renal failure, cardiac dysrhythmias, or esophageal or intestinal obstruction or perforation. There is no specific treatment and progression of the disease is variable. Fifty percent of individuals die within 5 years from onset of scleroderma.

Suitable clothing and warm environment are essential to protecting the hands. Trauma and smoking should be avoided. Vasodilator drugs or sympathectomy rarely has lasting effects. Symptomatic treatment is required for

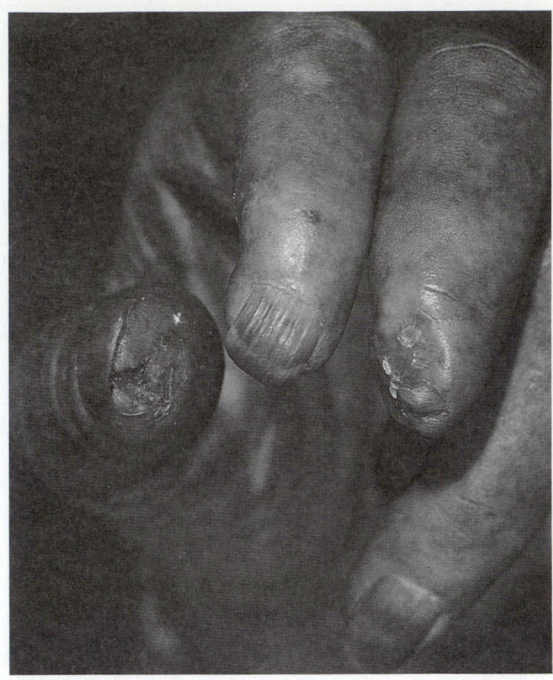

FIG. 41-19. Scleroderma (acrosclerosis). Fingertips are narrowed and the fingers are shortened as a result of distal bone resorption. (From Habif, 1985.)

involved organs (i.e., intestinal resection for obstruction, antibiotics for pneumonitis, and regulation of hypertension).

Insect Bites
Ticks

Ticks are significant vectors of transmitted diseases, including Rocky Mountain spotted fever and other rickettsial diseases, tularemia, and Lyme disease. Ticks vary in size from 1 cm to about the size of a comma on this printed page. They embed their head in the skin to obtain blood. As they gorge themselves on blood, they enlarge to many times their normal size and may release toxins or transmit microorganisms during feeding. In most instances, there is no consequence from a tick bite with the exception of a papular urticaria at the site of the bite. If mouth parts remain in the skin when the tick is removed, a persistent nodule remains that may require excision; the tick should be removed completely intact. Irritant substances, such as camphor, gasoline, soft wax, or heat from a match, may stimulate the tick to withdraw its head. Applying tick repellant, such as diethyltoluamide (DEET), butopryonoxyl (Indalone), or benzylbenzoate, helps to prevent tick bites.

Mosquitoes and Flies

There are thousands of species of **mosquitoes** throughout the world. Species from the Culicada family are responsible for malaria, yellow fever, dengue fever, filariasis, and St. Louis encephalitis. Mosquitoes can bite through thin, loose clothing and are attracted by warmth and sweat. The edema, pruritus, and papular lesions of the mosquitoe bite are caused by the disruption of the skin from the insertion of a blood tube by a female mosquitoe. Irritating salivary secretions also contain anticoagulants. Reactions vary depending on the sensitivity of the victim.

Several species of flies are blood suckers. The black fly (Simuliidae) is usually found in swarms, near moving bodies of water in the late spring and early summer, and is a vicious biter. The initial bite is painless because the fly injects an anesthetic with the bite. The subsequent lesions are painful and accompanied by significant swelling of surrounding tissues. Systemic reactions, such as fever, headache, and nausea, are common.

Very small flies of the Ceratopogonidae family, also known as "no-see-ums," "midges," "punkies," or sand fleas, are also blood suckers. The bite of the female is particularly miserable and produces immediate pain, erythema, and vesicles. Itching and vesicular reactions may persist for weeks.

The fiercest bloodsucking flies are the Tabanidae, or horseflies, deerflies, gadflies, greenheads, and clegs. These flies vary in size from 1 to 5 cm and produce painful, bleeding bites because of their large mouth parts. The bites produce urticaria that may be accompanied by weakness, dizziness, and wheezing.

Wounds produced by biting insects should be cleansed with soap and water and a local antiseptic should be applied. Local applications of steroid creams or antihistamine will reduce symptoms. Systemic reactions may require more specific medical care.

Benign Tumors

Most benign tumors of the skin are associated with aging. Benign tumors include seborrheic keratosis, keratoacanthoma, actinic keratosis, and moles.

Seborrheic Keratosis

Seborrheic keratosis is a benign proliferation of basal cells that produces elevated lesions that may be smooth or warty in appearance. They are usually seen in older people and occur as multiple lesions on the chest, back, and face. The color varies from tan to waxy yellow, flesh-colored, or dark brown-black. Lesion size varies from a few millimeters to several centimeters, and they are often oval and greasy appearing with a hyperkeratotic scale (Fig. 41-20). Cryotherapy with liquid nitrogen is effective treatment, and the lesions usually slough 2 to 3 weeks after treatment.

Keratoacanthoma

A keratoacanthoma is a benign, self-limiting tumor that arises from hair follicles. It usually occurs on sun-exposed surfaces and develops between 60 and 65 years of age. The most commonly affected sites are the face, back of the hands, forearms, neck, and legs. The lesion develops in stages. The proliferative stage produces a rapid growing dome-shaped nodule with a central crust. In the mature stage, the lesion is filled with whitish colored keratin (Fig. 41-21). The involution stage usually occurs over a 3- to 4-month period with regression of the lesion. The mature lesion requires differentiation

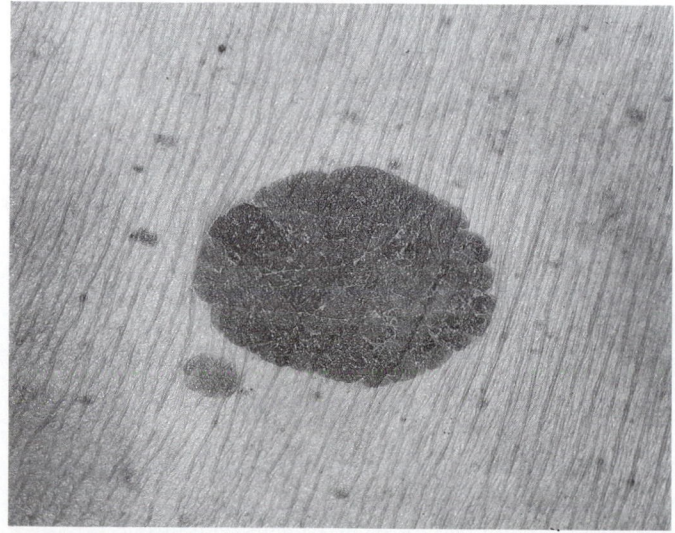

FIG. 41-20. Seborrheic keratosis. Typical distal extremity lesion that is broad, flat, and comparatively smooth surfaced. (From Habif, 1985.)

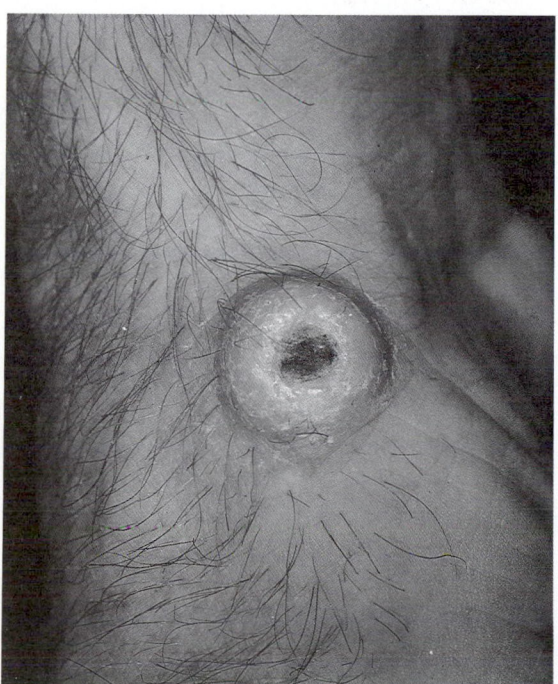

FIG. 41-21. Keratoacanthoma. Classic presentation of a fully developed tumor. Round smooth dome-shaped mass with a central keratin-filled crater.

from squamous cell carcinoma. Although the lesions will resolve spontaneously, they can be removed by curettage or excision to improve cosmetic appearance.

Actinic Keratosis

Actinic keratosis is a premalignant lesion found on skin surfaces exposed to the ultraviolet radiation of the sun. The prevalence is highest in individuals with unprotected, light-colored skin. Actinic keratosis is rare in black skin. The lesions appear as pigmented patches of rough, adherent scale. Surrounding areas may have telangiectasias. Freezing with liquid nitrogen provides quick, effective treatment. Excisions may also be performed providing tissue for cellular analysis. The lesions should continue to be evaluated for progression to squamous cell carcinoma. Protection from the sun with clothing or a sun-blocking agent to prevent lesions from developing elsewhere is advised.

Nevi (Moles)

Nevi are pigmented or nonpigmented lesions that form from melanocytes beginning at ages 3 to 5 years. During the early stages of development, the cells accumulate at the junction of the dermis and epidermis and are macular lesions. Over time the cells move down into the dermis and the nevi become nodular and palpable. Nevi may appear on any part of the skin and they vary in size. They occur singly or in groups and are not disfiguring. Nevi may undergo transition to malignant melanoma (see p. 1420). Nevi irritated by clothing can be excised.

Cancer

Since many cancerous skin lesions are treated and not reported, statistics on the incidence of skin cancer are difficult to obtain. It is estimated that skin cancers are the more prevalent form of cancer and nearly all persons

---

Important Trends for Skin Cancer

Incidence	Approximately 500,000 cases a year with the majority being the highly curable **basal** or **squamous** cell cancers. Not as common is the most serious **malignant melanoma** with an estimated 27,000 cases a year.
Mortality	Total estimated deaths in 1989 were 8200; 6000 from malignant melanoma and 2000 from other skin cancers.
Risk factors	Excessive exposure to ultraviolet radiation from the sun; fair complexion; occupational exposure to coal tar, pitch, creosote, arsenic compounds, and radium. Skin cancer is neglible in blacks because of heavy skin pigmentation.
Warning signals	Any unusual skin condition, especially a change in the size or color of a mole or other darkly pigmented growth or spot.
Prevention and early detection	Avoidance of sun when ultraviolet light is strongest (e.g., 10:00 A.M. and 3:00 P.M.). Use sunscreen preparations, especially those containing ingredients such as PABA (para-aminobenzoic acid). Basal and squamous cell skin cancers often form a pale, waxlike, pearly nodule, or a red, scaly, sharply outlined patch. Melanomas are usually dark brown or black pigmentation. They start as small molelike growths that increase in size, change color, become ulcerated, and bleed easily from a slight injury.
Treatment	There are four methods of treatment: surgery, electrodessication (tissue destruction by heat), radiation therapy, or cryosurgery (tissue destruction by freezing). For malignant melanomas, wide and often deep excisions and removal of nearby lymph nodes are required.
Survival	For basal cell and squamous cell cancers, cure is virtually assured with early detection and treatment. Malignant melanoma, however, metastasizes quickly. This accounts for a lower 5-year survival rate for white patients with this disease.

living beyond age 65 will have had at least one skin cancer. The most common types of skin cancer are basal cell carcinoma and squamous cell carcinoma. These carcinomas are 50% greater in men than in women and incidence increases steadily with age. Malignant melanoma is the most serious skin cancer affecting 27,000 people per year and is increasing at a rate of 3.4% per year (American Cancer Society, 1988, 1989). An estimated 8200 people die of skin cancer each year, 6000 from malignant melanoma (American Cancer Society, 1989).

Solar radiation causes most skin cancers. Areas widely exposed to the sun's rays; the face, neck, and hands, are highly vulnerable for such lesions. Outdoor workers (farmers, sailors, fishermen) are high-risk skin cancer populations. For other risk factors, refer to the box on p. 1418.

Basal Cell Carcinoma

Basal cell carcinoma is a surface epithelial tumor of the skin originating from undifferentiated basal or germinative cells. The tumors grow upward and laterally or downward to the dermal epidermal junction (Fig. 41-22). Early tumors are so small they are not clinically apparent. Generally, these tumors do not invade blood or lymph vessels; thus, they do not metastasize beyond the skin. However, basal cell carcinoma can cause severe local destruction.

Basal cell carcinoma, as the most common type of skin cancer, is thought to be caused by sunlight expo-

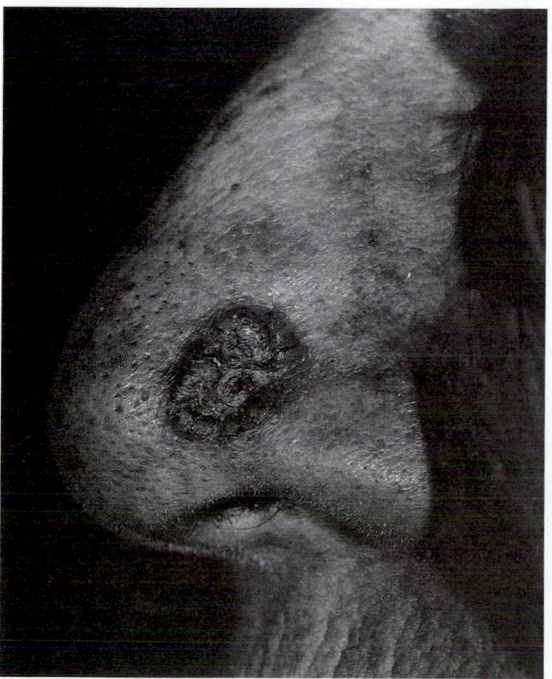

FIG. 41-22. Nodular basal cell carcinoma. Center has ulcerated and is covered with a crust. (From Habif, 1985.)

sure. These lesions are seen most frequently in regions with intense sunlight and on those areas most exposed, the face and neck. Dark-skinned persons and those avoiding sunlight are significantly less prone to develop these malignant tumors. In dark-skinned persons, basal cells contain the pigment melanin, a protective factor against sun exposure. Whereas ultraviolet radiation seems to be the primary etiologic agent, other factors are implicated: arsenic and genetic factors. The use of arsenic in insecticides has recently diminished; however, arsenic is found in drinking water from ground wells. Genetic factors are displayed in the less common nevoid basal cell carcinoma syndrome.

These tumors arise in consequence to a defect that prevents the cells from being shed by the normal keratinization process. The maturing process of epidermal cells is called keratinization; however, the process of keratinization specifically means the synthesis of fibrous protein or keratin. Basal cell tumors lack the normal keratin proteins; however, this may be reversible. Transplantation of basal cell and in vitro cultures shows the property of keratinization can be restored.

The growth rate for these tumors is quite slow. The lesion starts as a nodule (greater than 5 mm across) "pearly" or "ivory" in appearance, slightly elevated above the skin surface with small blood vessels on the surface. As the lesion grows, it often ulcerates, develops crusting, and is firm to the touch. If left untreated, basal cell lesions invade surrounding tissues and, over months or years, can destroy a nose, eyelid, or an ear (for treatment see the box on p. 1418).

Squamous Cell Carcinoma

Squamous cell carcinoma is a tumor of the epidermis characterized by two types: in situ and invasive. Because of the invasive nature of some tumors, squamous cell carcinoma is significantly more malignant if left untreated.

Both epidemiologic and experimental approaches have demonstrated sunlight as a cause of squamous cell carcinoma. Areas affected are the head and neck (75%), and the hands (15%), with 10% elsewhere on the body. In countries where arsenic is higher in drinking water, these tumors are more predominant. X-rays and gamma rays are also associated wtih squamous cell carcinoma. Patients who are immunosuppressed also experience a greater occurrence.

The exact mechanism for producing squamous cell carcinoma is unknown. Again, the initiator-promoter model can be applied to conceptually understand the cancer process (see Chapter 11). It is unclear whether ultraviolet light produces its harmful effects because of problems in DNA, synthesis, repair, or replication.

Invasive squamous cell carcinoma can arise from premalignant lesions of the skin. It rarely arises from nor-

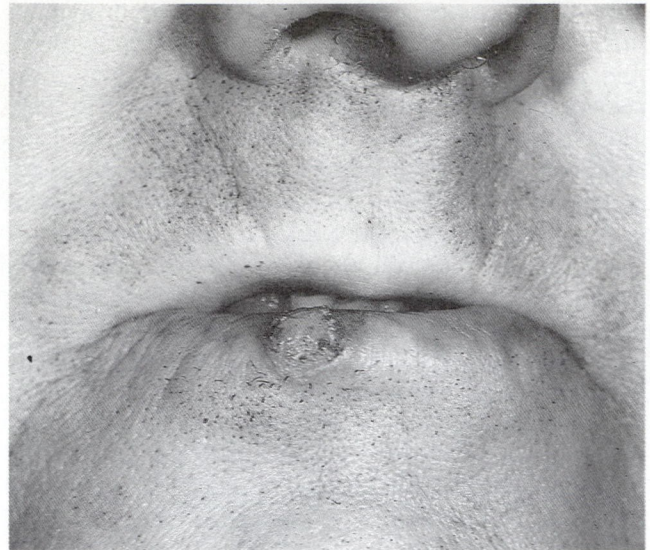

FIG. 41-23. Squamous cell carcinoma. The sun-exposed lower lip is a common site for squamous cell carcinoma. (From Habif, 1985.)

mal appearing skin or "de novo." The premalignant lesions include sun-damaged skin or dysplasias (actinic dermatitis); leukoplakia, or whitish discolored areas; scars; radiation-induced keratosis, tar and oil keratosis; and chronic ulcers and sinuses. The invasive type grows more rapidly than basal cell carcinomas and can spread to regional lymph nodes. These tumors are firm and increase in both elevation and diameter. The surface may be granular and bleed easily (Fig. 41-23).

In situ squamous cell carcinoma is usually confined to the epidermis (intraepidermal) but may extend into the dermis. Common premalignant skin lesions associated with in situ squamous cell carcinomas are actinic (solar) keratosis and Bowen disease. Actinic keratosis is a white, scaly, keratotic (horny) lesion on the exposed areas of the body. Bowen disease is a dysplasia of the basal layer of the dermis or carcinoma in situ. It often is found on unexposed areas of the body and is demonstrated by flat, reddish, scaly patches. These lesions may enlarge to more than a centimeter in diameter, rarely invading surrounding tissue and almost never metastasizing. Other cellular components in the skin (sweat glands, hair follicles, etc.) can give rise to skin cancer, but these are relatively uncommon.

Malignant Melanoma

Melanoma is a malignant tumor of the skin originating from melanocytes, or cells that synthesize the pigment melanin. Epidemiologists report the incidence of melanoma is doubling every 10 to 20 years (Bellet, Mastrangelo, & Maguire, 1983). Early recognition of cutaneous melanomas can have a major impact on surgically curing this disease.

Etiologic factors implicated in melanoma induction include genetic predisposition, solar radiation, and steroid hormone activity. There is strong evidence that sunlight is an important promotional factor. Melanomas arise as a result of malignant degeneration of melanocytes located either along the basal layer of the epidermis or in a benign melanocytic nevus. A nevus, or mole, is an aggregation of melanocytes (Fig. 41-24). These clusters of cells may not be apparent until puberty, when the pigmentation process is initiated by steroid

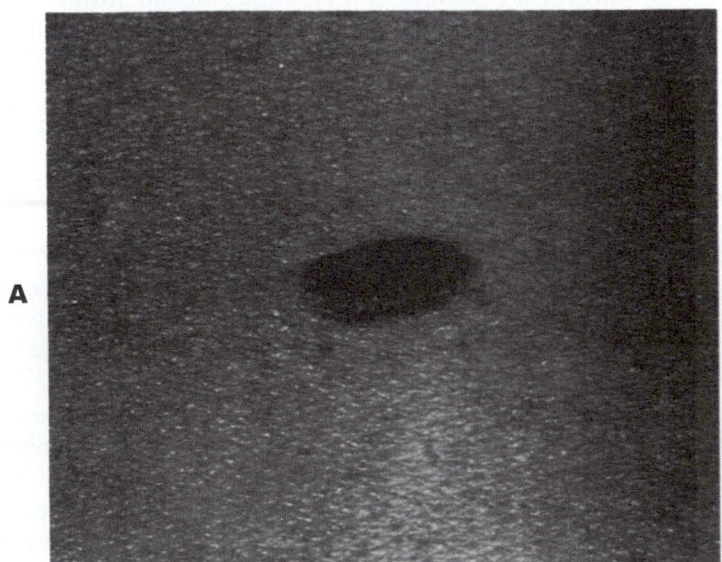
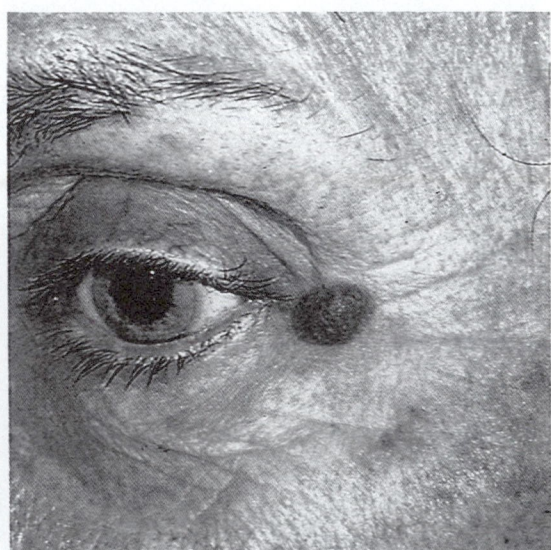

FIG. 41-24. Nevi. **A,** Junctional nevus. Color and shape of this black lesion are uniform. **B,** Dermal nevus. Dome shaped. (From Habif, 1985.)

TABLE 41-7 Classification of nevi

Type	Common characteristics
Junctional nevus	Flat, well-circumscribed, vary in size up to 2 cm, color is dark, hairs may be present. Originate in basal layer of epidermis and can eventually reach the cutaneous surface. This nevus is most likely to develop into a melanoma.
Compound nevus	Most common in adolescents and are the majority of pigmented lesions in children. Rarely does this lesion develop to melanoma. Usually 1 cm in size, hairs may be present. The surface is elevated and smooth.
Intradermal nevus	These are small, less than 1 cm, with regular edges and bristle-like hairs. The color ranges from skin tone to light brown. This type has a slight likelihood of developing into a melanoma.

hormones. The relationship between nevi and melanoma makes it important for the clinician to understand the various neval forms (Table 41-7). Most nevi never become suspicious; however, suspicious pigmented nevi need removal. Indications for biopsy include color change, size change, irregular notched margin, itching, bleeding or oozing, nodularity, scab formation, and ulceration. The clinical varieties of cutaneous melanoma include lentigo malignant melanoma (LMM) (Fig. 41-25), superficial spreading melanomas (SSM) (Fig. 41-26), and primary nodular melanoma (PNM). Clinical characteristics are summarized in the box below.

Treatment of melanoma with no evidence of metastatic disease involves surgical excision to the primary lesion site and regional lymph nodes. The extent of surgery is determined by the staging of disease. Lesions of the extremities have the best prognosis, next head and neck lesions, and trunk lesions the poorest. Only 20% to 40% of patients with regional lymph node involement are alive and cured at 5 years.

Kaposi Sarcoma

Kaposi sarcoma (KS) is a vascular malignancy with different types of presentation. It is associated with immune deficiency states and occurs among kidney transplant recipients taking immunosuppressive drugs. A rapidly progressive form of KS appears with acquired immunodeficiency syndrome (AIDS) (see Chapter 21). KS is also common among middle-aged, black males in equatorial Africa and those of Mediterranean or Jewish descent. Two forms of the disease have been described, classic and epidemic (Safai, 1987). Individuals with AIDS are immunosuppressed, and this allows for opportunistic infection and malignancy.

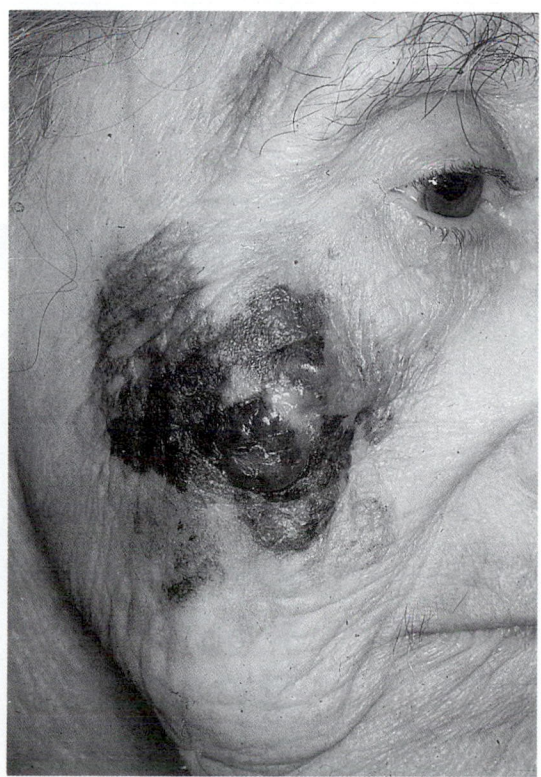

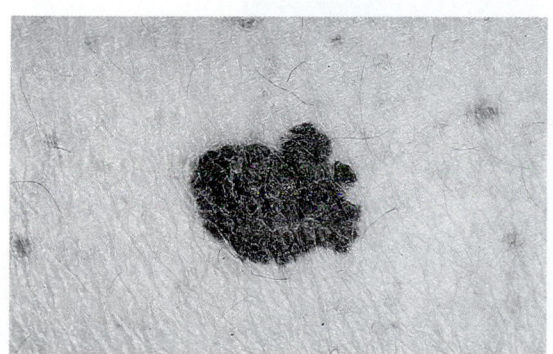

FIG. 41-25. Lentigo malignant melanoma. (From Haibf, 1985.)

FIG. 41-26. Superficial spreading melanoma. (From Habif, 1985.)

Clinical Characteristics of Varieties of Cutaneous Melanoma

LENTIGO MALIGNANT MELANOMA

Frequency	10% to 15% of cutaneous melanomas
Age at diagnosis	50 to 80 years old
Primary location	Head, neck, dorsum of hands
Pigmentation according to thickness	
<1.5 mm (level I, II)	Tan and brown
>1.5 mm (level III)	Tan, brown, and blue-black
>1.5 mm (level IV, V)	Nodule formation

SUPERFICIAL SPREADING MELANOMAS

Frequency	70% of cutaneous melanomas
Age at diagnosis	20 to 60 years old
Primary location	Legs of females; upper back of both sexes
Pigmentation according to thickness	
<1.5 mm (levels I and II)	Tan and brown
>1.5 mm (levels III)	Tan, brown, and blue-black
>1.5 mm (levels IV and V)	Nodule formation

NODULAR MELANOMA

Frequency	12% of cutaneous melanomas
Age at diagnosis	20 to 60 years old
Primary location	No specific site preference
Pigmentation according to thickness	
>1.5 mm (levels III)	Small nodule (any hue)
>1.5 mm (levels IV and V)	Large nodule (any hue)

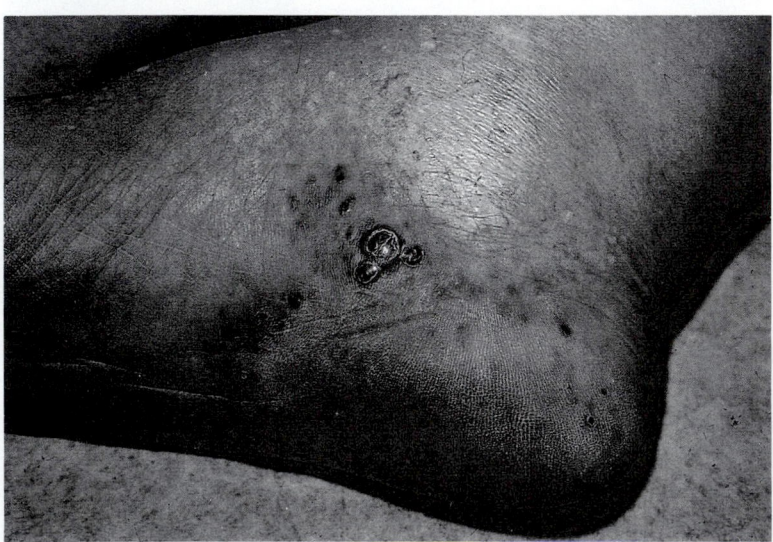

FIG. 41-27. Kaposi sarcoma. Purple nodules are most commonly seen on the lower legs. (From Habif, 1985.)

TABLE 41-8 American Burn Association classification of burn injury

Minor burn injury	Moderate, uncomplicated burn injury	Major burn injury
Second-degree burns of less than 15% TBSA in adults or less than 10% TBSA in children	Second-degree burns of 15% to 25% TBSA in adults or 10% to 20% TBSA in children	Second-degree burns of greater than 25% TBSA in adults or 20% TBSA in children
Third-degree burns of less than 2% TBSA not involving special care areas (eyes, ears, face, hands, feet, perineum)	Third-degree burns of less than 10% TBSA not involving special care areas	All third-degree burns of 10% TBSA burn of greater
Excludes electrical injury, inhalation injury, complicated injury (fractures), all poor-risk individuals (extremes of age, intercurrent disease, etc.)	Excludes electrical injury, complicated injury (fractures), inhalation injury, all poor-risk individuals (extremes of age, intercurrent disease, etc.)	All burns involving hands, face, eyes, ears, feet, perineum All inhalation injury, electrical injury, complicated burn injury involving fractures or other major trauma All poor-risk individuals

TBSA: Total body surface area.

The human immunodeficiency virus and cytomegalovirus have been proposed as cofactors in the development of KS (Goopman, 1987). The endothelial cell is thought to be the progenitor of KS. The lesions emerge as purplish brown macules and develop into plaques and nodules. They tend to be multifocal rather than spreading by metastasis. The lesions initially appear over the lower extremities in the classic form (Fig. 41-27). The rapidly progressive form associated with AIDS tends to spread symmetrically over the upper body, particularly the face and oral mucosa. The lesions are often pruritic and painful. About 75% of individuals with epidemic KS have involvement of lymph nodes, particularly in the gastrointestinal tract and lungs. Organ involvement is much less common in the classic form. The rapidly progressive form has a poor prognosis and shorter survival rates than the classic form. (See Chapter 21 for further discussion on AIDS.)

Diagnosis is by skin biopsy with a high index of suspicion for those with immune deficiency. Local lesions can be excised. Multiple disseminated lesions may be treated with a combination of α-interferon, radiotherapy, and cytotoxic drugs. Clinical trials for new treatments are in progress. General response to treatment is poor, but a 2-year survival rate is better in individuals with KS alone than in those with KS and an opportunistic infection.

Thermal Injury

It is estimated that about 2 million people are burned in the United States each year and about 20% of these individuals will require hospitalization (McManus & Pruitt, 1988). Most significant burns occur in the home

and the highest percentage of deaths (75%) are from home fires, usually in the kitchen (Maley & Wright, 1982).

Burns

Burns may be caused by thermal, chemical, or electrical injury. Thermal injuries result from exposure to direct flames, hot liquids, or radiation. Direct contact, inhalation, or ingestion of acids, alkalies, or blistering agents cause chemical burns. Electrical burns occur with the passage of electrical current through the body to the ground. Associated electrical flames or flashes can also burn the skin.

The physiologic consequences of major **thermal injury** center around the profound, life-threatening hypovolemic shock that occurs in conjunction with cellular and immunologic disruption within a few minutes of the injury. In contrast, the effects of minor and moderate burn injuries are limited to the localized destruction of the skin. Individuals with minor and moderate burn injuries will experience discomfort until healing or skin grafting is accomplished, but these burns are not life threatening. With a major burn injury, a systematic pathophysiology ensues that requires therapeutic intervention to sustain life. The American Burn Association (1976) defines the severity of burn injury according to the depth of injury and extent of injury (Table 41-8). The depth of injury identifies the level of tissue destruction; the extent of the injury determines the mortality rate.

Pathophysiology

First-Degree Burns The depth of injury is divided into

TABLE 41-9 Depth of burn injury

Characteristic	First degree	Second degree Superficial partial-thickness	Deep partial-thickness	Third degree Full-thickness
Morphology	Destruction of epidermis only	Destruction of epidermis and some dermis	Destruction of epidermis and dermis, leaving only skin appendages	Destruction of epidermis, dermis, and underlying subcutaneous tissue
Skin function	Intact	Absent	Absent	Absent
Tactile and pain sensors	Intact	Intact	Intact but diminished	Absent
Blisters	Present only after first 24 hr	Present within minutes, thin-walled and fluid-filled	May or may not appear as fluid-filled blisters; often is layer of flat, dehydrated "tissue paper" that lifts off in sheets	Blisters rare; usually is a layer of flat, dehydrated "tissue paper" that lifts off easily
Appearance of wound after initial debridement	Skin peels at 24 to 48 hr, normal or slightly red underneath	Red to pale ivory, moist surface	Mottled with areas of waxy white, dry surface	White, cherry red, or black; may contain visible thrombosed veins; dry, hard leathery surface
Healing time	3 to 5 days	21 to 28 days	30 days to many months	Will not heal, may close from edges as secondary healing if wound is small
Scarring	None	May be present, low incidence influenced by genetic predisposition	Highest incidence because of slow healing rate increasing scar tissue development, also influenced by genetic predisposition.	Skin graft; scarring minimized by early excision and grafting, influenced by genetic predisposition.

four categories (Table 41-9). First-degree burns are not included in estimates of the extent of total body surface area (TBSA) burn. The skin does not lose its ability to function as a water vapor and bacterial barrier with **first-degree burns**. The most common example of a first-degree burn is a sunburn, which results from indirect exposure to the heat of the sun. Initially there is local pain and erythema, but no blisters appear for about 24 hours. An extensive first-degree burn may cause systemic responses such as chills, headache, localized edema, and nausea or vomiting. No treatment of extensive first-degree burns is required unless the person is elderly or an infant, in which case severe nausea and vomiting may lead to inadequate fluid intake and dehydration. Therapy consists of intravenous hydration until the nausea and vomiting subside at 24 to 72 hours after burn injury. Comfort measures for previously healthy children or adults with extensive first-degree burns consist of aspirin for adults or acetaminophen for children,

every 4 hours in age-appropriate dosage, and the frequent application of a water-soluble lotion. First-degree burns heal in 3 to 5 days without scarring.

Second-Degree Burns **Second-degree burns** are classified as either superficial or deep partial-thickness injury (Table 41-9). The hallmark of **superficial partial-thickness injury** is the appearance of thin-walled, fluid-filled blisters that develop within just a few minutes after the injury. Another dominant characteristic of superficial injury is pain. As the blisters break or are removed, nerve endings are exposed to the air (Fig. 41-28). Tactile and pain sensors remain intact throughout the healing process, with each wound care procedure causing extreme pain. The wounds heal in 3 to 4 weeks, provided the individual is adequately nourished and no complications develop (Fig. 41-29). The amount of scarring that develops is a genetically determined trait and is not predictable during the early course of treatment. The tendency to scar is extremely high in black people and peo-

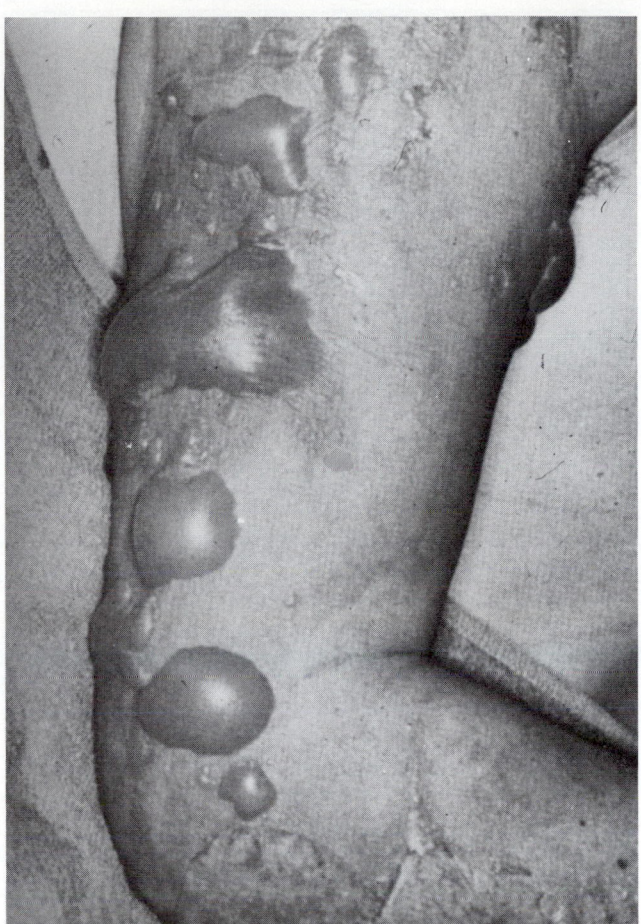

FIG. 41-28. Second-degree burn (superficial partial thickness). (Courtesy Intermountain Burn Center, University of Utah Health Sciences Center.)

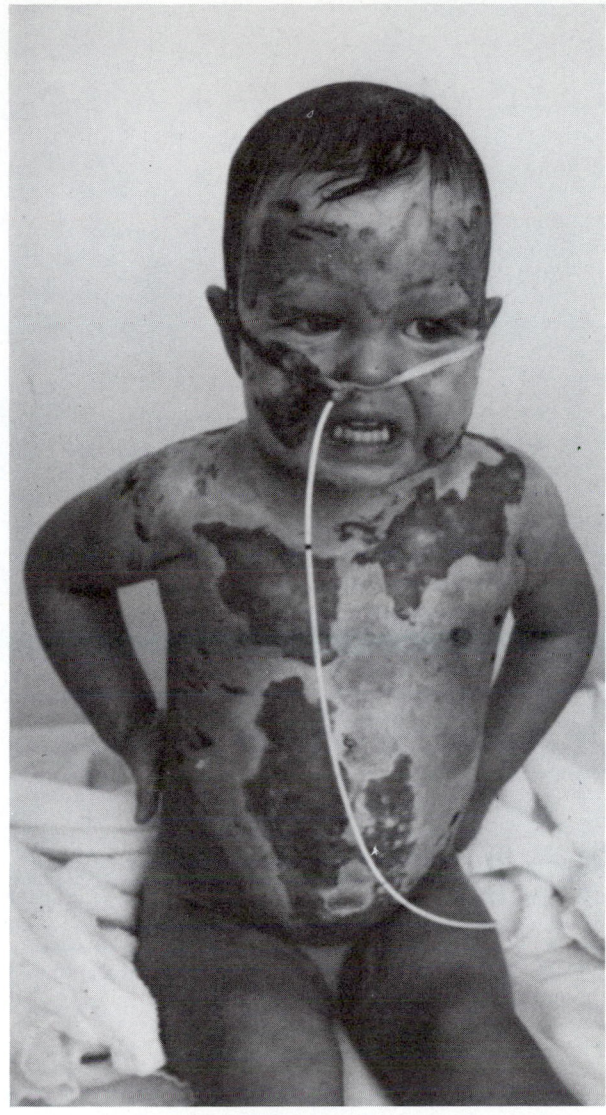

FIG. 41-29. Healing second-degree burn (superficial partial thickness). (Courtesy Intermountain Burn Center, University of Utah Health Sciences Center.)

ple with red hair and extremely low in Asian and American Indian Populations, although there is also great variation within these groups.

Deep partial-thickness burns may involve the entire dermis, leaving only the epidermal skin appendages located in the hair follicles (Table 41-9). The burn tends to be waxy white and is often surrounded by margins of superficial partial-thickness injury. The injury is initially clinically indistinguishable from a full-thickness injury (Fig. 41-30). By 7 to 10 days after burn injury, hair will appear from the hair follicles, indicating that epidermal appendages remain. These wounds take weeks to heal, and current therapy indicates the surgical removal of the burn wound (excision) followed by the application of the person's own unburned skin from another body area (autograft). Wounds that heal slowly produce more scar tissue and continue to be a potential source of infection until closed. However, in the presence of extensive wounds or a previously debilitating concomitant disease state, such as cardiopulmonary failure, deep partial-thickness wounds are not surgically treated but are primarily allowed to heal.

Third-Degree Burns

Third-degree, or full-thickness, burns involve the destruction of the entire epidermis, dermis, and some underlying subcutaneous tissue (Table 41-9). On occasion, all underlying subcutaneous tissue is destroyed and muscle or bone may be involved. Some classification systems designate burns to muscle, tendon, or bone as fourth-degree injury. In burn care facilities, fourth-degree injury is usually a term describing damage from electrical injury. Visible thrombosed veins may be present in some areas of the full-thickness injury, with the most common location being the dorsum of the hand. Full-thickness wounds often appear relatively innocuous when their color is white, and the delineation

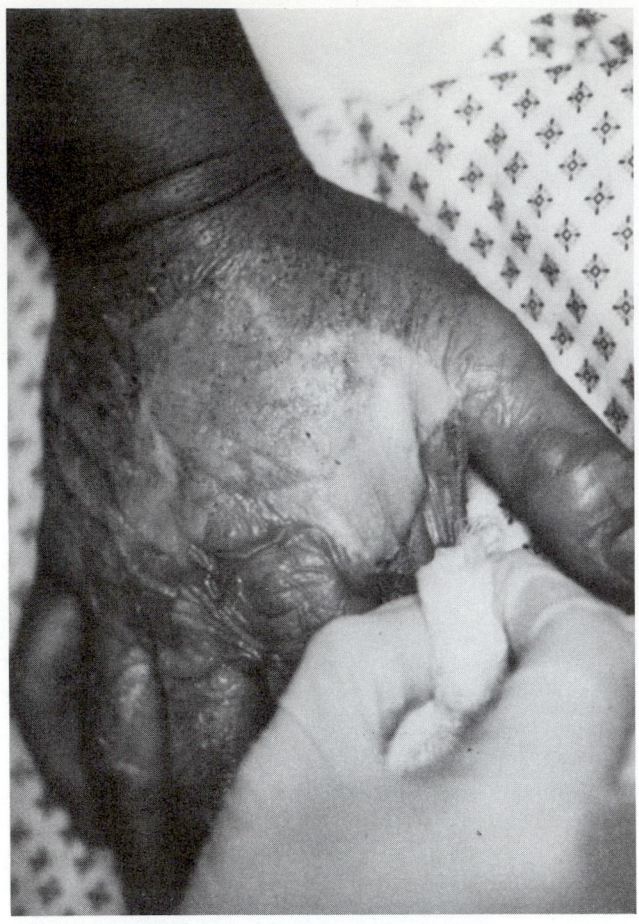

FIG. 41-30. Second-degree burn (deep partial thickness injury to dorsum of hand). (Courtesy Intermountain Burn Center, University of Utah Health Sciences Center.)

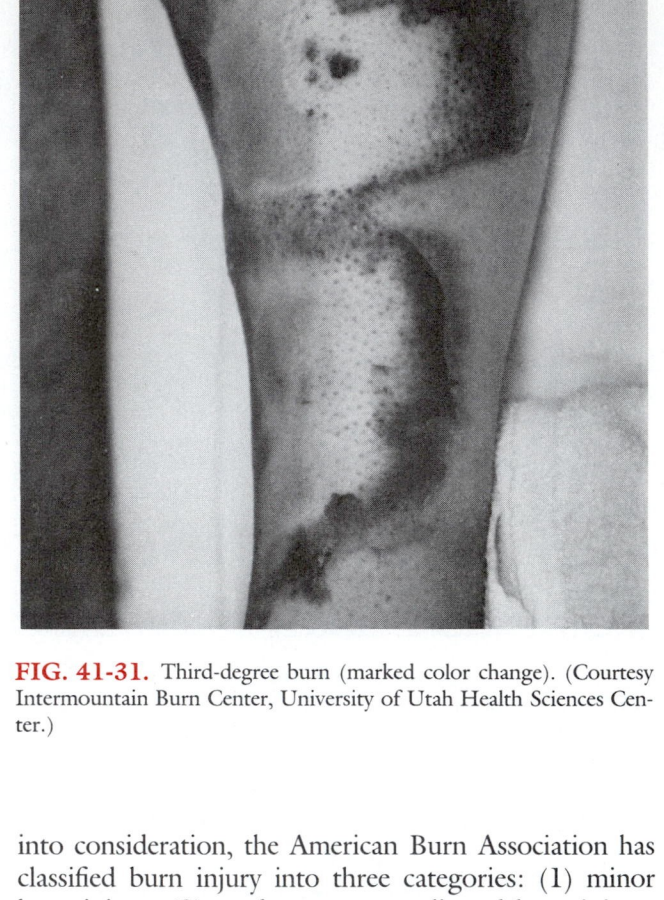

FIG. 41-31. Third-degree burn (marked color change). (Courtesy Intermountain Burn Center, University of Utah Health Sciences Center.)

between normal and burned skin is not accompanied by a marked color change. The elasticity of the dermis is destroyed giving the wound a dry, hard, leathery appearance (Fig. 41-31). As marked edema forms, distal circulation may be compromised in areas of circumferential burns. Full-thickness burns are painless because all nerve endings have been destroyed by the heat.

Clinical Manifestations

The extent of the total body surface area (TBSA) burn is estimated using either the "Rule of nines" (Fig. 41-32) or the Lund and Browder chart (Fig. 41-33). By convention, burn areas assessed as full-thickness injury are colored in red; areas of superficial or deep partial thickness are colored in blue; and areas of first-degree burn are omitted from the burn diagram and from the TBSA percent burn totals.

The severity of burn injury is a combination of many factors, including age, medical history, extent and depth of injury, and body area involved. Taking these factors

into consideration, the American Burn Association has classified burn injury into three categories: (1) minor burn injury; (2) moderate, uncomplicated burn injury; and (3) major burn injury (Table 41-8). In general, people with minor burn injury are expected to be treated as outpatients and those with moderate, uncomplicated burn injury are expected to be treated in a nearby hospital facility, although transfer to a burn care facility may be accomplished at the discretion of the health care provider. In both of the previously mentioned categories, treatment is aimed at promoting healing through wound cleansing and nutritional support. Tetanus toxoid is administered prophylactically.

With a major burn injury, a systemic pathophysiology ensues that requires therapeutic intervention to sustain life. The immediate physiologic consequences of major burn injury center around the profound, life-threatening hypovolemic shock, which occurs in conjunction with cellular and immunologic disruption within a few minutes of the injury. Burn shock is a phenomenon consist-

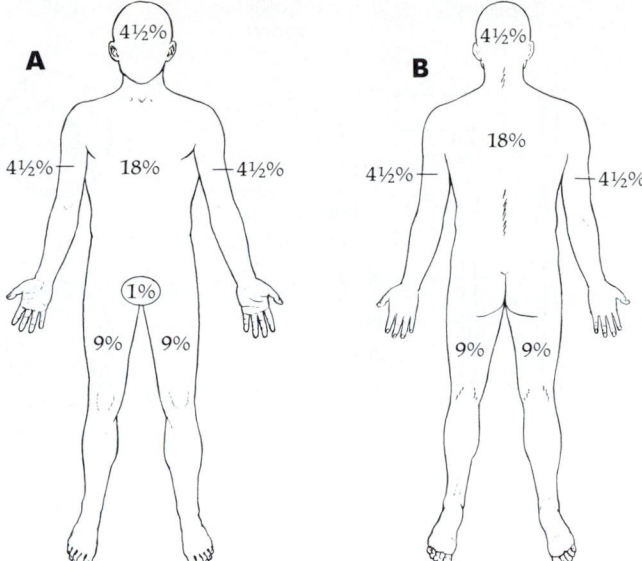

FIG. 41-32. Estimation of burn injury: rule of nines. **A,** Adults (anterior view). **B,** Adults (posterior view). (From Thompson et al., 1986.)

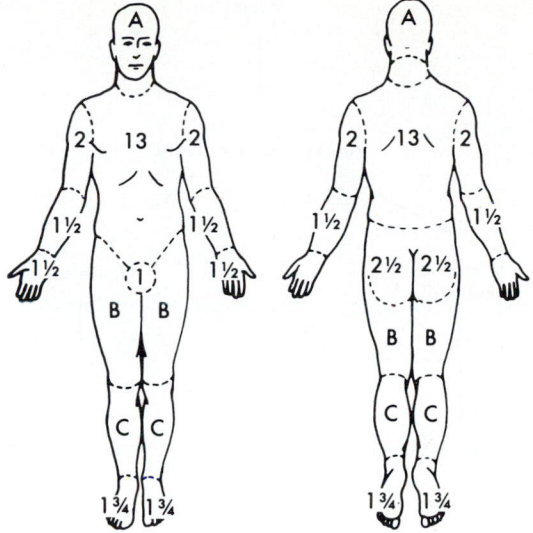

Relative percentages of areas affected by growth
(age in years)

	0	1	5	10	15	Adult
A: half of head	9½	8½	6½	5½	4½	3½
B: half of thigh	2¾	3¼	4	4¼	4½	4¾
C: half of leg	2½	2½	2¾	3	3¼	3½

Second degree _____ and

Third degree _____ =

Total percent burned____

FIG. 41-33 Estimation of burn injury: Lund and Browder chart. Areas designated by letters (*A, B,* and *C*) represent percentages of body surface area that vary according to age. Accompanying table indicates relative percentages of these areas at various stages in life. (From Sabiston, 1977.)

ing of both a hypovolemic cardiovascular component and a cellular component. The hypovolemic shock results from an increase in capillary permeability, which begins with the onset of burn injury and persists for approximately 24 hours after burn injury, even when adequate resuscitation fluid is given. Researchers have documented the release of many mediators (prostaglandins, thromboxanes, histamine, and serotonin) of the inflammatory response that may play a role in the cardiovascular response to burns (Zimmerman & Krizek, 1984). Evidence has also accumulated suggesting that cellular metabolism is disrupted with onset of the burn wound, resulting in altered membrane permeability and loss of normal electrolyte homeostasis. This cellular defect may be the pathophysiologic process responsible for the genesis of burn shock. Also, the many circulating factors demonstrated in burn serum may play a role in the generation of the cellular abnormalities known to occur. Although it is recognized that the cardiovascular and systemic response is intricately interwoven into the cellular response, they are presented here as separate entities for the purpose of describing their components.

Cardiovascular Response to Burn Injury

The end result of a major burn injury is hypovolemic shock. The severity of burn shock is directly proportional to the extent of the TBSA burn. Burns involving 25% to 40% TBSA in adults, or 15% to 25% TBSA in children, require cardiovascular support through intravenous fluid, but the treatment is usually tolerated in a fairly predictable manner. Burns involving larger TBSA

are potentially lethal injuries that are often accompanied by a stormy clinical course.

The cardiovascular system is normally a closed system with controlled movement of fluid and electrolytes occurring across selected areas, including the capillaries. However, within minutes of a major burn injury, the capillary bed opens not only in the burn area but also in the entire capillary system. This dilation of capillaries is referred to as a loss of capillary seal and is the mechanism for the ensuing hypovolemic shock. The mechanism of burn shock is not understood, but the sequence is known (Fig. 41-34). As the capillary seal is lost, leakage of intravascular fluid into the interstitial spaces occurs throughout the body with extravasation of water, electrolytes, and proteins (Fig. 41-35). The red and white blood cells remain in the circulation because their relatively larger size does not permit them to leak. Thus an elevated hematocrit and white blood cell count occur. The capillary leak quickly develops into profound hypovolemic shock which, if not treated, quickly leads

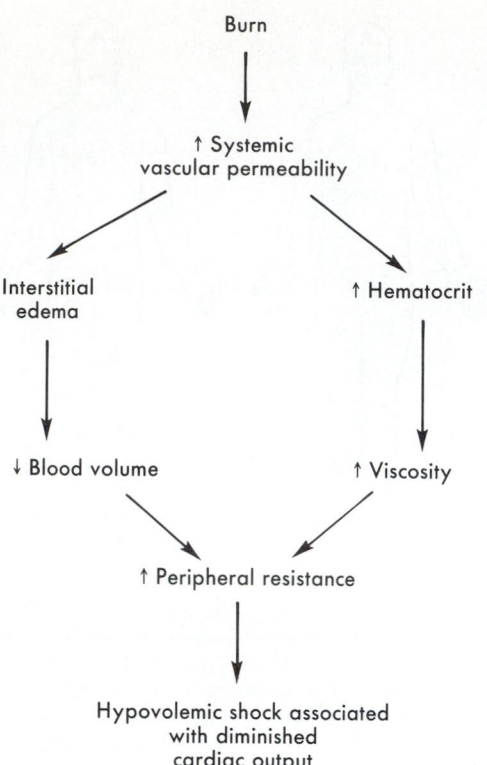

FIG. 41-34. Cardiovascular effects of major burn injury during burn shock. (Courtesy Intermountain Burn Center, University of Utah Health Sciences Center.)

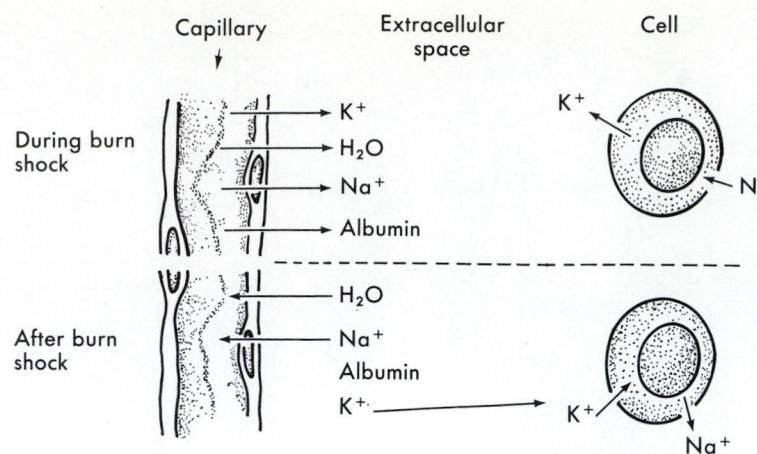

FIG. 41-35. Direction of fluid and electrolyte shifts associated with burn shock. (Courtesy Intermountain Burn Center, University of Utah Health Sciences Center.)

to irreversible shock and death within a few hours. Burn shock continues for about 24 hours after burn injury, at which time the capillary seal is restored by an unknown mechanism.

Burn shock resuscitation involves the infusion of intravenous fluid at a rate faster than the rate of the leak of circulating volume fluid for the 24 hours after burn shock. Resuscitation for burn shock can be accomplished using one of several available fluid regimens. The most frequently used fluid resuscitation protocol is the Parkland formula (Baxter, 1974). Lactated Ringer solution is the fluid of choice for burn shock because it most closely approximates the fluid being lost from the circulatory system (Table 41-10). Severe electrolyte imbalances will occur if fluid resuscitation is accomplished with electrolyte-free intravenous fluid (i.e., D_5W).

The massive edema associated with burn shock is an iatrogenic complication, but failure to deliver the resuscitation fluid results in irreversible hypovolemic shock and death. The edema occurs over the entire body, not just the burn area (Fig. 41-36). This often leads to mechanical airway obstruction, necessitating tracheal intubation, and increased severity of the interstitial pulmonary edema associated with inhalation injury.

The most reliable criterion for adequate resuscitation of burn shock is urine output. The individual is in hypovolemic shock and will, as a compensatory mechanism, decrease or cease urine output in an effort to preserve circulating volume. The adult receiving sufficient intravenous fluid will excrete 30 to 50 ml of urine/hour: children will excrete 1 ml/kg/hour. If the individual does not have adequate urine output, sufficient fluid is not being administered. The massive amount of intravenous fluid required by burned individuals during the shock phase is often intimidating to the person delivering the fluid. One common concern is that 30 L of intravenous fluid over 24 hours will result in pulmonary edema. It should be remembered that the individual is in hypovolemic shock and that the fluid is leaking out almost as fast as it is infused. Unless the individual is in cardiac failure as a result of a preexisting disease state, the fluid is distributed evenly throughout the body and does not

TABLE 41-10 Electrolyte content of lactated Ringer solution and extracellular fluid

Electrolyte	Extracellular fluid* (mEq/L)	Lactated Ringer† (mEq/L)
Sodium	135 - 145	130
Potassium	3.2 - 4.5	4
Chloride	95 - 105	109
Lactate (bicarbonate)	24 - 28	28

*Normal values may vary slightly between laboratories.
†Plus 80 to 100 ml free water per liter.

Estimation of Resuscitation Fluid Requirements Using the Parkland Formula

PARKLAND FORMULA
4 ml lactated Ringer solution/kg
   body weight/% TBSA burn = Fluid requirements
   in first 24 hours after burn
      ½ administered first 8 hr
      ¼ administered second 8 hr
      ¼ administered third 8 hr

EXAMPLE
A 70 kg man with a 50% TBSA burn

Parkland formula: 4 ml/kg/% TBSA burn

4 ml/70kg/50% TBSA burn = 14,000 ml or 14 L of
   Ringer lactate
      ½ in first 8 hr = 7000 ml or 875 ml/hr
      ¼ in second 8 hr = 3500 ml or 437 ml/hr
      ¼ in third 8 hr = 3500 ml or 437 ml/hr

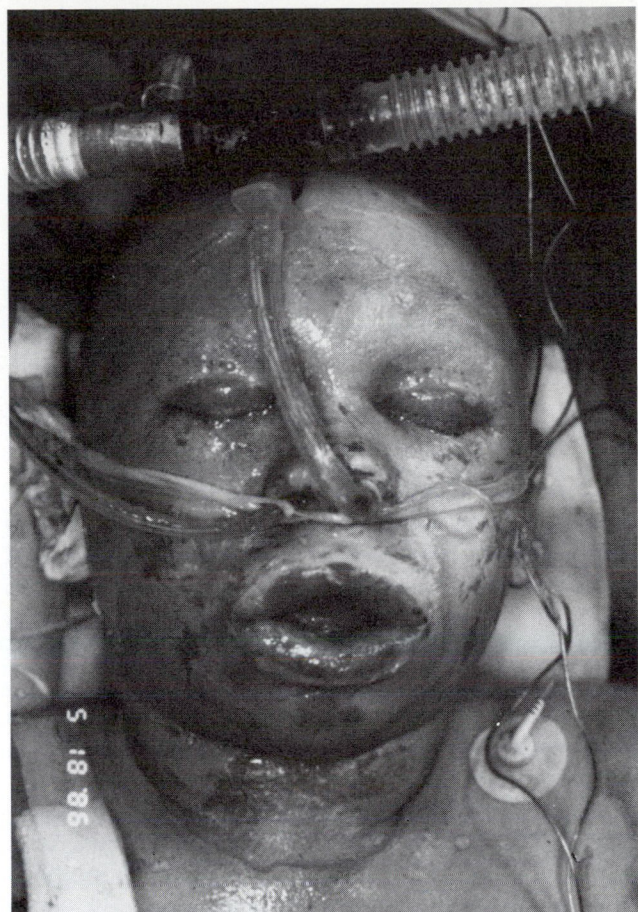

FIG. 41-36. Edema of burn shock. (Courtesy Intermountain Burn Center, University of Utah Health Sciences Center.)

accumulate in the lungs. If the individual is in cardiac failure, there is little chance of survival, because without the ability to circulate the administered fluid, hypovolemic shock cannot be resolved. If the fluid is administered, cardiac failure occurs; if the fluid is not administered, irreversible hypovolemic shock occurs. In either case, death is usually inevitable, although cardiac support drugs, such as dopamine, may help if the cardiac disease is not too severe.

The end point of burn shock is defined as the time when the individual is able to maintain adequate urine output for 2 hours with the hourly fluid administration rate at the person's maintenance rate (see box). As burn shock ends, the volume of fluid administered remains in the circulating volume and is reflected as increased urine output. The mechanism whereby capillary integrity is restored is unknown but usually occurs about 24 hours after burn injury. After the individual has reached the end point of burn shock, the term used to describe the person's condition is *sealed*. On completion of resuscitation, an infusion of type-specific, fresh frozen plasma, equal to 20% of the calculated blood volume, is administered.

Cardiac dysfunction is also a component of major burn injury. Burn shock is accompanied by a sudden precipitous drop in cardiac output, which does not parallel the gradual reduction of blood volume. Furthermore, the infusion of intravenous fluids in amounts to restore the circulating volume does not return the cardiac output to preburn levels (Aikawa, Martyn, & Burke, 1978; Dobson & Warner, 1957). The consistent burn shock finding of inappropriately low cardiac output in the presence of vigorous intravenous fluid resuscitation and massive catecholamine release led to the suggestion of a specific myocardial depressant factor (Baxter, Cook, & Shires, 1966; Lefer & Martin, 1970; Rosenthal, Hawley, & Hakin, 1972). Although there is agreement that myocardial dysfunction is present with all major burn injuries, the cause of the depression remains to be described except in the most general terms. It is accepted that there is no simple specific myocardial depressant factor, but rather a cascade of events that is generally termed the cellular response to burn and includes both metabolic and immunologic factors. These factors initiate the cardiovascular sequence of loss of capillary seal and subsequent hypovolemic shock.

Cellular Response to Burn Injury Major burn injury affects the entire physiologic system; however, survival depends on its ultimate impact at the cellular level. The cellular response to burn injury falls into two categories: (1) metabolic response and (2) immunologic response. The basic syndrome is referred to as the "sick cell syndrome." Welt and colleagues (1967) were among the first to describe this phenomenon as a cell membrane transport defect related to an alteration in the steady state composition characterized by high intracellular concentrations of sodium. Trunkey, Illner, Wagner, and Shires (1973) found a marked decrease in primate muscle extracellular water and an increase in both intracellular sodium and water during hypovolemic shock. In addition, other researchers demonstrated an associated decrease in resting membrane potential, a decrease in amplitude of the action potential, and a prolongation of both the repolarization and depolarization time in association with a decreased intracellular potassium concentration (Cunningham, Shires, & Wagner, 1971; Rosenthal & Tabor, 1945). The cellular dysfunction of burn injury extends beyond the transmembrane potential disruption and the sodium-potassium pump impairment to include a loss of intracellular magnesium and phosphate (Turinsky, Gonnerman, & Loose, 1981) and elevated serum lactic dehydrogenase (LDH) levels (Deets & Glaviano, 1973). This suggests impairments of basic cellular function as the underlying cause of the diminished membrane potentials. The data suggest a decrease in the efficiency of the pump—a change that can be reversed by adequate fluid resuscitation of burn shock over time.

Metabolic reactions to the stress of a major burn injury involve the response of the sympathetic nervous system and other homeostatic regulators. Catecholamines are found in elevated amounts in both the serum and urine of burned individuals. Changes in lipid metabolism are reflected as an elevation in plasma free fatty acids (FFA) and a decrease in plasma cholesterol and phospholipids (Okamoto, Glaviano, & Pindok, 1971).

Burn injury induces an almost immediate hypermetabolic state that persists until wound closure. Wilmore, Long, Mason, Skreen, and Pruitt (1974) described the hypermetabolic state of 20 burned individuals as unrelated to ambient temperatures with persistent elevation of core body temperatures. The metabolic rate increased with burn size in a curvilinear relationship with oxygen consumption rarely exceeding 2½ times basal levels. Evaporative water loss and surface cooling are not the primary stimulus for the hypermetabolic state; rather, the hypermetabolism is related to an increase and resetting of the thermal regulatory set point. A core body temperature of 38.5° C is typical. A reflex arc mobilizes neural and/or hormonal afferent stimuli to the hypothalamus, producing a catecholamine response clinically manifested as hypermetabolism, hyperthermia, and hyperglycemia.

Evidence also exists that the burn wound itself directly mediates the response to injury at both the local and systemic level. The body's priority response to injury is the wound itself, and the general systemic events observed may occur in response to the burn tissue inflammation (Gump, Price, & Kinney, 1970; Wilmore et al., 1977; Wilmore et al., 1980). That is, vasodilation, increased capillary permeability, and edema occur to facilitate healing of the local area. The distribution of the peripheral circulation following burn injury transports both heat and glucose preferentially to the wound. The energy cost of these reparative and transport processes is reflected in the increased metabolism and hyperdynamic circulation.

The extensive evaporative water loss that occurs in burn tissue is a heat-consuming process and the energy need is met, at least in part, by increased visceral heat production. The signal for the response is unknown because individuals whose wounds have been denervated continue to have posttraumatic metabolic response. Hypothalamic function alterations result in the elevation of human growth hormone (HGH) serum levels in the presence of hyperglycemia, a finding opposite normal states (Wilmore et al., 1975). Furthermore, the hypermetabolic rate is not decreased during rest, sleep, or warmth. Since the increased oxygen consumption cannot be accounted for on the basis of the elevated body temperature alone, an elevated metabolic state, not a thermoregulatory drive, is responsible for the increased heat production (Aulick et al., 1979).

Glucose and lactate kinetics are also altered after burn injury. Although tissue hypoxia produces lactic acidosis, its persistence in the presence of adequate tissue perfusion suggests an increased rate of glycogenolysis (Wilmore, Aulick & Goodwin, 1979). An absolute or relative insulin deficiency in combination with an excess of glucocorticoid, glucagon, and/or catecholamine are the signals that promote gluconeogenesis. Evidence of hepatic response to burn injury is characterized by alterations in the clotting factors. A **hypercoagulable** state develops as manifested by an elevated plasma fibrinogen concentration in the presence of shortened prothrombin (PT) and activated partial thromboplastin (PTT) times (McManus, Eurenius & Pruitt, 1973).

In summary, extensive burn injury initiates the most marked alterations in body metabolism associated with any illness. Much of the work explaining this response has been conducted by Wilmore and Aulick (1978), who reported the persistent tachycardia, hyperpnea, hyperpyrexia, and marked body wasting seen in burn injury reflect heightened metabolic activity and accelerated body catabolism. These systemic alterations occur as a result of the cutaneous inflammatory process and are thought to facilitate wound repair. The neural component of this alteration is in response to a sympathetic reaction that releases catecholamines in large amounts.

The immunologic response to burn injury is immediate, prolonged, and severe. The end result in individuals surviving burn shock is immunosuppression with increased susceptibility to potentially fatal systemic burn wound sepsis. The role of circulating factors has been intensely studied, and the findings clearly show that serum from burned animals will induce burn shock in an unburned animal and that burn serum has immunosuppressive qualities in vitro. Leukocyte chemotactic studies in vitro revealed a decrease in leukocyte migration with the decrease inversely correlated with burn size (Warden, Mason & Pruitt, 1974). Placing the burn-suppressed leukocytes into serum obtained from normal donors returned the levels to 107% of normal activity (Warden, Mason & Pruitt, 1975). Ninnemann (1980) reports the participation of both a serum-borne factor and a specific subset of B lymphocytes in the generation of suppressor cells.

A host of chemicals found in burn plasma in altered concentrations may also play a role in burn shock. These include vasoactive amines (histamine, serotonin), products of complement activation (C3a, C5a), prostaglandins, kinins, endotoxin, and the metabolic hormones (catecholamines, glucocorticoids). A decrease in the complement components C3a and C5a in the circulation after burn injury suggests a nonspecific activation of the complement system (Heideman, Kaijser & Gelin, 1978). Activation of the complement system in the injured tissue results in an inflammatory response caused by the release of histamine and serotonin by C3a and C5a. Since both histamine and serotonin alter capillary permeability, some investigators propose this cause for burn shock, since these vasoactive amines initiate the inflammatory response along with kinin polypeptides and other chemical mediators. As a result of these vascular changes, fluid and fibrinogen leave the dilated, permeable vessels. Prostaglandins function in the inflammatory process by regulating the metabolism of the cells of inflammation (see Chapter 7).

The white blood cells are also altered at this time when their need to inhibit sepsis is vital. Normally, opsonin renders bacteria susceptible to phagocytosis, but the burn injury triggers a consumptive opsoninopathy. Burn serum contains an inhibitor of C3 conversion that leads to decreased opsonization and polymorphonuclear (PMN) neutrophil dysfunction (Alexander et al., 1976; Bjornson, Altemeier & Bjornson, 1977).

Evaporative Water Loss One of the major purposes of intact skin is to serve as a barrier to evaporative water loss (EWL) from the body. With major burn injury, this ability of the skin to regulate evaporative water loss is totally disrupted. In a classic study done in 1962, Moncrief and Mason (1962) attempted to determine the magnitude of such a loss and determined that daily evaporative water loss was in the range of 20 times normal in the early phase of injury with gradual decreases as wound closure is achieved. Further studies revealed that the insensible water loss through the burned skin is not from evaporation of water from sweat glands but rather from water vapor formed within the body and lost through the skin (Moncrief, 1974; Roe & Kinney, 1964).

Calculation of the amount of fluid lost by evaporative water loss includes losses from all sources. Normally, the skin is the major source of insensible loss (75%) and the lungs are minor sources (25%), with a total loss of only about 600 to 800 ml/day. This changes dramatically with burns because not only does skin loss increase but lung loss also increases by hypermetabolism and hyperventilation, especially in an intubated individual. Total evaporative losses may be up to 1500 ml/day. Replacement of the loss is mandatory to prevent volume deficit.

Evaluation and Treatment

There are three essential elements of survival of major burn injury: (1) meticulous wound management, (2) adequate nutrition, and (3) early surgical excision and grafting of full-thickness wounds. Burn recovery is long and stormy, with complications the rule rather than the exception. The goal of burn management is wound closure in a manner that promotes survival. Recovery from a major burn injury is never assured but will usually occur once the burn wound is reduced to less than 20% TBSA. Scar formation with contractures is often a consequence of healing in deep partial-thickness and third degree burns (Fig. 41-37).

Frostbite

Frostbite is injury to the skin caused by exposure to extreme cold. The most common areas affected are fingers, toes, ears, nose, and cheeks. The mechanism of injury is complex but appears to be related to direct cold injury to cells, indirect injury from ice crystal formation, and impaired circulation to the exposed area. Frozen skin becomes white or yellowish and is waxy. There is numbness and no sensation of pain.

The extent of skin damage can range from mild to severe. There is redness and discomfort with mild frostbite with warming and a return to normal in a few hours. Cyanosis and mottling develops followed by redness, swelling, and burning pain on rewarming in more severe cases. Within 24 to 48 hours, vesicles and bullae appear that resolve into crusts that eventually slough off, leaving thin, newly formed skin. The most severe cases result in gangrene with loss of the affected part. Frostbite may be classified by depth of injury: superficial, including partial skin freezing (first degree) and full-thickness skin freezing (second degree); and deep, including full-thickness skin and subcutaneous freezing (third degree); and deep tissue freezing (fourth degree) (Fisher, Souba, & Ford, 1988).

Immediate treatment of frostbite is to cover affected areas with other body surfaces and warm clothing. The

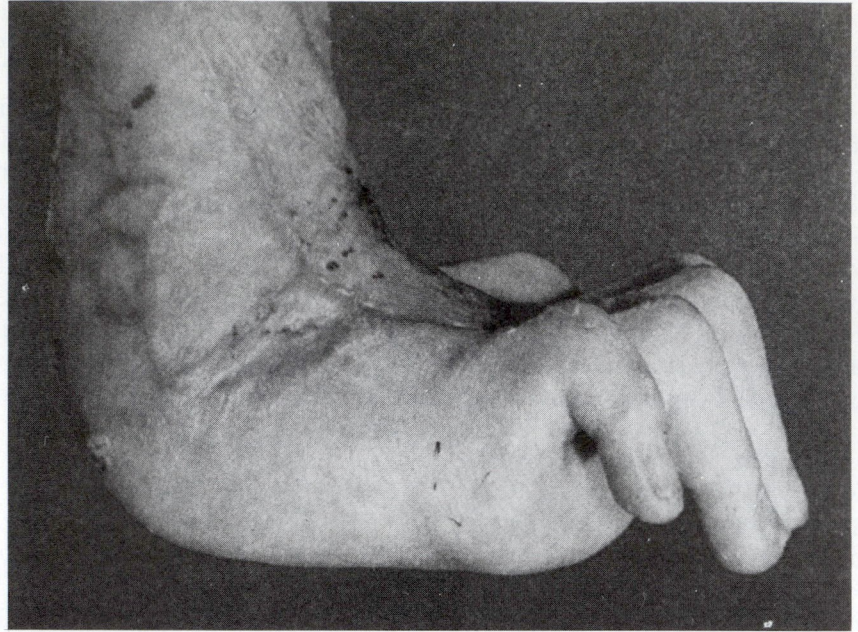

FIG. 41-37. Scar formation with contractures to the dorsum of the hand after deep partial-thickness burn. (Courtesy Intermountain Burn Center, University of Utah Health Sciences Center.)

area should not be rubbed or massaged. Local, dry heat should be avoided. Immersion in a warm water bath (40° C to 44° C) until frozen tissue is thawed is the best treatment. Pain during the thawing period is severe and should be treated with potent analgesics. Gentle cleansing and avoidance of pressure on the skin should be maintained during healing. Amputation of necrotic tissue is delayed until a clear line of demarcation is established.

DISORDERS OF THE HAIR

Alopecia

Male-Pattern Alopecia

Alopecia means loss of hair. Localized hair loss in men is not a disease but a genetically predisposed response to androgens. The mechanism of inheritance is unknown. Within the distribution of hair over the scalp, androgen-sensitive hair follicles are on top and androgen-insensitive follicles are on the sides and back. In genetically predisposed men, the androgen-sensitive follicles are transformed into vellus follicles. The normal hair is shed and replaced by fine, light, short hair. Male-pattern baldness begins with frontotemporal recession and progresses to loss of hair over the top of the scalp. There is no treatment to reverse the balding process. Affected men may choose to wear wigs, have hair transplants, or plastic surgery.

Female-Pattern Alopecia

Some women in their 20s and 30s experience progressive thinning and loss of hair over the central part of the scalp. Contrary to male-pattern baldness, there is no loss of hair along the frontal hairline. Many of these women have elevated levels of serum adrenal androgen dehydroepiandrosterone-sulfate (DHEAS) (Kasik et al., 1983). In rare instances a male-pattern baldness develops. Laboratory evaluation of serum androgenic hormones will show elevations and some women will have decreased hair loss when treated with daily doses of spironolactone (Kasik et al., 1983).

Alopecia Areata

Alopecia areata is rapid onset of hair loss in multiple areas of the scalp, usually in round patches. The eyebrows, eyelashes, beard, and other areas of body hair are rarely involved. The cause is unknown, but stressful events often occur before hair loss. Metabolic disorders, such as Addison disease, thyroid disease, and lupus erythematosus, are also associated with alopecia areata (Friedman, 1981).

The affected areas of skin are smooth or may have short shafts of hair. The hair shaft is poorly developed and breaks at the surface. Regrowth occurs within 1 to 3 months, but there may be recurrent hair loss at the same site. There is usually permanent regrowth of hair. There is total loss of hair (alopecia totalis) in some young people, and the long-term prognosis for total hair regrowth is poor.

Diagnosis is made by observation of the pattern of hair loss. Biopsy may reveal a lymphocytic infiltrate around the follicle. Intralesional steroids may be used to stimulate hair growth when there are a few small areas of hair loss. Systemic steroids are used for larger areas of alopecia. Topical applications of anthralin are also used to stimulate hair growth. Minoxidil has been tested for use in resistant cases and has been found effective in about 18% of cases with severe alopecia areata (Feidler-Weiss et al., 1987).

Hirsutism

Hirsutism is the growth and distribution of hair on the face, body, and pubic area in a male pattern. There is also frontotemporal hair recession. These areas of hair growth are androgen sensitive. Variations of hair growth in women are great and a male pattern may be normal. Women who develop hirsutism may be secreting hormones associated with ovarian or adrenal disease, and such women should be evaluated for polycystic ovaries, adrenal hyperplasia, or adrenal tumors. If no normonal pathologic conditions exist, treatment may include cosmetic removal of hair, oral contraceptives, glucocorticoids, or cimetidine (Vigersky et al., 1980).

DISORDERS OF THE NAIL

Paronychia

Paronychia is an acute or chronic infection of the cuticle. Acute paronychia is manifest by the rapid onset of painful inflammation of the cuticle, usually following minor trauma. An abscess may develop requiring incision and drainage for relief of pain. The most common causative organisms are staphylococci and streptococci. Occasionally *Candida* will be present.

Chronic paronychia develops slowly with tenderness and swelling around the proximal or lateral nail folds. One or more fingers or toes may be involved. Individuals whose hands are exposed to frequent moisture are at greatest risk. Manipulation of the cuticle can be predisposing because it opens the space between the proximal nail fold and nail plate leaving a moist, warm medium for the incubation of pathogenic organisms. The skin around the nail becomes more edematous and painful with progressive infection. Pus may be expressed from the proximal nail fold. The nail plate is usually not affected, although it can become discolored with ridges.

Treatment includes keeping the hands dry. Oral antibiotics are not very effective because they do not penetrate the affected tissues. Topical application of thymol is usually effective.

Onchyomycosis

Onchyomycosis is a fungal or dermatophyte infection of the nail plate. The most common pattern is a nail plate that turns yellow or white and becomes elevated with the accumulation of hyperkeratotic debris within the plate. Fungal infections of the nail are differentiated from psoriasis by the absence of pitting on the nail surface, which is characteristic of psoriasis. Treatment is difficult because topical or systemic antifungal agents do not penetrate the nail plate readily. Surgical excision of the nail may be required.

SUMMARY REVIEW

Structure and Function of the Skin

1 Skin is the largest organ of the body and equals 20% of body weight.
2 The skin has two layers, the dermis and epidermis.
3 The underlying epidermis contains a basal and spinous layer with melanocytes, Langerhans cells, and Merkel cells.
4 The dermis is composed of connective tissue elements, hair follicles, sweat glands, sebaceous glands, blood vessels, nerves, and lymphatic vessels.
5 The papillary capillaries provide the major blood supply to the skin, arising from deeper arterial plexuses.
6 Heat loss and heat conservation are regulated by arteriovenous anastomoses that lead to the papillary capillaries.
7 Older skin is thinner, dryer, and has fewer capillary loops with changes in pigmentation.
8 Loss of melanocytes and hair follicles leads to gray and thinner hair.
9 The skin is more permeable, there is decreased sweating, and loss of thermal regulation with decreased protective functions.
10 Pressure ulcers develop from pressure and shearing forces that occlude capillary blood flow with resulting ischemia and necrosis. Areas at greatest risk are pressure points over bony prominences, such as the greater trochanter, sacrum, ischia, and heels. Immobilized individuals with fractures and neurologic deficits are most prone to develop pressure ulcers.
11 Pruritus is itching and is associated with many skin disorders. The exact neurologic mechanism is unknown, but pain receptors with low-intensity stimulation is one theory of irritation. Scratching with skin trauma, potential infection, and scarring are associated with itching.

Disorders of the Skin

1 Contact dermatitis is a form of delayed hypersensitivity that develops with sensitization to allergies, such as metal, chemicals, or poison ivy.
2 Irritant contact dermatitis develops from prolonged exposure to chemicals, such as acids or soaps.
3 Atopic or allergic dermatitis is associated with a family history of allergies, hay fever, elevated IgE levels, and

increased histamine sensitivity. Pruritus and scratching predipose the skin to infection, scaling, and thickening.

4 Stasis dermatitis occurs on the legs and results from venous stasis and edema.

5 Seborrheic dermatitis involves scaly, yellowish, inflammatory plaques of the scalp, eyebrows, eyelids, ear canals, chest, axillae, and back. The cause is unknown.

6 Papulosquamous disorders are characterized by papules, scales, plaques, and erythema.

7 Psoriasis is a chronic skin disease with thickening of both the epidermis and dermis, characterized by scaly, erythematous, pruritic plaques.

8 Pityriasis rosea is a self-limiting disease characterized by oval lesions with scales around the edges located along skin lines of the trunk.

9 Lichen planus is a papular, violet-colored inflammatory lesion of unknown origin manifest by severe pruritus.

10 Acne vulgaris is an inflammation of the pilosebaceous follicle with the primary lesion being the comedo, which may become inflamed, forming pustules or nodules.

11 Acne rosacea develops on the middle third of the face with hypertrophy and inflammation of the sebaceous glands.

12 Lupus erythematosus can affect only the skin (discoid) or have a systemic presentation. The inflammatory lesions usually occur in sun-exposed areas with a butterfly distribution over the nose and cheeks.

13 Pemphigus is a chronic, autoimmune, blistering disease that begins in the mouth or on the scalp and spreads to other parts of the body, often with a fatal outcome. There are two forms, pemphigus vulgaris and bullous pemphigus.

14 Erythema multiforme is an acute inflammation of the skin and mucous membranes with lesions that appear targetlike with alternating rings of edema and inflammation, often associated with allergic reactions to drugs. Stevens-Johnson syndrome is a severe form that also involves the mucous membranes.

15 Folliculitis is a bacterial infection of the hair follicle.

16 A furuncle is an infection of the hair follicle that extends to the surrounding tissue.

17 A carbuncle is a collection of infected hair follicles that forms a draining abscess.

18 Cellulitis is a diffuse infection of the dermis and subcutaneous tissue.

19 Erysipelas is a superficial streptococcal infection of the skin commonly affecting the face, ears, and lower legs.

20 Impetigo may have a bullous or an ulcerative form and is caused by *Staphylococcus* or *Streptococcus*.

21 Herpes simplex virus type I (HSV-1) causes cold sores but can infect the cornea, mouth, and labia. HSV-2 causes genital lesions and is usually spread by sexual contact.

22 Herpes zoster and varicella are both caused by the same herpesvirus.

23 Warts are benign, rough, elevated lesions caused by papillomavirus. Condylomata accuminata, or venereal warts, are spread by sexual contact.

24 Tinea infections (fungal infections) can occur anywhere on the body and are classified by location (i.e., tinea pedis, tinea corporis, tinea capitis.)

25 Candidiasis is a yeastlike fungal infection occurring on skin, mucous membranes, and gastrointestinal tract.

26 Cutaneous vasculitis is an inflammation of skin blood vessels with purpura, ischemia, and necrosis resulting from vessel necrosis.

27 Urticarial lesions are associated with hypersensitivity responses and appear as wheals, welts, or hives.

28 Scleroderma is a sclerosis of the skin that may also affect systemic organs and cause renal failure, bowel obstruction, or cardiac dysrhythmias.

29 Ticks cause a local reaction and can cause systemic disease when mouth parts pierce the skin and remain embedded in the tissue.

30 Mosquitoes can transmit infectious diseases and the saliva from their bite produces the characteristic itching and wheal formation.

31 Bloodsucking flies are represented by many species, including Ceratopogonidae ("no-see-ums"), Tabandiae (horseflies), or Simulidiae (blackflies). Their bites are usually painful and produce bleeding, and the itching and local reactions may last for days with systemic symptoms of fever and malaise.

32 Seborrheic keratosis is a proliferation of basal cells that produce elevated, smooth, or warty lesions of varying size. They are most common among the elderly.

33 Keratoacanthoma arises from hair follicles on sun-exposed areas. Three stages of development characterize the lesion, which results in a dome-shaped, crusty lesion filled with keratin that resolves in 3 to 4 months.

34 Actinic keratosis is a pigmented scaly lesion that develops in sun-exposed individuals with fair skin. The lesion may become malignant in the form of a squamous cell carcinoma.

35 Nevi arise from melanocytes and may be pigmented or fleshy pink. They occur singly or in groups and may undergo transition to malignant melanoma.

36 Basal cell carcinoma is the most common skin cancer and occurs most frequently on sun-exposed areas.

37 Squamous cell carcinoma is a tumor of the epidermis and can be localized (in situ) or invasive

38 Malignant melanoma arises from melanocytes, and if not excised early, metastasis occurs through the lymph nodes.

39 Kaposi sarcoma is a vascular malignancy associated with immune deficiency states.

40 Burns are classified according to depth and extent of injury.

41 First-degree burns involve the superficial skin without loss of protective function.

42 Second-degree burns are superficial (blister formation) or superficial partial thickness with a waxy white appearance and no involvement of dermal appendages.

43 Third-degree burns involve full skin thickness and often underlying tissues. They are painless and can be life threatening from hypovolemic shock and metabolic and immunologic responses.

44 Keloids are sharply elevated scars that extend beyond the border of traumatized skin.

45 Frostbite usually occurs on cheeks and digits with direct injury to cells and impaired circulation.

Disorders of the Hair

1 Male-pattern alopecia is an inherited form of irreversible baldness with hair loss in the central scalp and recession of the temporo frontal hairline.

2 Female-pattern alopecia is a thinning of the central hair of the scalp beginning in women at 20 to 30 years of age.

3 Alopecia areata is patchy loss of hair usually associated with stress or metabolic diseases; it is usually reversible.

4 Hirsutism is a male pattern of hair growth in women that may be normal or the result of excessive secretion of androgenic hormones.

Disorders of the Nails

1 Paronychia is an inflammation of the cuticle that can be acute or chronic and is usually caused by staphylococci or streptococci.

2 Onchyomycosis is a fungal infection of the nail plate.

KEY TERMS

Acne rosacea, 1407

Acne vulgaris, 1406

Allergic contact dermatitis, 1402

Alopecia, 1432

Alopecia areata, 1432

Apocrine sweat gland, 1393

Atopic dermatitis, 1402

Basal cell carcinoma, 1419

Basal layer, 1392

Bullous pemphigoid, 1410

Candidiasis, 1414

Carbuncle, 1411

Cellulitis, 1411

Claw-like prolongations, 1401

Comedo, 1406

Condylomata acuminata, 1413

Cutaneous vasculitis, 1415

Deep partial-thickness burn, 1425

Dermal appendage, 1392

Dermis, 1391

Discoid lupus erythematosus (DLE), 1408

Eccrine sweat gland, 1393

Eczema, 1402

Epidermis, 1391

Erysipelas, 1411

Erythema multiforme, 1410

First-degree burn, 1424

Folliculitis, 1411

Frostbite, 1431

Furuncle, 1411

Hair, 1392

Herold patch, 1405

Herpes simplex virus (HSV), 1411

Herpes zoster, 1412

Hirsutism, 1433

Hypercoagulable, 1430

Hyphae, 1414

Hypodermis, 1391

Impetigo, 1411

Inflammatory acne, 1407

Integumentary system, 1391

Irritant contact dermatitis, 1402

Kaposi sarcoma, 1421

Keloid, 1400

Keratin, 1391

Keratinocyte, 1391

Langerhans cell, 1392

Lichen planus, 1405

Lupus erythematosus, 1408

Merkel cell, 1392

Melanocyte, 1392

Melanoma, 1420

Mosquitoe, 1416

Myofibroblast , 1400

Nail, 1392

Noninflammatory acne, 1406

Onchyomycosis, 1433

Papillary capillary, 1393

Papulosquamous disorder, 1404

Paronychia, 1433

Pemphigus, 1409

Pemphigus erythematosus, 1409

Pemphigus foliaceus, 1409

Pemphigus vulgaris, 1409

Pityriasis rosea, 1405

Propionibacterium acnes, 1407

Proteoglycan, 1400

Psoriasis, 1404

Scleroderma, 1416

Sebaceous gland, 1392

Seborrheic dermatitis, 1403

Second-degree burn, 1424

Spinous layer, 1392

Squamous cell carcinoma, 1419

Stasis dermatitis, 1403

Stevens-Johnson syndrome, 1410

Stratum corneum, 1391

Superficial partial-thickness injury, 1424

Sweat gland, 1392

Systemic lupus erythematosus (SLE), 1409

Thermal injury, 1423

Third-degree burn (full-thickness burn), 1425

Tinea capitis, 1414

Tinea corporis, 1414

Tinea infection, 1414

Tinea pedis, 1414

Urticarial lesion, 1415

Varicella, 1412

Warts, 1413

REFERENCES

Ahmed, A. R., Graham, J., Jordon, R. E., & Provost, T. T. (1980). Pemphigus: Current concepts. *Annals of Internal Medicine, 92,* 396-405.

Aikawa, N., Martyn, J. A. J., & Burke, J. F. (1978). Pulmonary artery catheterization and thermodilution cardiac output determination in the management of critically burned patients. *American Journal of Surgery, 135,* 811-817.

Alexander, J. W., McClellan, M. A., Ogle, C. K., & Ogle, J. D. (1976). Consumptive opsoninopathy: Possible pathogenesis in lethal and opportunistic infections. *Annals of Surgery, 184,* 672-678.

American Burn Association. (1976). American burn association committee on specific optimal criteria for hospital resources for care of patients with burn injury. San Antonio: The Association.

American Cancer Society. (1988). *Cancer facts and figures 1988.* New York: The Society.

American Cancer Society. (1989). Cancer statistics. *Ca-A Cancer: Journal for Clinicians, 39*[1].

Aulick, L. H., Hander, E. H., Wilmore, D. W., Mason, A. D. Jr., & Pruitt, B. A. Jr. (1979). The relative significance of thermal and metabolic demands on burn hypermetabolism. *Journal of Trauma, 19,* 559-556.

Balfour, H. H. Jr. (1984). Intravenous acyclovir therapy for varicella in immunocompromised children. *Journal of Pediatrics, 104,* 134.

Baxter, C. R. (1974). Fluid volume and electrolyte changes of the early postburn period. *Clinical Plastic Surgery, 1,* 693-709.

Baxter, C. R., Cook, W. A., & Shires, G. T. (1966). Serum myocardial depressant factor of burn shock. *Surgical Forum, 17,* 1-4.

Bellet, R. E., Mastrangelo, D. B., & Maguire, H. C. (1983). Primary cutaneous melanoma. In B. S. Kahn, R. R. Love, C. Sherman, R. Chakravorty (Eds.), *Concepts in cancer medicine.* New York: Grune & Stratton.

Bjornson, A. B., Altemeier, W. A., & Bjornson, H. S. (1977). Changes in humoral components of host defense following burn trauma. *Annals of Surgery, 186,* 96.

Buschard, K., Dabelsteen, E., & Bretlau, P. (1981). A model for the study of autoimmune diseases applied to pemphigus: Transplants of human oral mucosa to athymic nude mice binds pemphigus antibodies in vivo. *Journal of Investigative Dermatology, 76,* 171.

Callen, J. P. (1986). Subsets of lupus erythematosus: Clinical, serologic, and immunologic considerations. In J. P. Callen, M. V. Dahl, L. E. Golitz, J. E. Rasmussen, & S. J. Stegman (Eds.), *Advances in dermatology (volume I.)* Chicago: Yearbook Medical.

Crumpacker, C. S. (1987). Herpes simplex. In T. B. Fitzpatrick, A. Z. Eisen, K. Wolff, I. M. Freedberg, & K. F. Austen (Eds.), *Dermatology in general medicine* (3rd ed.). New York: McGraw-Hill.

Cunningham, J. N., Jr., Shires, G. T., & Wagner, Y. (1971). Changes in intracellular sodium and potassium content of red blood cells in trauma and shock. *American Journal of Surgery, 122,* 650-654.

Deets, D. K., & Glaviano, V. V. (1973). Plasma and cardiac lactic dehydrogenase activity in burn shock. *Proceedings of the Society of Experimental Biological Medicine, 142,* 412-416.

Dobson, E. L., & Warner, G. F. (1957). Factors concerned in the early stages of thermal shock. *Circulatory Research, V,* 69-74.

Dobson, R. L., & Abele, D. C. (1985). *The practice of dermatology.* Philadelphia: Harper & Row.

Ebertz, J. M., Hirshman, C. A., Kettlkamp, N. S., Uno, H., & Hanifin, J. M. (1987). Substance P-induced histamine release in human cutaneous mast cells. *Journal of Investigative Dermatology, 88,* 682-685.

Feidler-Weiss, V. C., Rumsfield, J., Cunera, B. M., West, D. P., & Wendrow, A. (1987). Evaluation of oral minoxidil in the treatment of alopecia areata. *Archives of Dermatology, 123,* 1488-1490.

Fisher, R. P., Souba, W. W., & Ford, E. G. (1988). Temperature associated injuries and syndromes. In K. L. Mattox, E. E. Moore, & D. V. Feliciano (Eds.), *Trauma* (p. 662). Norwalk, CT: Appleton-Lange.

Fitzpatrick, T. B., Eisen, A. Z., Wolff, K., Freedberg, I. M., & Austen, K. F. (1987). *Dermatology in general medicine* (3rd ed.). New York: McGraw-Hill.

Forstrom, L. (1980). The influence of sex hormones on acne. *Acta Dermato-Venereologica Supplementum (Stockholm), 89,* 27.

Friedman, P. S. (1981). Alopecia areata and autoimmunity. *British Journal of Dermatology, 105,* 153.

Gilchrist, B. A. (1984). *Skin and aging processes.* Boca Raton, FL: CRC Press.

Goopman, J. (1987). Neoplasms in the acquired immune deficiency syndrome: The multidisciplinary approach. *Seminars in Oncology, 14*(2) (Suppl. 3), 1-6.

Gump, F. E., Price, J. B. Jr., & Kinney, J. M. (1970). Blood flow and oxygen consumption in patients with severe burns. *Surgical Gynecology and Obstetrics, 130,* 23-28.

Habif, T. P. (1985). *Clinical dermatology: A color guide to diagnosis and therapy.* St Louis: C. V. Mosby.

Heideman, J., Kaijser, B., & Gelin, L. (1978). Complement activation and hematologic, hemodynamic, and respiratory reactions early after soft tissue injury. *Journal of Trauma, 18,* 696-700.

Huckbody, E. (1980). Dermatology throughout the dark ages. *International Journal of Dermatology, 6,* 344-347.

Johnson, M. L. (1977). Prevalence of dermatologic disease among persons 1-74 years of age: United States. *Advance Data From Vital and Health Statistics of the National Center for Health Statistics* (January 26), 4.

Kasik, J. M., Bergfeld, W. F., Steck, W. D., & Gupta, M. K. (1983). Adrenal androgenic female-pattern alopecia: Sex hormones and the balding woman. *Cleveland Clinic Journal of Medicine, 50,* 111.Q

Kragballe, K., & Voorhees, J. J. (1985). Arachidonic acid and leukotrienes in pathogenesis and treatment. In H. H. Roenick & H. I Maibach (Eds.), *Psoriasis* (pp. 255-264). New York: Marcel Dekker.

Lefer, A. M., & Martin, J. (1970). Origin of myocardial depressant factor in shock. *American Journal of Physiology, 218,* 1423-1427.

Majno, G. (1975). *The healing hand.* Cambridge, MA: Harvard University Press.

Maley, M. P., & Wright, J. (Eds.). (1982). *Clinical burn therapy* (p. 510). Boston: PSG Inc.

McManus, W. F., & Pruitt, B. A. Jr. (1988). Thermal injuries. In K. L. Mattox, E. E. Moore, & D. V. Feliciano (Eds.), *Trauma* (p. 675). Norwalk, CT: Appleton & Lange.

McManus, W. F., Eurenius, K., & Pruitt, B. A., Jr. (1973). Disseminated intravascular coagulation in burned patients. *Journal of Trauma, 13,* 416-422.

Moncrief, J. A. (1974). Burns. In S. I. Schwartz, R. C. Lillehei, G. T. Shires, F. C. Spencer, & E. H. Storer (Eds), *Principles of surgery* (2nd ed., (pp. 253-274). New York: McGraw-Hill.

Moncrief, J. A., & Mason, A. D. (1962). Water vapor loss in the burned patient. *Surgical Forum, 13,* 38-41.

Monk, B. E., Graham-Brown, R. A. C., and Sarkany, I. (1988). *Skin disorders in the elderly.* Oxford: Blackwell Scientific.

Ninnemann, J. L. (1980). Immunosuppression following thermal injury through a B cell activation of suppressor T cells. *Journal of Trauma, 20,* 206-213.

Okamoto, R., Glaviano, V. V., & Pindok, M. (1971). Myocardial lipases and catecholamines in burn shock. *Proceedings of the Society of Experimental Biological Medicine, 137,* 347-353.

Paget, J. (1873). Clinical lecture on bedsores. *Student Journal and Hospital Gazette, 1,* 144. Reprinted in: J. H. Gibbon & L. W. Freeman. (1946). Primary closure of decubitus ulcers. *American Journal of Surgery, 124,* 1149.

Puhvel, S. M., & Sakamoto, M. A. (1980). Cytotoxin production by comedonal bacteria (*Propionibacterium acnes, Propionibacterium granulosum, and Staphylococcus epidermidis*). *Journal of Investigative Dermatology, 74,* 36.

Ragozzino, M. W., Melton, L. J., Kurland, L. T., Chu, C. P., & Perry, H. O. (1982). Population based study of herpes zoster and its sequelae. *Medicine, 5*(61), 310.

Ramsey, D. L., & Hurley, H. J. (1985). Papulosquamous eruptions and exfoliative dermatitis. In S. L. Moschella & H. J. Hurley (Eds.), *Dermatology (vol. I,* p. 522). Philadelphia: W. B. Saunders.

Roe, C. F., & Kinney, J. M. (1964). Water and heat exchange in third-degree burns. *Surgery, 56,* 212-220.

Rosenthal, S. M., & Tabor, H. (1945). Electrolyte changes and chemotherapy in experimental burn and traumatic shock and hemorrhage. *Archives of Surgery, 51,* 244-252.

Rosenthal, S. R., Hawley, P. L., & Hakin, A. A. (1972). Purified burn toxic factor and its competition. *Surgery, 71,* 527-536.

Sabiston, D. C. Jr., (Ed.). (1977). *Textbook of surgery: the biological basis at modern surgical practice* (11th ed.). Philadelphia: W. B. Saunders.

Safai, B. (1987). Pathophysiology and epidemiology of epidemic Kaposi's sarcoma. *Seminars in Oncology, 14*(2) (Suppl. 3), 7.

Shelley, W. B., & Arthur. R. P. (1957). The neurohistology and neurophysiology of the itch sensation in man. *Archives of Dermatology, 76,* 296-323.

Singh, G., Marples, B. M., & Klingman, A. M. (1971). Staphylococcus infections in humans. *Journal of Investigative Dermatology, 57,* 149.

Stewart, W. D., Danto, J. L., & Maddin, S. (1978). *Dermatology: diagnosis and treatment of cutaneous disorders.* (4th ed.) St. Louis: Mosby.

Stone, S. P., Muller, S. A., & Glech, G. J. (1973). IgE levels in atopic dermatitis. *Archives of Dermatology, 108,* 806.

Strauss, J. (1985). Acne. In T. T. Provost & E. R. Farmer (Eds.), *Current therapy in dermatology 1985-1986* (p. 116). St. Louis: C. V. Mosby.

Theirs, B. H., & Dobson, R. L. (1986). *Pathogenesis of skin disease.* New York: Churchill Livingstone.

Thibodeau, G. A. (1987). *Anatomy and physiology.* St. Louis: Times Mirror/Mosby.

Thompson, J. M., McFarland, G. K., Hirsch, J. E., Tucker, S. M., & Bowers, A. C. (1986). *Clinical nursing.* St. Louis: C. V. Mosby.

Trunkey, D. D., Illner, H., Wagner, I. Y., & Shires, G. T. (1973). The effect of hemorrhagic shock on intracellular muscle action potentials in the primates. *Surgery, 74,* 241-250.

Turinsky, J., Gonnerman, W. A., & Loose, L. D. (1981). Impaired mineral metabolism in postburn muscle. *Journal of Trauma, 21,* 417-423.

Versluysen, M. (1986). How elderly patients with femoral fracture develop pressures sores in hospital. *British Medical Journal, 292,* 1311-1313.

Vigersky, R. A., Mehlman, I., Glass, A. R., & Smith, C. E. (1980). Treatment of hirsute women with cimetidine. *New England Journal of Medicine, 303,* 1042.

Warden, G. D., Mason, A. D. Jr., & Pruitt, B. A. Jr. (1975). Suppression of leukocyte chemotaxis *in vitro* by chemotherapeutic agents used in the management of thermal injuries. *Annals of Surgery, 181,* 363-369.

Warden, G. D., Mason, A. D. Jr., & Pruitt, B. A. Jr. (1974). Evaluation of leukocyte chemotaxis *in vitro* in thermally injured patients. *Journal of Clinical Investigation, 54,* 1001-1004.

Welt, L. G., Smith, E. K. M., Dunn, M. J., Czersinski, A., Proctor, H., Cole, C., Balfer, J. W., & Gitelman, H. J. (1967). Membrane transport defect: The sick cell. *Transactions of the Association of American Physicians, 80,* 217-226.

White, J. W. (1985). Hypersensitivity and miscellaneous inflammatory disorders. In S. L. Moschella & H. J. Hurley (Eds.), *Dermatology: (vol. I,* p. 468). Philadelphia: W. B. Saunders.

Whitely, R. J., Soong, S. J., Dolin, R., Betts, R., Linneman, C., & Alford, C. A. (1982). Early vidarabine therapy to control the complications of herpes zoster in immunosuppressed patients. *New England Journal of Medicine, 307*(16), 971.

Wilmore, D. W. Aulick, H. L., & Goodwin, C. W. (1979). Glucose metabolism following severe injury. *Acta Chirurgica Scandinavica, 498,* 43-47.

Wilmore, D. W., & Aulick, L. H. (1978). Metabolic changes in burned patients. *Surgical Clinics of North America, 58,* 1173-1187.

Wilmore, D. W., Aulick, H. L., Mason, A. D., Jr. & Pruitt, B. A. Jr. (1977). Influence of the burn wound on local and systemic responses to injury. *Annals of Surgery, 186,* 444-458.

Wilmore, D. W., Goodwin, C. W., Aulick, L. H., Powanda, M. C., Mason, A. D. Jr., & Pruitt, B. A. Jr. (1980). Effect of injury and infection on visceral metabolism and circulation. *Annals of Surgery, 192,* 491-500.

Wilmore, D. W., Long, J. M., Mason, A. D. Jr., Skreen, R. W., & Pruitt, B. A. Jr. (1974). Catecholamines: Mediator of the hypermetabolic response to thermal injury. *Annals of Surgery, 180,* 653-668.

Wilmore, D. W., Orcutt, T. W., Mason, A. D., & Pruitt, B. A. Jr. (1975). Alterations in hypothalamic function following thermal injury. *Journal of Trauma, 15,* 697-703.

Zimmerman, T. J., & Krizek, T. J. (1984). Thermally induced dermal injury: A review of pathophysiologic events and therapeutic intervention. *Journal of Burn Care & Rehabilitation, 5,* 193-201.

CHAPTER 42

Alterations of the Integument in Children

Sue E. Huether
Margaret M. Andrews

Dermatitis, 1439
  Atopic dermatitis, 1439
  Diaper dermatitis, 1440
Infections of the skin, 1440
  Bacterial infections, 1440
    Impetigo, 1440
      Bullous impetigo, 1440
      Vesicular impetigo, 1441
    Scalded skin syndrome, 1441
      Staphylococcal toxic epidermal necrolysis
        (staphylococcal scaled skin syndrome), 1441
      Nonstaphylococcal toxic epidural necrolysis, 1441
  Fungal infections, 1441
    Tinea corporis, 1442
    Tinea capitis, 1442
    Thrush, 1443
  Viral infections, 1443
    Mulloscum contagiosum, 1444
    Rubella (german or 3-day measles), 1444
    Rubeola (red measles), 1444
    Roseola (exanthem subitum), 1445
    Chickenpox and herpes zoster, 1445
      Chickenpox, 1445
      Herpes zoster, 1446
    Smallpox, 1446
Insect bites and parasites, 1446
  Scabies, 1446
  Pediculosis (lice), 1447
  Fleas, 1448
  Bedbugs, 1448
Vascular disorders, 1448
  Strawberry hemangioma, 1448
  Cavernous hemangiomas, 1448
  Salmon patches, 1449
  Port-wine stain, 1449
Other skin disorders, 1449
  Miliara, 1449
  Erythema toxicum neonatorum, 1449

The development of alterations in the skin frequently occurs in children. The lesions may be minor or severe and localized or generalized, and often there are no prodromal symptoms. Skin diseases in children may have different manifestations than in adults, although the etiologic mechanisms may be similar. Many diseases resolve spontaneously and require no treatment. Diagnosis is commonly made from the history, appearance, and distribution of the lesion or lesions. The most common skin diseases of childhood are presented here.

DERMATITIS

Atopic Dermatitis

Atopic dermatitis is the most common cause of eczema in children. It is usually associated with elevated IgE levels and a family history of asthma or allergic rhinitis (hay fever). The exact pathogenesis is unknown, but theories include cellular immunodeficiencies, abnormal β-adrenergic receptors, antibody deficiencies, and food allergies.

Manifestations of dry and red scaling areas usually develop by 2 years of age. Skin dryness and itching are the outstanding features of atopic dermatitis. The affected areas are located primarily on the face and cheeks (Fig. 42-1). The extensor surfaces of the extremities and the trunk may also be involved. Irritation from drooling, repeated washing, or scratching leads to weeping, crusting lesions. Itching can be severe and scratching can result in trauma and infection with thickening of the skin, fissures, and hypopigmentation or hyperpigmentation. The itching is often exacerbated by sweating or contact with wool or detergents. Mild cases usually resolve by 2 years of age, although lesions may persist in the flexures

A

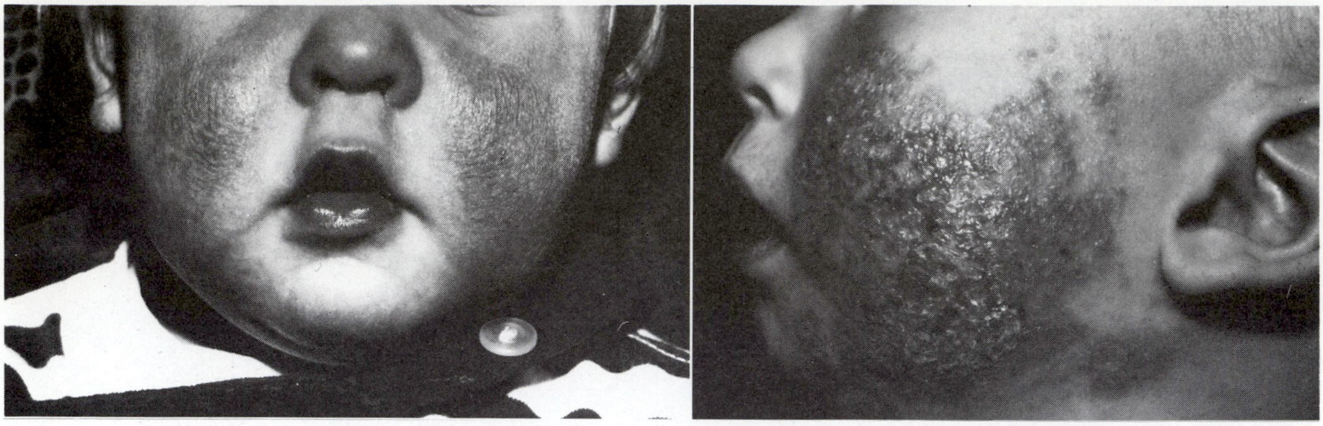

B

FIG. 42-1. Atopic dermatitis affecting the cheeks. (Courtesy Alfred T. Lane, M.D., Division of Dermatology, University of Rochester, School of Medicine and Dentistry; from Hoekelman et al., 1987.)

of the extremities in some children. Periods of remission occur more frequently as the child grows older.

Treatment is aimed at relieving pruritus and inflammation. Approaches include lubrication and hydration of the skin; avoidance of overheating, which produces sweating; and avoidance of tight clothing, wool, or anything that irritates the skin. Foods known to cause skin lesions should be avoided. Antihistamines may be used to control itching, and topical steroids reduce inflammation.

Diaper Dermatitis

Diaper dermatitis is a form of contact dermatitis that develops from prolonged exposure and irritation of the perineal skin to urine and feces. Detergents used to wash diapers are occasionally the irritant source. The skin becomes macerated by airtight plastic diaper covers.

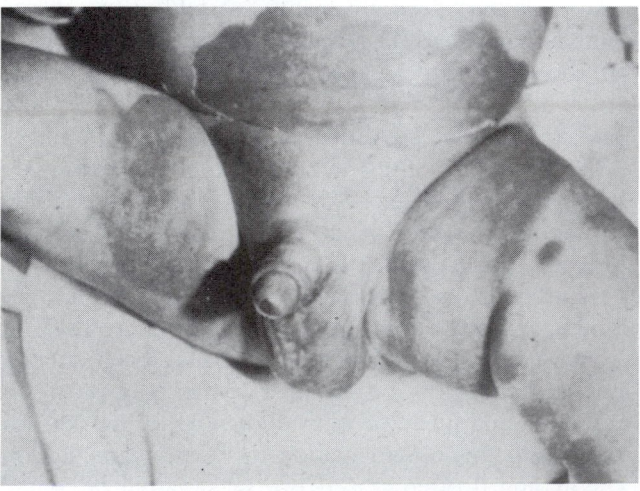

FIG. 42-2. Diaper dermatitis caused by primary irritation. (From Stewart, Danto, & Maddin, 1978.)

The lesions appear as erythematous papular lesions or ulcerations over the perineum and buttocks (Fig. 42-2). Invasion by *Candida albicans* is common. Treatment is frequent diaper changes to keep the area clean and dry or frequently exposing the perineal area to air. Changing detergents may be helpful. Topical nystatin cream is used to treat *Candida albicans*.

INFECTIONS OF THE SKIN

Infectious diseases caused by bacteria, viruses, and fungi constitute the major forms of skin disease. Most infections tend to occur superficially; however, systemic signs and symptoms develop occasionally and rarely are life threatening.

Bacterial Infections
Impetigo

Impetigo is a common bacterial skin infection in infants and children. The disease is more common in mid- to late summer, with a higher incidence in hot, humid climates. Impetigo is particularly infectious among those living in crowded conditions with poor sanitary facilities. It affects children in good health, but conditions such as anemia and malnutrition are predisposing factors. There are two types of impetigo, bullous and vesicular. Both start as vesicles with a very thin covering layer of stratum corneum.

Bullous Impetigo

Bullous impetigo is caused by *Staphylococcus aureus*. The staphylococci produce an exfoliative toxin that stimulates the formation of vesicles, which enlarge or coalesce to form bullae. There may be a few localized lesions or many lesions scattered over the skin. As the bullae rupture, a thin, flat, honey-colored crust appears.

The crust is the hallmark of impetigo. A moist, inflamed, serum weeping base is revealed when the crust is removed. Removal of crusts prevents extension of the vesicles to adjacent areas of the stratum corneum. The lesions are often located on the face around the nose and mouth, but the hands and other exposed areas are also frequently involved. The staphylococci may colonize in the nose and then spread to normal skin. Regional lymphadenitis is uncommon.

The Staphylococcus is identified by culture and treated with systemic antibiotics or locally applied antibiotic creams. Crusts should be carefully removed and the lesions washed with antibacterial soap. The entire body should be washed with antibacterial soap at least once a day to prevent spread to normal skin. Because the disease is contagious, handwashing and protection against direct contact with others is necessary. Treated lesions usually resolve in 2 to 3 weeks.

Vesicular Impetigo

Vesicular impetigo is caused by streptococci. The streptococci are disseminated by direct physical contact from other infected individuals or through insect bites. The lesions begin as small vesicles with a honey-colored serum. Yellow to white-brown crusts form as the vesicles rupture and extend radially (Fig. 42-3). Untreated lesions may last for weeks and extend to cover a large area. The lesions frequently become infected with staphylococci. Regional lymphadenitis is common.

Evaluation and treatment are the same as for bullous impetigo. Nephritis develops secondarily in about 2% of infected children, usually between the ages of 2 and 4 years (Fison, 1956).

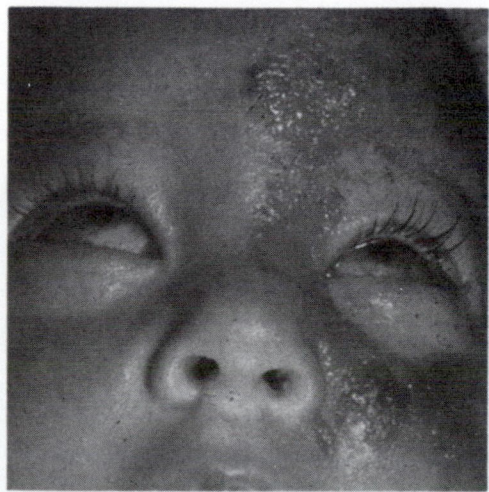

FIG. 42-3. Impetigo. Note characteristic crusting. (Courtesy Antoinette Hood, M. D., Department of Dermatology, School of Medicine, The Johns Hopkins University, Baltimore, MD., From Seidel et al., 1987.)

Scalded Skin Syndrome

Staphylococcal Toxic Epidermal Necrolysis (Staphylococcal Scalded Skin Syndrome)

Toxic epidermal necrolysis (TEN) caused by staphylococcal infection is also known as staphylococcal scalded skin syndrome. The toxin produced by group II staphylococci is an epidermolysin that causes a separation of the skin just below the granular layer of the epidermis. The syndrome is more common in children less than 10 years of age than in adults because adults have developed antistaphylococcal antibody and they are better able to metabolize and excrete the toxin.

The clinical symptoms begin with fever, malaise, rhinorrhea, and irritability followed by generalized erythema with exquisite tenderness of the skin. There may be an associated impetigo, but the infection may begin in the throat or chest. The erythema spreads from the face and trunk to cover the entire body. Separation of the epidermis occurs within 12 to 24 hours, and the outer layer of skin has a wrinkled appearance and slides over the underlying skin when pressure is applied (Nikolsky sign). Blisters and bullae may form and the pain is severe (Fig. 42-4). Fluid loss from ruptured blisters and evaporation may cause dehydration. Perioral and nasolabial crusting and fissures develop. In severe cases the skin of the entire body may slough. When secondary infection can be prevented, healing of the involved skin occurs in 10 to 14 days, usually without scarring.

Treatment with systemic antibiotics is required; topical antibiotics are ineffective. The skin should be treated the same as a severe burn with meticulous aseptic technique. Special care is required when there is involvement of the lips and eyelids.

Nonstaphylococcal Toxic Epidural Necrolysis

Nonstaphylococcal TEN is more common in adults but is increasing in children. Hypersensitivity to drugs (sulfonamides, penicillin, phenylbutazone, barbiturates) and vaccinations (polio, diphtheria, tetanus, and measles). The onset of skin eruptions is preceded by malaise, anorexia, fever, and mild inflammation of the eyelids, conjuctiva, mouth, or genitalia. Erythema with tenderness is first described in the axillae and groin, extending over the body surface. Blisters and bullae form and the entire epidermis may shed, leaving open, weeping, painful areas of underlying skin. With diffuse sloughing there is a 30% to 50% mortality within the first 7 days (Rook, Parish, & Beare, 1986) as a result of septicemia or shock. Treatment is the same as for staphylococcal TEN. Healing is usually complete, although there can be permanent loss of fingernails and toenails.

Fungal Infections

Fungal disorders are known as mycoses and, when caused by dermatophytes (fungi that thrive on keratin),

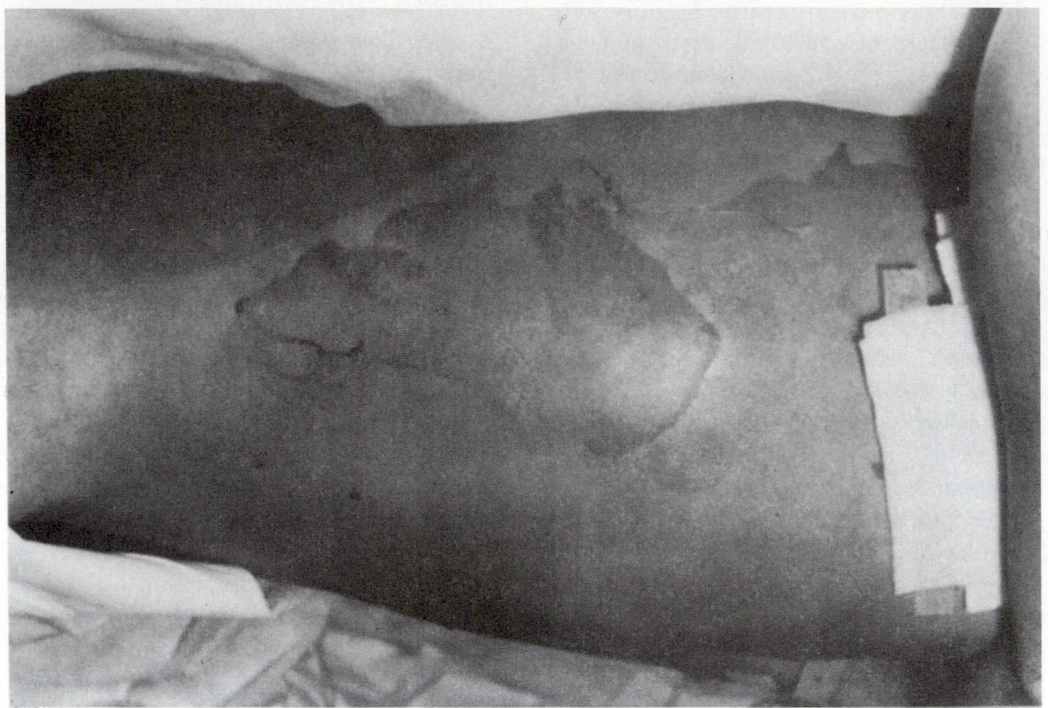

FIG. 42-4. Staphylococcal scalded-skin syndrome (Toxic epidermal necrolysis). The skin lesions, showing desquamation and wrinkling of the skin margins, appeared 1 day after drainage of a staphylococcal abscess. (From Levine & Norden, 1972.)

the mycoses are termed tinea (dermatophytosis or ringworm). Tinea pedis (a chronic, superficial fungal infection of the skin of the foot) occurs in children but is rare. Most scaling disorders of the toes and feet in prepubertal children are eczema (see Chapter 41). Tinea corporis (ringworm) and tinea capitis (a fungal infection of the scalp) are much more common in children than adults. (The different types of tinea are described in Chapter 41.)

Tinea Corporis

Tinea corporis is most common in children and has a predilection for the nonhairy parts of the face, trunk, and limbs. The lesions are distributed assymetrically, and multiple lesions, when present, overlap. Contact with young kittens and puppies is a common cause of the disorder. Most lesions respond to topical applications or a fungacide (Lotromin, Halotex, or Tinactin).

Tinea Capitis

Tinea capitis, a fungal infection of the scalp, is the most common fungal infection of childhood. It rarely affects infants and is seen in children between 2 and 10 years of age. The lesions are circular and manifest by broken hairs 1 to 3 mm above the scalp, leaving a partial alopecia from 1 to 5 cm in diameter (Fig. 42-5). A slight erythema and scaling with raised borders can be

observed. Unlike other fungal infections, tinea capitis may be contagious by direct contact with infected clothing.

Diagnosis is best made by preparing loose hairs with wet potassium hydroxide and observing them micro-

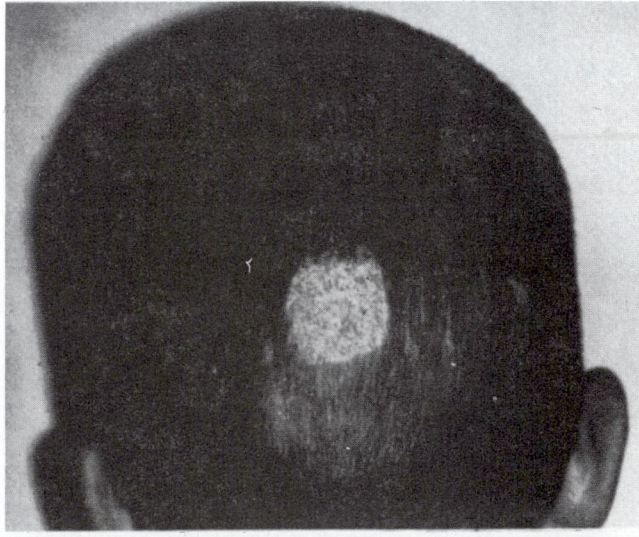

FIG. 42-5. Tinea capitis. (From Stewart, Danto, & Maddin, 1978.)

scopically with an ultraviolet light (Wood lamp). The spores are easily seen around the hair shaft. Oral griseofulvin is the best treatment; topical fungacides do not penetrate to the hair bulb.

Thrush

Candidiasis albicans infection is a superficial fungal infection that commonly occurs in children. **Thrush** is the term used to describe the presence of *Candida* in the mucous membranes of the mouth of infants and, less commonly, adults. Thursh is characterized by the formation of white plaques or spots in the mouth that are followed by shallow ulcers. The tongue may have a dense, white covering. The underlying mucous is red

and tender and may bleed when the plaques are removed. The disease is often accompanied by fever and gastrointestinal irritation. The infection commonly spreads to the groin, buttocks, and other parts of the body. Treatment is difficult and may include oral washes with Nystatin oral suspension or painting the inside of the mouth with gentian violet. Feeding bottles and nipples should be sterilized to prevent reinfection. The diaper area should be kept clean and dry.

Viral Infections

Viral infections of the skin in children are caused by poxvirus, papovavirus, and herpesvirus. The most common infections are described here.

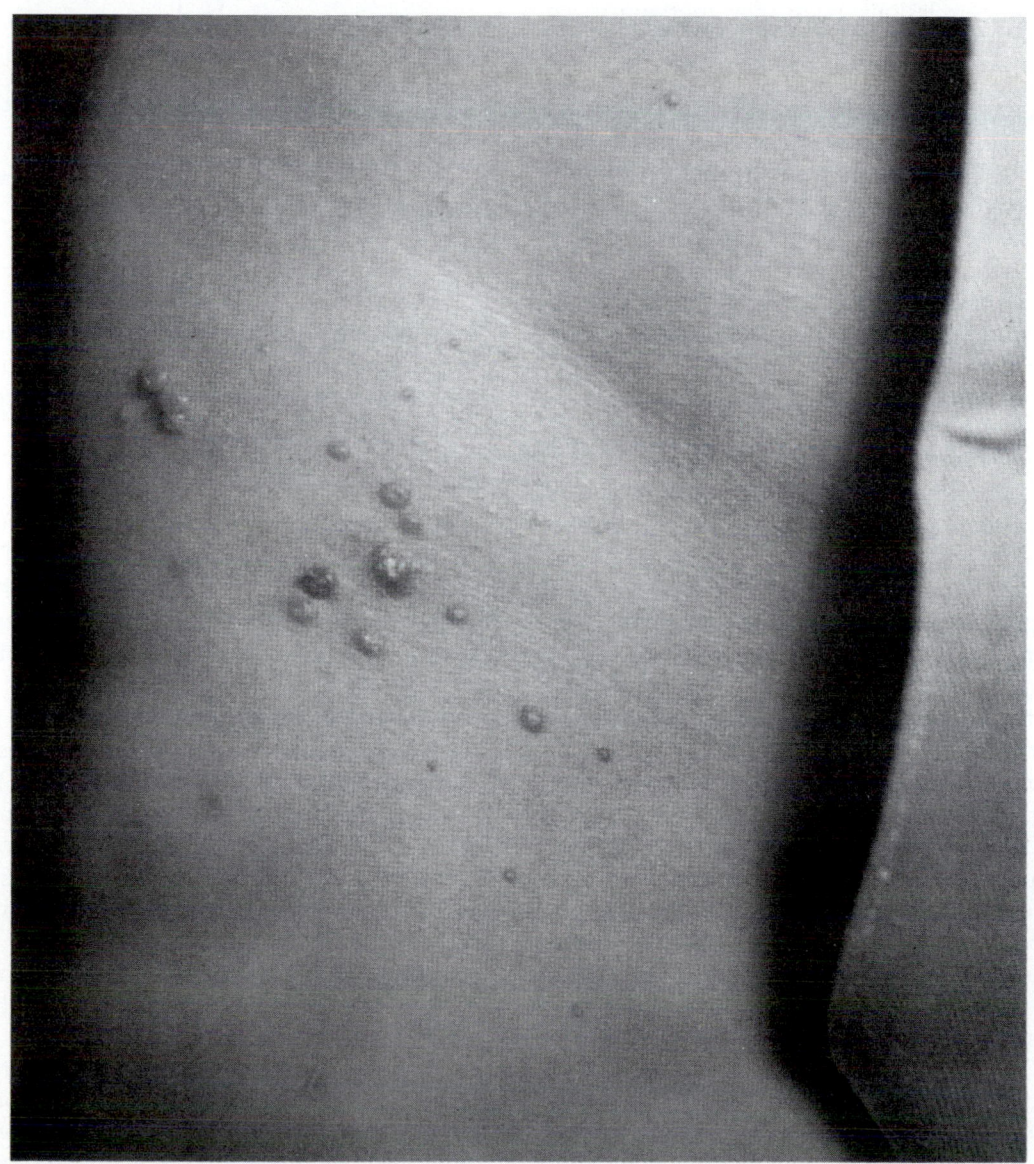

FIG. 42-6. Molluscum contagiosum. Waxy pink globules with umbilicated centers. (From Stewart, Danto, & Maddin, 1978.)

Mulloscum Contagiosum

Mulloscum contagiosum is a common poxvirus infection of the skin and, occasionally, of the conjunctiva that primarily affects children. The well-demarcated molluscum lesion is pear shaped with a base in the upper dermis. The epidermis grows down into the dermis to form saccules containing clusters of virus. The characteristic molluscum body is composed of mature, immature, and incomplete viruses, and cellular debris.

The lesions of molluscum are discrete, slightly umbilicated, dome shaped papules 1 to 5 cm in diameter that appear anywhere on the skin or conjunctiva. The distribution in children is mainly on the trunk, face, extremities, and, sometimes, the conjunctiva (Fig. 42-6). The pubic, genital, and perineal areas are favored in adults (see Chapter 21). There is usually no inflammation surrounding molluscum lesions unless they are traumatized or secondary infection occurs. Scarring occurs with healing.

The best three diagnostic procedures are (1) staining smears of the expressed molluscum body, (2) examining a biopsy, or (3) inoculating a molluscum suspension into cell cultures to demonstrate the cytotoxic reactions. The papule can be punctured with a needle or curette and the contents expressed with a comedone extractor. Most lesions are self-limiting and clear in 6 to 9 months. Freezing the papule with liquid nitrogen is usually effective. Painful or prolonged treatment is not justified because the lesions eventually resolve spontaneously.

Rubella (German or 3-day Measles)

Rubella is a common communicable viral disease of children and young adults. The disease has an incubation period of 14 to 21 days and is spread through the respiratory tract. Prodromal symptoms include enlarged cervical and postauricular lymph nodes, low-grade fever, headache, sore throat, runny nose, and cough. A pink to red coalescing maculopapular rash develops on the face with spread to the trunk and extremities 1 to 4 days after the onset of initial symptoms (Fig. 42-7). The rash subsides after 2 to 3 days, usually without complication. Children are usually not contagious after development of the rash. There is lifelong immunity to rubella, measles, chickenpox, and roseola after the disease (see Table 42-1 for differential presentations).

Vaccination for rubella is usually combined with vaccines for mumps and measles (rubeola). Women of childbearing age are immunized if their rubella hemagglutination-inhibition titer is low. Pregnancy should be avoided for 3 months after vaccination because the attenuated virus in the vaccine may remain for this period. Pregnant women, who have rubella early in the first trimester, may have a fetus that develops congenital defects.

There is no specific treatment. Recovery is spontaneous, although lymph nodes may remain enlarged for weeks. Supportive therapy includes rest, fluids, and use of a vaporizer. In rare cases a mild encephalitis or peripheral neuritis may follow rubella.

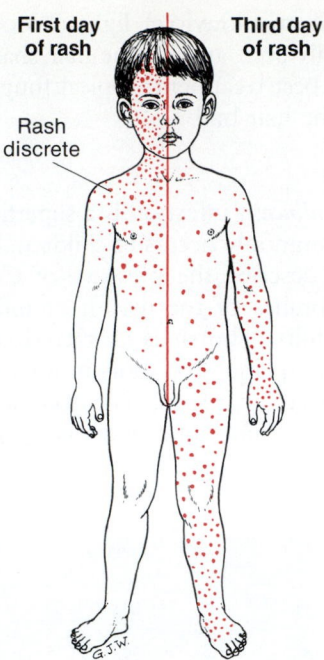

FIG. 42-7. Measles. Full-blown maculopapular rash with tendency to coalesce. (From Wehrle & Top, 1981.)

Rubeola (Red Measles)

Rubeola is a highly contagious, acute viral disease of children. The incubation period is 7 to 12 days during which there are no symptoms. Prodromal symptoms include high fever up to 40.5° C, malaise, enlarged lymph nodes, runny nose, conjunctivitis, and cough. Within 3 to 4 days, a erythematous maculopapular rash develops over the head and spreads distally over the trunk, extremities, hands, and feet. Early lesions blanch with pressure, followed by a brownish hue that does not blanch as the rash fades. Characteristic pinpoint red spots with a central white speck develop over the buccal mucosa and are known as Koplik spots. These spots precede the rash by 1 to 2 days. The rash then subsides within 3 to 5 days.

Complications associated with measles may be due to the primary infection or to a secondary bacterial infection. Measles encephalitis occurs in about 1 of 800 cases and most children recover completely. Only a small minority develop permanent brain damage or die. Bacterial complications include otitis media and pnemonia, usually caused by group A hemolytic streptococcus, *Hemophilus influenza,* or *Staphylococcus aureus* infection.

Measles is prevented by a single vaccination of live at-

TABLE 42-1 Differential presentation of viral diseases producing rashes

Viral disease	Incubation	Prodromal symptoms	Duration/ characteristics	Clinical symptoms
Rubella (German measles)	14-21 days	1-2 days Mild fever Malaise Respiratory symptoms	1-3 days Pink-red maculopapular Face and trunk	Enlarged and tender occipital and periauricular nodes
Rubeola (measles)	7-12 days	2-5 days Fever Cough Respiratory symptoms	3-5 days Purple-red to brown maculopapular Face, trunk, extremities	Koplick spots 1-3 days before rash
Roseola (exanthema subitum	5-15 days	2-5 days High fever	1-3 days Red macular Neck and trunk	Rash develops when fever subsides
Varicella (chickenpox)	11-20 days	1-2 days Low-grade fever Cough May be asymptomatic	7-14 days Red papules, vesicles, pustules in clusters	Eruption of new lesions for 4-5 days Occasional ulcerative lesion in the mouth

tenuated measles virus. Vaccination is usually given after 15 months of age so there will not be interference from maternal measles antibody. There is no specific treatment for measles and supportive therapy is the same as for rubella. Antibiotic therapy is initiated if secondary bacterial infections develop.

Roseola (Exanthem Subitum)

Roseola is a disease of infants beween 6 months and 2 years of age and can be seen up to 4 years of age. The exact cause of the disease is unknown (Brunell, 1987). The incubation period is 5 to 15 days, followed by the sudden onset of fever (38.9° to 40.5° C) that lasts for 3 to 5 days. After the fever, an erythematous macular rash that lasts about 24 hours develops primarily over the trunk and neck. Children usually feel well, eat normally, and have few other symptoms. There is usually no treatment.

Chicken pox and Herpes Zoster

Chickenpox (varicella) and herpes zoster (shingles) are both produced by the varicella-zoster virus. Varicella results from contact of the nonimmune host by the virus, whereas herpes zoster occurs in partially immune individuals who have had varicella.

Chickenpox

Chickenpox is a disease of early childhood, with 90% of children contracting the disease during the first de-

cade of life. Highly contagious, chickenpox is spread by close person-to-person contact and by airborne droplets. Introduction of an infected person into a household results in 90% possibility of susceptible persons developing the disease within the incubation period, usually 14 days. The incubation period can be as early as 11 days or as late as 20 days. Children are contagious for at least 1 day before development of the rash. Transmission of the virus may occur until approximately 5 days after the onset of the first skin lesions in normal children. In immunocompromised children the virus is recoverable for a longer period of time, but they must be considered contagious for at least 7 to 10 days. Chickenpox occurs most commonly in the late winter and early spring. Transmission occurs more readily in temperate climates than in tropical climates.

The vesicular lesions are in the epidermis or dermis where an inflammatory infiltrate is present. Pathologically, zoster and varicella lesions form intraepidermal bullae. Infected cells degenerate, swell, and become acantholytic, often containing inclusions surrounded by a clear halo and a circle of darkly staining chromatin. As the lesion evolves, polymorphnuclear cells enter the vesicle that ruptures and causes crust formation. On mucous membranes, the initial vesicles rupture and leave superficial, transient ulcers.

Normal children who develop chickenpox have no prodromal symptoms. The first sign of illness may be itching or the appearance of vesicles, usually on the trunk, scalp, or face. The rash later spreads to the extremities. Characteristically, lesions can be seen in various stages of maturation with macules, papules, and vesicles present in a particular area at the same time (Fig. 42-8). The vesicular lesions are superficial and can be easily ruptured. A red base can be observed surrounding the vesicle later in the course of the disease; this is particularly prominent in adults. New lesions will erupt for 4 to 5 days until there are about 100 to 300. The vesicles become crusted with only the crust remaining with an occasional vesicle on the palm later in the disease. Although uncommon, ulcerative lesions are sometimes seen in the mouth and, less commonly, on the conjunctiva and pharnyx. Fever usually lasts 2 to 3 days and ranges from 38.5° C to 40° C.

Complications are rare in children but more common in adults. They can include transient hematuria (from rupture of vesicles in the bladder), epistaxis, laryngeal edema, and varicella pneumonia. One case of chickenpox produces almost complete immunity against a second attack. The fetus may be malformed if chickenpox develops in the first trimester of pregnancy (Wheller, 1983). Infants whose mothers have chickenpox at any stage of pregnancy have a higher risk of developing herpes zoster during the first few years of life.

Uncomplicated chickenpox requires no specific therapy. Systemic or topical antipruritic agents are occasionally helpful to relieve itching and to prevent secondary infection from developing as a result of scratching. Hyperimmunogammaglobulin may be administered to immunodeficient individuals after exposure to chickenpox.

Herpes Zoster

Although herpes zoster (shingles) occurs mainly in adults, about 5% are children less than 15 years of age. The course of the disease in children with an immune defect is more complicated. The eruption of **shingles** consists of groups of vesicles situated on an inflammatory base and arranged along the course of a sensory nerve. The base of the lesions frequently appears hemorrhagic and some of the lesions may become necrotic and ulcerative. In addition to the localized eruption, there are frequently a few scattered lesions resembling chickenpox.

In immune individuals with impaired cellular immunity the incidence and severity of lesions are greatly increased. The incidence is particularly high in persons having Hodgkin disease, who are receiving chemotherapy and radiation (Sokal & Firat, 1965). In children, as in adults, the incidence in this high-risk group is about 50% and the eruption is either localized or disseminated. Children with disseminated lesions and a serious associated illness have a good prognosis; however, those with impaired cellular immunity may develop widespread, fatal systemic manifestations (pneumonia, gastroenteritis, or encephalitis) (Kain, Feldman, & Cohn, 1962).

Smallpox

Smallpox (variola) is a highy contagious and deadly but preventable disease. It is caused by poxvirus variolae. Because of worldwide mass immunizations, the world is now virtually free of smallpox.

INSECT BITES AND PARASITES

Insect bites and infestations are common causes of skin disorders in children and adults. Skin damage occurs by various mechanisms including trauma of bites and stings, allergic reactions, transmission of disease, injection of substances that cause local or systemic reactions, and inflammatory reactions from retained mouth parts.

Scabies

Scabies is a contagious disease caused by the itch mite, *Sarcoptes scabiei* (Fig. 42-9, *A*). It is transmitted by close personal contact (see Chapter 21) and by infected clothing and bedding. Scabies is frequently epidemic in areas of overcrowded housing and poor sanitation. Infestation is initiated by a female mite that tunnels into the skin creating a burrow several millimeters to a centimeter long in the stratum corneum.

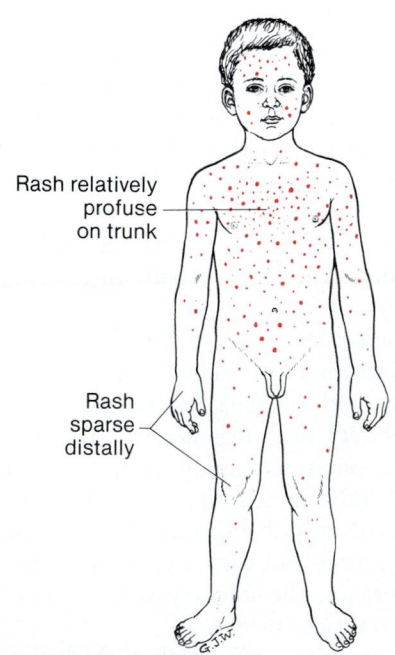

Rash relatively profuse on trunk

Rash sparse distally

FIG. 42-8. Chickenpox. Generalized, polymorphous eruption. (From Wehrle & Top, 1981.)

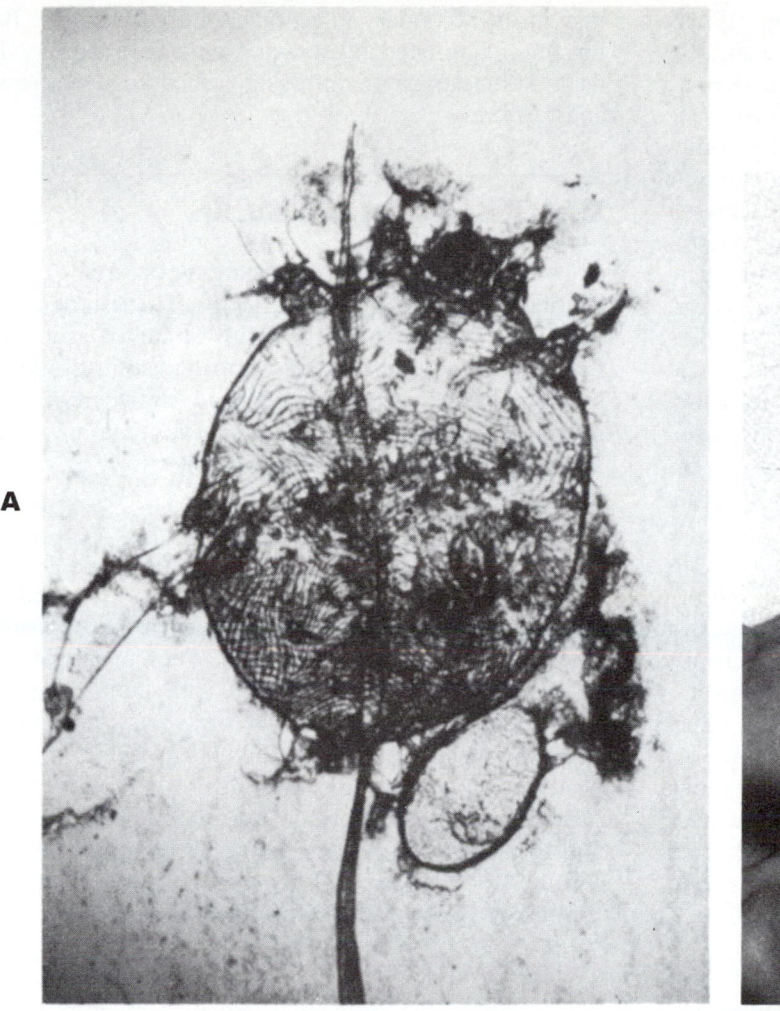
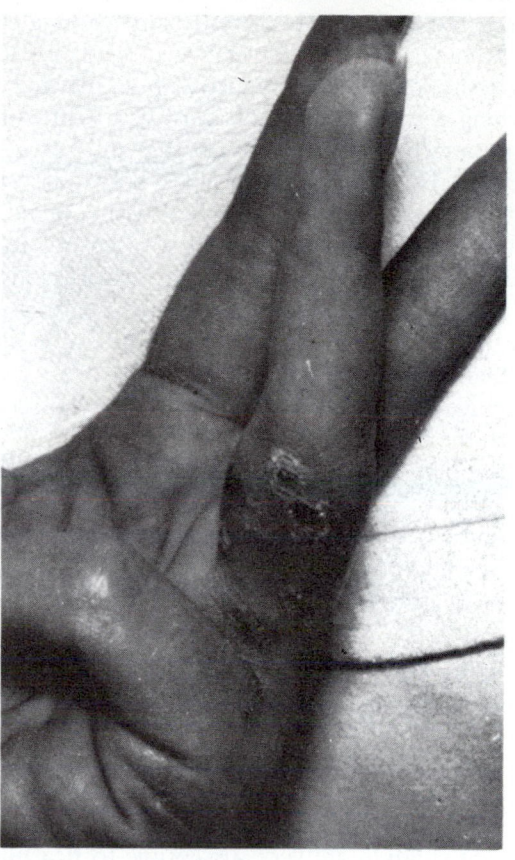

FIG. 42-9. **A,** Scabies mite, as seen clinically when removed from its burrow. **B,** Scabies. A characteristic location, often secondarily infected. (From Stewart, Danto, & Maddin, 1978.)

Symptoms appear 3 to 5 weeks after infestation. The primary lesions are burrows, papules, and vesicular lesions with severe itching that worsens at night. Itching is thought to be related to sensitization to the larval stages of the parasite. In older children and adults the lesions occur in the webs of fingers; axillae; creases of the arms and wrists; along the belt line; and around the nipples, genitals, and lower buttocks. Infants and young children have a different pattern of distribution with involvement of the palms, soles, head, neck, and face (Fig. 42-9, *B*). Secondary infections and crusting develop from scratching and eczematous changes.

Nodular scabies is the development of reddish brown pruritic nodules that resist treatment and persist for months. The nodules are located in the axillae, groin, buttocks, and genital areas. Histologically, they appear as forms of lymphoma or histiocytosis.

Crusted scabies is relatively rare with an affinity for the mentally retarded, particular those with Down syn-

drome. It is highly contagious and is characterized by heavily crusted lesions on the scalp, elbows, knees, palms, soles, and buttocks.

Diagnosis of scabies is made by observation of the tunnels and burrows and scraping of the skin with microscopic examination of the mite. Treatment is the application of 1% Lindane cream or lotion for 12 hours and washing of clothes and bedding. Lindane cream may cause neurotoxicity from systemic absorption through the skin (Solomon, Fahrner, & Dennis, 1977). Crotamiton has been recommended as a safe alternative (Cubela & Yawalkar, 1978). The mites rarely survive off the body for more than 8 hours.

Pediculosis (Lice)

There are three known types of human lice: (1) the head louse, (3) the body louse, and (3) the crab or pubic louse. They are parasites and survive by sucking blood. The mouth parts are shaped for piercing and sucking and attach to the skin while feeding. When piercing the skin, the louse secretes a toxic saliva and the mechanical trauma and toxin produce a pruritic dermatitis. Head and body lice are acquired by personal contact, combs, or brushes. Crab lice are spread by bodily contact (see Chapter 21) or toilet seats. Young children may become infected with crab lice on their eyebrows or eyelashes or by close contact with an infected adult.

Itching is the major symptom of lice. With head lice, the ova attach to hairs above the ears and in the occipital region. The primary lesion of the body louse is a pinpoint red macule, papule, or wheal with a hemorrhagic pucture site. The primary lesion is often not seen, because it is disrupted by scratching, wheals, and crusts. The crab louse is found on pubic hairs but may also involve other body hair such as eyelashes, moustache, beard, and axillae.

The live louse, 2 to 3 mm long, is rarely observed, although the ova, or nits, can be observed as oval, yellowish, pinpoint specks fastened to a hair shaft. The ova will fluoresce under an ultraviolet light (Wood lamp) and can be best observed with a microscope. Use of lindane shampoo (Kwell) for 2 consecutive days is effective for treating head lice. Lindane lotion left on for 12 hours, with retreatment in a week if ova are still visable, is used for body and crab lice. All clothes, towels, bedding, combs, and brushes should be washed and dried in hot air, boiled, or clothes ironed. Individuals who have close personal contact should also be treated.

Fleas

Young children are very susceptible to **flea bites** and the most common are the bites of cat, dog, and human fleas. Bites occur in clusters along the arms, legs, or where there are tight-fitting clothes. The bite produces an urticarial wheal with a central hemorrhagic puncture. Application of antihistamines, calamine lotion, or topical steroids relieves symptoms. Carpets, crevices, and furniture are sprayed with malathion or lindane powder. Infected animals should be treated, and clothes and bedding should be washed in hot water.

Bedbugs

Bedbugs live in the crevices and cracks of floors, walls, furniture, and in bedding or furniture stuffing. They are 3 to 5 mm long and reddish brown. Bedbugs emerge to feed in darkness and attach to the skin to suck blood. Feeding occurs for 5 to 15 minutes and the bedbug then leaves. It will move long distances to search for food and can travel from house to house.

Two or three bites usually appear in a line on exposed areas of the skin. If the host has not been previously sensitized, the only symptom is a red macule that develops into a nodule, lasting up to 14 days. In sensitized children and adults pruritic wheals, papules, and vesicles may form. Secondary infections require treatment. Bedbugs are eliminated by spraying with chlordane or lindane and cleaning or disposing of bedding, mattresses, and furniture.

VASCULAR DISORDERS

Congenital vascular malformations occur in 10% of all infants (Jacobs & Watson, 1976). The lesions are developmental in origin with islands of angioblastic tissue failing to communicate with normal adjacent blood vessels. The most common disorders are strawberry hemangioma, cavernous hemangioma, nevus flammeus, and salmon patches. They are known collectively as vascular nevi.

Strawberry Hemangioma

The **strawberry hemangioma** is a distinct, raised vascular lesion that may be present at birth but usually emerges 3 to 5 weeks after birth. They proliferate and become bright red and elevated with minute capillary projections that give them a strawberry appearance. There is usually only one lesion and it is located on the head and neck or trunk (Fig. 42-10). After the initial growth, the lesion grows at the same rate as the child and then starts to involute at 12 to 16 months of age. About 90% of strawberry hemangiomas will involute by 5 to 6 years of age, usually without scarring.

Cavernous Hemangiomas

Cavernous hemangiomas are present at birth and have larger and more mature vessels within the lesion than strawberry hemangiomas. They appear primarily on the head and neck and have a bluish red color with less distinct borders. Cavernous hemangiomas grow rapidly up to 6 months of age and mature by 1 year of age. A period of involution begins and proceeds for 6 to 12 months with complete involution by 2 to 3 years. Some lesions are a mixture of both strawberry and cavernous hemangiomas. The hemangioma has disappeared by 9 years of age in 90% of children.

Hemangiomas that require treatment are those located near structures such as the eye, nares, auditory canal, or pharynx, or those that grow rapidly and are susceptible to trauma or secondary infection. No form of treatment is entirely satisfactory; however, surgery, liquid nitrogen, or laser ablation can control bleeding or reduce the size of the lesion. The best cosmetic results are obtained when there is spontaneous involution. Ulceration, bleeding, and infection are relatively rare, but cleansing and use of topical antibiotics are effective when they do occur. Open lesions do better when left open to the air; Telfa dressings are recommended if bandages are required.

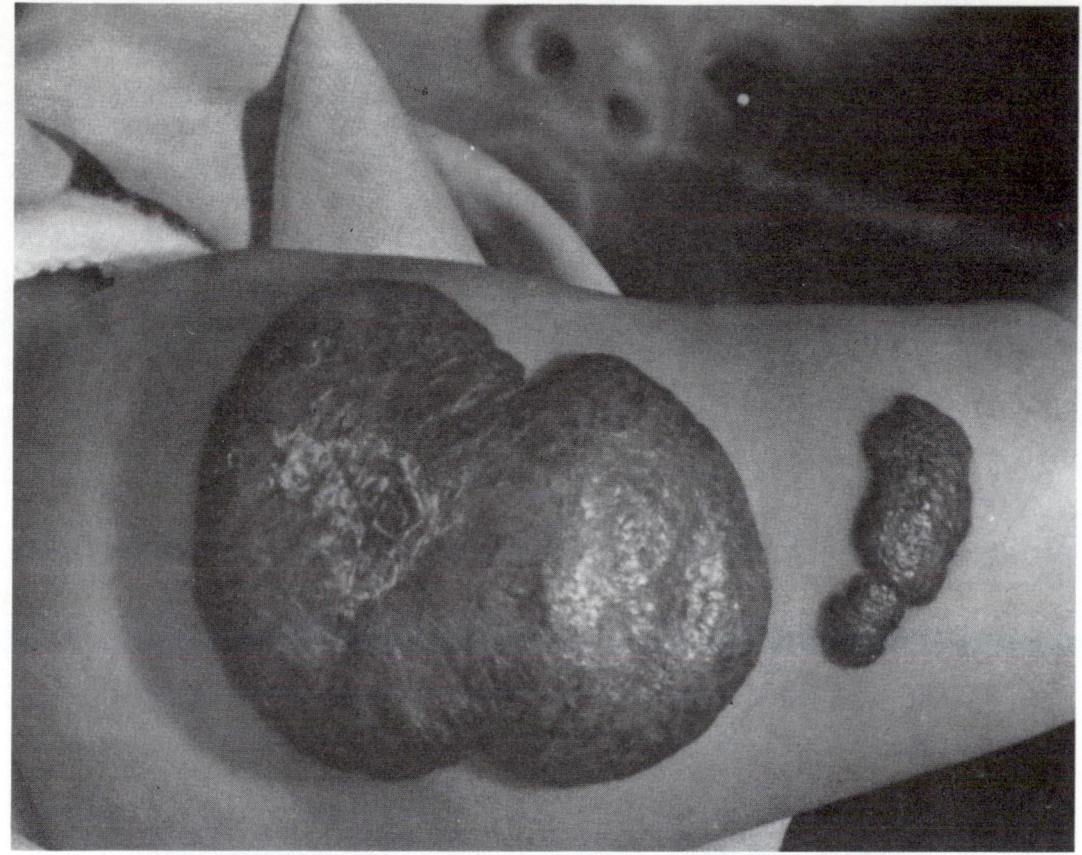

FIG. 42-10. Strawberry hemangioma. (From Stewart, Danto, & Maddin, 1978.)

Salmon Patches

Salmon patches are macular, pink lesions present at birth and located on the nape of the neck (stork bites), forehead, upper eyelids, or nasolabial fold region. The pink color results from distended dermal capillaries and 95% fade by 1 year of age. They generally do not present a cosmetic problem.

Port-Wine Stain

Port-wine stain (nevus flammeus) is a congenital malformation of the dermal capillaries. The lesions are flat and their color ranges from pink to dark reddish purple. They are present at birth or within a few days after birth and do not fade with age. Involvement of the face and other body surfaces is common and the lesions may be large (Fig. 42-11). During adolescence and later adult years, the port-wine stain may become papular and cavernous. Treatments using cryosurgery or tattooing are not very satisfactory. The argon ion laser has been used more recently to successfully lighten the color and flatten the more nodular and cavernous lesions (Rotteleur et al., 1988). Waterproof cosmetics may be used to cover the lesions.

OTHER SKIN DISORDERS

Miliara

Miliara (prickly heat) is a dermatosis commonly seen in infants. It is characterized by a vesicular eruption after prolonged exposure to perspiration. The immature sweat ducts of infants result in closure of the duct opening and sweat retention. The lesions may appear as clear, pinpoint vesicles or as small, red pruritic papules or vesicles. The lesions are usually located in skin folds or where cothing rubs against the skin. Avoidance of heat and humidity and light loose clothing prevent formation of the lesions. Cetaphil lotion may be used to treat the skin after formation of the lesions.

Erythema Toxicum Neonatorum

Erythema toxicum neonatorum (toxic erythema of the newborn) is a benign, erythematous accumulation of macules, papules, or pustules that appear at birth or 3 to 4 days after birth. The lesions first appear as a blotchy, macular erythematous rash. The macules vary from 1 mm to 1 cm. When papules or pustules develop, they are light yellow or white and 1 to 3 mm in diame-

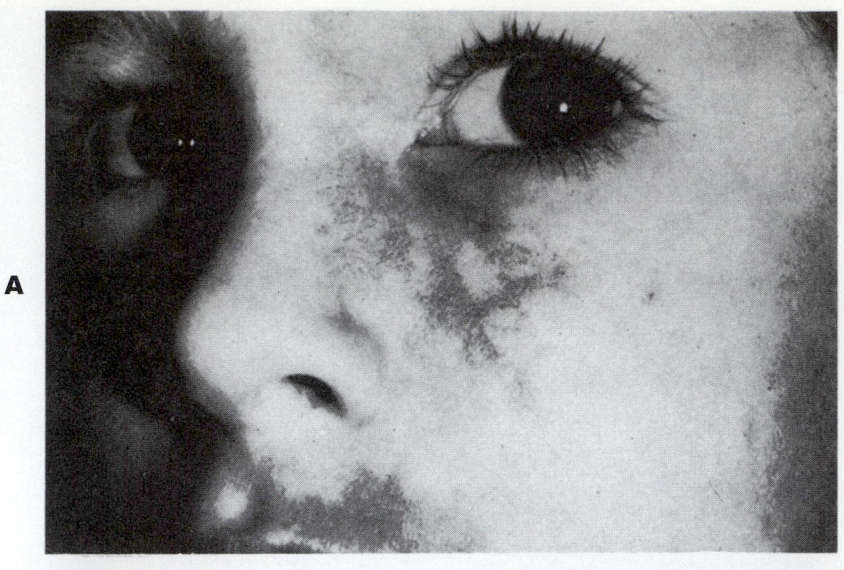

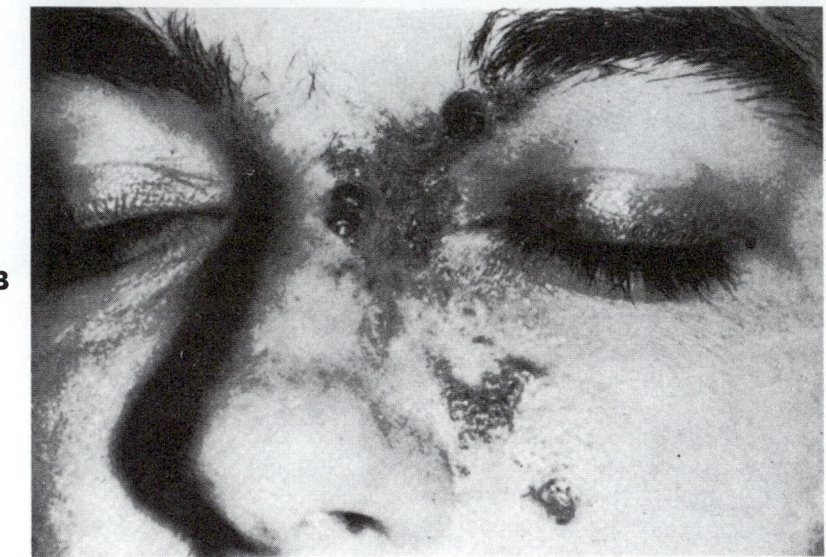

FIG. 42-11. Port-wine hemangioma in an infant, **A,** and adult, **B.** (From Stewart, Danto, Maddin, 1978.)

ter. There may be few lesions or several hundred and any body surface can be affected with the exception of the palms and soles where there are no pilosebaceous follicles. The cause of the lesion is unknown, and it is self-limiting. No treatment is required.

SUMMARY REVIEW

Dermatitis

1 Atopic dermatitis is associated with elevated IgE levels and a family history of asthma and hay fever. Red, scaly lesions commonly occur on the face, cheeks, and flexor surfaces of the extremities.

2 Diaper dermatitis is a type of contact dermatitis developing from prolonged exposure of urine and feces or diapers washed in detergent.

Infections of the Skin

1 Impetigo is a contagious bacterial disease occuring in two forms, bullous *(Staphylococcus)* and vesicular *(Streptococcus)*. The toxins from the bacteria produce a weeping lesion with a honey-colored crust.

2 Staphylococcal toxin epidural necrolysis (STEN) is a staphylococcal skin infection that occurs more commonly in young children with low titers of antistaphylococcal antibody. Painful blisters and bullae form over large areas of the skin requiring systemic antibiotics for treatment.

3 Nonstaphylococcal toxic epidermal necrolysis is similar to STEN, but the causative agent is usually a drug or a vaccination.

4 Thrush is a fungal infection of the mouth caused by *Candida albicans*.

5 Tinea corporis and tinea capitis are fungal infections of the scalp and body. The lesions are erythematous with a raised border and are commonly known as ringworm.

6 Mulloscum contagiosum is a poxvirus of the skin that produces pale papular lesions filled with viral and cellular debris.

7 Rubella (3-day measles) is a communicable disease characterized by fever, sore throat, enlarged cervical and postauricular nodes, and a generalized maculopapular rash that lasts from 1 to 4 days.

8 Rubeola is a contagious disease with symptoms of high fever, enlarged lymph nodes, conjunctivitis, and a red rash that begins on the head, spreads to the trunk and extremities, and lasts from 3 to 5 days. Both bacterial and viral complications may accompany rubeola.

9 Roseola is a benign disease of infants with a sudden onset of fever that lasts 3 to 5 days, followed by a rash that lasts for 24 hours.

10 Chickenpox (varicella) is a highly contagious disease caused by the varicella-zoster virus. Vesicular lesions occur on the skin and mucous membranes and individuals are contagious from 1 day before the development of the rash until about 5 days after the rash develops.

11 Herpes zoster (shingles) is a viral eruption of vesicles on the skin along the distribution of a sensory nerve. Children with immune suppression develop more serious complications.

12 Smallpox (variola) is a highly contagious, deadly disease that has been eradicated worldwide by vaccination.

Insect Bites and Parasites

1 Scabies is an itching lesion caused by the itch mite, which burrows into the skin forming papules and vesicles. The mite is very contagious and is transmitted by direct contact.

2 Pediculosis (lice) are blood-sucking parasites that secrete a toxic saliva and damage the skin to produce a pruritic dermatitis. Lice are spread by direct contact and are recognized by the ova or nits that attach to the shaft of body hairs.

3 Flea bites produce a pruritic wheal with a central puncture site and occur as clusters in areas of tight-fitting clothing.

4 Bedbugs are blood-sucking parasites that live in cracks of floors, furniture, or bedding and feed at night. They produce pruritic wheals and nodules.

Vascular Disorders

1 A strawberry hemangioma is a vascular lesion present at birth that proliferates in size and then grows at the same rate as the child. Most lesions resolve spontaneously by 5 years of age.

2 A cavernous hemangioma is present at birth with larger vessels than a strawberry hemangioma and is bluish red. They usually involute by 9 years of age and may require surgical removal if located near the eyes, nares, or genitalia.

3 Salmon patches are macular pink lesions with dilated capillaries that usually resolve by 1 year of age.

4 Port-wine stains are congenital malformations of dermal capillaries that do not fade with age.

Other Skin Disorders

1 Miliara are small pruritic papules or vesicles that result from closure of the sweat duct opening in infants.

2 Erythema toxicum neonatorum is a benign accumulation of macules, papules, and pustules that spontaneously resolves within a few weeks of birth.

KEY TERMS

Atopic dermatitis, 1439

Bedbug, 1448

Bullous impetigo, 1440

Cavernous hemangioma, 1448

Chickenpox, 1445

Crusted scabies, 1447

Diaper dermatitis, 1440

Erythema toxicum neonatorum, 1449

Flea bite, 1448

Impetigo, 1440

Miliara, 1449

Mulloscum contagiosum, 1444

Nodular scabies, 1447

Nonstaphylococcal TEN, 1441

Port-wine stain, 1449

Roseola, 1445

Rubella, 1444

Rubeolla, 1444

Salmon patch, 1449

Scabies, 1446

Shingles, 1446

Strawberry hemangioma, 1448

Smallpox, 1446

Thrush, 1443

Tinea capitis, 1442

Tinea corporis, 1442

Toxic epidural necrolysis (TEN), 1441

Vesicular impetigo, 1441

REFERENCES

Brunnel, P. A. (1987). In T. B. Fitzpatrick, et al. (Eds.), *Dermatology in general medicine* (p. 2296). New York: McGraw-Hill.

Cubela, V., & Yawalkar, S. J. (1978). Clinical experience with chromatin cream and lotion in treatment of infants with scabies. *British Journal of Clinical Practice, 32,* 229.

Demis, D. J. (Ed.). (1985). *Clinical dermatology* (12th ed.). Philadelphia: Harper & Row.

Fison, T. N. (1956). Acute glomerulonephritis in infancy. *Archives of Diseases in Children, 31,* 101.

Hoeckelman, R. A., Blatman, S., Friedman, S. B., Nelson, N. M., & Seidel, H. M. (Eds.). (1987) *Primary pediatric care.* St. Louis: C.V. Mosby.

Jacobs, A. H., & Watson, R. G. (1976). The incidence of birthmarks in the neonate. *Pediatrics, 58,* 218.

Kain, H. K., Feldman, C. A., & Cohn, L. H. (1962). Herpes zoster generalisatus pneumonia. *Archives of Internal Medicine, 110,* 98-101.

Larsen, W. G., & Maibach, H. I. (1985). Contact dermatitis. In S. L. Moschella & H. J. Hurley (Eds.), *Dermatology* (2nd ed.). Philadelphia: W. B. Saunders.

Lever, W. F., & Schaumburg-Lever, G. (1983). *Histopathology of the skin* (6th ed.). Philadelphia: J. B. Lippincott.

Levine, G., & Norden, C. (1972). *New England Journal of Medicine, 287,* 1339.

Moschella, S. L., & Hurley, H. J. (Eds.). (1985). *Dermatology* (2nd ed.). Philadelphia: W. B. Saunders.

Polak, L. (1980). Immunological aspects of contact sensitivity. In P. Dukor (Ed.), *Monographs in allergy* (vol. 15). Philadelphia: Basel S. Karger.

Rook, A., Parish, L. C., & Beare, J. M. (1986). *Practical mangement of the dermatologic patient.* Philadelphia: J. B. Lippincott.

Rotteleur, G., Mordon, S., Buys, B., Sozanski, J. P., & Brunetaud, J. M. (1988). Robotized scanning laser handpiece for the treatment of port wine stains and other angiodysplasias. *Laser Surgery and Medicine, 8,* 283-287.

Seidel, H., Ball, J., Dains, J., & Benedict, G.W. (1987). *Mosby's guide to physical examination.* St. Louis: C. V. Mosby.

Sokal, J. E., & Firat, D. (1965). Varicella-zoster infection in Hodgkin's disease. *American Journal of Medicine, 39,* 452-463.

Solomon, L. M., Fahrner, L., & Dennis, P. W. (1977). Gamma benzene hexachloride toxicity: A review. *Archives of Dermatology, 113,* 353.

Stewart, W. D., Danto, J. L., & Maddin, S. (1978). *Dermatology: diagnosis and treatment of cutaneous disorders* (4th ed.) St. Louis: C. V. Mosby.

Wehrle, P.F., & Top, F. H., Sr. (1981). *Communicable and infectious diseases* (9th ed.). St. Louis: C. V. Mosby.

Wheller, T. H. (1983). Varicella and herpes zoster: Changing concepts of the natural history, control, and importance of a not-so-benign virus. *New England Journal of Medicine, 309,* 1434.

Zaynoun, S. T. (1974). Topical antibodies in pyoderma. *British Journal of Dermatology, 90,* 331-334.

Index

A

A antigen, 200
A bands, 1309, 1310
  heart and, 875
A peptide, 580
Abdomen, undifferentiated lymphoma of, 852
Abdominal aortic aneurysm, 927, 928
Abdominal pain, 1216-1217
  cancer and, 305
  mesenteric insufficiency and, 1236
Abducens nerves, 375
Abduction, foot abnormality and, 1366
Aberrant conduction in heart disease, 967
Aberrations, chromosome, 121, 131-132
  prenatal diagnosis of, 127-128
ABO blood group, 199-200
ABO isoimmunization, 263, 832
ABO nail-patella linkage, 143
Abortion, spontaneous, 126
Abscess
  central nervous system and, 506-507
  inflammation and, 239
  lung, 1064-1065
Absolute refractory period, 28
Absorption, intestinal, 1184
  impairment of, in child, 1276-1280
Absorption atelectasis, 1060, 1061
Acalculia, 462
Accelerated junctional rhythm, 964
Accelerated ventricular rhythm, 965
Accessory organs of digestion, cancer of, 1259-1261
Accident
  cerebrovascular, 493-494
  motor vehicle, 477
  temperature and, 405, 406-408
Accidental hyperthermia, 405
Accidental hypothermia, 406-407
Accommodation, alterations in, 416-417
Accumulations, cellular injury and, 66-70
Acetabulum, 1363
Acetaldehyde, 12
Acetazolamide, 1128
Acetyl coenzyme A, 18
Acetylcholine, 253, 378
  Alzheimer disease and, 443
  IgE-mediated hypersensitivity and, 357
  Parkinson disease and, 510
Achalasia, 1219
Achondroplasia, 135, 136
Acid; see also Acid-base balance; Cellular environment
  disturbance of; see Acidosis; Alkalosis
  gastric, 1180-1181
    aspiration of, 1060
  loss of, 107

Acid—cont'd
  renal excretion of, 104
  volatile or nonvolatile form of, 101
Acid-base balance, 100-110
  buffer systems and, 101-104
  disturbance of, 96, 104-110
  hydrogen ion and pH in, 100-101
  primary and compensatory changes and, 105
  protein buffering in, 104
  renal failure and, 1155
Acid maltase deficiency, 1353
Acid phosphatase, tumor cell markers and, 300
Acidemia, 104-105
Acidosis, 93, 98, 105
  hyperkalemia and, 96
  metabolic, 102, 105-107
  pulmonary artery constriction and, 1042
  respiratory, 105, 108-109
  respiratory distress syndrome of newborn and, 1104, 1105
Acinus, 666, 1030
Acne rosacea, 1407
Acne vulgaris, 1406-1407
Acoustic nerves, 375
Acoustic trauma, 65
Acquired immune deficiencies, 265, 268-274; see also Acquired immunodeficiency syndrome
Acquired immunity, 194
Acquired immunodeficiency syndrome, 269-274
  Kaposi sarcoma and, 339-340, 1421-1423
Acquired immunodeficiency syndrome vaccine, 274
Acrania, 538
Acrocephaly, 539
Acromegaly, 602-603
Acrosclerosis, 1416
Actin, 875, 1310
Actin filaments, 10
Actinic keratosis, 1418
Actinomycetes, thermophilic, 254
Actinomycin D, 309
Action potentials, 28, 868-869, 871-873
Activated macrophages, 343
Activated partial thromboplastin time, 845
Active acquired immunity, 194
Active transport, 19, 22-24, 27
Acute leukemia, 803-805
Acute lymphoblastic leukemia, 803, 847-848, 850
  categories of, 847-848
  prognosis in, 850
  treatment of, 850
Acute myelogenous leukemia, 803

Acute nonlymphoblastic leukemia, 803, 847
Acute-phase reactants, 237
Acute renal failure, 1151-1153
Acute respiratory failure, 1067-1069
Acute tubular necrosis, 1151, 1151-1153
Acute undifferentiated leukemia, 847
Acute urethral syndrome, 737, 1142
Acyanotic heart defects, 999
  pulmonary blood flow and, 1003-1007
Adaptation, general syndrome of, 282
Addison disease, 634
  genetics and, 170
  hyperkalemia and, 97
  idiopathic, 634
  immunity and, 250
  manifestations of, 635
  melanin and, 68
  pathophysiologic mechanisms of, 635
Adduction, foot, 1366
Adenine, 117
Adenocarcinoma, 296
  colorectal, 1257
  ductal, 1261
  lung and, 1088, 1089
Adenohypophysis, 570
Adenoma, 296
  bronchial, 1088-1090
  pituitary, 600-601
  primary, 600-601
  renal, 1139
Adenosine deaminase deficiency, 275-276
Adenosine diphosphate, 17
  heart and, 877
  platelets and, 771, 772
Adenosine monophosphate, cyclic, 569
Adenosine triphosphate, 16-17, 18, 97
  active transport and, 23
  cellular metabolism and, 17
  chemical injury and, 56
  heart and, 876, 877
  hypoxic injury and, 53
  muscle contracture and, 1351
  myoadenylate deaminase deficiency and, 1353-1354
  shock and, 983
  skeletal muscle and, 1312
  transient neonatal thrombocytopenia and, 846
Adenoviruses, 334
Adherence, inflammation and, 230
Adipose tissue, 39
Adjuvants, immunity and, 198, 310
Adolescent, 649
  osteomyelitis in, 1372
Adrenal androgen hypersecretion, 633
Adrenal catecholamine release, 586

Adrenal cortex, 580-586, 587
  disorders of, 628-635
    child with secondary hypertension and,
      1017
  stress and, 282
  virilizing tumor of, 634
Adrenal estrogens, 586
  hypersecretion of, 633
Adrenal glands, 580-586
  aging and, 589
  alterations of function of, 628-637
  general adaptation syndrome and, 282
  stress response and, 283
Adrenal medulla, 580, 586
  disorders of, 635-637
    hyperfunction in, 636-637
    hypofunction in, 635-636
  stress response and, 283
Adrenalectomy, bilateral, 635
Adrenalitis, organ-specific autoimmune, 634
Adrenarche, premature, 678
Adrenergic blockers, hypertension and, 926
Adrenergic receptors, 283, 284
  heart and, 873-874
Adrenergic transmission, 378
Adrenocorticotropic hormone, 571, 575, 580
  deficiency of, 599-600
  effects of, 584
  hypercortisolism and, 629
  hypocortisolism and, 633-634
  melanin and, 68
  multiple sclerosis and, 517
  stress and disease and, 283, 286, 287, 288
  tumors and, 299, 300
    lung cancer in, 1088
Adriamycin, 309
Adult respiratory distress syndrome,
  1067-1069
Aerobic glycogen, 1312
Afferent loop obstruction, 1230
Afferent lymphatic vessel, 901
Afferent neuron, 364
Afferent pathways, 352
  pain and, 394-395
Aflatoxin, 328
African Burkitt lymphoma, 851
Afterload, 879, 881, 969
Agammaglobulinemia, 266, 274
  Bruton, 267
  childhood cancer and, 318
Aganglionic megacolon, congenital, 1273
Age; *see also* Aging
  cancer sites and, 301
  pain and, 393
Age pigment, 10
Agenesis, renal, 1163
Ageusia, 423
Agglutination, 200, 205, 668
Aggregated immunoglobulins, 274
Aging
  altered cellular and tissue biology and,
    73-77
  cardiovascular system and, 907-908
  cellular, 49, 75-76
  disorders related to, 168
  endocrine system and, 588-589
  familial diseases and, 166-168
  gastrointestinal system and, 1206-1207
  hearing and, 420, 421
  hematologic system and, 780
  inflammation and, 246
  of joints, 1315
  of muscles, 1315-1316

Aging—cont'd
  musculoskeletal system and, 1315-1316
  nervous system and, 380-383
  olfaction and, 422
  pulmonary system and, 1050
  renal function and, 1131-1132
  reproductive function and, 671-673
  skin integrity and, 1393-1394
  sleep patterns and, 410-411
  taste and, 422
  temperature regulation and, 404
  theories and mechanisms of, 74-75
  tissue and systems of, 76
  vision and, 415
Agnosia, 462-464
Agonal rhythm, 965
Agonist, muscle, 1314
Agranulocyte, 760
Agranulocytosis, 802
Agraphia, 462
AIDS dementia complex, 273
AIDS-related complex, 273
Air blast, 63
Air embolism, 931
Air pollution, 329-330
Air trapping
  chronic obstructive pulmonary disease
    and, 1073
  emphysema and, 1074
Airway
  caliber of, 1041-1042
  conducting, 1026-1030
  gas exchange and, 1030-1031
  hyperreactivity of, 1070
  lower, 1030
    disorders of, 1101-1107
  upper, 1028
    disorders of, 1098-1101
Airway obstruction
  acute respiratory acidosis and, 108
  asthma and, 1070
  chronic bronchitis and, 1073
Airway resistance, 1039-1040
Akathisia, 455
Akathitic movements, 455
Akinesia, 452-453, 512
Alar plate, 533
Alarm stage of general adaptation syndrome,
  282
Albinism, 68
Albumin, 755, 756
  bilirubin and, 69
  bone and, 1295
  cachexia and, 306
  hormones and, 566
  nephrotic syndrome and, 1149, 1150
Albuminuria, history of, 1111
Alcohol
  breast cancer and, 715
  carcinogenesis and, 329, 715
  coronary artery disease and, 937
  hypertension and, 921
  hypoglycemia and, 618, 620
Alcoholic cirrhosis, 1249-1252
Alcoholic hepatitis, 1250
Alcoholic myopathy, 1355-1356
Alcoholism, 170, 183
  fatty liver and, 67
Aldosterone, 584-586
  adrenocorticotropic hormone deficiency
    and, 600
  cardiovascular system and, 896
  hormonal regulation of secretion of, 631

Aldosterone—cont'd
  potassium regulation and, 93, 633
  sodium balance and, 87, 88
Aldosterone antagonists, 1128
Alexia, 462
Algor mortis, 76
Alimentary hypoglycemia, 620; *see also*
  Gastrointestinal system
Alkalemia, 105
Alkaline phosphatase, tumor cell markers
  and, 300
Alkaline reflux gastritis, 1230
Alkaline smoke, 326
Alkaline tide, 1181
Alkalosis, 93
  metabolic, 107
  respiratory, 109-110
Alkylating agents, 309
Alleles, 133
Allergens, 253
  shock and, 979-980
Allergy
  alveolitis and, 1067, 1070
  asthma and, 1069-1070
  conjunctivitis and, 413
  contact dermatitis and, 1402
  gastrointestinal, 254
  genetics and, 169, 171
  immunity and, 194, 249, 250, 260-261
  purpura and, 846
  vasculitis and, 1415
Alopecia
  discoid lupus erythematosus and, 1408
  female-pattern, 1432
  male-pattern, 1432
Alopecia areata, 1432-1433
Alpha cells, islets of Langerhans and, 578
Alpha-fetoprotein, 300, 339, 1260
Alpha motor neuron, 458
Alpha receptors, 378
Alpha-thalassemia, 841
Alpha trait, thalassemia and, 841
Alphaglycoprotein, 1295
Altered cellular and tissue biology; *see*
  Cellular and tissue biology alterations
Altered consciousness, 443
Aluminum hydroxide, 100
Alveolar-arterial-oxygen gradient, 1048
Alveolar hypoxia, 1042
Alveolar macrophages, 1031
Alveolar oxygen tension, 1045
Alveolar pressures, pulmonary blood flow
  and, 1043-1044
Alveolar surface tension, 1038
Alveolar ventilation, 1036, 1038
Alveolar wall, 1033
Alveolitis, allergic, 1067, 1070
Alveolocapillary membrane, 970
  diffusion across, 1044-1045
Alveolus, 1031
Alzheimer disease, 444-445
  acetylcholine and, 443
  genetics and, 183
  neurofibrillary tangles and, 382
Amblyopia, 415, 416
Amebiasis, 746
Amenorrhea
  primary, 680-681
  secondary, 681-682
American Burn Association classification of
  burn injury, 1423
American Rheumatism Association, 1339,
  1345

Amiloride, 1128
Amines, 566
  degranulation of vasoactive, 220-222
Amino acids, 117
  erythropoiesis and, 766, 767
  metabolism defects and, 544-546
  neurotransmitters and, 357
γ-Aminobutyric-acid–secreting neurons, 513
υ-Aminocaproic acid, 229
Aminopeptidases, 300
Aminopterin, 145, 314
Ammonia, renal buffering and, 104
Amnesic-confabulatory psychosis, 509
Amnestic dementia, 443
Amniocentesis, 127
Amniotic fluid embolism, 931
Amphiarthrosis, 1298
Amphipathic molecule, 13
Ampulla
  of fallopian tube, 653
  of Vater, 1200
Amputation, diabetes mellitus and, 627, 628
Amusia, 462
Amygdalin, 57
Amylase, pancreatic, 1202, 1254-1255
Amyotrophic lateral sclerosis, 517-519
Amyotrophy, 459-460
Anabolic steroids, 580
  childhood cancers and, 319
Anabolism, 16
Anaerobic glycolysis, 18, 19
Anal agenesis, 1274
Anal membrane atresia, 1274
Anal sphincter, 1190
Anal stenosis, congenital, 1274
Anaphase, 30
Anaphylatoxin, 223
Anaphylaxis, 252, 268, 979-980
  eosinophil chemotactic factor of, 221, 233
  slow-reacting substances of, 221
Anaplasia, 295
Anastomosis, 242, 1230
Androgen replacement therapy, 673
Androgen-secreting tumor, 633
Androgens, 586, 657, 665-666
  carcinogenesis and, 333
  hypersecretion of, 633
Anemia, 784-796
  aplastic, 791-792
    childhood cancers and, 318
  cancer and, 306-307
  child and, 318, 830-834, 836, 841
  of chronic disease, 794-796
  classification of, 784-785
  clinical manifestations of, 785-788
  Cooley, 841
  Fanconi, 318
  folate deficiency, 789
  gastrectomy and, 1231
  hemolytic, 170, 173, 792-794
    autoimmune, 251, 792
    congenital, 835
    drug-induced, 173
    prosthetic heart valve and, 786
  hypochromic-microcytic, 786
  of infectious disease, 834
  iron deficiency, 786, 789-790, 830-834
    history of, 789
  laboratory findings for, 787
  leukemia and, 806
  macrocytic, 786
  macrocytic-normochromic, 785, 788-789
  microangiopathic, 786

Anemia—cont'd
  microcytic-hypochromic, 785, 789-791
  normocytic-normochromic, 785, 791-796
  pernicious, 251, 786, 788-789
    history of, 753
  posthemorrhagic, 792
  sickle cell, 786, 836
  sideroblastic, 786, 790-791
Anencephaly, 535, 536, 538
Aneuploidy, 126-128
  autosomal, 128-129
  sex chromosome, 129-131
Aneurysm, 927-930
  intracranial, 494-497
  myocardial infarction and ventricular, 946
  types of, 929
Angiitis, 1415
Angina pectoris, 939
Angiogenesis, 302
Angiography
  cerebral, 385
  coronary, 907, 940
Angioma, 500
Angioneurotic edema, 229
Angioplasty, percutaneous transluminal
    coronary, 941
Angiotensin, 88, 584, 896
  renal blood flow and, 1121
Angiotensin inhibitors, 926
Angular stomatitis, 790
Angulation, fracture, 1322
Anion gap, 106
Anions, 19
Aniridia, 318
Anisocytosis, 785
Anistropy, 875
Ankylosing spondylitis, 251, 1346-1347
Anomalous viscosity, 890
Anomia, 468
Anomic dysphasia, 467
Anorectal gonorrhea, 728
Anorectal lymphogranuloma venereum, 738
Anorectal malformations, 1273-1274
Anorectal stenosis, 1274
Anorexia, 1214
  cancer and, 306
  leukemia and, 804, 807
Anorexia nervosa, 1237
Anosmia, 422
Anosognosia, 462
Anovulation, 680, 681
Anoxia, 52
Antacids, 1220
  constipation and, 1215
Antagonist, muscle, 1314
Anterior cerebral artery, 495
Anterior chamber, 415
Anterior fossa, 366
Anterior horn cell, 459
Anterior-inferior cerebellar artery, 495
Anterior interventricular artery, 868
Anterior midline defects, 535, 536
Anterior pituitary
  aging and, 589
  diseases of, 599-603
  hormones of, 571, 574
  menstrual cycle and, 659
Anterior-posterior diameter of thorax, 1037
Anterior spinal arteries, 371
Anti-tumor immune rejection response, 310
Antibiotics
  AIDS and, 274
  cancer and, 309

Antibody, 191, 202-207
  ABO blood group and, 200
  antisperm, 670
  blocking, 255, 343
  cortisol and, 285
  function of, 205
  hemorrhagic disease mediated by, 845-847
  maternal, 212-213
    hemolytic disease in newborn and, 832
  molecular structure of, 203
  monoclonal, 207
    cancer treatment and, 312-316
  plasma cells and, 757
  primary and secondary immune responses
    and, 194
  tests of production of, 275
  viral hepatitis and, 1245
Antibody binding, 257
Antibody-dependent, cell-mediated
    cytotoxicity, 256-257, 341, 342
Antibody marker, reproductive function and,
    668, 669
Antibody screen, 778
Anticholinergics, 523
Anticoagulant, circulating, 779
Anticodon, 122, 123
Antidiuretic hormone, 87, 573-574
  elevated, 597
  heart failure and, 973
  renal failure and, 1155
  syndrome of inappropriate secretion of,
    92, 597-598
  tumor cell markers and, 300
  urine and, 1127-1128
Antigen, 193, 194, 196-198
  A, 200
  B, 200
  blood group, 198-200
  carcinoembryonic, 330, 339, 1258
  cytoplasmic organelles and, 6
  foreign, 261
  histocompatibility; *see* Histocompatibility
    antigens
  immunotherapy and, 310
  leukemia, 848
  oncofetal, 339
  sequestered, 261
  tolergenic, 197
  tumor, 300, 301, 311-312, 337-338,
    340-343
  tumor-specific transplantation, 337-338
  viral, 338-339
Antigen-antibody complex, 205, 206, 223
  reproductive function and, 668, 669
Antigen-binding fragments, 202
Antigen processing, 211
Antigen receptors, 16
Antigenic compatibility, 193
Antigenic determinant, 197, 200, 205,
    209-210
Antigenic modulation, 342
Antiglobulin test, direct, 778
Antigravity posture, 452
Antihemophilic factor, 774
Antimetabolites, 309
Antiport, 22
Antipyretics, endogenous, 405
Antisperm antibody, 670
Antistreptolysin O antibody titer, 959
Antithyroid drugs, 604
Antitoxin, 191
α_1-Antitrypsin, 231, 1074
Antrectomy, 1230

Antrum of stomach, 1178
Anus, gonococcal infection of, 728
Anvil, 419
Anxiety, 392
Anxiety attacks, dream, 412
Aorta, 864
  aneurysm of abdominal, 927, 928
  coarctation of, 1001-1003
  hypertension and, 925
Aortic regurgitation, 955, 956-957
Aortic semilunar valve, 864
Aortic stenosis, 954-955
Aortic valve calcification, 70
Aphasia, 464
Aplastic anemia, 791-792
  childhood cancers and, 318
Aplastic crisis, 840
Apnea, 1054
  posthyperventilation, 434, 435
  sleep, 411
  sudden infant death syndrome and,
    1100
Apneusis, 435
Apoproteins, 55
Apoptosis, 72-73
Appendicitis, 1235, 1258
Appendicular skeleton, 1296
  development of, 1362
Apudoma, 1261
Aqueduct of Sylvius, 367
Aqueous humor, 415
Arachnoid membrane, 366
Arachnoid villi, 367
Arachnoiditis, inflammatory, 520
Arcuate artery, 1116
Areflexia, 458
Arenaviruses, 61
Areola, 666
Areolar connective tissue, loose, 37
Arginine vasopressin, 405
Armed macrophages, 342
Arnold-Chiari malformation, 538
Arousal
  level of, 432
  night terrors and, 412
  partial, 412
Arrhenoblastoma, 297
Arrhythmia, 174, 963
  sinus, 964
Arterial baroreceptor, 893
Arterial blood gases, 1049
  carbon dioxide and, 433-434
  oxygen and, 1045-1046
    hemoglobin concentration and, 1046
Arterial blood vessels, 886-889
Arterial chemoreceptors, 894
Arterial hypertension, 156
Arterial plasma components, 756
Arterial pressure, 895-896
Arterial pulse waveforms, 904
Arteries, 860, 884, 886
  brain and, 369
  collateral, 868
  diseases of, 917-947
    aneurysm and, 927-930
    arteriosclerosis and, 917
    atherosclerosis and, 917-920
    coronary artery disease and, 934-938
    embolism and, 930-931
    hypertension and, 920-926
    myocardial infarction and, 942-947
    myocardial ischemia and, 938-942
    orthostatic hypotension and, 927

Arteries—cont'd
  diseases of—cont'd
    peripheral arterial disease and,
      931-932
      thrombus formation and, 930
    lower extremity, hypertension and, 925
    narrowing of, 52
Arteriography, 907
Arteriole, 886
Arteriosclerosis, 52, 917
  thrombotic stroke and, 493
Arteriovenous malformation, 497
Arthritis, 1341-1350
  gouty, 1347, 1349
  rheumatoid, 251, 1342-1346
    diagnostic criteria for, 1346
    juvenile, 1373
    pathogenesis of, 1343
  secondary suppurative, 1371
Arthropathy, 1339
Arthropod-borne encephalitis, 508
Arthroscopy, 1314
Arthus reaction, 258
Articular capsule, 1300
Articular cartilage, 1301-1302
Articulation, joint, 1298
Aryl sulfatase B, 221
Arytenoid, 1027
Asbestosis, 1067
Ascending colon, 1190
Ascites, 1240, 1241-1242
Ascorbic acid
  collagen synthesis and, 244
  erythropoiesis and, 767
Aseptic meningitis, 505-506
Aspartate aminotransferase, 944
Aspergillus fumigatus, 254
Asphyxia, cerebral palsy and, 543
Asphyxiants, toxic, 56
Aspiration, 1060
Aspirin
  portal hypertension and, 1284
  Reye syndrome and, 548
Association fibers, 360
Astereognosia, 462
Asterixis, 454
Asthma, 1069-1071
  child and, 1101-1102
  genetics and, 169, 171
  immunity and, 255
Astigmatism, 417
Astrocytes, 355
Astrocytoma, 500, 501-502, 553, 555
  cerebellar, 555
  cerebral, 555
Asymmetric septal hypertrophy, 953
Asystole, 965
Ataxia-telangiectasia, 318
Ataxic breathing, 435
Atelectasis, 1060
  respiratory distress syndrome of newborn
    and, 1104
Atherogenesis, 919
Atherosclerosis, 917-920
  coronary, 907
  diabetes mellitus and, 627
  hypoxic injury and, 53, 55
  myocardial ischemia and, 938
  progression of, 918
Athetosis, 453
Atmospheric pressure, 1034
  cellular injury and, 63
Atomic bomb exposure, 331-332, 848

Atonic seizure, 450
Atopic dermatitis, 255, 260, 1402-1403
  child and, 1439-1440
Atrial contractions, premature, 963
Atrial fibrillation, 964
Atrial flutter, 964
Atrial natriuretic hormone, 1129
Atrial septal defect, 1006-1007
Atrial tachycardia, 964
Atrioventricular bundle electrocardiography,
  905-906
Atrioventricular dissociation, 966
Atrioventricular node, 870
Atrioventricular valve, 864
  cusp of, 864
Atrium, 862
Atrophic gastritis, 1224
Atrophy, 451
  aging and, 74
  cellular adaptation and, 50
  disuse, 1351-1352
  progressive spinal muscular, 460
  skin, 1398
  thymic, 214
Attentional dementia, 443
Atypical hyperplasia, 51
Auditory agnosia, 462
Auditory canal, external, 419
Auditory changes in aging, 420
Auditory dysfunction, 420
Auerbach plexus of stomach, 1178
Aura, 447
  seizure and, 448
Auscultation of heart sounds, 901-902
Australian antigen, 1247
Autoantibodies, 252
Autodigestion, 9, 70
Autoimmune adrenalitis, 634
Autoimmune diseases, 170, 250-251, 263
Autoimmune hemolytic anemia, 251, 792
Autoimmune purpura, 846-847
  thrombocytopenic, 251
Autoimmune thyroiditis, 250, 608
Autoimmunity, 250-251, 261-262
Autolysis, 70
Autolysosomes, 9
Autolyzed brain, 440
Automatic cells, 873
Automaticity, heart and, 873
Automobile accidents, 477
Autonomic hyperreflexia, 486-488
Autonomic nervous system, 353, 372-380
  allergic response and, 253
  coronary circulation and, 898
  functions of, 378-380
  immune system and, 288
  lung and, 1040-1042
Autophagic vacuoles, 50
Autophagy, 9
Autoprothrombin, 774
Autoregulation
  coronary circulation and, 898
  hypertension and, 922
  intracranial pressure and, 468
  kidney and, 1119-1120
Autosomal aneuploidy, 128-129
Autosomal dominant inheritance, 134-137
Autosomal recessive inheritance, 137-139
Autosomes, 124
Autotopagnosia, 462
Avascular diseases of bone, 1373-1376
Avulsion, 520
  tendon and, 1325

Axial skeleton, 1296
  development of, 1362
  malformations of, 538-541
Axon, 43, 353, 365
  degeneration of, 520
  of motor nerve, 1306
  myelin sheath and, 533
  neuropathy and, 461
Axon hillock, 353
Azidothymidine, 274
Azotemia, 1150, 1151, 1153

B

B antigen, 200
B cells, 193, 195, 200-202, 211
  acquired immune deficiency and, 268
  cancer treatment and, 314
  carcinogenesis and, 341
  cellular interactions and, 211
  cortisol and, 285
  dermatomyositis and, 1354
  immune deficiency and, 265, 268
  immune system and, 288
  immunity and, 193, 195, 200-202,
    211
  infection of, 802
  multiple myeloma and, 809
  protein accumulations in, 68
  rheumatoid arthritis and, 1342
  steroid receptors and, 288
  tests of numbers of, 275
B-endorphins, 286
B peptide, 580
Bachmann bundle, 870
Bacillus Calmette-Guérin vaccine, 311
Back pain, 399
  low, 489-491
Bacteremia, 59
Bacteria, 3
  conjunctivitis and, 413
  embolism and, 931
  endocarditis and, 931, 962
  gastroenteritis and, 1281
  immunotherapy and, 310
  infectious injury and, 58-59
  intestinal, 1192-1193
  macrophages and, 233
  meningitis and, 505
    child with, 549-551
  myositis and, 1354-1355
  opsonization of, 206
  pneumonia and
    child with, 1102
    pathophysiology of, 1078
  prostatitis and, 708-709
  sexually transmitted urogenital infections
    and, 727-736
  skin and, 1411, 1440-1441
  vaginosis and, 735-736
Bacterial plasmids, 118
Bacterial toxins, neutralization of, 204,
  205-206
Bacteroides species, 59
Bainbridge reflex, 882
Balanitis, 663, 700, 701, 1415
Ball valving in air trapping, 1073
Ballism, 453
Balloon pump, intra-aortic, 975
Balloon septostomy, 1010
Balloon-tipped catheter, 930
Baltimore Longitudinal Study on Aging,
  907-908
Band, 759

Barium studies
  cardiovascular function and, 905
  esophageal function and, 1219, 1220
Barometric pressure, 1034
Baroreceptors, 87, 882, 893-894
Barr bodies, 125
Bartholin glands, 650
  chlamydial infection of, 738
  inflammation of, 687
    gonorrhea and, 728
Bartter syndrome, 633
Basal body, 12
Basal body temperature
  menstrual cycle and, 660
  reproductive function test and, 670
Basal cell carcinoma, 296, 1419
  ultraviolet radiation and, 330
Basal ganglia, 359, 360
  Huntington disease and, 513
  Parkinson disease and, 509, 510, 513
Basal ganglia motor syndromes, 457-458
Basal layer of skin, 1392
Basal metabolic rate, 980, 981
  cancer and, 306
Basal plate, 533
Base pair substitution mutation, 121
Basement membrane, 37, 1308
  diabetes mellitus and, 624
Bases, 109-110; *see also* Alkalosis
Basilar artery, 368
Basilar skull fracture, 483
Basophil, 220, 757, 760
  hypersensitivity and, 253
  stippling of, 786, 801
Basophil count, 778
Basophilia, 786, 801
BAT gene, 180-182
Battle sign, 483
Becker muscular dystrophy, 1378
Beckwith-Wiedemann syndrome, 318
Bedbugs, 1448
Bedwetting, 412, 1168-1169
Bee venom, 254
Beef insulin, 616
Behavior
  carcinogenesis and, 326-329
  pain and, 399
Bell phenomenon, 437
Bellini, duct of, 1118
Bence Jones protein, 810
Bends, 63
Benign breast disorders, 714
Benign febrile seizure, 547
Benign ovarian cysts, 690
Benign prostatic hyperplasia, 707
Benign tumors, 294, 296
  skin and, 1417-1418
Benzene, 848
Benzo
  pyrene, 293, 328
Beriberi, 976
Berry aneurysm, 494
Beta-adrenergic blocking agents, 941
Beta cells, 578
Beta receptors, 378
Beta-thalassemia, 841
Bicarbonate, 88, 107
  carbonic acid and, 102
  pancreas and, 1201, 1202
  saliva and, 1176
  urine and, 1124-1125
Biceps, 1314
Bilateral adrenalectomy, 635

Bilateral renal agenesis, 1163
Bile, 1195-1197, 1253
  obstruction of flow of, 1249
Bile acid pool, 1196
Bile acid–dependent fraction, 1196
Bile canaliculi, 1195
Bile salts, 1195
  deficiency of, 1231-1232
Biliary atresia, 1282
Biliary cirrhosis, 1249, 1252
  primary, 251
Biliary colic, 1253
Biliary metabolism, disorders of, 1282
Biliary transport, disorders of, 1282
Bilirubin, 69, 1197-1198
  child and, 1282
  conjugated, 1198
  hemolytic disease in newborn and, 834
  metabolism of, 770, 1197
    liver and, 1205
  unconjugated, 1198
Billroth operation, 1230
Binding proteins, 566
Binge eating, 1237
Bioassay, 588
Biologic exposure, familial diseases and,
  162
Biologic response modifiers, 310
Biological response modifiers, 310
Biopsy
  bone marrow, 776-777
    anemia and, 791
  chorionic villi, 127
  endometrial, 670
  muscle, 1353
  reproductive function test and, 669
Bipolar neurons, 355
Birth control pills
  carcinogenesis and, 332
  history of, 645
Birth defects, 168
Bites, insect, 1446-1448
Biventricular heart failure, 972
Black fly, 1417
Black lung, 1066-1067
Blackhead, 1399
Bladder, 1118-1119
  acute bacterial prostatitis and, 708
  carcinogenesis and, 327
  carcinoma staging and, 1141
  control of, 1168
  distended
    benign prostatic hyperplasia and, 707
    spinal cord injury and, 488
  exstrophy of, 1163
  inflammation of, 1141-1142
  irritable, 1142
  male urinary, 1118
  multiple sclerosis and dysfunction of, 516
  neurogenic, 1138, 1139
  rhabdomyosarcoma and, 1384
  tumor of, 1139-1141
Bladder stones, history of, 1111
Blast cell, 317, 803, 850
Blast injury, 63
Bleb, 1062-1063
Bleeder syndrome, 140
Bleeding
  cerebral palsy and, 543
  cerebrovascular disorders and, 482, 493,
    494, 498
  disorders of
    antibody-mediated, 845-847

Bleeding—cont'd
  disorders of—cont'd
    inherited, 842-845
    manifestations of, 817
  dysfunctional uterine, 682-683
  epidural, 480
  hemoproteins and, 69
  hypertensive, 494
  intracerebral, 482, 498
  iron deficiency anemia and, 792, 831
  leukemia and, 806
  menstrual, 657
  occult, 831
  subarachnoid, 366, 497-498
  tumors and, 307
Bleeding time, 778
Bleomycin, 309
Blepharitis, 413
Blindness
  color, 418
  ipsilateral, 418
  word, 462
Blister, fever, 1411
Blocking antibody, 255, 343
Blood
  ancient Greeks and, 753
  cellular components of, 757-760
  composition of, 755-760
  history of study of, 857
  pleural effusion and, 1064
  postnatal changes in, 826-829
Blood-brain barrier, 370-371
Blood cells, 759
  development of, 763-771
  pathways of differentiation of, 764
  plasma, 202
  red; *see* Red blood cells
  white; *see* White blood cells
Blood circulation; *see* Circulation
Blood clot, 772-773
  lysis of, 776
Blood clotting, liver and, 1205
Blood flow, 890-895; *see also* Blood supply
  cardiac cycle and, 864-865
  renal, 1119-1121, 1130
Blood gases
  arterial; *see* Arterial blood gases
  mixed venous, 1049
Blood glucose, 615
Blood group antigens, 198-200
Blood loss; *see* Bleeding
Blood pressure, 895-897
  child and, 1018, 1019-1021
  familial diseases and, 178
  high; *see* Hypertension
Blood smears, normal, 786
Blood sucker, 1417
Blood supply; *see also* Blood flow
  brain and, 368-370
  central nervous system and, 368-371
  reduced, 52
  skin and, 1393
  spinal cord and, 371
Blood tests, 777-780
  renal function and, 1130
Blood transfusions; *see* Transfusions
Blood urea nitrogen, 1130
Blood velocity, 894
Blood vessels, 886-898
  arterial, 886-889
  blood flow and; *see* Blood flow
  blood pressure and; *see* Blood pressure
  coronary circulation and, 897-898

Blood vessels—cont'd
  of kidney, 1116-1117
  lumen of, 886
  tumors of, 500
  veins and, 889
Bloom syndrome, 318
Blunt trauma, 478
BMR; *see* Basal metabolic rate
Body of stomach, 1178
Body fluids, distribution of, 83-85
Body image agnosia, 462
Body louse, 1447
Body temperature, 400-408
  menstrual cycle and, 660
  reproductive function test and, 670
  somatic death and, 76
Body water, total, 83
Bohr effect, 1047
Boils, 1411
Bomb exposure, 331-332, 848
Bone, 40
  albumin and, 1295
  avascular disease of, 1373-1376
  carcinogenesis and, 327
  characteristics of, 1296-1297
  disorders of, 1328-1339
    infectious, 1332-1334
    metabolic, 1328-1332
    osteomalacia and, 1330
    osteomyelitis and, 1332-1334
    osteoporosis and, 1328-1330
    Paget disease and, 1331-1332
    renal failure and, 1155, 1156
    tumors and, 1334-1339
  endochondral formation in, 1361
  erosion of, 1315
  formation of, 1361-1362
  fracture types and, 1320
  function tests and, 1314
  growth of, 1362
  healing of, 1323
  infection of, 1370-1373
  leukemia and, 849-850
  loss of mass of, after menopause, 672
  maintenance of integrity of, 1297-1298
  matrix of, 1293, 1294-1295
  metastasis to, 305
  minerals and, 1295
  ossification centers in, 1361
  pain in, 807
  structure and function of, 1292-1298
  tissue types of, 1293, 1295-1296
Bone cells, 1293-1295
Bone marrow, 764
  aplasia of, 791
  aspiration of, 776-777
  biopsy of, 776-777
    anemia and, 791
  function tests and, 776-777
  hypoplasia of, 791
  radiation of, 308
  red, 1296
  stem cells and, 266
  transplantation of, 275
  tumors and, 307
Bone tumors, 317, 1334-1339, 1380-1382
  bone destruction in, 1335
  derivation of, 1334
  types of, 1335-1339
Botryoides subclass of rhabdomyosarcoma, 1383
Botulism, 521-522
Bowel diseases, inflammatory, 179

Bowen disease, 700, 701
  squamous cell carcinoma and, 1420
Bowing fracture, 1321
Bowman capsule, 1113
Bowman space, 1113
Brachial plexus, 372
Brachycephaly, 539
Bradycardia
  hyperkalemia and, 97
  junctional, 964
  sinus, 963
  ventricular, 965
Bradykinesia, 452, 512
Bradykinin, 225, 227
Brain
  abscess of, 506
  autolyzed, 440
  blood supply to, 368-370
  carcinogenesis and, 327
  cardiovascular control centers in, 881-882
  hypertension and, 925
  injury to, 477
  meninges of, 366
  pain and, 394
Brain death, 77, 437-440
Brain scan, 385
Brain tumor, 317, 500
  metastatic, 504
  pain and, 305
  types of, 552-555
Brainstem, 456
  breathing patterns and, 435
  glioma of, 553, 554, 555
  injury to, 436
  multiple sclerosis and, 516
  neurilemmoma and, 504
  supratentorial mass lesions and, 434
Brainstem syndromes, 459, 516
Breast
  disorders of, 711-719
    benign, 712, 713, 714
    carcinoma in; *see* Breast carcinoma
    proliferative, 713
  estrogen and, 657
  female, 666-668
    disorders of, 711-717
    lymphatic drainage of, 667
  growth of, 668
  lymphoid tissue and, 208
  male, 668
    disorders of, 717-719
  menopause and, 671
  menstrual cycle and, 668
  progesterone and, 657
  structure and function of, 666-668
Breast carcinoma, 715-719
  carcinogenesis and, 327, 333
  clinical manifestations of, 718
  estrogens and, 333
  familial diseases and, 169, 171-172
  male, 719
  progesterone and, 333
  staging of, 719
  tumor biology and, 301
  types of, 716
Breathing
  abnormal pattern of, 1055
  consciousness and pattern of, 433-435
  intermittent positive pressure, 1073
  mechanics of, 1037
  pattern of, 433-435
  work of, 1040

Brenner tumor, 297
Brittle bone disease, 1367-1368
Broca dysphasia, 466
Broca speech area, 360
Brodie abscess, 1334
Bromocriptine, 712
Bronchi, 1029
  adenoma of, 1088-1090
  circulation of, 1031-1034
  metaplasia and, 52
Bronchial-associated lymphoid tissue, 208
Bronchial asthma, 1070
Bronchiectasis, 1060-1061
Bronchiole, 1030
  terminal, 1032
Bronchiolitis, 1062
  child and, 1103-1104
Bronchiolitis obliterans, 1103-1104
Bronchitis, 1080
  acute, 1080
  child and, 1103
  chronic, 1070, 1072-1074
    pathogenesis of, 1072
Bronchoconstriction, 228
Bronchogenic carcinoma, 296, 1085-1090
Bronchopneumonia, 1078
Bronchopulmonary dysplasia, 1106
Bronchospasm, 1069
Brown adipose tissue, 180, 182, 402, 1236
Brudzinski sign, 498, 551
Bruise, 817
  hemoproteins and, 69
Brush border of small intestine, 1184
Bruton agammaglobulinemia, 267
Bubo, 735, 738
Buerger disease, 931-932
Buffering, acid-base balance and, 101-104
Bulbar myasthenia, 522
Bulbar palsy, 456, 460
Bulimarexia, 1238
Bulimia, 1237-1238
Bulla, 1396
Bullous impetigo, 1440-1441
Bullous pemphigoid, 250, 1410
Bumetanide, 1128
Bundle of His, 870
Bundle branch, 870
Burkitt lymphoma, 338-339, 815-816
  Epstein-Barr virus and, 319
Burn, 1423-1431
  American Burn Association classification
    of, 1423
  cellular response to, 1429-1431
  depth of, 1424
  keloid and, 1400-1401
  thermal, 408
    acquired immune deficiency and, 269
Burn blister, 63
Burn shock, 1426-1429
Burr cells, 1166
Burrow skin lesion, 1399
Burrow solution, 1403
Bursa of Fabricius, 191, 200
Bursal equivalent, 200
Bursitis, 1326
Burton disease, 318
Bypass graft, coronary artery, 941-942

C

C cells, 575
C1 esterase inhibitor, 228-229
C neurons, 395
c-onc, 335

C peptide, 580
C protein, 1310
c-src, 336
C wave, 865
Cachexia, 306
Café-au-lait patches, 137
Caisson disease, 63
Calcaneovalgus, 1366
Calcaneovarus, 1366
Calcaneus, 1366
Calcification
  bones and, 1294
  dystrophic, 69-70
  metastatic, 70
Calcitonin, 98, 575, 576
Calcium; *see also* Calcium ions
  bones and, 1295
  cellular environment and, 92-100
  hormones and, 98, 570
  hypertension and, 177
  injury and
    cellular, 69-70
    hypoxic, 55
  kidney function and, 1129
  menopause and, 672
  metabolism of, 578
  muscle contraction and, 1312
    myocardial, 878
  myocardial ischemia and, 941
  osteoporosis and, 1328
  renal failure and, 1155-1156
  renal stones and, 1137, 1138
  small intestine and, 1188-1189
  tumor cell markers and, 300
Calcium-calmodulin, 570
Calcium gluconate, 97
Calcium ions, 774; *see also* Calcium
  mitochondria and, 10
Calcium-protein complex, 1188-1189
Calculi, 1137
  staghorn, 1137-1138
Calices, 1113
California virus encephalitis, 508
Callosal dyspraxia, 463
Callus, 1298
  formation of, 51
  osteogenesis imperfecta and, 1368
Caloric ice water test, 439
Caloric intake
  acquired immunodeficiency syndrome and,
    268
  dietary, 182
  excessive, 1236-1237
  renal failure and, 1156-1158
Calymmatobacterium granulomatis, 735
Calyx, major or minor, 1113
Campylobacter, 745-746
Canaliculae, 1295
Cancellous bone, 1295
Cancer, 292-347; *see also* Carcinoma
  age and sites of, 301
  carcinogenesis in; *see* Carcinogenesis
  in child, 316-320
  clinical manifestations of, 305-308
  immune mechanisms and, 340-342
  immunobiology of, 337-343
  immunodeficiency and risk of, 339
  immunotherapy and, 314, 315
  monoclonal antibodies and, 314, 315
  therapy for, 308-316
    site-specific, 308
  tumor biology and, 293-322; *see also*
    Tumor biology

Cancer cells
  autonomy and, 295
  cell surface changes in, 299
  characteristics of, 295-301
  fused, 314
  hybridized, 314
Cancer tests, reproductive function and,
  668-669
Candidiasis, 268, 1414
  chronic mucocutaneous, 268
  diaper dermatitis and, 1440
  skin and, 1414-1415
  thrush in child and, 1443
  vaginitis and, 686, 687
Capillaries, 860, 886
  coronary, 868
Capillary basement membrane, 624
Capillary blood glucose, 615
Capillary flow, 896
Capillary net filtration forces, 85
Capillary network, 888
Caplan syndrome, 1345
Captopril, 926
Caput medusae, 1241
Caput succedaneum, 543
Carbohydrates
  acid-base balance and, 101
  cellular injury and, 66-67
  hypertriglyceridemia induced by, 935
  liver and, 1198
  metabolism of
    cancer and, 306
    cortisol and, 286
  plasma membranes and, 13, 14
  small intestine and, 1186-1187
Carbon dioxide, 1037
  arterial, 433-434
  respiratory acidosis and, 108
  transport of, 1047-1048
Carbon monoxide, 56, 57
Carbon tetrachloride poisoning, 54, 55
Carbonic acid, 101
  bicarbonate and, 102
Carbonic anhydrase inhibitors, 1128
Carboxyhemoglobin, 56
Carboxypeptidase, 1187
Carbuncle, 1411
Carcinoembryonic antigen, 300, 339, 1258
Carcinogenesis, 301, 324-347
  history of study of, 293
  indirect and direct-acting agents in, 328
  ionizing radiation and, 332
  prenatal exposure to, 319
  theories of, 324-347
    carcinogenic pathogens and, 333-337
    immunobiology of cancer and, 337-343
    multistage theory and, 324-333
    viral, 337
Carcinoma, 295, 296, 297; *see also* Cancer
  of accessory organs of digestion,
    1259-1261
  basal cell, 1419
    ultraviolet radiation and, 330
  bladder, staging of, 1141
  breast; *see* Breast carcinoma
  bronchogenic; *see* Lung cancer
  cervical, 693-696
    carcinogenesis of, 329
    FIGO staging of, 694
  cholangiocellular, 1259, 1260
  colon, 327, 1257-1259
    familial diseases and, 155, 169, 172-173
  of digestive system, 1255-1261

Carcinoma—cont'd
  endometrial, 696-697
  of esophagus, 1255-1256
  familial diseases and, 171-173
  female reproductive system and, 693-699
  of gallbladder, 1259, 1260
  of gastrointestinal tract, 1255-1261
  hepatocellular, 1259
  in situ, 295
    cervical, 693
    penile, 700, 701
  laryngeal, 1084-1085
  lip, 1083-1084
  liver, 1259-1260
  metastatic, to brain, 504
  nasopharyngeal, 338-339
  oral, 326
  ovarian, 697-699
    FIGO staging of, 698
  pain and, 400
  of pancreas, 1260-1261
  papillary, of renal pelvis, 1140
  penile, 700-701
  prostate, 332, 333, 709-710
  rectal, 327, 1257-1259; *see also*
    Carcinoma, colon
  renal cell, 1139
    lymphokines and, 312
    staging of, 1140
  scrotal, 293
  skin, 68, 155, 1418-1423
    trends for, 1418
  squamous cell, 1419-1420
    lung and, 1087
    ultraviolet radiation and, 330
  of stomach, 327, 1256-1257
  of testis, 704-705
  thyroid, 608-609
  vaginal, 696
Cardiac action potential, 868-869,
    871-873
Cardiac catheterization, 906-907
Cardiac cycle
  blood flow during, 864-865
  phases of, 866
Cardiac dysrhythmia, 162
Cardiac excitation, 869, 870-871
Cardiac function
  assessment of
    invasive, 905-907
    noninvasive, 901-905
  combined indicators of, 907
Cardiac index, 906
Cardiac innervation, 873-874
Cardiac metabolism, 866-867
Cardiac muscle, 42, 875
Cardiac orifice, 1177
Cardiac output, 883, 906
  arterial pressure and, 896
Cardiac performance, 879-886
  exercise, 908
  resting, 907-908
Cardiac plexus, 873
Cardiac septa, development of, 994
Cardiac vein, 866
Cardioexcitatory center, 881
Cardiogenic shock, 976-977
Cardiography, 902
Cardioinhibitory center, 881
Cardiomyopathy, 251, 950-953
  congestive, 951-952
  hypertrophic, 953
  morphologic characteristics of, 950

Cardiomyopathy—cont'd
  pathophysiology of, 952
  restrictive, 953
Cardiovascular control centers in brain,
    881-882
Cardiovascular function alterations, 916-991
  aneurysm and, 927-930
  arteriosclerosis and, 917
  atherosclerosis and, 917-920
  burn injury and, 1427-1429
  cardiomyopathy and, 950-953
  child and, 992-1023
    acquired disorders in, 1015-1019, 1020,
      1021
    congenital heart defects in, 996-1015;
      see also Congenital heart defects
  coronary artery disease and, 934-938
  diabetes mellitus and, 626-627
  dysrhythmia and, 963
  embolism and, 930-931
  endocardial disorders and, 953-962
  familial diseases and, 173-178
  heart failure and, 963-976; *see also* Heart
    failure
    child with, 1015-1017
  hypertension and, 920-926
    child with primary, 1017-1021
    child with secondary, 1017
  hypothyroidism and, 606
  myocardial infarction and, 942-947
  myocardial ischemia and, 938-942
  orthostatic hypotension and, 926-927
  pericardial disorders and, 947-951
  peripheral arterial disease and, 931-932
  rheumatic heart disease and, 1017
  shock and, 976-984
  stress-related, 287
  thrombus formation and, 930
  uremia and, 1157
  venous diseases and, 932-933
Cardiovascular system; *see also* Cardiovascular
    function alterations
  autonomic innervation of, 874
  development of, 993-996
  structure and function of, 859-915
    aging and, 907-908
    circulatory system and, 860
    heart and, 860-886; *see also* Heart
    systemic circulation and, 886-898; *see
      also* Systemic circulation
  tests of function of, 901-907
Carditis, 958
  acute rheumatic fever and, 959
Carina, 1029
Carnitine palmityl transferase, 1354
Carotenoid pigments, 69
Carotid arteries, internal, 368
Carriers, 134, 138
Cartilage
  articular, 1301-1302
  degenerative joint disease and, 1339
  development of, 1361
  elastic, 40
  fibrous, 40
  hyaline, 40, 1298
Cartilage cell, 1301
Cartilage-forming tumor, 1337
Cartilaginous joints, 1298
Caseous necrosis, 71
Cast, urinalysis and, 1131
Catabolism, 16, 18
Cataract, 416
Catastrophic theory of aging, 74, 75

Catecholamines, 586
  myocardial infarction and, 943
  pheochromocytoma and, 636
  stress response and, 283-284
Catheter
  balloon-tipped, 930
  cardiac, 857, 906-907
  cerebral angiography and, 385
Cation pump, 835
Cations, 19
Cat's eye reflex, 558
Cauda equina, 362
Causal risk factors, 159, 160, 162
Causalgia, 399
Cavernous hemangioma, 1448
Cavernous sinus, 368
Cavitation, lung, 1065
Cavus foot abnormality, 1366
CD4 antigen, 272-273
cDNA, 119
Cecum, 1190
Celiac disease, 251
Celiac ganglia, 377
Celiac sprue, 179, 1277
Cell, 2-113
  adaptation of, 49-51
  aging of, 75-76
  alpha, 578
  aneuploid, 126
  anterior horn, 459
  automatic, 873
  B; *see* B cells
  beta, 578
  blast, 803, 850
  blood; *see* Blood cells
  body of, 353
  bone marrow stem, 266
  burr, 1166
  C, 575
  cancer, 295-301
    cell surface changes in, 299
    hybridized, 314
  cartilage, 1301
  cellular biology and, 4-47; *see also* Cellular
    biology
    altered, 48-81; *see also* Cellular and
      tissue biology alterations
  chief, 1180
  clue, 736
  columnar, 35, 36, 37, 51, 52
  cuboidal, 35, 37
  cytotoxic, 209
  daughter, 132, 771
  death of, 48-49
    cellular and tissue biology and, 70-73
    inflammation and, 239
    myocardial infarction and, 943-944
  delta, 578
  diploid, 124
  division rates of, 30-31
  effector, 310
  ependymal, 355, 356
  epithelioid, 238
  euploid, 126
  F, 578
  fluids and electrolytes, acids and bases
    and, 82-113; *see also* Cellular
    environment
  fusion of, 145
  G, 1181
  gastrin-secreting, 1181
  giant, 238
  goblet, 1030

Cell—cont'd
granulosa, 655
hair, 419
haploid, 124
helper, 209
host, 59
hybrid, 144
hybridoma, 314
immunocompetent, 193
intake and output and, 19-28
junctions of, 32-33
K, 342
killer, 342
Kupffer, 769, 1195, 1198
Langerhans, 1392
Leydig, 661
liver
    carbon tetrachloride and, 55
    chemical injury of, 54, 55
    fatty change and, 67
lymphokine-producing, 209
mast, 220-222
    inflammation and, 218
mastoid air, 419
memory, 193, 202, 209, 310
Merkel, 1392
mesangial, 1113
mouse tumor, 144, 145, 314
myocardial, 874-876, 938-939
natural killer, 342
neuroglial, 353
null, 848
P, 870
parafollicular, 575
parietal, 1179-1180
plasma, 194
polyploid, 126
responder, 199
S, 1202
Schwann, 353, 356, 533
secretin-producing, 1202
Sertoli, 665
sickle, 836-841
somatic, 124
sperm, 646, 665
spleen, 314
squamous, 33, 34, 37, 51, 52
stem, 763-764
Sternberg-Reed, 812
stimulator, 199
synovial, 1300
T; see T cells
target, 568, 786
Tc, 209, 342
Th, 209
theca, 655
Ts, 209
Cell cycle, 28-31
Cell-derived proteins in immunotherapy, 311
Cell-mediated cytotoxicity, 337, 341, 342
    hypersensitivity and, 258-260
Cell-mediated immunity, 195-196, 209
Cell theory, 3
Cell transformation, oncogenic viruses and, 334
Cellular accumulations, 66
Cellular and tissue biology alterations, 48-81
    aging and, 73-77
        nervous system and, 382
    cellular adaptation and, 49-51
    cellular death and, 70-73
    cellular injury and, 51-66; see also Cellular injury

Cellular and tissue biology alterations—cont'd
    manifestations of cellular injury and, 66-70
    somatic death and, 76-77
Cellular biology, 4-47
    cell components in, 5-16
        cellular receptors and, 16
        cytoplasmic organelles and, 5-12
        nucleus and, 5
        plasma membranes and, 12-16
    cell functions in, 5
    cellular intake and output and, 19-28
    cellular metabolism and, 16-19
    cellular reproduction and, 28-31
    tissues and, 31-43
        connective, 37-41
        epithelial, 37
        intracellular communication and, 32-33
        muscle, 41
        neural, 41-43
        tissue formation and, 31-32
        types of, 33-43
Cellular components, 5-16
    cellular receptors and, 16
    cytoplasmic organelles and, 5-12
    of inflammation, 229-235
    nucleus and, 5
    plasma membranes and, 12-16
Cellular energy, 17-18
Cellular environment, 82-113
    acid-base balance and, 100-110
        buffer system and, 101-104
        disturbances in, 104-110
        hydrogen ion and pH and, 100-101
        protein buffering and, 104
        renal buffering and, 104
    body fluid distribution in, 83-85
    potassium, calcium, phosphate, and magnesium balance alterations in, 92-100
    sodium, chloride, and water balance and, 87-88
        alterations in, 88-92
    water movement alterations in, 85-87
Cellular functions
    cellular biology and, 5
    immunology and, 191, 209-212
    tests for, 275
Cellular injury, 51-66
    chemical, 54, 55-57
    genetic factors in, 62
    hypoxic, 52-55
    immunological and inflammatory, 61-62
    infectious, 57-61
    manifestations of, 66-70
        accumulations and, 66-70
        carbohydrates and, 66-67
        glycogen and, 67-68
        lipids and, 66-67
        systemic, 71
        water and, 66
    myocardial infarction and, 942-943
    nutritional imbalances in, 62
    physical agents in, 62-66
Cellular ion exchange mechanism, 104
Cellular metabolism, 16-19
    shock and, 980, 981-984
Cellular products, inflammation and, 235-236
Cellular proliferation, 292-347
    theories of carcinogenesis and, 324-347; see also Carcinogenesis

Cellular proliferation—cont'd
    tumor biology and, 293-322; see also Tumor biology
Cellular receptors, 16
Cellular reproduction, 28-31
    contact inhibition and, 30-31
Cellular self-digestion, 9
Cellular swelling, 66
    chemical injury and, 55-56
    hypoxic injury and, 53
Cellulitis, 1411
Centers for Disease Control, 727
Central canal, 362-364
Central chemoreceptor, 1042
Central fever, 408
Central herniation, 470
Central nervous system, 352, 357-371
    blood supply of, 368-371
    brain in, 357-362
    carcinogenesis and, 327
    disorders of; see Central nervous system disorders
    division of, 359
    human immunodeficiency virus and, 273
    pain and, 395
    protective structures of, 365-368
    spinal cord in, 362-365
Central nervous system disorders
    cerebrovascular disorders in, 493-498
    childhood tumors in, 317
    degenerative diseases and, 509-519
        amyotrophic lateral sclerosis and, 517-519
        Huntington disease and, 513-514
        multiple sclerosis and, 514-517
        Parkinson disease and, 509-513
    infection and inflammation in, 505-509
    inherited metabolic, 544-546
    intoxication in child and, 549
    leukemia and, 849
    malformations and, 532
    motor syndromes in, 455-458
    stress-related, 287
    trauma and, 477-493
        closed-head, 477-482
        fever in, 408
        herniated intervertebral disk and, 491-493
        low back pain and, 489-491
        open-head, 482-483
        spinal cord, 483-489
    tumors and, 498-505
    vomiting and, 435
Central neurogenic hyperventilation, 435
Central venous pressure, 970
Centriacinar emphysema, 1074
Centriole, 12
Centromere, 30
Cephalohematoma, 543
Ceratopogonidae, 1417
Cerebellar astrocytoma, 555
Cerebellar syndromes, 458
    multiple sclerosis and, 516-517
Cerebellar tonsil, 470
Cerebellar tremor, 454
Cerebellopontine angle neurilemmoma, 503
Cerebellum, 362
Cerebral aneurysm, leaking, 930
Cerebral angiography, 385
Cerebral aqueduct, 362, 367
Cerebral astrocytoma, 555
Cerebral atherosclerosis, diabetes mellitus and, 627

Cerebral cortex, 359
  agnosia and, 463
  consciousness and dysfunction of, 437
  Huntington disease and, 513
  unifocal alterations in, 462-465
Cerebral death, 77, 437-440
Cerebral edema, 469-470
Cerebral functions, cognitive, 432
Cerebral hemisphere
  dysphasia and, 465
  functional subdivisions of, 358
Cerebral homeostasis, alterations in, 465-470
Cerebral impulses, contralateral control and, 360
Cerebral infarction, 470
Cerebral palsy, 542-544
Cerebral peduncles, 362
Cerebral syndrome, multiple sclerosis and, 517
Cerebral thrombosis, 493
Cerebrospinal fluid, 367
  analysis of, 384, 385
  hydrocephalus and, 519, 541
  intracranial pressure and, 465
Cerebrovascular accidents, 493-494
Cerebrovascular disorders, 493-498
  child and, 551-552
Cerebrum, 359
  venous drainage of, 368-370
Cervical carcinoma, 693-696
  carcinogenesis and, 329
  FIGO staging of, 694
  in situ, 693
Cervical intraepithelial neoplasia, 693, 694
Cervical lymph node in Hodgkin disease, 813
Cervical mucus, 657
  menstrual cycle and, 660
  postcoital, 670
Cervicitis, 687
  chlamydial, 738
Cervix, 651, 652
  carcinogenesis and, 327
  carcinoma of; see Cervical carcinoma
Cesarean section, 846
Chancre, 730
Chancroid, 733-735
Chemical thermogenesis, 402
Chemicals
  cancer and, 293
  cellular injury and, 55-57
  familial diseases and, 162-163
  mutations and, 121
  toxic myopathy and, 1356
Chemoreceptors, 355, 1042
  arterial, 894
Chemotactic factors, 32, 221
  mast cell and degranulation of, 220-222
Chemotherapy, 307, 308
  classes of drugs in, 309
  combination, 850
  mechanisms of action of, 309
  ovarian cancer and, 698
  pain and, 400
Chest, flail, 1065, 1066
Chest cavity, 1033
Chest muscle retraction, 1099
Chest pain, central, 1056
Chest wall, 1034
  child and, 1097, 1098
  elastic properties of, 1038-1039
  restriction of, 1065
Chest x-ray, 1049
  cardiovascular function and, 905

Cheyne-Stokes respirations, 434, 435, 1055
Chickenpox, 1412, 1445-1446
Chief cells, 1180
Child
  anemia in, 830
  bacterial meningitis in, 549-551
  cancer in, 316-320
  cardiovascular function alterations in, 992-1023
    acquired, 1015-1019, 1020, 1021
    congenital, 996-1015; see also Congenital heart defects
    development and, 993-996
  cerebrovascular disease in, 551-552
  digestive function in, 1267-1289
    gastrointestinal tract disorders and, 1268-1282; see also Gastrointestinal system disorders, child and
    liver disorders and, 1282-1286
  hematologic function in, 825-855
    coagulation disorders and, 842-845
    erythrocyte disorders and, 829-842; see also Erythrocytes
    fetal and neonatal hematopoiesis and, 826
    leukemia and, 847-850
    lymphoma and, 851-852
    platelet disorders and, 845-847
    postnatal changes in blood and, 826-829
  lead absorption in, 550
  musculoskeletal function alterations in, 1360-1387
    bone formation and, 1361-1362
    bone growth and, 1362
    congenital defects and, 1363-1367
    congenital disease and, 1366-1367
    congenital dysplasia of hip joint and, 1363-1364
    development and, 1361-1363
    juvenile rheumatic arthritis and, 1373
    muscle growth and, 1362-1363
    muscular dystrophy and, 1376-1380
    osteochondrosis and, 1373-1376
    osteogenesis imperfecta and, 1367-1368
    osteomyelitis and, 1370-1373
    rickets and, 1368-1369
    scoliosis and, 1369-1370
    skeletal density and modelling and, 1367-1370
    skeletal development and, 1362
    syndactyly and, 1363
    talipes and, 1364-1366
    tumors and, 1380-1384
  neurologic dysfunction in, 531-561
    cerebrovascular disease and, 551-552
    encephalopathy and, 542-551
    malformations and, 535-541
    normal structure and function and, 532-535
    tumors and, 552-558
  pulmonary function alterations in, 1098-1107
    asthma and, 1101-1102
    bronchopulmonary dysplasia and, 1106
    croup syndrome and, 1098-1101
    cystic fibrosis and, 1106-1107
    infection and, 1102-1104
    normal structure and function and, 1096-1098
    respiratory distress syndrome of newborn and, 1104-1106
    stenosis in, 1000-1001

Child—cont'd
  seizure disorders in, 546-548
  skin disorders of, 1439-1452
    dermatitis and, 1439-1440
    infection and, 1440-1446
    insect bites and, 1446-1448
    parasites and, 1446-1448
    vascular disorders and, 1448-1449
  sleep dysfunctions and, 412
  sleep patterns and, 410
  tumors in, 552-558
    brain, 552-555
  urinary tract function in, 1160-1171
    enuresis and, 1168-1169
    glomerular disorders and, 1163-1166
    obstructive disorders and, 1166-1167
    renal system and, 1160-1161
    structural abnormalities and, 1161-1163
    Wilms' tumor and, 1167-1168
Chilling of cells, 63
Chlamydial infections, 736
  Bartholin glands and, 738
  cervicitis and, 738
  clinical syndromes caused by, 737
  conjunctivitis and, 413-414
    infant with, 738
  epididymitis and, 706
  lymphogranuloma venereum and, 738
  pneumonia in infant and, 738
  proctitis and, 737
  sexually transmitted urogenital infections and, 736-739
  smears and, 669
  urethritis and, 699
Chloride, 88
  cellular environment and, 87-88
  hypertension and, 177
  saliva and, 1176
  urine and, 1126-1127
    reabsorption of, 1128
Chloroquine, 1356
Chlorosis, 789
Cholangiocellular carcinoma, 1259
Cholangiography, 1206, 1252
Cholangitis, 1252
Cholecalciferol, 98
Cholecystectomy, 179
Cholecystitis, 1253, 1254
Cholecystogram, 1206
Cholecystokinin, 1178, 1179, 1202
Cholecystosonography, 1206
Cholelithiasis, 1253-1254
Cholera, 153
Choleresis, 1197
Cholescintigraphy, 1206
Cholesterol, 13, 175
  carcinogenesis and metabolites of, 328
  coronary artery disease and, 934
  gallstones and, 1253
  hypertension and, 1019
  receptor-mediated endocytosis and, 26
Choline acetyltransferase, 444
Cholinergic crisis, 523
Cholinergic transmission, 378
  Parkinson disease and, 510
Chondrocyte, 1301
Chondrogenic tumors, 1337
Chondroma, 296
Chondrosarcoma, 296, 1337
Chordae tendineae, 864
Chordee, 1162
Chorea, 453, 454, 513
  Huntington, 137

Chorea—cont'd
  rheumatic fever and, 959
Choreoathetosis, 453, 454
Choriocarcinoma, 297
  testicular, 705
Chorionic villi biopsy, 127
Choroid, 414
Choroid plexus, 366
Choroid plexus tumor, 500
Christmas disease, 842
Christmas factor, 774
Chromatids, 30
  sister, 128
Chromatin, 30, 116
Chromophil, 574
Chromophobe, 574
Chromosomal mosaic, 128
Chromosome, 5, 7, 28, 30, 124-133
Chromosome abnormalities, 121, 126-133
  childhood cancers and, 317
  prenatal diagnosis of, 127-128
  radiation and, 332
Chromosome bands, 124
Chromosome breakage, 131
Chromosome theory of inheritance, 134
Chronic obstructive pulmonary disease,
    1069
  sleep-provoked disorders and, 413
Chvostek sign, 99
Chyle, 1064
Chylomicron, 934, 1188
Chylothorax, 1064
Chyme, 1177
Chymotrypsin, 1187
Cigarette smoking, 330
  carcinogenesis and, 326
  coronary artery disease and, 936
  disease risk and, 158, 159
  hypertension and, 920
  lung cancer and, 164, 1086
  thromboangiitis obliterans and, 932
Cigars, 1086
Cilia, 10, 37
Cimetidine, 179
Cingulate gyrus herniation, 470
Circadian rhythm, 400
Circle of Willis, 368, 369
Circulating anticoagulant, 779
Circulating plasma proteins, 236
Circulation, 860, 884-885; *see also*
    Cardiovascular system
  at birth, 995-996
  cardiomyopathy and, 950
  coronary, 866, 897-898
  development of, 994-995
  elderly and, 404
  enterohepatic, 1195
  pulmonary, 860, 1032
    control of, 1042
  systemic, 860, 886
  thrombus formation and, 930
Circumcision, 663
Circumflex artery, 868
Circumlocution, 468
Cirrhosis, 67, 1248-1249
  alcoholic, 1249-1252
  ascites and, 1240
  biliary, 251, 1252
  child and, 1283
  clinical manifestations of, 1251
  postnecrotic, 1252
Cisternae, 6
Cisternal puncture, 385

Cisternography, isotope, 385
Citric acid cycle, 18
Clasp-knife phenomenon, 457
Clastogens, 131
Clearance, renal, 1129-1130
  renal failure and, 1154-1155
Cleft lip and cleft palate, 1268-1269
Climate, adaptation to, 403
Clitoris, 650
Clonal selection, 202
Clonal senescence, 919
Clones, 118
  hybrid, 144
    cancer treatment and, 314
Clonic seizure, 447, 448, 450, 453
Clonic-tonic seizure, 445
Closed-head trauma, 477-482
Closed reduction of fracture, 1323
Clostridium botulinum, 58, 521-522
Clostridium parvum, 311
Clostridium perfringens, 58
Clostridium tetani, 58
Clot lysis, 776
Clot retraction, 776, 779
Clotting factors, 218, 222, 225, 227, 755,
    757
  burn injury and, 1430
  coagulation disorders and, 818-819
  hemostasis and, 772-776
  tests for, 778-780
Clouding of consciousness, 440
Clubbing, 1056
Clubfoot, 1364-1365
Clue cells, 736
Clumping of erythrocytes, 200
Cluster breathing, 435
Coagulation, 218, 222, 225, 227; *see also*
    Clotting factors
  disorders of, 818-822, 843, 845
    child and, 842-845
Coagulation cascade, 225, 773, 775
Coagulative necrosis, 71
Coal tar, 293
Coal worker pneumoconiosis, 1066-1067
Coarctation of aorta, 1001-1003
Coated pits, 26
Cobalamin, 767
Cocarcinogens, 324
Cochlea, 419
Codominance inheritance, 134
Codons, 120
Coenzyme, 18
Cofactor deficiency, 544
Cognitive cerebral functions, 432
  pain and, 391
Cognitive dementia, 443
Cold, stress and, 282; *see also* Hypothermia
Cold antibody disease, 792
Cold sore, 739, 1411
Cold spots, 905
Colic
  biliary, 1253
  chronic mesenteric insufficiency and, 1236
Coliform bacteria, 708
Colitis
  granulomatous, 1258
  ulcerative, 251, 1232-1233, 1258
Collagen
  bones and, 1294
  dysfunctional synthesis of, 245
  immature, 243
  inflammation and, 244-245
  scar tissue and, 242, 1400

Collagen—cont'd
  skin and, 1394
  tissue repair and, 243
  tumors and, 1337-1338
Collagen fibers, 38, 39, 40, 41
  in articular cartilage, 1301
  bone and, 1294
Collagen theory of aging, 74
Collateral arteries, 868
Collateral ganglia, 377
Colliculi, 361
Colloid osmotic pressure, 21
Colon, 1190, 1192
  cancer of, 327, 1257-1259
    familial diseases and, 155, 169, 172-173
Colonoscopy, 1203
Colony-stimulating factor, 762
Color agnosia, 462
Color blindness, 418
Color vision, alterations in, 417-418
Colorectal cancer, 1258, 1259
  Duke classification for, 1258
Colorectal polyp, 1257
Columnar cells, 35, 36, 37, 51, 52
Coma, 433, 434
  hyperosmolar hyperglycemic nonketotic,
      622-623
  irreversible, 437-440
  myxedema, 608
Comedomastitis, 714
Comedone, 1399
Comminuted fracture, 1320, 1321
Common acute lymphoblastic leukemia
      antigen, 848
Common bile duct, 1195
Communicating hydrocephalus, 519
Compact bone, 1295
Compartment syndrome, 1327, 1328
Compensatory hyperplasia, 51, 243
Competitive inhibitors, 22
Complement, 62, 218, 222-225, 227
  burn injury and, 1431
  components of, 223, 224
  glomerulonephritis and, 1148
  immune deficiency and defects of, 265
Complement cascade, 222, 223
Complement fixation test, 748
Complement-mediated lysis, 256
Complementary DNA, 119, 120
Completed stroke, 493
Complex febrile seizure, 547
Compliance, lung, 1040
Compound fracture, 1320
  of skull, 483
Compression atelectasis, 1060
Compression injury of spine, 484
Compressive syndrome, 505
Computed tomography
  gastrointestinal tract and, 1203
  nervous system and, 383
Concentration gradient, 20
Concentric isotonic contraction, 1313
Concentric lamellae, 1296
Concussion, 478
Condoms, 645, 727
Conducting airways, 1026-1030
Conducting arteries, 368
Conduction, heart, 402, 869-873
  disorders of, 966-967
Conductive dysphasia, 467
Conductive hearing loss, 420-421
Condylomata acuminata, 741-742, 1413
Condylomata lata, 731

Cones, 414
Confabulation, 509
Confusion, 434, 440, 442
  right-left, 462
Congenital defects, 168
  childhood cancers and, 317-318
  of musculoskeletal system, 1363-1367
Congenital dysplasia of hip joint, 1363-1364
Congenital heart defects, 996-1015
  acyanotic, with increased pulmonary blood
      flow, 1003-1007
  classification of, 999
  congestive heart failure and, 1016
  cyanotic, pulmonary blood flow and
      decreased, 1012-1015
      increased, 1007-1012
  familial diseases and, 174
  ventricular outflow restriction and,
      999-1003
Congenital syphilis, 731, 732
Congestive cardiomyopathy, 951-952
Congestive heart failure, 971-975
  child and, 1002, 1008, 1015-1017
Conjugated bilirubin, 1198
Conjunctivitis, 255, 413-414
  chlamydial, 738
Connective tissue, 37-41
  autoimmunity and, 251
  cortisol and, 286
  diseases of, 1373
      congenital heart defects and, 998
      stress-related, 287
Consanguinity, 138-139
Consciousness
  alterations in, 432-451
      breathing pattern in, 433-435
      clinical manifestations and evaluation of,
          433-440
      content of thought and, 440-442
      level of consciousness in, 433, 434
      motor responses and, 437
      oculomotor responses and, 436-437
      outcomes of, 437-440
      pathophysiology of, 432
      pupillary changes in, 435-436
      seizures and, 445-451
      subacute and chronic, 442-445
  clouding of, 440
  full, 437
  levels of, 433, 434
Constipation, 1214-1215
Constitutional delay, 678
Constrictive pericarditis, 949-951
Constructional dyspraxia, 463
Contact dermatitis, 254, 260, 261, 1402
Contact factors, 774
  hypersensitivity and, 254
Contact guidance, tissue formation and, 32
Content of thought, 432
  alterations in, 440-442
Contraceptives, oral; *see* Oral contraceptives
Contracoup injury, 477, 478
Contraction alkalosis, 107
Contractions
  inflammation and, 243, 245-246
  muscle, 1311-1312
  myocardial, 876-878
      heart failure and, 963-969
  premature junctional, 964
  premature ventricular, 965
  wound, 243
Contracture
  muscle, 1351

Contracture—cont'd
  wound, 245
Contusion, 480
Conus
  coronary artery and, 868
  heart valves and, 1009
Conus medullaris, 362
Convection, 402
Convergence, 354
Convulsions; *see* Seizures
Cooley anemia, 841
Coombs test, 778, 834
COPD; *see* Chronic obstructive pulmonary
      disease
Coping process, 288-289, 289
Copper
  erythropoiesis and, 767
  Wilson disease and, 1285-1286
Cor pulmonale, 969-971, 1082-1083
Core temperature, 401, 404, 406, 407
Cornea, 414
Corniculate cartilage, 1027
Cornification, 660
Coronary angiography, 907, 940
Coronary angioplasty, percutaneous
      transluminal, 941
Coronary arteries, 866-867, 897-898
  hypertension and, 925
Coronary artery bypass graft, 941-942
Coronary artery disease, 155, 162, 169, 175,
      934-938
  development of, 934
  diabetes mellitus and, 626-627
  familial diseases and, 174-176
  menopause and, 672
  personality and, 163, 937-938
  sleep-provoked disorders and, 412
Coronary atherosclerosis, 163, 907
Coronary capillaries, 868
Coronary ostia, 866
Coronary perfusion pressure, 897
Coronary sinus, 866
Coronary sulcus, 868
Coronary veins, 868
Coronaviruses, 61
Corpora cavernosa, 663
Corpora quadrigemina, 361
Corpus callosum, 360
Corpus luteum, 654
Corpus luteum cyst, 690
Corpus spongiosum, 663
Corpus striatum, 360
  Parkinson disease and, 509
Cortex
  adrenal; *see* Adrenal cortex
  of bone, 1295, 1296
  cerebral; *see* Cerebral cortex
Corti, organ of, 65, 419
Cortical bone, 1295, 1296
Cortical nephron, 1113
Corticospinal syndrome, 516
Corticosteroid-binding globulin, 284, 566
Corticosteroids; *see* Steroids
Corticotropin-releasing hormone, 287, 288,
      573, 596
Cortisol, 583-584, 587
  Cushing syndrome and, 629-631
  ectopic adrenocorticotropic hormone and,
      299
  low levels of, 633-634
  stress response and, 284-286
Corynebacterium diphtheriae, 58, 1098
Corynebacterium vaginale, 735-736

Cosmic radiation, 331
Cough, 1055
  smoker's, 1073
Countercurrent exchange system, 1126,
      1127
Coup injury, 477, 478
Coupling, muscle contraction and, 1312
Cow's milk, iron deficiency anemia and, 831
Cowper's glands, 664
Cowpox, 61
Coxa plana, 1374
Crab louse, 745, 1447
Cracked-pot sign, 541
Cramps, heat, 405
Cranial meningocele, 536
Cranial nerves, 352, 374-375
  tumors of, 500
Craniopharyngioma, 553, 555
Craniostenosis, 539
Craniosynostosis, 538-540
Cranium, 365-366
  deformities of, 538-541
  development of, 535
  tumors in, 498
Creatine, 944, 1311, 1314
Creatinine, 1130
  renal failure and, 1154
Cretin, 609
CRH; *see* Corticotropin-releasing hormone
Cri-du-chat syndrome, 132, 998
Crib death, 1100
Cricoid cartilage, 1027
Crista supraventricularis, 865
Cristae, 10
Cristae ampullaris, 420
Critical micelle concentration, 1196
Crohn disease, 1233-1234, 1258
Cross-linking theory of aging, 74
Crossbridge theory of muscle contraction,
      876-878
Croup, 1098-1101
  types of, 1100-1101
Crush syndrome, 1327
Crust, skin, 1397
  bullous impetigo and, 1440-1441
  scabies and, 1447
Cryoprecipitate, 845
Cryptorchidism, 660, 702-703
Crypts of Lieberkühn, 1184
Crystalline fragment, 202
Crystals
  in synovial fluid, 1347
  urinalysis and, 1131
Cuboidal cells, 35, 37
Culdoscopy, 670
Cultures, 668
Cuneiform bone, 1027
Curettage, 670, 683
Cushing disease, 629
Cushing syndrome, 629, 630
  hypernatremia and, 89
Cushing ulcer, 1228-1229
Cutaneous vasculitis, 1415
Cuticle infection, 1433
Cyanide, 57
Cyanosis, 999, 1056
  congenital heart disease and, 999,
      1007-1015
Cyanothymidine, 274
Cyanotic heart defects, 999
  pulmonary blood flow and
      decreased, 1012-1015
      increased, 1007-1012

Cyclic adenosine monophosphate, 569
Cyclic guanosine monophosphate, 569
Cyclophosphamide, 711
Cylindroma, 1090
Cyst
  Bartholin, 687
  corpus luteum, 690
  follicular, 690
  Giardia lamblia, 746
  inflammation and, 239
  ovarian, 690
  pancreatic, 1255
  rheumatoid arthritis and, 1344
  skin and, 1397
Cystic fibrosis, 1106-1107, 1276-1277
  pedigree for, 138
Cystic mastitis, 713
Cystine, collagen synthesis and, 244
Cystitis, 1141-1142
Cystocele, 688, 689
Cystorchidism, 318
Cystosarcoma phyllodes, 296, 716
Cytochromes, 18, 69
Cytokinesis, 28, 124
  immunotherapy and, 310
  mitosis and, 30
Cytomegalovirus, 747-748
  reproductive function test and, 669
Cytoplasm, 5, 28
  cancer cells and, 297-298
Cytoplasmic organelle, 5-12
Cytosine, 117
Cytosine arabinoside, 309
Cytoskeleton, 10-12
Cytosol, 5
Cytotoxic cells, 209
Cytotoxic edema, cerebral, 469-470
Cytotoxic T lymphocytes, 342, 692
Cytotoxicity
  antibody-dependent, cell-mediated,
    256-257, 341, 342
  childhood cancers and, 319
Cytotropic antibody, 253
Cytoxan, 523

D

Damage-accumulation theories of aging, 74
Danazol, 714
Dandy-Walker malformation, 541
Dane particle, 1247
Dantrolene sodium, 406
Dark adaptation, 416
Dark-field microscopy, 732
Daughter cells, 30, 132, 771
Dawn phenomenon, 623-624
Dead hand, 65
Dead space, physiologic, 1058
Dead-space ventilation, 1036, 1058
Deafferentiation pain, 400
Deafness
  music, 462
  word, 462, 466
Deamination, 1198
Death
  brain, 440
  cellular, 70-73
  cerebral, 437-440
  somatic, 76-77
Débridement, 242
Decerebrate response, 439, 441, 451-452
Decompression, spinal cord injury and, 489
Decompression sickness, 63
Decornification, 660

Decorticate response, 439, 441, 452
Decubitus ulcer, 1400
Defecation reflex, 1192
Deficiencies in immunity and inflammation,
    265-276; *see also* Acquired immune
    deficiencies
  congenital, 265, 266-268
Degeneration, 490, 509-519
  aging and, 167
  disc, 490
  joint, 1340-1341
  Parkinson disease and, 509-513
  Wallerian, 356
Degranulation, 220
  inflammation and, 233
  mast cell, 220-222
  platelet, 772
Dehiscence, 245
Dehydration, 90
  edema and, 87
Dehydration test, 598
Delayed age of onset, 136-137
Delayed hypersensitivity, 252, 259, 275
Delayed puberty, 678
Deletions, genetic, 132
  mapping of, 145
Delirium, 440, 441
Delta cells, 578
Delusions, 442
Dementia, 442-443
  Parkinson disease and, 513
Demyelinating polyradiculopathy, acute
    inflammatory, 521
Demyelination, central nervous system, 514
  multiple sclerosis and, 515, 516
Dendrites, 43, 353
Dendritic zone, 353
Denervated muscle, 459
Deoxyhemoglobin, 766
Deoxyribonucleic acid, 4, 5, 7, 115,
    116-124
  aging and, 74, 75, 76
  anemia and, 788
  carcinogenesis and, 325
  crossing-over and, 141-142
  as genetic code, 116-120
  human immunodeficiency virus and, 271,
    272
  radiation and, 64, 309, 332
  recombinant, 118-119
  replication of, 120-121
  systemic lupus erythematosus and, 263
  viral replication and, 59
Dependent edema, 86
Depolarization, 28, 871, 965
  diastolic, 873
Depression, 170
  constipation and, 1214-1215
  secondary sleep disorders and, 412
Dermal appendages, 1392-1393
Dermatitis
  atopic, 255, 260, 1402-1403
    child and, 1439-1440
  child and, 1439-1440
  contact, 254, 260, 261, 1402
  diaper, 1440
  seborrheic, 1403-1404
  stasis, 1403
  substances causing, 1403
  of vulva, 687
Dermatomes, 372
  herpes zoster and, 1413
Dermatomyositis, 251, 1354-1355

Dermatophyte, 1414
Dermis, 1392
DES; *see* Diethylstilbestrol
Descending colon, 1190
Desensitization to allergens, 255
Desmosomes, 32, 33
Detoxification, metabolic, 1198-1199
Detrusor muscle, 1118
Diabetes insipidus, 598-599
Diabetes mellitus, 612-628
  acute complications of, 618-624
  autoimmunity and, 250
  characteristics of, 613
  chronic complications of, 624-628
  classification of, 613
  coronary artery disease and, 936
  epidemiology of, 614
  familial diseases and, 155, 163, 169, 170,
    173
  glycogen accumulation and, 67
  obesity and, 1236
  types of, 612-618
Diabetic ketoacidosis, 94, 619-622
Diabetic microangiopathy, 624
Diabetic neuropathy, 624, 625
Diabetic retinopathy, 625
Dialysis, 100, 1153, 1158
Diapedesis, 229, 230, 759
Diaper dermatitis, 1440
Diaphragm, 1037
Diaphysis, 1295, 1296
Diarrhea, 94, 1215-1216
  child with, 1280-1282
  gastric surgery and, 1230
Diarthrosis, 1298
Diascopy, 1394
Diastole, 864
  child and, 1020-1021
Diastolic depolarization, 873
DIC; *see* Disseminated intravascular
    coagulation
Dicalcium phosphate dihydrate, 1295
Diencephalic syndrome of infancy, 554
Diencephalon, 360-361
  unconsciousness and, 434
Diet
  atherosclerosis and, 920
  breast cancer and, 715
  calorie intake and, 182
  carcinogenesis and, 326-329
  constipation and, 1214
  diabetes mellitus and, 616
  fiber in, 329
  iron in, 831
  renal failure and, 1156
Diethylstilbestrol, 319, 333, 696
Differential white cell count, 778
Differentiation
  cellular functions and, 5
  hematopoiesis and, 763
Diffusing capacity of lung, 1049
Diffusion
  facilitated, 22, 23
  passive transport and, 19, 20
DiGeorge syndrome, 266-267
Digestion, 18; *see also* Digestive function
    alterations; Gastrointestinal system
  accessory organs of, 1193-1202
  cancer of, 1259-1261
  child and, 1267-1289
    gastrointestinal tract disorders in,
      1268-1282; *see also* Gastrointestinal
      system disorders, child and

Digestion—cont'd
  child and—cont'd
    liver disorders in, 1282-1286
    cortisol and, 286
    history of study of, 1173
    hormones and, 1179
    intestinal, 1184
Digestive enzymes, 578
Digestive function alterations, 1212-1266
  cancer and, 301, 1255-1261
  child and, 1276-1280
  familial diseases and, 179
  gallbladder disorders and, 1253-1254
  gastrointestinal tract and, 1213-1238; *see
      also* Gastrointestinal system
  liver disorders and, 1245-1252
    manifestations of, 1238-1245
  pancreas disorders and, 1254-1255
  tests for, 1202-1206
Digestive system
  alterations of; *see* Digestive function
      alterations
  structure and function of, 1174-1211
    accessory organs of digestion and,
        1193-1202
      cancer of, 1259-1261
    aging and, 1206-1207
    gastrointestinal tract and, 1175-1193;
        see also Gastrointestinal system
    tests and, 1202-1206
Digestive vacuoles, 9
Digoxin, 711
Dihydrotestosterone, 332, 333
Diiodotyrosine, 577
Dilation and curettage, 670, 683
Dilutional hyponatremia, 91
Dimethylnitrosamine, 328
Dinitrochlorobenzene, 311, 312
Diphtheria, 1099
Diploid cells, 124
Diplopia, 415, 435
Dipogenic hypothesis, 919
Direct antiglobulin test, 778
Discoid lupus erythematosus, 1408-1409
Disease
  aging and, 73
  factors causing, 155-158
  general adaptation syndrome and, 282
  occurrence of, 158
  risk 0f, 158-162
  stress and, 279-291; *see also* Stress
Disease rates, 158
Disk, intervertebral, 368
  degenerative disease of, 490
  herniated, 491-493
Dislocation, joint, 1323-1325
  hip, 1363-1364
Disorientation, 442
  consciousness and, 434
Disse space, 1195
Dissecting aneurysm, 929-930
Disseminated gonococcal infection, 728
Disseminated intravascular coagulation,
    819-821
  leukemia and, 806
Distal tubule, 1116, 1121, 1125-1126
  potassium concentration and, 93
  renal buffering and, 104
Distention
  alveolar, 1038
  gastric, 1224
  spinal cord injury and bladder, 488
Disulfiram, 711

Disuse atrophy, 50, 1351-1352
Diuresis, 1152
  postobstructive, 1137
  water, 1128
Diuretics, 107
  gout and, 1348
  hearing loss and, 421
  hypertension and, 926
  potassium-sparing, 96
  renal failure and, 1153
  urine flow and, 1128
Diverticulitis, 1234, 1258
Diverticulosis, 1234-1235
  intestinal obstruction and, 1222
DNA polymerase, 120, 122
Dolichocephaly, 539
Doll's eyes phenomenon, 437, 438
Dominance of genes, 134
Donor, universal, 200
Donovan bodies, 735
Donovania granulomatis, 735
Dopamine, 357, 362
  motor function and, 452
  Parkinson disease and, 510, 511
Dopaminergic nigrostriatal pathway, 509
Dopaminergic synaptic activity, 510
Doppler study, 904-905
Doriden; *see* Glutethimide
Dorsal column, 364, 516
Dorsal horn, 364
Dorsal root ganglion, 364
Dorsiflexion, foot, 1366
Dorsolateral funiculus, 395
Dose-equivalent rate, radiation and, 331
Double-helix, 117
Doubling time of tumor growth, 302
Down syndrome, 128-129
  childhood cancers and, 318
  congenital heart defects and, 998
Dream anxiety attacks, 412
Dressing dyspraxia, 463
Dressler postinfarction syndrome, 946
Drop attacks, 447
Drug abusers, intravenous, 270
Drug-induced hemolytic anemia, 173, 792
Drug-induced sexual dysfunction, 710
Drugs
  acquired immune deficiency and, 268, 274
  antithyroid, 604
  cancer treatment and, 308-309
  cellular receptors and, 16
  gynecomastia and, 718
  hypersensitivity and, 254
  hypertension and, 924
  prenatal exposure to, 319
Dry gangrene, 72
Duchenne muscular dystrophy, 1376-1377
  gamma-aminobutyric acid and, 1291
Duct of Bellini, 1118
Ductal adenocarcinoma, 1261
Ductus arteriosus, 994
Ductus venosus, 994
Duffy blood group locus, 144
Duke classification for colorectal cancer
    staging, 1258
Dumping syndrome, 1229-1230
Duodenal ulcer, 1226, 1227, 1229
Duodenoscopy, 1203
Duodenum, 1182
  obstruction of, 1272
Duplications
  chromosomes and, 132
  genetic mapping and, 145

Dupuytren contracture, 699-700
Dura mater, 366
Dust
  coal, 1066-1067
  hypersensitivity and, 254
Dwarfism, 600, 601
Dynamic steady state, 287
  stress and, 283
Dynorphin, 397
Dysbetalipoproteinemia, 935
Dyschezia, 692
Dysfunctional uterine bleeding, 682-683
Dyskinesia, 453-455
Dyslipoproteinemia, familial, 935
Dysmenorrhea, primary, 680
Dyspareunia, 672
Dysphagia, 704, 1219
  esophageal carcinoma and, 1256
  ocular myopathy and, 1355
Dysphasia, 464, 466-468
  left cerebral hemisphere and, 465
Dysplasia, 51
  congenital hip joint, 1363-1364
Dyspnea, 1054
  congestive heart failure and, 1016
  on exertion, 1054
Dyspraxia, 464
Dysreflexia, 486-488
Dysrhythmia, 162, 901, 946, 963
Dystonia, 451
Dystrophic calcification, 69-70

E

Ear
  normal, 419-420
  rhabdomyosarcoma and, 1384
Eastern equine encephalitis, 508
Eaton-Lambert syndrome, 461
Ecchymosis, 817
Eccrine sweat glands, 1393
Echocardiography, 904
  infective endocarditis and, 962
Echoencephalography, 385
Echolalia, 465
*eco*RI, 119
Ectopic hormones, tumors and, 299, 300
Eczema, 1402
Edema
  asthma and, 1101
  of burn shock, 1428-1429
  congestive heart failure and, 1016
  croup and, 1098
  hypothyroidism and, 607, 608
  inflammation and, 228
  localized, 86
  mechanisms of formation of, 86
  nephrotic syndrome and, 1144, 1149,
      1150
    child and, 1164
  pneumococcal pneumonia and, 1077
  pulmonary, 1058-1060
    heart failure and, 972
    high-altitude, 63, 1059
    pathogenesis of, 1059
    starvation and interstitial, 62
  spinal cord injury and, 485
  water movement and, 85-87
Edrophonium chloride, 522, 523
Edwin Smith papyrus, 351
Effective osmolality, 21
Effective renal blood flow, 1130
Effector cells, 310, 312
Effector organs, 353

Efferent fibers
  gamma, 459
  parasympathetic, 873
  sympathetic, 873
Efferent lymphatic vessel, 901
Efferent neuron, 364
Efferent pathways, 352-353
  consciousness and, 437
  pain and, 395
Efferent tubules, 661
Ehlers-Danlos syndrome, 244
Einthoven triangle, 902
Ejaculation, 663
Ejaculatory duct, 664
Ejection fraction, 883
Elastic artery, 886
Elastic cartilage, 40
Elastic connective tissue, 39
Elastic fibers, 38, 39, 40, 41
Elastic recoil, 1038
Elastin, 1394
Elbow dislocation, 1324
Elderly; *see also* Aging
  auditory changes and, 420
  immune function in, 213-214
  inflammation and, 246
  isolated systolic hypertension and, 923
  pressure ulcer and, 1400
  sleep patterns and, 410-411
  temperature regulation and, 404
Electrical impulse
  heart and, 871
  movement of, 28
  muscle and, 1311, 1313
  nervous system and, 354
Electrical systole, 873
Electrocardiography, 902
  atrioventricular bundle, 905-906
  myocardial infarction and, 945
  myocardial ischemia and, 940
  normal, 872-873
Electrocerebral silence, 440
Electroencephalography, 385
Electrolysis; *see* Cellular environment
Electrolytes, 19, 757
  burn shock and, 1428
  child and, 1161
  concentration of, 93
  distribution of, 88, 89
  ketoacidosis and, 621
  leukemia and, 807
  myocardial infarction and disturbance of, 943
  small intestine and, 1184
Electromechanical dissociation, 965
Electromyography, 1315, 1351
  myasthenia gravis and, 523
Electron-transport chain, 18
Elliptocytosis, hereditary, 786
Ellis–van Creveld syndrome, 998
Embolism, 930-931
  air, 931
  amniotic fluid, 931
  bacterial, 931
  fat, 931
  pulmonary, 1080-1082
  stroke and, 493-494
Embryo, hematopoiesis and, 826
Embryonal tumors, 555-558, 705
Embryonic development
  of external genitalia, 648
  of internal genitalia, 647
  of nervous system, 533

Embryonic development—cont'd
  oncofetal antigens and, 339
Embryonic hemoglobin, 826
Emotional control, 461-465
Emotional disorders, familial diseases and, 163
Emotional stress; *see* Stress
Emotions, alterations in, 461-465
Emphysema, 1070, 1074-1076
  centriacinar, 1074
  panacinar, 1074, 1076
  pathogenesis of, 1072
  types of, 1075
Empiric risks, 148
Empyema, 1064
Emulsification, 1187
Encephalitis, 251, 507-508
Encephalocele, 536
Encephalopathy, 542-551
  child and, 548-551, 1284
  hepatic, 1240, 1242
    child and, 1284
    tremor of, 454
  lead, 549
  portal-systemic, 1242
  static, 542-548
  Wernicke, 509
End-diastolic pressure, 881, 970, 971
End-diastolic volume, 879
End-stage renal failure, 1150
Endocarditis
  infective, 960-962
  nonbacterial thrombotic, 960
  subacute, 931
Endocardium, 862
  disorders of, 953-962
Endocervical canal, 652
  gonococcal infection and, 727
Endochondral bone formation, 1361
Endocrine disorders; *see also* Hormones
  familial diseases and, 173
  hypertension and, 924
  hyperthyroidism and, 604
  hypoglycemia and, 620
  hypothyroidism and, 606
  metabolic muscle diseases and, 1352-1353
  pancreatic dysfunction and, 612-628; *see also* Diabetes mellitus
  sexual dysfunction and, 710
  stress-related, 287
Endocrine feedback loops, 567
Endocrine glands, 562-643
  aging and, 588-589
  autoimmunity and, 250
  hormonal regulation and
    alterations of, 594-643; *see also* Hormones, alterations of
    mechanisms of, 564-593; *see also* Hormones, mechanisms of
  regulation of, 565
  structure and function of, 570-588
    adrenal glands and, 580-586
    hypothalamic-pituitary system and, 570-573
    neuroendocrine response to stressors and, 586-587
    pancreas and, 578-580
    posterior pituitary hormones and, 573-574
    tests and, 587-588
    thyroid and parathyroid glands and, 574-578
Endocrine theory of aging, 74

Endocytosis, 19, 25-26
Endolarynx, 1027
Endolymph, 419
Endometriosis, 691-693
Endometrium, 652
  biopsy of, 670
  carcinogenesis and, 327
  carcinoma of, 333, 696-697
  estrogen and, 657
  pathologic hyperplasia and, 51
  polyps of, 690
  progesterone and, 657
Endomysium, 1305
Endoneurium, 353
Endonucleases, restriction, 119
Endoplasmic reticulum, 5, 6
  rough, 8
Endorphins, 397, 398
  cellular receptors and, 16
  stress response and, 286
Endoscopy
  gastrointestinal tract and, 1203
  pelvic, 670
Endosteum, 1296
Endotoxins, 58-59
Energy
  muscle diseases and, 1353-1354
  oxidative phosphorylation and, 18-19
Enkephalin, 397
Entamoeba histolytica, 746
Enteritis, *Campylobacter*, 745-746
Entero-oxyntin, 1179
Enterobacter aerogenes, 59
Enterocolitis, 1273, 1280-1281
Enterogastrone, 1179
Enterohepatic circulation, 1195
Enterokinase, 1202
Enteropathy, gluten-sensitive, 1277-1279
Enthesis, 1346
Enuresis, 412, 1168-1169
Environmental factors, 162-163
  breast cancer and, 715
  carcinogenesis and, 325-332
  childhood cancer and, 319
  congenital heart defects and, 997
  genes and, 153-189; *see also* Genes
  interaction among, 163-168
Enzyme-linked immunosorbent assay, 588, 669
Enzymes
  amino acid metabolism defects and, 544
  cancer and, 299-300
  cellular metabolism and, 16-17
  cystic fibrosis and deficiency of, 1276
  degenerative joint disease and, 1340
  digestive, 578
  gene dosage analysis and, 145
  hydrolytic
    atrophy and, 50
    cellular death and, 70-71
  liver and, 1205
  lysosomal, 221
  severe combined immunodeficiency disease and, 275-276
  single-gene defects and, 178-179
Eosinophil chemotactic factor of anaphylaxis, 221, 233
Eosinophilia, 801
Eosinophils, 757, 760
  count of, 778
  infant and, 829
  inflammation and, 233-235
Ependymal cell, 355, 356

Ependymoma, 500, 502-503
  child and, 553, 555
Epidemic, 154
Epidemiology, 153-154
Epidermal necrolysis, staphylococcal toxic,
    1441
Epidermis, 1391-1392
Epidermodysplasia verruciformis, 1414
Epididymis, 662
Epididymitis, 706-707
Epidural hematoma, 367, 480
Epidural space, 366
Epiglottis, 1027
Epiglottitis, 1098, 1100
  acute, 1100
Epilepsy, 445; *see also* Seizures
  fluorescent lighting and, 65
  international classification of seizures and,
    447
Epileptogenic focus, 447
Epimysium, 1305
Epinephrine, 402
  cardiovascular system and, 874, 896, 973
  emotions and, 462
  immunity and, 253
  stress response and, 283-284
Epiphyseal plate, 1295, 1297
  osteomyelitis and, 1372
  rickets and, 1368
Epiphysis, 1295, 1296
Epispadias, 1162
Epithalamus, 360
Epithelial ovarian neoplasm, 697
Epithelial tissues, 37
Epithelialization, 243
  impaired, 245
Epithelioid cells, 238
Epithelium, 34, 35, 36
Epitope, 197
Epstein-Barr virus, 338-339
  childhood cancers and, 319
  infectious mononucleosis and, 802
  non-Hodgkin lymphoma and, 851
Equatorial plate, 30
Equilibrium, 419, 512
Equinovalgus, 1366
Equinovarus, 1366
Equinus, 1366
Erectile reflex, 663
Erection, 663
Erosion, skin, 1399
Error-catastrophe theory of aging, 74, 75
Erysipelas, 1411
Erythema, psoriasis and, 1404
Erythema marginatum, 959
Erythema multiforme, 1410-1411
Erythema toxicum neonatorum, 1449-1450
Erythroblast, 764-765
Erythroblastosis fetalis, 829, 832
Erythrocyte osmotic fragility test, 777
Erythrocyte plasma membranes, 199
Erythrocyte protoporphyrin, 790
Erythrocyte sedimentation, 237
Erythrocytes, 757-758, 784-785
  ABO system and, 200
  alterations of, 784-799
    anemia and, 784-796; *see also* Anemia
    myeloproliferative red cell disorders and,
      796-797
  biconcavity of, 758
  child and, 829, 830-834
  clumping of, 200
  development of, 764-770

Erythrocytes—cont'd
  fetal, 832
  history of, 753
  inherited disorders and, 834-842
  phagocytosis of, 770
  rouleaux formation and, 237
  senescent, 769-770
  sickled, 836
  tests and, 777
  transfusions of, 276
Erythrocytosis, 796, 797
Erythron, 765
Erythroplasia of Queyrat, 700, 701
Erythropoiesis, 764
  nutritional requirements for, 766-767
  regulation of, 769
Erythropoietin, 762
  kidney function and, 1129
  tumors and, 299
Escape mechanisms
  hyperaldosteronism and, 632
  immune surveillance, 342-343
Escherichia coli, 59
  empyema and, 1064
  orchitis and, 703
  prostatitis and, 708
Esophageal atresia, 1270
Esophageal malformations, 1270-1271
Esophageal sphincter
  lower, 1177, 1219
  upper, 1176-1177
Esophagitis, reflux, 1220, 1255
Esophagoscopy, 1203
Esophagus, 1176-1177
  carcinogenesis and, 327
  carcinoma of, 1255-1256
    alcohol and, 329
Essential hypertension, 177, 920
Essential tremor, 454
Estradiol, 333, 655
  fertility and, 671
Estrogen replacement therapy, 333
  coronary artery disease and, 937
Estrogen-secreting tumor, 633
Estrogens, 586, 657
  carcinogenesis and, 328, 332, 333
  endometrial cancer and, 696, 697
  gynecomastia and, 718
  hormonal hyperplasia and, 51
  hyperaldosteronism and, 631
  hypersecretion of adrenal, 633
  mammary cancer and, 293
  menopause and, 672
  osteoporosis and, 1330
  reproductive system and, 645, 649,
    655-656
  sexual dysfunction and, 711
Estrone, 333
Ethacrynic acid, 1128
Eucaryotes, 4-5, 6
  RNA and, 123
Eugenics, 115
Euploid cells, 126
Eupnea, 1055
Eustachian tube, 419
Evaporation
  heat reduction and, 403
  water loss in burns and, 1431
Eversion, foot, 1366
Evoked potentials, 385
Ewing sarcoma, 1382
Exanthem subitum, 1445
Excitable tissues, 23

Excitation
  cardiac, 869, 870-871, 878
  muscle contraction and, 1311
Excitatory postsynaptic potentials, 357
Excoriation, 1399
Excretion, urine; *see also* Urine
Exercise
  asthma induced by, 1070
  cardiac activity and, 905
  cardiac performance and, 908
  constipation and, 1214
  diabetes mellitus and, 616, 618
  hypoglycemia and, 618
  skeletal muscle and, 1312-1313
Exhaustion
  general adaptation syndrome and, 282
  heat, 405
Exocrine glands, 578
  cystic fibrosis and, 1277
Exocrine pancreas, 1193, 1200-1202
  tests of, 1203-1206
Exocytosis, 19
  vesicle formation and, 25-26
Exons, 123
Exophytic lower lip cancer, 1083
Exotoxins, bacterial, 58-59
  neutralization of, 204
Expiration, 1055
Expiratory flow rate, 1071
Expiratory reflex, Hering-Breuer, 1041
Expiratory reserve volume, 1036
Expiratory volume, forced, 1071
Expression, movement of, 452
Expressive dysphasia, 465, 466
Expressivity, autosomal dominant
    inheritance and, 137
Exstrophy of bladder, 1163
Extensor tone, 451
External anal sphincter, 1190
External auditory canal, 419
External ear, 419
External genitalia
  female, 650
  fetal development of, 648
  male, 660-663
Extinction, agnosia and, 464
Extracellular cations, 87-88
Extracellular fluid, 14, 19, 83, 84
  electrolytes and, 93, 94
  hypertonic imbalances and, 90
  hypotonic imbalances and, 91
Extracellular matrix, 31, 32, 41
Extracerebral disorders, 432
Extracerebral tumors, primary, 503-504
Extracorporeal shock-wave lithotripsy, 1138
Extradural brain abscess, 506
Extradural hematoma, 480-481
Extradural tumor, 504
Extrahepatic obstruction, 1249
  jaundice and, 1242
Extrahepatic portal hypertension, 1283
Extramedullary hematopoiesis, 763
Extramedullary tumor, 504
Extraocular muscles, 414
  paralysis of, 416
Extrapancreatic neoplasms, 619
Extrapyramidal motor syndromes, 457-458
Extrapyramidal system, 360
Extrinsic asthma, 1069-1070
Extrinsic pathway, 225
Exudate, 217, 239
  fibrinous, 229, 239
  hemorrhagic, 239

Exudate—cont'd
pleural effusion and, 1064
purulent, 229, 239
serous, 239
Exudative effusion, 1063
Eye
autoimmunity and, 251
external, 413-414
hypertension and, 925
normal, 414-415
Eye muscles, myasthenia gravis and, 522
Eyebrow, seborrheic dermatitis of, 1404

F

F cells, 578
Fabricius, bursa of, 191, 200
Facial expression, pain and, 393
Facial nerves, 375
taste dysfunction and, 423
Facial nuclear palsy, 460
Facilitated diffusion, 22, 23
Facilitation, 357
Facioscapulohumeral muscular dystrophy, 1377, 1378-1379
Factor, clotting; *see* Clotting factors
Factor VIII deficiency, 844
Factor XI deficiency, 843-844
Failure to thrive, 1279-1280
Fallopian tubes, 647, 653-654, 657
False aneurysm, 927-928
False joint, 1323
False vocal cords, 1027
carcinoma of, 1084
Falx cerebri, 366
Familial disease aggregation, 163-166
Familial disease tendency, 163-166
Familial diseases, 168-183; *see also* Genes
allergy and, 255
autoimmunity and, 262
carcinoma in, 171-173
breast, 715
cardiovascular disorders in, 173-178
congenital heart defects and, 997, 998
contingency tables and, 160-161, 163
coronary artery disease and, 936
correlation coefficient and, 161-162, 163
diabetes mellitus and, 616, 617
dyslipoproteinemia in, 935
endocrine disorders in, 173
erythrocytes and, 834-842
gastrointestinal disorders in, 179-183
hematologic disorders in, 173
hypokalemic periodic paralysis in, 94
immunologic disorders in, 168-171
neuromuscular disorders in, 183
psychiatric disorders in, 183
renal disorders in, 178-179
Familial tendency, 168
Familial tremor, 454
Family history, 184
Fanconi anemia, 62, 318
Fascia, 1305
Fascicle, 371, 1305
Fasciculata of adrenal gland, 580
Fasciculations, 453
Fasting, 1238
Fasting blood glucose, 615
Fat
acid-base balance and, 101
carcinogenesis and, 328
homeostasis and, 283
hypertriglyceridemia induced by, 935
liver and, 1198

Fat—cont'd
small intestine and, 1187-1188
Fat-cell theory of obesity, 1236
Fat embolism, 931
Fat necrosis, 71-72, 714
Fat-soluble vitamins, 1189
Fatty cirrhosis, 67, 1249
Fatty liver of alcoholic, 67
Fatty streak, 919
Favism, 835
Febrile seizures, 547-548
Fecal mass, 1192
Feces, 1192
Feedback, hormones and, 565
Fellatio, 728
Felty syndrome, 251
Female birth control pill; *see* Oral contraceptives
Female genitalia, 650-655
Female gonads, 654
Female hormonal alterations, 680-684
Female-pattern alopecia, 1432
Female pelvic organs, 652
Female reproductive system, 650-660
aging and, 671-673
disorders of, 680-699
benign growths and, 690-693
cancer and, 301, 693-699
hormonal alterations and, 680-684
infection and, 684-687
inflammation and, 684-687
malignant tumors in, 693
menstrual alterations and, 680-684
pelvic relaxation disorders in, 687-690
proliferative conditions and, 690-693
genitalia in, 650-655
cancer of, 301
history and, 645
menopause and, 672
menstrual cycle in, 657-660
sex hormones and, 655-657
Female urethra, 1119
Feminization, 633
Femoral head, 1363
Femur
giant cell tumor of, 1338
rheumatoid arthritis and, 1344
Fenestration, 888-889
Ferritin, 69
serum, 777
Fertility, 705; *see also* Infertility
Fertility control, history of, 645
Fertility tests, 670-671
Fetal circulation, 995
Fetal development
of genitalia, 647, 648
heart defects and, 994
radiation and, 332
Fetal erythropoiesis, 829
Fetal hematopoiesis, 826
Fetal hemoglobin, 826
Fetal immune function, 212-213
Fetoprotein, 300, 339, 1260
Fetus; *see also* Infant
amniocentesis and, 127
genital herpes and, 739-740
gonorrhea and, 727
isoimmunity and, 262
oncofetal antigens and, 339
syphilis and, 730
Fever
benefits of, 405
central, 408

Fever—cont'd
leukemia and, 849
pathogenesis of, 404-405
physiology of, 404-405
seizure and, 547
substances producing, 404
Fever blister, 1411
Fiber, dietary, 329
Fibril, 1294, 1306, 1310, 1314
Fibrillation, 459
atrial, 964
degenerative joint disease and, 1340
ventricular, 965
Fibrin, 227, 242, 773
Fibrin degradation product, 776, 819
Fibrin-fibrinogen degradation products, 780
Fibrin stabilizing factor, 774
Fibrinase, 774
Fibrinogen, 227, 757, 774
assay of, 780
Fibrinoligase, 774
Fibrinolytic system, 776
Fibrinopeptides, 225, 227
Fibrinous exudate, 229, 239
Fibroadenoma, 296, 714
Fibroadenomatosis, 713
Fibroblasts, 127, 144, 243
Fibrocartilage, 1298
Fibrocystic disease
of breast, 712-714
of pancreas, 1276
Fibroids, uterine, 691
Fibroma, 296, 1382
Fibrosarcoma, 296, 1337-1338
breast, 716
Fibrous cartilage, 40
Fibrous cortical defect, 1382
Fibrous joint capsule, 1300
Fibrous joints, 1298
Fibrous plaque, 919
Fibrous skeleton of heart, 863-864
Fibula, osteogenesis imperfecta in, 1368
Fight or flight response, 586
FIGO staging of cervical carcinoma, 694, 698
Filtration, 21
Filtration slit, 1114
Fimbriae, 653
Finger
clubbing of, 1056
webbing and, 1363
Finger agnosia, 462
First-degree burns, 1423-1424
First-degree heart block, 966
Fissure
of Rolando, 360
skin, 1399
sylvian, 360
Fistula
potassium losses and, 94
radiation and, 308
rheumatoid arthritis and, 1344
Flaccid paralysis, 452, 458
amyotrophic lateral sclerosis and, 518
Flagella, sperm, 12
Flail chest, 1065, 1066
Flat bones, 1297
Flavin adenine nucleotide, 18
Flavor, 422
Fleas, 1448
Flexion injury of spine, 484
Flexion-rotation injury of spine, 485
Flexor spasm, 486, 547

Flexor tone, 451
Flies, 1417
Flight or fight action, 282, 284
Flocculation test, 668
Fluids; *see also* Cellular environment
    burn shock and, 1428
    capillary filtration of, 85
    child and, 1161
    excess of, 85
    ketoacidosis and, 621
    leukemia and, 807
    renal failure and, 1156
    retention of; *see* Edema
Fluorescein, 668
Fluorescent lighting, 65
Fluorescent treponemal antibody absorption
        test, 732
Fluoroscopy, 907
Flush, vasomotor, 671
Flutter, atrial, 964
Focal seizures, 446, 447
Folate deficiency anemias, 789
Folic acid
    anemia and, 789
    erythropoiesis and, 767
Follicle-stimulating hormone
    alterations in production of, 596, 649
    deficiency of, 600
    fertility and, 671
    menstrual cycle and, 659
    production of, 571, 575
    reproductive system function and, 666
Follicular cyst, 690
Follicular phase of menstrual cycle, 657
Folliculitis, 1411
Fomite, 727
Fontan procedure, 1015
Fontanelle, 533, 535
Food
    absorption of, 1185
    carcinogenesis and, 326-329
    digestion of, 1185
    hypersensitivity and, 254
Food preservatives, 328
Foot
    congenital deformity of, 1364-1366
    diabetes mellitus and, 628
Foramen
    of Luschka, 367
    of Magendie, 367
    of Monro, 367
Foramen ovale, 994
Forbidden clone, 261
Forced expiratory volume, 1071
Forced vital capacity, 1071
Forearm ischemic exercise test, 1315
Forebrain, 359-361
Foreign antigens; *see* Antigen
Foreign matter in bloodstream, 931
Foreign proteins, 76
Foreskin, 663, 699
Fornix, 651
Fossa, cranial, 366
Founder cells, 31
Fovea centralis, 415
Fracture, 1320-1323
    classification of, 1320-1322
    complete, 1320
    overriding of, 1322
    skull, 480, 483
    vertebral, 485
Frameshift mutation, 121
Frank-Starling law, 879-880

Freckles, 68
Free erythrocyte protoporphyrin, 790
Free-radical theory of aging, 74
Freezing
    bradykinesia and, 453
    of cells, 63
French disease, 645
Frontal lobe, 360
    emotions and, 461
    hematoma in, 482
Frostbite, 1431-1432
Fructosemia, 1285
FSH; *see* Follicle-stimulating hormone
Full-thickness burn, 1425
Functional confusion, 442
Functional hearing loss, 421
Functional residual capacity, 1036, 1071
Fundus
    gastric, 1178
        plication of, 1276
    of uterus, 652
Fungal infection
    meningitis and, 506
    of skin, 1414-1416, 1441-1443
Furosemide, 1128
Furuncle, 1411
Fusiform aneurysm, 494
Fusiform muscles, 1305
Fusion, cell, 145

G

G cells, 1181
G_1 of G_2 phase of cellular reproduction, 29,
        30
GABAnergic neurons, 513
Gait, shuffling, 512
Gait dyspraxia, 463
Galactorrhea, 711-712
Galactosemia, 1284-1285
Galactosyl transferase, 300
Galea aponeurotica, 365
Gallbladder, 1193, 1199-1200
    cancer of, 1260
    disorders of, 1253-1254
    tests of, 1203, 1206
Gallop heart sounds, 903
Gallstones, 170, 1253
    familial diseases and, 179
Galvanometer, string, 857
Gametes, 28, 124
Gamma-aminobutyric acid, 357
Gamma globulin, 274, 756
Gamma glutamyl transpeptidase, 300
Gamma motor neuron, 458
Gamma neuropathy, 458
Ganglia, 353
    basal, 359, 360
    collateral, 377
Ganglioneuroblastoma, 556
Ganglioneuroma, 556
Gangrene, 72
    diabetes mellitus and, 627
    thromboangiitis obliterans and, 932
Gangrenous necrosis, 72
Gap junctions, 32, 33
Gardnerella, 735-736
Gas, inhalation of toxic, 1065-1066
Gas emboli, 63
Gas exchange, 1030-1031
    inadequate, 1067
Gas gangrene, 72
Gas pressure, measurement of, 1034-1036
Gas transport, 1043-1048

Gasping breathing pattern, 435
Gastrectomy, 1230
Gastric acid, 1180-1181
    history of study of, 1173
    stimulation of, 1204
Gastric cancer, 1256
Gastric distention, 1224
Gastric emptying, 1179
Gastric glands, 1179, 1180
Gastric motility, 1178-1179
Gastric mucus, 1181
Gastric phase of secretion, 1181-1182
Gastric pit, 1179
Gastric secretion, 1179-1182
Gastric surgery, 182, 1230
Gastric ulcer, 1226-1228, 1229
Gastrin, 1178, 1179
    tumor cell markers and, 300
Gastrin-secreting cells, 1181
Gastritis, 1224-1225
    alkaline reflux, 1230
    atrophic, 251
Gastrocolic reflex, 1192
Gastroenteritis, 1281
Gastroesophageal reflux, 1219-1220
    child and, 1275-1276
Gastroileal reflex, 1190
Gastrointestinal allergy, 254
Gastrointestinal bleeding, 1217-1219
Gastrointestinal system, 1175-1193
    autoimmunity and, 251
    cortisol and, 285-286
    disorders of; *see* Gastrointestinal system
        disorders
    esophagus in, 1176-1177
    intestinal bacteria in, 1192-1193
    large intestine in, 1190-1192
    mouth in, 1175
    small intestine and, 1182-1190
    stomach in, 1177-1182
    structural layers of, 1178
    tests for, 1202, 1204
    uremia and, 1157
Gastrointestinal system disorders, 1213-1238
    abdominal pain and, 1216-1217
    anorexia and, 1214
    appendicitis and, 1235
    bleeding and, 1217-1219
    cancer in, 1255-1259
    child and, 1268-1282
        absorption in, 1276-1280
        acquired motility impairment in,
            1274-1276
        anorectal malformations in, 1273-1274
        cleft lip and cleft palate in, 1268-1282
        congenital motility disorders in,
            1268-1274
        cystic fibrosis in, 1276-1277
        diarrhea in, 1280-1282
        digestion in, 1276-1280
        duodenal, jejunal, or ileal obstructions
            in, 1272-1273
        esophageal malformations in,
            1270-1271
        failure to thrive in, 1279-1280
        gastroesophageal reflux in, 1275-1276
        gluten-sensitive enteropathy in,
            1277-1279
        intussusception in, 1274-1275
        malrotation in, 1271-1272
        meconium ileus in, 1272
        nutrition in, 1276-1280
    constipation and, 1214-1215

Gastrointestinal system disorders—cont'd
  diarrhea and, 1215-1216, 1280-1282
  dysphagia and, 1219
  familial, 179-183
  gastritis and, 1224-1225
  gastroesophageal reflux and, 1219-1220, 1275-1276
  hiatal hernia and, 1220-1221
  history of study of, 1173
  hyperthyroidism and, 604
  hypothyroidism and, 607
  intestinal obstruction and, 1222-1224
  liver and, 1282-1286
  malabsorption syndromes and, 1231-1235
  manifestations of, 1214-1219
  nutrition and, 1236-1238, 1276-1280
  peptic ulcer disease and, 1225-1231
  potassium losses and, 94
  pyloric obstruction and, 1221-1223
  sexually transmitted infections and, 745-747
  stress-related, 287
  vascular insufficiency and, 1235-1236
  vomiting and, 1214
Gastrojejunostomy, 1230
Gastroscopy, 1203
Gate control theory of pain, 396-397
Gating, 33
Gay bowel syndrome, 745
Gene dosage analysis, 145
Gene mapping, 141-147
  cell fusion and, 145
Gene markers, 144
Gene splicing, 123
Gene therapy, 117, 119-120
General adaptation syndrome, 279-282
Genes
  autoimmunity and, 262
  BAT, 180-182
  cellular injury and injurious, 62
  childhood cancer and, 317-319
  environmental interaction and, 153-189
    analyzing disease risk and, 158-162
    carcinogenesis in, 332
    combined effects and, 163-168
    factors causing disease and, 155-158
    familial diseases and, 168-183; *see also* Familial diseases
    family history and, 183-184
    risk factors and, 162-163
  genetic diseases and, 114-152
    chromosomes and, 124-133
    DNA, RNA, and proteins and, 116-124
    linkage analysis and gene mapping and, 141-147
    multifactorial inheritance and, 147-148
    population genetics and, 133-134
    transmission of, 134-141
  immune response, 198
  marker, 143
  regulatory, 116
  structural, 116
  tooth, 181-182
Genetic code, 116-120
Genetic counseling
  muscular dystrophy and, 1380
  sickle cell disease and, 841
Genetic engineering, 118-119
Genetic probes, 157
Genetics
  new, 118-119
  population, 133-134
Genital warts, 741

Genitalia
  diabetes mellitus and pruritus of, 617
  female
    cancer and, 301
    external, 650
    internal, 650-655
  fetal development of, 647, 648
  herpes and, 739-741
  lymphoid tissue associated with, 208
  male
    cancer and, 301
    external, 660-663
    internal, 663-666
  ulcers of, 734
Genitourinary system; *see also* Reproductive system; Urinary tract function
  childhood cancers and anomalies of, 318
  rhabdomyosarcoma and, 1384
  stress-related diseases of, 287
Genome, 143
Genotype, 133-134
  obesity and, 180-181
Germ cell therapy, 119
Germ cell tumor, 697
  testicular, 704, 705
German measles, 1444, 1445
Germinoma, testicular, 705
Gertsmann syndrome, 462
Gestation, hematopoiesis and, 826
Gestational diabetes, 613, 618
Giant aneurysm, 494
Giant cell tumor, 1338-1339
Giant cells, 238
  Langhans'-type, 238
Giants, 601
Giardiasis, 746
Gibbs-Donnan equilibrium, 21
Giemsa stain, 124
Gilbert disease, 1243
Glands
  Bartholin, 650
  endocrine; *see* Endocrine glands
  exocrine, 578
  of Montgomery, 666
  parathyroid, 563, 577-578
  pituitary, 570
  Skene, 650
  thyroid, 574-577
Glandular epithelial carcinoma in situ, 295
Glans, 663
Glass factor, 774
Glaucoma, 416, 417
Glioblastoma multiforme, 500, 501
Gliomas, 295, 296, 499, 500
  brainstem, 553, 554, 555
  infiltrating, 553
  optic nerve, 553, 554, 555
Gliosis, 516
Glisson capsule, 1194
Global dysphasia, 467
Globin, 765
Globulin, 755, 757
Glomerular capillary, 1116
Glomerular disorders, 1144-1150
  child and, 1163-1166
Glomerular filtration, 1122-1126; *see also* Glomerular filtration rate
Glomerular filtration membrane, 1114
Glomerular filtration pressures, 1123, 1124
Glomerular filtration rate, 1119, 1124, 1129-1130
  child and, 1161
  plasma creatinine and, 1154

Glomerulonephritis, 1144-1149
  child and, 1164-1165
  chronic, 1145, 1147
  immune-complex, 251
  immunologic pathogenesis of, 1147
  membranoproliferative, 1148
  poststreptococcal, 261, 1146
  rapidly progressive, 1147
  types of, 1145
Glomerulosclerosis, diabetes mellitus and, 625
Glomerulotubular balance, 1126
Glomerulus, 1113, 1121, 1146; *see also* Glomerular filtration rate
  anatomy of, 1116
  types of lesions of, 1144
Glossopharyngeal nerves, 375
Glottis, 1027
Glucagon, 578, 580
Glucocorticoids, 582-583
  inflammatory response and, 285
Gluconeogenesis, 580, 1238
  cortisol and, 284
Glucose
  adenosine triphosphate and, 17
  burn injury and, 1430
  capillary, 615
  fasting blood, 615
  homeostasis and, 283
  nutritional imbalances and, 62
  oxidative phosphorylation and, 19
  shock and, 983-984
  small intestine and, 1186
  venous, 615
Glucose intolerance, 613
  coronary artery disease and, 936
  hypercortisolism and, 629
Glucose tolerance test, 612
Glucose-6-phosphate dehydrogenase deficiency, 173, 830, 834-835
  test for, 777
Glucuronide, 770
Glutamic acid, 836, 837
Gluten-sensitive enteropathy, 179, 251, 1277-1279
Glutethimide, 436
Glycerol, 1128
Glycogen
  aerobic, 1312
  cellular injury and, 67-68
  muscle disease and, 1353
Glycogenolysis, 580
Glycolipids, plasma membranes and, 13
Glycolysis, 18, 19
Glycolytic pathway, 1315
Glycoprotein, 14, 566, 1294-1295
  plasma membranes and, 13
Glycoprotein hormones, 575
Glycosaminoglycan, 1301
Glycosuria, 623
Glycosylated hemoglobin, 612
GM_2 ganglioside, 9
Goblet cell, 1030
Goiter, nodular, 605
Golgi complex, 6-8
Golgi tendon organs, 1306
Gomphosis, 1298
Gonadal dysgenesis, 318
Gonadal failure, premature, 250
Gonadotropin-releasing hormone
  hormonal alteration and, 596
  hormonal regulation and, 573
  menstrual cycle and, 659

Gonadotropin-releasing hormone—cont'd
   reproductive system and, 649, 666
Gonadotropins, 649
   aging and, 673
   secondary amenorrhea and, 682
Gonorrhea, 645, 727-729
   cultures and, 669
   urethritis and, 699
Gonorrheal warts, 741
Goodpasture syndrome, 251, 1145
Gout, 9, 1138, 1347-1350
   familial diseases and, 170
   tophaceous, 1350
Gouty arthritis, 1347, 1349
Gower sign, 1377
Grading of tumor, 301
Graft
   coronary artery bypass, 941-942
   rejection of, 264
Graft-versus-host disease, 266, 275
Gram-negative bacteria, 58
Gram staining, 668
Grand mal seizure, 447
Granulation tissue, 242
Granulocyte-releasing factor, 770-771
Granulocytes, 758, 801
   cancer and, 308
   inflammation and, 229
Granulocytic leukemia, 296
Granulocytopenia, 802
Granulocytosis, 801
Granuloma, chronic inflammation and, 238
Granuloma inguinale, 735
Granulomatous colitis, 1258
Granulomatous reaction, bacteria and, 59
Granulopoietin, 771
Granulosa cells, 655
Granulosa–theca cell tumors, 297
Graves disease, 170, 250, 263, 604-605
Gray, radiation and, 331
Gray matter, 359
Great vessels, 864
   transposition of, 1009-1010
Greeks, ancient, 351, 753, 857
Greenstick fracture, 1320, 1321
Ground substance, 41, 1293
Growth
   bone, 1362
   muscle, 1362-1363
   nervous system and, 533-535
Growth hormone, 336, 575
   hypersecretion of, 602-603
   stress response and, 286
Growth hormone-releasing factor, 573
Growth plate, rickets and, 1368
G-6-PD deficiency; *see* Glucose-6-phosphate
      dehydrogenase deficiency
Guanethidine, 711
Guanine, 117
Guanosine monophosphate, cyclic, 569
Guanosine triphosphate, 569
Guillain-Barré syndrome, 461, 521
Gumma, 730
Gustation, 421-423
Gut-associated lymphoid tissue, 208
Guttate psoriasis, 1405
Gynandroblastoma, 297
Gynecomastia, 130, 668, 717-719
Gyrus, 359
   postcentral, 360

H

H band, 1309, 1310
H2 receptors, 253

Haemophilus ducreyi, 733
Haemophilus influenzae, 1098
   bacterial meningitis and, 549
Haemophilus vaginalis, 735-736
Hageman factor, 773, 774
   coagulation and, 225, 226, 227, 228
Hair, 1392
   disorders of, 1432-1433
   loss of, 1432-1433
      discoid lupus erythematosus and, 1408
Hair cells, hearing and, 419
Hair follicle, 1393
Hallucinations, 442
   olfactory, 422-423
Hamartoma, 318
Hammer, 419
Hand
   dislocation of, 1324
   rheumatoid arthritis of, 1342
Haploid cells, 124
Haplotype, 198
Haptens, 197
   hypersensitivity and, 260
Hard chancre, 731
Hashimoto thyroiditis, 170, 608
HAT medium, 144, 314
Haustra, 1190, 1192
Haversian system, 1295
Hay fever, 250
Head
   circumference of, 541
   development of, 535
   rhabdomyosarcoma and, 1384
   veins of, 371
Head lice, 1447
Head trauma, open, 482-483
Headache, 396
   brain tumor and, 553-554
   subarachnoid hemorrhage and, 498
Healing, dysfunctional wound, 244-246
Hearing, 419-421
Hearing loss
   conductive, 420-421
   functional, 421
   mixed, 421
   noise-induced, 65
   sensorineural, 421
Hearing receptors, 419
Heart, 860-886
   actin and, 875
   action potentials and, 871-873
   adrenergic receptor function and, 873-874
   afterload and, 881
   beats per minute of, 869
   biochemicals and, 882
   blood flow during cardiac cycle and,
      864-865
   chambers of, 862-863
   conduction system and, 402, 869-873
      disorders of, 966-967
   congenital defects of, 174, 996-1015; *see
      also* Congenital heart defects
   coronary vessels in, 866-867
   development of, 993-994
   excitation and, 869, 870-871
   fibrous skeleton of, 863-864
   Frank-Starling law and, 879-880
   great vessels in, 864
   history of, 857
   hypertension and, 925
   hypokalemia and, 95
   innervation and, 873-874
   intracardiac pressures and, 865-866
   Laplace law and, 880-881

Heart—cont'd
   metabolism and, 866-867, 876
   myocardial cells and, 874-876
   myocardial contraction and, 876-878,
      882-883
   myocardial relaxation and, 878-879
   myosin and, 875
   output and, 883
   parasympathetic nerves and, 873
   performance and, 879-886
   preload and, 881
   rate of, 869, 881-882, 906
   structures that direct circulation and,
      860-866
   suction-pump theory of action of,
      883-886
   sympathetic nerves and, 873
   troponin-tropomyosin complex and,
      875-876
   valves of, 70, 169, 173, 863, 864
      prosthetic, 786
   wall of; *see* Heart wall
Heart attack, 934
Heart disease
   congenital; *see* Congenital heart defects
   coronary, 155, 169, 175
   manifestations of, 963-976
      dysrhythmia and, 963
      heart failure and, 963-976; *see also*
         Heart failure
   pulmonary, 1082-1083
   pulmonary edema and, 1059
   rheumatic, 169, 173
      aortic valve calcification and, 70
Heart failure, 963-976
   biventricular, 972
   congestive, 971-975
      child and, 1015-1017
   left, 971-975
   mechanisms of, 963-969
   right, 969-971
   types of, 969-975
Heart murmur, 903, 955
   tetralogy of Fallot and, 1014
Heart sounds
   abnormal, 902-903
   auscultation of, 901-902
   normal, 902
Heart transplantation, 857-858
Heart valves, 70, 169, 173, 863, 864
   prosthetic, 786
Heart wall, 860-862
   disorders of, 947-962
      cardiomyopathy and, 950-953
      endocardium and, 953-962
      pericardium and, 947-951
Heartbeat, irregular, 901
Heartburn, 1256
Heat
   conservation of, 400, 403
   loss of, 400
      mechanisms of, 402
   production of, 400, 402
   stress and, 282
Heat cramps, 405
Heat exhaustion, 405
Heatstroke, 405-406
Heavy chains, 202, 203
Heavy metals, 56
Height, multifactorial trait and, 157
Helper cells, 209
Hemangioblastoma, 500
Hemangioma, 296
   cavernous, 1448

Hemangioma—cont'd
strawberry, 1448, 1449
Hemangiosarcoma, 296
Hemarthrosis, 817
Hematemesis, 1217
Hematochezia, 1217
Hematocrit determination, 777
Hematogenous osteomyelitis, 1332
Hematologic function
autoimmunity and, 251
child and, 825-855
clinical evaluation of, 776-780
disorders of
blood tests for, 777-780
coagulation, 842-845
erythrocyte, 829-842; *see also*
Erythrocytes
familial diseases and, 173
platelet, 845-847
fetal hematopoiesis and, 826
hypothyroidism and, 606
leukemia and, 847-850
liver and, 1198
lymphoma and, 850-852
neonatal hematopoiesis and, 826
platelet disorders and, 845-847
postnatal changes in blood and, 826-829
structure and, 755-783
aging and, 780
blood cell development and, 763-771
blood tests and, 777-780
bone marrow function tests and, 776-777
composition of blood and, 755-760
hemostasis and, 771-776
lymphoid organs and, 760-761
mononuclear phagocyte system and, 761-763
uremia and, 1157
Hematology, history of study of, 753
Hematoma, 480-482, 817
bone repair and, 1297, 1298
Hematopoiesis, 763-764
fetal, 826
Hematuria, 1131
Heme, 765, 766
Hemiagnosia, 400
Hemianopia, 418, 554
Hemihypertrophy, 318
Hemiparesis, 451
Hemiplegia, 451
Hemiplegic posture, 452
Hemispheric breathing patterns, 435
Hemizygous male, 139
Hemochromatosis, 143, 170, 173
Hemoglobin, 758
arterial oxygenation and, 1046
carbon monoxide and, 56
determination of, 777
electrophoresis and, 777
embryonic, 826
fetal, 826
glycosylated, 612
hemoproteins and, 69
metabolism of, tests for, 777-778
molecular structure of, 765, 766
sickle cell, 837
synthesis of, 765-766
Hemoglobin A, 766
Hemoglobin buffer system, 103, 104
Hemoglobin desaturation, 1046
Hemoglobin F, 766
Hemoglobin Gower 1 and Gower 2, 766
Hemoglobin H disease, 841

Hemoglobin Portland, 766
Hemoglobin S, 836
Hemoglobin saturation, 1046
Hemolipin, 795
Hemolytic anemia, 792-794
autoimmune, 792
cancer and, 307
causes of, 793
congenital, 835
drug-induced, 173
familial diseases and, 170, 173
prosthetic heart valve and, 786
Hemolytic disease of newborn, 829, 831-834
Hemolytic jaundice, 1243
Hemolytic streptococci, 958
Hemolytic uremic syndrome, 1165-1166
Hemophilia, 173, 842-845
Hemophilia A, 140, 842
Hemophilia B, 842
Hemophilia C, 843-844
Hemoproteins, 69
Hemoptysis, 704, 1055-1056
Hemorrhage; *see* Bleeding
Hemorrhagic exudate, 239
Hemorrhagic pancreatitis, 1254
Hemorrhagic shock, 408
Hemorrhagic stroke, 494
Hemorrhagic thrombocythemia, 818
Hemorrhoids, thrombosed, 1258
Hemosiderin, 69
Hemosiderosis, 69
Hemostasis, 771-776
alterations in, 816-822
control of, 773-776
Hemothorax, 1064
Henderson-Hasselbalch equation, 102
Heparin, 773-776, 821
Heparin-neutralizing factor, 772
Hepatavax-B vaccine, 747
Hepatic encephalopathy, 1240, 1242
child and, 1284
tremor of, 454
Hepatitis
alcoholic, 1250
child and, 1282-1283
chronic active, 251, 1248
fulminant, 1248
history of, 1173
icteric phase of, 1248
non-A, non-B, 1247
viral, 1245-1248
Hepatitis A, 1245-1246
Hepatitis B, 1246-1247
sexually transmitted, 746-747
Hepatitis D, 1247
Hepatocellular carcinoma, 1259
Hepatocellular jaundice, 1244
Hepatocytes, 51, 1195
Hepatolenticular degeneration, 1285
Hepatomegaly, 66
congestive heart failure and, 1016
Hepatorenal syndrome, 1244-1245
Hereditary elliptocytosis, 786
Hereditary spherocytosis, 786, 835-836
Heredity, genes and; *see* Genes
Hering-Breuer expiratory reflex, 1041
Heritability; *see* Genes
Hernia
hiatal, 1220-1221
intestinal obstruction and, 1222
Herniated intervertebral disk, 490, 491-493
Herniation
brain tissue and, 469

Herniation—cont'd
tentorial, 470
Herpes, genital, 739-741
Herpes simplex encephalitis, 507, 508
Herpes simplex labialis, 1412
Herpes simplex virus, 739, 1411-1412
cervical cancer and, 329
in utero, 740
Herpes virus 5, 669
Herpes zoster, 1412-1413
child and, 1446
Herpesviruses, 61, 334
Heterogeneity, 163
Heterogeneous nuclear RNA, 123
Heterokaryote, 144
Heterozygosity, genes and, 133
Hiatal hernia, 1220-1221
Hiccup, 453
High-altitude pulmonary edema, 63, 1059
High blood pressure, 161
High-density lipoproteins, 626, 934, 937
High-molecular weight kininogen, 775
High-output failure, 975-976
Hilar cell tumor, 297
Hilus, 1029, 1113
Hindbrain, 362
Hip dislocation, 1324
Hip dysplasia, congenital, 1363-1364
Hirschsprung disease, 1273
Hirsutism, 681, 1433
His bundle electrocardiography, 905-906
Histaminase, 221
Histamine, 220, 226, 253
Histamine receptors, 253
Histocompatibility, 193
Histocompatibility antigens, 198
ankylosing spondylitis and, 1346, 1347
detection of, 199
diabetes mellitus and, 613
familial diseases and, 173
graft rejection and, 264
hypersensitivity and, 262
transplants and, 275
Histones, 4, 5, 7
History, medical family, familial diseases and, 184
Hives, 254-255
hnRNA, 123
Hodgkin disease, 811-814
carcinogenesis and, 327
child and, 852
contiguity theory of, 813
history of study of, 753
staging classification of, 814
tumor biology and, 303, 305
Holt-Oram syndrome, 998
Homeostasis, 282
cerebral, 465-470
immunologic, 252, 261
stress and, 283
Homologous chromosomes, 124
Homonymous hemianopia, 418-419
Homosexuality, AIDS and, 269, 270
Homozygosity, 133, 139
Hormonal hyperplasia, 51
Hormone replacement therapy
coronary artery disease and, 937
osteoporosis and, 1330
Hormones, 563, 564
adrenal, 628-637
general adaptation syndrome and, 282
aging and, 75, 588-589, 673
alterations of, 594-643
adrenal function and, 628-637

Hormones—cont'd
  alterations of—cont'd
    diabetes mellitus and, 612-628; *see also*
        Diabetes mellitus
    female, 680-684
    hypothalamic-pituitary system and,
        596-603
    parathyroid function and, 609-612
    thyroid function and, 603-609
  of anterior pituitary, 571, 574
  antidiuretic, 573-574
  arterial pressure and, 896
  breast cancer and, 715
  calcium balance and, 98
  cancer treatment and, 309
  carcinogenesis and, 332-333
  cellular mechanisms of, 568-570
  cellular receptors and binding of, 16
  chemical classification of, 566
  of digestive system, 1179
  ectopic, tumor cell markers and, 300
  female, 655-657
    alterations of, 680-684
  gonads and, 649
  gynecomastia and, 718
  heart and, 882
  hypothalamic, 573
  kidney and, 1121
  lipid-soluble, 569, 570
  male, 665-666
    aging and, 673
  mechanisms of, 564-593
    aging and, 588-589
    cellular mechanisms in, 568-570
    endocrine glands and, 570-588; *see also*
        Endocrine glands, structure and
        function of
    regulation of release in, 565
    transport in, 565-568
  menopause and, 671
  menstrual cycle and, 659
  osteoporosis and, 1328-1329
  of posterior pituitary, 573-574
  of pregnancy, 657
  regulation of release of, 565
  serum, fertility and, 671
  sex, 646
    female, 655-657
    history of, 645
    male, 665-666
  steroid, 570, 655
  stress response and, 283-287
  thymic epithelium and, 209
  transport of, 565-568
  tumors and, 299
  water-soluble, 568-570
Horseshoe kidney, 1162
Hospital-acquired pneumonia, 1077
Hospital-related infections, 308
Host cell, permissive, 59
Host tissue, tumor cells and, 303
Host-tumor relationship, 342
Hot flash, 671
Hot spots, myocardial infarction and, 905,
    945
Howell-Jolly bodies, 786
Howship lacunae, 1294
Human bursal equivalent, 200
Human chorionic gonadotropin, 299, 300,
    703
Human immunodeficiency virus, 270-273
Human leukocyte antigens; *see*
        Histocompatibility antigens

Human papillomavirus, 329, 741
Humoral immunity, 191, 195-196, 200-209
  leukemia and, 809
  tests of, 275
Hunner ulcer, 1142
Huntington disease, 136-137, 513-514
Hyaline cartilage, 40, 1298
Hyaline membrane disease, 1104
Hyalinization
  cellular injury and, 70
  of islets in diabetes mellitus, 616
Hyaluronate, 1300
Hybrid cells, 144, 314
Hybrid clones, 144
Hybridization
  in situ, 146
  somatic cell, 145-146
Hybridoma, 207, 314
Hydatiform mole, 297
Hydrocele, 701-702
Hydrocephalus, 519, 540
  acute, 519
  congenital, 541
  ex vacuo, 519
  noncommunicating, 470
  obstructive, 541
Hydrochloric acid, 1181
Hydrogen
  acid-base balance and, 100-101
  renal buffering and, 104
  renal tubular transport and, 1126
Hydrogen cyanide, 57
Hydrogen ion concentration, 93, 100-101
Hydrogen peroxide
  peroxisomes and, 10
  phagocytosis and, 231
Hydrogen sulfide, 57
Hydrolases, 8, 303
Hydrolytic enzymes
  atrophy and, 50
  cellular death and, 70-71
Hydronephrosis, 1136, 1137
Hydropic degeneration, 66
Hydrops fetalis, 832, 842
Hydrostatic pressure
  of fluid within capillaries, 85
  passive transport and, 19, 20-21
Hydrothorax, 1064
Hydroureter, 1136
Hydroxyapatite, 97, 1295
Hydroxylation
  calcium and, 69
  vitamin D and, 1129
Hyperaldosteronism, 107, 631-633
Hyperbaric chamber, 72
Hyperbilirubinemia, 69, 1242
  child and, 832, 1282
Hypercalcemia, 70, 99, 610, 611
Hypercapnia, 108, 1055, 1057
Hyperchloremia, 90-91
Hyperchloremic metabolic acidosis, 106
Hypercholesterolemia, 175, 935
  familial, 176
Hyperchromic erythrocyte, 784-785
Hypercoagulable state, 1430
Hypercortical function, 629-631
Hypercortisolism, 629-631
Hyperemia, 896
Hyperesthesia, 399
Hyperextension injury of spine, 483
Hyperglycemia, 62
  stress response and, 283-284
Hyperglycemic nonketotic coma, 622-623

Hyperhemolytic crisis, 840
Hyperinsulinemia, 617
Hyperkalemia, 96-97
  renal failure and, 1153
Hyperkeratosis of skin, 51
Hyperkinesia, 453-455
Hyperlipidemia, 62, 934-936
  nephrotic syndrome and, 1149
Hypermagnesemia, 100
Hypernatremia, 89-90
  leukemia and, 807
Hyperopia, 417
Hyperosalpingogram, 670
Hyperosmolality, hypernatremia and, 89
Hyperosmolar hyperglycemic nonketotic
    coma, 622-623
Hyperosmotic interstitium, 1126
Hyperparathyroidism, 609-611
Hyperphenylalaninemia, 545
Hyperphosphatemia, 100, 577
  hypoparathyroidism and, 611
Hyperpigmentation, Cushing syndrome and,
    629
Hyperpituitarism, 600-601
Hyperplasia
  cellular adaptation and, 50-51
  compensatory, 243
Hyperpnea, 1055
Hyperpolarization, 28, 871
Hyperprolactinemia, 681
  nonpuerperal, 711
Hyperreflexia, autonomic, 486-488
Hypersecretion of adrenal hormones, 633
Hypersensitivity, 249-264
  autoimmune and isoimmune diseases and,
    263-264
  IgE-mediated, 253-254
    tests of, 255
  mechanisms of, 252-260
  skin and, 1402
  targets of, 260-263
Hypersomnia, 442, 443
Hypersplenism, 816
Hypertension, 161, 169, 920-926, 936
  arterial, 156
  black child and, 1019
  classification of, 926
  complicated, 923-925
  essential, 177
  familial diseases and, 176-177
  hemorrhage and, 494
  hyperaldosteronism and, 633
  intracranial, 468
  isolated systolic, 920, 923
  left heart failure and, 971
  malignant, 925
  portal, 1238-1241
    child and, 1283-1284
  primary, 921-923
    child and, 1017-1019
    risk factors for, 920-921
  pulmonary, 1082, 1083
  salt-induced, 177, 178
  secondary, 920, 923
    child and, 1017
  pathogenesis of, 923-924
Hyperthermia, 63, 401, 405
Hyperthyroidism, 603-606
  heart failure and, 976
  hormonal regulation and, 563
  immunity and inflammation and, 250
Hypertonia, 89-91, 452
Hypertonic hyponatremia, 91

Hypertonic solution, 22
Hypertriglyceridemia, 935
Hypertrophic cardiomyopathy, 953
Hypertrophic scar, 245
Hypertrophy, 50, 451
Hyperuremia, 849
Hyperuricemia, 1348
Hyperventilation, 1055
  asthma and, 1071
Hypoalbuminemia
  cachexia and, 306
  nephrotic syndrome and, 1149
Hypocalcemia, 97, 98-99
  renal failure and, 1155
Hypocapnia, 109, 1055
Hypochloremia, 92
Hypochloremic alkalosis, 107
Hypochlorhydria, 1207
Hypochromic erythrocyte, 785
Hypochromic-microcytic anemia, 786
Hypocomplementemia, 258
Hypocortical function, 633-635
Hypocortisolism, 633-634
Hypodermis, 1392-1393
Hypogammaglobulinemia, 213, 266, 274
Hypogeusia, 423
Hypoglossal nerves, 375
Hypoglossal nuclear palsy, 460
Hypoglycemia, 618-619
  alimentary, 620
  endogenous causes of, 619
  exogenous causes of, 618
  functional causes of, 620
  organic, 619
  Somogyi effect and, 624
Hypoglycemic agents, oral, 618
Hypokalemia, 93, 94-96
  hyperaldosteronism and, 633
  leukemia and, 807
Hypokalemic periodic paralysis, 94, 1352
Hypokinesia, 452, 512
Hypolipidemia, 62
Hypomagnesemia, 100, 577, 611
Hyponatremia, 91-92, 597
Hypoparathyroidism, 611-612
  idiopathic, 250
Hypophosphatemia, 99-100
Hypopituitarism, 599-600, 601
Hypopolarized cell membrane, 97
Hyporeflexia, 458
Hyposmia, 422
Hypospadias, 1162
Hypotension, orthostatic, 926-927
Hypothalamic hormones, 573
  absence of, 596
Hypothalamic-pituitary-adrenal system, 288
Hypothalamic-pituitary-gonadal axis, 649
  disruption of, 678
Hypothalamic-pituitary-ovarian axis,
    amenorrhea and, 680
Hypothalamic-pituitary system, 570-573
  alterations of, 596-603
Hypothalamus, 360, 361
  emotional control and, 462
  menstrual cycle and, 659
  temperature control and, 401-404
Hypothermia, 401, 406
  accidental, 406-407
  injury and, 63
  therapeutic, 407
Hypothyroidism, 563, 606-609
  congenital, 608
  galactorrhea and, 712

Hypotonia, 91-92, 452
  causes and consequences of, 91
Hypotonic solution, 21
Hypoventilation, 1042, 1055
Hypovolemia, 89
  inflammation and, 244
Hypovolemic shock, 977, 978
  burns and, 1427
Hypoxanthines, 145, 314
Hypoxemia, 1057-1058, 1073
  respiratory distress syndrome of newborn
    and, 1104, 1105
Hypoxia, 52, 1057
  anemia and tissue, 787
  cellular injury and, 52-55
  cerebral palsy and, 543
  myocardial infarction and, 942
  tetralogy of Fallot and, 1013
Hypoxic vasoconstriction, 1042
Hysterectomy, 691
  first, 645
Hysteria, 645

I

I bands, 1309, 1310
  heart and, 875
Iatrogenic deficiencies, 268-269
Iatrogenic infections, 308, 1077
Icterus; *see* Jaundice
Icterus gravis neonatorum, 834
Icterus neonatorum, 833, 1282
Ideational dyspraxia, 463
Ideomotor dyspraxia, 463
Idiojunctional rhythm, 964
Idiopathic Addison disease, 634
Idiopathic hypertension, 920
Idiopathic hypertrophic subaortic stenosis,
  953
Idiopathic hypoparathyroidism, 250
Idiopathic lymphopenia, 251
Idiopathic neutropenia, 251
Idiopathic orthostatic hypotension, 927
Idiopathic polyneuritis, 521
Idiopathic pulmonary fibrosis, 1065
Idiopathic respiratory distress syndrome,
  1104
Idiopathic scoliosis, 1369
Idiopathic thrombocytopenic purpura, 170,
  818, 845-846
Idioventricular rhythm, 965
IF; *see* Intrinsic factor
IgE-mediated hypersensitivity, 252-254
  tests of, 255
Ileocecal valve, 1182, 1190
Ileocolic intussusception, 1274, 1275
Ileogastric reflex, 1190
Ileum, 1182
  obstruction of, 1272-1273
Ileus, paralytic, 1222
Illusions, 442
Immediate hypersensitivity reactions, 252
Immediate recall, loss of, 443
Immersion blast, 63
Immobility
  muscle, 1351-1352
  pressure ulcer and, 1400
Immune complex, 205
Immune-complex disease, 258
Immune-complex glomerulonephritis, 251
Immune-complex—mediated injury,
    hypersensitivity and, 257-258
Immune deficiencies, 265
  childhood cancers and, 318

Immune deficiencies—cont'd
  congenital, 265, 266-268
  laboratory evaluation of, 275
  replacement therapies for, 274-276
Immune memory cells, 310
Immune reserve, cortisol and, 286
Immune response; *see* Immunity
Immune response genes, 198
Immune surveillance theory of
    carcinogenesis, 337-343
Immune system
  autonomic nervous system and, 288
  burn injury and, 1430-1431
  cortisol and, 587
  elderly and, 213-214
  fetal, 212-213
  hypothalamic-pituitary-adrenal system and,
    288
  multiple sclerosis and, 515
  neonatal, 212-213
  neuroendocrine system and, 288
  secretory, 207-209
  stress response and, 287-288
  uremia and, 1157
Immune thrombocytopenic purpura, 263
Immunity, 192-216
  acquired, 194
  alterations in, 249-278
    deficiencies and, 265-276, 339; *see also*
      Acquired immune deficiencies
    hypersensitivity and, 249-264; *see also*
      Hypersensitivity
  cell-mediated, 195-196, 209
  cellular interactions in, 209-212
  characteristics of, 193-196
  clinical evaluation of, 274
  elderly and, 213-214
  exaggerated, 249
  fetal and neonatal, 212-213
  humoral, 195-196, 200-209
    leukemia and, 809
  inappropriate responses and, 249
  induction of, 196-200
  natural, 194
  primary, 194
  secondary, 194
Immunobiology of cancer, 337-343
Immunocompetent cells, 193
Immunocytes, 193, 758
Immunodiagnosis, tumor, 315
Immunofluorescent testing, 668
Immunogen, 196-198
Immunoglobulin A, 206, 208, 274
  deficiency of
    childhood cancers and, 318
    selective, 267
Immunoglobulin D, 207
Immunoglobulin E, 207
Immunoglobulin G, 206, 208, 212-213, 252
  blood test and, 779
  multiple sclerosis and, 515
Immunoglobulin G—coated fetal erythrocyte,
  832
Immunoglobulin M, 206-207, 208, 252, 274
  Wiskott-Aldrich syndrome and, 267
Immunoglobulins, 202-207, 755, 757
  aggregated, 274
  biologic properties of, 205
  classes of, 206-207
  familial diseases and, 194
  inflammation and, 218
  molecular structure of, 202-205
  physicochemical properties of, 202

Immunoglobulins—cont'd
rheumatoid arthritis and, 1342
thyroid-stimulating, 604
tumor cell markers and, 300
Immunologic exposure, 162
Immunologic homeostasis, 252, 261
Immunologic inflammatory injury, 61-62; *see also* Immunity
Immunologic stimulation, 343
Immunologic theory of aging, 74, 75
Immunologically privileged sites, 261
Immunology, 191; *see also* Immune response; Immunity
Immunomodulating agents, 310-311
Immunoreactive hormones, 287, 288
Immunostimulation, 311
Immunosuppressants, 342; *see also* Immunotherapy
childhood cancers and, 319
cortisol and, 285
Immunotherapy, 310-313, 316; *see also* Immunosuppressants
monoclonal antibodies and, 315
Immunotoxins, 313
Imperforate anus, 1274
Impetigo, 1411, 1440-1441
Implantation, metastasis by, 305
Impulse conduction, 356-357
heart disease and disorders of, 966-967
Impulse formation, heart disease and, 963-965
Inborn errors of metabolism
congenital heart defects and, 998
hypoglycemia and, 619
Incidence rate of disease, 158
Inclusion bodies, 61
Incontinence in child, 1169
Independent assortment, principle of, 134
Indirect Coombs test, 778
Indirect immunofluorescent antibody, 669, 748
Infant; *see also* Child; Neonate
chlamydial infection and, 736, 738
cytomegalovirus infection and, 747-748
diarrhea in, 1280
diencephalic syndrome of, 554
genital herpes and, 739-740
hematopoiesis and, 826
hepatitis B and, 747
hypoglycemia and, 620
hypothyroidism and, 608
osteomyelitis in, 1372
pneumonia and, 738
port-wine hemangioma in, 1450
reflexes of, 535
temperature regulation and, 404
Infantile microcytic disease, 1164
Infantile spasms, 450, 546-547
Infarction
cerebral, 470
myocardial, 934, 942-947
diabetes mellitus and, 627
pituitary, 599
Infection
anemia and, 834
bone, 1332-1334, 1370-1373
cancer and, 305, 307, 308
cellular injury and, 57-61
central nervous system and, 505-509
defenses against, 193
diabetes mellitus and, 617, 627-628
female reproductive system disorders and, 684-687

Infection—cont'd
fever and, 405
immune deficiency and, 265
leukemia and, 806
lower airway and, 1102-1104
reproductive function tests and, 668-669
sickle cell disease and, 840
skin, 1411-1415
bacterial, 1411, 1440-1441
child and, 1440-1446
fungal, 1414-1416, 1441-1443
tinea, 1414
viral, 1411-1415, 1443-1446
toe web, 1414
urinary tract, 1141-1144
vaginal, 651
viral replication and, 59
Infectious diarrhea in newborn, 1280
Infectious mononucleosis, 802-803
Infective endocarditis, 960-962
Inferior lateral pontine syndrome, 495
Inferior venae cavae, 864
Infertility
endometriosis and, 692
male, 250
Infiltrating glioma, 553
Infiltrations, cellular, 66
Infiltrative ophthalmopathy, 605
Inflammation, 192, 217-248
acute, 218-220
aging and, 246
alterations in, 249-278; *see also* Immunity
alternate pathway and, 223, 225
bacteria and, 59
cellular components of, 229-235
cellular products and, 235-236
central nervous system and, 505-509
chronic, 237, 238
classical pathway and, 223-225
cortisol and, 286
deficiencies in, 265-276; *see also* Acquired immune deficiencies
congenital immune, 265, 266-268
dysfunction during, 244
female reproductive system disorders and, 684-687
immunity and, 206
liver, in child, 1282-1283; *see also* Cirrhosis
local manifestations of, 238-239
mast cell and, 220-222
maturation phase of resolution and repair in, 242, 243-244
mononuclear phagocyte system and, 761-762
plasma protein systems and, 222-229
repair and, 239-246
resolution and, 239-246
skin and, 1402-1404
of spinal cord, 505
stomach, 1230
systemic manifestations of, 236-237
Inflammatory acne, 1407
Inflammatory arachnoiditis, 520
Inflammatory bowel diseases, 179
Inflammatory demyelinating polyradiculopathy, 521
Inflammatory joint disease, 1341-1350
Inflammatory muscle diseases, 1354-1355
Inflow tract of heart, 863
Influenza, 61
Influenza B, 548
Infratentorial herniation, 470

Infratentorial mass, coma and, 434
Infratentorial processes, 432
Infundibular process, 572
Infundibular stem, 570, 596
Infundibulum, 653
stenosis of, 1000
Ingestants
hypersensitivity and, 254
poisons and, 549
Inguinal canal, 660
Inhalants, hypersensitivity and, 254
Inhalation disorders, 1065-1067
Inheritance; *see also* Familial diseases; Genes
autosomal dominant, 134-137
autosomal recessive, 137-139
genetic; *see* Genes
multifactorial, 147-148
X-linked, 139-140
childhood cancers and, 319
Inherited hemorrhagic disease, 842-845
Inherited metabolic disorders of central nervous system, 544-546
Inhibin, 659
Inhibitory postsynaptic potentials, 357
Injury
aging and, 73
atherogenesis and, 919
cellular, 51-66; *see also* Cellular injury
chemical, 55-57
infectious, 57-61
musculoskeletal, 1320-1328
physical agents and, 62-66
Inner dura, 366
Inner ear, 419
Innervation; *see* Nerves
Inorganic phosphate, 17
Inotropic agents, 882
Insect bites, 1416-1417
child and, 1446-1448
Insertional mutagenesis, 337
Insomnia, 411
Inspiration, 1037
Inspiratory capacity, 1036
Inspiratory reserve volume, 1036
Insufficiency fracture, 1322
Insulin, 578, 580
deficiency of, 615
diabetic ketoacidosis and, 619
diabetes mellitus and, 616
gastric secretion and, 1181
glomerular filtration rate and, 1129
hypoglycemia and, 618
hypokalemia and, 94
recombinant DNA and, 119
tumors and, 299, 300
Insulin-dependent diabetes mellitus, 250, 613
Insulin receptors, 617
Insulin shock, 618
Intact nephron hypothesis, 1154
Integral membrane proteins, 14
Integration, viral replication and, 59
Integument; *see* Skin
Intellectual function, dementia and, 442-443
Intelligence quotient, 147
Intention, wound repair by primary or secondary, 240-241, 242
Intention tremor, 454
Intentional dementia, 443
Intercalated disk, 875
Intercostal muscles, 1037
Intercourse, cervical cancer and sexual, 329
Interdigestive myoelectric complex, 1190

Interferon inducers, 310
Interferons, 235-236, 310, 311
Interleukins, 312
  fever and, 404
  immune function and, 211, 288
  inflammation and, 236
Interlobar artery, 1116
Intermittent positive pressure breathing, 1073
Internal anal sphincter, 1190
Internal capsule of forebrain, 360
Internal carotid arteries, 368
  cerebrovascular aneurysm and, 495
Internal genitalia
  female, 650-655
  fetal development of, 647
  male, 663-666
Internal secretions, 563
International Federation of Gynecologists and Obstetricians, 694, 698
Interneurons, 355
Interphase, cellular reproduction and, 28, 30
Interspinous bursae, 490
Interstitial cell tumor, 297
Interstitial cystitis, 1142
Interstitial fluids
  cerebral, 469-470
  starvation and, 62
  water movement between plasma and, 84-85
Interstitial nephritis, chronic, 1143
Interstitium, hyperosmotic, 1126
Interventricular foramen, 367
Intervertebral disk, 368
  herniated, 491-493
Intestinal absorption, 1184
Intestinal bacteria, 1192-1193
Intestinal digestion, 1184
Intestinal disaccharidase deficiencies, 179
Intestinal drainage tubules, 94
Intestinal motility, 1190
Intestinal obstruction, 1222-1224
Intestine
  cystic fibrosis and, 1276
  large, 1190-1192
    carcinogenesis and, 327
  small, 1182-1190
Intestinointestinal reflex, 1190
Intima, 1300
Intoxication
  central nervous system, 549
  water, 92
Intra-aortic balloon pump, 975
Intracardiac catheterization, 857
Intracardiac pressures, normal, 865-866, 867
Intracellular communication, 32-33
Intracellular fluid, 14, 19, 83, 84
  electrolytes and, 93, 94
  imbalances and
    hypertonic, 90
    hypotonic, 91
Intracerebral brain abscess, 506
Intracerebral hemorrhage, 482, 498
Intracerebral tumors, primary, 499-503
Intracranial aneurysm, 494-497
Intracranial brain tumor, 498
Intracranial hemorrhage, 482, 493, 494, 498
Intracranial hypertension, 468
Intracranial pressure, 465-469
Intraductal papilloma, solitary, 714
Intradural tumor, 504
Intrahepatic obstruction, 1243, 1249
Intrahepatic portal hypertension, 1283

Intramedullary spinal cord abscess, 506
Intramedullary tumor, 504
Intramembranous bone formation, 1361
Intramuscular injection, toxic myopathy and, 1356
Intrarenal acute renal failure, 1151
Intrauterine radiation, 319
Intravenous drug abuse, AIDS and, 270
Intrinsic asthma, 1070
Intrinsic factor, 766, 788
Intrinsic pathway for coagulation, 225, 227
Introns, 123
Intussusception, 1274-1275
  intestinal obstruction and, 1222
Invasion, tumor, 302-303
Inversions, chromosomes and, 132
Involucrum, 1333
Involuntary movement, abnormal, 453
Iodide, thyroid hormone and, 566, 576-577
Iodine, radioactive, 604
Iodothyronines, 566, 576-577
Iodotyrosine, 577
Ion exchange mechanism, cellular, 104
Ionizing radiation, 331
  acquired immune deficiency and, 268
  cancer treatment and, 308-309
  carcinogenesis and, 332
  cellular injury and, 63-65
  leukemia and, 848
  prenatal exposure to, 319
Ions, 19
  potassium, 28
  sodium, 28
Ipsilateral blindness, 418
Ir genes; *see* Immune response genes
Ir hormones; *see* Immunoreactive hormones
Iris, 414
Iron
  blood cell development and, 767-769
  erythropoiesis and, 767
  hemoproteins and, 69
  small intestine and, 1189
Iron binding
  in anemia of chronic disease, 795
  total, 778
Iron chelation therapy, thalassemia and, 842
Iron deficiency anemia, 786, 789-790
  child and, 830-834
  history of, 789
Iron replacement therapy, 790
Irregular bones, 1297
Irreversible coma, 437-440
Irritable bladder, 1142
Irritant receptor, 1041
Irritants, contact dermatitis and, 1402
Irritative syndrome, 505
Ischemia, 52
  cerebrovascular disorders and, 493
  myocardial, 934, 938-942
Ischemic edema, cerebral, 469-470
Ischemic ulcer, 1228
Islet cell antibodies, 612
Islets of Langerhans, 578, 612
  hyalinization of, 616
Isoenzymes, 944
  tumor cell markers and, 300
Isohemagglutinins, 200
Isoimmune diseases, 252, 263-264
Isoimmune neutropenia, 263
Isoimmune thrombocytopenic purpura, 846
Isoimmunity, 250, 252, 262-263
Isometric contraction, 1313
Isosexual precocious puberty, 678, 679

Isotonic alterations, 89
Isotonic contraction, 1313
Isotonic solution, 21
Isotope cisternography, 385
Isotropic bands, 875, 1309, 1310
Isovolumic contraction, 865
Isthmus, 652
Itch mite, 1446
Itching, 1401

J

J-receptor, 1041
Jacksonian seizure, 447, 448
Jaundice, 1242-1244
  bilirubin and, 69
  congenital, 833, 834, 835
  mechanisms of, 1243
  of newborn, 834, 1282
Jejunal atresia, 1272
Jejunum, 1182
  obstruction of, 1272
Jerk nystagmus, 415
Jet-lag syndrome, 411
Joint capsule, 1300
Joint cavity, 1300
Joint mice, 1340
Joint space, 1300
Joints
  cartilaginous, 1298
  congenital dysplasia of hip, 1363-1364
  disorders of, 1339-1350
    ankylosing spondylitis and, 1346-1347
    degenerative disease and, 1339-1341
    gout and, 1347-1350
    inflammatory disease and, 1341-1350
    noninflammatory disease and, 1339-1341
    rheumatoid arthritis and, 1342-1346
  false, 1323
  fibrous, 1298
  function tests of, 1314
  history of disease of, 1291
  knee, 1300
  leukemia and, 849-850
  structure and function of, 1298-1304
  synovial, 1298-1304
    body movements and, 1303
    movements of, 1302-1303
    structure of, 1298-1302
  types of, 1299
Junctional bradycardia, 964
Junctional complex, 32, 33
Junctional contractions, premature, 964
Junctional rhythm, accelerated, 964
Junctional tachycardia, 965
Juvenile rheumatoid arthritis, 1373
Juxtaglomerular apparatus, 1116
Juxtamedullary nephron, 1113

K

K cells, 342
Kallidin, 225
Kallikrein, 225, 227
Kaposi sarcoma, 340, 1421-1423
Kartagener syndrome, 998
Karyolysis, 70
Karyotype, 124
Kasai procedure, 1282
Keloid, 245, 1400-1401
Keratin, 1391
Keratinocyte, 68, 1391
Keratitis, 414
Keratoacanthoma, 1417-1418

Keratosis
   actinic, 1418
   seborrheic, 1417
Kernicterus, 833
Kernig sign, 498
Ketoacidosis, diabetic, 94, 615, 619-622
Ketogenesis, 580
Ketogenic diet, 546
Ketone bodies, excretion of, 62
Kidney, 1111, 1112-1117; *see also* Kidney
      function
   blood vessels of, 1116-1117
   damage of, 1154
   distal tubule of; *see* Distal tubule
   horseshoe, 1162
   parathyroid glands and, 578
   permanent, 1160
   sodium and, 88
   tumor of, 1167
Kidney-based renin-angiotensin system, 896
Kidney failure; *see* Renal failure
Kidney function, 1121-1131
   erythropoiesis and, 769
   gout and, 1348
   hypertension and, 925
   nephron and, 1121-1126
   renal failure and, 1156
   renal hormones and, 1129
   tests of, 1129-1131
   urine and; *see* Urine
Kidney stones, 170, 179
Killer cells, 342
Kimmelstiel-Wilson nodule, 625
Kinetics, saturation, 22
Kinin system, 218, 222, 225, 227
Kininogen, 227
   high-molecular weight, 775
Kissing disease, 802
Klebsiella pneumoniae
   empyema and, 1064
   orchitis and, 703
Klinefelter syndrome, 126, 130-131
Knee
   dislocation of, 1324
   gout and, 1350
Knee joint, 1300
Kohn pores, 1030, 1060, 1061
Koilocytosis, 741-742
Koplik spots, 1444
Korsakoff psychosis, 509
Krebs cycle, 18
Kupffer cells, 769, 1195, 1198
Kussmaul respirations, 106, 619, 1055
Kwashiorkor, 306, 1279

L

Labia, 650
Labile factor, 774
Laceration, 480
Lacrimal glands, 208
Lactase deficiency, 179, 1231
   diarrhea and, 1216
Lactate dehydrogenase, 1203, 1205
Lactated Ringer solution, 1428
Lactation, 668
   inappropriate, 711
Lacteal, 1184
Lactic acid deficiency, 1353
Lactic acidosis, 1430
Lactic dehydrogenase, 944
Lactobacillus acidophilus, 651, 686
Lactoferrin, 795
Lactose intolerance, 170, 179, 1281-1282

Lactulose, 1242
Lacuna, 1294
Laennec cirrhosis, 1249
Laetrile, 57
LAK-cell therapy; *see* Lymphokine-activated
      killer cell therapy
Laki-Lorand factor, 774
Lamellae, 1295
Lamina propria, 1184
Laminar flow, 894-895
Laminectomy, 505
Langerhans cells, 1392
Langhans-type giant cells, 238
Language comprehension, 464
Language disturbances, 468
Laparoscopy, 670, 692
Laparotomy, 1261
Laplace law, 880-881
Large cell cancer, anaplastic, 1088
Large cell carcinoma, lung and, 1088, 1089
Large intestine, 1190-1192
   carcinogenesis and, 327
Laryngeal box, 1027
Laryngeal cancer, 1084-1085
Laryngeal papilloma, 741
Laryngitis, 1098
Laryngotracheobronchitis, 1098, 1100
Larynx, 1027, 1028
   cancer of, 329
   child and, 1098
   in quiet respiration, 1029
Lassa fever, 61
Late dumping syndrome, 1229-1230
Latent syphilis, 730
Lateral column, 364
Lateral horn, 364
Laurence-Moon-Biedl syndrome, 998
Laxative abuse, 94
Lead absorption, 550
Lead poisoning, 549
Lee-White coagulation time, 779
Left-to-right shunt, 999
Left ventricle, 862
   aneurysm of, 946
   myocardial infarction and, 942
Left ventricular afterload, 881
Left ventricular end-diastolic pressure, 971
Left ventricular preload, 881
Legg-Calvé-Perthes disease, 1374-1375
Legionella, 1077
Leiomyoma, 296, 691
Leiomyosarcoma, 296
   mixed mesodermal, 297
Lennox-Gastaut syndrome, 547
Lens, 415
Lentigo malignant melanoma, 1421
Lethal injury to cell, 72
Lethargy, 434
Leukemia, 295, 296, 301, 327, 803-809
   acute, 803-805
   atomic bomb exposure and, 332
   child and, 317, 847-850
   childhood, 317
   chronic, 803, 805-809
   chronic granulocytic, 803, 847
   chronic lymphocytic, 803, 847
   chronic myelocytic, 803
   classification of, 803
   clinical manifestations of, 806-807
   history of, 753, 803
   types of, 847-848
Leukemia antigen, common acute
      lymphoblastic, 848

Leukemia-associated inhibitory activity, 804
Leukemoid reaction, 801
Leukocyte endogenous mediator, 795
Leukocytes, 757, 758-760
   alterations of, 800-810
      infectious mononucleosis and, 802-803
      leukemias and, 803-809
      multiple myeloma and, 809-810
      qualitative, 800
      quantitative, 801-802
   child and, 829
   development of, 770-771
   glucocorticoids and, 285
   history of study of, 753
   hypophosphatemia and, 100
   inflammation and, 218, 229
   rheumatoid arthritis and, 1342-1343
   tests and, 778
Leukocytosis, 801
   inflammation and, 236, 237
Leukocytosis-inducing factor, 771
Leukoencephalopathy, 60
Leukokinin, 396
Leukokoria, 558
Leukopenia, 307, 308, 801
Leukorrhea, 672, 687
Leukotrienes, 221-222
Levodopa, 513
Lewis phenomenon, 406
Lewy bodies, 382
Leydig cells, 661
Lhermitte sign, 517
Libido, aging and, 672
Lice; *see* Louse
Lichen planus, 1405-1406
Lichenification, 1397
Licorice, 924
Lieberkühn crypts, 1184
Life changes, 279; *see also* Stress
Life expectancy, 73-74
Life span, normal, 73-74
Lifestyle
   carcinogenesis and, 326
   coronary artery disease and, 936-937
   familial diseases and, 162
Ligament, strain and, 1325-1326
Ligamentum teres of liver, 1194
Ligands, 16, 19
   internalization of, 26
Light
   fluorescent, 65
   ultraviolet, 68
Light chains, 202, 203
Limb girdle muscular dystrophy, 1377,
      1379
Limb kinetic dyspraxia, 463
Limbic system, 360
   emotions and, 461
Lindane cream, 1447
Linear-energy-transfer radiations, 331
Linear fracture, 1321
Link protein, 1302
Linkage analysis, 141-147
Lip
   cancer of, 1083-1084
   cleft, 1268-1269
Lipases, 72
   pancreatic, 1202
Lipid-acceptor proteins, 55
Lipid bilayer, 13-14, 16, 20
Lipid peroxidation, 55
Lipid-soluble hormones, 569, 570
Lipid-soluble molecules, 14

Lipids
  atherogenesis and, 919
  cellular injury and, 66-70
  coronary artery disease and, 934
  deficiency of, 62
    muscle metabolism and, 1354
  in liver cells, 67
  metabolism of
    cortisol and, 286
    defects in, 546
  plasma membranes and, 13-14, 16, 20
Lipiduria, 1149, 1150
Lipofuscin, 10, 50, 382
Lipolysis, 580, 1187
Lipoma, 296
Lipophilic molecules, 20
Lipoprotein, 757, 934
  high-density, 626
Lipoprotein-lipase theory of obesity, 1236
Liposarcoma, 296
Lipostatic theory of obesity, 1236
Liquefactive necrosis, 71
Literal paraphasia, 468
Lithotripsy, extracorporeal shock-wave, 1138
Liver, 1193, 1194-1199
  disorders of, 819, 1244, 1245-1252
    alcoholism and, 67
    cancer and, 1259-1260
    child and, 1282-1286
    cirrhosis in, 1248-1249
    clinical manifestations of, 1238-1245
    cystic fibrosis and, 1276
    diabetes mellitus and, 616
    hepatitis and, 746-747
    hypoglycemia and, 620
    leukemia and, 807
    metabolic, 1284-1286
    Reye syndrome and, 548
  history of study of, 1173
  lipid accumulation in, 67
  lobule of, 1195
  metabolic detoxification and, 1198-1199
  risk factors for cancer of, 1259
  tests of, 1202-1203, 1205
Liver cells, chemical injury of, 54, 55
Livor mortis, 76
Lobar pneumonia, 1078
Locked-in syndrome, 442
Locomotion, 452
Locus of chromosomes, 133, 144
Long bones, 1296, 1361
Long-term memory loss, 443
Long-term starvation, 1238
Loop diuretics, 1153
Loop of Henle, 1116, 1121, 1125-1126
Loose areolar connective tissue, 37
Lou Gehrig disease, 518
Louse, 1447-1448
  pubic, 745
Low back pain, 399, 489-491
Low-density lipoproteins, 26, 934
  coronary artery disease and, 937
Low-flow oxygen, 1073
Low-output failure, heart failure and, 975
Lower airway, 1030
  disorders of, 1101-1107
Lower esophageal sphincter, 1177, 1219
Lower extremities, hypertension and, 925
Lower motor neuron syndromes, 458-459
Lower motor neurons, 365
Lown-Ganog-Levine preexcitation
  syndrome, 967
Lumbar nucleus pulposus, herniated, 492

Lumbar plexus, 372
Lumbar puncture, 367
Lumbar spine spondylolysis, 490
Lumen, vessel, 891
Lumpectomy, 717
Lung, 1031
  allergic diseases of, 255
  black, 1066-1067
  cancer of; *see* Lung cancer
  child and disease of, 1101
  collapse of, 1060
  cystic fibrosis and, 1276
  elastic properties of, 1038-1039
  right heart failure and, 970
Lung cancer, 326, 327, 1085-1090
  characteristics of, 1089
  cigarette smoking and, 164
  familial diseases and, 155, 158, 162, 169,
    171
  large cell, 1088
  lifetime risk of, 165
  oat cell, 1087
  radon and, 330
  small cell, 1087-1088
  squamous cell, 1087
  staging of, 1090
  TNM classification of, 1089
  trends for, 1085
  types of, 1086-1088
Lung capacity, 1036-1037
  total, 1071
Lung receptors, 1041-1042
Lung volume, 1036-1037
Lupus erythematosus, 1408-1410
Luschka, foramina of, 367
Luteal/secretory phase of menstrual cycle,
  657-658
Luteinizing hormone, 571, 575, 596, 649,
  666
  deficiency of, 600
  estradiol and, 656
  fertility and, 671
  menstrual cycle and, 659
Lymph, 898
Lymph nodes, 761
  Hodgkin disease and, 813
  leukemia and, 807
Lymph theory of cancer, 293
Lymphadenopathy, 810-811
Lymphangitis, 59
Lymphatic system
  cancer and, 301
  history of study of, 857
  metastasis by, 303-305
  structure and function of, 898-901
Lymphatic vessels, 868, 900
Lymphoblast, 847
Lymphoblastic leukemia, 296
Lymphocyte reaction, mixed, 199
Lymphocytes, 757, 760, 802
  B; *see* B cells
  count of, 778
  immune deficiency and, 265
  immunity and, 191, 192, 195
  infection and cancer and, 308
  inflammation and, 229
  secretory immune system and, 207, 208
  T; *see* T cells
Lymphocytic leukemia, 296
Lymphocytic thyroiditis, 608
Lymphocytopenia, 802
Lymphocytosis, 802
Lymphogranuloma venereum, 738-739

Lymphoid organs, 760-761
Lymphoid tissue, 196, 208
  alterations in functions of, 810-816
Lymphokine-activated killer cell therapy,
  312
Lymphokine-producing cells, 209
Lymphokines, 209
  cancer treatment and, 312
  immunotherapy and, 310
  inflammation and, 233, 235
Lymphoma, 295, 296
  Burkitt, 338-339, 815-816
    Epstein-Barr virus and, 319
  childhood, 317, 851-852
  malignant, 811-816
  non-Hodgkin, 814-815
Lymphopenia, 802
  idiopathic, 251
Lymphoreticular cancer, childhood, 317
Lymphosarcoma, 296
Lymphotoxin, 235
Lyon hypothesis, 125
β-Lypotrophin, 397
Lysis
  complement-mediated, 256
  transfusion reactions and, 200
Lysosomal enzymes, 221
Lysosomal storage diseases, 9, 546
Lysosome, 5
  cellular organelle and, 8-10
  endocytosis and fusion with, 25
  gout and, 1348
  primary, 9
  secondary, 9
Lysylbradykinin, 225
Lytic enzymes, 303

M

M line, 1309, 1310
  myocardial cells and, 876
M phase of cellular reproduction, 29, 30
M protein, 1310
Ménière disease, 423
Macewen sign, 541
Macrocytic anemia, 786
Macrocytic erythrocyte, 784
Macrocytic-normochromic anemia, 785,
  788-789
Macromolecules, 19
  transport of, 25
Macrophage, 757, 760
  activated, 343
  alveolar, 1031
  armed, 342
  endometriosis and, 692
  immunity and, 191, 195, 209, 288
  inflammation and, 218, 229, 232-233,
    242
Macrophage-activating factor, 235
Macrostone, gallbladder, 1253
Macrovascular disease in diabetes mellitus,
  626-627
Macula, 416, 420
Macula adherens, 32, 33
Macula densa, 1116
Macule, 1395
Maculopathy, 625
Magendie, foramen of, 367
Magnesium
  cellular environment and, 92-100
  hypertension and, 177
  parathyroid glands and, 577
  renal stones and, 1137

Magnetic resonance imaging
  gastrointestinal tract and, 1203
  multiple sclerosis and, 517
  nervous system and, 383
Major histocompatibility complex, 198
Malabsorption, 1231-1235
  familial diseases and, 179
Malaria, 155
Maldigestion, 1231
Male breast, 668
  disorders of, 717-719
Male genitalia; *see also* Male reproductive
      system
  cancer and, 301
  external, 660-663
  internal, 663-666
Male infertility, 250
Male-pattern alopecia, 1432
Male reproductive system, 660-666
  aging and, 672-673
  disorders of, 699-711
    epididymis and, 706-707
    penis and, 699-701
    prostate gland and, 707-710
    scrotum and, 701-702
    sexual dysfunction and, 710-711
    testis and, 702-706
    urethra and, 699
  history of study of, 645
  organs of, 661
Male sex hormones, 665-666
  carcinogenesis and, 332
Male sexual dysfunction, 710-711
Male urethra, 1119
Male urinary bladder, 1118
Malformations
  axial skeleton and, 538-541
  childhood cancers and congenital,
      317-318
  neurological function alterations and,
      535-541
Malignant hypertension, 925
Malignant hyperthermia, 406
Malignant lymphoma, 811-816
Malignant melanoma, 296, 1420-1421
Malignant tumors, 294
  of female reproductive system, 693
  nomenclature and classification of, 296
Malnutrition
  cancer and, 306
  child and, 1279
  protein-calorie, 62
Malrotation of cecum, 1271-1272
Maltase, acid, 1353
Malunion of bone fracture, 1323
Mammary-associated lymphoid tissue, 208;
      see also Breast
Mammary ducts
  carcinoma of, 716
  ectasia of, 714
Mammary dysplasia, 713
Mammary lobules, carcinoma of, 716
Mammography, 669, 714
Manic-depressive disorders, 170, 183
Mannitol, 1128
Manometry, 1204
Mapping of gene, 141-147
Marasmus, 306, 1279
Margination, 229
Marker genes, 143
Markers, tumor cell, 298-301
Marrow; *see* Bone marrow
Marrow cavity, 1296

Masculinizing adrenogenital syndrome, 634
Mass reflex, spinal cord injury and, 486
Mast cell, 218, 220-222
Mastectomy, 717
Mastitis, cystic, 713
Mastoid air cells, 419
Mastoid process, 419
Maternal antibodies, 212-213
  hemolytic disease in newborn and, 832
Maternal autoimmune diseases, 262
Maturation, sexual, 678-680
Maximal life span, 73
McArdle disease, 1353
Mean arterial pressure, 895, 896
Mean corpuscular hemoglobin, 777
Mean corpuscular volume, 777
Measles, 61, 1444-1445
Mechanical factors in cellular injury, 65
Mechanoreceptors, 355
Meconium ileus, 1272
Median eminence, 570
Mediastinum, 860
  neuroblastoma and, 556
Mediated transport, 22-24
Medical family history, 184
Medulla, adrenal, 580, 586
Medulla oblongata, 362
Medullary hematopoiesis, 763
Medulloblastoma, 500, 553, 554
  treatment of, 555
Medusa head, 1241
Megacolon, congenital aganglionic, 1273
Megakaryoblast, 771
Megaloblast, 765
Megaloblastic anemias, 788
  cancer and, 307
Meiosis, 28, 124
Meissner corpuscles, 395
Meissner plexus of stomach, 1178
Melancholic women, 279
Melanin, 1392
  cellular injury and, 68-69
Melanin-stimulating hormone, 68
  tumor cell markers and, 300
Melaninogenesis, 68
Melanocyte, 68, 1392
Melanocyte-stimulating hormone, 571, 575,
      1392
Melanoma, 68, 297, 331
  characteristics of, 1422
  lymphokines and, 312
  malignant, 296, 1420-1421
Melanophores, 68
Melanosomes, 68
Melena, 1217
Membrane excitability, 95
Membrane proteins, 14
Membranoproliferative glomerulonephritis,
      1148
Memory cells, 193, 202, 209
Memory impairment, 441, 442
Menarche, 657
Mendelian traits, 133
Mendel's experiments with breeding, 116
Meningeal sarcoma, 296
Meninges, 366-367
Meningioma, 296, 500, 503, 504
  parasagittal, 503
Meningitis, 505-506
  bacterial, 549-551
Meningocele, 536
  cranial, 536
Meningococcus, 505

Meningomyelocele, 536-537
Menopause, 657, 671
  osteoporosis and, 1328
Menstruation, 657-660
  alterations in, 680-684
  retrograde, 691-692
Mental retardation, 134, 541
Merkel cells, 1392
Mesangial cells, 1113
Mesencephalon dysfunction, 437
Mesenteric artery occlusion, 1235-1236
Mesenteric ganglia, 377
Mesenteric insufficiency, 1235-1236
Mesentery, 1183
Mesodermal tissue tumor, 500
Mesothelioma, 1090
Metabolic acidosis, 102, 105-107
Metabolic alkalosis, 94, 105, 107, 108
Metabolic bone disease, 1328-1332
Metabolic cirrhosis, 1249
Metabolic coma, 434
Metabolic disorders, 179
  central nervous system inherited, 544-546
  of muscle, 1352-1354
Metabolic hypothesis of autoregulation, 898
Metabolic pathway, 16
Metabolic rate, basal, 980, 981
Metabolic theory of aging, 74
Metabolic tremor, 454
Metabolism, 182
  amino acid, 544-546
  biliary, 1282
  bilirubin, 1197
    liver and, 1205
  burn injury and, 1430
  calcium, 578
  cancer and carbohydrate, 306
  cardiac, 866-867
  chemical reactions of, 402
  diseases of, 1353-1354
  inborn errors of
    congenital heart defects and, 998
    hypoglycemia and, 619
  lipid, 546
  muscle, 1312-1313
    glycogen and, 1353
  myocardial, 876
  shock and, 981-984
  septic, 980
Metals, hypersensitivity and, 254
Metaphase in cellular reproduction, 30
Metaphase spread of chromosomes, 124
Metaphysis, 1296
Metaplasia, 51
  cervical cancer and, 693
Metarteriole, 888
Metastasis, 294, 303-305
  brain tumor and, 504
  breast cancer and, 715-716
  calcification and, 70
  pathogenesis of, 304
  prostatic cancer and, 709
  spinal cord tumor and, 504
Metencephalon, 362
Methadone, 711
Methemoglobin, 766, 768
Methotrexate, 307
Methyldopa, 711
3-Methylhistidine, 1310
Metronidazole, 736, 743
Micelle, 1187, 1196
Microangiopathic anemia, 786
Microangiopathy, diabetic, 624

Microbodies, 10
Microcephaly, 539, 540-541
Microcytic erythrocyte, 784
Microcytic hypochromic anemia, 785, 789-791
Microfilaments, 10, 353
Microglia, 355, 356
Micrographia, 3
Microhemagglutination assay, 732
Microinsults, 73
Microorganisms
  cancer and, 308
  pneumonia and, 1076
Microspherocyte, 835
Microstone, gallbladder, 1253
Microtubules, 10, 353
Microvascular disease in diabetes mellitus, 624-626
Microvilli, 10, 37
  in small intestine, 1184
Micturition, 1118, 1119
Midbrain, 361-362
Middle cerebral artery aneurysm, 495
Middle ear, 419
  rhabdomyosarcoma and, 1384
Middle fossa, 366
Migration, tissue formation by, 31, 533
Migration-inhibitory factor, 235
Miliaria, 1449
Milk
  breast, 668
  iron deficiency anemia and, 831
Milk sugar, 1281-1282
Milliequivalents, 19
Millirad, 331
Mineralocorticoid excess syndromes, 632
Mineralocorticoids, 584-586
Minerals
  bone, 1295
  erythropoiesis and, 766, 767
  homeostasis and, 1294
  liver and, 1199
  small intestine and, 1188-1190
Minor calyx, 1113
Mite, 1446, 1447
Mitochondria, 10
  atrophy and, 50
  DNA code and, 120
  oxidative phosphorylation and, 18
Mitomycin, 309
Mitosis, 12, 28, 124
  cancer treatment and, 309
  phases of, 30
  tissue formation by, 31
Mitral regurgitation, 955, 957
Mitral stenosis, 955-956
  left atrial failure and, 973
Mitral valve, 864
  prolapse of, 174, 957-958
Mitral and tricuspid complex, 864
Mixed connective tissue disease, 251
Mixed hearing loss, 421
Mixed hyperlipidemia, 935
Mixed lymphocyte reaction, 199
Mixed mesodermal leiomyosarcoma, 297
Mixed nerves, 372
Mixed transcortical dysphasia, 465
Mixed venous blood gas, 1049
Mobitz heart block, 966
Mode of inheritance, 134; *see also* Inheritance
  sex-linked, 139
Modified radical mastectomy, 717

Molds, hypersensitivity and, 254
Mole, 296, 1418
  hydatiform, 297
  pigmented, 331
Molecular genetics, 115, 117
Molecular oxygen, phosphorylation and, 18
Molluscum contagiosum, 742-743, 1443, 1444
Mongolism, 128-129
Monoamine oxidase inhibitors, 924
Monoclonal antibodies, 207
  cancer treatment and, 310, 312-316
Monoclonal hypothesis of atherogenesis, 919
Monocytes, 757, 760, 801
  count of, 778
  immune system and, 288
  inflammation and, 218, 229, 232-233
Monocytosis, 801
Monoiodotyrosine, 577
Mononuclear phagocyte system, 760, 761-763
  bilirubin and, 1197
Mononucleosis, infectious, 802-803
Monosodium urate crystals, 1348
Monosomy, 126
Monospot agglutination test, 803
Monozygous twins, 319
Monro, foramen of, 367
Mons pubis, 650
Montgomery, glands of, 666
Morbid obesity, 179-182
Morphine sulfate, 975
Mortality rate, 158
  cancer and, 327
Mosaic, chromosomal, 128
Mosquito, 1416-1417
Motilin, 1179
Motility impairment of gastrointestinal tract
  acquired, 1274-1276
  congenital, 1268-1274
Motion, range of, 1341
Motor cortex, 456
Motor dysfunction, 451-455
  cerebral palsy and, 542
Motor dysphasia, 466
Motor dyspraxia, 463
Motor function, 452
  aging and, 382
  alterations in, 451-461
    clinical manifestations and, 451-455
    motor syndromes and, 455-461, 517-519
Motor neurons, 355, 365
Motor neuropathy, 520
Motor outflow, feedback cycles of, 511
Motor pathway, primary voluntary, 360
Motor responses
  abnormal, 440
  consciousness and, 437
  unconscious states and, 439
Motor syndromes, 455-461
  basal ganglia, 457-458
  cerebellar, 458
  extrapyramidal, 457-458
  lower, 458-459
  paralysis of Guillain-Barré syndrome and, 521
  pyramidal, 455-457
  sporadic, 517-519
Motor unit, 365
  of skeletal muscle, 1306-1311
Motor unit syndromes, 458-461
Motor vehicle accident, 477

Mouse tumor cells, 144, 145, 314
Mouth, 1175
  cancer of, 329
  candidiasis and, 1415
Movement, 452; *see also* Motor function
mRNA, 119
Mucin, 1314
  metastasis and, 305
Mucocutaneous candidiasis, 268
Mucopurulent cervicitis, 687
Mucosa of stomach, 1178, 1181
Mucosal-associated lymphoid tissue, 208
Mucous membranes
  cardiovascular function tests and, 901
  hypersensitivity and, 255
Mucoviscidosis, 1276
Mucus
  chronic obstructive pulmonary disease and, 1073
  gastric, 1178, 1181
Multifactorial diseases, 148
Multifactorial inheritance, 147-148, 157
Multihaustral propulsion, colon and, 1192
Multiple myeloma, 296, 809-810
Multiple papilloma, 714
Multiple sclerosis, 514-517
  familial diseases and, 170, 183
  immunity and, 251
Multipolar neurons, 355
Multistage theory of carcinogenesis, 324-333
Mumps, 61
Murmur, heart, 903, 955
  tetralogy of Fallot and, 1014
Muscle; *see also* Skeletal muscles
  biopsy of, 1353
  congenital disease of, 1366
  denervated, 459
  function of, 1311-1314
  function tests for, 1314-1315
  growth of, 1362-1363
  history of study of, 1291
  malignant hyperthermia and, 406
  mechanics of, 1313
  metabolism of, 1312-1313
  movement of groups of, 1306, 1310, 1314
  myasthenia gravis and, 523
  nonprotein constituents of, 1311
  protein of, 1310-1311
  repetitive discharge and, 1313
  strength of, dysfunction and, 451
  stress-related diseases of, 287, 1351
  striated, 1309
  tissues of, 41
  tumors of, 1356, 1382-1384
  wasting of, 984
Muscle cells, 5
Muscle contraction, 1311-1312
  crossbridge theory of, 876-878
  heat and, 402
  types of, 1313-1314
Muscle fibers, 1306-1310
  action potential and, 1311
  characteristics of, 1308
  history of study of, 1291
Muscle fibrils, contractile proteins of, 1310
Muscle membrane, 1308
  abnormalities of, 1352
Muscle pump, 889
Muscle strain, 1326-1327
Muscle tension, stress-induced, 287, 1351
Muscle tone
  abnormalities in, 452

Muscle tone—cont'd
  heat production and decreased, 403
  motor dysfunction and, 451, 452
  neuropathy and, 461
Muscular artery, 886
Muscular atrophy, progressive spinal, 460
Muscular dystrophy, 1376-1380
  oculopharyngeal, 1355
Muscular exercise, prolonged, 620
Muscular subaortic stenosis, 953
Muscularis mucosa of stomach, 1178
Musculoskeletal system
  alterations of, 1319-1359
    bone disorders and, 1328-1339; *see also*
      Bone
    child and, 1360-1387; *see also* Child,
      musculoskeletal function alterations in
    injuries and, 1320-1328
    joint disorders and, 1339-1350; *see also*
      Joints
    skeletal density and, 1367-1370
    skeletal modeling and, 1367-1370
    skeletal muscle disorders and,
      1350-1356
    tumors and, 1380-1384
  bone formation and, 1361-1362
  bone growth and, 1362
  development of, 1361-1363
  function tests of, 1314-1315
  history of, 1291
  hypothyroidism and, 607
  muscle growth and, 1362-1363
  skeletal development and, 1362
  structure and function of, 1292-1318
    aging and, 1315-1316
    bones and, 1292-1298
    joints and, 1298-1304
    skeletal muscles and, 1304-1314; *see also*
      Skeletal muscles
    tests and, 1314-1315
Music deafness, 462
Mustarde procedure, 1010
Mutagenesis, insertional, 337
Mutagens, 121
Mutant sperm, 693
Mutation, 121, 337
Myasthenia gravis, 251, 263, 522-523
Myasthenic crisis, 523
Mycobacterium bovis, 311
Mycobacterium smegmatis, 700
Mycobacterium tuberculosis, 58, 71, 1079
Mycoplasma pneumoniae, 1077, 1078, 1102
Mycoses, 1414; *see also* Fungal infection
  aneurysm and, 494-496
  child and, 1441-1442
Myelencephalon, 362
Myelin, 353
  embryonic development and, 533
  multiple sclerosis and, 514
Myelin sheath, 353, 533
Myelocytic leukemias, 296
Myelodysplasia, 535-536
Myelofibrosis, 786
Myelogenic tumors, 1338-1339
Myelogenous leukemias, 296, 803
Myelography, 385
Myeloid, 753, 764
Myeloma, 1339
  multiple, 296, 809-810
Myeloma cells, tumor, 144, 145, 314
Myelomeningocele, 536-538
Myeloperoxidase, 231
Myeloproliferative red cell disorders, 796-797

Myenteric plexus of stomach, 1178
Myoadenylate deaminase deficiency,
  1353-1354
Myoblast, 1306
Myocardial cells, 874-876, 938-939
Myocardial contraction, 876-878, 882-883
Myocardial infarction, 934, 942-947
  diabetes mellitus and, 627
  hypoxic injury and, 52-53
  incidence rate of, 166
  left heart failure and, 973
  tissue changes after, 943
  zones of, 945
Myocardial ischemia, 938-942
Myocardial oxygen consumption, 876
Myocardium, 862
  contractility of, 876-878, 882-883
  disorders of, 950-953
  hypertension and, 925
  hypertrophy of, 50
  ion concentrations in, 871
  metabolism and, 876
  relaxation of, 878-879
Myoclonic seizure, 449, 546
Myoclonus, 453
Myocutaneous flap, 1400
Myofascial pain syndromes, 399-400
Myofibril, 1306, 1310
Myofibroblast, 243
  keloid and, 1400
Myofilament, 1310
Myogenic hypothesis of autoregulation, 898
Myoglobinuria, 1327-1328, 1356
Myoglobulin, 898
Myomectomy, 691
Myometrium, 652
Myoneural junction, 355
Myopathy, 461, 1355-1356
Myopia, 417
Myosin, 875, 1310
Myositis, 1354-1355
Myositis ossificans, 1326
Myotonia, 1352
Myotonic muscular dystrophy, 1377,
  1379-1380
Myxedema, 250, 607, 608
  pretibial, 605
Myxedema coma, 608
Myxoviruses, 61

N

Nail, 1392, 1393
  disorders of, 1433
Nail-patella syndrome, 142-143
Nasal wall, 1028
Nasopharynx, 1027
  carcinoma of, 338-339
  rhabdomyosarcoma and, 1384
Natriuretic hormone, 88, 1129
Natural immunity, 194
Natural killer cells, 342
Nausea, 1214
Neck, rhabdomyosarcoma and, 1384
Necrosis, 70-72
Necrotizing enterocolitis, 1280-1281
Necrotizing vasculitis, 251
Needle
  AIDS and contamination of, 270
  biopsy with, 669
Negative feedback, 565
Neglect syndrome, 464
Neisseria gonorrhoeae, 727
  clinical syndromes from, 737

Neisseria gonorrhoeae—cont'd
  epididymitis and, 706
  pelvic inflammatory disease and, 686
  penicillinase-producing, 729
  urethritis and, 699
Neisseria meningitidis, 549
Neoantigen, 260, 261
Neocyte transfusion, 842
Neologism, 468
Neonatal hematopoiesis, 826
Neonatal immune function, 212-213, 262
Neonatal thrombocytopenia, transient, 846
Neonate
  hemolytic disease of, 829, 831-834
  inflammation and, 246
  physiologic jaundice of, 1282
  reflexes of, 533
  respiratory distress syndrome of,
    1104-1106
  toxic erythema of, 1449-1450
Neoplasm, 294
Neospinothalamic tract, 396
Nephritic sediment, 1144
Nephritis, chronic interstitial, 1143
Nephroblastoma, 297, 1167
  host factors with, 318
Nephron, 1113-1116
  components of, 1114
  functions of, 1121-1126
  renal failure and, 1154
Nephropathy, diabetic, 598, 625-626
Nephrotic sediment, 1144
Nephrotic syndrome, 1149-1150
  child and, 1163-1164
Nerve impulse, 356-357
Nerves
  cranial, 374-375
  injury to, 356
  regeneration of, 356
  skin and, 1393
  spinal, 371-372
    pain and, 394
Nervous system
  aging and, 380-383
  autonomic, 372-380
    allergic response and, 253
    functions of, 378-380
  cells of, 353-356
  central, 357-371; *see also* Central nervous
    system
  in child, 532-535
  organization of, 533
  parasympathetic, 377-378
  peripheral, 371-372
  structure and function of, 352-353
  sympathetic, 376-377
  tests of, 383-385
Net filtration pressure, 1123
Neural crest, 533
Neural fold, 532
Neural groove, 532
Neural noise, 383
Neural plate, 532
Neural reflex, 882
Neural regulation
  of kidney, 1120
  of vasoconstriction, 922
Neural tissues, 41-43
Neural tube, 532
  defects of, 535-538
Neuralgia, 399
Neurilemic sarcoma, 296
Neurilemma, 353, 356

Neurilemmoma, 296, 500, 503-504
Neuritic plaques, 445
Neuritis, 460, 520
   retrobulbar, 416
Neuroanatomy of pain, 393-397
Neuroblastoma, 296
   child and, 317, 555-557
Neurocytoma, 296
Neuroendocrine system; *see also* Endocrine
   glands
   immune system and, 288
   Parkinson disease and, 512-513
   stress response and, 283-287, 586-587
Neuroendocrine theory of aging, 75
Neurofibrillary tangles, 382, 444, 445
Neurofibrils, 353
Neurofibromas, 137, 500, 504
   childhood cancers and, 318
Neurogenic bladder, 1138, 1139
Neurogenic shock, 977-979
Neuroglia, 355-356
Neuroglial cells, 353
Neuroglioma, 296
Neurohypophysis, 570
Neuroimmunomodulation, 279
Neurologic dysfunction, 431-529
   central nervous system disorders and,
       477-519; *see also* Central nervous
       system disorders
   cerebral homeostasis and, 465-470
   cerebrovascular disease and, 551-552
   child and, 531-561; *see also* Child,
       neurologic dysfunction in
   consciousness and, 432-451
      clinical manifestations and evaluation of,
       433-440
      content of thought and, 440-442
      pathophysiology of, 432
      seizures and, 445-451
      subacute and chronic, 442-445
   emotions and, 461-465
   encephalopathies and, 542-551
   history of treatment of, 351
   hypertension and, 924
   hypothyroidism and, 606
   motor function and, 451-461
      clinical manifestations of, 451-455
      motor syndromes in, 455-461
   peripheral nervous system and
      neuromuscular junction disorders
      and, 519-523
   sexual dysfunction and, 710
   structural malformations and, 535-541
   structure and function of nervous system
      and, 532-535
   unifocal cortical function and, 462-465
   uremia and, 1157
   visual dysfunction and, 418-419
Neurologic system, structure and function
   of, 352-389; *see also* Neurologic
   dysfunction
   aging and, 380-383
   autonomic nervous system in, 372-380
   central nervous system in, 357-371; *see*
      also Central nervous system
   nerve impulse in, 356-357
   nervous sytem cells in, 353-356
   peripheral nervous system in, 371-372
   tests and, 383-385
Neuroma, 296, 503
Neuromodulation, pain and, 397
Neuromuscular disorders
   familial diseases and, 183

Neuromuscular disorders—cont'd
   hypokalemia and, 95
Neuromuscular junction, 355, 365
   disorders of, 461, 521-523
   myasthenia gravis and, 522
Neuromuscular tissue, autoimmunity and,
   251
Neuron, 41, 43, 353-355
   epileptogenic, 447
   GABAnergic, 513
   motor, 365, 458
   pain and C, 395
   postganglionic, 372
   preganglionic, 372
Neuron axon, 365
Neuronal cell tumor, 500
Neuronal transmission, 354
Neuropathology, 351
Neuropathy, 460-461, 520-521
   diabetic, 624, 625
   gamma, 458
Neuroreceptors, 378
   autonomic nervous system and, 379-380
Neurosyphilis, 508-509, 731
Neurotransmitters, 15, 43, 357, 378
Neutralization, immunity and, 204, 205-206
Neutropenia, 801
   idiopathic, 251
   isoimmune, 263
Neutrophil, 757, 759
   gout and, 1348
   hypersensitivity and, 257
   infant and, 829
   inflammation and, 218, 229, 231-232
Neutrophil chemotactic factors, 221
Neutrophil count, 778
Neutrophilia, 801
Nevus, 296, 1418, 1420
   child and, 1449
   classification of, 1421
Newborn; *see* Neonate
Niacin, 767
Nicotinamide adenine dinucleotide, 18
Nicotine, 326; *see also* Smoking
Nidus, 1137
Night terrors, 412
Nigrostriatal disorders, 509
Nipple, 666
   retraction of, 717
Nipride; *see* Nitroprusside
Nissl substances, 353
Nitrates
   myocardial ischemia and, 941
   stomach cancer and, 1256
Nitrogen in blood, 1130
Nitroprusside, 57
Nitrosamines, 328
Nitrosoureas, 309
Nociceptors, 355, 394, 395
Nocturnal enuresis, 1168
Nodes
   heart and, 869, 963
   of Ranvier, 353
Nodular goiter, 605
Nodular scabies, 1447
Nodules of skin, 1396
Noise, cellular injury and, 65
Non-A, non-B hepatitis, 1247, 1283
Non-Hodgkin lymphoma, 811, 814-815
   child and, 851-852
Non-REM sleep, 409
   enuresis and, 1169
Nonbacterial cystitis, 1142

Nonbacterial prostatitis, 709
Nonbacterial thrombotic endocarditis, 960
Noncausal risk factors, 158, 159
Noncommunicating hydrocephalus, 470, 519
Nondisjunction, 128
Nongonococcal urethritis, 699, 737
Noninflammatory joint disease, 1339-1341
Nonpuerperal hyperprolactinemia, 711
Nonpurulent meningitis, 505-506
Nonsense codons, 120
Nonshivering thermogenesis, 402
Nonspecific diarrhea, child and, 1281-1282
Nonstaphylococcal toxic epidural necrolysis,
   1441
Nonunion of bone fracture, 1323
Nonvolatile body acids, 101
Norepinephrine, 357, 378, 873
   stress response and, 283
Normal anion gap, 106
Normal life span, 73-74
Normal-pressure hydrocephalus, 519
Normoblast, 765
Normocytic-normochromic anemia, 785,
   791-796
Normokalemia, 96
Nosocomial infections, 308, 1077
Nuclear envelope, 5, 7
Nuclear imaging, 905
Nuclear membrane, cancer cells and,
   297-298
Nuclear palsy syndromes, 459-460
Nuclear pores, 7
Nuclei, 358
Nucleolus, 5, 7
Nucleoplasm, 7
Nucleoproteins, 6
Nucleotide, 117
Nucleus, 5
Nucleus pulposus, 368
   herniated, 490
Null cell, 848
Nutrient arteries, 368
Nutrition
   disorders of, 1236-1238
      cellular injury and, 62
      child and, 1276-1280
      immune function and, 268
   liver and, 1198
Nystagmus, 415, 554

O

Oat cell carcinoma, 1087, 1089
O'Beirne sphincter, 1190
Obesity, 1236-1237
   carcinogenesis and, 328
   coronary artery disease and, 936
   diabetes mellitus and, 617
   familial diseases and, 155, 161, 170,
      179-183
   hypertension and, 1019
Obligate carriers, 137
Oblique fracture, 1320, 1321
Obstruction, airway, 108, 1069-1076
Obstructive hydrocephalus, 541
Obstructive jaundice, 1242
Obstructive pulmonary disease, 1069-1076
Obtundation, 434
Occipital lobe, 360
   tumor of, 554
Occult bleeding, 1217
   iron deficiency anemia and, 831
Occupational exposure
   AIDS and, 270

Occupational exposure—cont'd
  carcinogenesis and, 330
Occurrence of disease, 158
  genetics and, 136
Ocular myasthenia, 522
Ocular myopathy, 415-416, 1355
Ocular nuclear palsy, 460
Oculocephalic reflex, 436, 438
Oculomotor nerves, 374
Oculomotor responses, consciousness and, 436-437
Oculopharyngeal muscular dystrophy, 1355
Oculovestibular reflex, 436, 439
Oddi, sphincter of, 1199
Odor, sensitivity to, 422
Odynophagia, 1256
Olfaction, 421-423
Olfactory dysfunction, 422-423
Olfactory hallucinations, 422-423
Olfactory mucosa, 422
Olfactory nerves, 374
Oligodendrocytoma, 500
Oligodendroglia, 355-356
Oligodendroglioma, 502
Oliguria, 1127
  hepatic failure and, 1244
  potassium and, 96
  renal failure and, 1152
Onchyomycosis, 1433
Oncofetal antigens, 339
Oncogenes, 333-337
  cancer and, 293
Oncotic pressure, 21
Oophrectomy, 684
Oophritis, 685
Open reduction of fracture, 1323
Ophthalmia neonatorum, 729
Ophthalmopathy, infiltrative, 605
Ophthalmoplegia, 1355
  chronic progressive external, 1355
Opiates
  endogenous, 286
  receptors for, 397
Opioids in toxic myopathy, 1356
Opsonization, 206, 229-230
Optic chiasma, 418
Optic disk, 415
Optic nerve, 374
Optic nerve glioma, 553, 554, 555
Oral cancer, 326, 327
Oral contraceptives
  carcinogenesis and, 332, 693
  dysmenorrhea and, 680
  history of use of, 645
  hyperaldosteronism and, 631
  myocardial infarction and, 937
Orbit, rhabdomyosarcoma and, 1384
Orchitis, 703-704
Organ of Corti, 65, 419
Organ transplantation; *see* Transplantation
Organelles
  cytoplasmic, 5
  cytoskeletal, 11
Organic brain syndrome, 440
  myocardial infarction and, 946
Organic confusion, 442
Organic dust, inhalation of, 1067
Organic molecules, adenosine triphosphate and, 17
Orogenital sexual contact, 728, 739
Oropharynx, 1027
  rhabdomyosarcoma and, 1384
  swallowing and, 1177

Orthochromatic erythroblast, 765
Orthopnea, 1054
Orthostatic hypotension, 927
Osgood-Schlatter disease, 1375-1376
Osmolality, 21
Osmolarity, 21
Osmoreceptors, 87
Osmosis, 19, 21-22
Osmotic diarrhea, 1215-1216
Osmotic equilibrium, 84
Osmotic pressure, 21
Osseous tissue, 1295
Ossification centers, 1361
Osteitis deformans, 1331
Osteoarthritis, 1339
Osteoblast, 1293-1294
Osteocalcin, 1294-1295
Osteochondritis dissecans, 1322
Osteochondrosis, 1373-1376
Osteoclast, 1294
Osteocyte, 1294
Osteogenesis imperfecta, 1367
Osteogenic tumors, 1335-1336
Osteoid, 1293
Osteoma, 296
Osteomalacia, 1330
Osteomyelitis, 1332-1334, 1370-1373
Osteoporosis, 1328-1330
  menopause and, 672, 1328
Osteosarcoma, 296, 1335-1336
  child and, 1380-1381
Otolith, 420
Outflow tract of heart, 863
Oval window, 419
Ovarian cancer, 697-699
  FIGO staging of, 698
Ovarian cycle, 654, 659-660
Ovarian cysts, 690
Ovarian follicle, 654, 655
Ovarian hormone secretion, 682
Ovariotomy, 645
Ovary, 653, 654-655
  carcinogenesis and, 327
  menopause and, 671
  polycystic, 683
Overflow incontinence, 1169
Overnutrition, 1236-1237
Ovulation, 654
  lack of, 681
Ovum, 646
Oxidation, 18
Oxidative cellular metabolism, 18
Oxidative phosphorylation, 10, 18-19
Oxycephaly, 539
Oxygen
  heart failure and, 969
  lack of, 52
  low-flow, 1073
  oxidative phosphorylation and, 18
  shock and, 981-983
  toxicity of, 1065-1066
Oxygen consumption index, 906
Oxygen debt, 1313
Oxygen-dependent killing mechanism, 231
Oxygen deprivation, myocardial infarction and, 943
Oxygen molecule, 1045
Oxygen radicals, 75
Oxygen saturation, 1046
Oxygen transport, 1044-1047
Oxygenation, arterial, 1045-1046
  sickle cell disease and, 838

Oxyhemoglobin, 766, 1046-1047
Oxytocin, 573, 574

P

P cells, 870
P wave, 872
Pacinian corpuscles, 395
Paget disease, 716, 1331-1332
Pain, 391-400
  abdominal, 1216-1217
    colicky, 1236
  acute, 392
    clinical manifestations of, 397-399
  age and, 393
  bone fracture and, 1322-1323
  cancer and, 305
  chronic, 392, 397-400, 399-400
  degenerative joint disease and, 1341
  duodenal ulcer and, 1226
  endorphins and, 286
  insomnia and, 412
  low back, 399, 489-491
  motivational/affective system and, 391
  neuroanatomy of, 393-397
  neurophysiology of, 396-397
  pancreatitis and, 1254
  perception of, 393
  psychogenic, 391
  pulmonary disorders and, 1056
  radicular, 520
  referred, 397-399
  renal stone and, 1138
  skeletal trauma and, 1324-1325
  somatic, 397
  somatogenic, 391
  theories of, 396-397
  visceral, 397
Pain receptors, 396
Pain threshold, 392
Pain tolerance, 392-393
Palate, cleft, 1268-1269
Paleospinothalamic tract, 396
Palliative surgery for cancer, 309
Palsy, nuclear, 459-460
Panacinar emphysema, 1074, 1076
Pancreas, 578-580, 1193, 1200-1202
  cancer of, 1260-1261
  carcinogenesis and, 327
  cystic fibrosis and, 1276
  disorders of, 612-628, 1254-1255; *see also* Diabetes mellitus
  tests of, 1203-1206
Pancreatectomy, 1261
Pancreatic α-amylase, 1202
Pancreatic cyst, 1255
Pancreatic duct, 1200
Pancreatic insufficiency, 1231
Pancreatic lipase, 1202
Pancreatic tissue transplant, 616
Pancreatitis, 1254-1255
  hypocalcemia and, 98-99
Pancytopenia, 791, 804
Panhypopituitarism, 599
Pannus, 1344
Pantothenic acid, 767
Papanicolaou test, 669, 670
Papilla, renal, 1118
Papillary capillary of dermis, 1393
Papillary carcinoma of renal pelvis, 1140
Papillary layer of dermis, 1392
Papillary muscle, 864

Papilloma, 61, 296, 500
  colorectal, 1257
  multiple, 714
  solitary intraductal, 714
Papillomavirus, 741
Papovaviruses, 61, 334
Papule, 1395
Papulosquamous skin disorders, 1404-1409
Paraaminohippurate, 1130
Paracentesis, 1242
Paradox incontinence, 1169
Paraesophageal hiatal hernia, 1221
Parafollicular cells, 575
Parageusia, 423
Paralysis, 451
  of extraocular muscles, 416
  flaccid, 458
    amyotrophic lateral sclerosis and, 518
    Guillain-Barré syndrome and, 521
  periodic, 94, 1352
    familial hypokalemic, 94
  pyramidal motor syndrome and, 457
  upper motor neuron syndrome of spastic, 518
Paralysis agitans, 512
Paralytic ileus, 1222
Paralytic poliomyelitis, 459
Paramyxoviruses, 61
Paranasal structures
  cystic fibrosis and, 1276
  rhabdomyosarcoma and, 1384
Paraphimosis, 699
Paraplegia, 451
Parasagittal meningioma, 503
Parasites
  child and, 1446-1448
  myositis and, 1354-1355
  sexually transmitted urogenital infections and, 743-745
Parasympathetic nerves
  anatomy of, 377-378
  heart and, 873
Parasympathetic receptor, 1042
Parathormone; *see* Parathyroid hormones
Parathyroid glands, 563, 577-578; *see also*
    Hyperparathyroidism;
    Hypoparathyroidism
  aging and, 589
  alterations of function of, 609-612
  hyperplasia of, 610
Parathyroid hormones
  calcium and phosphate balance and, 98
  tumors and, 299, 300
Paratope, 197
Paravertebral ganglia, 376
Parenchyma, 41
Paresis; *see* Paralysis
Paresthesias
  diabetes mellitus and, 617
  radicular, 520
Parietal cells, 1179-1180
Parietal lobe, 360
Parietal pain, abdominal, 1216
Parietal pericardium, 860
Parkinson disease, 445, 455, 509-513
  autonomic symptoms of, 512-513
  tremor in, 454, 511
Parkland formula for fluid requirements in burn shock, 1429
Parlodel; *see* Bromocriptine
Paronychia, 1433
Parosmia, 423

Paroxysmal attacks in multiple sclerosis, 517
Paroxysmal choreoathetosis, 454
Paroxysmal dyskinesia, 454
Paroxysmal dystonia, 454
Paroxysmal nocturnal dyspnea, 1054
Pars distalis, 572
Pars interarticularis, 490
Pars intermedia, 572
Pars tuberalis, 572
Partial mastectomy, 717
Partial seizures, 446, 448-449
  child and, 547
Partial thromboplastin time, 779
Partial trisomy, 128
Passive acquired immunity, 194
Passive transport, 19, 20-22
Patch test, 1394, 1395
Patent ductus arteriosus, 1005-1006
Pathologic fracture, 1321
Pathologic hyperplasia, 51
Pattern theory of pain, 396
Pavementing, 229
Pediculosis, 745, 1447-1448
Pedigree
  autosomal dominant inheritance and, 134-136
  autosomal recessive inheritance and, 137-138
  coronary death and, 175
  for cystic fibrosis, 138
  evaluation of, 134, 140-143
  for hypertension, 177
  for Queen Victoria descendants, 140
  for retinoblastoma, 137
  symbols in, 135
  X-linked inheritance and, 139
Pelvic bone, chondrosarcoma of, 1337
Pelvic endoscopy, 670
Pelvic inflammatory disease, 685-686
Pelvic nerve, 378
Pelvic organs, female, 652
Pelvic relaxation disorders, 687-690
Pelvis, renal, 1113
  papillary carcinoma of, 1140
PEM; *see* Protein-energy malnutrition
Pemphigoid, bullous, 1410
Pemphigus, 1409-1410
Pemphigus erythematosus, 1409
Pemphigus foliaceus, 1409
Pemphigus vulgaris, 250, 1409
Pendular nystagmus, 415
Penetrance, 137
Penicillin allergy, 260
Penicillinase-producing *Neisseria gonorrhoeae*, 729
Penis, 661, 663
  candidiasis and, 1415
  disorders of, 699-701
    cancer in, 700-701
    syphilitic chancre in, 730
Pennate muscles, 1305
Pepsin, 1180
  history of study of, 1173
  secretion of, 1181
Pepsinogen, 1180
Peptic ulcers, 170, 1225-1231
  familial diseases and, 179
  surgery for, 1229
Peptides, 580
  small, 566
Perceptual dominance, 392
Percutaneous transluminal coronary angioplasty, 941

Perfusion
  blood pressure and tissue, 895
  distribution of pulmonary, 1043-1044
Periaqueductal gray, 395
Pericardial cavity, 862
Pericardial effusion, 948-949
Pericardial fluid, 862
Pericardial knock, 949
Pericardiocentesis, 948
Pericarditis
  acute, 947-948
  constrictive, 949-951
Pericardium, 860
  disorders of, 947-951
Perichondrium, 1361
Periduodenal band, 1271
Perilymph, 419
Perimetrium, 652
Perinatal trauma, 543
Periodic paralysis, hypokalemic, 1352
Periosteal collar, 1361
Periosteum, 366
Peripartum cardiomyopathy, 951
Peripheral arterial disease, 931-932
Peripheral chemoreceptor, 1042
Peripheral membrane proteins, 14
Peripheral nervous system, 352, 371-372
  disorders of, 519-521
  injury of, 399
  proprioceptive dysfunctions and, 424
  trunk of, 373
Peripheral thermoreceptors, 401
Peripheral vascular system, 886
  diabetes mellitus and, 627
  hypertension and, 1019
Peripheral vasodilation, 402
Peristalsis, 1177
  swallowing and, 1176
Peritoneal cavity, 1182
Peritoneum, 1182
Peritonitis, ascites and, 1241, 1242
Peritubular capillary, 1117
Permanent kidneys, 1160
Permissive effects
  cortisol and, 284, 285
  target cells and, 568
Permissive host cell, 59
Pernicious anemia, 786, 788-789
  history of study of, 753
  immunity and, 251
Peroxidation, lipid, 55
Peroxisomes, 10
Pes foot abnormality, 1366
Pessary, 690
Petechiae, 817, 1399
Petit mal seizure, 447
Peyronie disease, 699-700
pH, 100, 101, 105
  compensatory adjustment in, 102
  urinary, 1130
  vaginal, 686, 736
Phagocytes, 758
  inflammation and, 229-231
Phagocytosis, 9, 12, 25
  congenital defects of, 265
  of erythrocyte, 770
  hypersensitivity and, 256
  immunity and, 206
  inflammation and, 229
  phases of, 231, 232
  of sperm, 692
Phagolysosome, 230
Phakomatosis, 998

Phantom limb pain, 400
Pharynx, 1028
    cancer of, 329
    gonorrhea and, 728
Phenomena
    Bell, 437
    Lewis, 406
    Raynaud, 65, 258, 1408
Phenotypes, 133-134
    obesity and, 180-181
Phenylalanine, 544
Phenylalanine hydroxylase, 119, 544
Phenylketonuria, 119, 544
Phenyoxybenzamine, 488
Pheochromocytoma, 296, 636
Philadelphia chromosome, 298, 808
Phimosis, 699
Phlebitis, 930
Phonocardiogram, 904
Phosphate
    bones and, 1295
    cellular environment and, 92-100
    hypoparathyroidism and, 611
    inorganic, 17
    kidney function and, 1129
    parathyroid glands and, 577
    renal failure and, 1155-1156
Phosphocreatine, 448
Phospholipids, 13
Phosphorus
    hypoparathyroidism and, 611
    radioactive, 797
Phosphorylation, oxidative, 10
Photochemical receptors, 355
Phototoxins, 313
Phren sign, 707
Phthirus pubis, 745
Physical agents
    cellular injury and, 62-66
    familial diseases and, 162-163
Physiologic dead space, 1058
Physiologic jaundice of newborn, 1282
Physiologic stress, 279; *see also* Stress
    components of, 282
Pica, 549
Pickwickian syndrome, 411
Picornaviruses, 61
Pigment
    carotenoid, 69
    cellular injury and, 68
Pigmented gallstone, 1253
Pigmented mole, 68, 331
Pigmented nevus, 297
Pili, 727
Pilomatrixoma, 296
Pineal region tumor, 500
Pinkeye, 413
Pinna, 419
Pinocytosis, 25, 26
Pitting edema, 86
Pituitary giant, 601
Pituitary gland, 570
    adenoma of, 600-601
    anterior
        aging and, 589
        diseases of, 599-603
        hormones of, 571
        menstrual cycle and, 659
    infarction of, 599
    partial deficiency of, 250
    posterior
        aging and, 589
        diseases of, 597-599

Pituitary gland—cont'd
    posterior—cont'd
        hormones of, 573-574
    stress and, 282, 283
    tumor of, 500
        galactorrhea and, 712
Pityriasis rosea, 1405
pK value, 101, 102
Placental alkaline phosphatase, 300
Plagiocephaly, 539
Plantar flexion foot abnormality, 1366
Planus foot abnormality, 1366
Plaque
    Alzheimer disease and, 445
    atherosclerosis and, 919
    multiple sclerosis and, 515
    senile, 444
    skin and, 1395
Plasma, 755-757
    albumin in, 1150
    arterial, 756
    creatine in, 1311
    creatinine in, 1130, 1154
    glucose in venous, 615
    lipids in, 1150
    proteins in; *see* Plasma proteins
    quick-frozen, 845
    renal failure and, 1156
    water movement and, 84-85
Plasma cells, 194, 202, 778
Plasma kinin cascade, 225, 226
Plasma membranes, 5
    of cancer cells, 298
    cellular components and, 12-16
    composition of, 13
    fluidity of, 15-16
    hydrophilic region of, 14
    hydrophobic region of, 14
    immune surveillance theory and, 337
    passive diffusion and, 20
    receptors and, 16
    resting potential across, 27
Plasma proteins, 755-757
    immunity and, 191
    inflammation and, 222-229, 236
Plasma thromboplastin antecedent, 774,
        842
Plasma thromboplastin component, 774,
        842
Plasma transglutaminase, 774
Plasmalemma, 5
Plasmapheresis, 1145
Plasmids, recombinant DNA and bacterial,
        118
Plasmin, 227, 228
Plasminogen, 227
Platelet-activating factor, 229
Platelet adhesion study, 779
Platelet aggregation, 779
    myocardial infarction and, 942
Platelet cofactors, 774
Platelet count, 778
Platelet factor 4, 772
Platelet plug, 772
Platelet-release reaction, 772
Platelet-stimulating factor, 771
Platelets, 757, 760, 771
    alterations of function of, 818
    child and, 829
    degranulation of, 772
    development of, 771
    disorders of, 816-818, 845-847
    hemostasis and, 771-772

Platelets—cont'd
    hypophosphatemia and, 100
    inflammation and, 218, 229
    tests and, 778-779
    thrombocytopenia and, 818
Pleomorphism, 297, 1383
Pleura, 1034
    abnormalities of, 1062-1064
    pain and, 1056
Pleural effusion, 1063-1064
Pleural space, 1034
Pleurisy, 1064
Pleuritis, 1064
Plexus, 372
    injury of, 520
Pluripotential stem cell, 763
Pneumococcal pneumonia, 1077
Pneumoconiosis, 1066-1067
Pneumonia, 1076-1079
    aspiration-caused, 1060
    child and, 1102-1103
    chlamydial infection and, 738
    community-acquired, 1076-1077
    microorganism and, 1076
    pathophysiology of bacterial, 1078
    pneumococcal, 1077
    viral, 1077
Pneumothorax, 1062-1063
Podocyte, 1114
Podophyllin, 742
Poikilocytosis, 785
Poiseuille formula and law, 890
Poison ivy, 254, 260, 1402
Poisons, child and, 549
Polarity, 19
Poliomyelitis, 61, 459, 508
Pollens, 254, 260
Pollution, carcinogenesis and, 329-330
Polyarteritis nodosa, 251
Polyarthritis, 959
Polycyclic hydrocarbons, 293, 328
Polycystic ovarian syndrome, 683
Polycythemia, 784, 796-797
    tetralogy of Fallot and, 1014
Polydipsia, 95, 598, 615
Polygenic traits, 147, 156
Polymorphonuclear neutrophils, 231-232,
        759
Polymyositis, 251, 1354-1355
Polyneuritis, 251
    idiopathic, 521
    postinfectious, 521
    psychosis, 509
Polyp
    colorectal, 1257
    endometrial, 690
Polypeptides, 117, 123, 202
Polyphagia, 615
Polyploidy, 126
Polyradiculopathy, demyelinating, 521
Polyuria, 598
    diabetes mellitus and, 615
    hyperosmolar hyperglycemic nonketotic
        coma and, 623
    potassium deficiency and, 95
Pompe disease, 9, 1353
Pons, 362
    astrocytoma of, 501
Population genetics, 133-134
Pork insulin, 616
Porphyrins, 313, 778
Port-wine stain, 1449
Portal cirrhosis, 1249

Portal hypertension, 1238-1241
  child and, 1283-1284
Portal-systemic encephalopathy, 1240, 1242
Portal vein, 1239
Positive end-expiratory pressure, 1060
Positron emission tomography scan, 385
Postcentral gyrus, 360
Postcoital cervical mucus test, 670
Postconcussive syndrome, 478
Postductal coarctation of aorta, 1001-1002
Posterior cerebral artery aneurysm, 495
Posterior fossa, 366
Posterior horn, 364
Posterior-inferior cerebellar artery aneurysm, 495
Posterior pituitary
  aging and, 589
  diseases of, 597-599
  hormones of, 573-574
Posterior spinal arteries, 371
Postganglionic neuron, 372
Posthemorrhagic anemia, 792
Posthyperalimentation hypoglycemia, 620
Posthyperventilation apnea, 434, 435
Postictal state, 446
  seizure and, 447
Postinfectious polyneuritis, 521
Postmortem autolysis, 77
Postmortem change, 76
Postnecrotic cirrhosis, 1249, 1252
Postobstructive diuresis, 1137
Postoperative respiratory failure, 1069
Postrenal acute renal failure, 1152
Poststreptococcal glomerulonephritis, 1146
Postsynaptic neuron, 356
Postural hypotension, 926-927
Postural tremor, 454
Posture
  motor dysfunction and, 451-452
  Parkinson disease and, 512
Potassium
  aldosterone-stimulated loss of, 633
  cellular environment and, 92-100
  in distal tubular cells, 93
  electrocardiogram and, 96
  hyperaldosteronism and, 633
  hypertension and, 177, 178
  mineralocorticoids and, 584, 585
  renal failure and, 1155, 1156
  saliva and, 1176
Potassium ions, 28
Potter syndrome, 1163
Poxvirus, 61
PR interval, 872
Precapillary sphincter, 888
Precentral gyrus, 360, 456
Precipitation, 205
Precipitin, 191
Precocious puberty, 678-680
Prednisone, 517
Preductal coarctation of aorta, 1001, 1002
Preexcitation syndrome, 967
Prefrontal area of cerebral hemisphere, 360
Preganglionic neurons, 372, 377
Pregnancy
  hormone of, 657
  hyperaldosteronism and, 631
  macrocytic anemia in, 786
Prekallikrein, 775
Prekallikrein activator, 225, 227
Preload, 879, 881, 968-969
Premature contractions
  atrial, 963

Premature contractions—cont'd
  junctional, 964
  ventricular, 965
Premenstrual syndrome, 683-684, 685
Premotor area of cerebral hemisphere, 360
Prenatal cerebral hypoxia, 543
Prenatal diagnosis of chromosome abnormalities, 127-128
Prenatal exposure, childhood cancer and, 319
Prepuce, 699
Prerenal acute renal failure, 1151
Presbycusis, 421
Presbyopia, 416-417
Pressoreceptor, 882
Pressure, blood flow, 890-892
  arterial, 895-896
  venous, 897
Pressure ulcer, 1400
Pressurized chamber, 72
Presynaptic neuron, 356
Pretibial myxedema, 605
Prevalence rate of disease, 158
Preventive efficiency, disease risk and, 160
Priapism, 700, 710
Prickly heat, 1449
Primary intention, wound repair by, 240-241, 242
Principle
  of independent assortment, 134
  of segregation, 134
Prinzmetal angina, 939
Prions, 444
Proaccelerin accelerator globulin, 774
Proband, 134
Probe, genetic, 146, 157
Procainamide, 406
Procallus formation, 1297
Procaryotes, 4, 5
Procollagen, 243
Proconvertin, 774
Proctitis, chlamydial, 737
Prodromal phase of hepatitis, 1248
Prodromal symptoms, 447, 448
Proenzymes, 222
Proerythroblast, 765
Progastrectomy syndrome, 1229-1230
Progesterone, 656-657
  carcinogenesis and, 333
  endometrial cancer and, 696, 697
  fertility and, 671
  history of study of, 645
  osteoporosis and, 1330
  sleep disorders and, 411
Programmed senescence theory of aging, 74
Progressive bulbar palsy, 460
Progressive dementia, 513
Progressive relaxation training, 1351
Progressive spinal muscular atrophy, 460
Progressive systemic sclerosis, 251
Proinsulin, 580
Projectile vomiting, 1214
Prolactin, 575
  carcinogenesis and, 332
  fertility and, 671
  lactation and, 668
  stress response and, 286-287
  tumor cell markers and, 300
Prolactin-inhibiting factor, 573
  galactorrhea and, 712
Prolapse
  mitral valve, 174, 957-958
  uterine, 689-690

Proliferation
  embryonic development of nervous system and, 533
  hematopoiesis and, 763
Proliferative breast disease, 713
Pronormoblast, 765
Prophase of cellular reproduction, 30
Propionibacterium acnes, 1407
Propositus, 134
Propranolol, 711
Proprioception, 423-424
Prosopagnosia, 462
Prostacyclin$_2$, 772
Prostaglandins, 342, 772
  dysmenorrhea and, 680
  mast cell and synthesis of, 221-222
  renal blood flow and, 1121
Prostate gland, 664
  cancer of, 327, 332, 333, 709-710
  disorders of, 707-710
  rhabdomyosarcoma and, 1384
Prostatic hyperplasia, benign, 707
Prostatitis, 705-709
Prostatodynia, 708
Prosthetic heart valve, 786
Protein
  acquired immune deficiency and, 268
  Bence Jones, 810
  binding of, 566
  cellular injury and, 68
  cellular metabolism and, 16
  cortisol and, 285, 286
  DNA and, 120
  erythropoiesis and, 766, 767
  genes and, 121-124
  homeostasis and, 283
  immunotherapy and cell-derived, 311
  injurious nutritional inbalances and, 62
  lipid-acceptor, 55
  lipid bilayer of, 14
  liver and, 1198, 1205
  muscle, 1310-1311
  plasma, 222-229, 755-757
  plasma membranes and, 14
  shock and depletion of, 983-984
  small intestine and, 1187
Protein buffering, 104
Protein-calorie malnutrition, 62
Protein-energy malnutrition
  cancer and, 306
  child and, 1279
Protein hormones, 565, 566
Protein link, 1302
Protein wasting, 629
Proteinaceous globin, 765
Proteinuria, 68, 1150
  diabetes mellitus and, 625-626
  nephrotic syndrome and, 1149, 1164
Proteoglycan, 1294
Proteolysis, 580
Proteus mirabilis, 59
Prothrombin, 227, 774, 844
Prothrombin consumption, 845
Prothrombin time, 779, 845
Proto-oncogene, 336
Protoporphyrin, 765, 778
  free erythrocyte, 790
Proximal tubule, 1114, 1121, 1124-1125
Pruritus, 672, 1401
  diabetes mellitus and, 617
  scabies and, 744
Psammoma bodies, 70
Pseudoarthrosis, 1323

Pseudogout, 1347
Pseudohypertrophic muscles, 1376
Pseudomonas aeruginosa, 59, 1078
  orchitis and, 703
Pseudoprecocious puberty, 678
Pseudostratified epithelium, 37
Psoriasis, 1404-1405
Psychiatric disorders, 170
  familial diseases and, 183
Psychogenic pain, 391
Psychologic factors
  familial diseases and, 163
  pain and, 399
Psychologic mediators, stress and, 282-283
Psychologic stress, 279
Psychological stress; *see also* Stress
Psychomotor seizure, 447
Psychoneuroimmunology, 279
Psychosis, Korsakoff, 509
Ptosis, 522
  ocular myopathy and, 1355
Ptyalin, 1175
Puberty, 649-650
  delayed, 678
  precocious, 678-680
Pubic hair, 650
Pubic louse, 745, 1447
Pulmonary abbreviations, 1035
Pulmonary artery, 864, 1045
Pulmonary blood flow
  acyanotic heart defects with increased,
    1003-1007
  cyanotic heart defects and, 1007-1015
Pulmonary circulation, 860, 1031-1034
  control of, 1042
Pulmonary defense mechanisms, 1027
Pulmonary disease
  child and, 1098-1107
  history of, 1025
  obstructive, 1069-1076
    sleep-provoked disorders and, 413
Pulmonary edema, 1058-1060
  heart failure and, 972
  high-altitude, 63, 1059
Pulmonary embolism, 930, 1080-1082
Pulmonary fibrosis, 1065
Pulmonary function alterations, 1053-1095;
    see also Pulmonary disease; Pulmonary
    edema
  abscess formation and, 1064
  acute respiratory failure and, 1067-1069
  aspiration and, 1060
  atelectasis and, 1060
  breathing pattern and, 1055
  bronchiectasis and, 1060-1061
  bronchiolitis and, 1062
  cavitation and, 1065
  chest wall restriction and, 1065
  child and, 1096-1109; *see also* Child,
    pulmonary function alterations in
  clubbing and, 1056
  cough and, 1055
  cyanosis and, 1056
  dyspnea and, 1054
  embolism and, 930, 1058-1060
  flail chest and, 1065
  hemoptysis and, 1055-1056
  history of study of, 1025
  hyperventilation and, 1055
  hypoventilation and, 1055
  hypoxemia and, 1057-1058
  inhalation disorders and, 1065-1067
  laryngeal cancer and, 1084-1085

Pulmonary function alterations—cont'd
  lip cancer and, 1083-1084
  lung cancer and, 1085-1090
  obstructive pulmonary disease and,
    1069-1076
  pain and, 1056
  pleural abnormalities and, 1062-1064
  pulmonary edema and, 1058-1060
  pulmonary fibrosis and, 1065
  pulmonary vascular disease and,
    1080-1083
  respiratory tract infection and, 1076-1080
  signs and symptoms of, 1054-1057
  sputum and, 1057
  systemic disorders and, 1067
  tests of, 1048-1050
Pulmonary heart disease, 1082-1083
Pulmonary hypertension, 1082, 1083
Pulmonary pain, 1056
Pulmonary right-to-left shunt, 1058
Pulmonary system
  hypothyroidism and, 607
  stress-related diseases of, 287
  structure and function of, 1026-1052
    aging and, 1050
    alterations in; *see* Pulmonary function
      alterations
    bronchial circulation and, 1031-1034
    chest wall and, 1034
    child and, 1096-1098
    conducting airways and, 1026-1030
    control of pulmonary circulation and,
      1042
    gas-exchange airways and, 1030-1031
    gas transport and, 1043-1048
    neurochemical control of ventilation
      and, 1040-1042
    pleura and, 1034
    pulmonary circulation and, 1031-1034
    tests and, 1048-1050
    ventilation and, 1034-1040
Pulmonary thromboembolism, 1080
Pulmonary vascular disease, 1080-1083
Pulmonary vascular resistance, 906, 969
Pulmonary vein, 864
Pulmonic semilunar valve, 864
Pulse, manually palpated, 901
Pulse tracing, 904
Pulse waveforms, arterial, 904
Pulsus paradoxus, 948
Punnett square, 134, 135, 141
Pupil, 414
  consciousness and, 435-436
Pupillary reflex, white, 557, 558
Pure red cell aplasia, 791
Purines, 117
Purkinje fiber, 870
Purpura, 816, 817, 1399
  allergic, 846
  thrombocytopenic, 251, 263
Purulent exudate, 229, 239
Pus, 229, 239
  pleural effusion and, 1064
Pustule, 1396
Putrefaction, 77
Pyelonephritis, 1142-1144
Pyknosis, 64
Pyloric obstruction, 1221-1223
Pyloric sphincter, 1177
Pyloric stenosis, 147-148, 1271
Pyloromyotomy, 1271
Pyloroplasty, 1230
Pylorus, 1177

Pyramidal motor syndrome, 455-457
Pyramidal system, 360
Pyridoxine, 767
Pyrimidines, 117
Pyrogen, endogenous, 236, 404
Pyrogenic bacteria, 58
Pyrosis, 1256
Pyruvate, 18, 19
Pyuria, 1131

Q

Q wave, 944-945
QRS complex, 873
QT interval, 873
Quadrant excision, 717
Quadriplegia, 451
Queyrat, erythroplasia of, 700, 701
Quick-frozen plasma, 845

R

Rabies, 508
Rad, 331
Radiation, 308-309, 402
  bone marrow, 308
  cosmic, 331
  familial diseases and, 163
  intrauterine, 319
  ionizing, 331
    acquired immune deficiency and, 268
    carcinogenesis and, 293, 332
    cellular injury and, 63-65
    leukemia and, 848
  ovarian cancer and, 698
  solar, 330, 1419
  sources of, 331
  ultraviolet, carcinogenesis and, 330-332
Radical mastectomy, 717
Radicular pain, 520
Radicular paresthesia, 520
Radiculitis, 520
Radiculopathy, 460, 520
Radioactive iodine, 604
Radioactive phosphorus, 797
Radioactive probe, DNA, 146
Radioallergosorbent testing, 255
Radiography
  cardiovascular function and, 905, 945
  chest, 1049
  skull, 383
  spine, 383
Radioimmunoassay, 587
Radioimmunosorbent testing, 255
Radionuclide imaging, 940
  cardiovascular function and, 905, 945
  monoclonal antibodies and, 313
Radon, 330
Range of motion, 1341
Ranvier, nodes of, 353
Rapid eye movement sleep, 408
Rapid plasmin reagin test, 732
Rapidly progressive glomerulonephritis,
  1145, 1147
Rash in child, 1445
Rate of living theory of aging, 74
Raynaud disease, 932
Raynaud phenomenon, 258, 932
  discoid lupus erythematosus and, 1408
  prolonged vibration and, 65
Reactions
  anaphylactic, 268
  hypersensitivity, 194, 250, 252-253
  mixed lymphocyte, 199
Reagin, 253

Recall, loss of, 443
Receptive dysphasia, 466
Receptor-associated disorders, 595
Receptor-mediated endocytosis, 19, 26
Receptor molecules, 15
Receptors
  α, 378
  β, 378
  equilibrium, 419
  hearing, 419
  hormones and, 568
  opiate, 397
  pain, 396
  skeletal muscle and sensory, 1306
Recessiveness of genes, 134
Recipient, universal, 200
Reciprocal translocation, 133
Recombinant DNA, 118-119
Recombination, chromosomes and, 141
Reconstructive phase of resolution and
    repair, 242-243
  dysfunction during, 244-245
Recovery phase of hepatitis, 1248
Rectal examination, 710
Rectal reflex, 1192
Rectocele, 688, 689
Rectoperineal fistula, 1274
Rectovaginal fistula, 1274
Rectum, 1192
  atresia of, 1274
  cancer of, 327, 1257-1259
  gonococcal infection of, 728
Recurrence risks, 136, 138, 139
Red blood cells, 13, 753, 757, 786
  ABO system and, 200
  count of, 777
  history of study of, 753
  myeloproliferative disorders of, 796-797
  urinalysis and, 1131
Red bone marrow, 1296
Red measles, 1444-1445
Red muscle, 1308
Red nucleus, 361-362
Reduction of fracture, 1323
Reed-Sternberg cell, 812
Referred pain, 397-399
  abdominal, 1217
Reflex
  aging and, 382
  cat's eye, 558
  defecation, 1192
  erectile, 663
  expiratory, Hering-Breuer, 1041
  gastrocolic, 1192
  gastroileal, 1190
  ileogastric, 1190
  intestinointestinal, 1190
  micturition, 1119
  neonatal, 533
  rectal, 1192
  spinal cord injury and, 486
  white pupillary, 557, 558
Reflex arc, 364
Reflex areas, 364
Reflex sympathetic dystrophy, 399
Reflux
  gastroesophageal, 1219-1220
    child and, 1275-1276
  vesicoureteral, 1166-1167
Reflux esophagitis, 1220, 1255
Refraction, 417
Refractory period
  cardiac action potential and, 872

Refractory period—cont'd
  plasma membrane and, 28
Regeneration
  inflammation and, 239
  nerve, 356
Regional osteoporosis, 1329
Regulatory genes, 116
Regurgitation
  aortic, 955, 956-957
  mitral, 955, 957
  tricuspid, 955, 957
  valvular, 953, 954, 955
Rejection, transplant, 262, 263
Relaxation, muscle contraction and, 1312
Releasing factors, hormonal, 573
Rem radiation dose, 331
Remission, multiple sclerosis and, 516
Remodeling of bone, 1297
Renal adenocarcinoma, 296
Renal adenoma, 1139
Renal agenesis, 1163
Renal artery, 1116
Renal autoregulation, 1119-1120
Renal blood flow, 1119-1121
  alterations in, 1152
  renal clearance and, 1130
Renal buffering
  acid-base balance and, 104
  chronic respiratory acidosis and, 109
Renal capsule, 1113
Renal cell carcinoma, 296, 1139
  lymphokines and, 312
  staging of, 1140
Renal clearance, 1129-1130
Renal cortex, 1113
Renal disease
  hyperkalemia and, 97
  secondary hypertension and, 1017
Renal disorders
  familial diseases and, 178-179
  hypertension and, 923
  potassium losses and, 94
Renal excretion of acid, 104
Renal failure, 1150-1158
  acute, 1151
  chronic, 1153-1158
  end-stage, 1150
  hyperphosphatemia and, 100
  leukemia and, 849
  types of, 1150-1158
Renal fascia, 1113
Renal function
  alterations in; *see* Urinary tract function
  diabetes mellitus and, 625
  tests of, 1129-1131
Renal hormones, kidney function and, 1129
Renal insufficiency, 1132, 1150
Renal medulla, 1113
Renal papilla, 1118
Renal pelvis, 1113
  papillary carcinoma of, 1140
Renal plasma flow, 1130
Renal pyramid, 1113
Renal stones, 1137-1139
  gout and, 1350
Renal system; *see also* Renal function;
    Urinary tract function
  autoimmunity and, 251
  development of, 1160-1161
  hypothyroidism and, 607
  structure of, 1112-1119
    child and, 1160-1161
Renal tubular escape phenomenon, 632

Renal tubular transport, 1124-1126
Renal tumor, 1139-1140
Renin, 896
  secretion of, 631
Renin-angiotensin system, 88, 584, 585, 631
  renal blood flow and, 1120, 1121
Reoviruses, 61
Repair
  of bone, 1297-1298
  inflammation and, 239-246
  myocardial infarction and, 944
Replicases, 59
Replication of DNA, 120-121
Repolarization, 28, 871
Reproductive factors
  breast cancer and, 715
  carcinogenesis and, 329
Reproductive system
  alterations of, 677-724
    breast disorders and, 711-719
    female reproductive system and,
      680-699; *see also* Female reproductive
      system
    male reproductive system and, 699-711;
      see also Male reproductive system
    sexual maturation and, 678-680
  cystic fibrosis and, 1276
  development of, 646-650
  hyperthyroidism and, 604
  hypothyroidism and, 606
  male, 661
  malignant tumors of, 693
  structure and function of, 646-676
    aging and, 76, 671-673
    breast and, 666-668
    female reproductive system and,
      650-660; *see also* Female reproductive
      system
    male reproductive system and, 660-666
    tests of, 668-671
  tests for, 670
  uremia and, 1157
Residual bodies, 9
Residual volume, 1036
Resistance
  blood flow and, 890-892
  general adaptation syndrome and, 282
  innate or native, 194
  total peripheral, 896
Resolution, inflammation and, 218, 239-246
Resonance, 65
Respirations
  body temperature and, 403
  Cheyne-Stokes, 1055
  Kussmaul, 1055
Respiratory acidosis, 105, 108-109
Respiratory alkalosis, 94, 99, 105
  acid-base imbalance and, 109-110
  with compensation and correction, 110
Respiratory bronchiole, 1030
Respiratory control system, 1041
Respiratory disease; *see* Pulmonary function
    alterations
Respiratory distress syndrome of newborn,
    1104-1106
Respiratory failure, 1067-1069
Respiratory pump, venous pressure and, 897
Respiratory rate, 1034
Respiratory system
  autoimmunity and, 251
  cancer and, 301
  infections of, 1076-1080
  uremia and, 1157

Responder cells, 199
Resting cardiac performance, 907-908
Resting heart rate, 882
Resting membrane potential, 27, 28
Restrictive cardiomyopathy, 953
Retardation, mental, 134
Retching, 1214
Rete testis, 661
Reticular activating system, 357, 358
 consciousness and, 432
Reticular dysgenesis, 266
Reticular fibers, 41
Reticular formation, 358
Reticular layer of dermis, 1392
Reticularis, 580
Reticulocytes, 765
 count of, 777
Reticuloendothelial system, 762
 bilirubin and, 1197
Reticulum, 41
Retina, 414
 hypertension and, 925
Retinoblastoma, 296
 child and, 317, 557-558
 pedigree for, 137
Retinopathy, diabetic, 625, 626
Retrobulbar neuritis, 416
Retroperitoneal region
 neuroblastoma and, 556
 rhabdomyosarcoma and, 1384
Retropulsion, 1179
Retroviruses, 61, 334
 human immunodeficiency virus and, 272
 oncogenes and, 336
Reverse transcriptase, 119, 334
Rewarming
 frostbite and, 1431-1432
 hypothermia and, 407
Reye syndrome, 548-549
Rh-immune globulin, 834
Rh system, 198-199, 263
 hemolytic disease in newborn and,
 831-832, 833, 834
Rhabdomyolysis, 1327, 1356
Rhabdomyoma, 296, 1356
Rhabdomyosarcoma, 296, 1356
 alveolar subclass of, 1383
 child and, 317, 1383, 1384
Rheumatic fever, 251, 261
 acute, 958-960
 child and, 1017
Rheumatic heart disease, 169, 958-960
 aortic valve calcification and, 70
 child and, 1017
 valvular, 173
Rheumatoid arthritis, 170, 251, 1342-1346
 juvenile, 1373
Rheumatoid factors, 1342
Rheumatoid nodule, 1345
Rhinitis, 255
Rhinovirus, 61
Rhodopsin, 416
Rhythm, heart and, 873, 964, 965
Riboflavin, 767
Ribonuclease
 Alzheimer disease and, 444
 tumor cell markers and, 300
Ribonucleic acid, 5, 6, 7, 121-122
 aging and, 76
 muscle, 1315
 human immunodeficiency virus and, 271,
 272
 viral replication and, 59

Ribosomal RNA, 123
Ribosomes, 6, 123-124
Ricin, 313
Rickets, 1330, 1367-1368
Right-to-left shunt, 999, 1048, 1058
Right ventricle, 862
Right ventricular end-diastolic pressure, 970
Righting, disorders of, 512
Rigidity, 452
 Parkinson disease and, 512
Rigor mortis, 77
Ringer's solution, lactated, 1428
Risk factors
 analyzing, 158-162
 empiric, 148
 environmental, 163-168
 familial diseases and, 159-162
 genetic diseases and, 136
 inheritance and, 136, 138, 139
 for primary hypertension, 920-921
RNA polymerase, 122
Rods, 414
Roentgen, 331
Rolando, fissure of, 360
Roseola, 1445
Rotation of fracture, 1322
Rotation injury of spine, 485
Rough endoplasmic reticulum, 6, 8
Round ligament of liver, 1194
Rubella, 1444, 1445
Rubeola, 1444-1445
Rubins test, 670
Rubral tremor, 454
Ruga, 651
Rule of nines, 1426, 1427
Ruptured intracranial aneurysm, 496-497
Russell bodies, 68

S

S cells, 1202
S phase of cellular reproduction, 29, 30
Sabin vaccine, 208
Saccharin, 328
Saccular aneurysm, 494, 927-928
Saccular bronchiectasis, 1061
Sacral plexus, 372
Sagittal suture, premature closure of, 539
St. Louis encephalitis, 508
St. Vitus dance, 959
Salicylates, 548
Salivary α-amylase, 1175
Salivary glands, 208, 1175
 cystic fibrosis and, 1276
 tumor of, 1090
Salivation, 1175-1176
Salk vaccine, 208
Salmon patch, 1449
Salpingitis, 685
Salt, dietary
 carcinogenesis and, 328, 1256
 hypertension and, 177, 178
Saltatory conduction, 354
Sarcolemma, 1308
Sarcoma, 293, 295
 of breast, 716
 Ewing, 1382
 Kaposi, 340, 1421-1423
 meningeal, 296
 soft tissue, 317
Sarcomere, 875, 1309, 1310
 myocardial, 968
Sarcoplasm, 1308
Sarcoplasmic reticulum, 874, 875, 1309

Sarcoptes scabiei, 744, 1446
Sarcotubule, 1309
Saturation kinetics, 22
Scabies, 743-744, 1446-1447
Scalded skin syndrome, 1441
Scales of skin, 1397
Scalp, fungal infection of, 1442
Scalp electrodes, 385
Scaphocephaly, 539
Scapuloperoneal muscular dystrophy,
 1379
Scar, 242, 245, 1398
 hypertrophic, 245
Scarlet fever, 959
Schilling test, 789
Schizophrenia, 170, 183
Schwann cells, 353, 356, 533
 diabetic neuropathy and, 624
Schwann sheath, 353
Schwannoma, 503
Sclera, 414
Scleroderma, 251, 1416
Scoliosis, 1368-1370
Scotoma, 416
Scratch test, 1394
Scrotum, 662
 disorders of, 701-702
 cancer and, 293
Scurvy, 244
Sebaceous glands, 1392, 1393
Seborrhea, 513
Seborrheic dermatitis, 1403-1404
Seborrheic keratosis, 1417
Second-degree heart block, 966
Second messenger, 569-570
Secondary intention, wound repair by,
 240-241, 242
Secretin, 1178, 1179
 cells producing, 1202
Secretory diarrhea, 1216
Secretory granules, 8
Secretory immune system, 207-209
Secretory vesicles, 8
Sedentary life-style
 constipation and, 1214
 coronary artery disease and, 936-937
Segmental demyelinating neuropathy, 520
Segmented neutrophil, 759
Segregation, principle of, 134
Seizures, 445-451, 547
 child and, 546-548
 clinical manifestations of, 448-450
 generalized, 449-450
 child and, 546-547
 partial, 448-449
Selective IgA deficiency, 267
Selective vagotomy, 1230
Selenium, 329
Self-antigens, 197, 259, 261
Self-defense mechanisms
 immunity and, 192-216; *see also* Immunity
 inflammation and, 217-248; *see also*
 Inflammation
 stress and, 279-291; *see also* Stress
Self-digestion, 9
Sella turcica tumors, 554
Semen, 664, 706
 analysis of, 670
Semicircular canals, 419
Semilunar valve, 864
Seminal vesicle, 664
Seminiferous tubules, 661, 664-665
Seminoma, 297, 705

Sendai virus, 59, 144
Senescent erythrocytes, 769-770
Senile plaque, 382, 444, 445
Senses, 391, 413-423
  aging and, 382
  hearing and, 419-421
  olfaction and, 421-423
  taste and, 421-423
  vision and, 413-419
Sensitization, 253
Sensorimotor neuropathy, 520
Sensorineural hearing loss, 421
Sensory function, 391
  hyperthyroidism and, 604
  pain and, 391
Sensory inattentiveness, 464
Sensory-motor dysphasia, 467
Sensory neurons, 355
Sensory neuropathy, 520
Sensory receptors, skeletal muscle and,
  1306
Sepsis, wound, 244
Septic shock, 980-981
Septicemia, 59, 237
  heart failure and, 976
  shock and, 980
Septostomy, balloon, 1010
Sequestra, 1371
Sequestration crisis, 840
Serology, 668, 669
Serosa of stomach, 1178
Serotonin, 220, 357
  tumor cell markers and, 300
Serous exudate, 239
Serratia marcescens, 59
Sertoli cells, 665
Serum, 755
  enzymes in, 1205
  estradiol in, 671
  ferritin in, 777
  follicle-stimulating hormone in, 671
  glutamic oxaloacetic transaminase in, 944
  hormones in
    fertility and, 671
    immunology and, 191
  hypersensitivity and, 254
  luteinizing hormone in, 671
  magnesium in, 100
  phosphate in, 100
  potassium in, 94, 96
  progesterone in, 671
  prolactin in, 671
  prothrombin conversion factor in, 774
  sodium in, 89, 92
  testosterone in, 671
Serum colloid osmotic pressure, 306
Serum-free testosterone, 671
Serum proteins, 1205
Serum sickness, 258
Severe combined immune deficiencies, 266
Sex characteristics, secondary, 650
Sex chromosomes, 124, 128, 129-131
Sex cord mesenchyme, 297
Sex hormone–binding globulin, 566
Sex hormones, 646
  carcinogenesis and, 332, 333
  female, 655-657
  history of, 645
  male, 665-666
    aging and, 673
    carcinogenesis and, 332
Sex-linked inheritance, 139-140
Sexual behavior, carcinogenesis and, 329

Sexual differentiation in utero, 646-648
Sexual dysfunction
  male, 710-711
  pharmacologic agents and, 710
Sexual maturation, 678-680
Sexual stimulation, 663
Sexually transmitted diseases, 725-751
  diagnosis of, 669
  gastrointestinal infections in, 745-747
  hepatitis B and, 1246
  herpes simplex virus and, 1411-1412
  history of study of, 645
  systemic diseases and, 747-748
  urogenital infections in, 727-745
    bacterial, 727-736
    chlamydial, 736-739
    parasitic, 743-745
    viral, 739-743
  warts and, 741, 1413
Sharpey fibers, 1300
Sheehan syndrome, 599
Shigellosis, 745-746
Shingles, 1412, 1445
Shivering, 402, 406
Shock
  anaphylactic, 979-980
  burn, 1426-1429
  cardiovascular system and, 976-984
  hemorrhagic, 408
  hypovolemic, 977, 978
  insulin, 618
  neurogenic, 977-979
  septic, 980-981
  spinal, 457, 485-487
  thrombus formation and, 930
  treatment for, 984
  vasogenic, 977
Shock-wave lithotripsy, 1138
Short bones, 1297
Short-term memory loss, 443
Shunts, blood, 893, 999
  left-to-right, 999, 1006
  right-to-left, 999, 1048, 1058
Sialoprotein, 1294
Sialyl transferase, 300
Sick cell syndrome, 1429-1430
Sickle cell disease, 786, 830, 836-841
  clinical manifestations of, 839
  inheritance of, 837
Sickle cell hemoglobin, 837
Sickle cell test, 777
Sickle cell trait, 836, 840
Sickle cell–Hb C disease, 836, 840
Sickle cell–thalassemia, 836, 840
Sickled erythrocyte, 836
Sideroblast, 790
Sideroblastic anemia, 786, 790-791
Sigmoid colon, 1190
Sigmoidoscopy, 1203
Silent substitution mutation, 121
Silicosis, 1066
Sims-Hunher test, 670
Simuliidae, 1417
Single-gene defects, 178-179
  childhood cancers and, 317, 318
Sinoatrial node, 869, 963
Sinus arrhythmia, 964
Sinus block, 966
Sinus bradycardia, 963
Sinus tachycardia, 963
Sinusoids in liver, 1195
Sister chromatids, 30, 128
Sjögren syndrome, 251

Skeletal muscle disorders, 1350-1356
  metabolic muscle diseases and, 1352-1354
  muscle membrane abnormalities and, 1352
  muscle tumors and, 1356
  myositis and, 1354-1355
  ocular myopathies and, 1355
  secondary muscular dysfunction and,
    1351-1352
  toxic myopathies and, 1355-1356
Skeletal muscle pump, 897
Skeletal muscles
  contractile proteins of fibril of, 1310
  disorders of; *see* Skeletal muscle disorders
  heat and contraction of, 402
  history of study of, 1291
  structure and function of, 1304-1314
    contraction at molecular level and,
      1311-1312
    mechanics and, 1313
    metabolism and, 1312-1313
    movement of muscle groups and, 1314
    types of contraction and, 1313-1314
    whole muscle and, 1304-1311
Skeleton
  abnormal modeling or density of,
    1367-1370
  appendicular, 1296
  axial, 1296
    malformations of, 538-541
  development of, 1362
  trauma to, 1320-1325
  uremia and, 1157
Skene glands, 650
Skin
  autoimmunity and, 250
  biopsy of, 1394
  child and, 1439-1452; *see also* Child, skin
    disorders of
  diabetes mellitus and, 628
  diagnostic procedures and, 1394
  disorders of, 1402-1432
    benign tumors and, 1417-1418
    cancer and, 68, 155, 327, 1418-1423
    infection and, 1411-1415
    inflammatory, 1402-1404
    insect bites and, 1416-1417
    papulosquamous, 1404-1409
    thermal injury and, 1423-1432
    vascular, 1415-1416
    vesiculobullous, 1409-1411
    vulva and, 684-685
  history of study of, 1389
  hyperkeratosis of, 51
  hyperthyroidism and, 604
  hypothyroidism and, 607
  scraping of, 1394
  spinous layer of, 1392
  stress-related diseases of, 287
  structure and function of, 1391-1401
    aging and, 1393-1394
    dermis and, 1392
    epidermis and, 1391-1392
    hypodermis and, 1392-1393
    keloid and, 1400-1401
    layers of, 1391-1394
    lesions and, 1394-1399
    manifestations of skin dysfunction and,
      1394-1401
    pressure ulcer and, 1400
    pruritus and, 1401
    tests and, 1394
  uremia and, 1157
Skin tests, hypersensitivity, 255, 275

Skull
  asymmetric growth of, 538
  fracture of, 480, 483
  Paget disease and, 1331
  roentgenograms of, 383
Sleep, 391, 408-413
  deprivation of, 408
  disease and, 412-413
  disorders of, 411-412
  dysfunctions of, 412
  non-rapid-eye-movement, 409
    enuresis and, 1169
  patterns of, 410-411
  rapid eye movement, 408
  stages of, 409-411
Sleep apnea, 411
Sleep-provoked disorders, 412-413
Sleep-wake schedule, 411-412
Sleepwalking, 412
Sliding filament theory of muscle
    contraction, 878, 1311
Sliding hiatal hernia, 1221
Slow-reacting substances of anaphylaxis, 221
Slow-wave sleep, 408
Small cell carcinoma, 1087-1088, 1089
Small intestine, 1182-1190
Small motor neuron, 458
Smallpox, 191, 1446
Smell, 421-423
Smog, 329-330
Smokeless tobacco, 326
Smoking, 171, 330
  carcinogenesis and, 326
  coronary artery disease and, 936
  cough and, 1073
  disease risk and, 158
  hypertension and, 920, 1019
  lung cancer and, 164, 1086
  thromboangiitis obliterans and, 932
Smooth endoplasmic reticulum, 6
Smooth muscle, 42
Snuff, 326
Sodium, 28
  cellular environment and, 87-92
  deficits of, 91
  hypertension and, 922, 1019
  inadequate intake of, 91
  mineralocorticoids and, 584, 585
  pancreas and, 1201, 1202
  renal failure and, 1155, 1156
  saliva and, 1176
  shock and, 983
  small intestine and, 1184, 1186
  third factor in regulation of, 88
  urine and, 1124, 1126-1127, 1128
Sodium-potassium pump, 92
  hypertension and, 922-923
  hypoxic injury and, 53, 56
  obesity and, 1236
Soft chancre, 733
Soft spot in skull, 535
Soft tissue sarcoma, 317
Soft tissue tumor, 317, 1382-1383
Solar radiation, 330, 1419
Solid tumors
  avascular phase of, 302
  radiation and, 332
Solitary intraductal papilloma, 714
Solutes, 19
  concentration of, 20
  imbalances of, 89
  movement of, 19-24
Soma, 353

Somatic cells, 124
  hybridization of, 145-146
  therapy and, 119
Somatic death, 76-77
Somatic mutation theory of aging, 74-75
Somatic nervous system, 353
Somatic pain, 397
Somatogenic pain, 391
Somatomedins, 603
Somatomotropic hormones, 286, 575
Somatosensory function, 423-424
Somatostatin, 573, 578
Somatotropin, 286, 575
Somite, 533
Somnambulism, 412
Somnolence, 411
Somogyi effect, 623, 624
Sore
  cold, 1411
  pressure; *see* Decubitus ulcer
Sound waves, 419
Spasm, 453
  flexor, 547
  infantile, 450, 546-547
Spastic paresis, amyotrophic lateral sclerosis
    and, 518
Spasticity, 452
Spatial agnosia, 462
Spatial summation, 357
Specific gravity of urine, 1131
Specificity
  pain and, 396
  stress and, 282-283
Speech dyspraxia, 463
Sperm, 705-706
  cervical cancer and mutant, 693
  flagella of, 12
  phagocytosis and, 692
Sperm cell, 665
Spermatic cord, 660
Spermatid, 665
Spermatocele, 702
Spermatogenesis, 661, 664-665, 705
  impaired, 705-706
Spermatogonium, 665
Spermatozoan, 646
Spherocyte, 786
Spherocytosis, hereditary, 786, 835-836
Sphincter
  anal, 1190
  of Oddi, 1199
  urethral, 1118-1119
Spina bifida, 538
Spina bifida cystica, 536-537
Spina bifida occulta, 538
Spinal accessory nerves, 375
Spinal cord, 362-365, 456
  abscess of, 506
  blood supply to, 371, 372
  defective formation of, 536
  inflammation of, 505
  injury to, 483-489
    clinical manifestations of, 487
  pain and, 395-396
  tracts of, 364
  tumors of, 500, 504-505
    metastatic, 504
Spinal nerve root tumor, 500
Spinal nerves, 352, 371-372
  pain and, 394
Spinal shock, 457, 485-487
Spinal tracts, 364
Spindle fibers, 30

Spine
  epidural abscess of, 506
  injury of, 483, 484, 485
  progressive muscular atrophy of, 460
  reflex arc in, 1119
  roentgenogram of, 383
  scoliosis and, 1369, 1370
  stenosis in, 491
Spinothalamic tract, 364
  pain and, 395-396
Spiral fracture, 1320, 1321
Spirometry, 1048, 1071
Spironolactone, 96
  sexual dysfunction and, 711
  urine and, 1128
Splanchnic nerves, 377
Spleen, 760-761
  alterations in functions of, 816
  cancer treatment and, 314
  Hodgkin disease and, 814
  leukemia and, 807
  metastasis and, 305
Splenectomy, 816
  target cells after, 786
  thalassemia major and, 842
Splenic leukemia, history of, 753
Splenic pulp, 760
Splenomegaly, 66, 816, 1240
  iron deficiency anemia and, 831
Splicing, gene, 123
Split heart sounds, 903
Spondylolisthesis, 491
Spondylolysis, 490-491
Spongy bone, 1295
Spontaneous abortion, 126
Spontaneous mutation, 121
Spontaneous pneumothorax, 1062
Spontaneous reactive hypoglycemia, 620
Sporadic motor neuron disease, 517-519
Sprains, tendon, 1325-1326
Sputum, 1057
Squamous cell carcinoma, 296, 1419-1420
  lung and, 1087, 1089
  ultraviolet radiation and, 330
Squamous cells, 33, 34, 37, 51, 52
Squamous papilloma, 296
ST segment, 873, 944-945
Stab, 759
Staghorn calculi, 1137-1138
Staging, tumor, 301
Stains
  Giemsa, 124
  Gram, 668
  triacid, 753
Staphylococci, 1077
  cellulitis and, 1411
  orchitis and, 703
  scalded skin syndrome and, 1441
  toxic epidermal necrolysis and, 1441
Staphylococcus aureus, 1078
  bullous impetigo and, 1440
  empyema and, 1064
  folliculitis and, 1411
  hematogenous osteomyelitis and, 1332
  myositis and, 1354
  toxic shock syndrome and, 981
Starling hypothesis, 85
Starvation, 62, 1238
Stasis dermatitis, 1403
Static encephalopathy, 542-548
Status asthmaticus, 1071, 1102
Status epilepticus, 446
Steatorrhea, 1232, 1277

Stem cells, 266, 763-764
Stem tumor, 596
Stenosis
aortic, 954-955
mitral, 955-956
pulmonary, 1000-1001
spinal, 491
valvular, 953, 954, 955
Sternberg-Reed cell, 812
Steroidogenesis, 580
Steroids, 570, 655
anabolic, 319, 580
carcinogenesis and sex, 332, 333
fat-soluble, 566
inflammatory response and, 285
nephrotic syndrome and, 1164, 1165
Stevens-Johnson syndrome, 1410
Stiffness, joint, 1341
Stimulator cells, 199
Stimuli
nociceptors and, 396
stress and, 288
Stirrup, 419
Stomach, 1177-1182
cancer of, 327, 1256-1257
inflammation of, 1230
interior of, 1177
muscle layers of, 1177
Stomatitis, angular, 790
Stomatocyte, 786
Stone, renal, 1137-1139
gout and, 1350
history of study of, 1111
Stool studies, 1204
Storage diseases
lysosomal, 9
manifestations of, 66
Strabismus, 415
Strains
ligament, 1325-1326
muscle, 1326-1327
Stratified epithelium, 37, 1392
Strawberry hemangioma, 1448, 1449
Streptococci
orchitis and, 703
prostatitis and, 708
rheumatic fever and, 958, 1017
Streptococcus pneumoniae, 1077, 1078
child and, 1102
bacterial meningitis in, 549
Stress, 279
acquired immune deficiency and, 269
disease and, 279-283, 279-291
concepts of, 279-283
coping and illness in, 288-289
response and, 283-288
galactorrhea and, 712
hypertension and, 924
muscle tension and, 1351
response to, 280-281, 283-288, 586-587
Stress fracture, 1321
Stress incontinence, 1169
Stress testing, cardiac activity and, 905
Stress ulcer, 1228-1229
Stressors, 280, 288, 289
response to, 280-281, 283-288, 586-587
Stretch receptor, 1041
Stretch reflex, 451
Striated muscle, 1309
String galvanometer, 857
Stroke, 169
diabetes mellitus and, 627
embolic, 493-494

Stroke—cont'd
familial diseases and, 176-177
hemorrhagic, 494
hypoxic injury and, 52-53
thrombotic, 493
Stroke-in-evolution, 493
Stroke volume
cardiac function and, 906
heart and, 882
Stroke work index, 906
Struvite renal stone, 1137
Stuart factor, 774
Stuart-Prower factor, 773, 774
Stupor, 434
Subacute bacterial endocarditis, 931
Subacute thyroiditis, 608
Subarachnoid hemorrhage, 366, 497-498
Subarachnoid space, 366
Subcutaneous layer of skin, 1392-1393
Subdural hematoma, 481-482
Subdural space, 366
Subintima, 1300
Subluxation, joints and, 1323-1325
Submucosa of stomach, 1178
Subserosal plexus of stomach, 1178
Substance P, 573
Substantia gelatinosa, 364
pain and, 396-397
Substantia nigra, 361-362
Parkinson disease and, 510-511
Substrate, 17
Substrate phosphorylation, 18
Subthalamus, 360
Sudden infant death syndrome, 413, 1100-1101
Sudden unexplained nocturnal death syndrome, 413
Sulci, 359
Sulcus limitans, 533
Sunlight
melanin and, 68
skin cancer and, 330, 1419
vitamin D deficiency and, 99
Sunset sign, 541
Superior colliculi, 361
Superior mesenteric ganglia, 377
Superior vena cava, 864
Superior vena cava syndrome, 933
Superoxide dismutase-1, 145
Suppressor cells; *see* T suppressor cells
Supraglottis, 1027
Supratentorial herniation, 470
Supratentorial processes, 432
Supratentorial tumor, 554
unconsciousness and, 434
Supravalvular stenosis, 1000
Surface tension, alveolar, 1038
Surfactant, 1030, 1038, 1097
Suture
joints and, 1298
skull and, 533, 535
Swallowing, 1176-1177
difficult, 1219
Sweat glands, 1392, 1393
cystic fibrosis and, 1276
Sweating, 403
Swelling, cellular, 66; *see also* Edema
Sydenham chorea, 959
Sylvian fissure, 360
Sylvius, aqueduct of, 367
Sympathetic ganglia, 376
Sympathetic nervous system, 381
anatomy of, 376-377

Sympathetic nervous system—cont'd
endocrine system and, 587
heart and, 873
stress response and, 283
Sympathogonia, 555
Symphysis, 1298
Symport, 22
Synapses, 41, 356-357
Synaptic cleft, 354, 357
Synaptic terminal, 357
Synarthrosis, 1298
Synchondrosis, 1298
Syndactyly, 1363, 1364
Syndesmophyte, 1347
Syndesmosis, 1298
Syndrome of inappropriate antidiuretic hormone secretion, 92, 597-598
Synovial cavity, 1300
Synovial fluid, 1300-1301
analysis of, 1314
Synovial joints, 1298-1304
Synovial membrane, 1300
Synovitis, rheumatoid arthritis and, 1342
Synovium, 1300
Syphilis, 508-509, 729-733
history of study of, 645
serology for, 669
false-positive tests and, 733
Syringomyelic syndrome, 505
Syrinx, 505
Systemic circulation, 860, 886
Systemic lupus erythematosus, 170, 251, 263, 1409-1410
Systemic vascular resistance, 906, 969
left heart failure and, 972
Systole, 864
Systolic blood pressure in child, 1020-1021
Systolic compressive effect, 897

T

T cells, 193, 195-196, 209, 288
acquired immune deficiency and, 268
cancer immunotherapy and, 312
cortisol and, 285
cytotoxic, 342
endometriosis and, 692
dermatomyositis and, 1354
graft-versus-host disease and, 275
hypersensitivity and, 258
immune deficiency and, 265
immunity and, 193, 195-196, 288
rheumatoid arthritis and, 1342
tests of, 275
T helper cells, human immunodeficiency virus and, 272
T-independent antigen, 211
T suppressor cells, 197, 209, 212, 343
hypersensitivity and, 261-262
T wave, 944-945
Tabes dorsalis, 509
Tachycardia
atrial, 964
junctional, 965
simple sinus, 963
ventricular, 965
Tactile agnosia, 462
Tactile perception, 423
Talipes, 1364-1365
Tamponade, 948
Tardive dyskinesia, 454-455
Target cells, 568, 595
cell-mediated tissue destruction and, 259

Target cells—cont'd
  hormonal alterations and, 595
  pharmacologic effects and, 568
  splenectomy and, 786
Taste, 421-423
  aging and, 422
  dysfunction and, 423
Tay-Sachs disease, 9, 546
Technetium pyrophosphate, 905
Tegmentum, 361
Telangiectasia, 1399
Telencephalon, 359-360
Telophase in cellular reproduction, 30
Temperature
  cellular injury and, 63
  menstrual cycle and, 660
  regulation of, 391, 400-408
    disorders of, 405-408
  somatic death and, 76
Temporal fossa, 366
Temporal lobe, 360
Temporal lobe seizure, 447
Temporal summation, 357
Tendon reflex, neuropathy and, 461
Tendonitis, 1326
Tendons, 1305
  sprain of, 1325-1326
Teniae coli, 1190
Tenosynovitis, 728
Tensilon; *see* Edrophonium chloride
Tension pneumothorax, 1062, 1063
Tentorium cerebelli, 366
Teratocarcinoma, testicular, 705
Teratoma, testicular, 705
Terminal bronchiole, 1032
Terminal respiratory unit, 1031
Termination codons, 120
Testes, 660-662
  aging and, 672
  cancer of, 704-705
  carcinogenesis and, 327
  descent of, 662
  disorders of, 702-706
  enlargement of, 704
  rhabdomyosarcoma and, 1384
  torsion of, 703
  tumor of, 704, 705
Testosterone, 646, 665-666
  aging and, 673
  carcinogenesis and, 332, 333
  fertility and, 671
  history of study of, 645
  stress response and, 287
Tetanus, muscle and, 1313
Tetany, 98
Tetrahydroaminoacridine, 445
Tetralogy of Fallot, 1012-1014
Tetraploidy, 126
Thalamus, 360, 361
Thalassemia, 155, 830, 841-842
Thallium, 905, 940, 945
Theca cells, 655
Thelarche, 668
  premature, 678
Thermal injury, 408, 1423-1432
  acquired immune deficiency and, 269
  burns and, 1423-1431
  frostbite and, 1431-1432
Thermogenesis
  chemical, 402
  nonshivering, 402
Thermography, 669
Thermophilic actinomycetes, 254

Thermoreceptors, 355
  peripheral, 401
Thiamine
  heart failure and, 976
  Wernicke disease and, 509
Thiazides, 1128
Third-degree burns, 1425-1427
Third-degree heart block, 966
Thirst, regulation of, 87
Thomsen disease, 1365
Thoracic compliance, 1038
Thoracic duct, 900
Thoracolumbar division, 376
Thorax, 1034, 1098
  anterior-posterior diameter of, 1037
Thought content, 432
  alterations in, 440-442
Three-day measles, 1444
Threshold potential, 28
Threshold trait, 147
Thrombin, 227, 844
Thrombin time, 779, 845
Thromboangiitis obliterans, 931-932
Thrombocyte, 771
Thrombocytopenia, 307, 804, 817-818
  neonatal transient, 846
Thrombocytopenic purpura
  autoimmune, 251
  idiopathic, 170, 845-846
  immune, 263, 846
Thrombocytosis, 817, 818
Thromboembolism, 816, 819, 821-822,
    930, 930-931
  myocardial infarction and, 947
  pulmonary, 1080
Thrombogen, 774
  atherogenesis and, 919
Thrombokinase, 774
Thrombophlebitis, 930
Thromboplastin, 844
  tissue, 774
Thromboplastin generation test, 845
Thromboplastin time, partial, 779
Thromboplastinogen, 774
Thrombopoietin, 771
Thrombosed hemorrhoids, 1258
Thrombosis, 52, 821, 930; *see also*
    Thromboembolism
  venous, 933
Thrombotic stroke, 493
Thrombotic thrombocytopenic purpura, 818
Thromboxane A_2, 772, 938
Thrombus; *see* Thromboembolism;
    Thrombosis
Thrush, 1443
Thymidine, 314
Thymidine kinase, 145
Thymine, 117
Thymoma, 297
Thymosins, 276, 310
Thymus, 191, 209
  atrophy of, 214
  immune deficiencies and, 275
Thyrocalcitonin, 575
Thyroglobulin, 577
Thyroid-binding globulin, 566
Thyroid gland, 574-577, 1027; *see also*
    Hyperthyroidism; Hypothyroidism
  aging and, 588-589
  alterations of function of, 603-609
  carcinogenesis and, 327
  carcinoma of, 608-609
  dysgenesis of, 608

Thyroid hormone
  regulation of, 576
  secondary sleep disorders and, 412
  synthesis of, 576-577
Thyroid-stimulating hormone, 571, 575,
    576, 604
  deficiency of, 600
  tumor cell markers and, 300
Thyroid storm, 605-606
Thyroidectomy, 604
Thyroiditis
  acute, 608
  autoimmune, 250, 608
  chronic lymphocytic, 608
  Hashimoto, 170
  subacute, 608
Thyrotoxic crisis, 605-606
Thyrotropin-releasing hormone, 573, 576,
    596-597
Thyrotropin-stimulating hormone—releasing
    hormone, 401
Thyroxine, 401, 576, 577, 608
Tibia
  fibrosarcoma of, 1337
  osteogenesis imperfecta in, 1368
Ticks, 1416
Tics, 453
Tight junctions
  intercellular communication and, 32, 33
  small intestine and, 1184
Time-zone change, 411
Tinea capitis, 1414, 1442-1443
Tinea corporis, 1414, 1442
Tinea pedis, 1414
Tinnitus, 65, 421
Tissue factor, 774
Tissue-specific antigens, hypersensitivity and,
    255-257
Tissue thromboplastin, 774
Tissues, 31-43
  aging and, 76
  altered cellular biology and; *see* Altered
    cellular and tissue biology
  cell-mediated hypersensitivity and,
    258-260
  connective, 37-41
  epithelial, 37
  formation of, 31-32
  hypothermia of, 406
  hypoxia of, 787
  immunologic mechanisms and, 252
  intracellular communication and, 32-33
  muscle, 41
  neural, 41-43
  perfusion of, 895
  reproductive function test and biopsy of,
    669
TNM classification of lung cancer, 1090
Tobacco
  carcinogenesis and; *see* Smoking
  smokeless, 326
Toe
  clubbing of, 1056
  gout and, 1350
Toe web infection, 1414
Toilet training, 1168
Tolerance, immunity and, 197, 261-262
Tolergenic antigen, 197
Tonic-clonic seizure, 546
Tonic phase of seizure, 447
Tonicity, 21
Tonsil, cerebellar, 470
Tophi, 1350

TORCH test, 669
Torsion
  intestinal obstruction and, 1222
  of testis, 703
Torus fracture, 1321
Total anomalous pulmonary venous
    connection, 1010-1012
Total body surface area, burns and, 1424
Total body water, 83
  sodium and, 91
Total iron-binding capacity, 778
Total lung capacity, 1036, 1071
Total peripheral resistance, 892-895, 896
Touch, 423
Toxic epidermal necrolysis, 1441
Toxic epidural necrolysis, 1441
Toxic erythema of newborn, 1449-1450
Toxic gas inhalation, 1065-1066
Toxic myopathy, 1355-1356
Toxic nodular goiter, 605
Toxic shock syndrome, 981
Toxin-antitoxin complex, 206
Trabeculae, 1296
  sexual dysfunction and fibrosis of, 710
Trabeculae carneae, 865
Trachea, 1028, 1029
  bifurcation of, 1096
Tracheobronchial cartilaginous rings, 1098
Tracheoesophageal fistula, 1270
Trachoma, 413-414
Traction, bone fracture and, 1323
Traits
  continuous, 161
  familial aggregation of, 167
  mendelian, 133
  multifactorial, 157
  penetrance of, 137
  polygenic, 147, 156
  sex-influenced, 139-140
  threshold, 147
Transchondral fracture, 1322
Transcortical dysphasia, 465, 467
Transcortin, 284
Transcription, DNA, 122-123
Transfer factor, 276
  lymphokines and, 235
Transfer reactions, 18
Transfer RNA, 122, 123
Transferrin, 767, 778
  cachexia and, 306
  liver and, 1205
Transferrin saturation, 778
Transformation, cancer cells and, 297, 337
Transformation zone, 693, 695
  uterus and, 653
Transfusion reactions, isoimmunity and, 262
Transfusions, 199
  immune deficiency and, 275-276
  thalassemia major and, 842
Transient ischemic attack, 493
Transient neonatal thrombocytopenia, 846
Translation, RNA, 123-124
Translocations, 133
Transmembrane proteins, 14
Transplantation
  childhood cancers and, 318, 319
  diabetes mellitus and, 616
  heart, 857-858
  immune deficiency and, 275
  isoimmunity and, 262, 263, 264
Transplantation antigens, 337-338
Transport
  active or passive, 19

Transport—cont'd
  cellular injury and, 52
  nephron and maximum, 1124
  by vesicle formation, 25-27
Transport protein, 22
Transporter, 22
Transudative effusion, 1063, 1064
Transverse colon, 1190
Transverse tubule, 875, 1309
Trauma
  acquired immune deficiencies and, 269
  blunt, 478
  fever and central nervous system, 408
  head
    closed, 477-482
    open, 482-483
  perinatal, 543
  skeletal, 1320-1325
  spinal cord, 483-489
  temperature regulation and, 407
Traumatic aneurysm, 496
Travel, sleep disorders and, 411-412
Treitz ligament, 1182
Tremor, 453-454
  parkinsonian, 511
  at rest, 454
Trephination, 351
Treponema pallidum, 508, 730
  nephrotic syndrome and, 1164
Triacid stain, 753
Triad of Virchow, 821
Triamterene, 1128
Tricarboxylic acid cycle, 18
Triceps, 1314
Trichinosis, 1354
Trichomoniasis, 743
Tricuspid valve, 864
  atresia of, 1014-1015
  regurgitation of, 955, 957
Trigeminal nerves, 374
Trigger points, 400
Triglycerides, 934
Trigone, 1118
Triiodothyronine, 576, 577
Triploidy, 126
Trisomies, 126, 128-129
  childhood cancers and, 318
  congenital heart defects and, 998
Trochlear nerves, 374
Trophoblast, IgG and, 213
Tropomyosin, 1310
Troponin, 876, 1310
Troponin-tropomyosin complex, 875-876
Trousseau sign, 99
Truncus arteriosus, 1007-1009
Trypsin, 1187, 1202
  history of study of, 1173
Trypsin inhibitor, 1202
Tuberculosis, 191, 1079-1080
  Addison disease and, 634-635
  history of study of, 1025
Tuberous sclerosis, 318
Tubular obstruction theory, 1152
Tubule of kidney
  acute necrosis of, 1151
  distal, 1116, 1121, 1125-1126
    renal buffering and, 104
  proximal, 1114, 1121, 1124-1125
  reabsorption in, 1122
  secretion from, 1122
  transport and, 1124-1126
Tubulus rectus, 661
Tumor angiogenesis factor, 302

Tumor-associated antigens, 301, 337-338,
    340-343
  cross-reactive, 337-338
Tumor biology, 293-322
  cancer cell characteristics and, 294-300
  cancer in children and, 316-319
  cancer manifestations and, 304-307
  cancer treatment and, 307-315
  classification and nomenclature in, 294,
    295, 296
  tumor development in, 300-304
Tumor cell markers, 298-301
Tumor cells, mouse, 144, 145, 314
Tumor-immune surveillance, 310
Tumor-specific antigens; *see*
    Tumor-associated antigens
Tumors; *see also* Tumor biology
  bladder, 1139-1141
  bone, 1334-1339
    bone destruction in, 1335
    child and, 1380-1382
    derivation of, 1334
    types of, 1335-1339
  brain, 500
    child and, 552-555
    metastatic, 504
  breast, male, 719
  central nervous system and, 498-505
  child and, 552-558
  chondrogenic, 1337
  development of, 301-305
    multistage theory of, 325
  embryonal, 555-558
  extracerebral primary, 503-504
  of female reproductive system, 693
  germ cell, 697
  giant cell, 1338-1339
  growth rates for, 302
  immunodiagnosis of, 315
  immunologic defense against, 339-340
  initiation of, 326
  intestinal obstruction and, 1222
  muscle, 1356
    child and, 1382-1384
  musculoskeletal, 1380-1384
  myelogenic, 1338-1339
  osteogenic, 1335-1336
  pain and, 400
  pituitary, 712
  primary, 303
    intracerebral, 499-503
  promotion of, 326
  regression of, 311
  renal, 1139-1140
  skin, 1398
    benign, 1417-1418
  solid, radiation and, 332
  spinal cord, 500, 504-505
    metastatic, 504
  supratentorial, 554
  testicular germ cell, 704, 705
  uterine, 691
Tunica albuginea, 661
Tunica dartos, 662
Tunica externa, 886
Tunica intima, 886
Tunica media, 886
Tunica muscularis of stomach, 1178
Tunica vaginalis, 660
Turbulent blood flow in heart, 894-895
Turner syndrome, 126, 130, 681
  congenital heart defects and, 998
Twelve-lead electrocardiogram, 902

Twins, leukemia and monozygous, 319
Twitch, 1313
Tylectomy, 717
Tympanic cavity, 419
Tympanic membrane, 419
Type A personality, 163, 937-938
Tyrosine, 544, 545
Tyrosine kinase, 336

U

Ulcer
  Cushing, 1228-1229
  decubitus, 1389, 1398, 1400
  duodenal, 1226, 1227, 1229
  gastric, 1226-1228
  genital, 734
  Hunner, 1142
  ischemic, 1228
  peptic, 170, 1225-1231
  stress, 1228-1229
  venous stasis, 933
Ulcerative colitis, 251, 1232-1233
  chronic, 1258
Ultrafiltration, 1121
Ultraviolet radiation
  carcinogenesis and, 330-332
  melanin and, 68
Uncal herniation, 470
Unconsciousness, 433, 434
  motor responses and, 439
Unipolar neurons, 355
Uniport, 22, 23
Universal donor or recipient, 200
Unstable angina, 939
Upper airway, 1028
  child with disorders of, 1098-1101
Upper esophageal sphincter, 1176-1177
Upper motor neuron syndrome, 518
Upper motor neurons, 365
Uracil, 121-122
Urea, 1127, 1128
Urea clearance, 1154-1155
Urea nitrogen, 1130
Uremia, 1150, 1156, 1157
Ureter, 1118
Urethra, 663, 1118-1119
  disorders of, 699, 737, 1142
    urethrocele in, 688, 689
Urethral stricture, 699
Urethral syndrome, 737, 1142
Urethritis, 699
  nongonococcal, 737
Urethrocele, 688, 689
Urge incontinence, 1169
Uric acid
  gout and, 1348
  leukemia and, 807, 849
  stones and, 1138
Urinalysis, 1130-1131
Urinary bladder, male, 1118
Urinary meatus, 650
Urinary system, 1113, 1118-1119
  cancer and, 301
  function of; *see* Urinary tract function
  structural abnormalities in child and, 1161-1163
Urinary tract function
  alterations in, 1135-1159
    bacterial prostatitis and, 708
    glomerular disorders and, 1144-1150
    infection and, 1141-1144
    obstruction and, 1136-1141
    renal failure and, 1150-1158

Urinary tract function—cont'd
  child and, 1160-1171; *see also* Child, urinary tract function in
Urine
  burn shock and, 1428-1429
  child's output of, 1161
  concentration of, 1126-1128
  diabetes insipidus and, 598
  diabetes mellitus and testing of, 612
  epididymitis and reflux of, 706
  formation and excretion of, 1112-1134
    aging and, 1131-1132
    decreased, 92
    kidney function and, 1121-1131; *see also* Kidney function
    renal blood flow and, 1119-1121
    renal system and, 1112-1119
  history of study of, 1111
  pH of, 1130
  protein in, 68, 1149
  sediment in, 1131
Urobilinogen, 770, 1198
Urogenital infections, sexually transmitted, 727-745
  bacterial, 727-736
  chlamydial, 736-739
  parasitic, 743-745
  viral, 739-743
Urogenital sinus, 646
Urticaria, 254-255, 1415-1416
Uterine bleeding, dysfunctional, 682-683
Uterotubal insufflation, 670
Uterus, 651-653
  carcinogenesis and, 327
  estrogens and progesterone and, 657
  fibroids of, 691
  prolapse of, 689-690
Uveitis, 251

V

v-*onc*, 335
v-*src*, 335-336
V wave, 865
Vaccines, 191
  AIDS, 274
  cancer and, 312
  hypersensitivity and, 254
  Sabin, 208
  Salk, 208
Vaccinia, 61
Vacuolation, 66
Vacuoles, 9, 25, 50
Vagal nuclear palsy, 460
Vagina, 650-651
  cancer of, 696
  candidiasis and, 1415
  endothelium of, 660
  mucosa of, 657
  pH of, 686, 736
    menopause and, 672
  rhabdomyosarcoma and, 1384
  trichomoniasis and, 743
Vaginal mucosa, 657
Vaginal odor, 736
Vaginitis, 686-687
Vagotomy, 1230
Vagus nerves, 375
Valence, 19
Valgus foot abnormality, 1366
Valine, 836, 837
Valsalva maneuver, 1192
Valves
  heart, 863, 864

Valves—cont'd
  heart—cont'd
    dysfunction of, 953-958
    regurgitation or stenosis of, 953, 954, 955
  of vein, 889
  and varicose veins, 932
Variant angina, 939
Varicella, 1412-1413, 1445
  Reye syndrome and, 548
Varices, 1240
Varicocele, 701
Varicose bronchiectasis, 1061
Varicose veins, 932-933
Variola, 61, 1446
Varus foot abnormality, 1366
Vas deferens, 662
Vasa recta, 1117
Vasa vasorum, 886
Vascular compliance, 895
Vascular disorders
  congenital heart defects and, 998
  diabetes mellitus and, 627
  gastrointestinal tract and, 1235-1236
  hypertension and, 924
  liver and, 1198
  pulmonary, 1080-1083
  sexual dysfunction and, 710
  skin and, 1415-1416, 1448-1449
Vascular-leak syndrome, 316
Vascular phase of development of solid tumor, 302
Vascular resistance
  pulmonary, 969
  systemic, 969
    left heart failure and, 972
Vascular smooth muscle relaxants, 926
Vasculitis
  cutaneous, 1415
  necrotizing, 251
Vasoactive amines, degranulation of, 220-222
Vasoconstriction, 403, 888
  hypoxic, 1042
  inflammation and, 218
Vasodilation, 402-403, 888
  inflammation and, 218
  shock and, 979
Vasogenic edema, 469
Vasogenic shock, 977
Vasomotor flush, 671
Vasoocclusive crisis, 840
Vasopressin, 87, 573
Vasospasm
  angina and, 939
  intracranial aneurysm and, 497
Vater, ampulla of, 1200
Vectorcardiogram, 902
Vegetative states, 442, 443
Veins, 860, 885, 886, 889
  chronic insufficiency of, 932-933
    varicose veins and, 932
  diseases of, 932-933
  of head, 368-370, 371
  metastasis and, 303-305
  thrombus in, 821, 933
  varicose, 932-933
Velocity, blood, 894
Venereal diseases; *see* Sexually transmitted diseases
Venezuela equine encephalitis, 508
Venous blood gases, mixed, 1049
Venous pressure, 897
  central, 970

Venous sinus, 761
Venous stasis
  pulmonary embolism and, 1080
  skin ulcer and, 933
Ventilation, 1034-1040
  alveolar, 1036, 1038
  dead-space, 1036
  distribution of, 1043-1044
  muscles of, 1037
  neurochemical control of, 1040-1042
  spirometry and, 1048
Ventilation-perfusion ratio, 1058
Ventral column, 364
Ventral induction, embryonic development
    and, 533
Ventricle
  cerebral, 367
  left, 862
    aneurysm of, 946
    myocardial infarction and, 942
  right, 862
Ventricular activation, 870-871
Ventricular block, 967
Ventricular bradycardia, 965
Ventricular contractions, premature, 965
Ventricular fibrillation, 965
Ventricular outflow restriction, 999-1003
Ventricular rhythm, accelerated, 965
Ventricular septal defect, 1003-1005
Ventricular standstill, 965
Ventricular tachycardia, 965
Ventriculogram, 907
Venule, 886
Verbal paraphasia, 468
Vermiform appendix, 1190
Vermis, 362
Verrucae, 1413
Vertebra
  dislocation reduction and, 351
  fracture of, 485
  injury of, 485
  spina bifida occulta and, 538
Vertebral arteries, 368
Vertebral-basilar system, 495
Vertebral column, 362, 367-368
Vertigo, 423
Very low-density lipoproteins, 934
Vesicle, 1396
  formation of, 25-27
Vesicoureteral reflux, 1166-1167
Vesiculobullous skin disorders, 1409-1411
Vessels, blood; *see* Blood vessels
Vestibular nystagmus, 423
Vestibule, 419, 650
Vestibulocochlear nerves, 375
Vestigial tabs, 1363
Vibration, prolonged, 65-66
Villi
  biopsy of chorionic, 127
  in small intestine, 1184
Vinca alkaloids, 400
Viral carcinogenesis, 293, 319, 337,
    338-339
Viral conjunctivitis, 413
Viral croup, 1100
Viral encephalitis, 508
Viral gastroenteritis, 1281
Viral hepatitis, 1245-1248
Viral infections
  sexually transmitted urogenital infections
      and, 739-743
  of skin, 1411-1415
    in child, 1443-1446

Viral myositis, 1354-1355
Viral particles, 59
Viral pneumonia, 1077, 1102
Viral replication, 59-61, 274
Virchow triad, 821
Virilization, 633
Virions, 59
Viruses
  AIDS, 273
  cancer and, 293, 333-337, 338-339
    childhood, 319
  infectious injury and, 59
  leukemia and, 848
  neutralization of, 206
Visceral muscle, 42
Visceral pain, 397
  abdominal, 1217
Visceral pericardium, 860
Vision
  aging and, 415
  alterations in, 415-419
    color, 417-418
  diabetes mellitus and, 617, 628
Visual agnosia, 462
Visual cortex, 418
Visual pathway, 418
Vital capacity, 1036
Vitamins
  B_1, 509
  B_2, 767
  B_6, 767
  B_{12}
    erythropoiesis and, 767
    gastrectomy and, 1231
    pernicious anemia and, 788
    small intestine and, 1190
  C, 767
  D
    calcium and phosphate balance and, 98-99
    kidney function and, 1129
    nephrotic syndrome and, 1149, 1150
    osteomalacia and, 1330
    renal failure and, 1155-1156
    deficiency of, 62
  E, 767
  K
    deficiency of, 819
    liver and, 1198
    liver and, 1199
    small intestine and, 1188-1190
Vitiligo, 250
Vitreous humor, 415
Vocal cords, 1027
Voiding, precipitate, 1169; *see also* Urinary
    tract function
Volatile body acids, 101
Volkmann canals, 1296
Voltage-regulated channels, 28
Volume of solution, 21
Volume-pressure curve, lungs and, 1040
Volume-sensitive receptors, 87
Voluntary movement
  primary motor pathway and, 360
  slowness of, 452
Volvulus, 1222, 1271
Vomiting, 1214
  central nervous system disorders and, 435
  projectile, 1214
von Recklinghausen disease, 137
von Willebrand disease, 844
Vulva, 650
  condylomata lata of, 731
  skin disorders and, 684-685

Vulvitis, 687
Vulvovaginitis, 1415

W

Waking state, 409
Wallerian degeneration, 356
Warm antibody disease, 792
Warm climate, adaptation to, 403
Warming, frostbite and, 1431-1432
Warts, 1413-1414
  genital, 741, 1413
Waste product theory of aging, 74
Water
  burns and evaporative loss of, 1431
  cellular environment and, alterations in,
      85-87
  cellular injury and, 66
  deficits of, 87, 90
  diabetes insipidus and restriction of, 598
  drinking of, 87, 92
  movement of, 19-24
    alterations in, 85-87
    cellular environment and, 87-88, 90
    between plasma and interstitial fluids,
        84-85
    osmosis and, 21
    retention of, 85
    syndrome of inappropriate antidiuretic
        hormone secretion and, 597
  small intestine and, 1184
  total body, 83
  urine and, 1126-1127
Water balance
  cellular environment and, 87-88, 99
  renal failure and, 1155
Water deficit, 87, 90
Water deprivation test, 598
Water diuresis, 1128
Water-drinking behavior, 87, 92
Water imbalances, 89, 92
  burns and, 1431
Water intoxication, 92
Water retention, 85; *see also* Edema
  syndrome of inappropriate antidiuretic
      hormone secretion and, 597
Water-soluble hormones, 568-570
Water-soluble vitamins, intestinal absorption
    of, 1189
Waveforms, arterial pulse, 904
Wear-and-tear theory of aging, 74, 75
Webbing of fingers, 1363
Weight loss
  cancer and, 306
  diabetes mellitus and, 615
  gastric resection and, 1230-1231
  voluntary, 1237
Wenckebach heart block, 966
Wernicke area, 360
Wernicke disease, 509
Wernicke sensory dysphasia, 466
Western blot, 669
Western equine encephalitis, 508
Wet gangrene, 72
Wet mount, 736
Wheal, 255, 1396
Wheat, digestive system and, 179
Wheezing, 1055
White blood cells, 266, 757
  burn injury and, 1431
  congenital immune deficiencies and, 266
  differential count of, 778
  urinalysis and, 1131
White fast-motor fiber, 1306

White graft, 264
White matter, 359-360
White pupillary reflex, 557, 558
Whiteheads, 1399
Willis, circle of, 368, 369
Wilms' tumor, 297, 317, 1167-1168
Wilson disease, 1285-1286
Wind-chill factor, 402
Wirsung duct, 1200
Wiskott-Aldrich syndrome, 267, 318
Wolf-Parkinson-White syndrome, 967
Wood's lamp examination, 1394
Word blindness, 462
Word deafness, 466
Work of breathing, 1040
Wounds
    contraction of, 243

Wounds—cont'd
    disruption of, 245-246
    dysfunctional healing of, 244-246
    myocardial infarction healing and, 944
    sepsis of, 244
Wrist dislocation, 1324

X

X inactivation, 125-126
X-linked inheritance, 139-140
    childhood cancers and, 319
X-rays
    discovery of, 293
    exposure to, 331
        acquired immune deficiency and, 268
        fetal damage and, 319

Xeroderma pigmentosum, 331
D-Xylose absorption, 1204

Y

Y chromosome, 126
Yellow marrow, 1296
Yolksac tumor, 297

Z

Z line, 1309, 1310
    myocardial cells and, 876
Zinc deficiency, 268
Zona glomerulosa, 580
Zonula occludens, 32, 33
Zygote, 128, 132

ALSO AVAILABLE!

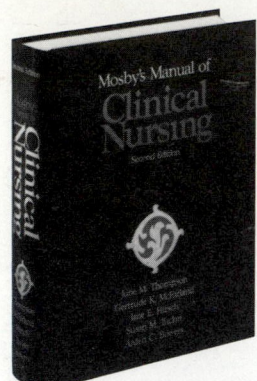

MOSBY'S MANUAL OF CLINICAL NURSING
2nd Edition
June M. Thompson, R.N., M.S.
Gertrude K. McFarland, R.N., D.N.Sc., F.A.A.N.
Jane E. Hirsch, R.N., M.S.
Susan M. Tucker, R.N., B.S.N.
Arden C. Bowers, R.N., M.S.
1989
ISBN 0-8016-5157-3

The new second edition of MOSBY'S MANUAL OF CLINICAL NURSING provides nurses and students with everything they need to plan and implement high-quality nursing care. The book presents complete care planning information, including rationales for over 300 conditions, diseases, and disorders, and over 90 nursing diagnoses. Don't start your career without it!

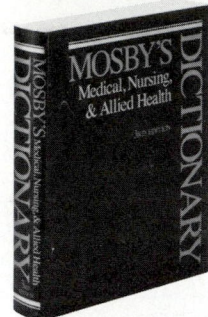

MOSBY'S MEDICAL, NURSING, AND ALLIED HEALTH DICTIONARY
3rd Edition
Kenneth Anderson
Lois Anderson
Walter D. Glanze
1990
ISBN 0-8016-3227-7

The third edition of this respected and widely used dictionary offers in-depth definitions of specialized terms currently used by physicians, nurses, and allied health professionals. Featuring comprehensive and easy-to-read definitions, this dictionary is an indispensable reference for all nurses.

PATHOPHYSIOLOGY CASEBOOK
Sharon Sims, R.N., Ph.D.
Donna Boland, R.N., Ph.D.
February 1990
ISBN 0-8016-0622-3

This practical new casebook complements McCance-Huether: PATHOPHYSIOLOGY: THE BIOLOGICAL BASIS FOR DISEASE IN ADULTS AND CHILDREN but can be used in conjunction with any pathophysiology book. This book demonstrates how nurses can apply their knowledge of pathophysiology to make clinical decisions affecting patient care. Each case study includes detailed presentations of past history, clinical manifestations, and evaluation and treatment. These case studies have been written by nurse experts from a variety of practice settings and have all been reviewed by clinical specialists.

To order, ask your bookstore manager or call toll-free 1-800-426-4545.
We look forward to hearing from you.   NMA-029